III. RESPIRATORY GAS TRANSPORT

Oxygen delivery ($\dot{Q}_{O_2}$)	$= \dot{Q}_T \times Ca_{O_2}$
Arterial oxygen content (Ca_{O_2})	$= 1.39 \times Sa_{O_2} \times [Hgb] + .0031 \times Pa_{O_2}$
Mixed venous oxygen content ($C\bar{v}_{O_2}$)	$= 1.39 \times S\bar{v}_{O_2} \times [Hgb] + .0031 \times P\bar{v}_{O_2}$
Arterio-venous oxygen content difference	$= Ca_{O_2} - C\bar{v}_{O_2}$
Oxygen consumption ($\dot{V}_{O_2}$)	$= \dot{Q}_T (Ca_{O_2} - C\bar{v}_{O_2})$
Extraction fraction	$= \dfrac{Ca_{O_2} - C\bar{v}_{O_2}}{Ca_{O_2}}$
Respiratory quotient (RQ)	$= \dfrac{\dot{V}_{CO_2}}{\dot{V}_{O_2}}$
CO_2 production ($\dot{V}_{CO_2}$)	$= f \cdot V_T \cdot F_{E_{CO_2}}$
O_2 consumption ($\dot{V}_{O_2}$)	$= f \cdot V_T \cdot (F_{I_{O_2}} - F_{E_{O_2}})$, when RQ = 1.0

IV. CIRCULATORY PARAMETERS AND CALCULATIONS

Systemic systolic pressure (SP)	100–140 mmHG
Systemic diastolic pressure (DP)	60–90 mmHG
Pulse pressure (SP – DP)	30–50 mmHg
Mean arterial pressure (BP, mmHg)	$\dfrac{(SP + 2DP)}{3}$ at normal heart rate
Heart rate (HR)	60–90/min
Stoke volume (SV)	50–100 mL
Stroke index (SI)	SV/Body surface area (BSA) $= 35$–50 mL/m^2
Right atrial pressure (Pra)	2–8 mmHg
Pulmonary systolic pressure	16–24 mmHg (15) - (30)
Pulmonary diastolic pressure	(4)5–12 mmHg
Pulmonary pulse pressure	8–15 mmHg
Mean pulmonary artery pressure ($P\bar{pa}$)	9–16 mmHg
Mean pulmonary capillary wedge pressure (Ppw)	5–12 mmHg
Cardiac output ($\dot{Q}_T = SV \times HR$)	4–6 L/min
Cardiac index (CI $= \dot{Q}_T$/BSA)	2.5–3 L/min/m^2
Systemic vascular resistance $$SVR = \frac{\overline{BP} - Pra}{\dot{Q}_T}$$	10–15 mmHg/L/min (to convert to c.g.s. units, multiply $\times 80$) (900–1200 dyne $\cdot$ s/cm^5)
Pulmonary vascular resistance $$PVR = \frac{Ppa - Ppw}{\dot{Q}_T}$$	1.5–2.5 mmHg/L/min (120–200 dyne $\cdot$ s/cm^5)
Venous return (VR) $= \dfrac{Pms - Pra}{Rvr}$	4–6 L/min
where Pms = mean systemic pressure	10–15 mmHg
Rvr = resistance to venous return	1–2 mmHg/L/min

PRINCIPLES OF
CRITICAL CARE

Editors

Jesse B. Hall, MD
Director of Critical Care Services
Professor of Medicine and of Anesthesia and Critical Care
Section of Pulmonary and Critical Care
University of Chicago
Chicago, Illinois

Gregory A. Schmidt, MD
Director, Critical Care Services
Professor of Medicine and of Anesthesia and Critical Care
Section of Pulmonary and Critical Care
University of Chicago
Chicago, Illinois

Lawrence D. H. Wood, MD, PhD
Faculty Dean of Medical Education
University of Chicago Pritzker School of Medicine
Professor of Medicine and of Anesthesia and Critical Care
Section of Pulmonary and Critical Care Medicine
University of Chicago
Chicago, Illinois

Associate Editors

Jameel Ali, MD, M Med Ed, FRCS[C], FACS
Professor of Surgery, University of Toronto
Toronto, Ontario, Canada
National ATLS faculty and Educator
American College of Surgeons Committee on Trauma
Toronto, Ontario, Canada
Chapters 87, 88, 92, 95

Keith R. Walley, MD
Associate Professor of Medicine
University of British Columbia
Pulmonary Research Laboratory
Vancouver, British Columbia, Canada

PRINCIPLES OF CRITICAL CARE

THIRD EDITION

Editors

JESSE B. HALL, MD
Director of Critical Care Services
Professor of Medicine and of Anesthesia and Critical Care
Section of Pulmonary and Critical Care
University of Chicago
Chicago, Illinois

GREGORY A. SCHMIDT, MD
Director, Critical Care Services
Professor of Medicine and of Anesthesia and Critical Care
Section of Pulmonary and Critical Care
University of Chicago
Chicago, Illinois

LAWRENCE D.H. WOOD, MD PHD
Faculty Dean of Medical Education
University of Chicago, Pritzker School of Medicine
Professor of Medicine and of Anesthesia and Critical Care
Section of Pulmonary and Critical Care Medicine
University of Chicago
Chicago, Illinois

Cora D. Taylor

Editorial Assistant

McGRAW-HILL
Medical Publishing Division

New York   Chicago   San Francisco   Lisbon
London   Madrid   Mexico City   Milan   New Delhi
San Juan   Seoul   Singapore   Sydney   Toronto

Principles of Critical Care, 3/e

1234567890   KGPKGP   098765

ISBN: 0-07-141640-4

This book was set in Palatino by TechBooks.
The editors were Jim Shanahan, Shelley Reinhardt, Karen G. Edmonson, and Patrick Carr.
The production supervisor was Catherine H. Saggese.
The cover designer was Mary McKeon.
The indexer was Kathrin Unger.
Quebecor World was printer and binder.

This book is printed on acid-free paper.

Library of Congress Cataloging-in-Publication Data

Principles of critical care / editors, Jesse B. Hall, Gregory A. Schmidt, Lawrence D.H.
    Wood; Cora D. Taylor, editorial assistant.—3rd ed.
      p.;   cm.
    Includes bibliographical references and index.
    ISBN 0-07-141640-4 (alk. paper)
    1. Critical care medicine.   I. Hall, Jesse B.   II. Schmidt, Gregory A.   III. Wood, Lawrence
D.H.
    [DNLM: 1. Critical Care. 2. Intensive Care Units. WX 218 P9573 2005]
    RC86.7.P752 2005
    616.02′8—dc22
                                                                    2004061086

We dedicate this edition to:

Larry Wood, who, through his guidance, clarity, and wisdom,
revealed to us the beauty of critical care;

Change, which excites and refreshes us;

and Karin and Barbara, who remind us of balance.

NOTICE

Medicine is an ever-changing science. As new research and clinical experience broaden our knowledge, changes in treatment and drug therapy are required. The authors and the publisher of this work have checked with sources believed to be reliable in their efforts to provide information that is complete and generally in accord with the standards accepted at the time of publication. However, in view of the possibility of human error or changes in medical sciences, neither the editors nor the publisher nor any other party who has been involved in the preparation or publication of this work warrants that the information contained herein is in every respect accurate or complete, and they disclaim all responsibility for any errors or omissions or for the results obtained from use of the information contained in this work. Readers are encouraged to confirm the information contained herein with other sources. For example and in particular, readers are advised to check the product information sheet included in the package of each drug they plan to administer to be certain that the information contained in this work is accurate and that changes have not been made in the recommended dose or in the contraindications for administration. This recommendation is of particular importance in connection with new or infrequently used drugs.

CONTENTS

CONTRIBUTORS

BENJAMIN S. ABELLA, MD, MPhil
Department of Medicine
Section of Emergency Medicine
University of Chicago
Chicago, Illinois
Chapters 15, 16

VENKATESH AIYAGARI, MD
Assistant Professor of Neurology and
Neurological Surgery
Washington University School of
Medicine
St. Louis, Missouri
Chapter 63

RICHARD K. ALBERT, MD
Professor
Department of Medicine
University of Colorado
Health Sciences Center
Chief of Medicine
Denver Health Medical Center
Denver, Colorado
Chapter 41

JAMEEL ALI, MD, M Med Ed, FRCS[C], FACS
Professor of Surgery, University of Toronto
Toronto, Ontario, Canada
National ATLS faculty and Educator
American College of Surgeons
    Committee on Trauma
Toronto, Ontario, Canada
Chapters 87, 88, 92, 95

JASON ALVARADO, BA
Department of Medicine
Section of Emergency Medicine
University of Chicago
Chicago, Illinois
Chapter 15

DEREK C. ANGUS, MD, MPH
Professor and Vice Chair
Department of Critical Care Medicine
Director, The CRISMA Laboratory
University of Pittsburgh
School of Medicine
Pittsburgh, Pennsylvania
Chapter 2

FRED Y. AOKI, MD
Professor of Medicine
Medical Microbiology, Pharmacology
and Therapeutics
University of Manitoba
Winnipeg, Manitoba, Canada
Chapter 45

JOSEPH J. AUSTIN, MD
Cardiothoracic Surgery
Overlake Hospital Medical Center
Bellevue, Washington
Chapter 30

GEORGE BALTOPOULOS, MD
Professor of Critical Care and
Pulmonary Diseases
University of Athens School of Nursing
Director
Athens University School of Nursing Intensive
Care Unit at KAT Hospital
Athens, Greece
Chapter 23

JOSEPH M. BARON, MD
Section of Hematology/Oncology
University of Chicago
Chicago, Illinois
Chapter 69

BEVERLY W. BARON, MD
Department of Pathology
Blood Banking/Transfusion Medicine
University of Chicago
Chicago, Illinois
Chapter 69

WALTER G. BARR, MD
Professor of Medicine
Director
Training Program
Division of Rheumatology
Northwestern University Feinberg
School of Medicine
Chicago, Illinois
Chapter 104

SARICE L. BASSIN, MD
  Neurointensivist
  Neuroscience Institute
  Critical Care Neurology and Stroke
  Queen's Medical Center
  Honolulu, Hawaii
  Chapter 64

LANCE B. BECKER, MD
  Professor of Clinical Medicine
  Section of Emergency Medicine
  University of Chicago
  Chicago, Illinois
  Chapters 15, 16

ISRAEL BELENKIE, MD
  Professor of Medicine
  Departments of Medicine and Cardiac Sciences
  Libin Cardiovascular Institute of Alberta
  University of Calgary
  Calgary, Alberta, Canada
  Chapter 28

THOMAS P. BLECK, MD
  The Louise Nerancy Eminent Scholar in Neurology and
  Professor of Neurology, Neurological Surgery,
  and Internal Medicine
  Director, Neuroscience Intensive Care Unit
  The University of Virginia
  Charlottesville, Virginia
  Chapter 64

IRA J. BLUMEN, MD
  Professor, Section of Emergency Medicine
  Department of Medicine
  University of Chicago
  Chicago, Illinois
  Program and Medical Director
  University of Chicago Aeromedical
  Network (UCAN)
  University of Chicago Hospitals
  Chicago, Illinois
  Chapter 7

JOHN BOHNEN, MD, FRCSC, FACS
  Director
  Postgraduate Surgical Education
  Associate Professor
  Department of Surgery
  University of Toronto
  Toronto, Ontario, Canada
  Chapter 89

ERIC J. BOW, MD
  Sections of Infectious Diseases and
  Haematology/Oncology
  Professor and Head,
  Section of Haematology/Oncology
  Department of Internal Medicine
  University of Manitoba
  Head, Department of Medical Oncology
  and Haematology
  Director, Infection Control Services, Cancer Care
  Manitoba
  Winnipeg, Manitoba, Canada
  Chapter 47

MICHAEL BRESLOW, MD
  Executive Vice President, Research and
  Development
  VISICU, Inc.
  Baltimore, Maryland
  Chapter 8

LAURENT BROCHARD
  Professor of Intensive Care Medicine
  Medical Intensive Care Unit
  Hôpital Henri Mondor
  Assistance Publique
  Hôpitaux de Paris
  Université Paris
  Créteil, France
  Chapter 33

STEVEN D. BROWN, MD
  Professor and Chief Medical Officer
  University of Texas Health Center at Tyler
  Tyler, Texas
  Chapter 112

JOHN B. BUSE, MD, PhD
  Associate Professor of Medicine
  Chief, Division of General Medicine
  and Clinical Epidemiology
  Director, Diabetes Care Center
  University of North Carolina
  School of Medicine
  Chapel Hill, North Carolina
  Chapter 78

MARK B. CARR, MD
  Baptist Hospital
  Nashville, Tennessee
  Chapter 49

SHANNON S. CARSON, MD
  Assistant Professor
  Division of Pulmonary and
  Critical Care Medicine
  University of North Carolina
  Chapel Hill, North Carolina
  Chapter 18

JEAN CHASTRE, MD
  Reanimation Medicale
  Groupe Hospitalier Pitie Salpetriere
  Institut de Cardiologie
  Paris, France
  Chapter 43

ANTHONY W. CHOW, MD
  Professor of Medicine
  Division of Infectious Diseases
  Department of Medicine
  University of British Columbia
  And Vancouver Hospital
  Health Sciences Center
  Director, MD/PhD Program, University of British
  Columbia
  Vancouver, British Columbia
  Chapter 54

JASON D. CHRISTIE, MD, MS
Assistant Professor of Medicine
Division of Pulmonary, Allergy, and
Critical Care Medicine
Assistant Professor of Epidemiology
Department of Biostatistics and Epidemiology
University of Pennsylvania
School of Medicine
Philadelphia, Pennsylvania
Chapter 38

GLENN C. COBBS, MD
Professor Emeritus of Medicine
University of Alabama at Birmingham
Birmingham, Alabama
Chapter 49

JOHN M. CONLY, MD
Head
Department of Medicine
University of Calgary
Calgary Health Region
Foothills Medical Centre
Calgary, Alberta, Canada
Chapters 50, 55

DEBORAH COOK, MD
Professor of Medicine and Clinical Epidemiology
and Biostatistics
Chair
Critical Care Medicine
McMaster University
Hamilton, Ontario, Canada
Chapter 10

THOMAS CORBRIDGE, MD
Associate Professor of Medicine
Director, Medical Intensive Care
Northwestern Scholl of Medicine
Chicago, Illinois
Chapters 40, 42, 102, 103

MICHAEL T. COUGHLIN, MA
Project Manager, The CRISMA Laboratory
Department of Critical Care Medicine
University of Pittsburgh School of Medicine
Pittsburgh, Pennsylvania
Chapter 2

DAVID C. CRONIN II, MD, PhD
Assistant Professor of Surgery
Section of Transplantation
University of Chicago
Chicago, Illinois
Chapter 83

STEPHEN W. CRAWFORD, MD
United States Navy Medical Corps
Pulmonary Medicine
Naval Medicine Center San Diego
San Diego, California
Chapter 73

FRANK D'OVIDIO, MD, PhD
Thoracic Surgery and Lung Transplantation
Toronto General Hospital
University of Toronto
Toronto, Ontario, Canada
Chapter 91

ROBERT H. DEMLING, MD
Burn Center
Brigham and Women's Hospital
Boston, Massachusetts
Professor of Surgery
Harvard Medical School
Boston, Massachusetts
Chapters 98, 99, 100

APURVA A. DESAI, MD
Assistant Professor of Medicine
Section of Hematology/Oncology
The University of Chicago Medical Center
Chicago, Illinois
Chapter 74

LESLIE DeSANTI, RN
Burn Research
Brigham & Women's Hospital
Boston, Massachusetts
Chapter 98, 99, 100

MICHAEL N. DIRINGER, MD
Associate Professor of Neurology, Neurosurgery
and Anesthesiology
Washington University School of Medicine
Director, Neurology/Neurosurgery
Intensive Care Unit
Barnes-Jewish Hospital
Department of Neurology
St. Louis, Missouri
Chapter 63

IVOR S. DOUGLAS, MD, MRCP (UK)
Assistant Professor
Pulmonary and Critical Care Medicine
Director
Medical Intensive Care
Denver Health
University of Colorado Health Sciences Center
Denver, Colorado
Chapter 39

TONY T. DREMSIZOV
Senior Research Specialist
CRISMA Laboratory
Department of Critical Care Medicine
University of Pittsburgh
Pittsburgh, Pennsylvania
Chapter 2

ELI D. EHRENPREIS, MD
Assistant Professor of Medicine
Rush Presbyterian St. Luke's Medical Center
Adult Care Specialists
Chicago, Illinois
Chapter 81

E. WESLEY ELY, MD, MPH
Associate Professor of Medicine
Division of Allergy, Pulmonary, and Critical Care
Vanderbilt University Medical Center
Associate Director of Research
Tennessee Valley Veterans Administration Geriatric
Research Education and Clinical Center
Nashville, Tennessee
Chapter 46, 62

JEAN-YVES FAGON, MD, PhD
Professor of Medicine
Service de Réanimation Médicale
Hôpital Européen Georges Pompidou
Paris, France
Chapter 43

J. CHRISTOPHER FARMER, MD
Professor of Medicine
Division of Pulmonary and Critical Care Medicine
Program in Translational Immunovirology and
Biodefense
Mayo Clinic
Rochester, Minnesota
Chapter 9

SUSAN FISHER-HOCH, MD
Professor
Division of Epidemiology
University of Texas School of Public Health at Brownsville
Brownsville, Texas
Chapter 60

GERASIMOS S. FILIPPATOS, MD
Critical Care Unit and Heart Failure Unit
Evangelismos General Hospital
Chairman
Working Group on Acute Cardiac Care
European Society of Cardiology
Athens, Greece
Chapter 23

GINI F. FLEMING, MD
Associate Professor, Department of Medicine
Section on Hematology, Oncology
The University of Chicago Medical Center
Chicago, Illinois
Chapter 74

RODNEY J. FOLZ, MD, PhD
Associate Professor of Medicine
Assistant Research Professor of Cell Biology
Division of Pulmonary, Allergy, and Critical Care
Medicine
Duke University Medical Center
Durham, North Carolina
Chapter 73

NATHAN B. FOUNTAIN, MD
Associate Professor of Neurology
Director
FE Dreifuss Comprehensive Epilepsy Program
University of Virginia
Charlottesville, Virginia
Chapter 64

JEFFREY I. FRANK, MD, FAAN, FAHA
Director
Neuromedical/Neurosurgical Intensive Care
Associate Professor
Neurology and Surgery
University of Chicago
Chicago, Illinois
Chapter 65, 67

JOHN C. GALBRAITH, MD
Medical Director
Dynacare Kasper Medical Laboratories
Edmonton, Alberta, Canada
Chapter 53

ALLAN GARLAND, MD
Associate Professor of Medicine
Case Western Reserve University School of Medicine
Director, Medical Intensive Care Unit
Division of Pulmonary and Critical Care Medicine
MetroHealth Medical Center
Cleveland Ohio
Chapter 3

BRIAN GEHLBACH, MD
Assistant Professor of Medicine
Section of Pulmonary and Critical Care
University of Chicago
Chicago, Illinois
Chapters 14, 34, 109

ANNE M. GILLIS, MD, FRCPC
Professor of Medicine
University of Calgary
Medical Director of Pacing and Electrophysiology
Department of Cardiac Sciences
Calgary Health
University of Calgary
Calgary, Alberta, Canada
Chapter 24

MARK T. GLADWIN, MD
Chief
Vascular Therapeutics Section
Cardiovascular Branch
National Heart, Lung, and Blood Institute
Critical Care Medicine Department
Clinical Center
National Institutes of Health
Bethesda, Maryland
Chapter 108

LAWRENCE TIM GOODNOUGH, MD
Department of Pathology and Medicine
Stanford University
Stanford, California
Chapter 70

LAWRENCE J. GOTTLIEB, MD
Professor of Surgery
Director of Burn and Complex Wound Center
University of Chicago
Chicago, Illinois
Chapter 97

JENNIFER E. GOULD, MD
  Assistant Professor of Radiology
  Washington University School of Medicine
  St. Louis, Missouri
  Chapter 101

RICHERT E. GOYETTE, MD
  Consultant
  Knoxville, Tennessee
  Chapter 46

JOHN T. GRANTON, MD
  Program Director
  Critical Care Medicine
  University of Toronto
  Director, Pulmonary Hypertension Program
  University Health Network
  Toronto, Ontario, Canada
  Chapter 37, 90

PERRY R. GRAY, MD
  Critical Care Site Manager
  Director
  SICU
  Health Sciences Center
  Winnipeg, Manitoba, Canada
  Chapter 59

GENEVIÈVE GRÉGOIRE, MD, FRCPC
  Assistant Professor of Medicine
  University of Montreal
  Intensivist
  Department of Medicine
  Hôpital du Sacre-Couer de Montreal
  Montreal, Quebec, Canada
  Chapter 6

JESSE B. HALL, MD
  Professor, Medicine, Anesthesia and
  Critical Care
  Section of Pulmonary and Critical Care Medicine
  Department of Medicine
  University of Chicago
  Chicago, Illinois
  Chapters 1, 36, 40, 44, 105

MICHAEL J. HALL, MD
  Section of Hematology and Oncology
  Department of Medicine
  University of Chicago
  Chicago, Illinois
  Chapter 71

NICOLA A. HANANIA, MD
  Assistant Professor of Medicine
  Pulmonary and Critical Care Medicine
  Director, Asthma Clinical Research Center
  Baylor College of Medicine
  Houston, Texas
  Chapter 110, 111

DENIS W. HARKIN, MD, FRCS
  Vascular Fellow
  Department of Surgery
  University of Toronto
  Toronto, Ontario, Canada
  Chapter 86

MARGARET S. HERRIDGE, MSc, MD, FRCPC, MPH
  Pulmonary and Critical Care Medicine
  University Health Network
  Assistant Professor of Medicine
  Interdepartmental Division of Critical Care
  University of Toronto
  Toronto, Ontario, Canada
  Chapter 19

DAREN K. HEYLAND, MD, MSc, FRCPC
  Associate Professor
  Kingston General Hospital
  Kingston, Ontario, Canada
  Chapter 11

PHILIP C. HOFFMAN, MD
  Professor of Medicine
  Section of Hematology/Oncology
  The University of Chicago
  Chicago, Illinois
  Chapter 72

STEVEN M. HOLLENBERG, MD
  Director
  Coronary Care Unit
  Cooper University Hospital
  Professor of Medicine
  Robert Wood Johnson Medical School/
  University of Medicine and Dentistry
  of New Jersey
  Camden, New Jersey
  Chapter 25

CHERYL L. HOLMES, MD
  Clinical Instructor
  Department of Medicine
  University of British Columbia
  Vancouver, British Columbia
  Director, Critical Care Medicine
  Department of Medicine
  Kelowna General Hospital
  Kelowna, British Columbia, Canada
  Chapter 6

RAMONA O. HOPKINS, PhD
  Psychology Department and
  Neuroscience Center
  Brigham Young University
  Provo, Utah
  and Department of Medicine
  Pulmonary and Critical Care Divisions
  LDS Hospital
  Salt Lake City, Utah
  Chapter 19

GARTH JOHNSON, MD
  Professor of Surgery
  University of Ottawa
  Division of Orthopedic Surgery
  Ottawa Hospital
  Ottawa, Ontario, Canada
  Chapter 94

MARSHALL B. KAPP, JD, MPH
Arthur W. Grayson Distinguished Professor of Law
and Medicine
Southern Illinois University
School of Law
Carbondale, Illinois
Chapter 5

ELIAS KARAMBATSOS, MD
Physician
Cellular and Molecular Biology
Naxos, Greece
Chapter 23

MANOJ KARWA, MD
Assistant Professor of Medicine
Critical Care Medicine
Montefiore Medical Center
Albert Einstein College of Medicine
Bronx, New York
Chapter 61

GREGORY J. KATO, MD
Investigator
Critical Care Medicine Department
Clinical Center
Vascular Therapeutics Section
Cardiovascular Branch
National Heart, Lung, and Blood Institute
National Institutes of Health
Bethesda, Maryland
Chapter 108

DAVID C. KAUFMAN, MD
Associate Professor
Department of Surgery
Strong Memorial Hospital
University of Rochester
Rochester, New York
Chapter 77

JOHN A. KELLUM, MD
Associate Professor
Departments of Critical Care Medicine
and Medicine
University of Pittsburgh
Pittsburgh, Pennsylania
Chapter 77

SHAF KESHAVJEE, MD, MSc, FRCSC, FACS
Head
Division of Thoracic Surgery
Director
Toronto Lung Transplant Program
Professor and Chair
Division of Thoracic Surgery
University of Toronto
Toronto General Hospital
Toronto, Ontario, Canada
Chapter 91

ANDREW J. KITCHING, MB, ChB
Consultant Anaesthetist
Royal Berkshire Hospital
London Road
Reading, United Kingdom
Chapter 77

MARIN H. KOLLEFF, MD
Associate Professor of Medicine
Washington University School of Medicine
Director
Medical Intensive Care Unit
Director
Respiratory Care Services
Barnes-Jewish Hospital
St. Louis, Missouri
Chapter 4

JOHN P. KRESS, MD
Assistant Professor of Medicine
Section of Pulmonary and Critical Care
University of Chicago
Chicago, Illinois
Chapters 12, 14, 109

VIDYA KRISHNAN
Pulmonary and Critical Care Division
Johns Hopkins University School of Medicine
Baltimore, Maryland
Chapter 103

SANJAY KULKARNI, MD
Assistant Professor
Section of Organ Transplantation and immunology
Yale University School of Medicine
New Haven, Connecticut
Chapter 83

VLADIMIR KVETAN, MD
Professor of Anesthesiology and Clinical Medicine
Associate Professor of Surgery
Director of Critical Care Medicine Service and Fellowship,
Critical Care Medicine
Montefiore Medical Center
Albert Einstein Medical Center
Bronx, New York
Chapter 61

MARIO E. LACOUTRE, MD
Resident, Dermatology Section University of
Chicago
University of Chicago
Chicago, Illinois
Chapter 107

ELIZABETH B. LAMONT, MD, MS
Assistant Professor of Medicine
Massachusetts General Hospital Cancer Center
Harvard Medical School
Boston, Massachusetts
Chapter 72

PAUL N. LANKEN, MD
Professor of Medicine
Pulmonary, Allergy, and Critical Care Division
Hospital of the University of Pennsylvania
Philadelphia, Pennsylvania
Chapter 38

RICHARD A. LARSON, MD
Professor of Medicine
Section of Hematology and Oncology
Department of Medicine
Cancer Research Center
University of Chicago
Chicago, Illinois
Chapter 71

ANNE E. LAUMANN, MBChB, MRCP (UK)
Associate Professor of Dermatology
Northwestern University
Chicago, Illinois
Chapter 107

JAMES W. LEATHERMAN, MD
Associate Professor of Medicine
University of Minnesota
Division of Pulmonary and
Critical Care Medicine
Hennepin County Medical Center, Minneapolis
Chapters 13, 66

RAPHAEL C. LEE, MD, ScD
Professor of Surgery, Dermatology,
Molecular Medicine, and Organismal Biology
and Anatomy
Director, Electrical Trauma Program
Director, Program for Research in Cellular Repair
University of Chicago
Chicago, Illinois
Chapter 97

ALLAN S. LIEW, MD, FRCSC
Division of Orthopedic Surgery
Ottawa Hospital
Ottawa, Ontario, Canada
Chapter 96

R. BRUCE LIGHT, MD
Professor of Medicine and Medical Microbiology
University of Manitoba
Winnipeg, Manitoba, Canada
Chapter 51

THOMAS F. LINDSAY, MD, FRCSC, FACS
Chair
Division of Vascular Surgery
Associate Professor of Surgery
University of Toronto
Toronto, Ontario, Canada
Chapter 86

RAGHU S. LOGANATHAN, MD
Fellow in Critical Care Medicine
Montefiore Medical Center
Albert Einstein College of Medicine
Bronx, New York
Chapter 61

JOHN M. LUCE, MD
Professor of Medicine and Anesthesia
University of California–San Francisco
Associate Medical Director, Medical and Surgical
Intensive Care Units
Medical Director, Quality, Utilization, and Risk
Management
San Francisco General Hospital
San Francisco, California
Chapters 17, 68

JUDITH A. LUCE, MD
Clinical Professor of Medicine
University of California–San Francisco
Director
Oncology Services
San Francisco General Hospital
Chapter 68

CONSTANTINE A. MANTHOUS, MD
Director, Medical Intensive Care
Bridgeport Hospital
Associate Clinical Professor of Medicine
Yale University School of Medicine
Bridgeport, Connecticut
Chapter 44

PAUL MARIK, MD, FCCM, FCCP
Director
Pulmonary and Critical Care
Professor of Medicine
Thomas Jefferson University
Philadelphia, Pennsylvania
Chapter 79

WILLIAM A. MARINELLI, MD
Associate Professor of Medicine
University of Minnesota
Medical Director, Respiratory Care
Hennepin County Medical Center
Minneapolis, Minnesota
Chapter 66

JOHN J. MARINI, MD
Professor of Medicine
University of Minnesota
Director of Translational Research
HealthPartners Medical Group
Minneapolis/St. Paul, Minnesota
Chapter 13

TIMOTHY M. McCASHLAND, MD
Associate Professor of Medicine
Section of Gastroenterology and Hepatology
University of Nebraska
Omaha, Nebraska
Chapter 82

STEVE A. McCLAVE, MD
Professor of Medicine
Division of Gastroenterology/Hepatology
Director of Clinical Nutrition
University of Louisville School of Medicine
Louisville, Kentucky
Chapter 11

JOHN F. McCONVILLE, MD
Assistant Professor of Medicine
University of Chicago
Chicago, Illinois
Chapter 12

DONNA I. McRITCHIE, MD, MSc, FRCSC
Assistant Professor of Surgery
University of Toronto
Medical Director
Clinical Care
North York General Hospital
Toronto, Ontario, Canada
Chapter 91

PAUL MICHEL MERTES, MD, PhD
Professor and Chair
Service d'Anésthesie-réanimation
CHU de Nancy
Hôpital Central
Nancy, France
Chapter 106

NUALA J. MEYER, MD
Fellow
Pulmonary and Critical Care
University of Chicago
Chicago, Illinois
Chapter 27

BABAK MOKHLESI, MD
Assistant Professor of Medicine
Division of Pulmonary and Critical Care Medicine
John H. Striger Jr. Hospital of Cook County/Rush
University Medical Center
Chicago, Illinois
Chapter 102

JULIO S. G. MONTANER, MD
Professor of Medicine & Chair in AIDS Research
St. Paul's Hospital/University of British Columbia
Vancouver, British Columbia, Canada
Chapter 48

BUSI MOOKA, MD, MRCPI
Specialist Registrar
Department of Infectious Diseases
Mater Hospital
Dublin, Ireland
Chapter 56

JONATHAN MOSS, MD, PhD
Professor and Vice Chairman for Research
Dept. of Anesthesia & Critical Care
Professor of the College
Chairman, Institutional Review Board
University of Chicago
Chicago, Illinois
Chapter 106

RICHARD J. MOULTON, MD, FRCSC
Medical Director
Trauma and Neurosurgery Program
St. Michael's Hospital
Associate Professor of Surgery
University of Toronto
Toronto, Ontario, Canada
Chapter 93

PATRICK MURRAY, MD
Associate Professor of Anesthesia, Critical Care
and Medicine
(Nephrology)
University of Chicago
Chicago, Illinois
Chapters 75, 76, 102, 103

ROBERT MUSTARD, MD
Assistant Professor of Surgery
St. Michael's Hospital
Toronto, Ontario, Canada
Chapter 89

MARKKU S. NIEMINEN, MD
Professor and Chief
Division of Cardiology
University Central Hospital
Chairman
Task Force on Acute Heart Failure
European Society of Cardiology
Helsinki, Finland
Chapter 23

MICHAEL F. O'CONNOR, MD
Associate Professor
Department of Anesthesia and Critical Care
Department of Medicine
Section of Pulmonary and Critical Care
University of Chicago
Chicago, Illinois
Chapters 35, 105

ANDRANIK OVASSAPIAN
Professor
Department of Anesthesia and Critical Care
The University of Chicago
Chicago, Illinois
Chapter 35

JOSEPH E. PARRILLO, MD
Professor of Medicine
Robert Wood Johnson Medical School
University of Medicine and Dentistry of New Jersey
Head
Division of Cardiovascular Disease and Critical Care
Medicine
Director
Cooper Heart Institute
Director
Cardiovascular and Critical Care Services
Cooper University Hospital
Camden, New Jersey
Chapter 25

CLAUDE A. PIANTADOSI, MD
Professor of Medicine
Duke University Medical Center
Durham, North Carolina
Chapter 112

DANIEL PICUS, MD
Professor of Radiology and Surgery
Department of Radiology
Washington University School of Medicine
St. Louis, Missouri
Chapter 101

LAWRENCE H. PITTS, MD
Professor of Neurosurgery
University of California–San Francisco
San Francisco, California
Chapter 93

PETER PHILLIPS, MD
Head, Infectious Diseases
St. Paul's Hospital
Vancouver, British Columbia, Canada
Chapter 48

WILLIAM J. POWERS, MD
Professor of Neurology, Neurological Surgery
and Radiology
Head, Cerebrovascular Section
Department of Neurology
Washington University School of Medicine
St. Louis, MO
Chapter 63

KENNETH S. POLONSKY, MD
Adolphus Busch Professor
Head
Department of Internal Medicine
Washington University School of Medicine
St. Louis, Missouri
Chapter 78

STEVEN M. RANKIN, MD
Department of Nephrology
St. Joseph Hospital
Pontiac, Michigan
Chapter 76

BHARATHI REDDY, MD
Assistant Professor of Medicine
Section of Nephrology
University of Chicago
Chicago, Illinois
Chapter 75

SAMUEL REFETOFF, MD
Frederick H. Rawson Professor Emeritus
Endocrinology Section
Department of Medicine and Pediatrics
Director
Endocrinology Laboratory
University of Chicago
Chicago, Illinois
Chapter 80

JOHN A. ROBINSON, MD
Professor of Medicine and Microbiology
Director
Therapeutic Apheresis
Stritch School of Medicine
Loyola University Medical Center
Chicago, Illinois
Chapter 104

GRAEME ROCKER, MD
Professor of Medicine
Dalhousie University
Halifax, Nova Scotia, Canada
President, Canadian Critical Care Society
Halifax, Nova Scotia, Canada
Chapter 10

AXEL J. ROSENGART, MD, PhD
Assistant Professor
Departments of Neurology and Surgery
Assistant Director
Neuromedical/Neurosurgical Intensive Care
University of Chicago
Chicago, Illinois
Chapters 65, 67

JAMES A. RUSSELL, MD
Intensivist, St. Paul's Hospital
Principal Investigator, James Hogg Centre
for Cardiovascular & Pulmonary Research
Professor of Medicine, Critical Care Medicine
University of British Columbia
Vancouver, British Columbia, Canada
Chapters 6, 48

DAMON C. SCALES, MD, FRCPC
Clinical Associate
Department of Critical Care
St. Michael's Hospital
Toronto, Ontario, Canada
Chapter 90

WILLIAM MICHAEL SCHELD, MD
Bayer-Gerald N. Mandell Professor of Infectious Diseases
Professor of Internal Medicine
Clinical Professor of Neurosurgery
Co-Director of the Center for Global Health
University of Virginia School of Medicine
Charlottesville, Virginia
Chapter 52

THOMAS D. SCHIANO, MD
Associate Professor of Medicine
Division of Liver Diseases
Mount Sinai Medical Center
New York, New York
Chapter 81

GREGORY A. SCHMIDT, MD
Section of Pulmonary and Critical Care Medicine
Department of Medicine
University of Chicago
Chicago, Illinois
Chapters 1, 36

B.D. SCHOUTEN, MD
  Sepsis Critical Care Research Office
  The Wellesley Hospital
  Toronto, Ontario, Canada
  Chapter 89

GERARD J. SHEEHAN, MB
  Consultant Physician in Infectious Diseases
  Mater Misericordiae Hospital
  Dublin, Ireland
  Chapter 56

JAMES M. SIZEMORE, JR., MD, MSPH
  Assistant Professor of Medicine
  Division of Infectious Diseases
  University of Alabama–Birmingham
  Birmingham, Alabama
  Chapter 49

ARTHUR S. SLUTSKY, MD
  Professor of Medicine
  Surgery and Biomedical Engineering Division
  Director, Interdepartmental Division of
  Critical Care Medicine
  University of Toronto
  Vice President, Research
  St. Michael's Hospital
  Queen Wing
  Toronto, Ontario, Canada
  Chapter 37

MATTHEW J. SORRENTINO, MD
  Associate Professor of Medicine
  University of Chicago Prtizker
  School of Medicine
  Department of Medicine
  Section Cardiology
  Chicago, Illinois
  Chapter 29

MARY E. STREK, MD
  Associate Professor of Medicine and Clinical
  Pharmacology
  Section of Pulmonary and Critical Care Medicine
  University of Chicago
  Chicago, Illinois
  Chapter 105

RAM M. SUBRAMANIAN, MD
  Fellow, Sections of Pulmonary & Critical Care
  Medicine and Gastroenterology
  Department of Medicine
  University of Chicago
  Chicago, Illinois
  Chapter 82

KEITH M. SULLIVAN, MD
  James B. Wyngaarden Professor of Medicine
  Director, Long-Term Follow-up and
  Information Research Program
  Division of Cellular Therapy
  Duke University Medical Center
  Durham, North Carolina
  Chapter 73

BRYCE TAYLOR, MD, FRCSC, FACS
  Surgeon-in-Chief
  University Health Network
  Professor and Chair
  Department of Surgery
  University of Toronto
  Toronto, Ontario, Canada
  Chapter 85

FRANK THOMAS, MD, MBA
  Medical Director IHC Life Flight, Adult Services
  Co-Director Shock Trauma ICU, LDS Hospital
  Clinical Professor of Medicine
  University of Utah School of Medicine
  Critical Care Medicine
  LDS Hospital
  Salt Lake City, Utah
  Chapter 7

JOEL M. TOPF, MD
  Department of Nephrology
  St. John's Hospital
  Detroit, Michigan
  Chapter 76

ALLAN R. TUNKEL, MD, PhD
  Professor of Medicine
  Associate Dean for Admissions
  Drexel University College of Medicine
  Philadelphia, Pennsylvania
  Chapter 52

JOHN V. TYBERG, MD, PhD
  Professor of Medicine and Physiology & Biophysics
  Departments of Medicine and Cardiac Sciences
  Libin Cardiovascular Institute of Alberta
  University of Calgary
  Calgary, Alberta, Canada
  Chapter 28

D. LORNE TYRRELL, MD, PhD
  Professor
  Department of Medical Microbiology and Immunology
  University of Alberta
  Edmonton, Alberta, Canada
  Chapter 53

TERRY VANDEN HOEK, MD
  Associate Professor of Clinical Medicine
  Section of Emergency Medicine
  University of Chicago
  Chicago, Illinois
  Chapters 15, 16

ROBERT VERITY, MD
  Dynacare Kasper Medical Laboratories
  Edmonton, Alberta, Canada
  Chapter 53

KEITH R. WALLEY, MD
  Professor of Medicine
  University of British Columbia
  Vancouver, Canada
  Chapters 21, 22

JEFFREY G. WALLS, MD
Staff Physician
Pulmonary and Critical Care
Presbyterian Hospital
Charlotte, North Carolina
Chapter 9

FERGUS WALSH
Consultant Anesthetist
Cork University Hospital
Clinical Lecturer
University College Cork
Cork, Ireland
Chapter 88

DAVID A. WARRELL, MA, DM, DSc
Professor of Tropical Medicine and Infectious Diseases
Founding Director of the Centre of Tropical Medicine
(Emeritus)
University of Oxford
Oxford
United Kingdom
Chapter 58

DAVID K. WARREN, MD
Assistant Professor
Division of Infectious Diseases
Department of Medicine
Washington University School of Medicine
Hospital Epidemiologist
Barnes-Jewish Hospital
Saint Louis, Missouri
Chapter 4

STEPHEN G. WEBER, MD, MS
Assistant Professor of Medicine
Section of Infectious Diseases
Hospital Epidemiologist
Director, Infection Control Program
The University of Chicago
Chicago, Illinois
Chapter 57

ROY E. WEISS, MD, PhD, FACP
Professor of Medicine
Director
Clinical Research Center
Department of Medicine
University of Chicago
Chicago, Illinois
Chapter 80

MICHAEL JUDE WELSCH, MD
Resident
Section of Dermatology
University of Chicago
Chicago, Illinois
Chapter 107

DAVID WILLIAMS, MD
Emergency Physician
Intermountain Health Care
Salt Lake City, Utah
Chapter 7

LAWRENCE D.H. WOOD, MD, PhD
Professor of Medicine
Section of Pulmonary and Critical Care
Medicine
Department of Medicine
University of Chicago
Chicago, Illinois
Chapters 1, 20, 42

GARY P. ZALOGA, MD
Medical Director, Methodist Research Institute
Clinical Professor of Medicine
Indiana University
Indianapolis, Indiana
Chapter 79

JANICE L. ZIMMERMAN, MD
Professor of Medicine
Baylor College of Medicine
Director, Medicine Emergency Services
Associate Chief, Medicine Service
Ben Taub General Hospital
Houston, Texas
Chapters 110, 111

PREFACE

The field of critical care has exploded since we last revised this textbook in 1998. In particular, the large number of high-quality clinical trials performed to elucidate mechanisms of critical illness and to guide clinical care has reverberated through ICUs around the world and generated tremendous excitement. A decade ago, intensivists managed patients based largely on an in-depth understanding of cardiopulmonary pathophysiology, coupled with a broad understanding of internal medicine, surgery, and a few related fields. The last decade has added to this a wealth of evidence revealing that there are better and worse ways to manage our patients. The modern intensivist must both master a complex science of pathophysiology and be intimately familiar with an increasingly specialized literature. No longer can critical care be considered the cobbling together of cardiology, nephrology, trauma surgery, gastroenterology, and other organ-based fields of medicine. In the 21st century, the specialty of critical care has truly come of age.

Why have a textbook at all in the modern era? Whether at home, in the office, or on the road, we can access electronically our patients' vital signs, radiographs, and test results; at the click of a mouse we can peruse the literature of the world; consulting experts beyond our own institutions is facilitated through email, listserves, and web-based discussion groups. Do we still have time to read books?

We believe the answer is a resounding yes. Indeed, the torrent of complex—and, at times, conflicting—data can be overwhelming for even the most diligent intensivist. We have challenged our expert contributors to deal with controversy, yet provide explicit guidance to our readers. Experts can evaluate new information in the context of their reason and experience to develop balanced recommendations for the general intensivist who may have neither the time nor inclination to do it all himself.

A definitive text of critical care must achieve two goals: the explication of the complex pathophysiology common to all critically ill patients, and the in-depth discussion of procedures, diseases, and issues integral to the care of the critically ill. The exceptional response to the first two editions of *Principles* showed us that we succeeded in meeting these goals. In this third edition, we have made numerous changes in line with the tremendous evolution in our field. We have deleted the illustrative cases and their discussion to make room for exciting new chapters dealing with catastrophe-preparedness,

therapeutic hypothermia, interpreting ventilator waveforms, adrenal dysfunction, telemedicine, biowarfare, intravascular devices, angioedema, massive hemoptysis, and evidence-based prophylactic strategies, among others. The changing nature of our patients and increasing recognition of complications following critical illness by weeks, months and years spawned chapters on obesity in critical illness, chronic critical illness, long-term outcomes, delirium, and economics of critical care. We have completely revised many chapters to keep pace with changing concepts in nutrition, myocardial ischemia, airway management, ARDS, severe sepsis, cardiac rhythm disturbances, pericardial disease, status epilepticus, intracranial hypertension, blood transfusion, acute renal failure, acid-base disorders, electrolyte disturbances, gastrointestinal hemorrhage, fulminant hepatic failure, cirrhosis, mesenteric ischemia, gastrointestinal infections, coma, care of the organ donor, toxicology, dermatologic conditions, sickle cell disease, hypothermia, and hyperthermia. Finally, a former colleague, Dr. V. Theodore Barnett, an intensivist with extensive experience in the melting pot of Hawaii, has contributed an introduction that reminds all of us of the challenges and opportunities we face when dealing with our multicultural patients and their families.

We have collected up front many of the issues of organization which provide the foundation for excellent critical care as well as topics germane to almost any critically ill patient. The remainder of the text follows an organ system orientation for in-depth, up-to-date descriptions of the unique presentation, differential diagnosis, and management of specific critical illnesses. While we have made many changes, we have preserved the strengths of the first two editions: a solid grounding in pathophysiology, appropriate skepticism based in scholarly review of the literature, and user-friendly chapters beginning with "Key Points."

We attempted to preserve our vision and approach in the third edition of *Principles of Critical Care* by contributing approximately one fourth of the total chapters ourselves and recruiting associate editors and colleagues who share our vision concerning academic critical care. In general, we are convinced that clinical scholarship in critical care is conferred by balanced involvement in both management and investigation of critical illness, so we invited two associate editors who actively deliver intensive care and publish about it. Our selection of associate editors having a shared spirit was considerably aided by our having practiced, researched, published, or taught with both.

Dr. Jameel Ali is a Canadian trauma surgeon actively involved in providing and teaching ATLS and critical care in North America. His wide range of publications on critical care topics addresses mechanisms in basic science journals such as the *Journal of Applied Physiology* and clinical investigations in the best surgical and medical journals. From this base in surgical critical care and its considerable overlap with anesthesiology and medicine, Dr. Ali coordinated most of the chapters aimed at essential surgical aspects of critical care and those related to the gastrointestinal system, while authoring (or co-authoring) four chapters himself. Dr. Keith Walley is another Canadian intensivist who combines basic and clinical investigation with his practice and teaching of critical care. He helped organize the sections covering general management and cardiovascular diseases and contributed two chapters himself.

We have encouraged our contributors to state cautiously and with experimental support their diagnostic and therapeutic approaches to critical illness, and to acknowledge that each approach has adverse effects, in order to define the least intervention required to achieve its stated therapeutic goal. With the help of our associate editors, our review process was closer to that enforced by excellent peer-reviewed journals than that encountered by most contributors of invited book chapters. We hope the attendant frustrations and revisions of the authors provide a better learning experience for the readers.

Our approach to patient care, teaching, and investigation of critical care is energized fundamentally by our clinical practice. In turn, our practice is informed, animated, and balanced by the information and environment arising around learning and research. Clinical excellence is founded in careful history taking, physical examination, and laboratory testing. These data serve to raise questions concerning the mechanisms for the patient's disease, upon which a complete, prioritized differential diagnosis is formulated and treatment plan initiated. The reality, complexity, and limitations apparent in the ICU drive our search for better understanding of the pathophysiology of critical care and new, effective therapies.

We enjoy teaching principles of critical care! We came to our affection for teaching the diagnosis and treatment of critical illness through internal medicine, albeit by different tracks. Two of us (JH, GS) were educated at the University of Chicago's Pritzker School of Medicine and Internal Medicine Residency before serving as chief medical residents in 1981 and 1985, respectively. The other (LW) graduated in medicine from the University of Manitoba in Winnipeg, Canada, completed a PhD program at McGill University in Montreal in the course of his internal medicine residency, then joined the critical care faculty in Winnipeg in 1975. There, critical care had a long tradition of effective collaboration among anesthesiol-

ogists, internists, and surgeons in the ICU and in the research laboratories. When we three began to work together at the University of Chicago in 1982, our experience in programs emphasizing clinical excellence combined with our questioning, mechanistic approach to patients' problems to help establish a robust and active clinical critical care service with prominent teaching and research activities. Our teaching program was built upon the components of: 1) an understanding of underlying pathophysiology; 2) a state-of-the-art knowledge of current diagnosis and management of problems in the ICU; 3) a familiarity and experience with the tools and results of basic and clinical investigation in critical care; and 4) an appreciation of the issues and methods of ICU organization and management. We have attempted to make this text incorporate just these components in its explication of the principles of critical care, and hope that the text continues to be a well-received and valued extension of our teaching methodology beyond the confines of the University of Chicago.

In addition to our associate editors and individual authors, others too numerous to mention facilitated the completion of this book. We are especially indebted to our own students of critical care at the University of Chicago who motivate our teaching – our critical care fellows; residents in anesthesia, medicine, neurology, obstetrics and gynecology, pediatrics, and surgery; and the medical students at the Pritzker School of Medicine. Our colleagues in providing critical care within the section, Edward Naureckas, John Kress, Brian Gehlbach, John McConville, Imre Noth, and Kyle Hogarth, combine with others in our institution such as Michael O'Connor, Avery Tung, Axel Rosengart, Jeffrey Frank, Michael Woo, Patrick Murray, and Lawrence Gottlieb, to make our practice of interdisciplinary critical care at the University of Chicago interesting and exciting.

Even with all this help, we could not have completed the organization and editing of this book without the combined efforts of many at McGraw-Hill. Our editors have guided this group of academic physicians through the world of publishing to bring our skills and ideas to a wide audience, and we are thankful for their collaboration.

Finally, the revision of a book such as this one is a major adventure that could not succeed simply through the efforts of its senior authors, nor the considerable contributions of our many colleagues, nor the meticulous work of its publisher. This book would never have seen the light of day without the untiring support of Cora D. Taylor, our editorial assistant, a remarkable colleague who guided all of our efforts through the day-to-day difficulties of writing this text. To this task she brought organization, persistence, and a sense of humor that delighted and aided all who were fortunate enough to work with her. We especially acknowledge her contributions, without which we would not likely have overcome the innumerable impediments during the three years of revising this book.

INTRODUCTION

"An elderly Hindu in a British hospital was found lying on the floor, so, thinking that he had fallen out of bed, the nurses placed him back. Shortly afterwards he was found on the floor again. He could not speak English to explain that he thought he was dying and wanted to die on the floor where he would be near Mother Earth, so that his soul could leave more freely than in a bed. Like many Hindus, he had a clear model of how he should die, yet he died alone, before his family could be summoned to perform the final rituals."

Shirley Firth, *Dying, Death and Bereavement in a British Hindu Community*

Caring For Critically Ill Patients and Their Families: Culture Matters

The probability of any two random persons in America being of the same ethnicity is 0.49; 58% of medical critical care fellows are graduates of foreign medical schools. These two facts are enough to explain why a discussion of cross-cultural medicine should be placed at the front of a critical care text. Diversity and cultural sensitivity are concepts which are much in the forefront of recent conversations regarding medicine. However, much of what is done with these concepts and realties is simplistic, and many of the tools purporting to help cultural sensitivity do little more than reinforce prejudgment and stereotypes.

Practitioners struggling to deal with the bewildering array of ethnicities, religions and cultures with which they are confronted and must interact could be forgiven for being overwhelmed. Learning the nuances of even one culture takes years of study. When that culture is confronted with an entrenched biomedical culture the complications multiply. It is therefore not possible to state in detail the proper way to approach any particular type of patient or family. The best that can be done is to learn what some of the fundamental issues are, and how to sensibly and practically approach them in the daily care of patients in the intensive care unit. Although there is some evidence of higher satisfaction when the patient and provider are similar in demographics, matching patients and physicians by demographics is neither reasonable nor desirable.

A look at the basic language and terms involved can illustrate the complexity of the situation and begin a process of coming to terms with this challenge. Culture has been described in many ways, but for purposes of simplicity can be defined as a system of beliefs and a learned and ingrained worldview that goes beyond surface belief to patterns of core values and meaning.

Culture should not be confused with either ethnicity or race. Race is a term which has no biological validity. The concept of race as a valid biological categorization has been refuted by the American Anthropological Association, and in general the term has no scientific meaning. Ethnicity refers to the ethnic background into which a person was born. It is generally similar to culture but can be very different (as in cross-ethnic adoption); although often used as a marker for culture, "ethnicity" and "culture" are not synonymous and cannot simply be used as such.

Acculturation modifies the effects of culture. This has long been recognized by immigrants themselves. The Japanese in America classify themselves as Issei, Nisei, Sansei, and Yonsei for successive generations after immigration. This is a tacit recognition that worldview and interaction with the dominant culture changes with increasing exposure to, and assimilation of pieces of, that culture. The rate of acculturation varies tremendously among immigrants, in part due to the degree to which cultural continuity is maintained in a specific locale as opposed to integration into the larger community.

A textbook discussion of specific issues and table of possible solutions does not remove the complexity of cultural diversity. What must be appreciated is the enormous variation in human belief and desires regarding health, illness, and dying. A realization and admission of lack of knowledge and beliefs is the first step. The one specific piece of information regarding your patient from whatever culture, ethnicity, nationality and religion that can be given is this: You do not know what they believe until you ask them, and that asking opens a dialogue of extraordinary value to all concerned.

Specific Considerations

COMMUNICATION

The ideal person to act as an interpreter in these situations is a cultural interpreter. This person can not only translate the words and conversation but interpret the appropriate social customs and mores and help in dealing with areas of cultural incongruity by interpreting the worldview and resultant

TABLE I-1 Communication During Critical Care

Subject	Possible Issue	Mechanism of Improving Care
Language	Miscommunication	Interpreter, translator second choice
Decision-Making	Alternate models	Clear delineation of decision maker early
Religion	Need for rituals	Trained chaplains, connections with sectarian clergy
Autonomy	No desire for autonomy	Clarify decision making with patient and family on admission
Visitation	Entire family with children	Allow maximal family interactions as possible including children

desire for care on each side of the physician/patient relationship. Unfortunately, cultural interpreters are uncommon and difficult–if not impossible–to obtain for all cultures that an intensivist may come into contact with. Many persons who act as interpreters can, although not trained, act as a valuable cultural resource. This, however, requires the practitioner to understand their limitations and the potential problems, and to ask the interpreter the proper questions about approach to the family and patient, and manner of dealing with them. A true interpreter, as opposed to a translator, will perform some of these tasks. They may say, for example, that in a particular culture the phrase "we'll think about it" generally means "we have decided to proceed but must wait a respectable period of time." That is the difference between a strict translator of words and an interpreter of meaning. An interpreter is the least that is required for true understanding; but again, this is not possible in many hospitals and in many situations, e.g., in the middle of the night where decisions are crucial and the abilities and resources at hand must be used. All too often a family member is recruited to translate. To make matters worse this is often a minor who knows English by virtue of school. Only under extreme circumstances should a family member be used to translate. Conscious and unconscious filtering are common in this situation. Almost as bad, a person who is available but untrained in either communication skills or medical interpreting is drafted into service. Hospitals have lists of translators but these persons have generally received little or no formal training. If these persons must be used (and realistically it cannot be avoided), training should be mandatory. It should not be forgotten, however, as with any other tool in the ICU, that using a strict translator is not using the optimal resource and obtaining the optimal information, and that inaccurate information may well be transmitted.

ETHICS

Many of the precepts of western biomedical ethics which are taken as undeniable truths in much of American medicine are simply cultural constructs which are subject to the same intercultural variability as all other cultural constructs. Three of these of primary importance in the ICU are autonomy, truth-telling, and beneficence.

Autonomy, as it regards decision making, becomes an issue as patients are admitted to the ICU and end-of-life discussions are begun. They often become a moot point by the time decisions occur concerning the pursuit of very aggressive care or withdrawal of care, as the patient is no longer capacitated for medical decision making. However, it must be noted from the beginning of the patient's admission that multiple models of decision making are possible. In many cultures, the concept that a patient would have the autonomy to bankrupt their family and put enormous strains on their community

without input from those larger entities would simply be unacceptable. Therefore, it is important to identify the mode of family communication and the decision-making processes of the family, as much as possible. Simply asking the family who will make the decisions and how is important. Truth-telling enters into the autonomy equation. Many cultures consider it potentially harmful to tell a patient they have a terminal illness, because telling a person they are dying may make that likelihood a certainty.

What is therefore needed at times is a hybrid. We are unwilling to give up our ethics as we feel we must practice them, and yet we are ethically obliged to respect the wishes of the patient. At times we have to respect the autonomy of a patient to make the decision to not be autonomous. Discussions with the patient regarding whom they feel should make the decisions, whether it should be them or another member of the family, are necessary in many cultural contexts. In addition, along with that discussion, a discussion concerning whether the patient wants to know their diagnosis and prognosis is important. It would seem, if autonomy is to be respected fully, that a patient should have the right to say "I do not want to know and please give my family the medical information and allow them to make the decisions." It is sometimes helpful to have a discussion with patients who are ambiguous about full knowledge in a third person way. "What would you think about a person who had this diagnosis or who had this happening to them or was going to have this happen to them?" "How do you feel this type of situation should be handled?" Those kinds of discussions with some degree of individual dissociation can be helpful in allowing a patient of any culture to discuss subjects that would otherwise not be acceptable, or emotionally or intellectually possible, topics of discussion.

FAMILY AND VISITATION

Intensive care units have traditionally had very restrictive visitation policies. These have, in general, become less stringent in recent years. They still clash with the feeling of many families regarding family presence at a sick bed. In many cultures it is regarded as a familial obligation for at least one member of the family to be present at the sick bed of a gravely ill person at all times. Although this is at times inconvenient for the medical staff, it is only rarely contraindicated and at these times having a family member wait outside the room is generally acceptable for all. Visitation by children and the presence of children in the rooms of the gravely ill also varies. Whether children are capable of handling visitation in the ICU is a decision best left to those family members who know them best. Their presence should be allowed unless there is a significant contraindication, particularly in end-of-life situations. In many cultures it is seen as quite normal to expose children to all aspects of life and death, and their exclusion leads to a sense of lacking a full family presence. This is particularly true in withdrawal of care situations.

PAIN CONTROL

The question of pain control has been addressed in several recent discussions regarding end-of-life care. It is generally taken as a tenet of end-of-life care that pain should be abolished if possible and maximally controlled if removal of pain is not possible. There are beliefs, particularly religious beliefs, regarding the redemptive value of pain. This exists in several religious traditions including the Catholic and Islamic traditions. It should not, however, be presumed that a member of these religions wishes to suffer, or that members of other religions do not. The presence of multiple meanings of pain simply needs to be realized. Our beliefs must be checked with the those of the patient, and their wishes followed.

RELIGION

Religion is often closely tied to culture and ethnicity. In many tribal societies, prior to western contact, religion was not defined as separate from the rest of life. Most commonly, however, we are dealing with patients with specific religious beliefs. Virtually all hospitals have chaplains or ministers of specific denominations. It is best to make an institutional relationship with religious leaders of any denomination with which significant contact is likely given the population of intensive care patients. In general, a chaplain trained in hospital chaplaincy can deal with most contingencies in helping the family cope. There are, however, specific rites and rituals which do require the presence of a practitioner with knowledge and credentials of the religion in question.

Treatises on specific religious beliefs regarding health and end-of-life issues can be found, but given the extraordinary proliferation of subgroups within any religion, generalities should be avoided and specific guidance sought from the family and their spiritual counselor.

END-OF-LIFE AND WITHDRAWAL OF CARE

Death is where the effects of culture impact most strongly in the ICU. Biomedicine often views death as a simple physiologic concept which all staff know can be confirmed by a rapid exam. It is, in reality, a complex and mutable concept. As illness is culturally defined, even death is subject to cultural definition. There are persons in the mainstream of American culture who believe death is the final event of a physical body with nothing further. There are those who know with equal assurance that there is a soul which lives on after the body and goes to one of a number of different fates. To the individuals involved these are less beliefs than truths and ways of defining existence. It is important to realize that this same tremendous diversity of ethical certainty and potential incompatibility of beliefs occurs in many situations. Regarding death, there has also been a long tradition in several cultures of regarding persons as being in the category of the dead before what we would consider physiologic death. Lest this seem ridiculous, it is worth remembering that within the last few decades biomedicine has changed the definition of death to now include persons whose brain function has irreversibly ceased. The full import of this change in a definition of death which has existed for the entire history of mankind can be felt at times when dealing with families who have not kept up with the pace of our changing medical beliefs, or whose faith does not allow them to acknowledge brain death. There are places in America and throughout the world where religion determines whether a person is deemed dead or not–a remarkable example of the influence of culture and religion on what we often believe are definitive medical concepts.

The events surrounding end-of-life are of particular interest to clinicians and researchers today. We should in no way believe, however, that we have created the concepts of the dying, the near-dead, and persons who are for most purposes dead although physiologically alive. Each of those concepts exists in multiple cultures throughout the world and has for millennia. It would be extreme hubris on our part to believe that we have somehow discovered dying and can now somehow manage it. We must learn from the billions of human beings who have already faced this situation with their families and communities. To do otherwise would be a disservice to our humanity.

TRUST

Patients and families from traditionally underprivileged ethnicities and poorer socioeconomic classes may have issues with trust in the dominant biomedical structure. The legacy of grievous breaches of ethics, and even currently documented inequality in care, leave a cloud of suspicion over recommendations to withdraw care in some patients. Families, with some historical justification, have suspicions of the medical establishment and the motives for recommendations which are made. It is also a concern among some minority patients and families that recommendations, particularly regarding limitation of expensive technology or withdrawal of care, are potentially being made for economic and not medical reasons. These are very difficult situations to resolve once mistrust has arisen. Clear communication from the beginning can help avoid such situations. Once a situation arises, involvement of medical personal of similar cultural background and the involvement of community resources in the dialogue can be helpful.

Recommendations

Several articles have examined some of the specific issues addressed here in more depth and have resources and additional suggestions for approaches to cross-cultural care.

What we must focus on when faced with a culture and belief system different than our own is attempting to understand how that person or persons knows the world. We must ask and listen to their answers regarding how they know disease, life and death. We must learn how to discern what is important to our patients and families, not try to focus on any specific belief of any group. It is impossible to know all of the answers. The best we can hope for is knowing what questions to ask.

V. Theodore Barnett, MD
Division of Pulmonary and Critical Care Medicine
Medical College of Wisconsin
Milwaukee, Wisconsin

PRINCIPLES OF CRITICAL CARE

PART I

AN OVERVIEW OF THE APPROACH TO AND ORGANIZATION OF CRITICAL CARE

Chapter 1

AN APPROACH TO CRITICAL CARE

JESSE B. HALL
GREGORY A. SCHMIDT
LAWRENCE D. H. WOOD

KEY POINTS

- *Thoughtful clinical decision making often contributes more to the patient's outcome than dramatic and innovative interventions or cutting-edge technology.*
- *Formulate clinical hypotheses, then test them.*
- *Define therapeutic goals and seek the least intensive intervention that achieves each.*
- *Novel treatments require objective clinical trials before they are implemented, and traditional therapies require clarification of goals and adverse effects in each patient before their use can be optimized.*
- *Determine daily whether the appropriate therapeutic goal is treatment for cure or treatment for palliation.*
- *Critical care is invigorated by a scholarly approach, involving teaching, learning, and performing research.*

Intensive care has its roots in the resuscitation of dying patients. Exemplary critical care provides rapid therapeutic responses to failure of vital organ systems, utilizing standardized and effective protocols such as advanced cardiac life support and advanced trauma life support. Other critically ill patients in less urgent need of resuscitation are vulnerable to multiple organ system failure, and benefit from prevention or titrated care of each organ system dysfunction according to principles for reestablishing normal physiology. This critical care tempo differs from the time-honored rounding and prescription practiced by most internists and primary care physicians. Furthermore, the critical care physicians providing resuscitation and titrated care often have little firsthand familiarity with their patients' chronic health history, but extraordinary tools for noninvasive and invasive description and correction of their current pathophysiology. Though well prepared for providing cure of the acute life-threatening problems, the intensivist is frequently disappointed to be the bearer of bad news when recovery is impossible, and increasingly must develop and use compassionate pastoral skills to help comfort dying patients and their significant others, using clinical judgment to help them decide to forego further life-sustaining treatment. Accordingly, experienced intensivists develop ways to curb their inclination toward action in order to minimize complications of critical care, while organizing the delivery of critical care to integrate and coordinate the efforts of many team members to help minimize the intrinsic tendency toward fragmented care. In academic critical care units, teaching and investigation of critical care are energized by the clinical practice; in turn, the practice is informed, animated, and balanced by the information and environment arising from and around teaching and research

programs. Yet the vast majority of critical care is delivered in community-based ICUs not affiliated with universities, where critical care physicians rely on their penchant for lifelong learning to update their knowledge and skills through informed reading and attending continuing medical education critical care conferences. These activities in providing, teaching, and investigating critical care contribute to a unique perspective on and approach to medicine among critical care physicians.

Providing Exemplary Care

DEVELOP AND TRUST YOUR CLINICAL SKILLS

Clinical excellence is founded in careful history taking, physical examination, and laboratory testing. These data serve to raise questions concerning the mechanisms for the patient's disease, on which a complete prioritized differential diagnosis is formulated and treatment plan initiated. The reality, complexity, and limitations apparent daily in the ICU present several pitfalls on the path to exemplary practice. By its very nature, critical care is exciting and attracts physicians having an inclination toward action. Despite its obvious utility in urgent circumstances, this proclivity can replace effective clinical discipline with excessive unfocused ICU procedures. This common approach inverts the stable pyramid of bedside skills, placing most attention on the least informative source of data, while losing the rational foundation for diagnosis and treatment.

FORMULATE CLINICAL HYPOTHESES AND TEST THEM

An associated problem is that ICU procedures become an end in themselves rather than a means to answer thoughtful clinical questions. Too often these procedures are implemented to provide monitoring, ignoring the fact that the only alarm resides in the intensivist's intellect. Students of critical care benefit from the dictum: "Don't just do something, stand there." Take the time to process the gathered data to formulate a working hypothesis concerning the mechanisms responsible for each patient's main problems, so that the next diagnostic or treatment intervention can best test that possibility. Without this thoughtful clinical decision making, students of critical care are swept away by the burgeoning armamentarium of the ICU toward the unproductive subspecialty of critical care technology. So often in the ICU thoughtful compilation of the patient's health evaluation preceding the acute event is more helpful than acquiring new data defining the current pathophysiologic state. Accordingly, attention to this search for meaningful collateral history and the retrieval of prior radiologic studies and laboratory values often should precede the next invasive ICU procedure. The next intervention should be chosen to test a diagnostic hypothesis formulated by thoughtful processing of the available data.

Testing a therapeutic hypothesis requires knowing the goal of the intervention and titrating the therapy toward that end point. Too often students of initial care employ too little too late during resuscitation. For example, the patient with hypovolemic shock receives a bolus of 250 mL of crystalloid solution followed by 200 mL/h infused through two 18-gauge needles in peripheral veins, while the mean blood pressure (bp) rises from 50 to 60 mm Hg over 2 hours. A far better volume resuscitation protocol targets urgent restoration of a normal bp and perfusion, so it establishes central venous access for a bolus of 3 L of warmed crystalloid and colloid in 20 minutes, to continue at that rate until the bp exceeds 90 mm Hg without inducing pulmonary edema. As another example, a patient requires intubation and ventilation with 100% oxygen for acute hypoxemic respiratory failure. Positive end-expiratory pressure (PEEP) is increased from 0 to 5 to 10 cm H_2O overnight, while arterial O_2 saturation (Sa_{O_2}) increases from 70% to 80% to 90% and bp remains at 95 mm Hg. A better PEEP resuscitation protocol targets an Sa_{O_2} of >90% on an inspired O_2 fraction ($F_{I_{O_2}}$) of <0.6, so it increases PEEP by 5-cm-H_2O increments from 0 to 20 cm H_2O at 5-minute intervals, dropping $F_{I_{O_2}}$ as tolerated until the end point is achieved unless bp falls. If bp does fall unacceptably, positive inotropic therapy or volume infusion corrects the hypotension, allowing further PEEP increments toward the end point. In each of the better protocols, a clinical hypothesis about the mechanism of the critical illness—(1) the patient is hypovolemic, so rapid volume infusion will correct the hypotension, or (2) the hypoxemia is due to airspace flooding, so PEEP will correct the shunt—can be tested by titration of therapy toward a thoughtful end point without causing common adverse effects (Fig. 1-1). The results are more timely correction of life-threatening conditions.

LIBERATE FROM INTERVENTIONS SO THERE ARE NOT MORE TREATMENTS THAN DIAGNOSES

One of the consequences of protocol-driven resuscitations is that the recovered patient now has more treatments than diagnoses. An effective approach to the adverse outcome of excess therapeutic interventions is the mindset that liberates the patient from these potentially harmful interventions as rapidly as their removal is tolerated. For example, the patient with hemorrhagic shock treated with volume resuscitation and blood products also received intravenous vasoconstricting agents to maintain perfusion pressure while hemostasis

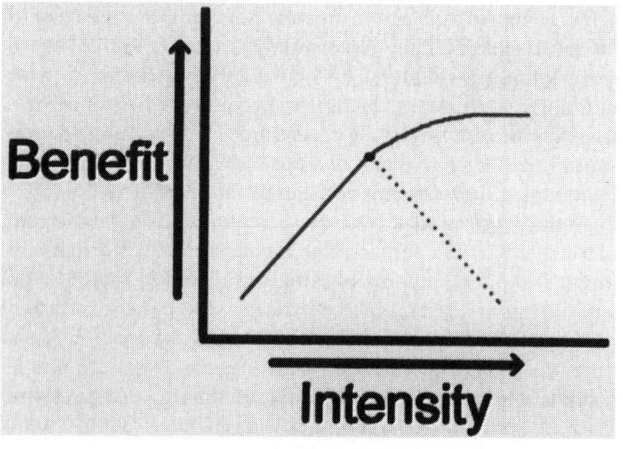

FIGURE 1-1 A schematic diagram relating therapeutic intensity (*abscissa*) to the benefit of therapy (*ordinate*). For many interventions in critical illness, there is a monotonic increase in benefit as treatment intensity increases (*solid line*), but concomitant adverse effects of the intervention cause harm at higher intensity (*interrupted line*) (for examples, see text). This leads to an approach to critical care that defines the overall goal of each intervention and seeks the least intense means of achieving it.

and volume resuscitation were achieved. Once a stable blood pressure and hemostasis are achieved, what is the time course for discontinuing the β-agonist therapy?

One answer is to wean the vasoconstrictor slowly (e.g., decrease the norepinephrine infusion rate from 30 μg per minute by 5 μg per minute each hour). Another approach is to liberate the patient from the vasoconstrictor by reducing the norepinephrine infusion rate by half every 15 minutes. The difference between these two approaches is more than the time taken to discontinue the agent, for if in the second approach the bp were to fall after reducing the norepinephrine to 15 μg per minute, the critical care physician learns that the patient remains hypovolemic and needs more volume infusion; the first approach would mask the hypovolemic hypoperfused state by the prolonged use of vasoconstrictor agents, leading to the adverse consequences of multiple organ hypoperfusion. Words convey meaning, and to *wean* connotes the removal of a nurturing, even friendly life-support system from a dependent, deprived infant, a process that should proceed slowly; by contrast, *liberation* is the removal of an unnecessary and potentially toxic intervention from an otherwise independent adult, a process that should proceed urgently.[1]

DEFINE THERAPEUTIC GOALS AND SEEK THE LEAST INTENSIVE INTERVENTION THAT ACHIEVES EACH

The principle from this example applies to many other critical care therapies, such as liberation from the ventilator, vasoactive drugs, and sedative and muscle-relaxing agents. Of course, the difficulty in all these examples is that the therapeutic intervention is initially life-saving, but how long the intervention needs to continue for the patient's benefit versus the patient's harm depends on a critical evaluation of the goal of therapy.

Figure 1-1 indicates the intensity-benefit relationship of many of these interventions (e.g., the continued use of high-dose norepinephrine in the hypotensive patient with hemorrhagic shock discussed earlier). During the initial resuscitation, the benefit of increasing the norepinephrine dose along the *x* axis (intensity) was demonstrated by the rising bp during hemostasis, volume resuscitation, and norepinephrine infusion. Yet bp is not the appropriate benefit sought in the hypoperfused patient, but rather adequate perfusion of all organs. Even without measuring cardiac output, an adequate perfusion state could be inferred from an adequate bp when the vasoconstrictor agent is diminished. However, with continued infusion of the vasoconstrictor, the adverse effect of a prolonged hypoperfusion state, even with an adequate bp, is indicated by the interrupted line, which illustrates a decreasing benefit as the intensity of the intervention and the shock it masks continues. Armed with this rationale, the intensivist should progressively reduce the intensity of norepinephrine infusion over a relatively short period to determine whether the volume resuscitation is adequate.

A second example is the use of fluid restriction and diuresis in the treatment of pulmonary edema. In Fig. 1-1 the intensity of the intervention is the reduction of the pulmonary capillary wedge pressure (PCWP), while the benefit would be the reduction of pulmonary edema. Considerable data suggest a monotonic relationship between the intensity of these therapeutic interventions and the benefit of reduced pulmonary edema.[2] Yet, if the PCWP is reduced too much, there is a consequent reduction in the cardiac output, so the benefit to the patient is more than offset by the attendant hypoperfusion state. The thoughtful intensivist recognizes that the goal of reducing PCWP and pulmonary edema should not induce a hypoperfusion state, so the targeted intensity is the lowest PCWP associated with an adequate cardiac output and oxygen delivery to the peripheral tissues. Similarly, for PEEP therapy, considerable data suggest that the higher the PEEP intensity, the greater will be the reduction in intrapulmonary shunt as the benefit to the patient. Yet the thoughtful intensivist recognizes that PEEP has adverse effects, as indicated by the interrupted line in Fig. 1-1 showing decreasing benefit as the intensity increases due to pulmonary barotrauma and decreased cardiac output. Accordingly, the goals of PEEP therapy should be the least PEEP that provides the end points of PEEP therapy—90% saturation of an adequate circulating hemoglobin on a nontoxic F_{IO_2}. Of course, the adverse effects of PEEP can be diminished by concomitant decreases in tidal volume, as currently practiced in "lung-protective ventilation" (see Chaps. 37 and 38).[2]

FIRST DO NO HARM

Beyond enhancing the clinical scholarship of critical care, this approach maximizes another hallowed principle of patient care—"First do no harm." Despite excited opinions to the contrary, effective critical care is rarely based on brilliant, incisive, dramatic, and innovative interventions, but most often derives from meticulously identifying and titrating each of the patient's multiple problems toward improvements at an urgent but continuous pace. This conservative approach breeds skepticism toward innovative strategies: Novel treatments require objective clinical trials before they are implemented, and traditional therapies require clarification of goals and adverse effects in each patient before their use can be optimized. Accordingly, intensivists should carefully consider the experimental support for each diagnostic and therapeutic approach to critical illness and acknowledge that each approach has adverse effects in order to define the least intensive intervention required to achieve its stated therapeutic goal.

ORGANIZE THE CRITICAL CARE TEAM

The ICU is no longer simply a room in which ventilators are used. Instead, in a well-functioning ICU, the physical plant and technology are planned to facilitate the delivery of care, while also responding to new opportunities in this rapidly evolving field. The physician director, the nurse manager, and the respiratory therapist must build a mutually supportive environment conducive to teaching, learning, and care. Intensivists must be aware of the economic and legal concerns as ICUs capture the interest of politicians, ethicists, and the courts. Furthermore, the managers of ICUs should build on experience. Quality assurance, triage and severity scoring, and infection surveillance are essential to the continued smooth running of ICUs and indeed to their improvement over time.[3]

Managing Death and Dying in the Intensive Care Unit

Perhaps no critical care issue is more emotionally charged and time-consuming than the decision to withhold and/or withdraw life-sustaining therapy (see Chap. 17). Practition-

ers and students of critical care are frequently called on to guide patients and their families through this new, complex decision-making process without much prior personal experience or literature on which to rely. Accordingly, we discuss an approach to managing death and dying in the ICU meant to minimize one current adverse outcome of modern critical care—our patients die alone in pain and distress because maximal care aimed at cure proceeds despite little chance of success.

DECIDE WHETHER THE PATIENT IS DYING

In a recent analysis of 6110 deaths in 126 ICUs between January and July of 1996, approximately half were associated with the decision to withhold or to withdraw ICU care, as distinguished from deaths after CPR or with full ICU care but no CPR.[4] One interesting feature of this study was the heterogeneity among different units, with some units reporting 90% of deaths associated with withholding and withdrawing ICU care, and others reporting less than 10% associated with this decision. Considerable discussion in the recent literature focuses on the definition of medical futility, and many intensive care physicians are perplexed regarding how to utilize the vagaries of survivorship data to be confident that continuing therapy would be futile.[5]

Yet many of these same physicians have a clear answer to another formulation of the question "Is this patient dying?"[6] An increasing number of critical care physicians are answering "yes" to this question based on their evaluation of the patient's chronic health history, the trajectory of the acute illness, and the number of organ systems currently failing. When the physician concludes that the patient is dying, this information needs to be communicated to the patient, or as so often happens in the ICU, to the significant other of the dying patient who is unable to communicate and has not left advance directives. This communication involves two complex processes: **1.** helping the patient or the significant others with the decision to withhold or withdraw life-sustaining therapy, and **2.** helping them process the grief this decision entails (Table 1-1).

CHANGE THE GOAL OF THERAPY FROM CURE TO COMFORT

In our view, this decision is best aided by a clear, brief explanation of the patient's condition and why the physician believes the patient is dying. When the patient or significant other has had the opportunity to challenge or clarify that explanation, the physician needs to make a clear recommendation that continued treatment for cure is most unlikely to be successful, so therapeutic goals should be shifted to treatment for comfort for this dying patient. In our experience, about 90% of such patients or their families understand and agree with the recommendation, most expressing considerable relief that they

TABLE 1-1 The Intensivist's Roles in Deciding to Forego Life-Sustaining Treatment

Guiding the Decision	Managing the Grief
Explanation	Patient's advocate
Recommendation	Empathic listening
Patient's response	Assemble support
Implementation	Acknowledge the loss

TABLE 1-2 Reconsdering the Goals of Therapy

Cure	Comfort
Ventilation	Treat pain
Perfusion	Relieve dyspnea
Dialysis	Allay anxiety
Nutrition	Minimize interventions
Treat infection	Family access
Surgery	Support
Differential diagnosis	Grieving

do not have to make a decision, but rather follow the recommendation of the physician. It is important to provide time and support for the other 10% while they process their reasons for disagreement with the physician's recommendation, but this remains a front-burner issue to be discussed again within 24 hours in most cases.

At this point, patients or their significant others who agree with the recommendation to shift goals from cure to comfort benefit from understanding that comfort care in the ICU constitutes a systematic removal of the causes of patient discomfort, together with the incorporation of comforting interventions of the patient's choice (Table 1-2). For example, treatment for cure often consists of positive-pressure ventilation associated with posturing, chest pummeling and tracheal suctioning, the infusion of vasoactive drugs to enhance circulation, dialysis for renal failure, aggressive intravenous or alimentary nutrition, antibiotics for multiple infections, surgery where indicated, and daily interruption of sedative infusions to allow ongoing confirmation of CNS status. Each of these components of treatment for cure includes uncomfortable interventions that need to be explicitly described so that patients or their significant others do not maintain the misconception that continued ICU care is a harmless, comfortable course of action. By contrast, treatment for comfort consists of intravenous medication effective at relieving pain, dyspnea, and anxiety. It also consists of withholding interventions that cause the patient pain or irritation, and of replacing both interventions and electronic monitoring of vital signs with free access of the family and friends to allow the intensive care cubicle to become a safe place for grieving and dying with psychospiritual support systems maximized. Once an orderly transition from treatment for cure to treatment for comfort has been effected in the ICU, timely transfer out of the unit to an environment that permits death and grieving with privacy and dignity is often appropriate. Whenever possible, continuity of care for the dying patient outside the ICU should be effected by the ICU physician-house staff team to minimize fragmentation of comfort measures and to keep the patient from feeling abandoned.

MANAGE GRIEF

The second process that is ongoing during this decision making allows the dying patient or the family and friends to begin to express their grief (see Table 1-1). The very best care of the patient is care for the patient, and the critical care physician's demeanor during the decision making process goes a long way toward demonstrating that he or she is acting as the patient's advocate. The urgent pursuit of an agenda that care should be withdrawn does not help the patient or family to trust in the physician's desire to help the patient. Instead, pas-

toral skills such as empathic listening, assembling the family and other support systems, and acknowledging and sharing in the pain while introducing the vocabulary of grief processing are constructive ways to help the patient and family reconsider the goals of therapy. This is not an easy task when the physician knows the patient and family well, but it is even more difficult in the modern intensive care environment, when the physician may have met the patient for the first time within hours to days preceding the reconsideration of therapeutic goals. Yet the critical care physician needs to establish his or her position as a credible advocate for the patient by being a source of helpful information, by providing direction, and by listening empathically. Because the critical care physician is often a stranger, all efforts should be made at the time of reconsidering the goals of therapy to assemble support helpful to the patient, including family friends, the primary physician, the bedside nurse, house staff and students caring for the patient, appropriate clergy, ethics specialists, and social services.

COMBINE EXCELLENCE AND COMPASSION

Since up to 90% of patients who die in modern ICUs do so with the decision to withhold and withdraw life-sustaining therapy, exemplary critical care should include a commitment to make this transition to treatment for comfort a humane and compassionate process, conducted with the same expertise and excellence sought during treatment for cure. In our view, the physician's conclusion that the patient is dying is the starting point. Thereafter, the physician's recommendation to shift treatment goals from cure to comfort is essential so that the patient and the family have no illusions that full ICU care will produce a cure. Third, understanding that comfort care is extensive and effective allows the ICU to become a safe place for grieving and dying. This is a distinctly different approach from that of many physicians who feel they have failed their dying patients by not providing cure; all too often this fear of failure leads to abandoning dying patients without providing effective comfort care. Since death is not an option but an inevitability for all of us, critical care physicians can bring their expertise and understanding to help patients decide when to forego life-sustaining therapy and to replace it with effective comfort care, making the ICU a safe and supporting space for the dying patient and his or her significant others. Note that the ministerial skills and attitudes required to implement this approach are more in the province and curriculum of social workers, psychologists, and clerical pastoral associates than critical care physicians. To the extent that experienced intensivists find this approach helpful, teaching it to students of critical care becomes an important contribution to a curriculum of critical care.

The Scholarship of Teaching and Discovery in Critical Care

The process of providing exemplary critical care is magnified and refined by learning interactions with students of critical care at all levels—from freshmen to senior medical students through residents in anesthesia, medicine, and surgery, to critical care fellows and practicing intensivists seeking continuing medical education. In such teaching sessions, these students always question the principles of critical care and how best to impart them, thereby helping direct a search for better teaching methods. Of course, any active ICU is a classroom for learning the principles of critical care. Yet teachers of critical care need to avoid the pitfalls to learning when there is little time for the student to process the reasons for the formulations of differential diagnostic and treatment plans in each patient. There can develop a "shoot from the hip" pattern recognition of critical illness that often misses the mark and perpetuates a habit of erroneous interventions that delay a more rational, mechanistic, questioning approach to each patient's problem.

IMPLEMENT A CRITICAL CARE CURRICULUM IN THE INTENSIVE CARE UNIT

One helpful teaching technique is to implement a schedule providing students of critical care with the luxury of time to think. This priority provides a counterpoint to the work rounds and clinical problem-solving activities that unfettered, tend to dominate the daily activities of the unit. A good start is to ritualize a curriculum for critical care learning. In many academic centers, house staff and fellows rotate through the ICU on monthly intervals. Accordingly, a monthly series of well-planned seminars addressing the essential topics that house staff and fellows need to know can incorporate medical students and nursing staff, and lay the foundations of conceptual understanding necessary to approach the critically ill patient effectively. In our teaching program, we emphasize a conceptual framework based on the pathophysiology of organ system dysfunction shared by most types of critical illness (Table 1-3).

This approach complements the specific etiology and therapy of individual illnesses, because the opportunity for favorably treating many concurrent organ system failures in each patient occurs early in the critical illness, when the specific diagnosis and focused therapy are less important than resuscitation and stabilization according to principles of organ system pathophysiology. Critically ill patients present many diagnostic and therapeutic problems to their attending physicians and so to the students of critical care. Recent advances in intensive care management and monitoring technology facilitate early detection of pathophysiology of vital functions, allowing the potential for prevention and early treatment. However, this greater volume of diagnostic data and possible therapeutic interventions occasionally can create "information overload" for students of critical care, confounding rather than complementing clinical skills. The purpose of a syllabus addressing the pathophysiology of critical illness is to provide students with an informed practical approach to integrating established concepts of organ system dysfunction with conventional clinical skills. New duty hour regulations for U.S. house officers have made it difficult to include all members of the team in these teaching sessions, an issue we have not been able to fully solve. A syllabus of reading material that follows the seminar topics closely is helpful to students.[7]

ENCOURAGE INDEPENDENT INTERPRETING OF IMAGING TECHNIQUES, BIOPSIES, AND OTHER INTERVENTIONS

A second forum for teaching critical care is to review essential imaging procedures. Accordingly, we set aside about 45 minutes at 11:00 AM each day to systematically review the diagnostic radiology imaging procedures conducted in the last

TABLE 1-3 Critical Care Curriculum: The Pathophysiology of Critical Illness

1. O_2 delivery and the management of life-threatening hypoxia
2. Pulmonary exchange of CO_2, Vd/Vt and ventilatory (type II) failure
3. Pulmonary exchange of O_2, shunt, and acute hypoxemic (type I) respiratory failure
4. Respiratory mechanics and ventilator-lung model demonstration
5. Perioperative (type III) respiratory failure and liberation of the patient from mechanical ventilation
6. Right heart catheter, central hemodynamics, and lung liquid flux
7. Cardiovascular management of acute hypoxemic respiratory failure
8. Ventilatory management of acute hypoxemic respiratory failure, including ventilator-induced lung injury
9. Ventilator waveforms to guide clinical management
10. Status asthmaticus and acute-on-chronic respiratory failure
11. Control of the cardiac output and bedside differential diagnosis of shock
12. Volume and vasoactive drug therapy for septic, hypovolemic, and cardiogenic shock
13. Left ventricular mechanics and dysfunction in critical illness—systolic versus diastolic
14. Acute right heart syndromes and pulmonary embolism
15. Acid-base abnormalities
16. Severe electrolyte abnormalities
17. Nutrition in critical illness
18. Sedation, analgesia, and muscle relaxation in critical illness
19. Evaluation and management of CNS dysfunction in critical illness
20. The physician on the other end of the ET tube—audiotape and discussion
21. Managing death and dying in the ICU—videotape and discussion
22. Miscellaneous additional topics: noninvasive ventilation, heat shock, rhabdomyolysis, acute renal failure, hypothermia, and critical illness in pregnancy

Vd/Vt, dead space/tidal volume ratio.

24 hours on each of our patients, including computer-assisted tomograms, magnetic resonance images, and ultrasonography. This formal review allows faculty and fellows to teach medical students and house staff a systematic review of the chest radiograph and special features of ICU radiology, including identification and positioning of diverse diagnostic and therapeutic instruments (e.g., the endotracheal tube, intravascular catheters, feeding tubes, pacemakers, and others). We also set aside one day per week to review the echocardiographic studies performed during the previous week. Of course, these have been reviewed online when the procedures were done, but this forum allows students of critical care to become more comfortable with the types of diagnostic information we seek from these imaging techniques. Encouraging students of critical care to be active participants in bedside diagnostic and therapeutic procedures such as endoscopy, and to follow-up on all biopsy specimens by direct observation with the pathologist are other ways to encourage active learning concerning the interpretation of ICU procedures and their integration with the patient's clinical evaluation in a timely manner.

TEACH HOW TO TEACH

An essential component of the critical care fellowship is learning how to teach. It is common in academic medical environments to assume that completing medical school and residency confers the ability to teach,[8] but most critical care fellows value the opportunity for supervised and guided enhancement of their teaching abilities by effective teaching faculty. The critical care syllabus outlined earlier gives the opportunity for fellows to observe faculty teaching during their first rotation through the unit and during subsequent months to organize and present selected topics from the syllabus with the help of their faculty preceptor. Our target is that our fellows have mastery of the complete syllabus by the time they complete their fellowship, an exercise that confers confidence and credibility on their teaching skills, and undoubtedly enhances their learning of the concepts they teach. Just as bench researchers go elsewhere and establish their laboratories, our clinical scholars have created the same learning programs elsewhere, exporting this approach and content rather than evolving it over years. A second forum is our daily morning report, where three to five new pulmonary and critical care patients are presented in a half-hour conference. One fellow provides a brief analysis and solution to each clinical problem, and suggestions or affirmations of the analysis by faculty and other fellows help develop the skill of processing and presenting complex patients.

LEARN AND USE A QUESTIONING APPROACH

Another important forum for encouraging active learning of critical care is the daily teaching round led by the intensive care faculty and critical care fellows. The format we have found most useful is to encourage the most junior member of the team responsible for the patient to provide a complete, systematic review of the patient, concluding with a differential diagnosis and treatment plan, while the attending faculty member provides an active listening presence. When the presentation is complete, the faculty member questions or confirms directly the essential points from the history, physical examination, and laboratory results, and provides any clarification helpful to the rest of the team on generic or specific teaching issues, integrating the input of more senior members of the team to encourage participation in the bedside decision making as a learning exercise.

Often the case discussions can be led to formulate questions not yet answered concerning the patient's problems. It is less important to provide answers to the questions formed than to point the students of critical care in the direction of how to find the answers, beginning with their reading of appropriate topics in a critical care text available in the ICU. This continues to the appropriate use of medical informatics to search the critical care literature electronically for answers expected in a short interval. Whenever the answer is not available, it is the teaching responsibility of the faculty and critical care fellows to help students of critical care formulate the clinical investigation that could answer the question. In this way, the rounds in the ICU become intellectually charged, and active participation of all members of the team is encouraged. A spin-off of this questioning approach to active learning in the ICU is much more informed cross-coverage between critical care teams. In units with active clinical investigation programs, this questioning approach stimulates interaction between the personnel delivering care and those conducting the research.

AFFIRM LEARNING

Students of critical care learn in a charged environment where some patients do not improve or actually deteriorate despite thoughtful, focused, and timely care. Teachers of critical care can diffuse the angst among students by appropriate, well-placed affirmation of the care being delivered. For example, exemplary case presentations, thoughtful and complete differential diagnoses, focused and insightful treatment plans, and well-formulated questions appropriately researched in the available literature are all targets for faculty approbation. When praised appropriately and without flattery, students of critical care respond with energy and enthusiasm, allowing them to learn to the limit of their potential.

TEACH CRITICAL CARE IN THE CURRICULA OF MEDICAL SCHOOLS AND RESIDENCY PROGRAMS

In many academic institutions, critical care faculty are well known among medical students and house staff as outstanding teachers. This can allow diverse outlets for teaching scholarship in the medical school curriculum and in residency training programs. In our medical school, freshmen students learn the physiology of the cardiovascular and respiratory systems during the winter quarter and have time for elective courses during the spring quarter. This created the opportunity for a freshman spring elective entitled "An Introduction to the Pathophysiology of Critical Illness," which attracts about a quarter of the freshman class each year. During two $2^1/_2$-hour sessions each week for the 10-week quarter, we review in detail with the students extensions of their cardiopulmonary physiology as it is deranged in critical illness, utilizing a core curriculum similar to the topics shown in Table 1-3. These students are stimulated by finding that their hard work in learning physiology has practical applications in treating critically ill patients, and are enthusiastic to apply this new knowledge of pathophysiology during preceptored visits on four occasions to patients with respiratory failure or hypoperfusion states. Utilizing clinically real teaching aids like a ventilator-lung model, an echocardiography teaching tape, and a heart sound simulator provides freshmen students with a vision of patient care at an early stage in their clinical exposure. During sophomore year, focused topics related to critical care are taught during our clinical pathophysiology course, including asthma and acute respiratory distress syndrome. In the junior year, students rotate twice through the ICU for 2-hour preceptored visits to patients illustrating manifestations of respiratory failure or hypoperfusion states. As described earlier, most senior medical students in our school spend a month as members of the critical care teams in our medical or surgical ICU.

In the medical ICU, medical residents and interns rotate for a least three 1-month periods during their 3-year residency program. To refresh and maintain the knowledge base acquired during these rotations, our critical care faculty leads two medicine morning reports per month, during which they review a syllabus of critical care meant to allow residents not on the ICU to utilize their critical care knowledge to process cases representing a specific aspect of critical care. Our faculty members are also regular participants in the house staff teaching conferences conducted by the departments of anesthesia and critical care, pediatrics, obstetrics and gynecology, and surgery, and this interaction fosters a collegial approach to critically ill patients among these different departments. Finally, the participation of academic critical care faculty in city, regional, national, and international critical care conferences helps to fine-tune and update teaching approaches that can then enhance the scholarship of teaching critical care at one's home institution.

INVESTIGATE MECHANISMS AND MANAGEMENT OF CRITICAL ILLNESS

Clinical investigation of critical illness is essential for the continued growth of effective critical care. Indeed, one of the hallmarks of critical care in the last decade has been the large number of high-quality clinical studies leading to better care. Yet the practice of critical care is often so demanding that the intensivist's time is consumed with providing state-of-the-art care. Accordingly, clinical investigation in the ICU requires an organized program that is parallel to and integrated with the practice and teaching of exemplary critical care. Such a program allows an outlet for the creative formulation of hypotheses arising at the bedside of critically ill patients. It also enhances the morale of the critical care physician–nurse–respiratory therapist team by developing shared confidence that new concepts are being regularly learned during delivery of critical care.

An effective critical care research team consists of a research director, critical care nurse research coordinator, and several critical care fellows. Regular scheduled communications about ongoing research protocols, their significance, and their need for patient recruitment need to be maintained between the research team and the critical care team. The research team needs to meet on a regular basis to interpret and update data in each of its protocols, and to consider and discuss new hypotheses for testing. Ideally, the clinical investigation of critical illness should interface with a basic science research program to allow bench or animal extensions of hypotheses that are difficult to test in the intensive care environment. Together the basic and clinical investigative teams implement the essential steps in clinical research in critically ill patients: formulate a hypothesis, prepare a protocol, obtain institutional review board approval, obtain funding, perform the study, and communicate the results.[9]

Many challenges exist in conducting studies in the environment of the ICU. These include the unpredictable and unscheduled nature of events, the need to maintain complex schedules related to routine care in parallel with schedules for study protocols, and the very heterogeneous nature of patient populations. In the view of many, the greatest challenge is conducting studies of promising therapies for which the precise risks and benefits are unknown, yet doing so in patients in whom informed consent is not possible because of their critical illness. Some would say that such studies simply cannot be done without consent, but we find this an undesirable acceptance of the current state of our ignorance. We believe that true equipoise exists in the interface between many clinical problems and their potential treatments (i.e., a realization on the one hand that our understanding of an existing treatment for a disease process is inadequate, yet no secure knowledge that a new approach or therapy is completely safe and efficacious).[10] In this circumstance we believe that prospective, randomized trials offer the only hope of informing our practice of medicine, and that studies in the ICU, even if conducted with proxy or under some circumstances waived consent, are justified. The function of the institutional review board is to foster careful deliberation of the merits of each situation and proposed study to ensure that these balances are struck.

References

1. Hall JB, Wood LDH: Liberation of the patient from mechanical ventilation. *JAMA* 257:1621, 1987.
2. Acute Respiratory Distress Syndrome (ARDS) Network: Ventilation with lower tidal volumes as compared with traditional tidal volumes for acute lung injury and the acute respiratory distress syndrome. *N Engl J Med* 342:1301, 2000.
3. Ralph DB, Gleason DH: Staffing and management of the intensive care unit, in Hall JB, Schmidt GA, Wood LDH (eds): *Principles of Critical Care.* New York, McGraw-Hill, 1992, p 465.
4. Prendergast TJ, Claessens MT, Luce JM: A national survey of end-of-life care for critically ill patients. *Am J Respir Crit Care Med* 158:1163, 1998.
5. Fine RL, Mayo TW: Resolution of futility by due process: Early experience with the Texas Advance Directives Act. *Ann Intern Med* 138:743, 2003.
6. Karlawish JHT, Hall JB: Managing death and dying in the intensive care unit. *Am J Respir Crit Care Med* 155:1, 1997.
7. Wood LDH, Schmidt GA, Hall JB: The pathophysiology of critical illness, in Hall JB, Schmidt GA, Wood LDH (eds): *Principles of Critical Care.* New York, McGraw-Hill, 1992, p 3.
8. Wipf JE, Pinsky LE, Burke W: Turning interns into senior residents: Preparing residents for their teaching and leadership roles. *Acad Med* 70:591, 1995.
9. Murray JF, Rodriguez-Roisin R: Clinical investigation in critically ill patients, in Hall JB, Schmidt GA, Wood LDH (eds): *Principles of Critical Care.* New York, McGraw-Hill, 1992, p 2269.
10. Karlawish JT, Hall J: Clinical commentary: The controversy over emergency research: A review of the issues and suggestions for a resolution. *Am J Respir Crit Care Med* 153:499, 1996.

Chapter 2 _____

ASSESSING COST EFFECTIVENESS IN THE INTENSIVE CARE UNIT

MICHAEL T. COUGHLIN
DEREK C. ANGUS

KEY POINTS

- *The care of critically ill patients in the modern ICU results in a large societal burden in terms of both manpower and monetary cost.*

- *The high cost of critical care can largely be attributed to high overhead costs (e.g., need for experienced staff and expensive equipment), high resource utilization (e.g., drugs, lab tests, and complex imaging procedures), and an ever-growing demand for ICU services.*

- *Complex economic analysis of health care decision making can be reduced to two fundamental questions that need to be answered: First, "Is a therapy worth using when compared with the alternatives?" The second question is broader and asks "Should a portion of available health care resources be allocated to a given therapy or program?"*

- *Routine incorporation of Cost Effectiveness studies is important to the conduct of high quality clinical trials research in the intensive care unit. Inclusion of cost effectiveness gives the clinician the opportunity to fully assess the effect of a new therapy in the ICU.*

The care of critically ill patients in the modern ICU results in a large societal burden in terms of both manpower and monetary cost. The high cost of critical care can largely be attributed to: high overhead costs (e.g., need for experienced staff and expensive equipment), high resource utilization (e.g., drugs, lab tests, and complex imaging procedures), and an ever-growing demand for ICU services. With the continuing rise in health care costs, there is an ever-increasing need to establish whether new therapies are not only efficacious, but also cost effective. The need for cost-effectiveness evaluations is spread throughout medicine, but the issue of cost effectiveness is especially important in critical care medicine. While ICU beds account for only about 10% of all inpatient hospital beds, ICU costs in the U.S. exceed $60 billion annually, and consume up to one third of all hospital costs.[1] Furthermore, attempts to reduce ICU costs by other mechanisms, such as reduction in length of stay, have proved to be difficult.[2] While access to new therapies is being tied increasingly to cost, physicians continue to be skeptical and suspicious of cost analyses. In large part, this skepticism is prompted by the variable quality of earlier cost analyses. However, skepticism is also due to the lack of familiarity many physicians have with the general principles of health economics. The U.S. Public Health Service (USPHS) attempted to set standards for the conduct of rigorous cost-effectiveness analyses in medicine.[3–5] In critical care medicine, the American Thoracic Society (ATS) established specific guidelines for the conduct of cost-effectiveness analyses based on the USPHS recommendations.[6] These standards have the potential to greatly improve the quality of future cost-effectiveness studies. However, if clinicians do not understand and embrace the principles of cost effectiveness, it is likely that such studies will continue to be viewed simply as ammunition for nonclinician administrators in the battle to restrict physician freedom of choice and to control clinical decision making.

In this chapter, we will cover many of the principal aspects of cost-effectiveness analyses and consider how such studies ought to be conducted on potential new therapies. We will use drotrecogin alfa (activated) as a working example of the type of therapy often utilized in the modern ICU that is expensive, but has potentially life-saving effects. The overall goal of this chapter is to encourage all of us to familiarize ourselves with cost analyses and to consider cost-effectiveness analysis as simply another tool in our evaluation toolkit, along with case reports, animal studies, and randomized clinical trials of potential new therapies. We have previously reviewed this topic,[7] and here will further describe the utility of economic analyses in critical care. For a more detailed in-depth discussion of economic analysis in health care, the reader is referred to the excellent text by Gold and associates.[8]

Economic Evaluations in Health Care

One can compress all of health economics down to two main questions. First, "Is a therapy worth using when compared with alternatives?" For example, what is the worth of a new antisepsis agent like drotrecogin alfa (activated) that has recently demonstrated a beneficial effect in a large randomized clinical trial? We can consider that worth represents some trade-off of cost and benefit (or effect). The second question is broader and asks "Should a portion of available health care resources be allocated to a given therapy or program?" This is principally a social policy issue and requires considering the worth of new therapies not only within a given disease, but also in comparison to other therapies in other diseases. For example, although drotrecogin alfa (activated) might be deemed worthwhile in the treatment of sepsis, a state Medicaid agency might be forced to compare its value to that of a hepatitis B vaccination program for newborns, or to influenza vaccinations for the elderly. These types of choices are becoming increasingly common in situations in which health care resources are limited and must be equitably distributed among multiple programs. In other words, we would wish to know if drotrecogin alfa (activated) is not only cost effective with respect to standard management for sepsis, but also whether we can afford it as a society.

There are a variety of different analytic approaches that address all or some part of these two questions. Though the approaches appear similar, and have similar names, there are key differences. In order to understand the strengths and weaknesses of each approach, we must first describe the various methodologies used to evaluate health care costs. There are essentially four types of cost analyses: cost minimization, cost benefit, cost effectiveness, and cost utility. The fourth, cost utility, is best viewed as a special case of cost effectiveness. In addition, there are situations in which a cost-effectiveness analysis can produce a cost-minimization statement.

COST-MINIMIZATION ANALYSIS

The cost studies that are most familiar to clinicians are cost minimization studies, and these consider only how much a drug costs to stock in the pharmacy. They are essentially studies of drug acquisition cost, and are most frequently conducted by hospital pharmacy departments. When comparing different products (e.g., two sulfonamides), each product is assumed to have equal efficacy and to equally impact all other aspects of treatment (although this may or may not be true). Drug effects such as shortened length of stay, reduced need for other therapies, and improved quality of life after illness are not considered in cost-minimization analyses. The preferred therapy is simply the one that costs the hospital less money per unit of treatment (e.g., per day of therapy, or per dose).

Additionally, a cost-minimization analysis can result when a formal cost-effectiveness analysis (CEA, see below) with sophisticated assessment of all potential changes in costs and effects between two programs demonstrates no difference in effect. However, in the situation in which there is no difference in effect, there may be significant differences in cost between the programs. This result does not produce a cost-effectiveness ratio (since one would be dividing the change in costs by zero), but does allow accurate assessment of the true differences in cost between two programs with comparable treatment effects. This explicit evaluation of costs and effects, as opposed to an assumption of no difference in effect, is in contrast to traditional cost-minimization studies done in the past.

COST-BENEFIT ANALYSIS

The term "cost benefit" is frequently confused with cost effectiveness.[9] In fact, a cost-benefit analysis is a very specific analysis, rarely conducted today, that expresses all costs and effects in monetary units. This means that a dollar value must be placed on all effects. For example, a life saved must be converted into a monetary value. This conversion of life into economic terms can be problematic and very nonintuitive. After conversion of all effects into monetary units, one then adds up all the costs (expressed in dollars) and subtracts them from all the benefits (effects, expressed in dollars). If the final total is negative, the costs outweigh the benefits, and vice versa. Although the final output is attractive in its simplicity, the manipulations required to convert all effects into dollar values are often very controversial. Because of this controversy concerning the "value" of effects, this type of analysis has largely fallen out of favor for health economic evaluations.

COST-EFFECTIVENESS ANALYSIS

Cost effectiveness is simply a ratio of the net change in costs (dollars) associated with two different programs or therapies divided by the net change in effects (health outcome). The denominator represents the gain in health (life-years gained, number of additional survivors, or cases of disease averted), while the numerator reflects the cost (in dollars) of affecting the gain in health. Since the units used are different for the numerator and denominator, the typical cost-effectiveness expression will take a form such as cost (dollars) per year of life saved. Cost-effectiveness analyses are the current dominant form of cost evaluation, and were endorsed by both the USPHS Panel on Cost-Effectiveness in Health and Medicine (PCEHM), and more recently by the ATS as the primary method by which to measure the costs and effects of health care programs and medical therapies.[4,6]

Deciding whether a therapy is cost effective is a subjective evaluation of the cost-effectiveness ratio. If $100,000 per year of life gained is deemed the threshold for effectiveness, then a new therapy with a cost-effectiveness ratio of $82,000 per year of life gained is viewed as cost effective. Though there is no absolute cut-off, there is general consensus that a level somewhere between $50,000 and $100,000 per year of life gained is acceptable in the U.S. today. However, the way in which both costs and effects are calculated can have profound effects on the resulting ratio, and therein lies much of the controversy over CEA.

The typical CEA requires the collection of a significant amount of information on costs and effects, much of which may be gathered from widely varying sources. Interpretation of this information is often difficult, and a decision analysis model is usually constructed that mimics the key clinical decisions and events. This model can most easily be represented by a tree in which each branch point is calibrated with a probability of occurrence and a cost. At its simplest, the tree will contain only branches for treatment allocation (e.g., drotrecogin alfa [activated] or standard therapy) and outcome (e.g., alive or dead). To calibrate such a tree, we would need to know only the probability of living or dying, depending on whether a given patient received the new therapy or not, and the average cost of care for survivors and nonsurvivors in the two treatment arms (Fig. 2-1).

Alternatively, we may be interested in understanding the key events that drive either morbidity or cost (e.g., mechanical ventilation or hemodialysis). This could be important for a variety of reasons; there may be evidence that the study population has a far lower rate of mechanical ventilation than is expected for septic patients in general. Therefore, the extent to which differences in cost are the result of the number of

FIGURE 2-1 Simple decision tree comparing outcome for patients treated with drotrecogin alfa (activated) versus standard care. In order to calibrate the tree, we must estimate: (1) the probability for a given patient to live or die, given whether they received the new therapy or not; and (2) the average costs associated with each of the four branches.

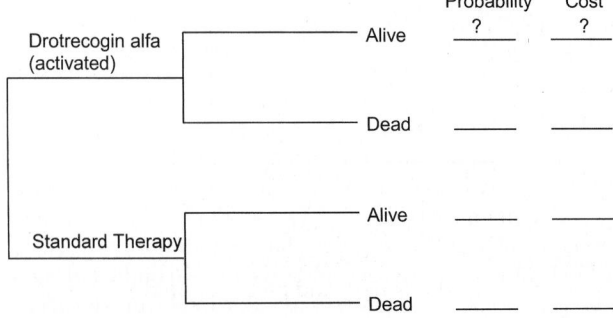

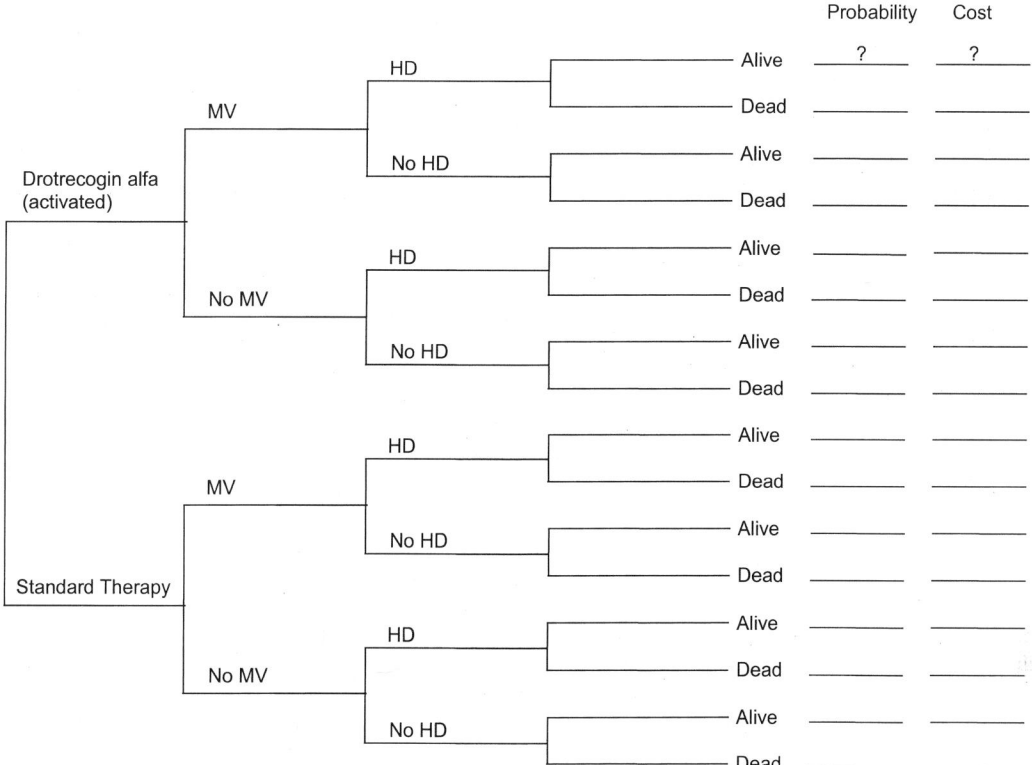

FIGURE 2-2 Decision tree comparing outcomes for patients treated with drotrecogin alfa (activated) versus standard care that incorporates the potential to undergo mechanical ventilation and receive hemodialysis. In order to calibrate the tree, we must estimate the probabilities and average costs for 16 separate trees. MV, mechanical ventilation; HD, hemodialysis.

patients undergoing mechanical ventilation may be important when estimating the cost effectiveness of the new therapy in the real world. Similarly, need for hemodialysis can be a significant cost driver. A new therapy that reduces the need for mechanical ventilation or hemodialysis may be expensive, but the cost of the therapy can be offset by the reduced need for supportive care, and hence deemed cost effective by CEA. In contrast, cost-benefit analysis would take into account only the expense of the new therapy, without considering the reduction in supportive care. However, considering changes in other care modalities leads to the addition of branch points for mechanical ventilation and hemodialysis, and thereby expands the model dramatically, creating 16 branches to consider. For each branch, we must know a patient's likelihood of entering such an arm and the average costs (Fig. 2-2).

COST-UTILITY ANALYSIS

A cost-utility analysis is a form of CEA in which the effects are converted into common units of utility. Typically, this approach involves adjusting the number of years of survival for the "quality" of that survival, in which a person living for one year with a quality-of-life score of 80% would be "awarded" 0.8 years of quality-adjusted survival. The advantage of this approach is that it allows comparison of different programs across different diseases. In this way we can compare the number of quality-adjusted life years (as opposed simply to the number of lives saved), and perhaps can more equitably compare drotrecogin alfa (activated) for critically ill adults to a hepatitis B vaccination program in newborns.

Methodologic Considerations in Cost-Effectiveness Analysis

Good cost-effectiveness analysis design requires consideration of multiple elements in order to both adequately explore the relationship between costs and effects, and to determine the robustness of the conclusions and the comparability of the results to those of other studies. Each of these elements is outlined in Table 2-1 with reference to both the PCEHM and ATS guidelines, and discussed individually in more detail below.

PERSPECTIVE

The costs considered in a CEA can vary depending on whose perspective is considered. As an example, consider the issue of early discharge from the hospital after childbirth. From the hospital's or managed care organization's perspective, cost may be reduced by early discharge. In contrast, from a societal perspective, the cost savings for the health care system may be offset by additional costs to the patient, such as extra time off work for the husband who must stay home to care for the new mother. Cost studies conducted to date have often been hampered by a lack of consistent perspective either within or among studies. Failure to maintain a consistent perspective hampers comparison of results across studies and threatens the validity of the study itself. Both the PCEHM and ATS

TABLE 2-1 Methodologic Considerations in Cost-Effectiveness Analysis

| Aspect | METHODOLOGIC PROBLEMS | | | PCEHM Recommendations (Rationale) | SECOND ATS WORKSHOP ON OUTCOMES RESEARCH | |
	Individual CEA	Comparing CEAs	ICU-Specific		Position	Comment
Perspective	Not defined	Different		Societal (ethical, pragmatic)	Agree	• May be instances when provider perspective is useful
Outcomes (effects)	Data are inadequate or difficult to evaluate	Different outcomes	Long-term follow-up is rare	QALYs (pragmatic, conventional)	Agree	• Require better natural history of ICU conditions and modeling or longer follow-up; other outcomes may be useful depending on perspective
				Best-designed, least biased source (pragmatic)	Agree	• Consider modeling reduced efficacy in sensitivity analysis
Costs	Data are inadequate or difficult to evaluate	Different costs	Only hospital costs are usually measured; no international standard	Costs to include: health care services; patient time; caregiving; nonhealth impacts (theoretical)	Agree	• Standard approach to measuring these costs not yet developed; estimating units of resource use and multiplying by standard costs probably most practical approach currently; detail with which resource use is tracked should be tailored to nature of intervention and likely effects on costs
				Include or exclude other disease costs and test in sensitivity analysis (theoretical, pragmatic, user needs and accounting)	Include costs of other diseases (too hard to disentangle)	
Comparators (standard care)	Choice distorts results	—	Determining standard often difficult	Existing practice (conventional)	Agree	
				If existing practice is suspect, consider best-available, viable low-cost, or "do nothing" (conventional)	Agree	• Many existing ICU practices may be ineffective or cost-ineffective; therefore, consider comparison to "best practice" rather than standard practice
Discounting	Inadequate representation of the effect of time	Different rates	Not usually done	Discount costs and effects to present value (theoretical)	Agree	
				Use a 3% discount rate (theoretical, pragmatic)	Agree	
Uncertainty	Inadequate representation of uncertainty on results	—	Not usually done	Sensitivity analysis essential; multi-way sensitivity analysis preferred (user needs)	Agree	• Multi-way sensitivity analyses probably essential given high likelihood that several key assumptions will be necessary to generate reference case from critical care trials
Reporting	—	Not standard		Reference case (user needs)	Agree	• But, also present "data-rich" case
				Compare to available ratios (user needs)	Agree	• Also file (e.g., on internet) intended analysis plan prior to unblinding when concurrent with randomized clinical trial
				Journal and technical report (user needs)	Agree	

Abbreviations: CEA, cost-effectiveness analysis; ICU, intensive care unit; PCEHM, Panel on Cost-effectiveness in Health and Medicine; ATS, American Thoracic Society; QALY, quality-adjusted life years.
Reproduced with permission from Angus et al.[6]

recommend adoption of the societal perspective when conducting cost-effectiveness studies.

OUTCOMES (EFFECTS)

This is an exceedingly difficult problem for CEA for a variety of reasons. First, information on outcomes usually comes from randomized clinical trials (RCTs), which often do not reflect the actual clinical practice of medicine. Conversely, the implications of a CEA are intended for real-world practice. A cost-effectiveness ratio is intended to capture the expected relationship between the costs incurred and the effects gained in actual practice. Conversely, an RCT is usually designed to maximize the likelihood of finding an effect. As such, an RCT can represent a rather idealized situation, which is quite distinctly different from the real world. For example, only specific patients may be selected, the dosage and timing of therapy will likely be optimized, and other aspects of care may be protocolized and carefully controlled. The effect size generated under such rigorous situations is termed a therapy's *efficacy* (or maximal effect). In the real world, the effect of a new therapy is likely diluted by less appropriate patient selection, changes in dosing and timing, and increased variability in other aspects of patient care. The effect of a new therapy under these real-world conditions is termed a therapy's *effectiveness*. The more RCTs are refined, the further removed they are from the reality of using a therapy in clinical practice.[10] Thus, the relationship between cost and effect in some RCTs becomes increasingly distorted.

A cost analysis conducted using efficacy from an RCT might better be termed a cost-efficacy study, rather than a cost-effectiveness study. However, there are no clear guidelines on how to reduce the bias introduced by using efficacy data instead of effectiveness data. One possibility is to consider adding an open-label, open-enrollment arm to clinical trials in which a CEA is being conducted.[11] However, this presents both many logistic and ethical problems. The more accepted alternative is to expose the cost model to varying estimates of reduced effect from those seen in the RCT during sensitivity analysis (see below).

Another problem encountered when determining effect or outcome is that the outcome measure evaluated in the RCT may not be directly relevant in the cost analysis. The PCEHM recommends, and the ATS agrees, that quality-adjusted life years (QALYs) be used as the units of effect, or utility. However, most RCTs in critical care use short-term (day 28 or hospital) mortality as the primary end point, and still others use indices such as "organ failure–free days" as outcome measures.[12] Although short-term survival likely correlates with long-term quality-adjusted survival, the relationship is not explicitly clear. Whether there is any relationship between organ failure–free days and long-term quality of life is even less clear. A recent study by Clermont and associates showed that patients who develop acute organ dysfunction are at risk for poor long-term quality of life (QOL), but that the risk is largely due to poor baseline health status, and not directly to organ failure in the ICU.[13]

This problem is only slowly evolving. While the PCEHM recommends long-term outcome, a National Institutes of Health (NIH)–sponsored workshop on sepsis studies recommended day 28 mortality.[12] More recently, the United Kingdom Medical Research Council workshop still recommended that day 28 mortality was an appropriate primary end point, but recommended follow-up to ≥90 days, and whenever possible to ≥6 months.[14] Recent successful trials in sepsis reported mortality at widely varying time points: 28 days (drotrecogin alfa [activated]),[15] 28 days and one year (steroids),[16] 60 days (early-goal directed therapy),[17] and a recent study of ARDS (Low Tidal Volume)[18] reported mortality to 180 days.

Proponents of short-term outcome state that longer follow-up is too expensive and not necessarily related to the therapy being studied. Advocates of longer follow-up state that short-term survival, of indeterminate quality of life, and possibly with death a short time thereafter, is of little utility to society.[8] They further argue that the ability to prioritize health care spending on the basis of value requires that we compare the long-term value of alternative programs for alternative disease processes. Many health care programs are administered, and/or have effects lasting, over a long period of time, making long term follow-up of patients enrolled in these programs essential.

There is currently relatively little long-term follow-up information on ICU patients. However, the available evidence does suggest that there is considerable mortality and morbidity beyond hospital discharge, supporting the notion that we should consider longer follow-up.[19–21] Quartin and colleagues showed that continuing mortality occurs in sepsis patients for many months after discharge from the hospital.[19] Studies exploring quality of life after ICU care have yielded conflicting results, but certainly several suggest considerable diminution of quality of life that appears to be sustained over time.[22]

Thus, until more evidence is available, studies of new ICU therapies upon which CEAs are to be performed should have some mechanism (e.g., a subset study or parallel cohort) to incorporate mortality follow-up for 6 to 12 months with an accompanying quality-of-life assessment.

COSTS

Which costs should be included? Debates over this subject can be very contentious and can resemble debates over whether to give colloids or crystalloids to hypotensive patients. The subject is further complicated by economic terms such as direct versus indirect costs and tangible versus intangible costs. We will attempt to avoid using too many accounting terms and to suggest alternative ways to understand this issue.

Let us reconsider the cost-effectiveness ratio. It is a ratio of *net costs* divided by *net effects*. Thereby, regardless of whether the costs of any given element seem important, if they are distributed equally in both comparison groups, the net difference will be zero and we therefore need not worry about them. In other words, we need consider only those costs we believe to be relevant *and* likely to differ between the treatment groups. As an example, the PCEHM believed that the intangible costs of pain and suffering were relevant costs that should be measured in CEAs, but we have never measured these costs in any critical care CEA. Therefore, if a new therapy is unlikely to cause either more or less pain, then we can continue to ignore such intangible costs, even though they are considered relevant. The caveat here is that we have now made the important assumption of no difference in pain, which may or may not be true.

We have of course glossed over the term "relevant." Which costs are relevant? All costs to society could be considered relevant from the societal perspective. Utilizing this perspective, one could argue that the costs of lost wages while a patient is sick are relevant. In response to this issue, the PCEHM recognized there are no correct answers. However, in order to promote standardization of CEA methodologies, they recommend inclusion of all health-related costs, and the ATS concurs that this is the current best approach. They also recommended including opportunity costs, and suggested that lost wages, not only as a postdischarge consequence of the illness but also during hospitalization, represents an example of an opportunity cost. Direct application of these guidelines to critical care is not easy. But one way to consider them is to think about a health care system without drotrecogin alfa (activated) and a health care system with the new therapy. We then need to include all possible cost elements that could differ between these two health care worlds.

ESTIMATING, MEASURING, OR GUESSING COSTS

Not all costs included in a CEA are necessarily measured empirically. The CEA is a model that is often calibrated using estimates. Some of these estimates come from measurements. For example, the estimate of differences in the mortality rate between a drug and placebo often is derived from the effect of size in an RCT. Other estimates can be based on expert opinion, or some combination of measurement and opinion. For example, the cost of the actual therapy is usually unknown since the therapy is often not yet approved, and no price has been set by the company that manufactures the therapy. One is therefore forced to estimate on the basis of an educated "best guess," perhaps with some knowledge of preliminary pricing from the company. While one might be alarmed at this notion of educated guesswork, it is important to appreciate that such estimates can be wildly erroneous, yet have minimal impact on the cost-effectiveness ratio. In order to test how sensitive a CEA ratio is to various estimates in the cost model, the completed CEA model is exposed to a rigorous sensitivity analysis (see below). In this way, we can decide to include many costs in a CEA, yet only measure specifically some portion of that total. As long as the estimated costs have little impact on the overall final CEA conclusions, the strategy regarding which costs to measure and which to estimate can be considered robust.

FOR HOW LONG DO WE MEASURE COSTS?

When the cost of therapy is computed, the duration of the costs attributed to the therapy must also be considered. For example, if our new therapy allows more people to leave the ICU, but causes a higher incidence of renal failure requiring long-term dialysis, shouldn't all the costs of dialysis be attributed to that therapy? The answer is yes.

Although most intensivists do not accept this concept of blaming therapy received in the ICU for incurred long-term costs, it is difficult to argue to the contrary. In producing a survivor, one must also take responsibility for the cost of maintaining survival, which means following the cost streams for a significant length of time. Furthermore, if chronic renal failure leads to a lower quality of life, the new therapy will be doubly penalized, both for the cost of the dialysis and for the reduced quality-adjusted survival.

HOW SHOULD COSTS BE MEASURED?

For those costs that we choose to measure, we must decide what represents true cost. When we consider hospital costs, true costs are generally assumed to be those generated by formal cost-accounting mechanisms. For example, the cost of a complete blood count includes the wage rate for and time spent by the employee who drew the blood, the cost of the tube, and some tiny amortized fraction of the cost of the equipment upon which the test is run. However, detailed information such as this is rarely available as part of a CEA. Another frequently used approach is to collect hospital charges and adjust them by the hospital- or department-specific cost-to-charge ratios. The relationship between hospital charges and costs has long been a source of skepticism for physicians. However, recent work by Shwartz and associates comparing department-specific cost-to-charge ratio-adjusted charges to estimates generated from a formal cost-accounting system, found good correlation when assessing patients in groups.[23] Agreement was much worse when comparing individual patients and when using hospital-specific ratios. However, CEAs rely on average grouped estimates of costs, and therefore department-specific cost-to-charge ratios appear adequate for estimating hospital costs.

Other proxy measures of cost, such as the Therapeutic Intervention Scoring System (TISS) or length of stay, can also be used.[24,25] As stated above, their value will depend on how sensitive the conclusions are to variations in the relationship between these measures and true costs.

DEFINING STANDARD CARE (COMPARATORS)

When comparing a new therapy, the choice of comparator, or standard therapy, is also critical. For example, the cost-effectiveness ratio of a 1-year cervical cancer screening program is quite different than that of 2-year or 3-year programs. Similarly, a tissue thromboplastin activator has a different cost-effectiveness ratio when compared to standard acute myocardial infarction therapy with no thrombolytic therapy as opposed to standard therapy with streptokinase. The PCEHM recommended that the control therapy used for comparative purposes be the least expensive available standard therapy. However, in the field of critical care this view is currently changing. In the treatment of sepsis, should standard care include early goal-directed therapy, steroids, and/or drotrecogin alfa (activated), even though these may be expensive? If so, do we consider all treatments to be standard therapy, or just one or two? The ATS Guidelines recommend that standard care isn't always "best practice," and that best practice should be the comparator of choice in critical care.

DISCOUNTING (TIME)

Discounting costs due to time is another important factor to consider when conducting a CEA. When we borrow money, we must pay it back with interest. This is because money is worth more now than it will be in the future. Therefore, $10 is more valuable now than $10 delivered at a rate of $1 per year for the next ten years. Thus, to pay back $10 that we just received over the next 10 years, we would be required to pay back more than $1 per year. Worldwide economic growth is occurring at approximately 3% per year, and therefore the PCEHM has recommended that all costs be discounted at a

3% rate per annum, and the ATS has agreed with this recommendation.

But what about effects; should they also be discounted? Are ten people living for one year more valuable than one person living for ten years? Although this issue may seem inhumane, consideration of this point is vital. Discounting costs without discounting effects will incur the Keeler-Cretin procrastination paradox wherein we would forever favor health care programs that take place some time in the future.[26] This situation would have us forever putting off until tomorrow that which could be done today, and therefore we also discount effects at 3%, the same rate as costs.

ROBUSTNESS AND UNCERTAINTY

When we perform an RCT, our primary conclusion is a statement of effect: did the new therapy change the outcome of interest? While it is highly likely that the outcome rates will be different (rarely would the mortality rates in both trial arms be identical), we rely on statistical significance to tell us whether the observed difference is due to a true effect of the therapy and not chance alone. We traditionally infer statistical significance when the p-value is <0.05. In this instance, we are 95% certain that the observed difference did not occur by chance alone. If we are interested only in effect, then we care only about which therapy arm is better, not how much better.

It is important to appreciate, however, that the p-value does not confirm the magnitude of effect. Consider the case of drotrecogin, for which a recent large RCT found a mortality rate in the treatment arm of 25%, as opposed to a placebo rate of 31%, with a $p = 0.006$.[15] This does not mean that six lives are saved per 100 persons treated. Rather, it tells us that our best estimate is that six lives are saved. If we presume a binomial distribution around the mortality rates, we can generate confidence intervals around the two estimates. These confidence intervals might now tell us that new therapy saves between 2 and 10 lives per 100 persons treated, but cannot tell us where the true value falls within that range. The p-value simply confirms the likelihood that there are lives saved by the new therapy, not how many lives.

In CEAs, however, we must quantify the magnitude of effect (and cost) so that we can generate a ratio. The general principle is to first take our best point estimates of cost and effect to generate a base case. Thereafter, we vary all our measures and estimates across their range of probabilities (e.g., 95% CI) in order to determine the extent to which the cost-effectiveness ratio varies. This is a *sensitivity analysis* and can be done either with one or multiple variables simultaneously. In one respect, the sensitivity analysis can be considered analogous to the p-value in that it allows us to explore the robustness of our conclusions. In other words, if, despite varying several or all variables across their stochastic distributions, there is minimal change in the final ratio, then one can have considerable confidence in the CE ratio estimate.

Another aspect of the sensitivity analysis is that it can be used to determine which model estimates must be the most accurate. For example, the CE ratio may be exquisitely sensitive to the estimate of ICU costs, but relatively insensitive to the expected costs of postdischarge health care resource use. In this situation, one might need to measure ICU costs very carefully, yet rely only on approximate estimates of postdischarge resource use. A comprehensive sensitivity analysis

can in fact often be considered more powerful than a p-value, because it can be used to graphically show all of the uncertainties inherent in the underlying assumptions of the CEA model.

Figure 2-3 shows the base case cost effectiveness and reference case cost-effectiveness ratio estimates for drotrecogin alfa (activated) generated by running 1000 simulations.[27] This is a common graphic representation of the output from a rigorously conducted CEA. The x axis shows incremental effects and the y axis incremental costs. Quadrants to the right of the y axis represent where treatment with drotrecogin alfa (activated) was associated with a net gain in effect. Quadrants above the x axis represent a net increase in cost. The majority of the simulation estimates fall within the upper right hand quadrant, indicating a net gain in effect with an associated increase in cost (more costly, more effective). The dashed lines represent thresholds of cost, with regions below and to the right of the thresholds being more cost effective than regions above and to the left.

Reporting and the PCEHM Reference Case

The PCEHM also recommended that all future CEAs produce a *reference case*. This is accomplished by generation of the CE ratio by a standardized approach to estimating and measuring each of the important elements of the CEA (see Table 2-1). This includes the perspective chosen, determination of costs and effects, study time horizon, and measurement of uncertainty and sensitivity analyses. Use of this standardized approach allows for comparison of CEA results across studies. Comparison of reference cases between CEAs allows us to make inferences about the cost effectiveness of a new sepsis therapy like drotrecogin alfa (activated) vs. a therapy used to fight breast cancer. It allows us to compare apples to oranges and bananas and not just apples to apples. Figure 2-4 shows comparisons of costs for a variety of treatments in different diseases. These include both interventions against specific disease states (e.g., myocardial infarction, stroke),[28,29] and interventions designed to prevent injury or illness (e.g., airbags).[30] The ATS Guidelines also recommend the generation of a reference case, and further recommend the presentation of a data-rich case from the results of the randomized trial. This case would be generated using a minimal number of model assumptions and the maximum amount of available data from the clinical trial.

Policy Implications

Decision making based on the results of a CEA is founded on the idea of social utilitarianism. This valuation is in turn based on the assumptions that: (1) good is determined by consequences at the community level, these consequences being the sum of individual utilities (health and happiness); (2) all utilities are equal within the metric used to measure them; and (3) loss of benefit to some individuals is balanced by benefit to others. As a simple example, consider the decision to fund a childhood immunization program rather than a radical chemotherapy program to treat a rare cancer. This decision assumes that spending resources on immunizations will maximize the community's utility (health) more than money spent on treating a rare cancer. Social utilitarianism acts to

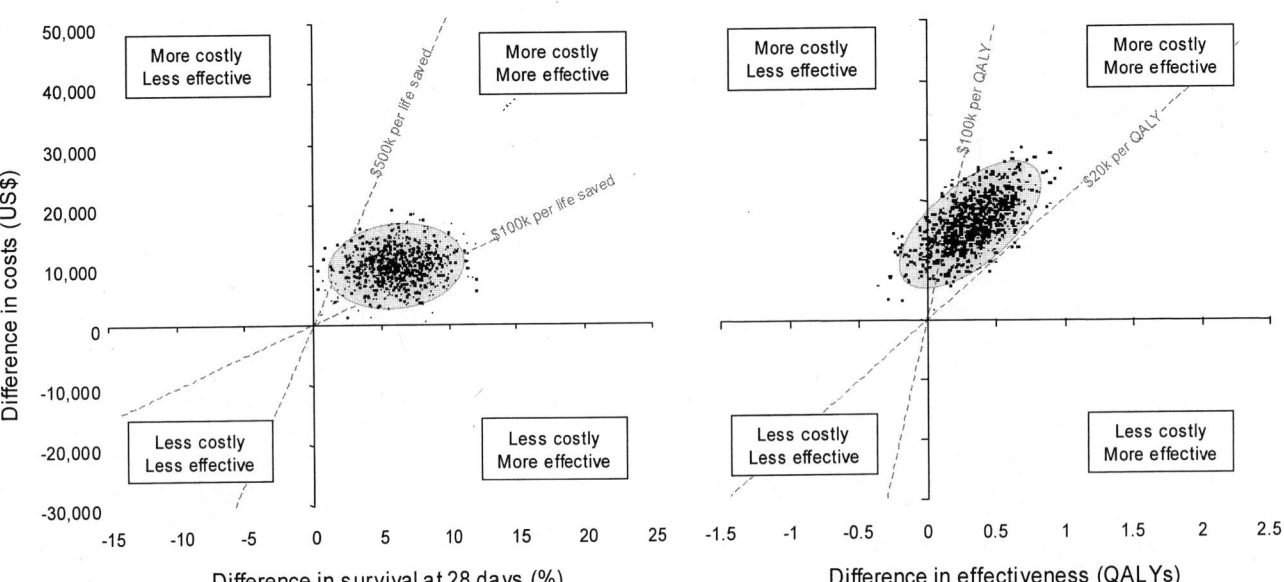

BASE CASE
Cost per survivor at 28 days

REFERENCE CASE
Lifetime cost per QALY

FIGURE 2-3 Cost effectiveness of drotrecogin alfa (activated) in severe sepsis. The figure shows the CE_{base} (*left panel*) and $CE_{reference}$ (*right panel*) distributions of cost-effectiveness ratios of the 1000 simulations with the corresponding 95% confidence ellipses generated by Fieller's method.[31] Incremental effects are shown on the *x* axes and incremental costs are shown on the *y* axes. Quadrants to the right of the *y* axes represent regions where treatment with drotrecogin alfa (activated) is associated with a net gain in effects. Quadrants above the *x* axes represent regions where treatment is associated with a net increase in costs.

The dotted lines are illustrative thresholds. Regions below and to the right of the thresholds are more cost effective than regions above and to the left of the thresholds. The ellipses are the smallest areas containing the average incremental costs and effects, with 95% confidence. Both distributions are predominantly in the "more costly, more effective" upper right quadrant, with the majority of simulations falling below the $500,000 per life saved and $100,000 per quality-adjusted life year thresholds. (*Reproduced with permission from Angus et al.*[27])

Cost-effectiveness ratio

Intervention	More favorable scenario	$/QALY		Less favorable scenario	$/QALY
Statins[32]	For secondary prevention with stepped care vs. niacin	1,600		For primary and secondary prevention vs. secondary only	48,000
Neonatal intensive care[33]	Vs. standard neonatal care for infants 1–1.5 kg	7,100		Vs. standard neonatal care for infants 0.5–1 kg	49,000
CABG[34]	For left main vessel disease vs. medical management of angina	7,100		For one-vessel disease vs. medical management of angina	56,000
tPA for AMI[28]	For anterior myocardial infarction vs. streptokinase	18,000		For inferior myocardial infarction vs. streptokinase	60,000
Drotrecogin alfa (activated)[27]	For severe sepsis with APACHE II ≥25 vs. standard therapy	27,000		For all severe sepsis vs. standard therapy	49,000
Air bags[30]	For driver side only vs. no air bags	28,000		Dual air bags vs. driver-side air bag only	72,000
Implantable defibrillators[35]	ICD-only regimen vs. amiodarone to ICD regimen	40,000		Amiodarone to ICD regimen vs. amiodarone only	157,000
Lung transplantation[36]	Vs. standard care, assuming 10-year survival	44,000		Vs. standard care, assuming 5-year survival	204,000

$0/QALY $20,000s/QALY $100,000/QALY

FIGURE 2-4 League table showing the range of cost-effectiveness ratios for a variety of medical or preventive interventions.[27,28,30,32–36] The vertical lines show the $20,000/quality-adjusted life year and $100,000/quality-adjusted life year levels. The range of values within an intervention indicates differences in conditions or assumptions included in the model.

maximize the health and happiness (utility) of the community, and consequently leads to maximum efficiency in use of health care resources for community benefit. CEA is designed to result in a ranked list of community benefits resulting from given cost outlays. While CEAs can inform us about where to spend money to improve utility, they cannot inform about how much money should be spent to improve health care overall.

The overall goal of CEAs is to provide decision makers with information that can be used to choose between medical care options when all options are not financially feasible. If monies are unlimited, the relevant question becomes "what treatment options minimize patient morbidity and mortality?" and CEAs are unnecessary. If funds are limited, the question becomes "what provides the best value?" and CEAs can help to answer this question. This was the overall conclusion of the ATS and the workshop further recommended that critical care researchers utilize the PCEHM Guidelines and conduct reference case cost-effectiveness analyses as part of the evaluation of ICU interventions. The rigorous application of this CEA methodology will allow more informative health care policy in the care of the critically ill.

Conclusion

The conduct of a rigorous CEA is clearly challenging. There are many methodologic complexities to consider within the study, and the analysis is likely to be highly dependent on the availability and quality of information from other studies (e.g., a phase III RCT). Much of the information required for thorough conduct of a CEA may in fact be missing, and therefore the analysis will require sophisticated modeling techniques to explore the impact of various assumptions and estimates. In order for the reader to be confident in the results of a CEA, the analysis must not only be robust, but must also be perceived as such. Accomplishing this requires clear reporting from the analyst and a commitment on the part of the reader to embrace cost-effectiveness analyses as a legitimate approach to determining the value of new therapies in the treatment of the critically ill.

References

1. Halpern NA, Bettes L, Greenstein R: Federal and nationwide intensive care units and healthcare costs: 1986–1992. *Crit Care Med* 22:2001, 1994.
2. Angus DC, Linde-Zwirble WT, Sirio CA, et al: The effect of managed care on ICU length of stay: Implications for Medicare. *JAMA* 276:1075, 1996.
3. Russell LB, Gold MR, Siegel JE, et al: The role of cost-effectiveness analysis in health and medicine. Panel on Cost-Effectiveness in Health and Medicine. *JAMA* 276:1172, 1996.
4. Weinstein MC, Siegel JE, Gold MR, et al: Recommendations of the Panel on Cost-Effectiveness in Health and Medicine. *JAMA* 276:1253, 1996.
5. Siegel JE, Weinstein MC, Russell LB, et al: Recommendations for reporting cost-effectiveness analyses. *JAMA* 276:1339, 1996.
6. Angus DC, Rubenfeld GD, Roberts MS, et al: Understanding costs and cost-effectiveness in critical care: Report from the Second American Thoracic Society Workshop on Outcomes Research. *Am J Respir Crit Care Med* 165:540, 2002.
7. Coughlin MT, Angus DC: Pharmacoeconomics of new therapies in critical illness. *Crit Care Med* 31(Suppl):S7, 2003.
8. Gold MR, Russell LB, Seigel JE, et al: *Cost-Effectiveness in Health and Medicine*. New York, Oxford University Press, 1996.
9. Doubilet P, Weinstein MC, McNeil BJ: Use and misuse of the term "cost effective" in medicine. *N Engl J Med* 314:253, 1986.
10. Linden PK, Angus DC, Chelluri L, et al: The influence of clinical study design on cost-effectiveness projections for the treatment of gram-negative sepsis with human anti-endotoxin antibody. *J Crit Care* 10:154, 1995.
11. Freemantle N, Drummond M: Should clinical trials with concurrent economic analyses be blinded? *JAMA* 277:63, 1997.
12. Dellinger RP: From the bench to the bedside: The future of sepsis research. Executive summary of an American College of Chest Physicians, National Institute of Allergy and Infectious Disease, and National Heart, Lung, and Blood Institute Workshop. *Chest* 111:744, 1997.
13. Clermont G, Angus DC, Linde-Zwirble WT, et al: Does acute organ dysfunction predict patient-centered outcomes? *Chest* 121:1963, 2002.
14. Cohen J, Guyatt G, Bernard GR, et al: New strategies for clinical trials in patients with sepsis and septic shock. *Crit Care Med* 29:880, 2001.
15. Bernard GR, Vincent JL, Laterre PF, et al: Efficacy and safety of recombinant human activated protein C for severe sepsis. *N Engl J Med* 344:699, 2001.
16. Annane D, Sebille V, Charpentier C, et al: Effect of treatment with low doses of hydrocortisone and fludrocortisone on mortality in patients with septic shock. *JAMA* 288:862, 2002.
17. Rivers E, Nguyen B, Havstad S, et al: Early goal-directed therapy in the treatment of severe sepsis and septic shock. *N Engl J Med* 345:1368, 2001.
18. The Acute Respiratory Distress Syndrome (ARDS) Network authors for the ARDS Network: Ventilation with lower tidal volumes as compared with traditional tidal volumes for acute lung injury and the acute respiratory distress syndrome. *N Engl J Med* 342:1301, 2000.
19. Quartin AA, Schein RM, Kett DH, et al: Magnitude and duration of the effect of sepsis on survival. *JAMA* 277:1058, 1997.
20. Angus DC, Carlet J, on behalf of the 2002 Brussels Roundtable Participants: Surviving intensive care: A report from the 2002 Brussels Roundtable. *Intensive Care Med* 29:368, 2003.
21. Angus DC, Carlet J (eds): *Surviving Intensive Care: Update in Intensive Care and Emergency Medicine*, No. 39. Berlin, Springer-Verlag, 2003.
22. Chelluri L, Grenvik AN, Silverman M: Intensive care for critically ill elderly: Mortality, costs, and quality of life. Review of the literature. *Arch Intern Med* 155:1013, 1995.
23. Shwartz M, Young DW, Siegrist R: The ratio of costs to charges: How good a basis for estimating costs? *Inquiry* 32:476, 1995.
24. Keene AR, Cullen DJ: Therapeutic Intervention Scoring System: update 1983. *Crit Care Med* 11:1, 1983.
25. Rapoport J, Teres D, Lemeshow S, et al: A method for assessing the clinical performance and cost-effectiveness of intensive care units: A multicenter inception cohort study. *Crit Care Med* 22:1385, 1994.
26. Keeler EB, Cretin S: Discounting of life-saving and other non-monetary effects. *Management Sci* 29:300, 1983.
27. Angus D, Linde-Zwirble WT, Clermont G, et al: Cost-effectiveness of drotrecogin alfa (activated) in the treatment of severe sepsis. *Crit Care Med* 31:1, 2003.
28. Kalish SC, Gurwitz J, Krumholz HM, et al: A cost-effectiveness model of thrombolytic therapy for acute myocardial infarction. *J Gen Intern Med* 10:321, 1995.
29. Gage BF, Cardinalli AB, Albers GW, et al: Cost-effectiveness of warfarin and aspirin for prophylaxis of stroke in patients with nonvalvular atrial fibrillation. *JAMA* 274:1839, 1995.

30. Graham JD, Thompson KM, Goldie SJ, et al: The cost-effectiveness of air bags by seating position. *JAMA* 278:1418, 1997.

31. Fieller EC: Some problems in interval estimation. *J R Stat Soc Ser B Methodological* 16:175, 1954.

32. Stinnett AA, Mittleman MA, Weinstein MC: The cost-effectiveness of dietary and pharmacologic therapy for cholesterol reduction in adults, in Gold MR, Siegel JE, Russell LB, et al (eds): *Cost-Effectiveness in Health and Medicine.* New York, Oxford University Press, 1996, p 349.

33. Boyle MH, Torrance GW, Sinclair JC, et al: Economic evaluation of neonatal intensive care of very-low-birth-weight infants. *N Engl J Med* 308:1330, 1983.

34. Weinstein MC, Stason WB: Cost-effectiveness of coronary artery bypass surgery. *Circulation* 66:III56, 1982.

35. Owens DK, Sanders GD, Harris RA, et al: Cost-effectiveness of implantable cardioverter defibrillators relative to amiodarone for prevention of sudden cardiac death. *Ann Intern Med* 126:1, 1997.

36. Ramsey SD, Patrick DL, Albert RK, et al: The cost-effectiveness of lung transplantation. A pilot study. *Chest* 108:1594, 1995.

Chapter 3

IMPROVING THE QUALITY OF CARE IN THE INTENSIVE CARE UNIT

ALLAN GARLAND

KEY POINTS

- *Improving ICU performance demands a systems-oriented approach embodied in total quality management (TQM).*
- *In most ICUs this requires a major paradigm shift away from the discredited notion that most omissions, errors, and other problems are the fault of individuals, and embraces the idea that meaningful and sustained improvement comes from transforming structures and processes into those that make it hard for people to make mistakes.*
- *Creating an effective program of TQM is much easier in an ICU having the resources to hire personnel and purchase information systems.*
- *The most difficult, labor-intensive, and expensive part of TQM is data collection, but there are ways to make this less burdensome.*
- *Every ICU should implement a system of TQM that is multidisciplinary and inclusive, has the vigorous support of hospital and ICU leadership, and has sufficient personnel and economic support to succeed.*

Intensive care units (ICUs) are an important component of modern health care. This importance derives from large costs that are both human and economic. Approximately one third of adult deaths in the U.S. occur in acute care hospitals,[1] and as many as half of these occur in ICUs.[2,3] An even greater fraction of people spend time in an ICU during the final 6 months of life.[3] Among patients admitted to ICUs, 8% to 17% die there, though for some diagnoses the ICU mortality rate is much higher.[4–6]

Beyond death rates, suffering is common among ICU patients. Half or more of ICU patients endure substantial pain.[7–9] Bergbom-Engberg and Haljamae found that 30% of patients surviving mechanical ventilation recall agony, panic, or both.[10] Among oncology patients in an ICU, 30% to 75% experienced dyspnea, hunger, anxiety, insomnia, or thirst, with increased suffering during even such innocuous procedures as turning.[9] Substantial dissatisfaction among relatives and friends of ICU patients[11–13] indicates that suffering in critical illness is not limited to the patients themselves.

To go along with these human costs, the economic costs of ICU care are staggering. Comprising just 8% of acute hospital beds,[14,15] ICU care consumes 20% of total inpatient expenditures,[15–17] equivalent to 0.9% of the gross domestic product of the United States, or $91 billion in 2001.[18] ICUs are a smaller portion of the health care systems in other industri-

alized countries, but still represent an important segment of medical care and its costs.[16,19–23]

A necessary starting point for improving ICUs is to recognize that problems of quality are common and serious. A recent Institute of Medicine Roundtable[24] stated that:

> Serious and widespread quality problems exist throughout American medicine. These … occur in small and large communities alike, in all parts of the country and with approximately equal frequency in managed care and fee-for-service systems of care. Millions of Americans are not reached by proven effective interventions that can save lives and prevent disability. Perhaps an equal number suffer needlessly because they are exposed to the harms of unnecessary health services. Large numbers are injured because preventable complications are not averted…. Quality of care is the problem, not managed care.

The U.S. health care system is by far the most expensive in the world, while ranking thirty-seventh in overall performance, and seventy-second in population health.[25] Canadian health care is the tenth most expensive, ranking thirtieth and thirty-fifth on these measures, respectively. This poor performance is not explained by society's violence, poor health habits, or high cholesterol levels.[26]

There are many factors contributing to this poor performance. Inappropriate use of medical interventions is common throughout the health care system,[26–29] with nonadherence to established standards of care being related to poor outcomes.[30,31] Medical errors are prevalent, often leading to disability and resulting in 27,000 to 98,000 deaths/year.[26,32,33] A study in Veterans Administration hospitals found that 6% to 34% of deaths there may be preventable.[34] A study limited to certain subsets of patients with iatrogenic complications in ICUs observed them to occur in 31% of patients, and to be severe in 13%.[35] Errors were observed to occur in 1% of all the interventions done each day to patients in an Israeli ICU.[36]

Another problem is variation in practice and outcomes not explained by patient or illness characteristics. Since wide and widespread variation could not exist if most practitioners practiced optimally, and such variation is evidence that suboptimal care is common. Variation has been found for many outcomes in a broad range of settings, with important differences by geographic region,[3,37,38] hospital,[39–41] physician,[40,42–48] and insurance status or payer system.[42,49–53] Such variation occurs in ICUs as well.[45,49,51,54–56] Lest one think otherwise, such variation is not just an American phenomenon.[48,57–62]

Given the primary function of ICUs, it is particularly troubling that they suffer from serious deficiencies regarding palliative and end-of-life care. In addition to the high prevalence of suffering discussed above, caregivers often don't ask about their patients' end-of-life preferences, with consequent discordance between the care desired and that received.[7,63] The conversations that do occur are often much delayed.[63–66] Communication between caregivers and ICU patients or their surrogates is frequently poor. Azoulay and associates found that 20% to 43% of surrogates did not understand what they had been told about diagnosis, prognosis, and therapeutic options, and that these problems correlated with family-doctor meetings that were too brief.[67] In other studies families expressed dissatisfaction with the amount and nature of communication, and many experienced actual conflict with the caregivers.[12,68] Even more worrisome was that 24% of patients said they were not aware of the current approach to care, and 47% of those who preferred a palliative approach felt the care they were receiving was inconsistent with that wish.[63] In addition, the variation in practice present in other aspects of ICU care is also present in end-of-life and palliative care.[3,4,62,64,65,69,70]

The data above demonstrate that ICUs are an important, expensive, and problematic component of health care. Therefore, vigorous efforts are needed to critically examine and improve every aspect of how well and how efficiently they perform their functions. Because "quality" is an extremely vague term often used to encompass various, often equally vague, concepts, this chapter will instead refer to the more tangible concept of ICU performance, and use the term performance improvement (PI) in place of the various alternatives.

Since it would require us to believe that ICU care is different than every other area of human endeavor, it is implausible that all ICUs perform equally well, or even that any given ICU is performing optimally. To identify how well a given ICU performs requires quantitation of relevant indices of performance. However, ICUs are complex organizations, and it is difficult to clearly define or measure such indices. In fact, the meaning, scope, and measurement of performance in health care have evolved and broadened over the past two decades. Some of the most widely used approaches to improving performance in health care have proved inadequate. This chapter will discuss both the conceptual basis and practical aspects of a superior method of evaluating and improving ICU performance.

Defining Intensive Care Unit Performance

Defining ICU performance is a difficult exercise that embraces diverse elements such as medical knowledge, ethics, economics, systems engineering, sociology, and philosophy. Efforts to measure ICU performance should follow two essential principles: (1) evaluate a variety of measures that span the dimensions of ICU performance; and (2) use performance measures that are directly relevant, or have an unequivocal relationship to measures that possess such relevance.

There are a number of domains within which an ICU should be judged (Table 3-1). While ultimately an ICU exists to serve the medical needs of critically ill patients, it also provides important services for families and friends of patients, health care workers in the ICU, the hospital, and society. Rating ICUs only on narrowly defined measures of health outcomes fails to recognize the larger social value associated with expert care of these patients. In addition, no single metric is adequate to address all of the categories of outcomes listed in Table 3-1.

Assessing performance requires direct measurement of end points that are relevant—to patients, society, and the hospital. Table 3-1 lists relevant measures of ICU performance. Because they are usually easier to measure, surrogate parameters are often used in PI efforts. While assessing surrogate end points is often a component of PI, this should not substitute for measuring and addressing the truly important parameters. For example, errors in drug administration have a proven association with detrimental outcomes,[32] and therefore the rate of such errors is a relevant performance measure. Processes instituted within the pharmacy to try and reduce errors, such as

TABLE 3-1 Domains and Measures of Intensive Care Unit Performance

Medical outcomes

- Survival rates: ICU, hospital, and long-term
- Complication rates related to care
- Medical errors
- Adequacy of symptom control

Economic outcomes

- Resource consumption: ICU, hospital, and posthospital
- Cost effectiveness of care

Psychosocial and ethical outcomes

- Patient satisfaction
- Family satisfaction
- Concordance of desired and actual end-of-life decisions
- Appropriateness of medical interventions provided
- Long-term functioning and quality of life among survivors

Institutional outcomes

- Staff satisfaction and turnover rate
- Effectiveness of ICU bed utilization
- Satisfaction of others in the hospital with the care and services supplied by the ICU
- Efficiency of the processes, procedures, and functions involved in ICU care

altered drug labeling or direct communication with nurses, represent surrogates for the relevant index. While addressing such processes is in fact the necessary means to the end, changing a given process may or may not result in improvement in the rate of such errors, and does not obviate the need to measure it.

The ICU readmission rate is not listed in Table 3-1 because it is at best a questionable indicator of ICU performance. Its potential value derives from observations that readmitted patients have a higher mortality rate and longer length of stay.[71] However, for it to be a meaningful surrogate requires that: (1) premature ICU discharge was the cause of a subsequent detrimental outcome due to a problem that was already present in the ICU, and (2) it would not have occurred if the patient had remained longer in the ICU. There are no data that have demonstrated this.[71,72] The optimal readmission rate is unknown, and a low one could indicate that on average, patients are inappropriately remaining in the ICU too long, when they could be adequately cared for in less expensive venues.

All of the performance parameters listed in Table 3-1 have limitations. ICU or hospital mortality rates are commonly used measures of ICU performance that are relatively simple to collect. While some data indicate that hospitals with higher death rates have more preventable deaths,[30] short-term survival tells us nothing about the things that are much more important to people, long-term survival and quality of life (QOL).[73–75] Also, certain attitudes about death and dying can mean that higher short-term mortality represents superior care by virtue of being more concordant with patients' end-of-life wishes.[76,77]

The laborious nature of collecting data on posthospital survival and QOL undoubtedly contributes to low usage of these important measures.[78] It is even more work to combine these into a quality-adjusted measure of long-term survival, such as quality-adjusted life years.[79] A variety of questionnaire-based tools have been developed for quantifying patients' QOL.[80–83] The most commonly used is SF-36.[84] These generally gauge health-related QOL on multiple domains, with heavy emphasis on functioning.[80,85] Indeed, ICU survivors often have demonstrated poor QOL.[86–88] Assessment of cognitive functioning, depression, and posttraumatic stress disorder also shed light on the long-term consequences of ICU care[89,90] (see Chap. 19).

Complication and error rates are often used as measures of ICU performance. These are relevant because of potential causal relationships of such adverse events with increased mortality, morbidity, or costs.[32] However, such adverse events do not necessarily lead to clinically relevant consequences, and some studies have found little effect.[34,35] Therefore, care must be taken to ensure that an established relationship to relevant outcomes exists for any medical error or complication whose rate is used as a surrogate for ICU performance. Since only a fraction of medical practices have been rigorously proved to be efficacious,[91] many deviations from recommended practice may have no such relationship.

Symptom control and end-of-life decision making are important aspects of ICU care. As discussed above, there is much room for improvement in this area. Use of these outcomes as measures of ICU performance has been limited by lack of training and orientation among physicians,[92,93] a paucity of pre-existing tools to measure them,[94] and other factors.[69]

Because of the enormous costs of ICU care, resource consumption should be part of every institution's assessment of ICU performance. The best measure that balances simplicity and information content is ICU length of stay. Others that require much effort to acquire include total monetary charges or costs,[95] usage of various diagnostic and/or therapeutic procedures, and Therapeutic Intervention Scoring System (TISS) score.[96] TISS is a relatively comprehensive attempt to measure resource utilization for ICU patients that works well for cohorts.[97,98] However, because spending a lot of money is justifiable if the benefits are commensurately large, while even small expenditures that generate no benefits are wasted, resource use is most relevant in combination with the noneconomic outcomes in Table 3-1. While the formalism associated with this concept, cost effectiveness, is well beyond the scope of local attempts to improve ICU performance,[99] it would be a powerful tool to assist society in clarifying the value of ICUs, as well as to assess the performance of individual ICUs. A simpler approach to assessing cost effectiveness that could be adapted within a single ICU depends on case-mix adjustment of short-term mortality and length of stay (see below).[100]

Effective use of ICU beds is important for a number of reasons. The ICU is an expensive and limited resource.[101,102] Moving patients out of the ICU prematurely due to limited availability has serious negative consequences.[103] But ICU triage decisions are often inefficient, and can be made more effective without adverse medical consequences.[104] Arguing that rationing of critical care is common but often inequitable, Kalb and Miller published a thoughtful framework for consideration of ICU triage in which they propose that the use of critical care be limited to clinical settings in which it has been demonstrated, or at least is presumed, to be cost effective.[105] They and others[106,107] provide arguments for using medical suitability as the primary determinant of such triage decisions, proposing that a low priority for ICU beds be assigned to those too healthy to require such care and to those too hopelessly ill to benefit. While rates of adherence to written or published admission and discharge standards is a common means of measuring ICU bed utilization, such information is not likely to result in much useful information, as such standards have not been subjected to scientific validation of whether they affect relevant outcomes.[108] Possible measures of utility include: (1) the percentage of ICU patients who only receive care that could be provided elsewhere in the hospital, (2) the fraction of patients for whom ICU care represents an exercise in medical futility,[109–111] and (3) patients who remain in an ICU for longer than they need its special capabilities.

The importance of satisfaction among patients and their families as measures of ICU performance is highlighted by data documenting that poor communication and dissatisfaction are common.[12,13,67,68] Unfortunately, at the local level there is usually more talk than action on this topic. This is partly because unfamiliar survey instruments, questionnaires, or interviews that are time-consuming to administer and analyze, are utilized to gather this data. There are numerous potential dimensions to such surveys in ICU care, including satisfaction with: (1) level of care from physicians, nurses, and other ancillary health care personnel; (2) involvement in decisions regarding care; (3) amount and quality of communications with health care and administrative personnel; (4) outcomes of care; (5) administrative hospital functions such as admissions, discharge, and billing; (6) food; and (7) housekeeping. While there are doubts about the validity of currently used methods,[112,113] a variety of tools exist to measure these aspects of satisfaction, including some created specially for use in ICUs.[11,13,68,114–117]

The satisfaction of all those who work in an ICU should likewise be considered a component of ICU performance. Job dissatisfaction contributes to higher rates of staff turnover,[118] which: (1) wastes training time and money;[119,120] (2) diminishes the ability of the ICU to perform as an experienced, highly functioning team;[121] and (3) further degrades staff morale while increasing stress on managers and remaining staff. The nursing shortage is already substantial, especially in ICUs.[122–125] That of respiratory therapists is not far behind,[126] and a shortage of ICU physicians is looming.[127] Problems related to dissatisfaction and turnover are obviously worse if those who quit cannot be replaced. In fact, dissatisfaction and burnout is common among nurses,[128–131] respiratory therapists,[132] and ICU physicians.[133–136] While staff retention rates are easily obtained from personnel records, data about job satisfaction are collected from questionnaires or interviews. Many survey tools exist to assess job satisfaction, burnout, and related constructs.[128,133,136–144]

A large class of performance measures quantifies problems in the processes, procedures, and functions occurring within the ICU, or that link the ICU to the rest of the hospital. This group of measures is strongly related to many of the other outcomes in Table 3-1, but possesses independent importance because of its relationship to the quality of interpersonal interactions, and the staff's perceptions of their workplace. An example is inefficiency or conflict in the course of interactions between the ICU and the pharmacy. Even in the absence of identified errors in drug administration resulting from such incidents, they have the potential to lead to errors, waste, or rework, and in any case generate negative feelings among the staff.

Measuring and Interpreting Intensive Care Unit Performance

The effectiveness of PI efforts depends on the type and quality of performance data collected. If that information is irrelevant, inaccurate, incomplete, or otherwise misleading, the effort expended may be wasted. This is a real problem, in part because in many hospitals PI efforts are primarily an exercise in analyzing individual adverse events (AE), such as complications, errors, or deaths.[145] Unfortunately, this inclination has been augmented by recent publicity about medical errors[32] and the response of regulatory entities toward such sentinel events.[146]

Though every performance measure can be phrased in terms of an AE that occurs in relation to individuals, *it is fundamental that detection of individual AEs cannot be used to measure performance*. This does not mean that analysis of individual AEs has no role in PI, but knowing that any given number of deaths, or even potentially avoidable errors occurred cannot inform us about performance without determining the rate of AEs. The number of individual events must be pooled and expressed as the rate of events by dividing by the aggregate number of at-risk patients, patient-days, or other appropriate denominator. This rate then is compared to some standard. The benchmark for comparison could be some accepted norm, the rate in other ICUs, the rate derived from analyses of databases, or the prior rate in that same ICU. It is this form of cumulative information—rates of death, errors, complications, family dissatisfaction, or others—that truly represents ICU performance.

There are multiple reasons that simply accumulating information about AEs, without their rates, is inadequate and potentially misleading. First, not all AEs are due to poor care. Even with implementation of every known beneficial practice, it is not plausible that AEs will disappear; rather the goal is to reduce their rate to an acceptable level, or below what they were previously. Second, an individual AE does not necessarily cause harm or increase costs (e.g., administering the incorrect dose of a drug often does no harm). Third, even an AE apparently caused by human error that led to harm is not proof that overall performance is poor; for example, it is entirely plausible that a surgeon who once amputated the wrong leg could have a superior overall complication rate. Fourth, the usual methods for identifying AEs, incident reports or chart review, are inefficient, inaccurate, and subject to significant disagreement.[34,36,147–150] This last point highlights the necessity of creating reliable methods of systematically collecting accurate data on the performance parameter being surveyed. Both the denominator and numerator must be accurate. This topic is beyond our scope, but a few guidelines are: (1) prospectively collected data are superior to retrospective data; (2) information collected by computerized information systems is superior to that collected by humans, especially if they are specifically programmed to acquire the desired information; and (3) identification of AEs should be based on objective, predefined criteria rather than subjective human judgment.

Measuring ICU performance using variables such as those in Table 3-1 is effected by calculating the rate for binary variables such as survival or complications, and the mean, median, or interquartile range for continuous variables, such as

a 0- to 100-point patient satisfaction scale. Whatever the data type, care must be taken to collect a sample size that is large enough to allow reliable statistical comparisons.[77,151,152] This point is illustrated by the example of a complication that occurs in approximately 3% of patients, with monthly tracking showing rates that fluctuate between 0% and 6%. If the rate jumps from 1% to 3% from January to February, this cannot be taken as indicative of anything other than statistical variation unless the confidence intervals are narrower than these fluctuations. In this example, there would have to be 1120 patients at risk per month to reduce the 95% confidence interval to ±2%.[153] Fewer are needed if the AE rate under consideration is higher, and if wider confidence intervals will suffice to convince oneself that the observed changes are real. A related issue in interpretation of comparative statistical performance data is the phenomenon of regression to the mean.[154] This principle tells us that if a performance indicator is either high or low at one time, due to innate statistical fluctuation it will tend on the next measurement to be more intermediate. Thus it is important not to overinterpret short-term changes in performance measurements.

A very important issue is that all these parameters are strongly influenced by patient demographics, comorbidities, and type and severity of acute illness, cumulatively referred to as case-mix. This may be true even for institutional outcomes such as staff satisfaction.[155] While raw data are "correct," they are problematic for comparing ICU performance between different time periods (a primary element of PI) if there have been important changes in case-mix. For example, an increase in ICU mortality over time may not represent worse care if sicker patients were admitted in the second epoch. Even the seasonal differences that occur in some critical illnesses[156–158] can create this problem. Case-mix differences are even more important in comparing performance between different ICUs.[76,159,160] Thus it is important for PI efforts to collect at least some case-mix data.

Within a single ICU the simplest way to handle this potential problem is to collect and compare case-mix data for the separate time periods under consideration. When appropriate to the performance issue being surveyed, comparisons might be made in the same season of successive years. If the case-mix variables are similar in the different intervals, then it is reasonable to believe that the performance comparisons are valid. The argument against this simple approach is that finding similarity among any given number of case-mix variables cannot exclude the possibility that there are other differences between the cohorts that remain undetected. While the point is valid, this simple approach is reasonable and the only practical one in many institutions having limited resources for PI efforts.

The case-mix variables chosen for assessment should follow the purpose of the PI project. For general purposes it is straightforward to record patient age, gender, race, the presence or absence of important comorbid states, and the organ system most responsible for ICU admission. With more data collection resources one should consider collecting socioeconomic variables such as insurance category (e.g., private or Medicare vs. Medicaid vs. none),[161–163] and measures of severity of illness such as the Acute Physiology and Chronic Health Evaluation (APACHE) score, TISS score, or Multiple Organ Dysfunction Score (MODS).[96,152,164] Special case-mix variables should be chosen for special purposes. For example, measuring outcomes of mechanically ventilated patients might lead one to record each patient's initial Pa_{O_2}/FI_{O_2} ratio as a measure of the severity of respiratory failure.

When the case-mix is not similar across time periods, it is best to make adjustments for the observed differences. A common method is to use one of the available ICU risk prediction systems.[100,165,166] Some of these, such as APACHE, the Mortality Probability Model (MPM), the Simplified Acute Physiology Score (SAPS), and IMPACT are for general adult ICU patients,[164,167] the Pediatric Risk of Mortality (PRISM) score is for general pediatric ICUs,[168] and others have been developed for specialized subsets of critically ill patients such as trauma or cardiac surgery patients.[169,170] These systems use equations derived from multivariable linear modeling of demographic and clinical data that predict one or more outcome variables for each patient by comparison with the large inception cohort of ICU patients used to create the equations (see Chap. 6). Nonlinear models achieve similar predictive power.[171] This approach is, in effect, an application of benchmarking against the outcomes in the inception cohort.[146,172] Most of these systems explicitly generate scores reflecting the severity of illness that are used within the equations. These scores should not be confused with the predictions, but are themselves good and convenient tools for evaluating case-mix as described above.

Unfortunately, these systems are very limited, and most of them only predict short-term mortality. This can be used to measure performance using the standardized mortality ratio (SMR). The SMR is calculated as the observed mortality rate of an ICU cohort divided by the average mortality rate predicted by the equations. The SMR is thus a death rate that is case-mix–adjusted by comparison with the original inception group.[77,165,166] Though unable to predict individual outcomes with sufficient accuracy to evaluate care for a given patient,[173,174] these perform reasonably well for groups of patients.[6,165,167,175–177] Other than short-term mortality, the list of performance measures for which validated prediction equations allow case-mix adjustments is short. The proprietary APACHE III system predicts ICU length of stay, days on mechanical ventilation, and the likelihood of receiving "active" intervention, though there has been published validation only for length of stay.[54] Similarly, in pediatrics the PRISM investigators have published a prediction of ICU length of stay.[55] Validated, ready-made tools to case-mix adjust the other important ICU performance measures do not yet exist.

Even for the few performance parameters included in these systems, there are problems related to calibration,[159,160,173] accuracy within some diagnostic subsets,[173,178] generalizability to other countries,[179,180] aging of the inception data set,[166,181] and even their utility in measuring performance.[176,182] In addition, none of these systems adjusts for nonphysiologic parameters that may be important determinants of outcomes, such as socioeconomic factors. While the older versions of these systems are in the public domain, some of the most current and usable ones, such as APACHE III and Project IMPACT, are proprietary and expensive.[183,184] It should be noted, however, that updating to the latest version often produces only modest increases in predictive power over earlier versions in the public domain.[177,185,186]

All of the prognostic systems mentioned are prospective. Predictions are generated from data available at the outset of the ICU admission, representing the clinical situation be-

fore ICU care was provided. However, use of commercially available, retrospective prognostic systems based on administrative or claims data is growing, in some cases mandated by governmental regulatory agencies. Many of these methodologies factor information about events that occurred during the course of care into the predictions. This represents a fundamentally flawed approach to evaluating performance and should not be used for this purpose. Not only is the accuracy of administrative databases problematic,[187–189] but such an approach is not capable of distinguishing whether poor outcomes are due to bad care or to pre-existing severity of illness.[76,187,190] Thus an ICU where many patients die due to avoidable complications could fail to be identified as a poor performer by a system that incorporated those complications into its prediction of the risk of death.

A more flexible approach that allows customized case-mix adjustment of any numerical performance parameter is to create your own multivariate regression analysis.[152,191] With the performance measure as the dependent variable, the case-mix variables as covariates, and an indicator variable to represent the different time periods, this avoids many of the disadvantages of the ready-made systems. The magnitude and statistical significance of the coefficient for the time period indicator variable then informs whether there has been a change in performance after adjusting for case-mix. A relatively simple implementation might include covariates of age, gender, race, important comorbid states, the organ system most responsible for ICU admission, and a measure of severity of illness. This approach requires some expertise in computer applications and statistical methods, but can be implemented within individual ICUs.[192]

Special comments must be made discouraging the use of diagnosis-related groups (DRGs) in PI efforts. In most hospitals, the DRG choices are not made by clinicians, and contain significant inaccuracies.[193] In addition, the DRG on hospital discharge is generally chosen to maximize reimbursement, and need not bear any relationship to the reason for ICU admission. Indeed, it may reflect a potentially avoidable complication of care.[194] Likewise, the admission DRG may not represent the reason for transfer to ICU.

In summary, every ICU should collect cumulative data on a variety of relevant measures of ICU performance. Efforts must be made to ensure the accuracy and completeness of the data collected. The data should be used to calculate summary measures, such as rates or means, for the patient cohort being assessed. Sufficient data must be accumulated to make these rates meaningful. At least some case-mix parameters should be collected as well. If there are substantial differences in case-mix between cohorts being compared, then some adjustment should be made for these differences. However, in the real world, the resources needed to collect and adjust for case-mix may exceed those available, requiring dependence on unadjusted data. In addition, the methodologies used for case-mix adjustment are not perfect. Such limitations should not lead to nihilism and inaction. Though unadjusted data could be misleading, it cannot possibly be more misleading than having no performance data at all. Similarly, adjustments made with the best available, though imperfect, methodologies are better than raw data.[195] Since the most common kind of performance comparison done in a single ICU is between two or more time intervals that are contiguous or nearly so, most of the potential difficulties in data interpretation mentioned above (except for the issue of seasonal variation) are probably of little significance.

Improving Intensive Care Unit Performance: Conceptual Framework

Improving ICU performance in a given area involves sequential steps of: (1) measuring indices of ICU performance relevant to that area, (2) making one or more interventions aimed at improving those measures, and then (3) remeasuring the indices to document the effect of the intervention.[196] Measurement is discussed above. This section will develop a framework for understanding the scope and nature of change.

There are two main domains of change for improving ICU performance. These are the technical components of ICU care, and the organizational features of the ICU. Both medical training and literature almost exclusively emphasize the technical. Thus the attention of clinicians is dominated by choices such as ventilator settings, vasopressors, imaging modalities, and the angle of the bed during tube feeding. While these are important, changes to ICU structures and processes are given little attention, but are at least as significant.[194] Indeed, it requires extensive organizational change to ensure effective, uniform application of the technical choices.

A useful framework for addressing technical interventions to improve care in individual ICUs is adapted from Berwick.[197] He tells us that we must: (1) know what works, (2) use what works, and (3) do what works adeptly. Knowing what works amounts to reading and understanding the literature. This includes recognizing the limits of current knowledge. With estimates that only 10% to 20% of medical practices are supported by rigorous studies,[91] many diagnostic and therapeutic interventions are used in the absence of clearly demonstrated efficacy. Many studies focus narrowly on physiologic efficacy instead of relevant outcomes.[198] Also, understanding and correctly interpreting the literature is impeded because many physicians lack the statistical and logical skills needed for such critical evaluation.[198,199]

As problematic as is our state of knowledge, the single most important deficiency in health care today is ensuring that we use what works, and do it well.[3,24,200] Even seminal studies in the most widely read journals often do not change practice.[201] To understand this deficiency, it is necessary to recognize that these things do not happen by themselves. Ensuring that all patients uniformly receive every applicable evidence-based "best practice" requires a paradigm shift. The historical, physician-centered paradigm holds individual physicians entirely responsible and free to guide care as they see fit, regardless of whether their choices concur with best practices, and independent of outside oversight except the risk of malpractice suits. Kassirer states that "...when it comes to setting standards of accountability and ethical behavior, our professional organizations and medical institutions have often faltered. In the guise of accountability, their efforts have often yielded lax standards that were intentionally and flagrantly self-serving."[202] Such a system, in which patients are entirely dependent on the knowledge and memory of their physicians, is not rational, and is not in the best interests of the patients or the clinicians. As Wennberg states: "the 'system' of care in the United States is not a system at all, but a largely unplanned and irrational sprawl of resources."[107] There are too many important things to know and remember to reasonably expect that any individual physician will always do all the right things. Even simple, universally accepted practices such as giving aspirin and β-adrenergic blockers to patients with acute myocardial infarction are often forgotten, leading to many unnecessary deaths.[203] This is not an indictment of physicians—it is unreasonable to harbor such expectations in the modern medical environment. Instead, it is necessary to create structures and implement processes that ensure that every ICU patient, every time, receives all applicable evidence-based practices. Doing so will ensure, for example, that no mechanically ventilated patient receiving tube feedings will fail to have the head of the bed elevated to reduce the risk of nosocomial pneumonia because their physician forgot to write that order among the dozens that were written.[204]

But ensuring the uniform application of beneficial medical practices is not the only reason we need to re-engineer ICU organization. ICUs are complex systems, and it has been known for many decades in the industry that "the structure of a system significantly determines the performance of the system."[205] By emphasizing that most opportunity for improving performance derives from altering the system itself, Deming, Juran, and others created the most effective method known of improving the performance of complex systems.[206,207] This methodology of PI, called total quality management (TQM), applies equally well to service industries such as health care,[205,208–210] and tells us that making changes in ICU organization offers opportunities to improve performance that are equal to or greater than the gains from purely technical improvements.[211–213] Though the systems approach of TQM is largely alien to health care, it is the recommended method of PI.[146]

The concept of TQM began with the seminal recognition that only 15% of errors and problems are a result of inadequate performance by individuals. Rather, 85% of the opportunities for performance improvement relate to flaws in institutional systems and processes that hinder the ability of individuals to perform their jobs well.[206] As stated by Berwick,[209] these original thinkers understood that problems had:

> ...been built directly into the complex production processes they studied, and that defects in quality could only rarely be attributed to a lack of will, skill, or benign intention among the people involved with the processes. Even when people were at the root of the defects, they learned, the problem was generally not one of motivation or effort, but rather of poor job design, failure of leadership, or unclear purpose. Quality can be improved much more when people are assumed to be trying hard already, and are not accused of sloth.

TQM is about improving the *systems* that are used to deliver ICU care. It is a continuous and relentless process of examining and improving *structures* and *processes*[194] for the purpose of improving relevant outcomes. It is driven by systematically collected and appropriately interpreted data on outcomes.[208,210,214] In TQM *every* structure, process, activity, function, and relationship, clinical and nonclinical, that influences the ICU in any way is open to scrutiny and change. Table 3-2 contains an illustrative list of areas for scrutiny.

Examples will aid in making these concepts more concrete. Evans and colleagues developed a computerized antibiotic

TABLE 3-2 Potential Areas for Improvement in the Intensive Care Unit

- The need for a function
- How a function is performed
- Which personnel perform a function
- The functional relationship between personnel
- How personnel communicate with each other
- The existence, frequency, and nature of ICU rounds
- The role of equipment (including computers)
- The interactions between personnel and equipment (including computers)
- The administrative, medical, and functional structures of the ICU
- The administrative, medical, and functional structures of personnel who provide care in, or support to, the ICU
- The rules governing responsibilities, practice privileges, etc
- The training, skills, competence, knowledge, and experience of personnel
- The scheduling of personnel, including shift coverage, night coverage, and weekend coverage
- Workload per worker
- The availability of supportive technology in the hospital (e.g., advanced imaging)
- The choice of products and services used in the ICU
- The number of ICU beds
- The physical layout of the ICU
- Availability of intermediate care and ward beds
- Availability of outcomes data to the ICU and hospital community
- Availability of outcomes data to public

consultant, available from every hospital workstation, to assist physicians in the selection of appropriate empiric antibiotics.[215] They found that this increased the adequacy of the initial antibiotic choice from 77% to 94%, and that the delay in ordering adequate antibiotics was reduced. Leape and coworkers altered the structure of morning work rounds in an ICU to include the participation of a senior pharmacist.[216] This simple structural change reduced avoidable drug errors by 65%. Bernstein found that what at first glance seemed like the ultimate in individual human error, surgery on the wrong side of the body, actually represented inadequacy of the procedures that should have been in place to prevent this problem.[217]

TQM views performance as a moving target that can be improving all the time, even in the absence of identified problems. Benchmarking, most simply against performance in the same ICU at earlier time period, allows for realization of this goal. TQM does not respect existing professional standards; rather it continually demands development of new ones that are more effective and efficient.[210] The purpose is to reduce waste, rework, and complexity, while improving relevant outcomes, reducing costs, generating loyalty, and creating a climate of teamwork.[208,209]

Shifting the focus from identifying and remediating defective workers, to identifying and re-engineering defective structures and processes is necessary to correct "the defects that we have built into our complex medical systems . . . the waste we encounter in outmoded habits, the rework we pay for when things fail to work correctly the first time, complexity we build into our processes for no good reasons at all, the random and unpredictable variation from our predicted aims."[197] One result of TQM is that it becomes easier for people to do their jobs right, and harder for mistakes to occur.

An important tenet of systems engineering is that organizational performance inevitably deteriorates unless the structures and processes of the organization evolve along with the needs they must serve. The most natural way to cope with a changing environment is to supplement the structures and processes already in existence; as demand grows, the system gets multiplied to scale. However, such growth by accretion inevitably leads to a cumbersome, inefficient system. What is needed instead is evolution of new systems and processes that match the new environment. Obviously, the nature of ICU patients and ICU care, as well as the size of ICUs, has changed dramatically over the years, and projections show that this growth will continue.[127] But the organization of many ICUs is not the result of thoughtful planning driven by improving outcomes, but rather reflects their historical origins and subsequent growth by accretion. As a result, their organization is inadequate to support the current demands.

The systems-oriented strategy of TQM is very different from the quality assurance/quality improvement (QA/QI) method that is still used in many ICUs. QA/QI responds to adverse events, errors, or other problems that are found. Obviously, problems are found only after they occur, and so QA/QI is reactive, instead of proactive. Leadership then convenes a group, usually composed of supervisory-level personnel, to do "root cause analysis." Most commonly, this takes the form of trying to identify the errors made by individuals who allowed the problem to occur. The morbidity and mortality conference held regularly in most institutions is an example of such a flawed approach to improving quality.

In fact, both components of QA/QI, identification of problems and errors, and root cause analysis, are fundamentally deficient. QA/QI relies on occurrence screening to identify problems.[145,218] This can take the form of medical record reviews, incident reporting, or use of prospective indicators. An example of an indicator is a document that bedside nurses complete when a mechanically ventilated patient is inadvertently extubated. Retrospective occurrence screening using the medical record is limited by the many inadequacies of that document as a window into actual events.[187] Incident reporting is also an inadequate method of identifying adverse events in hospitals. Only a small fraction of adverse drug events are identified by incident reports,[147,148] and a study of direct observation in an ICU estimated that only about half of errors were reported.[36] So-called audit filters, groups of prospectively defined and collected occurrence screens, are of low sensitivity.[219,220] Even prospective occurrence screening can obscure the magnitude of a problem, due to the changes individuals make in their behavior when they know that they are being watched, known as the Hawthorne effect.[221] In addition, medical care is so complex and variable that screening for even a large list of specific occurrences is unlikely to have much impact on overall performance.

Root cause analysis is a process in which medical professionals who are knowledgeable in the area under consideration perform a detailed review of an adverse event to identify its causes. As stated by Berwick:[222]

> Even when hospitals find ways to notice the injuries to their patients, their theories of cause often remain scientifically Neanderthal. They cling to unsound but deeply entrenched beliefs. They believe that bad people cause bad errors. . . . They believe that retrospection will allow them to find a single root cause,

even though in fact the very idea of a "root cause" is misleading, since most system failures result from complex interactions between latent failures . . . and specific actions; conclusions about root causes are often illusions created by hindsight bias.

One reason for the ineffectiveness of root cause analysis is that there is very poor agreement among experts about the causes, and even the occurrence, of adverse events.[34,149,150] The poorest agreement is for identifying management errors or negligence as the cause of adverse events.

QA/QI is about meeting minimum standards, detecting poor performance by individuals, and taking punitive actions. It is "at best inefficient, and at worst a formula for failure."[209] Despite prolonged and extensive use, there are almost no published data showing that health care is improved or behavior changed by PI methods that target individuals rather than structures and processes.[223] Chassin concludes that there is a "paucity of evidence that, as a whole, previous quality-assurance programs actually did anything to improve outcomes for patients."[224]

Implementing a Total Quality Management Program in the Intensive Care Unit

The ICU is an opportune place to establish a TQM program. ICUs are usually physically localized, well-defined entities that often already possess high degrees of organization. Compared with many other parts of the health care system, there are fewer people working there, making it easier to effect the necessary indoctrination into TQM concepts and to include a substantial fraction of personnel directly in the TQM process. Also, compared to other areas of health care, there are fewer confounding variables, with a relatively high degree of control over them. Methods to adjust for case-mix variation are more highly developed for ICUs than almost any other area of medical care.

TQM is a complex process. Implementing it in a hospital or ICU requires substantial commitments of leadership, resources, and time. It is estimated that 3 to 5 years are needed to adopt and fully institutionalize a new TQM program.[210] Outside assistance can be helpful. This can come from a similar institution that has been successful in creating a TQM program, or by contracting with a consulting firm. Specific training is needed for those who will lead the effort. While a complete delineation of its methods is beyond our scope, this section will outline important issues in the implementation of TQM.

Meaningful participation of every type of ICU personnel in TQM is needed because both performance and improvement are recognized to be shared responsibilities. Since the best people to identify and solve problems are those directly involved in them, the basic functional unit of TQM is the multidisciplinary quality team. Unlike most other PI efforts used in health care, TQM is not controlled by clinicians, though obviously they are included in it. Thus for PI purposes, TQM replaces managerial authority with a participatory approach that emphasizes collective rather than individual responsibility.[210]

Initiating a TQM program within an ICU is difficult, though not impossible, without the existence of a hospital-wide TQM program. In the following five-step outline for implementing TQM in an ICU, it is assumed to be part of such a larger effort.

The first step is that top leadership must take the lead. Those at the top of the administrative and medical hierarchy must make an overt and highly visible commitment that TQM is a clear priority. They demonstrate this by providing the leadership, encouragement, and economic and political support necessary for the institution to evolve into a "TQM culture." It has been observed that TQM is more readily assimilated in hospitals with corporate cultures that emphasize teamwork and development of human potential, are willing to take risks, and seize on opportunities as they arise.[225]

Second, investments must be made in education and training. Key administrative and medical managers undergo specialized education and training in the methods of TQM that they then bring back to the institution. Those who will act as facilitators for quality teams also require training. Subsequently the entire ICU staff needs to be familiarized with TQM concepts and the blueprint for improvement. Their involvement at all levels is necessary for TQM to succeed, and it is vital to elicit their support. An element of the human equation is that there must not be fear on the part of personnel that TQM is a smoke screen for downsizing, or that the discovery of problems, even of human error, will lead to retaliation.[214,224] The TQM environment must be one of trust. Everyone, from the top to the bottom, must become convinced of the central truth of TQM, that the problems are due to faulty systems, not faulty people. More informed personnel will be more motivated and better participants. Part of the framework for success is that the institutional leadership finds ways to encourage, recognize, and reward individuals who participate effectively.

Third, investments must be made in data gathering and analysis capabilities. As discussed in detail above, TQM requires extensive measurement and statistical analysis of performance parameters. Therefore these functions must be given the necessary institutional support, and often require the acquisition of additional personnel and/or information systems. This is the most costly part of a TQM program, and must be accepted as the price of becoming serious about PI. Some measures of ICU performance should be constantly gathered as surveillance for commonly recognized problems. Examples include rates of major nosocomial infections and overall ICU length of stay. Others are collected for limited times related to a specific PI project. Caution is indicated regarding use of existing clinical personnel to collect data. Because they are in the best positions to accurately collect certain types of data, bedside nurses, respiratory therapists, and physicians can be involved in this part of TQM. However, it is necessary to resist the cost-saving impulse of placing the major burden for data collection on clinical personnel who are already overloaded with work, and who lack special training in this area. Resentment and failure of the program can result if the hospital's top leadership does not provide adequate economic support for TQM.

Fourth, a TQM leadership team for ICU performance is formed. Made up of a multidisciplinary group of administrative, clinical, and nonclinical personnel, this group coordinates TQM activities. It (1) solicits, develops, and prioritizes proposals for areas to be surveyed; (2) selects and supports the individual quality teams created to work on areas of interest; (3) contributes to the choice of primary and surrogate performance measures used to assess ICU performance; and (4) facilitates implementation of proposals for change. Areas given priority often are those that represent high volume, possess high risk, or are perceived to be a problem.

Last, and most importantly, TQM quality teams (QTs) are created and trained. An appropriately constituted QT addresses the area of concern assigned to it by the leadership team. QTs must be of manageable size, usually no more than 8 to 10 individuals representing different departments and different levels. Each QT must be constructed to include all the expertise and experience needed for thorough understanding of the inner workings of the area or topic under consideration. This dictates that the teams be heavily weighted with lower level personnel who actually do the work. No group of ICU workers should be omitted when relevant to the performance issue at hand. For example, housekeepers are an important component of infection control efforts. They, as well as unit clerks and other nonprofessional personnel play important roles that must be addressed within QTs. QTs comprised primarily of managers and physicians are usually doomed to fail because they lack truly intimate knowledge of the systems that make the ICU work.

An ICU may have one or more QTs. A QT may be permanent, or it may be constituted to address a given area, then disband. In smaller ICUs there is often nearly complete overlap between the membership of the leadership team and the quality team.

One person who has undergone TQM training functions as the QT's facilitator. The facilitator guides the group in its central functions: (1) brainstorming to break down the topic of concern into its component structures and processes,[208,226-228] and (2) identifying practicable ways to modify or replace those components to improve the relevant outcomes. This procedure typically requires measurement of the relevant outcome parameter of interest, and of surrogate measures related to the structures and/or processes. With institutional support, data are collected, case-mix adjusted if necessary, statistically analyzed, and displayed to illuminate important relationships.[228] Following implementation of changes, the performance parameters are remeasured to document improvement.

The focus of a QT can range from big to small. One may be convened to deal with an unusually high rate of death among mechanically ventilated patients. The death rate is the primary, relevant end point, but this team's scope and range will include a large number of structures, processes, and procedures used in the care of such patients. Data collection will be a formidable task for this team. Another team may be asked to find ways to decrease conflict about roles between nurses and respiratory therapists on the night shift.

QTs are potent tools for improvement. In the process of their assigned task they often identify other cumbersome or otherwise deficient processes, even if no obvious error has been related to them. Such proactive problem solving should be encouraged by endowing the QTs with considerable latitude of scope. When embarking on an assigned task, QTs should be encouraged to think expansively. No arbitrary limitations should be placed on what may be altered to improve performance.

In starting their work, QTs should perform a literature review to identify what is already known about the topic under consideration. Practices of proven effectiveness should be incorporated into the structures and processes of every ICU. For many major topics there have been systematic reviews of the literature that can serve as a starting point. However, it is often necessary for one or more members of the QT to review the original studies and summarize the findings for the entire team.

The role in TQM of analyzing individual adverse events deserves mention. As discussed above, such analysis cannot serve as the primary method of PI. However, within an active QT, discussion and analysis of individual events can effectively focus the attention of the group, and assist in identifying the structures and processes that require alteration.[229] For this reason, it is still important that ICUs work to identify individual errors and other problems. Morbidity and mortality conference reviewing of each death and major adverse event is recommended, but its limited place within the larger context of TQM must be explicitly understood. There has been much discussion recently of improving error reporting in health care by creating a nonpunitive environment based on the systems and principles of TQM.[230] Such approaches have proved successful in the airline industry and elsewhere.[231]

There are significant challenges to implementing a TQM system in the ICU. These include substantial time commitments, financial investments, and commitment of top leadership in the ICU and hospital. Often the largest impediment to successful implementation of TQM is resistance from physicians. Physicians frequently respond to objective results about performance by insisting that the data are inaccurate, and usually resist proposals perceived as abridging their professional autonomy.[200] One contributor to this resistance is that their training and work experience generally do not instill physicians with the concepts of systems engineering. While there are a number of ways to try and change physicians' habits and performance,[232] the evidence amply demonstrates that this is difficult.[233-235] Nonetheless, gaining physician acceptance and participation in any TQM effort is necessary. Various strategies to achieve this goal have been discussed elsewhere.[208,228] One particular experience of note was the effort of the Cleveland Health Quality Choice consortium to gain provider and purchaser confidence for its hospital quality efforts.[236] Adapting its approach to the problem of gaining physician confidence in TQM would emphasize: (1) a large-scale effort to incorporate large numbers of physicians in the process from the start, especially those considered opinion leaders; and (2) sensitivity to physicians' concerns about presentation of data in ways that could be perceived as dangerous or threatening to their practices. The role of vigorous physician leadership in this regard cannot be overstated.[237]

Despite the difficulties, successful examples of implementing TQM in the ICU are there for emulation. Investigators at Intermountain LDS hospital in Utah described TQM implementation in their medical/surgical ICU, with extensive utilization of information systems support.[211] They reported improved cost effectiveness, comprised of an 18% reduction in costs, with no change in case-mix adjusted mortality or length of stay. A regional TQM initiative in New England reduced hospital mortality after coronary artery bypass surgery by 24%.[213]

Specific Strategies to Improve Performance

Improving ICU performance requires making organizational changes. A modest but growing body of research has studied strategies to improve performance via organizational changes in health care systems. These strategies range from simple to complex, and address widely differing aspects of change. They fall loosely into two categories: (1) strategies to increase use of evidence-based best practices, and (2) changes in structures and processes that are *not* directly related to the technical aspects of medical care. The former include education, clinical practice guidelines, reminders, audit with feedback, ordering policies, and combinations of these individual interventions. The latter are a diverse group of interventions. This section reviews much of that literature as it is applicable to ICUs. Strategies found to be effective in research studies are convenient, ready-made tools that individual ICUs can adopt, and are likely to be effective within their own TQM efforts. Of course, interventions that were effective in one setting may not be so in a different setting; as in all changes made under TQM, it is best if their local efficacy is demonstrated by local data.

STRATEGIES TO INCREASE USE OF EVIDENCE-BASED BEST PRACTICES

Didactic educational interventions are the traditional method of teaching health care practitioners how to optimally care for patients. Continuing medical education (CME) is a requirement for health professionals in most venues. Recently, Davis and coworkers published a systematic analysis of studies assessing the efficacy of traditional didactic CME methods, such as conferences, rounds, meetings, and symposia.[238] They found that the quality of these data is poor, that any benefit present was small and apparently limited to CME interventions having interactive elements. Another review of the topic also concluded that passive educational methods did not improve physician performance or patient outcomes.[233] One must be careful in reading this literature, because in fact the analyses that seem to show more impressive gains from CME have mixed together didactic education with other modalities such as reminders and audit with feedback.[239]

Practice guidelines represent attempts to increase use of evidence-based best practices by making available to clinicians a set of recommendations for care. The concept is born of the belief that these practices are omitted because clinicians are not aware of them. They can be simple, or complex and comprehensive. They have been promulgated by professional organizations, governments, consulting firms, HMOs, hospitals, and other groups. Many physicians harbor negative attitudes about practice guidelines.[240] In evaluating this body of literature, it is important to distinguish studies that assess clinically relevant outcomes from those that evaluate the surrogate of compliance with recommended patterns of care. This is especially important because many or most published guidelines fall short of the desirable features of practice guidelines.[241–244] While some studies of guidelines have demonstrated improvement in outcomes, most have found that the guidelines are of limited effectiveness without concomitant use of other strategies.[233,243] Numerous factors have been shown to influence acceptance, use, and effects of practice guidelines. These include their complexity, manner of dissemination, local input into their construction, characteristics of the targeted practitioners, and the ease with which they are accessible at the bedside.[233,242–243,249] Nonetheless, it is quite reasonable that practice guidelines be used as tools of ICU TQM, with attention to these acceptance factors, and in conjunction with other strategies.

Because the number of best practices that modern clinicians are expected to remember and implement is prohibitively large, automatic reminders could be a powerful tool to improve ICU performance. The bulk of evidence identifies reminders as one of the most effective methods of improving adherence to best practices.[233,242] The major limitation of this concept is effecting reliable and timely delivery of reminder messages to clinicians. Reminders can be delivered to clinicians in a number of ways. The most promising is via computers, as discussed below.

Audit with feedback can be defined as any summary of clinical performance of health care over a specified period of time that is communicated back to practitioners. These may or may not include recommendations for clinical action. Recent systematic reviews have concluded that this body of literature is of poor quality, and that while audit with feedback appears useful, the effects are small.[250,251] Isolated studies have, however, observed substantial benefits from audit with feedback. Eagle and associates reported that it led to economically relevant reductions in length of stay for patients admitted with chest pain, congestive heart failure, or syncope in three medical ICUs.[252] A review of 26 studies found that audit with feedback was less effective than reminders.[233]

Another potential method of ensuring best practices is to create groups of orders that have those practices built into them. The ICU is an opportune locale for such an approach by virtue of: (1) the relatively limited subset of diagnoses that gain a patient entry there, and (2) the applicability to many patients of a small set of proven safety practices. Sets of ICU admission orders can easily be created, either on paper or computer, to include by default orders such as prophylaxis against stress gastritis bleeding for patients who are mechanically ventilated.[253]

A recurrent theme seen in studies to improve use of best practices is that combining multiple strategies is more effective than the use of individual ones.[211,213,233,242,254]

CHANGES TO INTENSIVE CARE UNIT STRUCTURES AND PROCESSES NOT DIRECTLY RELATED TO TECHNICAL ASPECTS OF CARE

Table 3-3 summarizes a substantial portion of this literature. The interested reader who uses the listed references for further information will note that evidence-based information is sparse for some of these topics, with conflicting data for others.

The most prominent and best studied of these topics addresses whether the ICU is "closed" or "open." These terms refer to whether or not all the patients in the ICU at a given time are under the care of a single attending physician. Several groups of investigators have shown that outcomes are superior in closed ICU systems.[298–302] However, there are multitudinous organizational differences between different ICUs,[303] and the seemingly simple issue of closed vs. open is interrelated to considerations such as: (1) involvement of subspecialists in critical care medicine, (2) the relative roles

TABLE 3-3 Literature Assessing the Effect of Structures and Processes on Outcomes

Structure or Process	Reference Numbers
Open vs. closed ICU structure	255, 256
Telemedicine	257
24-Hour intensivist presence	258
Length of shifts for ICU physicians	259
Nighttime cross-coverage by house officers	260
Role of the ICU's medical director	261
Availability of an intermediate care unit	101, 102
Pharmacist participation in ICU rounds	262
Utilization of advanced nurse practitioners	263–266
Nurse:patient ratio	267–273
Formation of a ventilator team	274
Supplying cost information to ordering physicians	275–277
Disallowing standing orders	254, 277, 278
Infection control processes	279–281
Dissemination of performance data	262, 282, 284
Family visiting hours	285–288
Palliative and end-of-life care	7, 289–293
Nurse-physician communication and other aspects of ICU culture	254, 273, 294–297

TABLE 3-4 Benefits of Information Technology in Intensive Care Unit Performance Improvement

- Acquire, integrate, store, analyze, and display information
- More efficient and less error-prone entry of orders
- More efficient, available, and legible entry of progress notes and other patient information
- Make clinical data more readily available
- Make knowledge more readily accessible
- Facilitate availability and use of clinical practice guidelines
- Facilitate communication
- Provide clinical reminders
- Assist with calculations
- Assist with clinical monitoring
- Continuous, real-time monitoring for complications, adverse events, etc
- Provide decision support
- Automated assistance with technical aspects of care
- Verify correct administration of medications, blood products, etc (e.g., via bar coding with bedside scanning)
- Facilitate data collection and case-mix adjustment for total quality management purposes

of the intensivist and the primary attending physician, (3) the presence of residents and critical care fellows, (4) the existence and nature of daily rounds for ICUs having house staff, (5) the role of the ICU medical director, and (6) differences between daytime and nighttime physician coverage. Interpretation of this literature is problematic because: (1) intermixing of these interrelated topics leads to many gradations between open and closed ICU structures; (2) there is substantial variation in study design, outcome parameters assessed, and case-mix adjustments among published studies; (3) many of the individual investigations suffer from weak study design; and (4) the possibility of publication bias. A recent systematic review of these topics avoided restrictive definitions of open vs. closed, and instead analyzed 26 studies according to whether intensivists were involved in a fashion rated as high intensity (defined as a closed ICU staffed by intensivists, or a mandatory consultation by an intensivist) or low intensity (no intensivist involved in ICU care, or elective intensivist consultation).[255] High-intensity involvement of intensivists results in lower mortality rates and shorter lengths of stay. After case-mix adjustment, no individual study observed worse outcomes with more intensivist involvement in care. Another study concluded that high-intensity involvement by intensivists in care of all ICU patients in the U.S. would save almost 54,000 lives per year.[256] Trying to fill the evidence-based policymaking void present in U.S. health care, a consortium of large businesses, The Leapfrog Group, is attempting to improve hospital outcomes for its employees by making high-intensity involvement of intensivists in ICUs a requirement for any hospital to contract with their health plans.[304]

Information Systems in Intensive Care Unit Performance Improvement

Computers and other information technologies are powerful tools for improving ICU performance. Unlike people, computers can keep track of almost limitless amounts of information, never forget, and are essentially flawless in doing their assigned tasks. Table 3-4 lists some ways that computers can advance PI efforts in the ICU. Although there are as yet few studies evaluating whether such technologies improve ICU outcomes,[305] their further development and widespread diffusion will likely be necessary for improving health care.[200]

Computers have facilitated access to clinical data for several decades. In most hospitals clinicians can obtain laboratory and other test results on terminals throughout the hospital. More recently, many hospitals have bought picture archiving communications systems (PACS), making it possible to view radiologic images without leaving the ICU. Although there is conflicting evidence that PACS lead to more timely viewing of images by clinicians,[306,307] they do make viewing more convenient and save time.[308]

Keeping track of patient-related information is an ever-increasing challenge. Data about ICU patients originate from observations and manual measurements made by health care workers, bedside monitors, the laboratories, radiology, devices such as infusion pumps and ventilators, progress notes, clinical flowsheets, the hospital information system, and other sources. In most ICUs, collecting this mass of diverse information requires physicians to read paper records, use several different computer systems, and leave the ICU to obtain information residing elsewhere. This situation makes it difficult and inefficient for clinicians to acquire and integrate all the necessary data, and is obviously prone to oversight and error. Only highly competent computer systems can solve all of these problems.[309] Via various interfaces, such systems[311,312] can automatically acquire data from electronic connection to bedside devices and other computer systems in the hospital, and manual input via bedside workstations. They can display the data as customizable tables and graphs that people can understand and use at any enabled workstation, including those at remote locations via the internet. Because of these advantages, electronic, paperless medical records should become increasingly common.[312–314] The future likely includes use of hand-held devices for wireless remote access to clinical data, and more rapid communication to clinicians of problems such as critical laboratory values.[315]

Computer technologies have vastly improved access to sources of medical knowledge. Textbooks, databases such as MEDLINE, full text journals, and other authoritative sources are widely available around the clock from internet-ready terminals in ICUs. It no longer requires a time-consuming trip to the hospital library to learn state-of-the-art answers to clinical questions about the patient who just arrived in the ICU. An increasing amount of medical knowledge is even more conveniently accessible within software for hand-held devices.[316]

Errors in order writing are the most common sort of medical error.[32,317] Handwritten orders suffer from illegibility, mistakes in transcription, erroneous dosing, and other ills. Computerized order entry dramatically reduces such errors[319,320] and can reduce costs.[320] Computerized order entry is already relatively common and increasing in prevalence, driven by safety concerns of influential organizations such as the Leapfrog Group.[304]

As discussed above, reminders and clinical practice guidelines are strategies to increase use of evidence-based best practices. However, both are limited by problems making the information available to clinicians in a reliable, convenient, and timely way. Information systems can solve these problems. Each time a physician, nurse, or respiratory therapist logs on to the computer for any purpose is an opportunity to deliver a reminder message or offer up a relevant guideline. Having these occur during order entry makes it especially easy for the clinician to execute orders to act on the reminder or initiate the guideline's protocol. Simpler implementations of this concept would be triggered by the order being written.[322] For example, a computer-generated reminder could be displayed to order elevation of the head of the bed every time a clinician orders tube feedings.[204] Intelligent systems with access to other patient data residing in the electronic medical record are required to allow this concept to achieve its fullest potential. An integrated ICU information system linked to both the ventilator and the electronic medication administration record could identify that a patient is mechanically ventilated and not receiving prophylaxis for stress gastritis,[322] and automatically generate a reminder. If the patient was receiving sedatives, the computer could suggest use of the ICU's sedation protocol[323,324] and automatically generate the necessary orders for the clinician to implement. Currently, only sparse evidence exists about the effect of such systems. Computerized reminders have demonstrated benefit in most[321,325] but not all[326] studies. Studies of complex interventions that included computer-aided practice guidelines have observed improvements in care or reduced costs.[211,245,327]

Extending these uses of information systems is computer-aided decision support (CADS). In CADS, systems having electronic access to patient data provide clinicians with expert medical advice. Take the example of a physician doing computer entry of an order for gentamicin. Combining the latest creatinine value from the laboratory, the patient's weight from the daily nursing notes, and age from the admitting department's computer, the computer system estimates pharmacokinetic parameters and recommends a dosing regimen. When peak and trough levels become available, it would include those in the calculations, and the next time the clinician accessed that patient's electronic medical record, it would suggest revised dosing. These smart systems can help avoid incorrect dosing, and proactively identify drug interactions. Indeed, most studies of CADS have evaluated the effects on choice and dosing of pharmaceuticals. These have found an impressive variety of improvements in clinically relevant outcomes, including better empiric antibiotic choices, better dosing, reduced drug costs, reduction in adverse drug events, and others.[215,320,328–332]

The potential of computers to assist in management of ICU patients extends beyond providing technical advice. A computer linked to real-time monitoring can be programmed to automatically adjust devices such as ventilators and infusion pumps to maintain optimal parameters in a way that would be impossible for humans to accomplish.[333,334] In a recent study of computer control over ventilators in pressure support mode using ordinary closed-loop linear programming, a computer continuously monitoring respiratory rate, tidal volume, and end-tidal P_{CO_2} simultaneously maintained all three within desired limits 93% of the time, while humans did so 66% of the time.[333] Use of fuzzy logic controllers may have even wider ICU applications.[335] The ability of computers to tirelessly monitor and analyze the entire ICU data stream in real time makes them ideal, and superior to people, for tasks such as early detection of physiologic instability, adverse events,[148] and surveillance for care practices outside of established practice guidelines.[336]

In addition to assisting in care of individual patients, computer applications greatly facilitate implementation of TQM. Even within a single ICU, acquisition, analysis, and presentation of the information necessary for TQM is expensive and labor intensive.[194] Setting up the infrastructure for a comprehensive, electronic ICU patient database is an important step that will considerably ease the personnel demands for TQM. Likewise, collection of case-mix variables, and even adjustment for case-mix, can be automated. Manual calculation of scores for APACHE, SAPS, PRISM, or other prognostic systems is cumbersome and time consuming. Computer software linked to hospital information systems can compile, organize, calculate, and store these parameters automatically. Such databases are themselves potent tools for TQM. They can be queried to identify subtle relationships between variables that suggest opportunities for improving performance that are not obvious, even to those intimately involved in day-to-day operations. For example, an evaluation of database information identified laboratory ordering patterns in an ICU that led to policy changes and subsequent cost savings.[246] The best system for TQM purposes would be one that also serves as the electronic medical record and clinical information system for the ICU. Such systems do exist.[311]

Unfortunately, there are currently a number of barriers to widespread use of information technologies to improve ICU performance.[309,315,337] These include a paucity of user-friendly commercially available systems, high costs for those that do exist, a lack of interfacing standards leading again to high costs, and opposition from clinicians. Nonetheless, such highly capable systems do exist, and a few forward-looking institutions have invested in them, to their benefit.[311,338]

References

1. National Center for Health Statistics. http://www.cdc.gov/nchs.

2. Gleeson K, Wise S: The do-not-resuscitate order. Still too little too late. *Arch Intern Med* 150:1057, 1990.

3. Center for the Evaluative Clinical Sciences Staff: *The Dartmouth Atlas of Health Care 1999.* Chicago, American Hospital Publishing, 1999.

4. Prendergast TJ, Claessens MT, Luce JM: A national survey of end-of-life care for critically ill patients. *Am J Respir Crit Care Med* 158:1163, 1998.

5. Keenan SP, Busche KD, Chen LM, et al: A retrospective review of a large cohort of patients undergoing the process of withholding or withdrawal of life support. *Crit Care Med* 25:1324, 1997.

6. Knaus WA, Wagner DP, Draper EA, et al: The APACHE III prognostic system. *Chest* 100:1619, 1991.

7. The SUPPORT Principal Investigators: A controlled trial to improve care for seriously ill hospitalized patients. *JAMA* 274:1591, 1995.

8. Puntillo KA: Pain experiences of intensive care unit patients. *Heart Lung* 19(5 Pt 1):526, 1990.

9. Nelson JE, Meier DE, Oei EJ, et al: Self-reported symptom experience of critically ill cancer patients receiving intensive care. *Crit Care Med* 29:277, 2001.

10. Bergbom-Engberg I, Haljamae H: Assessment of patients' experience of discomforts during respiratory therapy. *Crit Care Med* 17:1068, 1989.

11. Azoulay E, Pochard F, Chevret S, et al: Meeting the needs of intensive care unit patient families: A multicenter study. *Am J Respir Crit Care Med* 163:135, 2001.

12. Abbott KA, Sago JG, Breen CM, et al: Families looking back: One year after discussion of withdrawal or withholding of life-sustaining support. *Crit Care Med* 29:197, 2001.

13. Malacrida R, Molo Bettelini C, Degrate A, et al: Reasons for dissatisfaction: A survey of relatives of intensive care patients who died. *Crit Care Med* 26:1187, 1998.

14. Groeger JS, Strosberg MA, Halpern NA, et al: Descriptive analysis of critical care units in the United States. *Crit Care Med* 20:846, 1992.

15. Halpern NA, Bettes L, Greenstein R: Federal and nationwide intensive care units and healthcare costs: 1986–1992. *Crit Care Med* 22:2001, 1994.

16. Jacobs P, Noseworthy TW: National estimates of intensive care utilization and costs: Canada and the United States. *Crit Care Med* 18:1282, 1990.

17. Berenson R: Health Technology Case Study 28. Intensive Care Units (ICUs): Clinical outcomes, costs, and decision-making. Washington, Office of Technology Assessment, 1984.

18. Health, United States, 2003. Hyattsville, MD: National Center for Health Statistics, 2003, p 306.

19. Dragsted L, Qvist J: Epidemiology of intensive care. *Int J Technol Assessment Health Care* 8:395, 1992.

20. Rapoport J, Teres D, Barnett R, et al: A comparison of intensive care unit utilization in Alberta and western Massachusetts. *Crit Care Med* 23:1336, 1995.

21. Sirio CA, Tajimi K, Tase C, et al: An initial comparison of intensive care in Japan and the United States. *Crit Care Med* 20:1207, 1992.

22. Sirio CA, Tajimi K, Taenaka N, et al: A cross-cultural comparison of critical care delivery: Japan and the United States. *Chest* 121:539, 2001.

23. Thompson LA, Goodman DC, Little GA: Is more neonatal intensive care always better? Insights from a cross-national comparison of reproductive care. *Pediatrics* 109:1036, 2002.

24. Chassin MR, Galvin RW: The urgent need to improve health care quality. Institute of Medicine National Roundtable on Health Care Quality. *JAMA* 280:1000, 1998.

25. World Health Staff: The World Health Report 2000—Health Systems: Improving Performance. World Health Organization; 2000. http://www.who.int/whr2001/2001/archives/2000/en/statistics.htm

26. Starfield B: Is US health really the best in the world? *JAMA* 284:483, 2000.

27. Chassin MR, Kosecott J, Park RE, et al: Does inappropriate use explain geographic variations in the use of health care services? *JAMA* 258:2533, 1987.

28. Schuster MA, McGlynn EA, Brook RH: How good is the quality of health care in the United States? *Milbank Q* 76:517, 1998.

29. McNeil BJ: Shattuck Lecture—hidden barriers to improvement in the quality of care. *N Engl J Med* 345:1612, 2001.

30. Dubois RW, Rogers WH, Moxley JH, Brook RH: Hospital inpatient mortality. *N Engl J Med* 317:1674, 1987.

31. Ashton CM, Kuykendall DH, Johnson ML, et al: The association between the quality of inpatient care and early readmission. *Ann Intern Med* 122:415, 1995.

32. Kohn LT, Corrigan JM, Donaldson MS (eds): *To Err Is Human.* Washington: National Academies Press, 2000.

33. Brennan TA, Leape LL, Laird NM, et al: Incidence of adverse events and negligence in hospitalized patients. Results of the Harvard Medical Practice Study I. *N Engl J Med* 324:370, 1991.

34. Haywood RA, Hofer TP: Estimating hospital deaths due to medical errors. *JAMA* 286:415, 2001.

35. Giraud T, Dhainaut J, Vaxelaire J, et al: Iatrogenic complications in adult intensive care units: A prospective two-center study. *Crit Care Med* 21:40, 1993.

36. Donchin Y, Gopher D, Olin M, et al: A look into the nature and causes of human errors in the intensive care unit. *Crit Care Med* 23:294, 1995.

37. Wennberg JE, Freeman JL, Culp WJ: Are hospital services rationed in New Haven or over-utilised in Boston? *Lancet* 23:1185, 1987.

38. Welch HG, Miller ME, Welch WP: Physician profiling: An analysis of inpatient practice patterns in Florida and Oregon. *N Engl J Med* 330:607, 1994.

39. Thomas EJ, Orav EJ, Brennan TA: Hospital ownership and preventable adverse events. *J Gen Intern Med* 15:211, 2000.

40. Burns LR, Wholey DR: The effects of patient, hospital, and physician characteristics on length of stay and mortality. *Med Care* 29:251, 1991.

41. Hartz AJ, Krakauer H, Kuh EM, et al: Hospital characteristics and mortality rates. *N Engl J Med* 219:1720, 1989.

42. Greenfield S, Nelson EC, Zubkoff M, et al: Variations in resource utilization among medical specialties and systems of care: Results from the Medical Outcomes Study. *JAMA* 267:1624, 1992.

43. Burns LR, Chilingerian JA, Wholey DR: The effect of physician practice organization on efficient utilization of hospital resources. *Health Sci Res* 29:583, 1994.

44. Tu JV, Austin PC, Chan BTB: Relationship between annual volume of patients treated by admitting physician and mortality after acute myocardial infarction. *JAMA* 285:3116, 2001.

45. Garland A, Kilkenny TM, Anderson MA, Paz HL: Physician-attributable differences in care of ICU patients. *Am J Respir Crit Care Med* 155(4, Part 2):A766, 1997.

46. Feinglass J, Martin GJ, Sen A: The financial effect of physician practice style on hospital resource use. *Health Sci Res* 26:183, 1991.

47. DeMott RK, Sandmire HF: The Green Bay cesarean section study: The physician factor as a determinant of cesarean birth rates. *Am J Obstet Gynecol* 162:1593, 1990.

48. Roos NP: Predicting hospital utilization by the elderly. *Med Care* 27:905, 1989.

49. Angus DC, Linde-Zwirble WT, Sirio CA, et al: The effect of managed care on ICU length of stay. *JAMA* 276:1075, 1996.

50. Canto JG, Rogers WJ, French WJ, et al: Payer status and the utilization of hospital resources in acute myocardial infarction. *Arch Intern Med* 160:817, 2000.

51. Rapoport J, Gehlbach S, Lemeshow S, Teres D: Resource utilization among intensive care patients: Managed care vs. traditional insurance. *Arch Intern Med* 152:2207, 1992.

52. Weissman J, Epstein AM: Case mix and resource utilization by uninsured hospital patients in the Boston Metropolitan Area. *JAMA* 261:3572, 1989.

53. Stern RS, Juhn PI, Gertler PJ, Epstein AM: A comparison of length of stay and costs for health maintenance organization and fee-for-service patients. *Arch Intern Med* 149:1185, 1989.

54. Knaus WA, Wagner DP, Zimmerman JE, Draper EA: Variations in mortality and length of stay in intensive care units. *Ann Intern Med* 118:753, 1993.

55. Ruttimann UE, Pollack MM: Variability in duration of stay in pediatric intensive care units: A multi-institutional study. *J Pediatr* 128:35, 1996.

56. Rapoport J, Teres D, Steingrub J, et al: Patient characteristics and ICU organizational factors that influence frequency of pulmonary artery catheterization. *JAMA* 283:2559, 2000.

57. Long MJ: Variation in outpatient procedure rates in Canadian teaching hospitals. *Clin Perform Qual Health Care* 2:16, 1994.

58. Jin Y, Marrie TJ, Carriere KC, et al: Variation in management of community-acquired pneumonia requiring admission to Alberta, Canada hospitals. *Epidemiol Infect* 130:41, 2003.

59. Chen E, Naylor CD: Variation in hospital length of stay for acute myocardial infarction in Ontario, Canada. *Med Care* 32:420, 1994.

60. Feasby TE, Quan H, Ghali WA: Geographic variation in the rate of carotid endarterectomy in Canada. *Stroke* 32:2417, 2001.

61. Ferrand E, Robert R, Ingrand P, et al: Withholding and withdrawal of life support in intensive-care units in France: A prospective survey. *Lancet* 357:9, 2001.

62. Cook DJ, Guyatt GH, Jaeschke R, et al: Determinants in Canadian health care workers of the decision to withdraw life support from the critically ill. *JAMA* 273:703, 1995.

63. Teno JM, Fischer E, Hamel MB, et al: Decision-making and outcomes of prolonged ICU stays in seriously ill patients. *J Am Geriatrics Soc* 48(5 Suppl):S70, 2000.

64. Hall RI, Rocker GM: End-of-life care in the ICU. *Chest* 118:1424, 2000.

65. Faber-Langendoen K, Bartels DM: Process of forgoing life-sustaining treatment in a university hospital: An empirical study. *Crit Care Med* 20:570, 1992.

66. Garland A, Anderson M, Kilkenny T, et al: Characteristics of length of stay outliers in a medical intensive care unit. *Am J Respir Crit Care Med* 157(3, Part 2):A302, 2998.

67. Azoulay E, Chevret S, Leleu G, et al: Half the families of intensive care unit patients experience inadequate communication with physicians. *Crit Care Med* 28:3044, 2000.

68. Johnson D, Wilson M, Cabanaugh B, et al: Measuring the ability to meet family needs in an intensive care unit. *Crit Care Med* 26:266, 1998.

69. Nelson JE, Danis M: End-of-life care in the intensive care unit: Where are we now? *Crit Care Med* 29(2 Suppl):N2, 2001.

70. Kollef MH: Private attending physician status and the withdrawal of life-sustaining interventions in a medical intensive care unit population. *Crit Care Med* 24:968, 1996.

71. Rosenberg AL, Watts C: Patients readmitted to ICUs: A systematic review of risk factors and outcomes. *Chest* 118:492, 2000.

72. Angus DC: Grappling with intensive care unit quality—Does the readmission rate tell us anything? *Crit Care Med* 26:1779, 1998.

73. Frankl D, Oye RK, Bellamy PE: Attitudes of hospitalized patients towards life support: A survey of 200 medical inpatients. *Am J Med* 86:645, 1989.

74. Ebell MH, Smith MA, Seifert DK, Polsinelli K: The do-not-resuscitate order: Outpatient experience and decision-making preferences. *J Fam Pract* 31:630, 1990.

75. Fried TR, Bradley EH, Towle VR, Allore H: Understanding the treatment preferences of seriously ill patients. *N Engl J Med* 346:1061, 2002.

76. Wu AW: The measure and mismeasure of hospital quality: Appropriate risk-adjustment methods in comparing hospitals. *Ann Intern Med* 122:149, 1995.

77. Randolph AG, Guyatt GH, Carlet J: Understanding articles comparing outcomes among intensive care units to rate quality of care. *Crit Care Med* 26:773, 1998.

78. Heyland DK, Guyatt G, Cook DJ, et al: Frequency and methodologic rigor of quality-of-life assessments in the critical care literature. *Crit Care Med* 26:591, 1998.

79. Kerridge RK, Glasziou PP, Hillman KM: The use of "quality-adjusted life years" (QALYs) to evaluate treatment in intensive care. *Anaesth Intensive Care* 23:322, 1995.

80. Testa MA, Simonson DC: Assessment of quality-of-life outcomes. *N Engl J Med* 334:835, 1996.

81. Barr JT: The outcomes movement and health status measures. *J Allied Health* 24:13, 1995.

82. Ebrahim S: Clinical and public health perspectives and applications of health-related quality of life measurement. *Soc Sci Med* 41:1383, 1995.

83. Ware JE: The status of health assessment 1994. *Annu Rev Pub Health* 1995;16:327–54.

84. Ware JE, Snow KK, Kosinski M, Gandek B: *SF-36 Health Survey Manual & Interpretation Guide.* Boston, Health Institute, New England Medical Center, 1993.

85. Wilson IB, Cleary PD: Linking clinical variables with health-related quality of life. A conceptual model of patient outcomes. *JAMA* 273:59, 1995.

86. Vazquez Mata G, Rivera Fernandez R, Gonzalez Carmona A, et al: Factors related to quality of life 12 months after discharge from an intensive care unit. *Crit Care Med* 20:1257, 1992.

87. Konopad E, Noseworthy TW, Johnston R, et al: Quality of life measures before and one year after admission to an intensive care unit. *Crit Care Med* 23:1653, 1995.

88. Angus DC, Musthafa AA, Clermont G, et al: Quality-adjusted survival in the first year after the acute respiratory distress syndrome. *Am J Respir Crit Care Med* 163:1389, 2001.

89. Schelling G, Stoll C, Haller M, et al: Health-related quality of life and posttraumatic stress disorder in survivors of the acute respiratory distress syndrome. *Crit Care Med* 26:651, 1998.

90. Hopkins RO, Weaver LK, Pope D, et al: Neuropsychological sequelae and impaired health status in survivors of severe acute respiratory distress syndrome. *Am J Respir Crit Care Med* 160:50, 1999.

91. Institute of Medicine: *Assessing Medical Technologies.* Washington, National Academy Press, 1985, p 5.

92. Stevens L, Cook D, Guyatt G, et al: Education, ethics, and end-of-life decisions in the intensive care unit. *Crit Care Med* 30:290, 2002.

93. Block SD, Sullivan AM: Attitudes about end-of-life care: A national cross-sectional study. *J Palliat Med* 1:347, 1998.

94. Brown University Center for Gerontology and Health Care Research. Toolkit of instruments to measure end of life. http://www.gwu.edu/~cicd/toolkit/toolkit.htm.

95. Shwartz M, Young DW, Siegrist R: The ratio of costs to charges: how good a basis for estimating costs? *Inquiry* 32:476, 1995.

96. Keene AR, Cullen DJ: Therapeutic Intervention Scoring System: Update 1983. *Crit Care Med* 11:1, 1983.

97. Dickie H, Vedio A, Dundas R, et al: Relationship between TISS and ICU cost. *Intensive Care Med* 24:1009, 1998.

98. Alzola C, Lynn J, Wagner D, Wu AW: Length of stay and therapeutic intervention allow estimation of in-hospital resource

use independent of site and inflation. *J Am Geriatr Soc* 48(5 Suppl):S162, 2000.

99. Weinstein MC, Stason WB: Foundations of cost-effectiveness analysis for health and medical practices. *N Engl J Med* 296:716, 1977.

100. Rapoport J, Teres D, Lemeshow S, Gehlbach S: A method for assessing the clinical performance and cost-effectiveness of intensive care units: A multicenter inception cohort study. *Crit Care Med* 22:1385, 1994.

101. Byrick RJ, Mazer CD, Caskennette GM: Closure of an intermediate care unit: Impact on critical care utilization. *Chest* 104:876, 1993.

102. Franklin CM, Rackow EC, Mamdani B, et al: Decreases in mortality in a large urban medical service by facilitating access to critical care. An alternative to rationing. *Arch Intern Med* 148:1403, 1988.

103. Goldfrad C, Rowan K: Consequences of discharges from intensive care at night. *Lancet* 355:1138, 2000.

104. Strauss MJ, LoGerfo MP, Yaltatzie JA, et al: Rationing of intensive care services: An everyday occurrence. *JAMA* 255:1143, 1986.

105. Kalb PE, Miller DH: Utilization strategies for intensive care units. *JAMA* 261:2389, 1989.

106. Task Force on Guidelines, Society of Critical Care Medicine: Recommendations for intensive care unit admission and discharge criteria. *Crit Care Med* 16:807, 1988.

107. Wennberg JE: Dealing with medical practice variations: A proposal for action. *Health Aff* 3:6, 1984.

108. Task Force of the American College of Critical Care Medicine, Society of Critical Care Medicine: Guidelines for intensive care unit admission, discharge, and triage. *Crit Care Med* 27:633, 1999.

109. Atkinson S, Bihar B, Smithies M, et al: Identification of futility in intensive care. *Lancet* 344:1203, 1994.

110. Spielman B: Collective decisions about medical futility. *J Law Med Ethics* 22:152, 1994.

111. Luce JM, Alpers A: End-of-life care: What do American courts say? *Crit Care Med* 29(2 Suppl.):N40, 2001.

112. Williams B: Patient satisfaction: A valid concept? *Soc Sci Med* 38:509, 1994.

113. Avis M, Bond M, Arthur A: Satisfying solutions? A review of some unresolved issues in the measurement of patient satisfaction. *J Adv Nurs* 22:316, 1995.

114. Leske JL: Internal psychometric properties of the Critical Care Family Needs Inventory. *Heart Lung* 20:236, 1991.

115. Guyatt GH, Mitchell A, Molloy DW, et al: Measuring patient and relative satisfaction with level or aggressiveness of care and involvement in care decisions in the context of life threatening illness. *J Clin Epidemiol* 48:1215, 1995.

116. Heyland DK, Rocker FM, Dodek PM, et al: Family satisfaction with care in the intensive care unit: Results of a multiple center study. *Crit Care Med* 30:1413, 2002.

117. Larson CO, Nelson EC, Gustafson D, Batalden PB: The relationship between meeting patients' information needs and their satisfaction with hospital care and general health status outcome. *Int J Qual Health Care* 8:447, 1996.

118. Steel RP, Ovalle NK: A review and meta-analysis of research on the relationship between behavioral intentions and employee turnover. *J Appl Psychol* 69:673, 1984.

119. Mann EE: A human capital approach to ICU nurse retention. *J Nurs Admin* 19:8, 1989.

120. Mann EE, Jefferson KJ: Retaining staff: Using turnover indices and surveys. *J Nurs Admin* 18:17, 1988.

121. Morrison AL, Beckmann U, Durie M, et al: The effects of nursing staff inexperience (NSI) on the occurrence of adverse patient experiences in ICUs. *Aust Crit Care* 14:116, 2001.

122. Projected Supply, Demand, and Shortages of Registered Nurses: 2002–2020. Washington, U.S. Department of Health and Human Services, Health Resources and Services Administration, Bureau of Health Professions, National Center for Health Workforce Analysis, 2002.

123. Buerhaus PI, Stainger DO, Auerbach DI: Implications of an aging registered nurse workforce. *JAMA* 283:2948, 2000.

124. Kimball B, O'Neil E: *Health Care's Human Crisis: The American Nursing Shortage.* Princeton, Robert Wood Johnson Foundation, 2002, p 41.

125. Buerhaus PI, Staiger DO, Auerbach DI: Why are shortages of hospital RNs concentrated in specialty care units? *Nurs Econ* 18:111, 2000.

126. The AARC Respiratory Therapist Human Resources Study—2000. Dallas, American Association of Respiratory Care, 2000.

127. Angus DC, Kelley MA, Schmitz RJ, et al: Current and projected workforce requirements for care of the critically ill and patients with pulmonary disease. *JAMA* 284:2762, 2000.

128. Aiken LH, Clarke SP, Sloane DM, et al: Hospital nurse staffing and patient mortality, nurse burnout, and job satisfaction. *JAMA* 288:1987, 2002.

129. Aiken LH, Clarke SP, Sloane DM, et al: Nurses' reports on hospital care in five countries. *Health Aff* 20:43, 2001.

130. Chen SM, McMurray A: "Burnout" in intensive care nurses. *J Nurs Res* 9:152, 2001.

131. Stechmiller JK, Yarandi HN: Job satisfaction among critical care nurses. *Am J Crit Care* 1:37, 1992.

132. Shelledy DC, Mikles SP, May DF, Youtsey JW: Analysis of job satisfaction, burnout, and intent of respiratory care practitioners to leave the field or the job. *Respir Care* 37:46, 1992.

133. Coomber S, Todd C, Park G, et al: Stress in UK intensive care unit doctors. *Br J Anaesth* 89:873, 2002.

134. Gay PC, Dellinger RP, Shelhamer JH, et al: The practice of critical care medicine: A national survey report. *Chest* 104:271, 1993.

135. Guntupalli KK, Fromm RE: Burnout in the internist-intensivist. *Intensive Care Med* 22:625, 1996.

136. Fields AI, Cuerdon TT, Brasseux CO, et al: Physician burnout in pediatric critical care medicine. *Crit Care Med* 23:1425, 1995.

137. Warr P, Cook J, Wall T: Scales for the measurement of some work attitudes and aspects of psychological well-being. *J Occup Psychol* 52:129, 1979.

138. Williams ES, Konrad TR, Linzer M, et al: Refining the measurement of physician job satisfaction: Results from the Physician Worklife Survey. *Med Care* 37:1140, 1999.

139. Landon BE, Reschovsky D, Blumenthal D: Changes in career satisfaction among primary care and specialist physicians, 1997–2001. *JAMA* 289:442, 2003.

140. Linn LS, Yager J, Cope D, Leake B: Health status, job satisfaction, job stress, and life satisfaction among academic and clinical faculty. *JAMA* 254:2775, 1985.

141. Shields MA, Ward M: Improving nurse retention in the National Health Service in England: The impact of job satisfaction on intentions to quit. *J Health Econ* 20:677, 2001.

142. LeBlanc PM, deJonge J, deRijk AE, Schaufeli WB: Well-being of intensive care nurses (WEBIC): A job analytic approach. *J Adv Nurs* 36:460, 2001.

143. Maslach C, Schaufeli WB, Leiter MP: Job burnout. *Annu Rev Psychol* 52:397, 2001.

144. Fenwick R, Taussig M: Scheduling stress: Family and health outcomes of shift work and schedule control. *Am Behav Sci* 44:1179, 2001.

145. Kapner P: Occurrence screening in critical care. *AACN Clin Issues* 2:15, 1991.

146. Joint Commission on Accreditation of Healthcare Organizations: *Improving Organization Performance. 2002 Comprehensive Accreditation Manual for Hospitals.* Oakbrook Terrace, IL, 2002.

147. Cullen DJ, Bates DW, Small SD, et al: The incident reporting system does not detect adverse drug events: A problem for quality improvement. *J Qual Improve* 21:541, 1995.

148. Classen DC, Pestotnik SL, Evans RS, Burke JP: Computerized surveillance of adverse drug events in hospital patients. *JAMA* 266:2847, 1991.

149. Localio AR, Weaver SL, Landis JR, et al: Identifying adverse events caused by medical care: Degree of physician agreement in a retrospective chart review. *Ann Intern Med* 125:457, 1996.

150. Thomas EJ, Studdert DM, Brennan TA: The reliability of medical record review for estimating adverse event rates. *Ann Intern Med* 136:812, 2002.

151. Gastmeier P, Sohr D, Geffers C, et al: Are nosocomial infection rates in intensive care units useful benchmark parameters? *Infection* 28:346, 2000.

152. Richardson D, Tarnow-Mordi WO, Lee SK: Risk adjustment for quality improvement. *Pediatrics* 103(1 Suppl E):255, 1999.

153. Simon R: Confidence intervals for reporting results of clinical trials. *Ann Intern Med* 105:429, 1986.

154. Morton V, Torgerson DJ: Effect of regression to the mean on decision making in health care. *BMJ* 326:1083, 2003.

155. Leveck JL, Jones CB: The nursing practice environment, staff retention, and quality of care. *Res Nurs Health* 19:331, 1996.

156. Garfield M, Ridley S, Kong A, et al: Seasonal variation in admission rates to intensive care units. *Anaesthesia* 56:1136, 2001.

157. Pell JP, Cobbe SM: Seasonal variations in coronary heart disease. *QJM* 92:689, 1999.

158. Kawai K, Nonaka K, Suzuki H, et al: Differential effects of activity and climate on onset of subarachnoid hemorrhage. *Neurologia Medico-Chirurgica* 41:229, 2001.

159. Glance LG, Osler T, Shinozaki T: Effect of varying the case mortality mix on the standardized mortality ratio and W statistic: A simulation study. *Chest* 117:1112, 2000.

160. Patel PA, Grant BJB: Application of mortality prediction systems to individual intensive care units. *Intensive Care Med* 25:977, 1999.

161. Rapoport J, Teres D, Steingrub J, et al: Patient characteristics and ICU organizational factors that influence frequency of pulmonary artery catheterization. *JAMA* 283:2559, 2000.

162. Aday LA: Indicators and predictors of health services utilization, in Williams SJ, Torrens PR (eds): *Introduction to Health Services*, 4th ed. Albany, NY, Delmar Publishers, 1993, p 46.

163. Freeman HE, Corey CR: Insurance status and access to health services among poor persons. *Health Serv Res* 28:531, 1993.

164. Rosenberg AL: Recent innovations in intensive care unit risk-prediction models. *Curr Opin Crit Care* 8:321, 2002.

165. Schuster DP: Predicting outcome after ICU admission. *Chest* 102:1861, 1992.

166. Teres D, Lemeshow S: Using severity measures to describe high performance intensive care units. *Crit Care Unit Manage* 9:543, 1993.

167. Cook SF, Visscher WA, Hobbs CL, et al: Project IMPACT: Results from a pilot validity study of a new observational database. *Crit Care Med* 30:2765, 2002.

168. Pollack MM, Ruttimann UE, Getson PR: Pediatric risk of mortality score. *Crit Care Med* 16:1110, 1988.

169. O'Connor GT, Plume SK, Olmstead EM, et al: Multivariate prediction of in-hospital mortality associated with coronary artery bypass graft surgery. *Circulation* 85:2110, 1992.

170. Champion HR, Copes WS, Sacco WJ, et al: A new characterization of injury severity. *J Trauma* 30:539, 1990.

171. Clermont G, Angus DC, DiRusso SM, et al: Predicting hospital mortality for patients in the intensive care unit: A comparison of artificial neural networks with logistic regression models. *Crit Care Med* 29:291, 2001.

172. Paz HL, Livingston J: Using a benchmarking system to improve patient care and assist in technology assessment. *Physician Exec* 22:10, 1996.

173. Schafer JH, Maurer A, Jochimsen F, et al: Outcome prediction models on admission in a medical intensive care unit: Do they predict individual outcome? *Crit Care Med* 18:1111, 1990.

174. Rogers J, Fuller HD: Use of daily Acute Physiology and Chronic Health Evaluation (APACHE) II scores to predict individual patient survival rate. *Crit Care Med* 22:1402, 1994.

175. Knaus WA, Draper EA, Zimmerman JE: APACHE II: A severity of disease classification system. *Crit Care Med* 13:818, 1995.

176. Glance LG, Osler TM, Dick A: Rating the quality of intensive care units: Is it a function of the intensive care unit scoring system? *Crit Care Med* 30:1976, 2002.

177. Castella X, Artigas A, Bion J, Kari A: A comparison of severity of illness scoring systems for intensive care unit patients: Results of a multicenter, multinational study. The European/North American Severity Study Group. *Crit Care Med* 23:1327, 1995.

178. Dart R, Patel B, Perez-Alard J, et al: Prognosis of oncology patients receiving intensive care using the APACHE II system. *Maryland Med J* 40:273, 1991.

179. Pappachan JV, Millar B, Bennett ED, Smith GB: Comparison of outcome from intensive care admission after adjustment for case mix by the APACHE III prognostic system. *Chest* 115:802, 1999.

180. Woods AW, MacKirdy FN, Livingston BM, et al: Evaluation of predicted and actual length of stay in 22 Scottish intensive care units using the APACHE III system. Acute Physiology and Chronic Health Evaluation. *Anaesthesia* 55:1058, 2000.

181. Teres D, Lemeshow S: As American as apple pie and APACHE. *Crit Care Med* 26:1297, 1988.

182. Iezzoni LI: The risks of risk adjustment. *JAMA* 278:1600, 1997.

183. APACHE Medical Systems, Inc. http://www.apache-msi.com/.

184. Project IMPACT, CCM, Inc. http://www.projectimpacticu.cc/default.html.

185. Barie PS, Hydo LJ, Fischer E: Comparison of APACHE II and III scoring systems for mortality prediction in critical surgical illness. *Arch Surg* 130:77, 1995.

186. Markgraf R, Deutschinoff G, Pientka L, Scholten T: Comparison of acute physiology and chronic health evaluations II and III and simplified acute physiology score II: A prospective cohort study evaluating these methods to predict outcome in a German interdisciplinary intensive care unit. *Crit Care Med* 28:26, 2000.

187. Iezzoni LI: Assessing quality using administrative data. *Ann Intern Med* 128(8 Pt 2):666, 1997.

188. Romano PS, Roos LL, Luft HS, et al: A comparison of administrative versus clinical data: Coronary artery bypass surgery as an example. *J Clin Epidemiol* 47:249, 1994.

189. Weissman C: Can hospital discharge diagnoses be used for intensive care unit administrative and quality management functions? *Crit Care Med* 25:1320, 1997.

190. Hannan EL: The relation between volume and outcome in health care. *N Engl J Med* 340:1677, 1999.

191. Hair JF, Anderson RE, Tatham RL, Black WC: *Multivariate Data Analysis*. Upper Saddle River, NJ, Prentice-Hall, 1998, p 141.

192. Gilbert J, Schoolfield J: The outcome index and system outcome score: a method of quality assurance through outcome analysis in the special care area. *Int J Clin Mon Comput* 8:85, 1991.

193. Hsia CD: Diagnosis related group coding accuracy of the peer review organizations. *J AHIMA* 63:56, 1992.

194. Sivak ED, Perez-Trepichio A: Quality assessment in the medical intensive care unit: Evolution of a data model. *Cleveland Clin J Med* 57:273, 1990.

195. Rafkin HS, Hoyt JW: Objective data and quality assurance programs. Current and future trends. *Crit Care Clin* 10:157, 1994.

196. Berwick DM: Developing and testing changes in delivery of care. *Ann Intern Med* 128:651, 1998.

197. Berwick DM: Health services research and quality of care. *Med Care* 27:763, 1989.

198. Eddy DM, Billings J: The quality of medical evidence: implications for quality of care. *Health Aff* 7:19, 1988.

199. Berwick DM, Fineberg HV, Weinstein MC: When doctors meet numbers. *Am J Med* 71:991, 1981.

200. McGlynn EA, Brook RH: Keeping quality on the policy agenda. *Health Aff* 20:82, 2001.

201. Weinert CR, Gross CR, Marinelli WA: Impact of randomized trial results on acute lung injury ventilator therapy in teaching hospitals. *Am J Respir Crit Care Med* 167:1304, 2003.

202. Kassirer JP: Pseudoaccountability. *Ann Intern Med* 134:587, 2001.

203. Chen J, Radford MJ, Wang Y, et al: Do "America's Best Hospitals" perform better for acute myocardial infarction? *N Engl J Med* 340:286, 1999.

204. Collard HR, Saint S, Matthay MA: Prevention of ventilator-associated pneumonia: An evidence-based systematic review. *Ann Intern Med* 138:494, 2003.

205. Nolan TW: Understanding medical systems. *Ann Intern Med* 128:293, 1998.

206. Deming WE: *Out of Crisis*. Cambridge, MA, M.I.T. Press, 1986.

207. Walton M: *The Deming Management Method*. New York, Perigee Books, 1986.

208. Buccini EP: Total quality management in the critical care environment. *Crit Care Unit Manage* 9:455, 1993.

209. Berwick DM: Continuous improvement as an ideal in health care. *N Engl J Med* 320:53, 1989.

210. McLaughlin CP, Kaluzny AD: Total quality management in health: Making it work. *Health Care Manage Rev* 15:7, 1990.

211. Clemmer TP, Spulher VJ, Oniki TA, Horn SD: Results of a collaborative quality improvement program on outcomes and costs in a tertiary critical care unit. *Crit Care Med* 27:1768, 1999.

212. Koska MT: Adopting Deming's quality improvement ideas: A case study. *Hospitals* 64:58, 1990.

213. O'Connor GT, Plume SK, Olmstead EM, et al: A regional intervention to improve the hospital mortality associated with coronary artery bypass graft surgery. *JAMA* 275:841, 1996.

214. Milakovich ME: Creating a total quality health care environment. *Health Care Manage Rev* 16:9, 1991.

215. Evans RS, Classen DC, Pestotnik SL, et al: Improving empiric antibiotic selection using computer decision support. *Arch Intern Med* 154:878, 1994.

216. Leape LL, Cullen DJ, Clapp MD, et al: Pharmacist participation on physician rounds and adverse drug events in the intensive care units. *JAMA* 282:267, 1999.

217. Bernstein M: Wrong-side surgery: systems for prevention. *Can J Surg* 46:144, 2003.

218. Hall IJ: Quality assurance: Monitors in special care. *AACN Clin Issues* 2:49, 1991.

219. Rhodes M, Sacco W, Smith S, Boorse D: Cost effectiveness of trauma quality assurance audit filters. *J Trauma* 30:724, 1990.

220. Copes WS, Staz CF, Konvolinka CW, Sacco WJ: American College of Surgeons audit filters: Associations with patient outcome and resource utilization. *J Trauma* 38:432, 1995.

221. Campbell JP, Maxey VA, Watson WA: Hawthorne effect: Implications for prehospital research. *Ann Emerg Med* 28:590, 1995.

222. Berwick DM: Errors today and errors tomorrow. *N Engl J Med* 348:2570, 2003.

223. Robinson MB: Evaluation of medical audit. *J Epidemiol Comm Health* 48:435, 1994.

224. Chassin MR: Quality of health care part 3: Improving the quality of care. *N Engl J Med* 335:1060, 1996.

225. Shortell SM, O'Brien JL, Carman JM: Assessing the impact of continuous quality improvement/total quality management: concept versus implementation. *Health Serv Res* 30:377, 1995.

226. Volden CM, Monnig R: Collaborative problem solving with a total quality model. *Am J Med Qual* 8:181, 1993.

227. Shortell SM, Zimmerman JE, Gillies RR, et al: Continuously improving patient care: Practical lessons and an assessment tool from the national ICU study. *Qual Rev Bull* 18:150, 1992.

228. Merry MD: Total quality management for physicians: Translating the new paradigm. *Qual Rev Bull* 16:101, 1990.

229. Mawji Z, Stillman P, Laskowski R, et al: First do no harm: Integrating patient safety and quality improvement. *Joint Comm J Qual Improve* 28:373, 2002.

230. Joshi MS, Anderson JF, Marwaha S: A systems approach to improving error reporting. *J Healthc Inf Manage* 16:40, 2002.

231. Spencer FC: Human error in hospitals and industrial accidents: Current concepts. *J Am Coll Surg* 191:410, 2000.

232. Greco PJ, Eisenberg JM: Changing physicians' practices. *N Engl J Med* 329:1271, 1993.

233. NHS Centre for Reviews and Dissemination: Getting evidence into practice. *Eff Health Care* 5:1, 1999.

234. Smith WR: Evidence for the effectiveness of techniques to change physician behavior. *Chest* 118(2 Suppl):8S, 2000.

235. Paz HL, Garland A, Weinar M, et al: Effect of clinical outcomes data on intensive care unit utilization by bone marrow transplant patients. *Crit Care Med* 26:66, 1998.

236. Rosenthal GE, Harper DL: Cleveland health quality choice: a model for collaborative community-based outcomes assessment. *J Qual Improve* 20:425, 1994.

237. Reinersten JL. Physicians as Leaders in the Improvement of Health Care Systems. *Ann Intern Med* 1998;128(10):833–38.

238. Davis D, O'Brien MA, Freemantle N, et al: Impact of formal continuing medical education: Do conferences, workshops, rounds, and other traditional continuing education activities change physician behavior or health care outcomes? *JAMA* 282:867, 1999.

239. Davis DA, Thomson MA, Oxman AD, Haynes RB: Changing physician performance. A systematic review of the effect of continuing medical education strategies. *JAMA* 274:700, 1995.

240. Tunis SR, Hayward RS, Wilson MC, et al: Internists' attitudes about clinical practice guidelines. *Ann Intern Med* 120:956, 1994.

241. Selker HP: Criteria for adoption in practice of medical practice guidelines. *Am J Cardiol* 71:339, 1993.

242. Davis DA, Taylor-Vaisey A: Translating guidelines into practice. A systematic review of the theoretic concepts, practical experience and research evidence in the adoption of clinical practice guidelines. *Can Med Assoc J* 157:408, 1997.

243. Gundersen L: The effect of clinical practice guidelines on variations in medical care. *Ann Intern Med* 133:317, 2000.

244. Pestotnik SL, Classen DC, Evans RS, Burke JP: Implementing antibiotic practice guidelines through computer-assisted decision support: Clinical and financial outcomes. *Ann Intern Med* 124:884, 1996.

245. Price J, Elkeberry A, Grover A, et al: Evaluation of clinical practice guidelines on outcome of infection in patients in the surgical intensive care unit. *Crit Care Med* 20:2118, 1999.

246. Roberts DE, Bell DD, Ostryzniuk T, et al: Eliminating needless testing in intensive care—an information-based team management approach. *Crit Care Med* 21:1452, 1993.

247. Ely EW, Baker AM, Dunagan DP, et al: Effect on the duration of mechanical ventilation of identifying patients capable of breathing spontaneously. *N Engl J Med* 335:1864, 1996.

248. Grimshaw JM, Russell IT: Effect of clinical guidelines on medical practice: A systematic review of rigorous evaluations. *Lancet* 342:1317, 1992.

249. Grilli R, Lomas J: Evaluating the message: The relationship between compliance rate and the subject of a practice guideline. *Med Care* 32:202, 1994.

250. Thomson-O'Brien MA, Oxman AD, Davis DA, et al: Audit and feedback: Effects on professional practice and health care outcomes. *Cochrane Database Sys Rev* 2:CD000259, 2000.

251. Balas EA, Boren SA, Brown GD, et al: Effect of physician profiling on utilization. Meta-analysis of randomized clinical trials. *J Gen Intern Med* 11:584, 1996.

252. Eagle KA, Mulley AG, Skates SJ, et al: Length of stay in the intensive care unit. Effects of practice guidelines and feedback. *JAMA* 264:992, 1990.

253. Cook DJ, Fuller HD, Guyatt GH, et al: Risk factors for gastrointestinal bleeding in critically ill patients. Canadian Critical Care Trials Group. *N Engl J Med* 330:377, 1994.

254. Civetta JM, Hudson-Civetta JA: Maintaining quality of care while reducing charges in the ICU. *Ann Surg* 202:524, 1985.

255. Pronovost PJ, Angus DC, Dorman T, et al: Physician staffing patterns and clinical outcomes in critically ill patients: A systematic review. *JAMA* 288:2151, 2002.

256. Young MP, Birkmeyer JD: Potential reduction in mortality rates using an intensivist model to manage intensive care units. *Eff Clin Pract* 6:284, 2000.

257. Rosenfeld BA, Dorman T, Breslow MJ, et al: Intensive care unit telemedicine: Alternative paradigm for providing continuous intensivist care. *Crit Care Med* 28:3925, 2000.

258. Blunt MC, Burchett KR: Out-of-hours consultant cover and case-mix-adjusted mortality in intensive care. *Lancet* 356:735, 2000.

259. Bollschweiler E, Krings A, Fuchs K, et al: Alternative shift models and the quality of patient care: An empirical study in surgical intensive care units. *Langenbecks Archiv fur Chirurgie* 386:104, 2001.

260. Petersen LA, Brennan TA, O'Neil AC, et al: Does housestaff discontinuity of care increase the risk for preventable adverse events? *Ann Intern Med* 121:866, 1994.

261. Mallick R, Strosberg M, Lambrinos J, Groeger JS: The intensive care unit medical director as manager. *Med Care* 33:611, 1995.

262. Rosenthal GE, Hammar PJ, Way LE, et al: Using hospital performance data in quality improvement: The Cleveland Health Quality Choice Experience. *Joint Comm J Qual Improve* 24:347, 1998.

263. Mitchell-DiCenso A, Guyatt G, Marrin M, et al: A controlled trial of nurse practitioners in neonatal intensive care. *Pediatrics* 98(6 Pt 1):1143, 1996.

264. Derengowski SL, Irving SY, Koogle PV, Englander RM: Defining the role of the pediatric critical care nurse practitioner in a tertiary care center. *Crit Care Med* 28:2626, 2000.

265. VanSoeren MH, Kirby AS, Andrusyszyn M: Lessons learned during implementation of an acute-care nurse practitioner role in adult critical care in Ontario. *Annals RCPSC* 35:556, 2002.

266. Snyder JV, Sirio CA, Angus DC, et al: Trial of nurse practitioners in intensive care. *New Horiz* 2:296, 1994.

267. Tarnow-Mordi WO, Hau C, Warden A, Shearer AJ: Hospital mortality in relation to staff workload: A 4-year study in an adult intensive-care unit. *Lancet* 356:185, 2000.

268. Amaravadi RK, Dimick JB, Pronovost PJ, Lipsett PA: ICU nurse-to-patient ratio is associated with complications and resource use after esophagectomy. *Intensive Care Med* 26:1857, 2000.

269. Vicca AF: Nursing staff workload as a determinant of methicillin-resistant *Staphylococcus aureus* spread in an adult intensive care unit. *J Hosp Infect* 43:109, 1999.

270. Beckmann U, Baldwin I, Durie M, et al: Problems associated with nursing staff shortage: An analysis of the first 3600 incident reports submitted to the Australian Incident Monitoring Study (AIMS-ICU). *Anaesth Intensive Care* 26:396, 1998.

271. The UK Neonatal Staffing Study Group: Patient volume, staffing, and workload in relation to risk-adjusted outcomes in a random stratified sample of UK neonatal intensive care units: A prospective evaluation. *Lancet* 359:99, 2002.

272. Bastos PG, Knaus WA, Zimmerman JE, et al: The importance of technology for achieving superior outcomes from intensive care. *Intensive Care Med* 22:664, 1996.

273. Shortell SM, Zimmerman JE, Rousseau DM, et al: The performance of intensive care units: Does good management make a difference? *Med Care* 32:508, 1994.

274. Cohen IL, Bari N, Strosberg MA, et al: Reduction in duration and cost of mechanical ventilation in an intensive care unit by use of a ventilatory management team. *Crit Care Med* 19:1278, 1991.

275. Sachdeva RC, Jefferson LS, Coss-Bu J, et al: Effects of availability of patient-related charges on practice patterns and cost containment in the pediatric intensive care unit. *Crit Care Med* 24:501, 1996.

276. Seguin P, Bleichner JP, Grolier J, et al: Effect of price information on test ordering in an intensive care unit. *Intensive Care Med* 28:332, 2002.

277. Blackstone ME, Miller RS, Hodgson AJ, et al: Lowering hospital charges in the trauma intensive care unit while maintaining quality of care by increasing resident and attending physician awareness. *J Trauma* 39:1041, 1995.

278. Price MB, Grant MJ, Welkie K: Financial impact of elimination of routine chest radiographs in a pediatric intensive care unit. *Crit Care Med* 27:1588, 1999.

279. Raymond DP, Pelletier SJ, Crabtree TD, et al: Impact of a rotating empiric antibiotic schedule on infectious mortality in an intensive care unit. *Crit Care Med* 29:1101, 2001.

280. Maury E, Alzieu M, Baudel JL, et al: Availability of an alcohol solution can improve hand disinfection compliance in an intensive care unit. *Am J Respir Crit Care Med* 162:324, 2000.

281. Eggimann P, Pittet D: Infection control in the ICU. *Chest* 120:2059, 2001.

282. Hannan EL, Kilburn H, Racz M, et al: Improving the outcomes of coronary artery bypass surgery in New York State. *JAMA* 271:761, 1994.

283. Baker DW, Einstadter D, Thomas CL, et al: Mortality trends during a program that publicly reported hospital performance. *Med Care* 40:879, 2002.

284. Marshall MN, Shekelle PG, Leatherman S, Brook RH: The public release of performance data. What do we expect to gain? A review of the evidence. *JAMA* 283:1866, 2000.

285. Henneman EA, McKenzie JB, Dewa CS: An evaluation of interventions for meeting the information needs of families of critically ill patients. *Am J Crit Care* 1:85, 1992.

286. Roland P, Russell J, Richards KC, Sullivan SC: Visitation in critical care: processes and outcomes of a performance improvement initiative. *J Nurs Care Qual* 15:18, 2001.

287. Simpson T, Wilson D, Mucken N, et al: Implementation and evaluation of a liberalized visiting policy. *Am J Crit Care* 5:420, 1996.

288. Krapohl GL: Visiting hours in the adult intensive care unit: using research to develop a system that works. *Dimens Crit Care Nurs* 14:245, 1995.

289. Hanson LC, Tulsky JA, Danis M: Can clinical interventions change care at the end of life? *Ann Intern Med* 126:381, 1997.

290. Morrison RS, Siu AL, Leipzig RM, et al: The hard task of improving the quality of care at the end of life. *Arch Intern Med* 160:743, 2000.

291. Lilly CM, DeMeo DL, Sonna LA, et al: An intensive communication intervention for the critically ill. *Am J Med* 109:469, 2000.

292. Knaus WA, Rauss A, LeGall AAJ, et al: Do objective estimates of chances for survival influence decisions to withhold or withdraw treatment? The French Multicentric Group of ICU Research. *Med Decis Making* 10:163, 1990.

293. Pollack MM, Getson PR: Pediatric critical care cost containment: combined actuarial and clinical program. *Crit Care Med* 19:12, 1991.

294. Baggs JG, Schmitt JH, Mushlin AI, et al: Association between nurse-physician collaboration and patient outcomes in three intensive care units. *Crit Care Med* 27:1991, 1999.

295. Shortell SM, Rousseau DM, Gillies RR, et al: Organizational assessment in intensive care units: Construct development, reliability, and validity of the ICU nurse-physician questionnaire. *Med Care* 29:709, 1991.

296. Mitchell PH, Shannon SE, Cain KC, Hegyvary ST: Critical care outcomes: Linking structures, processes, and organizational and clinical outcomes. *Am J Crit Care* 5:353, 1996.

297. Zimmerman JE, Shortell SM, Rousseau DM, et al: Improving intensive care: Observations based on organizational case studies in nine intensive care units: A prospective, multicenter study. *Crit Care Med* 21:1443, 1993.

298. Carson SS, Stocking C, Podsadecki R, et al: Effects of organizational change in the medical intensive care unit of a teaching hospital. *JAMA* 276:322, 1996.

299. Multz AS, Chalfin DB, Samson IM, et al: A "closed" medical intensive care unit (MICU) improves resource utilization when compared with an "open" MICU. *Am J Respir Crit Care Med* 157(5 Pt 1):1468, 1998.

300. Cowen JS, Matchett SC, Kaufman JH, et al: Progressive reduction in severity-adjusted mortality after implementation of a critical care program. *Crit Care Med* 27:A35, 1999.

301. Tai DYH, Goh SK, Eng PCT, Wang YT: Impact of quality of patient care and procedure use in the medical intensive care unit (ICU) following reorganization. *Ann Acad Med Singap* 27:309, 1998.

302. Ghorra S, Reinert SE, Cioffi W, et al: Analysis of the effect of conversion from open to closed surgical intensive care unit. *Ann Surg* 229:163, 1999.

303. Rubenfeld GD: The structure of intensive care: If you've seen one ICU, you've seen one ICU. *Crit Care Alert*, 2000.

304. The Leapfrog Group. Patient Safety. http://www.leapfroggroup.org/safety1.htm#IPS.

305. Adhikari N, Lapinsky SE: Medical informatics in the intensive care unit: Overview of technology assessment. *J Crit Care* 18:41, 2003.

306. Redfern RO, Kundel HL, Polansky M, et al: A picture archival and communication system shortens delays in obtaining radiographic information in a medical intensive care unit. *Crit Care Med* 28:1006, 2000.

307. Watkins J, Weatherburn G, Bryan S: The impact of a picture archiving and communication system (PACS) upon an intensive care unit. *Eur J Radiol* 34:3, 2000.

308. Reiner BI, Siegel EL, Hooper F, Protopapas Z: Impact of filmless imaging on the frequency of clinician review of radiology images. *J Digit Imaging* 11(3 Suppl 1):149, 1998.

309. Imhoff M: Acquisition of ICU data: Concepts and demands. *Int J Clin Monit Comput* 9:229, 1992.

310. Gardner RM, Maack BB, Evans RS, Huff SM: Computerized medical care: the HELP system at LDS Hospital. *J AHIMA* 63:68, 1992.

311. General Electric Medical Systems. QS Critical Care Clinical Information System. http://www.gemedicalsystems.com/monitor/products/info_sys/qscc_info.html.

312. Mahoney ME: Transforming health information management through technology. *Top Health Inf Manage* 23:52, 2002.

313. Greene ZB: Creating and managing a paperless health information management department. *Top Health Inf Manage* 23:26, 2002.

314. Langenberg CJ: Implementation of an electronic patient data management system (PDMS) on an intensive care unit (ICU). *Int J Bio-Med Comput* 42:97, 1996.

315. Bates DW, Gawande AA: Improving safety with information technology. *N Engl J Med* 348:2526, 2003.

316. Gillingham W, Holt A, Gillies J: Hand-held computers in healthcare: what software programs are available? *N Z Med J* 115:U185, 2002.

317. Dean B, Schachter M, Vincent C, Barber N: Prescribing errors in hospital inpatients: Their incidence and clinical significance. *Qual Saf Health Care* 11:340, 2002.

318. Mekhjian MS, Kumar RR, Kuehn L, et al: Immediate benefits realized following implementation of physician order entry at an academic medical center. *J Am Med Inform Assoc* 9:529, 2002.

319. Kaushal R, Shojania KG, Bates DW. Effects of computerized physician order entry and clinical decision support systems on medication safety: A systematic review. *Arch Intern Med* 163:1409, 2003.

320. Tierney WM, Miller ME, Overhage M, McDonald CJ: Physician inpatient order writing on microcomputer workstations. *JAMA* 269:379, 1993.

321. Overhage JM, Tierney WM, Zhou XH, McDonald CJ: A randomized trial of "corollary orders" to prevent errors of omission. *J Am Med Inform Assoc* 4:364, 1997.

322. Mutlu GM, Mutlu EA, Factor P: GI complications in patients receiving mechanical ventilation. *Chest* 119:1222, 2001.

323. Brook AD, Ahrens TS, Schaiff R, et al: Effect of a nursing-implemented sedation protocol on the duration of mechanical ventilation. *Crit Care Med* 27:2609, 1999.

324. Kress JP, Pohlman AS, O'Connor MF, Hall JB: Daily interruption of sedative infusions in critically ill patients undergoing mechanical ventilation. *N Engl J Med* 342:1471, 2000.

325. Larsen RA, Evans RS, Burke JP, et al: Improved perioperative antibiotic use and reduced surgical wound infections through use of computer decision analysis. *Infect Control Hosp Epidemiol* 10:316, 1989.

326. Overhage JM, Tierney WM, McDonald CJ: Computer reminders to implement preventive care guidelines for hospitalized patients. *Arch Intern Med* 156:1551, 1996.

327. Shiffman RN, Liaw Y, Brandt CA, Corb GJ: Computer-based guideline implementation systems: A systematic review of functionality and effectiveness. *J Am Med Inform Assc* 6:104, 1999.

328. Teich JM, Merchia PR, Schmiz JL, et al: Effects of computerized physician order entry on prescribing practices. *Arch Intern Med* 160:2741, 2000.

329. Bates DW, Leape LL, Cullen DJ, et al: Effect of computerized physician order entry and a team intervention on prevention of serious medication errors. *JAMA* 280:1311, 1998.

330. Johnston ME, Langton KB, Haynes RB, Mathieu A: Effects of computer-based clinical decision support systems on clinician performance and patient outcome. *Ann Intern Med* 120:135, 1994.

331. Hunt DL, Haynes RB, Hanna SE, Smith K: Effects of computer-based clinical decision support systems on physician performance and patient outcomes: A systematic review. *JAMA* 280:1339, 1998.

332. Walton R, Dovey S, Harvey E, Freemantle N: Computer support for determining drug dose: Systematic review and meta-analysis. *BMJ* 318:984, 1999.

333. Dojat M, Harf A, Touchard D, et al: Clinical evaluation of a computer-controlled pressure support mode. *Am J Respir Crit Care Med* 161(4 Part 1):1161, 2000.

334. Mason DG, Ross JJ, Edwards ND, et al: Self-learning fuzzy control with temporal knowledge for atracurium-induced neuromuscular block during surgery. *Comput Biomed Res* 32:187, 1999.

335. Bates JHT, Young MP: Applying fuzzy logic to medical decision making in the intensive care unit. *Am J Respir Crit Care Med* 167:948, 2003.

336. Evans RS, Pestotnik ST, Burke JP, et al: Reducing the duration of prophylactic antibiotic use through computer monitoring of surgical patients. *DICP* 24:351, 1990.

337. Teach RL, Shortliffe EH: An analysis of physician attitudes regarding computer-based clinical consultation systems. *Comput Biomed Res* 14:542, 1981.

338. Burke JP, Classen DC, Pestotnik SL, et al: The HELP system and its application to infection control. *J Hosp Infect* 18(Suppl A):424, 1991.

Chapter 4

INFECTION CONTROL AND SURVEILLANCE IN THE INTENSIVE CARE UNIT

DAVID K. WARREN
MARIN H. KOLLEF

KEY POINTS

- *Focused surveillance for nosocomial infections is the cornerstone of infection control activities in the ICU.*

- *Commonly used invasive devices such as central venous and urinary catheters and endotracheal tubes are significant risk factors for nosocomial infection. Evidence-based ICU policies and procedures and staff education can reduce the risk of device-related infections.*

- *Antibiotic resistance is an increasing problem, and its containment and prevention require a multifactorial approach, including adequate hand hygiene, surveillance for resistant pathogens, enforced infection control precautions, and prudent use of antibiotics.*

- *Standard infection control precautions should be applied to all ICU patients. Precautions for contagious or epidemiologically significant pathogens are based on modes of transmission.*

Nosocomial, or hospital-acquired, infections result in significant morbidity and mortality. Nosocomial infections have been reported to affect approximately 2 million hospitalized patients in the United States annually, at an estimated cost of $57.6 billion in 2000.[1,2] ICU beds, while only accounting for 5% to 10% of all hospital beds, are responsible for 10% to 25% of health care costs generated.[3] Patients admitted to the ICU have been shown to be at particular risk for nosocomial infections, with a prevalence rate as high as 30%.[4] Given the increasing strain on health care resources in the United States and other countries and the personal impact that these infections have on patients, the prevention of nosocomial infections in the ICU should be an important goal of any critical care clinician.

A likely explanation to account for the observation that ICU patients are more vulnerable to acquiring a nosocomial infection compared with other hospitalized patients is that critically ill patients frequently require invasive medical devices, such as urinary catheters, central venous and arterial catheters, and endotracheal tubes. Data on a sample of ICUs from the Centers for Disease Control and Prevention (CDC) show that adult ICU patients have central venous catheters in place and receive mechanical ventilation an average of 53% and 42% of their total time spent in the ICU, respectively.[5] These devices result in infection by compromising the normal skin and mucosal barriers and serving as a nidus for the development of biofilms, which provide a protected environment for bacteria and fungi. In a survey of cases of ICU-acquired

primary bacteremia, 47% were catheter-related.[6] While the increased severity of illness of ICU patients makes intuitive sense as a potential risk factor for nosocomial infection, few studies have shown a consistent relationship.[7] This may be explained, however, by the fact that scoring systems were developed primarily to predict mortality and may not adequately capture markers for nosocomial infection, such as the need for prolonged parenteral nutrition.

Infection control in the ICU arose from hospital-wide infection control programs developed in response to the staphylococcal pandemic of the late 1950s and early 1960s. In 1976, the CDC initiated the Study on the Efficacy of Nosocomial Infection Control (SENIC) to better understand the impact of infection control programs on nosocomial infection rates in a random sample of 338 U.S. hospitals.[8] Programs that had the greatest impact in reducing nosocomial infection rates had the following components: organized surveillance and active intervention in patient care by infection control staff to reduce the risk of infection, a physician trained in infection control methods, a fixed ratio of infection control specialists to patient beds, and a system for reporting surgical infection rate to surgeons. In hospitals that implemented infection control programs meeting these criteria, the incidence of nosocomial infections decreased hospital-wide by 32%, whereas in hospitals with ineffectual programs, infections increased by 18% over a 5-year period. These findings led to regulations requiring that hospitals demonstrate that their infection control programs meet the preceding criteria in order to maintain accreditation.

Surveillance

Surveillance for nosocomial infection is the cornerstone of effective infection control activity in the ICU. Surveillance activity serves several key functions, including the early detection of potential nosocomial outbreaks, the identification of high endemic rates of infection as targets for intervention, and evaluation of the effectiveness of efforts to prevent infection. The process of surveillance itself involves the continuous and systematic collection, tabulation, analysis, and dissemination of information on the occurrence of nosocomial infections within the ICU. It was noted early in the development of infection control programs that feedback of nosocomial infection rates to clinicians, along with active intervention, is a necessary element to a successful program and that collection of surveillance information without this feedback is ineffectual at reducing infection rates.[8] Nosocomial infection surveillance in the ICU involves the cooperation of both infection control and ICU personnel for both exchange of data and developing effective infection control measures.

Infection control surveillance, particularly when it involves chart review, can be labor-intensive. Because of the reality that limited resources are available for infection control surveillance and intervention, a practice known as *focused* or *targeted surveillance* is commonly employed. This involves both hospital infection control and ICU personnel making determinations of the particular nosocomial infections to be monitored routinely. The factors involved in making the decision include the degree of morbidity or mortality that results from the infection, the frequency that the infection is known or perceived to occur in the ICU, the proportion of ICU patients at risk of becoming infected, the extent to which effective interventions can be implemented by the ICU team, and finally, the perception by both infection control and ICU personnel that a particular infection represents a significant problem for that unit.

Infection control surveillance data in the ICU typically are reported as the occurrence of a particular infection over a defined time period at risk (e.g., cases of ventilator-associated pneumonia per total number of patient days spent on mechanical ventilation per month), also known as an *incidence density*. For infections that result from a point exposure (e.g., the number of tracheostomy site infections per total number of tracheotomies performed in one quarter), a *cumulative incidence* can be determined. Cumulative incidence is reported less commonly in the ICU owing to the observation that infections in the ICU result primarily from invasive devices that are in place for days to weeks.

In order for the information collected for infection surveillance to be interpretable, a case definition for infection has to be developed. Criteria for the diagnosis of nosocomial infections have been developed by the CDC[9] and are widely accepted. It is important to note that greater accuracy is required on the part of the infection control practitioner in determining if an episode represents a true nosocomial infection compared with the critical care physician, who may initiate antibiotic therapy in the case of a presumptive diagnosis.

Several methods exist for performing surveillance in the ICU, including the traditional methods of medical chart review and review of microbiology, radiology, and autopsy reports. More recently, the use of computerized expert systems and medical informatics in nosocomial infection surveillance has reduced the need for manual chart review, improved case ascertainment, and allowed for more resources to be used for intervention and prevention.[10]

Structural/Organizational Factors That Affect ICU Infection Control

ICU DESIGN AND LAYOUT

While published architectural guidelines require that isolation rooms be included in the layout of critical care units, few data are available to address the impact of ICU design on prevention of nosocomial infection. Mulin and colleagues[11] demonstrated a lower rate of bronchopulmonary colonization with *Acinetobacter baumannii* among mechanically ventilated patients in a surgical ICU after the unit was converted from one with a mixture of enclosed isolation rooms and open rooms to all enclosed rooms with hand washing facilities. Another study demonstrated a reduction in the incidence of ventilator-associated pneumonia and urinary tract infections in a pediatric ICU after it was converted from an open ward to separate isolation rooms, without a significant change in patient to staff ratios.[12] Despite the lack of data, it would seem prudent to ensure that adequate access to hand hygiene exists for ICU personnel.

NURSING STAFFING RATIOS

Much attention has been given recently to the issue of nurse staffing levels and the impact that this has on patient outcomes and complications, including infection. With increased workloads for registered nurses and the reliance on less trained health care personnel for the delivery of care, there is concern that lapses in infection control will occur, resulting in nosocomial infections. In a pediatric cardiac ICU over a 1-year period, a decrease in nurse-to-patient staffing ratios correlated significantly with an increase in nosocomial infections.[13] In a multicenter, retrospective cohort study among 2606 patients admitted to an ICU after abdominal aortic surgery, patients cared for in ICUs that reported nurse-to-patient ratio of 1:3 or greater on either day or night shifts were at greater risk of respiratory complications, including postoperative pneumonia.[14] This relationship was independent of patient age, comorbidity, level of surgical urgency, ICU size, and hospital procedure volume.

These studies, along with several others, have limitations, including retrospective design, no determination of nursing experience or level of training, and no comment on the role that other types of health care worker staffing levels, such as respiratory therapists, have on nosocomial infections rates. Despite these limitations, a direct association between increased nursing workload and the occurrence of nosocomial infections among ICU patients appears to exist. The optimal level of both nursing staffing and experience needed to minimize the risk of infection in ICUs remains to be determined but is unlikely to be uniform for every type of unit.

INFECTION CONTROL POLICIES AND PROCEDURES

Given the complexity of delivering care to critically ill patients, policies and procedure are a necessary part of the organization of any ICU. These policies ensure that personnel perform certain procedures, such as central venous catheter insertion and care, in a consistent manner. Written ICU policies should incorporate evidence-based infection control practices. For policies to be effective, they should be clear, concise, and shared with the staff. Policies that are complex or unrealistic either will be ignored or will result in even wider variation in how care is delivered owing to individual interpretation. Most private and state hospital accreditation programs base their review of ICUs not only on whether ICUs have required policies but also on whether they actually follow them. Therefore, it is important that ICU physician and nursing staff review these policies on a routine basis in consultation with infection control practitioners or the hospital infection control committee and revise these policies when needed.

Invasive Devices and ICU-Acquired Infections

CENTRAL VENOUS CATHETERS/PULMONARY ARTERIAL CATHETERS

Catheter-associated bloodstream infection is one of the most common nosocomial infections seen in ICU patients. Approximately 80,000 of these infections have been estimated to occur annually in ICUs in the United States (excluding insertion-site infection and septic thrombophlebitis).[15] These infections are associated with increased ICU length of stay, health care costs, and use of broad-spectrum antibiotics.

Risk factors for catheter-associated bloodstream infections include the anatomic catheter insertion site, type of catheter used, and the patient population. The pathogenesis includes microbial colonization of the subcutaneous catheter tract by skin flora with subsequent colonization of the catheter and biofilm formation, as well as colonization of the catheter hub from microbes introduced during use of the catheter. While intravascular catheters can result in bloodstream infections by other means, such as the infusion of contaminated fluids, the mechanisms just mentioned are the primarily methods by which nontunneled central venous catheters in place for less than 2 to 4 weeks cause bloodstream infections.

Numerous infection control practices have been effective in preventing intravascular catheter-related infections (Table 4-1). Meticulous hand hygiene before and after handling intravascular catheters, along with maintaining an intact, nonsoiled dressing at the catheter insertion site, are essential to preventing device-related infections. Maximal sterile barrier precautions (i.e., sterile gowns, gloves, surgical mask and hat, and a large surgical drape) during insertion reduce the incidence of infection.[16] In one randomized trial, subclavian vein insertion was associated with a lower incidence

TABLE 4-1 Specific Recommendations for Preventing Intravascular Catheter–Related Infections

- Proper hand hygiene before and after manipulation of intravascular catheter or catheter insertion site
- Aseptic technique during catheter insertion and care
- Use of hat, mask, sterile gowns and gloves, and large sterile drape during central venous catheter (CVC) insertion
- Use of 2% chlorhexidine or other skin antiseptic (tincture of iodine, iodophor, or 70% alcohol) for insertion-site antisepsis
- Use of sterile gauze or transparent semipermeable dressing to cover insertion site
- Prompt removal of catheters that are no longer essential
- Routine replacement of intravascular catheters to prevent infection:
  - Peripheral catheters—(adult) every 72 to 96 hours; (pediatric) remove if complication occurs
  - Central venous catheters—routine replacement not recommended
  - Pulmonary artery catheters—routine replacement not recommended
  - Arterial catheters—routine replacement not recommended
  - Umbilical catheters—routine replacement not recommended
- Do not replace catheters suspected of being infected over a guidewire
- Replace IV administration sets and tubing no more frequently than every 72 hours unless infection is suspected or blood products or lipid emulsions are used
- Antimicrobial/antiseptic-coated CVC should be used only after staff can demonstrate proper CVC care and insertion techniques
- Subclavian insertion site should be used when possible to reduce infection risk
- Avoid using arterial or venous cutdown procedures to insert catheters
- Replace catheter-site dressing when loose, damp, or soiled
- Use sterile sleeve for pulmonary artery catheters
- Pressure transducer systems:
  - Use disposable systems when possible with a sterile, closed flush system
  - Replace transducer, tubing, flush solution, and flush device every 96 hours

SOURCE: Adapted from O'Grady et al.[62]

of infectious complications and complete vessel thrombosis when compared with femoral insertion.[17] Structured educational programs incorporating the use of maximal sterile precautions have reduced the incidence of catheter-associated bloodstream infections by 27% to 66%.[18,19] Antibiotic-coated catheters are also effective.[20] The unexplored issue of emerging resistance associated with the use of these catheters makes their role in an overall infection control strategy unclear.

ARTERIAL CATHETERS AND PRESSURE TRANSDUCERS

Compared with central venous catheters, the incidence of catheter-associated bloodstream infection attributable to arterial catheters has not been as well studied but is estimated to be roughly 1.5% per device or 2.9 cases per 1000 catheter-days.[21] Pressure transducer systems have been a common source of epidemic outbreaks of nosocomial infection. From 1977 to 1987, these devices were the most common source of epidemic bloodstream infection investigated by the CDC.[22] These outbreaks were prolonged (mean 11 months) and involved large numbers of patients (mean 24 patients). In each case, reusable transducers were either improperly disinfected or fitted with improperly sterilized domes. Recommendations for the proper care and use of both arterial catheters and pressure transducer systems are shown in Table 4-1.

URINARY CATHETERS

Urinary catheter use is the primary cause of urinary tract infections among critically ill patients. A survey of 112 medical ICUs in the National Nosocomial Infection Surveillance System found urinary tract infections to be responsible for 31% of all ICU-acquired infections, making urinary tract infections the most common nosocomial infection.[23] Most of these infections are asymptomatic, but between 0.4% to 3.6% of patients with a nosocomial urinary tract infection develop a secondary bloodstream infection.[24,25] Potentially modifiable risk factors for infections with urinary catheters include the use of open urinary drainage systems or breaks in closed drainage systems, prolonged or unnecessary urinary tract catheterization, and retrograde flow from collection bags into the bladder. Infection control measures for urinary catheters should include proper hand hygiene when caring for these devices and prompt removal of catheters when they are no longer needed (Table 4-2).

RESPIRATORY THERAPY EQUIPMENT AND NASOGASTRIC TUBES

Respiratory failure requiring mechanical ventilation is one of the most common indications for ICU admission. Nasogastric tubes are used often for both gastric decompression and to permit feeding of ICU patients. Both mechanical ventilation and nasogastric intubation bypass the normal mucosal defenses of the upper and lower respiratory tract, which leaves patients at risk for nosocomial sinusitis and pneumonia.

Among ICU patients, the vast majority of nosocomial pneumonias are ventilator-associated pneumonias. Ventilator-associated pneumonia is most likely the result of aspiration of contaminated oropharyngeal and gastric secretions and contaminated condensate in the ventilator circuit. Risk factors include the supine position, sedation or impaired

TABLE 4-2 Recommendations for Preventing Urinary Catheter–Related Infections

- Urinary catheters should not be used solely for the convenience of health care personnel and should be removed when no longer necessary.
- Personnel should be trained on proper aseptic insertion and maintenance of urinary catheters.
- Proper hand hygiene should be performed before and after manipulating catheters.
- Insertion of catheters should be performed using aseptic technique and sterile equipment.
- A sterile, continuously closed system should be maintained.
- If necessary, perform closed continuous irrigation of catheter with sterile irrigant.
- Urine samples from catheter and collecting bag should be collected aseptically.
- Urine collection bags always should be below the level of the bladder.
- Maintain unobstructed urinary flow.

SOURCE: Adapted from Wong.[63]

TABLE 4-3 Selected Guidelines for the Prevention of Nosocomial Pneumonia

- Educate health care workers regarding nosocomial pneumonia and infection control and prevention methods.
- Use hand hygiene before and after contact with patient, respiratory devices, or objects contaminated with respiratory secretions.
- Do not routinely change ventilator breathing circuit components more frequently than every 48 hours.
- Periodically drain condensate from mechanical ventilator tubing; avoid draining of condensate toward the patient.
- Use sterile water to fill bubbling humidifiers and nebulizers.
- Do not use large-volume room-air humidifiers unless they undergo daily high-level disinfection; use sterile water in device.
- Devices used on multiple patients (e.g., portable respirators, oxygen sensors, Ambu bags) should undergo sterilization or high-level disinfection between patients.
- Thoroughly clean respiratory equipment prior to disinfection or sterilization.
- Use aseptic technique when changing a tracheostomy tube.
- Use only sterile fluid to remove secretions from respiratory suction catheter.
- Keep head of bed elevated at an angle of 30 to 45 degrees for patients on a ventilator or receiving enteral tube feedings, if possible.
- Discontinue mechanical ventilation and enteral tube feedings as soon as clinically feasible.

SOURCE: Adapted from Tablan et al.[64]

consciousness, and reduced gastric acidity.[25a] Contaminated respiratory equipment has been implicated as the source of outbreaks of nosocomial pneumonia. Devices that generate aerosols, such as nebulizer reservoirs used for humidification[26] and multidose medication nebulizers,[27] have been associated with outbreaks caused by hydrophilic bacteria. Bronchoscopes also have been a source of nosocomial pneumonia in the ICU, usually as a result of an incomplete or compromised disinfection between procedures.[28]

Guidelines for the prevention of ventilator-associated pneumonia focus on proper hand hygiene when handling respiratory equipment, nursing ventilated patients in a semirecumbent position (30 to 45 degrees), and maintaining a closed ventilator circuit (Table 4-3). The use of noninvasive ventilation in selected ICU patients results in a lower risk of nosocomial pneumonia when compared with endotracheal mechanical ventilation. In a randomized, clinical trial, patients ventilated noninvasively had a significantly lower rate of both pneumonia (3% versus 25%) and sinusitis (0% versus 6%).[29] Subglottic suctioning of oropharyngeal secretions using a specially designed endotracheal tube has been shown to reduce the incidence of ventilator-associated pneumonia and holds promise as another method to reduce the risk of nosocomial pneumonia among ventilated patients.[30]

The presence of a foreign body in the nasopharynx, such as a nasogastric feeding tube, predisposes to upper airway infections, particularly sinusitis. Nosocomial sinusitis is often difficult to diagnose. First, the classic signs and symptoms of sinusitis (i.e., sinus tenderness, pain, and fever) often are masked in the intubated and sedated patient. Also, sinus aspiration to determine if a sinus fluid collection is infected is performed only rarely. In a prospective study, paranasal sinus computed tomographic (CT) scans were obtained on all ICU patients with purulent nasal discharge and fever not attributable to another source, followed by sinus aspiration and culture of any fluid observed on CT scan.[31] Using this method, sinusitis was identified in 7.7% of patients. Risk factors for nosocomial sinusitis include nasotracheal intubation, feeding via nasogastric tube, and impaired mental status. These infections frequently are polymicrobial, with *Pseudomonas*

aeruginosa and *Staphylococcus aureus* being the most common organisms identified.[31,32] Prevention involves avoiding nasotracheal intubation, placing feeding tubes through the mouth rather than through the nose, and minimizing sedative use.

INTRACRANIAL PRESSURE MONITORING DEVICES

Several infectious complications can result from the use of intracranial pressure monitoring devices, including scalp exit-site and tunnel infections, osteomyelitis of the calvarium, meningitis, and ventriculitis. The rate of infectious complications has been reported at 7.4% to 14.1% per procedure.[33,34] Intracerebral or intraventricular hemorrhage, cerebrospinal fluid leaks, open head injuries, monitors in place for greater than 5 days, breaks in the pressure transducer system, and use of intraventricular versus intraparenchymal monitors have been associated with increased risk of infection. Coagulase-negative *Staphylococcus* spp. are the most common cause of intracranial pressure monitor–related infections, but gram-negative bacilli, such as *Acinetobacter baumannii*, *Klebsiella pneumoniae*, and *Proteus mirabilis*, have been reported in up to 50% of cases.[35] The role of prophylactic antibiotic therapy is unclear. Several cohort studies showed no impact on the incidence of infection among patients who received antibiotics during or after insertion of the devices,[34,36] but no randomized, controlled trials of sufficient sample size exist to address the question.

Interventions to Prevent Nosocomial Infections

Interventions designed to reduce nosocomial infections typically focus on device-related infection, are evidence-based, and often employ physician and nursing education or introduce a change in the process of care. An intervention consisting of a self-study module on risk factors for catheter-associated infections, a pre- and posttest assessment of knowledge, posters and handouts on the infection control practices related to central venous catheters, and didactic teaching were given to the nursing staff of a surgical ICU.[19] The authors reported a 66% reduction in the incidence of ICU-acquired bloodstream infections in the 18-month period after the intervention compared with the 18 months preintervention ($p < 0.001$), without a significant change in the patient population. This study demonstrates that focused intervention in ICUs can reduce nosocomial infections, possibly through changes in ICU practice and staff behavior.

Another practice designed to prevent nosocomial infection is selective digestive decontamination. The hypothesis behind this practice is that colonization of the oropharynx and gastrointestinal tract by flora acquired while a patient is in the ICU serves as a source of nosocomial infection, particularly in patients requiring prolonged ICU stays and mechanical ventilation. By administering oral, nonabsorbable antibiotics, selective digestive decontamination seeks to prevent the overgrowth of gram-negative aerobic bacteria and yeast while maintaining anaerobic flora. The method has been useful in controlling outbreaks of resistant gram-negative bacteria.[37] Studies of its routine use have had conflicting results, with more methodologically rigorous studies tending to show no benefit in terms of preventing nosocomial pneumonia or mortality.[38,39] These observations, plus the concern of selective digestive decontamination leading to increased antibiotic resistance, leave the role of this practice unclear.

Antibiotic Resistance in the ICU

Intensive care units have long been associated with an increased prevalence of antibiotic-resistant organisms compared with other areas of the hospital. The frequent use of broad-spectrum antibiotics, a patient population with prolonged lengths of stay and the need for invasive devices, and the close interactions between health care workers and critically ill patients all contribute to the propagation of antibiotic-resistant microorganisms within the ICU. The recent emergence of highly resistant virulent organisms, such as vancomycin-resistant *S. aureus*, highlights the importance of understanding and controlling antibiotic resistance within the ICU.

THE EPIDEMIOLOGY OF ANTIBIOTIC RESISTANCE

The resistant organisms seen most commonly in the ICU include methicillin-resistant *S. aureus* (MRSA), vancomycin-resistant *Enterococcus faecium* or *E. faecalis* (VRE), and multi-drug–resistant gram-negative bacilli, such as *P. aeruginosa*, *Stenotrophomonas maltophilia*, and extended-spectrum β-lactamase–producing Enterobacteriaceae. While each of these organisms has individual differences that affect how it is transmitted in the ICU, patients who are colonized or infected with these organisms tend to share common characteristics (Table 4-4).

Patients either can enter the ICU with endogenous resistant bacteria already present or can become colonized during their ICU stay owing to cross-contamination from other

TABLE 4-4 Factors Associated with Colonization or Infection with Multi-Drug–Resistant Microorganisms

- Extended length of hospitalization
- Interhospital or nursing home transfer
- Immunocompromised host
- Invasive devices (i.e., central venous catheters, mechanical ventilation)
- Advanced age
- Severity of illness
- Exposure to broad spectrum antibiotics

SOURCE: Adapted from Safdar and Maki.[65]

colonized patients. Bruin-Buisson and colleagues[40] demonstrated through serial rectal swabs that 90% of all patients subsequently found to be colonized with multi-drug–resistant Enterobacteriaceae were negative on admission to a medical ICU and had a mean time to colonization of 14 days.[40] The primary mechanism by which patient-to-patient transmission of resistant microorganisms occurs within the ICU is on the hands of health care workers. Resistant bacteria can be carried on health care workers' hands and clothing.[41] Another source of transmission of antibiotic-resistant microorganisms is the ICU environment itself. This is particularly true for hydrophilic gram-negative bacilli, such as *Pseudomonas* spp., *Stenotrophomonas* spp., and *Acinetobacter* spp., as well as VRE. These organisms are particularly resistant to the effects of drying; therefore, they can survive on inanimate objects in the environment for extended periods of time. Outbreaks of nosocomial infections associated with these bacteria can persist if the environmental source is not addressed.[42]

Preventing Antibiotic Resistance in the ICU

SURVEILLANCE

Understanding the extent to which ICU patients are colonized or infected with antibiotic-resistant microorganisms is important for identifying outbreaks or high endemic rates of particular pathogens and targeting methods for control. Strategies include both passive and active surveillance. Passive surveillance is employed most frequently in ICUs within the United States and consists of identifying patients colonized with resistant microorganisms by review of clinical specimens. While this strategy requires the least amount of labor and supplies, it fails to identify a significant proportion of colonized patients.[43] In active surveillance, cultures are obtained for the specific purpose of identifying colonized patients. These cultures can be performed on every patient or on selected high-risk subsets (see Table 4-4). Selective screening of high-risk patients, combined with other infection control interventions, reduced the prevalence of ICU-acquired MRSA infections in a medical ICU and was cost-effective.[44] Whether this approach is cost-effective for ICUs to use for other pathogens is an area of further study.

ANTIBIOTIC USE AND CONTROL

Inadequate initial antibiotic therapy of infections has been associated with increased mortality among ICU patients. This observation argues for the use of broad-spectrum antibiotics. However, the increasing use of broad-spectrum antibiotics has been associated with the acquisition of antibiotic-resistant pathogens. Exposure to broad-spectrum antibiotics can alter the normal flora of patients and can facilitate colonization with resistant organisms or expansion of populations of already-existing organisms. The dilemma created by these competing pressures has shaped efforts to control the use of antibiotics within the ICU, particularly drugs with a broad-spectrum of activity.

Antibiotic use in the ICU can be divided into empirical use against a suspected community-acquired or nosocomial infection, targeted use against a specific pathogen, and prophylactic use. There is considerable overlap between these concepts. For example, critically ill patients often are started empirically on broad-spectrum antibiotics and then switched to an antibiotic with a more targeted spectrum once the pathogen causing infection is known. Selective digestive decontamination as a method to prevent nosocomial infections is an example of the prophylactic use of antibiotics in the ICU, which was discussed earlier in this chapter. Strategies that have been applied to control antibiotic use include closed or restricted pharmacy formularies, rapid narrowing of antibiotic spectrum of activity once a pathogen is known, discontinuation of empirical antibiotic therapy based on set clinical parameters, cycling or rotation of empirical antibiotics with gram-negative activity, and decision-support systems for physician prescribing.

Often, antibiotic therapy that is started empirically in a critically ill patient is continued even after evidence suggests that infection is not present. In a study by Singh and colleagues,[45] patients suspected of having ventilator-associated pneumonia were scored using a validated clinical pulmonary infection score. Patients suspected clinically to be at risk for pneumonia but not meeting a predetermined threshold score were randomized to two groups. The experimental group received a single antibiotic for 3 days, with re-evaluation at that time. If this group still did not meet the threshold criteria, antibiotics were discontinued. The type and duration of antibiotic used in the control group were at the treating physicians' discretion. Antibiotic use was continued after 3 days in only 28% of the experimental group versus in 90% of the controls ($p < 0.001$). Mortality and ICU length of stay did not differ between the two groups, but compared with controls, patients in the experimental group had significantly shorter durations of antibiotic use and a lower incidence of antimicrobial-resistant isolates and nosocomial infections during their ICU stay. This study suggests that basing decisions to discontinue antibiotic therapy on formal clinical criteria is an effective and safe method of reducing antibiotic use and resistance.

Cycling empirical antibiotics usually requires the use of only a single antibiotic for the empirical treatment of suspected nosocomial infection, followed by a switch to another agent after a predetermined time period. Raymond and colleagues[46] compared a period of non-protocol–driven antibiotic prescribing with a set quarterly empirical antibiotic rotation and demonstrated a reduction in the occurrence of infections owing to resistant gram-negative and gram-positive bacteria along with a significant reduction in mortality owing to infection during the rotation period. While antibiotic cycling appears promising, questions remain regarding the impact that this strategy has on bacteria with multi-drug–

resistant plasmids and its applicability outside of a research setting.

Increased interest in computer-assisted physician order entry has allowed for the development of physician ordering support systems. A prospective study of a computerized antibiotic management program in one ICU found that patients treated using the computerized support system had a lower incidence of mismatches between antibiotics prescribed and the susceptibility of isolated bacteria.[47] The computerized support system also was associated with shorter durations of antibiotic use. Further studies need to be performed to see if the reduction in overall antibiotic use by this method can reduce the prevalence of antibiotic-resistant bacteria.

Hand Hygiene

Proper hand hygiene has been known to be fundamental in preventing nosocomial infections since the studies of puerperal fever by Semmelweis in the mid-nineteenth century. After contact with patients, health care workers' hands can become transiently colonized with pathogenic and antibiotic-resistant bacteria, which are then transferred to other patients. Hand soaps containing an antiseptic agent, such as chlorhexidine, or alcohol-based hand rubs have been shown to effectively reduce bacterial counts on hands when used properly.

Despite the known benefit of proper hand hygiene in preventing nosocomial infections and the transmission of antibiotic-resistant bacteria, observed compliance with hand hygiene among ICU personnel is poor, typically between 22% and 40% for each episode of patient contact.[48,49] The greatest barriers to compliance with hand hygiene are time and accessibility. An outbreak of *Enterobacter cloacae* infections in a neonatal ICU coincided with a period of patient overcrowding and short staffing of nurses.[50] During this time, adherence to hand hygiene was 25% and subsequently increased to 70% when staffing and patient census returned to normal levels. Accessibility to sinks in the ICU is often limited, particularly in older units. When personnel do wash their hands with antiseptic soap, it is often for a shorter period of time than the duration used to test the product's effectiveness.

Waterless alcohol-based hand rubs improve health care workers' compliance with hand hygiene in the ICU.[51] Compared with using traditional antiseptic soap and water, alcohol-based products require less time to use and are more convenient. Antiseptic soap and water should still be used, however, when hands are visibly soiled.

Other recommendations for ICU personnel concerning proper hand hygiene include avoiding the wearing of artificial fingernails owing to high periungual bacterial counts and outbreaks of nosocomial infections associated with these products, washing hands before and after using gloves, and providing staff with hand lotions to minimize the risk of irritant contact dermatitis.

Preventing Transmission of Pathogens between ICU Personnel and Patients

Health care workers in the ICU are potentially at risk of being exposed to infectious agents during the course of caring for patients. Likewise, the same health care workers potentially can spread infectious agents, particularly antibiotic-resistant bacteria, to patients. A primary goal of infection control is to prevent both. Transmitting infectious agents in the ICU currently is prevented by what has been termed by the CDC as *standard precautions* and *transmission-based precautions* (i.e., airborne, droplet, and contact precautions).[52]

STANDARD PRECAUTIONS

The concept of standard precautions arose primarily from attempts to prevent patient-to-health-care-worker transmission of blood-borne pathogens, particularly HIV. The concept of standard precautions is based on the assumption that all body substances (i.e., blood and other body fluids, secretions, and excretions) and certain body sites (e.g., nonintact skin and mucous membranes) are potential sources of infectious agents. Therefore, health care workers should use the same basic precautions, regardless of whether a patient is known to have a particular infection. Standard precautions are designed to minimize the risk of transmission of both recognized and unrecognized sources of infection in hospitals and include (1) wearing clean gloves when there is the potential for contact with blood, body fluids, secretions, excretions, contaminated items, mucous membranes, or nonintact skin, (2) washing hands immediately after gloves are removed or when body fluids are inadvertently contacted, (3) wearing a gown, mask, and eye protection or a face shield when there is the potential for splashing or spraying with bodily substances, (4) avoiding practices that increase the risk of exposures and injuries, such as recapping or removing used needles from syringes.

TRANSMISSION-BASED PRECAUTIONS

A change in the CDC guidelines in the mid-1990s was the elimination of multiple levels of isolation categories found in previous recommendations and a simplification of isolation precautions based on what is currently known of the modes of transmission of either highly contagious or epidemiologically significant pathogens (Table 4-5). Institution of transmission-based isolation for an ICU patient should occur when infection or carriage of one of these pathogens is either confirmed or suspected. Transmission-based categories of isolation include airborne, droplet, and contact isolation.[52] The transmission-based isolation precautions require that patients be placed in either a private room or be cohorted with patients who have the same infection, if necessary. Transport of the patient out of the room should be limited to procedures that are medically necessary and cannot be performed in the room. When patients must be transported out of the room, the area receiving the patient should be notified of their isolation status, and special precautions (such as a surgical mask being placed on the patient for airborne and droplet precautions) should be taken to minimize infection risk during transport.

Airborne precautions are for agents transmitted by airborne droplet nuclei (generally less than 5 μm in size) or other similarly sized particles. These small particles can remain suspended in the air currents in a room for hours and may be dispersed widely. Examples of pathogens spread in this manner include *Mycobacterium tuberculosis* and rubeola virus. Patients with an infection caused by a pathogen transmitted via airborne particles should be housed in a private room that has negative-pressure ventilation or other special air handling relative to the outside hallway. In addition, susceptible persons who enter the room should wear an N95 respirator or other respiratory equipment capable of filtering small airborne particles; a standard surgical mask is not protective. Negative-pressure systems and other special air handling systems should be tested regularly to ensure that they function properly.

Droplet precautions are for infectious agents that are spread by larger respiratory droplets that can be generated during coughing, sneezing, talking, or performing procedures. These larger droplets do not remain suspended in the air and travel only short distances, usually 1 m or less. Examples of pathogens transmitted primarily via large respiratory droplets include influenza virus and *Neisseria meningitidis*. Patients who are known or suspected to be infected with an agent spread by large respiratory droplets should be placed in a private room, and all individuals should wear a surgical mask (at least) when entering within 1 m of the patient (for practical purposes, most hospitals require a mask when entering the patient's room).

Contact precautions should be employed for agents capable of spread through direct contact with the patient or contact with contaminated environmental surfaces or equipment. This is the most frequently employed transmission-based precaution in the ICU setting, typically used to prevent the spread of antibiotic-resistant bacteria. Contact precautions generally are defined as the use of gloves by all personnel entering the patient's room and the use of a gown when contact with the patient or environmental surfaces is anticipated. The use of dedicated equipment (e.g., stethoscopes, thermometers) is recommended to prevent this equipment from transmitting the infectious agent to others. Equipment should be cleaned and disinfected properly before it is used on other patients. The risk of nosocomial transmission of MRSA in a neonatal ICU was reduced 16-fold by the use of contact precautions.[53] Once the patient on contact precautions is discharged from a room, environmental surfaces must be cleaned thoroughly to eliminate organisms that might persist.

OCCUPATIONAL HEALTH AND THE ICU

Occupational or employee health plays an important role in preventing the spread of highly infectious agents among health care workers. The hospital's occupational health department is responsible for screening employees for contagious diseases and offering employees vaccination for preventable infections related to health care, particularly hepatitis B virus and varicella-zoster virus. In the case of an exposure to an infectious agent from a patient, occupational health's role is to evaluate and, if necessary, treat exposed employees. For particular infectious agents, such as exposure of a nonimmune health care worker to varicella-zoster virus, occupational health has the authority to remove a worker from direct patient care. In smaller hospitals, often a single individual will be responsible for both infection control and occupational health, but most large hospitals have two separate departments. The role of infection control is to determine which health care workers were exposed to a contagious agent and refer exposed workers to occupational health for follow-up.

TABLE 4-5 Isolation Precautions Required for Selected Infections and Conditions

Infection/Condition	Type[a]	Precautions, Duration[b]
Anthrax, cutaneous or pulmonary	S	
Clostridium difficile–associated diarrhea	C	DI
Conjunctivitis, acute viral (acute hemorrhagic)	C	DI
Corona virus (SARS)	D,C	DI
Diphtheria		
Cutaneous	C	CN
Pharyngeal	D	CN
Epiglottitis due to *Hemophilus influenzae*	D	U (24 hrs)
Hepatitis A virus, diapered or incontinent patients	C	F[c]
Herpes simplex virus		
Encephalitis	S	
Mucocutaneous, disseminated or primary, severe	C	DI
Influenza	D	DI
Measles (rubeola), all presentations	A	DI
Meningitis		
Hemophilus influenzae, known or suspected	D	U (24 hrs)
Neisseria meningitidis, known or suspected	D	U (24 hrs)
Other diagnosed bacterial	S	
Meningococcal pneumonia	D	U (24 hrs)
Meningococcemia (meningococcal sepsis)	D	U (24 hrs)
Multi-drug–resistant organisms, infection or colonization		
Gastrointestinal	C	CN
Respiratory	C	CN
Pneumococcal	S	
Skin, wound, or burn	C	CN
Mycoplasma pneumonia	D	DI
Parovirus B19	D	F[d]
Pertussis (whooping cough)	D	U (5 days)
Plague		
Bubonic	S	
Pneumonic	D	U (72 hrs)
Infant and young children	D	U (72 hrs)
Rabies	S	
Respiratory syncytial virus infection, infants, young children, or immunocompromised adults	C	DI
Streptococcal disease (group A streptococcus), skin, wound, or burn		
Major (no dressing or uncontained drainage)	C	U (24 hrs)
Minor or limited (contained drainage)	S	
Tuberculosis		
Extrapulmonary, draining lesion (including scrofula)	S	
Extrapulmonary, meningitis	S	
Pulmonary or laryngeal disease, confirmed or suspected	A	F[e]
Skin-test–positive with no evidence of current pulmonary disease	S	
Varicella-zoster virus[f]		
Varicella (chickenpox)	A,C	F[g]
Zoster		
Localized in immunocompromised patient, disseminated	A,C	F[g]
Localized in normal patient	S	
Wound infections		
Major (no dressing or uncontained drainage)	C	DI
Minor or limited (contained drainage)	S	

SOURCE: Adapted from Garner.[55]

[a] Type of precautions: A = airborne; C = contact; D = droplet; S = standard.

[b] Duration of precautions: CN = until off antibiotics and culture-negative; DI = duration of illness; U = until time specified after initiation of effective therapy; F = see footnote.

[c] Maintain precautions in infants and children younger than 3 years of age for duration of hospitalization; in children 3 to 14 years of age, for 2 weeks after onset of symptoms; for children over 14 years of age, for 1 week after onset of symptoms.

[d] Maintain precautions for duration of hospitalization when chronic disease occurs in an immunodeficient patient. For patients with transient aplastic crisis, maintain precautions for 7 days.

[e] Discontinue precautions *only* when patient is on effective therapy, is improving clinically, and has three consecutive negative sputum smears collected on different days or tuberculosis is ruled out.

[f] Persons susceptible to varicella are at risk of varicella when exposed to patients with herpes zoster lesions or varicella and should not enter the room.

[g] Maintain precautions until all lesions are crusted; see text.

Infection Control Issues Related to Specific Pathogens

SEVERE ACUTE RESPIRATORY SYNDROME (SARS)

The recent experience with the spread of infection related to a corona virus producing a severe form of the acute respiratory distress syndrome (ARDS) with significant morbidity and mortality has highlighted the challenges presented by emerging infectious diseases requiring controlling exposures in the health care environment by rapidly implementing effective infection control measures.[53a–53c] The outbreak of this viral illness in 2003 resulted in infection in more than 8000 people and more than 900 deaths. SARS is predominantly a respiratory illness, spread by large droplets which are inspired, and possibly by the fecal-oral route as well. Important lessons from the experience with outbreaks in Taiwan and Toronto include early identification of the epidemic, institution of strict isolation and control measures, careful screening of health care workers and others exposed to active cases, quarantine of individuals early in the course of the epidemic, and limitation of exposures to high risk interventions in the intensive care unit such as intubations or other airway manipulations. Effective responses to outbreaks such as this, which are predicted to increase in our complex and interconnected world, can only be achieved by a high degree of integration of critical care clinicians, infection control staff, and public health officials. Anticipating such problems and working to solutions in advance is a better approach than attempting to implement solutions ad hoc.

BLOOD-BORNE PATHOGENS: HIV, HEPATITIS C VIRUS, AND HEPATITIS B VIRUS

Because of the need for frequent invasive procedures, the often-urgent nature of these procedures, and the patient population that is served, critical care personnel are at risk of exposure and infection with blood-borne pathogens. The most common mechanism by which ICU personnel are exposed is by a percutaneous injury, usually an inadvertent needle stick. The risk of infection after a percutaneous exposure varies significantly depending on the virus. The risk of infection with HIV after a percutaneous exposure to infected blood or bloody fluids has been estimated to be 0.3%. The risks associated with occupational mucous membrane and cutaneous exposures to HIV-infected blood appear to be substantially smaller. For hepatitis C virus, the risk of infection after percutaneous exposure is between 0% and 7%, and for hepatitis B virus, the risk of developing serologic evidence of infection in a nonimmune person is 23% to 62%, depending on whether the source patient is positive for the hepatitis B e antigen.[54]

Infection control efforts against these viruses focus primarily on preventing exposure to blood and, in the case of hepatitis B virus, offering vaccination on employment. Practices that minimize the risk of percutaneous injury (e.g., discarding disposable sharp devices in puncture-resistant containers immediately after use) are key aspects of prevention. Precautions also should be applied to other body fluids containing visible blood and to cerebrospinal, synovial, pleural, peritoneal, pericardial, and amniotic fluids and vaginal secretions and semen.[55] Protective equipment (i.e., gloves, gowns, masks, and eyewear) should be used when there is a potential for exposure to these fluids. Following an exposure, the affected skin should be cleaned immediately with soap and water, and mucous membranes should be rinsed with copious amounts of water. Zidovudine chemoprophylaxis following needlestick exposure to HIV-1 decreases transmission risk by 80%.[56] Current guidelines recommend 4 weeks of combination antiretroviral therapy with either a two- or three-drug regimen for postexposure prophylaxis, taking into consideration degree of exposure, level of viremia in the source patient, and the potential for resistant virus. For hepatitis C virus, no prophylaxis is currently available; exposed workers generally are monitored for 6 months for evidence of infection. For hepatitis B virus exposure, the immune status of the employee should be determined, and hepatitis B immunoglobulin and vaccination should be offered to nonimmune employees.

VARICELLA-ZOSTER VIRUS

Patients with evidence of disseminated varicella-zoster virus (VZV) infection (e.g., chickenpox, varicella pneumonia, disseminated zoster) or immunocompromised patients with localized zoster are capable of transmitting VZV via respiratory droplets and shedding virus from noncrusted skin lesions. These patients should be placed on airborne precautions with negative-pressure ventilation and contact precautions until all skin lesions are crusted. Immunocompetent hosts with localized zoster can be cared for using standard precautions. Health care workers without a history of chickenpox or documented evidence of immunity should not enter the room of a patient with an active VZV infection. If a potentially nonimmune health care worker or patient is exposed, VZV serology should be obtained on that individual. Seronegative personnel should be removed from direct patient contact between 10 to 21 days after the exposure occurred. Likewise, if a seronegative patient is exposed to a patient with VZV infection, he or she should be placed in the appropriate precautions between 10 and 21 days after the exposure. The use of VZV vaccine and varicella-zoster immunoglobulin should be considered in both nonimmune exposed ICU patients and personnel when not contraindicated.

TUBERCULOSIS

Tuberculosis is frequently unsuspected in hospitalized patients, including those admitted to ICUs. This failure of diagnosis has emerged as an important contributor to mortality[57] and also may increase the risk of transmission to hospital personnel. ICU personnel who perform procedures that generate respiratory aerosols (e.g., endotracheal intubation, fiberoptic bronchoscopy, and ventilator management) may be at particular risk for acquisition of tuberculosis. It should be noted that a negative acid-fast smear does not eliminate the possibility of transmission to medical personnel. ICU physicians must maintain a high level of suspicion for tuberculosis and initiate airborne precautions whenever the diagnosis is considered. Health care workers must wear National Institute of Occupational Safety and Health (NIOSH)–approved 95% (N95) particulate respirator masks or high-efficiency particulate air (HEPA)–filtered respirator masks when caring for patients with known or suspected tuberculosis.[58] In addition, all ICU personnel should undergo tuberculin skin testing on hire and at regular intervals.

RESPIRATORY SYNCYTIAL VIRUS

Respiratory syncytial virus (RSV) is a leading cause of bronchiolitis and pneumonia in infants and small children and is a frequent cause of nosocomial outbreaks of lower respiratory tract infections in pediatric wards. While RSV has been long recognized as a cause of seasonal infection in children, transmission has been reported in adult patients, with significant morbidity and mortality in immunocompromised hosts.[59] The primary mode of transmission of RSV is inoculation of the eyes and nasal mucosa by the hands after handling objects or touching surfaces contaminated by respiratory secretions. Infants have been shown to shed high titers of RSV in respiratory secretions for up to several weeks, and the virus is stable in the environment for up to 24 hours. Health care workers in pediatric wards have been infected themselves and have transmitted the virus to other patients via contaminated hands or equipment. Infection control measures for RSV include placing infected young children, infants, and immunocompromised adults on contact precautions. Personnel with respiratory illnesses during RSV outbreaks should not care for children and immunocompromised adults at risk for severe RSV infection.[60]

MENINGOCOCCUS

Patients with meningitis and bacteremia caused by *N. meningitidis* frequently require admission to the ICU for circulatory collapse and airway management. Often the diagnosis is suspected but not confirmed until the organism is isolated in culture. Patients with known or suspected meningococcal infection should be handled using droplet precautions because this organism typically is carried in the nasopharynx and spread by large respiratory droplets. Personnel should wear a surgical mask when caring for infected patients and either goggles or a face shield when performing procedures capable of generating droplets. Precautions can be discontinued after the patient has been on effective antibiotic therapy for at least 24 hours.

The admission of a patient with suspected or known meningococcal disease can generate a significant amount of anxiety among personnel. Cases of meningococcal nosocomial infection in health care workers have been associated with close contact with respiratory secretions without the use of precautions.[61] However, transmission resulting in disease in health care workers is rare, and the risk of transmission from casual contact with a patient is likely negligible. The incubation period for meningococcal disease after exposure can range between 2 to 10 days but is commonly 3 to 4 days; therefore, whether antibiotic prophylaxis is warranted does not need to be determined emergently. Infection control and occupational health staff should evaluate all potential employee exposures, educate staff on the risk of infection, and determine if antibiotic prophylaxis is needed on a case-by-case basis.

References

1. Public health focus: Surveillance, prevention, and control of nosocomial infections. *MMWR* 41:783, 1992.
2. *Consumer Price Index for Medical Care.* United States Department of Labor, Bureau of Labor Statistics; accessed on November 9, 2001 at *http://data.bls.gov/cgi-bin/dsrv?cu.*
3. Bryan-Brown CW: Pathway to the present: A personal view of critical care, in Civetta JM, Taylor RW, Kirby RR (eds): *Critical care,* 2nd ed. Philadelphia, Lippincott Williams & Wilkins, 1992, p 5.
4. Craven DE, Kunches LM, Lichtenberg DA, et al: Nosocomial infection and fatality in medical and surgical intensive care unit patients. *Arch Intern Med* 148:1161, 1988.
5. National Nosocomial Infections Surveillance (NNIS) System report: Data summary from January 1992 to June 2002, issued August 2002. *Am J Infect Control* 30:458, 2002.
6. Renaud B, Brun-Buisson C: Outcomes of primary and catheter-related bacteremia: A cohort and case-control study in critically ill patients. *Am J Respir Crit Care Med* 163:1584, 2001.
7. Keita-Perse O, Gaynes RP: Severity of illness scoring systems to adjust nosocomial infection rates: A review and commentary. *Am J Infect Control* 24:429, 1996.
8. Haley RW, Culver DH, White JW, et al: The efficacy of infection surveillance and control programs in preventing nosocomial infections in US hospitals. *Am J Epidemiol* 121:182, 1985.
9. Garner JS, Jarvis WR, Emori TG, et al: CDC definitions for nosocomial infections, in Olmsted RN (ed): *APIC Infection Control and Applied Epidemiology: Principles and Practice.* St. Louis, Mobsy, 1996, p A1.
10. Kahn MG, Steib SA, Dunagan WC, et al: Monitoring expert system performance using continuous user feedback. *J Am Med Inform Assoc* 3:216, 1996.
11. Mulin B, Rouget C, Clement C, et al: Association of private isolation rooms with ventilator-associated *Acinetobacter baumanii* pneumonia in a surgical intensive-care unit. *Infect Control Hosp Epidemiol* 18:499, 1997.
12. Ben Abraham R, Keller N, Szold O, et al: Do isolation rooms reduce the rate of nosocomial infections in the pediatric intensive care unit? *J Crit Care* 17:176, 2002.
13. Archibald LK, Manning ML, Bell LM, et al: Patient density, nurse-to-patient ratio and nosocomial infection risk in a pediatric cardiac intensive care unit. *Pediatr Infect Dis J* 16:1045, 1997.
14. Dang D, Johantgen ME, Pronovost PJ, et al: Postoperative complications: Does intensive care unit staff nursing make a difference? *Heart Lung* 31:219, 2002.
15. Mermel LA: Prevention of intravascular catheter-related infections. *Ann Intern Med* 132:391, 2000 (erratum in *Ann Intern Med* 133:5, 2000).
16. Raad II, Hohn DC, Gilbreath BJ, et al: Prevention of central venous catheter-related infections by using maximal sterile barrier precautions during insertion. *Infect Control Hosp Epidemiol* 15:231, 1994.
17. Merrer J, De Jonghe B, Golliot F, et al: Complications of femoral and subclavian venous catheterization in critically ill patients: A randomized, controlled trial. *JAMA* 286:700, 2001.
18. Sherertz RJ, Ely EW, Westbrook DM, et al: Education of physicians-in-training can decrease the risk for vascular catheter infection. *Ann Intern Med* 132:641, 2000.
19. Coopersmith CM, Rebmann TL, Zack JE, et al: Effect of an education program on decreasing catheter-related bloodstream infections in the surgical intensive care unit. *Crit Care Med* 30:59, 2002.
20. Veenstra DL, Saint S, Saha S, et al: Efficacy of antiseptic-impregnated central venous catheters in preventing catheter-related bloodstream infection: A meta-analysis. *JAMA* 281:261, 1999.
21. Crnich CJ, Maki DG: The promise of novel technology for the prevention of intravascular device-related bloodstream infection: I. Pathogenesis and short-term devices. *Clin Infect Dis* 34:1232, 2002.
22. Beck-Sague CM, Jarvis WR: Epidemic bloodstream infections associated with pressure transducers: A persistent problem. *Infect Control Hosp Epidemiol* 10:54, 1989.

23. Richards MJ, Edwards JR, Culver DH, et al: Nosocomial infections in medical intensive care units in the United States. National Nosocomial Infections Surveillance System. *Crit Care Med* 27:887, 1999.

24. Saint S: Clinical and economic consequences of nosocomial catheter-related bacteriuria. *Am J Infect Control* 28:68, 2000.

25. Laupland KB, Zygun DA, Davies HD, et al: Incidence and risk factors for acquiring nosocomial urinary tract infection in the critically ill. *J Crit Care* 17:50, 2002.

25a. Bonten JM, Kollef MH, Hall JB: Risk factors for ventilator-associated pneumonia: From epidemiology to patient management. *Clin Inf Dis* 38:1141, 2004.

26. Craven DE, Lichtenberg DA, Goularte TA, et al: Contaminated medication nebulizers in mechanical ventilator circuits: Source of bacterial aerosols. *Am J Med* 77:834, 1984.

27. Mastro TD, Fields BS, Breiman RF, et al: Nosocomial Legionnaires' disease and use of medication nebulizers. *J Infect Dis* 163:667, 1991.

28. Srinivasan A, Wolfenden LL, Song X, et al: An outbreak of *Pseudomonas aeruginosa* infections associated with flexible bronchoscopes. *N Engl J Med* 348:221, 2003.

29. Antonelli M, Conti G, Rocco M, et al: A comparison of noninvasive positive-pressure ventilation and conventional mechanical ventilation in patients with acute respiratory failure. *N Engl J Med* 339:429, 1998.

30. Smulders K, van der HH, Weers-Pothoff I, et al: A randomized clinical trial of intermittent subglottic secretion drainage in patients receiving mechanical ventilation. *Chest* 121:858, 2002.

31. George DL, Falk PS, Umberto MG, et al: Nosocomial sinusitis in patients in the medical intensive care unit: A prospective epidemiological study. *Clin Infect Dis* 27:463, 1998.

32. Salord F, Gaussorgues P, Marti-Flich J, et al: Nosocomial maxillary sinusitis during mechanical ventilation: A prospective comparison of orotracheal versus the nasotracheal route for intubation. *Intensive Care Med* 16:390, 1990.

33. Aucoin PJ, Kotilainen HR, Gantz NM, et al: Intracranial pressure monitors: Epidemiologic study of risk factors and infections. *Am J Med* 80:369, 1986.

34. Rebuck JA, Murry KR, Rhoney DH, et al: Infection related to intracranial pressure monitors in adults: Analysis of risk factors and antibiotic prophylaxis. *J Neurol Neurosurg Psychiatry* 69:381, 2000.

35. Mayhall CG, Archer NH, Lamb VA, et al: Ventriculostomy-related infections: A prospective epidemiologic study. *N Engl J Med* 310:553, 1984.

36. Clark WC, Muhlbauer MS, Lowrey R, et al: Complications of intracranial pressure monitoring in trauma patients. *Neurosurgery* 25:20, 1989.

37. Taylor ME, Oppenheim BA: Selective decontamination of the gastrointestinal tract as an infection control measure. *J Hosp Infect* 17:271, 1991.

38. van Nieuwenhoven CA, Buskens E, van Tiel FH, et al: Relationship between methodological trial quality and the effects of selective digestive decontamination on pneumonia and mortality in critically ill patients. *JAMA* 286:335, 2001.

39. Zwaveling JH, Maring JK, Klompmaker IJ, et al: Selective decontamination of the digestive tract to prevent postoperative infection: A randomized, placebo-controlled trial in liver transplant patients. *Crit Care Med* 30:1204, 2002.

40. Brun-Buisson C, Legrand P, Rauss A, et al: Intestinal decontamination for control of nosocomial multiresistant gram-negative bacilli: Study of an outbreak in an intensive care unit. *Ann Intern Med* 110:873, 1989.

41. Boyce JM, Potter-Bynoe G, Chenevert C, et al: Environmental contamination due to methicillin-resistant *Staphylococcus aureus*: Possible infection control implications. *Infect Control Hosp Epidemiol* 18:622, 1997.

42. Gerner-Smidt P: Endemic occurrence of *Acinetobacter calcoaceticus biovar anitratus* in an intensive care unit. *J Hosp Infect* 10:265, 1987.

43. Coello R, Jimenez J, Garcia M, et al: Prospective study of infection, colonization and carriage of methicillin-resistant *Staphylococcus aureus* in an outbreak affecting 990 patients. *Eur J Clin Microbiol Infect Dis* 13:74, 1994.

44. Chaix C, Durand-Zaleski I, Alberti C, et al: Control of endemic methicillin-resistant *Staphylococcus aureus*: A cost-benefit analysis in an intensive care unit. *JAMA* 282:1745, 1999.

45. Singh N, Rogers P, Atwood CW, et al: Short-course empiric antibiotic therapy for patients with pulmonary infiltrates in the intensive care unit: A proposed solution for indiscriminate antibiotic prescription. *Am J Respir Crit Care Med* 162:505, 2000.

46. Raymond DP, Pelletier SJ, Crabtree TD, et al: Impact of a rotating empiric antibiotic schedule on infectious mortality in an intensive care unit. *Crit Care Med* 29:1101, 2001.

47. Evans RS, Pestotnik SL, Classen DC, et al: A computer-assisted management program for antibiotics and other anti-infective agents. *N Engl J Med* 338:232, 1998.

48. Simmons B, Bryant J, Neiman K, et al: The role of handwashing in prevention of endemic intensive care unit infections. *Infect Control Hosp Epidemiol* 11:589, 1990.

49. Zimakoff J, Stormark M, Larsen SO: Use of gloves and handwashing behaviour among health care workers in intensive care units: A multicentre investigation in four hospitals in Denmark and Norway. *J Hosp Infect* 24:63, 1993.

50. Harbarth S, Sudre P, Dharan S, et al: Outbreak of *Enterobacter cloacae* related to understaffing, overcrowding, and poor hygiene practices. *Infect Control Hosp Epidemiol* 20:598, 1999.

51. Hugonnet S, Perneger TV, Pittet D: Alcohol-based handrub improves compliance with hand hygiene in intensive care units. *Arch Intern Med* 162:1037, 2002.

52. Garner JS. Guideline for isolation precautions in hospitals. The Hospital Infection Control Practices Advisory Committee *Infect Control Hosp Epidemiol* 17:53, 1996 (published erratum appears in *Infect Control Hosp Epidemiol* 17:214, 1996).

53. Jernigan JA, Titus MG, Groschel DH, et al: Effectiveness of contact isolation during a hospital outbreak of methicillin-resistant *Staphylococcus aureus*. *Am J Epidemiol* 143:496, 1996.

53a. Svoboda T, Henry B, Shulman L, et al: Public health measures to control the spread of Severe Acute Respiratory Syndrome during the outbreak in Toronto. *N Engl J Med* 350:2352, 2004.

53b. Weinstein RL: Planning for epidemics—the lessons of SARS. *N Engl J Med* 350:2332, 2004.

53c. Lapinsky SE, Granton JT: Critical care lessons from severe acute respiratory syndrome. *Clin Opin Crit Care* 10:53, 2004.

54. Werner BG, Grady GF: Accidental hepatitis-B-surface-antigen-positive inoculations: Use of e antigen to estimate infectivity. *Ann Intern Med* 97:367, 1982.

55. Garner JS: Guideline for isolation precautions in hospitals. The Hospital Infection Control Practices Advisory Committee. *Infect Control Hosp Epidemiol* 17:53, 1996.

56. Case-control study of HIV seroconversion in health-care workers after percutaneous exposure to HIV-infected blood—France, United Kingdom, and United States, January 1988–August 1994. *MMWR* 44:929, 1995.

57. Greenway C, Menzies D, Fanning A, et al: Delay in diagnosis among hospitalized patients with active tuberculosis—predictors and outcomes. *Am J Respir Crit Care Med* 165:927, 2002.

58. Guidelines for preventing the transmission of *Mycobacterium tuberculosis* in health-care facilities, 1994. Centers for Disease Control and Prevention. *MMWR Recomm Rep* 43:1, 1994.

59. Takimoto CH, Cram DL, Root RK: Respiratory syncytial virus infections on an adult medical ward. *Arch Intern Med* 151:706, 1991.

60. Garcia R, Raad I, Abi-Said D, et al: Nosocomial respiratory syncytial virus infections: Prevention and control in bone marrow transplant patients. *Infect Control Hosp Epidemiol* 18:412, 1997.

61. Gehanno JF, Kohen-Couderc L, Lemeland JF, et al: Nosocomial meningococcemia in a physician. *Infect Control Hosp Epidemiol* 20:564, 1999.

62. O'Grady NP, Alexander M, Dellinger EP, et al: Guidelines for the prevention of intravascular catheter-related infections. *Infect Control Hosp Epidemiol* 23:759, 2002.

63. Wong ES: Guideline for prevention of catheter-associated urinary tract infections. *Am J Infect Control* 11:28, 1983.

64. Tablan OC, Anderson W, Besser R, et al: Guidelines for preventing health-care–associated pneumonia, 2003: Recommendations of the CDC and the Healthcare Infection Control Practices Advisory Committee. *MMWR Recomm Rep* 53:1, 2004.

65. Safdar N, Maki DG: The commonality of risk factors for nosocomial colonization and infection with antimicrobial-resistant *Staphylococcus aureus*, enterococcus, gram-negative bacilli, *Clostridium difficile*, and *Candida*. *Ann Intern Med* 136:834, 2002.

Chapter 5

LEGAL ISSUES IN CRITICAL CARE

MARSHALL B. KAPP

KEY POINTS

- *In order to be considered legally effective, consent to medical treatment must meet three tests: (1) it must be voluntary; (2) it must be adequately informed or knowing; and (3) it is given by an individual with adequate mental capacity and legal authority.*

- *Whereas a variety of state laws in the United States pertain to decisional capacity and surrogate decision making, in most cases the physician relies on family members as the surrogate decision makers for an incapacitated patient, even in the absence of a specific statute, advance directive, or court order empowering the family.*

- *An increasing percentage of patients, especially as the population ages, lack available, willing relatives or friends to act as surrogate decision makers. In such cases physicians should seek guidance from living wills or other forms of advance directives, when these exist.*

- *Neither a patient nor his or her family has a legal right to, nor does the physician have the obligation to provide, medical treatment that would be futile—that is, nonbeneficial—for that patient.*

- *As directors of critical care units, critical care physicians should participate in creating institutional protocols that delineate operational principles of the critical care team and the individual physician's supervisory responsibilities.*

The making, implementation, and documentation of treatment decisions in the practice of critical care medicine raise a host of potential legal implications. This chapter briefly outlines some of the more salient issues and suggests avenues for their management and further exploration. Figure 5-1 depicts these issues as they arise within and impact upon the physician–patient relationship in ICUs.

It must be noted that what is described here are the evolving legal ramifications particular to critical care practice in the United States. For comparison, in critical care as practiced outside the United States, legal issues may impact much less on day-to-day decision making. It may be argued that the U.S. approach encourages greater sensitivity to and protection of the rights of patients. In contrast, the legal systems of many other countries, explicitly or by default, have elevated the role of the critical care physician as unquestioned advocate for the critically ill patient. A tangible outcome of this difference is that intensivists in the United States usually are more cautious in giving medical advice—especially advice with difficult ethical connotations—to their patients or surrogates compared to Australasian, European, or even Canadian intensivists, all of whom assume a more commanding presence at the physician–patient interface regarding critical

care decision making. It is not uncommon to encounter U.S. critical care decision making suspended, awaiting the input of family or an institutional ethics committee that has yet to be apprised of the patient's condition or need for a decision; in contrast, quite similar situations are decided autocratically by the attending intensivist in other countries. Because critical care is evolving rapidly throughout the world, the contributions of the legal system—positive and negative—to health care and to society as a whole are not yet clear. It is clear, however, that legal issues become less dominating and intrusive, and ethical concerns become more central, when intensivists and their critical care teams initiate and continue sensitive, complete, consistent, and honest communication with their critically ill patients and significant others.

Informed Consent[1]

The well-established legal doctrine of informed consent is based on the ethical principles of autonomy (personal self-determination) and beneficence (doing good for the patient).[2] Early lawsuits growing out of medical interventions conducted in the absence of informed consent were predicated on a battery theory (i.e., touching the person without their consent). But most such cases today are framed as negligence actions, in which the alleged unintentional wrong is the physician's violation of the fiduciary or trust duty to inform the patient adequately as part of the permission process.

In order to be considered legally effective, consent to medical treatment must meet three tests (in the absence of an exception such as an unforeseeable emergency). First, consent must be voluntary—that is, not coerced—in nature. The patient (or surrogate decision maker) must retain the ultimate power to accept or reject the available interventions.

Second, consent must be adequately informed or knowing. A slight majority of U.S. jurisdictions still enforce a physician-oriented standard of information disclosure, inquiring whether the amount of information shared by the physician with the patient or surrogate was consistent with the usual practice of other prudent, competent physicians in similar circumstances. Almost half the states, however, have adopted a more patient-oriented standard, requiring physicians to disclose all the information that a reasonable patient would want to know under the circumstances. This latter approach is also termed the *materiality standard,* since it compels the disclosure of information that would be material—that is, information that might affect the decision making—for a reasonable patient.

Under either a physician- or patient-oriented approach, several particular kinds of information need to be disclosed in understandable lay language. These include: the nature of the patient's medical problem; prognosis with and without treatment; nature of the suggested intervention; likely benefits of treatment; reasonable alternatives; and foreseeable risks of the various alternatives. Additionally, many people today are interested in knowing the probable financial ramifications of their medical decisions.

Third, informed consent is sufficient only when it is given by an individual with adequate mental capacity and

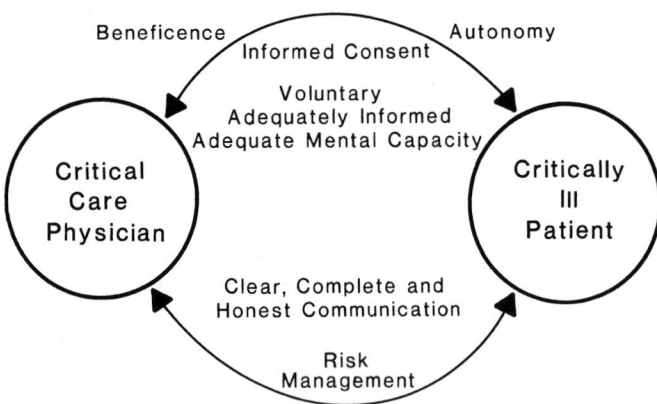

FIGURE 5-1 Outline of legal issues in critical care. The communication and interaction between critical care physician and critically ill patient involves areas (e.g., informed consent and risk management) with legal issues and precedents.

legal authority. This element of consent may be especially problematic in critical care and is discussed in the next section.

A note of caution regarding the legal value of written consent forms must be added here. Contrary to the usual mistake that health care providers make of treating the two things as synonymous, a written consent form is not the equivalent of legally effective informed consent. Informed consent is the process of mutual communication and ultimate patient or surrogate choice[3] as described earlier. The written form is only tangible documentation or evidence that the communication process occurred. This evidence may be very important to the physician in defending against a lawsuit claiming medical intervention in the absence of informed consent, by creating a legal presumption that consent was properly obtained. However, where inadequate communication actually took place, the presumption created by the consent form may be successfully rebutted or overcome by the plaintiff. While broad, blanket consent forms used in many hospitals are sufficient to authorize routine noninvasive medical treatments, more specifically tailored and informative forms are preferable for interventions that are nonroutine or invasive, and certainly for treatments that might be characterized as experimental or innovative.[4] One recent study[4a] of informed consent in critically ill patients suggested that early identification of patients at risk for needing invasive procedures facilitates an earlier discussion of risk-benefit relationships, fewer procedures performed as "emergent," and a possible reduction in surrogate consent.

Application of these general principles is somewhat complicated in critical care by the fact that in the ICU, interventions can be nearly continuous for the most unstable patients. Informed consent is necessary any time the doctor proposes doing anything to a patient (i.e., any "intervention"). For quasi-continuous interventions, informed consent must certainly be obtained at the initiation of the intervention, and the patient or surrogate must be afforded the opportunity to withdraw that consent at any later point.

Most interventions in critical care may be categorized as risky or invasive, that is, an intervention involving a higher degree of risk or intrusion for the patient than he or she would ordinarily face in normal, everyday life. However, this categorization is relevant only to the question of the extent of advisable documentation; the requirement of an informed consent process itself applies regardless of an intervention's level of risk or invasiveness.

Decisional Capacity and Surrogate Decision Making

Minor children (defined in almost every state for medical purposes as those younger than 18 years old) are presumed legally to be incapable of making their own medical decisions, and in the absence of an exception based on the minor's "emancipated" or "mature" status, the natural parent or court-appointed guardian is legally empowered as the medical decision maker. Adults, however, are presumed legally to be decisionally capable.[5] In critical care, many (although certainly not all) patients will be so ill and debilitated that they are not presently capable of making and expressing treatment choices resulting from a rational thought process of digesting and weighing information about the benefits and risks of different alternatives.[6]

Although in theory the same degree of mental capacity is necessary whether the patient is accepting or declining the recommended medical intervention, in practice, a formal inquiry into patient capacity usually occurs only in the case of patient refusal. Ideally, a judgment about patient decisional capacity, which may fluctuate widely over time because of a variety of natural and iatrogenic factors, is being made at least implicitly by the attending physician each time the patient is seen. Such an inquiry ought to be inherently built into every physician–patient encounter. Where decisional capacity is seriously questioned, a more focused examination needs to be conducted. In especially ambiguous cases, documentation in the patient's medical record by consultants who have evaluated the patient's decisional capacity is good risk management for the physician proposing an intervention, who is the one ultimately responsible for ensuring informed consent; the legal system affords psychiatrists a great deal (arguably an excessive amount) of deference as consultant capacity assessors.

For patients who in fact lack the ability to engage in a rational decision making process, the presumption of capacity is rebutted or overcome. This does not, however, mean that the physician may dispense with informed consent prior to initiating particular interventions. Consent remains necessary for treatment of incapacitated patients, but the consent must be obtained from a surrogate or proxy acting on the patient's behalf. Several approaches to surrogate medical decision making have developed.

Over half the states in the past three decades have enacted "family consent statutes," which specify relatives (ordinarily in a priority order) who may legally make medical decisions for an incapacitated family member.[7] Advance proxy directives (see next section), especially the durable power of attorney, may be used by currently capable persons to designate their own surrogates in the event of subsequent incapacity. A formal guardianship or conservatorship (precise terminology varies among jurisdictions) proceeding may be initiated, in which a probate court finds the patient (the ward) to be decisionally incapacitated (the legal term usually employed is *incompetent*) and appoints someone else (the guardian or conservator of the person) as the surrogate decision maker.

In most cases, however, the physician relies on family members as the surrogate decision makers for an incapacitated patient, even in the absence of a specific statute, advance directive, or court order empowering the family. This informal process of making do using next of kin, even without explicit legal authority, works well in the vast majority of situations in which the family members agree on a course of conduct both among themselves and with the physician, and where they appear to act consistently with the patient's values and preferences (the "substituted judgment" standard) or with the patient's best interests.

Decisions to Limit Treatment[8,9]

Some patients retain a sufficient degree of capacity to make and express their own medical decisions even after admission to a critical care unit (CCU). Legal precedent is very clear that, except in cases in which the welfare of a third party such as a minor dependent is jeopardized, a properly informed, capable patient has the right to make personal medical decisions, including a decision to refuse even life-prolonging treatment.

If the patient is decisionally incapacitated, a more difficult scenario may confront the physician. A surrogate decision maker may be identified (see previous section) under a state family consent statute, the patient's prior execution of a durable power of attorney (see Appendix 1 for a model) naming a surrogate or health care agent, a court appointment of a guardian/conservator, or informally relying on available, willing family members.

The surrogate is legally expected in most states to make decisions consistent with what the patient would choose if he or she were presently able to make and express choices personally (substituted judgment standard, or "donning the mental mantle" of the incapacitated person). If there is no reliable indication (some states, e.g., Missouri[10] and New York,[11] require proof by "clear and convincing evidence") of the patient's preference under the circumstances, the surrogate must act in the patient's best interests, considering—from the patient's perspective—the proportionality of likely benefits and burdens associated with available medical alternatives.

An increasing percentage of patients, especially as the population ages, lack available, willing relatives or friends to act as surrogate decision makers.[12] In such cases, there are several potential sources of guidance for the physician.

The patient may have executed a living will document while still decisionally capable. This type of advance directive, which is authorized by statute (frequently called a natural death act) in almost every jurisdiction, permits a capable adult to make a record of personal preferences regarding future medical treatment in the event of subsequent incapacity and critical illness (see Appendix 2 for a model). Although usually this directive is used to indicate a preference for the limitation of future medical intervention, the directive could be employed to request maximum medical intervention if there is any likelihood of benefit to the patient. However, neither a patient nor his or her family have a legal right to, nor does a physician have the obligation to provide, medical treatment that would be futile—that is, nonbeneficial—for that patient.[13,14]

A physician who complies in good faith with the patient's expressed voluntary, informed wishes to limit life-prolonging treatment is on firm legal ground.[15] For the physician who for ethical reasons chooses not to follow a living will's directive to limit treatment, there is an ethical and legal obligation to notify the patient or surrogate (if one is present), and to make a reasonable attempt to transfer the patient to another physician who is willing to comply with the living will, or at least not to prevent such a transfer.

In many states, a public guardianship system has been created to make surrogate decision makers available, either through a government agency or through a private agency under government contract, for incapacitated patients who lack available, willing relatives or friends.[16] There are also demonstration projects in some locales that use privately funded agencies to act as surrogate medical decision makers for incapacitated patients.[17] The physician should consult hospital legal counsel to determine acceptable sources of surrogate decision making for the incapacitated patient without relatives or friends.

The most controversial and complicated issue in the treatment limitation arena is the status of artificial feeding and hydration.[18] The courts have been unanimous in holding that feeding tubes are merely another form of medical intervention, which could be withheld or withdrawn under the same circumstances that would apply to the withholding or withdrawal of any other type of medical intervention.[19] The American Medical Association[20] and other groups[21] endorse this analysis. However, some argue that feeding and hydration, even where accomplished through tubes surgically or forcibly inserted in the patient's body, are fundamentally different and more elemental than medical treatment, and therefore ought to be continued as long as they can keep the patient alive.[22] A number of state legislatures have embodied this argument in living will or durable power of attorney statutes that purport to severely restrict the ability of surrogate decision makers to authorize the removal of feeding tubes. Both the wisdom and the constitutionality of these purported restrictions are extremely questionable.[23,24]

The case of Nancy Cruzan remains the only case decided by the U.S. Supreme Court, on June 25, 1990, that sheds light on the issue of discontinuing life-prolonging treatment. Cruzan was an automobile accident victim who was kept alive in a permanent vegetative state within a state-operated (Missouri) long-term care facility, through the use of feeding and hydration tubes. Her parents asked that this intervention be discontinued, a request they claimed was consistent with the patient's previously expressed (although not documented) wishes. The physicians refused this request, and the Missouri Supreme Court upheld the lower court decision and refused the parents' request to discontinue treatment.

The U.S. Supreme Court held that a mentally capable person has a fundamental constitutional right, under the liberty provision of the Fourteenth Amendment's due process clause, to make personal medical decisions, even regarding life-prolonging treatments, including artificial feeding and hydration. For incompetent patients, though, the court ruled that a state's interest in preserving life was strong enough to permit a state, if the state so chooses, to require "clear and convincing" evidence of the treatment preference the patient would hold if currently able to make and express an autonomous choice, before the state must comply with a surrogate's instructions to withdraw life-prolonging medical care. Presumably, a written declaration made while the patient was competent would suffice as evidence of treatment preference in the event of subsequent incapacity. Under the Cruzan decision, states are also free to set lower standards of proof than "clear and convincing" evidence for incapacitated patients, such as proof by a preponderance of the evidence (i.e., greater than 51% likelihood). In the Cruzan case itself, Missouri by statute imposed the "clear and convincing" evidentiary standard, and since Cruzan had never clearly documented her treatment wishes while still competent, the proof was inconclusive, and the state was permitted to err on the side of continued treatment.

One form of treatment limitation around which there is a high degree of current consensus is the do-not-resuscitate (DNR) or no code order, which instructs caregivers to refrain from initiating cardiopulmonary resuscitation (CPR) for a patient who suffers an anticipated cardiac arrest. There have been very few legal cases in this arena, but the well-accepted rule is that a decisionally capable patient has the right to refuse CPR, and that surrogates may elect to forego CPR for a patient if the likely burdens of this intervention to the patient would be disproportionate to any benefits (e.g., mere continued existence until the next arrest) that might be derived.[25] As is true for all medical decisions, a DNR order should be made only after a thorough consultation with the patient or surrogates and should be clearly documented in the medical record.

Where the patient or surrogate has declined aggressive, technologically oriented interventions, the physician still retains the legal obligation to continue basic palliative (comfort and pain control) and hygiene measures. Failure to do so could constitute negligence or form the basis for professional disciplinary action.[26]

The other side of the coin on treatment decision making is presented when the patient, or more usually the family, insists on initiation or continuation of medical treatment ("doing everything possible") that the clinician judges to be futile in terms of benefit to the patient.[27] On the very rare occasions that courts have been involved prospectively with the futility issue, their holdings have been confusing, inconsistent, and often poorly reasoned.[28] No court has ever imposed liability for failure to begin or perpetuate futile interventions for a critically ill patient, even in the face of family insistence on doing everything possible. In practice, clinicians usually seem to take the path of least resistance in such circumstances and "treat the family," often out of misapprehension of potential liability exposure. In the vast majority of cases, better physician–family communication, in which the realistic implications of "doing everything possible" are spelled out clearly, can obviate serious disagreement over how to proceed.[29]

Institutional Protocols and Institutional Ethics Committees

Most hospitals have adopted written policies and procedures concerning patient admission to, retention in, and discharge from CCUs. The ability of physicians to consult institutional guidelines generally leads to better, more consistent decisions that are easier to defend against later claims of impropriety.[30] Clear protocols facilitate communication and cooperation among members of the health care team, decreasing both inadvertent mistakes and interpersonal tension. Institutional protocols are also essential as inevitable discussions of health care rationing take on increasing urgency.[31]

The development and dissemination of institutional protocols regarding critical care, especially DNR orders, is required by the federal Patient Self-Determination Act (PSDA)[32] and by some states.[33] It is also required for approval by the Joint Commission on Accreditation of Healthcare Organizations (JCAHO).[34]

Critical care physicians must be completely familiar with their own institutions' formal policies and procedures, and must assure familiarity with them on the part of nurses and other staff members. Ideally, members of the medical staff should contribute to the drafting, continuing re-evaluation, and revision of institutional protocols.[35] Questions regarding the meaning or implementation of these protocols should be addressed in a timely fashion (i.e., before a crisis erupts) to hospital legal counsel.

Similarly, the physician must be knowledgeable about the operation of his or her hospital's institutional ethics committee (IEC). The past three decades have seen a proliferation within health care institutions of entities designed to provide education, formulate policies and procedures, and offer advice regarding particular cases and issues with serious bioethical implications.[36] JCAHO standards require that hospitals have in place a mechanism for carrying out these functions.[37] Although the emphasis of IECs is, and ought to be, on better ethical decision making, salutary legal by-products may also result from their activities. Effective use of an IEC may preclude resorting to the judicial system, initiated either by the family or by a health care team member who feels his or her opinion has been inadequately taken into account, for definitive resolution of a case. Furthermore, in the relatively unlikely event of the informal decision making process breaking down and court involvement being invoked, utilization of an IEC may act as powerful evidence of the provider's good faith and appropriate concern for patient autonomy and welfare.[38]

Determinations of Death

One inescapable aspect of critical care medicine with important legal implications is the determination and declaration of when a patient has died. Traditional standards of death based on cessation of cardiorespiratory functioning are no longer sufficient by themselves in light of modern medical technology that frequently can maintain the human organism almost indefinitely. Questions relating to the discontinuation of medical intervention and the harvesting of organs for transplantation have demanded new approaches to the legal definition of death.

In response to these questions, almost all states have adopted, either by statute or court decision, a version of "brain death." This definition provides, either as an alternative to or a replacement for the traditional heart-lungs approach, that a person is legally dead when there is irreversible cessation of all (including brain stem) brain function.[39] Brain death should be confirmed clinically according to the Harvard criteria,[40] as they have been periodically updated.[41,42] Once a patient has been declared dead, there are no longer any treatment decisions to be made (although autopsy and organ donation issues may remain). There is neither a legal duty nor a right to continue medical intervention on a patient who has become a corpse.[43]

Legal Responsibility and Vicarious Liability

Critical care medicine is an interdisciplinary team enterprise, and the manner in which members of the team relate to each other and to the patient and family carries legal consequences. Under the old doctrine of "captain of the ship," a physician in charge of a critical care unit automatically was held legally responsible for any negligently caused patient injury occurring in the unit, regardless of the physician's personal ignorance of or lack of involvement with the particular error or omission. The captain-of-the-ship doctrine has been abandoned by the courts over the past several years in recognition of the increasing complexity of health care delivery.

However, a physician still may be held responsible, under a vicarious liability rationale, for patient injuries proximately (directly) caused by negligent errors or omissions committed by nurses or other providers over whom the physician has supervisory power. The key inquiry in potential vicarious liability situations is not whether the physician actually was exercising supervisory power at the time of the supervisee's negligence, but whether he or she had the authority and opportunity to supervise properly if he or she had chosen to exercise that power.[44]

Thus, the vicarious liability doctrine has significant legal ramifications for the interdisciplinary team's conduct in rendering critical care. The physician and other team members must understand their legal relationships to each other, and their implications with regard to assignment of tasks, oversight, reporting, communication, and problem resolution. The physician must take their obligations as legal leader of the team seriously, without acting autocratically and thereby negating the benefits of broad interdisciplinary contributions to patient care.

Institutional protocols should delineate operational principles of the team and the individual physician's supervisory responsibilities. Where there are multiple consultants on a particular case (as is the norm), medical staff bylaws must spell out the continuing coordination and monitoring obligations of an identified attending or primary care physician; failure to do so unambiguously will increase the liability exposure of all involved clinicians and the hospital in the event of a bad clinical outcome. Consultants who are not hospital employees must be credentialed to practice within the hospital according to criteria contained in the bylaws. Hospital policies and procedures must designate their ICUs as either "closed" (in which case the patient is transferred to an intensivist who functions as the primary care physician) or "open" (in which case the original primary care physician retains ultimate authority and responsibility, but is permitted or required to consult with a critical care physician on the hospital's staff).

Similarly, methods of triaging patients into and out of the ICU should be delineated within the hospital's written policies and procedures. Included should be a specification of ultimate responsibility for a patient's admission or discharge.

As a general principle, when there is a question concerning allocation of responsibility for decisions or actions, development of an institutional policy may be advisable. Courts ordinarily grant hospitals broad leeway in the development and enforcement of the sort of institutional protocols discussed in this chapter, as long as policies and procedures appear to ensure patient care within currently acceptable medical standards. As noted earlier, accreditation standards of the JCAHO also set permissible parameters for internal institutional protocols.

For physicians who function as clinical instructors in teaching programs, residents and medical students may expose the attending physician to vicarious liability for negligent acts or omissions done in the course of the educational activity. The exercise of due care in the monitoring, supervision, task assignment, and evaluation of residents and students who are supposed to be under the physician's supervision cannot be overlooked.[45]

Documentation

The courts have held that creating and maintaining accurate records of patient care is an integral part of the duty that a health care provider owes to a patient. Good documentation is imperative to providing competent patient care, and since avoiding unexpected bad outcomes is the best legal prophylaxis, is therefore wise legal practice. Furthermore, in the event of accusations of substandard care, the physician's best (and often only) defense will lie in the quality of documentation created to explain and justify decisions made and actions taken. In addition, institutional accreditation and third-party reimbursement turn heavily on information drawn from medical records.

The quality of medical records is especially important in critical care, where patient conditions are subject to rapid change, many different professionals may be involved in treating the patient, cost considerations are ever present,[46] and decisions (such as limiting the application of life-prolonging technology) may be controversial. The watchwords of documentation are the same from the legal and medical perspectives: completeness, legibility (dictation is preferable, but dictated entries should be read and corrected before being signed), accuracy or truthfulness, timeliness, corrections should be made in a clear and unambiguous fashion, and objectivity.

A corollary to the subject of medical record keeping is confidentiality. In light of common law privacy principles and federal regulations effective in 2003 to implement the Health Insurance Portability and Accountability Act (HIPAA),[47] the physician must guard against unauthorized disclosures of personal information about the patient. The party who has authority to give or refuse consent for medical treatment (i.e., the patient or her or his surrogate) ordinarily controls the release of identifiable medical information to third parties, absent a court order or countervailing government regulation. All questions about the release of medical information to third parties in specific cases should be directed to the institution's medical records department or legal counsel.

The counterpart to the right of the patient or surrogate to control the release of information to others is the patient's own right of access to the information contained in the medical record. This right of access is guaranteed, at least for in-hospital care, by the federal Privacy Act for federal facilities, and by the HIPAA regulations, state statutes, and JCAHO standards in most private and public institutions. Patients or their surrogates request access to records for a variety of reasons, ranging from curiosity to serious questioning of quality of care. A physician who is informed of a patient's or surrogate's request for access to records should offer to go through the record with the patient or surrogate, explain matters, and answer questions. In short, treating this circumstance as an opportunity to bolster or correct existing but perhaps unnoticed deficiencies in communication between the physician and patient or surrogate, rather than as a personal affront calling for defensive posturing, often can pay risk management dividends by preventing at an early stage potential misunderstandings that would otherwise eventually manifest themselves as legal action.

Risk Management Program

The hospital's overall program to identify, mitigate, and avoid potential problems that could result in legal, and therefore financial, loss to the institution (i.e., the risk management program), should incorporate specific activities designed to address legal risks prevalent in the delivery of critical care.[48] Particular areas of attention in a critical care–sensitive risk management program should include the organization and administration of CCUs, the roles and responsibilities of the different professionals having contact with patients in those units, medical records, equipment maintenance, equipment modification, equipment records, analysis of equipment malfunctions, incident reporting, and trend analysis of unexpected incidents.

The physician should be knowledgeable about the institution's risk management program and cooperate with it to ensure appropriate sensitivity to critical care practices and potential problems and their avoidance or mitigation. The physician should view the risk manager as a partner in pursuit of the common goal of providing, and if necessary proving after the fact, quality patient care.

Perhaps the single most influential aspect of effective risk management is the fostering of a positive relationship between the critical care team, led by the physician, and the patient and his or her family. There is a demonstrated correlation between patient (or family) psychologic satisfaction with the quality of the physician–patient (or –family) relationship, and the propensity to file a lawsuit if a bad outcome occurs.[49] Communicating openly and compassionately, especially acknowledging the vast uncertainty that pervades much of critical care medicine, is as important a tool in the malpractice prophylaxis arsenal as being proficient, up to date, and conscientious in knowing and applying technologic information and skills.[50]

References

1. Rozovsky FA: *Informed Consent: A Practical Guide,* 3rd ed. Gaithersburg, MD, Aspen, 2000.
2. President's Commission for the Study of Ethical Problems in Medicine & Biomedical and Behavioral Research: *Making Health Care Decisions.* Washington, Government Printing Office, 1982.
3. Merz JF: On a decision-making paradigm of medical informed consent. *J Legal Med* 14:231, 1993.
4. Kinderman KL: *Medicolegal Forms with Legal Analysis.* Chicago, American Medical Association, 1999.
4a. Davis N, Pohlman A, Gehlbach B, et al: Improving the process of informed consent in the critically ill. *JAMA* 289:1963, 2003.
5. Kapp MB: Geriatrics and the Law, 3rd ed. New York, Springer Publishing, 1999, p 31.
6. Prendergast TJ, Luch JM: Increasing incidence of withholding and withdrawal of life support from the critically ill. *Am J Resp Crit Care Med* 155:15, 1997.
7. Furrow DB, Greanery TL, Johnson SH, et al: *Bioethics-Health Care Law and Ethics,* 4th ed. St. Paul, MN, West Publishing, 2001, p 264.
8. Meisel A: *The Right to Die,* 2nd ed. New York, John Wiley & Sons, 1995.
9. Cantor NL: Twenty-five years after Quinlan: A review of the jurisprudence of death and dying. *J Law Med Ethics* 29:182, 2001.
10. *Cruzan v. Director, Missouri Department of Health,* 110 S.Ct. 2841 (1990).
11. *In re Mary O'Connor,* 534 N.Y.S.2d 886, 531 N.E. 2d 697 (1988).
12. Gillick MR: Medical decision-making for the unbefriended nursing home resident. *J Ethics Law Aging* 1:87, 1995.
13. National Conference of Commissioners on Uniform State Laws: Health Care Decisions Act 7(f), in *Uniform Laws Annotated.* St. Paul, MN, West Publishing, 2003 Supplement, p 143.
14. Ethics Committee of the Society of Critical Care Medicine: Consensus statement regarding futile and other possibly inadvisable treatments. *Crit Care Med* 25:887, 1997.
15. Meisel A: Legal myths about terminating life support. *Arch Intern Med* 151:1497, 1991.
16. Schmidt WC, Jr (ed): *Guardianship: The Court of Last Resort for the Elderly and Disabled.* Durham, NC, Carolina Academic Press, 1995.
17. Teaster PB, Schmidt WC, Abramson H, Almeida R: Staff service and volunteer staff service models for public guardianship and "alternative" services: Who is served and with what outcomes? *J Ethics Law Aging* 5:131, 1999.
18. Finucane TE, Christman C: More caution about tube feeding. *J Am Geriatr Soc* 48:1167, 2000.
19. *Cruzan v. Director, Missouri Department of Health,* 110 S. Ct. 2841 (1990).
20. American Medical Association, Council of Ethical and Judicial Affairs: Code of Medical Ethics: *Critical Care Medicine.* Chicago, AMA Press, 2002, p E-2.20.
21. Ethics Committee of the Society of Critical Care Medicine: Recommendations for end-of-life care in the intensive care unit. *Crit Care Med* 29:2332, 2001.
22. Hildebrand AJ: Masked intentions: The masquerade of killing thoughts used to justify dehydrating and starving people in a "persistent vegetative state" and people with other profound neurological impairments. *Issues Law Med* 16:143, 2000.
23. Sieger CE, Arnold JF, Ahronheim JC: Refusing artificial nutrition and hydration: Does statutory law send the wrong message? *J Am Geriatr Soc* 50: 44, 2002.

24. Kapp MB: Regulating the foregoing of artificial nutrition and hydration: First, do some harm. *J Am Geriatr Soc* 50:586, 2002.

25. American Medical Association, Council of Ethical and Judicial Affairs: Code of Medical Ethics: *Current Opinions with Annotations.* Chicago, AMA Press, 2002, p E-2.22.

26. Furrow BR: Pain management and provider liability: No more excuses. *J Law Med Ethics* 29:28, 2001.

27. Kapp MB: Anxieties as a legal impediment to the doctor-proxy relationship. *J Law Med Ethics* 27:69, 1999.

28. Wiener RL, Eton D, Gibbons VP, et al: A preliminary analysis of medical futility decision making: Law and professional attitudes. *Behav Sci Law* 16:497, 1998.

29. The Ethics Committee of the Society of Critical Care Medicine: Consensus statement of the Society of Critical Care Medicine's Ethics Committee regarding futile and other possibly inadvisable treatments. *Crit Care Med* 25:887, 1997.

30. Berger AS: *When Life Ends: Legal Overviews, Medicolegal Forms, and Hospital Policies.* Westport, CT, Greenwood Publishing Group, 1995.

31. Kapp MB: Healthcare rationing affecting older persons: Rejected in principle but implemented in fact. *J Aging Social Policy* 14:27, 2002.

32. Omnibus Budget Reconciliation Act of 1990, Public Law No. 101-508, secs. 4206, 4751.

33. New York State Public Health Law secs. 2960–78 (1988).

34. Joint Commission on Accreditation of Healthcare Organizations: *Accreditation Manual for Hospitals.* Chicago, JCAHO, 2003, Standard RI. 1, 1.2.2–1.2.7.

35. Curtis JR, Rubenfeld GD: Managing death in the ICU: The transition from cure to comfort. New York, Oxford University Press, 2001, p 231.

36. Minogue B: Bioethics: A committee approach. Boston, Jones and Bartlett, 1996.

37. Joint Commission on Accreditation of Healthcare Organizations: *Accreditation Manual for Hospitals.* Chicago, JCAHO, 1997, Standard RI. 1, 1.2.2.–1.2.7.

38. Fletcher JC, Hoffmann DE: Ethics committees: Time to experiment with standards. *Ann Intern Med* 120:335, 1994.

39. Youngner SJ, Arnold M, Shapiro R (eds): *The Definition of Death: Contemporary Controversies.* Baltimore, Johns Hopkins University Press, 1999.

40. Ad Hoc Committee of the Harvard Medical School to Examine the Definition of Brain Death: A definition of irreversible coma. *JAMA* 206:337, 1968.

41. Swash M, Beresford R: Brain death: Still-unresolved issues worldwide. *Neurology* 58:9, 2002.

42. Wijdicks EFM: Brain death worldwide. *Neurology* 58:20, 2002.

43. *Strachan v. John F. Kennedy Memorial Hospital,* 109 N.J. 523, 538 A.2d 346 (1988).

44. Boumil MM, Elias CE, Moes DB: *The Law of Medical Liability in a Nutshell.* St. Paul, MN, West, 2003, p 179.

45. Helms LB, Helms CM, Biggs SE: Litigation in medical education: Retrospect and prospect. *J Contemp Health Law Policy* 11:317, 1995.

46. Noseworthy TW, Jacobs P: Economics of critical care, in Hall JB, Schmidt GA, Wood LDH (eds): *Principles of Critical Care*, 2nd ed. New York, McGraw-Hill, 1992, p 17.

47. 67 Federal Register 53182 (Aug. 14, 2002), codified at 45 CFR parts 160 and 164.

48. Balsamo RR, Brown MD: Risk management, in Sanbar SS and American College of Legal Medicine Textbook Committee (eds): *Legal Medicine*, 6th ed. St. Louis, Mosby, 2004, p 187.

49. Hickson GB, Clayton EW, Entman SS, et al: Obstetricians' prior malpractice experience and patients' satisfaction with care. *JAMA* 272:1583, 1994.

50. Way J, Back AL, Curtis JR: Withdrawing life support and resolution of conflict with families. *Br Med J* 325:1342, 2002.

APPENDIX 1

Florida Designation of Health Care Surrogate

Name: _____
          (Last)   *(First)*   *(Middle Initial)*

In the event that I have been determined to be incapacitated to provide informed consent for medical treatment and surgical and diagnostic procedures, I wish to designate as my surrogate for health care decisions:

Name: _____

Address: _____

_____ Zip Code: _____

Phone: _____

If my surrogate is unwilling or unable to perform his duties, I wish to designate as my alternate surrogate:

Name: _____

Address: _____

_____ Zip Code: _____

Phone: _____

I fully understand that this designation will permit my designee to make health care decisions and to provide, withhold, or withdraw consent on my behalf; to apply for public benefits to defray the cost of health care; and to authorize my admission to or transfer from a health care facility.

Additional instructions (optional):

I further affirm that this designation is not being made as a condition of treatment or admission to a health care facility. I will notify and send a copy of this document to the following persons other than my surrogate, so they may know who my surrogate is:

Name: _____

Address: _____

Name: _____

Address: _____

Signed: _____

Date: _____

Witness 1:

    Signed: _____

    Address: _____

Witness 2:

    Signed: _____

    Address: _____

NOTE: Legal requirements of individual states may vary and should be consulted.

APPENDIX 2

Florida Living Will

Declaration made this _____ day of _____ , 19 _____ .

I, _____ , willfully and voluntarily make known my desire that my dying not be artificially prolonged under the circumstances set forth below, and I do hereby declare:

If at any time I have a terminal condition and if my attending or treating physician and another consulting physician have determined that there is no medical probability of my recovery from such condition, I direct that life-prolonging procedures be withheld or withdrawn when the application of such procedures would serve only to prolong artificially the process of dying, and that I be permitted to die naturally with only the administration of medication or the performance of any medical procedure deemed necessary to provide me with comfort care or to alleviate pain.

It is my intention that this declaration be honored by my family and physician as the final expression of my legal right to refuse medical or surgical treatment and to accept the consequences for such refusal.

In the event that I have been determined to be unable to provide express and informed consent regarding the withholding, withdrawal, or continuation of life-prolonging procedures, I wish to designate, as my surrogate to carry out the provisions of this declaration:

Name: _____

Address: _____

_____ Zip Code: _____

Phone: _____

I wish to designate the following person as my alternate surrogate, to carry out the provisions of this declaration should my surrogate be unwilling or unable to act on my behalf:

Name: _____

Address: _____

_____ Zip Code: _____

Phone: _____

Additional instructions (optional):

I understand the full import of this declaration, and I am emotionally and mentally competent to make this declaration.

Signed: _____

Witness 1:

    Signed: _____

    Address: _____

Witness 2:

    Signed: _____

    Address: _____

NOTE: Legal requirements of individual states may vary and should be consulted.

APPENDIX 3

2.2 WITHHOLDING OR WITHDRAWING LIFE-PROLONGING TREATMENT.

The social commitment of the physician is to sustain life and relieve suffering. Where the performance of one duty conflicts with the other, the preferences of the patient should prevail. If the patient is incompetent to act in his own behalf and did not previously indicate his preferences, the family or other surrogate decisionmaker, in concert with the physician, must act in the best interest of the patient.

For humane reasons, with informed consent, a physician may do what is medically necessary to alleviate severe pain, or cease or omit treatment to permit a terminally ill patient to die when death is imminent. However, the physician should not intentionally cause death. In deciding whether the administration of potentially life-prolonging medical treatment is in the best interest of the patient who is incompetent to act in his own behalf, the surrogate decisionmaker and physician should consider several factors, including: the possibility for extending life under humane and comfortable conditions; the patient's values about life and the way it should be lived; and the patient's attitudes toward sickness, suffering, medical procedures, and death.

Even if death is not imminent but a patient is beyond doubt permanently unconscious, and there are adequate safeguards to confirm the accuracy of the diagnosis, it is not unethical to discontinue all means of life-prolonging medical treatment.

Life-prolonging medical treatment includes medication and artificially or technologically supplied respiration, nutrition or hydration. In treating a terminally ill or permanently unconscious patient, the dignity of the patient should be maintained at all times. (I,II,IV,V)

2.21 WITHHOLDING OR WITHDRAWING LIFE-PROLONGING MEDICAL TREATMENT—
PATIENTS' PREFERENCES.

A competent, adult patient may, in advance, formulate and provide a valid consent to the withholding or withdrawal of life-support systems in the event that injury or illness renders that individual incompetent to make such a decision. The preference of the individual should prevail when determining whether extraordinary life-prolonging measures should be undertaken in the event of terminal illness. Unless it is clearly established that the patient is terminally ill or permanently unconscious, a physician should not be deterred from appropriately aggressive treatment of a patient. (I,III,IV,V)

SOURCE: Reprinted by permission from 1995 Current Opinions of the Council on Ethical and Judicial Affairs of the American Medical Association.

Chapter 6 _____

ASSESSMENT OF SEVERITY OF ILLNESS

CHERYL L. HOLMES
GENEVIEVE GREGOIRE
JAMES A. RUSSELL

KEY POINTS

- *In the last three decades, intensive care units (ICUs) and critical care researchers have amassed a body of pathophysiologic knowledge that has advanced the care of critically ill patients. Severity of illness scoring systems are tools that have been designed both to predict and to evaluate, from multiple perspectives, the outcomes of critically ill patients.*

- *Most of these scoring systems have evolved from multivariate regression analysis applied to large clinical databases to identify the most relevant factors for prediction of mortality. Scoring systems are then validated by prospective application to other patient populations.*

- *The ideal components of a scoring system are data collected during the course of routine patient management that are easily measured, objective, and reproducible.*

- *The most widely applied scoring systems in adults at the present time are the Acute Physiology and Chronic Health Evaluation (APACHE), the Mortality Probability Models (MPM), Simplified Acute Physiology Score (SAPS), and Sequential Organ Failure Assessment (SOFA).*

- *The potential uses of severity-of-illness scoring systems as applied to patient groups include clinical investigation (to standardize or compare study groups), ICU administration (to guide resource allocation and budget), and assessment of ICU performance (to compare performance over time or between health care settings).*

- *The use of scores in the delivery of care to individual patients is controversial; in some studies the accuracy of prediction of outcomes of scoring systems is not greater than that of the individual clinician's judgment.*

Severity-of-illness scoring systems were developed to evaluate the delivery of care and provide prediction of outcome of groups of critically ill patients who are admitted to intensive care units (ICUs). The purpose of this chapter is to review the scientific basis for these scoring systems and to make recommendations for their use. While there is a growing recognition that when properly administered, these tools are useful in assessing and comparing patient populations with diverse critical illnesses, their use for predicting individual patient outcome is controversial and unresolved.

Purposes of Scoring Systems

There are five major purposes of severity-of-illness scoring systems (Table 6-1). First, scoring systems have been used in randomized controlled trials (RCTs) and other clinical investigations.[1-5] The second purpose of severity-of-illness scoring systems is to quantify severity of illness for hospital and health care system administrative decisions such as resource allocation. The third purpose of these scoring systems is to assess ICU performance and compare the quality of care of different ICUs and within the same ICU over time. For example, severity-of-illness scoring systems could be used to assess the impact on patient outcomes of planned changes in the ICU, such as changes in bed number, staffing ratios, and medical coverage.[6] The fourth purpose of these scoring systems is to assess the prognosis of individual patients in order to assist families and caregivers in making decisions about ICU care. Finally, scoring systems are now being used to evaluate suitability of patients for novel therapy (e.g., the use of the APACHE II assessment for prescription of recombinant human activated protein C [drotrecogin alfa]).

The general hypothesis underlying the use of severity-of-illness scoring systems is that clinical variables that can be assessed on ICU admission predict survival and other outcomes of critically ill patients. This hypothesis is based on observations that increasing age, presence of underlying chronic disease, and increasingly severe abnormalities of the physiology of critically ill patients are associated with increased mortality. Scoring systems that have evolved combine relevant clinical variables to yield prediction of risk of mortality. Early in this evolution, severity-of-illness scores calculated at ICU admission or in the 24 hours following ICU admission predicted hospital mortality. More recently, scores have been calculated over the course of the ICU stay to provide updated prediction of hospital mortality. This dynamic approach uses change in organ dysfunction over time to add further accuracy and precision to outcome prediction.[7-11]

It is important to note that scoring systems have been developed using databases from patients already admitted to ICUs and not from the pool of patients outside the ICU, where the triage decision to admit a patient to the ICU is made. While severity-of-illness scoring systems in theory could be used to increase the accuracy of triage decisions regarding appropriateness of ICU admission, reformulation of the scoring methods would likely be necessary to better reflect the patient population outside the ICU, in whom triage occurs. Obviously, ICU resources should be focused on patients who are most able to benefit from ICU care. However, to date there are no reports regarding the use of scoring systems to assist in decisions regarding appropriateness of ICU admission.

Development of Scoring Systems

The major scoring systems that are the focus of this chapter were designed specifically to predict outcome of critical illness. Initially, clinical and physiologic variable selection was based on subjective judgment of clinicians, review of the literature, and development of consensus. Subsequently, logistic regression modeling techniques were used to select predictive variables from a derivation data set. Ideal variables are simple, well-defined, reproducible, and widely available measurements or data that are collected routinely in the course of patient care. A large number of clinical and physiologic

TABLE 6-1 Potential Uses of Severity-of-Illness Scoring Systems

Uses of scoring systems in randomized controlled trials (RCTs) and clinical research
  To compare different RCTs and clinical studies
  To determine sample size
  To do stratified randomization (to determine subgroup identification and stratification for severity of illness)
  To assess success of randomization
  To assess treatment effects in subgroups (posttreatment subgroup identification)
  To compare study patients to patients in clinicians' practices
Uses of scoring systems for administrative purposes
  To describe resource utilization of ICU
  To describe acuity of illness
  To relate resource utilization to acuity of care
  To guide reimbursement and budget of ICU
Uses of scoring systems to assess ICU performance
  Quality assurance
    To assess performance of an ICU in general or for a specific disease category
    To assess performance of an ICU over time
    To compare individual intensivists' performances
    To assess the performance of a therapeutic intervention
  Comparison of ICU performance in different categories of hospitals, countries, etc.
  To assess performance for different ICU administrative characteristics (open/closed unit, communication, ICU director task, etc.)
  Effectiveness
Uses of scoring systems to assess individual patient prognosis and to guide care
  Triage of patients
  Decisions regarding intensity of care
  Decisions to withhold and withdraw care

variables were collected on many patients, and their survival status at ICU and hospital discharge was recorded. Multiple logistical regression identifies the specific variables that best predicted survival and assigns relative weights to each variable. This set of variables is then tested prospectively for accuracy of prediction in another sample of patients to validate the selection process and appropriate weighting of variables.[12]

The sampling frequency and the period of measurements of physiologic variables are additional methodologic considerations that are important in the development of scoring systems. Most scoring systems use the most abnormal measurement of a physiologic variable in the 24 hours prior to ICU admission. More recently, scoring systems have used the most abnormal value of a physiologic variable for each successive 24-hour period while a patient is in the ICU, and have then correlated physiologic variables during this period with subsequent ICU outcome. Therefore prediction prognosis could be adjusted daily based on the patient's course and response to treatment. Furthermore, the change in organ dysfunction could be used to improve outcome prediction.[7–11] Studies have shown that the change in organ dysfunction from day 0 to day 1, from day 0 to day 3,[9] and indeed from day to day,[13] can be used to accurately predict outcome of the critically ill.

Another important consideration in the development of severity-of-illness scoring systems is the patient sample used to derive the scoring system. For example, it is relevant to know whether scoring systems were derived in medical, surgical, or medical-surgical ICUs, whether community or tertiary care teaching hospital ICUs were used, whether ICUs were selected from one country or from many countries, and how many different ICUs were used to establish the scoring system. Furthermore, scoring systems derived from the sample of patients involved in a clinical trial may be biased and may not represent a general population of critically ill patients.

METHODOLOGIC CONSIDERATIONS

Critical appraisal of severity-of-illness scoring systems involves the measurement of accuracy (calibration and discrimination), reliability, content validity, and methodological rigor.[14]

Discrimination describes the ability of a model to distinguish between a patient who will live and one who will die. If discrimination is perfect, there is no overlap in probability estimates between patients who live and those who die.[15] Discrimination is described by the area under the receiver operating characteristic (ROC) curve[15,16] (Fig. 6-1). The ROC curve shows the relation between the true-positive rate (sensitivity) and the false-positive rate (100%-specificity). Because sensitivity and specificity are computed from independent columns in the decision matrix, and are therefore independent of sample mortality, the area under the ROC curve represents the proportion of patients who not only died, but who also had a higher probability of death than the patients who lived.[14]

The area under the ROC curve ranges from the lower limit of 0.5 for chance performance to 1.0 for perfect prediction. A model is considered to discriminate well when this area is greater than 0.8. An area of 0.9 means that a randomly selected actual nonsurvivor will have a more severe score than a randomly selected survivor 90% of the time.[12] It does not mean that a prediction of nonsurvival occurs with probability 0.9, nor does it mean that a prediction of death is associated with observed nonsurvival 90% of the time. The area under the ROC curve illustrates the discriminating ability over the entire range of prediction scores.[15]

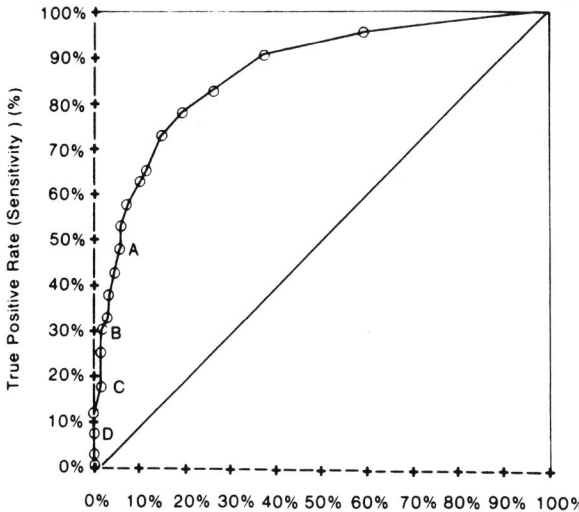

**FIGURE 6-1 The receiver operating characteristic (ROC) curve.
The diagonal line indicates an index that operates no better than
chance and has an area under the ROC curve of 0.5. Points *A, B, C,*
and *D* correspond to decision criteria of 50%, 70%, 80%, and 90%
predicted risk of death, respectively. A decision criterion of 0.5
(point A) means that every patient with a risk greater than 0.50 is
predicted to die. The overall correct classification rate was 86%,
with a sensitivity of 47% and a specificity of 92%. A decision
criterion of 0.80 (point C) had an overall correct classification rate
of 83%, with a sensitivity of 19% and a specificity of 93%. For a
90% predicted mortality, a scoring system has low sensitivity but
high specificity. It is most specific for minimizing the prediction
of a positive outcome (survival) when it actually does not occur,
and poorly sensitive to predict the outcome (survival) when it
actually occurs. (*Reproduced with permission from Knaus et al.*[18])**

②   *Calibration* compares the observed mortality with that predicted by the model within the severity strata. Patients are
placed into subgroups according to predicted risk. Typically,
10 strata are formed, called *deciles* of risk.[15] Calibration is evaluated using goodness-of-fit tests; the most commonly used is
the Hosmer-Lemeshow χ^2 statistic.[17] Typically, a $2 \times 10\chi^2$
table is created, with 10 strata of probabilities. The lower the
overall χ^2, the better the fit. The calibration test must be interpreted with care, as it is very sensitive to sample size.

③   *Reliability* refers to inter- (between) and intra- (within) observer agreement in the use of any severity of illness score, and
represents the agreement in the data collection.[14] The greater
the subjectivity involved in the scoring system (i.e., choosing
a primary diagnosis or assessing the level of consciousness
in a sedated, intubated patient), the poorer the reliability of
the system. Intraobserver reliability can be measured using a
variety of techniques, and is expressed on a range between 0
(measurement involves nothing but error) and 1 (no variable
error). A reliability coefficient of greater than 0.7 (suggesting that no more than 30% of the score is due to error) has
been used as a statistical standard.[14] The kappa statistic is a
measure of interobserver reliability.

Content validity reflects the comprehensiveness of the
model.[14] Mortality is dependent not only on measured physiologic derangements and underlying health status, but may
also be influenced by factors that are difficult to quantify, such

as duration of organ system failure before treatment was instituted, and whether the admission was planned or unplanned,
among others. However, as the number of variables increase
in a scoring system, the reliability and ease of capturing the
data decrease. The inclusion of many variables (overfitting)
may actually reduce the performance of the model because
some of these variables will be correlated with the outcome
by chance alone. It has been proposed that stepwise regression should not be used unless there are at least 10 outcome
events for each potential predictor.

Methodologic rigor refers to the avoidance of bias in development of a model. It is important that any severity-of-illness
scoring system is based on a large database of all consecutive eligible patients in order to avoid bias.[14] Several ICUs
should be involved in data collection to avoid local bias in
interpretation of coding or scoring rules. Clinical and laboratory variables should be those that are routinely collected,
because collection of unusual data (such as serum ammonia)
may bias treatment (treatment effect). Rigor must be applied
in the consistency of data collection, and rules for dealing
with missing data need to be uniformly applied. Validation
using a second independent patient population is important
in assessing the reliability of the model. Finally, the usefulness of a rigorously developed and validated scoring system
can be degraded by poor application.

Severity-of-Illness Scoring Systems in Clinical Use

SCORES ESTABLISHED AT ADMISSION

The scoring systems most commonly used in critically ill
adults are APACHE II,[18] APACHE III,[19] MPM II,[20] SAPS II,[21]
and SOFA.[7,22] The variables included in each of these scoring
systems are summarized in Table 6-2. The Pediatric Risk of
Mortality (PRISM) score[23] is the most widely used scoring
system in pediatric critical care.

Some clinical variables are common to APACHE II,
APACHE III, MPM II, SAPS II, and SOFA, probably because
these variables measure specific clinical and physiologic functions that are major determinants of mortality. Specifically,
each of these scoring systems uses age, type of admission,
heart rate, blood pressure, assessment of renal function (blood
urea nitrogen, creatinine, and/or urine output), assessment
of neurologic function (Glasgow Coma Scale or presence of
coma), assessment of respiratory function (mechanical ventilation, Pa_{O_2}/FI_{O_2}, or alveolar-arterial oxygen gradient), and assessment of chronic health status. In contrast, other variables
are not uniformly shared: serum potassium in APACHE II,
glucose and albumin in APACHE III, and serum bicarbonate
in SAPS II. These unique variables exist because of differences
in the derivation of each scoring system, such as patient sample size, types of patients included, and statistical methods
used to derive each score. An important difference between
severity of illness scoring systems is how the predictor variables were chosen.[24] For instance, in the APACHE II model,
the developers selected those variables they thought relevant
to patient outcome and then arbitrarily weighted each variable. In the development of MPM II, SAPS II, and APACHE
III, statistical techniques were applied to identify those variables that were independently associated with death. These

variables were then further refined by use of linear discriminant function and stepwise logistic regression analysis, and the final set of variables were then weighted by statistical methods and analyzed and presented as a cumulative score to predict mortality.

The Acute Physiology and Chronic Health Evaluation II (APACHE II) system[18] is the most commonly used clinical severity-of-illness scoring system in North America. APACHE II is a disease-specific scoring system. It uses age, type of admission, chronic health evaluation, and 12 physiologic variables (acute physiology score or APS) to predict hospital mortality (see Table 6-2). The 12 physiologic variables are defined as the most abnormal values during the 24 hours after ICU admission.

The predicted hospital death rate is computed from the weighted sum of APACHE II score, a variable determined by whether the patient had emergency surgery, and the specific diagnostic category weight. APACHE II score was validated in 5815 ICU admissions from 13 hospitals. The correct classification rate for a 50% predicted risk of death was 85%. APACHE III[19] extended APACHE II by improving calibration and discrimination through the use of a much larger derivation and validation patient sample. However, at this time, APACHE III is a proprietary commercial product.

The main disadvantages of the APACHE II system are its failure to compensate for lead-time bias,[25] the requirement to select only one clinical diagnosis, and inaccuracies in clinical subsets, which produce poor interobserver reliability. In spite of these shortcomings, APACHE II remains the most well known and most widely used severity of illness scoring system.[24]

APACHE III is a disease-specific score that was developed from 17,440 admissions in 40 U.S. hospitals. Eighteen variables (see Table 6-2) were included, and their respective weights were derived by logistic regression modeling. To improve the accuracy of assessment of neurologic function, the Glasgow Coma Scale (GCS) score was changed, because reliability testing suggested the need to eliminate similar GCS scores that could occur in patients who had different neurologic presentations. The APACHE III score is a sum of physiology, age, and data from seven potential comorbid conditions. The final APACHE III score can vary between 0 and 300. Risk estimate equations for hospital mortality are calculated from the weighted sum of disease category (78 diagnostic categories are included), a coefficient related to prior treatment location, and the APACHE III score. In the original derivation sample, estimates of mortality for the first day in the ICU had an area under the ROC curve of 0.90, and the correct classification at 50% mortality risk level was 88%. Although APACHE III scores can be calculated from published information, weights to convert the score to probability of death are proprietary, therefore the APACHE III system has not been widely accepted or used.

The Mortality Probability Model (MPM II)[20] was developed from 19,124 ICU admissions in 12 countries. MPM II is not disease specific. MPM_0 is the only severity-of-illness scoring system that was derived at ICU admission and can therefore be used at ICU admission. MPM II does not yield a score, but rather a direct probability of survival. Burn, coronary care, and cardiac surgery patients are excluded. MPM_0 includes three physiologic variables, three chronic diagnoses, five acute diagnoses, and three other variables: cardiopulmonary resuscitation prior to admission, mechanical ventilation, and medical or unscheduled surgery admission (see Table 6-2). Each variable is scored as absent or present and is allocated a coefficient. The sum of these coefficients constitutes the logit that is used to calculate the probability of hospital mortality.

The MPM_{24}[20] was designed to be calculated for patients who remained in the ICU for 24 hours or longer. MPM_{24} includes 13 variables, 5 of which are used in the MPM_0. In the validation data set, the area under the ROC curve was 0.82 and 0.84 for the MPM_0 and MPM_{24}, respectively.

The most recent version of the Simplified Acute Physiology Score II (SAPS II)[21] was developed from a sample of 13,152 admissions from 12 countries, based on a European/North American multicenter database. SAPS II is not disease specific. SAPS II uses 17 variables (see Table 6-2) that were selected by logistic regression: 12 physiology variables, age, type of admission (scheduled surgical, unscheduled surgical, or medical), and three underlying disease variables (acquired immunodeficiency syndrome, metastatic cancer, and hematologic malignancy). The area under the ROC curve was 0.86 in the validation sample. The probability of hospital mortality is calculated from the score.

The Sequential Organ Failure Assessment (SOFA) was originally developed as a descriptor of a continuum of organ dysfunction in critically ill patients over the course of their ICU stay.[22] The SOFA score is composed of scores from six organ systems, graded from 0 to 4 according to the degree of dysfunction/failure. The score was primarily designed to describe morbidity; however, a retrospective analysis of the relationship between the SOFA score and mortality was developed using the European/North American Study of Severity System database.[7,21] Subsequently, SOFA was evaluated as a predictor of outcome in a prospective Belgium study.[13] SOFA score on admission was not a good predictor of mortality (area under the ROC curve 0.79); however, mean SOFA score and highest SOFA score had better discrimination (area under the ROC curve 0.88 and 0.90, respectively). Independent of the initial value, an increase in the SOFA score during the first 48 hours of ICU admission predicts a mortality rate of at least 50%.

DYNAMIC SEVERITY OF ILLNESS SCORING SYSTEMS

All severity-of-illness scoring systems at ICU admission have a relatively high rate of misclassification of survivors and nonsurvivors. Misclassifications may be caused by the following: (1) exclusion of strong outcome risk factors that cannot be measured or have not been measured at ICU admission, (2) exclusion of complications that occur during ICU stay[26], and/or (3) exclusion of treatment effects that modify outcome. Scoring systems applied over the course of the ICU stay can diminish the impact of these factors. However, discrimination of scoring systems applied during the ICU course is lower than discrimination of scoring systems evaluating outcome at the time of initial admission to the ICU.

MPM_{48} and MPM_{72}[27] were developed to estimate the probability of hospital mortality at 48 and 72 hours in the ICU. MPM_{48} and MPM_{72} have the same 13 variables and

TABLE 6-2 Variables Included in Severity-of-Illness Scoring Systems in Clinical Use

	APACHE II	APACHE III	MPM II$_0$ ADM	MPM II$_{24}$ 24 Hours	SAPS II	SOFA
Age	X	X	X	X	X	
Prior treatment location		X				
Type of admission	X	X	X	X	X	
CPR prior to ICU admission			X			
Mechanical ventilation			X	X		
Vasoactive drug therapy				X		
Acute diagnoses						
Acute renal failure			X			
Cardiac dysrhythmias			X			
Cerebrovascular incident			X			
Gastrointestinal bleeding			X			
Confirmed infection				X		
Intracranial mass effect			X	X		
Select one of 50 diagnoses	X					
Select one of 78 diagnoses		X	⊢ NOT DISEASE SPECIFIC ⊣			
Physiology						
Temperature	X	X			X	
Heart rate	X	X	X		X	
Respiratory rate	X	X				
Blood pressure	X	X	X		X	X
Pressor dose						X
Hematocrit	X	X				
White blood cell count	X	X			X	
Platelet count						X
Albumin		X				
Bilirubin		X			X	X
Glucose		X				
Serum sodium	X	X			X	
Serum potassium	X				X	
Serum bicarbonate					X	
Blood urea nitrogen		X			X	
Creatinine	X	X		X	X	
Urine output		X		X	X	X
Pa$_{O_2}$ or (A–a)D$_{O_2}$ or F$_{IO_2}$	X	X		X	X	X
Pa$_{O_2}$/F$_{IO_2}$						X
pH and P$_{CO_2}$	X	X				
Prothrombin time				X		
GCS or modified GCS	X	X			X	X
Coma or deep stupor			X	X		
Chronic health status						
AIDS	X	X			X	
Immunosuppression	X	X				
Lymphoma	X	X			*a*	
Leukemia/mult. myeloma	X	X			*a*	
Metastatic cancer		X	X	X	X	
Hepatic failure	X	X				
Cirrhosis	X	X	X	X		
Chronic renal insufficiency	X	X				
Chronic coronary insufficiency	X					
Chronic respiratory insufficiency	X					

(handwritten: 0 à 4 × 6)

"In SAPS II, these two criteria are grouped into one entity called "hematologic malignancy."
ABBREVIATIONS: APACHE II, Acute Physiology and Chronic Health Evaluation II; APACHE III, Acute Physiology and Chronic Health Evaluation III; MPM II$_0$, Mortality Probability Models II, assessment at ICU admission; MPM II$_{24}$, Mortality Probability Models II, assessment 24 hours after ICU admission; SAPS II, Simplified Acute Physiology Score II; SOFA, Sequential Organ Failure Assessment; CPR, cardiopulmonary resuscitation; (A–a)D$_{O_2}$, alveolar-arterial oxygen difference; F$_{IO_2}$, fraction of inspired oxygen; GCS, Glasgow Coma Scale; AIDS, acquired immunodeficiency syndrome; mult. myeloma, multiple myeloma; insuff, insufficiency.

coefficients that are used in MPM_{24}, but the models differ in the constant terms, which reflect the increasing probability of mortality with increasing length of ICU stay, even if physiologic parameters are constant. In the validation group, the areas under the ROC curves of MPM_{48} and MPM_{72} were 0.80 and 0.75, respectively.

APACHE III also can be used to calculate a daily risk of hospital mortality.[28] A series of multiple logistic regression equations was developed for ICU days 2 to 7. The APACHE III daily risk estimate of mortality includes the acute physiology score (APS) on day 1, APS on current day, change in APS since the previous day, the indication for ICU admission, the location and length of treatment before ICU admission, whether the patient was an ICU readmission, age, and chronic health status.

The SOFA score has been used to describe increasing accuracy of outcome prediction when used over the first 7 days of the ICU course.[13] More recently, the changes in SOFA score in cardiovascular, renal, and respiratory dysfunction from day 0 to day 1 of sepsis were significantly correlated with 28-day mortality in two large cohorts of patients who had severe sepsis.

COMPARISON OF THE DIFFERENT SCORING SYSTEMS

Comparing the accuracy of the different scoring systems is difficult because of differences in populations used to derive these scores and different statistical methods. Thus there have been few head-to-head comparisons of different scoring systems. A multinational study[29] compared different generations of the three main severity-of-illness scoring systems in 4685 ICU patients. APACHE III, SAPS II, and MPM II all showed good discrimination and calibration in this international database and performed better than did APACHE II, SAPS, and MPM. APACHE II and APACHE III have been compared in 1144 patients from the United Kingdom.[30] APACHE II showed better calibration, but discrimination was better with APACHE III. Both scoring systems underestimated hospital mortality, and APACHE III underestimated mortality by a greater degree.

COMPARISON OF CLINICAL ASSESSMENT WITH SCORING SYSTEMS

Clinical judgment to predict outcome has been criticized because it is not very reproducible, it has a tendency to overestimate mortality risk, and bias is introduced by the ability to recall particularly memorable, rare, and recent events.[15] Three studies compared APACHE II with physicians' mortality predictions in the first 24 hours of ICU admission,[31–33] and one study evaluated physicians' predictions only.[34] Discrimination by physicians had ROC curve areas ranging between 0.85 and 0.89, which were similar to[32,34] and even significantly better than those of APACHE II.[31,33] In contrast to ability to discriminate, calibration rate of physicians' predictions of mortality versus APACHE II differed. For high-risk patients, APACHE II and physicians had similarly correct predictions for mortality, ranging from 71% to 85%. However, for estimated mortality risks below 30%, rates of correct classification of physicians' predictions were 39% to 69%, compared with 51% and 67% for APACHE II.[31]

CUSTOMIZATION OF SCORING SYSTEMS FOR SPECIFIC DISEASES

Severity-of-illness scoring systems have been developed, derived, and validated for specific diseases to improve the accuracy of general scoring systems. APACHE III uses 74 disease classifications and derives a unique mortality risk prediction for each of these disease classifications. New scoring systems have been introduced to better predict mortality for patients with multiple organ failure and sepsis. The original models of SAPS II and MPM II did not perform well in patients who had severe sepsis, because mortality in severe sepsis was higher than mortality in patients with other diagnoses. Both models subsequently were customized[5] for sepsis by using the original data to derive coefficients unique for sepsis to calculate predicted mortality. Furthermore, severity-of-illness scoring systems specifically designed for sepsis have been developed.

Prediction of mortality in sepsis will likely benefit from a dynamic approach that is based on evolution of multiple organ dysfunction. Commonly used organ failure–based systems that have been studied include the Sequential Organ Failure Assessment (SOFA) score,[22] the Multiple Organ Dysfunction Score (MODS),[35] and the Logistic Organ Dysfunction System (LODS).[36]

All three systems attribute points for organ dysfunction in six different organ systems. MODS,[35] which applies to surgical patients, differs from SOFA and LODS in the cardiovascular assessment. MODS scores the cardiovascular system based on the "pressure-adjusted heart rate," defined as the product of the heart rate multiplied by the ratio of the right atrial pressure to the mean arterial pressure. LODS and MODS have excellent discrimination, with ROC curve areas of 0.85 and 0.93, respectively.[35,36]

APACHE II, MODS, and SOFA were recently used to compare outcome prediction in and prospective study of 949 ICU patients.[37] There were no significant differences between MODS and SOFA in terms of mortality prediction. The area under the ROC curves for APACHE II, SOFA, and MODS were 0.880, 0.872, and 0.856, respectively. In patients with shock, the MODS and SOFA scores were slightly better mortality predictors than APACHE II score (area under ROC curve 0.852 and 0.869 vs. 0.825).

Some have suggested that organ failure–based scoring systems could provide an outcome measure to be used as a surrogate for the end point of mortality.[38] Thus, for large (and expensive) randomized clinical trials such as those recently conducted in the treatment of sepsis or acute lung injury, could a reduction in some score of organ failure be taken as a measure of reduced morbidity and hence high drug efficacy?

Many randomized controlled trials in critical care have successfully evaluated organ dysfunction as secondary outcome variables by using scoring systems. Important recent examples include the ARDS Network study of 6 mL/kg vs. 12 mL/kg of ideal body weight tidal volume in patients who had acute lung injury.[39] The use of a protocol of 6 mL/kg ideal body weight, positive end-expiratory pressure (PEEP), and guidelines for respiratory rate and minute ventilation decreased mortality from 40% (with 12 mL/kg tidal volume) to 30%. In addition, the 6 mL/kg tidal volume strategy significantly increased the number of days patients were alive and free of respiratory, hepatic, cardiovascular, coagulation, and renal dysfunction[39] as assessed using the Brussels scoring system.[9] The randomized controlled trial of recombinant human activated protein C (rhAPC; drotrecogin alfa) showed that rhAPC decreased mortality of severe sepsis from 31% to 25% compared to placebo.[40] The SOFA score was used in this study to evaluate organ dysfunction and rhAPC improved markers of organ dysfunction.

SCORING SYSTEMS SPECIFIC FOR TRAUMA PATIENTS

Scoring systems have been developed to improve triage of trauma patients and to predict their mortality (see Chap. 92). Trauma scoring systems were developed using general trauma patient samples, not specifically critically ill trauma patients. The initial scores were either anatomic (Injury Severity Score or ISS[1,41]) or physiologic (Trauma Score or TS[42] and Revised Trauma Score or RTS[43]). Recently, trauma scoring systems have been expanded to include age, anatomy, and physiology, including the Trauma and the Injury Severity Score or TRISS methodology,[2] and A Severity Characterization of Trauma or ASCOT.[44] Large trauma registries facilitated implementation and validation of trauma scoring systems in large samples of patients. Table 6-3 summarizes the main trauma scoring systems.

The accuracy of TRISS and APACHE II have been compared in critically ill trauma patients.[45] APACHE II classifies trauma patients under only four diagnostic categories: postoperative multiple trauma, postoperative head trauma, nonoperative multiple trauma, and nonoperative head trauma. In APACHE II, patients with combined head and other injuries were assigned to multiple trauma, which was given a lower weight than the isolated head trauma category in predicting mortality.[46] The number of derivation patient samples of APACHE II were much smaller than the samples used for the trauma scores. TRISS tends to perform better than APACHE II. APACHE II significantly overestimates the risk of mortality in the lower ranges of predicted risk and underestimates the risk of mortality in the higher ranges. APACHE III attempted to improve prediction of mortality for head-injured patients by revising the definition for head trauma, allowing assignment of patients with isolated head trauma as well as head trauma and other injuries to the head trauma category. This resulted in a higher predicted mortality that more closely reflected the actual mortality.

TABLE 6-3 Characteristics of the Major Trauma Scoring Systems

Name	Purpose and Main Characteristics	Variables Included	Comments
ISS	Description of the severity of injury Anatomic description Blunt trauma	Anatomic variables: 3 highest scoring body regions from the AIS are squared and summed Value 3–75	Developed for MVA (blunt) trauma victims
TS	Triage Survival probability Physiologic score Blunt and penetrating trauma	Respiratory rate Respiratory effort Systolic blood pressure Capillary refill GCS Range 1–16[a]	Immediately available for triage Determination of respiratory effort and capillary refill are subjective
RTS	Triage Survival probability Physiologic score Blunt and penetrating trauma	Respiratory rate Systolic blood pressure GCS Each coded 0–4 Range 0–12[b]	Value of each variable empirical, but weight of variables for probability of survival by regression analysis. Better goodness of fit than TS
TRISS	Survival probability Considers anatomy, physiology, age, blunt and penetrating trauma	RTS ISS (with revised AIS-85) Age < or >55 years Blunt/penetrating trauma	Coefficients by regression analysis Different values for blunt or penetrating trauma
ASCOT	Survival probability Considers anatomy, physiology, age, blunt and penetrating trauma	RTS Anatomy profile component—ICD/AIS-85 Age (5 subclasses) Blunt/penetrating trauma Set aside: very severe or very minor injury	More variables for calculation of survival probability Better performance than TRISS for blunt and penetrating trauma

[a] A score of 1 is the worst prognosis.
[b] A score of 0 is the worst prognosis.
ABBREVIATIONS: AIS, Abbreviated Injury Scale; AIS-85, the fifth review of the Abbreviated Injury Scale; ASCOT, A Severity Characterization of Trauma[44]; GCS, Glasgow Coma Scale; ICD, International Classification of Diseases; ISS, Injury Severity Score[1,41]; MVA, motor vehicle accident; RTS, Revised Trauma Score[43]; TRISS, Trauma and the Injury Severity Score; TS, Trauma Score.[42]

Clinical, Administrative, and Management Uses of Scoring Systems

SCORING SYSTEMS IN RANDOMIZED CONTROLLED TRIALS AND OTHER CLINICAL RESEARCH

Clinical research in critical care often includes heterogeneous samples of critically ill patients. Severity-of-illness scores are commonly used to describe the acuity of illness so that readers can compare different studies and so that studies can be compared with a clinician's practice. Scoring systems are used in randomized controlled trials (RCTs) to describe severity of illness, to assess comparability at baseline of control and treatment groups, to assess the expected mortality, to determine sample size, and to perform stratified randomization. The success of randomization is often assessed by using scoring systems to confirm that the baseline characteristics of control and treatment groups were not significantly different.

In a randomized controlled trial, if the randomization is not balanced, then outcomes may be altered by the imbalance in baseline characteristics. In that instance, severity of illness scoring systems may be used to do an adjusted analysis (i.e., by adjusting groups for differing severity of illness and then calculating adjusted mortality). For example, very recently a large multicenter RCT of two different PEEP regimens in patients who have acute lung injury was reported. There was no difference in mortality between groups, but unfortunately age was significantly higher in the high PEEP group. Therefore, an adjusted analysis using age and severity of illness was done to adjust for differences in baseline characteristics and found no difference in adjusted mortality. Scoring systems are also used to determine the effect of the therapeutic intervention across different disease severity and mortality risk strata. In a study with no positive drug effect, finding efficacy in a subgroup of patients (e.g., in the sickest patients[47]) can be hypothesis-generating for new studies involving these sicker patients only. Finally, the clinicians reading the results of an RCT can compare the severity of disease of patients in the study with the severity of disease of patients in their practices to decide whether to use the new treatment.

SCORING SYSTEMS FOR ADMINISTRATIVE PURPOSES

The major purposes of scoring systems in administration are to describe utilization of ICU beds and resources, to describe acuity of illness, and to relate resource utilization (e.g., funding, drug utilization, and/or personnel) to acuity of care in an ICU. Resource utilization can be described, for example, by the Therapeutic Intervention Scoring System (TISS) score,[48,49] developed at the Massachusetts General Hospital in 1974. The purpose of TISS was to provide quantitative data to determine the severity of illness in individual patients, in order to determine appropriate utilization of intensive care facilities. TISS quantifies the amount of critical care provided to patients by measuring 76 nursing activities, monitoring techniques, resuscitation procedures, and technology. Each intervention is given 1 to 4 points. Therefore, TISS assesses severity of illness indirectly by the level of services provided to the patient. TISS was designed as a descriptor of the intensity of care, and was not designed specifically to predict outcome.

TISS scores have been used to categorize the level of care that patients require.[49,50] Beck and coworkers used TISS scores at ICU discharge as an objective assessment of the risk of premature discharge, and investigated the relationships of discharge time, TISS scores, and discharge destination on post-ICU mortality.[51] There was a significant association between increasing TISS scores and post-ICU mortality at ICU discharge (χ^2 for trend $= 0.90$, $p = 0.028$). Patients with high TISS scores (>30) who were treated in hospital wards had significantly increased severity-adjusted mortality risks compared with a comparable group of patients who were discharged to high-dependency units.

In addition, acuity of care can be correlated with indices of resource utilization.[52] Furthermore, reimbursement can be guided by assessment of severity of illness. For example, planning for ICU bed allocation, staffing, and budget can be aided by measures of admission numbers, diagnoses (e.g., diagnosis-related groups [DRGs] and case-mix groups [CMGs]), and severity of illness.

SCORING SYSTEMS TO ASSESS INTENSIVE CARE UNIT PERFORMANCE

Scoring systems can be used by ICUs to evaluate quality of care (quality assurance; see Chap. 3), to assess performance of an ICU over time, to assess performance of different intensivists, and to assess performances of different ICUs (see Table 6-1). The scoring systems provide a tool to normalize for differences in severity of illness of different samples of patients. Although quality assurance has largely been supplanted by newer approaches such as continuous quality improvement, severity-of-illness scoring systems nonetheless can be used to assess predicted and actual mortality. ICUs can review the outcomes of patients in general, or for specific disease categories, and compare the actual outcomes with predicted mortality. The performance of an ICU also can be followed over time. Evaluation of new technologies or new treatment modalities in an ICU also can be the object of continuous quality improvement evaluations.

There are potential problems associated with the use of scoring systems to compare actual with expected mortality in an ICU. For example, biases in the regression techniques used to calculate the risks of mortality can lead to situations in which hospitals providing care to more severely ill patients will tend to have actual mortality rates above predicted, and thus will appear to be giving suboptimal care. This occurs because most scoring systems underestimate mortality of high-risk patients. Also, medical and nursing interventions can improve physiologic data, leading to a lower estimated risk of mortality for the same patient.[53] The outcomes of individual intensivists can be adjusted for severity of illness to better assess performance. This is controversial for several reasons. First, patient sample size of the intensivist may be insufficient to draw legitimate conclusions regarding performance.[54] Second, ICU care is team care, including house officers and other caregivers, so outcomes are less influenced by the behavior of individual physicians.

Scoring systems can be used to compare ICUs in different hospital settings (tertiary care, community, academic, etc) and to compare ICUs of different countries. A comparison of New Zealand and U.S. hospitals demonstrated different patient selection and fewer admissions to ICUs in New Zealand, and yet hospital mortality rates were comparable.[55] A similar comparison between hospitals in Canada and in the United States revealed similar results.[56] However, important differences in mortality have been observed between pediatric ICUs in the United Kingdom and Australia. For comparable severity of illness, the mortality rates of critically ill children were higher in the United Kingdom than in Australia.[57]

Severity-of-illness scoring systems also can be used to assess ICU performance in different models of organization. For example, Carson and coworkers[58] evaluated the effects of changing from an "open" to a "closed" model of ICU care by dedicated intensivists by using a "before/after" study design. Patient severity of illness as assessed by APACHE II was greater, yet care costs were similar, and the ratio of actual to predicted mortality was lower after converting a medical ICU from open to closed care. Similar studies involving patients with sepsis demonstrated that changing ICU staffing to include physicians formally trained in critical care medicine reduced mortality.[59,60] Other examples of the use of scoring systems to assess ICU performance include studies of availability of ICU technology and studies of organizational practices and outcomes.[61]

Rapoport and coworkers[62] described a method to assess cost effectiveness of ICUs. A clinical performance index was defined as the difference between actual and MPM II predicted mortality. The economic performance (resource use) used a surrogate for costs: the "weighted hospital days," a length-of-stay index that weights ICU days more heavily than non-ICU days. Predicted resource use was calculated by a regression including severity of illness and percentage of surgical patients. The actual and predicted survival and actual and predicted resource use of hospitals were compared with the mean. A scatterplot illustrated which units were more than one standard deviation off for clinical and economic performance.

The cost effectiveness of ICUs should include nonmortality measures of effectiveness such as quality of life, return to independent living, and patient/family satisfaction.[63] These nonmortality measures of outcome need to be adjusted for ICU severity of illness by using severity-of-illness scoring systems.

SCORING SYSTEMS TO ASSESS INDIVIDUAL PATIENT PROGNOSIS AND TO GUIDE CARE

The assessment of individual patient prognosis is complex. Moreover, the use of severity-of-illness scoring systems for assessment and prediction of individual patient prognosis is controversial. We believe that management decisions cannot be based solely on prognosis as evaluated by the scoring systems. Assessment of individual patient prognosis influences decisions regarding triage of patients (i.e., ICU admission), decisions regarding intensity of care, and decisions to withhold and withdraw care.

Theoretically, a very accurate estimate of patient prognosis could be used to triage patients who have such a good prognosis that ICU admission would be unnecessary and inappropriate, and to identify patients who are so hopelessly ill that ICU admission would be futile and inappropriate. Scoring systems may complement physician judgment regarding appropriateness of ICU admission. However, it is important to emphasize that most scoring systems were derived from

patients already admitted to an ICU using data from the first 24 hours of ICU admission. The Mortality Probability Model (MPM II) might be more accurate and appropriate because MPM_0 used variables available immediately at ICU admission rather than the worst values of variables over the first 24 hours in the ICU. However, none of the commonly used scoring systems were validated for the purpose of triage of ICU patients.

Scoring systems have been used to assist in triage of patients to intermediate care (monitoring) or to intensive care (life support). Recently, APACHE III was modified to estimate the probability of need for life support of patients admitted for ICU monitoring.[64] Among 8040 ICU admissions for monitoring, 79% were predicted to have a low probability (<10%) for active treatment during their ICU stay. These patients were admitted to an intermediate care unit and 96% received no subsequent active treatment. The predictive equation had a ROC curve area of 0.74. There are scoring systems designed specifically for triage of trauma patients. The Triage Index[65] for trauma patients assesses injury severity and predicts an outcome using physiologic variables available before admission. The Trauma Score[42] and the Revised Trauma Score[43] are derived from the Triage Index. In the part of the Revised Trauma Score used for triage, the T-RTS, specific decision rules are proposed to indicate appropriate transfer to a trauma center.[43] These rules are based on the score and the GCS score. There are at least two caveats regarding use of scoring systems to guide ICU triage decisions. First, a patient who could be admitted to the ICU who has a very low probability of mortality estimated by the MPM_0, might in fact have a higher actual probability of mortality if ICU admission were denied,[20] because outcome could be adversely affected by ward admission and the associated lower intensity of monitoring and treatment. Second, physicians tend to underestimate mortality in low-risk patients. Thus scoring systems can be more accurate than clinician judgment for risk estimate of low-risk patients.[31]

A novel use of severity of illness scoring systems is in patient selection for specific therapies. The advent of a new therapy for severe sepsis, recombinant human activated protein C (rhAPC; drotrecogin alfa), is an example. In a multicenter RCT (the PROWESS trial), rhAPC significantly decreased mortality compared to placebo in treatment of severe sepsis.[40] Treatment with rhAPC activated was associated with a reduction in the relative risk of death of 19.4% (95% confidence interval [CI], 6.6 to 30.5) and an absolute reduction in the risk of death of 6.1% (31% vs. 25%, $p = 0.005$). The number needed to treat (NNT) with rhAPC was 16 to save 1 life. A post-hoc analysis of the study data performed by the FDA reported a differential benefit according to APACHE II score (Fig. 6-2); among patients with an APACHE II score of 25 or more, the relative risk of death among patients treated with rhAPC, as compared with those given placebo, was 0.71 (95% CI, 0.59 to 0.85), whereas among those with a score of 24 or less, the relative risk of death was 0.99 (95% CI, 0.75 to 1.30). Consequently, the FDA concluded, "efficacy of drotrecogin alfa has not been established in patients with lower risk of death (e.g., APACHE II scores <25),"[66] and the drug has not been approved for use in patients with lower severity of illness. Therefore, in the U.S. and in some other countries, regulatory and payer groups permit use of rhAPC only in patients who have severe sepsis and a high risk of death as defined by an APACHE II score greater

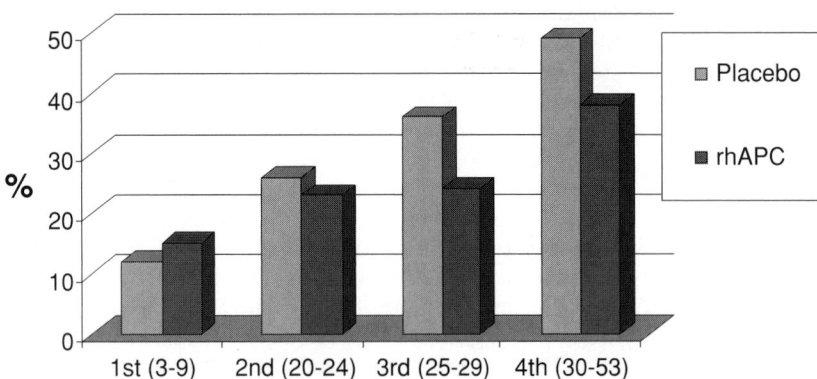

Mortality according to APACHE II Quartile

FIGURE 6-2 Data from PROWESS. Differential mortality benefit of rhAPC according to APACHE II quartile. In a subgroup analysis conducted by the U.S. Food and Drug Administration, the use of human recombinant activated protein C (rhAPC; drotrecogin alfa) was associated with a mortality benefit only in patients in the highest two quartiles of APACHE II. (*Data used by permission from Warren et al.*[123]).

than 25. In contrast, in Europe rhAPC was approved for use in patients who have severe sepsis and two or more organ dysfunctions *or* an APACHE II score greater than 25. These differing regulatory approvals and clinical practices likely reflect differences in how APACHE II scores can be used to make individual patient therapeutic decisions.

In support of this approach (i.e., use of APACHE II to identify high-risk patients), a cost-effectiveness analysis by Manns and coworkers[67] found that rhAPC is relatively cost effective when targeted to patients with severe sepsis, greater severity of illness (an APACHE II score of 25 or more), and a reasonable life expectancy if they survive the episode of sepsis. In a second cost-effectiveness analysis by Angus and coworkers, rhAPC cost $27,400 per quality-adjusted life-year when limited to patients with an APACHE II score ≥25, and was cost-ineffective when limited to patients with a score <25.[68] Clearly, the results of this subgroup analysis are dependent on the validity of the post hoc reanalysis performed by the FDA. Manns and coworkers concluded, "given the discrepancy between the published study results and the reanalysis, it would be reasonable to restrict the use of activated protein C to patients with an APACHE II score of 25 or more until convincing evidence of effectiveness and cost effectiveness in patients with less severe illness becomes available."[67]

There are several criticisms of using baseline APACHE II scores in individual patients to guide therapy.[69] First, the PROWESS trial was not powered to determine an efficacy difference among APACHE II subgroups. Even more importantly, the APACHE II disease severity scoring system was not designed and has not been validated for use to discriminate any parameter in the individual patient. Furthermore, the interobserver and intraobserver variability in the determination of APACHE II scores among experienced intensive care physicians may be as high as 10% to 15%.[70] To our knowledge, this is the only example of a proven therapy in critical care that is allocated based on an individual patient's APACHE II score.

Ethical Issues Relevant to Use of Scoring Systems to Guide Management

Use of severity-of-illness scoring systems to assist in decision making regarding withholding and withdrawal of care is

controversial for several reasons. First, scoring systems are designed to describe severity of illness and probability of death in groups of patients, not individual patients. Second, even in groups of patients, no system is perfectly calibrated and such systems cannot perfectly discriminate survivors from nonsurvivors. Third, scoring systems can guide care decisions only in the context of appropriate understanding of the ethical principles relevant to withholding and withdrawal of care.[71] Nonetheless, scoring systems could assist in deciding that ICU care is futile. Schneiderman and coworkers[72] proposed that "when physicians conclude (either through personal experience, experiences shared with colleagues, or considerations of published empirical data) that in the last 100 cases a treatment has been useless, they should regard that treatment as futile." Using this definition of futility, let us consider use of scoring systems and physician judgment to help predict futility. Calibration of APACHE III found that for an estimated mortality rate above 90%, the rate of correct classification was 85%, with a specificity of 99.8%. By comparison, for the same estimated mortality rate above 90% strata, physicians' predictions yield a correct classification of 70% to 76% and a specificity of 97% to 99%.[31,32] Thus APACHE III may be more accurate than physicians in predicting that a group of patients have a 90% chance of mortality. However, at a quantitative threshold of futility of less than 1% chance of survival, scoring systems are not precise enough. The highest precision of any scoring system to date was a 95% probability of death, meaning that 5% of patients with that score would survive[28] (Fig. 6-3). Therefore, severity-of-illness scoring systems may not accurately identify patients in whom ICU care is futile if futility is defined as less than 1% chance of survival. The SUPPORT study[73] (Study to Understand Prognoses and Preferences for Outcomes and Risks of Treatments) is important because it was designed to determine whether providing physicians with accurate predictions of death would change physician behavior, patient satisfaction, and decisions regarding care. SUPPORT was designed to estimate survival of seriously ill hospitalized patients who were not necessarily in an ICU. The SUPPORT[73] prognosis model includes nine diagnostic groups and the following 15 prognostic factors: disease group, 11 physiologic variables, age, history of malignancy, and the number of days the patient was hospitalized before study entry. In phase I of the study, the investigators noted shortcomings in communication, variability in frequency of aggressive treatment,

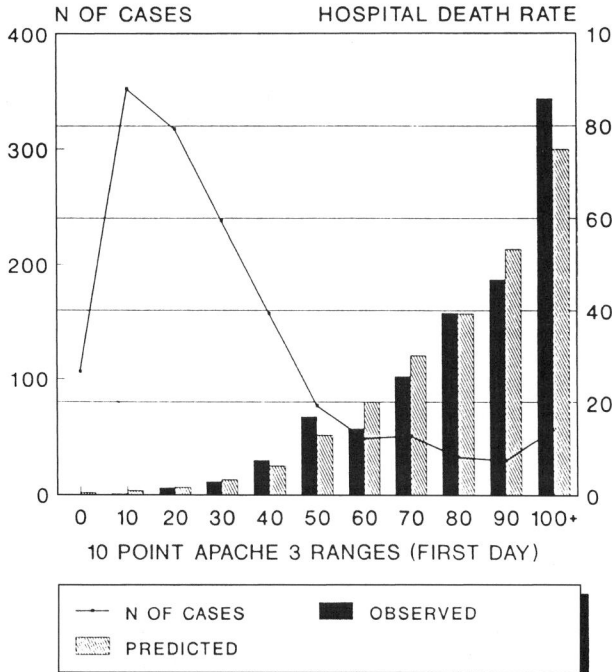

FIGURE 6-3 Relationship between first-day APACHE III score and risk of hospital mortality for trauma admissions to APACHE III study. With distribution of the sample into specific disease categories, the number of high risk of mortality patients used in the validation set is fairly low. In the highest score subset of patients, the mortality for these groups remains much lower than 99%. Also, severity-of-illness scoring systems are prone to underestimating the risk of mortality in high-risk patients. (*Reproduced with permission from Watts and Knaus.*[122])

and variability in care at the time of death (CPR, comfort care, pain management, etc). In phase II of the study[74] physicians in the intervention group received probability estimates of 6-month survival, outcome of cardiopulmonary resuscitation, and incidence of functional disability at 2 months. Specifically trained nurses made multiple contacts with the patients, families, physicians, and hospital staff to elicit preferences, improve understanding of outcomes, encourage attention to pain control, and facilitate advance care planning and patient-physician communication. Importantly, the phase II intervention did not improve care or patient outcomes. Patients experienced no improvement in patient-physician communication. Also, there was no change in the incidence or timing of written DNR (do not resuscitate) orders, physicians' knowledge of their patients' preferences not to be resuscitated, number of days spent in the ICU before death, or use of hospital resources. Thus the SUPPORT study showed that providing physicians with objective outcome predictions did not change physicians' attitudes and behavior.

Several observations suggest that there is a gap between scoring system predicted outcome and decisions to withhold and withdraw ICU care. Patients in whom care was withdrawn in a medical ICU had APACHE II predicted mortality on the day of ICU admission of only 61% ± 22%.[75] Furthermore, patients with prolonged multiorgan system failure who continue to require life support generally do not have very abnormal physiologic parameters[54] and thus have

relatively low APS scores. Finally, an increasing proportion of critically ill patients in ICUs die without CPR (cardiopulmonary resuscitation),[76] and many die after withholding or withdrawal of care.

A major portion of ICU resources is spent on patients who have minimal chances of survival. However, until a public consensus is reached about dealing with these very difficult issues,[77] broad ethical principles of beneficence, nonmalfeasance, and autonomy are likely to be more important components of end-of-life decisions than quantitative data provided by scoring systems. Broader social and economic policy issues should be separate concerns.

Sources of Error and Bias in Scoring Systems

Severity-of-illness scoring systems are not perfect, partially because of error and bias. Error and bias limit the reproducibility of scoring systems outside the original sample of patients, and thus limit the applicability of scoring systems to different clinical situations. Specifically, bias of scoring systems can be related to the selection of included variables, to the collection of data, to the lead time before the onset of the acute disease and admission of the patient to the ICU, to the imprecision in choosing a principal admission diagnosis, to the inaccuracy of certain scoring systems for specific disease categories, and finally to the use of scoring systems for purposes they were not meant to accomplish.

BIAS RELATED TO THE SELECTION OF VARIABLES AND TO THE COLLECTION OF DATA

Variables can be included in a severity-of-illness score by a multivariate analysis that shows that each variable is a statistically independent predictor of mortality. Alternatively, variables can be selected by consensus of experts. Consensus panel selection of variables is subjective, and variables can be interrelated.[15] The problem with interrelated variables is that two such variables are not independent of each other as predictors of mortality. Noncontinuous variables increase error in the computation of risk of mortality. Noncontinuous variables are classified as present or absent, so a single misclassification results in a large error in outcome prediction.[15]

Detection bias is another cause of bias of the included variables. *Detection bias* means that variables are only detected if measured. However, because scoring systems use variables measured in clinical practice, not all variables will be measured on all patients on all days. Therefore, in several scoring systems, unmeasured (undetected) variables are assigned a normal value. The assumption that unmeasured physiologic variables are normal can underestimate the risk of mortality. APACHE II, APACHE III, and SAPS II contain some variables that are not used routinely in daily care, such as albumin and bilirubin levels.

Use of the worst value of a variable in 24 hours also causes errors. Most scoring systems use the worst value of a variable in a 24-hour period. However, selection of the worst value can be subjective. There are other errors associated with collection of data, including temperature conversion from Fahrenheit to Celsius, creatinine conversion to the international system, use of the Glasgow Coma Scale on deeply sedated patients,[54]

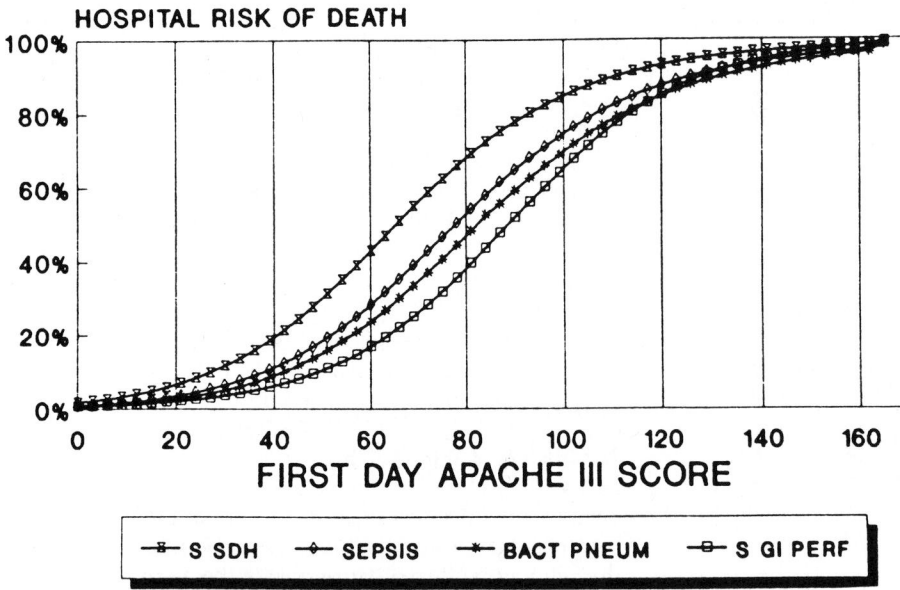

FIGURE 6-4 The influence of the choice of a single disease category for the prediction of hospital risk of death in APACHE III. Relationship between APACHE III score and predicted risk of hospital death for patients with postoperative subdural hematomas (S SDH), sepsis (other than urinary tract), bacterial pneumonia (BACT PNEUM), and postoperative gastrointestinal perforation (S GI PERF). The same APACHE III score can lead to different estimated hospital risk of death, depending on the choice of main diagnosis. (*Reproduced with permission from Knaus et al.[19]*)

transcription errors, and errors in analysis of data. Direct computer data entry may decrease transcription error.

BIAS RELATED TO POOR CALIBRATION

Statistical regression in scoring systems has a propensity for poor calibration. Regression techniques tend to underpredict the likelihood of death of more severely ill patients, and tend to overpredict the likelihood of death of patients with less severe illness (Fig. 6-3). These errors can create a pernicious bias. For example, hospitals providing care to more severely ill patients will tend to have actual mortality rates above predicted, and thus will appear to be giving poor care. On the other hand, hospitals with less severely ill patients will tend to have actual mortality rates lower than predicted, and will appear to be giving better than average care.[78]

LEAD-TIME BIAS

Lead-time bias refers to the different lengths of time that patients are ill prior to ICU care and scoring. Lead-time differences also influence mortality. Acute physiology scores do not assess previous treatments. Thus, for the same score, a patient hypoxemic in the emergency room can improve rapidly and have a better outcome than a patient referred from another hospital for persistent hypoxemia. Because of lead-time bias, APACHE II underestimates the mortality of patients referred from other ICUs,[25] other hospitals, or even within other parts of the same hospital.[15] APACHE III contains a variable to assess patient location and treatment prior to ICU admission in an attempt to minimize lead-time bias.

Therapies provided prior to and immediately after ICU admission change physiologic variables and thus influence physiologic scores. Rapid and successful resuscitation in the emergency department prior to ICU admission or early in the ICU will hide abnormally low values of variables that would have been recorded as the worst over 24 hours. Theoretically, poor care would increase physiologic scores and increase predicted mortality rate, whereas good care would decrease scores and reduce predicted mortality rate.[78] The ef-

fects of treatment can be minimized and mortality prediction might be enhanced by using hospital presentation data.

IMPRECISE PRINCIPAL DIAGNOSIS

Inaccurate diagnosis is another source of error in many scoring systems. Some scoring systems (e.g., APACHE III) adjust for the differing prognoses of patients who have different diseases but similar physiologic abnormalities. Accurate diagnosis can be difficult in the critically ill for several reasons. First, patients in the ICU often suffer from several conditions. APACHE II and APACHE III require identification of one diagnosis or organ failure that prompted ICU admission. Consider a patient with bacterial pneumonia and sepsis who is admitted to the ICU. In APACHE III, patients who have bacterial pneumonia and patients who have sepsis who have similar physiologic scores have different predicted mortality (see Fig. 6-4). Thus the assignment of appropriate diagnosis is very important in making an accurate mortality prediction.[15] The principal diagnosis could differ between prospective identification versus retrospective chart review.[54]

SEVERITY-OF-ILLNESS SCORING SYSTEMS FOR SPECIFIC DISEASE CATEGORIES

For patients with specific disease processes, it is debated whether specific severity scoring systems are better than general ones. Because inaccuracy of diagnosis can cause error, we recommend that scoring systems be tested for different diagnostic categories. Both disease-specific systems (APACHE II and APACHE III) and non–disease-specific systems (SAPS II and MPM II) need to be compared in external validating patient samples.[15]

APACHE II, APACHE III, and SAPS II have performed well in several disease-specific categories, including liver failure,[79,80] malignancy,[81–83] cardiac bypass surgery,[84–86] sepsis,[87] peritonitis,[88–90] pancreatitis,[91–97] acute myocardial infarction,[98–101] HIV patients,[102,103] obstetric patients,[104] and stroke.[105] APACHE III performed well in head-injured patients.[106,107] In general, the performance of APACHE II,

APACHE III, and SAPS II for these disease processes was similar to that reported for heterogeneous ICU patients.

APACHE II and III have consistently performed poorly in trauma,[46,108,109] in postoperative patients,[110,111] and in women with eclampsia.[112]

INACCURACY OF SCORING SYSTEMS FOR CERTAIN TYPES OF INTENSIVE CARE UNITS OR DIFFERENT GEOGRAPHIC REGIONS

The patient sample used to derive and validate a scoring system can influence the mortality predictions. There are potentially important differences in outcomes of comparable patients in community versus teaching hospitals, in different regions of a country, and in different countries because of the influence of health care funding and policy. For example, a comparison of New Zealand and U.S. hospitals demonstrated different patient selection and fewer ICU admissions in New Zealand, and yet found similar hospital mortality.[55]

Some investigators have used scoring systems to compare critical care in different countries but came to sharply different conclusions. For example, Sirio and coworkers[113] used APACHE II to compare Japan and the United States. Despite an ROC curve area of only 0.78 in the Japanese patient sample, they concluded that APACHE II performs well in Japan. In contrast, the Intensive Care Society APACHE II study[114] examined 8724 critically ill patients and reported that crude death rates in hospital varied more than twofold between intensive care units in Britain and Ireland. Application of the APACHE II equation produced an ROC value of 0.83 and failed to explain outcome in four intensive care units. They concluded that the American APACHE II equation did not fit their data uniformly, and cited systematic differences in medical definitions and diagnostic labeling, diagnostic mix, measurement of physiologic variables, effectiveness of treatment, and differences in age-specific health status between the two countries.

The performance of APACHE III has been assessed in several countries including Brazil,[115] the United Kingdom,[116] Korea,[117] and Australia.[118] In most countries, the observed hospital mortality was significantly higher than the APACHE III predicted mortality rate. In the Australian study, when the model was corrected for hospital characteristics, the observed hospital mortality rate was not different. The area under the ROC curve was 0.92. The APACHE III mortality model, when adjusted for hospital characteristics had good discrimination and calibration in the Australian adult ICU population.

Recommendations for Clinical Use

There has been rapid growth in the number and types of severity-of-illness scoring systems in critical care, and they are increasingly used for clinical research, administrative tasks, quality assurance, and individual patient prognosis. Therefore, physicians and administrators must understand the principles underlying development and testing of these systems, as well as the sources of errors in their development, to interpret the literature and to decide how and which system to use. We recommend four uses of severity-of-illness scoring systems. First, scoring systems are useful in clinical trials and in clinical research. The scoring system used must be validated and published in peer-reviewed literature.

When researchers and clinicians have a common language for description of severity of illness, clinicians can compare the patients in studies with the patients in their own practices to decide how the results of the studies influence their own practices.

Second, scoring systems may be used for administrative purposes, to describe resource utilization relative to acuity of illness, and to assist with resource-allocation decisions.

The third potential use of scoring systems is to assess ICU performance. However, several biases limit this application because very little is known about accuracy of generalizations of scoring systems to different categories of hospitals, hospitals from different countries with different health care systems, or even different ICUs in the same hospital. Therefore, we believe that use of scoring systems to compare ICU performance is limited and requires further evaluation.

The fourth potential use of scoring systems is to assess individual patient prognosis and to guide care. We believe that scoring systems have limited use for individual patient prognosis and care decisions. At best, they can guide physicians, families, and patients in difficult decisions. Patients' preferences and patients' quality of life prior to ICU admission cannot be integrated into mathematical models. Severity-of-illness scoring systems predict probability of mortality, but they are not helpful in assessing probability of death in the 6 months following discharge from the ICU. Finally, scoring systems do not predict quality of life or return to independent living of patients.

References

1. Baker SP, O'Neill B, Haddon W Jr, et al: The injury severity score: a method for describing patients with multiple injuries and evaluating emergency care. *J Trauma* 14:187, 1974.
2. Boyd CR, Tolson MA, Copes WS: Evaluating trauma care: The TRISS method. Trauma Score and the Injury Severity Score. *J Trauma* 27:370, 1987.
3. Feller I, Tholen D, Cornell RG: Improvements in burn care, 1965 to 1979. *JAMA* 244:2074, 1980.
4. Fowler AA, Hamman RF, Zerbe GO, et al: Adult respiratory distress syndrome. Prognosis after onset. *Am Rev Respir Dis* 132:472, 1985.
5. Le Gall JR, Lemeshow S, Leleu G, et al: Customized probability models for early severe sepsis in adult intensive care patients. Intensive Care Unit Scoring Group. *JAMA* 273:644, 1995.
6. Schwartz S, Cullen DJ: How many intensive care beds does your hospital need? *Crit Care Med* 9:625, 1974.
7. Vincent JL, de Mendonca A, Cantraine F, et al: Use of the SOFA score to assess the incidence of organ dysfunction/failure in intensive care units: Results of a multicenter, prospective study. Working group on "sepsis-related problems" of the European Society of Intensive Care Medicine. *Crit Care Med* 26:1793, 1998.
8. Antonelli M, Moreno R, Vincent JL, et al: Application of SOFA score to trauma patients. Sequential Organ Failure Assessment. *Intensive Care Med* 25:389, 1999.
9. Russell JA, Singer J, Bernard GR, et al: Changing pattern of organ dysfunction in early human sepsis is related to mortality. *Crit Care Med* 28:3405, 2000.
10. Cryer HG, Leong K, McArthur DL, et al: Multiple organ failure: By the time you predict it, it's already there. *J Trauma* 46:597, 1999; discussion 604.
11. Hutchinson C, Craig S, Ridley S: Sequential organ scoring as a measure of effectiveness of critical care. *Anaesthesia* 55:1149, 2000.

12. Ruttimann UE: Statistical approaches to development and validation of predictive instruments. *Crit Care Clin* 10:19, 1994.

13. Ferreira FL, Bota DP, Bross A, et al Serial evaluation of the SOFA score to predict outcome in critically ill patients. *JAMA* 286:1754, 2001.

14. Ridley S: Severity of illness scoring systems and performance appraisal. *Anaesthesia* 53:1185, 1998.

15. Cowen JS, Kelley MA: Errors and bias in using predictive scoring systems. *Crit Care Clin* 10:53, 1994.

16. Hanley JA, McNeil BJ: The meaning and use of the area under a receiver operating characteristic (ROC) curve. *Radiology* 143:29, 1982.

17. Lemeshow S, Hosmer DW Jr: A review of goodness of fit statistics for use in the development of logistic regression models. *Am J Epidemiol* 115:92, 1982.

18. Knaus WA, Draper EA, Wagner DP, et al: APACHE II: A severity of disease classification system. *Crit Care Med* 13:818, 1985.

19. Knaus WA, Wagner DP, Draper EA, et al: The APACHE III prognostic system. Risk prediction of hospital mortality for critically ill hospitalized adults. *Chest* 100:1619, 1991.

20. Lemeshow S, Teres D, Klar J, et al: Mortality Probability Models (MPM II) based on an international cohort of intensive care unit patients. *JAMA* 270:2478, 1993.

21. Le Gall JR, Lemeshow S, Saulnier F. A new Simplified Acute Physiology Score (SAPS II) based on a European/North American multicenter study. *JAMA* 270:2957, 1993.

22. Vincent JL, Moreno R, Takala J, et al: The SOFA (Sepsis-related Organ Failure Assessment) score to describe organ dysfunction/failure. On behalf of the Working Group on Sepsis-Related Problems of the European Society of Intensive Care Medicine. *Intensive Care Med* 22:707, 1996.

23. Pollack MM, Ruttimann UE, Getson PR: Pediatric risk of mortality (PRISM) score. *Crit Care Med* 16:1110, 1988.

24. Marik PE, Varon J: Severity scoring and outcome assessment. Computerized predictive models and scoring systems. *Crit Care Clin* 15:633, viii, 1999.

25. Dragsted L, Jorgensen J, Jensen NH, et al: Interhospital comparisons of patient outcome from intensive care: Importance of lead-time bias. *Crit Care Med* 17:418, 1989.

26. Lemeshow S, Teres D, Avrunin JS, et al: Refining intensive care unit outcome prediction by using changing probabilities of mortality. *Crit Care Med* 16:470, 1988.

27. Lemeshow S, Klar J, Teres D, et al: Mortality probability models for patients in the intensive care unit for 48 or 72 hours: A prospective, multicenter study. *Crit Care Med* 22:1351, 1994.

28. Wagner DP, Knaus WA, Harrell FE, et al: Daily prognostic estimates for critically ill adults in intensive care units: Results from a prospective, multicenter, inception cohort analysis. *Crit Care Med* 22:1359, 1994.

29. Castella X, Artigas A, Bion J, et al: A comparison of severity of illness scoring systems for intensive care unit patients: Results of a multicenter, multinational study. The European/North American Severity Study Group. *Crit Care Med* 23:1327, 1995.

30. Beck DH, Taylor BL, Millar B, et al: Prediction of outcome from intensive care: A prospective cohort study comparing Acute Physiology and Chronic Health Evaluation II and III prognostic systems in a United Kingdom intensive care unit. *Crit Care Med* 25:9, 1997.

31. Brannen AL 2nd, Godfrey LJ, Goetter WE: Prediction of outcome from critical illness. A comparison of clinical judgment with a prediction rule. *Arch Intern Med* 149:1083, 1989.

32. Kruse JA, Thill-Baharozian MC, Carlson RW: Comparison of clinical assessment with APACHE II for predicting mortality risk in patients admitted to a medical intensive care unit. *JAMA* 260:1739, 1988.

33. McClish DK, Powell SH: How well can physicians estimate mortality in a medical intensive care unit? *Med Decis Making* 9:125, 1989.

34. Poses RM, Bekes C, Winkler RL, et al: Are two (inexperienced) heads better than one (experienced) head? Averaging house officers' prognostic judgments for critically ill patients. *Arch Intern Med* 150:1874, 1990.

35. Marshall JC, Cook DJ, Christou NV, et al: Multiple organ dysfunction score: A reliable descriptor of a complex clinical outcome. *Crit Care Med* 23:1638, 1995.

36. Le Gall JR, Klar J, Lemeshow S, et al: The Logistic Organ Dysfunction system. A new way to assess organ dysfunction in the intensive care unit. ICU Scoring Group. *JAMA* 276:802, 1996.

37. Peres Bota D, Melot C, Lopes Ferreira F, et al: The Multiple Organ Dysfunction Score (MODS) versus the Sequential Organ Failure Assessment (SOFA) score in outcome prediction. *Intensive Care Med* 28:1619, 2002.

38. Dellinger RP, Opal SM, Rotrosen D, et al: From the bench to the bedside: the future of sepsis research. Executive summary of an American College of Chest Physicians, National Institute of Allergy and Infectious Disease, and National Heart, Lung, and Blood Institute Workshop. *Chest* 111:744, 1997.

39. Ventilation with lower tidal volumes as compared with traditional tidal volumes for acute lung injury and the acute respiratory distress syndrome. The Acute Respiratory Distress Syndrome Network. *N Engl J Med* 342:1301, 2000.

40. Bernard GR, Vincent JL, Laterre PF, et al: Efficacy and safety of recombinant human activated protein C for severe sepsis. *N Engl J Med* 344:699, 2001.

41. Baker SP, O'Neill B: The injury severity score: An update. *J Trauma* 16:882, 1976.

42. Champion HR, Sacco WJ, Carnazzo AJ, et al: Trauma score. *Crit Care Med* 9:672, 1981.

43. Champion HR, Sacco WJ, Copes WS, et al: A revision of the Trauma Score. *J Trauma* 29:623, 1989.

44. Champion HR, Copes WS, Sacco WJ, et al: A new characterization of injury severity. *J Trauma* 30:539, 1990; discussion 545.

45. Vassar MJ, Wilkerson CL, Duran PJ, et al: Comparison of APACHE II, TRISS, and a proposed 24-hour ICU point system for prediction of outcome in ICU trauma patients. *J Trauma* 32:490, 1992; discussion 499.

46. Vassar MJ, Holcroft JW: The case against using the APACHE system to predict intensive care unit outcome in trauma patients. *Crit Care Clin* 10:117, 1994; discussion 127.

47. Knaus WA, Harrell FE Jr, LaBrecque JF, et al: Use of predicted risk of mortality to evaluate the efficacy of anticytokine therapy in sepsis. The rhIL-1ra Phase III Sepsis Syndrome Study Group. *Crit Care Med* 24:46, 1996.

48. Cullen DJ, Civetta JM, Briggs BA, et al: Therapeutic intervention scoring system: A method for quantitative comparison of patient care. *Crit Care Med* 2:57, 1974.

49. Keene AR, Cullen DJ: Therapeutic Intervention Scoring System: update 1983. *Crit Care Med* 11:1, 1983.

50. Malstam J, Lind L: Therapeutic intervention scoring system (TISS)—a method for measuring workload and calculating costs in the ICU. *Acta Anaesthesiol Scand* 36:758, 1992.

51. Beck DH, McQuillan P, Smith GB: Waiting for the break of dawn? The effects of discharge time, discharge TISS scores and discharge facility on hospital mortality after intensive care. *Intensive Care Med* 28:1287, 2002.

52. Noseworthy TW, Konopad E, Shustack A, et al: Cost accounting of adult intensive care: methods and human and capital inputs. *Crit Care Med* 24:1168, 1996.

53. Boyd O, Grounds RM: Physiological scoring systems and audit. *Lancet* 341:1573, 1993.

54. Teres D, Lemeshow S. Why severity models should be used with caution. *Crit Care Clin* 10:93, 1994; discussion 111.

55. Zimmerman JE, Knaus WA, Judson JA, et al: Patient selection for intensive care: A comparison of New Zealand and United States hospitals. *Crit Care Med* 16:318, 1988.

56. Rapoport J, Teres D, Barnett R, et al: A comparison of intensive care unit utilization in Alberta and western Massachusetts. *Crit Care Med* 23:1336, 1995.

57. Pearson G, Shann F, Barry P, et al: Should paediatric intensive care be centralised? Trent versus Victoria. *Lancet* 349:1213, 1997.

58. Carson SS, Stocking C, Podsadecki T, et al. Effects of organizational change in the medical intensive care unit of a teaching hospital: a comparison of 'open' and 'closed' formats. *JAMA* 276:322, 1996.

59. Reynolds HN, Haupt MT, Thill-Baharozian MC, et al: Impact of critical care physician staffing on patients with septic shock in a university hospital medical intensive care unit. *JAMA* 260:3446, 1988.

60. Brown JJ, Sullivan G: Effect on ICU mortality of a full-time critical care specialist. *Chest* 96:127, 1989.

61. Zimmerman JE, Shortell SM, Rousseau DM, et al: Improving intensive care: Observations based on organizational case studies in nine intensive care units: a prospective, multicenter study. *Crit Care Med* 21:1443, 1993.

62. Rapoport J, Teres D, Lemeshow S, et al: A method for assessing the clinical performance and cost-effectiveness of intensive care units: A multicenter inception cohort study. *Crit Care Med* 22:1385, 1994.

63. Sherck JP, Shatney CH: ICU scoring systems do not allow prediction of patient outcomes or comparison of ICU performance. *Crit Care Clin* 12:515, 1996.

64. Zimmerman JE, Wagner DP, Knaus WA, et al: The use of risk predictions to identify candidates for intermediate care units. Implications for intensive care utilization and cost. *Chest* 108:490, 1995.

65. Champion HR, Sacco WJ, Hannan DS, et al: Assessment of injury severity: The triage index. *Crit Care Med* 8:201, 1980.

66. Xigris package insert. Indianapolis, Eli Lilly and Company, 2001.

67. Manns BJ, Lee H, Doig CJ, et al: An economic evaluation of activated protein C treatment for severe sepsis. *N Engl J Med* 347:993, 2002.

68. Angus DC, Linde-Zwirble WT, Clermont G, et al: Cost-effectiveness of drotrecogin alfa (activated) in the treatment of severe sepsis. *Crit Care Med* 31:1, 2003.

69. Morris PE, Light RB, Garber GE: Identifying patients with severe sepsis who should not be treated with drotrecogin alfa (activated). *Am J Surg* 184:S19, 2002.

70. Polderman KH, Jorna EM, Girbes AR: Inter-observer variability in APACHE II scoring: Effect of strict guidelines and training. *Intensive Care Med* 27:1365, 2001.

71. Luce JM, Wachter RM: The ethical appropriateness of using prognostic scoring systems in clinical management. *Crit Care Clin* 10:229, 1994.

72. Schneiderman LJ, Jecker NS, Jonsen AR: Medical futility: its meaning and ethical implications. *Ann Intern Med* 112:949, 1990.

73. Knaus WA, Harrell FE Jr, Lynn J, et al: The SUPPORT prognostic model. Objective estimates of survival for seriously ill hospitalized adults. Study to understand prognoses and preferences for outcomes and risks of treatments. *Ann Intern Med* 122:191, 1995.

74. The SUPPORT Principal Investigators for the SUPPORT Project; A controlled trial to improve care for seriously ill hospitalized patients: The study to understand prognoses and preferences for outcomes and risks of treatments (SUPPORT). *JAMA* 274:1591, 1995.

75. Lee DK, Swinburne AJ, Fedullo AJ, et al: Withdrawing care. Experience in a medical intensive care unit. *JAMA* 271:1358, 1994.

76. Prendergast TJ, Luce JM: Increasing incidence of withholding and withdrawal of life support from the critically ill. *Am J Respir Crit Care Med* 155:15, 1997.

77. Youngner SJ: Who defines futility? *JAMA* 260:2094, 1988.

78. Selker HP: Systems for comparing actual and predicted mortality rates: Characteristics to promote cooperation in improving hospital care. *Ann Intern Med* 118:820, 1993.

79. Zauner CA, Apsner RC, Kranz A, et al: Outcome prediction for patients with cirrhosis of the liver in a medical ICU: A comparison of the APACHE scores and liver-specific scoring systems. *Intensive Care Med* 22:559, 1996.

80. Chatzicostas C, Roussomoustakaki M, Notas G, et al: A comparison of Child-Pugh, APACHE II and APACHE III scoring systems in predicting hospital mortality of patients with liver cirrhosis. *BMC Gastroenterol* 3:7, 2003.

81. Sculier JP, Paesmans M, Markiewicz E, et al: Scoring systems in cancer patients admitted for an acute complication in a medical intensive care unit. *Crit Care Med* 28:2786, 2000.

82. Staudinger T, Stoiser B, Mullner M, et al: Outcome and prognostic factors in critically ill cancer patients admitted to the intensive care unit. *Crit Care Med* 28:1322, 2000.

83. Guiguet M, Blot F, Escudier B, et al: Severity-of-illness scores for neutropenic cancer patients in an intensive care unit: Which is the best predictor? Do multiple assessment times improve the predictive value? *Crit Care Med* 26:488, 1998.

84. Shaughnessy TE, Mickler TA: Does Acute Physiologic and Chronic Health Evaluation (APACHE II) scoring predict need for prolonged support after coronary revascularization? *Anesth Analg* 81:24, 1995.

85. Becker RB, Zimmerman JE, Knaus WA, et al: The use of APACHE III to evaluate ICU length of stay, resource use, and mortality after coronary artery by-pass surgery. *J Cardiovasc Surg (Torino)* 36:1, 1995.

86. Kern H, Redlich U, Hotz H, et al: Risk factors for prolonged ventilation after cardiac surgery using APACHE II, SAPS II, and TISS: comparison of three different models. *Intensive Care Med* 27:407, 2001.

87. Pittet D, Thievent B, Wenzel RP, et al: Bedside prediction of mortality from bacteremic sepsis. A dynamic analysis of ICU patients. *Am J Respir Crit Care Med* 153:684, 1996.

88. McLauchlan GJ, Anderson ID, Grant IS, et al: Outcome of patients with abdominal sepsis treated in an intensive care unit. *Br J Surg* 82:524, 1995.

89. Ohmann C, Hau T: Prognostic indices in peritonitis. *Hepatogastroenterology* 44:937, 1997.

90. Bosscha K, Reijnders K, Hulstaert PF, et al: Prognostic scoring systems to predict outcome in peritonitis and intra-abdominal sepsis. *Br J Surg* 84:1532, 1997.

91. Gates LK Jr: Severity scoring for acute pancreatitis: Where do we stand in 1999? *Curr Gastroenterol Rep* 1:134, 1999.

92. Soran A, Chelluri L, Lee KK, et al: Outcome and quality of life of patients with acute pancreatitis requiring intensive care. *J Surg Res* 91:89, 2000.

93. Halonen KI, Pettila V, Leppaniemi AK, et al: Multiple organ dysfunction associated with severe acute pancreatitis. *Crit Care Med* 30:1274, 2002.

94. Chatzicostas C, Roussomoustakaki M, Vlachonikolis IG, et al: Comparison of Ranson, APACHE II and APACHE III scoring systems in acute pancreatitis. *Pancreas* 25:331, 2002.

95. Khan AA, Parekh D, Cho Y, et al: Improved prediction of outcome in patients with severe acute pancreatitis by the APACHE II score at 48 hours after hospital admission compared with the APACHE II score at admission. Acute Physiology and Chronic Health Evaluation. *Arch Surg* 137:1136, 2002.

96. Liu TH, Kwong KL, Tamm EP, et al: Acute pancreatitis in intensive care unit patients: Value of clinical and radiologic prognosticators at predicting clinical course and outcome. *Crit Care Med* 31:1026, 2003.

97. Imrie CW: Prognostic indicators in acute pancreatitis. *Can J Gastroenterol* 17:325, 2003.

98. Ludwigs U, Hulting J: Acute Physiology and Chronic Health Evaluation II scoring system in acute myocardial infarction: A prospective validation study. *Crit Care Med* 23:854, 1995.

99. Reina A, Vazquez G, Aguayo E, et al: Mortality discrimination in acute myocardial infarction: Comparison between APACHE III and SAPS II prognosis systems. PAEEC Group. *Intensive Care Med* 23:326, 1997.

100. Ludwigs U, Csatlos M, Hulting J: Predicting in-hospital mortality in acute myocardial infarction: Impact of thrombolytic therapy on APACHE II performance. *Scand Cardiovasc J* 34:371, 2000.

101. Chiang HT, Lin SL, Hsu HC, et al: Prediction of in-hospital mortality in patients with myocardial infarction using APACHE II system. *Zhonghua Yi Xue Za Zhi (Taipei)* 64:501, 2001.

102. Brown MC, Crede WB: Predictive ability of acute physiology and chronic health evaluation II scoring applied to human immunodeficiency virus-positive patients. *Crit Care Med* 23:848, 1995.

103. Casalino E, Mendoza-Sassi G, Wolff M, et al: Predictors of short- and long-term survival in HIV-infected patients admitted to the ICU. *Chest* 113:421, 1998.

104. el-Solh AA, Grant BJ: A comparison of severity of illness scoring systems for critically ill obstetric patients. *Chest* 110:1299, 1996.

105. Navarrete-Navarro P, Rivera-Fernandez R, Lopez-Mutuberria MT, et al: Outcome prediction in terms of functional disability and mortality at 1 year among ICU-admitted severe stroke patients: A prospective epidemiological study in the south of the European Union (Evascan Project, Andalusia, Spain). *Intensive Care Med* 29:1237, 2003.

106. Cho DY, Wang YC, Lee MJ: Comparison of APACHE III, II and the Glasgow Coma Scale for prediction of mortality in a neurosurgical intensive care unit. *Clin Intensive Care* 6:9, 1995.

107. Cho DY, Wang YC: Comparison of the APACHE III, APACHE II and Glasgow Coma Scale in acute head injury for prediction of mortality and functional outcome. *Intensive Care Med* 23:77, 1997.

108. Muckart DJ, Bhagwanjee S, Neijenhuis PA: Prediction of the risk of death by APACHE II scoring in critically ill trauma patients without head injury. *Br J Surg* 83:1123, 1996.

109. Muckart DJ, Bhagwanjee S, Gouws E: Validation of an outcome prediction model for critically ill trauma patients without head injury. *J Trauma* 43:934, 1997; discussion 938.

110. Lertakyamanee J, Somprakit P, Vorakitpokaton P, et al: APACHE II in a postoperative intensive care unit in Thailand. *J Med Assoc Thai* 80:169, 1997.

111. McNelis J, Marini C, Kalimi R, et al: A comparison of predictive outcomes of APACHE II and SAPS II in a surgical intensive care unit. *Am J Med Qual* 16:161, 2001.

112. Bhagwanjee S, Paruk F, Moodley J, et al: Intensive care unit morbidity and mortality from eclampsia: An evaluation of the Acute Physiology and Chronic Health Evaluation II score and the Glasgow Coma Scale score. *Crit Care Med* 28:120, 2000.

113. Sirio CA, Tajimi K, Tase C, et al: An initial comparison of intensive care in Japan and the United States. *Crit Care Med* 20:1207, 1992.

114. Rowan KM, Kerr JH, Major E, et al: Intensive Care Society's APACHE II study in Britain and Ireland—II: Outcome comparisons of intensive care units after adjustment for case mix by the American APACHE II method. *BMJ* 307:977, 1993.

115. Bastos PG, Sun X, Wagner DP, et al: Application of the APACHE III prognostic system in Brazilian intensive care units: a prospective multicenter study. *Intensive Care Med* 22:564, 1996.

116. Pappachan JV, Millar B, Bennett ED, et al: Comparison of outcome from intensive care admission after adjustment for case mix by the APACHE III prognostic system. *Chest* 115:802, 1999.

117. Ihnsook J, Myunghee K, Jungsoon K: Predictive accuracy of severity scoring system: A prospective cohort study using APACHE III in a Korean intensive care unit. *Int J Nurs Stud* 40:219, 2003.

118. Cook DA: Performance of APACHE III models in an Australian ICU. *Chest* 118:1732, 2000.

119. Warren HS, Suffredini AF, Eichacker PQ, et al: Risks and benefits of activated protein C treatment for severe sepsis. *N Engl J Med* 347:1027, 2002.

120. Watts CM, Knaus WA: The case for using objective scoring systems to predict intensive care unit outcome. *Crit Care Clin* 10:73, 1994; discussion 91.

Chapter 7

TRANSPORTATION OF THE CRITICALLY ILL PATIENT

IRA J. BLUMEN
FRANK THOMAS
DAVID WILLIAMS

KEY POINTS

- *The objective of critical care transport is to provide an equivalent or higher degree of monitoring and medical care than the patient was receiving prior to transport.*
- *Each contemplated transport requires an evaluation of the risks and benefits of the transport.*
- *The risks to the patient during interhospital and intrahospital transport can be minimized through careful planning, use of appropriately qualified personnel, selection of appropriate transport equipment, and proper patient evaluation and stabilization.*
- *For interfacility transport, the referring physician is responsible for the transport-related decisions. It is common and appropriate for the receiving physician or critical care transport specialist to make recommendations regarding the mode of transport or need for specialty personnel or equipment.*

In recent years, advances in bedside capabilities, diagnostics, and therapeutic interventions have dramatically improved care for critically ill and injured patients. In addition, comprehensive critical care units are no longer limited to academic and urban tertiary care centers, and have expanded to other clinical settings in suburban and rural areas. Despite these advances, the movement of critical patients may still be required for optimal patient care.

Transport of critically ill patients may be divided into two categories: transport within the hospital (intrahospital) and transport between hospitals (interhospital). Despite the evolution in the bedside management of critical patients, it is anticipated that the number of critical patients who will need to be moved from one location to another will not diminish. Patients in outlying hospitals will need to be transferred to critical care centers, and patients in critical care units may require transfer to intermediate or special care units. Also, with continued advances in medical technology, it is expected that more critically ill patients will require transport for sophisticated diagnostic studies and therapeutic interventions, such as magnetic resonance imaging (MRI), computed tomography (CT), nuclear medicine imaging, angiography, and gastrointestinal contrast studies.

From a historical perspective, the United States government began to pay a great deal of attention to highway-related accidents and fatalities with the passage of the 1966 National Highway Safety Act. By the early 1970s, civilian medical helicopters were being used in the prehospital transport of trauma victims and in the interhospital transport of critically ill and injured patients.

In contrast, despite these advances in prehospital and interhospital transport, very little attention had been paid to the transport of patients within a facility. Intrahospital transports of critically ill patients are more likely to occur and require the same comprehensive and systematic approach as the interfacility transports.

The focus of this chapter is on the transport of the critically ill or injured patient. These transports can originate from a number of locations that include the various intensive care units, the emergency department (ED), the operating room (OR), and so forth. Patients may go into the operating room with nothing more than a peripheral IV, but leave the OR intubated, with chest tubes, an arterial line, and various drainage tubes. More important than where the patient comes from is the patient's condition and the need for comprehensive monitoring and highly skilled medical personnel in attendance during the patient transport.

It has been well documented that critically ill or injured patients can be transported safely, without evidence of major complications and without adverse impact on clinical outcome.[1-6] These studies support the transport of critical patients if the benefits outweigh the possible harm of the transport. The goal of critical care transport must be to minimize these risks and provide necessary ongoing care.

Risk Analysis and Prevention

The movement of any critically ill or injured patient is not without hazard. Though these patients may be considered "stable," their physiologic reserve is often limited. Even minor adverse physiologic changes in these patients during transport may cascade into life-threatening complications.

It is essential for everyone involved in the care of critical patients to have a basic understanding regarding the transport environment, personnel, equipment, and vehicles. Current technology makes it possible to nearly replicate the critical care environment during transport. Even with the best planning, personnel, and equipment, there may be times during transport when monitoring may be difficult and the capability to manage emergencies may be limited. As a result, ongoing therapy may be interrupted and a patient's clinical condition may be compromised.

While there are distinct differences between interhospital and intrahospital transport, there are numerous common concerns and considerations. To reduce transport-related risks, an appropriate level of monitoring and clinical support is necessary before departing the point of origin. It is not uncommon for these complex patients to have a variety of lines, tubes, and mechanical support devices that must be addressed before any patient movement is possible. Transport represents a period of potential cardiopulmonary instability for these critical patients. Central to a safe transport is the avoidance of any inadvertent interruption in the monitoring or maintenance of the patient's vital functions. Therapeutic modalities that are in place prior to transport must be continued to support the patient's airway, breathing, circulation, and disability, and to prevent physiologic complications.

AIRWAY

Intubated patients are at risk for accidental extubation during transport. This is especially true during multiple transfers between beds, carts, and vehicles. Endotracheal tubes are to be secured and placement documented before the transport begins. It is also recommended that the placement be verified following the movement of the patient from bed to cart, cart to CT table, vehicle to vehicle, and so forth. Physical restraints or sedation may be applied as needed to prevent accidental extubation.

Securing and maintaining a patent airway is considered the highest priority of medical transport personnel. Making the head of the bed or stretcher easily accessible will facilitate airway control. Patients with an unstable or potentially unstable airway should be accompanied during transport by personnel who have the skill and necessary equipment to reintubate.[7,8]

BREATHING

It is essential that adequate oxygenation and ventilation be maintained throughout the transport. Improper ventilation (overventilation or underventilation) may result in hypoxemia, hypocarbia, hypercarbia, or undesirable acid-base changes.

Some transport teams routinely use a portable transport ventilator, while others favor the bag-valve-mask (BVM) and manual ventilation. Weg and Haas[9] concluded that manual ventilation during intrahospital transport is safe if the person doing the manual ventilation can approximate the pretransport inspired oxygen fraction and minute ventilation. In a prospective study by Braman and colleagues involving 36 critically ill, ventilator-dependent patients transported outside the ICU, a rise in P_{CO_2} of at least 10 mm Hg during transport occurred in 14 of 20 patients manually bagged.[10] Of the 16 patients transported using a portable mechanical ventilator, six patients showed significantly fewer changes in their arterial blood gases. Braman and colleagues concluded that the use of portable mechanical ventilators during transport might reduce the incidence of acid-base changes, cardiac arrhythmias, and hypotension. Nakamura and coworkers[11] studied spontaneously breathing patients who needed ventilatory support during transport out of the ICU. They concluded that although both manual and mechanical ventilation could be used safely, the use of a transport ventilator with a patient-triggering function provided more consistent ventilation and less deterioration in the Pa_{O_2}/FI_{O_2} ratio.

Regardless of whether a portable transport ventilator or BVM ventilation is used, adequate oxygenation and ventilation must be assured. It is essential to establish an appropriate FI_{O_2}, tidal volume, rate of ventilation, and level of positive end-expiratory pressure (PEEP). While there are many transport ventilators that can perform comparably to traditional ICU ventilators, not all transport ventilators are created equal.[12] Pressure limitations may make some transport ventilators incapable of providing high minute ventilation, airway pressures, or PEEP when these are required. In these types of patients, manual bagging for long periods of time may prove to be impractical.

There are many monitoring devices that may be helpful to the transport team, including a spirometric device (for bag ventilation), end-tidal CO_2 monitors, transcutaneous P_{O_2} monitoring, and pulse oximetry. Transport personnel should also assess for and document the symmetric rise and fall of the chest wall.

In recent years, the therapeutic options available to treat respiratory failure have advanced to include noninvasive mask ventilation (NIMV), inhaled nitric oxide (iNO), and heliox. Without portable delivery systems to continue treatment, patients may be severely compromised or transports may be impossible. Patients who require positive pressure ventilation via NIMV to treat their acute respiratory failure may quickly deteriorate if taken off the ventilator. Discontinuation of iNO, which may be used in the treatment of acute hypoxemic respiratory failure, may result in a rebound phenomenon, with worsened gas exchange and cardiovascular instability.[13] The discontinuation of inhaled heliox may raise the work of breathing in obstructed patients, causing respiratory decompensation.[14]

CIRCULATION

Cardiovascular and hemodynamic complications may be a direct result of patient transport. The severity of these changes during transport generally corresponds with the patient's status before movement out of the protective critical care environment. Complications commonly include hypotension, hypertension, and cardiac dysrhythmia. To reduce the risk of these preventable complications, vasoactive agents are continued, and electrolyte abnormalities should be corrected.

During the movement of patients, there is the possibility of dislodging intravascular lines or inadvertently disconnecting lines carrying drug infusions. Battery-powered infusion pumps can also fail. It is essential that there is careful attention and supervision to prevent these problems.

DISABILITY

Neurologic compromise may be a direct result of the potentially life-threatening complications already identified, including hypoxia, hypotension, hypertension, hypoxemia, and hypercarbia. Cerebral ischemia and secondary brain injury yield a significant rise in mortality that may be preventable.

Andrews[15] found that the most common complications during intrahospital transports that led to secondary brain injury included systemic hypotension and hypertension, increased intracranial pressure (ICP), decreased cerebral perfusion pressure, and arterial desaturation. It was determined that adequate resuscitation and stabilization before transport may have prevented some of these secondary injuries. Bekar[16] observed that an increase in ICP might have been prevented by appropriate pretransport ventilation, sedation, and analgesia. If possible, patients with increased ICP should be transported with the head elevated. If a transducer and ventricular drain are in place, their heights are best kept at the pretransport level to prevent inaccurate readings or major cerebrospinal fluid shifts.

Transport Coordination—An Overview

Minimum standards for intrahospital and interhospital transport of critically ill patients were developed by a committee from the Society of Critical Care Medicine, the American Col-

TABLE 7-1 Guidelines for Safe Patient Transport

- Plan in advance for patient transfer and transport
- Prevent delays through comprehensive coordination and detailed communication
- Make appropriate selection and utilization of available resources (personnel, vehicles, and equipment)
- Ensure patient stabilization prior to transport
- Verify that all tubes and lines are functional and well secured
- Provide a safe transport environment for patient and staff
- Continuously monitor the patient during transport for any change in condition
- Treat as indicated for any changes in status
- Safely deliver the patient to a critical care unit for further monitoring, evaluation, and management

lege of Critical Care Medicine, and the American Association of Critical Care Nurses.[7] These guidelines list the minimum requirements for personnel, equipment, and medication to facilitate the movement of critical patients. Other associations and publications have also written standards and guidelines to ensure the appropriate and safe transfer of critically ill patients.[17–20]

While there are unique considerations for interhospital transport (e.g., vehicle selection), many issues regarding preplanning, equipment, and personnel are similar for both categories of transport (Table 7-1). Written hospital policies provide consistency and reduce the likelihood of intrahospital or interhospital transport errors.

TRANSPORT PERSONNEL

The transport of critically ill or injured patients is not a benign endeavor. Critical care transports, both intrahospital and interhospital, should be performed by specially trained transport personnel.[7] Whether it is a dedicated transport team, unit-based personnel, or on-call staff, it is essential for them to have the necessary training and experience for the unique transport environment. The medical personnel must also have the clinical abilities and equipment to adequately evaluate the critical patient and initiate appropriate treatment promptly.

TRANSPORT EQUIPMENT

For both interhospital and intrahospital transport, it is necessary that all equipment be appropriate for both the specific critical care patient and the transport environment. The basic equipment requirements are essentially the same whether you are transporting a patient several floors, several miles, or several hundred miles. Monitoring during the transport of critically ill patients should be similar to that received in the ICU. However, portable monitors have limited capabilities when compared with bedside monitors.[21] In addition, monitoring during transport may be compromised by vibration, motion artifacts, electromagnetic interference, and limited visibility.

Critically ill or injured patients require real-time monitoring. Pulse oximetry and electrocardiographic (ECG) monitoring can provide continuous oxygenation and cardiac assessment. The blood pressure can be measured using an automatic noninvasive blood pressure device if continuous measurements via arterial line are not indicated.

Suitable transport monitors and equipment are portable, durable, lightweight, and battery powered. The capability to be plugged directly into a power source helps prevent unnecessary battery consumption. Audible and visible alarms for monitors, infusion pumps, and ventilators are necessary in quickly assessing important patient changes or equipment failures. It is also important to be certain that transport equipment will be compatible with the lines, fittings, and power outlets at the destination unit or in the transport vehicle.

All transport equipment should fit into elevators and transport vehicles, while leaving enough room for transport personnel to function. The ability to secure the equipment within the transport vehicle or to the patient's bed improves visibility while protecting it from accidental damage. Some ICU, ED, and OR beds have footboards that can double as equipment trays. Some institutions have designed trays or carts that can attach directly to the patient bed.

Limiting the number of bed-to-bed transfers will further reduce the likelihood of an inadvertent equipment disconnect. Several military and commercially available self-contained stretcher-based miniature ICUs or modified beds have been designed for adults, children, and neonates. They are equipped with ventilators, cardiac monitors, blood pressure monitors, and infusion pumps, and some are compatible with radiologic equipment. These devices may result in a more efficient use of resources necessary to safely transport a critically ill patient and reduce movement from cart to cart.

Besides the equipment used for monitoring and physiologic support, airway (intubation) and IV equipment and medications must also be available and transportable. Transport medications include the standard resuscitation drugs, analgesics, sedative/hypnotic agents, and neuromuscular blocking agents as indicated. Commercially available carrying cases that contain these essentials help to efficiently organize these supplies.[22] Numerous organizations and publications provide lists of suggested equipment and medication for in-house transport or interfacility transport.

A failure in oxygen supply can have disastrous consequences when caring for the critically ill. Therefore it is important for the oxygen source to be sufficient to exceed, by a substantially safe margin, any patient transport time.

Transport equipment often differs from routine bedside equipment. Dedicated transport personnel, working in a familiar environment, may better test, maintain, and troubleshoot complex equipment than those who only occasionally are called to accompany a patient during transport. All personnel must assure properly functioning equipment before departure.

Interhospital Transport

Most commonly, interhospital transfers occur when a referring facility lacks sufficient resources, equipment, personnel, or expertise to meet the needs of the critically ill or injured patient. The patient may require further diagnosis, specialized care, or timely treatment that is not available at the referring hospital. There are data supporting the value of regional referral centers, as well as the organized systems and specialized teams to bring patients safely to them.[23,24] Nevertheless, there remain common misconceptions among many physicians that some patients are too ill to transfer. This generally stems from a lack of knowledge regarding sophisticated patient transport systems.[25]

In the past decade, changes in how decisions regarding patient transfers are made have occurred due to changes in government regulations, methods of reimbursement to hospitals, and third-party managed care providers.[26,27] It is not uncommon for patients (or their designees), their personal physicians, or managed care providers to request transfers to a specific hospital that may have similar critical care capabilities to those at the referring facility. These lateral transfers may be motivated by many factors, including continuity of care, patient (or family) preference, or insurance plan requirements, and their appropriateness is often controversial.

There are three essential participants in a successful interfacility transport that can be viewed as a "transfer triangle." This 3-cornered approach has the referring and receiving physicians/facilities at the bottom corners of the triangle, creating the foundation for the patient transfer. Direct physician-to-physician contact and exchange of patient information is optimal, but in many situations physicians may rely on a designee to coordinate a transfer between facilities. At the apex of the triangle are the transport personnel, in contact with both the referring and receiving facility, and serving as a vital link between them. Working together, these collaborators should assure that each patient transfer results in the appropriate utilization of available resources, which include vehicles, personnel, and equipment.

RESPONSIBILITIES OF THE REFERRING PHYSICIAN AND FACILITY

If a treating physician recognizes that hospital capabilities are inadequate to safely care for a critical patient, or if specialized treatment or expertise is indicated but not available, the patient will need to be transferred to a facility capable of providing these services. Knowing the services a referring hospital provides is best addressed prospectively in hospital policy so that all hospital physicians, administrators, and staff have the same information readily available.

In addition to the above medical responsibilities during interfacility patient transfers within the United States, referring facilities and physicians face several legal obligations. The interhospital transport of critical patients may be initiated from referring emergency departments, inpatient units, and other various locations. When the transfer is from an emergency department within the United States, the Emergency Medical Treatment and Active Labor Act (EMTALA)[28] requires that all unstable patients be transported by qualified personnel and transportation equipment. Transport decisions are no longer merely a patient care issue, but also a federal requirement for EMTALA compliance.

EMTALA was established in 1986 and created patient stabilization and transfer requirements for hospitals and physicians. The law applies to any individual who "comes to the emergency department," but interpretation by the Centers for Medicare & Medicaid Services (CMS) has clearly expanded this to include other areas of the hospital campus. The original EMTALA regulations did not specifically address the interfacility transfer of unstable admitted patients. As a result, varying conclusions had been reached in different federal courts and regional CMS offices. However, in September 2003, CMS published new regulations to resolve this issue. CMS concluded that "the transfer and stability issues for a patient, once he or she is admitted, are governed by the Medicare hospital conditions of participation, State law, and professional considerations, not EMTALA requirements."[29] While CMS has clarified its position regarding the admitted patient, the basic EMTALA transfer provisions seem to be in the best interest of the patient and therefore warrant careful consideration.

If an individual presents to the ED with an "emergency medical condition," a hospital cannot transfer the patient unless specific requirements are met. The referring hospital is to examine the patient and "provide the medical treatment within its capacity which minimizes the risks to the individual's health." If the hospital cannot stabilize a patient, then the patient may be transferred (an "appropriate transfer" under EMTALA) only after complying with the remaining provisions of the law. EMTALA does not allow for an "automatic transfer" from one hospital to another based on established referral patterns or affiliations (e.g., managed care, trauma systems, and perinatal networks, among others).

The referring physician determines which receiving facility and physician is most appropriate for the patient. The most appropriate hospital may not always be the closest. A more distant facility may be preferable, but not practical due to a lack of time or means of transport. In addition, a specific institution may be deemed more appropriate if they have a specialized transport team that can provide an appropriate level of care during the transport.

Ideally, in consultation with the receiving physician, the referring physician verifies that the receiving facility has the available space, can provide the appropriate medical treatment, and agrees to accept the transfer. Finally, it is also the referring physician's responsibility under EMTALA to be certain that "the transfer is effected through qualified personnel and transportation equipment, as required including the use of necessary and medically appropriate life support measures during the transfer."

It is necessary for the referring physician to explain to the patient (or family) the reasons for transfer, the receiving facility and physician, and the method of transport. Considerable time may be lost if a transfer is set into motion only to have family members refuse the selected receiving hospital or mode of transport. Written, signed consent for transfer is to be obtained by the referring hospital. Many transport teams use their own supplemental consent forms as well.

A summary of the risks and benefits of a transfer are to be included in the patient records. It is no longer adequate to simply state that the benefits of transfer outweigh the risks. EMTALA requires that specific risks and benefits be considered and explained to the patient or the "legally responsible person acting on the individual's behalf." Some hospitals have prepared forms with checklists to facilitate completion of the necessary transfer documents. All medical records (or copies) related to the emergency condition, preliminary diagnosis, treatment provided, results of any tests, and the informed written consent for transfer are to be sent by the referring hospital to the receiving facility.

For patients transferred from the inpatient setting, the medical records should include copies of the physicians' and nurses' notes, consultations, medication sheets, order sheets, flow sheets, ECGs, radiology reports, lab results, and pertinent x-rays. Whenever possible, a discharge summary or transfer note is included. This document summarizes the major events in the patient's hospital course, and should be readily available for the transport team to review. With appropriate planning, the medical records and x-rays are copied and available at the patient's bedside before the transport team departs.

RESPONSIBILITIES OF THE RECEIVING PHYSICIAN AND FACILITY

Any hospital that strives to be a regional resource and receiving hospital for critical care referrals should have a system in place to facilitate communications and transfers. Communications can be enhanced through a designated communications or transfer center, dedicated telephone lines, or the hospital operator. The most efficient tertiary care centers have a consulting/receiving physician available 24 hours a day who has the authority to accept transfers and experience in off-site patient management.

Being familiar with hospital resources, bed availability, and transport options will expedite transfer decisions. Once the patient is accepted for transfer, the referring and receiving physicians should agree on the mode of transport, the transport team composition, and the equipment that may be necessary during the transport.

Federal law also has implications for receiving institutions. EMTALA identifies "obligations of hospitals with specialized services," and specifies that "participating hospitals with specialized facilities shall not refuse to accept an appropriate transfer if they have the capacity to treat the individual." Receiving hospitals should document in hospital policy which of their services are "specialized," addressing the capabilities and capacities of these services. Under EMTALA, a receiving hospital cannot refuse to accept the transfer of a patient who is unstable or has an emergency medical condition if they have the capacity and ability to care for a patient.

COORDINATION OF THE INTERHOSPITAL TRANSFER

It is the referring physician who is ultimately held accountable to coordinate the transfer of a critical patient. Formal transfer policies and transport agreements between the referring and receiving hospitals and physicians can greatly facilitate patient transfers while minimizing EMTALA violations and preventable delays. Regional tertiary and specialty care centers (ICUs, trauma centers, burn units, and transport services) are best listed in these resource documents.

Patient transfer agreements identify the available specialty areas at potential receiving hospitals and the admission criteria for each of these services. Including the point(s) of contact, key telephone numbers, and procedures to secure patient acceptance are also helpful. Transfer agreements with multiple facilities for the various specialty services may be needed, as an individual hospital may at times be unable to accommodate a patient.

Patient *transport* procedures and agreements may also be incorporated into patient *transfer* agreements, or may be separate contracts with independent third-party transport services. Third-party transport providers may be independent or hospital transport services. Many transport agreements delineate the availability and composition of transport teams, medical crew capabilities, and resource availability (medical equipment and transport vehicles). When appropriate, this document may also address issues of billing and payment, and clarify questions pertaining to medical control during transport. Transport agreements streamline patient transfer by minimizing delays in processing a transport request. A resource directory that includes phone numbers, specific capabilities of each air or ground transport service, and receiving medical facilities should be readily available in the ICUs and ED.

A timely and accurate initial contact with a receiving physician will minimize delays, facilitate decision making, and promote transfer arrangements. Ideally, to assure a smooth and safe transfer, the referring and receiving physician discuss the patient directly. Without this interaction, significant gaps in the transfer of essential patient information may occur, resulting in missed or delayed diagnoses and treatment. It is often helpful for the referring and receiving physicians to use a systematic checklist to review and fill out while discussing the patient.

To begin the process, the referring physician provides his or her name and easy access callback number, which may be a specific telephone number, pager number, or mobile phone. The name and phone numbers of the referring hospital and unit should be logged by the receiving institution to facilitate follow-up phone calls. The patient's name, age, nature of illness or injury, vital signs, physical findings, results of pertinent diagnostic studies, treatment, current condition, and reason for transfer are described in detail to the receiving physician. This same information will need to be relayed to the transport team by physicians and eventually to the nursing staff at the receiving facility.

Once the patient is accepted for transfer, it is appropriate for the accepting physician to make recommendations regarding ongoing patient management. Both the referring and receiving physicians should document these recommendations.

In addition, the receiving physician or a specialist who is frequently involved in the transport of critically ill or injured patients may make recommendations regarding the mode of transportation, composition of the transport team, and preparation of the patient prior to transport. This happens most often when the receiving facility has its own critical care transport team. However, a receiving hospital cannot insist that their own transport team undertake a transport in order for them to accept the patient in transfer.

Critical transport decisions are often made under adverse conditions with limited information and limited time. The emphasis is on protecting the patient from further injury or medical deterioration, and optimizing the patient's chances for survival. Individuals with the most experience in transport should be a part of the transport decision making process. However, despite external recommendations of others, it remains the responsibility of the physician caring for the patient at the referring institution to make the transport-related decisions.

TRANSPORT DECISION MAKING

Anticipating patient care requirements prior to and during transport determines the method of transport. EMTALA states that the transfer is "effected through qualified personnel and transportation equipment." However, the law does not define "qualified." This leaves the interpretation and responsibility primarily up to the referring physician. In practical terms, the skills of the transport personnel include the ability to care for the patient's current condition and any reasonable foreseeable complications that could arise during transport. It is not possible to predict all the potential complications that may occur during any given transfer. However, it is imperative for referring facilities and physicians to have a reasonable understanding of the capabilities of transport services within their service area, even if that service is provided by the receiving hospital or a third party.

There are several key decisions to consider when making arrangements for a patient transport, including the personnel, the type of vehicle, and the proper equipment or medications to have on hand. The referring physician must accurately assess the patient's real and potential illnesses or injuries and anticipate complications that might occur during transport. He must also estimate the pace of illness in order to judge whether "team or time" represents the greater opportunity to improve outcome.

Level-of-care options for interfacility transport include basic life support (staffed by EMTs), advanced life support (staffed by two paramedics), and critical care/specialty care (staffed by a minimum of a nurse and a second crew member). The special requirements of high-risk neonates, complex obstetric patients, and those needing complex ventilator or hemodynamic management may dictate the transport personnel and equipment. However, for time-dependent disorders, urgent transfer may be more crucial than specialty transfer. For example, because a patient with a dissecting aortic aneurysm may require immediate surgical intervention, delaying the transport for a critical care transport team may be inadvisable. A dilemma arises when the patient's medical condition is both time-dependent *and* team configuration–dependent. Specialists experienced in transport medicine can greatly assist in making these complex judgments.

VEHICLE SELECTION

In determining the most appropriate method of transport, several considerations are addressed, including the availability of local resources (referring hospital, receiving hospital, and ambulance services, among others); speed of the transport vehicle; weather considerations (inclement weather, snow, or fog); ground traffic, construction, or accessibility of roads and landing areas (helipads or airports); and the total distance to travel to deliver the patient (one-way vs. round trip or two legs of a three-legged transport). A vehicle dispatched directly from the referring hospital to the receiving hospital constitutes a one-way transport. More commonly, the transfer will be two-way, with the vehicle and crew being sent from the receiving hospital to the referring hospital to pick up the patient. Three-legged transports describe those in which a third party (hospital-sponsored program or independent ambulance company) provides the vehicle and team from a location other than the receiving or referring hospital. Options for transport include ground and air ambulances (helicopter and airplane).

GROUND AMBULANCES

Ground ambulances are the most common vehicles used for interfacility transport and continue to be the primary means of prehospital patient transport. A major advantage is availability, since most geographic areas have ground ambulances. They also provide door-to-door service, without the need for a runway, helipad, or landing zone. Once placed on the stretcher and secured in the ambulance, the patient can be transported directly to the receiving facility without movement from one vehicle to another, limiting the most dangerous aspect of transport. The patient compartment of a ground ambulance tends to be larger than those found in helicopters and airplanes, accommodating up to four medical crew members and one to two patients. In addition, fewer restrictions apply to the size, weight, and amount of equipment that can be taken by ground transport when compared to flying. It is also easier to stop a ground ambulance to facilitate patient assessment and intervention. If necessary, ground ambulances can also be easily diverted to alternate destinations as dictated by patient condition or the need for an unanticipated intervention. Finally, ground ambulances operate in most weather conditions that restrict safe air operations.

There are also disadvantages to using ground ambulances, the most important being the increased amount of time required to transfer a patient from one facility to a distant facility in comparison to air transport. Ground vehicles are subject to delays imposed by poorly maintained roads, traffic congestion, construction, and inclement weather. In addition, ground ambulances may not be able to gain access to patients who are located in remote areas with limited road availability. In rural areas with limited numbers of ground ambulances, the dispatch of one unit on a distant transport may cause other areas to be temporarily without service. Finally, tight vehicle suspensions, narrow wheelbases, and high centers of gravity predispose ground vehicles to rough and turbulent rides, which may be detrimental or excessively painful to patients with spinal cord injury, intracerebral hemorrhage, or orthopedic injuries.

ROTOR-WING AIR AMBULANCE (HELICOPTER)

The use of the air ambulance has grown significantly over the past 30 years. Speed of travel is an important consideration for helicopter transport and the primary reason it is chosen over ground ambulances. Depending on the type of aircraft, weather conditions, flight altitude, and total load, helicopters may travel at speeds of 120 to 180 miles per hour. This speed and the fact that helicopters can make direct point-to-point transfers may reduce transport time to one third to one fourth that required by ground transport. The helicopter needs only a small (100-by-100-foot), flat area that is clear of obstructions to take off and land. In addition, the helicopter has the ability to fly into locations inaccessible to other modes of travel. This capability becomes extremely valuable when traffic is delayed or roads are impassable after snowstorms, floods, tornadoes, and other disasters, or when a patient is located in rural or wilderness areas. With a service area that generally ranges between 50 to 200 radial miles from its base, helicopters cover a much greater service area than would a ground ambulance, but less than a fixed-wing aircraft. Helicopters are often the fastest mode of transport for distances of 25 to 150 miles.

Helicopters also have inherent disadvantages. If an appropriate landing area is not readily available, the time needed to identify and secure a landing zone, in addition to the time needed to transport the patient to and from the distant landing site, may erode the helicopter's speed advantage. The patient cabin is typically smaller than in ground ambulances, and even in larger helicopters, patient access may be limited.

Weight restrictions may also prevent transport of some obese patients.

Fog, sleet, heavy snowfall and rain, low clouds, high winds, and lightning may significantly limit the utility of helicopter transport. Most helicopter programs operate under visual flight rules (VFRs), but travel under instrument flight rules (IFRs) is becoming more common. The majority of IFR flights are conducted airport-to-airport, but newer Global Positioning System (GPS) technology makes possible IFR missions directly to precertified hospital helipads.

Helicopters are unpressurized and a basic knowledge of flight physiology is important to understanding the effects of a changing altitude are essential. While airplane travel is clearly impacted by flight physiology and the stresses of flight, helicopter transport is also susceptible. It is often thought that only altitudes above 8000 feet impact the patient or crew, but this is not always the case. Boyle's law states that, as altitude increases and atmospheric pressure decreases, gas volumes expand (and vice versa on descent). As a result, crew members or patients flying with sinus problems, ear problems, or upper respiratory infections may feel the effects of barometric pressure changes with an altitude change of as little as 1000 to 2000 feet.

Henry's Law is another important gas law affecting air medical transport. According to this law, the amount of gas dissolved in liquid is determined by the partial pressure and the solubility of the gas. The *bends*, a decompression sickness, is a clinical condition affected by this law. When a scuba diver ascends too quickly, nitrogen gas bubble formation in the blood can occur. Special precautions should be taken for decompression victims who must be transported by helicopter. In some cases, even a minimal gain in altitude can cause significant gas bubble formation. It is advised that patients suffering from decompression illness be transported in nonpressurized aircraft at an altitude of not more that 1000 feet about the diver's ascent.

Patients, medical personnel, and pilots may all be impacted by the stresses of flight. Vibration, noise, and turbulence are generally more severe in helicopters than in other forms of transportation, and they may interfere with patient assessment or the function of medical equipment. Flight crew members wear headsets or helmets to facilitate in-flight communication and to minimize the long-term effects of working in a loud environment. Awake patients are commonly given headsets or earplugs.

FIXED-WING AIR AMBULANCE (AIRPLANE)

Fixed-wing transports usually lose their speed advantage at distances of less than 100 miles because of ground delays during airport transfers. Furthermore, these additional patient transfers to and from ground ambulances expose the patient to possible dislodgment of vital equipment. Despite these disadvantages, fixed-wing aircraft offer several advantages. Airplanes often have sufficient space to accommodate more than one patient, patient family members, and additional crew members or equipment. In addition, weight restrictions, weather, noise, and turbulence are less of a factor when compared to rotary-wing transport. Smaller unpressurized airplanes offer no benefit over the helicopter in combating the effects of the gas laws, and therefore are generally limited to altitudes under 10,000 feet. Pressurized fixed-wing aircraft, however, can fly higher while counteracting the neg-

TABLE 7-2 Effects of Altitude on Oxygenation When Breathing Ambient Air

Altitude, Feet	Barometric Pressure, mm Hg	PA_{O_2}, mm Hg	Pa_{O_2}, mm Hg	Pa_{CO_2}, mm Hg	Oxygen Saturation
Sea level	760	159.2	103.0	40.0	98%
8000	565	118.4	68.9	36.0	93%
10,000	523	109.6	61.2	35.0	87%
15,000	429	89.9	45.0	32.0	84%
18,000	380	79.6	37.8	30.4	72%
20,000	349	73.1	34.3	29.4	66%
22,000	321	67.2	32.8	28.4	60%

ative effects of altitude. At flight altitudes of 30,000 to 40,000 feet, pressurized aircraft can often create an internal cabin altitude of 7000 to 8000 feet. Flying at lower altitudes, aircraft with a high differential cabin pressure have the ability to create a cabin pressure that exceeds ground altitude pressures, a feature that may aid in transport of victims with decompression illness.

Due to the impact of Boyle's Law, on ascent a simple pneumothorax may expand to become hemodynamically significant or intestinal gas may expand to rupture a hollow viscus. Medical equipment that has an enclosed air space can also be affected, including endotracheal tube cuffs, intravenous lines (whose flow may be driven by air-filled pressure bags), and air-containing splints.

Hypoxia represents the greatest risk associated with high-altitude transport. Dalton's law states that the total pressure of a gaseous mixture is equal to the sum of the partial pressure of the gases. Therefore, any change in barometric pressure directly affects the partial pressure of oxygen (Table 7-2).

During fixed-wing transport, the most threatening concern with hypoxia is its insidious onset. The medical crew may not notice the early onset of signs or symptoms in the patient or themselves.[30] No one is exempt from the effects of hypoxia, even though the onset and severity of symptoms may vary with individuals. While altitude-related patient hypoxia is a concern, the routine use of pulse oximetry and supplemental oxygen minimizes this hazard. In the setting of hypoxemia, increasing $F_{I_{O_2}}$ levels or adding PEEP easily compensates for the hypoxic effects of altitude. However, in the rare patient who is on maximal oxygen support, flight at lower altitudes may allow the artificial cabin pressure to approach sea level, in this manner increasing the partial pressure of oxygen.

Hypoxia is more of a concern for the pilots and crew members who generally are not monitored. The Federal Aviation Administration (Federal Aviation Regulations [FAR], Part 135, which applies to on-demand air taxis) requires pilots to use supplemental oxygen if they are flying at cabin altitudes above 10,000 feet for more than 30 minutes and any time above 12,000 feet.[31] At cabin pressure altitudes above 15,000 feet each occupant of the aircraft must use supplemental oxygen.[32] During high-altitude transport, periodic assessment of the pulse oximetric saturation of medical crew members is prudent.

The medical crew must be prepared to deal with the effects of a malfunction of the pressurization equipment or aircraft structural damage. During a rapid decompression, the sudden drop in temperature causes the aircraft to fill with fog. A

Patient: _____ Transport Date: _____ Flight # _____

Referring Hospital: _____ City/State: _____ Loaded Miles: _____

General Criteria for Air Medical Transport

☐ Distance to the closest appropriate facility was too great for safe and timely transport by ground ambulance.
☐ Patient's clinical condition required that the time spent in transport be as short as possible.
☐ Patient's condition was time critical, requiring specific/timely treatment, not available at the referring hospital.
☐ Potential for transport delay associated with ground transport was likely to worsen the patient's clinical condition.
☐ Patient required critical care life support during transport, not available from the local ground ambulance service.
    ☐ Monitoring _____ ☐ Personnel _____
    ☐ Medication _____ ☐ Special equipment _____
☐ Patient was located in an area inaccessible to regular ground traffic, impeding ambulance egress or access due to
    ☐ Road obstacles and/or conditions   ☐ Wilderness rescue or geographic considerations
☐ Local ground units were not available for long distance transport.
☐ Use of a local ground transport service would have left the local area without adequate EMS coverage.

Indications for Transfer to an Appropriate Receiving Facility

☐ Patient required further diagnosis, specialized care and/or timely treatment, not available at the referring hospital.
☐ Patient required care by physician(s) at a receiving hospital where the patient had previously undergone specialized treatment and where medical records were located which were likely to significantly influence patient care.
☐ Patient's attending physician requested transport to a specific hospital based on medical needs/continuity of care.

Medical/Surgical Criteria for Critical Care Transfer

☐ Patient has unstable vital signs represented by:
    ☐ Respiratory Rate: <10 or >30
    ☐ Heart Rate: <50 or >150
    ☐ Systolic BP: <90 or >200 mm Hg
☐ Respiratory arrest within the past 12 hours
☐ Unstable or potentially unstable airway
☐ Patient required mechanical ventilator support or any constant positive airway pressure (CPAP)
☐ Patient has an indwelling pulmonary artery catheter, intra-aortic balloon pump, arterial line, or intracranial pressure monitor
☐ Patient required diagnostic procedures, specific therapy, or intensive care not available at the referring hospital, for any of the following critical conditions
    ☐ Acute respiratory failure
    ☐ Acute deterioration in mental status
    ☐ Acute cerebrovascular accident in evolution
    ☐ Acute neurologic or neurosurgical emergency
    ☐ Severe hypothermia requiring active therapy
    ☐ Acute hemodialysis
    ☐ GI bleeding
    ☐ Severe poisonings or overdoses
    ☐ Significant acidosis
    ☐ Status epilepticus
    ☐ Complications of cancer and chemotherapy
    ☐ Decompression sickness
    ☐ Life threatening infectious process
    ☐ Dissecting or leaking aneurysm
    ☐ Organ transplantation or procurement

☐ _____

Cardiac Criteria for Critical Care Transfer

☐ Cardiac arrest within the past 12–48 hours
☐ Patient had an acute myocardial infarction requiring therapy or diagnostic procedures not available at the referring institution
    ☐ Thrombolytic therapy
    ☐ Cardiac catheterization
    ☐ Intra-aortic balloon pump
☐ Patient required continuous intravenous vasoactive medications or mechanical ventricular assist to maintain a stable cardiac output
☐ Uncontrolled life threatening dysrhythmia
☐ Patient required continuous intravenous anti-dysrhythmia medications or a cardiac pacemaker to maintain a stable cardiac rhythm
☐ Any unstable cardiac conditions requiring urgent cardiac catheterization or cardiac surgery

Obstetrical Criteria for Critical Care Transfer

☐ Patient required urgent transport to a perinatal center for a high risk obstetrical condition
    ☐ Placenta previa
    ☐ Abruptio placenta
    ☐ Eclampsia
    ☐ Pre-eclampsia
    ☐ Premature labor
    ☐ Abnormal fetal lie
    ☐ Uncontrolled maternal diabetes
    ☐ Severe maternal medical illness

Other Criteria/Comments

_____
_____

Transfer Diagnosis   *Physician Signature*

FIGURE 7-1 Medical necessity for air medical transport for adult patients. *(Used with permission from the University of Chicago Hospitals Aeromedical Network [UCAN]).*

rapid drop in the cabin P_{O_2} quickly leads to hypoxia in crew members. Supplemental oxygen for the pilot, medical crew, and patient is essential. Any chest or nasogastric tube should then be unclamped to allow decompression of any gas subject to expansion.

EFFICACY OF AIR MEDICAL TRANSPORT

Despite over 30 years of air medical transport, definitive data indicating which types of patients should be flown are generally lacking. Questions regarding the triage of patients to air or ground transport, the efficacy of aeromedical care, and the effects of air medical transport on morbidity and mortality in both medical and surgical conditions remain controversial. To assist programs and physicians in determining the appropriateness of air medical transport, the Medical Advisory Committee of the Association of Air Medical Services has established criteria for the proper utilization of air medical transport.[33] These time, distance, and logistical indicators have been adopted by many air medical programs and EMS systems to aid in the appropriate triage of patients. An example of these general criteria for the adult nontrauma patient is summarized in the form reproduced as Figure 7-1.

Trauma patients have been the most studied with regard to helicopter EMS transport. Studies have shown that patients transported by aeromedical services may exhibit improved survival.[34–36] When patients are transported from rural areas, the higher level of care aboard the medical helicopter and the timely arrival to a trauma center were felt to be the main contributing factors to decreased mortality. The helicopter appears to provide no advantage for patients transported from an urban area.[37,38]

Transport of cardiac patients has raised concern because altitude raises heart rate and myocardial oxygen demand. Studies of patients with acute myocardial infarction and unstable angina revealed that complications such as hypotension, dysrhythmias, and exacerbation of chest pain occurred during transport and that most were managed effectively en route.[39,40] In one study, complications were more frequent in the group transported by air when compared to those transported by ground.[41] In general, it was found that major inflight events were uncommon.[40–42]

Aeromedical transport of the gravida is felt to be generally safe for both mother and fetus. If the fetus is at risk, the mother should be given supplemental oxygen during flight.[43] Another concern is the transport of women in active labor, since in-flight delivery is best avoided. It may be wise to defer transport of the patient whose cervix is dilated greater than 4 cm on preflight assessment.[44]

SAFETY OF TRANSPORT

Accidents occur with all modes of patient transport. Generally speaking, ground ambulances have a higher probability of being involved in an accident, but offer a better chance of survival than aircraft mishaps. A safety report published by the Air Medical Physician Association researched accident data for ground and helicopter EMS (HEMS).[45]

Since 1972, HEMS has flown an estimated 3 million hours while transporting approximately 2.75 million patients. In 31 years (through September 2002) there were 162 HEMS accidents in the United States, 67 of them fatal, with 183 deaths including 21 patients. From 1987 to 1997, HEMS averaged 4.9 accidents per year, but this has risen since 1998 to 10.75 accidents per year. Over the course of the 22 years reviewed, the death rate for HEMS patients was 0.76 per 100,000.

EMS experts estimate that 15,000 ground ambulance crashes occur each year, with as many as 10,000 injuries annually, 10 serious injuries daily, and 1 fatal ambulance crash each week. "Emergency vehicle passengers," which includes patients, medical personnel, and patient's family members account for 22% of the fatalities, with most deaths being occupants of the other vehicles.

MEDICAL PERSONNEL FOR INTERHOSPITAL TRANSPORT

Air and ground transport present many unique challenges to its medical personnel. Numerous associations and many state EMS agencies have developed training requirements for critical care transport. In addition to the appropriate clinical components, knowledge of altitude physiology and the stresses of transport, vehicle safety, stress management, and appropriate survival training are included.

Factors other than direct patient needs may determine the composition of the transport team. Since critical care transport teams are expensive, financial considerations may affect crew composition and availability. Utilizing in-house or on-call staff to transport patients may reduce the cost of transport, but this may result in crew members being unfamiliar with the transport environment and could deprive the home institution of adequate physician or nurse coverage. Receiving or referring physicians may also request the presence of a transport physician to ameliorate a perceived decrease in the level of care provided during a transport.

Medical personnel for interfacility transport represent the broad spectrum of health care providers. EMS ground ambulances are commonly staffed with paramedics who function at advanced life support (ALS) level, or emergency medical technicians (EMTs) who provide basic life support (BLS). Referring physicians must carefully evaluate the needs of critical care patients and the capabilities of ground EMS providers to determine if optimal patient care can be accomplished by these caregivers.

The majority of fixed-wing (61%) and rotor-wing (71%) programs in the United States staff their critical care transport teams with a nurse/paramedic crew. Nurse/nurse is the next most common medical crew configuration for both helicopter and airplane transport (8%). Other team combinations of registered nurses, EMTs, doctors, and EMT-paramedics (RN/EMT, RN/MD, and EMT-P/EMT-P) each account for 5% or less of the totals.[46]

Flight nurses generally have extensive experience in intensive care units or EDs. Paramedics often make their greatest contribution in the transport of critical patients from accident scenes since most of their training revolves around being first responders. Respiratory therapists bring expertise in airway and ventilator management and oxygen delivery systems.

The benefit of physicians on medical transport teams, as is common in Europe, remains unclear. Studies are conflicting on the subject of whether physician attendance improves patient outcome.[47–50] Optimal transport systems have the flexibility to send a physician on a case-by-case basis. Flight physicians are often residents in emergency medicine or surgery, and on occasion they may be attending physicians or medical directors of flight programs.

In some regions, transport services provide specialty care teams for specific patient populations, most commonly for pediatric critical care patients, high-risk neonates, or high-risk obstetric patients. Some nonspecialty teams may replace a team member or provide additional personnel for certain missions, such as intra-aortic balloon pump transports. A limited number of studies compare specialty teams to nonspecialty teams. Edge and colleagues found that adverse events occurred in only 1 of 49 (2%) pediatric transports by a specialized team compared to 18 of 92 (20%) of transports by nonspecialized personnel.[51] In another study comparing 1030 transports by a pediatric specialty care team to 55 transports by a nonspecialty care team, children were 22 times more likely to have an unplanned event and 2.4 times more likely to die when transported by a nonspecialty care team.[52] The most common unplanned events identified were airway problems (specialty, 0.4%, nonspecialty, 18%) and hypotension (specialty, 0.1%, nonspecialty, 10.9%).

THE TRANSPORT

Once the transport team arrives at the referring location, it is essential that a thorough but expeditious patient assessment be completed. Considerations include taking the time to perform stabilizing interventions prior to departing the referring unit. Gebremichael and colleagues[6] concluded that patients with profound respiratory failure benefited when stabilized prior to transport. However, with trauma patients[53,54] and cardiac patients,[55] it has been shown that rapid transport with minimal stabilization prior to transport may be beneficial, since the delay in getting to definitive care or therapeutic intervention is minimized.

Decisions regarding airway management are critical when it comes to interfacility transport. While patients can be intubated in the various transport vehicles—sometimes with extreme difficulty—it may be preferable to intubate in the more controlled environment of the referring unit. The threshold to intubate for transport may be appropriately lower compared to a patient who would otherwise not be leaving the in-hospital setting.

In preparing a patient for transport, other anticipated therapeutic changes are also best handled initially in the referring unit in order to determine the patient's response. Changing to a portable ventilator or to manual ventilation within the controlled ICU, ED, or OR setting will enable the transport team to identify any ventilation or oxygenation complications that arise and correct them before leaving the unit. A change in any medication to support the patient's blood pressure or cardiac rhythm is also best handled initially in the referring unit. It is often preferable to simplify transport by limiting the number of continuous IV infusions to necessary vasoactive agents and volume expanders. Paralytics and sedatives may be given by IV bolus during transport rather than by continuous infusion.

MEDICAL DIRECTION AND MEDICAL CONTROL

All medical transports require some form of medical direction and medical control. ALS ground ambulances are generally under the direction and control of an EMS system. Individual transports would generally be under the direction of an EMS resource hospital or standing medical orders (SMOs). Hospital-sponsored or independently operated air medical services or mobile intensive care programs generally have their own medical direction and medical control physicians.

While EMTALA leaves the transferring physician responsible for patients in transfer until they physically arrive at the receiving facility,[56,57] the law does not make any reference to the transport service, its medical director, or medical control. Out-of-hospital medical transport is regulated state by state, with all states requiring some type of physician medical direction and medical control.[58]

There are three options for medical control. On-line medical control represents direct real-time voice communication between the medical control physician and the transport team. With off-line medical control there is no direct contact between the transport team and the medical control physician. Written medical protocols or standing orders provided by the medical director, medical control physician, referring physician, or receiving physician will direct patient management. Visual medical control occurs when a physician is physically present during the transport.

Medical control during interfacility transport may be assumed by the transferring physician, receiving physician, EMS base station, or the medical director/designee of the transport service. The National Association of EMS Physicians (NAEMSP) has concluded that medical direction of the interfacility transport is a shared responsibility,[58] stating that the referring physician, transport service medical director, and accepting physician should agree on the responsibility of medical direction prior to the transport. The Air Medical Physician Association (AMPA), however, believes that medical control during transport should remain the responsibility of the air medical director or his or her designee.[59] AMPA states that any variation from this standard should be specified in a patient transfer agreement or at the time of request for air medical transport.

It is important to note that despite having interfacility transfer and transport agreements in place, the requirements of EMTALA are still in effect. Some physicians believe that the presence of a physician on the transport team relieves the referring physician of his or her liability and obligations. Others feel that when a transport team from the receiving hospital arrives at the referring facility and assumes patient care, the patient is considered to be admitted to the receiving hospital and that the responsibility shifts completely to the receiving institution. While these shifts of authority and liability may be implied or incorporated into transfer agreements or hospital policies, nothing in EMTALA can be interpreted to endorse these beliefs. The transferring physician and hospital may only decrease their liability and accountability by prospectively addressing these issues in transport agreements and hospital policies, but the responsibility for an "appropriate transfer" remains with the referring hospital and physician. Ideally the transferring physician is available and continues to assist in patient care until the patient has physically left the facility. The medical control physician, however, is responsible for the care provided by transport personnel during patient stabilization and preparation for transport. If a difference of opinion occurs regarding options for care, the referring physician and the medical control physician must reach an accord. This is when knowledge and experience regarding the transport environment is most important to ensure the quality of medical care and the safety of transport.

Intrahospital Transport

For the critically ill patient, it may be preferable for diagnostic studies and therapeutic or surgical procedures to be done at the bedside in the ICU or ED. This avoids the inherent hazards of transport outside of the unit and provides the patient with the additional benefits of the ICU environment, including advanced monitoring capabilities, and presence of additional critical care personnel who may provide additional assistance as needed. However, critical patients may require procedures that cannot be performed in the ICU or ED itself. Patients may need to be transported to the radiology department, operating room, or other locations within the hospital to receive specialized diagnostic or therapeutic procedures. In addition, many patients now leave the ICU for intermediate care units while still marginally stable and often with multiple indwelling catheters and other devices.

Intrahospital transport of critical patients has been associated with significant clinical complications. Braman and colleagues[10] found that 75% (15 of 20) of ventilator-dependent ICU patients had an increase in P_{CO_2}, with corresponding hypotension or cardiac dysrhythmias. These patients were transported using manual ventilation. Indeck and associates[60] reported a total of 113 serious physiologic changes of at least 5-minute duration during intrahospital transport. Of the 103 patients in the study, 68% experienced complications, including a change in systolic or diastolic blood pressure of at least 20 mm Hg (40% of the patients), a change in pulse by 20 beats per minute or more (21%), and a decrease of 5% or more in the arterial oxygen saturation (17%). Rutherford and Fisher[61] reviewed the transport of 31 critical ICU patients and reported 14 life-threatening complications. This study identified hypotension in four patients, severe respiratory distress in another four patients including an extubation, disconnection of central lines in three patients, and treatment for ventricular dysrhythmias in two patients. Szem and coworkers[1] identified an overall occurrence rate of complications of 5.9% in a study of 203 surgical ICU patient transports. A total of 12 complications included: marked hypoxemia (4), cardiac arrest (3), hypotension (2), cerebral infarction (1), pneumothorax requiring chest tube placement (1), and rupture of an infected arteriovenous fistula (1). Waddell[62] identified three transport-related deaths in a study of 86 intrahospital transports, with an overall complication rate of 8.1%. Complications seen were hypotension (3), cardiopulmonary arrest (1), airway obstruction (1), hypertension (1), and rebleeding from a pelvic fracture (1).

RESPONSIBILITIES OF THE ATTENDING PHYSICIAN

Any decision to transport a critical patient within a facility necessitates careful consideration. Physicians who transfer patients to other facilities generally understand the importance and responsibility of reviewing the risks and benefits of each transfer with a patient (or their designee). Similarly, physicians are also familiar with their obligation to explain the risks and benefits and obtain an informed consent prior to procedures or diagnostic testing. However, the risk of in-

trafacility transport may not be considered with the same significance or may be overlooked altogether.

With advances in medical technology, more diagnostic and therapeutic options can be brought to the ICU bedside, avoiding inherent risks of intrahospital transport. Bedside ultrasonography may provide valuable information, avoiding transport to a CT scanner. Some surgical procedures may also be done at the bedside. A percutaneous dilational tracheostomy can provide for a long-term airway while avoiding transport to the operating room. A bedside diagnostic peritoneal lavage or focused abdominal sonography for trauma (FAST exam) may avert the need for abdominal imaging.

The need for transport is best weighed against the outcome of the test and how it would impact patient care. If a positive or negative test will result in a timely change in therapy, the transport may be justified. However, if no immediate change is anticipated based on the results, or if the transport is considered high risk, then the transport is best avoided. Numerous studies have examined the impact of diagnostic testing outside of the ICU and its influence on patient management. Indeck and colleagues[60] evaluated 103 patient transports for radiographic tests and identified 113 physiologic complications. Only 24% of these transports resulted in therapeutic changes within 48 hours. In a study by Hurst and associates,[63] 66% of the ICU patients who were transported experienced physiologic deterioration, while only 39% of these transports yielded a change in patient management.

COORDINATION OF THE INTRAHOSPITAL TRANSPORT

Hospitalwide guidelines for the transport of patients within the facility can greatly assist in assuring patient safety for transport. Proper planning, training, and equipment minimizes risk. Communication and coordination are keys to the success of a safe intrahospital transport. Hospital security, transport personnel, or ancillary staff should be available to secure elevators as needed. Prior to departing the ICU, ED, or other point of origin, notification given to the destination (e.g., radiology, operating room, etc) will verify the availability to immediately accept the patient upon arrival. If multiple diagnostic studies are required, it may be preferable to undertake one prolonged trip outside the unit rather than several shorter trips. An immediate review of diagnostic studies is also beneficial to facilitate additional films or procedures as needed, while avoiding a second transport.

TRANSPORT DECISION MAKING

In the ideal situation, a dedicated in-hospital transport team with dedicated monitoring equipment and routine medications for resuscitation, intubation, and sedation provides intrafacility transfers. The reality, however, is that in most situations the physicians and nurses managing the patient will need to anticipate patient care requirements during transport to determine the qualified personnel and transport equipment that will be necessary for safety. Except for the vehicle-related considerations found in the decision making for interhospital transport, the process is similar for in-house transport: evaluate the patient, evaluate the medical care required, assess for special requirements (equipment and medication), and consider the personnel (availability, critical care capabilities, and training).

RISQUES DE TRANSPORT

MEDICAL PERSONNEL FOR INTRAHOSPITAL TRANSPORT

In 1993, the Transfer Guidelines Task Force Committee of the Society of Critical Care Medicine, the American College of Critical Care Medicine, and the American Association of Critical Care Nurses recommended that all critical care transports, both intrahospital and interhospital, should be performed by dedicated, specially trained transport teams. While some hospitals have developed dedicated in-house (intrafacility) critical care transport teams, other facilities are utilizing specially trained ICU or ED transport personnel. Similarly to their interhospital counterparts, these individuals have the training and experience for the transport environment, and have the clinical capabilities, transport equipment, and medications to perform these necessary and often complicated transports efficiently and safely. The use of these specialty teams can prevent many transport-related complications, improve patient flow, and reduce delays.[64] Unit-based ICU or ED nurses can remain on their units to continue care for their other patients rather than transporting patients throughout the hospital.

Whether or not a dedicated transport team exists, developing hospital policies and procedures helps to identify what constitutes an appropriate level of transport personnel. The guidelines developed by the Transfer Guidelines Task Force recommend that all transported critically ill patients be accompanied by a minimum of two people, one of whom should be a critical care nurse. They suggest that an accompanying physician is necessary only for unstable patients. Many teaching hospitals will use the patient's primary nurse and a resident physician. The transport may also use a combination of the primary nurse, one or more patient transporters, and a respiratory therapist. Even when the primary providers accompany the patient, it is advantageous for them to have formal transport-related training in order to avoid unnecessary risk to the patient.

Physicians are more often present than for interfacility transport. Smith and associates reported that a physician was present during 40% of the transports, using varied transport personnel depending on the severity of illness.[65] Szem and colleagues followed a standard regimen for transports, regardless of severity of illness, and had a physician present on every transport.[1] These researchers felt that this was an important contributing factor in their low number (5.9%) of transport-related complications. Smith and coworkers[65] on the other hand reported that one third of 125 transports sustained at least one mishap.

References

1. Szem JW, Hydo LJ, Fischer E, et al: High-risk intrahospital transport of critically ill patients: Safety and outcome of the necessary "road trip." *Crit Care Med* 23:1660, 1995.
2. Kaplan L, Walsh D, Burney RE: Emergency aeromedical transport of patients with acute myocardial infarction. *Ann Emerg Med* 16:55, 1987.
3. Stenbach G, Sumchai AP: Is aeromedical transport of patients during acute myocardial infarction safe? *J Emerg Med* 7:73, 1989.
4. Bellinger RL, Califf RM, Mark DB, et al: Helicopter transport of patients during acute myocardial infarction. *Am J Cardiol* 61:718, 1988.
5. Selevan JS, Fields WW, Chen W, et al: Critical care transport: Outcome evaluation after interfacility transfer and hospitalization. *Ann Emerg Med* 33:33, 1999.
6. Gebremichael M, Borg U, Habashi N, et al: Interhospital transport of the extremely ill patient: The mobile intensive care unit. *Crit Care Med* 28:179, 2000.
7. Guidelines Committee of the American College of Critical Care Medicine, Society of Critical Care Medicine and American Association of Critical-Care Nurses Transfer Guidelines Task Force: Guidelines for the transfer of critically ill patients. *Crit Care Med* 21:931, 1993.
8. AARC Clinical Practice Guideline: In-Hospital Transport of the Mechanically Ventilated Patient—2002 Revision & Update. *Respir Care* 47:721, 2002.
9. Weg J, Haas C: Safe intrahospital transport of critically ill ventilator-dependent patients. *Chest* 96:631, 1989.
10. Braman SS, Dunn SM, Amico CA, et al: Complications of intrahospital transport of critically ill patients. *Ann Intern Med* 107:469, 1987.
11. Nakamura T, Fujino Y, Uchiyama A, et al: Intrahospital Transport of critically ill patients using ventilator with patient-triggering function. *Chest* 123:159, 2003.
12. Miyoshi E, Fujino Y, Mashimo T, et al: Performance of transport ventilator with patient-triggered ventilation. *Chest* 118:1109, 2000.
13. Lavoie A, Hall JB, Olson D, Wylam ME: Life-threatening effects of discontinuing inhaled nitric oxide in severe respiratory failure. *Am J Resp Crit Care Med* 153:1985, 1996.
14. Manthous CA, Hall JB, Caputo MA, et al: The effect of heliox on pulsus paradoxus and peak flow in non-intubated patients with severe asthma. *Am J Resp Crit Care Med* 151:310, 1995.
15. Andrews P, Piper I, Dearden N, et al: Secondary insults during intrahospital transport of head-injured patients. *Lancet* 335:327, 1990.
16. Bekar A, Ipekoglu Z, Tureyen K, et al: Secondary insults during intrahospital transport of neurosurgical intensive care patients. *Neurosurg Rev* 21:98, 1998.
17. Commission on Accreditation of Medical Transport Systems: *2002 Accreditation Standards*, 5th ed. Anderson, SC, Commission on Accreditation of Medical Transport Systems, 2002.
18. American Academy of Pediatrics, Subcommittee for Revision of Interhospital Transport Guidelines, Section on Transport Medicine: *Guidelines for Air and Ground Transport of Neonatal and Pediatric Patients*. Elk Grove Village, IL, American Academy of Pediatrics, 1999.
19. James S, ed. *Standards for Critical Care and Specialty Ground Transport*. Denver, CO, Air & Surface Transport Nurses Association, 2002.
20. Arndt K (ed): *Standards for Critical Care and Specialty Rotor-wing Transport*. Denver, CO, Air & Surface Transport Nurses Association, 2003.
21. Haupt MT, Rehm CG: Bedside procedures. Solutions to the pitfalls of intrahospital transport. *Crit Care Clin* 16:1, 2000.
22. Thomas F: Evaluating medical equipment carrying cases. *Emerg Care Q* 1:33, 1986.
23. Thompson DR, Clemmer TP, Applefeld JJ, et al: Regionalization of critical care medicine: Task force report of the American College of Critical Care Medicine. *Crit Care Med* 22:1306, 1994.
24. Ehrenwerth J, Sorbo S, Hackel A: Transport of critically ill adults. *Crit Care Med* 14:543, 1986.
25. Clemmer TP, Thomas F: Transport of the critically ill (editorial). *Crit Care Med* 28:265, 2000.
26. Fromm RE, Varon J: Critical care transport. *Crit Care Clin* 16:695, 2000.
27. Thomas F, Larsen K, Clemmer TP, et al: Impact of prospective payments on a tertiary care center receiving large numbers of critically ill patients by aeromedical transport. *Crit Care Med* 14:227, 1986.

28. Congressional Omnibus Budget Reconciliation Act (COBRA) of 1985 (42 USCA 1395 DD), as amended by the Omnibus Budget Reconciliation Acts (OBRA) of 1987, 1989, and 1990.

29. 42 CFR Parts 413, 482, and 489. Medicare Program; Clarifying Policies Related to the Responsibilities of Medicare-Participating Hospitals in Treating Individuals With Emergency Medical Conditions. *Federal Register*, September, 9, 2003.

30. Thomas F, Blumen IJ: Assessing oxygenation in the transport environment. *Air Med J* 18:79, 1998.

31. FAR Part 135—Operating Requirements: Commuter and On-Demand Operations and Rules Governing Persons on Board Such Aircraft. Title 14 of the Code of Federal Regulations (CFR). *Federal Register*, September, 2000. http://www1.faa.gov/asd/international/TSO_FAR_AC/far-135%20-%20Notepad.pdf

32. FAR Part 91—General Operating and Flight Rules. Title 14 of the Code of Federal Regulations (CFR). *Federal Register*, September, 2000. http://www.airweb.faa.gov/Regulatory_ and _Guidance_Library/rgFAR.nsf/MainFrame?OpenFrameSet

33. Medical Advisory Committee, The Association of Air Medical Services: *Position Paper on the Appropriate Use of Air Medical Services. J Air Med Transport* 9:9, 29, 1990.

34. Baxt WG, Moody P: The impact of a rotorcraft aeromedical emergency care service on trauma mortality. *JAMA* 249:3047, 1983.

35. Baxt WG, et al: Hospital-based rotorcraft aeromedical emergency care services and trauma mortality: A multicenter study. *Ann Emerg Med* 14:859, 1985.

36. Urdaneta LF, et al: Evaluation of an emergency air transport service as a component of a rural EMS system. *Am Surg* 50:183, 1984.

37. Schiller WR, et al: Effect of helicopter transport of trauma victims on survival in an urban trauma center. *J Trauma* 28:1127, 1988.

38. Fischer RP, et al: Urban helicopter response to the scene of injury. *J Trauma* 24:946, 1984.

39. Kaplan L, Walsh D, Burney RM: Emergency aeromedical transport of patients with acute myocardial infarction, *Ann Emerg Med* 16:55, 1987.

40. Bellinger RL, et al: Helicopter transport of patients during acute myocardial infarction. *Am J Cardiol* 61:719, 1988.

41. Schneider S, Borok Z, Heller M: Critical cardiac transports: air versus ground? *Am J Emerg Med* 6:449, 1988.

42. Fromm RE, et al: Bleeding complications following imitation of thrombolytic therapy for acute myocardial infarction: A comparison of helicopter-transported and non transported patients. *Ann Emerg Med* 20:892, 1991.

43. Parer JT: Effects of hypoxia on the mother and fetus with emphasis on maternal air transport. *Am J Obstet Gynecol* 142:957, 1982.

44. Low RB, Martin D, Brown C: Emergency air transport of pregnant patients: The national experience. *J Emerg Med* 6:41, 1988.

45. Blumen IJ, Lemkin DL, Scott G, et al: A safety review and risk assessment in air medical transport, in *Air Medical Physician Handbook*. Salt Lake City, Air Medical Physician Association, 2002.

46. Rau W: 2000 Medical crew survey. *AirMed* 6(September/October):17, 2000.

47. Burney R, Passini L, Hubert D, et al: Comparison of aeromedical crew performance by patient severity and outcome. *Ann Emerg Med* 21:375, 1992.

48. Rubenstein J, Gomez M, Rybicki L, et al: Can the need for a physician as part of the pediatric transport team be predicted? *Crit Care Med* 20:1657, 1992.

49. van Wijngaarden M, Kortbeek J, Lafreniere R, et al: Air ambulance trauma transport: A quality review. *J Trauma* 41:26, 1996.

50. Baxt WG, Moody P: Impact of a physician as part of the aeromedical prehospital team in patients with blunt trauma. *JAMA* 257:3246, 1987.

51. Edge W, Kanter R, Weigle C, et al: Reduction of morbidity in interhospital transport by specialized pediatric staff. *Crit Care Med* 22:1186, 1994.

52. Orr R, et al: Pediatric specialty care teams are associated with reduced morbidity during pediatric interfacility transport. Presented at the 2000 Conference on Neonatal and Pediatric Critical Care Transport, American Academy of Pediatrics, Chicago, IL, June, 2000.

53. Valenzuela TD, Criss EA, Copass MK, et al: Critical care air transportation of the severely injured: Does long distance transport adversely affect survival? *Ann Emerg Med* 19:169, 1990.

54. Schwartz RJ, Jacobs LM, Yaezel D: Impact of pre-trauma center care on length of stay and hospital charges. *J Trauma* 29:1611, 1989.

55. Rubenstein DG, Treister NW, Kapoor AS, et al: Transfer of acutely ill cardiac patients for definitive care. *JAMA* 259:1695, 1988.

56. Bitterman RA: Providing Emergency Care Under Federal Law: Emergency Medical Treatment and Active Labor Act (EMTALA). Dallas, TX, American College of Emergency Physicians, 2000.

57. 42 USC 1395 dd(b)(2)(D), HCFA Interpretive Guideline, V-32.

58. Shelton SL, Swor RA, Domeier RM, et al: Medical direction of interfacility transports. Position Statement: National Association of EMS Physicians, Lenexa, KC, 2002. http://www.naemsp.org/Position%20Papers/MedDirInterfacility.html

59. Medical Direction and Medical Control of Air Medical Services. Position Statement of The Air Medical Physician Association. Salt Lake City, UT, 1998, revised 2002. http://ampa.org/medical_direction.pdf

60. Indeck M, Peterson S, Smith J, et al: Risk, cost, and benefit of transporting ICU patients for special studies. *J Trauma* 28:1020, 1988.

61. Rutherford WF, Fisher CJ: Risks associated with in-house transportation of the critically ill. *Clin Res* 34:414A, 1986.

62. Waddell G: Movement of critically ill patients within hospital. *Br Med J* 2:417, 1975.

63. Hurst J, Davis K, Johnson D, et al: Cost and complications during in-hospital transport of critically ill patients: A prospective cohort study. *J Trauma* 33:582, 1992.

64. Stearley HE: Patients and outcomes: Intrahospital transportation and monitoring of critically ill patients by a specially trained ICU nursing staff. *Am J Crit Care* 7:282, 1998.

65. Smith I, Flemming S, Cernaianu A: Mishaps during transport from the intensive care unit. *Crit Care Med* 18:278, 1990.

Chapter 8 ———————————
TELEMEDICINE
MICHAEL BRESLOW

KEY POINTS

- *Creating a centralized ICU care system provides a mechanism for implementing 24-hour 7-day intensivist oversight of critically ill patients throughout a network of hospitals.*

- *A major goal of centralizing ICU care is to spread intensivist care over larger numbers of patients, thereby extending both the number of patients managed by an intensivist and the hours of intensivist care. Creating a multidisciplinary remote care team in which ICU nurses and ancillary personnel work in support of the remote intensivist is central to maximizing operating efficiency.*

- *Available data suggest that implementing a remote intensivist management program that supplements on-site physician care can improve clinical outcomes and economic performance. We speculate that dedicated off-site intensivists improve outcomes by closely monitoring patient status when there is no on-site intensivist, thereby ensuring that care plans are adhered to and that new problems are detected and addressed promptly.*

- *The requisite technology includes 2-way audio and high-resolution video links to each patient room, a robust clinical information system that allows off-site physicians to access patient data, technology tools for performing routine care tasks (e.g., creating notes and orders), and a robust and secure broadband wide area network.*

- *Clear definition of roles and responsibilities, detailed elucidation of operating procedures, including how the remote program integrates with on-site physician activities, and ensuring compliance with standard inpatient care policies (e.g., licensure, credentialing, quality assurance, and the Health Insurance Portability and Accountability Act) are essential for a smoothly functioning and effective program.*

- *Centralized ICU care programs as part of a system-wide view of ICU care ensuring consistent 24-hour 7-day intensivist oversight and the use of an information technology backbone, create unique opportunities to standardize care practices, enhance operating effectiveness, and improve outcomes.*

There is wide variation in intensive care unit (ICU) care across U.S. hospitals. Despite data showing improved clinical outcomes with dedicated intensivist staffing[1] and the institution of a variety of best practices,[2] few ICUs are able to implement these care practices broadly and consistently. Fundamental problems in our current health care system make the goal of optimal ICU care nearly unobtainable for most hospitals. Considerable attention has been devoted to the current shortage of intensivists[3] and the high cost of 24-hour 7-day staffing models. Similar focus has been devoted to the difficulty of getting physicians to adopt best practices. While there are behavioral and managerial components to this problem, the lack of real-time prompts and data-based feedback represent equally important obstacles. Even where hospital leadership appreciates the clinical and financial impact of improved ICU care, the path is both costly and difficult. This chapter presents an alternate care paradigm—one that addresses many of the most serious barriers to improving ICU care. There are three core concepts central to this new care model. First, ICU care is viewed as a system-wide problem, where care across multiple institutions is addressed comprehensively, resources are shared across a network of facilities, and care practices are systematically standardized. Second, technology tools and alternate staffing patterns are used to allow intensivists to care for greater numbers of patients. Third, computer applications assist physicians in problem detection, guide their decision making, and provide feedback that helps drive quality improvement initiatives. The vision is for ICU care to become an integrated service across a network of hospitals, to be delivered in a consistent manner, and to achieve the highest level of care possible with existing resources.

Telemedicine and Early Intensive Care Unit Applications

Telemedicine can be defined broadly as the provision of health care services to patients by care providers that are not in physical proximity to the patient. Telemedicine was initially envisioned as a means of providing geographically isolated patients access to quality health care. Early applications, including military and rural health initiatives, focused on establishing adequate connectivity, developing tools that could be used remotely, and demonstrating clinical feasibility. Costs were high and usage was low—primarily because of low population densities in the target locales—and most projects were abandoned when external funding disappeared. One exception was the use of telemedicine for care of prison inmates. There savings of the high cost of patient transport helped to underwrite infrastructure costs. Over the past decade telecommunication costs have fallen markedly and several new uses of telemedicine have appeared, including teleradiology and telepathology. Both employ store-and-forward technology, in which images from multiple sites are transported to a centralized reading facility. Teleradiology probably represents the leading telemedicine application in use today, almost certainly because work volume is high and these centers can be profitable. This application, although potentially representing a more cost-effective way to deliver a service, does not fundamentally improve the quality of health care. While a variety of new programs are being evaluated, most telemedicine initiatives have failed to deliver on the promise of improved access to health care and better outcomes that spawned the concept 20 years ago.

The use of telemedicine for provision of ICU services dates back to the early 1980s. Grundy and associates established an ICU consultative program, in which intensivists provided advice to clinicians at a remote hospital lacking intensivists.[4] While short lived, the clinical teams at both sites subjectively cited value in the program. Almost 15 years later, a team of academic intensivists reported improved outcomes during a 17-week program of continuous intensivist oversight of ICU patients in a 10-bed surgical ICU that did not have dedicated intensivists.[5] This program operated 24 hours 7 days a week and the intensivists had real-time access to bedside monitor and laboratory data, as well as two-way audio-video connectivity. The remote intensivists worked in support of the on-site team but were credentialed at the remote hospital and had order-writing privileges. Detailed data were collected on all patients cared for during the pilot program and compared to similar data from patients cared for during two 4-month periods 6 and 12 months prior to the program. The Acute Physiology and Chronic Health Evaluation (APACHE) III methodology was used to adjust for changes in disease severity among the study periods. Actual-to-predicted mortality and length-of-stay (LOS) ratios both decreased by 30% during the intervention period, and the incidence of major complications decreased by 40%. A detailed financial analysis showed decreases in the cost of care that paralleled the shortening of ICU LOS. Although only a pilot project, the results suggested that a 24-hour 7-day remote intensivist care program might provide benefits similar to those reported with dedicated on-site intensivist staffing models.

In 1998, following completion of the continuous ICU telemedicine study described above, two of the investigators (including the author of this chapter) started a company to provide remote intensivist monitoring systems to hospitals. The first ICU telemedicine program using this technology was begun in 2000 in two hospitals at Sentara Healthcare, an integrated delivery network (IDN) in Virginia. A total of 36 ICU beds, representing 3 ICUs, were monitored initially. The remote care center was located in commercial office space 8 to 10 miles from the two hospitals, and staffed around the clock by an intensivist, an ICU nurse, and a clerical assistant. This off-site team worked in support of on-site physicians, actively monitored all patients, ensured that care plans were executed, and assisted with management of new problems. The technology infrastructure was provided and installed by the telemedicine vendor and intensivists from the IDN staffed the remote center. A detailed study of clinical and financial outcomes showed a 27% reduction in hospital mortality and decreases in ICU and hospital LOS of 17% and 13%, respectively.[5a] Costs of care decreased by 19%, hospital revenue for ICU patients increased by 7.5% as a result of an increase in ICU throughput, and contribution margin rose by $6 million annually. Of note, the decrease in ICU LOS was attributable to a reduction in the number of long-stay patients, an effect that may indicate fewer complications as a result of improved monitoring and earlier intervention.

The Sentara program has expanded over the past 24 months, and currently includes seven ICUs in four hospitals. Similar systems are in place in two large East Coast academic medical centers, a 29-hospital IDN in California, an eight-hospital system in the Midwest, and in several military facilities (including a 4000 mile remote link from Hawaii to Guam).

Rationale for Intensive Care Unit Telemedicine

Over the past 5 to 10 years, multiple studies have documented superior clinical outcomes in hospitals with dedicated intensivist staffing models.[1] Mortality rate reductions in these studies average >20%. Many of these reports also describe decreases in ICU LOS and resource utilization. Based on the strength of these data, the Leapfrog Group, an organization formed by Fortune 500 companies to establish health care purchasing standards, has called for all nonrural hospitals to implement dedicated intensivist staffing models within the next 1 to 2 years.[6] They project that adoption of this staffing model will result in 50,000 to 170,000 fewer ICU deaths annually in the U.S.[7] A number of other health care quality groups have issued similar recommendations for dedicated-intensivist staffing.[8,9]

Despite compelling evidence that dedicated intensivist staffing models result in better clinical outcomes, fewer than 15% of U.S. hospitals have this staffing in place.[3] The two most commonly cited obstacles to implementing this model are cost and the unavailability of intensivists. A common financial analysis places the salary cost of 4 to 5 intensivists (required for 24-hour 7-day staffing for 1 ICU) at >$1,000,000 annually, a number that exceeds projected professional services reimbursement. However, even when hospitals recognize the financial benefits of improved ICU clinical outcomes and management, a severe national shortage of intensivists makes recruitment difficult. A recently completed manpower study estimates that there are approximately 5500 practicing intensivists in the U.S.[10] Since the overwhelming majority of these intensivists also participate in other clinical and/or academic activities, the number of full-time equivalents (FTEs) is considerably smaller. When viewed in relation to the 30,000 FTEs required for 24-hour 7-day intensivist staffing in all U.S. ICUs, the shortfall is quite daunting. Moreover, projections based on the current pool of trainees suggest that the problem will worsen for many years.

By permitting a single intensivist-led team to provide care to patients in multiple sites simultaneously, telemedicine offers a potential means of leveraging the current pool of intensivists over larger numbers of patients. Central to this model is the creation of a network of ICUs and other high-acuity beds (e.g., stepdown, ED holding, and postanesthetic care unit) and the use of a dedicated team of intensivists and other care providers to supplement on-site care and thereby achieve 24-hour 7-day intensivist care. Viewing the delivery of critical care services from a system-based perspective, rather than the traditional model in which each individual ICU functions autonomously, represents a major shift in how we conceptualize the care of critically ill patients. This change in perspective (and execution) allows resources to be allocated more efficiently, ensures a more uniform level of service across facilities, and it also creates a platform for practice standardization. The use of a centralized intensivist team for the provision of physician services traditionally provided by on-site physicians creates a mechanism for increasing operating efficiency. By using physician extenders and technology tools to increase operating efficiency, this physical redeployment can enable intensivists to care for considerably larger numbers of patients than with traditional on-site physician staffing. Both staffing models and technology tools are covered later in this chapter.

When evaluating the potential for remote ICU care to permit more efficient provision of intensivist services, several important questions arise. Some of these are technology-related—connectivity, reliability, data access, and security—and are addressed in the next section. Others are more operational in nature. How does remote care integrate with on-site activities and how is continuity of care ensured across multiple care providers? This question is not unique to remote care, but one that assumes greater importance given that 24-hour 7-day intensivist care becomes feasible with this model. These operational issues require new processes and operating procedures. Several solutions developed by early adopters of this new technology are described in a later section of this chapter. The most important questions, however, concern the extent to which intensivist activities can be provided effectively by off-site intensivists. The improvement in clinical and economic outcomes reported with remote care trials suggest a level of efficacy comparable to that reported in studies examining the impact of implementing a dedicated daytime intensivist care model. However, understanding the strengths and weaknesses of this alternate care paradigm will be essential to defining the optimal balance between on-site and remote activities, and optimizing ICU care models moving forward.

At this time there are insufficient data to answer these important questions. However, considering the likely reasons for superior clinical outcomes with dedicated intensivist staffing may provide some useful insights and identify areas for future study. First, intensivists, as a result of their training and clinical activities, have greater familiarity and expertise in managing critically ill patients. This expertise presumably leads to more accurate and timely problem recognition and better management decisions, regardless of whether these activities are provided on-site or remotely. Second, dedicated ICU physicians coordinate the diverse tasks of the care team (consultants, nursing, pharmacy, respiratory, nutrition, etc.), establish priorities, and create a comprehensive care plan. This important activity, setting the care plan, usually occurs at the beginning of each day. Because it is time consuming and entails integrating large amounts of data (including physical exam findings) and communicating with multiple care providers and the patient's family, one might hypothesize that this activity is better performed by on-site physicians. Third, dedicated intensivists monitor each patient's progress throughout the day (altering therapies as needed to ensure that care objectives are met), and detect and respond to new problems promptly. This constant adjustment of care can only occur when intensivists monitor patients continuously, analyze new data as they become available, and respond immediately when changes in therapy become necessary. It is this continuous monitoring of patient status that is at the heart of the dedicated intensivist model. Because of their inherent physiologic instability, ICU patients sustain adverse events and develop complications at rates far exceeding those of other patients. Only through continuous monitoring by highly trained physicians can we ensure that patients progress according to plan and receive appropriate and timely treatment of all problems. We hypothesize that this continuous care function, which requires 24-hour 7-day physician vigilance, can be performed effectively by intensivists regardless of their location, and represents the optimal use of this new technology.

Technology

Effective telemedicine applications must provide off-site care providers with access to the key data required for monitoring clinical status, reliable mechanisms for communicating with on-site personnel, and tools to perform routine tasks such as generating notes and orders. Many of the tools used to enable off-site care will also be deployed in the ICU in order to facilitate integration of remote and on-site activities.

Key ICU telemedicine components include:

- *Two-way audio-video*: Audio-video equipment is used for visual monitoring of patient status and communicating with on-site personnel. Individual connections to each patient room are preferred, although portable devices may be useful in some low-use settings. Desired functionality includes full-motion video (>25 frames per second), remote camera control, automatic aperture control, zoom capability, and synchronization of audio and video switching.

- *Real-time viewing of bedside monitor waveforms and digital readouts*: Vital signs and other physiologic data provide essential information used for monitoring patient status. In addition to digital readouts of heart rate, vascular pressures, and other data, waveform displays are necessary for evaluation of rhythm disturbances and other cardiac anomalies.

- *Radiography and other image viewing*: Although on-site staff will read most radiographic studies, emergency viewing capability is important. High-resolution medical grade scanners can be used for this purpose in hospitals that have not changed over to digitized radiographs.

- *Access to detailed clinical data*: A wide variety of clinical data must be available to the care team, including laboratory, culture, and other test results; medications; vital signs; and other physiologic data (e.g., invasive hemodynamics and input and output, among others). Aggregating these diverse data can be a formidable undertaking, as can organizing and displaying them in user-friendly formats. Successful applications provide considerable value to on-site caregivers and can serve as a platform for knowledge-based applications, such as those described below.

- *Physician notes and orders*: Off-site care providers must be able to both generate notes and orders (the products of their work), and view physician documents created on-site. While many hospitals are evaluating the feasibility of system-wide computerized physician order entry systems, few have these in place. Some system for creating orders and printing them in the ICU is required, preferably one that captures key medication information and provides screening for allergies and drug interactions. Similar tools must be available for creating and viewing physician notes, as these contain key patient data not available elsewhere. The use of computer-based note writing tools is highly recommended, since traditional handwritten notes are very inefficient for information transfer (due to wide variations in content/organization, poor legibility, and lack of portability).

- *Communication tools*: The primary rationale for introducing a centralized care team is to expand intensivist coverage to both greater numbers of patients and more hours of the day (24 hours 7 days a week is optimal). Because of both geographic separation and expanded hours of physician coverage, specific tools to ensure rapid and effective communication between care teams is essential. Dedicated phone lines ensure that on-site personnel can access the remote team rapidly during emergencies, while the audio-video system allows effective in-room communication. Efficient and effective physician-to-physician communication is equally important. Although traditional verbal sign-out rounds can be used to outline treatment goals, delineate

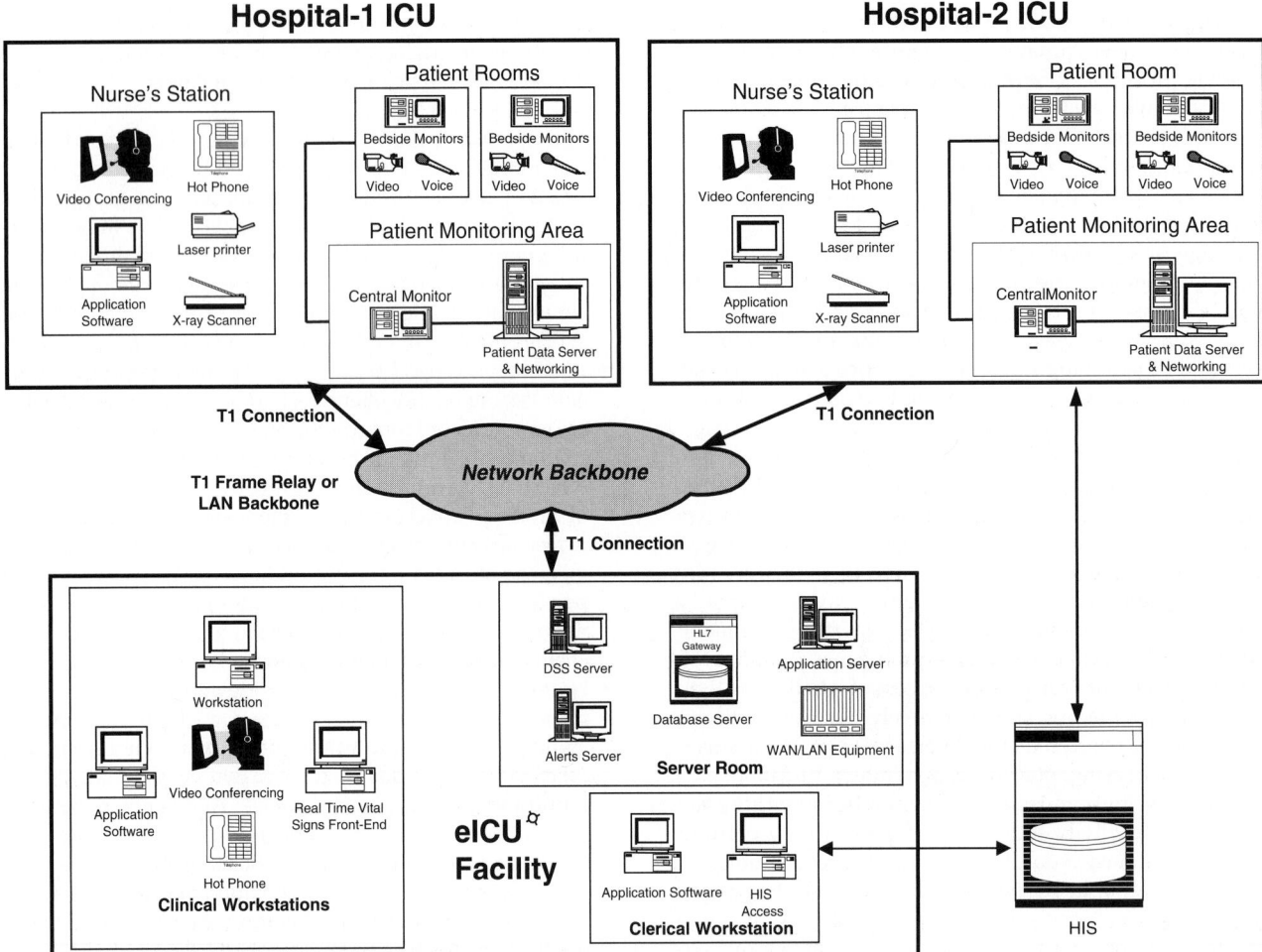

FIGURE 8-1 Schematic diagram showing remote care architecture.

key tasks, and communicate ideas and clinical information not appropriate for inclusion in traditional physician notes, they are time-consuming and difficult to coordinate. The use of computer-based applications for transmission of these data offers clear advantages.

- *A wide area network*: A wide area network that connects each ICU (or other high-acuity site) to the centralized monitoring center is necessary to support all the above applications. This network must be reliable (redundancy is desirable), secure, and have sufficient bandwidth to support full-motion video.

Commercial systems in use today also include computer-based decision-support tools and an alerting system that evaluates new clinical data (e.g., labs, physiologic data, and medications) and flags potential problems. These tools facilitate problem recognition and assist both remote and on-site physicians with decision making. Figure 8-1 shows a schematic representation of a remote care system.

Establishing the technology platform to support a centralized ICU care center is a complex undertaking. While some required functionality may be available in existing ICU or hospital applications, the entire system must function as an integrated whole. The diverse components must be simple to use and support routine ICU care processes. A dysfunctional technology infrastructure will limit the number of patients the remote care team can manage, thus undermining one of the key reasons for centralizing this function. On the other hand, installing a comprehensive patient care system that supports physician workflow, facilitates problem detection, standardizes practice patterns, and improves decision making can provide real benefits. Such systems can also bring value to on-site intensivists and help improve the safety and efficiency of their activities.

Operational Considerations

Establishing a remote ICU management program changes the care paradigm at several different levels. First, a host of new procedures must be introduced to support off-site care. Areas that must be addressed include credentialing, clinical processes, communication, documentation, training, and quality review. However, implementing a remote ICU program entails fundamental changes in ICU management—adopting a system-wide approach to ICU care, moving to 24-hour 7-day intensivist oversight, and standardizing care processes. Migrating to this alternate care paradigm provides substantial benefits, but requires strong institutional leadership and experience in implementing new clinical programs. Establishing clear goals, identifying champions and local leaders, creating appropriate incentives, and aggressively managing the change process are essential to achieving high levels of success.

Although centralized ICU care programs are still relatively new, the accumulated experience of the sites in current operation have generated considerable useful information. A brief summary of their experience in several key areas follows.

- *Staffing*: All programs to date have targeted reaching 35 to 50 networked beds within a short time frame. This represents a comfortable number of monitored patients for a physician/nurse team, and it also is of sufficient scale to justify the operating expenses of the remote center. As additional beds are added, more staff are required. Although experience is limited, it appears that a second physician will be needed when the number of networked beds approaches 100. Nonintensivists may be able to function as the second physician since they will be working in tandem with the intensivist. ICU fellows and acute care nurse practitioners may prove to be valuable additions to the care team. Because the remote care program supplements, rather than replaces, on-site clinical activities, the program will require the addition of new physicians and nurses. Although some individuals may prefer to work in the remote center exclusively (or may need to because of disabilities, such as latex allergy), most physicians and nurses prefer to divide their time between on-site and remote care. Many hospital systems have multiple groups of intensivists, sometimes representing different private practice teams, and other times representing different medical specialties (e.g., medical intensive care unit, surgical intensive care unit, or neurologic intensive care unit). Creating a structure in which all groups are able to participate in the remote care program simplifies staffing of the remote center and helps to build support for the project. It also increases the breadth of experience, fosters collaboration, and helps with standardizing practice patterns. Where ICU care is highly specialized, open discussion of care practices for different populations and formal back-up procedures for complex specialty cases are important.
- *Financial structure*: Third party reimbursement for telemedicine professional services is very limited at this time. As a result, all current ICU telemedicine programs are funded by the participating hospitals. Hospitals recognize cost savings from reduced ICU and hospital LOS and lower daily ancillary cost expenditures, and they also are able to create additional ICU capacity as a result of the decrease in ICU LOS. Initial data suggest that these financial benefits exceed the implementation and operating costs of the program, including the salary costs of the intensivists and other care team members. Salary levels must be appropriate for the market and sufficient to entice physicians to work nights and weekends.
- *Remote center operations*: The remote team consists of physicians, nurses, and clerical personnel, as well as dedicated administrators. It is important to clearly define the roles and responsibilities of each member of the team. This requires developing procedures for how all key tasks are to be performed (e.g., rounding, data gathering, and communications). Assembling a multidisciplinary team consisting of hospital administrators, program administrators, ICU team members (physicians and nurses), and stakeholders from other areas that interface with the ICU (e.g., pharmacy and ED) ensures broad representation and is recom-

mended. Once remote care processes have been defined, they need to be documented and understood by all. Formal training programs must be developed so that each participant is familiar with the technology and the clinical procedures. Back-up plans must be developed in the event of technical problems (e.g., network failure) and to deal with common problems. The more effective the planning process, the smoother the operation will be.

- *Integration with on-site activities*: The remote care team functions in support of the on-site physicians. In most ICUs the attending of record (or on-site intensivist) will review all data at least once a day, coordinate communication with all members of the team (nurses, consultants, respiratory therapy, etc), and establish the care plan. When that individual leaves the ICU (the time of day will vary depending on the staffing model), the remote team assumes responsibility for executing the care plan, making adjustments to ensure that goals are met, monitoring patients for new problems, and intervening where needed. The smooth transfer of responsibility embodied in this model requires effective communication between the on-site and remote teams. The computer-based applications required for off-site care, if deployed in the ICU, can provide a convenient forum for this information transfer. In this way the thoughts and plans of the attending of record are available to the remote intensivist, and the assessments and interventions of the off-site intensivist are immediately apparent to the on-site physicians when they return to the ICU. However, in order to get the requisite buy-in from busy ICU clinicians, effort must be devoted to ensuring that the on-site care team understands both the value provided by the remote team and the importance of effective communication. It is similarly important that the remote intensivist notify the attending of record when important decisions arise during off hours.
- *Oversight*: As should be evident from the above discussion, implementing a system-wide remote ICU care program is a major undertaking. A new operating center must be established, staff must be hired/recruited and trained, and a complex set of operating procedures need to be developed. ICU staff will need to be trained and physicians that admit to the ICU will require education as well. Assembling an experienced leadership team is essential to the success of the program. Senior hospital executives must clearly enunciate the rationale and vision of the program. Dedicated project leaders must be appointed, usually an intensivist physician and a remote center manager. These individuals should have the requisite skills for the job and have protected time to devote to the project. In addition, a broad-based program oversight committee should meet regularly to review problems, modify operating procedures, and track program progress. This committee, in conjunction with senior hospital leadership, should establish yearly goals for the program and track progress against these.

Regulatory Issues

There are a number of regulatory issues that must be considered when implementing a remote ICU care program. First, off-site intensivists are providing patient care. Although most remote care programs cover a limited geographic region, some may cross state lines, and physicians in the remote center must be licensed to practice medicine in each state that has hospitals within the network. Physicians also will need to be credentialed at each participating hospital. A few hospitals have developed special credentials for this purpose. The second important area concerns ensuring patient confidentiality. The recently issued federal security guidelines (part of the Health Insurance Portability and Accountability Act; HIPAA) outline general principles for protecting patient data and confidentiality. These have clear implications for remote ICU care, including keeping transmitted data secure, and instituting appropriate security policies at the remote site. Most hospitals include consent for remote care as part of their hospital admission consent process.

The Leapfrog Group has indicated that hospitals may use remote intensivist monitoring in order to meet their intensivist standard. They suggest that this may increase the feasibility of implementing dedicated intensivist coverage. They have defined several key features for a remote management program,[11,12] including:

- An on-site intensivist must review patient data and set the daily care plan.
- The tele-intensivist must provide care during all hours that there is not an intensivist on-site. He or she must be physically at the remote care site and have no concurrent responsibilities.
- Clinical data must be available to the remote intensivist, including laboratory results, medications, and notes, among others.
- The remote care system must be robust (>98% uptime) and secure (HIPAA compliant).
- The remote intensivist must be able to visualize the patient and communicate with on-site personnel, so camera resolution and bandwidth must be sufficient to assess breathing.
- The program must adhere to written standards, including at a minimum: (1) critical care certification, (2) state medical licensure, (3) hospital credentialing, (4) quality review of the program, (5) explicit policies defining roles and responsibilities, and (6) a program to educate staff about the program.
- Remote intensivist care must be proactive and include routine review of all patients.
- The workload of the tele-intensivist should not be excessive; he or she should be available within 5 minutes of a request from ICU personnel.
- There should be written procedures to ensure effective communication between the tele-intensivist and the on-site personnel.
- Actions performed by the remote intensivist should be documented and included in the medical record.

Future Directions, Broader Visions

Implementing a remote care program represents a major change in the patient care paradigm. The rationale for this change, as discussed above, is to improve clinical outcomes in our most vulnerable patients. However, there are several intriguing consequences of this new model. First, critical care is viewed as a system-wide priority and intensivists are viewed as the key resource. By elevating both the prominence of critical care and the importance of intensivists, cen-

tralized care programs should have a beneficial impact on the specialty. Second, conceptualizing critical care at the system level should facilitate practice standardization, which will further improve clinical outcomes. Third, the program aspires to continuous intensivist oversight, regardless of time of day. This care model accepts the need for 24-hour 7-day dedicated physician care, and as a result, requires a move to fixed shifts of clinical responsibility. While this change in staffing requires increased focus on processes to ensure continuity of care, it should improve quality of life for intensivists and address a major factor contributing to early burnout and choosing alternate career options. Fourth, remote care depends on the introduction of technology systems that are actually used to care for patients. This technology infrastructure creates opportunities to use information systems to improve the care process. Automated alerts can reduce errors, detailed information on practice patterns can be used to drive performance improvement initiatives, computerized decision support tools can ensure ready access to current knowledge, and time-saving computer applications can improve physician efficiency and effectiveness. It is worth noting that the promise of these smart systems can be realized because there is a physician monitoring all critically ill patients at all times, in contrast to other monitoring paradigms, because the physician doing the monitoring has the clinical skills to analyze the incoming alerts, and he or she is empowered to initiate a response. Finally, because the program views critical care as a system-wide service, operating efficiency can be optimized and resources can be used more effectively. As a result, this re-engineering of ICU patient care can both save lives and have major financial benefits for the hospital.

Centralized ICU care is still in its infancy. As experience increases we can look forward to an improved understanding of which elements of the program have the greatest effect on outcomes, and which functions are best performed by on-site physicians. Efficacy needs to be confirmed in different environments (academic, community, and rural) and with different on-site staffing models. Considerable uncertainty exists regarding preferred off-site staffing models, particularly as the size of the ICU network increases. Operating procedures need to be refined and new systems developed for training both on-site personnel and the remote team. Almost certainly the technology infrastructure will evolve, and this should both simplify establishing a remote program and increase operating efficiency. Like many new technologies, increased experience will enhance efficacy and expose weaknesses. It is important to recognize that the supporting technology enables new systems of care. As such, the success in different sites will depend on the diligence of the clinicians responsible for providing patient care. The potential looks promising and it should be exciting to follow the evolution of this care model moving forward.

References

1. Pronovost PJ, Angus DC, Dorman T, et al: Physician staffing patterns and clinical outcomes in critically ill patients. *JAMA* 288:2151, 2002.
2. Holcomb BW, Wheeler AP, Ely EW: New ways to reduce unnecessary variation and improve outcomes in the intensive care unit. *Curr Opin Crit Care* 7:304, 2001.

3. Angus DC, Kelley MA, Schmitz RJ, et al: Committee on Manpower for Pulmonary and Critical Care Societies (COMPACCS). Caring for the critically ill patient. Current and projected workforce requirements for care of the critically ill and patients with pulmonary disease: Can we meet the requirements of an aging population? *JAMA* 284:2762, 2000.

4. Grundy BL, Jones PK, Lovitt A: Telemedicine in critical care: Problems in design, implementation, and assessment. *Crit Care Med* 10:471, 1982.

5. Rosenfeld BA, Dorman T, Breslow MJ, et al: Intensive care unit telemedicine: Alternate paradigm for providing continuous intensivist care. *Crit Care Med* 28:3925, 2000.

5a. Breslow MJ, Rosenfeld BA, Doerfler M, et al: Effect of a multiple-site intensive care unit telemedicine program on clinical and economic outcomes: An alternative paradigm for intensivist staffing. *Crit Care Med* 32:31, 2004.

6. Milstein A, Galvin RS, Delbanco SF, et al: Improving the safety of health care: The Leapfrog Initiative. *Eff Clin Pract* 6:313, 2000.

7. Young MP, Birkmeyer JD: Potential reduction in mortality rates using an intensivist model to manage intensive care units. *Eff Clin Pract* 6:284, 2000.

8. *Safe Practices for Better Healthcare,* National Quality Forum, 2002. Washington. Available online at http://www.qualityforum.org/safe_practices_report.html. Accessed May 15, 2003.

9. Evidence Report/Technology Assessment No. 43, *Making Health Care Safer: A Critical Analysis of Patient Safety Practices.* Agency for Healthcare and Quality (AHRQ) Publication No. 01-E058, July 20, 2001. Available online at http://www.ahrq.gov/clinic/ptsafety/index.html#toc. Accessed May 15, 2003.

10. Pronovost PJ, Waters H, Dorman T: Impact of critical care physician workforce for intensive care unit physician staffing. *Curr Opin Crit Care* 7:456, 2001.

11. http://www.leapfroggroup.org/FactSheets/ICU_FactSheet.pdf. Accessed May 15, 2003.

12. https://leapfrog.medstat.com/content/FAQ.pdf. Accessed May 15, 2003.

Chapter 9 _____

PREPAREDNESS FOR CATASTROPHE

JEFFREY G. WALLS
J. CHRISTOPHER FARMER

KEY POINTS

- *The intensive care unit medical director should play an active role in each hospital's disaster planning.*
- *The Joint Commission on Accreditation of Healthcare Organizations requires that each hospital develop, implement, and regularly test a disaster plan.*
- *A hazard vulnerability analysis should be conducted by each hospital to identify threats to care of patients specific to its region.*
- *Preparation should coordinate all community resources and not be focused on a single ICU or hospital.*
- *Each ICU medical director should identify his or her role within the emergency command structure (typically the hospital emergency incident command system).*
- *Back-up methods of communication such as walkie-talkies should be acquired and tested to ensure reliable communication between the ICU and the hospital command center.*
- *A pool of potential volunteer ICU medical personnel should be identified prior to a disaster and mechanisms put into place to provide emergency credentialing.*
- *An active disaster education program should be created to keep all ICU personnel up to date.*
- *Participation in realistic disaster exercises is important to identify problems within each hospital's plan and to reinforce education.*

Hospitals today are faced with a daunting task: to prepare for community disasters that could bring a large number of injured or ill patients to their doorsteps. Since September 11, 2001, the threats to a community and its hospitals seem endless. In addition to the terrible events surrounding the World Trade Towers collapse, a more insidious attack occurred in the form of anthrax delivered through the mail. Health care workers have died as a result of severe acute respiratory syndrome (SARS), which represents an emerging, highly contagious infectious disease. Natural disasters have wreaked havoc on numerous health care facilities, and have jeopardized patient well-being.

During a disaster, hospitals serve as a refuge for the injured and ill. Unfortunately, the ability of health care organizations to prepare for these would-be crises is jeopardized by current financial constraints. To many hospital administrators, maintaining facility solvency at their current rate of reimbursement is the real threat, while expending funds for disaster preparedness seems less essential. Hospitals must operate in a fiscally efficient manner, operating near full capacity. The ability of a typical hospital system to absorb large numbers of injured patients during an emergency either acutely, or over a more prolonged period of time, is extremely limited. More importantly, there has been little outside financial support to fund hospital disaster preparedness efforts.

First responders (police, fire department, and EMS) remain the primary focus for most ongoing disaster preparedness efforts. However, as mandated by the Joint Commission on Accreditation of Healthcare Organizations (JCAHO), all hospitals must have a functional disaster plan. As we learned during the recent SARS dilemma, the intensive care unit (ICU) is a key element of a hospital's response to large-scale incidents. In addition to emerging infectious diseases, trauma, bioterrorism, chemical attack, and radiation-induced injury are possible occurrences. Unfortunately, there is little written in the medical literature about the effects on structure and function of an ICU during a disaster.[1,2] As one example, during a biological weapons attack or an outbreak of a highly contagious disease, the ICU physician will be called on to recognize the syndrome and initiate the appropriate investigation and therapy. Therefore, the ICU medical director must be intimately involved with the hospital disaster committee to ensure the optimal use of this limited resource, and to ensure that the proper training and equipment are accomplished and available. The purpose of this chapter is to educate the intensivist on the general components of a hospital disaster plan, to detail where an intensive care unit fits into the hospital preparedness plan, and to review what predisaster preparation initiatives an ICU should conduct.

Definitions

The definition of a *disaster* is imprecise. Many different definitions are published, and an appropriate definition should be broad enough to be applicable to most situations. Frederick C. Cuny defines disaster as "a situation resulting from an environmental phenomenon or armed conflict that produced stress, personal injury, physical damage, and economic disruption of great magnitude."[3] By this definition, a disaster includes a wide range of events and outcomes. A disaster can occur outside the hospital or inside the facility, and can be the result of a naturally-occurring phenomenon, an unintentional accident, or an intentional act. A mass casualty incident (MCI) occurs when the requirements to care for multiple casualties overwhelm the normal capacity of the health care system.

Hospital Requirements for Disaster Preparedness

Given recent events, it is self-evident that hospitals must be prepared for an MCI. In the U.S., the standards for hospital accreditation as set forth by the JCAHO[4] (revised standards effective January 1, 2001) serves as a foundation for understanding the minimal components required in disaster preparation. The JCAHO standards include three components:

1. Environment of care (EC) standard EC.1.4 requires a hospital to develop a management plan that addresses the response to emergencies affecting the EC.
2. EC standard EC.2.4 requires the hospital to implement the emergency management plan.
3. EC standard EC.2.9.1 requires the hospital to execute the plan by participating in emergency management drills.

The development of a hospital disaster plan must address four phases of emergency management: mitigation, preparedness, response, and recovery. *Mitigation* refers to the identification of potential emergencies that could affect a hospital, and implementing a plan to support the most vulnerable areas. The JCAHO also requires that a hazard vulnerability analysis (HVA) be conducted. An HVA is a formal assessment of the potential threats to the normal delivery of health care. This analysis should include plans for internal disasters such as fire and loss of power, as well as external disasters that could result in large numbers of patients coming to a hospital. To assist a hospital to evaluate their vulnerabilities, the American Society for Healthcare Engineering has developed a hazard vulnerability assessment tool that is available through their website.[5]

Preparedness is self-explanatory, and includes obtaining supplies and equipment, making arrangements with vendors and outside medical facilities to enable the urgent acquisition of supplies, and educating and preparing the hospital staff through literature, lectures, and drills. *Response* includes the predetermined actions of the medical staff in the event of a disaster, and the actions that management takes to initiate the plan, set up the command structure, and initiate communications with first responders. *Recovery* focuses on returning to normal operations and restoring needed services.

Coordinating Intensive Care Unit and Hospital Plans with the Community

A hospital emergency response plan must be coordinated with community emergency management planning. After the HVA has been accomplished for both the hospital and the community, there should be coordination between organizations regarding which potential hazards are given hierarchical planning priority. The flooding disaster of the Texas Medical Center (TMC) in Houston in June 2001 underscores the need for specific plans for operations and evacuation of hospitals at risk, and the need for a coordinated community response. This was especially true for all critical care functions within the TMC complex. JCAHO standard EC.1.4 highly recommends that hospitals within a geographic area know and share the names, roles, and contact numbers of all leaders in their local/regional emergency command structure. Resources such as hospital personnel staffing should be closely coordinated so that no person is committed to two facilities at one time.

The incident command system (ICS) is a leadership structure that was envisioned to alleviate the traditional problems of poor communications and poor planning during a disaster. It was originally developed in 1970 in response to problems experienced in the management of wildfires in Southern California. During a multiple casualty event, every hospital must be closely linked with the community's command structure. It is helpful for the hospital and ICU leadership to understand the basic premises of the ICS in order to function within it more effectively. The ICS is built on the following basic principles:

1. Common terminology.
2. Modular organization with a unified command structure starting with an incident commander. The incident commander will delegate duties to different functional areas as the situation unfolds. These functional areas will have written consolidated action plans following established strategic objectives.
3. Integrated communications.
4. Manageable span-of-control in which the number of individuals that report to a supervisor is established at a range of three to seven.
5. Predesignated incident facilities with areas for command post, search and rescue, decontamination, transport, and the press.
6. Comprehensive resource management.[6]

During a disaster, the subordinate leaders/representatives under the incident commander would likely include the fire department, emergency medical systems, public health organizations, law enforcement, and environmental agencies. Each of these functions is expected to keep a representative at the central command center. The on-site grouping of each of these liaison representatives dramatically improves communication and coordination of responders. A hospital should know in advance who to contact within the community command structure in order to obtain information about incoming casualties, who to convey information to regarding available hospital capabilities, and who to communicate with about the ongoing needs of their facility. The official point of contact for most hospitals will likely be the emergency medical systems commander.

Developing a Hospital Command Structure

A version of the ICS has been adapted for hospitals and is called the hospital emergency incident command system (HEICS).[7] Utilizing this system provides a seamless interface with the community command structure. Many hospitals are utilizing some form of the HEICS, and the HEICS document contains a proposed hospital command structure (Fig. 9-1). Job action sheets are provided that clearly define the responsibilities for each team member within the command structure. An intensivist may be asked to fill one of several roles. One proposed responsibility for the medical director of the ICU during a time of mass casualties would be as the medical care director. The medical care director coordinates patient care throughout the hospital and would optimize utilization of ICU beds and capability that becomes such a limited resource during surges in numbers of high acuity patients. The HEICS also defines the role of the critical care unit leader, who may be a nursing supervisor or a physician. An example of the associated job action sheet is provided (Fig. 9-2).

Finally, it is important to develop plans for maintaining ICU security during a disaster, as well as a means of communicating the status of patients with families and members of the media. Plans for securing the ICU should be made in cooperation with the safety and security officer identified within the HEICS. Ideally, a single point of entry into the ICU should be established with security present to control access. ICU personnel should be instructed to communicate with the media only with the approval of the public information officer or liaison officer. The public information officer should be consistently updating the media and families of victims and provide appropriate accommodations for them as they

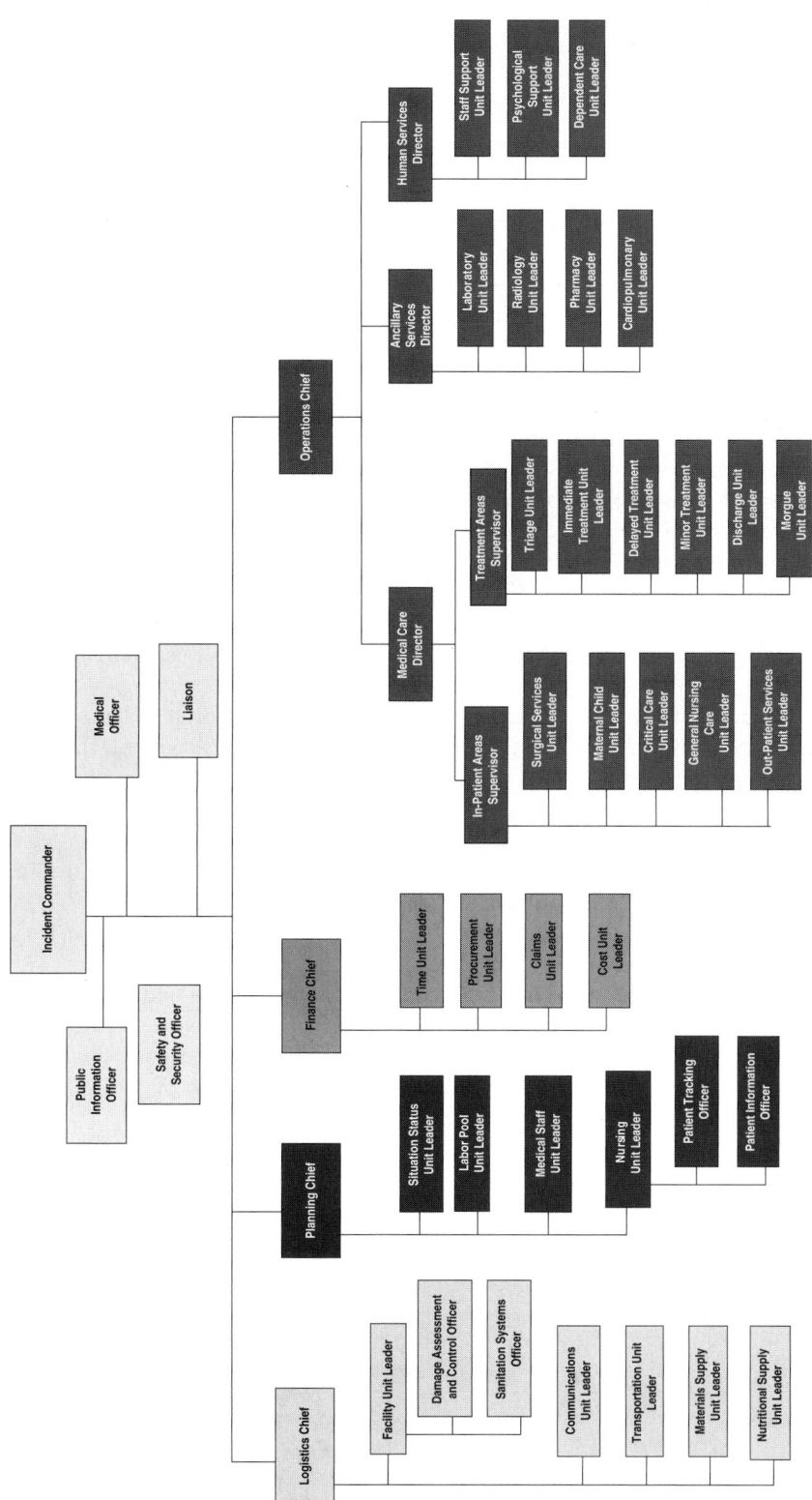

FIGURE 9-1 The hospital emergency incident command system (HEICS) proposed organizational chart. (*Courtesy of the California Emergency Medical Services Authority.*)

CRITICAL CARE UNIT LEADER

Positioned Assigned To:

You Report To: _____(In-Patient Areas Supervisor)

OperationsCommand Center: _____ Telephone: _____

Mission: Supervise and maintain the critical care capabilities to the best possible level to meet the needs of in-house and newly admitted patients.

Immediate
- ____ Receive appointment from In-Patient Areas Supervisor.
- ____ Read this entire Job Action Sheet and review organizational chart on back.
- ____ Put on position identification vest.
- ____ Receive briefing from In-Patient Areas Supervisor with other In-Patient Area unit leaders.
- ____ Assess current critical care patient capabilities. Project immediate and prolonged capabilities to provide services based on known resources.   Obtain medical staff support to make patient triage decisions if warranted.
- ____ Develop action plan in cooperation with other In-Patient Area unit leaders and the In-Patient Areas Supervisor.
- ____ Request the assistance of the In-Patient Areas Supervisor to obtain resources if necessary.
- ____ Assign patient care teams as necessary; obtain additional personnel from Labor Pool.

Intermediate
- ____ Identify location of Discharge Area; inform patient transportation personnel.
- ____ Contact Safety & Security Officer of security and traffic flow needs in the critical care services area(s). Inform In-Patient Areas Supervisor of action.
- ____ Report equipment/material needs to Materials Supply Unit Leader. Inform In-Patient Areas Supervisor of action.

Extended
- ____ Ensure that all area and individual documentation is current and accurate. Request documentation/clerical personnel from Labor Pool if necessary.
- ____ Keep In-Patient Areas Supervisor, Immediate Treatment, and Delayed Treatment Unit Leaders apprised of status, capabilities, and projected services.
- ____ Observe and assist any staff who exhibit signs of stress and fatigue. Report concerns to In-Patient Areas Supervisor. Provide for staff rest periods and relief.
- ____ Review and approve the area document's recordings of actions/decisions in the Critical Care Area(s). Send copy to the In-Patient Areas Supervisor.
- ____ Direct non-utilized personnel to Labor Pool.
- ____ Other concerns:

FIGURE 9-2 Critical care unit leader job action sheet. (*Courtesy of the California Emergency Medical Services Authority.*)

wait. This will maximize patient confidentiality and avoid intrusiveness due to lack of information or curiosity.

Communications with the Hospital Command Structure

During a disaster, traditional forms of communication between the various departments of the hospital may become useless. Traditional telephone lines, cellular communications, and pager systems may fail or become overburdened during a time of community crisis. The hospital disaster plan should include an alternative form of communication within the hospital between vital departments and the hospital command center. An ICU must be able to relay bed and personnel availability to the hospital incident commander and must be able to receive information about incoming critically ill patients. Several hospitals now have dedicated walkie-talkie units to facilitate communication during a disaster.[8,9] These backup communication systems should be tested as part of any disaster exercise and must be properly maintained.

Determining Intensive Care Unit Capacity for Care

If a mass casualty event occurs, hospital leaders must be able to calculate the current capacity of their facility, and the

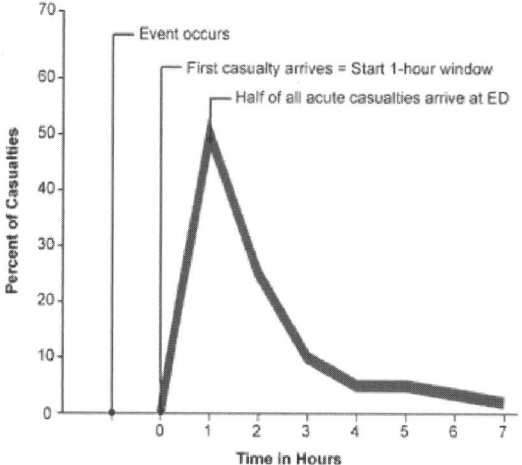

Predicted Emergency Department Casualties

- Event occurs
- First casualty arrives = Start 1-hour window
- Half of all acute casualties arrive at ED

Percent of Casualties / *Time in Hours*

FIGURE 9-3 The expected total number of casualties can be predicted by the number arriving within the first hour. (*Courtesy of the Centers for Disease Control and Prevention.*)

incremental number of patients that can be accepted for care. It is estimated that the capacity of a hospital to care for an emergency patient load is approximately 20% of the total bed capacity.[10] However, this may represent an overestimation of the ability to care for severely injured patients requiring critical care in a sudden mass casualty event. The actual number of trauma teams needed to resuscitate and stabilize critically injured patients may be a truer determinant of capacity. The total number of patients that can be accepted can then be ascertained, once the percentage of critically injured patients is known.[11] The Centers for Disease Control and Prevention (CDC) offers a webpage that provides a mass trauma casualty predictor and predictor of hospital capacity to care for critical casualties. Generally, 50% of all casualties will arrive within the first hour (Fig. 9-3). Of those patients, approximately 33% will be critical casualties. The hospital's capacity to care for these casualties will be determined by the number of available operating rooms staffed with surgery teams.[12]

In some circumstances, the requirement for medical care during an emergency response outstrips availability. In this circumstance, a form of disaster care rationing may be needed. The process of *triage,* a word coming from the French *trier* (to sort, to select), may be required to manage many casualties, and has been incorporated as part of the ICS. Triage sorts the patients, following established guidelines, in order to prioritize their initial management, as well as their evacuation to other facilities, according to the available resources and the type of incident.

Few hospitals maintain a sufficient number of empty beds for "surge capacity" due to cost constraints and the efficiency requirement to operate at or near full capacity. In the event of an emergency, a hospital plan should be in place to define a process for transferring existing ICU patients to other facilities. Agreements with neighboring hospitals should be established to accept predisaster ICU patients in transfer. Restrictions on out-of-ICU vasopressors or mechanical ventilation may need to be temporarily suspended to allow more stable ICU patients to be transferred to a hospital ward.

Not all disasters involve multiple traumas arriving at the hospital over a defined period of time. A bioterrorist act or an epidemic of an emerging infectious disease such as SARS would likely place strain on an ICU's capacity for care over a much more prolonged period. An infectious disease outbreak may mandate that a hospital protect its own employees and other patients first, thereby potentially limiting the capacity to care for all patients requiring critical care. It would be prudent to designate one hospital and ICU in a community or region as the isolation hospital where all confirmed or suspected contagious patients are admitted. This would both consolidate resources in one facility and limit exposure of other patients. The requirements for isolation will depend on the organism involved. Both smallpox and SARS patients would optimally be placed in isolation rooms with negative pressure relative to the surrounding area.[13] In most hospitals this resource is limited, and should be considered in determining capacity for care.

The vaccination of health care workers against smallpox has been controversial due to concerns about side effects from the vaccine and reimbursement of health care costs for those workers who become ill. There are many obvious benefits of having ICU and ancillary personnel who have been vaccinated taking care of patients with smallpox. Hospital personnel safety, limitation of the potential spread of the disease, and confidence of the health care team all would greatly benefit by a pre-exposure vaccine program.

Augmenting Resources During a Disaster

Previously, hospitals planned for a disaster assuming that outside assistance would not be available for up to 72 hours postevent.[1] This remains true in many countries; therefore appropriate supplies should be stockpiled in hospitals, pharmacies, and ICUs to sustain relief efforts until help is projected to arrive. As a response to this concern, in 1999 the CDC and the Department of Health and Human Services (HHS) established the National Pharmaceutical Stockpile. The purpose of this program is to resupply essential medical materiel such as drugs, antidotes, and surgical supplies, to any area of the country within 12 hours in the event of a national emergency. Included in these supplies are critical care-related materials such as mechanical ventilators. These assets were successfully deployed during the World Trade Center disaster. Effective in March 2003, the program became known as the Strategic National Stockpile (SNS), and is managed jointly by the Department of Homeland Security (DHS) and the HHS. To receive supplies from the SNS, the affected state's governor must directly request them from the DHS or the CDC.[14]

Professional organizations are also organizing volunteer personnel to help augment local staffing in the event of a disaster. As one example, the Society of Critical Care Medicine is cataloging the skills that each of its members possesses, and whether these individuals are willing to volunteer to help in times of disaster. In addition, the federal government has responded by creating the USA Freedom Corps as a way to organize volunteers. As a part of the USA Freedom Corps, the Medical Reserve Corps (MRC) is a group of locally organized medical volunteers that would serve in a time of disaster to augment existing medical staff. This program is sponsored by the HHS, and its primary role is to facilitate the establishment of these local organizations.[15] Provisions should be made by hospitals to establish a process for emergency credentialing of professional volunteers during times of crisis. State or national licensure bodies could also improve access to help by allowing physicians and nurses who are licensed in one state or region to practice medicine in another under emergency conditions.[16]

Education

A vital component of ICU preparedness is ongoing medical education that emphasizes clinical situations likely to be seen during a disaster. However, for busy clinical professionals, medical preparedness training does not compete favorably with traditional continuing medical education requirements. Clinicians have limited time and budgets to accomplish these training demands. External funding sources are negligible at this time. As a result, most clinicians lack sufficient knowledge of disaster response. To address this shortfall, the Society of Critical Care Medicine has developed a succinct disaster medicine course that is designed to either accompany their Fundamentals of Critical Care Support Course, or the material can be taught as a separate 5- to 6-hour course. The course is entitled Fundamentals of Disaster Management, and will be accompanied by a seven-chapter handbook. The American Medical Association has recently endorsed two multiday course offerings called Basic Disaster Life Support and Advanced Disaster Life Support. These courses will offer a more substantial exposure to medical disaster training.

It is beyond the scope of this chapter to provide details on the care of patients who may present to a hospital after a disaster. In today's environment, this can be overwhelming due to the large number of different threats that can face a community. The local hazard vulnerability analysis (HVA) will serve as an initial assessment of which topics should be emphasized. In this way, medical communities can target specific educational goals and then limit training to these highest priorities/risks, at least as a starting point.

The American College of Emergency Physicians has issued an executive summary from their task force on the education and training of its members on the care of casualties of nuclear, biological, or chemical incidents.[17] This summary includes a review of six available training courses, and found that none met all the objectives established by the task force. The primary barriers identified to obtaining the educational goals outlined were access to adequate training and ability to retain the knowledge once learned. Therefore the only acceptable method of improving educational retention is to conduct exercise training that involves a broad cross-section of health care professionals in the community.

Training

JCAHO (EC.2.9.1) currently requires a hospital's disaster plan to be tested twice a year, with the tests occurring at least 4 months apart, but not more than 8 months apart. Furthermore, they suggest that if a hospital is formally designated in the community as a disaster receiving station, then at least one drill per year should include simulated patients. One of these drills should also be conducted as part of a community-wide exercise that addresses likely emergencies, again using the HVA as a guide.[4]

The federal government has assigned a more imminent priority to disaster exercises since the terrorist attacks of September 11, 2001. As one example, the Department of Homeland Security conducted a week-long, $16 million dollar exercise in both Seattle and Chicago in May 2003. This exercise involved a simulated chemical, biologic, and "dirty bomb" attack. The scope of those involved in the exercise ranged from elected civic leaders and other decision makers, to hospitals and health care professionals. Unfortunately, these exercises tend to rediscover the same medical lessons. Specifically, elected civic leader decision making substantially impacts observed medical outcomes. Education and training of civic leaders regarding medical issues can be insufficient. Because of the common focus of these activities on prehospital events, critical care professionals should become actively involved in the planning and participate in these exercises. All medical personnel should know their roles within the HEICS, and then train for disaster in those roles.

In summary, several points should be repeated for emphasis:

1. The current breadth and depth of health care professional education in disaster response has much room for improvement.
2. Our current health care system is underfunded to improve disaster educational standards to optimal levels.
3. Health care professionals are very busy, and have limited time available to devote to disaster medical education.
4. Numerous high-quality courses and training programs are currently available. Further improvement is desirable.
5. Much of our current medical educational focus is on prehospital issues; critical care is required to ensure an effective response to disaster.
6. Effective medical training and education must include elected civic leaders.
7. JCAHO standards and a sensible HVA can be used to target and prioritize the most pressing disaster medical educational needs of a community.

References

1. Roccaforte JD, Cushman JG: Disaster preparation and management for the intensive care unit. *Curr Opin Crit Care* 8:607, 2002.
2. Angus DC, Kvetan V: Organization and management of critical care systems in unconventional situations. *Crit Care Clin* 9:521, 1993.
3. Al-Madhari AF, Keller AZ: Review of disaster definitions. *Prehospital Disaster Med* 12:17, 1997.
4. Joint Commission on Accreditation of Healthcare Organizations: Revised Environment of Care Standards for the Comprehensive Accreditation Manual for Hospitals (CAMH). Standards EC.1.4, EC.2.4, EC.2.9.1, EC.2.9.2. *Jt Comm Perspect* 21: 2001. http://www.jcrinc.com/subscribers/printview.asp?durki=1018.
5. Hazard Vulnerability Analysis. American Society for Healthcare Engineering. http://www.hospitalconnect.com/ashe/resources/hazvulanalysis.html.
6. Londorf D: Hospital application of the incident management system. *Prehospital Disaster Med* 10:184, 1995.
7. San Mateo County Health Services Agency, Emergency Medical Services: *The Hospital Emergency Incident Command System*, 3rd ed. June 1998. http://www.emsa.ca.gov/Dms2/heics3.htm
8. Klein JS, Weigelt JA: Disaster management: Lessons learned. *Surg Clin North Am* 71:257, 1991.

9. Bar-Joseph G, Michaelson M, Halberthal M: Managing mass casualties. *Curr Opin Anaesthesiol* 16:193, 2003.

10. Levi L, Michaelson M, Admi H, et al: National strategy for mass casualty situations and its effects on the hospital. *Prehospital Disaster Med* 17:12, 2002.

11. Hirshberg A, Holcomb J, Mattox K: Hospital trauma care in multiple-casualty incidents: A critical view. *Ann Emerg Med* 37:647, 2001.

12. Mass Trauma Preparedness and Response: Centers for Disease Control's Injury Center. http://www.cdc.gov/masstrauma/preparedness/predictor.htm

13. SARS Infection Control and Exposure Management. Centers for Disease Control and Prevention. http://www.cdc.gov/ncidod/sars/ic.htm

14. Strategic National Stockpile. Centers for Disease Control and Prevention. http://www.bt.cdc.gov/stockpile/index.asp

15. Medical Reserve Corps. http://www.medicalreservecorps.gov/

16. Hospital Preparedness for Mass Casualties. Summary of an Invitational Forum. American Hospital Association. August 2000. http://www.hospitalconnect.com/ahapolicyforum/resources/disaster.html

17. Waeckerle JF, Seamans S, Whiteside M, et al: Executive summary: Developing objectives, content, and competencies for the training of emergency medical technicians, emergency physicians, and emergency nurses to care for casualties resulting from nuclear, biological, or chemical (NBC) incidents. *Ann Emerg Med* 37:587, 2001.

PART II

GENERAL MANAGEMENT OF THE PATIENT

Chapter 10 ──────────
PREVENTING MORBIDITY IN THE ICU

DEBORAH COOK
GRAEME ROCKER

KEY POINTS

- *Effective preventive health care interventions based on evidence from rigorous randomized trials are increasing.*
- *Nonetheless, preventive strategies are applied suboptimally in many settings, particularly in the intensive care unit (ICU).*
- *Potential reasons such strategies are not more broadly employed include clinician habit, lack of awareness of (or resistance to) new information, reliance on physiologic outcomes rather than on clinically important outcomes when interpreting evidence, and lack of self-efficacy of physicians who question whether the benefits observed in the research setting will be realized in the practice setting.*
- *Another important, but underappreciated, reason for insufficient or delayed uptake of effective preventive strategies is the absence of reinforcements for preventive behavior in general.*
- *A working environment that facilitates the implementation of preventive strategies is a powerful facilitator of change. A crucial first step in trying to improve preventive care in the ICU is to do an environmental scan to understand the practice of the unit and to characterize the culture of the unit.*
- *The most effective strategies to implement behavioral change are interactive education rather than passive education, audit and feedback, reminders (manual or computerized), and involvement of local opinion leaders.*

Importance of Preventive Interventions in the ICU

Effective preventive health care interventions based on evidence from rigorous randomized trials are increasing. Application of such randomized trial evidence in practice has great potential to decrease the morbidity and mortality rates of inpatients and outpatients. However, preventive strategies are applied suboptimally in many settings, particularly in the intensive care unit (ICU). This poses a serious problem because critically ill patients are at high risk of death not only from the condition that necessitated their admission to the ICU but also from the complications of critical illness.

Examples of well-documented underuse of interventions that have been demonstrated to decrease morbid complications of critical illness in randomized trials include prevention of venous thromboembolism,[1] prevention of hyperglycemia,[2] and prevention of pneumonia.[3] Other interventions proved to prevent ICU mortality in patients with acute lung injury and sepsis such as lung protective ventilation strategies, use of corticosteroids, and activated protein C are also variably applied in practice, although mortality-reducing interventions are not the focus of this chapter.

In this chapter, we (a) present key clinical and behavioral issues relevant to preventive care for critically ill medical and surgical patients, (b) illustrate the gap between the evidence and its practical application, (c) underscore lost opportunities for prevention of morbidity by using several study designs, and (d) suggest strategies for improved analysis of, and increased attention to, prevention in the ICU.

Reasons for Inattention to Prevention in the ICU

The reasons clinicians fail to attend to prophylactic strategies supported by randomized trials may mirror those reasons that clinicians fail to apply valid evidence in practice, and the reasons that clinicians do not follow high-quality practice guidelines. Assuming that the evidentiary basis for the preventive strategy is valid and thus worth considering, there are many potential reasons for underuse of primary, secondary, or tertiary prevention, including clinician habit, lack of awareness of (or resistance to) new information, reliance on physiologic outcomes rather than on clinically important outcomes when interpreting evidence,[4] and lack of self-efficacy of physicians who question whether the benefits observed in the research setting can be realized in the practice setting.[5]

Another important, but underappreciated, reason for insufficient or delayed uptake of effective preventive strategies is the absence of reinforcements for preventive behavior in general. This is true particularly in comparison to treatment strategies. Clinicians do not experience direct and immediate feedback about the benefit of prophylactic interventions because they are designed to prevent the occurrence of future adverse events. In contrast, therapeutic interventions usually result in short-term, ongoing feedback about treatment responsiveness. In behavioral terms, the reinforcement for clinicians applying preventive strategies, as distinct from treatment strategies, is often covert and delayed, rather than overt and immediate.[6]

In addition, a factor recently recognized to contribute to inattention to preventive care, which is unrelated to cognitive or behavioral attributes of clinicians, is the lack of systems support to facilitate prevention. The ICU setting poses unique but not insurmountable barriers to preventive care, due to the multidisciplinary complex care of critically ill patients, and the need for fast-paced decision making. Multidisciplinary care has been postulated to result in improved outcomes for critically ill patients, but it can also lead to lack of clarity about responsibility for ministration of preventive care.[7] We discuss these ICU environmental factors in more detail below with respect to prevention of venous thromboembolism and hyperglycemia.

Effective Prevention in the ICU: Do an Environmental Scan

A working environment that facilitates the implementation of preventive strategies is a powerful facilitator of change. A crucial first step in improving preventive care in the ICU is to do an environmental scan. The ICU environment can be scanned quantitatively and qualitatively to help understand which preventive strategies require attention.

A recent qualitative study examining environmental factors that increase β-blocker use to prevent mortality for patients with myocardial infarction illustrates this.[8] Investigators conducted semi-structured interviews with eight cardiologists, four internists, two emergency physicians, 15 nurses, 11 quality-management staff, and five senior administrators in eight U.S. hospitals. Six factors were found to increase β-blocker use: setting goals, administrative support, clinician support, design and implementation of improvement initiatives, use of data, and contextual factors. From this study, we learn which environmental influences encourage the prescription of β blockers, and we may emulate successful strategies in our own environment for other preventive strategies. Investigations of this genre have been conducted to understand pneumonia-prevention strategies.[7]

Other approaches such as self-administered surveys can help us to understand the use of preventive strategies for care of acute lung injury and acute respiratory distress syndrome.[9] Surveys can indicate the information sources in the environment that are considered to inform practice, the availability of specific preventive interventions, and perceived reasons for local practice patterns.

Effective Prevention in the ICU: Understand Current Behavior

The second step toward optimal prevention of morbidity in the ICU is to take a scientific approach to evaluating whether effective prophylactic strategies are being applied in practice, and whether they are achieving the desired patient outcome. Casual interviews rarely provide valid data about preventive care. More credible data about compliance with effective preventive interventions can be obtained through formal surveys of stated practice and structured personal interviews.

However, surveys of stated practice have a universal limitation that must be kept in mind: they do not necessarily reflect actual practice. For example, in a self-administered survey, Canadian ICU clinicians stated that patients of older age with severe illness acuity and serious chronic comorbidity were most likely to undergo withdrawal of life support.[10] Subsequently, however, an observational study of actual practice demonstrated that rather than age, illness severity, and organ dysfunction, the four strongest determinants of ventilator withdrawal were inotrope or vasopressor dependency, perceived patient preferences to limit life support, and physician predictions of ICU survival rate and future cognitive function.[11] There are no substitutes for comprehensive audits, rigorous surveillance strategies, and observational studies to document practice patterns. To be valid, these strategies should be blinded so that clinicians remain unaware that their management is being observed, to avoid the inevitable practice change associated with this awareness (the Hawthorne effect). Although the foregoing example concerns end-of-life care, the design feature of blinding is very important for observational studies evaluating whether optimal prevention is being applied in the ICU.

 Qualitative research methods such as focus groups, document analysis, and in-depth interviews, as we found when exploring pneumonia prevention strategies in the ICU, are even more powerful for their insights about *when, where, why, how,*

and by whom preventive care is administered[7] than *whether* it is administered.[12]

Effective Prevention in the ICU: Adopt Effective Behavior-Change Strategies

It is now well understood that knowing the research evidence about health care interventions that decrease rates of morbidity and mortality does not ensure that it is used in practice. The research evidence about effective behavior-change strategies can be extremely helpful to improve preventive care. The behavior-change strategies that are most likely to enhance the faithful application of diagnostic, preventive, and therapeutic interventions have been summarized in the Cochrane Collaboration Systematic Review by Bero and colleagues,[13] which has been comprehensively updated by Grimshaw and associates.[14] Although few studies in these reviews focused exclusively on preventive interventions, there are useful signals from this literature. For example, the Cochrane Review clearly shows that passive dissemination of information is generally ineffective; it seems necessary to use specific strategies to encourage implementation of research-based recommendations and to ensure changes in practice. The most effective strategies are interactive education rather than passive education, audit and feedback, reminders (manual or computerized), and involvement of local opinion leaders.

To ensure that preventive care interventions are applied in practice, a behavioral program could be instituted that is specifically adapted to the ICU setting. A portfolio of behavior-change strategies may be desirable, some of which could be common and some of which may be different, to promote each preventive intervention. Further research on the relative effectiveness of different strategies specifically for preventive care and specifically for the ICU setting is needed. Studies on the cost effectiveness of behavioral-change strategies to promote prevention would also be useful. In the following sections of this chapter, we illustrate some behavior-change strategies using two examples in the ICU setting: prevention of venous thromboembolism and prevention of hyperglycemia.

PREVENTION OF VENOUS THROMBOEMBOLISM IN THE ICU

Venous thromboembolism (VTE) is a common complication of serious illness, conferring considerable morbidity and mortality in hospitalized patients. Patients with deep venous thrombosis (DVT) are at risk of subsequently developing pulmonary embolism (PE), which may be fatal if untreated. In the ICU setting, patients with DVT are significantly more likely to have PE,[15] and patients with DVT have a longer duration of mechanical ventilation ($p = 0.02$), ICU stay ($p = 0.005$), and hospitalization ($p < 0.001$) than do patients without DVT.[16] Critically ill patients can rarely communicate their symptoms, making it unlikely that patient self-reported symptoms will prompt intensivists to pursue the diagnosis of VTE; moreover, the physical examination is insensitive to detect DVT. Clinically unsuspected DVT and PE are frequently found at autopsy on critically ill patients.[17] In summary, VTE is a good example of an ICU-acquired morbidity that can be silent but potentially deadly.

There are only two published randomized trials testing heparin for VTE prophylaxis in medical and surgical ICU patients.[18,19] One double-blind single-center trial allocated 119 medical-surgical ICU patients at least 40 years of age to unfractionated heparin 5000 U twice daily or placebo subcutaneous injections.[18] Using serial fibrinogen leg scanning for 5 days, the rates of DVT were 13% in the heparin group and 29% in the placebo group (relative risk = 0.45, $p < 0.05$). Rates of bleeding and PE were not reported. This trial demonstrated that unfractionated heparin is better than no prevention (the number of patients needed to prophylax with 5000 U twice daily of subcutaneous heparin to prevent one DVT is four). A multicenter trial by Fraisse and colleagues randomized 223 patients with an acute exacerbation of chronic obstructive pulmonary disease requiring mechanical ventilation for at least 2 days to 3800 or 5700 IU of the low-molecular-weight heparin nadroparin once daily or placebo.[19] Patients were screened with weekly duplex ultrasounds and after clinical suspicion of DVT, and venography was attempted in all patients. Rates of DVT were 16% in the nadroparin group and 28% in the placebo group (relative risk = 0.67, $p < 0.05$). A similar number of patients bled in each group (25 vs. 18 patients, respectively; $p = 0.18$). Although patients were not screened for PE, no patients developed PE during the trial. This trial demonstrated that nadroparin is better than no prevention (the number of patients needed to prophylax with nadroparin to prevent one DVT is eight).

Although there are only two published randomized trials of thromboprophylaxis in medical-surgical ICU patients, randomized trials have been conducted in other populations for three decades and have clearly shown the effectiveness of anticoagulant VTE prophylaxis. Accordingly, anticoagulant thromboprophylaxis is universally recommended for critically ill patients except those with contraindications.[20] However, compliance with this recommendation for thromboprophylaxis is not what it should be.

COMPLIANCE WITH THROMBOPROPHYLAXIS

Several prospective single-center utilization reviews of VTE prophylaxis have provided evidence about the use of VTE prophylaxis in ICU practice. For example, thromboprophylaxis was prescribed in 33% of 152 medical ICU patients in one study[21] and in 61% of 100 medical ICU patients in another.[22] In contrast, in a medical-surgical ICU in which a clinical practice guideline was in place, VTE prophylaxis was prescribed for 86% of 209 patients.[23] In medical-surgical ICU patients, after excluding those receiving therapeutic anticoagulation and for whom heparin was contraindicated, only 63% of 96 received unfractionated heparin.[24]

In a multicenter 1-day cross-sectional utilization review of surgical ICU patients, unfractionated heparin was the predominant choice, and two methods of VTE prophylaxis were prescribed in 23% of patients.[25] Prophylaxis with unfractionated or low-molecular-weight heparin was significantly less likely for postoperative ICU patients requiring mechanical ventilation than for patients weaned from mechanical ventilation later in their ICU course (odds ratio = 0.36). Use of intermittent pneumatic compression devices was significantly associated with current hemorrhage (odds ratio = 13.5) and risk of future hemorrhage (odds ratio = 19.3).

In summary, the use of effective VTE prophylaxis ranges widely, according to the foregoing utilization reviews. One inference from this health services research is that insufficient attention is paid to thromboprophylaxis in the ICU setting. However, when prophylaxis is prescribed, clinicians appear to risk stratify, that is, patients with more VTE risk factors are more likely to receive prophylaxis than are patients with fewer risk factors. The dynamic competing risks of bleeding and thrombosis during critical illness underscore the individual risk:benefit ratios in critically ill patients.

Two studies evaluating implementation strategies to enhance appropriate VTE prophylaxis are relevant to the ICU setting. One three-armed multicenter randomized trial of 3158 surgical patients requiring VTE prophylaxis evaluated the impact of education versus education plus quality improvement.[26] Both interventions significantly improved appropriate VTE prophylaxis rates compared to the control group. In a time series study of 1971 orthopedic patients, a computer-decision support system significantly increased the rate of appropriate VTE prophylaxis prescribing from 83% to 95%.[27] Interestingly, each time that the computer-decision support was removed, practice patterns reverted to those observed previously. In a before-after single-center study, our group demonstrated how appropriate anticoagulant thromboprophylaxis increased from 65%[24] to 95%[28] after the introduction of a thromboprophylaxis practice guideline implemented by using interactive multidisciplinary educational in-services, ongoing verbal reminders to the ICU team, daily computerized nurse recordings of thromboprophylaxis, weekly graphic feedback to individual intensivists on prophylaxis adherence, and publically displayed graphic feedback on group performance. However, no randomized trials have formally tested individual behavior-change strategies for thromboprophylaxis in the ICU, in contrast with this multimethod approach. Fortunately, published thromboprophylaxis rates for critically ill patients appear to be increasing over time.[1]

PREVENTION OF HYPERGLYCEMIA IN THE ICU

The adverse consequences of acute hyperglycemia have been highlighted in numerous observational studies. A meta-analysis of 15 observational studies showed that, after myocardial infarction, diabetic patients with glucose values of 6.1 to 8.0 mmol/L had a fourfold higher risk of death than did patients without diabetes who had lower glucose values.[29] Among diabetic patients with glucose values of 10.0 to 11.0 mmol/L, the risk of death was increased twofold. After stroke, a meta-analysis of 32 observational studies among nondiabetic patients found that acute hyperglycemia with values of 6.1 to 8.0 mmol/L was associated with a threefold relative risk increase in hospital mortality and an increased risk of poor functional recovery in nondiabetic patients after stroke.[30]

To test the hypothesis that outcomes could be improved in patients with lower blood glucose during acute illness, the Insulin Glucose Followed by Subcutaneous Insulin Treatment in Diabetic Patients with Acute Myocardial Infarction (DIGAMI) study randomized 620 patients with diabetes and myocardial infarction to two different intervention strategies. Patients were allocated to intensive metabolic treatment with insulin plus glucose infusion followed by multidose insulin treatment or to standard treatment. Investigators found a significantly lower mortality rate in the intensive treatment group at 1 year[31] and at 3 years.[32] In diabetic patients, the adverse consequences of chronic hyperglycemia are well known. The Diabetes Control and Complications Trial (DCCT), which enrolled 1441 patients with type 1 diabetes, demonstrated that patients who had intensive insulin management had significantly less retinopathy, nephropathy, and neuropathy than did those managed conventionally.[33] Similarly, the UK Prospective Diabetes Study (UKPDS) of 3867 patients with type 2 diabetes showed that intensive glucose control with oral hypoglycemic agents or insulin to achieve a target fasting glucose level below 6 mmol/L resulted in significantly fewer microvascular complications than did conventional management.[34]

In addition to the foregoing findings, emerging evidence suggests that acute hyperglycemia has adverse consequences for ICU patients. During critical illness, stress hyperglycemia occurs due to production of excessive counter-regulatory hormones (glucocorticoids, catecholamines, growth hormones, and glucagon), effects of cytokines, insulin resistance, and pre-existing diabetes. Building on the results of the DCCT[33] and UKPDS[34] in diabetic patients and those of the DIGAMI trial in patients with and without diabetes,[31] a recent landmark randomized trial of 1548 critically ill patients demonstrated that patients allocated to a target of euglycemia (4.4 to 6.1 mmol/L) as compared with higher glucose values (10.0 to 11.1 mmol/L) had a significantly lower infectious morbidity rate, less renal failure, less polyneuropathy of the critically ill, and lower ICU and hospital mortality rates regardless of whether they had diabetes.[35]

Compliance with Euglycemia

Human behavior is partly determined by beliefs and attitudes. To determine the beliefs and attitudes held by ICU clinicians about prevention of hyperglycemia, we recently conducted a multicenter survey of ICU physicians and nurses.[2] The goals were to understand (a) perceived thresholds for clinically important hyperglycemia and hypoglycemia in ICU patients, (b) glucose measurement concerns in the critical care setting, and (c) strategies that clinicians would find most useful to help achieve optimal glucose management in the ICU.

ICU clinicians reported their perception that the clinically important threshold for hyperglycemia was 10 mmol/L for diabetic and nondiabetic ICU patients. Avoidance of hyperglycemia was judged most important for diabetic patients (88%), patients with acute brain injury (85%), a recent seizure (74%), advanced liver disease (64%), and acute myocardial infarction (64%). Physicians expressed more concern than nurses about avoiding hyperglycemia in patients with acute myocardial infarction ($p = 0.0004$). We conclude that randomized trial evidence showing the benefit of euglycemia in preventing morbidity and mortality in critically ill patients has not decisively influenced practice in these centers.

In summary, a recent randomized trial in critically ill patients associated euglycemia with lower morbidity and mortality rates than with higher glucose values. This work follows a consistent body of evidence about the importance of euglycemia to achieve optimal patient outcomes in other acute settings. Nevertheless, clinicians in our multicenter survey[2] did not consistently report application of this ev-

Evidence	Semirecumbency	Stress Ulcer Prophylaxis
quantity	small	large
quality	good	very good
currency	recent	remote
awareness	minimal	widespread

FIGURE 10-1 Preventing VAP and stress ulcer bleeding: Comparing the evidence for two interventions.

idence in practice. Lack of clinician awareness of the ICU trial[35] is unlikely; however, other plausible explanations include the short time since publication of this trial, uncertainty about the application of these results to noncardiac surgery patients or patients with short ICU stays, the challenge of achieving euglycemia in the ICU, concern about unrecognized hypoglycemia in critically ill patients, and a desire for more confirmatory evidence. Principles of behavior change mentioned earlier, and worth repeating, are that changing clinician behavior does not follow passive dissemination of information. The most effective strategies are interactive education, reminders, audit and feedback, and actively implemented, locally developed guidelines and protocols.[14] Further, in the ICU, strategies to improve glycemic control may be more effective by using a collaborative and interdisciplinary approach, rather than relying on a physician-led initiative. Meanwhile, pending the completion of future randomized trials in heterogeneous ICU populations, a shift toward tighter glucose control requires being aware of ICU clinicians' beliefs and attitudes. Addressing these beliefs and attitudes could enhance the success of future clinical, educational, and research efforts to modify practitioner behavior and thereby improve the outcomes for critically ill patients.

Conceptual Analysis of Two Preventive Interventions in the ICU

A different way to reflect on the preventive care that we have used is an analysis of three domains: (a) the evidence

FIGURE 10-2 Preventing VAP and stress ulcer bleeding: Comparing the characteristics of the intervention.

Intervention	Semirecumbency	Stress Ulcer Prophylaxis
characteristics	behaviour	drug
frequency	continuous	discrete
cointerventions	many	few
dimensions	complex	simple
familiarity	moderate	high

Uptake Strategies	Semirecumbency	Stress Ulcer Prophylaxis
publications	+	+++
CME	+	++
practice guidelines	+	++
industry detailing	0	+++
academic detailing	+	++
opinion leaders	+	++
audit & feedback	0	+
CDSS	0	+
multifaceted	0	++

FIGURE 10-3 Preventing VAP and stress ulcer bleeding: Comparing common evidence uptake strategies.

supporting the preventive interventions, (b) attributes of the preventive interventions themselves, and (c) existing strategies to enhance their uptake. We illustrate this analytic approach by comparing and contrasting two preventive interventions for mechanically ventilated patients: semirecumbency for pneumonia prevention (vs. supine positioning),[36] and stress ulcer prophylaxis with histamine-2 receptor antagonists (vs. other drugs or placebo).[37]

Figure 10-1 illustrates how the evidentiary basis for these two preventive interventions differs. The body of research in support of histamine-2 receptor antagonists for stress ulcer prophylaxis is much larger in terms of number of randomized trials, and the data are older and better known[38] than the body of evidence supporting semirecumbency for pneumonia prevention.[36,39–41] Figure 10-2 illustrates how the interventions themselves differ. Whereas semirecumbency is a complex, continuous, behavioral intervention potentially influenced by many alternative body positions, stress ulcer prophylaxis is a discrete, twice- or thrice-daily, simple pharmacologic intervention. Figure 10-3 illustrates that existing uptake strategies supporting stress ulcer prophylaxis are multiple, including publications, educational documents, presentations, computer-decision supports, and practice guidelines; in addition, the most powerful uptake strategy is operant: the well-oiled machine of industry detailing. In contrast, uptake strategies for semirecumbency are more limited in scope and effectiveness.

Although we cannot prove a causal relation between this conceptual analysis and the high penetrance of stress ulcer prophylaxis[42,43] as compared with a low penetrance of semirecumbency,[7,12] such a relation may be deduced.

Conclusions

In this chapter, we have emphasized preventive strategies that are grounded in evidence from randomized controlled trials and acknowledged that not all clinical questions in the ICU are best answered using the randomized controlled-trial approach. As we have illustrated, several other study designs can provide high-quality data that inform clinicians about preventive interventions that benefit patients, families, and staff.

Decreasing preventable morbidity (and, of course, mortality) should be among our top priorities in the ICU. Achieving these goals requires a multifaceted approach. It begins with an understanding of why clinicians fail in practice to use prophylactic strategies that are supported by valid evidence. Next, a scientific environmental scan can help to identify which preventive strategies are underused and require attention. An array of effective behavior-change strategies is desirable in the ICU setting. The ICU may be ideally suited to approaches such as population-specific practice guidelines, academic detailing by ICU pharmacists, and computer-assisted reminders. We must be mindful that these behavior-change strategies may require adaptation to the structure, function, and culture of each ICU. By adopting, yet locally adapting, effective behavior-change strategies, we can take essential steps to minimize lost opportunities for effective prevention in the ICU setting. If we fail, the commitment to research made by patients and their families in prior prevention trials will not be honored and will not benefit patients currently under our care.

References

1. Geerts W, Cook DJ, Selby R, Etchells E: Venous thromboembolism and its prevention in critical care. *J Crit Care* 17:95, 2002.
2. McMullin J, Brozek J, Jaeschke R, et al: Glycemic control in ICU: A multicenter survey. *Intensive Care Med* 30:798, 2004.
3. Cook DJ, Ricard JD, Reeve BK, et al: Ventilator circuit and secretion management strategies: A Franco-Canadian survey. *Crit Care Med* 28:3547, 2000.
4. McMullin J, Cook DJ, Meade M, et al: Clinical estimation of trunk position among mechanically ventilated patients. *Intensive Care Med* 28:304, 2002.
5. Cabana MD, Rand CS, Powe NR, et al: Why don't physicians follow clinical practice guidelines? *JAMA* 282:1458, 1999.
6. Cook DJ, Montori VM, McMullin JP, et al: Improving patients' safety locally: changing clinician behaviour. *Lancet* 363:1224, 2004.
7. Cook DJ, Meade M, Hand L, McMullin J: Semirecumbency for pneumonia prevention: A developmental model for changing clinician behaviour. *Crit Care Med* 30:1472, 2002.

8. Bradley EH, Holmboe ES, Mattera JA, et al: A qualitative study of increasing β-blocker use after myocardial infarction: Why do some hospitals succeed? *JAMA* 285:2604, 2001.

9. Meade MO, Jacka MJ, Cook DJ, et al, for The Canadian Critical Care Trials Group: Survey of interventions for the prevention and treatment of acute respiratory distress syndrome. *Crit Care Med* 32:946, 2004.

10. Cook D, Guyatt G, Jaeschke R, et al, for the Canadian Critical Care Trials Group: Determinants in Canadian health care workers of the decision to withdraw life support from the critically ill. *JAMA* 273:703, 1995.

11. Cook DJ, Rocker G, Marshall J et al, for the Level of Care Study Investigators and the Canadian Critical Care Trials Group: Withdrawal of mechanical ventilation in anticipation of death in the intensive care unit. *N Engl J Med* 349:1123, 2003.

12. Reeve BK, Cook DJ: Semirecubency among mechanically ventilated ICU patients: A multicenter observational study. *Clin Intensive Care* 10:241, 1999.

13. Bero LA, Grilli R, Grimshaw JM, et al, for the Cochrane Effective Practice and Organization of Care Review Group: Closing the gap between research and practice: An overview of systematic reviews of interventions to promote the implementation of research findings. *BMJ* 317:465, 1998.

14. Grimshaw JM, Shirran L, Thomas R, et al: Changing provider behaviour. An overview of systematic reviews of interventions. *Med Care* 39(suppl 2):II2, 2001.

15. Ibrahim EH, Iregui M, Prentice D, et al: Deep vein thrombosis during prolonged mechanical ventilation despite prophylaxis. *Crit Care Med* 30:771, 2002.

16. Cook DJ, Crowther M, Meade M, et al: Deep Venous thrombosis in medical-surgical ICU patients: Prevalence, incidence and risk factors. *Crit Care* 7(suppl 2):S54, 2003.

17. Stein PD, Henry JW: Prevalence of acute pulmonary embolism among patients in a general hospital and at autopsy. *Chest* 108:978, 1995.

18. Cade JF: High risk of the critically ill for venous thromboembolism. *Crit Care Med* 10:448, 1982.

19. Fraisse F, Holzapfel L, Couland JM, et al: Nadroparin in the prevention of deep vein thrombosis in acute decompensated COPD. *Am Rev Resp Crit Care Med* 161:1109, 2000.

20. Geerts WH, Heit JA, Clagett P, et al: Prevention of venous thromboembolism. Sixth ACCP Antithrombotic Consensus Conference on Antithrombotic Therapy. *Chest* 119:132S, 2001.

21. Keane MG, Ingenito EP, Goldhaber SZ: Utilization of venous thromboembolism prophylaxis in the medical intensive care unit. *Chest* 106:13, 1994.

22. Hirsch DR, Ingenito EP, Goldhaber SZ: Prevalence of deep venous thrombosis among patients in medical intensive care. *JAMA* 274:335, 1995.

23. Ryskamp RP, Trottier SJ: Utilization of venous thromboembolism prophylaxis in a medical-surgical ICU. *Chest* 113:162, 1998.

24. Cook DJ, Attia J, Weaver B, et al: Venous thromboembolic disease: An observational study in medical-surgical ICU patients. *J Crit Care* 15:127, 2000.

25. Cook DJ, Laporta D, Skrobic Y, et al, for the Canadian ICU Directors Group: Prevention of venous thromboembolism in critically ill surgery patients: A cross-sectional study. *J Crit Care* 16:161, 2001.

26. Anderson DR, O'Brien BJ, Levine MN, et al: Efficacy and cost of low-molecular weight heparin compared with standard heparin for the prevention of deep vein thrombosis after total hip arthroplasty. *Ann Intern Med* 119:1105, 1993.

27. Durieux P, Nizard R, Ravaud P, et al: A clinical decision support system for prevention of venous thromboembolism: Effect on physician behaviour. *JAMA* 283:2816, 2000.

28. McMullin J, Landry F, McDonald E, et al: Changing behavior in the ICU by optimizing thromboprophylaxis. *Am J Resp Crit Care Med* 167:A250, 2003.

29. Capes SE, Hunt D, Malmberg K, Gerstein HC: Stress hyperglycemia and increased risk of death after myocardial infarction in patients with and without diabetes: A systematic overview. *Lancet* 355:773, 2000.

30. Capes SE, Hunt D, Malberg K, et al: Stress hyperglcyemia and prognosis of stroke in nondiabetic and diabetic patients: A systematic overview. *Stroke* 32:2426, 2001.

31. Malmberg K, Ryden L, Efendic S, et al: Randomized trial of insulin-glucose followed by subcutaneous insulin treatment in diabetic patients with acute myocardial infarction (DIGAMI Study): Effects on mortality at one year. *J Am Coll Cardiol* 26:57, 1995.

32. Malmberg K: Prospective randomized study of intensive insulin treatment on long term survival after acute myocardial infarction in patients with diabetes mellitus (DIGAMI). *BMJ* 314:1512, 1997.

33. Diabetes Control and Complications Trial Research Group: The effect of intensive treatment of diabetes on the long term complications in insulin dependent diabetes mellitus. *N Engl J Med* 329:977, 1993.

34. UK Prospective Diabetes Study Group: Intensive blood glucose control with sulphonylureas or insulin compared with conventional treatment and risk of complications in patients with type 2 diabetes (UKPDS 33). *Lancet* 352:837, 1998.

35. Van den Berghe G, Wouters P, Weekers F, et al: Intensive insulin therapy in critically ill patients. *N Engl J Med* 345:1359, 2001.

36. Drakulovic MB, Torres A, Bauer TT, et al: Supine body position as a risk factor for nosocomial pneumonia in mechanically ventilated patients: A randomized trial. *Lancet* 354:1851, 1999.

37. Cook DJ, Guyatt GH, Marshall J, et al, for the Canadian Critical Care Trials Group: A comparison of sucralfate and ranitidine for prevention of upper gastrointestinal bleeding in patients requiring mechanical ventilation. *N Engl J Med* 338:791, 1998.

38. Cook DJ, Reeve BK, Guyatt GH, et al: Stress ulcer prophylaxis in critically ill patients: Resolving discordant meta-analyses. *JAMA* 275:308, 1996.

39. Torres A, Serra-Batiles J, Ros E, et al: Pulmonary aspiration of gastric contents in patients receiving mechanical ventilation: The effect of body position. *Ann Intern Med* 116:540, 1992.

40. Ibanez J, Penafiel A, Raurich JM, et al: Gastroesophageal reflux in intubated patients receiving enteral nutrition: effect of supine and semirecumbant positions. *JPEN* 16:419, 1992.

41. Orozco-Levi M, Torres A, Ferrer M, et al: Semirecumbant position protects from pulmonary aspiration but not completely from gastroesophageal reflux in mechanically ventilated patients. *Am J Respir Crit Care Med* 152:1387, 1995.

42. Erstad BL, Barletta JF, Jacobi J, et al: Survey of stress ulcer prophylaxis. *Crit Care Med* 3:145, 1999.

43. Lam NP, Le PD, Crawford SY, Patel S: National survey of stress ulcer prophylaxis. *Crit Care Med* 27:98, 1999.

Chapter 11 _____

NUTRITION IN THE CRITICALLY ILL

DAREN K. HEYLAND
STEVE A. MCCLAVE

KEY POINTS

- *Nutrients and gastrointestinal structure and function are linked to the pathophysiology of infection, organ dysfunction, and survival in critically ill patients.*

- *Nutrition support may both positively and negatively influence the morbidity and mortality of critically ill patients.*

- *When considering nutrition support in critically ill patients, enteral nutrition (EN) should be used in preference to parenteral nutrition (PN).*

- *Strategies to optimize delivery of EN (e.g., starting EN early, use of a feeding protocol with a high threshold of gastric residual volume, use of prokinetic agents, and use of small bowel feeding) and minimize the risks of EN (e.g., elevation of the head of the bed) should be considered.*

- *When initiating EN, PN should not be used in combination with it.*

- *For most patient populations in critical care in whom EN is not possible or feasible, standard therapy (IV fluid resuscitation without artificial nutrition support) is preferable to PN for the first 7 to 10 days.*

- *When PN is indicated, strategies that maximize the benefit (e.g., supplementing with glutamine) and minimize the risks of PN (e.g., hypocaloric dose, withholding lipids, continued use of EN, and the use of intensive insulin therapy to achieve tight glycemic control) should be considered.*

POURQUOI ???

Nutrition support is considered an integral component of standard supportive care in the critically ill patient. In humans, during stress associated with trauma, sepsis, or other critical illness, there is high consumption of various nutrients by the gastrointestinal tract, immune cells, kidneys, and other organs. Requirements for and losses of these nutrients may outstrip synthetic capacity, leading to an erosion of body stores and depletion of proteins and other key nutrients. Historically, in an attempt to mitigate such deficiencies and preserve lean body mass, traditional nutrition (protein, calories, vitamins, etc) has been provided to critically ill patients. The relative merits of nutrition were evaluated in the context of protein-calorie economy (weight gain, nitrogen balance, muscle mass and function, etc). In this chapter we take a broader view of the benefits and risks of nutrition support. The benefits of nutrition support in general include improved wound healing, a decreased catabolic response to injury, enhanced immune system function, improved GI structure and function, and improved clinical outcomes, including a reduction in complication rates and length of stay with accompanying cost savings.[1] Independent of their effects on nutritional status of the patients, key nutrients such as glutamine, arginine, and omega-3 fatty acids may also have favorable direct effects on organ function and clinical outcomes of critically ill patients. Thus nutrition support may be considered a specific therapeutic intervention by which the critically ill patient's disease course may be altered, leading to a more favorable outcome.

There is considerable evidence linking nutrition (and lack thereof) and GI function to the pathogenesis of infection and organ failure in critical illness.[2] Failure to obtain enteral access and to provide nutrients via the enteral route results in a proinflammatory state mediated by macrophages and monocytes. Oxidative stress is increased, severity of illness is exacerbated, and the likelihood of infectious morbidity, multi-organ failure, and prolonged length of stay is increased.[3-5] In contrast, the provision of enteral nutrition results in higher levels of secretory IgA in biliary tract secretions, greater preservation of gut-associated lymphoid tissue, less bacterial translocation, and greater preservation of upper respiratory tract immunity, all of which translates into improved clinical outcomes for critically ill patients.[1]

However, providing nutrients and nutrition support is not without adverse effects or risks. Acquired infection, particularly ventilator-associated pneumonia (VAP), is a major problem for critically ill patients, resulting in increased morbidity, mortality, and health care costs.[6,7] Gastric atony and the use of intragastric enteral feeds appear to increase the risk of gastric colonization and subsequent pneumonia.[8,9] Gastric colonization plays a significant role in the contamination of tracheal secretions and in the development of nosocomial pneumonia via a mechanism of gastroesophageal regurgitation and pulmonary microaspiration.[10] Parenteral nutrition has been associated with gut mucosal atrophy, overfeeding, hyperglycemia, adverse effects on immune function, an increased risk of infectious complications, and increased mortality in critically ill patients.[11] While providing supplemental glutamine to seriously stressed critically ill patients may increase their chances of survival,[12] depending on the circumstances, providing arginine to the same patients may increase their mortality.[13] Therefore, nutrition support must be viewed as a double-edged sword, and strategies that maximize the benefits of nutrition support while minimizing the associated risks need to be considered in formulating clinical recommendations.

In developing such recommendations, the patient populations to which these recommendations will be applied must also be considered. Studies of nutrition support in non–critically ill patient populations may not be generalizable to critically ill patients. For example, the treatment effect of PN in elective surgery patients is significantly different than the treatment effect of PN in critically ill patients.[11]

Even within subpopulations of critically ill patients, differences in outcome between the two routes of providing nutrition support are more likely to be seen with greater severity of illness. For example, the correlation between the importance of maintaining gut integrity and greater disease severity was demonstrated by a study evaluating septic complications in trauma patients, randomized at the time of surgery, to PN or to enteral tube feeding.[14] In patients with high Abdominal Trauma Index (ATI) scores (>24), the incidence of septic complications was greater in the PN group than the group on enteral tube feeding (47.6% vs. 11.1%, p <0.05). For those patients with moderate illness and lower ATI scores (<24), there was no significant difference in the incidence of septic complications between the parenteral and enteral groups (29.2% vs. 20.8%, p = NS).[14] Furthermore, in studies of EN versus PN in acute pancreatitis, faster resolution of the inflammatory response and significant differences in clinical outcomes (reduced septic morbidity and overall complications in the EN group) were seen in studies in which there were more patients with severe pancreatitis compared to studies with a lower proportion of patients with severe pancreatitis.[15–17]

In this chapter, we will discuss the relationships among nutrition, GI structure and function, immune function, and outcomes in critical illness. Upon this theoretical foundation, we will propose recommendations favoring the use of enteral nutrition over parenteral nutrition. Whereas PN may be life-sustaining in patients with a disrupted GI tract, PN has only a minor role in the ICU patient population with an intact GI tract. In most patient populations in the critical care setting when EN is not feasible, standard therapy (IV fluid resuscitation without artificial nutritional support) is actually preferable to PN for the first 7 to 10 days. Regardless of the route of nutrition support, we will suggest strategies that maximize the benefits and minimize the risks of both PN and EN.

Relationship of the Gastrointestinal Tract, Immune System, and Ischemia/Reperfusion Injury

The GI tract is the largest immune organ in the body, containing 65% of immune tissue overall and up to 80% of the immunoglobulin-producing tissues of the body.[4,5] In the fed state, the normal motility, villous microanatomy, rich blood supply, and epithelial intercellular tight junctions contribute to the overall integrity and barrier function of the GI tract. In response to luminal nutrients, propulsive contractions assist in controlling the concentration of luminal bacteria and the secretion of bile salts, mucus glycoproteins, and secretory IgA retard bacterial adhesion to gut epithelial cells and subsequent translocation.[18,19] The healthy gut acts as an important antigen-sensing organ, in which bacterial antigen is sampled and processed by the M cells, ultimately stimulating the release and maturation of a population of pluripotential stem cells or naïve CD4 helper T lymphocytes.[20,21] These cells will migrate out from the Peyer patches, through the mesenteric lymph nodes and thoracic duct, and into the systemic circulation as a mature line of B- and T-cell lymphocytes. A proportion of these cells generated in the maturation of the pluripotential stem cells migrate out as mucosal-associated lymphoid tissue (MALT) to distant sites such as the lungs, genitourinary tract, breast, and lacrimal glands.[18–21] Those that return to the enteric mucosa are known as gut-associated lymphoid tissue (GALT).[19–21] In some situations, instead of seeing an increase in aspiration pneumonia in response to enteral feeding of critically ill patients, clinicians may instead see a reduced incidence of pneumonia[14] due to maintenance of MALT in the lung by the trophic effects of luminal nutrients on the intestinal immune components.[19–21]

In a situation of even brief disuse, gut integrity may deteriorate. In contrast to the fed state, fasting leads to villous atrophy, diminished blood flow, and loss of intercellular tight junctions. This opens paracellular channels, allowing translocation of bacteria or other gut-derived factors such as endotoxin.[18] Without nutrient-induced stimulation of secretory IgA and bile salts, bacteria are more easily able to adhere to epithelial cells, promoting even greater translocation of bacteria and entry of their secretory products (e.g., endotoxin).[18] Lack of enteral nutrients may result in a reduction in the mass of GALT and antigen-processing and buildup of MALT at distant sites.

The most important aspect of gut disuse may be the diminished blood supply to the gut, which predisposes to regional ischemia/reperfusion injury.[22] The generation of superoxide radicals in response to ischemia/reperfusion may promote mucosal macrophage activation.[22,23] Macrophages, primed and activated at the level of the gut, may migrate to distant sites such as the liver, lung, and kidney. In such sites they may mediate tissue injury, resulting in the generation of oxidative species.[23] Macrophage activation is a key step linking gut functional compromise with more systemic factors that adversely affect patient outcome.[23,24] Activated macrophages also initiate the arachidonic acid cascade. Generation of prostaglandin E_2 suppresses delayed hypersensitivity reaction, generates superoxide radicals, and leads to an increased susceptibility to sepsis. Generation of leukotriene B_4 leads to chemotaxis and edema and the systemic inflammatory response syndrome (SIRS). Thromboxane A_2, another product of this cascade, leads to vasoconstriction and thrombosis. This event, in turn, promotes physiologic shunts and multiple organ failure.[23,25]

The overall tone of the systemic immune response may be modulated at the level of the gut. The dendritic macrophage cells act as antigen-presenting cells (APCs), which release cytokines and activate the naïve CD4 T cells (Th0). The specific cytokines that are generated ultimately affect the differentiation pathway of these lymphocytes[26] (Fig. 11-1). With gut disuse and fasting, contractility is decreased, which promotes bacterial overgrowth. Bacteria or viruses tend to generate a Th1 inflammatory response (while chronic parasitic infections are more likely to generate Th2 responses).[27] As bacterial antigen passes through M cells across the epithelium of the intestine, an initial response is elicited from the macrophages and dendritic cells,[26,28] (Fig. 11-2) releasing interleukin-12 (IL-12) and stimulating the naïve T cells to differentiate into the Th1 subset. This Th1 response represents cellular immunity, and results in the further release of other inflammatory cytokines, such as interleukin-2 (IL-2), interferon-γ (IFN-γ), and tumor necrosis factor-α (TNF-α). Th1 responses are associated with increased inflammation and are essential for a successful defense against infections. However, uncontrolled Th1 responses can result in self-injury. Feeding, on the other hand, may generate a different cytokine response and thus a different immune environment. Feeding is associated with oral tolerance, which represents a Th3 subset and is generated in the presence of interleukin-4 (IL-4), IL-10, and transforming growth factor-β (TGF-β), which tend to have immunosuppressive effects.[26] This immune environment allows ingestion of protein antigen from food without eliciting an inflammatory response. The production of IL-4 also stimulates a change in naïve T cells (Th0) into the Th2 subset.[26] Differentiation into Th2 lymphocytes represents humoral immunity, and causes further release of IL-4, interleukin-6 (IL-6), and interleukin-10 (IL-10). The Th2 response tends to curb or check the Th1 inflammatory response. Th2 responses are essential to prevent self-injury caused by inflammation.

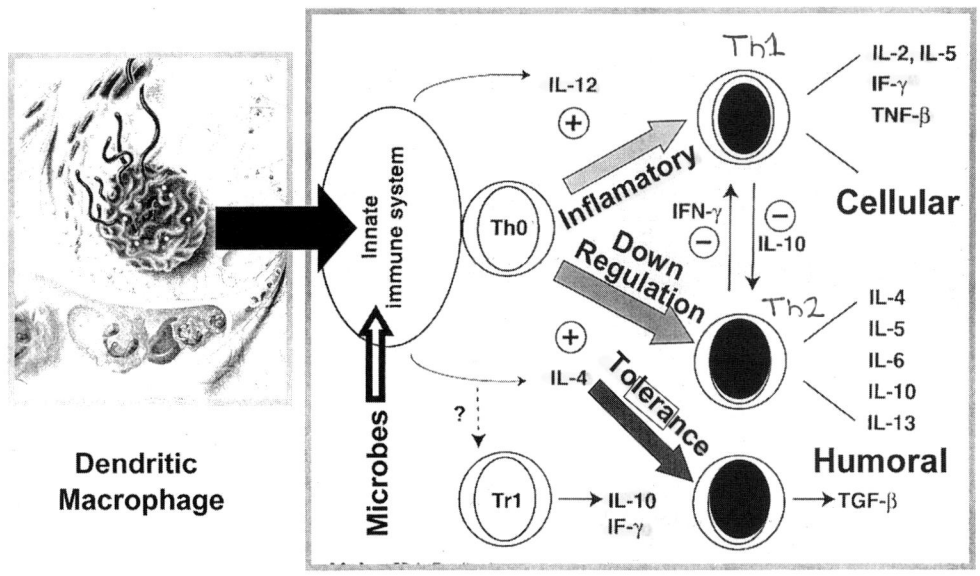

FIGURE 11-1 Antigen processing immune function by the gut.

Jeûne = Th1 >> Th2
EN = Th2 >> Th1

However, excessive regulation of inflammatory responses by Th2 cytokines can lead to increased immune suppression. This may cause anergy to skin test antigens, impaired antibody production, and diminished phagocytosis, rendering patients susceptible to additional infectious morbidity and mortality.[29]

These immune responses usually occur simultaneously, in effect competing with each other to set the overall immune environment, and may be responsible for the pattern of clinical response seen in critical illness. Initially the Th1 inflammatory response predominates, the intensity of which is determined in part by the injury itself. Almost immediately, the compensatory Th2 response is stimulated. At the point at which this compensatory Th2 response predominates over the initial Th1 response, the patient may pass into a period of relative immune suppression, characterized by anergy, hyporesponsiveness of T lymphocytes, and a diminished overall immune responsiveness.[1] Theoretically, any feeding by the enteral route early in the patient's disease process helps maintain gut integrity, promote motility, and minimize bacterial overgrowth in the small bowel, all of which may diminish the early gut-derived Th1 inflammatory response. As the patient progresses into the period of moderate immunosuppression, they are particularly at risk for late complications arising from aspiration or bacterial translocation, such as multiorgan failure and sepsis.[30] It is during this period of moderate immunosuppression that immune-enhancing formulas may have their greatest role in supporting the immune response, improving bactericidal activity, and reducing deleterious outcomes.

The Importance of Maintaining Gastrointestinal Integrity

Loss of gut structural integrity has been documented in humans, but it probably occurs as a late complication only with protracted disuse. A prospective study evaluating the effects of enteral feeding versus PN in patients with pancreatitis compared these patients against a control group without pancreatitis.[31] A segment of jejunum was resected at surgery to evaluate the effect of enteral feeding on mucosal integrity and architecture.[31] The control group maintained on enteral feeding had essentially normal villi. Pancreatitis was associated with villous atrophy in the experimental arm, but the effect was minimized in the enteral nutrition group. Those patients with pancreatitis placed on PN had the greatest villous atrophy. Longer periods of gut disuse completely transformed the mucosal architecture, resulting in a flattened featureless surface.[31]

Much more clinically important is the loss of functional integrity, which in some patients occurs over a very short period of time. With loss of functional integrity, the tight junctions between the intestinal epithelial cells open up, the gut becomes "leaky," and the patient experiences systemic bacterial challenge (through release of endotoxin and other gut-derived factors) and an exaggerated stress response with increased severity of disease.[18] In a prospective randomized trial, Windsor and colleagues showed that patients with pancreatitis maintained on enteral tube feeding had no change in IgM antibodies to endotoxin over a week of enteral feeding.[16] In contrast, controls placed on PN and gut disuse demonstrated a significant increase in IgM antibodies to endotoxin of 25% in response to a week of parenteral feeding ($p < 0.05$).[16] In a second study, increased gut permeability (measured by enteric absorption and urinary excretion of polyethylene glycol) and systemic endotoxemia correlated significantly with greater disease severity in patients with acute pancreatitis.[32] In a prospective randomized trial, normal healthy volunteers randomized to PN and gut disuse for 7 days demonstrated an exaggerated stress response to a standard IV challenge of E. coli endotoxin, as evidenced by higher glucagon, epinephrine, tumor necrosis factor, and C-reactive protein levels and greater muscle catabolism compared to a study group receiving a week of enteral feeding.[33] In two studies in patients with acute pancreatitis, significantly faster resolution of the SIRS response and "resolution of the disease process" (resolution of pain, decreasing amylase, and successful advancement to oral diet) was seen in patients randomized to EN compared to those placed on PN.[16,34]

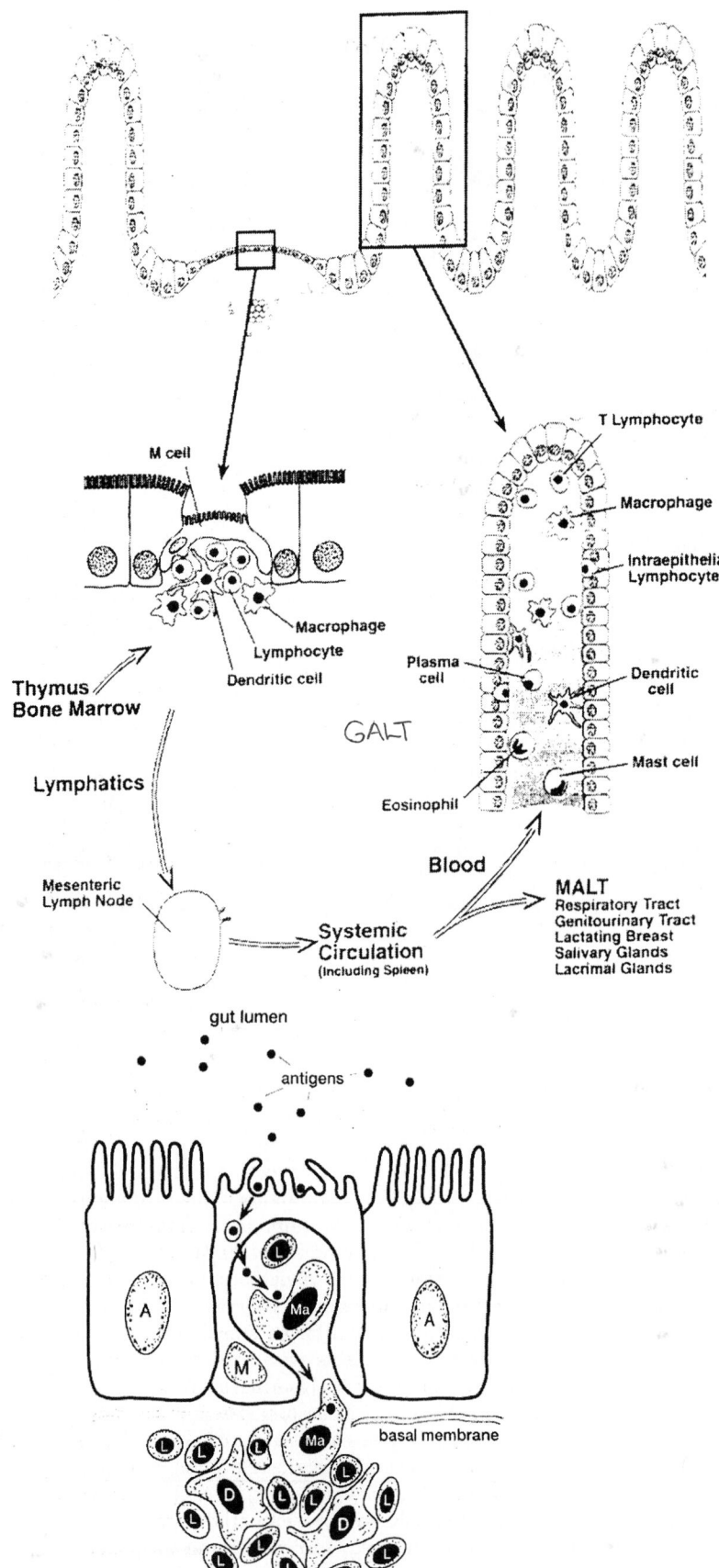

FIGURE 11-2 Pattern of immune response involving CD4 helper T cells.

Consistent with the theoretical evidence presented, there are 13 studies of critically ill patients with surgery, trauma, and medical illnesses, that evaluated the benefits of EN compared to PN. Compared to PN, EN was associated with a significant reduction in infectious complications (RR 0.61; 95% confidence intervals [CIs] 0.44, 0.84; $p = 0.003$).[35] No significant differences were seen in mortality between groups. *Thus in general, by feeding via the enteral route, we can expect to reduce the infectious complications associated with nutrition support in critically ill patients without adversely affecting survival.*

READINESS FOR ENTERAL NUTRITION

At the bedside, clinicians fail to recognize the relationship between gut structure and function and adverse patient outcome, primarily because there is significant delay in the development of complications that arise from poor management decisions related to enteral therapy. If mistakes are made with oxygen delivery, hypoxemia ensues immediately and the patient may deteriorate within minutes. If mistakes are made with volume resuscitation, there is a degree of delay, and problems arising from decreased vascular volume, hypoperfusion, and increasing azotemia may not develop for 12 to 24 hours. If no effort is made to maintain gut integrity, the complications that arise as a result may not develop for 3 to 5 days. At that point, when nosocomial infections occur or organs begin to fail, the clinician does not connect the development of these complications with management decisions made 5 days before with regard to enteral nutrition. In fact, only in prospective randomized trials can it be determined that had gut integrity been maintained, there might have been a decrease in the number of nosocomial infections, the number of organs failing, and the overall length of stay in the ICU prior to discharge.

COMBIEN ?

Initial Bedside Evaluation

The initial nutritional assessment that leads to the initiation of enteral tube feedings differs from the sequential monitoring that takes place as the patient continues to receive feeding. Low visceral proteins (such as albumin, transferrin, and prealbumin) on initial evaluation provide valuable prognostic information, accurately identifying those patients with the greatest degree of physiologic stress, severity of illness, and highest mortality.[36] Weight as percentage of ideal body weight, usual body weight, or as degree of recent weight lost, identify patients with possible underlying malnutrition that was present prior to the event causing the current hospital admission.[36] Determining risk for deterioration in nutrition status on initial evaluation may be facilitated by use of current scoring systems designed for certain patient populations. An Acute Physiology and Chronic Health Evaluation (APACHE) II score ≥10 in critically ill patients, an ATI score ≥24 in trauma patients, and presence of ≥3 Ranson criteria in patients with pancreatitis identify those patients with severe degrees of critical illness who are at high risk for rapid deterioration in nutritional status, with low likelihood for early advancement to oral diet, and in greatest need for aggressive enteral nutritional support.[14,37–39]

Determination of caloric requirements is very important on the initial nutritional evaluation, helping to set the goal (number of required calories) of nutritional support. Caloric requirements are best determined using simple equations (25 to 30 kcal/kg per day) or by specific measurement via indirect calorimetry. A dose-response effect in which the provision of 55% to 60% of the required number of calories *over the first 48 to 72 hours* to achieve a therapeutic effect has been suggested by several studies.[40–43] In a prospective study, burn patients who consumed an average of 64% of their goal calories showed no increased gut permeability and remained uninfected throughout their hospital course. In contrast, those who became infected consumed an average of only 40% of their goal calories, and showed evidence of significantly increased gut permeability.[40] Therefore, prolonged use of "trickle or trophic feeds," providing 10 to 30 mL/h, may be insufficient to adequately maintain gut integrity and translate into improved clinical outcomes.

COMMENT ?

ACHIEVING ACCESS

Unfortunately, obtaining enteral access early in the course of the critical illness may be very difficult. With greater severity of illness, patients become more prone to ileus with gastroparesis, high residual volumes, and intolerance of gastric feeds. Early on, the hypermetabolic response, SIRS, high doses of narcotic analgesics, and electrolyte abnormalities may potentiate gastroparesis. Compounding the problem is the fact that disuse of the gut reduces the secretion of prokinetic hormones such as gastrin, bombesin, and motilin.[18,19]

The ability to obtain enteral access may be vital to the success of nutritional support in the critically ill patient. Each institution needs specialists who have the skills to place tubes at the appropriate levels of the GI tract, with techniques that can usually be done at the bedside with minimal or no sedation. A number of techniques have been described for blind postpyloric placement at the bedside, which in the hands of a dedicated nurse, dietitian, or intensivist should be successful in >85% of cases.[44] In cases in which blind bedside placement is unsuccessful or deeper jejunal placement is required (such as in patients with severe acute pancreatitis), enteral access to the small bowel may require endoscopic or fluoroscopic placement. For these latter patients, transport out of the ICU should be avoided to prevent an increased risk of mishaps (e.g., cardiopulmonary arrest, new dysrhythmias, or loss of central IV line access) and pulmonary aspiration.[45–47]

ASSESSING TOLERANCE

Physical examination by the clinical nutritionist may be the most important element of monitoring the patient on enteral tube feeding. Abnormalities on physical exam usually reflect segmental abnormalities in contractility of the GI tract. Bloating, abdominal distention, hyperresonance, and increased residual volumes may signify delayed gastric emptying. In patients placed on nasogastric drainage, output of >1200 mL/d may indicate relative gastroparesis. Contractility of the colon may be assessed by passage of stool and gas. The presence of bowel sounds is a poor indicator of contractility in the small bowel, as evidenced by the fact that nasogastric suction will reduce its detection. Studies performed on the postoperative return of bowel function or contractility have provided valuable findings for the clinician. Invariably, contractility in the stomach stops initially, followed next by colonic contractility. Small bowel function or contractility appears to be retained the longest.[48] In most critically ill patients (particularly patients with trauma), who on baseline evaluation have grossly abnormal physical exams, tolerance to enteral tube feeding may be defined by slight decreases in abdominal distention and abdominal discomfort in the absence of high gastric residual volumes, metabolic acidosis, third-spacing of fluids, or a worsening clinical condition. These findings on serial physical examinations determine whether the position of the feeding tube needs to be changed (i.e., placing the tip of the tube lower down in the GI tract at or below the ligament of Treitz), whether a tube with simultaneous aspirating and feeding capabilities needs to be added, or whether the feeds need to be temporarily discontinued.

Strategies to Maximize the Benefits and Minimize the Risks of Enteral Nutrition

TIMING OF ENTERAL NUTRITION

While enteral feeding is the preferred route of nutrient administration, how soon it should be started after an acute injury or insult is not clear. In critically ill patients, there were eight randomized controlled trials comparing early EN (i.e., that started within 24 to 48 hours of admission to the ICU) to some form of delayed nutrient intake (i.e., delayed EN or oral diet).[49] When results from these studies were aggregated, early EN was associated with a trend towards a reduction in mortality (RR 0.52; 95% CIs 0.25, 1.08; $p = 0.08$) when compared to delayed nutrient intake. Three studies reported infectious complications.[50–52] When these were aggregated, early EN was associated with a trend towards a reduction in infectious complications (RR 0.66; 95% CIs 0.36, 1.22; $p = 0.19$) when compared to delayed nutrient intake. No differences in length of stay were observed between groups. All seven studies that reported nutritional end points showed a significant improvement in the groups receiving early EN (e.g., improvements in calorie intake, protein intake, percentage of goal achieved, and better nitrogen balance achieved). There were no differences in other complications between the groups.

Although the results lack statistical significance, they do suggest a large improvement in clinical outcome and a significant increase in nutrient delivery associated with early enteral feeding. However, before endorsing the concept of early enteral feeding, one must consider the potential risks of such a strategy. Two recent nonrandomized studies suggest that early enteral feeds delivered into the stomach may be associated with increased complications.[53,54] In contrast, Taylor and colleagues combined an aggressive early feeding protocol with the use of small bowel feedings and documented that head-injured patients fed aggressively, compared to standard (slower) provision of EN, not only had better nutritional status, but also had fewer complications and a more rapid recovery from their illness.[42]

Synthesizing these discordant results, it would seem that early EN may be associated with improved clinical outcomes when done in such a way that maximizes the benefits and minimizes the risks (see below). Furthermore, it should be noted that the goal of early EN, while critically ill patients are still early in the acute phase of their illness, is to provide enough critical nutrients to the gut to modulate the disease process and enhance gut barrier structure and function, not

to meet their caloric requirements as soon as possible. Thus for some patients with evidence of inadequate oxygen delivery, specific nutrients (e.g., glutamine and antioxidants) may be required in the first few days of critical illness. If patients are still on high-dose inotropes to maintain adequate blood pressure, the risk of providing EN may outweigh the benefits, and EN should be held until patients are weaning off pressor agents. As the patient enters the more stable, chronic phase of their illness (after 7 to 10 days), preserving lean body mass, stimulating protein synthesis, and minimizing nutritional deficits, rather than maintaining GI structure and function, become the primary goals.

REDUCING RISK OF ASPIRATION

It is important on initial evaluation to assess the patient's risk for aspiration on EN. Aspiration may occur from the antegrade passage of contaminated oropharyngeal secretions or the retrograde passage of contaminated gastric contents into the larynx. Regurgitation occurs more frequently than aspiration.[55] A number of risk factors have been identified that increase risk of aspiration in the ICU.[56] While it is difficult to quantify or stratify degree of risk among these factors, a simple categorization differentiates major risk factors for which change in management strategy may be needed, versus additional minor risk factors that may not warrant specific change in therapeutic course. *Major risk factors* include documented previous episode of aspiration, decreased level of consciousness (including sedation or increased intracranial pressure), neuromuscular disease, structural abnormalities of the aerodigestive tract, need for endotracheal intubation, overt vomiting or regurgitation, need for prolonged supine position, and persistently high gastric residual volumes.[56] *Additional risk factors* include presence of a nasoenteric tube, noncontinuous or bolus intermittent feeding, abdominal/thoracic surgery or trauma, delayed gastric emptying, poor oral care, advanced age, inadequate nursing staff, large bore feeding tube, malpositioned enteral tube (back into the esophagus), or transport out of the ICU.[1,56] Strategies to prevent aspiration in patients receiving nutrition support who have significant risk factors, as outlined below, should be utilized to minimize the risks associated with EN in this setting.

ROLE OF SMALL BOWEL FEEDING

A number of strategies may be employed to maximize the delivery of EN while minimizing the risks of gastric colonization, gastroesophageal regurgitation, and pulmonary aspiration (Table 11-1). By delivering enteral feeds into the small bowel, beyond the pylorus, the frequency of regurgitation and aspiration, as well as the risk of pneumonia, is decreased while at the same time nutrient delivery is maximized.[57] There are seven randomized trials that evaluated the effect of route of feeding on rates of ventilator-associated pneumonia (VAP).[58] When these results were aggregated, there was a significant reduction in VAP associated with small bowel feedings (RR 0.76; 95% CIs 0.59, 0.99) compared to gastric feeding. Therefore, the converse is also true. In some patients intragastric feeding may be associated with inadequate delivery of nutrition, increased regurgitation, pulmonary aspiration, and pneumonia, particularly if patients are cared for in the supine position.

TABLE 11-1 Summary of Strategies to Optimize the Benefits and Minimize the Risks of Enteral Nutrition and Total Parenteral Nutrition

Enteral Nutrition	Total Parenteral Nutrition
Initiate early, within 24–48 hours of admission	Hypocaloric dose
Use small bowel feedings	Do not use lipids for short term use (<10 days)
Elevate head of the bed	
Use motility agents	Tight control of blood sugars
Use feeding protocol that enables consistent evaluation of gastric residual volumes and specifies when feeds should be interrupted	Supplement with glutamine
	Continue to trickle concentrated amounts of enteral nutrition if able
Use concentrated feeding formulae in cases of intolerance	
Consider formulae with immune additives	

The clinical implications of these findings are influenced by the inherent difficulties in obtaining small bowel access. Given that some patients will tolerate intragastric feeds, it seems more prudent to reserve small bowel feeds for patients at high risk for intolerance to EN (due to use of inotropes, continuous infusion of sedatives, paralytic agents, high gastric residual volumes, or patients with high nasogastric drainage) or at high risk for regurgitation and aspiration (nursed in prolonged supine position).

BODY POSITION   1 RCT

While several studies document that elevation of the head of the bed is associated with less regurgitation and pulmonary aspiration, only one randomized controlled trial compared the frequency of pneumonia in critically ill patients assigned to semirecumbent or supine position.[59] Drakulovic and colleagues demonstrated that providing EN into the stomach in patients kept in the supine position was associated with a much higher risk of pneumonia compared to feeding patients with the head of the bed elevated to 45° (23% vs. 5%, $p < 0.05$). Thus, a simple maneuver (i.e., elevating the head of the bed to 30° to 45°) can reduce the risks associated with enteral feedings.

MOTILITY AGENTS   O RCT

Gastrointestinal prokinetic agents improve gastric emptying, improve tolerance to enteral nutrition, reduce gastroesophageal reflux and pulmonary aspiration, and therefore may have the potential to improve outcomes in critically ill patients.[60] While no study has demonstrated an impact from use of these agents on clinical outcomes, their low probability of harm and favorable feasibility and cost considerations warrant their use as a strategy to optimize nutritional intake and minimize regurgitation. Since cisapride is no longer available and due to the concerns of bacterial resistance with the use of erythromycin, metoclopramide is probably the drug of choice. It can be prescribed with the initiation of enteral feeds or reserved for patients who experience persistently high gastric residuals. It can be discontinued after four doses if there is no benefit observed, or after tolerance to EN is no longer

a problem clinically. Reducing narcotic dosages and potentially reversing their effect at the level of the gut by infusing naloxone through the feeding tube, and switching from bolus intermittent feeds to continuous infusion may also be effective in improving gastric function and tolerance to EN, while reducing risk of aspiration.[56] Methods not recommended solely to reduce risk of aspiration include switching to PN, adding acid to the enteral formula, switching from a large bore to a small bore nasoenteric tube, or converting a nasogastric tube to a percutaneous endoscopic gastrostomy tube.[56]

FEEDING PROTOCOLS

Several observational studies document that EN is frequently interrupted for high gastric residual volumes, procedures, nausea and vomiting, and other miscellaneous reasons.[61] Over the duration of ICU stay, this may result in inadequate delivery of EN to a critically ill patient and the associated complications of inadequate nutrition. Nurse-directed feeding protocols or algorithms have been shown to increase the amount of EN delivered on a daily basis.[62] Instituting a feeding protocol in ICUs that provides specific instructions on the patient's management related to EN to the bedside nurse has the potential to improve nutrient delivery and decrease complications.

ROLE OF IMMUNE STIMULANTS AND ANTIOXIDANTS

An additional strategy to maximize the benefits of enteral nutrition is to consider using products supplemented with specific nutrients that modulate the immune system, facilitate wound healing, and reduce oxidative stress. Enteral formulas developed to such an extent contain selected substrates such as glutamine, arginine, and omega-3 fatty acids, as well as selenium, vitamins E, C, and A, and beta-carotene in supraphysiologic concentrations. Unfortunately, with the possible exception of glutamine, the nutrients by themselves have not been adequately studied in critically ill patients, so their individual efficacy remains unknown. Nevertheless, these nutrients have been combined together and marketed as an immune-enhancing diet. We use the term *immunonutrition* as a general term to describe all these enteral products, but attempt to make summary recommendations based on the specific nutrients by themselves.

ARGININE

Supplementing arginine in the diet has a variety of biologic effects on the host[63,64] (Fig. 11-3). L-arginine is an active secretagogue that stimulates the release of growth hormone, insulin growth factor, and insulin, all of which may stimulate protein synthesis and promote wound healing. Conversion of arginine to ornithine by arginase provides two further functions. This pathway enables shuttling of nitrogen to urea, and ornithine is utilized in polyamine synthesis (which is involved in deposition of hydroxyproline, collagen, and the laying down of connective tissue to heal wounds). Arginine has also been shown to have significant immunostimulatory effects. Arginine has a trophic effect on the thymus gland that promotes the production and maturation of T lymphocytes. In the nitric oxide synthase pathway, the precursor arginine may contribute to improved bacterial killing.[63]

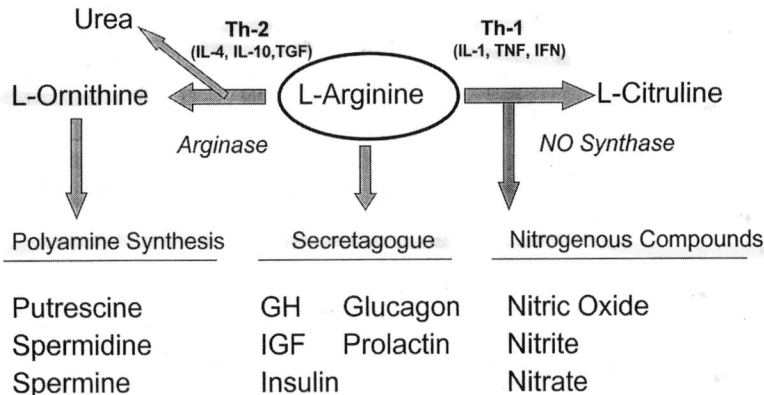

FIGURE 11-3 Arginine metabolic pathways.

Of interest is the fact that the arginase pathway is driven by a Th2 cytokine profile, mediated by further release of IL-4, IL-10 and TGF-β.[64] The Th2 cytokine profile has the effect of reducing the overall inflammatory immune response. In contrast, the nitric oxide synthase pathway is mediated by a Th1 cytokine profile, and is perpetuated by further release of IL-1, TNF, and IFN-γ.[64] This pathway has the capability of promoting the inflammatory response and inducing the formation of nitric oxide. Increased levels of nitric oxide may exert a negative inotropic and chronotropic effect on the cardiovascular system, and promote vasodilation (which may contribute to the hypotension and shock associated with sepsis syndrome). Nitric oxide in larger amounts may act as a mitochondrial toxin and inhibit several steps in the oxidative phosphorylation chain. Nitric oxide may also damage gut epithelium, increasing bacterial translocation and reducing overall gut integrity.[63] Nitric oxide can also have nonspecific cytotoxic effects of inhibiting growth or killing cells indiscriminately.[63]

Clinical Review

There are no randomized studies of pure arginine supplementation in critically ill patients that evaluate clinically important outcomes. All studies in critically ill patients have combined arginine with other immune-modulating nutrients. When the results of these 15 trials were aggregated, there was no effect on mortality (RR 1.05; 95% CIs 0.82, 1.35; $p = 0.7$), no overall effect on infectious complications (RR 0.94; 95% CIs 0.76 to 1.16; $p = 0.6$), and a trend towards reduction in hospital length of stay (weighted mean difference −3.5; 95% CIs −8.8, 1.9; $p = 0.20$). The presence of significant statistical heterogeneity across studies weakens the estimate of effect on length of stay.

Concerns have been expressed that based on the scientific rationale presented above, arginine-containing products may worsen outcomes in critically ill septic patients.[65] There are now three reports in the literature of excess mortality associated with critically ill septic patients who received arginine-supplemented diets.[66–68] In contrast, Galban and colleagues[69] demonstrated an increase in survival associated with arginine-supplemented diets in critically ill patients with infection. However, in this study, it was apparent that all the treatment benefit was in the least sick patients (baseline APACHE II score <15). The effect of arginine-containing products on critically ill patients with a high severity of illness remains unanswered. To the extent that in sepsis endotoxin exposure and cytokine activation have led to elevated levels of inducible nitric oxide synthesis, supplemental arginine may lead to the production of excessive amounts of nitric oxide, shock, and early death. Thus arginine-supplemented specialized diets should not be used in critically ill patients who are clearly septic. If a critically ill patient receiving an arginine-supplemented diet develops sepsis, the arginine-containing diet should be discontinued. Which subpopulations of critically ill patients benefit from these diets remains to be elucidated.

OMEGA-3 FATTY ACIDS

Omega-3 fatty acids may be provided in the form of fish oil or canola oil. These agents do not have direct stimulatory effects, but instead have an indirect effect by modifying phospholipids in cell membranes throughout the body.[70] Omega-6 fatty acids are involved in the cyclooxygenase pathway, generating prostaglandin E_2 (PGE_2) and leukotriene B_4 (LTB_4) from arachidonic acid. These are proinflammatory cytokines that lead to immune suppression and nosocomial infection, SIRS, and organ dysfunction. Through diet supplementation, omega-3 fatty acids compete with the omega-6 fatty acids for incorporation into cell membranes. Upon activation of the cyclooxygenase pathway, omega-3 fatty acids instead lead to the formation of PGE_3 and LTB_5. These compounds have $1/10$ the biologic activity of the PGE_2 and LTB_4 series, and as a result have a much less immunosuppressive effect.[70] Borage oil is unique as an omega-6 fatty acid, because it is metabolized to the PGE_1 series. PGE_1 possesses both anti-inflammatory and antiproliferative (reduced thrombosis) properties, and will attenuate the biosynthesis of arachidonic acid metabolites.[71]

Clinical Review

The only study of omega-3 fatty acids was conducted in patients with acute lung injury (ALI)/acute respiratory distress syndrome (ARDS).[72] The pathophysiology of this syndrome is thought be related to the release of arachidonic acid–related metabolites from inflammatory cells. Gadek and colleagues performed a multicenter, randomized, double-blind, clinical trial to evaluate whether a diet supplemented with eicosapentaenoic acid, docosahexaenoic acid (DHA), borage oil, and antioxidants (Oxepa, Ross Products, Columbus, OH) would have a favorable effect on markers of inflammation in the lung and an improvement in clinical outcomes.[72] In this study, 146 patients meeting the standard definition of ARDS with evidence of active pulmonary inflammation as indicated by fluid from a bronchoalveolar lavage (BAL) that contained a

PN → ↓ mortalité   EN ⟨ burn — ↓ mortalité / trauma — ↓ infections

neutrophil count >10%, were randomized to the experimental diet or a high-fat, low carbohydrate control feed.

In the subset of "evaluable" patients, those who received the experimental diet had higher plasma levels of dihomo-gamma linolenic acid, eicosapentaenoic acid, and an increased eicosapentaenoic/arachidonic acid ratio. With respect to the clinically important outcomes, patients fed the experimental diet experienced a reduction in days receiving supplemental oxygen (13.6 vs. 17.1; $p = 0.078$), required significantly fewer days of ventilatory support (9.6 vs. 13.2; $p = 0.027$), and less time in the ICU (11.0 vs. 14.8; $p = 0.016$), and had fewer new organ failures (10% vs. 25%; $p = 0.018$). There was also a trend towards a reduction in mortality associated with the experimental diet (16% vs. 25%; $p = 0.17$).

This study confirms that short-term administration of dietary lipids in critically ill patients can modify fatty acid levels with a resultant favorable effect on neutrophil recruitment in the lung and subsequent clinical outcomes. However, given that a high-fat diet in itself may be harmful,[73] the use of a high-fat control formula and the requirement for a BAL to identify patients with a high degree of neutrophils limits the applicability of these findings to clinical practice. Furthermore, it is difficult to attribute the beneficial effects of the experimental diet to fatty acid composition when it was combined with antioxidants as well.

GLUTAMINE

The amino acid glutamine plays a central role in nitrogen transport within the body, is a fuel for rapidly dividing cells (particularly lymphocytes and gut epithelial cells), is a precursor to glutathione, and has many other essential metabolic functions. As noted previously, plasma glutamine levels drop during critical illness, and lower levels of glutamine have been associated with immune dysfunction[74] and increased mortality.[75] Human studies suggest that glutamine supplementation maintains gastrointestinal structure[76] and is associated with decreased intestinal permeability compared to standard PN.[77,78] In humans, glutamine-supplemented formulas have resulted in improved nitrogen balance,[79] and higher intramuscular glutamine levels.[80] Glutamine plays a crucial role in enhancing immune cell function[81] with no elevation in proinflammatory cytokine production.[82,83]

There have been several randomized trials of perioperative or critically ill adults reporting on clinically important outcomes.[84] When the results of these trials were aggregated, a significant reduction in mortality (RR 0.78; 95% CIs 0.61 to 0.99; $p = 0.04$), a trend towards a reduction in infectious complications (RR 0.89; 95% CIs 0.73 to 1.08; $p = 0.2$), and no overall effect on length of stay (LOS in days –1.30; 95% CIs – 4.77, 2.17; $p = 0.5$) were observed.[85] Subgroup analysis suggested that with respect to mortality and infectious complications, the majority of the treatment effect observed was associated with parenteral glutamine in patients receiving PN compared to enteral glutamine supplementation. The majority of glutamine provided enterally will be metabolized in the gut and liver, and therefore may not have a systemic effect. The only study that demonstrated a mortality effect with enteral glutamine was a small study in burn patients.[86] In a study of trauma patients, enteral feeds supplemented with glutamine were associated with a trend towards a reduced rate of infection compared to control feeds (20/35 [57%] vs. 26/37 [70%], $p = 0.24$).[87]

Therefore, for critically ill patients requiring PN, we recommend parenteral glutamine supplementation as long as the patient remains on PN. For patients with major burns or trauma, enteral diets supplemented with glutamine could be considered. Recommendations about glutamine supplementation (enteral or parenteral) in other critically ill patient populations fed enterally are premature and warrant further study.

ANTIOXIDANT VITAMINS AND TRACE MINERALS

While there is a putative beneficial role of reactive oxygen species in modulating cell signaling (redox signaling), and thus regulating proliferation, apoptosis, and cell protection, oxygen-derived radicals may cause cellular injury by numerous mechanisms, including destruction of cell membranes through the peroxidation of fatty acids, disruption of organelle membranes such as those covering lysosomes and mitochondria, degradation of hyaluronic acid and collagen, and disruption of enzymes like Na^+,K^+-ATPase or alpha$_1$-proteinase inhibitor.

To protect tissues from oxygen free radical–induced injury, the body maintains a complex endogenous defense system that consists of a variety of extra- and intracellular antioxidant defense mechanisms. The first line of intracellular defense is comprised of a group of antioxidant enzymes such as superoxide dismutase, catalase, glutathione peroxidase, and glutathione reductase, including their metal cofactors selenium, copper, and zinc. When these enzymatic antioxidants are overwhelmed, oxygen free radicals (OFRs) are free to react with susceptible target molecules within the cell (i.e., unsaturated fatty acids of the cell membrane). Thus there is a need for a second line of defense scavenging OFRs by means of nonenzymatic antioxidants that are either water soluble, such as glutathione and vitamin C, or lipid soluble, such as vitamin E and beta-carotene.[88]

In critical illness, oxidative stress arises when the balance between protective antioxidant mechanisms and the generation of reactive oxygen species (ROS) is disturbed. This imbalance may be caused by excess generation of ROS by means of ischemia/reperfusion injury, inflammation, infection, and toxic agents (chemotherapy or drugs), or by low antioxidant capacity (secondary to comorbid illnesses, malnutrition, and excessive losses such as in the case of burns). Many studies have demonstrated low plasma and intracellular concentrations of the various antioxidants in critically ill patients, and the clinical consequence of these low endogenous stores of antioxidant levels is increased morbidity and mortality.[89–91]

Most of the immune formulas are fortified with vitamins and minerals that have increased antioxidant capabilities. Vitamins A, E, and C, and the trace mineral selenium have antioxidant capabilities and are added in different amounts to the various formulas. The exact doses of these components have not been standardized.

Single Antioxidant Nutrients

SELENIUM ALONE Selenium is an important co-factor in glutathione enzymatic function and has favorable effects on cellular immune function. In critically ill patients, there have been only a few randomized controlled trials looking at the effects of selenium supplementation alone.[92–95] In a poorly designed trial of 17 patients with acute necrotizing pancreatitis, parenteral supplementation of 500 μg of selenium was

STRESS OXIDATIF

associated with a significant reduction in ICU mortality (0% vs. 89%).[93] In a prospective randomized trial, Zimmermann and colleagues reported a reduction in mortality (15% vs. 40%) after IV administration of 1000 μg of sodium selenite for 28 days in patients with SIRS compared to placebo.[94] However, no difference in mortality or pneumonia was seen in critically ill trauma/surgical patients given IV selenium supplementation (2.9 μmol/d) compared to placebo.[92] In a trial of 42 patients with SIRS, subjects that received a higher dose of parenteral selenium (535 μg/d × 3 days, 285 μg/d × 3 days, 155 μg/d × 3 days, and 35 μg/d thereafter) versus a lower dose (35 μg/d) had a trend towards reduced hospital mortality (33% vs. 52%; $p = 0.13$).[95] When the results from the four trials that compared supplementation of selenium alone to standard were aggregated,[92–95] selenium was associated with a trend towards a reduction in mortality (RR 0.52; 95% CIs 0.21, 1.30; $p = 0.16$).[85]

ZINC ALONE   Zinc is an essential trace element necessary for normal protein metabolism, membrane integrity, and the function of more than 200 metalloenzymes including enzymes involved in oxidative capacity. In a randomized, prospective, double-blinded controlled trial in severely head injured, ventilated patients, those receiving a higher zinc supplement (12 mg elemental zinc via PN for 15 days, then progressing to 3 months of oral zinc) had a trend towards a reduction in mortality ($p = 0.09$) when compared to those receiving a placebo (2.5 mg elemental zinc).[96]

Combined Antioxidant Nutrients

Many randomized controlled trials have chosen to administer a combination of antioxidants via various routes of administration, thereby making it impossible to attribute the outcomes to a specific nutrient. When 11 trials of single and combined antioxidants were aggregated, overall antioxidants were associated with a trend towards a reduction in mortality (RR = 0.73; 95% CIs 0.47, 1.12; $p = 0.15$) and no effect on infectious complications (RR = 0.94; 95% CIs 0.63, 1.40; $p = 0.8$).[97] Thus, for critically ill patients, selenium supplementation in combination with other antioxidants (vitamin E/alpha tocopherol, vitamin C, N-acetylcysteine, and zinc) may be beneficial, but insufficient data currently exist to support clinical recommendations.

ROLE OF PARENTERAL NUTRITION

Several trials and meta-analyses have evaluated the treatment effect of parenteral nutrition in the last few years, and none has shown a positive result, while some have suggested increased harm associated with PN in the critically ill patient.[11,98,99] We have already stated that EN is used preferentially to PN. However, to optimize the delivery of nutrients, some prescribe PN at the same time EN is initiated, to provide nearly all required calories and protein immediately. Then, as EN becomes successfully established, PN is reduced and eliminated. There are five randomized trials that address the clinical benefits of such a strategy in critically ill patients.[100] All five studies reported on mortality and the aggregated results demonstrated a trend towards an increased mortality associated with the use of combination EN and PN (RR 1.27; 95% CIs 0.82 to 1.94; $p = 0.3$). In one study, there was a significant increase in mortality associated with supplemental PN.[101] Supplemental PN was not associated with a difference in the incidence of infections

(RR 1.14; 95% CIs 0.66 to 1.96; $p = 0.6$), had no effect on hospital stay (standardized mean difference 0.12; 95% CIs 0.45, 0.2; $p = 0.5$), and had no effect on ventilator days. Thus there appears to be no clinical evidence to support the practice of supplementing EN with PN when EN is initiated. If anything, there appears to be a signal of excess harm.

What about the patient who has been started on EN, and after several days is only tolerating inadequate amounts of EN? Does PN have a role in this patient population? The preferred approach is to continue with EN and standard IV therapy. However, at some point (probably between 7 and 14 days postinjury) the risk from further deterioration of nutritional status outweighs the risk of providing PN, due to the cumulative effect on immune function, continued losses to the lean body mass, and development of specific key nutrient deficiencies in the critically ill patient receiving inadequate nutritional support by EN. This time frame may be considerably shortened in patients at tremendously increased risk for deterioration of nutritional status due to the presence of large open wounds, enteric fistula, or short bowel syndrome. Unfortunately, there are no randomized trials to guide practitioners as to when PN should be initiated in patients tolerating inadequate amounts of EN. While the results of our previous reviews suggest that PN is associated with no clinical benefit or increased harm, prolonged starvation (more than 14 days) is equally associated with poor outcomes.[102]

In summary, PN has a very limited role in the critical care setting. PN should not be started in critically ill patients until all strategies to maximize EN delivery (such as the use of small bowel feeding tubes and motility agents) have been attempted. Waiting 2 weeks in someone tolerating inadequate amounts of EN is probably too long, but practitioners will have to weigh the safety and benefits of initiating PN in patients not tolerating EN on an individual case-by-case basis.

MAXIMIZING THE BENEFITS AND MINIMIZING THE RISKS OF PARENTERAL NUTRITION

If PN is associated with harm in critically ill patients, it may be due to a variety of potentially avoidable pathophysiologic mechanisms, including overfeeding, the immunosuppressant effects of lipids, hyperglycemia, absence of key nutrients like glutamine, and the association of gut disuse and systemic inflammation. Understanding these potential mechanisms can guide practitioners when they use PN to use it in such a way that its benefits are maximized and its risks are minimized.

Role of Hypocaloric Parenteral Nutrition

Because of the degree of insulin resistance so commonly observed in stressed critically ill patients, providing large amounts of dextrose intravenously results in hyperglycemia and predisposes critically ill patients to risk of infection. Other attendant complications associated with overfeeding carbohydrates include hepatic steatosis, hypertriglyceridemia, and hypercapnia. This has given rise to the notion of hypocaloric or hypoenergetic PN as a strategy to minimize complications associated with PN. There are only two small studies that have evaluated the effect of hypocaloric feeding in critically ill patients. To achieve a hypocaloric dose of PN, Choban and associates[103] reduced both carbohydrates and lipids in morbidly obese critically ill patients, while McCowen and colleagues[104] withheld lipids in a heterogeneous group of patients, including critically ill patients. Only one study reported infectious complications, and in that study[104] hypocaloric feeding was associated with a trend toward a reduction in infectious complications ($p = 0.2$). There were no significant differences in mortality or length of stay between groups in either study. Given the lack of positive treatment effect from standard PN, minimizing the dose of PN seems reasonable until further data emerge to prove the contrary.

Parenteral Lipids

2 studies { ↓ infections (mixts) / ↓ infections / LOS (Trauma)

There are several reports that demonstrate that intravenous lipids may adversely affect immune status and clinical outcomes.[105,106] The results of previously described meta-analysis of PN[11] suggest that the adverse effects of lipids may negate any beneficial effect of nonlipid parenteral nutritional supplementation. There are two studies reviewed that compared the use of lipids to no lipids in parenteral nutrition.[104,107] A significant reduction in pneumonia (48% vs. 73%; $p = 0.05$), catheter-related sepsis (19% vs. 43%; $p = 0.04$), and a significantly shorter stay in both ICU (18 vs. 29 days; $p = 0.02$) and hospital (27 vs. 39 days; $p = 0.03$) was observed in trauma patients not receiving lipids compared to those receiving lipids.[107] In the McCowen study mentioned previously, the group that received no lipids (hypocaloric group) showed a trend towards a reduction in infections (29% vs. 53%; $p = 0.2$). No difference in length of stay was seen in this study, and it did not report on ventilator days. Combining these two studies, the meta-analysis done showed a significant reduction in infections in the group that received no lipids (RR 0.63; CIs 0.42 to 0.93; $p = 0.02$) and no difference in mortality (RR 1.29; CIs 0.16 to 10.7; $p = 0.8$).

It is unknown what the effects of long-term fat-free parenteral nutrition would be, and there is a paucity of data in malnourished patients. Given these caveats, lipid-free PN is probably best indicated for those patients requiring PN for a ✳ short time (<10 days), where the risk of fatty acid deficiency would be minimal. This recommendation cannot be extrapolated to those who have an absolute contraindication to EN and need PN for a longer duration.

Tight Glycemic Control

Hyperglycemia, which occurs more often with PN than EN, is associated with increased infectious complications. Van den Berghe and associates[108] compared intensive insulin therapy (target range 4.4 to 6.1 mmol/L) vs. conventional treatment (10.0 to 11.1 mmol/L) in critically ill patients receiving nutrition support. This was a large study (n = 1548) of surgical ICU patients (predominantly elective cardiovascular surgery) with a relatively low APACHE II score (median 9). Study patients were started on a glucose load (200 to 300 g/d) and then were advanced to PN, combined PN/EN, or EN after 24 hours of admission. Intensive insulin therapy was associated with a lower incidence of sepsis ($p = 0.003$), a trend towards a reduction in ventilator days, and a reduced ICU ($p < 0.04$) and hospital mortality ($p = 0.01$), compared to conventional insulin therapy. From this study, one can infer that intensive insulin therapy to achieve tight glycemic control may be associated with improved clinical outcomes in critically ill patients. The corollary to this is that high glucose loads in patients who are insulin resistant is associated with excess complications and increased mortality, which can be reduced

by insulin. Whether insulin has any therapeutic effects in patients who do not receive such high glucose loads, or whether these results apply to other medical, sicker ICU patients is unknown. Despite these limitations, in the absence of further studies, patients prescribed PN should receive intensive insulin therapy to obtain tight glycemic control. This can best be accomplished by using an insulin protocol or nomogram.[109]

Supplementation with Glutamine

Perhaps the lack of treatment effect of PN relates to the lack of key nutrients necessary for repair and recovery following critical illness. As noted previously, there are data that suggest that PN supplemented with glutamine is associated with increased survival in seriously ill hospitalized patients.[12] It is difficult to provide high-dose free glutamine intravenously to critically ill patients due to problems with limited solubility and stability, especially in critically ill patients with volume-restricted conditions. However, recent advances in parenteral glutamine delivery have overcome some of these challenges, making the provision of bioavailable glutamine practical, even at higher doses.[110] The treatment effect is likely greatest when high-dose (>0.2 g/kg per day) glutamine is given parenterally to patients with gastrointestinal failure (and thus prescribed PN). Whether parenteral glutamine has a beneficial effect on patients receiving enteral nutrition is unknown.

Use of Enteral Nutrition in Patients on Parenteral Nutrition

The adverse effect of PN may be related to the absence of nutrients in the bowel. The gastrointestinal mucosa is metabolically very active and the lack of enteral nutrients (as in the case of PN) would result in mucosal atrophy, increased permeability, bacterial overgrowth, translocation of bacteria and/or gut-derived factors that activate the immune system, atrophy of the gut-associated lymphoid tissue, and increased production of proinflammatory cytokines.

An observational study suggested that low-volume EN is associated with less toxicity compared to PN alone.[111] Clearly our recommendation is that EN is used preferentially to PN, but in the patient who is not tolerating adequate amounts of EN over a prolonged period of time, if PN is going to be used, we suggest that attempts to provide EN be continued until EN is successful and the PN can be discontinued.

Summary and Conclusions

An opportunity exists for aggressive enteral nutritional support to favorably alter a patient's course through critical illness. The window of time to start enteral feeding and/or key nutrients to resuscitate the metabolically active gastrointestinal tract is variable in duration depending on the specific disease process; the opportunity may involve a time frame as limited as several hours or as long as 2 to 3 days. During this period, provision of enteral nutrients in a way that maximizes the benefits and minimizes the risks (see Table 11-1) has the capability to maintain gut integrity, minimize permeability, reduce oxidative stress and macrophage activation, and ultimately improve patient outcome through reduced infectious morbidity, organ failure, length of hospitalization, and even mortality. There is a limited role for PN, and when it is used it should similarly be used in a way that maximizes the benefits and minimizes the risks (see Table 11-1).

References

1. Heyland DK: Nutritional support in the critically ill patient, a critical review of the evidence. *Crit Care Clin* 14:423, 1998.
2. Heyland DK: A review of gut-specific strategies to reduce ICU-acquired infections. *Curr Opin Crit Care* 5:132, 1999.
3. Carrico CJ: The elusive pathophysiology of the multiple organ failure syndrome (editorial). *Ann Surg* 218:109, 1993.
4. Bengmark S: Gut microenvironment and immune function. *Curr Opin Clin Nutr Metab Care* 2:1, 1999.
5. Brandtzaeg P, Halstersen TS, Kett K, et al: Immunobiology and immunopathology of the human gut mucosa: Humoral immunity and intraepithelial lymphocytes. *Gastroenterology* 97:1562, 1989.
6. Girou E, Stephan F, Novara A, et al: Risk factors and outcome of nosocomial infections: Results of a matched case-control study of ICU patients. *Am J Resp Crit Care Med* 157:1151, 1998.
7. Bueno-Cavanillas A, Delgado-Rodriguez M, Lopez-Luque A, et al: Influence of nosocomial infection on mortality rate in an intensive care unit. *Crit Care Med* 22:55, 1994.
8. Atherton ST, White DJ: Stomach as source of bacteria colonising respiratory tract during artificial respiration. *Lancet* 2:968, 1978.
9. Pingleton SK, Hinthorn DR, Liu C: Enteral nutrition in patients receiving mechanical ventilation. *Am J Med* 80:827, 1986.
10. Heyland DK, Mandell LA: Gastric colonization and nosocomial pneumonia: Evidence for causation. *Chest* 101:187, 1992.
11. Heyland DK, MacDonald S, Keefe L, et al: Total parenteral nutrition in the critically ill patient: A meta-analysis. *JAMA* 280:2013, 1998.
12. Novak F, Heyland DK, Avenell A, et al: Glutamine supplementation in serious illness: A systematic review of the evidence. *Crit Care Med* 30:2022, 2002.
13. Heyland DK, Samis A: Does immunonutrition in septic patients do more harm than good? *Intensive Care Med* 29:669, 2003.
14. Kudsk KA, Croce MA, Fabian TC, et al: Enteral versus parenteral feeding—Effects on septic morbidity after blunt and penetrating abdominal trauma. *Ann Surg* 215:503, 1992.
15. McClave SA, Greene LM, Snider HL, et al: Comparison of the safety of early enteral versus parenteral nutrition in mild acute pancreatitis. *JPEN* 21:14, 1997.
16. Windsor ACJ, Kanwar S, Li AGK, et al: Compared with parenteral nutrition, enteral feeding attenuates the acute phase response and improves disease severity in acute pancreatitis. *Gut* 42:431, 1998.
17. Kalfarentzos F, Kehagias J, Mead N, et al: Enteral nutrition is superior to parenteral nutrition in severe acute pancreatitis: Results of a randomized prospective trial. *Br J Surg* 84:1665, 1997.
18. DeWitt RC, Kudsk KA: The gut's role in metabolism, mucosal barrier function, and gut immunology. *Infect Dis Clin North Am* 13:465, 1999.
19. Kagnoff MF: Immunology of the intestinal tract. *Gastroenterology* 105:1275, 1993.
20. Targan SR, Kagnoff MF, Brogan MD, Shanahan F: Immunologic mechanisms in intestinal diseases. *Ann Intern Med* 106:853, 1987.
21. Dobbins WO: Gut immunophysiology: A gastroenterologist's view with emphasis on pathophysiology. *Am J Physiol* 242:G1, 1982.
22. Frost P, Bihari D: The route of nutritional support in the critically ill: Physiological and economical considerations. *Nutrition* 13:58S, 1997.
23. Moore EE, Moore FA: The role of the gut in provoking the systemic inflammatory response. *J Crit Care Nutr* 2:9, 1994.
24. Fink MP: Why the GI tract is pivotal in trauma, sepsis, and MOF. *J Crit Illness* 6:253, 1991.
25. Moore FA, Feliciano DV, Andrassy RJ, et al: Early enteral feeding, compared with parenteral, reduces postoperative septic complications. *Ann Surg* 216:172, 1992.
26. Elson CO: The immunology of inflammatory bowel disease, in Kirsner JB (ed): *Inflammatory Bowel Disease*. Philadelphia, WB Saunders, 2000, p 208.
27. Jankovic D, Liu Z, Gause WC: Th1- and Th2-cell commitment during infectious disease: Asymmetry in divergent pathways. *Trends Immunol* 22:450, 2001.
28. Fujimura Y, Owen RL: The intestinal epithelial M cell: Properties and functions, in Kirsner JB (ed): *Inflammatory Bowel Disease*. Philadelphia, WB Saunders, 2000, p 33.
29. Astiz ME, Rackow EC: Septic shock. *Lancet* 351:1501, 1998.
30. Moore F: Effects of immune-enhancing diets on infectious morbidity and multiple organ failure. *JPEN* 25(2 Suppl):S36, 2001.
31. Groos S, Hunefeld G, Luciano L: Parenteral versus enteral nutrition: morphological changes in human adult intestinal mucosa. *J Submicrosc Cytol Pathol* 28:61, 1996.
32. Ammori BJ, Leeder PC, King RF, et al: Early increase in intestinal permeability in patients with severe acute pancreatitis: Correlation with endotoxemia, organ failure, and mortality. *J Gastrointest Surg* 3:252, 1999.
33. Fong YM, Marano MA, Barber A, et al: Total parenteral nutrition and bowel rest modify the metabolic response to endotoxin in humans. *Ann Surg* 210:449, 1989.
34. Abou-Assi S, Craig K, O'Keefe SJ: Hypocaloric jejunal feeding is better than total parenteral nutrition in acute pancreatitis: Results of a randomized comparative study. *Am J Gastroenterol* 97:2255, 2002.
35. Gramlich L, Kichian G, Pinilla J, et al: Does enteral nutrition compared to parenteral nutrition result in better outcomes in the critically ill adult? A systematic review of the literature. *Nutrition* 2004 (in press).
36. Stack JA, Babineau TJ, Bistrian BR: Assessment of nutritional status in clinical practice. *Gastroenterologist* 4:S8, 1996.
37. Larvin M, McMahon MJ: APACHE-II score for assessment and monitoring of acute pancreatitis. *Lancet* 2:201, 1989.
38. Corfield AP, Cooper MJ, Williamson RCN, et al: Prediction of severity in acute pancreatitis: Prospective comparison of three prognostic indices. *Lancet* ii:403, 1985.
39. Sax HC, Warner BW, Talamini MA, et al: Early total parenteral nutrition in acute pancreatitis: Lack of beneficial effects. *Am J Surg* 153:117, 1987.
40. Ziegler TR, Smith RJ, O'Dwyer ST, et al: Increased intestinal permeability associated with infection in burn patients. *Arch Surg* 123:1313, 1988.
41. Demeo MT: (personal communication).
42. Taylor SJ, Fettes SB, Jewkes C, Nelson RJ: Prospective, randomized, controlled trial to determine the effect of early enhanced enteral nutrition on clinical outcome in mechanically ventilated patients suffering head injury. *Crit Care Med* 27:2525, 1999.
43. Atkinson S, Sieffert E, Bihari D: A prospective, randomized, double-blind, controlled clinical trial of enteral immunonutrition in the critically ill. *Crit Care Med* 26:1164, 1998.
44. Zaloga GP: Bedside method for placing small bowel feeding tubes in critically ill patients. A prospective study. *Chest* 100:1643, 1991.
45. Evans A, Winslow EH: Oxygen saturation and hemodynamic response in critically ill, mechanically ventilated adults during intrahospital transport. *Am J Crit Care* 4:106, 1995.
46. Smith I, Fleming S, Cernaianu A: Mishaps during transport from the intensive care unit. *Crit Care Med* 18:278, 1990.
47. Gutierrez ED, Balfe DM: Fluoroscopically guided nasoenteric feeding tube placement: Results of a one-year study. *Radiology* 178:759, 1991.
48. Nachlas MM, Younis MT, Roda CP, et al: Gastrointestinal motility studies as a guide to postoperative management. *Ann Surg* 175:510, 1972.

49. Drover JW, Mackenzie S, Dhaliwal R, Heyland DK: Early enteral nutrition in critically ill patients: Is there a positive effect on patient outcomes? *Can J Gastroenterol* 17:394, 2003.

50. Minard G, Kudsk KA, Melton S, et al. Early versus delayed feeding with an immune-enhancing diet in patients with severe head injuries. *JPEN* 24:145, 2000.

51. Moore EE, Jones TN: Benefits of immediate jejunostomy feeding after major abdominal trauma—A prospective, randomized study. *J Trauma* 26:874, 1986.

52. Singh G, Ram RP, Khanna SK: Early postoperative enteral feeding in patients with nontraumatic intestinal perforation and peritonitis. *J Am Coll Surg* 187:142, 1998.

53. Ibrahim EH, Mehringer L, Prentice D, et al: Early versus late enteral feeding of mechanically ventilated patients: Results of a clinical trial. *JPEN* 26:174, 2002.

54. Mentec H, Dupont H, Bocchetti M, et al: Upper digestive intolerance during enteral nutrition in critically ill patients: Frequency, risk factors, and complications. *Crit Care Med* 29:1955, 2001.

55. Lukan JK, McClave SA, Stefater AJ, et al: Poor validity of residual volumes as a marker for risk of aspiration. *Am J Clin Nutr* 75:417, 2002.

56. McClave SA, Demeo MT, Delegge MH, et al: North American Summit on Aspiration in the Critically Ill Patient: Consensus Statement. *JPEN* 26:S80, 2002.

57. Heyland DK, Drover JW, MacDonald S, et al: Effect of postpyloric feeding on gastroesophageal regurgitation and pulmonary microaspiration: Results of a randomized controlled trial. *Crit Care Med* 29:1495, 2001.

58. Heyland DK, Drover JD, Dhaliwal R, Greenwood J: Optimizing the benefits and minimizing the risks of enteral nutrition in the critically ill: Role of small bowel feeding. *JPEN* 26:S51, 2002.

59. Drakulovic MB, Torres A, Bauer TT, et al: Supine body position as a risk factor for nosocomial pneumonia in mechanically ventilated patients: A randomised trial. *Lancet* 354:1851, 1999.

60. Booth CM, Heyland DK, Paterson WG: Gastrointestinal promotility drugs in the critical care setting: A systematic review of the evidence. *Crit Care Med* 30:1429, 2002.

61. Heyland DK, Konopad E, Alberda C, et al: How well do critically ill patients tolerate early, intragastric enteral feeding? Results of a prospective multicenter trial. *Nutr Clin Pract* 14:23, 1999.

62. Spain DA, McClave SA, Sexton LK, et al: Infusion protocol improves delivery of enteral tube feeding in the critical care unit. *JPEN* 23:288, 1999.

63. Suchner U, Heyland DK, Peter K: Immune-modulatory actions of arginine in the critically ill. *Br J Nutr* 87(Suppl 1):S121, 2002.

64. Ochoa JB, Bernard AC, O'Brien WE, et al: Arginase I expression and activity in human mononuclear cells after injury. *Ann Surg* 233:393, 2001.

65. Heyland DK, Novak F: Immunonutrition in the critically ill patient: More harm than good? *JPEN* 25:S51, 2001.

66. Bertolini G, Iapichino G, Radrizzani D, et al: Early enteral immunonutrition in severely septic patients: Results of an interim analysis of a randomized multicenter trial. *Intensive Care Med* 29:834, 2003.

67. Bower RH, Cerra FB, Bershadsky B, et al: Early enteral administration of a formula (Impact) supplemented with arginine, nucleotides, and fish oil in intensive care unit patients: results of a multicenter, prospective, randomized, clinical trial. *Crit Care Med* 23:436, 1995.

68. Dent, DL, Heyland DK, Levy H, et al: Immunonutrition may increase mortality in critically ill patients with pneumonia: Results of a randomized trial. *Crit Care Med* 30:A17, 2003.

69. Galban C, Montejo JC, Mesejo A, et al: An immune-enhancing enteral diet reduces mortality rate and episodes of bacteremia in septic intensive care unit patients. *Crit Care Med* 28:643, 2000.

70. Schloerb PR: Immune-enhancing diets: products, components, and their rationales. *JPEN* 25(2 Suppl):S3, 2001.

71. Fan Y, Chapkin RS: Importance of dietary γ-linoleic acid in human health and nutrition. *J Nutr* 128:1411, 1998.

72. Gadek JE, DeMichele SJ, Karlstad MD, et al: Effect of enteral feeding with eicosapentaenoic acid, gamma-linolenic acid, and antioxidants in patients with acute respiratory distress syndrome. *Crit Care Med* 27:1409, 1999.

73. Garrel D, Razi M, Lariviere F, et al: Improved clinical status and length of care with low-fat nutrition support in burns patients. *JPEN* 19:482, 1995.

74. Oehler R, Pusch E, Dungel P, et al: Glutamine depletion impairs cellular stress response in human leucocytes. *Br J Nutr* 87:S17, 2002.

75. Roth E, Funovics J, Muhlbacher F, et al: Metabolic disorders in severe abdominal sepsis: Glutamine deficiency in skeletal muscle. *Clin Nutr* 1:25, 1982.

76. Tremel H, Kienle B, Weilemann LS, et al: Glutamine dipeptide-supplemented parenteral nutrition maintains intestinal function in the critically ill. *Gastroenterology* 107:1595, 1994.

77. Buchman AL, Moukarzel AA, Bhuta S, et al: Parenteral nutrition is associated with intestinal morphologic and functional changes in humans. *JPEN* 19:453, 1995.

78. van der Hulst RR, van Kreel BK, von Meyenfeldt , et al: Glutamine and the preservation of gut integrity. *Lancet* 341:1363, 1993.

79. Hammarqvist F, Wernerman J, Ali R, et al: Addition of glutamine to total parenteral nutrition after elective abdominal surgery spares free glutamine in muscle, counteracts the fall in muscle protein synthesis, and improves nitrogen balance. *Ann Surg* 209:455, 1989.

80. Stehle P, Zander J, Mertes N, et al: Effect of parenteral glutamine peptide supplements on muscle glutamine loss and nitrogen balance after major surgery. *Lancet* 1:231, 1989.

81. Ogle CK, Ogle JD, Mao JX, et al: Effect of glutamine on phagocytosis and bacterial killing by normal and pediatric burn patient neutrophils. *JPEN* 18:128, 1994.

82. O'Riordain MG, De Beaux A, Fearon KC: Effect of glutamine on immune function in the surgical patient. *Nutrition* 12:S82, 1996.

83. Aosasa S, Mochizuki H, Yamamoto T, et al: A clinical study of the effectiveness of oral glutamine supplementation during total parenteral nutrition: Influence on mesenteric mononuclear cells. *JPEN* 23:S41, 1999.

84. Novak F, Heyland DK, Avenell A, et al: Glutamine supplementation in serious illness: A systematic review of the evidence. *Crit Care Med* 30:2022, 2002.

85. Heyland DK, Dhaliwal R, Suchner U: Immunonutrition, in *Clinical Nutrition: Enteral and Tube Feeding*. Ed, Rolandelli, 2003, (in press).

86. Garrel D, Nedelec B, Samson L, et al: Decreased mortality and infectious morbidity in adult burn patients given enteral glutamine supplementation. *Clin Nutr* 22:S78, 2003.

87. Houdijk AP, Rijnsburger ER, Jansen J, et al: Randomised trial of glutamine-enriched enteral nutrition on infectious morbidity in patients with multiple trauma. *Lancet* 352:772, 1998.

88. Tanswell AK, Freeman BA: Antioxidant therapy in critical care medicine. *New Horiz* 3:330, 1995.

89. Goode HF, Cowley HC, Walker BE, et al: Decreased antioxidant status and increased lipid peroxidation in patients with septic shock and secondary organ dysfunction. *Crit Care Med* 23:646, 1995.

90. Cowley HC, Bacon PJ, Goode HF, et al: Plasma antioxidant potential in severe sepsis: A comparison of survivors and non-survivors. *Crit Care Med* 24:1179, 1996.

91. Forceville X, Vitoux D, Guazit R, et al: Selenium, systemic immune response syndrome, sepsis and outcomes in critically ill patients. *Crit Care Med* 26:1536, 1998.

92. Berger MM, Recmond MJ, Shenkin A, et al: Influence of selenium supplements on the post-traumatic alterations of the thyroid axis: a placebo-controlled trial. *Intensive Care Med* 27:91, 2001.

93. Kuklinski B, Buchner M, Schweder R, Nagel R: Akute Pancreatitis-eine "Free Radical Disease": Letalitatssenkung durch Natriumselenit (Na₂SeO₃)-Therapie. *Z Gestamte Inn Med* 46:S145, 1991.

94. Zimmermann T, Albrecht S, Kühne H, et al: [Selenium administration in patients with sepsis syndrome. A prospective randomized study.] *Med Klin* 92:(Suppl III):3, 1997 (article in German).

95. Angstwurm MW, Schottdorf J, Schopohl J, Gaertner R: Selenium replacement in patients with severe systemic inflammatory response syndrome improves clinical outcome. *Crit Care Med* 27:1807, 1999.

96. Young B, Ott L, Kasarskis E, et al: Zinc supplementation is associated with improved neurologic recovery rate and visceral protein levels of patients with severe closed head injury. *J Neurotrauma* 13:25, 1996.

97. Heyland DK, Dhaliwal R, Berger M, et al: Antioxidant nutrients: A systematic review of vitamins and trace elements in the critically ill patients. *Crit Care Med* 31:A8, 2003.

98. Braunschweig CL, Levy P, Sheean PM, Wang X: Enteral compared with parenteral nutrition: A meta-analysis. *Am J Clin Nutr* 74:534, 2001.

99. Koretz RL, Lipman TO, Klein S: American Gastroenterological Association. AGA technical review on parenteral nutrition. *Gastroenterology* 121:970, 2001.

100. Dhaliwal R, Jurewitsch B, Harrietta D, Heyland DK: Combination enteral nutrition and parenteral nutrition in critically ill patients: harmful or beneficial? A review of the evidence. *Intensive Care Med* 2004 (in press).

101. Herndon DN, Barrow RE, Stein M, et al: Increased mortality with intravenous supplemental feeding in severely burned patients. *J Burn Care Rehabil* 10:309, 1989.

102. Sandstrom R, Drott C, Hyltander A, et al: The effect of postoperative intravenous feeding (PN) on outcome following major surgery evaluated in a randomized study. *Ann Surg* 217:185, 1993.

103. Choban PS, Burge JC, Scales D, et al: Hypoenergetic nutrition support in hospitalized obese patients: A simplified method for clinical application. *Am J Clin Nutr* 66:546, 1997.

104. McCowen KC, Friel C, Sternberg J, et al: Hypocaloric total parenteral nutrition: Effectiveness in prevention of hyperglycemia and infectious complications. A randomized clinical trial. *Crit Care Med* 28:3606, 2000.

105. Seidener DL, Mascioli EA, Istfan NW, et al: Effects of long-chain triglyceride emulsions on reticuloendothelial system function in humans. *JPEN* 13:614, 1989.

106. Freeman J, Goldmann DA, Smith NE, et al: Association of intravenous lipid emulsion and coagulase-negative staphylococcal bacteremia in neonatal intensive care units. *N Engl J Med* 323:301, 1990.

107. Basttistella FD, Widergren JT, Anderson JT, et al: A prospective, randomized trial of intravenous fat emulsion administration in trauma victims requiring total parenteral nutrition. *J Trauma* 43:52, 1997; discussion 58.

108. Van den berghe G, Wouters P, Weekers F, et al: Intensive insulin therapy in critically ill patients. *N Engl J Med* 345:1359, 2001.

109. Brown G Dodek P: Intravenous insulin nomogram improves blood glucose control in the critically ill. *Crit Care Med* 29:1714, 2001.

110. Furst P: New advances in glutamine delivery. *J Clin Nutr* 131:2562S, 2001.

111. Marik PE, Karnack C, Varon J: The addition of trickle feeds reduces the complications associated with parenteral nutrition. *Crit Care Shock* 5:165, 2002.

Chapter 12 _____

INTRAVASCULAR DEVICES

JOHN F. McCONVILLE
JOHN P. KRESS

KEY POINTS

- *The subclavian approach is preferred for placement of central venous catheters (CVCs).*
- *Real-time ultrasound may reduce the mechanical complications associated with CVC insertion.*
- *Chlorhexidine-based skin antiseptic solutions reduce the incidence of catheter-related bloodstream infections as compared with povidone-iodine.*
- *Almost 50% of hospital-acquired bloodstream infections are caused by staphylococcal species.*
- *CVCs should not be replaced nor exchanged over a guidewire on a routine basis.*

Central venous catheters (CVCs) have become an integral part of delivering care in the modern ICU. In fact, the Centers for Disease Control and Prevention (CDC) estimates that in U.S. ICUs there are 15 million CVC days per year (total number of days patients are exposed to CVCs).[1] Indications for placement of CVCs include invasive hemodynamic monitoring, administration of vasoactive drugs, administration of caustic agents (e.g., chemotherapy), administration of parental nutrition, renal replacement therapy, large-bore venous access for rapid administration of fluids, and long-term venous access. This chapter focuses on the use of CVCs in the ICU setting. Thus long-term tunneled catheters used for hemodialysis and peripherally inserted central catheters (PICCs) will not be discussed.

Placement of CVCs

The clinical presentation often dictates the type of catheter to be inserted. For example, a patient with a hemodynamically significant gastrointestinal hemorrhage may require only a single-lumen, large-bore CVC for volume resuscitation in addition to a peripheral IV, whereas a neutropenic patient with septic shock may require a triple-lumen CVC in order to administer vasoactive drugs and antibiotics simultaneously. Importantly, most evidence suggests that the number of catheter lumens does not affect the rate of CVC infectious complications.[2,3] Once the type of catheter has been selected, an anatomic site for insertion needs to be determined. The optimal anatomic location for insertion of CVCs has been a matter of debate for many years. In 2001, Merrer and colleagues[4] published a study of 289 patients who were randomized to have their CVCs inserted in either the femoral or subclavian vein. Patients with femoral vein catheters had a dramatically higher incidence of infectious complications (19.8% versus 4.5%; $p < 0.001$) and thrombotic complications (21.5% versus 1.9%; $p < 0.001$) as compared with patients with subclavian

catheters. The overall sum of mechanical complications (i.e., arterial puncture, pneumothorax, hematoma or bleeding, and air embolism) was similar between the two groups. To date, there are no randomized trials comparing subclavian versus internal jugular catheters with regard to infectious complications, although observational studies suggest a lower rate of infectious complications with subclavian catheters and a similar rate of mechanical complications.[5,6] As a result of these and other studies,[7] the CDC recommends that, if not contraindicated, the subclavian vein should be used for the insertion of nontunneled CVCs in adult patients in an effort to minimize infection risk.

Approaches to Insertion of CVCs

INFRACLAVICULAR SUBCLAVIAN APPROACH

Prior to the insertion of an infraclavicular subclavian CVC, a small rolled-up towel should be placed between the shoulder blades to move the vascular structures to a more anterior position. After the subclavian area has been sterilely prepped and draped (see below) and local anesthesia has been administered, the patient should be placed in the Trendelenburg position. The arm should be positioned at the patient's side so that the shoulder, clavicle, and sternal notch are aligned and perpendicular to the sternum. The subclavian vein arises from the axillary vein and travels beneath the clavicle and inferior to the subclavian artery prior to joining the internal jugular vein and forming the brachiocephalic vein. Thus the clavicle provides a good anatomic landmark for the insertion of a subclavian CVC. The skin and periosteum of the clavicle should be infiltrated with a local anesthetic (e.g., lidocaine 1%). Following administration of local anesthesia, the skin should be entered with a 16-gauge introducer needle 1 to 2.5 cm below the inferior edge of the clavicle and 2 to 4 cm lateral to the midpoint of the clavicle. Once the needle is directly underneath the clavicle, it should be advanced toward the sternal notch, making sure that the needle remains in the plane immediately below the clavicle. If no blood return is obtained, then the needle should be pulled back and directed more cephalad. Slight backpressure should be placed on the plunger of the syringe any time the needle is advanced or withdrawn so that blood return can be visualized when the vessel is cannulated. After the vessel has been accessed, the modified Seldinger technique is used to complete the insertion of the CVC. Inexperienced operators often have difficulty knowing when the needle is directly underneath the clavicle and are appropriately fearful of puncturing the visceral pleura. Thus we often use a slightly different approach when supervising an inexperienced operator. Once the skin is entered, the operator is instructed to find the clavicle with the tip of the introducer needle. After the edge of the clavicle is reached and more local anesthesia is given in the area, the introducer needle is removed slightly (1 cm) and redirected in a more posterior direction by pushing down on the syringe and needle as a unit with the nondominant hand. This prevents the inexperienced operator from advancing the needle at a steep angle toward the underlying visceral pleura of the lung while attempting to locate the posterior border of the clavicle. Once the needle is "walked down" the bone and is positioned underneath the clavicle, it is then redirected toward the sternal

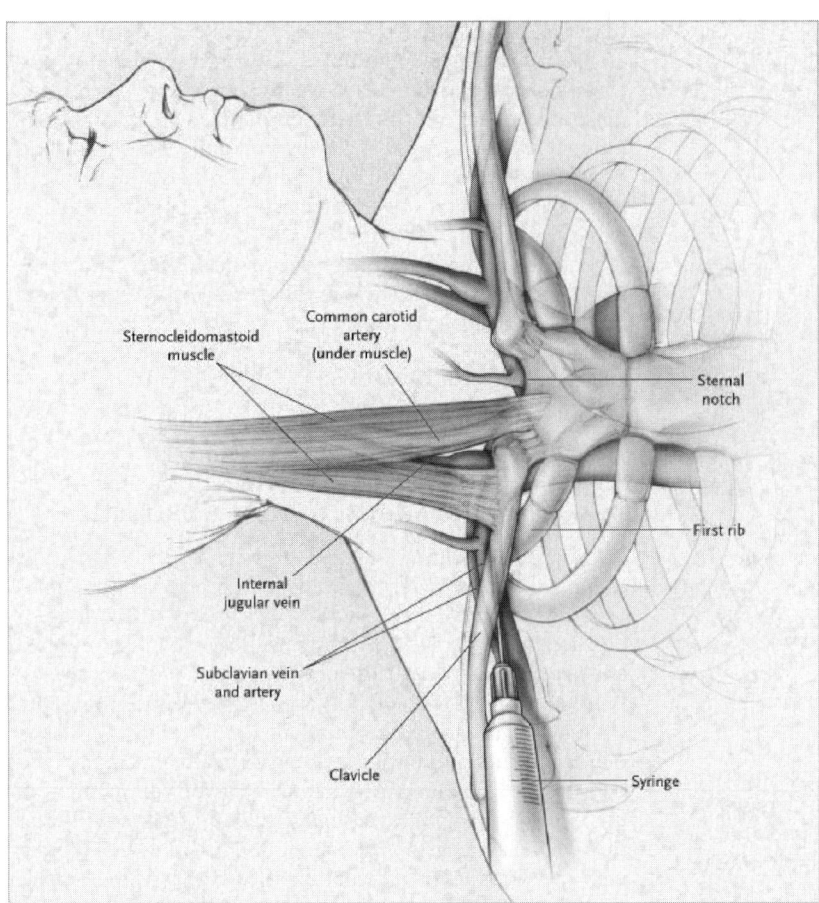

FIGURE 12-1 Insertion of a subclavian CVC.
See text for description. *(Used with permission
from McGee and Gould.[6] Copyright © 2003
Massachusetts Medical Society. All rights
reserved.)*

notch and advanced slowly while applying backpressure to the syringe (Fig. 12-1).

INTERNAL JUGULAR APPROACH

If the patient's anatomy (e.g., scar from previous vascular access) or a coagulation disorder prevents use of the subclavian vein, then the internal jugular vein should be used for placement of a CVC. The central approach to placing an internal jugular catheter uses the triangle formed by the two heads of the sternocleidomastoid muscle and the medial portion of the clavicle as the anatomic landmark. Typically, the internal jugular vein is lateral to the carotid artery, and both vessels run through the triangle beneath the sternocleidomastoid muscle. After the patient has been sterilely prepped and draped and local anesthesia has been administered, the patient is placed in the Trendelenburg position, and the head is rotated slightly toward the contralateral side such that carotid artery can be palpated in the apex of the triangle. The nondominant hand is used to lightly palpate the carotid artery, with careful attention paid to not place too much pressure on the skin because this can alter the position of the internal jugular vein. An 18- or 20-gauge "finder needle" often is used to locate the vessel prior to using the introducer needle (16 gauge). This finder needle should enter the skin at the apex of the triangle and be advanced at an angle of 60 degrees above the plane of the skin. If the nondominant hand is able to delineate the course of the common carotid artery, then the needle should

be advanced along a similar line just lateral to the carotid artery because both vessels are contained within the carotid sheath. If the carotid artery cannot be palpated with the nondominant hand, then the needle should enter the skin at the apex of the triangle at a 60-degree angle to the skin and be advanced in the direction of the ipsilateral nipple. If the needle is inserted 3 cm without achieving good blood return, then it should be pulled back slowly while applying constant backpressure to the plunger of the syringe and redirected more medially before being slowly advancing again. After the vessel has been cannulated, the modified Seldinger technique is used to complete insertion of the CVC (Fig. 12-2).

POSTERIOR INTERNAL JUGULAR APPROACH

The posterior internal jugular approach is an alternative to the central internal jugular approach that may be used if there is concern that the patient will not be able to tolerate a procedure-related pneumothorax (high positive endexpiratory pressure and/or high F_{IO_2} requirements). The puncture site is posterolateral to the sternocleidomastoid muscle and immediately cephalad to where the sternocleidomastoid is crossed by the external jugular vein. The needle should be directed beneath the muscle and advanced in an anterior and inferior direction toward the sternal notch. If blood return is not obtained, the needle should be pulled back and redirected slightly more posterior until venous blood is obtained. Because unintentional carotid artery puncture is more

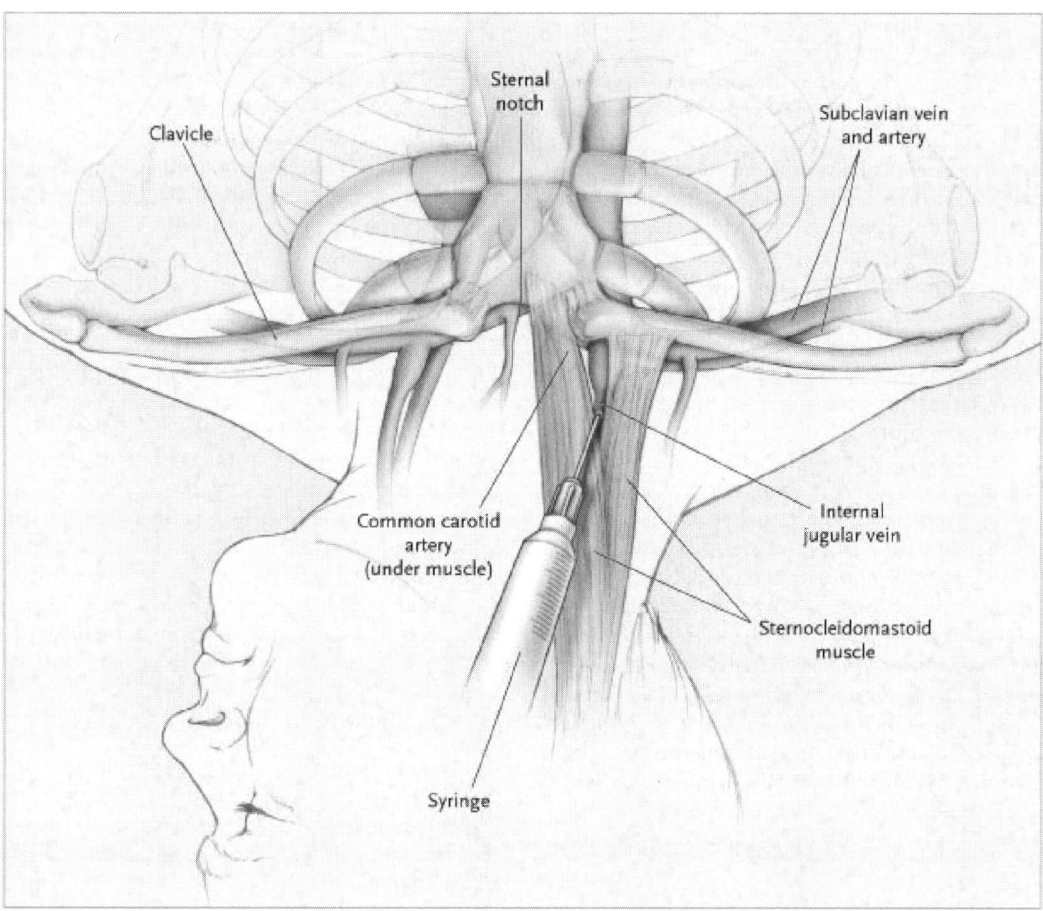

FIGURE 12-2 Insertion of an internal jugular CVC. See text for description. (*Used with permission from McGee and Gould.*[6]

likely with this approach, a "finder needle" should be used prior to cannulation with a large-bore needle.

ULTRASOUND-GUIDED PLACEMENT

Ultrasound guidance to assist in the placement of CVCs is a subject of controversy. Mansfield and colleagues[29] reported that ultrasound guidance did not affect the rate of complications or failures in 821 patients randomized to standard insertion procedures with anatomic landmark guidance versus ultrasound guidance for subclavian vein catheterization. It is noteworthy that this study used ultrasonography to locate the subclavian vein but did not use real-time ultrasound guidance for the actual venipuncture. In contrast, several studies have compared the use of real-time ultrasound with the use anatomic landmarks during the insertion of both subclavian and internal jugular CVCs. These studies showed decreased failure rates, decreased complication rates, and an increased rate of successful catheter placement on the first attempt with the use of real-time ultrasound.[30,31] A recent review of CVC complications reported a 6% to 10% incidence of mechanical complications with the insertion of subclavian and internal jugular CVCs.[6] Given the frequent use of CVCs in the ICU and the risk of mechanical complications, it seems prudent to use real-time ultrasound during the insertion of CVCs if

it is available, especially for patients with coagulation disturbances or unclear anatomic landmarks.

Infectious Complications of CVCs

Catheter-related infections (e.g., bloodstream infection, catheter colonization, or an exit-site infection) are thought to arise via several different mechanisms: Skin flora from the insertion site can migrate down the external surface of the catheter, the catheter hub can become infected with repeated manipulation, or hematogenous seeding of the catheter tip can result from a distant source of bacteremia.[22] CVC-related infections are the most common cause of nosocomial bacteremia in critically ill patients.[14] The incidence of hospital-acquired CVC-associated bloodstream infections is collected by the CDC's National Nosocomial Infection Surveillance System (NNIS) and is expressed as the number of bloodstream infections (BSI) per 1000 CVC-days. From 1992 to 2001, the rate of CVC-related bloodstream infections in adult ICUs ranged from 2.9 to 5.9 per 1000 catheter-days.[15] Diagnosis of a CVC-related BSI requires clinical symptoms of bacteremia (fever >38°C, chills, or hypotension) without another apparent source and isolation of an organism from a peripheral blood culture with either a semiquantitative or quantitative culture of a catheter segment that yields the same organism and

CRITERES DX

(handwritten) 6 – 10% complications mécaniques

antibiotic sensitivities as the organism cultured from blood. In the semiquantitative culture method, the catheter segment is rolled on a culture plate and considered positive if there are greater than 15 colony-forming units (CFUs) of an organism. In the quantitative method, the catheter is processed in broth and sonicated, followed by plating the broth on a culture plate. A positive culture requires growth of greater than 10^3 CFUs.[16] CVC-related BSI should be distinguished from catheter colonization, which only requires a positive semiquantitative or quantitative culture from a catheter segment. In addition to BSI and catheter colonization, a CVC can develop an exit-site infection, defined as erythema, tenderness, induration, or purulence within 2 cm of the catheter exit site.[16]

The majority of pathogens causing CVC-related bloodstream infection are skin flora, which suggests migration of bacteria down the catheter as the mechanism of infection. A study of 297 pulmonary artery catheters found that 80% of infected catheters showed concordance with organisms cultured from the skin at the insertion site.[5] According to NNIS data from 1992 to 1999, approximately 50% of hospital-acquired bloodstream infections were caused by staphylococcal species. The most common organisms isolated were coagulase-negative staphylococci (37%), *Staphylococcus aureus* (13%), enterococcus (13%), gram-negative rods (14%), and *Candida* spp. (8%).[15] Given the frequency and cost associated with treating catheter-related infections, there has been a great deal of research into reducing the rate of these infections. Several interventions implemented at the time of catheter insertion have been shown to reduce the rate of catheter-associated infections.

SKIN PREPARATION

The use of antiseptic skin preparations prior to sterile draping and percutaneous placement of CVCs is a routine part of the procedure. Although povidone-iodine is the most commonly used skin antiseptic agent in the United States, a recent meta-analysis reported a 50% reduction in catheter-related bloodstream infections with the use of chlorhexidine-based solutions rather than povidone-iodine (risk ratio 0.49, 95% confidence interval [CI] 0.28–0.88).[19] This meta-analysis included several different types of chlorhexidine gluconate solutions for the insertion of central venous, peripheral venous, peripheral arterial, and pulmonary artery catheters. Subset analysis indicated that most of the benefit appeared to come from the chlorhexidine gluconate alcohol solutions rather than chlorhexidine gluconate aqueous solutions. Additionally, a subsequent meta-analysis determined that the use of chlorhexidine for central catheter site care resulted in a 0.23% decrease in the incidence of death and savings of $113 per catheter used.[20] Finally, it should be noted that there are little data about whether antibiotic resistance emerges with the use of antiseptic solutions.

MAXIMAL STERILE BARRIERS

Meticulous attention to sterile technique is of paramount importance during the placement of CVCs. The use of maximal sterile barriers likely decreases the incidence of inadvertent contamination of gloves, guidewires, and other equipment in the CVC kit. The technique of employing maximal sterile barriers, including a full body sterile drape, sterile gloves and long-sleeved gown, and nonsterile cap and mask, has been shown to reduce the incidence of CVC-related infections. Mermel and colleagues[5] found that pulmonary artery catheters (PACs) placed in the ICU with the use of maximal sterile barrier precautions developed fewer infections (15.1% versus 24.6%, $p < 0.01$) when compared with PACs placed in the operating room without maximal sterile barrier precautions. Raad and colleagues[21] found that the time to occurrence of catheter-related bloodstream infection was lengthened in cancer patients who had CVCs and peripherally inserted CVCs inserted with maximal sterile barriers as compared with patients who had catheters inserted with sterile gloves and a small sterile field ($p < 0.05$). Another study investigated the impact of a 1-day course taken by first-year resident physicians on infection control practices and hands-on instruction for several common procedures (arterial puncture and placement of arterial lines and CVCs). Subsequently, the documented use of full-size sterile drapes increased from 44% to 65%, and the rate of catheter-related infections decreased from 4.51 infections per 1000 patient-days before the first course to 2.92 infections per 1000 patient-days 18 months after the course. This decrease in catheter-related infections was associated with an estimated cost savings of $63,000.[22]

ANTIMICROBIAL CATHETER TREATMENT

Another approach to reducing the incidence of catheter-related infections is the use of catheters treated with antimicrobial agents. Catheters coated with chlorhexidine and silver sulfadiazine and minocycline and rifampin are currently available for clinical use. Compared with conventional catheters, these antimicrobial-treated catheters are associated with significant reductions in catheter-related bacteremia.[23,24] A study by Maki and colleagues[25] comparing conventional triple-lumen polyurethane catheters with catheters coated with chlorhexidine and silver sulfadiazine reported both a reduction in catheter colonization and a nearly fivefold reduction in bloodstream infection. A recent randomized trial of minocycline and rifampin versus chlorhexidine and silver sulfadiazine catheters, however, found a significant decrease in the incidence of catheter-related BSI in the group of patients using minocycline and rifampin (0.3% versus 3.4%, $p < 0.002$).[26] There are several possible reasons for the differences between the two catheters. The minocycline and rifampin catheters had antibacterial substances both outside and inside the catheters, as opposed to the chlorhexidine catheters, which were only externally coated. Importantly, neither study reported hypersensitivity reactions to the catheters, and neither reported the occurrence of infections by organisms with resistance to the antimicrobial agents. A newer chlorhexidine and silver sulfadiazine catheter with antiseptic located on both the internal and external surfaces is now available, and studies comparing this new catheter with the minocycline and rifampin catheter are underway. While the exact role of the catheters remains the subject of some debate, a cost-benefit analysis suggests that antiseptic catheters are beneficial if an institution's rate of catheter-related bacteremia is 3 infections per 1000 catheter-days.[25]

CATHETER EXCHANGE OVER A GUIDEWIRE

In order to avoid mechanical complications of placing a new CVC, a strategy of inserting a sterile guidewire through an existing catheter, removing the catheter, and inserting a new sterile CVC over the guidewire is employed frequently. Since the existing catheter is not sterile, contamination of the new catheter is a concern with this technique. There have been several studies comparing scheduled catheter exchange over a guidewire and scheduled replacement of a CVC at a new site every 2 days, 3 days, 7 days, or as needed. In a meta-analysis, Cook and colleagues[27] found trends toward higher catheter colonization (relative risk [RR] 1.26, 95% CI 0.87–1.84) and catheter-related bacteremia (RR 1.72, 95% CI 0.89–3.33) associated with exchange over a guidewire. Additionally, prophylactic catheter replacement was not found to reduce catheter colonization or catheter-related bacteremia as compared with replacement of the catheter on an as-needed basis. In fact, the CDC strongly recommends that CVCs should *not* be replaced or exchanged over a guidewire on a routine basis[15] (category 1B recommendation: strongly recommended for implementation and supported by some experimental, clinical, or epidemiologic studies and a strong theoretical rationale). However, most authorities recommend wire exchange for suspicion of infection or mechanical catheter dysfunction. If infection is suspected, the catheter should be cultured on removal, and the new catheter should be removed if the culture of the old catheter is positive (>15 CFUs by the roll-plate method). Catheters with inflamed or purulent entry sites should be removed, and a new catheter should be inserted into a new site[6,28] (Fig. 12-3).

Mechanical Complications of CVCs

Lefrant and colleagues[32] reported their experience with subclavian vein catheterization over a 5-year period. Seven hundred and seven patients in a surgical critical care unit had subclavian vein catheterization attempted, with 562 successful procedures (79.5%). For the remaining 145 catheterizations, there were 67 failed procedures (overall failure rate of 9.5%). By multivariate analysis, more than one attempted venipuncture was the only independent risk factor for failed catheterization and immediate complications (e.g., arterial puncture, pneumothorax, misplacement of catheter). Elderly patients (>77 years of age) were more likely to have immediate complications but not failed catheterization. It is noteworthy that the operator's level of training and experience (junior, but not senior, residents were supervised by a critical care anesthesiologist) did not affect outcomes in the study, suggesting that adequately supervised physicians in training can perform CVC placement safely. Based on their observations, the authors recommended no more than two attempts at subclavian vein catheterization before aborting the procedure, with consideration of attempting at a different anatomic site. Contralateral attempts to cannulate the internal jugular or subclavian vein should be preceded by a chest radiograph to rule out pneumothorax, however, prior to proceeding.

ARTERIAL PUNCTURE/BLEEDING

Accidental arterial puncture is a well-recognized complication of CVC placement. The incidence of this complication in published reports ranges from 0% to 15%.[8–10] Complications arising from accidental arterial puncture include mediastinal hematoma formation, hemothorax, tracheal compression and possible asphyxiation, and retroperitoneal hemorrhage. A re-

cent meta-analysis comparing internal jugular versus subclavian catheter placement noted a higher incidence of arterial puncture with internal jugular catheter attempts.[10] Although arterial puncture occurs more frequently with internal jugular attempts, the carotid artery is more readily compressible compared with the subclavian artery, which makes this approach more attractive in patients with coagulation disturbances. Most complications of accidental arterial puncture occur with dilation and subsequent placement of large-bore catheters into an artery. Several case reports and small series have acknowledged this important complication.[11–13] Traditional means of confirming arterial versus venous puncture of a blood vessel (e.g., bright red color, pulsatile blood return) may be unreliable in hypotensive, hypoxemic patients frequently encountered in the ICU. Transduction of the pressure waveform with intravenous extension tubing before dilation and placement of a large-bore catheter may reduce the occurrence of this complication. One may use tubing filled with sterile saline and attached to a three-way stopcock. After a vessel is entered, this tubing is connected to the needle while it is in the vessel, the tubing is elevated, and movement of the column of saline is analyzed to reflect either a venous or arterial waveform. Alternatively, the guidewire can be placed through the needle into the vessel using the modified Seldinger technique. Subsequently, a small, short catheter (e.g., 18- or 20-gauge 2-in intravenous catheter) can be placed over the wire into the vessel and the wire removed. The saline-filled, intravenous extension tubing can be attached to the catheter in the vessel to confirm a venous or arterial waveform. After confirmation of a venous waveform, the guidewire is replaced through this small intravenous catheter, the catheter is removed, and the procedure is finished. If unintentional arterial cannulation occurs, the small catheter is removed from the artery, and pressure is held at the site. Such a small catheter is much less likely to cause serious complications compared with a dilator and large-bore catheter. In our teaching hospital, we stress the importance of placing sterile intravenous extension tubing on the sterile field before the procedure is started so that a venous waveform can be confirmed prior to dilation and insertion of the catheter.

Bleeding complications from both arterial and venous punctures are exacerbated dramatically in patients who are thrombocytopenic or in those with coagulation disturbances. Unfortunately, such problems are common in critically ill patients. Those with platelet counts below $50,000/\mu L$ or those with an international normalized ratio (INR) above 2 probably should have catheters placed at a site with compressible vessels (e.g., internal jugular or femoral vein) unless the clotting problem can be corrected. The external jugular vein is an alternative that should be considered in those with clotting disturbances because it is a superficial vein that is easily compressible.

PNEUMOTHORAX

Pneumothorax is another important mechanical complication of CVC placement. The reported incidence of this complication ranges from 0% to 4.5%. Although some studies have reported a higher incidence of pneumothorax with subclavian catheter placement, a recent meta-analysis did not describe differences in the incidence of this complication when

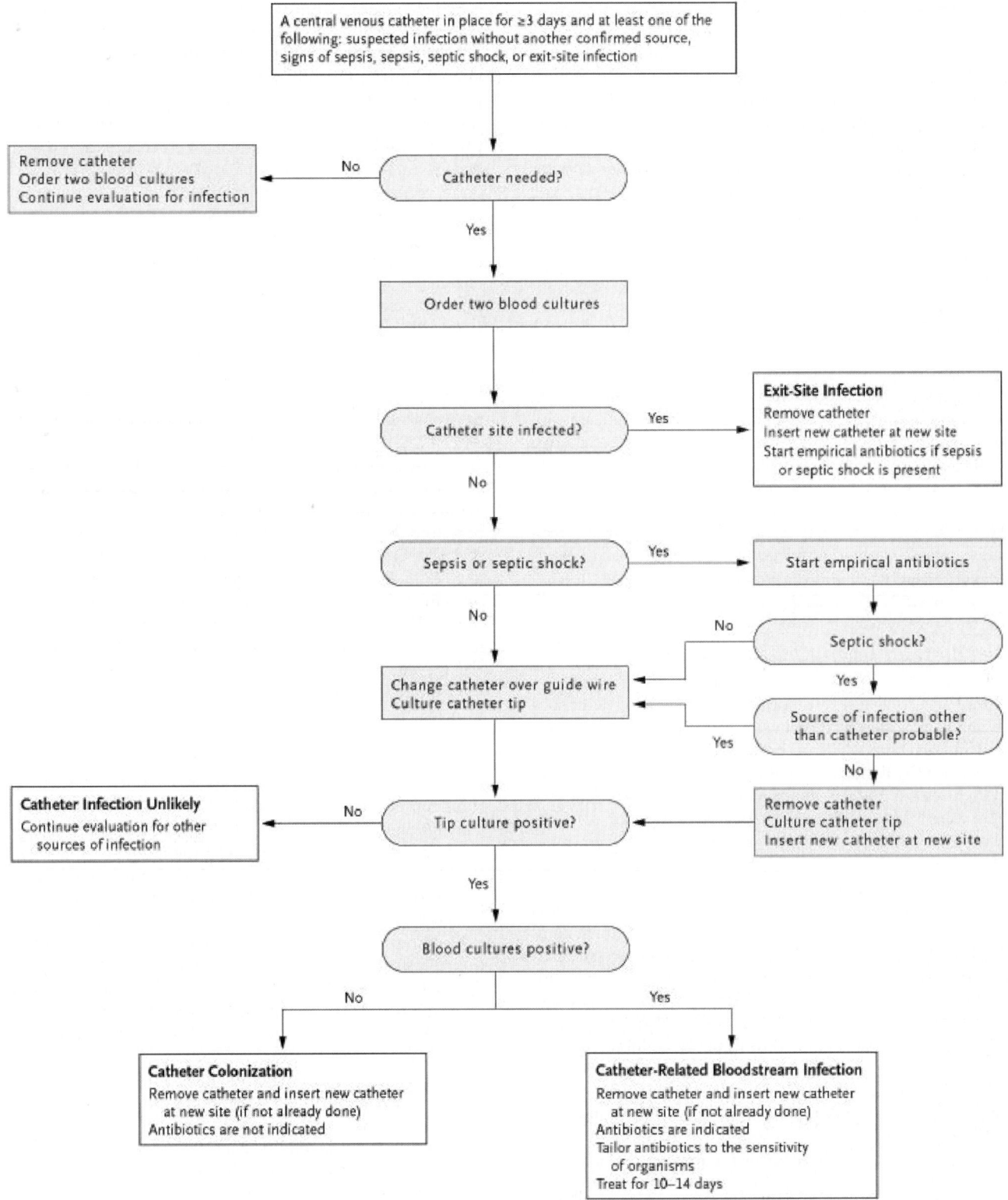

FIGURE 12-3 Management of suspected CVC infection. See text for description. (*Used with permission from McGee and Gould.*[6]

internal jugular and subclavian approaches were compared.[10] Although many pneumothoraces occurring after CVC placement may not require treatment,[33] patients undergoing positive-pressure ventilation should have the pneumothorax evacuated. The use of small-caliber pleural catheters is ef-

fective as an alternative to conventional tube thoracostomy in evacuating simple iatrogenic pneumothoraces[34]; however, since this therapy has not been tested extensively in patients undergoing positive-pressure ventilation, tube thoracostomy remains the treatment of choice in this situation.

THROMBOTIC COMPLICATIONS

Catheter-related venous thrombosis is a relatively common complication, occurring in between 2% to 66% of catheters.[5,39] Catheter-related venous thrombosis may manifest as either a fibrin sleeve around the catheter or a thrombus that adheres to the wall of the vein that is typically asymptomatic. Because CVCs injure the endothelium and expose the venous intima, the coagulation system can become activated, resulting in thrombus formation. Difficulty with insertion of the line appears to increase the incidence of thrombosis, presumably owing to a greater degree of local venous trauma.[40] There is some evidence that *in an ICU setting* a subclavian vein CVC is less likely to develop a catheter-related thrombosis than an internal jugular vein CVC.[41] Timsit and colleagues[41] used color Doppler ultrasound just before or within 24 hours of catheter removal to determine the frequency of catheter-related thrombosis associated with 208 CVCs placed in the ICU (catheters in place for 9.35 ± 5.4 days). A catheter-related internal jugular or subclavian vein thrombosis occurred in 42% (95% CI 34–49) and 10% (95% CI 3–18), respectively. The overall rate of thrombus formation was 33%, and an internal jugular CVC increased the risk of thrombus formation by a factor of four (RR 4.13 [95% CI 1.72–9.95]). Importantly, this study also determined that the risk of catheter-related sepsis was 2.62-fold higher when thrombosis occurred ($p = 0.011$). These findings contradict two studies that examined the incidence of complications in more *permanent tunneled catheters* and found a decreased incidence of venous stenosis and thrombus formation in the internal jugular group as compared with the subclavian group.[42,43] Finally, the femoral vein is the least desirable anatomic location with regard to the risk of venous thrombosis. Merrer and colleagues[4] reported that 25 of 116 (21.5%) patients randomized to femoral vein catheterization had ultrasound-detected venous thrombosis. This differed dramatically from those randomized to subclavian vein catheterization, in whom 2 of 107 (1.9%) had venous thrombosis ($p < 0.001$).[4]

CATHETER OCCLUSION

Occlusion of a CVC is another mechanical complication that occurs, particularly when catheters have been in place for extended periods of time. Thrombosis at the tip of the catheter may lead to this problem. Other reasons for CVC occlusion include precipitation of incompatible medications, a problem that can be avoided by careful attention to medication compatibility. Patients may suffer occasionally from the "pinch-off syndrome," in which a subclavian catheter is compressed between the clavicle and the first rib.[17] This complication usually occurs in long-term indwelling catheters; however, a narrow space between the clavicle and the first rib sometimes can interfere with successful placement of subclavian catheters, particularly those of large bore. CVCs placed for extended time periods have been reported to break and embolize to the right side of the heart or pulmonary artery, requiring radiologic or surgical removal.[17,33]

CATHETER MISPLACEMENT

Most CVC placements in critically ill patients are performed without direct real-time visualization of the catheter. Typically, a chest radiograph is obtained after the procedure to ensure proper catheter position and to assess for evidence of a pneumothorax. Malpositioned catheters can then be repositioned correctly. Ideally, thoracic CVCs should terminate in the superior vena cava. Catheters occasionally may terminate in subclavian or jugular vein, as well as in the azygous, internal mammary, or pericardiophrenic vein, which may result in vascular injury and even perforation. When the tip of a catheter is positioned in the right atrium or right ventricle, perforation and subsequent cardiac tamponade may result.[35,36] In order to avoid complications when CVCs are positioned in cardiac chambers, it is recommended that the tip of the catheter lie proximal to the angle between the trachea and the right mainstem bronchus.[37] Ultrasonic examination after CVC placement may provide an alternative means of assessing adequacy of catheter placement.[44]

AIR EMBOLISM

When there is a communication between the great veins and the atmosphere, air may enter into the venous system. This potential complication is particularly relevant when considering the large-bore venous catheters used frequently in critically ill patients. Dysfunctional one-way valves or uncapped catheters may allow air to enter the venous system when intrathoracic pressure is subatmospheric during inspiration. Another problem is the possibility of venous air embolism during catheter removal, when a communication from the skin to a great vein may occur temporarily. Use of the Trendelenburg position and biooclusive dressings may prevent this problem.[38]

Conclusion

In conclusion, intravascular catheters are necessary routinely for the management of critically ill patients. Mechanical, infectious, and thrombotic complications contribute considerable morbidity and mortality to these vulnerable patients. Recent evidence suggests that the subclavian vein may be the most desirable anatomic location for CVC placement; however, thrombocytopenia or coagulation disturbances—common problems in critically ill patients—may preclude this approach in some patients. It is encouraging that evidence to guide the appropriate management of CVCs is accumulating. Such evidence should allow clinicians to use these potentially lifesaving devices effectively while minimizing complications associated with their use.

References

1. O'Grady NP, Alexander M, Dellinger EP, et al: Guidelines for the prevention of catheter-related infections. *MMWR* 51:1, 2002.
2. Farkas JC, Liu N, Bleriot JP, et al: Single- versus triple-lumen central catheter-related sepsis: A prospective, randomized study in a critically ill population. *Am J Med* 93:277, 1992.
3. Ma TY, Yoshinaka R, Banaag A, et al: Total parenteral nutrition via multilumen catheters does not increase the risk of catheter-related sepsis: A randomized, prospective study. *Clin Infect Dis* 27:500, 1998.
4. Merrer J, DeJonghe B, Golliot F, et al: Complications of femoral and subclavian venous catheterization in critically ill patients: A randomized, controlled trial. *JAMA* 286:700, 2001.

5. Mermel LA, McCormick RD, Springman SR, et al: The pathogenesis and epidemiology of catheter-related infection with pulmonary artery Swan-Ganz catheters: A prospective study utilizing molecular subtyping. *Am J Med* 91:S197, 1991.

6. McGee DC, Gould MK: Preventing complications of central venous catheterization. *N Engl J Med* 348:1123, 2003.

7. Goetz AM, Wagener MM, Miller JM, Muder RR: Risk of infection due to central venous catheters: Effect of site placement and catheter type. *Infect Control Hosp Epidemiol* 19:842, 1998.

8. Jobes DR, Schwartz AJ, Greenhow DE, et al: Safer jugular vein cannulation: Recognition of arterial puncture and preferential use of the external jugular route. *Anesthesiology* 59:353, 1983.

9. Mansfield PF, Hohn DC, Fornage BD, et al: Complications and failures of subclavian vein catheterization. *N Engl J Med* 331:1735, 1994.

10. Ruesch S, Walder B, Tramer MR: Complications of central venous catheters: Internal jugular versus subclavian access—a systematic review. *Crit Care Med* 30:454, 2002.

11. Todd MR, Barone JE: Recognition of accidental arterial cannulation after attempted central venipuncture. *Crit Care Med* 19:1081, 1991.

12. Silverman S, Olson KW: Avoidance of unintentional arterial cannulation. *Anesthesia* 44:1003, 1989.

13. Ricci M, Puente AO, Gusmano F, et al: Central venous access: Accidental arterial puncture in a patient with right-sided aortic arch. *Crit Care Med* 27:1025, 1999.

14. Richards MJ, Edwards JR, Culver DH, et al: Nosocomial infections in combined medical-surgical intensive care units in the United States. *Infect Control Hosp Epidemiol* 21:510, 2000

15. CDC: National Nosocomial Infections Surveillance (NNIS) System report: Data summary from January 1992–June 2001, issued August 2001. *Am J Infect Control* 6:404, 2001.

16. Pearson, ML, Hierholzer WJ, Garner JS, et al: Guideline for prevention of intravascular device-related infections: I. Intravascular device-related infections: An overview. *Am J Infect Control* 24:262, 1996.

17. Polderman KH, Girbes ARJ: Central venous catheter use: 1. Mechanical complications. *Intensive Care Med* 28:1, 2002.

18. Mimoz O, Pieroni L, Lawrence C, et al: Prospective, randomized trial of two antiseptic solutions for prevention of central venous or arterial catheter colonization and infection in intensive care unit patients. *Crit Care Med* 24:1818, 1996.

19. Chaiyakunapruk N, Veentra DL, Lipsky BA, et al: Chlorhexidine versus povidone-iodine solution for vascular catheter site care: A meta-analysis. *Ann Intern Med* 136:792, 2002.

20. Chaiyakunapruk N, Veenstra DL, Lipsky BA, et al: Vascular catheter site care: The clinical and economic benefits of chlorhexidine gluconate compared with povidone iodine. *Clin Infect Dis* 37:764, 2003.

21. Raad II, Hohn DC, Gilbreath BJ, et al: Prevention of central venous catheter–related infections by using maximal sterile barrier precautions during insertion. *Infect Control Hosp Epidemiol* 15:231, 1994.

22. Sherertz RJ, Ely EW, Westbrook DM, et al: Education of physicians-in-training can decrease the risk for vascular catheter infection. *Ann Intern Med* 132:641, 2000.

23. Veenstra DL, Saint S, Saha S, et al: Efficacy of antiseptic-impregnated central venous catheters in preventing catheter-related bloodstream infection: A meta-analysis. *JAMA* 281:261, 1999.

24. Raad II, Darouiche R, Dupuis J, et al: Central venous catheters coated with minocycline and rifampin for the prevention of catheter-related colonization and bloodstream infections: A randomized, double-blind trial. *Ann Intern Med* 127:267, 1997.

25. Maki DG, Stolz SM, Wheeler S, et al: Prevention of central venous catheter-related bloodstream infection by use of an antiseptic-impregnated catheter: A randomized, controlled trial. *Ann Intern Med* 127:257, 1997.

26. Darouiche RO, Raad II, Heard SO, et al: A comparison of two antimicrobial-impregnated central venous catheters. Catheter Study Group. *N Engl J Med* 340:1, 1999.

27. Cook DJ, Randolph A, Kernerman P, et al: Central venous catheter replacement strategies: A systematic review of the literature. *Crit Care Med* 25:1417, 1997.

28. Safdar N, Kluger DM, Maki DG: A review of risk factors for catheter-related bloodstream infection caused by percutaneously inserted, noncuffed central venous catheters. *Medicine* 81:466, 2002.

29. Mansfield PF, Hohn DC, Fornage BD, et al: Complications and failures of subclavian vein catheterization. *N Engl J Med* 331:1735, 1994.

30. Gualtieri E, Deppe S, Sipperly ME, et al: Subclavian venous catheterization: Greater success rate for less experienced operators using ultrasound guidance. *Crit Care Med* 23:692, 1995.

31. Randolph AG, Cook DJ, Gonzales CA, et al: Ultrasound guidance for placement of central venous catheters: A meta-analysis of the literature. *Crit Care Med* 24:2053, 1996.

32. Lefrant JY, Muller L, De La Coussaye JE, et al: Risk factors of failure and immediate complication of subclavian vein catheterization in critically ill patients. *Intensive Care Med* 28:1036, 2002.

33. Funaki B: Central venous access: A primer for the diagnostic radiologist. *AJR* 179:309, 2002.

34. Martin T, Fontana G, Olak J, et al: Use of a pleural catheter for the management of simple pneumothorax. *Chest* 110:1169, 1996.

35. Collier PE, Blocker SH, Graff DM, et al: Cardiac tamponade from central venous catheters. *Am J Surg* 176:212, 1998.

36. Booth SA, Norton B, Mulvey DA: Central venous catheterization and fatal cardiac tamponade. *Br J Anaesth* 87:298, 2001.

37. Rutherford, JS, Merry AF, Occleshaw CJ: Depth of central venous catheterization: An audit of practice in a cardiac surgical unit. *Anaesth Intensive Care* 22:267, 1994.

38. Ely EW, Hite RD, Baker AM, et al: Venous air embolism from central venous catheterization: A need for increased physician awareness. *Crit Care Med* 27:2113, 1999.

39. Chastre J, Cornud F, Bouchama A, et al: Thrombosis as a complication of pulmonary artery catheterization via the internal jugular vein: Prospective evaluation by phlebography. *N Engl J Med* 306:278, 1982.

40. Koksoy C, Kuzu A, Erden I, et al: The risk factors in central venous catheter-related thrombosis. *Aust NZ J Surg* 65:796, 1995.

41. Timsit JF, Farkas JC, Boyer JM, et al: Central vein catheter-related thrombosis in intensive care patients: Incidence, risk factors, and relationship with catheter-related sepsis. *Chest* 114:207, 1998.

42. Trerotola SO, Kuhn-Fulton J, Johnson MS, et al: Tunneled infusion catheters: Increased incidence of symptomatic venous thrombosis after subclavian versus internal jugular venous access. *Radiology* 217:89, 2000.

43. Macdonald S, Watt AJ, McNally D, et al: Comparison of technical success and outcome of tunneled catheters inserted via the jugular and subclavian approaches. *J Vasc Interv Radiol* 11:225, 2000.

44. Maury E, Guglielminotti J, Alzieu M, et al: Ultrasound examination: An alternative to chest radiography after central venous catheter insertion. *Am J Respir Crit Care Med* 164:403, 2001.

Chapter 13

CLINICAL USE OF THE PULMONARY ARTERY CATHETER

JAMES W. LEATHERMAN
JOHN J. MARINI

KEY POINTS

- *Recent randomized trials found that use of a pulmonary artery catheter (PAC) did not influence the mortality of high-risk surgical patients or critically ill patients with shock or acute respiratory distress syndrome (ARDS).*

- *Insertion of a PAC is associated with a low incidence of serious complications. Of potentially greater risk to the patient than insertional complications are errors in recording and interpreting hemodynamic data that lead to faulty clinical decisions. Several studies have shown that there are serious deficiencies in the understanding of basic aspects of hemodynamic monitoring among physicians and nurses who use the PAC.*

- *Incomplete wedging can lead to marked overestimation of the actual pulmonary artery wedge pressure (Ppw) and always should be suspected when the measured Ppw exceeds the pulmonary artery diastolic pressure (Ppad). However, with pulmonary hypertension, incomplete wedging may be present despite a positive Ppad–Ppw gradient and should be suspected when the latter markedly narrows in comparison with previous values.*

- *Careful inspection of the PAC waveforms may be helpful in the diagnosis of underlying cardiac disorders: Acute mitral regurgitation results in prominent v waves in the Ppw tracing, pericardial tamponade is characterized by equalization of the Ppw and right atrial pressure (Pra) and by blunting of the y descent in the atrial waveform, tricuspid regurgitation often leads to a broad cv wave and a prominent y descent, and both constrictive pericarditis and restrictive cardiomyopathy result in prominence of both the x and y descents in the atrial waveform.*

- *Over the range of values most often seen in the ICU, neither the Pra nor the Ppw provides a reliable indicator of the adequacy of preload and of fluid responsiveness. However, the change in Pra with a spontaneous breath may be a useful indicator of fluid responsiveness in that failure of the Pra to fall with inspiration predicts that the patient is unlikely to benefit from a fluid challenge.*

- *Positive end-expiratory pressure (PEEP) causes the measured Ppw to overestimate transmural left atrial pressure; the effect of PEEP on transmural pressure can be quantified by calculating the percentage of alveolar pressure that is transmitted to the pleural space during a positive-pressure breath. Active expiration also causes the measured Ppw to overestimate transmural pressure and usually results in much greater errors than does applied PEEP.*

- *Thermodilution cardiac output ($\dot{Q}T$) can be measured by the intermittent bolus method or continuously with a modified*

catheter. Several noninvasive and minimally invasive methods of measuring $\dot{Q}T$ are also available.

- *Venous oxygen saturation in the pulmonary artery (Sv_{O_2}) or superior vena cava (Scv_{O_2}) serves as a global indicator of the adequacy of O_2 delivery relative to tissue O_2 demands.*

Although the pulmonary artery catheter (PAC) has been in use for more than 30 years,[1] its value in management of critically ill patients remains controversial. Different studies have concluded that use of the PAC is associated with increased mortality,[2,3] has no effect on mortality,[4,5] or decreases major morbidity.[6,7] Several prospective, randomized studies have been initiated within the last few years in an effort to better define the impact of the PAC on patient outcome.[8] Three trials have been completed, and none found an impact of the PAC on mortality.[9–11] The appropriateness of these trials has been questioned,[8,12,13] and it has been suggested that efforts instead should be directed toward improvement of the standard of practice through intensive educational efforts, institution of more stringent accreditation policies, and evaluation of newer monitoring techniques before proceeding with expensive and time-consuming randomized clinical trials.[8,12,13] The latter view is based in part on evidence that ICU nurses and physicians who use the PAC may have significant deficiencies in knowledge about some of the most fundamental aspects of hemodynamic monitoring,[14,15] raising concern that the value of the PAC may be difficult to assess if data are not collected and interpreted optimally.[16]

We believe that carefully designed prospective clinical trials may provide some guidance regarding appropriate use of the PA catheter but are unlikely to clarify with certainty whether an individual patient who is critically ill and hemodynamically unstable will benefit from the information available from a PAC. At least for the time being, ICU physicians should continue to assess the benefits and risks of catheterization on a case-by-case basis, including in the decision analysis the applicability of alternative, less invasive methods of hemodynamic assessment.[17,18] We share the view that the PAC is an "occasionally useful tool" that can be of value in guiding therapy of selected critically ill patients, especially when empirical therapeutic trials have proven unsuccessful or are considered hazardous.[19] Implicit in this view, however, is the understanding that hemodynamic data must be collected accurately by ICU nurses and must be interpreted by physicians who are knowledgeable about cardiopulmonary pathophysiology. Faulty clinical decisions based on inaccurate or misinterpreted data may be a greater risk to the patient than the procedure per se. This chapter reviews clinical use of the PAC in the ICU, with particular emphasis on principles of data acquisition and interpretation and on the practical application of PAC-derived data in guiding therapy. Where appropriate, comparisons between the PAC and alternative methods of hemodynamic assessment will be discussed.

Indications

There are no absolute indications for PA catheterization. However, a PAC sometimes may aid in the diagnosis and management of a number of common clinical conditions (Table 13-1). These include cardiogenic and distributive

TABLE 13-1 Clinical Uses of Bedside Pulmonary Artery Catheterization

Condition	Primary Data Sought
DIAGNOSTIC USES	
Pulmonary edema	Ppw
Shock	$\dot{Q}T$ and SVR; Ppw; Sv_{O_2}
Oliguric renal failure	Ppw, $\dot{Q}T$
Perplexing lactic acidemia	$\dot{Q}T$, Sv_{O_2}
Pulmonary hypertension	Ppa and PVR, Ppad versus Ppw
Cardiac disorders:	
Ventricular septal defect	Step-up in O_2 saturation (RA to PA)
RV infarction	Pra ≥ Ppw
Pericardial tamponade	Pra = Ppw; blunted *y* descent
Tricuspid regurgitation	Broad *cv* wave, Kussmaul's, deep *y* descent
Constrictive pericarditis	Pra = Pw, Kussmaul's; deep *y* descent
Narrow-complex tachyarrhythmia	Mechanical flutter waves (Pra waveform)
Wide-complex tachyarrhythmia	Cannon *a* waves (Pra waveform)
Lymphatic carcinoma	Aspiration cytology
Caloric requirements	V_{O_2} (by Fick equation)
MONITORING USES	
Assess adequacy of intravascular volume:	
Hypotension	
Oliguria	
High-risk surgical patient	
Assess effect of change in Ppw on pulmonary edema	
Assess therapy for shock	
Cardiogenic (vasodilator, inotrope)	
Septic (volume, vasopressor, inotrope)	
Hypovolemic (volume)	
Assess effects of PEEP or $\dot{Q}T$ in ARDS	

shock, severe acute respiratory distress syndrome (ARDS), pulmonary edema of uncertain etiology, oliguric renal failure, perplexing lactic acidosis, and unexplained pulmonary hypertension. Preoperative insertion of a PAC also has been advocated for patients undergoing cardiac surgery and for high-risk patients undergoing major noncardiac operations. However, one large prospective study found no benefit to routine placement of a PAC before cardiac surgery and concluded that catheterization should be deferred until there was a clear indication for invasive monitoring.[20] A large prospective, randomized trial involving high-risk surgical patients found no benefit to the use of a goal-oriented hemodynamic approach based on data obtained from a PAC.[10] Anticipatory placement of a PAC because a patient *might* become unstable would not seem to be justified in most instances. Rather, placement of a PAC usually should be reserved for circumstances in which important questions about underlying pathophysiologic derangements cannot be answered confidently by less invasive means. In this regard, it is interesting to note that the controversial study linking PAC use to increased mortality found that the risk of the PAC appeared to be greatest in less critically ill patients who had the highest likelihood of survival on entry into the ICU.[2]

Patients for whom a PAC might be considered often can be managed effectively with alterative methods for assessing preload, cardiac output ($\dot{Q}T$), and cardiac contractility.[17,18,22] The decision to proceed with invasive hemodynamic monitoring should be influenced by a variety of factors, including an assessment of procedural risk, the level of confidence in clinical assessment, and especially by the availability and expertise with alternative noninvasive techniques. For example, the etiology of unexplained hypotension may become obvious when echocardiography reveals severe depression of left ventricular contraction, acute pulmonary hypertension with right ventricular failure, hypovolemia with inspiratory collapse of the vena cava, or pericardial tamponade, potentially obviating the need for insertion of a PAC to establish a diagnosis.[22] On the other hand, patients with multiple and complex hemodynamic derangements that are likely to change over time, e.g., septic shock with multiorgan dysfunction, potentially may benefit from continuous hemodynamic monitoring with a PAC.

Complications

Complications of PAC insertion include those related to achieving vascular access and those resulting from the catheter itself (Table 13-2). Only catheter-related complications will be considered here.

Both atrial and ventricular tachyarrhythmias can develop as a result of catheter insertion.[23–25] Ventricular ectopy during passage through the right ventricle (RV) is not uncommon but almost always ceases as soon as the catheter tip passes through the pulmonic valve. Sustained ventricular tachycardia is unusual, and ventricular fibrillation is rare; in two large series, only 1.3% and 1.5% of patients required antiarrhythmic therapy, chest thump, or cardioversion.[23,24] Given the low incidence of sustained ventricular tachycardia, prophylactic administration of lidocaine is not recommended. Ongoing ischemia, shock, hypoxemia, electrolyte disturbances, acidosis, and/or high endogenous catecholamine levels may increase the risk of ventricular tachycardia. Arrhythmogenic factors should be eliminated before catheter insertion, when possible, and time in the RV should be kept to a minimum.

Transient right bundle branch block has been reported to occur in 0.05% to 5% of catheterizations.[25] Although generally of little consequence, even transient right bundle branch block is obviously of major concern if the patient already has left bundle branch block. However, a study of 82 patients with

TABLE 13-2 Complications of Pulmonary Artery Catheterization

Complications related to central vein cannulation
Complications related to insertion and use of the PAC
Tachyarrhythmias
Right bundle branch block *ad 5%*
Complete heart block (pre-existing left bundle branch block)
Cardiac perforation
Thrombosis and embolism *(0 - 1.5 %)*
Pulmonary infarction due to persistent wedging
Catheter-related sepsis
Pulmonary artery rupture and pseudoaneurysm
Knotting of the catheter
Endocarditis, bland and infective
Pulmonic valve insufficiency
Balloon fragmentation and embolization

left bundle branch block found no episodes of complete heart block during PAC insertion, and the two episodes of complete heart block that occurred while the catheters were in place were ascribed to the underlying disease rather than to the catheter.[26] It is not necessary to place a prophylactic transvenous pacemaker when a PAC is inserted into patients with left bundle branch block, but an external pacemaker should be at the bedside.

Clinically silent thromboses occur commonly at the site of PAC insertion, and PAC-associated clots can form occasionally in the heart or pulmonary artery.[23,27] In a recent prospective, randomized study, pulmonary emboli occurred more often in patients randomized to a PAC, but the incidence of pulmonary embolism in the PAC group was only 1.6%.[10] In a second large study, none of the 335 patients randomized to a PAC developed clinically evident pulmonary embolism.[11] Pulmonary infarction related to peripherally placed catheters is also infrequent, with an incidence of 0% to 1.4% in a large series.[25] Even when infarction does occur, it is often evidenced only by a new radiographic abnormality beyond the catheter tip without apparent clinical deterioration. In brief, clinically significant thromboembolism and infarction attributable to the PAC appear to be quite uncommon.

Pulmonary artery rupture and pseudoaneurysms can occur as a direct result of PAC-induced vascular injury. Pulmonary artery rupture, the most serious complication of pulmonary artery catheterization, usually is heralded by the abrupt onset of frank hemoptysis and carries a mortality rate of up to 50%.[25] Fortunately, this complication is rare, being observed in 0.06% and 0.2% of catheterizations in two large series.[23,24] Pulmonary hypertension, cardiopulmonary bypass, and anticoagulation place the patient at increased risk for morbidity and mortality from pulmonary artery rupture.[25] It has been suggested that pulmonary hypertension may favor distal migration of the catheter tip on balloon deflation, permitting

vascular rupture when the balloon is reinflated.[28] In some cases, rupture occurs with the first reinflation. Avoidance of distal catheter placement and of balloon overinflation may reduce the risk of pulmonary artery rupture. Pseudoaneurysms can develop as a result of nonlethal pulmonary artery rupture, posing a significant risk of subsequent hemorrhage that may prove fatal.[29] The possibility of a false aneurysm should be considered whenever self-limited hemoptysis occurs after manipulation of the PAC. The diagnosis can be made by dynamic computed tomographic (CT) scanning or by angiography. Prompt treatment by coil embolization may prevent subsequent aneurysm rupture.[29]

A number of unusual complications of pulmonary artery catheterization have been reported (see Table 13-2). However, a review of nine large series found that major complications are quite uncommon.[25] A different "complication" associated with use of the PAC—erroneous recording and interpretation of hemodynamic data that results in bad clinical decisions and adverse patient outcome—may be much more frequent than these procedural risks. The remainder of this chapter will focus on the principles of data acquisition and their physiologic relevance to caring for the critically ill.

Pressure Monitoring

PRESSURE MONITORING SYSTEM

Essential system components required for pressure monitoring include a fluid-filled catheter and connecting tubing, a transducer to convert the mechanical energy from the pressure wave into an electrical signal, and a signal-processing unit that conditions and amplifies this electrical signal for display (Fig. 13-1). Two primary features of the pressure monitoring system determine its dynamic response properties: natural resonant frequency and damping coefficient.[30,31] Once

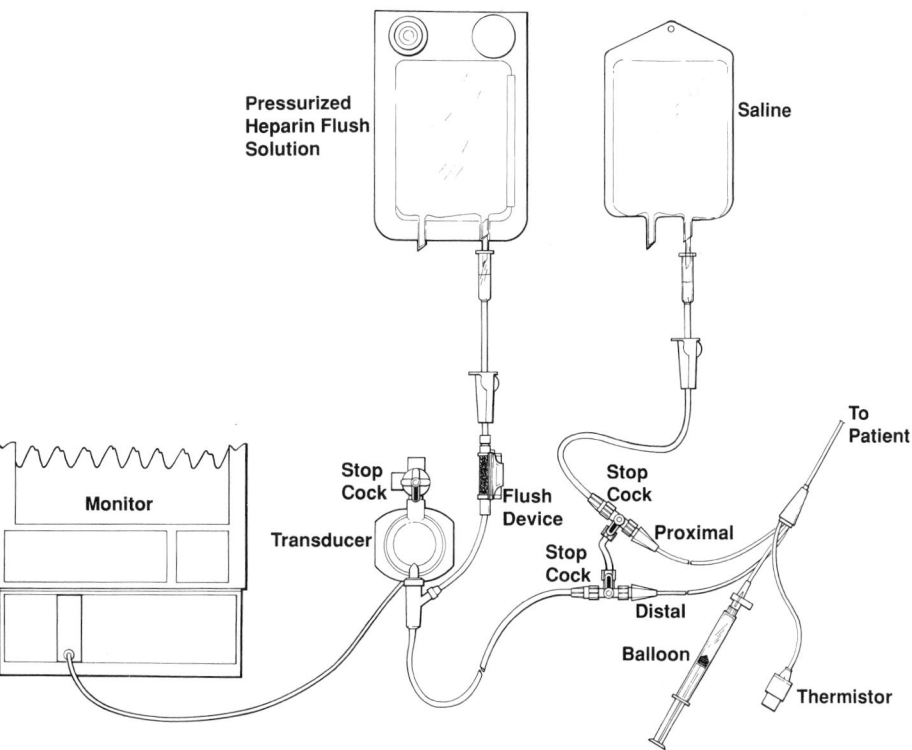

FIGURE 13-1 Standard four-lumen pulmonary artery catheter with pressure tubing, heparinized flush, transducer, and signal-processing unit (monitor). Pulmonary arterial or right atrial pressure can be displayed by stopcock adjustment.

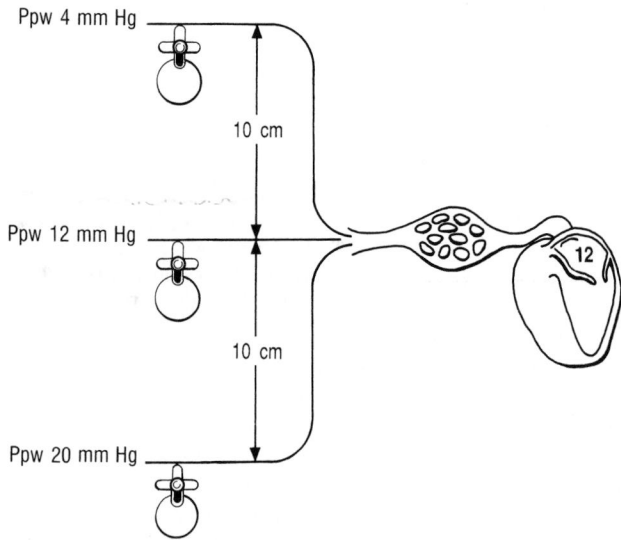

FIGURE 13-2 Effect of transducer malposition on pressure measurement. In this example, left atrial and wedge pressures are 12 mm Hg. Once the transducer has been zeroed at the left atrial level (see text), movement of the transducer above or below the left atrial plane will result in erroneous pressure measurement (10 cm $H_2O \sim$ 8 mm Hg).

perturbed, each catheter-transducer system tends to oscillate at a unique (natural resonant) frequency determined by the elasticity and capacitance of its deformable elements. An undamped system responds well to the low-frequency components of a complex waveform, but it exaggerates the amplitude of components near the resonant value. Modest damping is desirable for optimal fidelity and for suppression of unwanted high-frequency vibration (*noise*); however, excessive damping smoothes the tracing unnaturally and eliminates important frequency components of the pressure waveform (see below).

For the hydraulic monitoring system to display accurate pressures, it is essential that the system be *zeroed* (balanced) at the phlebostatic axis (i.e., midaxillary line, fourth intercostal space). Body angle is not crucial, so one can zero the transducer with the orthopneic patient upright or semiupright. Once the transducer has been zeroed, however, movement of the transducer relative to the heart will cause the recorded pressure to underestimate or overestimate, respectively, the true value (Fig. 13-2). Because the pulmonary circuit is a low-pressure vascular bed, small errors in transducer position

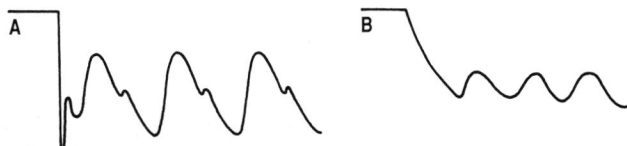

FIGURE 13-3 Rapid-flush test. *A.* Appropriately damped system. *B.* Overdamped system.

may be clinically significant. The transducer converts mechanical energy from the fluid-filled tubing into an electrical signal that is then amplified and displayed. The quality and cost of transducers vary considerably. The plastic disposable transducers used in the ICU are sufficiently accurate for routine clinical purposes.[32]

CATHETER INSERTION

The standard 7F PAC includes four essential elements: (1) a distal lumen for measurement of pressure in the pulmonary artery and for sampling of blood to determine mixed venous oxygen saturation (Sv_{O_2}), (2) a proximal lumen whose orifice is 30 cm from the catheter tip for measuring right atrial pressure (Pra) and infusing fluids, (3) a lumen to introduce air for balloon inflation, and (4) a thermistor at the catheter tip to enable estimation of $\dot{Q}T$ by thermodilution (see Fig. 13-1). Various catheter modifications are available, including an additional lumen for infusion of fluids, a fiberoptic system to continuously assess Sv_{O_2}, a heating coil and modified thermistor to allow continuous measurement of $\dot{Q}T$, a rapid-response thermistor that permits measurement of right ventricular ejection fraction, and a pacing electrode.

In the ICU, the PAC usually is inserted via the internal jugular or subclavian vein. A femoral approach may require fluoroscopy, although one study reported a surprisingly high success rate of 90% with nonfluoroscopic insertion via the femoral vein.[33] Before insertion, the proximal and distal lumens are connected to the appropriate pressure tubing, balloon integrity is tested, and a rapid-flush test is performed to assess the dynamic responsiveness of the pressure monitoring system (Figs. 13-3 and 13-4). Although the proximal and distal ports can be connected to separate transducers, more often a single transducer is connected to the distal port, and the proximal port is connected to a separate infusion of intravenous fluid (see Fig. 13-1). Use of a "bridge" and stopcocks permits monitoring of Pra when desired. The stopcocks should be checked before insertion to be sure that the monitor

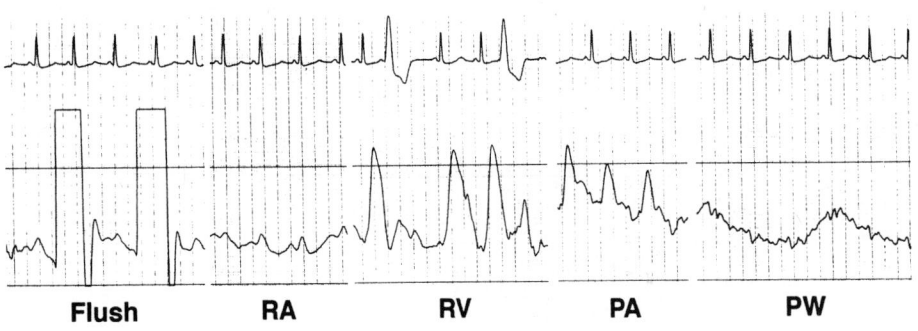

Flush   RA   RV   PA   PW

FIGURE 13-4 Waveform transition as catheter is advanced from the right atrium (RA) to the wedge (PW) position. The rapid flush test before insertion reveals good dynamic responsiveness. Passage from the right ventricle (RV) into the pulmonary artery (PA) is evidenced by a rise in diastolic pressure, and catheter wedging is evidenced by a fall in pressure and the appearance of an atrial waveform. Note the ventricular ectopy when the catheter is in the RV.

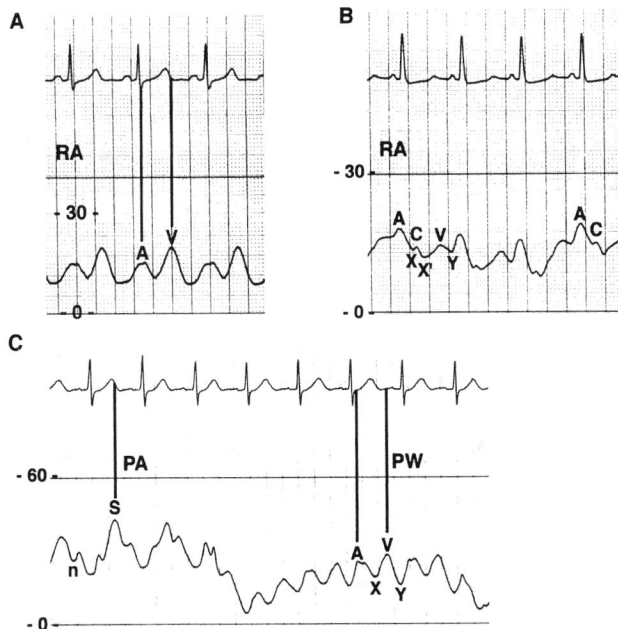

FIGURE 13-5 Pressure waveforms recorded simultaneously with an electrocardiographic lead. *A.* Right atrial (RA) tracing showing timing of *a* and *v* waves and *x* and *y* descents. *B.* RA tracing with visible *c* wave. *C.* Pulmonary artery (PA) tracing showing systolic wave (*s*); wedge (PW) tracing showing *a* and *v* waves and *x* and *y* descents. Note the difference in timing of the PA and PW pressure waves with respect to the electrocardiogram. (Scale is in millimeters of mercury.)

sive catheter while the tip is in the RV should be avoided to prevent coiling and possible knotting within the RV. Entry into the pulmonary artery is reflected by an abrupt rise in diastolic pressure (see Fig. 13-4). The catheter is then advanced gradually until a pulmonary artery occlusion (wedge) pressure (Ppw) is signaled by a transition to an atrial waveform and a fall in mean pressure (Figs. 13-4 and 13-5).

A number of factors may interfere with recognition of characteristic waveforms during catheter insertion. Severe hypovolemia or other causes of decreased stroke volume reduces the pulmonary artery pulse pressure and the difference between mean pulmonary artery pressure (Ppa) and Ppw, potentially creating difficulties in determining whether a valid Ppw tracing has been achieved. With pericardial tamponade or RV infarction, the right ventricular end-diastolic pressure (RVEDP) approaches pulmonary artery diastolic pressure (Ppad), making the transition from RV to pulmonary artery sufficiently difficult to appreciate that fluoroscopy may be required to confirm catheter position.[34] Large swings in intrathoracic pressure may create major problems with waveform interpretation. If the patient is mechanically ventilated, elimination of large respiratory excursions with sedation (or temporary paralysis) may aid in delineation of the tracing and will enhance reliability of the measurements obtained.[35] Another problem is excessive catheter "whip" caused by "shock transients" being transmitted to the catheter during RV contraction in hyperdynamic states (Fig. 13-6). Overdamping occurs when air bubbles, clots, fibrin, or kinks diminish transmission of the pulsatile pressure waveform to the transducer, resulting in a decrease in systolic pressure and an increase in diastolic pressure. An overdamped Ppa tracing may be mistaken for a Ppw, leading to unnecessary retraction of a properly positioned catheter. A simple bedside test for overdamping is the "rapid flush" test[30] (see Fig. 13-3). Because of the length and small gauge of the catheter, very high pressures are generated near the transducer when the flush device is opened. An appropriately damped system will show a rapid fall in pressure with an "overshoot" and prompt return to a crisp pulmonary artery tracing on sudden closure of the flush device. In contrast, an overdamped system will generate a tracing that demonstrates a gradual return to the baseline pressure without an overshoot (see Fig. 13-3).

displays pressure from the distal lumen. Inadvertent recording from the proximal lumen will result in an unusually long length of catheter being inserted without achieving an RV tracing. This pitfall also should be suspected if the displayed pressure is initially near zero and then suddenly increases (proximal lumen enters the introducer) or if ventricular ectopy (tip in RV) is noted while the monitor displays a Pra waveform.

The RV should be reached within 30 to 40 cm from the internal jugular or subclavian entry sites. After entering the RV, insertion of an additional 10 to 15 cm of catheter is usually sufficient to reach the pulmonary artery. Feeding exces-

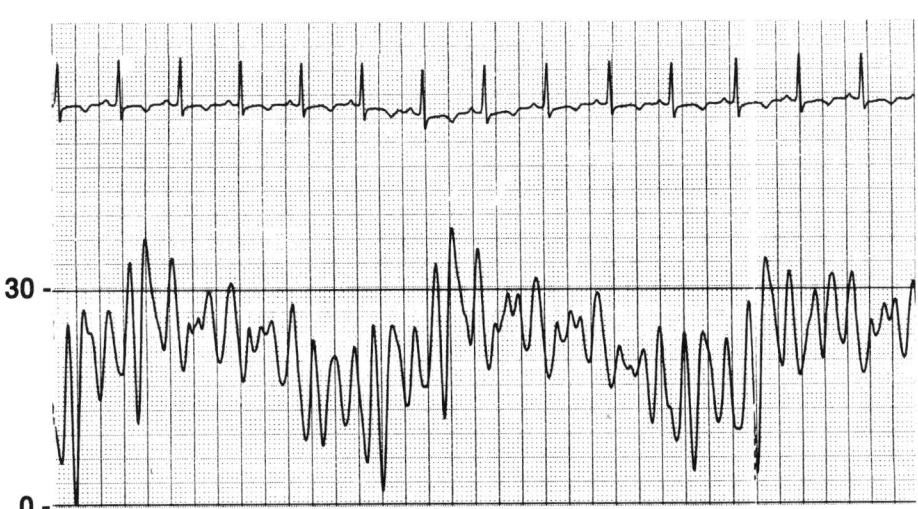

FIGURE 13-6 Catheter whip. Prominent excursions in the pulmonary artery tracing are due to "shock transients" transmitted directly to the catheter from the contracting right ventricle. (Scale is in millimeters of mercury.)

PAC-DERIVED PRESSURES

The properly positioned PAC provides access to pressures from three sites: right atrium (Pra), pulmonary artery (Ppa), and pulmonary vein (Ppw). Each of these pressures will be discussed sequentially in relationship to its determinants, waveform characteristics, and factors that commonly confound its interpretation. Subsequently, clinical use of PAC-derived pressure data will be discussed.

RIGHT ATRIAL PRESSURE (Pra)

In sinus rhythm, the Pra waveform is characterized by two major positive deflections (a and v waves) and two negative deflections (x and y descents) (see Fig. 13-5). A third positive wave, the c wave, is sometimes seen. The a (atrial) wave is due to atrial systolic contraction. The a wave is followed by the x descent as the atria undergo postsystolic relaxation and the atrioventricular junction moves downward during early ventricular systole. When visible, a c wave due to closure of the atrioventricular valves interrupts the x descent. When a c wave is seen, standard nomenclature dictates that the initial descent is termed x and the second descent is termed x'[34] (see Fig. 13-5). After the x descent, the v (ventricular) wave is generated by passive filling of the atria during ventricular systole. The y descent reflects the reduction in atrial pressure as the tricuspid valve opens (see Fig. 13-5).

In order to evaluate pressure waveforms adequately, it is essential to use a two-channel recorder that allows simultaneous recording of cardiac electrical activity and pressure. An electrocardiographic lead that clearly demonstrates atrial electrical activity should be chosen. Analysis of the atrial pressure tracing begins with identification of the electrical P wave. The first positive-pressure wave to follow the P wave is the a wave. The right atrial a wave usually is seen at the beginning of the QRS complex, provided that atrioventricular conduction is normal (see Fig. 13-5). When visible, the c wave follows the a wave by an interval equal to the electrocardiographic PR interval (see Fig. 13-5). The peak of the right atrial v wave normally occurs simultaneously with the T wave of the electrocardiogram, provided that the QT interval is normal (see Fig. 13-5).

Normal Pra is approximately 2 to 8 mm Hg.[34] In the absence of left ventricular (LV) dysfunction, the Pra is typically 2 to 5 mm Hg lower than the Ppw.[36] However, the Ppw may be markedly higher than the Pra in patients who have either systolic or diastolic LV dysfunction.[37] Conversely, the Pra may exceed the Ppw in patients with RV failure due to increased pulmonary vascular resistance (PVR) or RV infarction. In the absence of tricuspid stenosis or regurgitation, mean Pra approximates RVEDP. However, there is only a modest correlation between Pra and right ventricular end-diastolic volume (RVEDV), and the Pra required for optimal filling varies among patients.[38,39] Besides being an indicator of RV filling pressure, Pra also represents the downstream pressure for venous return. Normally, the decrease in intrathoracic pressure during a spontaneous breath produces a reduction in Pra, increasing the gradient for venous return from extrathoracic veins. When the right atrium is at its limits of distensibility, however, Pra will not fall with inspiration and may even rise (Kussmaul's sign). The response of Pra to a spontaneous breath may provide insight into the adequacy of volume expansion (see below).[39]

PULMONARY ARTERY PRESSURE (Ppa)

The pulmonary artery waveform has a systolic pressure wave and a diastolic trough (see Fig. 13-5). A dicrotic notch due to closure of the pulmonic valve may be seen on the terminal portion of the systolic pressure wave, and the pressure at the dicrotic notch closely approximates mean Ppa.[40] Like the right atrial v wave, the pulmonary artery systolic wave typically coincides with the electrical T wave (see Fig. 13-5). The pulmonary artery diastolic pressure (Ppad) is recorded as the pressure just before the beginning of the systolic pressure wave.

Ppa is determined by the volume of blood ejected into the pulmonary artery during systole, the resistance within the pulmonary vascular bed, and the downstream (left atrial) pressure. Normal values for Ppa are as follows: systolic, 15 to 30 mm Hg; diastolic, 4 to 12 mm Hg; and mean, 9 to 18 mm Hg.[34] The normal pulmonary vascular network is a low-resistance circuit with enormous reserve, so large increases in cardiac output ($\dot{Q}T$) do not cause pressure to rise significantly. This large capillary reserve normally offers such slight resistance to runoff during diastole that the difference between the Ppad and the Ppw (the Ppad–Ppw gradient) is 5 mm Hg or less. Increased pulmonary vascular resistance (PVR) causes the Ppad–Ppw gradient to widen, whereas an increase in left atrial pressure results in a proportional rise in the Ppad and Ppw.[41,42] Therefore, the Ppad–Ppw gradient is used to differentiate pulmonary hypertension due to increased PVR from pulmonary venous hypertension.

An increased $\dot{Q}T$ alone will not cause pulmonary hypertension. However, in the setting of increased vascular resistance, the degree to which Ppa increases will be influenced by the $\dot{Q}T$. Pulmonary hypertension may result from the combination of a modest increase in vascular resistance and a major increase in $\dot{Q}T$ due to sepsis, cirrhosis, agitation, fever, or other factors. The relative contributions of blood flow and the pulmonary vasculature to the increase in Ppa can be assessed by measuring $\dot{Q}T$ by thermodilution and calculating PVR (PVR $= [P_{pa} - P_{pw}]/\dot{Q}T$). It should be appreciated, however, that interpretation of the PVR is confounded by the fact that the pulmonary vascular bed behaves like a Starling (variable) resistor; PVR increases as flow ($\dot{Q}T$) decreases, and the calculated PVR must be interpreted with respect to the $\dot{Q}T$ at the time the measurement is made.[43] For example, a fall in $\dot{Q}T$ owing to hemorrhage may produce a rise in calculated PVR even though the pulmonary vascular bed has not been affected directly; the PVR then may normalize once the $\dot{Q}T$ returns to its baseline value. Conversely, calculated PVR may decrease solely due to an increase in $\dot{Q}T$. The latter may be particularly relevant when assessing the response to vasodilators that affect both the pulmonary and systemic vascular beds. With decreased $\dot{Q}T$, a rise in calculated PVR that is accompanied by an increase in driving pressure within the pulmonary circuit (Ppa–Ppw) would clearly indicate active pulmonary vasoconstriction, whereas a reduction in driving pressure at increased $\dot{Q}T$ would provide unequivocal evidence of vasodilation.[44]

PULMONARY ARTERY WEDGE PRESSURE (Ppw)

The Ppw tracing contains the same sequence of waves and descents as the right atrial tracing. However, when the atrial waveform is referenced to the electrocardiogram, the mechanical events arising in the left atrium will be seen later than

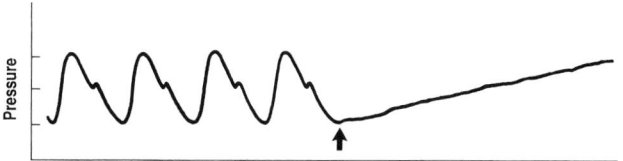

FIGURE 13-8 **Overwedging. Arrow indicates time of balloon inflation.**

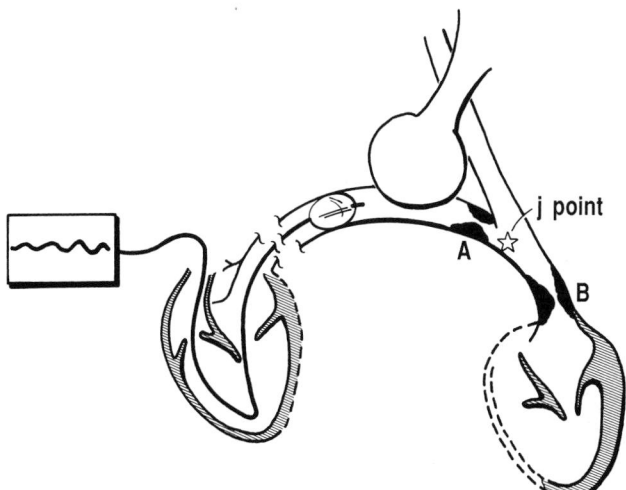

FIGURE 13-7 **Principle of the wedge pressure (Ppw) measurement. When the inflated balloon obstructs arterial inflow, the catheter will record the pressure at the junction of the static and flowing venous channels, the j point. An obstruction distal (*B*) to the j point will cause the Ppw to overestimate left atrial pressure (Pla). With obstruction proximal (*A*) to the j point (e.g., veno-occlusive disease), the Ppw accurately reflects Pla but greatly underestimates pulmonary capillary pressure. (*Used with permission from O'Quinn and Marini.*[30])**

those in the right atrium because the left atrial pressure waves must travel back through the pulmonary vasculature and a longer length of catheter. Therefore, in the Ppw tracing, the *a* wave usually appears after the QRS complex, and the *v* wave is seen after the T wave (see Fig. 13-5). Thus the systolic pressure wave in the pulmonary artery tracing *precedes* the *v* wave of the Ppw tracing when referenced to the electrocardiogram. An appreciation of the latter relationship is critical when tracings are being analyzed to ensure that balloon inflation has resulted in a transition from an arterial (Ppa) to an atrial (Ppw) waveform and to detect the presence of a "giant" *v* wave in the Ppw tracing (see below).

The Ppw is obtained when the inflated catheter obstructs forward flow within a branch of the pulmonary artery, creating a static column of blood between the tip of the catheter and the point (junction, or j point) in the pulmonary venous bed where it intersects with flowing blood (Fig. 13-7). Since the fully inflated catheter impacts in segmental or lobar pulmonary arteries, the j point is usually located in medium to large pulmonary veins. If the catheter were to be advanced with the balloon only partially inflated (or uninflated), obstruction to flow would occur in a much smaller artery, and the j point accordingly would move upstream to the smaller pulmonary veins. Since there is normally a resistive pressure drop across the small pulmonary veins, the Ppw recorded with a distal uninflated catheter will be slightly higher than the Ppw obtained with a fully inflated catheter.[45] Owing to resistance in the small pulmonary veins, the Ppw will underestimate the pressure in the pulmonary capillaries (see below), but the absence of any appreciable resistive pressure drop across the larger pulmonary veins dictates that the Ppw will reliably reflect left atrial pressure (Pla).

For the Ppw to accurately represent Pla, it is essential that the tip of the inflated catheter lie free within the vessel lumen,

OVERWEDGING

and the inflated balloon must completely interrupt forward flow within the obstructed artery. Obstruction to flow at the catheter tip can lead to *overwedging*, whereas failure of the balloon to seal the vessel lumen results in a *partial* or *incomplete* Ppw. Overwedging is recognized by a progressive rise in pressure during balloon inflation and usually results from the balloon trapping the tip against the vessel wall. In such cases, the continuous flow from the flush system results in a steady buildup of pressure at the catheter tip, or at least as high as required to cause compensatory leakage from the trapped pocket (Fig. 13-8). If overwedging occurs, the deflated catheter should be retracted before reinflating the balloon to achieve a more suitable Ppw tracing and to prevent possible vessel injury.

An incomplete Ppw tracing occurs when the inflated balloon does not completely interrupt forward flow, resulting in a recorded pressure that is intermediate between mean Ppa and Ppw. As a result, the measured Ppw will overestimate the true value, potentially leading to serious errors in patient management. In the absence of pulmonic valve insufficiency or prominent *a* or *v* waves that increase its mean value, the Ppw should be equal to or less than the Ppad. Therefore, incomplete wedging always should be suspected if the Ppw exceeds the Ppad.[46] However, incomplete wedging also can occur despite the presence of a positive Ppad–Ppw gradient. Incomplete wedging occurs often in patients with pulmonary hypertension whose increased pulmonary vascular resistance results in a marked increase in the Ppad–Ppw gradient. In this setting, the measured Ppw can increase significantly above the true value owing to incomplete wedging yet still remain less than the Ppad, giving the impression that a reliable Ppw has been obtained[47] (Fig. 13-9). When this occurs, the measured Ppad–Ppw gradient will decrease in comparison with previous values. With pulmonary hypertension, incomplete wedging should be suspected when the Ppad–Ppw narrows unexpectedly or when at the time of insertion a normal Ppad–Ppw gradient is found when a widened gradient would be suspected (e.g., severe ARDS)[47] (Fig. 13-10). Another clue to incomplete wedging is provided by a pressure waveform that is more consistent with Ppa than Ppw (see Fig. 13-9). Incomplete wedging can result from a catheter that is too proximal, in which case advancement of the inflated catheter may be corrective. Alternatively, a catheter that is too distal, perhaps with its tip at a vascular branch point, also can lead to incomplete wedging. This circumstance is suggested by measuring a lower (more accurate) Ppw when the balloon is only partially inflated.[47] In this case, retraction of the deflated catheter before full balloon inflation may yield a more accurate Ppw and potentially reduce the risk of vessel injury due to distal catheter placement.

One method that has been suggested to confirm the reliability of the Ppw is aspiration of highly oxygenated

UNDERWEDGING

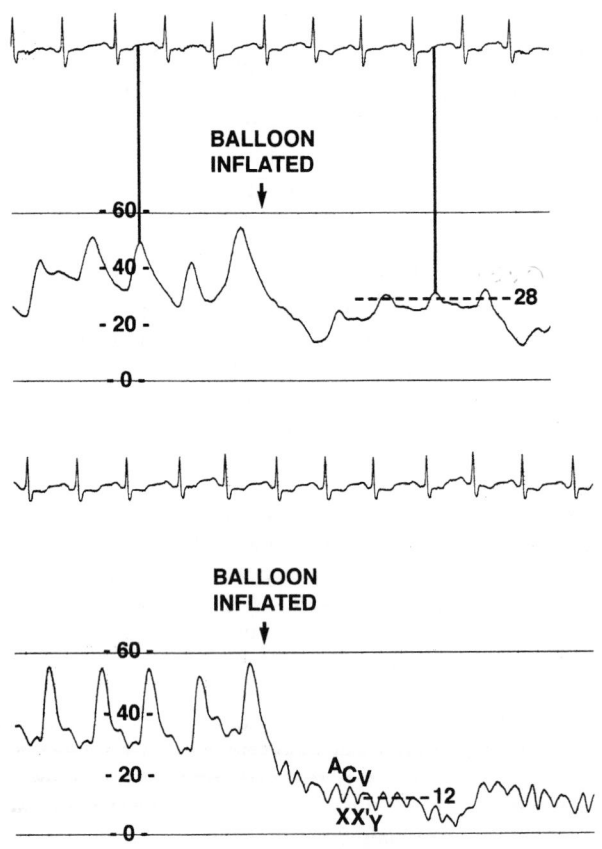

FIGURE 13-9 Incomplete wedge pressure (Ppw). (*Above*) With balloon inflation, there is a fall in pressure to a value that approximates pulmonary artery diastolic pressure (Ppad). However, the clinical setting (severe ARDS) is usually associated with a large Ppad–Ppw gradient. Review of the tracings reveals that there is a single positive wave coinciding with the electrocardiographic T wave after balloon inflation, a pattern inconsistent with a left atrial waveform. (*Below*) Waveforms after catheter has been retracted and balloon reinflated. Now there is a large Ppad–Ppw gradient, and the tracing after balloon inflation is consistent with a left atrial waveform. (Scale is in millimeters of mercury.)

blood from the distal lumen of the inflated catheter.[48] However, there are several important considerations when using the Pa_{O_2} of aspirated blood to confirm a wedge position. First, failure to obtain highly oxygenated blood in the Ppw

position could occur if the catheter tip is located in a vessel whose capillary bed supplies an area of markedly reduced alveolar ventilation.[30,49] Second, it is recommended that an initial 15 to 20 mL of "dead space" blood be withdrawn and discarded before the sample for analysis is obtained so as to reduce the likelihood of obtaining a false-negative result when the inflated catheter has truly wedged.[49] Finally, a false-positive result (i.e., high O_2 saturation in aspirated blood when the catheter is not wedged) can occur if the sample is aspirated too quickly. It is recommended that the sample be aspirated at a rate no faster than 3 mL/min.[49]

RESPIRATORY INFLUENCES ON THE Ppw

The Ppw is an intravascular pressure, but it is the *transmural* pressure (intravascular minus pleural, Ppw − Ppl) that represents the distending pressure for cardiac filling and the hydrostatic component of the Starling forces that govern transcapillary fluid movement. During normal breathing, the lung returns to its relaxed volume at end expiration, with alveolar pressure being atmospheric and Ppl being slightly negative. The Ppw therefore should be measured at end expiration, the point in the respiratory cycle when juxtacardiac (pleural) pressure can be estimated most reliably (Fig. 13-11). Either a strip recording or the cursor method should be used to record the end-expiratory Ppw because digital readouts that average over the respiratory cycle may overestimate or underestimate Ppw.

Even when strip recordings are used, there may be inaccuracies in identifying the end-expiratory Ppw.[14] In one study, agreement among a group of critical care physicians who interpreted the same pressure recordings was only moderate.[50] A recent study found considerable interobserver variability among ICU nurses and physicians who were asked to record the Ppw from the same strip recordings. The most important factor contributing to interobserver variability was the presence of a large amount of respiratory variation.[51] Furthermore, a brief educational program did not improve the agreement among observers.[52] These data highlight some of the ongoing educational deficiencies among ICU physicians and nurses regarding some of the most basic aspects of hemodynamic monitoring and support the need for more intensive instruction, as proposed in the recent report by the Pulmonary Artery Consensus Conference Organization (PACCO).[53]

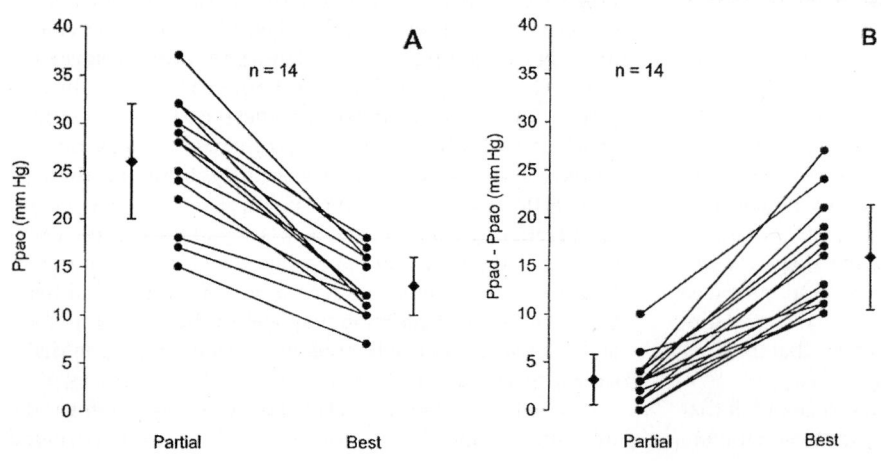

FIGURE 13-10 Effect of partial wedging on the measured pulmonary artery occlusion (wedge) pressure (Ppao) (*A*) and the pulmonary artery diastolic pressure (Ppad)–Ppao gradient (Ppad–Ppao) (*B*) in patients with pulmonary hypertension. These patients initially had a large Ppad–Ppao gradient that narrowed unexpectedly, leading to suspicion of partial wedging. Catheter repositioning to obtain a lower, more reliable ("best") Ppao resulted in a marked fall in the measured Ppao and a simultaneous increase in the Ppad–Ppao gradient. (*Used with permission from Leatherman and Shapiro.*[47])

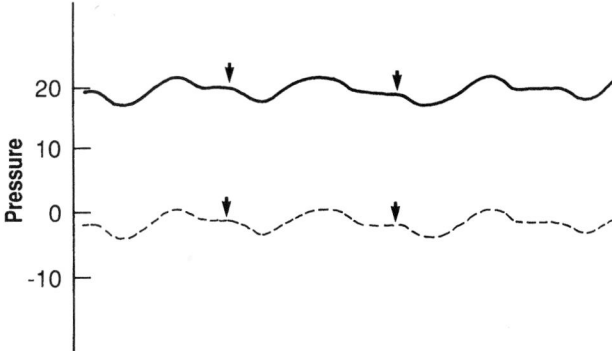

FIGURE 13-11 Effect of varying intrathoracic pressure on the wedge pressure (Ppw). (*Above*) Ppw tracing. (*Below*) Intrapleural pressure (Ppl). In this example, the patient is receiving assisted mechanical ventilation. Arrows indicate end-expiratory pressures. Negative deflections in Ppl and Ppw result from inspiratory muscle activity, and subsequent positive deflections represent lung inflation by the ventilator. At end expiration (*arrow*), the respiratory system has returned to its relaxed state, and Ppl is back to baseline (22 cm H_2O). Transmural wedge pressure remains approximately constant throughout the ventilating cycle. Since Ppl usually is not measured simultaneously with Ppw, however, it is necessary that the Ppw be recorded at a point where Ppl can be estimated reliably (i.e., end exhalation, assuming no active expiratory muscle activity). A digital scan may under- or overestimate transmural pressure depending on whether the pressure is sampled during a period of negative or positive change in Ppl.

A frequent error in identifying end expiration is the false assumption that during mechanical ventilation the lowest point in the Ppw tracing reflects end expiration. While this may be true during controlled ventilation, inspiratory efforts that trigger mechanical breaths will produce a nadir in the Ppw tracing immediately after end expiration[54] (see Fig. 13-11). Identification of end expiration in the Ppw tracing is aided by the knowledge that expiration is usually longer than inspiration, two exceptions being marked tachypnea and inverse-ratio ventilation. In reality, identification of end expiration in the Ppw tracing should not be difficult so long as the respiratory influences on the Ppw are interpreted in relationship to the patient's ventilatory pattern. When confusion occurs, a simultaneous airway pressure tracing may help to identify the end of expiration.

Even when the Ppw is reliably recorded at end expiration, the measured value will overestimate the transmural pressure if intrathoracic pressure is positive at that point in the respiratory cycle. Positive juxtacardiac pressure at end expiration may result from the increase in lung volume that results from applied positive end-expiratory pressure (PEEP) or auto-PEEP or from increased intraabdominal pressure due to active expiration or the abdominal compartment syndrome. In the latter two circumstances, lung volume is not increased. Whatever the cause, increased juxtacardiac (pleural) pressure at end expiration should be taken into account when Ppw is used in clinical decision making.

APPLIED PEEP AND AUTO-PEEP

PEEP may influence the Ppw in one of two ways. First, the positive alveolar pressure conceivably could compress the pulmonary microvasculature sufficiently that there is no

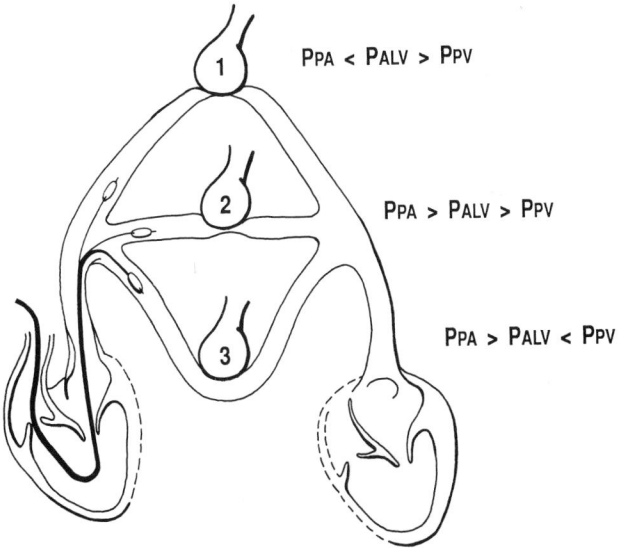

FIGURE 13-12 Physiologic lung zones based on the relationship between pressures in the pulmonary artery (Ppa), alveolus (Palv), and pulmonary vein (Ppv). (*Used with permission from O'Quinn and Marini.*[30])

longer a continuous column of blood between the catheter tip and left atrium, resulting in a Ppw that reflects *alveolar* rather than pulmonary venous pressure. Second, even when PEEP does not interfere with the reliability of the Ppw as an indicator of pulmonary venous pressure, it nonetheless may result in increased juxtacardiac pressure so that the measured Ppw overestimates transmural pressure (Pla – Ppl).

In theory, the lung can be divided into three physiologic zones based on the relationship of pressures in the pulmonary artery (Ppa), alveolus (Palv), and pulmonary vein (Ppv)[30] (Fig. 13-12). This model would predict that the catheter tip must be in zone 3 (Ppv > Palv) at end expiration for the Ppw to provide a reliable estimate of left atrial pressure (Pla), and this would not be the case if PEEP was greater than Pla. However, in the great majority of instances the Ppw will reflect Pla reliably even when PEEP exceeds the latter.[55–58] Several factors may help to explain this apparent paradox. First, regardless of the values of PEEP and Pla, as long as there is a patent vascular channel between the catheter tip and the left atrium, the Ppw should reflect Pla. Since flow-directed catheters often place themselves below the level of the left atrium, local Ppv will be higher than Pla, encouraging vascular patency.[59] Even when the catheter tip lies at or above the atrial level, there may still be a branch of the occluded artery extending below the left atrium that prevents the wedged catheter from recording Palv[60] (Fig. 13-13). Finally, damaged lungs may not transmit Palv as fully to the capillary bed as normal lungs. In a dog model of unilateral lung injury, agreement between Ppw and Pla in the injured lung was excellent up to a PEEP of 20 cm H_2O, whereas Ppw overestimated Pla in the uninjured lung at a PEEP above 10 cm H_2O[55] (Fig. 13-14). A clinical study involving patients with ARDS found good agreement between the Ppw and left ventricular end-diastolic pressure (LVEDP) even at a PEEP of 20 cm H_2O.[56] Since high levels of applied PEEP generally are restricted to patients with ARDS, the Ppw is likely to reflect Pla reliably even when high-level PEEP is required.

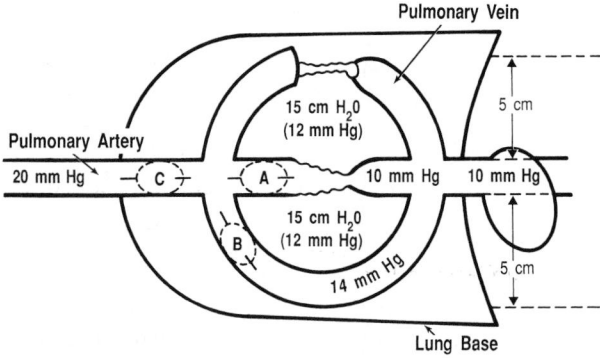

FIGURE 13-13 Reliability of the end-expiratory wedge pressure (Ppw) as a measure of pulmonary venous pressure (Ppv) during application of positive end-expiratory pressure (PEEP). With the balloon inflated, forward flow into the vessel is interrupted, and the catheter will record the higher of the two downstream pressures, Ppv or Palv. In this example, Ppv at the left atrial level is less than Palv. In catheter position *A*, the downstream Ppv is less than Palv, and the latter will be recorded. In position *B*, the catheter is below the left atrium, and local Ppv in this channel exceeds Palv, preserving vascular patency. Thus a reliable Ppw (10 mm Hg) will be recorded. In position *C*, the catheter is located at left atrial level, but it is situated more proximally than in *A*. Since a branch of the occluded vascular segment remains patent, an accurate Ppw (10 mm Hg) will be recorded. *(Used with permission from Culver.[60])*

Although uncommon, a non-zone 3 condition should be considered when the Ppw tracing does not possess characteristics of an atrial waveform and the end-expiratory Ppw approximates PEEP. In this circumstance, a simple bedside method of ensuring a zone 3 condition may be useful.[57] This technique involves a comparison of the change in pulmonary artery systolic pressure (ΔPpas) and change in Ppw (ΔPpw)

FIGURE 13-14 Effect of lung injury on accuracy of the wedge pressure (Ppw) as an estimate of left atrial pressure (Pla). At high levels of PEEP, Ppw overestimates Pla in the uninjured lung but accurately predicts Pla in the injured lung. Thus lung injury favors a zone 3 condition, even though PEEP may exceed Pla significantly. *(Used with permission from Hassan et al.[55])*

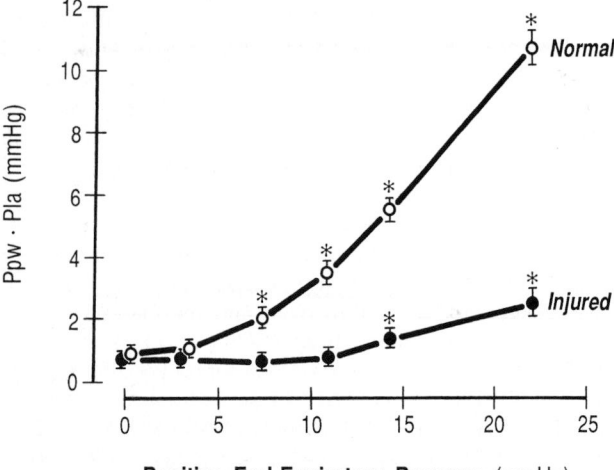

Positive End-Expiratory Pressure (mmHg)

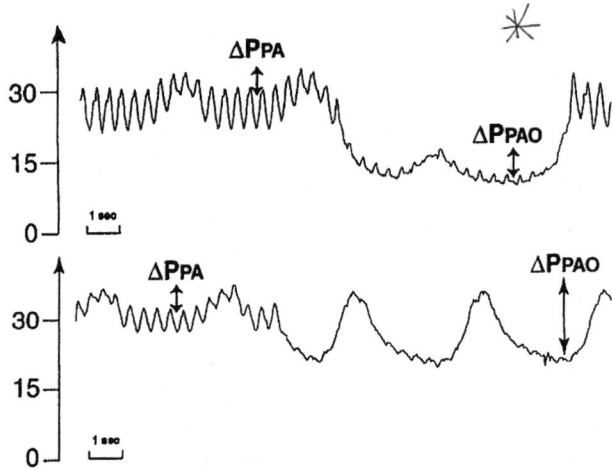

FIGURE 13-15 Changes in pulmonary artery systolic pressure (Ppas) and pulmonary artery occlusion (wedge) pressure (Ppao) during a positive-pressure breath. In the top figure, Ppao tracks with changes in pleural pressure, ensuring a zone 3 condition. In the bottom figure, the Ppao tracks the larger change in alveolar pressure, indicating that a zone 3 condition may not be present. *(Used with permission from Teboul et al.[57])*

during a controlled ventilator breath (Fig. 13-15). Since the former reflects the increment in Ppl during a positive-pressure breath, a ratio of ΔPpas/ΔPpw close to unity would indicate that the ventilator-induced rise in Ppw also results from change in Ppl, thereby ensuring a zone 3 condition. In contrast, ΔPpw will exceed ΔPpas if the Ppw tracing tracks the larger pressure change within the alveoli, in which case a zone 3 condition may not be present.[57] Over 90% of patients with ARDS have a ΔPpas/ΔPpw close to unity (0.7 to 1.2), even at a PEEP of 20 cm H_2O.[57] In those few instances when Ppw tracks Palv during inspiration, a zone 3 condition could still be present at end expiration, when alveolar pressures are lowest. In brief, data from several sources strongly indicate that the end-expiratory Ppw nearly always will represent the downstream vascular pressure (Ppv, Pla) in ARDS, even when high levels of PEEP are required. Concern that the Ppw instead may be representing Palv should be limited to those rare instances in which the Ppw tracing has an unnaturally smooth appearance that is uncharacteristic of an atrial waveform, the end-expiratory Ppw is close to 80% of the applied PEEP (because mm Hg ~ 0.8 × cm H_2O), and the ΔPpw is significantly greater than ΔPpas during a controlled ventilator breath.

Even though PEEP seldom interferes with the reliability of the Ppw as a measure of Pla, it does cause the Ppw to overestimate the actual *transmural* pressure by increasing Ppl at end expiration (Fig. 13-16). The effect of PEEP on Ppl is determined by two factors: the PEEP-induced increase in lung volume and chest wall compliance. The degree to which lung volume increases in response to PEEP is inversely related to lung compliance.[30,61] Decreased chest wall compliance (e.g., increased intraabdominal pressure or morbid obesity) enhances the fraction of PEEP transmitted to the pleural space, whereas reduced lung compliance (e.g., ARDS) may blunt PEEP transmission. One study found that the percentage of PEEP transmitted to the pleural space (as estimated

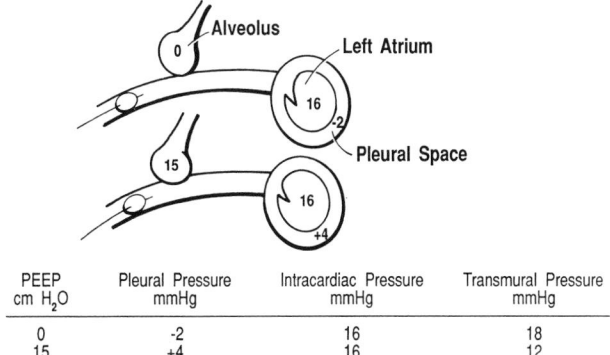

PEEP cm H_2O	Pleural Pressure mmHg	Intracardiac Pressure mmHg	Transmural Pressure mmHg
0	-2	16	18
15	+4	16	12

FIGURE 13-16 The effect of positive end-expiratory pressure (PEEP) on transmural pressure. In this example, 50% of PEEP is transmitted to the juxtacardiac space (15 cm H_2O $\sim$ 12 mm Hg). The same wedge pressure of 16 mm Hg corresponds to greatly different effective transmural filling pressures.

with an esophageal balloon) in ARDS varied from 24% to 37%.[62] However, changes in esophageal pressure may underestimate the actual changes in juxtacardiac pressure when the heart and lungs are both expanded.[63,64] Thus in individual patients it may be difficult to estimate the actual juxtacardiac pressure reliably and hence the transmural pressure (Ppw − Ppl) with PEEP.   NIVEAU PEEP TRANSMIS

Two methods for measuring transmural pressure on PEEP have been described. The first employs a brief ventilator disconnection, during which time the Ppw falls rapidly to a nadir and then subsequently rises due to altered ventricular loading conditions. It has been shown that the nadir Ppw within 2 to 3 seconds of PEEP removal closely approximates the transmural pressure while on PEEP.[65] Although this technique potentially yields a more accurate estimate of transmural pressure, it may encourage alveolar derecruitment and hypoxemia in patients with severe ARDS. In addition, the nadir method will not be reliable in patients with auto-PEEP owing to airflow obstruction because their intrathoracic pressure falls very slowly after ventilator disconnection. The second technique, which does not require ventilator disconnection, uses the *transmission ratio* of ΔPpw/ΔPalv during a controlled ventilator breath to calculate the percent of alveolar pressure that is transmitted to the pleural space.[66] (In zone 3, ΔPpw should reflect the change in pleural pressure, and ΔPalv is defined as plateau pressure-PEEP.) The Ppl on PEEP is then estimated by multiplying PEEP by the transmission ratio, allowing calculation of transmural pressure (Ppw − Ppl)[66] (Fig. 13-17A). In one study, estimates of transmural pressure using the latter technique were virtually identical to those obtained by the nadir method in patients on PEEP who did not have dynamic hyperinflation[66] (see Fig. 13-17B). As noted earlier, the nadir method is unreliable for estimating transmural pressure in patients with airflow obstruction and auto-PEEP, whereas the technique involving calculation of the transmission ratio retains its validity in this patient population.[66] Even though these techniques may provide valid estimates of transmural pressure, it is unclear whether they contribute positively to patient management. In clinical decision making, use of the Ppw should not focus excessively on its absolute value. Rather, *change* in the Ppw with therapeutic interventions and

their correlation with relevant end points (e.g., blood pressure, Pa_{O_2}, $\dot{Q}_T$, and urine output) are of greater importance, and such changes can be assessed without correcting the measured Ppw for the effects of PEEP.

Auto-PEEP may create greater difficulties in use of the Ppw than applied PEEP for several reasons. First, hemodynamically significant auto-PEEP may be occult. Second, because auto-PEEP usually occurs in the setting of chronic obstructive pulmonary disease (COPD) with normal or increased lung compliance, a larger component of the alveolar pressure may be transmitted to the juxtacardiac space. Third, the absence of parenchymal lung injury may promote non-zone 3 conditions. As noted earlier, estimates of transmural pressure based on the ΔPpw/ΔPalv ratio are more reliable than the nadir Ppw technique in patients with auto-PEEP owing to airflow obstruction.[66] From a practical standpoint, the potential hemodynamic significance of auto-PEEP can be determined easily by assessing whether a 30- to 45-second interruption of positive-pressure ventilation leads to an increase in blood pressure and $\dot{Q}_T$.[67] Although this maneuver usually also results in a lower Ppw, an unchanged Ppw does not exclude the presence of hemodynamically significant auto-PEEP because a large increase in venous return could offset the reduction in juxtacardiac pressure.

ACTIVE EXPIRATION

When the abdominal expiratory muscles remain active throughout expiration, the resulting increase in juxtacardiac pressure causes the end-expiratory Ppw to overestimate transmural pressure[35,68–70] (Fig. 13-18). Although initially described in spontaneously breathing patients with COPD, this problem also occurs in the absence of obstructive lung disease and in mechanically ventilated patients.[35,70] Since the pressure generated by the abdominal expiratory muscles is transmitted directly to the pleural space and is not "buffered" by the lungs, active exhalation typically causes the end-expiratory Ppw to overestimate transmural pressure to a much greater extent than does the application of PEEP.[70] With active exhalation, it is common for the end-expiratory Ppw to overestimate transmural pressure by more than 10 mm Hg.[35,70] Failure to appreciate the effect of active exhalation on the measured Ppw may result in inappropriate treatment of hypovolemic patients with diuretics or vasopressors on the basis of a misleadingly elevated Ppw.

When respiratory excursions in the Ppw tracing are due entirely to inspiratory muscle activity, the end-expiratory Ppw will remain unaffected. However, respiratory excursions that exceed 10 to 15 mm Hg increase the likelihood of active expiration.[35] Inspection of the Ppw tracing may provide a clue to active expiration if pressure rises progressively during exhalation. However, an end-expiratory plateau in the Ppw tracing does not exclude positive intrathoracic pressure due to tonic expiratory muscle activity.[69,70] Abdominal palpation may be useful in detecting muscle activity that persists throughout expiration. In mechanically ventilated patients, sedation (or even paralysis) may be used to reduce or eliminate expiratory muscle activity.[35,70] In the nonintubated patient, recording the Ppw while the patient sips water through a straw sometimes helps to eliminate large respiratory fluctuations. An esophageal balloon also can be used to

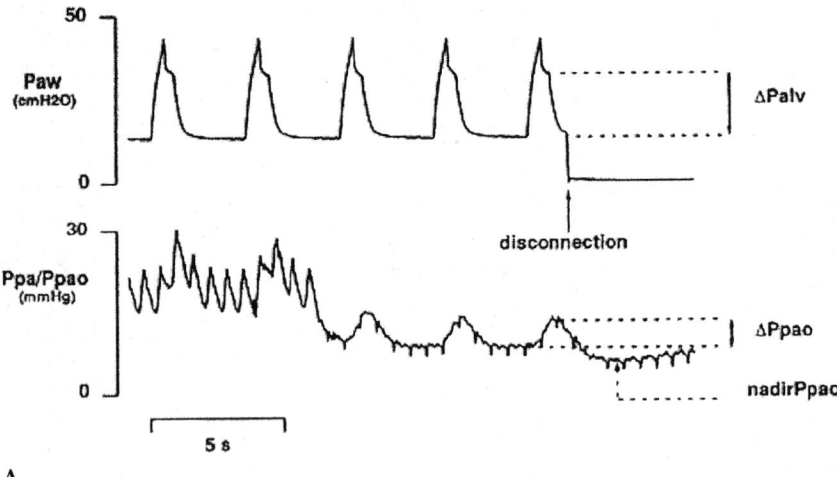

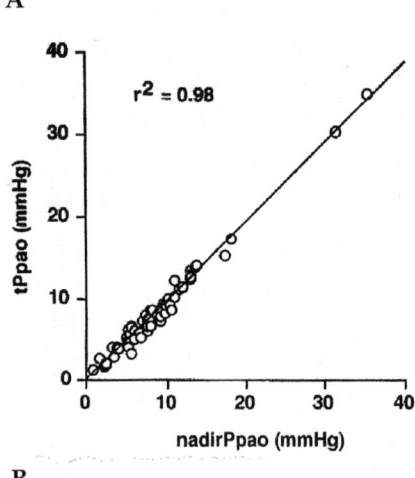

FIGURE 13-17 A. (*Above*) Airway pressure (Paw) during volume-cycled ventilation with an inspiratory pause. The change in alveolar pressure (ΔPalv) resulting with each tidal breath is the plateau pressure minus PEEP. (*Below*) There is an identical change in pulmonary artery pressure (Ppa) and pulmonary artery occlusion (wedge) pressure (Ppao) with each tidal breath, indicating that the catheter is in zone 3, and the ΔPpao therefore reflects the change in pleural pressure. Transmural Ppao is calculated by the transmission-ratio method as transmural pressure = measured Ppao − 0.8 (ΔPpao/ΔPalv) × PEEP. (PEEP, in cm H_2O, is converted to mm Hg by multiplying by 0.8.) B. Also shown is the nadir Ppao measured 2 to 3 seconds after ventilator disconnection. Correlation between determinations of the on-PEEP transmural Ppao by the transmission-ratio method (tPpao) and the nadir method (nadir Ppao). (*Used with permission from Teboul et al.*[66])

FIGURE 13-18 Effect of vigorous respiratory muscle activity on end-expiratory wedge pressure (Ppw). *A.* Patient on mechanical ventilation is observed at the bedside to be making vigorous inspiratory and expiratory efforts. The Ppw measured at end exhalation (*arrow*) is 25 mm Hg. *B.* In order to obtain a reliable Ppw, respiratory muscle activity is temporarily eliminated with a short-acting paralyzing agent. The Ppw is now measured at 8 mm Hg.

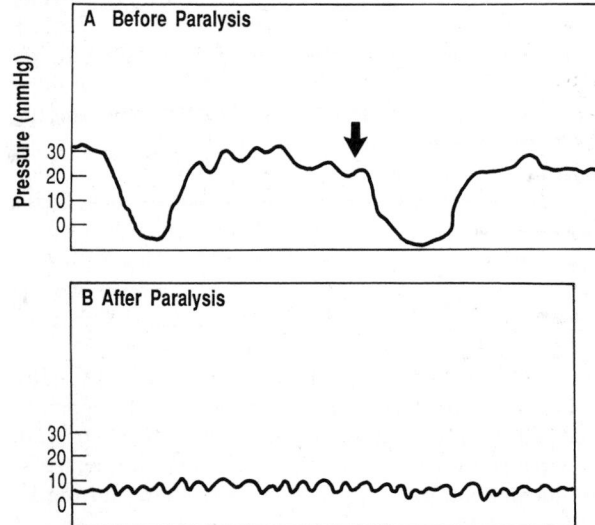

provide a better estimate of transmural pressure.[68] In circumstances where prominent respiratory muscle activity cannot be eliminated and esophageal pressure is unavailable, transmural pressure often is better estimated by the Ppw measured midway between end inspiration and end expiration.[70] However, the latter is not true in all instances,[70] and it may be most appropriate simply to recognize that an accurate estimate of transmural pressure may not be possible in this situation.

CLINICAL USE OF PRESSURE MEASUREMENTS

There are three principal uses of PAC-derived pressures in the ICU: (1) diagnosis of cardiovascular disorders by waveform analysis, (2) diagnosis and management of pulmonary edema, and (3) evaluation of preload.

ABNORMAL WAVEFORMS IN CARDIAC DISORDERS

Unfortunately, physicians and nurses sometimes focus solely on the numbers generated by the pressure monitoring system without carefully assessing the pressure waveforms. Analysis of pressure waveforms may prove valuable in the diagnosis of certain cardiovascular disorders, including mitral regurgitation, tricuspid regurgitation, RV infarction, pericardial tamponade, and limitation of cardiac filling due to constrictive pericarditis or restrictive cardiomyopathy.

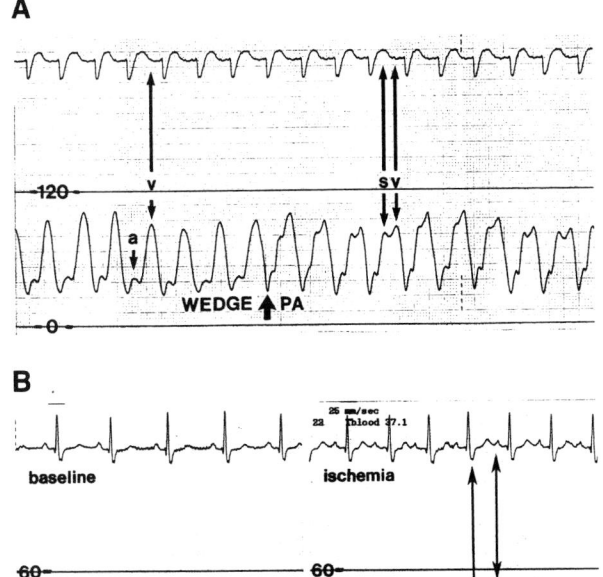

FIGURE 13-19 *A. Acute mitral regurgitation with a giant v wave in the pulmonary wedge tracing. The pulmonary artery (PA) tracing has a characteristic bifid appearance due to both a PA systolic wave and the v wave. Note that the v wave occurs later in the cardiac cycle than the PA systolic wave, which is synchronous with the T wave of the electrocardiogram. B. Intermittent giant v wave due to ischemia of the papillary muscle. Wedge tracings are from the same patient at baseline and during ischemia. (Scale is in millimeters of mercury.) (Used with permission from Sharkey.[34])*

Acute mitral regurgitation most often is due to papillary muscle ischemia or rupture. When the mitral valve suddenly becomes incompetent, an unaccommodated left atrium accepts blood from the left ventricle during systole, producing a prominent v wave (Fig. 13-19). A large v wave gives the Ppa tracing a bifid appearance owing to the presence of both a pulmonary artery systolic wave and the v wave (see Fig. 13-19). When the balloon is inflated, the tracing becomes monophasic as the pulmonary artery systolic wave disappears (see Fig. 13-19). A giant v wave is confirmed most reliably with the aid of a simultaneous recording of the electrocardiogram during balloon inflation. Although the pulmonary artery systolic wave and the left atrial v wave are generated simultaneously, the latter must travel back through the pulmonary vasculature to the catheter tip. Therefore, when the pressure tracing is referenced to the electrocardiogram, the v wave will be seen later in the cardiac cycle than the pulmonary artery systolic wave (see Fig. 13-19). In the presence of a giant v wave, the Ppad is lower than the mean Ppw, and the mean pressure may change only minimally on transition from Ppa to Ppw, giving the impression that the catheter has failed to wedge. This impression may lead to insertion of excess catheter, favoring distal placement that could lead to pulmonary infarction or to rupture of the artery on balloon inflation.

A large v wave leads to an increase in pulmonary capillary pressure, often with resulting pulmonary edema. When mitral insufficiency is due to intermittent ischemia of the papillary muscle, giant v waves may be quite transient (see Fig. 13-19). Failure to appreciate these intermittent giant v waves may lead to a mistaken diagnosis of noncardiogenic pulmonary edema because the Ppw will be normal between periods of ischemia.

Large v waves are not always indicative of mitral insufficiency. The size of the v wave depends on both the volume of blood entering the atrium during ventricular systole and left atrial compliance.[71,72] Decreased left atrial compliance may result in a prominent v wave in the absence of mitral regurgitation. Conversely, when the left atrium is markedly dilated, severe valvular regurgitation may give rise to a trivial v wave, especially when there is coexisting hypovolemia.[72] The important effect of left atrial compliance on the size of the v wave was demonstrated by a study that simultaneously evaluated the height of the v wave and the degree of regurgitation, as determined by ventriculography.[72] One-third of patients who had large v waves (>10 mm Hg) had no valvular regurgitation, and a similar percentage of patients with severe valvular regurgitation had trivial v waves.[72]

Hypervolemia is a common cause of a prominent v wave. When the left atrium is overdistended, it operates on the steep portion of its compliance curve; i.e., small changes in volume produce large changes in pressure (Fig. 13-20). As a result, passive filling from the pulmonary veins can lead to a prominent v wave, and the latter may be quite large if $\dot{Q}\text{T}$ is increased. With hypervolemia or intrinsic reduction in left atrial compliance, the a wave also may be prominent, provided that the underlying rhythm is not atrial fibrillaton. Following diuresis, the a and v waves become less pronounced. Another cause of a large v wave is an acute ventricular septal defect because the increased pulmonary blood flow enhances filling of the left atrium during ventricular systole. Thus both papillary muscle rupture (or dysfunction) and acute ventricular septal defect (VSD) can be associated with prominent v waves, and these two complications of myocardial infarction usually must be differentiated by other means (see below).

Tricuspid regurgitation most often is due to chronic pulmonary hypertension with dilation of the right ventricle. With tricuspid regurgitation, there is often a characteristically broad v (or cv) wave in the central venous (right atrial) tracing (Fig. 13-21). The v wave of tricuspid regurgitation generally is less prominent than the v wave of mitral regurgitation, probably because the systemic veins have a much greater capacitance than do the pulmonary veins. One of the most consistent findings in the Pra tracing of patients with tricuspid regurgitation is a steep y descent. The latter often becomes more pronounced with inspiration (see Fig. 13-21). Kussmaul's sign, an increase in Pra with inspiration, also is observed commonly in patients with severe tricuspid regurgitation.

RV infarction may complicate an inferoposterior myocardial infarction. Common findings include hypotension with clear lung fields, Kussmaul's sign, positive hepatojugular reflux, and a Pra that equals or even exceeds the Ppw. The Pra tracing in RV infarction often reveals prominent x and y descents, and these deepen with inspiration or volume loading.[34] With RV infarction, the RV and pulmonary artery pulse pressures narrow, and with RV failure, the RVEDP may approximate the Ppad (Fig. 13-22). This, together with the frequent presence of tricuspid regurgitation, may lead to difficulties in bedside insertion of the PAC, and fluoroscopy may be required.[34] In the setting of a patent foramen ovale,

A

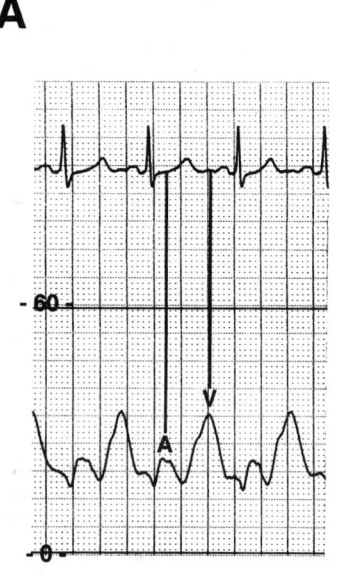

B

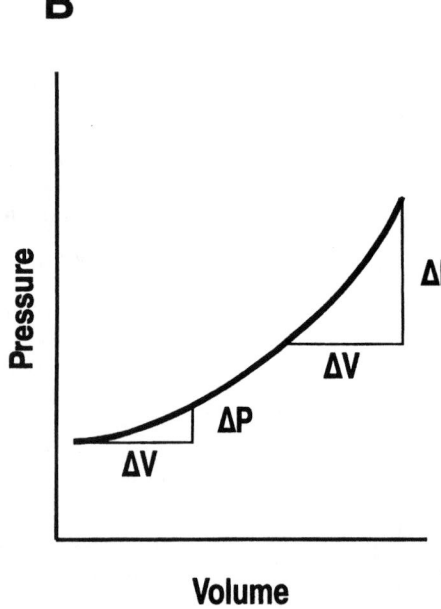

FIGURE 13-20 *A.* Prominent *v* wave. The echocardiogram showed only trace mitral regurgitation. *B.* Left atrial pressure-volume relationship. The same degree of passive filling during diastole (ΔV) produces a much larger change in pressure (ΔP) when the left atrium is overdistended and is operating on the steep portion of the compliance curve. This explains the presence of a large *v* wave with hypervolemia.

patients with RV infarction may develop significant hypoxemia due to a right-to-left atrial shunt. Profound hypoxemia with a clear chest radiograph and refractory hypotension also would be consistent with major pulmonary embolus. The hemodynamic profiles of these two disorders are different, however, in that massive pulmonary embolism is characterized by a significant increase in the Ppad–Ppw gradient, whereas the latter is unaffected by RV infarction.[41]

Pericardial tamponade is characterized by an increase of intrapericardial pressure that limits cardiac filling in diastole. With advanced tamponade, intrapericardial pressure becomes the key determinant of cardiac diastolic pressures,

resulting in the characteristic *equalization* of the Pra and Ppw. Intrapericardial pressure is a function of the amount of pericardial fluid, pericardial compliance, and total cardiac volume. The *x* descent is preserved in tamponade because it occurs in early systole when blood is being ejected from the heart, thereby permitting a fall in pericardial fluid pressure. In contrast, the *y* descent occurs during diastole when blood is being transferred from the atria to the ventricles, during which time total cardiac volume and intrapericardial pressure are unchanged. As a result, there is little (if any) change in Pra during diastole, accounting for the characteristically blunted *y* descent of pericardial tamponade[73] (Fig. 13-23). Attention to the *y* descent may prove to be quite useful in the differential diagnosis of a low Q̇T with near equalizaton of pressures. An absent *y* descent dictates that echocardiography be performed to evaluate for possible pericardial tamponade, whereas a well-preserved *y* descent argues against this diagnosis.

Constrictive pericarditis and restrictive cardiomyopathy have similar hemodynamic findings. Both disorders may be associated with striking increases in Pra and Ppw due to limitation of cardiac filling. In restrictive cardiomyopathy the Ppw usually is greater than the Pra, whereas in constrictive pericarditis the right and left atria exhibit similar pressures. In contrast to pericardial tamponade, the *y* descent is prominent and often is deeper than the *x* descent. The prominent *y* descent is due to rapid ventricular filling during early dias-

FIGURE 13-21 Tricuspid regurgitation. A broad *v* (or *cv*) wave and prominent *y* descent are apparent in the right atrial tracing. Note that inspiration leads to accentuation of the *y* descent and that mean right atrial pressure increases slightly (Kussmaul's sign).

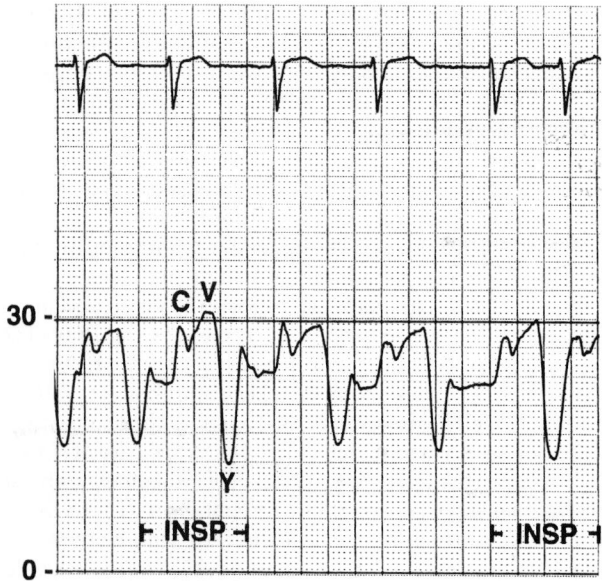

FIGURE 13-22 Right ventricular infarction. Note the similarity of the tracings from different chambers. Fluoroscopy may be required during insertion to confirm catheter position. (*Used with permission from Sharkey.[34]*)

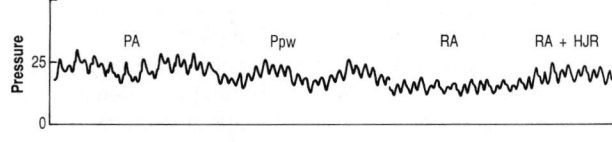

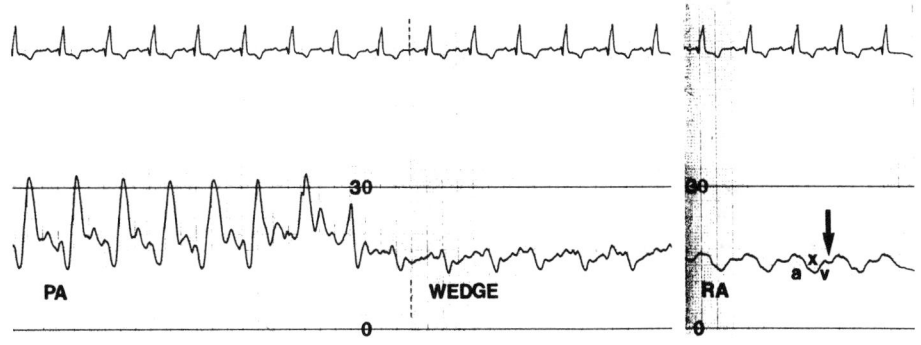

FIGURE 13-23 Pericardial tamponade. Tracings show characteristic equalization of wedge and right atrial pressures and blunting of the *y* descent (*arrow*). (*Used with permission from Sharkey.*[34])

tole, with sharp curtailment of further filling during the later portion of diastole (Fig. 13-24).

DIAGNOSIS AND MANAGEMENT OF PULMONARY EDEMA

The Ppw is used commonly to aid in the differentiation of cardiogenic and noncardiogenic pulmonary edema. For un-injured lungs, the expected Ppw threshold for hydrostatic pulmonary edema is approximately 22 to 25 mm Hg. (A higher threshold is common if the Ppw has been chronically elevated.) When capillary permeability is increased, how-ever, pulmonary edema occurs at a much lower Ppw. Indeed, one generally accepted criterion for ARDS has been a Ppw < 18 mm Hg. It is important to appreciate, how-ever, that an isolated Ppw reading does not reliably pre-dict whether pulmonary edema occurred on the basis of in-creased capillary pressure (Pcap) alone or on the basis of altered permeability, especially when recorded after a ther-apeutic intervention. Acute hydrostatic pulmonary edema occurs frequently despite normal intravascular volume on the basis of an acute decrease in LV compliance resulting from ischemia or accelerated hypertension. By the time a PAC is placed, the acute process often has resolved, re-sulting in a normal or even reduced Ppw, depending in

part on what type of therapy (e.g., diuretics or vasodilators) has been given. In this circumstance, maintaining the Ppw ≤ 18 mm Hg over the next 24 hours should lead to marked clinical and roentgenographic improvement if pulmonary edema had been due to elevated Pcap prior to catheter inser-tion. Conversely, lack of improvement or worsening would suggest altered permeability as the etiology of pulmonary edema. One must be careful, however, when hydrostatic pul-monary edema is due to intermittent elevations in Ppw due to myocardial ischemia. Transient ischemia-related elevations in Ppw may be missed by intermittently recording Ppw (see Fig. 13-19), potentially leading to an erroneous diagnosis of ARDS. Some bedside monitors store pressure data from the previous 12 to 24 hours, and inspection of a graphic display of the stored data may be useful in detecting transient elevations in Ppa that occur during periods of intermittent ischemia. Just as patients with hydostatic pulmonary edema may have a nor-mal Ppw, patients whose pulmonary edema is due primarily to increased permeabililty may have an increased Ppw due to volume expansion.[74] In brief, the pathogenesis of pulmonary edema formation should not be based solely on Ppw, and clar-ification of the underlying mechanism may require a period of careful clinical and radiologic observation.

Ppw, the pressure in a large pulmonary vein, represents a very low-end estimate of the average pressure across the fluid-permeable vascular bed. Normally, about 40% of the re-sistance across the pulmonary vascular bed resides in the small veins[75] (Fig. 13-25). When pulmonary arterial and ven-ous resistances are normally distributed, the Gaar equation

FIGURE 13-24 Constrictive pericarditis. Right atrial tracing (obtained in the cardiac catheterization laboratory) reveals a very prominent *y* descent. Lack of a prominent *x* descent may be due to atrial fibrillation. Paper speed is 50 mm/s.

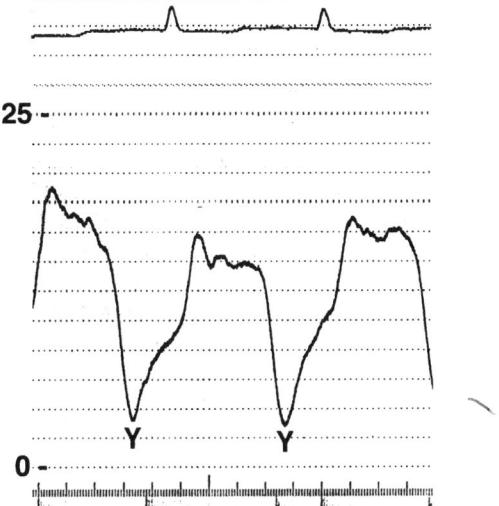

FIGURE 13-25 Pulmonary vascular resistance (PVR) is due to precapillary arteriolar resistance (Ra) and postcapillary venous resistance (Rv). Normally, it is estimated that 60% of total PVR is due to Ra and 40% is due to Rv. The inflection point during decay from the pulmonary artery (mean) to the wedge tracing approximates capillary pressure (Pcap).

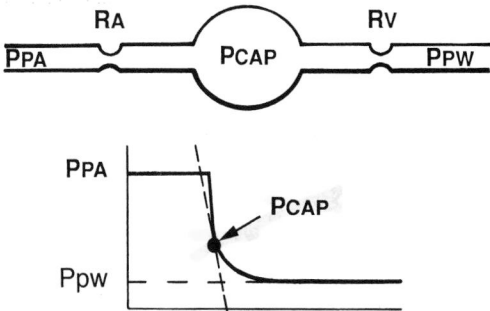

predicts Pcap by the formula $Pcap = Ppw + 0.4(Ppa - Ppw)$.[75] Since the driving pressure $(Ppa - Ppw)$ across the vascular bed is normally very low, Pcap will be only a few millimeters of mercury above Ppw. However, a significant pressure drop from Pcap to Ppw could occur under conditions of increased venous resistance, increased $\dot{Q}_T$, or both. For example, the markedly increased venous resistance of pulmonary veno-occlusive disease results in clinical evidence of increased Pcap (e.g., pulmonary edema, Kerley B lines) despite a normal Ppw.[76] Other clinical conditions that selectively increase venous resistance are not well defined.

A number of techniques for determining Pcap have been described.[77-79] The transition from a Ppa to a Ppw waveform after balloon occlusion includes an initial rapid decay and a subsequent slower decay (see Fig. 13-25). In experimental animals, the inflection point between the rapid and slow components has been shown to represent Pcap, as measured by isogravimetric or simultaneous double-occlusion (arterial and venous) techniques.[77] Estimates of Pcap from visual inspection of pressure tracings after balloon occlusion has been used in humans.[78,79] One study concluded that Pcap was on average 7 mm Hg higher than the measured Ppw in patients with ARDS.[78] In this study, the estimated Pcap and the calculated Pcap by the Gaar equation were highly correlated, implying that arterial and venous resistances are increased equally in ARDS.[78] It should be appreciated, however, that it may be difficult to determine Pcap confidently by inspection of the pressure tracing following balloon occlusion.[80] Furthermore, even if an accurate estimate of Pcap can be obtained, it is unclear how this would have any practical advantage over the Ppw in guiding fluid management. The important point is that Ppw is a low-range estimate of Pcap; the true value of the latter lies somewhere between Ppa and Ppw. It follows that increases in the driving pressure across the microvasculature caused by increases in $\dot{Q}_T$ have the potential to exacerbate edema formation.

Downward manipulation of Ppw by diuresis or ultrafiltration will reduce Pcap and may benefit gas exchange markedly in patients with ARDS. There is no minimum value for Ppw below which removal of intravascular volume is contraindicated, provided that $\dot{Q}_T$ is adequate. If the clinical problem is severely impaired gas exchange requiring high F_{IO_2} or high PEEP, then a trial of Ppw reduction is reasonable as long as $\dot{Q}_T$ and blood pressure remain within acceptable limits. As with all therapeutic manipulations, clinically relevant end points (e.g., Pa_{O_2}, blood pressure, and $\dot{Q}_T$) should be assessed before and after Ppw reduction.

ASSESSMENT OF PRELOAD

When afterload and intrinsic contractility are held constant, the forcefulness of ventricular contraction is determined by end-diastolic fiber length (preload).[81] The most commonly used indicators of preload are Ppw and Pra.[82] Indeed, one of the principal reasons for developing the PAC was to have a bedside method of assessing LV preload.[1] In order to assess preload reliably, the Ppw must accurately reflect LVEDP, and LVEDP must correlate well with left ventricular end-diastolic volume (LVEDV). Under most circumstances, the Ppw provides a close approximation of LVEDP. Exceptions include an overestimation of LVEDP by the mean Ppw with mitral stenosis or mitral regurgitation with a very large v wave and

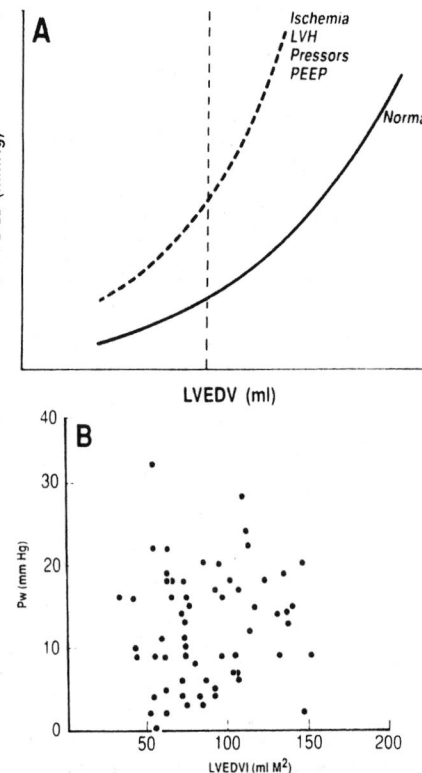

FIGURE 13-26 *A.* Pressure-volume (compliance) relationship of the left ventricle (LV). Ischemia, LV hypertrophy, and high doses of pressors may decrease LV compliance. Positive end-expiratory pressure (PEEP) increases juxtacardiac pressure and may increase ventricular interdependence owing to an increased right ventricular afterload. These factors result in a lower left ventricular end-diastolic volume (LVEDV) at a given left ventricular end-diastolic pressure (PLVED), necessitating a higher PLVED (and thus a higher wedge pressure, Pw) to achieve optimal preload (as compared with normal individuals). *B.* Simultaneous measurements of LVEDV index (LVEDVI) and Pw in a diverse group of critically ill patients. The poor correlation between LVEDVI and Pw is apparent. (*Adapted from Raper and Sibbald, Chest 89:427, 1986.*)

underestimation of LVEDP by the mean Ppw when diastolic dysfunction or hypervolemia causes the LVEDP to increase markedly with atrial systole ("atrial kick").[30] (With a large v wave, LVEDP is best estimated by the pressure just before the onset of the v wave; with a prominent a wave, LVEDP is best estimated by the pressure at the z point, just after the peak of the a wave.)[81] Unfortunately, even though the mean Ppw is usually equivalent to LVEDP, factors that alter LV compliance (e.g., hypertrophy or ischemia) or change juxtacardiac pressure (e.g., PEEP or active exhalation) may profoundly influence the relationship between LVEDP and LVEDV (Fig. 13-26A). It is not surprising, therefore, that among different patients, an equivalent LVEDV may be associated with widely varying Ppw[83] (see Fig. 13-26B).

The optimal Ppw (for preload) can be defined as the Ppw above which there is minimal increase in stroke volume. In normal individuals, optimal Ppw is often 10 to 12 mm Hg.[84] During resuscitation from hypovolemic or septic shock, the optimal Ppw is usually ≤ 14 mm Hg,[85] whereas in acute myocardial infarction it is often between 14 and 18 mm Hg.[86] However, these target values certainly are not valid in all cases. By measuring stroke volume at different Ppw values, a cardiac function curve can be constructed, thereby defining optimal Ppw for an individual patient. This may be particularly useful in patients who also have established or incipient ARDS because a Ppw above the optimal value will increase the risk of worsening oxygenation without offering any benefit with regard to Q̇т. It should be appreciated, however, that the relationship between Ppw and Q̇т may change as a consequence of alterations in LV compliance, myocardial contractility, or juxtacardiac pressure and therefore may need to be redefined if clinical status changes.

A clinically relevant test of the utility of the Ppw is its ability to predict the hemodynamic response to a fluid challenge when hypotension, oliguria, or tachycardia leads to uncertainty about the adequacy of preload. Studies that have examined the utility of the Ppw in predicting fluid responsiveness have been reviewed recently.[18] Seven of nine studies found that the Ppw was no different in fluid responders and nonresponders, and analysis by receiver operating characteristic (ROC) curves in two studies indicated that the Ppw was not particularly useful as a predictor of fluid responsiveness.[87,88] One study did find a significant inverse relationship between Ppw and fluid-induced change in stroke volume, but the degree of correlation was only moderate.[89] Although these data suggest a major limitation of the Ppw as an indicator of preload, it is clear that there must be a Ppw above which volume expansion almost always would be futile and a Ppw below which a positive response to fluid virtually is certain. To define these cutoff Ppw values confidently, however, would require a large study in which individual values for Ppw and fluid-induced change in stroke volume are reported for each patient, with a wide range of Ppw values being examined. Individual values for Ppw and fluid-induced change in stroke volume were reported in two studies.[89,90] Although no patient with a Ppw >18 mm Hg had a positive response to fluid and all patients with a Ppw <8 mm Hg were fluid responders, the number of patients within these Ppw domains was too small to draw any firm conclusions about the usefulness of these cutoff values.[89,90] Furthermore, in the great majority of patients who had a Ppw between 8 and 18 mm Hg there was no apparent relationship between Ppw and fluid response. In brief, while the Ppw is used often in clinical practice as an indicator of the adequacy of preload, most of the evidence to date would suggest that it has limited utility in predicting fluid responsiveness, at least over the range of values encountered most often in the ICU.

Overall, the data for Pra were quite similar to those described for the Ppw, in that three of five studies found no difference between the Pra values of responders and nonresponders,[18] and in one of the studies that did find a difference, there was only a modest inverse correlation between Pra and the fluid-induced change in stroke volume.[89] Although there does not appear to be an appreciable difference in the predictive value of the Pra and the Ppw with regard to fluid response for most patients, it might be anticipated that the Pra would be inferior to the Ppw in a population of patients with severe isolated LV dysfunction related to acute myocardial infarction or other causes.[37] Conversely, in patients with

severe RV dysfunction and preserved LV function, the Pra may be more relevant than the Ppw.[91]

Although Ppw and Pra are used most widely in guiding fluid therapy in the ICU,[18,82] measurements of cardiac volumes also have been used to predict fluid responsiveness.[89,92–94] A modified PAC with a rapid-response thermistor permits simultaneous measurement of RV ejection fraction (RVEF) and stroke volume, from which RV end-diastolic volume (RVEDV) can be calculated. Several studies have compared the Ppw and RVEDV as predictors of fluid responsiveness.[89,92,93] One study found the RVEDV to be superior to the Ppw and suggested that either a positive or negative response to fluid could be predicted reliably when the RVEDV index was less than 90 or greater than 138 mL/m², respectively.[93] However, a subsequent study found that these threshold values for RVEDV index were unreliable and that both the Ppw and Pra predicted the response to fluid better than RVEDV.[89] It is not clear that the RVEDV is any better than the Ppw (or Pra) at predicting fluid responsiveness.

Left ventricular end-diastolic area (LVEDA), measured by transesophageal echocardiography, is another potential indicator of fluid responsiveness. Two studies found that LVEDA was significantly lower in responders than in nonresponders and that LVEDA was superior to Ppw as a predictor of fluid responsiveness.[87,90] However, there was considerable overlap in the LVEDA values between groups, and analysis using ROC curves demonstrated minimal utility of LVEDA in predicting the fluid response of individual patients.[87] Another study found that the Ppw was a better predictor of fluid response than LVEDA during cardiac surgery.[95] In addition, a recent study of patients in septic shock also found the LVEDA to be of minimal value in predicting the response to volume expansion.[96]

In contrast to the static indicators of preload mentioned earlier, methods that rely on the dynamic response to respiratory changes in intrathoracic pressure have performed somewhat better at predicting fluid response. One method is based on the presence or absence of a reduction in Pra during a spontaneous breath.[39] When Pra decreased with inspiration, a positive response to fluid was likely (although not inevitable). Conversely, when a spontaneous breath did not produce a fall in Pra, Q̇т remained unchanged or decreased after a fluid challenge.[39] In this study, neither the Ppw nor the Pra discriminated responders from nonresponders.[39] A follow-up study confirmed that patients with an inspiratory decrease in Pra had a much greater probability of responding to fluid than did patients whose Pra did not change with inspiration.[97] A second method is based on the change in arterial pressure from inspiration to expiration during controlled positive-pressure ventilation.[88] In a study involving septic patients with circulatory failure, the respiratory variation in arterial pulse pressure was much greater in responders than in nonresponders, and a threshold value was found that discriminated these two groups with a high degree of accuracy.[88] A second study that used a modification of this technique also found the respiratory variation in arterial pressure to predict the response to fluid much better than the Ppw or LVEDA in patients with sepsis.[87] Although more investigations are needed to confirm these studies, methods that rely on the dynamic response to respiratory changes in intrathoracic pressure ultimately may prove to be better indicators of the adequacy of preload than static indicators such as the Ppw, Pra, RVEDV, and LVEDA.[18]

Cardiac Output

PRINCIPLES OF MEASUREMENT

The thermodilution technique for measuring $\dot{Q}T$ is an indicator-dilution method in which the indicator is thermal depression (cold). Cold fluid is injected through the proximal lumen of the PAC and, after mixing thoroughly in the RV with venous blood returning from the periphery, passes into the pulmonary artery, where a thermistor at the tip of the catheter senses dynamic changes in temperature. The Stewart-Hamilton formula relates $\dot{Q}T$ to temperature change over time:

$$\dot{Q}T = \frac{V(TB - TI) \times K_1 \times K_2}{\int TB(t)dt}$$

where V is injected volume, TB is blood temperature, TI is injectate temperature, $\int TB(t)dt$ is change in blood temperature as a function of time, and K_1 and K_2 are computational constants. The numerator contains known constants or measured values, whereas the denominator is the area beneath the time-temperature curve derived by computer integration of the thermistor signal. Although it would seem that increasing the strength of the signal by cooling the injectate should enhance the accuracy and reproducibility of thermodilution $\dot{Q}T$ ($\dot{Q}T_{td}$), studies have shown that iced and room-temperature injectates usually are similar in effect as long as careful attention to technique is employed.[98]

Errors may occur if the wrong computational constant is entered into the computer or if either the volume or the recorded temperature of the injectate is incorrect. In addition, the temperature-time curve should be inspected for irregularities. A valid curve shows a rapid early ascent to a peak value and then smoothly returns to the thermal baseline within 10 to 15 seconds of injection (Fig. 13-27). Inadequate blending of injectate with blood, prolonged (>4 s) or uneven injection, thermistor contact with the vessel wall, or abrupt changes in heart rate may result in a grossly irregular curve, and the

data should be discarded. The measured $\dot{Q}T_{td}$ may vary significantly depending on the phase of the respiratory cycle at which the injection is begun.[99] Timing of injection may be less important when the respiratory rate is high because the duration of injection will span the entire respiratory cycle. The average of three to five randomly spaced injections probably gives the best overall measure of $\dot{Q}T$.

Certain conditions can render $\dot{Q}T_{td}$ an unreliable estimate of net systemic $\dot{Q}T$. Since individual measurements are made over a few cardiac cycles, major irregularities in cardiac rhythm during the period of injection could affect the extent to which $\dot{Q}T_{td}$ reflects average $\dot{Q}T$ over a longer period. Left-to-right shunts (e.g., atrial septal defect or ventricular septal defect) increase the ratio of pulmonary to systemic $\dot{Q}T$, causing $\dot{Q}T_{td}$ to seriously overestimate systemic $\dot{Q}T$. The effect of tricuspid regurgitation on the reliability of $\dot{Q}T_{td}$ is controversial. In two studies, $\dot{Q}T_{td}$ significantly underestimated $\dot{Q}T$ measured by the Fick method or continuous-flow Doppler in patients with severe tricuspid regurgitation.[100,101] In contrast, other investigators found that tricuspid regurgitation had no discernible impact on the agreement between simultaneous measurements of $\dot{Q}T_{td}$ and Fick-derived $\dot{Q}T$.[102,103] Given the uncertainty regarding accuracy of $\dot{Q}T_{td}$ in individual patients with significant tricuspid regurgitation, it may be advisable to measure $\dot{Q}T$ with an alternative method (see below) when significant tricuspid regurgitation is diagnosed by inspection of the Pra tracing (see above), by echocardiography, or by a characteristically attenuated time-temperature thermodilution curve (see Fig. 13-27).

Continuous monitoring of $\dot{Q}T_{td}$ is possible with a modified PAC that contains a 10-cm-long thermal filament that transfers heat directly to the blood using a pseudorandom binary sequence.[104] The amount of heat applied is safe, and the upper limit of temperature attained within the filament is 44°C. Temperature change is detected at the catheter tip and is cross-correlated with the input sequence to produce a thermodilution washout curve. The displayed $\dot{Q}T$ value is an average of the last 10 separate determinations over the previous 6 to 8 minutes.[104] Several studies have compared measurements of $\dot{Q}T_{td}$ by the continuous and bolus injection methods.[104–106] Reported agreement between methods appears good, with observed differences of little clinical significance. An in vitro study in which flow was controlled found both the bolus

FIGURE 13-27 Thermodilution curves in patients with (A) low $\dot{Q}T$, (B) normal $\dot{Q}T$, (C) high $\dot{Q}T$, and (D) tricuspid regurgitation. The notch on each curve represents the end of data processing. The remainder of the curve is extrapolated. (*Used with permission from Sharkey.[34]*)

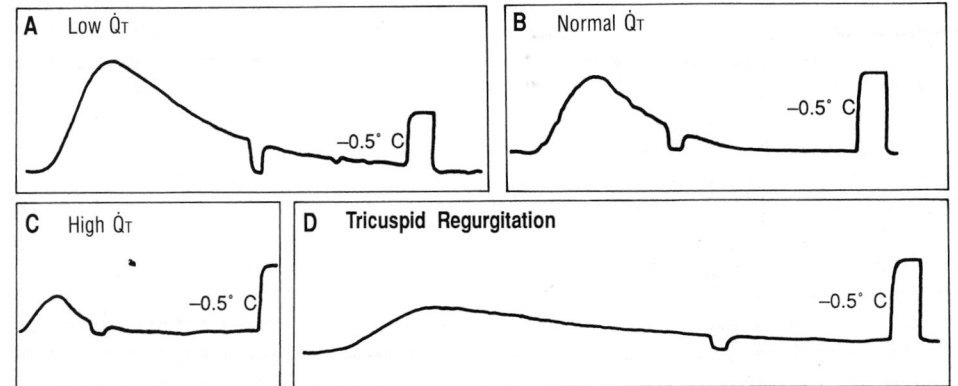

and continuous thermodilution methods to be reliable, but the continuous method was more accurate when flow was very low (<3 L/min).[106] A recent study of patients with a left ventricular assistance device that allowed an independent intravascular measurement of $\dot{Q}_T$ also found the continuous cardiac output to be reasonably accurate.[107] Although the clinical impact of continuous $\dot{Q}_{T_{td}}$ monitoring is uncertain, it could have potential utility when $\dot{Q}_T$ is likely to undergo marked fluctuations either spontaneously or in response to therapy. From a practical standpoint, it may be more convenient to use the continuous thermodilution method when frequent assessments of $\dot{Q}_T$ are desired during titration of inotropic or vasodilator agents or with incremental application of PEEP.

ALTERNATIVE METHODS OF MEASURING $\dot{Q}_T$

cf Blue Book 2004

Several noninvasive or minimally invasive alternatives to the thermodilution technique for measuring $\dot{Q}_T$ have been introduced to clinical practice recently. These methods include pulse contour analysis of the arterial pressure waveform, esophageal Doppler analysis of aortic blood flow, thoracic electrical bioimpedance, the indirect Fick method employing partial carbon dioxide rebreathing, and a transpulmonary thermodilution technique.[17] Because all methods have limitations, there is no "gold standard" for measuring $\dot{Q}_T$. However, for logistic reasons, assessment of these less invasive methods generally has been done by comparison with the PAC-based bolus thermodilution technique as the reference technique. The partial CO_2 rebreathing technique, a method applicable to intubated patients, is entirely noninvasive and has shown good agreement with the bolus thermodilution method in some studies. However, although the issue currently remains unsettled, there has been some concern regarding accuracy of this technique in the setting of severe lung injury (where CO_2 shunting occurs) or when there is variability in tidal volume due to spontaneous breaths, potentially limiting its general applicability in the ICU.[17,108] Esophageal Doppler measurements of $\dot{Q}_T$ generally have shown good concordance with those obtained by bolus thermodilution, including investigations performed in critically ill patients with sepsis.[109,110] To achieve reliable results with this method, it is important that nurses who perform the procedure receive sufficient training to achieve proficiency.[111] Thoracic electrical bioimpedance has been evaluated in numerous studies. A meta-analysis of over 150 studies concluded that while it may be useful for trend analysis, this method is probably not reliable enough for diagnostic purposes.[112] Bioimpedance methodology may be less accurate when there is significant pulmonary or peripheral edema or in the setting of large pleural effusions, possibly limiting its utility in the ICU.[17] A recent study suggested that advances in technology have made the current systems more reliable than earlier versions.[113] In contrast to the standard bolus thermodilution technique using a PAC, which measures right-sided $\dot{Q}_T$, the transpulmonary thermodilution technique measures left-sided $\dot{Q}_T$ by injection of a cold injectate intravenously and detection of the change in temperature in the arterial system.[17,114,115] The agreement between these two methods has been reasonably good, with the transpulmonary technique values being somewhat higher, possibly due to loss of indicator (cold) in the lung.[17] Pulse contour analysis of the arterial pressure waveform to measure stroke volume was developed 20 years ago.[17] Most studies comparing the pulse contour and bolus thermodilution methods of measuring $\dot{Q}_T$ have shown excellent correlation.[17,116] The standard pulse contour device must be calibrated with a $\dot{Q}_T$ value measured independently, such as by the transpulmonary thrermodilution technique. An alternative method of calibration is an indicator dilution technique in which lithium chloride is the indicator.[117] The lithium pulse contour method has been shown to correlate very well with the bolus thermodilution technique, and in one study the coefficient of variation for multiple measurements was significantly less for the former method.[118]

CLINICAL USE OF $\dot{Q}_{T_{td}}$

Combining $\dot{Q}_{T_{td}}$ with measurement of systemic and pulmonary pressures allows calculation of vascular resistances: systemic vascular resistance (SVR) = (Pa − Pra)/$\dot{Q}_T$ and pulmonary vascular resistance (PVR) = (Ppa − Ppw)/$\dot{Q}_T$. To assess the appropriateness of $\dot{Q}_T$ to body mass, $\dot{Q}_{T_{td}}$ is divided by body surface area (BSA) to calculate cardiac index. Unlike flow ($\dot{Q}_T$), pulmonary and systemic pressures are not dependent on body size. Therefore, to avoid misinterpretation due to variation in body mass, it is also appropriate to compute indices of systemic and pulmonary vascular resistance by using cardiac index rather than $\dot{Q}_T$ in the resistance calculations.

Assessment of $\dot{Q}_{T_{td}}$ and SVR may be particularly helpful in the assessment of hypotension, oliguria, and unexplained lactic acidosis. Measurement of $\dot{Q}_{T_{td}}$ is of particular value in the management of septic shock and ARDS. Septic hypotension often is due primarily to excessive arterial vasodilation, but decreased venous return and myocardial dysfunction may contribute to the hemodynamic derangement. By assessing the relative contribution of $\dot{Q}_T$ and SVR to systemic hypotension, the clinician may be able to apply fluid, vasopressor, and inotropic therapy more rationally. In ARDS, a fall in blood pressure could result from hypovolemia, LV dysfunction, pneumothorax, pulmonary emboli, increasing PVR from ARDS, a change in applied PEEP, or dynamic hyperinflation, all of which produce hypotension through a decrease in $\dot{Q}_T$. Evaluation would consist of measurement of intravascular and airway pressures, perhaps along with obtaining a chest x-ray, electrocardiogram, or echocardiogram. On the other hand, these conditions would be of little concern if it were known that $\dot{Q}_T$ remained unchanged, indicating that the fall in blood pressure was due entirely to a reduction in SVR.

Sepsis is the most common cause of hypotension with a low SVR, but other conditions may produce a similar hemodynamic profile. Severe hypotension resulting from excessive arterial vasodilation can occur as a result of acute adrenal insufficiency, thiamine deficiency (beriberi), severe pancreatitis, or poisoning with a variety of drugs or toxins (e.g., nitrates, calcium channel blockers, aspirin, and tricyclic antidepressants). Systemic arteriovenous fistulas, as occur with cirrhosis, also lead to a high $\dot{Q}_T$–low SVR hemodynamic profile, albeit usually with normal blood pressure. Failure to include noninfectious processes in the differential diagnosis of a high $\dot{Q}_T$–low SVR state may result in misdiagnosis of life-threatening, treatable conditions.[119]

The hemodynamic response to a fluid challenge, inotropes, vasodilators, or alterations in PEEP is often assessed in part by measuring changes in $\dot{Q}_{T_{td}}$. Critically ill patients may undergo significant spontaneous fluctuations in tissue O_2 demand and $\dot{Q}_T$ throughout the day. Therefore, determinations of $\dot{Q}_{Ttd}$ ideally should be made immediately before and after a specific intervention. Even when assessment is optimal, the normal variability in measured $\dot{Q}_{Ttd}$ may confound the response to an intervention. A study involving hemodynamically stable patients found that measured $\dot{Q}_{Ttd}$ varied by an average of 7.7% over a period of 1 hour.[120] Therefore, the clinician must observe a change in measured $\dot{Q}_{Ttd}$ of at least 10% to 15% before concluding that the observed response was actually due to a specific intervention.[120,121]

Mixed Venous Oxygen Saturation

Mixed venous oxygen saturation (Sv_{O_2}) is the O_2 saturation of blood in the pulmonary artery after the venous effluent from various organs has been mixed thoroughly in the RV. The Sv_{O_2} can be measured intermittently by slowly withdrawing a sample of blood from the distal port of the unwedged PAC or continuously with a fiberoptic PAC that measures O_2 saturation by reflectance oximetry.[122] Intermittent sampling of Sv_{O_2} is accomplished by discarding the initial 3 mL of blood and then withdrawing a sample very slowly so as to avoid contamination with capillary blood. The Sv_{O_2} should be measured by co-oximetry because the steep slope of the O_2 dissociation curve in the venous range means that small errors in measurement of Pv_{O_2} may result in substantial errors in calculation of Sv_{O_2}.

Ordinarily, the O_2 saturation is lower in the superior vena cava than in the inferior vena cava, but the reverse is true in shock due to redistribution of blood flow away from splanchnic, renal, and mesenteric beds.[123,124] Thus the oxygen saturation of blood obtained from a central venous catheter in the superior vena cava (Scv_{O_2}) will overestimate Sv_{O_2} in shock. Although the absolute values of Sv_{O_2} and Scv_{O_2} may differ, they tend to track together with changing hemodynamic conditions.[124] Furthermore, it has been argued that a low Scv_{O_2} in the setting of shock may be clinically relevant because it implies an even lower Sv_{O_2}.[124]

Oxygen delivery is the product of $\dot{Q}_T$ and arterial O_2 content, the latter being determined by the hemoglobin and arterial O_2 saturation (Sa_{O_2}). The body's O_2 consumption (V_{O_2}) is determined by the underlying metabolic activity of tissues and normally is independent of O_2 delivery.[125] Thus, as O_2 delivery falls, so too will Sv_{O_2} (Fig. 13-28). Therefore, measurement of Sv_{O_2} helps to assess the adequacy of O_2 delivery in relationship to tissue O_2 requirements. Under normal conditions, the $Sa_{O_2} - Sv_{O_2}$ difference is 20% to 25%, yielding an Sv_{O_2} of 65% to 75% when arterial blood is well oxygenated. An Sv_{O_2} in the normal range may be associated with very different levels of $\dot{Q}_T$ depending on underlying aerobic metabolism. For example, a "low" $\dot{Q}_T$ of 3 L/min may be entirely appropriate if metabolic activity is reduced, in which case the Sv_{O_2} would be normal. However, the same $\dot{Q}_T$ in association with a decrease in Sv_{O_2} would suggest inadequacy of either intravascular volume or cardiac function. Similarly, a low Sv_{O_2} despite a normal (or increased) $\dot{Q}_T$ indicates that the latter is inadequate to meet increased metabolic demands for O_2. In essence, the Sv_{O_2} helps to define the appropriateness of measured $\dot{Q}_T$.

Increased Sv_{O_2} may be seen in a variety of conditions. In sepsis, Sv_{O_2} is often normal, but in some cases there is extreme

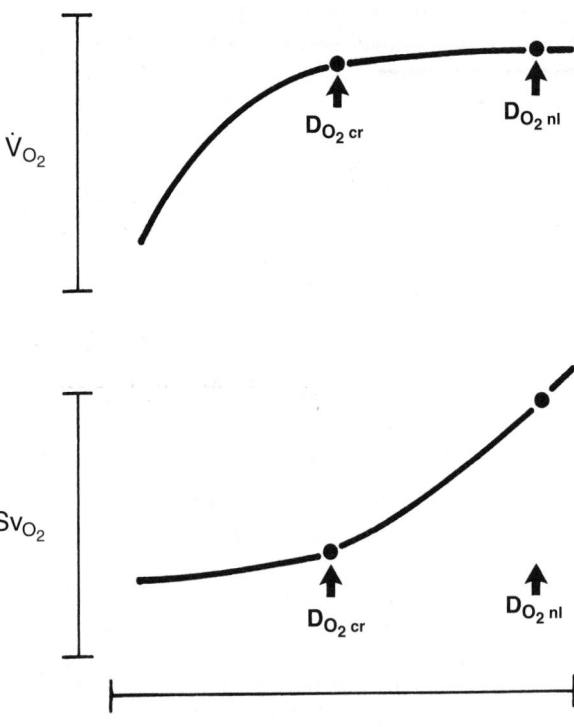

FIGURE 13-28 (*Upper panel*) Relationship between oxygen delivery (D_{O_2}) and oxygen consumption ($\dot{V}_{O_2}$). (*Lower panel*) Relationship between D_{O_2} and mixed venous O_2 saturation (Sv_{O_2}). Normally, $\dot{V}_{O_2}$ is independent of D_{O_2} until D_{O_2} falls to a critical value (D_{O_2cr}), at which point further reductions in D_{O_2} lead to reduced $\dot{V}_{O_2}$. Above D_{O_2cr}, the Sv_{O_2} and D_{O_2} are linearly related, but below D_{O_2cr}, the Sv_{O_2} does not change markedly as D_{O_2} falls (as long as Sa_{O_2} does not change).

peripheral vasodilation, and $\dot{Q}_T$ increases disproportionately to metabolic demands, resulting in an increase in Sv_{O_2}. Cirrhosis is one of the more common causes of a markedly increased Sv_{O_2}, with values occasionally in excess of 85%. A number of vasodilating agents and left-to-right cardiac shunts also result in an increase in Sv_{O_2}. Lastly, agents that interfere with mitochondial cytochrome activity (e.g., cyanide) may produce striking elevations in Sv_{O_2} owing to the inability of tissues to use O_2.

Continuous measurement of Sv_{O_2} with a fiberoptic PAC has been advocated as a useful technique for early detection of inadequate $\dot{Q}_T$ relative to tissue O_2 demand. If hemoglobin and Sa_{O_2} remain unchanged, then a reduction in Sv_{O_2} would predict either a primary reduction in $\dot{Q}_T$ or a rise in tissue O_2 requirement that is unmet by a compensatory increase in $\dot{Q}_T$. Theoretically, continuous Sv_{O_2} monitoring could lead to more rapid detection of hemodynamic instability than simple monitoring of blood pressure and heart rate, but it is unclear whether it has a significant impact on patient care.[126–128] Perhaps the most rational use of the fiberoptic PAC is in the management of patients with cardiac dysfunction, in whom rapid changes in $\dot{Q}_T$ may be expected to occur on the basis of the underlying disease process or in response to pharmacologic interventions. This would be particularly true when measurement of $\dot{Q}_{Ttd}$ has been documented to be erroneous in the setting of significant tricuspid regurgitation or as a result of markedly variable heart rhythm. In the latter circumstances, Sv_{O_2} assumes primary importance as an indicator of $\dot{Q}_T$, and continuous monitoring might prove more convenient than intermittent sampling from the catheter's distal lumen.

CLINICAL USE OF Sv_{O_2}

Use of the Sv_{O_2} may be a pivotal indicator of the adequacy of hemodynamic support. A low Sv_{O_2} in the absence of severe hypoxemia often indicates a deficiency of oxygen delivery relative to tissue O_2 needs and the need for augmentation of $\dot{Q}_T$ with volume loading or inotropic support or with red blood cell transfusion if anemia is present.[129] In contrast, a normal or high Sv_{O_2} does not necessarily indicate adequacy of oxygen delivery (as in sepsis), but the need to further augment $\dot{Q}_T$ in this setting is controversial.[129] A number of studies have evaluated the use of Sv_{O_2} in critical illness, but few have addressed important end points such as mortality or major morbidity. One randomized study reported decreased morbidity after cardiac surgery when therapy was targeted to achieve an Sv_{O_2} greater than 70% and a lactate level of less than 2 mg/dL.[130] In contrast, another study involving a more heterogeneous group of critically ill patients in the ICU found no clear benefit to goal-directed hemodynamic therapy based on the Sv_{O_2}.[131] However, it has been argued that the potential benefits of Sv_{O_2}-based hemodynamic resuscitation may be greater during the *early* management of critically ill patients.[124] While placement of a PAC to measure Sv_{O_2} is impractical during initial resuscitation, a recent study evaluated the use of vena caval O_2 saturation (Scv_{O_2}) obtained from central venous catheters placed in the emergency department in the early management of patients with severe sepsis.[132] Patients whose resuscitation was targeted to achieve an Scv_{O_2} of greater than 70% had significantly lower mortality than those randomized to conventional therapy based on mean arterial pressure and central venous pressure.[132]

Miscellaneous Diagnostic Applications of the PAC

Although the PAC is used primarily to aid in the management of fluids and vasoactive drug therapy during critical illness, it has additional applications that may be useful occasionally. These include microvascular cytology,[133] evaluation of arrhythmias,[34] detection of intracardiac shunts,[34] and determination of caloric requirements.[134,135]

Microvascular cytology of blood drawn through the distal port of the wedged PAC has been used to diagnose lymphangitic carcinoma.[133] It is unlikely that this technique will replace transbronchial biopsy as the initial diagnostic approach for this condition. However, very breathless patients with suspected lymphangitic carcinoma may tolerate insertion of a PAC better than bronchoscopy, and those with bleeding tendencies cannot undergo transbronchial biopsy safely.

Narrow-complex, regular tachyarrhythmias at a rate of 140 to 180 beats per minute are common in the ICU. It is sometimes difficult to differentiate atrial flutter from sinus tachycardia and paroxysmal supraventricular tachycardia, even with the aid of a 12-lead electrocardiogram. Although the response to adenosine is often the best way to define the underlying atrial rhythm, in some cases atrial flutter also may be diagnosed by

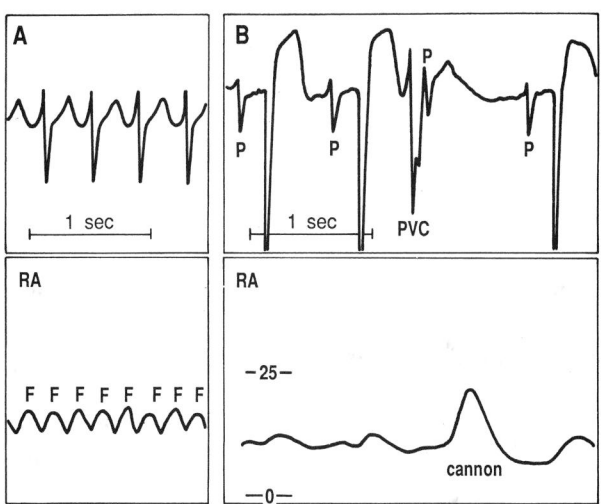

FIGURE 13-29 *A.* Surface electrocardiogram indicates a narrow-complex tachycardia (*top*) of uncertain nature. Simultaneous right atrial (RA) pressure tracing (*bottom*) shows mechanical flutter waves (*F*) at a rate exactly twice that of the ventricular response, indicating atrial flutter with a 2:1 block. *B.* Premature wide complex (PVC) beat (*top*) is defined as ventricular in origin by the presence of a cannon *a* wave in a simultaneous RA pressure tracing. (*Used with permission from Sharkey.*[34])

inspection of the Pra tracing[34] (Fig. 13-29*A*). The Pra tracing also may be of value in defining wide-complex premature beats as ventricular in origin if clear-cut cannon *a* waves are seen[34] (see Fig. 13-29*B*).

Intracardiac left-to-right shunts can occur between atria or ventricles. One of the more serious complications of myocardial infarction is acute perforation of the ventricular septum. Postinfarction ventricular septal defect is not diagnosed reliably by clinical examination. A ventricular septal defect is associated with a step-up in O_2 saturation from the right atrium to the pulmonary artery. In addition, the patient may be in shock despite a normal (or elevated) $\dot{Q}_{Ttd}$ because the latter measures right-sided rather than systemic flow. Both a ventricular septal defect and acute mitral regurgitation may present as postinfarction pulmonary edema with a new systolic murmur. A step-up in O_2 saturation from the right atrium to the pulmonary artery occasionally occurs in acute mitral regurgitation due to reflux of pulmonary venous blood into the pulmonary artery, and a ventricular septal defect occasionally produces a large *v* wave.[34] Differentiation of ventricular septal defect from acute mitral regurgitation by pressure waveform and O_2 saturation criteria could prove difficult, but Doppler echocardiography should clarify the diagnosis.

Fick-derived measurement of the volume of oxygen consumed (V_{O_2}) may be used to help guide nutritional support. Caloric needs are a function of overall metabolic activity, which in turn can be assessed by measuring V_{O_2}. Resting energy expenditure (REE) is the caloric intake required to meet ongoing metabolic demands. The Fick-derived estimate of REE is as follows: REE (kcal/d) = $V_{O_2} \times 7.0$, or REE = $\dot{Q}_T \times$ Hb $\times (Sa_{O_2} - Sv_{O_2}) \times 95$.[134] Prediction of REE by the Fick method, using PAC-derived data while assuming a respiratory quotient of 0.85, has been shown to correlate reasonably well with measurement of REE by indirect calorimetry.[135] While placement of a PAC solely for the purpose of assessing caloric needs would be inappropriate, it may be reasonable to use the available data to help guide nutritional support when a catheter is already in place.

References

1. Swan HJ, Ganz W, Forrester J, et al: Catheterization of the heart in man with use of a flow-directed balloon-tipped catheter. *N Engl J Med* 283:447, 1970.

2. Connors AF Jr, Castele RJ, Farhat NZ, et al: Complications of right heart catheterization: A prospective autopsy study. *Chest* 88:567, 1985.

3. Gore JM, Goldberg RJ, Spodick DH, et al: A community-wide assessment of the use of pulmonary artery catheters in patients with acute myocardial infarction. *Chest* 92:721, 1987.

4. Murdoch SD, Cohen AT, Bellamy MC: Pulmonary artery catheterization and mortality in critically ill patients. *Br J Anaesth* 85:611, 2000.

5. Vieillard-Baron A, Girou E, Valente E, et al: Predictors of mortality in acute respiratory distress syndrome: Focus on the role of right heart catheterization. *Am J Respir Crit Care Med* 161:1597, 2000.

6. Ivanov R, Allen J, Calvin JE: The incidence of major morbidity in critically ill patients managed with pulmonary artery catheters: A meta-analysis. *Crit Care Med* 28:615, 2000.

7. Mimoz O, Rauss A, Rekik N, et al: Pulmonary artery catheterization in critically ill patients: A prospective analysis of outcome changes associated with catheter-prompted changes in therapy. *Crit Care Med* 22:573, 1994.

8. Williams G, Grounds M, Rhodes A: Pulmonary artery catheter. *Curr Opin Crit Care* 8:251, 2002.

9. Rhodes A, Cusack RJ, Newman PJ, et al: A randomized controlled trial of the pulmonary artery catheter in critically ill patients. *Intensive Care Med* 28:256, 2002.

10. Sandham JD, Hull RD, Brant RF, et al: A randomized, controlled trial of the use of pulmonary-artery catheters in high-risk surgical patients. *N Engl J Med* 348:5, 2003.

11. Richard C, Warszawski J, Anguel N, et al: Early use of the pulmonary artery catheter and outcomes in patients with shock and acute respiratory distress syndrome: A randomized, controlled trial. *JAMA* 290: 2713, 2003.

12. Vincent JL, Dhainaut JF, Perret C, et al: Is the pulmonary artery catheter misused? A European view. *Crit Care Med* 26:1283, 1998.

13. Weil MH: The assault on the Swan-Ganz catheter: A case history of constrained technology, constrained bedside clinicians, and constrained monetary expenditures (comment).*Chest* 113:1379, 1998.

14. Gnaegi A, Feihl F, Perret C: Intensive care physicians' insufficient knowledge of right-heart catheterization at the bedside: Time to act? *Crit Care Med* 25:213, 1997.

15. Squara P. Bennett D. Perret C: Pulmonary artery catheter: Does the problem lie in the users? *Chest* 121:2009, 2002.

16. Papadakos PJ, Vender JS: Training requirements for pulmonary artery catheter utilization in adult patients. *New Horiz* 5:287, 1997.

17. Chaney JC. Derdak S: Minimally invasive hemodynamic monitoring for the intensivist: Current and emerging technology. *Crit Care Med* 30:2338, 2002.

18. Michard F, Teboul JL: Predicting fluid responsiveness in ICU patients: A critical analysis of the evidence. *Chest* 121:2000, 2002.

19. Layon AJ: The pulmonary artery catheter: Nonexistential entity or occasionally useful tool? *Chest* 115:859, 1999.

20. Tuman KJ, McCarthy RJ, Spiess BD, et al: Effect of pulmonary artery catheterization on outcome in patients undergoing coronary artery surgery. *Anesthesiology* 70:199, 1989.

21. Boyd O, Grounds RM, Bennett ED: A randomized clinical trial of the effect of deliberate perioperative increase of oxygen delivery on mortality in high-risk surgical patients. *JAMA* 270:2699, 1993.

22. Kaul S, Stratienko AA, Pollock SG, et al: Value of two-dimensional echocardiography for determining the basis of hemodynamic compromise in critically ill patients: A prospective study. *J Am Soc Echocardiogr* 7:598, 1994.

23. Boyd KD: A prospective study of complication of pulmonary artery catheterizations in 500 consecutive patients. *Chest* 84:245, 1983.

24. Shah KB, Rao TLK, Laughlin S, et al: A review of pulmonary artery catheterizations in 6245 patients. *Anesthesiology* 61:271, 1984.

25. Putterman CE: The Swan-Ganz catheter: A decade of hemodynamic monitoring. *J Crit Care* 4:127, 1989.

26. Morris D, Mulrihill D, Lew WYW: Risk of developing complete heart block during bedside pulmonary artery catheterization in patients with left bundle-branch block. *Arch Intern Med* 147:2005, 1987.

27. Chastre J, Corund F, Bouchoma A, et al: Thrombosis as a complication of pulmonary artery catheterization: Prospective evaluation by phlebography. *N Engl J Med* 306:278, 1982.

28. Fletcher EC, Mihalick MJ, Siegel CO: Pulmonary artery rupture during introduction of the Swan-Ganz catheter: Mechanism and prevention of injury. *J Crit Care* 3:116, 1988.

29. Poplausky MR, Rozenblit G, Rundback JH, et al: Swan-Ganz catheter-induced pulmonary artery pseudoaneurysm formation: Three case reports and a review of the literature. *Chest* 120:2105, 2001.

30. O'Quinn R, Marini JJ: Pulmonary artery occlusion pressure: Clinical physiology, measurement and interpretation. *Am Rev Respir Dis* 128:319, 1983.

31. Gardner RM: Direct blood pressure measurement-dynamic response requirements. *Anesthesiology* 54:227, 1981.

32. Gardner RM: Accuracy and reliability of disposable pressure transducers coupled with modern pressure monitors. *Crit Care Med* 24:879, 1996.

33. Findling R, Lipper B: Femoral vein pulmonary artery catheterization in the intensive care unit. *Chest* 105:874, 1994.

34. Sharkey SW: Beyond the wedge: Clinical physiology and the Swan-Ganz catheter. *Am J Med* 83:111, 1987.

35. Shuster DP, Seeman MD: Temporary muscle paralysis for accurate measurement of pulmonary artery occlusion pressure. *Chest* 84:593, 1983.

36. Marinelli WA, Weinert CR, Gross CR, et al: Right heart catheterization in acute lung injury: An observational study. *Am J Respir Crit Care Med* 160:69, 1999.

37. Forrester JS, Diamond G, McHugh TJ, Swan HJC: Filling pressures in the right and left sides of the heart in acute myocardial infarction. *N Engl J Med* 285:190, 1971.

38. Reuse C, Vincent JL, Pinsky MR: Measurements of right ventricular volumes during fluid challenge. *Chest* 1990:1450, 1990.

39. Magder S, Georgiadis G, Cheone T: Respiratory variations in right atrial pressure predict the response to fluid challenge. *J Crit Care* 7:76, 1992.

40. Thyrault M, Teboul JL, Richard C, et al: Relation between dicrotic notch and mean pulmonary artery pressure studied by using a Swan-Ganz catheter in critically ill patients. *Intensive Care Med* 24:77, 1998.

41. Cozzi PJ, Hall JB, Schmidt GA: Pulmonary diastolic-occlusion pressure gradient increased in acute pulmonary embolism. *Crit Care Med* 23:1481, 1995.

42. Enson Y, Schmidt DH, Ferrer MI, et al: The effect of acutely induced hypervolemia on resistance to pulmonary blood flow and pulmonary arterial compliance in patients with chronic obstructive lung disease. *Am J Med* 57:395, 1974.

43. Zapol WM, Snider MT, Rie MA, et al: Pulmonary circulation during adult respiratory distress syndrome, in Zapol WM, Falke

KJ (eds): *Acute Respiratory Failure*. New York, Marcel Dekker, 1985, p 241.

44. Naeije R: Pulmonary vascular resistance: A meaningless variable? *Intensive Care Med* 29:526, 2003.

45. Teboul J-L, Andrivet P, Ansquer M, et al: Bedside evaluation of the resistance of large and medium pulmonary veins in various lung diseases. *J Appl Physiol* 72:998, 1992.

46. Wilson RF, Beckman SB, Tyburski JG, et al: Pulmonary artery diastolic and wedge pressure relationships in critically ill and injured patients. *Arch Surg* 123:933, 1988.

47. Leatherman JW, Shapiro RS: Overestimation of pulmonary artery occlusion pressure in pulmonary hypertension due to partial occlusion. *Crit Care Med* 31:93, 2003.

48. Morris AH, Chapman RH: Wedge pressure confirmation by aspiration of pulmonary capillary blood. *Crit Care Med* 13:756, 1985.

49. Suter PM, Lindauer JM, Fairley HB, Schlobolym RM: Errors in data derived from pulmonary artery blood gas values. *Crit Care Med* 3:175, 1975.

50. Komadina KH, Schenk DA, LaVeau P, et al: Interobserver variability in the interpretation of pulmonary artery catheter pressure tracings. *Chest* 100:1647, 1991.

51. Al-Kharrat T, Zarich S, Amoateng-Adjepong Y, Manthous CA: Analysis of observer variability in measurement of pulmonary artery occlusion pressures. *Am J Respir Crit Care Med* 160:415, 1999.

52. Zarich S, Pust-Marcone J, Amoateng-Adjepong Y, et al: Failure of a brief educational program to improve interpretation of pulmonary artery occlusion pressure tracings. *Intensive Care Med* 26:698, 2000.

53. Bernard GR, Sopko G, Cerra F, et al: Pulmonary artery catheterization and clinical outcomes: National Heart, Lung, and Blood Institute and Food and Drug Administration workshop report. Consensus statement. *JAMA* 283:2568, 2000.

54. Silverman HJ, Eppler JH, Pitman AP, Patz D: Pulmonary artery wedge pressure measurements in patients on assisted ventilation. *J Crit Care* 2:115, 1987.

55. Hassan FM, Weiss WB, Braman SS, Hoppin FG: Influence of lung injury on pulmonary wedge-left atrial pressure correlation during positive end-expiratory pressure ventilation. *Am Rev Respir Dis* 131:246, 1985.

56. Teboul JL, Zapol WH, Brun-Buisson C, et al: A comparison of pulmonary artery occlusion pressure and left ventricular end-diastolic pressure during mechanical ventilation with PEEP in the patients with severe ARDS. *Anesthesiology* 70:266, 1989.

57. Teboul JL, Besbes M, Andrivet P, et al: A bedside index assessing the reliability of pulmonary artery occlusion pressure measurements during mechanical ventilation with positive end-expiratory pressure. *J Crit Care* 7:22, 1992.

58. Albert RK, Lamm WJ: Left atrial pressure can be accurately transmitted to the pulmonary artery despite zone 1 conditions. *Am J Respir Crit Care Med* 167:1016, 2003.

59. Shasby DM, Dauber JM, Pfister S, et al: Swan-Ganz location and left atrial pressure determine the accuracy of the wedge pressure when positive pressure, end-expiratory pressure is used. *Chest* 80:666, 1981.

60. Culver BH: Hemodynamic monitoring: Physiologic problems in interpretation, in Fallat RJ, Luce JM (eds): *Clinics in Critical Care Medicine*, Vol 14: *Cardiopulmonary Critical Care Management*. New York, Churchill Livingstone, 1988, p 165.

61. Cassidy SS, Schweip F: Cardiovascular effects of positive end-expiratory pressure, in Scharf SM, Cassidy SS (eds): *Heart-Lung Interaction in Health and Disease*. New York, Marcel Dekker, 1989, p 463.

62. Jardin F, Genevisy B, Brun-Ney D, Bourdarais JP: Influence of lung and chest wall compliances on transmission of airway pressure to the pleural space in critically ill patients. *Chest* 86:653, 1985.

63. Cassidy SS, Robertson CH, Pierce AK, et al: Cardiovascular effects of positive end-expiratory pressure in dogs. *J Appl Physiol* 44:743, 1978.

64. Pharnant JF, Devaux JY, Monsallier JF, et al: Mechanisms of decreased left ventricular preload during continuous positive pressure ventilation in ARDS. *Chest* 90:74, 1986.

65. Pinsky M, Vincent J-L, DeSmet J-M: Estimating left-ventricular filling pressure during positive end-expiratory pressure in humans. *Am Rev Respir Dis* 143:25, 1991.

66. Teboul JL, Pinsky MR, Mercat A, et al: Estimating cardiac filling pressure in mechanically ventilated patients with hyperinflation. *Crit Care Med* 28:3631, 2000.

67. Pepe PE, Marini JJ: Occult positive end-expiratory pressure in mechanically ventilated patients with airflow obstruction. *Am Rev Respir Dis* 126:166, 1982.

68. Rice DL, Chon KE, Gaasch WN, et al: Wedge pressure measurements in obstructive pulmonary disease. *Chest* 66:628, 1974.

69. Lessard MR, Lofaso F, Brochard L: Expiratory muscle activity increases intrinsic positive end-expiratory pressure independently of dynamic hyperinflation in mechanically ventilated patients. *Am J Resp Crit Care* 151:562, 1995.

70. Hoyt JD, Leatherman JW: Interpretation of the pulmonary artery occlusion pressure in mechanically ventilated patients. *Intensive Care Med* 23:1125, 1997.

71. Pichard AD, Kay R, Smith H, et al: Large *v* waves in the pulmonary wedge pressure tracing in the absence of mitral regurgitation. *Am J Cardiol* 50:1044, 1982.

72. Fuchs RM, Heuser RR, Yin FC, Brinker JA: Limitations of pulmonary wedge *v* waves in diagnosing mitral regurgitation. *Am J Cardiol* 49:849, 1982.

73. Sharkey SW: *A Guide to the Interpretation of Hemodynamic Data in the Coronary Care Unit*. Philadelphia, Lippincott-Raven, 1997, p 161.

74. Ferguson ND, Meade MO, Hallett DC, Stewart TE: High values of the pulmonary artery wedge pressure in patients with acute lung injury and acute respiratory distress syndrome. *Intensive Care Med* 28:1073, 2002.

75. Gaar KA, Taylor AI, Owens LJ, Guyfon AC: Pulmonary capillary pressure and filtration coefficient in the isolated perfused lung. *Am J Physiol* 213:910, 1967.

76. Palevsky HI, Pietra GG, Fishman AP: Pulmonary veno-occlusive disease and its response to vasodilator agents. *Am Rev Respir Dis* 142:426, 1990.

77. Cope DK, Grimbert F, Downey JM, Taylor AE: Pulmonary capillary pressure: A review. *Crit Care Med* 20:1043, 1992.

78. Collee GG, Lynch KE, Hill RD, Zapol WM: Bedside measurement of pulmonary capillary pressure in patients with acute respiratory failure. *Anesthesiology* 66:614, 1987.

79. Takala J: Pulmonary capillary pressure. *Intensive Care Med* 29:890, 2003.

80. Oppenheimer L, Goldberg HS: Pulmonary circulation and edema formation, in Scharf SM, Cassidy JS (eds): *Heart-Lung Intersection in Health and Disease*. New York, Marcel Dekker, 1987, p 93.

81. Braunwald E, Ross J Jr: Control of cardiac performance, in Berne RM, Sperelakis N, Geiger SR (eds): *Handbook of Physiology*, Sec 2: *The Cardiovascular System*, Vol. 1: *The Heart*. Bethesda, MD, American Physiological Society, 1979, p 533.

82. Boldt J, Lenz M, Kumle B, et al: Volume replacement strategies on ICUs: Results from a postal survey. *Intensive Care Med* 24:147, 1998.

83. Sibbald WJ, Driedger AA, Myers ML, et al: Biventricular function in the adult respiratory distress syndrome: Hemodynamic and radionuclide assessment, with special emphasis on right ventricular function. *Chest* 84:126, 1983.

84. Parker J, Case R: Normal left ventricular function. *Circulation* 60:4, 1979.

85. Packman MI, Rackow EC: Optimum left heart filling pressure during fluid resuscitation of patients with hypovolemic and septic shock. *Crit Care Med* 11:165, 1983.

86. Crexalls C, Chatterjee R, Forrester J, et al: Optimal level of filling pressure in the left side of the heart in acute myocardial infarction. *N Engl J Med* 289:1064, 1973.

87. Tavernier B, Makhotine O, Lebuffe G, et al: Systolic pressure variation as a guide to fluid therapy in patients with sepsis-induced hypotension. *Anesthesiology* 89:1313, 1998.

88. Michard F, Boussat S, Chemla D, et al. Relation between respiratory changes in arterial pulse pressure and fluid responsiveness in septic patients with acute circulatory failure. *Am J Respir Crit Care Med* 162:134, 2000.

89. Wagner JC, Leatherman JW: Right ventricular end-diastolic volume as a predictor of the hemodynamic response to a fluid challenge. *Chest* 113:1048, 1998.

90. Tousignant CP, Walsh F, Mazer CD: The use of transesophageal echocardiography for preload assessment in critically ill patients. *Anesth Analg* 90:351, 2000.

91. Magder S: More respect for the CVP. *Intensive Care Med* 24:651, 1998.

92. Reuse C, Vincent JL, Pinsky MR: Measurements of right ventricular volumes during fluid challenge. *Chest* 98:1450, 1990.

93. Diebel LN, Wilson RF, Tagett MG, et al: End-diastolic volume: A better indicator of preload in the critically ill. *Arch Surg* 127:817, 1992.

94. Schneider AJ, Teule GJJ, Groeneveld ABJ, et al: Biventricular performance during volume loading in patients with early septic shock, with emphasis on the right ventricle: A combined hemodynamic and radionuclide study. *Am Heart J* 116:103, 1988.

95. Bennett-Guerrero E, Kahn RA, Moskowitz DM, et al: Comparison of arterial systolic pressure variation with other clinical parameters to predict the response to fluid challenges during cardiac surgery. *Mt Sinai J Med* 69:96, 2002.

96. Feissel M, Michard F, Mangin I, et al: Respiratory changes in aortic blood velocity as an indicator of fluid responsiveness in ventilated patients with septic shock. *Chest* 119:867, 2001.

97. Magder S, Lagonidis D: Effectiveness of albumin vs normal saline as a test of volume responsiveness in post-cardiac surgery patients. *J Crit Care* 14:164, 1999.

98. Elkayam U, Berkley R, Azen S, et al: Cardiac output by thermodilution technique: Effect of injectate's volume and temperature on accuracy and reproducibility in the critically ill patient. *Chest* 84:418, 1981.

99. Stevens JH, Raffin TA, Milum FG, et al: Thermodilution cardiac output measurement: Effects of the respiratory cycle on its reproducibility. *JAMA* 253:2240, 1985.

100. Cigarroa RG, Lange RA, Williams RH, et al: Underestimation of cardiac output by thermodilution in patients with tricuspid regurgitation. *Am J Med* 86:417, 1989.

101. Balik M Effect of the degree of tricuspid regurgitation on cardiac output measurements by thermodilution. *Intensive Care Med* 28:1117, 2002.

102. Hoeper MM, Maier R, Tongers J, et al: Determination of cardiac output by the Fick method, thermodilution, and acetylene rebreathing in pulmonary hypertension. *Am J Respir Crit Care Med* 160:535, 1999.

103. Gonzalez J, Delafosse C Fartoukh M, et al: Comparison of bedside measurement of cardiac output with the thermodilution method and the Fick method in mechanically ventilated patients. *Crit Care* 7:171, 2003.

104. Yelderman ML, Ramsay MA, Quinn MD, et al: Continuous thermodilution cardiac output measurement in intensive care unit patients. *J Cardiothorac Vasc Anesth* 6:27, 1992.

105. Haller M, Zollner C, Briegel J, Forst H: Evaluation of a new continuous thermodilution cardiac output monitor in critically ill patients: A prospective criterion standard study. *Crit Care Med* 23:860, 1995.

106. Mihaljevic T, von Segesser LK, Tonz M, et al: Continuous versus bolus thermodilution cardiac output measurements: A comparative study. *Crit Care Med* 23:944, 1995.

107. Mets B, Frumento RJ, Bennett-Guerrero E, Naka Y: Validation of continuous thermodilution cardiac output in patients implanted with a left ventricular assist device. *J Cardiothorac Vasc Anesth* 16:727, 2002.

108. Gama de Abreu M, Quintel M, Ragaller M, et al: Partial carbon dioxide rebreathing: A reliable technique for noninvasive measurement of nonshunted pulmonary capillary blood flow. *Crit Care Med* 25:675, 1997.

109. Bernardin G, Tiger F, Fouche R, et al: Continuous noninvasive measurement of aortic blood flow in critically ill patients with a new esophageal echo-Doppler system. *J Crit Care* 13:177, 1998.

110. Valtier B, Cholley BP, Belot JP, et al: Noninvasive monitoring of cardiac output in critically ill patients using transesophageal Doppler. *Am J Respir Crit Care Med* 158:77, 1998.

111. Lefrant JY, Bruelle P, Aya AGM, et al: Training is required to improve the reliability of esophageal Doppler to measure cardiac output in critically ill patients. *Intensive Care Med* 24:347, 1998.

112. Raaijmakers E, Faes JC, Scholten RJ, et al: A meta-analysis of three decades of validating thoracic impedance cardiography. *Crit Care Med* 27:1203, 1999.

113. Van De Water JM, Miller TW, Vogel RL, et al: Impedance cardiography: The next vital sign technology? *Chest* 123:2028-33, 2003.

114. Sakka SG, Reinhart K, Wegscheider K, et al: Is the placement of a pulmonary artery catheter still justified solely for the measurement of cardiac output? *J Cardiothorac Vasc Anesth* 14:119, 2000.

115. Zollner C, Briegel J, Kilger E, et al: Retrospective analysis of transpulmonary and pulmonary arterial measurement of cardiac output in ARDS patients. *Anaesthesist* 47:912, 1998.

116. Zollner C, Haller M, Weis M, et al: Beat-to-beat measurement of cardiac output by intravascular pulse contour analysis: A prospective criterion standard study in patients after cardiac surgery. *J Cardiothorac Vasc Anesth* 14:125, 2000.

117. Jonas MM, Tanser SJ: Lithium dilution measurement of cardiac output and arterial pulse waveform analysis: An indicator dilution calibrated beat-by-beat system for continuous estimation of cardiac output. *Curr Opin Crit Care* 8:257, 2002.

118. Kurita T, Morita K, Kato S, et al: Comparison of the accuracy of the lithium dilution technique with the thermodilution technique for measurement of cardiac output. *Br J Anaesth* 79:770, 1997.

119. Leatherman JW, Schmitz PG: Fever, hyperdynamic shock, and multiple-system organ failure: A pseudo-sepsis syndrome associated with chronic salicylate intoxication. *Chest* 100:1391, 1991.

120. Sasse SA, Chen PA, Berry RB, et al: Variability of cardiac output over time in medical intensive care unit patients. *Crit Care Med* 22:225, 1994.

121. Stetz CW, Miller RG, Kelly GE, et al: Reliability of the thermodilution method in the determination of cardiac output in clinical practice. *Am Rev Respir Dis* 126:1001, 1982.

122. Sperinte JM, Senelly KM: The oximetrix opticath system: Theory and development, in Fahey PJ (ed): *Continuous Measurement of Blood Oxygen Saturation in the High Risk Patient,* Vol 2. San Diego, Beach International, 1985, p 59.

123. Lee J, Wright F, Barber R, Stanley L: Central venous oxygen saturation in shock. *Anesthesiology* 36:472, 1972.

124. Rivers EP, Ander DS, Powell D: Central venous oxygen saturation monitoring in the critically ill patient. *Curr Opin Crit Care* 7:204, 2001.

125. Russell JA, Phang TP: The oxygen delivery/consumption controversy: Approaches to management of the critically ill. *Am J Respir Crit Care Med* 149:533, 1994.

126. Jastremski MS, Chelluri L, Beney KM, Bailly RT: Analysis of the effects of continuous on-line monitoring of mixed venous

oxygen saturation on patient outcome and cost-effectiveness. *Crit Care Med* 17:148, 1989.

127. Vaugh S, Puri VK: Cardiac output changes and continuous mixed venous oxygen saturation measurement in the critically ill. *Crit Care Med* 16:495, 1988.

128. Rajput MA, Richey HM, Bush BA, et al: A comparison between a conventional and a fiberoptic flow-directed thermal dilution pulmonary artery catheter in critically ill patients. *Arch Intern Med* 149:83, 1989.

129. Vincent JL, De Backer D: Cardiac output measurement: Is least invasive always the best? *Crit Care Med* 30(10):2380, 2002.

130. Polonen P, Ruokonen E, Hippelainen M, et al: A prospective, randomized study of goal-oriented hemodynamic therapy in cardiac surgical patients. *Anesth Analg* 90:1052, 2000.

131. Gattinoni L, Brazzi L, Pelosi P, et al: A trial of goal-oriented hemodynamic therapy in critically ill patients: Sv_{O_2} Collaborative Group. *N Engl J Med* 333:1025, 1995.

132. Rivers EP, Nguyen HB: Goal-directed therapy for severe sepsis. *N Engl J Med* 345:1368, 2001.

133. Masson RG, Krikorian J, Luke P, et al: Pulmonary vascular cytology in the diagnosis of lymphangitic carcinomatosis. *N Engl J Med* 321:71, 1989.

134. Liggett SB, St John RE, Lefrak SS: Determination of resting energy expenditure utilizing the thermodilution pulmonary artery catheter. *Chest* 91:562, 1987.

135. Smithies MN, Royston B, Makita K, et al: Comparison of oxygen consumption measurements: Indirect calorimetry versus the reversed Fick method. *Crit Care Med* 19:1401, 1991.

Chapter 14 _____

PAIN CONTROL, SEDATION, AND USE OF MUSCLE RELAXANTS

BRIAN GEHLBACH

JOHN P. KRESS

KEY POINTS

- *Sedatives and analgesics used commonly in the care of critically ill patients often exhibit pharmacokinetics and pharmacodynamics that are significantly different when compared with studies of their use in other arenas, such as the operating room. Knowledge of these differences is crucial to designing a sedation protocol for the critically ill patient.*

- *While the administration of sedatives and analgesics to the critically ill patient is indicated for a variety of conditions ranging from relief of suffering to facilitation of lung protective strategies of mechanical ventilation, continued reassessment of the need for and means of providing sedation is necessary to prevent the prolongation of mechanical ventilation.*

- *Intravascular catheters, endotracheal intubation, suctioning, immobility, and underlying illnesses all may cause pain in the critically ill patient. While physical remedies always should be tried—e.g., repositioning a patient to alleviate arthritic pain—most patients require intravenous narcotics at least initially. Thus adequate sedation begins with adequate analgesia.*

- *Regional pain control techniques, such as with epidural catheter–administered anesthetics or opiates, can be highly effective at achieving pain control in the postoperative patient. The placement and removal of such catheters require correction of any underlying coagulation abnormalities in order to reduce the risk of epidural hematoma.*

- *The evaluation of sedation adequacy can only be performed at the bedside and is facilitated by the use of a validated sedation scale, such as the Richmond Agitation-Sedation Scale, along with a protocol for the systematic assessment and administration of sedatives and analgesics.*

- *Although both continuous and intermittent bolus strategies for sedative administration have been advocated, the two strategies have not been compared directly in a large, randomized, controlled trial. Regardless of the approach used, most patients require larger doses of sedatives—sometimes in excess of drug manufacturer guidelines—in the initial 48 hours than subsequently. Thus the level of sedation must be reassessed continuously and a protocol for downward titration of sedation applied.*

- *If continuous administration is used, daily sedative interruption is recommended to prevent drug accumulation, allow the performance of a neurologic examination, and permit reassessment of the need for sedation. If resedation is required, restarting the infusion at half the previous dose, with subsequent titration as necessary, is a useful strategy for systematic downward titration.*

- *Prolonged (>24 h) neuromuscular blockade should be used as a last resort owing to the high incidence of neuromuscular complications associated with this practice in critically ill patients. In particular, the administration of these agents in combination with high-dose corticosteroids is discouraged.*

Administration of analgesics and sedatives is commonplace in the ICU. Unfortunately, many early studies of analgesic and sedative medications were performed in the operating room, a setting very different from the ICU. The clinician must recognize the diverse and often unpredictable effects of critical illness on the pharmacokinetics and pharmacodynamics of sedatives and analgesics. Failure to recognize these effects may lead to inadequate or excessive sedation. Sedatives and analgesics may cause prolonged alterations in mental status and may mask the development of coincident complications of critical illness. Data studying the effects of analgesia and sedation in the ICU have accumulated in the last decade and have had important influences on this aspect of critical care. As outcomes data have become available, analgesia and sedation practices driven by protocol guidelines have emerged.

Indications for Sedation and Analgesia

Analgesia and sedation needs vary widely in ICU patients. Although nonpharmacologic means such as comfortable positioning in bed and verbal reassurance should be considered initially, treatment with analgesic and sedative agents frequently is needed. An effective approach to the use of analgesics and sedatives in critically ill patients begins with an understanding of the various indications for their use in this setting. Effective *analgesia* is extremely important and is discussed in detail in a later section of this chapter. *Dyspnea* is common in ICU patients and may be a source of distress. Excessive coughing may contribute to patient-ventilator dyssynchrony. Opiates may alleviate dyspnea and coughing, particularly in intubated patients. *Excessive oxygen consumption* (V_{O_2}) and related *carbon dioxide production* (V_{CO_2}) may be detrimental in patients with respiratory failure or shock, and restoration of the delicate balance of oxygen delivery and consumption is important in the management of these patients. Oxygen consumption in intubated patients who are agitated can be reduced by 15% after administration of sedatives and opiates.[1] For those with shock or severe hypoxemic respiratory failure, this reduction in oxygen consumption may be important for cardiopulmonary stability. The importance of *amnesia* during critical illness is not well understood. Although it may seem intuitive that amnesia for the period of critical illness is desirable, data supporting this notion are lacking. Certainly it seems logical that amnesia for short periods (e.g., during unpleasant interventions such as bronchoscopy) may be desirable; however, there are some data suggesting that complete amnesia for prolonged periods (e.g., for the entire period of mechanical ventilation) may be detrimental.[2–4] As discussed later, it is certain that complete amnesia is mandatory during the administration of neuromuscular blocking agents. *Delirium*—an acutely changing or fluctuating mental status, inattention, disorganized thinking, and an altered level of consciousness that may or may not be accompanied by agitation—is common in ICU patients.[5] Some patients may manifest an aggressive type of delirious behavior. This delirium may occur as a result of medications, sepsis, fevers, encephalopathy (e.g., hepatic or renal), paranoia, or withdrawal syndromes (alcohol, tobacco, or illicit drugs). Agitated delirium often responds well to neuroleptic medications such as haloperidol.[6] More commonly, ICU patients exhibit a hypoactive, quiet form of delirium. There is no currently established pharmacologic therapy for hypoactive delirium, although sedative medications are likely to exacerbate rather than alleviate the problem.

Analgesia

It is undeniable that pain is a common experience for most ICU patients.[7–9] Failure to recognize that pain frequently leads to agitation may lead to inappropriate administration of nonanalgesic sedatives. Accordingly, an aggressive approach to managing pain has been strongly recommended by published consensus opinions regarding sedation in the ICU.[6,10] Addressing analgesic needs frequently poses a challenge to the critical care clinician. The ability to discern pain accurately may be difficult because many clinical parameters such as changes in vital signs are sensitive but not specific indicators. There are numerous reasons for pain in the ICU patient. While causes such as surgical incisions or trauma may be obvious, other causes such as endotracheal suctioning or invasive catheters may be less apparent. Other causes of pain include pain from preexisting diseases (e.g., vertebral compression fractures from multiple myeloma), endotracheal tubes, and prolonged immobility during bed rest.[7,11]

Pain may result in many adverse effects, including increased endogenous catecholamine activity, myocardial ischemia, hypercoagulability, hypermetabolic states, sleep deprivation, anxiety, and delirium.[12] Adequate analgesia may diminish some of these detrimental effects.[13]

It is sobering to note that pain is treated inadequately in many different medical care settings,[14] including the critical care unit.[15,16] Ineffective communication with patients is sometimes at the root of this problem because delirium in the ICU is a common occurrence.[5] Concern over addiction to opiates,[17] adverse cardiopulmonary effects of analgesics, and arbitrary limits placed on drug doses may be other reasons for inadequate analgesia in the ICU.

Certainly, the assessment of pain in critically ill patients can be challenging. As mentioned earlier, even the recognition of pain in these patients may be impaired by communication problems because many are intubated and/or delirious. Tools to categorize pain, such as scales or scoring systems, may be beneficial. In general, simpler scales are more effective because communication for many ICU patients is limited. The Visual Analogue Scale (VAS) has been found to have very good reliability and validity,[18,19] although it has not been evaluated specifically in critically ill patients. This scale is a self-report measure of pain intensity that typically consists of a 10-cm line on paper with verbal anchors ("no pain" and "severe pain") on the ends. A similar scale is the Numeric Rating Scale. This scale also consists of a horizontal line with numeric markings 1 and 10 anchoring either extreme of the pain intensity scale.[20,21] It may be preferred because it can be completed by writing, speaking, or hand gestures and may be better across various age groups.[6]

Previous studies have shown that benzodiazepines may enhance the analgesic effects of opiates[22,23] and that opiate requirements are decreased in patients sedated with benzodiazepines rather than propofol.[1,24] Notwithstanding this interesting observation, it is imperative that sedative agents are not used in the place of analgesics.

Although nonpharmacologic analgesic strategies are worth considering, they are frequently ineffective in dealing with pain in ICU patients. Nevertheless, malpositioning of invasive catheters (e.g., endotracheal tube impinging on the main carina) is a problem that may be remedied easily. Likewise, optimal patient positioning in bed may relieve at least in part low back pain, pain from chest tubes, etc. Despite appropriate attention to nonpharmacologic approaches, most patients require administration of some pharmacologic agents, with opiates being the mainstay of therapy. Strategies for administration include continuous infusions and intermittent dosing strategies. Among the intermittent dosing strategies are scheduled intermittent opiate administration, administration on an "as needed" or prn basis, and patient-controlled analgesic (PCA) strategies. Strategies given "as needed" are discouraged because of fluctuations between inadequate and excessive analgesia that are seen frequently. Intravenous rather than intramuscular injection is the preferred route of administration because intramuscular injections themselves may be painful, and absorption of a drug given intramuscularly is frequently sporadic in critically ill patients. Patients alert enough to respond to their own pain needs may benefit from PCA strategies. Transdermal opiates may be continued in patients who are chronically receiving such medications; however, absorption is often unreliable during critical illness. Therefore, this route should not be used for treating acute pain in the ICU; conversion to transdermal medications toward the end of a bout of critical illness is sometimes a reasonable approach. Clearly, intravenous injection remains the preferred route.

Opiate withdrawal can be seen in patients receiving opiates for extended periods when the drugs are discontinued suddenly. Patients who abuse opiates are at risk for this when hospitalized during critical illness. The signs and symptoms seen in withdrawal are mostly nonspecific and include pupillary dilation, sweating, lacrimation, rhinorrhea, piloerection, tachycardia, vomiting, diarrhea, hypertension, yawning, fever, tachypnea, restlessness, irritability, increased sensitivity to pain, nausea, cramps, muscle aches, dysphoria, insomnia, symptoms of opioid craving, and anxiety.[25] The lack of specificity for many of these signs and symptoms may make it difficult to establish a diagnosis of opiate withdrawal in critically ill patients. Patients without previous illicit drug use also may experience opiate withdrawal when pharmacologically administered opiates given for extended periods are stopped suddenly. Whether downward titration of opiate doses or regular interruption of opiate administration can prevent this is not known. One study of trauma/surgical ICU patients reported a 32% incidence of withdrawal in patients receiving opiates and/or sedatives who were in the ICU for more than 1 week.[25] Those manifesting withdrawal received higher opiate and benzodiazepine drug doses than their counterparts who did not experience withdrawal. The role of long-acting opiates such as methadone to overcome this problem has not been studied.

REGIONAL TECHNIQUES FOR ANALGESIA

EPIDURAL ANALGESIA

Regional analgesic techniques may be effective strategies, particularly for postoperative analgesia. Epidural administration of pharmacologic agents is an alternative approach to systemic administration. Local anesthetics may be used to block sensory nerve transmission. Autonomic nerves are more sensitive to local anesthetics than sensory nerves. Therefore, loss of sympathetic vascular tone is common with epidural local anesthetics. Motor nerves are most resistant to epidural local anesthetics.   *autonomic nerves > sensitive > motor*

Ideally, an epidural catheter is placed at the spinal level that is at the same level as the pain source. For example, thoracic epidural catheters frequently are used for patients undergoing thoracic surgical procedures to optimize the ability to cough and deep breathe after surgery. Although any local anesthetic may be used, bupivacaine is the most commonly used drug because of its long duration of action and preferential blockade of sensory over motor neurons. A relatively dilute, high-volume concentration of local anesthetic is preferred (e.g., bupivacaine 0.125% to 0.25%) because of spread over a wider dermatomal distribution. However, recent studies have reported that high-concentration, low-volume dosing regimens may produce similar analgesia and patient satisfaction but less profound motor block and improved hemodynamic stability.[26] Continuous infusions of local anesthetic are typically used, which may provide effective analgesia for days.

Side Effects

Although central neuroaxial blockade is an extremely effective analgesic technique, side effects such as hypotension may limit its use in critically ill patients. Inevitably, there is some sympathetic blockade with administration of local anesthetics for central neuroaxial block. The resulting venodilation and increase in venous capacitance produces a relative hypovolemia. Accordingly, patients are routinely given crystalloid prior to administration of epidural (or spinal) local anesthetics. Obviously, patients with hemodynamic instability (e.g., septic or hemorrhagic shock) may not tolerate decreases in sympathetic tone. Sympathetic blockade at a high level may block outflow from the so-called cardiac accelerator fibers at the T1–T4 levels. The resulting bradycardia may further compromise hemodynamic stability. Drugs for treating hemodynamic instability after central neuroaxial blockade include ephedrine (alpha and beta agonist, 5 to 10 mg), epinephrine (10 to 100 μg), and atropine (0.4 mg). Genitourinary blockade (parasympathetic S2–S4) with resulting urinary retention is problematic occasionally in patients without bladder catheters.

Complications

Epidural hematoma formation is a rare but potentially devastating complication of central neuroaxial blockade. Although exact cutoff values precluding this approach in patients with coagulation disturbances are not known, platelet counts less than 50,000/μL or international normalized ratios above 2 generally are considered absolute contraindications. There is controversy regarding lesser degrees of coagulation abnormalities because of the lack of outcomes data; however, a conservative approach—where a normal coagulation state is required—is typically adhered to by most clinicians. The use of prophylactic heparin has been linked to epidural or spinal hematoma formation.[27] Such case reports have led to recommendations that when prophylactic or low-molecular weight heparin (LMWH) is used perioperatively, neuroaxial block should be delayed for 10 to 12 hours after the last dose.[28] Indeed, most recommend leaving existing epidural catheters in place in patients with coagulation abnormalities until these problems are corrected. In 1997, the Food and Drug Administration (FDA) issued a public health advisory regarding reports of epidural or spinal hematomas with the concurrent use of LMWH and spinal-epidural anesthesia or lumbar puncture.[29] Fortunately, the incidence of complications from epidural anesthesia is extremely low. A study of over 4000 patients scheduled for abdominal or abdominothoracic surgery reported a predicted maximum risk for permanent neurologic complications from epidural placement of 0.07%.[30] An epidural hematoma may be difficult to detect in a critically ill patient. New motor deficits and back pain are the most common early signs. Ideally, an awake, interactive patient is preferred so that serial neurologic examinations can be performed, facilitating early detection.

Epidural catheter infection is another rare complication. Avoiding placement of catheters through inflamed or infected skin is mandatory and certainly will reduce this complication risk. Careful, frequent assessments of skin entry sites and catheter dressings are an important part of the care of these catheters. Some clinicians advise against placement of these catheters in patients with bacteremia or sepsis, although there is some controversy surrounding this recommendation owing to a paucity of outcomes data. Exact guidelines for the use of epidural analgesia in critical illness have not been established. Indeed, it is clear that there is wide practice variation regarding the use of this technique in critically ill patients.[31]

NEUROAXIAL OPIATE ANALGESIA   *Morphine vs fentanyl*

Opiates also are used frequently for neuroaxial analgesia. The presence of opiate receptors in the spinal cord was noted over 25 years ago,[32,33] and spinal opiate-mediated analgesia is currently a mainstay of regional anesthesia. Opiate receptors found on the dorsal region of the spinal cord (substantia gelatinosa) mediate analgesia. Analgesia is profound and prolonged with water-soluble opiates such as morphine. Lipid-soluble opiates such as fentanyl have a more rapid onset than morphine but a shorter duration. A single dose of epidural fentanyl may last 2 to 4 hours, whereas a single dose of epidural morphine typically lasts 16 to 24 hours. Accordingly, fentanyl usually is given by continuous infusion through epidural catheters. Neuroaxial opiates also can be given by intrathecal routes. Much smaller doses are needed when opiates are given intrathecally—typically 10 percent of the epidural dose is adequate. Opiates given by neuroaxial routes produce effective analgesia with less alteration in mental status than systemic opiates. The analgesia tends to be distributed dermatomally in the region of the spinal cord where the drug is administered when lipid-soluble drugs such as fentanyl are used. On the other hand, water-soluble drugs such as morphine tend to move rostrally regardless of the spinal cord level of injection. Importantly, when lipid-soluble neuroaxial opiates are used, the injection site must be at the same level as the pain source (e.g., thoracic epidural after thoracic surgery). There is controversy over the benefits of epidural versus intravenous fentanyl analgesia. Some studies have reported similar outcomes when these two strategies are compared,[34] whereas others have reported more effective analgesia with thoracic epidural fentanyl.[35,36] In thoracic surgery patients, epidural fentanyl has been associated with better preservation of respiratory function compared with intravenous fentanyl. These salutary effects may be related to the catheter being located near the source of pain.

Sedation

While pain is certainly a cause for anxiety in most ICU patients, many patients suffer from anxiety despite adequate analgesia. It is obvious that a state of critical illness and dependence on others for care can invoke anxiety. Accordingly, sedation strategies must recognize and respond to this problem.

ASSESSING ADEQUACY OF SEDATION

Assessing adequacy of sedation can be difficult because of its subjective nature. Several sedation scales such as the Ramsay Sedation Score[37] (Table 14-1), the Sedation Agitation Scale (SAS),[38] and most recently, the Richmond Agitation-Sedation Scale (RASS)[39] (Table 14-2) have been developed. The Ramsay scoring system is the most frequently referenced in clinical investigations of sedation. While it has the benefit of simplicity, it does not effectively measure quality or degree of sedation with regard to the goals outlined earlier[40] and has never been validated objectively.[41] Sedation scales such as the Sedation Agitation Scale and the Richmond Agitation-Sedation Scale have been tested extensively for validity and reliability.[38,39,42] The RASS is perhaps the most extensively evaluated scale. It has been validated for ability to detect changes in sedation status over consecutive days of ICU care, as well as against constructs of level of consciousness and delirium. Furthermore, this scale has been shown to correlate with doses of sedative and analgesic medications administered to critically ill patients. As such, the RASS and SAS are preferable over the traditional Ramsay Sedation Score.

The evaluation of sedation adequacy remains an individual bedside maneuver. The nurse's input is critical because

TABLE 14-1 Ramsay Sedation Score

1. Patient anxious and agitated or restless or both
2. Patient cooperative, oriented, and tranquil
3. Patient responds to commands only
4. Patient asleep, shows brisk response to light glabellar tap or loud auditory stimulus
5. Patient asleep, shows sluggish response to light glabellar tap or loud auditory stimulus
6. Patient asleep, shows no response to light glabellar tap or loud auditory stimulus

SOURCE: Adapted with permission from Ramsay et al.[37]

TABLE 14-2 Richmond Agitation-Sedation Scale

Score	Term	Description
+4	Combative	Overtly combative/violent; danger to staff
+3	Very agitated	Pulls/removes tubes or catheters; aggressive
+2	Agitated	Nonpurposeful movement; not synchronous with ventilator
+1	Restless	Anxious, but movements not aggressive/violent
0	Alert and calm	
−1	Drowsy	Sustained awakening (>10 s) with eye contact, to voice
−2	Light sedation	Briefly awakens (<10 s) with eye contact, to voice
−3	Moderate sedation	Movement to voice, but no eye contact
−4	Deep sedation	No response to voice; movement to physical stimulation
−5	Unarousable	No response to voice or physical stimulation

Procedure:
Observe patient. Calm? (score zero) Does patient have restless or agitated behavior? (1 to 4)

SOURCE: Adapted with permission from Sessler et al.[39]

he or she often will notice changes from an optimal level of sedation. Armed with validated sedation scales, clinicians may strive to administer sedatives and analgesics to more concrete, reportable levels. Ideally, one would prefer a patient whose indications for sedation as outlined earlier are met yet who remains fully communicative with bedside caregivers. Such a state of sedation correlates with a Ramsay score of 2 or 3, a Sedation Agitation Scale score of 3 or 4, or a RASS score of 0 or −1.[37–39] This state of being awake and communicative while sedatives are still infusing is achievable in some patients. However, in many patients the stress of critical illness precludes such a condition, and patients may require sedation and analgesia to a point where constant communication is not possible.

Recently, the Bispectral Index Monitor, a device that processes the raw electroencephalogram (EEG) signal into a discreet scaled number from 0 (absence of cortical activity) to 100 (fully awake), has been evaluated as a tool to monitor sedation in the ICU setting. Some have found this device to reliably detect a patient's level of consciousness under general anesthesia,[43] although others have questioned the overall utility of this device for preventing awareness.[44] Preliminary data suggest a reasonable correlation between the bispectral index and the sedation agitation scale,[45] as well as the RASS[42]; however, this device has not been evaluated extensively in the ICU and awaits more extensive validation before its role in the critical care setting is established.[6]

Recently, the occurrence of delirium in mechanically ventilated ICU patients has been shown to be associated with higher six-month mortality even after adjusting for severity of illness and the use of sedatives or analgesic medications.[45a] How to decrease the risk of delirium in critically ill patients, and the impact of such a strategy on overall outcome, is not known. The Confusion Assessment Method for diagnosing delirium has been modified for the ICU (the CAM-ICU) and has been validated (see chapter 62).[45b]

STRATEGIES FOR ADMINISTERING SEDATIVES IN THE ICU

Since no single drug can achieve all the indications for sedation and analgesia in the ICU, a combination of drugs, each titrated to specific end points, is a more effective strategy. This may allow lower doses of individual drugs and reduce problems of drug accumulation. In the ICU, sedatives and analgesics almost always are administered by the intravenous route. Both continuous infusion and intermittent bolus techniques have been advocated. While continuous infusions of sedatives may reduce rapid fluctuations in the level of sedation, accumulation of drugs resulting in prolongation of mechanical ventilation and ICU stay has been described.[46] Intermittent administration of sedatives and analgesics may increase demands on nursing time, potentially distracting attention away from other patient care issues. Other perceived benefits of continuous sedative infusions include a more consistent level of sedation with greater levels of patient comfort. The convenience of this strategy for both patients and caregivers is likely the greatest reason for its popularity.

Ideally, strategies for sedation and analgesia in critically ill patients should adhere to pharmacokinetic and pharmacodynamic principles. Unfortunately, ICU patients frequently exhibit unpredictable alterations in pharmacology,[47] so precise guidelines for drug administration are not possible. For instance, when "short acting" benzodiazepines[48,49] such as midazolam and lorazepam are administered in the ICU, these drugs accumulate in tissue (especially adipose) stores with a resulting prolonged clinical effect.[24,46,50–52] Other circumstances that confound prediction of the pharmacologic behavior of sedatives and analgesics include altered hepatic and/or renal function,[53] polypharmacy in the ICU with complex drug-drug interactions, altered protein binding, and circulatory instability. The multicompartmental pharmacokinetics typical in critically ill patients defy simple bedside pharmacokinetic profiling. As such, titration of sedatives and analgesics against discernible clinical end points, while imprecise, is the only tool available. Further confounding administration of sedatives in the ICU is the dramatic difference between extremes of sedation. Frequently, oversedated patients are easier to manage than undersedated patients, and in an effort to avoid unmanageable agitation, clinicians may be heavy handed when sedating agitated patients. In the initial stages of critical illness, such as the period immediately following intubation and mechanical ventilation, this may be appropriate; however, maintaining deep levels of sedation after patients are stabilized on mechanical ventilation can lead to the problems of prolonged sedation alluded to earlier.

It is not uncommon for some critically ill patients to require extraordinarily high doses of sedatives to achieve tranquility; such doses may be much greater than quoted in the literature and recommended by drug manufacturers.[54] Indeed, occasional patients may even require pharmacologic paralysis to achieve synchrony with mechanical ventilation.[55]

Recently, evidence-based treatment strategies for many common conditions seen in critical illness have emerged.

In the last decade, improved outcomes for critically ill patients with acute respiratory distress syndrome (ARDS),[56] sepsis,[57,58] acute renal failure,[59] status asthmaticus,[60] and cancer[61] all have been reported. As sicker patients continue to demonstrate improved outcomes in the ICU, more aggressive levels of sedation and analgesia may be necessary. This is particularly likely for patients managed with unconventional ventilator strategies (e.g., permissive hypercapnia, low tidal volumes, prone positioning, and pressure-controlled ventilation) because these strategies may be inherently distressing to many patients. For selected patients, deep sedation may be the only practical option.

The use of deep sedation carries a heavy price because the neurologic examination is severely limited in these patients. Ideally, a head-to-toe daily assessment for the presence of organ failure should be routine for every critically ill patient. This is particularly so during resuscitative phases of ICU care, when assessing the adequacy of end-organ perfusion and function is of paramount importance. The mental status examination is an important gauge of brain perfusion. Since brain injury is a devastating complication of critical illness, acute cerebral dysfunction must be detected quickly and corrected, if possible, before permanent injury takes place. The veil of sedation severely handicaps a clinician's ability to serially follow a patient's neurologic condition. Communication and thorough physical examination may detect problems early on and obviate urgent diagnostic studies and therapeutic interventions after a problem has advanced.

A protocol-driven approach to sedation has been shown to alleviate many of the problems mentioned earlier. A protocol directed by bedside nurses can shorten the duration of mechanical ventilation, ICU and hospital length of stay, and the need for tracheostomy[62] (Fig. 14-1). Such protocols ensure adequate analgesia and sedation using frequent assessments of patient needs with goal-directed titration of analgesics and sedatives. Alternatively, a routine protocol of daily interruption of continuous sedative infusions can reduce many of the complications of sedation in the ICU setting, including duration of mechanical ventilation and ICU length of stay[24,24a] (Figs. 14-2 and 14-3). Such a strategy allows patients to spend a substantial portion of their ICU time awake and interactive, potentially reducing the amount of sedative and opiate given, as well as reducing the need for diagnostic studies (e.g., brain CT scan) to evaluate unexplained alterations in mental status.

Such protocol-driven sedation strategies allow a focused downward titration of sedative infusion rates over time, streamlining administration of these drugs and minimizing the tendency for accumulation. Protocol-driven sedation may allow the depth of sedation to be decreased without compromising the stated goals of sedation. This strategy may allow clinicians to minimize sedative accumulation. Initially, the thought of decreasing or stopping sedatives in a critically ill patient who has been agitated may be unsettling. As such, clinicians may sedate patients aggressively early in their ICU course and maintain the same level of deep sedation indefinitely. A daily holiday from sedatives can eliminate the tendency to "lock in" to a high sedative infusion rate, which—while appropriate early in ICU care—may be unnecessary on subsequent days. When sedative infusions are decreased or stopped, tissue stores can redistribute drug

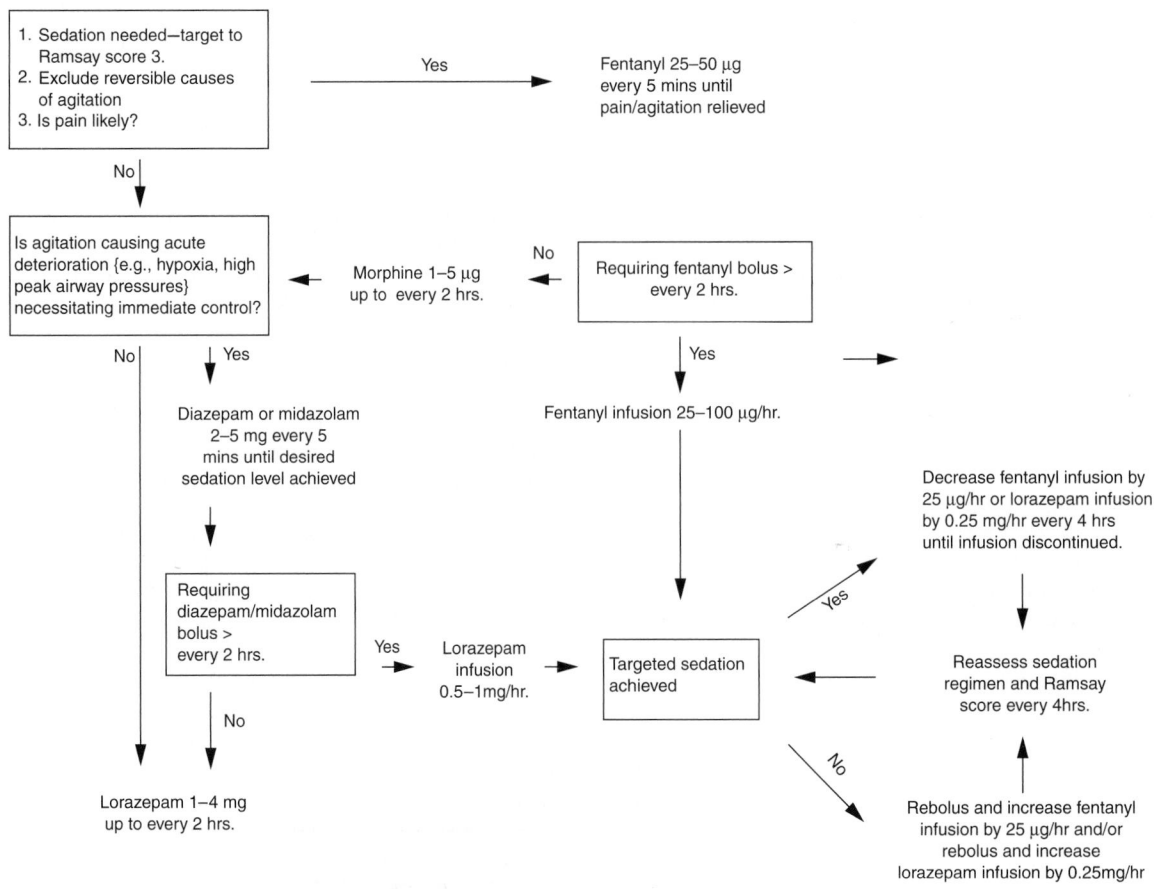

FIGURE 14-1 Protocol for nursing management of sedation during mechanical ventilation. (*Used with permission from Brook et al.*[62])

back into the circulation. The interruption of sedative infusions sometimes may lead to abrupt awakening and agitation. This must be anticipated by the ICU team to avoid complications such as patient self-extubation; if excessive agitation is noted, sedatives should be restarted. Although the attempt

at waking and communicating with a patient may fail on a given day, this does not portend inevitable failure on all subsequent days. When awakening patients from sedation, one need only bring patients to the brink of consciousness—able to follow simple commands (i.e., open eyes, squeeze hand,

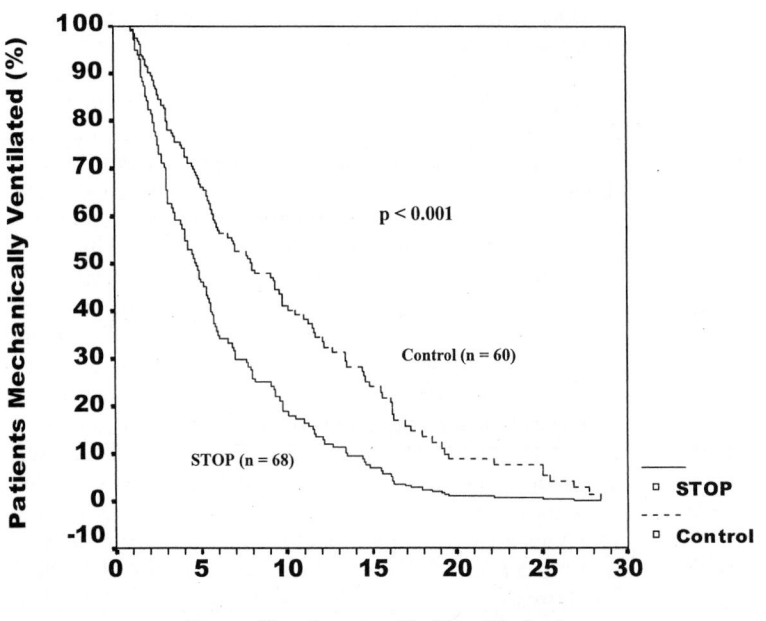

FIGURE 14-2 Kaplan–Meier analysis of the duration of mechanical ventilation, according to study group. After adjustment for base-line variables (age, sex, weight, APACHE II score, and type of respiratory failure), mechanical ventilation was discontinued earlier in the STOP group than in the control group (relative risk of extubation, 1.9; 95 percent confidence interval 1.3 to 2.7; $P < 0.001$).

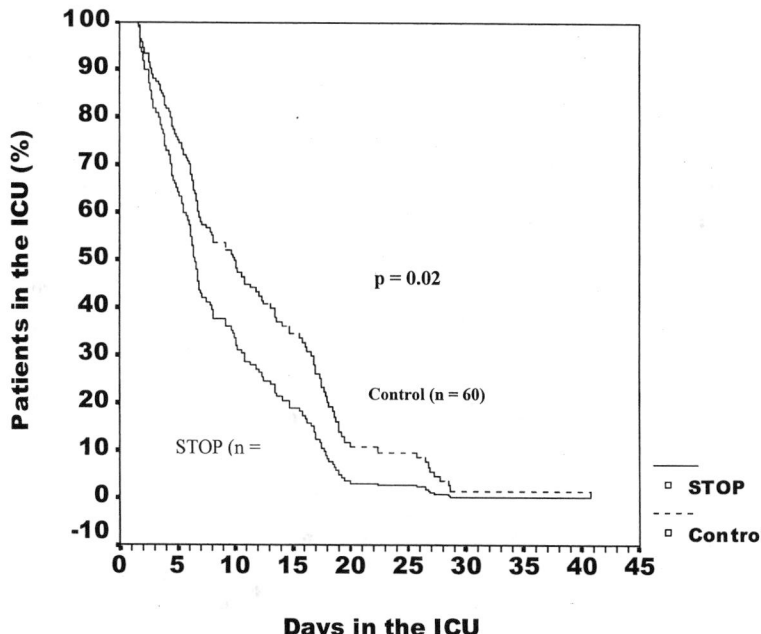

FIGURE 14-3 Kaplan–Meier analysis of the length of stay in the intensive care unit (ICU), according to study group. After adjustment for base-line variables (age, sex, weight, APACHE II score, and type of respiratory failure), discharge from the intensive care unit (ICU) occurred earlier in the STOP group than in the control group (relative risk of discharge, 1.6; 95 percent confidence interval, 1.1 to 2.3; $P = 0.02$).

track with eyes, open mouth/stick out tongue) without precipitating excessive agitation. Once objective signs of consciousness are demonstrated, restarting sedatives as needed is recommended. If after discontinuing the sedative infusion the patient requires resedation, we recommend restarting the infusion at 50 percent of the previous dose. Adjustments from this starting point can be individualized to patient needs.

It is clear that sedatives may have an impact on the duration of mechanical ventilation.[24,62] Protocolized sedation strategies may reduce the duration of mechanical ventilation by allowing earlier recognition of patient readiness to undergo a spontaneous breathing trial. Others have reported previously an important link between a successful spontaneous breathing trial and subsequent liberation from mechanical ventilation.[63,64] The use of a daily spontaneous waking trial, followed, when possible, by a daily spontaneous breathing trial, should be implemented widely in the care of critically ill patients requiring mechanical ventilation.

DRUGS FOR SEDATION OF MECHANICALLY VENTILATED PATIENTS

OPIATES
Opiate receptors are found in the central nervous system, as well as in peripheral tissues. There are several classes of receptors, but the two most clinically important are the mu and kappa receptors. The mu receptors have two subtypes, mu-1 and mu-2. Mu-1 receptors are responsible for analgesia, whereas mu-2 receptors mediate respiratory depression, nausea, vomiting, constipation, and euphoria. The kappa receptors are responsible for such effects as sedation, miosis, and spinal analgesia. Table 14-3 presents a summary of the pharmacologic properties of the opiates.

Pharmacokinetics
The following discussion applies to the intravenous opiates used most commonly in the ICU.

TABLE 14-3 Properties of Commonly Used Opiates

	Morphine	Meperidine	Fentanyl	Methadone
Typical starting dose	2–5 mg	20–50 mg	25–50 μg	5–10 mg
Onset	10 min	3–5 min	0.5–1 min	10–20 min
Duration after single dose	4 h	1–4 h	0.5–1 h	6–24 h
Metabolism	Hepatic	Hepatic	Hepatic	Hepatic
Elimination	Renal	Renal	Renal	Renal
Anxiolysis	+	++	++	+
Analgesia	++++	++++	++++	++++
Hypnosis	No reliable effect	No reliable effect	No reliable effect	No reliable effect
Amnesia	No reliable effect	No reliable effect	No reliable effect	No reliable effect
Sz threshold	No effect	May decrease	No effect	No effect
Reducing dyspnea	++++	++++	++++	++++
CV effect	Venodilation	Venodilation	Venodilation	Venodilation
Respiratory effect	Hypoventilation	Hypoventilation	Hypoventilation	Hypoventilation
Common side effects	N/V, ileus, itching	Seizure, N/V, ileus, itching	N/V, ileus, itching	N/V, ileus, itching

NOTE: + = minimal effect; ++ = mild effect; +++ = moderate effect; ++++ = large effect; N/V = nausea and vomiting.

MORPHINE   Intravenous morphine has a relatively slow onset of action (typically 5 to 10 minutes) owing to its relatively low lipid solubility, which delays movement of the drug across the blood-brain barrier. The duration of action after a single dose is approximately 4 hours. As the drug is given repeatedly, accumulation in tissue stores may prolong its effect. Morphine undergoes glucuronide conjugation in the liver and has an active metabolite, morphine-6-glucuronide. Elimination occurs in the kidney, so effects may be prolonged in renal failure.

MEPERIDINE   Meperidine's greater lipid solubility leads to more rapid movement across the blood-brain barrier and a more rapid onset of action, typically 3 to 5 minutes. Because of redistribution to peripheral tissues, its duration of action after a single dose is less than that of morphine (1 to 4 hours). Meperidine undergoes hepatic metabolism and renal elimination. A major problem with the use of meperidine is its metabolite normeperidine, a CNS stimulant that can precipitate seizures, especially with renal failure and/or prolonged use. Since meperidine offers no apparent advantage over other opiates, its side effect of CNS toxicity largely should preclude its use in critically ill patients.

FENTANYL   Fentanyl is very lipid soluble, thereby rapidly crossing the blood-brain barrier and exhibiting very rapid onset of action. Its duration of action after a single dose is short (0.5 to 1 hour) because of redistribution into peripheral tissues; however, as with all opiates, accumulation and prolongation of effect can occur when this drug is given for extended periods. Inactive products of hepatic metabolism are excreted by the kidney.

HYDROMORPHONE   The onset of action is similar to morphine. The duration of action is likewise similar to that of morphine when given as a single dose. However, the absence of active metabolites makes the duration of effect typically shorter than that of morphine when administered for extended periods.

REMIFENTANIL   Remifentanil is a lipid-soluble drug with a rapid onset of action. This drug is unique in that it is metabolized rapidly by hydrolysis by nonspecific blood and tissue esterases. As such, its pharmacokinetic profile is not affected by hepatic or renal insufficiency. It must be given by continuous infusion because of its rapid recovery time. This rapid recovery, typically minutes after cessation of the drug infusion, may prove useful in the management of critically ill patients. To date, the drug has not been studied extensively in the critical care setting. Most studies have been performed in neurosurgical and cardiac surgical settings, and little data are available regarding long-term use of this drug. Remifentanil as a component of general anesthesia may have a role in reducing the need for ICU admissions by allowing extubation in the operating room and preventing the need for postoperative ICU care.[65,66]

Pharmacodynamics

All opiates have similar pharmacodynamic effects and will be discussed without reference to individual drugs except where important differences are present.

CENTRAL NERVOUS SYSTEM   The primary effect of opioids is analgesia, mediated mainly through the mu and kappa receptors. Mild to moderate anxiolysis is also common, although less than with benzodiazepines. Opiates have no reliable amnestic properties.

RESPIRATORY SYSTEM   Opiates lead to a dose-dependent centrally mediated respiratory depression, one of the most important complications associated with their use. Respiratory depression, mediated by the mu-2 receptors in the medulla, typically presents with a decreased respiratory rate but preserved tidal volume. The CO_2 response curve is blunted, and the ventilatory response to hypoxia is obliterated. An important benefit of these drugs is the relief of the subjective sense of dyspnea frequently present in critically ill patients with respiratory failure.

CARDIOVASCULAR SYSTEM   Opiates have little hemodynamic effect on euvolemic patients whose blood pressure is not sustained by a hyperactive sympathetic nervous system. When opiates and benzodiazepines are given concomitantly, they may exhibit a synergistic effect on hemodynamics. The reasons for this synergy are not entirely clear. Meperidine has a chemical structure similar to atropine and may elicit a tachycardia, another reason its use is discouraged in the ICU. All other opiates usually decrease heart rate by decreasing sympathetic activity. Morphine and meperidine may cause histamine release, although it is rarely important in doses typically used in the ICU. Fentanyl does not release histamine.[67] Remifentanil may cause bradycardia and hypotension, particularly when administered concurrently with drugs known to cause vasodilation, such as propofol.

OTHER EFFECTS   Other side effects include nausea, vomiting, and decreased gastrointestinal motility. Methylnaltrexone, a specific antagonist of mu-2 receptors in the gut, has been reported recently to attenuate this side effect in humans.[68] The utility of methylnaltrexone in the ICU has not been tested. Other side effects include urinary retention and pruritus. Muscle rigidity occasionally occurs with fentanyl and remifentanil. This is seen typically when high doses of these drugs are injected rapidly and may affect the chest wall muscles, making ventilation impossible. Neuromuscular blockade, typically with succinylcholine, reverses this problem.

BENZODIAZEPINES

Benzodiazepines act by potentiating γ-aminobutyric acid (GABA) receptor complex–mediated inhibition of the CNS. The GABA receptor complex regulates a chloride channel on the cell membrane, and by increasing the intracellular flow of chloride ions, neurons become hyperpolarized, with a higher threshold for excitability. Flumazenil is a synthetic antagonist of the benzodiazepine receptor that may reverse many of the clinical effects of benzodiazepines. Table 14-4 presents a summary of the pharmacologic properties of the benzodiazepines.

Pharmacokinetics

The three available intravenous benzodiazepines, midazolam, lorazepam, and diazepam, are discussed below.

MIDAZOLAM   The onset of action of midazolam is rapid (0.5 to 5 minutes), and the duration of action following a

TABLE 14-4 Properties of Commonly Used Benzodiazepines

	Midazolam	Lorazepam	Diazepam
Typical starting dose	1–2 mg	0.5–1 mg	5–10 mg
Onset	0.5–2 min	3–5 min	1–3 min
Duration after single dose	2 h	6–10 h	1–6 h
Metabolism	Hepatic	Hepatic (less influenced by age and liver disease)	Hepatic
Elimination	Renal	Renal	Renal
Anxiolysis	++++	++++	++++
Analgesia	No effect	No effect	No effect
Hypnosis	++++	++++	++++
Amnesia	++++	++++	++++
Seizure threshold	+++	++++	+++
Reducing dyspnea	+	+	+
CV effect	Venodilation	Venodilation	Venodilation
Respiratory effect	Hypoventilation	Hypoventilation	Hypoventilation
Common side effects	Paradoxical agitation	Paradoxical agitation	Paradoxical agitation

NOTE: + = minimal effect; ++ = mild effect; +++ = moderate effect; ++++ = large effect.

single dose is short (~2 hours). All benzodiazepines are lipid soluble with a large volume of distribution and therefore are distributed widely throughout body tissues. For all benzodiazepines, the duration of action after a single bolus depends mainly on the rate of redistribution to peripheral tissues, especially adipose tissue. Midazolam undergoes hepatic metabolism and renal excretion. Alpha-hydroxy midazolam is an active metabolite but has a half-life of only 1 hour in the presence of normal renal function.

The kinetics of midazolam change considerably when it is given by continuous infusion to critically ill patients. After continuous infusion for extended periods, this lipid-soluble drug accumulates in peripheral tissues rather than being metabolized. On discontinuing the drug, peripheral tissue stores release midazolam back into the plasma, and the duration of clinical effect can be prolonged.[69] Obese patients with larger volumes of distribution and elderly patients with decreased hepatic and renal function may be even more prone to prolonged effects.

LORAZEPAM Intravenous lorazepam has a slower onset of action than midazolam (~5 minutes) because of its lower lipid solubility, which increases the time required to cross the blood-brain barrier. The duration of action following a single dose is long (6 to 10 hours) and is proportional to the dose given; however, most pharmacokinetic studies are done on healthy volunteers and may not apply to critically ill patients. Lorazepam's longer duration of action is due to lower lipid solubility with decreased peripheral tissue redistribution.

DIAZEPAM The onset of action of intravenous diazepam is short (~1 to 3 minutes). Duration of action following a single dose also is short (30 to 60 minutes) owing to high lipid solubility and peripheral redistribution. Diazepam rarely is given by continuous infusion because it has a long termination half-life. Once the peripheral tissue compartment is saturated, recovery can take several days. Diazepam has several active metabolites that themselves have prolonged half-lives. The metabolism of diazepam depends on hepatic function and is prolonged in liver disease and in the elderly.

Pharmacodynamics

The benzodiazepines have similar effects and will be discussed without reference to individual drugs except where important differences are present.

CENTRAL NERVOUS SYSTEM All benzodiazepines cause a dose-dependent suppression of awareness along a spectrum from mild depression of responsiveness to obtundation. They are potent amnestic agents;[70,71] lorazepam appears to produce the longest duration of antegrade amnesia. All are potent anxiolytic agents. A paradoxical state of agitation that worsens with escalating doses may occur occasionally, especially in elderly patients. All benzodiazepines have anticonvulsant properties.[72]

RESPIRATORY SYSTEM Benzodiazepines cause a dose-dependent, centrally mediated respiratory depression. This ventilatory depression is less profound than that seen with opiates; however, it may be synergistic with opiate-induced respiratory depression. In contrast to opiates (described earlier), the respiratory pattern of a patient receiving benzodiazepines is a decrease in tidal volume and an increase in respiratory rate. Even low doses of benzodiazepines can obliterate the ventilatory response to hypoxia.

CARDIOVASCULAR SYSTEM Benzodiazepines have minimal effects on the cardiovascular system in patients who are euvolemic. They may cause a slight decrease in blood pressure without a significant change in heart rate. Clinically important hypotensive responses usually are seen only in patients who are hypovolemic and/or those whose increased endogenous sympathetic activity is maintaining a normal blood pressure.

PROPOFOL

Propofol is an alkylphenol intravenous anesthetic. The exact mechanism of action is unclear, although it is thought to act at the GABA receptor. It is an oil at room temperature and is prepared as a lipid emulsion.

Pharmacokinetics

Propofol is highly lipid soluble and rapidly crosses the blood-brain barrier. Onset of sedation is rapid (1 to 5 minutes) and depends on whether or not a loading dose is given. Duration of action depends on dose but is usually very short (2 to 8 minutes) owing to rapid redistribution to peripheral tissues.[73,74] When continuous infusions are used, duration of action may be increased, but it is rare for the effect to last longer than 60 minutes after the infusion is discontinued. The drug is metabolized mainly in the liver with an elimination half-life of 4 to 7 hours. Propofol has no active metabolites. Because of its high lipid solubility and large volume of distribution, propofol can be given for prolonged periods without significant changes in its pharmacokinetic profile. The termination of its clinical effect depends solely on redistribution to peripheral fat tissue stores. When the infusion is discontinued, the fat tissue stores redistribute the drug back into the plasma, but usually not to clinically significant levels.

Pharmacodynamics

CENTRAL NERVOUS SYSTEM Propofol is a hypnotic agent that, like the benzodiazepines, provides a dose-dependent suppression of awareness from mild depression of responsiveness to obtundation. It is a potent anxiolytic as well as a potent amnestic agent.[75] Its effect on seizure activity is controversial. Animal studies suggest that it is neither pro- nor anticonvulsant; however, there are case reports of propofol being used to treat seizures, as well as being associated with seizure activity. Propofol has no analgesic properties and should be accompanied by a separate analgesic agent in most, if not all, patients. Failure to recognize this may lead to difficulty keeping patients comfortable, and excessive doses of propofol may be administered.

RESPIRATORY SYSTEM The CO_2 response curve is blunted, and apnea may be seen, especially after a loading dose is given. The respiratory pattern is usually a decrease in tidal volume and an increase in respiratory rate.

CARDIOVASCULAR SYSTEM Propofol can cause significant decreases in blood pressure, especially in hypovolemic patients. This is mainly due to preload reduction from dilation of venous capacitance vessels. A lesser effect is mild myocardial depression.[76,77] Care must be taken in giving this drug to patients with marginal cardiac function; however, since myocardial oxygen consumption is decreased by propofol and the myocardial oxygen supply-demand ratio is preserved, it may be useful in patients with ischemic heart disease.

OTHER EFFECTS Because it is delivered in an intralipid carrier, hypertriglyceridemia is a possible side effect.[78,79] Therefore, triglyceride levels should be checked frequently. If hypertriglyceridemia occurs, the drug should be stopped. Intralipid parenteral feedings should be adjusted according to the propofol infusion rate because there is a significant caloric load from propofol. Strict aseptic technique and frequent changing of infusion tubing are essential to prevent iatrogenic transmission of bacteria and fungi because propofol can support their growth.[80] Dysrhythmias, heart failure, metabolic acidosis, hyperkalemia, and rhabdomyolysis have been reported in both children and adults treated with propofol, especially at high doses (>80 μg/kg per minute in adults).[81]

BUTYROPHENONES (HALOPERIDOL AND DROPERIDOL)

Butyrophenones such as haloperidol and droperidol are used occasionally in the ICU for sedation. These drugs induce a state of tranquility such that patients often demonstrate a detached affect. Butyrophenones appear to antagonize dopamine, especially in the basal ganglia, although their exact site of action is not known.

Pharmacokinetics

HALOPERIDOL After an intravenous dose, onset of sedation usually occurs after 2 to 5 minutes. The half-life is approximately 2 hours but is dose dependent. Dose requirements vary widely, starting at 1 to 10 mg and titrating to effect. Haloperidol undergoes hepatic metabolism.

DROPERIDOL Onset of action is usually 2 to 5 minutes, with a typical starting dose of 0.625 to 2.5 mg. Half-life is approximately 2 hours but is longer when higher doses are used. Droperidol, like haloperidol, is metabolized in the liver.

Pharmacodynamics

CENTRAL NERVOUS SYSTEM Both haloperidol and droperidol produce CNS depression, resulting in a calm, often detached appearance. These drugs are used most commonly in critically ill patients who are acutely agitated and hyperactive. Patients may demonstrate a mental and psychiatric indifference to the environment.[82] Patients also may experience a state of cataleptic immobility. There is no demonstrable amnesia with these drugs. They have no effect on seizure activity. Analgesic effects are minimal with haloperidol; however, droperidol seems to have a significant potentiating analgesic effect when given concomitantly with an opiate. Indeed, droperidol and fentanyl are given occasionally in combination, producing a so-called neuroleptanesthesia. The butyrophenones are the drugs of choice for patients thought to be demonstrating psychotic behavior or agitation resistant to other pharmacologic interventions.

RESPIRATORY SYSTEM Neither haloperidol nor droperidol has any significant effect on the respiratory system when used alone. There are reports of attenuation of respiratory depression in the presence of opiates, but this effect is mild. Droperidol has been shown to maintain the hypoxic pulmonary drive.[83]

CARDIOVASCULAR SYSTEM Haloperidol and droperidol may result in mild hypotension secondary to peripheral α_1 blocking effects. Haloperidol also may decrease the neurotransmitter function of dopamine and lead to mild hypotension by this mechanism. Haloperidol may prolong the QT interval and has been reported to result in torsade de pointes,[84] although this problem is quite rare.

OTHER EFFECTS Extrapyramidal effects are seen occasionally with these drugs but are much less common with intravenous than with oral butyrophenones. When these complications occur, treatment with diphenhydramine or benztropine may be necessary. Neuroleptic malignant syndrome (NMS) occurs rarely and is characterized by "lead pipe" muscle rigidity, fever, and mental status changes. The mechanism of NMS is not fully understood, although some data suggest a central dopaminergic blockade that leads to extrapyramidal

TABLE 14-5 Properties of Other Sedative Agents

	Propofol	Haloperidol	Dexmedetomidine
Typical starting dose	1–2 mg/kg	0.5–1 mg	0.5–1.0 μg/kg over 10 min; 0.2–0.7 μg/kg/h infusion
Onset	0.5–1 min	2–5 min	5–10 min
Duration after single dose	2–8 min	2 h	30–60 min
Metabolism	Hepatic, renal, lungs?	Hepatic	Hepatic
Elimination	Renal	Renal	Renal
Anxiolysis	++++	+++	+++
Analgesia	No effect	No effect	++
Hypnosis	++++	++	+++
Amnesia	++++	No effect	+
Seizure threshold	??	No effect	No effect
Reducing dyspnea	+	No effect	No effect
CV effect	Venodilation, arteriolar dilation, myocardial depression	Venodilation, arteriolar dilation	Venodilation, arteriolar dilation, bradycardia, occasional hypertension
Respiratory effect	Hypoventilation	No effect	No effect
Common side effects	Increased triglycerides	Neuroleptic malignant syndrome (rare), extrapyramidal effects (rare)	Hypotension, bradycardia

NOTE: + = minimal effect; ++ = mild effect; +++ = moderate effect; ++++ = large effect.

side effects and muscle rigidity with excess heat generation. Bromocriptine, dantrolene, and pancuronium all have been used to treat NMS successfully.[85] Droperidol is a potent antiemetic and sometimes is used for nausea and vomiting associated with general anesthesia or chemotherapy.

OTHER DRUGS USED FOR SEDATION IN THE ICU

Dexmedetomidine[86–88] is a selective α_2 agonist approved for short-term use (<24 hours) in patients initially receiving mechanical ventilation. While patients remain sedated, when undisturbed, they arouse easily with stimulation. This drug is attractive because patients seem to transition from sedated to awake states rather easily, thus facilitating neurologic examinations. The drug has both analgesic and anxiolytic effects. Side effects include bradycardia and hypotension, especially with hypovolemia or high sympathetic tone. Unfortunately, dexmedetomidine has not been studied extensively as an agent for long-term administration to critically ill patients.

Ketamine has a molecular structure similar to phencyclidine. Patients given this drug experience a profound dissociative state. They may keep their eyes open and maintain a protective cough reflex but appear unaware of their surroundings. It is recommended to give this drug slowly over a period of approximately 1 minute. Ketamine causes minimal respiratory depression. There may be amnesia, but this is not a reliable property of the drug. Coordinated but seemingly purposeless movements are seen often. Profound analgesia is seen with ketamine. The common side effect of emergence delirium and severe hallucinations has limited its usefulness for sedation of adult patients in the ICU. This phencyclidine derivative has gained popularity recently as an illicit drug of abuse.

Barbiturates such as thiopental and pentobarbital are potent agents that cause amnesia and unconsciousness. They have little use as sedatives in critically ill patients because of a propensity to cause hemodynamic instability. In addition to this, they are lipid soluble and thus accumulate in periph-

eral tissues after long-term infusions, leading to prolonged recovery from sedation. These drugs may be used to induce a pharmacologic coma in patients with severe brain injury.

Inhalational anesthetics such as *isoflurane* have been studied in critically ill patients and shown to be safe and effective.[89] These drugs have analgesic, amnestic, and hypnotic properties and may be useful as single agents. Isoflurane undergoes only 0.2% metabolism, being eliminated almost exclusively through the lungs. Technical problems delivering the drug safely through the ventilator at accurate concentrations, as well as difficulty scavenging the exhaled gas, have limited the use of inhalational anesthetics for sedation in the ICU in the United States.

Table 14-5 summarizes pharmacologic properties of other commonly used sedative agents.

Neuromuscular Blocking Agents

The frequency with which neuromuscular blocking agents (NMBs) are used in critically ill patients has decreased significantly over the last 20 years. As reports of complications related to the use of NMBs continue to accrue, intensive care clinicians typically administer these agents only as a last resort. The usual indications for the use of NMBs in the ICU are to facilitate mechanical ventilation in patients with ventilator dyssynchrony despite optimal sedation, to manage tetanus with chest wall rigidity, and to facilitate redistribution of blood flow away from respiratory muscles in patients with acute hypoxemic respiratory failure accompanied by shock. It is mandatory that patients given NMBs be given agents to ensure amnesia while they are pharmacologically paralyzed.

Normally, at the neuromuscular junction, acetylcholine is released from synaptic vesicles at the terminal end of the motor nerve. The acetylcholine binds to the postsynaptic endplate, propagating an electrical signal through the muscle and leading to muscle contraction. Pharmacologic NMBs bind to the acetylcholine receptor at the terminal end of the motor nerve. These agents can activate the acetylcholine receptor (depolarizing agents) or competitively inhibit the receptor without activating it (nondepolarizing agents). Succinylcholine is the only available depolarizing NMB. In normal individuals, depolarization of skeletal muscle beds leads to release of intracellular potassium, typically resulting in an increase in the serum potassium level of approximately 0.5 mEq/L. Denervation of skeletal muscle from tissue injury as in burns or upper motor neuron lesions may result in more dramatic rises in serum potassium, which may precipitate malignant cardiac dysrrhythmias. Succinylcholine may be used to facilitate endotracheal intubation but is not indicated for ongoing neuromuscular blockade in critically ill patients and will not be discussed further in this chapter. Table 14-6 presents a summary of the pharmacologic properties of the neuromuscular blocking agents.

NONDEPOLARIZING NMBs

A number of nondepolarizing NMBs are available currently. The pharmacology of the ones more commonly used in the ICU will be discussed below.

PANCURONIUM

Pancuronium is an older NMB that is used during general anesthesia, as well as in the ICU. It has an aminosteroidal molecular structure. The drug has a long half-life, with a duration of action of between 60 and 90 minutes after a single intravenous bolus dose of 0.1 mg/kg. Its vagolytic side effect (typically results in an increase in heart rate of ~10 beats per minute), active metabolite (3-hydroxypancuronium), and reliance on renal clearance limit its attractiveness in critically ill patients.

VECURONIUM

Vecuronium also has an aminosteroidal molecular structure but a shorter half-life than pancuronium. After a bolus of 0.1 mg/kg, this drug typically lasts 30 minutes. Fifty percent of the drug is excreted in bile, so prolongation of effect may be seen in patients with liver dysfunction. In addition to this, one-third of the drug is excreted in the kidneys, so accumulation in the setting of renal insufficiency may be seen. The active metabolite 3-desacetylvecuronium may lead to prolongation of effect with repeated dosing, particularly in those with renal failure.[90]

ROCURONIUM

Rocuronium also has an aminosteroidal molecular structure. Unlike the other aminosteroidal nondepolarizing NMBs, rocuronium has a rapid onset of action. It may be used to facilitate endotracheal intubation as a substitute for succinylcholine when the latter is contraindicated (e.g. burns, muscle tissue injury, upper motor neuron lesions). The usual bolus dose is 0.6 to 1.0 mg/kg, with a duration of effect of 30 to 45 minutes, similar to vecuronium. The metabolite, 17-desacetylrocuronium, has minimal neuromuscular blocking activity.

DOXACURIUM

Doxacurium is a benzylisoquinolinium agent with a half-life lasting 60 to 90 minutes. The usual bolus dose is 0.5 to 1.0 mg/kg. The drug is eliminated by renal excretion and has no hemodynamic effects.

ATRACURIUM

Atracurium is a benzylisoquinolinium compound with a duration of action of between 20 and 45 minutes. The initial loading dose is 0.4 to 0.5 mg/kg. The drug usually is given by continuous infusion in the ICU at a dose of 10 to 20 μg/kg per minute. Atracurium is inactivated in plasma by ester hydrolysis and Hofmann elimination, so renal or hepatic dysfunction do not have an impact on its duration of blockade. This feature has made it attractive for use in ICU patients because most patients sick enough to require NMBs suffer from renal or hepatic dysfunction. Atracurium may cause histamine release, and its breakdown product, laudanosine, has been associated with central nervous system excitation and seizures in animal models.

CISATRACURIUM ✳

An isomer of atracurium is cisatracurium, which has a similar pharmacologic profile to atracurium. The initial loading dose is 0.1 to 0.2 mg/kg, and the duration of action is approximately 25 minutes. Like atracurium, this drug is inactivated in plasma by ester hydrolysis and Hofmann elimination. Cisatracurium does not cause histamine release. Because of its short half-life, it requires administration by continuous infusion. The usual dose is 2.5 to 3 μg/kg per minute. This drug is currently one of the most frequently used for neuromuscular blockade in ICU patients.

MONITORING THE LEVEL OF NEUROMUSCULAR BLOCKADE

The depth of neuromuscular blockade is monitored most accurately with use of a peripheral nerve stimulator. This device sends a current between electrodes placed on the skin along the course of a peripheral nerve, most commonly the ulnar nerve. With this setup, the twitches of the adductor pollicus muscle are evaluated to assess depth of neuromuscular blockade. The peripheral nerve stimulator is programmed to deliver four sequential stimuli at 2 Hz. Each stimulus causes release of acetylcholine from synaptic vesicles. In the absence of pharmacologic neuromuscular blockade, the fourth twitch of the adductor pollicus muscle is as strong as the first. However, when neuromuscular receptors are occupied by nondepolarizing NMBs, the strength of the fourth twitch is less than the first, until eventually the muscle does not twitch with the fourth stimulus. This phenomenon is known as *fade*. When 85% to 90% of the neuromuscular receptors are occupied by NMBs, only the first twitch in the train of four is visible. When 70% to 85% of the neuromuscular receptors are occupied by NMBs, between two and four twitches are visible. Typically, two or three of four twitches are sought, and dosing of NMBs is titrated to this goal. Peripheral nerve stimulator use in the ICU has been shown to reduce the amount of drug used and shorten recovery of neuromuscular function and spontaneous ventilation.[91] Another study showed a reduction in the incidence of persistent neuromuscular weakness.[92]

COMPLICATIONS OF NEUROMUSCULAR BLOCKADE

Prolonged weakness after the use of NMBs is the most concerning complication of their use. Categorically, two separate

TABLE 14-6 Properties of Commonly Used Neuromuscular Blocking Agents

	Succinylcholine	Pancuronium	Vecuronium	Rocuronium	Atracurium	Cisatracurium
Type	Depolarizing	Nondepolarizing	Nondepolarizing	Nondepolarizing	Nondepolarizing	Nondepolarizing
Typical loading/intubation	1.0–1.5 mg/kg	0.1 mg/kg	0.1 mg/kg	0.6–1.0 mg/kg	0.5 mg/kg	0.1–0.2 mg/kg
Continuous infusion? (Dose)	No	No	No	No	Yes (10–20 µg/kg/min)	Yes (2–3 µg/kg/min)
Onset	60 s	3–5 min	3–5 min	1–2 min	3–5 min	3–5 min
Duration after loading dose	7–9 min	60–90 min	30–40 min	30–45 min	20–45 min	25 min
Metabolism	Plasma cholinesterase	Hepatic	Hepatic/biliary	Hepatic	Ester hydrolysis/Hoffman elimination	Ester hydrolysis/Hoffman elimination
Elimination		Renal	Renal/biliary	Biliary clearance of parent molecule from plasma		
Active metabolite?	No	Yes	Yes	Yes (minimal)	No	No
CV effect	Supraventricular and ventricular rhythm disturbances with hyperkalemia	Vagolytic—tachycardia	None	None	Histamine release	No histamine release
Common side effects	Hyperkalemia	None	None	None	Histamine release	None

conditions may arise that lead to this problem. As mentioned earlier, accumulation of NMB parent drug or its metabolites is seen with several drugs, particularly with renal and/or hepatic insufficiency. This condition of prolonged recovery from NMBs is defined by an increase in the time to recovery of 50% to 100% longer than predicted by pharmacologic parameters after the drugs are stopped.[93] The second cause of weakness associated with NMBs is acute quadriplegic myopathy syndrome. Patients with this syndrome manifest acute paresis, myonecrosis with increased creatine phosphokinase (CPK) concentration, and abnormal electromyography (EMG). Findings on EMG are consistent with denervation of skeletal muscle (decreased compound motor action potential amplitudes). This may progress to muscle atrophy and even necrosis.

Concerns over complications of NMBs have led to a dramatic decrease in their use in the ICU.[94] This is particularly noteworthy when corticosteroids are used in conjunction with NMBs. Several studies have suggested that this combination is associated with a significant incidence of myopathy.[95,96]

Conclusions

Sedation is an important component of the treatment of critically ill patients who require mechanical ventilation. Directing treatment to specific and individualized goals will ensure that patient needs are met. All currently available sedatives for use in the ICU have limitations. Rather than seeking an ideal drug, strategies of drug administration that focus attention on principles of sedative pharmacology in critical illness should be used. Recognition of the goals of sedation in individual patients will allow rational administration strategies to be implemented in the care of these patients. The use of neuromuscular blocking agents should be reserved for those patients with extreme ventilator dyssynchrony despite optimal sedation, tetanus, and critically reduced oxygen delivery from hypoxemia with shock.

References

1. Kress JP, O'Connor MF, Pohlman AS, et al: Sedation of critically ill patients during mechanical ventilation: A comparison of propofol and midazolam. *Am J Respir Crit Care Med* 153:1012, 1996.
2. Jones C, Griffiths RD: Disturbed memory and amnesia related to intensive care. *Memory* 8:79, 2000.
3. Jones C, Griffiths RD, Humphris G, Skirrow PM: Memory, delusions, and the development of acute posttraumatic stress disorder–related symptoms after intensive care. *Crit Care Med* 29:573, 2001.
4. Kress JP, Gehlbach BK, Lacy M, et al: The long-term psychological effects of daily sedative interruption in critically ill patients. *Am J Respir Crit Care Med* (in press).
5. Ely EW, Inouye SK, Bernard GR, et al: Delirium in mechanically ventilated patients: Validity and reliability of the confusion assessment method for the intensive care unit (CAM-ICU). *JAMA* 286:2703, 2001.
6. Jacobi J, Fraser GL, Coursin DB, et al: Clinical practice guidelines for the sustained use of sedatives and analgesics in the critically ill adult. *Crit Care Med* 30:119, 2002.
7. Novaes MA, Knobel E, Bork AM, et al: Stressors in the ICU: perception of the patient, relatives and healthcare team. *Intensive Care Med* 25:1421, 1999.
8. Puntillo KA: Pain experiences of intensive care unit patients. *Heart Lung* 19:526, 1990.
9. Turner JS, Briggs SJ, Springhorn HE, Potgieter PD: Patients' recollection of intensive care unit experience. *Crit Care Med* 18:966, 1990.
10. Shapiro BA, Warren J, Egol AB, et al: Practice parameters for intravenous analgesia and sedation for adult patients in the intensive care unit: An executive summary. *Crit Care Med* 23:1596, 1995.
11. Desbiens NA, Wu AW, Broste SK, et al: Pain and satisfaction with pain control in seriously ill hospitalized adults: Findings from the SUPPORT research investigators. *Crit Care Med* 24:1953, 1996.
12. Epstein J, Breslow. The stress response of critical illness. *Crit Care Clin* 15:17, 1999.
13. Lewis KS, Whipple JK, Michael KA, et al: Effect of analgesic treatment on the physiological consequences of acute pain. *Am J Hosp Pharm* 51:1539, 1994.
14. World Health Organization Expert Committee Report: *Cancer Pain Relief and Palliative Care*. Technical report Series 804. Geneva: World Health Organization; 1990.
15. Carroll KC, Atkins PJ, Herold GR, et al: Pain assessment and management in critically ill postoperative and trauma patients: A multicenter study. *Am J Crit Care* 8:105, 1999.
16. Ferguson J, Gilroy D, Puntillo K: Dimensions of pain and analgesic administration associated with coronary artery bypass in an Australian intensive care unit. *J Adv Nurs* 26:1065, 1997.
17. Sun X, Weissman C: The use of analgesics and sedatives in critically ill patients: Physicians' orders versus medications administered. *Heart Lung* 23:169, 1994.
18. Price DD, Bush FM, Long S, et al: A comparison of pain measurement characteristics of mechanical visual analogue and simple numerical rating scales. *Pain* 56:217, 1994.
19. Price DD, McGrath PA, Rafii A, et al: The validation of visual analogue scales as ratio scale measures for chronic and experimental pain. *Pain* 17:45, 1983.
20. Jensen MP, Karoly P, Braver S: The measurement of clinical pain intensity: A comparison of six methods. *Pain* 27:117, 1986.
21. Meehan DA, RcRae ME, Rourke DA, et al: Analgesia administration, pain intensity, and patient satisfaction in cardiac surgical patients. *Am J Crit Care* 4:435, 1995.
22. Bianchi M, Mantegazza P, Tammiso R, et al: Peripherally administered benzodiazepines increase morphine-induced analgesia in the rat: Effect of RO 15-3505 and FG 7142. *Arch Int Pharmacodyn Ther* 322:5, 1993.
23. Sivam SP, Ho IK. GABA in morphine analgesia and tolerance. *Life Sci* 37:199, 1985.
24. Kress JP, Pohlman A, O'Connor MF, Hall JB: Daily interruption of sedative infusions in critically ill patients undergoing mechanical ventilation. *N Engl J Med* 342:1471, 2000.
24a. Schweickert WD, Gehlbach BK, Pohlman AS, et al: Daily interruption of sedative infusions and complications of critical illness in mechanically ventilated patients. *Crit Care Med* 32:1272, 2004.
25. Cammarano WB, Pittet JF, Weitz S, et al: Acute withdrawal syndrome related to the administration of analgesic and sedative medications in adult intensive care unit patients. *Crit Care Med* 26:676, 1998.
26. Dernedde M, Stadler M, Bardiau F, Boogaerts JG: Continuous epidural infusion of large concentration/small volume versus small concentration/large volume of levobupivacaine for postoperative analgesia. *Anesth Analg* 96:796, 2003.
27. Sandhu H, Morley-Forster P, Spadafora S: Epidural hematoma following epidural anesthesia in a patient receiving unfractionated heparin for thromboprophylaxis. *Reg Anesth Pain Med* 25:72, 2000.

28. Liu SS, McDonald SB: Current issues in spinal anesthesia. *Anesthesiology* 94:888, 2001.

29. Herbstreit F, Kienbaum P, Merguet P, Peters J: Conservative treatment of paraplegia after removal of an epidural catheter during low-molecular-weight heparin treatment. *Anesthesiology* 97:733, 2002.

30. Giebler RM, Scherer RU, Peters J: Incidence of neurologic complications related to thoracic epidural catheterization. *Anesthesiology* 86:55, 1997.

31. Low JH: Survey of epidural analgesia management in general intensive care units in England. *Acta Anaesthesiol Scand* 46:799, 2002.

32. Yaksh TL, Rudy TA: Analgesia mediated by a direct spinal action of narcotics. *Science* 192:1357, 1976.

33. Cousins MJ, Mather LE: Intrathecal and epidural administration of opioids. *Anesthesiology* 61:276, 1984.

34. Guinard JP, Carpenter RL, Chassot PG: Epidural and intravenous fentanyl produce equivalent effects during major surgery. *Anesthesiology* 82:377, 1995.

35. Salomaki TE, Leppaluoto J, Laitinen JO, et al: Epidural versus intravenous fentanyl for reducing hormonal, metabolic, and physiologic responses after thoracotomy. *Anesthesiology* 79:672, 1993.

36. Salomaki TE, Laitinen JO, Nuutinen LS: A randomized, double-blind comparison of epidural versus intravenous fentanyl infusion for analgesia after thoracotomy. *Anesthesiology* 75:790, 1991.

37. Ramsey MAE, Savege TM, Simpson BRJ, Goodwin R: Controlled sedation with alphalaxone-alphadolone. *Br Med J* 2:256, 1974.

38. Riker RR, Picard JT, Fraser GL: Prospective evaluation of the Sedation-Agitation Scale for adult critically ill patients. *Crit Care Med* 27:1325, 1999.

39. Sessler CN, Gosnell MS, Grap MJ, et al: The Richmond Agitation-Sedation Scale: Validity and reliability in adult intensive care unit patients. *Am J Respir Crit Care Med* 166:1338, 2002.

40. Crippen DW: Neurologic monitoring in the intensive care unit. *New Horizons* 2:107, 1994.

41. Hansen-Flaschen J, Cowen J, Polomano RC: Beyond the Ramsay scale: Need for a validated measure of sedating drug efficacy in the intensive care unit. *Crit Care Med* 22:732, 1994.

42. Ely EW, Truman B, Shintani A, et al: Monitoring sedation status over time in ICU patients: Reliability and validity of the Richmond Agitation-Sedation Scale (RASS). *JAMA* 289:2983, 2003.

43. Glass PS, Bloom M, Kearse L, et al: Bispectral analysis measures sedation and memory effects of propofol, midazolam, isoflurane, and alfentanil in healthy volunteers. *Anesthesiology* 86:836, 1997.

44. O'Connor MF, Daves SM, Tung A, et al: BIS monitoring to prevent awareness during general anesthesia. *Anesthesiology* 94:520, 2001.

45. Simmons LE, Riker RR, Prato BS, Fraser GL: Assessing sedation during intensive care unit mechanical ventilation with the Bispectral Index and the Sedation-Agitation Scale. *Crit Care Med* 27:1499, 1999.

45a. Ely EW, Shintani A, Truman B, et al: Delirium as a predictor of mortality in mechanically ventilated patients in the intensive care unit. *JAMA* 291:1753, 2004.

45b. Ely EW, Inouye SK, Bernard GR, et al: Delirium in mechanically ventilated patients: Validity and reliability of the confusion assessment method for the intensive care unit (CAM-ICU). *JAMA* 286:2703, 2001.

46. Kollef MH, Levy NT, Ahrens TS, et al: The use of continuous IV sedation is associated with prolongation of mechanical ventilation. *Chest* 114:541, 1998.

47. Bodenham A, Shelly MP, Park GR: The altered pharmacokinetics and pharmacodynamics of drugs commonly used in critically ill patients. *Clin Pharmacokinet* 14:347, 1988.

48. Wagner BKJ, O'Hara DA: Pharmacokinetics and pharmacodynamics of sedatives and analgesics in the treatment of agitated critically ill patients. *Clin Pharmacokinet* 33:426, 1997.

49. Michalk S, Moncorge C, Fichelle A, et al: Midazolam infusion for basal sedation in intensive care: absence of accumulation. *Intensive Care Med* 15:37, 1988.

50. Shelly MP, Mendel L, Park GR: Failure of critically ill patients to metabolise midazolam. *Anaesthesia* 42:619, 1987.

51. Byatt CM, Lewis LD, Dawling S, Cochrane GM: Accumulation of midazolam after repeated dosage in patients receiving mechanical ventilation in an intensive care unit. *Br Med J* 289:799, 1984.

52. Malacrida R, Fritz ME, Suter PM, Crevoisier C: Pharmacokinetics of midazolam administered by continuous intravenous infusion to intensive care patients. *Crit Care Med* 20:1123, 1992.

53. Bertz RJ, Granneman GR: Use of in vitro and in vivo data to estimate the likelihood of metabolic pharmacokinetic interactions. *Clin Pharmacokinet* 32:210, 1997.

54. Oldenhof H, de Jong, M, Steenhoek A, Janknegt R: Clinical pharmacokinetics of midazolam in intensive care patients: A wide interpatient variability? *Clin Pharmacol Ther* 43:263, 1988.

55. Gottlieb JE, Park P, Girod A, et al: Comparison of neuromuscular blocker and sedative use among patients with ARDS treated with low versus high tidal volume. *Am J Respir Crit Care Med* 161:A506, 2000.

56. The Acute Respiratory Distress Syndrome Network: Ventilation with lower tidal volumes as compared with traditional tidal volumes for acute lung injury and the acute respiratory distress syndrome. *N Engl J Med* 342:1301, 2000.

57. Bernard GR, Vincent JL, Laterre PF, et al; Recombinant human protein C Worldwide Evaluation in Severe Sepsis (PROWESS) study group: Efficacy and safety of recombinant human activated protein C for severe sepsis. *N Engl J Med* 344:699, 2001.

58. Rivers E, Nguyen B, Havstad S, et al: Early goal-directed therapy in the treatment of severe sepsis and septic shock. *N Engl J Med* 345:1368, 2001.

59. Schiffl H, Lang SM, Fischer R: Daily hemodialysis and the outcome of acute renal failure. *N Engl J Med* 346:305, 2002.

60. Tuxen DV, Williams T, Scheinkestel C: Limiting dynamic hyperinflation in mechanically ventilated patients with severe asthma reduces complications. *Anaesth Intensive Care* 21:718, 1993.

61. Rubenfeld GD, Crawford SW: Withdrawing life support from mechanically ventilated recipients of bone marrow transplants: A case for evidence-based guidelines. *Ann Intern Med* 125:625, 1996.

62. Brook AD, Ahrens TS, Schaiff R, et al: Effect of a nursing-implemented sedation protocol on the duration of mechanical ventilation. *Crit Care Med* 27:2609, 1999.

63. Ely EW, Baker AM, Dunagan DP, et al: Effect on the duration of mechanical ventilation of identifying patients capable of breathing spontaneously. *N Engl J Med* 335:1864, 1996.

64. Kollef MH, Shapiro SD, Silver P, et al: A randomized, controlled trial of protocol-directed versus physician-directed weaning from mechanical ventilation. *Crit Care Med* 25:567, 1997.

65. Park GR, Evans TN, Hutchins J, et al: Reducing the demand for admission to intensive care after major abdominal surgery by a change in anesthetic practice and the use of remifentanil. *Eur J Anaesthesiol* 17:111, 2000.

66. Cohen J, Royston D: Remifentanil. *Curr Opin Crit Care* 7:227, 2001.

67. Rosow CE, Moss J, Philbin DM, et al: Histamine release during morphine and fentanyl anesthesia. *Anesthesiology* 56:93, 1982.

68. Yuan CS, Foss JF, O'Connor MF, et al: Methylnaltrexone for reversal of constipation due to chronic methadone use: A randomized, controlled trial. *JAMA* 283:367, 2000.

69. Byatt CM, Lewis LD, Dawling S, et al: Accumulation of midazolam after repeated dosage in patients receiving mechanical ventilation in an intensive care unit. *Br Med J* 289:799, 1984.

70. Dundee JW, Wilson DB: Amnesic action of midazolam. *Anaesthesia* 35:459, 1980.

71. George KA, Dundee JW: Relative amnesiac actions of diazepam, flunitrazepam and lorazepam in man. *Br J Clin Pharmacol* 4:45, 1977.

72. Treiman DM: The role of benzodiazepines in the management of status epilepticus. *Neurology* 40:32, 1990.

73. Shafer SL: Advances in propofol pharmacokinetics and pharmacodynamics. *J Clin Anesth* 5:14S, 1993.

74. Bailie GR, Cockshott ID, Douglas EJ, et al: Pharmacokinetics of propofol during and after long-term continuous infusion for maintenance of sedation on ICU patients. *Br J Anesth* 68:486, 1992.

75. Veselis RA, Reinsel RA, Marino P, et al: Propofol in sedative doses is an amnestic agent. *Anesthesiology* 75:A1023, 1991.

76. Goodchild CS: Cardiovascular effects of propofol and relevance to use in patients with compromised cardiovascular function. *Semin Anesth* 11:S37, 1992.

77. Mouren S, Baron J, Albo C: Effects of propofol and thiopental on coronary blood flow and myocardial performance in an isolated rabbit heart. *Anesthesiology* 80:634, 1994.

78. Gottardis M, Khuenl-Brady KS, Koller W, et al: Effect of prolonged sedation with propofol on serum triglyceride and cholesterol concentrations. *Br J Anesth* 62:393, 1989.

79. Barrientos-Vega R, Mar Sanchez-Soria M, Morales-Garcia C, et al: Prolonged sedation of critically ill patients with midazolam or propofol: impact on weaning and costs. *Crit Care Med* 25:33, 1997.

80. Bennett SN, McNeil MM, Bland LA, et al: Postoperative infections traced to contamination of an intravenous anesthetic, propofol. *N Engl J Med* 333:147, 1995.

81. Cremer OL, Moons KGM, Bouman EAC, et al: Long-term propofol infusion and cardiac failure in adult head-injured patients. *Lancet* 357:117, 2001.

82. Riker RR, Fraser GL, Cox PM: Continuous infusion of haloperidol controls agitation in critically ill patients. *Crit Care Med* 22:433, 1994.

83. Ward DS: Stimulation of the hypoxic pulmonary drive by droperidol. *Anesth Analg* 63:106, 1984.

84. Zee-Cheng CS, Mueller CE, Seifert CF, et al: Haloperidol and torsades de pointes. *Ann Intern Med* 102:418, 1985.

85. Burke C, Fulda GJ, Castellano J: Neuroleptic malignant syndrome in a trauma patient. *J Trauma* 39:796, 1995.

86. Peden CJ, Cloote AH. Stratford N, et al: The effect of intravenous dexmedetomidine premedication on the dose requirement of propofol to induce loss of consciousness in patients receiving alfentanil. *Anaesthesia* 56:408, 2001.

87. Ebert TJ, Hall JE, Barney JA, et al: The effects of increasing plasma concentrations of dexmedetomidine in humans. *Anesthesiology* 93:382, 2000.

88. Venn RM, Bradshaw CJ, Spencer R, et al: Preliminary UK experience of dexmedetomidine, a novel agent for postoperative sedation in the intensive care unit. *Anaesthesia* 54:1136, 1999.

89. Spencer EM, Willatts SM: Isoflurane for prolonged sedation in the intensive care unit: efficacy and safety. *Intensive Care Med* 18:415, 1992.

90. Segredo V, Caldwell JE, Matthay MA, et al: Persistent paralysis in critically ill patients after long-term administration of vecuronium. *N Engl J Med* 27:524, 1992.

91. Frankel H, Jeng J, Tilly E, et al: The impact of implementation of neuromuscular blockade monitoring standards in a surgical intensive care unit. *Am Surg* 2:503, 1996.

92. Tavernier B, Rannou JJ, Vallet B: Peripheral nerve stimulation and clinical assessment for dosing of neuromuscular blocking agents in critically ill patients. *Crit Care Med* 26:804, 1998.

93. Murray M, Cowen J, DeBlock H, et al: Clinical practice guidelines for sustained neuromuscular blockade in the adult critically ill patient. *Crit Care Med* 30:142, 2002.

94. Hansen-Flaschen JH, Brazinsky S, Basile C, Lanken PN: Use of sedating drugs and neuromuscular blocking agents in patients requiring mechanical ventilation for respiratory failure: A national survey. *JAMA* 66:2870, 1991.

95. Leatherman JW, Fluegel WL, David WS, et al: Muscle weakness in mechanically ventilated patients with severe asthma. *Am J Respir Crit Care Med* 153:1686, 1996.

96. Behbehani NA, Al-Mane F, D'Yachkova Y, et al: Myopathy following mechanical ventilation for acute severe asthma: the role of muscle relaxants and corticosteroids. *Chest* 115:1627, 1999.

CARDIOPULMONARY RESUSCITATION

BENJAMIN S. ABELLA
TERRY L. VANDEN HOEK
JASON ALVARADO
LANCE B. BECKER

KEY POINTS

- *Most cardiac arrests in the community setting occur as a result of coronary artery disease and cardiac ischemia.*
- *Given the high mortality of cardiac arrest, prevention is crucial.*
- *Cardiopulmonary resuscitation and rapid defibrillation are the keys to successful resuscitation from cardiac arrest.*
- *Advanced Cardiopulmonary Life Support (ACLS) guidelines provide treatment algorithms for the different cardiac rhythms of arrest.*
- *Automatic external defibrillators provide a means for rapid defibrillation by the public.*

Cardiac arrest, defined as the sudden complete loss of cardiac output and therefore blood pressure, is the leading cause of death in the United States and much of the developed world, claiming at least 300,000 lives each year in the United States alone.[1] In the majority of cases, myocardial ischemia in the setting of coronary artery disease represents the underlying etiology of arrest. Conversely, cardiac arrest is the initial presentation of myocardial ischemia in approximately 20% of patients.[2] A wide variety of other processes can lead to cardiac arrest, including septic shock, electrolyte abnormalities, hypothermia, pulmonary embolism, and massive trauma (Table 15-1).

Survival from cardiac arrest remains dismal, even after the introduction of electrical defibrillation and cardiopulmonary resuscitation (CPR) over 50 years ago. In the best cases (witnessed ventricular fibrillation arrest with rapid defibrillation), survival to hospital discharge ranges from 30% to 46%,[3,4] although overall out-of-hospital arrest survival is usually much lower, ranging from 2% to 26%.[5] In large American cities, out-of-hospital arrest survival may be even worse—survival rates of 1.4% and 1.8% have been reported for New York and Chicago, respectively.[6–8] Even after successful resuscitation from cardiac arrest, most patients die within 24 to 48 hours despite aggressive intensive care treatment. Reperfusion injury, a subject of much basic science investigation, is thought to be involved in this postarrest deterioration.[9,10]

Demographic data from multiple studies demonstrate that the mean age of patients who suffer out-of-hospital cardiac arrest is approximately 68 to 70 years, with a slightly higher incidence in men than in women.[1,2,11] Over 70% of these patients experience arrest in the home or other residential location.[12,13] In-hospital cardiac arrest patients exhibit similar demographics, with one survey showing a mean age of 71 years and also somewhat higher incidence in males.[14] There do not ap-

pear to be significant survival differences between men and women.[2]

To standardize treatment during cardiac arrest, a number of treatment algorithms have been developed based on laboratory and clinical evidence. These have been compiled into the Basic Life Support (BLS) and Advanced Cardiopulmonary Life Support (ACLS) guidelines published and updated regularly by the American Heart Association's Emergency Cardiac Care Committee,[15] as well as other international resuscitation organizations (International Liaison Committee on Resuscitation).[15] For additional information about ACLS guidelines and their revisions, see the contact information listed in Table 15-2.

Pediatric Cardiac Arrest

The majority of discussion in this chapter pertains to adult cardiac arrest because cardiac arrest in children, fortunately, is much less common. When it occurs, pediatric cardiac arrest more often is secondary to trauma or pulmonary derangements, such as drowning, status asthmaticus, or foreign-body obstruction, rather than due to a primary cardiac arrhythmia.[16] However, ventricular fibrillation does occur in the pediatric population.[17] Guidelines for pediatric resuscitation have been established and are compiled in the Pediatric Advanced Life Support (PALS) manual. For neonates, in whom cardiac arrest is yet another specialized problem, the manual Neonatal Advanced Life Support (NALS) has been developed. While many of the general principles of this chapter also apply to children, readers should refer to these additional texts for more detailed information.[15]

Prevention of Cardiac Arrest

Given the poor prognosis of cardiac arrest, prevention remains the best hope to save lives. To this end, out-of-hospital and in-hospital cardiac arrests require different prevention strategies.

In the outpatient setting, careful attention to coronary artery disease risk factors such as smoking, hypertension, and hypercholesterolemia and aggressive treatment for these conditions can lower the risk of myocardial ischemia and therefore the risk of cardiac arrest. In consultation with their physicians, most patients with multiple cardiac risk factors should be treated with aspirin to lower the probability and severity of myocardial infarction. Patients otherwise at risk for sudden death, such as patients with bouts of ischemic ventricular tachycardia and/or a history of myocardial infarction with subsequently depressed ejection fraction, should be considered for implantable cardioverter defibrillator (ICD) placement (reviewed in refs. 18 and 19). The use of ICD devices remains an area of active investigation and likely will expand as smaller and less expensive devices are developed.

In the in-hospital setting, where sudden ventricular fibrillation/ventricular tachycardia (VF/VT) from coronary events is not the most common mechanism of arrest, prevention requires a different approach. Several studies have demonstrated that hospitalized patients who suffer cardiac arrest frequently exhibit signs and symptoms of destabilization up to 12 hours before they become pulseless.[20,21] These symptoms include vital sign changes such as progressive hypoten-

TABLE 15-1 Etiologies of Cardiac Arrest

Myocardial ischemia/infarction
Primary cardiac arrhythmia
Hypothermia
Septic shock
Trauma
Systemic inflammatory response syndrome
Tension pneumothorax
Myocardial pump failure
  Pulmonary embolism
  Cardiac tamponade
  Ventricular wall rupture
  Severe valvular disease
  Infiltrative cardiomyopathy
  Inflammatory cardiomyopathy
Massive hemorrhage
  Postoperative
  Trauma
  Gastrointestinal bleeding
Hypoxemia/respiratory failure
  Pneumonia
  Pulmonary embolism
  Status asthmaticus
  Suffocation, e.g., foreign-body aspiration
Electrolyte derangement
  Hyperkalemia
  Hypocalcemia
Drug toxicity/overdose
  Digoxin
  β Blockers
  Calcium channel blockers
  Tricyclic antidepressants

NOTE: This list is by no means exhaustive; a number of etiologies are grouped by mechanism, although some most likely involve multiple mechanisms (e.g., pulmonary embolism causing hypoxemia and right ventricular pump failure). Myocardial ischemia and primary cardiac arrhythmia are the most common underlying pathophysiologic mechanisms in cardiac arrest, especially in out-of-hospital arrest.

sion, tachycardia, hypothermia, or hypoxia. They also include clinical changes such as mental status deterioration or progressive shortness of breath. Therefore, nursing staff should be appropriately vigilant in monitoring for such changes, and physicians should be duly attentive to warning signs from patients and staff. Early stabilization by such measures as intubation, initiation of vasopressor therapy, and/or transfer to an intensive care unit are far more effective than treating cardiac arrest once it has occurred. In Europe, this concept has been formalized into the ALERT course, in which hospital staff and

TABLE 15-2 Contact Information for BLS and ACLS Training and Resources

American Heart Association (AHA)
  Web site: *www.americanheart.org*
  Telephone: (800) 242-8721

American Red Cross (ARC)
  Web site: *www.redcross.org*
  Telephone: (202) 303-4498

European Resuscitation Council (ERC)
  Web site: *www.erc.edu*
  Telephone: +32 3 821 36 16

physicians are trained to recognize and treat the early signs of destabilization that may lead to cardiac arrest.[22–24]

Resuscitation Team Organization

It is very important for hospitals, ICUs, and prehospital care systems to establish a clearly delineated team structure for cardiac arrest treatment. In-hospital studies have shown that a well-trained and organized arrest team is an important component in the resuscitation from sudden death.[25] Team members should be ACLS trained and have a specified team leader who will lead the resuscitation efforts. Training should emphasize the need for a hierarchical structure, with the team leader making most treatment decisions, to prevent the confusion that often occurs during cardiac arrest events. It also should be emphasized that response time is critical, such that a resuscitation team should be able to arrive on the scene of a cardiac arrest within minutes to initiate treatment. Recent data demonstrate that groups with best-practice survival from cardiac arrest have mean "call to shock" times (for VF/VT arrest) of 5 minutes or less,[26] and certainly the earlier the response, the more likely a better outcome will be obtained.

Resuscitation efforts during cardiac arrest require activities to be performed quickly, calmly, and in regimented fashion. Rescuer panic and disorganized efforts are counterproductive and can best be avoided by appropriate training before (and debriefing after) events take place. With the growth of medical simulation technology and sophisticated manikins for resuscitation training, it is possible for cardiac arrest teams to rehearse scenarios to supplement education and enhance preparedness.[27,28]

Basic Life Support

The first steps of resuscitation from cardiac arrest involve what is known as Basic Life Support (BLS). These fundamental skills are part of CPR training courses offered to the public by organizations such as the American Heart Association and the American Red Cross. Given the importance of early recognition and care for cardiac arrest, it is incumbent on all medical personnel from ward receptionists to radiology technicians to physicians to maintain BLS training. Health care workers also should encourage the public to obtain these skills, which are often summarized by the ABC's—airway, breathing, and circulation.

Initial Assessment

When a patient is first assessed, it must be determined if the patient is truly unresponsive. Stimulation by squeezing a shoulder or rubbing the sternum is reasonable, and if no movement, eye opening, or verbal response is noted, attention should be turned to the ABC's. The outdated BLS teaching that a patient should be shaken probably should be avoided given that the unresponsive state may be secondary to head and neck trauma. Care should be given to moving a patient as little as possible until this is determined. If a patient is deemed unresponsive, the initial observer immediately should call for help while assessing the ABC's.

Airway

To attempt optimal airway opening, the chin should be lifted, and the jaw should be thrust forward. A quick evaluation of the oropharynx should be performed to look for a foreign body, blood, or other occluding material. Any visualized foreign body should be removed by suction or by careful use of fingers or forceps. After this evaluation, several "rescue breaths" should be delivered via mouth-to-mouth or mask-to-mouth technique. If the chest wall does not rise with these breaths, it is possible that a complete airway obstruction exists, and abdominal thrusts should be performed to attempt airway clearance. If these fail, trained personnel may need to establish a surgical airway via cricothyrotomy.

Breathing

While holding the chin and jaw in the correct position, breaths should be delivered during initial efforts until a more definitive airway can be obtained. In cardiac arrest, this is performed via endotracheal intubation, which is performed routinely by anesthesiologists, emergency physicians, respiratory therapists, and paramedics. If possible, ventilation should be performed with maximal F_{IO_2} via bag-valve-mask until intubation is performed. Pulse oximetry can be used to monitor patient oxygen saturation during this process.

Circulation

The hemodynamic status of the patient should be assessed via palpation of arterial sites. As an approximate rule of thumb, the radial, femoral, and carotid pulses are lost at systolic pressures below 80, 70, and 60 mm Hg, respectively.[15] Therefore, the most sensitive site to assess is the carotid artery. If no pulse can be felt at the carotid, chest compressions should be initiated immediately. Compressions should be performed at a rate of 100 beats per minute and to a depth of at least 1 to 2 in.

Recent studies have demonstrated the importance of "good quality" chest compressions, partially defined by compressions performed at the appropriate rate and depth. This is important in light of the fact that an observational study has shown performance of chest compressions to be grossly suboptimal in practice.[29] Rescuers should pay particular attention to the performance of this skill. Future generations of resuscitation devices may aid this process by monitoring the quality of chest compressions and generating alarms during suboptimal performance. Exciting recent data have suggested that chest compressions may be more important than defibrillation in the initial treatment of cardiac arrest.[30,31] These observations, which might have been considered heretical just several years ago, lend support to an important new paradigm in cardiac arrest, that of the *three-phase model* of cardiac arrest (see discussion later in this chapter).[32] It has been proposed that 90 seconds of CPR be performed before defibrillation,[33] but this recommendation has not been evaluated fully for inclusion in the American Heart Association ACLS guidelines.

Monitoring the adequacy of the circulation during performance of CPR traditionally has been based on palpation of pulses. Capnography is an attractive adjunct to bedside clinical monitoring because the amount of carbon dioxide returned from peripheral tissues and then exhaled from the lung should be a measure of the adequacy of cardiac output. In one prospective, observational study,[33a] 150 consecutive cardiac arrests out of hospital were monitored by end-tidal carbon dioxide levels after intubation. After 20 minutes of advanced cardiac life support, end-tidal carbon dioxide levels averaged 4.4 ± 2.9 mm Hg in nonsurvivors and 32.8 ± 7.4 mm Hg in survivors ($p < 0.001$). A 20-minute end-tidal carbon dioxide value of 10 mm Hg or less successfully discriminated between the 35 patients who survived to hospital admission and the 115 nonsurvivors. While not yet routine, capnography may be useful for both judging the adequacy of resuscitative efforts and offering prognostic information.

While not strictly part of BLS, fluid resuscitation is a crucial adjunct to circulatory support in the initial phases of resuscitation. Intravenous access should be obtained rapidly if it is not already present, and adult patients should receive a rapid infusion of at least 500 to 1000 mL of 0.9% saline or lactated Ringer's solution. In children, the crystalloid infusion should be calculated at 20 mL/kg. The ideal IV access would include a peripheral large-bore (i.e., 14 to 18 gauge) catheter and/or large-bore central catheter (i.e., not a double- or triple-lumen catheter). The optimal site for central line placement in resuscitation is the femoral vein because the chest and neck are busy sites for chest compressions and ventilatory support, respectively, making subclavian or internal jugular approaches impractical unless already present. In children, an intraosseous line may be a convenient approach to initial access.

Ventricular Tachycardia with a Pulse

Ventricular tachycardia (VT) may or may not generate a pulse. Therefore, it is crucial to assess the hemodynamic status before ACLS resuscitative measures are begun. If the patient has a pulse, is conscious, and has only mild complaints of palpitations, mild chest discomfort, weakness, and/or anxiety, immediate electrical cardioversion is not required. On the other hand, if the patient exhibits signs of instability, including syncope, severe chest pain, or marked hypotension, then cardioversion should proceed immediately after appropriate sedation is delivered.

The treatment of VT with a pulse includes intravenous administration of lidocaine or amiodarone and supportive care (oxygen administration and preparation for electrical cardioversion). In cases in which both VT and supraventricular tachycardia with aberrancy cannot be distinguished with certainty, the use of procainamide can be considered because it is appropriate for both conditions. Recurrent VT often requires electrophysiologic evaluation and treatment, including the placement of an implantable cardioverter defibrillator (reviewed in ref. 34).

Ventricular Fibrillation/Ventricular Tachycardia without a Pulse

Ventricular fibrillation and ventricular tachycardia without a pulse (VF/VT) are grouped together because both require the same treatment—immediate defibrillation. In

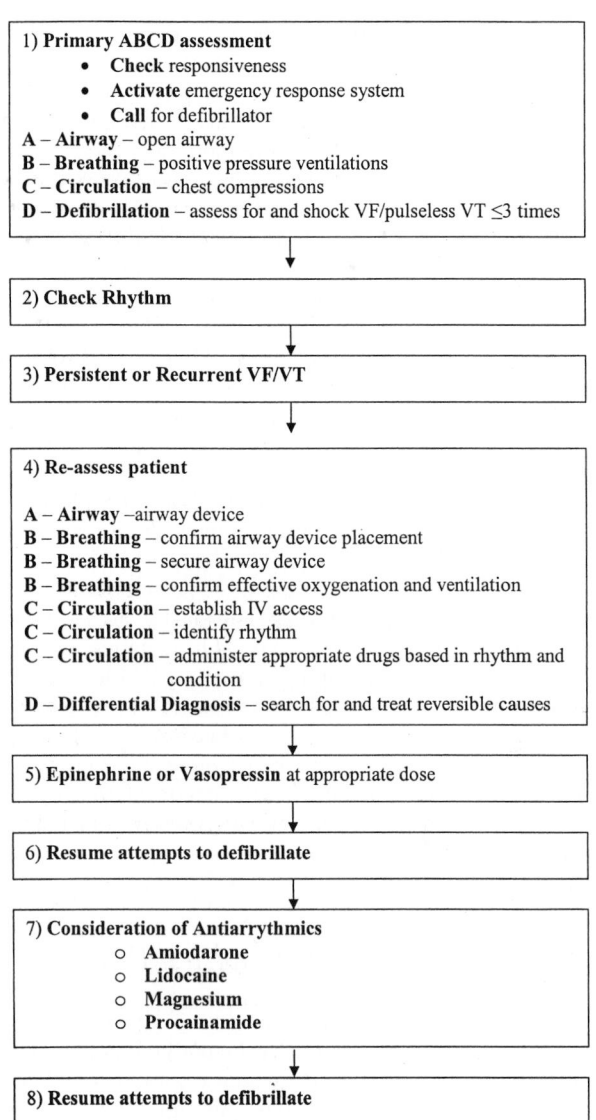

FIGURE 15-1 ACLS algorithm for VF/VT. Perhaps the most important aspect of this algorithm is the need for early defibrillation. *(Modified from American Heart Association ACLS Manual.)*

fact, defibrillation should precede any other assessment or treatment. Studies have shown consistently that the earlier a patient is defibrillated successfully, the better are the chances for survival.[35] This observation has stimulated the use of automatic external defibrillators (AEDs) in airports and other public locations (see the section on AEDs later in this chapter).

When a patient is found in VF/VT, up to three defibrillatory shocks should be delivered in rapid succession, with a brief pause between each shock to examine the cardiac monitor (see Fig. 15-1 for a VF/VT algorithm). There is no need to feel for a pulse between shocks unless the rhythm has changed. Using standard monophasic defibrillators, the first shock should be delivered at 200 J; the next two shocks can be delivered at 200 J or at 300 and 360 J, respectively, in the energy escalation proposed in the ACLS guidelines. Using biphasic defibrillators (see later in this chapter for a discussion of different defibrillator types), all shocks should be delivered at 150 J or at the energy suggested by the manufacturer.[4]

If a patient remains in pulseless VF/VT immediately after these three shocks, further treatments include assessment of the ABC's and pharmacologic adjuncts. Chest compressions should be initiated immediately, with care taken to ensure compression quality, as discussed previously. Patients should be intubated immediately and ventilated with 100% O_2, with care taken to ensure correct endotracheal tube placement by both auscultation and end-tidal CO_2 detection, if available. If not already performed, IV access should be established. Large-bore (not multilumen) central venous access by the femoral approach is most convenient and practical in this setting if skilled personnel are available. It is often useful to obtain an arterial blood gas sample at this point as well because it will take some time for the results to return to the team in any case. While these steps are taking place, the arrest team leader should rapidly obtain a very brief history from available sources, including nursing staff, family, or physicians caring for the patient. The most important details to obtain are when the patient was last seen with a pulse, what pertinent medical problems the patient has, and what has taken place in the last few hours of patient observation.

In VF/VT arrest, either epinephrine 1 mg IV or vasopressin 40 U IV should be given early, preferably within the first 5 minutes of resuscitation efforts. Vasopressin, a relatively new addition to the ACLS guidelines, has been shown to improve coronary perfusion pressure and possibly improve initial resuscitation compared with epinephrine.[36–38] However, despite some optimism regarding the theoretical advantages of vasopressin over epinephrine, conclusive data showing improved survival to hospital discharge are still lacking.[39] Additionally, high doses of epinephrine (e.g., 3 or 5 mg IV) previously had been hoped to have additional benefit over the standard 1 mg IV dose, but human trials have demonstrated no significant survival benefit.[40–42]

After the administration of epinephrine or vasopressin, another shock at 360 J should be delivered. If the patient remains in VF/VT after this, additional medications can be administered before additional defibrillation attempts. One such pharmacologic option is amiodarone, given as a 300-mg IV bolus. Two studies have shown clearly higher initial survival with amiodarone compared with lidocaine, although lidocaine and amiodarone have yet to show an effect on survival to hospital discharge.[43,44]

Pulseless Electrical Activity

Pulseless electrical activity (PEA) is a state defined by having no detectable pulse despite the appearance of an organized electrical rhythm on cardiac monitoring. This electrical activity may appear as so-called normal sinus rhythm or similar pattern but must be differentiated from pulseless VF/VT, which requires specific treatment (see above). PEA used to be described as "electromechanical dissociation" (EMD), based on the assumption that some pathophysiologic process had separated the normal electrical conduction of the heart from its ability to cause myocardial contraction. Echocardiographic studies of myocardium in PEA, however, demonstrate some degree of visible muscle activity.[45] Thus, the term *EMD* has fallen out of favor compared with the more appropriate PEA.

The initial approach to a patient in PEA is much the same as the approach to patients with other pulseless rhythms

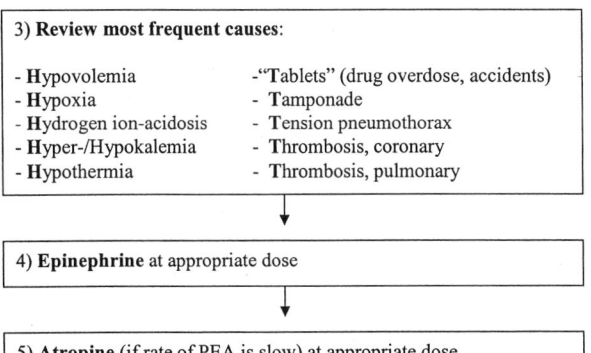

FIGURE 15-2 ACLS algorithm for PEA. Note that this algorithm really serves more as a prompt for differential diagnosis; see Table 15-3 for elaboration of PEA etiologies. (*Modified from American Heart Association ACLS Manual.*)

TABLE 15-3 PEA Differential Diagnosis and Possible Treatments

PEA Etiology	Possible Treatment
Cardiac temponade	Needle pericardiocentesis
Drug overdose	Specific antidotes as required
Hyperkalemia	Administration of calcium, insulin, glucose, bicarbonate
Hypothermia	Rewarming with warm IV fluids, warming blankets
Hypovolemia	Administration of IV fluids, blood, and/or blood products
Hypoxia	Ventilation with 100% O_2
Massive pulmonary embolism	tPA or other thrombolytic agent
Myocardial infarction	Thrombolytic agent or interventional catheterization
Tension pneumothorax	Needle thoracostomy on affected side of chest

NOTE: This list only covers the major common etiologies that might be considered in the treatment of PEA. Hypovolemia and hypoxia are probably the most likely in-hospital factors leading to PEA arrest; myocardial infarction and hypothermia are probably the most common out-of-hospital etiologies.

(see Fig. 15-2 for a PEA algorithm). CPR should be initiated immediately, a definitive airway should be established, and the patient should be ventilated with 100% O_2. Large-bore central venous access should be established. An arterial blood gas sample should be obtained early, with a request to check hemoglobin and potassium, if possible. A brief history should be taken from staff by the resuscitation team leader regarding the events leading up to the pulseless state. Neck veins should be examined to consider cardiac tamponade, lungs should be auscultated to rule out tension pneumothorax, and if appropriate, the patient's temperature should be taken to evaluate for hypothermia. All patients in PEA should receive epinephrine 1 mg IV early in the resuscitation efforts.

In contrast to VF/VT, there is no specific treatment for PEA per se. There are, however, a number of appropriate therapeutic options depending on the *cause* of PEA. Therefore, a differential diagnosis must be considered quickly (Table 15-3). Intravascular hypovolemia, through either hemorrhage or leakage of fluid from the vascular compartment, is a common cause of cardiac arrest in the hospital setting. A high suspicion for this etiology should be maintained for patients

who recently underwent surgery or for patients known to have a serious infectious process and now may be presenting in septic shock. Hypoxemia is another common cause of PEA, although ventilation with 100% O_2 renders this largely a diagnosis of exclusion. A third common process underlying PEA is hypothermia, which again may be common in postoperative and/or septic patients. Aggressive treatment with warm IV fluids and warming blankets should be undertaken in these patients during resuscitation. Resuscitative efforts should not be terminated until all efforts have been made to warm the patient to normothermia.

Tension pneumothorax also can lead to PEA arrest and should be considered especially in any patient who was mechanically ventilated prior to arrest. Lung auscultation during ventilatory cycles should help to identify this problem. If lung sounds are diminished unilaterally, the endotracheal tube should be pulled back several centimeters to determine if a main stem bronchus intubation was present. If decreased breath sounds persist after this maneuver, a needle thoracostomy should be performed with a 16- to 18-gauge IV catheter in the second intercostal space on the side exhibiting diminished lung sounds.

Another major cause of PEA arrest that deserves some discussion is massive pulmonary embolism, which can lead not only to hypoxemia but also to cardiogenic shock from sudden right ventricular (RV) dysfunction. If the resources are available, rapid echocardiography can be performed during resuscitation efforts to evaluate the size and function of the right ventricle. A markedly enlarged and poorly contracting right ventricle supports the diagnosis of pulmonary embolism. This diagnosis also should be considered for patients with known deep venous thrombosis or possible thrombophilia from disease processes such as malignancy or systemic lupus and for patients who have been hospitalized and/or immobile for at least several days. If pulmonary embolism is strongly suspected, treatment with tissue plasminogen activator (tPA) can be considered. The use of tPA in cardiac arrest remains controversial, however (see discussion of tPA later in this chapter).

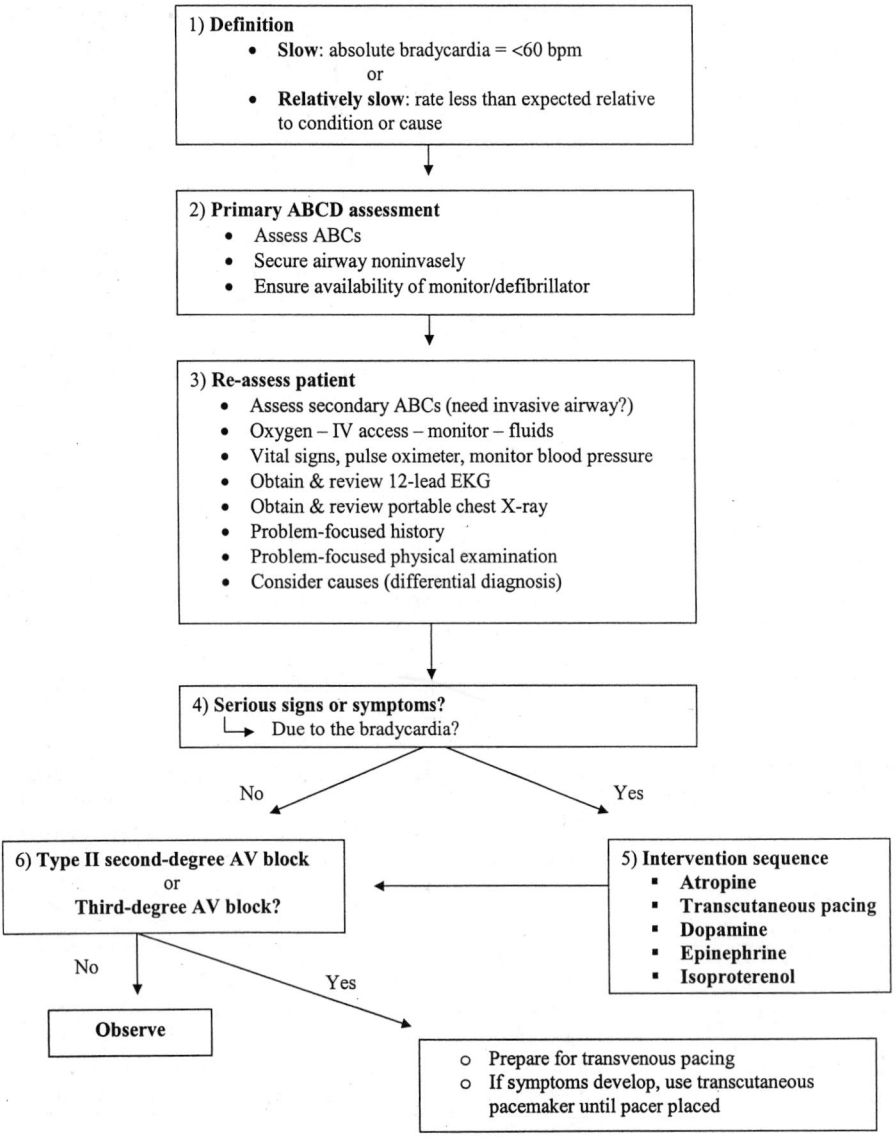

FIGURE 15-3 ACLS algorithm for bradycardia. *(Modified from American Heart Association ACLS Manual.)*

The patient should be evaluated for other causes of PEA. These include cardiac tamponade, for which pericardiocentesis with a long spinal needle can be lifesaving; hyperkalemia, requiring treatment with intravenous calcium, insulin, and glucose; and drug toxicity, which requires specific therapies depending on the drug in question.

Bradycardia

In some cases, a pulseless state can occur if the heart rate slows dramatically, e.g., to less than 30 to 40 beats per minute. This can occur in cases of complete heart block, hypoxemia, hypothermia, and toxic states from certain medications, especially β blockers and calcium channel blockers. In a sense, pulseless bradycardia is a subset of PEA arrest in which additional specific treatments may be attempted beyond that for PEA itself.

After standard ACLS maneuvers including CPR, intubation, and ventilation with 100% O_2 and administration of epinephrine (see preceding sections), treatment should be directed toward increasing the rate of electrical activity, which may be sufficient to generate a blood pressure (and therefore a pulse). If this increased rate does not generate a pulse, the patient truly can be considered to be in PEA arrest.

Methods to increase the heart rate include administration of atropine 1.0 mg IV, which may be repeated up to a total of 0.04 mg/kg, and a trial of electrical pacing (see Fig. 15-3 for a bradycardia algorithm). Transcutaneous electrical pacing, a standard capability of most hospital defibrillators, can be attempted as well, although no evidence-based recommendations exist regarding rate and current to be applied. We recommend starting at a rate of 80 impulses per minute and 50 mA current, ramping up the current as necessary to obtain capture, if possible at all.[46]

Asystole

All patients in cardiac arrest eventually converge into the rhythm of *asystole,* which is defined as no discernible electrical activity on cardiac monitoring (see Fig. 15-4 for an asystole algorithm). An occasional wide complex can be seen in asystole, which is known as an *agonal rhythm*—this carries the

```
1) Primary ABCD assessment
   • Check responsiveness
   • Activate emergency response system
   • Call for defibrillator
A – Airway – open airway
B – Breathing – positive pressure ventilations
C – Circulation – chest compressions
C – Confirm true asystole
D – Defibrillation – assess for and shock VF/Pulseless VT
```

⬇

```
2) Re-assess patient

A – Airway – airway device
B – Breathing – confirm airway device placement
B – Breathing – secure airway device
B – Breathing – confirm effective oxygenation and ventilation
C – Circulation – confirm true asystole
C – Circulation – establish IV access
C – Circulation – identify rhythm
C – Circulation – give medications appropriate for rhythm and
condition
D – Differential Diagnosis – search for and treat reversible causes
```

⬇

```
3) Transcutaneous pacing (perform immediately if considered)
```

⬇

```
4) Epinephrine at appropriate dose
```

⬇

```
5) Atropine at appropriate dose
```

⬇

```
6) Persistent Asystole; consider whether to withhold or cease
resuscitative efforts
   ○ Consider quality of resuscitation
   ○ Presence of atypical clinical features?
```

FIGURE 15-4 ACLS algorithm for asystole. (*Modified from American Heart Association ACLS Manual.*)

same grave prognosis as asystole itself. Unwitnessed cardiac arrest with the presenting rhythm of asystole has a dismal rate of survival, usually considered to be less than 1%.[47] There are very few treatment options for rescuers confronted with asystolic patients, and therefore, a rapid search for reversible causes combined with standard ACLS measures in most cases should not lead to lengthy resuscitation efforts.

Besides standard resuscitation techniques (described earlier), including chest compressions, intubation, ventilation with 100% O_2, and administration of epinephrine, atropine infusion and a trial of electrical pacing may be used. Atropine should be dosed intravenously in 1-mg increments every 3 to 5 minutes during arrest, up to 0.04 mg/kg. Transcutaneous electrical pacing may be attempted as well, following the same recommendations as those for bradycardia (see discussion on bradycardia above).

After three rounds of epinephrine and atropine administration, 10 to 15 minutes of chest compressions, and possibly transcutaneous pacing, the clinical situation should be reassessed. If the rhythm remains in asystole, efforts should be terminated, because survival after 10 to 15 minutes of

confirmed asystole despite pharmacologic intervention and intubation is essentially zero.[48,49] An important caveat in the assessment of asystole is that at least two cardiac monitoring leads should be examined for a rhythm—often what appears to be asystole in one lead actually represents a loose electrical connection, and one might find a treatable rhythm in another lead.

Ending Resuscitation Efforts

The subject of resuscitation team function and performance remains poorly studied, and usually ACLS training gives short shrift to team cooperation and leadership skills. The decision to terminate efforts represents a difficult moment for the resuscitation team and the team leader.[50] One simple recommendation to ease the tension of this moment and ensure that all reasonable effort has been given to save the life of the patient is to involve the entire team in the termination process. We recommend that the team leader, sensing that effort has become futile, should verbally summarize to the team all the treatment rendered so far, e.g., how long CPR has been performed, what drugs and shocks were given, and what underlying arrest etiologies were considered. The team leader then can ask if any team member has final recommendations or suggestions before efforts are halted. In this fashion, the decision to stop resuscitation procedures is made by the group, and staff will feel satisfied that resuscitation was not terminated prematurely. After termination, it is often useful to conduct a debriefing session among key team personnel before disbanding, especially to troubleshoot any technical or team function problems. Hospitals should establish CPR review committees to monitor the quality of resuscitations on a periodic basis and implement system changes as necessary to improve outcomes.

Aspects of Defibrillation

Modern electrical defibrillation, or the use of electric current applied directly to a patient's chest to restore a viable heart rhythm, grew out of research into electrocution deaths among maintenance workers at Consolidated Edison of New York. The first human defibrillation was performed intraoperatively by Claude Beck in 1947; the first external defibrillation was undertaken by Paul Zoll in 1955.[51] Since that time, defibrillation has become a cornerstone of cardiac resuscitation and has been used successfully by physicians, nurses, paramedics, police, and even the public at large.

The exact mechanism of defibrillation remains uncertain. Whether a critical number of myocardial cells require membrane depolarization to overcome ventricular fibrillation or whether certain regions of the heart must achieve a critical current density remains a subject of active study. Several mechanistic aspects are clear, however. The energy discharged (measured in joules, or watt-seconds) appears to have both dose-response and therapeutic window characteristics. That is, the chance of successful defibrillation rises with increasing energies delivered; however, as energy is increased further, functional myocardial injury predominates over useful resuscitative properties. With standard defibrillators, 200 J is the recommended energy for initial shock; 300 and 360 J are accepted levels for subsequent attempts to defibrillate. For children, the recommended initial dose is 2 J/kg, with a second shock at 4 J/kg if the first shock fails.

Technique of defibrillation is also important. Firm pressure must be applied with defibrillation paddles to ensure proper delivery of energy without electrical arc or skin burn. Similarly, defibrillation pads must be well applied to the chest. Positioning of paddles or pads must ensure that the imaginary line connecting the two electrodes runs through the heart. That is, in one standard approach, an electrode should be placed at the right upper sternal border and the other at the left midaxillary line near the apex of the heart.

Perhaps the most important observation regarding electrical defibrillation is that the longer the delay before a shock is delivered, the less chance there is for a successful resuscitation. Ventricular fibrillation or tachycardia should be defibrillated immediately; this is the fundamental principle underlying implantable cardioverter defibrillators (ICDs), a commonly placed device for patients with recurrent ventricular tachycardia or history of cardiac arrest.[18] If VF/VT persists for even 5 minutes without CPR or defibrillation, the chance for a successful outcome falls dramatically.

Given the need for early defibrillation, automatic external defibrillators (AEDs) have become an important tool for paramedics and the lay public. These devices, commonly found in airports and other heavily trafficked public locales, perform rhythm analysis and provide defibrillatory shocks if needed. In theory, no prior experience should be required to operate such a device. AEDs are discussed in more detail below.

Most defibrillators in use today generate monophasic waveform shocks. Over the past few years, biphasic defibrillators have become available commercially and likely will become the standard of care over the next decade. These defibrillators have been shown to be equally effective as monophasic devices at lower energies, which may optimize the benefits of the shock while minimizing myocardial injury.[4]

A New Three-Phase Time-Sensitive Model of Cardiac Arrest Therapy

There is hope that in the coming years resuscitation science will offer substantially improved survival for victims of cardiac arrest. With the success of early defibrillation programs in airports, casinos, and other public places, survival rates in these special locales have soared to greater than 50%.[52] However, a new paradigm has emerged in our understanding of sudden death. The three-phase time-sensitive model of cardiac arrest, based on data from the past several years, offers the hope of better survival with therapy tailored to the time after initial arrest.[32]

This model proposes that time in cardiac arrest can be divided into different phases: the electrical phase (the first 4 minutes after arrest), the circulatory phase (minutes 4 through 10), and the metabolic phase (after 10 minutes), with each requiring different therapeutic approaches (Fig. 15-5). The electrical phase calls for defibrillation as the first therapy for VF/VT and is currently our standard of care regardless of time spent in cardiac arrest. This fits well with national efforts to get more rapid defibrillation with AEDs—because the evidence suggests that defibrillation within the first few minutes is associated with a better than 50% chance of initial survival. However, a challenge during this electrical phase is the need to get defibrillators rapidly to victims at home, where over 70% of cardiac arrests take place. The circulatory phase appears to be best treated initially with chest compressions and ventilations and then followed by defibrillation after several minutes of CPR. Note that this is not the current standard of care according to the American Heart Association at the time of this writing. Using this "CPR first" algorithm, paramedic services in Norway have improved survival rates from 4% to 20% over standard advanced cardiac life support during this circulatory phase.[30] However, another challenge becomes apparent during this phase: our current quality of CPR remains unmeasured and poorly controlled. Recent studies would suggest that CPR quality in real resuscitation falls far short of the high quality required for survival—and new technology offers us the ability to markedly improve on this in the next few years.[29] This circulatory phase may be difficult to identify because we usually do not have accurate information on time of collapse and thus may not know in which phase a patient resides. The circulatory phase depends on very good CPR, so prioritizing good compression rate, compression depth, minimal pauses in compression, and proper ventilatory management all become critical priorities.

The third so-called metabolic phase is the most lethal and challenges our basic scientific understanding of ischemia and

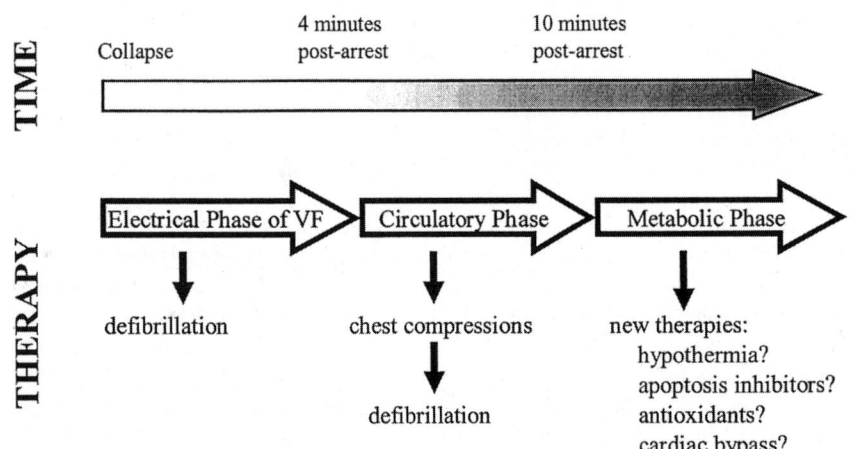

FIGURE 15-5 This three-phase model serves as a paradigm shift in the categorization and treatment of cardiac arrest. While some data have been published recently to support the model, it is still considered theoretical but likely will serve as a tool to think about future therapies.

reperfusion injury. Novel therapies, such as advanced cardioprotective pharmacologic agents, cardiopulmonary bypass, induced hypothermia (see Chap. 16), preconditioning pathways, inflammatory mediators, apoptosis signaling, and hibernation may offer promise in the understanding and treatment for this phase—but the need for new translational research in this area is vital. The tools of molecular biology, proteomics, and cellular physiology are likely to provide important insights and to create new biosensors that can guide clinical therapies. It is not unrealistic to believe that major improvements in survival rates will result as we change our current practices in the near future.[53]

Automatic External Defibrillators

Given the assumption that early defibrillation remains the best treatment for VF/VT cardiac arrest, a number of devices have been developed to allow inexperienced users to defibrillate victims before the arrival of medical personnel (reviewed in ref. 54). These devices, known as *automatic external defibrillators* (AEDs), have become ubiquitous in airports and other public locations. These simple-to-use defibrillators contain waveform analysis software that determines whether a shock is warranted when a layperson attaches sensing pads to the chest of a comatose individual. Appropriate shocks are then delivered. Audio prompts guide the user through the process.

The placement of AEDs in public places has been shown to affect survival from cardiac arrest, supporting the concept that earlier defibrillation correlates with improved outcomes.[52] However, the majority of cardiac arrests occur in the home, not in public. Data from Seattle suggest that as many as 70% of out-of-hospital cardiac arrests take place in residences, and only 21% occur in public locales.[1] Whether AEDs should be available for home installation, much like fire extinguishers, remains an active question. As AEDs become smaller, smarter, and cheaper, this debate may tip toward home availability.[55]

Whether AEDs should be placed in hospital wards remains another topic under current discussion.[56] Although hospital resuscitation teams include ACLS-trained personnel, most "first responders" in the hospital setting are nurses or other health care staff who may not be ACLS proficient and therefore unlikely to perform defibrillation. It has been argued that the availability of AEDs in the hospital would allow for rapid defibrillation attempts before the arrival of resuscitation teams. However, the presence of AEDs would not be sufficient—nurses and other health care workers would have to accept defibrillation as a possible primary responsibility. There are some data to suggest nurses would support such a role.[57]

Induced Hypothermia in Cardiac Arrest

In the search for novel cardiac arrest therapies, induced hypothermia has generated a great deal of recent interest, spurred by two well-conducted studies showing improved survival when patients were cooled to 32 to 34°C after resuscitation from cardiac arrest.[58,59] An international recommendation has been issued based on this evidence that patients should be cooled after out-of-hospital cardiac arrest; data on in-hospital cardiac arrest are still under discussion.[60] Much work remains to further define this treatment, regarding both depth and duration of hypothermia. Novel techniques for cooling patients are under development as well, including multiphase coolant fluids and cooling catheters. Chapter 16 of this book is devoted to this exciting field of induced hypothermia.

Pharmacologic Therapy of Cardiac Arrest

CPR and electrical defibrillation are the central treatment modalities for cardiac arrest in current practice. While medications such as epinephrine, atropine, lidocaine, and amiodarone have been incorporated into treatment algorithms for cardiac arrest, to this day they do not have any proven survival benefit.[61] A surge of interest in "high dose" epinephrine in recent years was quelled when a number of studies demonstrated no benefit from this approach.[42,62] Current interest in amiodarone as a treatment for VF/VT is based largely on one study that showed an improvement in initial resuscitation but did not demonstrate an improved survival to hospital discharge.[43] There are no definitive data to demonstrate a survival benefit from atropine or lidocaine. Similarly, bicarbonate, while widely administered during cardiac arrest, has not been proven to aid resuscitation. In fact, ACLS guidelines only recommend bicarbonate infusion in a small subset of cardiac arrest patients, namely, those known to be hyperkalemic.[15] Doses of standard ACLS medications are given in Table 15-4.

Thrombolytic therapy in cardiac arrest has received recent interest because a number of uncontrolled studies and cohort series have suggested a benefit from the use of urokinase or tPA.[63–65] A small but well-executed controlled study recently demonstrated no improvement in return of spontaneous circulation or survival with tPA in the treatment of PEA arrest.[66] A larger European study is currently ongoing and may help to resolve this controversy, and certain subsets of cardiac arrest patients may be found to benefit from this treatment modality. At this point, it is fair to say that thrombolytic therapy may be attempted if there is strong evidence to suspect pulmonary embolism as the cause of arrest.[61,67]

TABLE 15-4 Standard ACLS Medications and Doses

Medication	ACLS Dosing
Amiodarone	300 mg IV bolus, then 1 mg/min IV drip for up to 6 hours
Atropine (asystole)	1 mg IV bolus
Atropine (bradycardia)	0.5 mg IV bolus
Epinephrine	1 mg IV bolus (10 mL of a 1:10,000 solution)
Lidocaine	1.5 mg/kg IV bolus, then 1–4 mg/min (30–50 μg/kg/min) IV drip
Magnesium sulfate	1–2 g IV bolus
Sodium bicarbonate	1–2 mEq/kg IV bolus
Vasopressin	40 U IV bolus

NOTE: A more comprehensive list of ACLS medications and their dosing regimens can be found in the ACLS manual published by the American Heart Association. It is important to stress that very little data suggest that any of these medications actually improve survival to hospital discharge.

Limitations on Cardiac Arrest Efforts

The idea of a *chemical code,* i.e., performing resuscitation with pharmacologic agents only and not with chest compressions or defibrillation, is not controversial insofar as there is no disagreement among expert providers. Studies have demonstrated clearly that the concept lies much more in the realm of mythology or wishful thinking than in science. The only controversy is that the concept has persisted in hospitals and among health care workers across the world to this day.[68] It is important to stress the following point because the chemical code is often presented to family members as an option for care of their loved one: cardiac arrest is not a medical problem treatable by medications only.

In a similar vein, the *slow code,* in which efforts to resuscitate are intentionally delayed or limited by rescuers, is ethically unacceptable.[69] Patients who are *full code* should have every appropriate effort made to resuscitate them; decisions regarding appropriateness of resuscitation efforts should be made by patients and their primary physicians, not by a resuscitation team at the time of arrest.

Ethical Issues

The ethical dimensions of cardiac arrest treatment are complex and important for physicians to consider.[70,71] Decisions regarding termination of efforts and even the decision not to initiate efforts in the first place should be calibrated carefully depending on the individual case in question. The growing establishment of *do not resuscitate* (DNR) protocols has allowed patients and their families to avoid the traumatic and often futile efforts of resuscitation.

It cannot be stressed enough that physicians should initiate frank and truthful end-of-life discussions with patients early in their care, before hospitalization or cardiac arrest appear on the horizon. In this fashion, the use of cardiac arrest treatment can be judiciously tailored to the appropriate patients.[72] Physicians must emphasize the distinction to patients between DNR and *comfort care.* That is, a DNR order means that all curative measures could be employed except chest compressions and defibrillation. This distinction is also important for hospital personnel and physicians to understand, lest a DNR order influence other care decisions in the critically ill. In short, *do not resuscitate* should never mean *do not treat.*[73]

References

1. Eisenberg MS, Mengert TJ: Cardiac resuscitation. *N Engl J Med* 344:1304, 2001.
2. Engdahl J, Holmberg M, Karlson BW, et al: The epidemiology of out-of-hospital "sudden" cardiac arrest. *Resuscitation* 52:235, 2002.
3. White RD, Hankins DG, Atkinson EJ: Patient outcomes following defibrillation with a low energy biphasic truncated exponential waveform in out-of-hospital cardiac arrest. *Resuscitation* 49:9, 2001.
4. Schneider T, Martens PR, Paschen H, et al: Multicenter, randomized, controlled trial of 150-J biphasic shocks compared with 200- to 360-J monophasic shocks in the resuscitation of out-of-hospital cardiac arrest victims. Optimized Response to Cardiac Arrest (ORCA) Investigators. *Circulation* 102:1780, 2000.
5. Eisenberg MS, Horwood BT, Cummins RO, et al: Cardiac arrest and resuscitation: A tale of 29 cities. *Ann Emerg Med* 19:179, 1990.
6. Lombardi G, Gallagher J, Gennis P: Outcome of out-of-hospital cardiac arrest in New York. *JAMA* 271:678, 1994.
7. Becker LB, Han BH, Meyer PM, et al: CPR Chicago: Racial differences in the incidence of cardiac arrest and subsequent survival. *N Engl J Med* 329:600, 1993.
8. Becker LB, Ostrander MP, Barrett J, Kondos GT: Outcome of CPR in a large metropolitan area: Where are the survivors? *Ann Emerg Med* 20:355, 1991.
9. Abella BS, Becker LB: Ischemia-reperfusion and acute apoptotic cell death, in Vincent JL (ed): *Yearbook of Intensive Care and Emergency Medicine.* Berlin, Springer, 2002, p 3.
10. Vanden Hoek TL: Preconditioning and postresuscitation injury. *Crit Care Med* 30:S172, 2002.
11. Becker LB: The epidemiology of sudden death, in Paradis NA, Halperin HR, Nowak RM (eds): *Cardiac Arrest: The Science and Practice of Resuscitation Medicine.* Baltimore, Williams & Wilkins, 1996, p 28.
12. Herlitz J, Eek M, Holmberg M, et al: Characteristics and outcome among patients having out of hospital cardiac arrest at home compared with elsewhere. *Heart* 88:579, 2002.
13. Holmberg M, Holmberg S, Herlitz J: Effect of bystander cardiopulmonary resuscitation in out-of-hospital cardiac arrest patients in Sweden. *Resuscitation* 47:59, 2000.
14. Ornato JP, Peberdy MA, Tadler SC, Strobos NC: Factors associated with the occurrence of cardiac arrest during hospitalization for acute myocardial infarction in the second national registry of myocardial infarction in the US. *Resuscitation* 48:117, 2001.
15. Guidelines 2000 for cardiopulmonary resuscitation and emergency cardiovascular care: International consensus on science. *Circulation* 102(suppl):I-1, 2000.
16. Reis AG, Nadkarni V, Perondi MB, et al: A prospective investigation into the epidemiology of in-hospital pediatric cardiopulmonary resuscitation using the international Utstein reporting style. *Pediatrics* 109:200, 2002.
17. Mogayzel C, Quan L, Graves JR, et al: Out-of-hospital ventricular fibrillation in children and adolescents: causes and outcomes. *Ann Emerg Med* 25:484, 1995.
18. Moss AJ: MADIT-II and its implications. *Eur Heart J* 24:16, 2003.
19. Prystowsky EN: Screening and therapy for patients with nonsustained ventricular tachycardia. *Am J Cardiol* 86:K34, 2000.
20. Smith AF, Wood J: Can some in-hospital cardio-respiratory arrests be prevented? A prospective survey. *Resuscitation* 37:133, 1998.
21. Franklin C, Mathew J: Developing strategies to prevent inhospital cardiac arrest: Analyzing responses of physicians and nurses in the hours before the event. *Crit Care Med* 22:244, 1994.
22. Smith GB, Osgood VM, Crane S: ALERT: A multiprofessional training course in the care of the acutely ill adult patient. *Resuscitation* 52:281, 2002.
23. Hodgetts TJ, Kenward G, Vlachonikolis IG, et al: The identification of risk factors for cardiac arrest and formulation of activation criteria to alert a medical emergency team. *Resuscitation* 54:125, 2002.
24. Buist MD, Moore GE, Bernard SA, et al: Effects of a medical emergency team on reduction of incidence of and mortality from unexpected cardiac arrests in hospital: Preliminary study. *Br Med J* 324:387, 2002.
25. Hillman K, Parr M, Flabouris A, et al: Redefining in-hospital resuscitation: The concept of the medical emergency team. *Resuscitation* 48:105, 2001.
26. Pearn J: Improving survival: A multi-portal approach to improving cardiopulmonary resuscitation outcomes. *Resuscitation* 42:3, 1999.
27. Christensen UJ, Heffernan D, Andersen SF, Jensen PF: ResusSim 98: A PC advanced life support trainer. *Resuscitation* 39:81, 1998.

28. Gaba DM, Howard SK, Flanagan B, et al: Assessment of clinical performance during simulated crises using both technical and behavioral ratings. *Anesthesiology* 89:8, 1998.

29. Abella BS, Sandbo N, Vassilatos P, et al: Chest compression rates frequently fall below AHA recommendation during in-hospital cardiac arrest. *Circulation* 106:1832, 2002.

30. Wik L, Hansen TB, Fylling F, et al: Three minutes of basic cardiopulmonary resuscitation (CPR) of pre-hospital ventricular fibrillation (VF) patients increases the number of patients who restore spontaneous circulation (ROSC). *Circulation* (suppl II), 2001.

31. Cobb LA, Fahrenbruch CE, Walsh TR, et al: Influence of cardiopulmonary resuscitation prior to defibrillation in patients with out-of-hospital ventricular fibrillation. *JAMA* 281:1182, 1999.

32. Weisfeldt ML, Becker LB: Resuscitation after cardiac arrest: A three-phase time-sensitive model. *JAMA* 288:3035, 2002.

33. Berg RA, Cobb LA, Doherty A, et al: Chest compressions NON and basic life support: Defibrillation. *Ann Emerg Med* 37:S26, 2001.

33a. Levine RL, Wayne MA, Miller CC: End-tidal carbon dioxide and outcome of out-of-hospital cardiac arrest. *N Engl J Med* 337:301, 1997.

34. Weigner MJ, Buxton AE: Nonsustained ventricular tachycardia: A guide to the clinical significance and management. *Med Clin North Am* 85:305, 2001.

35. Cummins RO: From concept to standard-of-care? Review of the clinical experience with automated external defibrillators. *Ann Emerg Med* 18:1269, 1989.

36. Babar SI, Berg RA, Hilwig RW, et al: Vasopressin versus epinephrine during cardiopulmonary resuscitation: A randomized swine outcome study. *Resuscitation* 41:185, 1999.

37. Wenzel V, Lindner KH, Krismer AC, et al: Survival with full neurologic recovery and no cerebral pathology after prolonged cardiopulmonary resuscitation with vasopressin in pigs. *J Am Coll Cardiol* 35:527, 2000.

38. Stadlbauer KH, Wagner-Berger HG, Wenzel V, et al: Survival with full neurologic recovery after prolonged cardiopulmonary resuscitation with a combination of vasopressin and epinephrine in pigs. *Anesth Analg* 96:1743, 2003.

39. Stiell IG, Hebert PC, Wells GA, et al: Vasopressin versus epinephrine for inhospital cardiac arrest: A randomised, controlled trial. *Lancet* 358:105, 2001.

40. Callaham M, Madsen CD, Barton CW, et al: A randomized clinical trial of high-dose epinephrine and norepinephrine vs standard-dose epinephrine in prehospital cardiac arrest. *JAMA* 268:2667, 1992.

41. Brown CG, Martin DR, Pepe PE, et al: A comparison of standard-dose and high-dose epinephrine in cardiac arrest outside the hospital. The Multicenter High-Dose Epinephrine Study Group. *N Engl J Med* 327:1051, 1992.

42. Stiell IG, Hebert PC, Weitzman BN, et al: High-dose epinephrine in adult cardiac arrest. *N Engl J Med* 327:1045, 1992.

43. Kudenchuk PJ, Cobb LA, Copass MK, et al: Amiodarone for resuscitation after out-of-hospital cardiac arrest due to ventricular fibrillation. *N Engl J Med* 341:871, 1999.

44. Dorian P, Cass D, Schwartz B, et al: Amiodarone as compared with lidocaine for shock-resistant ventricular fibrillation. *N Engl J Med* 346:884, 2002.

45. Bocka JJ, Overton DT, Hauser A: Electromechanical dissociation in human beings: An echocardiographic evaluation. *Ann Emerg Med* 17:450, 1988.

46. Bern AI, Pane GA, Hamilton GC: Electrical interventions in cardiopulmonary resuscitation: Pacing. *Emerg Med Clin North Am* 1:541, 1983.

47. Engdahl J, Bang A, Lindqvist J, Herlitz J: Can we define patients with no and those with some chance of survival when found in asystole out of hospital? *Am J Cardiol* 86:610, 2000.

48. Pepe PE, Levine RL, Fromm RE Jr, et al: Cardiac arrest presenting with rhythms other than ventricular fibrillation: Contribution of resuscitative efforts toward total survivorship. *Crit Care Med* 21:1838, 1993.

49. Stratton SJ, Niemann JT: Outcome from out-of-hospital cardiac arrest caused by nonventricular arrhythmias: Contribution of successful resuscitation to overall survivorship supports the current practice of initiating out-of-hospital ACLS. *Ann Emerg Med* 32:448, 1998.

50. Larkin GL: Termination of resuscitation: The art of clinical decision making. *Curr Opin Crit Care* 8:224, 2002.

51. Eisenberg M: The quest to reverse sudden death: A history of CPR, in Paradis NA, Halperin HR, Nowak RM (eds): *Cardiac Arrest: The Science and Practice of Resuscitation Medicine.* Baltimore, Williams & Wilkens, 1996.

52. Caffrey SL, Willoughby PJ, Pepe PE, Becker LB: Public use of automated external defibrillators. *N Engl J Med* 347:1242, 2002.

53. Becker LB, Weisfeldt ML, Weil MH, et al: The PULSE initiative: Scientific priorities and strategic planning for resuscitation research and life saving therapies. *Circulation* 105:2562, 2002.

54. Marenco JP, Wang PJ, Link MS, et al: Improving survival from sudden cardiac arrest: The role of the automated external defibrillator. *JAMA* 285:1193, 2001.

55. Chen MA, Eisenberg MS, Meischke H: Impact of in-home defibrillators on postmyocardial infarction patients and their significant others: an interview study. *Heart Lung* 31:173, 2002.

56. Kenward G, Castle N, Hodgetts TJ: Should ward nurses be using automatic external defibrillators as first responders to improve the outcome from cardiac arrest? A systematic review of the primary research. *Resuscitation* 52:31, 2002.

57. Stewart AJ, Lowe MD: Knowledge and attitude of nurses on medical wards to defibrillation *J R Coll Phys Lond* 28:399, 1994.

58. The Hypothermia after Cardiac Arrest Study Group: Mild therapeutic hypothermia to improve the neurologic outcome after cardiac arrest. *N Engl J Med* 346:549, 2002.

59. Bernard SA, Gray TW, Buist MD, et al: Treatment of comatose survivors of out-of-hospital cardiac arrest with induced hypothermia. *N Engl J Med* 346:557, 2002.

60. Nolan JP, Morley PT, Vanden Hoek TL, et al: Therapeutic hypothermia after cardiac arrest: an advisory statement by the advanced life support task force of the International Liaison Committee on Resuscitation. *Circulation* 108:118, 2003.

61. Nolan JP, De Latorre FJ, Steen PA, et al: Advanced life support drugs: Do they really work? *Curr Opin Crit Care* 8:212, 2002.

62. Gueugniaud PY, Mols P, Goldstein P, et al: A comparison of repeated high doses and repeated standard doses of epinephrine for cardiac arrest outside the hospital. European Epinephrine Study Group. *N Engl J Med* 339:1595, 1998.

63. Böttiger BW, Padosch SA: Thrombolysis using recombinant tissue-type plasminogen activator during cardiopulmonary resuscitation in patients with out-of-hospital cardiac arrest. *Resuscitation* 52:308, 2002.

64. Böttiger BW, Bode C, Kern S, et al: Efficacy and safety of thrombolytic therapy after initially unsuccessful cardiopulmonary resuscitation: A prospective clinical trial. *Lancet* 357:1583, 2001.

65. Schreiber W, Gabriel D, Sterz F, et al: Thrombolytic therapy after cardiac arrest and its effect on neurological outcome. *Resuscitation* 52:63, 2002.

66. Abu-Laban RB, Christenson JM, Innes GD, et al: Tissue plasminogen activator in cardiac arrest with pulseless electrical activity. *N Engl J Med* 346:1522, 2002.

67. Bailen MR, Cuadra JA, Aguayo De Hoyos E: Thrombolysis during cardiopulmonary resuscitation in fulminant pulmonary embolism: A review. *Crit Care Med* 29:2211, 2001.

68. Holleran RS: When is dead, dead? The ethics of resuscitation in emergency care *Nurs Clin North Am* 37:11, 2002.

69. DePalma JA, Ozanich E, Miller S, Yancich LM: "Slow" code: Perspectives of a physician and critical care nurse. *Crit Care Nurs Q* 22:89, 1999.

70. Marco CA, Schears RM: Societal opinions regarding CPR. *Am J Emerg Med* 20:207, 2002.

71. Holmberg S, Ekstrom L: Ethics and practicalities of resuscitation: A statement for the Advanced Life Support Working Party of the European Resuscitation Council. *Resuscitation* 24:239, 1992.

72. Ghusn HF, Teasdale TA, Boyer K: Characteristics of patients receiving or foregoing resuscitation at the time of cardiopulmonary arrest. *J Am Geriatr Soc* 45:1118, 1997.

73. Marik PE, Zaloga GP: CPR in terminally ill patients? *Resuscitation* 49:99, 2001.

Chapter 16 _____

THERAPEUTIC HYPOTHERMIA

BENJAMIN S. ABELLA
TERRY L. VANDEN HOEK
LANCE B. BECKER

KEY POINTS

- *Induced hypothermia has been shown to reduce mortality when applied after resuscitation from cardiac arrest.*
- *While the ideal temperature for hypothermia is not known, most experts believe that cooling to 32 to 34°C is optimal.*
- *Induced hypothermia may have benefit for other disease processes such as myocardial infarction and stroke.*
- *The mechanisms by which hypothermia acts are multifaceted and a focus of much current investigation.*

The notion of cooling patients for medical benefit is quite old. In 1814, Baron Larrey, a French surgeon in the service of Napoleon's army, reflected on soldiers who suffered major injuries on the frozen battlefields in Russia by commenting that "cold acts on the living parts... the parts may remain... in a state of asphyxia without losing their life."[1] A belated resurgence of interest in hypothermia has taken place in the past decade, expanding the possible medical indications for its use. Induced hypothermia, the intentional lowering of body temperature, has been explored in a number of acute critical care settings, including myocardial infarction, stroke, head trauma, and after cardiac arrest. While the optimal depth and timing of hypothermia are not yet established for these uses, most experts advocate a temperature goal of 32 to 34°C because it seems to provide significant benefit while avoiding most of the adverse effects associated with the intervention. Timing of hypothermia, with respect to both time of induction and duration of therapy, is even more uncertain, although general consensus holds that cooling should be initiated as soon as possible after the morbid event and should be maintained for at least 12 to 24 hours. Regarding specific uses, there is particularly good evidence that hypothermia is protective for the resuscitated cardiac arrest patient after return of spontaneous circulation.[2,3] The use of hypothermia in other clinical scenarios remains promising but less clear at present.

This chapter addresses elements of the history of hypothermia, the laboratory and clinical data that have developed our understanding of its use, some of the various techniques used to cool patients, and the clinical syndromes for which hypothermia appears to offer the greatest advantage.

History of Induced Hypothermia

The protective effects of hypothermia induction have been suggested since the time of Hippocrates, who advocated packing bleeding patients in snow.[4] Hypothermic protection also was noted by Napoleon's battlefield surgeon, Baron Larrey, during the French invasion of Russia. He observed improved survival of injured soldiers left in the snow compared with those treated with warm blankets and heated drinks.[1] Induced hypothermia has been studied in a wide variety of illnesses, both ischemic and nonischemic in nature (reviewed in refs. 5 through 7). These include traumatic brain injury,[8–10] status epilepticus,[11] arrhythmia, sepsis, and the ischemic illnesses of myocardial infarction, stroke, and cardiac arrest.[7,12] Interestingly, the first reported use of induced hypothermia was in the setting of malignancy. In 1939, Fay and colleagues treated patients with metastatic carcinoma, with the goal of both pain reduction and retardation of tumor growth.[13] While hypothermia to 32°C for 24 hours did not prove effective for the stated goals, it was considered well tolerated.[13]

A decade later, Bigelow studied the induction of hypothermia in the setting of cardiac surgery, with the goal of cerebral protection.[14] Two other studies using hypothermia as therapy for cardiac arrest also were published. Both these early cardiac arrest studies used moderate hypothermia of 30 to 34°C in patients after resuscitation from cardiac arrest. One of these pioneering papers presented a series of four patients, all of whom were cooled and survived arrest.[15] In the other study, 12 patients were cooled with a survival rate of 50% compared with 14% survival in 7 normothermic control patients.[16]

During the 1960s and 1970s, the field of induced hypothermia lay relatively dormant for reasons that remain unclear. Some have suggested that more dramatic therapies were developed that overshadowed cooling as a possible therapy, such as controlled ventilation, monitored ICU management, and cardiopulmonary resuscitation (CPR).[5] Additionally, several adverse effects of hypothermia were described, which may have dampened enthusiasm.[17,18]

Interest in "resuscitative hypothermia" was rekindled by Safar and others at the University of Pittsburgh, who demonstrated in a ventricular fibrillation dog model of cardiac arrest that mild to moderate hypothermia could be induced to improve outcomes.[19,20] Trauma research also provided a motivation for the development of induced hypothermia. It was understood from military combat experience that definitive therapy for penetrating trauma was often delayed for practical reasons (e.g., transportation and access to surgical care) and that measures were needed to preserve exsanguinating soldiers until appropriate care could be delivered.[21] Given the animal data on exsanguination and cooling, it appeared that hypothermia might be a suitable approach.[22]

Safar went on further to describe "suspended animation," a process that allows "rapid preservation of viability of the organisms in temporarily unresuscitable cardiac arrest, which allows time for transport and repair during clinical death and is followed by delayed resuscitation, hopefully to survival without brain damage."[12] Hypothermia has been a primary component of this concept of *stasis*. In this paradigm, victims of cardiac arrest may be cooled to some target temperature and maintained at that temperature for a specific period of time. With advanced medical interventions, which may include cardiopulmonary bypass, metabolic correction, and controlled reperfusion, the patient is stabilized and rewarmed, and "reanimation" is initiated. While many methodologies have been studied under the rubric of suspended animation, including cardiopulmonary bypass and pharmacologic interventions,[23] these are used most often as adjuncts to the use of hypothermia.

Since these initial observations in the 1980s and early 1990s, much of the work pertaining to hypothermia and ischemic disease has focused on focal ischemia and reperfusion, e.g., animal stroke and myocardial infarction models. A number of ischemia-reperfusion (IR) model systems have been developed over the last two decades, including cellular,[24] isolated organ,[25] and whole-animal models in which arterial supply to the organ under study is temporarily occluded.[26,27] In this latter category are included experiences with human IR, for example, during coronary vascular procedures.[28] Recently, two seminal papers were published describing the use of hypothermia to successfully treat resuscitated cardiac arrest patients.[2,3] With these studies, hypothermia has moved from the laboratory to active clinical use.

Mechanisms of Hypothermic Protection

The mechanisms by which induced hypothermia protects against cellular and tissue injury are poorly understood. Given the importance of temperature in a wide range of physiologic processes, it is reasonable to conclude that multiple mechanisms may be involved in any given tissue (reviewed in refs. 5 and 6). Some mechanisms implicated in hypothermic protection include modulation of transcription and/or translation, suppression of reactive oxygen species (ROS) production, and inhibition of programmed cell death, or apoptosis. The mechanisms by which cooling protects tissues may overlap as well. For example, the effect of hypothermia on cellular metabolism may lead indirectly to modulation of programmed cell death, and cooling may have a direct effect on cell death machinery itself. Most of the data pertaining to mechanism of hypothermic protection comes from studies of IR injury in models of stroke and myocardial infarction.

A number of gross physiologic changes have been observed in the setting of hypothermia that may contribute to decreased injury. As early as 1954 it was noted that hypothermia induced by ice water immersion could lower cerebral oxygen consumption in dogs by approximately 7% per 1°C drop in temperature.[29] Other studies have demonstrated that mild hypothermia in rats improves postischemic cerebral blood flow disturbances.[30] Another marker of general physiologic injury after reperfusion, brain edema, also was found to be reduced by hypothermia in a rat model of global ischemia.[30,31] Finally, hypothermia has been shown to minimize damage to the blood-brain barrier, which in turn may protect against blood-borne toxic metabolites reaching brain tissues through the compromised barrier.[30,32]

Intracellular signaling can alter the array of gene transcription activity of a cell quickly and dramatically, and this, in turn, can trigger a variety of injury processes. In a cardiac arrest mouse model, a group of signaling pathway genes known as the *immediate early genes* was activated after resuscitation.[33] A study of liver IR demonstrated a drop in c-jun terminal kinase activity at 25°C when compared with normothermic controls.[34] An extracellular signaling molecule thought to protect against injury, BDNF, was increased in a rat model of cardiac arrest when animals were cooled to 33°C.[35]

A number of biochemical changes during IR can be modified by the induction of hypothermia. In a gerbil stroke model, animals subjected to mild hypothermia were found to have decreased arachidonic acid metabolism compared with normothermic controls.[36] In a rat brain ischemia model, hypothermia to 32°C reduced nitric oxide production, as measured in jugular blood.[37] Whether these attenuations are simply markers of hypothermic effects or actually relevant factors in reperfusion injury remains to be clearly established. Other biochemical phenomena seem more likely to be linked directly to damage processes, such as the observation that hypothermia slows ATP depletion during IR.[38] ROS production also appears to be attenuated by hypothermic conditions in a rat cerebral ischemia model.[39]

Programmed cell death is a complex yet ubiquitous process by which cells actively chose or are chosen to die. This cellular program can be activated as part of normal physiology, such as during embryonic development, or as an abnormal response in a wide variety of disease states.[40,41] Much evidence implicates the induction of apoptosis as a component of reperfusion injury.[42,43] A recent report showed that the apoptotic pathway enzyme caspase 3 was upregulated in brain tissue after resuscitation from cardiac arrest, as measured at autopsy in patients who died within days of undergoing resuscitative measures.[44] Widespread evidence from animals also supports the notion that apoptosis is activated after reperfusion.[25,45] Hypothermia may inhibit this process. Proteolysis of the cytoskeletal protein fodrin, a characteristic step in the apoptotic pathway, is inhibited by hypothermia to 32°C in a rat brain IR model.[46] The process of apoptosis is an active one, requiring protein synthesis and enzymatic activity, both of which may be inhibited by lower temperatures. While some data suggest that the degree of apoptosis can be reduced by hypothermia, the topic certainly deserves more investigation in animal models.

Hypothermia in Cardiac Arrest

Cardiac arrest is a highly mortal condition that leads to at least 300,000 deaths each year in the United States alone.[47] Survival from cardiac arrest remains dismal some 50 years after introduction of chest compressions and electrical defibrillation, with only 1% to 11% of patients surviving until hospital discharge after out-of-hospital cardiac arrest.[48–50] While initial survival from in-hospital cardiac arrest ranges from 25% to over 50%, subsequent survival until hospital discharge is much lower, from 5% to 22%, suggesting that a high mortality rate is seen shortly after initial return of spontaneous circulation. Some of this mortality after return of normal circulation may be due to events related to reperfusion injury. For further discussion of cardiac arrest and resuscitation therapies, see Chap. 15.

Cardiac arrest remains a major medical challenge despite research efforts over the past few decades. There is little time after arrest to defibrillate the heart and thereby stop ongoing ischemic injury to key organs such as the heart and brain, and few therapies are proven to be useful during the postresuscitation phase of cardiac arrest—when up to 90% of patients go on to die despite successful defibrillation. New approaches are desperately needed to improve cardiac arrest survival, and induced hypothermia may be one of the most promising new approaches.[51]

Hypothermia may be helpful during three periods of time in a cardiac arrest (Fig. 16-1): (1) prearrest, (2) intraarrest, and (3) postarrest. Prearrest cooling can only be used practically

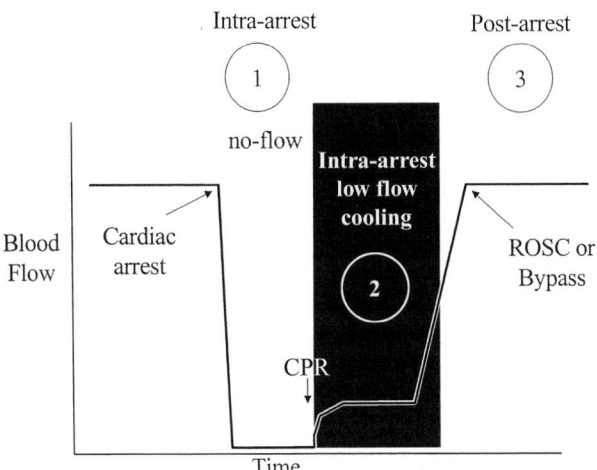

FIGURE 16-1 Time periods during which hypothermia may be used during an ischemia-reperfusion injury such as cardiac arrest or myocardial infaction.

as a preoperative intervention when the heart is stopped in a controlled fashion during cardiac surgery. Postarrest cooling to 32 to 34°C was found to be protective in recent human cardiac arrest trials, induced by applying cooling blankets or ice packing in the subset of cardiac arrest patients having return of spontaneous circulation (ROSC) who remained unresponsive.[2,3] The goal of this level of hypothermia was to prevent neurologic injury and decrease mortality while maintaining a temperature warm enough to prevent the other adverse effects of more profound cooling (e.g., cardiac arrhythmia, coagulopathy, and infection—see discussion of adverse effects later in this chapter). This cooling was protective despite taking 4 to 8 hours to reach target temperature after ROSC (Fig. 16-2). Intraarrest cooling, when cooling is induced after failed initial CPR, has the potential to induce a protective state long enough for more definitive circulation (e.g., cardiac bypass) to be established and life restored. Little is known about the optimal depth or clinical potential of such hypothermia owing in large part to the technical difficulties involved in inducing hypothermia during the low-flow states of sudden cardiac arrest.

Given the current data on hypothermia in cardiac arrest, guidelines for resuscitation likely will include hypothermia as a recommended intervention in the not too distant future. Recent large clinical trials support the use of hypothermia to 32 to 34°C in the successfully resuscitated patient with postarrest global neurologic dysfunction.

Cooling in these patients should be achieved as rapidly as possible using cooling blankets or ice. When ice is used, cloth or other material should be placed between the skin and the ice to avoid frostbite. Temperature should be measured via bladder probe, pulmonary artery catheter, or tympanic probe if invasive temperature monitoring is not available. Temperature should be taken every 15 to 30 minutes during the cooling protocol and until a stable cooled temperature state is achieved. Avoidance of temperatures below 32°C is important, and further temperature drops need to be addressed.

Cooling almost always will induce shivering and could result in discomfort. In the published studies of hypothermia after cardiac arrest, patients uniformly received neuromuscular blockade and sedation, and it is likely most patients will require such pharmacologic treatment. The disadvantages of this management strategy is that neurologic examination is not interpretable, and paralytic agents carry the risk of long-term neuromyopathy.

Rewarming often requires active intervention, which can include warmed intravenous fluids and warming blankets.

Although induced hypothermia has not been formally included in Advanced Cardiac Life Support (ACLS) guidelines at the time of this writing, it is recommended that ICU physicians and staff develop protocols for cooling after cardiac arrest because this recommendation likely will be forthcoming soon. Development of cooling protocols will require some time because a number of hospital-specific technical issues (e.g., how to cool, who will do the cooling, how to monitor temperature) will need to be established.

Induced Hypothermia in Myocardial Infarction

Induced hypothermia to 32 to 34°C has been shown in a variety of model systems to limit the size of a myocardial infarction in ischemia without reperfusion and to limit myocardial

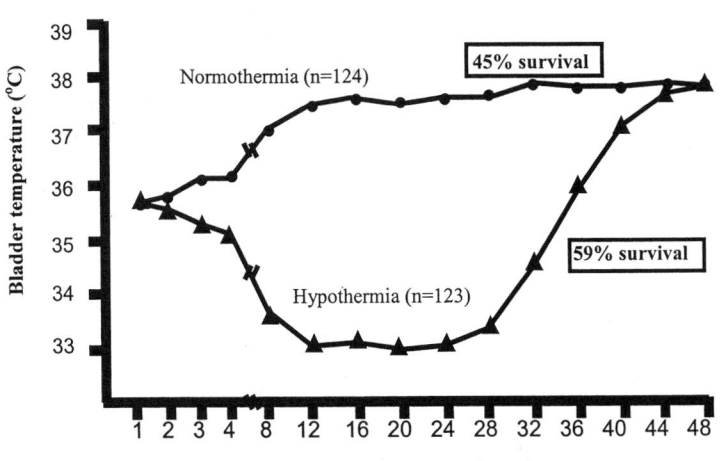

FIGURE 16-2 Data from the Hypothermia After Cardiac Arrest (HACA) study, in which hypothermia was induced via circulated-air cooling blankets. Temperatures shown are taken via bladder monitoring. Mortality differences between the hypothermia patient group and normothermic groups are shown at right. (*Adapted from the HACA study data.*[2])

injury when reperfusion is established. Given that current clinical practice is directed toward early reperfusion of myocardial tissue via thrombolytic therapy or percutaneous coronary intervention (PCI), it is the IR model that has received the most current attention. A recent trial in pigs used an endovascular cooling catheter to induce hypothermia during ischemia and after reperfusion of 60-minute coronary occlusions. Hypothermia to 34°C had a substantial protective effect, with smaller infarct size, better cardiac output, and improved microvascular flow.[52]

Endovascular cooling also has been studied to induce hypothermia during PCI in humans. In a pilot study, patients were randomized to cooled (34 to 35°C) or normothermic PCI. Cooling was maintained for 3 hours after intervention. No patients suffered adverse effects from cooling, and there was a trend toward smaller infarct size in the cooled patients.[53] Larger studies will be required to both confirm this finding and test the induction of hypothermia in the setting of thrombolytic therapy as well. Given that no major randomized studies have shown benefit from induced hypothermia in myocardial infarction, there is currently no clinical recommendation for its use. However, it is likely that hypothermia will become a standard technique to reduce infarct damage in the next decade.

Induced Hypothermia in Stroke

The rationale for the consideration of induced hypothermia in acute ischemic stroke is similar to that for cardiac arrest and myocardial infarction. Stroke is a difficult clinical problem with severe outcomes; not only is stroke the second most common cause of death in the world, but it is also the leading cause of disability in patients over 65 years of age.[54] Moreover, few improvements in acute stroke care have improved the general outcome of the disease.[55,56] Treatment with thrombolytic agents such as tissue plasminogen activator, while a powerful option when a patient presents within 3 hours of ischemic stroke onset, carries significant risks and has only demonstrated improvement in a subset of stroke patients.[57,58] In part, this is so because irreversible damage to brain tissue may have occurred already before restoration of blood flow. However, reperfusion of ischemic neuronal tissues also may produce additional damage via free radical production and induction of programmed cell death and the other so-called IR injury mechanisms described earlier[59] (reviewed in ref. 42).

The use of induced hypothermia in the setting of stroke remains experimental, although promising data exist to support its use (reviewed in refs. 60 and 61). In a variety of model systems, hypothermia reduces injury, as measured by biochemical and histologic markers. Cooling also appears to extend the time in which brain tissue can suffer ischemia without irreversible damage.[62,63] In several animal models, cooling to 32 to 34°C for greater than 24 hours provided significant benefit, whereas shorter periods of hypothermia provided more inconsistent results.[64,65] Several pilot studies have evaluated the feasibility and safety of cooling after ischemic stroke in humans. In one study, cooling to 33 to 34°C appeared to reduce intracranial pressure in patients with severe middle cerebral artery strokes.[66] In a trial of induced hypothermia after thrombolysis, cooling stroke patients to 32°C for at least 12 hours demonstrated a nonsignificant trend toward improved functional outcomes compared with normothermic

controls.[56] These pilot studies were limited by small sample size. Larger randomized trials of induced hypothermia in stroke are currently underway in Europe.

While the induction of hypothermia after ischemic stroke requires additional refinement before becoming the established standard of care, aggressive prevention of hyperthermia is clearly indicated. A number of epidemiologic and clinical studies have shown that even modest elevations in temperature increase stroke severity and patient mortality.[67,68] Antipyretic medications in combination with either forced-air cooling or cooling blankets are sufficient to maintain core temperatures below 37°C. A clinical investigation using such modest measures demonstrated significant mortality risk reduction.[69]

Additional Clinical Applications

The induction of hypothermia has been used experimentally in a number of other clinical scenarios from surgical to critical care applications. One such indication is traumatic brain injury, in which an extensive body of laboratory work suggests that hypothermia may improve outcomes for severe trauma.[70] In one clinical study of 87 patients, hypothermia to 33 to 35°C for at least 72 hours provided a significant functional benefit at 1 year after injury.[71] However, a larger randomized trial of 392 patients failed to find a significant benefit at 6 months after cooling to 33°C for 48 hours.[10] While this has been widely interpreted as a "negative study," the authors have pointed out that the likely reason for finding no benefit was that owing to technical challenges (including taking 4 hours to get informed consent), the average time to cooling was nearly 8 hours after injury. There are no animal studies that suggest any improvement in neurologic results at this late time—the longest delay in cooling that shows any positive effect is about 1 hour following injury. Another clue to these conflicting results was provided by a clinical trial in which hypothermia was found to have no benefit in patients who did not exhibit elevated intracranial pressure.[72] Thus hypothermia may be useful in only a subset of brain injury patients. Taken together with studies demonstrating worrisome electrolyte abnormalities and pneumonia in cooled head injury patients,[73,74] no definitive recommendations exist currently for treatment of traumatic brain injury with induced hypothermia, although it is likely that future work will establish a role for cooling in this disease entity.

Induced hypothermia also has been studied in the setting of acute liver failure, such as from acetaminophen toxicity.[75] As many as 50% of patients with acute liver failure succumb from complications of increased intracranial pressure,[76] and induced hypothermia to 32 to 33°C has been shown to reduce intracranial pressure as much as 20 to 30 mm Hg in patients awaiting orthotopic liver transplantation.[77] Cooling also lowers arterial ammonia concentration and ammonia delivery to the brain, which may be one of the mechanisms by which hypothermia acts, because ammonia delivery to the brain contributes to increased brain edema and intracranial pressure.[78] It remains an open question whether hypothermia could be used to treat the hepatic encephalopathy of cirrhosis, also felt to be mediated by ammonia or at least compounds for which ammonia acts as a surrogate marker.

Neonatologists have studied induced hypothermia in the setting of hypoxic-ischemic encephalopathy after perinatal asphyxia, an important cause of acute neurologic injury at the time of birth.[79] In a piglet model of brain ischemia, early cooling to 33 to 35°C improved neurologic outcomes by both functional and histologic criteria, whereas a delay in cooling by even 30 minutes negated this benefit.[80,81] Initial clinical trials have demonstrated the feasibility of selective head cooling in infants, with minimal differences in complications between cooled patients and normothermic controls.[82] Larger randomized clinical trials are in progress at the time of this writing.

A number of surgical applications of induced hypothermia have been evaluated, including aortic arch repair[83] and cardiac bypass surgery.[84] In these settings, hypothermia induction and rewarming can be controlled precisely and used for presumed important portions of the procedure in question. Unlike the clinical scenarios described earlier, surgical hypothermia does not attempt to treat a pathophysiologic problem but rather to prevent one from occurring. On a cautionary note, however, an extensive meta-analysis showed only a modest trend toward morbidity benefit in the setting of cardiac bypass surgery, with a trend toward decreased stroke rate offset by increased perioperative complications and myocardial injury.[84]

Risks of Hypothermia

Hypothermia is not without risk of adverse effects. As the body cools, a series of physiologic changes take place, including shivering, alterations in the clotting cascade, immunologic suppression, and cardiac membrane changes that increase the risk of arrhythmia (see Chap. 110). These effects are poorly characterized and depend on the extent and duration of cooling. Therefore, the optimal therapeutic window of hypothermia needs to be established.

Shivering, a common occurrence during the induction of hypothermia, can serve to counteract the mechanisms thought to be beneficial from the cooling itself, raising metabolic rates and myocardial oxygen demands. Pharmacologic options to control shivering include opioid and neuroleptic medications. Simply covering the arms and legs during central cooling has demonstrated some reduction in shivering as well, supporting the notion that an increase in peripheral to central temperature gradient may be responsible for triggering a shivering response.[85] A recent study demonstrated that meperidine and buspirone acted synergistically to reduce shivering,[86] and this technique has been used successfully with endovascular cooling in myocardial infarction.[53]

Hypothermia induces a poorly characterized diuresis in which patients may develop significant hypokalemia, hypomagnesemia, and/or hypophosphatemia.[74] Careful attention to electrolytes during the period of cooling and rewarming is required, and aggressive supplementation should be given when indicated.

A study of stroke patients demonstrated a risk of pneumonia with hypothermia, consistent with the cardiac arrest study results.[66] It is unclear whether the immune system is globally suppressed by hypothermia or whether some pulmonary-specific mechanism is the culprit for this increased pneumonia risk. Induced hypothermia does not seem to lead to a significantly increased risk of bacteremia, urinary tract infection, or other infectious complications. Whether patients undergoing induced hypothermia should be treated prophylactically with antibiotics remains to be determined.

While cardiac arrythmias are a theoretical risk of induced hypothermia, human studies in which target temperatures were above 32°C did not exhibit significant arrhythmia. It is possible that deeper cooling may provoke such electrical dysfunction. Therefore, no additional clinical precautions need be taken when hypothermia to 32 to 34°C is performed.

Unresolved Questions

There are a number of unresolved questions regarding the use of induced hypothermia. First, the optimal degree of cooling has yet to be established. As described earlier, hypothermia can have adverse effects such as shivering, reduced immune system function, and other possible complications.[87–89] Therefore, the therapeutic window of hypothermia must be defined to provide maximum benefit. Most clinical research has concentrated on the use of mild (34 to 36°C) or moderate (30 to 34°C) hypothermia. Evaluation of deep hypothermia has been confined largely to specific applications such as brain cooling during surgery and reduced cerebral perfusion.[90] Some animal investigations have compared different depths of cooling directly.[91] It is possible that different disease states may require different depths of cooling to provide optimal protection.

The timing of hypothermia is another crucial question. There are three general time periods in which hypothermia may be considered, although only two are realistic for clinicians. Preinsult hypothermia, or cooling some time before the onset of an ischemic process, is only possible in the setting of surgical intervention, in which ischemia is iatrogenic and controlled.[92,93] Induced hypothermia initiated immediately during an ischemic process, such as during stroke or myocardial infarction but before reperfusion has been initiated, is feasible but poorly studied in the clinical setting. A more dramatic example of this, the induction of hypothermia during CPR, is theoretically attractive and a promising area of current research but has not been attempted clinically. Postreperfusion hypothermia, or cooling after definitive treatment such as thrombolytic therapy or resuscitation, has been the most commonly attempted timing strategy and is certainly the most clinically convenient. Recent large-scale clinical trials have demonstrated significant benefit from induced hypothermia after resuscitation from cardiac arrest.[2,3] These studies raise a secondary timing question related to postreperfusion hypothermia: Is the delay in hypothermia initiation clinically important? Cooling to target core body temperatures may take several hours in clinical settings.[94,95] A variety of laboratory data suggests that earlier induction of hypothermia confers a greater benefit.[27,96]

The duration of the hypothermic state required for protection also remains to be clearly established. Clinical studies to date have all maintained mild hypothermic conditions for at least 12 hours.[2,3,87] However, animal studies have shown benefit from hypothermia lasting only 2 to 6 hours.[26,27] Certainly, a shorter duration of cooling would have a number of clinical advantages, including minimizing the logistical difficulties of maintaining a constant cooled state and also minimizing the potential adverse effects from hypothermia. This question has not been addressed directly in clinical studies at this time.

Finally, a number of other aspects of induced hypothermia remain to be examined. How quickly should patients be rewarmed at the end of a period of hypothermia? Would certain drugs serve as useful adjuncts to hypothermia, either to provide additional benefit or to protect against certain adverse effects of a cooled state? A number of pharmacologic strategies have been employed to protect against IR injury, including barbiturates, benzodiazepines, and gas anesthetic agents. These and other issues surrounding induced hypothermia await randomized clinical trials.

Future of Induced Hypothermia

Before induced hypothermia becomes a standard therapy for such critical illnesses as myocardial infarction, stroke, and cardiac arrest, many of the questions just posed will require resolution. It is also important to note that the optimal combination of these factors may be different for each disease state, and therefore, such principles may not be generalized easily. It is possible, for example, that adverse effects such as electrolyte abnormalities may limit the depth of cooling in the more critically ill state of resuscitated cardiac arrest compared with myocardial infarction or that cardiac arrest patients require a slower rewarming period.

One such parameter, the time between injury and the initiation of cooling, may be the most consistent between different disease states. That is, the sooner a patient is cooled after a given insult, the more likely it is to prevent tissue injury from that disease process. This has been shown in a large variety of IR models at the cellular, organ, and whole-animal levels.[20,52] Therefore, techniques to allow for early and rapid cooling will need to be developed. Current external cooling methods such as ice packing and cooling blankets take several hours to lower core body temperatures adequately in humans. Endovascular cooling catheters appear promising, especially for localized cooling in stroke or myocardial infarction. Additional techniques involving multiphase coolants are currently under development. One goal for induced hypothermia research in cardiac arrest would be to develop a cooling method that could be initiated in the prehospital setting by paramedics.

Hypothermia induction in cardiac arrest fits squarely within the metabolic phase of cardiac arrest, as part of the three-phase time-sensitive model of CPR (see further discussion of the three-phase model in Chap. 15).[97] With the failure of defibrillation and medications to restore viable hemodynamics, patients could be cooled rapidly to protect organs from ongoing ischemia and as a bridge to additional therapies such as establishment of cardiopulmonary bypass with controlled reperfusion.[98–103] Under such intensive control, further attention could be given to reversal of metabolic injury caused by reactive oxygen species, mediators of apoptosis, compromise of cell membrane integrity, and so forth. The limits for reversal of ischemic injury when treated under such a "suspended animation" paradigm remain to be determined.

References

1. O'Sullivan ST, O'Shaughnessy M, O'Connor TP: Baron Larrey and cold injury during the campaigns of Napoleon. *Ann Plast Surg* 34:446, 1995.
2. Hypothermia After Cardia Arrest Study Group. Mild therapeutic hypothermia to improve the neurologic outcome after cardiac arrest. *N Engl J Med* 346:549, 2002.
3. Bernard SA, Gray TW, Buist MD, et al: Treatment of comatose survivors of out-of-hospital cardiac arrest with induced hypothermia. *N Engl J Med* 346:557, 2002.
4. Adams F: *The Genuine Works of Hippocrates*. New York, William Wood, 1886.
5. Bernard S: Induced hypothermia in intensive care medicine. *Anaesth Intensive Care* 24:382, 1996.
6. Colbourne F, Sutherland G, Corbett D: Postischemic hypothermia: A critical appraisal with implications for clinical treatment. *Mol Neurobiol* 14:171, 1997.
7. Eisenburger P, Sterz F, Holzer M, et al: Therapeutic hypothermia after cardiac arrest. *Curr Opin Crit Care* 7:184, 2001.
8. Resnick DK, Marion DW, Darby JM: The effect of hypothermia on the incidence of delayed traumatic intracerebral hemorrhage. *Neurosurgery* 34:252, 1994; discussion 255.
9. Marion DW, Leonov Y, Ginsberg M, et al: Resuscitative hypothermia. *Crit Care Med* 24:S81, 1996.
10. Clifton GL, Miller ER, Choi SC, et al: Lack of effect of induction of hypothermia after acute brain injury. *N Engl J Med* 344:556, 2001.
11. Orlowski JP, Erenberg G, Lueders H, Cruse RP: Hypothermia and barbiturate coma for refractory status epilepticus. *Crit Care Med* 12:367, 1984.
12. Safar P, Tisherman SA, Behringer W, et al: Suspended animation for delayed resuscitation from prolonged cardiac arrest that is unresuscitable by standard cardiopulmonary-cerebral resuscitation. *Crit Care Med* 28:N214, 2000.
13. Fay T: Clinical report and evaluation of low temperature in treatment of cancer. *Proc Int St Postgrad Med Assoc North Am* 1941:292, 1941.
14. Bigelow WG, Lindsay WK, Greenwood WF: Hypothermia: Its possible role in cardiac surgery: an investigation of factors governing survival in dogs at low body temperature. *Ann Surg* 132:849, 1950.
15. Williams GR, Spencer FC: The clinical use of hypothermia following cardiac arrest. *Ann Surg* 148:462, 1958.
16. Benson DW, Williams GR, Spencer FC, et al: The use of hypothermia after cardiac arrest. *Anesth Analg* 38:423, 1959.
17. Steen PA, Milde JH, Michenfelder JD: The detrimental effects of prolonged hypothermia and rewarming in the dog. *Anesthesiology* 52:224, 1980.
18. Michenfelder JD, Terry HR, Daw EF, Uihlein A: Induced hypothermia: Physiological effects, indications and techniques. *Surg Clin North Am* 45:889, 1965.
19. Leonov Y, Sterz F, Safer P, Radovsky A: Moderate hypothermia after cardiac arrest of 17 min in dogs: Effect of cerebral and cardiac outcome. A preliminary study. *Stroke* 21:1600, 1990.
20. Leonov Y, Sterz F, Safer P, et al: Mild cerebral hypothermia during and after cardiac arrest improves neurologic outcome in dogs. *J Cereb Blood Flow Metab* 10:57, 1990.
21. Bellamy RF: The causes of death in conventional land warfare: Implications for combat casualty care research. *Milit Med* 149:55, 1984.
22. Bellamy R, Safar P, Tisherman SA, et al: Suspended animation for delayed resuscitation. *Crit Care Med* 24:S24, 1996.
23. Safar P: Cerebral resuscitation after cardiac arrest: Research initiatives and future directions. *Ann Emerg Med* 22:324, 1993.
24. Vanden Hoek TL, Shao Z, Li C, et al: Reperfusion injury in cardiac myocytes after simulated ischemia. *Am J Phys* 270:H1334, 1996.
25. Maulik N, Yoshida T, Das DK: Regulation of cardiomyocyte apoptosis in ischemic reperfused mouse heart by glutathione peroxidase. *Mol Cell Biochem* 196:13, 1999.
26. Markarian GZ, Lee JH, Stein DJ, Hong SC: Mild hypothermia: Therapeutic window after experimental cerebral ischemia. *Neurosurgery* 38:542, 1996; discussion 551.

27. Carroll M, Beek O: Protection against hippocampal CA1 cell loss by post-ischemic hypothermia is dependent on delay of initiation and duration. *Metab Brain Dis* 7:45, 1992.

28. Ferreira R, Burgos M, Llesuy S, et al: Reduction of reperfusion injury with mannitol cardioplegia. *Ann Thorac Surg* 48:77, 1989; discussion 83.

29. Rosomoff HL, Holaday DA: Cerebral blood flow and cerebral oxygen consumption during hypothermia. *Am J Physiol* 179:85, 1954.

30. Karibe H, Zarow GJ, Graham SH, Weinstein PR: Mild intrais- chemic hypothermia reduces postischemic hyperperfusion, de- layed postischemic hypoperfusion, blood-brain barrier disrup- tion, brain edema, and neuronal damage volume after tempo- rary focal cerebral ischemia in rats. *J Cereb Blood Flow Metab* 14:620, 1994.

31. Xiao F, Zhang S, Arnold TC, et al: Mild hypothermia induced before cardiac arrest reduces brain edema formation in rats. *Acad Emerg Med* 9:105, 2002.

32. Dietrich WD, Busto R, Halley M, Valdes I: The importance of brain temperature in alterations of the blood-brain barrier following cerebral ischemia. *J Neuropathol Exp Neurol* 49:486, 1990.

33. Böttiger B, Teschendorf P, Krumnikl J, et al: Global cerebral is- chemia due to cardiocirculatory arrest in mice causes neuronal degeneration and early induction of transcription factor genes in the hippocampus. *Mol Brain Res* 65:135, 1999.

34. Kato A, Singh S, McLeish KR, et al: Mechanisms of hypothermic protection against ischemic liver injury in mice. *Am J Physiol Gastrointest Liver Physiol* 282:G608, 2002.

35. D'Cruz BJ, Fertig KC, Filiano AJ, et al: Hypothermic reperfusion after cardiac arrest augments brain-derived neurotrophic factor activation. *J Cereb Blood Flow Metab* 22:843, 2002.

36. Kubota M, Nakane M, Narita K, et al: Mild hypothermia reduces the rate of metabolism of arachidonic acid following postis- chemic reperfusion. *Brain Res* 779:297, 1998.

37. Kumura E, Yoshimine T, Takaoka M, et al: Hypothermia sup- presses nitric oxide elevation during reperfusion after focal cere- bral ischemia in rats. *Neurosci Lett* 220:45, 1996.

38. Lundberg J, Elander A, Soussi B: Effect of hypothermia on the ischemic and reperfused rat skeletal muscle, monitored by in vivo ^{31}P-magnetic resonance spectroscopy. *Microsurgery* 21:366, 2001.

39. Kil HY, Zhang J, Piantadosi CA: Brain temperature alters hy- droxyl radical production during cerebral ischemia/reperfusion in rats. *J Cereb Blood Flow Metab* 16:100, 1996.

40. Hengartner MO: The biochemistry of apoptosis. *Nature* 407:770, 2000.

41. Jacobson MD, Weil M, Raff MC: Programmed cell death in ani- mal development. *Cell* 88:347, 1997.

42. Abella BS, Becker LB: Ischemia-reperfusion and acute apoptotic cell death, in Vincent JL (ed): *Yearbook of Intensive Care and Emer- gency Medicine*. Berlin, Springer, 2002, p 3.

43. Hearse DJ, Bolli R: Reperfusion induced injury: Manifestations, mechanisms, and clinical relevance. *Trends Cardiovasc Med* 1:233, 1991.

44. Love S, Barber R, Srinivasan A, Wilcock GK: Activation of caspase-3 in permanent and transient brain ischaemia in man. *Neuroreport* 11:2495, 2000.

45. Crack PJ, Taylor JM, Flentjar NJ, et al: Increased infarct size and exacerbated apoptosis in the glutathione peroxidase-1 (*Gpx-1*) knockout mouse brain in response to ischemia/reperfusion in- jury. *J Neurochem* 78:1389, 2001.

46. Harada K, Maekawa T, Tsuruta R, et al: Hypothermia inhibits translocation of CaM kinase II and PKC-alpha, beta, gamma isoforms and fodrin proteolysis in rat brain synaptosome during ischemia-reperfusion. *J Neurosci Res* 67:664, 2002.

47. Eisenberg MS, Mengert TJ: Cardiac resuscitation. *N Engl J Med* 344:1304, 2001.

48. Eisenberg MS, Horwood BT, Cummins RO, et al: Cardiac arrest and resuscitation: A tale of 29 cities. *Ann Emerg Med* 19:179, 1990.

49. Lombardi G, Gallagher J, Gennis P: Outcome of out-of-hospital cardiac arrest in New York. *JAMA* 271:678, 1994.

50. Becker LB, Han BH, Meyer PM, et al: CPR Chicago: Racial differ- ences in the incidence of cardiac arrest and subsequent survival. *N Engl J Med* 329:600, 1993.

51. Weil MH, Becker LB, Budinger T, et al: Workshop executive sum- mary report: Post-resuscitative and initial utility in life saving efforts (PULSE). *Circulation* 103:1182, 2001.

52. Dae MW, Gao DW, Sessler DI, et al: Effect of endovascular cool- ing on myocardial temperature, infarct size, and cardiac output in human-sized pigs. *Am J Physiol Heart Circ Physiol* 282:H1584, 2002.

53. Dixon SR, Whitbourn RJ, Dae MW, et al: Induction of mild sys- temic hypothermia with endovascular cooling during primary percutaneous coronary intervention for acute myocardial infarc- tion. *J Am Coll Cardiol* 40:1928, 2002.

54. Kaste M, Fogelholm R, Rissanen A: Economic burden of stroke and the evaluation of new therapies. *Public Health* 112:103, 1998.

55. DeGraba TJ, Pettigrew LC: Why do neuroprotective drugs work in animals but not humans? *Neurol Clin* 18:475, 2000.

56. Krieger DW, De Georgia MA, Abou-Chebl A, et al: Cooling for acute ischemic brain damage (cool aid): An open pilot study of induced hypothermia in acute ischemic stroke. *Stroke* 32:1847, 2001.

57. Hacke W: Advances in stroke management: Update 1998. *Neu- rology* 53:S1, 1999.

58. Kwiatkowski TG, Libman RB, Frankel M, et al: Effects of tissue plasminogen activator for acute ischemic stroke at one year. Na- tional Institute of Neurological Disorders and Stroke Recombi- nant Tissue Plasminogen Activator Stroke Study Group. *N Engl J Med* 340:1781, 1999.

59. Ambrosio G, Tritto I: Reperfusion injury: Experimental evidence and clinical implications. *Am Heart J* 138:S69, 1999.

60. Feigin VL, Anderson CS, Rodgers A, et al: The emerging role of induced hypothermia in the management of acute stroke. *J Clin Neurosci* 9:502, 2002.

61. Hanley DF: Review of critical care and emergency approaches to stroke. *Stroke* 34:362, 2003.

62. Yanamoto H, Hashimoto N, Nagata I, Kikuchi H: Infarct tol- erance against temporary focal ischemia following spreading depression in rat brain. *Brain Res* 784:239, 1998.

63. Huh PW, Belayev L, Zhao W, et al: Comparative neuroprotective efficacy of prolonged moderate intraischemic and postischemic hypothermia in focal cerebral ischemia. *J Neurosurg* 92:91, 2000.

64. Gunn AJ, Gunn TR: The "pharmacology" of neuronal rescue with cerebral hypothermia. *Early Hum Dev* 53:19, 1998.

65. Guan J, Gunn AJ, Sirimanne ES, et al: The window of opportu- nity for neuronal rescue with insulin-like growth factor-1 after hypoxia-ischemia in rats is critically modulated by cerebral tem- perature during recovery. *J Cereb Blood Flow Metab* 20:513, 2000.

66. Schwab S, Schwarz S, Spranger M, et al: Moderate hypothermia in the treatment of patients with severe middle cerebral artery infarction. *Stroke* 29:2461, 1998.

67. Wang Y, Lim L, Levi C, et al: Influence of admission body tem- perature on stroke mortality. *Stroke* 31:404, 2000.

68. Hajat C, Hajat S, Sharma P: Effects of poststroke pyrexia on stroke outcome: A meta-analysis of studies in patients. *Stroke* 31:410, 2000.

69. Kammersgaard LP, Jorgensen HS, Rungby JA, et al: Admis- sion body temperature predicts long-term mortality after acute stroke: The Copenhagen Stroke Study. *Stroke* 33:1759, 2002.

70. Marion DW: Moderate hypothermia in severe head injuries: The present and the future. *Curr Opin Crit Care* 8:111, 2002.

71. Jiang J, Yu M, Zhu C: Effect of long-term mild hypothermia ther- apy in patients with severe traumatic brain injury: 1-year follow- up review of 87 cases. *J Neurosurg* 93:546, 2000.

72. Shiozaki T, Hayakata T, Taneda M, et al: A multicenter prospective randomized controlled trial of the efficacy of mild hypothermia for severely head injured patients with low intracranial pressure. Mild Hypothermia Study Group in Japan. *J Neurosurg* 94:50, 2001.

73. Ishikawa K, Tanaka H, Shiozaki T, et al: Characteristics of infection and leukocyte count in severely head-injured patients treated with mild hypothermia. *J Trauma* 49:912, 2000.

74. Polderman KH, Peerdeman SM, Girbes AR: Hypophosphatemia and hypomagnesemia induced by cooling in patients with severe head injury. *J Neurosurg* 94:697, 2001.

75. Jalan R, Olde Damink SW: Hypothermia for the management of intracranial hypertension in acute liver failure. *Curr Opin Crit Care* 7:257, 2001.

76. Makin AJ, Wendon J, Williams R: A 7-year experience of severe acetaminophen-induced hepatotoxicity (1987–1993). *Gastroenterology* 109:1907, 1995.

77. Jalan R, Damink SW, Deutz NE, et al: Moderate hypothermia for uncontrolled intracranial hypertension in acute liver failure. *Lancet* 354:1164, 1999.

78. Master S, Gottstein J, Blei AT: Cerebral blood flow and the development of ammonia-induced brain edema in rats after portacaval anastomosis. *Hepatology* 30:876, 1999.

79. Gunn AJ: Cerebral hypothermia for prevention of brain injury following perinatal asphyxia. *Curr Opin Pediatr* 12:111, 2000.

80. Laptook AR, Corbett RJ, Sterett R, et al: Modest hypothermia provides partial neuroprotection when used for immediate resuscitation after brain ischemia. *Pediatr Res* 42:17, 1997.

81. Laptook AR, Corbett RJ, Burns DK, Sterett R: A limited interval of delayed modest hypothermia for ischemic brain resuscitation is not beneficial in neonatal swine. *Pediatr Res* 46:383, 1999.

82. Gunn AJ, Gluckman PD, Gunn TR: Selective head cooling in newborn infants after perinatal asphyxia: A safety study. *Pediatrics* 102:885, 1998.

83. Yokoyama H: Aortic arch aneurysm complicated with coronary artery disease: Still a surgical challenge? *Ann Thorac Cardiovasc Surg* 8:62, 2002.

84. Rees K, Beranek-Stanley M, Burke M, Ebrahim S: Hypothermia to reduce neurological damage following coronary artery bypass surgery. *Cochrane Database Syst Rev* CD002138, 2001.

85. Sund-Levander M, Wahren LK: Assessment and prevention of shivering in patients with severe cerebral injury: A pilot study. *J Clin Nurs* 9:55, 2000.

86. Mokhtarani M, Mahgoub AN, Morioka N, et al: Buspirone and meperidine synergistically reduce the shivering threshold. *Anesth Analg* 93:1233, 2001.

87. Yanagawa Y, Ishihara S, Norio H, et al: Preliminary clinical outcome study of mild resuscitative hypothermia after out-of-hospital cardiopulmonary arrest. *Resuscitation* 39:61, 1998.

88. Sessler DI: Complications and treatment of mild hypothermia. *Anesthesiology* 95:531, 2001.

89. Connor EL, Wren KR: Detrimental effects of hypothermia: A systems analysis. *J Perianesth Nurs* 15:151, 2000.

90. Saccani S, Beghi C, Fragnito C, et al: Carotid endarterectomy under hypothermic extracorporeal circulation: A method of brain protection for special patients. *J Cardiovasc Surg (Torino)* 33:311, 1992.

91. Weinrauch V, Safar P, Tisherman SA, et al: Beneficial effect of mild hypothermia and detrimental effect of deep hypothermia after cardiac arrest in dogs. *Stroke* 23:1454, 1992.

92. Cleveland JC Jr, Meldrum DR, Rowland RT, et al: Optimal myocardial preservation: Cooling, cardioplegia, and conditioning. *Ann Thorac Surg* 61:760, 1996.

93. Takaba T, Inoue K: Past and present in myocardial protection. *Ann Thorac Cardiovasc Surg* 6:3, 2000.

94. Bernard SA, Jones BM, Horne MK: Clinical trial of induced hypothermia in comatose survivors of out-of-hospital cardiac arrest. *Ann Emerg Med* 30:146, 1997.

95. Zeiner A, Holzer M, Sterz F, et al: Mild resuscitative hypothermia to improve neurological outcome after cardiac arrest: A clinical feasibility trial. Hypothermia After Cardiac Arrest (HACA) study group. *Stroke* 31:86, 2000.

96. Kuboyama K, Safar P, Radovsky A, et al: Delay in cooling negates the beneficial effect of mild resuscitative cerebral hypothermia after cardiac arrest in dogs: A prospective, randomized study. *Crit Care Med* 21:1348, 1993.

97. Weisfeldt ML, Becker LB: Resuscitation after cardiac arrest: A 3-phase time-sensitive model. *JAMA* 288:3035, 2002.

98. Younger JG, Schreiner RJ, Swaniker F, et al: Extracorpeal resuscitation of cardiac arrest. *Ann Acad Emerg Med* 6:700, 1999.

99. Beyersdorf F, Kirsch M., Buckberg GG, Allen BS: Warm glutamate/aspartate-enriched blood cardioplegic solution for perioperative sudden death. *J Thorac Cardiovasc Surg* 104:1141, 1992.

100. Buckberg GD: Substrate enriched warm blood cardioplegia reperfusion: An alternate view. *Ann Thorac Surg* 69:334, 2000.

101. Ihnken K, Morita K, Buckberg GD, et al: Controlling oxygen content during cardiopulmonary bypass to limit reperfusion/reoxygenation injury. *Transplant Proc* 27:2809, 1995.

102. Ihnken K, Morita K, Buckberg GD, et al: Prevention of reoxygenation injury in hypoxaemic immature hearts by priming the extracorporeal circuit with antioxidants. *Cardiovasc Surg* 5:608, 1997.

103. Allen BS, Hartz RS, Buckberg GD, Schuler JJ: Prevention of ischemic damage using controlled limb reperfusion. *J Card Surg* 13:224, 1998.

Chapter 17
WITHHOLDING OR WITHDRAWING OF LIFE-SUSTAINING THERAPY AND ADMINISTERING OF PALLIATIVE CARE

JOHN M. LUCE

KEY POINTS

- *Many, if not most, patients who die in intensive care units do so during the withholding or withdrawing of life-sustaining therapy and the administering of palliative care.*
- *Life-sustaining therapy usually is withheld or withdrawn and palliative care is administered because physicians and patients or their surrogates agree that further restorative care would not be beneficial.*
- *Cardiopulmonary resuscitation, mechanical ventilation, and vasoactive drugs are the therapies most commonly withheld or withdrawn.*
- *Palliative care involves attention to the physical, emotional, and spiritual needs of patients and their families.*
- *Withholding or withdrawing of life-sustaining therapy and administering of palliative care are well supported by ethical pronouncements and case law.*

Defining Withholding or Withdrawing of Life-Sustaining Therapy and Palliative Care

Withholding or withdrawing of life-sustaining therapy or life support is a process by which various medical interventions either are not given to or are taken away from patients with the expectation that they will die from their underlying illnesses. This process is carried out in many medical settings but is especially common in the ICU, which offers an array of therapies capable of sustaining life. An example of withholding life-sustaining therapy is to not provide mechanical ventilation to a patient with chronic obstructive pulmonary disease (COPD) and acute respiratory failure who probably will die without the ventilator but is thought to be unweanable once mechanical ventilation is begun. An example of withdrawing life-sustaining therapy is the removal of mechanical ventilation from a patient with COPD with the provision that he or she will neither be ventilated again if acute respiratory failure recurs nor receive cardiopulmonary resuscitation (CPR) in the event of cardiopulmonary arrest. This second patient is different from a patient with COPD who is being weaned from mechanical ventilation and will be ventilated again or resuscitated if he or she deteriorates during the weaning process.

Strictly speaking, all patients who die while receiving close medical attention in an ICU or elsewhere do so as a direct result of the withholding or withdrawal of life-sustaining therapy. This is either because a decision has been made not to resuscitate the patient in advance of decompensation or because even vigorous resuscitation will not be provided indefinitely. For example, the second patient described earlier would receive CPR if he or she were to suffer an unexpected cardiopulmonary arrest during weaning, but CPR would be discontinued if it were not of benefit in restoring a viable cardiac rhythm in, say, an hour. The withdrawal of life support in this second patient would be comparable to the withholding of CPR in the first patient but for the fact that deliberate planning was more possible for the first patient before cardiopulmonary arrest. It is this more deliberate form of withholding and withdrawing of life-sustaining therapy from critically ill adults that is focused on in this chapter, in which the ethical, legal, clinical, and practical aspects of limiting care are discussed.

Note that the only patients who die in the ICU during the withholding or withdrawing of life-sustaining therapy who are not expected to die are those who are dead already owing to complete and irreversible loss of function of the cerebral hemisphere and brain stem. These patients frequently receive mechanical ventilation and other forms of life support either because the diagnosis of brain death has not been confirmed by apnea testing (after which the ventilator will be removed) or because vital organs (excluding the central nervous system) are being preserved prior to transplantation. Indeed, if transplantation is accomplished, the withholding or withdrawing of mechanical ventilation and other therapies usually takes place in the operating room, where the patient's organs are harvested. Because in brain-dead patients interventions such as mechanical ventilation are removed after death, these interventions are better thought of as organ support than as life support. Nevertheless, because patients and surrogates may not appreciate this distinction, and because the decisions and practical steps preceding the removal of interventions are similar in brain-dead and non-brain-dead patients, mention is made of brain-dead patients in this chapter.

Palliative care may be described as the prevention or treatment of pain, dyspnea, anxiety, and other kinds of suffering in dying patients. Palliative care represents an attitude in addition to a series of actions that ideally bring symptomatic relief and comfort as patients die. This attitude includes an emphasis on the family as well as the patient as the focus of treatment, a commitment to clear and continuous communication between the critical care team and these parties, and a concern for the emotional and spiritual, as well as the physical, well-being of patients and families. As in the withholding or withdrawing of life-sustaining treatment, the administering of palliative care is prompted by the appreciation that further restorative treatment would no longer be beneficial to patients who are dying.

Ethical Aspects of Withholding or Withdrawing of Life-Sustaining Therapy and Administering of Palliative Care

Physicians who care for critically ill adults and are considering withholding or withdrawing life-sustaining therapy care can draw from several summaries of the ethical propriety of limiting care.[1–5] One of the most succinct group statements is the "Consensus Report on the Ethics of Foregoing Life-Sustaining Treatments in the Critically Ill," which was published by the Task Force on Ethics of the Society of Critical Care Medicine in 1990.[6] This report noted that it is ethically appropriate to withhold or withdraw therapy either because a patient or surrogate decides to forego treatment or because a physician judges that further treatment is not likely to be beneficial. A decision to withdraw a treatment should not be more problematic than a decision not to initiate a treatment, particularly because starting a therapy may be necessary to adequately evaluate a patient's condition. Any treatment derives its medical justification from the benefits that a patient and physician hope to achieve by employing it. When the treatment has achieved those benefits or can no longer be expected to do so, it loses its justification and may be withdrawn.

The Society of Critical Care Medicine Task Force consensus statement also noted that there are no intrinsic moral differences between categories of treatment, such as CPR, ventilatory support, medications such as vasopressors and antibiotics, and the provision of hydration and nutrition by artificial means. Each treatment should be considered from the patient's perspective in light of the overall benefit that it may offer and the burdens it may entail, as well as the professional duties that are involved. Treatments that serve only to prolong the dying process should not be employed, and the indefinite maintenance of patients in a persistent vegetative state raises ethical concerns both for the dignity of the patient and for the appropriate use of health care resources.

A basic provision of the consensus statement was that the wishes of an informed adult patient with decision-making capacity should be the primary consideration in almost all decisions regarding treatment. When the patient (or surrogate in the case of a patient who is incapable of making decisions) and the physician (and other members of the critical care team) agree that therapy should be limited, it usually should be. When the patient or surrogate requests therapy that the physician considers nonbeneficial, the physician should clarify the goals of treatment with the patient or surrogate and may accede to their wishes. However, the physician is not ethically obligated to provide therapy and may elect to transfer the patient's care.

In 2001, the Ethics Committee of the Society of Critical Care Medicine published a statement entitled "Recommendations for End-of-Life Care in the Intensive Care Unit" that explored the ethical aspects of administering palliative care.[7] The recommendations were based on recognition of the needs of patients, families, and providers during the dying process. The patients' needs are to receive adequate pain management, to avoid inappropriate prolongation of dying, to achieve a sense of control, to relieve themselves of burdens, and to strengthen their relationships with loved ones. The families' needs are to be with dying persons, to be helpful to them, to be informed of their changing condition, to understand what is being done to them and why, to be assured of the patients' comfort, to be comforted themselves, to express their own emotions, to be assured that their decisions regarding the patients were correct, to find meaning in the dying of their loved ones, and to be fed and rested. The needs of the critical care team are to establish consensus regarding the goals and strategies for

providing palliative care, to gain knowledge and skills in palliation, to be supported in their tasks by their institutions, and to have opportunities for grieving and bereavement after patients die. In addition to articulating these needs, the recent statement by the Society of Critical Care Medicine offers a number of helpful recommendations in delivering end-of-life care.

Legal Aspects of Withholding or Withdrawing of Life-Sustaining Therapy and Administering of Palliative Care

In the United States, withholding and withdrawing life support are legally justified primarily by the principles of informed consent and informed refusal. Both principles have strong roots in the common law and reflect the American regard for self-determination. The principles hold that treatment may not be initiated without the approval of patients or their surrogates, except in emergency situations, and that patients or surrogates may refuse any and all therapies.[8]

The right of competent patients to refuse therapy was established directly in *Bartling v. Superior Court*,[9] in which a California Court of Appeal held that a patient could be removed from a ventilator at his request over the objections of his physicians and the hospital where he was cared for. In *Bouvia v. Superior Court*,[10] the California Court of Appeal held that a conscious and competent hospitalized patient with severe pain could refuse nutrition and hydration even if by doing so she believed she would die. Currently, all American courts recognize a competent adult's right to refuse life-sustaining treatment, although the constitutional, statutory, and common-law bases of the right may vary by jurisdiction. Most of the cases concerning that right have arisen, however, from situations involving patients who cannot make medical decisions for themselves.

The application of the principles of informed consent and informed refusal to the care of decisionally impaired critically ill patients began with *In re Quinlan*.[11] In this case, the Supreme Court of New Jersey held that a patient had the right to refuse mechanical ventilation and that, because she was vegetative and could not exercise that right directly, her parents could act as surrogates and make a "substituted judgment" for her. The California Court of Appeal took a similar approach in *Barber v. Superior Court*,[12] in which it held that physicians charged with murder had not committed an unlawful act when, with permission from a patient's family, they removed nutrition and hydration from a comatose patient. In *Barber*, the court noted that medical interventions ranging from mechanical ventilation to nutrition and hydration should not be distinguished by terms such as *extraordinary* and *ordinary* that had been used previously. Rather, the court stated, medical interventions should be evaluated by the benefits and burdens they offer patients; if the burdens of a particular treatment outweigh the benefits it confers, the treatment can be foregone.

Although the principles of informed consent and refusal articulated in *Quinlan*, *Barber*, and other cases are well established, states vary in their processes and rules for vindicating these principles for decisionally impaired patients. In general, these variations fall into two categories: rules for selecting surrogate decision makers and rules determining what surrogates can decide. As for the latter rules, all states agree that medical decisions should be guided by the wishes of the patient whenever possible. Some states require a high level of certainty before a surrogate may refuse life-sustaining treatment. For example, in the *O'Conner* case,[13] a New York court ruled that treatment is obligatory unless evidence shows that it is almost certain that the patient would have refused treatment. Missouri also requires "clear and convincing evidence" of a decisionally impaired patient's wishes, a position that was contested in *Cruzan v. Director, Missouri Department of Health*,[14] as will be discussed.

In most other states, however, surrogates may consider other factors, such as the patient's "best interests," when a patient has not expressed a prior unequivocal preference. The most influential case to describe the best interests standard is the New Jersey Supreme Court's decision in *In re Conroy*,[15] which was made 9 years after that court decided *Quinlan*. The *Conroy* court would apply the best interests standard only when there was no reliable evidence of the patient's wishes. The test of this standard has two elements. First, the burdens of the patient's life with treatment must outweigh the benefits to the patient of continued life. Second, the recurring, unavoidable pain of the patient's life with treatment must be such that administering the treatment is inhumane.

The issue of withholding or withdrawing life-sustaining treatment was first addressed by the U. S. Supreme Court in the aforementioned *Cruzan* case,[14] which involved a request by parents to have a feeding tube removed from their daughter in a Missouri nursing home. In its decision, the Court allowed Missouri and other states to require "clear and convincing evidence" of patients' wishes and thereby potentially limited the role of surrogates in making decisions for decisionally impaired patients without advance directives. Nevertheless, the Court accepted the principle that a competent person's right to forego treatment, including nutrition and hydration, is a liberty interest protected under the Fourteenth Amendment to the Constitution. Thus, although *Cruzan* did not set a single standard for surrogate decision making for patients who cannot make decisions for themselves, it did affirm the legal principles of informed consent and refusal that are used in all the United States.

After *Cruzan*, the Supreme Court confirmed its approval of the foregoing of life-sustaining treatment in *Washington v. Glucksberg*[16] and *Vacco v. Quill*[17] and also furnished guidelines for administering palliative care. These last two cases dealt with the constitutionality of laws prohibiting physician-assisted suicide in Washington and New York. In *Glucksberg*, the court decided that terminally ill patients did not have a liberty interest in committing suicide or in receiving physician assistance in suicide because of both the long tradition of prohibiting suicide in the United States and the states' legitimate reasons for continuing to make suicide illegal. In *Vacco*, the court drew further distinctions between assisted suicide and withholding or withdrawing life-sustaining therapy. "Everyone, regardless of physical condition, is entitled, if competent, to refuse lifesaving medical treatment; no one is permitted to assist a suicide," the court wrote. "When a patient refuses life-sustaining medical treatment, he dies from an underlying fatal disease or pathology; but if a patient ingests lethal medication prescribed by a physician, he is killed by that medication."

In *Glucksberg* and *Vacco*, five justices of the Supreme Court reasoned in concurring opinions that Washington and New York could prohibit assisted suicide because these states had no legal barriers that prevented patients from obtaining medications to relieve pain and suffering and therefore had no need for assisted suicide. However, as Justice Breyer wrote in his opinion concurring in the judgment in the two cases, "Were state law to prevent the provision of palliative care, including the administration of drugs as needed to avoid pain at the end of life, an action against such law might be called for by the Supreme Court." Through this and other statements, a majority of Supreme Court justices suggested that the Constitution's guarantee of individual liberty included the liberty to be free of unnecessary pain during the dying process.[18] Indeed, the justices' opinions have been interpreted as indicating a willingness on the part of the Supreme Court to mandate patient access to palliative care.[19]

The Supreme Court distinguished assisted suicide from palliative care in *Glucksberg* and *Vacco* by accepting the principle of double effect. Under this principle, acts such as giving sedatives and analgesics that lead to morally good effects, such as the relief of pain, are permissible even if they produce morally bad effects, such as the hastening of death, provided that only the good effect is intended.[20] The Supreme Court's approval of palliative care included sanctioning the practice of terminal sedation, in which patients are rendered comatose and then may have nutrition and hydration withdrawn. The term *terminal sedation* appears only in a footnote concerning sedation while withdrawing ventilatory support or other treatment in the *Vacco* majority opinion. Nevertheless, under *Vacco*, a state may allow terminal sedation if it is "based on informed consent and the double effect. Just as a state may prohibit assisting suicide while permitting patients to refuse unwanted lifesaving treatment, it may permit palliative care related to that refusal, which may have the foreseen but unintended 'double effect' of hastening the patient's death."

Clinical Aspects of Withholding or Withdrawing Life-Sustaining Therapy

Information about the clinical aspects of withholding or withdrawing life support has come primarily from surveys of physicians and other health professionals and from observational studies of the limiting of life-sustaining care. For example, several surveys[21–23] have suggested that the great majority of critical care physicians have withheld or withdrawn life support at one time or another and that many have done so frequently. Similarly, retrospective studies[24–26] have revealed that approximately one-half of the patients who die in ICUs do so during the withholding or withdrawal of life-sustaining therapy. Prospective studies[27,28] conducted in two ICUs in hospitals affiliated with the University of California, San Francisco, revealed that withholding or withdrawal of life support preceded 90% of deaths in 1992 and 1993 compared with 51% of deaths in 1988 and 1989. To determine whether limiting care is as commonplace as suggested by the aforementioned studies, a prospective survey[29] was conducted in 1994 and 1995 of 107 ICUs associated with all U.S. training programs in critical care medicine or pulmonary and critical care medicine. It revealed that only 25% of deaths followed full ICU care and failed CPR.

Similar observations have been reported recently concerning the practice of critical care medicine in Europe.[29a] In a prospective observational study in 37 ICUs in 17 European countries from 1999–2000, of the patients who died, 72.6% had a limitation of therapy, although substantial intercountry variability in practice was noted. Limitation of therapy versus continuation of life-sustaining therapy was associated with patient age, acute and chronic diagnoses, number of days in the ICU, region, and religion.

Most surveys[21–23,30] and studies[24–28,30,31] have indicated that physicians recommend that life support be withheld or withdrawn either because patients or surrogates request this action or because physicians believe that further care is not beneficial. This belief stems from prognostication on the physicians' part. They generally arrive at estimates of prognosis through their personal experience and knowledge of the medical literature and not with the help of prognostic scoring systems such as the Acute Physiology and Chronic Health Evaluation (APACHE) system, although use of such systems is increasing in some ICUs. If present, brain death, persistent coma, other unacceptable neurologic prognoses, and multiple-organ-system failure are important rationales for care withdrawal. The need for ICU beds, patients' social worth, and financial cost-benefit analyses are not important rationales.

Most patients have not prepared medical directives in advance of suffering a critical illness, and most patients are too neurologically depressed by their disease or by therapeutic drugs to make medical decisions when they become critically ill. Surrogates usually were available and willing to take part in the decision-making process in the prospective studies[27,28] of withholding or withdrawing life support. When surrogates were not available, physicians were willing to make decisions for the patients. Although consultation from other physicians often was sought before deciding to limit care, hospital ethics committees were involved infrequently. Furthermore, probate courts or judicial hearings were never used.

The surrogates who were available in these studies[27,28] either recommended by themselves that support be withheld or withdrawn when patients were not improving or accepted physician recommendations to that effect. These recommendations were not always accepted immediately, but in most cases the surrogates agreed within a few days. Only rarely did surrogates insist on continued care against the advice of physicians, and in all cases care was continued. In certain instances, however, the physicians stopped short of providing CPR in patients who were otherwise supported.

Although differences between physicians and surrogates do occur over the issue of limiting care, their incidence is uncertain. In one survey[22] of self-identified members of the critical care section of the American Thoracic Society, 34% of respondents reported that they had refused surrogate requests to withdraw care either because they believed that the patient still had a reasonable chance of recovery or because they believed that the surrogates might not be acting in the best interest of the patient. At the same time, 83% of physicians reported that they had unilaterally withheld life-sustaining treatment on the basis of futility, often without patient or surrogate knowledge or consent, and 82% had withdrawn treatment on the same basis.

CPR probably is the therapy most often withheld from ICU patients, as suggested by the finding that do-not-resuscitate (DNR) orders preceded 60% of all in-unit deaths in a large observational study[32] in 40 U.S. hospitals. Antibiotics, vasoactive drugs, renal dialysis, and mechanical ventilation were withheld commonly in the two studies[27,28] from ICUs in hospitals affiliated with the University of California, San Francisco. Mechanical ventilation was the therapy most commonly withdrawn in these studies, followed by vasoactive drugs. In the survey[22] of American Thoracic Society members, 89% of the respondents had withdrawn mechanical ventilation, 88% had withdrawn vasoactive drugs, and 80% had withdrawn blood or blood products.

In a study[33] conducted in the two ICUs at hospitals affiliated with the University of California, San Francisco, analgesics and sedatives were given to 75% of non–brain-dead patients during the withholding or withdrawal of life support. Patients who did not receive medication were comatose and considered incapable of benefiting from the drugs. Physicians ordered analgesics and sedatives to decrease pain in 88% of patients, to decrease anxiety in 85%, to comfort families in 82%, to decrease air hunger in 76%, and to hasten death in 39%; in no instance was hastening death the only reason cited. The amounts of opiates and benzodiazepines averaged 3.3 mg/h of morphine and 2.2 mg/h of diazepam in the 24 hours before withholding or withdrawing of life support and 11.2 and 9.8 mg/h, respectively, in the 24 hours thereafter. The median time until death following the initiation of withholding or withdrawal of life support was 3.5 hours in the patients who received drugs and 1.3 hours in patients who did not. Thus the administration of sedatives and analgesics did not appear to hasten death in this study.

It would appear from these surveys and studies that withholding or withdrawal of life-sustaining therapy from adults occurs frequently in most U.S. ICUs and that these processes commonly follow a similar course. Furthermore, professional attitudes and behaviors on the part of physicians are consistent with ethical pronouncements and judicial decisions regarding the withholding or withdrawal of life support. The only major area in which consistency may be lacking concerns physician refusal to follow surrogate demands either to limit care in certain circumstances or to provide care that the physicians consider nonbeneficial. This finding is not surprising given the lack of ethical and legal clarification of the issue; hopefully, such clarification will occur over time.

Practical Aspects of Withholding or Withdrawing of Life-Sustaining Therapy

The surveys and studies discussed in the preceding section suggest that physicians, patients, and surrogates generally reach consensus regarding when and how withholding or withdrawal of life support should take place. Consensus is not reached in all cases, at least not initially, and the process of foregoing life-sustaining treatment can be quite strained. Most of the differences that exist between the parties involved in this process result from difficulties in communication and can be breached if communication is improved. There is much interest in the critical care community for enhancing the process of withholding or withdrawing care and providing palliative care, as well as enhancing communication generally in the ICU. Models for improved communication have been proposed and at least preliminarily tested.[34]

The following 12 suggestions are designed to facilitate communication inside and outside the ICU[34a]:

1. Regular meetings should be held with physicians and patients or their surrogates from the time of ICU admission to discuss all medical matters, including prognosis. The meetings should be held in a quiet, comfortable, and private place conducive to conversation. The timing of the meetings should allow the participation of the attending physician, the primary physician (if different from the attending), consultants, bedside nurses, and facilitators such as family counselors or clergy. House staff may be included, but a physician in training should not serve as a substitute for an experienced attending in directing the course of the meetings.

2. Consensus should be reached by the physicians regarding prognosis and other medical matters before they communicate with the patients or their surrogates. Although physicians may disagree privately among themselves, they should be prepared to present an opinion to the family that they can publicly agree on. This includes neurologists or neurosurgeons who may be asked to consult regarding functional outcome. Ideally, the viewpoints of all physicians can be summed up and communicated by the attending physician to patients or surrogates. Nurses and other caregivers should be included in the consensus-building process.

3. The role of surrogates in decision making should be clarified from the outset of ICU admission.[35] Surrogates should be informed that they can help the patient best by articulating his or her wishes and determining what he or she would want done in a given situation instead of expressing the surrogates' wishes and what the surrogates themselves would want done. If a certain family member carries a durable power of attorney for the patient or only one family member is available, this individual will act for the family as a whole. Otherwise, and especially if the family is divided in opinion, it should be asked to designate a spokesperson.

4. Discussions with surrogates should be frank, informative, and as consistent as possible. The major purpose should be a regular updating of the family about the patient's condition, including his or her chances of recovery. Physicians should be aware that the ICU is a foreign and often frightening place for most family members. Bedside explanations, drawings, radiographs, CT scans, and other visual aids may help families understand the patient's status and appreciate the full extent of supportive therapy.

5. Withholding or withdrawal of life support should be recommended, not merely listed as a therapeutic option, once physicians and nurses agree that life support should be withheld or withdrawn. This agreement should be based on disease-specific data, prognostic indices, and clinical experience, all of which should be explained to the family in detail. The family then should be asked to respond to the recommendation as the patient would if he or she were able to do so.

6. CPR should not be the focus of discussions regarding the withholding or withdrawing of life support. Some physicians who intend to recommend the forgoing of further life-sustaining therapy instead advise that the patient not be resuscitated in the event of cardiopulmonary arrest. Yet such events are uncommon in the ICU unless another form of life support such as mechanical ventilation is withheld or withdrawn. Furthermore, by focusing on CPR, the physician implies that the patient actually may benefit from the procedure despite medical evidence to the contrary[36] and puts surrogates in the uncomfortable position of having to refuse what is presented as a potentially beneficial therapy. A better approach is to recommend that all therapies considered incapable of benefiting the patient, including CPR, will be withheld or withdrawn.

7. Surrogates should be allowed to accept the recommendation to forgo life-sustaining therapy. Some families actually precede physicians in their realization that further care would be futile for and unwanted by a given patient. Others are willing to accept the recommendation to withhold or withdraw life support once they have accepted the prognosis offered them. Even if the patient is brain dead, surrogates may have difficulty realizing that the patient is not alive despite the presence of a heart beat and respiratory excursions caused by a mechanical ventilator. Such acceptance may take time, particularly if the patient was entirely well prior to a critical illness. Only a few surrogates are unwilling to accept the prognosis or demand that the patient be supported indefinitely because he or she would prefer life under any circumstances.

8. Physicians should inform surrogates that physicians are not obligated to provide nonbeneficial care if the issue arises. In general, a physician who cannot in good conscience continue therapy he or she considers nonbeneficial should transfer responsibility for the patient's care to another physician in the same or another institution. If transfer is not possible, life support may be withdrawn in accordance with institutional policies. However, such policies are uncommon, and the courts may require that life support be continued when a family insists that a patient would so desire.

9. Surrogates should be told that life support will be withheld or withdrawn as humanely and expeditiously as possible once they have accepted the recommendation to forgo further life-sustaining therapy. They should be given time to spend with the patient and may, if they wish, be present at the patient's death. For many ICU patients, death will come only after removal of supplemental oxygen, positive end-expiratory pressure (PEEP), and the mechanical ventilator. Terminal weaning of this sort should be long enough to allow the family to visit with the patient but should not be prolonged beyond several hours or, in rare cases, a few days. However, early extubation may produce signs of upper airway restriction that are uncomfortable to surrogates and caregivers alike and therefore should be avoided unless sedatives are provided.

10. Whatever process of withholding or withdrawing of life support is followed, surrogates should be assured that the patient will receive sedatives and analgesics to relieve pain and suffering but that death will not be hastened intentionally, in keeping with the principle of double effect. Drugs are best given unobtrusively by constant infusion

at doses sufficient to suppress grimacing and signs of air hunger. Formal protocols that dictate how sedatives and analgesics are to be given may help nurses who give the drugs feel that they are doing so properly and to avoid the impression of hastening death. Muscle relaxants should be avoided if at all possible because they provide no therapeutic benefit in the dying patient. The same is true for agents such as potassium chloride that do not relieve pain and suffering but merely hasten death.

11. Physicians, nurses, and other caregivers should meet after the patient dies to discuss how his or her death was managed. Discussions are particularly helpful to the ICU team when conflicts have existed with the patient and his or her surrogates. These discussions provide emotional support for the team and can generate ideas about how to improve the dying process for future patients. They may even inspire the development of guidelines and standing orders used during the dying process.

12. Physicians should be as available to surrogates after the patient dies as they were beforehand. In particular, the attending or primary physician should be accessible by telephone or in person to answer medical questions and report the results of an autopsy or other postmortem procedure. The bedside nurse or family counselor may have been helpful to the family in the ICU and may continue to be a source of emotional support. Through such actions, the caregivers communicate their ongoing concern for the patient and his or her family.

References

1. Council on Ethical and Judicial Affairs, American Medical Association: Decisions near the end of life. *JAMA* 267:2229, 1992.
2. Ruark JE, Raffin TA, Stanford University Medical Center Committee on Ethics: Initiating and withdrawing life support: Principles and practice in adult medicine. *N Engl J Med* 318:25, 1988.
3. Butler P, Carton RW, Elpern E, et al: Ethical and moral guidelines for the initiation, continuation, and withdrawal of intensive care. *Chest* 97:949, 1990.
4. American Thoracic Society: Withholding and withdrawing life-sustaining therapy. *Am Rev Respir Dis* 144:726, 1991.
5. Luce JM: Ethical principles in critical care. *JAMA* 263:696, 1990.
6. Task Force on Ethics of the Society of Critical Care Medicine: Consensus report on the ethics of foregoing life-sustaining treatments in the critically ill. *Crit Care Med* 18:1435, 1990.
7. Truog RD, Cist AFM, Brackett SE, et al: Recommendations for end-of-life care in the intensive care unit: The Ethics Committee of the Society of Critical Care Medicine. *Crit Care Med* 29:2332, 2001.
8. Luce JM, Alpers A: End-of-life care: What do the American courts say? *Crit Care Med* 29:N40, 2001.
9. *Bartling v. Superior Court*, 163 Cal. App. Ed 190, 209 Cal. Rptr. 220 (1984).
10. *Bouvia v. Superior Court*, 179 Cal. App. 3d 1127, 225 Cal. Rptr. 297 (1986).
11. *In re Quinlan*, 755 A2a 647 (NJ) cert. denied, 429 US 922 (1976).
12. *Barber v. Superior Court*, 147 Cal. App. 3d 1006 (Cal. App. 1983)
13. *In re O'Conner*, 72 N.Y. 2d 517, 531 N.E. 2d 607, 534 N.Y.S. 2d 886 (1988).
14. *Cruzan v. Director, Missouri Department of Health*, 497 DS 261 (1990).
15. *In re Conroy*, 486A:2d 1209 (N.J. 1985).
16. *Washington v. Glucksberg*, 521 US 702 (1997).
17. *Vacco v. Quill*, 521 US 793 (1997).
18. Gostin LO: Deciding life and death in the courtroom: From *Quinlan* to *Cruzan, Glucksberg,* and *Vacco*—A brief history and analysis of constitutional protection of the "right to die." *JAMA* 278:1523, 1997.
19. Burt RA: The Supreme Court speaks: Not assisted suicide but a constitutional right to palliative care. *N Engl J Med* 337:1234, 1997.
20. Quill TE, Dresser R, Brock DW: The rule of double efect: A critique of its role in end-of-life decision making. *N Engl J Med* 337:1768, 1997.
21. The Society of Critical Care Medicine Ethics Committee: Attitudes of critical care medicine professionals concerning forgoing life-sustaining treatments. *Crit Care Med* 20:320, 1992.
22. Asch DA, Hansen-Flaschen J, Lanken PN: Decisions to limit or continue life-sustaining treatment by critical care physicians in the United States: Conflicts between physicians' practices and patients' wishes. *Am J Respir Crit Care Med* 151:288, 1995.
23. Faber-Langendoen K: The clinical management of dying patients receiving mechanical ventilation: A survey of physician practice. *Chest* 106:880, 1994.
24. Koch KA, Rodeffer HD, Wears RL: Changing patterns of terminal care management in an intensive care unit. *Crit Care Med* 22:233, 1994.
25. Vincent JL, Parquier JN, Preiser JC, et al: Terminal events in the intensive care unit: Review of 258 fatal cases in one year. *Crit Care Med* 17:530, 1989.
26. Parker JM, Landry FJ, Phillips YY: Use of do-not-resuscitate orders in an intensive care setting. *Chest* 104:1592, 1993.
27. Smedira NG, Evans BH, Grais LS, et al: Withholding and withdrawal of life support from the critically ill. *N Engl J Med* 322:309, 1990.
28. Prendergast TJ, Luce JM: Increasing incidence of withholding and withdrawal of life support from the critically ill. *Am J Respir Crit Care Med* 155:15, 1997.
29. Prendergast TJ, Luce JM: A national survey of withdrawal of life support from critically ill patients. *Am J Respir Crit Care Med.* 156:A153, 1996.
29a. Sprung CL, Cohen SL, Sjokvist P, Baras M, et al. End-of-life practices in European Intensive Care Units. *JAMA* 290:790, 2003.
30. Lee DKP, Swinburne AJ, Fedullo AJ, Wahl GW: Withdrawing care: Experience in a medical intensive care unit. *JAMA* 271:1358, 1994.
31. Cook DJ, Guyatt GH, Jaeschke R, et al: Determinants in Canadian health care workers of the decision to withdraw life support from the critically ill. *JAMA* 273:703, 1995.
32. Jayes RL, Zimmerman JE, Wagner JP, et al: Do-not-resuscitate orders in intensive care units. *JAMA* 270:2213, 1993.
33. Wilson WC, Smedira NG, Fink C, et al: Ordering and administration of sedatives and analgesics during the withholding and withdrawal of life support from critically ill patients. *JAMA* 267:949, 1992.
34. Lilly CM, Sonna LA, Haley KJ, Massaro AF. Intensive communication: Four-year follow-up from a clinical practice study. *Crit Care Med* 31(suppl):S394, 2003.
34a. Campbell ML, Curtis JR: End-of-life care. *Crit Care Clin* 20: xiii, 2004.
35. Arnold RM, Kellum J. Moral justifcations for surrogate decision maing in the intensive care unit: Implications and limitations. *Crit Care Med* 31(suppl):S347, 2003.
36. Bedell SE, Delbanco TL, Cook EF, Epstein FH: Survival after cardiopulmonary resuscitation in the hospital. *N Engl J Med* 309: 569, 1983.

Chapter 18
CHRONIC CRITICAL ILLNESS
SHANNON S. CARSON

KEY POINTS
- *Chronically critically ill patients account for 5% to 10% of patients admitted to an adult ICU. They account for as many as 88,000 hospital discharges per year in the United States. Most chronically critically ill patients are over age 65. The burden of chronic critical illness is anticipated to increase dramatically in the next decade.*
- *Chronically critically ill patients have distinct physiology compared with more acutely ill patients, including suppressed levels of anterior pituitary hormones and severe depletion of protein stores with muscle wasting.*
- *Important principles of patient management include prevention of infection, protein repletion, aggressive physical therapy, and careful attention to treating symptoms.*
- *Liberation from mechanical ventilation usually is achieved with work-rest cycles that are guided by frequent assessments of readiness for weaning and careful monitoring to avoid fatigue.*
- *One-year survival for chronically critically ill patients is between 23% and 38% in most cohorts, but younger patients with few comorbidities have distinctly better chances of survival. Quality of life for survivors is similar to that of patients with shorter periods of critical illness.*
- *Costs of care for chronically critically ill patients are extreme during hospitalization and after discharge. Cost savings can be achieved by managing patients in dedicated wards or facilities outside of the acute ICU setting.*

Advances in medical management and technology have greatly enhanced patients' ability to survive critical illness and injury. For most critically ill patients, the clinical course is typified by liberation from organ support systems such as vasoactive drugs and mechanical ventilation after reversal of the acute process, followed by a short period of observation before transfer from the ICU to a medical/surgical ward or an intermediate care unit. For a significant number of patients however, this timely transition to a more stable condition does not occur, and they remain dependent on life support systems or other ICU services for prolonged periods. These patients often are referred to as the *chronically critically ill* (CCI). As larger proportions of patients are surviving episodes of severe sepsis, acute respiratory distress syndrome (ARDS), multiple trauma, or acute or chronic respiratory failure, CCI patients are becoming a significant component of the practice of critical care medicine.

CCI patients are recognized more easily than defined. Every clinician in the ICU is familiar with the patient who has been supported through the initial period of hemodynamic, neurologic, or respiratory instability that characterized their first few days in the ICU but whose continued recovery has been arrested by the persistence of the acute insult, new

complications, or decompensation of severe underlying comorbidities. The patient is weak and frequently dependent on mechanical ventilation. A tracheostomy is present or being contemplated. Such patients are often delirious, if not minimally responsive, and the more alert among them are troubled by significant discomfort. Their physical appearance is altered by muscle atrophy and diffuse edema. They are often cycling through recurring infections, multiple antibiotics, and evolving resistant organisms. Their families are distressed, frustrated, and exhausted. Finally, their physicians and nurses are equally frustrated and often are challenged to maintain enthusiasm for their care.

A specific definition for chronic critical illness is more elusive. For the purposes of epidemiologic studies and clinical trials, patients usually are identified by the requirement for prolonged mechanical ventilation, by number of days in the ICU, by presence of a tracheostomy for prolonged mechanical ventilation, or by transfer to a ventilator rehabilitation unit. The actual number of days of ventilation or ICU stay that is considered to meet a threshold of *prolonged* has varied from 5 to 28 days depending on restrictions of administrative databases used in studies or an investigator's intuitive sense of what is exceptional. Care must be taken to consider the actual population enrolled in any study describing CCI patients. For example, there may be significant differences between populations of patients who have been ventilated for 28 days compared with those ventilated for 5 days. Diagnosis, comorbidities, and severity of acute processes can vary considerably between CCI patients at different types of institutions or even within a single ICU. Despite this heterogeneity, a number of important clinical factors are common to CCI patients and require a different approach to management than for a typical patient in the ICU. These unique factors will be discussed in this chapter.

Incidence

Depending on the definition, between 5% and 10% of patients admitted to adult ICUs become chronically critically ill.[1,2] Using DRG 483 (tracheostomy for conditions other than face, neck, and mouth diagnoses) to identify patients requiring prolonged mechanical ventilation in the Nationwide Inpatient Sample, it was estimated that there were 88,000 such discharges in the United States in 1997[3] (Table 18-1). These represent 0.25% of the 35 million annual hospital discharges in the United States. Although this is a small fraction of all hospital admissions, these patients have a substantial impact on hospital resources owing to prolonged stays and high-intensity care. Importantly, 52% of patients in that sample were over age 65. This reflects an overall higher incidence of acute respiratory failure in elderly patients. As the baby boom generation approaches this age group in the next 10 years, the number of CCI patients in ICUs is expected to increase substantially. A trend toward increasing numbers of discharges under DRG 483 is already evident in the state of New York according to an analysis from 1992 to 1996.[4]

Risk Factors

Patients who are susceptible to chronic critical illness are as heterogeneous as the general ICU population (Table 18-2). Pa-

TABLE 18-1 Characteristics of DRG 483 in the United States, 1997 (Estimated $n = 88,000$)

Age Groups	Number (%)	In-Hospital Mortality	Length of Stay in Days (Median/Mean)	Charges in $1000s, Median (Range)
Age 0–21	5,280 (6%)	10%	30/53	$120 ($0.6–$2100)
Age 22–49	17,600 (20%)	17%	30/39	$120 ($1.2–$2870)
Age 50–64	19,360 (22%)	25%	32/40	$131 ($0.07–$2220)
Age 65–74	22,000 (25%)	31%	32/40	$135 ($1.9–$2553)
Age 75–84	19,360 (22%)	36%	32/41	$134 ($0.3–$5186)
Age 85 or older	4,400 (5%)	38%	32/40	$120 ($0.6–$977)

SOURCE: From Carson SS, Bach PB: The epidemiology and costs of chronic critical illness. *Crit Care Clin* 18:461, 2002. Reproduced by permission of W. B. Saunders Company.

tients with postoperative complications from cardiac or abdominal surgery are at risk, and trauma patients are common as well. Medical patients with acute lung disease with or without multiorgan failure and patients with chronic lung disease (especially COPD) or neurologic diseases as their primary diagnoses are also susceptible. Critically ill patients admitted to the ICU with significant comorbidities are at higher risk, especially those with underlying heart disease, chronic obstructive pulmonary disease (COPD), and kidney disease. For surgical patients, preoperative instability, COPD, prolonged operation, and in the case of cardiac surgery patients, increased bypass time are important risk factors for prolonged mechanical ventilation.[5] Development of nosocomial pneumonia, aspiration events, and failed extubations are additional proven risk factors for prolonged mechanical ventilation.[6] In one predictive model, primary disease, Acute Physiology and Chronic Health Evaluation survey (APACHE III) score, age, COPD, prior functional limitations, and length of hospital stay prior to ICU admission were significant risk factors for mechanical ventilation for greater than 7 days.[1] The acute physiology score and primary reason for ICU admission accounted for 0.66 of the explanatory power for the model. Of the variables

in the acute physiology score, pH, Pa_{CO_2}, Pa_{O_2}/FI_{O_2} ratio, albumin level, and respiratory rate were significant. Further development of clinically useful prediction models for prolonged mechanical ventilation would be of great benefit for resource planning in the ICU.

Perhaps one of the most important risk factors for chronic critical illness is neuromuscular abnormalities associated with acute critical illness. Critical illness polyneuropathy (CIP) is evident in up to 47% of patients who are ventilated for greater than 7 days[7] and in 95% of patients who are ventilated for more than 28 days.[8] The presence of the systemic inflammatory response syndrome (SIRS) or sepsis is the greatest risk factor. The use of aminoglycosides, neuromuscular blockers, and steroids also may contribute to the development of CIP in some patients. Abnormalities on neurophysiologic testing persist for up to 5 years, but functional deficits after that much time are unusual.[8] There is no specific therapy for this condition other than aggressive rehabilitation. In most cases, recovery is very slow.

Diaphragm paralysis from phrenic nerve injury is another neuromuscular condition that contributes to prolonged mechanical ventilation. It is difficult to diagnose, but it should be suspected in any patient who has had cardiothoracic or neck surgery and has difficulty with spontaneous breathing, especially in the supine position. An elevated hemidiaphragm on chest radiograph is suggestive, but it is often not present.

TABLE 18-2 Risk Factors and Predictors for Chronic Critical Illness

Preexisting factors:	Acute factors:
Advanced age	Primary disease
Prior functional limitations	Pneumonia
Length of hospital stay prior to ICU	ARDS
Poor nutrition	Neuromuscular disease
Comorbidities	Postoperative head trauma
COPD	Postoperative intracerebral hemorrhage
Renal failure	Abnormal acute physiology
Congestive heart failure	pH
Morbid obesity	Pa_{CO_2}
Surgical issues:	Pa_{O_2}/FI_{O_2} ratio
Preoperative instability	Serum albumin
Prolonged operation	Respiratory rate
Prolonged cardiopulmonary bypass time	
Hemidiaphragm paralysis	
Complications of critical illness:	
Nosocomial pneumonia	
Aspiration	
Failed extubation	
Critical illness polyneuropathy	

Pathophysiology of Chronic Critical Illness: The Neuroendocrine Model

Despite the varied definitions and nonspecific clinical findings that have been used to describe CCI patients, they appear to be a physiologically distinct subset of the overall ICU population. This has been best demonstrated by the work of Grete Van den Berghe and others who have examined neuroendocrine responses to critical illness. During the acute phase of critical illness, adrenocorticotropic hormone (ACTH), cortisol, and prolactin levels are elevated, whereas thyrotropic and gonadotropic hormone levels are reduced.[9] During the chronic phase of critical illness, hormonal responses are significantly different (Fig. 18-1). ACTH and other anterior pituitary hormone levels decrease, but hypercortisolism persists, suggesting an alternative pathway for cortisol release.[10] CCI patients lose thyroid-stimulating hormone (TSH) pulse amplitude, which results in typically low or low-normal TSH

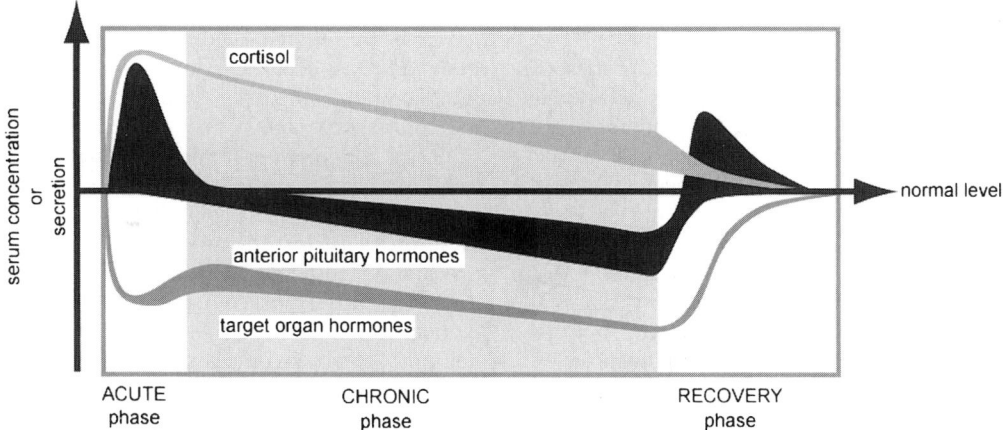

FIGURE 18-1 Simplified concept of the pituitary-dependent changes during the course of critical illness. In the acute phase of illness (first hours to a few days after onset), the secretory activity of the anterior pituitary is essentially maintained or amplified, whereas anabolic target-organ hormones are inactivated. Cortisol levels are elevated in concert with ACTH. In the chronic phase of protracted critical illness (intensive care–dependent for weeks), the secretory activity of the anterior pituitary appears uniformly suppressed in relation to reduced circulating levels of target-organ hormones. Impaired anterior pituitary hormone secretion allows the respective target-organ hormones to decrease proportionately over time, with cortisol being a notable exception, the circulating levels of which remain elevated through a peripheral drive, a mechanism that ultimately also may fail. The onset of recovery is characterized by restored sensitivity of the anterior pituitary to reduced feedback control. *(Used with permission from Van den Berghe G, de Zegher F, Bouillon R: Acute and prolonged critical illness as different neuroendocrine paradigms.* J Clin Endocrinol Metab *83:1827, 1998.)*

levels and low triiodothyroxine (T_4) and triiodothyronine (T_3) concentrations compared to acutely stressed patients.[11] This may be related to reduced expression of the thyrotropin-releasing hormone (TRH) gene in the hypothalamic paraventricular nuclei.[12]

The somatotropic axis also demonstrates important differences between acute and chronic critical illness. For patients who are in the acute phase of critical illness, the pituitary gland actively secretes growth hormone (GH) into the circulation in a pulsatile fashion that is regulated by hypothalamic growth hormone–releasing hormone (GHRH). GH levels and GH pulse frequency are increased compared with normal function. In contrast, for patients who have received mechanical ventilation for greater than 21 days, the pattern of GH secretion is less regular, and the amount that is released in pulses is greatly reduced.[9] Nocturnal secretion of GH is reduced relative to the acute stressed condition.

The hormonal changes that occur in acute illness may be positive adaptations that help divert energy away from anabolism and toward maintenance of vital tissues and immune function, for example. However, the hormonal responses to chronic critical illness may be maladaptive. CCI patients suffer from significant protein deficiencies owing to ongoing degradation and suppressed production. This hypercatabolic state likely contributes to the severe and prolonged muscle weakness that is characteristic of these patients. While protein is lost despite feeding, reesterification of free fatty acids allows fat stores to build up.[9] Hyperglycemia, insulin resistance, and hypertriglyceridemia are common. Prolonged hypercortisolism and low levels of GH and thyroid hormone may contribute significantly to these processes. In addition to prolonged wasting, immune function is also likely to be affected as well. As a clinical correlate, prolonged weakness associated with ventilator dependence and recurrent infectious complications are hallmarks of the CCI condition.

Management of the CCI Patient

INFECTION CONTROL

CCI patients are at very high risk for nosocomial infection. Perhaps their greatest risk factor is disruption of multiple infection barriers. Most patients have tracheostomies or endotracheal tubes that promote aspiration, inhibit cough, and greatly increase their risk of airway colonization with nosocomial organisms. Central venous catheters are common and remain in place for long periods, significantly increasing the risk of bloodstream infections. The presence of bladder catheters promotes urinary tract infections, and nasogastric tubes increase the risk of sinusitis. Weeks of immobility and edema predispose patients to skin breakdown, which provides another infection source.

The underlying comorbidities that make patients susceptible to chronic critical illness also make them susceptible to infections. COPD is often accompanied by bacterial colonization of lower airways and compromised airway clearance. Neurologic impairment increases aspiration risk and weakens cough response. Diabetes mellitus, renal failure, congestive heart failure, and hepatic dysfunction are all associated with compromised immune function and are important risk factors for pneumonia. Diabetes mellitus and hepatic dysfunction also increase the risk for fungemia. Immune function is further compromised by nutritional deficiencies, protein depletion, and ongoing catabolic processes.

Because CCI patients spend weeks in ICUs where multidrug-resistant bacteria are common, the incidence of infection or colonization with these organisms is quite high. This problem is compounded by multiple rounds of broad-spectrum antibiotics over the course of their hospitalization. This is a particularly important issue for ventilator rehabilitation hospitals, where patients are admitted from numerous different referring hospitals. Nearly every new admission brings unique strains of resistant organisms. Containing the spread of these organisms is a constant challenge.

Infectious complications were documented in a series of 100 patients admitted to a hospital unit dedicated to the care of patients with chronic critical illness.[13] All patients were receiving mechanical ventilation through a tracheostomy after at least 2 weeks of critical illness. During hospitalization on this unit, 61% of patients developed evidence of SIRS, and 11% developed septic shock. Line sepsis (11%), primary bacteremia (6%), tracheostomy-associated pneumonia (10%), and *Clostridium difficile* colitis (10%) were the most common infections. Urosepsis was less common in this series, but the authors were appropriately conservative in the diagnosis of urosepsis. This diagnosis required the presence of SIRS and pyuria or a positive urine culture without any other obvious source of infection.

The management of nosocomial infections in CCI patients begins with prevention. Elimination of all unnecessary compromise of barriers to infection is paramount. Venous catheters should be well maintained and removed as soon as possible. A patient who is hemodynamically stable with a functioning gastrointestinal tract may be able to receive all medications enterally. Continued maintenance of a venous catheter out of habit or ICU policy in a hemodynamically stable patient is inappropriate. When central venous catheters are necessary for long periods, tunneled catheters or chlorhexadine-, silver-, or antimicrobial-impregnated catheters should be considered. Bladder catheters should be removed as soon as possible. Strategies to prevent ventilator-associated pneumonia include semirecumbent positioning, removal of the nasogastric tube when possible, avoidance of gastric overdistention, and scheduled drainage of condensate from ventilator circuits.[14] As always, effective hand washing is essential. Judicious use of broad-spectrum antibiotics and effective isolation will decrease the incidence of *C. difficile* colitis and infections with multiresistant organisms. Routine surveillance for these organisms may be beneficial.

NUTRITION

Some of the hallmarks of chronic critical illness include low protein stores owing to impaired synthesis and persistent losses, muscle wasting and atrophy, and weight loss (unless volume overload persists). Adequate nutrition is essential if a patient is going to improve respiratory and skeletal muscle function and avoid life-threatening infectious complications. Clinical studies specifically addressing nutrition management for CCI patients are lacking. However, some systematic approaches have been developed based on principles derived from the literature for acutely critically ill patients and nonventilated long-term care patients. One approach attempts to replace protein stores in the hypoalbuminemic patient while trying to avoid the common complication of overfeeding.[15] Caloric overfeeding results in volume expansion, hyperglycemia, steatocholestasis, and possibly hypercapnea with increased ventilatory load. In a study of 213 CCI patients from 32 hospitals,[16] 58.2% of patients were receiving more than 110% of required calories according to indirect calorimetry, whereas only 12.2% were being underfed. To avoid this syndrome, one initially can provide lower total calories (20 to 25 kcal/kg per day) than is usually recommended for ICU patients with greater protein content

(1.2 to 1.5 g/kg per day). Adjustments to this balance can be made by following clinical parameters and biochemical measurements such as serum albumin and prealbumin levels, blood urea nitrogen levels, and urine urea nitrogen levels. Indirect calorimetry can be used if overfeeding remains a concern. For enteral formulas, a semielemental feed may be most appropriate for CCI patients with serum albumin concentrations of less than 2.5 g/dL to achieve better amino acid absorption and insulin response.[15]

Enteral feeding through a nasogastric tube or a gastrostomy tube is the most common route of nutrition for the CCI patient. Enteral feeding should be accompanied by careful attention to common complications. Aspiration may be reduced by head elevation, postpyloric tube placement, promotility agents, and avoidance of persistently increasing gastric residuals. Sinus infections and nasal complications can be reduced by using gastrostomy tubes placed with the help of interventional radiologists, endoscopists, or surgeons when enteral nutrition is expected to be prolonged. Frequent assessments should be made of a patient's swallowing capabilities to allow for as much oral feeding as possible. Oral feeding provides significant comfort to the patient and provides an important source of enjoyment and empowerment. Oral feeding may have to be supplemented, however, if it is limited by reduced stamina, nausea, or depression. Parenteral nutrition usually is reserved for situations where enteral feeding is not possible owing to issues with enteral access or function.

LIBERATION FROM MECHANICAL VENTILATION

Although prolonged mechanical ventilation is one of the defining characteristics of CCI patients, little data exist regarding optimal approaches to liberation from mechanical ventilation. Patients' generally weakened states usually dictate a slower pace of weaning than is recommended in the acutely critically ill patient. However, patients also can have an unnecessarily prolonged course when clinicians and therapists are not aggressive enough. By definition, most of these patients have failed early attempts at liberation. Subsequent efforts depend on continued maintenance of hemodynamic stability, avoidance of preventable complications, optimal nutrition, frequent assessments of readiness for weaning, and careful exercise of respiratory muscles to improve strength and function.

A standard approach to weaning usually involves work-rest cycles that include periods of "exercise" alternating with periods of "rest." What constitutes appropriate exercise and actual rest is debatable. Patients typically are maintained on mandatory ventilation with assist control or synchronized intermittent mandatory ventilation during the night. In the morning, the patient is placed on a setting requiring more patient effort using some degree of pressure-support ventilation. Alternatively, spontaneous breathing trials are performed using humidified oxygen via a tracheostomy collar. The degree of ventilatory support and length of exercise efforts depend on patient strength and endurance. Patients are monitored for early evidence of fatigue, as suggested by increased heart rate or blood pressure, increased respiratory rate, anxiety or diaphoresis, or oxygen desaturation. Frequent blood gas monitoring in slowly weaning CCI patients is not useful. While work-rest cycles is a common approach, there are no data to suggest that this is a more effective weaning method in

CCI patients compared with gradual decreases in continuous pressure-support ventilation, for example.

The advantage of exercising with spontaneous breathing trials is that rapid improvements in strength are recognized more easily, and earlier weaning may be accomplished. The disadvantage is that these patients are very weak and have limited ability to signal for help if they become acutely distressed. Acute respiratory distress is frequent in these patients owing to rapid fatigue, myocardial ischemia, and especially airway occlusion from mucous plugging or tracheostomy dysfunction. Therefore, spontaneous breathing trials require careful supervision and monitoring because ventilator alarms are not available.

As with liberating more acutely ill patients from the ventilator, some data support the use of formal weaning protocols in CCI patients. In one prospective cohort study using historical controls, a respiratory therapist–implemented weaning protocol decreased median time to wean from 29 days in historical control subjects to 17 days in the protocol group.[17] In the historical control group, weaning orders had been written by physicians on a daily or as-needed basis. Important components of this work-rest cycle–based therapist-driven protocol include (1) daily objective screens for readiness to wean, (2) regular assessments of how the patient tolerates decreases in respiratory support, and (3) acceleration steps for patients showing rapid progress to allow them to progress as fast as possible. This protocol was applied in a long-term acute care hospital where the respiratory therapist-to-patient ratio was 1:7. A therapist-implemented protocol such as this may be even more effective for CCI patients who are being managed in acute ICU settings where physician attention is often drawn to more severely ill patients. Success would be contingent on availability of enough experienced respiratory therapy staff.

AIRWAY MANAGEMENT

Most CCI patients who require prolonged mechanical ventilation are managed with a tracheostomy. Tracheostomies have many advantages, including improved comfort and communication, less sedation requirement, lower dead space, and better pulmonary toilet, and they allow for oral feeding in some patients. They require lower levels of monitoring than endotracheal tubes, and they facilitate transfer of the patient to lower levels of care. Despite their advantages, they are not without acute and long-term complications. Acute obstruction by mucous plugging or malfunction happens uncommonly, but consequences are devastating. Therefore, caregivers should not become complacent with regard to pulmonary toilet and monitoring, especially when patients are weak and unable to signal for assistance. Long-term complications and controversies regarding the timing of tracheostomies are discussed elsewhere.

An important question for CCI patients is timing of decannulation after liberation from the ventilator. Clinicians often are tempted to remove the tracheostomy tube quickly in order to simplify discharge planning and improve patient comfort. This can be hazardous, however, because patients remain diffusely weak after weaning and are at risk for recurrence of respiratory failure for at least several weeks. They are also at great risk for aspiration. Swallowing function remains compromised in many of these patients owing to muscle atrophy, pharyngeal edema, neurologic dysfunction, and

effects of the tracheostomy itself on swallowing mechanics. Upper airway obstruction is also common due to granulation tissue associated with the tracheostomy, vocal cord dysfunction, and upper airway edema. Therefore, decannulation should take place in a stepwise fashion with careful assessments of swallowing function and airway patency. Some clinicians advocate waiting at least 2 weeks before decannulation to help avoid common complications. For patients who demonstrate adequate ability to protect their airway but remain at high risk of respiratory failure for other reasons, the tracheostomy tract can be kept patent after the tracheostomy tube has been removed using a stoma stent.[18]

PHYSICAL THERAPY

Owing to their immobility, generalized edema, and poor nutrition, CCI patients are prone to skin breakdown, particularly in the regions of the sacrum, coccyx, and heels. Pressure ulcers become an important site of infection, protein loss, and discomfort. Courses of antibiotics, débridements, and diverting colostomies that are required for treatment of the ulcers further complicate a complex medical course. Frequent turning is essential for prevention, but care should be taken to avoid skin breakdown related to other positions, such as the ears, the greater trochanter, and the lateral malleoli. Specialty beds offer benefit and should be considered as soon as a persistent immobilized state becomes likely. Specialty beds should not, however, lead to relaxed vigilance toward skin condition in vulnerable sites.

Routine interventions typical of care on a general medical or surgical ward such as physical or occupational therapy often are overlooked for patients in an ICU setting, but critically ill patients are in great need of these services. Prolonged immobility can predispose patients to a range of organ dysfunctions, some of which can be prevented[19] (Table 18-3). While critical illness polyneuropathy is difficult

TABLE 18-3 Adverse Effects of Immobilization on Different Organ Systems

Organ Systems	Conditions
Muscles	Reduced strength, endurance, flexibility, and bulk
Joints	Reduced flexibility, joint contractures
Bones	Osteopenia and osteoporosis
Heart	Reduced stroke volume, cardiac output, and exercise capacity
Peripheral circulation	Reduced orthostatic tolerance and venous return, deep vein thrombosis
Lungs	Atelectasis and pneumonia, pulmonary embolism
Gastrointestinal tract	Reduced appetite and bowel motility, constipation
Urinary tract	Urolithiasis, infection
Skin	Pressure ulcers
Endocrine	Reduced endorphin production and insulin sensitivity, reduced lean body mass, obesity
Psychological	Reduced self-image and stress tolerance, anxiety and depression

SOURCE: From Thomas DC, Kreizman IJ, Melchiorre P, Ragnarsson KT: Rehabilitation of the patients with chronic critical illness. *Crit Care Clin* 18:695, 2002. Reproduced by permission of W. B. Saunders Company.

to prevent, disuse atrophy can be lessened in some patients, and joint contractures can be avoided in most. Range-of-motion exercises should begin as soon as a period of immobility exceeding 3 or 4 days is expected. While full range-of-motion exercises involving multiple joints can tax a busy ICU nurse, nursing aides and even family members can contribute to the effort with instruction from physical therapists. Once the patient is hemodynamically stable and alert, a mechanical ventilator should not prevent strengthening exercises against resistance, sitting in bed with legs dangling, or transfers to a bedside chair. These activities help patients to regain balance and overcome orthostatic hypotension, which can develop after only 4 to 7 days of bed rest.[20]

If a patient continues to require mechanical ventilation because of persistent respiratory muscle weakness or increased ventilatory load but is otherwise stable and free of multiple IV lines, many centers encourage CCI patients to ambulate while ventilation is provided via a bag-valve connection to their tracheostomy. This effort requires the help of at least two caregivers, and they must be careful to maintain the airway and IV lines and protect against falls. While this therapy is personnel-intensive, it can be managed if it is organized into the daily care plan and anticipated by the unit. It is also another opportunity to involve able family members. While there is little evidence that this type of advanced physical therapy decreases time on the ventilator or in the ICU, it may decrease overall length of stay in the hospital. It has other benefits, such as prevention of deep venous thrombosis (DVT), pressure ulcers, bone demineralization, and atelectasis. It also provides an important psychological benefit to the patient. Care must be taken not to push the patient beyond his or her physical capabilities. Muscle fatigue and injury should be carefully avoided.

PSYCHOLOGICAL SUPPORT

Common barriers to ventilator weaning and physical therapy include oversedation and delirium. While some patients with acute respiratory failure initially may require high doses of sedatives to decrease anxiety and facilitate mandatory ventilation, the clinician should decrease sedative usage as much as possible as soon as the patient achieves a more stable condition. Less sedative medication improves delirium, thus further decreasing the amount of sedating medications that are given. Alert patients are better able to participate in weaning efforts and physical therapy. Importantly, they are also able to communicate their symptoms, which can allow the clinician to formulate a more rational approach to anxiolysis, pain control, and diagnosis and management of depression.

Symptoms of depression are common in CCI patients.[21] Depression should be considered in patients who appear unmotivated despite gradual improvement in their condition or in patients with persistent symptoms of delirium despite simplification of their medical regimen. This should not be considered a "reactive depression" related to their difficult circumstances because there are usually other important contributors. Many patients, particularly the elderly, have preexisting depression that was either being treated or was undiagnosed. Changes in the neurohumoral axis described earlier may play a role, and other metabolic disturbances could contribute as well. After correcting medical factors, including control of pain and delirium, medical therapy with antidepressants can be started, especially when the depressive symptoms are interfering with the patient's participation in care. It should be remembered that clinical benefit from such medical therapies is slow to develop, and rapid escalation of doses should be avoided. Low doses of psychostimulants such as methylphenidate can be considered when a more immediate impact is desired.[22] Taking time to communicate with the patient, promoting family interactions, and general supportive care can be very effective and also will have an immediate impact.

Other common symptoms in CCI patients include dyspnea, pain, anxiety, and sleep disturbance.[21] These symptoms can elicit physiologic responses that will worsen the course of critical illness, such as increased oxygen consumption, immune dysfunction, protein catabolism, and electrolyte disturbance. Addressing these symptoms through appropriate medical and environmental interventions may improve patient outcome while providing humane care for a desperately ill patient. Frustration from inability to communicate is a particularly common problem that exacerbates other symptoms. Letter boards and writing pads should be easily accessible to patients. One-way valves on tracheostomies that allow for air passage through the vocal cords with cuff deflation should be used as soon as the patient is able to protect his or her airway. Regaining vocalization is a tremendous relief to the patient. Most of all, time should be taken to inform the patient of his or her condition and elicit responses and concerns.

ALTERNATIVE SITES OF CARE

In the 1980s, clinicians in the ICU began to understand the unique medical requirements of CCI patients, and they recognized that these needs often could be better accommodated in settings that are removed from the acute ICU. Otherwise stable CCI patients requiring prolonged mechanical ventilation can be managed safely outside the ICU setting. Patients should be off vasopressors, have simple fluid requirements, and have stable airways. Managing such patients outside the ICU allows for lower nurse-to-patient ratios, which results in substantial cost savings. At the same time, other essential services such as physical therapy, speech therapy, or occupational therapy can be provided more consistently, especially if they are managed in a dedicated unit whose focus is on the CCI patient. These dedicated units have taken a number of forms, including separate units in acute care hospitals, specialized units in acute rehabilitation hospitals or subacute care facilities, or free-standing long-term acute care hospitals designed specifically for the care of CCI patients. Units dedicated to CCI patients vary in the type and acuity of the patients they manage. This variation usually is driven by resource needs and goals of care. Some units exist primarily to offload the acute ICU of patients with prolonged courses and poor prospects of recovery. Other units restrict admissions to patients who have good rehabilitation potential and can benefit most from a multidisciplinary approach to weaning and comprehensive rehabilitation.

ICU physicians should familiarize themselves with the units and facilities that are available in their region. They should be aware of the resources that are available and general approaches to care in each facility so that they can make referrals according to patient needs and best possible outcome. Referrals to facilities outside the acute hospital setting should be made only when it is clear that complex diagnostic services are no longer required for the patient and that the receiving center can manage any active medical or surgical issues adequately. It also should be remembered that a seemingly stable patient in an acute ICU setting may become somewhat unstable with the stress of transportation. Studies have documented trends toward earlier discharge of CCI patients to post-ICU care settings. These earlier discharges have resulted in a high rate of urgent transfers back to the acute ICU.[23]

Only a minority of CCI patients will have access to specialized acute hospital units or long-term acute care hospitals. The rest will continue to receive care in the acute ICU setting until they are free of life-sustaining therapies. This should not be an impediment to excellent care. Physicians and nurses should adapt their approach to care of the patient according to the principles discussed earlier, and they should involve the essential ancillary services as soon as indicated. For hospitals that do not have access to specialized facilities, multidisciplinary care teams consisting of physicians, respiratory therapists, nutritionists, physical therapists, and social workers who have expertise in managing chronic critical illness can be helpful.[24]

Outcomes

SURVIVAL

The study of outcomes for CCI patients has generated a great deal of interest in recent years. Intuitively, many clinicians assume that their long-term outcomes are poor based on the many physical challenges that were discussed earlier. The clinicians witness a relatively high hospital mortality and a high degree of suffering on the part of patients and families. These observations raise the question, "Is this prolonged invasive care worth what the patient is going through?" A number of studies have been designed to try to address this type of question. Results of these studies have been informative, but much more remains to be learned. The greatest challenge in interpreting outcomes data in this population is the heterogeneity of patients and patient settings. There is tremendous variation in age, primary ICU diagnosis, comorbidities, complications, disease states prior to the acute illness, and care before and after hospital discharge. All these factors likely have some impact on long-term outcomes. The same holds true for more acute critically ill patients, but for that population there exist validated measures of illness severity such as APACHE II that can be used to standardize comparisons among different groups of ICU patients. No such measure exists for CCI patients. As discussed at the beginning of this chapter, there is not even a commonly accepted definition of chronic critical illness. For these reasons, any conclusions that are to be gained from outcomes studies in the CCI population need to be interpreted carefully based on the setting and methodology of the study and the predominant type of patient that is represented.

Population-based studies can overcome some of these problems by being inclusive of many types of hospitals, with all types of patients being represented. The Nationwide Inpatient Sample, described earlier, includes discharge data from a large probability sample of patients from general hospitals in the United States. Using DRG 483 (tracheostomy for conditions other than face, mouth, and neck diagnoses) to identify patients requiring prolonged mechanical ventilation, it was estimated that at least 88,000 patients in the United States suffered some degree of chronic critical illness in 1997.[3] Patients in all age groups are susceptible, but prevalence increases with age. Hospital mortality increases with age also. Average hospital mortality for the whole population is 27%, which does not differ substantially from hospital mortality for the general population of mechanically ventilated ICU patients. These mortality figures do not account for patients who were transferred alive on a ventilator to a long-term acute care hospital but died before final discharge.

Considering that CCI patients who survive hospitalization are discharged with a high degree of unresolved acute and chronic medical problems, 1-year outcomes are better indicators of overall outcome. Currently, long-term outcomes studies in this population are limited to single-institution cohort studies. Most of those studies represent patients who had been transferred to long-term acute care institutions. One-year survival in these studies ranges from 23% to 38% in relatively nonselective institutions, although survival can be as high as 76% for patients managed in institutions that select for likelihood of better outcomes. While these 1-year outcomes are not encouraging, it should be noted that long-term acute care hospitals generally select for older patients who have poorer long-term prognoses than younger patients. However, cohort studies following CCI patients from more general acute care hospitals before 1990 report 1-year survival to be in a similar range. It is possible that outcomes for the general population of CCI patients in acute care hospitals have improved since 1990 as clinicians have become more familiar with their unique problems and postdischarge care has improved, but this remains to be seen. Results of more recent studies are pending.

While long-term survival for the overall population of CCI patients is poor, a significant number of patients do survive. Investigators have been attempting recently to identify patients with better long-term prognoses. One study in a single long-term acute care population indicated that patients who were younger than age 65 or between the ages of 65 and 75 with good prior functional status had a 1-year survival rate of 56%.[25] In contrast, patients over age 75 or over age 65 with poor prior functional status had a 1-year survival rate of only 5% (Fig. 18-2). Another important risk factor for poor outcome is the requirement for hemodialysis in addition to prolonged mechanical ventilation. Underlying cardiac dysfunction or chronic pulmonary disease are significant risk factors as well. Further studies are underway in more general CCI populations to gain more specific information regarding long-term prognoses.

QUALITY OF LIFE

CCI patients experience considerable functional limitations in long-term follow-up. Cohort studies of patients discharged to long-term acute care hospitals or other post–acute care institutions indicate that only 40% to 50% of survivors, or 10% of total patients, are completely independent in activities of daily living after 1 year. Clearly, chronic critical illness combined with the patients' underlying comorbidities takes a heavy toll on physical functioning. However, overall quality of life is not as closely linked to functional limitations as

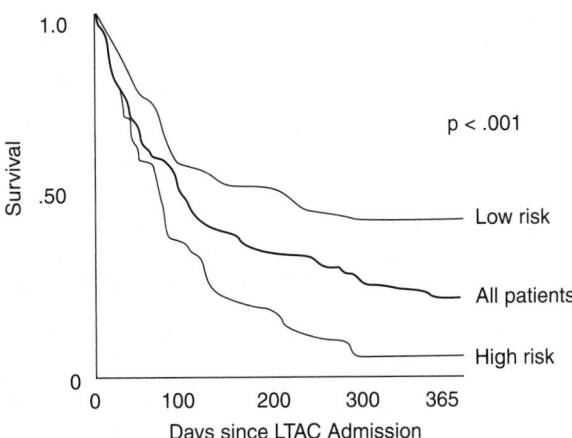

FIGURE 18-2 One-year mortality risk for 133 mechanically ventilated patients admitted to a long-term acute care hospital from 37 acute hospital ICUs. High risk: Age $\geq$ 75 or age $\geq$ 65 and poor functional status prior to illness. Low risk: Age < 65 or age < 75 with good functional status prior to illness.
SOURCE: From Carson SS, Bach PB: The epidemiology and costs of chronic critical illness. *Crit Care Clin* 18:461, 2002. Reproduced with permission of W.B. Saunders Company.

many people would believe. Patients who have experienced near-death events can be satisfied with living with physical limitations when death is the obvious alternative. This is especially true in the elderly, for whom physical limitations often were present before their critical illness. Recent assessments of quality of life in long-term survivors of chronic critical illness support these statements. Depending on the setting, between 50% and 80% of survivors report their quality of life to be fair, good, or excellent. In fact, quality-of-life outcomes do not differ significantly from those of other ICU patients.[3] It should be remembered, however, that the majority of patients in these studies do not survive to 1 year. Additionally, a significant proportion of those who do survive are not able to respond to quality-of-life surveys owing to cognitive deficits or severe physical limitations. For the majority of patients who die within the year, their terminal courses are characterized by long periods of invasive and institutionalized care, with accompanying symptoms of discomfort and emotional distress.

COSTS

The growing burden of chronic critical illness has significant cost implications for health care systems. Annual ICU costs for CCI patients in the United States have been estimated to be as high as $24 billion. Patients who require more than 7 days of mechanical ventilation consume as much as 37% of ICU resources, and 21% of ICU resources are consumed after their seventh day of mechanical ventilation.[2] Median hospital charges per patient with DRG 483 in the Nationwide Inpatient Sample range from $120,000 to $135,000 depending on age group (see Table 18-1). Actual hospital costs are lower than these figures, but the costs are still quite substantial. Since few of these patients are discharged home, additional costs are accrued from rehabilitation or long-term care charges. In a cohort of patients from three hospitals who received mechanical ventilation for more than 96 hours, the mean total charges for health care for the year after hospital

discharge was $131,190 for all patients and $178,516 per 1-year survivor.[26]

These high costs attract the attention of hospital administrators and third-party payers, and given the overall poor outcomes for many of these patients, clinicians often wonder about the appropriateness of some of these expenditures. Only one study has addressed the subject of cost-effectiveness of care for CCI patients. Heyland and colleagues[27] compared costs for patients who required ICU care for more than 14 days (mean ICU length of stay 24.5 ± 11.7 days) with costs for patients in the ICU who had life support withdrawn. In their analysis, the incremental cost-effectiveness ratio was Can$65,219 per life saved or Can$4350 per life-year saved. They concluded that continuing treatment for patients with prolonged ICU stays may be an efficient use of hospital resources. It should be noted, however, that their study did not account for costs associated with care after the acute hospitalization. While similar studies involving a broader range of patients will be helpful in the future, for now it appears that the high costs of care for CCI patients may not be out of line with that of other medical interventions. Clinicians should use good judgment, however, recognizing that continued aggressive care in individual patients who are unlikely to survive or have an acceptable quality of life is not an appropriate use of resources, nor is it in the patient's best interests. Clinicians also should remain cognizant of ways to decrease costs in this patient population.

Alternative sites of care are the most effective means of reducing costs for the care of CCI patients. These cost savings are largely related to lower-intensity nursing. In one study, CCI patients were randomized to receive continued care in the acute ICU versus further management in a specialized multidisciplinary unit in the same hospital.[28] Hospital mortality did not differ between the two groups, but mean hospital costs per survivor in the specialized unit were $109,220 compared with $138,434 in the ICU ($p = 0.0005$). There have been no direct cost comparisons between acute ICU care and offsite facilities, but costs likely decrease continuously as intensity of services decreases from acute hospital ICUs to long-term acute care hospitals to subacute care.[23] Limitations in acute hospital reimbursement, combined with potential for cost savings, have been a major factor driving the proliferation of post-ICU care facilities in the United States over the last decade.

References

1. Seneff MG, Zimmerman JE, Knaus WA, et al: Predicting the duration of mechanical ventilation: The importance of disease and patient characteristics. *Chest* 110:469, 1996.
2. Wagner DP: Economics of prolonged mechanical ventilation. *Am Rev Respir Dis* 140:S14, 1989.
3. Carson SS, Bach PB: The epidemiology and costs of chronic critical illness. *Crit Care Clin* 18:461, 2002.
4. Dewar DM, Kurek CJ, Lambrinos J, et al: Patterns in costs and outcomes for patients with prolonged mechanical ventilation undergoing tracheostomy: An analysis of discharges under diagnosis-related group 483 in New York State from 1992 to 1996. *Crit Care Med* 27:2640, 1999.
5. Thompson MJ, Elton RA, Mankad PA: Prediction of requirement for, and outcome of, prolonged mechanical ventilation following cardiac surgery. *Cardiovasc Surg* 5:376, 1997.

6. Kollef MH, Ahrens TS, Shannon W: Clinical predictors and outcomes for patients requiring tracheostomy in the intensive care unit. *Crit Care Med* 27:1714, 1999.

7. Leijten FS, Harinck de Weerd JE, Poortvliet DC, et al: The role of polyneuropathy in motor convalescence after prolonged mechanical ventilation. *JAMA* 274:1221, 1995.

8. Fletcher SN, Kennedy DD, Indrajit RG, et al: Persistent neuromuscular and neurophysiologic abnormalities in long-term survivors of prolonged critical illness. *Crit Care Med* 31:1012, 2003.

9. Van den Berghe G, de Zegher F, Bouillon R: Acute and prolonged critical illness as different neuroendocrine paradigms. *J Clin Endocrinol Metab* 83:1827, 1998.

10. Vermes I, Beishuizen A, Hampsink RM, Haanen C: Dissociation of plasma adrenocorticotropin and cortisol levels in critically ill patients: Possible role of endothelin and atrial natriuretic hormone. *J Clin Endocrinol Metab* 80:1238, 1995.

11. Van den Berghe G, de Zegher F, Veldhuis JD, et al: Thyrotropin and prolactin release in prolonged critical illness: Dynamics of spontaneous secretion and effects of growth hormone secretagogues. *Clin Endorinol* 47:599, 1997.

12. Fliers E, Guldenaar SEF, Wiersinga WM, et al: Decreased hypothalamic thyrotropin-releasing hormone gene expression in patients with non-thyroidal illness. *J Clin Endocrinol Metab* 82:4032, 1997.

13. Kalb TH, Lorin S. Infection in the chronically critically ill: Unique risk profile in a newly defined population. *Crit Care Clin* 18:529, 2002.

14. Kollef MH: The prevention of ventilator-associated pneumonia. *N Engl J Med* 340:627, 1999.

15. Mechanick JI, Brett EM: Nutrition support of the chronically critically ill patient. *Crit Care Clin* 18:597, 2002.

16. McClave SA, Lowen CC, Kleber MJ, et al: Are patients fed appropriately according to their caloric requirements? *J Parent Enteral Nutr* 22:375, 1998.

17. Scheinhorn DJ, Chao DC, Stearn-Hassenpflug M, Wallace WA: Outcomes in post-ICU mechanical ventilation-a therapist driven protocol. *Chest* 119:236, 2001.

18. Scheinhorn DJ, Stearn-Hassenpflug M: Provision of long-term mechanical ventilation. *Crit Care Clin* 14:819, 1998.

19. Thomas DC, Kreizman IJ, Melchiorre P, Ragnarsson KT: Rehabilitation of the patients with chronic critical illness. *Crit Care Clin* 18:695, 2002.

20. Greenleaf JE: Physiological responses to prolonged bed rest and fluid immersion in humans. *J Appl Physiol* 57:619, 1984.

21. Nelson JE: Palliative care of the chronically critically ill patient. *Crit Care Clin* 18:659, 2002.

22. Woods SW, Tesar G, Murray GB, et al: Psychostimulant treatment of depressive disorders secondary to medical illness. *J Clin Psychol* 47:12, 1986.

23. Nasraway SA, Button GJ, Rand WM, et al: Survivors of catastrophic illness: Outcome after direct transfer from intensive care to extended care facilities. *Crit Care Med* 28:19, 2000.

24. Burns SM, Dempsey E: Long-term ventilator management strategies: Experiences of two hospitals. *AACN Clin Issues* 11:424, 2000.

25. Carson SS, Bach PB, Brzozowski L, Leff A: Outcomes after long-term acute care: An analysis of 133 mechanically ventilated patients. *Am J Respir Crit Care Med* 159:1568, 1999.

26. Douglas AS, Daly BJ, Gordon N, Brennan PF: Survival and quality of life: Short-term versus long-term ventilator patients. *Crit Care Med* 30:2655, 2002.

27. Heyland DK, Konopad E, Noseworthy TW, et al: Is it "worthwhile" to continue treating patients with a prolonged stay (>14 days) in the ICU? *Chest* 114:192, 1998.

28. Rudy EB, Daly BJ, Douglas S, et al: Patient outcomes for the chronically critically ill: Special care unit versus intensive care unit. *Nurs Res* 44:324, 1995.

Chapter 19 _____

LONG-TERM OUTCOMES OF CRITICAL ILLNESS

MARGARET S. HERRIDGE
RAMONA O. HOPKINS

KEY POINTS

- *Survivors of critical illness experience decreased health-related quality of life due to physical limitations, depression and anxiety, and cognitive impairments.*

- *There may be irreversible long-term neuromuscular dysfunction (e.g., muscle weakness, critical illness polyneuropathy, and myopathy).*

- *Other organ dysfunction (e.g., pulmonary) is present following critical illness but does not appear to have the same impact on patients' self-reported quality-of-life outcomes as other morbidities.*

- *Hypoxia and delirium are risk factors for poor long-term outcome resulting from cognitive impairments.*

- *Approximately one-third to one-half of survivors of critical illness will develop long-term cognitive impairments.*

- *Recent reports suggest that exercise capacity and cognitive function plateau at a lower than normal level at 1 year with limited improvement 2 years following ICU discharge.*

- *Long-term physical and neuropsychological dysfunction may be remediable through the implementation of a multidisciplinary and family-centered rehabilitation program. This is currently being evaluated.*

Background

In the United States, 55,000 patients are hospitalized in the ICU on any given day,[1] and approximately one-half million Americans undergo protracted (>96 hours) mechanical ventilation in an ICU each year. Historically, outcome studies in adult critically ill patients have focused on mortality. Recently, survival in some of our highest-acuity patients (e.g., acute respiratory distress syndrome, sepsis) has improved significantly[2] through novel ventilation strategies,[3] early interventions for sepsis,[4,5] daily administration of renal replacement therapy,[6] tight glycemic control,[7] and other emerging therapeutic modalities. These dramatic improvements in ICU survival have reinvigorated interest in understanding the nature, determinants, and modifiers of long-term morbidity in ICU survivors.

Patients who survive critical illness are at risk for permanent physical, functional, emotional, and neurocognitive deficits, of which some or all may contribute to decreased health-related quality of life (HRQL). The reasons for this late morbidity after ICU care are multifactorial and include but are not limited to the following: (1) nature of and treatment for the inciting critical illness; (2) multiple-organ-dysfunction syndrome and hypoxemia; (3) physiologic and emotional stress in the ICU related to the illness itself, sleep fragmentation, psychoactive medications, and impaired drug metabolism owing to simultaneous administration of multiple medications; and (4) prolonged immobility and long ICU stay.

Patients with the acute respiratory distress syndrome (ARDS) represent some of the most complex, highest-acuity, and long-stay ICU patients (see Chap. 38). ARDS affects an estimated 150,000 people per year in the United States and is manifested by acute lung injury and severe hypoxemic respiratory failure.[8] ARDS is associated with a variety of insults, including, pneumonia, sepsis, trauma, massive transfusion, and other medical/surgical conditions.[9] It is a systemic illness involving inflammatory and coagulopathic disturbances that may induce dysfunction of multiple organ systems, including skeletal muscle and the peripheral and central nervous systems.[10,11] Because of the significant potential for morbidity, ARDS patients have been the focus in long-term outcome studies in survivors of critical illness. We are in the early stages of understanding the long-term impact of ARDS on physical, emotional, and cognitive functioning and how each contributes to the patients' HRQL. Most studies in ARDS survivors have focused on 6- to 12-month outcomes, and there is limited information on morbidity beyond this time point. Comprehensive 5- and 10-year follow-up data are not available for ARDS patients, and it is unclear whether all survivors of critical illness—even with a severe episode—will suffer from the same morbidity as observed in ARDS survivors. Despite these limitations, the ARDS survivor data are some of the most complete long-term outcome data available and represent the current state of the art in the critical care outcomes literature. As such, they will form the primary basis for this review.

Evolution of Outcomes Research in Survivors of Critical Illness

Historically, the assessment of outcome in critical care has focused largely on mortality and to a lesser extent on short-term physiologic and radiologic measures of impairment. As the focus has shifted to include the evaluation of longer-term outcomes, more investigators have moved toward patient-centered measures of functional status and HRQL. One advantage of these measures is that many are self-administered, and valuable information pertaining to physical, emotional, and cognitive well-being can be obtained without an in-person visit. This strength is also a limitation because these data will not facilitate understanding of the many and varied determinants of reported impairments in HRQL. This limitation is further compounded by heterogeneity across studies related to study sample, case mix, follow-up time for the population of interest, and difficulties comparing studies owing to the different HRQL measures administered. One potential solution to this dilemma is to focus on relatively homogeneous populations of patients, characterize their HRQL, and then proceed with in-person natural history cohort studies to identify and describe the specific determinants of reported morbidity. One example of data on a relatively homogeneous group is the ARDS long-term outcomes literature. Many recent publications describe decreased quality of life in ARDS survivors. Most studies suggest that physical and/or

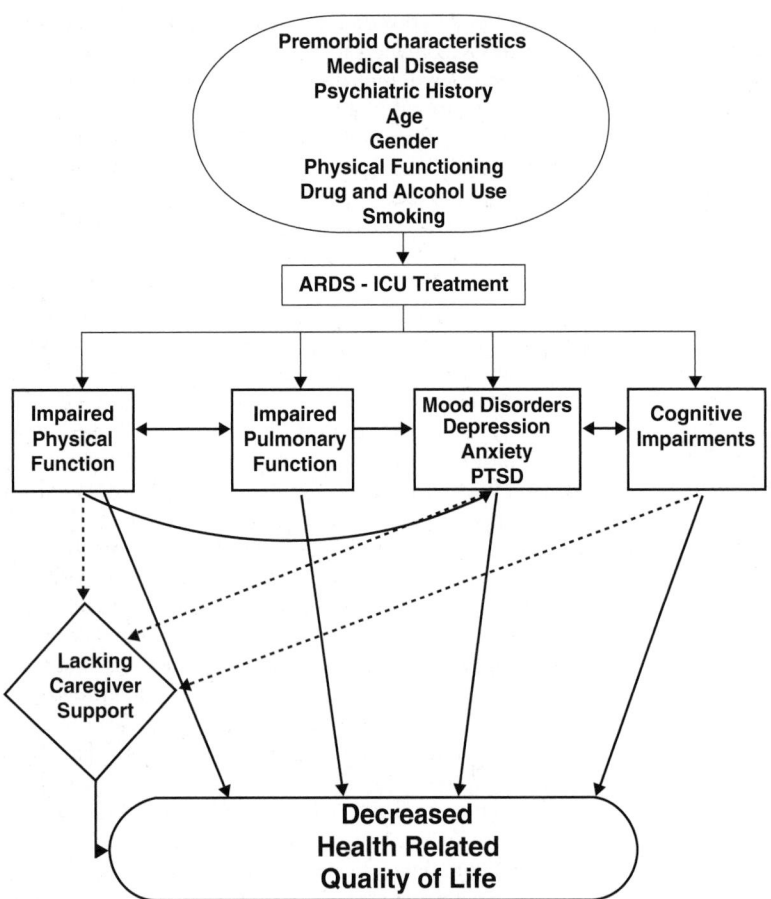

FIGURE 19-1 Determinants of health-related quality of life in ARDS survivors.

cognitive impairments are the main determinants of long-term disability. Through natural history cohort data in ARDS survivors, we have gained important insights into the heterogeneity of pulmonary, neuromuscular, and neuropsychological sequelae that contribute—to a greater or lesser extent in individual patients—to decreased HRQL. Ultimately, a detailed understanding of the spectrum of contributors to morbidity and their determinants will allow development, testing, and implementation of interventions that will lead to improved functional status and HRQL (Fig. 19-1).

Long-Term Outcome Measures in Critical Illness

HEALTH-RELATED QUALITY OF LIFE (HRQL)

HRQL can be defined as a set of causally linked dimensions of health, including biologic/physiologic, mental, physical, social function, cognitive, and health perception.[12] Measures of HRQL assess how disease and its treatment are related to physical, social, emotional, or cognitive functioning. HRQL has emerged as an important measure of recovery from a variety of disease states, including critical illness, and has been used to evaluate patient-centered outcomes.

Most studies indicate that a significant proportion of ICU survivors experience some impairment in HRQL; however, this can be quite variable.[13,14] Case mix may represent one important reason for these differences in reported HRQL. Criti-

cally ill patient populations are very diverse. The premorbid functional status of the patient and the etiology of the critical illness and its outcome represent important determinants of reported HRQL. Trauma patients with brain injury but normal cognitive function and intact social and work functioning reported a higher quality of life than trauma patients who were unemployed and had cognitive impairment.[15] Critically ill multiple-trauma survivors experience decreased quality of life associated with cognitive impairments and decreased income.[16] Elderly patients (>70 years) hospitalized in the ICU more than 30 days reported decreased physical functioning and poorer health and memory, but most were still functionally independent.[17] Survivors of sepsis[18] and prolonged mechanical ventilatory support (mean of 45 days) had compromised physical function, and the degree of dysfunction was related to premorbid functional status and the underlying disease.[19]

Although there is clearly some heterogeneity across different populations of ARDS patients, there appears to be less variability in reported HRQL compared with general populations of critically ill patients. In 1994, McHugh and her colleagues,[20] using a prospective cohort study, serially evaluated pulmonary function and quality of life to assess the relationship between pulmonary dysfunction and functional disability. These authors found that the Sickness Impact Profile (generic quality-of-life measure of the subject's self-perceived physical and psychological condition) scores were very low at extubation, rose substantially in the first 3 months, and then exhibited only slight improvement to 1 year. When quality of life was assessed using a lung-related Sickness Impact Profile score, only a modest proportion of the patients' overall dysfunction was attributed to residual pulmonary problems. Weinert and coworkers[21] identified functional impairment in a cohort of acute lung injury survivors. They administered the Medical Outcomes Study 36-item short-form health survey (SF-36), which yields scores in eight domains including physical and social functioning, role limitations because of emotional or physical problems, mental health, vitality, bodily pain, and general health perceptions.[22] While all domains of the SF-36 were reduced, the largest decrements were in physical ability to maintain their roles (role-physical) and physical functioning. While some decreased quality of life was attributed to pulmonary dysfunction, many more patients attributed this to global and generalized disability. Schelling and colleagues[23] made similar observations about impaired physical functioning and inferred that disability was due to pulmonary dysfunction; however, they did not assess this in their study. Davidson and colleagues[24] designed a study to determine if there were differences in health-related quality of life in ARDS survivors and comparably ill controls. They used the SF-36 and a pulmonary disease–specific measure (St. George's Respiratory Questionnaire [SGRQ]) to determine the degree to which perceived physical disability in ARDS survivors was related to pulmonary dysfunction. Similar to previous reports, all domains of the SF-36 were reduced, and the largest decrement was in the role-physical domain. ARDS survivors had significantly worse scores on the SGRQ compared with critically ill controls. There appeared to be an ARDS-specific degree of physical disability, but it was not clear whether this was solely related to pulmonary dysfunction or there were other important extrapulmonary contributors.

Angus and colleagues[25] used the quality-of-well-being (QWB) score in a prospective cohort of ARDS survivors to measure quality-adjusted survival in the first year after hospital discharge. The mean QWB scores for the ARDS cohort at 6 and 12 months were significantly lower than the scores of a control population of patients with cystic fibrosis. When QWB was disaggregated into its component subscores, post hoc analyses showed that the symptom-component scores of the QWB accounted for 70 percent of the decrement in perfect health at 6 and 12 months. Although respiratory symptoms were reported in almost half the patients, the most common complaints were musculoskeletal and constitutional.

In a prospective cohort study of 78 survivors of ARDS, Orme and coworkers[26] evaluated HRQL and pulmonary function outcomes in patients treated with higher tidal volume versus lower tidal volume ventilation strategies. Both groups (higher and lower tidal volumes) reported decreased HRQL in physical functioning, role-physical, bodily pain, general health, and vitality (energy) on the SF-36. The pulmonary function abnormalities correlated with decreased HRQL for domains reflecting physical function.

Not only is the observation of impaired physical functioning robust across studies and investigators, but it also appears to persist for long periods of time following ICU or hospital discharge. The paper by Davidson and coworkers[24] discussed earlier reported outcomes at 23 months after discharge, and Herridge and colleagues[27] also have reported persistent physical dysfunction at 2 years after ICU discharge.

Hopkins and colleagues[28] were the first to rigorously evaluate cognitive dysfunction in ARDS survivors and toreport the significant impact this had on reported HRQL outcomes. Fifty-five consecutive ARDS survivors completed detailed neuropsychological testing and questionnaires relating to health status and cognitive and psychological function at hospital discharge and 1 year after ARDS onset. These authors reported that decreased HRQL was related to cognitive dysfunction. Impaired cognitive function following ARDS also has been reported by others.[29]

Decreased HRQL has been associated with posttraumatic stress disorder (PTSD) and is manifest in the emotional domains of the SF-36 (e.g., role-emotional, mental health, and vitality). PTSD may represent yet another important contributor to subsequent disability and loss of employment.[30]

HRQL in ARDS survivors is affected by physical limitation, cognitive impairment, and emotional dysfunction. The HRQL data have had an enormous impact on the critical care community and have helped to focus attention on long-term morbidity after critical illness. However, these data provide limited insights into the specific determinants of morbidity. Natural history cohort data—evaluating both functional and cognitive long-term outcomes—have helped us to begin to understand the heterogeneous nature of reported morbidity and the complexity of interaction among physical, emotional, and cognitive domains in individual patients (see Fig. 19-1).

PHYSIOLOGIC AND FUNCTIONAL OUTCOMES IN ARDS SURVIVORS

Many authors have focused on residual pulmonary function abnormalities as a probable explanation for long-term functional impairment in ARDS patients. While most ARDS follow-up studies report pulmonary dysfunction, the pulmonary function abnormalities tend to be modest and may not fully explain functional limitation. More recently, neuromuscular dysfunction sustained as a result of the inciting critical illness and its attendant ICU care has been associated with ongoing physical impairment in ARDS survivors. These data have been gleaned from in-person prospective natural history cohort data.

PULMONARY FUNCTION ABNORMALITIES

The lung was the obvious focus of outcome studies early after the first description of ARDS in 1967. The studies of pulmonary function have suffered from several limitations, including a lack of consecutive patient recruitment and loss to follow-up, limited sample size, limited follow-up times, and studies of pulmonary function in isolation without any concurrent functional evaluation. Evaluation of pulmonary function on its own or coupled with HRQL measures has remained a dominant theme until recently.

Many ARDS survivors have persistent pulmonary function impairments that typically are mild to moderate, with restrictive changes and a reduction in diffusion capacity.[31–33] Orme and colleagues[26] reported that ARDS survivors had abnormal pulmonary function associated with decreased health-related quality of life 1 year following hospital discharge, and Schelling and colleagues[34] recently reported no additional improvement in pulmonary function after the first year following ARDS. In a recent publication, Neff and colleagues[35] reviewed 30 studies that evaluated pulmonary function in ARDS survivors. They reported significant variability in obstructive (0% to 33%) and restrictive (0% to 50%) defects, as well as compromised diffusion capacity (33% to 82%). This spectrum of pulmonary dysfunction may relate to population heterogeneity with respect to evolving definitions or severity of ARDS, severity of lung injury, ICU ventilatory strategy, prior history of lung disease or smoking, and the presence of other pulmonary processes that fulfill the ARDS definition but have a very different natural history (e.g., bronchiolitis obliterans organizing pneumonia).

Most outcome studies found that ARDS survivors frequently are unable to resume their prior lifestyle, but the degree of pulmonary dysfunction does not fully explain their functional limitation. This observation has led investigators to explore other possible contributors to physical disability.

LIMITATION IN PHYSICAL FUNCTIONING
One of the limitations in the ARDS morbidity literature has been an absence of data that objectively quantify functional disability. These data would be most useful in the context of in-person assessment in addition to concurrent physiologic and HRQL outcome measures. Multiple outcome measures may result in a better understanding of the determinants of functional morbidity and how this might be ameliorated. The Toronto ARDS Outcomes group evaluated exercise capacity (distance walked in 6 minutes with continuous oximetry) and pulmonary function and conducted an interview, physical examination, and HRQL measure in 109 ARDS survivors at 3, 6, and 12 months after ICU discharge.[36,37] Similar to other pulmonary function studies, the ARDS patients had mild restrictive disease and reduced diffusion capacity at 3 months following ICU discharge. By 6 and 12 months, they had normal to near-normal lung volumes and spirometric measures with a persistent mild reduction in carbon dioxide diffusion capacity—lung impairment similar to that noted by others. The ARDS survivors had profound muscle weakness and wasting and were only able to achieve 66% of their predicted exercise capacity 1 year after ICU discharge. This functional disability was reflected in the HRQL assessment, in which patients reported profound reduction in the physical functioning and role-physical domains of the SF-36. Impaired exercise capacity was related to burden of comorbid disease, exposure to systemic corticosteroid treatment during the ICU period and the rate of resolution of lung injury, and multiple-organ dysfunction during the ICU stay. The precise determinant(s) of the observed muscle wasting and weakness were not clear, but possibilities included critical illness polyneuropathy, ICU-acquired myopathy, and entrapment neuropathies.

Critical Illness Polyneuropathy
An acute polyneuropathy was described in the 1980s in association with multiple-organ dysfunction and sepsis. This was called *critical illness polyneuropathy* and has been characterized electrically and morphologically by a primary axonal degeneration of motor and sensory fibers.[38,39] The prevalence of critical illness polyneuropathy is 70 percent and has been documented in populations with sepsis, multiple-organ dysfunction, and ARDS.[40] The precise etiology is unknown, but it may represent ischemic nerve injury secondary

to a disturbance in the microcirculation. There has been a recent report that critical illness polyneuropathy may persist for years following ICU discharge and contribute to long-term physical limitation.[41]

ICU-Acquired Myopathy
The incidence of an ICU-acquired myopathy and its impact on disability and prolonged rehabilitation in the post-ICU period are uncertain. A recent report described a 25% incidence of ICU-acquired paresis in patients remaining on the mechanical ventilator for 7 or more days.[42] Myopathic changes have been documented both in the presence[43] and the absence[44] of corticosteroid and neuromuscular blockade use. Several patients from the Toronto ARDS Outcomes study underwent open muscle biopsy[45] in an attempt to better understand the nature of the observed muscle wasting and weakness. The median time to biopsy was almost 1 year after ICU discharge, and all patients had histopathologic evidence of a chronic myopathic process. Muscle injury is likely multifactorial, and it may represent an important determinant of long-term functional impairment.

Entrapment Neuropathy
The Toronto ARDS Outcomes study observed a 6% prevalence of peroneal and ulnar nerve palsies.[37] Although this represents only a small proportion of patients, these nerve palsies complicated rehabilitation therapy and precluded return to original work in some cases. Other studies also have found detrimental long-term consequences resulting from compression neuropathies.[46]

Heterotopic Ossification
Heterotopic ossification is the deposition of para-articular ectopic bone and has been associated previously with polytrauma, burns, pancreatitis, and ARDS.[47,48] It has been linked with paralysis and prolonged immobilization. There was a 5% prevalence of heterotopic ossification in the Toronto ARDS Outcomes study, with all patients having large joint immobilization, leading to important functional limitation (Fig. 19-2). Natural history cohort studies facilitate unexpected observations—such as heterotopic ossification—and

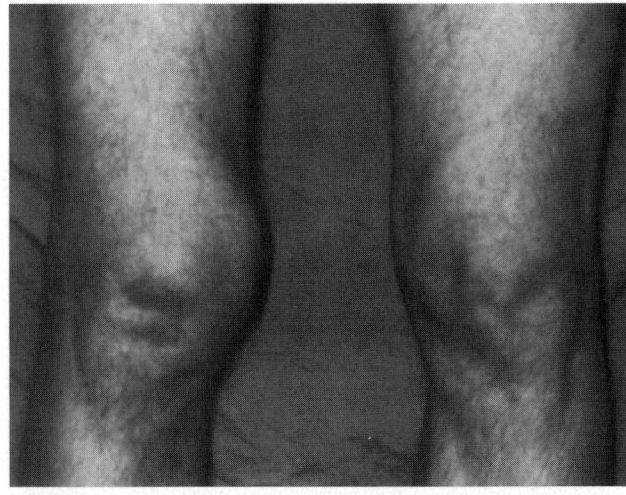

FIGURE 19-2 Heterotopic ossification involving the right knee of an ARDS survivor.

link them to functional disability. Heterotopic ossification is remediable with appropriate surgical intervention, and screening for this might be an important part of a multidisciplinary intervention to improve functional outcomes.

EMOTIONAL OUTCOMES
Emotional Function after ARDS
The relationship between critical illness and emotional (mood) disorders is being recognized increasingly. Mood disorders represent important contributors to long-term HRQL impairments in survivors of critical illness. However, it is unclear whether these disorders are a psychological reaction to extraordinary emotional and physiologic stress, sequelae of brain injury sustained due to a critical illness and its treatment, or both.

Individuals with critical illness have to cope with a disease or injury that is life threatening as well as very burdensome interventions. The combination of medications, physiologic changes, pain, altered sensory inputs, and an unfamiliar environment may contribute to emotional changes following critical illness.[49–51] Recent evidence suggests that mood disorders that occur secondary to medical illness may constitute discrete entities in which symptoms are similar to primary mood disorders, but there is a male predominance and earlier onset.[52]

The reported prevalence and severity of mood disorders including symptoms of depression, anxiety, and PTSD in survivors of critical illness are quite variable among patients following ICU hospitalization.[49,50,53–54] Rincon and colleagues[55] noted symptoms of depression and anxiety in 14% and 24%, respectively, of patients following critical illness. Similar prevalence rates of anxiety and depression have been reported by Scragg[56] and Orme and coworkers.[26] In contrast, Weinert and colleagues[21] found that 43% of patients with acute lung injury reported symptoms of depression, and Angus and coworkers[25] reported a 50% prevalence of depression and anxiety at 1 year in ARDS patients. The Toronto ARDS Outcomes study found that 58% of ARDS survivors reported depressive symptoms almost 2 years after ICU discharge.[57] By contrast, Hopkins and coworkers[28] found that ARDS patients reported minimal symptoms of depression or anxiety that were within the normal range in their natural history ARDS cohort study. The observed depression and anxiety after ICU treatment are likely multifactorial, and further study will be needed to better understand patient predisposition, illness, and treatment-specific determinants of affective morbidity.

PTSD is the development of characteristic symptoms that occur following a traumatic event(s) where triggers include a serious personal threat experienced with helplessness and intense fear.[58,59] The diagnostic criteria include a history of traumatic event(s) accompanied by symptoms from each of three symptom clusters: hyperarousal symptoms, intrusive recollections, and avoidant/numbing symptoms.[60] Schelling and colleagues[30] were the first to introduce the concept of PTSD resulting from critical illness and ICU treatment to the critical care community. These authors evaluated HRQL and PTSD in a cohort of 80 ARDS survivors 4 years following discharge from the ICU. Almost a third of the ARDS survivors reported impaired memory, bad dreams, anxiety, and sleeping difficulties after ICU discharge, with a prevalence rate of PTSD of 28%. PTSD was related to the number of adverse

ICU-related memories recalled by patients. Other authors[61,62] also have noted this relationship. Memory for nightmares or delusions while in the ICU, as well as a complete absence of any ICU memories, also has been perceived as a traumatic event.[63] The prevalence of PTSD has been reported to be as high as 38%[61] and is a persistent complaint for years after ICU discharge.[29,61,63a] We are just beginning to fully appreciate how long-standing and debilitating mood disorders are following critical illness and the important contribution they have to decreased HRQL.

COGNITIVE OUTCOMES
Cognitive Impairment in ARDS Survivors
Cognitive impairment represents the major threat to both recovery and quality of life following an acute illness.[29] Quality of life is largely determined by the ability to return to baseline level of cognitive performance.[24,28,56] Long-term cognitive dysfunction—even when modest—results in vastly increased medical and disability costs. For example, a 3-point decrease on the Mini Mental State Exam was associated with increased overall health care expenditures of $6000 per year.[29] The per-patient societal cost burden for even mild cognitive impairments is over $15,000 per year, and it is considerably higher ($34,515) for individuals with moderate to severe cognitive dysfunction.[64]

Cognitive impairments have been observed in a variety of patient populations with hypoxia.[65–73] Hypoxia-related cognitive impairments include memory deficits,[74] executive dysfunction,[74,75] visual-spatial deficits,[77] and intellectual decline.[73,77] Critical illness, including ARDS, is associated with significant cognitive dysfunction.[28,29,78,79] Approximately 33% of ICU survivors develop cognitive impairments that are similar to the cognitive dysfunction observed in mild dementia.[66] Cognitive impairments are a major determinant of the ability to return to work, work productivity, and life satisfaction following cardiac surgery,[80,81] traumatic brain injury,[82] and ARDS.[29] Even mild cognitive dysfunction results in clinically significant difficulties in driving, money management, and activities of daily living.[83–87] Data obtained from interviews with seriously ill patients indicate that 90 percent of these patients would rather die than survive with cognitive disability.[88]

Hopkins and colleagues[28] published the seminal long-term cognitive outcome study in ARDS survivors in 1999. In this natural history cohort, they found that 100% of ARDS survivors had cognitive impairments, including memory, attention, concentration, and decreased intellectual function, at the time of hospital discharge. At 1-year follow-up, 30% of the survivors had decreased intellectual function, and 78% had impaired memory, attention, concentration, and/or mental processing speed. ARDS survivors had significantly lower IQ than their estimated premorbid IQ ($p \leq 0.05$) and the measured IQ 1 year later.

Hopkins and colleagues[28] hypothesized that hypoxia may be an important contributor to cognitive dysfunction in ARDS survivors, and they undertook a detailed assessment of oximetry during the period of critical illness. The ARDS survivors' oximetry was measured for a total of 31,665 hours, with a mean of 609 ± 423 hours. The patients' mean oxygen saturations and their duration were outlined as follows: <90% = 122 ± 144 hours, <85% = 13 ± 18 hours, and <80% = 1 ± 3 hours. On average, these patients had 25 episodes of oxygen desaturation of less than 90% and 1 episode of desaturation of less than 85% for a duration of more than 2 hours. In this cohort, the degree of hypoxia was significantly correlated with neurocognitive sequelae (r^2 = 0.25–0.45, all $p < 0.01$).[28]

Since the Hopkins and colleagues report of cognitive impairments in ARDS survivors, other groups have confirmed their findings.[29,57,78] In a retrospective study of 33 ARDS survivors, Marquis and coworkers[78] reported impaired attention, visual processing, psychomotor speed, and cognitive flexibility compared with critically ill control subjects. Rothenhäusler and colleagues[29] retrospectively evaluated 46 ARDS survivors and found that 24% had cognitive impairments and 41% were disabled and could not return to work. Limitations of this study were low follow-up rate and the administration of one brief cognitive test that assessed only memory and attention. A study of self-reported memory problems in the Toronto ARDS Outcomes cohort found that 20% of ARDS survivors rated their memory as poor 18 months following their ICU discharge.[57]

Cognitive impairments occur in a significant number of ARDS survivors at 1 year, with little improvement at 2 years after hospital discharge.[89] In their recent prospective 2-year follow-up study, Hopkins and colleagues[28] assessed cognitive outcome in 71 consecutive ARDS survivors treated with higher and lower tidal volume strategies. The result was that 59% and 43% of patients had evidence of cognitive dysfunction (>1.5 SD below the mean) in at least two cognitive domains at 1- and 2-year follow-up, respectively. Cognitive performance at hospital discharge was significantly lower than at 1- and 2-year follow-up ($p < 0.001$). There were no significant differences between 1- and 2-year cognitive outcomes except improvement in performance IQ. Cognitive impairments at 1 and 2 years correlated with duration of hypoxemia, but they were not associated with gender, type of ventilator treatment, mean blood pressure, or time on sedative medications.

The recent report entitled, "Surviving Intensive Care: A Report from the 2002 Brussels Roundtable," indicated that future investigations should prioritize studies of cognitive impairments in survivors of critical illness.[90] Cognitive dysfunction in ARDS survivors is prevalent, with impairments reported in up to 78% of patients in some studies.[28] It represents significant morbidity and is a major obstacle to recovery in severely ill patients. The etiology of the cognitive impairments is likely multifactorial and the subject of ongoing debate, but the paper by Hopkins and colleagues[28] already has demonstrated a relationship to hypoxia, and several recent studies have demonstrated an association between delirium and cognitive impairments in critically ill patients.[91,92] For a detailed review of delirium in this book, see Chap. 62. Future investigations are required to further delineate etiology and to identify interventions that may improve or prevent cognitive impairment in ARDS survivors.

BRAIN TISSUE LOSS AFTER ARDS

Hypoxia and/or ischemia damage the hippocampus in humans,[74,93–95] rats,[96] and monkeys.[97] Research in humans using quantitative magnetic resonance imaging (MRI) analysis of neural structures shows significant reductions in hippocampus volume associated with hypoxia but not in the nearby areas of the parahippocampal gyrus or the temporal lobe.[75,94,95,98] Using quantitative MRI, brain morphologic changes, including ventricular enlargement, cerebral atrophy, and hippocampal atrophy, have been found in patients with pulmonary disorders following anoxia,[98] asthma,[99] carbon monoxide poisoning,[73,100] and obstructive sleep apnea.[68,69,101] Carbon monoxide poisoning and its concomitant hypoxia result in acute demyelination, generalized cortical atrophy,[73] and discrete lesions in the basal ganglia,[102] thalamus,[103] substantia nigra,[104] and white matter.[72] Hopkins and colleagues reported recently generalized atrophy[68] and atrophy of both gray and white matter structures, including the corpus callosum,[105] fornix,[106] and hippocampus,[74,94,95] following carbon monoxide poisoning.

In light of their prior work linking hypoxia to morphologic changes in the brain and cognitive dysfunction, Hopkins and colleagues sought to evaluate whether there was a structural correlate for hypoxia and impaired cognition in ARDS survivors. They compared computed tomographic (CT) brain scans of 15 ARDS patients with those of normal age- and gender-matched controls (with normal scans) using quantitative image analysis.[107] ARDS survivors exhibited brain atrophy, significantly enlarged ventricles, and an increased ventricle-to-brain ratio (another measure of generalized atrophy and an indirect index of white matter integrity) compared with the matched controls. The generalized brain atrophy, which was similar morphologically to that found in carbon monoxide poisoning, was associated with cognitive dysfunction.

Caregiver and Family Burden in Critical Illness

As more patients are surviving critical illness and are being discharged from hospital more quickly, the burden of caregiving has shifted to family members. It is important to note that in most cases the caregivers are the same individuals who have just completed a protracted bedside vigil in the ICU. They may be physically and emotionally spent and experiencing financial stress due to the cost of medical care and time spent at the hospital and away from their workplace. They are likely to have very little reserve and will now be responsible for all aspects of the patient's recovery.

It is surprising that there is such limited literature on caregiver and family burden in survivors of a severe episode of critical illness. Potential contributors to this paucity of information include the historic focus on mortality as the main outcome of interest in critical illness and exclusive focus on patient-centered care. Neonatologists and pediatric intensivists understand that critical illness disrupts families—not just the lives of their patients—and adult critical care physicians might do well to embrace the concept of family-centered care.

The following discussion has been excerpted from an excellent recent review on this subject by Levy.[108] In this review, Levy notes that Grad and Sainsbury first introduced the concept of family burden in 1966.[109] These authors defined *burden* as the cost or negative consequences sustained by the family or caregiver and whether these were of a subjective or objective nature. *Subjective* burden refers to the caregivers' attitude toward or emotional reaction to the caregiving experience, and *objective* burden relates to the nature or degree of family disruption that can be observed directly or verified.

Chou and colleagues[110] introduced a conceptual model of caregiver burden. The model includes four components: critical attributes and predisposing factors that influence the occurrence of burden, moderating/mediating factors, and consequences or outcomes. *Critical attributes* refer to the primary determinants of burden, including (1) the subjective burden as outlined earlier, (2) the multidimensional nature of demands that arise from caregiving, (3) the concept that illness is dynamic and therefore that the demands of caregiving also will be dynamic, and (4) the concept of overload, where the demands of caregiving exceed available resources. Predisposing factors relate to caregiver characteristics, including economic resources, race, and ethnicity. *Mediating* or *moderating factors* refer to elements that may alter the impact of burden, such as social or spiritual support. Consequences and outcome include the impact of the caregiving responsibilities on the caregiver and family.

Two recent papers highlight the burden of caregivers of ICU survivors. In a comprehensive review, Johnson and colleagues[111] indicated that a very high degree of caregiver burden is related to patient neuropsychological dysfunction as compared with severe physical disability. Caregiver stress is also related to lack of education about the demands of the caregiver role and the responsibility of managing complex medical treatments and technology in the home.

Pouchard and coworkers[112] conducted a prospective evaluation of anxiety and depression in 836 family members of critically ill patients. The prevalence of symptoms of anxiety and depression was almost 70% and 35%, respectively. It is still unclear whether or how long these symptoms persist and how they affect the care of the patient and the ability of the family to function normally.

CASE HISTORY FROM THE TORONTO ARDS OUTCOMES COHORT[37]

The following case history will help to emphasize the functional and neuropsychological morbidity in survivors of critical illness that has been the focus of this chapter.

- A 47-year-old previously healthy female teacher presented to the ICU with hypoxemic respiratory failure secondary to pneumococcal pneumonia complicated by ARDS.
- The patient was intubated and mechanically ventilated for 5 weeks in the ICU.
- Her ICU course was complicated by the development of multiple-organ dysfunction requiring pressor support and renal replacement therapy.
- Three chest tubes were inserted during the ICU stay for pneumothoraces resulting from her complicated ventilatory management.
- The patient underwent tracheostomy at 3 weeks into the ICU stay and had a protracted wean from the ventilator related to weakness and difficulty clearing secretions.
- The patient had received continuous sedation and analgesia during the first 3 ICU weeks to facilitate mechanical ventilation. She had been immobile and noncommunicative.

- At the time of ICU discharge, the patient had severe weakness and generalized muscle wasting. She was unable to sit up. She could not walk, bear weight, or even transfer on her own.
- Prior to transfer, she was confused and was only able to obey simple commands intermittently.
- On transfer to the medical ward, she complained of insomnia and disturbing and recurrent dreams that she had been physically and sexually assaulted during her ICU stay.
- After 2 weeks on the medical ward, she was able to stand and take a few steps and was transferred to a rehabilitation facility for ongoing physical therapy.
- At 4 weeks, she was decannulated and discharged to her friend's home.
- She did not return to her own home because she couldn't be left by herself, and her husband and children were at work/school for the entire day.
- At 3 months following ICU discharge, she continued to have significant proximal muscle weakness with inability to fully abduct her arms. She could not get in or out of cars nor climb stairs because of proximal leg weakness (Fig. 19-3).
- At 12 months following ICU discharge, she had regained her lost weight, had mild proximal muscle weakness, but now could abduct her arms and reported being quite functional (see Fig. 19-3). However, because of her need to stand most of the day as a teacher, she was unable to return to work because of residual weakness and fatigue.
- A more intensive physical rehabilitation program was organized for her, and she continued to experience slow and progressive improvement in her weakness.
- At 18 months following ICU discharge, she returned to her original job on a part-time basis. At that time, she found her tracheostomy scar stigmatizing and underwent scar revision by a plastic surgeon.
- She began to complain of very severe depression and inability to cope with the stressors in her workplace. She underwent formal neuropsychological and psychiatric assessments.
- At 20 months after ICU discharge, she was diagnosed with mild cognitive dysfunction and PTSD. She received psychiatric treatment.
- At 24 months—with modest residual weakness and mild cognitive dysfunction—she returned to full-time work as a teacher and is performing well in the workplace.
- Throughout her recovery period, her family has endured significant financial stress related to her inability to work, and her children have had significant behavioral and academic problems.

Multidisciplinary Intervention

The goal of this chapter was to review the current state of the art in the outcomes literature in survivors of critical illness. Another goal was to emphasize the importance of viewing critical illness as a continuum—from inciting illness through the ICU course and through recovery and rehabilitation. Understanding long-term outcome following critical illness is in

3
Months

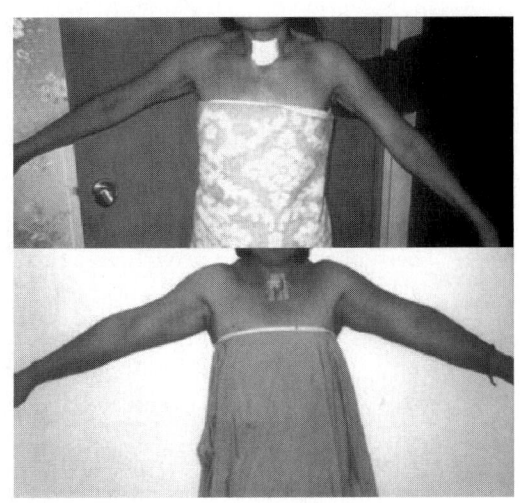

12
Months

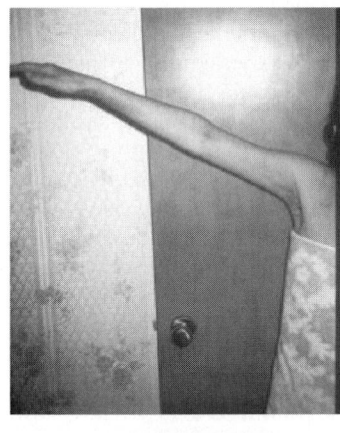

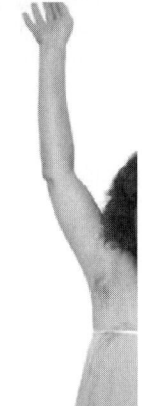

12
Months

3 Months

FIGURE 19-3 Resolution of muscle wasting and proximal muscle weakness from 3 to 12 months after ICU discharge in ARDS survivor.

its infancy. We are just beginning to understand the profound nature of functional and neuropsychological morbidity that may be sustained by the patients under our care every day in the ICU. In addition, we are only beginning to appreciate the caregiver and family burden experienced during and following the ICU stay.

A multidisciplinary model has been proposed[113] that identifies predictors and modifiers of morbidity outcomes in survivors of critical illness (Fig. 19-4). This model is centered on a longitudinal post–critical illness clinic in which the physician and his or her team provide a support network. The goal is to provide ongoing continuity of care as patients recover from the morbidity of critical illness and to facilitate patient access to appropriate diagnostic and treatment referrals.

The different components of this model reflect the different types of morbidity that we have described in this chapter. Given the burden of neuropsychological morbidity, one component of this intervention is to offer neuropsychological and psychiatric assessment and supportive counseling to survivors of critical illness *and* their family members. The determinants of muscle wasting and weakness would be further delineated through formal neurologic and physiatry assessments, and treatment programs would be organized through occupational and physical therapy. Social work supports also would facilitate return to work and management of other family or child-related concerns. Variations of this model are currently under study, and hopefully, we will soon be in a position to ameliorate the long-term morbidity of critical illness.

Summary

Survivors of critical illness experience decreased health-related quality of life due to physical limitations, depression and anxiety, and cognitive impairments. Neuromuscular dysfunction may represent an important—and potentially irreversible—determinant of long-term functional disability in these patients. Other organ impairment such as pulmonary dysfunction also has been documented following critical illness but does not appear to have the same impact on patients' health-related quality of life. We now understand that approximately one-third to one-half of survivors of critical illness will develop long-term cognitive impairments and that both this and functional capacity appear to plateau at a lower than normal level at 1 to 2 years following ICU discharge. Long-term physical and neuropsychological dysfunction may be remediable through the implementation of a multidisciplinary and family-centered rehabilitation program, and this hypothesis is currently being tested.

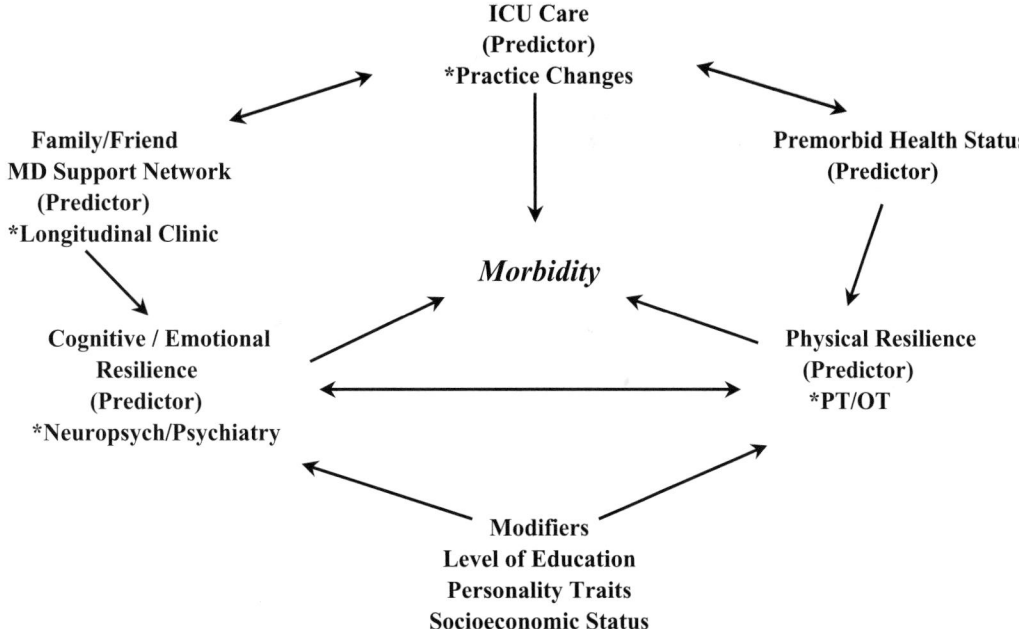

FIGURE 19-4 Model of predictors and modifiers of morbidity in survivors of critical illness. Asterisks mark components of Multidisciplinary Intervention.

References

1. Schmitz R, Lantin M, White A: *Future Workforce Needs in Pulmonary and Critical Care Medicine.* Cambridge, Mass., Abt Associates, 1999.

2. Milberg JA, Davis DR, Steinberg KP, et al: Improved survival of patients with acute respiratory distress syndrome (ARDS): 1983–1993. *JAMA* 273(4):306, 1995.

3. The Acute Respiratory Distress Syndrome Network: Ventilation with lower tidal volumes as compared with traditional tidal volumes for acute lung injury and the acute respiratory distress syndrome. *N Engl J Med* 342:1301, 2000.

4. Rivers E, Nguyen B, Havstad S, et al: Early goal-directed therapy in the treatment of severe sepsis and septic shock. *N Engl J Med* 345:1368, 2001.

5. Bernard GR, Vincent J-L, Laterre P-F, et al: Efficacy and safety of recombinant human activated protein C for severe sepsis. *N Engl J Med* 344:699, 2001.

6. Schiffl H, Lang SM, Fischer R: Daily hemodialysis and the outcome of acute renal failure. *N Engl J Med* 346:305, 2002.

7. Van den Berghe G, Wouters P, Weekers F, et al: Intensive insulin therapy in critically ill patients. *N Engl J Med* 345:1359, 2001.

8. Gross CH, Brower RG, Hudgon LD, et al: Incidence of acute lung injury in the United States. *Crit Care Med* 31:1607, 2003.

9. Bernard GR, Artigas A, Brigham KL, et al: The American-European Consensus Conference on ARDS: Definitions, mechanisms, relevant outcomes, and clinical trial coordination. *Am J Respir Crit Care Med* 149:818, 1994.

10. Ranieri VM, Giunta F, Suter PM, et al: Mechanical ventilation as a mediator of multisystem organ failure in ARDS. *JAMA* 284:43, 2000.

11. Imai Y, Paroda J, Kajikawa O, et al: Injurious mechanical ventilation and end-organ epithelial cell apoptosis and organ dysfunction in an experimental model of ARDS. *JAMA* 289:2104, 2003.

12. Weinert CR, Gross CR, Kangas JR, et al: Health-related quality of life after acute lung injury. *Am J Resp Crit Care Med* 156:1120, 1997.

13. Tian AM, Miranda DR: Quality of life after intensive care with the sickness impact profile. *Int Care Med* 21:422, 1995.

14. Konobad E, et al: Quality of life measures before and 1 year after admission to an intensive care unit. *Crit Care Med* 23:1653, 1995.

15. Warren L, et al: Factors associated with life satisfaction among a sample of persons with neurotrauma. *J Rehabil Res Dev* 33:404, 1996.

16. Thiagarajan J, Miranda DR: Quality of life after multiple trauma requiring intensive care. *Anaesthesia* 49:211, 1995.

17. Montuclard L, Garrouste-Orgeas M, Timsit J-F, et al: Outcome, functional autonomy, and quality of life of elderly patients with a long-term intensive care unit stay. *Crit Care Med* 28:3389, 2000.

18. Heyland DK, Hopman W, Coo H, et al: Long-term health-related quality of life in survivors of sepsis. Short Form 36: A valid and reliable measure of health-related quality of life. *Crit Care Med* 28:3599, 2000.

19. Chatila W, Kreimer DT, Criner GJ: Quality of life in survivors of prolonged mechanical ventilatory support. *Crit Care Med* 29:737, 2001.

20. McHugh, LG, Milberg JA, Whitcomb ME, et al: Recovery of function in survivors of the acute respiratory distress syndrome. *Am J Respir Crit Care Med* 150:90, 1994.

21. Weinert CR, Gross CR, Kangas JR, et al: Health-related quality of life after acute lung injury. *Am J Respir Crit Care Med* 156:1120, 1997.

22. Ware JE, Sherbourne CD: The MOS 36-item short form health survey (SF-36): I. Conceptual framework and item selection. *Med Care* 39:473, 1992.

23. Schelling G, Stoll C, Haller M, et al: Health-related quality of life and posttraumatic stress disorder in survivors of the acute respiratory distress syndrome. *Crit Care Med* 26:651, 1998.

24. Davidson, TA, Caldwell ES, Curtis JR, et al: Reduced quality of life in survivors of acute respiratory distress syndrome compared with critically ill control patients. *JAMA* 281:354, 1999.

25. Angus DC, Musthafa AA, Clermont G, et al: Quality-adjusted survival in the first year after the acute respiratory distress syndrome. *Am J Respir Crit Care Med* 163:1389, 2001.

26. Orme J, Romney JS, Hopkins RO, et al: Pulmonary function and health-related quality of life in survivors of acute respiratory distress syndrome. *Am J Respir Crit Care Med* 167:690, 2003.

27. Herridge MS, Cheung AM, Tansey CM, et al: Two-year outcomes in survivors of the acute respiratory distress syndrome. *Am J Respir Crit Care Med* 167:A736, 2003.

28. Hopkins RO, Weaver LK, Pope D, et al: Neuropsychological sequelae and impaired health status in survivors of severe acute respiratory syndrome. *Am J Respir Crit Care Med* 160:50, 1999.

29. Rothenhausler H-B, Ehrentraut S, Stoll C, et al: The relationship between cognitive performance and employment and health status in long-term survivors of the acute respiratory distress syndrome: Results of an exploratory study. *Gen Hosp Psychiatry* 23:90, 2001.

30. Schelling G, Stoll C, Haller M, et al: Health-related quality of life and posttraumatic stress disorder in survivors of the acute respiratory distress syndrome. *Crit Care Med* 26:651, 1998.

31. Lakshminarayam S, Hudson LD: Pulmonary function following the adult respiratory distress syndrome. *Chest* 74:489, 1978.

32. Elliott CG, Morris AH, Cengiz M: Pulmonary function and exercise gas exchange in survivors of adult respiratory distress syndrome. *Am Rev Respir Dis* 123:492, 1981.

33. Elliott CG, Rasmussen BY, Crapo RO, et al: Prediction of pulmonary function abnormalities after adult respiratory distress syndrome (ARDS). *Am Rev Respir Dis* 135:634,1987.

34. Schelling G, Stoll C, Vogelmeier C, et al: Pulmonary function and health-related quality of life in a sample of long-term survivors of the acute respiratory distress syndrome. *Intensive Care Med* 26:1304, 2000.

35. Neff TA, Stocker R, Frey H-R, et al: Long-term assessment of lung function in survivors of severe ARDS. *Chest* 23:845, 2003.

36. Herridge MS: Long-term outcomes after critical illness. *Curr Opin Crit Care* 8:331, 2002.

37. Herridge MS, Cheung AM, Tansey CM, et al: One-year outcomes in survivors of the acute respiratory distress syndrome. *N Engl J Med* 34:683, 2003.

38. Bolton CF, Gilbert JJ, Hajan AF, et al: Polyneuropathy in critically ill patients. *J Neurol Neurosurg Psychiatry* 47:1223, 1984.

39. Bolton CF, Laverty DA, Brown JD, et al: Critically ill polyneuropathy: Electrophysiological studies and differentiation from Guillain-Barré syndrome. *J Neurol Neurosurg Psychiatry* 49:563, 1986.

40. Zochodne DW, Bolton CF, Wells GA, et al: Critical illness polyneuropathy: A complication of sepsis and multiple organ failure. *Brain* 110:819, 1987.

41. Fletcher SN, Kennedy DD, Ghosh IR, et al: Persistent neuromuscular and neurophysiologic abnormalities in long-term survivors of prolonged critical illness. *Crit Care Med* 31:1012, 2003.

42. DeJonghe B, et al: Paresis acquired in the intensive care unit: A prospective multicenter study. *JAMA* 288:2859, 2002.

43. McFarlane IA, Rosenthal FD: Severe myopathy after status asthmaticus. *Lancet* 2:615, 1977.

44. Deconinck N, Van Parijs V, Beckers-Bleukx G, et al: Critical illness myopathy unrelated to corticosteroids or neuromuscular blocking agents. *Neuromusc Disord* 8:186, 1998.

45. Bril V, Nasir N, Cheung AM, et al: Long-term neuromuscular function in adult ARDS survivors. *Am J Respir Crit Care Med* 161:A381, 2000.

46. Wijdicks EF, Litchy WJ, Harrison BA, et al: The clinical spectrum of critical illness polyneuropathy. *Mayo Clin Proc* 70:198, 1995.

47. Clements NC, Camilli AE: Heterotopic ossification complicating critical illness. *Chest* 104:1526, 1993.

48. Jacobs JW, DeSonnaville PB, Hulsmans HM, et al: Polyarticular heterotopic ossification complicating critical illness. *Rheumatology* 38:1145, 1999.

49. Szokol JW, Vender JS: Anxiety, delirium, and pain in the intensive care unit. *Crit Care Clin* 17:821, 2001.

50. Skodol AE: Anxiety in the medically ill: Nosology and principles of differential diagnosis. *Semin Clin Neuropsychiatr* 4:64, 1999.

51. McCartney JR, Boland RJ: Anxiety and delirium in the intensive are unit. *Crit Care Clin* 10:673, 1994.

52. Clayton PJ, Lewis CE: The significance of secondary depression. *J Affect Disord* 3:25, 1981.

53. Milisen K, et al: A nurse-led interdisciplinary intervention program for delirium in elderly hip-fracture patients. *J Am Geriatr Soc* 49:523, 2001.

54. Michaels AJ, et al: PTSD in critical care. *J Trauma* 48:841, 2000.

55. Rincon HG, et al: Prevalence, detection and treatment of anxiety, depression, and delirium in the adult critical care unit. *Psychosomatics* 42:391, 2001.

56. Scragg P, Jones A, Fauvel N: Psychological problems following ICU treatment. *Anaesthesia* 56:9, 2001.

57. Al-Saidi F, Cheung AM, Tansey CM, et al: Neuropsychological sequelae in ARDS survivors. *Am J Respir Crit Care Med* 167:A737, 2003.

58. Horowitz MJ: Stress-response syndromes: A review of posttraumatic stress and adjustment disorders, in Wilson JP, Raphael B (eds): *International Handbook of Traumatic Stress Syndromes.* New York, Plenum Press, 1993, p 49.

59. Gersons BPR: Post-traumatic stress disorder: The history of a recent concept. *Br J Psychiatry* 161:742, 1992.

60. American Psychiatric Association Task Force on Nomenclature and Statistics: *Diagnostic and Statistical Manual of Mental Disorders,* 4th ed. Washington, American Psychiatric Association, 1996.

61. Jones C, et al: Memory, delusions, and the development of acute posttraumatic stress disorder-related symptoms after intensive care. *Crit Care Med* 29:573, 2001.

62. Stoll C, et al: Sensitivity and specificity of a screening test to document traumatic experiences and to diagnose post-traumatic stress disorder in ARDS patients after intensive care treatment. *Intensive Care Med* 25:697, 1999.

63. Perrins J, Keing N, Collings J: Assessment of long-term psychological well-being following intensive care. *Intensive Crit Care Nurs* 14:108, 1998.

63a. Kapfhammer HP, Rothenhausler HB, Krauseneck T, et al: Posttraumatic stress disorder and health-related quality of life in long-term survivors of acute respiratory distress syndrome. *Am J Psychiatry* 161:45, 2004.

64. Jonsson L, et al: Costs of Mini Mental State Examination–related cognitive impairment. *Pharmacoeconomics* 16:409, 1999.

65. Prigatano GE, Wright EC, Levin D: Quality of life and its predictors in patients with mild hypoxemia and chronic obstructive pulmonary disease. *Arch Intern Med* 144:1613, 1984.

66. Grant I, et al: Progressive neuropsychologic impairments and hypoxemia: Relationship in chronic obstructive pulmonary disease. *Arch Gen Psychiatry* 44:999, 1987.

67. Grant I, et al: Neuropsychological findings in hypoxemic chronic obstructive pulmonary disease. *Arch Intern Med* 142:1470, 1982.

68. Gale S, Hopkins R: Effects of hypoxia on the brain: Neuroimaging and neuropsychological findings following carbon monoxide poisoning and obstructive sleep apnea. *J Int Neuropsychol Soc* 10:60, 2004.

69. Gale S, et al: Hippocampal atrophy following sleep apnea and carbon monoxide poisoning: Similarities and differences. *J Int Neuropsychol Soc* 6:154, 2000.

70. Kales A, et al: Severe obstructive sleep apnea: II. Associated psychopathology and psychosocial consequences. *J Chron Dis* 38:427, 1985.

71. Weaver L, et al: Hyperbaric oxygen for acute carbon monoxide poisoning. *N Engl J Med* 347:1057, 2002.

72. Parkinson R, et al: White matter hyperintensities and neuropsychological outcome following carbon monoxide poisoning. *Neurology* 58:1525, 2002.

73. Gale S, et al: MRI, quantitative MRI, SPECT, and neuropsychological findings following carbon monoxide poisoning. *Brain Injury* 13:229, 1999.

74. Hopkins R, Kesner R: Item and order recognition memory in subjects with hypoxic brain injury. *Brain Cogn* 27:180, 1995.

75. Hopkins R, Kesner R, Goldstein M: Memory for novel and familiar spatial and linguistic temporal distance information in hypoxic subjects. *J Int Neuropsychol Soc* 1:454, 1995.

76. Barat M, Blanchard J, Carriet D: Les troubles neuropsychologiques des anozies cerebrales prolongees. *Ann Readapt Med Phys* 32:657, 1989.

77. Bigler E, Alfano M: Anoxic encephalopathy: Neuroradiological and neuropsychological findings. *Arch Clin Neuropsychol* 3:383, 1988.

78. Marquis K, et al: Neuropsychological sequelae in survivors of ARDS compared with critically ill control patients. *Am J Respir Crit Care Med* 161:A383, 2000.

79. Jackson JC, et al: Six-month neuropsychological outcome of medical intensive care unit patients. *Crit Care Med* 31:1226, 2003.

80. Newman M, et al: Report of the substudy assessing the impact of neurocognitive function on quality of life 5 years after cardiac surgery. *Stroke* 32:2874, 2001.

81. Newman M, et al: Longitudinal assessment of neurocognitive function after coronary-artery bypass surgery. *N Engl J Med* 344:395, 2001.

82. Streadman-Pare D, et al: Factors associated with perceived quality of life many years after traumatic brain injury. *J Head Trauma Rehabil* 16:330, 2000.

83. Withaar FK, Brouwer WH, Van Zomeren AH: Fitness to drive in older divers with cognitive impairment. *J Int Neuropsychol Soc* 6:480, 2000.

84. Tabert MH, et al: Functional deficits in patients with mild cognitive impairments: Prediction of AD. *Neurology* 58:758, 2002.

85. Nygard L: Instrumental activities of daily living: A stepping stone towards Alzheimer's disease diagnosis in subjects with mild cognitive impairment? *Acta Neurol Scand* 179:S42, 2003.

86. Griffith HR, et al: Impaired financial abilities in mild cognitive impairment: A direct assessment approach. *Neurology* 60:449, 2003.

87. Albert SM, et al: Functional significance of mild cognitive impairment in elderly patients without a dementia diagnosis. *Am J Geriatr Psychiatry* 7:213, 1997.

88. Fried T, et al: Understanding the treatment preferences of seriously ill patients. *N Engl J Med* 346:1061, 2002.

89. Hopkins RO, Collingridge D, Weaver LK, et al: Neuropsychological sequelae following acute respiratory distress syndrome: Two year outcome. *J Int Neuropsychol Assoc* 9:584, 2003.

90. Angus DC, Carlet J, on behalf of the 2002 Brussels Roundtable Participants: Surviving intensive care: A report from the 2002 Brussels Roundtable. *Intensive Care Med* 167:695, 2003.

91. Dolan MM, Hawkes WG, Zimmerman SI, et al: Delirium on hospital admission in aged hip fracture patients: Prediction of mortality and 2-year functional outcomes. *J Gerontol Med Sci* 55A:M527, 2001.

92. Katz IR, Curyto KJ, TenHave T, et al: Validating the diagnosis of delirium and evaluating its association with deterioration over a one-year period. *Am J Geriatr Psychiatry* 9:148, 2001.

93. Bayley PJ, Hopkins R, Squire L: Successful recollection of remote autobiographical memories by amnesic patients with medial temporal lobe lesions. *Neuron* 38:135, 2003.

94. Manns JR, Hopkins R, Squire L: Semantic memory and the human hippocampus. *Neuron* 38:127, 2003.

95. Manns JR, et al: Recognition memory and the human hippocampus. *Neuron* 37:171, 2003.

96. Davis H, Volpe B: Memory performance after ischemic or neurotoxin damage of the hippocampus. In Squire L, Lindlaub E: *The biology of memory. Symposia Medica Hoechst 23.* Stuttgart, New York: FK Schattauer Verlag.

97. Zola-Morgan S, Squire L: Neuropsychological investigations of memory and amnesia: Findings from humans and non human primates, in Diamond A (ed): *The Development and Neural Bases of Higher Cognitive Functions.* New York: New York Academy of Sciences, 1990, p 434.

98. Hopkins R, et al: evere anoxia with and without concomitant brain atrophy and neuropsychological impairments. *J Int Neuropsychol Soc* 1:501, 1995.

99. Hopkins R, Bigler E: Pulmonary disorders, in Tarter R, Butters M, Beers S (eds): *Medical Neuropsychology.* Boston: Kluwer Academic, 2001, p 25.

100. Hopkins R, Weaver L, Kesner R: Long term memory impairments and hippocampal magnetic resonance imaging in carbon monoxide poisoned subjects. *Abstr of the Undersea and Hyperbaric Society* 20:15, 1993.

101. Walker J, et al, Hippocampal atrophy and long-lasting neuropsychological deficits in patients with severe sleep apnea. *Am J Resp Crit Care Med* 159:A770, 1999.

102. Ferrier D, et al: Magnetic resonance features in carbon monoxide poisoning. *Can Assoc Radiol J* 45:466, 1994.

103. Tuchman R, Moser F, Moshe S: Carbon monoxide poisoning: Bilateral lesions in the thalamus on MR imaging of the brain. *Pediatr Radiol* 20:478, 1990.

104. Kawanami T, et al: The pallidorecticular pattern of brain damage on MRI in a patient with carbon monoxide poisoning. *J Neurol Neurosurg Psychiatry* 64:282, 1998.

105. Porter S, et al: Corpus callosum atrophy and neuropsychological outcome following carbon monoxide poisoning. *Arch Clin Neuropsychol* 17:195, 2002.

106. Kesler S, et al: Verbal memory deficits associated with fornix atrophy in carbon monoxide poisoning. *J Int Neuropsychol Soc* 7:640, 2001.

107. Hopkins R, et al: Ventricular enlargement in patients with acute respiratory distress syndrome. *J Int Neuropsychol Soc* 6:229, 2000.

108. Levy MM: The burden of caregiving on families of ICU survivors, in Angus D, Carlet J (eds): *Surviving Intensive Care.* New York: Springer-Verlag, 2003, p.63.

109. Grad J, Sainsbury P: Problems of caring for the mentally ill at home. *Proc R Soc Med* 59:20, 1966.

110. Chou KR, LaMontagne LL, Hepworth JT: Burden experienced by caregivers of relatives with dementia in Taiwan. *Nurs Res* 48:206, 1999.

111. John P, Chaboyer W, Foster M, et al: Caregivers of ICU patients discharged home: What burden do they face? *Intens Crit Care Nurs* 17:219, 2001.

112. Pouchard F, Azoulay E, Chevret S, et al: Symptoms of anxiety and depression in family members of intensive care unit patients: Ethical hypothesis regarding decision-making capacity. *Crit Care Med* 29:1893, 2001.

113. Herridge MS: Morbidity and functional limitation in survivors of ARDS, in Angus D, Carlet J (eds): *Surviving Intensive Care.* New York: Springer-Verlag, 2003, p. 21.

PART III

CARDIOVASCULAR DISORDERS

Chapter 20 —————————————————

THE PATHOPHYSIOLOGY OF THE CIRCULATION IN CRITICAL ILLNESS

LAWRENCE D. H. WOOD

KEY POINTS

- *Left ventricular (LV) stroke volume (SV) creates arterial pulse pressure (PP) by distending conducting vessels during systole, and systemic vascular resistance (SVR) preserves diastolic pressure (DP) by preventing SV from flowing through arterioles during diastole.*

- *This coupling of ventricular and vascular elements allows rapid clinical separation of hypotensive patients into those with increased SV and cardiac output ($\dot{Q}T$) demonstrating bounding pulses with large PP, low DP, and warm digits (low SVR, high $\dot{Q}T$ hypotension, or septic shock) from those who demonstrate thready pulses with small PP and cool digits signaling low SV and $\dot{Q}T$ with increased SVR, as in cardiogenic or hypovolemic shock.*

- *LV pumping function is described by relating LV end-DP as estimated by pulmonary wedge pressure (Ppw) to SV; LV dysfunction is signaled by increased Ppw and decreased SV and may be due to systolic or diastolic dysfunction.*

- *Systolic dysfunction, or decreased contractility, connotes increased LV end-systolic volume for a given LV end-systolic pressure that is approximately the mean blood pressure (BP); common causes of acute systolic dysfunction in critical illness are myocardial ischemia, hypoxia, acidosis, sepsis, intercurrent negative inotropic drugs (β or calcium blockers), and acute-on-chronic systolic dysfunction in cardiomyopathies.*

- *Diastolic dysfunction connotes decreased LV end-diastolic volume despite increased Ppw because the heart cannot fill normally; common causes of diastolic dysfunction in critical illness are pericardial tamponade or constriction, positive end-expiratory pressure (PEEP), or other causes of increased pleural pressure as in pneumothorax, pleural effusion, or abdominal distention, ventricular interdependence in acute right heart syndromes, and chronic LV stiffness as in LV hypertrophy.*

- *Early differentiation between diastolic and systolic dysfunctions in critical illness is aided by a questioning approach and dynamic imaging such as echocardiography; this avoids inappropriate and ineffective therapy for the wrong etiology of LV dysfunction.*

- *Venous return (VR) to the right atrium is controlled by mechanical characteristics of the systemic vessels (unstressed volume, vascular capacitance, vascular volume); together these determine the mean systemic pressure responsible for driving VR back to the right atrium (Pra) through the resistance to VR.*

- *For a given Pms, VR increases as Pra decreases to define the VR curve of the circulation, whereas SV and $\dot{Q}T$ from the heart increase as Pra and preload increase to define the cardiac*

function curve that intersects the VR curve at a unique value of Pra where $VR = \dot{Q}T$.

- *When $\dot{Q}T$ is insufficient, volume infusion, baroreceptors, or metabolic receptors can increase mean systemic pressure to increase VR and Pra; this effect is mimicked by venoconstricting drugs such as dopamine or epinephrine; alternatively, VR can be increased by positive inotropic (dobutamine) or afterload-reducing (sodium nitroprusside) drugs that decrease Pra by enhancing cardiac function.*

- *In hypovolemic shock, hemostasis and volume resuscitation are essential, whereas arteriolar constricting agents such as norepinephrine may be used briefly to provide a window of higher BP; in septic shock, considerable volume resuscitation is needed due to nitric oxide–mediated venodilation and decreased Pms, positive inotropic agents such as dobutamine treat the myocardial depression, and arterial vasoconstrictors such as norepinephrine may be needed to maintain BP despite high $\dot{Q}T$ due to very low SVR.*

- *In cardiogenic shock, preload reduction (morphine, nitroglycerin, furosemide) is effected by venodilation and decreased Pms, but VR often increases because cardiac function improves to decrease Pra; arterial dilating drugs often increase $\dot{Q}T$ from the injured LV, so BP may even increase despite impaired contractility and $\dot{Q}T$ without increasing myocardial O_2 consumption when heart rate does not increase.*

- *Early airway control and continuous mechanical ventilation decrease oxygen consumption and prevent respiratory acidosis but may decrease VR further in hypovolemic patients by raising pleural pressure and Pra; in cardiogenic shock, continuous mechanical ventilation and PEEP have less effect on VR and may increase $\dot{Q}T$ by decreasing LV afterload.*

- *Cardiogenic and low-pressure pulmonary edema are decreased by decreasing Ppw, and $\dot{Q}T$ and oxygen delivery can be maintained at low Ppw with vasoactive drugs and blood transfusion; arterial oxygenation can be supported with PEEP without decreasing $\dot{Q}T$ and oxygen delivery by affecting the least PEEP and tidal volumes that achieve 90% O_2 saturation of an adequate hematocrit on a nontoxic fraction of inspired O_2 without profound acidosis.*

This chapter reviews several essential concepts of normal cardiovascular function as a basis for approaching and correcting disturbed circulation in critical illness. It begins with a discussion of left ventricular (LV) pumping function and an approach to ventricular dysfunction. Then follows a review of the mechanisms by which the venous return (VR) to the heart is controlled by the systemic vessels as a basis for diagnosis and treatment of hypoperfusion states. The pulmonary circulation and factors governing lung liquid flux are described through measurements obtained by right heart catheterization to provide an approach to treating pulmonary edema without compromising adequate peripheral perfusion. Along this discussion pathway, common mechanical interactions between respiration and circulation are highlighted as a basis for understanding the cardiovascular diseases discussed in the following chapters in this section and in the next section on pulmonary disorders in critical illness.

A primary role of the cardiovascular system is to deliver energy sources from the gut and liver and oxygen from the lungs to all systemic organ systems for their aerobic metabolism; effluent from these tissues removes the waste products of

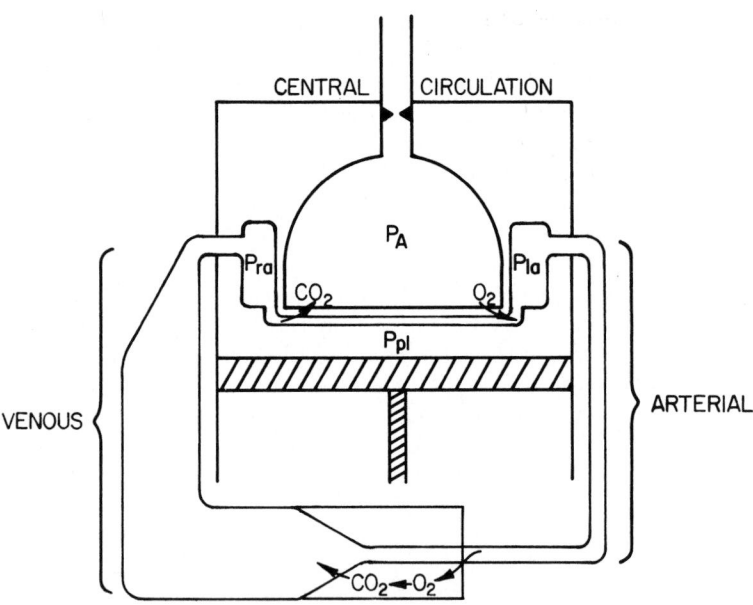

FIGURE 20-1 Schematic showing circulation proceeding from the left atrium (Pla, left atrial pressure) through a high-pressure arterial system (low volume, low compliance, high resistance) to peripheral tissues (where oxygen leaves the vessels to produce energy and CO_2, shown entering the vessels) and through the low-pressure venous system (high volume, high compliance, low resistance), which returns blood to the right atrium (Pra, right atrial pressure). The circuit is completed by perfusing the lung back to the left atrium; the pulmonary vessels are shown in close apposition with the alveoli (PA, alveolar pressure), facilitating gas exchange. This central circulation is enclosed in the thorax, the floor of which is the diaphragm (indicated by the piston). Between the lungs and the thorax is the pleural space (Ppl, pleural pressure). Ppl approximates the pressure on the outside of all extraalveolar vessels within the central circulation, including the heart, whereas PA is the pressure outside the alveolar vessels. The anatomic arrangement accounts for the many mechanical interactions between respiration and circulation in critical illness described throughout this chapter.

metabolism and delivers them to the lungs, kidney, and liver for excretion. This process is facilitated by return of the entire circulation through the lungs, where CO_2 is eliminated and O_2 is taken up to arterialize the blood. As depicted in Fig. 20-1, this central circulation is located within the thoracic cavity; movement of gas between the atmosphere and the alveolar space is done by the respiratory muscles, especially the diaphragm, depicted as a piston at the floor of the thoracic cavity. Beyond effecting ventilation to permit pulmonary gas exchange, spontaneous movement of the piston decreases the pleural pressure (Ppl), which approximates the pressure on the outside of extraalveolar vessels including the right and left heart (depicted as chambers labeled Pra [right atrial pressure] and Pla [left atrial pressure]); changes in alveolar pressure (PA) affect pressures within alveolar vessels. Once the blood leaves the lung and enters the left heart, the ventricular pumping function ejects blood into the stiff, high-resistance arterial circulation to perfuse the systemic capillary beds, where O_2 is consumed and CO_2 is taken up before the venous blood returns to the right heart through the large-volume, very compliant, low-resistance venous circuit.[1,2]

Ventricular Dysfunction in Critical Illness

VENTRICULAR–VASCULAR COUPLING

Figure 20-2 illustrates the typical events in the two phases of ventricular activity: active contraction (systole) and relaxation (diastole). In diastole, the left ventricle fills through the open mitral valve from the left atrium while the aortic valve is closed. After electrical stimulation and contraction of the left ventricle in systole, a stroke volume (SV) is ejected into the proximal arterial chamber. Because more blood is being ejected than runs off through the peripheral resistance located in the distal arterioles, the arterial walls are distended outward, thus raising the pressure (P) in inverse proportion to the capacitance $(C = \Delta V / \Delta P)$ of the walls of the larger arteries

FIGURE 20-2 During ventricular systole, the stroke volume ejected by the ventricle results in some forward capillary flow, but most of the ejected volume is stored in the elastic arteries. During ventricular diastole, the elastic recoil of the arterial walls maintains capillary flow through the remainder of the cardiac cycle. Accordingly, pulse pressure is proportional to stroke volume, and diastolic pressure increases with peripheral resistance, heart rate, and vascular capacitance, all of which reduce the diastolic runoff of the ejected volume. (*Reproduced with permission from Berne RM, Levy MN (eds): Physiology. St. Louis, Mosby, 1988, p 487.*)

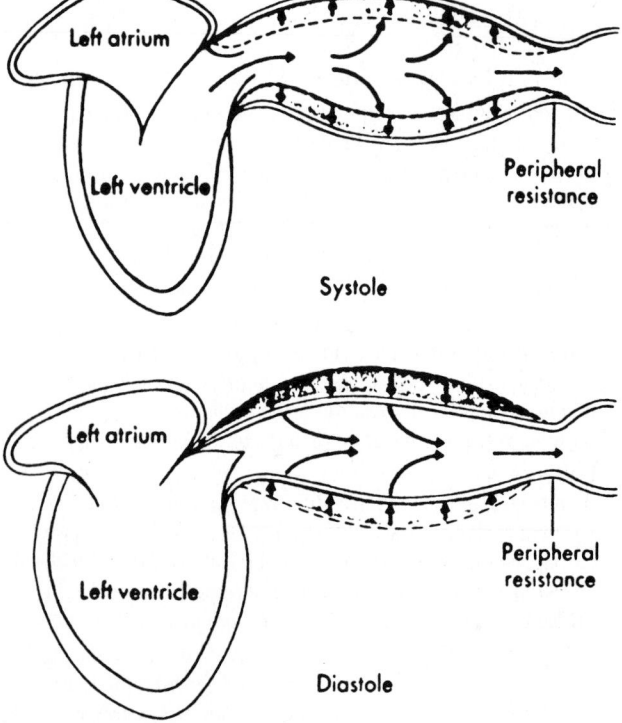

SHOCK-ARTERIAL PULSE

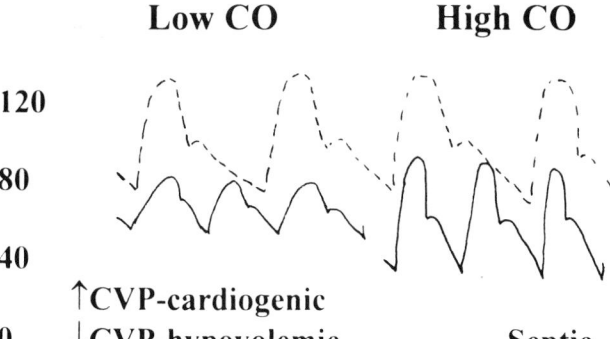

Low CO   High CO

↑CVP-cardiogenic
↓CVP-hypovolemic   Septic

FIGURE 20-3 Schematic illustrations of the normal arterial pressure waveform (interrupted pulse pressure); the continuous pressure waves in low cardiac output ($\dot{Q}T$) hypotension (*left*) and in high $\dot{Q}T$ hypotension (*right*) illustrate key differences from the normal pulse. Ordinate, arterial pressure (mm Hg); abscissa, time (seconds). The lower left panel illustrates the difference between cardiogenic shock (increased central venous pressure = 20 mm Hg) and hypovolemic shock (central venous pressure = 0 mm Hg). For discussion, see text.

proximal to the resistance vessels. As the ventricle's volume (V) decreases, its ability to generate pressure decreases, as dictated by the length-dependent activation of actin and myosin cross-bridges in the cardiac myocytes,[3] until ventricular systolic pressure (SP) falls below the simultaneous arterial pressure. Then the aortic valve closes, as indicated by the dicrotic notch on the arterial pressure pulse (Fig. 20-3). As the ventricle relaxes, the mitral valve opens, and the ventricle fills along its diastolic volume-pressure (V-P) curve; this diastolic filling is aided by atrial contraction and by suction by the ventricle relaxing from its low end-contraction volume. During diastole, the part of the SV stored in the distended arterial bed continues to run off through the peripheral resistance, associated with a progressive decrease in arterial pressure until the next contraction.

This ventricular–vascular coupling acts as a hydraulic filter to convert the intermittent ejection of an SV into a continuous organ flow, the cardiac output ($\dot{Q}T$). It also decreases the work of the heart by allowing some of the energy imparted by the systolic ventricle to the blood to be stored in distention of the arterial chamber and returned to the circulation by continued flow while the ventricle is resting in diastole. The systemic vascular resistance (SVR) is also essential to the control of blood pressure (BP = $\dot{Q}T \times$ SVR) and to the distribution of blood flow among, or within, organs according to tissue needs. For example, in conditions of hypovolemic or cardiogenic shock, reflex sympathetic output constricts arterioles, especially in the mesenteric, renal, and skin vascular beds, to preserve flow to vital organs such as the heart and brain by maintaining aortic BP; alternatively, during pyrexia and tachypnea, the increased metabolic need demands a high $\dot{Q}T$ associated with dilation of the coronary and respiratory muscle vessels induced by accumulation of anaerobic metabolites (e.g., adenosine, H^+, and K^+) to maintain adequate O_2 flow to these vital pumps.

Clinical evaluation of the cardiovascular system in patients with critical illness is much aided by interpretation of the diastolic pressure (DP), the pulse pressure (PP), and indices of SVR such as the rate of color return to the nail bed after releasing pressure on the fingernail and digital temperature. For example, a hypotensive patient with a heart rate (HR) of 110 beats/min, an SP/DP of 100/40 mm Hg, and warm extremities with good color return to the nail bed has a high $\dot{Q}T$ and a low SVR (see Fig. 20-3). This is because the large PP (60 mm Hg) signals a large SV, which, when multiplied by the increased HR, produces increased $\dot{Q}T$, and the low DP indicates rapid peripheral runoff through low SVR confirmed by digital examination and low mean BP (60 mm Hg) in the face of the high $\dot{Q}T$. In contrast, a second hypotensive patient with the same HR and mean BP but an SP/DP of 80/65 mm Hg and cold extremities with very slow return of color to the nail bed has a low $\dot{Q}T$ with increased SVR indicated by the small PP (hence, low SV and $\dot{Q}T$), preserved DP, and constricted digital vessels. As indicated in the lower left panel of Fig. 20-3, this low $\dot{Q}T$ hypotension is cardiogenic when the central venous pressure (CVP) is high and hypovolemic when the CVP is low. Of course, the relation between PP and SV is not quantitative, because it is proportioned by an unknown constant—the vascular capacitance. Nevertheless, in a given critically ill patient whose vascular capacitance changes minimally in a course of acute interventions, a change in PP is the earliest indicator of a change in SV.

THE STARLING CURVE OF THE HEART

Figure 20-4 presents Starling relations of the heart.[2,3] On the abscissa is plotted Pla, which approximates the filling pressure of the left ventricle. On the ordinate is plotted SV (in milliliters); this volume ejected per heartbeat is one measure of ventricular output. Another measure of output can be expressed by multiplying stroke volume by the pressure developed during each beat to obtain stroke work (SV × [BP − Pla]). As filling pressure of the heart increases, the ejected volume and the work done by the heart increase in a curvilinear manner; at higher filling pressures, there is less increase in SV per increase in Pla than at lower values of Pla. On the continuous Starling curve shown in Fig. 20-4B, the normal Pla (10 mm Hg) is associated with a normal SV (75 mL) calculated from $\dot{Q}T$ (6.0 L/min) divided by HR (80 beats/min). When hypovolemia decreases the Pla to 5 mm Hg, SV decreases to 40 mL, thus decreasing $\dot{Q}T$; if therapeutic expansion of the circulating volume increases Pla to 20 mm Hg, SV increases to 100 mL, thus increasing $\dot{Q}T$ above normal. These relations comprise a common framework for understanding ventricular function in critical illness. A shift up and to the left of the Starling curve generally indicates enhanced ventricular function, with greater SV for a given filling pressure (see interrupted curve in Fig. 20-4). Conversely, a shift down and to the right with reduced SV at a given filling pressure (see dotted Starling curve through points *A* and *B*) indicates depressed ventricular function. The lower SV for a Pla of 10 mm Hg at point *A* could be due to reduced contractility, to increased BP allowing the same stroke work to eject a smaller SV at point *A*, or to a stiffer ventricle allowing a smaller LV end-diastolic volume (LVEDV) at a Pla of 10 mm Hg. This variety of mechanisms to explain the same data is a limitation of the analysis of hemodynamics by the Starling curve, so a more complete description of ventricular function is helpful.

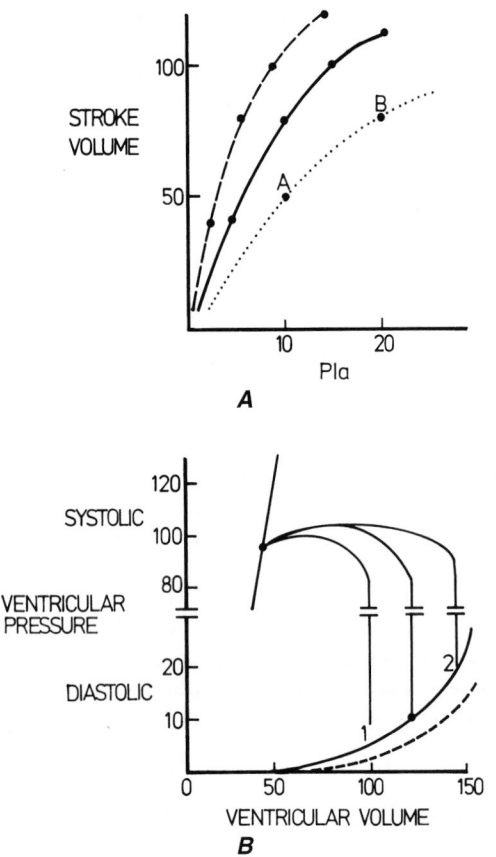

FIGURE 20-4 *A.* Starling function curves. Stroke volume (SV, in milliliters; *ordinate*) is plotted against left atrial pressure (Pla, in mm Hg; *abscissa*). The middle continuous line depicts a normal Starling function curve for comparison with a depressed curve (*dotted line AB*) and with a curve depicting enhanced ventricular function (*interrupted curve*); all three curves may have the same systolic function (contractility) if diastolic volume-pressure (V-P) relations or afterload differs from each other. *B.* Corresponding left ventricular volume (milliliters; *abscissa*) versus pressure (mm Hg; *ordinate*) relations; the break in the ordinate scale emphasizes the normal diastolic V-P relation (*continuous line 1,2*) and the end-systolic V-P relation (*continuous line up and to the left*). For discussion of the three V-P loops originating from the diastolic curve, see text. The interrupted diastolic V-P curve depicts a more compliant chamber such as the right ventricle, where there is less diastolic pressure for each volume.

The ventricular function shown by the Starling relation is based on the mechanical properties of the relaxed (diastolic) or contracting (systolic) V-P relations of the ventricle. This section reviews the factors that influence the diastolic and systolic mechanics in health and in critical illness and relates these mechanics to the corresponding Starling function curves of the heart. In Fig. 20-4B, LV end-diastolic pressure (LVEDP) and LV end-systolic pressure (LVESP) are plotted against the corresponding volumes (LVEDV and LV end-systolic volume [LVESV]). The continuous end-diastolic V-P curve is marked with a dot at an LVEDP of 10 mm Hg, where the normal LVEDV is 120 mL. When the ventricle contracts, pressure increases at the same volume until the aortic valve is opened, and blood is ejected until the valve closes at an LVESV of 45 mL. The SV (LVEDV − LVESV) is 75 mL, as plotted on the continuous Starling curve shown in Fig. 20-4A. When

hypovolemia decreases the LVEDV (1 in Fig. 20-4B), LVEDP and SV decrease along the Starling curve above; if volume expansion increases the LVEDV to position 2, SV and LVEDP increase along the Starling curve. Intracardiac pressures such as Pla are measured with respect to atmospheric pressure, so they do not represent true transmural, or filling, pressures of the heart chamber when the pressure on the outside of the heart is not atmospheric.[4,5] Pericardial pressure is most often equal to Ppl, which is subatmospheric during spontaneous breathing (−3 to −10 mm Hg) and can become very negative in airflow obstruction or very positive with mechanical ventilation and positive end-expiratory pressure (PEEP). For convenience, the following discussion refers to the intravascular pressures as transmural, or filling, pressures, and any cause for altered pericardial or pleural pressure is noted.

THE DIASTOLIC V-P CURVE AND VENTRICULAR FILLING DISORDERS

Figure 20-4B plots LVEDV against LVEDP. As ventricular volume increases from zero, the transmural pressure of the ventricle does not exceed zero until about 50 mL (the unstressed volume) is added. Then LVEDP increases in a curvilinear manner with ventricular volume (the stressed volume) first as a large change in volume for a small change in pressure and then as a small change in volume for a large change in pressure. If the pericardium is removed, these V-P characteristics are more linear such that the large change in LVEDP at higher values of LVEDV is no longer evident. Thus the pericardium acts like a membrane with a large unstressed volume loosely surrounding the heart up to a given ventricular volume, but at greater LVEDV the pericardium becomes very stiff. At higher heart volumes, most of the pressure across the heart is across the pericardium, accounting for the very steep rise in the diastolic V-P relation. In the presence of pericardial effusion, the volume at which the pericardium becomes a limiting membrane is reduced by the volume of the effusion. When the effusion is large enough, reduced end-diastolic volumes are associated with quite large end-DPs (see Chap. 28). In turn, pericardial pressure decreased VR by increasing Pra, thus keeping end-diastolic volume and Q̇T abnormally low. Tension pneumothorax, massive pleural effusions, high levels of PEEP, and greatly increased abdominal pressures can increase pressure outside the heart (Ppl) and thus reduce LVEDV and SV despite high values of LVEDP (Table 20-1). Intercurrent LV hypertrophy or infiltrative diseases (amyloidosis) occasionally stiffen the relaxed ventricle such that high filling pressures are needed to maintain an adequate SV, and inadequate filling time or poorly coordinated atrial contraction also impairs ventricular filling.[6]

A right-to-left shift of the interventricular septum also can restrict diastolic filling. Presumably, the distention of the right ventricle causes the interventricular septum to bulge from right to left, thereby reducing the unstressed volume and compliance of the left ventricle.[2,7] This effect of ventricular interdependence is much less marked when the pericardium is removed, perhaps because the limiting membrane of the pericardium restricts freedom of motion of the left ventricle, making it more vulnerable to displacements of the septum. Accordingly, conditions in which the right ventricle is abnormally loaded (e.g., acute pulmonary embolism or acute-on-chronic respiratory failure due to obstructive or restrictive

TABLE 20-1 Common Causes of Diastolic Dysfunction in Critically Ill Patients Signaled by High Left Atrial Pressure and Low Ventricular End-Diastolic Volume

External compression
  Pericardial effusion or construction
  Positive pressure ventilation with PEEP, auto-PEEP
  Tension pneumothorax, massive pleural effusions
  Greatly increased abdominal pressure
Myocardial stiffness
  LV hypertrophy—aortic stenosis, systemic hypertension
  Infiltrative diseases—amyloidosis
  Ischemic heart disease
Ventricular interdependence and right-to-left septal shift
  Pulmonary hypertension
  RV infarction
  High levels of PEEP
Intraventricular filling defects
  Tumor
  Clot
Rhythm or valvular impediments to filling
  Tachycardia
  Heart block
  Artial fibrillation, flutter
  Mitral stenosis

ABBREVIATIONS: V, left ventricular; PEEP, positive end-expiratory pressure; RV, right ventricular.

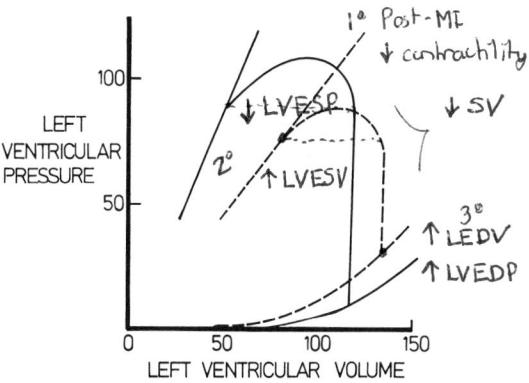

FIGURE 20-5 Schematic representation of left ventricular end-diastolic volume (LDEDV) and pressure (LVEDP) amd end-systolic (ES) volume and pressure relations before (*continuous curves*) and after (*interrupted curves*) acute myocardial infarction. The myocardial injury depresses the contractility to increase ES volume despite the decrease in pressure afterload; accordingly, LVEDV increases to accommodate venous return, whereas LVEDP increases even more due to the diastolic dysfunction of the myocardial injury. Accordingly, LV dysfunction is signaled by reduced stroke volume and cardiac output despite a large elevation in LVEDP; therapy aims to reduce preload, enhance contractility, and reduce afterload. For further discussion, see text.

lung disease) may impede the emptying of the right ventricle, causing it to work at a higher end-diastolic volume. Then LV filling pressures will be higher than expected for the end-diastolic volume. This provides one possible explanation for why PEEP is often associated with increased filling pressure to maintain a normal SV even when LVEDP is corrected to the true filling pressure by subtracting the increase in Ppl (ΔPpl) measured when PEEP is applied.[4,5,8,9] Acute myocardial ischemia also displaces the diastolic V-P curve of the left ventricle up and to the left (Fig. 20-5). Conceivably, myocardial injury alters the elastic properties of the relaxed ventricle.[6] Therefore, a higher ventricular filling pressure is required at each end-diastolic volume. This accounts in part for the often noted observation that patients with acute myocardial injury need values of LVEDP as high as 30 mm Hg to maintain adequate $\dot{Q}$T, whereas normal patients need filling pressures below 10 mm Hg.

THE END-SYSTOLIC V-P CURVE AND CONTRACTILITY

The normal diastolic V-P relation is demonstrated by the continuous line in the lower right-hand portion of Fig. 20-5. Consider the effects when the ventricle contracts during systole without ejecting any blood, as if the aortic valve could not open. A very large pressure is generated during this isovolumic contraction from a normal LVEDV, but when the LVEDV is reduced, the pressure generated during a similar isovolumic contraction is much less, as a manifestation of the force–length characteristics of the myocardium.[2,3,10,11] That is, the less the muscle is stretched, the less force it can generate, a manifestation of the length-dependent activation of actin–myosin cross-bridges. The units of force in the hollow sphere of myocardium are the units of pressure, or force per unit area. A line connecting the end-systolic V-P points is linear and

extrapolates toward the origin (see the continuous end-systolic V-P line in Fig. 20-5, upper left).

Of course, the aortic valve does open in early systole when the isovolumic pressure exceeds the aortic DP; then LV volume decreases as the SV is ejected (see Fig. 20-5). The contracting ventricle shortens against the aortic afterload pressure until its volume reaches the end-systolic volume; at that lower volume, the maximum pressure that can be generated is equal to the afterload pressure, so the aortic valve closes and ejection is over. If the afterload pressure were decreased, the ventricle could eject further to a lower end-systolic volume, where the maximum generated pressure equals the reduced afterload; hence, SV would increase.

The line connecting all end-systolic V-P points is an indicator of the pumping function or contractility of the heart because this line defines the volume to which the ventricle can shorten against each afterload for a given contractile state.[10–13] Agents that enhance contractility (e.g., epinephrine, calcium, dobutamine, and dopamine) shift the end-systolic V-P relation up and to the left; then the ventricle can shorten to a smaller end-systolic volume for each afterload, thereby increasing SV at a given LVEDV/LVEDP.[10,11] Conversely, negative inotropic agents such as propranolol, myocardial ischemia, hypoxia, and acidemia depress the end-systolic V-P relation down and to the right, as indicated by the interrupted end-systolic V-P line shown in Fig. 20-5.[12,13] Then end-systolic volume is increased for a given pressure afterload, thereby reducing the SV at a given filling pressure. Such a reduction in contractility is a common cause for the depressed Starling curve *AB* shown in in Fig. 20-4.

AN APPROACH TO ACUTE VENTRICULAR DYSFUNCTION

These concepts provide a framework for understanding the pathophysiology and therapy of acute myocardial infarction (see Chap. 25). Figure 20-5 depicts normal diastolic and systolic V-P relations and indicates a normal systolic ejection (continuous lines). From an LVEDV of 120 mL and an LVEDP of 10 mm Hg, the ventricle contracts isovolumically until the aortic valve opens at a DP of 80 mm Hg. Blood is then ejected as SP increases to 110 mm Hg and decreased toward an LVESP of 90 mm Hg and an LVESV of 50 mL, when the aortic valve closes to generate the dicrotic notch on the arterial pressure trace. Accordingly, SV is 70 mL at a Pla of 10 mm Hg and $\dot{Q}_T$ is 5.6 L/min when HR is 80 beats/min. Acute myocardial infarction depresses the end-systolic V-P relation so that the end-systolic volume is increased to 90 mL at a reduced LVESP of 75 mm Hg (interrupted lines). At the same time, the end-diastolic volume is increased to 130 mL to accommodate the VR, and end-DP is increased even more than expected (LVEDP = 30 mm Hg) due to the shift up and to the left of the end-diastolic V-P relation (interrupted line). Thus SV (40 mL) and $\dot{Q}_T$ (4.4 L/min) are reduced despite reflex tachycardia (HR = 110 beats/min) at an increased LV filling pressure, and BP is decreased (SP/DP = 90/70 mm Hg) despite the reflex increase in SVR.

Conventional therapy consists of preload reduction, inotropic agents, and afterload reduction, in addition to measures to reestablish and maintain coronary blood flow (see Chap. 25). Interventions such as morphine, furosemide, nitrates, and rotating tourniquets decrease VR by dilating venous capacitance beds to increase the unstressed volume and decrease mean systemic pressure (Pms; see below). These actions in turn decrease LVEDV and LVEDP. The reduction in end-diastolic volume tends to decrease LVEDP along the steep diastolic V-P curve so that there is a large reduction in LVEDP for a small reduction in LVEDV and SV. Further, the potential adverse effect of reduced SV is often offset by increased contractility and reduced afterload when myocardial wall stress is decreased by the reduction in LVEDV and LVEDP (see Chaps. 22 and 25). Reduced afterload and reduced myocardial O_2 consumption improve ventricular pumping function by shifting the end-systolic V-P relation up and to the left, so LVESV decreases and SV increases. Further, the decreased end-DP reduces the complication of cardiogenic pulmonary edema.

Positive inotropic agents such as dopamine and dobutamine act directly on the myocardium to reduce end-systolic volume at a given end-SP, thereby increasing SV (see Chaps. 22 and 25). Dopamine also causes venoconstriction by increasing Pms and VR, so the increase in SV is often associated with increased LVEDV, whereas dobutamine tends to increase SV and decrease LVEDV.[14] Afterload-reducing agents such as nitroprusside dilate peripheral arteries to decrease end-SP and afterload; in turn, end-systolic volume decreases along the depressed end-systolic V-P relation to increase SV.[14] Nitroprusside and other arteriolar vasodilating agents also decrease end-DP without changing end-diastolic volume; this effect appears to enhance ventricular function viewed on the Starling relation, as discussed above.[15] The decrease in LVEDP decreases pulmonary edema and may decrease myocardial oxygen demands by decreasing ventricular wall stress. To the extent that it decreases ventricular wall stress, end-systolic V-P relations may shift to the left due to enhanced contractility. In some patients with cardiogenic shock, vasodilator therapy appears to increase SV and $\dot{Q}_T$ without decreasing or even

increasing arterial BP, that is, arterial dilation appears to reduce end-systolic volume at a given end-SP as if contractility were enhanced.[14,15]

Noninvasive mechanical ventilation (or continuous positive airway pressure, CPAP) lowers both preload and afterload, in addition to beneficial effects on gas exchange and work of breathing.[16] $\dot{Q}_T$ is not reduced despite decreased transmural pressures, indicating improved pump function.

Other concomitant effects of critical illness cause ventricular dysfunction characterized by reduced SV at increased Pla (see Table 20-1). Arterial hypoxemia[12] and acidemia[13] depress the end-systolic V-P curve and increase diastolic stiffness, as shown by the interrupted curve in Fig. 20-5. Acute arterial hypertension raises the pressure afterload, so SV decreases as end-systolic volume increases along the continuous end-systolic V-P curve in Fig. 20-5. Then LVEDV increases to accommodate VR, so LVEDP increases, often more than expected, due to diastolic stiffness, in turn due to LV hypertrophy in the hypertensive patient. Accordingly, pulmonary edema is a common complication, and it responds to vasodilator therapy when BP is decreased. In some or all of these conditions, diastolic dysfunction merits special management.[6] When acute or acute-on-chronic congestive heart failure is present, decreasing LVEDP and LVEDV, maintaining atrial contraction, increasing the duration of diastole, and minimizing myocardial ischemia are helpful. Each of these therapeutic measures is also helpful in managing hypoperfusion states associated with diastolic dysfunction.[6]

Valvular dysfunction mimics systolic and diastolic dysfunctions such that LVEDV is much increased and the forward SV is reduced (see Chap. 29). With aortic regurgitation, after a vigorous systolic ejection, aortic blood runs off forward and backward in diastole such that LVEDP increases and arterial DP decreases toward equal values at 40 mm Hg. The large LVEDV then ejects a large SV to increase SP to 120 mm Hg, causing a bounding PP of 80 mm Hg, but the aortic regurgitation reduces forward SV and $\dot{Q}_T$ to a low value. Consider also mitral valve incompetence. During systole, a large fraction of the blood ejected from the ventricle regurgitates to the left atrium, thereby reducing forward SV and $\dot{Q}_T$ but increasing LVEDV and LVEDP when the left atrium fills the ventricle in diastole. In this circumstance, PP and BP are decreased. In both cases, the ventricular mechanics resemble the interrupted curves shown in Fig. 20-5 and improve toward the normal continuous curves when forward flow is increased by vasodilator therapy that lowers SVR to allow more peripheral runoff and less regurgitant flow (see Chap. 29).

Control of Cardiac Output by the Systemic Vessels

Ventricular pumping function generates the flow in the circulation but retains control of the VR, so $\dot{Q}_T$ resides in the systemic vessels.[1,2] The heart is best regarded as a mechanical pump having diastolic and systolic properties that determine how it accommodates the VR. This section reviews the mechanical characteristics of the systemic vessels as a basis for understanding control of $\dot{Q}_T$ in health and in critical illness.

MEAN SYSTEMIC PRESSURE

When the heart stops beating (see Fig. 20-1), pressure equalizes throughout the vascular system, and its new value is the Pms (10 to 15 mm Hg). This pressure is much lower than the arterial pressure and is closer to the Pra. When flow stops, blood drains from the high-pressure, low-volume arterial system into the high-volume, low-pressure venous system, which accommodates the displaced volume with little change in pressure. When the heart begins to beat again, the left heart pumps blood from the central circulation into the systemic circuit, thus increasing pressure there. At the same time, the right heart pumps blood into the lungs, thereby decreasing its pressure (Pra) with respect to Pms, so blood flows from the venous reservoir into the right atrium. Pressure on the venous side decreases slightly below Pms, whereas pressure on the arterial side increases considerably above Pms with succeeding heartbeats. This continues until a steady state is reached, when arterial pressure has increased enough to drive the whole SV of each succeeding heartbeat through the high arterial resistance into the venous reservoir. The Pms does not change between the state of no flow and the new state of steady flow because neither the vascular volume nor the compliance of the vessels has changed. What has changed is the distribution of the vascular volume from the compliant veins to the stiff arteries; this volume shift creates the pressure difference driving flow through the circuit.[1,2,17,18]

Pms is the driving pressure for VR to the right atrium when circulation resumes. It can be increased to increase VR by increasing the vascular volume or by decreasing the unstressed volume and compliance of the vessels.[17,18] The latter two mechanisms are mediated by baroreceptor reflexes responding to hypotension by increasing venous tone and usually occur together. The unstressed volume also may be reduced by raising the legs of a supine patient or applying military antishock trousers; both methods return a portion of the unstressed vascular volume from the large veins in the legs to the stressed volume, thereby increasing Pms and VR. When the heart has an improvement in inotropic state or a reduction in afterload, blood is shifted from the central compartment to the stressed volume of the systemic circuit, thereby increasing Pms and VR;[18] moreover, improved ventricular pumping function decreases Pra to increase VR further (see below).

VENOUS RETURN AND CARDIAC FUNCTION CURVES

Before the heart was started in the discussion above, Pra was equal to the pressure throughout the vascular system, Pms. With each succeeding heartbeat, Pra decreases below Pms and VR increases. This sequence is repeated in a more controlled, steady state by replacing the heart with a pump set to keep Pra at a given value while VR is measured.[17,18] Typical data are plotted in Fig. 20-6. As Pra is decreased from 12 to 0 mm Hg (indicated by the thin continuous line), VR is progressively increased with the driving pressure (Pms − Pra). The slope of the relation between VR and Pms − Pra is the resistance to VR (RVR = Δ[Pms − Pra]/ΔVR). When Pra falls below zero, VR does not increase further because flow becomes limited while entering the thorax. This occurs when the pressure in

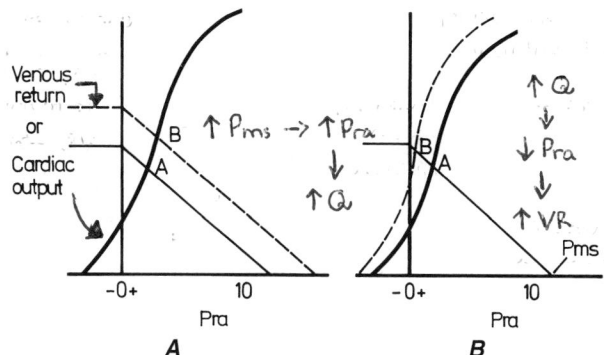

FIGURE 20-6 Control of cardiac output by systemic vessels. Venous return (VR) or cardiac output ($\dot{Q}_T$) is plotted on the ordinate against right atrial pressure (Pra) on the abscissa. *A, B.* The thin continuous VR curve shows that VR increases as Pra decreases below Pra equal to mean systemic pressure (Pms; where VR = 0), so the inverse of the slope of this VR curve ([Pms − Pra]/VR) is the resistance to VR (RVR). The thick continuous cardiac function curve shows that $\dot{Q}_T$ increases as Pra increases because ventricular end-diastolic volume increases. The intersection (shown in *A*) marks the unique value of Pra where VR equals $\dot{Q}_T$ in *A* and *B*. When this value of $\dot{Q}_T$ is insufficient, VR can be increased by increasing Pms without changing RVR, indicated by the interrupted VR curve intersecting the unchanged cardiac function curve at a higher $\dot{Q}_T$ and Pra (shown in *B, left panel*). In the *right panel,* VR is increased from point *A* to point *B* by increased cardiac function (see interrupted cardiac function curve intersecting the original VR curve at point *B*). Accordingly, inotropic agents that increase contractility (dobutamine) can produce modest increases in VR by lowering Pra, but further increases in VR are limited by compression of the great veins at lower values of Pra (*right panel*); such an enhanced cardiac function displaces central blood volume into the peripheral circulation, tending to increase Pms and thus promote further increases in VR (*left panel*). Often, other inotropic agents (dopamine, epinephrine) also raise Pms and VR by venoconstriction.

these collapsible great veins decreases below the atmospheric pressure outside the veins. Further decreases in Pra and CVP are associated with progressive collapse of the veins rather than with an increase in VR.

For a given stressed vascular volume and compliance, Pms is set and RVR is relatively constant. In the absence of pulmonary hypertension or right heart dysfunction, LV function will determine Pra and, hence, VR to the right heart, which must equal the $\dot{Q}_T$ from the left heart. $\dot{Q}_T$ is described by the cardiac function curve, drawn as a thick continuous line relating Pra (abscissa) to $\dot{Q}_T$ (ordinate), in Fig. 20-6. The heart is able to eject a larger SV and $\dot{Q}_T$ when the end-DP is greater because more distended ventricles eject to about the same end-systolic volume as less distended ventricles do. Accordingly, as Pra decreases, $\dot{Q}_T$ decreases along the cardiac function curve. However, VR increases as Pra decreases until VR equals $\dot{Q}_T$ at a unique value of Pra, indicated by the intersection of the cardiac function and VR curves in Fig. 20-6 (see point *A* in both panels).

When $\dot{Q}_T$ is insufficient, VR can be increased in several ways. A new steady state of increased VR is achieved by increasing Pms with no change in RVR, indicated by the interrupted VR curve in the left panel of Fig. 20-6. This new VR

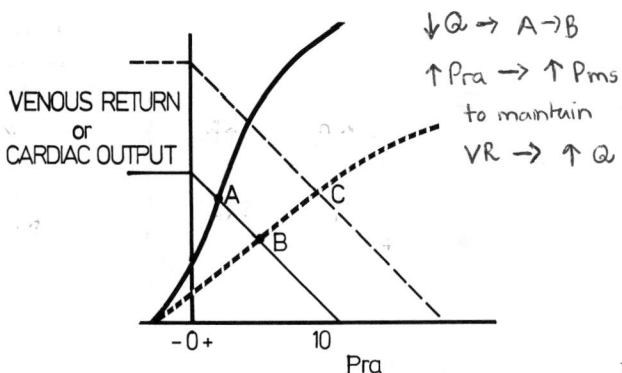

FIGURE 20-7 Reduced cardiac function (*interrupted curve BC*) decreases steady-state venous return from *A* to *B* because right atrial pressure (Pra) increases along the normal venous return curve (*continuous line AB*). In response, baroreceptor reflexes and/or vascular volume retention increase mean systemic pressure such that the new interrupted venous return curve intersects the depressed cardiac function curve at *C*, whereby caridac output has returned to normal at increased Pra. The new steady state can be produced by systolic or diastolic dysfunction of the left or right ventricle. For further discussion, see text.

curve intersects the same cardiac function curve at a higher value of $\dot{Q}_T$ at point *B*. This method of increasing VR is associated with an increase in Pra. Due to the steep slope of the cardiac function curve in normal hearts, large increases in VR occur with only small increases in Pra. Alternatively, VR can be increased by enhanced cardiac function by increasing contractility or decreasing afterload of the heart. This is depicted as an upward shift of the cardiac function curve, as in the right panel of Fig. 20-6, such that greater $\dot{Q}_T$ occurs at each Pra. The increase on each VR curve by this mechanism is associated with a reduction in Pra. Further, in the normal heart, only a small change in VR is possible (from point *A* to point *B* in the right panel), and greater reductions in Pra do not increase $\dot{Q}_T$ further because VR becomes flow limited as Pra decreases to below zero. This explains why inotropic agents that enhance contractility are ineffective in hypovolemic shock.

When cardiac pumping function is depressed, as depicted by the interrupted line in Fig. 20-7, VR is decreased from point *A* to point *B* for the same value of Pms as Pra increases. The patient must then retain fluid or initiate cardiac reflexes to increase Pms toward the new value required to maintain adequate $\dot{Q}_T$, as in chronic congestive heart failure. This is associated with a large increase in Pra from point *B* to point *C*, which in turn causes jugular venous distention, hepatomegaly, and peripheral edema. Diuretic reduction of vascular volumes will correct these cosmetic abnormalities at the expense of decreasing Pms and VR. In contrast, inotropic and vasodilator drugs, which improve depressed cardiac function by shifting the interrupted cardiac function curve upward, increase $\dot{Q}_T$ and decrease Pra more effectively than in patients with normal cardiac function.

EFFECTS OF PRESSURE OUTSIDE THE HEART ON CARDIAC OUTPUT

In the figures cited and the preceding discussions, values of Pms and Pra were expressed relative to atmospheric pressure. However, the transmural pressure of the right atrium exceeds

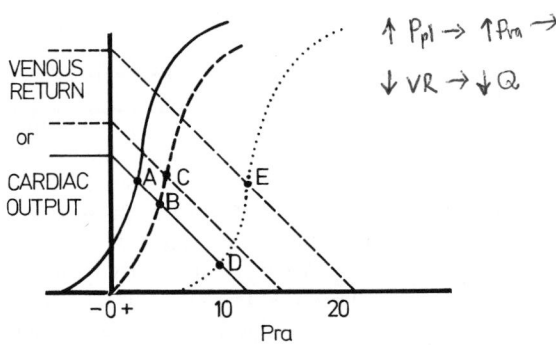

FIGURE 20-8 Schematic showing effects of increased pleural pressure (Ppl) on venous return (VR) and cardiac output ($\dot{Q}_T$). Compared with the normal steady state (*continuous VR and cardiac function curves*), increasing Ppl and right atrial pressure (Pra) by 4 mm Hg shifts the normal cardiac function curves to the right (*interrupted cardiac function curve BC*) so that venous return decreases from *A* to *B*. This accounts for the decrease in $\dot{Q}_T$ when thoracotomy exposes the right atrium to atmospheric pressure; similarly, the increase in Ppl and Pra when positive end-expiratory pressure (PEEP) is applied to a patient with an intact thorax decreases $\dot{Q}_T$. In both cases, baroreceptor reflexes or iatrogenic expansion of vascular volume increase Pms to allow the new interrupted VR curve to intersect the displaced cardiac function curve at *C*, thereby returning $\dot{Q}_T$ to normal. A much larger increase in PEEP increases Ppl and Pra even more so that the displaced normal cardiac function curve (*dotted curve DE*) intersects the normal VR curves at a very low value (*E*) required by a larger increase in mean systemic pressure to allow the new interrupted VR curve to intersect the dotted function curve at *E*. For further discussion, see text.

the Pra by the subatmospheric value (about −4 mm Hg) of the Ppl surrounding the heart. Consider the effect of opening the thorax, which raises Ppl from −4 to 0 mm Hg: VR decreases from point *A* to point *B* in Fig. 20-8 because Pra increases.[19] This is indicated by the interrupted cardiac function curve shifted to the right by the increase in pressure outside the heart but parallel to the normal cardiac function curve (continuous line through point *A*). Normal VR can be restored (point *B* to point *C*) by increasing Pms by an amount equal to the increase in Ppl and Pra induced by thoracotomy. Then transmural Pra will be the same as at point *A*, and Pra will have increased from point *A* to point *C* at the same $\dot{Q}_T$.

This mechanism for the decrease in $\dot{Q}_T$ with thoracotomy also partly explains the decrease in $\dot{Q}_T$ with PEEP. The Ppl within an intact thorax increases with passive positive-pressure ventilation, thereby increasing Pra and decreasing VR.[4,5,8,9,20] When 8 mm Hg of PEEP (10 cm H_2O) is added to the ventilator, the end-expiratory value of Ppl increases by about half that amount, e.g., from −4 to 0 mm Hg. Accordingly, VR decreases with PEEP from point *A* to point *B* in Fig. 20-8, with no change in cardiac function or Pms. $\dot{Q}_T$ is returned to normal by volume infusion or vascular reflexes that increase Pms by an amount equal to the increases in Ppl and Pra. Greater PEEP (20 cm H_2O, as in the dotted line shown in Fig. 20-8) decreases VR further (from point *A* to point *D*) and requires greater increases in Pms to return it to normal (from point *D* to point *E*). Alternatively, Pms increases as much as Pra when PEEP is added, so the decrease in VR must be due to an increase in RVR with PEEP.[20] In either event, VR can be restored on PEEP by increasing Pms.

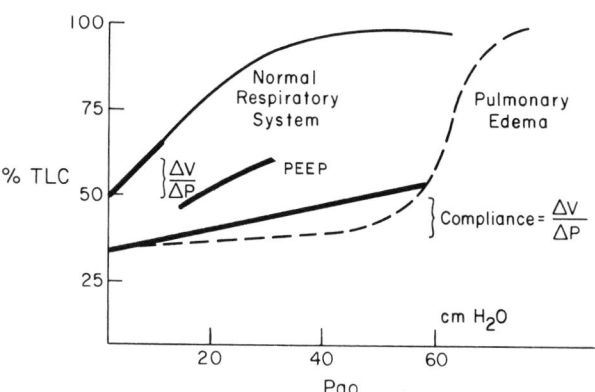

	Before edema	After edema
ΔV(litres) with PEEP (20 cm H_2O)	1.42±0.38	1.39±0.22
ΔPpl (cm H_2O) with PEEP	10.1±2.2	9.7±0.7
Lung Compliance (ml/cm H_2O)	102±28	47±17

FIGURE 20-9 Relations between lung volume (percent total lung capacity, TLC; *ordinate*) and pressure across the respiratory system (pressure airway opening [cm H_2O], Pao; *abscissa*). The thin continuous line represents the inflation volume-pressure (V-P) relation of the normal respiratory system, showing an end-expired lung volume (Pao = 0) of 50% TLC and inflation compliance (V-P) during a tidal volume of about 10% TLC (*thick part of line*). In contrast, the interrupted line shows the inflation V-P curve after pulmonary edema floods many lung units, thereby decreasing end-expired lung volume to about 30% TLC; then a tidal inflation of the same volume causes a much larger increase in Pao because there are many fewer airspaces to accommodate the tidal volume. Adding 15 cm H_2O positive end-expiratory pressure (PEEP) might be expected to produce a much smaller increase in end-expired lung volume in edematous lungs than in a normal respiratory system; however, when PEEP is effective in reducing shunted fraction of total pulmonary blood flow by redistributing alveolar edema, the increase in end-expired lung volume (and, hence, pleural pressure) is as large after pulmonary edema as in the normal respiratory system (*table at right of graph*). (*Reproduced with permission from Prewitt and Wood[4] and Hall and Wood.[24]*)

$\dot{Q}T$ is much less susceptible to the deleterious effects of PEEP when Pms is high. In patients with reduced circulatory volume, vascular reflexes are already operating to maintain VR and Pms by reducing unstressed volume or vascular compliance. Such patients have little vascular reflex reserve and poorly tolerate intubation and positive-pressure ventilation without considerable intravenous infusion to increase vascular stressed volume. In contrast, well-hydrated or overhydrated patients may tolerate even large amounts of PEEP with no reduction in $\dot{Q}T$ because their previously inactive vascular reflexes can increase Pms in well-filled systemic vessels by the amount that Ppl increases with PEEP. These considerations allow the physician to anticipate and treat the hypotension induced by ventilator therapy; the concept should not be interpreted as an indication for maintaining high circulatory volume in critically ill patients on ventilators because this often increases lung edema and provides even more $\dot{Q}T$ than was already deemed sufficient. Further, pressure outside the heart can be increased by a variety of other concomitant conditions and complications of critical illness; all these actions increase pressures measured in the heart chambers and decrease heart volume and, as a consequence, are often interpreted as diastolic dysfunction (see Table 20-1).

How much is the pressure outside the heart increased by PEEP, and is there a practical approach to relating the transmural wedge pressure to SV and $\dot{Q}T$? When PEEP increases end-expired lung volume, the inflated lungs push the thorax to an increased volume through greater pleural pressure, and this change in Ppl (ΔPpl) with PEEP is approximately equal to the change in pressure outside the right and left ventricles.[8] During mechanical ventilation, the ratio of ΔPpl to the change in static elastic pressure across the lung and chest wall (ΔPel) for each breath is given by the ratio of respiratory system compliance (Crs) to the compliance of the chest wall (Cw); that is, $\Delta Ppl/\Delta Pel = Crs/Cw$ (assuming no alveolar recruitment). When lung compliance (CL) is normal, CL = Cw, so $\Delta Ppl/\Delta Pel = 0.5$. When the lungs lose compliance in acute hypoxemic respiratory failure (AHRF), ΔPel increases because Crs decreases, but ΔPpl changes little (at constant tidal volume) because Cw is unaffected by the lung disease, and ΔPpl becomes much less than half of ΔPel. To the extent that the increase in lung volume (ΔVL) with PEEP is determined by Crs, $\Delta Ppl/PEEP = Crs/Cw$, and a decrease in Crs with AHRF would decrease Ppl for a given amount of PEEP well below the normal value of 0.5. However, ΔVL with PEEP is much greater than that predicted by Crs in AHRF because PEEP recruits many previously flooded airspaces,[21,22] so $\Delta Ppl/PEEP$ is as great after acute lung injury as before[4] (Fig. 20-9). Accordingly, the ΔPpl with PEEP is difficult to measure and hard to predict, so many approaches have been tested to estimate the transmural pressure of heart chambers on PEEP.[23] Because PEEP is used most often to decrease shunt in pulmonary edema and because accurate knowledge of transmural Pla shows that the value associated with an adequate $\dot{Q}T$ can differ between patients by 20 mm Hg according to the extent of LV dysfunction, a better approach is to seek the lowest pulmonary wedge pressure (Ppw) that provides adequate output on each level of PEEP. In this way, therapy to decrease Ppw and edema and maintain $\dot{Q}T$ is not confounded by erroneous estimates of transmural Ppw on PEEP.[24,25]

AN APPROACH TO HYPOPERFUSION STATES

A hypoperfusion state, or shock, is almost always signaled by systemic hypotension; commonly associated clinical features of multiple organ system hypoperfusion are tachycardia, tachypnea, prerenal oliguria (urine flow < 20 mL/h, urine Na^+ > 20 mEq/L, urine K^+ > 20 mEq/L, urine-specific gravity > 1.020), abnormalities of mentation and consciousness, and metabolic acidosis. The mean BP is determined by the product of $\dot{Q}T$ and SVR. A conceptual framework for the initial diagnosis and management of the hypotensive patient is outlined in Table 20-2. Utilization of this approach aims to categorize the patient's symptoms into one of the three common causes of shock (septic, cardiogenic, or hypovolemic) and to initiate early appropriate therapy of the presumed diagnosis (see Chap. 21). Response to the therapeutic intervention tests the accuracy of the initial diagnosis, so the hemodynamic response is reevaluated within 30 minutes. The diagnostic decision is aided by collating clinical data from the medical history, physical examination, and routine laboratory tests to answer three questions in sequence.

SEPTIC SHOCK

Is BP decreased because $\dot{Q}T$ is decreased? If not, SVR must be reduced, a condition almost always related to sepsis or sterile endotoxemia associated with severe liver disease. As indicated in Table 20-2 (right column), a low BP is often characterized by a large PP because the SV is large and by a very low DP because each SV has a rapid peripheral runoff through dilated peripheral arterioles (see Fig. 20-3). This produces warm, pink skin with rapid return of color to the nail bed and crisp heart sounds. As in other types of shock, tachycardia is evident due in part to baroreceptor reflex response to hypotension, but the arterial vasoconstriction response to reflex sympathetic tone is blocked by relaxation of arteriolar smooth muscle induced by endothelium-derived relaxing factor (or nitric oxide). The combination of tachycardia and large PP indicates a large $\dot{Q}T$ that is almost always present early unless concurrent hypovolemia or myocardial dysfunction precludes the hyperdynamic circulatory state of sepsis.

Initial therapy starts with appropriate broad-spectrum antibiotics (see Chap. 46) and expands the circulating volume by intravenous infusion of fluids to treat associated hypovolemia, which is due to venodilation decreasing Pms and VR lower than needed to maintain adequate perfusion pressure of vital organs. The end point of volume infusion is obscure because $\dot{Q}T$ and oxygen delivery (D_{O_2}) are already increased, and although $\dot{Q}T$ usually increases further with intravenous infusions, BP increases little with increased $\dot{Q}T$. Further, the need for an even greater $\dot{Q}T$ to increase D_{O_2} is questionable because the lactic acidosis of septic shock may not be due to anaerobic metabolism.[26-28] Accordingly, septic patients in whom $\dot{Q}T$ is maximized do not have improved survival.[29,30] Conversely, pulmonary vascular pressures always increase with volume infusion, thus increasing pulmonary edema when the septic process increases the permeability of lung vessels.[25,31-33] This coincidence of the acute respiratory

TABLE 20-2 Initial Approach to the Diagnosis and Management of the Hypotensive Patient

Blood pressure (BP) = Cardiac output ($\dot{Q}T$) × systematic vascular resistance (SVR)		
	IS $\dot{Q}T$ REDUCED?	
	Yes	No
BP	90/70 mm Hg	90/40 mm Hg
Skin	Cool, blue	Warm, pink
Nail bed return	Slow	Rapid
Heart sounds	Muffled	Crisp
History/lab	Hypervolemic or	↓ or ↑ WBC and/or temperature
	Cardiogenic etiology	Source of infection
		Immune compromise
		Severe liver disease
Working diagnosis	See next question	**Septic shock/endotoxemia**
	IS THE HEART TOO FULL?	
	Yes	No
Presentation	Angina, dyspnea	Hemorrhage, dehydration
Signs	Cardiomegaly	Dry mucous membranes
	Extra heart sounds	↓ tissue turgor
	↑ JVP	Stool, gastric blood
Lab	ECG, x-ray	↓ hematocrit
	Echocardiogram	↑ BUN/creatinine
Working diagnosis	**Cardiogenic shock**	**Hypovolemic shock**
	WHAT DOES NOT FIT?	
	Cardiac tamponade	Anaphylaxis
	Acute pulmonary hypertension	Spinal shock
	Right ventricular infarction	Adrenal insufficiency
	Overlapping multiple etiologies	

ABBREVIATIONS: BUN, serum urea nitrogen; ECG, electrocardiogram; JVP, jugular venous pressure; WBC, white blood cell count.

distress syndrome (ARDS) and septic shock has created an apparent dilemma concerning fluid therapy and cardiovascular management of these conditions. My approach is to ensure resuscitation from septic shock as the first priority by ensuring a large $\dot{Q}T$ with a Ppw that does not exceed 15 mmHg and add dobutamine to increase $\dot{Q}T$ and BP as necessary.[25] When early ARDS is not associated with septic shock, I seek the lowest circulating volume to provide adequate $\dot{Q}T$.[25]

The septic myocardium does not function normally,[34,35] but this dysfunction is often associated with SV values larger than 100 mL at normal values of LVEDP. Accordingly, it seems unlikely that systolic dysfunction contributes substantially to the shock, but infusion of dobutamine does increase $\dot{Q}T$ for a given high-normal LVEDP without increasing O_2 uptake or correcting lactic acidosis in septic shock.[36] Even when $\dot{Q}T$ and D_{O_2} are made adequate with fluid and dobutamine infusions, the perfusion pressure for vital organs such as the brain and heart may still be too low in some septic patients. In this case, norepinephrine infusion increases BP and splanchnic blood flow[37,38] without compromising renal function;[39] in contrast, dopamine and epinephrine infusions cause splanchnic hypoperfusion in septic shock.[37,38,40] Tachypnea and respiratory distress may be severe, so initial supportive therapy includes consideration of early intubation and mechanical ventilation and correction of hyperthermia with antipyretics, paralysis, and cooling (see Table 21-4). This prevents catastrophic respiratory muscle fatigue, respiratory acidosis, and the complications of emergent intubation and may improve tissue oxygenation by reducing O_2 requirements in patients with limited D_{O_2}.[41,42]

CARDIOGENIC SHOCK

In contrast to septic shock, low $\dot{Q}T$ is signaled by low PP indicating low SV (see Fig. 20-3), signs of increased systemic vascular resistance (e.g., cold, blue, damp extremities and poor return of color to the nail bed), and a history or presentation including features suggesting a cardiogenic or hypovolemic cause of hypotension. If $\dot{Q}T$ is reduced in the hypotensive patient, then the heart may be too full.

A heart that is too full (see Table 20-2) is often signaled by symptoms of ischemic heart disease or arrhythmia, signs of cardiomegaly, the third and fourth sounds or gallop rhythm of heart failure, new murmurs of valvular dysfunction, increased jugular or CVP, and laboratory tests suggesting ischemia (e.g., electrocardiogram [ECG] or creatine phosphokinase determination) or ventricular dysfunction (e.g., chest x-ray suggesting cardiomegaly, a widened vascular pedicle, or cardiogenic edema or echocardiogram showing regional or global systolic dyskinesia). The most common cause of hypotension associated with a circulation that is too full on initial evaluation is cardiogenic shock due to myocardial ischemia (see Chaps. 22 and 25). Initial therapy treats this presumptive diagnosis with inotropic drug therapy (dobutamine 3 to 10 μg/kg per minute) to assist the ejecting function of the ischemic heart. Such therapy does not directly address the coronary insufficiency and may increase the myocardial O_2 demand, especially if it causes tachycardia. Concurrent sublingual, dermal, or intravenous nitroglycerin ameliorates elements of coronary vasospasm to increase blood flow and reduces preload to decrease myocardial O_2 consumption. Morphine also decreases pain, anxiety, and preload.[43]

In this situation, even a cautious volume challenge (250 mL 0.9% NaCl over 20 minutes) may be risky because ventricular function and $\dot{Q}T$ are decreased as often as they are increased by this intervention, and the risk of pulmonary edema is increased. When signs of pulmonary edema are present on clinical and radiologic examinations of the thorax, diuretics, morphine, and nitroglycerin often reduce preload by relaxing the capacitance veins, associated with an increase in LV systolic performance. However, about 10% of patients with myocardial ischemia present with significant hypovolemia. Accordingly, the clinical assessment of hemodynamics should be supplemented as soon as possible with other means to exclude hypovolemia (e.g., right heart catheterization, empiric volume challenge, echocardiography, or dynamic tests of the adequacy of circulating volume) so that appropriate volume infusion or reduction can be titrated. When these measures are addressed adequately but the hypoperfusion state persists, early movement toward arteriolar vasodilator therapy or a balloon-assist device is indicated to reduce LV afterload and preserve coronary perfusion pressure (see Chap. 25). These latter interventions are not relegated to the last resort but are considered early in this initial stabilization of cardiogenic shock. Similarly, early elective intubation and mechanical ventilation allow effective sedation and reduce O_2 consumption,[41] and PEEP improves arterial oxygenation, often without reducing VR and with improvement of pumping function in the damaged left ventricle by reducing preload and afterload.[44]

HYPOVOLEMIC SHOCK

Beyond the absence of clinical features suggesting that the heart is too full in the hypotensive patient who is presenting reduced $\dot{Q}T$ (see Table 20-2), hypovolemic shock is distinguished from cardiogenic shock by several positive clinical features. Often there is an obvious source of external bleeding (e.g., multiple trauma, hemoptysis, hematemesis, hematochezia, or melena); internal bleeding is often signaled by blood aspirated from the nasogastric tube or on rectal examination, by increasing abdominal girth, or by clinical and radiologic examinations of the thoracic cavity for pleural, alveolar, retroperitoneal, or periaortic blood. Each of these signals is often associated with a new reduction in the hematocrit. Nonhemorrhagic hypovolemia often presents with recognizable excess gastrointestinal fluid losses (e.g., vomiting, diarrhea, suctioning, and stomas), excess renal losses (e.g., osmotic or drug diuresis and diabetes insipidus), or third-space losses as in extensive burns. Physical examination shows dry mucous membranes with decreased tissue turgor, and routine laboratory tests often show increased serum urea nitrogen out of proportion to a relatively normal creatinine level and increased hematocrit due to hemoconcentration.

The initial management of patients with presumed hypovolemic shock necessitates early vascular access with two large-bore (14-gauge) peripheral intravenous catheters for rapid infusion of large volumes of warmed blood and fluids for hemorrhagic shock and the appropriate crystalloid solution for dehydration. Central venous access ensures adequate volume resuscitation and allows early measurement of CVP. An immediate response of increased BP and pulse volume supports the presumed diagnosis, whereas no improvement in these hemodynamic measurements necessitates emergent repair of the site of blood loss or a reevaluation of the working diagnosis. Achieving hemostasis in hemorrhagic shock is a prerequisite for adequate volume resuscitation: urgent and simultaneous pursuit of hemostasis and fluid resuscitation is encouraged.[45] Vasoconstricting drugs such as norepinephrine should be used only as short-term antihypotensives to mobilize endogenous unstressed volume or enhance arteriolar vasoconstriction until the circulating volume is restored by transfusion; prolonged use of these drugs confounds the physician's assessment of the end point of volume resuscitation. Early endotracheal intubation and mechanical ventilation reduce the patient's work of breathing and allow respiratory compensation for lactic acidosis during volume resuscitation; warming the fluids and covering the patient with warm dry blankets prevent the complication of hypothermia, including cold coagulopathy and further bleeding (see Table 21-4).

OTHER COMMON CAUSES OF SHOCK: A SHORT DIFFERENTIAL DIAGNOSIS

The purpose of this initial schema is to formulate a working diagnosis for the most common presentations of shock so that early and rapid therapy can be initiated. The response to the initial therapy confirms or challenges the working diagnosis. When features of the initial clinical presentation or the response of the patient to appropriate management challenges the working diagnosis, early acquisition of more objective hemodynamic data is appropriate. In the interim, other features of the clinical presentation often suggest a cause of shock that falls outside this simplistic schema, or the possibility of overlapping or concurrent causes expands. This section briefly reviews several important differential diagnostic conditions for cardiogenic shock (e.g., tamponade or acute right heart syndromes) and hypovolemic shock (e.g., anaphylactic, neurogenic, or adrenal shock; (see Table 20-2, what does not fit?).

CARDIAC TAMPONADE

Pericardial effusion is often suggested early by the clinical setting (e.g., renal failure, malignancy, or chest pain), physical examination (e.g., elevated neck veins, systolic BP that decreases >10 mm Hg on inspiration, or distant heart sounds), or routine investigations (e.g., chest radiograph with "water bottle" heart, low voltage on the ECG, or electrical alternans). Such a constellation of clinical data requires early echocardiographic confirmation of pericardial effusion, and tamponade is signaled by right ventricular and right atrial collapse that worsens with inspiration, with a relatively small left ventricle (see Chap. 28). Tamponade requires urgent pericardiocentesis or operative drainage by pericardiostomy. While deciding on definitive treatment, one should remember that intravenous expansion of the circulating volume may produce small increases in BP, whereas reductions in circulating volume (e.g., diuretics, nitroglycerin, morphine, or intercurrent hemodialysis) are often associated with catastrophic reduction in $\dot{Q}_T$ by reducing the venous tone and volume necessary to maintain the Pms required to drive VR back to high Pra.

Right heart catheterization typically shows a Pra increased to about 16 to 20 mm Hg and equal to pulmonary arterial DP and the arterial Pwp; $\dot{Q}_T$ and SV are much reduced (see Chap. 28). This hemodynamic subset resembles that of cardiogenic shock (high Ppw and low SV). However, in the case of pericardial tamponade, Ppw is increased because pericardial pressure is increased, so the transmural pressure of the left ventricle approaches zero, a value consistent with the very low LVEDV accounting for the low SV. Other etiologies of hypotension associated with high cardiac pressures and small ventricular volumes include constrictive pericarditis, tension pneumothorax, massive pleural effusion, positive-pressure ventilation with high PEEP, and very high intraabdominal pressure (see Table 21-1). Up to 33% of patients presenting with cardiac tamponade have increased BP despite low $\dot{Q}_T$; this subset of patients has a high incidence of hypertension preceding the onset of tamponade.[46]

RIGHT VENTRICULAR OVERLOAD AND INFARCTION

Another clinical presentation that may fall outside the simplest scheme presented in Table 20-2 is the hypotension associated with acute or acute-on-chronic pulmonary hypertension. Shock after acute pulmonary embolism is often signaled by the clinical setting including risk factors (e.g., perioperative, immobilized, thrombophilia, or prior pulmonary embolisms); symptoms of acute dyspnea, chest pain, or hemoptysis; physical examination showing a loud P_2 with a widened and fixed split of the second heart sound; new hypoxemia without obvious radiologic explanation; and acute right heart strain on the ECG (see Chap. 27). Noninvasive Doppler studies of the veins in the lower extremities and helical computed tomographic angiography confirm the diagnosis. Anticoagulation or placement of a filter in the inferior vena cava reduces the incidence of subsequent emboli, and there may be some success with thrombolytic therapy (or, in some centers, surgical removal of the embolus) in patients with shock due to pulmonary embolism. Acute-on-chronic pulmonary hypertension causes shock in the setting of prior primary pulmonary hypertension, recurrent pulmonary emboli, progression of collagen vascular disease, or chronic respiratory failure (e.g., chronic obstructive pulmonary disease or pulmonary fibrosis) aggravated in part by hypoxic pulmonary vasoconstriction. In these circumstances, O_2 therapy and pulmonary vasodilator therapy combine to decrease pulmonary hypertension and increase $\dot{Q}_T$ in a small but significant proportion of patients (see Chap. 27).

Right heart catheterization shows a unique hemodynamic profile: a very high mean pulmonary artery pressure, pulmonary arterial DP considerably greater than the Pwp, and reduced $\dot{Q}_T$ and SV. Not uncommonly, arterial Pwp is normal or increased despite a small LVEDV on echocardiographic examination, which also shows a right-to-left shift of the interventricular septum; presumably, this causes stiffening of the diastolic V-P curve of the left ventricle. A complication of pulmonary vasodilator therapy is hypotension due to systemic arterial dilation unaccompanied by increased right heart output. Such effects aggravate the hypoperfusion state, perhaps by reducing coronary blood flow to the hypertrophied, dilated right ventricle. Some evidence suggests that shock associated with pulmonary hypertension is ameliorated by α-agonist therapy (e.g., norepinephrine or phenylephrine), which acts as a predominant systemic arteriolar constrictor to increase BP sufficiently to maintain right ventricular perfusion.[47,48]

Right ventricular infarction causes low pulmonary artery pressures and normal LV filling pressures because the dilated, injured right ventricle is unable to maintain adequate flow to the left heart.[49] Elevated neck veins and Pra tend to decrease with dobutamine infusion, perhaps because the enhanced contractility of the left ventricle improves systolic function of the mechanically interdependent right ventricle.[45,46] Volume expansion often aggravates right ventricular dysfunction, and systemic vasoconstriction may preserve right ventricular perfusion.[50]

ANAPHYLACTIC, NEUROGENIC, AND ADRENAL SHOCK

Other etiologies of shock having unique clinical presentations that usually lead to early diagnosis are anaphylactic shock and neurogenic shock. Beyond identifying the etiology early through their association with triggering agents and trauma, respectively, the physician should note that the pathophysiology of each is a dilated venous bed with greatly increased unstressed volume of the circulation leading to hypovolemic shock. Accordingly, the mainstay of therapy for both conditions is adequate volume infusion; adjunctive therapy for anaphylaxis includes antihistamines, steroids, and epinephrine to antagonize the mediators released in the anaphylactic reaction (see Chap. 106), whereas a careful search for sources of blood loss and hemorrhagic shock is part of the early resuscitation of spinal shock in the traumatized patient (see Chap. 94).

Not uncommonly, the presentation of patients with nonhemorrhagic hypovolemic shock raises the concern of acute adrenal cortical insufficiency. When this possibility is not obviously excluded, it is appropriate to draw a serum cortisol level, provide adequate circulating steroids with dexamethasone, and conduct a corticotropin stimulation test to confirm or refute the diagnosis. Characteristically, hypotension and hypoperfusion in such patients will not respond to adequate vascular volume expansion until dexamethasone is administered (see Chap. 79).

MULTIPLE ETIOLOGIES OF SHOCK

With this differential diagnosis and management evaluation in mind, the initial approach to patients with hypoperfusion states should be completed in less time than it takes to read about it. The target is to distinguish among patients with septic shock, cardiogenic shock, and hypovolemic shock and to initiate an appropriate therapeutic challenge—antibiotics, inotropic agents, or a volume challenge—within 30 minutes of presentation. By the response, the diagnosis is confirmed or challenged, with special regard to equivocal responses to therapy or to several other diagnostic categories of shock. Sorting out the primary etiology of the hypoperfusion state often requires considerable additional data. This process is rendered more complex by concurrent etiologies contributing to the shock, for example, the patient with septic shock unable to increase $\dot{Q}_T$ due to intercurrent myocardial dysfunction, the patient with acute myocardial infarction who is hypovolemic, or the patient with hemorrhagic shock who becomes septic. Other combinations of these major categories overlap with confounding effects of tamponade, positive-pressure ventilation, pneumothorax, and pulmonary hypertension—all to challenge ongoing diagnostic and management approaches.

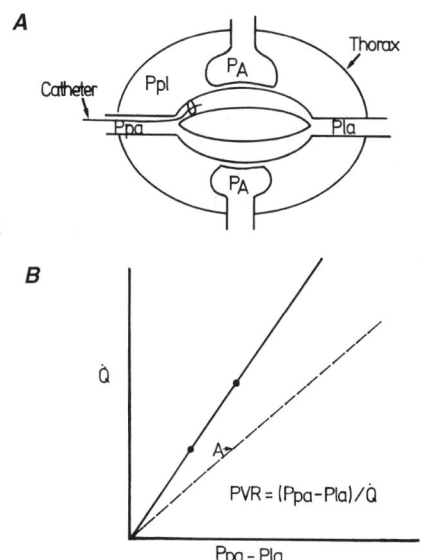

FIGURE 20-10 *A.* Schematic of the pulmonary circulation illustrates a simple view of pulmonary vascular resistance (PVR). Pulmonary blood flows from the pulmonary arteries (Ppa) through branching vessels to the left atrium (Pla). This central circulation is enclosed by the thorax, which contains airspaces (Pa) that abut alveolar vessels. Between the airspaces and thorax is the pleural (pl) space, so pleural pressure (Ppl) approximates the pressure outside extraalveolar vessels, including the heart. A balloon-tipped catheter occludes the upper branch of the pulmonary artery so that the catheter tip sits in a stagnant column of blood, continuous with Pla, to provide an estimate of pulmonary wedge pressure (Ppw), unless alveolar pressure (Pa) exceeds Pla, when occlusion pressure exceeds Pla because Pa closes the alveolar vessels; in either case, when the balloon is deflated, the catheter tip measures Ppa, and a thermistor near the tip can measure pulmonary blood flow ($\dot{Q}$) by thermodilution. *B.* Plots of $\dot{Q}$ (*ordinate*) against Ppa 2 Pla (*abscissa*); the inverse of the slope of the continuous line drawn through the two PQ̇ points is PVR; for a given $\dot{Q}$ at the lower point, Ppa 2 Pla increases to A on the interrupted PQ̇ line, indicating increased PVR.

The Pulmonary Circulation

PRESSURES, FLOW, AND RESISTANCE IN PULMONARY VESSELS

$\dot{Q}_T$ from the left heart is equal to VR to the right heart, so the entire $\dot{Q}_T$ traverses the pulmonary circulation in pulsatile fashion (Fig. 20-10). The right ventricle ejects blood into the pulmonary artery, thereby increasing its pressure (Ppa) to drive flow through a branching arteriolar system into the lung parenchyma, where a network of very small alveolar septal vessels or capillaries passes between the airspaces of the lung to effect pulmonary gas exchange. These septal vessels converge into pulmonary veins that empty into the left atrium, where the pressure (Pla) is often regarded as the outflow pressure of the pulmonary circulation. When this pressure gradient across the pulmonary circulation (Ppa − Pla) is divided by the pulmonary blood flow ($\dot{Q}$), the pulmonary vascular resistance is calculated (mm Hg/L per minute) and sometimes converted to metric units (dyn-s/cm[5]) by multiplying by 80. By this analysis, increasing blood flow from one level to another is associated with decreasing pressure across the pulmonary circulation (Ppa − Pla) along a unique pressure-flow relation given by the continuous line in Fig. 20-10B. Resistance to Q̇ may be increased by smooth muscle constriction within the pulmonary arterioles and alveolar vessels by hypoxia, by compression of the alveolar septal vessels by elevated PA, by obstruction of larger pulmonary vessels by thromboembolism, or by obliteration of many of the parallel vascular channels as they traverse the lung so that the same blood must flow through fewer channels. Such an increase in pulmonary vascular resistance would be calculated as at point *A* on the interrupted line in Fig. 20-10, where the pressure difference across the lung (Ppa − Pla) has increased for the same amount of Q̇. Pulmonary hypertension is a frequent abnormality in critical illness; its causes are listed in Table 22-4 and its treatment is discussed in Chaps. 22 and 26.

Figure 20-10 also depicts a common way to make these measurements with a pulmonary artery catheter (PAC) that is passed throurg systemic veins into the central circulation. When a small balloon near its tip is inflated, the balloon passes with the VR into the right atrium, right ventricle, and pulmonary artery until it wedges in a pulmonary artery branch, obstructing the flow there. Because there is no flow, the hole in the catheter tip is open to a stagnant column of blood extending through the pulmonary vessels to the left atrium. Accordingly, this Ppw approximates Pla, providing an estimate of LVEDP to evaluate ventricular function and an estimate of pulmonary microvascular pressure to help manage pulmonary edema (see below). When the balloon is deflated and flow resumes through that vessel, the pressure there is equal to pulmonary arterial pressure. Mixed venous blood drawn from the pulmonary artery provides a measure of O_2 content (C̄VO_2); when related to the simultaneous measurement of arterial O_2 content (CaO_2) and Q̇T, the patient's O_2 consumption (V̇O_2 = Q̇T[CaO_2 − C̄VO_2]) can be calculated and interpreted in the context of the patient's O_2 transport (D$_{O_2}$ = Q̇T × CaO_2). A sensitive thermistor at the tip of the catheter may be used to detect temperature changes after the injection of a cold saline bolus into the right atrium to allow estimation of Q̇T from the resulting thermodilution curve.

The pulmonary artery and the left atrium are surrounded by Ppl, so absolute values of Ppa and Pla change with respiration. When spontaneous active inspiration decreases Ppl, pulmonary arterial and left atrial pressures decrease, but the driving pressure of blood flow across the lung stays the same (Ppa − Pla); when positive-pressure inflation increases Ppl, Ppa and Pla increase. Accordingly, it is helpful to record pulmonary vascular measurements at end expiration when the mode of ventilation has minimally different effects; even this approach can be confounded when the patient exerts vigorous respiratory activity. When alveolar pressure (PA) exceeds Pla, the true driving pressure for pulmonary blood flow is Ppa − PA. One often overlooked adverse effect of positive-pressure ventilation with high PEEP or high tidal volume is the large increase in dead space (VD/VT) when pulmonary blood flow is interrupted by the high PA; not infrequently, alveolar ventilation can actually increase when tidal volume is reduced in these conditions, causing a paradoxical fall in PaCO_2. A second consequence of PA being greater than Pla is an overestimation of Ppw; this can be detected when the

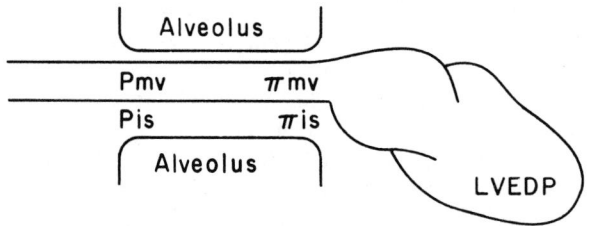

$$\text{Edema Flow} = [\,(Pmv - Pis) - (\pi mv - \pi is)\,\sigma\,]\,Kf$$

FIGURE 20-11 Schematic representation of Starling forces governing the flux of lung liquid from the intravascular to the extravascular space (for discussion, see text). is, interstitial space; LVEDP, left ventricular end-diastolic pressure; mv, microvessels of the lung; p, colloid osmotic pressure; s, reflection coefficient. (*Reproduced with permission from Hall and Wood.*[24])

respiratory fluctuation in Ppa is much less than that in Ppw.[51] Given these effects of respiration on measurements of Ppa and Ppw, it is not surprising that many physicians err in their interpretation of PAC data.[52,53] Further, PAC use is accompanied by complications, and it can be argued that the hemodynamic data obtained can be deduced by clinical examination, are not helpful in clinical decision making, or do not improve outcome.[54,55] However, physicians err in their clinical evaluations,[56–57] so it seems reasonable to encourage the informed use of PAC to obtain hemodynamic data when there is clinical uncertainty and when those data will be used to titrate aspects of the patient's management.

PULMONARY EDEMA

Figure 20-11 shows a schematic diagram depicting the circulatory factors governing the movement of edema (Q̇E) between the pulmonary vessels and the lung interstitial tissues; the Starling equation describing lung liquid flux is written beneath the figure. The hydrostatic pressure in the microvessels of the lung (Pmv = 12 mm Hg) lies about halfway between Ppa (normally about 15 mm Hg) and LVEDP (normally about 10 mm Hg). Hydrostatic pressure in the septal interstitial space (Pis = −4 mm Hg) is subatmospheric, in part because it drains into the peribronchovascular interstitium, which has a more negative pressure, and in part because lymph vessels, valved like veins for unidirectional flow, actively remove liquid from the interstitial spaces that have intrinsic structural stability to resist collapse.[58] Accordingly, there is a positive hydrostatic pressure (Pmv − Pis = 16 mm Hg) driving edema across the microvascular endothelium to the lung septal interstitium. The vascular wall presents a barrier to this bulk flow of liquid characterized by its permeability to water (K_f; mL edema/min per mm Hg); K_f includes surface area (S) and thus is heavily weighted by the characteristics of the alveolar vessels, where so much S resides.[58] The microvascular membrane is also characterized by its permeability to circulating proteins, dominated by albumin and globulin. If these plasma proteins were completely reflected ($\sigma = 1$), no protein would pass from lung blood to the interstitium; in contrast, if the microvascular membrane were freely permeable ($\sigma = 0$), interstitial protein concentration (CL), as measured in lung lymph, would equal that of plasma proteins (Cp). CL/Cp is about 0.6 in the normal steady-state edema flow in most mammals; when $\dot{Q}E$, as estimated from lung lymph flow ($\dot{Q}L$), is progressively increased by elevating Pmv, CL/Cp decreases to a plateau value of about 0.3. This plateau value indicates the microvascular protein reflection coefficient ($\sigma = 1\,2\,CL/Cp = 0.7$) measured in conditions of high edema flow; at lower $\dot{Q}E$ levels, water diffuses from the interstitium to the blood along the concentration gradient for water established by $Cp > CL$.[58]

In cardiogenic pulmonary edema, $\dot{Q}E$ is increased by increasing Pmv. Several factors act to keep the lungs from accumulating excess liquid: lymphatic flow increases, CL/Cp decreases, and Pis increases. The increased septal Pis drives edema through tissue planes toward the intraparenchymal peribronchovascular interstitium, where Pis is rendered even more subatmospheric (-10 mm Hg) by the outward pull of alveolar walls on the adventitia surrounding the relatively stiff bronchi and vessels.[58] This adventitial pull renders Pis even more negative with each inspiration, creating a cyclic suction to move edema from the alveolar septa toward the hilum of the lung, where peribronchovascular interstitial pressures are most negative, where the tissues have the largest capacity to accommodate the edema, and where the most dense accumulation of lymphatics is arranged to clear the edema to the systemic veins. This accounts for the Kerley lines, the bronchial cuffing, and the perihilar "butterfly" distribution of interstitial cardiogenic pulmonary edema on the chest radiograph. When edema genesis continues to fill these interstitial reservoirs, Pis rises at the alveolar septa, disrupting tight junctions between alveolar type I epithelium to flood the airspaces. Histologic morphometry of edematous lungs shows that flooded alveoli have about one-eighth the volume of unflooded alveoli, indicating that a relatively small volume of alveolar edema floods eight times that volume of airspace; for example, in a patient with an end-expired lung gas volume of 4 L, 250 mL of alveolar edema fills half the airspaces ($8 \times 250 = 2$ L), accounting for a large intrapulmonary shunt and for a large reduction in CL because only half the lung is ventilated.[22]

In the exudative phase of ARDS, a greater proportion of noncardiogenic edema accumulates in airspaces, so there is a much greater shunt per edema volume than in cardiogenic edema. Presumably, this different distribution of edema occurs because the lung injury that increases K_f and decreases S also damages the alveolar epithelial barrier, so increased $\dot{Q}E$ has access to a low-resistance pathway to a very large reservoir for edema—the airspaces of the lung.[59] Often, the hydrostatic pressure driving edema from vessels to airspace is normal or reduced; as $\dot{Q}E$ increases at normal Pmv after an acute lung injury, CL/Cp does not decrease as in cardiogenic edema but increases slightly to a value of about 0.8, so the reflection coefficient decreases ($\sigma = 1\,2\,CL/Cp = 0.2$ L). Accordingly, alveolar fluid protein concentration (CA) approaches Cp in ARDS but is much lower than Cp in cardiogenic edema.[56] When the vascular membrane is repaired, alveolar edema is cleared very slowly from noninjured lungs by active transport of sodium; water follows the osmotic gradient through an intact alveolar membrane, and this clearance raises CA above Cp as a clinical marker of recovery from ARDS.[60]

PEEP increases end-expired lung volume to decrease Pis and increase capacity in the peribronchovascular intersti-

TABLE 20-3 Therapeutic Goals in Acute Hypoxemic Respiratory Failure

1. Seek the least PEEP providing 90% saturation of an adequate hematocrit (>30%) on nontoxic FIO_2 (<.6)
2. Seek the least tidal volume providing adequate CO_2 elimination (pH > 7.2)
3. Seek the least circulatory volume or Ppw providing adequate CO and DO_2

ABBREVIATIONS: DO_2, O_2 delivery; FIO_2, fraction inspired O_2; PEEP, positive end-expiratory pressure.

tium; this in turn redistributes much of the alveolar edema into this interstitial reservoir, associated with the aeration of flooded airspaces at a much larger alveolar volume to reduce shunt and to increase CL without altering the amount of edema.[11,12,61] Because lung volume increases greatly when PEEP is effective in redistributing edema, Ppl must increase to push the chest wall to an equivalently higher volume (see Fig. 20-5). This raises Pra to reduce VR and BP[4,5,20] unless the patient's baroreceptor reflexes, iatrogenic infusions of fluid, or vasoactive drugs maintain Pms and $\dot{Q}T$.[25,62] As illustrated in Fig. 20-9, this recruitment of previously flooded airspaces occurs within the large P-V hysteresis of the edematous lung, so less PEEP is required than that indicated by the inflection point of the inflation P-V curve.[63]

AN APPROACH TO MANAGING ACUTE HYPOXEMIC RESPIRATORY FAILURE

As with many therapeutic interventions in critical illness, too much can cause harm, so it is helpful to define the goal of each intervention and then use the mildest intervention to achieve that goal. Ventilator management of pulmonary edema causing AHRF is summarized in Table 20-3. Because the aim of PEEP therapy is to maintain arterial saturation (>90%) of an adequate circulating hemoglobin (<12 g%) on a nontoxic fraction inspired O_2 (FIO_2; <0.6)—all to effect adequate DO_2 without aggravating the lung injury with oxygen toxicity—it is helpful to use the least PEEP to achieve these goals so as not to reduce $\dot{Q}T$. Because PEEP already increases end-expired lung volume, superimposed large tidal volumes cause pulmonary barotraumas, further reduce VR, and contribute to mortality; using the least tidal volume (e.g., 6 mL/kg ideal body weight) effecting adequate CO_2 elimination at an increased rate minimizes these complications. It is remarkable how rapidly PEEP redistributes edema to reduce hypoxemia (in minutes) and how rapidly the shunt returns when PEEP is removed. Accordingly, the informed physician can implement an effective, tolerable estimate of least PEEP in less than 15 minutes in ventilated patients in whom BP and pulse oximetry are being monitored continuously. Beginning with a small tidal volume (6 mL/kg), high respiratory rate (30 breaths/min), and FIO_2 of 1 in a well-sedated patient, PEEP is increased by 5 cm H_2O every minute from 0 to 20 minutes. If BP does not decrease and arterial O_2 saturation (SaO_2) remains 95%, FIO_2 is reduced to 0.8 for 5 minutes and then to 0.7 and 0.6 at 5-minute intervals. If SaO_2 still exceeds 95%, PEEP is reduced by 5 cm H_2O every 5 minutes until SaO_2 is greater than 90% and then increased by 2 to 3 cm H_2O to restore SaO_2 to less than 90%. A decrease in BP as PEEP is initially increased indicates relative circulatory hypovolemia, so PEEP must be reduced again until $\dot{Q}_T$ and BP are restored with volume infusion including packed red blood cells to achieve an adequate hematocrit or with an infusion of dobutamine titrated from 1 to 10 μg/kg per minute to maintain $\dot{Q}_T$ at a lower circulatory volume and Ppw. Similarly, if the initial F_{IO_2} reductions decrease Sa_{O_2} by less than 90%, PEEP should be increased in 2.5-cm H_2O increments above 20 cm H_2O until Sa_{O_2} is high enough to allow F_{IO_2} reduction; at this stage, it is prudent to reduce the tidal volume further. When PEEP is effective, plans to prevent its inadvertent removal, as during routine bedside suctioning, can prevent sudden hypoxemic cardiovascular catastrophe.

Cardiovascular management of cardiogenic and noncardiogenic edema aims to reduce edema formation and accumulation without inducing inadequate $\dot{Q}_T$ or D_{O_2} (see Table 20-3), thereby decreasing the duration and complications of intensive care.[62] Cardiogenic edema is caused by high Pmv, often related to acute or acute-on-chronic LV dysfunction that increases LVEDP. Reducing the central blood volume by venodilating agents (e.g., morphine, furosemide, or nitroglycerin) or procedures (e.g., rotating tourniquets, phlebotomy, or diuresis) reduces LVEDP and edema genesis, but excess preload reduction will adversely reduce $\dot{Q}_T$ from a poorly functioning ventricle that often requires a higher LVEDP (16 to 30 mm Hg) than normal (8 to 12 mm Hg). Where indicated, vasoactive drugs to enhance systolic function (e.g., dobutamine, milrinone, nitroglycerin, or oxygen) or reduce afterload (e.g., enalaprilat, calcium channel blockers, or nitroprusside) and measures to correct diastolic dysfunction (e.g., prolong filling time, maintain coordinated atrial contraction, or correct myocardial hypoxia and ischemia) act to reduce the LVEDP required for adequate $\dot{Q}_T$ and thus reduce cardiogenic edema formation by the Starling equation. Increasing π_{mv} by colloid infusion also reduces edema formation, provided Pmv is not increased; an albumin infusion that raises π_{mv} from 15 to 20 mm Hg and Pmv from 25 to 30 mm Hg causes more $\dot{Q}_E$ because $\sigma = 0.7$.

Colloid infusion is even less helpful in reducing noncardiogenic edema, where σ is much reduced. In one study of oleic acid-induced noncardiogenic edema in dogs, raising π_{mv} by 5 mm Hg had no effect on edema when Pmv was not allowed to change, but lowering Pmv by 5 mm Hg (when π_{mv} did not change) reduced edema by 50% over the same 4 hours of treatment.[57] Compelling evidence in other animal[64–67] and clinical studies[31–33] of acute lung injury supports the therapeutic effect of reducing pulmonary vascular pressures in reducing pulmonary edema (Fig. 20-12), and this is currently being tested prospectively in patients with acute lung injury and ARDS (ARDS Network Fluid and Catheter Treatment Trial). When noncardiogenic edema occurs at normal or low Pmv, the reduction of LVEDP by only 5 mm Hg reduces LVEDV, SV, and $\dot{Q}_T$ by as much as a 20 mm Hg reduction in LVEDP in cardiogenic edema. Accordingly, reducing the measured Ppw in a patient with acute lung injury must avoid causing inadequate $\dot{Q}_T$ and D_{O_2}. As in cardiogenic edema, Ppw can be reduced considerably without evidence of inadequate output and D_{O_2}, and vasoactive drugs and increased hematocrit are effective in restoring adequacy of D_{O_2} at low Ppw when indicated. This approach constantly seeks the least Ppw associated with an adequate $\dot{Q}_T$ and D_{O_2} during the early stage of edema formation in ARDS. Of course, this is only

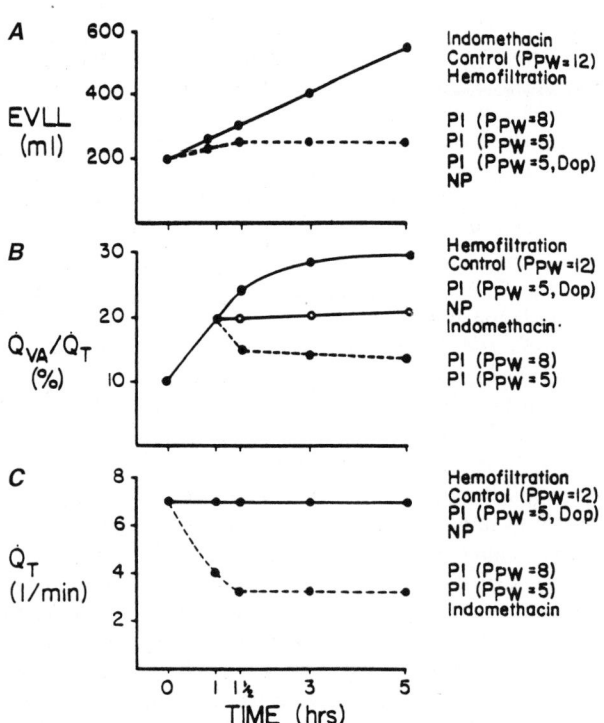

FIGURE 20-12 Schematic diagram illustrating the effects of reducing pulmonary wedge pressure (Ppw) 1 hour after hydrochloric acid or kerosene aspiration at time 0 hour (*abscissa*) on extravascular lung liquid (EVLL by thermal dilution; *A*), shunt ($\dot{Q}_{VA}/\dot{Q}_T$; *B*), and cardiac output ($\dot{Q}_T$; *C*). Data are compiled from six studies by the same group with similar experimental protocols. *A.* Edema increases linearly with time after injury in the control group (Ppw = 12 mm Hg, *continuous line*), but reduction of Ppw to 8 or 5 mm Hg at 1 hour by plasmapheresis (PI) or sodium nitroprusside (NP) attenuates or stops edema accumulation (*interrupted line*) such that EVLL is less than half that in the control group by 5 hours; all EVLL values were confirmed by gravimetric edema measures in the lungs excised at 5 hours. Hemofiltration to a Ppw of 5 mm Hg did not reduce edema, and indomethacin had no effect on edemagenesis when Ppw was kept the same as in the control group. *B.* Shunt increased in a curvilinear manner to about 30% as EVLL increased with time in the control group (*continuous line through closed circles*); when Ppw was reduced by plasmapheresis, $\dot{Q}_{VA}/\dot{Q}_T$ stopped increasing and actually decreased to about 15% owing in part to reduced edema. Dopamine and NP also decreased $\dot{Q}_{VA}/\dot{Q}_T$ and edema; moreover, dopamine and NP also decreased $\dot{Q}_{VA}/\dot{Q}_T$ when they reduced edema (*continuous line through open circles*), but $\dot{Q}_{VA}/\dot{Q}_T$ was greater in these groups than in plasmapheresis alone (*interrupted line*) because the vasoactive drugs increased $\dot{Q}_T$; similarly, indomethacin reduced $\dot{Q}_{VA}/\dot{Q}_T$ compared with the control group despite similar edema because $\dot{Q}_T$ decreased (see *C*). *C.* $\dot{Q}_T$ did not change with time when Ppw was maintained in the control group; when Ppw was reduced by plasmapheresis, $\dot{Q}_T$ was maintained equal to the control group by dopamine and NP (*continuous line*). Plasmapheresis reduced $\dot{Q}_T$ by decreasing Ppw (*interrupted line*) but reduced oxygen delivery less by increasing the hematocrit. Indomethacin reduced $\dot{Q}_T$ at the same Ppw (*interrupted line*) but reduced oxygen delivery less by increasing the hemocrit. Indomethacin reduced $\dot{Q}_T$ at the same Ppw, suggesting decreased ventricular function; as a consequence, $\dot{Q}_{VA}/\dot{Q}_T$ decreased with no change in edema.

symptomatic treatment; as yet there are no specific therapies for the acute lung injury that correct an increased K_f and a reduced S. The aim is to minimize the edema consequences of vascular injury and thereby shorten duration of ventilation and care in the intensive care unit.[31–33]

References

1. Goldberg HS, Rabson J: Control of cardiac output by systemic vessels. *Am J Cardiol* 47:696, 1981.

2. Wood LDH: The cardiovascular system, in Hall JB, Schmidt GA, Wood LDH (eds): *Principles of Critical Care*. New York, McGraw-Hill, 1992, p 26.

3. Sarnoff SJ: Myocardial contractility as described by ventricular function curves: Observations on Starling's law of the heart. *Physiol Rev* 35:107, 1955.

4. Prewitt RM, Wood LDH: The effect of positive end-expiratory pressure on ventricular function in dogs. *Am J Physiol* 45:H534, 1979.

5. Prewitt RM, Oppenheimer L, Sutherland JB, Wood LDH: The effects of positive end-expiratory pressure on left ventricular mechanics in patients with hypoxemic respiratory failure. *Anesthesiology* 55:409, 1981.

6. Spencer KT, Lang RM: Diastolic heart failure. *Postgrad Med* 101:63,1997.

7. Taylor RR, Coveld JW, Sonnenblick EH, Ross J: Dependence of ventricular distensibility on filling of the opposite ventricle. *Am J Physiol* 213:711, 1967.

8. Craven KD, Wood LDH: Extrapericardial and esophageal pressures with positive end expiratory pressure in dogs. *J Appl Physiol* 51:798, 1981.

9. Pinsky MR, Desmet J-M, Vincent J: Effect of positive end-expiratory pressure on right ventricular function in humans. *Am Rev Respir Dis* 146:681, 1992.

10. Sagawa K: End-systolic pressure-volume relationship in retrospect and prospect. *Fed Proc* 43:2399, 1984.

11. Kass DA, Maughn WL, Guo ZM, et al: Comparative influence of load versus inotropic states on indices of ventricular contractility. *Circulation* 76:1422, 1987.

12. Walley KR, Becker CJ, Hogan RA, et al: Progressive hypoxemia limits left ventricular oxygen consumption and contractility. *Circ Res* 63:849, 1988.

13. Walley KR, Lewis TH, Wood LDH: Acute respiratory acidosis decreases left ventricular contractility but increases cardiac output. *Circ Res* 67:628, 1990.

14. Carroll JD, Lang RM, Neuman AL, et al: The differential effects of positive inotropic and vasodilator therapy on diastolic properties in patients with congestive cardiomyopathy. *Circulation* 74:815, 1985.

15. Prewitt RM, Wood LDH: Effects of altered resistive load on left ventricular systolic mechanics in dogs. *Anesthesiology* 56:195, 1982.

16. Chadda K, Annane D, Hart N, et.al: Cardiac and respiratory effects of continuous positive airway pressure and noninvasive ventilation in acute cardiac pulmonary edema. *Crit Care Med* 30:2457, 2002.

17. Mitzner W, Goldberg HS: Effects of epinephrine on resistive and compliant properties of the canine vasculature. *J Appl Physiol* 39:272, 1975.

18. Mitzner W, Goldberg HS, Lichtenstein S: Effect of thoracic blood volume changes on steady state cardiac output. *Circ Res* 38:255, 1976.

19. Fermoso JD, Richardson QT, Guyton AC: Mechanism of decrease in cardiac output caused by opening the chest. *Am J Physiol* 207:1112, 1964.

20. Fessler HE, Brower RG, Wise RA, Permutt S: Effects of positive end-expiratory pressure on the gradient for venous return. *Am Rev Respir Dis* 19:143, 1991.

21. Pare PD, Warriner E, Baile M, Hogg JC: Redistribution of pulmonary extravascular lung water with positive end-expiratory pressure in canine pulmonary edema. *Am Rev Respir Dis* 127:590, 1983.

22. Malo J, Ali J, Wood LDH: How does positive end-expiratory pressure reduce intrapulmonary shunt in canine pulmonary edema? *J Appl Physiol* 57:1002, 1984.

23. Pinsky M, Vincent J-L, Desmet J-M: Estimating left ventricular filling pressure during positive end-expiratory pressure in humans. *Am Rev Respir Dis* 143:25, 1991.

24. Hall JB, Wood LDH: Acute hypoxemic respiratory failure. *Med Grand Rounds* 3:183, 1984.

25. Wood LDH, Hall JB: A mechanistic approach to providing adequate oxygenation in acute hypoxemic respiratory failure. *Respir Care* 38:784, 1993.

26. Siegal JH, Cerra FB, Coleman B, et al: Physiological and metabolic correlations in human sepsis. *Surgery* 186:163, 1979.

27. Vary TC: Increased pyruvate dehydrogenase kinase activity in response to sepsis. *Am J Physiol* 260:E669, 1991.

28. Curtis SE, Cain SM: Regional and systemic oxygen deliver/uptake relations and lactate flux in hyperdynamic, endotoxin treated dogs. *Am Rev Respir Dis* 145:348, 1992.

29. Hayes MA, Timmins AC, Yau EHS, et al: Elevation of systemic oxygen delivery in the treatment of critically ill patients. *N Engl J Med* 330:1717, 1994.

30. Gattinoni L, Brazzi L, Pelosi P, et al: A trial of goal-oriented hemodynamic therapy in critically ill patients. *N Engl J Med* 333:1025, 1995.

31. Humphrey H, Hall J, Sznajder F, et al: Improved survival in ARDS patients associated with a reduction in pulmonary capillary wedge pressure. *Chest* 97:1176, 1990.

32. Schuller D, Mitchell JP, Calandrino FS, Schuster DP: Fluid balance during pulmonary edema: Is fluid gain a marker or a cause of poor outcome? *Chest* 100:1068, 1991.

33. Mitchell JP, Schuller D, Calandrino FS, Schuster DP: Improved outcome based on fluid management in critically ill patients requiring pulmonary artery catheterization. *Am Rev Respir Dis* 145:990, 1992.

34. Parker MM, Shelhamer JH, Bacharach SL, et al: Profound but reversible myocardial depression in patients with septic shock. *Ann Intern Med* 100:483, 1984.

35. Granton JT, Goddard CM, Allard MF, et al: Leukocytes and decreased left ventricular contractility during endotoxemia in rabbits. *Am J Respir Crit Care Med* 155:1977, 1997.

36. Manthous CA, Schumacker PT, Pohlman A, et al: Absence of supply dependence of oxygen consumption in patients with septic shock. *J Crit Care* 8:203, 1993.

37. Marik PE, Mohedin M: The contrasting effects of dopamine and norepinephrine on systemic and splanchnic oxygen utilization in hyperdynamic sepsis. *JAMA* 272:1354, 1994.

38. Meir-Hellman A, Reinahrt K, Bredle D, et al: Epinephrine impairs splanchnic perfusion in septic shock. *Crit Care Med* 25:399, 1997.

39. Desjars P, Pinaud M, Brignon D, et al: Norephinephrine therapy has no deleterious renal effects in human septic shock. *Crit Care Med* 17:426, 1989.

40. Nevière R, Chagnon J-L, Vallet B: Dobutamine improves gastrointestinal mucosal blood flow in a porcine model of endotoxic shock. *Crit Care Med* 25: 1371, 1997.

41. Manthous CA, Hall JB, Kushner R, et al: The effect of mechanical ventilation on oxygen consumption in critically ill patients. *Am J Respir Crit Care Med* 151:210, 1995.

42. Manthous CA, Hall JB, Olson D, et al: Effect of cooling on oxygen consumption in febrile critically ill patients. *Am J Respir Crit Care Med* 151:10, 1995.

43. Levin TN: Acute congestive heart failure: The need for aggressive therapy. *Postgrad Med* 101:97, 1997.

44. Scharf SM, Bianco JA, Tow DD, et al: The effects of large negative intrathoracic pressure on left ventricular function in patients with coronary artery disease. *Circulation* 63:871, 1981.

45. Bicknell WH, Wall MJ, Pepe PE, et al: Immediate versus delayed fluid resuscitation for hypotensive patients with penetrating torso injuries. *N Engl J Med* 331:1105, 1994.

46. Brown J, MacKinnon D, King A, et al: Elevated arterial blood pressure in cardiac tamponade. *N Engl J Med* 327:463, 1992.

47. Ducas J, Prewitt RM: Pathophysiology and therapy of right ventricular dysfunction due to pulmonary embolism. *Cardiovasc Clin* 17:191, 1987.

48. Layish DT, Tapson VF: Pharmacologic hemodynamic support in massive pulmonary embolism. *Chest* 111:218, 1997.

49. Lorell B, Leinbach RC, Pohost GM: Right ventricular infarction: Clinical diagnosis and differentiation from cardiac tamponade and pericardial construction. *Am J Cardiol* 43:465, 1979.

50. Dell'Italia LJ, Starling MR, Blumhardt R, et al: Comparative effects of volume loading, dobutamine and nitroprusside in patients with predominant right ventricular infarction. *Circulation* 72:1327, 1985.

51. Teboul J-L, Besbes M, Andrivet P, et al: A bedside index assessing the reliability of pulmonary artery occlusion pressure measurements during mechanical ventilation with positive end-expiratory pressure. *J Crit Care* 7:22, 1992.

52. Connors AF, McCaffree DR, Gray BA: Evaluation of right heart catheterization in the critically ill patient without acute myocardial infarction. *N Engl J Med* 308:263, 1983.

53. Iberti TJ, Fischer EP, Leibowitz AB, et al: A multicentre study of physicians' knowledge of the pulmonary artery catheter. *JAMA* 264:2928, 1990.

54. Sandham JD, Hull RD, Brant RF, et.al: A randomized, controlled trial of the use of pulmonary-artery catheters in high-risk surgical patients. *N Engl J Med* 348: 5, 2003.

55. Richard C, Warszawski J, Anguel N, et.al: Early use of the pulmonary artery catheter and outcomes in patients with shock and acute respiratory distress syndrome: a randomized controlled trial. JAMA 290: 2713, 2003.

56. Connors AF, Dawson NV, Shaw PK, et al: Hemodynamic status in critically ill patients with and without acute heart disease. *Chest* 98:1200, 1990.

57. Steingrub JS, Celoria G, Vickers-Lahti M, et al: Therapeutic impact of pulmonary artery catheterization in a medical/surgical ICU. *Chest* 99:1451, 1991.

58. Taylor A, Parker J: Interstitial spaces and lymphatics, in Fishman AP, Fisher AB (eds): *Handbook of Physiology, Volume I, Section 3: The Respiratory System, Circulation and Nonrespiratory Function.* Bethesda, American Physiological Society, 1984, p 167.

59. Montaver JSG, Tsang J, Evans KG, et al: Alveolar epithelial damage: A critical difference between high pressure and oleic acid-induced low pressure edema. *J Clin Invest* 77:1786, 1986.

60. Matthay MA, Wiener-Kronish JP: Intact epithelial barrier functions is critical for the resolution of alveolar edema in humans. *Am Rev Respir Dis* 142:1250, 1990.

61. Prewitt RM, McCarthy J, Wood LDH: Treatment of acute low pressure pulmonary edema in dogs: Relative effects of hydrostatic and oncotic pressure, nitroprusside and PEEP. *J Clin Invest* 67:409, 1981.

62. Wood LDH, Prewitt RM: Cardiovascular management in acute hypoxemic respiratory failure. *Am J Cardiol* 47:963, 1981.

63. Amato MBP, Barbas CSV, Medeiros DM, et al: Beneficial effects of the "open lung approach" with low distending pressures in acute respiratory distress syndrome: A prospective randomized study on mechanical ventilation. *Am J Respir Crit Care Med* 152:1835, 1995.

64. Long GR, Breen PH, Mayers I, Wood LDH: Treatment of canine aspiration pneumonitis: Fluid volume reduction versus fluid volume expansion. *J Appl Physiol* 65:1736, 1988.

65. Sznajder JI, Zucker AR, Wood LDH, Long GR: Effect of plasmapheresis and hemofiltration on acid aspiration pulmonary edema. *Am Rev Respir Dis* 134:222. 1986.

66. Gottlieb SS, Wood LDH, Hansen DE, Long GR: The effect of nitroprusside on pulmonary edema, oxygen exchange, and blood glow in hydrochloric acid aspiration. *Anesthesiology* 67:47, 1987.

67. Mayers I, Breen PH, Gottlieb S, et al: The effects of indomethacin on edema and gas exchange in canine acid aspiration. *Respir Physiol* 69:149, 1987.

Chapter 21
SHOCK
KEITH R. WALLEY

KEY POINTS

- *Shock is present when there is evidence of multisystem organ hypoperfusion; it often presents as decreased mean blood pressure.*

- *Initial resuscitation aims to establish adequate airway, breathing, and circulation. Rapid initial resuscitation (usefully driven by protocol) is fundamental for improved outcome, since "time is tissue."*

- *A working diagnosis or clinical hypothesis of the cause of inadequate circulation should always be made immediately, while treatment is initiated, based on clinical presentation, physical examination, and by observing the response to therapy.*

- *Drug and/or definitive therapy for specific causes of shock must be considered and implemented early (e.g., thrombolysis for myocardial infarction, hemostasis for hemorrhage, appropropriate antibiotics, and activated protein C for severe sepsis, etc.).*

- *The most common causes of shock are high cardiac output hypotension, or septic shock; reduced pump function of the heart, or cardiogenic shock; and reduced venous return despite normal pump function, or hypovolemic shock. Overlapping etiologies can confuse the diagnosis, as can a short list of other less common etiologies, which are often separated by echocardiography and pulmonary artery catheterization.*

- *Shock has a hemodynamic component, which is the focus of the initial resuscitation, but shock also has a systemic inflammatory component (ameliorated by rapid initial resuscitation) that leads to adverse sequelae including subsequent organ system dysfunction.*

This chapter discusses shock with respect to the bedside approach: first with an early working diagnosis, then an approach to urgent resuscitation that confirms or changes the working diagnosis, followed by a pause to ponder the broader differential diagnosis of the types of shock and the pathophysiology of shock leading to potential adverse sequelae. Effective initial diagnosis and treatment at a rapid pace depend in large part on understanding cardiovascular pathophysiology.

Establishing a Working Diagnosis of the Cause of Shock

DEFINITION OF SHOCK

Shock is present if evidence of multisystem organ hypoperfusion is apparent. Evidence of hypoperfusion includes tachycardia, tachypnea, low mean blood pressure, diaphoresis, poorly perfused skin and extremities, altered mental status, and decreased urine output. Hypotension has special importance because it commonly occurs during shock, be-cause blood pressure is easily measured, and because extreme hypotension always results in shock. Important caveats are: (1) relatively low blood pressure is normal in some healthy individuals and (2) systolic blood pressure may be preserved in some patients in shock by excessive sympathetic tone. In the latter case, it is important to anticipate that sedation will unmask hypotension. Further, cuff blood pressure measurements may markedly underestimate central blood pressure in low flow states.[1] The focus of initial resuscitation is reversing the hemodynamic component of shock, which leads to tissue hypoxia and lactic acidosis. However, all types of shock are also associated with a systemic inflammatory component that is a key contributor to subsequent multisystem organ failure and death. The development of the systemic inflammatory component is minimized by rapid and adequate (usefully driven by protocol) initial resuscitation.[2]

A QUESTIONING APPROACH TO THE INITIAL CLINICAL EXAMINATION

Mean blood pressure is the product of cardiac output and systemic vascular resistance (SVR). Accordingly, hypotension may be caused by reduced cardiac output or reduced SVR. Therefore, initial examination of the hypotensive patient seeks to answer the question: Is cardiac output reduced? High cardiac output hypotension is most often signaled by a high pulse pressure, a low diastolic pressure, warm extremities with good nail bed return, fever (or hypothermia), leukocytosis (or leukopenia), and other evidence of infection; these clinical findings strongly suggest a working diagnosis of septic shock (Table 21-1), the initial treatment for which is thoughtful antibiosis combined with rapid expansion of the vascular volume and subsequent vasopressors, inotropes, and blood transfusion as necessary to achieve an adequate mean arterial pressure (MAP) and central venous oxygen saturation (Scv_{O_2}; see below).

In contrast, low cardiac output is signaled by a low pulse pressure, mottled cyanotic skin, and cool extremities with poor nail bed return. In this case, clinical examination turns to a second question: Is the heart too full? A heart that is too full in a hypotensive patient is signaled by elevated jugular venous pressure, peripheral edema, crepitations on lung auscultation, a laterally displaced precordial apical impulse with extra heart sounds (S_3, S_4), chest pain, ischemic changes on the electrocardiogram, and a chest radiograph showing a large heart with dilated upper lobe vessels and pulmonary edema.[3] These findings suggest cardiogenic shock, most often caused by ischemic heart disease, and are generally absent when low cardiac output results from hypovolemia (see Table 21-1). Clinical examination then shows manifestations of blood loss (hematemesis, tarry stools, abdominal distention, reduced hematocrit, or trauma) or manifestations of dehydration (reduced tissue turgor, vomiting or diarrhea, or negative fluid balance). This distinction between cardiogenic and hypovolemic shock allows initial therapy to focus on vasoactive drugs and on volume infusions, respectively.

Whenever the clinical formulation is not obvious after answering the first two questions, ask a third: What does not fit? Most often, the answer is that the hypotension is due to overlap of two or more of these common etiologies of

TABLE 21-1 Rapid Formulation of an Early Working Diagnosis of the Etiology of Shock

Defining features of shock	
Blood pressure	↓
Heart rate	↑
Respiratory rate	↑
Mentation	↓
Urine output	↓
Arterial pH	↓

	High-Output Hypotension Septic Shock	Low Cardiac Cardiogenic and Hypovolemic Shock
Is cardiac output reduced?	No	Yes
Pulse pressure	↑	↓
Diastolic pressure	↓	↓
Extremities/digits	Warm	Cool
Nail bed return	Rapid	Slow
Heart sounds	Crisp	Muffled
Temperature	↑ or ↓	↔
White cell count	↑ or ↓	↔
Site of infection	++	—

	Reduced Pump Function, Cardiogenic Shock	Reduced Venous Return, Hypovolemic Shock
Is the heart too full?	Yes	No
Symptoms clinical context	Angina on electrocardiogram	Hemorrhage dehydration
Jugular venous pressure	↑	↓
S₃, S₄, gallop rhythm	+++	—
Respiratory crepitations	+++	—
Chest radiograph	Large heart ↑ Upper lobe flow Pulmonary edema	Normal

What does not fit?
Overlapping etiologies (septic cardiogenic, septic hypovolemic, cardiogenic hypovolemic)
Short list of other etiologies

High-output hypotension	High right atrial pressure	Nonresponsive hypovolemia
Liver failure	hypotension	Adrenal insufficiency
Severe pancreatitis	Pulmonary hypertension	Anaphylaxis
Trauma with significant	(Most often pulmonary	Spinal shock
systemic inflammatory	embolus)	
response	Right ventricular infarction	
Thyroid storm	Cardiac tamponade	
Arteriovenous fistula		
Paget disease		

Get more information
Echocardiography, right heart
  catheterization

shock: septic shock complicated by myocardial dysfunction or hypovolemia, cardiogenic shock complicated by hypovolemia or sepsis, and hypovolemic shock masking sepsis or ischemic heart disease. At this time, more data are frequently needed, especially aided by echocardiography and pulmonary artery catheterization. Interpretations of the data and response to initial therapy frequently confirm the multiple etiologies or lead to a broader differential diagnosis of the etiologies of shock (see below). A short list of common etiologies other than septic, cardiogenic, or hypovolemic shock can be grouped as they present (see Table 21-1): high cardiac output hypotension that does not appear to be caused by sepsis, high right atrial pressure hypotension not caused by left ventricular ischemia, and poorly responsive hypovolemic shock.

Urgent Initial Resuscitation

PRIMARY SURVEY

Early institution of aggressive resuscitation improves a patient's chances of survival.[2,4] To improve efficiency at the necessarily rapid tempo, a systematic approach to initial evaluation and resuscitation is useful as it is during cardiac emergencies (advanced cardiac life support [ACLS]) and trauma (advanced trauma life support [ATLS]). In analogy to these systematic "ABC" approaches, a primary survey includes establishing an airway (*airway*), choosing a ventilator mode and small tidal volumes that minimize ventilator-induced lung injury (*breathing*), rapid (usefully protocol driven) resuscitation of the inadequate circulation

(*circulation*), and *drugs/definitive therapy* consisting of early consideration and implementation of definitive therapy for specific causes of shock (e.g., thrombolysis or angioplasty for myocardial infarction; hemostasis for hemorrhage; appropriate antibiotics, surgical drainage of abscess, activated protein C, and steroids for severe sepsis; etc.).

AIRWAY

Almost all patients in shock have one or more indications for airway intubation and mechanical ventilation (Table 21-2), which should be instituted early. Significant hypoxemia (based on blood-gas analysis, pulse oximetry, or high clinical suspicion) is one indication for airway intubation because external masks and other devices do not reliably deliver an adequate fraction of inspired O_2 ($F_{I_{O_2}}$). Initially, a high $F_{I_{O_2}}$ (100%) is used until blood-gas analysis or reliable pulse oximetry allows titration of the $F_{I_{O_2}}$ down toward less toxic concentrations.

Ventilatory failure is another indication for airway intubation and mechanical ventilation. Elevated and rising partial pressure of CO_2 in arterial blood reliably establishes the diagnosis of ventilatory failure but is often a late finding. In particular, young, previously healthy patients are able to defend partial pressure of CO_2 (P_{CO_2}) and pH up until a precipitous respiratory arrest. Therefore, clinical signs of respiratory muscle fatigue or subtle evidence of inadequate ventilation are more important early indicators.[5] Evidence of respiratory muscle fatigue, including labored breathing precluding more than rudimentary verbal responses, tachypnea greater than 40/minute or an inappropriately low and decreasing respiratory rate, abdominal paradoxical respiratory motion, accessory muscle use, and other manifestations of ventilatory failure such as inadequately compensated acidemia should lead to early elective intubation and ventilation of the patient in shock (see Chap. 31).

Obtundation, due to shock or other causes, resulting in inadequate airway protection is an important indication for intubation. In shock, airway intubation and mechanical ventilation should precede other complicated procedures, such as central venous catheterization, or complicated tests that require transportation of the patient because these procedures and tests restrict the medical staff's ability to continuously assess the airway and ensure adequacy of ventilation.

TABLE 21-2 Indications for Intubation in Shock Patients

Indication	Why
Hypoxemia	High $F_{I_{O_2}}$ is not guaranteed by oxygen masks; PEEP can be added
Ventilatory failure (inappropriately high P_{CO_2}, signs of ventilatory muscle fatigue)	Ensure adequate CO_2 removal Correct hypoxia due to hypoventilation Prevent sudden respiratory arrest
Vital organ hypoperfusion	Rest ventilatory muscles (and divert cardiac output to hypoperfused vital organs)
Obtundation	Protect and ensure an adequate airway

ABBREVIATIONS: $F_{I_{O_2}}$, fraction of inspired O_2; P_{CO_2}, partial pressure of CO_2; PEEP, positive end-expiratory pressure.

BREATHING

Initially, mechanical ventilation with sedation and, if necessary, paralysis are instituted to remove work of breathing as a confounding factor from the initial resuscitation and diagnostic pathway and to redistribute limited blood flow to vital organs.[6] The change from spontaneous breathing (negative intrathoracic pressure ventilation) to mechanical ventilation (positive intrathoracic pressure ventilation) leads to reduced venous return so that additional volume resuscitation must be anticipated when hypovolemia contributes to shock. Application of positive end-expiratory pressure (increases intrathoracic pressure) and administration of sedative or narcotic drugs (increases venous capacitance) similarly should be expected to reduce venous return and highlight the importance of aggressive volume resuscitation at the time of intubation and institution of mechanical ventilation in hypovolemic patients. Conversely, when hypovolemia is not a problem (e.g., cardiogenic shock), application of positive intrathoracic pressure may improve cardiac output and blood pressure.

A relatively small tidal volume (6 to 8 mL/kg) should be selected to minimize hypotension due to high intrathoracic pressures and, more importantly, to reduce ventilator-induced lung injury.[7] When arterial hypoxemia due to acute lung injury or frank adult respiratory distress syndrome (ARDS) complicates shock, adherence to tidal volumes of 6 mL/kg ideal body weight significantly decreases mortality rate and number of days on a ventilator in the intensive care unit.[8]

CIRCULATION

Just as low tidal volumes limit ongoing lung inflammation and injury, rapid resuscitation of the circulation limits ongoing generation of a systemic inflammatory response and multiple organ injury. Hence, rapid protocol-driven approaches with defined end points improve shock outcome.[4,9] For all types of shock, "time is tissue." Thus, for cardiogenic shock secondary to acute myocardial infarction, the early goal is immediate thrombolysis, angioplasty, or surgical revascularization.[3] For hypovolemic shock due to hemorrhage, the early goal is immediate hemostasis and rapid volume resuscitation. The early goals of volume resuscitation in hypovolemic or septic shock are incorporated in the Early Goal-Directed Therapy algorithm (Fig. 21-1), which was initially designed to aid resuscitation of septic shock.[2] This requires immediate monitoring (even before formal admission to the intensive care unit) of MAP (goal > 65 mm Hg), central venous pressure (CVP; goal 8 to 12 mm Hg), and Scv_{O_2} (goal > 70%).

Volume

Aggressive volume resuscitation up to the point of a heart that is too full is the first step in resuscitation of the circulation. The rate and composition of volume expanders must be adjusted in accord with the working diagnosis. The Early Goal-Directed Therapy algorithm for resuscitation of septic shock calls for 500 mL saline every 30 minutes, but this is much too slow in hypovolemic patients in whom 1 L every 10 minutes, or faster, is initially required. During volume resuscitation, infusions must be sufficient to test the clinical hypothesis that the patient is hypovolemic by effecting a short-term end point indicating benefit (increased blood pressure and pulse

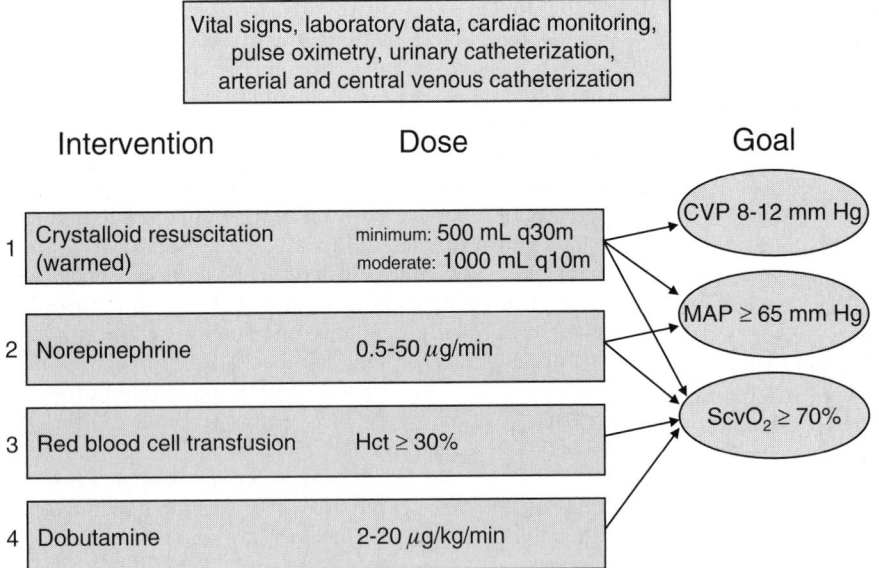

FIGURE 21-1 An approach to initial resuscitation of the circulation based on Early Goal-Directed Therapy. Cardiac monitoring, pulse oximetry, urinary catheterization, and arterial and central venous catheterizations must be instituted. Volume resuscitation is the initial step. If this is insufficient to raise mean arterial pressure (MAP) to 65 mm Hg, then vasopressors are the second step. Adequate tissue oxygenation (reflected by central venous O_2 saturation [Scv_{O_2}] > 70%) is a goal of all resuscitation interventions. If this Scv_{O_2} goal is not met by volume resuscitation and vasopressors, then red blood cell transfusion and inotrope infusion are the third and fourth interventions, respectively. When the goals of resuscitation are met, then reduction of vasopressor infusion, with further volume infusion if necessary, becomes a priority. CVP, central venous pressure; Hct, hematocrit. (*Adapted from Rivers et al.*[2])

pressure and decreased heart rate) or complication (increased jugular venous pressure and pulmonary edema). Absence of either response indicates an inadequate challenge, so the volume administered in the next interval must be greater than the previous one. In obvious hemorrhagic shock, immediate hemostasis is essential[10]; blood must be obtained early, warmed and filtered; blood substitutes are administered in large amounts (crystalloid or colloid solutions) until blood pressure increases or the heart becomes too full. At the other extreme, a working diagnosis of cardiogenic shock without obvious fluid overload requires a smaller volume challenge (250 mL NaCl in 20 minutes). In each case, and in all other types of shock, the next volume challenge depends on the response to the first; it should proceed soon after the first so that the physician does not miss the diagnostic clues evident only to the examining critical care team at the bedside during this urgent resuscitation (Table 21-3).

Role of Red Blood Cell Transfusion during Initial Resuscitation

Transfusion of red blood cells is a component of the initial volume resuscitation of shock when severe or ongoing blood loss contributes to shock. In addition, when anemia contributes to inadequate oxygen delivery so that mixed venous oxygen saturation or its surrogate Scv_{O_2} <70% despite an adequate CVP (8 to 12 mm Hg) and an adequate MAP (>65 mm Hg), then transfusion of red blood cells to hematocrit greater than 30% is a reasonable component of Early Goal-Directed Therapy and improves outcome.[2] After initial resuscitation and stabilization, transfusion of red blood cells to maintain a hemoglobin above 90 g/L is no more beneficial than maintaining a hemoglobin level above 70 g/L and only incurs additional transfusion risk.[11]

Is There a Role for Delayed Resuscitation of Hypovolemia?

During brisk ongoing hemorrhage, massive crystalloid or colloid resuscitation increases blood pressure and the rate of hemorrhage, so patient outcome may be worse.[12] This does not mean that resuscitation is detrimental; rather, control of active bleeding is more important than volume replacement. Preventing blood loss conserves warm, oxygen-carrying, protein-containing, biocompatible intravascular volume and is therefore far superior to replacing ongoing losses with fluids deficient in one or more of these areas. I and my colleagues believe that delayed or inadequate volume resuscitation, after blood loss is controlled, is a significant error that will have a detrimental effect on patient outcome.[10]

This approach of aggressive volume resuscitation avoids persistent hypovolemia as the cause for prolonged hypotension at the risk of causing pulmonary edema or aggravating the pumping dysfunction of the ischemic myocardium. We are not cavalier about fluid overload; just as soon as early resuscitation goals are met and as the heart becomes evaluated as too full, we shift goals to aim for the lowest circulating volume that provides adequate perfusion and O_2 delivery, but we emphasize that rational diagnosis and early resuscitation from shock require an adequate circulating volume before vasoactive drugs can be effective. Of course, the discerning intensivist is aware that the initial evaluation of some hypotensive patients demonstrates a heart that is too full, so vasoactive therapy starts immediately.

Vasopressors

Volume-resuscitated septic shock stands out as a challenging hemodynamic problem. Here the inflammatory component of shock is prominent; after vigorous volume resuscitation, right atrial pressure and cardiac output may be high, but MAP may be distressingly low and evidence of organ system hypoperfusion may persist (oliguria, impaired mentation, and lactic acidosis). Here there is a role for pressor agents. Whereas adequate cardiac output is more important than blood pressure (because adequate tissue oxygen delivery is the underlying issue), effective distribution of flow by the vascular system depends on an adequate pressure head. At pressures below an autoregulatory limit, normal flow distribution mechanisms are lost, so significant vital organ system hypoperfusion may persist in the face of elevated cardiac output

TABLE 21-3 Urgent Resuscitation of the Patient with Shock—Managing Factors Aggravating the Hypoperfusion State

Respiratory therapy
    Protect the airway—consider early elective intubation
    Prevent excess respiratory work—ventilate with small volumes
    Avoid respiratory acidosis—keep Pa_{CO_2} low
    Maintain oxygen delivery—FI_{O_2}, PEEP, hemoglobin
Infection in presumed septic shock (see Chap. 46)
    Empirical rational antibiosis for all probable etiologies
    Exclude allergies to antibiotics
    Search, incise, and drain abscesses (consider laparotomy)
Arrhythmias aggravating shock (see Chap. 24)
    Bradycardia
        Correct hypoxemia—FI_{O_2} of 1.0
        Atropine 0.6 mg, repeat × 2 for effect
        Increase dopamine to 10 mg/kg per minute
        Add isoproterenol (1–10 mg/min)
        Consider transvenous pacer
    Ventricular ectopy, tachycardia
        Detect and correct K^+, Ca^{2+}, Mg^{2+}
        Detect and treat myocardial ischemia
        Amiodarone for sustained ventricular tachycardia
    Supraventricular tachycardia
        Consider defibrillation early
        β blocker, digoxin for rate control of atrial fibrillation
    Sinus tachycardia 140/min
        Detect and treat pain and anxiety
            Midazolam fentanyl drip
            Morphine
        Detect and treat hypovolemia
Metabolic (lactic) acidosis
    Characterize to confirm anion gap without osmolal gap
    Rule out or treat ketoacidosis, aspirin intoxication
    Hyperventilate to keep Pa_{CO_2} of 25 mm Hg
    Calculate bicarbonate deficit and replace half if pH <7.0
    Correct ionized hypocalcemia
    Consider early dialysis
Hypothermia
    Maintain skin dry and covered with warmed blankets
    Warm vascular volume expanders
    Aggressive rewarming if temperature <35°C (95°F)

ABBREVIATIONS: FI_{O_2}, fraction of inspired O_2; P_{CO_2}, partial pressure of CO_2; PEEP, positive end-expiratory pressure.

due to maldistribution of blood flow. In this case, where inadequate pressure is the dominant problem, an assessment of organ system perfusion is made (urine output, mentation, and lactic acid concentration), and then a vasopressor agent such as noradrenaline is initiated to raise MAP.[13] The increased afterload will decrease cardiac output, so this intervention as single therapy is appropriate only when cardiac output is high. If cardiac output and oxygen delivery are inadequate, then combination of vasopressor therapy with inotropic agents should be considered (see below).

Too often, the blanket coverage of "pressor agents" is used early in all types of shock. Because some positive inotropic drugs can cause venoconstriction to increase cardiac output by endogenous volume shifts (dopamine and epinephrine), there is a rationale (like that of raising the patient's legs or applying military antishock trousers) for the common practice of starting these agents in some hypotensive patients while the volume resuscitation proceeds. However, this strategy often confounds the determination of an adequate circulating

volume and the diagnosis of the etiology of shock. Thus, vasopressor use as part of Early Goal-Directed Therapy must be reassessed during ongoing volume resuscitation. Even when the numerical MAP and CVP goals have been attained, additional rapid volume challenge generally should be used to test for further clinical improvement (increased MAP, decreased heart rate, increased Scv_{O_2}, and increased urine output) and to determine whether this will allow titration of vasopressor use down or off.

Assessment of organ system perfusion is the most important component of vasopressor therapy; increase in blood pressure by itself is insufficient and can distract from careful reassessment of adequacy of oxygen delivery. If urine output increases, mentation improves, and lactate levels decrease, then vasopressor therapy has achieved its goals, and there is no need to increase MAP further even if the MAP that reverses these signs of hypoperfusion is 55 mm Hg. If the measures of organ system perfusion are not improved by vasopressor therapy, then arbitrarily driving MAP much above 70 mm Hg is rarely useful in septic shock and usually detrimental because cardiac output will decrease further and excessive vasoconstrictor tone will impair blood flow distribution. If evidence of hypoperfusion persists, then inadequate volume resuscitation, cardiac output, hemoglobin, and oxygen saturation are more likely problems.

Inotropes
If evidence of inadequate perfusion persists (assessed by clinical indicators, by direct measurement of cardiac output, or by Scv_{O_2}, etc.) despite adequate circulating volume (Early Goal-Directed Therapy goal: CVP 8 to 12 mm Hg) and vasopressors (Early Goal-Directed Therapy goal: >65 mm Hg), then inotropic agents are indicated.[13] Inotropes are not effective when volume resuscitation is incomplete. In this case, the arterial vasodilating properties of inotropes such as dobutamine and milrinone result in a drop in arterial pressure that is not countered by an increase in cardiac output because venous return is still limited by the inadequate volume resuscitation. The corollary is, if initiation of inotropes results in a significant drop in blood pressure, then adequate volume resuscitation is not complete.

The objective of inotrope use is to increase cardiac output to achieve adequate oxygen delivery to all tissues. Of the many clinical and laboratory indicators that should be measured, mixed venous O_2 saturation (when a pulmonary artery catheter is placed) or Scv_{O_2} are useful surrogate measures of adequacy of O_2 delivery.[14] Rapidly achieving a goal Scv_{O_2} greater than 70% results in a substantial improvement in survival and limits the systemic inflammatory response so that the subsequent need for further volume, red blood cell transfusion, vasopressor use, and mechanical ventilation is reduced.[2]

Accordingly, we encourage early aggressive volume resuscitation, judicious use of vasopressors to aid in rapidly achieving an adequate MAP in septic shock, titration of a positive inotropic agent (dobutamine 2 to 20 μg/kg per minute) to enhance myocardial contractility, and blood transfusion to hematocrit greater than 30, if necessary, to achieve Scv_{O_2} greater than 70%. Resuscitation of the circulation is often usefully driven by protocol. When numerical resuscitation goals are met, additional rapid volume infusions can be used to determine whether volume resuscitation is complete and to help titrate vasopressor agents down and off. After a rapid and adequate resuscitation, timely reduction in vasopressor and inotrope use should be anticipated and is the next goal.

DRUGS/DEFINITIVE THERAPY

During the rapid initial assessment of the patient in shock and initial resuscitation aimed at supporting respiration and circulation, it is important to consider early institution of other definitive therapy for specific causes of shock and early input from consultant experts. When myocardial infarction is the cause of cardiogenic shock, immediate thrombolysis or angioplasty is considered, using intraaortic balloon pump support and coronary artery bypass surgery when necessary[3] (see Chap. 25). During resuscitation of hypovolemic shock, continuous and early application of techniques to anticipate, prevent, or correct hypothermia prevents secondary coagulopathy, coma, and nonresponsiveness to volume and pharmacologic resuscitation. Hemostasis is the immediate goal for hemorrhage[10] because it removes the cause of hypovolemic shock and lessens the need for further volume expanders, none of which are as effective as keeping the patient's own blood intravascular. Emergent radiologic and surgical consultation and intervention may be required. Similarly, when septic shock is secondary to a perforated viscus, an undrained abscess, or rapid spread of infection in devitalized tissue or in tissue planes (gas gangrene, necrotizing fasciitis, etc.), then immediate surgical intervention is fundamental to survival. Early institution of appropriate antibiotics has a profound effect on patient survival from septic shock.[15] Activated protein C decreases mortality for severe sepsis and is most effective when given early.[16] Low-dose steroid therapy of septic shock in patients who are unresponsive to corticotropin (ACTH) similarly improves survival in patients having septic shock.[17] Thus, an ACTH stimulation test should be conducted and low-dose steroid therapy should be initiated immediately thereafter. Steroid therapy can be discontinued as soon as the results of the ACTH stimulation test demonstrate adrenal responsiveness.[17]

CATHETERS AND FREQUENT MEASUREMENTS DURING INITIAL RESUSCITATION

After an airway is established and breathing ensured, correction of the circulatory abnormality always requires good intravenous access. For large-volume administration, two peripheral intravenous catheters of gauge 16 or larger or large-bore central venous access is required. Early Goal-Directed Therapy mandates immediate placement of a central venous catheter. Electrocardiographic monitoring is easily accomplished and usefully measures heart rate and rhythm for early detection and, hence, rational treatment of tachyarrhythmias or bradyarrhythmias aggravating the low-flow state.

The urinary bladder should be catheterized to measure urine output and to facilitate urine sampling. A nasogastric or orogastric tube to decompress the stomach and later to deliver medication and nutrition is generally required in the intubated patient. Measuring arterial pressure with a peripheral arterial or femoral arterial catheter is useful because, in the patient in shock with low cardiac output or low blood pressure, cuff pressures may be inaccurate.[1] Arterial blood-gas and other blood samples are then readily obtained.

Early echocardiography is a useful adjunct to Scv_{O_2} to distinguish poor ventricular pumping function from hypovolemia; a good study can exclude or confirm tamponade, right heart failure, pulmonary hypertension possibly due to pulmonary embolism, or significant valve dysfunction, all of which influence therapy, and can replace more invasive pulmonary artery catheterization.

Effective use and interpretation of Scv_{O_2} and echocardiography often obviate pulmonary artery catheterization when the clinical hypothesis of cardiogenic, hypovolemic, or septic shock is confirmed and corrected by initial therapeutic intervention. There is no role for pulmonary artery catheterization for routine monitoring or management of uncomplicated shock states.[18,19] Use of pulmonary artery catheterization should be restricted to circumstances in which the derived measurements will alter management or direct therapeutic interventions. For example, when confirmed septic shock does not respond fully, or as expected, to volume resuscitation and vasopressor use (e.g., persistent narrow pulse pressure, low Scv_{O_2}, and elevated lactate), then myocardial dysfunction contributes. When echocardiography excludes other causes (see above), then subsequent pulmonary artery catheterization guides the balance between vasopressor (to maintain an adequate MAP for blood flow distribution to vital organs) and inotrope use (to achieve an adequate cardiac output and oxygen delivery to maintain vital organ function).

TEMPO

One of the most important contributions the intensivist can make to the care of a shock patient is to establish an appropriately rapid management tempo. Rapid initial resuscitation improves survival ("time is tissue"). In many instances, resuscitation driven by protocol can achieve adequate resuscitation faster. Effective protocol-driven resuscitation requires significant preliminary discussion, buy in, and training of emergency room physicians, house staff, nurses, respiratory therapists, and others.

The mirror image of urgent implementation is rapid liberation of the resuscitated patient from excessive therapy. It is not uncommon for the patient with hypovolemic or septic shock to stabilize hemodynamically on positive-pressure ventilation with high circulating volume and several vasoactive drugs infusing at a high rate. Too often, hours or days of "weaning" pass, when a trial of spontaneous breathing, diuresis, and sequential reduction of the drug dose by half each 10 minutes can return the patient to a much less treated, stable state within the hour. Of course, this rapid discontinuation may be limited by intercurrent hemodynamic or other instability, but defining each limit and justifying ongoing or new therapy is the essence of titrated care in this postresuscitation period.

Types of Shock

We use cardiac function curves and venous return relations in the following discussion to compare and contrast cardiovascular mechanisms responsible for cardiogenic shock (Fig. 21-2), hypovolemic shock (Fig. 21-3), and septic shock (Fig. 21-4). The goal is to link pathophysiology of the circulation to the broader differential diagnosis of the types of shock

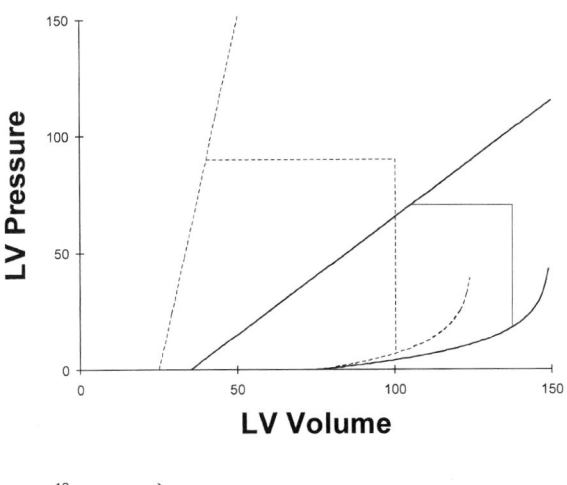

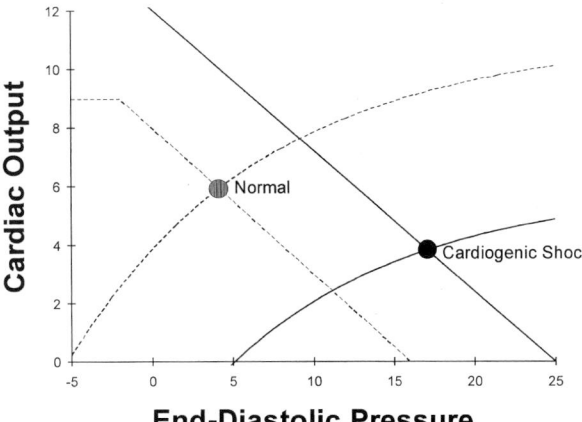

FIGURE 21-2 Cardiovascular mechanics in cardiogenic shock. *Upper panel.* Abnormalities of systolic and diastolic left ventricular (LV) pressure and volume (*ordinate and abscissa, respectively*) relations during cardiogenic shock (*continuous lines*) with normal pressure-volume relations (*dashed lines*). The primary abnormality is that the end-systolic pressure-volume relation (*sloped straight lines*) is shifted to the right mainly by a marked reduction in slope (decreased contractility). As a result, at similar or even lower systolic pressures, the ventricle is not able to eject as far, so end-systolic volume is greatly increased and stroke volume is therefore decreased. To compensate for the decrease in stroke volume, the curvilinear diastolic pressure-volume relation shifts to the right, which indicates decreased diastolic stiffness (increased compliance). To maximize stroke volume, diastolic filling increases even further, associated with an increase in end-diastolic pressure. *Lower panel.* Why end-diastolic pressure increases is determined from the pump function and venous return curves as a plot of cardiac output (*ordinate*) versus right atrial end-diastolic pressure (*abscissa*). The decrease in contractility (*upper panel*) results in a shift of the curvilinear cardiac function curve from its normal position (*dashed curve, lower panel*) down and to the right (*continuous curve, lower panel*). Because end-diastolic pressure and cardiac output are determined by the intersection of the cardiac function curve (*curvilinear relations, lower panel*) with the venous return curve (*straight lines, lower panel*), the shift of the cardiac function curve immediately results in a decrease in cardiac output and an increase in end-diastolic pressure. Compensatory mechanisms (fluid retention by the kidneys, increased sympathetic tone) act to maintain venous return by increasing mean systemic pressure (venous pressure when cardiac output = 0) from 16 to 25 mm Hg as indicated by the rightward shift from the *dashed straight line* to the *continuous straight line* in the *lower panel*. The effect is that end-diastolic pressure increases so that stroke volume (*upper panel*) and cardiac output (*lower panel*) are increased toward normal.

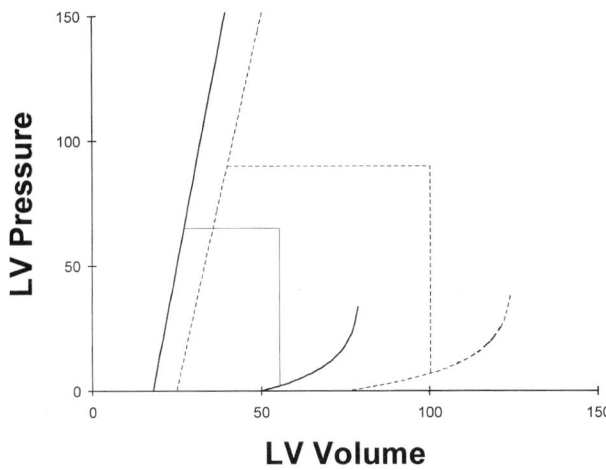

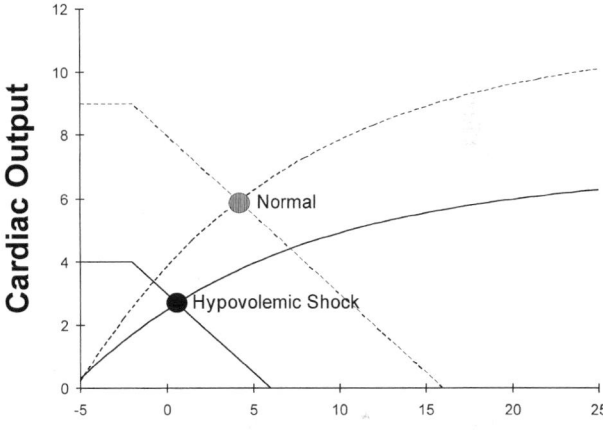

FIGURE 21-3 Cardiovascular mechanics in hypovolemic shock (axes as labeled as in Fig. 21-2). *Lower panel.* During hypovolemic shock, the primary abnormality is a decrease in the intravascular volume so that mean systemic pressure decreases as illustrated by a shift of the venous return curves from the normal relation (*straight dashed line*) leftward (*straight continuous line*). This hypovolemic venous return curve now intersects the normal cardiac function curve (*dashed curvilinear relation*) at a much lower end-diastolic pressure so that cardiac output is greatly reduced. *Upper panel.* The increased sympathetic tone accompanying shock results in a slight increase in contractility, as illustrated by the slight left shift of the left ventricular end-systolic pressure-volume relation (*from the dashed straight line to the solid straight line*). However, because the slope of the end-systolic pressure-volume relation is normally quite steep, the increase in contractility cannot increase stroke volume or cardiac output much and is therefore an ineffective compensatory mechanism in patients with normal hearts. If volume resuscitation to correct the primary abnormality is delayed for several hours, the diastolic pressure-volume relation shifts from its normal position (*dashed curve, upper panel*), resulting in increased diastolic stiffness (*continuous curve, upper panel*). Increased diastolic stiffness results in a decreased stroke volume and therefore a depressed cardiac function curve (*continuous curve, lower panel*) compared with normal (*dashed curve, lower panel*). This decrease in cardiac function due to increased diastolic stiffness probably accounts for irreversibility of severe prolonged hypovolemic shock. LV, left ventricular.

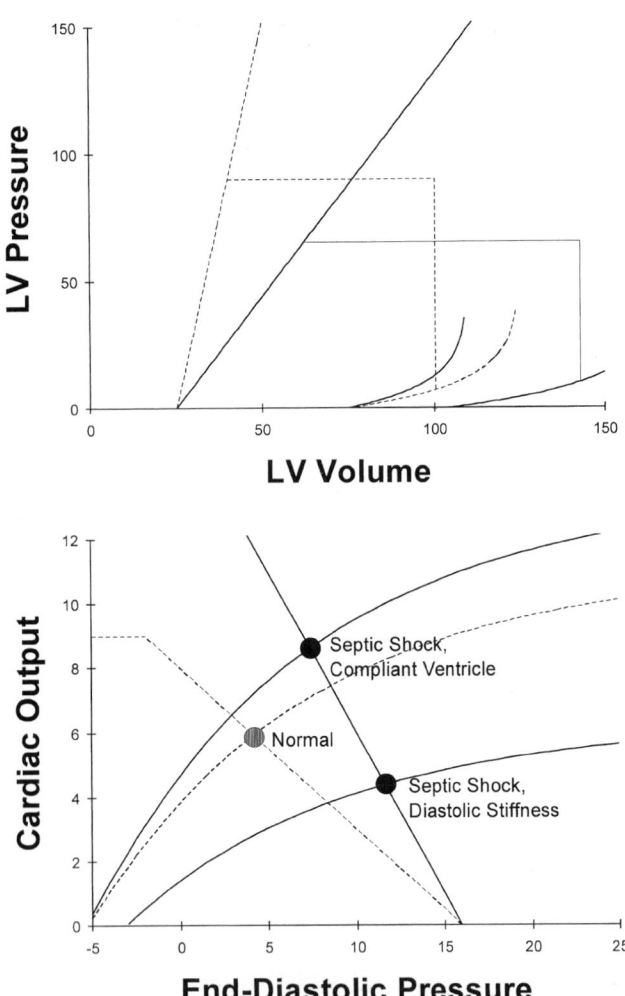

FIGURE 21-4 Cardiovascular mechanics in septic shock (axes as labeled as in Fig. 21-2). Septic shock has important independent effects on left ventricular (LV) pressure-volume relations, on the venous return curve, and on arterial vascular resistance. *Upper panel.* Depressed systolic contractility indicated by a decreased slope of the LV end-systolic pressure-volume relation from normal (*dashed sloped line*) to sepsis (*continuous sloped line*) is caused in part by a circulating myocardial depressant factor, but the end-systolic volume remains about normal owing to the reduced afterload. Survivors of septic shock have a large end-diastolic volume even at reduced diastolic pressure associated with dilation of their diastolic ventricles, indicated by a shift of the normal diastolic pressure-volume relation (*dashed curve*) to the right (*right-hand continuous curve*). As a result, stroke volume is increased. However, in nonsurvivors, stroke volume decreases because of a leftward shift of the diastolic pressure-volume relation (*left-hand continuous curve*), indicating increased diastolic stiffness and impaired diastolic filling. *Lower panel.* The cardiac function curve for survivors is normal (*dashed curvilinear relation*) or slightly increased (*continuous curvilinear relation* owing to reduced afterload). The peripheral *circulation* during septic shock is often characterized by high flows and low vascular pressures. It follows that the resistance to venous return is decreased as indicated by a steeper venous return curve (*continuous straight line*) compared with normal (*straight dashed lines*). This accounts for the high venous return and large end-diastolic volumes and stroke volumes. As with other interventions, resistance to venous return may be decreased in part by redistribution of blood flow to vascular beds with short time constants. However, the nonsurvivors may have significantly depressed cardiac function (*downward shifted continuous curve*) because of the additive effects of decreased systolic contractility and impaired diastolic filling. Depending on the relative contribution of the abnormalities of ventricular mechanics and peripheral vascular changes, cardiac output is usually normal or high even at relatively normal end-diastolic pressures until diastolic dysfunction limits cardiac output by reducing diastolic volume even at high diastolic pressures.

presented in Table 21-4 to facilitate the accurate etiologic diagnosis and management based on additional hemodynamic measures as required by the response to urgent resuscitation.

Shock caused by decreased pump function of the heart is commonly cardiogenic shock resulting from left ventricular ischemia. For high right atrial pressure hypotension not obviously caused by left ventricular ischemia, greatly elevated pulmonary arterial pressure (most commonly pulmonary embolism), right ventricular ischemia, and dysfunction of heart valves must be excluded. Of course, right atrial pressure may be increased by abnormal pressures surrounding the heart in the absence of ventricular dysfunction. Because of this clinical presentation, I have included cardiac tamponade in the category of high right atrial pressure hypotension. Tamponade and pulmonary embolism might have been classified as decreased venous return due to obstruction of the circulation (see Table 21-1). Decreased venous return despite normal pump function is most commonly due to hemorrhagic or dehydration hypovolemia, but I emphasize other mechanisms including decreased venous tone caused by drugs, neurologic injury, and adrenal insufficiency, particularly for nonresponsive hypovolemia. Septic shock is the most common cause of high cardiac output hypotension resulting from abnormal arterial tone and blood flow distribution, although other causes such as severe liver failure, severe pancreatitis, trauma

with tissue damage eliciting a significant inflammatory response, anaphylactic shock, thyroid storm, Paget disease, and other peripheral shunts share this mechanism. Defining shock as anaerobic metabolism of multiple organ systems, often signaled by lactic acidosis, allows classification of the shock state associated with metabolic poisons such as carbon monoxide that results in histotoxic hypoxia caused by inadequate uptake of oxygen by the mitochondria (see Table 21-4). Other shock states, in particular septic shock, may also involve an inability of tissues to extract delivered oxygen, but the lactic acidosis of sepsis is not necessarily caused by anaerobic metabolism.

DECREASED PUMP FUNCTION—CARDIOGENIC SHOCK

Pump function is measured as the output of a pump for a given input. The diagnosis of decreased pump function as the cause of shock is made by finding evidence of inappropriately low output (cardiac output) despite normal or high input (right atrial pressure). Cardiac output is the most important "output" of the heart and is clinically assessed in the same way that perfusion was assessed during the urgent initial examination. Better estimates are later obtained by thermodilution measurement using a pulmonary artery catheter, nuclear medicine scans, and Doppler echocardiographic

TABLE 21-4 Causes of and Contributors to Shock

Decreased pump function of the heart—cardiogenic shock	Constrictive pericarditis
Left ventricular failure	High intrathoracic pressure
Systolic dysfunction—decreased contractility	Tension pneumothorax
Myocardial infarction	Massive pleural effusion
Ischemia and global hypoxemia	Positive-pressure ventilation
Cardiomyopathy	High intraabdominal pressure
Depressant drugs: β blockers, calcium channel blockers,	Acites
antiarrhythmics	Massive obesity
Myocardial contusion	After extensive intra abdominal surgery
Respiratory acidosis	Intravascular hypovolemia (reduced mean systemic pressure)
Metabolic derangements: acidosis, hypophosphatemia,	Hemorrhage
hypocalcemia	Gastrointestinal
Diastolic dysfunction—increased myocardial diastolic stiffness	Trauma
Ischemia	Aortic dissection and other internal sources
Ventricular hypertrophy	Renal losses
Restrictive cardiomyopathy	Diuretics
Consequence of prolonged hypovolemic or septic shock	Osmotic diuresis
Ventricular interdependence	Diabetes (insipidus, mellitus)
External compression (see cardiac tamponade below)	Gastrointestinal losses
Greatly increased afterload	Vomiting
Aortic stenosis	Diarrhea
Hypertrophic cardiomyopathy	Gastric suctioning
Dynamic outflow tract obstruction	Loss via surgical stomas
Coarctation of the aorta	Redistribution to extravascular space
Malignant hypertension	Burns
Valve and structural abnormality	Trauma
Mitral stenosis, endocarditis, mitral aortic regurgitation	Postsurgical
Obstruction owing to atrial myxoma or thrombus	Sepsis
Papillary muscle dysfunction or rupture	Decreased venous tone (reduced mean systemic pressure)
Ruptured septum or free wall	Drugs
Arrhythmias	Sedatives
Right ventricular failure	Narcotics
Decreased contractility	Diuretics
Right ventricular infarction, ischemia, hypoxia,	Anaphylactic shock
acidosis	Neurogenic shock
Greatly increased afterload	Increased resistance to venous return
Pulmonary embolism	Tumor compression or invasion
Pulmonary vascular disease	Venous thrombosis with obstruction
Hypoxic pulmonary vasoconstriction, PEEP, high alveolar	PEEP
pressure	Pregnancy
Acidosis	High cardiac output hypotension
ARDS, pulmonary fibrosis, sleep disordered breathing,	Septic shock
chronic obstructive pulmonary disease	Sterile endotoxemia with hepatic failure
Valve and structural abnormality	Arteriovenous shunts
Obstruction due to atrial myxoma, thrombus, endocarditis	Dialysis
Arrhythmias	Paget disease
Decreased venous return with normal pumping	Other causes of shock with unique etiologies
function—hypovolemic shock	Thyroid storm
Cardiac tamponade (increased right atrial pressure—central	Myxedema coma
hypovolemia)	Adrenal insufficiency
Pericardial fluid collection	Hemoglobin and mitochondrial poisons
Blood	Cyanide
Renal failure	Carbon monoxide
Pericarditis with effusion	Iron intoxication

ABBREVIATIONS: ARDS, acute respiratory distress syndrome; PEEP, positive end-expiratory pressure.

techniques. Right atrial pressure or CVP is the most easily measured "input" of the whole heart and is initially assessed by examination of jugular veins. After catheter insertion, CVP can be measured accurately. Other outputs, such as stroke work or left ventricular ejection fraction, and other inputs, such as left ventricular end-diastolic pressure (LVEDP) or volume (LVEDV), are useful to determine the specific cause of decreased pump function. Left and right ventricular

dysfunction can be caused by decreased systolic contractility, increased diastolic stiffness, greatly increased afterload (including obstruction), valvular dysfunction, or abnormal heart rate and rhythm.

CAUSES OF LEFT VENTRICULAR FAILURE

Acute or acute-on-chronic left ventricular failure resulting in shock is the classic example of cardiogenic shock and is identified as a subset of decreased pump function by evidence of a low cardiac output in relation to high left ventricular filling pressures. Clinical findings of low cardiac output and increased left ventricular filling pressures include, in addition to assessment of perfusion, pulmonary crackles in dependent lung regions, a laterally displaced and diffuse precordial apical impulse, elevated jugular veins, and presence of a third heart sound.[20] These findings are not always present or unambiguous. Therefore, echocardiography or pulmonary artery catheterization is helpful and often essential in establishing the diagnosis and titrating therapy. Cardiogenic shock then is usually associated with a cardiac index lower than 2.2 L/m^2 per minute when the pulmonary artery occlusion pressure has been raised above 18 mm Hg.[21]

Systolic Dysfunction

Figure 21-2 illustrates the pathophysiologic abnormalities of cardiogenic shock resulting from decreased left ventricular contractility. The primary abnormality is that the relation of end-systolic pressure to volume is shifted down and to the right (see Fig. 21-2, upper panel) so that, at the same afterload, the ventricle cannot eject as far (decreased contractility). It follows that pump function is also impaired, indicated by a shift down and to the right (see Fig. 21-2, lower panel) so that at similar preloads cardiac output is reduced. Three mechanisms that counter the decrease in cardiac output are illustrated. The diastolic ventricle becomes more compliant, possibly from stress relaxation of the pericardium and myocardium, so that stroke volume increases at the same end-diastolic pressure (rightward shift of the diastolic pressure-volume relation in the upper panel). Afterload decreases, resulting in increased stroke volume (see Fig. 21-2, upper panel). Mean systemic pressure rises (see Fig. 21-2, lower panel), aided by avid fluid retention by the kidneys and by increased venous tone mediated by the sympathetic nervous system. Thus, the Frank-Starling mechanism of increasing cardiac output by increasing diastolic filling is used.

As a result of a decrease in contractility, the patient presents with elevated left and right ventricular filling pressures and a low cardiac output. Mixed venous oxygen saturation may be well below 50% because cardiac output is low. In the presence of physiologic pulmonary shunt that accompanies pulmonary edema, the low saturation of mixed venous blood shunting by the lung contributes to substantial arterial desaturation. Accordingly, arterial desaturation aggravates the low oxygen delivery due to reduced cardiac output, as does intercurrent anemia.

Acute myocardial infarction or ischemia is the most common cause of left ventricular failure leading to shock. The principal effect of myocardial infarction is to depress systolic contractility, which in completely infarcted areas becomes zero or even negative (paradoxical regional wall motion). Earlier series described shock occurring in 10% to 20% of patients with transmural myocardial infarction.[22] However, the recent use of fibrinolytic therapy and early angioplasty or surgical revascularization has reduced the incidence of cardiogenic shock to less than 5%.[23] Infarction greater than 40% of the myocardium is often associated with cardiogenic shock;[24] anterior infarction is 20 times more likely to lead to shock than is inferior or posterior infarction.[25] Details of the diagnosis and management of ischemic heart disease are discussed in Chap. 25; other causes of decreased left ventricular contractility in critical illness are discussed in more detail in Chaps. 22 and 23, and each may contribute to shock.

Diastolic Dysfunction

Increased left ventricular diastolic chamber stiffness contributing to cardiogenic shock occurs during myocardial ischemia and in a range of less common disorders including late stages of hypovolemic shock and septic shock (see Table 21-4); all causes of tamponade listed in Table 21-4 need to be considered in a systematic review of causes of diastolic dysfunction.[26] Cardiac function is depressed because stroke volume is decreased by decreased end-diastolic volume caused by increased diastolic chamber stiffness. Diastolic dysfunction in a hypotensive patient with low cardiac output and high filling pressures is often identified by a small (rather than large) LVEDV by bedside echocardiography. Conditions resulting in increased diastolic stiffness are particularly detrimental when systolic contractility is decreased because decreased diastolic stiffness (increased compliance; see Fig. 21-2, upper panel) is normally a compensatory mechanism. Increased diastolic chamber stiffness contributing to hypotension in patients with low cardiac output and high ventricular diastolic pressures is best identified echocardiographically by small diastolic volumes.

Treatment of increased diastolic stiffness is approached by first considering the potentially contributing reversible causes. Acute reversible causes include ischemia and the many causes of tamponade physiology listed in Table 21-4. Fluid infusion results in large increases in diastolic pressure without much increase in diastolic volume. Positive inotropic agents and afterload reduction are generally not helpful and may decrease blood pressure further. If conventional therapy of cardiogenic shock aimed at improving systolic function is ineffective, then increased diastolic stiffness should be strongly considered as the cause of decreased pump function. Cardiac output responsiveness to heart rate is another subtle clue suggesting impaired diastolic filling. Heart rate does not normally alter cardiac output (which is normally set by and equal to venous return) except at very low heart rates (maximally filled ventricle before end diastole) or at very high heart rates (incomplete ventricular relaxation and filling). However, if diastolic filling is limited by tamponade or a stiff ventricle, then very little further filling occurs late in diastole. In this case, increasing heart rate from 80 to 100 or 110 beats/min may result in a significant increase in cardiac output, which may be therapeutically beneficial and also a diagnostic clue.

Valvular Dysfunction

Acute mitral regurgitation, due to cordal or papillary muscle rupture or papillary muscle dysfunction, most commonly is caused by ischemic injury. The characteristic murmur and the presence of large V waves on the pulmonary artery occlusion pressure trace suggest significant mitral regurgitation, which is quantified by Doppler echocardiographic examination. Rupture of the ventricular septum with left-to-right shunt is detected by Doppler echocardiographic examination or by observing a step-up in oxygen saturation of blood from the right atrium to the pulmonary artery.[27] Rarely, acute obstruction of the mitral valve by left atrial thrombus or myxoma may also result in cardiogenic shock. These conditions are generally surgical emergencies.

More commonly, valve dysfunction aggravates other primary etiologies of shock. Aortic and mitral regurgitation reduces forward flow and raises LVEDP, and this regurgitation is ameliorated by effective arteriolar dilation and by nitroprusside infusion. Vasodilator therapy can effect large increases in cardiac output without much change in mean blood pressure, pulse pressure, or diastolic pressure, so pulmonary artery catheterization and repeat echocardiography, to confirm increased cardiac output and reduced valvular regurgitation, are essential to titrating effective vasodilator doses. In contrast, occasional patients develop decreased blood pressure and cardiac output on inotropic drugs such as dobutamine; in this case, excluding dynamic ventricular outflow tract obstruction by echocardiography or treating it by increasing preload, afterload, and end-systolic volume are essential.

Cardiac Arrhythmias

Not infrequently, arrhythmias aggravate hypoperfusion in other shock· states. Ventricular tachyarrhythmias are often associated with cardiogenic shock; sinus tachycardia and atrial tachyarrhythmias are often observed with hypovolemic and septic shock. Specific therapy of tachyarrhythmias depends on the specific diagnosis, as discussed in Chap. 24. Inadequately treated pain and unsuspected drug withdrawal should be included in the intensive care unit differential diagnosis of tachyarrhythmias; whatever their etiology, the reduced ventricular filling time can reduce cardiac output and aggravate shock. Bradyarrhythmias contributing to shock may respond acutely to atropine or isoproterenol infusion and then pacing; hypoxia or myocardial infarction as the cause should be sought and treated. Symptomatic hypoperfusion resulting from bradyarrhythmias, even in the absence of myocardial infarction or high-degree atrioventricular block, is an important indication for temporary pacemaker placement that is sometimes overlooked.

Treatment of Left Ventricular Failure

After initial resuscitation, which includes consideration of early institution of thrombolytic therapy in acute coronary thrombosis and revascularization or surgical correction of other anatomic abnormalities where appropriate,[3] management of patients with cardiogenic shock requires repeated testing of the hypothesis of "too little versus too much." Clinical examination is not accurate enough; when the response to initial treatment of cardiogenic shock is inadequate, a pulmonary artery catheter may be required. Therapy for cardiogenic shock follows from consideration of the pathophysiology illustrated in Fig. 21-2 and includes optimizing filling pressures, increasing contractility by improving the ratio of myocardial oxygen supply to demand, or by using inotropic drugs, and optimizing afterload. Temporary mechanical support using an intraaortic balloon pump is often extremely useful in cardiogenic shock and should be considered early as a support device in patients who may benefit from later surgical therapy.[28] Cardiac transplantation and mechanical heart implantation are considered when other therapy fails.

Filling pressures are optimized to improve cardiac output but avoid pulmonary edema. Depending on the initial presentation, cardiogenic shock frequently spans the spectrum of hypovolemia (so fluid infusion helps) to hypervolemia with pulmonary edema (where reduction in intravas-cular volume results in substantial improvement). If gross fluid overload is not present, then a rapid fluid bolus should be given. In contrast to patients with hypovolemic or septic shock, a smaller bolus (250 mL) of crystalloid solution should be infused as quickly as possible. Immediately after infusion, the patient's circulatory status should be reassessed. If there is improvement but hypoperfusion persists, then further infusion with repeat examination is indicated to attain an adequate cardiac output and oxygen delivery while seeking the lowest filling pressure needed to accomplish this goal. If there is no improvement in oxygen delivery and evidence of worsened pulmonary edema or gas exchange, then the limit of initial fluid resuscitation has been defined. Crystalloid solutions are used particularly if the initial evaluation is uncertain because crystalloid solutions rapidly distribute to the entire extracellular fluid compartment. Therefore, after a brief period only one-fourth to one-third remains in the intravascular compartment, and evidence of intravascular fluid overload rapidly subsides.

Contractility increases if ischemia can be relieved by decreasing myocardial oxygen demand, by improving myocardial oxygen supply by increasing coronary blood flow (coronary vasodilators, thrombolytic therapy, surgical revascularization, or intra-aortic balloon pump counterpulsation), or by increasing the oxygen content of arterial blood. Inotropic drug infusion attempts to correct the physiologic abnormality by increasing contractility (see Fig. 21-2). However, this occurs at the expense of increased myocardial oxygen demand. Afterload is optimized to maintain arterial pressures high enough to perfuse vital organs (including the heart) but low enough to maximize systolic ejection. When systolic function is reduced, vasodilator therapy may improve systolic ejection and increase perfusion, even to the extent that blood pressure rises.[29] In patients with very high blood pressure, end-systolic volume increases considerably so that stroke volume and cardiac output decrease unless LVEDV and LVEDP are greatly increased; this sequence is reversed by judicious afterload reduction.

Diagnosis and Management of Right Ventricular Failure

Right ventricular failure as a cause of cardiogenic shock is often identified by elevated right atrial pressure and low cardiac output not explained by left ventricular failure or cardiac tamponade. The most common causes of shock owing to right ventricular failure are right ventricular infarction and pulmonary embolism resulting in greatly increased right ventricular afterload.

Right ventricular infarction is found in approximately half of inferior myocardial infarctions and is complicated by shock only 10% to 20% of the time.[30] Isolated right ventricular infarction with shock is uncommon and has a mortality rate ~50% comparable to left ventricular infarction shock.[25] The hemodynamic findings of right ventricular infarction must be distinguished from cardiac tamponade and constrictive pericarditis and include Kussmaul sign, low cardiac output, high filling pressures, and often equalization of right atrial, right ventricular diastolic, pulmonary artery diastolic, and pulmonary artery occlusion pressures. Pulmonary crackles are classically absent. Early recognition of right versus left ventricular infarction as the cause of shock is important, so potentially dangerous therapy, including vasodilators, morphine, and β blockers, are avoided. Therapy includes infusion of dobutamine and volume expansion, although excessive volume can aggravate shock by shifting the intraventricular septum from right to left.[31] Because bradyarrhythmias are common and atrioventricular conduction is frequently abnormal, atrioventricular sequential pacing may preserve right ventricular synchrony and often dramatically improves cardiac output and blood pressure in shock caused by right ventricular infarction.[31] Afterload reduction using balloon counterpulsation may also be useful,[25] as are early fibrinolytic therapy and angioplasty when indicated (see Chap. 25).

Right ventricular ischemia, with or without coronary artery disease, probably is a more important cause of right ventricular dysfunction than generally recognized. In shock states systemic arterial pressure is often low, and right ventricular afterload (pulmonary artery pressure) may be high owing to emboli, hypoxemic pulmonary vasoconstriction, acidemic pulmonary vasoconstriction, sepsis, or ARDS. Therefore, right ventricular perfusion pressure is low leading to right ventricular ischemia and decreased contractility, which, in the face of normal or high right ventricular afterload, results in right ventricular dilation. Subsequent right-to-left shift of the interventricular septum limits left ventricular filling. Cardiac output is then limited by right ventricular systolic ejection and left ventricular diastolic filling.

Therapy of right ventricular failure caused by decreased right ventricular perfusion and increased afterload is evolving. Animal studies suggest that, acutely in right ventricular shock caused by pulmonary embolism, interventions such as norepinephrine infusion may increase systemic arterial pressure more than pulmonary arterial pressure, resulting in improved right ventricular perfusion. Improved right ventricular function and total cardiac function may result. This approach has not been carefully tested in patients in shock owing to right ventricular failure.[32] Established approaches include verifying that pulmonary emboli are present and initiating therapy with anticoagulation, fibrinolytic agents for submassive pulmonary embolism or shock, or surgical embolectomy as necessary.[33] Hypoxic pulmonary vasoconstriction may be reduced by improving alveolar and mixed venous oxygenation. More aggressive correction of acidemia should be considered in this setting. Pulmonary vasodilator therapy may be useful in some patients if pulmonary artery pressures can be lowered without significantly lowering systemic arterial pressures. Inhaled nitric oxide, prostaglandin E_1, and many other agents have been variably successful. Measurements of pulmonary artery pressure, systemic pressure, cardiac output, and oxygen delivery before and after a trial of a specific potential pulmonary vasodilator are essential (see Chap. 26).

Compression of the Heart by Surrounding Structures
Compression of the heart (cardiac tamponade) limits diastolic filling and can result in shock with inadequate cardiac output despite very high right atrial pressures. Diagnosis of cardiac tamponade is made physiologically by using pulmonary artery catheterization to demonstrate a low cardiac output in addition to elevated and approximately equal right atrial, right ventricular diastolic, pulmonary artery diastolic, and pulmonary artery occlusion pressures (particularly their waveforms). The diagnosis is often best confirmed anatomically by using echocardiographic examination to demonstrate pericardial fluid, diastolic collapse of the atria

and right ventricle, and right-to-left septal shift during inspiration. Septal shift during inspiration and increased afterload that accompany decreased intrathoracic pressure during inspiration account for the clinically observed pulsus paradoxus. Although pericardial tamponade by accumulation of pericardial fluid is the most common cause of cardiac tamponade, other structures surrounding the heart may also produce tamponade. Tension pneumothorax, massive pleural effusion, pneumopericardium (rarely), and greatly elevated abdominal pressures may also impair diastolic filling.

Decreasing the pressure of the tamponading chamber by needle drainage of the pericardium, pleural space, and peritoneum can rapidly and dramatically improve venous return, blood pressure, and organ system perfusion. Therefore, the goal of therapy is to accomplish this decompression as rapidly and safely as possible. In patients who are hemodynamically stable, fluid infusion is a temporizing therapy that increases mean systemic pressure so that venous return increases even though right atrial pressure is high. In hemodynamically stable patients, if it is safe to take the time needed to get ultrasonic guidance for needle aspiration or surgical drainage, then this should be done. Otherwise, in an emergency, blind needle drainage is necessary.

DECREASED VENOUS RETURN—HYPOVOLEMIC SHOCK

The pressure driving venous return to the right atrium is described as mean systemic pressure minus right atrial pressure, where the mean systemic pressure is determined by the vascular volume and by the unstressed volume and capacitance of the systemic vessels. Venous return to the heart when right atrial pressure is not elevated may be inadequate owing to decreased intravascular volume (hypovolemic shock), to decreased tone of the venous capacitance bed so that mean systemic pressure is low (e.g., drugs, neurogenic shock), and occasionally to increased resistance to venous return (e.g., obstruction of the inferior vena cava by abdominal compartment syndrome). In the presence of shock, decreased venous return is determined to be a contributor to shock by finding low left and right ventricular diastolic pressures, often in an appropriate clinical setting such as trauma or massive gastrointestinal hemorrhage.

HYPOVOLEMIC SHOCK
Hypovolemia is the most common cause of shock caused by decreased venous return and is illustrated in Fig. 21-3. Intravascular volume is decreased, so the venous capacitance bed is not filled, leading to a decreased pressure driving venous return back to the heart. This is seen as a left shift of the venous return curve in Fig. 21-3, lower panel, so that cardiac output decreases at a low end-diastolic pressure (intersection of the venous return curve and cardiac function curve). Endogenous catecholamines attempt to compensate by constricting the venous capacitance bed, thereby raising the pressure driving venous return back to the heart, so that 25% reductions in intravascular volume are nearly completely compensated for. Orthostatic decrease in blood pressure by 10 mm Hg or an increase in heart rate of more than 30 beats/min[34] may detect this level of intravascular volume reduction. When approximately 40% of the intravascular volume is lost, sympathetic stimulation can no longer maintain

mean systemic pressure, resulting in decreased venous return and clinical shock.

After sufficient time (>2 hours) and severity (>40% loss of intravascular volume), patients often cannot be resuscitated from hypovolemic shock.[35] This observation highlights the urgency with which patients should be resuscitated. A "no reflow" phenomenon is described in microvascular beds, gut ischemia with systemic release of inflammatory mediators,[36] and increased diastolic stiffness (see Fig. 21-3) contribute to the pathophysiology.[37]

Shock after trauma is a form of hypovolemic shock in which a significant systemic inflammatory response, in addition to intravascular volume depletion, is present. Intravascular volume may be decreased because of loss of blood and significant redistribution of intravascular volume to other compartments, i.e., "third spacing." Release of inflammatory mediators may result in pathophysiologic abnormalities resembling septic shock. Cardiac dysfunction may be depressed from direct damage from myocardial contusion, from increased diastolic stiffness, from right heart failure, or even from circulating myocardial depressant substances. Shock related to burns similarly is multifactorial with a significant component of intravascular hypovolemia and a systemic inflammatory response (see Chaps. 98 to 100).

Other causes of shock caused by decreased venous return include severe neurologic damage or drug ingestion resulting in hypotension caused by loss of venous tone. As a result of decreased venous tone, mean systemic pressure decreases, thereby reducing the pressure gradient driving blood flow back to the heart so that cardiac output and blood pressure decrease. Obstruction of veins owing to compression, thrombus formation, or tumor invasion increases the resistance to venous return and occasionally may result in shock.

The principal therapy of hypovolemic shock and other forms of shock caused by decreased venous return is rapid initial fluid resuscitation. Warmed crystalloid solutions are readily available. Colloid-containing solutions result in a more sustained increase in intravascular volume. However, in the setting of demonstrated or potential leaking endothelial surfaces (e.g., ARDS), the colloid rapidly redistributes into the entire extravascular water compartment. Pulmonary edema and tissue edema may be aggravated. Overall, no benefit of colloid over crystalloid has been convincingly demonstrated. The role of hypertonic saline and other resuscitation solutions is currently uncertain. Alternatively, transfusion of packed red blood cells increases oxygen-carrying capacity and expands the intravascular volume and is therefore a doubly useful therapy. In an emergency, initial transfusion often begins with type-specific blood before a complete cross-match is available. During initial resuscitation, the Early Goal-Directed Protocol suggests that achieving a hematocrit greater than 30% may be beneficial when Scv_{O_2} is less than 70%. However, after initial resuscitation, maintaining hemoglobin above 90 g/L does not appear to be better than maintaining hemoglobin above 70 g/L. After a large stored red blood cell transfusion, clotting factors, platelets, and serum ionized calcium decrease and therefore should be measured and replaced if necessary (see Chap. 68).

Recognizing inadequate venous return as the primary abnormality of hypovolemic shock alerts the physician to several commonly encountered and potentially lethal complications of therapy. Airway intubation and mechanical ventilation increase negative intrathoracic pressures to positive values and thus raise right atrial pressure. The already low pressure gradient driving venous return to the heart worsens, resulting in marked reduction in cardiac output and blood pressure. However, ventilation treats shock by reducing the work of respiratory muscle, so ventilation should be implemented early with adequate volume expansion. Sedatives and analgesics are often administered at the time of airway intubation, resulting in reduced venous tone because of a direct relaxing effect on the venous capacitance bed or because of a decrease in circulating catecholamines. Thus, the pressure gradient driving venous return decreases. Therefore, in the hypovolemic patient, these medications may markedly reduce cardiac output and blood pressure and should be used with caution and with ongoing volume expansion.

HIGH CARDIAC OUTPUT HYPOTENSION—SEPTIC SHOCK

Septic shock is the most common example of shock that may be caused primarily by reduced arterial vascular tone and reactivity, often associated with abnormal distribution of blood flow. Gram-negative bacilli account for half of all cases of sepsis and approximately 50% of these patients develop septic shock.[38] In contrast, shock accompanies only 5% to 10% of gram-positive or fungal bloodstream infections,[38] although candida infections are emerging as an important cause of attributable mortality.[39] Evidence of end-organ hypoperfusion and dysfunction may be present at low, normal, and high cardiac outputs and oxygen deliveries. During evaluation and resuscitation, normal or increased cardiac output with low SVR hypotension is manifested by a high pulse pressure, warm extremities, good nail bed capillary filling, and low diastolic and mean blood pressures. This high cardiac output hypotension is often accompanied by an abnormal temperature and white blood cell count and differential and an evident site of sepsis. However, the diagnosis is sometimes initially unclear when septic shock is combined with cardiogenic or hypovolemic shock, which limit the usual increase in cardiac output, oxygen delivery, and mixed-venous oxygen saturation.

Several pathophysiologic mechanisms contribute to inadequate organ system perfusion in septic shock. There may be abnormal distribution of blood flow at the organ system level, within individual organs, and even at the capillary bed level. The result is inadequate oxygen delivery in some tissue beds.

The cardiovascular abnormalities of septic shock (see Fig. 21-4) are extensive and include systolic and diastolic abnormalities of the heart, abnormal arterial tone, decreased venous tone, and abnormal distribution of capillary flow leading to regions of tissue hypoxia. In addition, there may be a cellular defect in metabolism so that even cells exposed to adequate oxygen delivery may not maintain normal aerobic metabolism. Depressed systolic contractility illustrated as a rightward shift of the end-systolic pressure-volume relation in Fig. 21-4, upper panel, occurs in septic shock[40] due to circulating proinflammatory cytokines and other mediators, nitric oxide production by activated endothelial cells and cardiomyocytes, and reactive oxygen intermediate generation by retained leukocytes and other cells.[41] Decreased systolic contractility associated with septic shock is reversible over 5 to 10 days as the patient recovers.[40] Systolic and diastolic dysfunctions during sepsis that progress to the point that high cardiac output (hyperdynamic circulation) is no longer maintained (normal or low cardiac output is observed) are associated with poor outcome.[40]

Decreased arterial resistance is almost always observed in septic shock. Early in septic shock, a high cardiac output state exists with normal or low blood pressure. The low arterial resistance is associated with impaired arterial and precapillary autoregulation and may be due to increased endothelial nitric oxide production and opening of potassium adenosine triphosphate channels on vascular smooth muscle cells. Redistribution of blood flow to low-resistance, short time-constant vascular beds (such as skeletal muscle) results in decreased resistance to venous return, as illustrated in Fig. 21-4 (lower panel) by a steeper venous return curve. As a result, cardiac output may be increased even when cardiac function is decreased (see Fig. 21-4, lower panel) because of decreased contractility (see Fig. 21-4, upper panel). Hypovolemia, caused by redistribution of fluid out of the intravascular compartment and to decreased venous tone, impedes venous return during septic shock.

Early institution of appropriate antibiotic therapy and surgical drainage of abscesses or excision of devitalized and infected tissue is central to successful therapy. Activated protein C and low-dose steroids therapy in patients with inadequate adrenal responses to ACTH stimulation improve outcome. Many other anticytokine and anti-inflammatory therapies and inhibition of nitric oxide production have not been successful in improving outcome.

OTHER TYPES OF SHOCK

As detailed in Table 21-4, there are many less common etiologies of shock, and the diagnosis and management of several causes of high right atrial pressure hypotension are discussed elsewhere in this book (see Chaps. 22, 26, and 28). A few other types of hypovolemic shock merit early identification by their characteristic features and lack of response to volume resuscitation including neurogenic shock and adrenal insufficiency. Anaphylactic shock results from the effects of histamine and other mediators of anaphylaxis on the heart, circulation, and the peripheral tissues (see Chap. 106). Despite increased circulating catecholamines and the positive inotropic effect of cardiac H_2 receptors, histamine may depress systolic contractility via H_1 stimulation and other mediators of anaphylaxis. Marked arterial vasodilation results in hypotension even at normal or increased cardiac output. Like septic shock, blood flow is redistributed to short time-constant vascular beds. The endothelium becomes more permeable, so fluid may shift out of the vascular compartment into the extravascular and intracellular compartments, resulting in intravascular hypovolemia. Venous tone and therefore venous return are reduced, so the mainstay of therapy of anaphylactic shock is fluid resuscitation of the intravascular compartment and includes epinephrine and antihistamines as adjunctive therapy.[42]

Neurogenic shock is uncommon. In general, in a patient with neurologic damage that may be extensive, the cause of shock is usually associated with blood loss. Patients with neurogenic shock develop decreased vascular tone, particularly of the venous capacitance bed, which results in pooling of blood in the periphery. Therapy with fluid will increase mean systemic pressure. Catecholamine infusion also will increase mean systemic pressure, and stimulation of α receptors will increase arterial resistance, but these are rarely needed once circulation volume is repleted.

Several endocrinologic conditions may result in shock. Adrenal insufficiency (Addison disease, adrenal hemorrhage and infarction, Waterhouse-Friderichsen syndrome, adrenal insufficiency of sepsis, and systemic inflammation) or other disorders with inadequate catecholamine response may result in shock or may be important contributors to other forms of shock.[17] Whenever inadequate catecholamine response is suspected, diagnosis should be established by measuring serum cortisol and conducting an ACTH stimulation test, whereas presumptive therapy proceeds using dexamethasone (see Chap. 79). Hypothyroidism and hyperthyroidism may in extreme cases result in shock; thyroid storm is an emergency requiring urgent therapy with propylthiouracil or other antithyroid drug, steroids, propranolol, fluid resuscitation, and identification of the precipitating cause[43] (see Chap. 80). Pheochromocytoma may lead to shock by markedly increasing afterload and by redistributing intravascular volume into extravascular compartments.[44] In general, the therapeutic approach involves treating the underlying metabolic abnormality, resuscitating with fluid to produce an adequate cardiac output at the lowest adequate filling pressure, and infusing inotropic drugs, if necessary, to improve ventricular contractility if it is decreased. Details of diagnosis and therapy of shock associated with poisons (carbon monoxide, cyanide) are discussed in Chap. 102.

Organ System Pathophysiology of Shock

INFLAMMATORY COMPONENT OF SHOCK

Shock has a hemodynamic component that has been the focus of much of the preceding discussion. In addition, shock is invariably associated with some degree of inflammatory response, although this component of shock varies greatly. A severe systemic inflammatory response (e.g., sepsis) can result primarily in shock. Conversely, shock results in an inflammatory response because ischemia-reperfusion injury[45] will be triggered to some extent after successful hemodynamic resuscitation of shock of any kind. Ischemia-reperfusion causes release of proinflammatory mediators, chemotactic cytokines, and activation of endothelial cells and leukocytes. Because of the multiorgan system involvement of shock, the inflammatory response of ischemia-reperfusion involves many organ systems. Rapid hemodynamic correction of hypovolemic or cardiogenic shock may result in a minimal systemic inflammatory response. However, trauma with significant tissue injury or prolonged hypoperfusion states usually elicit marked systemic inflammatory responses. Because the resolution and repair phases of the inflammatory response are complex and take time, this component of shock is important to recognize and characterize clinically because it has prognostic value with profound effects on the subsequent clinical course.

A systemic inflammatory response results in elevated levels of circulating proinflammatory mediators (tumor necrosis alpha, interleukins, prostaglandins, etc.) that activate endothelial cells and leukocytes. Subsequent production of nitric oxide by activated vascular endothelial cells via inducible nitric oxide synthase results in substantial vasodilation. Products of the arachidonic acid pathway generated during the systemic inflammatory response contribute to systemic vasodilation (prostaglandin I_2) and pulmonary hypertension (thromboxane A_2). Activated endothelial cells and leukocytes upregulate expression of cellular adhesion molecules and their corresponding ligands, resulting in accumulation of activated leukocytes in pulmonary and systemic capillaries and postcapillary venules. Expression of chemotactic cytokines by endothelial and parenchymal cells contributes to flow of activated leukocytes into the lungs and systemic tissues. Activated leukocytes release destructive oxygen free radicals, resulting in further microvascular and tissue damage. Damaged and edematous endothelial cells, retained leukocytes, and fibrin and platelet plugs associated with activation of the complement and coagulation cascades block capillary beds in a patchy manner, leading to increased heterogeneity of microvascular blood flow. As a result of the significant damage to the microvasculature, oxygen uptake by metabolizing tissues is further impaired.[46] A severe systemic inflammatory response leads to very high levels of circulating proinflammatory mediators, leukopenia, and thrombocytopenia owing to uptake in excess of production, disseminated intravascular coagulation owing to excessive activation of the coagulation cascades, diffuse capillary leak, marked vasodilation that may be quite unresponsive to high doses of vasopressors, and generalized organ system dysfunction.

Whereas the hemodynamic component of shock is often rapidly reversible, the resolution and repair phases of an inflammatory response follow a frustratingly slow time course: recruitment of adequate and appropriate leukocyte populations, walling off or control of the initial inciting stimuli, modulation of the subsequent inflammatory response toward clearance with apoptosis of inflammatory and damaged cells (T-helper 1 type of response), or, when the inflammatory stimulus is not as easily cleared, toward a more chronic response with recruitment of new populations of mononuclear leukocytes and fibrin and collagen deposition (T-helper 2 type of response). During this repair and resolution phase, current therapy involves vigilant supportive care of the patient to prevent and avoid the common multiple complications associated with multiple organ system dysfunction and mechanical ventilation.

INDIVIDUAL ORGAN SYSTEMS

Altered mental status, ranging from mild confusion to coma, is a frequently observed effect of shock on neurologic function, when brain blood flow decreases by approximately 50%.[47] Autoregulation of cerebral blood flow is maximal, and decreased neurologic function ensues, when MAP decreases to below 50 to 60 mm Hg in normal individuals. Elevated P_{CO2} transiently dilates and decreased P_{CO2} transiently constricts cerebral vessels. Profound hypoxia also results in markedly decreased cerebral vascular resistance. Patients recovering from shock infrequently suffer frank neurologic deficit unless they have concomitant cerebrovascular disease. However, subsequent subtle neurocognitive dysfunction is now increasingly recognized.

Systolic and diastolic myocardial dysfunction during shock have been discussed above. Myocardial oxygen extraction is impaired during sepsis and myocardial perfusion is redistributed away from the endocardium. This maldistribution is further aggravated by circulating catecholamines. Segmen-

tal and global myocardial dysfunction occur with ST and T-wave changes apparent on the electrocardiogram, and elevations in creatine kinase and troponin concentrations may be observed[48] in the absence of true myocardial infarction. In addition, the metabolic substrate for myocardial metabolism changes so that free fatty acids are no longer the prime substrate and more lactic acid and endogenous fuels are metabolized.

More than any other organ system, the lungs are involved in the inflammatory component of shock. ARDS is the acronym given to lung injury caused by the effect of the systemic inflammatory response on the lung and has aptly been called "shock lung." Inflammatory mediators and activated leukocytes in the venous effluent of any organ promptly affect the pulmonary capillary bed, leading to activation of pulmonary vascular endothelium and plugging of pulmonary capillaries with leukocytes. Ventilation perfusion matching is impaired and shunt increases. High tidal volume ventilation induces a further intrapulmonary inflammatory response and lung damage. Increased ventilation associated with shock results in increased work of breathing to the extent that a disproportionate amount of blood flow is diverted to fatiguing ventilatory muscles.

Early in shock, increased catecholamines, glucagon, and glucocorticoids increase hepatic gluconeogenesis leading to hyperglycemia. Later, when synthetic function fails, hypoglycemia occurs. Clearance of metabolites and immunologic function of the liver are also impaired during hypoperfusion. Typically, centrilobular hepatic necrosis leads to release of transaminases as the predominant biochemical evidence of hepatic damage, and bilirubin levels may be high. Shock may lead to gut ischemia before other organ systems become ischemic, even in the absence of mesenteric vascular disease. Mucosal edema, submucosal hemorrhage, and hemorrhagic necrosis of the gut may occur. Hypoperfusion of the gut has been proposed as a key link in the development of multisystem organ failure after shock, particularly when ARDS precedes sepsis[49]; that is, loss of gut barrier function results in entrance of enteric organisms and toxins into lymphatics and the portal circulation. Because the immunologic function of the liver is impaired, bacteria and their toxic products, particularly from portal venous blood, are not adequately cleared. These substances and inflammatory mediators produced by hepatic reticuloendothelial cells are released into the systemic circulation and may be an important initiating event of a diffuse systemic inflammatory process that leads to multisystem organ failure or to the high cardiac output hypotension of endotoxemia. Decreased hepatic function during shock impairs normal clearance of drugs such as narcotics and benzodiazepines, lactic acid, and other metabolites that may adversely affect cardiovascular function. In addition, pancreatic ischemic damage may result in the systemic release of a number of toxic substances including a myocardial depressant factor.

The glomerular filtration rate decreases as renal cortical blood flow is reduced by decreased arterial perfusion pressures and by afferent arteriolar vasoconstriction owing to increased sympathetic tone, catecholamines, and angiotensin. The ratio of renal cortical to medullary blood flow decreases. Renal hypoperfusion may lead to ischemic damage with acute tubular necrosis, and debris and surrounding tissue edema obstruct tubules. Loss of tubular function is compounded by loss of concentrating ability because medullary hypertonicity decreases. Impaired renal function or renal failure leads to worsened metabolic acidosis, hyperkalemia, impaired clearance of drugs and other substances; all contribute to the poor outcome of patients in shock with renal failure.

Shock impairs reticuloendothelial system function, leading to impaired immunologic function. Coagulation abnormalities and thrombocytopenia are common hematologic effects of shock. Disseminated intravascular coagulation occurs in approximately 10% of patients with hypovolemic and septic shock. Shock combined with impaired hematopoietic and immunologic function seen with hematologic malignancies or after chemotherapy is nearly uniformly lethal. Endocrine disorders, from insufficient or ineffective insulin secretion to adrenal insufficiency, adversely affect cardiac and other organ system function. Conceivably, impaired parathyroid function is unable to maintain calcium homeostasis. As a result, ionized hypocalcemia is observed during lactic acidosis or its treatment with sodium bicarbonate infusion.[50]

SHOCK AND THERAPEUTIC INTERVENTIONS

Hypoperfusion alters the efficacy of drug therapy by slowing delivery of drugs, altering pharmacokinetics once delivered, and decreasing the clearance of drugs. For example, subcutaneous injection of medications may fail to deliver useful quantities of a drug in the setting of decreased perfusion. When adequate perfusion is re-established, the drug may be delivered in an unpredictable way at an inappropriate time. Thus, parenteral medications should be given intravenously to patients with evidence of hypoperfusion. In marked hypoperfusion states, peripheral intravenous infusion also may be ineffective, and central venous administration may be necessary to effectively deliver medications. Once the drug is delivered to its site of action, it may not have the same effect in the setting of shock. For example, catecholamines may be less effective in an acidotic or septic state. Because there may be significant renal and hepatic hypoperfusion, drug clearance is frequently greatly impaired. With these observations in mind, it is appropriate to consider, for each drug, necessary changes in route, dose, and interval of administration in shock patients.

Bicarbonate therapy of metabolic acidosis associated with shock may have adverse consequences.[50] Bicarbonate decreases ionized calcium levels further, with a potentially detrimental effect on myocardial contractility. Because bicarbonate and acid reversibly form carbon dioxide and water, a high P_{CO_2} is observed. Particularly during bolus infusion, acidotic blood containing bicarbonate may have a very high P_{CO_2}, which readily diffuses into cells, resulting in marked intracellular acidosis; recall that hypoperfusion increases tissue P_{CO_2} by carrying off the tissue CO_2 production at a higher mixed venous P_{CO_2} owing to reduced blood flow. Intracellular acidosis results in decreased myocardial contractility. These adverse consequences of bicarbonate therapy may account in part for the lack of benefit observed with bicarbonate therapy of metabolic acidosis.[50]

Outcome

Untreated, shock leads to death. Even with rapid, appropriate resuscitation, shock is associated with a high initial mortality rate, and tissue damage sustained during shock may lead to delayed sequelae. Several studies have identified important predictors. For cardiogenic shock, 85% of the predictive information is contained in age, systolic blood pressure, heart rate, and presenting Killip class.[3] A blood lactic acid level in excess of 5 mmol/L is associated with a 90% mortality rate in cardiogenic shock[51] and a high mortality rate in other shock states. These mortality rates have decreased during the past decade of interventional cardiology and aggressive antibiosis (see Chaps. 25 and 46). In septic shock, decreasing cardiac output predicts death, and high concentrations of bacteria in blood and a failure to mount a febrile response predict a poor outcome. Age and pre-existing illness are important determinants of outcome. Multisystem organ failure is an important adverse outcome, leading to a mortality rate in excess of 60%.

References

1. Cohn JN: Blood pressure measurement in shock. Mechanism of inaccuracy in ausculatory and palpatory methods. *JAMA* 199:118, 1967.
2. Rivers E, Nguyen B, Havstad S, et al: Early Goal-Directed Therapy Collaborative G. Early goal-directed therapy in the treatment of severe sepsis and septic shock. *N Engl J Med* 345:1368, 2001.
3. Menon V, Hochman JS: Management of cardiogenic shock complicating acute myocardial infarction. *Heart* 88:531, 2002.
4. Kern JW, Shoemaker WC: Meta-analysis of hemodynamic optimization in high-risk patients. *Crit Care Med* 30:1686, 2002.
5. Grassino A, Macklem PT: Respiratory muscle fatigue and ventilatory failure. *Annu Rev Med* 35:625, 1984.
6. Hussain SN, Roussos C: Distribution of respiratory muscle and organ blood flow during endotoxic shock in dogs. *J Appl Physiol* 59:1802, 1985.
7. Imai Y, Parodo J, Kajikawa O, et al: Injurious mechanical ventilation and end-organ epithelial cell apoptosis and organ dysfunction in an experimental model of acute respiratory distress syndrome. *JAMA* 289:2104, 2003.
8. Anonymous: Ventilation with lower tidal volumes as compared with traditional tidal volumes for acute lung injury and the acute respiratory distress syndrome. The Acute Respiratory Distress Syndrome Network. *N Engl J Med* 342:1301, 2000.
9. Shoemaker WC, Appel PL, Kram HB, et al: Prospective trial of supranormal values of survivors as therapeutic goals in high-risk surgical patients. *Chest* 94:1176, 1988.
10. de Guzman E, Shankar MN, Mattox KL: Limited volume resuscitation in penetrating thoracoabdominal trauma. *AACN Clin Issues* 10:61, 1999.
11. Hebert PC, Wells G, Blajchman MA, et al: A multicenter, randomized, controlled clinical trial of transfusion requirements in critical care. Transfusion Requirements in Critical Care Investigators, Canadian Critical Care Trials Group. *N Engl J Med* 340:409, 1999.
12. Bickell WH, Wall MJ Jr, Pepe PE, et al: Immediate versus delayed fluid resuscitation for hypotensive patients with penetrating torso injuries. *N Engl J Med* 331:1105, 1994.
13. Ruokonen E, Parviainen I, Uusaro A: Treatment of impaired perfusion in septic shock. *Ann Med* 34:590, 2002.
14. Reinhart K, Rudolph T, Bredle DL, et al: Comparison of central-venous to mixed-venous oxygen saturation during changes in oxygen supply/demand. *Chest* 95:1216, 1989.
15. Vincent JL, Abraham E, Annane D, et al: Reducing mortality in sepsis: new directions. *Crit Care* 6:S1, 2002.
16. Bernard GR, Vincent JL, Laterre PF, et al: Recombinant human protein CWEiSSsg. Efficacy and safety of recombinant human

activated protein C for severe sepsis. *N Engl J Med* 344:699, 2001.

17. Annane D, Sebille V, Charpentier C, et al: Effect of treatment with low doses of hydrocortisone and fludrocortisone on mortality in patients with septic shock. *JAMA* 288:862, 2002.

18. Connors AF Jr, Speroff T, Dawson NV, et al: The effectiveness of right heart catheterization in the initial care of critically ill patients. SUPPORT Investigators. *JAMA* 276:889, 1996.

19. Sandham JD, Hull RD, Brant RF, et al: Canadian Critical Care Clinical Trials G. A randomized, controlled trial of the use of pulmonary-artery catheters in high-risk surgical patients. *N Engl J Med* 348:5, 2003.

20. Rame JE, Dries DL, Drazner MH: The prognostic value of the physical examination in patients with chronic heart failure. *Congest Heart Fail* 9:170, 2003.

21. Forrester JS, Diamond G, Chatterjee K, Swan HJ: Medical therapy of acute myocardial infarction by application of hemodynamic subsets (second of two parts). *N Engl J Med* 295:1404, 1976.

22. Scheidt S, Ascheim R, Killip T III: Shock after acute myocardial infarction. A clinical and hemodynamic profile. *Am J Cardiol* 26:556, 1970.

23. Lieu TA, Gurley RJ, Lundstrom RJ, Parmley WW: Primary angioplasty and thrombolysis for acute myocardial infarction: an evidence summary. *J Am Coll Cardiol* 27:737, 1996.

24. Page DL, Caulfield JB, Kastor JA, et al: Myocardial changes associated with cardiogenic shock. *N Engl J Med* 285:133, 1971.

25. Pfisterer M: Right ventricular involvement in myocardial infarction and cardiogenic shock. *Lancet* 362:392, 2003.

26. Zile MR, Brutsaert DL: New concepts in diastolic dysfunction and diastolic heart failure: Part II: Causal mechanisms and treatment. *Circulation* 105:1503, 2002.

27. David TE: Operative management of postinfarction ventricular septal defect. *Semin Thorac Cardiovasc Surg* 7:208, 1995.

28. Baskett RJ, Ghali WA, Maitland A, Hirsch GM: The intraaortic balloon pump in cardiac surgery. *Ann Thoracic Surg* 74:1276, 2002.

29. Lipkin DP, Frenneaux M, Maseri A: Beneficial effect of captopril in cardiogenic shock. *Lancet* 2:327, 1987.

30. Kinch JW, Ryan TJ: Right ventricular infarction. *N Engl J Med* 330:1211, 1994.

31. Jacobs AK, Leopold JA, Bates E, et al: Cardiogenic shock caused by right ventricular infarction: A report from the SHOCK registry. *J Am Coll Cardiol* 41:1273, 2003.

32. Layish DT, Tapson VF: Pharmacologic hemodynamic support in massive pulmonary embolism. *Chest* 111:218, 1997.

33. Konstantinides S, Geibel A, Heusel G, et al: Prognosis of Pulmonary Embolism-3 Trial I. Heparin plus alteplase compared with heparin alone in patients with submassive pulmonary embolism. *N Engl J Med* 347:1143, 2002.

34. McGee S, Abernethy WB III, Simel DL: The rational clinical examination. Is this patient hypovolemic? *JAMA* 281:1022, 1999.

35. Rush BF Jr: Irreversibility in the post-transfusion phase of hemorrhagic shock. *Adv Exp Med Biol* 23:215, 1971.

36. Reilly PM, Wilkins KB, Fuh KC, et al: The mesenteric hemodynamic response to circulatory shock: An overview. *Shock* 15:329, 2001.

37. Walley KR, Cooper DJ: Diastolic stiffness impairs left ventricular function during hypovolemic shock in pigs. *Am J Physiol* 260:H702, 1991.

38. Rangel-Frausto MS: The epidemiology of bacterial sepsis. *Infect Dis Clin North Am* 13:299, 1999.

39. Angus DC, Wax RS: Epidemiology of sepsis: An update. *Crit Care Med* 29:S109, 2001.

40. Parker MM, Shelhamer JH, Bacharach SL, et al: Profound but reversible myocardial depression in patients with septic shock. *Ann Intern Med* 100:483, 1984.

41. Walley KR: Many roles of nitric oxide in regulating cardiac function in sepsis. *Crit Care Med* 28:2135, 2000.

42. Ellis AK, Day JH: Diagnosis and management of anaphylaxis. *Can Med Assoc J* 169:307, 2003.

43. Cooper DS: Hyperthyroidism. *Lancet* 362:459, 2003.

44. Bravo EL: Pheochromocytoma. *Curr Ther Endocrinol Metab* 6:195, 1997.

45. Hochman JS: Cardiogenic shock complicating acute myocardial infarction: expanding the paradigm. *Circulation* 107:2998, 2003.

46. Walley KR: Heterogeneity of oxygen delivery impairs oxygen extraction by peripheral tissues: Theory. *J Appl Physiol* 81:885, 1996.

47. Harper AM: Autoregulation of cerebral blood flow: Influence of the arterial blood pressure on the blood flow through the cerebral cortex. *J Neurol Neurosurg Psychiatry* 29:398, 1966.

48. Spies C, Haude V, Fitzner R, et al: Serum cardiac troponin T as a prognostic marker in early sepsis. *Chest* 113:1055, 1998.

49. Aranow JS, Fink MP: Determinants of intestinal barrier failure in critical illness. *Br J Anaesth* 77:71, 1996.

50. Cooper DJ, Walley KR, Wiggs BR, Russell JA: Bicarbonate does not improve hemodynamics in critically ill patients who have lactic acidosis. A prospective, controlled clinical study. *Ann Intern Med* 112:492, 1990.

51. Weil MH, Afifi AA: Experimental and clinical studies on lactate and pyruvate as indicators of the severity of acute circulatory failure (shock). *Circulation* 41:989, 1970.

Chapter 22

VENTRICULAR DYSFUNCTION IN CRITICAL ILLNESS

KEITH R. WALLEY

KEY POINTS

- *Understanding cardiovascular dysfunction in a critically ill patient requires consideration of cardiac function and systemic vascular factors controlling venous return.*
- *Compression by surrounding structures (cardiac tamponade) and increased afterload must be considered as external causes or contributors to cardiac dysfunction.*
- *Decreased ventricular pump function may be due to decreased systolic contractility, increased diastolic stiffness, abnormal heart rate and rhythm, or valvular dysfunction.*
- *Management of ventricular dysfunction aims to reverse the cause by optimizing preload and afterload and correcting abnormalities in heart rhythm, valve function, and contractility.*
- *Acute reversible contributions to depressed contractility result from ischemia, hypoxemia, acidosis, ionized hypocalcemia and other electrolyte abnormalities, myocardial depressant factors, and hypo- and hyperthermia.*
- *Management of acute-on-chronic heart failure progressively includes oxygen; optimizing preload with diuretics, morphine, and nitrates or fluid infusion for hypovolemia; afterload reduction; increasing contractility using catecholamines or phosphodiesterase inhibitors; antiarrhythmic drugs and resynchronization using biventricular pacing; intraaortic balloon counterpulsation; and cardiac transplantation.*

This chapter reviews the etiology and management of circulatory disturbances arising in critically ill patients whose primary cause for ventricular dysfunction is more related to complications of other multisystem organ failures without diminishing the possibility that occult ischemic heart disease (see Chap. 25) might be unmasked by the stress imposed by multisystem organ failure or its diverse treatments. I emphasize how critical illness disturbs ventricular function and the systemic factors governing venous return and refer the reader to Chap. 25 for the detailed diagnosis and management of ischemic heart disease. To avoid redundancy, I refer liberally to other chapters in this book that discuss mechanisms for ventricular dysfunction in the context of other diseases (see Chaps. 20, 21, 26, 28, and 29).

Assessment of Cardiovascular Dysfunction

Cardiac pump function can be defined by the relation of the heart's output to its input.[1] Cardiac output is the most important output of the entire heart, and right atrial pressure (Pra) is an easily measured input of the entire heart. Cardiac output is initially assessed as high, adequate, or inadequate by cardiovascular examination and by clinical evaluation of perfusion. Later, after placement of a central venous catheter to allow measurement of central venous pressure (CVP) and central venous oxygen saturation, after placement of a pulmonary artery catheter, or after echocardiography, cardiac output can be more accurately quantitated. Pra is initially evaluated by clinical examination of distention of the jugular veins and later may be more accurately measured as the CVP. Other outputs, such as stroke work, and other inputs, such as pulmonary artery occlusion (or wedge) pressure (Ppw), serve to quantitate cardiac dysfunction and to determine the specific cause of cardiac dysfunction.

Depressed cardiac function may be due to left ventricular dysfunction, right ventricular dysfunction, external compression (cardiac tamponade), or excessively elevated right or left ventricular afterload. I focus on left ventricular and right ventricular dysfunction because cardiac tamponade is discussed in Chap. 28 and pulmonary embolism in Chap. 27. Yet in every case one should consider whether the pericardium and other structures surrounding the heart or right- and left-side afterloads are affecting cardiac function. The specific causes of ventricular dysfunction, right and left, are decreased contractility (a shift down and to the right of the end-systolic pressure-volume relation), increased diastolic stiffness (a shift up and to the left of the diastolic pressure-volume relation), a change in heart rhythm and rate, and abnormal valvular function. How can one determine the presence of depressed ventricular pump function, distinguish between right and left ventricular dysfunction, and then identify the specific cause?

THE CLINICAL EXAMINATION

Left ventricular dysfunction is characterized by high left ventricular filling pressures in relation to cardiac output. Likewise, right ventricular dysfunction is characterized by high right ventricular filling pressures in relation to cardiac output. Importantly, there is a close interaction between the left and right ventricles so that, most commonly, left and right ventricular dysfunction coexist. Initially, clinical examination attempts to identify the presence and severity of depressed cardiac pump function and to distinguish the contributions of right and left ventricular dysfunction. Evaluation of perfusion and mean blood pressure, pulse pressure, and heart rate provide a clinical estimate of whether or not cardiac output is decreased (see Table 21-1). Right ventricular filling pressure may be judged by distention of jugular veins. Evidence of dependent pulmonary crackles on physical examination due to heart failure suggests that left ventricular filling pressure is elevated, usually above 20 to 25 mm Hg. However, in chronic congestive heart failure, where pulmonary lymphatic drainage increases, crackles may not be present even at filling pressures as high as 30 mm Hg. Interstitial edema clearance lags decreases in left atrial pressure (Pla) by hours, so rapid decreases in Pla are not accurately reflected by pulmonary auscultation. An audible third heart sound suggests an elevated Pla in the presence of a dilated left ventricle.[2]

CENTRAL VENOUS AND RIGHT HEART CATHETERS

In severe ventricular dysfunction or in critical illness, where even mild ventricular dysfunction contributes significantly to severity of illness, more accurate measures of ventricular function than can be determined by clinical examination are required to test and titrate therapy. Important tools in the intensive care unit (ICU) are central venous catheterization, pulmonary artery catheterization, and echocardiographic evaluation (see Chap. 13). Central venous catheterization allows measurement of right ventricular filling pressure (CVP) and central venous oxygen saturation, which can be used to estimate cardiac output by using the Fick equation. Pulmonary artery catheterization, using a thermistor-tipped catheter with a distal port at the tip and a proximal port 30 cm from the tip, can accurately determine cardiac output by using the thermodilution technique. Right ventricular filling pressure (CVP) can be measured with the proximal port. Left ventricular filling pressure may be estimated as the Ppw (with important limitations discussed in Chap. 13). Therefore, the separate contributions of right ventricular and left ventricular dysfunction can be distinguished. Right ventricular afterload can be measured as pulmonary artery pressure (Ppa) by using the distal port of the pulmonary artery catheter, and left ventricular afterload is reflected by measuring systemic arterial pressure. Uncritical use of a pulmonary artery catheter may be associated with no benefit or even an increased mortality rate.[3,4] Nonetheless, thoughtful use of a pulmonary artery catheter in the most severely ill may decrease mortality rate.[5]

INTEGRATING HEMODYNAMICS
WITH IMAGING STUDIES

The distinction between decreased contractility and increased diastolic stiffness cannot be determined by right heart catheterization alone. Accordingly, techniques that image ventricular diastolic and systolic volumes contribute substantially to the information obtained from pulmonary artery catheterization. The presence of enlarged v waves on the Pra trace or on the Ppw trace indicates tricuspid and mitral regurgitation, respectively. However, the size of the v waves depends on a number of factors, including compliance of the atria and ventricles so that accurate assessment of valvular dysfunction using a pulmonary artery catheter alone is impossible. Thus, additional imaging techniques are required to assess valvular function.

The most readily available and useful imaging technique is echocardiography, which can be used to evaluate ventricular function and valvular function (see Chap. 29). An estimated ejection fraction smaller than 0.4 is generally an excellent indicator of decreased contractility in hemodynamically stable patients. However, ejection fraction and related fractional shortening measurements are sensitive to changes in preload and afterload.[6,7] In the hemodynamically unstable patient, ejection fraction must be interpreted in conjunction with hemodynamic measurements from systemic and pulmonary artery catheters. Alternatively, echocardiography can be used to estimate ventricular diastolic and systolic volumes and filling of surrounding venous structures. Two distinctions are evident: a small end-diastolic volume (EDV) when filling pressures are normal or high indicates that increased diastolic stiffness contributes to decreased ventricular pump function,[8] and a large end-systolic volume (ESV) when afterload is normal or low indicates that depressed contractility contributes to decreased ventricular pump function. Therefore, end-diastolic and end-systolic diameters should be determined separately and interpreted in the light of measured pressures and flows.

Doppler echocardiographic examination allows measurement of the pressure gradient across valves, which is proportional to four times velocity squared, because blood flow across valves is turbulent. For example, it is usually possible to estimate Ppa from the tricuspid regurgitation velocity and CVP. Valvular insufficiency is also identified using Doppler and color Doppler echocardiographic imaging of blood velocities. The major limitation of conventional transthoracic echocardiographic examinations is that critically ill patients frequently are on positive-pressure mechanical ventilation and have lung disease, so lung shadows obscure echocardiographic views, thus making accurate examination difficult. Transesophageal echocardiographic examination circumvents this problem and is therefore an important tool for evaluating ventricular pump function in critically ill patients.[9–11]

DEFINITION OF CARDIAC FUNCTION AND ITS RELATION TO VENOUS RETURN

The pump function curve of the entire heart is illustrated as the relation between cardiac output and Pra over a range of values (Fig. 22-1A). Sometimes this relation is called a *Starling function curve*, although this term has been applied historically to a pump function curve where stroke work is the output.[12] The relation between cardiac output and Pra importantly illustrates that increasing Pra is more effective in increasing cardiac output at low values than at high values of Pra.

Most physicians are aware that increased contractility improves cardiac and ventricular pump function by shifting the pump function curve upward and to the left so that, at the same filling pressure, an increased cardiac output is generated. It is equally important to realize that abnormalities in diastolic stiffness, afterload, valve function, and heart rate can shift this relation, and these factors are often more important than changes in systolic function in modulating ventricular dysfunction encountered in the noncoronary care ICU.

CONTROL OF VENTRICULAR PUMPING FUNCTION

The ventricular pump function curve can be altered by changes in contractility, preload, afterload, heart rate and rhythm, and valvular function. Consider the pressure-volume relation of the left ventricle shown in Fig. 22-2. All end-systolic pressure-volume points lie along a line, the end-systolic pressure-volume relation (ESPVR). All ejections from different diastolic volumes end on the ESPVR.[13] The ESPVR shifts to the left when contractility increases, resulting in increased ejection at any given afterload; conversely, a shift to the right of the ESPVR indicates decreased contractility. Because of these characteristics, the ESPVR is a good index of ventricular contractility independent of changes in preload and afterload; because this slope is maximal at end systole and has the units of elastance ($E = \Delta P / \Delta V$), it has been denoted E_{max} or E_{es}.[13]

This pressure-volume representation of ventricular function is related to the ventricular pump function curve in a straightforward manner (Fig. 22-3). If the diastolic pressure-volume relation is constant, afterload is constant and if heart rate is constant, an increase in contractility decreases ESV and results in an increased stroke volume and cardiac output at the same filling pressure. Accordingly, an increase in

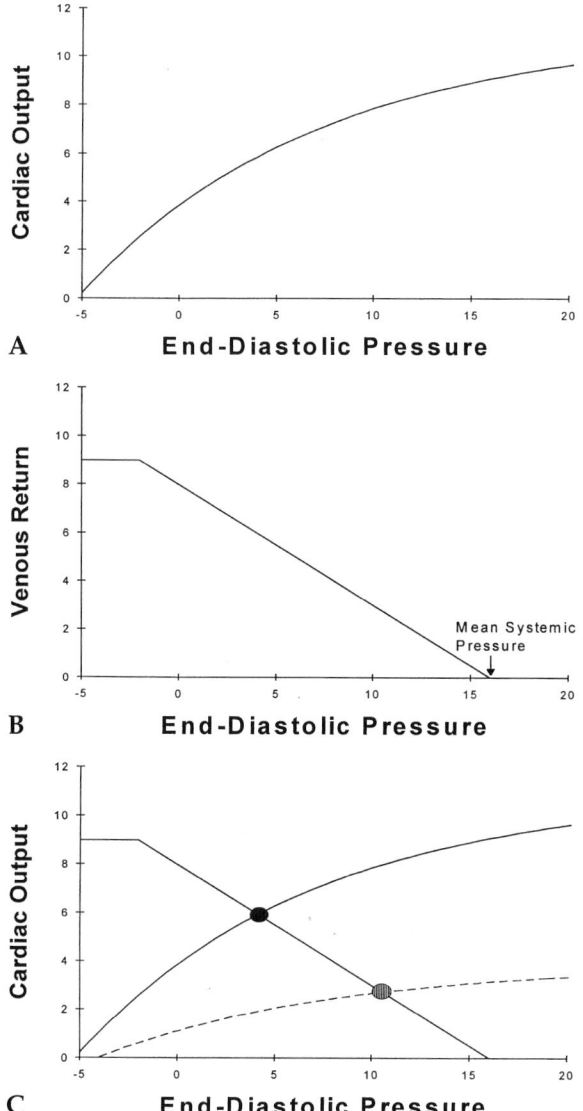

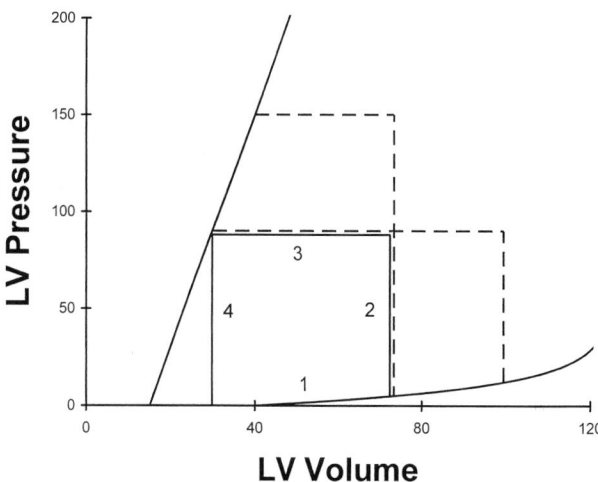

FIGURE 22-2 Left ventricular pressure-volume relations. The continuous thick lines represent a single cardiac cycle as a pressure-volume loop. During diastole, the ventricle fills along a diastolic pressure-volume relation (1). At the onset of systole, left ventricular pressure rises with no change in volume (2). When left ventricular pressure exceeds aortic pressure, the aortic valve opens, and the left ventricle ejects blood (3) to an end-systolic pressure-volume point. The ventricle then relaxes isovolumically (4). At a higher-pressure afterload, the left ventricle is not able to eject as far (*short interrupted lines*). Conversely, at a lower afterload, the left ventricle is able to eject farther, so that all end-systolic points lie along and define the end-systolic pressure-volume relation (ESPVR or E_{max}, *sloped solid line*). Increased diastolic filling (*long interrupted lines*) results in increased stroke volume from the larger end-diastolic volume to an endsystolic volume that lies on the same ESPVR; accordingly, increased afterload reduces stroke volume unless preload increases to compensate.

FIGURE 22-1 *A*. The cardiac function curve relates right atrial pressure (Pra) or end-diastolic pressure (EDP; *abscissa*) to cardiac output (*ordinate*). As EDP increases, cardiac output increases; however, at high EDPs, further increases cause less increase in cardiac output. *B*. The relation between EDP (Pra, *abscissa*) and venous return (*ordinate*) is illustrated. When EDP equals mean systemic pressure (Pms), there is no pressure gradient (Pms-Pra) driving the blood flow back to the heart, so venous return is zero. As EDP (Pra) decreases, the gradient from the veins to the heart to drive blood flow back to the heart increases, so venous return increases. At very low EDPs (Pra 0 mm Hg), central veins collapse and act as Starling resistors, so further decreases in EDP do not increase venous return. *C*. The cardiac function curve and the venous return curve are drawn on the same axes (*continuous lines*). The intersection of the cardiac function curve and the venous return curve defines the operating point of the circulation, here at an EDP (Pra) of approximately 5 mm Hg and a cardiac output of approximately 5 L/min. The interrupted cardiac function curve illustrates decreased cardiac function, causing decreased cardiac output (~3 L/min) at a higher EDP (Pra = 10 mm Hg).

ventricular contractility results in a leftward and upward shift of the ventricular pump function curve. An increase in contractility from a normal steep ESPVR does not decrease ESV much and therefore does not improve the ventricular pump

function much (Fig. 22-4). This explains why increased contractility is only a minor contributor to regulation of ventricular function in normal human beings. In contrast, when ventricular contractility is decreased, as indicated by a decrease in slope of the ESPVR, an increase in contractility significantly decreases ESV to improve ventricular pump function (see Fig. 22-4), thereby explaining why positive inotropic agents are useful in acute treatment of dilated cardiomyopathies.

A decrease in pressure afterload will result in a decrease in ESV, so stroke volume and cardiac output increase when contractility, the diastolic pressure-volume relation, and heart rate are constant.[13] Thus, decreased afterload also improves ventricular pump function by shifting the function curve up and to the left. Analogous to the effects of changing contractility, normal hearts with steep ESPVRs do not eject substantially further with a decrease in afterload because ESV does not decrease much (Fig. 22-5). This explains the observation that decreasing afterload in normal patients does not substantially increase cardiac function and output but leads to hypotension. However, in patients with depressed contractility, as signaled by a decreased slope of the ESPVR, a small decrease in afterload causes greater ejection to a smaller ESV so that stroke volume and cardiac output are substantially increased at the same ventricular filling pressure (see Fig. 22-5). Therefore, in patients with depressed systolic contractility, afterload reduction is an effective means for improving ventricular pump function.[14,15]

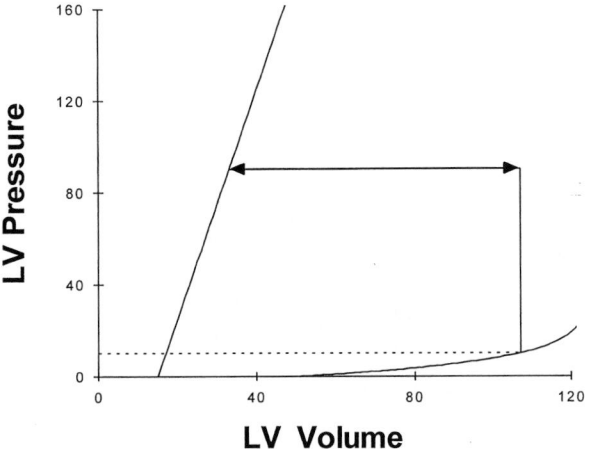

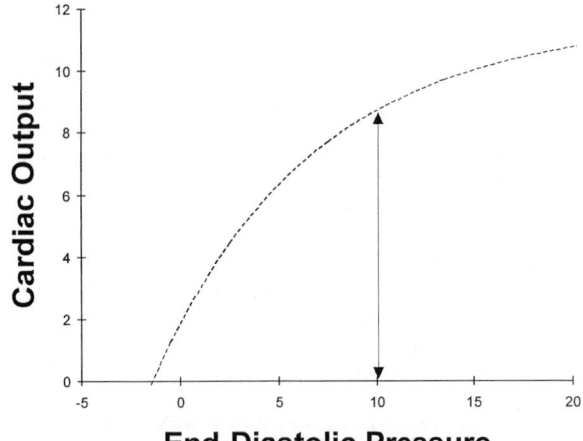

FIGURE 22-3 The cardiac function curve (*bottom*) is related to the left ventricular pressure-volume relations (*top*). *Top.* Stroke volume (*double-headed arrow*) is the difference between end-systolic volume (ESV) and end-diastolic volume (EDV). EDV at end-diastolic pressure (EDP = 10 mm Hg) is illustrated on the diastolic pressure-volume relation; ESV is determined by the end-systolic pressure (ESP) and the end-systolic pressure-volume relation (ESPVR or E_{max}). Therefore, for any EDP, cardiac output can be calculated if heart rate is known. *Bottom.* An increase in EDP increases EDV and cardiac output. At an EDP of 510 mm Hg, an increase in contractility would result in an increased stroke volume because the ESPVR shifts to the left; therefore, cardiac output increases at the same EDP and the cardiac function curve shifts up.

Increased stiffness of the diastolic pressure-volume relation reduces stroke volume because EDV is decreased at the same ventricular filling pressure independent of contractile state, afterload, and heart rate (Fig. 22-6). Therefore, an increase in stiffness of the diastolic left ventricle leads to a rightward and downward shift of the ventricular pump function curve.[16] This may be erroneously interpreted as decreased ventricular contractility when, in this case, depressed ventricular function is completely accounted for by increased ventricular diastolic stiffness. An increase in heart rate also may shift the ventricular pump function curve to the left and upward. However, when heart rate increases, stroke volume often decreases because there is less time for the ventricle to fill during diastole, so EDV decreases. Ultimately, when there is no

other change in the factors driving venous return, heart rate increases cardiac output only slightly at heart rates slower than 100 beats/min and has essentially no effect on cardiac output at faster heart rates.[17] At very fast heart rates exceeding 150 beats/min, diastolic filling becomes markedly impaired, and cardiac output decreases as heart rate quickens further. When control of heart rate is abnormal due to abnormal pacemaker function or abnormal cardiac rhythm, inappropriately slow heart rates become important and can limit cardiac output. For example, if a patient is hypotensive and critically ill to the extent that heart rate is expected to be 100 beats/min but the patient is able to generate a heart rate of only 50 beats/min, then artificially increasing heart rate will substantially improve cardiac output.

CONTROL OF VENOUS RETURN BY THE SYSTEMIC VESSELS

Cardiac function is tightly coupled to venous return, and many patients with presumed cardiac dysfunction instead have abnormalities of the factors driving venous return.[18] Pra and cardiac output define the cardiac function curve and define the venous return relation.[19] Figure 22-1B shows that, as Pra is decreased, venous return increases, because the pressure driving venous return back to the heart, mean systemic pressure (Pms) minus Pra, increases. The factors that determine venous return are Pms, Pra, and resistance to venous return (RVR).

$$\text{Venous return (VR)} = \frac{\text{Pms} - \text{Pra}}{\text{RVR}}$$

In steady state, the cardiac function curve and the venous return curve are necessarily coupled because cardiac output must equal venous return. Thus the operating point of the heart is not defined by the cardiac function curve or by the venous return curve but by the intersection of these two curves (see Fig. 22-1C). Accordingly, patients with cardiovascular dysfunction having abnormal values of heart rate, Pra, aortic pressure, and cardiac output may have cardiac dysfunction that accounts for these abnormalities or may have abnormalities of venous return. It follows that, in every patient with suspected abnormal cardiovascular function, one should consider cardiac function and venous return in attempting to understand the abnormality.[18,20]

In health, cardiac output is controlled by mechanical properties of the systemic vessels adjusted by neurohumoral reflexes; when output and blood pressure decrease, baroreceptor reflexes act to increase flow by raising Pms by sympathetic nervous and humoral output. The importance of factors driving venous return is evident during exercise or even during the act of standing up. Without increased venous tone (as can occur with some spinal cord injuries) or increased muscle activity aided by venous valves, cardiac output and therefore blood pressure decrease precipitously in changing from a recumbent to an upright position. As an extension of normal physiology, in critically ill patients without a previous history of cardiac dysfunction, the major factor limiting cardiac output is often limited venous return. Only in patients with marked ventricular dysfunction is cardiac output limited by decreased pump function. Knowing this avoids incorrect diagnosis and treatment. For example, positive inotropic drugs (dopamine and epinephrine) increase cardiac output even in

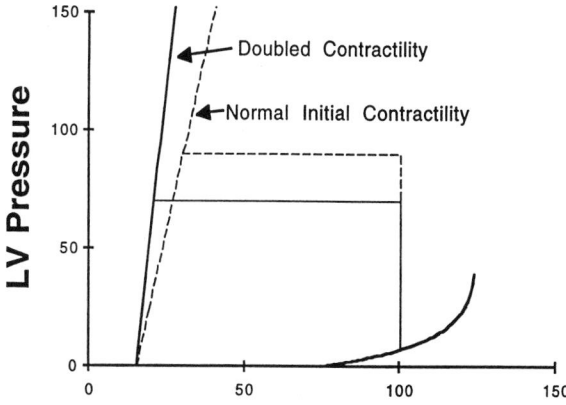

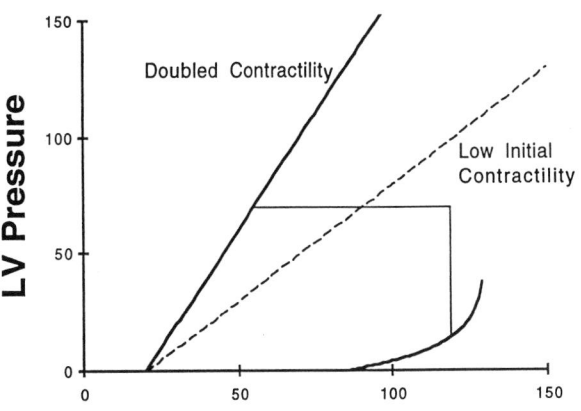

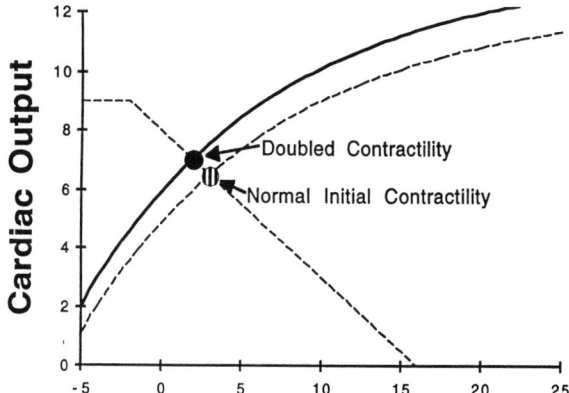

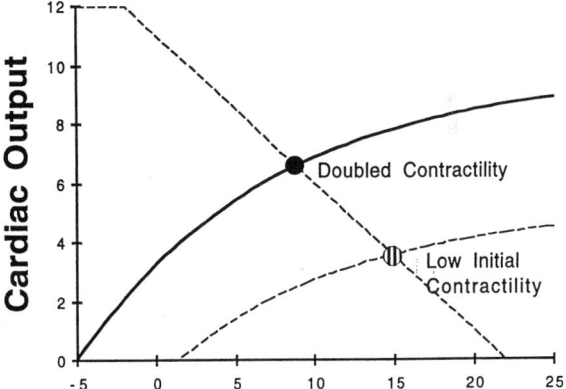

FIGURE 22-4 The *bottom two panels* show cardiac function curves derived (see Fig. 22-3 for derivation) from the pressure-volume relations illustrated in the *top panels*. The *left-hand panels* show that, when contractility is initially normal, then greatly increasing it does not improve cardiac function very much (*dashed and solid cardiac function curves* in the *lower left-hand panel* are similar). Flogging a normal heart with inotropic agents is ineffective, although vasoactive agents with effects on the venous circulation can increase venous return

without correcting underlying pathophysiology. Conversely, the *right-hand panels* show that, when contractility is initially low, then inotropic agents substantially improve cardiac function (from the *dashed cardiac function curve to the solid cardiac function curve* in the *lower right-hand panel*). For the same venous return curve (*dashed biphasic line* in the *lower right-hand panel*), cardiac output increases at a lower left ventricular end-diastolic pressure (*black dot* versus *striped dot* in *lower right-hand panel*).

patients with no ventricular dysfunction by increasing venous return due to increased Pms and decreased resistance to venous return (by redistributing blood flow to vascular beds with short transit times). This improvement in cardiovascular function is often attributed to improved cardiac function. Yet this interpretation is often incorrect and may delay therapy aimed at correcting factors governing venous return, such as plasma volume expansion, whereas the vasoactive drugs ineffectively flog the empty heart.

In summary, a complete evaluation of the contribution of ventricular dysfunction to cardiovascular performance in critical illness acknowledges that cardiac output and ventricular filling pressures depend as much on factors driving venous return as on cardiac function. Most critically ill patients without a history of cardiac disease have abnormalities of venous return in excess of abnormalities of cardiac function. Accordingly, cardiac output is limited by the heart only in patients with marked ventricular dysfunction, and the ventricular pump function curve is dependent not only on contractility but also on afterload, the diastolic ventricular pressure-volume relation, and heart rate.

Mechanisms and Management of Left Ventricular Dysfunction

This section addresses the diverse acute and chronic etiologies of left ventricular dysfunction and concludes with principles of management for each.

DECREASED LEFT VENTRICULAR SYSTOLIC FUNCTION

CHRONIC CAUSES
Dilated cardiomyopathies are the best-known chronic causes of decreased left ventricular contractility.[21] Dilated cardiomyopathy is often idiopathic with evidence that genetic, viral, and immune factors contribute. Dilated cardiomyopathy may also be associated with coronary artery disease, presumably due to previous ischemic events and subsequent adverse remodeling and apoptosis of cardiomyocytes leading to a dilated, poorly functional left ventricle.[22] Alcoholic cardiomyopathy is an important cause of chronic dilated ventricular

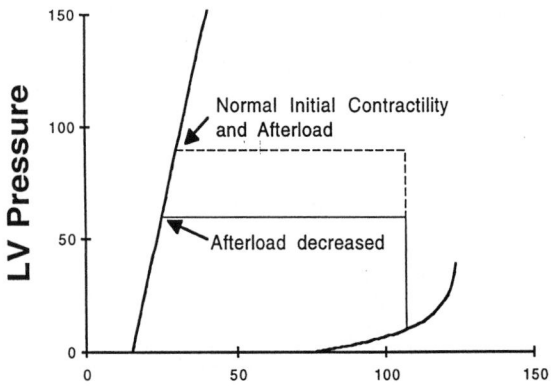

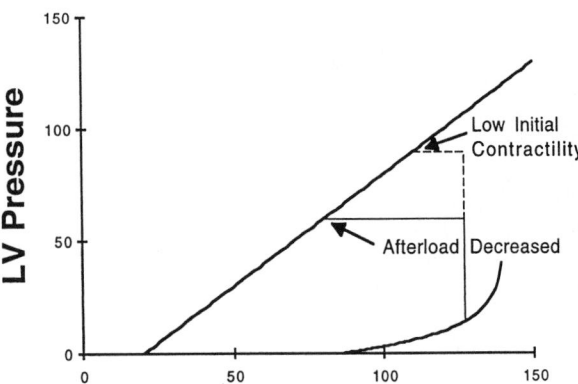

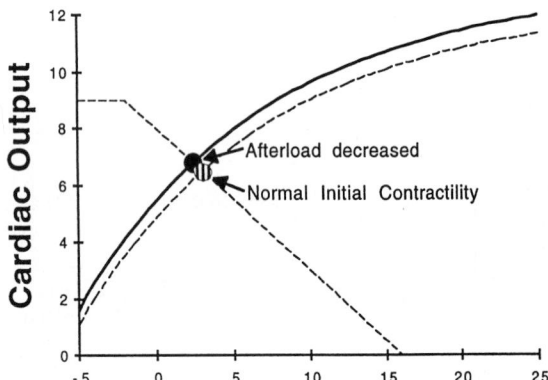

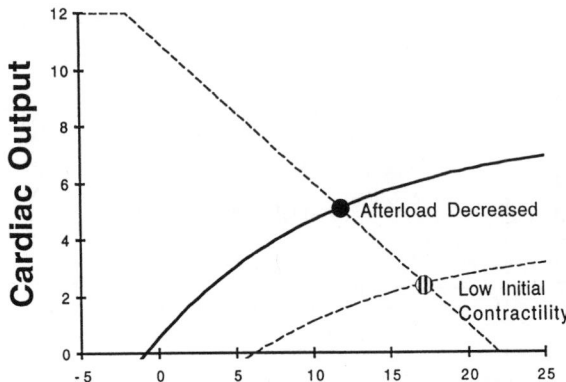

FIGURE 22-5 The *bottom two panels* show cardiac function curves derived (see Fig. 22-3 for derivation) from the pressure-volume relations illustrated in the *top panels*. The *left-hand panels* show that, when contractility is initially normal, then afterload reduction does not improve cardiac output or cardiac function (*dashed and solid cardiac function curves* in the *lower left-hand panel* are similar) and serves only to produce hypotension. Conversely, the *right-hand panels* show that, when contractility is initially reduced (*dashed cardiac function curve* in the *lower right-hand panel*), then afterload reduction substanially improves cardiac function (*solid cardiac function curve* in the *lower right-hand panel*). For the same venous return curve (*dashed biphasic line* in the *lower right-hand panel*), cardiac output increases at a lower left ventricular end-diastolic pressure (*black dot versus striped dot* in the *lower right-hand panel*).

dysfunction to be considered in critically ill patients.[21] Particularly in younger patients, inflammatory cardiomyopathy (myocarditis), usually viral, is an important cause of acute dilated cardiomyopathy that may lead to a chronic dilated cardiomyopathy in 10% of cases. Evidence of familial occurrence of similar disease is common, suggesting a genetic contribution in up to 25% of cases.[21,23] Rare causes such as the glycogen storage diseases also may be found in young patients. Multiple, less common causes may be encountered (Table 22-1).

These multiple, different etiologies of dilated cardiomyopathy lead to decreased ventricular contractility in a number of ways. Loss of myocardium with degradation of the normal collagen architecture by matrix metalloproteinases and replacement with fibrous connective tissue leads to remodeling and decreased contractility.[24] Increased levels of circulating renin, angiotensin II, endothelin, and norepinephrine promote cardiomyocyte hypertrophy, apoptosis, myocardial fibrosis, and vascular cell hypertrophy. Myocardial norepinephrine stores are depleted and β-receptor density is reduced in chronic dilated cardiomyopathy.[24,25] Biochemical changes that may contribute to decreased contractility include decreased efficiency of the sarcoplasmic reticulum calcium pump, decreased actin-myosin adenosine

triphosphatase activity, and change in myosin isoenzyme composition.

ACUTE CAUSES
In the ICU, acute causes of decreased left ventricular contractility are important because the acute causes are potentially reversible (Table 22-2). Acute causes of depressed left ventricular contractility include ischemia, hypoxemia, respiratory acidosis, metabolic acidosis, ionized hypocalcemia, hypo- and hyperthermia, exogenous toxins such as alcohol and drugs, endogenous toxins such as circulating depressant factors of sepsis, inflammatory cytokines, and increased nitric oxide (NO) production.

Myocardial Ischemia
Transient ischemic episodes occur frequently in critically ill patients. The onset of ischemia is due to myocardial oxygen demand exceeding the ability of the myocardium to extract oxygen from the oxygen supply (coronary blood flow multiplied by arterial oxygen content). Myocardial oxygen demand is increased by increasing heart rate, contractility, afterload, preload, and the basal metabolic rate of the myocardium (which increases with increased sympathetic

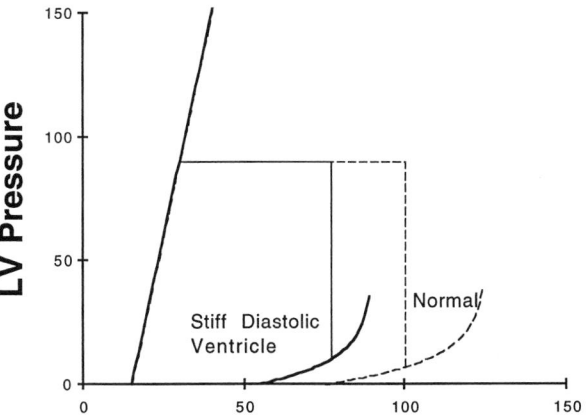

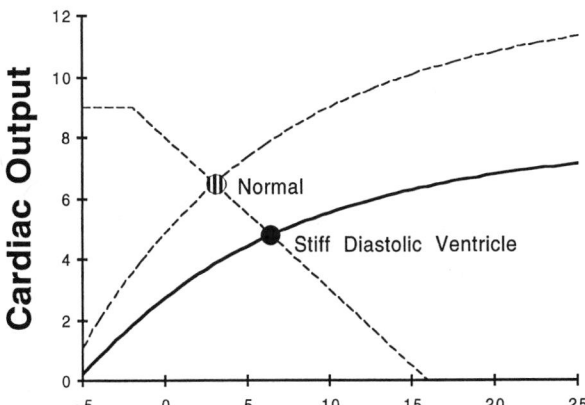

FIGURE 22-6 The *bottom panel* shows a cardiac function curve derived (see Fig. 22-3 for derivation) from the pressure-volume relations illustrated in the *top panel*. An increase in diastolic stiffness results in a decrease in end-diastolic volume (EDV) and in stroke volume at the same EDP, end-systolic pressure, and end-systolic pressure-volume relation, so increased diastolic stiffness shifts the cardiac function curve down and to the right (*dashed cardiac function curve* to the *solid cardiac function curve* in the *bottom panel*).

tone and catecholamines).[26] Many of the underlying illnesses encountered in the critically ill and many of the therapies, including fluid and inotropic or vasoactive drug infusion, contribute to markedly increased oxygen demand. Because of the prevalence of coronary artery disease in older patient popu-

TABLE 22-1 Chronic Causes of Decreased Contractility (Dilated Cardiomyopathies)

Coronary artery disease
Idiopathic
Inflammatory (viral, toxoplasmosis, Chagas disease)
Alcoholic
Infection with the human immunodeficiency virus
Postpartum
Uremic
Diabetic
Nutritional deficiency (selenium deficiency)
Metabolic disorder (Fabry disease, Gaucher disease)
Toxic (Adriamycin, cobalt)

TABLE 22-2 Acute Reversible Contributors to Decreased Contractility

Ischemia
Hypoxia
Respiratory acidosis
Metabolic acidosis
Hypocalcemia
Hypophosphatemia
Possibly other electrolyte abnormalities (Mg^{2+}, K^+)
Exogenous substances (alcohol, β blockers, calcium channel blockers, antiarrhythmics)
Endogenous substances (endotoxin, histamine, tumor necrosis factor, interleukin 1, platelet-activating factor)
Hypo- and hyperthermia

lations, ischemia in the ICU is frequently regional with associated wall motion abnormalities. Accordingly, a high index of suspicion and an early aggressive diagnostic approach are indicated and facilitate the early treatment of ischemic coronary artery disease, as discussed in more detail in Chap. 25.

Myocardial Hypoxia
In the absence of coronary artery disease, critically ill patients with sepsis also may manifest global heterogeneous left ventricular hypoxia with increased creatine kinase MB and troponin levels. The heart consumes less lactic acid and may produce lactic acid.[27] If inadequate oxygen delivery in relation to demand is not corrected quickly, then the heart may enter a detrimental positive-feedback loop of decreasing contractility, decreasing cardiac output and coronary perfusion, and, hence, decreasing contractility leading to precipitous cardiac arrest.[28] In the canine model, this vicious cycle occurred when arterial O_2 saturation decreased below 75% (arterial partial pressure of $O_2 = 40$ mm Hg) when hemoglobin concentration was 14 g/dL. Accordingly, aggressive measures to prevent this level of hypoxemia by keeping arterial O_2 saturation above 85% to 90% are indicated; maintaining a reasonable hematocrit in hypoxic critically ill patients with risks for myocardial ischemia is part of this therapy.

Myocardial Acidosis
Respiratory acidosis results in myocardial intracellular acidosis, and intracellular acidosis decreases the effect of intracellular calcium on the contractile proteins so that contractility is decreased.[29] In critically ill patients, respiratory acidosis may significantly contribute to depressed contractility and reduced cardiac output at partial pressure of CO_2 (P_{CO_2}) levels of 60 mm Hg and certainly by P_{CO_2} levels of 90 mm Hg.[30] Whether long-term elevations in P_{CO_2} have the same myocardial depressant effect is uncertain because intracellular pH will normalize, despite high P_{CO_2}, over time. These considerations may be particularly important in patients in whom the clinician actually seeks a high P_{CO_2} during mechanical ventilation (permissive hypercapnia) to minimize ventilator-associated lung injury (see Chaps. 37, 38, and 40).

Metabolic acidosis also may decrease left ventricular contractility, but its effects are less marked. Arterial blood gas measurement identifies metabolic acidosis in the extracellular compartment. The intracellular compartment is affected to the extent that the metabolic acid anion permeates the cell. Common organic acids such as lactic acid and ketoacids have anions that do not easily cross into the intracellular compartment, so a severe metabolic acidosis may not be associated with significant intracellular acidosis and therefore may not depress ventricular contractility much. For example, lactic acidosis at a normal P_{CO_2} begins to depress contractility at pH 7.1 to 7.2, but even at a pH of 7.0 the depression in contractility remains quite small.[31]

Ionized Hypocalcemia

During septic shock and in patients critically ill from diverse causes, serum ionized calcium levels are often low.[32] Further acute reductions may result in a substantial decrease in left ventricular contractility. Decreased extracellular ionized calcium concentration results in decreased calcium flux during systole and decreased contractility.[33] After transfusion of red blood cells stored in standard citrated media, serum ionized calcium levels can decrease dramatically because calcium is bound by citric acid. During shock and other conditions, lactic acid, like citric acid, also appears to bind ionized calcium.[34] Bicarbonate infusion also can rapidly decrease ionized calcium levels and, as a result, may depress ventricular contractility.[35] In addition to ionized hypocalcemia, other electrolyte abnormalities, including hypophosphatemia, hypomagnesemia, and hypokalemia or hyperkalemia, may contribute to decreased contractility or, more importantly, to arrhythmias.

Side Effects of Common Drugs

Exogenous toxins may result in acutely depressed myocardial contractility. Ethanol is a commonly encountered substance that acutely depresses contractility. Drugs commonly used in the ICU that significantly depress contractility include β blockers, calcium channel blockers, and antiarrhythmics such as disopyramide and procainamide.

Septic Shock and Systemic Inflammatory Responses

Many inflammatory pathways triggered by bacterial endotoxins and sepsis have been suggested to contribute to myocardial dysfunction of sepsis. A number of proinflammatory cytokines, including tumor necrosis factor α (TNF), interleukin (IL)–1, IL-2, and IL-6, decrease myocardial contractility in humans and in animal models of sepsis.[36,37] Proinflammatory cytokines trigger increased NO production. NO is normally an important regulator of beat-to-beat contractility and, in the setting of enhanced NO production, becomes an important myocardial depressant factor.[37] Reactive oxygen intermediates released by leukocytes and cardiomyocytes contribute directly, and by formation of peroxy nitrite radicals, to myocardial damage and dysfunction. Coronary capillary endothelial activation, damage, and dysfunction also contribute, in part due to impaired regulation of coronary microvascular blood flow, which impairs myocardial oxygen extraction.[38] Thus, multiple pathways of the intramyocardial inflammatory response may contribute to myocardial dysfunction of systemic inflammation and sepsis.

During hyperdynamic sepsis, the etiology of the hypoperfusion state likely resides in the septic paralysis of arteriolar (and in part venular) smooth muscle, with a minor contribution from decreased contractility, because cardiac output is maintained or elevated. However, the late decrease in cardiac output leading to death involves significant decreases in systolic contractility and increases in diastolic stiffness.

During anaphylactic shock, histamine depresses left ventricular contractility in human beings,[39] although the primary cause of hypoperfusion is hypovolemia (see Chap. 106). Hyperthermia and hypothermia may decrease myocardial contractility and contribute to depressed left ventricular function observed during sepsis and other critical illnesses associated with marked abnormalities of body temperature (see Chaps. 110 and 111).

MANAGEMENT OF DECREASED LEFT VENTRICULAR CONTRACTILITY IN CRITICAL ILLNESS

Identify and Correct Acute Reversible Causes

It is important to identify the multiple, different potentially reversible causes for depressed contractility in critically ill patients because, although alone they may be insufficient to account for the left ventricular dysfunction, together they may significantly depress function. For example, if ischemia or hypoxemia is present, aggressive attempts to correct it should be instituted. In the presence of coronary artery disease, standard care including heparin, antiplatelet therapy (when indicated), β blockade, and coronary vasodilation using nitrates may be helpful. Thrombolytic therapy within 4 to 6 hours of acute coronary thrombosis or emergency angioplasty decreases the incidence of congestive heart failure and improves outcome (see Chap. 25). Correction of hypoxemia and anemia may result in substantial improvement in ventricular function. Attention should be paid to decreasing factors that increase myocardial oxygen demand. Therefore, when β blockade is not feasible, choosing the lowest level of inotropic and vasoactive drugs that produces the desired therapeutic effect will minimize their contribution to myocardial oxygen demand. Likewise, alleviating pain is important to diminish the associated tachycardia and increased sympathetic tone.

In ventilated patients with left ventricular dysfunction, the detrimental effects of acute respiratory acidosis should be considered; mixed venous and, hence, tissue P_{CO_2} is much higher than the arterial partial pressure of CO_2 when the cardiac output is low. In general, metabolic acidosis should be treated by reversing its etiology. Alkali therapy for increased anion gap metabolic acidosis is of no benefit and may be dangerous even at pH values as low as 7.0 for a number of reasons.[35] Bicarbonate infusion results in an increase in P_{CO_2} due to chemical equilibrium of HCO_3^- with H_2O and CO_2 unless compensatory hyperventilation is also instituted. Particularly during rapid bolus injection, local P_{CO_2} may climb to extremely high values so that myocardial intracellular acidosis transiently may be severe, leading to decreased ventricular contractility.[30] Bicarbonate therapy is associated with an increase in lactic acid production because bicarbonate increases the rate-limiting step of glycolysis. Bicarbonate therapy also decreases blood levels of ionized calcium.[34,35]

Decreased contractility due to ionized hypocalcemia can be corrected with an intravenous infusion of calcium. After approximately 6 U of transfusion, ionized hypocalcemia should be measured and corrected, if necessary. Hypophosphatemia, hypomagnesemia, hypokalemia, hyperkalemia, and other metabolic disturbances also should be corrected because they may lead directly or indirectly to altered cardiovascular function.

Treatment of myocardial depression due to circulating myocardial depressant factors has been attempted with antibodies to endotoxin and TNF, naloxone, and dialysis, but these

TABLE 22-3 Effect of Direct-Acting Vasodilators

Drug	Route of Administration	Dosage	Onset of Effect	Duration of Effect	Large Arteries	Arterioles	Veins
Sodium nitroprusside (Nipride)	Intravenous	25–400μg/min	Immediate	—	+	+ + +	+ + +
Nitroglycerin (Tridil)	Intravenous	10–200μg/min	Immediate	—	+ +	+	+ + +
Isosorbide dinitrate (Isordil; Sorbitrate, Isobid; Isotrate; Sorate, Sorbide; Dilatrate)	Oral	20–60 mg	30 min	4–6 h	+ +	+	+ + +
Hydralazine (Apresoline)	Oral	50–100 mg	30 min	6–12 h	0	+ + +	±
Hydralazine (Apresoline)	IV or IM	5–40 mg	15 min	4–8 h	0	+ + +	±
Minoxidil (Loniten)	Oral	10–30 mg	30 min	8–12 h	0	+ + +	0
Diazoxide (Hyperstat)	IV bolus	100–300 mg	Immediate	4–12 h	0	+ + +	±
Nifedipine (Procardia)	Oral	10–20 mg	20–30 min	2–4 h	+ +	+ + +	±
	Sublingual	10–20 mg	15 min	2–4 h	+ +	+ + +	±

ABBREVIATIONS: IM, intramuscular; IV, intravenous.
SOURCE: Reproduced with permission from Cohn JN: Drugs used to control vascular resistance and capacitance, in Hurst JW, et al (eds): *The Heart*. New York, McGraw-Hill, 1990, p 1675.

investigational treatments have not led to improved clinical outcomes. Inhibitors of circulating inflammatory mediators appear to be beneficial in severe sepsis but are limited in less severe sepsis,[40] possibly because circulating factors (endotoxin, TNF, and IL-1) are present for only limited periods early in the course of sepsis. Naloxone administered over short periods is not consistently effective, but longer-duration infusions of 1 or more days may result in improvement of hemodynamic measurements. Dialysis, hemofiltration, and plasmapheresis have not been tested adequately in human septic shock, but preclinical evidence suggests that depressed left ventricular contractility due to a myocardial depressant factor of sepsis can be reversed with these treatments.[41]

Managing the Depressed Heart

Having reversed the acute contributors to depressed left ventricular contractility, standard therapy of decreased left ventricular contractility includes optimizing ventricular filling pressure, decreasing afterload using angiotensin-converting enzyme inhibitors or alternatives when arterial pressure is adequate, increasing contractility using inotropic agents, resynchronization therapy using biventricular pacing,[42,43] and, when appropriate, using intraaortic balloon counterpulsation followed by surgical correction of coronary artery stenosis or other surgically correctable lesions[24,44] (see Chap. 23).

The ventricular pump function curve illustrates the Frank-Starling mechanism, which shows that increased ventricular filling results in increased ejection even when contractility is depressed. The limit to increased ventricular filling is generally set by the onset of pulmonary edema. Pulmonary edema fluid enters the lung interstitium according to the Starling equation. At normal protein osmotic pressures (largely due to albumin) and normal permeability of the pulmonary endothelium, pulmonary edema starts to develop at Ppw values of at least 20 to 25 mm Hg.[45] In the presence of decreased oncotic pressure due to decreased albumin or in the presence of a leaky pulmonary endothelium, pulmonary edema may form at considerably lower Ppw values; in acute respiratory distress syndrome (ARDS) or pneumonia, pulmonary edema may form at very low Ppw values. With this in mind, it is appropriate to search for the Ppw that produces the highest cardiac output without resulting in substantial pulmonary

edema. Most often, this search necessitates preload reduction using diuretics and vasodilating agents (Table 22-3). However, when pulmonary edema does not limit oxygenation, it is appropriate to consider increasing cardiac output by intravascular fluid expansion.

Further management of decreased ventricular contractility then proceeds with afterload reduction[14] and inotropic agents.[46,47] These therapies are considered in detail below (Acute on Chronic Heart Failure). When vasodilator and inotropic therapy is insufficient, temporary support using intraaortic balloon counterpulsation is appropriate when damaged myocardium is expected to recover or as supportive therapy leading to surgical correction of an anatomic abnormality.[24,44] Balloon inflation during diastole improves diastolic perfusion of the coronary and systemic arterial beds. During systole, deflation of the balloon reduces afterload, allowing for increased ejection by a ventricle with markedly decreased contractility (see Chap. 25). Stem cell transplantation is a promising new approach under investigation to repair damaged myocardium.[48]

INCREASED DIASTOLIC STIFFNESS

In normal hearts and in hearts with depressed ventricular function, increasing preload is an important mechanism of increasing cardiac output. For hearts with normal systolic function, left ventricular end-diastolic filling pressures are often in the range of 0 to 10 mm Hg and result in an adequate cardiac output. For hearts with depressed contractility, higher filling pressures are usually required for an adequate cardiac output. Therefore, there is no uniformly optimal filling pressure. Left ventricular function may be substantially impaired by increased diastolic stiffness of the left ventricle—a shift up and to the left of the diastolic pressure-volume relation.[16,49] This is a problem whose importance is equal at least to depressed contractility in the critically ill patient.[8] Depressed systolic function reduces stroke volume because ESV increases; in contrast, increased diastolic stiffness reduces stroke volume because EDV decreases. Increased diastolic stiffness is a relatively frequent problem encountered in critically ill patients. It differs from depressed ventricular contractility because it is much more difficult to treat and does not respond to conventional therapy of decreased left ventricular pump function.[50] In fact, in the absence of an imaging study that demonstrates increased diastolic stiffness (small EDV in relation to the end-diastolic pressure [EDP]), the diagnosis of increased diastolic stiffness is suggested by finding depressed ventricular pump function unresponsive to fluid loading, afterload reduction, and inotropic agents. Occasionally, the diagnosis of increased diastolic stiffness is suggested by the observation that cardiac output is unusually sensitive to changes in heart rate.

CHRONIC CAUSES

Chronic diseases that increase diastolic stiffness include concentric left ventricular hypertrophy due to hypertensive cardiovascular disease, hypertrophic cardiomyopathy, and restrictive myocardial diseases. In addition, diseases of the pericardium, including constriction and effusion, and other processes that increase intrathoracic pressure result in increased diastolic stiffness, as discussed in Chap. 28. Concentric hypertrophy due to chronic hypertension is very common; although it seldom primarily accounts for severe depression in ventricular pump function, it may be an important contributor in combination with acute diseases depressing systolic function. Hypertrophic cardiomyopathy results in increased diastolic stiffness and, in the setting of hypovolemia, may also result in greatly increased afterload due to dynamic aortic outflow obstruction. Over a period of days and months, β blockers and calcium channel blockers, in particular verapamil, may reduce evidence of increased diastolic stiffness. More rapidly, these agents alleviate dynamic outflow obstruction in patients with hypertrophic cardiomyopathy due to their negative inotropic effect.[51] Restrictive cardiomyopathies include amyloidosis, hemochromatosis, sarcoidosis, endomyocardial fibrosis, some glycogen storage diseases, and restriction because of surgical correction of acquired and congenital abnormalities. Amyloidosis is uncommon at age 40 but by age 90 has a prevalence of 50%.

Clinical examination may show a Kussmaul sign, rapid x and y descents in the jugular venous pressure waveform so that a and v waves are prominent, and a fourth heart sound. Hepatojugular reflux may be prominent because the increased venous return produced by this maneuver cannot be accommodated by the stiff heart. Diastolic ventricular pressure measurements may show a square root sign, which is a rapid early rise in diastolic pressure to a relatively constant plateau. Echocardiographic evaluation may demonstrate rapid early diastolic filling to a relatively fixed diastolic diameter similar to the square root sign, and increased myocardial echogenicity may be observed in amyloidosis.[52,53]

ACUTE CAUSES

As with diseases resulting in depressed left ventricular systolic function, it is important to consider the acute, potentially reversible causes of increased diastolic stiffness.[8] Regional or global ischemia results in delayed systolic relaxation, contributing to increased diastolic stiffness. This change in diastolic stiffness usually precedes depressed contractility because the sarcoplasmic reticulum calcium pump has a lower affinity for adenosine triphosphate than do the contractile proteins. In addition, ischemia may result in increased diastolic stiffness by increasing pericardial pressure as a result of increased CVP.[54] Therefore, in the setting of increased diastolic stiffness, any ischemia should be treated aggressively.[55] Nitrates increase coronary blood flow and decrease tone in the venous capacitance bed, thereby reducing pericardial pressure; nitroprusside also decreases diastolic stiffness.

Increased intrathoracic or intrapericardial pressure is a common reversible cause of apparent increased diastolic stiffness in critical illness. Intrathoracic pressure is increased by positive-pressure mechanical ventilation and more so by the addition of positive end-expiratory pressure (PEEP). Positive airway pressures and PEEP are variably transmitted to the heart, depending on the distensibility of the lungs and chest wall. If the lungs are very distensible and the chest wall is relatively rigid (as with a tense abdomen), then most of an increase in airway pressure will be transmitted to the heart; to maintain the same chamber volumes, the atrial and ventricular pressures have to increase as much. This accounts for part of the reduction in venous return and cardiac output if and when Pms does not increase by a similar amount. A common misconception is that, if the lungs are very stiff, as in the early exudative phase of ARDS, then less of an increase in airway pressures will be transmitted to the heart. However, because PEEP reduces shunt by re-aerating flooded lung regions, the chest wall volume and pleural pressure increase as much or more in ARDS, so the increase in Pra with PEEP may be just as much as in patients with normal lungs. Increased intrathoracic pressure due to pneumothorax or massive pleural effusion may tamponade the heart and thereby result in apparent increased diastolic stiffness. Greatly increased intraabdominal pressure may elevate the diaphragm and similarly increase diastolic stiffness. Pericardial pressure may be increased by pericardial effusion and rarely by massive pneumopericardium. Because all these causes of increased intrathoracic or intrapericardial pressure leading to apparent increased diastolic stiffness are treatable, they must be identified or excluded early in critically ill patients.

Hypovolemic shock and septic shock may result in increased diastolic stiffness.[56] The increased diastolic stiffness associated with these kinds of shock is associated with irreversibility of the shock state and increased mortality rate. In septic shock, when depressed left ventricular systolic contractility occurs, the response of surviving patients is that of decreased diastolic stiffness or increased diastolic ventricular compliance.[57] This is the usual response to decreased left ventricular systolic contractility seen with other dilated cardiomyopathies.[58] However, in patients with septic shock who do not survive, the diastolic left ventricles do not dilate to increase EDV and, hence, do not compensate normally for decreased systolic contractility. The diastolic ventricles of those who do not survive are therefore much stiffer than the ventricles of those who do survive.[59] Infusion of catecholamines and calcium may further contribute to increased diastolic stiffness by contraction band formation.

Hypothermia with body temperature falling below 35.8°C (95.8°F) also results in increased left ventricular diastolic stiffness. This is a reversible phenomenon as temperature is increased. This is an important consideration during massive fluid resuscitation and mandates resuscitation with warmed infusions.

MANAGEMENT OF DIASTOLIC DYSFUNCTION

Whereas acute diastolic stiffness due to ischemia, tamponade, and tension pneumothorax are readily treated, acute therapy to reverse diastolic stiffness in the critical care setting is limited. Therefore, searching for an optimal filling pressure that maximizes ventricular diastolic filling without resulting in substantial pulmonary edema is a critically important component of care in these patients. In addition, hypovolemia and sepsis should be treated aggressively and promptly, inotropic agents should be avoided or used at the smallest dose that results in the desired systolic or vascular effect, hypothermia should be prevented and treated, and tachycardia or atrioventricular arrhythmias should be treated early (see below). Intrathoracic pressure is minimized by appropriate ventilator management and by decompressing surrounding compartments (pericardial, pleural, and abdominal) when these cause cardiac tamponade.

SPECIAL EFFECTS OF ALTERED AFTERLOAD ON VENTRICULAR FUNCTION IN CRITICAL ILLNESS

An increase in afterload decreases left ventricular pump function because stroke volume is reduced as a result of increased ESV (see Fig. 22-2). In malignant hypertension, elevated aortic pressure results in decreased cardiac output and elevated left ventricular filling pressures leading to pulmonary edema even if contractility is normal. Antihypertensive therapy results in rapid improvement. When contractility is depressed, increased afterload may worsen cardiac function even more. This is particularly important in dilated cardiomyopathies, in which increased afterload may be observed due to increased sympathetic tone, activation of the renin-angiotensin-aldosterone axis, and abnormally increased vascular smooth muscle tone.

Aortic valvular stenosis or dynamic obstruction of the aortic outflow tract also may increase afterload and contribute to decreased left ventricular pump function[14] (see Chap. 29). Dynamic outflow tract obstruction is most commonly due to hypertrophic cardiomyopathy. However, patients with preexisting concentric hypertrophy due to chronic hypertension who have a decrease in intravascular volume may develop dynamic aortic outflow tract obstruction with the classic findings of systolic anterior motion of mitral valve leaflet, increased ejection velocities signifying increased gradients across the aortic outflow tract, and cavity obliteration at end systole. This appears to occur most commonly in elderly patients with previously treated hypertension. Volume infusion to reverse intravascular hypovolemia may prevent left ventricular cavity obliteration and outflow tract obstruction and thereby reduce ventricular afterload. It is important to identify outflow tract obstruction as the cause of increased afterload because this cause of increased afterload is worsened by conventional afterload reduction therapy.

When afterload is reduced dramatically, or when intravascular volumes are expanded, the resulting high cardiac output state is sometimes called *high-output cardiac failure.* Actually, cardiac function still lies on a normal cardiac function curve, but the greatly increased venous return associated with low afterload results in high right- and left-side filling pressures with the appearance of right- and left-side congestion. This is particularly apparent in the presence of atrioventricular valvular stenosis, which previously may have been occult. Causes of high-output failure include anemia, arteriovenous fistulas, hepatic failure, Paget disease, thyrotoxicosis, pregnancy, carcinoid syndrome, and renal cell carcinoma.

ABNORMAL HEART RATE AND RHYTHM

Normally, heart rate and contractile states are matched to venous return and afterload to maximize the efficiency of the cardiovascular system. Even though heart rate is often of lesser importance in trying to increase cardiac output, excessively fast or excessively slow heart rates may limit cardiac output. Bradycardia is an important abnormal rhythm in a critically ill patient. Primarily, it is important to determine whether hypoxemia, drugs such as acetylcholinesterase inhibitors, or other reversible insults are the cause of bradycardia. In these cases, treatment consists of rapid reversal of the cause. In other cases in which bradycardia is due to primary cardiac disease, including myocardial infarction with involvement of the conducting system, therapy is directed at increasing heart rate by other means. Acutely, bradycardia may be treated with atropine and, if necessary, by isoproterenol or epinephrine infusion titrated to heart rate response. These temporizing measures allow placement of temporary or permanent pacemakers. In addition to the well-known indications for temporary pacing after myocardial infarction, it should be recognized that symptomatic bradycardia from any cause is an indication for pacing.

Tachycardia at sufficiently high rates results in an inadequate diastolic filling time, so stroke volume is reduced because adequate diastolic filling does not occur and the contribution to ventricular diastolic filling by the atria is less efficient, particularly in atrial fibrillation. An end-diastolic gradient across the mitral valve develops at fast heart rates. Hypoxemia and acidosis encountered in critically ill patients are frequently associated with ventricular and, even more commonly, supraventricular tachyarrhythmias. Hyperkalemia and hypokalemia, hypocalcemia, and hypomagnesemia are common electrolyte disturbances associated with increased incidence of ventricular arrhythmias. Accordingly, management of atrial and ventricular tachyarrhythmias involves correcting these potential contributing abnormalities.

Cardiac resynchronization therapy using biventricular pacing appears to improve cardiac function in patients having a decreased ejection fraction, bundle branch block, and New York Heart Association class III or IV heart failure.[42,43] The role for resynchronization therapy in the critical care setting has not been fully defined.

Arrhythmias including atrial fibrillation, atrial flutter, and ventricular tachycardia should be immediately cardioverted if they are contributing to a shock state. Otherwise, rapid heart rate due to atrial fibrillation is slowed using β blockers or second-line agents including calcium channel blockers. Adenosine, verapamil, and maneuvers to increase vagal tone may be useful in the diagnosis of tachyarrhythmias and in treating paroxysmal supraventricular tachycardia.[60] Multifocal atrial tachycardia responds to correction of underlying pulmonary disease and to verapamil.[61] Ventricular dysrhythmias contributing to altered hemodynamic function must be treated. Specific management of ventricular arrhythmias is detailed in Chap. 24.

VALVULAR DYSFUNCTION

The valves regulate preload and afterload and are therefore important determinants of left ventricular pump function (see Chap. 29). In critically ill patients, the effect of preexisting valvular disease may change with altered hemodynamics, or the extent of valvular disease may change primarily. For example, aortic and mitral insufficiencies contribute to low cardiac output at high ventricular filling pressures in critical illness, and both respond quickly to afterload reduction. Moreover, mitral regurgitation may worsen acutely due to increased EDV and expansion of the mitral annulus. In contrast, mitral valve prolapse may worsen at low ventricular volumes due to hypovolemia. In high cardiac output states, previously insignificant mitral stenosis may result in a high Pla and pulmonary edema. The gradient across the stenotic aortic valve may increase in high-flow states and conversely decrease in low-flow states, so that, without considering the flow across the valve, an incorrect judgment of the functional significance of the valvular disease may be made. Dysfunction of prosthetic valves is important to identify and may be a surgical emergency.

Mechanisms and Management of Right Ventricular Dysfunction

Right ventricular pump function also depends on contractility, afterload, preload (the diastolic pressure-volume relation), heart rhythm, and valve function. However, the right ventricle differs from the left ventricle, so the relative importance of each of these components is different. The left ventricle is well designed to generate high pressures. Its thick walls and small chamber volume result in manageable levels of wall stress despite high intracavitary pressures. The helical arrangement of muscle fibers changing from endocardium to epicardium in concentric layers results in a strong wall with an efficient distribution of wall stress.[62] In contrast, the right ventricle is a thin-walled pump whose surface has a large radius of curvature and it is not suited as a high-pressure generator. Instead, the right ventricle functions as an excellent flow generator at low pressures. Right ventricular contraction moves sequentially from the apex to the pulmonary outflow tract, giving it features of a peristaltic volume pump. During diastole, the right ventricle at normal diastolic pressure lies below its stressed volume, a feature that allows it to accommodate a large filling volume without an elevation in EDP. Because of these features, volume preload and, most importantly, pressure afterload become even more important determinants of right ventricular function than they are in the left ventricle.

DECREASED RIGHT VENTRICULAR SYSTOLIC FUNCTION

Contractility of the right ventricle is decreased approximately to the same extent as in the left ventricle by the many causes listed for the left ventricle (see Tables 22-1 and 22-2). Occasionally, right ventricular contractility is disproportionately reduced as in right ventricular infarction, right ventricular dysplasia, Uhl anomaly, isolated right ventricular myopathy, and myopathy associated with uncorrected atrial septal defect. Right ventricle ischemia in the absence of coronary artery disease is very important during critical illness. When afterload is elevated, the right ventricle responds along a preload-dependent right ventricular systolic pressure-volume relation, so right ventricular ESV increases.[63] Right ventricular chamber pressures are increased, the radius of curvature is

increased, and, hence, the wall stress in the thin right ventricular wall increases dramatically. Therefore, right ventricular myocardial oxygen demand increases proportionately. At increased right ventricular pressures, the right ventricular intramural pressure increases, and hence, the gradient for right ventricular coronary blood flow decreases. Oxygen supplied to the right ventricular myocardium may not meet oxygen demand, so contractility decreases, further worsening right ventricular function.[64]

DISORDERS OF RIGHT VENTRICULAR PRELOAD, AFTERLOAD, RHYTHM, AND VALVES

Increasing right ventricular EDV results in an increase in right ventricular stroke volume, even though right ventricular EDP may not increase much because normally EDV is below the right ventricular diastolic stressed volume. Because of this, and because Pra is heavily influenced by intraabdominal, intrathoracic, and intrapericardial pressures, Pra (CVP) is probably a poor indicator of right ventricular preload.

The afterload of the right ventricle is the Ppa (Table 22-4). This may be elevated long term by emphysematous destruction of small pulmonary vessels, chronic hypoxic pulmonary vasoconstriction due to obstructive pulmonary disease and restrictive chest wall diseases, recurrent pulmonary embolism, chronically elevated Pla due to mitral stenosis or left ventricular congestive failure, primary pulmonary hypertension, and several connective tissue and inflammatory diseases that involve the pulmonary vasculature. The acute pulmonary vasodilator response to nitroglycerin infusion is useful for predicting which patients will do well.[15] Acute causes of pulmonary hypertension are also important to identify because they are more often reversible. In addition, whereas the right ventricle may hypertrophy and accommodate severe chronically increased afterload, moderate acute pulmonary hypertension may rapidly lead to right ventricular decompensation. Important causes of acute pulmonary hypertension in critically ill patients include pulmonary embolism, hypoxic pulmonary vasoconstriction, acidemic pulmonary vasoconstriction, pulmonary infection, ARDS, sepsis, and acutely elevated Pla (see Chap. 26).

As with the left ventricle, the right ventricle depends on normal rate and rhythm to attain optimal function. Right ventricular valvular disease is less common and less important

TABLE 22-4 Causes of Elevated Right Ventricular Afterload

Chronic
　Chronic hypoventilation
　Recurrent pulmonary emboli
　Primary pulmonary hypertension
　Associated with connective tissue diseases
　Chronically elevated left atrial pressure (mitral stenosis, left ventricular failure)
Acute
　Pulmonary embolus
　Hypoxic pulmonary vasoconstriction
　Acidemic pulmonary vasoconstriction
　ARDS
　Sepsis
　Acute elevation in left atrial pressure
　Positive-pressure mechanical ventilation

ABBREVIATION: ARDS, acute respiratory distress syndrome.

than left ventricular valvular disease because right ventricular pressures are much less than left ventricular pressures, so gradients across the valves are considerably less. In critically ill patients, tricuspid valve disease with endocarditis is common as a preexisting condition such as endocarditis or as a result of instrumentation with a pulmonary artery catheter or other right heart catheters.

VENTRICULAR INTERACTION

DIAGNOSIS OF VENTRICULAR INTERDEPENDENCE

Combined pump dysfunction of the right and left ventricles is more common than isolated right or left ventricular pump dysfunction. Part of the explanation is that the diseases resulting in decreased pump function more commonly involve both ventricles. However, the right and left ventricles interact in important ways that, when recognized, may lead to a more effective therapeutic approach. The right and left ventricles are contained inside the same pericardial cavity within the chest wall, and the right and left ventricles share the interventricular septum. Accordingly, much of the interaction between the right and left ventricles is mediated by the parallel coupling produced by the pericardium and septal shift. The right ventricle is also connected in series with the left ventricle so that a substantial rise in Pla is transmitted back through the pulmonary vasculature and results in an increase in right ventricular afterload. In addition, the left ventricle is the pump that perfuses the right and left coronary circulations; hence, decreased systemic pressure combined with elevated right ventricular pressures may result in hypoperfusion of the right ventricle.

Detrimental ventricular interaction is generally only a problem when right heart and pulmonary circulation pressures are high. Table 22-4 lists a number of important and common causes in critically ill patients. Pulmonary embolus is a common and often missed diagnosis requiring helical computed tomography or pulmonary angiography. Right ventricular pressure and Pra rise. Elevated right ventricular pressure shifts the interventricular septum from right to left during diastole, resulting in increased left ventricular diastolic stiffness. During systole, left ventricular pressure usually is sufficiently greater than right ventricular pressure, so the septum shifts back. This change in systolic shape means that the myocardium of the left ventricular free wall must shorten even more for less of an ejected stroke volume. The rise in Pra is transmitted through the compliant right atrium to the pericardial space. The increase in pericardial pressure tamponades all other cardiac chambers. When pericardial effusion is present, these effects are magnified. When Pla is high due to mitral stenosis or decreased left ventricular pump function, Ppa values rise. In the long term, this also may result in increased pulmonary vascular resistance. The resulting right ventricular failure with right-to-left septal shift impairs left ventricular filling, which may be a critical insult in these diseases.

TREATMENT OF VENTRICULAR INTERDEPENDENCE

Management aims to decrease Ppa values and to decrease parallel coupling of the left and right ventricles. Reversible contributions to pulmonary hypertension are treated as outlined in the discussion of right ventricular afterload. Parallel coupling by elevated pericardial pressure is decreased by relieving pericardial tamponade, if present; by decreasing intrathoracic pressures by decompressing thoracic and abdominal fluid and air collections; by airway management to reduce Ppa; in select patients by surgically opening or removing the pericardium; and in patients after sternotomy, by leaving a sternal incision open and closing only the overlying skin.

Unresuscitatable cardiac arrest is a common outcome when perfusion of the right ventricle is threatened because right ventricular pressures are high relative to left ventricular pressures. This happens in massive pulmonary embolism and in cases of severe pulmonary hypertension. Thrombolytic therapy and pulmonary vasodilator therapy attempt to reverse the cause. Animal models of massive pulmonary embolism suggest that successful acute cardiovascular management attempts to raise systemic pressures more than right-side pressures.[64] Therefore, norepinephrine or epinephrine, both of which have a substantial α-agonist effect, improves right ventricular perfusion and is more successful in immediate resuscitation than is isoproterenol or fluid infusion.

Acute on Chronic Heart Failure

Heart failure affects almost 5 million Americans, with more than half a million new cases each year. Seventy-five percent of heart failure hospitalizations involve patients older than 65 years. Heart failure carries a poor prognosis, with a survival rate of less than 50% after 5 years.[24] Mortality rate is often related to episodes of acute decompensation that punctuate the course of heart failure. Important precipitating causes of acute decompensation are listed in Table 22-5. A review of these causes shows why chronic heart failure is often exacerbated in the course of critical illness, so early detection and management of acute-on-chronic heart failure are essential components of critical care.[65]

PRECIPITATING FACTORS

Poor compliance with medications and new medications are common precipitating events. Dietary indiscretions with increased sodium load and alcohol ingestion leading to a further acute depression in systolic contractility are seen frequently. Intercurrent illness such as a urinary tract infection or viral

TABLE 22-5 Common Precipitating Factors of Acute on Chronic Heart Failure

Poor compliance with medications
Dietary indiscretion (salt load, alcohol)
Infection
Fever
High environmental temperature
Effect of a new medication (β blocker, calcium channel blocker, antiarrhythmic, nonsteroidal anti-inflammatory)
Arrhythmia (typically, new atrial fibrillation)
Ischemia or infarction
Valve dysfunction (endocarditis, papillary muscle dysfunction)
Pulmonary embolism
Surgical abdominal event (cholecystitis, pancreatitis, bowel infarct)
Worsening of another disease (diabetes, hepatitis, hyperthyroidism, hypothyroidism)

syndrome, fever, or high ambient temperatures may make greater demands on cardiac output than can be met. Onset may be slow, and patients complain of decreased exercise tolerance, dyspnea, paroxysmal nocturnal dyspnea, and swelling of ankles and abdomen worsening over days and weeks. Rapid onset suggests that ischemia or arrhythmia may be the cause. Cardiac output may be depressed, so the kidneys are hypoperfused. The response of the kidneys is to avidly retain sodium and water, which may further worsen volume overload. Volume overload leads to elevated venous pressures with subsequent pulmonary edema due to elevated Pla and peripheral edema due to elevated systemic venous pressures. There is an excessive reflex release of catecholamines leading to tachycardia and increased arterial tone, so arterial resistance rises. Increased arterial resistance as afterload may be detrimental to left ventricular pump function. Activation of the renin-angiotensin axis accounts for avid renal absorption of sodium. Vasopressin release increases water retention. Coronary artery disease is common in this population, so decompensation may have followed an acute ischemic coronary event or coronary ischemia may be precipitated by worsened congestive heart failure.

CLINICAL FEATURES

Patients are often anxious, tachycardic, and tachypneic, with evidence of hypoperfused extremities and possibly cyanosis. Jugular veins are distended, and hepatojugular reflux may be demonstrable on physical examination. Typically the sternal angle is approximately 5 cm above the right atrium when the patient's torso is at a 30- to 45-degree angle. Jugular venous distention is usually no higher than 1 to 3 cm above the sternal angle in normal patients, but it is elevated during acute heart failure. An apical impulse lateral to the midclavicular line or farther than 10 cm from the midsternal line is a sensitive but not specific indicator of left ventricular enlargement, whereas an apical diameter larger than 3 cm indicates left ventricular enlargement.[66] A sustained apical impulse suggests left ventricular hypertrophy or aneurysm. A third heart sound or summation gallop is often present but may be obscured by increased respiratory sounds. Pulse pressure is often reduced, so peripheral pulses are "thready." Crackles are heard in dependent lung fields but in severe cardiac failure are heard in all zones. Wheezes and a prolonged expiratory phase may be noted, suggesting edema surrounding the airways. Hepatomegaly, which may be pulsatile particularly with tricuspid valve insufficiency, may be present, and there is evidence of dependent edema in the lower extremities and over the sacrum.

Chest radiographic findings suggesting elevated left ventricular filling pressures include upper zone redistribution of vascular markings, septal lines (Kerley B lines), loss of pulmonary vascular definition, perivascular and peribronchial cuffing, perihilar interstitial and then alveolar filling patterns, and pleural effusions. The cardiopericardial silhouette may be enlarged, suggesting enlarged cardiac chambers, and the azygos vein may be enlarged, suggesting elevated Pra.

MANAGEMENT

Therapy of acute-on-chronic heart failure initially aims to treat intravascular overload and improve gas exchange. Therefore, the patient is positioned with the torso elevated at least 45 degrees, and oxygen is administered. Good intravenous access, optimally central venous, is established. Furosemide (20 to 40 mg initially, followed by increasing doses as required) induces a rapid diuresis. Even before diuresis is established, furosemide reduces Pla by a venodilation effect and also reduces intrapulmonary shunt.[67] Titrated morphine doses decrease venous tone and thereby decrease left ventricular filling pressures and improve pulmonary edema. In addition, morphine may make the patient less anxious, thereby decreasing whole-body oxygen demand. Nitrates are venodilators that serve to decrease left ventricular filling pressure and mild arterial vasodilators, resulting in decreased afterload. Nitrates have the additional benefit of being coronary vasodilators.

Afterload reduction is an important therapeutic intervention in patients with depressed left ventricular systolic contractility[14] due to a decrease in the slope of the ESPVR. Because there is a decrease in the slope of this relation, small reductions in pressure afterload can result in improved ejection to smaller ESVs. The reduction in ESV results in increased stroke volume and in substantially decreased end-systolic wall stress because, by the Laplace relation, wall stress is proportional to the product of cavity pressure and radius. The decrease in wall stress reduces myocardial oxygen demand. Afterload reduction in some critically ill patients may result in unacceptable hypotension. For this reason, it is best to start with an easily titratable medication with a very short half-life such as nitroprusside or, in the setting of ischemia, intravenous nitroglycerin (see Chap. 25). Nitroprusside is infused at an increasing dose while the response of cardiac output and blood pressure is measured repeatedly, so that an optimal dose resulting in maximum cardiac output with adequate perfusing pressures is chosen. Nitroprusside and other nitrates are direct or indirect NO donors that cause vascular smooth muscle relaxation. Nitroprusside at larger doses can result in significant toxicity, with cyanide formation and methemoglobinemia. When circulatory stability is achieved, other, longer-acting agents are substituted; angiotensin-converting enzyme inhibitors are particularly useful,[21,24] as are alternative drugs (see Table 22-3).

Inotropic or vasoactive agents are extremely useful in reversing depressed systolic contractility, but routine use of inotropes is not indicated for heart failure because inotropic use may increase mortality rate.[47,68] Dobutamine acts mainly on β_1 receptors and results primarily in increased ventricular contractility and in mild peripheral vasodilation. Doses from 2 to 15 μg/kg per minute are infused through a central venous line. Particularly in the presence of intravascular hypovolemia, the vasodilating effect of dobutamine may exceed its effect on increasing cardiac output, so blood pressure may decrease unacceptably. Dopamine has significant adverse effects that should limit its use. Low-dose dopamine has been clearly shown not to be beneficial. Dopamine is predominantly a β agonist in doses of 5 to 10 μg/kg per minute; at doses exceeding 10 μg/kg per minute, dopamine is an α agonist and therefore increases arterial resistance. Dopamine increases Pms and, hence, venous return increases, resulting in increased left ventricular filling pressures. The increased afterload at large doses and increased filling pressures associated with dopamine are often undesirable in treating decreased contractility. Milrinone and enoximone are phosphodiesterase inhibitors that increase contractility by increasing intracellular calcium during systole. These agents also may result in afterload reduction and therefore may be particularly beneficial in short-term treatment of depressed contractility. The use of digoxin to increase contractility is not generally helpful in the acute setting.[69]

In general, although positive inotropic agents improve contractility, they do so at the cost of increased myocardial oxygen demand and decreased efficiency of oxygen use and therefore may precipitate ischemia, arrhythmias, and other adverse outcomes. Dobutamine and milrinone are superior to dopamine, epinephrine, and isoproterenol for minimizing this adverse effect. If acute decompensation leads to cardiogenic shock and recovery is anticipated after medical or surgical intervention, then intraaortic balloon counterpulsation should be instituted when afterload reduction and inotropic therapy are insufficient.

References

1. Elzinga G, Westerhof N: How to quantify pump function of the heart. The value of variables derived from measurements on isolated muscle. *Circ Res* 44:303, 1979.
2. Joshi N: The third heart sound. *South Med J* 92:756, 1999.
3. Connors AF Jr, Speroff T, Dawson NV, et al: The effectiveness of right heart catheterization in the initial care of critically ill patients. SUPPORT Investigators. *JAMA* 276:889, 1996.
4. Sandham JD, Hull RD, Brant RF, et al, for the Canadian Critical Care Clinical Trials G: A randomized, controlled trial of the use of pulmonary-artery catheters in high-risk surgical patients. *N Engl J Med* 348:5, 2003.
5. Chittock DR, Dhingra VK, Ronco JJ, et al: Severity of illness and risk of death associated with pulmonary artery catheter use. *Crit Care Med* 32:911, 2004.
6. Burger W, Jockwig B, Rucker G, Kober G: Influence of right ventricular pre- and afterload on right ventricular ejection fraction and preload recruitable stroke work relation. *Clin Physiol* 21:85, 2001.
7. Kass DA, Maughan WL, Guo ZM, et al: Comparative influence of load versus inotropic states on indexes of ventricular contractility: experimental and theoretical analysis based on pressure-volume relationships. *Circulation* 76:1422, 1987.
8. Andrew P: Diastolic heart failure demystified. *Chest* 124:744, 2003.
9. Colreavy FB, Donovan K, Lee KY, Weekes J: Transesophageal echocardiography in critically ill patients. *Crit Care Med* 30:989, 2002.
10. Vieillard-Baron A, Prin S, Chergui K, et al: Echo-Doppler demonstration of acute cor pulmonale at the bedside in the medical intensive care unit. *Am J Respir Crit Care Med* 166:1310, 2002.
11. Bossone E, DiGiovine B, Watts S, et al: Range and prevalence of cardiac abnormalities in patients hospitalized in a medical ICU. *Chest* 122:1370, 2002.
12. Sarnoff SJ, Berglund E: Ventricular function. I. Starling's law of the heart studied by means of simultaneous right and left ventricular function curves in the dog. *Circulation* 9:706, 1954.
13. Sagawa K: The ventricular pressure-volume diagram revisited. *Circ Res* 43:677, 1978.
14. Khot UN, Novaro GM, Popovic ZB, et al: Nitroprusside in critically ill patients with left ventricular dysfunction and aortic stenosis. *N Engl J Med* 348:1756, 2003.
15. Gavazzi A, Ghio S, Scelsi L, et al: Response of the right ventricle to acute pulmonary vasodilation predicts the outcome in patients with advanced heart failure and pulmonary hypertension. *Am Heart J* 145:310, 2003.
16. Mandinov L, Eberli FR, Seiler C, Hess OM: Diastolic heart failure. *Cardiovasc Res* 45:813, 2000.
17. Cowley AW Jr, Guyton AC: Heart rate as a determinant of cardiac output in dogs with arteriovenous fistula. *Am J Cardiol* 28:321, 1971.
18. Jacobsohn E, Chorn R, O'Connor M: The role of the vasculature in regulating venous return and cardiac output: Historical and graphical approach. *Can J Anaesth* 44:849, 1997.
19. Goldberg HS, Rabson J: Control of cardiac output by systemic vessels. Circulatory adjustments to acute and chronic respiratory failure and the effect of therapeutic interventions. *Am J Cardiol* 47:696, 1981.
20. Brengelmann GL: A critical analysis of the view that right atrial pressure determines venous return. *J Appl Physiol* 94:849, 2003.
21. Elliott P: Cardiomyopathy. Diagnosis and management of dilated cardiomyopathy. *Heart* 84:106, 2000.
22. Cohn JN, Ferrari R, Sharpe N: Cardiac remodeling—Concepts and clinical implications: A consensus paper from an international forum on cardiac remodeling. Behalf of an international forum on cardiac remodeling. *J Am Coll Cardiol* 35:569, 2000.
23. Shaw T, Elliott P, McKenna WJ: Dilated cardiomyopathy: a genetically heterogeneous disease. *Lancet* 360:654, 2002.
24. Wu AH, Cody RJ: Medical and surgical treatment of chronic heart failure. *Curr Prob Cardiol* 28:229, 2003.
25. Cohn JN: Structural basis for heart failure. Ventricular remodeling and its pharmacological inhibition. *Circulation* 91:2504, 1995.
26. Suga H, Yamada O, Goto Y: Energetics of ventricular contraction as traced in the pressure-volume diagram. *Fed Proc* 43:2411, 1984.
27. Dhainaut JF, Huyghebaert MF, Monsallier JF, et al: Coronary hemodynamics and myocardial metabolism of lactate, free fatty acids, glucose, and ketones in patients with septic shock. *Circulation* 75:533, 1987.
28. Walley KR, Becker CJ, Hogan RA, et al: Progressive hypoxemia limits left ventricular oxygen consumption and contractility. *Circ Res* 63:849, 1988.
29. Endoh M: Acidic pH-induced contractile dysfunction via downstream mechanism: Identification of pH-sensitive domain in troponin I [comment]. *J Mol Cell Cardiol* 33:1297, 2001.
30. Walley KR, Lewis TH, Wood LD: Acute respiratory acidosis decreases left ventricular contractility but increases cardiac output in dogs. *Circ Res* 67:628, 1990.
31. Teplinsky K, O'Toole M, Olman M, et al: Effect of lactic acidosis on canine hemodynamics and left ventricular function. *Am J Physiol* 258:H1193, 1990.
32. Carlstedt F, Lind L, Rastad J, et al: Parathyroid hormone and ionized calcium levels are related to the severity of illness and survival in critically ill patients. *Eur J Clin Invest* 28:898, 1998.
33. Lang RM, Fellner SK, Neumann A, et al: Left ventricular contractility varies directly with blood ionized calcium. *Ann Intern Med* 108:524, 1988.
34. Cooper DJ, Walley KR, Dodek PM, et al: Plasma ionized calcium and blood lactate concentrations are inversely associated in human lactic acidosis. *Intens Care Med* 18:286, 1992.
35. Cooper DJ, Walley KR, Wiggs BR, Russell JA: Bicarbonate does not improve hemodynamics in critically ill patients who have lactic acidosis. A prospective, controlled clinical study. *Ann Intern Med* 112:492, 1990.
36. Cunnion RE, Parrillo JE: Myocardial dysfunction in sepsis. Recent insights. *Chest* 95:941, 1989.
37. Kumar A, Haery C, Parrillo JE. Myocardial dysfunction in septic shock. *Crit Care Clin* 16:251, 2000.
38. Herbertson MJ, Werner HA, Russell JA, et al: Myocardial oxygen extraction ratio is decreased during endotoxemia in pigs. *J Appl Physiol* 79:479, 1995.
39. Cooper DJ, Thompson CR, Walley KR, et al: Histamine decreases left ventricular contractility in normal human subjects. *J Appl Physiol* 73:2530, 1992.
40. Minneci P, Deans K, Natanson C, Eichacker PQ: Increasing the efficacy of anti-inflammatory agents used in the treatment of sepsis. *Eur J Clin Microbiol Infect Dis* 22:1, 2003.

41. Stegmayr BG: The presence of superantigens and complex host responses in severe sepsis may need a broad therapeutic approach. *Ther Apheresis* 5:111, 2001.

42. Adamson PB, Kleckner KJ, VanHout WL, et al: Cardiac resynchronization therapy improves heart rate variability in patients with symptomatic heart failure. *Circulation* 108:266, 2003.

43. Kalinchak DM, Schoenfeld MH: Cardiac resynchronization: a brief synopsis part II: Implant and followup methodology. *J Interv Card Electrophysiol* 9:163, 2003.

44. Westaby S, Banning AP, Saito S, et al: Circulatory support for long-term treatment of heart failure: experience with an intraventricular continuous flow pump. *Circulation* 105:2588, 2002.

45. Stein L, Beraud JJ, Morissette M, et al: Pulmonary edema during volume infusion. *Circulation* 52:483, 1975.

46. Klein L, O'Connor CM, Gattis WA, et al: Pharmacologic therapy for patients with chronic heart failure and reduced systolic function: Review of trials and practical considerations. *Am J Cardiol* 91:18F, 2003.

47. Stevenson LW: Clinical use of inotropic therapy for heart failure: looking backward or forward? Part I: Inotropic infusions during hospitalization. *Circulation* 108:367, 2003.

48. Tang GH, Fedak PW, Yau TM, et al: Cell transplantation to improve ventricular function in the failing heart. *Eur J Cardiothorac Surg* 23:907, 2003.

49. de Simone G, Greco R, Mureddu G, et al: Relation of left ventricular diastolic properties to systolic function in arterial hypertension. *Circulation* 101:152, 2000.

50. Aggarwal A, Brown KA, LeWinter MM: Diastolic dysfunction: pathophysiology, clinical features, and assessment with radionuclide methods. *J Nuclear Cardiol* 8:98, 2001.

51. Nishimura RA, Holmes DR Jr: Clinical practice. Hypertrophic obstructive cardiomyopathy. *N Engl J Med* 350:1320, 2004.

52. Koyama J, Ray-Sequin PA, Falk RH: Longitudinal myocardial function assessed by tissue velocity, strain, and strain rate tissue Doppler echocardiography in patients with AL (primary) cardiac amyloidosis. *Circulation* 107:2446, 2003.

53. Ammash NM, Seward JB, Bailey KR, et al: Clinical profile and outcome of idiopathic restrictive cardiomyopathy. *Circulation* 101:2490, 2000.

54. Smiseth OA, Manyari DE, Lima JA, et al: Modulation of vascular capacitance by angiotensin and nitroprusside: a mechanism of changes in pericardial pressure. *Circulation* 76:875, 1987.

55. Miller RR, DeMaria AN, Amsterdam EA, et al: Improvement of reduced left ventricular diastolic compliance in ischemic heart disease after successful coronary artery bypass surgery. *Am J Cardiol* 35:11, 1975.

56. Walley KR, Cooper DJ: Diastolic stiffness impairs left ventricular function during hypovolemic shock in pigs. *Am J Physiol* 260:H702, 1991.

57. Parrillo JE, Parker MM, Natanson C, et al: Septic shock in humans. Advances in the understanding of pathogenesis, cardiovascular dysfunction, and therapy. *Ann Intern Med* 113:227, 1990.

58. Forrester JS, Diamond G, Parmley WW, Swan HJ: Early increase in left ventricular compliance after myocardial infarction. *J Clin Invest* 51:598, 1972.

59. Russell JA, Ronco JJ, Lockhat D, et al: Oxygen delivery and consumption and ventricular preload are greater in survivors than in nonsurvivors of the adult respiratory distress syndrome. *Am Rev Respir Dis* 141:659, 1990.

60. Trohman RG: Supraventricular tachycardia: Implications for the intensivist. *Crit Care Med* 28:N129, 2000.

61. Scher DL, Arsura EL: Multifocal atrial tachycardia: mechanisms, clinical correlates, and treatment. *Am Heart J* 118:574, 1989.

62. Streeter DD Jr, Spotnitz HM, Patel DP, et al: Fiber orientation in the canine left ventricle during diastole and systole. *Circ Res* 24:339, 1969.

63. Dell'Italia LJ, Walsh RA: Right ventricular diastolic pressure-volume relations and regional dimensions during acute alterations in loading conditions. *Circulation* 77:1276, 1988.

64. Layish DT, Tapson VF: Pharmacologic hemodynamic support in massive pulmonary embolism. *Chest* 111:218, 1997.

65. Poppas A, Rounds S: Congestive heart failure. *Am J Respir Crit Care Med* 165:4, 2002.

66. Eilen SD, Crawford MH, O'Rourke RA: Accuracy of precordial palpation for detecting increased left ventricular volume. *Ann Intern Med* 99:628, 1983.

67. Braunwald E: ACE inhibitors—A cornerstone of the treatment of heart failure. *N Engl J Med* 325:351, 1991.

68. Felker GM, O'Connor CM: Inotropic therapy for heart failure: an evidence-based approach. *Am Heart J* 142:393, 2001.

69. Almeda FQ, Hollenberg SM: Update on therapy for acute and chronic heart failure. Applying advances in outpatient management. *Postgrad Med* 113:36, 2003.

Chapter 23 _____

DIAGNOSTIC AND MANAGEMENT STRATEGIES FOR ACUTE HEART FAILURE IN THE INTENSIVE CARE UNIT

GERASIMOS S. FILIPPATOS
GEORGE BALTOPOULOS
ELIAS KARAMBATSOS
MARKKU S. NIEMINEN

KEY POINTS

- *Patients are admitted to the intensive care unit (ICU) with manifestations of acute heart failure (AHF) that arise in three general contexts: decompensation of chronic heart failure, as a complication of a cardiac process such as ischemia or valve incompetence, and when cardiomyopathy complicates other critical illness.*

- *Determining which of the contexts of AHF is present is invaluable to guide therapy.*

- *Predominant signs and symptoms arise from venous congestion after elevation of ventricular end-diastolic pressure and hypoperfusion; in a given patient, different contributions of these processes may be present.*

- *Measurement of brain natriuretic peptide has been a useful addition to the diagnostic armamentarium to determine whether heart failure is a cause of acute dyspnea; this measurement is most useful when obtained acutely and before initiation of therapies and, hence, has a limited role for assessing patients after admission to the ICU.*

- *Echocardiography is an extremely useful tool to assess ventricular function and define cardiac anatomy; on occasion, information from invasive measurement of intravascular pressure or venous oxygen saturation is also required to guide therapy.*

- *Many patients will exhibit respiratory distress and different degrees of impaired oxygenation; whereas many, if not most, patients can be managed with oxygen for this component of AHF, ventilatory support in the form of continuous positive airway pressure or bilevel airway support (BiPAP) should be considered for patients not responding adequately to oxygen therapy alone or whose respiratory symptoms and findings are severe from the onset.*

- *Diuretics are useful for treating venous congestion and inotropes for inadequate perfusion, but each carry risk of excessive dosing; the mainstay of therapy for most patients should be afterload reduction and search for the underlying causes of ventricular dysfunction and decompensation.*

- *Vasoconstrictive agents should be used only when and as long as truly life-threatening hypotension is present*

Acute heart failure (AHF) is the primary or an underlying diagnosis in many patients admitted to the intensive care unit

(ICU), but its exact incidence is unknown. The cause of heart failure (HF) in 60% to 70% of hospitalized patients is ischemic heart disease,[1–3] but many diagnoses, including arrhythmias, idiopathic dilated cardiomyopathy, systemic or pulmonary hypertension, congenital and valvular heart disease, or myocarditis, should be considered (see Chap. 24). HF is complicated by diabetes in 27% of hospitalized patients, renal dysfunction in 17%, and respiratory disease in 32%, and the vast majority of individuals hospitalized for AHF are older than 70 years.[3]

AHF may present with left or right HF or the combination of these conditions. The cardiac dysfunction may be systolic or "diastolic" (with preserved ejection fraction), and the underlying pathogenetic mechanism may be cardiac or extracardiac and may induce transient or permanent cardiac damage.[4] Especially in the ICU, multiple extracardiac pathologies may result in AHF by changing preload, afterload, or contractility, including pericardial disease, renal failure, endocrinopathy, sepsis, thyrotoxicosis, anemia, end-stage liver disease, and central nervous system lesions. Some rare cardiac pathologies also may be responsible for AHF, such as tumors of the heart and cardiac contusion.

Mortality rate is high, with as many as 13.5% of patients succumbing in the first 3 months after an episode of AHF in some series.[3] The incidence of hospitalizations for HF as a primary diagnosis have increased recently, and 24% of patients will be rehospitalized within 90 days. Most patients hospitalized for management of HF represent cases of decompensation of chronic HF.[3,5–7]

This chapter offers a definition of the clinical syndrome of HF and then describes the underlying pathophysiology. Diagnostic and therapeutic approaches to patients admitted to the ICU with HF are described. The definitions and diagnostic and management strategies described in this chapter have been recently formulated as Guidelines of the Task Force on Acute Heart Failure by the European Society of Cardiology.[1]

Definition

The clinical syndrome of AHF may occur with or without previous cardiac disease. The time needed to characterize HF as acute has not been defined. The different clinical presentations of AHF are:[1,8]

1. Pulmonary edema: AHF accompanied by severe respiratory distress and O_2 saturation (Sa_{O_2}) less than 90% with room air before treatment.
2. Cardiogenic shock: Tissue hypoperfusion, after correction of preload, induced by cardiac disease. There is no simple and precise definition for cardiogenic shock. It is characterized by decreased systolic blood pressure (<90 mm Hg; or a drop of mean arterial blood pressure >30 mm Hg) and/or low urine output (<0.5 mL/kg per hour) with a pulse rate faster than 60 beats/min with or without evidence of organ congestion.
3. Hypertensive AHF: Signs and symptoms of HF accompanied by extremely high blood pressure and relatively preserved left ventricular systolic function.
4. Acute decompensation of heart function, occurring de novo or as deterioration of chronic HF: Signs and symptoms of AHF that do not fulfill criteria for cardiogenic shock, pulmonary edema, or hypertensive HF.

5. High-output failure: Characterized by warm periphery, pulmonary congestion, and sometimes low blood pressure, as seen in thyrotoxicosis.
6. Right HF: Characterized by low-output syndrome with increased jugular venous pressure, peripheral edema, and sometimes hypotension. It is often associated with left HF but may occur in isolation as a result of lung or pulmonary vascular disease or ischemia largely limited to the right ventricle.

Many other classifications for AHF have been used in the ICU. The most widely recognized are the Killip and the Forrester classifications originally designed to provide a clinical estimate of prognosis in acute myocardial infarction.[9,10] The Forrester classification categorizes patients by clinical and hemodynamic criteria to four different subsets:

1. No evidence of pulmonary congestion or peripheral hypoperfusion (normal cardiac index and pulmonary capillary pressure).
2. Pulmonary congestion only (elevated pulmonary capillary wedge pressure [PCWP]).
3. Hypoperfusion only (depressed cardiac index).
4. Pulmonary congestion and hypoperfusion (depressed cardiac index and elevated PCWP).

These definitions have been used to classify AHF patients in an attempt to improve prognostic information and management. However, AHF is a continuum, and this should be taken into consideration during the diagnostic and therapeutic assessments.

Practical Issues in the Pathophysiology of Acute Heart Failure

AHF is characterized by a relatively sudden inability of the heart to maintain cardiac output adequate for the demands of the circulation. Cardiac output is reduced with associated tissue hypoperfusion, usually with increased cardiac filling pressures (as reflected by an elevated PCWP) and associated tissue congestion. The primary response to this state is neuroendocrine activation, such as the renin-angiotensin-aldosterone axis, sympathetic system activation, cytokine and endothelin release, and peptide release, including vasopressin and natriuretic peptides.[11,12] Natriuretic peptides cause vasodilation, inhibit endothelin release, and counterbalance the effects of the sympathetic and renin-angiotensin-aldosterone systems. Moreover, they have diuretic, lusitropic (ventricular relaxation), and antifibrotic properties.[13,14]

Although activation of these pathways is no doubt an attempt to maintain homeostasis, the final result of neuroendocrine activation is vasoconstriction leading to retention of sodium and water, increased left ventricular filling pressures, and increased ventricular wall tension. This in turn causes myocardial oxygen demand to increase, unfortunately in a circumstance in which coronary blood flow cannot be increased in a commensurate fashion because of associated coronary artery disease or primary myocardial dysfunction and pump failure. In addition to renal and vascular effects, neurohormonal activation and hypoperfusion exert direct effects on the cardiac cells, leading to further deterioration of myocardial function within hours by induction of apoptosis and necrosis.[15–17] The significance of myocardial cell regeneration, which has been recently described in humans, is not known.[18] Large-dose catecholamine treatment can further induce cell death and desensitization of the β-adrenergic system,[19] leading to tolerance to inotropic stimulation by therapeutic catecholamines.[20] Oxygen free radical formation and endothelial injury have been implicated in AHF pathophysiology and may not only lead to abnormalities in the peripheral circulation but may also contribute to the pathogenesis of myocardial stunning and hibernation.

In patients with ischemic heart disease and acute coronary syndromes, the AHF syndrome may persist for hours to days after the restoration of coronary blood flow. This transient reduction in myocardial function, which may occur also after cardiac arrest, is called *myocardial stunning*.[21] A mechanism of depressed myocardial function that is also important in the ICU is *myocardial hibernation*. This impaired myocardial function is a result of severe chronic hypoperfusion and decreased coronary blood flow due to coronary artery stenosis. It appears to be a protective mechanism aimed at limiting myocardial cell injury and death under conditions of excessive load and inadequate perfusion.[22] These mechanisms may be particularly important in the ICU patient with a history of ischemic heart disease and myocardial dysfunction, even when AHF is not the primary admission diagnosis. Patients with stunned and hibernating myocardium can return to normal cardiac function when appropriately treated. Hibernating myocardium improves when coronary blood flow is restored, whereas stunned myocardium responds to inotropic stimulation.[23,24] However, the exact role of treatment on the outcome of critically ill patients with coexisting coronary artery disease is unknown.

Diagnosis of Heart Failure

Etiologic diagnosis of AHF based on history and on clinical findings is difficult in the ICU. A 12-lead electrocardiogram is useful to identify acute myocardial infarction. It may also help in the diagnosis of acute right ventricular strain; ST elevation of the V4R lead is characteristic of right ventricular myocardial infarction, which is present in 30% to 50% of patients with an inferior myocardial infarction.

Chest radiography is necessary to evaluate cardiac size and shape and to assess pulmonary congestion. Blood count and biochemical tests, including calcium and thyroid function, are necessary in the initial evaluation of AHF patients. Troponin and creatinine kinase MB fractions have been used to evaluate acute myocardial injury, but these standard markers often lose sensitivity and specificity in complex ICU patients with confounding effects of renal failure, trauma, and recent surgery.[25,26] Arterial blood gas analysis is extremely helpful to identify oxygenation abnormalities associated with pulmonary edema and metabolic acidosis resulting from hypoperfusion. Pulse oximetry and end-tidal CO_2 are helpful monitoring tools but are less reliable in shock states.

Natriuretic peptides and especially B-type natriuretic peptide (BNP) play a significant role as adaptive mechanisms in AHF. BNP is released from the cardiac ventricles in response to increased wall stretch resulting from pressure and volume overload.[27] BNP and NT-BNP (the product of the posttranslational processing of the pro-BNP molecule) have been used for the diagnosis of decompensated HF in patients with dyspnea in the emergency department[1,28] and increased levels of plasma BNP and NT-BNP carry important prognostic information in patients with decompensated HF.[29,30] Moreover, it has been suggested that increased BNP level is a strong predictor for cardiac dysfunction in ICU patients.[31] However, the exact time of BNP rise in patients with AHF is not known, and BNP levels may be normal at the time of admission. BNP has a half-life of 22 minutes and NT-BNP has a half-life of 120 minutes, suggesting that meaningful hemodynamic changes could be reflected after 2 to 12 hours.[32] Many of the interventions used to treat AHF no doubt rapidly influence BNP levels, thus making use of this test questionable once the patient has had treatment initiated. Moreover, BNP concentration increases in patients with chronic renal failure, pulmonary embolism, pulmonary hypertension, and chronic obstructive pulmonary disease with right heart strain. Thus, an elevated level cannot be taken as unequivocal evidence of left HF, and patients with findings consistent with acute right heart strain require further diagnostic workup.[33–38] The effect of acute lung injury or ARDS with or without right HF upon BNP serum levels has not been evaluated. Plasma BNP is also increased after acute myocardial infarction[39] and is a predictor of major adverse events independent of ejection fraction.[40,41]

Although it has been suggested that increased plasma BNP concentrations are a useful marker for predicting cardiac rupture after acute myocardial infarction, the exact role of BNP in patients with cardiogenic shock or pulmonary edema from a mechanical complication after an acute myocardial infarction has not been extensively evaluated.[42]

Echocardiography is essential for the evaluation of the patient with AHF. Transthoracic echocardiography can be used to evaluate left and right ventricular functions, valvular integrity, pericardial pathology, and mechanical complications of acute myocardial infarction and is useful to identify intracavitary lesions. An echo Doppler study can be used for the hemodynamic evaluation of the HF patient, although in the ICU transesophageal echocardiography is often used because of the limited quality of the transthoracic images, particularly in patients undergoing mechanical ventilation.[43–45] Echocardiography has not been compared with right heart catheterization in patients with AHF, but the information from these two tools would likely be complementary by providing pressure and volume assessments of ventricular function.

Insertion of a pulmonary artery catheter for the diagnosis of AHF is usually unnecessary but can be helpful in complex patients with concurrent cardiac and pulmonary disease.[45] The measurement of mixed venous saturation or even of superior vena caval blood saturation as a surrogate measure (obtainable from a standard central venous catheter) is very useful to determine the adequacy of the cardiac output; saturations less than 60% strongly suggest inadequate tissue perfusion apart from the cardiac output measured by other means.

Monitoring the Patient with Acute Heart Failure

There are no prospective randomized clinical trials assessing the efficacy of different monitoring devices in AHF patients. However, as in all critically ill patients, temperature, respiratory rate, heart rate, electrocardiogram, and blood pressure should be monitored. The frequency with which these observations need to be taken depends on the severity of decompensation. Blood pressure should be checked regularly until the patient has demonstrated stability on a given dosage of vasodilators, diuretics, or inotropes. Noninvasive blood pressure monitoring is usually sufficient. An arterial catheter is sometimes used in shock states or when continuous analysis of arterial blood pressure or multiple arterial blood analyses are necessary. The Sa_{O2} of hemoglobin should be checked by pulse oximetry, continuously, or at regular intervals in any patient receiving oxygen therapy for AHF. The Sa_{O2} estimate by pulse oximetry is of limited value when the patient is in cardiogenic shock.

Many different noninvasive hemodynamic monitoring devices have been used in the ICU, but their exact role in the management of an AHF patient has not been definitively determined. Central venous lines can be used for the delivery of fluids and drugs to the central venous circulation and for monitoring right atrial pressure. However, right atrial pressure correlates poorly to preload in HF patients.

Pulmonary artery catheters (PACs) can measure intracardiac pressures, cardiac output, right ventricular end-diastolic volume and ejection fraction, and mixed venous saturation (see Chap. 13). Several retrospective studies have demonstrated an increased mortality rate associated with the use of this technology, including in patients with acute myocardial infarction.[46,47] These observations have been ascribed to limitations of the retrospective study, but the consistency of this association in other patient groups raises concern regarding the value of this mode of monitoring.[48–50] Recently, a prospective study randomized critically ill patients to a PAC group or to treatment without the use of data from a PAC. In this study, management with the PAC led to increased fluid resuscitation within the first 24 hours but no long-term differences in patient outcome.[51] Other studies evaluating the utility of PAC monitoring in patients with AHF and other causes of critical illness are currently underway.

Treatment of Acute Heart Failure

AHF is a complex and heterogeneous syndrome, with only a few randomized controlled trials that have assessed treatment approaches. The comorbidities that are common in ICU patients make management more difficult and complicated. The immediate goals of treatment include improvement of tissue perfusion and oxygenation, correction of underlying hemodynamic abnormalities and the causes of cardiac decompensation, and control of symptoms. These short-term goals should then be linked to longer-term management strategies that ideally improve morbidity and mortality rates.

RESPIRATORY THERAPY AND VENTILATORY SUPPORT

A priority in treating patients with acute cardiac failure is the maintenance of arterial oxygen saturation (SaO_2) within the normal range to improve tissue oxygenation. This can be achieved by using supplemental oxygen in most patients and by the use of noninvasive (see Chap. 33) or invasive (see Chap. 36) ventilatory strategies for patients with greater degrees of respiratory compromise.

Several trials have suggested a benefit of continuous positive airway pressure (CPAP) in patients with AHF, in particular a reduction in the need for endotracheal intubation.[52–56] These investigations have been criticized for their small size and a failure to demonstrate a difference in mortality rate, but a recent meta-analysis showed a trend to decreased hospital mortality rate when CPAP was used as a routine measure for patients with AHF.[57]

Other forms of noninvasive ventilatory support have been studied, most often bilevel support delivered by nasal or full-face mask. Three randomized trials compared this approach with conventional oxygen therapy, large-dose nitrate therapy, or CPAP,[58–60] with mixed results. A recent multicenter study of treatment of patients in pulmonary edema secondary to AHF showed no benefit for the general population of patients but did show a trend toward improvement by subset analysis of the more severely compromised patients.[61]

Analysis of these studies suggests that benefit is likely to be seen in more severely ill patients not stabilized with oxygen therapy alone. One approach is to use CPAP or other forms of support in patients with pulmonary edema, an elevated arterial partial pressure of CO_2 (suggesting impending ventilatory failure) and a low pH even when an arterial pressure of CO_2 is normal (suggesting more severe hypoperfusion).

MEDICAL TREATMENT

Vasodilators are the first line therapy in patients with pulmonary congestion and adequate blood pressure. Nitrates relieve pulmonary congestion by reducing left ventricular preload and afterload. The highest tolerable dose of nitrates with low dose furosemide should be administered since it is more effective than furosemide treatment alone in acute pulmonary edema.[62] However, close monitoring during intitiation of therapy is necessary because excessive vasodilation may induce a steep reduction in blood pressure, ischemia, sometimes shock and renal failure. Moreover, rapid development of tolerance to nitrates, especially when they are given intravenously, limits their effectiveness after 16 to 24 hours.

Sodium nitroprusside (SNP) has been also used for patients with acute heart failure and has found its widest application in patients with hypertensive crisis and ventricular decompensation. Controlled trials of its use are lacking in heart failure per se. Use of SNP requires close blood pressure monitoring. Prolonged administration can be associated with thiocyanate and/or cyanide toxicity and patients should be converted early to alternative agents to avoid these problems, particularly when renal and/or hepatic dysfunction are present.

Diuretics are indicated in patients with symptoms secondary to fluid retention. Diuretics increase the urine volume by enhancing the excretion of water and sodium chloride leading to decreased plasma and extracellular fluid volume and a decrease in peripheral and pulmonary edema. The acute hemodynamic effect of the intravenous administration of loop diuretics is vasodilation manifested by a reduction in ventricular filling pressures and in pulmonary vascular resistance.[63] With high doses reflex vasoconstriction has been reported. In acutely decompensated heart failure the use of diuretics normalizes loading conditions and may reduce neurohormonal activation in the short term.[64,65]

Intravenous administration of loop diuretics (furosemide, bumetanide, torasemide) is preferred in acute heart failure. The dose should be titrated according to the diuretic response and relief of congestive symptoms. Administration of a loading dose followed by continuous infusion has been shown to be more effective than bolus alone with a lower incidence of toxicity.[65–69] Diuretic resistance has been described and when present alternative means of fluid removal by dialysis or ultrafiltration should be considered.

Morphine can be used in the treatment of patients with pulmonary edema although its effectiveness has not been studied in clinical trials. Morphine induces venodilation and mild arterial dilation, reduces heart rate[70] and relieves breathlessness in patients with acute pulmonary edema.

There is no evidence from clinical trials to support the use of anticoagulants in critically ill patients with AHF without myocardial ischemia or atrial flutter/fibrillation. However, the morbidity and mortality from thromboembolic disease in the ICU warrants the consideration of prophylactic anticoagulation in patients with AHF. A placebo controlled study evaluating enoxaparine in acutely ill patients, which included patients with AHF, demonstrated a reduction in the incidence of complicating venous thromboembolism but no improvement in survival or duration of hospitalization.[71]

Nesiritide, a recombinant human BNP, has been used for the treatment of AHF. Nesiritide reduces right atrial pressure, pulmonary capillary wedge pressure and increases stroke volume. Additional beneficial actions include coronary artery vasodilation, diuresis, natriuresis and neurohormonal suppression.[72] The drug has been shown to be more efficacious than placebo in symptom improvement without a pro-arrhythmic effect. When compared to intravenous nitroglycerin neseritide results in a more rapid improvement in hemodynamic profile in patients with AHF.[73] In an open-label randomized trial of nesiritide and standard care versus standard care alone, patients treated with nesiritide exhibited a trend toward decreased readmissions and six-month mortality.[74] Nesiritide is administered as a 2 μg/kg bolus followed by a fixed dose infusion of 0.01 μg/kg per minute. The dose can be increased every three hours, to a maximum of 0.03 μg/kg/min, if the pulmonary capillary wedge pressure is more than 20 mm Hg and systolic blood pressure is more than 100 mm Hg (using a 1 μg/kg bolus followed by an increase of 0.005 μg/kg/min over the previous infusion rate). If hypotension occurs, the infusion should be discontinued and restarted after blood pressure stabilization, at a 30% lower infusion rate without bolus. Hypotension is a significant adverse effect of the drug, and may persist despite immediate cessation of infusion. Accordingly, nesiritide should not be employed in patients with extremely labile blood pressure dipping below a level of 90 mm Hg systolic.

In the near future, therapies directed at potentiating the beneficial effects of endogenous natriuretic peptides by reducing their degradation may find clinical application. A target under current investigation is neutral endopeptidase, the primary enzyme involved in their degradation. However, preliminary studies of inhibitors of neutral endopeptidase showed increased neurohormonal activation with increased levels of angiotensin II and endothelin-1 after enzyme inhibition.[75] Thus, vasopeptidase inhibitors, which could provide simultaneous inhibition of angiotensin converting enzyme and neutral endopeptidase have been developed. Early use of such agents has been confounded by a high incidence of angioedema.[76,77]

Beta-blocking agents are contraindicated in patients with AHF, at least if it is clear that systolic dysfunction of the left ventricle is significant. Among patients in whom ischemia and tachycardia per se are felt to contribute significantly to their deterioration, beta blockade may be required; under such circumstances a short acting agent such as esmolol or metoprolol may given intravenously to permit cessation of therapy if adverse effects are encountered. Patients admitted to the ICU with AHF already receiving beta blockers should be continued on this therapy unless inotropic support is needed or excessive dosages is suspected.

In the initial management of the patient with acute heart failure, ACE inhibitors are not recommended and calcium antagonists are contraindicated. ACE inhibitors have an important role in the patient with systolic heart failure early after stabilization. Some new compounds with diuretic effect and vasodilating properties are under investigation, including vasopressin receptor antagonists.

Inotropic agents are indicated in the presence of hypotension and low cardiac output, with or without pulmonary congestion, refractory to optimal doses of diuretics and vasodilators (see Table 23-1). Inotropes are potentially harmful in chronic HF as they increase oxygen demand and calcium loading and should be used with caution.[78–80] However, in patients with AHF, symptom relief and prognosis appear dependent on correction of grossly deranged hemodynamics. Only a few controlled trials assessing specific inotropic regimens have been performed and thus rigid guidelines for drug administration do not exist.[80]

Dopamine is an endogenous cathecolamine and a precursor of norepinpehrine. Its effects differ according to dosage. At low doses ($\leq$2 to 3 μg/kg/min) activation of dopaminergic DA1 and DA2 receptors predominates with vasodilation in renal, mesenteric, coronary and cerebral vascular beds. The activation of DA2 receptors inhibits norepinephrine release from nerve terminals, activates the emetic center, decreases prolactin release and inhibits angiotensin II mediated aldosterone secretion. In the past, dopamine was widely used in the ICU to improve renal blood flow and diuresis in AHF patients with hypotension and low urine output. However,

administration of low-dose dopamine to critically ill patients at risk of renal failure does not confer clinically significant protection from renal dysfunction.[81,82] Small trials suggested some benefit of dopamine at low doses in patients with AHF but this general practice is not strongly supported by existing literature.[83] In AHF with hypotension dopamine can be used at higher doses for both inotropic and vasoconstrictive purposes but adverse effects of increased afterload or mismatch of oxygen supply to myocardial demand should be anticipated.

Dobutamine is a synthetic, sympathomimetic agent with substantial beta agonist activity resulting in significant inotropic and chronotropic effects on the heart.[84] It is usually initiated with a 2 to 3 μg/kg/min infusion rate without a loading dose. The infusion rate may be progressively titrated according to symptoms, diuretic response or assessments of hemodynamics (cardiac output, mixed venous oxygen saturation). The dose may be initially increased to 20 μg/kg/min as required. When undesirable side effects are encountered (tachycardia, hypotension, chest pain, arrhythmia), discontinuation of the drug is usually associated with reversal of effect due to short half life. Dobutamine may have an additive effect when given concurrently with phosphodiesterase inhibitors (see below). Prolonged infusion of dobutamine (above 48 hours) is associated with tolerance effects.[85,86]

Type III phosphodiesterase inhibitors (PDEI) are drugs with hemodynamic activity intermediate between that of a pure vasodilator and that of an inotrope.[85] They are mainly used in patients with AHF and peripheral hypoperfusion, refractory to optimal diuretic and vasodilating therapy. Milrinone and enoximone are the PDEIs used in clinical practice. They act by inhibiting the breakdown of cyclic-AMP (cAMP) into AMP in both the vascular and myocardial smooth muscle. As a result, contractility improves in cardiomyocytes and relaxation in the smooth muscle cells. Because their site of action is distal to the beta-adrenergic receptors PDEIs maintain their effects even during concomitant beta-blocker therapy. When administered to patients with advanced HF, milrinone improves hemodynamics without tolerance development.[86] Hypotension may be caused by excessive peripheral venodilation and is observed mainly in the patients with low intravascular volume. Therefore PDEIs are used in patients with preserved systemic blood pressure. Outcome data

TABLE 23-1 Inotropic Agents

	Indication	Bolus	Infusion Rate
Dobutamine	Hypotension, hypoperfusion	No	2 to 20–40 μg/kg per minute (predominant β-agonist effect throughout this range)
Dopamine	Hypotension, hypoperfusion	No	<3 μg/kg per minute: dopaminergic effect 3–5 μg/kg per minute: β-agonist effect predominant >5 μg/kg per minute: α agonist, vasoconstriction predominant
Milrinone	Hypoperfusion with preserved blood pressure, patients on β blockers	25–75 μg/kg per minute over 10–20 min	0.375–0.75 μg/kg per minute
Norepinephrine	Severe hypotension refractory to dobutamine		0.2–1.0 μg/kg per minute

regarding PDE-I administration in patients with acute HF are limited but not encouraging especially in patients with ischemic cardiomyopathy. Based on hemodynamic data alone, the combination of milrinone and dobutamine has a greater positive inotropic effect than each drug alone. However, the pharmacokinetic profile of milrinone is not optimal for ICU patients because individual responses to milrinone vary considerably.

A new class of medications which enhance calcium sensitization of the contractile proteins has found application in Europe and agents are in survival clinical trials in Europe and North America. Levosimendan is such an agent, and has been used in patients with symptomatic low cardiac output secondary to cardiac systolic dysfunction without severe hypotension. Levosimendan improves cardiac contractility by increasing the sensitivity of troponin C to calcium although is also type III PDE inhibitor.[87–91] Activation of adenosine triphosphate (ATP) sensitive potassium channels are responsible for its vasodilatory properties. Levosimendan has an active, potent, acetylated metabolite with half-life of approximately 80 hours, which probably explain the prolonged hemodynamic effects of a 24-hours levosimendan infusion.[88–91] Levosimendan has not been used extensively in patients with AHF. In patients with decompensated chronic systolic HF increases cardiac output, heart rate and stroke volume and decreases the pulmonary capillary wedge pressure and systemic and pulmonary vascular resistance.[88–91] An improvement in symptoms and decreased mortality has been shown in trials comparing levosimendan with dobutamine in patients with advanced chronic HF.[91] The hemodynamic effect of levosimendan is maintained in heart failure patients on concomitant beta-blocker therapy. Tachycardia and hypotension are its main side effects and levosimendan is not recommended in patients with low systolic blood pressure.

When the combination of inotropic agent and fluid challenge fails to restore organ perfusion and blood pressure, therapy with vasoconstrictors may be needed. Since this treatment may result in excessive afterload applied to a failing ventricle, it should be used as an emergency measure to sustain life and maintain perfusion in the face of life-threatening hypotension. Recent data indicate that if a vasopressor is needed, norepinephrine may be used because epinephrine has more negative effects on splanchnic circulation and on lactate metabolism.[92,93]

Cardiac glycosides inhibit sodium-potassium ATPase, thereby increasing calcium-sodium exchange with resulting positive inotropic effects. In AHF, cardiac glycosides produce a small increase in cardiac output and a reduction of filling pressures.[94,95] However, in patients with heart failure following myocardial infarction, increase of creatine kinase was more pronounced in patients receiving cardiac glycosides,[96,97] and in some studies a proarrhythmic effect and an adverse effect on outcome have been described. Accordingly, cardiac glycosides are not recommended for the acute management of AHF especially after acute myocardial infarction.

MECHANICAL ASSIST DEVICES

Mechanical circulatory support may be used in patients with AHF without permanent end-organ dysfunction, non-responding to conventional therapy, as a bridge to recovery or as a bridge to heart transplant. In clinical trials left ventricular assist devices have been used as destination therapy for patients with advanced chronic heart failure but device related complications limit their use for this indication.

INTRAAORTIC BALLOON PUMP (IABP)

IABP is most frequently used in patients with cardiogenic shock or ongoing severe myocardial ischemia, refractory to initial medical therapy, in preparation for revascularization. It is also useful in patients with acute myocardial infarction complicated by significant mitral regurgitation or rupture of the interventricular septum, to obtain hemodynamic stabilization for definitive diagnostic studies and treatment or after cardiac surgical procedures for patients with low cardiac output states.[98] The IABP has obvious advantages over other cardiac assist devices because of the rapidity and ease of insertion, accomplished through a femoral artery and performed at the bedside of the ICU patient. However, IABP does not augment forward flow to the extent achieved with ventricular assist devices (see below).

IABP operation is based on the principle of counterpulsation. A balloon is positioned in the descending aorta just distal to the left sublavian artery. The balloon deflates at the onset of systole immediate prior to the ejection of blood from the left ventricle. Thus reduces afterload, thereby decreasing left ventricular work and myocardial oxygen consumption. It inflates in diastole, increasing diastolic pressure resulting in increased coronary artery perfusion. In the setting of non-ischemic heart failure the afterload reduction may be still useful but the benefits of increased coronary flow are not clear. Vascular complications are common and careful monitoring of lower extremity perfusion is necessary. Intraabdominal (mesenteric ischemia, pancreatitis, splenic infarction), neurologic (stroke, paraplegia) and infectious complications have been described. Balloon rupture with helium embolization and balloon entrapment has been also reported. IABP is contraindicated in patients with aortic dissection or significant aortic insufficiency and its use should be restricted to patients with a correctable underlying condition.

VENTRICULAR ASSIST DEVICES

AHF patients not responding to conventional treatment including intra-aortic balloon pumping are candidates for mechanical circulatory support with ventricular assist devices (VAD).[99–101] This situation should be understood as one of bridging the patient ventricular function is expected to improve or transplantation is planned. VAD has been used after acute myocardial infarction, in post cardiac surgery low cardiac output syndrome and in acute myocarditis. Specific hemodynamic criteria have been used for patient selection in decompensated chronic heart failure but patient selection is more difficult in AHF. Patients with right heart failure are candidates for biventricular support, patients with aortic valve prosthesis are at increased risk for thromboembolism with some systems and aortic regurgitation is exaggerated after left VAD insertion because of the lowered left ventricular end diastolic pressure. An incompetent aortic valve may need repair or replacement before VAD insertion.

Many VAD are currently available and can be categorized in several different ways including: (a) left versus right VAD; (b) pulsatile versus non pulsatile flow; (c) internal versus external placement. No current single VAD is appropriate for the management of all AHF patients. Selection of the device is determined by the expected duration of support, the specific cardiac pathology, type of support needed (right, left or biventricular), the device availability and surgical team experience. It is not possible for all cardiac surgery centers to use all available systems. Ideally, a center should have access to a short term support system for AHF, a long term support system and a system capable of providing support to the right ventricle.[101]

The patient with a VAD is a challenge for the ICU team because thromboembolism, bleeding, infection, hemolysis and device malfunction are common complications associated with the use of these systems.

Management of Specific Diseases in Acute Heart Failure

ACUTE MYOCARDIAL INFARCTION

In all patients with acute myocardial infarction and signs and symptoms of heart failure echocardiography is necessary for assessment of ventricular function and mechanical complications (see Table 23-2). In acute myocardial infarction complicated by cardiogenic shock emergency percutaneous intervention or surgery improves prognosis and should be considered at an early state. If neither of these are available, or can be only provided after long delay, fibrinolytic therapy should be considered.[102,103] Temporary stabilization of the patient can be achieved by adequate fluid and pharmacological support, intra aortic balloon pump and mechanical ventilation.

Acute right heart failure after myocardial infarction is usually related to acute right ventricular infarction with a typical electrocardiogram and echocardiogram. Early revascularization of the culprit coronary artery may improve prognosis.

FREE WALL RUPTURE

The incidence of cardiac wall rupture after an acute myocardial infarction is 0.8–6.2%.[104–107] Recent studies have shown that percutaneous intervention decreased the incidence of cardiac rupture, compared with the thrombolytic era. Older age, female gender, anterior location of the infarct and longer time to reperfusion carry an increased risk of cardiac rupture. Usually, death occurs within minutes due to cardiac tamponade and the diagnosis is established in autopsy. However, in around 30% of cases thrombus seals the rupture giving an opportunity for intervention, if the condition is recognized. Most of these patients have signs of hemodynamic collapse

TABLE 23-2 Cardiac Disorders with Acute Heart Failure that Require Surgical Treatment

After Acute Myocardial Infarction
    Cardiogenic shock and multi-vessel coronary artery disease
    Ventricular septal defect
    Free wall rupture
    Acute mitral regurgitation
Valvular Disease
    Acute decomposition of preexisting heart valve disease
    Prosthetic valve failure or thrombosis
    Acute mitral regurgitation (myxomatous degenerative lesions, endocarditis, trauma)
    Acute aortic regurgitation (endocarditis, aortic dissection, trauma)
    Ruptured sinus of Valsalva aneurysm
Acute heart failure requiring support by mechanical assist devices

Modified from Nieminen MS, Bohm M, Drexler H, et al.[1]

and in some patients rupture is preceded by chest pain, nausea and T wave changes or new ST segment elevation in the infarct related leads. All these patients should undergo immediate echocardiography. The clinical presentation, pericardial effusions more than 10 mm and intrapericardial echo densities consistent with thrombus confirm the diagnosis. Pericardiocentesis, fluids and positive inotropes have been used for temporary hemodynamic stabilization. However, the patients should be immediately transferred to the operating room for surgical repair of the rupture. Free wall rupture has been also described during dobutamine stress echocardiography after acute myocardial infarction.[107]

POST-INFARCTION VENTRICULAR SEPTAL RUPTURE (VSR)

Acute rupture of the interventricular septum occurs in 1–2% of all infarcts. VSR usually occurs in the first 5 days after an acute myocardial infarction. However, in the thrombolytic era the incidence has decreased and the median time of VSR is 1 day.[108–111] Septal rupture is more frequent in patients with transmural anterior myocardial infarction but in these patients VSR is generally apical and simple. In patients with an inferior myocardial infarction ruptures are in the basal inferoposterior septum and are more complex. The VSR is typically presented as acute pulmonary edema or cardiogenic shock in a patient with right-sided ventricular failure and a harsh, loud, holosystolic murmur usually at the left lower sternal border. With low output state the murmur is difficult to identify. Echocardiography is generally diagnostic. It will identify the site of the ventricular rupture, the size of the left to right shunt, left and right ventricular function and the existence of mitral incompetence. Severe mitral regurgitation coexists in 20 percent of patients with VSR. Pulmonary artery catheterization can be helpful if echocardiography is not diagnostic. It will document the increase in oxygen saturation in the right ventricle and the pulmonary to systemic blood flow ratio (usually more than 2). Temporary medical therapy consists of diuretics, vasodilators, inotropes, intraaortic balloon pump, oxygen and in some patients positive pressure ventilation. However, surgical repair should be performed soon after the diagnosis in most patients.[108] The timing of the surgical repair has been an issue of debate. It was believed that in the acute phase of the myocardial infarction the myocardium was too fragile for the safe repair of the VSR. However, current Guidelines recommend immediate surgical repair, regardless of the clinical status of the patient, because the rupture can abruptly expand even in stable patients.[1,111]

In some small, retrospective clinical studies has been supported that concomitant coronary artery bypass grafting improves late functional status and survival.[109] Thus, revascularization is usually performed although the number of patients in these studies was too small to draw any firm conclusions.[109] Percutaneous closure of the VSR has been used to stabilize selected patients but more experience is needed before it can be recommended. VSR has been also described in patients with normal coronary arteries and myocardial bridge.

Moreover, a new systolic murmur and cardiogenic shock have been described in some patients with anterior myocardial infarction.[112] In these patients with apical anterior myocardial infarction compensatory hyperkinesis of the basal segments of the heart induces left ventricular outflow tract (LVOT) obstruction. The syndrome persists until appropriate therapy decreases the LVOT obstruction.

ACUTE MITRAL REGURGITATION (MR)

Mild MR is common after an acute myocardial infarction and is not usually associated with hemodynamic compromise. However, acute severe MR is the cause of shock in approximately 10% of patients with cardiogenic shock after an acute myocardial infarction.[113,114] It occurs 1–10 days after the infarction. Successful reperfusion by thrombolytic therapy or percutaneous intervention probably reduces the incidence of acute MR and is associated with an earlier occurrence (median 1 day). Several different mechanisms are responsible for acute MR after an acute myocardial infarction. The most dramatic is complete papillary muscle rupture where most of the non operated patients die in the first 24 hours. Cordae tendineae rupture, partial papillary muscle rupture or dysfunction of the papillary muscle are more common and with better survival. In most patients posteromedial papillary muscle is involved because of its single blood supply from the posterior descending coronary artery.

Acute severe MR is manifested by flash pulmonary edema and shock. The characteristic apical systolic murmur may be absent, due to the acute elevation of pressure in the non compliant left atrium and the rapid pressure equalization between left atrium and left ventricle. Moreover, auscultatory finding of pulmonary edema may mask the MR murmur. Chest radiograph shows pulmonary edema (might be unilateral). Echocardiography is the standard diagnostic tool for detecting the presence and severity of mitral regurgitation. The left atrium is usually small or slightly enlarged. Transesophageal echocardiography may be needed to establish the diagnosis in some patients with not adequate transthoracic images. However, when the mitral valve is not well visualized, the demonstration of preserved systolic function in a patient with acute myocardial infarction and pulmonary edema is helpful. A pulmonary artery catheter is rarely needed for diagnostic purposes but it may be useful in monitoring the effects of therapy.

The patients with severe acute MR and pulmonary edema or shock from papillary muscle or chordal rupture require emergency surgical repair. Even if medical therapy and intra aortic balloon pumping result in hemodynamic stabilization operation should be done early because many patients deteriorate suddenly.

MANAGEMENT OF ACUTE HEART FAILURE FROM PROSTHETIC VALVE THROMBOSIS

The incidence of prosthetic valve thrombosis depends on valve location and type and the adequacy of anticoagulation. It is from 0.2–6% per patient year in patients with mitral or aortic valve prostheses up to an overall 20% in patients with prostheses in the tricuspid valve.[115–121] Clinical presentation of patients with prosthetic valve thrombosis (PVT) includes patients with clinically silent PVT, patients with stroke or peripheral embolism and patients with hemodynamic compromise and signs and symptoms of heart failure. All patients with a prosthetic valve and heart failure symptoms should undergo immediately a transthoracic and/or transesophageal echocardiographic study. Thrombolytic therapy is considered the treatment of choice for tricuspid valve thrombosis. The ideal therapy for left sided PVT remains controversial.[116–118] Surgical mortality is high for emergency operations in critically ill patients with hemodynamic instability (New York Heart Association functional class III or IV

symptoms, pulmonary edema, hypotension). Thus, thrombolytic therapy was recommended for high risk surgical candidates.[116] However, thrombolysis takes several hours to be effective and this delay may lead to further deterioration in critically ill patients. The recommended dose of rtPA is 10 mg intravenous bolus followed by 90 mg infused over 90 min or 250–500,000 IU of streptokinase infused over 30 min followed by 100.000 IU per hour for 10 hours. Urokinase can be also used in a dose of 4,400 IU/kg/h for 12 hours without heparin or 2000 IU/kg/h with heparin for 24 hours. Echocardiography should be repeated in all patients after thrombolytic therapy. Thrombolysis is ineffective in approximately 18% and in these patients surgical intervention is indicated, although repeated infusions of thrombolytic therapy have been used in some studies.[118,119] Moreover, mortality is 6% and the risk of thromboembolism is 12%. Patients with aortic PVT and patients with large or mobile thrombi have a higher risk for thromboembolic complications after thrombolytic therapy and surgical intervention should be considered in these patients. Moreover, thrombolysis is not effective when fibrous tissue ingrowth (pannus) is implicated in the obstruction of the prosthetic valve. Clinical history, presentation and transesophageal echocardiography are helpful in the differential diagnosis but sometimes the distinction is still difficult.[120] Patients who are in stable clinical condition usually are not admitted in the ICU. Their management is also controversial. Small retrospective studies suggest that fibrinolytic therapy may be equally effective and in these patients.[116,118]

In conclusion, the clinical presentation of the individual patient, the characteristics of the PVT and the expertise at each center should be used to arrive at a therapeutic decision.

References

1. Nieminen MS, Böhm M, Drexler H, et al: Task force members on the treatment of acute heart failure, European Society of Cardiology: Guidelines for the diagnosis and treatment of acute heart failure. *Eur Heart J* 2004, in press.
2. Fox KF, Cowie MR, Wood DA, et al: Coronary artery disease as the cause of incident heart failure in the population. *Eur Heart J* 22:228, 2001.
3. Cleland JFG, Swedberg K, Follath F, et al: The Euroheart Heart Failure programme—A survey on quality of care among patients with heart failure in Europe. *Eur Heart J* 36:442, 2003.
4. Krumholz MH, Parent EM, Tu N, et al: The treatment target in acute decompensated heart failure. *Rev Cardiovasc Med* 2 (suppl 2):S7, 2001.
5. Angeja BG, Grossman W: Evaluation and management of diastolic heart failure. *Circulation* 107:659, 2003.
6. Roguin A, Behar D, Ben Ami H, et al: Long-term prognosis of acute pulmonary oedema—An ominous outcome. *Eur J Heart Fail* 2:137, 2000.
7. Fonarow GC: Strategies to improve the use of evidence-based heart failure therapies: OPTIMIZE-HF. *Rev Cardiovasc Med* 5(suppl 1):S45, 2004.
8. Cotter G, Moshkovitz Y, Milovanov O, et al: Acute heart failure: A novel approach to its pathogenesis and treatment. *Eur J Heart Fail* 4:227, 2002.
9. Killip T, Kimball JT: Treatment of myocardial infarction in a coronary care unit. *Am J Cardiol* 20:457, 1967.
10. Forrester JS, Diammond GA, Swan HJC: Correlative classification of clinical and hemodynamic function after acute myocardial infarction. *Am J Cardiol* 39:137, 1977.

11. Bartling B, Holtz J, Darmer D: Contribution of myocyte apoptosis to myocardial infarction? *Basic Res Cardiol* 93:71, 1998.

12. Filippatos G, Leche J, Sunga R, et al: Expression of FAS by surviving myocardial cells adjacent to fibrotic foci in the failing human heart is not associated with increased apoptosis. *Am J Physiol* 277:H455, 1999.

13. Tamura N, Ogawa Y, Chusho H, et al: Cardiac fibrosis in mice lacking brain natriuretic peptide. *Proc Natl Acad Sci USA* 97:4239, 2000.

14. Dhingra H, Roongsritong C, Kurtzman NA: Brain natriuretic peptide: Role in cardiovascular and volume homeostasis. *Semin Nephrol* 22:423, 2002.

15. Kajstura J, Cigola E, Malhotra A, et al: Angiotensin II induces apoptosis of adult ventricular myocytes in vitro. *J Mol Cell Cardiol* 29:859, 1997.

16. Communal C, Singh K, Sawyer DB, Colucci WS: Opposing effects of β_1- and β_2-adrenergic receptors on cardiac myocyte apoptosis. Role of a pertussis toxin-sensitive G-protein. *Circulation* 100:2210, 1999.

17. Filippatos GS, Gangopadhyay N, Lalude O, et al: Regulation of apoptosis by vasoactive peptides. *Am J Physiol Cell Mol Physiol* 281:L749, 2001.

18. Beltrami AP, Urbanek K, Kaystura J, et al: Evidence that human cardiac myocytes divide after myocardial infarction. *N Engl J Med* 244:1750, 2002.

19. Böhm M, Kouchi I, Schnabel P, Zolk O: Transition from hypertrophy to failure—β-Adrenergic desensitization of the heart. *Heart Fail Rev* 4:329, 1999.

20. Gilbert ME, Hershberger ER, Wiechmann JR, et al: Pharmacologic and hemodynamic effects of combined β-agonist stimulation and phosphodiesterase inhibition in the failing human heart. *Chest* 108:1524, 1995.

21. Patel B, Kloner RA, Przyklenk K, et al: Postischemic myocardial "stunning": A clinically relevant phenomenon. *Ann Intern Med* 108:626, 1988.

22. Rahimtoola SH: The hibernating myocardium. *Am Heart J* 117:211, 1989.

23. Bolli R: Basic and clinical aspects of myocardial stunning. *Prog Cardiovasc Dis* 40:477, 1988.

24. Wijns W, Vatner SF, Camici PG: Hibernating myocardium. *N Engl J Med* 339:173, 1998.

25. Lovis C, Mach F, Unger PF, et al: Elevation of creatine kinase in acute severe asthma is not of cardiac origin. *Intensive Care Med* 27:528, 2001.

26. Arlati S, Brenna S, Prencipe L, et al: myocardial necrosis in ICU patients with acute non-cardiac disease: a prospective study. *Intensive Care Med* 26:31, 2000.

27. Yasue H, Yoshimura M, Sumida H, et al: Localization and mechanism of secretion of B-type natriuretic peptide in comparison with those of A-type natriuretic peptide in normal subjects and patients with heart failure. *Circulation* 90:195, 1994.

28. Maisel AS, Krishnaswamy P, Nowak RM, et al: Breathing Not Properly Multinational Study Investigators. Rapid measurement of B-type natriuretic peptide in the emergency diagnosis of heart failure. *N Engl J Med* 347:161, 2002.

29. Morrison LK, Harrison A, Krishnaswamy P, et al: Utility of a rapid B-natriuretic peptide assay in differentiating congestive heart failure from lung disease in patients presenting with dyspnea. *J Am Coll Cardiol* 39:202, 2002.

30. Morrison KL, Harrison A, Krishnaswamy P, et al: Utility of a rapid B-natriuretic peptide (BNP) assay is differentiating CHF from lung disease in patients presenting with dyspnea. *J Am Coll Cardiol* 39:202, 2002.

31. McLean AS, Tang B, Nalos M, et al: Increased B-type natriuretic peptide (BNP) level is a strong predictor for cardiac dysfunction in intensive care unit patients. *Anaesth Intensive Care* 31:21, 2003.

32. McCullough PA, Omland T, Maisel AS: B-type natriuretic peptides: A diagnostic breakthrough for clinicians. *Rev Cardiovasc Med* 4:72, 2003.

33. Nagaya N, Nishikimi T, Uematsu M, et al: Plasma brain natriuretic peptide as a prognostic indicator in patients with primary pulmonary hypertension. *Circulation* 102:865, 2000.

34. Morrison LK, Harrison A, Krishnaswamy P, et al: Utility of a rapid B-natriuretic peptide assay in differentiating congestive heart failure from lung disease in patients presenting with dyspnea. *J Am Coll Cardiol* 39:202, 2002.

35. Tulevski II, Hirsch A, Sanson BJ, et al: Increased brain natriuretic peptide as a marker for right ventricular dysfunction in acute pulmonary embolism. *Thromb Haemost* 86:1193, 2001.

36. ten Wolde M, Tulevski II, Mulder JW, et al: Brain natriuretic peptide as a predictor of adverse outcome in patients with pulmonary embolism. *Circulation* 107:2082, 2003.

37. Ando T, Ogawa K, Yamaki K, et al: Plasma concentrations of atrial, brain, and C-type natriuretic peptides and endothelin-1 in patients with chronic respiratory diseases. *Chest* 110:462, 1996.

38. Ishii J, Nomura M, Ito M, et al: Plasma concentration of brain natriuretic peptide as a biochemical marker for the evaluation of right ventricular overload and mortality in chronic respiratory disease. *Clin Chim Acta* 301:19, 2000.

39. Morrow DA, de Lemos JA, Sabatine MS, et al: Evaluation of B-type natriuretic peptide for risk assessment in unstable angina/non–ST-elevation myocardial infarction: B-type natriuretic peptide and prognosis in TACTICS-TIMI 18. *J Am Coll Cardiol* 41:1264, 2003.

40. Richards AM, Nicholls MG, Espiner EA, et al: B-type natriuretic peptides and ejection fraction for prognosis after myocardial infarction. *Circulation* 107:2786, 2003.

41. Omland T, Persson A, Ng L, et al: N-terminal pro–B-type natriuretic peptide and long-term mortality in acute coronary syndromes. *Circulation* 106:2913, 2002.

42. Arakawa N, Nakamura M, Endo H, et al: Brain natriuretic peptide and cardiac rupture after acute myocardial infarction. *Ann Intern Med* 40:232, 2001.

43. Tousignant CP, Walsh F, Mazer CD: The use of transesophageal echocardiography for preload assessment in critically ill patients. *Anesth Analg* 90:351, 2000.

44. Nagueh SF, Kopeen HA, Zoghbi WA: Feasibility and accuracy of Doppler echocardiographic estimation of pulmonary catheter occlusive pressure in the intensive care unit. *Am J Cardiol* 75:1256, 1995.

45. Marik PE: Pulmonary artery catheterization and esophageal Doppler monitoring in the ICU. *Chest* 116:1085, 1999.

46. Gore JM, Goldberg RJ, Spodick DH, et al: A community-wide assessment of the use of pulmonary artery catheters in patients with acute myocardial infarction. *Chest* 92:721, 1987.

47. Zion MM, Balkin J, Rosenmann D, et al: Use of pulmonary artery catheters in patients with acute myocardial infarction. Analysis of experience in 5,841 patients in the SPRINT Registry. SPRINT Study Group. *Chest* 98:1331, 1990.

48. Connors AF Jr, Speroff T, Dawson NV, et al: The effectiveness of right heart catheterization in the initial care of critically ill patients. SUPPORT Investigators. *JAMA* 276:889, 1996.

49. Ivanov R, Allen J, Calvin JE: The incidence of major morbidity in critically ill patients managed with pulmonary artery catheters: a meta-analysis. *Crit Care Med* 28:615, 2000.

50. Sandham JD, Hull RD, Brant RF, et al: A randomized, controlled trial of the use of pulmonary artery catheters in high risk surgical patients. *N Engl J Med* 348:5, 2003.

51. Rhodes A, Cusack RJ, Newman PJ, et al: A randomised controlled trial of the pulmonary artery catheter in critically ill patients. *Intensive Care Med* 28:256, 2002.

52. Rasanen J, Heikkila J, Downs J et al: Continuous positive airways pressure by face mask in acute cardiogenic pulmonary edema. *Am J Cardiol* 55:296, 1985.

53. Berstan AD, Holt AW, Vedig AE, et al: Treatment of severe pulmonary edema with continuous positive airways pressure delivered by face mask. *N Engl J Med* 325:1825, 1991.

54. Lin M, Yang YF, Chiang HT, et al: Reappraisal of continuous positive airways pressure therapy in acute cardiogenic pulmonary edema: short-term results and long-term follow-up. *Chest* 107:1379, 1995.

55. Takeda S, Nejima J, Takano T, et al: Effect of nasal continuous positive airways pressure on pulmonary edema complicating acute myocardial infarction. *Jpn Circ J* 62:553, 1998.

56. Kelly CA, Newby DE, McDonagh TA, et al: Randomised controlled trial of continuous positive airway pressure and standard oxygen therapy in acute pulmonary oedema: Effects on plasma brain natriuretic peptide concentrations. *Eur Heart J* 23:1326, 2002.

57. Pang D, Keenan SP, Cook DJ, et al: The effect of positive airway support on mortality and the need for intubation in cardiogenic pulmonary edema: A systematic review. *Chest* 114:1185, 1998.

58. Masip J, Betbese AJ, Paez J, et al: Non-invasive pressure support ventilation versus conventional oxygen therapy in acute cardiogenic pulmonary oedema: A randomised trial. *Lancet* 356:2126, 2000.

59. Sharon A, Shpirer I, Kaluski E, et al: High dose intravenous isosorbide dinitrate is safer and better than Bi-PAP ventilation combined with conventional treatment forn severe pulmonary oedema. *J Am Coll Cadiol* 36:832, 2000.

60. Sangeeta M, Gregory J, Woolard W, et al: Randomized, prospective trial of bilevel versus continuous positive airway pressure in acute pulmonary oedema. *Crit Care Med* 25:620, 1997.

61. Nava S, Carbone G, DiBattista N, et al: Noninvasive ventilation in cardiogenic pulmonary edema. *Am J Respir Crit Care Med* 168:1432, 2003.

62. Cotter G, et al: Randomised trial of high-dose isosorbide dinitrate plus low-dose furosemide versus high-dose furosemide plus low-dose isosorbide dinitrate in severe pulmonary oedema. *Lancet* 351:389, 1998.

63. Wilson JR, Reichek N, Dunkman WB, Goldberg S: Effect of diuresis on the performance of the failing left ventricle in man. *Am J Med* 70:234, 1981.

64. Johnson W, Omland T, Hall C, et al: Neurohormonal activation rapidly decreases after intravenous therapy with diuretics and vasodilators for class IV heart failure. *J Am Coll Cardiol* 39:1623, 2002.

65. Pivac N, Rumboldt Z, Sardelic S, et al: Diuretic effects of furosemide infusion versus bolus injection in congestive heart failure. *Int J Clin Pharmacol Res* 18:121, 1998.

66. van Meyel JJ, Smits PT, Gerlag PG, et al: Continuous infusion of furosemide in the treatment of patients with congestive heart failure and diuretic resistance. *J Intern Med* 235:329, 1994.

67. Dormans TP, Gerlag PG: Combination of high-dose furosemide and hydrochlorothiazide in the treatment of refractory congestive heart failure. *Eur Heart J* 12:1867, 1996.

68. Kramer BK, Schweda F, Riegger GA: Diuretic treatment and diuretic resistance in heart failure. *Am J Med* 106:90, 1999.

69. Dormans TP, van Meyel JJ, Gerlag PG, et al: Diuretic efficacy of high dose furosemide in severe heart failure: Bolus injection versus continuous infusion. *J Am Coll Cardiol* 28:376, 1996.

70. Lee G, DeMaria A, Amsterdam E, et al: Comparative effects of morphine, meperidine and pentazocine on cardiocirculatory dynamics in patints with acute myocardial infarction. *Am J Med* 60:949, 1976.

71. Samama MM, Cohen AT, Darmon J-Y, et al: Comparison of enoxaparin with placebo for the prevention of venous thromboembolism in acutely ill medical patients. *N Engl J Med* 341:793, 1999.

72. Colucci WS, et al: Intravenous nesiritide, a natriuretic peptide, in the treatment of decompensated congestive heart failure. *N Engl J Med* 343:246, 2000.

73. Publication Committee for the VMAC Investigators: Intravenous nesiritide vs nitroglycerin for treatment of decompensated congestive heart failure. *JAMA* 287:1531, 2002.

74. Silver MA, Horton DP, Ghali JK, Elkayam U: Effect of nesiritide versus dobutamine on short term outcomes in the treatment of patients with acutely decompensated heart failure. *J Am Coll Cardiol* 39:798, 2002.

75. Brunner-La Rocca HP, Kiowski W, Ramsay D, Sutsch G: Therapeutic benefits of increasing natriuretic peptide levels. *Cardiovasc Res* 51:510, 2001.

76. Packer M, Califf RM, Konstam MA, et al: Comparison of omapatrilat and enalapril in patients with chronic heart failure: The Omapatrilat Versus Enalapril Randomized Trial of Utility in Reducing Events (OVERTURE). *Circulation* 106:920, 2002.

77. Gheorghiade M, Gattis WA, O'Connor CM, et al: Effects of tolvaptan, a vasopressin antagonist, in patients hospitalized with worsening heart failure: A randomized controlled trial. *JAMA* 291:1963, 2004.

78. Katz AM: Potential deleterious effects of inotropic agents in the therapy of chronic heart failure. *Circulation* 73:III184, 1986.

79. O'Connor CM, Gattis WA, Uretsky BF, et al: Continuous intravenous dobutamine is associated with an increased risk of death in patients with advanced heart failure: Insights from the Flolan International Randomized Survival Trial (FIRST). *Am Heart J* 138:78, 1999.

80. Thackray S, Easthaugh J, Freemantle N, Cleland J: The effectiveness and relative effectiveness of intravenous inotropic drugs acting through the adrenergic pathway in patients with heart failure-a meta-regression analysis. *Eur J Heart Fail* 4:51, 2002.

81. Chatterjee K, De Marco T: Role of nonglycosidic inotropic agents: indications, ethics, and limitations. *Med Clin North Am* 87:391, 2003.

82. Bellomo R, Chapman M, Finfer S, et al: Low-dose dopamine in patients with early renal dysfunction: a placebo-controlled randomised trial. Australian and New Zealand Intensive Care Society (ANZICS) Clinical Trials Group. *Lancet* 356:2139, 2000.

83. Varriale P, Mossavi A: The benefit of low dose dopamine during vigorous diuresis for congestive heart failure associated with renal insufficiency: Does it protect renal function? *Clin Cardiol* 20:627, 1997.

84. Colucci WS, Wright RF, Jaski BE, et al: Milrinone and dobutamine in severe heart failure: differing hemodynamic effects and individual patient responsiveness. *Circulation* 73(suppl III):III175, 1986.

85. Metra M, Nodari S, D'Aloia A, et al: Beta-blocker therapy influences the hemodynamic response to inotropic agents in patients with heart failure: A randomized comparison of dobutamine and enoximone before and after chronic treatment with metoprolol or carvedilol. *J Am Coll Cardiol* 40:1248, 2002.

86. Leier CV, Binkley PF: Parenteral inotropic support for advanced congestive heart failure. *Prog Cardiovasc Dis* 41:207, 1998.

87. Kivikko M, Lehtonen L, Colucci WS: Sustained hemodynamic effects of intravenous levosimendan. *Circulation* 107:81, 2003.

88. Nieminen MS, Akkila J, Hasenfuss G, et al: Hemodynamic and neurohumoral effects of continuous infusion of levosimendan in patients with congestive heart failure. *J Am Coll Cardiol* 36:1903, 2000.

89. Slawsky MT, Colucci WS, Gottlieb SS, et al: Acute hemodynamic and clinical effects of levosimendan in patients with severe heart failure. Study Investigators. *Circulation* 102:2222, 2000.

90. Follath F, Cleland JG, Just H, et al: Efficacy and safety of intravenous levosimendan compared with dobutamine in severe low-output heart failure (the LIDO study): A randomised double-blind trial. *Lancet* 360:196, 2002.

91. Cleland JG, McGowan J: Levosimendan: A new era for inodilator therapy for heart failure? *Curr Opin Cardiol* 17:257, 2002.

92. Koreny M, Karth GD, Geppert A, et al: Prognosis of patients who develop acute renal failure during the first 24 hours of

cardiogenic shock after myocardial infarction. *Am J Med* 112:115, 2002.

93. Ratshin RA, Rackley CE, Russel RO Jr: Hemodynamic evaluation of left ventricular function in shock complicating myocardial infarction. *Circulation* 45:127, 1972.

94. Lee DC-S, Johnson RA, Bingham JB, et al: Heart failure in outpatients: A randomized trial of digoxin versus placebo. *N Engl J Med* 306:699, 1982.

95. Rahimtoola SH, Sinno MZ, Chuquimia R, et al: Effect of ouabain on impaired left ventricular function in acute myocardial infarction. *N Engl J Med* 287:527, 1972.

96. Spargias SK, Hall SA, Ball GS: Safety concerns about digoxin after acute myocardial infarction. *Lancet* 354:391, 1999.

97. Varonkow Y, Shell WE, Smirnov V, et al: Augmentation of serum CPK activity by digitalis in patients with acute myocardial infarction. *Circulation* 55:719, 1977.

98. Mehlhorn U, Kroner A, de Vivie ER: 30 Years clinical intraaortic balloon pumping: Facts and figures. *Thorac Cardiovasc Surg* 47(suppl 2):298, 1999.

99. Delgado DH, Vivek Rao V, Ross HJ, et al: Mechanical circulatory assistance. State of the art. *Circulation* 106:2046, 2002.

100. Mielniczuk L, Mussivand T, Davies R, et al: Patient selection for left ventricular assist devices. *Artif Organs* 28:152, 2004.

101. Hirsch DJ, Cooper JR Jr: Cardiac failure and left ventricular assist devices. *Anesthesiol Clin North Am* 21:625, 2003.

102. Bertrand ME, Simoons ML, Fox KFA, et al: Management of acute coronary syndromes in patients presenting without persistent ST-segment elevation. *Eur Heart J* 23:1809, 2002.

103. Van De Werf F, Ardissino D, Betriu A, et al: Management of acute myocardial infarction with ST segment elevation. Task force report. *Eur Heart J* 24:28, 2003.

104. Pohjola-Sintonen S, Muller JE, Stone PH, et al: Ventricular septal and free wall rupture complicating acute myocardial infarction: Experience in the Multicenter Investigation of Limitation of Infarct Size. *Am Heart J* 117:809, 1989.

105. London RE, London SB: The electrocardiographic signs of acute hemopericardium. *Circulation* 25:780, 1962.

106. Lopez-Sendon J, Gonzalez A, Lopez de Sa E, et al: Diagnosis of subacute ventricular wall rupture after acute myocardial infarction: Sensitivity and specificity of clinical, hemodynamic and echocardiographic criteria. *J Am Coll Cardiol* 19:1145, 1992.

107. Zamorano J, Moreno R, Almeria C, et al: Left ventricular free wall rupture during dobutamine stress echocardiography. *Rev Esp Cardiol* 55:312, 2002.

108. Moreno R, Lopez-Sendon J, Garcia E, et al: Primary angioplasty reduces the risk of left ventricular free wall rupture compared with thrombolysis in patients with acute myocardial infarction. *J Am Coll Cardiol* 39:598, 2002.

109. Deja MA, Szostec J, Widenka K, et al: Post infarction ventricular septal defect—Can we do better? *Eur J Cardiothorac Surg* 18:194, 2000.

110. Dalrymple-Hay MJR, Monro JL, Livesey SA, Lamb RK: Postinfarction ventricular septal rupture: The Wessex experience. *Semin Thorac Cardiovasc Surg* 10:111, 1998.

111. Crenshaw BS, Granger CB, Birnbaum Y, et al, for the GUSTO-1 Trial Investigators: Risk factors, angiographic patterns, and outcomes in patients with ventricular septal defect complicating acute myocardial infarction. *Circulation* 101:27, 2000.

112. Ryan TJ, Antman EM, Brooks NH, et al: 1999 Update: ACC/AHA guidelines for the management of patients with acute myocardial infarction. A report of the American College of Cardiology/American Heart Association task force on practice guidelines (committee on management of acute myocardial infarction). *J Am Coll Cardiol* 34:890, 1999.

113. Thompson CR, Buller CE, Sleeper LA, et al, for the SHOCK Investigators: Cardiogenic shock due to acute mitral regurgitation complicating acute myocardial infarction: A report from the SHOCK Trial Registry. *J Am Coll Cardiol* 36(suppl A):1104, 2000.

114. Tavakoli R, Weber A, Brunner-La Rocca H, et al: Results of surgery for irreversible moderate to severe mitral valve regurgitation secondary to myocardial infarction. *Eur J Cardiothorac Surg* 21:818, 2002.

115. Horstkotte D, Follath F, Gutschik E, et al: Guidelines on prevention, diagnosis and treatment of infective endocarditis executive summary: The task force on infective endocarditis of the European Society of Cardiology. *Eur Heart J* 25:267, 2004.

116. Lengyel M, Fuster V, Keltai M, et al: Guidelines for management of left-sided prosthetic valve thrombosis: A role for thrombolytic therapy. *J Am Coll Cardiol* 30:1521, 1997.

117. Bonow RO, Carabelo B, de Leon AC Jr, et al: ACC/AHA guidelines for the management of patients with valvular heart disease: executive summary. A report of the American College of Cardiology/American Heart Association Task Force on Practice Guidelines. *Circulation* 98:1949, 1998.

118. Roudaut R, Lafitte S, Roudaut MF, et al: Fibrinolysis of mechanical prosthetic valve thrombosis: A single-center study of 127 cases. *J Am Coll Cardiol* 41:653, 2003.

119. Alpert JS: The thrombosed prosthetic valve. Current recommendations based on evidence from the literature. *J Am Coll Cardiol* 41:659, 2003.

120. Hering D, Piper C, Horstkotte D: Management of prosthetic valve thrombosis. *Eur Heart J* 3(suppl Q):Q22, 2001.

121. Ozkan M, Kaymaz C, Kirma C, et al: Intravenous thrombolytic treatment of mechanical prosthetic valve thrombosis: a study using serial transesophageal echocardiography. *J Am Coll Cardiol* 35:1881, 2000.

Chapter 24

CARDIAC ARRHYTHMIAS, PACING, CARDIOVERSION, AND DEFIBRILLATION IN THE CRITICAL CARE SETTING

ANNE M. GILLIS

KEY POINTS

- *Correct diagnoses and understanding of arrhythmia mechanisms are crucial to successful arrhythmia management.*
- *The hemodynamic effects of an arrhythmia are important in developing an appropriate treatment strategy.*
- *Predisposing conditions and reversible causes should be recognized and corrected.*
- *Knowledge of antiarrhythmic drug therapy, cardiac pacing, electrical cardioversion, and defibrillation are essential to successful arrhythmia management.*
- *The proarrhythmic potential of antiarrhythmic drugs must be recognized and preventive measures taken whenever possible.*
- *Knowledge of antiarrhythmic drug pharmacokinetics and pharmacodynamics and the effect of multisystem organ disease on these parameters are important in preventing drug toxicity.*
- *The intensivist should be skilled in the implantation of temporary pacing systems, external cardioversion, and defibrillation.*
- *The intensivist should recognize when temporary and implantable pacemakers or cardioverter defibrillators are not functioning appropriately.*
- *Not all arrhythmias require long-term prophylactic treatment.*

Cardiac arrhythmias are common in the critical care setting. Many arrhythmias detected are benign, may occur in healthy individuals, and require no investigation or treatment (e.g., sinus tachycardia, sinus bradycardia, Mobitz type I second-degree atrioventricular [AV] block, or premature atrial and ventricular beats). Correct diagnosis and understanding of arrhythmia mechanisms and knowledge of antiarrhythmic drug pharmacology and nonpharmacologic therapies of arrhythmias are crucial for successful arrhythmia management. This chapter focuses on the mechanisms, investigation, and management of the most common, clinically significant arrhythmias encountered.

Tachyarrhythmias

MECHANISMS

Tachycardia mechanisms have been classified as due to abnormalities of impulse formation or impulse conduction.[1–3] Abnormalities of impulse formation may be due to normal automaticity, abnormal automaticity, or triggered activity occurring within atrial or ventricular muscle tissue or the specialized conduction system (Fig. 24-1A).[1,2] Natural pacemaker cells are found in the sinus node, parts of the atria, the atrioventricular node, and the His-Purkinje system. These cells exhibit phasic spontaneous depolarization during diastole, resulting in an action potential when the threshold potential is reached.[1] Although the sinus node is the dominant pacemaker in the normal heart, subsidiary pacemakers may become dominant under certain conditions, such as sympathetic stimulation or digitalis toxicity (see Fig. 24-1). Normal atrial and ventricular muscles maintain a high negative resting potential (−90 mV) and only depolarize when stimulated. Under certain pathophysiologic conditions, including electrolyte abnormalities and ischemia, the resting membrane potential may decrease (−60 mV) and cells may depolarize spontaneously.

Triggered activity is caused by after-depolarizations that occur early in repolarization (early after-depolarizations) or after repolarization is complete (delayed after-depolarizations; see Fig. 24-1B).[1,2] Early after-depolarizations may reach threshold to activate the slow inward current generating a new action potential, and this cycle may repeat, generating a sustained tachycardia. Early after-depolarizations are believed to be the mechanism of torsade de pointes ventricular tachycardia (VT).[2] Delayed after-depolarizations initiate a triggered response only when their amplitude reaches a critical threshold (see Fig. 24-1C). Increasing the heart rate or the prematurity of an extrastimulus increases the amplitude of a delayed after-depolarization, thus increasing the probability of inducing a tachycardia. Delayed after-depolarizations are thought to cause arrhythmias secondary to digitalis toxicity.

Abnormalities of impulse conduction are due primarily to reentry (see Fig. 24-1).[3] Reentry requires an area of fixed or functional unidirectional block in one pathway, slow conduction in an alternate pathway, and return of the impulse along the original path after this tissue has recovered excitability (see Fig. 24-1D). Reentry is the mechanism of many types of supraventricular tachycardias (SVTs; atrioventricular node reentry or in the Wolff-Parkinson-White syndrome) and VT that occur after a myocardial infarction. Table 24-1 summarizes the mechanisms of common tachyarrhythmias.

Antiarrhythmic Drug Therapy

Antiarrhythmic drug therapy may be required for the termination of tachyarrhythmias and prevention of recurrence. Knowledge of the potential mechanisms of an arrhythmia and of the pharmacology of antiarrhythmic drugs are important in selecting appropriate drug therapy. Because the critical care patient often has multisystem disease, special attention to factors that influence drug absorption, protein binding, drug

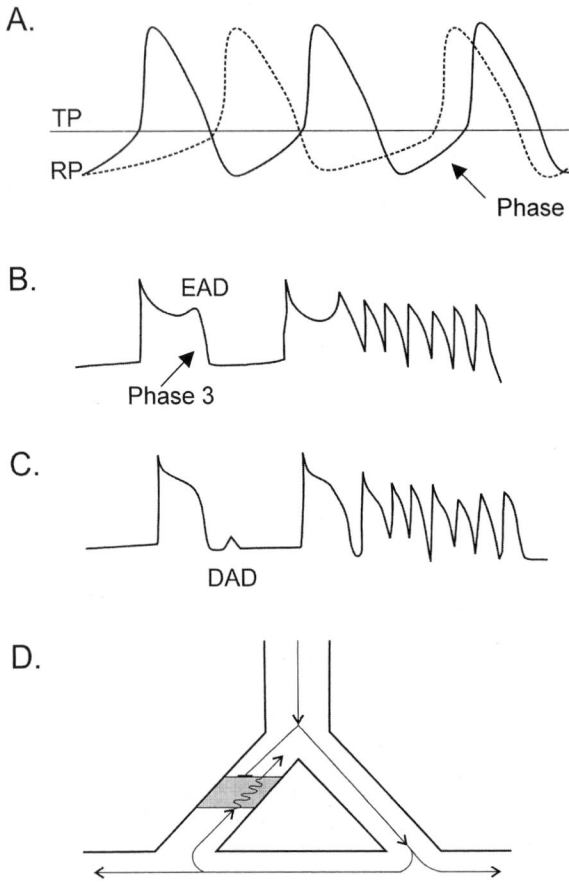

FIGURE 24-1 Mechanisms of cardiac arrhythmias: enhanced or abnormal automaticity and triggered activity or reentry. *A.* The rate of phase 4 depolarization may increase, causing the myocardial cell to reach the threshold potential (TP) sooner and spontaneously depolarize. In diseased tissue, the resting potential (RP) may be elevated and the time to reach TP may then be shortened (not shown). *B.* Early afterdepolarizations (EADs) develop late on phase 3 of repolarization of the action potential and, if they reach threshold, may trigger a depolarization. This is the mechanism of torsade de pointes ventricular tachycardia. *C.* Delayed afterdepolarizations (DADs) occur in diastole after repolarization is complete. If they reach threshold, they may trigger a depolarization. This is the mechanism associated with digitalis toxicity. *D.* Reentry is associated with an area of anatomic or functional unidirectional block (*speckled area*) and a region of slow conduction (*zigzag arrow*). A propagated impulse blocks in one area of tissue, passes through an area of slow conduction, and then conducts retrogradely through the original area of conduction block, which has now repolarized.

metabolism and excretion and knowledge of potential drug interactions are essential (see Chap. 103).[4]

The cardiac action potential varies strikingly in duration and morphology in specific regions of the heart, reflecting differences in ion channel expression or differences in modulators of ion channel function.[4] Antiarrhythmic drugs may therefore exert different effects on these various cardiac cells. Moreover, the effects of antiarrhythmic drugs may be modified in diseased cardiac tissue. For example, the effects of sodium channel blockers may be exaggerated in ischemic myocardium, and the effects of potassium channel blockers may

TABLE 24-1 Mechanisms of Common Tachycardias

Arrhythmia	Mechanism(s)
Supraventricular tachycardia	
AV node	Reentry
Accessory pathway	Reentry
Atrial tachycardia	Enhanced automaticity or reentry
Atrial flutter	Reentry
Atrial fibrillation	Onset: triggered activity
	Maintenance: multiple wavelet reentry
Ventricular tachycardia	
Monomorphic after MI	Reentry
Catecholamine-sensitive	Triggered activity
Torsade de pointes	Triggered activity
Ventricular fibrillation	Multiple wavelet reentry

ABBREVIATIONS: AV, atrioventricular; MI, myocardial infarction.

be exaggerated in the setting of left ventricular hypertrophy.[4] Antiarrhythmic drugs are classified most commonly by their dominant mechanism of action.[4–6] However, this drug classification scheme is imperfect because many of these drugs have effects on multiple ion channels or cell membrane receptors (Table 24-2). Efficacy of one drug does not predict the efficacy of another drug in the same class.

Class I drugs block the inward sodium current, resulting in slowing of conduction in atrial and ventricular muscles.[6] Their subclassification is based on the rate of recovery from sodium channel block. Class Ia antiarrhythmic drugs have an intermediate rate of recovery of sodium channel block and may cause prolongation of the QRS duration at physiologic heart rates. Class Ib drugs have a rapid recovery from sodium channel block and thus slow ventricular conduction only at very rapid heart rates. Class Ic drugs have a slow rate of recovery from sodium channel block and may cause significant prolongation of the QRS duration at resting heart rates. Class Ia and Ic drugs also block different potassium channels that cause prolongation of the atrial and ventricular action potential durations. This may manifest as prolongation of the QT interval. Class II drugs are β-adrenergic receptor blocking drugs.[7] Some of these agents are selective β_1-receptor blockers (see Table 24-2). Class III drugs are predominantly potassium channel blockers and prolong repolarization in atrial and ventricular muscle.[8] They can cause significant prolongation of the QT interval. Class IV drugs are calcium channel blocking drugs that decrease intracellular calcium concentrations.[7]

The mechanisms of action of commonly used antiarrhythmic drugs are listed in Table 24-2. Many of these agents are used to treat supraventricular and ventricular arrhythmias. Perhaps the most serious adverse response to antiarrhythmic drugs is the risk of proarrhythmia.[9,10] Proarrhythmia is defined as provocation of a new arrhythmia or worsening of an existing arrhythmia during therapy with a drug at concentrations not considered to be toxic. Class Ia and Ic drugs may cause excessive slowing of conduction in diseased atrial or ventricular muscle tissue that may exacerbate the clinical arrhythmia (e.g., atrial flutter or VT). These drugs increase the risk of sudden cardiac death in patients after myocardial infarction. Thus, class I antiarrhythmic drugs are contraindicated in patients with ischemic heart disease and a prior myocardial infarction because of the risk of

TABLE 24-2 Pharmacodynamics of Antiarrhythmic Drugs

	Recovery From Sodium Channel Block	K^+ Channels	Receptors
Class I			
Sodium channel blockers			
Class Ia			
Disopyramide	Intermediate	$\downarrow I_{to}, \downarrow I_{Kr}$ $\downarrow I_{K(ATP)}$	Inhibits muscarinic receptors
Quinidine	Intermediate	$\downarrow I_{to}, \downarrow I_{Kr}$	Inhibits α and muscarinic receptors
Procainamide	Intermediate		
N-acetyl procainamide	—	$\downarrow I_{Kr}$	
Class Ib			
Lidocaine	Rapid	—	—
Mexiletine	Rapid	—	—
Class Ic			
Flecainide	Slow	$\downarrow I_{Kr}, \downarrow I_{Kur}$	
Propafenone	Slow	$\downarrow I_{Kr}, \downarrow I_{Kur}$	Inhibits β receptors
Class II			
β-Adrenergic receptor blockers			
Atenolol	—		β_1-Receptor blocker
Bisoprolol	—		β_1-Receptor blocker
Carvedilol	—		β_1-Receptor blocker, α-receptor blocker
Metoprolol	—		β_1-Receptor blocker
Nadolol	—		Nonselective β blocker
Propranolol	Rapid		Nonselective β blocker
Class III			
Drugs that prolong repolarization			
Amiodarone	Rapid	$\downarrow I_{Kr}$	Inhibits α and β receptors, calcium channel blocker
Dofetilide	—	$\downarrow I_{Kr}$	
Sotalol	—	$\downarrow I_{Kr}$	Nonselective β blocker
Class IV			
Calcium channel blockers			
Diltiazem	—	—	—
Verapamil	Rapid	—	—
Digoxin	—	—	Blocks Na^+, K^+ ATPase

ABBREVIATIONS: $I_{K(ATP)}$, ATP-sensitive K^+ channel sensitive to adenosine triphosphate; I_{Kr}, rapidly activating component of delayed rectifying current; I_{Kur}, ultra rapidly activating delayed rectifying current in atrial tissue; I_{to}, transient outward current.

ventricular proarrhythmia. Drugs that cause excessive prolongation of the QT interval may cause torsade de pointes VT.[4,9,10] Torsade de pointes VT may occur in 1% to 8% of patients exposed to QT interval prolonging antiarrhythmic drugs.[4]

The pharmacokinetic characteristics of commonly used antiarrhythmic drugs are summarized in Table 24-3.[6,11–14] Drug dosing, adverse effects, and potential interactions are listed in Table 24-4.[4,6–8,11,15,16] Adverse effects may develop from pharmacokinetic or pharmacodynamic drug interactions. Pharmacokinetic drug interactions develop when one drug modifies the absorption, distribution, metabolism, or elimination of a second drug, such as warfarin with amiodarone or digitalis with quinidine.[4,11] Pharmacodynamic interactions occur when a drug or condition increases or decreases the pharmacologic effect of a drug without changing plasma drug concentrations, such as increased protein binding of propafenone, verapamil, or lidocaine secondary to elevated α_1-acid glycoprotein after myocardial infarction.[11] Several enzymes in the cytochrome P450 family are responsible for drug metabolism. Some drugs may inhibit or induce these enzymes, resulting in important drug interactions (see Table 24-4).[4,11,12]

Ventricular Tachyarrhythmias

VENTRICULAR TACHYARRHYTHMIA CLASSIFICATION AND MECHANISMS

Sustained ventricular arrhythmias including monomorphic VT, polymorphic VT, and ventricular fibrillation (VF) usually occur in the setting of structural heart disease, most frequently in the setting of coronary artery disease, previous myocardial infarction, and poor left ventricular function.[17] However, any form of structural heart disease may be associated with ventricular arrhythmias. In addition, some individuals have primary electrical disease, usually associated with a mutation affecting one or more ion channels or proteins that regulate ion channels, as in the long QT syndrome and Brugada syndrome.[18]

The QRS complexes are uniform in monomorphic VT, whereas the QRS complexes change continuously in polymorphic VT. In VF, the surface electrocardiogram is disorganized without discernible QRS complexes. VT frequently precedes the development of VF, particularly in patients with a prior history of myocardial infarction. These arrhythmias are considered to be sustained if they last longer

TABLE 24-3 Pharmacokinetic Characteristics of Antiarrhythmic Drugs

Drug	Bioavailability (%)	Binding to Plasma Proteins (%)	Renal Elimination of Unchanged Drug (%)	Plasma Half-life (h)	Active Metabolites	Hepatic Metabolism
Class Ia						
Disopyramide	83 ± 11	$28–68^a$	55 ± 6	6.0 ± 1.0	Racemic mixture	
Quinidine	70–80	87 ± 3	18 ± 5	6.2 ± 1.8	3-Hydroxy quinidine	CYP3A4
Procainamide	83 ± 16	16 ± 5	67 ± 8	3.0 ± 0.6	NAPA	NAT2 acetylation^b
Class Ib						
Lidocaine	Parenteral administration only	70 ± 5	2 ± 1	1.8 ± 0.4	Monoethyl-glycyl-xylidide	CYP3A4
Mexiletine	87 ± 13	63 ± 3	4–15	9.2 ± 2.1	—	CYP1A2, CYP2D6
Class Ic						
Flecainide	70 ± 11	61 ± 10	43 ± 3	11 ± 3	—	CYP2D6
Propafenone	$5–50^a$	85–95	<1	5.5 ± 2.1	5-Hydroxy-propafenone	CYP2D6
Class II						
Atenolol	50–60	<5	85–100	5–7	Racemic mixture	—
Bisoprolol	90	30	50	11–17	Racemic mixture	CYP3D6
Carvedilol	25	95	<2	2.2 ± 0.3	Racemic mixture	—
Metoprolol	38 ± 1.4	11 ± 1	10 ± 3	3.2 ± 0.2	Racemic mixure	CYP2D6
Propranolol	26 ± 10	87 ± 6	<0.5	3.9 ± 0.4	Racemic mixture, hydroxy propranolol	CYP2D6, CYP1A2
Class III						
Amiodarone	46 ± 22	99.9 ± 0.1	0	25 ± 12 d	Desethyl amiodarone	CYP3A4
Dofetilide	96 (83–108)	64	52 ± 2	7.5 ± 0.4		CYP3A4
Sotalol	90–100	None	>90	8 ± 3	Racemic mixture	—
Class IV						
Diltiazem	38 ± 11	78 ± 3	<4	4.4 ± 1.3	Desacyldiltiazem, N-desmethyl diltiazem	CYP3A4
Verapamil	22 ± 8	90 ± 2	<3	4.0 ± 1.5	Racemic mixture	CYP3A4, CYP2C9
Digoxin	7.0 ± 13	25 ± 5	60 ± 11	39 ± 13	—	

^{a} Concentration dependent.
^{b} Depends on acetylation phenotype.
ABBREVIATIONS: CYP, cytochrome P-450; NAPA, N-acetyl procainamide; NAT, N-acetyltransferase.
SOURCE: Data printed with permission from Gillis,[6] Roden,[11] Wilkinson,[12] Wadworth et al,[13] and McGavin and Keating.[14]

than 30 seconds or if they require acute intervention for termination.[14,19]

Multiple mechanisms contribute to VT. Monomorphic VT that develops in patients with a prior myocardial infarction is due to reentry near the border of the scar. In patients with dilated cardiomyopathy and an underlying intraventricular conduction delay, monomorphic VT usually with a left bundle branch block pattern may develop due to bundle branch reentry. In patients without structural heart disease, catecholamine-sensitive VT may originate in the right ventricular outflow tract due to triggered activity initiated by cyclic adenosine monophosphate. A verapamil-sensitive monomorphic VT that originates in the region of the left posterior fascicle is thought to be due to triggered activity.[18]

Polymorphic VT in the setting of a normal QT interval usually occurs in the setting of acute ischemia or significant hemodynamic instability,[20] although it may also occur in otherwise healthy individuals due to a mutation of the ryanodine receptor.[21] Torsade de pointes VT is a polymorphic, pause-dependent VT that develops in association with drugs or pathophysiologic conditions that excessively prolong the QT interval (Fig. 24-2 and Table 24-5).[7,8] Torsade de pointes VT is initiated by focal triggered activity and maintained by ventricular reentry. Risk factors for the development of

torsade de pointes VT include female sex, baseline QT interval prolongation, excessive QT interval prolongation on drug therapy (>550 ms), bradycardia/pauses, hypokalemia, hypomagnesemia, congestive heart failure, cardiac hypertrophy, prior history of VT or VF, and renal impairment. The drugs and pathophysiologic conditions associated with torsade de pointes VT are listed in Table 24-5.[9] In addition to QT interval prolongation, electrocardiographic features that are harbingers of torsade de pointes VT include QT prolongation and T-wave morphology changes after an extrasystolic pause, T-wave alternans, late-coupled polymorphic ventricular premature beats, and repetitive polymorphic beats.[9]

VF is frequently associated with acute myocardial ischemia, or sustained VT may degenerate into VF. VF may be initiated by a triggered focus or reentrant mechanism and is maintained by multiple reentrant wavelets in the ventricles.

EVALUATION OF THE PATIENT WITH VT/VF

The initial evaluation of the patient with sustained VT or VF should be directed at detecting underlying reversible causes.[22] This evaluation should include a thorough history (if the patient is able to communicate) and physical examination. A 12-lead electrogram of VT is extremely valuable, as is

TABLE 24-4 Antiarrhythmic Drug Dosing and Adverse Effects

Drug	Dosage	Dosage Adjustment	Adverse Effects	Drug Interactions
Class Ia				
Quinidine gluconate (SR)	250 mg PO q 8 h ↑ By 250 mg doses if QTc <460 ms ↓ Dose if QTc ≥500 ms Discontinue if QTc ≥550 ms	↓ Initial dose 50% + ↑ dosing interval to q 12 h in renal failure	Diarrhea, stomach cramps, tinnitus; torsade de pointes VT	→ Digoxin dose by 50% monitor INR if on warfarin ↓ Dose of β blocker; amiodarone, cimetidine, diltiazem, propranolol, and verapamil may increase quinidine concentrations
Procainamide SR	250 mg PO q 6 h ↑ By 250 mg increments if QTc <460 ms Maximum dose 1 g PO 1 6 h ↓ Dose if QTc ≥500 ms Discontinue if QTc >550 ms	Metabolism depends on rate of acetylation; the active metabolite NAPA accumulates in fast acetylators and in renal failure; monitor procainamide + NAPA levels and keep sum <80 μM: monitor ECG intervals	Agranulocytosis, rash, fever, SLE syndrome, torsade de pointes VT	Amiodarone, cimetidine, propranolol may increase procainamide concentrations
Procainamide IV	750–1000 mg loading 15–17 mg/kg at 20 mg/min; maintenance 1–4 mg/min		Hypotension	
Disopyramide	100 mg PO q 8 h SR 150–250 mg q 12 h ↑ By 100-mg increments if QTc <460 ms Maximum dose 300 mg PO q 8 h ↓ Dose if QTc ≥500 ms Discontinue if QTc ≥550 ms	↓ Initial dose 50% and ↑ dosing interval q 12 h in renal failure	Urinary retention, blurred vision constipation, dry month, worsening heart failure, torsade de pointes VT	
Class Ib				
Lidocaine IV	1.5 mg/kg loading; 1–4 mg/min maintenance	↓ dose in CHF		
Mexiletine	150 mg–300 mg PO q 8 h		Numbness, paresthesia, slurred, speech, altered consciousness. Nausea, stomach cramps, tremor, blurred vision, ataxia, confusion.	Propranolol, metoprolol, cimetidine increase lidocaine concentrations Cimetidine, quinidine, increase mexiletine concentrations
Class Ic				
Flecainide	50 mg PO q 12 h ↑ by 25–50-mg increments Maximum dose 200 mg PO q 12 h ↓ Dose if QRS prolonged >20% from baseline	↓ Initial dose 50% in renal failure; titrate dose based on QRS intervals.	Tremor, blurred vision, headache, ataxia, CHF, VT proarrhythmia	Amiodarone, cimetidine, propranolol, quinidine increase flecainide concentrations
Propafenone	150 mg PO q 8–12 h Maximum dose 300 mg PO q 8 h ↓ Dose if QRS prolonged >20% from baseline	↓ Initial dose 50% in renal and hepatic failure and ↑ dosing interval to q 12 h Active metabolites accumulate in rapid metabolizers; monitor QRS duration carefully	Constipation, dizziness, headache, metallic taste, exacerbation of asthma, VT proarrhythmia	↓ Digoxin dose by 25%–50%; cimetidine and quinidine increase propafenone concentrations
Class II				
Atenolol	50–200 mg PO daily	Caution in patients with CHF or bronchiospastic lung disease Monitor carefully in diabetic patients ↓ Dose in moderate to severae renal insufficiency	Bradycardia, hypotension, dyspnea, fatigue, depression	With digoxin, Ca²⁺ channel blockers, amiodarone ↓ Dose 25%–50% Hypoglycemic agents

(continued)

TABLE 24-4 Antiarrhythmic Drug Dosing and Adverse Effects (*continued*)

Drug	Dosage	Dosage Adjustment	Adverse Effects	Drug Interactions
Bisoprolol	2.5–10 mg PO bid	As per atenolol	As per atenolol	As per atenolol
Carvedilol	3.25–50 mg PO bid	As per atenolol	As per atenolol	As per atenolol
		Titrate dose every 1–2 wk to achieve maximum tolerated dose		
Metoprolol	5–15 mg IV	As per atenolol	As per atenolol	As per atenolol
	25–400 mg PO bid			
Nadolol	20–160 mg PO daily	As per atenolol and ↓ dose in moderate to sever renal insufficiency	As per atenolol	As per atenolol
Propranolol	1–2 mg IV q 2–4 min PRN × 4–5 doses	As per atenolol	As per atenolol	As per atenolol
	20–80 mg PO bid/tid			
Class III				
Amiodarone	For AF: 200 mg PO tid × 2 wk, then 200 mg/d	Avoid high loading dose in setting of sinus bradycardia (HR <50 beats/min)	Pulmonary toxicity, CNS effects, hyper-/hypothyroidism, photosensitivity, corneal deposits, hepatic toxicity.	↑ Quinidine/procainamide dose by 50%
	For VT: accelerated loading dose in hospital 400 mg PO tid × 10–14 d, then 400 mg PO bid × 7 d, then 300–400 mg PO daily			↓ Digoxin dose by 50%
				↓ β-blocker dose by 50%
				↓ Warfarin dose by 50%
Amiodarone IV	150–300 mg IV over 20–30 min, then 0.5–1 mg/min; repeat boluses may be required	May cause hypotension		
Dofetilide	125–500 μg PO bid	↓ Dose if QT interval prolongs after first dose by 15%; discontinue if QTc ≥550 ms	Headache; torsade de pointes VT	Cimetidine, verapamil, ketoconazole, trimethoprim alone or in combination with sulfamethoxazole
Sotalol	80 mg PO q 12 h	↓ Initial dose in renal failure	Torsade de pointes VT, hypotension, bradycardia, wheezing; caution in CHF and bronchospastic lung disease	Digoxin/verapamil/other β blockers may cause AV block, bradycardia
	↑ By 80-mg increments if QTc <460 ms Maximum dose 240 mg PO q 12 h	↓ Initial dose to 40 mg PO q 12 h in the elderly		
	↓ Dose if QTc ≥500 ms; discontinue if QTc ≥550 ms			
Class IV				
Diltiazem	0.25–0.35 mg/kg IV	Caution in patients with CHF	Bradycardia, hypotension, peripheral edema	β Blockers, digoxin, amiodarone
	120–480 mg PO daily/bid			
Verapamil	5–15 mg IV	Caution in patients with CHF	Bradycardia, hypotension, constipation, flushing	β Blockers, digoxin, amiodarone
	80 mg PO tid; maximum dose 120 mg qid or 240 mg bid			
Digoxin	0.0625–0.25 mg PO daily	↓ Dose in renal failure	Arrhythmias, visual disturbance, nausea, vomiting	β Blockers; calcium channel blockers, quinidine, propafenone, procainamide, amiodarone.
Digoxin IV	0.25–1.0 mg IV over 20–30 min			

ABBREVIATIONS: AF, atrial fibrillation; AV, atrioventricular; bid, twice daily; CHF, congestive heart failure; CNS, central nervous system; ECG, electrocardiographic; INR, international ratio; IV, intravenous; NAPA, N-acetylprocainamide; PO, per os; PRN, as needed; SLE, systemic lupus erythematosus; SR, sustained release; tid, three time daily; VT, ventricular tachycadia.

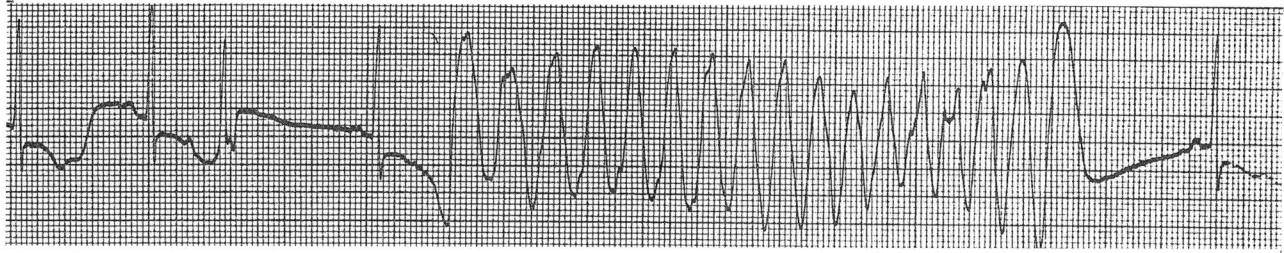

FIGURE 24-2 Example of torsade de pointes ventricular tachycardia (VT). There is significant QT interval prolongation before the onset of polymorphic nonsustained VT.

a review of rhythm strips documenting the onset of VT/VF. Laboratory tests should include cardiac enzymes (creatine kinase or troponin), creatinine, and serum electrolytes including K^+ and Mg^{2+}. An echocardiogram should be performed to determine the presence of structural heart disease and to assess ventricular function. Cardiac hemodynamic data should be reviewed. A drug screen may be required if drug toxi-

TABLE 24-5 Drugs and Conditions Associated with Torsade de Pointes Ventricular Tachycardia

Drug Class	Specific Drugs
Antiarrhythmic drugs	
Class Ia	Disopyramide
	Procainamide
	Quinidine
Class Ic	Propafenone
Class III	Amiodarone
	Dofetilide
	Ibutilide
	d, l-Sotalol
Antifungal	Ketoconazole
	Fluconazole
	Itraconazole
Antihistamines	Diphenhydramine
	Terfenadine
	Astemizole
Antimicrobial	Erythromycin
	Clarithromycin
	Trimethoprim-sulfamethoxazole
	Pentamidine
Diuretics	Furosemide
	Hydrochlorothiazide
	Indapamide
	Metolazone
Psychotropic	Haloperidol
	Phenothiazines
	Risperidone
	Tricyclic antidepressants
	Tetracyclic antidepressants
Other conditions	Pathophysiologic condition
Bradycardia	Complete heart block, sinus pauses, or profound sinus bradycardia
Congenital long QT syndrome	Mutations of potassium or sodium channels
Electrolyte abnormalities	Hypokalemia
	Hypomagnesemia
	Hypocalcemia
Nervous system injury	Subarachnoid hemorrhage
Starvation	Anorexia nervosa, liquid protein diets

city is suspected (e.g., digitalis or tricyclic antidepressants). Some electrocardiographic features that allow discrimination of VT from SVT with aberrant conduction are summarized in Table 24-6.

MANAGEMENT OF VENTRICULAR TACHYARRHYTHMIAS

GENERAL PRINCIPLES OF TREATMENT
Sinus rhythm should be restored as soon as possible in sustained VT or cardiac arrest.[22–24] Treatment of underlying cardiovascular disease should be initiated and any reversible causes should be identified and corrected (Table 24-7).[22–24] Serum potassium should be maintained 4.0 mmol/L or higher, and serum magnesium should be maintained above 0.7 mmol/L. Beta blockers should be prescribed unless contraindicated (see Table 24-4). Management of ischemic heart disease, left ventricular dysfunction, and hypertension must be optimized. If ongoing ischemia is present despite medical therapy, the patient should be considered for urgent coronary artery revascularization.

NONSUSTAINED VT
Beta blockers should be prescribed unless contraindicated, and doses should be titrated to suppress nonsustained VT (see Table 24-4).[16,22,25–27] If frequent, hemodynamically significant nonsustained VT persists, amiodarone may be initiated for suppression.[16,22,24,28] Patients with mild to moderate left ventricular dysfunction (left ventricular ejection fraction [LVEF] >0.30) may be considered for risk stratification electrophysiology study to determine the risk of sudden cardiac death.[16,29] Patients with severe left ventricular dysfunction in the setting of ischemic heart disease (LVEF ≤0.30) should be considered for an implantable cardioverter defibrillator (ICD) for prophylaxis of sudden cardiac death.[19,30]

MONOMORPHIC VENTRICULAR TACHYCARDIA
The acute management algorithm for sustained monomorphic VT is shown in Fig. 24-3. This algorithm is based on

TABLE 24-6 Electrocardiographic Criteria Consistent With Ventricular Tachycardia During Wide QRS Complex Tachycardia

Atrioventricular dissociation
Fusion beats
Extreme left-axis deviation
QRS duration >160 ms
Different QRS morphology during tachycardia compared to baseline in patient with preexisting bundle branch block
R-wave duration ≥60 ms in V_1

TABLE 24-7 Management of Ventricular Tachycardia due to Reversible Causes

Acute ischemia/myocardial infarction	Amiodarone and/or β blockers, revascularization
CHF	Optimize therapy of CHF, ACE inhibitors, β blockers; consider ICD
Electrolyte abnormalities (usually torsade de pointes VT)	MgSO₄ I–4 g IV, KC1, atrial overdrive pacing
Drug toxicity/long QT (torsade de pointes VT)	MgSO₄ 1–4 g IV, atrial overdrive pacing (80–100 beats/min), discontinue class I/III drugs
Drug toxicity (incessant monomorphic VT, e.g., flecainide/propafenone/ tricyclic antidepressants)	Sodium bicarbonate (50–200 mEq IV), lidocaine (0.5–0.75 mg/kg)
Catecholamine sensitive VT	β Blockers

ABBREVIATIONS: ACE, angiotensin-converting enzyme; CHF, congestive heart failure; ICD, implantable cardioverter defibrillator; IV, intravenously; VT, ventricular tachycardia.

the recommendations of the American Heart Association in collaboration with the International Liaison Committee on Resuscitation.[22–25] Synchronized cardioversion with 50 to 150 J of biphasic shock or 50 to 200 J of monophasic shock is the initial approach for the patient with hemodynamically unstable VT. The higher energy shocks should be used if the patient is unconscious. If the patient is hemodynamically stable and has normal or only mild left ventricular dysfunction, intravenous procainamide or sotalol may promote conversion. Beta-blocker therapy should be initiated to prevent recurrence. The patient with hemodynamically stable VT in the setting of significant left ventricular dysfunction should be treated with intravenous amiodarone (see Table 24-4 and Fig. 24-3).[22–25,28] If VT does not convert with pharmacologic therapy, synchronized electrical cardioversion may be required.

Long-term antiarrhythmic drug therapy in addition to long-term β-blocker therapy may be required to prevent VT recurrence. This decision is made after treatment of underlying

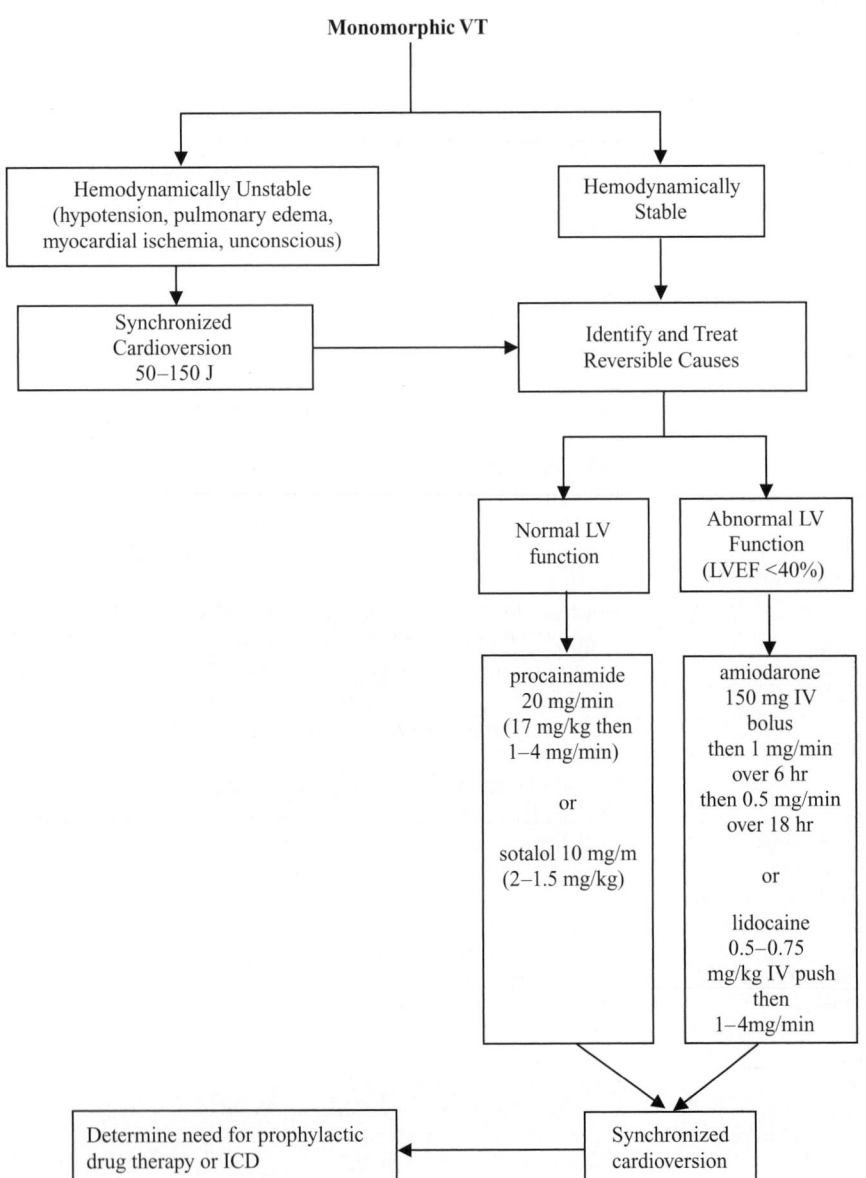

FIGURE 24-3 Management algorithm for sustained monomorphic ventricular tachycardia. ICD, implantable cardioverter defibrillator; LV, left ventricular.

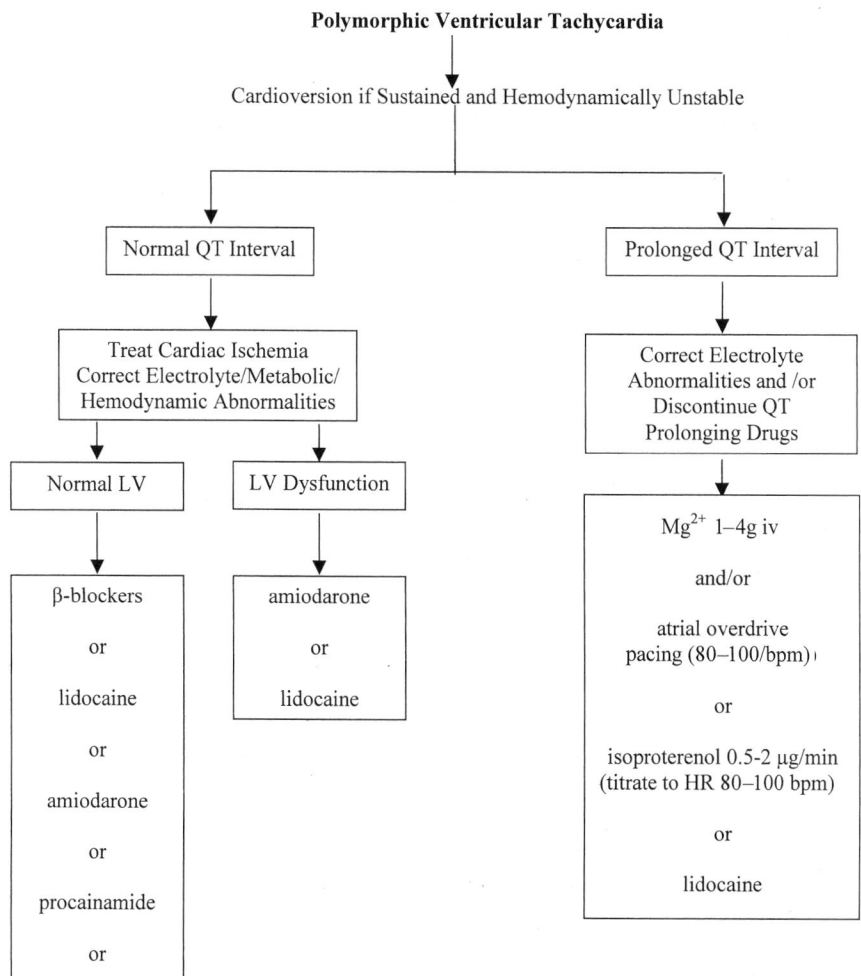

FIGURE 24-4 Management algorithm for sustained polymorphic ventricular tachycardia. LV, left ventricular.

causes has been achieved and coronary artery revascularization, if required, has been accomplished. Class I antiarrhythmic drugs are contraindicated in patients with coronary artery disease and prior myocardial infarction, and class I drugs and sotalol are relatively contraindicated in patients with left ventricular dysfunction because of the risk of ventricular proarrhythmia.[9,10] Patients with sustained VT in the absence of a reversible, correctable cause and in the setting of moderate to severe left ventricular dysfunction (LVEF ≤ 0.35) should be considered for an ICD. In this setting, the ICD has been shown to decrease cardiovascular mortality rate as compared with amiodarone therapy.[31–33] In patients with less severe left ventricular dysfunction, amiodarone appears to be as efficacious as the ICD, and long-term therapy with amiodarone or an ICD may be individualized.[33]

POLYMORPHIC VENTRICULAR TACHYCARDIA IN THE SETTING OF A NORMAL QT INTERVAL

The acute management algorithm for sustained polymorphic VT is shown in Fig. 24-4.[22,24] This algorithm is based on the recommendations of the American Heart Association in collaboration with the International Liaison Committee on Resuscitation.[24] Synchronized cardioversion with 50 to 150 J of biphasic shock or 50 to 200 J of monophasic shock is the initial approach for a patient with hemodynamically unstable sustained VT. Polymorphic VT in the absence of QT interval prolongation often is associated with myocardial ischemia.[20] Catecholaminergic polymorphic VT also has been described in patients without structural heart disease who have mutations of cardiac ryanodine receptors.[21] A patient with ischemia should be considered for urgent coronary angiography and revascularization, if required. This arrhythmia is frequently recurrent and intravenous β blockers or amiodarone should be administered to prevent recurrence. If a reversible cause, such as acute ischemia, is identified, long-term prophylactic antiarrhythmic drug therapy may not be required. Patients with significant left ventricular dysfunction should be considered for an ICD in the absence of a reversible, correctable cause.[29–33]

TORSADE DE POINTES VT

This arrhythmia frequently terminates spontaneously. However, cardioversion/defibrillation may be required if the patient develops sustained VT or VF. Magnesium, 1 to 4 g intravenously, is the initial treatment followed by cardiac overdrive pacing at 80 to 100 beats/min, which shortens the QT interval and prevents long pauses after premature beats (see Fig. 24-4).[22,34] Atrial overdrive pacing is preferred to ventricular overdrive pacing. An isoproterenol infusion may be

Ventricular Fibrillation

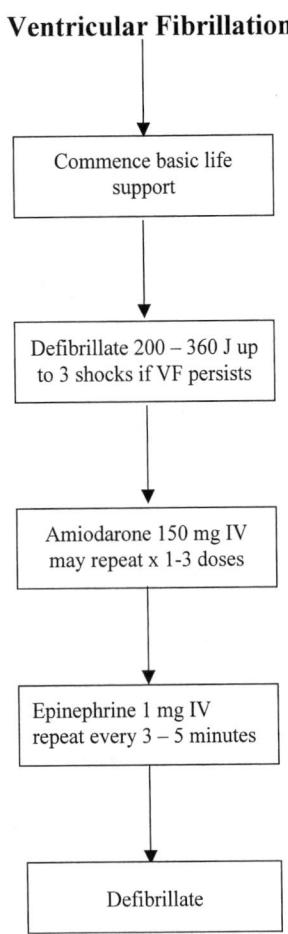

FIGURE 24-5 Management algorithm for ventricular fibrillation.

started until a temporary pacemaker is inserted. Drugs causing QT interval prolongation should be stopped and any electrolyte imbalances corrected. Temporary pacing should be continued until the VT has subsided and the QT interval returns to normal. If the patient has congenital long QT syndrome, long-term prophylactic therapy with β blockers or permanent cardiac pacing will prevent torsade de pointes VT.[18,35] An ICD is the treatment of choice in patients with congenital long QT syndrome who have sustained a cardiac arrest or who have a significant family history of sudden cardiac death.[18]

VENTRICULAR FIBRILLATION
Advanced life support should be initiated for VF, followed by prompt defibrillation (Fig. 24-5).[22–24] If defibrillation is unsuccessful at least three times, amiodarone and adrenaline should be administered before repeat defibrillation.[36] Intravenous amiodarone has been shown to improve resuscitation rates and overall survival rate if initial defibrillation is unsuccessful. If acute myocardial ischemia is the cause of VF, coronary angiography and percutaneous coronary intervention should be considered in the patient with recurrent VF. In the absence of a reversible cause, long-term therapy for prevention of sudden cardiac death should be prescribed. Patients with VF should be considered for an ICD, although in patients with well-preserved left ventricular dysfunction, amiodarone may also be a reasonable treatment option.[29–33]

VT/VF ELECTRICAL STORM
This is defined as multiple recurrent episodes of sustained VT or VF within a 24-hour period. Reversible causes should be identified and treated (see Table 24-7). Beta blockers are effective in suppressing some episodes of VT/VF storm.[22,26] Even in the setting of congestive heart failure (except cardiogenic shock), intravenous β blockers can be administered safely. Amiodarone is very effective in suppressing VT/VF, although multiple boluses may be required in some patients.[28] Combination β-blocker and amiodarone therapy is likely synergistic in suppressing recurrent VT/VF.[22] In the patient with an ICD and VT electrical storm who is receiving frequent, painful shock therapies, the VT cardioversion or defibrillation therapies may need to be temporarily programmed off until pharmacologic therapy suppresses the frequency of VT.

Supraventricular Tachyarrhythmias

SUPRAVENTRICULAR ARRHYTHMIA CLASSIFICATION AND MECHANISMS

Atrial fibrillation (AF) is the most common sustained arrhythmia observed, and its frequency increases with advancing age.[37] AF is believed to be triggered by spontaneous depolarizations that originate most commonly in the pulmonary veins. These often fire repetitively, initiating an atrial tachycardia that degenerates into AF through the development of multiple wavelets of reentry in the atria. AF is characterized by the absence of distinct P waves on the electrogram and an irregular ventricular response. The ventricular response during AF is usually very rapid (120 to 170 beats/min) unless the patient is on AV node blocking drugs or the patient has coexisting AV conduction system disease. Atrial flutter is characterized by atrial rates of approximately 300 beats/min and is usually due to reentry in the atrium, most commonly in the right atrium involving the isthmus between the inferior vena cava and tricuspid annulus. AF and atrial flutter often occur in the same patient. In atrial flutter, distinct P waves are observed on the electrogram; these are often inverted in leads II, III, and aVF. In the absence of AV node blocking drugs or coexisting AV conduction disease, 2:1 AV conduction with ventricular rates of 150 beats/min is the most common pattern observed. Class I antiarrhythmic drugs in the absence of adequate AV node blocking drugs may slow the atrial rate during atrial flutter such that 1:1 AV conduction occurs. This may be misdiagnosed as VT because an intraventricular conduction delay may develop at rapid ventricular rates.[9]

The most common type of SVT is due to AV node reentry.[38] This is characterized by swiftly and slowly conducting pathways in the AV node.[3] The electrogram is characterized by a regular narrow complex tachycardia with a short RP interval; usually P waves, if visible, are observed in the early part of the ST segment. Reciprocating tachycardia is secondary to macro reentry involving an accessory atrioventricular connection, characterized by a narrow complex tachycardia with a longer RP interval. Most patients have overt ventricular preexcitation (Wolff Parkinson White syndrome); however, in some patients, ventricular preexcitation is not manifest on the electrogram and retrograde conduction through the accessory connection is concealed. True atrial tachycardia is most commonly due to enhanced or abnormal atrial automaticity or triggered activity. P waves usually precede each QRS complex unless there is AV conduction block. Multifocal atrial tachycardia is characterized by variation in P-wave morphology on a beat-to-beat basis.

EVALUATION OF THE PATIENT WITH SUPRAVENTRICULAR TACHYARRHYTHMIA

The initial evaluation of a patient with a sustained supraventricular tachyarrhythmia should include a thorough history (if the patient is able to communicate) and physical examination with special attention to detecting structural heart disease.[15] A 12-lead electrogram of the arrhythmia and during sinus rhythm should be obtained. Rhythm strips documenting onset and termination of the arrhythmia should be reviewed. Laboratory tests should include cardiac enzymes (creatine kinase or troponin), complete blood count, international normalized ratio, and thyroid-stimulating hormone. An echocardiogram should be made to determine the presence of structural heart disease and to assess ventricular function. In some instances, a transesophageal echocardiogram may be required to assess valve function or to determine whether intracardiac thrombus is present. Cardiac hemodynamic data during the arrhythmia, if available, should be reviewed.

MANAGEMENT OF SUPRAVENTRICULAR TACHYARRHYTHMIAS

GENERAL PRINCIPLES OF TREATMENT
Sinus rhythm should be restored as soon as possible if the patient is symptomatic. In the case of AF, therapy aimed at controlling the ventricular rate may be the initial approach. Any reversible causes should be identified and corrected. Underlying structural heart disease should be treated, in particular ischemic heart disease, left ventricular dysfunction, or hypertension. The probability of recurrence and the need for chronic prophylactic therapy should be determined.

ATRIAL FIBRILLATION OR FLUTTER
The therapeutic approach for the management of sustained AF or atrial flutter is illustrated in Fig. 24-6.[15,37] Synchronized electrical cardioversion may be required if the patient is

Acute Therapy of Recent Onset Sustained Paroxysmal Atrial Fibrillation/Flutter

FIGURE 24-6 Management algorithm for atrial fibrillation (AF) or flutter.

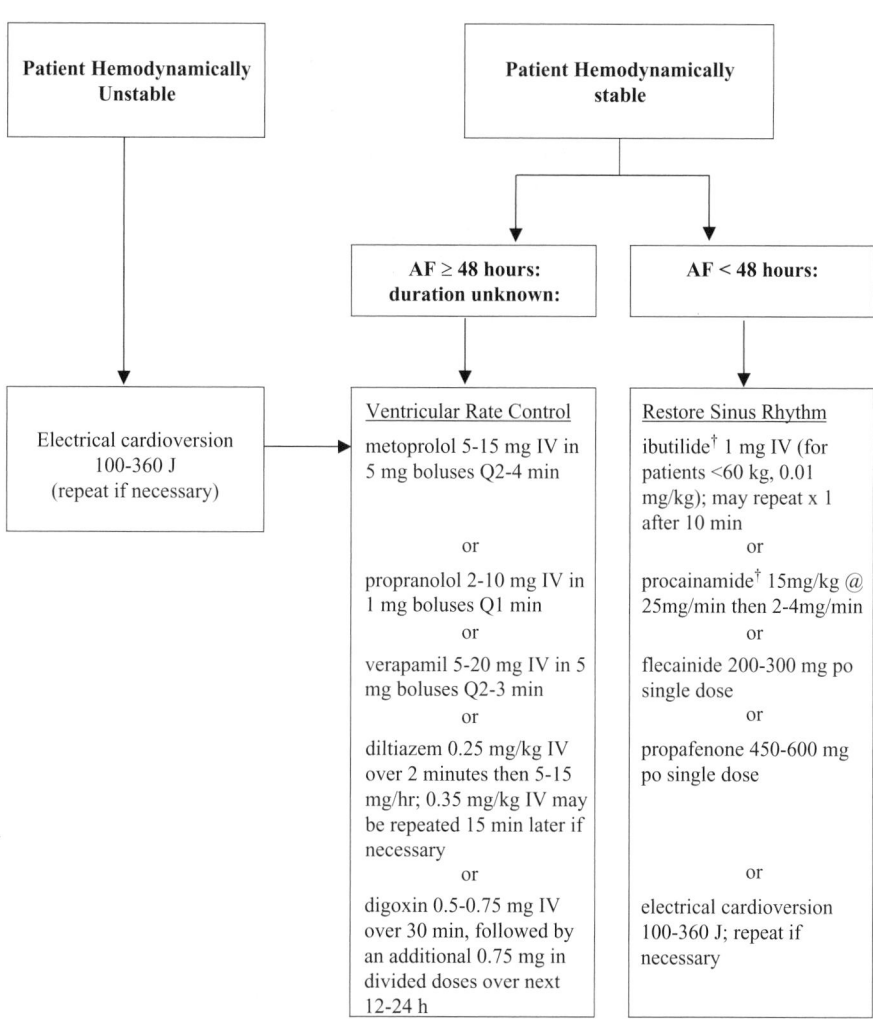

† Procainamide or ibutilide is the drug of choice for Wolff-Parkinson-White Syndrome.

hemodynamically unstable. Atrial flutter is frequently terminated with low-energy cardioversion (50 J), whereas higher energies may be required for AF (≥100 J). Since the incorporation of biphasic waveforms into external defibrillators, it is rare for cardioversion to fail to convert recent onset AF. Atrial flutter may be terminated by rapid atrial overdrive pacing. Some dual-chamber pacemakers and implantable defibrillators have atrial antitachycardia pacing therapies for pace termination of atrial flutter.

If AF or flutter has persisted for at least 48 hours in the absence of effective anticoagulation, therapy should be aimed at achieving ventricular rate control (heart rate < 90 beats/min). Pharmacologic cardioversion to sinus rhythm can be considered if the patient has been in AF no longer than 48 hours. Anticoagulant therapy with heparin or low-molecular-weight heparin must be initiated. If cardioversion is performed, anticoagulant therapy should be continued for at least 3–6 weeks after cardioversion.[15,37] Ibutilide or procainamide can be administered intravenously to promote pharmacologic conversion for recent onset AF or flutter or in patients who have been on effective long-term anticoagulation (Table 24-8).[15] The electrogram must be monitored for significant QT interval prolongation because both drugs may cause torsade de pointes VT.[9,15] Intravenous amiodarone is less effective in promoting conversion to sinus rhythm, although it may facilitate improved rate control.[39] One important principle in the management of AF is that each patient deserves at least one attempt at restoration of sinus rhythm.[37]

The decision to initiate class I or III antiarrhythmic drug therapy to maintain sinus rhythm should be based the patient's symptoms and the hemodynamic significance of the arrhythmia. In the relatively asymptomatic patient, rate control is a reasonable first approach.[40,41] Beta blockers, verapamil, or diltiazem should be prescribed in doses to achieve a ventricular rate at rest or with minimal activity at rates slower than 90 beats/min (see Table 24-4).[15,37] Digoxin alone is frequently ineffective in achieving rate control of AF or atrial flutter, although it may be synergistic with class II or IV antiarrhythmic drugs. Rhythm control with class I or III antiarrhythmic drugs may be desirable in the very symptomatic patient or when these arrhythmias cause adverse hemodynamic effects.[40–42] AV node blocking drugs are required in conjunction with class I or III antiarrhythmic drugs because AF or atrial flutter is usually paroxysmal in nature and these drugs are rarely 100% effective at suppression. The dosages, potential side effects, and drug interactions of these drugs are summarized in Table 24-4. Class I drugs are contraindicated for chronic prophylaxis in patients with a prior myocardial infarction, and class I drugs and sotalol are relatively contraindicated in those with significant left ventricular dysfunction because of the risk of ventricular proarrhythmia.[9,10,37,43,44] Long-term antiarrhythmic drug therapy for prevention of AF or atrial flutter may not be required if the episode is thought to be due to a reversible cause, such as pneumonia or perioperative stress.

Catheter ablation for cure of atrial flutter is an effective therapy.[45] Pulmonary vein isolation can be considered for long-term cure of AF in selected patients.[46] AV junction ablation and ventricular pacing is an effective option in patients in whom effective ventricular rate control of AF cannot be achieved pharmacologically.[47]

The patient with AF or atrial flutter is at risk of thromboembolism, particularly if the patient is older or has structural heart disease.[37] Aspirin is indicated for prevention of thromboembolism in low-risk patients, whereas anticoagulation with heparin and then warfarin is required in high-risk patients (see Table 24-8).[37,48] If the patient has not been on anticoagulant therapy, electrical or pharmacologic cardioversion should be deferred for at least 3 weeks if the patient has been in AF or atrial flutter for at least 48 hours or if the duration is unknown. Alternatively, a transesophageal echocardiogram can be performed to demonstrate the absence of intracardiac thrombus if restoration of sinus rhythm is desired urgently. Patients should be maintained on oral anticoagulation for at least 6 weeks after electrical cardioversion.

SUPRAVENTRICULAR TACHYCARDIA

The therapeutic approach to the management of SVT is illustrated in Fig. 24-7.[15,24] Vagal maneuvers (carotid sinus massage or Valsalva maneuver) may terminate AV node reentry or reciprocating tachycardia involving a bypass tract. Adenosine is the initial drug of choice for regular narrow complex SVT, although β blockers, verapamil, and diltiazem are also effective. Oral antiarrhythmic drug therapy may be required to prevent recurrent SVT (see Table 24-4). Infrequently, synchronized electrical cardioversion may be required; 25 to 50 J is usually sufficient. Catheter ablation is an effective cure for AV node reentrant tachycardias secondary to accessory pathways or atrial tachycardias.[49] Multifocal atrial tachycardias may be difficult to suppress or to achieve rate control pharmacologically. In this case, implantation of a ventricular pacemaker followed by a total AV junction ablation is an effective treatment option.[47]

Bradyarrhythmias

Disorders of impulse formation or conduction may cause bradyarrhythmias. Sinus node dysfunction characterized by sinus bradycardia, sinoatrial exit block, or sinus arrest causing symptomatic bradycardia is the most common indication for permanent cardiac pacing.[50] AV block, permanent or

TABLE 24-8 Antithrombotic Treatment for Paroxysmal and Chronic Atrial Fibrillation

Medical Condition	Drug
Patient with no risk factors and age <65 ys	ASA 325 mg/d
Age 65–75 y with any one of the following risk factors	
Congestive heart failure	Warfarin (INR 2.0–3.0)
Left ventricular dysfunction	
Mitral valve disease	
Hypertension	
Diabetes mellitus	
Previous stroke or embolism	
Left atrial enlargement	
Age ≥75 y	Warfarin (INR 2.0–2.5) unless high risk of hemorrhage

ABBREVIATIONS: ASA, aspirin; INR, international ratio.

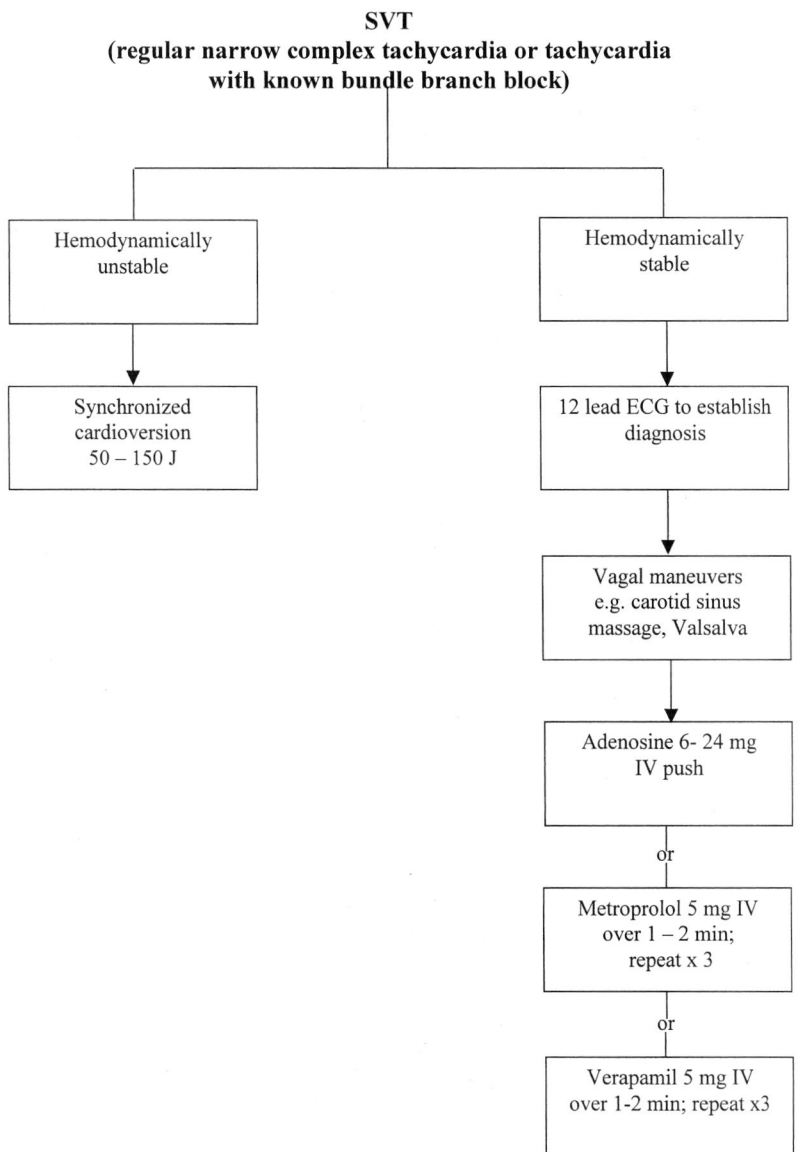

FIGURE 24-7 Management algorithm for regular narrow complex supraventricular tachycardia (SVT).

intermittent, is the second most common cause for permanent cardiac pacing.

EVALUATION OF THE PATIENT WITH BRADYARRHYTHMIAS

The initial evaluation of the patient with a documented bradyarrhythmia should include a thorough history (if the patient is able to communicate) and physical examination with a focus on detecting structural heart disease. A 12-lead electrogram and rhythm strips documenting the bradyarrhythmia should be reviewed. Carotid sinus massage should be performed to look for carotid sinus hypersensitivity unless contraindicated (carotid bruits or prior stroke). Cardiac hemodynamic data during the arrhythmia should be reviewed. Any drugs likely to contribute to the bradyarrhythmia should be identified and drug levels should be determined, if appropriate. Laboratory tests should include cardiac enzymes (creatine kinase or troponin). Echocardiography should be per-

formed to determine the presence of structural heart disease and to assess ventricular function.

GENERAL PRINCIPLES OF TREATMENT

In a patient in the intensive care unit (ICU) with hemodynamically significant persistent bradycardia, transcutaneous pacing should be commenced until a temporary pacemaker can be inserted. A transvenous electrode catheter usually can be placed at the bedside and inserted through the internal jugular or subclavian route by using a flotation pacing catheter. Fluoroscopy may be required for positioning the pacing electrode if adequate pacing thresholds cannot be achieved. If the bradyarrhythmia is transient, temporary pacing may not be required and the risk/benefit of this intervention needs to be considered. Any reversible causes should be identified and corrected. Drugs contributing to bradycardia should be discontinued. Second-degree AV block or complete heart block after an inferior myocardial infarction may not be persistent.

TABLE 24-9 Indications for Cardiac Pacing

Acquired AV block
  Class I
    Symptomatic permanent or intermittent AV block
    Symptomatic second-degree AV block
    Atrial flutter or fibrillation with advanced symptomatic AV block
  Class II
    Asymptomatic complete AV block with ventricular rate >40 beats/min
    Asymptomatic type II second-degree AV block
After myocardial infarction
  Class I
    Persistent complete heart block
    Persistent type II second-degree AV block
  Class II
    Newly acquires bundle branch block with transient high-grade AV or complete heart block
    Newly acquired bundle branch block with first-degree AV block
    Newly acquired bifascicular bundle branch block
Chronic bifascicular block
  Class I
    Symptomatic patients with fascicular block and intermittent high-grade AV or complete heart block
    Symptomatic patients with bifascicular block and HV interval prolongation (>100 ms) or block distal to the His bundle at rates <100 beats/min
  Class II
    Symptomatic patients with bifascicular block and no identifiable cause of syncope
    Asymptomatic patients with bifascicular block and intermittent type II second-degree AV block.
Sinus node dysfunction
  Class I
    Sinus node dysfunction with symptoms of bradycardia with or without required drug therapy
    Symptomatic sinus bradycardia
    Symptomatic chronotropic incompetence
  Class II
    Sinus bradycardia <40–50 beats/min or asystole >3 s and suggested symptoms not documented to be due to bradycardia
Hypersensitive carotid sinus
  Class I
    Recurrent syncope and asystole or heart block >3 s during carotid sinus massage or clearcut clinical situation suggestive of a vasoinhibitory response
  Class II
    Recurrent syncope without clear clinical setting but abnormal response to carotid sinus massage

ABBREVIATIONS: AV, atrioventricular; class I, general consensus that a pacing system is indicated; class II, consensus that a pacing system might be beneficial.
SOURCE: Printed with permission from Yee et al.[49]

If the bradyarrhythmia does not resolve, permanent cardiac pacing may be required. The indications for permanent cardiac pacing are summarized in Table 24-9.[50]

TEMPORARY PACING

Transcutaneous pacing may be achieved by delivering a high current (40 to 100 mA) through defibrillation pads on most ex-

TABLE 24-10 Pacing System Code

Chamber Paced	Chamber Sensed	Response
A	A	O/I/T
V	V	O/I/T
D	D	O/I/T/D

ABBREVIATIONS: A, atrium; D, dual chamber; I, inhibited; O, off; T, triggered; V, ventricle.

ternal cardioverters. Because this is painful for the conscious patient, the current should be decreased to the lowest setting that achieves continuous pacing. The rate programmed should be 60 to 70 beats/min and may need to be adjusted based on the patient's hemodynamic status. A temporary transvenous pacing lead should be inserted as quickly as possible. The initial current should be 3 to 5 mA. The current should then be reduced every five beats until there is failure to capture. The selected current for pacing should be twice the lowest current that effectively captured the atrium or ventricle.

PACING MODALITIES

The codes that are frequently used to describe the functions of a pacing system are summarized in Table 24-10.[51] The first letter describes the chamber paced, the second describes the chamber sensed, and the third describes how the chamber responds to a paced or intrinsic event. AAI indicates that the pacemaker paces and senses in the atrium and inhibits when an intrinsic cardiac signal is sensed in the atrium. DDD indicates that the pacemaker paces and senses in the atrium and ventricle and that there are dual responses to sensed events (e.g., the system inhibits in response to sensed events in both chambers, but a sensed or paced event in the atrium triggers a paced event in the ventricle after a programmed delay). The code R denotes a rate adaptive feature. VVIR indicates that the pacemaker paces and senses in the ventricle, inhibits when an intrinsic cardiac signal is sensed in the ventricle, and has the ability to change the pacing rate within a programmed range, for example, 60 to 130 beats/min, based on the programmable rate sensor settings.

CHOICE OF PACING MODALITY

Atrially based pacing (AAI/R or DDD/R systems) has been shown to prevent the development of paroxysmal and permanent AF as compared with ventricular pacing systems.[52–54] In patients with sinus node dysfunction, atrially based pacing has been reported to reduce symptomatic heart failure in comparison with ventricular pacing.[54] Atrially based pacing optimizes cardiac hemodynamics by preserving the atrial contribution to cardiac output, which is particularly important in patients with heart failure and patients with diastolic dysfunction. However, atrially based pacing therapies have not been shown to be associated with substantial improvements in quality of life, exercise tolerance, or overall survival rate when compared with ventricular pacing in several large, prospective, randomized, clinical trials.[52–54] Thus, the choice of pacing modality should be individualized based on the patient's long-term prognosis, associated comorbidities, and expected functional status.

CARDIAC PACING ISSUES IN THE ICU

The pacing system consists of an implantable pulse generator, which contains the battery and integrated circuits that control pacing function, and one or more leads. The programming of a pacemaker is determined by the patient's underlying intrinsic rhythm. If the patient has only transient episodes of bradycardia, the pacemaker may be programmed to VVI at a low backup rate of 40 beats/min. If the patient has complete heart block, the pacemaker is usually programmed to a lower physiologic rate of 60 to 70 beats/min and an upper rate of 120 to 150 beats/min depending on age, type of heart disease, and activity level.

The most common problems related to a pacing system are capture failure, undersensing, oversensing, and triggered pacing. Capture failure may be due to pacing lead dislodgement, lead perforation, lead fracture, disconnection of the pacing lead from the power source, power source failure, or pacing thresholds higher than programmed. Pacing threshold may increase secondary to myocardial infarction, fibrosis, antiarrhythmic drug use, electrolyte abnormalities (hyperkalemia), and acidosis. Failure to sense may occur due to lead dislodgment or perforation, changes in intracardiac electrograms due to underlying disease state, electromagnetic interference causing reversion to asynchronous pacing, or spontaneous occurrence of a spontaneous ventricular event in the pacemaker blanking period. Oversensing may occur due to myopotential inhibition (more common with unipolar leads), sensing extraneous signals (usually due to lead insulation failure), or P- or T-wave oversensing. Triggered pacing may occur inappropriately when the patient with a dual-chamber pacemaker develops AF or atrial flutter or the pacemaker senses retrograde P waves causing pacemaker-mediated tachycardia. Most of these problems can be identified by interrogation and evaluation of the pacing system by using the pacemaker programmer. Many of these problems can be solved by reprogramming the pacemaker.[55]

Cardioversion and Defibrillation

Electrical shocks delivered transcutaneously, transvenously, or epicardially induce changes in the transmembrane potential of myocardial cells.[56] These stimuli may interrupt reentrant circuits by prolonging tissue refractoriness or by producing new excitation waves. Synchronized cardioversion effectively terminates most supraventricular tachyarrhythmias and monomorphically sustained VT. Biphasic waveforms have been incorporated into ICDs and the most recent generations of external defibrillators. These biphasic

FIGURE 24-8 Example of ventricular antitachycardia pacing (ATP) for ventricular tachycardia (VT). The *upper trace* is an intracardiac ventricular electrogram; the *middle trace* is the electrographic signal recorded from the intracardiac lead and the ICD can; and the *lower trace* indicates the marker channel annotations (how the device classifies each beat) and the interval between successive beats (in milliseconds).

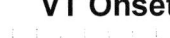

VT Onset

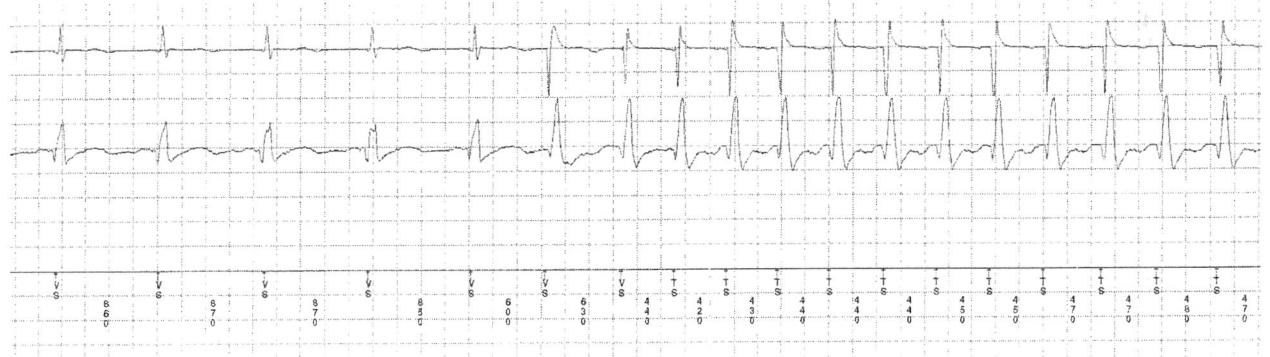

ATP Terminates VT

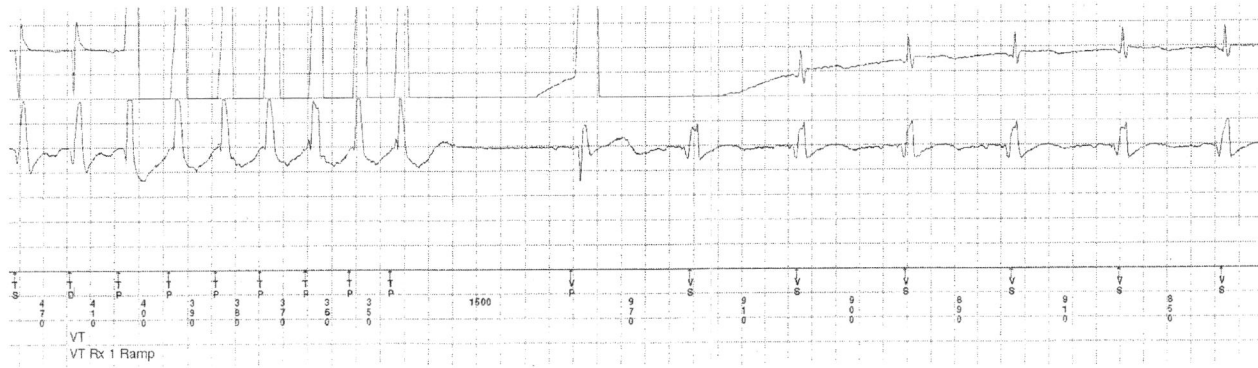

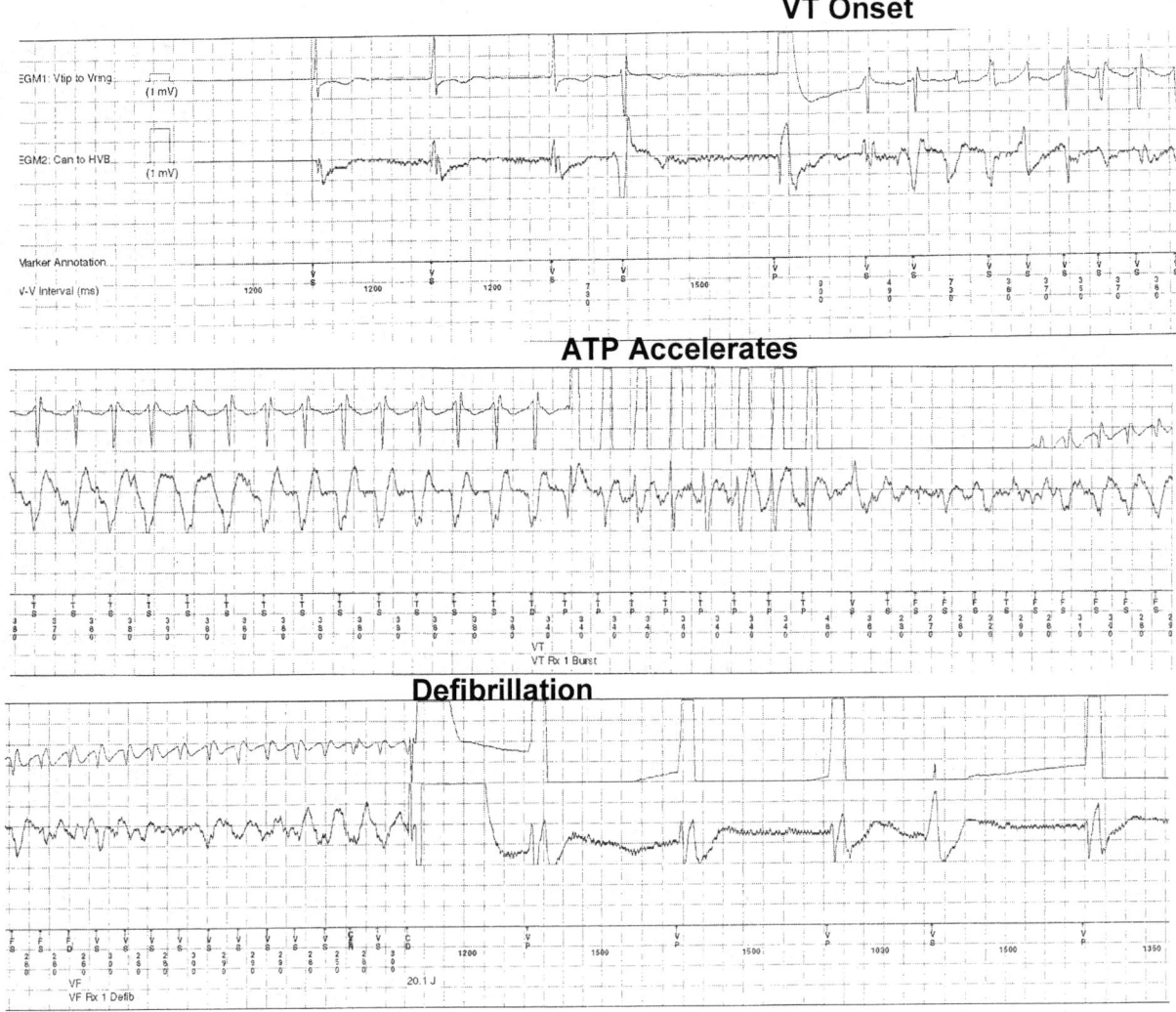

FIGURE 24-9 Example of ventricular antitachycardia pacing therapy that accelerates the ventricular tachycardia. A 20-J shock converts the arrhythmia to sinus rhythm. The format is similar to that shown in Fig. 24-8.

waveforms have been demonstrated to reduce cardioversion and defibrillation energy requirements.[57] If an electrical shock is not synchronized to the QRS complex, the shock may be delivered during the vulnerable repolarization phase and initiate VF. External pads rather than handheld paddles improve tissue contact, decrease overall system impedance, and reduce the energy required for cardioversion or defibrillation.

Implantable Cardioverter Defibrillators

Three major secondary prevention trials have demonstrated the superiority of the ICD over pharmacologic therapy for the prevention of sudden cardiac death in patients presenting with a life-threatening episode of VT or VF in the absence of a reversible cause.[31–33] In several clinical trials, the ICD also has been shown to prevent sudden cardiac death in patients with coronary heart disease and no history of spontaneous, sustained VT/VF.[29,30,58] As a consequence, more and more patients will receive ICDs, and knowledge of their functioning is important to the critical care physician.

ICD THERAPIES

ICDs provide antitachycardia pacing therapies for termination of sustained VT, internal cardioversion therapies for VT if pacing therapies are ineffective, and defibrillation therapies for VF and very rapid VT.[59] In addition, pacing therapy for bradycardia may be programmed. The ICD is usually programmed to back up VVI pacing at 40 beats/min unless the patient has significant bradycardia at baseline. VT detection is based on rate and sometimes on onset characteristics, regularity of rhythm, or duration of the intracardiac electrogram. An example of effective antitachycardia pacing therapy for sustained VT is shown in Fig. 24-8. Occasionally, the antitachycardia pacing therapy accelerates the VT to a more rapid VT or VF for which a shock is delivered (Fig. 24-9). One of the most frequent complications associated with the ICD is the delivery of an inappropriate shock for sinus tachycardia or a rapid atrial tachyarrhythmia. This can be minimized by programming a high tachycardia-detection interval (the rate that the device classifies as VT), programming a sudden rate onset feature to eliminate detection of sinus tachycardia that is rarely abrupt in onset, or programming a rate regularity feature to prevent AF being detected as VT. Newer ICDs may discriminate between VT and atrial tachyarrhythmias by using ventricular electrographic morphologic changes. Dual-chamber ICDs enhance discrimination of AF or SVT from VT by comparing atrial activity relations with ventricular activity.

ICD ISSUES IN THE ICU SETTING

Device malfunctions similar to those described in the section on cardiac pacing may occur in the ICD patient. If the patient experiences AF or atrial flutter or other SVT, this may be classified by the ICD as VT resulting in inappropriate ICD therapies. Transthoracic cardioversion or defibrillation in the region of, or over, an ICD or pacemaker may damage the electronic circuits. If performed, the device should be interrogated after the procedure to ensure that the device is functioning appropriately. If a patient is experiencing frequent incessant VT, cardioversion and defibrillation therapies may need to be programmed "off" until pharmacologic therapy has been initiated to suppress the frequency of episodes. If surgery is urgently required, precautions must be implemented to minimize the likelihood that electrocautery signals will be detected by the ICD.[60]

References

1. Vos MA, Lerman BB: Automaticity and triggered activity, in Spooner PM, Rosen MR (eds): *Foundations of Cardiac Arrhythmias: Basic Concepts and Clinical Approaches.* Basel, Switzerland, Marcel Dekker Inc, 2001, p 425.
2. Zipes DP: Mechanisms of clinical arrhythmias. *J Cardiovas Electrophysiol* 14:902, 2003.
3. Janse MJ, Dorinar E: Reentry, in Spooner PM and Rosen MR (eds): *Foundations of Cardiac arrhythmias: Basic Concepts and Clinical Approaches.* Basel, Switzerland, Marcel Dekker Inc, 2001, p 449.
4. Roden DM: Antiarrhythmic drugs: from mechanisms to clinical practice. *Heart* 84:339, 2000.
5. Members of the Sicilian Gambit: New approaches to antiarrhythmic therapy. Part 1. *Circulation* 104:2865, 2001.
6. Gillis AM: Class I antiarrhythmic drugs: Quinidine, procainamide, disopyramide, lidocaine, mexiletine, flecainide, propafenone, in Zipes D, Jalife J (eds): *Cardiac Electrophysiology: From Cell to Bedside,* 4th ed. Philadelphia, WB Saunders, 2004, p 911.
7. Singh B: Beta-blockers and calcium channel blockers as antiarrhythmic drugs, in Zipes DP, Jalife J (eds): *Cardiac Electrophysiology: From Cell to Bedside,* 3rd ed. Philadelphia, WB Saunders, 1995, p 1317.
8. Dorian P: Mechanisms of action of class III agents and their clinical relevance. *Europace* 1:C6, 2000.
9. Gillis AM: Proarrhythmia syndromes, in Saksena S, Camm AJ (eds): *Electrophysiological Disorders of the Heart,* 1st ed. Philadelphia, WB Saunders, in press.
10. Roden DM: Mechanisms and management of proarrhythmia. *Am J Cardiol* 82:491, 1998.
11. Roden DM: Antiarrhythmic drugs, in Hardman JG, Limberg LE (eds): *Goodman and Gilman's The Pharmacological Basis of Therapeutics,* 10th ed. New York, McGraw-Hill, 2001, p 933.
12. Wilkinson GR: Pharmacokinetics, in Hardman JG, Limberg LE (eds): *Goodman and Gilman's The Pharmacological Basis of Therapeutics,* 10th ed. New York, McGraw-Hill, 2001, p 3.
13. Wadworth AN, Murdoch D, Brogden RN: Atenolol. A reappraisal of its pharmacological properties and therapeutic use in cardiovascular disorders. *Drugs* 42:468, 1991.
14. McGavin JK, Keating GM: Bisoprolol: A review of its use in chronic heart failure. *Drugs* 62:2677, 2002.
15. Gillis AM, Wyse DG: Supraventricular tachycardia, in Gray JD (ed): *Therapeutic Choices,* 4th ed. Ottawa, Canada, Canadian Pharmacists Association, 2003, p 330.
16. Dorian P: Ventricular Tachyarrhythmias, in Gray JD (ed): *Therapeutic Choices,* 4th ed. Ottawa, Canada, Canadian Pharmacists Association, 2003, p 346.
17. Myerburg RJ: Scientific gaps in the prediction and prevention of sudden cardiac death. *J Cardiovasc Eelctrophysiol* 13:709, 2002.
18. Gillis AM, Hamilton RM, LeFeuvre CA: Unusual causes of sudden cardiac death due to ventricular tachyarrhythmias. *Can J Cardiol* 16:34C, 2000.
19. Connolly SJ, Krahn A, Klein G: Long term management of the survivor of ventricular fibrillation or sustained ventricular tachycardia. *Can J Cardiol* 16:20C, 2000.
20. Grogin HR, Scheinman MM: Evaluation and management of patients with polymorphic ventricular tachycardia. *Cardiol Clin* 11:39, 1993.
21. Priori SG, Napolitano C, Memmi M, et al: Clinical and molecular characterization of patients with catecholaminergic polymorphic ventricular tachycardia. *Circulation* 106:69, 2002.
22. Gillis AM: Intractable ventricular tachyarrhythmias: immediate evaluation and management, role of pharmacological therapy. *Card Electrophysiol Rev* 5:354, 2001.
23. The American Heart Association in collaboration with the International Liaison Committee on Resuscitation: Advanced cardiac life support. Section I: Introduction to ACLS 2000: Overview of recommended changes in ACLS from the Guidelines 2000 Conference. *Circulation* 102: I-86, 2000.
24. The American Heart Association in Collaboration with the International Liaison Committee on Resuscitation: The tachycardia algorithms. *Circulation* 102: I-158, 2000.
25. The American Heart Association in collaboration with the International Liaison Committee on Resuscitation: Pharmacology I: Agents for Arrhythmias. *Circulation* 102: I-112, 2000.
26. Nadamanee K, Taylor R, Bailey WE, et al: Treating electrical storm. Sympathetic blockade versus advanced cardiac life support–guided therapy. *Circulation* 102:742, 2000.
27. Credner SC, Klingenheben T, Mauss, et al: Electrical storm in patients with transvenous implantable cardioverter-defibrillators: incidence, management and prognostic implications. *J Am Coll Cardiol* 32:1909, 1998.
28. Kowey PR, Levin JH, Herre JM, et al, for the Intravenous Amiodarone Multicenter Investigators Group: Randomized, double-blind comparison of intravenous amiodarone and bretylium in the treatment of patients with recurrent, hemodynamically destabilizing ventricular tachycardia or fibrillation. *Circulation* 92:3266, 1995.
29. Buxton AE, Lee KL, Fisher JD, et al: A randomized study of the prevention of sudden death in patients with coronary artery disease. Multicenter Unsustained Tachycardia Trial Investigators. *N Engl J Med* 341:1882, 1999.
30. Moss AJ, Zareba W, Hall WJ, et al: Prophylactic implantation of a defibrillator in patients with myocardial infarction and reduced ejection fraction. *N Engl J Med* 346:877, 2002.
31. The Antiarrhythmics Versus Implantable Defibrillators (AVID) Investigators: A comparison of antiarrhythmic-drug therapy with implantable defibrillators in patients resuscitated from near-fatal ventricular arrhythmias. *N Engl J Med* 337:1576, 1997.
32. Connolly SJ, Gent M, Roberts RS, et al: Canadian implantable defibrillator study (CIDS): A randomized trial of the implantable cardioverter defibrillator against amiodarone. *Circulation* 101:1297, 2000.
33. Connolly SJ, Hallstrom AP, Cappato R, et al: Meta-analysis of the implantable cardioverter defibrillator secondary prevention trials. AVID, CASH and CIDS studies. Antiarrhythmics vs

Implantable Defibrillator study. Cardiac Arrest Study Hamburg. Canadian Implantable Defibrillator Study. *Eur Heart J* 21:2071, 2000.

34. Tzivoni D, Banai S, Schuger C, et al: Treatment of torsade de pointes with magnesium sulfate. *Circulation.* 77:392, 1988.

35. Viskin S: Cardiac pacing in the long QT syndrome: review of available data and practical recommendations. *J Cardiovasc Eelectrophysiol* 11:593, 2000.

36. Dorian P, Cass D, Schwartz B, et al: Amiodarone as compared with lidocaine for shock-resistant ventricular fibrillation. *N Engl J Med* 346:884, 2002.

37. Fuster V, Ryden LE, Asinger RW, et al: ACC/AHA/ESC guidelines for the management of patients with atrial fibrillation: Executive summary. A report of the American College of Cardiology/American Heart Association Task Force on Practice Guidelines and the European Society of Cardiology Committee for Practice Guidelines and Policy Conferences (Committee to Develop Guidelines for the Management of Patients With Atrial Fibrillation) developed in collaboration with the North American Society of Pacing and Electrophysiology. *Circulation* 104:2118, 2001.

38. Chauhan VS, Kran AD, Klein GJ, et al: Supraventricular tachycardia. *Med Clin North Am* 85:193, 2001.

39. Kochiadakis GE, Igoumenidis NE, Simantirakis EN, et al: Intravenous propafenone versus intravenous amiodarone in the management of atrial fibrillation of recent onset: a placebo-controlled study. *Pacing Clin Electrophysiol* 21:2475, 1998.

40. Wyse DG, Waldo AL, DiMarco JP, et al: A comparison of rate control and rhythm control in patients with atrial fibrillation. *N Engl J Med* 347:1825, 2002.

41. Van Gelder IC, Hagens VE, Bosker HA, et al: A comparison of rate control and rhythm control in patients with recurrent persistent atrial fibrillation. *N Engl J Med* 347:1834, 2002.

42. Newman D, Gillis AM, Gilbert M, Dorian P: Chronic drug therapy to prevent the recurrence of atrial fibrillation. Canadian Cardiovascular Society Consensus Conference Report. *Can J Cardiol* 12:24A, 1996.

43. The Cardiac Arrhythmia Suppression Trial Investigators: Preliminary report: Effect of encainide and flecainide on mortality in a randomized trial of arrhythmia suppression after myocardial infarction. *N Eng J Med* 321:406, 1989.

44. Waldo AL, Camm AJ, deRuyter H, et al: Effect of d-sotalol on mortality in patients with left ventricular dysfunction after recent and remote myocardial infarction. The SWORD Investigators. Survival with oral d-sotalol. *Lancet* 348:7, 1996.

45. Cosio FG: Atrial flutter update. *Cardiol Electrophysiol Rev* 6:356, 2002.

46. Weerasooriya R, Shah DC, Hocini, et al: Ablation therapy for atrial fibrillation (AF): Past, present and future. *Cardiovasc Res* 54:337, 2002.

47. Wood MA, Brown-Mahoney C, Kay GN, Ellenbogen KA: Clinical outcomes after ablation and pacing therapy for atrial fibrillation: A meta-analysis, *Circulation* 101:1138, 2000.

48. Hart RG, Benavente O, McBride R, Pearce LA: Antithrombotic therapy to prevent stroke in patients with atrial fibrillation: a meta-analysis. *Ann Intern Med* 131:492, 1999.

49. Yee R, Connolly S, Noorani H: Clinical review of radiofrequency catheter ablation for cardiac arrhythmias. *Can J Cardiol* 19:1273, 2003.

50. Gregoratos G, Abrams J, Epstein AE, et al: ACC/AHA/NASPE 2002 guideline update for implantation of cardiac pacemakers and antiarrhythmia devices: Summary article. A report of the American College of Cardiology/American Heart Association Task Force on Practice Guidelines (ACC/AHA/NASPE Committee to Update the 1998 Pacemaker Guidelines). *J Cardiovasc Electrophysiol* 13:1183, 2002.

51. Bernstein AD, Daubert JC, Fletcher RD, et al: The revised NASPE/BPEG generic code for antibradycardia, adaptive-rate, and multisite pacing. North American Society of Pacing and Electrophysiology/British Pacing and Electrophysiology Group. *Pacing Clin Electrophysiol* 25:260, 2002.

52. Gillis AM, Kerr CR: Whither physiologic pacing? Implications of CTOPP. *PACE* 23:8:1193, 2000.

53. Connolly SJ, Kerr CR, Gent M, et al, for the CTOPP Investigators: Effects of physiologic pacing versus ventricular pacing on the risk of stroke and death due to cardiovascular causes. *N Engl J Med* 342:1385, 2000.

54. Lamas GA, Lee K, Sweeney M, et al: The mode selection trial (MOST) in sinus node dysfunction: design, rationale, and baseline characteristics of the first 1000 patients. *Am Heart J* 140:541, 2000.

55. Fraser JD, Gillis, AM, Irwin ME, et al, for the Canadian Working Group on Cardiac Pacing: Guidelines for pacemaker follow-up in Canada: A consensus statement of the Canadian Working Group on Cardiac Pacing. *Can J Cardiol* 16:355, 2000.

56. Gillis AM, Fast VG, Rohr S, et al: Spatial changes in transmembrane potential during extracellular electrical shocks in cultured monolayers of neonatal rat ventricular myocytes. *Circ Res* 79:676, 1996.

57. Bardy GH, Marchlinski FE, Sharma AD, et al: Multicenter comparison of truncated biphasic shocks and standard damped sine wave monophasic shocks for transthoracic ventricular defibrillation. Transthoracic Investigators. *Circulation* 15:2507, 1996.

58. Moss AJ, Hall WJ, Cannom DS, et al: Improved survival with an implanted deibrillator in patients with coronary disease at high risk for ventricular arrhythmia. Multicenter Automatic Defibrilltor Implantation Trial Investigators. *N Engl J Med* 335:1933, 1996.

59. Swygman C, Wang PJ, Link MS, et al: Advances in implantable cardioverter defibrillators. *Curr Opin Cardiol* 17:24, 2002.

60. Gillis AM, Philippon F, Cassidy MR, et al, for the Canadian Working Group on Cardiac Pacing: Guidelines for ICD follow-up in Canada: A consensus statement of the Canadian Working Group on Cardiac Pacing. *Can J Cardiol* 19:21, 2003.

Chapter 25 _____

MYOCARDIAL ISCHEMIA

STEVEN M. HOLLENBERG
JOSEPH E. PARRILLO

KEY POINTS

- *Myocardial ischemia results from an imbalance between myocardial oxygen demand and supply.*
- *The major determinants of myocardial oxygen requirements are heart rate, contractility, and wall stress (afterload).*
- *Patients with myocardial ischemia are categorized by presentation with or without ST elevation, in accordance with treatment strategies. Patients with ST elevation benefit from immediate reperfusion with thrombolytic agents or direct angioplasty.*
- *All patients with suspected myocardial ischemia should be given aspirin at presentation.*
- *Myocardial infarction is diagnosed by a compatible clinical history, evolution of characteristic electrocardiographic changes, and an increase and subsequent decrease in cardiac enzymes.*
- *Acute reperfusion of the occluded coronary artery is the key to achieving a good outcome. The promptness of reperfusion is more important than the mode by which it is accomplished.*
- *Prognosis after myocardial infarction is most closely related to the degree of left ventricular impairment.*
- *Risk stratification is the key to initial management of patients with non–ST-elevation acute coronary syndromes.*
- *In patients with high-risk non–ST-elevation acute coronary syndromes, use of low-molecular-weight heparin, glycoprotein IIb/IIIa inhibition, and an early invasive approach is preferred.*
- *Aspirin, β blockers, angiotensin-converting enzyme inhibitors, and statins have been shown to decrease mortality rate after myocardial infarction.*
- *Echocardiography is extremely useful for the diagnosis of complications after myocardial infarction.*
- *Patients with cardiogenic shock should be stabilized with an intra-aortic balloon pump and promptly revascularized, if possible, by angioplasty or bypass surgery.*

Myocardial ischemia can go unrecognized in an intensive care unit (ICU). Signs of myocardial ischemia may be obscured by other illnesses in the critically ill patient. Physical examination in these patients often is limited, or its results altered, by the presence of other disease processes.

Myocardial ischemia and attendant left ventricular dysfunction may complicate the course and treatment of a particular illness. Conversely, multisystem illness may set the conditions for increased oxygen demand, often accompanied by diminished delivery of oxygen to the heart. For these reasons, the critical care physician must maintain a high index of suspicion for myocardial ischemia in the ICU setting, especially in the patient with a history of or multiple risk factors for coronary artery disease (CAD).

Terminology

Myocardial ischemia results from an imbalance of oxygen supply and oxygen demand. The heart is an aerobic organ with only a limited capacity for anaerobic glycolysis, and it makes use of oxygen avidly and efficiently, extracting 70% to 80% of the oxygen from coronary arterial blood.[1] Because the heart extracts oxygen nearly maximally, independent of demand, increases in demand must be met by commensurate increases in coronary blood flow.

Classically, myocardial ischemia has been divided into categories such as stable angina, unstable angina, and myocardial infarction (MI). Typical angina is exertional and is relieved promptly by rest or nitroglycerin. Stable angina occurs reproducibly with a similar level of exertion, in a pattern that is unchanged over the previous 6 months. Acute coronary syndromes comprise unstable angina and MI. Unstable angina consists of ischemic symptoms that are more frequent, severe, or prolonged than the patient's usual angina, are more difficult to control with drugs, or are occurring at rest or with minimal exertion. Cardiac biomarkers are not elevated. MI has been classified as "transmural" and "nontransmural," but this division has been largely abandoned due to the recognition that electrocardiographic (ECG) criteria are neither sensitive nor specific enough to make this distinction.

Acute coronary syndromes have traditionally been classified into Q-wave MI, non–Q-wave MI, and unstable angina. More recently, classification has shifted and has become based on the initial electrocardiogram: patients are categorized into three groups: those with ST-elevation MI (STEMI), those without ST elevation but with enzyme evidence of myocardial damage (non–ST-elevation MI, or NSTEMI), and those with unstable angina. Classification according to the presenting electrocardiogram coincides with current treatment strategies because patients presenting with ST elevation benefit from immediate reperfusion and should be treated with thrombolytic therapy or urgent revascularization, whereas fibrinolytic agents are not effective in other patients with acute coronary syndromes. The discussion of MI in this chapter follows this schematization.

Pathophysiology

Myocardial ischemia results from an imbalance between oxygen supply and demand. The myocardial requirement for oxygen and, hence, for oxygenated blood is affected by three major variables: heart rate, myocardial wall stress, and contractility. Myocardial wall stress is a function of the radius and the transmural ventricular pressure, which is highly dependent on ventricular afterload (Fig. 25-1).

Coronary blood flow depends on coronary perfusion pressure and filling time. Because coronary perfusion occurs primarily in diastole, the relevant pressure gradient is aortic diastolic pressure minus left ventricular diastolic pressure. Filling time is directly related to heart rate.

Myocardial ischemia usually develops in the setting of an obstructive atherosclerotic left ventricle, which limits blood supply. The pathophysiology of unstable coronary syndromes and MI usually involves dynamic partial or complete occlusion of an epicardial coronary artery because of acute intracoronary thrombus formation.[2]

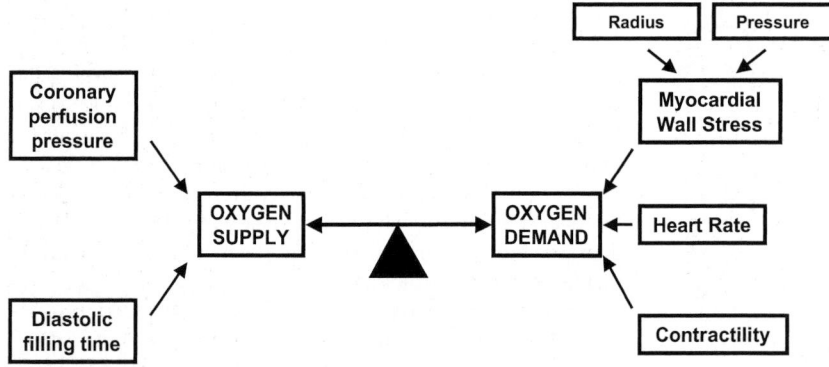

FIGURE 25-1 Determinants of myocardial oxygen supply and demand.

Different factors in critically ill patients can increase myocardial oxygen demand, including tachycardia, hypertension, and increased catecholamines. Similarly, many factors may contribute to limitation of oxygen supply, particularly in the setting of hemodynamic instability. These factors include hypotension (decreasing coronary perfusion pressure) and tachycardia (limiting diastolic filling time). In addition, anemia and hypoxemia can limit the amount of oxygen delivered to the heart. Coronary vasospasm may also play a role in some patients. Elevation of left ventricular pressures by heart failure can increase demand and decrease coronary perfusion pressure.

Thus, critically ill patients, usually those with at least some component of obstructive coronary artery disease, may develop myocardial ischemia on a hemodynamic basis, with variable contributions of increased demand and decreased supply. On the other hand, catecholamine surges, hemodynamic changes, and inflammatory processes may predispose to rupture of preexisting atherosclerotic plaques. Making the distinction is vital because the treatment is completely different. In the former case, treatment is aimed at decreasing the oxygen requirement of the myocardium by eliminating provocative stimuli and controlling heart rate and blood pressure and on optimizing oxygenation and hemoglobin concentration. Relief of myocardial ischemia by these measures usually results in prompt restoration of left ventricular function without significant cellular damage because the obstruction to flow is ordinarily fixed and not total. If plaque rupture is playing a role, then simply removing or lessening stimuli that increase myocardial oxygen requirements may not be sufficient to increase the ratio of myocardial oxygen supply to demand, and, unless attempts are made to reestablish coronary blood flow, significant myocardial damage may ensue. Antithrombotic and anticoagulant strategies should be instituted, and consideration of coronary revascularization may be indicated.

RECOGNITION OF MYOCARDIAL ISCHEMIA

SIGNS AND SYMPTOMS

Myocardial ischemia is most commonly manifested as constant substernal chest tightness or pressure. The pain typically is on the left side and may radiate to the throat and jaw or to the left shoulder and left arm and is often accompanied by acute onset of dyspnea and diaphoresis. Angina occasionally may be right-sided, interscapular, or perceived in the epigastrium.

Because other syndromes may mimic angina, it is important to consider them in the differential diagnosis. These include dissecting aortic aneurysm; pericarditis; pleuritis; pulmonary processes such as pulmonary embolism, pneumonia, and pneumothorax; gastrointestinal processes such as esophageal or peptic ulcer disease and cholecystitis; musculoskeletal pain; and costochondritis. Other heart diseases (valvular heart disease, cardiomyopathies, and myocarditis) not attributable to coronary artery stenosis may also cause substernal chest tightness and should be included in the differential diagnosis. The presentation of ischemia in postsurgical patients may be subtle. Aftereffects of surgery and medication can mimic or mask the classic features of MI such as substernal chest pain radiating to the arm, neck, or jaw, and dyspnea, nausea, and diaphoresis. The vigilant clinician must therefore maintain a high index of suspicion and a low threshold for obtaining a 12-lead electrocardiogram.

The physical examination, although sometimes insensitive and nonspecific, especially in the patient with multisystem illness or preexisting left ventricular dysfunction, may be helpful in confirming the diagnosis. Elevated jugular veins signal right ventricular diastolic pressure elevation, and the appearance of pulmonary crackles (in the absence of pulmonary disease) indicates elevated left ventricular filling pressures secondary to depressed left ventricular function. A systolic bulge occasionally can be palpated on the precordium in the area of the apex of the heart, representing contact of an ischemic dyskinetic segment of the left ventricle with the chest wall. During the ischemic episode, auscultation of the precordium may demonstrate the presence of a fourth heart sound, indicative of a noncompliant left ventricle. With extensive myocardial dysfunction, a third heart sound may be present. A murmur of mitral regurgitation attributable to papillary muscle dysfunction may also emerge.

THE ELECTROCARDIOGRAM

The ECG abnormalities in myocardial ischemia vary widely and depend in large part on the extent and nature of coronary stenosis and the presence of collateral blood flow to ischemic zones. With acute total occlusion of a coronary artery, the first demonstrable ECG changes are peaked T-wave changes in the leads reflecting the anatomic area of myocardium in jeopardy. As total occlusion continues, there is elevation of the ST segments in the same leads. With continued occlusion, there is an evolution of ECG abnormalities, with biphasic and then inverted T waves. If enough myocardium is infarcted, q waves may appear, representing unopposed initial depolarization forces away from the mass of infarcted myocardium, which has lost electrical activity and no longer contributes to the mean QRS voltage vector. The formation of q waves is accompanied by a decrease in the magnitude of the R waves in the same leads, representing diminution of voltage in the mass of infarcted myocardium. Loss of R-wave voltage, visualized by comparison with previous ECG tracings, may be the only ECG evidence for the presence of permanent myocardial damage. It is important to note that QRS voltage can be affected by multiple factors, such as lead placement, body position, QRS axis shifts, and pericardial and thoracic abnormalities that may shield the electrical activity of the heart. These conditions are frequently encountered in patients in the ICU and should be taken into consideration in interpretation of q and R waves.

Extension of an inferior MI to the posterior segment can be detected by enhancement of R waves in the anterior chest leads because these forces are now less opposed by posterior forces. True posterior infarction can be subtle because the only signs may be prominent R waves, tall upright T waves, and depressed ST segments in leads V_1 and V_2. Involvement of the right ventricle in inferior MI also is not readily detected on the standard 12-lead electrocardiogram because of the small mass of the right ventricle relative to the left ventricle and because of the positioning of the standard precordial leads away from the right ventricle. Right ventricular infarction may be detected by ST elevation in recordings from right precordial leads, in particular V_{4R}.[3]

Subtotal occlusion of an epicardial coronary artery may not result in ST elevation but in T-wave changes or ST depression in the leads reflecting the involved myocardium. These findings are less specific than ST elevation for myocardial ischemia because they may also be caused by a myriad of factors other than ischemia, including cardioactive drugs, in particular digoxin, and electrolyte disorders, in particular hypokalemia. Left ventricular hypertrophy and acute left ventricular pressure overload, as might occur in hypertensive crisis, may also result in ST depression—the so-called strain pattern. Supraventricular tachycardias have also been shown to cause ST depression, even in the absence of left ventricular pressure. In the presence of preexisting T-wave abnormalities, ST-segment or T-wave changes are even less specific for ischemia. Ischemia may also be indicated by previously flattened or inverted T waves that revert to upright—the so-called pseudonormalization of T waves.

The clinician also must be careful not to be fooled by ECG "imposters" of acute infarction, which include pericarditis, J-point elevation, Wolff-Parkinson-White syndrome, and hypertrophic cardiomyopathy. In pericarditis, ST segments may be elevated, but the elevation is diffuse and the morphology of the ST segments tends to be concave upward, whereas that of ischemia is convex. Pericarditis also may be distinguished from infarction by the presence of PR-segment depression in the inferior leads (and also by the PR segment in lead aVR).[4]

SILENT ISCHEMIA

Recent interest has focused on "silent" myocardial ischemia, that is, objective ECG evidence of myocardial ischemia that is not associated with angina or with anginal equivalents.[5] Silent myocardial ischemia may be an incidental observation on a cardiac monitor or on a routine electrocardiogram and consists of transient ST-segment depression that may last several minutes or even hours. The frequency of episodes of ST-segment depression correlates with the severity of coronary artery disease in patients with known left ventricular pressure or a history of angina.

Decreased left ventricular function is associated with episodes of silent ST depression.[6,7] In patients monitored with pulmonary artery catheters (PACs), silent ischemia may be manifested by increased pulmonary artery occlusion pressures, reflecting increased left ventricular end-diastolic pressure. Echocardiography may demonstrate transient wall motion abnormalities and diminished diastolic compliance. These signs of left ventricular dysfunction may precede ST-segment changes.[6,7]

Not all episodes of transient ST-segment depression are attributable to silent ischemia. Nevertheless, should this finding be observed on the cardiac monitor, especially in association with transient elevation of left ventricular filling pressures, it is prudent to consider the possibility of myocardial ischemia as a potential factor complicating the course of the critically ill patient.

CARDIAC BIOMARKERS

Measurement of enzymes released into the serum from necrotic myocardial cells after infarction can aid in the diagnosis of MI.[8,9] The classic biochemical marker of acute MI is elevation of creatine phosphokinase (CPK) levels. The CPK-MB isoenzyme is found primarily in cardiac muscle, and only small amounts are present in skeletal muscle and brain. CK released from the myocardium begins to appear in the plasma 4 to 8 hours after onset of infarction, and its level peaks at 12 to 24 hours and returns to baseline at 2 to 4 days. The magnitude of the increase in serum CK level and the rate at which it rises and falls are a function of the total mass of myocardium affected, the extent and nature of coronary occlusion (e.g., total or subtotal occlusion), the rate of washout from the infarcted myocardium, and the clearance from the body. To be diagnostic for MI, the total plasma CK value must exceed the upper limit of normal, and the fraction consisting of the MB isoenzyme must exceed a certain value (which depends on the CK-MB assay used, usually >5%).

A newer serologic test for the detection of myocardial damage uses measurement of cardiac troponins.[10] Troponins T and I are constituents of the contractile protein apparatus of cardiac muscle. Whereas CPK-MB may arise from other tissues, troponins originate only from cardiac muscle, rendering them more specific than the conventional CPK-MB assays for the detection of myocardial damage. Their use is becoming more widespread and has superseded the use of CPK-MB in many settings.[11] Troponins are also more sensitive for the detection of myocardial damage, and troponin elevation in patients without ST elevation (or without elevation of CPK-MB) identifies a subpopulation at increased risk for complications. Rapid point-of-care troponin assays, which have become available in the past few years, have extended the clinical utility of this marker. Troponins may not be elevated until 6 hours after an acute event, so critical therapeutic interventions should not be delayed pending assay results. Once elevated, troponin levels can remain high for days to weeks, thereby limiting their utility to detect late reinfarction.

Lactate dehydrogenase (LDH) is also released from necrotic myocardial tissue after infarction, although elevation of this enzyme is relatively nonspecific for MI because LDH is present in many other tissues. LDH levels peak at 72 to 96 hours and may be used to detect recent infarction, which is associated with an increase in the LDH_1 isoenzyme.

ECHOCARDIOGRAPHY

To the physician confronted with a critically ill patient, echocardiography can be a key element in successful differential diagnosis.[12] Echocardiography is simple, safe, and permits systemic interrogation of cardiac chamber size, left and right ventricular functions, valvular structure and motion, atrial size, and the anatomy of the pericardial space. The presence of segmental left ventricular wall motion abnormalities suggests compromise of blood flow to those segments.[13] Doppler interrogation can be used for noninvasive assessment of right and left ventricular filling pressures, pulmonary artery pressures, stroke volume, and cardiac output.

Echocardiography is particularly useful in the evaluation of patients with acute heart failure or suspected cardiogenic shock, and early echocardiography should be performed routinely.[14] Expeditious evaluation of global and regional left ventricular performance is crucial for management of congestive heart failure, with or without suspected myocardial ischemia.

Echocardiography is also extremely valuable for the rapid diagnosis of mechanical causes of shock after MI such as papillary muscle rupture and acute mitral regurgitation, acute ventricular septal defect, and free wall rupture and tamponade.[14] In some cases, echocardiography may demonstrate findings compatible with right ventricular infarction. Echocardiography can also show alternative diagnoses, such as valvular abnormalities, pericardial tamponade, or hypertrophic cardiomyopathy. Acute right heart failure, manifested by a dilated and hypokinetic right ventricle without hypertrophy suggestive of chronic pulmonary hypertension, can suggest pulmonary embolism (see Chap. 26).[15]

Transthoracic echocardiographic images may be suboptimal due to a poor acoustic window in critically ill patients, in particular those who are obese, have chronic lung disease, or are on positive pressure ventilation. Contrast echocardiography may be used to improve image quality.[16] Transesophageal echocardiography also can provide better visualization, particularly of valvular structures, and can be performed safely at the bedside.

RADIONUCLIDE STUDIES

Technetium pyrophosphate is deposited in irreversibly damaged regions of myocardium.[17] The regions of radioactivity are detected by scintigraphy and appear as "hot spots" on imaging. The period during which technetium pyrophosphate scanning is most sensitive for the detection of infarcted myocardium is approximately 1 to 3 days after MI; if a scan performed then is positive, scans may remain positive for weeks to months thereafter. Whereas the sensitivity and specificity for detection of a transmural infarct are high with this technique, they are low to moderate for a non–Q-wave or subendocardial infarct. Therefore, the usefulness of this test is limited for the diagnosis of MIs, especially non–Q-wave infarcts, because it offers little information unavailable by other means.[18]

Thallium 201 is transported into viable myocardial tissue by processes dependent on adenosine triphosphate via Na/K-ATPase. It is distributed to the myocardium on the basis of blood flow. Necrotic or scarred myocardial tissue from a new or previous MI will appear as a "cold spot" on scintigraphy. Technetium 99 sestamibi is a newer isotope preparation widely used to assess myocardial perfusion. Sestamibi also distributes to the myocardium on the basis of blood flow. The major advantage of using sestamibi instead of thallium is that the photons produced by the technetium 99 radionuclide have higher energy and therefore more readily penetrate the fat and other tissues that overlie the heart, resulting in fewer attenuation artifacts than seen with thallium 201. In addition, unlike thallium, sestamibi does not undergo significant redistribution, so perfusion defects seen on scintigraphic images do not reverse over time. Sestamibi scans at rest can be used in patients presenting to the emergency department with chest pain of unclear cause. Patients without perfusion defects do not have evidence of ongoing myocardial underperfusion and can be safely discharged, with follow-up stress testing as needed.[19] A positive scan does not differentiate between new and old perfusion defects, so hospital admission and further evaluation are necessary.

HEMODYNAMIC MONITORING

In patients with hemodynamic instability that does not improve relatively quickly with simple therapeutic maneuvers, pulmonary artery catheterization should be considered (see Chap. 13). Pulmonary artery catheterization provides simultaneous assessment of filling pressures and cardiac output and can be quite useful for differential diagnosis in critically ill patients. In patients with hypoxemia and pulmonary infiltrates on chest radiogram, a frequent dilemma in ICU patients, pulmonary artery catheterization may be used to differentiate cardiac from pulmonary causes. Right heart catheterization is also quite useful in the differential diagnosis of shock. Hemodynamic profiles of patients with different forms of shock are presented in Table 25-1. It is important to recognize the possibility of mixed forms of shock in the critically ill patient (see Chap. 21). For example, even in the presence of significant left ventricular dysfunction and suspected cardiogenic shock, patients with cardiogenic shock can be relatively depleted of volume, perhaps due to diaphoresis or vomiting.[20,21]

Hemodynamic monitoring also can be useful in the diagnosis of mechanical complications of infarction. Right heart catheterization may show a step up in hemoglobin oxygen saturation diagnostic of ventricular septal rupture. The waveform of the pulmonary artery occlusion pressure tracing may show a prominent V wave (10 mm Hg above the mean pulmonary artery occlusion pressure is regarded as significant), suggesting severe mitral regurgitation, although V waves also may be present in acute ventricular septal rupture. Equalization of diastolic filling pressures may suggest pericardial tamponade. The hemodynamic profile of right ventricular infarction includes high right-side filling pressures in the presence of normal or low occlusion pressures.[22]

Perhaps more importantly, pulmonary artery catheterization may be used to guide therapy in hemodynamically unstable patients. Infusions of vasoactive agents need to be titrated carefully in patients with myocardial ischemia to maximize coronary perfusion pressure with the least possible increase in myocardial oxygen demand. Invasive hemodynamic monitoring is often considered useful in guiding therapy in these unstable patients because clinical estimates of filling pressure can be unreliable;[23] in addition, changes in myocardial performance and compliance and therapeutic interventions can

TABLE 25-1 Use of Right Heart Catheterization to Diagnose the Etiology of Shock

Diagnosis	PAOP	$\dot{Q}_T$	SVR	Miscellaneous Comments
Cardiogenic shock				
Cardiogenic shock due to myocardial dysfunction	↑↑	↓↓	↑↑	Usually extensive infarction (>40% of left ventricle), severe cardiomyopathy, or myocarditis
Cardiogenic shock due to mechanical defects				
Acute ventricular septal defect	↑	↓↓	↑↑	Oxygen "step-up" at RV level
Acute mitral regurgitation	↑↑	Forward $\dot{Q}_T$ ↓↓	↑	V waves in Paop tracing
RV infarction	Normal or ↓	↓↓	↑↑	Elevated RA and RV filling pressures with low or normal Paop
Extracardiac obstructive forms of shock				
Pericardial tamponade	↑	↓ Or ↓↓	↑↑	RA mean, RV end-distolic pulmonary capillary wedge mean pressures are elevated and within 5 mm Hg of one another
Massive pulmonary embolism	Normal or ↓	↓↓	↑↑	Usual finding is elevated right-side pressures
Hypovolemic shock	↓↓	↓↓	↑↑	
Distributive forms of shock				
Septic shock	↓ Or normal	↑ Or normal, rarely ↓	↓↓	
Anaphylactic shock	↓ Or normal	↑ Or normal	↓↓	

ABBREVIATIONS: ↑↑ or ↓↓, moderate to severe increase or decrease; ↑ or ↓, mild to moderate increase or decrease; $\dot{Q}_T$, cardiac output; PAOP, pulmonary artery occlusion pressure; RA, right atrial; RV, right ventricular; SVR, systemic vascular resistance.

change cardiac output and filling pressures precipitously. Optimization of filling pressures and serial measurements of cardiac output (and other parameters such as mixed venous oxygen saturation) allow for titration of the dosage of inotropic agents and vasopressors to the minimum dosage required to achieve the chosen therapeutic goals. This minimizes the increases in myocardial oxygen demand and arrhythmogenic potential.[24]

The PAC provides hemodynamic data not easily inferred from physical examination or laboratory evaluation, but whether its use translates into definable benefits for patients has long been questioned.[25] Despite the many theoretical advantages to the PAC, retrospective analyses in patients with acute myocardial ischemia have found no benefit,[26] and some have found associations between catheter use and adverse outcomes. Prospective trials have shown PAC to be practical in high-risk surgical patients and in patients with septic shock and acute respiratory distress syndrome; such a trial would be interesting in patients with cardiac ischemia. Lacking prospective trials to answer the question of efficacy, we nevertheless believe the benefits of more rapid diagnosis are clear and find the catheter essential to guide supportive therapy.[21] Prudence should be exercised in choosing a site for central venipuncture because many will have received or are candidates for thrombolytic and intravenous heparin therapy. Insertion sites that can be compressed easily should significant bleeding occur are preferred.

MANAGEMENT OF ANGINA

Patients with a history of stable angina who develop chest pain while in the critical care setting are best treated by removal of provocative stimuli that increase myocardial oxygen consumption or lead to compromised coronary blood flow, if these factors can be identified. For example, correction of hypoxia, anemia, hypovolemia, tachycardia, or labile hypertension may be sufficient to control anginal episodes. Often overlooked are fever, infection, anxiety, stress, activity, and the work of breathing. Antianginal medications the patient was receiving before hospitalization should be continued, and the doses may have to be increased.

In instances of refractory angina or when provocative stimuli cannot be ameliorated, it may be necessary to perform coronary angiography and revascularization of the culprit vessels (preferably percutaneously), especially if the myocardial ischemia is complicating further management of the patient.

ASPIRIN

Aspirin is the best known and most widely used of the antiplatelet agents because of its low cost and relatively low toxicity. Use of salicylates to treat coronary artery disease in the United States was first reported in 1953.[27] Aspirin inhibits the production of thromboxane A_2 by irreversibly acetylating the serine residue of the enzyme prostaglandin H_2 synthetase.

Reduction of death or nonfatal MI in patients with unstable angina and NSTEMI has been well established in several large randomized clinical trials.[28,29] In addition to its use in acute clinical settings, aspirin has been shown to be beneficial in preventing cardiovascular events when administered as secondary prevention in patients after acute MI and as primary prevention in subjects with no prior history of vascular disease.[30]

The most widely used and effective dose of aspirin in cardiovascular disease is 81 to 325 mg/d. Despite the fact that small-dose aspirin preferentially blocks the conversion of thromboxane to prostacyclin and thus has a more profound antiplatelet effect, large-dose aspirin has been found to be as effective as small-dose aspirin in prevention of cardiovascular death, MI and stroke,[31] which suggests that anti-inflammatory effects of aspirin also play a role.[32] Once begun, aspirin likely should be continued indefinitely. Toxicity with aspirin is mostly gastrointestinal; enteric-coated preparations may minimize these side effects.

NITRATES

Nitroglycerin is a mainstay of therapy for angina because of its efficacy and rapid onset of action. The most important antianginal effect of nitroglycerin is preferential dilation of venous capacitance vessels. Myocardial oxygen consumption is reduced as left ventricular volume and arterial pressure decrease.[33] At larger doses, nitroglycerin also may relax arterial smooth muscle, causing a modest decrease in afterload.[33] In addition, nitroglycerin can dilate epicardial coronary arteries and redistribute coronary blood flow to ischemic regions by dilating collateral vessels. Nitroglycerin also has antithrombotic and antiplatelet effects.

The quickest route of administration of nitroglycerin is sublingual. Sublingual doses of 0.4 mg may be administered every 5 to 10 minutes to a total of three doses, if required to control pain. Topical or oral nitrates may be used for long-term therapy.

In patients with unstable angina, if sublingual nitroglycerin does not cause chest pain to resolve completely, intravenous nitroglycerin should be administered, starting at a dose of 10 to 20 $\mu g/min$. This dose may be titrated upward as tolerated in increments of 10 to 20 $\mu g/min$ every 5 to 10 minutes until pain resolves. An upper limit of 400 $\mu g/min$ is usually accepted as maximal; above this dose, usually there is no further clinical response. Excessive lowering of blood pressure can compromise perfusion of the coronary vascular bed.

Because of its hemodynamic actions, systemic blood pressure may fall after nitroglycerin administration, so frequent blood pressure checks are required. Hypotension typically responds to the Trendelenburg-position and to fluid boluses.

β BLOCKERS

The rationale for administering β blockers during ischemic episodes derives from their negative chronotropic and inotropic properties. Heart rate and contractility are two of the three major determinants of myocardial oxygen consumption. By altering these variables, myocardial ischemia can be attenuated significantly.[34] These agents are particularly effective in patients with angina who remain tachycardic or hypertensive (or both) and in patients with supraventricular tachycardia complicating myocardial ischemia. Rapid control can be achieved by intravenous administration of metoprolol, a β_1-selective blocker, in 5-mg increments every 5 minutes up to 15 mg. Thereafter, 25 to 50 mg every 6 hours can be given orally.

Beta blockers should be used with caution in patients with marginal blood pressure, preexisting bradycardia, atrioventricular nodal conduction disturbances, or evidence for left ventricular failure and in those with bronchospastic disease. A short-acting intravenous β blocker, such as esmolol, may be the preferred agent in patients who have the potential for hemodynamic instability or who have relative contraindications.

CALCIUM CHANNEL BLOCKERS

Nondihydropyridine calcium channel blockers (verapamil and diltiazem) also have negative chronotropic and inotropic effects and can be used to control myocardial oxygen demand in patients with ischemia. Both can be given as intravenous boluses, starting with small doses (diltiazem 10 to 20 mg, verapamil 2.5 mg), and then infused continuously.

Calcium channel blockers are particularly useful in the setting of coronary vasospasm because they cause direct dilation of coronary vascular smooth muscle. Vasospasm can produce variant angina in patients with mild or no coronary artery disease (Prinzmetal's angina) or aggravate ischemia in patients with atherosclerotic coronary stenoses that are subcritical but serve as sites of vasospasm, possibly as a consequence of abnormalities of the underlying smooth muscle or derangements in endothelial physiology.[35] The illicit use of cocaine is increasingly being recognized as a cause of coronary vasospasm leading to angina and myocardial ischemia. Coronary vasospasm usually presents with ST elevation associated with chest pain and can be difficult to differentiate from vessel closure due to coronary thrombosis. Consideration of the clinical setting, rapid fluctuation of ST segments, and prompt resolution with nitrates can provide useful clues. Variant angina attributable to vasospasm responds well to treatment with calcium channel blockers.

ANGIOTENSIN-CONVERTING ENZYME INHIBITORS

Angiotensin-converting enzyme (ACE) generates angiotensin II from angiotensin I and catalyzes the breakdown of bradykinin. Thus ACE inhibitors can decrease circulating levels of angiotensin II and increase levels of bradykinin, which in turn stimulates production of nitric oxide by endothelial nitric oxide synthase. In the vasculature, ACE inhibition promotes vasodilation and tends to inhibit smooth muscle proliferation, platelet aggregation, and thrombosis.

The major hemodynamic effect of ACE inhibition is afterload reduction, which is most important as an influence of myocardial oxygen demand in patients with impaired left ventricular function. A recent study, however, has demonstrated that ACE inhibition may be beneficial to prevent recurrent events in high-risk patients. The HOPE trial randomized 9297 patients with documented vascular disease or at high risk for atherosclerosis (diabetes plus at least one other risk factor) in the absence of heart failure to treatment with the tissue-selective ACE inhibitor ramipril (target dose 10 mg/d) or placebo.[36] An impressive 22% reduction in the combined end point of cardiovascular death, MI, and stroke was observed, and the number of patients and effect size were sufficient so that the reduction in individual end points was significant.[36] Patients were normotensive at the start of the trial, and the magnitude of benefit observed was not explained by the modest reduction in blood pressure (2 to 3 mm Hg).[36] On the basis of this study, the latest American College of Cardiology/American Heart Association guidelines recommend the use of ACE inhibitors in most cases as routine secondary prevention for patients with known CAD, particularly in diabetics without severe renal disease.[37]

LIPID-LOWERING AGENTS

There is extensive epidemiologic, laboratory, and clinical evidence linking cholesterol and coronary artery disease. Total cholesterol level has been linked to the development of

CAD events with a continuous and graded relation.[38] Most of this risk is due to low-density lipoprotein (LDL) cholesterol. Different large primary and secondary prevention trials have associated decreasing LDL cholesterol with a decreased risk of coronary disease events. Earlier lipid-lowering trials used bile-acid sequestrants (cholestyramine), fibric acid derivatives (gemfibrozil and clofibrate), or niacin in addition to diet. The reduction in total cholesterol in these early trials was 6% to 15% and was accompanied by a consistent trend toward a reduction in fatal and nonfatal coronary events.[39]

More impressive results have been achieved by using 3-hydroxy-3-methylglutaryl coenzyme A reductase inhibitors (statins). Statins have been demonstrated in several trials to decrease the rate of adverse ischemic events in patients with documented CAD.[40–42] The goal of treatment has conventionally been an LDL cholesterol level below 100 mg/dL,[37] but a recent study has shown that more aggressive LDL lowering has significantly greater protective effects. Patients were randomized within 10 days of an acute coronary syndrome to pravastatin (40 mg/d, standard therapy) or atorvastatin (80 mg/d, intensive therapy). Atorvastatin lowered LDL cholesterol more (to 62 mg/dL compared with 95 mg/dL) and significantly reduced the composite end point of death, MI, unstable angina, revascularization, and stroke.[42] Maximum benefit may require management of other lipid abnormalities (elevated triglycerides and low high-density lipoprotein cholesterol) and treatment of other atherogenic risk factors.

REFRACTORY ANGINA

Intraaortic Balloon Pump Counterpulsation

When angina remains refractory to maximal medical therapy, intraaortic balloon pump (IABP) counterpulsation may be considered. The IABP is a device that is inserted through the femoral artery into the descending thoracic aorta just distal to the aortic arch. A 40-mL balloon at the tip of the catheter is inflated in diastole by a pneumatic pump in synchrony with closure of the aortic valve and is deflated on opening of the aortic valve. Inflation and deflation are gated to the R and T waves on the electrocardiogram or to the arterial pressure recording. By deflating during ventricular systole, ventricular afterload is reduced, resulting in significant decreases in myocardial wall stress and significant decreases in myocardial oxygen requirements.[43] Further, inflation during diastole augments coronary blood flow by increasing coronary perfusion pressure. The main way in which an IABP relieves myocardial ischemia is by decreasing oxygen demand through afterload reduction.[44]

Use of an IABP is indicated in unstable angina when the angina and attendant ECG abnormalities are persistent and refractory to maximal pharmacologic therapy. Insertion of an IABP may improve hemodynamics and control symptoms so that coronary angiography can be performed safely. An IABP also may be inserted in patients who are stable and have undergone angiography but in whom precarious coronary lesions (e.g., left main coronary artery stenosis) have been identified. Typically, these patients are maintained on the device while awaiting surgery or angioplasty.

Although insertion of an IABP can result in immediate and dramatic relief of myocardial ischemia, placement of this device can be associated with significant complications.[43] These include aortic dissection, femoral artery lacerations, hematomas, femoral neuropathies, renal failure from renal artery occlusion, arterial thrombi and emboli, limb ischemia, and line sepsis. These potential complications must be weighed in determining whether an IABP should be inserted. Once one is inserted, the patient should be maintained on full anticoagulating doses of intravenous heparin by constant infusion. Frequent checks of peripheral pulses and surveillance for other complications should be performed routinely.

Coronary Angiography

If anginal symptoms persist despite maximal medical therapy, coronary angiography with an aim toward possible revascularization should be considered. One must keep in mind that coronary angiography is not a therapeutic intervention but a diagnostic test. Angiography is of little tangible value if there are no viable revascularization options.

Recommendations for the timing of angiography in patients with unstable ischemic syndromes are controversial. Early angiography can identify patients with left main or severe three-vessel disease, in whom early coronary artery bypass surgery can be lifesaving. The decision to perform angiography early should be based on the frequency and severity of angina episodes and the nature and extent of ECG changes. For example, extensive ST depression in the anterior chest leads suggests stenosis of the proximal left anterior descending artery or left main coronary artery, total occlusion of which might result in sudden death. Frequent anginal episodes or episodes that are difficult to control with conventional antianginal medications also point to impending infarction. Under these circumstances, early angiography is indicated. Otherwise, in cases in which the patient is stabilized readily with pharmacologic agents, including aspirin and heparin, there is no need for early angiography. Under these circumstances, one option is to forego coronary angiography altogether and then to evaluate patients several days to weeks later when they are completely stabilized and ambulatory. That can be accomplished by exercise stress testing, which can stratify patients according to their risk for subsequent cardiac events. Our usual approach, however, is to perform coronary angiography in all patients who are appropriate candidates after they have been stabilized but before hospital discharge.

ST-ELEVATION MYOCARDIAL INFARCTION

Symptoms suggestive of MI are usually similar to those of ordinary angina but are greater in intensity and duration. Nausea, vomiting, and diaphoresis may be prominent features, and stupor and malaise attributable to low cardiac output may occur. Compromised left ventricular function may result in pulmonary edema with development of pulmonary bibasilar crackles and jugular venous distention; a fourth heart sound can be present with small infarcts or even mild ischemia, but a third heart sound is usually indicative of more extensive damage.

Patients presenting with suspected myocardial ischemia should undergo a rapid evaluation and should be treated with oxygen, sublingual nitroglycerin (unless systolic pressure < 90 mm Hg), adequate analgesia, and aspirin (160 to 325 mg orally).[45] Narcotics should be used to relieve pain and anxiety, the salutary effects of which have been known for decades and must not be underestimated. It is also important to provide reassurance to the patient. A 12-lead electrocardiogram should be made and interpreted expeditiously.

ST-segment elevation of at least 1 mV in two or more contiguous leads provides strong evidence of thrombotic coronary occlusion: the patient should be considered for immediate reperfusion therapy. The diagnosis of STEMI can be limited in the presence of preexisting left bundle branch block or permanent pacemaker. Nonetheless, new left bundle branch block with a compatible clinical presentation should be treated as acute MI and treated accordingly. Recent data have suggested that patients with STEMI and new left bundle branch block may gain greater benefit from reperfusion strategies than those with ST elevation and preserved ventricular conduction.[46]

THROMBOLYTIC THERAPY

Early reperfusion of an occluded coronary artery is indicated for all eligible candidates. Overwhelming evidence from multiple clinical trials has demonstrated the ability of thrombolytic agents administered early in the course of an acute MI to reduce infarct size, preserve left ventricular function, and decrease short-term and long-term mortality rates.[47,48] Patients treated early derive the most benefit. Indications and contraindications for thrombolytic therapy are listed in Table 25-2. Because of the small, but nonetheless significant, risk of a bleeding complication, most notably intracranial hemorrhage, the decision to give a thrombolytic agent should be undertaken with prudence and caution. That is of special importance in ICU patients who may have a predisposition to bleeding complications because of multiple factors. Contraindications can be regarded as absolute or relative. In the surgical patient, thrombolysis may pose a prohibitive risk and emergent coronary angiography (with percutaneous coronary intervention as clinically indicated) may be preferable.

In contrast to the treatment of STEMI, thrombolytics have shown no benefit or even increased risk of adverse events when used for the treatment of unstable angina or NSTEMI.[49] Based on these findings, there is currently no role for thrombolytic agents in these latter syndromes.

Thrombolytic Agents

Streptokinase (SK) is a single-chain protein produced by α-hemolytic streptococci. SK is given as a 1.5 million U intravenous infusion over 1 hour, which produces a systemic lytic state for approximately 24 hours. Hypotension with infusion usually responds to fluids and a decreased infusion rate, but allergic reactions are possible. Hemorrhagic complications are the most feared side effect, with a rate of intracranial hemorrhage of approximately 0.5%. SK produces coronary arterial patency approximately 50% to 60% of the time and has been shown to decrease mortality rate by 18% compared with placebo.[47]

Tissue plasminogen activator (t-PA) is a recombinant protein that is more fibrin selective than SK and produces a higher early coronary patency rate (70% to 80%). The Global Utilization of Streptokinase and Tissue Plasminogen Activator for Occluded Coronary Arteries (GUSTO) was a large (41,021 patients) clinical trial comparing SK with t-PA in patients with STEMI and demonstrated a small but significant survival benefit for t-PA (1.1% absolute, 15% relative reduction).[50] The GUSTO angiographic substudy showed that the difference in patency rates explains the difference in clinical efficacy between these two agents.[51] t-PA is usually given in an accelerated regimen consisting of a 15-mg bolus, with 0.75 mg/kg (up to 50 mg) intravenously over the initial 30 minutes and 0.5 mg/kg (up to 35 mg) over the next 60 minutes. Allergic reactions do not occur because t-PA is not antigenic, but the rate of intracranial hemorrhage may be slightly higher ($\sim$0.7%) than that with SK.

Reteplase is a deletion mutant of t-PA with an extended half-life and is given as two 10-mg boluses 30 minutes apart. Reteplase was originally evaluated in angiographic trials that demonstrated improved coronary flow at 90 minutes compared with t-PA, but subsequent trials showed similar 30-day mortality rates.[52] Why enhanced patency with reteplase did not translate into lower mortality is uncertain.

Tenecteplase (TNK-tPA) is a genetically engineered t-PA mutant with amino acid substitutions that result in prolonged half-life, resistance to plasminogen-activator inhibitor 1, and increased fibrin specificity. TNK-tPA is given as a single bolus adjusted for weight. A single bolus of TNK-tPA has been shown to produce coronary flow rates identical to those seen with accelerated t-PA, with equivalent 30-day mortality and bleeding rates.[53] Based on these results, single-bolus TNK-tPA is an acceptable alternative to t-PA.

Because these newer agents have equivalent efficacy and side effect profiles at no additional cost compared with t-PA, and because they are simpler to administer, they have gained popularity. The ideal thrombolytic agent has not been developed. Newer recombinant agents with greater fibrin specificity, slower clearance from the circulation, and more resistance to plasma protease inhibitors are being studied.

TABLE 25-2 Indications for and Contraindications to Thrombolytic Therapy in Acute Myocardial Infarction

Indications
    Symptoms consistent with acute myocardial infarction
    Electrocardiogram showing 1-mm (0.1-mV) ST elevation in ≥2
        contiguous leads or new left bundle branch block
    Presentation within 12 h of symptom onset
    Absence of contraindications
Contraindications
    Absolute
        Active internal bleeding
        Intracranial neoplasm, aneurysm, or AV malformation
        Stroke or neurosurgery within 6 wk
        Trauma or major surgery within 2 wk, which may be a
          potential source of serious rebleeding
        Aortic dissection
    Relative
        Prolonged (>10 min) or clearly traumatic cardiopulmonary
          resuscitation[a]
        Noncompressible vascular punctures
        Severe uncontrolled hypertension (>200/110 mm Hg)[a]
        Trauma or major surgery within 6 wk (but >2 wk)
        Preexisting coagulopathy or current use of anticoagulants with
          INR >2–3
        Active peptic ulcer
        Infective endocarditis
        Pregnancy
        Chronic severe hypertension

[a] May be an absolute contraindication in low-risk patients with myocardial infarction.
ABBREVIATIONS: AV, atrioventricular; INR, international normalized ratio.

PRIMARY PERCUTANEOUS CORONARY INTERVENTION IN ACUTE MI

As many as 50% to 66% of patients presenting with acute MI may be ineligible for thrombolytic therapy, and these patients should be considered for primary percutaneous coronary intervention (PCI). The major advantages of primary PCI over thrombolytic therapy include a higher rate of normal (Thrombolysis In Myocardial Infarction [TIMI] grade 3) flow,[48] lower risk of intracranial hemorrhage, and the ability to stratify risk based on the severity and distribution of coronary artery disease. Data from several randomized trials have suggested that PCI is preferable to thrombolytic therapy for patients with acute MI at higher risk, including those older than 75 years, those with anterior infarctions, and those with hemodynamic instability.[54] The largest of these trials is the GUSTO-IIb angioplasty substudy, which randomized 1138 patients. At 30 days, there was a clinical benefit in the combined primary end points of death, nonfatal reinfarction, and nonfatal disabling stroke in the patients treated with percutaneous transluminal coronary angioplasty (PTCA) as opposed to t-PA, but there was no difference in the "hard" end points of death and MI at 30 days.[55]

These trials were performed in institutions in which a team skilled in primary angioplasty for acute MI was immediately available, with standby surgical backup, allowing for prompt reperfusion of the infarct-related artery. More important than the method of revascularization is the time to revascularization.[56] Procedural volume also is important.[57] A recent meta-analysis comparing direct PTCA with thrombolytic therapy found lower rates of mortality and reinfarction among those receiving direct PTCA.[58,59] Thus, direct angioplasty, if performed in a timely manner (ideally within 60 minutes) by highly experienced personnel, may be the preferred method of revascularization because it offers more complete revascularization with improved restoration of normal coronary blood flow and detailed information about coronary anatomy. There are certain subpopulations in which primary PCI is preferred. These subsets are listed in Table 25-3.

Coronary Stenting and Glycoprotein IIb/IIIa Antagonists

Primary angioplasty for acute MI results in a significant decrease in mortality rate but is limited by the possibility of abrupt vessel closure, recurrent in-hospital ischemia, reocclusion of the infarct-related artery, and restenosis. The use of coronary stents has been shown to decrease restenosis and adverse cardiac outcomes in routine and high-risk PCI.[60]

TABLE 25-3 Situations in Which Primary Angioplasty Is Preferred in Acute Myocardial Infarction

Situations in which PTCA is clearly preferable to thrombolytics
  Contraindications to thrombolytic therapy
  Cardiogenic shock
  Patients in whom uncertain diagnosis prompted cardiac
    catherization which revealed coronary occlusion
Situations in which PTCA *may be* preferable to thrombolytics
  Elderly patients (>75 y)
  Hemodynamic instability
  Patients with prior coronary artery bypass grafting
  Large anterior infarction
  Patients with a prior myocardial infarction

ABBREVIATION: PTCA, percutaneous transluminal coronary angioplasty.

The Primary Angioplasty in Myocardial Infarction Stent Trial tested the hypothesis that routine implantation of an intracoronary stent in the setting of MI would reduce angiographic restenosis and improve clinical outcomes compared with primary balloon angioplasty alone. This large, randomized, multicenter trial involving 900 patients did not show a difference in mortality rate at 6 months but did show improvement in ischemia-driven target vessel revascularization and less angina in the stented patients compared to PTCA alone.[61]

Glycoprotein (GP) IIb/IIIa receptor antagonists inhibit the final common pathway of platelet aggregation by blocking cross linking of activated platelets, and their use in percutaneous intervention has become routine.[62] The benefits of GP IIb/IIIa inhibition and coronary stenting appear to be additive.[63,64] Thus, combining GP IIb/IIIa antagonism and stenting in acute MI makes theoretical sense and has been tested in two large clinical trials. The ADMIRAL trial evaluated abciximab as an adjunct to primary PTCA and stenting in 300 patients with acute MI. Abciximab used in conjunction with stenting improved coronary patency before stenting and resulted in a nearly 50% relative risk reduction in the incidence of death, recurrent MI, and urgent revascularization at 30 days, although this was associated with an increased incidence of minor bleeding.[65] The CADILLAC trial randomized 2082 patients to angioplasty alone, angioplasty plus abciximab, stenting alone, or stenting plus abciximab. The composite end point of death, reinfarction, disabling stroke, and repeat revascularization was reduced with addition of abciximab to angioplasty, and outcomes were better with stenting (but abciximab added to stenting alone did not improve outcomes, although the event rate was low).[66] Based on the results of these trials, stenting has become routine for patients with PCI in the setting of acute MI, usually with the addition of GP IIb/IIIa inhibition.

In patients who fail thrombolytic therapy, salvage PTCA is indicated, although the initial success rate is lower than that of primary angioplasty, reocclusion is more common, and mortality is higher. The RESCUE trial focused on a subset of patients with acute MI and anterior infarction and showed a reduction in the combined end point of death and congestive heart failure at 30 days in the group receiving salvage PTCA.[67]

There is no convincing evidence to support empirical delayed PTCA in patients without evidence of recurrent or provocable ischemia after thrombolytic therapy. The TIMI IIB trial and other studies have suggested that a strategy of "watchful waiting" allows for identification of patients who will benefit from revascularization.[68]

ADJUNCTIVE THERAPIES IN STEMI

Aspirin

Aspirin has been shown to decrease mortality rate in acute infarction to the same degree as thrombolytic therapy, and its effects are additive to thrombolytics.[69] In addition, aspirin reduces the risk of reinfarction. Unless contraindicated, all patients with a suspected acute coronary syndrome (STEMI, NSTEMI, or unstable angina) should be given aspirin as soon as possible.

Heparin

Administration of full-dose heparin after thrombolytic therapy with t-PA is essential to diminish reocclusion after successful reperfusion.[47,69] Dosing should be adjusted to weight, with a bolus of 60 U/kg up to a maximum of 4000 U and an initial infusion rate of 12 U/kg per hour up to a maximum of 1000 U/hr, with adjustment to keep the partial thromboplastin time between 50 and 70 seconds. Heparin should be continued for 24 to 48 hours.

Nitrates

Nitrates have several beneficial effects in acute MI. They reduce myocardial oxygen demand by decreasing preload and afterload and may improve myocardial oxygen supply by increasing subendocardial perfusion and collateral blood flow to the ischemic region. Occasional patients with ST elevation due to occlusive coronary artery spasm may have dramatic resolution of ischemia with nitrates. In addition to their hemodynamic effects, nitrates also reduce platelet aggregation. Despite these benefits, the Third Gruppo Italiano per lo Studio della Streptochinasi nell'Infarto Miocardico (GISSI-3) and Fourth International Study of Infarct Survival (ISIS-4) trials found no significant decrease in mortality rate from routine short- and long-term nitrate therapies.[70,71] Nonetheless, nitrates remain first-line agents for the symptomatic relief of angina pectoris and when MI is complicated by congestive heart failure.

β Blockers

Beta blockers are beneficial in the early management of MI and as long-term therapy. In the era before thrombolysis, early intravenous atenolol was shown to significantly decrease reinfarction, cardiac arrest, cardiac rupture, and death.[72] In conjunction with thrombolytic therapy with t-PA, immediate β blockade with metoprolol resulted in a significant reduction in recurrent ischemia and reinfarction, although mortality rate was not decreased.[68]

Intravenous β blockade should be considered for all patients presenting with acute MI, especially those with continued ischemic discomfort and sympathetic hyperactivity manifested by hypertension or tachycardia. Therapy should be avoided in patients with moderate or severe heart failure, hypotension, severe bradycardia or heart block, and severe bronchospastic disease. Metoprolol can be given intravenously as a 5-mg bolus, repeated every 5 minutes for a total of three doses. Because of its brief half-life, esmolol may be advantageous in situations in which precise control of heart rate is necessary or rapid drug withdrawal may be needed if adverse effects occur.

Oral β blockade has been clearly demonstrated to decrease mortality rate after acute MI[73,74] and should be initiated in all patients who can tolerate it, even if they have not been treated with intravenous β blockers. Diabetes mellitus is not a contraindication.

Angiotensin-Converting Enzyme Inhibitors

ACE inhibitors have been shown unequivocally to improve hemodynamics, functional capacity and symptoms, and survival in patients with chronic congestive heart failure.[75,76] Moreover, ACE inhibitors prevent the development of congestive heart failure in patients with asymptomatic left ventricular dysfunction.[77] This information was the spur for trials evaluating the benefit of prophylactic administration of ACE inhibitors in the period after MI. The Survival and Ventricular Enlargement trial showed that patients with left ventricular dysfunction (ejection fraction < 40%) after MI had

a 21% improvement in survival rate after treatment with the ACE inhibitor captopril.[78] A smaller but still significant reduction in mortality rate was seen when all patients were treated with captopril in the ISIS-4 study.[71] The HOPE study demonstrated that the ACE inhibitor ramipril improves survival rate when added to aspirin and β blockers.[36] The mechanisms responsible for the benefits of ACE inhibitors probably include limitation in the progressive left ventricular dysfunction and enlargement (remodeling) after infarction, but a reduction in ischemic events also is seen.

ACE inhibition should be started early, preferably within the first 24 hours after infarction. Immediate intravenous ACE inhibition with enalaprilat has not been shown to be beneficial.[79] Patients should be started on small doses of oral agents (captopril 6.25 mg three times daily) and rapidly increased to the range demonstrated to be beneficial in clinical trials (captopril 50 mg three times daily, enalapril 10 to 20 mg twice daily, lisinopril 10 to 20 mg once daily, or ramipril 10 mg once daily).

Calcium Channel Blockers

Randomized clinical trials have not demonstrated that routine use of calcium channel blockers improves survival rate after MI. Meta-analyses have suggested that large doses of the short-acting dihydropyridine nifedipine increase mortality rate in MI. Adverse effects of calcium channel blockers include bradycardia, atrioventricular block, and exacerbation of heart failure. The relative vasodilating, negative inotropic effects, and conduction system effects of the various agents must be considered when they are used in this setting. Diltiazem is the only calcium channel blocker that has been proven to have tangible benefits by reducing reinfarction and recurrent ischemia in patients with non–Q-wave infarctions who do not have evidence of congestive heart failure.[80]

Calcium channel blockers may be useful for patients whose postinfarction course is complicated by recurrent angina because these agents not only reduce myocardial oxygen demand but also inhibit coronary vasoconstriction. For hemodynamically stable patients, diltiazem can be given starting at 60 to 90 mg orally every 6 to 8 hours. In patients with severe left ventricular dysfunction, a long-acting dihydropyridine without prominent negative inotropic effects such as amlodipine, nicardipine, or the long-acting preparation of nifedipine may be preferable; increased mortality rate with these agents has not been demonstrated.

Antiarrhythmic Therapy

A major purpose for admitting patients with MI to the ICU is to monitor for and prevent malignant arrhythmias. Ventricular extrasystoles are common after MI and are a manifestation of electrical instability of peri-infarct areas. The incidence of sustained ventricular tachycardia or fibrillation is highest in the first 3 to 4 hours, but these arrhythmias may occur at any time. Malignant ventricular arrhythmias may be heralded by frequent premature ventricular contractions (more than five or six per minute), closely coupled premature ventricular contractions, complex ectopy (couplets, multiform premature ventricular contractions), and salvos of nonsustained ventricular tachycardia. However, malignant arrhythmia may occur suddenly without these "warning" arrhythmias.

Based on these pathophysiologic considerations, prophylactic use of intravenous lidocaine has been advocated, even

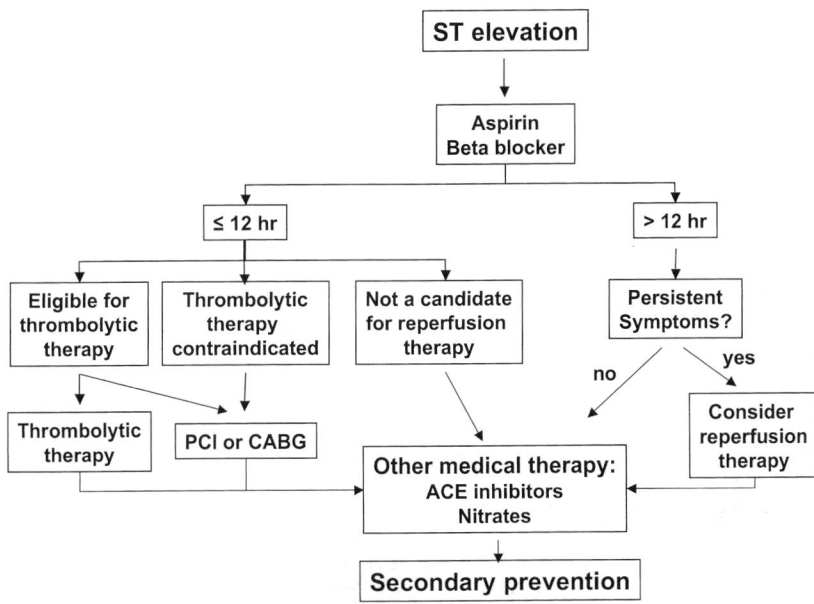

FIGURE 25-2 Possible treatment algorithm for patients presenting with ST-elevation myocardial infarction. ACE, angiotensin-converting enzyme; CABG, coronary artery bypass grafting; PCI, percutaneous coronary intervention.

in the absence of ectopy. Even though lidocaine decreases the frequency of premature ventricular contractions and of early ventricular fibrillation, overall mortality rate is not decreased. Meta-analyses of pooled data have demonstrated increased mortality rate from the routine use of lidocaine.[81] Therefore, routine prophylactic administration of lidocaine is no longer recommended.

Nonetheless, lidocaine infusion is clearly indicated after an episode of sustained ventricular tachycardia or ventricular fibrillation and should be considered in patients with nonsustained ventricular tachycardia. Lidocaine is administered as a bolus of 1 mg/kg (not to exceed 100 mg), followed by a second bolus of 0.5 mg/kg 10 minutes later, and an infusion at 1 to 3 mg/min. Lidocaine is metabolized by the liver, so smaller doses should be given in the presence of liver disease, in the elderly, and in patients who have congestive heart failure severe enough to compromise hepatic perfusion. Toxic manifestations primarily involve the central nervous system and can include confusion, lethargy, slurred speech, and seizures. Because the risk of malignant ventricular arrhythmias decreases after 24 hours, lidocaine is usually discontinued after this point. For prolonged infusions, monitoring of lidocaine levels (therapeutic between 1.5 and 5 μg/mL) is sometimes useful.

Intravenous amiodarone is an alternative to lidocaine for ventricular arrhythmias. Amiodarone is given as a 150-mg intravenous bolus over 10 minutes, followed by 1 mg/min for 6 hours, and then 0.5 mg/min for 18 hours.

Perhaps the most important points in the prevention and management of arrhythmias after acute MI are correcting hypoxemia and maintaining normal serum potassium and magnesium levels. Serum electrolytes should be followed closely, particularly after diuretic therapy. Magnesium depletion is another frequently overlooked cause of persistent ectopy.[82] The serum magnesium level may not reflect myocardial concentrations. Routine administration of magnesium has not been shown to decrease mortality rate after acute MI,[71] but empiric administration of 2 g of intravenous magnesium in patients with early ventricular ectopy is probably a good idea.

One possible treatment algorithm for treating patients with STEMI is shown in Fig. 25-2.

NON–ST-ELEVATION MYOCARDIAL INFARCTION

The key to initial management of patients with acute coronary syndromes who present without ST elevation is risk stratification. The overall risk of a patient is related to the severity of preexisting heart disease and the degree of plaque instability. Risk stratification is an ongoing process, which begins with hospital admission and continues through discharge.

Braunwald proposed a classification for unstable angina based on severity of symptoms and clinical circumstances for risk stratification.[83] The risk of progression to acute MI or death in acute coronary syndromes increases with age. ST-segment depression on the electrocardiogram identifies patients at higher risk for clinical events.[83] Conversely, a normal electrocardiogram confers an excellent short-term prognosis. Biochemical markers of cardiac injury are also predictive of outcome. Elevated levels of troponin T are associated with an increased risk of cardiac events and a higher 30-day mortality rate and are more strongly correlated with 30-day survival rate than is ECG category or CPK-MB level.[84] Conversely, low levels are associated with low event rates, although the absence of troponin elevation does not guarantee a good prognosis and is not a substitute for good clinical judgment.

ANTIPLATELET THERAPY

Aspirin is a mainstay of therapy for acute coronary syndromes. The Veterans Administration Cooperative Study Group[28] and the Canadian Multicenter Trial[85] showed that aspirin reduces the risk of death or MI by approximately 50% in patients with unstable angina or non–Q-wave MI. Aspirin also reduces events after resolution of an acute coronary syndrome and should be continued indefinitely.

Clopidogrel or ticlopidine, thienopyridines that inhibit platelet activation induced by adenosine diphosphate and are more potent than aspirin, can be used in place of aspirin, if necessary. They are used in combination with aspirin when intracoronary stents are placed. Clopidogrel is generally better tolerated than ticlopidine because the risk of neutropenia is much lower.

In the CURE trial, 12,562 patients were randomized to receive clopidogrel or placebo in addition to standard therapy with aspirin within 24 hours of unstable angina symptoms.[86] Clopidogrel significantly reduced the risk of MI, stroke, or cardiovascular death from 11.4% to 9.3% ($p < 0.001$).[86] It should be noted that this benefit included a 1% absolute increase in major, non–life-threatening bleeds ($p = 0.001$) and a 2.8% absolute increase in major or life-threatening bleeds associated with coronary artery bypass graft (CABG) within 5 days ($p = 0.07$).[86] These data have raised concerns about giving clopidogrel before obtaining information about the coronary anatomy.

Clopidogrel has also been tested for secondary prevention of events. The Clopidogrel Versus Aspirin in Patients at Risk of Ischaemic Events trial, a multicenter trial of 19,185 patients with known vascular disease (prior stroke, MI, or peripheral vascular disease), randomized patients to 75 mg/d of clopidogrel or 325 mg/d aspirin.[87] After an average follow-up period of 1.6 years, patients treated with clopidogrel had significantly fewer cardiovascular events than did patients treated with aspirin (5.8% vs. 5.3%, a relative risk reduction of 8.7%).[87]

ANTICOAGULANT THERAPY

Heparin is an important component of primary therapy for patients with unstable coronary syndromes without ST elevation. When added to aspirin, heparin has been shown to reduce refractory angina and the development of MI,[29] and a meta-analysis of the available data has indicated that addition of heparin reduces the composite end point of death or MI.[88]

Heparin can be difficult to administer because the anticoagulant effect is unpredictable in individual patients; this is due to heparin binding to heparin-binding proteins, endothelial and other cells, and heparin inhibition by several factors released by activated platelets. Therefore, the activated partial thromboplastin time must be monitored closely. The potential for heparin-associated thrombocytopenia is another safety concern.

Low-molecular-weight heparins (LMWHs), which are obtained by depolymerization of standard heparin and selection of fractions with lower molecular weights, have several advantages. Because they bind less avidly to heparin-binding proteins, there is less variability in the anticoagulant response and a more predictable dose-response curve, so the need to monitor activated partial thromboplastin time is eliminated. The incidence of thrombocytopenia is lower (but not absent, and patients with heparin-induced thrombocytopenia with anti-heparin antibodies cannot be switched to LMWH). Moreover, LMWHs have longer half-lives and can be given by subcutaneous injection. These properties make treatment with LMWH at home after hospital discharge feasible. Because evidence suggests that patients with unstable coronary syndromes may remain in a hypercoagulable state for weeks or months, the longer duration of anticoagulation possible with LMWH may be desirable.

Several trials have documented beneficial effects of LMWH therapy in unstable coronary syndromes. The Efficacy and Safety of Subcutaneous Enoxaparin in Non-Q-Wave Coronary Events trial showed that the LMWH enoxaparin reduces the combined end point of death, MI, or recurrent ischemia

at 14 days and at 30 days when compared with heparin.[89] Similar results were found in the TIMI 11B trial comparing enoxaparin with heparin.[90] A meta-analysis of these two very similar trials demonstrated a 23% 7-day and an 18% 42-day reduction in death or MI.[91] Dalteparin, another LMWH, is also available, but the evidence for its efficacy is not nearly as compelling as that for enoxaparin.

Although LMWHs are substantially easier to administer than standard heparin and long-term administration can be contemplated, they are more expensive. Specific considerations with the use of LMWHs include decreased clearance in renal insufficiency and the lack of a commercially available test to measure the anticoagulant effect. LMWH should be given strong consideration in high-risk patients, but whether substitution of LMWH for heparin in all patients is cost effective is uncertain.

GLYCOPROTEIN IIB/IIIA ANTAGONISTS

Given the central role of platelet activation and aggregation in the pathophysiology of unstable coronary syndromes, attention has focused on platelet GP IIb/IIIa antagonists, which inhibit the final common pathway of platelet aggregation. Three agents are currently available. Abciximab is a chimeric murine-human monoclonal antibody Fab fragment that binds with relatively high affinity to platelet receptors, giving it a short plasma half-life (10 to 30 minutes) but a long duration of biologic action by virtue of the strength of the bond formed with the surface of the activated platelet. Because there is a relatively low ratio of abciximab molecules to platelets (i.e., limited plasma pool of unbound drug), platelet transfusions may be helpful in the event of a major bleeding complication. Abciximab is currently approved for elective PCI or unstable coronary syndromes with planned PCI. Tirofiban is a synthetic nonpeptide agent with a half-life of approximately 2.5 hours and a lower receptor affinity than abciximab. This drug is approved for the medical management of unstable angina or NSTEMI with or without planned PCI. Given the large ratio of drug to platelet (i.e., large plasma pool of free drug) seen with this agent and with eptifibatide, platelet transfusions are generally not regarded as helpful in the event of a major bleed. It is recommended that the drug simply be stopped and supportive therapy instituted during the relatively short biologic activity period. Eptifibatide is a cyclic heptapeptide with a 2-hour half-life. Like tirofiban, it is approved for the medical management of unstable angina with or without subsequent PCI; however, it may also be used as adjunctive therapy in elective PCI.

The benefits of GP IIb/IIIa inhibitors as adjunctive treatment in patients undergoing percutaneous intervention have been substantial and consistently observed. Abciximab has been most extensively studied, but a benefit for eptifibatide has also been demonstrated. In acute coronary syndromes, the evidence supporting the efficacy of GP IIb/IIIa inhibitors is somewhat less impressive. Five major trials have been completed (the "4 P's" and GUSTO-IV). In the Platelet Receptor Inhibition in Ischemic Syndrome Management trial, tirofiban decreased death rate, MI, or refractory ischemia when compared with heparin, from 5.6% to 3.8% ($p < 0.01$) at 48 hours, but there was no difference at 30 days (7.1% vs. 5.8%, $p = 0.11$).[92] In the subsequent Platelet Receptor Inhibition in Ischemic Syndrome Management in Patients Limited by Unstable Signs and Symptoms trial, tirofiban added to heparin decreased death rate, MI, or refractory ischemia at 30 days, from 11.9% to 8.7% ($p = 0.03$).[31] In the PURSUIT trial, eptifibatide decreased the rate of death or MI, from 15.7% to 14.2% ($p = 0.04$) at 30 days.[93] The PARAGON trial with lamifiban did not show a significant benefit with GP IIb/IIIa inhibition.[94] In the GUSTO-IV ACS trial, however, abciximab did not produce an improvement; death rate or MI was slightly higher in the treatment group.[95] This trial included patients for whom percutaneous intervention was not planned; when patients with refractory angina and planned angioplasty were randomized to receive abciximab or placebo from 24 hours before the procedure through 1 hour after PTCA in the CAPTURE trial, the primary end point—death, MI, or urgent revascularization at 30 days—was decreased by GP IIb/IIIa inhibition, and the rate of MI before PTCA also was decreased.[96] When patients were categorized as those with or without increased troponin, the benefit was confined to the positive troponin group.[96]

Recent meta-analyses have found a relative risk reduction of 40% for GP IIb/IIIa therapy adjunctive to PCI, and a reduction of 11% for GP IIb/IIIa inhibitors in NSTEMI acute coronary syndromes.[62] Additional analysis has suggested that GP IIb/IIIa inhibition is most effective in high-risk patients (those with ECG changes or elevated troponin).[62] The benefits appear to be restricted to patients undergoing percutaneous intervention.

INTERVENTIONAL MANAGEMENT

Cardiac catheterization may be undertaken in patients presenting with symptoms suggestive of unstable coronary syndromes for one of several reasons: to assist with risk stratification, as a prelude to revascularization, and to exclude significant epicardial coronary stenosis as a cause of symptoms when the diagnosis is uncertain.

An early invasive approach has been compared with a conservative approach in several prospective studies. Two earlier trials were negative. The TIMI IIIb study randomized 1473 patients to early angiography or conservative management with angiography and revascularization only for recurrent chest pain or provocable ischemia.[49] No significant difference was found in the combined end point of death, MI, or positive treadmill test at 6 weeks. However, there was a high (64%) cross-over rate from the conservative to the invasive arm, and hospital stays were shorter with the early invasive approach.[49] The VANQWISH trial of 920 patients with non–Q wave MI showed an increase in the primary end point of death rate or MI with an invasive strategy, although overall mortality was not significantly different.[97] Difficulties with this trial included the fact that only 44% of patients randomized to the invasive arm actually underwent revascularization, compared with 33% in the conservative arm, and the entire trial had a very high surgical mortality rate (11.6%).[97] It is important to realize that these trials were performed before widespread use of coronary stenting and platelet GP IIb/IIIa inhibitors, both of which have been shown to improve outcomes after angioplasty.

More recently, a substudy of the Second Fragmin and Fast Revascularisation during Instability in Coronary Artery Disease study, which used the LMWH dalteparin, randomized 2457 patients to an early invasive or a noninvasive strategy and found a significantly lower mortality rate in the invasive group at 30 days, which was maintained at 1 year.[98] The TACTICS TIMI-18 trial used aspirin, heparin, and tirofiban in 2220 patients and found a significant reduction in the combined end point of death rate, MI, or readmission for acute coronary syndrome with invasive management.[99] It is important to recognize that these trials selected high-risk patients (identified on the basis of ECG changes or enzyme elevations) for inclusion. Addition of antiplatelet therapy (beyond the use of aspirin alone) to reperfusion also may have contributed to the improved outcomes with invasive strategies in these more recent trials.

Risk stratification is the key to managing patients with NSTEMI acute coronary syndromes. One possible algorithm for managing patients with NSTEMI is shown in Fig. 25-3. An initial strategy of medical management with attempts at stabilization is warranted in patients with lower risk, but patients at higher risk should be considered for cardiac catheterization. Pharmacologic and mechanical strategies are intertwined in the sense that selection of patients for early revascularization will influence the choice of antiplatelet and anticoagulant medication. When good clinical judgment is used, early coronary angiography in selected patients with acute coronary syndromes can lead to better management and lower morbidity and mortality rates.

COMPLICATIONS OF ACUTE MYOCARDIAL INFARCTION

POSTINFARCTION ISCHEMIA

Causes of ischemia after infarction include decreased myocardial oxygen supply due to coronary reocclusion or spasm, mechanical problems that increase myocardial oxygen demand, and extracardiac factors such as hypertension, anemia, hypotension, or hypermetabolic states. Nonischemic causes of chest pain, such as postinfarction pericarditis and acute pulmonary embolism, should also be considered.

Immediate management includes aspirin, β blockade, intravenous nitroglycerin, heparin, consideration of calcium channel blockers, and diagnostic coronary angiography. Postinfarction angina is an indication for revascularization. PTCA can be performed if the culprit lesion is suitable. CABG should be considered for patients with left main disease, three-vessel disease, or unsuitable for PTCA. If the angina cannot be controlled medically or is accompanied by hemodynamic instability, an IABP should be inserted.

VENTRICULAR FREE WALL RUPTURE

Ventricular free wall rupture typically occurs during the first week after infarction. The classic patient is elderly, female, and hypertensive. Early use of thrombolytic therapy decreases the incidence of cardiac rupture, but late use may actually increase the risk. Free wall rupture presents as a catastrophic event with shock and electromechanical dissociation. Salvage is possible with prompt recognition, pericardiocentesis to relieve acute tamponade, and thoracotomy with repair.[100] Emergent echocardiography or pulmonary artery catheterization can help make the diagnosis.

VENTRICULAR SEPTAL RUPTURE

Septal rupture presents as severe heart failure or cardiogenic shock, with a pansystolic murmur and parasternal thrill. The hallmark finding is a left-to-right intracardiac shunt ("step up" in oxygen saturation from the right atrium to the right

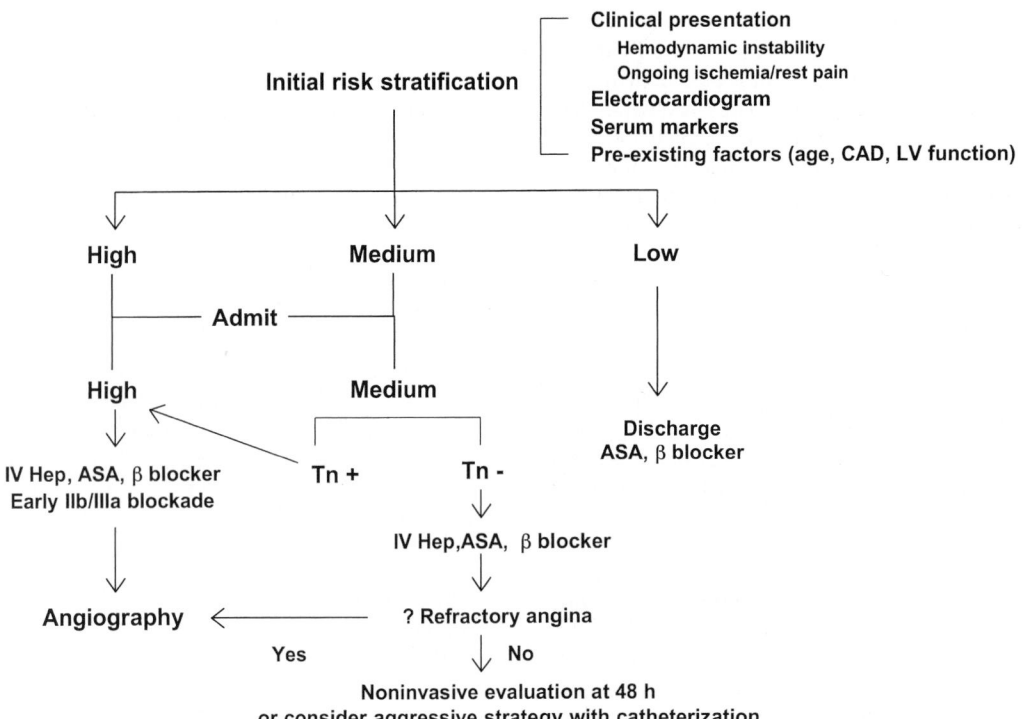

FIGURE 25-3 Possible treatment algorithm for patients with non–ST-elevation acute coronary syndromes. ASA, aspirin; Hep, heparin; IV, intravenous; Tn, troponin.

ventricle), but the diagnosis is most easily made with echocardiography.

Rapid institution of an IABP and supportive pharmacologic measures is necessary. Operative repair is the only viable option for long-term survival. The timing of surgery has been controversial, but most authorities currently suggest that repair should be undertaken early, within 48 hours of the rupture.[101]

ACUTE MITRAL REGURGITATION

Ischemic mitral regurgitation is usually associated with inferior MI and ischemia or infarction of the posterior papillary muscle, although anterior papillary muscle rupture can also occur. Papillary muscle rupture typically occurs 2 to 7 days after acute MI and presents dramatically with pulmonary edema, hypotension, and cardiogenic shock. When a papillary muscle ruptures, the murmur of acute mitral regurgitation may be limited to early systole because of rapid equalization of pressures in the left atrium and left ventricle. More importantly, the murmur may be soft or inaudible, especially when cardiac output is low.[102]

Echocardiography is extremely useful in the differential diagnosis, which includes free wall rupture, ventricular septal rupture, and infarct extension with pump failure. Hemodynamic monitoring with pulmonary artery catheterization may also be helpful. Management includes afterload reduction with nitroprusside and an IABP as temporizing measures. Inotropic or vasopressor therapy also may be needed to support cardiac output and blood pressure. Definitive therapy is surgical valve repair or replacement, which should be undertaken as soon as possible because clinical deterioration can be sudden.[102,103]

RIGHT VENTRICULAR INFARCTION

Right ventricular infarction occurs in up to 30% of patients with inferior infarction and is clinically significant in 10%.[104] The combination of a clear chest radiograph with jugular venous distention in a patient with an inferior wall MI should lead to the suspicion of a coexisting right ventricular infarct. The diagnosis is substantiated by demonstration of ST-segment elevation in the right precordial leads (V_{3R} to V_{5R}) or by characteristic hemodynamic findings on right heart catheterization (elevated right atrial and right ventricular end-diastolic pressures with normal to low pulmonary artery occlusion pressure and low cardiac output). Echocardiography can demonstrate depressed right ventricular contractility.[22] Patients with cardiogenic shock on the basis of right ventricular infarction have a better prognosis than do those with left-side pump failure.[104] This may be due in part to the fact that right ventricular function tends to return to normal over time with supportive therapy.[105]

In patients with right ventricular infarction, hypovolemia should be avoided because it can seriously compromise perfusion. However, most patients have elevated central venous pressures after initial resuscitation, and fluid loading is ineffective in raising perfusion further. Continued fluid loading can compromise left ventricular filling and cardiac output.[105] Inotropic therapy with dobutamine is often more effective in increasing cardiac output. Serial echocardiograms may be useful to detect right ventricular overdistention.[105] Maintenance of atrioventricular synchrony is also important in these patients to optimize right ventricular filling.[22] For patients with continued hemodynamic instability, using an IABP may be useful, particularly because elevated right ventricular pressures and volumes increase wall stress and oxygen consumption and decrease right coronary perfusion pressure, exacerbating right ventricular ischemia.

Reperfusion of the occluded coronary artery is also crucial. A study using direct angioplasty found that restoration of normal flow can result in dramatic recovery of right ventricular function and a mortality rate of only 2%, whereas unsuccessful reperfusion was associated with persistent hemodynamic compromise and a mortality rate of 58%.[106]

CARDIOGENIC SHOCK

Epidemiology and Pathophysiology

Cardiogenic shock, resulting from left ventricular pump failure or from mechanical complications, represents the leading cause of in-hospital death after MI.[20] Despite advances in the management of heart failure and acute MI, clinical outcomes in patients with cardiogenic shock have been frustratingly poor, with reported mortality rates ranging from 50% to 80%.[107] Patients may have cardiogenic shock at initial presentation, but shock often evolves over several hours.[108,109] This is important because it suggests that early treatment may potentially prevent shock.

Cardiac dysfunction in patients with cardiogenic shock is usually initiated by MI or ischemia. The myocardial dysfunction resulting from ischemia worsens that ischemia, creating a downward spiral (Fig. 25-4). Once a critical mass of ischemic or necrotic left ventricular myocardium (usually about 40%)[110] fails to pump, stroke volume and cardiac output begin to diminish significantly. Systolic dysfunction leads to decreased systemic perfusion and hypotension, which reduces coronary perfusion pressure and induces compensatory peripheral vasoconstriction and fluid retention. These compensatory mechanisms create a vicious cycle that further worsens the systolic dysfunction. Likewise, myocardial ischemia increases myocardial stiffness, thus increasing left ventricular end-diastolic pressure and myocardial wall stress at a given end-diastolic volume. Increased left ventricular stiffness limits diastolic filling and may result in pulmonary congestion, causing hypoxemia and worsening the imbalance of oxygen delivery and oxygen demand in the myocardium, resulting in further ischemia and myocardial

dysfunction. The compensatory mechanisms that retain fluid to maintain cardiac output may add to the vicious cycle and further increase diastolic filling pressures. The interruption of this cycle of myocardial dysfunction and ischemia forms the basis for the therapeutic regimens for cardiogenic shock.

Initial Management

Maintenance of adequate oxygenation and ventilation is critical. Many patients require intubation and mechanical ventilation, if only to reduce the work of breathing and facilitate sedation and stabilization before cardiac catheterization. Electrolyte abnormalities should be corrected, and morphine (or fentanyl, if systolic pressure is compromised) should be used to relieve pain and anxiety, thus decreasing excessive sympathetic activity and oxygen demand, preload, and afterload. Arrhythmias and heart block may have major effects on cardiac output and should be corrected promptly with antiarrhythmic drugs, cardioversion, or pacing.

The initial approach to the hypotensive patient should include fluid resuscitation unless frank pulmonary edema is present. Patients are commonly diaphoretic and relative hypovolemia may be present in as many as 20% of patients with cardiogenic shock. Fluid infusion is best initiated with predetermined boluses titrated to clinical end points of heart rate, urine output, and blood pressure. Ischemia produces diastolic and systolic dysfunctions; hence, elevated filling pressures may be necessary to maintain stroke volume in patients with cardiogenic shock. Patients who do not respond rapidly to initial fluid boluses or those with poor physiologic reserve should be considered for invasive hemodynamic monitoring. Optimal filling pressures differ from patient to patient; hemodynamic monitoring can be used to construct a Starling curve at the bedside to identify the filling pressure at which cardiac output is maximized. Maintenance of adequate preload is particularly important in patients with right ventricular infarction.

When arterial pressure remains inadequate, therapy with vasopressor agents may be required to maintain coronary perfusion pressure. Dopamine increases blood pressure and

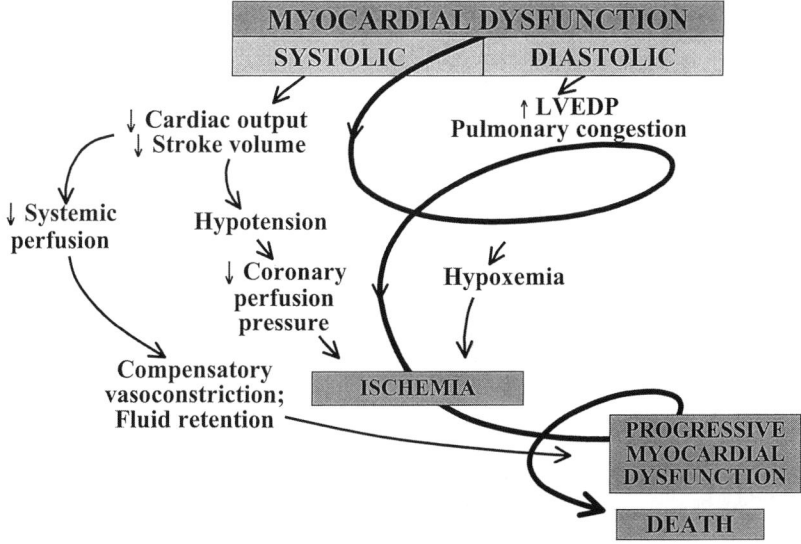

FIGURE 25-4 The 'downward spiral' in cardiogenic shock. Stroke volume and cardiac output fall with left ventricular (LV) dysfunction, producing hypotension and tachycardia that reduce coronary blood flow. Increasing ventricular diastolic pressure reduces coronary blood flow, and increased wall stress elevates myocardial oxygen requirements. All of these factors combine to worsen ischemia. The falling cardiac output also compromises systemic perfusion. Compensatory mechanisms include sympathetic stimulation and fluid retention to increase preload. These mechanisms can actually worsen cardiogenic shock by increasing myocardial oxygen demand and afterload. Thus, a vicious circle can be established. LVEDP, left ventricular enddiastolic pressure. (*Adapted with permission from Hollenberg and colleagues.*[20])

cardiac output and is usually the initial choice in patients with systolic pressures below 80 mm Hg. When hypotension remains refractory, norepinephrine may be necessary to maintain organ perfusion pressure. Phenylephrine, a selective α_1-adrenergic agonist, may be useful when tachyarrhythmias limit therapy with other vasopressors. Vasopressor infusions need to be titrated carefully in patients with cardiogenic shock to maximize coronary perfusion pressure with the least possible increase in myocardial oxygen demand. Hemodynamic monitoring, with serial measurements of cardiac output and filling pressures (and other parameters such as mixed venous oxygen saturation), allows for titration of the dosage of vasoactive agents to the minimum dosage required to achieve the chosen therapeutic goals.[24]

After initial stabilization and restoration of adequate blood pressure, tissue perfusion should be assessed. If tissue perfusion remains inadequate, inotropic support or use of an IABP should be initiated. If tissue perfusion is adequate but significant pulmonary congestion remains, diuretics may be used. Vasodilators also can be considered, depending on the blood pressure.

In patients with inadequate tissue perfusion and adequate intravascular volume, the circulation should be supported with inotropic agents. Dobutamine, a selective β_1-adrenergic receptor agonist, can improve myocardial contractility and increase cardiac output and is the initial agent of choice in patients with systolic pressures above 80 mm Hg. Dobutamine may exacerbate hypotension in some patients, especially when hypovolemia has not been corrected, and can precipitate tachyarrhythmias. Dopamine may be preferable if systolic pressure is below 80 mm Hg, although tachycardia and increased peripheral resistance may worsen myocardial ischemia. In some situations, a combination of dopamine and dobutamine can be more effective than either agent used alone. Phosphodiesterase inhibitors such as milrinone increase intracellular cyclic adenosine monophosphate by mechanisms not involving adrenergic receptors, have positive inotropic and vasodilatory actions, and are less arrhythmogenic than catecholamines. Milrinone, however, has the potential to cause hypotension and has a long half-life; in patients with tenuous clinical status, its use is often reserved for situations in which other agents have proven ineffective. Standard administration of milrinone calls for a bolus loading dose followed by an infusion, but many clinicians eschew the loading dose (or halve it) in patients with marginal blood pressure.

Counterpulsation with an IABP reduces afterload and augments diastolic perfusion pressure, thereby increasing cardiac output and improving coronary blood flow.[111] These beneficial effects, in contrast to those of inotropic or vasopressor agents, occur without an increase in oxygen demand. However, IABP does not produce a significant improvement in blood flow distal to a critical coronary stenosis and has not been shown to improve mortality when used alone, that is, without reperfusion therapy or revascularization. In patients with cardiogenic shock and compromised tissue perfusion, IABP can be an essential support mechanism to stabilize patients and allow time for definitive therapeutic measures.[111,112] In appropriate settings, more intensive support with mechanical assist devices may also be implemented.

Reperfusion Therapy

Although thrombolytic therapy reduces the likelihood of subsequent development of shock after initial presentation,[109] its role in the management of patients who have already developed shock is less certain. The number of patients in randomized trials is small because most fibrinolytic trials have excluded patients with cardiogenic shock at presentation, but the available trials (GISSI, ISIS-2, and GUSTO-1)[47,50,69,113] have not demonstrated that fibrinolytic therapy decreases mortality rate in patients with established cardiogenic shock. In contrast, in the Should We Emergently Revascularize Occluded Coronaries for Cardiogenic Shock? (SHOCK) Registry,[114] patients treated with fibrinolytic therapy had a lower in-hospital mortality rate than did those who were not (54% vs. 64%, $p = 0.005$), even after adjustment for age and revascularization status (odds ratio, 0.70; $p = 0.027$).

Fibrinolytic therapy is clearly less effective in patients with cardiogenic shock than in those without. The explanation for this lack of efficacy appears to be the low reperfusion rate achieved in this subset of patients. The reasons for decreased thrombolytic efficacy in patients with cardiogenic shock likely include hemodynamic, mechanical, and metabolic factors that prevent achievement and maintenance of infarct-related artery patency.[115] Attempts to increase reperfusion rates by increasing blood pressure with aggressive inotropic and pressor therapies and counterpulsation with an IABP make theoretical sense, and two small studies have supported the notion that vasopressor therapy improves thrombolytic efficacy.[115,116] The use of an IABP to augment aortic diastolic pressure also may increase the effectiveness of thrombolytics.

To date, emergency percutaneous revascularization is the only intervention that has been shown to reduce mortality rates consistently in patients with cardiogenic shock. Use of angioplasty in patients with cardiogenic shock grew out of its use as primary therapy in patients with MI. An analysis of the first 1000 patients treated with primary angioplasty at the Mid America Heart Institute showed a mortality rate of 44% in the subgroup of 79 patients presenting with cardiogenic shock, which was substantially lower than the 80% to 90% mortality rate in historical controls.[117] Most other reported case series also showed results with percutaneous intervention that were superior to those with fibrinolytic therapy or conservative medical management (mortality rates of approximately 40% to 50%).[20] Observational studies from registries of randomized trials have also reported improved outcomes in patients with cardiogenic shock selected for revascularization. Notable among these are the GUSTO-1 trial, in which patients treated with an "aggressive" strategy (coronary angiography performed within 24 hours of shock onset with revascularization by PTCA or CABG) had a significantly lower mortality rate (38% vs. 62%).[118] This benefit was present even after adjustment for baseline characteristics[118] and persisted to 1 year.[119]

The National Registry of Myocardial Infarction 2 (NRMI-2), which collected 26,280 patients with cardiogenic shock in the setting of MI between 1994 and 1997, similarly supported the association between revascularization and survival.[120] Improved short-term mortality rate was noted in those who underwent revascularization during the reference hospitalization by PTCA (12.8% vs. 43.9% mortality rate) or CABG (6.5%

vs. 23.9%).[120] These data complement the GUSTO-1 substudy data and are important, not only because of the sheer number of patients from whom these values are derived but also because NRMI-2 was a national cross-sectional study that more closely represents general clinical practice than carefully selected trial populations.

This extensive body of observational and registry studies showed consistent benefits from revascularization but could not be regarded as definitive due to their retrospective design. Two randomized controlled trials have evaluated revascularization for patients with MI.

The SHOCK study was a randomized, multicenter international trial that assigned patients with cardiogenic shock to receive optimal medical management, including IABP and thrombolytic therapy, or cardiac catheterization with revascularization using PTCA or CABG.[121,122] The trial enrolled 302 patients and was powered to detect a 20% absolute decrease in 30-day all-cause mortality rates. Mortality rates at 30 days were 46.7% in patients treated with early intervention and 56% in patients treated with initial medical stabilization, but this difference did not quite reach statistical significance ($p = 0.11$).[121] It is important to note that the control group (patients who received medical management) had a lower mortality rate than that reported in previous studies; this may reflect the aggressive use of thrombolytic therapy (64%) and IABP (86%) in these controls. These data provide indirect evidence that the combination of thrombolysis and IABP may produce the best outcomes when cardiac catheterization is not immediately available. At 6 months, the absolute risk reduction with early invasive therapy in the SHOCK trial was 13% (50.3% vs. 63.1%, $p = 0.027$),[121] and this risk reduction was maintained at 12 months (53.3% vs. 66.4% mortality rate, $p < 0.03$).[122] Subgroup analysis showed a substantial improvement in mortality rates in patients younger than 75 years at 30 days (41.4% vs. 56.8%, $p = 0.01$) and 6 months (44.9% vs. 65.0%, $p = 0.003$).[121]

The Swiss Multicenter Trial of Angioplasty for Shock (SMASH trial) was independently conceived and had a very similar design, although a more rigid definition of cardiogenic shock resulted in enrollment of sicker patients and a higher mortality rate.[123] The trial was terminated early due to difficulties in patient recruitment and enrolled only 55 patients. In the SMASH trial, a similar trend in 30-day absolute decrease in mortality rate similar to that in the SHOCK trial was observed (69% mortality rate in the invasive group vs. 78% in the medically managed group; relative risk, 0.88; 95% confidence interval, 0.6 to 1.2; $p = $ NS).[123] This benefit was also maintained at 1 year.

When the results of the SHOCK and SMASH trials are put into perspective with results from other randomized, controlled trials of patients with acute MI, an important point emerges: despite the moderate decrease in *relative* risk (0.72 for the SHOCK trial, with a 95% confidence interval of 0.54 to 0.95; and 0.88 for the SMASH trial, with a 95% confidence interval of 0.60 to 1.20), the *absolute* benefit is important, with nine lives saved for 100 patients treated at 30 days in both trials, and 13.2 lives saved for 100 patients treated at 1 year in the SHOCK trial. This latter figure corresponds to a number needed to treat of 7.6, one of the lowest figures ever observed in a randomized, controlled trial of cardiovascular disease.

On the basis of these randomized trials, the presence of cardiogenic shock in the setting of acute MI is a class I indication for emergency revascularization by PCI or CABG.[45]

INDICATIONS FOR TEMPORARY PACING IN ACUTE MYOCARDIAL INFARCTION

Damage to the impulse formation and conduction system of the heart from MI can result in bradyarrhythmias and conduction disturbances that do not respond reliably to conventional pharmacologic agents such as atropine or isoproterenol. These disturbances may lead to further hemodynamic compromise and coronary hypoperfusion. Disturbances of conduction distal to the atrioventricular node and the bundle of His are particularly worrisome, even if they are tolerated well hemodynamically. Ventricular escape rhythms in the setting of acute MI are unstable and unreliable; their discharge rate may vary widely, with abrupt acceleration to ventricular tachycardia or deceleration to asystole. It is this characteristic of subsidiary ventricular pacemakers that guides the indication for prophylactic placement of temporary transvenous pacing in acute MI (see Chap. 24). Table 25-4 lists these indications, which are based on studies documenting the progression to high-grade atrioventricular block when the indicated conduction disturbances are present. Any bradyarrhythmia unresponsive to atropine that results in hemodynamic compromises requires pacing.

TABLE 25-4 Indications for Temporary Transvenous Pacing in Acute Myocardial Infarction[a]

Class I
  Asystole
  Complete heart block
  Mobitz type II second-degree heart block
  Bilateral BBB (alternating BBB or RBBB with alternating LAFB/LPHB)
  New bifascicular block (RBBB with LAFB or LPHB or with LBBB) with first-degree AV block
  Symptomatic bradycardia
Class IIa
  New bifascicular block
  RBBB with first-degree AV block
  Incessant VT, for atrial or ventricular overdrive pacing
  Recurrent sinus pauses (>3 s) not responsive to atropine
  New LBBB[b]
Class IIb
  Bifascicular block of indeterminate age
  New isolated RBBB
Class III
  First-degree AV block
  Type I second-degree AV block
  Accelerated idioventricular rhythm

[a] Class I, general agreement that treatment is effective; class IIa, weight of evidence favors efficacy; class IIb, efficacy less well established by evidence or opinion; class III, general agreement treatment is not useful and in some cases may be harmful.
[b] Controversial.
ABBREVIATIONS: AV, atrioventricular; BBB, bundle branch block; LAFB, left anterior fascicular block; LPFB, left posterior fascicular block; LBBB, left bundle branch block; RBBB, right bundle branch block; VT, ventricular tachycardia.
SOURCE: Printed with permission from Ryan et al.[45]

References

1. Braunwald E: Control of myocardial oxygen consumption. Physiologic and clinical considerations. *Am J Cardiol* 27:416, 1971.

2. Sherman CT, Litvack F, Grundfest W, et al: Coronary angioscopy in patients with unstable angina pectoris. *N Engl J Med* 315:913, 1986.

3. Croft CH, Nicod P, Corbett JR, et al: Detection of acute right ventricular infarction by right precordial electrocardiography. *Am J Cardiol* 50:421, 1982.

4. Spodick DH: Diagnostic electrocardiographic sequences in acute pericarditis. Significance of PR segment and PR vector changes. *Circulation* 48:575, 1973.

5. Pepine CJ: Silent myocardial ischemia: Definition, magnitude, and scope of the problem. *Cardiol Clin* 4:577, 1986.

6. Upton MT, Rerych SK, Newman GE, et al: Detecting abnormalities in left ventricular function during exercise before angina and ST-segment depression. *Circulation* 62:341, 1980.

7. Sugishita Y, Koseki S, Matsuda M, et al: Dissociation between regional myocardial dysfunction and ECG changes during myocardial ischemia induced by exercise in patients with angina pectoris. *Am Heart J* 106(pt 1):1, 1983.

8. Rapaport E: Serum enzymes and isoenzymes in the diagnosis of acute myocardial infarction. Part II: Isoenzymes. *Mod Concepts Cardiovasc Dis* 46:47, 1977.

9. Lee TH, Goldman L: Serum enzyme assays in the diagnosis of acute myocardial infarction. Recommendations based on a quantitative analysis. *Ann Intern Med* 105:221, 1986.

10. Katus HA, Remppis A, Neumann FJ, et al: Diagnostic efficiency of troponin T measurements in acute myocardial infarction. *Circulation* 83:902, 1991.

11. Jaffe AS, Ravkilde J, Roberts R, et al: It's time for a change to a troponin standard. *Circulation* 102:1216, 2000.

12. Kaul S, Stratienko AA, Pollock SG, et al: Value of two-dimensional echocardiography for determining the basis of hemodynamic compromise in critically ill patients: A prospective study. *J Am Soc Echocardiogr* 7:598, 1994.

13. Feigenbaum H, Corya BC, Dillon JC, et al: Role of echocardiography in patients with coronary artery disease. *Am J Cardiol* 37:775, 1976.

14. Nishimura RA, Tajik AJ, Shub C, et al: Role of two-dimensional echocardiography in the prediction of in-hospital complications after acute myocardial infarction. *J Am Coll Cardiol* 4:1080, 1984.

15. Ribeiro A, Lindmarker P, Juhlin-Dannfelt A, et al: Echocardiography Doppler in pulmonary embolism: right ventricular dysfunction as a predictor of mortality rate. *Am Heart J* 134:479, 1997.

16. Reilly JP, Tunick PA, Timmermans RJ, et al: Contrast echocardiography clarifies uninterpretable wall motion in intensive care unit patients. *J Am Coll Cardiol* 35:485, 2000.

17. Parkey RW, Bonte FJ, Meyer SL, et al: A new method for radionuclide imaging of acute myocardial infarction in humans. *Circulation* 50:540, 1974.

18. Massie BM, Botvinick EH, Werner JA, et al: Myocardial scintigraphy with technetium-99m stannous pyrophosphate: an insensitive test for nontransmural myocardial infarction. *Am J Cardiol* 43:186, 1979.

19. Kontos MC, Jesse RL, Schmidt KL, et al: Value of acute rest sestamibi perfusion imaging for evaluation of patients admitted to the emergency department with chest pain. *J Am Coll Cardiol* 30:976, 1997.

20. Hollenberg SM, Kavinsky CJ, Parrillo JE: Cardiogenic shock. *Ann Intern Med* 131:47, 1999.

21. Hollenberg SM, Parrillo JE: Shock, in Longo DL (ed): *Harrison's Principles of Internal Medicine*, 14th ed. New York, McGraw-Hill, 1997, p 214.

22. Kinch JW, Ryan TJ: Right ventricular infarction. *N Engl J Med* 330:1211, 1994.

23. Hansen RM, Viquerat CE, Matthay MA, et al: Poor correlation between pulmonary arterial wedge pressure and left ventricular end-diastolic volume after coronary after bypass graft surgery. *Anesthesiology* 64:764, 1986.

24. Hollenberg SM, Hoyt JW: Pulmonary artery catheters in cardiovascular disease. *New Horizons* 5:207, 1997.

25. Connors AF Jr, Speroff T, Dawson NV, et al: The effectiveness of right heart catheterization in the initial care of critically ill patients. *JAMA* 276:889, 1996.

26. Zion MM, Balkin J, Rosenmann D, et al: Use of pulmonary artery catheters in patients with acute myocardial infarction. Analysis of experience in 5,841 patients in the SPRINT registry. *Chest* 98:1331, 1990.

27. Craven L: Experience with aspirin (acetylsalicylic acid) in the non-specific prophylaxis of coronary thrombosis. *Miss Valley Med J* 75:38, 1953.

28. Lewis HD Jr, Davis JW, Archibald DG, et al: Protective effects of aspirin against acute myocardial infarction and death in men with unstable angina. Results of a Veterans Administration cooperative study. *N Engl J Med* 309:396, 1983.

29. Theroux P, Ouimet H, McCans J, et al: Aspirin, heparin, or both to treat acute unstable angina. *N Engl J Med* 319:1105, 1988.

30. Steering Committee of the Physicians' Health Study Research Group: Final report on the aspirin component of the ongoing physicians' health study. *N Engl J Med* 321:129, 1989.

31. Platelet Receptor Inhibition in Ischemic Syndrome Management in Patients Limited by Unstable Signs and Symptoms (PRISM-PLUS) Study Investigators: Inhibition of the platelet glycoprotein IIb/IIIa receptor with tirofiban in unstable angina and non–Q-wave myocardial infarction. *N Engl J Med* 338:1488, 1998.

32. Ridker PM, Cushman M, Stampfer MJ, et al: Inflammation, aspirin, and the risk of cardiovascular disease in apparently healthy men. *N Engl J Med* 336:973, 1997.

33. Cohn PF, Gorlin R: Physiologic and clinical actions of nitroglycerin. *Med Clin North Am* 58:407, 1974.

34. Frishman WH: Multifactorial actions of beta-adrenergic blocking drugs in ischemic heart disease: current concepts. *Circulation* 67(pt 2):I11, 1983.

35. Oliva PB, Potts DE, Pluss RG: Coronary arterial spasm in Prinzmetal angina. Documentation by coronary arteriography. *N Engl J Med* 288:745, 1973.

36. Yusuf S, Sleight P, Pogue J, et al: Effects of an angiotensin-converting-enzyme inhibitor, ramipril, on cardiovascular events in high-risk patients. *N Engl J Med* 342:145, 2000.

37. Gibbons RJ, Abrams J, Chatterjee K, et al: ACC/AHA 2002 guideline update for the management of patients with chronic stable angina—summary article: a report of the American College of Cardiology/American Heart Association Task Force on Practice Guidelines (Committee on the Management of Patients With Chronic Stable Angina). *Circulation* 107:149, 2003.

38. Lipid Research Clinics Program: The lipid research clinics coronary primary prevention trial results. II. The relationship of reduction in incidence of coronary heart disease to cholesterol lowering. *JAMA* 251:365, 1984.

39. Frick MH, Elo O, Haapa K, et al: Helsinki heart study: primary-prevention trial with gemfibrozil in middle-aged men with dyslipidemia. Safety of treatment, changes in risk factors, and incidence of coronary heart disease. *N Engl J Med* 317:1237, 1987.

40. Sacks FM, Pfeffer MA, Moye LA, et al: The effect of pravastatin on coronary events after myocardial infarction in patients with average cholesterol levels. *N Engl J Med* 335:1001, 1996.

41. Long-Term Intervention with Pravastatin in Ischaemic Disease (LIPID) Study Group: Prevention of cardiovascular events and death with pravastatin in patients with coronary heart disease and a broad range of initial cholesterol levels. *N Engl J Med* 339:1349, 1998.

42. Cannon CP, Braunwald E, McCabe CH, et al: Intensive versus moderate lipid lowering with statins after acute coronary syndromes. *N Engl J Med* 350:1495, 2004.

43. Ferguson JJ III, Cohen M, Freedman RJ Jr, et al: The current practice of intra-aortic balloon counterpulsation: Results from the Benchmark Registry. *J Am Coll Cardiol* 38:1456, 2001.

44. Gewirtz H, Ohley W, Williams DO, et al: Effect of intraaortic balloon counterpulsation on regional myocardial blood flow and oxygen consumption in the presence of coronary artery stenosis: Observations in an awake animal model. *Am J Cardiol* 50:829, 1982.

45. Ryan TJ, Antman EM, Brooks NH, et al: 1999 update: ACC/AHA guidelines for the management of patients with acute myocardial infarction. A report of the American College of Cardiology/American Heart Association Task Force on Practice Guidelines (Committee on Management of Acute Myocardial Infarction). *J Am Coll Cardiol* 34:890, 1999.

46. Go AS, Barron HV, Rundle AC, et al: Bundle-branch block and in-hospital mortality in acute myocardial infarction. National Registry of Myocardial Infarction 2 Investigators. *Ann Intern Med* 129:690, 1998.

47. Gruppo Italiano per lo Studio della Streptochinasi nell'Infarto Miocardico (GISSI): Effectiveness of intravenous thrombolytic treatment in acute myocardial infarction. *Lancet* 1(8478):397, 1986.

48. TIMI Study Group: The Thrombolysis in Myocardial Infarction (TIMI) trial. Phase I findings. *N Engl J Med* 312:932, 1985.

49. TIMI Investigators: Effects of tissue plasminogen activator and a comparison of early invasive and conservative strategies in unstable angina and non–Q-wave myocardial infarction. Results of the TIMI IIIB Trial. *Circulation* 89:1545, 1994.

50. GUSTO Investigators: An international randomized trial comparing four thrombolytic strategies for acute myocardial infarction. *N Engl J Med* 329:673, 1993.

51. GUSTO Angiographic Investigators: The effects of tissue plasminogen activator, streptokinase, or both on coronary-artery patency, ventricular function, and survival after acute myocardial infarction. *N Engl J Med* 329:1615, 1993.

52. Global Use of Strategies to Open Occluded Coronary Arteries (GUSTO III) Investigators: A comparison of reteplase with alteplase for acute myocardial infarction. *N Engl J Med* 337:1118, 1997.

53. Assessment of the Safety and Efficacy of a New Thrombolytic Investigators: Single-bolus tenecteplase compared with front-loaded alteplase in acute myocardial infarction: The ASSENT-2 double-blind randomised trial. *Lancet* 354(9180):716, 1999.

54. Grines CL, Browne KF, Marco J, et al: A comparison of immediate angioplasty with thrombolytic therapy for acute myocardial infarction. The Primary Angioplasty in Myocardial Infarction Study Group. *N Engl J Med* 328:673, 1993.

55. GUSTO IIb Investigators: A comparison of recombinant hirudin with heparin for the treatment of acute coronary syndromes. *N Engl J Med* 335:775, 1996.

56. Cannon CP, Gibson CM, Lambrew CT, et al: Relationship of symptom-onset-to-balloon time and door-to-balloon time with mortality in patients undergoing angioplasty for acute myocardial infarction. *JAMA* 283:2941, 2000.

57. Canto JG, Every NR, Magid DJ, et al: The volume of primary angioplasty procedures and survival after acute myocardial infarction. National Registry of Myocardial Infarction 2 Investigators. *N Engl J Med* 342:1573, 2000.

58. Grines C, Patel A, Zijlstra F, et al: Primary coronary angioplasty compared with intravenous thrombolytic therapy for acute myocardial infarction: Six-month follow up and analysis of individual patient data from randomized trials. *Am Heart J* 145:47, 2003.

59. Keeley EC, Boura JA, Grines CL: Primary angioplasty versus intravenous thrombolytic therapy for acute myocardial infarction: A quantitative review of 23 randomised trials. *Lancet* 361(9351):13, 2003.

60. Rankin JM, Spinelli JJ, Carere RG, et al: Improved clinical outcome after widespread use of coronary-artery stenting in Canada. *N Engl J Med* 341:1957, 1999.

61. Stone GW, Brodie BR, Griffin JJ, et al: Clinical and angiographic follow-up after primary stenting in acute myocardial infarction: The Primary Angioplasty in Myocardial Infarction (PAMI) stent pilot trial. *Circulation* 99:1548, 1999.

62. Chew DP, Moliterno DJ: A critical appraisal of platelet glycoprotein IIb/IIIa inhibition. *J Am Coll Cardiol* 36:2028, 2000.

63. Lincoff AM, Califf RM, Moliterno DJ, et al: Complementary clinical benefits of coronary-artery stenting and blockade of platelet glycoprotein IIb/IIIa receptors. Evaluation of Platelet IIb/IIIa Inhibition in Stenting Investigators. *N Engl J Med* 341:319, 1999.

64. EPISTENT Investigators: Randomised placebo-controlled and balloon-angioplasty-controlled trial to assess safety of coronary stenting with use of platelet glycoprotein-IIb/IIIa blockade. *Lancet* 352(9122):87, 1998.

65. Montalescot G, Barragan P, Wittenberg O, et al: Platelet glycoprotein IIb/IIIa inhibition with coronary stenting for acute myocardial infarction. *N Engl J Med* 344:1895, 2001.

66. Stone GW, Grines CL, Cox DA, et al: Comparison of angioplasty with stenting, with or without abciximab, in acute myocardial infarction. *N Engl J Med* 346:957, 2002.

67. Ellis SG, da Silva ER, Heyndrickx G, et al: Randomized comparison of rescue angioplasty with conservative management of patients with early failure of thrombolysis for acute anterior myocardial infarction. *Circulation* 90:2280, 1994.

68. TIMI Study Group: Comparison of invasive and conservative strategies after treatment with intravenous tissue plasminogen activator in acute myocardial infarction. Results of the Thrombolysis In Myocardial Infarction (TIMI) phase II trial. *N Engl J Med* 320:618, 1989.

69. ISIS-2 (Second International Study of Infarct Survival) Collaborative Group: Randomised trial of intravenous streptokinase, oral aspirin, both, or neither among 17,187 cases of suspected acute myocardial infarction: ISIS-2. *Lancet* 2(8607):349, 1988.

70. Gruppo Italiano per lo Studio della Sopravvinza nell'Infarto Miocardico (GISSI): GISSI-3: Effects of lisinopril and transdermal glyceryl trinitrate singly and together on 6-week mortality and ventricular function after acute myocardial infarction. *Lancet* 343:1115, 1994.

71. ISIS-4 (Fourth International Study of Infarct Survival) Study Group: ISIS-4: A randomised factorial trial assessing early oral captopril, oral mononitrate, and intravenous magnesium sulphate in 58,050 patients with suspected acute myocardial infarction. *Lancet* 345:669, 1995.

72. First International Study of Infarct Survival Collaborative Group: Randomised trial of intravenous atenolol among 16 027 cases of suspected acute myocardial infarction: ISIS-1. *Lancet* 2(8498):57, 1986.

73. MIAMI Trial Research Group: Metoprolol in acute myocardial infarction (MIAMI). A randomised placebo-controlled international trial. *Eur Heart J* 6:199, 1985.

74. The International Collaborative Study Group: Reduction of infarct size with the early use of timolol in acute myocardial infarction. *N Engl J Med* 310:9, 1984.

75. CONSENSUS Trial Study Group: Effects of enalapril on mortality in severe congestive heart failure. Results of the Cooperative North Scandinavian Enalapril Survival Study (CONSENSUS). *N Engl J Med* 316:1429, 1987.

76. SOLVD Investigators: Effect of enalapril on survival in patients with reduced left ventricular ejection fractions and congestive heart failure. *N Engl J Med* 325:293, 1991.

77. SOLVD Investigators: Effect of enalapril on mortality and the development of heart failure in asymptomatic patients with

reduced left ventricular ejection fractions. *N Engl J Med* 327:685, 1992.

78. Pfeffer MA, Braunwald E, Moye LA, et al: Effect of captopril on mortality and morbidity in patients with left ventricular dysfunction after myocardial infarction. Results of the Survival and Ventricular Enlargement Trial. *N Engl J Med* 327:669, 1992.

79. Edner M, Bonarjee VV, Nilsen DW, et al: Effect of enalapril initiated early after acute myocardial infarction on heart failure parameters, with reference to clinical class and echocardiographic determinants. CONSENSUS II Multi-Echo Study Group. *Clin Cardiol* 19:543, 1996.

80. Gibson RS, Boden WE, Theroux P, et al: Diltiazem and reinfarction in patients with non–Q-wave myocardial infarction. Results of a double-blind, randomized, multicenter trial. *N Engl J Med* 315:423, 1986.

81. MacMahon S, Collins R, Peto R, et al: Effects of prophylactic lidocaine in suspected acute myocardial infarction. An overview of results from the randomized, controlled trials. *JAMA* 260:1910, 1988.

82. Lauler DP: Magnesium—Coming of age. *Am J Cardiol* 63:1g, 1989.

83. Braunwald E: Unstable angina. A classification. *Circulation* 80:410, 1989.

84. Ohman EM, Armstrong PW, Christenson RH, et al: Cardiac troponin T levels for risk stratification in acute myocardial ischemia. *N Engl J Med* 335:133, 1996.

85. Cairns JA, Gent M, Singer J, et al: Aspirin, sulfinpyrazone, or both in unstable angina. Results of a Canadian multicenter trial. *N Engl J Med* 313:1369, 1985.

86. Yusuf S, Zhao F, Mehta SR, et al: Effects of clopidogrel in addition to aspirin in patients with acute coronary syndromes without ST-segment elevation. *N Engl J Med* 345:494, 2001.

87. CAPRIE Steering Committee: A randomised, blinded, trial of clopidogrel versus aspirin in patients at risk of ischaemic events (CAPRIE). *Lancet* 348:1329, 1996.

88. Oler A, Whooley MA, Oler J, Grady D: Adding heparin to aspirin reduces the incidence of myocardial infarction and death in patients with unstable angina. A meta-analysis. *JAMA* 276:811, 1996.

89. Cohen M, Demers C, Gurfinkel EP, et al: A comparison of low-molecular-weight heparin with unfractionated heparin for unstable coronary artery disease. Efficacy and Safety of Subcutaneous Enoxaparin in Non–Q-Wave Coronary Events Study Group [see comments]. *N Engl J Med* 337:447, 1997.

90. Antman EM, McCabe CH, Gurfinkel EP, et al: Enoxaparin prevents death and cardiac ischemic events in unstable angina/non–Q-wave myocardial infarction. Results of the thrombolysis in myocardial infarction (TIMI) 11B trial. *Circulation* 100:1593, 1999.

91. Antman EM, Cohen M, Radley D, et al: Assessment of the treatment effect of enoxaparin for unstable angina/non–Q-wave myocardial infarction. TIMI 11B-ESSENCE meta-analysis. *Circulation* 100:1602, 1999.

92. Platelet Receptor Inhibition in Ischemic Syndrome Management (PRISM) Study Investigators: A Comparison of Aspirin plus Tirofiban with Aspirin plus Heparin for Unstable Angina. *N Engl J Med* 338:1498, 1998.

93. The PURSUIT Trial Investigators: Inhibition of platelet glycoprotein IIb/IIIa with eptifibatide in patients with acute coronary syndromes. *N Engl J Med* 339:436, 1998.

94. PARAGON Investigators: International, randomized, controlled trial of lamifiban (a platelet glycoprotein IIb/IIIa inhibitor), heparin, or both in unstable angina. *Circulation* 97:2386, 1998.

95. Simoons ML: Effect of glycoprotein IIb/IIIa receptor blocker abciximab on outcome in patients with acute coronary syndromes without early coronary revascularisation: The GUSTO IV-ACS randomised trial. *Lancet* 357(9272):1915, 2001.

96. CAPTURE Investigators: Randomised placebo-controlled trial of abciximab before and during coronary intervention in refractory unstable angina: The CAPTURE Study. *Lancet* 349:1429, 1997.

97. Boden WE, Ra OR, Crawford MH, et al: Outcomes in patients with acute non–Q-wave myocardial infarction randomly assigned to an invasive as compared with a conservative management strategy. *N Engl J Med* 338:1785, 1998.

98. Fragmin and Fast Revascularisation during Instability in Coronary Artery Disease Investigators: Invasive compared with non-invasive treatment in unstable coronary-artery disease: FRISC II prospective randomised multicentre study. *Lancet* 354(9180):708, 1999.

99. Cannon CP, Weintraub WS, Demopoulos LA, et al: Comparison of early invasive and conservative strategies in patients with unstable coronary syndromes treated with the glycoprotein IIb/IIIa inhibitor tirofiban. *N Engl J Med* 344:1879, 2001.

100. Reardon MJ, Carr CL, Diamond A, et al: Ischemic left ventricular free wall rupture: prediction, diagnosis, and treatment. *Ann Thorac Surg* 64:1509, 1997.

101. Killen DA, Piehler JM, Borkon AM, et al: Early repair of postinfarction ventricular septal rupture. *Ann Thorac Surg* 63:138, 1997.

102. Khan SS, Gray RJ: Valvular emergencies. *Cardiol Clin* 9:689, 1991.

103. Bolooki H: Emergency cardiac procedures in patients in cardiogenic shock due to complications of coronary artery disease. *Circulation* 79:I137, 1989.

104. Zehender M, Kasper W, Kauder E, et al: Right ventricular infarction as an independent predictor of prognosis after acute inferior myocardial infarction. *N Engl J Med* 328:981, 1993.

105. Dell'Italia LJ, Starling MR, Blumhardt R, et al: Comparative effects of volume loading, dobutamine, and nitroprusside in patients with predominant right ventricular infarction. *Circulation* 72:1327, 1985.

106. Bowers TR, O'Neill WW, Grines C, et al: Effect of reperfusion on biventricular function and survival after right ventricular infarction. *N Engl J Med* 338:933, 1998.

107. Goldberg RJ, Samad NA, Yarzebski J, et al: Temporal trends in cardiogenic shock complicating acute myocardial infarction. *N Engl J Med* 340:1162, 1999.

108. Hochman JS, Boland J, Sleeper LA, et al: Current spectrum of cardiogenic shock and effect of early revascularization on mortality. Results of an international registry. *Circulation* 91:873, 1995.

109. Holmes DR Jr, Bates ER, Kleiman NS, et al: Contemporary reperfusion therapy for cardiogenic shock: the GUSTO-I trial experience. The GUSTO-I Investigators. Global Utilization of Streptokinase and Tissue Plasminogen Activator for Occluded Coronary Arteries. *J Am Coll Cardiol* 26:668, 1995.

110. Alonso DR, Scheidt S, Post M, Killip T: Pathophysiology of cardiogenic shock. Quantification of myocardial necrosis, clinical, pathologic and electrocardiographic correlations. *Circulation* 48:588, 1973.

111. Willerson JT, Curry GC, Watson JT, et al: Intraaortic balloon counterpulsation in patients in cardiogenic shock, medically refractory left ventricular failure and/or recurrent ventricular tachycardia. *Am J Med* 58:183, 1975.

112. Bates ER, Stomel RJ, Hochman JS, Ohman EM: The use of intraaortic balloon counterpulsation as an adjunct to reperfusion therapy in cardiogenic shock. *Int J Cardiol* 65(suppl 1):S37, 1998.

113. Gruppo Italiano per lo Studio Della Streptochinasi Nell'Infarto Miocardico (GISSI): Effectiveness of intravenous thrombolytic treatment in acute myocardial infarction. *Lancet* 2:397, 1986.

114. Sanborn TA, Sleeper LA, Bates ER, et al: Impact of thrombolysis, intra-aortic balloon pump counterpulsation, and their combination in cardiogenic shock complicating acute myocardial infarction: a report from the SHOCK Trial Registry. Should we

emergently revascularize occluded coronaries for cardiogenic shock? *J Am Coll Cardiol* 36(suppl A):1123, 2000.

115. Becker RC: Hemodynamic, mechanical, and metabolic determinants of thrombolytic efficacy: A theoretic framework for assessing the limitations of thrombolysis in patients with cardiogenic shock. *Am Heart J* 125:919, 1993.

116. Garber PJ, Mathieson AL, Ducas J, et al: Thrombolytic therapy in cardiogenic shock: effect of increased aortic pressure and rapid tPA administration. *Can J Cardiol* 11:30, 1995.

117. O'Keefe JH Jr, Bailey WL, Rutherford BD, Hartzler GO: Primary angioplasty for acute myocardial infarction in 1,000 consecutive patients. Results in an unselected population and high-risk subgroups. *Am J Cardiol* 72:107G, 1993.

118. Berger PB, Holmes DR Jr, Stebbins AL, et al: Impact of an aggressive invasive catheterization and revascularization strategy on mortality in patients with cardiogenic shock in the Global Utilization of Streptokinase and Tissue Plasminogen Activator for Occluded Coronary Arteries (GUSTO-I) trial. An observational study. *Circulation* 96:122, 1997.

119. Berger PB, Tuttle RH, Holmes DR Jr, et al: One-year survival among patients with acute myocardial infarction complicated by cardiogenic shock, and its relation to early revascularization: Results from the GUSTO-I trial. *Circulation* 99:873, 1999.

120. Rogers WJ, Canto JG, Lambrew CT, et al: Temporal trends in the treatment of over 1.5 million patients with myocardial infarction in the US from 1990 through 1999: The National Registry of Myocardial Infarction 1, 2 and 3. *J Am Coll Cardiol* 36:2056, 2000.

121. Hochman JS, Sleeper LA, Webb JG, et al: Early revascularization in acute myocardial infarction complicated by cardiogenic shock. *N Engl J Med* 341:625, 1999.

122. Hochman JS, Sleeper LA, White HD, et al: One-year survival following early revascularization for cardiogenic shock. *JAMA* 285:190, 2001.

123. Urban P, Stauffer JC, Bleed D, et al: A randomized evaluation of early revascularization to treat shock complicating acute myocardial infarction. The (Swiss) Multicenter Trial of Angioplasty for Shock-(S)MASH. *Eur Heart J* 20:1030, 1999.

Chapter 26 _____
ACUTE RIGHT HEART SYNDROMES

IVOR S. DOUGLAS
GREGORY A. SCHMIDT

KEY POINTS

- *Right heart syndromes (RHS) as a cause of shock are less common than left heart dysfunction, but recognizing them requires a high level of vigilance.*

- *Clues to recognizing RHS as a cause of shock include a history of a condition that is associated with pulmonary hypertension, elevated neck veins, peripheral edema greater than pulmonary edema, or a right-sided third heart sound, in addition to electrocardiographic, radiographic, and echocardiographic findings.*

- *Echocardiography is extremely valuable, not only for demonstrating the presence of RHS, but also for guiding hemodynamic management.*

- *Progressive right heart shock can be worsened by excessive fluid infusion, concomitant left ventricular failure, inappropriate application of extrinsic positive end-expiratory pressure (PEEP) and hypoxia.*

- *The drug of choice for resuscitation of patients with acute RHS is dobutamine, initially infused at 5 µg/kg per minute. Systemically-active vasoconstrictors may provide additional benefit.*

- *Prostacyclin and nitric oxide are often beneficial in improving pulmonary hemodynamics and oxygenation, but may not improve survival.*

In the majority of patients with shock due to "pump failure," assessment is focused appropriately on the left ventricle. However, in a substantial minority of patients, right heart dysfunction is the cause of shock. Examples include acute pulmonary embolism (PE), other causes of acute right heart pressure overload (e.g., acute respiratory distress syndrome [ARDS] treated with positive pressure ventilation), acute deterioration in patients with chronic pulmonary hypertension, and right ventricular infarction. Although right ventricular infarction differs from the other right heart syndromes (RHS) in that the pulmonary artery pressure is not high, in many other regards right ventricular infarction resembles the other syndromes, so we will consider them together. Failure to consider the right heart in the differential diagnosis of shock risks incomplete or inappropriate treatment of the shock. It would be hard to overemphasize the importance of echocardiography, both in aiding the recognition of the right heart syndromes and in guiding management. In this chapter we review the notable features that distinguish the right heart from the left, describe the themes that unify the acute RHS and allow their recognition, discuss the pathophysiology and differential diagnosis of RHS, and review their management.

Right Ventricular Physiology

The right ventricle (RV) has long been considered the "forgotten ventricle," because under normal pressure and volume loading conditions the RV is thought to function as a passive conduit for systemic venous return. When the pulmonary vasculature is normal, right ventricular performance has little impact on the maintenance of cardiac output. In animal models, complete ablation of the right ventricular free wall has little effect on venous pressures.

Despite the requirement for an equal, average cardiac output between the left and right ventricles, the bioenergetic requirement for RV ejection is approximately one fifth of the left ventricle (LV). This is in large part accounted for by the significant difference in downstream vascular resistance between the systemic and pulmonary circulations. In comparison with the LV, the RV ejects into a low-resistance circuit (normally only one tenth the resistance of the systemic arteries).

The pressure-volume relationship of the normal RV differs significantly from that of the LV. In contrast to the LV ejection, the RV ejects into the pulmonary outflow tract early during systole, continuing even after the maximal development of RV systolic pressure.[1] This exaggerated "hang out" period (ventricular outflow between the onset of right ventricular pressure decline and pulmonary valve closure) optimizes pump efficiency and results in a triangular pressure-volume relationship compared with the square wave pump of the LV.

Under conditions of increased RV impedance (e.g., pulmonary stenosis or pulmonary embolism) the RV pressure-volume relationship assumes a square wave appearance similar to that of the LV.[2] Unlike the LV, however, even modest acute increases in RV afterload may precipitate ventricular failure. This is not the case if volume and pressure loading develop more chronically. Significant contractile reserve is supported by RV myocyte hypertrophy and is regulated in part by increased expression of angiotensin II, insulin-like growth factor-I, and endothelin-1.[3] Ventricular hypertrophy is not uniform and is frequently associated with regional diastolic and systolic dysfunction.[4] Increased cardiac output is accommodated by recruitment of previously unperfused pulmonary vessels and by distention of vessels.

However, when pulmonary vascular resistance and pulmonary artery (PA) pressure rise, right ventricular systolic function deteriorates more readily than that of the left ventricle. Right ventricular ejection fraction falls as mean PA pressure rises and RV end-systolic and end-diastolic pressures rise. During acute PA hypertension, RV preload, afterload, and contractile state rise at the same time that heart rate rises. These features join to raise the RV myocardial oxygen consumption. At the same time, when an acute RHS is sufficiently severe to cause systemic hypotension, coronary perfusion of the RV may fall. The combination of rising oxygen demand and falling coronary oxygen supply subjects the RV to ischemia sufficient to reduce RV contractility and reduce systolic ejection against the increased PA pressure afterload (Fig. 26-1). The close anatomic approximation between the right and left ventricles confers a mechanical and functional interdependence in the face of right ventricular dysfunction.

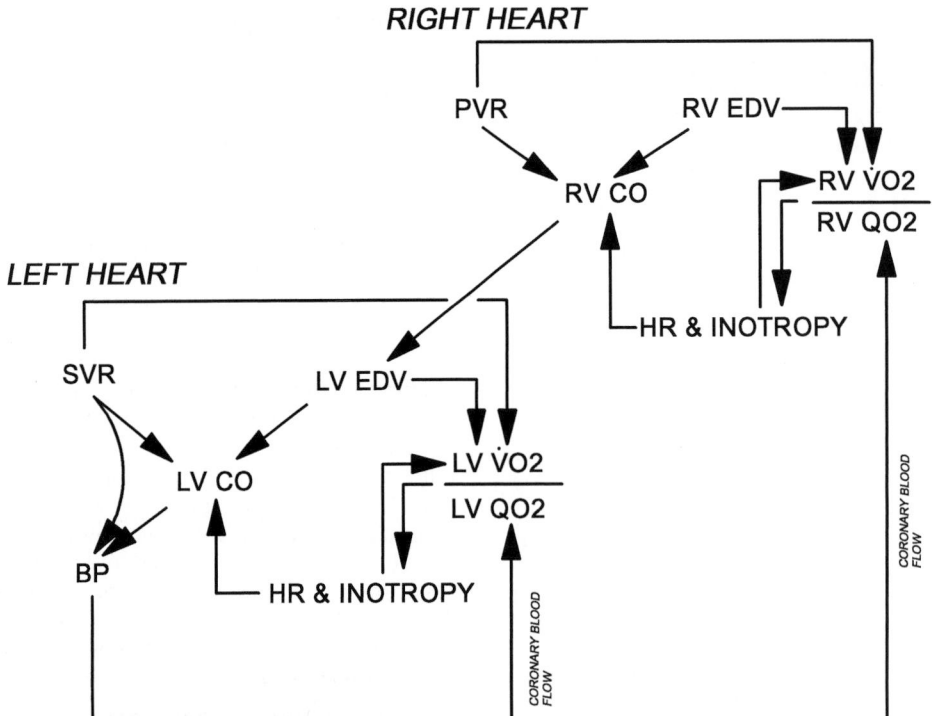

FIGURE 26-1 This figure illustrates the theory of right ventricular infarction in the right heart syndromes. A sudden rise in pulmonary artery pressure impedes right ventricular ejection. Right ventricular stroke volume falls, and end-diastolic and end-systolic volumes rise. Heart rate increases as the baroreceptors sense the fall in systemic blood pressure. These features of increased preload, afterload, and rate raise the right ventricular oxygen consumption. At the same time, the fall in aortic pressure lessens the driving gradient (roughly aortic pressure – right atrial pressure) for right coronary flow, reducing oxygen delivery to the right ventricle. If the rise in pulmonary artery pressure is sufficient, the right ventricle will fail. Vasoconstrictors have the potential to partially restore right ventricular function. Constriction of the systemic arteries raises left ventricular oxygen demands, but the normal left ventricle is operating with a margin of safety before the increased aortic pressure would be a problem. The higher aortic pressure drives more blood flow to the right ventricle without augmenting any of the components of right ventricular oxygen demand, thereby relieving ischemia and improving function.

Interdependence is influenced by (1) the cardiac fibroskeleton that limits acute annular distension, (2) the interventricular septum, and (3) the pericardium. As right heart pressures rise, the interventricular septum shifts progressively to the left, causing left ventricular diastolic dysfunction, further reducing systemic cardiac output and coronary perfusion pressure. Additionally, the pericardium restricts excessive acute ventricular distension while impairing diastolic filling of both the left and right heart. A vicious cycle ensues in which RV ischemia impairs right ventricular ejection, which leads to progressive dilation of the RV and septal displacement that causes more LV diastolic dysfunction, progressive systemic hypotension, and further impairment of RV perfusion.

This cycle has long been recognized in the acute inability of the RV to sustain a mean pulmonary artery pressure greater than about 40 mm Hg, based on studies of pulmonary hemodynamics in patients with acute PE without prior cardiopulmonary disease.[1,5]

There is significant evidence that RV ischemia underlies acute RV failure in settings of acute pulmonary hypertension. Indirect indications include the significantly increased load tolerance of the right ventricle when aortic pressure is raised,[6] and a beneficial hemodynamic response to infusion of norepinephrine.[7] These findings suggest, but do not establish, that greater coronary flow driven by the higher aortic pressure enhances RV function by relieving ischemia. More direct evidence comes from a biochemical analysis of the RV during PA constriction[8] (Table 26-1). In this experiment, constriction of the pulmonary artery led to both hemodynamic failure and to biochemical evidence of ischemia. Moreover, the infusion of a vasoconstrictor reversed the hemodynamic deterioration and reversed the biochemical evidence of ischemia. Additional support for the role of RV ischemia comes from the occasional patient with electrocardiographic evidence of RV infarction or elevated myocardium-derived enzymes (MB fractions of serum creatine phosphokinase and troponins). Significant troponin elevation may be an early and reliable marker of right ventricular dysfunction in acute pulmonary embolism, and has been shown to predict an adverse outcome.[9] Significant elevations of serum cardiac troponins T and I are thought to result from RV microinfarction.[10]

RECOGNIZING THE RIGHT HEART SYNDROMES: CLINICAL CLUES

In the hypoperfused patient, several clinical features should suggest the possibility of an acute right heart syndrome (Table 26-2). First, any history of pulmonary hypertension raises the possibility that the new shock state represents a (potentially minor) precipitant on top of preexisting right heart compromise (acute-on-chronic pulmonary hypertension; Table 26-3). When there is no antecedent history of pulmonary

TABLE 26-1 Right Ventricular Ischemia Due to Pulmonary Hypertension

Assay	Control	RV HTN	RV Failure	Phenylephrine
Creatine phosphate (mmol/g)	8.4	8.2	3.7	7.5
Lactate:pyruvate ratio	18	14	57	19

Simultaneous biopsies of the LV showed no change in creatine phosphate or lactate:pyruvate ratios at any stage of the experiment.
RV HTN, Right ventricular hypertension caused by pulmonary artery constriction; Phenylephrine, infusion at $1-3\mu g/kg$ per minute.
SOURCE: Data taken from Vlahakes et al.[8]

hypertension, elevated neck veins, a pulsatile liver, peripheral edema out of proportion to pulmonary edema, a right-sided third heart sound, or tricuspid regurgitation, these factors should alert the intensivist that she or he may be dealing with an RHS. The pulmonic component of the second heart sound may be loud, and the time interval between the aortic (A_2) and the pulmonary (P_2) components of the second heart sound (A_2-P_2 splitting) is increased in the presence of pulmonary hypertension. However, these findings are appreciable with a binaural stethoscope in only a minority of patients with acute pulmonary embolism,[11] and are probably too subjective to be useful. More sophisticated acoustic processing of digitally acquired heart sounds may provide an accurate estimation of pulmonary arterial pressures.[12]

Despite the insensitivity of individual clinical signs to detect and diagnose acute right heart syndromes, a combination of clinical features (symptoms of deep venous thrombosis [DVT]; an alternative diagnosis is less likely than PE; heart rate >100 bpm; immobilization or surgery in the previous 4 weeks; previous DVT or PE; hemoptysis; and cancer, being treated currently or within the previous 6 months) and laboratory results, especially serum D-dimer level, can be useful in excluding pulmonary embolism as a likely cause.[13]

Electrocardiographic (ECG) evidence of pulmonary hypertension includes right axis deviation or a rightward shift in axis, right atrial enlargement, right ventricular hypertrophy, right bundle-branch block (RBBB), right precordial T-wave inversions, and the $S_1Q_3T_3$ pattern. In the Prospective Investigation of Pulmonary Embolism Diagnosis (PIOPED) trial, fewer than 1 patient in 17 with proven pulmonary embolism had any of the patterns of acute right heart strain.[11] By contrast, the experience at a single Italian center of 160 cases of proven PE resulted in a higher rate of electrocardiographic abnormalities. Of all patients, 76% had at least one abnormality; RBBB in 47%, $S_1Q_3T_3$ in 37%, T-wave inversion in 32%, and an inferior distribution "pseudonecrosis pattern" in 11%.[14] This variation in detection between studies suggests relative insensitivity in the performance characteristics of the 12-lead ECG in broad groups of mixed severity right heart syndrome patients. However, in patients with hemodynamically signif-

icant pulmonary embolism, the likelihood of suggestive electrocardiographic findings is probably much higher. For example, among 49 patients with PE (all of whom had RV dilation and tricuspid regurgitation by echocardiography), 37 (76%) had electrocardiographic abnormalities strongly suggestive of PE, including at least three of the following: incomplete or complete RBBB; S waves greater than 1.5 mm in leads I and aVL; shift of the precordial transition zone to V_5; Q waves in leads III and aVF, but not lead II; right axis deviation or an indeterminate axis; low QRS voltage in the limb leads; or T-wave inversion in leads III and aVR or in leads V_1 to V_4.[15] The electrocardiographic signs of right ventricular infarction are described below in the section on right ventricular infarction.

TABLE 26-2 Clues to Recognition of Right Heart Syndromes

Elevated neck veins
Pulsatile liver
Peripheral >> lung edema
Right sided S_3, tricuspid regurgitation
Radiographic
Electrocardiographic
Echocardiographic

TABLE 26-3 Causes of the Acute Right Heart Syndrome

Acute pressure overload
  Pulmonary embolism
  ARDS
  Excessive PEEP, tidal volume, and alveolar pressure
  Air, amniotic, fat, or tumor microembolism
  Sepsis (rarely)
  Pulmonary leukostasis, leukoagglutination
  Extensive lung resection
  Drugs (e.g., heparin-protamine reaction) ✳
  Hypoxia
Acute-on-chronic PA hypertension
  Chronic lung diseases
    Emphysema, chronic bronchitis, bronchiectasis, cystic fibrosis
    Restrictive diseases of the lung
    Collagen vascular diseases of the lung
Thoracic cage deformities
  Kyphoscoliosis, thoracoplasty
Cardiovascular disorders
  Chronic thromboembolism
  Primary pulmonary hypertension
  Congenital heart diseases
  Pulmonary venoocclusive disease
Miscellaneous disorders
  Sleep disordered breathing
  Hyperviscosity syndromes
  Toxins and drugs
  Parasites
  End-stage liver disease
  HIV infection
Right ventricular systolic dysfunction
  RV infarction
  Sepsis
  Toxins

ABBREVIATIONS: ARDS, acute respiratory distress syndrome; HIV, human immunodeficiency virus; PA, pulmonary artery; PEEP, positive end-expiratory pressure; RV, right ventricular.

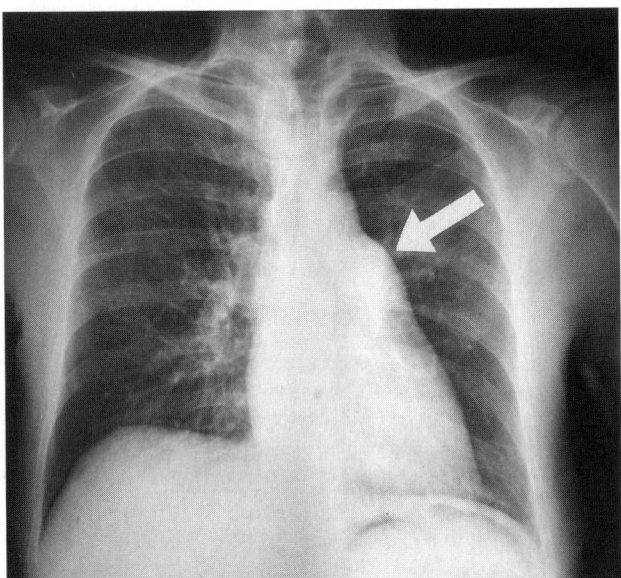

FIGURE 26-2 Chest radiograph demonstrating significant enlargement of the main pulmonary artery (*arrow*) in a young woman with chronic pulmonary hypertension due to recurrent pulmonary emboli.

Radiographic signs include an enlarged pulmonary artery or right ventricle, oligemia of a lobe or lung (Westermark's sign), and a distended azygos (or other central) vein (Figs. 26-2 and 26-3). Contrast-enhanced computed tomography of the pulmonary vasculature (helical CT angiography) has evolved as a central diagnostic tool in the evaluation of acute right heart syndromes, particularly pulmonary thromboembolism, as discussed in Chap. 27.[16–19] The sensitivities range from

53% to 89%, and specificities from 78% to 100% for single-slice helical CT diagnosis of acute PE.[20] Newer multi-row detector scanners should increase sensitivity to more than 90%.[21] In addition to detecting the presence of a pulmonary vascular clot, CT is able to detect RV dilatation and septal shift. In a small series of patients with acute PE, CT sensitivity was 78% for detecting RV dysfunction when compared with transthoracic echocardiography (TTE).[22]

Furthermore, TTE can be used to quantify pulmonary artery pressures and assess right ventricular function, thereby allowing for rapid initiation of appropriate therapeutic interventions. Echocardiography may also provide indirect evidence of pulmonary embolism by demonstrating a specific pattern of right ventricular dysfunction characterized by freewall hypokinesis with apical sparing, a finding possibly useful in differentiating pulmonary embolism from other causes of right ventricular dysfunction.[23–25] Finally, echocardiography can be used to visualize massive pulmonary embolism directly in many patients.[26] Therefore we believe that echocardiography is a practical and readily available diagnostic tool that should be considered in the evaluation of patients with suspected pulmonary embolism.

The typical echocardiographic findings include a normally contracting left ventricle, often with end-systolic obliteration of the LV cavity; a thin-walled, dilated, poorly contracting RV; right atrial enlargement; tricuspid insufficiency with a high-velocity regurgitant jet; increased estimated PA pressures; leftward shift of the interventricular septum causing the typical "D" shape of the LV on the short-axis view (Fig. 26-4); right PA dilation; or loss of respirophasic variation in the inferior vena cava.[27] RV infarction can usually be readily distinguished from acute pulmonary hypertension in that high PA pressures are lacking. Right ventricular diastolic dimensions can be obtained by measuring right ventricular end-diastolic area in the long axis, from an apical four-chamber view, or by a transesophageal approach in the volume-repleted patient.[28]

FIGURE 26-3 Chest radiograph showing a huge azygos vein (*arrow*) in an elderly man with shock due to acute massive pulmonary embolism. The normal vein measures less than 10 mm in transverse diameter, whereas this patient's azygos vein measures more than 22 mm. This film also demonstrates Westermark's sign (oligemia, here of all lung fields).

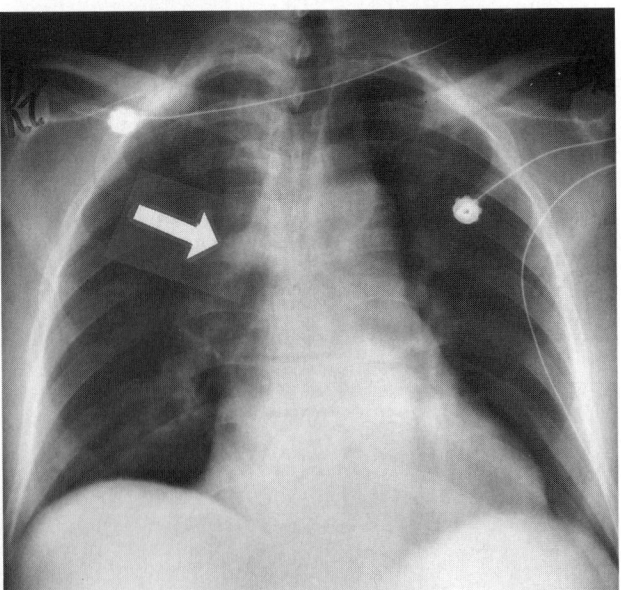

FIGURE 26-4 Echocardiographic short-axis view showing the obvious shift of the interventricular septum toward the left ventricle, changing the shape of the left ventricle from its normal circular cross-section to a "D" shape.

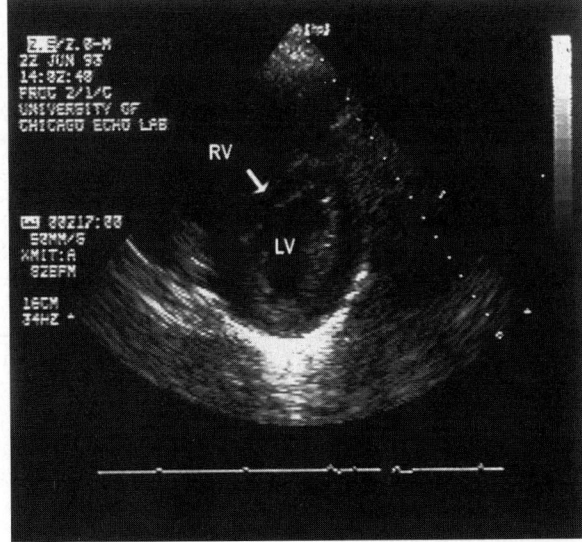

TABLE 26-4 Features of Right Heart Syndromes

Diagnosis not readily apparent: A high index of suspicion aids recognition
Routine therapy for congestive heart failure may be detrimental
Fluid loading may lower cardiac output
Vasodilators may cause abrupt deterioration
Vasoconstrictors may have a role in some patients
Echocardiography is extremely valuable

Echocardiography is of great utility in the detection of RHS and should be obtained early in the hypoperfused patient whenever one of the previously mentioned clinical indicators is present.[24] Of course, most of these signs are not specific for RHS, but their recognition is important because the treatment of RHS is unique in several regards (Table 26-4). TTE is particularly useful in differentiating at the bedside right ventricular pressure overload from myocardial infarction, aortic dissection, or pericardial tamponade, all of which may be clinically indistinguishable from PE.[29] Identification of a patent foramen ovale and free-floating right-heart thrombus are echocardiographic markers of particularly grave prognosis, including recurrent PE and death.[26,29,30]

Pulmonary artery catheterization can estimate pulmonary arterial pressures more accurately than echocardiography. However, interpretation of mean pulmonary pressures and measurement of tricuspid regurgitation by thermodilution are confounded by technical limitations. A pulmonary artery catheter (PAC) with a fast-response thermistor has been advocated for accurate measurement of right ventricular volume and hemodynamic parameters by thermodilution in the presence of tricuspid regurgitation. However, as is the case for PAC use in the management of ARDS and left heart shock, the fast-response thermistor PAC has not been demonstrated to confer an improvement in survival.

Severity of RV systolic failure is an independent determinant of serum levels of brain natriuretic peptide (BNP) in patients with severe heart failure.[31] Furthermore, BNP elevations have been demonstrated to predict RV dysfunction in patients with acute PE. In one study, the relative risk ratio for RV dysfunction was 28.4 (95% CI, 3.22 to 251.12) if the serum BNP >90 pg/mL.[32] A lower cut-off of 50 pg/mL might improve the specificity of BNP as a predictor of favorable outcome, but it remains unclear whether measurement of BNP has any role in these patients.[10,33]

Specific Right Heart Syndromes

ACUTE PULMONARY HYPERTENSION

Acute pulmonary hypertension is caused by an abrupt increase in pulmonary vascular resistance due to vascular obstruction or surgical resection. The prototype of acute pulmonary hypertension is acute pulmonary embolism (PE; see Chap. 27), but other forms of embolism (e.g., air or fat), microvascular injury (e.g., ARDS), drug effect, and inflammation can acutely raise pulmonary vascular resistance (see Table 26-3). For example, Zapol and Snider described the pulmonary hemodynamics in 30 patients with severe ARDS (20% survival; 8 had received extracorporeal membrane oxygenation).[34] Following correction of hypoxemia, the mean pulmonary artery pressure was about 30 mm Hg

and was abnormally elevated in all patients. Similar levels of pulmonary artery pressure were seen in a group of postsurgical patients with ARDS who were treated with nitric oxide (NO).[35] Mean pulmonary artery pressure fell from 33 ± 2 mm Hg to 28 ± 1 mm Hg when NO was inhaled at 18 ppm. Contributors to PA hypertension in ARDS include hypoxic pulmonary vasoconstriction, mediator release, high alveolar pressure during mechanical ventilation, and microthrombi.

The frequency of significant pulmonary hypertension in ARDS has not been clearly defined. In the patients studied by Zapol and Snider, right heart dysfunction was clinically significant, even when the change in PA pressures and pulmonary vascular resistance was small.[34] The large prospective European ARDS Collaborative Study evaluated pulmonary hemodynamic variables in 424 of 586 ARDS patients.[36] In most patients, PA pressure was modestly elevated on admission (26.1 ± 8.5 mm Hg) and was persistently elevated at 48 hours in nonsurvivors compared with survivors (28.4 ± 8.5 mm Hg versus 24.1 ± 6.7 mm Hg). The ratio of RV to LV stroke work was also significantly elevated in all patients, and along with the ratio of partial oxygen pressure to the fraction of inspired oxygen (OR 0.96 to 0.98), was identified as an independent predictor of survival (OR 20 to 85; $p = 0.0001$).

These findings would suggest an aggressive approach to lowering RV afterload in patients with ARDS by reducing alveolar pressures and administering inhaled nitric oxide or prostacyclin. However, despite reproducible reductions in PA pressure and improvements in oxygenation indices, randomized controlled studies using this approach have repeatedly failed to demonstrate a survival benefit, as discussed below.

Sepsis itself is probably capable of causing pulmonary hypertension, even in the absence of acute lung injury, based on animal models[37] and limited human studies.[38,39] Although common in patients with severe sepsis, it is our experience that acute pulmonary hypertension is only of clinical importance when ARDS (or another clear precipitant) is present. It seems likely that the systemic hypotension of septic shock makes the RV more vulnerable to ischemic systolic dysfunction when combined with modest increases in afterload.[40] It has been argued that this right ventricular perfusion gradient accounts for the differentially impaired perfusion and contractility of the RV compared with the LV in sepsis.[39] The sepsis-associated proinflammatory cytokines tumor necrosis factor-α and interleukin-1β have been demonstrated to have negative inotropic effects on the ventricular myocardium.

A notable insight into the complex role of endogenous nitric oxide in regulating pulmonary vascular tone in septic shock patients was derived from a randomized, placebo-controlled, double-blind study of the nitric oxide synthase inhibitor 546C88.[41] Patients who were randomized to the treatment arm had a 10% absolute higher mortality rate at 28 days than patients in the placebo arm. 546C88-treated patients had a greater incidence of pulmonary hypertension, with an initial increase in the pulmonary vascular resistance and a sustained reduction in the pulmonary venous admixture, possibly through augmented hypoxic pulmonary vasoconstriction. Three patients in the treatment arm developed right heart failure. It has been suggested that sepsis-associated NO production may have a partially protective effect on the pulmonary vasculature by optimizing pulmonary ventilation-perfusion relationships.

SICKLE CELL

Acute pulmonary hypertension in sickle chest syndrome results from pulmonary microvascular in-situ thrombosis, pulmonary fat embolism from infarcted long bone marrow, and hypoxic vasoconstriction. Recurrent episodes result in secondary chronic pulmonary hypertension and cor pulmonale. Inhaled NO, in addition to supplemental oxygen, blood transfusions, and bronchodilators, may provide some additional benefit for generalized vasoocclusive crises,[42] but has not been systematically studied for sickle-associated pulmonary hypertension.[43]

CPB

Acute right heart failure following cardiac surgery, especially in patients operated on for severe mitral valve disease, some congenital cardiac defects, acute pulmonary embolism, or following heart transplantation or institution of left ventricular mechanical assistance, continues to vex cardiac surgeons and surgical intensivists. The mechanisms underlying this are multifactorial[44] and include cardiopulmonary bypass–induced activation of pulmonary inflammatory pathways,[45] and impairment of nitric oxide production by pulmonary endothelial cells. A favorable response to inhaled NO has been demonstrated when used postoperatively[46,47] or perioperatively.[48] More recently, inhaled prostacyclin has been shown to improve PA hypertension and RV dysfunction.[49]

✱

In about 1.5% of CPB patients, reversal of heparin anticoagulation with protamine is accompanied by transient, at times intense, pulmonary vasoconstriction.[50] This phenomenon is thought to result from thromboxane B_2 generation.[50] Effective prophylaxis for this syndrome has not yet been reported. Inhibition of poly(ADP-ribose) polymerase, a terminal effector of oxidative stress injury, may offer future therapeutic opportunities for this syndrome.[51]

ACUTE-ON-CHRONIC PULMONARY HYPERTENSION

Many patients with acute RHS have preexisting pulmonary vascular disease, at times with clinically recognized pulmonary hypertension, but often without (see Table 26-3). In such patients, intercurrent critical illness may unmask pulmonary vascular disease when a higher-than-normal cardiac output is needed. For example, in 12 men with moderate to severe but stable chronic obstructive pulmonary disease (COPD), mean PA pressure was normal at rest (17 ± 6 mm Hg), and the systolic PA pressure ranged from 21 to 27 mm Hg.[52] During exercise (25 to 50 Watts), mean PA pressure rose significantly to 31 ± 11 mm Hg and systolic PA pressure to 20 to 55 mm Hg. At the same time, right ventricular end-diastolic volume increased, and right ventricular ejection fraction failed to rise.

When pulmonary hypertension is diagnosed during the course of critical illness, the potential for underlying chronic pulmonary vascular disease should be considered, especially when the history suggests chronic disease, the mean PA pressure is higher than 40 mm Hg, or echocardiography shows evidence of RV hypertrophy.

RIGHT VENTRICULAR INFARCTION

Right ventricular infarction is a well-recognized and fatal feature of inferior myocardial infarction.[53,54] It is also seen in anterior infarcts. Meta-analysis of six studies involving 1198 patients with RV myocardial involvement suggested an increased probability of death (OR 3.2; 95% CI 2.4 to 4.1) com-

pared with non RV MI.[55] In most cases RV free wall infarction or ischemia is accompanied by varying degrees of septal and posteroinferior left ventricular injury, but relatively isolated RV injury is occasionally seen. RV myocardial injury and dysfunction representing noninfarcted hibernating myocardium may be able to sustain long periods of low coronary oxygen delivery and ultimately recover substantial contractile function.[56]

RV dilation accompanies significant myocardial injury. Concomitant LV infarction involving the interventricular septum may lead to further hemodynamic deterioration in patients with RV infarction because of the loss of LV septal contraction which can assist RV ejection. Elevation of right atrial pressure on physical examination or direct measurement in a patient with an inferior myocardial infarction and clear lungs by exam and chest x-ray should lead to suspicion of RV infarction. When these features occur in a critically ill patient, the essential distinction is between RHS resulting from acute PA hypertension and RHS resulting from RV infarction. Confirmatory evidence includes a right precordial electrocardiogram or echocardiographic evidence of RV injury (see Chap. 25). The focus of management in RV infarction is on maintenance of optimal RV preloading to avoid worsened RV distension, preservation of RV synchrony, reduction in RV afterload (particularly when LV dysfunction is present), and inotropic and mechanical support of the RV.[57]

Early reperfusion with fibrinolytics or direct coronary intervention may have a role in many patients. Echocardiography can be highly useful in confirming RV infarction and in determining the response to therapeutic interventions.

Treatment

Some patients with acute RHS may benefit from specific therapies, such as thrombolysis for acute pulmonary embolism (see Chap. 27). In most patients, however, the two basic aims of treatment are supportive: to reduce systemic oxygen demand while improving oxygen delivery (Table 26-5). Oxygen demand can be lowered by treating fever, sedating the patient, instituting mechanical ventilation, and in severe cases, using therapeutic muscle relaxation. Oxygen delivery can be enhanced by correcting hypovolemia, transfusing red blood cells, relieving alveolar hypoxia, infusing vasoactive drugs, and avoiding detrimental ventilator settings. The goals of oxygen therapy in RHS are to enhance arterial saturation (Sa_{O_2}) and to block alveolar hypoxic vasoconstriction (AHV). Using a sufficient oxygen concentration to achieve 88% Sa_{O_2} is advocated in ARDS and other alveolar flooding diseases (see Chap. 38), but in RHS not associated with intrapulmonary

TABLE 26-5 Goals of Therapy in the Right Heart Syndromes

Correct hypoxemia

Find optimal volume

Exclude or treat concomitant left ventricular dysfunction

Minimize volume of oxygen utilization

Reduce intrinsic positive end-expiratory pressure and other causes of elevated alveolar pressure

Dobutamine, begin at 5 µg/kg per minute

Norepinephrine, begin at 0.4 µg/kg per minute

Nitric oxide, begin at 18 ppm

shunt, we target Sa_{O_2} to >96% to ensure alveolar oxygen values sufficient to block AHV (Pa_{O_2} >55 mm Hg). It may be useful to correct anemia with red blood cell transfusion, raising the arterial oxygen content, and reducing the necessary cardiac output. The resulting increased blood viscosity (and its tendency to raise pulmonary vascular resistance) probably does not outweigh the reduced demand for forward flow.

Fluid therapy, ventilator management, and vasoactive drug infusion are discussed below and have been the subject of a recent review.[58]

FLUID THERAPY

In most patients with shock it is appropriate to administer fluid, often in massive quantities, to restore left ventricular diastolic filling and boost cardiac output. Despite the recognition that the right heart becomes extremely preload dependent during ischemia and infarction,[56] excessive fluid administration is likely to worsen hemodynamic stability. In many of these patients the right-sided pressures are already well above normal, signaled by neck vein distention. Data from animal models of pulmonary embolism, as well as from studies of patients with right ventricular infarction, demonstrate that fluid therapy may be unhelpful or even detrimental.

In a canine autologous clot model of pulmonary embolism, the effects of fluid loading were studied before embolism, then following embolism.[59] Before embolism, fluid loading significantly raised the right atrial pressure, the transmural left ventricular end-diastolic pressure (LVEDP), and the left ventricular end-diastolic area index (a measure of left ventricular volume using sonomicrometry). Following multiple emboli, fluid loading raised right atrial pressure, but transmural LVEDP fell significantly as did the left ventricular end-diastolic area index. These findings indicate that fluid loading following embolism causes further leftward displacement of the interventricular septum, further compounding LV diastolic dysfunction. In a canine glass bead embolization model, fluid loading was found to precipitate right ventricular failure, even when relatively small volumes were infused.[60]

Similar results have been shown in human right ventricular infarction.[61,62] Despite raising the right atrial and wedge pressures, fluid loading failed to increase the cardiac index, blood pressure, or left and right ventricular stroke work. These findings should serve as a caution regarding fluid administration to patients with shock due to acute RHS. Since some patients may be volume depleted at presentation, a fluid challenge is reasonable, especially if the neck veins are flat or right heart filling pressures are low. Nevertheless, fluid should be given with a healthy degree of skepticism and careful attention to the consequences. We recommend that a discrete crystalloid fluid bolus of no more than 250 mL be administered while assessing relevant indicators of perfusion such as blood pressure, heart rate, pulsus paradoxus, cardiac output, central venous oxyhemoglobin saturation, or urine output. If no benefit can be detected, further fluids should not be given, and attention should shift to vasoactive drugs.

VASOACTIVE DRUG THERAPY

A wide variety of vasoactive drugs has been tried in patients or animal models for the treatment of acute RHS due to pulmonary embolism, ARDS, or right ventricular infarction, with variable success. These include nonspecific vasodilators (hydralazine[63] and nitroprusside[61,64,65]), vasoconstrictors (norepinephrine,[7,60,66] epinephrine,[67] phenylephrine,[8,68] dopamine,[69] and vasopressin[70,71]), inotropes (dobutamine,[61,62,72–74] amrinone,[75] milrinone,[76] isoproterenol,[7] epinephrine,[67] and levosimendan[77]), and pulmonary vasodilators (prostaglandin E_1,[78,79] prostaglandin I_2,[35] and nitric oxide[35,65,70,80–86]). Predicting the response to any of these drugs a priori is complicated by their tendency toward opposing effects. Conflicting data from studies of an agent in different animal models suggest that the interspecies variation and prevailing pulmonary vascular tone are important in determining if a particular agent has a predominantly pulmonary vasodilatory or vasoconstricting effect.[73,74] Thus the choice of vasoactive drugs cannot be based solely on the presumed pathophysiology, but also must be based on the results of human and animal studies summarized below. We contend that a vasoactive drug is effective in RHS when it significantly raises cardiac output without significantly worsening systemic hypotension, Sa_{O_2}, or RV ischemia. Dobutamine is our preferred positive inotrope, inhaled NO (and perhaps aerosolized prostacyclin) have salutary short-term physiologic effects as pulmonary vasodilators, and norepinephrine may provide added benefit as a systemic vasoconstrictor and positive inotrope by raising coronary perfusion pressure to an ischemic RV.

CATECHOLAMINES

In massive pulmonary embolism, dobutamine and norepinephrine appear superior to other vasoactive drugs.[7,72] In human PE, dobutamine has been most intensively studied. For example, of 10 patients with shock due to massive PE treated with dobutamine, 1 rapidly died, but 9 showed impressive hemodynamic improvement (Table 26-6). These results show that dobutamine improves cardiac output by improving right ventricular function or reducing pulmonary vascular resistance. Although fewer data are available regarding norepinephrine in human embolism, animal studies and limited human data support its use.[7,66,72] In a canine model of pulmonary embolism, dobutamine and dopamine had essentially identical hemodynamic effects.[69] Data from a separate canine study suggest that at doses less than 10 μg/kg per minute, dobutamine-induced pulmonary circulatory changes are exclusively flow dependent.[74] At higher doses, changes in pulmonary vascular resistance are variable and may depend on the prevailing pulmonary vascular tone. These drugs

TABLE 26-6 Dobutamine for Shock Due to Massive Pulmonary Embolism in 10 Patients

	Preinfusion	Dobutamine
Pao (mm Hg)	81	86
Ppa (mm Hg)	32	31
Pra (mm Hg)	13	11
Ppw (mm Hg)	12	11
CI (L/min per m²)	1.7	2.3
HR (beats/min)	108	86
$P\bar{v}_{O_2}$ (torr)	24	29

[a]Mean dobutamine dose 8.3 μg/kg per minute; values after 30 minutes.
CI, cardiac index; HR, heart rate; Pao, mean aortic pressure; Ppa, mean pulmonary artery pressure; Ppw, pulmonary artery wedge pressure; Pra, right atrial pressure; $P\bar{v}_{O_2}$, mixed venous oxygen pressure.
SOURCE: Data taken from Jardin et al.[72]

should be titrated according to clinical measures of the adequacy of perfusion, such as renal function, mentation, thermodilution cardiac output, or central venous oxyhemoglobin saturation, rather than to blood pressure alone. We begin dobutamine at 5 μg/kg per minute, raising the dose in increments of 5 μg/kg per minute every 10 minutes. If the patient fails to respond to dobutamine (or the response is incomplete), we substitute (or add) norepinephrine infused at 0.4 to 4 μg/kg per minute. In patients with hypoperfusion due to right ventricular infarction, dobutamine is superior to nitroprusside[61] (and to fluid infusion[61,62]), significantly improving right ventricular ejection fraction and cardiac output. Therefore dobutamine is the drug of first choice in all cases of RHS. We avoid the use of dopamine because of its highly variable pharmacokinetics and concern for disproportionate splanchnic vasoconstriction, even in relatively low doses.

VASOPRESSIN

The role of vasopressin (and its longer acting congener, terlipressin) remains controversial and incompletely evaluated. Vasopressin clearly functions as a systemic vasoconstrictor at high doses. In patients with septic shock, replacement of acutely depleted endogenous vasopressin with a low-dose infusion (0.04 U/min) is thought to improve catecholamine sensitivity via the functionally vasoconstricting V_1 receptor. The pulmonary vasculature has been shown by some investigators to express V_1 receptors, but that vasopressinergic stimuli may paradoxically mediate pulmonary vasodilation.[87,88] This might suggest a salutary potential for vasopressin therapy in acute right heart syndromes. In a canine model, however, vasopressin caused both systemic and pulmonary vasoconstriction while impairing RV contractility.[71] Our present practice is to avoid vasopressin for acute right heart syndromes unless catecholamine-dependent septic shock is present.

PROSTAGLANDINS

Prostaglandin E_1 (PGE$_1$) is a potent pulmonary vasodilator that exhibited promise in the treatment of ARDS. When infused at a dose of 0.02 to 0.04 μg/kg per minute to patients with severe ARDS and mean PA pressure greater than 20 mm Hg, PA pressure fell 15% despite an increase in cardiac output. At the same time, however, systemic blood pressure fell to a similar degree, and intrapulmonary shunting rose significantly.[78] In an oleic acid model of porcine ARDS, PGE$_1$ lowered pulmonary artery pressure, but stroke volume and stroke work did not improve significantly.[79] In patients with ARDS given prostacyclin (4 ng/kg per minute), pulmonary artery pressure fell, RV ejection fraction rose, and cardiac output increased significantly.[35] A small series of patients with chronic pulmonary hypertension have been given aerosolized prostacyclin, and they demonstrated pulmonary vasodilation, increased cardiac output, and improved arterial oxyhemoglobin saturation.[89] Systemic blood pressure fell somewhat, but to a much lesser degree than when prostacyclin was infused intravenously (for similar degrees of pulmonary vascular effect). When compared for acute hemodynamic effects in patients with primary pulmonary hypertension (PPH), aerosolized prostacyclin (approximately 14 ng/kg per minute over 15 minutes) was demonstrated to be a pharmacologically more potent acute vasodilator than inhaled NO (NO 40 ppm for 15 minutes).[90]

In a similar comparison in ARDS patients, gas exchange parameters were comparably improved when inhaled prostacyclin (7.5 $\pm$ 2.5 ng/kg per minute) was compared with inhaled NO at a dose lower than that in the PPH study (17.8 $\pm$ 2.7 ppm).[91] This may suggest that in patients with right heart syndromes and long-standing pulmonary hypertension, inhaled prostacyclin may afford greater efficacy.

Although not conclusively demonstrated, inhaled prostacyclin has been used with some success in perioperative acute RHS.

ADENOSINE

Adenosine is an endogenous vasodilator that has a very short half-life (less than 10 seconds) due to rapid metabolism by adenosine deaminase. When used following cardiac surgery, adenosine lowered pulmonary artery pressure, raised cardiac output, and did not cause hypotension.[46,92] Adenosine was infused centrally at a dose of 50 μg/kg per minute.

PHOSPHODIESTERASE INHIBITORS: AMRINONE, MILRINONE, DIPYRIDAMOLE, AND SILDENAFIL

Amrinone is an inotrope and vasodilator with potential in the acute right heart syndromes. In a canine model of massive embolism, amrinone (0.75 mg/kg bolus followed by 7.5 μg/kg per minute) lowered pulmonary artery pressure, raised cardiac output, and raised systemic blood pressure.[75] Limited data are available for the use of milrinone in acute RHS and its use is limited by a long half-life and limited ability of titration.[76] Additionally, milrinone has been shown to be less efficacious than inhaled NO in treating pulmonary hypertension post–cardiac surgery.[82] Another phosphodiesterase inhibitor, dipyridamole, has been evaluated as an adjunct to NO in pediatric patients with acute RHF, and shown to have some additional pulmonary vasodilatory effects.[93,94]

Significant interest has arisen in the therapeutic potential of the selective type 5 PDE inhibitor sildenafil, presently approved for male erectile dysfunction. Impressive acute reductions in pulmonary arterial pressures have been demonstrated with oral and intravenous administration in animal models of acute lung injury[95] and RHS, in patients with established pulmonary hypertension,[96] and in 93 patients with pulmonary hypertension complicating pulmonary fibrosis.[97] Additionally, synergistic effects of selective PDE inhibitors in combination with inhaled and intravenous vasodilators has been demonstrated in acute lung injury–associated right heart syndromes.[98–100]

NITRIC OXIDE

Nitric oxide brings together the potential for hemodynamic as well as gas exchange improvement. When patients with ARDS and pulmonary hypertension were given NO via endotracheal inhalation at a dose of 18 ppm, PA pressure fell, right ventricular ejection fraction rose, and RV end-systolic and end-diastolic volumes fell.[35] There was no detectable change in mean arterial pressure, and arterial oxygen pressure rose significantly. Increasing the dose of NO to 36 ppm had no incremental effect. These findings have been confirmed in similar patients with ARDS who were managed with permissive hypercapnia (mean arterial carbon dioxide pressure = 71 mm Hg) and given a lower dose of NO (5 ppm), although the effect was more modest.[80] Disappointingly, survival has not been improved in four large randomized controlled studies of NO in ARDS patients.[83–86]

ANTIPROLIFERATIVE AGENTS

Both prostacyclin and the newer nonselective endothelin receptor antagonists (ETRA) have been demonstrated to have antiproliferative activity on the pulmonary vasculature. This mechanism has been suggested to account for the modest functional improvement in patients with chronic pulmonary hypertension.[101,102] Although single case reports suggest beneficial effects of the orally administered nonselective ETRA bosentan, this agent has not been subjected to rigorous evaluation in patients with acute right heart syndromes, and it may have limited potential in critically ill patients because of significant associated hepatic toxicity.

VENTILATOR MANAGEMENT

Ventilator manipulation has the potential to dramatically affect the circulation in patients with shock, including those with acute RHS. For example, in animal models of shock, institution of mechanical ventilation significantly prolongs survival, an effect much greater than that seen with fluid therapy or vasoactive drugs. Of particular interest in patients with RHS is the maintenance of oxygenation, the role of hypercapnia (including permissive hypercapnia), and the effects of tidal volume and positive end-expiratory pressure (PEEP).

Hypercapnia increases pulmonary artery pressure. In patients with ARDS, reducing minute ventilation as part of the strategy of permissive hypercapnia leads to small but real increases in mean pulmonary artery pressure.[103–105] In most patients with ARDS who do not exhibit right heart limitation, this effect of hypercapnia is probably unimportant. However, in the subset of patients with severe pulmonary hypertension, permissive hypercapnia may lead to unacceptable hemodynamic deterioration.

The effect of PEEP on right ventricular function is complex, controversial, and highly variable from patient to patient.[106,107] Many studies are limited by the failure to correlate hemodynamic pressures to juxtacardiac pressure. The effect of PEEP can be expected to differ depending on whether atelectatic or flooded lung is recruited, or whether relatively normal lung is overdistended. In a study of patients with ARDS, PEEP had little effect on RV function when given in amounts up to that associated with improving respiratory system compliance.[106] At higher levels of PEEP, the dominant effect was to impair RV systolic function.

The dominant effect of mechanical ventilation is related to its effect on preload. Sustained airway pressure increases in volume-repleted patients with normal RV function result in a mild increase in right atrial pressure that is offset by increases in abdominal pressures that sustain venous return. However, it remains to be determined if this is true for patients with acute RHS and elevated right heart pressures.[108] Large-tidal-volume breathing impairs RV systolic function, presumably by increasing pulmonary vascular resistance in alveolar vessels. In a canine model with normal lungs, raising the tidal volume above 10 mL/kg caused a detectable rightward and downward shift of the RV function curve.[109]

These effects of mechanical ventilation on right ventricular function suggest the following strategy in patients with critical compromise of the RV: (1) give sufficient oxygen to reverse any hypoxic vasoconstriction; (2) avoid hypercapnia; (3) keep PEEP at or below a level at which continued alveolar recruitment can be demonstrated and seek to minimize self-controlled PEEP (Auto-PEEP); and (4) use the lowest tidal volume necessary to effect adequate elimination of carbon dioxide. Of course, the acute effects of each intervention should be measured to confirm that cardiac output increases. These principles are consonant with the goals of ventilation in most patients with ARDS, except that when there is an RHS, hypercapnia should be avoided if it leads to further hemodynamic deterioration.

MECHANICAL THERAPY

In contrast to the now well-defined role for mechanical assist devices in decompensated left heart failure,[110] there remains relatively little experience with mechanical therapy for the failing right heart. Notably, progressive right ventricular dysfunction complicates left ventricular assist device implantation or orthotopic heart transplantation for decompensated left heart failure[111,112] and is associated with progressive end-organ dysfunction.[113] The presently available approaches include extracorporeal and paracorporeal pulsatile and centrifugal pump ventricular assist systems.[75,76] An alternative approach uses a right atrial catheter to draw blood into a centrifugal pump and a percutaneously placed pulmonary artery catheter as the outflow cannula.[114] Small implantable centrifugal pumps are under development.

References

1. Redington AN, Gray HH, Hodson ME, et al: Characterisation of the normal right ventricular pressure-volume relation by biplane angiography and simultaneous micromanometer pressure measurements. *Br Heart J* 59:23, 1988.
2. Redington AN: Right ventricular function. *Cardiol Clin* 20:341, v, 2002.
3. Modesti PA, Vanni S, Bertolozzi I, et al: Different growth factor activation in the right and left ventricles in experimental volume overload. *Hypertension* 43:101, 2004.
4. Quaife RA, Lynch D, Badesch DB, et al: Right ventricular phenotypic characteristics in subjects with primary pulmonary hypertension or idiopathic dilated cardiomyopathy. *J Card Fail* 5:46, 1999.
5. McIntyre KM, Sasahara AA: The hemodynamic response to pulmonary embolism in patients without prior cardiopulmonary disease. *Am J Cardiol* 28:288, 1971.
6. Scharf S, Warner K, Josa M, et al: Load tolerance of the right ventricle: effect of increased aortic pressure. *J Crit Care* 1:163, 1986.
7. Molloy WD, Lee KY, Girling L, et al: Treatment of shock in a canine model of pulmonary embolism. *Am Rev Respir Dis* 130:870, 1984.
8. Vlahakes GJ, Turley K, Hoffman JI: The pathophysiology of failure in acute right ventricular hypertension: hemodynamic and biochemical correlations. *Circulation* 63:87, 1981.
9. Konstantinides S, Geibel A, Olschewski M, et al: Importance of cardiac troponins I and T in risk stratification of patients with acute pulmonary embolism. *Circulation* 106:1263, 2002.
10. Kucher N, Goldhaber SZ: Cardiac biomarkers for risk stratification of patients with acute pulmonary embolism. *Circulation* 108:2191, 2003.
11. Stein PD, Terrin ML, Hales CA, et al: Clinical, laboratory, roentgenographic, and electrocardiographic findings in patients

with acute pulmonary embolism and no pre-existing cardiac or pulmonary disease. *Chest* 100:598, 1991.

12. Xu J, Durand LG, Pibarot P: A new, simple, and accurate method for non-invasive estimation of pulmonary arterial pressure. *Heart* 88:76, 2002.

13. Wells PS, Anderson DR, Rodger M, et al: Derivation of a simple clinical model to categorize patients probability of pulmonary embolism: increasing the models utility with the SimpliRED D-dimer. *Thromb Haemost* 83:416, 2000.

14. Casazza F, Agostoni O, Mandelli V, Morpurgo M: [The cardiologist facing pulmonary embolism. The experience of 160 cases of acute cor pulmonale.] *Ital Heart J* 1:520, 2000.

15. Sreeram N, Cheriex EC, Smeets JL, et al: Value of the 12-lead electrocardiogram at hospital admission in the diagnosis of pulmonary embolism. *Am J Cardiol* 73:298, 1994.

16. Kanne JP, Lalani TA: Role of computed tomography and magnetic resonance imaging for deep venous thrombosis and pulmonary embolism. *Circulation* 109:I15, 2004.

17. Gulsun M, Goodman LR: CT for the diagnosis of venous thromboembolic disease. *Curr Opin Pulm Med* 9:367, 2003.

18. MacDonald SL, Mayo JR: Computed tomography of acute pulmonary embolism. *Semin Ultrasound CT MR* 24:217, 2003.

19. Enden T, Klow NE: CT pulmonary angiography and suspected acute pulmonary embolism. *Acta Radiol* 44:310, 2003.

20. Remy-Jardin M, Mastora I, Remy J: Pulmonary embolus imaging with multislice CT. *Radiol Clin North Am* 41:507, 2003.

21. Schoepf UJ, Costello P: Multidetector-row CT imaging of pulmonary embolism. *Semin Roentgenol* 38:106, 2003.

22. Contractor S, Maldjian PD, Sharma VK, Gor DM: Role of helical CT in detecting right ventricular dysfunction secondary to acute pulmonary embolism. *J Comput Assist Tomogr* 26:587, 2002.

23. Kasper W, Meinertz T, Kerstin F, et al: Echocardiography in assessing acute pulmonary hypertension due to pulmonary embolism. *Am J Cardiol* 45:567, 1980.

24. Vieillard-Baron A, Prin S, Chergui K, et al: Echo-Doppler demonstration of acute cor pulmonale at the bedside in the medical intensive care unit. *Am J Respir Crit Care Med* 166:1310, 2002.

25. Vieillard-Baron A, Qanadli SD, Antakly Y, et al: Transesophageal echocardiography for the diagnosis of pulmonary embolism with acute cor pulmonale: a comparison with radiological procedures. *Intensive Care Med* 24:429, 1998.

26. Chartier L, Bera J, Delomez M, et al: Free-floating thrombi in the right heart: diagnosis, management, and prognostic indexes in 38 consecutive patients. *Circulation* 99:2779, 1999.

27. Jardin F, Dubourg O, Bourdarias JP: Echocardiographic pattern of acute cor pulmonale. *Chest* 111:209, 1997.

28. Bommer W, Weinert L, Neumann A, et al: Determination of right atrial and right ventricular size by two-dimensional echocardiography. *Circulation* 60:91, 1979.

29. Goldhaber SZ: Pulmonary embolism. *N Engl J Med* 339:93, 1998.

30. Goldhaber SZ: Echocardiography in the management of pulmonary embolism. *Ann Intern Med* 136:691, 2002.

31. Troughton RW, Prior DL, Pereira JJ, et al: Plasma B-type natriuretic peptide levels in systolic heart failure: importance of left ventricular diastolic function and right ventricular systolic function. *J Am Coll Cardiol* 43:416, 2004.

32. Kruger S, Graf J, Merx MW, et al: Brain natriuretic peptide predicts right heart failure in patients with acute pulmonary embolism. *Am Heart J* 147:60, 2004.

33. Kucher N, Printzen G, Goldhaber SZ: Prognostic role of brain natriuretic peptide in acute pulmonary embolism. *Circulation* 107:2545, 2003.

34. Zapol WM, Snider MT: Pulmonary hypertension in severe acute respiratory failure. *N Engl J Med* 296:476, 1977.

35. Rossaint R, Slama K, Steudel W, et al: Effects of inhaled nitric oxide on right ventricular function in severe acute respiratory distress syndrome. *Intensive Care Med* 21:197, 1995.

36. Squara P, Dhainaut JF, Artigas A, Carlet J: Hemodynamic profile in severe ARDS: results of the European Collaborative ARDS Study. *Intensive Care Med* 24:1018, 1998.

37. Dehring DJ, Fader RC, Traber LD, Traber DL: Cardiopulmonary changes occurring with pulmonary intravascular clearance of live bacteria in sheep. *Circ Shock* 29:245, 1989.

38. Reuse C, Frank N, Contempre B, Vincent JL: Right ventricular function in septic shock. *Intensive Care Med* 14(Suppl 2):486, 1988.

39. Kumar A, Haery C, Parrillo JE: Myocardial dysfunction in septic shock: Part I. Clinical manifestation of cardiovascular dysfunction. *J Cardiothorac Vasc Anesth* 15:364, 2001.

40. Schneider AJ, Teule GJ, Groeneveld AB, et al: Biventricular performance during volume loading in patients with early septic shock, with emphasis on the right ventricle: a combined hemodynamic and radionuclide study. *Am Heart J* 116:103, 1988.

41. Lopez A, Lorente JA, Steingrub J, et al: Multiple-center, randomized, placebo-controlled, double-blind study of the nitric oxide synthase inhibitor 546C88: effect on survival in patients with septic shock. *Crit Care Med* 32:21, 2004.

42. Weiner DL, Hibberd PL, Betit P, et al: Preliminary assessment of inhaled nitric oxide for acute vaso-occlusive crisis in pediatric patients with sickle cell disease. *JAMA* 289:1136, 2003.

43. Sullivan KJ, Goodwin SR, Evangelist J, et al: Nitric oxide successfully used to treat acute chest syndrome of sickle cell disease in a young adolescent. *Crit Care Med* 27:2563, 1999.

44. Paparella D, Yau TM, Young E: Cardiopulmonary bypass induced inflammation: pathophysiology and treatment. An update. *Eur J Cardiothorac Surg* 21:232, 2002.

45. Khan TA, Bianchi C, Araujo EG, et al: Activation of pulmonary mitogen-activated protein kinases during cardiopulmonary bypass. *J Surg Res* 115:56, 2003.

46. Fullerton DA, Jones SD, Grover FL, McIntyre RC Jr.: Adenosine effectively controls pulmonary hypertension after cardiac operations. *Ann Thorac Surg* 61:1118, 1996; discussion 1123.

47. Beck JR, Mongero LB, Kroslowitz RM, et al: Inhaled nitric oxide improves hemodynamics in patients with acute pulmonary hypertension after high-risk cardiac surgery. *Perfusion* 14:37, 1999.

48. Miller OI, Tang SF, Keech A, et al: Inhaled nitric oxide and prevention of pulmonary hypertension after congenital heart surgery: a randomised double-blind study. *Lancet* 356:1464, 2000.

49. Theodoraki K, Rellia P, Thanopoulos A, et al: Inhaled iloprost controls pulmonary hypertension after cardiopulmonary bypass. *Can J Anaesth* 49:963, 2002.

50. Kreil EMG, Robinson DR, et al: Adverse heparin-protamine neutralization interactions and the lung, in Zapol W, Lemaire F (eds): *Adult Respiratory Distress Syndrome*. New York, Marcel Dekker, 1991, p 451.

51. Szabo G, Soos P, Bahrle S, et al: Role of poly(ADP-ribose) polymerase activation in the pathogenesis of cardiopulmonary dysfunction in a canine model of cardiopulmonary bypass. *Eur J Cardiothorac Surg* 25:825, 2004.

52. Mahler DA, Brent BN, Loke J, et al: Right ventricular performance and central circulatory hemodynamics during upright exercise in patients with chronic obstructive pulmonary disease. *Am Rev Respir Dis* 130:722, 1984.

53. Serrano CV, Ramires JA, Cesar LA, et al: Prognostic significance of right ventricular dysfunction in patients with acute inferior myocardial infarction and right ventricular involvement. *Clin Cardiol* 18:199, 1995.

54. Cohn JN, Guiha NH, Broder MI, Limas CJ: Right ventricular infarction. Clinical and hemodynamic features. *Am J Cardiol* 33:209, 1974.

55. Mehta SR, Eikelboom JW, Natarajan MK, et al: Impact of right ventricular involvement on mortality and morbidity in patients with inferior myocardial infarction. *J Am Coll Cardiol* 37:37, 2001.

56. Goldstein JA: Right heart ischemia: pathophysiology, natural history, and clinical management. *Prog Cardiovasc Dis* 40:325, 1998.

57. Jacobs AK, Leopold JA, Bates E, et al: Cardiogenic shock caused by right ventricular infarction: a report from the SHOCK registry. *J Am Coll Cardiol* 41:1273, 2003.

58. Mebazaa A, Karpati P, Renaud E, Algotsson L: Acute right ventricular failure—from pathophysiology to new treatments. *Intensive Care Med* 30:185, 2004.

59. Belenkie I, Dani R, Smith ER, Tyberg JV: Effects of volume loading during experimental acute pulmonary embolism. *Circulation* 80:178, 1989.

60. Ghignone M, Girling L, Prewitt RM: Volume expansion versus norepinephrine in treatment of a low cardiac output complicating an acute increase in right ventricular afterload in dogs. *Anesthesiology* 60:132, 1984.

61. Dell'Italia LJ, Starling MR, Blumhardt R, et al: Comparative effects of volume loading, dobutamine, and nitroprusside in patients with predominant right ventricular infarction. *Circulation* 72:1327, 1985.

62. Ferrario M, Poli A, Previtali M, et al: Hemodynamics of volume loading compared with dobutamine in severe right ventricular infarction. *Am J Cardiol* 74:329, 1994.

63. Bates ER, Crevey BJ, Sprague FR, Pitt B: Oral hydralazine therapy for acute pulmonary embolism and low output state. *Arch Intern Med* 141:1537, 1981.

64. Calvin J, Langlois S, Garneys G: Ventricular interaction in a canine model of acute pulmonary hypertension and its modulation by vasoactive drugs. *J Crit Care* 13:43, 1988.

65. Cockrill BA, Kacmarek RM, Fifer MA, et al: Comparison of the effects of nitric oxide, nitroprusside, and nifedipine on hemodynamics and right ventricular contractility in patients with chronic pulmonary hypertension. *Chest* 119:128, 2001.

66. Angle MR, Molloy DW, Penner B, et al: The cardiopulmonary and renal hemodynamic effects of norepinephrine in canine pulmonary embolism. *Chest* 95:1333, 1989.

67. Boulain T, Lanotte R, Legras A, Perrotin D: Efficacy of epinephrine therapy in shock complicating pulmonary embolism. *Chest* 104:300, 1993.

68. Hirsch LJ, Rooney MW, Wat SS, et al: Norepinephrine and phenylephrine effects on right ventricular function in experimental canine pulmonary embolism. *Chest* 100:796, 1991.

69. Ducas J, Stitz M, Gu S, et al: Pulmonary vascular pressure-flow characteristics. Effects of dopamine before and after pulmonary embolism. *Am Rev Respir Dis* 146:307, 1992.

70. Wasson S, Govindarajan G, Reddy HK, Flaker G: The role of nitric oxide and vasopressin in refractory right heart failure. *J Cardiovasc Pharmacol Ther* 9:9, 2004.

71. Leather HA, Segers P, Berends N, et al: Effects of vasopressin on right ventricular function in an experimental model of acute pulmonary hypertension. *Crit Care Med* 30:2548, 2002.

72. Jardin F, Genevray B, Brun-Ney D, Margairaz A: Dobutamine: a hemodynamic evaluation in pulmonary embolism shock. *Crit Care Med* 13:1009, 1985.

73. Bradford KK, Deb B, Pearl RG: Combination therapy with inhaled nitric oxide and intravenous dobutamine during pulmonary hypertension in the rabbit. *J Cardiovasc Pharmacol* 36:146, 2002.

74. Pagnamenta A, Fesler P, Vandinivit A, et al: Pulmonary vascular effects of dobutamine in experimental pulmonary hypertension. *Crit Care Med* 31:1140, 2003.

75. Wolfe MW, Saad RM, Spence TH: Hemodynamic effects of amrinone in a canine model of massive pulmonary embolism. *Chest* 102:274, 1992.

76. Kihara S, Kawai A, Fukuda T, et al: Effects of milrinone for right ventricular failure after left ventricular assist device implantation. *Heart Vessels* 16:69, 2002.

77. Leather HA, Ver Eycken K, Segers P, et al: Effects of levosimendan on right ventricular function and ventriculovascular coupling in open chest pigs. *Crit Care Med* 31:2339, 2003.

78. Melot C, Lejeune P, Leeman M, et al: Prostaglandin E1 in the adult respiratory distress syndrome. Benefit for pulmonary hypertension and cost for pulmonary gas exchange. *Am Rev Respir Dis* 139:106, 1989.

79. Bolliger C, Fourie P, Coetzee A: The effect of prostaglandin E1 on acute pulmonary artery hypertension during oleic acid-induced respiratory dysfunction. *Chest* 99:1501, 1991.

80. Fierobe L, Brunet F, Dhainaut JF, et al: Effect of inhaled nitric oxide on right ventricular function in adult respiratory distress syndrome. *Am J Respir Crit Care Med* 151:1414, 1995.

81. Kaisers U, Busch T, Deja M, et al: Selective pulmonary vasodilation in acute respiratory distress syndrome. *Crit Care Med* 31:S337, 2003.

82. Solina A, Papp D, Ginsberg S, et al: A comparison of inhaled nitric oxide and milrinone for the treatment of pulmonary hypertension in adult cardiac surgery patients. *J Cardiothorac Vasc Anesth* 14:12, 2000.

83. Lundin S, Mang H, Smithies M, et al: Inhalation of nitric oxide in acute lung injury: results of a European multicentre study. The European Study Group of Inhaled Nitric Oxide. *Intensive Care Med* 25:911, 1999.

84. Dellinger RP, Zimmerman JL, Taylor RW, et al: Effects of inhaled nitric oxide in patients with acute respiratory distress syndrome: results of a randomized phase II trial. Inhaled Nitric Oxide in ARDS Study Group. *Crit Care Med* 26:15, 1998.

85. Taylor RW, Zimmerman JL, Dellinger RP, et al: Low-dose inhaled nitric oxide in patients with acute lung injury: a randomized controlled trial. *JAMA* 291:1603, 2004.

86. Troncy E, Collet JP, Shapiro S, et al: Inhaled nitric oxide in acute respiratory distress syndrome: a pilot randomized controlled study. *Am J Respir Crit Care Med* 157:1483, 1998.

87. Eichinger MR, Walker BR: Enhanced pulmonary arterial dilation to arginine vasopressin in chronically hypoxic rats. *Am J Physiol* 267:H2413, 1994.

88. Evora PR, Pearson PJ, Schaff HV: Arginine vasopressin induces endothelium-dependent vasodilatation of the pulmonary artery. V1-receptor-mediated production of nitric oxide. *Chest* 103:1241, 1993.

89. Olschewski H, Walmrath D, Schermuly R, et al: Aerosolized prostacyclin and iloprost in severe pulmonary hypertension. *Ann Intern Med* 124:820, 1996.

90. Hoeper MM, Olschewski H, Ghofrani HA, et al: A comparison of the acute hemodynamic effects of inhaled nitric oxide and aerosolized iloprost in primary pulmonary hypertension. German PPH study group. *J Am Coll Cardiol* 35:176, 2000.

91. Walmrath D, Schneider T, Schermuly R, et al: Direct comparison of inhaled nitric oxide and aerosolized prostacyclin in acute respiratory distress syndrome. *Am J Respir Crit Care Med* 153:991, 1996.

92. Fullerton DA, Kirson LE, Jones SD, McIntyre RC Jr.: Adenosine is a selective pulmonary vasodilator in cardiac surgical patients. *Chest* 109:41, 1996.

93. Ziegler JW, Ivy DD, Wiggins JW, et al: Effects of dipyridamole and inhaled nitric oxide in pediatric patients with pulmonary hypertension. *Am J Respir Crit Care Med* 158:1388, 1998.

94. Kinsella JP, Torielli F, Ziegler JW, et al: Dipyridamole augmentation of response to nitric oxide. *Lancet* 346:647, 1995.

95. Wang L, Zhu du M, Su X, et al: Acute cardiopulmonary effects of a dual-endothelin receptor antagonist on oleic acid-induced pulmonary arterial hypertension in dogs. *Exp Lung Res* 30:31, 2004.

96. Mikhail GW, Prasad SK, Li W, et al: Clinical and haemodynamic effects of sildenafil in pulmonary hypertension: acute and mid-term effects. *Eur Heart J* 25:431, 2004.

97. Ghofrani HA Wiedemann R, Rose F, et al: Sildenafil for treatment of lung fibrosis and pulmonary hypertension: a randomised controlled trial. *Lancet* 360:895, 2002.

98. Schermuly RT, Leuchte H, Ghofrani HA, et al: Zardaverine and aerosolised iloprost in a model of acute respiratory failure. *Eur Respir J* 22:342, 2003.

99. Bigatello LM, Hess D, Dennehy KC, et al: Sildenafil can increase the response to inhaled nitric oxide. *Anesthesiology* 92:1827, 2000.

100. Atz AM, Wessel DL: Sildenafil ameliorates effects of inhaled nitric oxide withdrawal. *Anesthesiology* 91:307, 1999.

101. Rubin L, Badesch D, Barst R: Bosentan therapy for pulmonary arterial hypertension. *N Engl J Med* 346:896, 2002.

102. Galie N, Hinderliter AL, Torbicki A, et al: Effects of the oral endothelin-receptor antagonist bosentan on echocardiographic and doppler measures in patients with pulmonary arterial hypertension. *J Am Coll Cardiol* 41:1380, 2003.

103. Amato MB, Barbas CS, Medeiros DM, et al: Beneficial effects of the "open lung approach" with low distending pressures in acute respiratory distress syndrome. A prospective randomized study on mechanical ventilation. *Am J Respir Crit Care Med* 152:1835, 1995.

104. Puybasset L, Stewart T, Rouby JJ, et al: Inhaled nitric oxide reverses the increase in pulmonary vascular resistance induced by permissive hypercapnia in patients with acute respiratory distress syndrome. *Anesthesiology* 80:1254, 1994.

105. Rose CE Jr., Van Benthuysen K, Jackson JT, et al: Right ventricular performance during increased afterload impaired by hypercapnic acidosis in conscious dogs. *Circ Res* 52:76, 1983.

106. Jardin F, Brun-Ney D, Hardy A, et al: Combined thermodilution and two-dimensional echocardiographic evaluation of right ventricular function during respiratory support with PEEP. *Chest* 99:162, 1991.

107. Pinsky MR, Desmet JM, Vincent JL: Effect of positive end-expiratory pressure on right ventricular function in humans. *Am Rev Respir Dis* 146:681, 1992.

108. van den Berg PC, Jansen JR, Pinsky MR: Effect of positive pressure on venous return in volume-loaded cardiac surgical patients. *J Appl Physiol* 92:1223, 2002.

109. Pinsky MR: Determinants of pulmonary arterial flow variation during respiration. *J Appl Physiol* 56:1237, 1984.

110. Rose EA, Gelijns AC, Moskowitz AJ, et al: Long-term mechanical left ventricular assistance for end-stage heart failure. *N Engl J Med* 345:1435, 2001.

111. Reiss N, El-Banayosy A, Mirow N, et al: Implantation of the Biomedicus centrifugal pump in post-transplant right heart failure. *J Cardiovasc Surg (Torino)* 41:691, 2000.

112. Chen JM, Levin HR, Rose EA, et al: Experience with right ventricular assist devices for perioperative right-sided circulatory failure. *Ann Thorac Surg* 61:305, 1996; discussion 311.

113. Kavarana MN, Pessin-Minsley MS, Urtecho J, et al: Right ventricular dysfunction and organ failure in left ventricular assist device recipients: a continuing problem. *Ann Thorac Surg* 73:745, 2002.

114. Yano M, Onitsuka T, Shibata K, Koga Y: Efficacy and safety of a percutaneous right ventricular assist system. *Ann Thorac Surg* 61:1231, 1996.

Chapter 27 _____

PULMONARY EMBOLIC DISORDERS: THROMBUS, AIR, AND FAT

NUALA J. MEYER
GREGORY A. SCHMIDT

KEY POINTS

- *Pulmonary embolism (PE) is common, underdiagnosed, and lethal, yet readily treatable.*
- *Prophylaxis and accurate diagnosis are essential to improving outcome.*
- *The cause of death in PE is most often circulatory failure (acute cor pulmonale) due to right heart ischemia.*
- *There is no perfect diagnostic test for PE; accurate diagnosis requires both an informed clinical pretest probability and a stepwise application of tests including D-dimer, helical CT angiography, and lower extremity duplex.*
- *A careful risk assessment may identify patients ideal for outpatient therapy. Conversely, patients with hypotension, cancer, heart failure, hypoxemia, and present or prior deep vein thrombosis are at significantly higher risk for death, recurrence, or major bleeding from PE, and are best managed in an appropriately monitored setting.*
- *Low molecular weight heparin (LMWH) is approved and recommended as the initial therapy for PE, and should be used in most patients unless there exists a compelling reason to do otherwise. When LMWH is not used, unfractionated heparin is typically used to maintain the partial thromboplastin time at 1.5 to 2.5 times control. Numerous new anticoagulants are being tested and may soon be approved for the treatment of PE.*
- *Critically ill patients may especially benefit from aggressive use of vena caval interruption.*
- *Thrombolytic therapy is life-saving in patients with massive embolism and circulatory instability.*
- *Air and fat embolism usually present as acute respiratory distress syndrome, and are managed with mechanical ventilation, oxygen, and positive end-expiratory pressure.*

This chapter will cover diseases involving embolism to the pulmonary circulation, including pulmonary thromboembolism, as well as the less common conditions of venous air embolism and fat embolism. Thromboembolism is predominantly an acute circulatory insult, with important but less dramatic consequences for gas exchange. In contrast, both air and fat embolism usually present as acute hypoxemic respiratory failure (AHRF). All three of these forms of embolism may cause acute right heart failure, which is more fully discussed in Chap. 26.

Pulmonary Thromboembolism

Pulmonary embolism (PE) is a dramatic and life-threatening complication of underlying deep venous thrombosis (DVT). Therefore, much of the management of PE is grounded in the prophylaxis, diagnosis, and treatment of DVT. Much of our knowledge about DVT and PE is derived from patients who are not critically ill. When generalizations regarding clinical manifestations, utility of diagnostic tests, and efficacy of therapeutic approaches are extrapolated to the critically ill population, it is with some risk.

Pulmonary thromboembolism is a common yet underdiagnosed illness which accounts for substantial morbidity and mortality. It was estimated nearly 25 years ago that 630,000 persons each year suffer PE in the United States alone, with nearly 200,000 deaths (Fig. 27-1).[1] The incidence of PE over the past two decades may be decreasing[2] but this is controversial.[3,4] Recent hospital-based studies estimate an incidence of 1 case per 1000 persons per year, with 200,000 to 300,000 annual hospitalizations.[5,6] Data on mortality from PE are less problematic; a recent analysis of all U.S. death certificates between 1979 and 1998 found that PE mortality has decreased substantially over the past 20 years, from over 35,000 deaths in 1979 to fewer than 25,000 deaths in 1998.[7] Accurate estimates for its incidence and lethality are notoriously difficult to calculate, for reasons largely related to difficulties in diagnosis and data collection.[3,8] However, there is general consensus that venous thromboembolism is underdiagnosed. Failure to diagnose PE is a serious management error since 30% of untreated patients die, while only 8% succumb with effective therapy.

ICU patients are not a homogenous group of patients and the incidence of thromboembolism ranges widely across subsets of patients (Table 27-1). For example, in one study of medical ICU patients, 33 percent were found to have deep venous thrombosis, despite prophylaxis in more than half of them.[9] Among patients with DVT, half of them had thrombi in the proximal lower extremity, a site associated with a high risk of embolization. In addition, 15% of thrombi were catheter-associated thrombi in the upper extremities. One prospective study found that 33% of ICU patients with a central venous catheter had a sonographically detectable thrombus in the internal jugular or subclavian vein; of note, none of these patients were symptomatic, and none developed a symptomatic pulmonary embolus.[10] In trying to devise prophylactic and diagnostic plans, intensivists should take into account the patient mix in their own ICUs.

In spite of great strides in the understanding of venous thromboembolism, PE continues to cause substantial morbidity and mortality. Critically ill patients form a unique and challenging subset of those at risk. The presence of indwelling lines and forced immobility make these patients particularly susceptible to venous thromboemboli. Diagnosis, which is difficult even in ambulatory patients, is further impeded by barriers to communication and physical examination. Moreover, alternate explanations for hypoxemia, lung infiltrates, respiratory failure, and hemodynamic instability are readily available, such that a diagnosis of pulmonary thromboembolism may not be seriously considered. Finally, critically ill patients are likely to have limited cardiopulmonary reserve, so that pulmonary emboli may be particularly lethal.

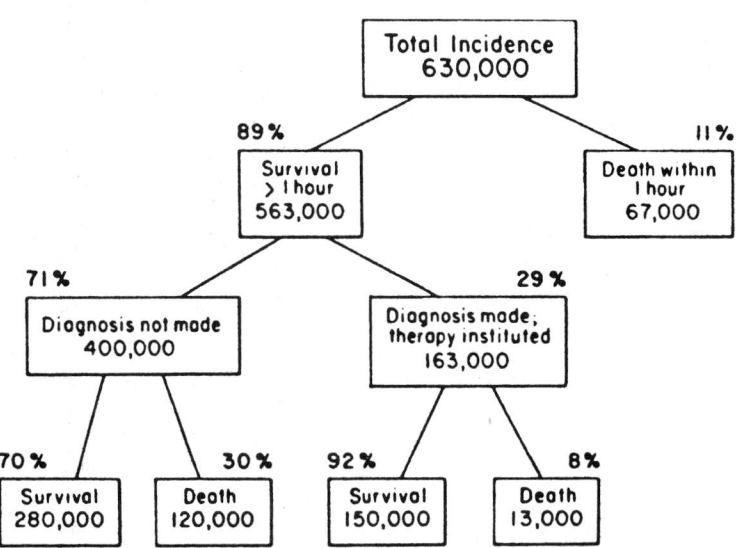

FIGURE 27-1 Natural history of pulmonary embolism based on reasonable extrapolations from known data. (*Reproduced with permission from Dalen et al.*[1])

PATHOPHYSIOLOGY

Venous thrombosis begins with the formation of microthrombi at a site of venous stasis or injury. Thrombosis impedes flow and generates further vascular injury, favoring progressive clot formation. In some patients, clot becomes substantial and propagates to a proximal vein where it has the potential to embolize to the pulmonary circulation. Most clinically relevant pulmonary emboli originate as proximal venous thrombi in the leg or pelvic veins. However, in the ICU, the routine placement of upper body catheters for vascular access, monitoring, drug administration, and nutrition raises the likelihood of important upper body sources of thrombi. How significantly these line-related upper body thrombi contribute to PE in critically ill patients is unknown, but they clearly have embolic potential.[15] Such upper extremity thrombi have important implications for diagnostic strategies based on detection of lower extremity thrombi and therapies such as inferior vena caval interruption which presume a lower extremity source.

PE occurs when thrombi detach and are carried through the great veins to the pulmonary circulation. Pulmonary vascular occlusion has important physiologic consequences which lead to the manifestations of illness as well as to clues to diagnosis. PE has an impact most notably on gas exchange and the circulation.

GAS EXCHANGE

Physical obstruction to pulmonary artery (PA) flow creates dead space in the segments served by the affected arteries. This creation of dead space has several effects on the partial pressure of carbon dioxide (P_{CO_2}) and end-tidal CO_2 (ET_{CO_2}), which can provide clues to diagnosis. If minute ventilation ($\dot{V}_E$) does not change, as occurs in a mechanically ventilated, muscle-relaxed patient, P_{CO_2} will rise. However, most patients augment $\dot{V}_E$ more than necessary to maintain elimination of CO_2, so that P_{CO_2} typically falls with PE. In health, the ET_{CO_2} is nearly the same as arterial CO_2. After pulmonary embolization, since end-tidal gas is a mixture of alveolar gas (in which the partial pressure of carbon dioxide [PA_{CO_2}] approximates Pa_{CO_2}) as well as the newly created physiologic dead space gas (in which P_{CO_2} approximates inspired P_{CO_2}, or is nearly zero), ET_{CO_2} falls in proportion to the degree of dead space and no longer approximates Pa_{CO_2} (Fig. 27-2). This principle of a fixed alveolar-to-arterial gradient for P_{CO_2} has been used to distinguish acute exacerbations of chronic obstructive pulmonary disease (COPD) from pulmonary embolism in patients with acute ventilatory failure.[16] While not yet studied in the critically ill population, the steady-state end-tidal alveolar dead space fraction—which can be easily derived once one has both an accurate Pa_{CO_2} and end-tidal pressure of carbon dioxide (ET_{CO_2})—has a sensitivity of 79.5% and a negative predictive value of 90.7% in hospitalized patients with PE.[17]

A widened alveolar-to-arterial gradient for oxygen [(A-a)P_{O_2}] is present in the majority of patients with PE. However, since in PE hyperventilation is the rule, Pa_{O_2} may not be low. In fact, only 63% of patients with proven PE demonstrate a $Pa_{O_2} <70$.[18] Therefore, a normal Pa_{O_2} does not conclusively exclude a diagnosis of PE. There have been several efforts to use various combinations of the Pa_{O_2}, the P_{CO_2}, and the

TABLE 27-1 Incidence of Venous Thromboembolism in Selected Groups of ICU Patients

	No.	Method	Either DVT or PE, %
"High-risk" trauma	57	Biweekly duplex exams	21
Head injury	32	Tc-venogram + $\dot{V}/\dot{Q}$ scan	25
MICU	100	Biweekly duplex	33
Spinal cord injury	198	[125]I scan; venogram	60
Class IV SICU	152	Autopsy	10
Central venous catheter	208	Jugular and subclavian vein duplex	33

ABBREVIATIONS: MICU, medical intensive care unit; SICU, surgical intensive care unit.
SOURCE: Some data for this table from Timsit et al,[10] Burns et al,[11] Gersin et al,[12] Merli et al,[13] and Byrick et al.[14]

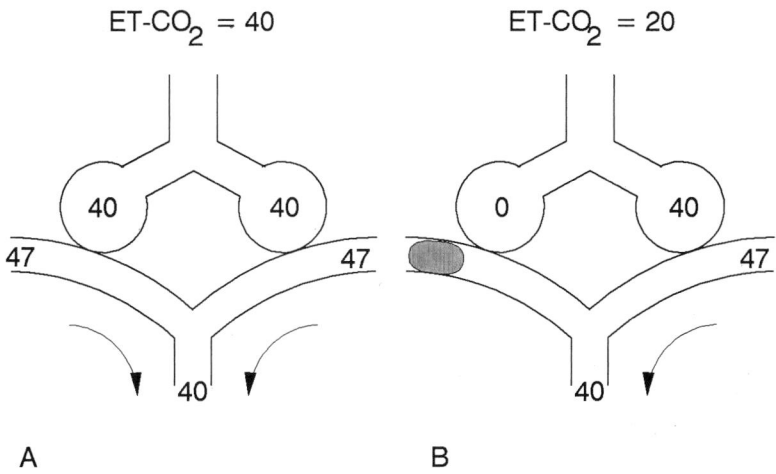

FIGURE 27-2 End-tidal CO_2 in PE. Panel *A* demonstrates the normal end-tidal CO_2, reflecting the alveolar CO_2 of 40. Panel *B* illustrates the effect of obstruction of blood flow to half of the ventilated alveoli. The end-tidal CO_2 falls in proportion to the fraction of ventilated alveoli that are no longer perfused. All numbers are P_{CO_2}, in millimeters of mercury.

$(A\text{-}a)P_{O_2}$ to predict the likelihood of (or adequately exclude) pulmonary embolism, but these have all been shown to have insufficient discriminant value, even in patients without antecedent cardiopulmonary disease.[19]

The mechanisms of hypoxemia have been elucidated by applying the multiple inert gas elimination technique (MIGET) to patients with PE.[20,21] Shunt is found in only a few patients. In some, this may be due to opening of a probe patent foramen ovale when right atrial pressure rises following PE (see below), with a consequent intracardiac right-to-left shunt. Since shunt is more likely to be found when patients are studied after some delay, atelectasis due to impaired surfactant production may contribute. In most patients, however, the most important pulmonary derangement is mismatching of ventilation and perfusion. In addition, the fall in cardiac output ($\dot{Q}T$) that accompanies most pulmonary emboli leads to a fall in mixed venous saturation. This lowered venous saturation magnifies any hypoxemia due to shunt or ventilation-perfusion ($\dot{V}/\dot{Q}$) mismatch (Fig. 27-3).

While impaired oxygenation is important and often provides a clue to the diagnosis of PE, it is typically responsive to modest oxygen enrichment of inspired gas. Severe hypoxemia is usually seen only in patients with profound shock. If oxygen-refractory hypoxemia is present without obvious hypoperfusion, a patent foramen ovale should be suspected. Ventilatory failure is usually not a significant problem either, since most patients are able to double or triple $\dot{V}E$ if necessary, in order to maintain a normal (or reduced) P_{CO_2}. In fact, the greatest impact of PE is on the circulation,

not on gas exchange. Although there are exceptions (e.g., some patients with severe COPD), morbidity and mortality from PE relate to cardiovascular compromise, not respiratory failure.

CIRCULATION

PE obstructs the pulmonary vascular bed mechanically as well as via humoral and other mechanisms. This increases right ventricular afterload, which when compounded by tachycardia, increases right ventricular oxygen consumption. The right ventricle dilates and thins, its wall tension rises, and coronary perfusion is impeded. At the same time, pulmonary vascular obstruction hinders $\dot{Q}T$ and contributes to hypoxemia. Therefore, just at the time when the right ventricle demands an increase in oxygen delivery, the left ventricle may not be able to supply it. The superimposition of increased right heart oxygen demand on decreased oxygen supply puts the right ventricle at risk for ischemia, precipitating failure of the right heart (cor pulmonale). Acute right heart dysfunction is the likely cause for sudden death in patients with massive PE. There are substantial animal and human data supporting this hypothesis, which is further discussed in Chapter 26.

Of particular interest to the intensivist is the patient with a sublethal, yet large, PE. With increased afterload, the right ventricle dilates to a larger end-diastolic volume. This is associated with elevated right atrial and ventricular pressures and abnormally low $\dot{Q}T$. One consequence of raised right atrial pressure is the potential for right-to-left shunting across a probe patent foramen ovale, causing oxygen-refractory

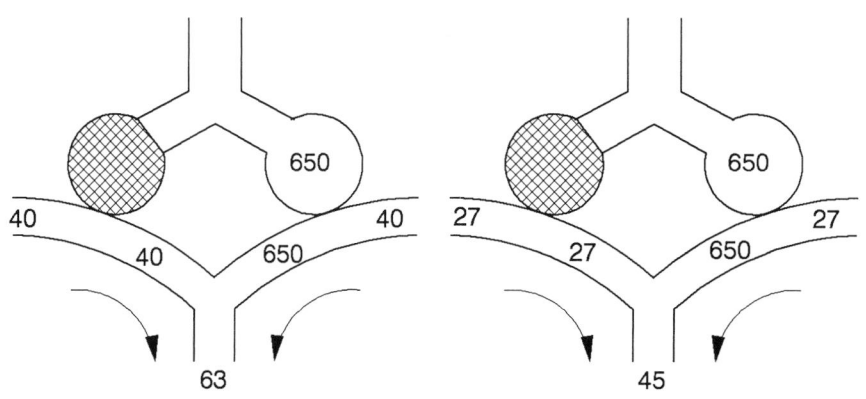

FIGURE 27-3 Effect of the mixed venous oxyhemoglobin saturation on arterial saturation in the setting of venous admixture. Panel *A* shows the effect of a 50% shunt on P_{O_2} in a patient breathing 100% oxygen who has a normal mixed venous P_{O_2} of 40 mm Hg (75% saturation). Panel *B* illustrates the same patient after the mixed venous P_{O_2} has fallen to 27 (50% saturation). Note that the P_{O_2} and saturation have fallen significantly despite the fact that the fraction of inspired oxygen ($F_{I_{O_2}}$) and the lungs have not changed at all. All numbers are P_{O_2} in millimeters of mercury.

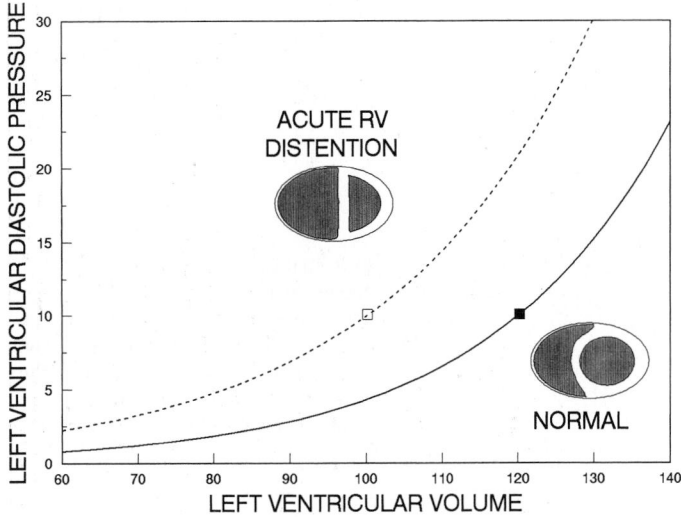

FIGURE 27-4 Left ventricular diastolic pressure-volume (PV) relationship before and after right ventricular dilation. The normal PV relationship (solid line) shows that large increments in diastolic volume are accompanied by small changes in pressure. With right ventricular distention (broken line), increments in volume are associated with relatively greater pressure changes. Note that at the same LV filling pressure of 10 mm Hg, the normal ventricle contains 20 mL more blood than following RV distention. This is associated with a correspondingly higher stroke volume and cardiac output. Pressures are in millimeters of mercury and volumes are in milliliters.

hypoxemia. This could allow paradoxical embolization of thrombus to the systemic arteries. The increase in right ventricular pressure and volume also affects the left heart. A change in shape of the right ventricle and corresponding shift of the interventricular septum from right to left alters the diastolic pressure-volume characteristics of the left ventricle (Fig. 27-4) and may be detected echocardiographically. The consequent reduction in left ventricular compliance impairs diastolic filling, thereby reducing left ventricular preload and creating yet another obstacle to cardiac output. An alternative explanation for the apparent decrease in left ventricular performance is reduced preload due to a fall in transmural filling pressure. Pericardial constraint might explain the fact that the left ventricular end-diastolic pressure (or wedge pressure) does not fall.[22]

Clinical Manifestations

HISTORY, EXAMINATION, AND LABORATORY DATA

Most patients with PE will complain of dyspnea, chest pain, and apprehension.[23] Less common symptoms are cough, diaphoresis, and hemoptysis. It is notable that most patients will not have symptoms of venous thrombosis. Syncope is uncommon but described in all large series of PE (Table 27-2).

The majority of patients will demonstrate tachypnea and tachycardia. Pleural rub and signs of DVT are seen only occasionally. Fever is more common than is generally appreciated and seen in half of patients,[23] but only rarely is the temperature >38.5°C. Patients with large emboli may have the typical findings of any patient with low output shock such as hypotension, narrow pulse pressure, and poor peripheral perfusion. Occasionally, unanticipated failure to come off mechanical ventilation or unexplained episodes of respiratory distress may be hints to a diagnosis of PE. Rare patients with PE have disseminated intravascular coagulation, systemic embolization, or acute respiratory distress syndrome (ARDS) as their presenting manifestation.

Most patients will demonstrate hypoxemia or at least a widened $(A-a)P_{O_2}$. However, since a small but significant fraction will have normal oxygenation,[18] the blood gas value should not dissuade a physician from considering the diagnosis when the rest of the clinical picture is suggestive. In fact, as described above, the blood gas does not provide data that are useful in discriminating patients with PE from those without. The chest x-ray may demonstrate areas of oligemia (Westermark's sign) and rare patients will develop a pleural based, truncated cone (Hampton's hump); however, most films have only nonspecific findings. In fact, the greatest utility of the chest film is in making (or excluding) alternative diagnoses such as pneumonia, pneumothorax, or aortic dissection. Nevertheless, the typical (albeit nonspecific) findings of basilar atelectasis, elevation of the diaphragm, and pleural effusion should always suggest PE when there is no apparent alternative explanation. Electrocardiography (ECG) may reveal signs of right heart strain such as rightward axis shift, right bundle-branch block, or right precordial strain, but often shows only sinus tachycardia.

TABLE 27-2 Symptoms and Signs of Pulmonary Embolism

	Incidence, %
Symptoms	
Dyspnea	80
Pleuritic pain	70
Apprehension	60
Cough	50
Symptoms of DVT	35
Hemoptysis	25
Central chest pain	10
Palpitations	10
Syncope	5
Signs	
Tachypnea	90
Fever	50
Tachycardia	50
Increased P_2	50
Signs of DVT	33
Shock	5

ABBREVIATIONS: DVT, deep venous thrombosis; P_2, pulmonic second sound.

SIGNS FROM MORE INVASIVE MONITORING

Valuable signs of PE may come from many of the devices used to monitor critically ill patients. The intensivist may derive clues from the ventilator, expired gas analysis, the PA catheter, or during echocardiography. The sensitivity and specificity of these monitors for the diagnosis of PE are not known. Nevertheless, wise physicians attempt to incorporate all available data into their synthesis of the patient. This is especially important in the ICU, where the history and physical examination are often difficult or impossible to obtain.

THE VENTILATOR

To maintain P_{CO_2}, the patient with PE must augment the $\dot{V}_E$. Therefore, any unexplained increase in $\dot{V}_E$ should prompt consideration of PE. Of course, any cause of rising dead space (airflow obstruction, hypovolemia, or positive end-expiratory pressure [PEEP]) or CO_2 production (anxiety, pain, fever, or sepsis) will also increase $\dot{V}_E$. However, when none of these conditions is apparent, especially when supporting clues are evident, PE becomes more likely.

EXPIRED CARBON DIOXIDE

As described above, the increment in dead space after PE causes a detectable fall in ET_{CO_2}. With technologic improvements in ventilators, noninvasive assessment of expired CO_2 is becoming increasingly practical in the ICU. A corollary of the fall in ET_{CO_2} with PE is that if $\dot{V}_E$ does not rise (e.g., in a muscle-relaxed patient), the total excretion of CO_2 (expired CO_2 concentration $\times \dot{V}_E$) must fall. Therefore Pa_{CO_2} will rise progressively until a new steady state is reached at a higher Pa_{CO_2}. This can be demonstrated numerically by the alveolar dead-space fraction (AVDSf) as follows:

$$AVDSf = (Pa_{CO_2} - ET_{CO_2})/Pa_{CO_2}$$

When combined with a negative D-dimer value, as will be discussed shortly, an AVDSf of less than 0.15 has been shown to exclude PE in hospitalized patients with a sensitivity of 97.8% and a negative predictive value of 98%.[17] In calculating the AVDSf, however, one must take care to ensure proper calibration of the blood gas analyzer, as even small changes in Pa_{CO_2} measurements will cause large differences in AVDSf. Again, in the muscle-relaxed patient there are many explanations for a rising arterial CO_2, but if no explanation is forthcoming, especially if the CO_2 production is known to be constant, consideration of PE is warranted.

PULMONARY ARTERY CATHETER

The most obvious clues from the pulmonary artery catheter (PAC) are the elevations in right atrial, right ventricular, and PA pressures and concomitant fall in $\dot{Q}_T$ that occur with PE. With the reduced $\dot{Q}_T$, one also sees a widening of the arterial-to-venous oxygen content difference [$(a-v)P_{O_2}$] (Fick principle) and a decrement in the mixed venous oxygen saturation ($S\bar{v}_{O_2}$) or the central venous oxygen saturation. An oximetric catheter may facilitate early recognition of the fall in venous oxygenation. A final clue from the PAC may lie in the difference between the PA diastolic pressure and the pulmonary capillary wedge pressure (Ppw). Normally, flow through the pulmonary circulation is pulsatile, so that by the end of diastole, there is no more flow from the PA to the left atrium.

Without flow, there can be no pressure gradient from the PA to the left atrium. Thus the end-diastolic PA pressure and the Ppw are nearly equal. However, when there is obstruction of the pulmonary vascular bed, flow is not completed by the end of diastole and a pressure gradient remains. A discrepancy between the PA diastolic pressure and Ppw may provide a clue to PA obstruction.[24]

Unfortunately, each of these observations is certainly nonspecific (and likely insensitive) so that only rarely do such changes indicate PE. For example, cardiac dysfunction (systolic or diastolic) causes a rise in right heart pressures and a fall in $\dot{Q}_T$; any cause of low $\dot{Q}_T$ causes a widened $(a-v)P_{O_2}$; and any cause of acute lung injury may raise the PA diastolic-to-Ppw gradient. A further layer of complexity is added by the recent observation in a trial of surgical patients that pulmonary embolism was disproportionately associated with the PAC compared with central venous catheters (0.8% vs. 0%).[25] Given the limitation of the PAC as a diagnostic tool and the risk of actually causing PE, it cannot be advocated for the diagnosis of PE.

ECHOCARDIOGRAPHY

The role of echocardiography in the evaluation of suspected PE is evolving, but seems most helpful in determining a patient's prognosis. While its attractions include portability—especially for the evaluation of critically ill patients—noninvasiveness, potential to elucidate competing diagnoses (such as myocardial infarction or pericardial disease), and rapid availability, echocardiography is insensitive, and should not be used to diagnose PE. In prospective trials of unselected patients, sensitivities of between 29% and 52% are reported for various echocardiographic criteria of right ventricular strain or dysfunction or tricuspid regurgitation.[26,27] Many patients with PE have normal echocardiograms. Occasionally, a study requested for evaluation of a low flow state may unexpectedly reveal findings strongly suggestive of PE.[28,29] These include a dilated, thin-walled, poorly contracting right ventricle, and bowing of the interventricular septum to the left. Very rarely, echocardiography may demonstrate a thrombus in the right atrium or right ventricle (Table 27-3), clinching the diagnosis of PE.

When echocardiography exhibits right ventricular dysfunction, it reliably predicts an increased risk of mortality from pulmonary embolism. One study examined 126 patients with PE with echocardiography on the day of diagnosis, and found moderate RV dysfunction to impart a sixfold increased risk of in-hospital death compared to normal RV function.[30] Even in patients assessed to be hemodynamically stable at presentation, right ventricular dysfunction portends a worse

---

TABLE 27-3 Echocardiographic Signs of Pulmonary Embolism

Dilated, thin-walled right ventricle
Poorly contracting right ventricle
Tricuspid regurgitation
Pulmonary hypertension estimated from the tricuspid regurgitation jet
Leftward shifting of the interventricular septum
Pulmonary artery dilation
Visualized thrombus in right atrium, right ventricle, or pulmonary artery
Loss of respirophasic variation in inferior vena caval diameter

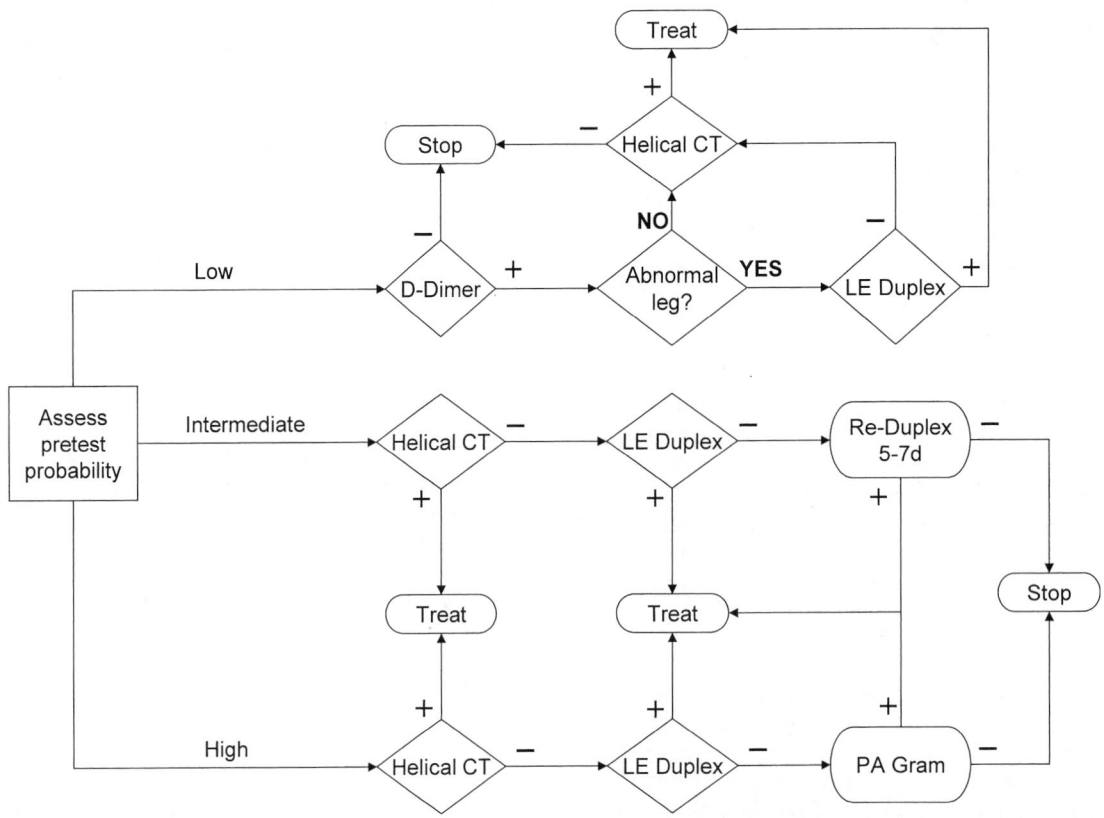

FIGURE 27-5 Algorithm for evaluation of a critically ill patient suspected of having a pulmonary embolus. If alternate diagnoses are not confirmed by examination, chest x-ray, and ECG, the pretest probability of pulmonary embolism should be assessed. D-dimer may be useful in some patients at low suspicion when this test is negative. Helical computed tomographic (CT) angiography may not be sufficiently sensitive to act as a screening test, and unless the clinical suspicion is low, negative studies should be followed by additional testing. Ventilation-perfusion scanning may be useful in occasional patients when CT angiography cannot be performed. Echocardiography is not sufficiently reliable for routine use, but it may greatly aid diagnosis in the patient with shock. "Treat" means treatment for PE is generally indicated; "STOP" means PE is very unlikely and an alternate explanation for the patient's symptoms or signs should be sought. These decisions hinge critically on clinical judgment and experience.

prognosis; one study found that 10% of such patients develop shock and 5% died in the hospital, compared to a 0% mortality among patients with normal RV function.[31] In another series of hemodynamically stable patients, recurrent embolism was strongly associated with baseline echocardiographic abnormalities in right ventricular wall motion.[32] A word of caution is prudent, however, in that the classic echocardiographic findings of PE are nonspecific, and are common to a number of causes of acute right ventricular pressure overload such as ARDS, other forms of severe hypoxemia, or status asthmaticus (see Chap. 26).

Diagnosis

SPECIAL PROBLEMS IN THE ICU

The typical critically ill patient is unable to complain of the usual symptoms of PE, has numerous explanations for tachycardia and tachypnea, is hemodynamically unstable, and is a poor candidate for transport for radiographic studies. For that reason, it is important to have a clear sense of the probability of PE in any given patient. Such a judgment is complex, and validated algorithms for determining prior probability in critically ill patients are not available. Synthesis of the patient's cardiopulmonary physiology, combined with an assessment of risk factors, is all the clinician has to go on. Obviously, there is no substitute for experience in managing these very difficult patients. In the following sections, the contribution of various tests in evaluating suspected PE is discussed. An approach to diagnosis is summarized in Fig. 27-5.

RISK FACTORS

Since the symptoms, signs, and laboratory findings of PE are usually nonspecific, delay before pursuing a diagnosis in a patient with classic, unmistakable clues risks missing this potentially lethal disease. However, since nonspecific indicators of potential PE are ubiquitous, indiscriminant pursuit of the diagnosis is prohibitively costly and dangerous. Most patients with PE have identifiable risk factors (Table 27-4). Absence of such risk factors should lead the physician to seek alternative explanations for the patient's findings other than thromboembolism. On the other hand, when numerous risk factors are present, the diagnosis should be more seriously considered.

TABLE 27-4 Risk Factors for Pulmonary Embolism

Epidemiologic factors: Obesity, prior thromboembolism, advanced age, malignancy (especially adenocarcinoma), chemotherapy (particularly thalidomide), estrogens
Venous stasis: Immobility, paralysis, leg casts, varicose veins, congestive heart failure, prolonged travel, and use of muscle relaxants
Injury: Postsurgical, posttrauma, postpartum
Hypercoagulable states: Proteins C and S and antithrombin III deficiency, activated protein C resistance, antiphospholipid antibody syndromes, polycythemia, macroglobulinemia
Indwelling lines: Central venous and pulmonary artery catheters

DIAGNOSTIC TESTS

The gold standard for the diagnosis of PE has long been the pulmonary angiogram. However, its use in critically ill patients is limited by invasiveness, expense, need for dye infusion, and the risks attendant to transport out of the ICU. In many patients, the pulmonary angiogram can be replaced by its noninvasive cousin, the helical computed tomography (CT) angiogram. Helical CT angiography is rapidly replacing both the ventilation-perfusion ($\dot{V}/\dot{Q}$) lung scan and pulmonary angiography in the diagnosis of PE. The limitations of pulmonary angiography and $\dot{V}/\dot{Q}$ scanning, combined with residual doubts regarding the reliability of helical CT angiography, have led to attempts to supplant or augment these tests with alternatives. These include noninvasive leg studies, MRI imaging of the thorax, and various blood tests such as the D-dimer assay. An integrated approach to the diagnosis of PE is described in Figure 27-5.

COMPUTED TOMOGRAPHY AND MAGNETIC RESONANCE IMAGING

Advances in CT and MR imaging have rekindled great interest in the potential for these relatively noninvasive studies to replace the $\dot{V}/\dot{Q}$ scan and pulmonary angiogram as diagnostic procedures of choice.

Magnetic resonance imaging and angiography (MRA) technology has progressed greatly in the past 10 years, with rapidly improving resolution and speed of image attainment. MR does not require iodinated contrast, making it ideal for patients with renal insufficiency, or for those who should not be exposed to ionizing radiation. Among initial reports in 1997, one study listed a sensitivity of 100% and specificity of 95% when MRA was performed in 30 patients undergoing pulmonary angiography for suspected PE.[33] Three of the 22 "negative" MRAs were also termed "poor quality," yet were considered negative readings for calculation of sensitivity and specificity. A larger (118 patients) study with an arguably less selected group of patients found the sensitivity of MRA to be 77% but with a wide 95% confidence interval; specificity was better, at 98%.[34] In both studies, MRA proved difficult either due to patient factors that made them ineligible for magnetic resonance (9% to 15% of eligible patients), or due to poor image quality (6% to 9%), which made the study uninterpretable. Thus while promising, MRA has not yet attained a sensitivity that allows one to rule out PE.

CT scanning has received even more attention and is widely used. Helical CT angiography produces a two-dimensional image of the lung and its vessels at very small collimator, or slice thickness. It has been shown to detect central emboli—

out to fourth-division vessels—with a high degree of reliability. Like MRI, helical CT angiography is minimally invasive and may provide alternative diagnoses in the work-up of PE. It does, however, require the injection of intravenous contrast, it is expensive (though less so than either MR or pulmonary angiography) to perform and interpret, and it can be difficult to perform in patients who are unable to hold their breath or are hemodynamically unstable. The most significant criticisms of this technique have been its inability to detect emboli to the level of subsegmental arteries and its variation in interobserver interpretation.

In a prospective trial of 42 patients with suspected PE who underwent helical CT angiography followed by pulmonary angiogram, all 23 patients with a normal CT were found to have a negative pulmonary angiogram, for a sensitivity of 100%.[35] The test likewise appeared to be extremely specific, with only one false-positive, for a reported specificity of 96%. However, with further studies, a range of sensitivity emerges of 53% to 100%, and of specificity between 81% and 100%. Two well-performed recent reviews[36,37] of the CT data came to similar conclusions: that the available literature on CT in the diagnosis of PE remains limited by small studies with incomplete use of a reference standard; that the sensitivity and specificity of CT in diagnosing PE are as yet undetermined; and that the safety of withholding anticoagulation based on a negative CT study is untested and unknown. Both studies raised concerns that interobserver variation and the potential inability of CT to reliably determine subsegmental PEs might preclude its usefulness as a diagnostic test. It is interesting to recall that in PIOPED, subsegmental PEs accounted for 6% of the PEs detected, and that the interobserver agreement for pulmonary angiograms among these small PEs was wider than that of larger PEs (66% for subsegmental PEs compared to 90% for segmental and 98% for lobar PEs).[38] It would appear that subsegmental PEs are challenging to diagnose even by pulmonary angiography, and that the clinical significance of such clots remains difficult to ascertain.

One recent study may shed some light on the safety of withholding anticoagulation following negative CT scan.[39] One hundred seventeen patients in whom PE was suspected but who were found to have a negative helical CT angiogram were followed for a mean duration of 21 months. The study population was elderly (mean = 65 years) and with frequent comorbidity; 70% of patients had known cardiac or respiratory disease. The recurrence rate for PE was 4.5%, based on three patients who died of unknown cause within 1 month of their initial suspected PEs, and two cases of repeat presentation with suspected PE which was confirmed by imaging. One of the patients who died was receiving anticoagulation for severe cardiac insufficiency; excluding his death yields a recurrence rate of 4.9%. If one were to consider the three unexplained deaths—two were older than 90 years with significant comorbidities—as not being due to recurrent PE, the recurrence rate would fall to 1.8%. For pulmonary angiogram, the reported rate of recurrence of PE following a negative study ranges from 0.6% to 4.9%. Thus it may be that helical CT angiography, while by no means a perfect test, has a PE recurrence rate similar to that of pulmonary angiography following a negative study, and is therefore adequate grounds for withholding anticoagulation. Further investigations to confirm or contrast the above findings are necessary to validate this claim.

Both CT and MRA have the advantage of being able to diagnose alternative conditions that may explain the patient's symptoms. Both are less invasive and less expensive than pulmonary angiography, and are probably easier than V̇/Q̇ scan to perform in a critically ill patient. Yet lacking comprehensive prospective studies using angiography as a gold standard—lacking PIOPED—both MRA and CT may remain suspect to some practitioners.

NONINVASIVE LEG STUDIES

Noninvasive leg studies include impedance plethysmography (IPG), phleborheography, venous Doppler, and B-mode ultrasound scanning of leg veins. The technical details of these procedures and differences between them are beyond the scope of this chapter, but which particular test to choose is largely a function of local expertise. Both IPG and venous ultrasonography are extremely helpful in assessing a patient with symptomatic proximal deep vein thrombosis. In this population, across numerous studies venous ultrasonography has a sensitivity of 97%, a positive predictive value (PPV) of 100%, and a negative predictive value (NPV) of 100%;[40] IPG was similar though slightly inferior, with a sensitivity of 92%, PPV of 78%, and NPV of 96%.[40] Falsely abnormal results on IPG can be seen with nonthrombotic compression of the vein, increased central venous pressure, and chronic obstructive pulmonary disease.[41] The troublesome aspect to both of these imaging modalities is their performance in asymptomatic patients, particularly asymptomatic patients with high clinical probability of thromboembolism. Patients with symptomatic DVT are far more likely to have a proximal than a distal, or isolated calf vein, DVT.[42,43] In contrast, among asymptomatic patients screened for thromboses, the majority—almost two thirds—are distal.[44,45] When the natural history of postoperative deep vein thrombosis was studied in 1969, approximately 20% of distal DVTs subsequently extended into the proximal veins, and while nonextending distal DVT caused no clinical cases of pulmonary embolism, 4 of 9 cases with proximal DVT did cause PE.[45] Subsequently, studies have observed that distal clots which subsequently progress tend to do so within a week of presentation,[46] and that proximal extension of distal DVT after more than a week is unusual,[40] spurring the evaluation of serial noninvasive leg studies for the diagnosis of proximal DVT. In evaluating the safety of withholding anticoagulation following a negative test, both IPG and venous duplex appear to have similar rates of subsequent DVT (1.5% to 2%) during the 6 months following a negative test.[40] However, pooling data from combined studies of IPG, 4 of 1625 patients (0.25%) with an initial negative IPG died from PE during serial testing or follow-up, whereas one of 1747 patients (0.06%) with initial negative venous ultrasound died of PE.[40]

Precisely because PE more commonly follows asymptomatic, rather than symptomatic, DVT,[38] noninvasive leg studies cannot make or exclude the diagnosis of PE. Moreover, the ultrasonic characteristics of any thrombus appear to predict poorly the likelihood of associated PE.[47] Nevertheless, the wide availability of accurate noninvasive leg studies provides a simple method for managing many patients who cannot be transported or who have nondiagnostic helical CT angiography. In patients with angiographically proven PE, 43% to 57% will have detectable DVT.[48,49] In some patients,

TABLE 27-5 Serial Leg Studies in Patients with Suspected Venous Thromboembolism

	N (%)
Initial negative IPG	1114
Positive IPG, days 2–5	23 (2.8)
Positive IPG, days 6–10	6 (0.7)
Thromboembolism at 3 mo	11 (1.0)
Fatal PE at 3 mo	1 (0.1)

ABBREVIATIONS: IPG, impedance plethysmography.
NOTE: 380 of these patients had suspected PE, the remainder having suspected DVT only. Patients were not critically ill. Anticoagulation was withheld while serial studies were performed. Data abstracted from references 46 and 50–52.

diagnostic testing can be avoided by performing serial noninvasive leg studies. Demonstration of venous thrombosis provides grounds for treatment (usually anticoagulation), so the question of PE may cease to be important. On the other hand, failure to detect DVT may sufficiently reassure the intensivist that neither further diagnostic measures nor empirical treatment is urgently needed. The rationale for this approach is that if deep venous thrombosis cannot be detected, the likelihood of re-embolism is very low. Furthermore, if deep venous thrombosis develops, or a subclinical thrombosis propagates to the proximal deep veins, serial testing will reveal it before it has much chance to embolize. In ambulatory patients, this strategy is effective (Table 27-5). It is important to note that this approach has not been validated in critically ill patients and does not take into account the role of upper extremity thrombosis.

VENTILATION-PERFUSION LUNG SCAN

V̇/Q̇ scanning traditionally was the initial test of choice in the evaluation of PE, but two important studies have led to a sobering reappraisal of this test.[38,48] V̇/Q̇ scans can be extremely helpful to the clinician when they provide either a high probability result—with an attendant specificity of 85%, confirming the diagnosis—or a normal result, when the diagnosis of PE is virtually excluded.[38] Although 15 of 100 patients with "high probability" V̇/Q̇ scans will not have PEs, the risk of treating them is felt to be less than the risk and cost of performing pulmonary angiography in all 100 patients. The frustration with V̇/Q̇ scanning stems from the large number of tests which yield either intermediate probability or indeterminate results. Scans of intermediate probability indicate a substantial likelihood of PE (about 40%) necessitating further evaluation to prove or exclude the diagnosis. Among patients with low probability scans, the prevalence of PE ranges from 16% to 40%, necessitating further diagnostic work-up in all but those deemed to have a low clinical likelihood of PE, among whom only 4% of patients had PE. Thus the V̇/Q̇ scan results, which are sufficient in themselves to terminate the evaluation (because PE is either highly likely or has been reliably excluded) include all normal scans, all high probability scans, and low probability scans in patients with a low clinical pretest probability of PE. Unfortunately, a minority of patients fall into these three categories, so that for the majority of patients undergoing V̇/Q̇ scan, it prompts further testing.

How useful the ventilation-perfusion scan is when applied to the subset of critically ill patients remains an open question. In a retrospective analysis of the PIOPED database, 223 patients were defined to be "critically ill" (room air Pa_{O_2} <50 [$n = 89$]; mechanically ventilated [$n = 46$]; hypotensive, but not ventilated [$n = 3$]; or physically in an ICU, but not ventilated [$n = 85$]).[53] While it is difficult to know precisely how ill these patients were (no severity of illness scores were reported), only 29 of 223 had a high probability result, and no critically ill patients had normal or near normal scans. Sixteen critically ill patients had the combination of low clinical pretest probability and low probability scan. Thus even in this group of ICU patients presumably stable enough to be enrolled in a clinical trial and in whom the scan could be performed, the test was definitive in only 20%. Although the investigators concluded that the sensitivity and positive predictive value of the $\dot{V}/\dot{Q}$ scan were similar in "critically ill" and "non–critically ill" patients, it is clear that the $\dot{V}/\dot{Q}$ scan is not helpful in the majority of patients. Given the surging popularity of CT scanning, combined with ever better CT and MR detectors, there seems to be little role for perfusion or ventilation-perfusion scanning in critically ill patients.

OTHER NONINVASIVE MEANS OF DIAGNOSIS

The most recent potentially useful blood test is the D-dimer assay. Very low levels of D-dimer argue against a diagnosis of PE, with a sensitivity of 95% and a negative likelihood ratio of 0.9 to 0.13 using the widely available quantitative rapid enzyme-linked immunosorbent assay (ELISA).[54] Essential to the use of a D-dimer test in diagnosing patients with thromboembolic disease is an assessment of clinical pretest probability; one clinical prediction rule for DVT found a prevalence of DVT of 6%, 9%, and 28% in patients whose clinical prediction rule was low, intermediate, or high, respectively.[55] Converting the prevalence to odds, and applying the D-dimer test with a 0.9 negative likelihood ratio, posttest probability is as low as 0.006 for the initial low-probability patients, whereas it is an order of magnitude greater (0.03%) in the high-probability patients. If one were to imagine extremely high-risk patients, with a pretest probability of 80%, the posttest probability of PE could be as high as 0.28 despite a negative D-dimer result. D-dimer assays can be considered unidirectional, in that a negative result can be extremely useful, yet a positive result has little effect on the likelihood of either DVT or PE.[54] This fact unfortunately limits the utility of the D-dimer test in the critically ill population, in whom so many patients will have a positive D-dimer level. For example, in a retrospective analysis of patients with severe sepsis randomized to undergo aspirin versus placebo, 100% of patients had an elevated D-dimer.[56] On the other hand, when D-dimer testing was applied to patients with cancer suspected of having deep vein thrombosis, it proved to be an effective test, with a 98% sensitivity, a 97% negative predictive value, and a negative likelihood ratio of 0.03.[57] Despite concern that the high prevalence of thromboembolic disease in a population with cancer would limit the utility of D-dimer, the test performed well and allowed outpatient evaluation in 29% of the patients studied.

The combination of pulse oximetry and static compliance of the respiratory system yielded a very high sensitivity and specificity for PE in critically ill trauma patients.[58] In patients with COPD, capnography during a prolonged passive exhalation had a negative predictive value of 100% when values of arterial P_{CO_2} and end-maximal expiratory P_{CO_2} were nearly equal.[16] Combining steady-state end-tidal alveolar dead space fraction and D-dimer was also quite sensitive in diagnosing PE in hospitalized, though not critically ill, patients, with a sensitivity and negative predictive value of 98%.[17] The proper place of each of these tests depends on further study.

PULMONARY ANGIOGRAPHY

Pulmonary angiography is considered the definitive test for the diagnosis of PE. Positive findings include an intraluminal filling defect or a cutoff of a 2-mm or larger vessel seen in more than one view. Experienced radiologists agree on 98% of studies showing lobar embolism.[59] However, agreement falls to 90% with segmental embolism, and only 66% in those with subsegmental clots. Thus even this test has limitations. Its sensitivity is sufficiently high to occasionally detect embolism even weeks to months after the acute episode. The earliest documented resolution of an angiogram to normal following a pulmonary embolus is 1 week, although faster resolution has been seen in animal studies.[60] Thus this test can reliably exclude embolism if a negative study is obtained even a week following the onset of symptoms.[61] Since it is invasive, costly, riskier than CT angiography, and requires the presence of an interventional radiologist (rather than a CT technician), it is usually reserved for patients in whom the diagnosis cannot be made or excluded by less invasive means. However, pulmonary angiography is safer than generally appreciated. Mortality is around 0.2% as shown in several large series.[62,63] Several patients who have died had severe pulmonary hypertension and cor pulmonale at the time of the procedure, leading some to conclude that pulmonary hypertension is a contraindication to pulmonary angiography. The degree of risk in such patients was directly addressed in one review of pulmonary angiography.[63] Elevated pulmonary systolic pressure (greater than 70 mm Hg) and elevated right ventricular diastolic pressure (greater than 20 mm Hg) were identified as risk factors. However, even in these sickest patients the mortality was only 2%. In patients with severe chronic pulmonary hypertension who are being considered for surgical endarterectomy (admittedly a different population) angiography has been performed quite safely.[64] Nonionic, low osmolality contrast agents improve image quality and may be able to reduce risk even further.

EMPIRICAL DIAGNOSIS

Occasionally, an empirical diagnosis of PE seems clear cut to the managing physician. No alternative diagnoses may seem plausible, or further diagnostic steps seem risky or unnecessary. Although this approach may appear attractive, it rarely proves correct. First, the clinical diagnosis is simply too unreliable, even for the most experienced clinician. Second, one can always expand the differential diagnosis to include alternative causes. Finally, the doubt that lingers after an empirical diagnosis too frequently haunts subsequent management. Progression of symptoms or signs despite therapy raises questions about failure of treatment or the need for alternative treatments. Complications of treatment (usually hemorrhage due to heparin, occasionally thrombocytopenia) create

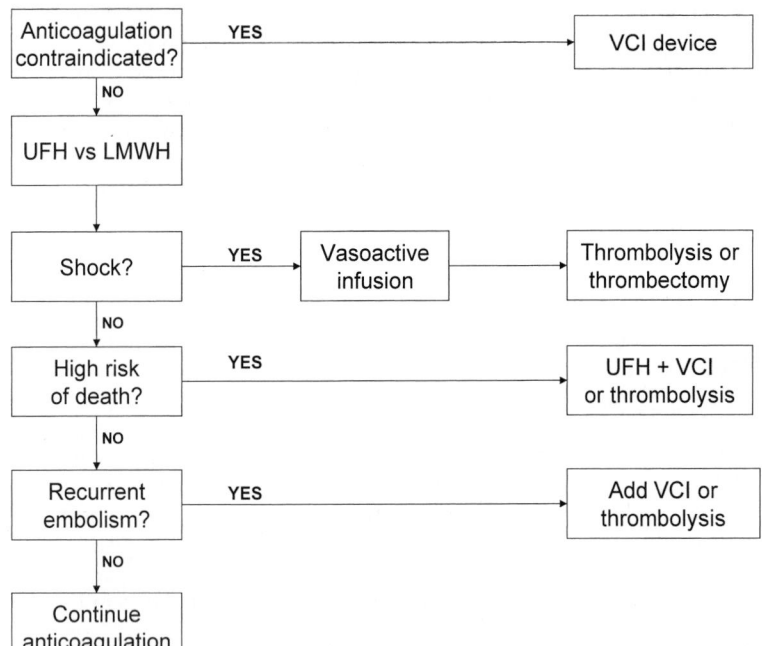

FIGURE 27-6 Treatment of PE in critically ill patients. UFH, unfractionated heparin; LMWH, low-molecular-weight heparin; VCI device, vena cava interrupting device.

uncertainty about the necessity of the toxic therapy, or precipitate more diagnostic interventions in a newly unstable state. Since critically ill patients are more likely to have complications of therapy, empiricism is rarely appropriate.

Treatment

The majority of patients with PE will not die from the clot that leads to diagnosis. As long as re-embolization is prevented, the patient will survive, while intrinsic fibrinolysis restores pulmonary blood flow. Therefore the primary goal of all therapies for PE is to prevent re-embolization. Some patients, however, survive the initial embolus yet remain in shock. These patients, who are overrepresented in ICU populations, may succumb to the initial embolus. Additional therapy to hasten clot resolution, aimed at more promptly restoring the circulation, is useful in such patients. Supportive care, anticoagulation, vena caval interruption, thrombolysis, fluid and vasoactive drug administration, and rarely surgical embolectomy all must be considered in the treatment of this disease. An integrated approach to the treatment of PE is presented in Figure 27-6.

RISK ASSESSMENT

Having made a diagnosis of PE, the clinician and patient face numerous potential therapies and outcomes. Pulmonary embolism is spectacularly inconsistent in its clinical presentation, and can range from asymptomatic or mildly symptomatic dyspnea to profound shock due to right ventricular dysfunction. Several characteristics of each presentation can allow the clinician to identify patients with the poorest prognosis, who almost certainly benefit from close observation in a monitored setting, and who may benefit from a more aggressive therapeutic approach. Equally important, the clinician may also identify those patients at low risk for complications, in

whom a strategy of anticoagulation alone, potentially as an outpatient, will suffice. The Geneva prognostic index, generated from a prospective study of 296 patients with PE admitted through the emergency room, identified six predictors of adverse outcome, defined as death, recurrent thrombotic event, or major bleeding.[65] Hypotension imparted an odds ratio of 15; cancer of 9.5; and prior DVT, DVT by ultrasound, heart failure, and hypoxemia odds ratios of between 2.6 and 3.8. Cardiac biomarkers have also become potential prognostic indicators; when elevated, both troponin T and troponin I portend a high risk for complications, and troponin I was significantly associated with increased overall mortality in one study.[66] Low brain natriuretic peptide (BNP) was positively associated with survival, and high BNP with higher mortality and PE-specific mortality in another study of 110 normotensive patients with PE.[67] As previously discussed, echocardiographic evidence of right ventricular dysfunction clearly identifies a subgroup of patients with PE at high risk of shock or death.[31] To date no data have shown a decreased mortality or decreased recurrence of thromboembolic events by adopting a more aggressive treatment strategy for patients deemed to be high risk, and we do not advocate basing therapeutic decisions, such as whether or not to use thrombolytic medications, on such criteria. However, it seems prudent to use a careful risk assessment of death, recurrence, or major bleeding when contemplating which patients may benefit from outpatient therapy, treatment on the general ward, or surveillance in an ICU.

SUPPORTIVE CARE

OXYGEN AND BED REST
Patients typically present with hypoxemia, which responds well to oxygen therapy since the underlying pathophysiology is usually $\dot{V}/\dot{Q}$ mismatch. Bed rest, once advocated as the standard of care in treating venous thromboembolic disease, has recently been called into question by two randomized

prospective studies.[68,69] Both studies found that allowing patients with DVT to ambulate on day 2—compared to imposed strict bed rest for between 4 and 10 days—failed to increase the incidence of PE as detected by $\dot{V}/\dot{Q}$ scanning. Ambulating patients wore thigh-length compression stockings and walked up to 4 hours per day. Admittedly, the applicability of these studies to an ICU population may be problematic, as patients were excluded if they had clinically overt PE, free floating thrombus, pregnancy, renal insufficiency, or were unable to ambulate. Many of our ICU patients, and all patients with symptomatic PE, would have failed to qualify for these studies. Bed rest may have advantages to the critically ill patient beyond the theoretical advantage of reducing clot dislodgment. By reducing oxygen consumption ($\dot{V}_{O_2}$) and thus $\dot{Q}_T$ to their absolute minimum, bed rest—combined with sedation and mechanical ventilation in selected patients—is indicated in the treatment of patients with PE and shock.

SPECIFIC THERAPIES

ANTICOAGULATION

Unfractionated Heparin (UFH)

Heparin has long been the mainstay of therapy for PE, although its pre-eminent role in treating thromboembolic disease has lately been challenged by newer medications. Unfractionated heparin is a mixture of acidic glycosaminoglycans typically extracted from porcine intestinal mucosa, with a variable molecular weight of between 5000 and 30,000 da, depending on its clinical preparation.[70,71] Along with a coumarin derivative, it was the first anticoagulant to be prospectively shown to decrease mortality and recurrent PE, decreasing mortality by 25%.[72] While it has proven effective, it requires monitoring of coagulation parameters as well as dose adjustment due to unpredictable plasma levels even within individuals. Although a recent study has shown that UFH given subcutaneously is as effective and safe as fixed dose nadroparin,[73] UFH is generally given by continuous intravenous infusion and we expect this practice to continue. These limitations functionally restrict the use of heparin to the hospital setting. Heparin essentially catalyzes the effect of antithrombin to rapidly inhibit several of the factors from the intrinsic and common coagulation pathways, factors Xa, IXa, XIa, and XIIa.[70] It also inhibits the activation of factors V and VIII by thrombin.[71] Heparin is cleared rapidly from the plasma by binding to cell surface receptors on endothelial cells and reticuloendothelial elements,[70] and its clearance is not affected by renal or hepatic insufficiency.

In dosing heparin, a singular concept emerges: one must give enough heparin to surpass a minimal level of anticoagulation in order to prevent further thromboembolism. This threshold level appears to be doses at which the activated partial thromboplastin time (aPTT) is at least 1.5 times control[74] (or alternatively at which a heparin level of 0.2 to 0.4 U/mL by the protamine sulfate assay or 0.3 to 0.6 IU/mL by amidolytic anti-Xa study is reached), and it should be reached as quickly as possible. When continuous intravenous heparin was compared with intermittent subcutaneous heparin in the treatment of proximal deep vein thrombosis, only 1 of 61 patients who achieved an aPTT of greater than 1.5 times control suffered recurrent venous thromboembolism (VTE). In contrast, 13 of 53 patients whose aPTT was below

1.5 times control for 24 hours had recurrence, independent of the method of administration of heparin (relative risk = 15:1).[74] Rapid, adequate anticoagulation is facilitated by a weight-based nomogram.[73,75] Heparin is typically initiated with a bolus of 80 U/kg followed by a continuous infusion of 18 U/kg per hour. For most patients, oral anticoagulation (coumadin) is begun within 3 days of initiating heparin.

While the evidence supporting a lower therapeutic limit for heparin of 1.5 times control as judged by the aPTT is quite strong, the conventional upper limit (2.5 times control) is arbitrary. For years it had been assumed that the risk of hemorrhage was significantly related to the level of the aPTT, but one trial has cast doubt on this assumption.[76] In this study, hemorrhagic complications were related to underlying predisposing factors (eg, recent surgery, ulcer disease, or cancer) rather than to supratherapeutic levels of the aPTT. Patients were initially treated with heparin plus warfarin or with heparin alone. Of 99 patients in the combined treatment group, 69 (69%) had aPTT levels greater than 2.5 times control for more than 24 hours. In contrast, in the heparin only group, 24 of 100 patients (24%) had supratherapeutic aPTT levels. Bleeding complications were similar in the two groups (combined therapy, 9.1%; heparin alone, 12.0%). In addition, bleeding complications were seen in only 8 of 93 patients with supratherapeutic aPTT regardless of therapeutic arm, compared with 13 of 106 patients without such elevation. These findings refute an association between modestly elevated aPTT and hemorrhage, and combined with the importance of prompt, adequate anticoagulation, suggest the value of an approach that aims to assure enough heparin in the first hours of treatment, rather than to avoid too much.

Complications of Heparin

Complications of heparin, in addition to hemorrhage, include heparin-induced thrombocytopenia (HIT), osteoporosis, hypersensitivity, and (rarely) hyperkalemia. The most important complication of heparin is bleeding. In a pooled analysis of its use in deep venous thrombosis, major bleeding (bleeding greater than 1 L, bleeding requiring blood transfusion, or intracerebral bleeding) was reported in 2 of 59 patients (3%).[77] In a group of 121 patients given heparin for all indications, 8% developed major hemorrhage (fatal, life-threatening, potentially life-threatening, or bleeding leading to reoperation or requiring at least three units of blood).[78] When heparin dosing is guided by nomogram as described above, the risk of hemorrhage was 9% to 12%.[76] Hemorrhage typically occurs from the gastrointestinal or urinary tract, or from surgical incisions. Less common sites of serious bleeding include the retroperitoneum, adrenal glands, soft tissues, nose, and pleural space. Intracranial hemorrhage is uncommon in patients anticoagulated with heparin.

The approach to treatment of the patient who bleeds on heparin depends on the severity of bleeding. When bleeding is minor, simply stopping the heparin may be sufficient. Bleeding related to needlesticks may respond to sustained direct pressure. When hemorrhage endangers life or organ function, a more aggressive approach is mandatory. Transfusion of fresh frozen plasma is usually ineffective since circulating heparin inhibits the function of transfused factors. Protamine sulfate is an antidote to heparin. The dose of protamine depends on heparin levels, and is therefore related to dose, route of administration, and time since the last dose. When hemorrhage immediately follows a bolus of heparin, sufficient protamine to completely neutralize the heparin (1 mg protamine per 100 U heparin) should be administered. In the more usual situation in which heparin therapy is ongoing, the dose of protamine should be based on the approximate half-life of heparin (90 minutes). Since protamine is also an anticoagulant, the dose should be calculated to only half-correct the estimated circulating heparin. Protamine has been known to cause hypotension, shock, dyspnea, and pulmonary hypertension upon intravenous injection. The incidence is reduced by giving the drug very slowly (no more than 50 mg in 10 minutes). When protamine is administered, a physician should be present in case of an anaphylactoid reaction. Alternatives for the treatment of underlying conditions should be considered once heparin is stopped. For example, the patient with pulmonary embolization should have vena caval interruption with a percutaneous filter (see below).

Thrombocytopenia is a relatively common complication of heparin administration, typically occurring after several days of therapy. In large series, roughly 1% to 3% of patients given full-dose intravenous heparin have developed thrombocytopenia.[79] Interestingly, in our experience at a tertiary care center where many of our patients are repeatedly exposed to heparin, the incidence of heparin-induced thrombocytopenia seems to be much higher. The mechanism in most patients is thought to be related to specific IgG directed against heparin. Thrombocytopenia is less commonly seen with highly purified low-molecular-weight heparins, suggesting that higher-molecular-weight components may be responsible. It is also rare in patients given prophylactic, minidose heparin, occurring in only one of 348 patients.[80] The onset of thrombocytopenia is usually on the third to fifteenth day (mean = day 10), but it can occur after several hours in patients previously sensitized. The severity of thrombocytopenia is variable (commonly to $50,000/mm^3$), but can be severe ($<5000/mm^3$). Most patients remain asymptomatic, but some suffer major arterial or venous thrombosis, or life-threatening hemorrhage. Rarely, this syndrome is associated with skin bullae that progress to necrosis ("heparin necrosis"). These may occur at sites of injection or at distant sites. Any time heparin is given, it is prudent to measure platelet counts on a daily basis. An otherwise unexplained drop in platelet count of 30% has been suggested as the threshold that should prompt discontinuation of heparin,[80] although there are few data upon which to base this. Heparin-dependent IgG should be sought in the patient's serum, since a positive result may simplify management decisions. None of the available assays are fully sensitive, so a negative test is no guarantee against recurrent thrombocytopenia or thrombosis if the patient is rechallenged with heparin.

Low Molecular Weight Heparin

The promise of low molecular weight heparins (LMWHs) is a simple, once or twice daily therapy for venous thromboembolism that does not require monitoring of anticoagulant effect. As a class, the LMWHs encompass a number of fragments of unfractionated heparin which are on average 5000 da in molecular weight. The different LMWHs have been depolymerized by various means, and thus differ in their pharmacokinetic and pharmacodynamic properties.[70] One LMWH may not be interchangeable with another. LMWHs

achieve excellent bioavailability when given subcutaneously (about 90% of that achieved with an equal intravenous dose), have a long half-life (2 to 4.4 hours), correlate well between anticoagulant response and body weight, and have equal or better antithrombotic effects than unfractionated heparin. There have now been numerous trials comparing LMWHs (subcutaneously or intravenously) with unfractionated heparin in both DVT and PE.[81–85] In an early meta-analysis pooling the results of over 2000 patients, LMWHs appeared superior with regard to venographic score improvement, recurrence rate of VTE, and hemorrhage. There is also a trend towards an all-cause mortality benefit for LMWHs.[81] Similarly, a recent meta-analysis of LMWH compared to unfractionated heparin for the treatment of PE found non–statistically-significant decreases in recurrent symptomatic VTE, PE, and bleeding complications.[86] With such data, groups such as the American College of Chest Physicians now recommend that clinicians use LMW heparin over unfractionated heparin.[71]

Aspects of caring for critically ill patients may limit the full implementation of such recommendations in the ICU. Many patients with critical illness have coincident renal failure, bleeding diatheses, or need for ongoing invasive procedures, all of which make unfractionated heparin, which can be quickly discontinued and rapidly cleared from the body, preferable. Conversely, certain situations appear to be ideally suited to the use of LMWH, such as in the long-term treatment of cancer patients with venous thromboembolism.[87,88] As stated, the incidence of HIT is lower with LMWH than with unfractionated heparin, although in many trials of LMWH for DVT or PE, the incidence of HIT was sufficiently low in both arms to preclude a statistical comparison. In orthopedic and surgical studies as well as the initial industry-sponsored trials of various LMWHs, the incidence of HIT varied between 0% and 0.8% of patients, compared with approximately 3% of patients treated with unfractionated heparin.[89] However, antibodies from patients with previous HIT cross-react with every commercially available LMWH, therefore LMWHs cannot be safely used in a patient known to have HIT.[89]

Alternatives to Heparin

Neither heparin nor low molecular weight heparin can be used in patients with HIT; furthermore, no safe dosing regimen has been approved for LMWH in the presence of renal failure. Current alternatives to heparin include selective factor Xa inhibitors, direct thrombin inhibitors, and oral anticoagulants.

Direct thrombin inhibitors include the hirudin family, first isolated from leeches, and the argatroban family of active-site inhibitors. The advantage of such agents over unfractionated heparin is their ability to inhibit fibrin-bound thrombin with a predictable dose response, and their inability to produce HIT.[70] Hirudin and its derivatives, especially lepirudin and bivalirudin, are potent anticoagulants which have been proven more effective than enoxaparin, a LMWH, in DVT prophylaxis of patients undergoing hip replacement.[90] The risk of life-threatening bleeds appears to be equal between hirudin and heparin,[90,91] although an increased risk of moderate bleeding was observed with hirudin.[91] aPTT must be monitored with hirudin agents (goal aPTT = 1.5 to 2.5 times control). Dosages must be adjusted for renal insufficiency. The agents are approved for use in patients with HIT, but they have not been extensively studied in prospective comparison to heparin or LMWH in treatment of pulmonary embolism.

Additional direct thrombin inhibitors are the class represented by argatroban, melagatran, and the new oral agent ximelagatran. Argatroban is an effective anticoagulant in patients with HIT, and has been licensed for use in this capacity.[70] Like the hirudins, argatroban has not been studied in any randomized trials in PE, but it appears to be as safe or safer than heparin when given to patients with myocardial infarction.[92] It is cleared principally by the biliary system and the dose needs no adjustment for renal failure. Monitoring of both the aPTT and the prothrombin time (PT) is recommended. Ximelagatran, an oral prodrug converted to melagatran, does not require monitoring. Having been proved favorable in preventing DVT following total knee replacement compared to both coumadin[93] and enoxaparin,[94] ximelagatran was tested for secondary prevention of DVT. In this study, the oral drug was compared to warfarin therapy for patients who had already received 6 months of oral anticoagulation with coumadin.[95] Recurrent thromboembolism was significantly reduced in the ximelagatran group (2.8% vs. 12.6% in the warfarin group, $p < 0.001$), with similar rates of major bleeding. Three cases of fatal pulmonary embolism were diagnosed in the warfarin group, compared to none in the ximelagatran group, though overall mortality was equivalent between groups. Ximelagatran has been shown to cause elevated liver aminotransferases, especially in the first 4 months of therapy; in this study, all cases of elevated alanine aminotransferase were transient, and no case (out of 600) progressed to hepatic failure.[95]

Among the newest of antithrombotic agents approved for the prophylaxis of DVT and pulmonary embolus is fondaparinux, a novel synthetic drug inhibiting factor Xa. By binding to antithrombin with tight affinity and inducing a conformational change, fondaparinux facilitates the binding of antithrombin with factor Xa, thus blocking the common pathway of coagulation.[70] It has been approved by the FDA as a subcutaneous injection of 2.5 mg once daily for use in DVT and PE prophylaxis in patients undergoing orthopedic surgery for hip fracture, hip replacement, or knee replacement, after several randomized controlled trials found superior reduction of DVT for fondaparinux compared to enoxaparin.[96] A study comparing fondaparinux and heparin for pulmonary embolism found the new agent to be as effective and safe as heparin, with a nonsignificant trend toward fewer recurrences of VTE in the fondaparinux group.[97] Bleeding events were similar, and no difference in mortality was detected. HIT has not been observed with fondaparinux use. A number of additional anti–factor Xa agents are in development, but they have not yet been widely tested in humans. While fondaparinux shows promise in the acute treatment of PE, more studies are necessary before recommending that factor Xa inhibition replace our traditional anticoagulant strategies.

Warfarin anticoagulation should be instituted in the first few days (5 mg PO qhs for the first 2 days, then adjust the dose to achieve an International Normalized Ratio [INR] between 2.0 and 3.0) and continued to overlap with heparin therapy for at least 5 days. If the patient is clinically unstable or likely to require ongoing invasive procedures, heparin or a rapidly adjustable agent such as lepirudin or argatroban should be used preferentially, to facilitate rapid adjustment of anticoagulation if necessary.

VENA CAVAL INTERRUPTION

Occasionally patients have compelling reasons that preclude anticoagulation, or continue to embolize despite adequate anticoagulation. As most thromboemboli originate in the legs, pelvis, or inferior vena cava (IVC),[98] inferior vena caval interruption (VCI) has the potential to prevent subsequent embolization. Conventional indications for the use of VCI in patients with venous thromboembolism have included contraindications to anticoagulation, hemorrhage following anticoagulation, failure of anticoagulation to prevent recurrent embolization, and prophylaxis of extremely high-risk patients. Only one randomized prospective trial has evaluated using VCI to prevent PE.[99] This trial randomized 400 patients with proximal DVT who were at risk for PE to receive a vena caval filter or standard anticoagulation. Over the first 12 days, the vena caval filter group had significantly fewer cases of PE (1.1% vs. 4.8%, $p < 0.03$). However, over the subsequent 2 years, during which all patients were anticoagulated for at least 3 months, the rates of PE, major bleeding, and death were similar in both groups. Moreover, the vena caval filter group actually had a significantly higher rate of recurrent DVT, with a nearly twofold increase in odds ratio for DVT compared to the no-filter group. Thus VCI appeared to be a successful short-term strategy to prevent PE, but came at the expense of increased long-term DVT and a trend toward increased thromboembolic disease. This landmark study prompted widespread discussion on two fronts: whether anticoagulation should be considered for all patients receiving a vena caval filter, and whether a temporary or retrievable filter might be more successful.[100] Unfortunately, no prospective trial evaluates either question. Progress has been made in the technology of retrievable filters, and small case series of several different types of temporary filters have been published.[101,102] Whereas initially, temporary filters had to be removed within a 2-week period in order to minimize the risk of endothelialization, newer filters have been retrieved after up to 134 days without complication.[101]

As VCI devices have evolved, they have become smaller and more easily placed. As physicians have become more experienced with them, they have become safer as well, although published complication rates have varied widely, from 2% to 19%.[101] Proposed indications for VCI continue to expand as the technology improves,[100] yet caval filters are probably underutilized in the sickest patients. Those with critical cardiopulmonary compromise may be least able to tolerate the admittedly low risk of heparin failure. Patients who survive sublethal embolism but remain hemodynamically compromised may benefit from VCI since recurrent embolism, while unlikely, will be fatal. In addition, some patients have such a predictably high risk of venous thromboembolism that VCI may be indicated even before any thrombosis is detected. For example, we have placed caval filters prophylactically in patients with severe COPD and proximal venous thrombosis and in a woman with Crohn's disease complicated by toxic megacolon and ARDS on her way to the operating room. Additional potential indications include extensive free-floating vena caval thrombus (since the efficacy of heparin in this setting is controversial), pre–pulmonary embolectomy, and as primary treatment in patients with malignancy (since anticoagulants seem less effective and less safe in this setting). The advent of safe, effective retrievable filters may greatly expand our use of VCI.

Complications include filter fracture (occasionally with embolization of fragments), improper placement of the filter, venous thrombosis at the insertion site (seen in 8% to 25%[103]), caval occlusion (which is now far less common than when the Mobin-Uddin "umbrella" filters were in use), inadvertent dislodgment by guidewires during central venous catheterization, and erosion or perforation of the caval wall and other viscera. A final point about VCI is that while it prevents most recurrent emboli, it does not treat the (presumed) leg source. Therefore, when these devices are used, concomitant anticoagulation is necessary (unless the indication for VCI is contraindication to anticoagulation). The significance of upper extremity sources of thromboemboli in ICU patients, who often have central catheters, is unknown but probably small. Nevertheless, inferior VCI would clearly be ineffective so that when the clinical presentation suggests an upper source, due consideration should precede placement of this device. Filters have been placed in the superior vena cava and in the suprarenal IVC with apparent safety, but the experience is limited.

THROMBOLYTIC THERAPY

It has been clear for more than three decades that thrombolytic therapy more rapidly lyses pulmonary emboli and improves hemodynamics.[104] However, 7 days after therapy, patients given thrombolytic therapy cannot be distinguished from those treated only with heparin on the basis of clinical findings or lung perfusion.[105] Combined with the clearly increased risk and cost of thrombolytic agents, this has led to a general skepticism about the value of thrombolytic therapy for the treatment of PE. In a survey of pulmonary physicians, only 11% would give thrombolytic therapy for a large PE without hypotension, severe hypoxemia, or right ventricular strain.[106] However, nearly all would give thrombolytics to a patient with shock due to PE, and there is now convincing data to support this approach. For example, when patients with massive PE were given alteplase (1 mg/kg over 1 hour) in an uncontrolled trial, there was significant clinical improvement in 11 of 15 with shock.[107]

In another study comparing alteplase (100 mg over 2 hours) and heparin, right ventricular function assessed echocardiographically improved more rapidly in patients given alteplase.[108] This more rapid hemodynamic improvement could translate into improved survival in critically compromised patients. Furthermore, of the 55 patients treated with heparin alone, 5 suffered recurrence (2 fatal) within 14 days, whereas none of 46 patients given alteplase recurred. Finally, one very small (eight patients) randomized clinical trial comparing thrombolysis (streptokinase, 1,500,000 U over 1 hour) with heparin in patients with massive embolism and hypoperfusion showed a mortality benefit for thrombolytic therapy; all four patients receiving heparin alone died, while there were no deaths in the streptokinase group.[109]

Recently, the debate over thrombolytic therapy has moved from discussion of massive PE to that of submassive PE: PE which has not yet provoked hypotension, but for which the risk for death is high. Data from echocardiographic studies show an indisputably higher mortality in patients with moderate RV dysfunction.[30] The utility of echocardiography in prognostication has led to great interest as to whether echocardiographic criteria should be used routinely to guide the use of thrombolytic therapy.[110,111] Two studies address this question. In a retrospective cohort study of patients with radiographically large emboli and right ventricular dilation (but without hypotension or shock), those who received thrombolytic therapy had better pulmonary perfusion on day one, but this advantage disappeared by day seven.[112] Mortality was 6% in the thrombolytic group compared to no deaths in the heparin group, and severe bleeding in the thrombolytic group approached 10%, with intracranial bleeds in 4% of patients. In a second, prospective study, patients with acute PE and right ventricular dysfunction (but without shock) were randomized to heparin plus alteplase or heparin plus placebo.[113] While there was no difference in mortality between groups, the alteplase group had a significantly lower rate of treatment escalation, mostly consisting of secondary thrombolysis for worsened symptoms. No significant difference in bleeding was found between groups, which was surprising, as previous studies have never failed to show an increased risk of major hemorrhage with thrombolytic therapy compared to heparin. In a large prospective registry of over 2400 patients with PE, the rate of major hemorrhage in patients receiving thrombolytics was almost 22%, and intracranial bleeds were noted in 3%.[114] The retrospective, nonrandomized nature of the first study raises concerns for its validity, but the latter has also been cited as potentially flawed in its design, both in its definition of "right heart dysfunction" and its use of secondary thrombolysis based on vague clinical criteria.[115] As no mortality benefit has yet been established for patients with submassive PE who receive thrombolysis, we advocate restricting thrombolytic therapy for those patients with clinically apparent shock.

The optimal regimen for thrombolytic therapy has not been established. A number of approaches are listed in Table 27-6.[104,107,109,116–118] There has been a general trend towards bolus, as opposed to long-duration, infusion, based on both animal studies and human trials in patients with myocardial infarction showing increased efficacy and reduced hemorrhage. Yet the increasing benefits of front-loaded regimens

TABLE 27-6 Alternative Thrombolytic Strategies in Acute Massive Pulmonary Embolism

[a] Urokinase, 4400 U/kg bolus, followed by 4400 U/kg per hour for 24 hours[104]

Urokinase, 1,000,000 U bolus over 10 minutes, followed by 2,000,000 U over 110 minutes[116]

Urokinase, 15,000 U/kg bolus over 10 minutes[117]

rt-PA, 0.6 mg/kg bolus over 2–15 minutes [118]

rt-PA, 1 mg/kg over 10 minutes [107]

[a] rt-PA, 100 mg over 2 hours [116]

Streptokinase, 1,500,000 U over 1 hour[109]

[a] Streptokinase, 250,000 U over 30 minutes, followed by 100,000 U/h for 24 hours

[a] Approved by the Food and Drug Administration.

ABBREVIATIONS: rt-PA, recombinant tissue plasminogen activator.

NOTE: Heparin is infused at 1300 U/h when the activated prothrombin time falls below twice normal, then adjusted to keep the aPTT between 1.5 and 2.5 times control.

TABLE 27-7 Contraindications to Thrombolytic Therapy

Absolute
  Recent puncture in a noncompressible site
  Active or recent internal bleeding
  Hemorrhagic diathesis
  Recent central nervous system surgery or active intracranial lesion
  Uncontrolled hypertension (BP >180/110 mm Hg)
  Known hypersensitivity, or for streptokinase, use of streptokinase
    within 6 months
  Diabetic hemorrhagic retinopathy
  Acute pericarditis
  Recent obstetric delivery
  History of stroke
Relative
  Trauma (including cardiopulmonary resuscitation) or major
    surgery within 10 days
  Pregnancy
  High likelihood of left heart thrombus
  Advanced age
  Liver disease

NOTE: See text for discussion about "absolute" contraindications.

has a limit as demonstrated in a comparison of alteplase, 0.6 mg/kg (maximum dose = 50 mg) over 15 minutes versus 100 mg over 2 hours, in which there was no significant difference in efficacy or rate of hemorrhage.[119–121] The particular thrombolytic agent is probably not of much importance. In a head-to-head comparison of alteplase (100 mg over 2 hours) and urokinase (1,000,000 U over 10 minutes followed by 2,000,000 over 110 minutes), the two regimens yielded similar efficacy and safety.[122] A powerful case can be made that streptokinase is the agent of choice since it is the one agent for which a mortality benefit has been shown,[109] and it is fourfold cheaper than any of the current alternatives. Careful attention should be given to selecting patients appropriately to reduce the rate of hemorrhagic complications (Table 27-7). Especially important is a concerted effort to avoid invasive procedures, including arterial blood gases, arterial catheters, central venous punctures, and pulmonary angiograms, where possible.[123]

Various measures of the lytic state correlate poorly with both efficacy and incidence of bleeding, so that outside of clinical research protocols, routine monitoring is not indicated. When streptokinase is given, the manufacturer recommends that the thrombin time be assayed at 4 hours to ensure that a lytic state is achieved. An adequate lytic state can be assumed if the thrombin time is prolonged above the normal limits of the laboratory, or if the fibrinogen level is reduced. Clinical monitoring should include serial neurologic examinations to detect central nervous system hemorrhage and frequent vital signs to detect gastrointestinal or retroperitoneal hemorrhage. Patients who have undergone catheterization should have the groin puncture examined, and preferably have repeated measurements of thigh girth. Huge volumes of blood can be lost into the thigh and groin, especially in obese patients, with little external evidence of bleeding.

After the thrombolytic agent is discontinued, heparin is typically begun (without a bolus) when the thrombin time or the aPTT falls to less than 2 times control. Heparin is begun as an intravenous infusion at 1300 U/h and titrated to a PTT of 1.5 to 2.5 times control.

No advantage to infusing the thrombolytic agent directly into the pulmonary artery has been shown in controlled trials despite claims of benefit in small case series.[124] Investigational approaches include pharmacomechanical thrombolysis[125] and augmentation of cardiac output to enhance thrombolysis.[126]

Thrombolytic Therapy following Surgery
Although recent surgery is generally included among the absolute contraindications to thrombolytic therapy, there is an evolving literature supporting its use. For example, 13 patients with angiographically confirmed embolism within 2 weeks of major surgery (mean = 9.6 days) were given a modified regimen of urokinase (2200 U/kg directly into the clot, followed by 2200 U/kg per hour for up to 24 hours).[127] Complete lysis was achieved in all and there were no deaths or bleeding complications. In another report, two patients in shock due to PE were given bolus regimens of urokinase (1,200,000 U) or alteplase (40 mg, followed by another 40 mg over 1 hour) only 2 days after lung resection.[128] There was prompt clinical improvement, although one patient had delayed hemorrhage. Finally, nine patients were treated with urokinase (1,000,000 U over 10 minutes, followed by 2,000,000 U over 110 minutes) following neurosurgery (mean = 19 days following surgery).[129] All of the patients survived their acute episode of PE and no intracranial hemorrhage occurred, although one patient developed a subgaleal hematoma. These reports suggest that recent surgery is a relative, not an absolute, contraindication, and that the risks and benefits should be considered on an individual basis.

Complications
The greatest limitation of the thrombolytic drugs, and the factor which has limited their acceptance for the treatment of venous thromboembolism, is the consequential incidence of bleeding. In patients treated for pulmonary embolism the risk of major hemorrhage is reported to be around 15%,[107] but these data were gathered in an era of frequent pulmonary angiography. As mentioned, intracranial bleeds have been observed in as many as 4.7% of patients,[112] although larger series report a 3% incidence.[114] When serious bleeding occurs, the lytic agent should be immediately discontinued, and reliable, multiple, large-bore catheters secured. Direct compression of bleeding vessels may stop or slow ongoing blood loss. If heparin has been given, it too should be stopped and consideration given to reversing heparinization with protamine. Most patients will be adequately managed without the transfusion of clotting factors. If it becomes necessary to reverse the lytic state, cryoprecipitate, which contains fibrinogen and factor VIII (both of which are consumed by plasmin) is the preferred blood product.[130] The initial dose is 10 units, after which the fibrinogen level should be assayed. Fresh frozen plasma (as a source of factors V and VIII), platelets, and fibrinolytic drugs (e.g., epsilon aminocaproic acid 5 g over 30 minutes) all may play a role in the critically bleeding patient.

Allergic Effects
Allergic reactions, including skin rashes, fever, and hypotension are rare except with streptokinase. Mild reactions can be treated with antihistamines and acetaminophen. More

severe reactions should prompt the addition of hydrocortisone. Hypotension usually responds to volume administration.

FLUID, VASOACTIVE DRUGS, AND NITRIC OXIDE

Volume administration with saline or colloid has generally been advocated in patients with PE and shock on the grounds that it will increase filling pressures and thereby augment $\dot{Q}_T$. However, in a patient with elevated right heart pressures and a grossly distended right ventricle, it is possible that further distention of the right ventricle during volume administration will increase myocardial oxygen consumption, yet fail to increase $\dot{Q}_T$ and oxygen supply. In addition, to the extent that fluids increase right ventricular end-diastolic volume, the interventricular septum will bulge further to the left, impede left heart filling, and further compromise $\dot{Q}_T$. Experimental studies to determine the effect of fluids have shown a detrimental effect on hemodynamics.[131] Therefore, volume administration should not be routine therapy unless the patient is clearly hypovolemic. When fluids are given, central venous catheterization (to measure venous oxyhemoglobin saturation and changes in right atrial pressure) and echocardiography may provide useful guidance. These issues are further discussed in Chapter 26.

There is also controversy regarding the use of vasoactive drugs to treat the hypoperfusion caused by PE. Successful use of vasoconstrictors, inotropes, and vasodilators has been reported. Since no controlled studies in patients have been performed, it is hard to give firm recommendations. However, the pathophysiology of this form of shock, the results of some animal experiments, and limited human data (all discussed in Chapter 26) provide some guidance. When any of these drugs are used, serial assessment of the effect of the intervention is mandatory. Any drug which does not result in the intended salutary effect should be discontinued promptly.

The vasoactive drug of choice, based on the largest published experience in patients, is dobutamine.[132] Dobutamine is infused beginning at 5 μg/kg per minute and increased to effect. If dobutamine is ineffective or incompletely effective, norepinephrine should be tried. The rationale for the use of this vasoconstrictor is based on the assumption that right ventricular ischemia is the fundamental problem leading to shock. A vasoconstrictor that increases systemic arteriolar tone could raise aortic pressure and augment coronary blood flow, without increasing right ventricular load. In animal models of sublethal PE, norepinephrine was shown to be superior to no therapy, to volume administration, and to isoproterenol in the maintenance of cardiac output as well as in survival time.[133] Infusion is initiated at 2 μg/min and adjusted (up to 30 μg/min) based on the hemodynamic response. In the clinical setting, hypoperfusion may have additional contributors such as left ventricular dysfunction or ischemic heart disease, so that a vasoconstrictor might be less beneficial than in controlled animal experiments. If dobutamine and norepinephrine fail to improve cardiac output, epinephrine may succeed.[134] Finally, nitric oxide, which can lower the pulmonary artery pressure, boost cardiac output, and improve oxygenation, can be tried if available.[135,136]

EMBOLECTOMY AND MECHANICAL THERAPIES

Surgical embolectomy is a major procedure rarely resorted to in most institutions. In part, this is related to the availability of other, more benign, therapies such as heparin and thrombolysis. Additionally, it takes time to organize a surgical team, operating room, cardiopulmonary bypass and so on, by which time the patient is often hemodynamically improved or moribund. Yet embolectomy has its advocates, who maintain that thrombolytic therapy is often contraindicated in patients who could benefit from it, the operative mortality for embolectomy is now acceptable, and chronic cor pulmonale can be averted.

In one institution's review of 87 patients with PE, 34 were treated with heparin, 28 with streptokinase, and 25 with embolectomy.[137] Pretreatment embolic scores were most severe in the embolectomy group. Hospital mortality in the heparin, streptokinase, and surgery groups was 6%, 21%, and 20%, respectively. However, cumulative survival at 5 years was 68%, 64%, and 80%, a trend favoring embolectomy. However, most late deaths were due to malignancy, not recurrent PE or chronic pulmonary hypertension. Although the authors recommended surgical embolectomy for all patients with emboli in the main pulmonary arteries based on their results, regardless of the hemodynamic impact, this study was not randomized and the possibility seems large that the long-term benefit for embolectomy was related to selection of patients. A more recent trial showed that surgical embolectomy was comparable to thrombolytic therapy in patients with massive PE.[138]

Mortality due to embolectomy appears to be in the range of 30% to 40%, but may be as low as 8% in those who have not sustained cardiac arrest preoperatively.[139,140] Even if this lower number reflects improvements in anesthetic or operative technique, this mortality is still comparable to that of patients with massive embolism treated less invasively.[141] The argument that embolectomy might reduce the long-term consequences of chronic pulmonary hypertension lacks force, even though this complication is more common than previously thought.[142] Thus it has never been demonstrated in a well-performed trial that embolectomy confers any advantage over thrombolytic therapy, or for that matter heparin. The population of patients who might benefit from embolectomy appears to be those who meet the following criteria: those with a hemodynamically significant embolism, in whom thrombolytic therapy is contraindicated; and in a center with a rapidly responding cardiopulmonary bypass team and a surgeon experienced in the technique of embolectomy.

Several new devices have been tested which aim to remove pulmonary emboli less invasively than the direct surgical approach. For example, a 10F suction catheter, inserted through a jugular or femoral venotomy and advanced into the pulmonary artery has been used to extract clot.[143] Eleven of eighteen patients improved immediately. Suction embolectomy was more likely to be successful in patients treated promptly after hemodynamic deterioration. More recently, patients with shock underwent mechanical fragmentation of their massive PE with a rotational pigtail catheter, followed by thrombolytic therapy.[144] Nine of ten patients survived, and 6 of the survivors achieved hemodynamic stability within 48 hours of the procedure. Alternative methods to re-establish pulmonary artery patency include endovascular stents,[145] but experience with all of these techniques is limited.

Special Considerations

PREGNANCY

The pregnant woman who may have PE presents unique challenges.[146] Pregnancy is thought to be a risk factor for venous thrombosis, and PE is the second leading cause of death among gravidas (next to trauma).[147] The addition of the fetus, as well as anatomic considerations, leads to several key differences in management.

DIAGNOSIS

Diagnosis can be more difficult because of reluctance to perform potentially risky procedures, particularly involving diagnostic radiology. However, it is important not to lose sight of the risk of failing to make the diagnosis. Thus when the diagnosis is seriously considered, it should be pursued. $\dot{V}/\dot{Q}$ scans probably pose little risk to the fetus. The estimated radiation dose is small, and the risk is clearly less than that of missing a diagnosis.[148] Impedance plethysmography is also less useful in pregnancy due to mechanical compression of the IVC by the enlarged uterus, especially in the third trimester. A positive result in the first two trimesters is sufficient basis on which to anticoagulate, but may not be in the last trimester unless the vascular laboratory has particular expertise in pregnancy.[149] The risk of helical CT angiography is not known, but when indicated, it should not be withheld out of concern for fetal radiation exposure. The maternal risks of undiagnosed and untreated PE are clear. A diagnosis of thromboembolism in pregnancy has serious implications for the mother, not just in the current pregnancy, but during any subsequent pregnancies. Because of the risk of heparin-induced osteoporosis and the remaining uncertainties about effective prophylaxis against recurrence during future pregnancies, the diagnosis of thromboembolism should never be made lightly in a gravida, but instead should be based on solid evidence.

TREATMENT

The use of heparin in pregnancy is no different than in the nonpregnant patient. Heparins do not cross the placenta, and pose a low risk to the fetus. However, warfarin, which is teratogenic, should not be instituted. Rather, long-term treatment should consist of subcutaneous heparin[150] or LMWH.[151] LMWHs are preferred in that they have a lower incidence of both bleeding and of heparin-induced thrombocytopenia.[151] Osteoporosis is a serious complication of full-dose heparin during pregnancy, with fractures occurring in 2% of women.[152] There are indications that bone mineral loss is reversible,[153] but several cases of debilitating back pain have been reported. Low molecular weight heparins, when prospectively studied, do not appear to accelerate bone mineral density loss.[154] Thrombolytic therapy risks spontaneous abortion and uterine bleeding. Nevertheless, several case reports of the successful use of thrombolytic treatment of PE have appeared. Vena caval interruption requires some modification as well. The left ovarian vein (a potential source of clot) drains into the left renal vein. Therefore, when a caval filter is placed, it should be inserted to a suprarenal position, rather than below the renal veins. Again, several cases of successful use of these devices have been described. Pregnancy may be an ideal situation for the temporary vena caval interruption device.

CHRONIC OBSTRUCTIVE PULMONARY DISEASE

Patients with COPD are at increased risk for PE. In addition, their preexisting respiratory compromise and abnormal pulmonary vasculature leave them particularly vulnerable to the cardiopulmonary consequences of PE. Ironically, diagnosis of PE in the setting of COPD is unusually difficult. Patients commonly complain of dyspnea, chest pain, cough, and anxiety, and occasionally note hemoptysis and leg swelling. Their examinations, chest radiograms, ECGs, and arterial blood gas values are usually abnormal at baseline. $\dot{V}/\dot{Q}$ scans are most often unhelpful. For example, in PIOPED 108 patients were identified as having COPD (although objective data were available in only 43).[155] Scans were intermediate probability in a full 60%. Only 20 patients (19%) had results which made pulmonary angiography unnecessary by being normal, high probability, or low probability paired with a low pretest clinical estimate. Nevertheless, for the occasional patient, $\dot{V}/\dot{Q}$ scanning obviated pulmonary angiography.

When patients with COPD present with symptoms that are atypical for their usual exacerbation, particularly when the Pa_{CO_2} is reduced from previously elevated values, it is worth considering the diagnosis.[156] Positive leg studies may provide a rationale for anticoagulation and obviate the need for further investigation, although this approach has been called into question.[41] CT angiography or pulmonary angiography may be necessary to establish a diagnosis. The physician and patient may be in the unfortunate position of having to repeatedly consider an invasive procedure or risk a missed diagnosis. In fact, it is in just this type of situation that PEs go undiagnosed. There is no simple answer to this problem and PEs will continue to be underdiagnosed until better, less invasive tests are available.

PATIENTS WITH COAGULATION OR PLATELET DISORDERS

The risk of venous thromboembolism in patients with chronic liver disease or marked thrombocytopenia is not known. While it seems sensible to conclude that the risk must be lower than if clotting and platelet function were normal, PEs occur even when the bleeding tendency is severe.[157,158] Therefore, when the clinical presentation strongly suggests PE, thrombocytopenia and coagulopathy should provide little reassurance, and diagnostic testing is indicated. Patients with chronic renal failure—excepting those with nephrotic syndrome—do seem to be at a remarkably low risk of venous thromboembolism, so alternative diagnoses should always be sought.

Prophylaxis against Venous Thromboembolism

A discussion of prophylaxis has been left to the end of the section on thromboembolism because here it is particularly easy to emphasize several points. PE is common, lethal, usually missed, difficult to evaluate, and costly to treat. Critical illness makes these statements especially true, therefore the goal must be to prevent this disease. A full treatment of prophylaxis is beyond the scope of this chapter, but a few points are worth making. Prophylaxis in the ICU is discussed further in Chapter 10.

Over the last 20 years, a large volume of information regarding the risks and benefits of numerous prophylactic strategies has been collected. The greatest accumulated experience is with low-dose heparin, typically 5000 U administered subcutaneously either bid or tid both in surgical and medical patients. Other methods of thromboprophylaxis are also available, and may have a role in special subsets of patients, patients in whom heparin is ineffective or contraindicated, or those who are at unusually high (or low) risk of VTE. These alternatives include low molecular weight heparins (LMWHs), adjusted-dose heparin, aspirin, warfarin, dextrans, antiembolism stockings, intermittent pneumatic (or sequential) compression cuffs, and vena caval interruption. In some patients combined prophylaxis is superior. For example, the combination of minidose heparin and intermittent pneumatic compression was more effective than minidose heparin alone in patients following cardiac surgery.[159] In trauma patients[160] and in patients suffering hip fracture, LMWH is superior to low-dose heparin. In many settings the optimal approach has not yet been clarified and there are far fewer data regarding medical patients than surgical patients. Nevertheless, for most patients at risk of VTE, some method which is both safe and effective is available. In one survey of 152 medical ICU patients, only 33% were given prophylaxis and there was a mean delay of 2 days before prophylaxis was prescribed, although risk factors were identified in 87% of patients.[161] In the absence of a contraindication, nearly all critically ill patients should receive minidose heparin. When heparin is unsafe (e.g., neurosurgical patients), alternative methods of prophylaxis, such as intermittent pneumatic compression cuffs, should be instituted. In some patients at very high risk of thromboembolism, such as those with acute spinal cord injury, minidose heparin is ineffective and LMWH is preferred.[83] In most patients, however, the increased cost of LMWHs is not matched by clearly incremental efficacy or improved safety.[83] Finally, although controversial, some patients at extremely high risk of PE should have consideration given to prophylactic insertion of vena caval filters (see above).

Air Embolism

The syndrome of air (or gas) embolism results when air enters the vasculature, travels to the pulmonary circulation, and causes circulatory or respiratory embarrassment. It is uncommonly recognized in critically ill patients, but is quite likely underdiagnosed.

PATHOPHYSIOLOGY

The syndrome is triggered when a gas, usually air, enters a vessel, typically a vein. It travels with the venous return to the right heart and lungs, where it may have circulatory or respiratory consequences. Occasionally, air reaches the arterial circulation leading to systemic manifestations. Although air embolism is often abrupt and short-lived, intriguing cases of continuous streaming of bubbles in mechanically ventilated patients have been reported.[162] At times, such embolism may persist over many days.

ENTRY OF AIR INTO THE VASCULATURE

Development of air embolism requires an abnormal communication between air and the blood vessel. In addition, there must be a pressure gradient to favor entry of air into the vessel, rather than bleeding from the vessel. Trauma, surgical incisions, and intravascular catheters create the most common sources of air entry. In addition, there are more subtle paths through which air can reach the vasculature, such as in damaged, mechanically ventilated lungs of patients with ARDS. The driving gradient for air entry may be provided by air under pressure, as during positive pressure ventilation or high pressure wound irrigation. Alternatively, the air may be at atmospheric pressure, but the intravascular pressure is subatmospheric. For example, any vein which is above the heart by an amount exceeding the right atrial pressure is likely to be at less than atmospheric pressure (and therefore appears collapsed). Table 27-8 lists some of the causes of the air embolism syndrome.

CIRCULATORY CONSEQUENCES

Massive air embolization can fill the right heart, impede venous return, and thereby stop circulation; thus sudden death is one of the possible outcomes. It is estimated that >100 mL of air must be acutely infused to arrest circulation. Most often, however, air passes through the right heart into the lungs. There it raises PA pressure, but has predominantly respiratory consequences. Since unilateral experimental air embolism causes pulmonary hemodynamic changes similar to bilateral embolism, humoral or reflex vascular changes

TABLE 27-8 Etiology of Air Embolism

Surgery and Trauma Related	Nonsurgical
Neurosurgery, especially upright	Cardiopulmonary resuscitation
Liver transplantation	Gastrointestinal endoscopy
Total hip replacement	Barotrauma
Harrington rod insertion	Positive pressure ventilation
Spinal fusion	Infusion computed tomography scan
Pulsed saline irrigation	Scuba diving
Removal of tissue expanders	Self-induced
Transurethral resection of prostate	Orogenital sex
Cesarean section	
Arthroscopy	
Open heart surgery	
Hysterectomy	
Head and neck trauma	
Dental implant surgery	
Pacemaker insertion	
Tenckhoff catheter placement	
Intra-aortic balloon pump	
Bone marrow harvest	
Epidural catheter placement	
Central line placement	
Central line removal	
Percutaneous lung biopsy	
Pulmonary contusion	
Laser bronchoscopy	
Retrograde pyelography	
Hemodialysis	
Percutaneous lithotripsy	

probably account for some of the increase in pulmonary vascular resistance. In an experimental canine model of massive air embolism, systemic hypotension and pulmonary hypertension were attenuated by pretreatment with an intravenous endothelin-receptor antagonist.[163] Such work suggests that the circulatory effects of air embolism may be due to cytokine release following release of endothelin—a potent pulmonary vasoconstrictor—and that the activation of the cyclooxygenase pathway may contribute. One case study described a patient with suspected air embolism who developed the systemic inflammatory response syndrome,[164] perhaps lending further credence to the idea that air in the circulation causes downstream humoral, not simply mechanical, consequences.

RESPIRATORY CONSEQUENCES

Air is carried into the pulmonary vasculature where it embolizes in pulmonary arterioles and capillaries. The abnormal air-blood interface is thought to denature plasma proteins, creating amorphous proteinaceous and cellular debris at the surface of air bubbles.[165] This debris attracts and activates white blood cells, facilitating injury to the pulmonary capillaries. Endothelial injury increases capillary permeability, which leads to alveolar flooding. The resulting noncardiogenic pulmonary edema accounts for the majority of symptoms and signs due to air embolism (see Chap. 38). In addition, air embolization leads to bronchoconstriction, a point which may be useful in diagnosis.[166]

Although the dominant gas exchange abnormality is hypoxemia, carbon dioxide elimination is impaired as well. As pulmonary vessels become occluded, alveoli subtended by them are ventilated, but unperfused. This increment in dead space may be signaled by a drop in end-tidal CO_2, if this is being monitored. In the patient with fixed minute ventilation (e.g., if the patient is on a muscle relaxant), P_{CO_2} will rise. Either of these may lead to suspicion of the diagnosis.

EXTRATHORACIC MANIFESTATIONS

Air embolism is occasionally accompanied by systemic findings. If air directly enters the pulmonary veins, as may occur in patients being mechanically ventilated with acute lung injury, bubbles pass directly to the arterial circulation. However, since air typically enters a systemic vein, the arterial circulation is protected from embolization by the filtering effect of the pulmonary circulation. Nevertheless, bubbles can pass to the left side of the heart via the foramen ovale, which is probe patent in up to 30% of people. This type of foramen ovale does not ordinarily allow right-to-left shunting, due to the higher pressures in the left atrium. However, after significant embolization to the pulmonary circulation, right heart pressures rise, reversing the interatrial gradient. This allows bubbles to pass directly from the right to left atrium, then to the systemic circulation. Even in the absence of a foramen ovale, air can reach the arterial circulation since the lungs do not fully filter air, especially when a large amount is embolized. Air may pass through large extra-alveolar vessels or through the pulmonary capillaries themselves. In animal experiments, the threshold rate of venous air infusion that overwhelms pulmonary filtering is 0.30 mL/kg per minute.[167] For a 70-kg man, this value translates to only 21 mL/min.

Once air reaches the arterial circulation, peripheral embolization leads to ischemic manifestations in the brain, heart, skin (livedo reticularis),[168] and other organs. Some of the

TABLE 27-9 Manifestations of Air Embolism

Dyspnea, hypoxemia
Confusion, stroke, or peripheral embolization
Hypotension and shock
Diffuse alveolar infiltrates
Increment in airway pressures
Increased dead space and rising minute ventilation
Abrupt fall in end-tidal CO_2
Detection of air by echocardiography, Doppler monitor, or radiography

ischemic manifestations in the periphery are probably mediated by polymorphonuclear leukocytes and oxygen radicals, as is the injury in the lung.[169]

PRESENTATION

Air embolism is usually recognized when it presents as acute hypoxemic respiratory failure. As noted above, it may also manifest as an acute hypoperfusion state or as peripheral embolization. The chest x-ray shows diffuse alveolar filling. We have seen one case in which intracardiac and intra-arterial air was grossly evident on the chest radiograph. Increased dead space may be indicated by increased $\dot{V}_E$, increased P_{CO_2}, or decreased ET_{CO_2}. Rarely, echocardiography will demonstrate residual air (or ongoing embolization) in the heart. Precordial Doppler monitoring during high-risk surgery is well suited for detecting air (Table 27-9).

A diagnosis of air embolism is usually considered when air is witnessed to enter an intravascular catheter. It is also likely to be considered in extremely high-risk settings such as upright neurosurgery. However, if air embolism is only considered when it is grossly apparent, many episodes will go unappreciated. It should also be included in the differential diagnosis of patients with hypoperfusion, systemic embolization, obtundation, and respiratory failure, especially when more likely causes are lacking. It is also worth emphasizing that many cases are related to central lines, not only during placement, but while the catheters are in place (catheter disconnection, hub fracture, or gas in the line), while being changed over a wire, and after they are removed (through a persistent cutaneous tract).

The differential diagnosis of air embolism includes other forms of noncardiogenic pulmonary edema, as well as cardiogenic edema. Thus volume overload, sepsis, and gastric acid aspiration must be excluded.

MANAGEMENT

The goals of treatment are to prevent re-embolization while supporting respiration and circulation. In most cases, resolution is prompt. The source of air entry should be identified and closed if possible. Alternatively, the gradient favoring air entry can be lessened, as for example by saline administration to raise intravascular pressures. When air embolism complicates positive pressure ventilation, it is advisable to lower airway pressures by lowering tidal volumes, reducing positive end-expiratory pressure (PEEP), or intentionally hypoventilating. Oxygen hastens the reabsorption of air from bubbles, so all patients with significant air embolism should receive 100% oxygen during the initial resuscitation.[170]

In certain situations, it may be possible to retrieve air from the venous circulation or right heart, especially intraoperatively when a catheter is in place for that purpose. However, this should not be routinely attempted in other settings because significant amounts of air cannot usually be removed. Positional maneuvers to prevent air from embolizing to the lungs (such as head down left decubitus) are largely unproved. Similarly, the distribution of arterial emboli seems little affected by the Trendelenburg position, since the force of arterial flow greatly outweighs the buoyancy of the bubbles.[171]

Standard treatment is similar to that of any patient with ARDS. Mechanical ventilation to reduce the work of breathing, with oxygen and PEEP to maintain arterial saturation are usually necessary. Although the pulmonary edema is not related to hypervolemia, the degree of lung leak is probably sensitive to filling pressures. Therefore we reduce filling pressures to the lowest value that allows an adequate $\dot{Q}T$ (see Chap. 38).

In animal experiments, corticosteroids given before embolization, or shortly following embolization, reduce the degree of lung injury. In high-risk neurosurgical patients on steroids, the incidence of the syndrome seems less than in similar patients who are not so treated, suggesting a prophylactic benefit in human beings as well. Nevertheless, no clear treatment role for these agents has been demonstrated, and they should not be routinely given. Potential future therapies include other anti-inflammatory drugs and agents directed against oxygen free radicals.

Hyperbaric treatment is of theoretical benefit since compression reduces the size of bubbles. This reduces the surface area for activation of white blood cells and can thereby limit pulmonary and systemic injury. Such therapy is standard when the mechanism of gas embolism is decompression, such as in professional and recreational divers. It is not routinely used in other critically ill patients, however. Since patients usually respond readily to standard supportive measures, and since the syndrome typically resolves in only 24 to 48 hours, it is unlikely that hyperbaric treatment will find a prominent role in treatment. It is probably better to keep patients in the ICU where they remain under the watchful eye of the health care team, rather than to risk transport for an unproven treatment. When such patients are transported by air, a pressurized craft flying at low altitude should be requested.

Fat Embolism

The fat embolism syndrome (FES) is associated with fat particles in the microcirculation of the lung. It consists typically of lung dysfunction, neurologic manifestations, and petechiae, usually following a latent interval. It is most common following long bone fractures, typically presenting as dyspnea and confusion. However, FES is seen after other forms of trauma and in several nontraumatic conditions as well. For example, FES has been proposed as a major cause of the acute chest syndrome in patients with sickle cell disease[172](see Chap. 108). After long bone or pelvic fracture, the incidence of the syndrome is at least 10% when evidence for it is prospectively sought,[173] although serious clinical manifestations are seen in only 1% to 3%. Since the clinical presentation is usually mild, FES is often unrecognized. Even when lung injury is

TABLE 27-10 Causes of Fat Embolism Syndrome

Traumatic fat embolism
   Long bone fracture (especially femur)
   Other fractures
   Orthopedic surgery
   Blunt trauma to fatty organs (e.g., liver)
   Liposuction
   Bone marrow biopsy
Nontraumatic fat embolism
   Pancreatitis
   Diabetes mellitus
   Lipid infusions
   Sickle cell crisis
   Burns
   Cardiopulmonary bypass
   Decompression sickness
   Corticosteroid therapy
   Osteomyelitis
   Alcoholic fatty liver
   Acute fatty liver of pregnancy
   Lymphangiography
   Cyclosporine infusion

obvious, its cause may be attributed to infection, aspiration, or traumatic ARDS, rather than to fat embolization. Some of the causes of FES are presented in Table 27-10.

PATHOPHYSIOLOGY

NONTRAUMATIC EMBOLISM

Fat globules are seen in pulmonary (and other) vessels at autopsy and can be found in venous blood. In contrast to traumatic embolism, the fat is probably not derived from bone marrow, but rather arises from lipids in the blood. Serum from acutely ill patients has the capacity to agglutinate chylomicrons and very low density lipoproteins, as well as liposomes of nutritional fat emulsions.[174] It has been proposed that C-reactive protein (CRP), which provokes the calcium-dependent agglutination of each of these lipid-containing substances, may underlie nontraumatic FES. Since CRP is dramatically elevated in trauma, sepsis, and inflammatory disorders, this provides a mechanism for fat embolization.

An alternative, but less attractive, hypothesis implicates the liberation of free fatty acids (FFAs) from fat stores. Although FFAs are known to injure the pulmonary vascular endothelium, their concentration in the systemic circulation during critical illness does not rise sufficiently to account for lung injury. An understanding of the pathophysiology is potentially valuable in the search for prophylactic and therapeutic approaches to these patients, since corticosteroids, for example, may ameliorate the toxic effect of embolized fat but act to mobilize FFA.

TRAUMATIC EMBOLISM

Fracture of bone releases neutral fat which embolizes into the pulmonary vasculature. The derivation of this fat from bone is supported by the finding of coincident particles of bone marrow at autopsy in patients with long bone fractures and by echocardiographic studies showing frequent, often dramatic embolism at the time of medullary reaming.[175] Local hydrolysis of fat by lung lipase releases toxic FFAs, which generate endothelial injury. Systemic findings in FES probably relate to passage of venous fat emboli across the pulmonary circulation, although serum-derived fat may play a role. Elevated right heart pressures following embolism may open a probe patent foramen ovale, causing severe, even fatal systemic embolism.[176] Further, fat can cross the pulmonary circuit even in the absence of a right-to-left shunt, as has been shown in experimental animals.[177] Fat was able to traverse the pulmonary microcirculation even though 15-micron radiolabeled microspheres could not, perhaps due to enhanced deformability of fat emboli.[177]

CLINICAL MANIFESTATIONS

Following injury, there is usually a latent interval of 12 to 72 hours before the syndrome becomes evident. The dominant findings are related to lung injury. Patients with FES present as ARDS, with dyspnea, hypoxemia, and a diffuse lung lesion. In addition, there is often confusion, obtundation, or coma, signs due to cerebral fat embolism rather than coincident hypoxemia. The typical neuropathologic findings include fat microemboli and diffuse petechial hemorrhagic infarcts. Petechiae are also seen on the skin, particularly over the upper chest, neck, and face. On funduscopic examination, embolized fat may be detected in retinal vessels (Purtscher's retinopathy). Often thrombocytopenia and anemia are present. Rare patients will develop a full blown acute right heart syndrome[176] (see Chap. 26).

The diagnosis is usually based on the clinical findings in a patient at risk for FES. Fat globules in the urine are neither sensitive nor specific for the diagnosis of FES. Attempts have been made to find alternative, objective means of diagnosis, since this might be useful in devising prophylactic or therapeutic strategies. Fat can be detected in bronchoalveolar lavage specimens in many patients following trauma, but this finding appears not to be a reliable means of diagnosis.[178] Fat can also be seen in spun samples of blood withdrawn from a wedged pulmonary artery catheter, but this finding is also not clinically useful.[179]

PROPHYLAXIS AND TREATMENT

The substantial incidence of the syndrome and the large number of patients with a well-defined risk factor (long bone fracture) have provided the opportunity to evaluate prophylactic approaches. The least controversial strategy has involved a shift toward early fixation of long bone fractures, even in patients with multiple trauma. Early fixation decreases the incidence of FES, as well as of ARDS and pneumonia, and reduces length of stay.[180–182] Orthopedic surgery, and particularly total hip arthroplasty, carries a high risk of fat embolism, which has been demonstrated by transesophageal echocardiography to occur during the preparation of the femur and insertion of the femoral component. Specific surgical techniques, such as using bone vacuum with the preparation of the femur,[183] have shown decreased fat emboli detected by transesophageal echocardiography, although the clinical significance of such of echo-detected emboli is less clear. More controversial is the use of prophylactic corticosteroids. Nearly all trials of methylprednisolone, in both high (7.5 mg/kg every 6 hours) or low dose (1.5 mg/kg every 8 hours), have shown a reduction in the incidence of the FES, as well as less severe hypoxemia.[184–186] Nevertheless, concerns regarding the risk of infection and impairment of wound healing

have limited the routine use of these drugs. Since most cases of FES are mild and the great majority of patients recover, an acceptable prophylactic regimen would have to be quite safe and inexpensive.

Once the syndrome becomes evident, treatment is that of ARDS (see Chap. 38). Prevention of re-embolization by fracture fixation should be attempted, and supportive management with oxygen and PEEP initiated. It has been suggested that corticosteroids may be of benefit even once the syndrome is established, but it is not clear that the benefits outweigh the risks, and we do not recommend them. No clear role has been established for glucose and insulin, heparin, ethanol, and albumin, despite studies seeking a useful therapy for FES.

References

1. Dalen JE, Alpert JS: Natural history of pulmonary embolism. *Prog Cardiovasc Dis* 17:4:259, 1975.
2. Lilienfeld DE, Chan E, Ehland J, et al: Mortality from pulmonary embolism in the United States: 1962–1984. *Chest* 98:1067, 1990.
3. Alpert JS, Dalen JE: Epidemiology and natural history of venous thromboembolism. *Prog Cardiovasc Dis* 36:417, 1994.
4. Stein PD, Henry JW: Prevalence of acute pulmonary embolism among patients in a general hospital and at autopsy. *Chest* 108:978, 1995.
5. Anderson FA, Wheeler HB, Goldberg RJ, et al: A population-based perspective of the hospital incidence and case-fatality rates of deep vein thrombosis and pulmonary embolism: The Worcester DVT Study. *Arch Intern Med* 151:933, 1991.
6. Silverstein MD, Heit JA, Mohr DN, et al: Trends in the incidence of deep vein thrombosis and pulmonary embolism: A 25-year population based study. *Arch Intern Med* 158:585, 1998.
7. Horlander KT, Mannino DM, Leeper KV: Pulmonary embolism mortality in the United States 1979–1999: an analysis using multiple-cause mortality data. *Arch Intern Med* 163:1711, 2003.
8. Carter CJ: The natural history and epidemiology of venous thrombosis. *Prog Cardiovasc Dis* 36:423, 1994.
9. Hirsch DR, Ingenito EP, Goldhaber SZ: Prevalence of deep venous thrombosis among patients in medical intensive care. *JAMA* 274:335, 1995.
10. Timsit J-F, Farkas JC, Boyer JM, et al: Central vein catheter-related thrombosis in intensive care patients: Incidence, risk factors, and relationship with catheter-related sepsis. *Chest* 114:207, 1998.
11. Burns GA, Cohn SM, Frumento RJ, et al: Prospective ultrasound evaluation of venous thrombosis in high-risk trauma patients. *J Trauma* 35:405, 1993.
12. Gersin K, Grindlinger GA, Lee V, et al: The efficacy of sequential compression devices in multiple trauma patients with severe head injury. *J Trauma* 37:205, 1994.
13. Merli GJ, Crabbe S, Paluzzi RG, Fritz D: Etiology, incidence, and prevention of deep vein thrombosis in acute spinal cord injury. *Arch Phys Med Rehabil* 74:1199, 1993.
14. Cullen DJ, Nemeskal AR: The autopsy incidence of acute pulmonary embolism in critically ill surgical patients. *Intensive Care Med* 12:399, 1986.
15. Monreal M, Lafoz E, Ruiz J, et al: Upper-extremity deep venous thrombosis and pulmonary embolism: A prospective study. *Chest* 99:280, 1991.
16. Chopin C, Fesard P, Mangalaboyi J, et al: Use of capnography in diagnosis of pulmonary embolism during acute respiratory failure of chronic obstructive pulmonary disease. *Crit Care Med* 18:353, 1990.
17. Rodger M, Jones G, Rasuli P, et al: Steady-state end-tidal alveolar dead space friction and D-dimer: Bedside tests to exclude pulmonary embolism. *Chest* 120:115, 2001.

18. D'Alonzo GE, Dantzker DR: Gas exchange alterations following pulmonary thromboembolism. *Clin Chest Med* 5:411, 1984.

19. Stein PD, Goldhaber SZ, Henry JW, et al: Arterial blood gas analysis in the assessment of suspected acute pulmonary embolism. *Chest* 109:78, 1996.

20. Manier G, Castaing Y, Guenard H: Determinants of hypoxemia during the acute phase of pulmonary embolism in humans. *Am Rev Respir Dis* 132:332, 1985.

21. Santolicandro A, Prediletto R, Fornai E, et al: Mechanisms of hypoxemia and hypocapnia in pulmonary embolism. *Am J Respir Crit Care Med* 152:336, 1995.

22. Belenkie I, Dani R, Smith ER, et al: Ventricular interaction during experimental acute pulmonary embolism. *Circulation* 78:761, 1988.

23. Stein PD, Willis PW, DeMets DL: History and physical examination in acute pulmonary embolism in patients without preexisting cardiac or pulmonary disease. *Am J Cardiol* 47:218, 1981.

24. Cozzi PJ, Hall JB, Schmidt GA: Pulmonary artery diastolic-occlusion pressure gradient is increased in acute pulmonary embolism. *Crit Care Med* 23:1481, 1995.

25. Sandham JD, Hull RD, Brant RF, et al: A randomized, controlled trial of the use of pulmonary-artery catheters in high-risk surgical patients. *N Engl J Med* 348:5, 2003.

26. Bova C, Greco F, Misuraca G, et al: Diagnostic utility of echocardiography in patients with suspected pulmonary embolism. *Am J Emerg Med* 21:180, 2003.

27. Miniati M, Simonetta M, Lorenza P, et al: Value of transthoracic echocardiography in the diagnosis of pulmonary embolism: Results of prospective study in unselected patients. *Am J Med* 110:528, 2001.

28. Patel JJ, Chandrasekaran K, Maniet AR, et al: Impact of the incidental diagnosis of clinically unsuspected central pulmonary artery thromboembolism in treatment of critically ill patients. *Chest* 105:986, 1994.

29. Come PC: Echocardiographic recognition of pulmonary arterial disease and determination of its cause. *Am J Med* 84:384, 1988.

30. Ribeiro A, Lindmarker P, Juhlin-Dannfelt A, et al: Echocardiography Doppler in pulmonary embolism: Right ventricular dysfunction as a predictor of mortality rate. *Am Heart J* 134:479, 1997.

31. Grifoni S, Olivotto I, Cecchini P, et al: Short-term clinical outcome of patients with acute pulmonary embolism, normal blood pressure, and echocardiographic right ventricular dysfunction. *Circulation* 101:2817, 2000.

32. Wolfe M, Lee RT, Feldstein ML, et al: Prognostic significance of right ventricular hypokinesis and perfusion lung scan defects in pulmonary embolism. *Am Heart J* 127:1371, 1994.

33. Meaney JFM, Weg JG, Chenevert TL, et al: Diagnosis of pulmonary embolism with magnetic resonance angiography. *N Engl J Med* 336:1422, 1997.

34. Oudkerk M, van Beek EJR, Wieloposki P, et al: Comparison of contrast-enhanced magnetic resonance angiography and conventional pulmonary angiography for the diagnosis of pulmonary embolism: A prospective study. *Lancet* 359:1643, 2002.

35. Remy-Jardin M, Remy J, Wattinne L, et al: Central pulmonary thromboembolism: diagnosis with spiral volumetric CT with the single-breath-hold technique—comparison with pulmonary angiography. *Radiology* 185:381, 1992.

36. Rathbun S, Raskob G, Whitsett T: Sensitivity and specificity of helical computed tomography in the diagnosis of pulmonary embolism: a systematic review. *Ann Intern Med* 132:227, 2000.

37. Mullins MD, Becker DM, Hagspiel KD, et al: The role of spiral volumetric computed tomography in the diagnosis of pulmonary embolism. *Arch Intern Med* 160:293, 2000.

38. PIOPED Investigators: Value of the ventilation/perfusion scan in acute pulmonary embolism: Results of the Prospective Investigation of Pulmonary Embolism Diagnosis (PIOPED). *JAMA* 263:2753, 1990.

39. Bourriot K, Couffinhal T, Bernard V: Clinical outcome after a negative spiral CT pulmonary angiographic finding in an inpatient population from cardiology and pneumology wards. *Chest* 123:359, 2003.

40. Kearon C, Julian J, Math M, et al: Noninvasive diagnosis of deep venous thrombosis. *Ann Intern Med* 128:663, 1998.

41. Prescott SM, Richards KL, Tikoff G, et al: Venous thromboembolism in decompensated chronic obstructive pulmonary disease. *Am Rev Respir Dis* 123:32, 1981.

42. Heijboer H, Buller HR, Lensing AWA, et al: A comparison of real-time compression ultrasonography with impedance plethysmography for the diagnosis of deep-vein thrombosis in symptomatic outpatients. *N Engl J Med* 329:1365, 1993.

43. Wells P, Hirsh J, Anderson D, et al: Accuracy of clinical assessment of deep-vein thrombosis. *Lancet* 345:1326, 1995.

44. Ginsberg JS, Caco CC, Brill-Edwards PA, et al: Venous thrombosis in patients who have undergone major hip or knee surgery: Detection with compression US and impedance plethysmography. *Radiology* 181:651, 1991.

45. Kakkar VV, Flanc C, Howe CT, et al: Natural history of postoperative deep-vein thrombosis. *Lancet* 2:230, 1969.

46. Huisman MV, Büller HR, ten Cate JW, et al: Serial impedance plethysmography for suspected deep venous thrombosis in outpatients. *N Engl J Med* 314:823, 1986.

47. Lusiani L, Visonà A, Bonanome A, et al: The characteristics of the thrombi of the lower limbs, as detected by ultrasonic scanning, do not predict pulmonary embolism. *Chest* 110:996, 1996.

48. Hull RD, Hirsh J, Carter CJ, et al: Pulmonary angiography, ventilation lung scanning, and venography for clinically suspected pulmonary embolism with abnormal perfusion lung scan. *Ann Intern Med* 98:891, 1983.

49. Hull RD, Hirsh J, Carter CJ, et al: Diagnostic value of ventilation-perfusion lung scanning in patients with suspected pulmonary embolism. *Chest* 88:819, 1985.

50. Wheeler HB, Anderson FA, Cardullo PA, et al: Suspected deep vein thrombosis: Management by impedance plethysmography. *Arch Surg* 117:1206, 1982.

51. Hull RD, Raskob GE, Coates G, et al: A new noninvasive management strategy for patients with suspected pulmonary embolism. *Arch Intern Med* 149:2549, 1989.

52. Hull RD, Raskob GE, Carter CJ: Serial impedance plethysmography in pregnant patients with clinically suspected deep-vein thrombosis: Clinical validity of negative findings. *Ann Intern Med* 112:663, 1990.

53. Henry JW, Stein PD, Gottschalk A, et al: Scintigraphic lung scans and clinical assessment in critically ill patients with suspected acute pulmonary embolism. *Chest* 109:462, 1996.

54. Stein PD, Hull RD, Patel KC, et al: d-Dimer for the exclusion of acute venous thrombosis and pulmonary embolism: A systematic review. *Ann Intern Med* 140:589, 2004.

55. Bates SM, Kearon C, Crowther M, et al: A diagnostic strategy involving a quantitative latex d-dimer assay reliably excludes deep venous thrombosis. *Ann Intern Med* 138:787, 2003.

56. Yan SB, Helterbrand J, Hartman DL, et al: Low levels of protein C are associated with poor outcome in severe sepsis. *Chest* 120:915, 2001.

57. ten Wolde M, Kraaijenhagen RA, Prins MH, et al: The clinical usefulness of D-dimer testing in cancer patients with suspected deep venous thrombosis. *Arch Intern Med* 162:1880, 2002.

58. Brathwaite CEM, O'Malley KF, Ross SE, et al: Continuous pulse oximetry and the diagnosis of pulmonary embolism in critically ill trauma patients. *J Trauma* 33:528, 1992.

59. Stein PD, Athanasoulis C, Alavi A, et al: Complications and validity of pulmonary angiography in acute pulmonary embolism. *Circulation* 85:462, 1992.

60. Fred HL, Axelrad MA, Lewis JM, et al: Rapid resolution of pulmonary thromboemboli in man. *JAMA* 196:13:1137, 1996.

61. Dalen JE, Banas JS, Brooks HL, et al: Resolution rate of acute pulmonary embolism in man. *N Engl J Med* 280:1194, 1969.
62. Mills SR, Jackson DC, Older RA, et al: The incidence, etiologies, and avoidance of complications of pulmonary angiography in a large series. *Radiology* 136:295, 1980.
63. Perlmutt LM, Braun SD, Newman GE, et al: Pulmonary arteriography in the high risk patient. *Radiology* 162:187, 1987.
64. Nicod P, Peterson K, Levine M, et al: Pulmonary angiography in severe chronic pulmonary hypertension. *Ann Intern Med* 107:565, 1987.
65. Wicki J, Perrier A, Perneger T, Bounameaux H, et al: Predicting adverse outcome in patients with acute pulmonary embolism: a risk score. *Thromb Haemost* 84:548, 2000.
66. Konstantinides S, Geibel A, Olschewski M, et al: Importance of cardiac troponins I and T in risk stratification of patients with acute pulmonary embolism. *Circulation* 106:1263, 2002.
67. ten Wolde M, Tulevski II, Mulder JWM, et al: Brain natriuretic peptide as a predictor of adverse outcome in patients with pulmonary embolism. *Circulation* 107:2082, 2003.
68. Aschwanden M, Engel H, Schwob A, et al: Acute deep vein thrombosis: early mobilization does not increase the frequency of pulmonary embolism. *Thromb Haemost* 85:42, 2001.
69. Schellong SM, Schwarz T, Kropp J, et al: Bed rest in deep vein thrombosis and the incidence of scintigraphic pulmonary embolism. *Thromb Haemost* 82:127, 1999.
70. Bauer KA: Selective inhibition of coagulation factors: advances in antithrombotic therapy. *Semin Thromb Hemost* 28:15, 2002.
71. Hyers TM, Agnelli G, Hull R, et al: Antithrombotic therapy for venous thromboembolic disease. *Chest* 119:176S, 2001.
72. Barrit DW, Lond MD, Jordan SC, et al: Anticoagulant drugs in the treatment of pulmonary embolism: A controlled trial. *Lancet* 275:1309, 2004.
73. Writing Committee for the Galilei Investigators: Subcutaneous adjusted-dose unfractionated heparin vs fixed-dose low-molecular-weight heparin in the initial treatment of venous thromboembolism. *Arch Intern Med* 164:1077, 2004.
74. Hull RD, Raskob GE, Hirsh J, et al: Continuous intravenous heparin compared with intermittent subcutaneous heparin in the initial treatment of proximal vein thrombosis. *N Engl J Med* 315:1109, 1986.
75. Raschke RA, Reilly BM, Guidry JR, et al: The weight-based heparin dosing nomogram compared with a "standard care" nomogram: a randomized controlled trial. *Ann Intern Med* 119:874, 1993.
76. Hull RD, Raskob GE, Rosenbloom D, et al: Heparin for 5 days as compared with 10 days in the initial treatment of proximal venous thrombosis. *N Engl J Med* 322:1260, 1990.
77. Goldhaber SZ, Buring JE, Lipnick RJ, et al: Pooled analyses of randomized trials of streptokinase and heparin in phlebographically documented acute deep venous thrombosis. *Am J Med* 76:393, 1984.
78. Landefeld CS, Cook EF, Flatley M, et al: Identification and preliminary validation of predictors of major bleeding in hospitalized patients starting anticoagulant therapy. *Am J Med* 82:703, 1987.
79. Schmitt BP, Adelman B: Heparin-associated thrombocytopenia: a critical review and pooled analysis. *Am J Med Sci* 305:208, 1993.
80. Warkentin TE, Kelton JG: Heparin and platelets. *Hematol Oncol Clin North Am* 4:243, 1990.
81. Leizorovicz A, Simonneau G, Decousus H, et al: Comparison of efficacy and safety of low molecular weight heparins and unfractionated heparin in initial treatment of deep venous thrombosis: a meta-analysis. *Br Med J* 309:299, 1994.
82. Hull R, Pineo GF: Low molecular weight heparin treatment of venous thromboembolism. *Prog Cardiovasc Dis* 37:71, 1994.
83. Green D, Hirsh J, Heit J, et al: Low molecular weight heparin: a critical analysis of clinical trials. *Pharmacol Rev* 46:89, 1994.
84. Simonneau G, Sors H, Charbonnier B, et al: A comparison of low-molecular-weight heparin with unfractionated heparin for acute pulmonary embolism. *N Engl J Med* 337:663, 1997.
85. Büller HR, Gallus AS, Ginsberg J, et al: Low-molecular-weight heparin in the treatment of patients with venous thromboembolism. *N Engl J Med* 337:657, 1997.
86. Quinlan DJ, McQuillan A, Elkelboom JW: Low-molecular-weight heparin compared with intravenous unfractionated heparin for treatment of pulmonary embolism. *Ann Intern Med* 140:175, 2004.
87. Meyer G, Marjanovic Z, Valcke J, et al: Comparison of low-molecular-weight heparin and warfarin for the secondary prevention of venous thromboembolism in patients with cancer. *Arch Intern Med* 162:1729, 2002.
88. Lee AYY, Levine MN, Baker RI, et al: Low-molecule-weight heparin versus a coumarin for the prevention of recurrent venous thromboembolism in patients with cancer. *N Engl J Med* 349:146, 2003.
89. Walenga JM, Jeske WP, Prechel MM, et al: Decreased prevalence of heparin-induced thrombocytopenia with low-molecular-weight heparin and related drugs. *Semin Thromb Hemost* 30:69, 2004.
90. Erikson BI, Willie-Jorgensen P, Kalebo P, et al: A comparison of recombinant hirudin with a low-molecular-weight heparin to prevent thromboembolic complications after total hip replacement. *N Engl J Med* 337:1329, 1997.
91. GUSTO IIb Investigators: A comparison of recombinant hirudin with heparin for the treatment of acute coronary syndromes. *N Engl J Med* 335:775, 1996.
92. Jang I-K, Brown DFM, Giugliano RP, et al: A multicenter, randomized study of argatroban versus heparin as adjunct to tissue plasminogen activator (TPA) in acute myocardial infarction: myocardial infarction with novastan and TPA (MINT) Study. *J Am Coll Cardiol* 33:1879, 1999.
93. Francis CW, Berkowitz SD, Comp PC, et al: Comparison of ximelagatran with warfarin for the prevention of venous thromboembolism after total knee replacement. *N Engl J Med* 349:1703, 2003.
94. Heit JA, Colwell CW, Francis CW, et al: Comparison of the oral direct thrombin inhibitor ximelagatran with enoxaparin as prophylaxis against venous thromboembolism after knee replacement. *Arch Intern Med* 161:2215, 2001.
95. Schulman S, Wahlander K, Lundstrom T, et al: Secondary prevention of venous thromboembolism with the oral direct thrombin inhibitor ximelagatran. *N Engl J Med* 349:1713, 2003.
96. Turpie AGG, Bauer KA, Erikson BI, et al: Fondaparinux vs enoxaparin for the prevention of venous thromboembolism in major orthopedic surgery: A meta-analysis of 4 randomized double-blind studies. *Arch Intern Med* 162:1833, 2002.
97. The Matisse Investigators: Subcutaneous fondaparinux versus intravenous unfractionated heparin in the initial treatment of pulmonary embolism. *N Engl J Med* 349:1695, 2003.
98. Moser KM: Venous thromboembolism. *Am Rev Respir Dis* 141:235, 1990.
99. Decousus H, Leizorovicz A, Parent F, et al: A clinical trial of vena caval filters in the prevention of pulmonary embolism in patients with proximal deep-vein thrombosis. *N Engl J Med* 338:409, 1998.
100. Streiff MB: Venal caval filters: A comprehensive review. *Blood* 95:3669, 2000.
101. Asch MR: Initial experience in humans with a new retrievable inferior vena cava filter. *Radiology* 225:835, 2002.
102. Millward SF, Bhargava A, Aquino JJ, et al: Gunther tulip filter: preliminary clinical experience with retrieval; venous thromboembolic disease. *J Vasc Intervent Radiol* 11:75, 2000.
103. Bergqvist D: The role of vena caval interruption in patients with venous thromboembolism. *Prog Cardiovasc Dis* 37:25, 1994.
104. Clagett GP, Anderson FA, Geerts W, et al: Prevention of venous thromboembolism. *Chest* 114:531S, 1998.

105. Dalla-Volta S, Palla A, Santolicandro A, et al: PAIMS 2: Alteplase combined with heparin versus heparin in the treatment of acute pulmonary embolism. Plasminogen activator Italian multicenter study 2. *J Am Coll Cardiol* 20:520, 1992.

106. Witty LA, Krichman A, Tapson VF: Thrombolytic therapy for venous thromboembolism: Utilization by practicing pulmonologists. *Arch Intern Med* 154:1601, 1994.

107. Diehl JL, Meyer G, Igual J, et al: Effectiveness and safety of bolus administration of alteplase in massive pulmonary embolism. *Am J Cardiol* 70:1477, 1992.

108. Goldhaber SZ, Haire WD, Feldstein ML, et al: Alteplase versus heparin in acute pulmonary embolism: Randomised trial assessing right-ventricular function and pulmonary perfusion. *Lancet* 341:507, 1993.

109. Jerjes-Sanchez C, Ramírez-Rivera A, García M, et al: Streptokinase and heparin versus heparin alone in massive pulmonary embolism: A randomized controlled trial. *J Thromb Thrombolysis* 2:227, 1995.

110. Goldhaber SZ: Thrombolysis for pulmonary embolism. *N Engl J Med* 347:1131, 2002.

111. Arcasoy SM, Kreit JW: Thrombolytic therapy of pulmonary embolism. *Chest* 115:1695, 1999.

112. Hamel E, Pacouret G, Vicentelli D, et al: Thrombolysis or heparin therapy in massive pulmonary embolism with right ventricular dilation. *Chest* 120:120, 2001.

113. Konstantinides S, Geibel A, Heusel G, et al: Heparin plus alteplase compared with heparin alone in patients with submassive pulmonary embolism. *N Engl J Med* 347:1143, 2002.

114. Goldhaber SZ, Visani L, De Rosa M: Acute pulmonary embolism: clinical outcomes in the International Cooperative Pulmonary Embolism Registry (ICOPER). *Lancet* 353:1386, 1999.

115. Kreit JW: The impact of right ventricular dysfunction on the prognosis and therapy of normotensive patients with pulmonary embolism. *Chest* 125:1539, 2004.

116. Goldhaber SZ, Heit J, Sharma GVRK, et al: Randomised controlled trial of recombinant tissue plasminogen activator versus urokinase in the treatment of acute pulmonary embolism. *Lancet* ii:293, 1998.

117. Petitpretz P, Simmoneau G, Cerrina J, et al: Effects of a single bolus of urokinase in patients with life-threatening pulmonary emboli: a descriptive trial. *Circulation* 70:861, 1984.

118. Levine MN, Weitz J, Turpie AGG, et al: A new short infusion dosage regimen of recombinant tissue plasminogen activator in patients with venous thromboembolic disease. *Chest* 97(Suppl):168S, 1990.

119. Sors H, Pacouret G, Azarian R, et al: Hemodynamic effects of bolus vs 2-h infusion of alteplase in acute massive pulmonary embolism: A randomized controlled multicenter trial. *Chest* 106:712, 1994.

120. Goldhaber SZ, Agnelli G, Levine MN, et al: Reduced dose bolus alteplase vs conventional alteplase infusion for pulmonary embolism thrombolysis: An international multicenter randomized trial. *Chest* 106:718, 1994.

121. Goldhaber SZ, Feldstein MD, Sors H: Two trials of reduced bolus alteplase in the treatment of pulmonary embolism: An overview. *Chest* 106:725, 1994.

122. Goldhaber SZ, Kessler CM, Heit JA, et al: Recombinant tissue-type plasminogen activator versus a novel dosing regimen of urokinase in acute pulmonary embolism: A randomized controlled multicenter trial. *J Am Coll Cardiol* 20:24, 1992.

123. Stein PD, Hull RD, Raskob G: Risks for major bleeding from thrombolytic therapy in patients with acute pulmonary embolism. *Ann Intern Med* 121:313, 1994.

124. Verstraete M, Miller GAH, Bounameaux H, et al: Intravenous and intrapulmonary recombinant tissue-type plasminogen activator in the treatment of acute massive pulmonary embolism. *Circulation* 77:353, 1988.

125. Tapson VF, Gurbel PA, Witty LA, et al: Pharmacomechanical thrombolysis of experimental pulmonary emboli: Rapid, low-dose, intraembolic therapy. *Chest* 106:1558, 1994.

126. Prewitt RM, Downes AMT, Gu S, et al: Effects of hydralazine and increased cardiac output on recombinant tissue plasminogen activator-induced thrombolysis in canine pulmonary embolism. *Chest* 102:677, 1992.

127. Molina JE, Hunter DW, Yedlicka JW, et al: Thrombolytic therapy for postoperative pulmonary embolism. *Am J Surg* 163:375, 1992.

128. Girard P, Baldeyrou P, Le Guillou J-L, et al: Thrombolysis for life-threatening pulmonary embolism 2 days after lung resection. *Am Rev Respir Dis* 147:1595, 1993.

129. Severi P, Lo Pinto G, Poggio R, et al: Urokinase thrombolytic therapy of pulmonary embolism in neurosurgically treated patients. *Surg Neurol* 42:469, 1994.

130. Sane DC, Califf RM, Topol EJ, et al: Bleeding during thrombolytic therapy for acute myocardial infarction: Mechanisms and management. *Ann Intern Med* 111:1010, 1989.

131. Belenkie I, Dani R, Smith ER, et al: Effects of volume loading during experimental acute pulmonary embolism. *Circulation* 80:178, 1989.

132. Jardin F, Genevray B, Brun-Ney D, et al: Dobutamine: A hemodynamic evaluation in pulmonary embolism shock. *Crit Care Med* 13:1009, 1985.

133. Molloy WD, Lee KY, Girling L, et al: Treatment of shock in a canine model of pulmonary embolism. *Am Rev Respir Dis* 130:870, 1984.

134. Boulain T, Lanotte R, Legras A, et al: Efficacy of epinephrine therapy in shock complicating pulmonary embolism. *Chest* 104:300, 1993.

135. Estagnasie P, Le Bourdelles G, Mier L, et al: Use of inhaled nitric oxide to reverse flow through a patent foramen ovale during pulmonary embolism. *Ann Intern Med* 120:757, 1994.

136. Böttiger BW, Motsch J, Dorsam J: Inhaled nitric oxide selectively decreases pulmonary artery pressure and pulmonary vascular resistance following acute massive pulmonary microembolism in piglets. *Chest* 110:1041, 1996.

137. Lund O, Nielsen TT, Schifter S, et al: Treatment of pulmonary embolism with full dose heparin, streptokinase or embolectomy—results and indications. *Thorac Cardiovasc Surg* 34:240, 1986.

138. Gulba DC, Schmid C, Borst HG, et al: Medical compared with surgical treatment for massive pulmonary embolism. *Lancet* 343:576, 1994.

139. Gray HH, Miller GAH, Paneth M: Pulmonary embolectomy: Its place in the management of pulmonary embolism. *Lancet* i:1441, 1988.

140. Yalamanchili K, Fleisher AG, Lehrman SG, et al: Open pulmonary embolectomy for treatment of major pulmonary embolism. *Ann Thorac Surg* 77:819, 2004.

141. Alpert JS, Smith RE, Ockene IS, et al: Treatment of massive pulmonary embolism: The role of pulmonary embolectomy. *Am Heart J* 89:413, 1975.

142. Pengo V, Lensing AWA, Prins MH, et al: Incidence of chronic thromboembolic pulmonary hypertension after pulmonary embolism. *N Engl J Med* 350:2257, 2004.

143. Timsit J-F, Reynaud P, Meyer G, et al: Pulmonary embolectomy by catheter device in massive pulmonary embolism. *Chest* 100:655, 1991.

144. Schmitz-Rode T, Janssens U, Schild HH, et al: Fragmentation of massive pulmonary embolism using a pigtail rotation catheter. *Chest* 114:1427, 1998.

145. Haskal ZJ, Soulen MC, Huettl EA, et al: Life-threatening pulmonary emboli and cor pulmonale: Treatment with percutaneous pulmonary artery stent placement. *Radiology* 191:473, 1994.

146. Toglia MR, Weg JG: Venous thromboembolism during pregnancy. *N Engl J Med* 335:108, 1996.

147. Kaunitz AM, Hughes JM, Grimes DA, et al: Causes of maternal mortality in the United States. *Obstet Gynecol* 65:605, 1985.

148. Ponto JA: Fetal dosimetry from pulmonary imaging in pregnancy: Revised estimates. *Clin Nuclear Med* 11:108, 1986.

149. Didolkar SM, Koontz C, Schimberg PI: Phleborrheography in pregnancy. *Obstet Gynecol* 61:363, 1983.

150. Ginsberg JS, Hirsh J: Use of anticoagulants during pregnancy. *Chest* 95:156S, 1989.

151. Ginsberg JS, Bates SM: Management of venous thromboembolism during pregnancy. *Thromb Haemost* 1:1435, 2003.

152. Dahlman TC: Osteoporotic fractures and the recurrence of thromboembolism during pregnancy and the puerperium in 184 women undergoing thromboprophylaxis with heparin. *Am J Obstet Gynecol* 168:1265, 1993.

153. Dahlmann TC, Sjöberg HE, Ringertz H: Bone mineral density during long term prophylaxis with heparin in pregnancy. *Am J Obstet Gynecol* 170:1315, 1994.

154. Carlin AJ, Farquharson RG, Topping J, et al: Prospective observational study of bone mineral density during pregnancy: Low molecular weight heparin versus control. *Hum Reprod* 19:1211, 2004.

155. Lesser BA, Leeper KV, Stein PD, et al: The diagnosis of acute pulmonary embolism in patients with chronic obstructive pulmonary disease. *Chest* 102:117, 1992.

156. Lippmann M, Fein A: Pulmonary embolism in the patient with chronic obstructive pulmonary disease. *Chest* 79:39, 1981.

157. Phillips B, Woodring J: Autoanticoagulation does not preclude pulmonary emboli. *Lung* 165:37, 1987.

158. Needleman SW, Stein MN, Hoak JD: Pulmonary embolism in patients with acute leukemia and severe thrombocytopenia. *West J Med* 135:9, 1981.

159. Ramos R, Salem BI, De Pawlikowski MP, et al: The efficacy of pneumatic compression stockings in the prevention of pulmonary embolism after cardiac surgery. *Chest* 109:82, 1996.

160. Geerts WH, Jay RM, Code KI, et al: A comparison of low-dose heparin with low-molecular-weight heparin as prophylaxis against venous thromboembolism after major trauma. *N Engl J Med* 335:701, 1996.

161. Keane MG, Ingenito EP, Goldhaber SZ: Utilization of venous thromboembolism prophylaxis in the medical intensive care unit. *Chest* 106:13, 1994.

162. Morris WP, Butler BD, Tonnesen AS, et al: Continuous venous air embolism in patients receiving positive end-expiratory pressure. *Am Rev Respir Dis* 147:1034, 1993.

163. Tanus-Santos J, Gordom WM, Udelsmann A, et al: Nonselective endothelin-receptor antagonism attenuates hemodynamic change after massive pulmonary air embolism in dogs. *Chest* 118:175, 2004.

164. Kapoor T, Gutierrez G: Air embolism as a cause of the systemic inflammatory response syndrome: A case report. *Crit Care* 7:R98, 2003.

165. Albertine KH: Lung injury and neutrophil density during air embolization in sheep after leukocyte depletion with nitrogen mustard. *Am Rev Respir Dis* 138:1444, 1998.

166. Sloan TB, Kimovec MA: Detection of venous air embolism by airway pressure monitoring. *Anesthesiology* 64:645, 1986.

167. Butler BD, Hills BA: Transpulmonary passage of venous air emboli. *J Appl Physiol* 59:543, 1985.

168. Marini JJ, Culver BH: Systemic gas embolism complicating mechanical ventilation in the adult respiratory distress syndrome. *Ann Intern Med* 110:699, 1989.

169. Dutka AJ, Kochanek PM, Hallenbeck JM: Influence of granulocytopenia on canine cerebral ischemia induced by air embolism. *Stroke* 20:390, 1989.

170. Annane D, Troché G, Delisle F, et al: Effects of mechanical ventilation with normobaric oxygen therapy on the rate of air removal from cerebral arteries. *Crit Care Med* 22:851, 1994.

171. Karuparthy VR, Downing JW, Husain FJ, et al: Incidence of venous air embolism during cesarean section is unchanged by the use of a 5 to 10 degree head up tilt. *Anesth Analg* 69:620, 1989.

172. Godeau B, Schaeffer A, Bachir D, et al: Bronchoalveolar lavage in adult sickle cell patients with acute chest syndrome: Value for diagnostic assessment of fat embolism. *Am J Respir Crit Care Med* 153:1691, 1996.

173. Fabian TC, Hoots AV, Stanford DS, et al: Fat embolism syndrome: Prospective evaluation in 92 fracture patients. *Crit Care Med* 18:42, 1990.

174. Hulman G: Pathogenesis of non-traumatic fat embolism. *Lancet* i:1366, 1998.

175. Christie J, Robinson CM, Pell ACH, et al: Transcardiac echocardiography during invasive intramedullary procedures. *J Bone Joint Surg* [Br] 77-B:450, 1995.

176. Pell ACH, Hughes D, Keating J, et al: Brief report: Fulminating fat embolism syndrome caused by paradoxical embolism through a patent foramen ovale. *N Engl J Med* 329:926, 1993.

177. Byrick RJ, Mullen JB, Mazer CD, et al: Transpulmonary systemic fat embolism: studies in mongrel dogs after cemented arthroplasty. *Am J Respir Crit Care Med* 150:1416, 1994.

178. Vedrinne JM, Guillaume C, Gagnieu MC, et al: Bronchoalveolar lavage in trauma patients for diagnosis of fat embolism syndrome. *Chest* 102:1323, 1992.

179. Gitlin TA, Seidel T, Cera PJ, et al: Pulmonary microvascular fat: The significance? *Crit Care Med* 21:673, 1993.

180. Bone LB, Johnson KD, Wiegelt J, et al: Early versus delayed stabilization of femoral fractures. *J Bone Joint Surg* 71A:336, 1989.

181. Johnson KD, Cadambi A, Seibert GB, et al: Incidence of adult respiratory distress syndrome in patients with multiple musculoskeletal injuries: Effect of early operative stabilization of fractures. *J Trauma* 25:375, 1985.

182. Behrman SW, Fabian TC, Kudsk KA, et al: Improved outcome with femur fractures: Early vs. delayed fixation. *J Trauma* 30:792, 1990.

183. Pitto RP, Hamer H, Fabiani R: Prophylaxis against fat and bone-marrow embolism during total hip arthroplasty reduces the incidence of postoperative deep-vein thrombosis. *J Bone Joint Surg* 84-A:39, 2002.

184. Kallenbach J, Lewis M, Zaltzman M, et al: "Low dose" corticosteroid prophylaxis against fat embolism. *J Trauma* 27:1173, 1987.

185. Lindeque BGP, Schoeman HS, Dommisse GF, et al: Fat embolism and the fat embolism syndrome: A double blind therapeutic study. *J Bone Joint Surg* 69-B:128, 1987.

186. Schonfeld SA, Ploysongsang Y, DiLisio R, et al: Fat embolism prophylaxis with corticosteroids: A prospective study in high-risk patients. *Ann Intern Med* 99:438, 1983.

Chapter 28 _____
PERICARDIAL DISEASE
ISRAEL BELENKIE

KEY POINTS

- *Accurate hemodynamic assessment of seriously ill patients requires an understanding of the concepts of transmural (effective) filling pressures and ventricular interaction.*

- *A systematic approach to the assessment of a patient with a low cardiac output and increased right atrial pressure will result in the correct determination when pericardial disease is a contributing factor.*

- *Echocardiography is the most important test for the initial evaluation of patients with pericardial disease.*

- *Pericardial drainage should be performed without delay in patients with cardiac tamponade. Volume loading or inotropic agents are not effective therapies for tamponade.*

- *Conditions such as localized tamponade and constrictive pericarditis must be considered in patients without a good alternative explanation for low cardiac output.*

- *Although rare, the possibility of purulent pericarditis should be considered in patients who are most susceptible.*

- *Anticoagulation is not contraindicated in pericarditis.*

A pericardial cause of otherwise unexplained low cardiac output should always be considered in critically ill patients. Pericardial inflammation or infection may also deserve consideration. This chapter focuses largely on the hemodynamic implications of constraint to ventricular filling and the approach to diagnosis and treatment of pericardial disease. The goals are to provide the reader with tools to assess the potential for suspected or known pericardial disease to relieve a patient's condition. The reader should refer to standard cardiology texts to learn the details of specific causes of pericardial disease (Table 28-1).

Physiology of Constraint

PERICARDIAL CONSTRAINT

The key to understanding pericardial physiology is to understand transmural pressure. The ventricles distend in proportion to transmural pressure, not to intracavitary pressure; this is frequently overlooked because changes in intracavitary pressure often (but not always) reflect changes in transmural pressure. Effective distending pressure is the *pressure difference* across the chamber wall, that is, transmural pressure.[1] This principle is rarely important with respect to systolic pressures[2] but may be critical with respect to diastolic pressures.[3] If left ventricular end-diastolic pressure (LVEDP) is 12 mm Hg, then LVEDP is 12 mm Hg greater than atmospheric pressure. However, if pericardial pressure is 4 mm Hg, then transmural LVEDP, the effective distending pressure, is 8 mm Hg. Further, if LVEDP increases to 15 mm Hg and pericardial pressure increases to 7 mm Hg, then transmural

LVEDP remains 8 mm Hg and left ventricular end-diastolic volume (LVEDV) does not change.

VENTRICULAR INTERACTION

Ventricular interaction can be defined as the complementary change in right ventricular (RV) and left ventricular (LV) volumes such that, when right ventricular end-diastolic volume (RVEDV) increases, LVEDV decreases, and vice versa. Ventricular interaction involves the septum moving toward the left or right ventricle and is modulated by external constraint that is pericardial or due to other mediastinal structures. The pericardium, in the short term, is effectively nondistensible; thus, the heart is surrounded by an effectively unyielding sac. Therefore, RVEDV can increase only "at the expense" of LVEDV. This interaction can occur because the septum is elastic and moves leftward or rightward with small decreases or increases in the difference between LVEDP and right ventricular end-diastolic pressure (RVEDP; i.e., the trans-septal gradient is equal to LVEDP minus RVEDP). When the pericardium is opened and the lungs are held back from the heart, ventricular interaction is substantially less; when pericardial pressure is very low, ventricular interaction is also diminished.[4]

EXPERIMENTAL OBSERVATIONS

It had been thought that the relation between LVEDP and LVEDV, the so-called diastolic compliance,[5] is practically invariant. This assumption was the basis for the Sarnoff ventricular function curve analysis in which LV filling pressure was used to reflect LVEDV, or LV preload.[6] However, diastolic compliance can be changed rapidly, for example, by giving nitroglycerin for heart failure.[7] It was suggested that this was due to unappreciated decreases in pericardial pressure,[8] but many thought this was unlikely because pericardial pressure had been shown to be negative and unchanging, even as RVEDP was increased to high values.[9] It was later shown that pericardial pressure is more accurately measured[10,11] with a flat, liquid-containing balloon transducer; an open

TABLE 28-1 Etiology of Pericardial Disease

Etiology	Effusive	Constrictive	Effusive/Constrictive
Idiopathic	X	X	X
Postirradiation			
Early	X	—	—
Late	X	X	X
Postinfarction			
Early	X	—	—
Late	X	X	—
Infection			
Early	X	—	—
Late	X	X	X
Collagen disease (SLE, MCTD, RA)	X	X	
Renal failure	X	X	—
Postoperative			
Early	X	—	—
Late		X	
Malignancy	X	—	X

ABBREVIATIONS: MCTD, mixed connective tissue disease; RA, rheumatoid arthritis; SLE, systemic lupus erythematosus.

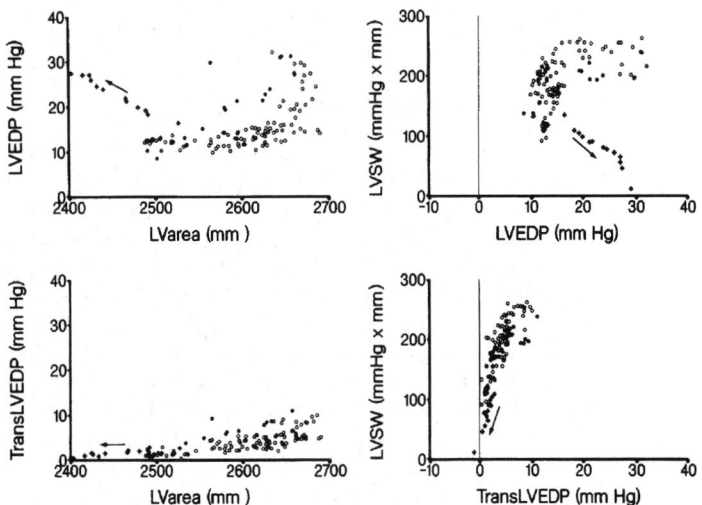

FIGURE 28-1 Pressure-dimension and stroke work-pressure relations after repeated pulmonary embolizations with autologous clots in a dog. *Top left.* This panel suggests that left ventricular compliance changes during volume loading after repeated embolism (*arrow* indicates changes in the relation between LVEDP and LVarea, in index of left ventricular end-diastolic volume). *Top right.* Similarly, this plot suggests that left ventricular contractibility is altered during volume load (*arrow*). *Bottom.* However, these panels clearly show that neither compliance nor contractility has changed during the volume load when left ventricular volume (LVarea) and transmural LVEDP (transLVEDP) are used to indicate changes in left ventricular preload. LVarea, left ventricular area; LVEDP, left ventricular end-diastolic pressure.

catheter seriously underestimates pericardial pressure unless there is sufficient fluid in the pericardial space. It is important to note that pericardial pressure is similar to mean right atrial (RA) pressure, and both increase (during volume loading) in parallel.[12] Thus, pericardial pressure is changeable acutely and is approximately equal to RVEDP in most circumstances.[13] Without an excess of liquid, pericardial pressure is fundamentally a compressive contact stress.[11]

An excellent demonstration of the importance of these concepts consists of the hemodynamic effects of acute pulmonary embolism and subsequent volume loading.[14–16] As shown in Figs. 28-1 and 28-2, with the pericardium intact, the relations between LVEDP and LVEDV and between LV stroke work and LVEDP suggest that pulmonary embolism and subsequent volume loading decrease LV compliance and contractility.[14] However, when diastolic compliance and contractility are evaluated with transmural LVEDP instead of intracavitary pressure, it is clear that LV compliance and contractility are unaffected by embolism.[17] Most importantly, despite increased LVEDP during volume loading after embolism, *transmural LVEDP and LVEDV may decrease* and result in decreased stroke work and worsening hypotension. In those circumstances, volume removal may *increase transmural LVEDP, LVEDV, and stroke work*, despite the decreased LVEDP. In the absence of constraint, this apparent paradoxical response to volume manipulation is not observed.[16]

The complementary change in RV and LV volumes occurs largely by septal shift, which is controlled by the transseptal gradient; therefore, changes in the trans-septal gradient are a convenient indicator of ventricular interaction. Mirsky and Rankin observed that the left ventricle is surrounded by the pericardium over approximately two-thirds of its surface and by the right ventricle over the remaining third.[18] Therefore, when changes in RV and pericardial pressures are not similar, it is best to modify the definition of transmural pressure to better account for those differences.[19]

VENTRICULAR INTERACTION DURING MECHANICAL VENTILATION

As intrathoracic pressure increases during positive-pressure inspiration, there are complex interactions between the heart and lung that are beyond the scope of this chapter. However, constraint to ventricular filling and ventricular inter-

action deserve consideration here. Positive end-expiratory pressure increases constraint to filling and thus decreases cardiac output. Therefore, if pericardial pressure is increased by an effusion or especially if tamponade is present, mechanical ventilation will increase constraint further and should be avoided. Some studies have suggested that leftward septal shift (perhaps due to increased pulmonary vascular resistance at larger lung volumes) may decrease LV filling more than that caused by constraint alone.[20] In addition, positive-pressure inspiration decreases venous return and RV output, with the reverse occurring during expiration.[21,22] The consequences of these complex changes on LV function appear to differ. In some circumstances, LVEDV and output decrease during positive-pressure inspiration; in others, both increase. A synthesis of available data suggests that, during mechanical ventilation, pulmonary vascular resistance increases more at lower LVEDPs (zone 2 conditions) and causes leftward septal shift during inspiration and that pulmonary vascular resistance increases little during inspiration at higher LVEDPs (zone 3 conditions) with little or no leftward septal shift; the decreased RVEDV that occurs during inspiration then allows for increased filling of the left ventricle (despite a decreased total volume of the ventricles) and, hence, output. The reverse occurs during expiration.

Clinical Manifestations of Pericardial Disease

Pericardial disease is most often manifested clinically as the pain syndrome caused by pericarditis or by the hemodynamic compromise caused by increased pericardial fluid (tamponade) or by a thickened or calcified pericardium (constrictive pericarditis). Other clinically important diseases of the pericardium are much less common (e.g., purulent or tubercular pericarditis) but also must always be considered, as discussed below.

PERICARDITIS

Pericarditis commonly presents with a characteristic syndrome that includes central, pleuritic chest pain that is worse when lying down and less severe when standing upright or leaning forward. Frequently, there is no pericardial friction

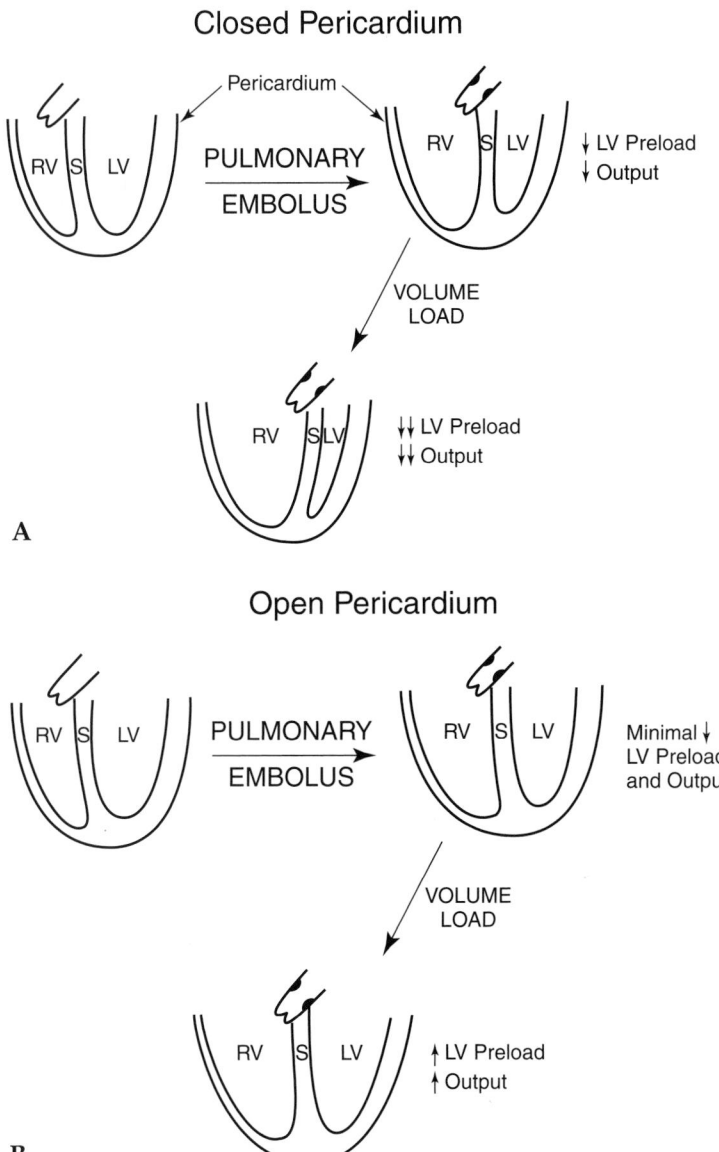

Closed Pericardium

Open Pericardium

FIGURE 28-2 *A.* This panel illustrates how pulmonary hypertension, such as after pulmonary embolism, may cause a substantial reduction in LV preload by direct ventricular interaction and how subsequent volume loading may aggravate the hemodynamic problem. There is decreased RV output with a consequent LV output decrease (series interaction). In addition, the increased RVEDP and the decreased LVEDP result in a decreased transseptal pressure gradient, which causes a leftward septal shift (decreased LVEDV) by direct interaction. Thus, decreased RV output and decreased LV filling because of septal shift contribute to the hemodynamic consequences of acute pulmonary hypertension. Subsequent volume loading increases the RVEDP more than the LVEDP; this decreases the transseptal pressure gradient further and shifts the septum even farther to the left. Thus, LVEDV is reduced even further despite the increased intracavitary LVEDP. Constraint by the pericardium prevents the free wall from distending, so RVEDV increases only at the expense of LVEDV (and therefore stroke volume). *B.* This panel illustrates the importance of external constraint in modulating direct ventricular interaction. Pulmonary embolism increases RVEDV, there is leftward septal shift, but the absence of external constraint allows the LV free wall to distend so that the hemodynamic effects of the embolism are less severe. The animal tolerated much greater amounts of infused clot than when the pericardium was intact. Furthermore, subsequent volume loading increases RV and LV preloads and outputs. LV, left ventricle/left ventricular; LVEDP, left ventricular end-diastolic pressure; LVEDV, left ventricular end-diastolic volume; RV, right ventricle/right ventricular; RVEDP, right ventricular end-diastolic pressure; RVEDV, right ventricular end-diastolic volume; S, septum.

rub; however, the presence of a friction rub or an abnormal electrocardiogram or echocardiogram may suggest pericarditis in patients without symptoms of pericarditis who are being assessed for other conditions such as cancer, myocardial infarction, uremia, or a collagen vascular disease. The pain associated with pericarditis may be atypical and difficult to differentiate from pain caused by myocardial ischemia. The electrocardiogram is often normal or not diagnostic; the characteristic type of diffuse ST elevation (concave upward), not restricted to leads reflecting a region supplied by one coronary artery, when present, may be difficult to distinguish from early repolarization (normal). PR-segment depression is very suggestive of pericarditis. Repolarization changes may evolve over hours to days; in contrast to changes due to ischemia or infarction, the ST segment returns to baseline before the T wave inverts. No Q waves develop, and cardiac enzymes usually are normal but may increase in some patients.

In general, it is not difficult to discriminate between myocardial ischemia and pericarditis. However, occasionally, this can be very difficult and the two may coexist. The classic symptoms of pericarditis, unassociated with symptoms, signs, or electrocardiographic changes (Fig. 28-3) suggesting ischemia or infarction, can be confidently attributed to acute pericarditis. This may be confirmed by the presence of classic ST changes on the electrocardiogram (frequently absent) and/or a pericardial friction rub (also frequently absent). If the patient has known or suspected chronic or acute coronary artery disease, the disease may coexist with pericarditis so that the potential for pericarditis after infarction should be considered. Other characteristics may be helpful in discerning the cause of the pain, such as its duration, the response to anti-ischemic or anti-inflammatory medications, or the results of laboratory tests. Minor elevations in cardiac enzymes including troponin T or I may not be indicative unless serial changes indicate either diagnosis. It is not rare for the dilemma to be resolved in the cardiac catheterization laboratory. The association of myocarditis with pericardial pain may make the diagnosis even more difficult to resolve.

Benign idiopathic pericarditis is appropriately named except for occasional cardiac tamponade[23] or refractory chest pain. Progression from clinically apparent idiopathic pericarditis to constrictive pericarditis is very uncommon.

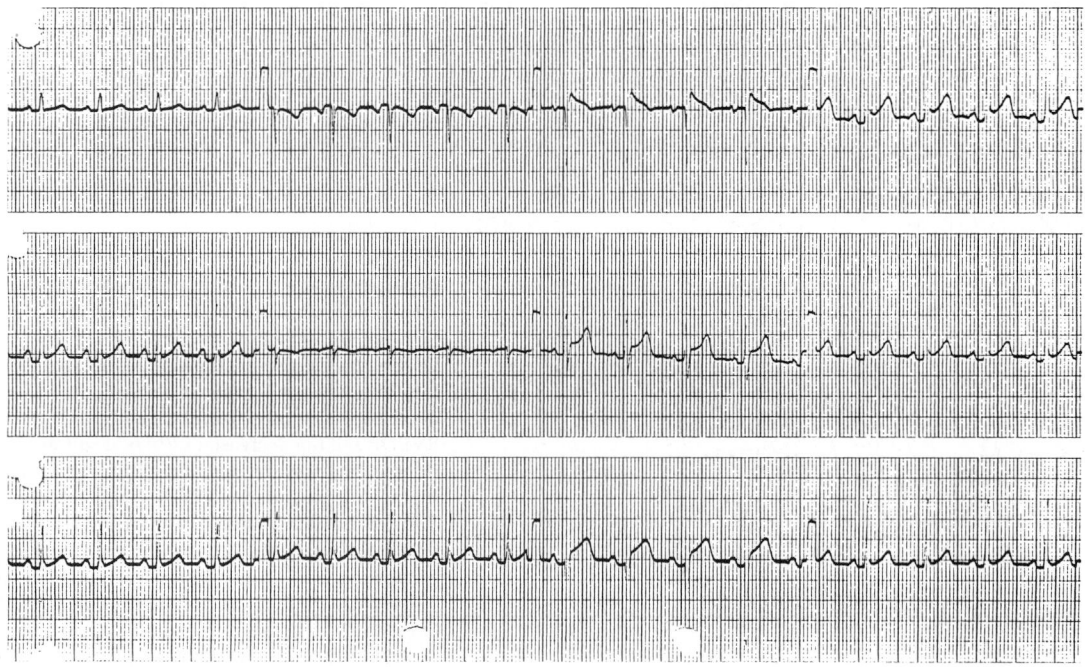

FIGURE 28-3 Twelve-lead electrocardiogram of a patient with acute pericarditis. Note PR segment depression prominent leads 2, 3, and aVF. ST-segment elevation is present globally (except in lead aVR) and is concave upward.

TREATMENT

Unless the clinical characteristics suggest a condition other than benign idiopathic pericarditis or there is a hemodynamically significant effusion, a conservative approach is generally appropriate and diagnostic pericardiocentesis is usually not indicated. Treatment is usually with nonsteroidal antiinflammatory drugs or colchicine; steroids should be reserved for only the most refractory symptoms, and pericardiectomy is only rarely indicated.[23] If the cause of the pericarditis is known, specific treatment for that disease is indicated.

CARDIAC TAMPONADE

Small pericardial effusions are relatively common in patients with heart disease or in critically ill patients. The presence or absence of a pericardial friction rub correlates poorly with the volume of fluid. Tamponade is caused by accumulated fluid usually distributed throughout the pericardial space over the ventricles and the right atrium and, to a lesser extent, behind the left atrium. Localized collections of fluid, particularly early after open heart surgery, may compress individual chambers with similar consequences. The rate of fluid accumulation is very important; if slow, the pericardium stretches over time and large volumes (up to several liters) may collect before causing hemodynamic difficulty. However, if the fluid accumulates quickly, the noncompliant pericardium does not stretch and tamponade can be caused by as little as 150 to 200 mL. As pericardial pressure increases, transmural ventricular pressures decrease despite increased intracavitary pressures.

Cardiac tamponade develops when constraint is sufficient to substantially reduce cardiac filling and, hence, output. When this happens, diastolic pressures equilibrate in all chambers so that RA and left atrial pressures, RVEDP, LVEDP and pulmonary artery diastolic pressures become equal or nearly equal (<3- to 5-mm Hg difference).[24] Commonly, cardiac tamponade is apparent at pericardial pressures of 15 to 20 mm Hg and with a jugular venous pressure usually greater than 10 cm of water above the sternal angle. It is characteristically associated with tachycardia, decreased cardiac output, and hypotension, although hypertension occasionally is present. The normal inspiratory decrease in arterial blood pressure (<10 mm Hg) is exaggerated (pulsus paradoxicus); this is not specific for tamponade and can occur in other circumstances, particularly when there is increased inspiratory effort. However, it is almost always present in cardiac tamponade (in the absence of aortic regurgitation, atrial septal defect, or severe LV dysfunction).[24] The normal inspiratory increase in venous return persists in tamponade; the resultant increase in RVEDV causes a decrease in LVEDV and output because the pericardium cannot expand to accommodate the increased RVEDV. The decrease in LVEDV causes blood to accumulate in the lungs during inspiration. Persistent constraint to filling throughout diastole is responsible for the decreased y descent (early diastole) in the jugular venous pulse and RA pressure tracing and the slowly rising RV early diastolic pressure (Figs. 28-4 and 28-5). The Kussmaul sign and the square root (dip-plateau) sign in the jugular venous pulse are not seen in tamponade.

Once considered, the diagnosis of cardiac tamponade is generally straightforward. In a critically ill patient, a pericardial infusion sufficiently large to cause hemodynamic problems may be discovered fortuitously when echocardiography is performed for various reasons. Increased right-sided filling pressures or pulsus paradoxicus should initiate a systematic hemodynamic assessment that will ultimately lead to the correct diagnosis. Physical examination may show an obvious cause for the increased right-sided filling pressure. However, causes of increased filling pressures are often best evaluated initially by transthoracic or transesophageal

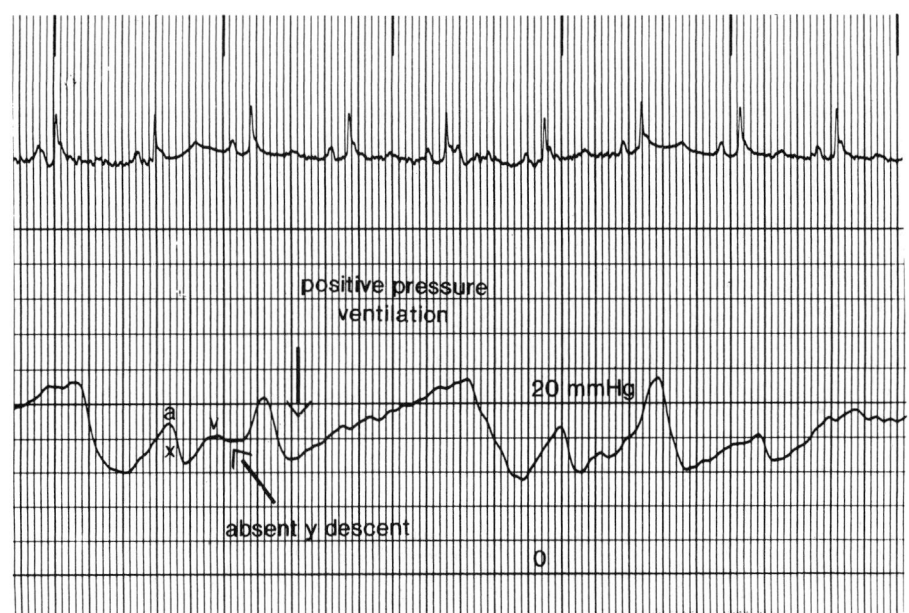

FIGURE 28-4 Right atrial pressure in a patient with cardiac tamponade during mechanical ventilation. Note the absent *y* descent and the blunting of the waveforms, especially during positive-pressure ventilation.

echocardiography. Either modality helps to detect valvular or myocardial disease and pericardial causes of increased RA pressure. The assessment may be complicated by the presence of other conditions. One may also be faced with the management of tamponade and the need to deal with the specific cause of the effusion, for example, tuberculosis or neoplasm.

The characteristic hemodynamic features of tamponade (equilibration of diastolic pressures) may be readily apparent in hemodynamically monitored patients. Electrocardiographic features of tamponade include low voltage and electrical alternans, but these findings need not be present. Electrical alternans suggests the presence of tamponade (Fig. 28-6); it is generally associated with swinging of the heart within the pericardium. Hemodynamically significant effusions are characterized echocardiographically[25–30] by the presence of moderate or large effusions (unless accumulated

rapidly), early diastolic RV collapse, right atrial collapse (Fig. 28-7), the presence of fluid behind the left atrium, a dilated inferior vena cava, and increased respiratory variation in tricuspid and mitral Doppler flow velocities. However, the diagnosis of tamponade remains a clinical diagnosis.[31] Differentiation from constrictive pericarditis is not an issue, although hemodynamic comparisons are interesting (see below). The chest x-ray can be useful in identifying patients with cardiac tamponade, especially when associated with a quiet precordium (Fig. 28-8). There may be a characteristic "water-bottle" appearance, with rapid tapering of the bulging pericardial silhouette. Pulmonary edema is almost never seen in uncomplicated tamponade. Decreased QRS voltage associated with an enlarged cardiac silhouette on radiography or electrical alternans may suggest the presence of a large effusion. Other radiographic signs are not relevant because of the greater sensitivities of other imaging modalities. Computed

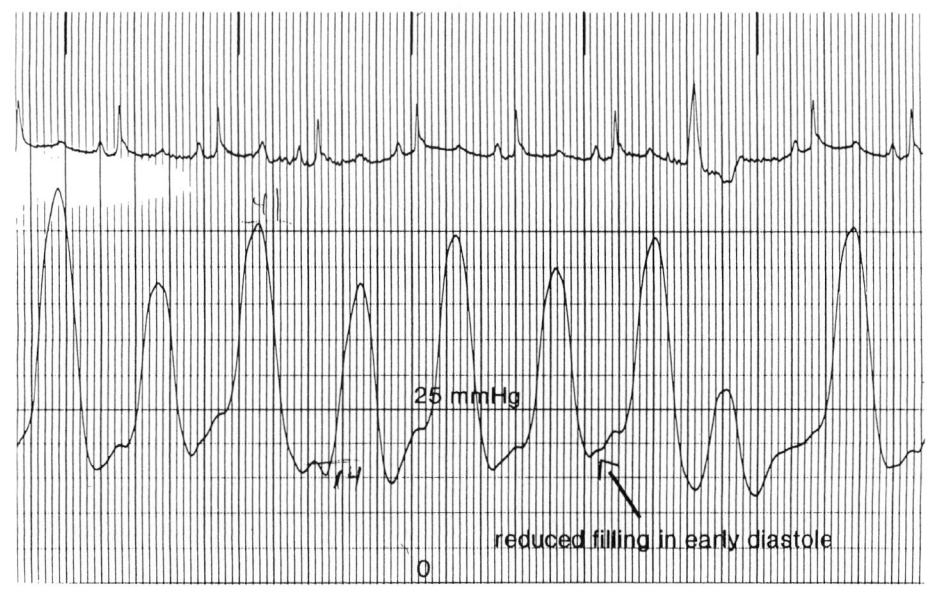

FIGURE 28-5 Right ventricular pressure in a patient with cardiac tamponade. Note the slow rise in ventricular pressure in early diastole, corresponding to decreased passive filling.

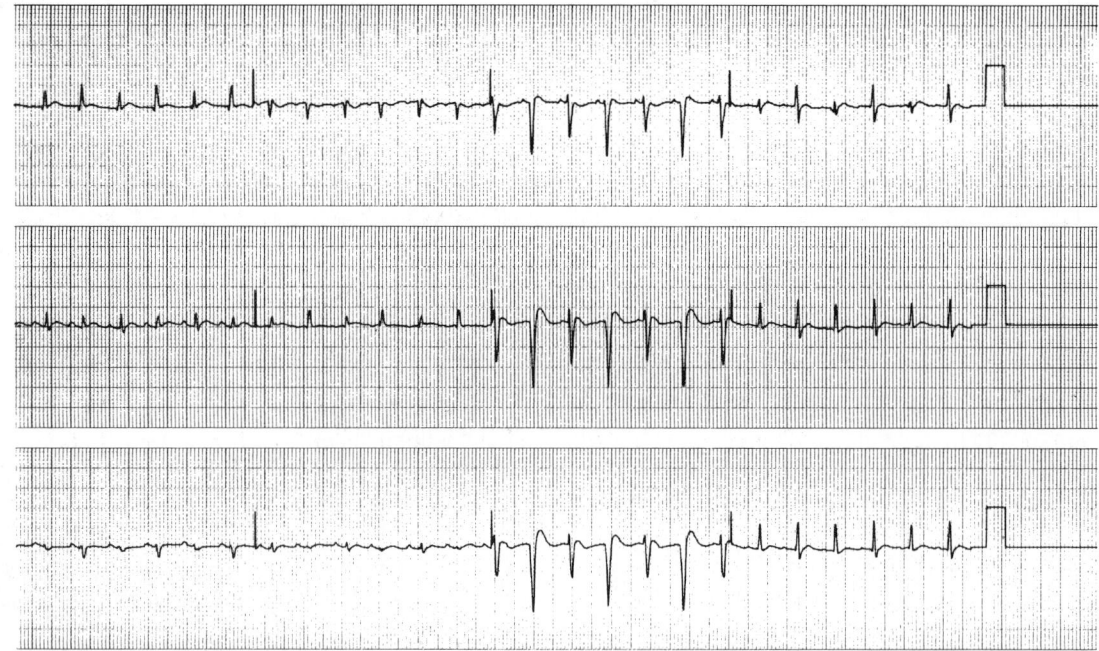

FIGURE 28-6 Electrocardiogram of a patient with cardiac tamponade demonstrates low voltages in the limb leads and marked electrical alternans.

tomography and magnetic resonance imaging are useful to diagnose effusions and may indicate the nature of the effusion.[32]

The contribution of a small effusion to a patient's condition may be difficult to ascertain and is based on the principles described above. Even a small effusion may be significant if it accumulated rapidly; examples include trauma, recent invasive cardiac procedures, and other conditions that may cause bleeding into the pericardium, such as aortic dissection.

FIGURE 28-8 Chest radiogram (anterior) of a patient with rapidly increasing pericardial effusion and hemodynamic evidence of cardiac tamponade. Note how the cardiac silhouette is rounded in its lower portion and tapers at the base of the heart, resembling a plastic bag filled with water sitting on a table.

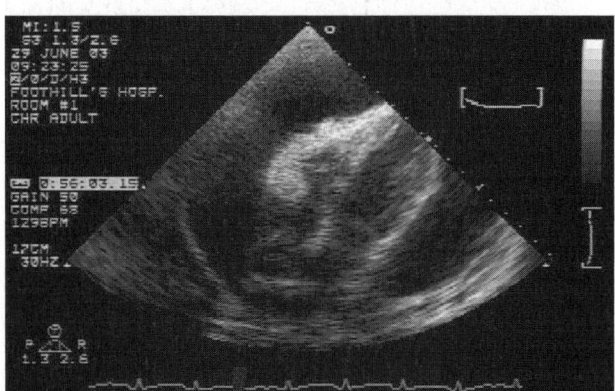

A

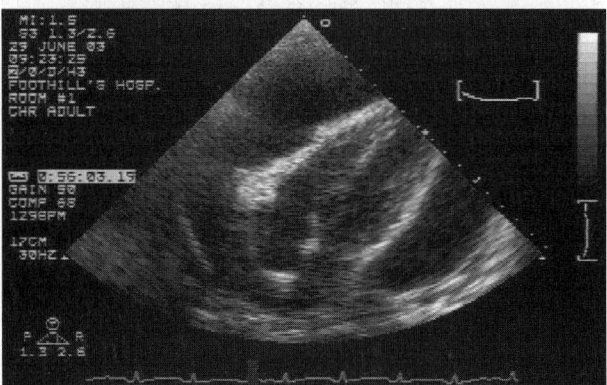

B

FIGURE 28-7 *Left.* An early diastolic frame of a two-dimensional echocardiogram in a patient with cardiac tamponade. There is a very large pericardial effusion and right atrial and right ventricular collapse. *Right.* A late diastolic frame from the same cardiac cycle; both ventricles are underfilled.

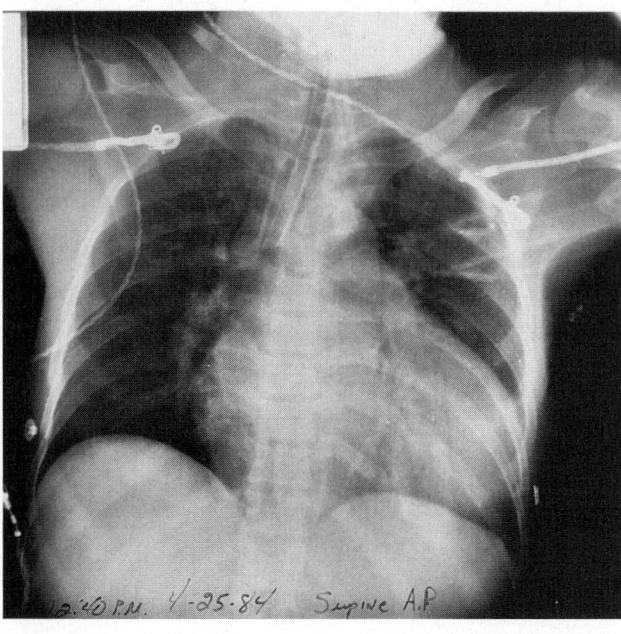

TREATMENT

In the absence of tamponade, even large effusions may not need to be drained.[33] If the effusion is believed to be benign, a careful conservative approach may be sufficient. The fundamental problem in cardiac tamponade is constrained ventricular filling, so removal of the fluid is central to effective treatment. Unless the patient's volume has been depleted, there is no potential benefit from volume loading because filling cannot be increased. There is also limited potential benefit from inotropic agents because there is already substantial neurohumoral stimulation in these patients. The method of pericardial drainage is not standardized.[34–38] Unless the etiology of the effusion indicates otherwise, needle drainage should be performed with echocardiographic guidance. Large effusions are usually safely drained, whereas small effusions are inherently associated with greater risk. Electrocardiographic monitoring with a lead connected to the needle (using ST-segment elevation on the electrocardiogram to indicate contact with the myocardium) is not as safe as echocardiographic monitoring. Drainage of the first 50 to 100 mL of fluid usually relieves much of the hemodynamic compromise. A catheter is usually left in place under suction to drain the pericardial space for at least 2 to 3 days. Clotting of the catheter may be prevented with a slow infusion of heparinized saline.[39] The drained fluid should be sent for appropriate diagnostic assessment even if the underlining etiology is known or suspected, despite a low diagnostic yield.[40] The presence of blood in the effusion is not helpful in establishing the cause of the effusion.[41] Recurrent effusions are not uncommon, particularly if the original effusion was large. Other different techniques are used initially or subsequently. These include balloon pericardiotomy,[42] thoracoscopic drainage (which improves diagnostic accuracy),[43,44] and a pericardial window.[35] Surgical drainage should be considered initially in patients with smaller effusions because of the higher risk when drained by needle. Long-term survival rate is dependent on the underlying disease rather than on the method of drainage.[34,35,45,46] Large effusions due to metastatic disease may be best treated surgically, whereas benign effusions may be adequately treated with a single-needle drainage procedure. Chemotherapeutic or sclerosing agents or steroids may be installed in the pericardium after drainage.[47]

ANTICOAGULATION

Whereas substantial pericardial effusions have been associated with anticoagulation, the presence of a friction rub or a very small amount of pericardial fluid detected by echocardiography should not deter the clinician from continuing anticoagulation when there is a clear indication for it. Examples include myocardial infarction and the presence of a prosthetic heart valve. Patients can be safely monitored clinically and echocardiographically for the unlikely development of tamponade. Anticoagulants should be discontinued in Dressler syndrome (which is increasingly rare after myocardial infarction).

RENAL FAILURE

Up to 40% of patients with chronic renal failure develop pericardial effusions during the course of their disease. Effusions may occur before dialysis and during maintenance dialysis.[48] There is some question as to whether heparin contributes to the development of effusion, but patients on dialysis using heparin-free solutions still develop effusions. Because preload is reduced during hemodialysis, the risk of rendering an asymptomatic effusion hemodynamically significant is real. The probability that dialysis will cause an effusion to clear is highest when the effusion predates the start of intensive hemodialysis or develops early in its course (within weeks).[49] The size of the effusion is the single most important determinant of need for surgical therapy. Hemodialysis is more effective than peritoneal dialysis for reducing effusions and should be initiated early if there is evidence of enlargement. Indomethacin and steroids are of uncertain value. Failure to resolve or progression of an effusion during the course of intense hemodialysis may dictate the need for drainage.

CARDIAC SURGERY

Pericardial abnormalities are common after cardiac surgery. Early after surgery, hemopericardium and hemomediastinum can cause tamponade, even though the pericardium is commonly left open. When there is postoperative hemodynamic compromise, it is necessary to consider the possibility of tamponade. Although echocardiography is often very helpful in this regard, tamponade is sometimes caused by a localized collection of fluid or blood that may be difficult to identify, even by transesophageal echocardiography. A careful synthesis of hemodynamic and echo data may require reoperation without a clear diagnosis beforehand. The presence of unexplained hemodynamic deterioration (e.g., with good ventricular function) suggests the possibility of localized tamponade, even if it is difficult to demonstrate echocardiographically.

The postpericardiotomy syndrome occurs several weeks postoperatively in 10% to 20% of patients and is characterized by fever, chest pain, and the presence of a friction rub.[50] In many ways, it is analogous to the Dressler syndrome, which occurs weeks after myocardial infarction. Good evidence supports an autoimmune pathogenesis, with anti-heart antibodies and circulating immune complexes present in many patients.[51] Electrocardiographic changes identical to those seen in acute pericarditis may or may not be present. Aspirin is the treatment of choice. Corticosteroids may be considered in patients who do not respond to aspirin or colchicine.

PURULENT PERICARDITIS

Pericardial effusions are much more likely to be sterile than infected. Purulent pericarditis is most often the result of local spread from empyema, mediastinitis, endocarditis, prior pericardiotomy, or burn injury.[52] It is rare, tends to occur in immunocompromised patients, and may be difficult to treat. Although drainage is necessary, it is not clear what the best approach is. It is commonly first discovered when pericardiocentesis is performed by needle; continuous catheter drainage should be initiated then, but surgery likely will be necessary. Patients with the human immunodeficiency virus may present with tamponade, and an infectious cause is frequent; this is associated with a very high mortality rate.[53]

Purulent pericarditis may develop in the setting of severe infectious disease with a wide variety of causative organisms. When pericardial fluid is evident on echocardiography in a patient who is at risk for purulent pericarditis, a definitive diagnostic procedure should be considered because its mortality rate is high. The best approach is removal of the fluid. Some centers perform a subxiphoid procedure and proceed to pericardiectomy, if infection is present. Thoracoscopic pericardiectomy also may be useful in such cases.

It is clearly important to discriminate between purulent and sterile effusions. Electrocardiography and echocardiography are not useful. Gallium 67 (^{67}Ga) uptake, when used with single-photon emission computed tomography, has been reported to have a resolution that can distinguish pericardial from myocardial inflammation and that may be able to detect inflammation associated with secondary infection of the pericardial space. There are several reports of tuberculous pericarditis diagnosed by planar ^{67}Ga imaging. In patients with complex disease who may have multiple areas of ^{67}Ga uptake in the region, simultaneous use of technetium 99 and ^{67}Ga with subtraction imaging may increase the specificity of the test.

CONSTRICTIVE PERICARDITIS

In constrictive pericarditis, the pericardium becomes thickened, may be calcified, and prevents normal ventricular filling. Signs of constriction may become evident as effusive pericarditis resolves, and normal hemodynamics may return spontaneously or with conservative treatment.[54,55] Forward output is compromised and the increased diastolic pressures cause edema. Early diastolic ventricular filling is rapid in constriction and is responsible for the classic dip-plateau configuration of atrial and ventricular pressure tracings; there is a rapid y descent with an early nadir and a sharp rise in pressure as the chamber reaches its limits of expansion (Fig. 28-9). After atrial systole, there is a rapid x descent so that an M-shaped jugular venous pulsation may be observed (Fig. 28-10). The fixed maximum volume of the pericardium results in equalization of end-diastolic pressures, similar to that in cardiac tamponade. If the central volume has been decreased, as might result from excessive diuresis, equalization of pressures may not be observed; volume expansion, however, will cause this to occur.

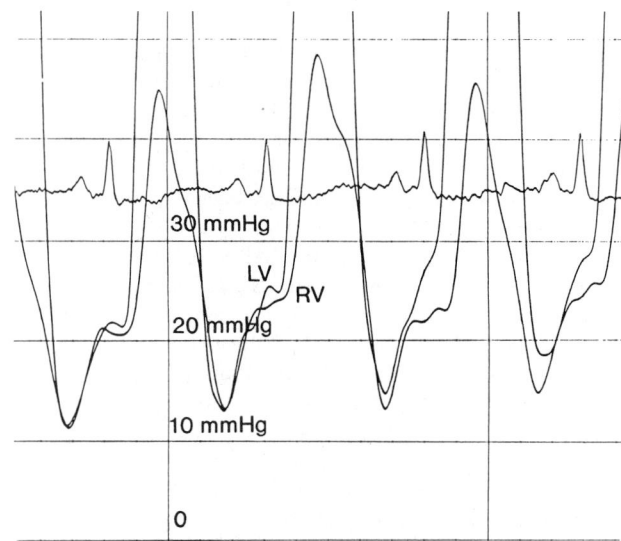

FIGURE 28-9 Simultaneous right ventricular and left ventricular pressures in a patient with constrictive pericarditis. The pressures are elevated and nearly equal, with little rise in right ventricular pressure during the last two-thirds of diastole. LV, left ventricle; RV, right ventricle.

The Kussmaul sign (inspiratory increase in the jugular venous pressure) is common[56] but not specific for constriction; it is seen most often in RV infarction and other conditions affecting the right ventricle. There are several echocardiographic findings associated with constrictive pericarditis (Fig. 28-11), none of which is pathognomonic.[29] The pericardium may appear thickened, but this usually cannot be discerned with confidence; transesophageal studies may be more accurate in defining pericardial thickness. Because rapid ventricular filling occurs early and stops abruptly, M-mode evidence of absent LV filling in the last half of diastole is common (flat posterior wall tracing); continued expansion of the left ventricle throughout diastole suggests that constriction is absent. During early rapid filling, there is a "septal bounce," and there may be premature opening of the pulmonary valve (Fig. 28-12). During inspiration, there is substantial leftward

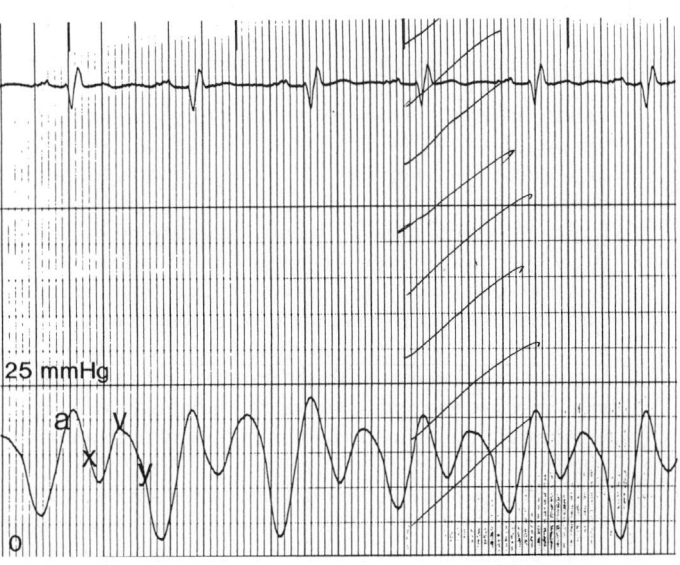

FIGURE 28-10 Right atrial pressure in a patient with constrictive pericarditis. Note the prominent x and y descents and the M shape. The a and v waves and the x and y descents are as described in text.

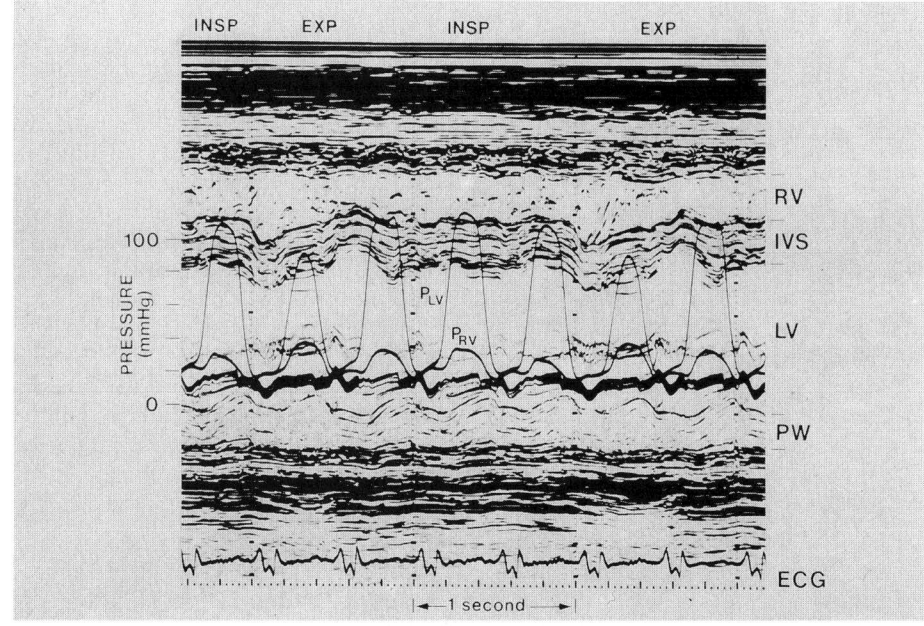

A

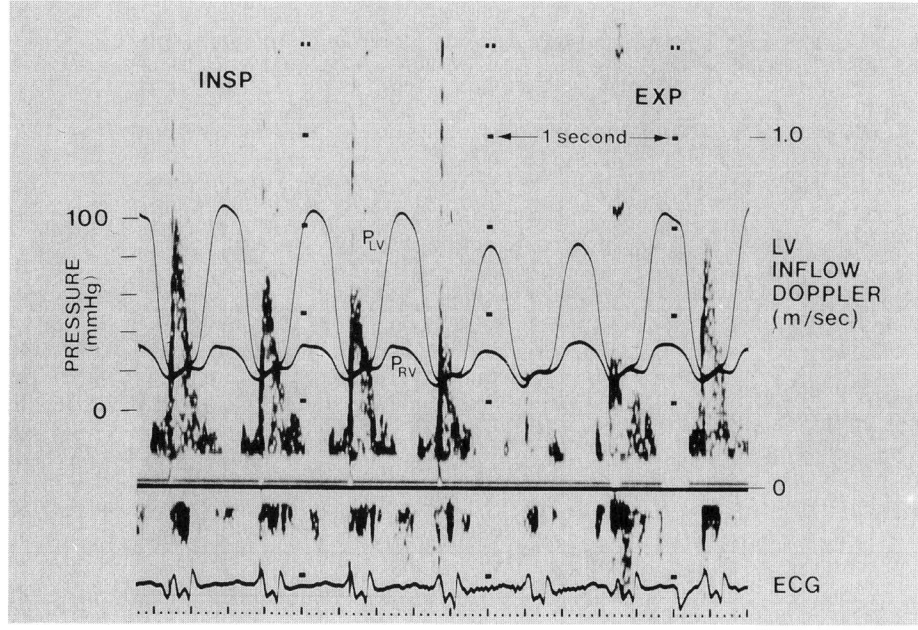

B

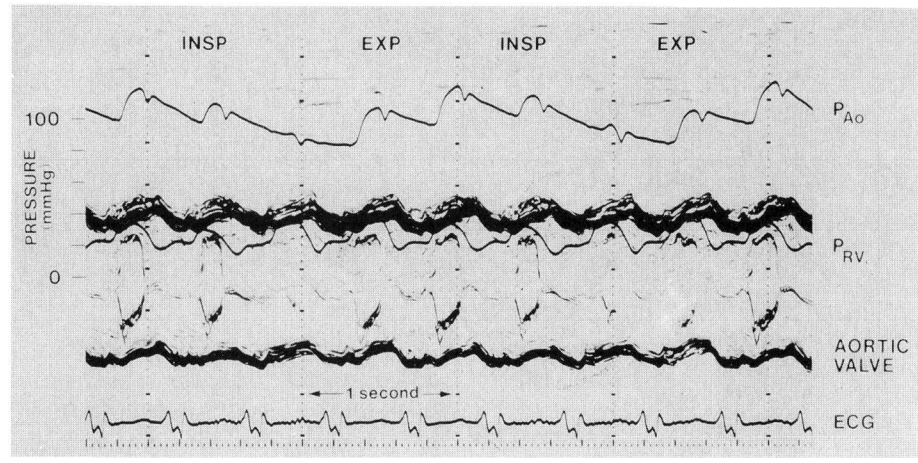

C

FIGURE 28-11 *A.* Simultaneous left and right ventricular pressures superimposed on an M-mode echocardiogram in a patient with constrictive pericarditis. At end inspiration, the interventricular septum shifts leftward, thereby enlarging the right ventricle and shrinking the left ventricle. Associated with this shift are increased right ventricular systolic pressure and decreased left ventricular systolic pressure. *B.* Simultaneous left and right ventricular pressures superimposed on the left ventricular inflow Doppler signal. Left ventricular inflow velocity decreases during inspiration, corresponding to the decrease in left ventricular filling noted in the top panel. This change is associated with a decrease in generated left ventricular pressure and an increase in right ventricular pressure. *C.* Aortic pressure superimposed on an M-mode echocardiogram through the aortic valve. At end inspiration, opening of the aortic valve is markedly reduced, as is aortic pressure. Ao, aorta; EXP, expiration; INSP, inspiration; IVS, interventricular septum; LV, left ventricle; PW, posterior wall; RV, right ventricle.

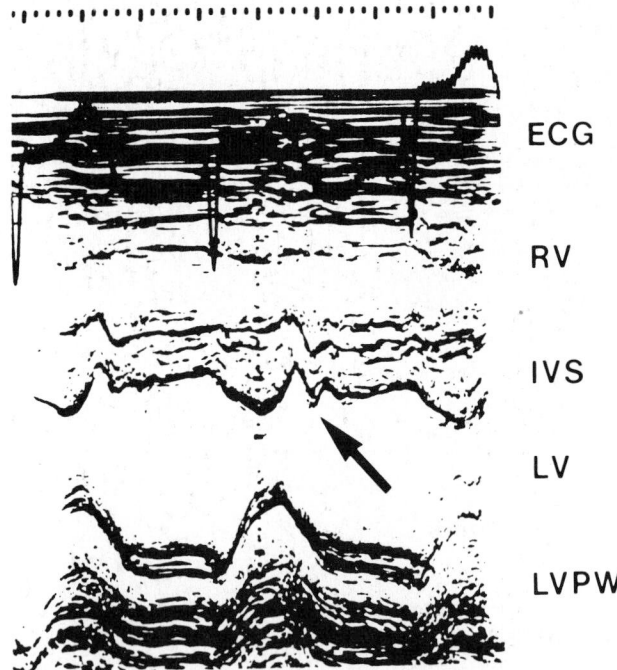

FIGURE 28-12 M-mode echocardiogram in a patient with constrictive pericarditis. Note the flattened posterior wall of the left ventricle during diastole, consistent with little ventricular filling. The early rush of blood into the ventricle results in a shuttering motion of the interventricular septum and creates a notch (*arrow*). ECG, electrocardiogram; IVS, interventricular septum; LV, left ventricle; LVPW, left ventricular posterior wall; RV, right ventricle.

septal shift in keeping with the unchanged or increased RVEDP and decreased LVEDP. Doppler echocardiography adds diagnostic accuracy but is not widely accepted as definitive.[57,58] Chest radiography is often helpful; the absence of signs of left heart failure in the presence of right heart failure helps to narrow the focus. The cardiac silhouette can be small or large, depending on antecedent heart disease. Egg shell–like calcification may be apparent, usually more easily seen in the lateral projection; the absence or presence of calcification is not useful to rule in or out constriction.[59] Nonspecific ST-T-wave abnormalities are often present on the electrocardiogram, but this is of little value.

Pericardial thickening is detected readily and with high sensitivity by computed tomography and magnetic resonance imaging;[32] however, in a large series, it was not present in almost one in five patients with constriction.[60] Because fast computed tomography and magnetic resonance imaging are capable of visualizing dynamic chamber processes and patterns of filling, they can also provide physiologic information.

The characteristic presentation of constrictive pericarditis is that of right heart failure, often severe, without another apparent cause. The diagnosis may be difficult to prove in the presence of other forms of heart disease; this is increasingly problematic because constriction after cardiac surgery is not rare. Hepatosplenomegaly sometimes incorrectly suggests the presence of metastases. The jugular venous pulse may suggest constriction; there may be a Kussmaul sign and the characteristic M-shaped pulsation highlighted by the rapid *y*

descent. A pericardial knock (an early diastolic, sometimes loud, sound) may be heard.

In some instances, it is difficult to distinguish constrictive pericardial disease from restrictive cardiomyopathy.[28,29,58] Cardiac catheterization is required for simultaneous measurement of right and left filling pressures; when low, these pressures may differ but will converge if fluid is administered (<5-mm Hg difference). In restrictive cardiomyopathy, diastolic pressures are generally different and pulmonary artery pressure is often higher than in constriction. Volume loading is suggested if the diagnosis is not evident from the initial hemodynamics.[61] Similar measurements can be obtained with a flow-directed pulmonary artery catheter. Doppler echocardiography also may be helpful but remains sufficiently unreliable to preclude it as the only diagnostic test.[62] Myocardial biopsy can be helpful.

Constrictive pericarditis may be a complication of cardiac surgery, occurring in fewer than 1% of patients.[63] The time to onset can be as short as 6 weeks or as long as years after surgery. In one series, almost 65% of patients with postoperative constriction were thought to have developed the postpericardiotomy syndrome earlier in their course.[64] Pericardiectomy is made more difficult by the presence of bypass grafts.

In constrictive pericarditis, pericardiectomy is the only effective treatment. This is often very difficult and sometimes results are poor. As a result, some patients will have persistently increased venous pressure, and others, after initial improvement, may have recurrent constriction.[65]

EFFUSIVE-CONSTRICTIVE PERICARDITIS

Effusive-constrictive pericarditis is a combination of a thickened, potentially constricting pericardium with a variable amount of pericardial fluid. It occurs most often in patients with malignancies.[66] The hemodynamic characteristics are similar to those of tamponade and may evolve into those due to constriction as the volume of fluid is decreased.

References

1. Henderson Y, Barringer TBJ: The relation of venous pressure to cardiac efficiency. *Am J Physiol* 13:352, 1913.
2. Haykowsky M, Taylor D, Teo K, et al: Left ventricular wall stress during leg-press exercise performed with a brief Valsalva maneuver. *Chest* 119:150, 2001.
3. Katz LN: Analysis of the several factors regulating the performance of the heart. *Physiol Rev* 35:91, 1955.
4. Gibbons-Kroeker CA, Shrive NG, Belenkie I, Tyberg JV: Pericardium modulates left and right ventricular stroke volumes to compensate for sudden changes in atrial volume. *Am J Physiol Heart Circ Physiol* 284:H2247, 2003.
5. Braunwald E, Ross J Jr: Editorial: The ventricular end-diastolic pressure. *Am J Med* 34:147, 1963.
6. Sarnoff SJ, Berglund E: Ventricular function. 1. Starling's law of the heart studied by means of simultaneous right and left ventricular function curves in the dog. *Circulation* 9:706, 1954.
7. Ludbrook PA, Byrne JD, Kurnik PB, McKnight RC: Influence of reduction of preload and afterload by nitroglycerin on left ventricular diastolic pressure-volume relations and relaxation in man. *Circulation* 56:937, 1977.
8. Tyberg JV, Misbach GA, Glantz SA, et al: A mechanism for the shifts in the diastolic, left ventricular, pressure-volume curve: The role of the pericardium. *Eur J Cardiol* 7(suppl):163, 1978.

9. Kenner HM, Wood EH: Intrapericardial, intrapleural, and intracardiac pressures during acute heart failure in dogs studied without thoracotomy. *Circ Res* 19:1071, 1966.

10. Smiseth OA, Frais MA, Kingma I, et al: Assessment of pericardial constraint in dogs. *Circulation* 71:158, 1985.

11. Hamilton DR, deVries G, Tyberg JV: Static and dynamic operating characteristics of a pericardial balloon. *J Appl Physiol* 90:1481, 2001.

12. Tyberg JV, Taichman GC, Smith ER, et al: The relation between pericardial pressure and right atrial pressure: An intraoperative study. *Circulation* 73:428, 1986.

13. Boltwood CM, Skulsky A, Drinkwater DC, et al: Intraoperative measurement of pericardial constraint: role in ventricular diastolic mechanics. *J Am Coll Cardiol* 8:1289, 1986.

14. Belenkie I, Dani R, Smith ER, Tyberg JV: Ventricular interaction during experimental acute pulmonary embolism. *Circulation* 78:761, 1988.

15. Belenkie I, Dani R, Smith ER, Tyberg JV: Effects of volume loading during experimental acute pulmonary embolism. *Circulation* 80:178, 1989.

16. Belenkie I, Dani R, Smith ER, Tyberg JV: The importance of pericardial constraint in experimental pulmonary embolism and volume loading. *Am Heart J* 123:733, 1992.

17. Glantz SA, Parmley WW: Factors which affect the diastolic pressure-volume curve. *Circ Res* 42:171, 1978.

18. Mirsky I, Rankin JS: The effects of geometry, elasticity, and external pressures on the diastolic pressure-volume and stiffness-stress relations. How important is the pericardium? *Circ Res* 44:601, 1979.

19. Baker AE, Belenkie I, Dani R, et al: Quantitative assessment of the independent contributions of the pericardium and septum to direct ventricular interaction. *Am J Physiol Heart Circ Physiol* 275:H476, 1998.

20. Jardin F, Gueret P, Prost JF, et al: Two-dimensional echocardiographic assessment of left ventricular function in chronic obstructive pulmonary disease. *Am Rev Respir Dis* 129:135, 1984.

21. Pinsky MR: Determinants of pulmonary arterial flow variation during respiration. *J Appl Physiol* 56:1237, 1984.

22. Pinsky MR: Instantaneous venous return curves in an intact canine preparation. *J Appl Physiol* 56:765, 1984.

23. Sagrista-Sauleda J, Angel J, Permanyer-Miralda G, Soler-Soler J: Long-term follow-up of idiopathic chronic pericardial effusion. *N Engl J Med* 341:2054, 1999.

24. Battle RW, LeWinter MM: The evaluation and management of pericardial disease. *Curr Sci* 5:331, 1990.

25. Singh S, Wann LS, Schuchard GH, et al: Right ventricular and right atrial collapse in patients with cardiac tamponade—A combined echocardiographic and hemodynamic study. *Circulation* 70:966, 1984.

26. Burstow DJ, Oh JK, Bailey KR: Cardiac tamponade: Characteristic Doppler observations. *Mayo Clin Proc* 64:312, 1989.

27. Merce J, Sagrista-Sauleda J, Permanyer-Miralda G, et al: Correlation between clinical and Doppler echocardiographic findings in patients with moderate and large pericardial effusion: implications for the diagnosis of cardiac tamponade. *Am Heart J* 138:759, 1999.

28. Hoit BD: Management of effusive and constrictive pericardial heart disease. *Circulation* 105:2939, 2002.

29. Asher CR, Klein AL: Diastolic heart failure: Restrictive cardiomyopathy, constrictive pericarditis, and cardiac tamponade: Clinical and echocardiographic evaluation. *Cardiol Rev* 10:218, 2002.

30. Zhang S, Kerins DM, Byrd BF: Doppler echocardiography in cardiac tamponade and constrictive pericarditis. *Echocardiography* 11:507, 1994.

31. Fowler NO: Cardiac tamponade—A clinical or an echocardiographic diagnosis? *Circulation* 87:1738, 1993.

32. Wang ZJ, Reddy GP, Gotway MB, et al: CT and MR imaging of pericardial disease. *Radiographics* 23:S167, 2003.

33. Merce J, Sagrista-Sauleda J, Permanyer-Miralda G, Soler-Soler J: Should pericardial drainage be performed routinely in patients who have a large pericardial effusion without tamponade? *Am J Med* 105:190, 1998.

34. McDonald JM, Meyers BF, Guthrie TJ, et al: Comparison of open subxiphoid pericardial drainage with percutaneous catheter drainage for symptomatic pericardial effusion. *Ann Thorac Surg* 76:811, 2003.

35. Dosis T, Theakos N, Angouras D, Asimacopoulos P: Risk factors affecting the survival of patients with pericardial effusion submitting to subxiphoid pericardiostomy. *Chest* 124:242, 2003.

36. Tsang TS, Enriquez-Sarano M, Freeman WK, et al: Consecutive 1127 therapeutic echocardiographically guided pericardiocenteses: Clinical profile, practice patterns, and outcomes spanning 21 years. *Mayo Clin Proc* 77:429, 2002.

37. Allen KB, Faber LP, Warren WH, Shaar CJ: Pericardial effusion: subxiphoid pericardiostomy versus percutaneous catheter drainage. *Ann Thorac Surg* 67:437, 1999.

38. Olson JE, Ryan MB, Blumenstock DA: Eleven years' experience with pericardial-peritoneal window in the management of malignant and benign pericardial effusions. *Ann Surg Oncol* 2:165, 1995.

39. Patel AK, Kosolcharoen PK, Nallasivan M: Catheter drainage of the pericardium. Practical method to maintain long term patency. *Chest* 92:1018, 1987.

40. Mueller XM, Tevaearai HT, Hurni M, et al: Etiologic diagnosis of pericardial disease: the value of routine tests during surgical procedures. *J Am Coll Cardiol* 184:645, 1997.

41. Atar S, Chiu J, Forrester JS, Siegel RJ: Bloody pericardial effusion in patients with cardiac tamponade: Is the cause cancerous, tuberculous, or iatrogenic in the 1990's? *Chest* 116:1564, 1999.

42. Wang HJ, Hsu KL, Chiang FT, et al: Technical and prognostic outcomes of double-balloon pericardiotomy for large malignancy-related pericardial effusions. *Chest* 122:893, 2002.

43. Seferovie PM, Ristie AD, Maksimovie R, et al: Diagnostic value of pericardial biopsy. *Circulation* 107:978, 2003.

44. Nugue O, Millaire A, Porte H, de Groote P: Pericardioscopy in the etiologic diagnosis of pericardial effusion in 141 consecutive patients. *Circulation* 94:1635, 1996.

45. Tsang TS, Barnes ME, Gersh BJ, et al: Outcomes of clinically significant idiopathic pericardial effusion requiring intervention. *Am J Cardiol* 91:704, 2003.

46. Retter AS: Pericardial disease in the oncology patient. *Heart Dis* 4:387, 2002.

47. Maisch B, Pankuweit S, Billa C, et al: Intrapericardial treatment of inflammatory and neoplastic pericarditis guided by pericardioscopy and epicardial biopsy—Results from a pilot study. *Clin Cardiol* 22:117, 1999.

48. Frommer JP, Young JB, Ayus JC: Asymptomatic pericardial effusion in uremic patients: Effect of long term dialysis. *Nephron* 39:296, 1985.

49. Rutsky EA, Rostand SG: Treatment of uremic pericarditis and pericardial effusion. *Am J Kidney Dis* 10:2, 1987.

50. Miller RH, Horneffer PJ, Gardner TJ: The epidemiology of the post pericardiotomy syndrome: A common complication of cardiac surgery. *Am Heart J* 116:1323, 1988.

51. De Scheerder I, Wulfrank D, Van Renterghem L: Association of anti-heart antibodies and circulating immune complexes in the post-pericardiotomy syndrome. *Clin Exp Immunol* 57:423, 1984.

52. Fowler NO: Infectious pericarditis. *Prog Cardiovasc Dis* 16:323, 1973.

53. Gowda RM, Khan IA, Mehta NJ, et al: Cardiac tamponade in patients with human immunodeficienty virus disease. *Angiology* 54:469, 2003.

54. Oh JK, Hatle LK, Mulvagh SL, Tajik AJ: Transient constrictive pericarditis: Diagnosis by two-dimensional Doppler echocardiography. *Mayo Clin Proc* 68:1158, 1993.

55. Sagrista-Sauleda J, Permanyer-Miralda G, Candell-Riera J, et al: Transient cardiac constriction: an unrecognized pattern of evolution in effusive acute idiopathic pericarditis. *Am J Cardiol* 59:961, 1987.

56. Meyer TESP, Marcus RH: Mechanisms underlying Kussmaul's sign in chronic constrictive pericarditis. *Am J Physiol* 238:H494, 1989.

57. Klodas E, Nishimura RA, Appleton CP, et al: Doppler evaluation of patients with constrictive pericarditis: Use of tricuspid regurgitation velocity curves to determine enhanced ventricular interaction. *J Am Coll Cardiol* 28:652, 1996.

58. Hatle LK, Appleton CP, Popp RL: Differentiation of constrictive pericarditis and restrictive cardiomyopathy by Doppler echocardiography. *Circulation* 79:357, 1989.

59. Ling LH, Oh JK, Breen JF, et al: Calcific constrictive pericarditis: Is it still with us? *Ann Intern Med* 132:444, 2000.

60. Talreja DR, Edwards WD, Danielson GK, et al: Constrictive pericarditis in 26 patients with histologically normal pericardial thickness. *Circulation* 108:1852, 2003.

61. Meaney E, Shabetai R, Bhargava V: Cardiac amyloidosis, constrictive pericarditis, and restrictive cardiomyopathy. *Am J Cardiol* 38:547, 1976.

62. Rajagopalan N, Garcia MJ, Rodriguez L, et al: Comparison of new Doppler echocardiographic methods to differentiate constrictive pericardial heart disease and restrictive cardiomyopathy. *Am J Cardiol* 87:86, 2001.

63. Cimino JJ, Kogan AD: Constrictive pericarditis after cardiac surgery: Report of three cases and review of the literature. *Am Heart J* 118:1292, 1984.

64. Killian DM, Furiasse JG, Scanlon PJ: Constrictive pericarditis after cardiac surgery. *Am Heart J* 118:563, 1989.

65. McCaughan BC, Schaff HV, Piehler JM: Early and late results of pericardiectomy for constrictive pericarditis. *J Thorac Cardiovasc Surg* 89:340, 1985.

66. Mann T, Brodie BR, Grossman W: Effusive-constrictive hemodynamic pattern due to neoplastic involvement of the pericardium. *Am J Cardiol* 41:781, 1978.

VALVULAR HEART DISEASE

MATTHEW J. SORRENTINO

KEY POINTS

- *Valvular heart disease may remain asymptomatic until an underlying serious illness causes rapid deterioration of health.*

- *Patients with valvular heart disease are at increased risk of bacterial endocarditis following invasive procedures.*

- *Aortic stenosis significantly increases the mortality of patients requiring noncardiac surgery.*

- *Aortic stenosis is a common comorbidity in elderly patients.*

- *Heart failure in a patient with hypertrophic cardiomyopathy should be treated with rate-slowing and negative inotropic agents.*

- *Acute regurgitant lesions are frequently medical emergencies and are not as well tolerated as chronic regurgitant lesions.*

- *Once left ventricular dysfunction occurs in a patient with mitral regurgitation, the lesion is severe and unlikely to improve with surgical correction; in fact, surgery may worsen left ventricular function.*

Valvular heart disease is a common cause of morbidity and mortality in the U.S. Although the incidence of rheumatic fever has declined, many patients that acquired the disease years ago are now presenting with valvular abnormalities. In addition, degenerative diseases of the valves are becoming increasingly common as the population ages. Recognition of valvular diseases is important for proper management of seriously ill patients.

The cardiac physical examination is the essential first step in making the diagnosis of valvular heart disease. Patients presenting with signs and symptoms of cardiac illness, such as shortness of breath, pulmonary edema, angina pectoris, or syncope, should have a detailed examination of the cardiovascular system to ascertain the presence of valvular lesions. Assessment of patients prior to noncardiac surgery should include an evaluation for valvular lesions. Once valvular heart disease is suspected, a diagnostic work-up can be completed to determine the severity of the abnormality and quantitate the risk to the patient.

Many patients with valvular abnormalities remain asymptomatic until the onset of an underlying medical illness precipitates heart failure. Tachycardia due to arrhythmias, pain, blood loss, or hypoxia can suddenly precipitate pulmonary edema or low-output states in patients with previously compensated valvular disease. In these instances, prompt treatment of the critical illness is essential to avoid complications of the valvular lesion.

The lesions of valvular heart disease can be broadly categorized as stenotic and regurgitant. The impact of these abnormalities on left or right ventricular function will determine the clinical presentation and risk to the patient at times of critical illness. Traditionally, cardiac catheterization has been used to diagnose and quantify valvular stenosis or regurgitation. Advances in echocardiography have made this imaging modality highly accurate in assessing valvular structure and function.

The degree of stenosis of a valve can be measured by the Gorlin formula.[1] The Gorlin formula uses the principle that flow equals area times velocity. The formula for calculating aortic valve stenosis can be stated as $A = F/(C \times V)$, where A is the valve area, F is aortic valve flow (calculated as cardiac output divided by the systolic ejection period in seconds multiplied by the heart rate), C is an empiric constant accounting for valvular energy loss and orifice contraction, and V is velocity. Velocity can be expressed as $V = \sqrt{2gh}$, where g is gravitational acceleration ($980 \ cm/s^2$), and h is the measured pressure gradient. The Gorlin equation for aortic valve area can then be written as $A = F/(C \times 44h)$.

Considering the empirical nature of the Gorlin formula, the calculated valve areas have been useful in predicting prognosis and risk. Recently formulas calculating valve resistance have been devised. Resistance is less flow dependent and therefore less variable than aortic valve areas.[2] Echocardiographic methods of calculating valve areas have shown good correlation with invasive methods.

Determination of the degree of valvular leakage by cardiac catheterization has depended on visualization of contrast opacifying the receiving chamber. Important determinants of the severity of regurgitation are the size and function of the receiving chamber, both of which can be estimated either by invasive or noninvasive means. Acute and chronic regurgitant lesions have markedly different presentations, in part owing to the inability of a receiving chamber to accommodate a sudden volume overload.

This chapter will review the etiology, pathophysiology, clinical presentation, diagnostic evaluation, and management of the major valvular lesions and hypertrophic cardiomyopathy. The physical examination will be highlighted, as it yields the first crucial clues to the presence of valvular disease. Management of prosthetic valve abnormalities will be covered as well.

Aortic Stenosis

ETIOLOGY AND PATHOPHYSIOLOGY

Over the past few decades, there has been a dramatic shift in the presentation of valvular aortic stenosis. The prevalence of rheumatic fever and rheumatic heart disease has decreased substantially in developed countries, and the advancing age of the population has increased the incidence of degenerative valvular lesions. At present, there are three major etiologies of valvular aortic stenosis: congenital malformations of the valve, which are usually suspected in younger patients; rheumatic aortic disease, which is usually accompanied by mitral valve disease; and calcific or degenerative changes of normal aortic valves, which are seen later in life.

Congenital aortic stenosis may present early in life when fusion of the valvular commissures is present at birth, or later in life after calcification of a congenitally bicuspid valve occurs. It is estimated that 1% to 2% of aortic valves are bicuspid, making this one of the most common congenital heart malformations.[3] A bicuspid valve functions normally in younger people, but the leaflets are prone to earlier calcific

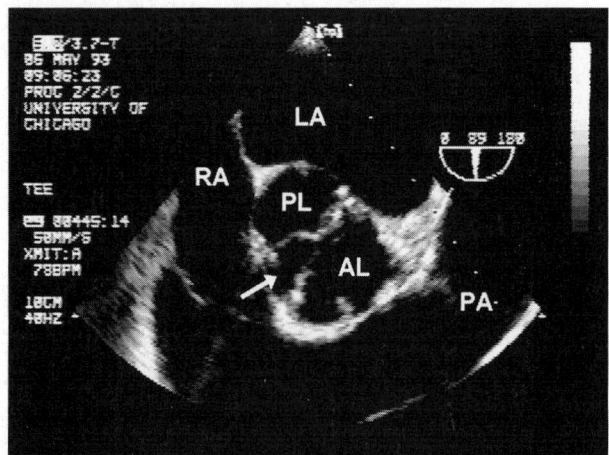

FIGURE 29-1 Bicuspid aortic valve with aortic stenosis. Cross-section transesophageal echocardiogram of a bicuspid aortic valve showing two leaflets. PL, posterior leaflet; AL, anterior leaflet. The valve leaflets are thickened and calcified, with decreased leaflet mobility. The *arrow* indicates the full extent of the opening of the stenotic valve. RA, right atrium; LA, left atrium; PA, pulmonary artery.

and degenerative changes because of increased stress on the valve compared to a normal tricuspid valve. Calcific aortic stenosis of a bicuspid valve usually develops in middle or late adult life (Fig. 29-1).

Senile calcification of normal three-leaflet valves is an increasingly common cause of aortic stenosis in the elderly. Surgical series have reported the incidence of degenerative aortic stenosis at 10% to 30% of surgical cases,[4] but this finding significantly underestimates the true prevalence of the condition in the elderly, since many patients are not referred for surgical correction. Because of its high prevalence, this disease represents a significant morbidity in patients presenting with life-threatening diseases.

As aortic stenosis progresses, the reduced orifice offers increased resistance to blood flow, represented by the transvalvular pressure gradient. The relationship between blood flow or cardiac output and the pressure gradient is not linear, but instead is related to the square root of the pressure gradient. Therefore small changes in cardiac output may have significant effects on the pressure gradient. Critical aortic stenosis is usually considered to exist when the mean pressure gradient exceeds 50 mm Hg or when the calculated orifice area is 0.75 cm^2 or less.

Left ventricular outflow is initially maintained by hypertrophy of the left ventricle. Left ventricular volumes remain normal until late in the disease. In calcific aortic stenosis in which not all of the commissures are fused, the increase in left ventricular systolic pressure may maintain or even augment cardiac output. A fall in cardiac output, however, may make aortic stenosis more severe by preventing adequate opening of the valve. In patients with a relatively fixed aortic orifice, any sudden reduction in blood pressure or systemic vascular resistance, such as that seen in sepsis or with the use of vasodilating drugs, can lead to a precipitous fall in cardiac output and cardiac arrest.

The early symptoms of aortic stenosis are usually related to the left ventricular outflow obstruction. Symptoms of angina or syncope may develop during the early stages. Angina may

be due to epicardial coronary artery disease or subendocardial ischemia. About 50% of patients with aortic stenosis and typical angina pectoris have normal coronary arteries. Syncope may be secondary to a vasodepressor response when an abrupt rise in left ventricular pressure with exertion is not accompanied by a corresponding rise in aortic pressure.[5]

Dyspnea is a late symptom of aortic stenosis and is frequently related to changes in left ventricular systolic or diastolic function. With the onset of left ventricular failure, cardiac output decreases, leading to a corresponding fall in the transvalvular pressure gradient. Left atrial, pulmonary, and right heart pressures all increase, presenting as pulmonary edema and heart failure. The left ventricle will then dilate to compensate for the falling output.

Correction of aortic stenosis brings about significant improvement in cardiac function and lowers elevated right heart pressures and left ventricular filling pressures. Left ventricular hypertrophy regresses early, sometimes eventually to a normal mass.[6]

CLINICAL PRESENTATION

Patients with aortic stenosis may present with angina, syncope, or dyspnea on exertion. Some patients complain of nonspecific symptoms such as fatigue, dizziness, or palpitations. Many elderly and sedentary patients remain asymptomatic despite having critical aortic stenosis; the stenosis only becomes life threatening when they develop other critical illnesses or require elective or emergent surgery.

The physical examination can suggest hemodynamically significant aortic stenosis that will likely cause complications in patients who have critical illnesses or require surgery. A loud systolic murmur heard throughout the precordium with radiation to the neck is characteristic. This murmur usually has a crescendo/decrescendo pattern, although in critical aortic stenosis in which there is a significant delay in outflow, the murmur may be late-peaking or holosystolic. The murmur may be loud at the apex of the heart, mimicking mitral regurgitation. Severe aortic stenosis murmurs may be palpable. The aortic component of the second heart sound is typically soft or absent. An absent aortic closing sound may be the most sensitive finding for critical aortic stenosis, but it is not a common auscultatory sign.[7] The carotid impulse is generally diminished in volume and has a delayed, slow-rising peak. The cardiac impulse is usually strong and is not significantly displaced unless the ventricle has dilated.

DIAGNOSTIC EVALUATION

The electrocardiogram (ECG) usually shows left ventricular hypertrophy with a repolarization abnormality or strain pattern. A normal ECG virtually rules out the presence of critical aortic stenosis. The chest x-ray can show calcification of the valve, although cardiac enlargement is present only in the most severe cases, when left ventricular dilation is present.

Echocardiography can reliably diagnose aortic stenosis. There is a high correlation between transvalvular gradients and calculated aortic valve areas derived from Doppler echocardiography and those derived from angiography.[8–10] Doppler methods permit direct noninvasive measurement of the pressure gradient across the aortic valve. The peak gradient is estimated by the modified Bernoulli equation, which states that the pressure drop in mm Hg is equal to four times the square of the velocity (Fig. 29-2). The aortic valve area can

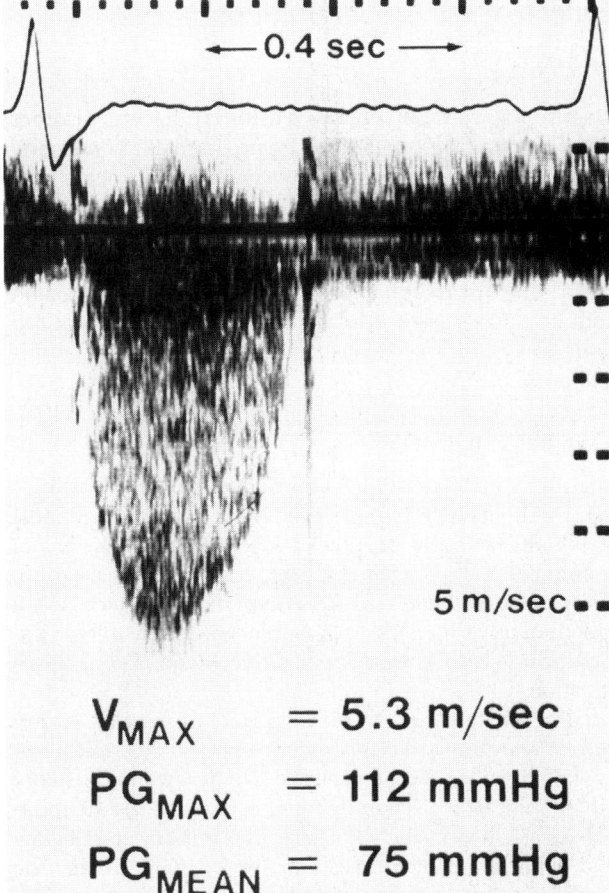

FIGURE 29-2 Doppler echocardiographic signal across a stenotic aortic valve. The peak instantaneous velocity (V_{max}) across the valve is 5.3 m/s. By the modified Bernoulli equation ($4v^2$), the peak instantaneous gradient (PG_{max}) is calculated to be 112 mm Hg. The mean velocity is determined as the mean of the squares of the instantaneous velocities. The mean pressure gradient (PG_{mean}) can then be calculated and is the value used for assessing the severity of aortic stenosis.

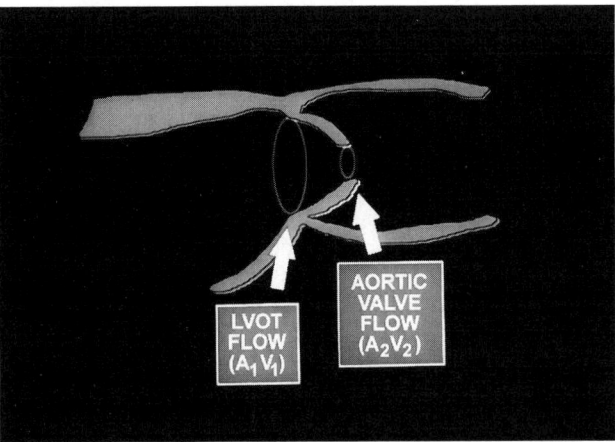

FIGURE 29-3 Continuity equation. The area of the left ventricular outflow tract (A_1) and the Doppler-measured velocities in the outflow tract (V_1) and across the stenotic aortic valve (V_2) can be determined. The aortic valve area (A_2) can then be calculated.

be visualized, because of the high incidence of concomitant coronary artery disease in elderly patients.

MANAGEMENT

Aortic stenosis is a mechanical problem, so the only effective long-term treatment is correction of the obstruction to outflow with surgery. The onset of symptoms is an indication for surgery. The development of heart failure with aortic stenosis is associated with a high mortality, especially if the left ventricular ejection fraction is reduced. Patients with severe aortic stenosis and left ventricular dysfunction have a mean survival of only one year.[11] Patients that present in heart failure must first have their symptoms stabilized and will then need an evaluation of the severity of the stenotic lesion and the degree of left ventricular dysfunction before proceeding with definitive aortic valve replacement surgery.

The left ventricular ejection fraction can be depressed in patients with aortic stenosis due to excessive systolic wall stress (afterload) seen in "true" aortic stenosis, or due to an intrinsic abnormality of myocardial contractility or cardiomyopathy referred to as "pseudo" or "relative" aortic stenosis.[12] Aortic valve replacement in true aortic stenosis can lead to a significant improvement in the ejection fraction once the afterload excess is relieved. Aortic valve replacement may have minimal benefit in pseudo aortic stenosis since the depressed ejection fraction is a muscle contractile abnormality that may not improve with valve replacement.

Patients with severe aortic stenosis and low cardiac output may present with only a modest increase in the transvalvular pressure gradient, referred to as "low-gradient" aortic stenosis. It can be difficult to distinguish true aortic stenosis causing low cardiac output from a low cardiac output state due to a cardiomyopathy in association with only mild or moderate aortic stenosis. In patients with abnormal myocardial contractility, the low-flow state and low pressure gradient can lead to a calculated aortic valve area in the severe range. The standard valve area formula is less accurate and will underestimate the valve area in low flow states.[13]

One method to determine whether a patient is presenting with true fixed aortic stenosis or pseudo aortic stenosis due to left ventricular dysfunction is to calculate the aortic valve

be calculated by the continuity equation, which is based on the law of conservation of mass, which states that for a fluid in a closed system, flow at all points must be equal. To calculate aortic valve area, flow is measured proximal to the aortic valve by calculating the area of the left ventricular outflow tract just below the valve, and the velocity at the same level. Velocity is also measured across the valve (Fig. 29-3). The continuity equation can be written as $A_1v_1 = A_2v_2$, where A_1 is the area of the outflow tract, v_1 is the velocity in the outflow tract, A_2 is the aortic valve area, and v_2 is the velocity at the aortic valve. A_2 is the unknown and is solved for from the known measurements.

Cardiac catheterization can confirm the severity of aortic stenosis. Most patients presenting with early symptoms of aortic stenosis will have a normal cardiac output, normal right heart and pulmonary capillary wedge pressures, and a normal ejection fraction. The left ventricular end-diastolic pressure will be increased, with a prominent A wave reflecting a stiff left ventricular chamber. In advanced states, the cardiac output and ejection fraction will be depressed, with a corresponding increase in left atrial and pulmonary pressures. In patients anticipating surgery, the coronary arteries should area at two different flow conditions by using dobutamine stress. Patients with true aortic stenosis will increase cardiac output and the transvalvular gradient with dobutamine, but the aortic valve area will remain unchanged.[14] Patients with pseudo aortic stenosis will have an increase in valve area that is frequently outside of the severe range (>1.0 cm^2) with dobutamine infusion. One protocol that has been used is intravenous dobutamine 5 μg/kg per minute and increased by 5 μg/kg per minute every 3 minutes until a maximal dose of 20 μg/kg per minute is obtained.[14] The presence of contractile reserve with dobutamine (increased stroke volume and ejection fraction) is associated with a low operative risk and a good long-term prognosis, whereas operative mortality is high in the absence of contractile reserve.[15]

The development of heart failure in patients with aortic stenosis is an indication for surgery, which should be performed as soon as possible after medical stabilization. Diuretics are frequently used to relieve pulmonary congestion, but need to be used cautiously so as not to decrease stroke volume. It has been thought that vasodilators are contraindicated in aortic stenosis because they may lead to a precipitous drop in blood pressure, causing cardiac arrest. Recent experience with nitroprusside in patients with true aortic stenosis and depressed ejection fraction has shown that afterload reduction with this agent can lead to a significant increase in cardiac output and can be used as a therapeutic bridge to surgery.[16] Therefore, current medical management of severe aortic stenosis with decreased cardiac function consists of the careful use of diuretics, with either positive inotropes (dobutamine) and/or afterload reduction (nitroprusside), being careful not to cause hypotension. Digitalis and angiotensin-converting enzyme inhibitors, as used in heart failure, can be carefully used as well.

The patient that presents with critical noncardiac disease and severe aortic stenosis is a challenging medical problem. The augmentation in cardiac output required for perfusion of tissues in disease states such as sepsis or profound anemia may not be adequate in patients with true fixed aortic stenosis. The need for urgent noncardiac surgery in patients with severe aortic stenosis puts a patient at a very high risk for cardiac complications, including myocardial infarction, congestive heart failure, and death.[17]

Percutaneous balloon aortic valvuloplasty is a procedure in which a balloon is placed across the stenotic valve and inflated, leading to stretching of the valve annulus and separation of the calcified and fused valve commissures. This can lead to an improvement in left ventricular function, a decrease in the transvalvular gradient, and an increase in the aortic valve area.[18] Because of a high complication rate and a high rate of restenosis within 6 months, this procedure is not recommended as definitive therapy. This procedure can be used as a temporizing solution in patients with cardiogenic shock,[19] or in the management of patients requiring major noncardiac surgery.[20] After recovery, definitive aortic valve replacement surgery can be performed at a later date.

Recently a percutaneous implantable prosthetic heart valve made of three bovine pericardial leaflets mounted in a balloon-expandable stent was developed and implanted in a critically ill patient with aortic stenosis and cardiogenic shock, and it led to immediate hemodynamic improvement.[21] Further studies are now in development for this promising new technology.

Hypertrophic Cardiomyopathy

ETIOLOGY

Hypertrophic cardiomyopathy (HCM) is a genetic disorder of cardiac muscle characterized by myocardial hypertrophy out of proportion to the hemodynamic stress. Patients classically present with dynamic obstruction to left ventricular outflow. Valvular aortic stenosis and hypertension are usually absent. Left ventricular diastolic dysfunction is invariably present. The disease is uncommon, estimated to be present in about 2 of 1000 young adults.[22] Because this condition can mimic valvular aortic stenosis, it will be considered in this section.

PATHOPHYSIOLOGY

The pattern and extent of left ventricular hypertrophy differs among patients with hypertrophic cardiomyopathy. In most patients, hypertrophy involves the septum and portions of the anterolateral free wall of the left ventricle. Rare morphologic forms include isolated apical hypertrophy, which is seen predominantly in patients of Japanese descent. Histologic features include cardiac muscle cell disarray and fibrous tissue formation.

In a subset of patients with the severe form of HCM, left ventricular outflow tract obstruction occurs at rest and worsens with exertion. The left ventricle is hyperdynamic, usually with an increased ejection fraction. A pressure gradient can be demonstrated in the left ventricular outflow tract below the aortic valve that at times may exceed 100 mm Hg. The gradient is augmented by factors that increase contractility (such as exercise or premature ventricular contractions) or by factors that decrease ventricular volume. The gradient may represent true obstruction to left ventricular ejection, resulting from portions of the mitral valve apparatus moving across the outflow tract and contacting the hypertrophied septum in midsystole. The displacement of the mitral valve occurs because of Venturi effects generated by the increased ejection velocities in the narrowed outflow tract. As the anterior mitral valve leaflet is drawn toward the septum by these Venturi effects, concomitant mitral regurgitation is produced.

Most patients with HCM have diastolic function abnormalities whether or not they are symptomatic.[23] Diastolic dysfunction is manifested by increased left ventricular filling pressures despite a normal ejection fraction. Isovolumic relaxation is prolonged, early diastolic filling is impaired, and atrial filling becomes an important component of cardiac output. Because of the importance of the atrial contribution to left ventricular filling, the acute onset of atrial fibrillation may cause clinical deterioration of patients with HCM.[24]

CLINICAL PRESENTATION

Classic symptoms of HCM include exertional chest pain, dyspnea, fatigue, and syncope.[24a,24b] Most patients with HCM, however, are asymptomatic until an unrelated illness causes deterioration. Tachycardia, sudden blood loss, or atrial or ventricular arrhythmias can suddenly precipitate pulmonary edema and hemodynamic collapse. As the outflow obstruction worsens, mitral regurgitation increases, leading to high left atrial and pulmonary venous pressures. Blood pressure may fall as cardiac output is impaired.

TABLE 29-1 Physical Examination Differences between Aortic Stenosis and Hypertrophic Cardiomyopathy

Feature	Aortic Stenosis	Hypertrophic Cardiomyopathy
Murmur location	Sternal border to neck	Sternal border to apex
Murmur with Valsalva maneuver	No change or decrease	Increase
Ejection click	Frequent in congenital stenosis	Rare
Regurgitant diastolic murmur	Common	Rare
Carotid pulse	Delayed upstroke	Brisk upstroke
A_2	Soft or absent	Normal

The diagnosis of HCM can be made definitively by careful cardiac physical examination. The carotid pulse has a characteristic brisk upstroke followed by sudden cutoff as obstruction occurs. The left ventricular impulse is vigorous and sustained. A large palpable A wave is present (easily felt in the left lateral decubitus position). A systolic thrill is commonly palpated. The first and second heart sounds are typically normal. The systolic murmur of outflow obstruction is harsh and has a crescendo/decrescendo configuration. The murmur radiates throughout the precordium, but not to the neck. A second murmur of mitral regurgitation can be heard at the apex, with radiation to the axilla. The murmur of HCM increases significantly in intensity with the Valsalva maneuver, a response that can be used to differentiate the murmur reliably from valvular aortic stenosis (Table 29-1).

DIAGNOSTIC EVALUATION

The electrocardiogram is almost always abnormal, with ST- and T-wave abnormalities, left ventricular hypertrophy, and predominant Q waves in the inferior or lateral leads. Giant negative T waves are characteristic of apical HCM of the Japanese type. The chest x-ray generally shows an enlarged cardiac silhouette. Echocardiography can make the diagnosis of HCM definitively and can quantitate the severity of the outflow tract obstruction. Classic features include a markedly hypertrophied interventricular septum, at times more than 20 mm thick (Fig. 29-4), systolic anterior motion of the mitral

valve into the left ventricular outflow tract, premature closure of the aortic valve at the time of obstruction, and mitral regurgitation. Doppler echocardiography can accurately measure the magnitude of the outflow tract gradient. The modified Bernoulli equation is used to calculate the gradient in millimeters of mercury by the equation $4v^2$, where v is the maximum velocity measured in the outflow tract.

Cardiac catheterization can demonstrate the systolic pressure gradient in the left ventricle. The arterial pressure tracing may show a "spike and dome" configuration, representing the brisk outflow and sudden obstruction (Fig. 29-5). The pulmonary capillary wedge pressure is usually elevated, with a prominent A wave indicative of diastolic noncompliance. A large V wave may be present if mitral regurgitation is significant. A pressure gradient may be present in the right ventricular outflow tract as well.

MANAGEMENT

It is important to recognize HCM in patients presenting with pulmonary congestion, because management is substantially different than for other forms of heart failure. Pulmonary edema should be treated initially with diuretics to relieve congestion, but excessive preload reduction may aggravate the situation by accentuating the left ventricular outflow tract gradient. β agonists are contraindicated, because they may worsen outflow tract gradients, cause ischemia, and

FIGURE 29-4 Hypertrophic cardiomyopathy. Short-axis two-dimensional echocardiographic view showing the left ventricle in cross-section. Note the thick (>20 mm) left ventricular septum (*top*) compared with the normal-thickness posterior wall (*bottom*).

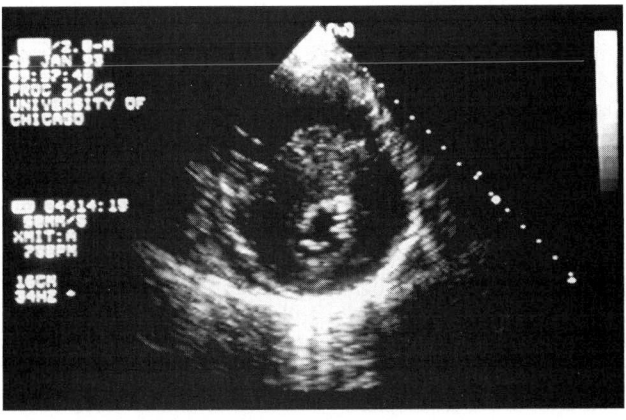

FIGURE 29-5 Carotid artery pulse tracing showing "spike and dome" configuration in the pressure tracing following the premature ventricular contraction, representing sudden obstruction to flow. In the figure, the first line is the surface ECG, the second line is a phonocardiogram, and the third line is the carotid artery pulse tracing.

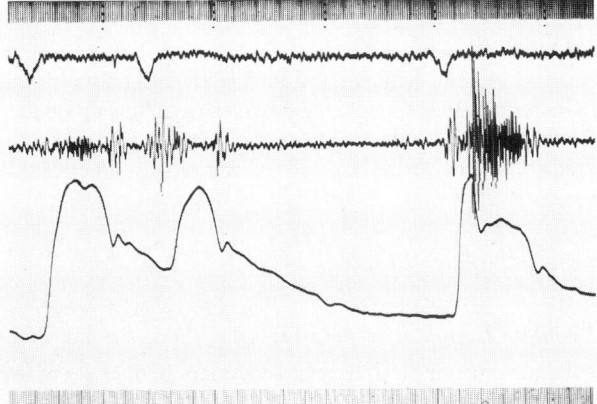

precipitate arrhythmias. Likewise, digitalis should be avoided unless used to treat atrial fibrillation.

The mainstay of treatment is use of β-adrenergic blockers and calcium channel blockers. β-receptor blockade slows the heart rate and blunts the chronotropic response to exercise or stress, thus preventing the increase in outflow tract obstruction. Patients presenting in pulmonary edema should be started on intravenous β blockers such as esmolol, which has the advantage of a short half-life. The heart rate should be slowed to the slowest tolerated rate that decreases the outflow tract gradient. Large doses of β blockers may be required. If the heart rate cannot adequately be slowed with β blockers, then calcium channel blockers such as verapamil may be added. Verapamil doses of 360 to 480 mg and higher are frequently used. Other negative inotropic agents such as disopyramide can also be used to limit the outflow tract gradient.[25] The antiarrhythmic drug amiodarone has β-blocking activity and may improve survival in some patients with HCM.[26]

Atrial fibrillation may cause sudden deterioration of patients with HCM, as a result of both the increased heart rate and the loss of the atrial contribution to ventricular filling. Electrical cardioversion may be necessary acutely. Pharmacologic treatment may then be started to prevent recurrence. Agents that block the atrioventricular (AV) node, such as β blockers and calcium channel blockers, may be used prophylactically to prevent the sudden increase in heart rate should atrial fibrillation recur.

Surgical techniques for HCM have been developed that are aimed at eliminating the outflow tract gradient and reducing the amount of mitral regurgitation. Septal myotomy-myomectomy performed through the ascending aorta removes a portion of the hypertrophied interventricular septum, and has been associated with a significant reduction in outflow tract gradients and with symptomatic relief.[27] Mitral valve replacement has also been found to reduce or eliminate the outflow tract gradient and to improve symptoms.[28] Valve replacement may be especially helpful in patients with severe mitral regurgitation. There has been interest in pacemaker therapy with dual-chamber pacing of the right heart to decrease outflow tract gradients by changing the timing of depolarization of the interventricular septum to improve symptoms in patients with refractory disease.[29] This therapy may be beneficial acutely with use of temporary pacing wires. Some studies have not shown any clinical benefit with pacing, and possible detrimental effects on ventricular filling and cardiac output.[30] A new procedure using percutaneous septal ablation by infusing ethanol into the septal perforator branches of the left anterior descending artery has been studied.[31–33] This technique causes infarction and thinning of the thickened proximal septum, reducing the outflow obstruction with improvement in symptoms. Long-term results of this procedure are under study. None of these techniques have been shown to reduce the incidence of sudden death associated with this disease.

Aortic Insufficiency

ETIOLOGY

Aortic insufficiency (AI) may be secondary to diseases of the valve leaflets or to abnormalities of the aortic root (Table 29-2).

TABLE 29-2 Etiologies of Aortic Insufficiency

Valvular
  Rheumatic fever
  Infective endocarditis
  Trauma
  Bicuspid aortic valve
  Myxomatous/prolapsing aortic valve
  Fenestrated valve
Aortic root dilation
  Aortic dissection
  Systemic hypertension
  Annuloaortic ectasia
  Connective tissue diseases (Marfan syndrome, Ehlers Danlos syndrome, and related disorders)
  Seronegative arthritides (ankylosing spondylitis, Reiter syndrome, and related disorders)
  Rheumatoid arthritis
  Syphilitic aortitis
  Discrete subaortic stenosis

AI can be classified as chronic or acute.[34] Chronic AI may remain indolent for years and not require treatment until left ventricular dysfunction becomes evident. Acute severe AI, however, is a medical emergency with a high mortality and frequently requires early operative intervention. The three most common causes of acute AI are (1) infective endocarditis, (2) aortic dissection, and (3) rupture or prolapse of an aortic valve leaflet.[35] The aortic valve is the valve most commonly involved after blunt chest trauma.[36]

PATHOPHYSIOLOGY

The cardiac performance of patients with aortic insufficiency depends on the ability of the left ventricle to adapt to the volume overload. In chronic AI, the left ventricle gradually dilates with a shift in the pressure-volume relationship, so that any change in volume is accommodated at a lower pressure. In acute AI, the left ventricle is suddenly subjected to a large regurgitant volume for which it is not prepared. Left ventricular dilation is limited by the compliance of the ventricle and by the constraining pericardium. Therefore in acute AI, a small rise in volume may lead to a dramatic increase in left ventricular diastolic pressure. As a consequence, patients with acute AI usually present with signs and symptoms of pulmonary congestion.

If the patient survives the acute insult, the left ventricle and pericardium may adapt to the volume overload by dilating. Left ventricular wall stress is diminished by left ventricular hypertrophy. The increase in chamber size and diastolic volume leads to an augmentation of forward stroke volume despite high regurgitant volumes. Afterload is reduced because of the rapid runoff of blood from the aorta into the ventricle. Cardiac performance can be maintained in the normal range for many years despite the presence of severe AI. However, decompensation can occur at any time, owing to ischemia or other factors for which the heart cannot accommodate. Once left ventricular dysfunction develops, the disease tends to progress rapidly. Left ventricular volumes (left ventricular end-systolic dimension >50 mm, left ventricular end-diastolic dimension >70 mm) can be used to predict which patients are more likely to have progressive disease and the development of left ventricular failure.[37]

TABLE 29-3 Clinical Features of Acute versus Chronic Aortic Insufficiency

Feature	Acute	Chronic
Presentation	Pulmonary edema	Gradual congestive heart failure
Systolic blood pressure	Normal to low	Increased
Pulse pressure	Normal	Wide
Heart rate	Tachycardia	Normal
Left ventricular impulse	Normal size	Dilated
S_1	Soft	Usually normal
S_2	P_2 loud	Normal
S_3 gallop	Usually present	May be present
AI murmur	Short	Long
Peripheral signs	Absent	Present

CLINICAL PRESENTATION

Patients that present with acute AI are usually critically ill, with signs of pulmonary edema, diaphoresis, cyanosis, and peripheral vasoconstriction. The left ventricular end-diastolic pressure is markedly increased, at times equaling the aortic diastolic pressure, shortening the aortic regurgitant murmur. Patients are typically tachycardic without a wide pulse pressure or prominent peripheral signs of aortic insufficiency. Systolic pressure may be normal or low. The heart is not enlarged. The first heart sound may be soft, owing to premature closure of the mitral valve caused by the aortic regurgitant jet. The pulmonic component of the second heart sound may be loud, reflecting pulmonary hypertension. A gallop rhythm is usually present. Table 29-3 compares the features of acute versus chronic aortic regurgitation.

DIAGNOSTIC EVALUATION

In acute AI, the electrocardiogram is usually normal, showing only sinus tachycardia. Left ventricular hypertrophy may be present in patients with chronic AI, and usually signifies severe regurgitation. The chest x-ray in acute AI usually shows pulmonary edema with a normal heart size. A widened mediastinum should raise the suspicion of acute aortic dissection as the cause of the aortic insufficiency. In chronic AI, the chest x-ray is likely to show cardiomegaly with a prominent left ventricle. The ascending aorta may be dilated.

Echocardiography is useful for detecting aortic insufficiency and determining its severity and for evaluating left ventricular performance. Aortic insufficiency may be suspected from the appearance of the valve leaflets on two-dimensional echocardiography, but Doppler techniques are the most sensitive for diagnosing AI and determining the severity of the leakage.[38] The presence of AI is confirmed by Doppler echocardiography when an abnormal, high-velocity turbulent jet is detected just below the aortic valve during diastole. Color flow mapping is used to depict the origin and size of the regurgitant jet. The severity of the regurgitation can be estimated from the size of the regurgitant jet, from the size of the regurgitant orifice, or by calculation of the regurgitant volume or fraction. In patients with severe AI, the consequences of a significant increase in left ventricular pressure can be noted by premature closure of the mitral valve, diastolic mitral regurgitation, and premature closure of the aortic valve if left ventricular pressure transiently exceeds aortic pressure.

Transesophageal echocardiography (TEE) should be considered when endocarditis or an acute aortic dissection is suspected as the cause of aortic insufficiency. TEE can better evaluate valvular structure and is more sensitive for the diagnosis of endocarditic lesions than transthoracic echocardiography (Fig. 29-6 and Color Plate 29-6). TEE has been shown to have a sensitivity comparable to that of magnetic resonance imaging (MRI) or computed tomography (CT) for detecting an acute aortic dissection,[39] and it is more easily performed in an intensive care unit on an unstable critically ill patient.

Cardiac catheterization can provide definitive information about the degree of regurgitation, and it can be used to evaluate the aortic root and the status of the coronary arteries if surgery is indicated. Pulmonary artery catheterization is indicated in acute AI to help with management. The pulmonary artery wedge pressure is usually elevated, and pulmonary hypertension may be present. Stroke volume may be normal or increased.

MANAGEMENT

Acute aortic insufficiency is a medical emergency. Fulminant pulmonary edema is a common presentation, because the left ventricle cannot handle the sudden large increase in volume. It is important to determine the cause of the lesion, especially if endocarditis or an acute aortic dissection is suspected. Aortic valve replacement is indicated when the regurgitation is severe. Early aortic valve replacement has been shown to decrease mortality in patients with endocarditis.[40] If heart failure can be medically managed, aortic valve replacement may be delayed until after completion of an antibiotic regimen.[41]

Patients presenting with acute pulmonary edema should be treated promptly with loop diuretics to relieve congestion. Inotropic agents are of limited value, because left ventricular function is usually hyperdynamic. Pressor agents are relatively contraindicated, because an increase in systemic vascular resistance will worsen the amount of regurgitation. Likewise, an intra-aortic balloon pump is absolutely contraindicated.[42] Vasodilators can improve forward stroke volume by inducing dilation of the arterial vessels. An agent such as nitroprusside is ideal, because it can be rapidly titrated to effect. This drug should be administered with pulmonary artery catheter guidance so that the response to therapy can be followed closely. Nitroprusside has been shown to improve cardiac performance, enhance forward stroke volume, reduce the amount of regurgitation, and lower left ventricular filling pressures.[43,44]

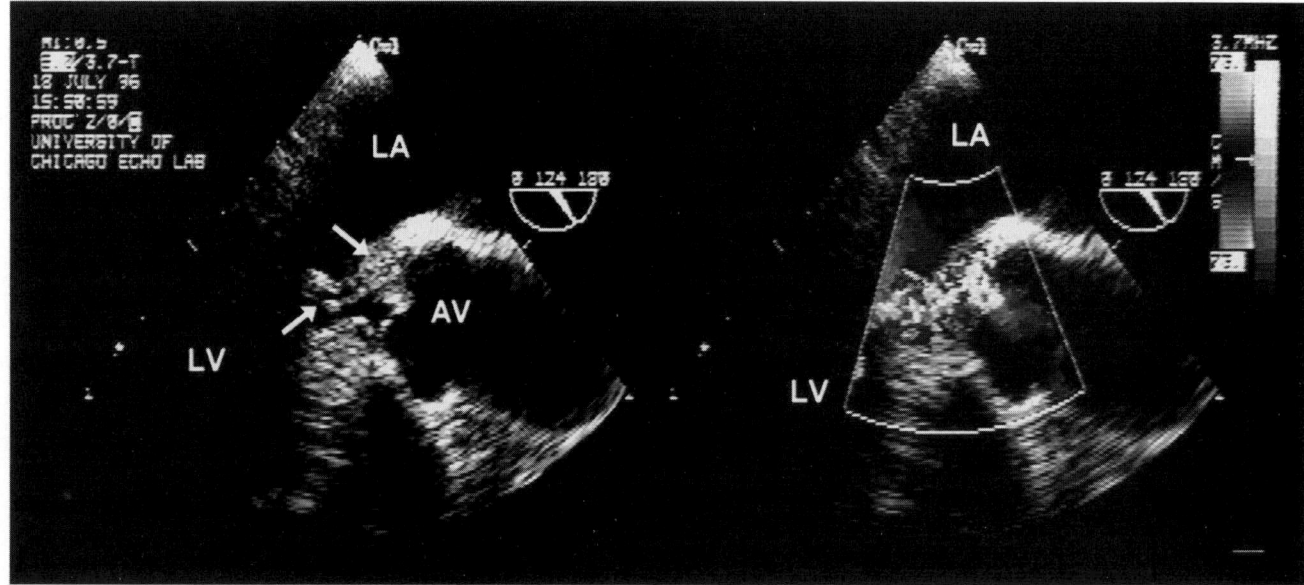

FIGURE 29-6 Acute aortic insufficiency secondary to endocarditis. Transesophageal echocardiogram showing a large mobile vegetation (*arrows*) extending from the aortic valve (AV) into the left ventricle (LV). Doppler echocardiography reveals significant regurgitation from the aorta into the LV. LA, left atrium. (See Color Plate 29-6.)

Patients that can be stabilized should be treated with long-term vasodilator therapy. Vasodilator agents such as hydralazine, angiotensin-converting enzyme inhibitors (ACEIs), β blockers, and calcium channel blockers have been used.[45] Recently, nifedipine has been shown to delay the need for aortic valve replacement in patients with asymptomatic chronic severe aortic insufficiency.[46] Aortic valve replacement should be performed before irreversible changes occur in the left ventricle. The end-systolic dimensions and shortening characteristics of the left ventricle can be used to determine the optimal time for operative intervention.[47] Aortic valve replacement for severe aortic insufficiency with a low left ventricular ejection fraction has a high perioperative mortality and an increased incidence of congestive heart failure after surgery, but many patients will sustain improvement in their cardiac function and a prolonged survival.[48]

Mitral Stenosis

ETIOLOGY

Rheumatic fever is the main cause of mitral stenosis, and in underdeveloped countries is a significant cause of morbidity and mortality in young people. Recent outbreaks of rheumatic fever and an influx of immigrants from countries where rheumatic fever is prevalent will ensure that this disease remains an important valvular condition in the United States as well.[49] Other forms of mitral stenosis may be encountered, such as calcification of the mitral annulus so extensive as to involve the submitral apparatus and the valvular leaflets. This rare cause of mitral stenosis is seen in elderly patients and patients with long-standing renal failure.

PATHOPHYSIOLOGY

Rheumatic mitral stenosis results from an inflammatory process that leads to fusion of the mitral commissures, chordae tendineae, or both. The disease tends to cause a slowly progressive degeneration of the valve, and many patients remain asymptomatic for decades after the initial infection. The normal mitral valve has an area of 4 to 6 cm^2. When the valve has narrowed to 2 cm^2, mild mitral stenosis is present. A valve area of 1 cm^2 is thought to represent critical mitral stenosis. At this orifice size, a transvalvular gradient of approximately 20 mm Hg is required to maintain a normal cardiac output. As a consequence, left atrial pressure rises, leading eventually to pulmonary hypertension.

Any increase in heart rate will shorten diastolic filling time and diminish the time for blood to flow across the stenosed mitral valve. Tachycardia will augment the transvalvular pressure gradient and further increase left atrial pressure. That is why patients may suddenly present with pulmonary edema and the onset of atrial fibrillation.[50] Patients with mild to moderate mitral stenosis may be asymptomatic at rest, but exercise may cause a dramatic rise in the transmitral gradient and left atrial pressure, leading to exertional dyspnea.[51] In addition, the atrial contribution to left ventricular filling may account for 20% or more of total cardiac output. Loss of the atrial filling component can significantly worsen symptoms in patients with mitral stenosis.

As mitral stenosis becomes more severe, resting pulmonary artery pressures begin to increase. In critical mitral stenosis, pulmonary pressures may exceed systemic pressures. Pulmonary pressures greater than 70 mm Hg lead to elevated right ventricular and right atrial pressures, eventually causing right ventricular dilation and failure.

CLINICAL PRESENTATION

Patients with rheumatic mitral stenosis may be asymptomatic for many years despite progressive narrowing of the valve. Symptoms initially occur with exercise. Patients may suddenly decompensate and present in pulmonary edema during an episode of respiratory infection, atrial fibrillation, or another condition associated with tachycardia.

Sudden, profuse hemorrhage may occur from disruption of bronchial veins. Thromboembolism can be a serious complication, occurring most often in patients with chronic atrial fibrillation.

The physical examination in critically ill patients with mitral stenosis can be difficult. The left ventricle is usually normal in size, although it may be displaced leftward owing to right ventricular enlargement. The first heart sound is usually accentuated if the mitral leaflets remain pliable. As pulmonary hypertension develops, the pulmonic closing sound (P_2) becomes accentuated. Other signs of pulmonary hypertension include a right ventricular heave, tricuspid regurgitation (a holosystolic murmur at the right or left sternal border with respiratory variation), and the Graham Steell murmur of pulmonic insufficiency. At the left ventricular apex, an opening snap may be heard, followed by the low-pitched rumbling murmur of mitral stenosis. In severe mitral stenosis, the murmur is heard throughout diastole, with presystolic accentuation of the murmur in patients who remain in sinus rhythm.

DIAGNOSTIC EVALUATION

The electrocardiogram will typically show left atrial enlargement and signs of right ventricular hypertrophy in severe mitral stenosis. Atrial fibrillation is a common rhythm disturbance. The chest x-ray can show left atrial enlargement with upward displacement of the left mainstem bronchus by the enlarged atrium. The left atrial appendage may appear as a bulge between the aortic knob and the left ventricular silhouette. With pulmonary hypertension, the pulmonary arteries will be prominent, and the right ventricle may be enlarged. Calcification of the mitral annulus can frequently be detected.

Echocardiography and Doppler techniques have been used to assess and quantify the severity of mitral stenosis noninvasively. Two-dimensional echocardiography can delineate the anatomy of the mitral valve (Fig. 29-7). As the valve leaflets begin to open during diastole, the leaflet tips appear to remain tethered while the body of the leaflet continues to show mobility (doming), producing a characteristic deformity that is classic for rheumatic mitral stenosis. Planimetry

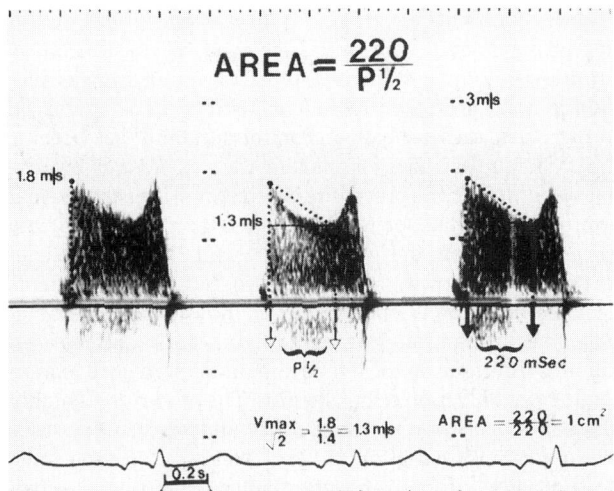

FIGURE 29-8 Pressure half-time method for calculating mitral valve area. Doppler echocardiography depicts an increased velocity across the stenotic mitral valve. The pressure half-time ($P^1/_2$) is the time required for the maximal velocity (Vmax) to fall to a value equal to the maximal velocity divided by the square root of 2. The mitral valve area is then 220 divided by the pressure half-time; in this example it is 1 cm^2.

of the cross-sectional valve area from the short axis view has correlated well with valve areas calculated invasively by the Gorlin formula.[52] Doppler echocardiographic methods have also been used to quantify mitral valve areas by using a pressure half-time method (Fig. 29-8). The time required for the diastolic gradient to drop to half its initial peak reflects the severity of mitral stenosis.[53] The noninvasively determined pressure half-time is defined as the time required for the early maximal inflow velocity to fall to a value equal to the maximum velocity divided by the square root of 2.[54] The mitral valve area is then calculated by dividing the empirically derived number 220 by the pressure half-time.

Cardiac catheterization is used to verify the severity of the valve lesion and to measure right heart pressures. Left atrial puncture via a transseptal approach can directly measure left atrial pressure. Pulmonary capillary wedge pressures may be used as well, but at times they exaggerate the left atrial pressure and overestimate the severity of the mitral stenosis.[55]

MANAGEMENT

Patients presenting with pulmonary edema should undergo initial diuretic treatment to decrease lung congestion and improve oxygenation. For patients presenting in atrial fibrillation, control of heart rate is crucial. A combination of digoxin, β blockers, and/or calcium channel blockers may be required to achieve rate control. Use of intravenous esmolol or diltiazem can quickly bring about rate control and is preferred over intravenous digoxin. Patients in sinus rhythm may also benefit from β blockers to slow the heart rate and allow more time for diastolic filling of the left ventricle. Anticoagulation should be started in patients with atrial fibrillation to prevent thromboembolism (IV heparin and warfarin with a goal International Normalized Ratio [INR] of 2 to 3).

FIGURE 29-7 Mitral stenosis. Cross-section echocardiogram of the mitral valve showing the severely stenotic mitral valve leaflets with a fish-mouth appearance. Planimetry of the fully opened valve yielded a valve area of less than 1 cm^2.

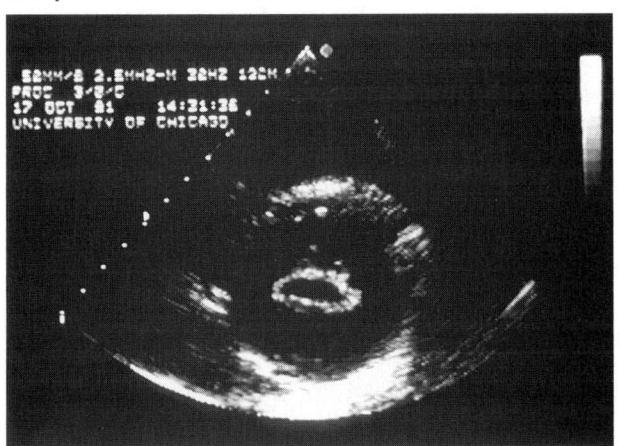

Once symptoms develop, mitral stenosis requires definitive management. That can be achieved by surgical mitral commissurotomy, mitral valve replacement, or catheter balloon commissurotomy. For patients with pure rheumatic mitral stenosis, catheter balloon commissurotomy has become the procedure of choice for relieving the stenosis and improving symptoms.[56] The procedure is performed via a transseptal approach, and a balloon is passed across the mitral valve from the left atrium into the left ventricle. A small atrial septal defect remains following the procedure, but in most patients it closes or becomes smaller. Contraindications to catheter balloon commissurotomy include significant mitral regurgitation, a thrombus in the left atrium, unfavorable valve morphology, or only mild mitral stenosis. The procedure is highly successful with low mortality rates and greater than 60% of patients improving to New York Heart Association functional class I.[57] If there are contraindications to catheter balloon commissurotomy, then surgical valvular repair would be necessary.

Mitral Regurgitation

ETIOLOGY

There are multiple conditions that can cause acute or chronic mitral regurgitation (MR) involving the mitral valve leaflets, mitral annulus, chordae tendineae, or papillary muscles (Table 29-4). Involvement of the leaflets is usually due to rheumatic disease leading to shortening or retraction of one or both leaflets. Infective endocarditis, trauma, or systemic lupus erythematosus with Libman-Sacks endocarditis can lead to significant MR (Fig. 29-9 and Color Plate 29-9). Finally, mitral valve prolapse can present with severe MR due to myxomatous change of the valve leaflets.

Abnormalities of the mitral annulus involve dilation and calcification. Severe dilation of the left ventricle, as seen in dilated cardiomyopathies, is associated with mitral regurgitation, although the amount of leakage tends to be less than that seen in primary valvular disorders. Calcification of the

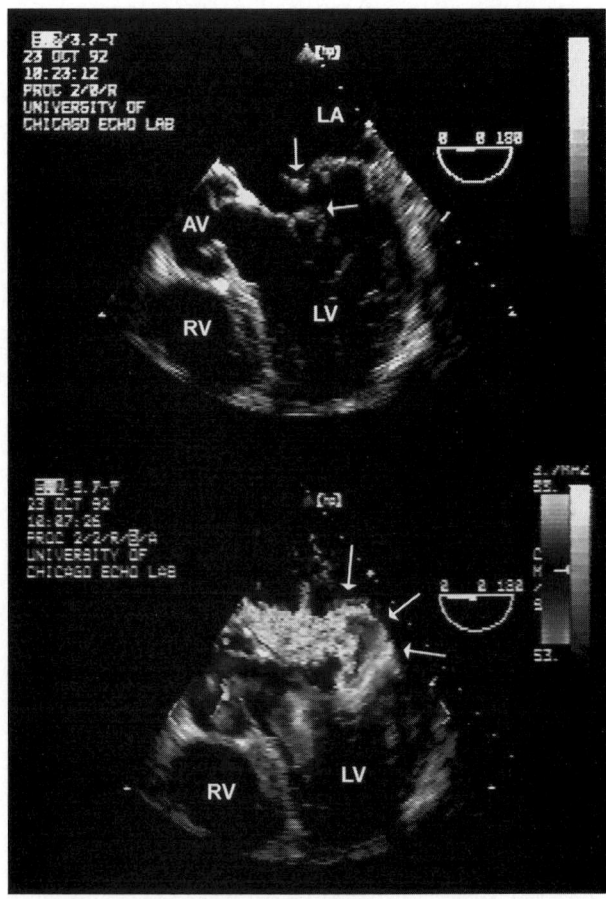

FIGURE 29-9 Mitral regurgitation secondary to endocarditis and a flail posterior mitral valve leaflet. Transesophageal echocardiogram showing thickened mitral valve leaflets with vegetations (*arrows*). The posterior leaflet has prolapsed from the left ventricle (LV) into the left atrium (LA). The second panel depicts severe mitral regurgitation by Doppler echocardiography (*arrows*). AV, aortic valve; RV, right ventricle. (See Color Plate 29-9.)

TABLE 29-4 Causes of Mitral Regurgitation

Disorders of the mitral leaflets
  Rheumatic heart disease
  Infective endocarditis
  Trauma
  Systemic lupus erythematosus
  Myxomatous mitral valve prolapse
  Congenital mitral valve clefts/fenestrations
  Parachute mitral valve
Disorders of the mitral annulus
  Left ventricular dilation
  Mitral annular calcification
Disorders of the chordae tendineae
  Myxomatous involvement in mitral valve prolapse
  Infective endocarditis
  Trauma
  Spontaneous rupture
Disorders of the papillary muscles
  Dysfunction (myocardial ischemia/infarction/infiltrative
    diseases)
  Rupture (infarction/trauma)

mitral annulus is a common degenerative change that when severe, may cause significant MR.

The chordae tendineae and papillary muscles may be involved in patients with ischemic heart disease. Myocardial ischemia or infarction may lead to papillary muscle dysfunction or frank rupture of the muscle head, causing acute severe MR. Ischemia of the papillary muscles may be transient, with improvement in the MR occurring after relief of the ischemia or revascularization therapy. On the other hand, patients with moderately severe to severe MR complicating an acute myocardial infarction have a high risk of mortality.[58] Chordae tendineae may rupture in patients with infective endocarditis and in patients with myxomatous mitral valve prolapse. Mitral valve prolapse is becoming the most common etiology for patients requiring valvular surgery for mitral regurgitation.

PATHOPHYSIOLOGY

In patients who develop acute MR, the left ventricle is initially unloaded, with the regurgitant volume ejected into the left atrium. The left ventricular wall tension is reduced, since

TABLE 29-5 Differential Diagnosis of Systolic Murmurs

Feature	Mitral Regurgitation	Tricuspid Regurgitation	Ventricular Septal Defect
Murmur	Holosystolic	Holosystolic	Holosystolic
Location	Apex	Left sternal border	Left sternal border
Radiation	Axilla	None	Left precordium
Thrill	At apex	Rare	Left sternal border
P_2	Normal	Increased	Normal, usually delayed
Murmur with inspiration	No change	Increased	No change
Apical impulse	Hyperkinetic	Normal	Hyperkinetic
Jugular venous pulse	Normal	Elevated, prominent V wave	Elevated, prominent A and V waves
Pulsatile liver	No	Yes	No

acute MR reduces systolic ventricular pressure and volume. Early diastolic filling of the left ventricle is enhanced, causing small elevations in myocardial contractility and ejection fraction. Following initial compensation, the left ventricle dilates rapidly. The increase in left ventricular end-diastolic volume increases wall tension. Ejection indices will eventually decline to normal, reflecting impairment of myocardial function. Ejection fractions of 40% to 50% already reflect severe impairment of myocardial contractility. Ejection fractions less than 40% represent advanced cardiac dysfunction and indicate a patient who has a high operative risk and is unlikely to experience any improvement in function following correction of the problem.[59]

The compliance of the left atrium and the pulmonary venous system will determine the hemodynamic and clinical manifestations of mitral regurgitation. In patients in whom MR occurs suddenly, as with rupture of a chorda tendineae, left atrial compliance is normal. Left atrial size remains normal, but there is a marked elevation of left atrial pressure (large V wave), and pulmonary congestion is predominant. In contrast, in patients with long-standing chronic MR, massive enlargement of the left atrium occurs with normal or only slightly elevated left atrial pressures. Pulmonary artery pressures and pulmonary vascular resistance are normal or only slightly elevated. Atrial fibrillation is almost invariably present.[60]

CLINICAL PRESENTATION

The symptoms of patients with mitral regurgitation depend on the acuity and severity of the disease. In patients with chronic MR, symptoms usually do not develop until the left ventricle begins to fail. By the time low-output symptoms, pulmonary congestion, or atrial fibrillation develops, permanent myocardial dysfunction may already be present. The onset of a critical illness may cause rapid deterioration in a previously stable patient if increased systemic vascular resistance augments the regurgitant fraction. Patients with acute MR may present with florid pulmonary edema and low cardiac output. Ischemic symptoms may also be present, since myocardial infarction with papillary muscle dysfunction and rupture is an important cause of acute MR.

On physical examination, the left ventricular impulse is usually dynamic and displaced, with a palpable early diastolic filling impulse (S_3). The systolic murmur of mitral regurgitation begins at the first heart sound (frequently obscuring it) and extends throughout systole and beyond the second heart sound to mitral valve opening. The murmur is constant in intensity, is high-pitched, is loudest at the apex, and radiates to the axilla. The intensity of the murmur does not correlate with severity. Patients with acute MR may have barely audible brief murmurs. Murmurs of mitral valve prolapse may begin in mid or late systole and vary in position and intensity depending on left ventricular volume.[61]

Mitral regurgitation murmurs need to be differentiated from other systolic murmurs (Table 29-5). Tricuspid regurgitation frequently exhibits respiratory variation and does not radiate to the axilla. Ventricular septal defect murmurs tend to be harsher, to be located at the sternal border, and to be heard less well in the axilla. Aortic stenosis murmurs may radiate to the apex, but they are usually accompanied by a delayed carotid upstroke and a decreased intensity of the aortic component of the second heart sound.

DIAGNOSTIC EVALUATION

The electrocardiogram in acute mitral regurgitation is usually normal, although it may show signs of acute myocardial infarction. Patients with chronic MR may have signs of left atrial enlargement, right ventricular hypertrophy, or atrial fibrillation. Chest x-ray shows cardiomegaly with left ventricular prominence, left atrial enlargement, and at times evidence of mitral annular calcification.

Two-dimensional echocardiography can help determine the etiology and severity of mitral regurgitation. The underlying cause of the regurgitation, such as rupture of a chorda tendineae, mitral valve prolapse with a flail leaflet, or valvular endocarditis, can readily be determined. Transesophageal echocardiography has improved the diagnostic acumen of echocardiographic studies, especially in determining the presence of valvular vegetations. Doppler echocardiography makes it possible to estimate the severity of MR from the distance the jet travels into the left atrium, the width of the jet at the mitral annulus, and the area of the color Doppler envelope in the left atrium.

Cardiac catheterization is useful in diagnosis and management. Left ventriculography showing opacification of the left atrium is used to quantify severity of the leakage. Effective or forward cardiac output is depressed in severe MR. The pulmonary wedge pressure will show a characteristically tall V wave, reflecting the filling of the left atrium by both pulmonary venous and regurgitant blood during ventricular systole. This tall V wave is frequently seen in the pulmonary artery tracing, and at times little difference between the pulmonary artery tracing and the wedge pressure tracing is evident. Successful treatment of MR will bring about a significant decline in the V wave.

MANAGEMENT

Patients presenting with acute mitral regurgitation should be treated with the same modalities used in patients who present with acute heart failure. Afterload reduction with vasodilators or noninvasive positive pressure ventilation[62] will reduce the impedance to ejection into the aorta, diminish the amount of mitral regurgitation, increase forward output, and reduce pulmonary congestion.[63] In acute presentations, nitroprusside can achieve these clinical goals and has the advantage of easy titration to blood pressure. If hypotension is present, positive inotropic agents such as dobutamine may need to be combined with the nitroprusside. Diuretics are used to relieve congestion. Digoxin may be useful if left ventricular dysfunction or atrial fibrillation is present. Chronic afterload reduction can then be initiated with ACEIs or other vasodilators.

Unless patients with acute severe MR are treated aggressively, death is almost certain. Emergency surgery should be considered in patients with acute pulmonary edema caused by acute MR due to myocardial infarction and papillary muscle rupture, rupture of a chorda tendineae with a flail mitral leaflet in the mitral valve prolapse syndrome, traumatic MR, or severe MR associated with valvular endocarditis.

Patients with chronic MR should be considered for surgery when they become symptomatic. Exercise testing can precipitate symptoms in patients that are asymptomatic at rest. Asymptomatic patients should be considered for surgical intervention when the ejection fraction falls below 50%, the end-systolic volume index exceeds 50 mL/m^2, or pulmonary hypertension develops.[64]

The decision of whether to replace the mitral valve or to perform valvular reconstruction will depend on the degree of deformity of the valve leaflets and support structures. Mitral valve repair appears to be associated with a lower surgical mortality than is mitral valve replacement, although the patient populations differ.[65] Mitral valve repair is most often used in patients with myxomatous mitral valve prolapse and a flail mitral leaflet or with papillary muscle rupture after an acute myocardial infarction. Repair procedures consist of annuloplasty with the use of a prosthetic ring or resection and repair of the valve. Replacement, reimplantation, or shortening of chordae tendineae is performed in selected patients. Patients who are not candidates for repair receive either a mechanical or bioprosthetic valve. Surgeons frequently leave the submitral apparatus in place, as doing so favors a return to a more normal cardiac function after surgery.[66]

PROSTHETIC VALVES

There are two major types of prosthetic heart valve: mechanical valves, which are made of synthetic material, and tissue valves, which are composed at least in part of biologic tissue. The first mechanical valves were ball valves, such as the Starr-Edwards prosthesis. These valves have largely been replaced by the tilting disk valves, which offer a greater orifice area and less resistance to blood flow. Common examples of the disk valves are the Bjork-Shiley and St. Jude Medical valves. The two major types of tissue valves are stented porcine aortic valves (the Carpentier-Edwards and Hancock valves) and a trileaflet valve made with bovine pericardium (Ionescu-

Shiley valve). Other tissue valves are under development, including ones that use cryopreserved aortic homografts.

The advantage of tissue valves is a lower risk of thromboembolism than with mechanical valves. Anticoagulation is frequently used during the first few months after implantation, until the sewing ring becomes endothelialized. Anticoagulation is not required after this time; the thromboembolism rate is estimated to be 1 to 2 episodes per 100 patient-years.[67]

The main problem with the tissue valves concerns durability. The tissue valves are prone to calcification, fibrosis, degeneration, fibrin deposition, and cuspal tears. Valve dysfunction is more common in younger patients and in patients with disordered calcium metabolism. Evidence of degeneration can usually be detected by 5 years after replacement.[68] By 15 years, over 50% of tissue valves will have failed.[69] Fortunately, valve failure is rarely sudden, and a second operation can frequently be done on an elective basis. Sudden cuspal tears can present as an acute regurgitant lesion.

Mechanical valves have the advantage of durability but require anticoagulation to prevent thromboembolism. Without anticoagulation, major systemic embolisms occur at a rate of about 2% to 3% per year.[70] The incidence is higher for valves in the mitral than in the aortic position. With adequate anticoagulation, however, the incidence of thromboembolism is similar to that for tissue valves. The use of a small dose of aspirin plus warfarin anticoagulation may decrease the risk of thromboembolism further, but increases the risk of a bleeding complication.[71]

For patients who require noncardiac surgery and have a mechanical prosthetic valve, the anticoagulation regimen may be stopped for a few days with minimal risk. Minimizing the time off anticoagulants is essential to avoid thromboembolism. Heparin or low-molecular-weight dextran is frequently administered up to the time of surgery, to protect the patient. Heparin should then be restarted after surgery until warfarin treatment increases the International Normalized Ratio (INR) to the target level of 2.5 to 3.5.

Mechanical valve thrombosis is a serious complication and is associated with a high mortality.[72] The tilting disk valves are particularly susceptible to this complication. Thrombosis of mechanical valves is especially common for valves in the tricuspid position, so tissue valves are usually used in this location.[73] Inadequate anticoagulation or withdrawal of anticoagulation for surgical procedures accounts for most instances of thrombotic obstruction.[74] Thrombosis of the valve may lead to leaflet entrapment with acute regurgitation and circulatory collapse. Some patients, however, may remain asymptomatic or develop gradually worsening symptoms.

Obstruction of a mechanical valve usually necessitates reoperation, although that may be associated with a high risk of operative mortality. Thrombolytic therapy has been used successfully for prosthetic valve obstruction, with a success rate of 73% reported for one series.[75] Recurrence rates, however, have averaged 18% regardless of valve position.[76]

Prosthetic valve obstruction may be difficult to detect. Abnormal auscultatory findings, such as muffled opening or closing sounds or the presence of a new murmur, may indicate thrombosis. Doppler echocardiography can diagnose obstruction by detecting an increased transvalvular gradient. Transesophageal echocardiography can frequently visualize thrombosed mechanical valves that are not well seen with transthoracic approaches owing to signal scatter from the valve structures.

Prosthetic valve endocarditis is a serious complication that occurs in 1% to 9% of patients.[77] Early prosthetic valve endocarditis occurs within 60 days of implantation and results from contamination during the perioperative period. Most contamination probably occurs intraoperatively from direct wound inoculation or via the cardiopulmonary bypass machine. Postoperative sources include intravenous lines, pacing wires, and chest tubes. *Staphylococcus epidermidis* and *Staphylococcus aureus* are the most common organisms. A preoperative diagnosis of native valve endocarditis represents an increased risk of prosthetic valve involvement following surgery. Mortality is high, with one survey reporting a 64% mortality.[77]

Late prosthetic valve endocarditis occurs owing to seeding of the valve by transient bacteremia arising from dental, gastrointestinal, or genitourinary tract procedures. Nosocomial bacteremia has been reported to cause prosthetic valve endocarditis in 11% of patients within 45 days after discovery of the bacteremia.[78] The bacteria responsible are similar to those found in native valve endocarditis, with viridans streptococci the most common isolates. The prognosis of late prosthetic valve endocarditis is worse than that of native valve endocarditis, with mortality rates between 36% and 53%.[79] Complications of prosthetic valve endocarditis include myocardial abscesses, dehiscence of the valve with perivalvular leakage, and embolization (Fig. 29-10 and Color Plate 29-10). Immediate surgery is indicated in patients who are unstable or have significant prosthetic valve dysfunction.[80]

Antibiotic prophylaxis for medical and dental procedures is recommended for all patients with prosthetic valves. Procedures in which prophylaxis is recommended include bronchoscopy, sclerotherapy for esophageal varices, urethral catheterization if a urinary tract infection is present, incision and drainage of infected tissue, and vaginal delivery in the presence of infection.[81] Antibiotic schedules are listed in Table 29-6.

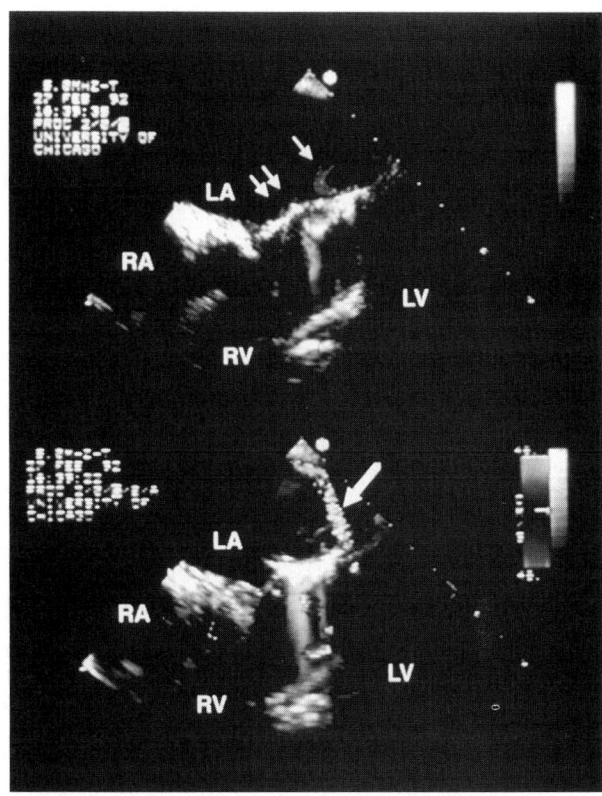

FIGURE 29-10 Endocarditis involving a St. Jude Medical mechanical valve in the mitral position. Transesophageal echocardiogram showing vegetations on the left atrial (LA) side of the mechanical valve (*small arrows*). Doppler echocardiography reveals perivalvular mitral regurgitation (*large arrow*). LV, left ventricle; RV, right ventricle; RA, right atrium. (See Color Plate 29-10.)

TABLE 29-6 Antibiotic Prophylaxis for Medical and Dental Procedures

Regimens for dental, oral, respiratory tract or esophageal procedures:	
Standard regimen:	
Amoxicillin	2 g orally 1 h before procedure
Regimen for amoxicillin/ampicillin/penicillin-allergic patients:	
Clindamycin	600 mg given orally 1 h before procedure, or
Cepahalexin or cefadroxil	2 g orally 1 h before procedure, or
azithromycin or clarithromycin	500 mg orally 1 h before procedure
Regimens for genitourinary/gastrointestinal procedures:	
Standard regimen: high-risk patients	
Ampicillin, gentamicin, and amoxicillin	2 g ampicillin plus 1.5 mg/kg gentamicin (120 mg maximum) IV or IM 30 min before procedure; amoxicillin, 1 g orally 6 h after first dose
For ampicillin/amoxicillin-allergic patients:	
Vancomycin and gentamicin	Vancomycin, 1 g IV over 1–2 h, plus gentamicin, 1.5 mg/kg (120 mg maximum) IV or IM; complete infusion 30 minutes before procedure
Moderate risk-patients	
Amoxicillin	Amoxicillin 2 g orally 1 h before procedure or ampicillin 2 g IV or IM within 30 min of starting procedure
Ampicillin/amoxicillin-allergic	Vancomycin 1 g over 1–2 h

SOURCE: Adapted with permission from Committee on Rheumatic Fever, Endocarditis, and Kawasaki Diseases.[81]

References

1. Gorlin R, Gorlin SG: Hydraulic formula for calculation of the area of the stenotic mitral valve, other cardiac valves, and central circulatory shunts. *Am Heart J* 41:1, 1951.

2. Ford LE, Feldman T, Chiu YC, et al: Hemodynamic resistance as a measure of functional impairment in aortic valvular stenosis. *Circ Res* 66:1, 1990.

3. Roberts WC: The congenitally bicuspid aortic valve. A study of 85 autopsy cases. *Am J Cardiol* 26:72, 1970.

4. Selzer A: Changing aspects of the natural history of valvular aortic stenosis. *N Engl J Med* 317:92, 1987.

5. Johnson AM: Aortic stenosis, sudden death, and the left ventricular baroreceptors. *Br Heart J* 33:1, 1971.

6. Monrad ES, Hess OM, Murakami T, et al: Time course of regression of left ventricular hypertrophy after aortic valve replacement. *Circulation* 77:1345, 1988.

7. Lombard JT, Selzer A: Valvular aortic stenosis. A clinical and hemodynamic profile of patients. *Ann Intern Med* 106:191, 1987.

8. Warth DC, Stewart WJ, Block PC, et al: A new method to calculate aortic valve area without left heart catheterization. *Circulation* 70:978, 1984.

9. Currie PJ, Seward JB, Reeder GS, et al: Continuous-wave doppler echocardiographic assessment of severity of calcific aortic stenosis: A simultaneous doppler-catheter correlative study in 100 adult patients. *Circulation* 71:1162, 1985.

10. Otto CM, Pearlman AS, Comess KA, et al: Determination of the stenotic aortic valve area in adults using doppler echocardiography. *J Am Coll Cardiol* 7:509, 1986.

11. Aronow WS, Ahn C, Kronzon I, Nanna M: Prognosis of congestive heart failure in patients aged greater than or equal to 62 years with unoperated severe valvular aortic stenosis. *Am J Cardiol* 72:846, 1993.

12. Zile MR, Gaasch WH: Heart failure in aortic stenosis—Improving diagnosis and treatment. *N Engl J Med* 348:18, 2003.

13. Bonow RO, Carabello B, de Leon AC Jr, et al: ACC/AHA guidelines for the management of patients with valvular heart disease: A report of the American College of Cardiology/American Heart Association Task Force on Practice Guidelines (Committee of Management of Patients with Valvular Heart Disease). *J Am Coll Cardiol* 32:1486, 1998.

14. deFilippi CR, Willett DL, Brickner ME, et al: Usefulness of dobutamine echocardiography in distinguishing severe from nonsevere valvular aortic stenosis in patients with depressed left ventricular function and low transvalvular gradients. *Am J Cardiol* 75:191, 1995.

15. Monin J-L, Monchi M, Gest V, et al: Aortic stenosis with severe left ventricular dysfunction and low transvalvular pressure gradients. *J Am Coll Cardiol* 37:2101, 2001.

16. Khot UN, Novaro GM, Popovic ZB, et al: Nitroprusside in critically ill patients with left ventricular dysfunction and aortic stenosis. *N Engl J Med* 348:1756, 2003.

17. Goldman L, Caldera DL, Nussbaum SR, et al: Multifactorial index of cardiac risk in noncardiac surgical procedures. *N Engl J Med* 297:845, 1977.

18. McKay RG, Safian RD, Lock JE, et al: Assessment of left ventricular and aortic valve function after aortic balloon valvuloplasty in adult patients with critical aortic stenosis. *Circulation* 75:192, 1987.

19. Moreno PR, Jang I-K, Newell JB, et al: The role of percutaneous aortic balloon valvuloplasty in patients with cardiogenic shock and critical aortic stenosis. *J Am Coll Cardiol* 23:1071, 1994.

20. Roth RB, Palacios IF, Block PC: Percutaneous aortic balloon valvuloplasty: Its role in the management of patients with aortic stenosis requiring major noncardiac surgery. *J Am Coll Cardiol* 13:1039, 1989.

21. Cribier A, Eltchaninoff H, Bash A, et al: Percutaneous transcatheter implantation of an aortic valve prosthesis for calcific aortic stenosis. *Circulation* 106:3006, 2002.

22. Maron BJ, Gaardin JM, Flack JM, et al: Prevalence of hypertrophic cardiomyopathy in a general population of young adults. Echocardiographic analysis of 4111 subjects in the CARDIA study. *Circulation* 92:785, 1995.

23. Maron BJ, Spirito P, Green KJ, et al: Noninvasive assessment of left ventricular diastolic function by pulsed doppler echocardiography in patients with hypertrophic cardiomyopathy. *J Am Coll Cardiol* 10:733, 1987.

24. Robinson K, Frenneaux MP, Stockins B, et al: Atrial fibrillation in hypertrophic cardiomyopathy: A longitudinal study. *J Am Coll Cardiol* 15:1279, 1990.

24a. Elliott P, McKenna WJ: Hypertrophic cardiomyopathy. *Lancet* 363:1881, 2004.

24b. Nishimura RA, Holmes DR Jr: Clinical practice: Hypertrophic obstructive cardiomyopathy. *N Engl J Med* 350:1320, 2004.

25. Pollick C: Muscular subaortic stenosis. Hemodynamic and clinical improvement after disopyramide. *N Engl J Med* 307:997, 1982.

26. McKenna WJ, Oakley CM, Krikler DM, et al: Improved survival with amiodarone in patients with hypertrophic cardiomyopathy and ventricular tachycardia. *Br Heart J* 53:412, 1985.

27. Fighali S, Krajcer Z, Leachman RD: Septal myomectomy and mitral valve replacement for idiopathic hypertrophic subaortic stenosis: Short- and long-term follow-up. *J Am Coll Cardiol* 3:1127, 1984.

28. Cooley DA, Leachman RD, Wukasch DC: Diffuse muscular subaortic stenosis: Surgical treatment. *Am J Cardiol* 31:1, 1973.

29. Fananapazir L, Epstein ND, Curiel RV, et al: Long-term results of dual-chamber (DDD) pacing in obstructive hypertrophic cardiomyopathy: Evidence for progressive symptomatic and hemodynamic improvement and reduction of left ventricular hypertrophy. *Circulation* 90:2731, 1994.

30. Spirito P, Seidman CE, McKenna WJ, et al: The management of hypertrophic cardiomyopathy. *N Engl J Med* 336:775, 1997.

31. Seggewiss H, Gleichmann U, Faber L, et al: Percutaneous transluminal myocardial ablation (PTSMA) in hypertrophic obstructive cardiomyopathy: Acute results and 3-month follow-up in 25 patients. *J Am Coll Cardiol* 32:252, 1998.

32. Lakkis NM, Nagueh SF, Kleiman NS, et al: Echocardiography-guided ethanol septal reduction for hypertrophic obstructive cardiomyopathy. *Circulation* 98:1750, 1998.

33. Faber L, Seggewiss H, Gleichmann U: Percutaneous transluminal septal myocardial ablation in hypertrophic obstructive cardiomyopathy. *Circulation* 98:2415, 1998.

34. Otto CM: Aortic valve insufficiency: Changing concepts in diagnosis and management. *Cardiologia* 41:505, 1996.

35. Morganroth J, Perloff JK, Zeldis SM, et al: Acute severe aortic regurgitation. Pathophysiology, clinical recognition, and management. *Ann Intern Med* 87:223, 1977.

36. Levine RJ, Roberts WC, Morrow AG: Traumatic aortic regurgitation. *Am J Cardiol* 10:752, 1962.

37. Siemienczuk D, Greenberg B, Morris C, et al: Chronic aortic insufficiency: Factors associated with progression to aortic valve replacement. *Ann Intern Med* 110:587, 1989.

38. Grayburn PA, Smith MD, Handshoe R, et al: Detection of aortic insufficiency by standard echocardiography, pulsed Doppler echocardiography, and auscultation. *Ann Intern Med* 104:599, 1986.

39. Nienaber CA, von Kodolitsch Y, Nicolas V, et al: The diagnosis of thoracic aortic dissection by noninvasive imaging procedures. *N Engl J Med* 328:1, 1993.

40. Mann T, McLaurin L, Grossman W, et al: Assessing the hemodynamic severity of acute aortic regurgitation due to infective endocarditis. *N Engl J Med* 293:108, 1975.

41. Aranki SF, Santini F, Adams DH, et al: Aortic valve endocarditis. Determinants of early survival and late morbidity. *Circulation* 90(Part 2):II-175, 1994.

42. Sorrentino M, Feldman T: Techniques for IABP timing, use—and discontinuance. *J Crit Illness* 7:597, 1992.

43. Bolen JL, Alderman EL: Hemodynamic consequences of afterload reduction in patients with chronic aortic regurgitation. *Circulation* 53:879, 1976.

44. Miller RR, Vismara LA, DeMaria AN, et al: Afterload reduction therapy with nitroprusside in severe aortic regurgitation: Improved cardiac performance and reduced regurgitant volume. *Am J Cardiol* 38:564, 1976.

45. Greenberg BH: Medical therapy for patients with aortic insufficiency. *Cardiol Clin* 9:255, 1991.

46. Scognamiglio R, Rahimtoola SH, Fasoli G, et al: Nifedipine in asymptomatic patients with severe aortic regurgitation and normal left ventricular function. *N Engl J Med* 331:689, 1994.

47. Grossman W: Aortic and mitral regurgitation. How to evaluate the condition and when to consider surgical intervention. *JAMA* 252:2447, 1984.

48. Chaliki HP, Mohty D, Avierinos J-F, et al. Outcomes after aortic valve replacement in patients with severe aortic regurgitation and markedly reduced left ventricular function. *Circulation* 106:2687, 2002.

49. Carroll JD, Feldman T: Percutaneous mitral balloon valvotomy and the new demographics of mitral stenosis. *JAMA* 270:1731, 1993.

50. Meisner JS, Keren G, Pajaro OE, et al: Atrial contribution to ventricular filling in mitral stenosis. *Circulation* 84:1469, 1991.

51. Leavitt JI, Coats MH, Falk RH: Effects of exercise on transmitral gradient and pulmonary artery pressure in patients with mitral stenosis or a prosthetic mitral valve. A Doppler echocardiographic study. *J Am Coll Cardiol* 17:1520, 1991.

52. Martin RP, Rakowski H, Kleiman JH, et al: Reliability and reproducibility of two dimensional echocardiographic measurement of the stenotic mitral valve orifice area. *Am J Cardiol* 43:560, 1979.

53. Libanoff AJ, et al: Atrioventricular pressure half-time. Measure of mitral valve orifice area. *Circulation* 33:218, 1968.

54. Hatle L: Noninvasive assessment of atrioventricular pressure half-time by Doppler ultrasound. *Circulation* 60:1096, 1979.

55. Feldman T, Carroll JD: Percutaneous transvenous balloon mitral commissurotomy: When? For whom? *J Crit Illness* 6:1009, 1991.

56. Reyes VP, Raju BS, Wynne J, et al: Percutaneous balloon valvuloplasty compared with open surgical commissurotomy for mitral stenosis. *N Engl J Med* 331:961, 1994.

57. Rahimtoola SH, Durairaj A, Mehra A, et al: Current evaluation and management of patients with mitral stenosis. *Circulation* 106:1183, 2002.

58. Tcheng JE, Jackman JD, Nelson CL, et al: Outcome of patients sustaining acute ischemic mitral regurgitation during myocardial infarction. *Ann Intern Med* 117:18, 1992.

59. Ross J: Afterload mismatch in aortic and mitral valve disease: Implications for surgical therapy. *J Am Coll Cardiol* 5:811, 1985.

60. Braunwald E, Awe WC: The syndrome of severe mitral regurgitation with normal left atrial pressure. *Circulation* 27:29, 1963.

61. Sorrentino MJ: Mitral valve prolapse. Avoiding complications of a progressive disease. *Postgraduate Med J* 93:63, 1993.

62. Bellone A, Barbieri A, Ricci C, et al: Acute effects of non-invasive ventilatory support on functional mitral regurgitation in patients with exacerbation of congestive heart failure. *Intensive Care Med* 28:1348, 2002.

63. Harshaw CW, Grossman W, Munro AB, et al: Reduced systemic vascular resistance as therapy for severe mitral regurgitation of valvular origin. *Ann Intern Med* 83:312, 1975.

64. Crawford MH, Souchek J, Oprian CA, et al: Determinants of survival and left ventricular performance after mitral valve replacement. *Circulation* 81:1173, 1990.

65. Sand ME, Naftel DC, Blackstone EH, et al: A comparison of repair and replacement for mitral incompetence. *J Thorac Cardiovasc Surg* 94:208, 1987.

66. Zile MR: Chronic aortic and mitral regurgitation. Choosing the optimal time for surgical correction. *Cardiology Clin* 9:239, 1991.

67. Atkins CW, Carroll DL, Buckley MJ, et al: Late results with Carpentier-Edwards porcine bioprosthesis. *Circulation* 82(IV):IV-65, 1990.

68. Cipriano PR, Billingham ME, Oyer PE, et al: Calcification of porcine prosthetic heart valves: A radiographic and light microscopic study. *Circulation* 66:1100, 1982.

69. Sugimoto JT, Karp RB: Homografts and cryopreserved valves, in Crawford FA (ed): *Cardiac Surgery: Current Heart Valve Prostheses*, Vol. 1. Philadelphia, Hanley & Belfus, 1987, p 295.

70. Bloomfield P, Wheatley DJ, Prescott RJ, et al: Twelve-year comparison of a Bjork-Shiley mechanical valve with porcine bioprostheses. *N Engl J Med* 324:573, 1991.

71. Turpie AGC, Gent M, Laupacis A, et al: A comparison of aspirin with placebo in patients treated with warfarin after heart-valve replacement. *N Engl J Med* 329:524, 1993.

72. Karp RB, Cyrus RJ, Blackstone EH, et al: The Bjork-Shiley valve. Intermediate-term follow-up. *J Thorac Cardiovasc Surg* 81:602, 1981.

73. Thorburn CW, Morgan JJ, Shanahan MX, et al: Long-term results of tricuspid valve replacement and the problem of prosthetic valve thrombosis. *Am J Cardiol* 51:1128, 1983.

74. Deviri E, Sareli P, Wisenbaugh T, et al: Obstruction of mechanical heart valve prostheses: Clinical aspects and surgical management. *J Am Coll Cardiol* 17:646, 1991.

75. Roudaut R, Labbe T, Lorient-Roudaut MF, et al: Mechanical cardiac valve thrombosis: Is fibrinolysis justified? *Circulation* 86(Suppl 2):II-8, 1992.

76. Hurrell DG, Schaff HV, Tajik AJ: Thrombolytic therapy for obstruction of mechanical prosthetic valves. *Mayo Clin Proc* 71:605, 1996.

77. Ivert TSA, Dismukes WE, Cobbs CG, et al: Prosthetic valve endocarditis. *Circulation* 69:223, 1984.

78. Fang G, Keys TF, Gentry LO, et al: Prosthetic valve endocarditis resulting from nosocomial bacteremia. *Ann Intern Med* 119:560, 1993.

79. Watanakunakorn G: Prosthetic valve endocarditis. *Prog Cardiovasc Dis* 22:181, 1979.

80. Dinubile MJ: Surgery in active endocarditis. *Ann Intern Med* 96:650, 1982.

81. Committee on Rheumatic Fever, Endocarditis, and Kawasaki Disease: Prevention of bacterial endocarditis: Recommendations of the American Heart Association. *JAMA* 277:1794, 1997.

Chapter 30

AORTIC DISSECTION

JOSEPH J. AUSTIN

KEY POINTS

- *Acute aortic dissection occurs more commonly than ruptured abdominal aortic aneurysm.*
- *The typical pain, poor peripheral perfusion, and evidence of aortic branch occlusion suggest the diagnosis.*
- *Early pharmacologic control of systolic blood pressure and the pulse wave (dP/dT) is imperative.*
- *Investigations must be undertaken urgently to confirm the diagnosis and direct definitive treatment.*
- *Emergency surgical repair is indicated for type A dissections.*
- *Control of hypertension is important to minimize complications and maximize survival both in the postoperative period and in the long term.*
- *Type B dissections may have a more ominous prognosis than previously thought and require very close long-term follow-up.*

Aortic dissection is the most common catastrophe affecting the aorta, occurring two to three times more commonly than acute abdominal aortic aneurysm rupture.[1] The reported incidence is approximately 10 to 20 per 1 million per year.[2] Rarely is the outcome of a cardiovascular disease so dependent on the skills and cooperation of the emergency room physician, the cardiac surgeon, and the intensivist as it is with acute dissections of the aorta. Maximal survival depends on a high index of suspicion of the diagnosis despite a myriad of different presentations, early pharmacologic intervention for control of hypertension, rapid diagnosis with definitive imaging, and then appropriate relegation to medical or surgical management depending on the dissection type. Without treatment, the 3-month mortality is 85% to 90%, but with the appropriate treatment, survival rates of over 80% can be expected.

Pathogenesis

Previously, aortic dissections were referred to as *dissecting aneurysms,* as originally coined by Laënnec. This is a misnomer in that the pathology is a dissecting hematoma that separates the intima and inner layers of the media from the outer medial and adventitial layers (Fig. 30-1). The intima is therefore not aneurysmal, and is if anything, narrowed. Blood invades the media through a tear in the intima and proceeds ante- or retrogradely through the aortic wall, forming a false lumen. The hematoma spirals around the right and posterior aspects of the ascending aorta, supraposteriorly along the arch, and then down the left and posterior aspects of the descending aorta.[3] The hematoma may then have several serious sequelae. It may rupture into the pericardial space causing tamponade, or into the pleural space with exsanguinating hemorrhage. This occurs less frequently than expected because the adventitial layer represents 66% of the overall strength of the aortic wall. It may also cause

occlusion of aortic branch arteries or prolapse of one or more of the aortic valve cusps, resulting in acute aortic insufficiency.

Generally the tear is due to either a weakening of the wall of the aorta, an increase in luminal shear stress, or both.[3] Weakening of the aortic wall occurs as the result of medial degeneration or iatrogenic injury. Medial degeneration (cystic medial degeneration or necrosis) is manifested by the loss of smooth muscle cells and accumulation of basophilic amorphous material with or without associated "cysts" in the aortic media. This is believed to be due to inborn errors of metabolism (Marfan's or Ehlers-Danlos syndrome). There is a reduction in the cohesiveness of the layers of the aortic wall as a result. Other causes of reduced wall strength causing aortic dissection include annuloaortic ectasia, bicuspid aortic valve, coarctation, and pregnancy (especially in the third trimester.)

Iatrogenic injuries occur during open heart surgical procedures at any point where the aorta is invaded, such as the aortotomy for an aortic valve replacement or the proximal anastomosis of an aortocoronary bypass graft.

Stresses applied to the aortic wall increase wall tension and lead to dissections. Most important are intraluminal shear stresses, which are related both to the level of the systolic blood pressure and to the steepness of the aortic pulse wave.[2] This is referred to as dP/dT_{max} and represents the speed with which the maximal systolic pressure is attained in the aortic root. As this increases, so too does the shear stress on the ascending aorta.

Classification

Dissections are classified by timing and location to identify the morbidity and mortality for the specific lesions.

TIMING

- Acute: <2 weeks
- Chronic: >2 weeks

Acute dissections are very high-risk lesions, with an estimated mortality of 50% for the first 48 hours (or 1% per hour).

LOCATION

- Type A: The ascending aorta is involved independent of the site of the intimal tear (since 15% of transverse arch and 5% of descending aortic tears will involve the ascending aorta), and may include the aortic arch and part of or all of the descending thoracic and abdominal aorta.
- Type B: Descending aorta (beyond the left subclavian artery).

This classification system, proposed by Daily and colleagues and popularized by the Stanford group, replaces the original system proposed by DeBakey (Fig. 30-2). Using this classification, 60% of all dissections are type A, and 40% are type B. The classification system is based on the risk of sudden death from the dissection, which is highest in type A. Here the dissection may cause tamponade or severe aortic insufficiency with congestive heart failure, as well as coronary thrombosis, especially involving the right coronary artery with acute myocardial infarction. Type B dissections do not have these risks and generally can be approached and managed

CAL ILLNESS

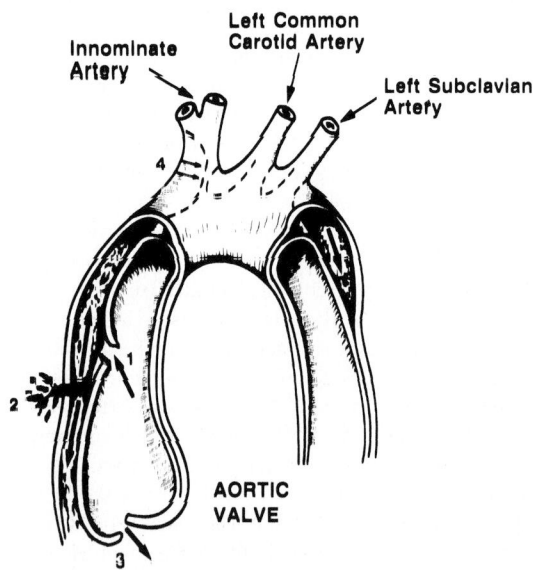

FIGURE 30-1 Aortic dissection begins with an intimal tear *(1)* leading to a hematoma that separates the layers of the aortic wall. The sequelae are rupture through the adventitia into the pericardium *(2)*, prolapse of the aortic valve cusps leading to aortic insufficiency *(3)*, compression of the aortic branch vessels *(4)*, and aneurysmal dilation of the ascending arch and descending aorta.

FIGURE 30-2 Classification of aortic dissection based on the presence or absence of ascending aortic involvement. Type A dissections involve the ascending aorta, and type B dissections do not. The intimal tear in type A dissections may be in the ascending aorta *(1)*, the arch *(2)*, or the descending aorta *(3)*. Type A includes DeBakey types I and II. In type B dissection the intimal tear is distal to the left subclavian artery origin. Type B dissections correspond to DeBakey's type III. *(Reprinted with permission from McGoon C: Cardiac Surgery, 2nd ed. Philadelphia, FA Davis, 1987, p 42.)*

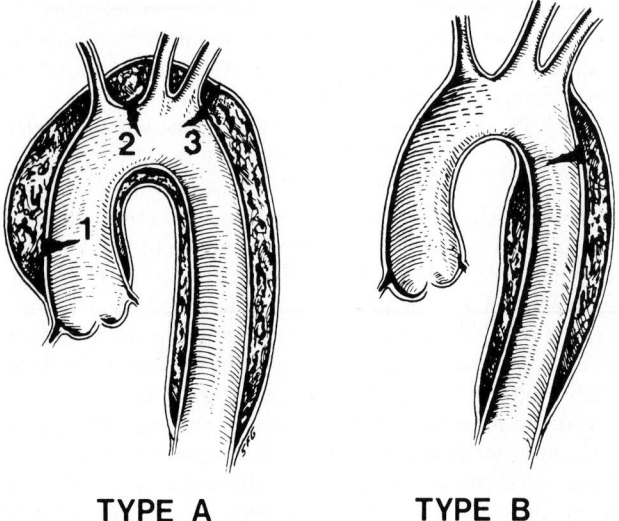

TYPE A   **TYPE B**

conservatively. As a result, therapeutic interventions are dependent on location, with almost all type A dissections requiring urgent operative intervention, whereas type B dissections are managed primarily pharmacologically, with surgery only for specific complications. However, recent evidence suggests that up to 40% of type B dissections can lead to late death, and there is great interest in endovascular stenting to improve long-term survival.[4–6]

Aortic Intramural Hematoma

Aortic intramural hematoma (IMH) results from hemorrhage within the aortic wall without disruption of the intima. It is likely due to rupture of the vasa vasorum and may progress to rupture through the intima to form a classic dissection in up to 33% of cases.[7] It is an entity that is frequently confused with aortic dissection whose diagnosis, management, and prognosis remain debatable. Most authors believe the clinical course is similar enough to warrant treatment of IMH the same as a classical dissection.[8–10] A high percentage (up to 80%) may completely resolve within 1 year, but up to 60% of the remaining patients can go on to develop saccular aneurysms within 45 days with a significant annular growth rate.[8,10] The diameter of the aorta is important in that if the aortic diameter is <45 mm at 1 month follow-up, then most will resolve. Complications appear to occur mainly in patients with an aortic diameter over 45mm.[9]

Clinical Picture

Men, particularly black men, are at two to three times the risk of developing an aortic dissection as women. More than 90% will have a history of hypertension requiring treatment. The presentation of an acute dissection can be subtle, demanding great attention to detail to make the diagnosis, or classic and obvious. A new murmur of aortic insufficiency is present in 50% to 66% of type A dissections[11] due to the loss of support of the valve at the commissures as the inner layer of the aorta collapses inward. A continuous murmur suggests rupture of the dissection into the right ventricle or atrium.[12] The signs and symptoms are related to the location of the tear and the extent of the hematoma dissection. These are manifested mainly by pain, poor peripheral perfusion despite an increased blood pressure, and signs and symptoms of aortic branch occlusion.

PAIN

Typically, the pain is either retrosternal, or central interscapular back pain, but it may be epigastric. Classically, it begins in the chest, moves to the back, and then moves down to the abdomen or lower extremities as the dissection progresses, but this pattern is rarely seen. Patients describe the pain as "sharp," "tearing," or "knife-like," and it is most often excruciating in intensity. To differentiate it from angina, the pain is maximal immediately upon onset, and it is difficult to obtain complete relief with opiates alone. Clinical diagnostic accuracy may approach 90% if three basic questions are asked regarding the pain's quality (tearing or ripping), radiation (beginning between the scapulae and radiating down the back), and the intensity at onset (abrupt onset of 10/10 pain).[13]

POOR PERFUSION

Patients frequently present with evidence of shock, with a cool, clammy periphery, ashen coloring, and depressed level of consciousness, and yet markedly elevated systolic blood pressure frequently exceeding 200 mm Hg. Most often this is due to reflex sympathetic discharge from the intense pain. It can occur, however, with myocardial infarction due to coronary artery occlusion by the dissection, or from severe aortic insufficiency with congestive heart failure, which is present in 30% to 60% of patients with type A dissections. If the blood pressure is depressed, the dissection may have ruptured into the pericardium with tamponade (as occurs in 30% of type A dissections) or into the pleural space (left more often than right) in type B dissections, with resulting hypovolemia.

SIGNS AND SYMPTOMS OF AORTIC BRANCH OCCLUSION

Approximately one third of all patients will present with compromised flow to a major branch of the aorta as part of their presentation.[14] The vessel may be sheared off or compressed, resulting in occlusion and/or thrombosis, or be perfused through the false channel (Fig. 30-3). Table 30-1 lists the vessels affected and the manifestations. The dissection usually travels in a spiral motion down the thoracic aorta such that the celiac axis, superior mesenteric artery, and right renal artery remain intact. In type A dissections the innominate artery (and thus blood flow to the right carotid artery to the brain, causing cerebrovascular insufficiency, and the right subclavian artery to the right upper extremity, causing a pulse deficit) are the most frequently affected. A measured brachial

TABLE 30-1 Aortic Branch Occlusion

Site	Manifestation
Iliofemoral (35%)	Lower extremity ischemia
Carotid (21%)	Cerebrovascular accident (CVA)
Subclavian (14%)	Upper extremity ischemia
Renal (14%)	Renal failure or hypertension
Mesenteric (8%)	Intestinal ischemia
Abdominal aorta (7%)	Aortic aneurysm

NOTE: Peripheral vascular complications are listed in decreasing frequency. Overall 8% to 56% of patients sustain aortic branch complications. Extensive dissections are at higher risk (49% to 56%) than if isolated to either the ascending or proximal descending aorta (8% to 13%).

pressure differential of greater than 20 mm Hg is an independent predictor of the presence of a dissection.[15] The dissection usually stops at the level of the iliac arteries, with the left iliac more often affected, leading to compromised blood flow to the left leg. Rarely is there only one tear in the aorta, and more commonly, the dissection has multiple re-entry sites along its path down the aorta. The common femoral arteries are seldom dissected, an important issue at surgery, since cannulation of the femoral artery is necessary for placing the patient on cardiopulmonary bypass.[16] Fortunately, the visceral and renal vessels are affected in less than 3% of patients, since their involvement denotes a much increased mortality rate of 41% versus 27%.[17]

Neurologic sequelae are of particular concern. Some neurologic dysfunction, such as depressed level of consciousness or dizziness, is said to occur in 30% to 50% of patients.[3] However, concrete focal neurologic deficits occur much less frequently (<10% overall), and may affect the central nervous system (CNS), spinal cord, or peripheral nerves. CNS deficits range from minor transient ischemic attacks to deep coma. Cerebrovascular accidents (CVAs) causing hemiparesis affect 5.5% to 6.7% of patients with type A dissections. They are primarily due to innominate–carotid artery occlusion, with the right side affected in two thirds of cases. They also can be caused by emboli or low flow with thrombosis due to previous carotid stenosis. Paraparesis and paraplegia fortunately are rare (2% of type A), because they portend a very poor prognosis.

Occasionally patients may present with vascular compromise foremost in their complaints and findings. A patient suffering an acute occlusion of blood flow into their lower extremity, particularly the left, with no definite clot or embolus found at surgery should be strongly suspected of having a dissection and investigated immediately. Unfortunately the physical findings classically associated with dissection are present in less than half of all cases, thereby necessitating a high index of suspicion to save these patients.[18]

Investigations and Diagnosis

LABORATORY

Laboratory data are usually within normal limits in patients with acute dissection. The white blood cell count may be slightly elevated to 12,000 to 20,000/μL, most likely as a stress response. Electrocardiogram (ECG) interpretation may show left ventricular hypertrophy due to chronic hypertension, but other changes are rare. Acute ischemic changes should raise

FIGURE 30-3 Aortic branch occlusion mechanisms. *A.* Compression of the true lumen by the false lumen with a patent true lumen. *B.* Complete occlusion of the true lumen by the false lumen with thrombosis. *C.* Complete avulsion of the intima from the origin of the branch vessel with blood flow provided both from the false lumen and the true lumen via distal re-entry. *D.* Complete occlusion of the true lumen by the false lumen beyond the branch orifice. *(Reprinted with permission from Cambria et al.[14])*

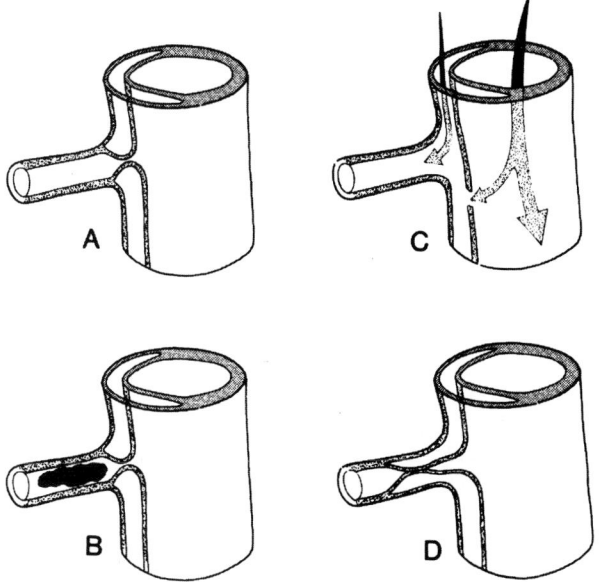

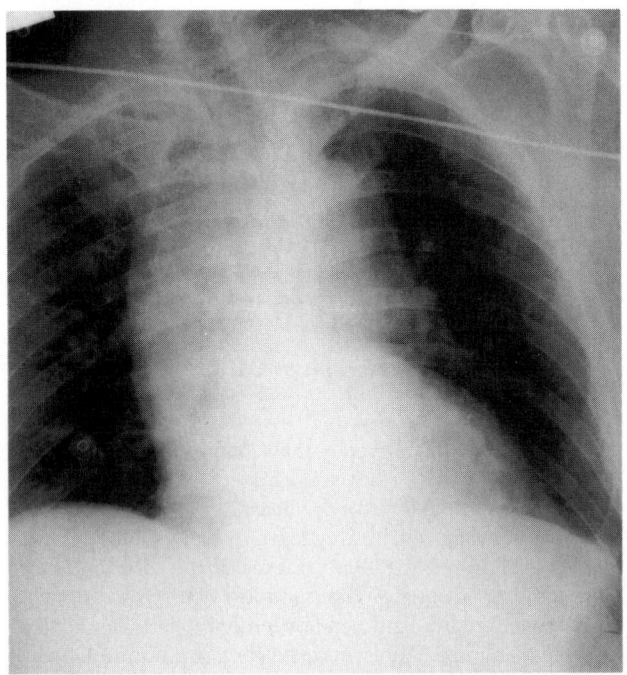

FIGURE 30-4 Chest x-ray illustrating widened mediastinum with blunting of the aortic knob.

the concern of coronary artery involvement by the dissection in the patient with a typical history. Conversely, to avoid the dire consequences of misdiagnosis, any patient presenting to the ER with ECG changes suggesting myocardial ischemia (especially with evidence of right coronary artery involvement) should have their history considered carefully before immediately moving to anticoagulation, thrombolytics, and

urgent cardiac catheterization to treat the more prevalent condition of atherosclerotic coronary artery disease.

DIAGNOSTIC IMAGING

Diagnostic imaging is the most important investigation for the diagnosis and classification of aortic dissections. Standard anteroposterior and upright lateral chest x-rays often reveal a widened mediastinum, although this may be absent in up to 40% of type A dissections (Fig. 30-4). Classically, the aorta bulges to the right with type A and to the left with type B dissections. Occasionally a double rim of calcification may be present in the distal aortic arch or a pleural effusion may be present (left more than right), due mainly to a serous sympathetic reaction rather than to frank blood from a rupture.

Significant debate exists as to the best imaging modality presently available for aortic dissections. The ideal modality would be readily available, easy to interpret, represent no risk to the patient, and provide all the information the surgeon requires. These needs include assessment of the ascending aorta, identifying the site of the intimal tear, the full extent of the dissection, existence of branch vessel involvement, presence of a pericardial effusion, and presence and severity of aortic valve insufficiency.[19] Several imaging techniques including aortography, computed tomographic (CT) scanning, magnetic resonance imaging (MRI), and echocardiography are highly accurate for the diagnosis and classification of dissections.[20] Controversy exists as to which of these is the most accurate.[19,20–24] In the past many authors believed that aortic angiography was the most definitive diagnostic method, with sensitivity and specificity of 88% to 90% and 90% to 95%, respectively.[2,25] In addition to confirming the diagnosis by illustrating the true and false channels, the aortogram could pinpoint the site of the intimal tear (Fig. 30-5),

FIGURE 30-5 *A.* Aortogram (lateral projection). Grossly dilated ascending aorta (*open arrow*) with visible intimal flap (*solid arrow*). Note normal descending aorta. *B.* Contrast-enhanced CT scan of the thorax of the same patient. Arrow identifies intimal flap. (*Reprinted with permission from Kotler N, Steiner RM: Cardiac Imaging: New Technologies and Clinical Applications. Philadelphia, FA Davis, 1986.*)

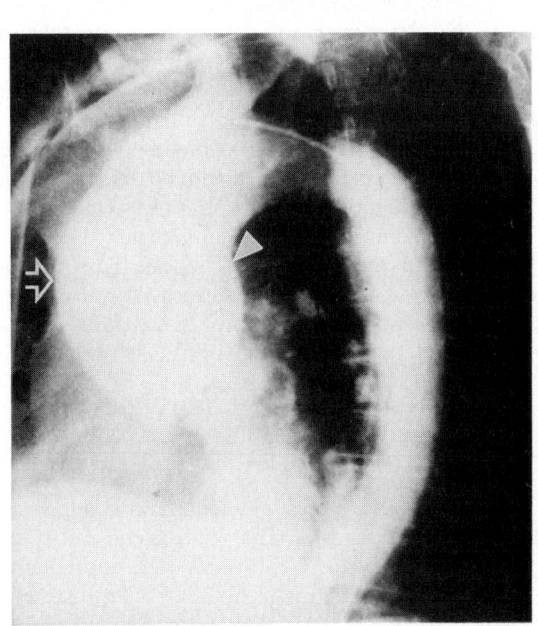

A

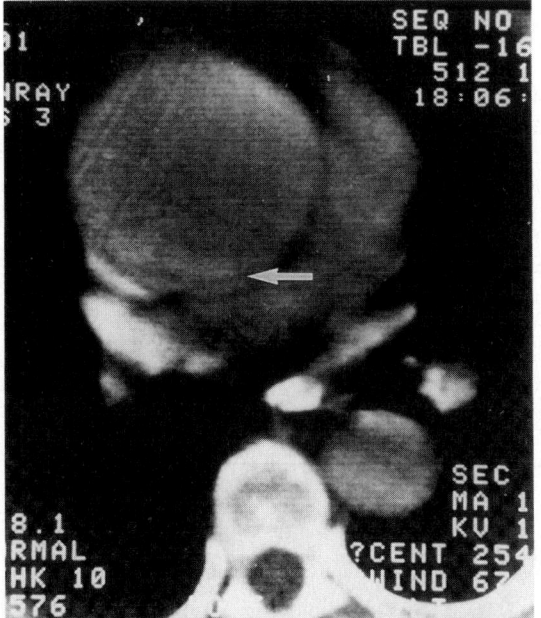

B

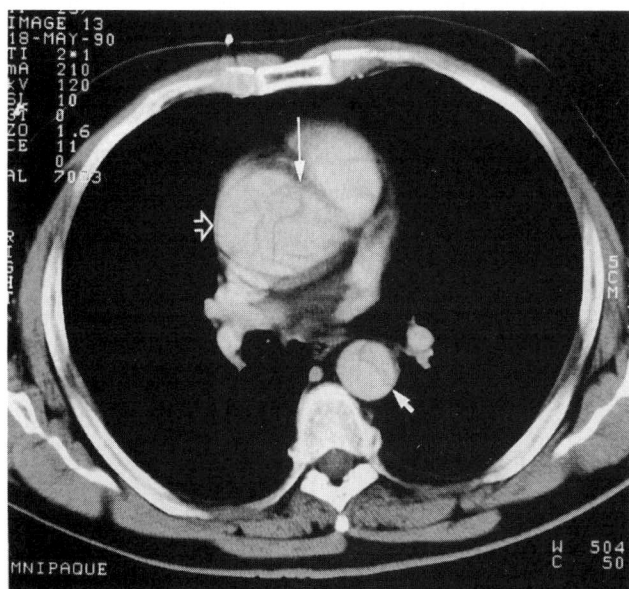

FIGURE 30-6 Contrast-enhanced CT scan of the thorax. Aneurysmal dilation of the aorta is clearly evident (*open arrow*). An intimal flap seen in the ascending aorta (*long arrow*) and continuing into the descending aorta (*short arrow*).

two and three dimensions (Fig. 30-8). CT is very specific and accurate (~100%) for the diagnosis of dissection,[18,25] and 96% accurate for the presence of aortic branch involvement.[19] CT scanning does not yield information regarding aortic insufficiency or left ventricular function, and requires both contrast administration and exposure to radiation. CT scanning is also inferior to aortography for identifying the site of the intimal tear. Recently, however, the site of the intimal tear has had debatable bearing on the type of dissection or surgical success. Since CT scanning lacks somewhat in sensitivity, if the CT scan is negative and the suspicion of aortic dissection remains high, other investigations should be done to rule out a dissection. Helical CT scanning is the author's recommended imaging technique for the long-term follow-up of the patient, given its low expense, high reproducibility, and minimal patient discomfort.

Echocardiography is likely the diagnostic modality of choice for acute aortic dissections. Both transthoracic and transesophageal two-dimensional echocardiography can accurately evaluate the most important issues of dissections; involvement of the ascending aorta, presence and severity of aortic insufficiency, the entry sites in the intimal flap, and presence of aortic arch dilation. Two lumens may be seen separated by a flap, or there may be central displacement of intimal calcification. The addition of color-coded Doppler allows better identification of the true and false lumens, even if the false lumen is thrombosed. The presence of a pericardial effusion and any left ventricular wall motion abnormalities also may be assessed accurately. Transesophageal echocardiography (TEE) was previously criticized for being unable to visualize the aortic arch, but current multiplanar TEE transducers have few blind areas. Its main limitation is inability to see the intra-abdominal aorta, but this can be assessed with simple ultrasound.[23]

Transthoracic echocardiography is less accurate than transesophageal echocardiography in the diagnosis of aortic dissections. It is also frequently technically limited due to chest wall abnormalities, chronic obstructive pulmonary disease, and obesity.

TEE[21,23] is the most efficient and accurate diagnostic modality available (Fig. 30-9). Its sensitivity and specificity are

establish the extent of the dissection, quantitate the severity of aortic insufficiency if present, and identify the presence and degree of aortic branch occlusions. Some authors, however, have expressed concerns over false-negative reports due to viewing the flap and both lumens en face, with the central beam missing a small localized dissection, and possibly missing the flap due to simultaneous opacification of both true and false lumens.[12] The procedure is also invasive and requires a contrast load, so less invasive investigations are preferred.

CT scanning is a noninvasive technique that yields excellent images of dissections, especially type B. Specific identification of true and false lumens with a flap is possible, as well as detection of pericardial effusions and accurate depiction of the extent of the dissection (Figs. 30-6 and 30-7). The new third-generation helical CT scanners yield excellent images both in

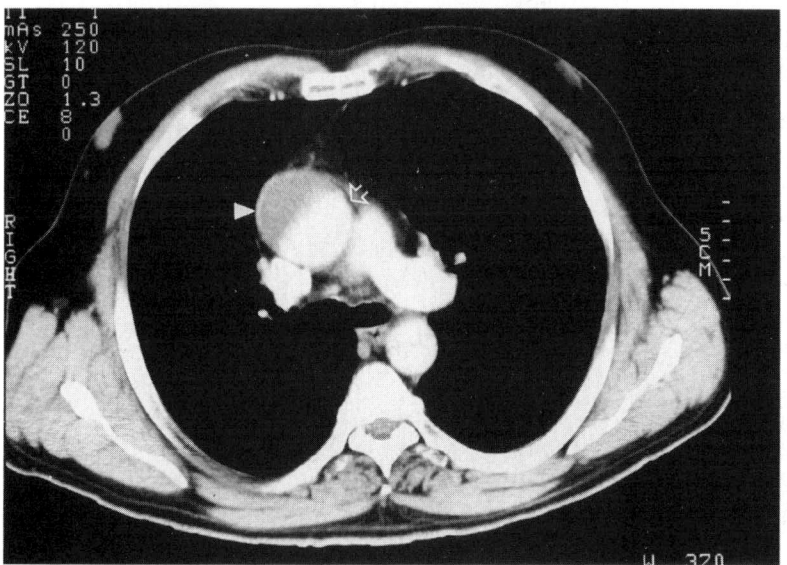

FIGURE 30-7 Contrast-enhanced CT scan of the thorax. A dilated aortic root and intimal tear are present. Contrast material fills the true lumen first (*open arrow*), while false-lumen filling is delayed (*solid arrow*).

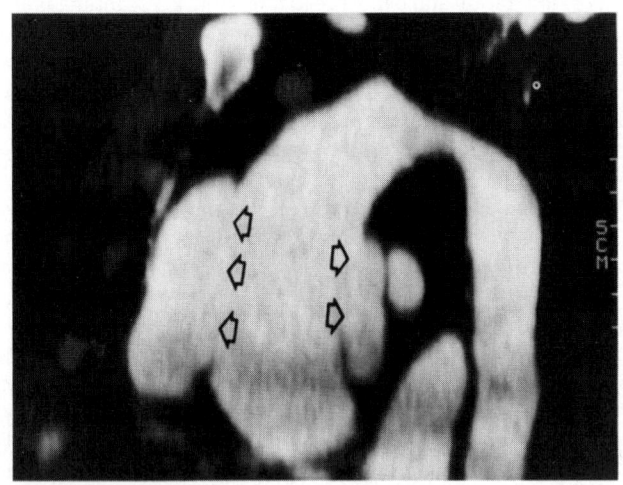

A

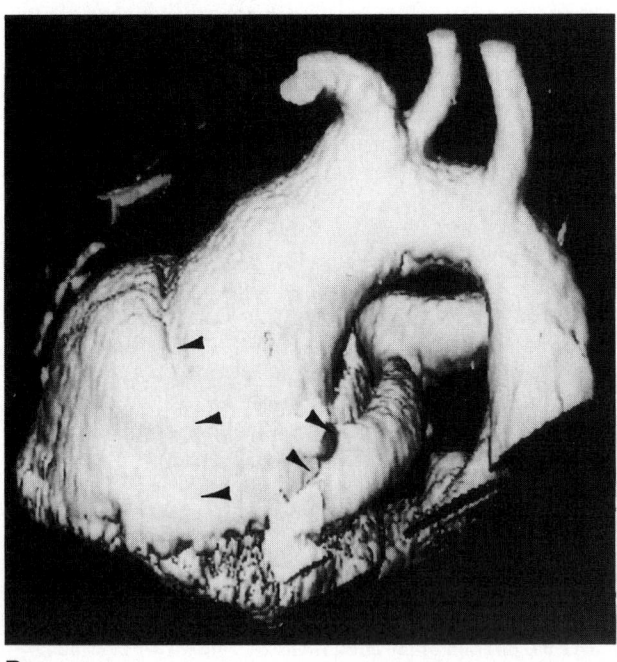

B

FIGURE 30-8 *A.* Two-dimensional images of a spiral CT scan from a patient with an acute type A aortic dissection. (Open arrows point to saccular dilation of the false channel outside the true one.) *B.* Three-dimensional image reconstruction of the spiral CT scan above. Observe the false channel (*solid arrows*) surrounding the true one. (*Reprinted with permission from Borst HG, Heinemann MK, Stone C: Surgical Treatment of Aortic Dissection. New York, Churchill-Livingstone, 1996, p 121.*)

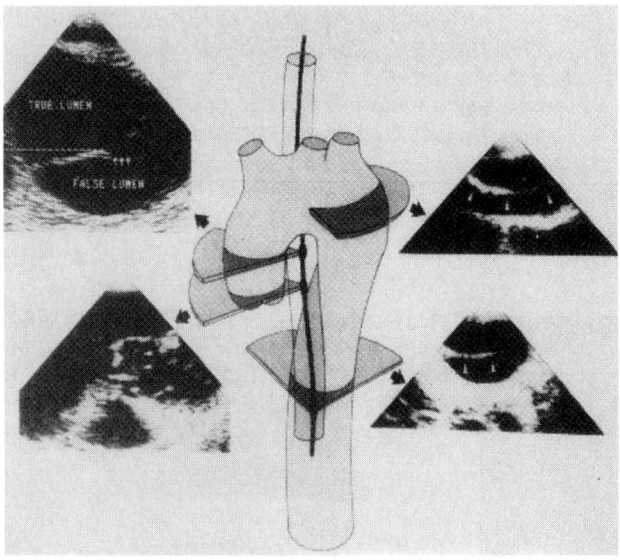

A

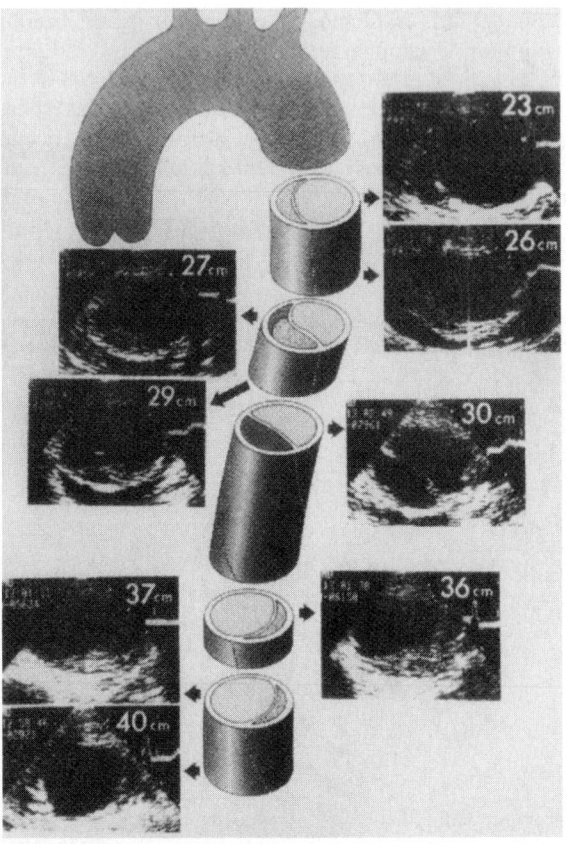

B

FIGURE 30-9 *A.* Transesophageal echocardiogram of type A dissection. Note clear depiction of true and false lumens as well as intimal flap originating in the ascending aorta (*two arrows* in bottom left image) and extending into the descending aorta. (*Reprinted with permission from Erbel et al.[21]*) *B.* Transesophageal echocardiogram of type B dissection. True and false lumens are illustrated with spiraling of the dissecting hematoma around the aorta. (*Reprinted with permission from Erbel et al.[21]*)

over 98%, so this technique very accurately identifies the presence or absence of a dissection. Notably, it can be performed in less than 30 minutes in an emergency room or intensive care unit. The efficiency and mobility are very important in the management of critically ill patients, who are best cared for in a well-monitored ICU rather than in the radiology suite. Occasional complications (<1%) have included transient arrhythmias (atrioventricular block, bradyarrhythmias, or premature ventricular contractions), reports of rupture of the dissection during the insertion of the probe, and esophageal perforation. Generally the procedure is well tolerated with appropriate control of pain and hypertension.[21,22,24]

MRI is very accurate, sensitive, and specific in dissections, but has been used sparingly as the procedure requires 45 minutes and can be difficult due to limited access to a critically ill patient.[19,23–25] It is, however, the only modality that provides all of the previously mentioned preoperative needs of the surgeon. It is noninvasive and does not require contrast material or ionizing radiation. Excellent contrast can be obtained between extraluminal structures, and it allows the visualization of vascular walls and both clotted and flowing blood. MR technology is advancing rapidly, with accuracy of 100% with phase-contrast cine MR angiography,[1–9] and new MRI sequences (such as the breath-hold gradient-echo) have been able to reduce the procedure time to less than 5 minutes without compromising accuracy.[26]

The author presently recommends TEE as the initial investigation. If this is not immediately available, then a helical CT scan of the thorax is performed. If this is negative and there is still a strong suspicion of dissection, then MR angiography may be performed in a stable patient. Of course, this approach should be modified by availability and the local expertise with these imaging techniques at each institution.

Natural History

Untreated acute type A aortic dissections have a uniformly poor prognosis. Fifty percent of patients die within the first 48 hours, and <10% will survive 1 month. Poor prognostic variables include aortic branch complications (particularly mesenteric and renal arteries), type A dissections, associated coronary artery disease (CAD), and neurologic deficits (CVA and paraplegia).[27]

Hemodynamic instability (systolic BP <90 mm Hg) represents a 32% mortality vs. 8.5% for those with stable hemodynamics.[28]

Treatment

To maximize survival, optimal treatment of acute dissections must include early pharmacologic control of blood pressure and pain, often before the definitive diagnosis is made, combined with appropriate surgical intervention. All patients with aortic dissections must have intensive monitoring in a critical care setting. The patient should be placed on a cardiac monitor, and have an intra-arterial catheter (for ongoing blood pressure control), and central venous pressure and urinary catheters inserted. Blood should be drawn for standard laboratory investigations as well as cross and typing for blood transfusion in case surgery is needed. The patient should be observed closely for any change in hemodynamic parameters or neurologic function and for evidence of organ ischemia.

Pharmacologic Control of Blood Pressure

Intravenous antihypertensive agents are used to reduce the level of systolic blood pressure and the pulse wave (dP/dT_{max}) to halt the progression of the dissecting hematoma. With the hematoma stabilized, pain usually can be controlled with intravenous opiates. Several agents are available for the ICU control of systolic blood pressure and dP/dT_{max}, and these are listed in Table 30-2 along with their suggested mechanism of action and duration of activity.

Labetalol remains the first choice in antihypertensive agents for aortic dissections. It is a selective α_1 nonselective β_1- and β_2-adrenoreceptor blocker, and so reduces dP/dT_{max} and systolic blood pressure by β-blockade and vasodilation. It can be delivered by bolus (as preferred by most authors) or continuous infusion, even in the ER setting. Its peak reduction in systolic blood pressure occurs within 5 minutes,

TABLE 30-2 Antihypertensive Agents in Acute Aortic Dissection

Drug	Mechanism	Administration (Intravenous)
Labetalol hydrochloride	α_1- And β_{1+2}- adrenergic blocker; decreases peripheral resistance without reflex increase in heart rate and myocardial contractility (dP/dT_{max}); action in 5–10 min; half-life 5–8 h	1. Bolus infusion: 0.25 mg/kg over 2 min; may repeat every 10 min 2. Continuous infusion: 1–2 mg/min
Esmolol hydrochloride	β-Blocker with β_1-selective blockade; decrease in heart rate and myocardial contractility (dP/dT_{max}); action in 2 min; half-life 9–10 min.	1. Bolus infusion: 500 μg/kg over 1 min 2. Continuous infusion: 25–200 μg/kg/min
Sodium nitroprusside	Direct vascular smooth muscle relaxant; decreased peripheral resistance and preload, may increase dP/dT_{max} when used alone; action in 1–2 min; half-life 3–4 min	Continuous infusion: 0.5–8.0 μg/kg per min
Propanolol hydrochloride	β-Adrenergic blocker; decreases myocardial contractility and peripheral resistance; action in 1–2 min; half-life 2–3 h	Bolus infusion: 1–3 mg over 2–3 min; may repeat in 2–3 min
Trimethaphan camsylate	Autonomic ganglion blocker; direct vascular smooth muscle relaxant; decreases peripheral resistance.	Continuous infusion: Begin with 3–4 mg/min

and its duration of action is 2 to 12 hours. It is suitable for long-term control of hypertension in oral form.

Esmolol, an ultra-short-acting β-blocker with β_1-selective adrenergic receptor blockade, is extremely useful for the acute control of hypertension in patients with dissections. Its very rapid onset (decrease in heart rate in less than 2 minutes) and short duration of action (half-life of 9 to 10 minutes) allow for tight control of blood pressure, especially in labile patents.

If labetalol and esmolol are not available, then sodium nitroprusside and propranolol hydrochloride may be used. Propranolol must be given because nitroprusside increases dP/dT_{max} through a sympathetic reflex from its peripheral vasodilatory effects when used alone.

Patients who cannot tolerate β-blockade (e.g., those with severe asthma, decompensated congestive heart failure, or bradycardia) may be treated with trimethaphan camsylate. In order to adequately reduce the systolic blood pressure, it may be necessary to elevate the head of the bed or dangle the patient's legs over the side of the bed. Occasionally, trimethaphan may need to be combined with reserpine or guanethidine. It has many sympathoplegic side effects and can drop the blood pressure quite precipitously. Tachyphylaxis occurs quickly.

Systolic blood pressure should be reduced to levels that will halt the progression of the dissection. Most authors agree that a systolic blood pressure of 90 to 100 mm Hg is desirable as long as the patient has adequate organ perfusion, as evidenced by a clear sensorium, good urine output, and the absence of lactic acidosis. If respiratory distress occurs that requires high doses of opiates and benzodiazepines, the patient should be intubated by an experienced cardiac anesthesiologist to minimize changes in heart rate and blood pressure.

Definitive Management

Acute aortic dissections, especially type A, are extremely dangerous lesions that may become complicated with rupture and death at any moment. Investigations should be performed expeditiously to determine the dissection type and the presence of aortic branch complications. Patients with type A dissections should be offered urgent surgical intervention for maximal survival. Relative contraindications to surgery include severe organ dysfunction such as diffuse coronary artery disease, end-stage chronic obstructive pulmonary disease, old age (for those over age 80 the risk rises markedly, perhaps as high as 80%),[29] moribund patient, paraplegia, and CVA. Whether an acute CVA represents a contraindication to surgery is controversial. CVA does represent an independent negative influence on survival. Surgery may make the neurologic deficit worse due to intraoperative bleeding from heparinization, embolization, or reperfusion injury when the occluded carotid is reopened. Without surgery, however, these patients have a near uniformly fatal prognosis. It has been shown that the presence of the CVA does not increase the risk of mortality with surgery. Shumway's group[30] found 85% of survivors to be improved or unchanged neurologically, and suggested that there is no way to predict neurologic outcome from the preoperative neurologic status. A CVA is therefore only a relative contraindication to surgery, and only deeply comatose or moribund patients should be refused definitive surgical repair.

Aortic branch complications in type A dissections are best managed by surgically restoring flow to the true lumen by definitive repair of the dissection and postoperative assessment for persistent ischemia.[14] Less than 10% of patients will require further procedures for persistent ischemia after definitive repair of the dissection. Rarely, organ hypoperfusion may continue, necessitating emergent fenestration (creating communication between the true and false lumina) of the abdominal aorta, ideally by an interventional radiologist with cutting balloons.[4]

Type B dissections are generally best managed by intensive medical treatment of blood pressure, with surgery reserved for complications of the disease. These complications are a result of progression of the dissection despite maximal medical therapy. Intervention is recommended if the aorta increases in size or if evidence of organ ischemia due to aortic branch occlusion (e.g., abdominal pain, renal dysfunction, or lower extremity ischemia) exists. Intractable pain, evidence of a new pleural or pericardial effusion, acute saccular aneurysms, or a rapid increase in size over a period of hours indicates impending or frank rupture, and emergent surgical repair (or endovascular stenting if available) is imperative for survival.

This conservative approach has been challenged.[27] The surgical mortality in acute type B dissections was reported to be reduced from 38% to 13% in a small group of patients. This would be an improvement over medical therapy alone, which incurs a 20% mortality. A larger experience is necessary before this aggressive approach is adopted for all type B dissections. Similarly, stent-grafts have been inserted in the acute setting with good early but unsatisfactory long-term results.[4–6]

Surgical Intervention

Dr. Michael DeBakey is credited with the initial surgical successes in the treatment of acute aortic dissections. The procedures can be considered as being separate for type A and type B dissections.

TYPE A

The surgical procedures for type A dissections are designed to treat the life-threatening complications in the ascending aorta. There are many factors that are important for deciding the appropriate surgical procedure for each patient. Many of these can be identified preoperatively, such as the presence of a preexisting abnormality and/or competency of the aortic valve, patency of the coronary arteries, size of the aortic arch, quality of the aortic tissue (e.g., Marfan's or Ehlers-Danlos syndrome), and presence or absence of associated aortic branch compromise (Figs. 30-10 and 30-11). The surgical options include simple graft interposition, resuspension of the aortic valve and graft interposition, replacement of the aortic valve and supra-sinus graft interposition, and valved-conduit graft insertion (Bentall procedure).

General preparation of the patient for the procedure includes continuous monitoring of arterial and central venous pressures and usually insertion of a pulmonary artery catheter and a transesophageal echocardiography probe. The patient is placed on cardiopulmonary bypass (CPB) by inserting the arterial cannula into either a femoral artery (usually the right) or the right axillary artery[31] to leave the ascending aorta and aortic arch clear for surgical repair. Through a

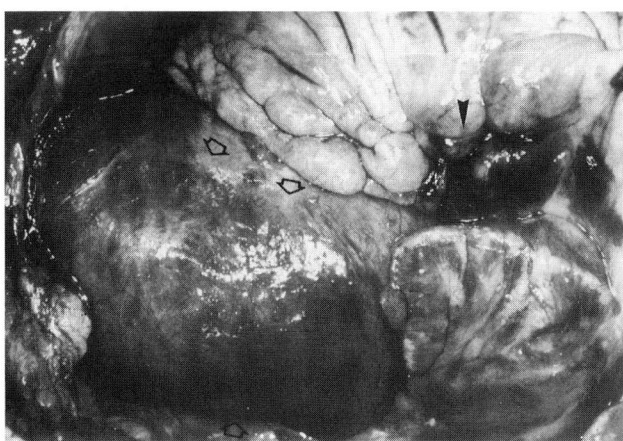

FIGURE 30-10 External appearance of the acutely dissected proximal aorta (*open arrows*). Note the "beefy" appearance as the hematoma spreads down to the origin of the right coronary artery (*solid arrow*), suggesting an ostial injury. (*Reprinted with permission from Borst HG, Heinemann MK, Stone C: Surgical Treatment of Aortic Dissection. New York, Churchill-Livingstone, 1996, p 86.*)

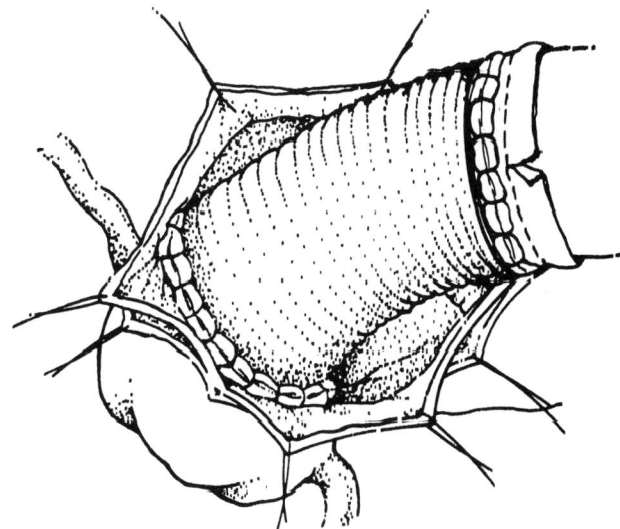

FIGURE 30-12 Suprasinus repair. The ascending aorta is replaced with a Dacron graft. The proximal anastomosis is above the aortic valve, and the suture lines are reinforced with felt strips. The distal anastomosis is proximal to the origin of the innominate artery.

median sternotomy, the patient undergoes continuous CPB and may require hypothermic cardiac arrest or deep hypothermia (15° to 18°C) and total circulatory arrest.[32]

Many surgeons feel it is important to resect the area of the tear in the aorta and thus use total circulatory arrest for all cases, especially for the distal anastomosis when replacing part or all of the aortic arch.[3–1] The time spent with the circulation arrested ideally should be kept to less than 45 minutes to minimize organ dysfunction. The brain is the most sensitive of the body's organs to prolonged circulatory arrest, so several methods have been proposed to improve cerebral protection. Selective antegrade perfusion of the innominate and left carotid arteries, as well as retrograde perfusion by cannulating the superior vena cava are utilized for periods of more prolonged arrest.[33–36]

FIGURE 30-11 Acute proximal aortic dissection opened demonstrating the aortic valve (*Ao*), the inner layer of the aorta (*white arrows*), and the outer layer (*black arrows*). The hematoma (*H*) lies in the false lumen separating them below. (*Reprinted with permission from Borst HG, Heinemann MK, Stone C: Surgical Treatment of Aortic Dissection. New York, Churchill-Livingstone, 1996, p 87.*)

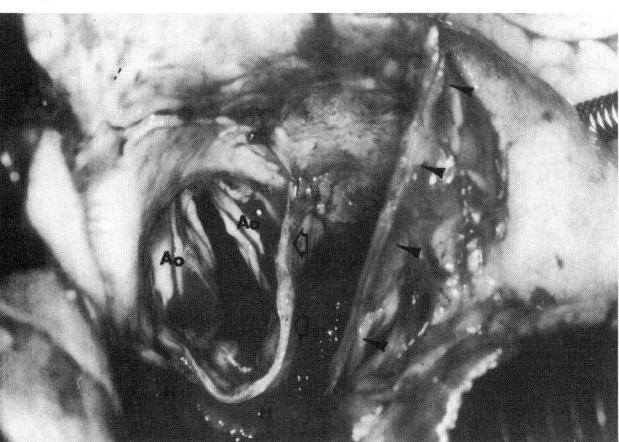

Suprasinus graft interposition is performed for dissections not involving the aortic valve and without gross dilatation of the aortic arch. It involves interposing a woven Dacron tube graft from just above the aortic valve (at the level of the sinotubular junction) to the innominate artery (Fig. 30-12). The aortic wall may be reinforced with fibrin glue and/or felt to increase the strength of these friable tissues.

Resuspension of the aortic valve with suprasinus tube graft replacement of the ascending aorta is indicated for aortic insufficiency in patients without connective tissue abnormalities. The aortic valve commissures are tacked back to the outer wall of the aorta (Fig. 30-13) so as to return the cusps to their normal position and restore competency to the valve. The patient's own aortic valve is preserved and is most often competent.[37] The ascending aorta is then replaced with a tube of Dacron. If the aortic arch is not frankly aneurysmal, the graft is sutured to the distal ascending aorta.

Valved-conduit grafts consist of a prosthetic valve attached to a Dacron tube graft (Fig. 30-14). This procedure was popularized by Bentall and requires replacement of the aortic valve and ascending aorta and insertion of the left and right coronary arteries into the graft. The Bentall procedure is indicated for underlying disease of the aortic wall where there is a high risk of later aneurysmal dilation of the aorta, as in Marfan's or Turner's syndrome and annuloaortic ectasia. It is also indicated for tears arising close to the coronary sinuses or if the native aortic valve is diseased. The prosthetic valve may be either mechanical or bioprosthetic. The most popular mechanical valves are bileaflet such as those made by St. Jude Medical. These are placed primarily in young patients (<60 years old) in whom there are no contraindications to anticoagulation, as they require lifelong warfarin therapy. Older patients or those with contraindications to anticoagulation may have a bioprosthetic-valved conduit inserted, such as the Carpentier-Edwards porcine valve.

Each of these procedures may involve extensive replacement of the aorta to include the aortic arch, in whole or in

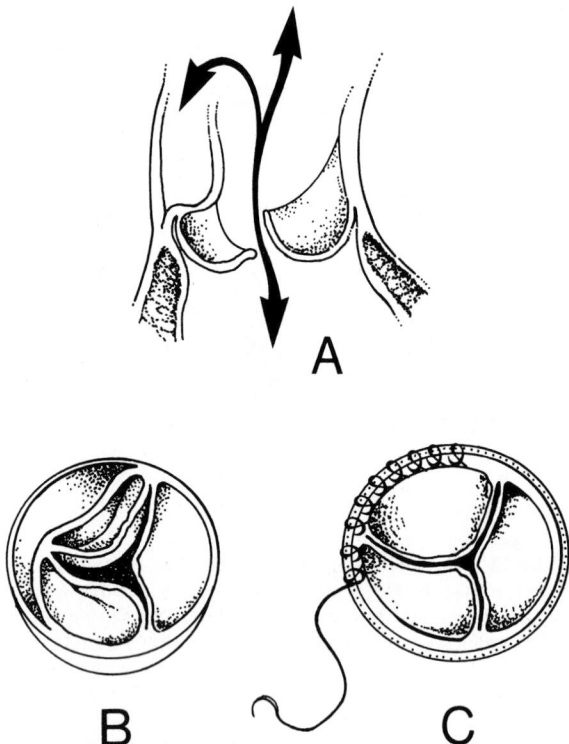

FIGURE 30-13 Resuspension of the aortic valve. *A.* and *B.* **The valve cusps are detached from the aortic wall, resulting in aortic insufficiency.** *C.* **The commissures of the aortic valve are sutured back to the outer wall of the aorta to restore the normal relationships of the valve. The ascending aorta is replaced with a suprasinus graft.**

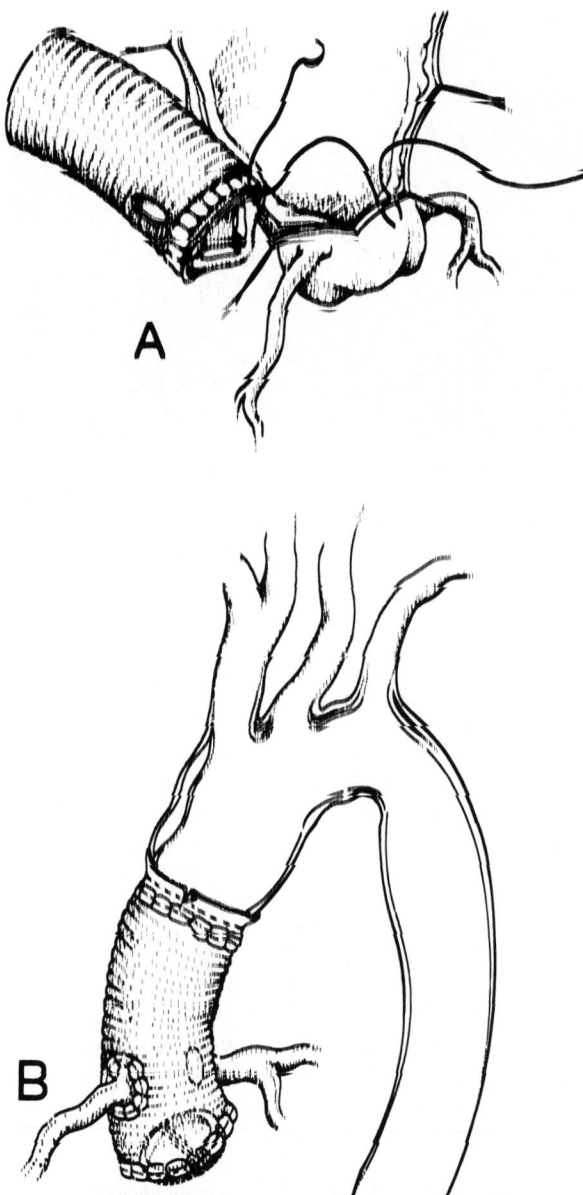

FIGURE 30-14 Composite graft replacement (Bentall). *A.* **The aortic valve is removed and replaced with a valved conduit.** *B.* **The left and right main coronary arteries are reimplanted into the graft.**

part. This adds to the risk of the operative procedure, but if the arch is grossly aneurysmal, freedom from late operation and overall survival are increased significantly with immediate repair.[38]

Rarely, in cases of extensive aneurysmal dissections involving the ascending aorta, arch, and descending portions of the thoracic aorta, an "elephant trunk" technique must be used.[39] This requires replacement of the ascending aorta and the arch with a graft (Fig. 30-15), with the addition of several inches of telescoping redundant graft beyond the distal anastomosis and down the descending aorta. At a later date the patient has the rest of the descending thoracic aorta replaced through a left thoracotomy utilizing the free end of the redundant, previously placed graft. Dr. Lars Svensson of the Cleveland Clinic has a novel and successful approach to these difficult cases, using stent-grafts to manage the descending thoracic portion of the dissection when aneurysmal. After the patient has recovered from the elephant trunk procedure they return to have a stent-graft placed endovascularly from below and attached to the free end of the "trunk," thereby avoiding the difficult and risky thoracic surgical procedure. Of great interest is that Dr. Svensson has utilized this procedure with excellent results for isolated type B dissections in patients who would not tolerate surgical repair.

The resolution of aortic branch complications should be assessed at the end of the procedure. Pulses should be checked over both carotids and the radial and femoral arteries. If concerns exist for the presence of ongoing ischemia, then imme-

diate surgical revascularization should be undertaken. This usually involves an extra-anatomic reconstruction such as axilloaxillary bypass for upper limb ischemia or femorofemoral bypass for unilateral lower limb ischemia. Aortic fenestration is necessary for bilateral lower extremity or renal ischemia. This can be done either surgically, or perhaps preferably by catheter-based techniques in the radiology department. Surgically this involves opening the abdominal aorta and resecting a portion of the inner wall (consisting of intima and part of the media) so as to allow flow through both the true and false lumens to restore blood flow. With the catheter-based technique, catheters are placed up both lumens and a cutting balloon creates the fenestration between the two.[4]

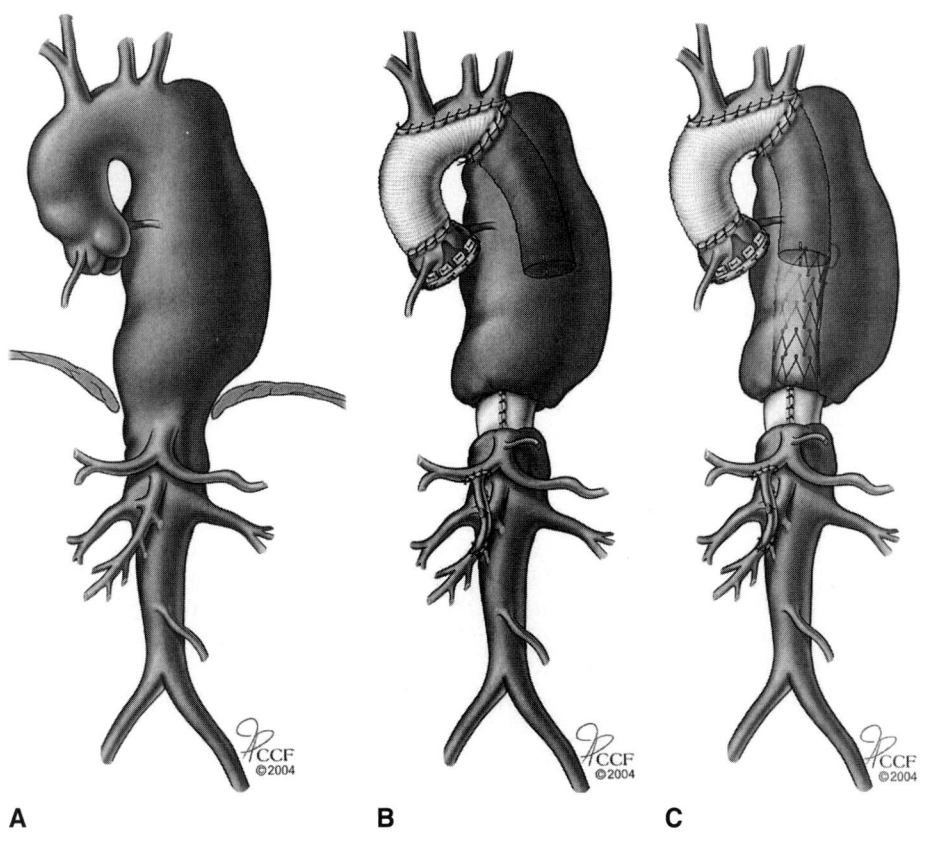

A B C

FIGURE 30-15 "Elephant trunk" procedure with stent-grafting of the descending thoracic aorta. *A.* The entire aorta is aneurysmal, but most notably the arch, descending thoracic, and proximal abdominal aorta. *B.* The aortic valve has been replaced. A suprasinus tube graft replaces the ascending aorta and the entire arch, with the terminal portion of the graft (the "elephant trunk") hanging free in the descending aorta. The abdominal aorta has been narrowed for the stent-graft "landing site." Incidental aortohepatic and aortosuperior mesenteric artery bypasses have been performed. *C.* The nitinol stent-graft has been placed endovascularly from the terminal portion of the elephant trunk to the landing site in the abdominal aorta. *(Reproduced with permission from Dr. Lars Svensson, Cleveland Clinic Foundation, 2004.)*

TYPE B

Repair of dissections involving the descending thoracic aorta is undertaken for failure of medical therapy to control the progress of the dissecting hematoma (i.e., rupture or aneurysm formation) and for aortic branch compromise. Replacement of the descending thoracic aorta is usually nec-essary from the left subclavian artery down to middle or lower thoracic levels (Fig. 30-16). The entire descending thoracic and abdominal aorta may require replacement if it is involved with the dissection and becomes diffusely aneurysmal. This requires the reimplantation of the arteries supplying

FIGURE 30-16 Repair of type B dissection. *A.* The intimal tear is just distal to the left subclavian artery. *B.* The descending aorta is replaced with a Dacron graft with felt reinforcement of the suture lines.

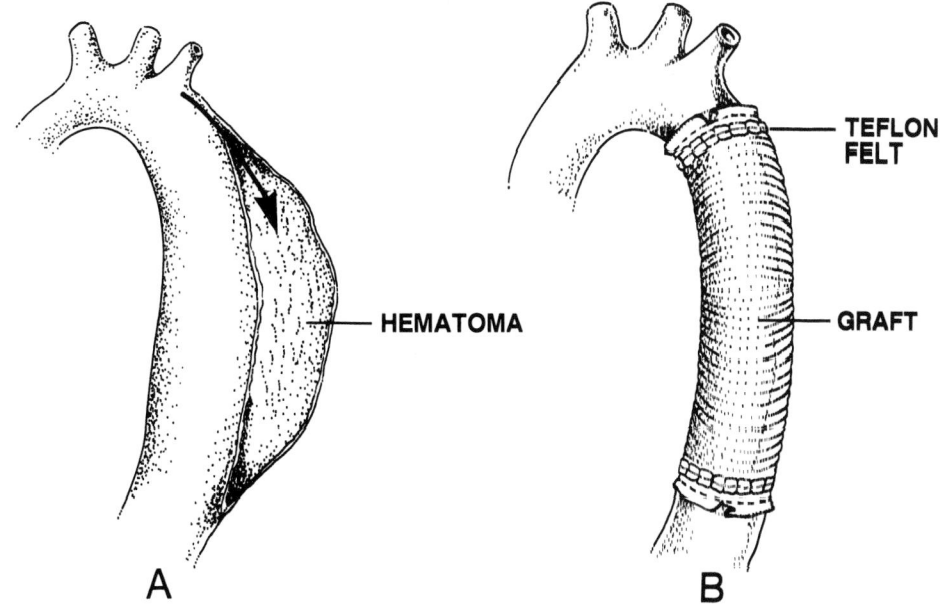

A B

the spinal cord, especially the artery of Adamkiewicz (usually arising between the ninth thoracic and second lumbar segments of the aorta), as well as the neighboring intercostal arteries. Even this does not ensure protection from spinal cord ischemia and resulting paralysis.[40] All renal and visceral vessels must be reimplanted into the graft as well. The surgery is performed through a left thoracotomy or thoracoabdominal incision and requires single-lung anesthesia and cross-clamping of the aorta at the level of the left subclavian artery. The aorta is opened and replaced with a long Dacron tube. Controversy exists as to protection of the spinal cord during aortic cross-clamping. The concern is to maintain blood flow to the distal aorta and so to the collateral vessels to the cord. Although many options exist, the most popular are some form of CPB (using femorofemoral or atriofemoral bypass), intraluminal shunt (Gott), partial drainage of cerebrospinal fluid,[41–43] and the simple clamp-and-sew technique. However, no technique has been shown to be superior to the others in reducing the high risk (~40%) of paraplegia with surgical repair of acute type B dissections.

Stent-grafting of the descending thoracic aorta has been experimented with in both acute and chronic dissections. Between 20% and 40% of patients who survive the acute phase will go on to aneurysm formation within 2 to 5 years, significantly impacting their survival.[44] Aortic stent-graft placement allows for occlusion of the intimal entry tear by implantation of a membrane-covered (Dacron), self-expanding (usually nitinol) stent (see Fig. 30-15C) to initiate progressive thrombus formation within the false lumen and resultant aortic remodeling.[4] Unfortunately, despite good initial procedural success with few complications, long-term results and complications have thus far limited enthusiasm for this approach until marked improvements are made in both the delivery system and the stent-grafts themselves.

Consideration should also be given to the management recommended by Dr. Svensson and illustrated in Fig. 30-15, which combines an elephant trunk procedure with stent-grafting of the descending aorta.

Results

MORBIDITY

Patients undergoing surgical repair of aortic dissections are subject to the same postoperative complications as with any open-heart procedure. Early complications include myocardial infarction, low-output syndrome (systolic BP <90 mm Hg with an elevated pulmonary wedge pressure requiring inotropic support), arrhythmia, bleeding, respiratory complications (prolonged ventilation, atelectasis, and effusion), stroke, and renal failure. Complications specific to repair of type B dissections include paraplegia/paraparesis (up to 40% with rupture), renal and intestinal ischemia, recurrent laryngeal nerve palsy, and chylothorax.[45] Important late complications of both type A and type B dissections include late aneurysm formation and redissection of the aorta. In type B dissections moderate to severe aortic insufficiency is present late in 5% to 20% of patients with insufficiency preoperatively. This is usually well tolerated, with over 80% of these patients not requiring valve replacement at 10 years follow-up.[46]

MORTALITY

Acute type A dissections have an approximate mortality risk of 20% with operation (range = 7% to 35%). The risk is increased with rupture, age >80 years old, and associated illnesses, especially coronary artery diseases and preoperative hemodynamic instability.

Patients with type B dissections survive with medical therapy in 80% of cases. If complications arise requiring surgery, then the mortality increases, reaching 75% if renal and visceral artery occlusion is present.

Follow-Up

Control of the patient's blood pressure and close observation for the development of late aneurysm are the most important variables determining the late complications and survival in type A and B dissections, whether they have undergone surgical repair or not.[2,46,47] The development and rupture of postdissection aneurysms account for 30% of all late deaths. In the postoperative period, the systolic blood pressure is maintained at the lowest level capable of sustaining normal organ function, as indicated by sensorium, urine output, and other parameters. When the patient is transferred to the ward and onto oral antihypertensives, the type and dose must be modified to prevent orthostatic hypotension and syncope. Some form of β-blocker must be used (unless contraindicated) to control dP/dT_{max} as well as systolic pressure. The blood pressure control must be maintained lifelong so as to minimize the risk of late aneurysmal development or redissection.[46] Follow-up must be performed regularly and over the long term, preferably with an easily available and reproducible imaging technique such as CT scanning.[47] New aneurysms form because in 85% of cases the false lumen remains patent, and so the wall of the aorta is permanently weakened. DeBakey's study[48] highlights the importance of long-term hypertension control. Five hundred twenty-seven patients were followed for 20 years after surgical repair of dissections. If hypertension was not controlled, 45.5% developed subsequent aneurysms, compared to 17.4% for those with proper control. Research is ongoing to improve stent-graft delivery and durability to improve long-term survival in these patients.[49,50]

References

1. Sorenson HR, Olsen H: Ruptured and dissecting aneurysms of the aorta: Incidence and prospects of surgery. *Acta Chir Scand* 128:644, 1964.
2. Wheat MW Jr: Acute dissection of the aorta, in Brest A (ed): *Cardiovascular Clinics,* Vol. 17, No. 3. Philadelphia, FA Davis, 1987, p 241.
3. Hirst AE, Gore I: The etiology and pathology of aortic dissection, in Doroghazi RM, Slater EE (eds): *Aortic Dissection.* New York, McGraw-Hill, 1983, p 291.
4. Eggebrecht H, Erbel R, et al: Interventional management of aortic dissection. *Herz* 27:539, 2002.
5. Greenberg RK, Haulon S, Khwaja J, et al: Contemporary management of acute aortic dissection. *J Endovasc Ther* 10:476, 2003.
6. Yada I, Shimono T, Kato N, et al: Transluminal stent-graft

placements for the treatments of acute onset and chronic aortic dissections. *Circulation* 106(Suppl I):I-241, 2002.

7. Sawhney NS, DeMaria AN, Blanchard DG: Aortic intramural hematoma. An increasingly recognized and potentially fatal entity. *Chest* 120:1340, 2001.

8. Sueyoshi E, Matsuoka Y, Sakamoto I, et al: Fate of intramural hematoma of the aorta: CT evaluation. *J Comput Assist Tomogr* 2:931, 1997.

9. Kang D, Song J, Song M, et al: Clinical and echocardiographic outcomes of aortic intramural hemorrhage compared with acute aortic dissection. *Am J Cardiol* 81:202, 1998.

10. Nishigami K, Tsuchiya T, Shono H, et al: Disappearance of aortic intramural hematoma and its significance to the prognosis. *Circulation* 102:III243, 2000.

11. Anagnostopoulos CE, Prabhakar MJ, Kittle CF: Aortic dissection and dissecting aneurysms. *Am J Cardiol* 30:263, 1972.

12. Slater EE: Aortic dissection: Presentation and diagnosis, in Doroghazi RM, Slater EE (eds): *Aortic Dissection*. New York, McGraw-Hill, 1983, p 61.

13. Rosman HS, Patel S, Borzak S, et al: Quality of history taking in patients with aortic dissection. *Chest* 114:793, 1998.

14. Cambria RP, Brewster DC, Gertler J, et al: Vascular complications associated with spontaneous aortic dissection. *J Vasc Surg* 7:199, 1988.

15. Pumphrey CW, Fat T, Weir I: Aortic dissection during pregnancy. *Br Heart J* 55:106, 1986.

16. Hirst AE, Johns VJ, Kime SW: Dissecting aneurysms of the aorta: A review of 505 cases. *Medicine* 37:217, 1958.

17. Heinemann M, Buhner B, Jurmann M, Borst HG: Thoracoabdominal malperfusion in aortic dissection. *J Cardiac Surg* 9:748, 1994.

18. Thorsen MK, San Dretto MA, Lawson TL, et al: Dissecting aortic aneurysms: Accuracy of computed tomographic diagnosis. *Radiology* 148:773, 1983.

19. Herfkens RJ, Silverman JM, Raissi S, et al: Phase-contrast cine MR angiography detection of thoracic aortic dissection. *Int J Card Imaging* 16:461, 2000.

20. Sommer T, Fehske W, Holzknecht N, et al: Aortic dissection: A comparative study of diagnosis with spiral CT, multiplanar transesophageal echocardiography, and MR imaging. *Radiology* 199:347, 1996.

21. Erbel R, Daniel W, Visser C, et al: Echocardiography in diagnosis of aortic dissection. *Lancet* 8636:458, 1989.

22. Pearson AC, Casteloo R, Labovitz AJ: Safety and utility of transesophageal echocardiography in critically ill patients. *Am Heart J* 119:1083, 1990.

23. Hartnell GG: Imaging of aortic aneurysms and dissection: CT and MRI. *J Thorac Imaging* 16:35, 2001.

24. Sommer T, Fehske W, Holzknecht N, et al: Aortic dissection: a comparative study of diagnosis with spiral CT, multiplanar transesophageal echocardiography and MR imaging. *Radiology* 199:347, 1996.

25. Wechsler RJ, Kotler MN, Steiner RM: Multimodality approach to thoracic aortic dissection, in Brest A (ed): *Cardiovascular Clinics*, Vol. 17, No. 1. Philadelphia, FA Davis, 1986, p 385.

26. Nair CK, Khan IA: Clinical, diagnostic and management perspective of aortic dissection. *Chest* 122:311, 2002.

27. Miller DC, Mitchell RS, Oyer PE, et al: Independent determinants of operative mortality for patients with aortic dissections. *Circulation* 70:153, 1984.

28. Estrera AL, Huynh EE, Miller CC III, et al: Is acute type A aortic dissection a true surgical emergency? *Semin Vasc Surg* 25:2, 75, 2002.

29. Neri E, Toscoano T, Massetti M, Capannini G, et al: Operation for acute type A dissection in octogenarians: Is it justified? *J Thorac Cardiovasc Surg* 121:259, 2001.

30. Fann JI, Sarris GE, Miller C, et al: Surgical management of acute dissection complicated by stroke. *Circulation* 80(Suppl I):257, 1989.

31. Bachet J: Acute type A dissection: Can we dramatically reduce the surgical mortality? *Ann Thorac Surg* 73:701, 2002.

32. Graham JM, Stinnett DM: Operative management of acute aortic arch dissection using profound hypothermia and circulatory arrest. *Ann Thorac Surg* 44:192, 1987.

33. Bachet J, Builmet D, Goudot B, et al: Replacement of the transverse aortic arch during emergency operations for type A acute aortic dissections: Report of 26 cases. *J Thorac Cardiovasc Surg* 96:878, 1988.

34. Deville C, Roques X, Fernandez G, et al: Should circulatory arrest with deep hypothermia be revised in aortic arch surgery? *Eur J Cardiothorac Surg* 2:185, 1988.

35. Coselli JS: Retrograde cerebral perfusion via the superior vena cava cannula for aortic arch aneurysm operations. *Ann Thorac Surg* 57:1668, 1994.

36. Bavaria JE, Woo YJ, Hall RA, et al: Circulatory management with retrograde cerebral perfusion for acute type A aortic dissection. *Circulation* 94(Suppl 9):II-173, 1996.

37. Koster JK Jr, Cohn LH, Mee RBB: Late results of operation for acute aortic dissection producing aortic insufficiency. *Ann Thorac Surg* 26:461, 1987.

38. Bachet J: Replacement of the transverse aortic arch during emergency operation or type A acute aortic dissection. *J Thorac Cardiovasc Surg* 98:310, 1989.

39. Crawford ES: Diffuse aneurysmal disease (chronic aortic dissection, Marfan and mega-aorta syndrome) and multiple aneurysms: Treatment by subtotal and total aortic replacement emphasizing elephant trunk technique. *Am Surg* 211:521, 1990.

40. Coselli JS: Thoracoabdominal aneurysms: Experience with 372 patients. *J Cardiac Surg* 9:638, 1994.

41. Crawford ES, Svensson LG, Hess KR, et al: A prospective randomized study of cerebral spinal fluid drainage to prevent paraplegia after high risk surgery on the thoracoabdominal aorta. *J Vasc Surg* 13:36, 1990.

42. Borst HG, Jurmann M, Buhner B, Laas J: Risk of replacement of descending aorta with a standardized left heart bypass technique. *J Thorac Cardiovasc Surg* 107:126, 1994.

43. Safi HJ, Bartoli S, Hess KR, et al: Neurological deficit in patients at high risk with thoracoabdominal aneurysms: The role of cerebral spinal drainage and distal aortic perfusion. *J Vasc Surg* 20:434, 1994.

44. Huynk TT, Porat EE, Miller CC III, et al: The effect of aortic dissection on outcome in descending thoracic and thoracoabdominal aortic aneurysm repair. *Semin Vasc Surg* 15:2, 108, 2002.

45. Jex RK, Schaff HV, Piehler JM, et al: Early and later results following repair of dissections of the descending thoracic aorta. *J Vasc Surg* 3:226, 1986.

46. Mazzucco A, Luciani GB: Aortic insufficiency after surgical repair of acute type A aortic dissection: Incidence, indications for reoperation and medical management. *J Heart Valve Dis* 10:12, 2001.

47. Doroghazi RM, Slater EE, DeSanctis RW, et al: Long-term survival of patients with treated aortic dissection. *J Am Coll Cardiol* 3:1026, 1984.

48. DeBakey ME, McCollum CH, Crawford ES, et al: Dissection and dissecting aneurysms of the aorta: Twenty-year follow-up of five hundred and twenty-seven patients treated surgically. *Surgery* 92:1118, 1982.

PART IV

PULMONARY DISORDERS

Chapter 31

THE PATHOPHYSIOLOGY AND DIFFERENTIAL DIAGNOSIS OF ACUTE RESPIRATORY FAILURE

LAWRENCE D.H. WOOD

KEY POINTS

- *Type I respiratory failure, characterized by severe, oxygen-refractory hypoxemia, is caused by shunting due to airspace filling.*

- *When blood transport of oxygen is inadequate, treatment includes optimizing cardiac output, hemoglobin concentration, and arterial saturation, and lowering oxygen consumption.*

- *Optimizing does not mean maximizing, and the end point of each therapeutic approach needs to be selected for the individual patient.*

- *Type II respiratory failure is characterized by alveolar hypoventilation and increased P_{CO_2}, caused by loss of CNS drive, impaired neuromuscular competence, excessive dead space, or increased mechanical load.*

- *Type III respiratory failure typically occurs in the perioperative period when factors that reduce functional residual capacity combine with causes of increased closing volume to produce progressive atelectasis.*

- *Type IV respiratory failure ensues when the circulation fails and resolves when shock is corrected, as long as one of the other types of respiratory failure has not supervened.*

- *Liberation from mechanical ventilation is enhanced by identifying and correcting the many factors contributing to increased respiratory load and decreased neuromuscular competence.*

Respiratory failure (RF) is diagnosed when the patient loses the ability to ventilate adequately or to provide sufficient oxygen to the blood and systemic organs. Urgent resuscitation of the patient requires airway control, ventilator management, and stabilization of the circulation, while effective ongoing care for the patient with RF necessitates a differential diagnosis and therapeutic plan derived from an informed clinical and laboratory examination supplemented by the results of special ICU interventions. Recent advances in ICU management and monitoring technology facilitate early detection of the pathophysiology of vital functions, with the potential for prevention and early titration of therapy for the patient's continual improvement. The purpose of this chapter is to provide an informed, practical approach to integrating established concepts of pathophysiology with conventional clinical skills. This chapter does not provide a course in pulmonary physiology nor a comprehensive review of how to treat respiratory failure. Rather, it attempts to provide a conceptual framework of principles useful in approaching the patient with RF, first by discussing an approach to tissue hypoxia, and then by describing the mechanisms causing four types of RF, showing how correcting each derangement allows the patient to resume spontaneous breathing effected by respiratory muscles that are not fatigued.

An Approach to Inadequate Blood Transport of Oxygen

Patients with RF are susceptible to anaerobic metabolism, either because they deliver inadequate O_2 to their systemic organs or because their tissues develop an abnormal inability to extract oxygen from the blood.[1] During air breathing, arterialized blood leaves the normal alveoli with a partial pressure of oxygen (Pa_{O_2}) of about 100 mm Hg. When the hemoglobin concentration is 15 g%, arterial O_2 content (Ca_{O_2}) is about 20 mL per 100 mL blood on the fully saturated hemoglobin and about 0.3 mL in physical solution. Accordingly, a cardiac output ($\dot{Q}T$) of 5.0 L/min transports approximately 1000 mL/min of O_2 to the tissues (transport of oxygen; $\dot{Q}_{O_2}$). There, tissue metabolism (oxygen consumption; $\dot{V}_{O_2}$) extracts 250 mL/min, so 5.0 L/min of mixed venous blood returns to the lungs with 750 mL/min of O_2, or a mixed venous O_2 content ($C\bar{v}_{O_2}$) of 15 mL per 100 mL blood. Accordingly, the normal extraction fraction [EF $= \dot{V}_{O_2}/\dot{Q}_{O_2} = (Ca_{O_2} - C\bar{v}_{O_2})/Ca_{O_2}$] is 0.25. Because this O_2 content corresponds to 75% O_2 saturation (15/20), mixed venous P_{O_2} ($P\bar{v}_{O_2}$) is 40 mm Hg, as determined by the oxyhemoglobin dissociation curve for normal venous pH, partial pressure of carbon dioxide (P_{CO_2}), and temperature. Figure 31-1 plots the relationships between $\dot{V}_{O_2}$ (left ordinate) and EF (right ordinate) with $\dot{Q}_{O_2}$ (abscissa) using these values normalized to a body size of about 65 kg: $\dot{V}_{O_2}$ is 4 mL/kg per minute and $\dot{Q}_{O_2}$ is 16 mL/kg per minute as plotted on the continuous lines.

In many patients with RF, the O_2 transport to the tissues is reduced by abnormally low cardiac output, hemoglobin, or O_2 saturation. Consider the effects of acute myocardial injury or hypovolemia that reduces $\dot{Q}T$ to 2.5 L/min and $\dot{Q}_{O_2}$ to 8 mL/kg per minute. To maintain the $\dot{V}_{O_2}$ necessary for aerobic metabolism, the tissues must extract 250 mL/min from half the blood flow, so $C\bar{v}_{O_2}$ decreases to 10 mL O_2 per 100 mL blood and EF increases to 0.50. Because this value corresponds to 50% saturation (10/20) of the normal hemoglobin concentration, $P\bar{v}_{O_2}$ is 27 mm Hg. When cardiac output is returned toward normal with vasoactive drug or volume therapy, $P\bar{v}O_2$ rises again. In another patient with normal cardiac output (5 L/min) but severe arterial hypoxemia ($PaO_2 = 40$ mm Hg, O_2 saturation $= 75\%$, $CaO_2 = 15$ mL O_2/100 mL blood), Cv_{O_2} must decrease to 10 mL per 100 mL blood to provide the tissues with 250 mL/min of O_2; again, $P\bar{v}_{O_2}$ decreases to 27 mm Hg. When cardiac output increases in response to hypoxia, $P\bar{v}_{O_2}$ increases again. In a third patient with normal $\dot{Q}T$ and PaO_2 but with reduced concentration of hemoglobin (7.5 g/100 mL blood), CaO_2 is reduced to 10 mL per 100 mL blood. Accordingly, $C\bar{v}_{O_2}$ and $P\bar{v}_{O_2}$ must decrease to 5 mL per 100 mL blood and 27 mm Hg, respectively, to maintain aerobic metabolism, and these venous values increase again with greater cardiac output or hemoglobin concentration. In

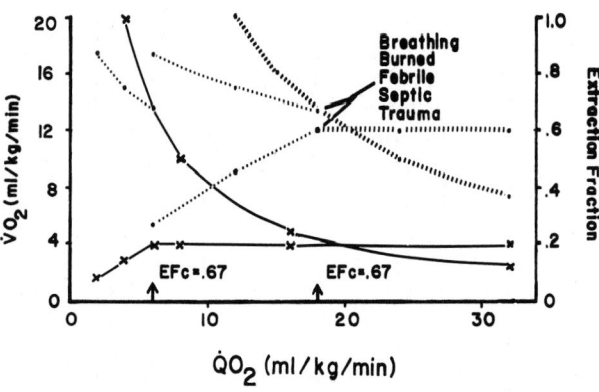

FIGURE 31-1 Oxygen consumption ($\dot{V}_{O_2}$, *left ordinate*) depends on oxygen delivery ($\dot{Q}_{O_2}$, *abscissa*) when low $\dot{Q}_{O_2}$ exceeds the limits of tissue oxygen extraction (EF, *right ordinate*). In patients with normal metabolism ($\dot{V}_{O_2} = 4$ mL/kg per minute), $\dot{V}_{O_2}$ is maintained as $\dot{Q}_{O_2}$ is progressively decreased from 16 to 6 mL/kg per minute (*continuous hyperbolic line drawn through x's*). Below this critical $\dot{Q}_{O_2}$ ($\dot{Q}_{O_2}c$), $\dot{V}_{O_2}$ decreases due to anaerobic metabolism, leading to lactic acidemia because tissue O_2 extraction cannot compensate for the low $\dot{Q}_{O_2}$ indicated by the dotted line departing from continuous hyperbolic EF line at the critical extraction fraction (EF$_c$ = 0.67). When $\dot{V}_{O_2}$ is increased threefold (*dotted lines drawn through closed circles*) by several common manifestations of critical illness (e.g., work of breathing, burns, fever, sepsis, and trauma), EF is tripled at each value of $\dot{Q}_{O_2}$, and supply dependence of O_2 consumption begins at a value of $\dot{Q}_{O_2}$ three times greater than for the patient with normal $\dot{V}_{O_2}$ despite normal EF$_c$ = 0.67. Accordingly, $\dot{Q}_{O_2}$ must increase with $\dot{V}_{O_2}$ to maintain aerobic metabolism, or $\dot{V}_{O_2}$ must be reduced. See text for discussion.

each case, $\dot{V}_{O_2}$ was maintained as $\dot{Q}_{O_2}$ decreased, creating the horizontal continuous line in Fig. 31-1 indicating that V_{O_2} is independent of O_2 delivery in this range; $\dot{V}_{O_2}$ was constant because EF increased in the hyperbolic manner indicated by the continuous line relating EF to $\dot{Q}_{O_2}$.

These considerations illustrate that one end point of reduced O_2 transport in the blood is reduced $P\bar{v}_{O_2}$. Since $P\bar{v}_{O_2}$ approximates the P_{O_2} adjacent to the exchange vessels in the tissues, it is the driving pressure for O_2 diffusion from the capillaries to the metabolizing cells. When $P\bar{v}_{O_2}$ falls too low, insufficient O_2 diffuses to maintain aerobic metabolism, and the cells begin to produce lactic acid as the end point of anaerobic metabolism.[2] This is illustrated in Fig. 31-1 by the decrease in $\dot{V}_{O_2}$ as $\dot{Q}_{O_2}$ is reduced below 6 mL/kg per minute; this supply dependency of V_{O_2} occurs when EF exceeds 0.67 and tissue O_2 extraction can no longer increase along the hyperbolic continuous line relating EF to $\dot{Q}_{O_2}$. Accordingly, reduced $P\bar{v}_{O_2}$ and increased serum lactate (or falling pH with unchanged partial pressure of arterial carbon dioxide [Pa$_{CO2}$]) are indications of tissue hypoxia. This improves with therapy increasing Ca$_{O_2}$ (by increasing hemoglobin or O_2 saturation) and increasing cardiac output. In many critically ill patients, two or three of these factors reducing O_2 transport to the tissues coexist, so attention to optimizing all these ($\dot{Q}$T , hemoglobin concentration, and O_2 saturation) is reasonable in the hypoxic patient. This description of the effects of diminished $\dot{Q}_{O_2}$ on $P\bar{v}_{O_2}$ and hence the utility of $P\bar{v}_{O_2}$ as a monitor of the adequacy of $\dot{Q}_{O_2}$ helps one understand the benefits of early goal-directed

therapy guided by this measurement in the treatment of patients with shock[3] (see Chap. 21).

OPTIMIZING $\dot{Q}_{O_2}$

Of course, optimizing does not mean maximizing, and the end point of each therapeutic approach needs to be selected for the individual patient. Patients with low cardiac output due to heart disease may not tolerate infusions of packed erythrocytes even though their tissue hypoxia is made worse by concurrent anemia. Yet thoughtful integration of packed cells within the therapy of plasma volume reduction is often helpful in such patients and may prevent anaerobic metabolism at a time when cardiac output cannot be increased to adequate levels. In other patients with severe arterial hypoxemia and O_2 desaturation due to acute hypoxemic respiratory failure, tissue hypoxia may be relieved by increasing cardiac output and hematocrit. Yet this is often associated with higher central blood volume and pulmonary vascular pressures that increase pulmonary vascular leakage unless vasoactive drugs, diuretics, and fluid restriction are used concurrently. Again, thoughtful integration of the three approaches to therapy of tissue hypoxia provides the optimal level of circulating hemoglobin and cardiac output while reducing rather than aggravating the pulmonary edema. Some patients with chronic severe anemia (e.g., chronic renal failure) become acutely ill with low cardiac output and/or hypoxemic respiratory failure. Their tissue hypoxia is often ameliorated by prompt, transient increases in their hemoglobin concentration without circulatory overload, as by plasmapheresis. Yet the institution of this therapy, like the others mentioned above, has complications that must be weighed against the likely benefit in that patient at that time. Accordingly, this approach to therapy of reduced blood O_2 transport implements early each of the three major interventions ($\dot{Q}$T , hematocrit, and arterial oxygen saturation [Sa$_{O_2}$]) in a combination best suited to the condition of each patient.[2,3]

Dissolved O_2 contributes a very small amount to $\dot{Q}_{O_2}$. Yet, in critical hypoxemia, raising the fraction of inspired oxygen (F$_{I_{O_2}}$) to maximal values may be effective.[2] Consider again the patient with acute myocardial infarction without lung disease in whom low cardiac output has lowered $P\bar{v}_{O_2}$ to 27 mm Hg during air breathing. Even though the hemoglobin is fully saturated, Ca$_{O_2}$ may be increased by 1.7 mL per 100 mL blood when Pa$_{O_2}$ is increased to 650 mm Hg by ventilation with O_2. Then C$\bar{v}_{O_2}$ increases from 10 to 11.7 mL O_2 per 100 mL blood, raising mixed venous saturations to 58% and $P\bar{v}_{O_2}$ to about 34 mm Hg; of course, if anaerobic metabolism existed before oxygen therapy, C$\bar{v}_{O_2}$ may not increase as much as Ca$_{O_2}$ because $\dot{V}_{O_2}$ increases with oxygen. These changes tend to diminish tissue hypoxia and the adverse consequences of anaerobic metabolism by an amount equivalent to that achieved by a 1 g% increase in hemoglobin or a 0.2 L/min increase in cardiac output and so complement a combined approach to hypoxia.[2] Increasing F$_{I_{O_2}}$ may be effected by nasal prongs to deliver O_2 at 1 to 5 L/min (F$_{I_{O_2}}$ .21 to 0.4), by rebreathing masks (F$_{I_{O_2}}$ .21 to 0.6), or by head tent (F$_{I_{O_2}}$ .21 to 0.8). The ranges of F$_{I_{O_2}}$ are to indicate that all methods frequently give no O_2 enrichment due to inadequate delivery to the patient (lower limit), and that the amount of O_2 delivered is often

TABLE 31-1 Intratracheal Oxygen Concentrations (%) Attained Using Various Delivery Systems

Oxygen Delivery System	Intended F_{IO_2}	TRACHEAL O_2 CONCENTRATION	
		Quiet Breathing	Hyperventilating
Nasal prongs			
3 L/min		22.4	22.7
10 L/min		46.2	30.5
15 L/min		60.9	36.2
Face mask			
10 L/min	60	53.4	41.0
15 L/min	100	68.1	50.2
Venturi mask			
4 L/min	28	24.2	21.4
8 L/min	40	36.4	29.4

SOURCE: Reproduced with permission from Gibson RL, Comer PB, Beckham RW, et al: Actual tracheal concentrations with commonly used oxygen equipment. *Anesthesiology* 44:71, 1976.

less than expected (upper limit), even when the O_2 delivery system is working properly (Table 31-1).

REDUCING $\dot{V}_{O_2}$

With its attendant risks, tracheal intubation ensures delivery of the highest possible F_{IO_2} and allows another approach to therapy of tissue hypoxia, namely to reduce $\dot{V}_{O_2}$ (Table 31-2). Normally, the work of breathing is very low, but in patients with acute hypoxemic respiratory failure and its associated tachypnea and lung stiffness, $\dot{V}_{O_2}$ of the respiratory muscles alone can approach 100mL/min.[4] Increased work of breathing may result in high $\dot{V}_{O_2}$ in other patients with other causes of restriction such as morbid obesity[5] (see Chap. 109). This is illustrated by the interrupted lines in Fig. 31-1 showing that supply dependence of $\dot{V}_{O_2}$ occurs at a high level of $\dot{Q}_{O_2}$ when $\dot{V}_{O_2}$ is tripled (12 mL/kg per minute) by common concomitants of critical illness, even when the tissue ability to extract O_2 is normal. Normally, cardiac output increases with $\dot{V}_{O_2}$, as in exercise, to keep $C\bar{v}_{O_2}$ and $P\bar{v}_{O_2}$ close to their resting values. Yet consider the effects of such work of breathing in the common circumstance of cardiogenic pulmonary edema when cardiac output may not increase much above 5.0 L/min. Then $C\bar{v}_{O_2}$ must fall toward 5 mL O_2 per 100 mL of blood to deliver the total $\dot{V}_{O_2}$ of 750 mL/min so that $P\bar{v}_{O_2}$ approaches 22 mm Hg, a level associated with tissue hypoxia and anaerobic metabolism. Relaxation of the respiratory muscles and

TABLE 31-2 Oxygen Cost ($\dot{V}_{O_2}$) of Breathing and Fever in 20 Critically Ill Patients

Mode	BREATHING (MEAN ± SD; REF. 4) $\dot{V}_{O_2}$	FEVER (MEAN ± SD, REF. 6) Body Temp.	$\dot{V}_{O_2}$
CPAP	255±92	39.4±0.8°C	359±65
AC/MR	209±79	37.0±0.5°C	295±57
$\dot{V}_{O_2}$ resp	46±21	$\dot{V}_{O_2}$/°C	27.5±8.1

NOTE: $\dot{V}_{O_2}$, oxygen consumption (mL/min) by spirometer (Deltatrac); CPAP, continuous positive airway pressure (spontaneous breathing); AC/MR, assist-control mode with muscle relaxation (full mechanical ventilation); $\dot{V}_{O_2}$ resp, O_2 cost of breathing equals CPAP − AC/MR; °C, body temperature in degrees centigrade; $\dot{V}_{O_2}$/°C, the change in $\dot{V}_{O_2}$ per °C change in body temperature.

positive pressure ventilation reduce $\dot{V}_{O_2}$ to 250 mL/min and raise $P\bar{v}_{O_2}$ to normal with no change in cardiac output.[4]

Another effect on tissue hypoxia in patients already ventilated is to reduce $\dot{V}_{O_2}$ by cooling the febrile hypoxic patient.[6] Consider the patient with pneumonia causing Pa_{O_2} of 40 mm Hg (Ca_{O_2} = 15 mL%). Then reduction of $\dot{V}_{O_2}$ from 500 to 250 mL/min by sedation, muscle relaxation, and cooling from 40° to 37°C raises $C\bar{v}_{O_2}$ from 5 to 10 mL O_2 per 100 mL of blood. This increase in mixed venous saturation from 25% to 50% would increase $P\bar{v}_{O_2}$ from 22 to 27 mm Hg in normothermic blood. The left shift of the oxyhemoglobin dissociation curve between 40° and 37°C does not limit oxygen extraction in canine studies of the limits of aerobic metabolism,[7] so cooling the febrile patient may be enough to relieve tissue hypoxia in critical situations.

DETECTING ANAEROBIC METABOLISM IN RESPIRATORY FAILURE

To illustrate how several clinical interventions have a beneficial effect on tissue hypoxia, this discussion emphasized how $P\bar{v}_{O_2}$ tracks the changes in $\dot{Q}_{O_2}$. Yet the value of $P\bar{v}_{O_2}$ at the onset of anaerobic metabolism might vary widely as a result of the $\dot{Q}_{O_2}/\dot{V}_{O_2}$ variance among peripheral tissues.[8,9] This is especially true in the septic patient when very high $\dot{Q}_T$ and $\dot{Q}_{O_2}$ are associated with very high values of $P\bar{v}_{O_2}$ and lactic acidosis. To the extent that such lactic acidosis arises from anaerobic metabolism, the rise in $P\bar{v}_{O_2}$ with increased $\dot{Q}_{O_2}$ in the septic patient confounds the utility of $P\bar{v}_{O_2}$ as a marker of tissue hypoxia. Furthermore, lactic acidosis at high levels of oxygen transport does not necessarily signal pathologic supply dependence of oxygen utilization; rather, the high O_2 demands of critical illness may exceed even normal extraction limits from the apparently high but insufficient O_2 transport.[1] An important observation complicating this problem is that lactic acidosis when $\dot{Q}_{O_2}$ is high does not necessarily indicate anaerobic metabolism, but instead accelerated aerobic glycolysis associated with sepsis-related disturbance of important glycolytic enzymes.[10,11] Clinical and experimental studies demonstrate that progressive reduction in $\dot{Q}_{O_2}$ due to hypovolemic or cardiogenic shock is associated with lactic acidemia having a high lactate-to-pyruvate ratio (L/P); yet, in septic shock, the frequently observed lactic acidemia, even at high levels of $\dot{Q}_{O_2}$, is not associated with an increased L/P ratio, for the pyruvate levels have risen in proportion to the lactate levels.[12] These observations raise the possibility that metabolic utilization of tissue protein stores in septic shock produces abundant pyruvate in excess of that required for generation of high-energy adenosine triphosphate (ATP) bonds through aerobic glycolysis; then excess pyruvate circulates in normal equilibrium with excess lactate, and clinicians mistake this lactic acidosis for anaerobic metabolism. To the extent that pathologic supply dependence does not occur in patients,[13,14] and that the lactic acidosis of sepsis is not anaerobic, the critical care practice of maximizing cardiac output and $\dot{Q}_{O_2}$ confers no benefit on oxygen utilization. Even in the apparent absence of sepsis, the value of $P\bar{v}_{O_2}$ at the onset of anaerobic metabolism varies widely, and some organs may be anaerobic when $P\bar{v}_{O_2}$ and $\dot{Q}_{O_2}$ are not worrisome.[15] Accordingly, measuring and following changes in $P\bar{v}_{O_2}$ and venous saturation in conjunction with acid-base status and lactic acid

TABLE 31-3 Mechanistic Approach to Respiratory Failure

	Type I, Acute Hypoxemic	Type II, Ventilatory	Type III, Perioperative	Type IV, Shock
Mechanism	$\dot{Q}s/\dot{Q}T$	$\dot{V}A$	Atelectasis	Hypoperfusion
Etiology	Airspace flooding	1. CNS drive 2. N-M coupling 3. Work/dead-space	1. FRC 2. CV	1. Cardiogenic 2. Hypovolemic 3. Septic
Clinical Description	1. ARDS 2. Cardiogenic pulmonary edema 3. Pneumonia 4. Alveolar hemorrhage	1. Overdose/CNS injury 2. Myasthenia gravis, polyradiculitis/ALS, botulism/curare 3. Asthma/COPD, pulmonary fibrosis, kyphoscoliosis	1. Supine/obese, ascites/peritonitis, upper abdominal incision, anesthesia 2. Age/smoking, fluid overload, bronchospasm, airway secretions	1. Myocardial infarct, pulmonary hypertension 2. Hemorrhage, dehydration, tamponade 3. Endotoxemia, bacteremia

ABBREVIATIONS: ALS, amyotrophic lateral sclerosis; ARDS, acute respiratory distress syndrome; CNS, central nervous system; COPD, chronic obstructive pulmonary disease; CV, cardiovascular; FRC, functional residual capacity; N-M, neuromuscular; $\dot{Q}s/\dot{Q}T$, intrapulmonary shunt; $\dot{V}A$ alveolar ventilation.

measurements allow deductions concerning the effects of altered $\dot{Q}_{O_2}$ on $\dot{V}_{O_2}$ and aerobic metabolism, but these are nonspecific and subject to errors and uncertainties. It seems reasonable to ensure sufficient $\dot{Q}_{O_2}$ to provide a normal $P\bar{v}_{O_2}$ in septic patients without maximizing $\dot{Q}_{O_2}$ to treat hypothetical tissue O_2 extraction defects,[13,14] except where measurement of organ acidosis demonstrates improvement with increased $\dot{Q}_{O_2}$.[15]

A Mechanistic Approach to Respiratory Failure

HYPOXEMIC VERSUS VENTILATORY FAILURE

A descriptive survey of patients requiring mechanical ventilation for respiratory failure reveals four patterns of pathophysiology, each having a predominant mechanism[1] (Table 31-3). Intrapulmonary shunt ($\dot{Q}s/\dot{Q}T$) causes hypoxemia refractory to O_2 therapy despite hyperventilation and reduced Pa_{O_2} in type I or acute hypoxemic respiratory failure (AHRF).[2,16] Primary failure of alveolar ventilation ($\dot{V}A$) leads to CO_2 retention and arterial hypercapnia associated with reduced Pa_{O_2}; this hypoxemia corrects easily with O_2 therapy in type II or ventilatory failure.[1,2,17] Figure 31-2 illustrates the different mechanisms for these two common abnormalities in pulmonary O_2 exchange.[2]

ABNORMALITIES IN PULMONARY GAS EXCHANGE

It is helpful to recall that the cause of hypocapnia (inadequate $\dot{V}A$) is often independent of the cause of hypoxemia,[1] so the treatment for hypercapnia (raising $\dot{V}A$) is different from the treatment for hypoxemia (raise $F_{I_{O_2}}$, positive end-expiratory pressure [PEEP]). When CNS depression of the drive to breathe or loss of neuromuscular coupling (see Chap. 66) reduces minute ventilation ($\dot{V}E$), the CO_2 produced at rest each minute ($\dot{V}_{CO_2} = 250$ mL/min) is added to the reduced $\dot{V}A$ (normally about 4 L/min), raising the alveolar and arterial partial pressures (P) of CO_2 ($PA_{CO_2} = Pa_{CO_2} = k \times \dot{V}_{CO_2}/\dot{V}A$); recall that the P of a gas in the lungs is the product of the gas fraction (F_g) and the dry barometric pressure ($Pbar2P_{H2O}$), so $PA_{CO_2} =$

$(250/4000) \times 713 \times 0.86$, or about 40 mm Hg. Mild alveolar hypoxia develops as the required oxygen uptake ($\dot{V}_{O_2}$) is absorbed from the reduced $\dot{V}A$ ($PA_{O_2} = PI_{O_2} - Pa_{CO_2}/R$, where $R = \dot{V}_{CO_2}/\dot{V}_{O_2}$), so the consequent arterial hypoxemia is corrected with small increments in inspired oxygen fraction ($F_{I_{O_2}}$). In diseases characterized by airflow obstruction[17-19] or lung restriction,[20] $\dot{V}A$ is reduced despite normal or increased $\dot{V}E$ because the dead space:tidal volume ratio [$V_{DS}/V_T = (Pa_{CO_2} - P_{ECO_2})/Pa_{CO_2}$] is increased when large numbers of poorly perfused alveoli are excessively ventilated (high $\dot{V}A/\dot{Q}$ units). Accordingly, when a patient requires an abnormally large $\dot{V}E$ to maintain a normal Pa_{CO_2}, the causes are an abnormally increased $\dot{V}_{CO_2}$, V_{DS}/V_T, or both. Hypoxemia develops with airflow obstruction or lung restriction when other alveoli are poorly ventilated in relation to their perfusion (low $\dot{V}A/\dot{Q}$ units), and the hypoxemia is made worse by low mixed venous oxygen content[2,17-20] (see Chap. 39); again, modest increments in $F_{I_{O_2}}$ correct this hypoxemia (see Fig. 31-2, panel A). By contrast, even an $F_{I_{O_2}}$ of 1.0 cannot correct the hypoxemia induced by increased $\dot{Q}s/\dot{Q}T$ (see Fig. 31-2, panel B), and this refractory hypoxemia of AHRF is often associated with increased $\dot{V}E$ and $\dot{V}A$ and so decreased Pa_{CO_2}[1] (see Chap. 38).

ABNORMALITIES IN RESPIRATORY MECHANICS

These two classic types of respiratory failure have distinctly different abnormalities in the mechanics of breathing (Fig. 31-3), while they share mechanisms leading to respiratory muscle dysfunction and fatigue.[1] The schematic illustration of the normal respiratory system (see Fig. 31-3A) indicates that spontaneous respiration is effected by the pressure (ΔP) generated by inspiratory muscles to expand the lung and chest wall (ΔV) against their elastance and to cause inspiratory flow ($\dot{V}I$) past the airways resistance (R). When R is increased in acute-on-chronic respiratory failure (ACRF) or in status asthmaticus,[1,22] the ΔP required to breathe often exceeds the strength of the respiratory muscles, resulting in fatigue of the muscles. When such a patient is mechanically ventilated, the peak pressure (Ppeak) generated at the airway opening increases well above the normal value (about 20 cm H_2O in Fig. 31-3B, upper left) to 60 cm H_2O (Fig. 31-3B, lower

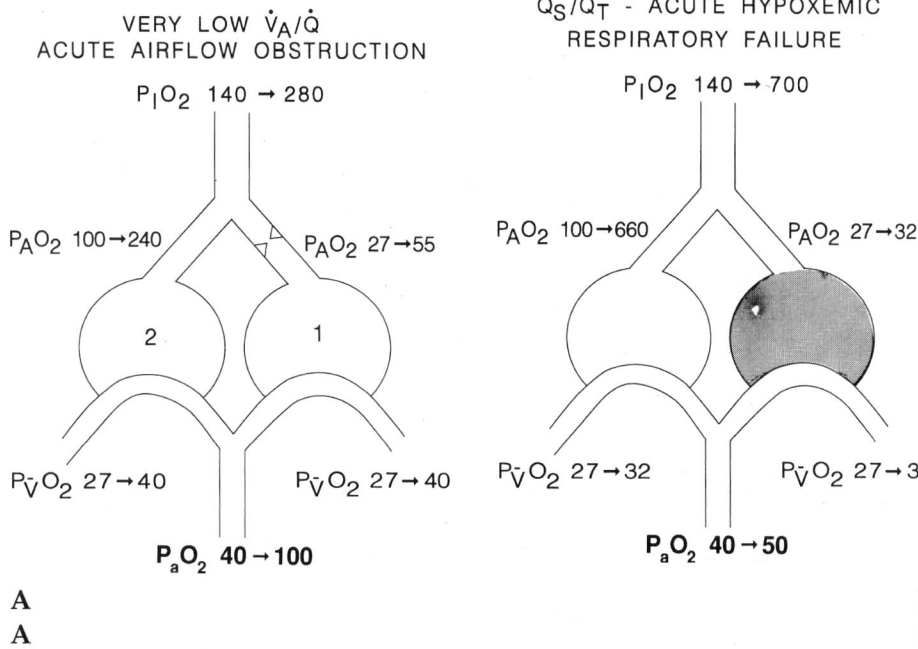

A

A

FIGURE 31-2 Schematic illustration showing the effects of oxygen therapy on arterial P_{O_2} (Pa_{O_2}) in two conditions: (*A*) acute airflow obstruction and (*B*) airspace flooding with acute hypoxemic respiratory failure (AHRF). Each panel depicts a two-compartment lung in which each airspace is perfused by half the mixed venous blood with a P_{O_2} ($P\bar{v}_{O_2}$) of 27 mm Hg while breathing room air, which has a fractional concentration of oxygen in the inspired gas ($F_{I_{O_2}}$) of 0.21. Acute airflow obstruction causes severe hypoxemia that is relatively easily corrected by breathing supplementary oxygen, but hypoxemia in AHRF is much more refractory to oxygen administration and so requires adjunctive therapies. *A*. Because the airspace distal to the obstruction is so poorly ventilated, all its inspired oxygen is absorbed and alveolar P_{O_2} values (PA_{O_2}) approach mixed venous P_{O_2} values (27 mm Hg). By contrast, because alveolar P_{O_2} in the well-ventilated alveolus is considerably higher (100 mm Hg), its effluent blood becomes fully saturated (oxygen saturation [S_{O_2}] = 100%); when this blood mixes with an equal amount of effluent blood from the obstructed unit (S_{O_2} = 50%), the resulting arterial blood (Sa_{O_2} = 75%) has a

B

B

very low P_{O_2} (40 mm Hg). Raising $F_{I_{O_2}}$ to 0.4 (P_{O_2} = 280 mm Hg) increases both the amount of oxygen ventilating the obstructed unit and the alveolar P_{O_2} (55 mm Hg). Accordingly, effluent blood from the obstructed airspace (S_{O_2} = 90%) mixes with fully saturated blood from the well-ventilated alveolus, which also contains more dissolved oxygen, causing arterial S_{O_2} to approach 100% and arterial P_{O_2} to approach 100 mm Hg. Note that this increased arterial oxygen transport is associated with increased mixed venous P_{O_2} (27 to 40 mm Hg). *B*. During room air breathing, the oxygen exchange is as described in *A*, because half the mixed venous blood traverses the flooded airspace from which no oxygen can be absorbed; accordingly, arterial P_{O_2} is 40 mm Hg and mixed venous P_{O_2} is 27 mm Hg. Raising $F_{I_{O_2}}$ to 1.0 increases the dissolved oxygen content in the fully saturated blood exiting the well-ventilated alveolus by about 2 mL/dL (because alveolar P_{O_2} increases from 100 to 660 mm Hg), but oxygen is still not absorbed from the flooded airspace. Accordingly, arterial P_{O_2} increases slightly (40 to 50 mm Hg), and the increased O_2 delivery allows mixed venous P_{O_2} to increase slightly (27 to 32 mm Hg).

right); yet end-inspiratory occlusion allows the airway pressure to return to the normal elastic pressure (Pel = 10 cm H_2O in these same panels), confirming that the resistive pressure (Pr = Ppeak − Pel) has increased fivefold from the normal Pr value of 10 cm H_2O. By contrast, when airspaces become flooded with edema, pus, or blood in AHRF, the tidal volume is delivered to a smaller number of aerated alveoli, overdistending them to increase Pel and Ppeak.[1,23,24] In the lower left panel of Fig. 31-3B, Ppeak is increased to 60 cm H_2O because end-inspiratory occlusion pressure has increased to 50 cm H_2O; in this instance of increased elastance, Pr (Ppeak − Pel) is normal. This large increase in the ventilator pressure mirrors the increased load on the respiratory muscles during spontaneous breathing; combined with the tachypnea, O_2 desaturation, and acidosis in AHRF, this leads to respiratory muscle fatigue.[1,21,23,24]

CLINICAL PRESENTATION AND TREATMENT GOALS

These mechanical and lung gas-exchange distinctions between AHRF and ventilatory failure are paralleled by sub-

stantial differences in the clinical description and presentation of patients with type I and type II respiratory failure (Table 31-3). In the second type, decreased $\dot{V}_A$ is caused by reduced drive to breathe (e.g., drug overdoses or head injuries), or by reduced coupling of the adequate or increased drive to breathe to the respiratory muscles (e.g., myasthenia gravis, Guillain-Barré syndrome, amyotrophic lateral sclerosis, botulism, or muscle-relaxing drugs); often the clinical and radiologic examinations of the chest are normal in these patients (see Chap. 66). Alveolar hypoventilation also occurs commonly in respiratory diseases characterized by airflow obstruction and wasted ventilation; Pa_{CO2} increases despite increased CNS drive to breathe, adequate neuromuscular coupling, and increased total ventilation (e.g., status asthmaticus, ACRF, or restrictive pulmonary disease). Wheezing, accessory muscle use, and hyperinflated lungs are common clinical and radiologic features in ACRF and asthma[17,18,25,26] (see Chaps. 39 and 40), while crackles and typical interstitial shadows without consolidated airspaces are observed in patients with RF due to pulmonary fibrosis.[20] The clinical

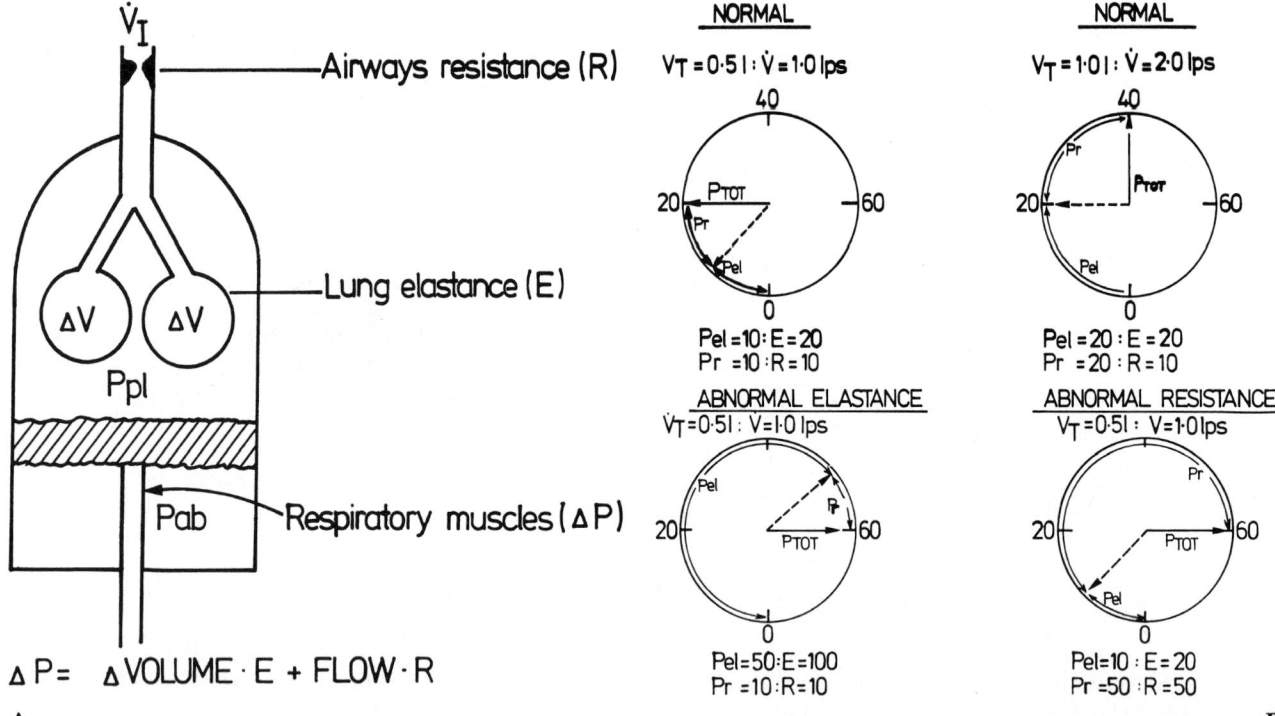

$$\Delta P = \Delta VOLUME \cdot E + FLOW \cdot R$$

A

B

FIGURE 31-3 *A.* Schematic depicts the mechanical characteristics of the respiratory system. Inspiratory flow ($\dot{V}_I$) is delivered through an airway with resistance (R) to a two-compartment lung model, the units of which have elastance (E) and are distended by the delivered volume (V). During positive pressure ventilation, lung distention raises the pressure between the lungs and chest wall (pleural pressure; Ppl) to increase the volume of the chest wall, in part by pushing the diaphragm downward (see piston at the floor of the thorax) to raise the abdominal pressure (Pab); during a spontaneous breath, the respiratory muscles (P) pull the piston down to lower Ppl and inspire V across R. In either case, ΔP = the elastic pressure (Pel = V x E) plus the resistive pressure (Pr = $\dot{V}_I$ x R). *B.* Schematic of the pressure dial on a mechanical ventilator illustrating the measurement of respiratory elastic pressure (Pel) and resistive pressures (Pr) and a calculation of E and R. The upper panels illustrate normal respiratory mechanics for a normal tidal volume and flow rate (*left*) and for a large tidal volume and flow rate (*right*). The lower panels illustrate abnormal elastance (*left*) and abnormal resistance (*right*). See text for discussion.

presentation of each of these categories of hypoventilating patients contrasts markedly with that of patients presenting with type I AHRF, where cyanosis, tachypnea, and refractory hypoxemia lead to early identification of airspace flooding by physical and radiologic examinations[3] (see Chap. 38). The differential diagnosis of the airspace flooding leading to $\dot{Q}s/\dot{Q}_T$ includes cardiogenic or permeability pulmonary edema,[27] pneumonia, and lung hemorrhage,[28] each having specific etiologies and therapy.

While specific diagnostic and treatment plans are being implemented, goals of supportive therapy for types I and II RF are quite different. Therapy for patients with AHRF includes four objectives: (1) stabilization of the patient on the ventilator with minimal respiratory work, (2) ventilation with the least tidal volume providing adequate CO_2 elimination, (3) addition of the least amount of PEEP effecting 90% saturation of an adequate circulating hemoglobin on a nontoxic F_{IO_2}, and (4) cardiovascular management to reduce airspace edema by seeking the lowest pulmonary vascular pressures compatible with an adequate cardiac output and oxygen transport to the peripheral tissues (see Chap. 38 for further discussion). Each of these goals of management of type I AHRF differs from the goals of management of type II ventilatory failure, where the patients with depressed CNS drive or reduced neuromuscular coupling receive adequate ventilation and require

minimal oxygen supplementation with careful attention to preventing atelectasis and correcting hypoperfusion until the abnormal neurologic condition resolves; the patients requiring ventilation for airflow obstruction are supported with bronchodilator therapy and ventilator settings that minimize intrinsic PEEP until the airways resistance is reduced sufficiently for the respiratory muscles to achieve adequate ventilation independent from the ventilator (see Chaps. 39 and 40 for further discussion). One reason for identifying the causes of increased respiratory load is to view liberation from mechanical ventilation for patients with type I or type II RF as the mirror image of the cause of RF (i.e., a systematic approach to reverse factors increasing the respiratory load and decreasing the respiratory muscle strength) (Table 31-4).

PERIOPERATIVE RESPIRATORY FAILURE

The physician frequently encounters patients in the perioperative period who are unusually susceptible to atelectasis as a primary mechanism causing type III or perioperative respiratory failure.[29,30] In general, abnormal abdominal mechanics reduce the end-expired lung volume ($\downarrow$FRC)[31–33] below the increased closing volume ($\uparrow$CV) in these patients,[31,34,35] leading to progressive collapse of dependent lung units (see Table 31-3). The end result can be type I AHRF, or type II ventilatory RF, or both. Yet identification of atelectasis as a distinct

TABLE 31-4 Liberation of the Patient from Mechanical Ventilation

Type I: AHRF	Type IV: Shock
Reduce edema production	Hypoperfusion
Enhance edema clearance	Hypotension
Treat pneumonia	Anemia
Drain pleural effusions	Hypoxia
Stabilize chest wall	Sepsis
Least PEEP	Fever
Minimize dead space	Acidosis
	Electrolytes (K^+, Ca^{2+}, Mg^{2+},
Type II; Airflow obstruction	$PO_4{}^{2-}$)
Hypoxemia—give O_2	Protein-calorie nutrition
Reverse sedation	Aminophylline
Bronchodilation	
Clear bronchial secretions	Common confounding
Treat bronchial infection	conditions
Pneumothorax—chest tube	Neuromuscular disease
Fractured ribs—nerve block	Muscle-relaxing drugs
Decrease intrinsic PEEP	Coma, sedation
Allow bicarbonate	Cerebrovascular accident
accumulation	Subclinical status epilepticus
Reduce CO_2 production	Hypothyroidism
	Phrenic nerve paralysis
Type III: Perioperative	
respiratory failure	Respiratory muscle fatigue
Posturize and pummel	
Ventilate 45° upright	Respiratory muscle exercise
Treat incisional/abdominal	program
pain	Tone
Drain ascites	Power
Re-expand atelectasis early	Coordination
Stop smoking 6 weeks	Animation
preoperatively	
Avoid overhydration	

ABBREVIATIONS: AHRF, acute hypoxemic respiratory failure; PEEP, positive end-expiratory pressure.

mechanism leading to this third type of respiratory failure can be harnessed to prevent lung collapse by reducing the adverse effects of common clinical circumstances promoting reduction in FRC, and of those conditions promoting abnormal airways closure at increased lung volume. Because many of these mechanisms are shared by patients with type I or type II respiratory failure, implementation of approaches to minimize atelectasis should be a part of the management of all patients with respiratory failure.

The principles of preventing or reversing type III perioperative respiratory failure are listed in Table 31-4. Bedside nurses in the ICU turn the patient every 1 to 2 hours from the supine position to the left or right lateral decubitus position; during this time, they provide vigorous chest physiotherapy with pummeling, chest vibration, and endotracheal suction. In patients vulnerable to atelectasis, a fourth position 30° to 45° upright is helpful by reducing the load imposed by the abdomen; also, the addition of sighs, continuous positive airway pressure (CPAP), or PEEP returns the end-expired lung volume to a position above the patient's closing volume.[34] Special attention to the treatment of incisional or abdominal pain (e.g., epidural anesthesia or transcutaneous electrical nerve stimulation) and to minimization of the intra-abdominal pressure of ascites or tight bandages helps to prevent atelectasis.[32,36] When lobe or lung collapse is detected by physical or radiologic examination, an early, aggressive approach to re-expansion includes placing the patient in the lateral decubitus position with the collapsed lobe uppermost for vigorous pummeling and suctioning, and then increasing the tidal volume progressively to a pressure limit of 40 cm H_2O with end inspiratory pauses. Re-expansion often occurs within 10 minutes and is signaled by a fall in the ΔPel associated with the normal tidal volume at the end of the re-expansion maneuver; if this re-expansion is not confirmed radiologically, repeating these maneuvers after bronchoscopy to clear endobronchial obstructions is indicated. Once re-expansion has occurred, the implementation of increased levels of PEEP and/or sighs often prevents further episodes of atelectasis. Discontinuation of smoking at least 6 weeks prior to elective operations reduces bronchorrhea and atelectasis,[37] and avoiding overhydration in perioperative patients especially vulnerable to atelectasis reduces this problem.

HYPOPERFUSION STATES CAUSE TYPE IV RESPIRATORY FAILURE

A significant number of ventilated patients fall outside the categories of type I, II, or III respiratory failure. These are the patients who have been intubated and stabilized with ventilatory support during resuscitation from a hypoperfusion state, so type IV RF is most commonly due to cardiogenic, hypovolemic, or septic shock without associated pulmonary problems (see Chaps. 21 and 46). The appropriate rationale for ventilator therapy in these patients who are frequently tachypneic with erratic respiratory patterns is to stabilize gas exchange and minimize the steal of a limited cardiac output by the working respiratory muscles until the mechanism for the hypoperfusion state is identified and corrected.[21,38,39] Note that liberation from the ventilator of the patient with type IV RF is simple: when shock is corrected, the patient resumes spontaneous breathing and is extubated. Note further that when patients with type I, II, or III RF suffer a concurrent hypoperfusion state, the causes of reduced blood flow, hypotension, anemia, acidosis, and sepsis need identification and correction as part of the liberation process (see Table 31-4). Accordingly, the physician managing RF frequently employs the principles of diagnosis and management of hypoperfusion states, as discussed in the next section.

Respiratory Muscle Exercise and Fatigue in Respiratory Failure

The respiratory muscles share with other major muscle groups of the body the characteristic that excessive work leads to fatigue.[21,40,41] This concept seems to explain why patients with severe airflow obstruction or airspace flooding ultimately stop breathing, and why patients requiring mechanical ventilation for these and other causes of respiratory failure are unable to breathe independent from the ventilator until the load on their respiratory muscles is reduced, the respiratory muscles become stronger, or both. Note, however, that while this is a useful paradigm with which to manage patients with RF, it is exceedingly difficult to identify fatigue under clinical conditions. Nonetheless, as a rough guide, spontaneous ventilation can be sustained indefinitely when the effort of each spontaneous breath is less than one third the maximal respiratory effort achievable.[40,41] In normal patients, the maximum negative inspiratory pressure (MIP) measured at FRC exceeds 100 cm H_2O, whereas the work of spontaneous breathing is less than 10 cm H_2O, providing considerable respiratory muscle reserve before the conditions of fatigue are approached. In contrast, patients with acute respiratory failure frequently have values of MIP <30 cm H_2O, while the load on the respiratory muscles, as measured by the pressure generated by the ventilator during each breath, exceeds 30 cm H_2O.[22–24] Such values predict that the patient's respiratory muscles will fatigue quickly if spontaneous ventilation were required, a hypothesis easily confirmed in such patients who breathe rapidly and insufficiently when taken off the ventilator.[42] Another measure of maximum respiratory effort in the conscious patient is vital capacity (VC). As a rough guideline, when VC is three times the tidal volume (VT) required to maintain eucapnia and normal pH, respiratory muscle fatigue is unlikely. A corresponding alternate measure of respiratory load is the minute ventilation required to maintain normal Pa_{CO_2} and pH. Factors that increase CO_2 production, dead space, or metabolic acidosis necessarily increase this ventilation and so promote respiratory muscle fatigue. Such fatigue is often signaled by increased respiratory rate (RR >35 breaths per minute), by paradoxical respiratory motion (the abdomen moves in with inspiration as the fatigued diaphragm is pulled craniad by the negative pleural pressure), and by the patient's unexplained somnolence or decreased responsiveness.[21,41] Accordingly, evaluation of the patient's ability to resume spontaneous ventilation includes measurements of MIP, VC, VT, RR, and V̇E, as well as direct observation of the respiratory motions during a period of spontaneous breathing[43,44] (see Chap. 44).

RESTING FATIGUED RESPIRATORY MUSCLES

Current evidence and common sense suggest that the treatment for respiratory muscle fatigue is respiratory muscle rest, a strategy that must be balanced in nearly all patients against a thoughtful respiratory exercise program. The timing of the move from respiratory muscle rest to an exercise program is not currently guided by objective criteria identifying fatigue. Accordingly, many physicians confronted with this problem develop empirical guidelines as to the likely presence of respiratory muscle fatigue integrated with the type of early ventilator management necessary for the patient's overall condition. For example, the cardiovascular stability and optimal ventilator management of patients with type I AHRF are frequently enhanced by respiratory muscle rest during the first 6 hours after elective intubation for severe hypoxemia. During this time, the acutely depleted glycogen stores of the resting respiratory muscle are repleted, and the accumulated lactic acid or other metabolites associated with fatigue are washed out;[38,39,45] then the patient is ready to move to a respiratory exercise program. By contrast, the patient with ACRF who has developed respiratory muscle fatigue over a longer period of time may require up to 72 hours of respiratory muscle rest before resuming an exercise program free from fatigue. Note that many patients being managed for respiratory muscle rest by mechanical ventilation are actually working as hard or harder than during spontaneous ventilation by breathing actively against the ventilator.[46] This is easily detected by clinical examination coupled with observation of the airway pressure, which should rise at the start of each ventilated breath.

In many patients, the airway pressure stays at or below zero during inspiration, indicating active inspiration by the patient; the amount and duration of inspiratory effort often can be assessed by the fall in central venous or pulmonary artery pressure with each inspiration. When respiratory rest is indicated, it can be achieved in these circumstances by increasing the inspiratory flow rate, by increasing the minute ventilation, or, if these measures of eliminating the patient's respiratory effort are inadequate, by sedating and paralyzing the patient to ensure respiratory rest.[40]

EXERCISING RESTED RESPIRATORY MUSCLES

As soon as the patient with respiratory failure is stabilized on the ventilator, the physician should make a decision whether to rest the fatigued respiratory muscles or to institute a program of respiratory muscle exercise in those patients in whom fatigue is neither evident nor expected. The objective of the respiratory exercise program is to increase the tone, power, and coordination of the respiratory muscles.[21,47] The efficacy of each program in increasing tone and power is evaluated by the daily MIP and vital capacity measurements. Coordination is evaluated by bedside observation confirming that the patient's respiratory efforts interact with the ventilator in a manner that is comfortable for the patient. Here the goal is to adjust the ventilator such that the patient receives a breath on demand at a volume and frequency within the ranges expected for that patient off the ventilator. Several different modes of ventilation seek to achieve these goals of increased tone, power, and coordination during the liberation process, and each is described in detail in Chaps. 32, 36, and 44.[39]

LIBERATING THE PATIENT FROM MECHANICAL VENTILATION

This aggressive approach attempts to liberate the patients as soon as possible from mechanical ventilation by using the mode as an exercise program. Then ventilator mode becomes a thoughtful part of a larger program addressing about 50 correctable factors constraining the patient's freedom to breathe (Table 31-4). This effective approach to liberating patients from the ventilator measures and attempts to increase the values of MIP and VC while simultaneously measuring and reducing the respiratory load.[47] The left column of Table 31-4 lists correctable factors to reduce the respiratory muscle load. As a general rule, these are the abnormal respiratory mechanics associated with the several types of acute respiratory failure. The right column of Table 31-4 lists correctable factors increasing respiratory muscle strength, first in the context of those many disturbances of the circulation or internal environment most common to patients with type IV respiratory failure. Attempting to liberate patients with hypoperfusion states or hypotension is almost never successful. Correction of these hemodynamic variables complements the correction of anemia, hypoxemia, and acidosis to provide dramatic increases in the objectively measured respiratory muscle strength by MIP and VC. Similarly, attempting to liberate patients who are septic or have body temperatures >38.5°C is often unsuccessful. While these systemic abnormalities are being corrected, it is also helpful to initiate adequate daily protein-calorie nutrition utilizing protein (0.8 g/kg) and nonprotein calories (about 30 kcal/g of protein), of which calories 20% to 50% should be supplied as lipid.[48] Elemental malnutrition is corrected by adjustments of serum potassium, calcium, magnesium, and phosphate levels; severe abnormalities of each of these electrolytes is sufficient to cause respiratory muscle fatigue,[49,50] so modest abnormalities in the patient already weakened by critical illness may converge to make the patient weaker than necessary. When each of these abnormalities has been corrected, there is some evidence that respiratory muscles may be strengthened by the infusion of aminophylline in doses that achieve serum concentrations associated with effective bronchodilation.[51] When all other factors are corrected but the patient remains weak, it is helpful to exclude clinical conditions that occasionally cause reduced respiratory muscle strength. Neuromuscular disease, muscle-relaxing drugs,[52] steroids,[53] sedatives, coma, and intercurrent cerebrovascular accidents cause obscure reductions in respiratory muscle strength. Often overlooked causes of inadequate respiratory muscle function are subclinical status epilepticus, hypothyroidism, and paralysis of the phrenic nerve on one or both sides after cardiac surgery with cold cardioplegia or other thoracic trauma.[47]

References

1. Wood LDH: The respiratory system, in Hall JB, Schmidt GA, Wood LDH (eds): *Principles of Critical Care.* New York, McGraw-Hill, 1992, p 3.

2. Hall JB, Wood LDH: Oxygen therapy in the critically ill patient, in Hall JB, Schmidt GA, Wood LDH (eds): *Principles of Critical Care.* New York: McGraw-Hill, 1992, p 165.

3. Rivers E, Nguyen B, Havstad S, Ressler J, et al: Early goal-directed therapy in the treatment of severe sepsis and septic shock. *N Engl J Med* 345:1368, 2001.

4. Manthous CA, Hall JB, Kushner R, et al: The effect of mechanical ventilation on oxygen consumption in critically ill patients. *Am J Respir Crit Care Med* 151:210, 1995.

5. Kress JP, Pohlman AS, Alverdy J, Hall JB: The impact of morbid obesity on oxygen cost of breathing at rest. *Am J Respir Crit Care Med* 160:883, 1999.

6. Manthous CA, Hall JB, Olson D, et al: Effect of cooling on oxygen consumption in febrile critically ill patients. *Am J Respir Crit Care Med* 151:10, 1995.

7. Schumacker PT, Rowland J, Saltz S, et al: Effects of hyperthermia and hypothermia on oxygen extraction by tissues in hypovolemia. *J Appl Physiol* 63:1246, 1987.

8. Walley KR: Heterogeneity of oxygen delivery impairs oxygen extraction by peripheral tissues: theory. *J Appl Physiol* 81:885, 1996.

9. Schumacker PT, Samsel RW: Analysis of oxygen delivery and uptake relationships in the Krogh tissue model. *J Appl Physiol* 67:1234, 1989.

10. Vary TC: Increased pyruvate dehydrogenase kinase activity in response to sepsis. *Am J Physiol* 260:E669, 1991.

11. Curtis SE, Cain SM: Regional and systemic oxygen deliver/uptake relations and lactate flux in hyperdynamic, endotoxin treated dogs. *Am Rev Respir Dis* 145:348, 1992.

12. Siegel JH, Cerra FB, Coleman B, et al: Physiologic and metabolic correlations in human sepsis. *Surgery* 86:163, 1979.

13. Ronco JJ, Fenwick JC, Wiggs JR, et al: Oxygen consumption is independent of increases in oxygen delivery by dobutamine in septic patients who have normal or increased plasma lactate. *Am Rev Respir Dis* 147:25, 1993.

14. Manthous CA, Schumacker PT, Pohlman A, et al: Absence of supply dependent of oxygen consumption in patients with septic shock. *J Crit Care* 8:203, 1993.

15. Gutierrez G, Bismar H, Dantzker DR, et al: Comparison of gastric intramucosal pH with measures of oxygen transport and consumption in critically ill patients. *Crit Care Med* 20:451, 1992.

16. Dantzker RM: Gas exchange in the adult respiratory distress syndrome. *Clin Chest Med* 3:57, 1982.

17. Wagner P, Dantzker D, Dueck D, et al: Ventilation-perfusion inequality in chronic obstructive pulmonary disease. *J Clin Invest* 59:203, 1977.

18. Torres A, Reyes A, Roca J, et al: Ventilation-perfusion mismatching in chronic obstructive pulmonary disease during ventilator weaning. *Am Rev Respir Dis* 140:1246, 1989.

19. Rodriquez-Roisin R, Ballester E, Roca J, et al: Mechanisms of hypoxemia in patients with status asthmaticus requiring mechanical ventilation. *Am Rev Respir Dis* 139:732, 1989.

20. Agusti AGN, Roca J, Gea J, et al: Mechanisms of gas exchange impairment in idiopathic pulmonary fibrosis. *Am Rev Respir Dis* 143:219, 1991.

21. Roussos C: Respiratory muscle fatigue and ventilatory failure, in Hall JB, Schmidt GA, Wood LDH (eds): *Principles of Critical Care.* New York, McGraw-Hill, 1992, p 1701.

22. Gottfried SB, Rossi A, Higgs BD, et al: Noninvasive determination of respiratory system mechanics during mechanical ventilation for acute respiratory failure. *Am Rev Respir Dis* 131:414, 1985.

23. Ranieri VM, Eissa NT, Corbeil C, et al: Effects of positive end-expiratory pressure on alveolar recruitment and gas exchange in patients with the adult respiratory distress syndrome. *Am Rev Respir Dis* 144:544, 1991.

24. Marini JJ: How to recruit the injured lung. *Minerva Anestiol* 69:193, 2003.

25. Palm KH, Decker WW: Acute exacerbations of chronic obstructive pulmonary disease. *Emerg Med Clin North Am* 21:331, 2003.

26. Rodrigo GJ, Rodrigo C, Hall JB: Acute asthma in adults: a review. *Chest* 125:1081, 2004.

27. Light RB, Mink SN, Wood LDH: The pathophysiology of gas exchange and pulmonary perfusion in pneumococcal lobar pneumonia in dogs. *J Appl Physiol* 50:524, 1981.

28. Rodriguez W, Hanania N, Guy E, Guntupalli J: Pulmonary-renal syndromes in the intensive care unit. *Crit Care Clin* 18:881, 2002.

29. Raju P, Manthous CA: The pathogenesis of respiratory failure: an overview. *Respir Care Clin North Am* 6:195, 2000.

30. Ali J: Special considerations in the surgical patient, in Hall JB, Schmidt GA, Wood LDH (eds): *Principles of Critical Care.* New York, McGraw-Hill, 1998, p 1289.

31. Alexander JL, Horton PW, Millar WT, et al: The effect of upper abdominal surgery on the relationship of airway closing point to end tidal position. *Clin Sci* 43:137, 1972.

32. Ali J, Weisel RD, Layug AB, et al: Consequences of postoperative alterations in respiratory mechanics. *Am J Surg* 128:376, 1974.

33. Ford GT, Whitelaw WA, Rosenal TW, et al: Diaphragm function after upper abdominal surgery in humans. *Am Rev Respir Dis* 127:431, 1983.

34. Craig DB, Wahba WM, Don HF, et al: "Closing volume" and its relationship to gas exchange in seated and supine positions. *J Appl Physiol* 31:717, 1971.

35. Hoeppner VH, Cooper DM, Zamel N, et al: Relationship between elastic recoil and closing volume in smokers and nonsmokers. *Am Rev Respir Dis* 109:81, 1974.

36. Ali J, Yaffe C, Serrette C: The effect of transcutaneous electric nerve simulation on postoperative pain and pulmonary function. *Surgery* 89:507, 1981.

37. Warner MA, Divertie MB, Tinker JH: Preoperative cessation of smoking and pulmonary complications in coronary artery bypass patients. *Anesthesiology* 60:380, 1984.

38. Gottfried SB, Rossi A, Higgs BD, et al: Noninvasive determination of respiratory system mechanics during mechanical ventilation for respiratory failure. *Am Rev Respir Dis* 131:414, 1985.

39. Ward ME, Magder SA, Hussain SNA: Oxygen delivery-independent effect of blood flow on diaphragm fatigue. *Am Rev Respir Dis* 145:1058, 1992.

40. Vassilakopoulos T, Petrof BJ: Ventilator-induced diaphragmatic dysfunction. *Am J Respir Crit Care Med* 169:336, 2004.

41. Respiratory Muscle Fatigue Workshop Group: NHLBI Workshop Summary: Respiratory muscle fatigue. *Am Rev Respir Dis* 142:474, 1990.

42. Mador MJ: Respiratory muscle fatigue and breathing pattern. *Chest* 100:1430, 1991.

43. Jabour ER, Rabil DM, Truwit JD, et al: Evaluation of a new weaning index based on ventilatory endurance and the efficiency of gas exchange. *Am Rev Respir Dis* 144:531, 1991.

44. Yang KL, Tobin MJ: A prospective study of indexes predicting the outcome of trials of weaning from mechanical ventilation. *N Engl J Med* 324:1445, 1991.

45. Viires N, Sillie G, Aubier A, et al: Regional blood flow distribution in dogs during induced hypotension and low cardiac output: Spontaneous breathing versus artificial ventilation. *J Clin Invest* 72:935, 1983.

46. Smith TC, Marini JJ: Impact of PEEP on lung mechanics and work of breathing in severe airflow obstruction. *J Appl Physiol* 65:1488, 1988.

47. MacIntyre NR, Cook DJ, Ely EW, Epstein SK, et al: Evidence based guidelines for weaning and discontinuing ventilatory support: a collective task force facilitated by the American College of Chest Physicians, the American Association for Respiratory Care, and the American College of Critical Care Medicine. *Chest* 120:375S, 2001.

48. Talpers SS, Romberger DJ, Bunce SB, Pingleton SK: Nutritionally associated increased carbon dioxide production. *Chest* 102:551, 1992.

49. Aubier M, Murciano D, Lecocguic Y, et al: Hypophosphatemia-associated respiratory muscle weakness in a general inpatient population. *Am J Med* 84:870, 1988.

50. Dhingra S, Solven F, Wilson A, et al: Hypomagnesemia and respiratory muscle power. *Am Rev Respir Dis* 129:497, 1984.

51. Murciano D, Aubier M, Lecocquic Y, et al: Effects of theophylline on diaphragmatic strength and fatigue in patients with chronic obstructive pulmonary disease. *N Engl J Med* 311:349, 1984.

52. Argov Z: Drug-induced myopathies. *Curr Opin Neurol* 13:541, 2000.

53. Lacomis D, Campellone JV: Critical illness neuromyopathies. *Adv Neurol* 88:325, 2002.

Chapter 32
VENTILATOR WAVEFORMS: CLINICAL INTERPRETATION

GREGORY A. SCHMIDT

KEY POINTS

- *Pressure and flow waveforms reveal a wealth of information regarding the patient's physiologic derangement.*
- *Distinguishing the contributions of resistive and elastic pressures allows tailoring and monitoring of therapy.*
- *Auto-PEEP should be sought in all mechanically ventilated patients.*
- *Ventilator waveforms show how adequately the physician has accommodated the ventilator to the patient.*
- *Patient effort confounds interpretation of pressures and flows.*
- *Attention to ventilator waveforms can improve the accuracy of hemodynamic interpretation.*

Intensive care ventilators generate tidal ventilation by applying to the endotracheal tube or mask a pressure higher than the alveolar pressure. This is true whether the mode of ventilation is volume-preset (volume assist-control ventilation [ACV] and synchronized intermittent mandatory ventilation [SIMV]); pressure-preset (pressure-support ventilation [PSV] and pressure-control ventilation [PCV]); or more complex modes (pressure-regulated volume control [PRVC], proportional assist ventilation [PAV], airway pressure release ventilation [APRV], and volume-support ventilation [VSV]). The capability to display waveforms turns modern ventilators into sophisticated probes of patient respiratory mechanics and of patient-ventilator interaction. Respiratory system mechanics and waveform analysis should be integrated into routine ventilator management of the critically ill patient. The fundamental aims are to (1) determine the nature of the mechanical derangement of the respiratory system; (2) assay the response to therapy; (3) reveal intrinsic positive end-expiratory pressure (auto-PEEP); and (4) determine the patient-ventilator interaction to guide adjustment of ventilator settings. In addition, respiratory muscle activity must be considered when measuring hemodynamic pressures such as the pulmonary artery occlusion pressure (pulmonary wedge pressure, Ppw) or the right atrial pressure (Pra), since these pressures are determined at end-expiration. The time point of end-expiration, as well as the presence of inspiratory and expiratory effort (both of which can greatly confound interpretation of hemodynamic pressures) can be readily discerned by analyzing ventilator waveforms.

It is easiest to derive clinically useful information about the patient's respiratory system when volume-preset modes such as ACV or SIMV are used. At least when the patient is passive, the pressure at the airway opening (Pao) and the pressure vs. time waveform reflect the mechanical properties of the respiratory system, yielding valuable clinical information. During pressure-preset modes, such as PSV and PCV, some information can be derived from the flow vs. time waveform, but this information is generally less readily interpreted than that obtained during volume-preset ventilation. Below we review the determinants of the pressure and flow versus time waveforms during volume-preset, then pressure-preset ventilation, including how to recognize and quantitate auto-PEEP as well as a method for using this information to adjust the ventilator. Volume-pressure loops are reviewed in terms of how they may aid management of the patient with acute lung injury (ALI) or acute respiratory distress syndrome (ARDS). The potentially confounding effect of patient effort on the pressure and flow waveforms is discussed. Finally, examples of problems revealed through careful interpretation of waveforms are presented.

Pressure at the Airway Opening

VOLUME-PRESET MODES

Gas is driven to and from the lung by a pressure difference between alveolus and airway opening. The majority of adult patients are ventilated, at least initially, with a volume-preset mode (i.e., ACV or intermittent mandatory ventilation [IMV]),[1] allowing ready determination of the respiratory system mechanics. When a muscle-relaxed patient is mechanically ventilated at constant inspiratory flow, the inspiratory Pao consists of three components: one to drive gas across the inspiratory resistance, the second to expand the alveoli against the elastic recoil of the lungs and chest wall, and the third equal to the alveolar pressure present before inspiratory flow begins (PEEP or auto-PEEP) (Fig. 32-1).

The contributions of each of these three components can be found by inserting a 0.3- to 0.5-second end-inspiratory pause,[2] briefly stopping flow and allowing the pressure to fall from its peak value (Ppeak) to a plateau pressure (Pplat), in order to quantitate the flow-related pressure, Pres (Pres = Ppeak − Pplat). At any point during passive inspiration, Pao reflects the sum of these three components, as follows:

$$Pao = Pres + Pel + Total\ PEEP\ or$$

$$Pao = Flow_I \times Rrs + \Delta V \times Ers + Total\ PEEP$$

where Pao is the airway opening pressure, Pres is the resistive pressure component, Pel (Pel = Pplat − Total PEEP) is the elastic pressure, Rrs is inspiratory resistance, ΔV is the increment in lung volume, Ers is elastance of the respiratory system, and total PEEP is applied PEEP or auto-PEEP, whichever is higher. Diagnostic and therapeutic information can be gleaned by distinguishing the individual components of the peak Pao (Ppeak) as follows. First, PEEP is set on the ventilator and this value can be used when auto-PEEP is absent. However, auto-PEEP is present in most ventilated critically ill patients,[3] and methods for quantitating it are described below. The Ppeak can be apportioned between its two remaining components, Pres and Pel, by stopping flow (end-inspiratory pause) and allowing the Pres to fall to 0. When flow is 0, Pao drops to a lower Pplat. Then:

$$Pres = Ppeak - Pplat$$

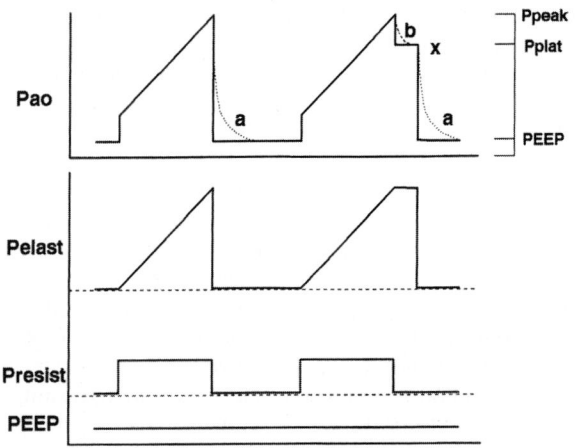

FIGURE 32-1 During constant flow, volume-preset ventilation of a passive patient, Pao is composed of resistive and elastic elements, the latter consisting of the end-expiratory pressure (PEEP or auto-PEEP) and a component proportional to the change in volume and the respiratory system compliance. The second breath includes an inspiratory pause allowing determination of the components of Pao.

The final component (Pel = Pplat − Total PEEP) is proportional to the elastance of the respiratory system and the tidal volume.

At normal inspiratory flow rates in the range of 1 L/s, Pres is typically between 4 and 10 cm H_2O. Elevated Pres is found with high inspiratory flow or increased inspiratory resistance. At constant flow, a rise in Pres may indicate, for example, increased bronchospasm or endotracheal tube obstruction. Conversely, falling Pres may correspond to a response to bronchodilators. Because the Pres depends on ventilator flow rate as well as inspiratory resistance, when interpreting its value one must be careful to take the set flow rate into consideration. The most dramatic example of potential error in this regard is when the inspiratory flow is set to a decelerating profile (Fig. 32-2).

Since Pel = $\Delta V \times$ Ers, elevated Pel indicates excessive tidal volume or increased elastic recoil of the lungs or chest wall, as in pulmonary fibrosis, acute lung injury, or abdominal distention. Respiratory system static compliance (Crs) is the inverse of Ers:

$$Crs = \Delta V / Pel$$

which is normally about 70 mL/cm H_2O. When the tidal volume is a typical 500 mL, Pel should be only about 7 cm H_2O (500 mL/70 mL per cm H_2O). Thus a ventilated healthy patient should have a Ppeak of roughly 17, consisting of Pres (5 cm H_2O), Pel (7 cm H_2O), and applied PEEP (5 cm H_2O). Often the cause of ventilatory failure has not been determined by the time of endotracheal intubation. If the Ppeak is not increased in a passive ventilated patient, the physician should suspect impaired drive, neuromuscular weakness, or a transient, now resolved, problem (e.g., upper airway obstruction bypassed by the endotracheal tube) as the cause for ventilatory failure. When the Ppeak is high, partitioning its components into the resistive pressure (Pres), the elastic pressure (Pel), and PEEP can aid the physician to narrow the differential diagnosis (Fig. 32-3 and Table 32-1).

In addition, such analysis may allow therapy to be tailored specifically to the cause of ventilatory failure. For example, in a patient with COPD and congestive heart failure who fails extubation following colon resection, bronchodilators will not be helpful if Pres is normal and auto-PEEP is 0. Similarly, if auto-PEEP is greatly elevated, measures to decompress the abdomen are not likely to get the patient off of the ventilator.

FIGURE 32-2 This is a passive patient with modest airflow obstruction ventilated with a volume-preset mode and square wave flow (*panel A*) at 60 liters per minute (lpm) or decelerating flow (*panel B*) beginning at 60 lpm. A 0.4-second end-inspiratory pause is set in order to allow determination of Pplat. Notice that there is a significant difference between Ppeak and Pplat (40 to 22) during square wave ventilation, but not during decelerating flow (27 to 22) because flow is so low during the later parts of the breath.

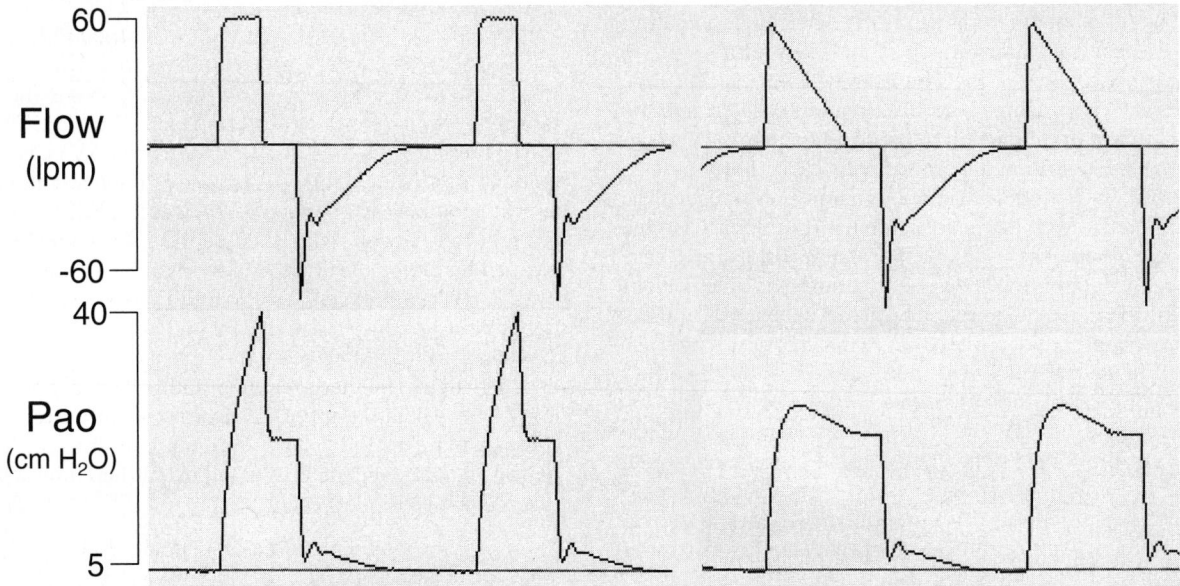

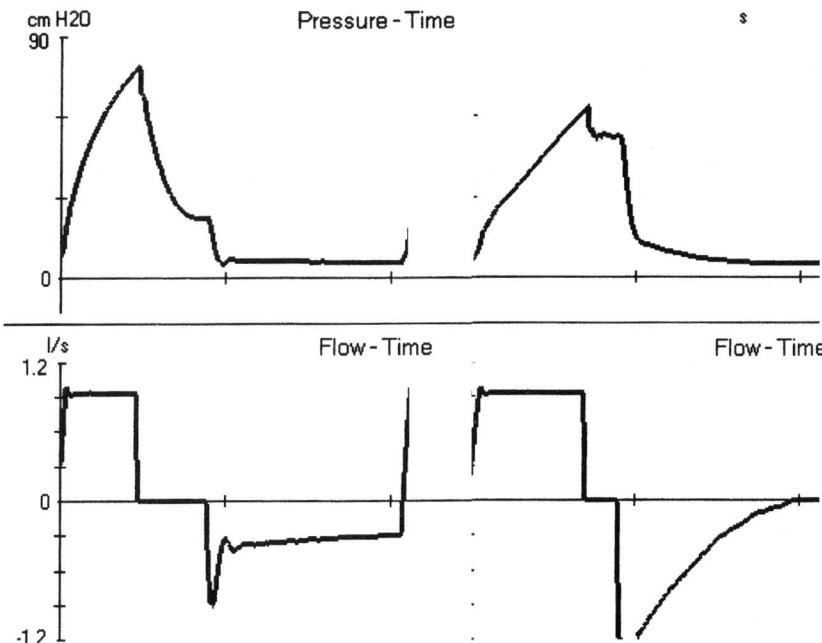

FIGURE 32-3 Both patients have elevated airway pressures. A brief pause inserted at end-inspiration reveals a striking difference between the two records: the left-hand tracing shows that Pao falls dramatically when flow is stopped, indicating elevated Pres (this patient had status asthmaticus); the right-hand tracing shows that Pao falls quite modestly, since Pel is elevated (this patient had a massively distended abdomen and abdominal compartment syndrome). Note also that expiratory flow differs substantially between the two, with low and prolonged expiratory flow in the left-hand tracing.

PRESSURE-PRESET MODES

The inspiratory pressure waveform during pressure-preset modes, such as PSV and PCV, reflects ventilator settings only and reveals nothing about the respiratory system physiology. These waveforms serve mostly to reveal the current ventilator settings as a snapshot (Fig. 32-4) or to demonstrate the impact of certain complex modes on ventilator actions (Fig. 32-5).

EXPIRATORY PRESSURE

During either volume-preset or pressure-preset ventilation, analyzing the expiratory pressure [Paw(ex)] is substantially less useful than the inspiratory pressure, since Paw(ex) is largely determined by characteristics of the mechanical ventilator, not the patient.

$$Paw(ex) = PEEP + Flow_E \times Rexlimb$$

where PEEP is the applied PEEP (not auto-PEEP), $Flow_E$ is expiratory flow rate, and Rexlimb is the resistance of the expiratory limb of the ventilator. It is important to realize that Paw(ex) does not reflect expiratory alveolar pressure or auto-PEEP, and relates to the patient's respiratory system only indirectly through the expiratory flow. Although some ventilators display inspiratory and expiratory pressure-volume plots, only the inspiratory segment gives useful information about the patient.

Flow Waveforms

EXPIRATORY FLOW

Expiratory flow depends largely on patient features, such as end-inspiratory lung volume, lung elastic recoil, and characteristics of the airways, rather than ventilator settings. For this reason, expiratory waveforms can be analyzed without respect to mode of ventilation. Look again at Fig. 32-3. Notice the striking difference in the expiratory flow between these two patients, the first having airflow obstruction, the second restriction.

The most valuable information to come from the expiratory flow tracing is evidence suggesting airflow obstruction, signaled by low or prolonged expiratory flow, often with flow at end-expiration. In addition, there may be two distinct components to the expiratory flow decay, rather a single exponential one (Fig. 32-6), in patients with airflow obstruction.

INSPIRATORY FLOW

PRESSURE-PRESET MODES

It is more difficult to infer the mechanical properties of the respiratory system during pressure-preset ventilation than when

TABLE 32-1 Differential Diagnosis of Elevated Peak Airway Pressure

Increased Pres	Increased Pel	Increased Total PEEP
High flow	High tidal volume	High applied Peep
Bronchospasm	Chest wall	Auto-PEEP
COPD	Kyphoscoliosis	Expiratory limb malfunction
Secretions	Rib deformity	
Kinked or obstructed tubing	Pleural disease	
Airway edema	Obesity	
Airway tumor/mass	Abdominal distention	
Airway foreign body	Lung	
	Interstitial lung disease	
	Lung resection	
	Atelectasis	
	Pulmonary edema	
	Pneumonia	

ABBREVIATIONS: Auto-PEEP; COPD, chronic obstructive pulmonary disease; PEEP, positive end-expiratory pressure; Pel, elastic pressure; Pres, flow-related pressure.

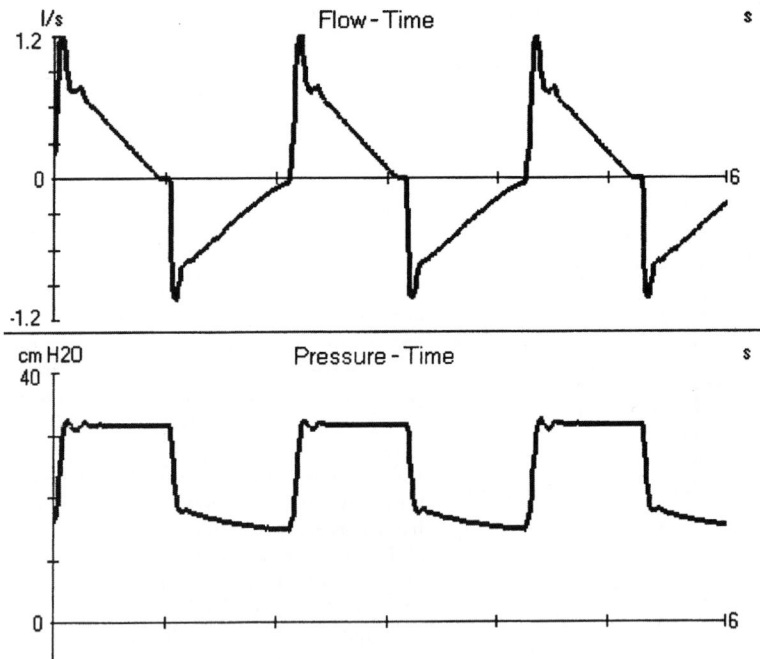

FIGURE 32-4 Flow and pressure waveforms during PCV, showing the typical linear fall in flow through the breath. The pressure tracing merely reflects the ventilator settings as pressure cycles between P_I (32 cm H_2O) and PEEP (14 cm H_2O).

using constant-flow volume-preset ventilation, since the Pao waveform becomes meaningless. Information regarding the combined respiratory resistance and elastance (or time constant) can be gained by examining the slope of the inspiratory flow waveform (Fig. 32-7). Assuming a passive patient, during PCV the flow falls throughout inspiration as the rising alveolar pressure reduces the driving pressure for flow (since the Pao is maintained constant by the ventilator). The rate of fall of the flow is related to how fast Palv rises, itself a function of the mechanical properties of the respiratory system. Because the slope of the flow decay cannot be measured readily at the bedside, and because the information it contains lumps features of elastance and resistance, it may be useful

to turn patients from PCV to ACV periodically to determine the respiratory mechanics.

Flow may or may not terminate before end-expiration depending on the inspiratory time (T_I) and the time constant of the respiratory system (Fig. 32-8). If inspiratory flow terminates in a passive patient, the peak alveolar pressure equals the ventilator inspiratory pressure (P_I). Flow waveform displays facilitate adjustments of T_I and respiratory rate as discussed below.

When patients are breathing spontaneously on PSV, thereby determining their own T_I and rate, waveform analysis aids the identification of patient-ventilator asynchrony. This may be especially important during noninvasive ventilation

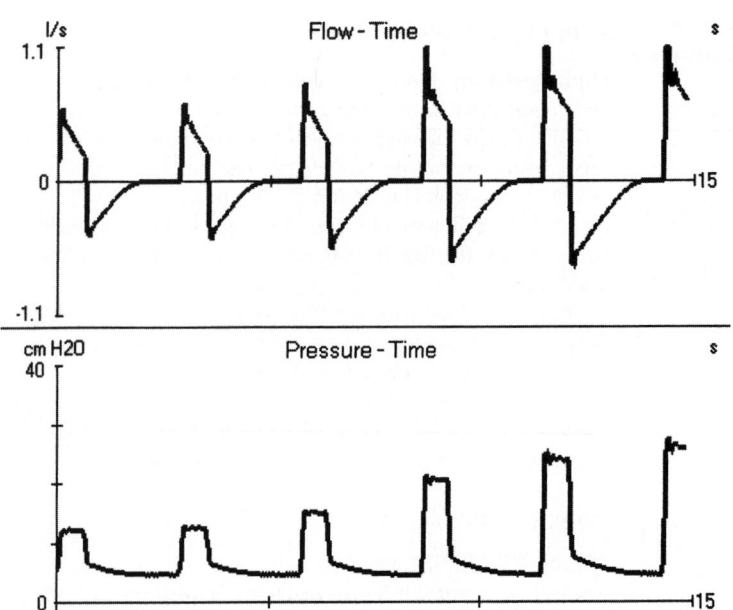

FIGURE 32-5 These waveforms of flow and pressure demonstrate the effect during pressure-regulated volume control mode of increasing the tidal volume. Over the course of several breaths, pressure gradually rises, driving more flow and increasing the tidal volume, until the new target tidal volume is reached.

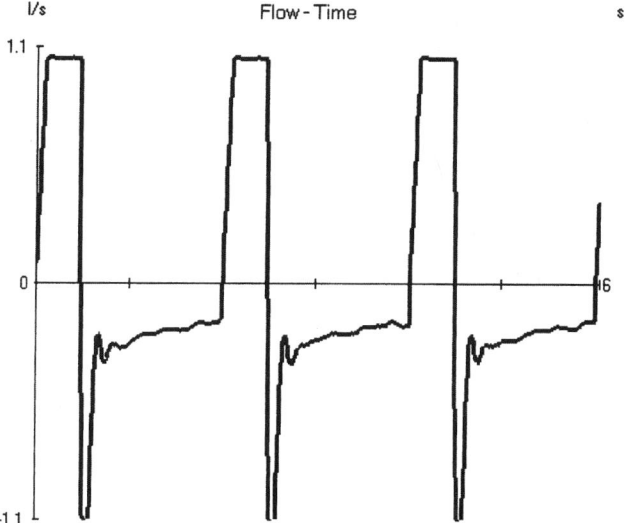

FIGURE 32-6 Flow waveform in a patient with emphysema. The initial expiratory flow is quite high, but quickly falls off to a much lower (and abnormally low) flow rate, persisting until the next breath. These two components reflect initial airway collapse at the onset of expiration (high flow) followed by much lower flow driven by the reduced elastic recoil of the emphysematous lung.

(NIV). Common problems during NIV include failure of the ventilator to recognize the onset of patient inspiration (generally due to auto-PEEP, as described below) and the onset of expiration (most often due to mask leaks).

VOLUME-PRESET MODES

During ACV and SIMV, flow is set by the physician either directly or indirectly through the choice of minute ventilation and rate. Flow may also be altered by changes in rise time, inspiratory plateau, inspiratory:expiratory ratios, and other settings, depending on the particular ventilator in use. Flow waveforms can reveal the effects on flow of other set-

ting changes, as discussed below, and also whether the flow profile (square, decelerating, or sine) has been inadvertently changed.

The Obstructed Patient

CLUES IN THE WAVEFORMS

The waveform indications of increased respiratory resistance are: (1) increased Pres when an end-inspiratory pause has been set; (2) a high shoulder on the early portion of the Pao versus time tracing (Fig. 32-9); (3) low and prolonged expiratory flow, often with persistent flow at end-expiration (see Fig. 32-9); (4) the presence of two components to the expiratory waveform (indicating early airway collapse; see Fig. 32-6); and (5) scooping of the expiratory flow-volume curve (Fig. 32-10).

DETERMINING AUTO-PEEP

The auto-PEEP effect occurs when there is insufficient time for the respiratory system to return to functional residual capacity by end-expiration.[4,5] Short expiratory times, high minute volumes, and increased expiratory resistance contribute to auto-PEEP, but all of these need not be present. Auto-PEEP is present in the majority of ventilated patients with asthma and COPD (and in many during spontaneous breathing[6,7]), but it is also seen in ARDS and other settings with high minute ventilation.[3] In many regards auto-PEEP acts like PEEP to impede venous return, heighten the risk of barotrauma, and improve oxygenation. In addition, auto-PEEP increases the work of breathing and impairs the patient's ability to trigger the ventilator. For these reasons, it is imperative to monitor routinely the presence and amount of auto-PEEP in mechanically ventilated patients.

Auto-PEEP is present when the expiratory flow tracing reveals persistent end-expiratory flow (Fig. 32-11). Additionally, when the Pres is lower than the height of the early step change in the Pao waveform, auto-PEEP is likely to be present.

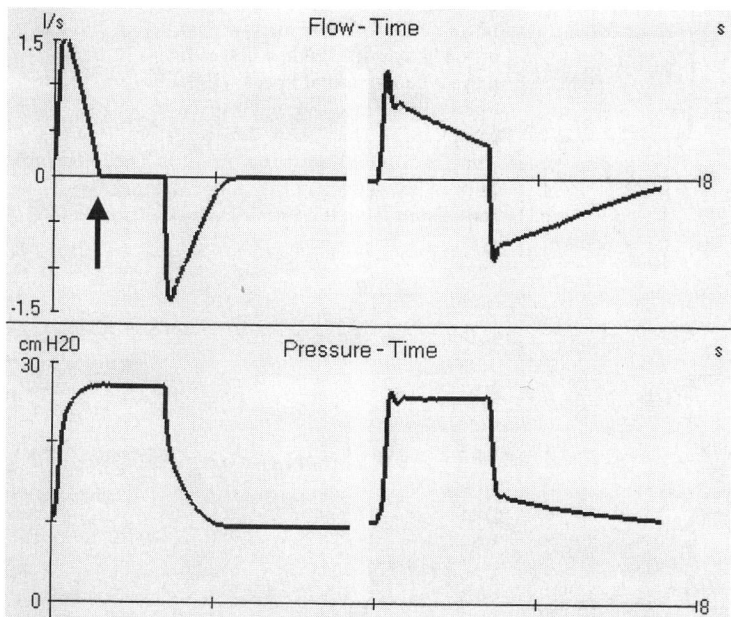

FIGURE 32-7 These two passive patients were ventilated with identical settings on PCV. The patient shown on the left had reduced lung compliance but normal airways, while the patient on the right had normal compliance and increased airways resistance. The slope of the flow waveform reveals these mechanical differences. Note that flow ceases completely in the first patient (*arrow*) well before the ventilator cycles to the expiratory pressure.

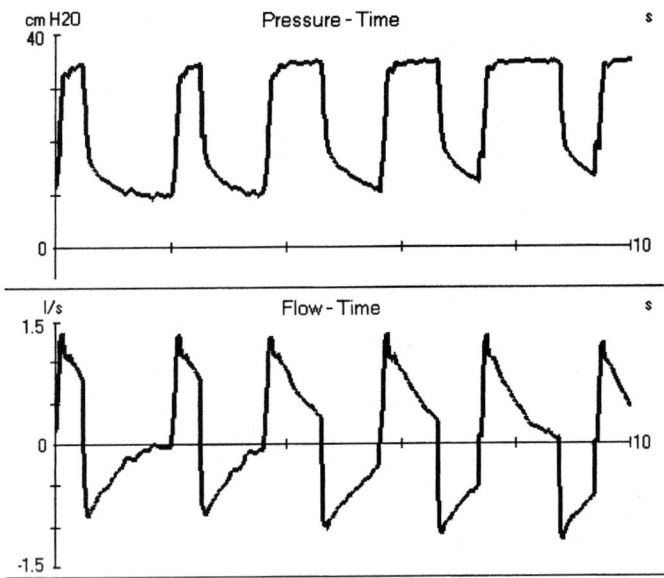

FIGURE 32-8 Pressure-control ventilation as T_I is progressively increased. The first two breaths are characterized by short T_I and cessation of inspiratory flow well before alveolar pressure (Palv) and P_I are equal. Expiratory flow ceases just before the subsequent breaths, showing that the lung has returned to functional residual capacity. Increasing T_I (second pair of breaths) lengthens the time of flow (thereby increasing tidal volume) but shortens exhalation time (T_E) sufficiently that there is now flow at end-expiration (i.e., there is dynamic hyperinflation or auto-PEEP). The final pair of breaths shows end-inspiratory cessation of flow (indicating that $P_I = Palv$), but now T_E is so short that dynamic hyperinflation worsens.

Several methods for quantifying auto-PEEP are available, but the one typically used clinically is the end-expiratory port occlusion method.[4] Several ventilators facilitate this determination by providing an expiratory pause switch. This method will not provide accurate estimation of auto-PEEP if there is a leak in the tubing or around the endotracheal tube cuff, there is gas flow into the circuit during expiration (as during continuous nebulization of bronchodilators), or the patient is not fully passive during the maneuver. In one survey of ventilated patients, quantitation of auto-PEEP was possible by the end-expiratory port occlusion technique in only one-third, because patient effort confounded the airway pressure.[3] Serial measurement of auto-PEEP may give information regarding the obstructed patient's response to bronchodilator therapy (if minute ventilation is constant).[8]

USING PEEP TO EASE TRIGGERING

Auto-PEEP presents an inspiratory threshold load to the spontaneously breathing patient, as discussed in Chap. 36 and Fig. 36-4.[9] The work of breathing due to this inspiratory threshold load is roughly equal in magnitude to the excessive resistive work of breathing in patients with COPD exacerbations,[10] contributing to distress even when on the ventilator. Thus therapy should be directed at reducing auto-PEEP when it is present. Meanwhile, PEEP can be applied externally, greatly easing the effort required to trigger the breath. In intubated patients with acute-on-chronic respiratory failure, continuous positive airway pressure (CPAP) has been demonstrated to reduce the work of breathing by nearly 50%.[11] In patients with COPD and acute respiratory failure, nasal CPAP immediately improves respiratory rate, sensation

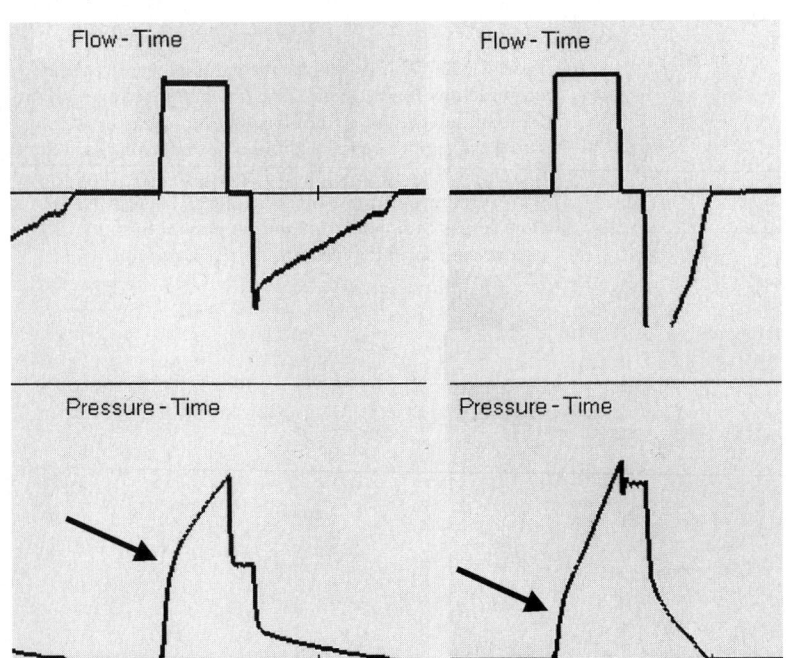

FIGURE 32-9 These two patients had elevated Ppeak to a similar degree but for differing reasons. The left-hand patient had airflow obstruction and an elevated Ppeak – Pplat, whereas the right-hand patient had a normal Ppeak – Pplat but an elevated Pplat (signaling abnormal respiratory system compliance). The Pao vs. time waveform changes slope at different pressures (*arrows*). The difference in pressure between PEEP and this "knee" is roughly equal to the Ppeak-to-Pplat difference.

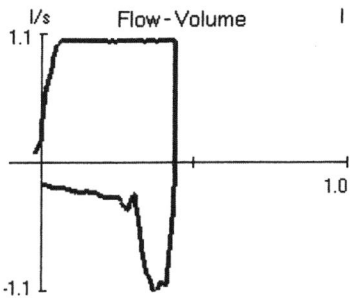

FIGURE 32-10 Flow-volume curve in a patient with airflow obstruction, showing the typical rapid decrement in expiratory flow as lung volume falls. Inspiratory flow is constant since this is set by the ventilator.

of dyspnea, and the partial pressure of carbon dioxide (P_{CO_2}).[12] The amount of auto-PEEP is largely independent of the set PEEP, since the airways of obstructed patients behave more like Starling resistors than like ohmic resistors, much as the rate of flow of water over a waterfall is unrelated to how far the water will fall into the pool below (Fig. 32-12). As long as the set PEEP is not higher than roughly 75% of the auto-PEEP, there is little effect on Palv, expiratory flow, or the magnitude of auto-PEEP,[13] although there are occasional exceptions.[14]

EFFECTS OF THERAPY

A reduction in airways resistance or a response to bronchodilators may be signaled by (1) reduced Pres (and lower Ppeak), (2) reduced auto-PEEP,[8] and (3) a more normal expiratory flow-volume curve. However, expiratory peak flow often does not increase with bronchodilators, because the lowered alveolar pressure (less auto-PEEP) reduces the driving pressure for exhalation.

Effect of Patient Effort

Flow and pressure waveforms are generally easy to analyze when patients are fully passive. On the other hand, an active

patient presents numerous challenges and pitfalls. The discussion above always assumed a passive patient, but this is often not the case.

INSPIRATORY EFFORT PRECEDING MACHINE INSPIRATION

The inspiratory threshold load presented by auto-PEEP sometimes leads to a striking delay between the initiation of the patient's inspiratory effort and the onset of machine inspiration, sometimes consisting of several hundred milliseconds (Fig. 32-13). This delay, which signals the presence of auto-PEEP, is often shortened markedly by the addition of externally applied PEEP, a feature that may aid the setting of PEEP in obstructed patients.

EFFORT DURING MACHINE INSPIRATION

It has long been known that patients perform inspiratory work throughout an assist control breath.[15] With modern ventilator management shifted to greater patient effort, lower tidal volumes, less sedation, and only rare use of therapeutic paralysis, most patients exhibit effort on most ventilator breaths, no matter the mode of ventilation. This effort may not be obvious despite careful examination of the patient unless measures of intrathoracic pressure (esophageal, central venous, or wedge pressures) are available. Inspiratory effort may alter Pao (volume-preset breaths), inspiratory flow (pressure-preset breaths), or expiratory flow (any mode). Effort at the end of a volume-preset breath will affect the Ppeak and Pplat, making determination of respiratory system mechanics unreliable. The magnitude of this problem is illustrated in Fig. 32-14, where the degree of patient effort is hidden until therapeutic paralysis reveals it. Some patients have extremely high drive, despite being connected to a ventilator. They may desire inspiratory flow rates much higher than are typically ordered (often in excess of 100 L/min). Since inspiratory flow is set by the physician and ventilator during typical volume-preset ventilation, no amount of patient effort can raise the flow. The effect of this is that Pao may not become positive during the breath or may even become negative (since the Pao reflects the competition between the ventilator,

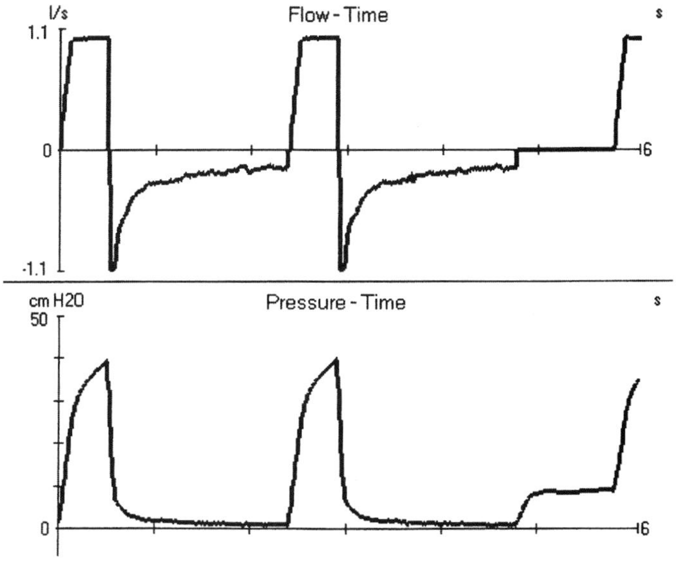

FIGURE 32-11 Auto-PEEP determined by the end-expiratory port occlusion technique. At the time a breath is due, the ventilator closes the inspiratory and expiratory ports and withholds the expected breath. The Pao during expiration of the second breath reflects the set PEEP (here zero) until the third breath is due, when the pressure suddenly rises, reflecting end-expiratory Palv, the auto-PEEP pressure. This patient has 10 cm H_2O auto-PEEP. The presence of auto-PEEP (but not its magnitude) is signaled by the presence of flow at end-expiration.

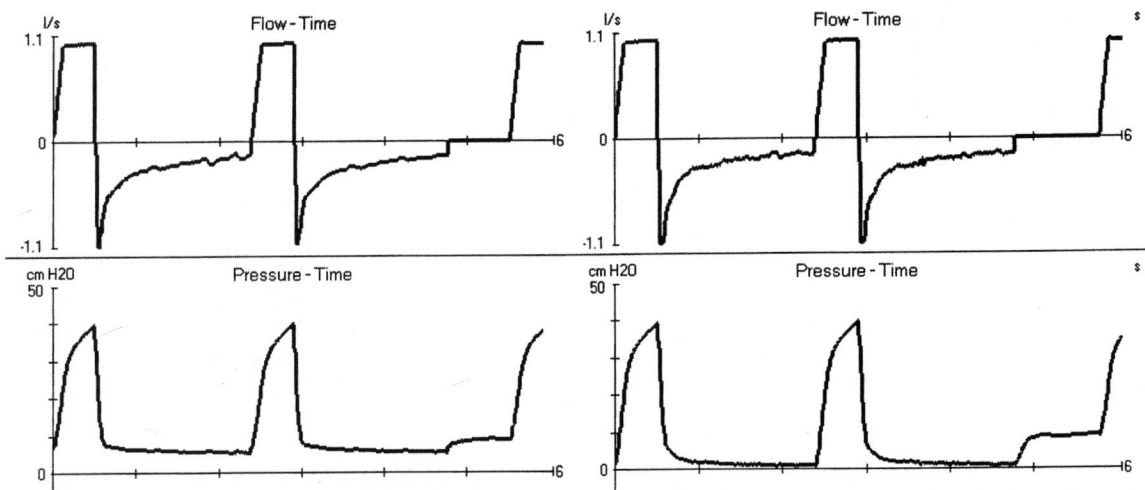

FIGURE 32-12 This is the same patient shown in Fig. 32-11, this time showing the measurement of auto-PEEP while the applied PEEP is 7 cm H_2O (*left panel*) or 0 cm H_2O (*right panel*). The measured auto-PEEP (10 cm H_2O) is identical.

tending to raise Pao, and the patient, tending to lower it). If Pao is not positive during inspiration, the ventilator is not doing work on the patient. That is, the patient's work of breathing would be no lower if the ventilator were disconnected. In extreme circumstances, the ventilator may even impede respiration. This represents a fundamental problem of ACV and SIMV: the greater the patient demand, the lower the Pao. One of the advantages of pressure-preset modes is that Pao is maintained, no matter how high the flow required, and these modes may be more comfortable for the patient with high drive (Fig. 32-15). It would even be sensible to augment pressure when the patient effort is high, and this rationale underlies PAV (see Chap. 36).

Clues to patient effort are often available from the airway pressure tracing when using a volume-preset mode, such as concavity of the rise in Pao, variability of Ppeak, and a dip in Pao before inspiration, indicating a triggering effort (Fig. 32-16). Since every breath of a passive patient should produce identical flow and pressure waveforms, an important clue to effort is simply a lack of uniformity of breaths.

EFFORT PERSISTING AFTER MACHINE INSPIRATION

One of the paradoxes of mechanical ventilation is that the patient's desired inspiratory duration (neural T_I) may bear no relationship to the ventilator inspiratory time (mechanical T_I). Mechanical T_I is set by the physician, either directly (as with PCV) or indirectly (as with ACV and SIMV), whereas neural T_I depends on arterial blood gases, the gas exchange efficiency of the lung, the impact of sedatives, and other central nervous system and patient features. In the usual setting, the patient desires a longer T_I than is set so that the patient's inspiratory effort persists, even while the ventilator has cycled to expiration. When neural and mechanical T_Is are dissimilar, patients may be uncomfortable. Pressure-support ventilation goes far toward solving this problem by switching off when

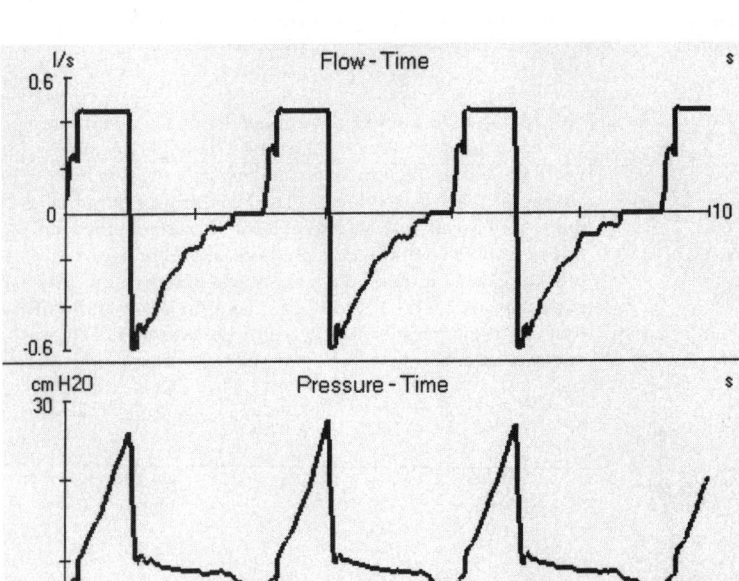

FIGURE 32-13 The pressure waveform in this patient shows a significant fall in Pao preceding each breath by several hundred milliseconds and lasting until the ventilator delivers a breath. This long delay was due to the difficulty experienced by the patient in overcoming a large amount of auto-PEEP. A casual inspection of the flow tracing might lead one to conclude that auto-PEEP was not present (since flow near end-expiration is zero), but flow has ceased only because the patient is making inspiratory effort. On other breaths (not shown) the patient failed to trigger at all, even while lowering Pao and stopping expiratory flow completely.

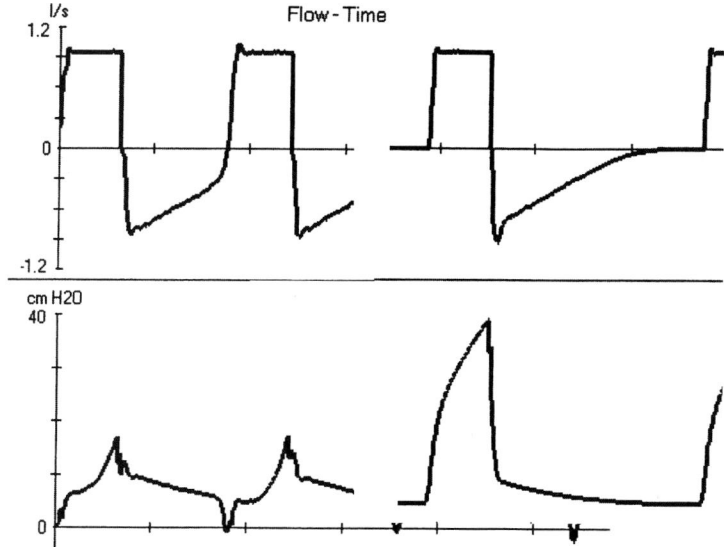

FIGURE 32-14 This patient had respiratory failure due to septic shock. Despite ACV at a high minute ventilation, the patient continued to work hard to breathe, lowering Pao during inspiration below the set PEEP level (*left panel*). Notice that Pao only rises at the termination of inspiration. Following therapeutic paralysis (*right panel*), Ppeak rises to 40 cm H_2O. The difference in Pao before and after paralysis reflects the very high work of breathing of this patient.

inspiratory flow falls, since reduced flow often correlates with the end of neural inspiration. In contrast, many patients ventilated with PCV or volume-preset modes rely on happenstance or sedatives to accommodate their neural T_I to the machine T_I (Fig. 32-17).

Postinspiratory effort can be recognized as loss of the usually rapid initial expiratory flow, as illustrated in Fig. 32-17, or by double- or triple-triggering. The patient shown in Fig. 32-18 was being ventilated with a lung-protective tidal volume (6 mL/kg ideal body weight [IBW]) for ARDS. Every breath actually consists of a double-triggered breath: exhaled total ventilation (V_T) alternated between 2 mL/kg and 10 mL/kg, showing that this patient was probably not receiving lung-protective ventilation, despite the set tidal volume. Ventilator T_I can be lengthened during volume-preset modes by increasing tidal volume (although this may conflict with lung-protective goals; see Chap. 37) or by reducing inspira-

tory flow (although this may prompt the patient to exert even more inspiratory effort).

A separate phenomenon is additional attempts to trigger the ventilator during expiration (Fig. 32-19). This is quite common, generally when there is auto-PEEP, and especially during PSV at high levels, and its clinical significance is not known.[16] When ventilator-dependent patients were subjected to increasing degrees of ventilator assistance (and demonstrated reduced inspiratory pressure-time product), the rate of ineffective triggering rose even while the total respiratory rate fell.[17] It is probably valuable to consider the impact of patient-ventilator asynchrony (PVA) in light of the patient's respiratory drive. When drive is high, PVA should be addressed by manipulation of the ventilator to improve the patient-ventilator interaction. If drive is low, however, PVA

FIGURE 32-15 This shows Pao as a function of patient effort during various modes of ventilation. Pressure-preset modes deliver a fixed pressure, whatever the effort, whereas volume-preset (constant flow) modes like ACV and IMV produce ever-decreasing pressure with increasing effort. IMV forces the patient to work even harder, since not all breaths are supported. PAV responds to increasing patient demand by augmenting flow.

FIGURE 32-16 Signs of patient effort during constant flow, volume-preset ventilation include concavity of the Pao versus time waveform during inspiration; a drop in Pao before the breath indicating triggering; and variability in the height of the Ppeak. Notice the first breath shows marked concavity, the second reveals obvious triggering, and during the third the patient is passive.

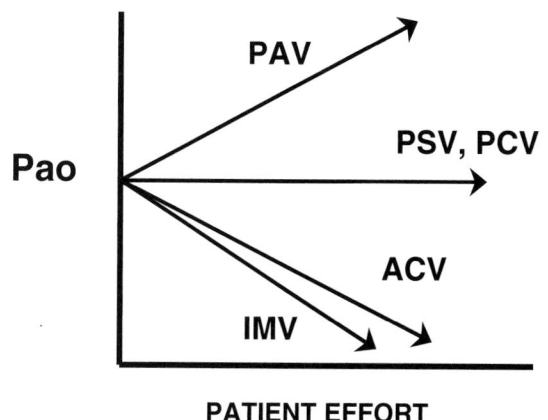

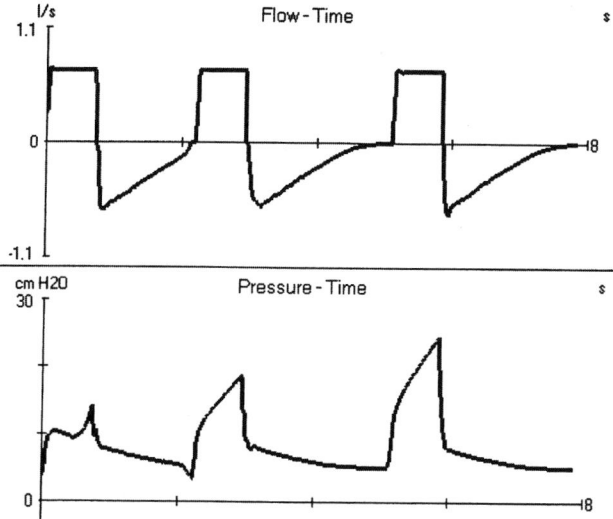

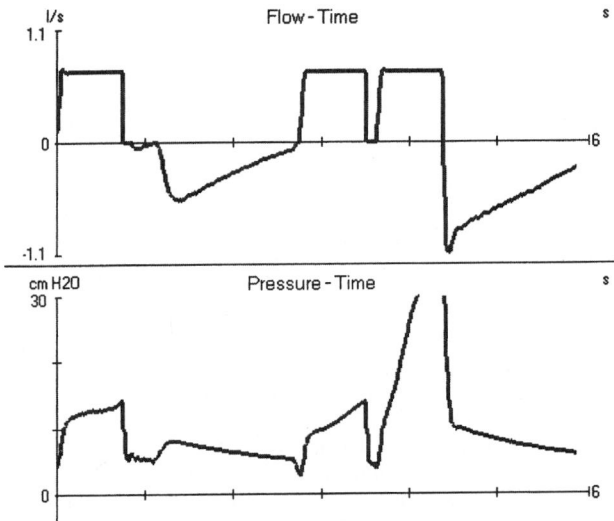

FIGURE 32-17 Volume assist controlled ventilation with a machine T_I of 0.7 second. Notice that expiratory flow does not follow the first breath until after a substantial delay because the patient is still contracting the inspiratory muscles. Only after a total neural T_I of about 1.2 seconds does the patient turn off the inspiratory muscles and begin to exhale. The same phenomenon is seen after the second breath, but this time the patient's continued inspiratory effort is sufficient to double-trigger the ventilator.

may simply indicate unloading of the respiratory system and no changes in ventilator settings are indicated.[18]

EXPIRATORY EFFORT

Patients may recruit expiratory muscles during machine inspiration or expiration. Expiratory effort during machine inspiration may raise Pao during ACV or SIMV, even setting off the pressure alarm, and reduce tidal volume on any mode. Expiratory effort at end-inspiration occasionally raises Pplat artifactually (Fig. 32-20). For this reason, it is prudent to view the waveform whenever measuring plateau pressure in order to confirm that there is a true plateau.

A more common problem is expiratory muscle recruitment throughout expiration, even to end-expiration, as is often seen in patients with severe airflow obstruction. Measured values of auto-PEEP may be artifactually elevated by expiratory effort[19] (as may hemodynamic pressures, as discussed below).

Patient-Ventilator Asynchrony

VENTILATION VIA ENDOTRACHEAL TUBE OR TRACHEOSTOMY

Patients vary greatly in their breathing pattern and desire for flow, tidal volume, rate, and T_I. Any particular initial ventilator settings are unlikely to coincide with the individual patient's needs.[16,17,20] Thus the initial settings should be considered a first approximation. Then, taking into account the patient-ventilator interaction, as judged by subjective patient comfort and waveform displays of flow and pressure, the settings can be tailored to the individual patient. At times, only modest adjustment will improve patient-ventilator synchrony or patient comfort (Fig. 32-21). The beneficial impact of such changes may be evident not just in the flow and pressure waveforms, but in hemodynamic waveforms as well (Fig. 32-22).

A stepwise approach to adjusting the ventilator to the patient during volume-preset ventilation involves changing (1) tidal volume, (2) rate, (3) inspiratory flow rate, (4) T_I, itself a consequence of tidal volume and flow rate, and (5) PEEP to counter auto-PEEP. Rarely, rise time may require consideration, as discussed below. For patients on PCV, the steps are to change (1) P_I, (2) T_I, (3) rate, and (4) PEEP. An example of this process is shown in Figure 32-23. Of course, any of these adjustments can cause problems or create conflict with other goals of ventilation. For example, raising rate (say to match

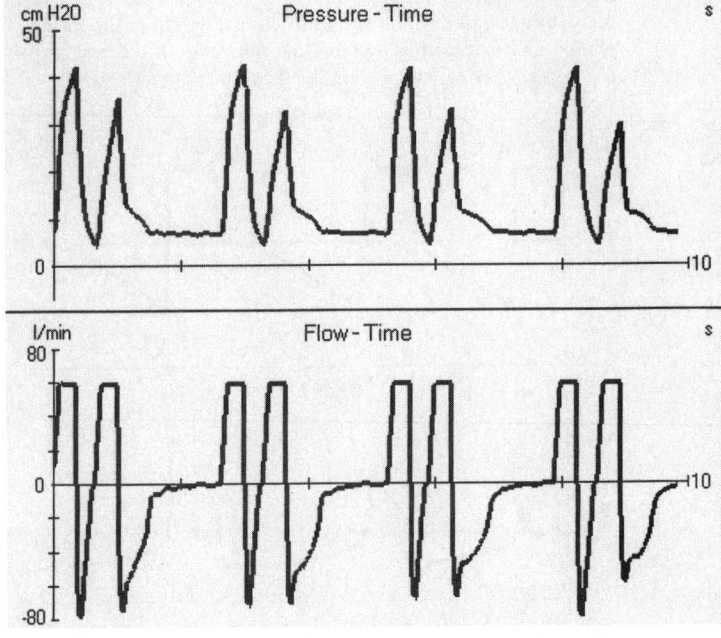

FIGURE 32-18 A patient with ARDS, ventilated with lung-protective settings of tidal volume of 6 mL/kg ideal body weight. Notice that every breath actually consists of two stacked breaths, effectively doubling the tidal volume, since only a trivial amount of each initial breath is exhaled before the next breath is triggered.

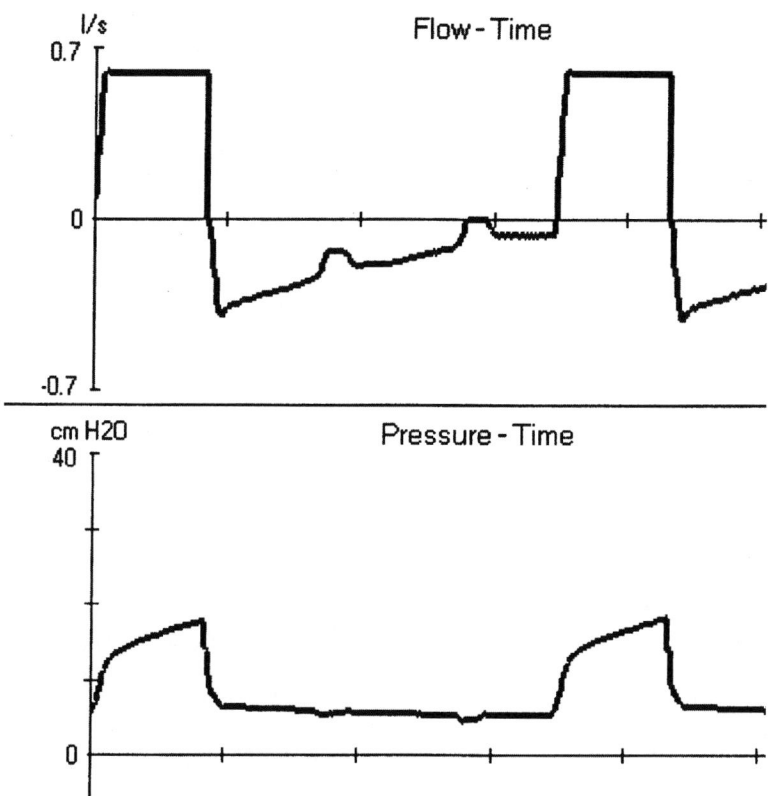

FIGURE 32-19 Patient with airflow obstruction ventilated with ACV. Notice the brief reductions in expiratory flow between the two ventilator breaths, both signaling failed attempts by the patient to trigger the ventilator. The presence of auto-PEEP contributes to the difficulty in triggering.

a patient's high drive) may cause undesired auto-PEEP or hypocapnia, or raising tidal volume to lengthen machine T_I may violate lung-protective goals. Often additional sedation is required to accommodate the patient to the ventilator, but this is appropriate only after steps have been taken to accommodate the ventilator to the patient.

FIGURE 32-20 An end-inspiratory pause is set in order to measure Pplat. Notice that there really is no "plateau," but rather that Pao rises during the pause. This effect is due to expiratory effort, artifactually raising Pao following inspiration.

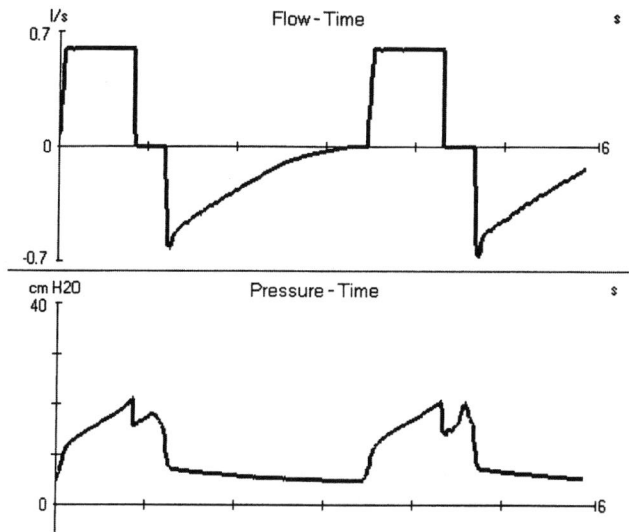

THE NONINVASIVELY VENTILATED PATIENT

During NIV, the patient and ventilator are coupled less tightly than when an endotracheal tube or tracheostomy is used. That is, the patient and ventilator are more easily asynchronous during NIV and it is even more important to carefully adapt ventilator to patient in order to improve the success of NIV.[18]

Two mechanisms of patient-ventilator asynchrony (PVA) are common. The first is failure of the patient to lower the proximal airway pressure (mask pressure) sufficiently to be able to trigger, due to the presence of auto-PEEP as discussed above. Adding PEEP is helpful to improve synchrony, but it is not generally practical to measure the amount of auto-PEEP in these patients, due to their effort. Rather, the clinician must adjust the machine PEEP upwards while assessing the patient's triggering effort. This modification can be greatly aided by the analysis of flow and pressure waveform displays. We begin routinely with the PEEP set at 2 or 3 cm H_2O and find that maximal benefit is reached between 4 and 10 cm H_2O.

The second common mechanism for PVA is failure of the ventilator to detect end-inspiration because the patient's subsiding effort is cloaked by a mask leak. Most PSV ventilators terminate inspiration when inspiratory flow falls to a preset threshold, often at an arbitrary low value of flow or at a fixed percentage of the peak inspiratory flow. Mask leaks prevent the flow from falling to this threshold, so the ventilator fails to switch off the inspiratory pressure, even while the patient is making active expiratory efforts. This serves to increase patient discomfort and the work of breathing. Using other methods for terminating inspiration, such as time-cycled pressure-support or ACV, can minimize this problem. Six patients with acute lung injury were studied during NIV with both conventional flow-cycled PSV and time-cycled PSV while the

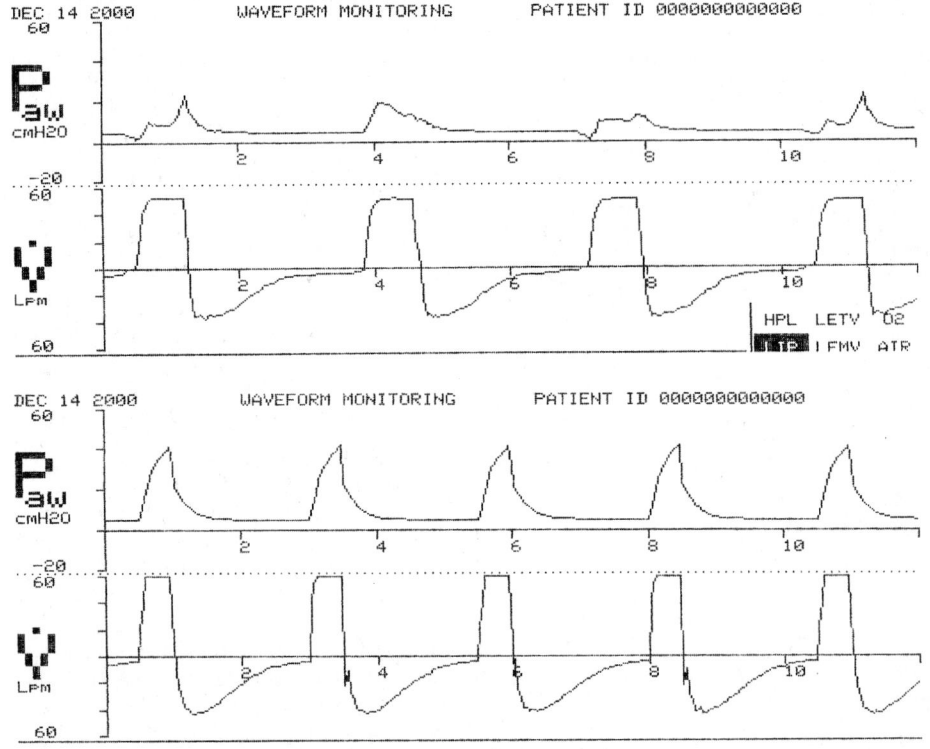

FIGURE 32-21 This patient was being ventilated for severe sepsis, yet Pao (*top panel*) was only slightly and inconsistently above PEEP during inspiration, indicating substantial patient effort. Increasing inspiratory flow rate modestly and raising the rate (at the same tidal volume) changed the pressure waveform greatly (*bottom panel*). Now all breaths are identical, each complex is convex upwards, and there are no signs of triggering (i.e., the patient appears passive).

masks were adjusted to facilitate leaks.[21] Time-cycled PSV significantly reduced the work of breathing (as judged by the esophageal pressure tidal swing and pressure-time product) and also more dramatically lowered the respiratory rate.

Displays of inspiratory and expiratory flows can be very valuable in detecting PVA and further assist the intensivist in modifying the mask or ventilator to improve synchrony and comfort. Carefully observing the patient-ventilator interaction and modifying the settings accordingly requires substantial time in the first hour on the part of the physician-respiratory therapist-nurse team.

FIGURE 32-22 Central venous pressure tracings in the patient shown in Fig. 32-21. Notice the periodic falls in pressure (coinciding with inspiration) in the top panel (before ventilator adjustment), which are replaced by positive deflections following ventilator adjustment (showing that pleural pressure is rising during inspiration in this now passive patient).

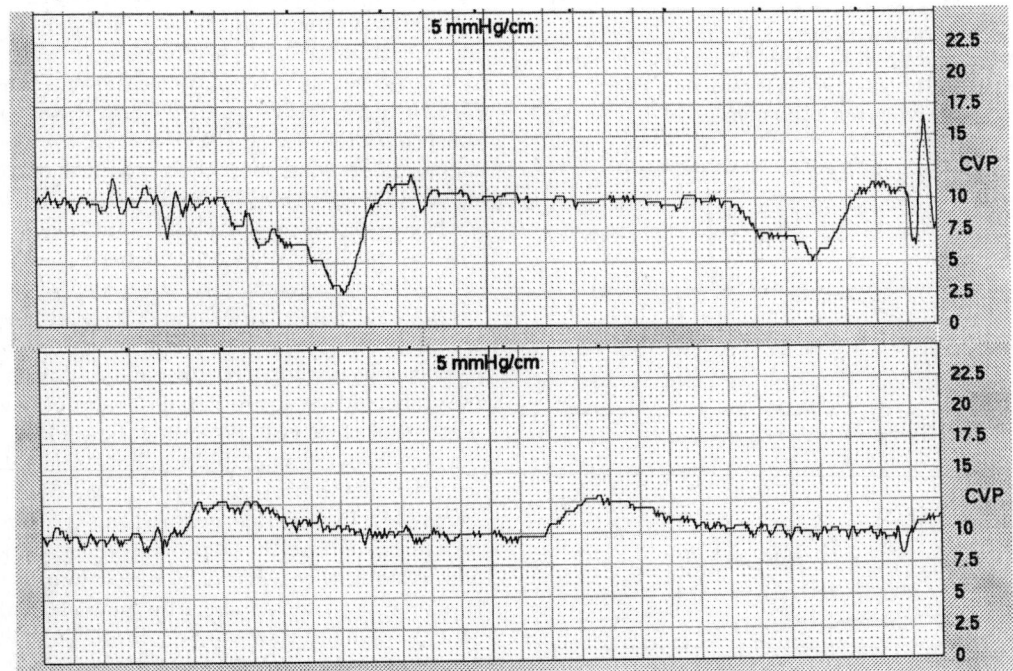

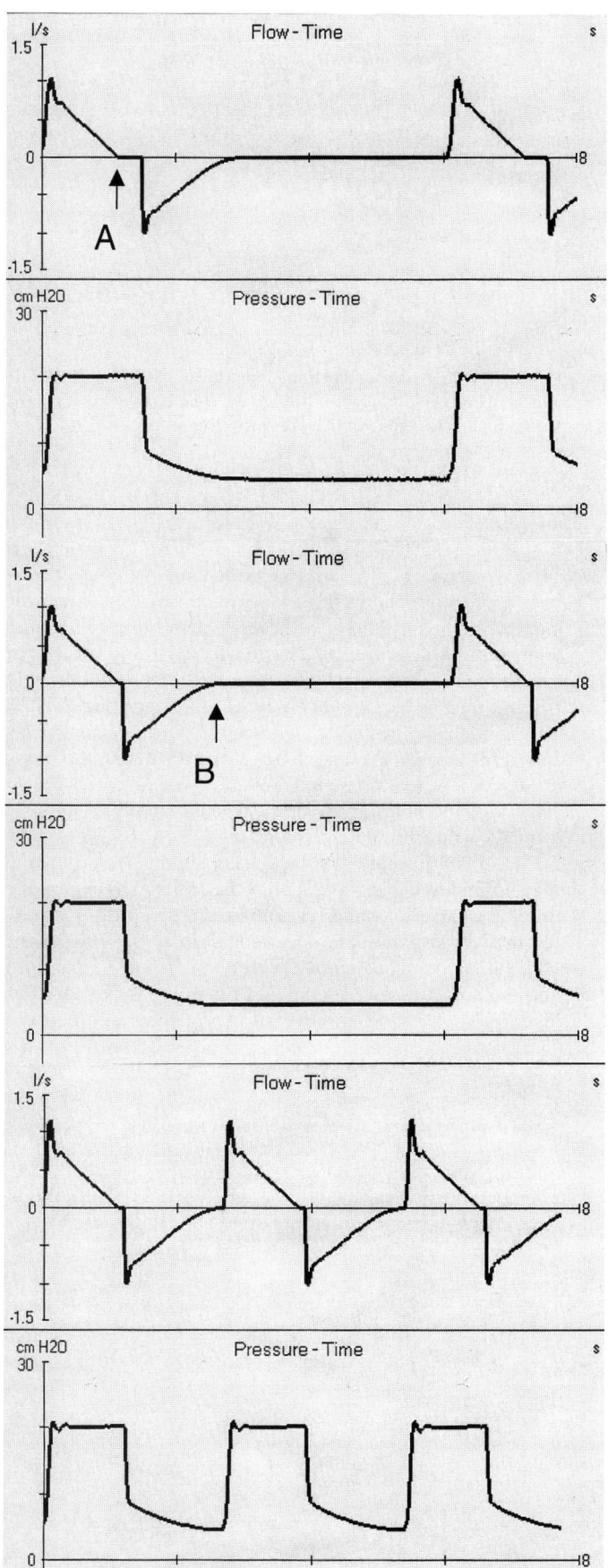

FIGURE 32-23 The settings on PCV are adjusted during ventilation of a passive, hypercapnic patient. The top two waveforms show flow and pressure with initial settings of $P_I = 20$; PEEP = 5; f = 10; T_I = 1.5 seconds. Note that flow ceases before the end of the set T_I (*arrow A*), indicating that T_I is set too long for this patient. The next two panels show T_I reduced to 1.2 seconds to match the patient's mechanics. Now expiratory flow ceases (*arrow B*) well before the subsequent breath, indicating that the rate can be raised without causing auto-PEEP. The final two panels show the flow and pressure waveforms after the rate is raised from 10 to 22. Any further increase in rate will create some degree of auto-PEEP.

Volume-Pressure Curves in Acute Respiratory Distress Syndrome

Some intensivists have recommended adjusting the ventilator based on the inspiratory volume-pressure (VP) curve.[22] Specifically, the upper end of the curve is examined for an upper inflection point (UIP), thought to signify alveolar overdistention (Fig. 32-24). If a UIP is present the tidal volume should be reduced, according to this view. The bottom part of the curve can be examined in an attempt to identify a lower inflection point (LIP), which may indicate recruitment during inspiration (Fig. 32-25). Such repeated recruitment (and during expiration derecruitment) has been shown in animal models of ARDS to be detrimental.[23] One must take care to reduce the inspiratory flow rate to a low level (e.g., 15 liters per minute or 0.25 liters per second) when displaying the VP curve in order to avoid a flow-related artifact. If the flow rate is not reduced, the VP curve appears to show a LIP regardless of whether there is alveolar recruitment (Fig. 32-26).

There remain multiple problems with using VP curves to guide ventilator management in patients with ALI and ARDS. First, obtaining the VP curve is tedious: it requires physician time; detection of inflection points requires very careful analysis; any inflection points probably change as the lung changes, so repeated measures might be needed to guide ventilator settings; any patient effort makes the curve uninterpretable; the flow rate must be greatly reduced during measurement, which in most patients requires a temporary reduction in breathing rate (in order not to drastically curtail T_E), during which the patient must remain fully passive; lower inflection points may not correlate with recruitment and derecruitment,[24] and most importantly, this method has not been shown to improve outcomes despite its theoretical elegance. A recent study by the ARDS Network failed to show a benefit to a PEEP level higher than "least PEEP" when applied in patients ventilated with tidal volumes of 6 mL/kg IBW.

FIGURE 32-24 During a slow inspiration, the Pao reflects mostly the respiratory system compliance. The falling slope of the inspiratory limb once the volume exceeds about 550 mL indicates alveolar overdistention. There is no lower inflection point in this patient on 10 cm H_2O PEEP.

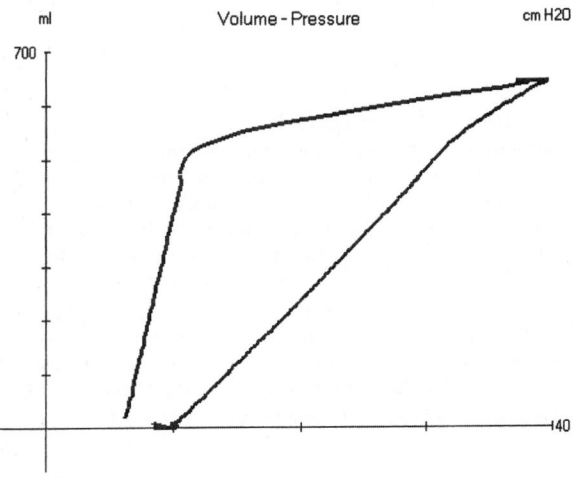

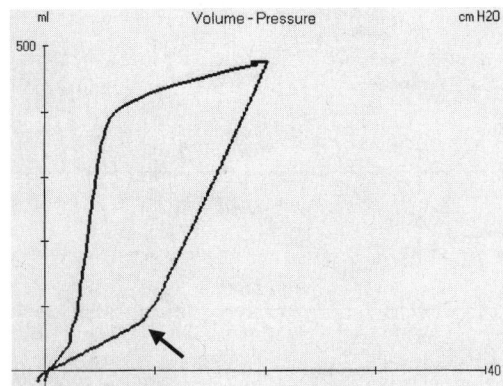

FIGURE 32-25 A pressure-volume loop during ACV, zero PEEP, and very low flow (12 L/min), showing a clear change in slope of the volume-pressure loop (a lower inflection point).

Measuring Hemodynamic Pressures

Respiratory muscle activity greatly affects intrathoracic pressure, which alters measured hemodynamic values. By convention, hemodynamic values such as Pra and Ppw are measured at end-expiration since the respiratory muscles are most likely to be passive at end-expiration. It can be quite difficult to determine the point of end-expiration from a hemodynamic tracing, mostly because of respiratory activity (Fig. 32-27). This can lead to incorrect measurement of important pressures, perhaps prompting incorrect treatments. In the modern era of low tidal volume ventilation, reduced reliance on sedatives, and sparing use of therapeutic paralysis, effort is more the rule than the exception.

End-expiration can often be detected in the hemodynamic waveforms by paying attention to inspiratory-to-expiratory ratios, the nature of the respiratory rise in pressure (which differs between the ventilator-induced rise in the passive patient and the spontaneous expiratory rise in the active patient), and the abruptness of the falls in pressure, as discussed in Fig. 32-27. Additional confidence can be gained at the bedside

FIGURE 32-26 Several volume pressure loops are superimposed while the inspiratory flow rate is reduced from 60 L/min (*largest loop*) to 45 L/min to 30 L/min, and finally to 12 L/min. Notice that what appears to be a LIP moves leftward and becomes progressively less evident as flow is reduced, showing that this is not a LIP but rather an artifact of the changing flow early in the breath.

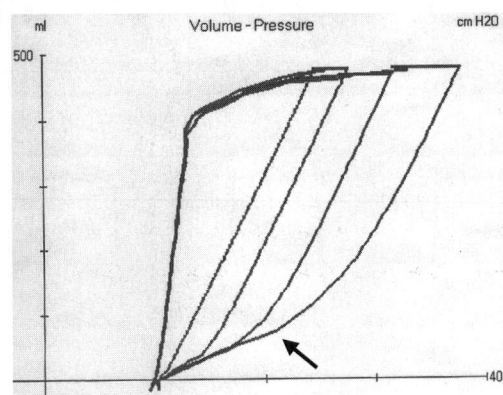

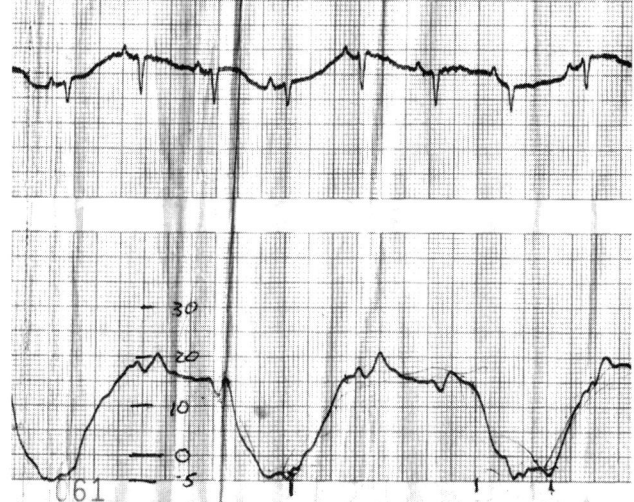

FIGURE 32-27 Wedge pressure (Ppw) tracing in this ventilated patient who was making strong respiratory efforts. Since the Ppw varies from 20 to −5 cm H_2O, reading the tracing properly (at end-expiration) is vitally important. If this patient were passive, one would expect the end-expiratory pressure to be roughly −5 cm H_2O, but then the inspiratory-to-expiratory (I:E) ratio would be 2:1 (inverse ratio ventilation), the fall in pressure during (presumed) expiration too abrupt, and the (presumed) inspiratory pressure would continue to rise (rather than plateauing) throughout the breath. Instead this ventilated patient is quite active and pulls the Ppw down during inspiration. The end-expiratory pressure is 15 cm H_2O.

by examining the patient and ventilator while simultaneously displaying the hemodynamic tracing in question. Perhaps the simplest and most accurate approach, however, is to connect the ventilator circuit to a pressure transducer and display this on the same time scale as the hemodynamic waveform. End-expiration is readily identified on the ventilator pressure waveform (Fig. 32-28). One then moves 200 milliseconds earlier on the time scale (since patient effort begins before machine inspiration, especially in the patient with auto-PEEP, as discussed above) and measures the hemodynamic pressure there.

Unusual Problems Revealed by Waveform Analysis

Modern ventilators allow remarkable control over many aspects of ventilation beyond those related to tidal volume, rate, and PEEP. The ability to adjust flow profiles, flow rates, and rise times gives the intensivist tools for improving patient-ventilator synchrony and patient comfort. At the same time, however, changing some of these parameters has unanticipated consequences, many of which are revealed by comparing flow or pressure waveforms before and after the intervention. For example, the first set of pressure and flow tracings shown in Fig. 32-29 were seen in a patient ventilated with ACV and a rise time of 10% (meaning that 10% of the total respiratory cycle is devoted towards raising flow towards its peak value). Pressure does not rise above the PEEP value for the first two-thirds of the breath. The basis for this is readily evident from the flow tracing, which shows that flow is

FIGURE 32-28 The least equivocal method for identifying end-expiration on a vascular waveform is to simultaneously display the vascular pressure (here the CVP; *top waveform*) and the Pao (PRS; *bottom waveform*). A point 200 milliseconds before the Pao rises (signaling inspiration) generally precedes the patient's inspiratory effort and is a good marker for end-expiration. Because the CVP varies during respiration in this patient, selecting end-expiration reproducibly is essential to getting reliable pressures. Here the CVP is 10 cm H_2O.

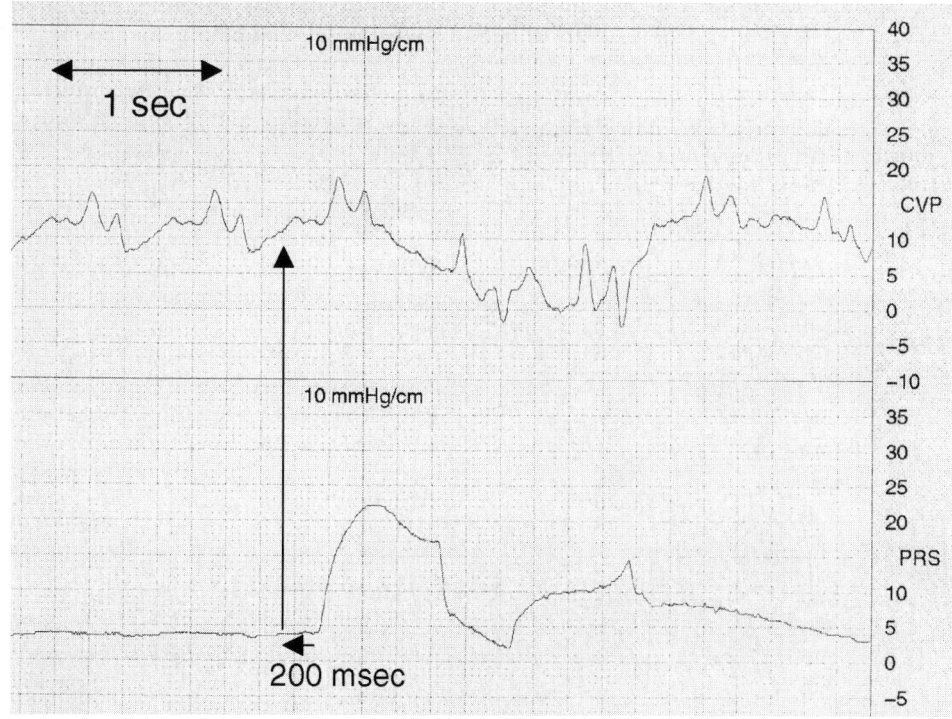

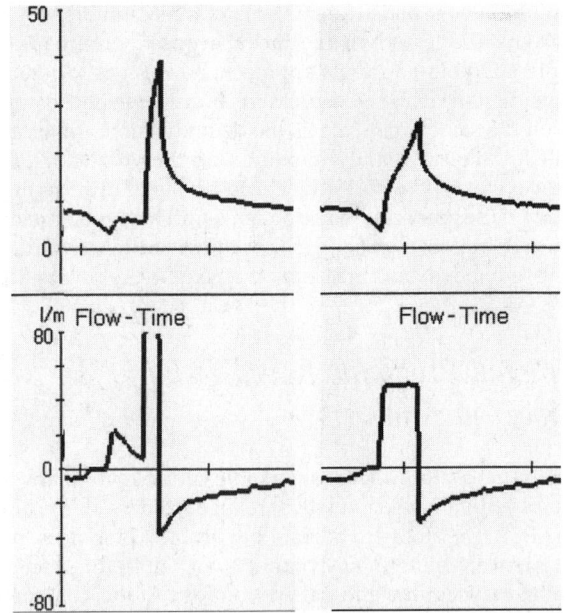

FIGURE 32-29 This patient was ventilated with ACV and a rise time of 10% (*left panel*). Notice that inspiratory flow and pressure are very low for the first two-thirds of the breath, then both rise abruptly. This occurs because the patient had somewhat increased drive and tried to pull inspiratory flow higher than that allowed if the rise time was to remain at 10%. The ventilator resists the patient's effort until finally allowing adequate flow once the 10% time has passed. This same phenomenon was apparent (although less dramatic) when the rise time was set at the default value of 5% (not shown). The right hand panel shows the same patient once the rise time was reduced to 1%. Notice that Pao rises sooner, flow is constant through the breath, and the ventilator is performing more work (although the patient is still not passive).

positive, but excruciatingly slow, for the first two-thirds of the breath. Flow is maintained low because the ventilator is not allowed to give the peak flow until 10% of the respiratory cycle has elapsed. If the patient tries to get more flow before this time, the ventilator simply throttles flow down further. Obviously, this is counterproductive, forcing the patient to

FIGURE 32-30 During ACV, the rise time was raised from 1% to 10%. Notice that peak airway pressure rises measurably despite no change in the patient's mechanics or tidal volume.

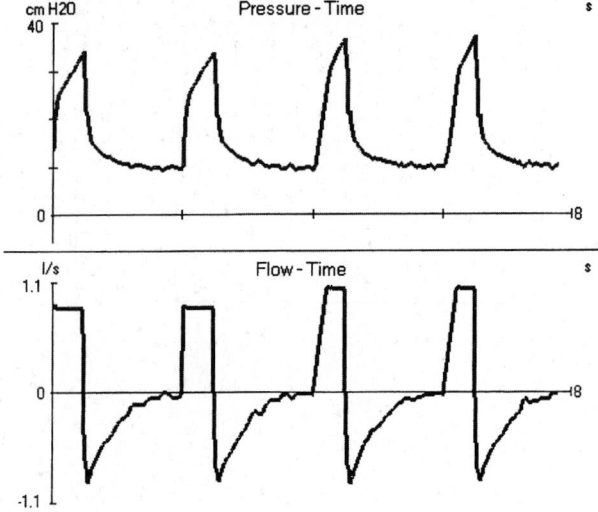

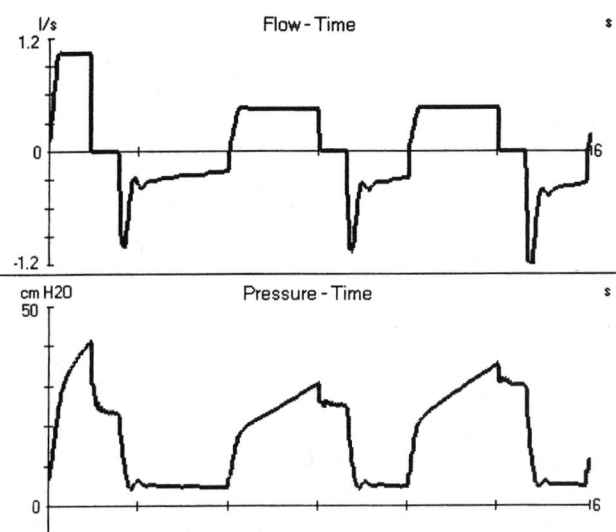

FIGURE 32-31 During ACV, the inspiratory flow was reduced from 1 L/s to 0.5 L/s. Notice that Ppeak falls with the second breath (as does Pres), but then begins to rise again by the third breath. This occurs because the shortened T_E worsens auto-PEEP, raising the Ppeak again. This process will continue to raise the auto-PEEP for several breaths until Palv rises sufficiently to drive the full tidal volume out during the shorter T_E.

work excessively. Yet no alarm will sound; the only clue to this problem is found in the ventilator waveforms. When the rise time was set appropriately (see Fig. 32-29), patient effort was reduced as the ventilator took on more of the burden of the work of breathing.

Lengthening the rise time also affects peak flow, since as the percentage of time at peak flow is reduced, the amount of flow must be raised in order to keep T_I constant (Fig. 32-30). Therefore changing rise time can alter Ppeak, potentially confounding assessment of the respiratory system mechanics or response to therapy.

Many ventilators are provided with an option during volume-preset modes to give constant flow (the standard approach) or a decelerating (or sine wave) flow profile. Although the decelerating flow profile most closely mimics the flow pattern seen with PSV and PCV, there is no evidence that this pattern is either better or more comfortable than constant flow. The decelerating profile is most often selected when Pao is very high and there is concern for barotrauma. The effect of this is to lower Ppeak since at end-inspiration, when lung recoil is greatest, flow is much reduced. Yet an unavoidable consequence of lowering the flow late in the breath is that T_I is lengthened (and T_E shortened). This almost always serves to cause or exacerbate auto-PEEP (see Fig. 32-2). We strongly discourage the use of any flow profile other than square.

Even when inspiratory flow is kept constant throughout the breath, lowering its value can have a marked impact on auto-PEEP (Fig. 32-31). There are few reasons to ever ventilate a patient with the inspiratory flow set lower than 50 L/min (0.83 L/s).

References

1. Esteban A, Anzueto A, Alia I, et al: How is mechanical ventilation employed in the intensive care unit? An international utilization review. *Am J Respir Crit Care Med* 161:1450, 2000.

2. Barberis L, Manno E, Guerin C: Effect of end-inspiratory pause duration on plateau pressure in mechanically ventilated patients. *Intensive Care Med* 29:130, 2003.

3. Kress JP, O'Connor MF, Schmidt GA: Clinical examination reliably detects intrinsic positive end-expiratory pressure in critically ill, mechanically ventilated patients. *Am J Respir Crit Care Med* 159:290, 1999.

4. Pepe PE, Marini JJ: Occult positive end-expiratory pressure in mechanically ventilated patients with airflow obstruction. *Am Rev Respir Dis* 126:166, 1982.

5. Rossi A, Gottfried SB, Zocchi L, et al: Measurement of static compliance of the total respiratory system in patients with acute respiratory failure during mechanical ventilation: The effect of intrinsic positive end-expiratory pressure. *Am Rev Respir Dis* 131:672, 1985.

6. Haluszka J, Chartrand DA, Grassino AE, et al: Intrinsic PEEP and arterial PCO2 in stable patients with chronic obstructive pulmonary disease. *Am Rev Respir Dis* 141:1194, 1990.

7. Aldrich TK, Hendler JM, Vizioli LD, et al: Intrinsic positive end-expiratory pressure in ambulatory patients with airways obstruction. *Am Rev Respir Dis* 147:845, 1993.

8. Gay PC, Rodarte JR, Tayyab M, et al: Evaluation of bronchodilator responsiveness in mechanically ventilated patients. *Am Rev Respir Dis* 136:880, 1987.

9. MacIntyre N, Kuo-Chen G, McConnell R: Applied PEEP during pressure support reduces the inspiratory threshold load of intrinsic PEEP. *Chest* 111:188, 1997.

10. Coussa ML, Guérin C, Eissa NT, et al: Partitioning of work of breathing in mechanically ventilated COPD patients. *J Appl Physiol* 75:1711, 1993.

11. Petrof BJ, Legaré M, Goldberg P, et al: Continuous positive airway pressure reduces work of breathing and dyspnea during weaning from mechanical ventilation in severe chronic obstructive pulmonary disease. *Am Rev Respir Dis* 141:281, 1990.

12. de Lucas P, Tarancón C, Puente L, et al: Nasal continuous positive airway pressure in patients with COPD in acute respiratory failure: a study of the immediate effects. *Chest* 104:1694, 1993.

13. Gay PC, Rodarte JR, Hubmayr RD: The effects of positive expiratory pressure on isovolume flow and dynamic hyperinflation in patients receiving mechanical ventilation. *Am Rev Respir Dis* 139:621, 1989.

14. Tuxen DV: Detrimental effects of positive end-expiratory pressure during controlled mechanical ventilation of patients with severe airflow obstruction. *Am Rev Respir Dis* 140:5, 1989.

15. Marini JJ, Capps JS, Culver BH: The inspiratory work of breathing during assisted mechanical ventilation. *Chest* 87:612, 1985.

16. Jubran A, Van de Graff W, Tobin MJ. Variability of patient-ventilator interaction with pressure support ventilation in patients with chronic obstructive pulmonary disease. *Am J Respir Crit Care Med* 152:129, 1995.

17. Leung P, Jubran A, Tobin MJ: Comparison of assisted ventilator modes on triggering, patient effort, and dyspnea. *Am J Respir Crit Care Med* 155:1940, 1997.

18. Hubmayr RD: The importance of patient/ventilator interactions during non-invasive mechanical ventilation. *Acta Anaesthesiol Scand* 109:46, 1996.

19. Zakynthinos SG, Vassilakopoulos T, Zakynthinois E: Accurate measurement of intrinsic positive end-expiratory pressure: How to detect and correct for expiratory muscle activity. *Eur Respir J* 10:522, 1997.

20. Parthasarathy S, Jubran A, Tobin MJ, et al: Cycling of inspiratory and expiratory muscle groups with the ventilator in airflow obstruction. *Am J Respir Crit Care Med* 158:1471, 1998.

21. Calderini E, Confalonieri M, Puccio PG, et al: Patient-ventilator asynchrony during noninvasive ventilation: The role of expiratory trigger. *Intensive Care Med* 25:662, 1999.

22. Amato MBP, Barbas CSV, Medeiros DM, et al: Beneficial effects of the "open lung approach" with low distending pressures in acute respiratory distress syndrome: A prospective randomized study on mechanical ventilation. *Am J Respir Crit Care Med* 152:1835, 1995.

23. Dreyfuss D, Saumon G: Ventilator-induced lung injury: Lessons from experimental studies. *Am J Respir Crit Care Med* 157:294, 1998.

24. Crotti S, Mascheroni D, Caironi P, et al: Recruitment and derecruitment during acute respiratory failure: A clinical study. *Am J Respir Crit Care Med* 164:131, 2001.

Chapter 33

NONINVASIVE VENTILATION

LAURENT BROCHARD

KEY POINTS

- *Many patients with ventilatory failure can be successfully managed with noninvasive positive pressure ventilation (NIPPV).*

- *NIPPV improves gas exchange, reduces the work of breathing, and relieves dyspnea.*

- *Patients most likely to benefit include those with acute hypercapnic exacerbations of chronic obstructive pulmonary disease (COPD) or hypercapnic forms of acute cardiogenic pulmonary edema.*

- *In selected patients with acute hypoxemic nonhypercapnic respiratory failure, NIPPV may obviate the need for endotracheal intubation. Selection may require exclusion of patients with hemodynamic instability, central neurologic dysfunction, or an inability to protect the upper airway.*

- *In severely hypoxemic patients, undiscerning use of NIPPV may inappropriately delay intubation. In these patients, the decision to switch to endotracheal intubation should be made early.*

- *The use of NIPPV to treat postextubation respiratory distress has not been found to be superior to conventional management.*

- *The first hour on NIPPV is crucial in predicting the outcome and requires that experienced physicians, nurses, or respiratory therapists spend considerable time at the bedside.*

- *A favorable response to NIPPV is usually apparent within the first hour. Absence of improvements in dyspnea, respiratory rate, and gas exchange within 1 hour strongly suggests a need for endotracheal intubation.*

- *Typical settings in a patient with COPD include pressure support of 10 cm H_2O above a positive end-expiratory pressure (PEEP) of 5 cm H_2O.*

- *In appropriately selected patients, NIPPV produces better outcomes than does endotracheal mechanical ventilation.*

Noninvasive positive pressure ventilation (NIPPV) has emerged as a valuable tool in the treatment of acute respiratory failure (ARF). NIPPV can substantially reduce the need for endotracheal intubation (ETI) and mechanical ventilation (MV). In selected patients, the benefits of NIPPV include decreased rates of adverse events associated with MV, shorter time spent in the ICU and hospital, and lower mortality rates. Patients with hypercapnic forms of ARF are most likely to benefit, but NIPPV may also improve outcomes of carefully selected patients with hypoxemic respiratory failure. This chapter reviews the evidence supporting NIPPV use in patients with ARF.

Rationale and Objective

When MV was first developed for widespread clinical use during the poliomyelitis epidemic, attention focused on replacing the failing respiratory muscles by a perithoracic pump. This led to the development of the "iron lung," the first form of noninvasive ventilation, which saved many lives.[1,2] However, the device was cumbersome and impeded patient care. In addition, the iron lung proved of limited efficacy in the treatment of parenchymal lung disease. Thus delivery of mechanical assistance through an endotracheal tube that provided access to the lower airway was considered a significant advance, and positive pressure ventilation became the standard for MV.

Soon after the introduction of endotracheal MV, many complications of positive pressure ventilation were identified.[3,4] These complications were found to be common and generated concern about the invasiveness of MV. ETI itself has been implicated in a large number of complications. Of these, some are directly related to the procedure, such as cardiac arrest following laryngospasm or difficult tube insertion and laryngeal or tracheal injury leading to long-term sequelae. Others are ascribable to the fact that the endotracheal tube bypasses the barrier of the upper airway: an important example is nosocomial pneumonia, which carries its own risk of mortality. Other complications are indirectly related to ETI, such as the need for sedation, which often prolongs weaning. These major safety considerations prompted efforts to develop noninvasive methods for delivering positive pressure ventilation. Thus, in patients with ARF, the main goal of NIPPV is to provide ventilatory assistance while lowering the risk of adverse events by reducing the need for invasive MV. Convincing evidence that NIPPV diminishes the risk of infectious complications has been obtained not only from pooled analyses of data from randomized controlled trials, but also from multivariate analyses of large cohort studies and from carefully performed case-controlled studies, all of which show large decreases in all categories of nosocomial infection.[5–7] The reason is that NIPPV is associated with a reduction in the overall invasiveness of patient management: sedation is given at lower levels or not at all, and the use of central venous lines, urinary catheters, and other invasive devices is considerably reduced, as compared to patients receiving endotracheal MV.[8]

Another important factor in promoting the use of NIPPV is the growing number of patients who are either unwilling to accept ETI or considered poor candidates for endotracheal MV because of their poor underlying health status.[9,10] In these patients, NIPPV can offer a chance of recovery with a low risk of complications. Further, by postponing ETI, NIPPV may provide a window of opportunity for the physician, family, and patient to make informed decisions about the goals of therapy.

EPIDEMIOLOGY

The use of NIPPV in the acute setting has increased markedly since the first small case-series were published in the last decade of the twentieth century.[11,12] A multicenter international study on MV was reported in 1998 by Esteban and colleagues.[13] In this study, NIPPV was used in about 5% of ICU patients who required MV. However, because only patients who received MV for longer than 12 hours were included, the study may have missed many patients treated with NIPPV. In a similar observational study performed in 42 ICUs in France in 1997, 16% of patients with ARF received NIPPV as the first-line method of ventilatory support.[14]

Importantly, among those patients who were not intubated before ICU admission, 35% received first-line NIPPV. In 2002, the same group did an identical study in 72 ICUs in France, including most of those in the previous study.[15] In the overall population of admitted patients, the percentage of patients who required some form of ventilatory support was the same in the two study periods. In 2002, the rates of NIPPV use among patients requiring ventilatory support had increased to 24% overall and 52% among patients who were not intubated before ICU admission. Although these results cannot be extrapolated to all countries, they indicate a strong trend toward increasing use of NIPPV in ICU patients with a variety of conditions, and they also reflect the current tendency to reduce the invasiveness of ICU management. Although many patients can be expected to benefit from this approach, great care should be taken to identify those patients who require immediate ETI, as delaying this procedure may reduce the chances of recovery in some patients.

EQUIPMENT

Several types of ventilator can be used to deliver NIPPV to patients with ARF. Turbine ventilators specifically designed for NIPPV have been developed, but standard ICU ventilators can be used as well. Turbine ventilators designed for NIPPV deliver two levels of positive airway pressure synchronized on patient trigger or time trigger, and reproducing pressure support ventilation or pressure control plus PEEP.[16] These ventilators are designed to compensate for air leakage, which is an important characteristic of NIPPV.[17] Although the meaning of "leak compensation" varies from one ventilator to the next, leakage compensation usually results in less triggering dysfunction than with standard ventilators. The main adverse effect of leakage on inspiratory triggering is auto-cycling. Auto-cycling is thought to be more common when high levels of PEEP are used. The cycling mechanism at end-inspiration can also be affected by leakage. When leakage is marked, the ventilator may be unable to recognize the end of inspiration based on flow rate deceleration, unless the unit is equipped with a special adaptive mechanism. This mechanism exists in turbine ventilators and in some ICU ventilators offering an NIPPV option. Adequate patient monitoring may be essential to assess patient-ventilator interaction, to detect leaks, and to fine-tune pressure levels. Bench comparisons assessing in vitro ventilator performance suggest that both turbine ventilators specially designed for NIPPV and late-generation standard ICU ventilators are satisfactory for delivering NIPPV to ICU patients with severe dyspnea.[16–19]

The use of an ICU ventilator that works from wall gas supply requires warming and humidification of the gas prior to airway delivery. With endotracheal MV, the gas temperature drops in the endotracheal tube. This does not occur with NIPPV, and in addition warm gas at the mouth may be difficult for the patient to tolerate. Therefore, lower gas temperatures are used for NIPPV than for endotracheal MV. One option is to use a heat and moisture exchanger. Unfortunately, the internal volume of these devices imposes an additional workload on the patient by generating CO_2 rebreathing. In patients with hypercapnic respiratory failure, this diminishes the effectiveness of NIPPV in reducing blood CO_2 levels and correcting respiratory acidosis.[20,21] A similar problem of CO_2 rebreathing occurs when turbine ventilators (using ambient room air) equipped with a one-line circuit are used with low levels of PEEP.[22,23] The expiratory flow generated to create the PEEP level is also used to flush the exhaled CO_2 from the circuit. With low PEEP levels, high minute ventilation, and/or a high respiratory rate, this can have adverse clinical effects that may require addition of a nonrebreathing valve to the circuit.

The interface used to connect the patient to the ventilator is usually a full face mask covering both the nose and the mouth. Although nasal interfaces are available, their use in ICU patients frequently results in major leakage through the mouth that diminishes the effectiveness of NIPPV and promotes patient-ventilator asynchrony and discomfort.[24,25] Full face masks are responsible for unwanted effects including skin breakdown over the nose, conjunctivitis related to leakage of air directed toward the eyes, rebreathing, claustrophobia, and overall discomfort.[12,26] These problems prompted efforts to design improved interfaces. The first improvement consisted in varying the pressure sites on the face to achieve better tolerance during prolonged use, and subsequently much larger masks enclosing the entire face or head were developed.[27,28] Use of a helmet has been suggested, primarily for patients with acute hypoxemic respiratory failure.[29–31] Because helmets may induce more rebreathing than other masks, they may be less suitable for patients with hypercapnic respiratory failure. The helmet probably markedly improves patient comfort and tolerance, at the price, however, of decreased effectiveness in unloading the respiratory muscles. This latter point is of importance since several studies have established that good clinical tolerance is crucial to successful NIPPV. In their large observational survey, Carlucci and colleagues identified two independent predictors of failure: the severity score (as assessed by the Simplified Acute Physiology Score [SAPS] II) and clinical tolerance.[14] Interestingly, recent physiologic studies with integral masks compared to standard full face masks seem to indicate comparable efficacy in terms of respiratory muscle unloading, suggesting that the theoretical risk of rebreathing associated with the large internal volume may be small or nonexistent in clinical practice.[32,33]

ACUTE EXACERBATION OF CHRONIC RESPIRATORY FAILURE

Many of the studies in the field of NIPPV have been performed in patients with obstructive disease, mainly chronic obstructive pulmonary disease (COPD).[12,34–38] All forms of acute or chronic ventilatory failure share several pathophysiologic pathways, but major differences exist as well. A few data suggest that NIPPV may be less effective in patients with chronic restrictive lung disease than in patients with COPD.[39]

PATHOPHYSIOLOGY

Exacerbation of COPD is a common cause of admission to the hospital and ICU. In addition to worsening of dyspnea and bronchitic symptoms and to development of right ventricular failure and encephalopathy, rapid and shallow breathing with hypoxemia and hypercapnia characterizes these exacerbations. The pathophysiologic pathway involves an inability of the respiratory system to maintain adequate alveolar ventilation in the presence of major abnormalities in respiratory mechanics. This can be modified by NIPPV, which allows the patient to take deeper breaths with less effort, thus reversing the clinical abnormalities resulting from hypoxemia, hypercapnia, and acidosis.[34,40] At baseline, the transdiaphragmatic pressure generated by these patients can be considerably higher than normal and represents a high percentage of their maximal diaphragmatic force, a situation that carries a major risk of respiratory muscle fatigue.[34,41,42] The main role of NIPPV is to offer the patient a way to increase the tidal volume at a lower work level. The use of ventilatory modalities working in synchrony with the patient's efforts allows larger breaths to be taken with less effort. As a result of the increased alveolar ventilation, arterial partial carbon dioxide pressure (Pa_{CO_2}) and pH values improve, and this in turn reduces the patient's ventilatory drive, thereby lowering the respiratory rate and improving the dyspnea.

CLINICAL EVIDENCE

The efficacy of NIPPV in patients admitted for acute exacerbation of COPD has been extensively studied. An international consensus conference recommended that NIPPV be considered a first-line treatment in these patients,[43] and the British Thoracic Society Guidelines indicate that every hospital should be able to deliver NIPPV on a 24-hour-per-day basis for this indication.[44] The first evidence that NIPPV markedly reduced the need for ETI came from case-control series reported in 1990.[34] Subsequently, several prospective randomized trials confirmed that NIPPV reduced the need for ETI and the rate of complications, shortened the length of stay, and improved survival in patients with COPD.[35,37,38,45–48] In a study by Kramer and associates, 74% of patients had COPD, and in this group NIPPV use was associated with a striking decrease in the ETI rate, from 67% to 9%.[38] Two studies conducted in the United Kingdom established that NIPPV was also effective in non-ICU settings.[35,48] Bott and coworkers[35] reported major improvements in dyspnea and gas exchange with a significant decrease in mortality when patients who refused NIPPV were excluded from the analysis. In the largest ICU study reported to date, Brochard and colleagues randomized 85 patients with COPD to treatment with or without face mask pressure-support ventilation.[37] The ETI rate was 74% in the controls given standard treatment and 26% in the NIPPV group. Benefits in the NIPPV group included a decreased rate of complications during the ICU stay, a shorter length of hospital stay, and more importantly, a significant reduction in mortality (from 29% to 9%). The overall decrease in mortality was ascribable to reductions in the need for ETI and in various ICU-related complications. In the United Kingdom, Plant and colleagues conducted a prospective multicenter randomized trial comparing standard therapy alone (control group) to NIPPV in 236 COPD patients admitted to general respiratory wards for ARF.[48] Treatment failure (defined as fulfillment of criteria for ARF) was more common in the control group (27%) than in the NIPPV group (15%), and NIPPV was associated with a lower in-hospital mortality rate. Because of admission policies in the United Kingdom, patients who failed NIPPV were not routinely transferred to the ICU, and consequently the findings may not be relevant to all health care institutions. The authors emphasized that the benefits of NIPPV out of the ICU were marginal in the most severely affected patients (pH <7.30 on admission), in whom the mortality rate was high. Those patients would probably have done better with early ICU admission for early NIPPV delivery in the ICU environment.

These studies indicate that early NIPPV to prevent further deterioration must become an important component of first-line therapy for COPD exacerbation.[49]

A very low pH, marked mental status alterations at NIPPV initiation, presence of comorbidities, and a high severity score are associated with early NIPPV failure[14] or late secondary failure after an initial improvement.[50] Several of these factors seem to indicate that a longer time from onset of the exacerbation to NIPPV initiation may reduce the likelihood of success. Every effort should be made to deliver NIPPV early, and close monitoring is in order when NIPPV is started late. In addition, a randomized controlled trial found that NIPPV was less effective when started late in the course of COPD exacerbation.[51] In this study, Conti and coworkers found a large reduction in the ETI rate, from 100% to 52%, contrasting with limited short-term benefits.[51] The patients stayed in the emergency ward for a mean of 14 hours before being admitted to the ICU because they met criteria for ETI, and NIPPV was initiated only at ICU admission. Interestingly, NIPPV was associated with significant long-term benefits such as a decrease in the readmission rate.

Whether the results of randomized controlled trials apply to everyday ICU practice must be evaluated. This is particularly important with NIPPV, since there is a learning curve, as shown in two studies. In a single-center study by Carlucci and colleagues, the NIPPV success rate remained stable over the study period, but the patients treated with NIPPV during the last few years of the study period had more severe disease with higher Pa_{CO_2} levels and lower pH values.[52] In an 8-year study performed in our institution, we found that NIPPV use increased gradually, in lockstep with a decline in conventional treatment with ETI.[53] In parallel with this gradual increase in NIPPV use, the nosocomial infection and mortality rates diminished. These important results were obtained in the group of patients with acute exacerbation of COPD and hypercapnic pulmonary edema.

LONG-TERM SURVIVAL

Several studies have suggested that NIPPV use may be associated with higher 1-year survival rates, as compared to standard ICU therapy or invasive MV.[51,54–56] Although these studies have a number of methodologic flaws, the consistency of their results suggests a major benefit of NIPPV, the mechanisms of which remain to be elucidated.

NEGATIVE PRESSURE VENTILATION

This technique is available in very few centers in the world. In acute exacerbations of COPD, it seems to provide better outcomes than conventional invasive MV and may be similar to face mask NIPPV.[57–60]

LOCATION

The study by Plant and associates cited above was performed in the respiratory wards, where the staff received 8 hours of training over the 3 months preceding the study.[48] During the study, it was estimated that maintaining the level of expertise provided by the prestudy training required on average 1 hour of additional training per month in each center. Wood and colleagues performed a study in the emergency ward, but the patients had very low severity, and few had COPD.[61] The results suggested that NIPPV use may have inappropriately delayed ETI. However, the small sample sizes, existence of several baseline differences across groups, and lack of accurate information on NIPPV settings make it difficult to draw conclusions from this study. The feasibility of treating patients with COPD out of the ICU has thus been demonstrated, but when evaluating whether this applies to a specific ward, the need to train the staff must be taken into account.

HELIUM-OXYGEN MIXTURE
The use of a helium-oxygen mixture for NIPPV seems very promising in patients with COPD.[62–64] Several randomized controlled trials are under way to determine whether this gas mixture increases the NIPPV success rate. Disappointingly, the first study found only modest benefits when helium was added to the gas mixture.

CARDIOGENIC PULMONARY EDEMA

PATHOPHYSIOLOGY
Continuous positive airway pressure (CPAP) elevates intrathoracic pressure, decreases shunting, and improves arterial oxygenation and dyspnea in patients with cardiogenic pulmonary edema. Interestingly, CPAP can both substantially lessen the work of breathing and improve cardiovascular function by decreasing the left ventricular afterload in non–preload-dependent patients.[65] Pressure support plus PEEP induces similar pathophysiologic benefits.

Most patients with cardiogenic pulmonary edema improve rapidly under medical therapy. A few, however, develop severe respiratory distress and/or refractory hypoxemia and require ventilatory support until the medical treatment starts to work. This is particularly common in elderly patients, who may also have a mild degree of chronic bronchitis.[66,67] Several NIPPV modalities have been used successfully, the goal being to avoid ETI.

CONTINUOUS POSITIVE AIRWAY PRESSURE OR PRESSURE SUPPORT PLUS POSITIVE END-EXPIRATORY PRESSURE
Randomized trials comparing either CPAP or pressure support plus PEEP to standard therapy found closely similar results with the two techniques in terms of improvement in arterial blood gases and breathing rate. Both CPAP and pressure support plus PEEP significantly reduced the rate of ETI.[67–71] Several studies, however, indicate a need for caution. One compared pressure support plus PEEP to CPAP.[72] Acute myocardial infarction was more common in the pressure support plus PEEP group than in the CPAP group. Although this difference may be ascribable to randomization bias rather than to a deleterious effect of pressure support plus PEEP, it invites caution in patients with coronary heart disease. No increases in the acute myocardial infarction rates were found in the NIPPV arm of a randomized controlled trial of pressure support and PEEP or in any of the observational studies, although the outcome of these patients may be worse than outcome in those with nonischemic causes of heart failure.[71,73,74] Another study compared intravenous bolus therapy with high-dose nitrates to conventional medical therapy (a different medical therapy) plus pressure support plus PEEP.[75] High-dose nitrate bolus therapy was far more effective clinically than NIPPV and resulted in better outcomes. These studies draw attention to the vulnerability of patients with cardiogenic pulmonary edema, particularly those with

coronary heart disease.[70,73] They indicate that both appropriate drug therapy and close monitoring are in order when using any form of NIPPV, especially in patients with coronary heart disease. In a randomized controlled trial, L'Her and associates showed that administration of CPAP to elderly patients with acute cardiogenic pulmonary edema in the emergency ward markedly improved physiologic parameters and 48-hour survival.[67] Unfortunately, there was no effect on hospital survival.

It is also important to draw attention to the fact that most of the studies demonstrating benefits of CPAP or pressure support plus PEEP included patients who, on average, had marked hypercapnia and acidosis indicating acute ventilatory failure.[67,70,71,73] A large multicenter study conducted by Nava and colleagues in patients with pulmonary edema found major benefits of NIPPV in the subgroup of hypercapnic patients, but no significant benefits in terms of ETI rate or outcome in the overall population, which included both hypercapnic and nonhypercapnic patients.[76]

In patients with hypercapnic pulmonary edema, ventilatory support with pressure support above PEEP is therefore a useful adjunct to medical treatment that reduces the ETI rate and improves outcomes. However, caution is needed when using NIPPV in patients with coronary heart disease.

HYPOXEMIC RESPIRATORY FAILURE

PATHOPHYSIOLOGY
Applying PEEP to the airway opening has been shown to increase functional residual capacity and to benefit respiratory mechanics and gas exchange.[77] These findings led intensivists to use CPAP as a means of preventing clinical deterioration and reducing the need for ETI.[70,78] Nevertheless, clinical data do not strongly support the use of CPAP in patients with acute lung injury (ALI),[79] and far better clinical outcomes have been reported with the combined use of pressure support ventilation and PEEP.[8,80,81] In patients with severe hypoxemia, ventilatory support should be able to relieve the dyspnea, improve oxygenation, and decrease the patient's effort to breathe. In a physiologic study, L'Her and coworkers confirmed the limited efficacy of CPAP alone in lessening the work of breathing.[82] They showed that addition of pressure support was crucial to reduce patient effort and dyspnea, whereas effects on oxygenation were dependent on the PEEP level.

CLINICAL EVIDENCE
CPAP
A recent investigation evaluated whether face mask CPAP produced physiologic benefits and reduced the need for ETI in patients with ALI.[79] Despite an early favorable physiologic response to CPAP in terms of comfort and oxygenation, no differences were found in the need for ETI, in-hospital mortality, or length of ICU stay. In addition, the use of CPAP was associated with a higher rate of complications including stress ulcer bleeding and cardiac arrest at the time of ETI. Therefore, CPAP alone cannot be recommended as a means of avoiding ETI in patients with ALI. Its use should be limited to a short initial period when no other method is available.

Pressure Support and PEEP
Until the late 1990s, the most convincing successes with NIPPV were obtained in patients with acute respiratory

acidosis in whom hypoxemia was not the main reason for respiratory failure. A randomized controlled trial by Wysocki and colleagues found no benefit of NIPPV in patients with no previous history of chronic lung disease, except in the subgroup of patients who developed acute hypercapnia.[83] However, NIPPV has now been proved beneficial in carefully selected patients with a variety of patterns of hypoxemic respiratory failure.[8,47,80,81,84–87] Recent studies suggest that in selected groups of patients NIPPV may reduce the need for ETI and improve outcomes.[86,88–90] Patient selection generally involves excluding patients who have shock, neurologic disorders with a need for upper airway protection, respiratory arrest, or any other concomitant organ failure. In a randomized controlled study by Antonelli and coworkers, NIPPV using pressure support and PEEP was highly beneficial in hypoxemic patients free from COPD, hemodynamic instability, or neurologic impairment, who were randomized when they reached predefined criteria for ETI.[81] Improvements in oxygenation were similar with the noninvasive and the invasive approach. Despite a 30% failure rate, patients treated with NIPPV had shorter durations of ventilation and ICU stay and experienced fewer complications. This study demonstrated that NIPPV could be effective in selected patients with hypoxemic respiratory failure but no hemodynamic or mental impairment. Other randomized controlled trials confirmed this beneficial effect.[80] The benefits seem greatest in specific subgroups, as discussed below. However, as indicated further on, patients with severe community-acquired pneumonia and profound hypoxemia or patients with acute respiratory distress syndrome (ARDS) may not always benefit from NIPPV, and in inexperienced hands the use of this technique may expose some patients to the risks associated with inappropriately delayed ETI.[15] Nevertheless, a recent study by Ferrer and colleagues indicates that NIPPV is effective in avoiding ETI and improving survival.[87] The study population comprised 105 patients admitted to the ICUs of three hospitals for acute non-hypercapnic hypoxemic respiratory failure due to community-acquired pneumonia, ARDS, cardiogenic pulmonary edema, or other diseases. Compared with oxygen therapy, NIPPV decreased the need for ETI (25% vs. 52%), the incidence of septic shock, and the ICU mortality rate (18% vs. 39%) and increased the cumulative 90-day survival rate.

SUBGROUPS

IMMUNOCOMPROMISED PATIENTS

Because one of the main benefits of NIPPV may be a decreased rate of infectious complications,[6,7,53] patients in whom MV carries a high risk for nosocomial infection may be particularly likely to benefit from NIPPV. Several trials have shown major benefits of NIPPV as a preventive measure during episodes of acute hypoxemic respiratory failure in solid organ-transplant patients or in patients with severe immunosuppression, particularly related to hematologic malignancies and neutropenia.[8,86,88] Significant reductions in ETI use, infectious complications, length of stay, and mortality occurred with NIPPV. Because of the high risk associated with ETI in patients with severe immunosuppression, NIPPV seems of particular interest in this group.[8,86,88,90] Similarly, patients experiencing *Pneumocystis carinii* pneumonia during the course of HIV infection seem to benefit from

NIPPV, as shown in a case-control study by Confalonieri and associates.[90]

In the population with immunosuppression, careful patient selection and early initiation of NIPPV are key factors in decreasing the need for ETI and in maximizing benefits to the patients.

LUNG SURGERY

Several studies looked at the use of NIPPV after surgery.[89,91,92] Auriant and associates conducted a randomized controlled trial in patients who experienced respiratory distress after lung resection.[89] Because reintubation shortly after lung surgery carries a very grim prognosis, avoiding ETI in this situation is a major goal. NIPPV was associated with lower ETI rates and higher hospital survival. Furthermore, an uncontrolled study found evidence supporting a beneficial effect of NIPPV in patients with respiratory distress after bilateral lung transplantation.[92] Thus, NIPPV seems useful in preventing reintubation after lung surgery.

COMMUNITY-ACQUIRED PNEUMONIA

A randomized controlled trial reported by Confalonieri and colleagues in patients with community-acquired pneumonia showed major benefits of NIPPV consisting of reductions in ETI rates, complication rates, and length of stay.[47] These favorable effects, however, were almost entirely ascribable to the subgroup of patients with COPD. In a case-control study done by the same group in patients with *Pneumocystis carinii* pneumonia, NIPPV reduced ETI rates, length of stay, and mortality.[90] Other studies found high rates of NIPPV failure in the subgroup of patients characterized by pneumonia with severe hypoxemia.[84,93–95] By contrast, the benefits found in the study by Ferrer and associates were marked in the subgroup of patients with pneumonia.[87] Therefore caution is necessary when using NIPPV in patients with severe community-acquired pneumonia. There is no consensus about recommendations for the use of NIPPV in this situation. The results of NIPPV in patients with severe community-acquired pneumonia may depend on the experience of the user and on the quality of patient monitoring.

POSTEXTUBATION RESPIRATORY FAILURE

The physiologic rationale for this approach in patients with COPD was recently demonstrated by Vitacca and coworkers.[96] A case-control study by Hilbert and associates suggested that NIPPV might prevent reintubation in patients with COPD.[97] A prospective randomized trial by Keenan and colleagues was performed in a population with postextubation respiratory distress that included only a few patients with COPD; no benefit of NIPPV was found.[98] Another prospective randomized trial did not find any evidence that NIPPV decreased reintubation rates.[99] By contrast, the preliminary results of another randomized trial provided indications of strong beneficial effects in COPD.[100] Lastly, a recent multicenter trial by Esteban and associates suggested that NIPPV used for postextubation respiratory distress may delay reintubation and increase mortality.[101]

Thus there is considerable doubt about the effectiveness of NIPPV in obviating the need for reintubation in all patients with postextubation respiratory distress. Using NIPPV in patients with postextubation respiratory distress may increase morbidity rates, and perhaps also mortality rates, by inappropriately delaying reintubation. The benefits of NIPPV in the treatment of postextubation respiratory distress may be limited to those patients with COPD. When NIPPV is used, the need for ETI should be evaluated early, within the first 2 hours of NIPPV, in order to avoid adverse outcomes related to delayed ETI.

WEANING

A number of patients with COPD require ETI because they fail NIPPV, have a contraindication to NIPPV (such as a need for surgery), or exhibit criteria for immediate ETI. However, when there is a need for prolonged ventilatory assistance, these patients can be switched to NIPPV after a few days of ETI.[102,103] This approach was shown in two randomized controlled trials to reduce the ETI time.[102,103] In a study by Nava and colleagues, complications were reduced and 60-day survival rates were higher with this approach.[102] This benefit was not found in the other study, in which the total length of ventilation was increased in the NIPPV arm.[103] A trial by Ferrer and coworkers suggested major benefits in COPD patients experiencing persistent weaning difficulties.[104] This study included 43 mechanically ventilated patients who had failed a weaning trial for 3 consecutive days. Compared with the conventional-weaning group, the NIPPV group had shorter times on invasive MV and in the ICU and hospital, as well as higher ICU and 90-day survival rates. Multicenter trials are needed to confirm the safety and efficacy of this approach.

PATIENTS WHO SHOULD NOT BE INTUBATED

Several reports have described the effects of NIPPV in patients with acute respiratory failure who were poor candidates for ETI because of advanced age, debilitation, or a "do not resuscitate" order.[9,10] The overall success rate in these reports approximated 60% to 70%. Gas exchange improved rapidly in successfully treated patients. Even when respiratory failure did not resolve, NIPPV provided symptomatic relief from dyspnea.

PATIENTS WITH SEVERE ACUTE ASTHMA

A few studies indicate that NIPPV can be used in asthmatic patients. Two cohort studies found beneficial short-term effects of NIPPV in asthmatic patients whose condition was deteriorating despite medical therapy.[105,106]

NEW MODES OF VENTILATION

Several studies used a new ventilatory mode known as proportional-assist ventilation, which is designed to improve the adjustment of ventilatory support to the patient's needs.[107–110] In several comparative studies with pressure-support ventilation in one of the arms, the efficacy of the two techniques seemed similar, although very few patients required ETI. Studies in patients with greater disease severity are needed. A prospective randomized trial by Fernandez-Vivas and associates in 117 patients with mixed causes of ARF again showed no difference in clinical outcomes between NIPPV delivered with pressure support or with proportional-assist ventilation.[110] Subjective comfort was better with proportional-assist ventilation, however, and intolerance was less common.

FIBEROPTIC BRONCHOSCOPY

Several studies have suggested or demonstrated that fiberoptic bronchoscopy can be performed under NIPPV (CPAP for hypoxemic patients or pressure support plus PEEP),[111–113] and that this approach resulted in better tolerance of the procedure and reduced complication rates and the need for ETI.[113]

References

1. Drinker P, McKhann CF: Landmark article May 18, 1929: The use of a new apparatus for the prolonged administration of artificial respiration. I. A fatal case of poliomyelitis. By Philip Drinker and Charles F. McKhann. *JAMA* 255:1473, 1986.
2. Drinker PA, McKhann CF 3rd: Landmark perspective: The iron lung. First practical means of respiratory support. *JAMA* 255:1476, 1986.
3. Stauffer JL, Olson DE, Petty TLE: Complications and consequences of endotracheal intubation and tracheotomy. A prospective study of 150 critically ill adult patients. *Am J Med* 70:65, 1981.
4. Pingleton SK: Complications of acute respiratory failure. *Am Rev Respir Dis* 137:1463, 1988.
5. Guérin C, Girard R, Chemorin C, et al: Facial mask noninvasive mechanical ventilation reduces the incidence of nosocomial pneumonia. A prospective epidemiological survey from a single ICU. *Intensive Care Med* 23:1024, 1997.
6. Nourdine K, Combes P, Carton M-J, et al: Does noninvasive ventilation reduce the ICU nosocomial infection risk? A prospective clinical survey. *Intensive Care Med* 25:567, 1999.
7. Girou E, Schortgen F, Delclaux C, et al: Association of noninvasive ventilation with nosocomial infections and survival in critically ill patients. *JAMA* 284:2361, 2000.
8. Antonelli M, Contin G, Bufi M, et al: Noninvasive ventilation for treatment of acute respiratory failure in patients undergoing solid organ transplantation. A randomized trial. *JAMA* 283:235, 2000.
9. Benhamou D, Girault C, Faure C, et al: Nasal mask ventilation in acute respiratory failure. Experience in elderly patients. *Chest* 102:912, 1992.
10. Meduri GU, Fox RC, Abou-Shala N, et al: Noninvasive mechanical ventilation via face mask in patients with acute respiratory failure who refused endotracheal intubation. *Crit Care Med* 22:1584, 1994.
11. Meduri GU, Conoscenti CC, Menashe P, Nair S: Noninvasive face mask ventilation in patients with acute respiratory failure. *Chest* 95:865, 1989.
12. Mehta S, Hill NS: Noninvasive ventilation. *Am J Respir Crit Care Med* 163:540, 2001.
13. Esteban A, Anzueto A, Frutos F, et al: Characteristics and outcomes in adult patients receiving mechanical ventilation: a 28-day international study. *JAMA* 287:345, 2002.
14. Carlucci A, Richard J-C, Wysocki M, et al, and the SRLF Collaborative Group on Mechanical Ventilation: Noninvasive versus conventional mechanical ventilation. An epidemiological survey. *Am J Respir Crit Care Med* 163:874, 2001.
15. Demoule A, Girou E, Taille S, Brochard L, and the SRLF Collaborative Group on Mechanical Ventilation: Current use of noninvasive ventilation. Results from a 2002 multicenter French survey. *Intensive Care Med* 29:S63, 2003.
16. Richard JC, Carlucci A, Breton L, et al: Bench testing of pressure support ventilation with three different generations of ventilators. *Intensive Care Med* 28:1049, 2002.
17. Mehta S, McCool FD, Hill NS: Leak compensation in positive pressure ventilators: a lung model study. *Eur Respir J* 17:259, 2001.

18. Stell IM, Paul G, Lee KC, et al: Noninvasive ventilator triggering in chronic obstructive pulmonary disease. A test lung comparison. *Am J Respir Crit Care Med* 164:2092, 2001.

19. Tassaux D, Strasser S, Fonseca S, et al: Comparative bench study of triggering, pressurization, and cycling between the home ventilator VPAP II and three ICU ventilators. *Intensive Care Med* 28:1254, 2002.

20. Lellouche F, Maggiore SM, Deye N, et al: Effect of the humidification device on the work of breathing during noninvasive ventilation. *Intensive Care Med* 28:1582, 2002.

21. Jaber S, Pigeot J, Fodil R, et al: Long-term effects of different humidification systems on endotracheal tube patency: evaluation by the acoustic reflection method. *Anesthesiology* 100:782, 2004.

22. Ferguson GT, Gilmartin M: CO$_2$ rebreathing during BiPAP ventilatory assistance. *Am J Respir Crit Care Med* 151:1126, 1995.

23. Lofaso F, Brochard L, Hang T, et al: Evaluation of carbon dioxide rebreathing during pressure support with BiPAP devices. *Chest* 108:772, 1995.

24. Carrey Z, Gottfried SB, Levy RD: Ventilatory muscle support in respiratory failure with nasal positive pressure ventilation. *Chest* 97:150, 1990.

25. Navalesi P, Fanfulla F, Frigerio P, et al: Physiologic evaluation of noninvasive mechanical ventilation delivered with three types of masks in patients with chronic hypercapnic respiratory failure. *Crit Care Med* 28:1785, 2000.

26. Schettino GP, Tucci MR, Sousa R, et al: Mask mechanics and leak dynamics during noninvasive pressure support ventilation: a bench study. *Intensive Care Med* 27:1887, 2001.

27. Criner GJ, Travaline JM, Brennan KJ, Kreimer DT: Efficacy of a new full face mask for noninvasive positive pressure ventilation. *Chest* 106:1109, 1994.

28. Gregoretti C, Confalonieri M, Navalesi P, et al: Evaluation of patient skin breakdown and comfort with a new face mask for non-invasive ventilation: a multi-center study. *Intensive Care Med* 28:278, 2002.

29. Antonelli M, Conti G, Pelosi P, et al: New treatment of acute hypoxemic respiratory failure: noninvasive pressure support ventilation delivered by helmet—a pilot controlled trial. *Crit Care Med* 30:602, 2002.

30. Antonelli M, Pennisi MA, Pelosi P, et al: Noninvasive positive pressure ventilation using a helmet in patients with acute exacerbation of chronic obstructive pulmonary disease: a feasibility study. *Anesthesiology* 100:16, 2004.

31. Chiumello D, Pelosi P, Carlesso E, et al: Noninvasive positive pressure ventilation delivered by helmet vs. standard face mask. *Intensive Care Med* 29:1671, 2003.

32. Fraticelli A, Lellouche F, Taillé S, et al: Comparison of different interfaces during NIV in patients with acute respiratory failure. *Am J Respir Crit Care Med* 167:A863, 2003.

33. Lellouche F, Fraticelli A, Taille S, et al: Physiological evaluation of five interfaces during non-invasive ventilation in healthy subjects. *Intensive Care Med* 28:S50, 2002.

34. Brochard L, Isabey D, Piquet J, et al: Reversal of acute exacerbations of chronic obstructive lung disease by inspiratory assistance with a face mask. *N Engl J Med* 323:1523, 1990.

35. Bott J, Carroll MP, Conway JH, et al: Randomised controlled trial of nasal ventilation in acute ventilatory failure due to chronic obstructive airways disease. *Lancet* 341:1555, 1993.

36. Vitacca M, Rubini F, Foglio K, et al: Non invasive modalities of positive pressure ventilation improve the outcome of acute exacerbations in COLD patients. *Intensive Care Med* 19:450, 1993.

37. Brochard L, Mancebo J, Wysocki M, et al: Noninvasive ventilation for acute exacerbations of chronic obstructive pulmonary disease. *N Engl J Med* 333:817, 1995.

38. Kramer N, Meyer TJ, Meharg J, et al: Randomized, prospective trial of noninvasive positive pressure ventilation in acute respiratory failure. *Am J Respir Crit Care Med* 151:1799, 1995.

39. Robino C, Faisy C, Diehl JL, et al: Effectiveness of non-invasive positive pressure ventilation differs between decompensated chronic restrictive and obstructive pulmonary disease patients. *Intensive Care Med* 29:603, 2003.

40. Appendini L, Patessio A, Zanaboni S, et al: Physiologic effects of positive end-expiratory pressure and mask pressure support during exacerbations of chronic obstructive pulmonary disease. *Am J Respir Crit Care Med* 149:1069, 1994.

41. Nava S, Ambrosino N, Rubini F, et al: Effect of nasal pressure support ventilation and external PEEP on diaphragmatic activity in patients with severe stable COPD. *Chest* 103:143, 1993.

42. Nava S, Bruschi C, Fracchia C, et al: Patient-ventilator interaction and inspiratory effort during pressure support ventilation in patients with different pathologies. *Eur Respir J* 10:177, 1997.

43. Evans TW: International Consensus Conferences in Intensive Care Medicine: Non-invasive positive pressure ventilation in acute respiratory failure. *Intensive Care Med* 27:166, 2001.

44. Baudouin S, Blumenthal S, Cooper B, et al: Non-invasive ventilation in acute respiratory failure. *Thorax* 57:192, 2002.

45. Angus RM, Ahmed AA, Fenwick LJ, Peacok AJ: Comparison of the acute effects on gas exchange of nasal ventilation and doxapram in acute exacerbations of chronic obstructive pulmonary disease. *Thorax* 51:1048, 1996.

46. Celikel T, Sungur M, Ceyhan B, Karakurt S: Comparison of noninvasive positive pressure ventilation with standard medical therapy in hypercapnic acute respiratory failure. *Chest* 114:1636, 1998.

47. Confalonieri M, Potena A, Carbone G, et al: Acute respiratory failure in patients with severe community-acquired pneumonia. A prospective randomized evaluation of non-invasive ventilation. *Am J Respir Crit Care Med* 160:1585, 1999.

48. Plant PK, Owen JL, Elliott MW: Early use of non-invasive ventilation for acute exacerbations of chronic obstructive pulmonary disease on general respiratory wards: a multicentre randomised controlled trial. *Lancet* 355:1931, 2000.

49. Brochard L: Non-invasive ventilation for acute exacerbations of COPD : a new standard of care. *Thorax* 55:817, 2000.

50. Moretti M, Cilione C, Tampieri A, et al: Incidence and causes of non-invasive mechanical ventilation failure after initial success. *Thorax* 55:819, 2000.

51. Conti G, Antonelli P, Navalesi P, et al: Noninvasive vs. conventional mechanical ventilation in patients with chronic obstructive pulmonary disease after failure of medical treatment in the ward: a randomized trial. *Intensive Care Med* 28:1701, 2002.

52. Carlucci A, Del Mastro M, Rubini F, et al: Changes in the practice of non-invasive ventilation in treating COPD patients over 8 years. *Intensive Care Med* 29:419, 2003.

53. Girou E, Brun-Buisson C, Taille S, et al: Secular trends in nosocomial infections and mortality associated with noninvasive ventilation in patients with exacerbation of COPD and pulmonary edema. *JAMA* 290:2985, 2003.

54. Confalonieri M, Parigi P, Scartabellati A, et al: Noninvasive mechanical ventilation improves the immediate and long-term outcome of COPD patients with acute respiratory failure. *Eur Respir J* 9:422, 1996.

55. Vitacca M, Clini E, Rubini F, et al: Non-invasive mechanical ventilation in severe chronic obstructive lung disease and acute respiratory failure: short-and long-term prognosis. *Intensive Care Med* 22:94, 1996.

56. Bardi G, Pierotello R, Desideri M, et al: Nasal ventilation in COPD exacerbations: early and late results of a prospective, controlled study. *Eur Respir J* 15:98, 2000.

57. Corrado A, Gorini M, Ginanni R, et al: Negative pressure ventilation versus conventional mechanical ventilation in the treatment of acute respiratory failure in COPD patients. *Eur Respir J* 12:519, 1998.

58. Corrado A, Confalonieri M, Marchese S, et al: Iron lung vs mask ventilation in the treatment of acute on chronic respiratory

failure in COPD patients: a multicenter study. *Chest* 121:189, 2002.

59. Corrado A, Ginanni R, Villella G, et al: Iron lung versus conventional mechanical ventilation in acute exacerbation of COPD. *Eur Respir J* 23:419, 2004.

60. Gorini M, Ginanni R, Villella G, et al: Non-invasive negative and positive pressure ventilation in the treatment of acute on chronic respiratory failure. *Intensive Care Med* 30:875, 2004.

61. Wood KA, Lewis L, Von Harz B, Kollef MH: The use of noninvasive positive pressure ventilation in the emergency department: results of a randomized clinical trial. *Chest* 113:1339, 1998.

62. Jolliet P, Tassaux D, Thouret JM, Chevrolet JC: Beneficial effects of helium:oxygen versus air:oxygen noninvasive pressure support in patients with decompensated chronic obstructive pulmonary disease. *Crit Care Med* 27:2422, 1999.

63. Jaber S, Fodil R, Carlucci A, et al: Noninvasive ventilation with helium-oxygen in acute exacerbations of chronic obstructive pulmonary disease. *Am J Respir Crit Care Med* 161:1191, 2000.

64. Jolliet P, Tassaux D, Roeseler J, et al: Helium-oxygen versus air-oxygen noninvasive pressure support in decompensated chronic obstructive disease: A prospective, multicenter study. *Crit Care Med* 31:878, 2003.

65. Lenique F, Habis M, Lofaso F, et al: Ventilatory and hemodynamic effects of continuous positive airway pressure in left heart failure. *Am J Respir Crit Care Med* 155:500, 1997.

66. L'Her E, Moriconi M, Texier F, et al: Non-invasive continuous positive airway pressure in acute hypoxaemic respiratory failure—experience of an emergency department. *Eur J Emerg Med* 5:313, 1998.

67. L'Her E, Duquesne F, Girou E, et al: Noninvasive continuous positive airway pressure in elderly cardiogenic pulmonary edema patients. *Intensive Care Med* 30:882, 2004.

68. Räsänen J, Heikkilä J, Downs J, et al: Continuous positive airway pressure by face mask in acute cardiogenic pulmonary edema. *Am J Cardiol* 55:296, 1985.

69. Lin M, Yang YF, Chiang HT, et al: Reappraisal of continuous positive airway pressure therapy in acute cardiogenic pulmonary edema. Short-term results and long-term follow-up. *Chest* 107:1379, 1995.

70. Bersten AD, Holt AW, Vedig AE, et al: Treatment of severe cardiogenic pulmonary edema with continuous positive airway pressure delivered by face mask. *N Engl J Med* 325:1825, 1991.

71. Masip J, Betbese AJ, Paez J, et al: Non-invasive pressure support ventilation versus conventional oxygen therapy in acute cardiogenic pulmonary oedema: a randomised trial. *Lancet* 356:2126, 2000.

72. Mehta S, Gregory DJ, Woolard RH, et al: Randomized, prospective trial of bilevel versus continuous positive airway pressure in acute pulmonary edema. *Crit Care Med* 25:620, 1997.

73. Masip J, Paez J, Merino M, et al: Risk factors for intubation as a guide for noninvasive ventilation in patients with severe acute cardiogenic pulmonary edema. *Intensive Care Med* 29:1921, 2003.

74. Hoffmann B, Welte T: The use of noninvasive pressure support ventilation for severe respiratory insufficiency due to pulmonary oedema. *Intensive Care Med* 25:15, 1999.

75. Sharon A, Shpirer I, Kaluski E, et al: High-dose intravenous isosorbide-dinitrate is safer and better than Bi-PAP ventilation combined with conventional treatment for severe pulmonary edema. *J Am Coll Cardiol* 36:832, 2000.

76. Nava S, Carbone G, DiBattista N, et al: Noninvasive ventilation in cardiogenic pulmonary edema: a multicenter randomized trial. *Am J Respir Crit Care Med* 168:1432, 2003.

77. Katz JA, Marks JD: Inspiratory work with and without continuous positive airway pressure in patients with acute respiratory failure. *Anesthesiology* 63:598, 1985.

78. Goldberg P, Reissmann H, Maltais F, et al: Efficacy of noninvasive CPAP in COPD with acute respiratory failure. *Eur Respir J* 8:1894, 1995.

79. Delclaux C, L'Her E, Alberti C, et al: Treatment of acute hypoxemic nonhypercapnic respiratory insufficiency with continuous positive airway pressure delivered by a face mask: A randomized controlled trial. *JAMA* 284:2352, 2000.

80. Martin TJ, Hovis JD, Costantino JP, et al: A randomized, prospective evaluation of noninvasive ventilation for acute respiratory failure. *Am J Respir Crit Care Med* 161:807, 2000.

81. Antonelli M, Conti G, Rocco M, et al: A comparison of noninvasive positive-pressure ventilation and conventional mechanical ventilation in patients with acute respiratory failure. *N Engl J Med* 339:429, 1998.

82. L'Her E, Taille S, Deye N, et al: Physiological response of hypoxemic patients to different modes of noninvasive ventilation. *Am J Respir Crit Care Med* 167:A863, 2003.

83. Wysocki M, Tric L, Wolff MA, et al: Noninvasive pressure support ventilation in patients with acute respiratory failure. A randomized comparison with conventional therapy. *Chest* 107:761, 1995.

84. Meduri GU, Turner RE, Abou-Shala N, et al: Noninvasive positive pressure ventilation via face mask. First-line intervention in patients with acute hypercapnic and hypoxemic respiratory failure. *Chest* 109:179, 1996.

85. Gregoretti C, Beltrame F, Lucangelo U, et al: Physiologic evaluation of non-invasive pressure support ventilation in trauma patients with acute respiratory failure. *Intensive Care Med* 24:785, 1998.

86. Hilbert G, Gruson D, Vargas F, et al: Noninvasive ventilation in immunosuppressed patients with pulmonary infiltrates, fever, and acute respiratory failure. *N Engl J Med* 344:481, 2001.

87. Ferrer M, Esquinas A, Leon M, et al: Noninvasive ventilation in severe hypoxemic respiratory failure: a randomized clinical trial. *Am J Respir Crit Care Med* 168:1438, 2003.

88. Azoulay E, Alberti C, Bornstain C, et al: Improved survival in cancer patients requiring mechanical ventilatory support: Impact of noninvasive mechanical ventilatory support. *Crit Care Med* 29:519, 2001.

89. Auriant I, Jallot A, Herve P, et al: Noninvasive ventilation reduces mortality in acute respiratory failure following lung resection. *Am J Respir Crit Care Med* 164:1231, 2001.

90. Confalonieri M, Calderini E, Terraciano S, et al: Noninvasive ventilation for treating acute respiratory failure in AIDS patients with *Pneumocystis carinii* pneumonia. *Intensive Care Med* 28:1233, 2002.

91. Aguilo R, Togores B, Pons S, et al: Noninvasive ventilatory support after lung resectional surgery. *Chest* 112:117, 1997.

92. Rocco M, Conti G, Antonelli M, et al: Non-invasive pressure support ventilation in patients with acute respiratory failure after bilateral lung transplantation. *Intensive Care Med* 27:1622, 2001.

93. Jolliet P, Abajo B, Pasquina P, Chevrolet J-C: Non-invasive pressure support ventilation in severe community-acquired pneumonia. *Intensive Care Med* 27:812, 2001.

94. Domenighetti G, Gayer R, Gentilini R: Noninvasive pressure support ventilation in non-COPD patients with acute cardiogenic pulmonary edema and severe community-acquired pneumonia: acute effects and outcome. *Intensive Care Med* 28:1226, 2002.

95. Antonelli M, Conti G, Moro M, et al: Predictors of failure of noninvasive positive pressure ventilation in patients with acute hypoxemic respiratory failure: a multi-center study. *Intensive Care Med* 27:1718, 2001.

96. Vitacca M, Ambrosino N, Clini E, et al: Physiological response to pressure support ventilation delivered before and after extubation in patients not capable of totally spontaneous autonomous breathing. *Am J Respir Crit Care Med* 164:638, 2001.

97. Hilbert G, Gruson D, Portel L, et al: Noninvasive pressure support ventilation in COPD patients with postextubation hypercapnic respiratory insufficiency. *Eur Respir J* 11:1349, 1998.

98. Keenan S, Powers C, McCormack D, Block G: Noninvasive positive-pressure ventilation for postextubation respiratory distress: a randomized controlled trial. *JAMA* 287:3238, 2002.

99. Jiang J, Kao SJ, Wang SN: Effect of early application of biphasic positive airway pressure on the outcome of extubation in ventilator weaning. *Respirology* 4:161, 1999.

100. Carlucci A, Gregoretti C, Squadrone V, et al: Preventive use of non-invasive mechanical ventilation to avoid post-extubation respiratory failure: a randomized controlled trial. *Eur Resp J* 18:29S, 2001.

101. Esteban A, Frutos-Vivar F, Ferguson ND, et al: Noninvasive positive-pressure ventilation for respiratory failure after extubation. *N Engl J Med* 350:2452, 2004.

102. Nava S, Ambrosino N, Clini E, et al: Noninvasive mechanical ventilation in the weaning of patients with respiratory failure due to chronic obstructive pulmonary disease. A randomized, controlled trial. *Ann Intern Med* 128:721, 1998.

103. Girault C, Daudenthun I, Chevron V, et al: Noninvasive ventilation as a systematic extubation and weaning technique in acute-on-chronic respiratory failure. *Am J Respir Crit Care Med* 160:86, 1999.

104. Ferrer M, Esquinas A, Arancibia F, et al: Noninvasive ventilation during persistent weaning failure: a randomized controlled trial. *Am J Respir Crit Care Med* 168:70, 2003.

105. Meduri UG, Cook TR, Turner RE, et al: Noninvasive positive pressure ventilation in status asthmaticus. *Chest* 110:767, 1996.

106. Fernandez M, Villagra A, Blanch L, Fernandez R: Non-invasive mechanical ventilation in status asthmaticus. *Intensive Care Med* 27:486, 2001.

107. Patrick W, Webster K, Ludwig L, et al: Noninvasive positive-pressure ventilation in acute respiratory distress without prior chronic respiratory failure. *Am J Respir Crit Care Med* 153:1005, 1996.

108. Gay P, Hess D, Hill N: Noninvasive proportional assist ventilation for acute respiratory insufficiency. Comparison with pressure support ventilation. *Am J Respir Crit Care Med* 164:1606, 2001.

109. Wysocki M, Richard J-C, Meshaka P: Noninvasive proportional assist ventilation compared with noninvasive pressure support ventilation in hypercapnic acute respiratory failure. *Crit Care Med* 30:323, 2002.

110. Fernandez-Vivas M, Caturla-Such J, Gonzalez de la Rosa J, et al: Noninvasive pressure support versus proportional assist ventilation in acute respiratory failure. *Intensive Care Med* 29:1126, 2003.

111. Antonelli M, Conti G, Riccioni L, Meduri GU: Noninvasive positive-pressure ventilation via face mask during bronchoscopy with BAL in high-risk hypoxemic patients. *Chest* 110:724, 1996.

112. Antonelli M, Conti G, Rocco M, et al: Noninvasive positive-pressure ventilation vs. conventional oxygen supplementation in hypoxemic patients undergoing diagnostic bronchoscopy. *Chest* 121:1149, 2002.

113. Maitre B, Jaber S, Maggiore S, et al: Continuous positive airway pressure during fiberoptic bronchoscopy in hypoxemic patients. A randomized double-blind study using a new device. *Am J Respir Crit Care Med* 162:1063, 2000.

Chapter 34
UPPER AIRWAY OBSTRUCTION

BRIAN GEHLBACH
JOHN P. KRESS

KEY POINTS

- Suspected upper airway obstruction (UAO) constitutes a medical emergency. The immediate bedside consultation of a clinician experienced in the management of this condition is indicated.

- The initial evaluation of UAO is focused on determining the severity and suspected site of the obstruction. Arterial desaturation is a late manifestation; better indicators of severity include stridor, poor air movement, accessory muscle use, abnormal mentation or agitation, tachycardia, hypertension, and pulsus paradoxus.

- Infections represent important causes of oropharyngeal and hypopharyngeal UAO and include Ludwig angina, peritonsillar abscess, and infections of the retropharyngeal and lateral pharyngeal spaces. Otolaryngology consultation is indicated. Depending on the initial site of infection, spread to other critical sites (e.g., the mediastinum) may occur.

- While intubation is not always required in adults with epiglottitis, management in an ICU is mandatory, and intubation equipment and a tracheostomy tray should be at the bedside.

- Bacterial infections of the larynx are life-threatening. Causative organisms include Staphylococcus aureus, Streptococcus pneumoniae, Haemophilus influenzae, and Corynebacterium diphtheriae.

- Laryngospasm and laryngeal edema are important causes of postextubation stridor. Prophylactic corticosteroids have not shown a benefit in preventing postextubation stridor. A short (48 hours) course of corticosteroids is reasonable to treat established cases of laryngeal edema.

- Long-term intubation may result in a variety of problems related to the upper airway, including endotracheal tube obstruction from secretions, vocal cord injury, subglottic stenosis, and tracheal stenosis.

- Risk factors for foreign body aspiration in adults include diminished level of consciousness; impaired swallowing mechanism or diminished upper airway sensation as a result of neuromuscular disorder, prior cerebrovascular accident, or advanced age; and inability to chew food properly because of poor dentition.

- All suspected traumatic laryngeal injuries should be evaluated promptly to reduce the immediate risk of UAO, as well as to prevent long-term sequelae such as subglottic stenosis.

- Early laryngoscopic examination of the upper airway is crucial in the evaluation of burn patients with suspected inhalation injury. The risk of UAO increases throughout the first 24 hours.

- Functional upper airway obstruction may occur in patients who exhibit abnormal glottic closure during inspiration and/or expiration. There is a high risk of coincident asthma, complicating the evaluation of such patients.

- Angioedema may result from allergy, hereditary or acquired disorders of the complement cascade, direct release of histamine from mast cells from nonallergic mechanisms (e.g., opiates), and from angiotensin-converting enzyme inhibitors.

- Angioedema from angiotensin-converting enzyme inhibitors may occur at any time during the course of therapy.

- Helium-oxygen mixtures reduce the density-dependent pressure required to drive airflow across obstructing upper airway lesions, and may stabilize patients with UAO pending definitive therapy.

- Prompt evaluation and management of suspected UAO may prevent subsequent complications including cardiac arrest, anoxic brain injury, and negative pressure pulmonary edema.

There are few medical conditions that are as rapidly and predictably lethal as the loss of upper airway patency. Because of the relative infrequency with which upper airway obstruction (UAO) is encountered by most physicians, opportunities to acquire significant clinical experience are limited. This, combined with the frequently subtle presentation of upper airway obstruction and the clinician's inability to visualize the upper airway in its entire extent through routine physical examination, may hamper diagnosis of this condition until a crisis results. This chapter describes an approach to diagnosing and treating UAO as it presents in adults. While certain infections of the head, neck, and upper respiratory tract are considered here as they relate to UAO, the specific approach to their management is considered in greater detail in Chap. 54. A high index of suspicion for UAO, combined with early consultation of anesthesia and otolaryngology services, is critical to the successful management of this condition.

Anatomy of the Upper Airway

The upper airway comprises air-conducting passages that begin at the mouth or nose and end at the mainstem carina.[1,2] The thoracic inlet divides the upper airway into the intrathoracic and extrathoracic airways. The extrathoracic airways are further divided into the nasopharynx, oropharynx, hypopharynx, larynx, and extrathoracic trachea. Air inspired through the nose passes through the nasal cavities and enters the nasopharynx after exiting the nose by way of the posterior nares. Airflow proceeds inferiorly through the nasopharynx, passes posterior to the soft palate, and enters the oropharynx. Closure of the soft palate allows inspiration of air through the mouth. Air passes inferiorly through the oropharynx to the hypopharynx, which begins just superior to the hyoid bone, and passes the epiglottis, thereby entering the larynx.

The larynx is constructed of a cartilaginous skeleton consisting of the thyroid, cricoid, and arytenoid cartilages (Fig. 34-1). This skeleton surrounds the vocal cords, the movements of which are controlled by the intrinsic muscles of the larynx, with their innervation arising from the left and right branches of the recurrent laryngeal nerve. An exception to this rule is the innervation of the cricothyroid muscle, which arises from the superior laryngeal nerve. This nerve also supplies sensation to the epiglottis and vestibular folds (false cords), which lie superior to the true vocal cords. The larynx is

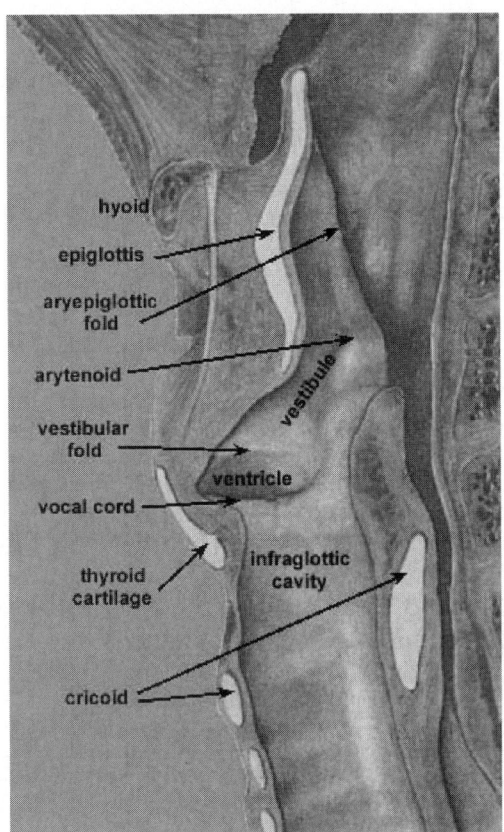

FIGURE 34-1 Laryngeal anatomy. *(Reproduced with permission from http://mywebpages.comcast.net/wnor/homepage.htm, author Wesley Norman, PhD, DSc.)*

divided into the supraglottic portion, the glottis, and the subglottic portion. The glottis contains the structures within the plane of the true vocal cords and is located at the midpoint of the thyroid cartilage. The supraglottic region extends from the epiglottis to just above the true vocal cords, while the subglottic region lies between the vocal cords and the lower border of the cricoid cartilage.

The trachea lies between the inferior border of the cricoid cartilage and the main carina, and is 10 to 13 cm in length in adults. The extrathoracic trachea is typically 2 to 4 cm long, and comprises the segment that lies between the cricoid cartilage and the thoracic inlet. The normal trachea has roughly the same coronal as sagittal diameter. Normal coronal tracheal diameter is 13 to 25 mm in men and 10 to 21 mm in women.

This chapter will focus on disorders of the extrathoracic upper airway because of this region's greater importance to the topic of UAO.

Pathophysiology of Upper Airway Obstruction

While obstruction may occur at any point in the upper airway, laryngeal obstruction is most problematic because the airway is narrowest at this point. The glottis is the narrowest region in adults, while the subglottic region is the narrowest in infants. The basis for which seemingly minor reductions in the cross-sectional area of the upper airway have important effects on airflow is presented below.

Alveolar ventilation is accomplished through the bulk flow of fresh gas down to the terminal bronchioles, at which point the cross-sectional area of the airways becomes so large that the forward velocity of gas molecules becomes negligible, and diffusive flow occurs.[3] Airflow may be laminar, transitional, or turbulent. Laminar flow consists of orderly streams of gas arranged in lines parallel to the airway. At higher flow rates and at branch points flow may become transitional, with gas eddies that break away from the parallel streams. Turbulent flow is the most disorganized pattern, and occurs at high flow rates. The Reynolds number (Re) is a dimensionless number that derives from the ratio of inertial to viscous forces and allows prediction of whether flow will be laminar or not:

$$Re = 2rvd/\mu$$

where r is the radius of the tube, v is the average gas velocity, d is the gas density, and μ is the gas viscosity. Values less than 2000 predict laminar flow, values between 2000 and 4000 predict transitional flow, and values greater than 4000 predict turbulent flow. The driving pressure for laminar flow is proportional to the flow rate and inversely related to the fourth power of the radius, among other factors. Thus a relatively minor decrease in the radius of a tube like the upper airway causes a large increase in the driving pressure necessary to achieve the same flow rate. Turbulent flow as occurs in a rough tube like the larynx and trachea requires greater driving pressure than laminar flow, being proportional to the density of the gas and the *square of the flow rate*. Inhalation of a low-density gas such as helium therefore decreases the driving pressure required for airflow through two mechanisms: reducing the Reynolds number, thereby increasing the proportion of flow that is laminar; and decreasing the density-dependent driving pressure where turbulent flow exists.[4]

The clinical implications of these principles are as follows: (1) Upper airway obstructing lesions, once symptomatic, can progress rapidly to a crisis with relatively small increases in size and consequent reduction in the size of the airway lumen; (2) while awaiting definitive treatment of the upper airway obstruction, inhalation of a low-density gas mixture such as helium-oxygen may stabilize the patient by decreasing the driving pressure required for a given airflow.

Upper airway obstructing lesions may limit inspiratory flow, expiratory flow, or both, depending on the site and nature of the lesion. Flow-volume loops obtained by spirometry are useful for understanding the physiology of different sites of upper airway obstruction.[5]

VARIABLE EXTRATHORACIC OBSTRUCTION

During normal inspiration the intrathoracic airways dilate, while the extrathoracic airways tend to collapse as the increase in gas velocity causes a fall in intraluminal pressure (Bernoulli effect). As gas velocity increases past an obstructing lesion, this effect is increased, causing flow limitation, with a reduction in peak inspiratory flow and a flattening of the inspiratory limb of the flow volume loop. In contrast, during forced expiration the intraluminal pressure is positive relative to the atmosphere, preserving expiratory flow. These lesions occur above the thoracic inlet and include bilateral vocal cord paralysis, paradoxical movement of the vocal cords, and tracheomalacia of the extrathoracic airway.

VARIABLE INTRATHORACIC OBSTRUCTION

During forced expiration the intrathoracic airways have a tendency to narrow as a result of airway compression and the Bernoulli effect. This leads to a reduction in peak expiratory flow and a flattening of the expiratory limb of the flow volume loop. Inspiratory flow, in contrast, is preserved as lung expansion increases the radius of the airway at the site of the obstructing lesion. Common causes of variable intrathoracic obstruction include low tracheal tumors and tracheomalacia of the intrathoracic airway.[6]

FIXED UPPER AIRWAY OBSTRUCTION

Fixed upper airway obstruction occurs when airflow at the site of obstruction is insensitive to the effects of the respiratory cycle because the lesion imparts rigidity to the walls of the affected area. Affected patients have reductions in peak inspiratory and expiratory flow, while the flow volume loop depicts flattening of the inspiratory and expiratory limbs. Examples of this disorder include subglottic stenosis and some tumors.

Clinical Presentation and Initial Evaluation

Patients presenting with upper airway obstruction may complain of a variety of symptoms including hoarseness, stridor, hemoptysis, dysphagia, odynophagia, drooling, and swelling of the neck or face. Dyspnea is typically exacerbated by exercise, and in the case of certain diseases—for example, anterior mediastinal tumors—by the supine position. In many cases prior evaluations have yielded a diagnosis of asthma or chronic obstructive pulmonary disease. While certain disorders such as epiglottitis have very acute presentations, at times symptoms have developed so insidiously that the patient has habituated to the condition, and has few or no complaints.

If time permits, initial evaluation should include a history of the present illness, focusing on the duration of symptoms and any associated oropharyngeal, gastrointestinal, or constitutional symptoms, along with a history of prior upper aerodigestive tract disorders, recent dental problems or procedures, and smoking. Physical examination is directed toward localizing the site of the lesion.[7] Inspiratory stridor generally indicates a lesion at or above the level of the glottis, while biphasic stridor (stridor present during both inspiration and expiration), which is usually higher in pitch, suggests a lesion at the subglottic or tracheal level. The presence of stridor indicates a severe degree of narrowing, typically to ≤6 mm. Supraglottic lesions may cause a muffling of the voice, while oral abscesses may cause a "hot potato voice" (i.e., the speech of someone who has a hot potato in his mouth). Hoarseness accompanies unilateral vocal cord paralysis. An oral examination should be performed, unless epiglottitis is suspected and skilled airway personnel are not present. The submental and submandibular regions should be palpated, along with the neck and cervical and supraclavicular lymph nodes.

The first priority in encountering a patient with suspected UAO is to determine the severity of obstruction. When the obstruction is severe and loss of the airway is feared, the airway should be secured by an experienced operator. Arterial desaturation is an extremely late sign of UAO in the patient with normal lungs, and often heralds a catastrophe. This is illustrated by the difficulty normal, untrained individuals have in achieving arterial desaturation during breath holding. Similarly, arterial blood gases provide little information beyond that obtained through the bedside assessment of an experienced clinician. Better indicators of severe airway obstruction include stridor, poor air movement, accessory muscle use, abnormal mentation or agitation, tachycardia, hypertension, and pulsus paradoxus. All patients with newly diagnosed UAO of more than trivial severity should be monitored in an ICU until treatment can be initiated or clinical stability can be determined.

If UAO is suspected but there is no immediate risk of losing the airway, further evaluation may employ a range of techniques, depending on the suspected diagnosis. Spirometry is useful in the elective evaluation of subacute to chronic UAO; however, because the airway must be narrowed to ≤8 mm in order to affect the flow volume loop, spirometry is relatively insensitive. Inspection of the flow volume loop for flattening of the inspiratory or expiratory limb is the most reliable spirometric indication of UAO, particularly when done by an experienced reader. Poor effort may mimic UAO. The report of patient effort by the technician and the reproducibility of the loops are useful in distinguishing poor effort from UAO. Spirometry may fail to detect even significant degrees of UAO in patients with severe chronic obstructive pulmonary disease.

Plain chest radiographs may demonstrate tracheal deviation from masses arising in the mediastinum or neck. Lateral neck films may suggest the diagnosis of croup or epiglottitis. Computed tomography (CT) is extremely useful in evaluating suspected tumors of the upper airway, and in characterizing the extent of upper airway soft tissue infections. Three-dimensional reconstruction is useful in identifying fixed anatomic abnormalities of the upper airway, such as tracheal stenosis, and in following the response to therapy.[8] However, dynamically determined disorders such as tracheomalacia require direct visualization.

Endoscopic evaluation may be flexible or rigid. Rigid endoscopy is useful in the management of suspected foreign body aspiration. Flexible endoscopy may be performed via the oropharyngeal or nasopharyngeal route.

Causes of Upper Airway Obstruction

NASAL AND NASOPHARYNGEAL CAUSES

Benign and malignant masses of the nose and nasopharynx constitute important sources of morbidity, and occasionally, mortality. However, because ventilation can usually be maintained via the oropharyngeal route in these cases, they will not be discussed here.

OROPHARYNGEAL CAUSES

INFECTIOUS CAUSES
Infectious etiologies represent relatively common causes of upper airway obstructing lesions. Ludwig angina is an infection of the submandibular space.[9] The source of infection is usually a second or third mandibular molar tooth, with causative organisms representing typical oral flora: streptococci, staphylococci, and anaerobes. Gram-negative

organisms should be considered as potential etiologies in patients with altered oral flora, such as immunocompromised patients and recipients of broad-spectrum antibiotics. Airway obstruction may result from elevation and posterior displacement of the tongue and supraglottic edema. The infection may extend to the lateral and retropharyngeal spaces, and subsequently along the carotid sheath and to the mediastinum.

Affected patients present with dysphagia, neck swelling ("bull neck") and stiffness, trismus, drooling, and brawny induration of the floor of the mouth. Occasionally, crepitus of the submandibular area is present. Tooth pain or a history of recent tooth extraction is usual, but not invariable. While not all patients with Ludwig angina need to undergo endotracheal intubation or tracheostomy, the decision to observe the airway rather than secure it should not be made lightly, and should be made after consultation with an otolaryngologist. If intubation is deemed necessary, placement via a flexible fiberoptic approach may be useful in decreasing the risk of laryngospasm during the procedure. Treatment consists of antibiotic therapy, and in some patients, surgical drainage. Obviously, any infected teeth should be extracted.

Lymphatic drainage from the oropharynx, teeth, maxillary sinuses, and ears passes through the retropharyngeal space, predisposing it to infections from the ear, nose, and throat.[10] While the space itself contains no vital structures, infection may extend into the mediastinum or epidural space, or provoke atlantoaxial dislocation. Whereas this condition usually follows an upper respiratory tract infection, pharyngitis, or otitis media in children, in adults the more common antecedent problems are odontogenic infection or procedures, or oral trauma. Patients present with throat and neck pain, and may have drooling or symptoms of upper airway obstruction. On occasion, infection may spread to the retropharyngeal space from the prevertebral space, such as with tuberculosis of the spine (Pott disease). The diagnosis may be made through a lateral neck radiograph; however, CT is advisable for helping define the boundaries of infection. Importantly, physical examination may fail to reveal any posterior pharyngeal swelling, highlighting the need for a high index of suspicion for this condition and further investigation via endoscopy or imaging. Treatment consists of antibiotics directed at oral flora (streptococci, staphylococci, anaerobes, and in some patients, gram-negative organisms), airway stabilization, and surgical exploration.

Because the lateral pharyngeal space is bounded by the retropharyngeal and submandibular spaces, it serves as a means of transmitting infections from diverse sources, as suggested previously. Again, infections in this space are typically treated with a combination of antibiotics and surgical drainage.

Peritonsillar abscesses are located between the tonsil and the superior constrictor muscle of the pharynx. Affected patients are typically young adults and have a history of prior tonsillitis; not surprisingly, *Streptococcus* species are most commonly isolated, along with other oral organisms. Presenting symptoms include sore throat, trismus, and voice change. Despite the prevalence of this disorder, there are several aspects of management that remain controversial.[11] While steroids are occasionally administered to patients with peritonsillar abscess, there are no studies to support or refute their efficacy. Both needle aspiration and open abscess drainage with tonsillectomy ("quinsy tonsillectomy") have been advocated as initial treatment, and both are effective.

Complications include UAO and rarely, thrombophlebitis of the internal jugular vein, a condition known as Lemierre syndrome. This condition is usually associated with *Fusobacterium necrophorum*, but other oral flora may be responsible. Bacteremia and septic emboli may result. The role of anticoagulation in Lemierre syndrome is controversial.

Occasionally, tonsillar enlargement from infectious mononucleosis may be so significant as to obstruct the airway. Management consists of close observation of the airway in a monitored setting, and the administration of corticosteroids.

OTHER CAUSES

Angioedema from a variety of causes can involve the tongue and hypopharynx and threaten airway patency both above and at the level of the larynx. This disorder is discussed below along with other disorders of the larynx. Stevens-Johnson syndrome and toxic epidermal necrolysis are rare vesiculobullous diseases that involve the skin and mucous membranes. Affected patients may develop bullae and edema of the upper airway mucosa, leading to obstruction. Causes typically include medications (with antibiotics, nonsteroidal anti-inflammatory medications, and anticonvulsants frequently being implicated), infections, and malignancies. Depending on their location, facial fractures may lead to UAO through local swelling and a loss of support for the tongue and/or facial skeleton. While oral neoplasms are common, patients typically present for evaluation before the airway can be compromised. Obstructive sleep apnea is a form of chronic UAO that is exhibited only during sleep, and is considered in greater detail in Chap. 109.

LARYNGEAL CAUSES

INFECTIOUS CAUSES

Supraglottitis, or infection of the supraglottic portion of the larynx, may cause life-threatening UAO primarily through involvement of the epiglottis. Vaccination against *Haemophilus influenzae* has successfully decreased the number of cases of epiglottitis in children caused by this organism. As a result, adults comprise a greater proportion of all cases of epiglottitis. In addition to *H. influenzae*, *Streptococcus pneumoniae*, *Staphylococcus aureus*, *Haemophilus parainfluenzae*, and anaerobes all have been implicated as causes of epiglottitis. Because most physicians who treat adults will work a lifetime without seeing a single patient with the acute onset of sore throat go on to develop UAO, the diagnosis may be missed. The classic presentation is that of a patient sitting upright and leaning forward, drooling; however, these signs may not be present initially. An additional clue is the rapid onset and severity of odynophagia. Signs of toxicity, such as fever and tachycardia, may be present. Otolaryngology and anesthesiology consultation should be obtained if the diagnosis is suspected, while an oral examination should be performed extremely carefully, if at all. The approach to diagnosis depends on the patient's overall clinical status. While lateral films of the neck may reveal the diagnosis, a negative examination does not exclude epiglottitis. A fiberoptic examination can often be performed carefully via the nasopharyngeal route, but should be performed only by a person experienced in treating this problem, preferably a seasoned otolaryngologist or anesthesiologist. Visualization of a swollen, cherry-red epiglottis confirms the diagnosis. This examination is preferentially performed in the operating room, or at a minimum with all necessary airway personnel and equipment available. Although many adults with epiglottitis may be managed with antibiotics and observation in the ICU, the potential for acute airway obstruction should always be considered to be extremely high.[12,13] A tracheostomy tray should be at the bedside, and all relevant airway personnel—anesthesia as well as otolaryngology—should be alerted to the patient's condition and location. At no time should the patient be sent unaccompanied to another location in the hospital. While blood cultures may on occasion reveal the etiology, in most cases the specific organism is not identified, and antibiotic treatment is empirical. The response to treatment is typically prompt.

Infections of the larynx may be caused by viruses, bacteria, or fungi. Laryngotracheitis in children (croup) is usually caused by a viral infection, and UAO may result. While viral infections of the larynx are rarely serious in adults, bacterial laryngotracheitis can be life-threatening. Because the causative organisms include *Staphylococcus aureus, Streptococcus pneumoniae,* and *Haemophilus influenzae,* pneumonia may be present as well. *Corynebacterium diphtheriae* should always be considered in the differential diagnosis despite the relative infrequency with which it is currently encountered in the United States. In particular, nonimmunized persons and those individuals who have not received a booster in the past 10 years are at risk. Diphtheria is also more frequently encountered in communities with low immunization rates, as in some Native American communities. Diphtheria commonly presents initially as tonsillitis and pharyngitis. Subsequent spread inferiorly may cause laryngitis, although occasionally the larynx is the only site of involvement. Clinical manifestations include fever, sore throat, malaise, headache, and vomiting. Physical examination may reveal a tenacious gray or black membrane overlying involved sites, and cervical lymphadenopathy may be present. Delays in treatment increase the likelihood of systemic complications from circulating toxin, such as myocarditis, neuritis, and nephritis. Death occurs in 5% to 10% of cases, either from systemic effects of diphtheria toxin or from UAO, the latter occurring more commonly in infants. Treatment includes antibiotics and equine antitoxin, which can be obtained through the Centers for Disease Control and Prevention. Sensitivity to horse serum should be assessed prior to administration of the antitoxin, and desensitization should be performed as necessary. Because infection does not ensure immunity, immunization is indicated after recovery.[14]

Fungal laryngotracheitis may be caused by *Candida albicans,* histoplasmosis, blastomycosis, and coccidioidomycosis. In addition to fever and sore throat, affected patients may develop dyspnea and voice change from vocal cord nodules and/or vocal cord fixation. The diagnostic approach depends on the presentation, as other sites of involvement—for example, pulmonary infiltrates—may be present. Respiratory papillomatosis is caused by human papillomavirus types 6 and 11, and is manifested by multiple—sometimes innumerable—papules in the larynx and trachea.

IATROGENIC AND TRAUMATIC CAUSES
Related to Endotracheal Intubation

A variety of upper airway problems can follow endotracheal intubation and are listed in Table 34-1. Several of these problems merit further discussion here. Laryngospasm consists of uncontrolled glottic closure, and respiratory distress with inability to ventilate the patient may result. It can be provoked

TABLE 34-1 Upper Airway Disorders Related to Endotracheal Intubation

Related to insertion
  Epistaxis (with nasotracheal intubation)
  Tooth avulsion and aspiration
  Hypopharyngeal trauma
    Laryngospasm (either from airway manipulation or medications)
    Laryngeal trauma
  Mucosal trauma
  Vocal cord paralysis and/or arytenoid dislocation
Related to long-term intubation
    Endotracheal tube obstruction from secretions or kinking
    Vocal cord injury: edema, ulceration, granuloma, and paralysis possible
    Laryngomalacia from ischemic cuff injury
    Subglottic stenosis
    Tracheal stenosis
Related to extubation
    Excess secretions
    Residual sedation
    Laryngospasm
    Previous undiagnosed laryngeal edema or other upper airway injury or disorder

by a variety of stimuli, including stimulation of the glottic aperture and/or superior laryngeal nerve during intubation, medications including general anesthetics and opioids, and the presence of secretions or blood in the upper airway. Careful suctioning of the mouth and endotracheal tube prior to extubation may reduce the likelihood of laryngospasm after extubation, in addition to improving pulmonary toilet. When laryngospasm occurs, gentle mask ventilation with 100% oxygen should be performed. If the laryngospasm fails to break and ventilation is not possible, the short-acting paralytic succinylcholine may be administered followed by mask ventilation or endotracheal intubation. It should be emphasized that in the ICU, laryngeal edema is a much more likely cause of postextubation stridor than laryngospasm.

Long-term endotracheal intubation may cause a variety of injuries to the upper airway. Fortunately, current endotracheal tube cuffs have a higher volume and lower pressure than were used a number of years ago, decreasing problems related to long-term intubation. Whether or not an individual patient will develop subglottic or tracheal stenosis is difficult to predict. While duration of intubation has been shown in some studies to be correlated with laryngeal or tracheal stenosis, the relationship is not strong. Similarly, while increased tube caliber, frequency of insertion, the severity of respiratory failure, female gender, and the presence of diabetes or immunocompromise have all been suggested as exacerbating factors, the data on this topic are inconsistent.[1] The decision to perform a tracheostomy therefore depends on the expected duration of need for an artificial airway, and the extent to which conversion to tracheostomy will facilitate other aspects of care; for example, liberation from mechanical ventilation, or recovery from more proximal upper airway injury or toxic therapy (e.g., surgery or irradiation for neoplasm). In general, the usual recommendation of considering tracheostomy for all patients intubated for 2 to 3 weeks who are not likely to recover soon is a prudent one. As mentioned previously, possibility of subglottic or tracheal stenosis should be considered when encountering breathless patients who have undergone long-term intubation previously. In such cases, the diagnosis of UAO may easily be overlooked. Voice change and stridor are clues to the diagnosis. CT of the upper airway with three-dimensional reconstruction can be very useful in such cases, if patient stability permits.

Endotracheal tube obstruction from secretions may be an insidious cause of UAO that may progress occasionally to a circumstance in which ventilation becomes impossible. Its occurrence may be prevented through frequent suctioning. The development of obstructed respiratory system mechanics—a high peak to plateau airway pressure gradient—in a patient without a history of obstructive lung disease, or in the absence of wheezing, suggests the diagnosis. While difficulty passing a suction catheter is highly suggestive, we have removed endotracheal tubes that are nearly completely occluded through which a suction catheter was able to be passed. If time permits, bronchoscopic examination quickly establishes the diagnosis. Chap. 36 outlines the approach to high peak airway pressures in further detail; here, we stress that prompt removal of the endotracheal tube, with manual mask ventilation of the patient while awaiting reintubation, can be lifesaving.

Stridor has been reported to occur following 2% to 16% of extubations in the ICU, with laryngeal edema most frequently responsible.[15] Limited investigations in adults do not support the prophylactic administration of corticosteroids in order to reduce the incidence of reintubation.[16] Even if corticosteroids are effective at reducing laryngeal edema, the low incidence of reintubation for this disorder in adults means that an extraordinary number of patients would have to be treated in order to demonstrate a benefit in reducing this occurrence. For this reason, a randomized controlled trial of corticosteroids to treat patients with postextubation stridor is not likely to be performed. Our practice is to administer a short (48 hours) course of parenteral corticosteroids such as dexamethasone in such cases. More important is notification of relevant airway personnel and close observation; aerosolized racemic epinephrine may be useful in decreasing laryngeal edema through local vasoconstriction.

Other Traumatic Injuries

Aspirated foreign bodies lodge in the upper airway much less commonly in adults than in children.[17] Still, asphyxiation may follow foreign body aspiration in adults, while large objects aspirated into the esophagus can occasionally obstruct the upper airway. Risk factors in adults include diminished level of consciousness; impaired swallowing mechanism or diminished upper airway sensation as a result of neuromuscular disorder, prior cerebrovascular accident, or advanced age; and inability to chew food properly because of poor dentition. Food particles and medical or dental appliances are most frequently aspirated. Symptoms include cough and dyspnea, and stridor may be present. Chest radiography or lateral films of the neck may reveal the diagnosis. In the case of impending respiratory arrest, the Heimlich maneuver may be lifesaving. Otherwise, the patient should undergo endoscopy in most cases with a rigid endoscope. Flexible fiberoptic endoscopy is generally inadvisable for foreign body removal because the airway cannot be protected if the object lodges in the glottis during removal; however, experienced operators may elect to attempt removal in carefully selected patients.

Upper airway injury may result from inhalation of toxic chemicals, or more commonly from thermal injury. Upper airway burn injury should be suspected whenever a patient has survived a fire or explosion in an enclosed space, and when chemicals or plastics have burned. Physical examination findings that suggest the presence of upper airway injury include the presence of burns or soot on the face, singed nasal hairs, erythema of the oropharynx, and hoarse voice. Sometimes the external signs are relatively mild despite significant inhalation injury. Thus any patient suspected of incurring inhalation injury should undergo fiberoptic laryngoscopy. Affected patients may experience life-threatening UAO from airway edema and mucosal sloughing anytime from initial presentation to 24 hours later. In addition, upper airway edema may be exacerbated by the considerable amount of fluids required to resuscitate patients with extensive burns.[18] When the airway needs to be secured, endotracheal intubation is preferred over tracheostomy because of the higher incidence of tracheal stenosis associated with the latter therapy when performed in burn patients. Because corticosteroids increase the incidence of infectious complications and may increase mortality when administered to burn patients, we do not recommend their use here.

Traumatic neck injury may directly injure the larynx.[7] Such an injury should be suspected whenever there are ecchymoses or tenderness over the thyroid or cricoid cartilages. In addition to pain, patients may have stridor, hoarseness, and hemoptysis. Cervical spine injury should be excluded, while endotracheal intubation must be done with care to avoid exacerbating any existing injury. Stabilization of the neck and avoidance of neck extension during airway manipulation are mandatory. In a crisis, tracheostomy may be necessary to establish an airway. The evaluation and treatment of laryngeal injury is beyond the scope of this review.

There are a number of iatrogenic causes of UAO. A hematoma in the neck may cause UAO through direct compression, as may rarely occur following surgery. Inadvertent carotid artery puncture during central line placement may cause a rapidly expanding hematoma with airway compromise, particularly if the patient has a bleeding diathesis. Recurrent laryngeal nerve injury may occur during neck dissection or cardiac surgery and cause vocal cord paralysis. While unilateral vocal cord paralysis does not by itself embarrass respiration because the contralateral cord has full mobility, bilateral vocal cord paralysis typically requires surgery.

MISCELLANEOUS CAUSES

Functional UAO may result from abnormal closure of the vocal cords during inspiration, expiration, or both. Affected patients often have a history of frequent treatment for severe "asthma" exacerbations, at times even undergoing intubation. We have witnessed patients with this condition who exhibit significant pulsus paradoxus and respiratory acidosis during attacks mimicking status asthmaticus. Physical examination is revealing in that stridor is heard. If the patient is intubated, the respiratory system mechanics are normal, and wheezing is not heard. Complicating the diagnosis is the fact that a significant portion of patients with this condition also have asthma, which may be severe.[19] Spirometry may show flattening of the inspiratory limb of the flow volume loop, indicating a variable extrathoracic obstruction. The diagnosis is confirmed when laryngoscopy reveals abnormal vocal cord closure, particularly during inspiration. Unfortunately, laryngoscopy may be normal, particularly between attacks, and frequently the diagnosis must be made on clinical grounds. While psychiatric disorders and a history of abuse have been reported to be present in a number of cases, these findings are not invariable, and a loss of regulation of normal reflexes controlling the laryngeal muscles has been postulated.[20] Treatment involves speech therapy and treatment of any underlying psychiatric disorder.

Neoplasms are important causes of laryngeal obstruction, with squamous cell carcinoma being the most common malignancy of the larynx. Risk factors include tobacco and alcohol use, and patients may present with hoarseness or hemoptysis.[21] The diagnosis is typically established through a combination of direct visualization and CT. The evaluation and management of tumors of the head and neck is beyond the scope of this review.

As mentioned previously, bilateral vocal cord paralysis invariably results in UAO, although the presentation is often delayed.[22] Previous thyroidectomy is often responsible for the condition, although malignancy, neck irradiation, neck trauma, and prior intubation are additional causes.

Several systemic diseases are associated with upper airway obstructing lesions.[23] Airway involvement in Wegener granulomatosis is common, although frequently subclinical. Manifestations include ulcerations, mass lesions from proliferating granulation tissue, and circumferential narrowing, particularly in the subglottic region. Treatment typically involves a combination of immunosuppression—usually prednisone and cyclophosphamide—and surgery. Tracheostomy is frequently necessary when subglottic stenosis is severe.

Rheumatoid arthritis presents several potential problems where the upper airway is concerned. Arthritis of the temporomandibular joint may limit the degree to which the mouth can be opened, frustrating attempts at oral intubation. Cervical spine arthritis, particularly of the atlantoaxial joint, should be considered a serious impediment to manipulation of the cervical spine. In particular, neck extension may lead to catastrophic cervical spinal cord injury when significant atlantoaxial disease is present. When patients with rheumatoid arthritis develop hoarseness, vocal cord nodules or cricoarytenoiditis are frequently responsible. The latter is often associated with significant pain. Over time, the vocal cords may fuse in the midline.[24] While treatment with systemic and intralesional corticosteroids is the rule, surgical removal of the arytenoids or tracheostomy may be necessary. Of note, cricoarytenoiditis occurs infrequently in patients with systemic lupus erythematosus, although in affected patients the presentation is more acute, and the response to steroid therapy is more gratifying.[25]

While pulmonary involvement in sarcoidosis is extremely common, laryngeal disease is relatively rare. When present, it is usually the supraglottic region that is affected, and on occasion upper airway patency may be threatened. Treatment includes a combination of intralesional and systemic steroids. Relapsing polychondritis is manifest as recurrent inflammation of the cartilages of the ears, nose, larynx, trachea, and joints. Half of affected patients have respiratory tract involvement. UAO may result initially from airway edema, subsequently from increased collapsibility from dissolution of cartilage, and later from fibrosis and fixed stenosis. Amyloidosis affecting the larynx and trachea is rare, and presents as firm nodules that may coalesce and cause UAO.

ANGIOEDEMA

Angioedema is a typically intense, painless swelling of a localized body area caused by leakage of plasma into the affected tissues, and preferentially involving the face, tongue, larynx, gastrointestinal tract, and extremities. Except in the case of angiotensin-converting enzyme inhibitor–associated angioedema, this leakage typically derives either from mast cell–stimulated histamine release or from activation of the complement system. Mast cell histamine release may occur following IgE-mediated hypersensitivity reactions such as those due to severe food allergies, as well as in response to certain substances—such as codeine, aspirin, and iodinated contrast media—that directly stimulate histamine release. Treatment of histamine-mediated angioedema includes histamine blockade (both H_1- and H_2-receptor blockers are given), corticosteroids, and if the airway is compromised or hemodynamic instability is present, epinephrine.

There are several diseases of the complement cascade that result in angioedema. They can be generally classified according to whether they are hereditary or acquired. Hereditary angioedema (HAE) is an autosomal dominant disease characterized by recurrent episodes of angioedema of the skin, upper airway, and gastrointestinal tract.[26] Attacks may be provoked by dental surgery or general anesthesia. Type I HAE is the most common form and is caused by decreased production of C1 esterase inhibitor. Patients with type II HAE have functionally impaired C1 esterase inhibitors. Corticosteroids, antihistamines, and epinephrine are generally considered to be ineffective in acute attacks in patients with HAE, but should not be withheld until the diagnosis is secured. Purified C1 esterase inhibitor concentrate seems to be both effective and safe in treating exacerbations of HAE, but is not widely available outside of Europe.[27] Fresh frozen plasma infusion may be considered as a means of administering C1 esterase inhibitor, but carries the potential risk of paradoxical worsening of angioedema through C4-mediated tissue damage. Generally, this treatment is reserved as a means of preventing angioedema in patients undergoing major surgical or dental procedures, when C1 esterase inhibitor is not available. Attenuated androgens and antifibrinolytic agents are used as prophylactic therapy. Although the latter is somewhat less effective, they are useful alternatives to androgens in children.

Acquired angioedema (AAE) is associated with autoimmune disorders, lymphoproliferative diseases, various carcinomas, and a number of chronic infections such as those caused by human immunodeficiency virus and hepatitis B and C viruses. Affected patients have circulating antibodies directed either against specific immunoglobulins expressed on B cells or against C1 esterase inhibitor. There is some evidence that antihistamines, corticosteroids, and epinephrine are somewhat more effective in treating AAE than HAE.

Immunosuppressive therapy may prevent attacks by decreasing autoantibody production. Some patients respond to attenuated androgens, although usually not if antibodies to C1 esterase inhibitor are present. Antifibrinolytic agents may be tried if androgens are ineffective.

Some patients experience recurrent angioedema, yet have no known cause. Most such patients also have urticaria. The evaluation of these patients is beyond the scope of this review.

Angioedema occurs in a small fraction (0.1% to 0.5%) of patients receiving angiotensin-converting enzyme inhibitors

(ACEIs). Still, because of the widespread use of these agents, a significant percentage of all cases of UAO are caused by ACEIs. Attacks typically occur shortly after initiation of therapy, but may occur years later. The angioedema seems to respond poorly if at all to treatment with corticosteroids, antihistamines, and epinephrine; although studies demonstrating the efficacy of these agents are lacking, they are frequently administered anyway. The pathophysiology is unclear; although accumulation of bradykinin has been implicated as the cause, the occurrence of angioedema in some patients who have been switched from ACE inhibitors to angiotensin receptor antagonists, which do not inhibit the catabolism of bradykinin, raises questions about the mechanisms by which each agent causes angioedema.[28] We believe that angiotensin receptor antagonists should be used in patients who have had a prior episode of angioedema attributed to ACEI therapy only when there is no other reasonable alternative.

Treatment of Upper Airway Obstruction

The most important aspect of managing a patient with suspected UAO is to immediately summon to the bedside a clinician experienced in the management of such patients. Once a significant UAO has been diagnosed, early involvement of anesthesia and otolaryngology services is crucial. The approach to management varies considerably depending on the site, severity, and tempo of UAO; while patients with slowly progressive or easily treatable causes of UAO may be managed expectantly, signs of impending respiratory arrest dictate that the airway be secured immediately. The presence of an experienced clinician is also important in ensuring that inappropriately aggressive interventions do not take place, such as attempts at intubation by an inexperienced operator with inadequate equipment and backup. In such cases, attempts to secure the airway may in fact precipitate a catastrophe. Because each patient requires an individual approach to management, explicit recommendations are difficult. Following is a discussion of available techniques for treating patients with UAO.

GENERAL STABILIZING MEASURES

If the patient has normal mentation and is able to speak, attempts can be made at stabilizing a severe UAO with noninvasive means pending definitive treatment. Because the pressure required to drive airflow across the upper airway depends in part on the density of the gas, the inhalation of a low-density inert gas such as helium in combination with oxygen has the effect of reducing the work of breathing. In fact, helium-oxygen mixtures have been shown to decrease the transdiaphragmatic pressure swings and the pressure-time index of the diaphragm, as well as improve comfort, in a group of patients with postextubation stridor.[29] The proportion of inhaled gas that can be administered as helium is obviously limited by the need to maintain an adequate arterial saturation. On the other hand, mixtures comprising less than 70% helium are of little to no benefit.

We have used noninvasive positive pressure ventilation in some patients with UAO, particularly those who have postextubation stridor and significantly increased work of breathing. While no controlled trials exist to support its use, we believe this therapy may have a role in preventing respiratory

muscle fatigue, and occasionally reintubation in this setting. Conceivably, inspiratory positive airway pressure reduces the work of breathing by unloading the inspiratory muscles, while expiratory positive airway pressure may help to "splint" any collapsible segment of the upper airway in a manner similar to that seen in its use in obstructive sleep apnea.[30] We caution that this treatment should only be used in carefully selected patients. In particular, the decision to defer intubation in favor of noninvasive ventilation may allow the UAO an opportunity to progress to a point at which intubation becomes more difficult, if not impossible. Similarly, this approach should not take the place of intubation when the UAO is critical and expected to progress (e.g., in the case of an upper airway infection or tumor awaiting definitive therapy, such as surgery or radiation). We believe an additional role for noninvasive ventilation is in the stabilization of the patient with UAO while relevant airway personnel and equipment can be assembled, and a consensus reached among the medical team—anesthesia, otolaryngology, and the critical care service—as to the best approach to securing the airway.

SECURING THE AIRWAY

When time permits, and the UAO is known to be severe, the opportunity to perform awake fiberoptic intubation in a controlled manner is invaluable. The unconscious patient with UAO who is unable to be ventilated should first undergo a head-tilt or jaw thrust maneuver to advance the mandible and relieve any obstruction from the tongue base in the hypopharynx. In patients with suspected cervical spine injury, the jaw thrust may be performed without the head-tilt maneuver. Placement of an oral airway also facilitates ventilation when the UAO is proximal. If these measures are unsuccessful, the obstruction is likely to be more distal. Direct laryngoscopy with an anterior commissure laryngoscope and gum bougie introducer often permits successful passage of a small endotracheal tube over the bougie introducer and through the glottis. In situations in which the glottis cannot be well visualized, placement of a laryngeal mask airway may be useful. Subsequent fiberoptic tube placement can then be performed through this device. Depending on operator experience, the esophagotracheal Combitube, which is a dual-lumen tube with an open tracheal cannula and a blind esophageal end that is designed for emergency resuscitation by personnel lacking advanced airway management skills, may serve a similar purpose. Ventilation is performed between two inflated balloons, one in the oropharynx and one in the esophagus. This device should not be used when there is known hypopharyngeal or esophageal pathology, or when time permits an attempt to secure the airway by an experienced otolaryngologist or anesthesiologist. Depending on the level of obstruction, ventilation may still not be possible despite successful insertion of either the laryngeal mask airway or the esophagotracheal Combitube.[31]

If the airway cannot be effectively secured with an endotracheal tube, a surgical airway is indicated. Emergency cricothyrotomy is performed by first making a 1-cm horizontal incision just above the superior border of the cricoid, which can be found 2 to 3 cm below the thyroid notch.[32] The cricothyroid membrane is then slit in the midline with the blade directed inferiorly so as to avoid damaging the vocal cords. If the blade is passed too deeply, entry into the esophagus is possible. The hole is then widened with a blunt instrument to allow passage of a small tube or cannula for ventilation. Complications include vocal cord injury, esophageal perforation, and later, subglottic stenosis. While jet ventilation via needle cricothyrotomy utilizing a 14-gauge angiocath may allow adequate ventilation of the patient pending definitive therapy, the frequency of complications is high and operator experience with this technique is typically limited.

The best approach to securing an obstructed upper airway is best determined through a multidisciplinary approach involving the critical care team, anesthesia, and otolaryngology. Available techniques for securing the airway are discussed in greater detail in Chap. 35.

THE DECISION TO EXTUBATE

Deciding when to extubate a patient with an UAO is often difficult. The presence of the endotracheal tube makes an assessment of upper airway patency difficult. Sometimes improvement in the UAO is suggested by the overall clinical course; for example, if a patient was intubated for a borderline indication in the setting of a soft tissue infection, a significant reduction in facial and neck swelling may indicate that the UAO has improved to the point where extubation is safe. Similarly, complete resolution of lip, tongue, and hypopharyngeal swelling from angioedema is often accompanied by resolution of laryngeal edema. However, care must be taken in such circumstances. It is frequently useful to perform a "cuff leak" test. After scrupulous oral and endotracheal suction, the endotracheal tube cuff is deflated. If a patient is unable to pass air around the tube, its removal may not be tolerated, particularly if the tube is small (i.e., 6.0 or 6.5 mm). When the patency of the airway is in question, it is useful to pass a tube changer through the endotracheal tube prior to its removal. The tube changer allows repassage of an endotracheal tube through the glottis and into the trachea if reintubation is required. Careful consultation with anesthesia and otolaryngology services prior to making a decision to extubate is important, and all necessary equipment and personnel should be at the bedside in marginal cases.

Some studies have suggested that quantification of the cuff leak, either by volume or by percentage of total tidal volume, may predict the occurrence of postextubation stridor in patients not intubated for UAO. Because the rate of reintubation in such cases is low and the benefit of steroids uncertain, it is not clear whether this practice should be generally employed, particularly if it results in more patients remaining intubated for longer periods.

Complications of Upper Airway Obstruction

Short of cardiac arrest, the most feared complication of UAO is anoxic brain injury. Negative-pressure pulmonary edema may also occur.[33] This condition typically occurs in patients with severe UAO, in whom several mechanisms act synergistically to promote its development. First, the patient generates extremely negative pleural pressures during inspiration attempting to overcome the UAO. This promotes venous return and a shift of the interventricular septum to the left, decreasing left ventricular preload. At the same time, left

ventricular afterload is dramatically increased by the fall in intrathoracic pressure, as well as by catecholamine-induced systemic hypertension. These events cause a transfer of blood volume from the systemic to the pulmonary circulation. Here, pulmonary capillary transmural pressure is elevated because of reduced interstitial pressure and possibly elevated capillary pressure, the latter from increased blood volume and pulmonary vascular tone from hypercapnia and hypoxia. This rise in capillary transmural pressure causes pulmonary edema. On occasion, the edema fluid in such patients has been noted to be pink or blood-tinged, possibly from red blood cell leakage caused by high transmural pressures across disrupted alveolar-capillary membranes.

References

1. Aboussouan LS, Stoller JK: Diagnosis and management of upper airway obstruction. *Clin Chest Med* 15:35, 1999.
2. Rosen CA, Anderson D, Murry T: Evaluating hoarseness: keeping your patient's voice healthy. *Am Fam Physician* 57:2775, 1998.
3. West JB: *Respiratory Physiology: The Essentials*, 6th ed. Baltimore, Lippincott Williams & Wilkins, 2000, p 4.
4. Jolliet P, Tassaux D: Usefulness of helium-oxygen mixtures in the treatment of mechanically ventilated patients. *Curr Opin Crit Care* 9:45, 2003.
5. Miller RD, Hyatt RE: Evaluation of obstructing lesions of the trachea and larynx by flow-volume loops. *Am Rev Respir Dis* 108:475, 1973.
6. Lunn WW, Sheller JR: Flow volume loops in the evaluation of upper airway obstruction. *Otolaryngol Clin North Am* 28:721, 1995.
7. Khosh MM, Lebovics RS: Upper airway obstruction, in Parrillo J, Dellinger RP (eds): *Critical Care Medicine*, 2nd ed. St. Louis, Mosby, 2002, p 808.
8. Grenier PA, Beigelman-Aubry C, Fétita C, et al: New frontiers in CT imaging of airway disease. *Eur Radiol* 12:1022, 2002.
9. Marple BF: Ludwig angina: a review of current airway management. *Arch Otolaryngol Head Neck Surg* 125:596, 1999.
10. Tannebaum RD: Adult retropharyngeal abscess: a case report and review of the literature. *J Emerg Med* 14:147, 1996.
11. Johnson RF, Stewart MG, Wright CC: An evidence-based review of the treatment of peritonsillar abscess. *Otolaryngol Head Neck Surg* 128:332, 2003.
12. Chan ED, Hodges TN, Parsons PE: Sudden respiratory insufficiency in a previously healthy 47-year-old man. *Chest* 112:1419, 1997.
13. Frantz TD, Rasgon BM, Quesenberry Jr CP: Acute epiglottitis in adults. Analysis of 129 cases. *JAMA* 272:1358, 1994.
14. http://www.cdc.gov/nip/publications/pink/dip.pdf. Accessed September 28, 2003.
15. Jaber S, Chanques G, Matecki S, et al: Post-extubation stridor in intensive care unit patients: risk factors evaluation and importance of the cuff-leak test. *Intensive Care Med* 29:69, 2003.
16. Markovitz BP, Randolph AG: Corticosteroids for the prevention and treatment of post-extubation stridor in neonates, children and adults. *Cochrane Library* Vol. 1, 2003.
17. Baharloo F, Veyckemans F, Francis C, et al: Tracheobronchial foreign bodies: presentation and management in children and adults. *Chest* 115:1357, 1999.
18. Haponik EF, Meyers DA, Munster AM, et al: Acute upper airway injury in burn patients. *Am Rev Respir Dis* 135:360, 1987.
19. Newman KB, Mason UG 3rd, Schmaling KB: Clinical features of vocal cord dysfunction. *Am J Resp Crit Care Med* 152:1382, 1995.
20. Elshami AA, Tino G: Coexistent asthma and functional upper airway obstruction: case reports and review of the literature. *Chest* 110:1358, 1996.

21. Bradley PJ: Treatment of the patient with upper airway obstruction caused by cancer of the larynx. *Otolaryngol Head Neck Surg* 120:737, 1999.

22. Schwartz AR, Smith PL, Kashima HK, et al: Disorders of the upper airways, in Murray J, Nadel J (eds): *Textbook of Respiratory Medicine*, 3rd ed. Philadelphia, WB Saunders, 2000, p 1343.

23. Lerner DM, Deeb Z: Acute upper airway obstruction resulting from systemic diseases. *South Med J* 86:623, 1993.

24. Lawry GV, Finerman ML, Hanafee WN, et al: Laryngeal involvement in rheumatoid arthritis. A clinical, laryngoscopic, and computerized tomographic study. *Arthritis Rheum* 27:873, 1984.

25. Karim A, Ahmed S, Siddiqui R, et al: Severe upper airway obstruction from cricoarytenoiditis as the sole presenting manifestation of a systemic lupus erythematosus flare. *Chest* 121:990, 2002.

26. Nzeako UC, Frigas E, Tremaine WJ: Hereditary angioedema. *Arch Intern Med* 161:2417, 2001.

27. Waytes AT, Rosen FS, Frank MM: Treatment of hereditary angioedema with a vapor-heated C1 inhibitor concentrate. *N Engl J Med* 334:1630, 1996.

28. Howes LG, Tran D: Can angiotensin receptor antagonists be used safely in patients with previous ACE inhibitor-induced angioedema? *Drug Saf* 25:73, 2002.

29. Jaber S, Carlucci A, Boussarsar M, et al: Helium-oxygen in the postextubation period decreases inspiratory effort. *Am J Respir Crit Care Med* 164:633, 2001.

30. Sundaram RK, Nikolic G: Successful treatment of post-extubation stridor by continuous positive airway pressure. *Anaesth Intensive Care* 24:392, 1996.

31. Sofferman RA, Johnson DL, Spencer RF: Lost airway during anesthesia induction: alternatives for management. *Laryngoscope* 107:1476, 1997.

32. Gabrielli A, Layon AJ, Wenzel V, et al: Alternative ventilation strategies in cardiopulmonary resuscitation. *Curr Opin Crit Care* 8:199, 2002.

33. Schwartz DR, Maroo A, Malhotra A, Kesselman H: Negative pressure pulmonary hemorrhage. *Chest* 115:1194, 1999.

Chapter 35 _____

AIRWAY MANAGEMENT

MICHAEL F. O'CONNOR
ANDRANIK OVASSAPIAN

KEY POINTS

- *The choice between noninvasive ventilation via mask versus ventilation via translaryngeal tracheal intubation is an increasingly critical branch point in the management of patients with respiratory failure.*

- *Shock, a failed trial of extubation, inability to protect and maintain one's own airway, need for larger minute ventilations or larger transpulmonary pressures, and transport of an unstable patient all remain indications for tracheal intubation.*

- *Assessment and adequate preparation of the patient prior to intubation are crucial to ensuring successful and safe intubation.*

- *Awake tracheal intubation with topical anesthesia remains the preferred technique, although skilled operators can perform rapid sequence induction and intubation with a high degree of success. General anesthesia and paralysis are associated with substantial risks in critically ill, hemodynamically unstable patients.*

- *The appropriate timing of tracheostomy remains poorly defined. Improved endotracheal tubes allow for prolonged intubation with a low risk of associated traumatic injury.*

- *Percutaneous tracheostomy and conventional tracheostomy are increasingly performed at the bedside to minimize the hazards associated with transporting a critically ill patient.*

Tracheal intubation remains one of the most common and important procedures performed in the intensive care unit (ICU). When done well, tracheal intubation can be a lifesaving procedure. When done poorly, it may initiate a cascade of events that can lead directly or indirectly to trauma, severe complications, and death. The widespread adoption of noninvasive ventilation in the management of patients with type II acute-on-chronic respiratory failure (ACRF) and high-pressure pulmonary edema has created a population of patients who have failed moderate levels of ventilatory support and require emergent airway management (see Chap. 33). It is imperative that those who manage the airways in these patients have a high degree of knowledge, skill, and comfort in managing patients with little physiologic reserve. It is imperative that ICU physicians have knowledge and understanding of the indications for tracheal intubation, the assessment of the patient for tracheal intubation, the devices and techniques available for tracheal intubation, and the consequences and complications of tracheal intubation.[1]

Indications for Intubation

The decision about whether to intubate a critically ill patient requires that a practitioner at the bedside synthesize all of the information they have at their disposal about a patient, compare it to their institutional practice patterns and resources, and decide how to proceed. These decisions are rarely clear-cut; reasonable practitioners can arrive at different decisions in identical circumstances. Patients who require intubation as part of the initial management of their respiratory failure include but are not limited to those with cardiopulmonary arrest, respiratory arrest, acute respiratory distress syndrome (ARDS) of almost any cause, and any patient who is unlikely to respond to noninvasive ventilation (Table 35-1). The decision to intubate a patient after noninvasive ventilation is even more difficult to make. Triggers to convert to an invasive airway include progressive hypercapnia in spite of adequate levels of support (such as a patient with sleep apnea who is worsening on biphasic positive airway pressure [BIPAP]), unacceptably high airway pressure, hypoxemia which persists in spite of moderate levels of continuous positive airway pressure (CPAP) and high fraction of inspired oxygen (F_{IO_2}), diminishing mental status, patterns of respiration which suggest evolving respiratory muscle fatigue or impending respiratory arrest, and unfavorable anatomy (which is present at the start of treatment, or which evolves) (Table 35-2).

In patients with airway compromise, two decisions need to be made at the time the patient is evaluated: (1) Does this patient require an artificial airway? and (2) Does this patient require a tracheostomy? It may be difficult or impossible to translaryngeally intubate the trachea in patients with an unstable cervical spine, airway tumor, unfavorable anatomy, or significant facial trauma. Preparation for tracheostomy should occur concurrently with preparation for translaryngeal tracheal intubation in such high-risk patients.

The decision to intubate patients in cardiopulmonary arrest is a simple one, as intubation is the safest and most effective way to both ensure adequate ventilation in these patients and to protect their airway. The goal of intubating the trachea in the patient in shock is to decrease the proportion of cardiac

TABLE 35-1 Indications for Tracheal Intubation

Airway support
  Diminished mental status or decreased ability to maintain airway and clear secretions
  Compromised airway anatomy
  Diminished airway reflexes, full stomach, or fluctuating consciousness
  Requirement for sedation where airway control may be difficult to establish
  Pharyngeal instability
Pulmonary disease
  Acute respiratory distress syndrome
  High pressure pulmonary edema unlikely to respond to noninvasive ventilation, or which has not responded to a reasonable trial of noninvasive ventilation
  Hypoventilation (including central nervous system causes and weakness)
  Hypercapneic respiratory failure that has failed noninvasive ventilation
  Failed trial of extubation
  Forseeable protracted course of respiratory failure
Circulatory
  Cardiopulmonary arrest
  Shock
Other situations
  Elevated intracranial pressure requiring hyperventilation (increasingly rare)
  Transport to less monitored situations

TABLE 35-2 Indications for Converting Noninvasive Ventilation to Intubation and Mechanical Ventilation

Patient inability to tolerate noninvasive ventilation
Unfavorable anatomy and poor mask fit or large leak
Progressive hypercapnia in spite of adequate levels of support (typically over 1 hour)
Requirement for unacceptably high airway pressure (typically total delivered pressures >20 cm H_2O)
Hypoxemia in spite of appropriate levels of continuous positive airway pressure and high F_{IO_2}
Diminished mental status and inability to protect the airway
Respiratory pattern consistent with evolving fatigue or impending respiratory arrest

output devoted to perfusing their respiratory muscles, allowing this blood flow to be diverted to other vital organs.

Assessing the Patient Prior to Intubation

All patients being evaluated for tracheal intubation should be treated with the highest F_{IO_2} available. Oxygen saturation, blood pressure, heart rate, electrocardiography (ECG), and the frequency and strength of respiration should be closely monitored. Blood gas analysis may be helpful in facilitating the decision to intubate the patient, but has been largely supplanted by pulse oximetry, which is also essential for monitoring during intubation.

Patients requiring urgent intubation benefit from an expeditious but thorough assessment of their underlying medical conditions and airway anatomy (Tables 35-3 and 35-4). The possibility of increased intracranial pressure (ICP) or increased risk of intracranial hemorrhage is important to ascertain, since the presence of elevated ICP changes the emphasis in airway management from the maintenance of an adequate airway to the avoidance of further increases in ICP. Whereas most airway manipulation in the ICU can be done safely with patients awake, patients with elevated ICP and increased risk of intracranial hemorrhage (from unstable arteriovenous malformations or aneurysms) are best managed with intravenous general anesthesia for intubation. Laryngoscopy and tracheal intubation reliably produce myocardial ischemia in patients with coronary artery disease. Adequate anesthesia—topical and intravenous—can attenuate or prevent the myocardial ischemia associated with laryngoscopy and intubation. Inadequate anesthesia can elicit ischemia and associated arrhythmias. The use of intravenous agents in this setting is fraught with hazard. Too little intravenous agent can be associated with ischemia, while too much can cause hypotension, ischemia, hypoperfusion of vital organs, and a decreased rate of redistribution of the offending agent, prolonging its cardiovascular effects. The use of intravenous agents in these patients is thus best avoided if possible.

Intubation and positive pressure ventilation (PPV) will magnify the shock associated with intravascular hypovolemia. In hypovolemic patients, reflex sympathetic tone usually decreases venous capacitance, increases mean systemic pressure, and maintains venous return. Administration of sedative or anesthetic agents blunts this physiologic compensation. PPV increases intrathoracic pressure and therefore decreases the pressure gradient driving venous return. Singly or

TABLE 35-3 Medical Evaluation for Intubation

Neurologic factors
  Elevated intracranial pressure
  Presence of intracranial bleeding, arteriovenous malformation, or aneurysm
  Cervical spine disease
Cardiovascular factors
  Ischemia
  Hypovolemia
  Myocardial infarction (especially within the past 6 months)
  Cardiomyopathy
  Dysrhythmias
Drug allergies
Pulmonary factors
  Severity of hypoxemia, airway obstruction, or lung restriction
Aspiration risk
  Nothing by mouth (NPO) status
  Morbid obesity
  Impaired gastric emptying or gastroparesis
  Ileus
  Obstruction
  Pregnancy
Coagulation factors
  Thrombocytopenia
  Anticoagulant therapy
  Coagulopathy
  Recent or anticipated therapy with thrombolytics
  Current therapy with activated protein C for sepsis
Contraindications to succinylcholine
  Major burn within the past year
  Crush injuries
  Stroke or spinal cord injury resulting in denervation of a significant portion of the body
  Malignant hyperthermia
  Hyperkalemia

in combination, these effects can substantially reduce venous return, blood pressure, and tissue perfusion. In the setting of suspected hypovolemia, intravascular volume expansion may be desirable before intubation. In any case, preparation for rapid volume infusion should be made prior to intubation.

TABLE 35-4 Anatomic Evaluation for Intubation

Obesity
Pregnancy
Short neck
Large tongue
Inadequate mouth opening or temporomandibular joint dysfunction
Small or recessed mandible (short thyromental distance)
Limited flexion at the base of the neck or extension at the base of the skull
Cervical instability
Prominent incisors
Dentures
Loose teeth
Tumor (e.g., adenoma, carcinoma, or abscess)
Large epiglottis
Lingual tonsil hyperplasia
Copious secretions or blood
Trauma
History of prior intubations
Mallampati 3 and 4
Lip bite test

Patients with respiratory failure require thoughtful assessment of their shunt, V/Q mismatch, and bronchospasm prior to airway manipulation. The more severe their pathology, the more rapidly they will become hypoxic or hypercarbic during airway manipulation. Patients with acute hypoxemic respiratory failure are usually hypoxemic in spite of a high F_{IO_2}, and frequently desaturate further during airway manipulation. Patients with type II respiratory failure may become hypoxemic, hypercapneic, or both during airway manipulation. The more severe the lung disease, the less likely it is that ventilation with a mask or laryngeal mask airway (LMA) will be successful. Patients with severe pulmonary edema or severe bronchospasm cannot generally be ventilated successfully with a mask or LMA because the pressures and flows required to maintain an acceptable minute ventilation cannot be generated with these systems.

Manipulation of the airway in the ICU is accompanied by a substantial risk of aspiration. Unlike patients undergoing airway manipulation in an elective setting, such as the bronchoscopy suite or operating room, patients in the ICU typically are at high risk of aspiration. Stomach contents may include enteral feedings, blood (from gastrointestinal hemorrhage), acid, and bacteria. Conditions that decrease emptying, such as diabetic gastroparesis, morbid obesity, and perhaps critical illness itself, require management as if the patient has a full stomach, even during elective airway management. Cricoid pressure (the Sellick maneuver) should be performed whenever possible on patients undergoing tracheal intubation in the ICU.[1–4]

The presence of a coagulopathy is a relative contraindication to nasal intubation and techniques that are associated with a risk of bleeding, such as transtracheal injection of anesthesia, superior laryngeal nerve blocks, and retrograde intubation techniques.

Finally, contraindications to the use of succinylcholine (see Table 35-3), the most commonly used muscle relaxant for airway management in the ICU, should be considered prior to any airway manipulation.

A variety of anatomic conditions are associated with increased difficulty of intubation by rigid laryngoscopy (see Table 35-4).[5] A history of difficult intubation is perhaps one of the most important but least available elements of a patient's history. The presence of many anatomic conditions makes attempts at rigid laryngoscopy and intubation in the awake or asleep patient more difficult. This in turn increases the attractiveness of techniques which allow for the patient to be awake and spontaneously breathing, and that do not require direct laryngoscopy, such as fiberoptic intubation, blind nasal intubation, and techniques which utilize an intubating laryngeal airway. Patients with severely compromised airway anatomy may be best managed by either awake fiberoptic intubation or tracheostomy. When a difficult airway is anticipated, it is best to have equipment for performing a tracheostomy immediately available, and physicians skilled at performing the procedure at hand.

Equipment

In spite of the vast array of available equipment, most tracheal intubation can be accomplished using a very small subset of the equipment and a very simple checklist (Table 34-5). A

TABLE 35-5 Equipment List for Intubation

Cardiac arrest
Two laryngoscopes with functioning lights (ideally one with a short handle)
Macintosh no. 3 and 4 and Miller no. 3 blades
Small, medium, and large face masks
Laryngeal airways (e.g., laryngeal mask airway [LMA], cuffed oropharyngeal airway [COPA], Proseal, Combitube)
Suction with Yankauer tip
6.5, 7.0, 7.5, 8.0, 8.5, and 9.0 mm endotracheal tubes with cuffs checked
Malleable metal stylet
10-mL syringe for inflation of endotracheal tube cuff
Oxygen supply
Ambubag or other circuit (e.g., Mapleson D) to ventilate patient
Stethoscope
Gloves and eye protection
Portable end-tidal CO_2 monitoring device (e.g., EZ-Cap, capnograph)
Cricothyroidotomy kit
Urgent and elective intubation
Functioning IV line
Monitors: pulse oximeter, blood pressure, electrocardiograph
Resuscitation cart
Drugs
   Atropine
   IV lidocaine
   Ephedrine
   Epinephrine
   Glycopyrrolate
   Succinylcholine
   Rocuronium
   Topical anesthetics (lidocaine jelly, benzocaine spray)
   Topical phenylephrine spray
Controlled substances
   Propofol
   Thiopental
   Etomidate
   Midazolam
   Fentanyl
   Ketamine
Tape
Magill forceps
Size 7, 8, 9, and 10 oral airways
28, 30, 32, and 34 French nasal trumpets
Full variety of endotracheal tubes, including 7.0 and 8.0 mm Endotrol tubes, armored tubes
Fiberoptic bronchoscope
Jet ventilator

cart that is fully stocked with all of the equipment required to manage a difficult airway should be available to airway managers, but need not be brought to the bedside of every patient in crisis.[6]

Ideally, bags or boxes containing the equipment on the basic list for cardiac arrest are readily available to airway managers and can be brought by them to any situation in which they may be asked to manage an airway. The more complete equipment set for urgent and elective intubation can be kept in a cart stocked specifically for this purpose. Equipment should be checked at least daily and should be stored so that it is readily accessible. It is important that the equipment is checked by the person who will use it. This procedure ensures that the airway manager can focus on the patient during airway manipulation, and is not distracted by equipment failures, equipment checks, or preparation.

PHARMACOLOGIC PREPARATION AND USE

The goals of pharmacologic preparation of the patient include creating conditions that allow safe intubation, providing relief from the discomfort and hemodynamic consequences associated with airway manipulation and tracheal intubation, and decreasing the hormonal and neurologic consequences of the procedure. The spectrum of pharmacologic preparation ranges from topical to intravenous general anesthesia. In the hands of experienced operators, most airway manipulations can be accomplished with topical anesthesia alone. Intravenous general anesthesia is indicated in the setting of elevated ICP and favorable airway anatomy (Table 35-6). There are many institutions where an intravenous general anesthetic is routinely administered for tracheal intubation, but this practice should be strongly discouraged. The majority of the literature suggests that the use of intravenous general anesthesia to facilitate airway management may be associated with a higher rate of failure and need for emergency tracheostomy/cricothyroidotomy.

Patients who require urgent intubation benefit from pharmacologic preparation when circumstances allow. The administration of 0.2 mg IV glycopyrrolate will dry the mouth and facilitate direct laryngoscopy or fiberoptic laryngoscopy. The oropharynx can be anesthetized topically with 4% lidocaine spray, followed by approximately 1 to 2 mL of 2% lidocaine jelly on an oral airway of appropriate size for the patient. The oral airway can also be used to direct topical anesthetic at the vocal cords. The use of lidocaine for topical anesthesia is preferable to benzocaine, as the latter can cause methemoglobinemia. Care should be taken to avoid giving high doses (>6 mg/kg) of lidocaine for topical anesthesia, since lidocaine is readily absorbed by the mucosa of the pharynx. Some practitioners routinely perform transtracheal and superior laryngeal nerve blocks to facilitate awake intubation, but these procedures add little or nothing to topical anesthesia, and can cause significant bleeding in coagulopathic patients. Topical/local anesthesia schemes that avoid anesthetizing the trachea have several advantages in the ICU setting. They allow the patient to retain some ability to protect themselves from aspiration, and they also allow confirmation of tracheal intubation when the patient coughs in response to introduction of the tube into the trachea.

The use of intravenous agents to facilitate tracheal intubation in the ICU is hazardous. The degree of hypovolemia, myocardial dysfunction, and shock that often exists in these patients is difficult to ascertain prior to manipulating the airway in an urgent situation. Doses of intravenous agents that are well tolerated or even subtherapeutic in healthy patients can precipitate respiratory arrest or circulatory collapse in critically ill patients, converting a serious situation into a desperate one. Intravenous lidocaine in a dose of 100 mg is frequently sufficient to induce general anesthesia in patients with shock. The use of intravenous agents such as midazolam, fentanyl, thiopental, etomidate, propofol, and ketamine should be restricted to experienced practitioners. When indicated, these agents may be used to either titrate up to an acceptable level of sedation (which will be accompanied by a corresponding decline in both hemodynamics and minute ventilation, with associated worsening of hypoxia and hypercapnia), or to deliberately induce brief general anesthesia.

MUSCLE RELAXANTS AND AIRWAY MANAGEMENT IN THE INTENSIVE CARE UNIT

The use of muscle relaxants to facilitate airway management in the ICU remains controversial. Although these agents are routinely administered to facilitate airway management in the operating room, their use in ICU patients is not essential. The use of intravenous induction agents to initiate general anesthesia is motivated by the desire to produce intubating conditions quickly and to minimize unpleasant recall. Most patients undergoing elective surgery tolerate the hemodynamic consequences of intravenous anesthetic agents well and can be readily oxygenated and ventilated with a bag and mask. When anesthesiologists are confronted with patients who have abnormal airway anatomy or who may be impossible to oxygenate or ventilate with a bag and mask, they tend to opt for awake intubation strategies, as outlined in this chapter. Muscle relaxants, including succinylcholine, vecuronium, mivacurium, rocuronium, and cisatracurium should be used only by those who are experienced in managing the airway with an Ambu bag and mask, and who are thoroughly versed in techniques used to manage the difficult airway. The reason for this stipulation is that once these agents are administered, it is imperative that a definitive airway be obtained within minutes. Attempts at ventilating most patients in respiratory failure with an Ambu bag and mask are often difficult and frequently futile, since the decreased compliance of the lungs and/or increased airway resistance makes it difficult to maintain adequate minute ventilation. Among muscle relaxants available to facilitate airway management, succinylcholine remains the agent of first choice in ICU and ER patients for whom it is not contraindicated.[7]

There is an evolving literature about the use of intravenous anesthetic agents and muscle relaxants to facilitate airway management in both the field and the emergency department.[8–18] This literature suggests that the use of intravenous agents can both improve intubating conditions and cause hypotension, although brain-injured trauma patients have worse outcomes.[19,20] Airway management utilizing muscle relaxants in these reports is associated with a

TABLE 35-6 Steps for Tracheal Intubation in the Presence of Elevated Intracranial Pressure and an Anatomically Favorable Airway

1. Administer 1 mg vecuronium or pancuronium (if available)
2. Preoxygenate for 3 minutes
3. Apply cricoid pressure
4. Administer 0.03 mg/kg midazolam (if available)
5. Administer 1–2 µg/kg fentanyl (if available)
6. Administer 100 mg lidocaine (optional, but generally desirable)
7. Administer 3–5 mg/kg thiopental or 2 mg/kg propofol
8. Administer 1.5 mg/kg succinylcholine or 0.2 mg/kg vecuronium or 1 mg/kg rocuronium
9. Hyperventilate for 45 seconds with Ambu bag/mask following succinylcholine administration, or for 2 minutes following vecuronium administration
10. Perform laryngoscopy/intubation
11. Confirm intubation with auscultation or capnography
12. Elevate head of bed and ventilate to goals for patient

success rate in the range of 94% to 99%, with 1% of patients requiring a surgical airway of some kind. At first glance, this appears to be conspicuous success, but compared to airway management in the operating room, it is a very high rate of failure, and a very high rate of requirement for a surgical airway. No doubt some of the need for surgical airways in these patients is a consequence of their pathology, their anatomy, and the circumstances surrounding their airway management. Nevertheless, it seems plausible if not certain that the requirement for a surgical airway in some of these patients is a consequence of the use of either intravenous anesthetics or muscle relaxants as part of their airway management.

Procedures for Intubation

Compared to the operating room environment, arterial oxygen desaturation occurs quite rapidly in most patients undergoing intubation in the ICU, even if the patient has been preoxygenated with 100% oxygen. Factors that contribute to desaturation include an increased alveolar-arterial gradient, decreased functional residual capacity (FRC), and increased metabolic rate. Nevertheless, all patients undergoing airway management in the ICU should be preoxygenated.

The presence and help of well-trained assistants increases safety and success of intubation. Assistants might include other physicians, ICU nurses, respiratory therapists, and others trained in airway management and routinely engaged in the bedside care of critically ill patients. Ideally, the person managing the airway in the ICU has several helpers, one to help position the patient and apply cricoid pressure, one to hand off equipment, and one to monitor the patient and administer IV drugs as necessary.

Patients in cardiopulmonary arrest are relatively straightforward to intubate, as they are typically unconscious and flaccid. No drug therapy is necessary to facilitate airway management in these patients. Direct laryngoscopy should be attempted immediately, and the largest possible appropriate-sized endotracheal tube (ETT) should be inserted into the trachea. Many patients will have aspirated oral secretions or gastric contents prior to or after their cardiopulmonary arrest, and the necessity of suctioning using a rigid catheter (Yankauer) to achieve adequate visualization should be anticipated. Patients receiving cardiopulmonary resuscitation (CPR) do not typically deliver much carbon dioxide to their lungs, and attempts to confirm endotracheal intubation with CO_2 monitors may therefore be futile. The ability to detect carbon dioxide in the exhaled gases of such patients is usually a sign of the recovery of a spontaneous circulation. Cervical instability is the only coexisting condition that requires serious consideration during the intubation of a patient receiving CPR. All other medical and anatomic considerations are secondary in this situation.

In the past few years, there have been several clinical studies that have demonstrated an association between nasal intubation and the evolution of sinusitis, and between sinusitis and the development of ventilator-associated pneumonia (VAP) (see Chap. 43). Given this, it is probably the case that the oral route of intubation is preferable in most critically ill patients. Nasal intubation may still be desirable in a select population of patients with normal immunity, normal coagulation status, and relative contraindications to oral intubation.

OROTRACHEAL INTUBATION

Advantages of oral intubation include the requirement for less equipment (a laryngoscope), less trauma and bleeding, a lower incidence of sinusitis and VAP, and a high success rate independent of patient respiratory effort.[21,22] The disadvantages of oral intubation include the substantial stimulus associated with direct laryngoscopy, risk of dental and cervical trauma, difficulty securing the tube, difficulty of maintaining oral hygiene, and the occasional problem of a patient biting the tube. Patients must generally be supine to undergo orotracheal intubation. Orotracheal intubation is far more difficult to accomplish than it appears to the casual observer, especially in the less-than-ideal conditions that are typical of airway management in the ICU.

Most patients can be successfully intubated with topical anesthesia alone. Most patients will benefit from treatment with 0.2 mg of glycopyrrolate as a drying agent, and topical anesthesia using a combination of lidocaine spray (4%) and jelly (2% to 4%). Topical anesthesia usually begins with spraying the oropharynx with lidocaine, obtaining as much coverage of the oro- and hypopharynx as possible to obliterate the gag reflex. An appropriately sized oral airway (9 mm is a good default) is then covered with lidocaine liquid or jelly and inserted into the pharynx. The patient is instructed to suck on the airway. Lidocaine can also be sprayed through the oral airway directly towards the larynx. The importance of the oral airway as a mechanism to administer topical lidocaine requires emphasis, as it is the quality of the hypopharyngeal anesthesia that allows direct laryngoscopy to be performed. An adequately prepared patient will permit placement of a laryngoscope blade or even a more uncomfortable device such as an intubating LMA. Once the operator is assured that the airway has been adequately prepared, laryngoscopy (direct or fiberoptic) is performed, and intubation is attempted. Direct laryngoscopy in adults is usually performed using a Macintosh no. 3 or 4 blade, although straight blade designs (such as the Miller) are popular with some operators. The curved blades are generally easier to use, but the straight blades may be more useful in the event of difficulty obtaining an adequate view. It is desirable for those who manage airways in the ICU to be comfortable with both designs. Although circumstances are frequently less than ideal, the operator should do everything possible to ensure successful laryngoscopy. If possible, the head of the bed should be removed, and the bed moved away from the wall. The patient should be positioned in the sniffing position using pillows and rolled blankets as necessary. Failure to adequately position the patient is a common cause of repeated intubation attempts in the ICU setting. Once the patient has been intubated, it is imperative that the airway manager hold the tube firmly in place until the tube has been secured. Oral ETTs must be secured at least with tape; they may be wired to secure teeth in circumstances in which the use of tape is undesirable or impossible. Importantly, the pressure in the cuff of the tracheal tube should be maintained at 20 to 22 cm H_2O pressure from the time it is inserted to minimize the risk of VAP.[23]

Successful tracheal intubation can be confirmed by a variety of techniques in the spontaneously breathing patient, including the appearance of humidified gases in the tube, audible breath sounds at the end of the tube, breath sounds synchronous with Ambu bag ventilation, and carbon dioxide detected via capnography or capnometry.

NASOTRACHEAL INTUBATION

The disadvantages of nasal intubation are the increased risk of associated purulent sinusitis, VAP, and bleeding.[24,25] Advantages of nasal intubation include ease of securing the tube, free access to the mouth, greater stability relative to oral intubation, and absence of biting-associated obstruction. Nasal intubation can be accomplished with the head in a neutral position (or in traction) and with the patient sitting upright in bed. Nasally intubated patients are less likely to self-extubate than orally intubated patients.[26,27] Blind nasal and fiberoptic nasal intubation are readily accomplished in patients with air hunger. Other disadvantages include the greater length of the ETT and trauma to the nasal mucosa, septum, and turbinates. Relative contraindications to nasal intubation include coagulopathy, compromised immune function, and suspected or known skull-base trauma.

Nasal intubation can be performed either blindly, with direct laryngoscopy, or fiberoptically. Larger-bore tubes, such as 8.0 mm ETTs, should be used in nasal intubation, as they can be inserted as readily as smaller tubes in most patients, present substantially less resistance to air movement than do smaller tubes, and are large enough to allow fiberoptic bronchoscopy to be performed.[28]

Nasal intubation can be successfully performed without sedation, provided that adequate topical anesthesia is used. Many experienced operators prepare both nares simultaneously, so if an anatomic complication arises in attempts to use the first one, the second one can be used without delay. Those who desire to vasoconstrict the nasal mucosa prior to manipulating it can do so with 0.5% phenylephrine spray.[29] Topical anesthesia such as 4% lidocaine can then be sprayed into both nostrils. Following this step, a nasal trumpet lubricated with 2% lidocaine jelly is introduced into one of the nares. Successful introduction of the trumpet confirms the presence of a passage patent enough to allow an ETT to be passed. If the operator encounters any difficulty in passing the nasal trumpet, the attempt to intubate the trachea through that nostril should be abandoned. Once the trumpet is successfully inserted, lidocaine is then sprayed through the trumpet onto the vocal cords. It is best to use ETTs intended for use in the nose (such as the Endotrol tube) when performing nasal tracheal intubation, as conventional tubes may be too short and too rigid to be used safely for this purpose. The ETT is lubricated with 2% lidocaine jelly and passed into the nasopharynx. If any resistance is encountered as the tube is advanced, the operator should stop immediately. Attempts to advance the tube past substantial resistance are associated with mucosal tears, polypectomies, turbinatectomies, crushed and perforated nasal septa, and tunneling of the ETT underneath the mucosa, all of which can be associated with exuberant bleeding and other major complications. If fiberoptic intubation is planned, the bronchoscope is introduced through the tube into the nasopharynx and is advanced into the trachea. The bronchoscope is used as a stylet to advance the ETT into the trachea. Tracheal intubation can be confirmed by observing the carina and presence of tracheal rings beyond the tip of the ETT. If the plan is to perform nasal intubation under direct laryngeal visualization with a rigid laryngoscope, the oropharynx should be anesthetized concurrently with the nose. Direct laryngoscopy is then performed, and a Magill forceps may be used to guide the tube into the trachea. If blind nasal intubation is planned, then the ETT is advanced slowly, with inspiration, while the operator listens at the end of the tube for breath sounds. As the end of the tube gets close to the glottis, the breath sounds become louder. The tube is advanced into the trachea while the patient is instructed to take a deep breath. The sensation of the tube popping through the cords followed by efforts at a cough by the patient suggest successful introduction of the tube into the trachea. The disappearance of breath sounds suggests that the esophagus has been intubated. If this occurs, the tube should be withdrawn until breath sounds are heard again. The patient's head should then be repositioned and another attempt made to pass the ETT. If an Endotrol tube is being used, tension should be applied to the ring to redirect the tip of the tube more anteriorly before another attempt is made.

FIBEROPTIC INTUBATION

Fiberoptic tracheal intubation is increasingly performed in critical care units.[6] There are a variety of explanations for this, including the proliferation of fiberoptic bronchoscopes, increased familiarity and comfort with their use, and increased recognition of their utility as the technique of first choice in the patient with an anticipated difficult airway. Because the technique can be made difficult or impossible by the presence of blood or secretions, it requires meticulous preparation of the airway with drying agents, suctioning of secretions, and careful avoidance of any trauma which might cause bleeding. The technique is more successfully performed in awake patients, because their airway muscle tone maintains airway patency, which is important for good viewing conditions.[30]

Preparation for performing fiberoptic intubation consists of warming the ETT, if possible, to soften it and make it easier to advance through the vocal cords. The ETT is then placed on the fiberoptic scope in position to be slid forward when the scope is advanced into the trachea. The airway is prepared with topical anesthesia as discussed previously. Specialized oral airways, such as the Ovassapian airway are very useful, as they keep the tube midline, displace the tongue anteriorly, and prevent biting on the bronchoscope (Fig. 35-1). For optimal viewing conditions, it is imperative that a competent assistant either provide a vigorous jaw thrust or pull on the tongue, delivering it anteriorly. The fiberoptic bronchoscope is then passed through the vocal cords, down the trachea to the carina. The tube is then threaded into the trachea, over the scope with a smooth twisting motion. Tracheal intubation is confirmed with the bronchoscope as it is withdrawn from the trachea. The distance from the carina to the tip of the tube is determined by measuring how far the bronchoscope must be withdrawn from the carina before the tip of the tube becomes visible. Difficulty advancing the tube is usually from the tube catching laryngeal structures, and can be corrected by pulling the tube back and advancing with a twisting motion. Rarely, the tube may be too large for the glottic opening, requiring the bronchoscope to be withdrawn and a smaller tube to be placed instead. Of note, cricoid pressure may decrease the time and difficulty of fiberoptic intubation.[30]

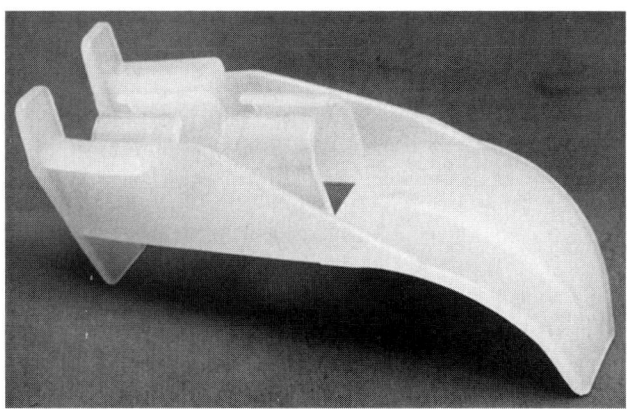

FIGURE 35-1 Ovassapian fiberoptic intubating airway. It keeps the tongue forward and the fiberscope midline, provides open air space in the hypopharynx, protects the fiberscope from the patient's bite, and is removed from the mouth without disconnecting the endotracheal tube adapter.

The technique for nasal fiberoptic intubation is similar in most regards. Most operators will introduce the tube through the nose and into the nasopharynx, thus proving patency of the nose and allowing the tube to be used as a guide through the nose for the bronchoscope. Viewing conditions for the nasal approach are also improved by either the jaw thrust or the tongue-tug, especially in unconscious or sedated patients.

INTUBATING WITH A LARYNGEAL MASK AIRWAY

Laryngeal mask airways in their various forms have become a critical component of airway management, especially in difficult-to-intubate patients (Fig. 35-2).[31] A variety of LMAs (e.g., the classic, Fastrach, and ProSeal) have been designed to facilitate ventilation and intubation under the most difficult conditions. As with most airway management skills, the use of such devices appears to be deceptively easy and unskilled practitioners will have a high rate of failure.[32,33]

The intubating LMA is designed to facilitate tracheal intubation with a large size ETT. It has a rigid anatomically curved tube made of stainless steel with a standard 15-mm connector, and an epiglottic elevating bar (EEB). The caudal end of the EEB is not fixed, allowing it to elevate the epiglottis when an ETT is passed through the aperture. The tube is large enough to accept a cuffed 8-mm ETT, and is short enough to ensure passage of the ETT cuff beyond the vocal cords. The Fastrach is fitted with a rigid handle to facilitate one-handed insertion, removal, and adjustment of the device's position.

The device permits single-handed insertion from any position without moving the head and neck from a neutral position and without placing fingers in the mouth. Ventilation and oxygenation may be continued during intubation attempts, lessening the likelihood of desaturation. Prior to insertion of the LMA-Fastrach, the cuff should be tightly deflated using a syringe so that it forms a smooth spoon shape without any wrinkles on the distal edge. Lubricant is applied to the posterior surface of the LMA before insertion. The LMA cuff is inflated with 20, 30, and 40 mL of air for size 3, 4, and 5 tubes, respectively.

The application of cricoid pressure reduces the chances of successfully positioning the LMA and intubating the trachea by 30%.[34] For this reason, and because LMAs do not protect against aspiration, the intubating laryngeal mask airway is more properly used as a rescue device than an approach of first choice in any ICU patient who may have a full stomach. In the settings of upper airway bleeding or copious secretions and failed rigid laryngoscopy, it is reasonable to attempt to use an intubating LMA.

THE DIFFICULT AIRWAY

The difficult airway is far more commonly encountered in the ICU and emergency room than in the operating room. Under these emergent conditions of airway management, multiple attempts at laryngoscopy are common (25% to 35%), and between 0.5% and 2% of patients require a surgical airway. Copious secretions and inadequate positioning are common obstacles encountered in the ICU, but not in the operating room. The American Society of Anesthesiologists' Difficult Airway Algorithm outlines the options available to practitioners faced with a difficult airway (Fig. 35-3).[31] Choices for proceeding include: ventilate with the bag and mask, summon help in the form of another operator, reposition, attempt laryngoscopy with a different blade, and apply other techniques as appropriate. Ideally, a competent operator will ventilate the patient with an Ambu bag as the operator prepares for their next attempt to secure the airway. If the patient can be adequately oxygenated with mask ventilation, then the operator has a variety of options for how to proceed. Changing the operator or laryngoscope blade will sometimes permit successful intubation where previous attempts have failed. Straight blades, such as the Miller blade, are especially useful in patients with prominent maxillary teeth, a small mandible, an anterior larynx, a floppy epiglottis, or trismus.

LMAs are useful as a bridge to oxygenate patients who cannot be intubated, but cannot be counted on to do so in the presence of abnormal lung mechanics or very abnormal anatomy.[35]

Care must be taken when using classic LMAs in such situations; a malpositioned LMA can insufflate the esophagus and increase the risk of aspiration. Even when properly inserted, inflation pressures over 20 cm H_2O can cause both leaks and esophageal and gastric insufflation. The LMA-ProSeal is a better option than a classic LMA under these conditions.

The LMA-ProSeal is an advanced form of the classic LMA and has four components: cuff, inflation line with pilot balloon, airway tube, and drain tube (see Fig. 35-2). The drain tube communicates with the upper esophageal sphincter and permits blind insertion of gastric tubes and venting of the stomach. The LMA-ProSeal introducer is provided to aid insertion of the LMA-ProSeal without the need to place fingers in the mouth. The technique of LMA-ProSeal placement with the introducer is similar to LMA-Fastrach placement.

The features of the LMA-ProSeal provide more patient management options. While the classic LMA may be used with low-pressure PPV, the LMA-ProSeal has been designed for use with PPV at higher airway pressures. The drain tube will direct the regurgitated fluid to the outside, avoiding aspiration of gastric contents; however, it is not as effective as an ETT in preventing aspiration.

If the patient cannot be either intubated or oxygenated with less invasive means, then a surgical airway is indicated. This decision cannot be made lightly, as emergency surgical airways (such as tracheostomy) have a complication rate

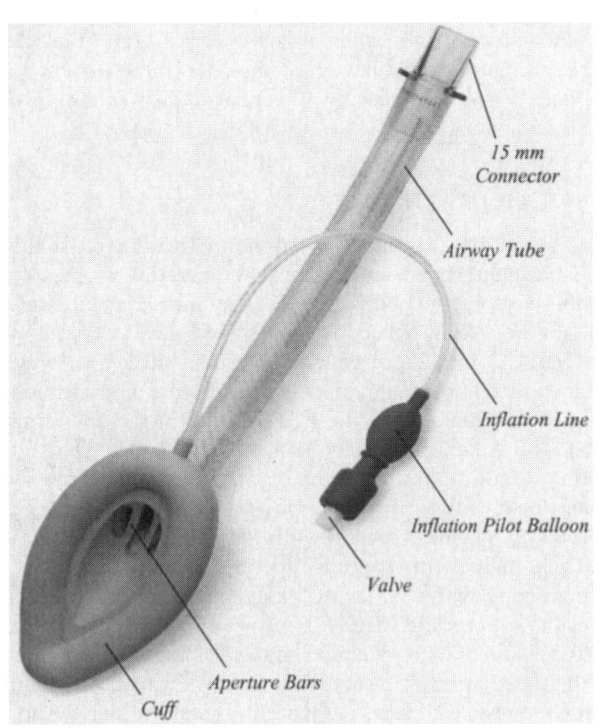

A

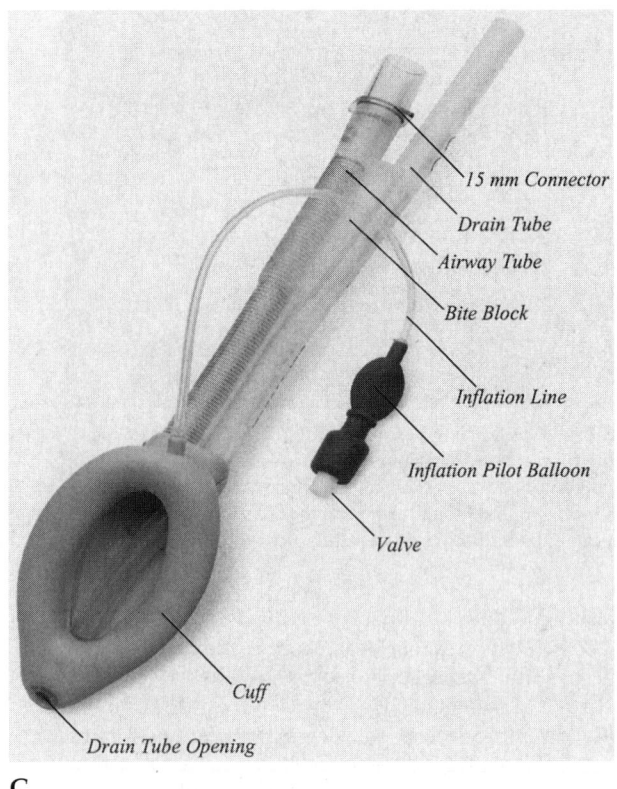

C

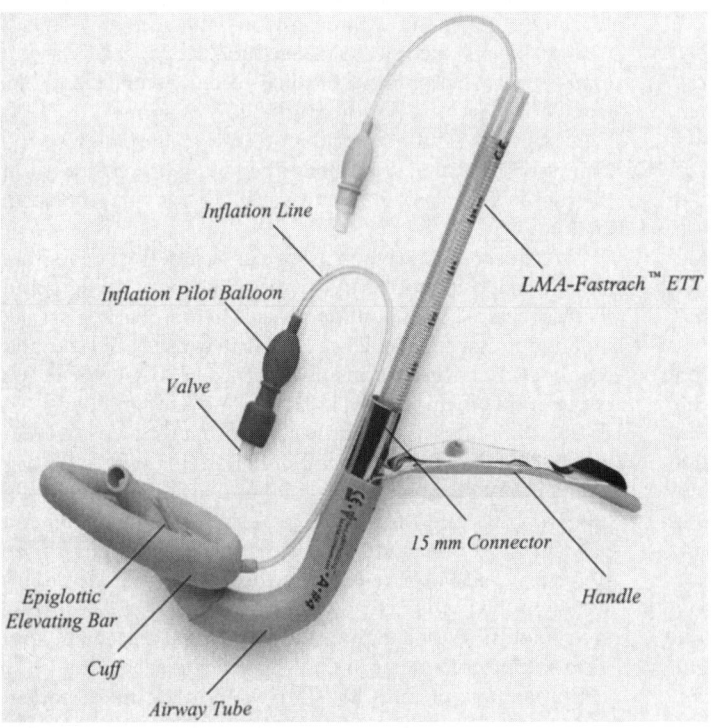

B

FIGURE 35-2 *A*. Classic laryngeal mask airway is available in eight sizes (1, 1$^{1}/_{2}$, 2, 2$^{1}/_{2}$, 3, 4, 5, and 6) that can be used in patients ranging from neonates to large adults. Its role in difficult or failed face mask ventilation is well established, and it has multiple applications in the American Society of Anesthesiologists' Practice Guidelines for Management of the Difficult Airway algorithm published in 1993 and revised in 2003. *B*. Intubating LMA (Fastrach) is available in sizes 3, 4, and 5, and is designed to facilitate tracheal intubation with endotracheal tubes up to 8-mm inside diameter. Intubation can be performed blindly or in case of difficulty with the help of flexible bronchoscope. Like the classic LMA, the Fastrach establishes ventilation when face mask ventilation has failed, and permits oxygenation and ventilation during intubation, which is useful when large amounts of secretions and blood are present in the airway following failed intubation attempts. *C*. LMA-ProSeal is an advanced version of the classic LMA with more airway management options. It provides higher seal pressure and therefore is more suitable for positive pressure ventilation. The drain tube communicates with the upper esophagus and permits passage of a nasogastric tube and decompression of the stomach, which is very valuable in patients with failed intubation and a distended stomach. ProSeal will establish ventilation and allow decompression of the stomach. *(Courtesy of LMA North America, Inc.)*

of 30%.[36] Tracheostomy is preferable to cricothyroidotomy, but requires the timely availability of both skilled personnel and appropriate equipment. Tracheostomy provides a large-bore cuffed airway that both protects against aspiration and can be used for mechanical ventilation. A wide variety of kits are commercially available for these procedures, and are preferable to ad-hoc kits because they contain all of the necessary equipment and supplies, are sterile, and have a variety of training aids. Individuals who anticipate the possibility of using such kits as part of their airway management practice should obtain training in their use. Needle cricothyroidotomy and jet ventilation is increasingly viewed as the approach

1. Assess the likelihood and clinical impact of basic management problems:
    A. Difficult Ventilation
    B. Difficult Intubation
    C. Difficulty with Patient Cooperation or Consent
    D. Difficult Tracheostomy
2. Actively pursue opportunities to deliver supplemental oxygen throughout the process of difficult airway management
3. Consider the relative merits and feasibility of basic management choices:

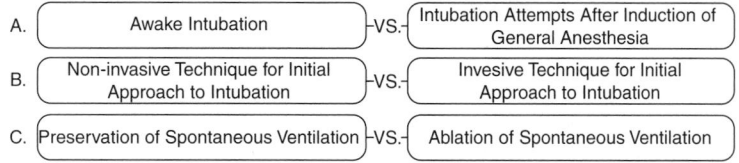

4. Develop primary and alternative strategies:

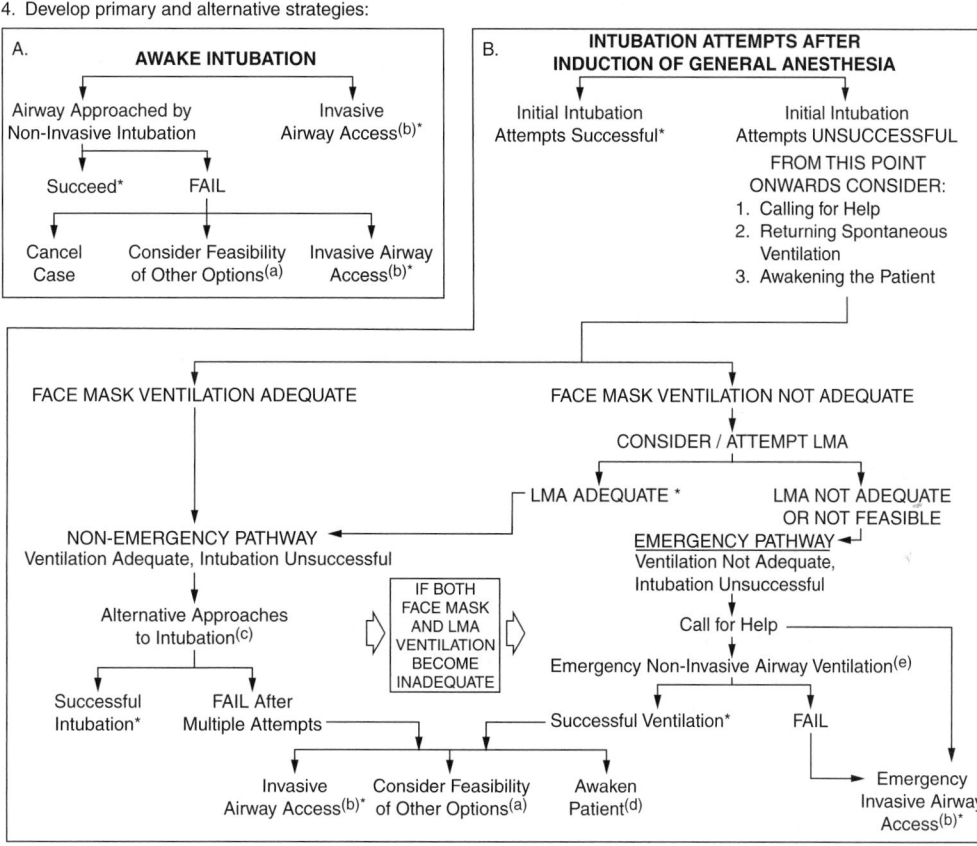

* Confirm ventilation, tracheal intubation, or LMA placement with exhaled CO2

FIGURE 35-3 The American Society of Anesthesiologists' Difficult Airway Algorithm provides a simple general guideline for management of an anticipated and unanticipated difficult airway. *Confirm ventilation, tracheal intubation, or LMA placement with exhaled CO2. (a) Other options include (but are not limited to): surgery utilizing face mask or LMA anesthesia, local anesthesia infiltration or regional nerve blockade. Pursuit of these options usually implies that mask ventilation will not be problematic. Therefore, these options may be of limited value if this step in the algorithm has been reached via the Emergency Pathway. (b) Invasive airway access includes surgical or percutaneous tracheostomy or cricothyrotomy. (c) Alternative non-invasive approaches to difficult intubation include (but are not limited to): use of different laryngoscope blades, LMA as an intubation conduit (with or without fiberoptic guidance), fiberoptic intubation, intubating stylet or tube changer, light wand, retrograde intubation, and blind oral or nasal intubation. **(d) Consider re-preparation of the patient for awake intubation or** canceling surgery. (e) Options for emergency non-invasive airway ventilation include (but are not limited to): rigid bronchoscope, esophageal-tracheal combitube ventilation, or transtracheal jet ventilation.

that is most likely to succeed when attempts to ventilate and secure an airway via laryngoscopy fail.[37]

CHANGING THE ENDOTRACHEAL TUBE

Changing the endotracheal tube is frequently more hazardous than original insertion, because the patient may have evolved significant facial and airway edema, and may require both very high $F_{I_{O_2}}$ and positive end-expiratory pressure (PEEP). The most common indications for changing ETTs include failure of the cuff to retain volume and pressure, occlusion of the tube by inspissated secretions and clots, and the requirement for a different tube than the one originally inserted (e.g., one of a larger diameter, or a different type such as a single- rather than a double-lumen tube). Tube changes motivated by complete occlusion or cuff rupture in the face of high PEEP may be dire emergencies; most other endotracheal tube changes are not.

Practitioners called on to change an endotracheal tube have the advantage that the patient already has an artificial airway, and hence the ease or difficulty of obtaining an airway has been discovered at least once for the patient. If laryngoscopy was easily accomplished before, and the patient's airway anatomy has not changed appreciably (e.g., as a result of edema), many practitioners elect to perform endotracheal tube changes with direct laryngoscopy under deep sedation and paralysis. This practice is safe when the old tube is withdrawn simultaneously with the introduction of the new tube into the trachea. Many operators prefer to perform endotracheal tube changes with the patient breathing spontaneously, reasoning that attempts at ventilation by the patient will delay the onset of hypoxia and hypercarbia in the event of difficulty in inserting the new airway. Withdrawing the old tube prior to attempting laryngoscopy, or when the view is difficult, can produce a cannot-intubate, cannot-ventilate situation, which can quickly become a crisis.

A variety of semirigid catheters are available for use as tube changers. Although they can be helpful in difficult circumstances, they can become dislodged from the trachea, and in some cases it is impossible to thread the new tube over them. Such tube changers may be best used in combination with direct laryngoscopy when the anatomy is challenging. Tube changers with a central lumen may be used to attempt to jet ventilate patients in the event that a more permanent airway cannot be established immediately. In patients with substantial facial and neck edema or burns, several assistants will be required for successful tube changes. Fiberoptic-guided exchange of tracheal tubes requires both excellent preparation of the airway (including treatment with drying agents such as glycopyrrolate and aggressive suctioning), and a high degree of skill by the operator, but can produce success where most or all other approaches would yield failure.[38]

Physiologic Changes Associated with Intubation and Mechanical Ventilation

Tracheal intubation has a range of important physiologic consequences. These are not complications of the procedure per se, but are consequences of the presence of an artificial airway and mechanical ventilation.

Tracheal intubation and the institution of positive pressure ventilation can cause a variety of changes in circulatory physiology. Laryngoscopy and tracheal intubation are frequently accompanied by hypertension and tachycardia.

Endotracheal tubes may cause an increase in airway resistance. An 8.0-mm endotracheal tube causes a 20% increase in airway resistance in the normal airway, all of it in the central airways and nonresponsive to therapy with inhaled bronchodilators. Smaller tubes have exponentially higher resistances.[39] A 7.0-mm endotracheal tube has twice the resistance of an 8.0-mm tube, whereas a 9.0-mm tube has one-third the resistance of an 8.0-mm tube. The airways resistance associated with a particular tube increases as inspissated secretions accumulate in the tube, decreasing its diameter and increasing the turbulence of flow. Tracheal intubation can also

precipitate bronchospasm in susceptible individuals, which can further increase airways resistance.

Hypotension frequently evolves after the establishment of tracheal intubation and mechanical ventilation, and has many contributing factors.[40] First, these usually entail a change in mean intrathoracic pressures from large negative pressures to large positive pressures, with a corresponding fall in venous return and cardiac output. Mechanical ventilation is also frequently associated with a resolution of hypoxia, hypercapnia, and dyspnea, and a proportionate decline in circulating catecholamines.[41] Patients with obstructive lung disease can develop high levels of auto-PEEP very quickly during vigorous ventilation with an Ambu bag, which can be associated with hypotension.[42,43] Finally, high levels of PEEP can increase the pulmonary vascular resistance, with an associated shift of the interventricular septum into the left ventricle.[44,45]

Complications

Airway manipulation in critically ill patients is a necessarily hazardous undertaking (Table 35-7). Death, circulatory collapse, arrhythmias, hypoxia, airway trauma, aspiration, and failed intubation can all occur, even when the airway is managed flawlessly.

Right mainstem intubation is a common consequence of intubation in the ICU. It can be avoided in many cases by

TABLE 35-7 Complications of Intubation

Immediate
  Right mainstem intubation
  Esophageal intubation
  Gastric aspiration
  Dental injury, tooth aspiration
  Mucosal laceration or tear
  Hypertension/tachycardia
  Myocardial ischemia
  Elevated intracranial pressure
  Hypotension
  Arrhythmias
    Ventricular premature beats
    Ventricular tachycardia
    Ventricular fibrillation
    Atrial fibrillation
    Bradycardia (in young patients)
  Bronchospasm
  Vocal cord trauma
  Dislocation of arytenoid cartilage
  Pain
Chronic
  Serous or purulent otitis
  Sinusitis
  Mucosal ulceration
  Necrosis of lip or nose
  Granulomas
  Dental damage from biting
  Tracheal mucosal injury
  Tracheoesophageal fistula, tracheoinnominate fistula
  Laryngeal stricture
  Vocal cord synechiae/paralysis
  Tracheomalacia, cricoarytenoid edema, subluxation and
    fracture
  Tracheal stenosis

taping tubes at 23 cm at the lip in males and 21 cm at the lip in females of average stature (using the average tooth-to-carina distance, which is 28 cm in the average male and 24 cm in the average female).[46] Tooth-to-carina distance varies; a tube taped at 24 cm at the lip might be in perfect position for the average 180-cm male, but might not even be in the trachea of a very tall patient. Correct positioning of the endotracheal tube is difficult to verify clinically and requires fiberoptic bronchoscopy or a chest radiograph for confirmation.[47,48]

In spite of assertions that it should never happen, esophageal intubation remains an inevitable complication of airway management. In theory, it should be quickly recognized and the offending tube removed expeditiously. In practice, it will occur in circumstances in which auscultation of the breath sounds is difficult and where endotracheal intubation cannot be confirmed with capnography, including patients with severe bronchospasm (especially children), and in adults in full cardiopulmonary arrest.[49]

Gastric aspiration that occurs around the time of intubation in the ICU can cause pneumonia and precipitate acute respiratory distress syndrome; it occurs approximately 4% of the time.[10] In less controlled settings, such as in trauma patients, aspiration may occur in up to 30% of patients around the time they are intubated.[50] The application of cricoid pressure and manipulation of the airway with the patient awake are the two most effective strategies to avoid this problem.

A variety of tissue injuries are associated with airway management in the ICU setting.[51–54] These injuries are more likely to occur in uncooperative patients, seizing patients, and patients with anatomically difficult airways.[55] Dental injury and tooth fragment aspiration remain a complication of airway management. Tracheal and esophageal lacerations can also occur. At least some bleeding is likely to occur in coagulopathic patients and in patients with friable tissues. The vocal cords and arytenoid cartilages can also be traumatized during intubation. Prolonged tracheal intubation can also impair swallowing, which increases the risk of aspiration in these patients after extubation.[56] Residual muscle paralysis is an important risk factor for aspiration in perioperative patients, and perhaps in critically ill patients as well.[57]

A variety of cardiac complications may occur around the time of airway manipulation. Myocardial ischemia can be precipitated by the stress response to airway manipulation. The amount of ischemia precipitated can be minimized with adequate topical anesthesia and by matching the sedation given to the degree of stimulation created. Ventricular premature beats are a common consequence of the stress response in the setting of airway manipulation. Ventricular tachycardia and ventricular fibrillation can occur in patients susceptible to these arrhythmias. Bradycardia can also occur, particularly in young patients with high vagal tone.

Death occurs around the time of endotracheal intubation in approximately 3% of critically ill patients.[10] In some patients, issues of airway management will contribute to the sequence of events that result in death; an expeditious intubation averts death in the vast majority of patients.

Tracheostomy

The role of tracheostomy continues to evolve in critically ill patients. The improved design of endotracheal tubes and

careful attention to sedation has minimized the traumatic consequences of intubation, making translaryngeal intubation for weeks both safe and tractable. On the other side, the improved techniques for performing tracheostomy, and the increasing ability to perform tracheostomy at the bedside has made tracheostomy safer and more available than it has been previously. Tracheostomy continues to have immediate and long-term complications that intensivists manage.

INDICATIONS FOR TRACHEOSTOMY

The least controversial indication for tracheostomy is upper airway obstruction, especially long-term or permanent airway obstruction. Tracheostomy is also widely accepted as preferable to transglottic intubation for long-term mechanical ventilation. Tracheostomy is also indicated when a patient will be unable to clear their airway secretions for a long period of time. Finally, tracheostomy is frequently used to facilitate liberation from mechanical ventilation.

Tracheostomy has several benefits in patients who will require long-term mechanical ventilation. It allows easier and safer access to the mouth, which allows improved oral hygiene. It is substantially more comfortable than translaryngeal intubation, so the need for both analgesics and sedation may be significantly reduced. Specially designed tracheostomy tubes allow for speech and even normal eating in patients who are either continuously or intermittently ventilated. There was a time when patients underwent tracheostomy after only very brief periods of translaryngeal intubation and mechanical ventilation (e.g., 7 to 10 days). The decision to perform a tracheostomy on a patient in these circumstances should not be motivated as much by the time that has already elapsed on mechanical ventilation, but rather by the amount of time it can be foreseen that they will require mechanical ventilation. If the patient will obviously require ventilation for the coming weeks, then it is quite reasonable to perform a tracheostomy for both their safety and comfort.[58,59] Patients at high risk of the complications of translaryngeal intubation, such as diabetics, may benefit from earlier tracheostomy.

Tracheostomy has the great benefit of reducing the anatomic dead space, resulting in substantially greater alveolar ventilation for any given minute ventilation. This benefit may be of critical importance in patients whose strength is very closely matched to their requirement for minute ventilation, and who might not otherwise be easy to liberate from the ventilator. The ease of reinstituting mechanical ventilation, and the wide bore and short length of tracheostomy tubes are also of benefit in these circumstances.

PERCUTANEOUS VERSUS SURGICAL TRACHEOSTOMY

There is a large and growing literature which clearly demonstrates that percutaneous and surgical tracheostomy are equally successful and safe in competent hands.[60–62] Interestingly, the sum of the patients in all of the prospective studies published thus far is less than 600, limiting the statistical power of inferences about rare complications, such as death, pneumothorax, and posterior tracheal wall perforation, but certainly allowing the conclusion that the success rates and overall complication rates of the two procedures are very similar. Mortality of either procedure is now less than 1%, which is significantly lower than that reported in older literature. When performed at the bedside in the ICU, both percutaneous and surgical tracheostomy are significantly less expensive and easier to arrange than tracheostomy in the operating room. The difference in cost between the two procedures performed at the bedside is small, and likely to be outweighed by other institutional factors and considerations.

A variety of techniques for percutaneous tracheostomy have been described and are in widespread use. Briefly, after appropriate sedation, the patient's neck is extended to open the tracheal interspaces. The skin over tracheal interspaces below the cricoid cartilage is then anesthetized, prepped with an appropriate cleansing agent, and draped in the usual sterile fashion. A 2-cm horizontal incision is made, and the neck is bluntly dissected down to the trachea. The existing tracheal tube is then withdrawn to a position just below the vocal cords. A needle is then inserted into the trachea (usually under bronchoscopic guidance), and a wire threaded into the tracheal lumen. The tract is then mechanically dilated, and an appropriately sized tube inserted into the trachea. Commercially available kits are now available that replace multiple dilators with a single dilator (e.g., Blue Rhino PDT from Cook Critical Care, Bloomington, IN), which may save time and reduce the risk of the procedure as well. Two of the advantages of the percutaneous technique are the minimal sharp dissection involved, and the use of dilation to create the tract for the tracheostomy tube, both of which limit the bleeding associated with the procedure.

The literature about percutaneous tracheostomy clearly documents that it can be accomplished successfully and safely in the hands of competent practitioners. Some techniques incorporate bronchoscopic guidance, incurring additional expense, time delay, and need for additional operators to provide some increase in the safety of the procedure. Although simultaneous bronchoscopy is advocated by some authorities, many more experienced operators rarely if ever use it to facilitate the procedure. The speed with which percutaneous tracheostomy without the use of a bronchoscope can be accomplished is impressive, making it attractive as a procedure to emergently secure the obstructed airway in institutions with readily available kits and highly skilled operators. Morbid obesity and previous tracheostomy are frequently cited contraindications to percutaneous tracheostomy, but there are case series which suggest that the procedure can be performed safely in select patients with either diagnosis.[63,64] There is no doubt that as with any other procedural skill, there is and will be significant variation across practitioners and institutions, which makes prescriptions about percutaneous tracheostomy inappropriate.

MINITRACHEOSTOMY

Minitracheostomy is a procedure that is sometimes performed in select critically ill patients to facilitate clearance of bronchial secretions.[65] Minitrach allows repeated suctioning of the trachea below the cords without passing a tube through them at the cost of undergoing the procedure (which is generally performed at the bedside) with its attendant complications. The procedure itself is very similar to that described for percutaneous tracheostomy, except that it does not result in an airway. Minitracheostomy has been demonstrated to reduce the incidence of radiographic collapse, but has not otherwise

been proven to improve outcomes.[66,67] Minitracheostomy is commonly done at some centers, rarely done at most, and never done at others. This is unlikely to change unless studies demonstrating more dramatic benefit to the procedure are published.

COMPLICATIONS OF TRACHEOSTOMY

The immediate complications of tracheostomy include hemorrhage, malpositioning of the tracheostomy tube, and pneumothorax/pneumomediastinum. Hemorrhage can occur as a consequence of bleeding from subcutaneous vessels, neck veins, and the thyroid gland. Most postoperative bleeding is venous in origin, and it may take hours for a noticeable hematoma to form. A hematoma in the neck can compress the trachea or cause it to deviate, resulting in increased airway pressures, a sensation of dyspnea on the part of the patient, and hypoventilation. Airway obstruction caused by a hematoma is best treated by decompression/evacuation, as all other therapies will fail to interrupt the cascade of events leading to deterioration and will allow the underlying process to progress.

Rarely, tracheostomy tubes may be placed into tissue planes in the neck instead of the trachea. Monitoring end-tidal carbon dioxide concentrations after the tube is inserted will aid in the timely recognition of this problem, allowing it to be quickly corrected. Tracheal positioning of the tracheostomy tube can be verified with auscultation, capnography, and fiberoptic bronchoscopy.

Pneumothorax and pneumomediastinum are consequences of invasion of these tissue planes, which can extend superiorly into the neck in some patients (particularly those with chronic obstructive pulmonary disease or on high amounts of PEEP). These complications are more likely to occur in situations in which the anatomy is difficult, such as patients with morbid obesity, previous neck surgery, or goiter. These complications are usually recognized on the routine chest radiograph taken postoperatively in these patients to confirm adequate positioning of the new tracheostomy tube.

LONG-TERM COMPLICATIONS OF TRACHEOSTOMY

Tracheostomy tubes are frequently left in patients for months and occasionally years. This situation puts the patient at risk of complications due to chronic irritation or erosion of the trachea, including tracheoesophageal fistula, tracheoinnominate fistula, tracheomalacia, and tracheal stenosis.

The absence of a large epidemiologic database, the heterogeneity of patient populations undergoing tracheostomy in the ICU, and the high mortality in some patient populations that undergo the procedure make discussion of the complications of tracheostomy difficult.[68] Tracheal stenosis is diagnosed in 40% to 60% of patients who have undergone tracheostomy, but it is unclear if this is a complication of their tracheostomy or their prior transglottic tracheal intubation.[69,70] The high cuff pressures thought to be the major cause of the tissue injury that drives this process are more likely to be present during the early, acute phase of critical illness, when high airway pressures are present.[71] On the other hand, the disruption of the tracheal cartilages caused by the presence of the tracheostomy tube may lead to instability, which may in turn cause tissue injury, which may be worsened by the immune response to both the tracheostomy tube and the purulent secretions that contaminate its tract. Given this, it is unsurprising that a majority of the tracheal stenoses attributed to tracheostomy occur at the level of entry into the trachea.

Tracheoinnominate fistula occurs in less than 1% of patients, typically within 1 month of undergoing insertion of a low-lying tracheostomy. Either the tip of the tube or its cuff erodes through the wall of the trachea and into the vessel, causing life-threatening bleeding which requires immediate surgical repair. Tracheoesophageal fistula occurs via the same mechanism, but entails erosion through the posterior wall of the trachea into the esophagus. Tracheoesophageal fistula is frequently difficult to diagnose, as it can present as recurrent pneumonia in a ventilated patient. Other more obvious symptoms include cuff leak refractory to inflation, aspiration of large quantities of tube feeds in spite of an appropriately inflated tracheostomy cuff, and gastric distention with large quantities of air. The diagnosis of a tracheoesophageal fistula can be established with either barium swallow or computed tomography scan. Treatment is usually surgical, although a variety of stents have been employed as an alternative.[72]

Teaching Airway Management Skills

The place to learn basic airway management skills is the operating room, not the ICU. Basic airway management skills, although apparently very simple, in fact take a great deal of time and experience to master. These basics are best learned in an environment in which patients will generally have normal anatomy, circulation, and lung mechanics. Elective procedures in the operating room present ideal opportunities to learn the basics of mask ventilation, laryngoscopy, fiberoptic laryngoscopy, nasal intubation, and insertion of laryngeal mask airways. Outpatient bronchoscopies present excellent opportunities to learn how to adequately topically anesthetize the nasopharynx and oropharynx. Literature from a wide variety of fields supports the contention that most practitioners tasked with managing the airway are either inadequately trained, or will predictably benefit from more training.[73,74] Once the basics of airway management have been mastered in the elective setting, they can be applied in airway management under adequate supervision in the ICU. Attempts to teach the basics of airway management at the bedside in the ICU should be discouraged, as critically ill patients do not tolerate the high rates of failure that typically occur as practitioners learn these skills. Participating in airway management workshops and the practice of various airway management techniques in models and simulators is extremely valuable, especially for procedures such as fiberoptic bronchoscopy, which requires hours of practice to attain facility manipulating the bronchoscope. The wide variety of things that skillful airway managers take into account at the bedside or consider as they proceed are given in Table 35-8.

References

1. O'Connor MF, Ovassapian A: Management of the airway and tracheal intubations, in Murray MJ, Coursin DB, Pearl RG, Prough DS (eds): *Critical Care Medicine Perioperative Management.* Philadelphia, Lippincott, Williams & Wilkins, 2002, p 89.
2. Sellick BA: Cricoid pressure to control regurgitation of stomach contents during induction of anaesthesia. *Lancet* 2:404, 1961.
3. Fanning GL: The efficacy of cricoid pressure in preventing regurgitation of gastric contents. *Anesthesiology* 32:553, 1970.
4. Salem MR, Joseph NJ, Heyman HJ, et al: Cricoid compression is effective in obliterating the esophageal lumen in the presence of a nasogastric tube. *Anesthesiology* 63:443, 1985.
5. Frerk CM: Predicting difficult intubation. *Anaesthesia* 46:1005, 1991.
6. Ovassapian A (ed): *Fiberoptic Endoscopy and the Difficult Airway,* 2nd ed. Philadelphia, Lippincott-Raven, 1996, p 201.
7. Perry JJ, Lee J, Wells G: Are intubation conditions using rocuronium equivalent to those using succinylcholine? *Acad Emerg Med* 9:813, 2002.
8. Siviloiit ML, Ducharme J: Randomized, double-blind study on sedatives and hemodynamics during rapid sequence intubation in the emergency department: the SHRED study. *Ann Emerg Med* 31:313, 1998.
9. Smith DC, Bergen JM, Smithline H, et al: A trial of etomidate for rapid sequence intubation in the emergency department. *J Emerg Med* 18:13, 2000.
10. Schwartz DE, Matthay MA, Cohen NH: Death and other complications of emergency airway management in critically ill adults. *Anesthesiology* 82:367, 1995.
11. Wayne MA, Friedland E: Prehospital use of succinylcholine: a 20 year review. *Prehosp Emerg Care* 3:107, 1999.
12. Tayal VS, Riggs RW, Marx JA, et al: Rapid sequence intubation at an emergency medicine residency: success rate and adverse events during a two-year period. *Acad Emerg Med* 3:107, 1999.
13. Sakles JC, Laurin EG, Rantapaa AA, et al: Airway management in the emergency department: a one year study of 620 tracheal intubations. *Ann Emerg Med* 31:326, 1998.
14. Adnet F, Jouriles NJ, Le Toumelin P, et al: Survey of out-of-hospital emergency intubations in the French prehospital medical system: a multi-center study. *Ann Emerg Med* 32:454, 1998.
15. Vijaykumar E, Bosscher H, Renzi FP, et al: The use of neuromuscular blocking agents in the emergency department to facilitate tracheal intubation in the trauma patient: help or hindrance? *J Crit Care* 13:1, 1998.
16. Bernard S, Smith K, Foster S, et al: The use of rapid sequence intubation by ambulance paramedics for patients with severe head injury. *Emerg Med* 14:406, 2002.
17. Bulger EM, Copass MK, Maier RV, et al: An analysis of advanced prehospital airway management. *J Emerg Med* 23:183, 2002.
18. Bair AE, Filbin MR, Kulkarni RG, et al: The failed intubation attempt in the emergency department: analysis of prevalence, rescue techniques, and personnel. *J Emerg Med* 23:131, 2002.
19. Davis DP, Hoyt DB, Ochs M, et al: The effect of paramedic rapid sequence intubation on outcome in patients with severe traumatic brain injury. *J Trauma-Injury Infect Crit Care* 54:444, 2003.

TABLE 35-8 Some Practical Bedside Rules of Thumb

1. Save the brain
2. Save the circulation
3. A spontaneously breathing patient has at least one vital sign; an apneic patient may soon have none
4. Mask ventilation is better than esophageal intubation
5. The worst time for a patient to aspirate is when it's time to intubate
6. If you don't give any IV anesthetics, the CODE can't be blamed on you
7. The patient who asks for a tube needs one
8. A patient who doesn't mind a tube needs one
9. The best procedure for a patient may be the one that you know how to do best
10. The place to learn basic airway management skills is the operating room, not the ICU

20. Bochicchio GV, Ilahi O, Joshi M, et al: Endotracheal intubation in the field does not improve outcome in trauma patients who present without an acutely lethal traumatic brain injury. *J Trauma-Injury Infect Crit Care* 54:307, 2003.

21. Holzapfel L, Chevret S, Madinier G, et al: Influence of long-term oro- or naso-tracheal intubation on nosocomial maxillary sinusitis and pneumonia: results of a prospective, randomized clinical trial. *Crit Care Med* 21:1132, 1993.

22. Holzapfel L, Chastang C, Demingeon G, et al: A randomized study assessing the systematic search for maxillary sinusitis in nasotracheally mechanically ventilated patients. Influence of nosocomial maxillary sinusitis on the occurrence of ventilator-associated pneumonia. *Am J Resp Crit Care Med* 159:965, 1999.

23. Rello J, Sonora R, Jubert P, et al: Pneumonia in intubated patients: role of respiratory airway care. *Am J Resp Crit Care Med* 154:111, 1996.

24. Rouby JJ, Laurent P, Gosnach M, et al: Risk factors and clinical relevance of nosocomial maxillary sinusitis in the clinically ill. *Am J Resp Crit Care Med* 150:776, 1994.

25. Heffner JE: Nosocomial sinusitis: den of multiresistant thieves? *Am J Resp Crit Care Med* 150:608, 1994.

26. Tindol GA Jr, DiBenedetto RJ, Kosciuk L: Unplanned extubations. *Chest* 105:1804, 1994.

27. Chevron V, Menard J, Richard J, et al: Unplanned extubation: risk factors for the development and predictive criteria for reintubation. *Crit Care Med* 26:1049, 1998.

28. Sims WS, Chung IS, Chin JU, et al: Risk factors for epistaxis during nasotracheal intubation. *Anesth Intensive Care* 30:449, 2002.

29. Sessler CN, Vitaliti JC, Cooper KR, et al: Comparison of 4% lidocaine/0.5% phenylephrine with 5% cocaine: Which dilates the nasal passages better? *Anesthesiology* 64:274, 1986.

30. Ovassapian A, Krejcie TC, Yelich SJ, et al: Awake fiberoptic intubation of the patient at high risk of aspiration. *Br J Anesth* 62:13, 1989.

31. American Society of Anesthesiologists Task Force on Management of the Difficult Airway, Caplan RA, Benumof JL, Berry FA, et al: Practice guidelines for management of the difficult airway. An updated report by the American Society of Anesthesiologists Task Force on Management of the Difficult Airway. *Anesthesiology* 98:1269, 2003.

32. Levitan RM, Ochroch EA, Stuart S, et al: Use of the intubating laryngeal mask airway by medical and non-medical personnel. *Am J Emerg Med* 18:12, 2000.

33. Avidan MS, Harvey A, Chitkara N, et al: The intubating laryngeal mask airway compared with direct laryngoscopy. *Br J Anaesth* 83:615, 1999.

34. Harry RM, Nolan JP: The use of cricoid pressure with the intubating laryngeal mask. *Anesthesia* 54:656, 1999.

35. Martin SE, Ochsner MG, Jarman RH, et al: Use of the laryngeal mask airway in air transport when intubation fails. *J Trauma* 47:352, 1999.

36. Gillespie MB, Elise DW: Outcomes of emergency surgical airway procedures in a hospital wide setting. *Laryngoscope* 109:1766, 1999.

37. Patel RG: Percutaneous transtracheal jet ventilation: a safe, quick, and temporary way to provide oxygenation and ventilation when conventional methods are unsuccessful. *Chest* 116:1689, 1999.

38. Ovassapian A: Fiberoptic airway endoscopy in critical care, in Ovassapian A (ed): *Fiberoptic Endoscopy and the Difficult Airway*. Philadelphia, Lippincott-Raven, 1996, p 157.

39. Habib MP: Physiologic implications of artificial airways. *Chest* 96:180, 1989.

40. Franklin C, Samuel J, Hu T-C: Life-threatening hypotension associated with emergency intubation and the initiation of mechanical ventilation. *Am J Emerg Med* 12:425, 1994.

41. Dripps RD, Comroe JH: The respiratory and circulatory response of normal man to inhalation of 7.6 and 10.4% CO_2 with a

42. Pepe PE, Marini JJ: Occult positive end-expiratory pressure in mechanically ventilated patients with airflow obstruction: The auto-PEEP effect. *Am Rev Respir Dis* 126:166, 1982.

43. Rogers PL, Schlichtig R, Miro A, Pinsky M: Auto-PEEP during CPR: An "occult" cause of electromechanical dissociation? *Chest* 99:492, 1991.

44. Jardin F, Farcot J-C, Boisante L, et al: Influence of positive end-expiratory pressure on left ventricular performance. *N Engl J Med* 304:387, 1981.

45. Baigorri F, de Monte A, Blanch L, et al: Hemodynamic responses to external counterbalancing of auto-positive end-expiratory pressure in mechanically ventilated patients with chronic obstructive pulmonary disease. *Crit Care Med* 22:1782, 1994.

46. Owen RL, Cheney F: Endobronchial intubation: A preventable complication. *Anesthesiology* 67:255, 1987.

47. Schwartz DE, Lieberman JA, Cohen NH: Women are at greater risk than men for malpositioning of the endotracheal tube after emergent intubation. *Crit Care Med* 22:1127, 1994.

48. Brunel W, Coleman DL, Schwartz DE, et al: Assessment of routine chest roentgenograms and the physical examination to confirm endotracheal tube position. *Chest* 96:1043, 1989.

49. Bagshaw O, Gillis J, Schell D: Delayed recognition of esophageal intubation in a neonate: Role of radiologic diagnosis. *Crit Care Med* 22:2020, 1994.

50. Lockey DJ, Coats T, Parr JM: Aspiration in severe trauma: a prospective study. *Anesthesia* 54:1097, 1999.

51. Whited RE: Posterior commissure stenosis post long-term intubation. *Laryngoscope* 93:1314, 1983.

52. Belson TP: Cuff induced tracheal injury in dogs following prolonged intubation. *Laryngoscope* 93:549, 1983.

53. Rashkin MC, Davis T: Acute complications of endotracheal intubation: Relationship to reintubation, route, urgency, and duration. *Chest* 89:165, 1986.

54. Kastanos N, Miró RE, Perez AM, et al: Laryngotracheal injury due to endotracheal intubation: Incidence, evolution, and predisposing factors. A prospective long-term study. *Crit Care Med* 11:362, 1983.

55. Thomas R, Kumar EV, Kameswaran M, et al: Post intubation laryngeal sequelae in an intensive care unit. *J Laryngol Otol* 109:313, 1995.

56. de Larminat V, Montravers P, Dureuil B, Desmonts JM: Alteration in swallowing reflex after extubation in intensive care unit patients. *Crit Care Med* 23:486, 1995.

57. Kopman AF, Yee PS, Neuman GG: Relationship of the train-of-four fade ratio to clinical signs and symptoms of residual paralysis in awake volunteers. *Anesthesiology* 86:765, 1997.

58. Marsh HM, Gillespie DJ, Baumgartner AE: Timing of tracheostomy in the critically ill patient. *Chest* 96:190, 1989.

59. Heffner JE: Medical indications for tracheotomy. *Chest* 96:186, 1989.

60. Angel LF, Simpson CB: Comparison of surgical and percutaneous dilational tracheostomy. *Clin Chest Med* 24:423, 2003.

61. Freeman BD, Isabella K, Lin N, Buchman TG: A meta-analysis of prospective trials comparing percutaneous and surgical tracheostomy in critically ill patients. *Chest* 118:1412, 2000.

62. Dulguerov P, Gysin C, Perneger TV, Chevrolet JC: Percutaneous or surgical tracheostomy: a meta-analysis. *Crit Care Med* 27:69, 1999.

63. Mansharamani NG, Koziel H, Garland R, et al: Safety of bedside percutaneous dilational tracheostomy in obese patients in the ICU. *Chest* 117:1426, 2000.

64. Meyer M, Critchlow J, Mansharamani N, et al: Repeat bedside percutaneous dilational tracheostomy is a safe procedure. *Crit Care Med* 30:986, 2002.

65. Wright C: Minitracheostomy. *Clin Chest Med* 24:431, 2003.

66. Issa MM, Healy DM, Maghur HA, Luke DA: Prophylactic mini-tracheostomy in lung resections. *J Thorac Cardiovasc Surg* 101:895, 1991.

67. Randell TT, Tierala EK, Lepantalo MJ, et al: Prophylactic mini-tracheostomy after thoracotomy: a prospective, random control, clinical trial. *Eur J Surg* 157:501, 1991.

68. Stauffer JL, Olson DE, Petty TL: Complications and consequences of endotracheal intubation and tracheostomy. *Am J Med* 70:65, 1981.

69. Walz MK, Peitgen K, Thurauf N, et al: Percutaneous dilatational tracheostomy—early results and long-term outcome of 326 critically ill patients. *Intensive Care Med* 24:685, 1998.

70. Dollner R, Verch M, Schweiger P, et al: Laryngotracheoscopic findings in long-term follow-up after Grigg's tracheostomy. *Chest* 122:206, 2002.

71. Arola MK, Puhakka H, Makela P: Healing of lesions caused by cuffed tracheostomy tubes and their late sequelae. *Acta Anaesthesiol Scand* 24:169, 1980.

72. Macchiarini P, Verhoye JP, Chapelier A, et al: Evaluation and outcome of different surgical techniques for post-intubation tracheoesophageal fistulas. *J Thorac Cardiovasc Surg* 119:268, 2000.

73. Mulcaster JT, Mills J, Hung OR, et al: Laryngoscopic intubation: learning and performance. *Anesthesiology* 98:23, 2003.

74. Swanson ER, Fosnocht DE: Effect of an airway education program on prehospital intubation. *Air Med J* 21:28, 2002.

Chapter 36

MANAGEMENT OF THE VENTILATED PATIENT

GREGORY A. SCHMIDT
JESSE B. HALL

KEY POINTS

- *Effective preventive measures in ventilated patients include raising the head of the bed during enteral feeding, using measures to prevent venous thromboembolism, avoiding unnecessary changes of the ventilator circuit, and reducing the amount of sedation.*

- *Ventilator parameters should be determined by the pathophysiology underlying the particular form of respiratory failure; this approach facilitates stabilization and comfort of the patient on the ventilator, prevention of common complications, and early liberation from this supportive therapy.*

- *Although some patients may require sedation and muscle relaxation for initial stabilization on the ventilator, these agents should not be used to routinely adapt the patient to the machine; rather, ventilator adjustments should be used to stabilize and comfort the patient. This latter approach is facilitated by a careful analysis of airway pressure and flow waveforms.*

- *Whenever the adequacy of oxygen exchange is in question, the initial fraction of inspired oxygen (F_{IO_2}) should be 1.0; this will be diagnostic and therapeutic because failure to achieve full arterial hemoglobin saturation identifies a significant right-to-left shunt.*

- *Typical ventilator settings for the patient with normal lung mechanics and gas exchange include an F_{IO_2} of 0.5, tidal volume of 8 to 12 mL/kg, and respiratory rate of 8 to 12 breaths/min; if mechanical ventilation has been instituted to rest fatigued respiratory muscles, deep sedation may be necessary to minimize respiratory muscle activity.*

- *The patient with severe airflow obstruction often develops hypoperfusion after institution of positive-pressure ventilation as a result of occult positive end-expiratory pressure (autoPEEP); this responds to temporary cessation of ventilation and vigorous volume resuscitation while measures are used to reduce airflow obstruction.*

- *The goals of ventilator management in severe airflow obstruction include a plateau airway pressure below 30 cm H_2O, an autoPEEP below 10 cm H_2O, or an end-inspired lung volume smaller than 20 mL/kg even if this results in hypercapnia; short expiratory times must be avoided.*

- *The patient with acute hypoxemic respiratory failure resulting from pulmonary edema benefits from lung-protective ventilation (6 mL/kg ideal body weight and rate approximately 30 breaths/min). The initial F_{IO_2} of 1.0 can be lowered to nontoxic levels by raising PEEP, which is guided by pulse oximetry.*

Too often, the management of the patient on a ventilator is guided by (a) a standard protocol applied to diverse patients regardless of the underlying pulmonary derangement or (b)

mode-dominated thinking on the part of the physician, by which various microprocessor-controlled machine functions are hoped to have a salutary effect on patient outcome. This chapter offers an alternative approach, in which ventilator parameters are tailored to the patient's mechanical and gas exchange abnormalities. This facilitates early stabilization of the patient on the ventilator in such a way as to optimize carbon dioxide removal and oxygen delivery within the limits of abnormal neuromuscular function, lung mechanics, and gas exchange and limit complications of barotrauma, lung injury, and cardiovascular depression.

Other chapters of this book are complementary to the information presented here. The pathophysiology of respiratory failure is broadly reviewed in Chap. 31; monitoring the respiratory system is delineated in Chap. 32; noninvasive ventilation is covered in Chap. 33; ventilator-induced lung injury is discussed in Chap. 37; and several chapters (e.g., Chap. 38, "Acute Respiratory Distress Syndrome"; Chap. 39, "Acute on Chronic Respiratory Failure"; Chap. 40, "Status Asthmaticus"; Chap. 42, "Restrictive Disease of the Respiratory System") discuss ventilatory support for specific problems.

The fundamental purpose of mechanical ventilation is to assist in elimination of carbon dioxide and inspiration of adequate oxygen when the patient is unable to do so or should not be allowed to do so. Such patients fall into two main groups: those in whom full rest of the respiratory muscles or permissive hypercapnia is indicated (e.g., during shock, severe acute pulmonary derangement, or with deep sedation or anesthesia) and those in whom some degree of respiratory muscle use is desired (e.g., to strengthen or improve the coordination of the respiratory muscles, to assess the ability of the patient to sustain the work of breathing, or to begin spontaneous ventilation). It is important for the intensivist to be explicit about whether the respiratory muscles should be rested or exercised because the details of ventilation (mode and settings) usually follow logically from this fundamental point.

We discuss the various conventional modes of ventilation practiced in most intensive care units (ICUs). If full rest of the respiratory muscles is desired, it is incumbent on the physician to ensure that this is achieved. Although some patients are fully passive while being ventilated (those with deep sedation, some forms of coma, metabolic alkalosis, sleep-disordered breathing), most patients will make active respiratory efforts, even on volume assist-control ventilation (ACV),[1] at times performing extraordinary amounts of work. Unintended patient effort can be difficult to recognize but, aside from obvious patient effort, may be signaled by an inspiratory decrease in intrathoracic pressure (as noted on central venous or pulmonary artery pressure tracings or with an esophageal balloon), by triggering of the ventilator, or by a careful analysis of real-time flow and pressure waveforms, discussed more fully in Chap. 32. When there is evidence of unwanted patient effort, ventilator adjustments, psychological measures, pharmacologic sedation, and therapeutic paralysis can be useful, as discussed later in this chapter. Ventilator strategies to decrease the patient's work of breathing include increasing the minute ventilation to decrease arterial partial pressure of CO_2 (Pa_{CO_2}; although this may run counter to other goals of ventilation, especially in patients with acute respiratory distress syndrome [ARDS] or severe obstruction), increasing the inspiratory flow rate, and changing the mode to pressure-preset ventilation, as in pressure-support (PSV) or pressure-control

(PCV) mode. Adjusting the ventilator to the patient's demand is described more fully below.

If some work of breathing on the patient's part is desired, this can be achieved through any of the existing ventilatory modes. The amount of work done may be highly variable, however, and depends on the specific mode, the settings chosen within each mode, and the interaction between the patient and the ventilator. A recurring question during the time when a patient can carry some of the work of breathing is, "Can this patient breathe without ventilatory assistance?" This issue is more fully developed in Chap. 44, "Liberation from Mechanical Ventilation."

Choosing a ventilatory mode and settings appropriate for each patient depends not only on the physician's goals (rest versus exercise) but also on knowledge of the mechanical properties of the patient's respiratory system. Determining respiratory system mechanics is an integral part of ventilator management and a routine part of examination of the critically ill patient, discussed fully in Chap. 32 ("Ventilator Waveforms") and reviewed extensively in the literature.[2,3] The intensivist can combine clinical information, chest radiography, and respiratory system mechanical properties (as described in Chap. 32) to categorize the patient into one of four prototypes: (a) normal gas exchange and mechanics, (b) significant airflow obstruction (as in status asthmaticus or acute exacerbations of chronic obstructive pulmonary disease (COPD), (c) acute lung injury and ARDS, and (d) restriction of the lung or chest wall.

Appropriate initial ventilator settings and subsequent adjustments for each of these four states is discussed later in this chapter. We emphasize the use of pressure and flow waveforms to further adjust the ventilator to meet the physician's goals and maximize the patient's comfort. We discuss the role of sedation of the ventilated patient and describe how to respond to "crises" on the ventilator. This chapter concludes with a brief review of novel modes of ventilation, such as high-frequency ventilation, followed by a summary of preventive measures appropriate to all ventilated patients.

General Preventive Measures

Mechanically ventilated patients are at risk of numerous complications related to the presence of the endotracheal tube, most notably ventilator-associated pneumonia (VAP), and complications of the sedatives and paralytics that are often given. Effective preventive measures are more fully discussed in Chaps. 4, 10, and 14, but are briefly summarized here.

Noninvasive ventilation should be used in appropriate candidates because this decreases the risk of VAP in COPD patients and perhaps those in an immunocompromised state.[2,3] For intubated patients, the head of the bed should be elevated to 30 to 45 degrees during enteral feeding, a simple but effective step for decreasing the risk of VAP.[4] Ventilator tubing should be changed only when the tubing is visibly soiled or malfunctioning, rather than on a time-based schedule.[5] Heat and moisture exchangers should not be changed more than every 48 hours. Sedative use should be limited and patients should be allowed to wake up daily, as discussed below and in Chap. 14. Prophylaxis against venous thromboembolism is indicated in most patients. There is no consensus regarding the effectiveness of selective decontamination of the digestive tract, the use of lateral rotation therapy, or postpyloric placement of feeding tubes, so these measures should not be routinely applied.

Modes of Mechanical Ventilation

Technologic innovations have provided a plethora of different modes by which a patient can be mechanically ventilated. Various modes have been developed with the hope of improving gas exchange, patient comfort, or speed of return to spontaneous ventilation. Aside from minor subtleties, nearly all modes allow full rest of the patient, on the one hand, or substantial exercise, on the other. Thus, in the great majority of patients, choice of mode is merely a matter of patient or physician preference. Noninvasive ventilation should be considered before intubation and ventilation in many patients who are hemodynamically stable and do not require an artificial airway, especially those with acute-on-chronic respiratory failure, postoperative respiratory failure, and cardiogenic pulmonary edema. Management of the patient ventilated noninvasively is discussed thoroughly in Chap. 33.

PRESSURE-PRESET VERSUS VOLUME-PRESET MODES OF VENTILATION

The terminology describing modes of ventilation can be very confusing and may vary from one manufacturer to another. In this chapter, we refer to volume-preset modes as those in which the physician sets a desired tidal volume (V_T) that the ventilator delivers, using whatever pressure required, and pressure-preset modes, in which the physician sets a desired pressure that the ventilator maintains, delivering a volume that depends on the settings, respiratory mechanics, and patient effort. These two fundamental types of mode are compared in Table 36-1. Some modern modes (dual-control modes, see below) attempt to blend pressure and volume presets.

Historically, most adult patients have been ventilated using volume-preset modes (ACV and synchronized intermittent mandatory ventilation [SIMV]), but pressure-preset modes have several theoretical advantages. Few studies have compared these modes except with respect to comfort, a measure generally favoring pressure-preset modes.[6,7] The only mode of ventilation shown to affect mortality rate was the application of ACV to patients with acute lung injury and ARDS when physiologic V_T is used (6 mL/kg ideal body weight [IBW] compared with 12 mL/kg), but pressure-preset modes were not employed in that trial.[8]

The differences between volume-preset and pressure-preset modes are fewer than is often appreciated, because volume and pressure are related through the mechanical properties of the patient's respiratory system, most notably the respiratory system compliance (C_{rs}). For example, a passive patient with a static C_{rs} of 50 mL/cm H_2O ventilated on ACV at a V_T of 500 mL with no positive end-expiratory pressure will have a plateau airway pressure (Pplat; see Chap. 32) of about 10 cm H_2O, whereas the same patient ventilated on PCV at 10 cm H_2O can be expected to have a V_T close to 500 mL. The difference to the patient between these modes may be quite trivial, often amounting to small differences in inspiratory flow profile. Thus, although the physician's comfort level with volume-preset and pressure-preset

TABLE 36-1 Volume-Preset and Pressure-Preset Modes

	Volume-Preset Modes	Pressure-Preset Modes
Examples	ACV, SIMV	PSV, PCV
Set (independent) parameter	Volume	Pressure
Dependent parameter	Pressure	Volume
Potential advantages	1. Greater control over ventilation	1. Greater patient comfort
	2. Evidence-based benefit in ALI, ARDS	2. Greater protection against VILI
	3. Easier to measure mechanical properties of the respiratory system	3. PSV facilitates weaning compared with SIMV
		4. More effective support for some patients

ABBREVIATIONS: ACV, volume assist-control; ALI, acute lung injury; ARDS, acute respiratory distress syndrome; PCV, pressure control ventilation; PSV, pressure support ventilation; SIMV, synchronized intermittent mandatory ventilation; VILI, ventilator-induced lung injury.

modes may be very different, the modes can be similar because they are tied to each other through the patient's Crs.

CONVENTIONAL MODES OF VENTILATION

In the following descriptions, each mode is first illustrated for a passive patient, such as after muscle paralysis, and then for the more common situation in which the patient plays an active role in ventilation. On some ventilators, V_T can be selected by the physician or respiratory therapist; on others, minute ventilation and respiratory rates (f) are chosen, secondarily determining the V_T. Similarly, on some machines, an inspiratory flow rate ($\dot{V}$) is selected, whereas on others $\dot{V}$ depends on the ratio of inspiratory time to total respiratory cycle time (T_I/T_T) and f, on an inspiratory-expiratory (I:E) ratio and f, or on rise time and other parameters.

PRESSURE-PRESET MODES

In pressure-preset modes, a fixed inspiratory pressure (P_I) is applied to the patient, whatever the resulting V_T. Depending on the particular ventilator, the physician may have to specify the actual level of P_I or the increment in pressure over the expiratory pressure (PEEP). Ventilators designed primarily for noninvasive ventilation often require setting P_I and PEEP independently, whereas most ICU ventilators require setting the PEEP and an inspiratory pressure increment. For example, the following settings are identical: $P_I = 20$ cm H_2O and PEEP = 5 cm H_2O (noninvasive ventilator) versus pressure increment (e.g., "pressure-support" or "pressure-control") = 15 cm H_2O and PEEP = 5 cm H_2O. In this chapter, we specify inspiratory (P_I) and expiratory (PEEP) pressures to avoid confusion.

In pressure-preset modes, the V_T is predictable (for the passive patient) when the Crs is known:

$$V_T = (P_I - PEEP) \times Crs$$

assuming time for equilibration between P_I and alveolar pressure (P_A) and the absence of autoPEEP (these assumptions are often not true in patients in the ICU: see below).

Compared with volume-preset modes, a potential advantage of pressure-preset ventilation is greater physician control over the peak airway pressure (Ppk; because Ppk = P_I) and

the peak P_A, which could lessen the incidence of ventilator-induced lung injury (see Chap. 37). However, this same reduction in volutrauma risk should be attainable during volume-preset ventilation if a V_T appropriate to the lung derangement is chosen, as has been shown in patients with acute lung injury and ARDS.[8] Nevertheless, pressure-preset modes make such a lung protection strategy easier to carry out by obviating repeated determinations of Pplat and periodic adjustment of V_T.

Pressure-preset modes also allow the patient greater control over inspiratory flow rate and therefore potentially increased comfort. A disadvantage of pressure-preset modes is that changes in respiratory system mechanics (e.g., increased airflow resistance or lung stiffness) or patient effort may decrease the minute ventilation, necessitating alarms for adequate ventilation. Further, the mechanics cannot be determined readily and partitioned as described in Chap. 32 without switching modes or inserting an esophageal balloon.

Pressure-Control Ventilation

In the passive patient, ventilation is determined by f, the inspiratory pressure increment (P_I − PEEP), the I:E, and Crs. In patients without severe obstruction given a sufficiently long T_I, there is equilibration between the ventilator-determined P_I and P_A, so that inspiratory flow ceases (Fig. 36-1A). In this situation, V_T is highly predictable, based on $P_I (= P_A)$ and the mechanical properties of the respiratory system (Crs). In the presence of severe obstruction or if T_I is too short to allow equilibration between the ventilator and alveoli, V_T will decrease below the value predicted based on P_I and Crs (see Fig. 36-1A). One of the advantages of PCV is that it may facilitate ventilation with a lung protective strategy. For example, alveolar overdistention can be prevented by ensuring that P_A never exceeds some threshold value (this is often taken to be 30 cm H_2O, but a truly safe level is unknown) by simply setting P_I (alternatively, PEEP + PSV) to the desired upper limit. During PCV, T_I and f are set by the physician and may not approximate the patient's desired T_I and f.

When the patient is active, the V_T reflects patient effort, and the patient may trigger additional breaths. When the patient makes inspiratory efforts synchronized with machine inspiration, the V_T is generally greater than that predicted from the Crs and P_I. However, dyssynchrony or expiratory

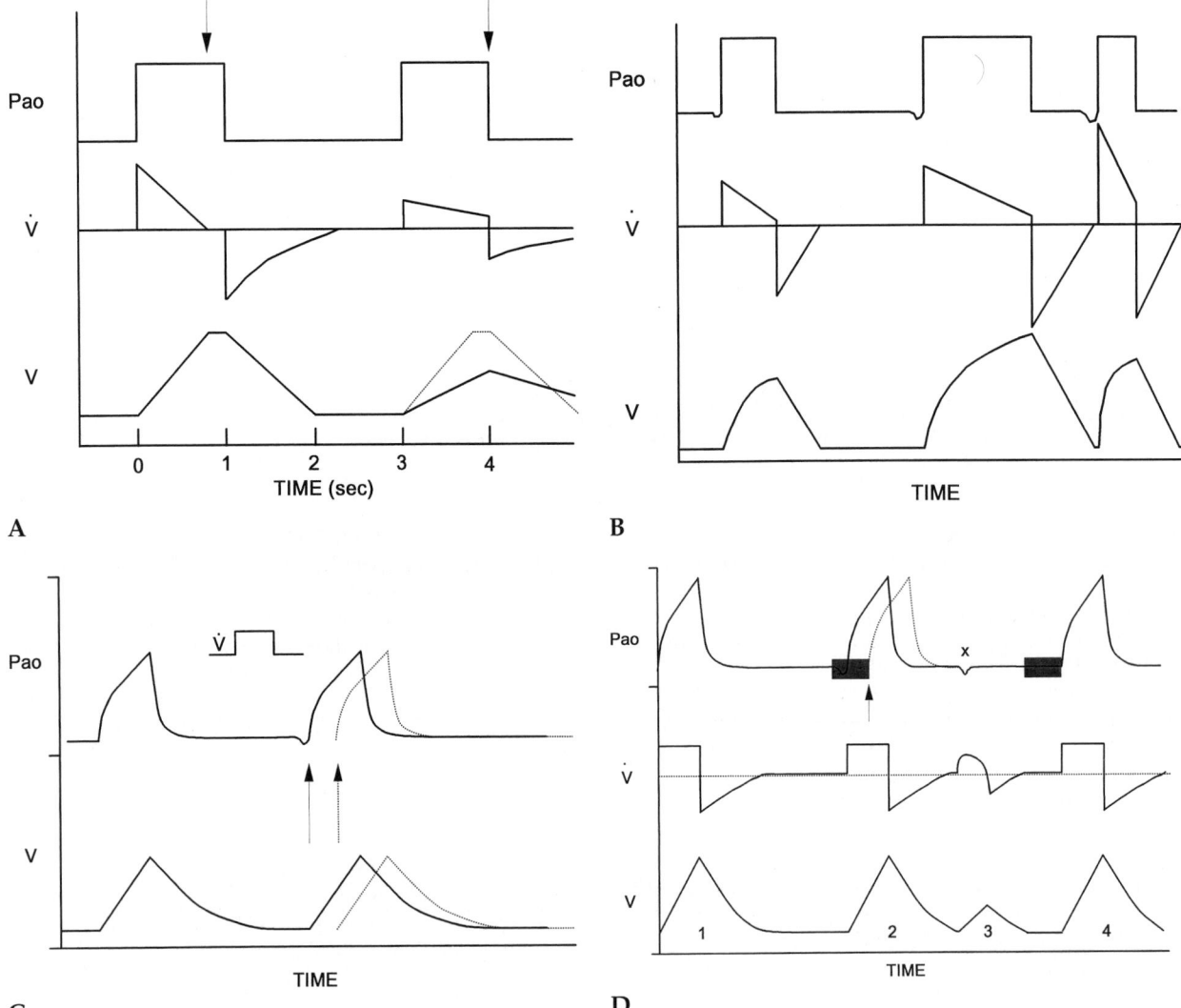

FIGURE 36-1 *A.* Pressure-control ventilation of a muscle-relaxed patient showing the effects of changed inspiratory resistance. The *left-hand panel* shows a pressure-control breath with normal resistance, during which inspiratory pressure (PI) equilibrates with alveolar pressure (PA) before the inspiratory cycle is terminated (*left arrow*), flow ceases, and tidal volume (VT) can be predicted from the PI and Cst (VT = Cst × PI− positive end-expiratory pressure [PEEP]). In the *right-hand panel*, inspiratory resistance is elevated. At the same PI, inspiratory flow is reduced, the VT is not reached until the inspiratory phase is terminated (*right arrow*), and the VT (*solid line*) falls below that predicted by Cst and PI minus PEEP (*dotted line*). *B.* Pressure-support ventilation. When a breath is triggered pressure-airway opening (Pao) rises to the set level (PI) with flow and VT depending on the PI minus PEEP, respiratory system mechanics, and patient effort. The first breath shown represents a patient who triggers the ventilator and then remains fully passive (a hypothetical circumstance used here for contrast with the usual patient efforts shown in the next two breaths). As long as there is no significant airflow obstruction, VT nearly reaches the volume that would be predicted based on the compliance of the respiratory system (Crs; VT = Crs × PI − PEEP). During the middle breath shown, the patient makes a moderate but prolonged inspiratory effort. The Pao remains at the set inspiratory level as long as patient effort maintains flow, and a much longer inspiratory time (TI) and VT result. In the final breath, a more powerful but briefer inspiratory effort is made, shortening the TI but generating a larger Vt than during the passive breath. *C.* Pao and lung volume (V) during assist-control ventilation of a patient who is periodically triggering the ventilator. The second breath was set to be delivered at the time marked by the *second arrow;* instead, the patient lowers the Pao, triggering the ventilator at the time marked by the *first arrow*, thereby increasing the respiratory rate above the default value, decreasing the expiratory time (TE), and increasing the inspiratory-expiratory (I:E) ratio. *D.* Pao, flow (V̇), and V during synchronized intermittent mandatory ventilation. Breath 1 (a mandatory breath) is not triggered by the patient, who remains fully passive. V and V̇ are determined by the ventilator, whereas the Pao reflects the passive mechanical characteristics of the respiratory system. The *shaded rectangle* near the second breath denotes the interval during which the ventilator is programmed to synchronize with the patient's inspiratory effort by delivering the mandatory breath slightly ahead of schedule. At the end of this time interval (*arrow*), a mandatory breath would have been delivered (*dotted tracing*) if the patient had not triggered the ventilator. The synchronized breath (breath 2) has the same volume and flow as a mandatory breath. The Pao may not be the same as during a passive breath because of continued patient effort throughout inspiration. Breath 3 is initiated before the synchronization interval at *x* and is therefore not assisted. Flow and VT are totally determined by the patient's effort and mechanics. These breaths are typically shorter and smaller (as indicated) than the mandatory breaths. When the patient fails to trigger another breath within the next synchronization window, another mandatory breath (breath 4) is delivered.

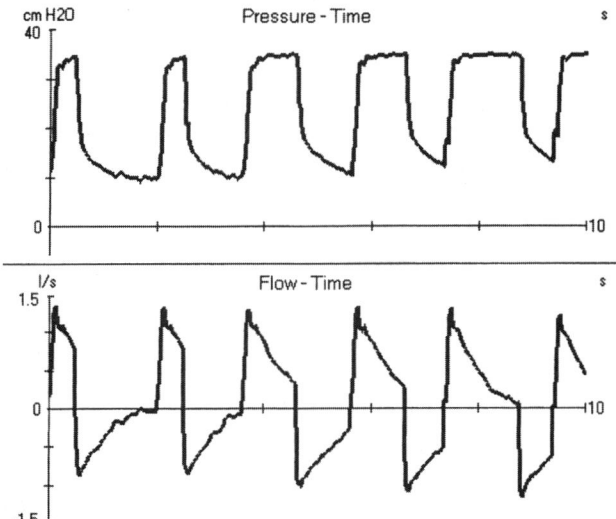

FIGURE 36-2 The effect of changing inspiratory time (TI) on ventilation in the passive patient during pressure-control ventilation. As TI is raised from an initial value of 0.5 second (first two breaths) to 1.0 second (middle breaths) to 1.5 seconds (last breaths), tidal volume increases; expiratory time decreases so much that no positive end-expiratory pressure is created (once TI reaches 1.0 second) and end-inspiratory alveolar pressure increases (signaled by the lower flow at end inspiration, essentially 0 at a TI of 1.5 seconds).

TABLE 36-2A Reducing the Work of Breathing of the Ventilated Patient

Identify source of pain, anxiety, discomfort
Treat the derangement in gas exchange or respiratory mechanics
Decrease CO_2 production
Reassurance ("vocal anesthesia")
Increase tidal volume
Increase respiratory rate
Increase inspiratory flow rate
Use flow triggering
Try pressure support ventilation
Sedation
Therapeutic paralysis

TABLE 36-2B Increasing the Work of Breathing of the Ventilated Patient

T-piece or trach collar trials
CPAP trials
Lower the level of pressure-support ventilation
Change the sensitivity on ACV, PSV, or IMV
Decrease the rate of IMV

ABBREVIATIONS: ACV, assist-control ventilation; CPAP, continuous positive airway pressure; IMV, intermittent mandatory ventilation; PSV, pressure-support mode.

effort during machine inspiration may decrease VT below the value expected. Special care must be taken to adjust TI to the individual patient (Fig. 36-2); otherwise, heavy sedation is typically needed. When unphysiologic settings are intentionally chosen, as when the physician desires an unusually long TI (TI longer than TE results in inverse ratio ventilation [IRV], described later), deep sedation or therapeutic paralysis is often given.

Pressure-Support Ventilation

The patient must trigger the ventilator to activate this mode, so PSV is not applied to passive patients. Ventilation is determined by PI − PEEP, patient-determined f, patient effort, and the patient's mechanics. Once a breath is triggered, the ventilator attempts to maintain PI by using whatever flow is necessary. Eventually, flow begins to decrease due to cessation of the patient's inspiratory effort or to increasing elastic recoil of the respiratory system as lung volume rises. The ventilator maintains PI until inspiratory flow decreases an arbitrary amount (e.g., to 20% of initial flow) or below an absolute flow rate (depending on the ventilator).

It is useful to first consider what happens if the patient were to trigger the ventilator and then remain passive (an artificial situation). VT would be determined by PI and the (largely static) mechanical properties of the respiratory system, as during PCV (see Fig. 36-1B). More typically, the patient makes an effort throughout inspirations, in which case VT is determined in part by the degree of effort (see Fig. 36-1B). At a constant minute ventilation, the patient's work of breathing can be increased by decreasing PI or making the trigger less sensitive (Table 36-2) and can increase inadvertently if respiratory system mechanics change despite no change in ventilator settings. Respiratory system mechanical parame-

ters cannot be determined readily on this mode because the ventilator and patient contributions to VT and V̇ are not distinguishable from analysis of the ventilator airway opening pressure (Pao); accordingly, the important measurements of Pplat, Ppk minus Pplat, and autoPEEP are measured during a brief daily switch from PSV to ACV at the corresponding values of VT, V̇, and I:E observed during PSV.

A potential advantage of PSV is improved patient comfort.[6,7] An important caution about PSV is that it can account for a large fraction of total minute ventilation, even when set at rather low levels, as in patients with normal respiratory system mechanics. For example, in a patient with myasthenia gravis, 10 cm H_2O of PSV may represent full mechanical ventilation. A "successful" spontaneous breathing trial with these settings should not be used to judge the patient's readiness for extubation.

VOLUME-PRESET MODES

During volume-preset ventilation, a volume is delivered to the patient at the required pressure (within the limits of the high pressure alarm). The physician generally also sets a V̇ (indirectly determining the TI) and f. In volume-preset modes, the Pplat is predictable (in a passive patient) when the Crs is known:

$$Pplat = VT/Crs + PEEP$$

where PEEP includes autoPEEP.

Compared with pressure-preset modes, a potential advantage of volume-preset ventilation is greater control over the total minute ventilation because VT does not depend on potentially changing patient effort or respiratory system mechanical properties. Another advantage of volume-preset modes was reported by ARDS Network Tidal Volume Trial, which demonstrated an advantage with respect to mortality rate when using ACV. Moreover, it is easy to characterize the respiratory system mechanics by measuring Ppk and Pplat, thereby simplifying follow-up of the patient's progress or response to therapies.

Assist Control Ventilation

The set parameters of the assist-control mode are the $\dot{V}$, f, and V_T (on some ventilators, one must set the total minute ventilation and rate, thereby determining V_T and indirectly determining $\dot{V}$). In the passive patient, the ventilator delivers f (f = 60 seconds/[$T_I + T_E$]) equal breaths per minute, and V_T or $\dot{V}$ setting determine the T_I, T_E, and the I:E. Pplat is related to the V_T and the Crs, whereas Ppk minus Pplat includes contributions from $\dot{V}$ and inspiratory resistance (see Fig. 36-1C).

The active patient can trigger extra breaths by exerting an inspiratory effort exceeding the preset trigger sensitivity at the set V_T and $\dot{V}$ and thereby change T_I, T_E, and I:E and (potentially) create or increase autoPEEP. Typically, each patient will display a preferred rate for a given V_T and will trigger all breaths when the controlled ventilator frequency is set a few breaths per minute slower than the patient's rate; in this way, the control rate serves as an adequate support should the patient stop initiating breaths. When high inspiratory effort continues during the ventilator-delivered breath, the patient may trigger a second, superimposed ("stacked") breath (and, rarely, a third breath). The total V_T of this breath is determined by the point in the first breath at which the second was triggered, so the total V_T can range from the set V_T to twice the V_T.

Typically, the patient performs inspiratory work during an assist-control breath.[1,9] This may not be obvious despite careful examination of the patient unless measures of intrathoracic pressure (esophageal pressure and central venous pressure) are available, or the inspiratory pressure waveform is examined carefully (Chap 32). Effort at the end of the breath will affect the Ppk and Pplat, making determination of respiratory system mechanics unreliable. When the patient is assisting every breath, the work of breathing can be increased by increasing the magnitude of the trigger or by lowering V_T (which increases the rate of assisting; see Table 36-2). Decreasing f at the same V_T generally has no effect on the work of breathing (in contrast to SIMV, discussed below) when the patient is initiating all breaths.

Synchronized Intermittent Mandatory Ventilation

In the passive patient, intermittent mandatory ventilation (IMV) cannot be distinguished from controlled ventilation in the ACV mode. Ventilation is determined by the mandatory f, V_T, and $\dot{V}$ values. However, if the patient is not truly passive, he or she may perform respiratory work during the mandatory breaths. More to the point of the SIMV mode, the patient can trigger additional breaths by decreasing Pao below the trigger threshold (see Fig. 36-1D). If this triggering effort comes in a brief, defined interval before the next mandatory breath is due, the ventilator will deliver the mandatory breath ahead of schedule to synchronize (SIMV) with the patient's inspiratory effort. If a breath is initiated outside the synchronization window, V_T, $\dot{V}$, and I:E are determined by patient effort and respiratory system mechanics (see Fig. 36-1D), not by ventilator settings. The spontaneous breaths tend to be of small volume, as depicted in Fig. 36-1D, and are highly variable from breath to breath. The SIMV mode is often used to gradually augment the patient's work of breathing by lowering the mandatory breath f (or V_T), thereby driving the patient to breathe more rapidly to maintain adequate ventilation, but this approach appears to prolong "weaning"[10,11] (see Table 36-2). Although this mode continues to be used widely, there is little rationale for it and SIMV is falling out of favor.

MIXED MODES

Some ventilators allow combinations of modes, most commonly SIMV plus PSV. There is little reason to use such a hybrid mode, although some physicians use the SIMV mode as a means to add sighs to PSV, an option not otherwise generally available. Because SIMV plus PSV guarantees some backup minute ventilation (which PSV does not), this mode combination may have value in occasional patients at high risk for abrupt deterioration in central drive.

DUAL-CONTROL MODES

The sophisticated microprocessors included with modern ventilators allow remarkably complex modes of ventilation. These modes typically try to meld the best features of volume- and pressure-preset modes. Some cause a switch of modes between breaths (e.g., pressure-regulated volume control [PRVC] and volume support) or within a breath (e.g., volume-assured pressure support). In general, these modes are complex, and their effects may vary greatly depending on the details of the patient's effort. None has been shown to be safer or more useful than more conventional modes. The greatest problem with such newer modes is that they are very complex, the algorithm describing their function is not usually understood by practitioners, and they change during a breath or from breath to breath, depending on patient effort, sometimes in ways that can provoke unanticipated effects.

Pressure-Regulated Volume Control

This is a pressure-preset mode with a set T_I (i.e., it is time cycled) in which the ventilator compares the V_T with a physician-set V_T and automatically and gradually adjusts P_I of subsequent breaths to deliver the desired V_T. A downside of PRVC is that, as patient effort increases, the ventilator decreases support. Proponents argue that this mode provides the benefits of pressure-preset modes and simultaneously guarantees V_T; whether this guarantee makes the mode better or worse for the patient is debated.

Volume Support

Volume support is a pressure-preset mode in which P_I is automatically changed to gradually bring V_T in line with the desired V_T over several breaths, differing from PRVC in that T_I is not set but rather depends on patient effort as in PSV. It is unknown whether this mode speeds or impedes weaning.

Volume-Assured Pressure Support

This mode begins as PSV, but, if a desired V_T is not met, the ventilator switches to ACV within the same breath to guarantee V_T. As with many dual-control modes, the physician delegates decision making to the ventilator. Complex adjustments and their potentially detrimental effects on the patient may come into play at any time of day or night, depending on changes in the mechanical properties of the respiratory system or changes in the patient's level of consciousness, comfort, or neuromuscular competence.

CONTINUOUS POSITIVE AIRWAY PRESSURE

Continuous positive airway pressure (CPAP) is not a mode of ventilation but a means of increasing functional residual capacity and allowing the patient to breathe spontaneously. This approach is frequently used when assessing the patient's ability to breathe without ventilatory assistance. Advantages of CPAP over T-piece breathing is that oxygenation may be increased, ventilator alarms (e.g., low minute ventilation and apnea) remain in place, the patient's spontaneous V_T and rate can be easily read from the ventilator panel, and the work of breathing is decreased if autoPEEP is present.[12,13] Disadvantages include the loss of mobility and independence that comes with being tethered to the ventilator and the sometimes increased work of breathing attributed to triggering ventilator valves and driving flow through excess tubing and flow meters. A potentially misleading feature of some ventilators is that the display may show the mode as "CPAP" when it is "PSV." This could lead health care providers to draw erroneous conclusions about the patient's ability to sustain spontaneous ventilation.

EFFECT OF INSPIRATORY FLOW PROFILE

With most ventilators, the physician can choose one of several inspiratory waveforms, most commonly square or decelerating. The rationale for the use of decelerating flow is the possible improvement in the distribution of ventilation and minimization of Ppk. This rationale works because maximal flow (and therefore flow-related pressure) occurs early in the breath when lung volume (and elastic recoil pressure) is minimal; in addition, near the end of the breath, lung volume is maximal but flow is minimal. However, an inescapable consequence of the overall lower $\dot{V}$ (assuming equal peak inspiratory $\dot{V}$ and a passive patient) is a shorter T_E. Thus, in patients who have obstruction or high minute ventilations (those in whom a decelerating flow pattern will most decrease Ppk), autoPEEP is likely to be caused or increased (Fig. 36-3). Although the relative contributions of Ppk and PEEP (or autoPEEP) to barotrauma risk are not clearly defined, it seems likely that, in most patients, barotrauma risk will be worsened rather than improved with a decelerating profile. A sine waveform similarly lowers Ppk and shortens T_E.

When a square waveform is used, the flow-related pressure near end inspiration is nearly the same as at the beginning of the breath and adds to the elastic recoil pressure to produce a higher Ppk than during sine wave or decelerating flow. However, this higher Ppk is largely borne by the robust proximal airways and not by the alveoli; by contrast, greater autoPEEP means greater P_A and risk of alveolar disruption. Because the peak pressure is visibly decreased by decelerating and sine wave profiles and increased autoPEEP is typically occult, such flow patterns can be insidiously threatening. Accordingly, we believe that there is little reason to use anything other than the conventional square wave inspiratory flow profile, except when IRV is desired (see below). When a decelerating flow profile is used, autoPEEP should be measured diligently and the hidden complexities of this phenomenon made clear to all caring for the patient.

A peak $\dot{V}$ of 1 L/s (60 L/min) is a common initial setting, but this may require adjustment upward (for patient comfort or to lengthen T_E) or downward (to create IRV). Increased

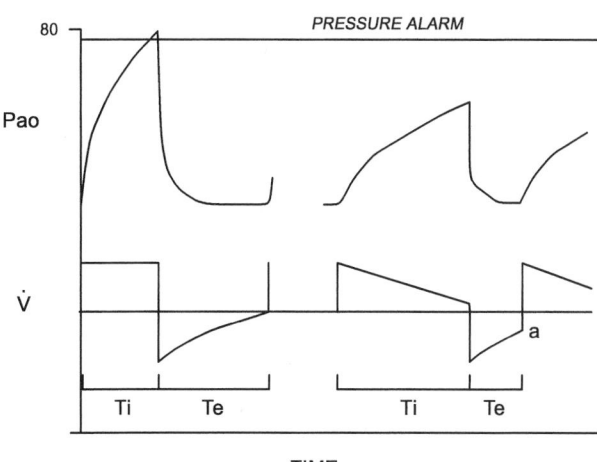

FIGURE 36-3 Effect of flow profile on pressure-airway opening (Pao) and inspiratory-expiratory (I:E) ratio in a patient with status asthmaticus during assist-control or mandatory intermittent mandatory ventilation breaths. The *left-hand tracings* show the typical high peak airway pressure (Ppk) and slow expiratory flow in a patient with severe obstruction ventilated with a square wave inspiratory flow profile. Expiratory flow just reaches zero before the next breath is delivered. The Ppk can be dramatically reduced by changing to a decelerating flow profile (*right-hand tracing*) because much of the high Pao is related to flow. However, to deliver the same tidal volume at the now lower mean inspiratory flow, the inspiratory time (T_I) must increase. At the same respiratory rate, the expiratory time (T_E) decreasing, thereby increasing the I:E ratio. With the now shortened T_E, there is insufficient time for the respiratory system to reach functional residual capacity, expiratory flow is still detected at the onset of inspiratory flow (*a*), and no positive end-eexpiratory pressure (auotPEEP) is present. Therefore, the lower (but not "improved") Pao comes at the cost of new (or higher) autoPEEP and a higher mean alveolar pressure. $\dot{V}$, flow.

$\dot{V}$ may have a stimulatory effect on respiratory rate in active patients,[14] paradoxically shortening T_E, although the impact on respiratory rate and work of breathing after the first few seconds has not been studied. Decreasing the peak $\dot{V}$ will decrease Ppk when there is significant resistance to airflow but, in this setting, will usually worsen autoPEEP, as described above. One often overlooked adverse consequence of setting peak $\dot{V}$ at less than the patient wishes is that the patient will actively inspire against the ventilator, thereby increasing the respiratory work. This occurs frequently when patients having low ventilatory requirements are placed on volume-preset ventilators on which $\dot{V}$ cannot be set directly but rather is determined by V_T and T_I (e.g., the Siemens 900C).

TRIGGERED SENSITIVITY

In the ACV, SIMV, and PSV modes, the patient must decrease the Pao below a preset threshold to "trigger" the ventilator. In most situations this is straightforward because a more negative sensitivity increases the effort demanded of the patient. This can be used intentionally to increase the work of breathing when the goal is to strengthen the inspiratory muscles. In contrast, when autoPEEP is present, the patient must decrease P_A by the autoPEEP amount to have any effect on Pao and then by the trigger amount to initiate a breath. This can dramatically increase the required

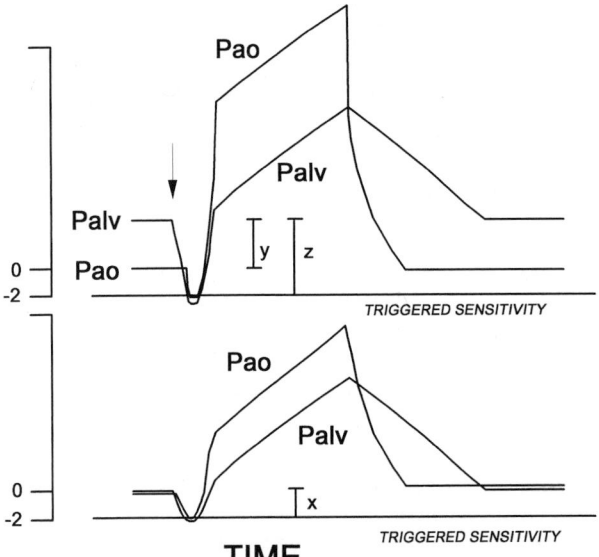

FIGURE 36-4 Effect of occult positive end-expiratory pressure (autoPEEP) on triggering. The *lower tracings* of pressure-airway opening (Pao) and alveolar pressure (PA) represent a patient who is triggering volume-preset ventilator breaths and who does not have autoPEEP. The *upper tracing* shows a patient similarly ventilated and with the same triggered sensitivity (-2 cm H_2O) but who has 4 cm H_2O of autoPEEP. The patient without autoPEEP must decrease PA by x (~2 cm H_2O) to lower the Pao by the same amount, thereby triggering a breath. In contrast, the patient with autoPEEP must lower the PA by y (~4 cm H_2O) before there is any impact on Pao and then by another 2 cm H_2O to trigger the ventilator. In the patient with autoPEEP, the total reduction in PA (z) required to trigger the ventilator rises as autoPEEP rises and is occult. In the extreme, autoPEEP may be so elevated that a weak patient is unable to trigger the ventilator despite great effort.

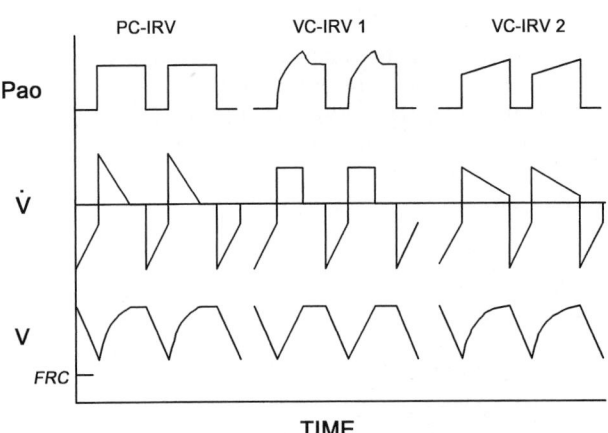

FIGURE 36-5 Inverse ratio ventilation (IRV). The *first panel* shows pressure-controlled IRV (PC-IRV) in which pressure-airway opening (Pao) during inspiration is held constant and expiration time (TE) is shortened to invert the inspiratory-expiratory (I:E) ratio. Flow and tidal volume (VT) can be predicted from the passive elastic properties of the respiratory system (assuming inspiration time [TI] is sufficiently long for equilibration of inspiration pressure [PI] and alveolar pressure [PA]). The very short TE is insufficient for lung volume (V) to return to functional residual capacity (FRC), and there is persistent expiratory flow at end expiration (i.e., no positive end-expiratory pressure [autoPEEP] is present). The *second panel* shows volume-controlled IRV (VC-IRV) with a square wave flow pattern in which an end-inspiratory pause is used to invert the I:E ratio. Peak pressure is higher than during equivalent PC-IRV because flow remains high at end inspiration (when elastic recoil is maximal). AutoPEEP is also present. In the *third panel*, IRV is created by using a decelerating flow profile. The peak airway pressure (Ppk) is midway in between the other two modes because end-inspiratory flow is present but small. The short TE does not allow expiration to FRC, causing autoPEEP. In all three cases, the mean V and, hence, mean PA would be increased compared with ventilator modes having normal I:E ratios. V̇, flow.

effort for breath initiation (Fig. 36-4). In several instances, we have seen physicians suspect machine malfunction and even change the ventilator when they are confronted with an obviously struggling patient seemingly unable to get a breath despite a "minimal" trigger threshold. The solution for this problem is to eliminate the cause for autoPEEP, sedate the patient, or use externally applied PEEP to counterbalance the autoPEEP (which only occasionally increases autoPEEP, risking barotrauma and hypotension)[15–17] (see Chap. 39).

Flow-triggering systems ("flow-by") have been used to further decrease the work of triggering the ventilator. In contrast to the usual approach, in which the patient must open a demand valve to receive ventilatory assistance, continuous-flow systems maintain a continuous high flow and then augment flow when the patient initiates a breath. These systems can decrease the work of breathing below that encountered when using conventional demand valves,[18,19] in part by shortening the time to pressurization of the inspiratory circuit,[20] but they do not solve the problem of triggering when autoPEEP is present.

UNCONVENTIONAL VENTILATION MODES

INVERSE RATIO VENTILATION
IRV is defined as a mode in which the I:E is greater than 1. Like PEEP, it was introduced as an empirical variation to salvage

lung oxygen exchange in patients with severe acute hypoxemic respiratory failure. There are two general ways to apply IRV: pressure-controlled IRV (PC-IRV), in which a preset airway pressure is delivered for a fixed period at an I:E greater than 1, or volume-controlled IRV (VC-IRV), in which a VT is delivered at a slow (or decelerating) V̇ (or an end-inspiratory pause is inserted) to yield an I:E greater than 1[21] (Fig. 36-5). For PC-IRV, the physician must specify the inspiratory airway pressure, f, and I:E, and VT and flow profile are determined by respiratory system impedance as discussed for PCV (see Fig. 36-5). Commonly, the initial PI is 20 to 40 cm H_2O (or 10 to 30 cm H_2O above the PEEP), f is 20/min, and the I:E is 2:1 to 4:1. For VC-IRV, the operator selects a VT, f, V̇ (typically a low value), flow profile, and, possibly, an end-inspiratory pause (see Fig. 36-5). The chosen values result in an I:E greater than 1:1 and as high as 5:1.

Compared with conventional modes of ventilation, lung oxygen exchange is often improved on IRV owing to increased mean PA and volume consequent to the longer time above functional residual capacity (FRC)[22,23] or owing to creation of autoPEEP.[24,25] Conceivably, this decreases shunt as PEEP does by redistributing alveolar edema into the pulmonary interstitium.[26] It is remotely possible that IRV causes better ventilation of lung units with long time constants, but these are so short in normal lungs[27] (and shorter in ARDS) that such redistribution is unlikely to occur with slower flow and could not reduce shunt even if it did. Because autoPEEP is a common consequence of IRV, serial determination of its magnitude is essential for safe use of this mode. PC-IRV and VC-IRV generally require heavy sedation with or without muscle paralysis.

AIRWAY PRESSURE-RELEASE VENTILATION

Airway pressure-release ventilation (APRV) consists of CPAP that is intermittently released to allow a brief expiratory interval.[28] Conceptually, this mode is pressure-controlled IRV, during which the patient is allowed to initiate spontaneous breaths. It has been applied to patients with acute lung injury[29,30] and has proved effective in maintaining oxygenation and assisting ventilation. A potential advantage of APRV is that mean P_A is lower than it would be during positive-pressure ventilation from the same amount of CPAP, possibly decreasing the risks of barotrauma and hemodynamic compromise. It has been claimed that the most important clinical advantage of APRV is that, compared with conventional ventilation, peak airway pressure can be decreased dramatically.[29] In these studies, however, conventional positive-pressure ventilation was delivered by using excessive V_T (10 to 15 mL/kg).[29,30] Disadvantages of APRV include hypoxemia due to the interruption of CPAP, atelectasis,[30] and patient discomfort that sometimes mandates sedation. Another concern relates to the fact that, because the lung cycles tidally below rather than above the volume determined by CPAP, this mode probably encourages repeated recruitment and de-recruitment of flooded and collapsed alveoli. Although this point is controversial, the weight of evidence suggests that this may amplify ventilator-induced lung injury. Whether this mode provides any benefit over modern low-V_T ventilation remains to be shown.

PROPORTIONAL-ASSIST VENTILATION

Proportional-assist ventilation is intended only for spontaneously breathing patients. The goal of this novel mode is to attempt to normalize the relation between patient effort and the resulting ventilatory consequences.[31,32] The ventilator adjusts P_I in proportion to patient effort throughout any given breath and from breath to breath. This allows the patient to modulate the breathing pattern and total ventilation. This is implemented by monitoring instantaneous $\dot{V}$ and volume (V) of gas from the ventilator to the patient and changing the P_I as follows:

$$P_I = f_1 \times V + f_2 \times \dot{V}$$

where f_1 and f_2 are selectable functions of volume (elastic assist) and flow (resistive assist), respectively, values that can be estimated from the patient's respiratory mechanics. Potential advantages of this method are greater patient comfort, lower P_{pk}, and enhancement of the patient's reflex and behavioral respiratory control mechanisms. In contrast, proportional-assist ventilation can amplify instabilities in the patient's breathing rhythm, as in the common instance of periodic (Cheyne-Stokes) respiration.

HIGH-FREQUENCY VENTILATION

Several modes of ventilation have in common the use of V_T smaller than the dead space volume.[33] Gas exchange does not occur through convection as during conventional ventilation but through bulk flow, Taylor diffusion, molecular diffusion, non-convective mixing, and possibly other mechanisms. These modes include high-frequency oscillatory ventilation and high-frequency jet ventilation. Theoretical benefits of high-frequency ventilation (HFV) include lower risk of barotrauma due to smaller tidal excursions, improved gas exchange through a more uniform distribution of ventilation, and improved healing of bronchopleural fistulas.[34] Animal studies have suggested that HFV may be superior to lung protective ACV with respect to ventilator-induced lung injury, hemodynamic compromise, and inflammation.[35,36] Delivered V_T is affected mostly by rate but also by I:E and frequency amplitude. In an animal model of severe lung injury, settings of 4 Hz, an I:E of 1:1, and a pressure amplitude of 60 cm H_2O, the V_T was 4.4 mL/kg, a value approaching conventional V_T values.[37] A substantial risk is that dynamic hyperinflation is the rule, and P_A is greatly underestimated by monitoring P_{ao}.[38] A controlled trial of HFV found no clinically relevant benefit, but the approach was shown to be safe, at least in the context of a clinical trial.[39] Nevertheless, HFV is the natural extension of reducing the V_T as a means to prevent volutrauma, and there is renewed interest in this old technique.[39a]

Management of the Patient

INITIAL VENTILATOR SETTINGS

Initial ventilator settings depend on the goals of ventilation (e.g., full respiratory muscle rest versus partial exercise), the patient's respiratory system mechanics, and minute ventilation requirements. Although each critically ill patient presents myriad challenges, it is possible to identify four subsets of ventilated patients: the patient with normal lung mechanics and gas exchange, the patient with predominant airflow obstruction, the patient with acute hypoxemic respiratory failure, and the patient with restrictive lung or chest wall disease. Specific recommendations regarding ventilator settings are detailed more fully in Chaps. 38, 39, 40, and 42 but are reviewed here briefly, in addition to guidelines for ventilating patients with normal respiratory system mechanics.

In all patients, the initial $F_{I_{O_2}}$ should usually be 0.5 to 1.0 to ensure adequate oxygenation, although usually it can be decreased within minutes when guided by pulse oximetry and, in the appropriate setting, applying PEEP. In the first minutes after institution of mechanical ventilation, the physician should remain alert for several common problems, most notably, airway malposition, aspiration, and hypotension. Positive-pressure ventilation may decrease venous return and, hence, cardiac output, especially in patients with a low mean systemic pressure (e.g., hypovolemia, venodilating drugs, decreased sympathetic tone from sedating drugs, or neuromuscular disease) or a very high ventilation-related pleural pressure (e.g., chest wall restriction, large amounts of PEEP, or airway obstruction causing autoPEEP). If hypotension occurs, intravascular volume should be expanded rapidly while steps are taken to decrease the pleural pressure (a smaller V_T and less minute ventilation). Meanwhile, the

F_{IO_2} should be raised to 100%. If these steps do not rapidly restore the circulation, another complicating event (pneumothorax or myocardial ischemia) should be considered while the patient is taken off the ventilator and bagged manually to assess respiratory load and to observe the response of blood pressure to a brief suspension of positive-pressure ventilation.

THE PATIENT WITH NORMAL RESPIRATORY MECHANICS AND GAS EXCHANGE

Patients with normal lung mechanics and gas exchange may require mechanical ventilation because of loss of the central drive to breathe (e.g., drug overdose or structural injury to the brain stem), because of neuromuscular weakness (e.g., high cervical cord injury, acute idiopathic myelitis, or myasthenia gravis), as an adjunctive therapy in the treatment of shock,[40,41] or to achieve hyperventilation (e.g., in the treatment of elevated intracranial pressure after head trauma). After intubation, initial ventilator orders should be an F_{IO_2} of 0.5 to 1.0, a V_T of 8 to 12 mL/kg, a respiratory rate of 8 to 12 breaths/min, and a $\dot{V}$ of 50 to 60 L/min (Table 36-3). Alternatively, if the patient has sufficient drive and is not profoundly weak, PSV can be used. The level of pressure support is adjusted (usually to the range of 10 to 20 cm H_2O above PEEP) to bring the respiratory rate down into the low 20s, usually corresponding to a V_T of about 500 mL. It is important to realize that PSV is mechanically supported but entirely spontaneous, with no machine "backup" unless mixed with a mode such as SIMV. Thus, hypoventilation may occur despite the use of PSV, if there is further deterioration of muscle strength or blunting of drive by disease or drugs. If gas exchange is entirely normal, the F_{IO_2} likely can be decreased further based on pulse oximetry or arterial blood gas determinations. However, because right mainstem intubation, aspiration, and bronchospasm are relatively common complications of intubation, it is wise to initiate ventilation with the F_{IO_2} at 0.5 or higher. Should hyperventilation be desired, the initial respiratory rate should be increased to the range of 16 to 20 breaths/min. The $\dot{V}$ can be increased if the patient complains of air hunger, but 50 to 60 L/min is often sufficient.[1] Even in most tachypneic patients with underlying lung disease and certainly in those individuals with normal lung mechanics, a $\dot{V}$ greater than 60 L/min is rarely necessary or useful.

Soon after the initiation of ventilation, airway pressure and flow waveforms should be inspected for evidence of dyssynchrony between the patient and the ventilator or undesired patient effort (see Chap. 32). If the goal of ventilation is full rest, the patient's drive often can be suppressed by increasing the $\dot{V}$, f, or V_T.[42,43] The latter two changes may induce respiratory alkalemia. If such adjustments do not diminish breathing effort, despite normal blood gases, to an undetectable level, sedation may be necessary. If this does not abolish inspiratory efforts and full rest is essential (as in shock), muscle paralysis can be considered.

Measures to prevent atelectasis should include sighs (6 to 12 per hour at 1.5 to 2 times the V_T) or small amounts of PEEP (5 to 7.5 cm H_2O). This is particularly important in patients with neuromuscular diseases during protracted ventilation because atelectasis is common. In these patients, we use the upper limit of V_T (12 mL/kg). Three-point turning and chest physiotherapy are desirable in all patients unless other conditions preclude their use. Rotating beds may be effective in some patients for preventing atelectasis and pneumonia.[44]

PATIENTS WITH DOMINANT AIRFLOW OBSTRUCTION

Two general types of patients require mechanical ventilation for significant airflow obstruction; those with status asthmaticus (see Chap. 40) and those with exacerbations of chronic airflow obstruction (see Chap. 39). Rare alternative causes are inhalation injury or central airway lesions, such as tumor or foreign body, not bypassed with the endotracheal tube. In isolated upper airway injuries, assessment of the extent of damage is often possible by bronchoscopy shortly before or at the time of intubation. Bronchoscopy should not be performed routinely in patients with asthma.

STATUS ASTHMATICUS

Because the gas exchange abnormalities of airflow obstruction are largely limited to ventilation-perfusion mismatch, an F_{IO_2} of 0.5 suffices in the vast majority of patients.[45] Requirements for a higher F_{IO_2} should prompt a search for an alveolar filling process or for lobar atelectasis. We have had success ventilating these patients with PSV by setting P_I at 25 to 30 cm H_2O. Because these patients are typically anxious, we often give large doses of narcotics to suppress drive, an approach that, when combined with high-level PSV, often leads to an unusual but stable pattern of breathing, with a V_T larger than 900 mL and an f of 3 to 7. This approach appears to minimize autoPEEP by allowing such a long T_E. Alternatively, ventilation can be initiated using the ACV mode with a normal V_T (5 to 7 mL/kg) and respiratory rate of 12 to 15 breaths/min (see Table 36-3). A peak flow of 60 L/min is recommended, and higher flow rates do little to increase

TABLE 36-3 Initial Ventilator Settings

	Mode	F_{IO_2}	PEEP (cm H_2O)	V_T (mL/kg)	RR (min[21])	Flow (L/min)	Sighs
Normal	ACV[a]	0.5	5	8–12	10	60	Yes
Asthma	ACV	0.5	0[b]	5–7	10–18	60	No
ACRF	ACV[a]	0.5	5	5–7	24	60	Yes
AHRF	ACV	1.0	15[c]	4–6, using IBW	24	60	No
Restriction	ACV	0.5	5	5–7	20	60	Yes

[a] PSV is an alternative.

[b] Assumes that the patient is deeply sedated or therapeutically paralyzed.

[c] Adjust promptly based on pulse oximetry; may not be helpful in focal lung lesions; monitor for hypotension.

ABBREVIATIONS: ACV, assist-control ventilation; ACRF, acute-on-chronic respiratory failure ; AHRF, acute hypoxemic respiratory failure; F_{IO_2}, fraction of inspired oxygen; IBW, ideal body weight; PEEP, positive end-expiratory pressure; RR, respiratory rate; V_T, tidal volume.

T_E. For example, if the V_T is 500 mL, the respiratory rate is 15 breaths/min, and the $\dot{V}$ 60 L/min, the T_E is 3.5 seconds. Raising $\dot{V}$ (dramatically) to 120 L/min increases the T_E to only 3.75 seconds, a trivial improvement. In contrast, a small reduction in respiratory rate to 14 breaths/min increases the T_E to 3.8 seconds. This example emphasizes not only the relative lack of benefit of raising the flow rate but also the importance of minimizing minute ventilation when the goal is to reduce autoPEEP. If the patient is triggering the ventilator, it is essential that some PEEP be added to reduce the work of triggering. This does not generally worsen the hyperinflation as long as PEEP is not higher than about 85% of the autoPEEP.[16,46–48] Ventilatory goals are to minimize alveolar overdistention (keep Pplat<30) and to minimize dynamic hyperinflation (keep autoPEEP<10 cm H_2O or end-inspiratory lung volume <20 mL/kg), a strategy that largely prevents barotrauma.[49] Reducing minute ventilation to achieve these goals generally causes the partial pressure of CO_2 to rise above 40 mm Hg, often to 70 mm Hg or higher. Although this requires sedation, such permissive hypercapnia is quite well tolerated except in patients with increased intracranial pressure and perhaps in those with ventricular dysfunction or pulmonary hypertension.

Patients with status asthmaticus requiring mechanical ventilation are usually extremely anxious and distressed, especially when ventilated using a volume-preset mode. Deep sedation is usually necessary and supplemented in rare patients by therapeutic paralysis. The frequent occurrence of postparalytic myopathy in patients with asthma[50–52] has led us to greatly decrease our use of paralytics, an approach facilitated by the use of high-level PSV.

Sighs are undesirable because they may lead to lung rupture. Because peak proximal airway pressure is so high in this patient group, upper-limit alarms of 75 cm H_2O (and sometimes higher) are often required. Careful attention should be paid to the $\dot{V}$ and flow profile. Changes in flow that have little effect in the patient without airflow obstruction can have a dramatic impact in obstructed patients. Specifically, reducing the inspiratory flow or changing to a decelerating flow profile reduces the airway pressures and the amount of ventilator alarming but, by prolonging inspiration, actually worsens autoPEEP. Although the ventilator looks "better," the patient is worse, but this is only recognized if autoPEEP is regularly sought or if the expiratory flow profile is examined (see Fig. 36-3). Aggressive chest physiotherapy is advised because many patients mobilize mucous plugs during their recovery phase; often these plugs are so large and tenacious that they compromise endotracheal tube patency.

ACUTE-ON-CHRONIC RESPIRATORY FAILURE

Acute-on-chronic respiratory failure is a term used to describe exacerbations of chronic ventilatory failure usually occurring in patients with COPD[53] (see Chap. 39). Many of these patients are successfully (and preferably) ventilated noninvasively (see Chap. 33). When intubated, they are found to have relatively smaller increases in inspiratory resistance (compared with asthma), with their expiratory flow limitation arising largely from loss of elastic recoil.[54] As a consequence, in the patient with COPD, peak airway pressures tend to be only modestly elevated (e.g., 30 cm H_2O), but autoPEEP and its consequences are common.[55] At the time of intubation, hypoperfusion is common, as manifested by tachycardia and

relative hypotension, and typically responds to briefly ceasing ventilation combined with fluid loading.

Because most of these patients are ventilated after days to weeks of progressive deterioration, the goal is to rest the patient (and respiratory muscles) completely for 36 to 48 hours, although excessive rest and ventilatory support may contribute to atrophy and weakness of the diaphragm.[56] Also, because the patient typically has an underlying compensated respiratory acidosis, excessive ventilation risks severe respiratory alkalosis and, over time, bicarbonate wasting by the kidney. The goals of rest and appropriate hypoventilation usually can be achieved with initial ventilator settings of a V_T of 5 to 7 mL/kg and a respiratory rate of 16 to 24 breaths/min, with an ACV mode set on minimal sensitivity (see Table 36-3). Because gas exchange abnormalities are primarily those of ventilation-perfusion mismatch, supplemental oxygen in the range of an F_{IO_2} of 0.4 should achieve better than 90% saturation of arterial hemoglobin. Gas exchange abnormalities requiring an F_{IO_2} greater than 0.5 should prompt a search for complicating alveolar filling processes, such as left ventricular failure with pulmonary edema, pneumonia, or lobar collapse. $\dot{V}$ may be adjusted for patient comfort but usually is in the range of 50 to 60 L/min. Measures to prevent atelectasis and its complications (e.g., three-point turning, chest physiotherapy, or sighs) are necessary. PEEP should be used in this phase when the patient is triggering the ventilator because autoPEEP is universally present.

Most patients with COPD appear exhausted at the time when mechanical support is instituted and will sleep with minimal sedation. To the extent that muscle fatigue has played a role in a patient's functional decline, rest and sleep are desirable. Two days of such rest presumably will restore biochemical and functional changes associated with muscle fatigue, but 24 hours is probably not sufficient.[57] Small numbers of patients are difficult to rest on the ventilator and they continue to demonstrate effortful breathing. Examination of airway pressure and flow waveforms can be very helpful in identifying this extra work and in suggesting strategies for improving the ventilator settings (Fig. 36-6). In many patients, this is the result of autoPEEP-induced triggering difficulty, as discussed in Chap. 32 and shown in Fig. 36-4.[58] Frequently, adding extrinsic PEEP to nearly counterbalance the autoPEEP dramatically improves the patient's comfort.[59] An alternative approach is to increase minute ventilation to drive down the partial pressure of CO_2, but this will worsen autoPEEP and waste bicarbonate. This can be a difficult management problem. We advise a careful search for processes that might drive the patient to a respiratory rate higher than is desirable (e.g., hypoperfusion, pleural effusion or pain). If the patient continues to make significant inspiratory efforts—especially if these efforts are ineffective in actually triggering a machine breath or generating a V_T—judicious sedation is in order.

Once the patient improves and the respiratory muscles are rested, the patient should assume some of the work of breathing and be evaluated for liberation. During this phase, some extrinsic PEEP is typically useful to reduce the work of triggering.[59]

PATIENTS WITH ACUTE HYPOXEMIC RESPIRATORY FAILURE

Acute hypoxemic respiratory failure is caused by alveolar filling with blood, pus, or edema, the end results of which are

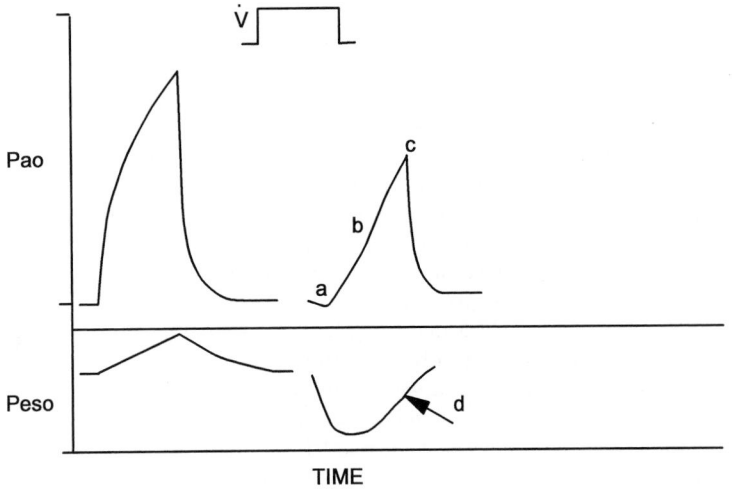

N.B.: VT CONSTANT

FIGURE 36-6 Signs of patient effort during volume-preset ventilation (assist-control ventilation [ACV] or intermittent mandatory ventilation [IMV] breaths). In these two breaths of equal tidal volume, the *left tracing* represents a muscle-relaxed patient, and the *right tracing* indicates a patient making inspiratory effort. The change in esophageal pressure (Peso) is shown in the *bottom tracings*. Signs of patient effort in the tracing of the pressure-airway opening (Pao) include a decrease in Pao just before the ACV or synchronized IMV breath (triggering; *a*), a concave upward rise in Pao during inspiration (*b*), and a peak airway pressure that is less than it would be if the patient made no effort (*c*). *d*. During the triggered breath, Peso (as an indicator of the pleural pressure) remains more negative than baseline throughout the breath and even after end inspiration (*arrow*).

impaired lung mechanics and gas exchange (see Chap. 31). The gas exchange impairment results from intrapulmonary shunt that is largely refractory to oxygen therapy. In ARDS (see Chap. 38), the significantly reduced FRC due to alveolar flooding and collapse leaves many fewer alveoli to accept the VT, making the lung appear stiff and dramatically increasing the work of breathing. The ARDS lung should be viewed as a small lung rather than as a stiff lung. In line with this current conception of ARDS, it is clearly established that excessive distention of the ARDS lung compounds lung injury and may induce systemic inflammation.[8,60] Ventilatory strategies have evolved markedly in the past decade and have changed clinical practice and generated tremendous excitement.

The goals of ventilation are to reduce shunt, avoid toxic concentrations of oxygen, and choose ventilator settings that do not amplify lung damage. The initial F_{IO_2} should be 1.0 in view of the typically extreme hypoxemia (see Table 36-3). PEEP is indicated in patients with diffuse lung lesions but may not be helpful in patients with focal infiltrates, such as lobar pneumonia. In patients with ARDS, PEEP should be instituted immediately, beginning with 15 cm H_2O, and then rapidly adjusted to the least PEEP necessary to produce an arterial saturation of 88% on an F_{IO_2} no higher than 0.6 (the "least PEEP approach"). An alternative approach (the "open-lung approach"[61]) sets the PEEP at a value 2 cm H_2O higher than the lower inflection point of the inflation pressure-volume curve (see Chap. 32), but this has not been shown to confer benefit. The VT should be 6 mL/kg IBW on ACV because a higher VT is associated with a higher mortality rate.[8] Some have speculated that unstudied VT values, such as 9 or 3 mL/kg IBW, might be even more beneficial than 6 mL/kg. It seems likely that there is a dose-response relation, with lower VT values being superior, and this explains the resurgence in interest in HFV in which VT can be very small. Nevertheless, because 6 mL/kg IBW has been conclusively shown to be safe and effective, this represents the standard of care to which other (potentially better, potentially worse) ventilator strategies should be compared. There is little doubt that lung protection can be achieved with pressure-preset ventilation, but safe settings are unknown. Some have extrapolated from the 30 cm H_2O plateau pressure limit in the ARDS Network study that a PI of 30 cm H_2O ought to be safe; however, because the mean

Pplat in those ventilated with 6 mL/kg IBW was only 26 cm H_2O, 30 cm H_2O may be too high. Whatever the mode, the respiratory rate should be set at 24 to 36 breaths/min as long as there is no autoPEEP. An occasional consequence of lung protective ventilation is hypercapnia. This approach of preferring hypercapnia to alveolar overdistention ("permissive hypercapnia") is discussed further in Chaps. 37 and 40.[61–63] Alternative modes of ventilation for ARDS, such as IRV, HFV, and tracheal gas insufflation, may have a role as salvage therapies but are of unproven benefit.

Once specimens have been collected from the airway for microbiologic and other studies, PEEP generally should not be disconnected to suction patients or to measure hemodynamic values because alveoli readily re-flood, provoking extreme hypoxemia. This supports multiple observations that PEEP does not reduce lung water but rather redistributes it into the lung interstitium to improve gas exchange.[26] Several modified suction adapters are available to provide a route to the airway and maintain PEEP, although most tend to leak at PEEP levels above 15 cm H_2O.

Sighs and other measures to prevent atelectasis are not necessary during the acute phases of acute hypoxemic respiratory failure, when PEEP levels are typically in excess of 10 cm H_2O. It should be remembered that these patients are at risk of atelectasis as they improve and PEEP levels are lowered. This is probably due in part to surfactant deficiency during the recovery from diffuse alveolar damage and certainly will be aggravated by the use of small VT.

THE PATIENT WITH RESTRICTION OF THE LUNGS OR CHEST WALL

Several restrictive diseases of the lungs or chest wall can lead to respiratory failure, especially when there is a superimposed ventilatory challenge (e.g., pneumonia). These conditions are fully discussed in Chaps. 42 and 66 and include lung disease (e.g., advanced pulmonary fibrosis or late-stage ARDS), abdominal disease (e.g., massive ascites), and other chest wall abnormalities (e.g., kyphoscoliosis). We describe ventilator management.

Small VT (5 to 7 mL/kg) and rapid rates (18 to 24 breaths/min) are especially important to minimize the hemodynamic consequences of positive-pressure ventilation and to reduce the likelihood of barotrauma (see Table 36-3). The

$F_{I_{O_2}}$ is usually determined by the degree of alveolar filling or collapse, if any. Rarely, we have encountered patients with enormous restrictive loads from intraabdominal catastrophes (e.g., massive intraperitoneal bleeding) who have a large intrapulmonary shunt but lack signs of alveolar flooding on the chest radiograph. We speculate that, in such patients, large numbers of alveolar units may be subserved by airways forced below their closing volume throughout tidal ventilation, so that these nonventilated alveoli comprise a large intrapulmonary shunt (see Chap. 42). Reversible contributors to restriction (e.g., circumferential burn eschar or tense ascites) should be identified and treated. Sitting the patient up in bed or on a chair may reduce the abdominal pressure, thereby easing the work of breathing.

The high P_A values typically generated in these patients may lead to increased physiologic dead space (when P_A exceeds the pulmonary artery pressure), especially when large V_T values are used. When the restrictive abnormality involves the chest wall (including the abdomen), the large ventilation-induced rise in pleural pressure has the potential to compromise cardiac output. This in turn will lower the mixed venous partial pressure of O_2 and, in the setting of ventilation-perfusion mismatch or shunt, the arterial partial pressure of O_2. If the physician responds to this decreasing arterial partial pressure of O_2 by augmenting PEEP or increasing the minute ventilation, further circulatory compromise ensues. A potentially catastrophic cycle of worsening gas exchange, increasing ventilator settings, and progressive shock is begun. This circumstance must be recognized because treatment is to reduce dead space (e.g., by lowering minute ventilation or correcting hypovolemia).

FACILITATING PATIENT COMFORT AND COMMUNICATION

THE ROLE OF SEDATION

Ideally, the mechanically ventilated patient should be alert, comfortable, and capable of communicating with the health care team. These desirable goals must be weighed against the need to heavily sedate and even therapeutically paralyze some patients with cardiovascular instability, severely compromised oxygen delivery to peripheral tissues, or severely deranged respiratory system mechanics.[64]

Much excessive sedation can be avoided by frequent communication, reassurance, and identification of sources of pain, anxiety, and agitation. Often, ventilator adjustment is more effective than drug therapy for calming the patient (see Table 36-1). Patients should be maximally alert during the day, with sedation limited to the evening, if possible. Short-acting benzodiazepines or haloperidol may facilitate sleep, thereby ensuring that the patient is maximally rested for efforts at spontaneous breathing during the day. Many patients must be deeply sedated to ensure comfort or to stabilize them hemodynamically during acute illness. A daily "wake up" during which sedatives are withheld until the patient awakens and is able to follow commands (or becomes agitated) is safe and effective in shortening time on the ventilator and in the ICU.[65] We advocate such a wake up in essentially all patients, even those who are hemodynamically unstable and unlikely to be breathing spontaneously for days.

Whenever neuromuscular blockers are used, the agent should be withdrawn on a daily basis until neuromuscular function returns to prevent excessive drug accumulation.[63] It

also may be useful to monitor the degree of neuromuscular blockade with a nerve stimulator (aiming for a train-of-two out of four), although this has not been shown to decrease the incidence of postparalytic myopathy. In patients with impaired renal and hepatic function, continuous infusion of *cis*-atracurium is preferred because pancuronium may accumulate and lead to protracted paralysis. During muscle paralysis, careful assessment of the level of sedation is essential because individuals differ widely in their response to sedatives and narcotics.

When the patient is optimally alert, it is important that the caretakers provide brief, clear explanations of all interventions proposed, especially changes in ventilator settings, to evaluate the patient's perception of beneficial effect. This allows the patient to be a part of the decision making concerning the optimal ventilator settings.

PATIENT-VENTILATOR SYNCHRONY

The initial ventilator settings should be reassessed promptly to assess their appropriateness for the individual patient. Such fine tuning of the ventilator often means the difference between a patient who rests on the ventilator or who continues to perform fatiguing efforts, who is calm yet awake, or who requires deep sedation or therapeutic paralysis. Assessing the patient-ventilator interaction requires substantial skill and experience. In part, the adequacy of ventilator settings is judged by the appearance of the patient (comfortable and resting versus diaphoretic and fighting) and arterial blood gas analysis. Tremendously valuable additional information comes from examination of waveforms, as elaborated in Chap. 32.

The intensivist should ensure that the patient and ventilator are synchronized, that is, that each attempt by the patient to trigger the ventilator generates a breath. The most common situation in which the patient fails to trigger breaths occurs in severe obstruction when autoPEEP is present (see Fig. 36-4). This is recognized at the bedside when the patient makes obvious efforts that fail to produce a breath. Using waveforms, these ineffective efforts cause a temporary slowing of expiratory flow, sometimes halting it completely (Fig. 36-7).

As an example, a patient was newly ventilated for septic shock and ARDS. His physicians found very high Pplat

FIGURE 36-7 Ventilation of an obstructed patient with assist-control or intermittent mandatory ventilation. A failed attempt to trigger can be detected in the expiratory flow waveform, where the expiratory flow briefly ceases (due to the patient's inspiratory effort) but the effort is insufficient to initiate a breath. Often the patient can be seen to make obvious inspiratory efforts between ventilator breaths. $\dot{V}$, flow.

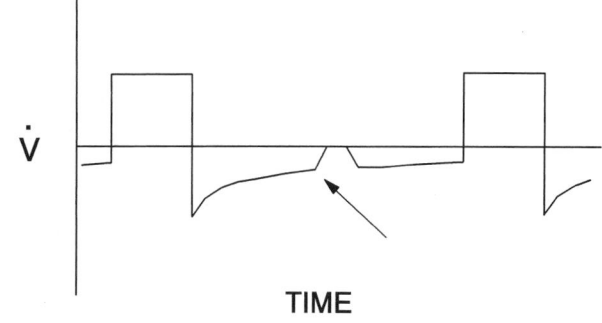

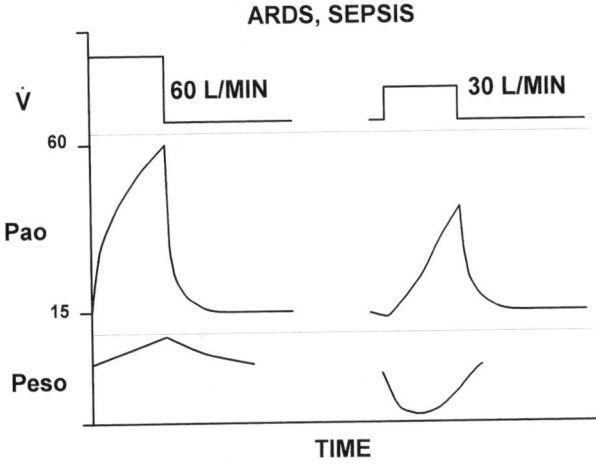

ARDS, SEPSIS

N.B.: VT CONSTANT

FIGURE 36-8 Ventilated patient with acute respiratory distress syndrome and sepsis. The first breath, at an inspiratory flow rate of 60 L/min, shows no signs of patient effort in the pressure-airway opening (Pao) waveform or the esophageal pressure (Peso) tracing. After the inspiratory flow is reduced to 30 L/min, the Pao decreases, but at the cost of greater patient effort, as reflected in the Pao waveform and the Peso. V̇, flow.

(38 cm H_2O) on the following settings: ACV mode, VT of 480 mL, an f of 28/min, and V̇ of 60 L/min. By reducing the V̇ to 30 L/min, Pplat was newly measured at 28 cm H_2O, which the physicians interpreted as an improvement (Fig. 36-8). However, the airway pressure decreased only at the cost of greatly increased efforts on the patient's part, efforts that can consume a remarkable fraction of the cardiac output (>30% in animal models[40,66,67]). Moreover, the transpulmonary pressure remained excessive because the VT was not reduced.

RESPONSE TO "CRISES" IN THE VENTILATED PATIENT

A vast array of sudden and potentially catastrophic changes in clinical condition can occur in the course of mechanical ventilation (Table 36-4). We focus on high- and low-pressure alarms, worsened oxygenation, and hypercapnia. Whenever the function of the ventilator or the position and patency of the airway are in question, the patient should be removed from the ventilator and hand bagged with 100% oxygen. This point is extremely important because this maneuver immediately circumvents the ventilator (and any malfunction of it), provides the clinician with a direct assessment of respiratory system mechanics, and focuses attention on the patient and not on the machine.

HIGH-PRESSURE ALARM

Aside from alarm or gauge malfunction, increased airway pressure indicates obstruction of the airway, obstruction to gas flow through the ventilator circuit, patient effort against the ventilator, or a change in the mechanics of the respiratory system. If manual bag ventilation is difficult, a suction catheter should be passed immediately through the endotracheal tube. If the catheter cannot be advanced 25 cm or farther, obstruction of the airway is likely. If repositioning of the head does not relieve kinking, and if the patient is not biting the

TABLE 36-4 Ventilator Crises

Increased peak airway pressure
  Endotracheal tube obstruction, kink, malposition
  Airway obstruction (e.g., bronchospasm, mucous plug)
  Reduced lung compliance (e.g., pulmonary edema)
  Reduced chest wall/abdomen compliance (e.g., pneumothorax, abdominal distention)
  Patient effort, agitation (e.g., coughing, biting, fighting)
Reduced oxygen saturation
  Ventilator/mixer malfunction
  Endotracheal tube malposition, leak
  New lung derangement (e.g., atelectasis, aspiration, edema)
  New cardiovascular derangement (e.g., shock, pulmonary embolism, fall in hemoglobin concentration)
  Increased oxygen consumption
  Change in body position, increasing shunt
Rising partial pressure of CO_2
  Ventilator malfunction
  Endotracheal tube malfunction, leak
  New patient mechanical derangement (e.g., bronchospasm, edema)
  Increased dead space
  Increased CO_2 production
Patient distress
  Pain, discomfort unrelated to the ventilator or respiratory system (e.g., myocardial ischemia)
  Endotracheal tube malposition
  Rising work of breathing
  Rising partial pressure of CO_2 (see above)
  Oxyhemoglobin desaturation (see above)
  Shock, pulmonary embolism
  Inadequate sedation
  Alcohol or other drug, withdrawl

airway, reintubation is necessary. If the patient is biting an endotracheal tube, a bite block should be placed; if this cannot be done, a short-acting neuromuscular blocking drug should be administered.

If the airway is patent but manual ventilation is difficult and the patient is struggling, a sedative should be given. If the patient can be easily ventilated (implicating vigorous respiratory muscle activity), the cause of the patient's distress should be sought. Possibilities include hypoxemia, hypercapnia, shock, or a new central nervous system process.

If ventilation remains difficult after deep sedation or muscle paralysis of a patient with a patent endotracheal tube, a new lower airway, pleural, lung, or chest wall process should be sought. Auscultation, palpation, and percussion often identify pneumothorax, collapse, or consolidation. Early portable chest radiography confirms these diagnoses or identifies an alternative cause of the crisis. Placing the patient back on the ventilator and measuring peak and plateau pressures and autoPEEP will further delineate the problem, as described above.

LOW-PRESSURE ALARM

Low-pressure alarms signal machine malfunction, a leak, or inspiratory effort by the patient (usually obvious). Large persistent leaks can occur within the ventilator itself, in the inspiratory limb, at the connection to the Y adaptor and endotracheal tube, around the endotracheal tube cuff, or through a bronchopleural fistula. If normal resistance to ventilation is noted during manual ventilation, the problem lies with the ventilator or tubing. If hand bagging shows minimal resistance, an endotracheal tube cuff leak is likely. This can be confirmed by listening over the neck or by placing a hand over the mouth. A large bronchopleural fistula can be identified by inspection of the chest tube and pleural drainage system.

WORSENED OXYGENATION

When a patient develops hypoxemia, sufficient oxygen should be given immediately to return the saturation to 88%. However, this must be followed by a search for the cause of deterioration. Progression of the primary cause of respiratory failure (ARDS, pneumonia, or lung hemorrhage) will impair gas exchange, but this should not be assumed to be the case. Also possible is a new lesion (e.g., nosocomial pneumonia) that may be identified by physical examination or chest radiograph. However, a systematic approach is useful to identify the myriad (including nonpulmonary) causes of hypoxemia.

From a pathophysiologic perspective, new hypoxemia implies a reduced F_{IO_2} (including ventilator malfunction), hypoventilation, ventilation-perfusion mismatching, shunt, or a decrease in the mixed venous oxygen saturation. Hypoventilation is usually obvious, being signaled by hypercapnia. Ventilation-perfusion mismatch typically causes mild hypoxemia that is easily corrected with supplemental oxygen. Bronchospasm, airway secretions, and airway plugging are common contributors in intubated patients. Inhaled bronchodilators may acutely worsen ventilation-perfusion relations,[68] as will vasodilators.[45] The combination of worsened ventilation-perfusion matching and an increase in dead space should prompt consideration of pulmonary embolism. Most often, when new hypoxemia develops in a mechanically ventilated patient, shunt or a decrease in mixed venous oxygenation can be found. A new shunt (e.g., pulmonary edema, pneumonia, or atelectasis) typically can be found on the chest radiograph, whereas mixed venous desaturation is detected by analyzing a venous blood sample or performing venous oximetry. The causes of venous desaturation include reduced cardiac output or hemoglobin concentration or increased systemic oxygen consumption. These nonpulmonary causes of hypoxemia are particularly common in patients with severe shunt lung disease and may herald life-threatening crises (e.g., pneumothorax).

HYPERCAPNIA

A rising Pa_{CO_2} often elicits a change in the ventilator orders (increased frequency or V_T). However, a pathophysiologic approach is useful in this situation. From the equation for Pa_{CO_2}:

$$Pa_{CO_2} = (V_{CO_2} \times k)/(V_T \times f \times [1 - V_D/V_T])$$

where V_{CO_2} is CO_2 production, k is a constant, and V_D is the dead space, it can be seen that, in addition to a decrease in minute ventilation, rising CO_2 production (e.g., fever, shivering, or agitation) or increasing dead space (e.g., hypovolemia, pulmonary embolism, PEEP) may account for new hypercapnia. Responding to hypercapnia by simply raising the minute ventilation is dangerous because causes of increased CO_2 production and dead space may be important to diagnose in their own right. In addition, augmenting minute ventilation has the potential to (paradoxically) decrease alveolar ventilation if the increase in V_T or f worsens dead space (such as when autoPEEP is present). In this setting, the Pa_{CO_2} may *rise* when minute ventilation is increased and *fall* when minute ventilation is reduced. These issues are further discussed in Chap. 40.

LIBERATION OF THE PATIENT FROM MECHANICAL VENTILATION

We refer to the discontinuation of mechanical ventilation not as *weaning* (which implies the withdrawal of a nurturing life-support system) but as *liberation* (connoting freedom from a confining, noxious, and dangerous circumstance[69]). Because liberation from the ventilator is fully discussed in Chap. 44, we make only a few points relevant to all ventilated patients. Patients recover the ability to breathe spontaneously because central drive is regained, neuromuscular competence is restored, and respiratory system load is reduced. Once these are achieved, the ventilator is no longer needed. Gradual adjustments of IMV rates or pressure-support levels that are too slow for the patient's needs simply serve to prolong the duration of mechanical ventilation, as shown in large trials of weaning strategies,[10,11] and do not facilitate the recognition of evolving ventilatory failure.[70] However, if drive, strength, and load are not repaired, no amount of ventilator technology will allow the patient to breathe on his or her own. Most often, when physicians believe they are "weaning" the patient, they are simply allowing time for their other therapies to treat the respiratory failure; ventilator changes are prescribed coincidentally but are irrelevant. Accordingly, effective liberation of each patient begins with intubation and stabilization on the ventilator, with the measurement of respiratory mechanics to assist in evaluating the reversible features of the patient's abnormally increased load; as soon as is clinically relevant, the respiratory muscle strength is evaluated for reversible causes of weakness.

Before an acceptable balance between neuromuscular competence and load is attained, different methods for exercising the patient may be useful because disuse causes muscles to weaken[56] (see Table 36-3). These include T-piece sprints with which the patient is allowed to breathe without ventilatory assistance for progressively longer periods as ventilatory function improves. Alternatively, the pressure-support mode can be adjusted to allow a reasonably spontaneous V_T (e.g., 300 to 500 mL H_2O) and respiratory rate (<30 breaths/min) but at a level that demands some work from the patient. The physician should be familiar with a number of different modes because patient preference can then dictate which is used in a particular circumstance. SIMV appears to prolong the period of ventilator dependency and should no longer be used for weaning. Aside from this, the method of exercise chosen is not clearly important and certainly secondary to the main goals of restoring drive, improving neuromuscular competence, and reducing load.

Of overriding importance is an approach that asks on a daily basis, "Can this patient breathe on his or her own?" In several studies of methods of weaning, 75% of patients assessed at entry into the trial were extubated successfully.[10,11] The use of interdisciplinary weaning teams or respiratory therapist–driven protocols may expedite successful liberation by actively addressing this question each day.[71,72]

CONVERSION TO A TRACHEOSTOMY

A tracheostomy provides easier tracheobronchial toilet, enhances communication, and is more comfortable for the patient than translaryngeal intubation (TLI). In contrast, endotracheal intubation is less invasive and, in the short run, less likely to cause complications. The timing of tracheostomy involves balancing its complications[73] against the (typically) more delayed complications of TLI. The major complication of TLI is laryngeal damage with resulting postextubation upper airway obstruction or dysphonia.[74] Injuries likely arise from abrasion and compression of laryngeal structures, with sequelae including posterior commissural stenosis, posterior cordal synechiae, arytenoid fixation, and subglottic stenosis. The precise contributions of insertion trauma, duration of TLI, and movement during ICU management to these injuries is not clear, but all are likely important. Some clinicians have suggested that women and patients with diabetes mellitus, rheumatoid arthritis, and ankylosing spondylitis are at increased risk of laryngeal injury during TLI. The incidence of cuff-induced injury to the trachea itself is probably similar between tracheostomy and TLI, at least in the critical care environment.[75]

Our own approach is to begin with TLI in most critically ill patients. Those with an immediate indication for tracheostomy, such as upper airway obstruction or severe sleep apnea, are scheduled for this procedure at the earliest opportunity. Patients who are extremely restless, have copious pulmonary secretions, or are likely to require more than 2 weeks of mechanical ventilation are also considered for early tracheostomy. All other patients are reassessed on a daily basis for these indications for tracheostomy. If extubation seems likely within the first 2 to 3 weeks, TLI is maintained. Occasionally, this approach provides TLI for 3 weeks or longer; however, even with soft cuffs and careful monitoring, the complications of this prolonged TLI begin to outweigh its advantages, and tracheostomy becomes indicated for its greater comfort and potential for enhanced communication. Percutaneous tracheostomy has several advantages in the critically ill patient. Performance of tracheostomy in the ICU provides a safely monitored environment for the procedure and obviates the risks of transporting the patient.

EXTUBATION

Extubation after prolonged (>5 days) intubation should be approached cautiously. In addition to demonstrating freedom from mechanical ventilatory support, as discussed in Chap. 44, the patient must be capable of maintaining airway patency, have sufficient airway reflexes to avoid aspiration, and have adequate cough to mobilize secretions. Laryngeal injury causing postextubation upper airway obstruction should be anticipated.

The most common cause of postextubation stridor is posterior commissure edema, arising from direct mechanical injury to these soft tissues, and impaired vocal cord abduction. Before extubation, the degree of upper airway edema may be assessed by direct laryngoscopy or by deflating the tube cuff, obstructing its lumen, and measuring the amount of airflow around it. Alternatively, the airway can be inspected by fiberoptic laryngoscopy immediately after extubation. Despite these precautions, progressive airway edema with stridor will be encountered in 1% to 5% of patients after prolonged TLI. The initial management should include bag-mask ventilation synchronized to augment the patient's efforts. Noninvasive positive-pressure ventilation is generally considered to be useful, although one clinical trial showed no benefit,[76] and another trial has called into use its general application for respiratory failure emerging shortly after extubation.[76a] Racemic epinephrine by inhalation and intravenous corticosteroids are usually recommended but have not been rigorously studied. A helium-oxygen gas mixture (heliox) also can be useful in this setting.[77] Administration of this low-density gas mixture reduces the large pressure drop associated with turbulent flow across the obstruction, thus reducing the work of breathing. Heliox (21% oxygen and 79% helium) can be delivered by a mask connected to an H tank, supplemented by nasal cannula oxygen, to maintain an arterial hemoglobin saturation of 90%. Heliox and noninvasive positive-pressure ventilation should be used only to temporize while awaiting more definitive therapy of the critical airway narrowing.

If stridor fails to respond to initial measures or reemerges while on therapy, reintubation is usually necessary. The usual approach is to use a small endotracheal tube (6.0 or 6.5 mm) through the nasal route to minimize further injury to the posterior commissure. The managing team should be prepared to perform cricothyrotomy or tracheostomy, if necessary. After reintubation, edema resolves in most patients over 48 to 72 hours. During this time, corticosteroid therapy should be continued (e.g., dexamethasone 4 mg every 6 hours), and the airway should be viewed directly to confirm resolution of edema.

Extubation failure is a marker for prolonged ventilation and ICU stay, increased hospital costs and mortality rate, and greater likelihood of tracheostomy.[78] Risk factors include age, longer duration of ventilation, continuous sedative infusion, and anemia.

AIRWAY DURING SPLIT-LUNG VENTILATION

The lungs may be separated for purposes of differential ventilation by two major means: blocking the bronchus of a lobe or whole lung while ventilating with a standard endotracheal tube or passing a double-lumen tube. Different devices have been used to obstruct a bronchus, but experience is greatest with the Fogarty embolectomy catheter. Double-lumen tubes carry the advantages of allowing each lung to be ventilated, collapsed, reexpanded, or inspected independently.

Split-lung ventilation is only rarely useful in the critical care unit, but occasionally its benefits are dramatic. Large bronchopleural fistulas severely compromise ventilation and may not respond to HFV.[79] A double-lumen tube will maintain ventilation of the healthy lung and facilitate closure of the bronchopleural fistula.[80] During massive hemoptysis, lung separation may be lifesaving by minimizing blood aspiration, maintaining airway patency, and tamponading the bleeding site while awaiting definitive therapy.[81] Patients with focal causes of acute hypoxemic respiratory failure, such as lobar pneumonia or acute total atelectasis, may benefit from differential ventilation and application of PEEP.[82]

Complications with these devices are common because they are difficult to maintain in ideal position during a protracted period of respiratory failure and tend to directly injure the trachea and main bronchi. A clear protocol for airway assessment and repositioning should exist, and routine input from senior anesthesiology staff is required.

References

1. Marini JJ, Capps JS, Culver BH: The inspiratory work of breathing during assisted mechanical ventilation. *Chest* 87:612, 1985.
2. Brochard L, Mancebo J, Wysocki M, et al: Noninvasive ventilation for acute exacerbations of chronic obstructive pulmonary disease. *N Engl J Med* 333:817, 1995.
3. Hilbert G, Gruson D, Vargas F: Noninvasive ventilation in immunosuppressed patients with pulmonary infiltrates, fever, and acute respiratory failure. *N Engl J Med* 344:481, 2001.
4. Drakulovic MB, Torres A, Bauer TT, et al: Supine body position as a risk factor for nosocomial pneumonia in mechanically ventilated patients: A randomised trial. *Lancet* 354:1851, 1999.
5. Fink JB, Krause SA, Barrett L, et al: Extending ventilator circuit change interval beyond 2 days reduces the likelihood of ventilator-associated pneumonia. *Chest* 113:405, 1998.
6. Girault C, Richard JC, Chevron V, et al: Comparative physiologic effects of noninvasive assist-control and pressure support ventilation in acute hypercapnic respiratory failure. *Chest* 111:1639, 1997.
7. Macintyre NR: Respiratory function during pressure support ventilation. *Chest* 89:677, 1986.
8. Acute Respiratory Distress Syndrome Network: Ventilation with lower tidal volumes as compared with traditional tidal volumes for acute lung injury and the acute respiratory distress syndrome. *N Engl J Med* 342:1301, 2000.
9. Marini JJ, Rodriguez RM, Lamb V: The inspiratory workload of patient-initiated mechanical ventilation. *Am Rev Respir Dis* 134:902, 1986.
10. Esteban A, Frutos F, Tobin MJ, et al: 1995. A comparison of four methods of weaning patients from mechanical ventilation. *N Engl J Med* 332:345, 1995.
11. Brochard L, Rauss A, Benito S, et al: Comparison of three methods of gradual withdrawal from ventilatory support during weaning from mechanical ventilation. *Am J Respir Crit Care Med* 150:896, 1994.
12. Shivaram U, Miro AM, Cash ME, et al: Cardiopulmonary responses to continuous positive airway pressure in acute asthma. *J Crit Care* 8:87, 1993.
13. Appendini L, Purro A, Patessio A, et al: Partitioning of inspiratory muscle workload and pressure assistance in ventilator-dependent COPD patients. *Am J Respir Crit Care Med* 154:1301, 1996.
14. Corne S, Gillespie D, Roberts D, et al: Effect of inspiratory flow rate on respiratory rate in intubated ventilated patients. *Am J Respir Crit Care Med* 156:304, 1997.
15. Marini JJ: Should PEEP be used in airflow obstruction? *Am Rev Respir Dis* 140:1, 1989.
16. Tuxen DV: Detrimental effects of positive end-expiratory pressure during controlled mechanical ventilation of patients with severe airflow obstruction. *Am Rev Respir Dis* 140:5, 1989.
17. Smith TC, Marini JJ: Impact of peep on lung mechanics and work of breathing in severe airflow obstruction. *J Appl Physiol* 65:1488, 1988.
18. Marini JJ: Strategies to minimize breathing effort during mechanical ventilation. *Crit Care Clin* 6:635, 1990.
19. Beydon L, Chasse M, Harf A, et al: Inspiratory work of breathing during spontaneous ventilation using demand valves and continuous flow systems. *Am Rev Respir Dis* 138:300, 1988.
20. Cox D, Tinloi SF, Farrimond JG: Investigation of the spontaneous modes of breathing of different ventilators. *Intensive Care Med* 14:532, 1988.
21. Marcy TW, Marini JJ: Inverse ratio ventilation in ARDS: Rationale and implementation. *Chest* 100:494, 1991.
22. Modell HI, Cheney FW: Effects of inspiratory flow pattern on gas exchange in normal and abnormal lungs. *J Appl Physiol* 46:1103, 1979.
23. Boysen PG, McGough E: Pressure-control and pressure support ventilation: Flow patterns, inspiratory time, and gas distribution. *Respir Care* 33:126, 1988.
24. Duncan SR, Rizk NW, Raffin TA: Inverse ratio ventilation: PEEP in disguise. *Chest* 92:390, 1987.
25. Cole AGH, Weller SF, Sykes MK: Inverse ratio ventilation compared with PEEP in adult respiratory failure. *Intensive Care Med* 10:227, 1984.
26. Malo J, Ali J, Wood LDH: How does positive end-expiratory pressure reduce intrapulmonary shunt in canine pulmonary edema? *J Appl Physiol* 57:1002, 1984.
27. Macklem PT, Mead J: Resistance of central and peripheral airways measured by a retrograde catheter. *J Appl Physiol* 22:395, 1967.
28. Downs JB, Stock MC: Airway pressure release ventilation: a new concept in ventilatory support. *Crit Care Med* 15:459, 1987.
29. Rasanen J, Cane RD, Downs JB, et al: Airway pressure release ventilation during acute lung injury: A prospective multicenter trial. *Crit Care Med* 19:1234, 1991.
30. Cane RD, Peruzzi WT, Shapiro BA: Airway pressure release ventilation in severe acute respiratory failure. *Chest* 100:460, 1991.
31. Younes M: Proportional assist ventilation, a new approach to ventilatory support: Theory. *Am Rev Respir Dis* 145:114, 1992.
32. Younes M, Puddy A, Roberts D, et al: Proportional assist ventilation: results of an initial clinical trial. *Am Rev Respir Dis* 145:121, 1992.
33. Drazen JM, Kamm RD, Slutsky AS, et al: High-frequency ventilation. *Physiol Rev* 64:505, 1984.
34. Turnbull AD, Carlon G, Howland WS, et al: High-frequency jet ventilation in major airway or pulmonary disruption. *Ann Thorac Surg* 32:468, 1981.
35. Imai Y, Nakagawa S, Ito Y, et al: Comparison of lung protection strategies using conventional and high-frequency oscillatory ventilation. *J Appl Physiol* 91:1836, 2001.
36. Rotta AT, Bunnarsson B, Fuhrman BP, et al: Comparison of lung protective ventilation strategies in a rabbit model of acute lung injury. *Crit Care Med* 29:2176, 2001.
37. Sedeek KA, Takeuchi M, Suchodolski K, et al: Determinants of tidal volume during high-frequency oscillation. *Crit Care Med* 31:227, 2003.
38. Breen PH, Ali J, Wood LDH: High frequency ventilation in lung edema: Effects on gas exchange and perfusion. *J Appl Physiol* 56:187, 1984.
39. Derdak S, Mehta S, Stewart TE, et al: High-frequency oscillatory ventilation for acute respiratory distress syndrome in adults: A randomized, controlled trial. *Am J Respir Crit Care Med* 166:801, 2002.
39a. Mehta S, Granton J, MacDonald RJ, et al. High frequency oscillatory ventilation in adults: The Toronto experience. *Chest* 126:518, 2004.
40. Aubier M, Trippenbach T, Roussos C: Respiratory muscle fatigue during cardiogenic shock. *J Appl Physiol* 51:499, 1981.
41. Viires N, Sillie G, Aubier A, et al: Regional blood flow distribution in dogs during induced hypotension and low cardiac output: Spontaneous breathing versus artificial ventilation. *J Clin Invest* 72:935, 1983.
42. Marantz S, Patrick W, Webster K, et al: Response of ventilator-dependent patients to different levels of proportional assist. *J Appl Physiol* 80:397, 1996.
43. Tobert DG, Simon PM, Stroetz RW, et al: The determinants of respiratory rate during mechanical ventilation. *Am J Respir Crit Care Med* 155:485, 1997.
44. Choi SC, Nelson LD: Kinetic therapy in critically ill patients: Combined results based on meta-analysis. *J Crit Care* 7:57, 1992.

45. Rodriguez-Roisin R, Ballester E, Roca J, et al: Mechanisms of hypoxemia in patients with status asthmaticus requiring mechanical ventilation. *Am Rev Respir Dis* 139:732, 1989.

46. Gay PC, Rodarte JR, Hubmayr RD: The effects of positive expiratory pressure on isovolume flow and dynamic hyperinflation in patients receiving mechanical ventilation. *Am Rev Respir Dis* 139:621, 1989.

47. Tobin MJ, Lodato RF: PEEP, auto-PEEP, and waterfalls. *Chest* 96:449, 1989.

48. Ranieri VM, Giuliani R, Cinnella G, et al: Physiologic effects of positive end-expiratory pressure in patients with chronic obstructive pulmonary disease during acute ventilatory failure and controlled mechanical ventilation. *Am Rev Respir Dis* 147:5, 1993.

49. Tuxen DV, Williams TJ, Scheinkestel CD, et al: Use of a measurement of pulmonary hyperinflation to control the level of mechanical ventilation in patients with acute severe asthma. *Am Rev Respir Dis* 146:1136, 1992.

50. Coakley JH, Nagendran K, Ormerod IEC, et al: Prolonged neurogenic weakness in patients requiring mechanical ventilation for acute airflow limitation. *Chest* 101:1413, 1992.

51. Giostra E, Magistris MR, Pizzolato G, et al: Neuromuscular disorder in intensive care unit patients treated with pancuronium bromide. *Chest* 106:210, 1994.

52. Leatherman JW, Fluegel WL, David WS, et al: Muscle weakness in mechanically ventilated patients with severe asthma. *Am J Respir Crit Care Med* 153:1686, 1996.

53. Schmidt GA, Hall JB: Acute on chronic respiratory failure: Assessment and management of patients with COPD in the emergent setting. *JAMA* 261:3444, 1989.

54. Coussa ML, Guérin C, Eissa NT, et al: Partitioning of work of breathing in mechanically ventilated COPD patients. *J Appl Physiol* 75:1711, 1993.

55. Pepe PE, Marini JJ: Occult positive end-expiratory pressure in mechanically ventilated patients with airflow obstruction. *Am Rev Respir Dis* 126:166, 1982.

56. Vassilakopoulos T, Petrof BJ: Ventilator-induced diaphragmatic dysfunction. *Am J Respir Crit Care Med* 169:336, 2004.

57. Laghi F, D'Alfonso N, Tobin MJ: Pattern of recovery from diaphragmatic fatigue over 24 hours. *J Appl Physiol* 79:539, 1995.

58. Fleury B, Murciano D, Talamo C, et al: Work of breathing in patients with chronic obstructive pulmonary disease in acute respiratory failure. *Am Rev Respir Dis* 131:822, 1985.

59. Petrof BJ, Legaré M, Goldberg P, et al: Continuous positive airway pressure reduces work of breathing and dyspnea during weaning from mechanical ventilation in severe chronic obstructive pulmonary disease. *Am Rev Respir Dis* 141:281, 1990.

60. Ranieri VM, Suter PM, Tortoella C, et al: Effects of mechanical ventilation on inflammatory mediators in patients with acute respiratory distress syndrome: a randomized controlled trial. *JAMA* 282:54, 1999.

61. Amato MBP, Barbas CSV, Medeiros DM, et al: Beneficial effects of the "open lung approach" with low distending pressures in acute respiratory distress syndrome: A prospective randomized study on mechanical ventilation. *Am J Respir Crit Care Med* 152:1835, 1995.

62. Roupie E, Dambrosio M, Servillo G, et al: Titration of tidal volume and induced hypercapnia in acute respiratory distress syndrome. *Am J Respir Crit Care Med* 152:121, 1995.

63. Hickling KG, Walsh J, Henderson S, et al: Low mortality rate in adult respiratory distress syndrome using low-volume, pressure-limited ventilation with permissive hypercapnia: A prospective study. *Crit Care Med* 22:1568, 1994.

64. Gehlbach BK, Kress JP: Sedation in the intensive care unit. *Curr Opin Crit Care* 8:290, 2002.

65. Kress JP, Pohlman AS, O'Connor MF, et al: Daily interruption of sedative infusions in critically ill patients undergoing mechanical ventilation. *N Engl J Med* 342:1, 2000.

66. Hussain SNA, Graham R, Ruthledge F, et al: Respiratory muscle energetics during endotoxic shock in dogs. *J Appl Physiol* 60:486, 1986.

67. Hussain SNA, Simkus G, Roussos C: Respiratory muscle fatigue: a cause of ventilatory failure in septic shock. *J Appl Physiol* 58:2033, 1985.

68. Ballester E, Reyes A, Roca J, et al: Ventilation-perfusion mismatching in acute severe asthma: Effects of salbutamol and 100% oxygen. *Thorax* 44:258, 1989.

69. Hall JB, Wood LDH: Liberation of the patient from mechanical ventilation. *JAMA* 257:1621, 1987.

70. Stroetz RW, Hubmayr RD: Tidal volume maintenance during weaning with pressure support. *Am J Respir Crit Care Med* 152:1034, 1995.

71. Anton WR, Wilhelm P, Jordan T: Reduction of length of time on mechanical ventilation by use of a multidisciplinary weaning protocol. *Respir Care* 37:1279, 1992.

72. Ely EW, Baker AM, Dunagan DP, et al: Effect on the duration of mechanical ventilation of identifying patients capable of breathing spontaneously. *N Engl J Med* 335:1864, 1996.

73. Myers EN, Carrau RL: Early complications of tracheotomy: Incidence and management. *Clin Chest Med* 12:589, 1991.

74. Colice GL, Stukel TA, Dain B: Laryngeal complications of prolonged intubation. *Chest* 96:877, 1989.

75. Stauffer JL, Olson DE, Petty TL: Complications and consequences of endotracheal intubation and tracheostomy. *Am J Med* 70:65, 1981.

76. Keenan SP, Powers C, McCormack DG, et al: Noninvasive positive-pressure ventilation for postextubation respiratory distress: A randomized controlled trial. *JAMA* 287:3238, 2002.

76a. Esteban A, Frutos- Vivar F, Ferguson ND, et al. Noninvasive positive pressure ventilation for respiratory failure after extubation. *N Engl J Med* 350:2452, 2004.

77. Orr JB: Helium-oxygen gas mixtures in the management of patients with airway obstruction. *Ear Nose Throat J* 67:866, 1988.

78. Rothaar RC, Epstein SK: Extubation failure: magnitude of the problem, impact on outcomes, and prevention. *Curr Opin Crit Care* 9:59, 2003.

79. Bishop MJ, Benson MS, Sato P, et al: Comparison of high-frequency jet ventilation with conventional mechanical ventilation for bronchopleural fistula. *Anesth Analg* 66:833, 1987.

80. Pierson DJ, Horton CA, Bates PW: Persistent bronchopleural air leak during mechanical ventilation: A review of 39 cases. *Chest* 90:321, 1986.

81. Garzon AA, Cerrutt MM, Golding ME: Exsanguinating hemoptysis. *J Thorac Cardiovasc Surg* 84:829, 1982.

82. Stow PJ, Grant I: Asynchronous independent lung ventilation: Its use in the treatment of acute unilateral lung disease. *Anesthesia* 40:163, 1985.

Chapter 37 _____

VENTILATOR-INDUCED LUNG INJURY

JOHN T. GRANTON
ARTHUR S. SLUTSKY

KEY POINTS

- *Ventilator-induced lung injury may occur with both lung volumes that lead to overdistention of lung units (volutrauma) or with low distending pressures that lead to the development of atelectasis (atelectrauma).*

- *Ventilator-induced lung injury may cause injury in previously healthy regions of lung, and may also lead to multiorgan dysfunction.*

- *To reduce the risk of ventilator-induced lung injury, low tidal volumes of 6 mL/kg should be used in treating most patients with acute respiratory distress syndrome.*

- *The appropriate level of positive end-expiratory pressure remains to be determined, but levels of PEEP that minimize atelectrauma may be beneficial.*

- *Permissive hypoventilation (hypercapnia) may be a necessary component of a lung-protective ventilatory strategy.*

There is consistent and convincing experimental evidence that mechanical ventilation, particularly in the setting of lung injury, can contribute to functional and structural alterations in the lung. The experimental evidence has led to the notion that mechanical ventilation not only perpetuates the lung injury, but also contributes to both the morbidity and mortality of the acute respiratory distress syndrome (ARDS). Concern surrounding ventilator-induced lung injury (VILI) culminated in a consensus conference in 1993 that made (based solely on studies in animal models of ARDS) the empirical recommendation to limit tidal volumes to the range of 5 to 7 mL/kg and plateau pressures less than 35 cm H_2O.[1] It would be 8 years until the recommendations of the consensus group were affirmed by a randomized controlled trial demonstrating that a lung-protective strategy designed to limit VILI would lead to an improvement in patient outcome.[2] Unfortunately, it seems that it may take even longer until there is incorporation of these concepts into widespread clinical practice.[3]

The objectives of this chapter are to develop the concept of VILI and provide the rationale for the shift in ventilation philosophy for patients with ARDS. First, the relevant features of ARDS as it pertains to VILI will be reviewed, since most of the studies evaluating VILI have focused on ARDS. Then, the concept of lung-protective ventilation strategies will be discussed, and pertinent studies evaluating these newer strategies in patients with ARDS will be presented. Recommendations based on current clinical evidence, and when this is lacking best experimental evidence, will also be presented (Table 37-1).

Acute Respiratory Distress Syndrome

ARDS is characterized by endothelial and epithelial cellular injury. This loss of integrity of the alveolar-capillary membrane results in a high-permeability pulmonary edema and formation of hyaline membranes. Injury to type II pneumocytes also occurs, and there are alterations in surfactant function. Plain chest radiographs are frequently misleading, in that they suggest that the lung damage is uniformly distributed. However, evaluation of patients with ARDS using computed tomography (CT) of the thorax has demonstrated that the airspace disease is patchy.[4,5] Marked heterogeneity and regional differences in lung injury exist in the lungs of these patients. Regions of lung with airspace disease are contrasted to adjacent areas with normal-appearing alveoli. In addition, an exaggerated vertical gradient of lung inflation has been demonstrated in ARDS, with compression of alveoli and a decrease in aerated lung as one progresses from nondependent to more dependent lung regions.[6] Indeed as emphasized by Mead and coworkers in the early 1970s it is likely this degree of heterogeneity of the lung injury that makes the lung uniquely susceptible to the effects of ventilator-induced injury.[7] The heterogeneity of the lung injury is also responsible for the decrease in lung compliance that characterizes ARDS. It is worth emphasizing that this loss of compliance is due to a functional reduction in alveolar units and not due to the development of "stiff" lungs. Indeed the recognition that ARDS is characterized by a loss of functional lung units with preservation of other alveoli with normal lung compliance (specific lung compliance) is central to the current notion of lung protection strategies.[8] In many respects owing to the reduction in effective lung volume, the 70-kg adult patient with ARDS must be treated from the pulmonary point of view as a 30-kg pediatric patient. Consequently the use of traditional tidal volumes of 10 to 15 mL/kg (700 to 900 mL in our 70-kg patient) would be inappropriate and will simply result in overdistention of lung units with relatively normal compliance. The need to modify the approach to mechanical ventilation in ARDS is further emphasized by three decades of investigations that demonstrate that the overdistention of lung units may in itself lead to lung injury identical to that seen in ARDS. ARDS is also a syndrome characterized by inflammation of the lung with various cytokines and other mediators thought to play a major role. In recent years, there has been a large body of evidence indicating that mechanical ventilation may have an impact on this aspect of the pathophysiology of ARDS, and indeed there is the suggestion that the improvement in mortality with lung-protective strategies may be partly due to a reduction in release of various mediators by these strategies.

Ventilator-Induced Lung Injury

MACROSCOPIC INJURY

Recent evidence suggests that mechanical ventilation may have both regional and systemic effects. VILI may be broadly classified into macroscopic and microscopic injury (Table 37-2). Macroscopic injury consists of what has been classically described as barotrauma. Pneumothorax, pneumomediastinum, pneumoperitoneum, and subcutaneous

TABLE 37-1 Goals of Mechanical Ventilation Modified to Reduce the Risk of Ventilator-Induced Lung Injury

Oxygenation
    Maintain saturation >90% (may only require >85%)
    Ensure adequate oxygen delivery
Avoid overdistention
    Limit tidal volumes to 6 mL/kg PBW
    Limit peak inspiratory pressure to <35 cm H_2O
    Peak lung inflation less than upper inflection point?
Recruit alveoli
    Recruitment maneuver with a sustained inflation?
    Pressure-preset ventilation waveform?
Keep alveoli patent
    End-expiratory volume greater than lower inflection point?
    Titrate end-expiratory volume to best lung compliance?
    Keep total positive end-expiratory pressure generally above
       15 cm H_2O?
Ventilation
    Accept pH to 7.15?

emphysema are recognized complications of mechanical ventilation, and are characterized by the presence of extra-alveolar air.[9] The mechanism of the development of extra-alveolar air was elegantly demonstrated by Macklin and Macklin in 1944.[10] During positive-pressure ventilation (PPV), alveoli rupture at the point where the alveolar base meets the bronchovascular sheath. Air then dissects along the vascular sheaths towards the mediastinum and into the hilum and mediastinal soft tissues. If sufficient gas accumulates, the mediastinal parietal pleura ruptures, and a pneumothorax develops.

Macroscopic barotrauma correlates with a variety of factors. In a retrospective study in 139 intubated patients, barotrauma occurred in 34 patients.[11] Peak airway pressure, level of positive end-expiratory pressure (PEEP), tidal volume, and minute ventilation correlated with the development of barotrauma. However, in a subsequent prospective study of

TABLE 37-2 The Scope of Ventilator-Induced Lung Injury

Oxygen toxicity
Tracheal and upper airway injury
Alterations in venous return and pulmonary vascular resistance
    and in turn cardiac output
    Macroscopic
        Pneumothorax
        Pneumomediastinum
        Pneumopericardium
        Pneumoperitoneum
        Subcutaneous emphysema
        Parenchymal emphysema
        Cystic lung spaces
    Microscopic
        Regional
            Epithelial injury
            Endothelial injury
            Damage to the alveolar-capillary barrier
            Surfactant dysfunction
            Bronchiolar injury
            ? Late phase of ARDS (fibrosis)
        Systemic
            Multisystem organ injury

168 patients over a 1-year period, only the presence of ARDS was associated with the development of barotrauma.[12] Gas trapping has also been associated with the development of extra-alveolar air leakage. In a study in mechanically ventilated asthmatics, an elevation in end-inspiratory lung volume above 1.4 L was associated with macroscopic barotrauma.[13] The relationship of PEEP to the development of extra-alveolar air is inconsistent.[12,14] Patients with severe underlying lung disease often require higher levels of PEEP to maintain oxygenation, and it is possible that it is the underlying lung disease in such patients that explains the correlation between air leaks and PEEP levels. More recently Eisner and colleagues, using data from the ARDS Network trial, reported that higher PEEP was associated with an increased risk of barotrauma (relative risk = 1.5; 95% confidence interval [CI] 0.98 to 2.3).[15] The strength of the association in this trial was the ability to control for other potentially relevant risk factors and uniformity of the ventilation methodology. One will have to see how this observation is born out by clinical trials that are currently underway to evaluate higher PEEP strategies in patients with ARDS. Patients with underlying lung damage are particularly prone to the development of macroscopic barotrauma. Asthma, chronic obstructive pulmonary disease (COPD), and pneumonia have all been identified as risk factors.[11] ARDS has consistently been associated with a very high risk for the development of extra-alveolar air, with an incidence in some series of 40%.[11,12,16] In addition to the immediate hemodynamic consequences, the development of macroscopic barotrauma in patients receiving mechanical ventilation portends a worse prognosis. CT studies of patients with ARDS have expanded the scope of macroscopic injury. Gattinoni and coworkers have described the appearance of bullae and cystic parenchymal lesions located predominantly in the dependent (dorsal) lung regions.[4] These lesions are often occult and are not readily detected on plain chest radiographs. In a histologic study in patients with severe respiratory failure, airspace enlargement with alveolar distention in aerated lungs or intraparenchymal pseudocysts in nonaerated regions were identified in 87% of the lungs examined. Importantly, patients with severe airspace enlargement were ventilated with higher airway pressures and higher levels of inspired oxygen and had a higher rate of pneumothoraces. One reasonable hypothesis is that the cystic changes observed in aerated lungs occur because of the high airway pressures causing overdistention of alveoli. The etiology of the cystic lesions observed in nonaerated, more dependent lung regions remains speculative. Since they occur in dependent regions of the lung, their appearance is not explained by lung overdistention. Possibly they are caused by repetitive opening and closing of nonrecruited alveoli (see below). Alternatively, because perfusion is greater in dependent regions, the cystic lesions may be caused by blood-borne factors such as cytokines and inflammatory cells.

The importance of lung perfusion was emphasized by Broccard and coworkers, who used an isolated rabbit lung preparation and demonstrated that an increase in lung perfusion lead to more severe hemorrhage, an increase in filtration coefficient, and heavier lungs.[17] Injury to conducting airways could also potentially lead to an increase in regional airways resistance, with resultant gas trapping and progressive downstream regional lung distention. Regions of local superinfection and resultant inflammation may intensify the bronchiolar injury. Goldstein and associates used a piglet model and found cystic lung changes and areas of bronchiolectasis in animals that received intrabronchial inoculation with *Escherichia coli*.[18] The importance of bronchiolectasis in the pathogenesis of VILI is further highlighted by observations that the dead space (a potential prognostic marker in ARDS[19]) correlated with the presence and severity of bronchiolar injury and dilation.[20] In summary, macroscopic lung injury represents a continuum from airspace enlargement through interstitial emphysema and eventually to radiographically apparent extra-alveolar air.

MICROSCOPIC INJURY

More recent investigations have centered on the development of microscopic lung injury related to mechanical ventilation. Shortly after the institution of invasive positive pressure ventilation as a therapeutic modality, the development of lung damage was observed in animals ventilated for prolonged periods. The term "respirator lung" was coined to describe the functional and histologic features.[21] Subsequent investigations have demonstrated that mechanical ventilation, even at modest airway pressures, is capable of producing functional impairment of the lung with loss of integrity of the alveolar-capillary barrier, surfactant dysfunction, and parenchymal damage that mimics the histologic appearance of ARDS. These observations have led some investigators to speculate that mechanical ventilation itself could be contributing to some of the lung injury, morbidity, and mortality in patients with acute respiratory failure.

In 1974, Webb and Tierney graphically illustrated the deleterious effects of mechanical ventilation in rats using varying levels of peak airway pressure and PEEP.[22] Animals ventilated using low peak airway pressures (14 cm H_2O and no PEEP) had no pathologic or physiologic changes. In contrast, rats ventilated with peak pressures of 30 cm H_2O and no PEEP had perivascular edema and no alveolar edema. These findings were magnified in rats ventilated with peak pressures of 45 cm H_2O. Alveolar and perivascular edema developed, along with severe hypoxemia, decreased dynamic compliance, and obvious gross anatomic changes (Fig. 37-1). Interestingly, rats ventilated using 10 cm H_2O of PEEP and peak pressures of 45 cm H_2O had no alveolar edema (see Fig. 37-1, center). This latter finding led to the concept of a protective effect of PEEP, which will be discussed later.

HIGH AIRWAY PRESSURES AND LUNG INJURY

High airway pressures themselves are not responsible for lung injury. As anyone who has seen Dizzy Gillespie play the horn knows, high airway pressures do not produce alveolar disruption. Trumpet players are capable of generating large increases in airway pressure, up to 150 cm H_2O, without pulmonary sequelae.[23] The key factor causing lung injury is an increase in lung stretch that is best assessed in the pressure domain by the transpulmonary pressure (alveolar minus pleural pressure). For Dizzy Gillespie to generate such high airway pressures, he had to generate a high pleural pressure so the transpulmonary pressure was not elevated. Recently the emphasis has shifted away from the concept of pressure-induced injury (barotrauma) to lung overdistension (volutrauma). In this regard, peak inspiratory pressure (PIP) is often used at the bedside as a surrogate marker for the degree of lung inflation.

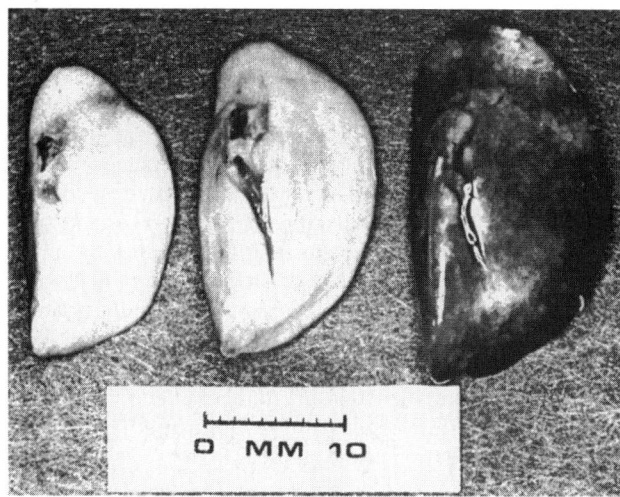

FIGURE 37-1 The effects of high distending pressures in rats and the protective effect of PEEP on the development of VILI. Rats ventilated using low airway pressures (14 cm H_2O and no PEEP) had no pathologic or physiologic changes (*left*). In contrast, rats ventilated with high airway pressures (45 cm H_2O and no PEEP) developed severe perivascular edema, hypoxemia, decreased dynamic compliance, and obvious gross anatomic changes (*right*). Importantly, the use of 10 cm H_2O of PEEP with peak pressures of 45 cm H_2O reduced the amount of lung injury (*center*). (*Reproduced with permission from Webb and Tierney.[22]*)

However, PIP is dependent on the resistive pressure drop arising from flow across the endotracheal tube and conducting airways, and is also dependent on the compliance of the respiratory system. Consequently, PIP may not be indicative of the degree of lung inflation; plateau pressure obtained after occlusion of the airway following inspiration more accurately reflects alveolar pressure, but is also hampered by the compliance of the respiratory system, and thus is also an inaccurate surrogate of lung distension. In normal individuals, full inspiration to total lung capacity (TLC) occurs at a transpulmonary pressure of 20 to 25 cm H_2O. Patients with hypoxic respiratory failure, however, are commonly ventilated with very high inspiratory pressures, producing transpulmonary pressures greater than 20 to 25 cm H_2O.[11] Plateau pressures in excess of 30 cm H_2O occur frequently and are often beyond the level expected to produce full inspiration.[24] The development of such high airway pressures in patients with ARDS could in turn lead to high transpulmonary pressures, and consequently to overdistention of lung units and lung injury.

Direct evidence for volutrauma stems from several observations in animals. To separate the effects of pressure and changes in lung volume, excursion of the chest (and hence tidal volume) was limited by binding the thorax during PPV.[25] Open-chest animals whose lungs were ventilated with peak pressures of 15 cm H_2O for 15 minutes had an 850% increase in their filtration coefficient. In contrast, the filtration coefficients of closed-chest animals increased by 31% with a PIP of 30 cm H_2O, and by 450% with a PIP of 45 cm H_2O. Animals in which lung expansion was limited did not develop lung edema during ventilation with peak airway pressures up to 45 cm H_2O. The concept of volutrauma as opposed to a pure pressure-related effect was further supported in a study that compared the development of edema with the use of negative-pressure ventilation and high tidal volumes, to that with the use of PPV to achieve similar tidal volumes.[26] The amount of edema obtained using negative-pressure ventilation was comparable to that in the animals ventilated with PPV at the same tidal volumes. These studies are important for two reasons. First, they established the importance of lung inflation, and second they demonstrated a dose-response relationship, with larger transpulmonary pressures and tidal volumes producing an incremental increase in lung injury and edema.[27] Theoretically, overdistention of lung units may lead to mechanical disruption of the alveolar-capillary barrier and the development of pulmonary edema.[28] In a very illustrative histologic study using electron microscopy, overdistention of the lung increased the number of endothelial and epithelial breaks and contributed to rupture of the blood-gas barrier and separation of the epithelium from its underlying basement membrane (Fig. 37-2).

Patients with patchy regions of lung injury may be particularly susceptible to the development of VILI. A nonuniform distribution of lung injury with regional differences in lung compliance may lead to regional differences in lung inflation. The importance of regional overdistention of lung units was emphasized in a study in dogs that compared the effect of delivering a PIP of 40 cm H_2O to the entire lung and delivering the same PIP to an isolated lung segment. Inflation of the entire lung did not result in edema.[29] However, distention of a small area for 20 minutes produced a protein-permeable epithelium. Thus inflation limited to a subsection of lung resulted in overdistention as the surrounding lung was compressed and allowed for greater expansion for a given PIP. This observation is particularly germane to the discussion of potential VILI in patients with inhomogeneous lung compliance, such as that described in ARDS. Consequently, the notion of a "safe" level of peak airway pressure in these patients must take into account the heterogeneous nature of the disease.

In addition to a time effect, there appear to be species- and age-specific differences in susceptibility to VILI. Younger and smaller animals seem more susceptible to the injurious effects of high airway pressures.[22,29–31] It has been postulated that this finding is due to immaturity of the alveolar-capillary barrier. Importantly, injured lungs also appear to be especially susceptible to the development of VILI. In rabbits with mild oleic acid–induced lung injury, the effects on lung edema of mechanical ventilation using high airway pressures were greater than those of either lung injury or mechanical ventilation alone.[32] Consequently, patients with underlying acute lung injury secondary to ARDS or pneumonia may be exquisitely sensitive to the adverse effects of mechanical ventilation, and predisposed to the development of VILI.

Gas flow rate may also be important in the development of lung injury. In one study, high flow rates were associated with an increase in filtration coefficient despite similar peak inspiratory pressures, although end-inspiratory lung volume was not accounted for.[33]

In summary, there is persuasive experimental evidence to support the concept of lung overdistention as a major component of VILI. Studies have demonstrated a dose-response relationship, in which both higher inflation pressures and tidal volumes administered over progressively longer periods of time produce a graded severity of lung injury. Second,

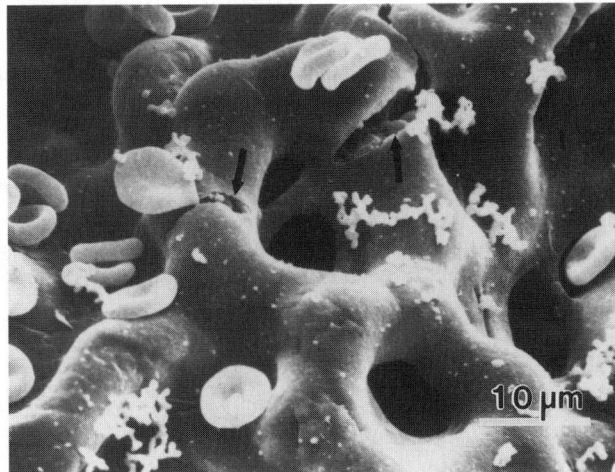

A

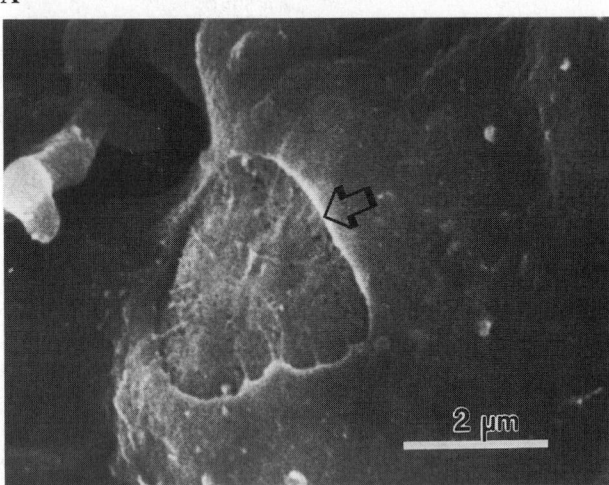

B

FIGURE 37-2 Scanning electron micrographs illustrating disruptions of the blood-gas barrier in rabbit lungs perfused at 20 cm H_2O transpulmonary pressure and 52.5 cm H_2O capillary transmural pressure. Examples of both endothelial (*a*) and epithelial stress failure (*b*) are shown. *A.* Adjacent capillaries with several areas of complete rupture of the blood-gas barrier (*arrows*) can be seen at various angles relative to the capillary axis; they have resulted in red blood cells and proteinaceous material accumulating on the alveolar surface. *B.* Round rupture involving only the epithelial layer (*arrow*). (*Reproduced with permission from Fu et al.*[28])

VILI has been demonstrated in many animal models, negating the possibility that these observations were due to a species-specific effect.

THE ROLE OF END-EXPIRATORY LUNG VOLUME

In addition to lung overdistention, it is becoming increasingly apparent that ventilation at low lung volumes may also lead to lung injury. Webb and Tierney[22] demonstrated that when animals were ventilated using high airway pressures without PEEP, significant edema and lung injury resulted. These effects were not seen when PEEP of 10 cm H_2O was used, even though the peak airway pressures were identical (see Fig. 37-1). Subsequent studies have confirmed these findings. For example in a canine aspiration model, low levels of PEEP during mechanical ventilation were associated with an increase in edema compared to ventilation with higher PEEP levels.[34] The precise mechanism of the effect of PEEP on VILI is controversial and potentially multifactorial. The application of PEEP is known to have effects on distribution of lung water, pulmonary hemodynamics, and pulmonary compliance. In patients with ARDS, providing PEEP may have one of three effects on the state of lung inflation. First, lung units that are already aerated may show increased distention, which could contribute to VILI. Second, partially aerated lung units or those that collapse at the end of a tidal breath may be kept patent during the entire respiratory cycle. Third, previously closed alveoli may be recruited, leading to an increase in functional lung and resulting in an increase in total lung compliance. The latter two points deserve further emphasis. In addition to an upper inflection point, a lower inflection point has been described in patients with ARDS. With a progressive increase in end-expiratory pressure, there is a gradual increase in end-expiratory lung volume or functional residual capacity (FRC), until a point is reached at which compliance improves.[35,36] This finding was supported in studies using CT, in which PEEP was found to reduce the vertical gradient of lung density and increase the amount of aerated lung.[6] Consequently, in patients with ARDS, the application of PEEP appears to result in the opening of nonventilated or poorly ventilated alveoli.

In addition to serving as a purely mechanical stent, PEEP may keep alveoli patent by preserving surfactant function (which has been observed to be functionally altered in ARDS), and in so doing may reduce surface tension and reduce the tendency of alveoli to close.[37,38] In a study evaluating the effect of PEEP, eight patients with ARDS initially underwent a lung recruitment procedure involving a period of sustained inflation.[39] When PEEP was decreased below the inflection point, a decay in lung compliance occurred. Interestingly, this study found a decelerating waveform to be more beneficial in producing an improvement in compliance than a constant-flow waveform. It was hypothesized that the decelerating waveform produced an initial high airway pressure that was maintained throughout the respiratory cycle, allowing recruitment of alveoli.[40] This concept is important and raises the possibility that peak airway pressures may in fact lead to alveolar recruitment, and that PEEP maintains the level of recruitment.

The relative importance of maintaining airway patency and using relatively high levels of PEEP is emphasized by recent observations that lung underdistention may be as injurious as lung overdistention and may contribute to the development of VILI. Ventilation without PEEP or at levels of PEEP that did not result in lung recruitment has been shown to cause respiratory and membranous bronchiolar injury, a reduction in lung compliance, and hyaline membrane formation.[41,42] In theory, ventilation at low lung volumes causes repetitive opening and closure of alveoli. This in turn may lead to the development of shear stress along the bronchial and alveolar walls. Repetitive stress is known to disrupt surfactant and is speculated to disrupt epithelial structures and contribute to failure of the alveolar-capillary barrier.

PEEP also improves gas exchange and lung mechanics, potentially by redistributing lung water from the alveolar to the extra-alveolar interstitial space.[43] Finally, PEEP also has significant hemodynamic effects and typically results in a reduction in ventricular preload and a reduction in cardiac output. Dreyfuss and Saumon postulated that the benefits of PEEP in ARDS stem from its effect on pulmonary perfusion, and demonstrated that the reduction of lung edema produced by PEEP was negated when dopamine was administered to keep arterial blood pressure constant.[26] They concluded that it was end-inspiratory volume, and not end-expiratory volume (FRC), that was important in the development of VILI. A recent study by Duggan and coworkers has highlighted the importance of atelectasis.[44] They evaluated the effects of a lung recruitment maneuver on lung and cardiac function. Animals whose lungs were not recruited (and presumably remained atelectatic) had a higher mortality, increased microvascular leak, worse oxygenation, and worse pulmonary vascular resistance. The increase in pulmonary vascular resistance may have led to the decrease in right ventricular function and increase in serum lactate in these animals.

In summary, in patients with ARDS, PEEP may improve lung compliance and oxygenation by recruiting alveoli and maintaining patency throughout the respiratory cycle (Fig. 37-3). Furthermore a ventilation strategy that fails to optimize end-expiratory volume with PEEP may contribute to VILI through the development of shear stress during repetitive opening and closing of lung units. Consequently, the notion of *best* PEEP needs to be extended to include an end-expiratory pressure level that will minimize lung injury.

BIOTRAUMA

It is becoming increasingly clear that mechanical stretch or shear injury leads to inflammatory mediator release and cellular activation. Mechanotransduction—whereby a physical stimulus produces cellular signaling—has been an area of active investigation, and in the setting of mechanical ventilation this effect has been termed *biotrauma*.[45,46] The notion that VILI may be responsible for the production of inflammatory mediators was highlighted in a study by Tremblay and associates in an isolated perfused rat model.[47] They demonstrated that the use of an injurious ventilation strategy (zero PEEP, high tidal volume, or both) had a dramatic influence on lung inflammatory mediators. Since this study, mechanical ventilation has been shown to be capable of causing the regional production of a variety of proinflammatory mediators, including tumor necrosis factor-α (TNF-α), interleukin-1β (IL-1β), interleukin-6 (IL-6), interleukin-10 (IL-10), macrophage inflammatory protein-2 (MIP-2), and interferon-γ (IFN-γ).[48–55] Indeed both overdistention (volutrauma) and underdistention (atelectrauma) may be equally important in inducing inflammatory mediator release.[51,56] However, as emphasized in an excellent review by Uhlig, it is important to differentiate the effects of cellular stretch– or shear stress–induced necrosis from true mechanotransduction, in which intracellular signaling occurs.[46] Cellular necrosis would potentially lead to the release of preformed cellular inflammatory mediators, while stimulation of intact cells would potentially lead to the release of preformed mediators via alterations in the cellular cytoskeleton, and from stimulation of mRNA and production of new proteins. The fact that production and release of inflammatory mediators does occur was illustrated by Tremblay and colleagues in an isolated perfused rat model of VILI, whereby injurious patterns

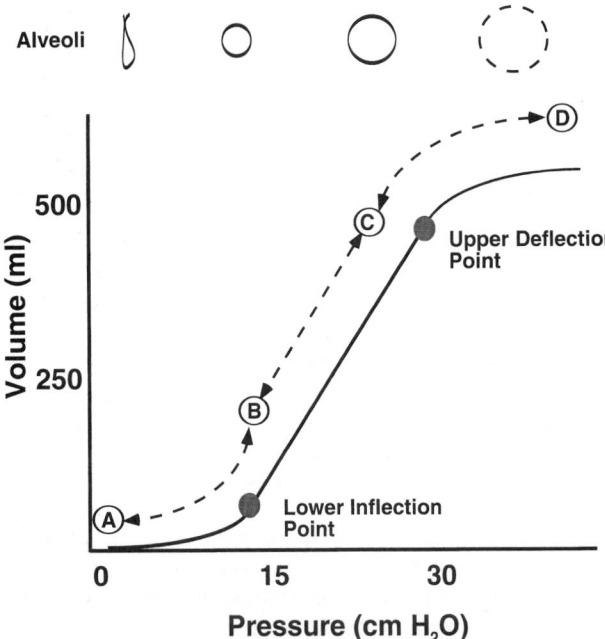

FIGURE 37-3 The sigmoidal shape of the pressure-volume curve of the respiratory system in a patient with ARDS. The outlines across the top of the graph indicate the relative state of inflation of alveoli. At airway pressures above the upper inflection point C (30 cm H_2O), the curve flattens as the limits of lung compliance are reached, and there is progressive overdistention of alveoli. Airway pressures below the lower inflection point B are also associated with lower compliance and result in alveolar collapse. A typical ventilation strategy using 15 cm H_2O of PEEP and a PIP of 40 cm H_2O (points B to D) would lead to repetitive inflation above the upper inflection point, and potentially to disruption of alveoli and the alveolar-capillary barrier (see text). A strategy that attempts to reduce lung distention by reducing PIP (points A to C) would still lead to repetitive opening and closure of alveoli (also associated with lung injury). An optimal ventilation strategy should consider both the lower and upper inflection points of the pressure-volume curve (points B to C). Note also that for the same driving pressure (the segments from A to B, B to C, or C to D), a change in pressure from points B to C is associated with the largest change in lung volume. Thus an optimal ventilation strategy should aim for volume excursions along the steepest portion of the pressure-volume curve (maximal compliance).

of mechanical ventilation led to an increase in production of c-fos mRNA.[50]

The concept of ventilator-induced mechanotransduction and subsequent inflammation is evolving and the cellular source of inflammatory mediators and subsequent lung injury is an area of active research.[57,58] Both inflammatory cells and pulmonary epithelial cells appear to be capable of responding to mechanical stresses. Earlier workers attributed the increase in lung lavage cytokines predominantly to production by neutrophils and macrophages.[59,60] More recent attention has focused on mesenchymal cells. Mechanical stretch of cultured fetal rat lung cells increased the expression of MIP-2, a potent neutrophil chemokine.[58] Interestingly stretch alone did not lead to an increase in MIP-2 mRNA expression while stretch in addition to LPS did. This finding and the rapid increase in MIP-2 following stretch suggested that stretch alone leads to secretion and not synthesis of MIP-2. The same group

later demonstrated increased expression of TNF-α and IL-6 mRNA in pulmonary epithelial cells following the application of an injurious ventilatory strategy, in an ex-vivo rat model.[50] Importantly, they demonstrated that the epithelial cells were a major source of TNF-α. These findings are extremely relevant as they support the notion that mechanical stretching or injury to the lung epithelium is sufficient to stimulate an inflammatory response and potentially recruit neutrophils to the lung.[59]

In addition to epithelial cells, endothelial cellular stretch may also lead to the development of a proinflammatory state. Using a novel method of cellular recovery and evaluation of endothelial cells, Bhattacharya and coworkers demonstrated that lung stretch was capable of inducing P-selectin expression on the cell surface through a tyrosine phosphorylation signaling pathway.[61] Indeed the importance of endothelial expression of cell surface receptors may be critical to the development of neutrophil accumulation in the lungs.[62] Bhattacharya and coworkers also observed that lung stretch lead to the development of focal adhesions, suggesting that endothelial cells actively respond to the adverse mechanical milieu, and that the matrix proteins participated in this response. Several investigations have suggested that stretch-induced release of matrix proteins is an important mediator of VILI.[63,64] In particular, the release of matrix metalloproteinases (a group of enzymes that are capable of damaging the extracellular matrix and stimulating fibroblasts) and fibronectin have been reported to be upregulated in models of VILI.[58,65]

The inflammatory effects induced by injurious ventilatory strategies may be attenuated by pretreatment with corticosteroids or heat stress (presumably by induction of heat shock proteins).[48,66,67] Ohta and colleagues demonstrated that 250 mg/kg of methylprednisone suppressed markers of neutrophil activation in rats subjected to high-tidal-volume ventilation.[66] Similarly Held and coworkers[48] demonstrated that administration of dexamethasone blocked the release of nuclear factor-κB (NF-κB), cytokines, and chemokines in an isolated perfused mouse model of endotoxin-mediated acute lung injury and VILI. From a clinical perspective these observations are enticing. They also raise the possibility that the late phase of ARDS, characterized by fever and persistent airspace disease, in some patients may be mediated by ongoing ventilator-induced lung injury.[68–70] Thus the experimental observation that corticosteroids are capable of modifying the inflammatory response from VILI *may* also account for the observed improvement in these patients with persistent ARDS following the administration of glucocorticoids.[71]

In summary mechanotransduction due to lung distention during mechanical ventilation appears to be capable of stimulating signaling pathways with secretion of inflammatory mediators in a variety of cells including neutrophils, macrophages, epithelial and endothelial cells, and the extracellular matrix. However, in the face of these observations, the notion that VILI contributes to mortality in patients with ARDS presents somewhat of a paradox, as most patients with ARDS do not typically succumb to progressive hypoxic respiratory failure from worsening lung injury. Rather, death in these patients is caused by the development of multiple organ dysfunction.[72,73] However, recent experimental and clinical studies suggest that ongoing VILI is capable of causing nonpulmonary organ injury through the translocation of regional inflammatory mediators and bacteria into the systemic circulation.

DECOMPARTMENTALIZATION

Damage to the alveolar-capillary barrier from mechanical ventilation may be central to several important pathophysiologic mechanisms in the development of VILI. First, loss of membrane integrity is key to the development of the pulmonary edema and hyaline membrane formation—the hallmarks of ARDS. The loss of barrier function may also allow for entry of inflammatory cells into the lung, in turn promoting the perturbation of lung structure and function. More recently, however, the loss of the integrity of the alveolar-capillary membrane has been proposed to be central to the spread of lung inflammation (partially produced by mechanical injury) to nonpulmonary organs, and thus may lead to their subsequent dysfunction.

The development of increased edema fluid during mechanical ventilation is in part due to an increase in filtration of fluid into the interstitial space.[74,75] With progressive lung inflation, a decrease in interstitial pressure occurs.[76] In addition, lung inflation causes dilation of extra-alveolar vessels. The net effect of progressive lung inflation, therefore, is an increase in the hydrostatic gradient for fluid to move from the capillaries into the interstitial space.[76–78] In addition to an increase in filtration, ventilation with high lung volumes may also cause an increase in permeability of the alveolar-capillary barrier to proteins. Several studies have demonstrated an increase in filtration coefficient during mechanical ventilation.[29,79] This effect is thought to be due to a reduction in the integrity of the alveolar-capillary barrier. During mechanical ventilation, injury has been demonstrated to occur to both the epithelial and endothelial membranes. Both edema and injury to the alveolar-capillary barrier can develop rapidly, with transient alterations in filtration coefficient occurring in animals ventilated for only 2 minutes.[80] Subsequent studies have demonstrated that ventilation for more prolonged periods is associated with progressively worse edema, which becomes irreversible. In rats ventilated for 5 to 20 minutes, extravascular fluid accumulation increased with time of ventilation, progressing from perivascular edema to interstitial edema, and eventually to alveolar edema. Damage to type I cells, denudation of the basement membrane, and hyaline membrane formation were seen at 20 minutes. Thus mechanical ventilation appears to have a cumulative effect, with increased exposure to high airway pressures resulting in progressive and eventually sustained lung injury.

It seems logical that the movement of proteins would not be unidirectional from circulation to lung. Indeed recent evidence suggests that translocation of proteins occurs from lung to circulation as well. Using a rat model of VILI, Lesur and associates demonstrated an increase in total protein in lung lavage fluid with lung overdistention.[81] Furthermore they demonstrated that Clara cell protein (found in high concentrations in Clara cells located in terminal bronchioles) decreased in lung lavage fluid with time, but increased in the serum of the rats. These observations are highly relevant and demonstrate that mechanical ventilation can lead to bidirectional translocation of proteins. Promotion of translocation of endotoxin and bacteria from the lungs to the circulation has also been demonstrated to be a feature of VILI.[82–84] This loss

of compartmentalization and resultant translocation of proteins, potential inflammatory mediators, and bacteria may be central to the development of more distal organ damage. The concern then is that the lung may become the machinery for multiple-organ dysfunction syndrome (MODS). Indeed Choi and associates recently demonstrated that large tidal volumes produced both pulmonary and renal microvascular leakage of protein and Evans blue dye.[85] Interestingly, endothelial nitric oxide synthase (eNOS) expression was significantly increased in the affected lung and kidney samples. Their observation that inhibition of eNOS attenuated the degree of microvascular leakage supported the notion that eNOS contributed to the loss of the integrity of the membrane barrier. These observations were extended in a recent study by Imai and associates.[86] They demonstrated that serum from rabbits that were ventilated with an injurious ventilation strategy was capable of increasing the rate of apoptosis in cultured epithelial cells from the kidney and villi of the small intestine (Fig. 37-4). Functionally this correlated with biochemical evidence of worsened renal function when intact animals were studied.

That distal organ injury in humans may be mediated by mechanical ventilation is supported by two observations. First, studies in humans have shown that an injurious ventilator strategy leads to an increase in circulating cytokine levels. Ranieri and coworkers randomized 44 patients to receive either mechanical ventilation to maintain normal blood gases (n = 19), or a lung-protective strategy attentive to both lung distention and maintenance of an adequate end-expiratory lung volume (above the lower inflection point; see below).[53] Despite similar levels of circulating cytokines at baseline, patients in the control group had an increase in plasma concentrations of TNF-α, IL-6, and TNF-α receptors over a period of 36 hours. Conversely, patients in the lung-protective strategy group had a reduction in plasma concentrations of IL-6, soluble TNF-α receptor 75, and IL-1 receptor antagonist. Additionally they found that the concentration of the inflammatory mediators 36 hours after randomization was significantly lower in the lung-protective strategy group than in the control group. In a subsequent analysis of the serum in 11 of the controls and 9 of the lung-protective strategy group, levels of soluble Fas ligand (shown to induce apoptosis in human epithelial cells in vitro[87,88]) and creatinine were found to be elevated in the controls.[89]

Lung-Protective Strategies: Do No Harm

Traditionally, the goals of mechanical ventilation have been to maintain adequate tissue oxygenation (generally accepted as a saturation greater than 90%, with a reasonable cardiac output) and adequate ventilation to achieve normocarbia and maintain normal blood pH. To achieve these goals, patients with acute respiratory failure were often ventilated using a standard ventilation cocktail consisting of variable levels of PEEP and oxygen, and a tidal volume in the range of 10 to 15 mL/kg. This strategy was often employed with little regard for the underlying cause of respiratory failure. However, based on the forgoing discussion, adopting such a strategy may be deleterious. Consequently clinical trials and experimental endeavors have focused on the development of lung-protective strategies. The principal objectives of a lung-protective strategy are to limit alveolar distention and

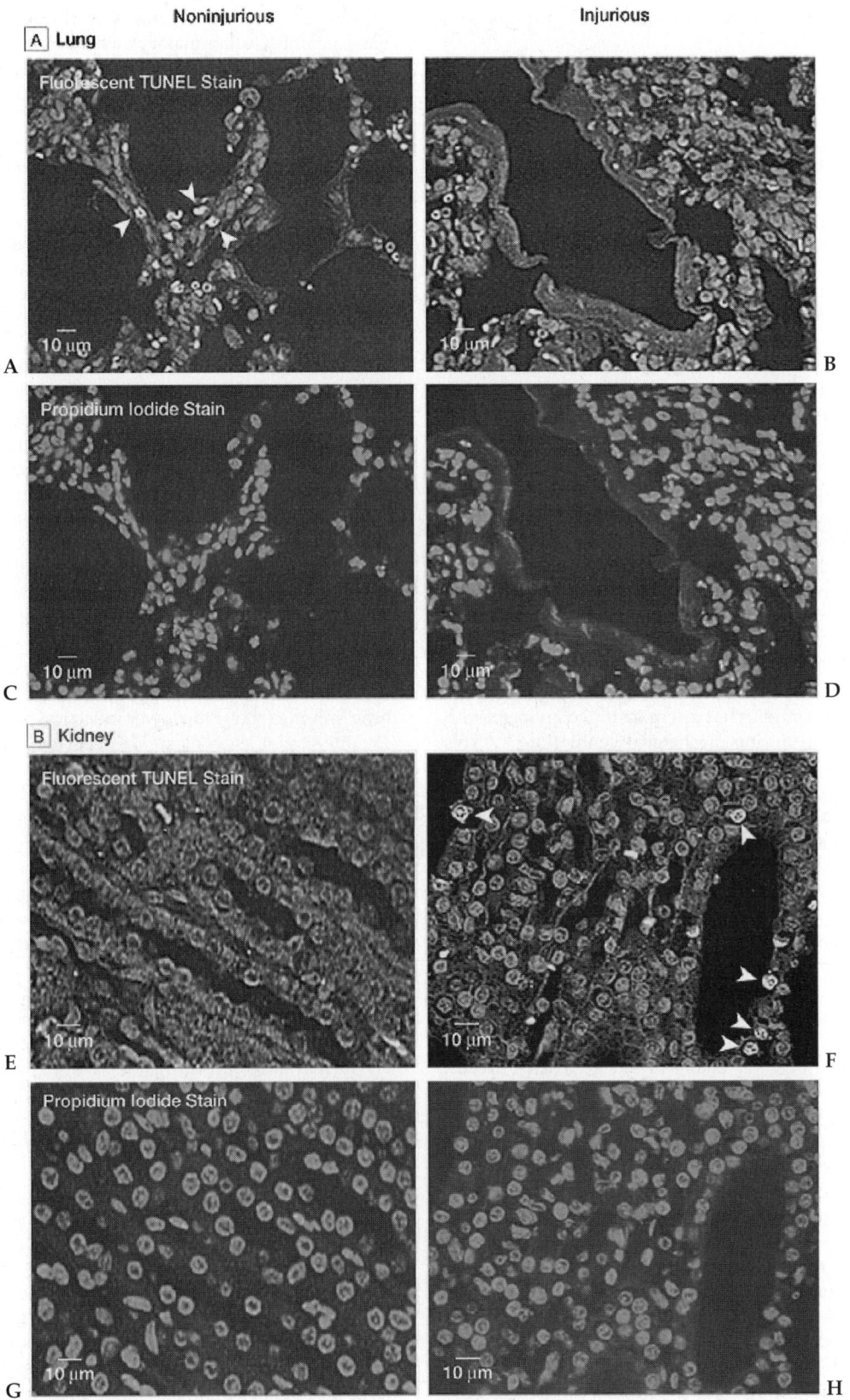

FIGURE 37-4 There was greater apoptosis of renal tubular epithelial cells in the group that received injurious mechanical ventilation compared to the group that received the noninjurious strategy, as evidenced by the greater number of TUNEL-positive cells (*arrowheads*) in the injurious group. Terminal deoxynucleotidyltransferase-mediated dUTP nick end-labeling (TUNEL) staining identifies the apoptotic cell, and propidium iodide staining identifies nuclei and helps ensure that noncellular background staining is not inadvertently identified as a TUNEL-positive cell (original magnification ×400). (*Reproduced with permission from Imai et al.[89]*) (See Color Plate 37-4.)

maintain alveolar patency. A lung-protective strategy should be implemented early in the course of respiratory failure to prevent the development of VILI.

There are four potential strategies, none of which are mutually exclusive, to reduce alveolar overdistention. The first strategy is to limit inflation pressure. Current opinion and recommendations from a consensus conference on mechanical ventilation in ARDS recommend that plateau pressure be kept below 35 cm H_2O in patients with ARDS. However, as emphasized in a review by Brower,[90] a strategy that focuses on plateau pressure alone may still produce potentially injurious tidal volumes. Conversely, another limitation of using airway pressure as an indicator of lung inflation is that this method assumes that chest wall (including abdominal) compliance is normal. Patients with ARDS and conditions such as obesity or ascites may have a significantly reduced abdominal compliance. Consequently, high airway pressures may not be a reflection of overdistention. A second strategy to prevent lung overdistention is to limit tidal volume. This strategy is attractive because it is simple and eliminates concerns about changes in thoracic or abdominal compliance. In addition, this method was shown to be effective in decreasing mortality compared to conventional lung volumes.[2] The potential difficulty with limiting volume is that the tidal volume used is still rather arbitrary and does not take into account the severity of lung injury. In fact, the ARDS Network study[2] used a protocol that limited tidal volume to 6 mL/kg predicted body weight (PBW) *and* limited plateau pressures to less than 30 cm H_2O. It is clear based on this study that tidal volumes of 12 mL/kg are excessive. What is not known at present is whether 6 mL/kg PBW volumes are superior to larger volumes (8 to 10 mL/kg). Whether 6 mL/kg is superior or inferior to 8 mL/kg remains a matter of debate. However, until evidence to support the contrary emerges, 6 mL/kg PBW should be considered the standard of care. It is worth emphasizing that the ARDS Network trial based tidal volumes on the patient's PBW, and not measured body weight. In this study a tidal volume of 6 mL/kg based on predicted body weight was on average equivalent to a tidal volume of 5 mL/kg measured body weight.

THE PRESSURE-VOLUME CURVE IN ACUTE RESPIRATORY DISTRESS SYNDROME

Some argue that ventilator settings should be individualized based on the pressure-volume (P-V) curve (see Fig. 37-3).[24] Examination of the P-V relationship of the lungs of patients with ARDS provides a good conceptualization of the changes that occur during ARDS, and has been instrumental in the development of strategies of mechanical ventilation to reduce lung injury in these patients. Indeed one approach to optimize ventilation in patients with ARDS makes use of the shape of the P-V curve, in order to maintain lung inflation between the upper and lower inflection points. With a progressive increase in static airway pressure, there is a gradual increase in lung volume, which depends on the compliance of the respiratory system. As lung inflation approaches total lung capacity, a similar increase in airway pressure produces less lung inflation, and the P-V curve begins to flatten. This is often referred to as the *upper inflection point*. Continued inflation beyond this point results in overdistention of alveoli and increases the risk for macroscopic and microscopic lung injury. Similarly (although more controversial a notion) the lower inflection point is felt to reflect opening of atelectatic regions of

the lung. It has been suggested that the level of PEEP be maintained above this level to avoid cyclic injury (atelectrauma) to the lung. However, this attractive approach has a number of problems. First, use of PEEP a few cm H_2O above the lower inflection curve does not ensure that the lung is recruited; indeed recruitment takes place over the entire steep portion of the P-V curve.[91–93] Secondly, the upper inflection point may indicate the completion of recruitment, rather than the development of overdistension.[93] Furthermore, for the practicing intensivist, determining the lower inflection point may not be practical. Some guidance is provided by studies that suggest that in most patients with ARDS, PEEP levels above 15 cm H_2O are generally required to maintain lung inflation above the lower inflection point.[24,94]

PERMISSIVE HYPERCAPNIA

Permissive hypercapnia was first described in patients with asthma who were being mechanically ventilated. In an attempt to reduce dynamic hyperinflation and gas trapping, minute ventilation was decreased to allow sufficient expiratory time for the lung to empty via the obstructed airways. Relative to historical controls, patients managed in this manner had much better outcomes, with less barotrauma and less time spent receiving mechanical ventilation.[95,96] The concept of permissive hypercapnia was extended to the management of patients with ARDS, and follows occasionally from a mechanical ventilation strategy that demands a restriction in tidal volume. It should be emphasized that permissive hypercapnia does not represent a method of mechanical ventilation per se. Rather, it is the consequence of a strategy that limits lung volume excursions in an attempt to minimize alveolar overdistention and hence VILI. In an uncontrolled study, Hickling and associates described the use of a pressure-limited strategy and permissive hypercapnia in patients with advanced ARDS. Mortality was significantly lower than that which would have been predicted from the APACHE II score alone.[97] This was subsequently confirmed by some of the same authors in a prospective uncontrolled study in patients with ARDS.[98] These were landmark studies, but used historical controls, the method of ventilation was not well defined, and efforts were made concurrently to limit oxygen toxicity. Therefore, these studies suggested, but did not conclusively prove, that a pressure-limited strategy and disregard for the partial arterial pressure of carbon dioxide (Pa_{CO_2}) improved outcome. Importantly, serious side effects of an elevation of Pa_{CO_2} were not observed in either study.

The physiologic consequences of hypercapnia and respiratory acidosis have been reviewed extensively.[99,100] At present, the only absolute contraindication to a rise in Pa_{CO_2} is increased intracranial pressure, although acute hypercarbia may have adverse effects on the fetus in gravid individuals. In patients with critical illness and impaired oxygen delivery, there have been concerns about effects on cardiovascular performance. However, the potential myocardial depressant effects are usually short-lived owing to the buffering capacity of myocytes and the increase in sympathetic activity and decrease in afterload that accompany hypercapnia.[101] Caution, however, is warranted in patients with evidence of myocardial dysfunction. A final concern surrounds the increase in pulmonary arterial pressures that develops with hypercapnic acidosis. This response is likely mediated by a reduction in nitric oxide and has been shown to be reversible with nitric oxide inhalation.[102] In the face of these concerns hypercapnia has been shown to be protective in a variety of settings.[103–106] Indeed it has been postulated that hypercapnia may attenuate the severity of acute lung injury, or at the very least that the development of hypocapnia may be harmful.[100,103,107,108] Hypercapnic acidosis has been shown to attenuate protein leakage, lung edema, lung lavage inflammatory mediators, and lung injury score, and preserve oxygenation and lung compliance in several models of lung injury (Fig. 37-5).[1,108–110]

More controversial is whether the resulting respiratory acidosis should be corrected by the infusion of a buffer solution. Although some advocate the use of a bicarbonate

FIGURE 37-5 A representative micrograph of lung tissue from a hypercapnic animal. The alveoli are free of edema and cellular infiltrate (*A*), normal parenchymal architecture is maintained, and only a small number of macrophages are present in the alveoli (*arrow*). *B*. A comparable micrograph from the eucapnic group. There is marked cellular infiltration in the interstitium and alveoli (*arrows*), which also fills the lumen of a bronchiole (BR). Alveolar and interstitial edema, as well as hyaline membrane formation (*arrowheads*) are also present (hematoxylin and eosin stained; 120× magnification; scale indicates 100 μm). (*Reproduced with permission from Sinclair et al.*[125]) (See Color Plate 37-5.)

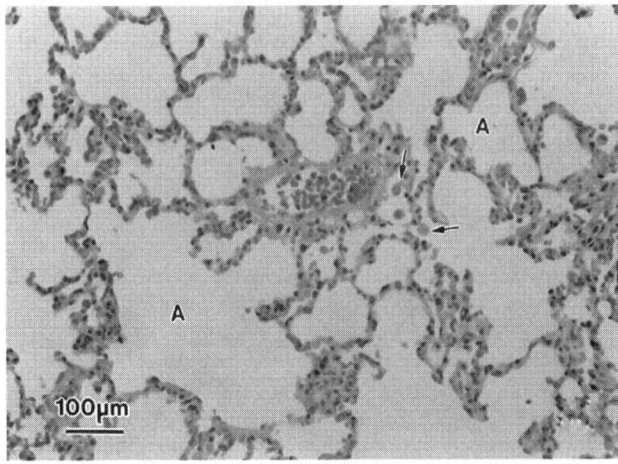

A

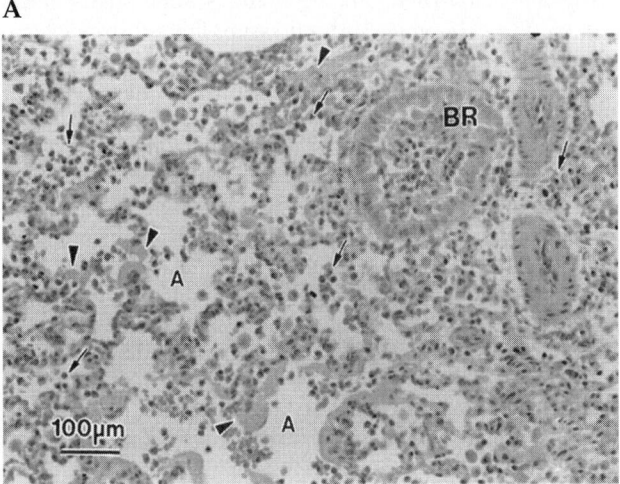

B

infusion, in the setting of impaired ventilation the additional CO_2 generated during the buffering of H^+ with bicarbonate might worsen intracellular pH. Second, as pointed out by Feihl and Perret, very large doses of bicarbonate are required to produce a significant improvement in pH during hypercapnia, owing to the large volume of distribution of the bicarbonate ion, to renal bicarbonate losses, and to conversion of bicarbonate to CO_2.[99] In addition, although extracellular pH is low, intracellular pH is rapidly corrected and seldom becomes critical. Consequently, the slow bicarbonate infusion recommended by some studies is not likely to be of benefit, and the routine administration of bicarbonate during permissive hypercapnia remains controversial. Indeed Laffey and coworkers demonstrated that correction of hypercapnic acidosis worsened lung function in an ischemia-reperfusion lung injury model.[107] Other buffers such as Carbicarb may theoretically be more efficacious in the setting of hypercapnia.[99,111]

CLINICAL TRIALS

Based on the foregoing discussions several controlled clinical trials have evaluated the effects of a lung protective strategy on outcome in ARDS (Table 37-3). However, initial randomized clinical trials evaluating the effect of lower tidal volumes on outcome were disappointing.[112–114] There was even a suggestion that tidal volume restriction was harmful, as it was associated with a greater use of neuromuscular blockers, a greater need for dialysis (perhaps related to the lower pH from a higher Pa_{CO_2}), and a trend toward higher mortality. In the study by Stewart and associates, the mortality in the tidal volume restriction arm was 50% compared to the control arm mortality of 47%, while in the study by Brochard and colleagues, the mortality was 47% and 39%, respectively.[112,114] However, the NIH-sponsored multicenter study of patients with ARDS has vindicated many of the earlier animal studies and clinical trials.[2] In this trial patients were randomized to receive either "conventional" tidal volumes (12 mL/kg PBW; tidal volume was reduced if plateau pressure was greater than 50 cm H_2O), or a lower tidal volume (6 mL/kg PBW, and maintenance of a plateau pressure between 25 and 30 cm H_2O). The trial was stopped early after an interim analysis demonstrated a survival benefit in the group with low tidal volume (Fig. 37-6). Mortality was reduced by 22% from 40% in the conventional arm to 31% in the low-lung-volume arm (CI 2.4 to 15.3 percent difference between the groups). The benefit of a lung-protection strategy seemed to be independent of the severity of the lung compliance at baseline. In addition to a mortality effect, the number of days alive and free of mechanical ventilation was lower in the intervention arm. However, this effect was solely due to the reduction in mortality, as the median duration of mechanical ventilation was 8 days for survivors in both groups. The benefit did not appear to differ when patients were stratified based on their risk factor for ARDS.[115] Interestingly the number of days with nonpulmonary organ failure was lower in the intervention arm, and the plasma interleukin-6 concentration was decreased compared to the control group. This again supported the notion that a lung protection strategy achieved its benefit through a reduction in the systemic release of inflammatory mediators

TABLE 37-3 Clinical Trials Evaluating the Effects of Different Lung-Protective Strategies on Outcome in Acute Respiratory Distress Syndrome

Study	Intervention Used	TIDAL VOLUMES USED, mL/kg		PEEP, cm H_2O		RECRUITMENT		Outcome
		Intervention	Control	Intervention	Control	Intervention	Control	
Brower (n = 52)	Low stretch	7.3 ± 0.1 (day 5)	10.2 ± 0.1 (day 5)	8 (day 3)	8 (day 3)	None	—	No differences
Amato (n = 53)	Low stretch, lung open; using P-V curve[a]	Not reported Goal <6	Not reported Goal >12	Not reported P-Flex	Not reported P-Flex	Yes	None	A, B, E
Brochard (n = 116)	Low stretch	7.1 ± 1.3 (day 1)	10.3 ± 1.7 (day 1)	—	—	None	None	No differences
Stewart (n = 120)	Low stretch	7.2 ± 0.8 (day 3)	10.8 ± 1.0 (day 3)	8.7 ± 3.6 (day 3)	8.4 ± 3.8 (day 3)	None	None	C
ARDS Network (n = 861)	Low stretch	6.2 ± 0.8 (day 3)	11.8 ± 0.8 (day 3)	9.2 ± 3.6 (day 3)	8.6 ± 4.2 (day 3)	None	None	A, D
ALVEOLI trial (n = 550) stopped early	Low stretch, lung open	Goal was 6	Goal was 6	Goal of 2–6 cm H_2O> controls	Same as ARDSNet trial	Yes	None	No differences in mortality; unpublished
LOVS trial (ongoing)	Low stretch, lung open; present PEEP levels depending on FI_{O_2}	Ongoing goal is 6	Ongoing goal is 10	High	Same as ARDSNet trial	Yes	None	Ongoing

ABBREVIATIONS: [a]PEEP was adjusted in the intervention arm to 2 to 4 cm H_2O greater than the lower inflection point (P-Flex). PEEP, positive end-expiratory pressure; FI_{O_2}, fraction of inspired oxygen. A = Reduction in mortality compared to conventional group. B = Improvement in physiological parameters (oxygenation and compliance). C = Suggestion of worse outcome in the lung protection group. D = Reduction in inflammatory mediators. E = Reduction in barotrauma.

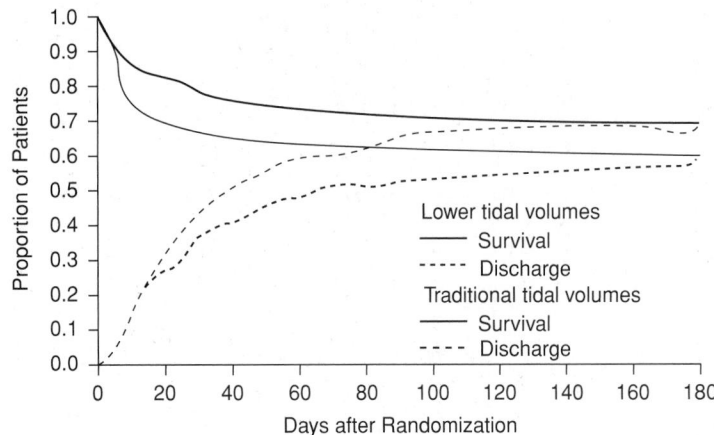

FIGURE 37-6 Probability of survival, being discharged home, and breathing without assistance during the first 180 days after randomization in patients with acute lung injury and ARDS randomized to either the 12 mL/kg PBW or 6 mL/kg PBW treatment arms. *(Reproduced with permission from the ARDS Network Group.[2])*

and reduction in severity of multiple system organ failure. Unlike previous studies, however, there was no difference in the use of neuromuscular blockers.

It is difficult to reconcile the difference in the results of the ARDSNet study with earlier clinical trials evaluating a lung volume restriction strategy, because the ARDSNet study differed in several ways, making direct comparisons difficult.[116] First, the method of determining predicted body weight (and hence tidal volume) was different from earlier trials. Second, patients in the low-tidal-volume arm had higher respiratory rates that may have led to significant auto-PEEP, in turn leading to improved alveolar patency or recruitment. Third, the respiratory acidosis was more likely to be corrected with bicarbonate. This may have reduced the number of patients dialyzed, and could have reduced some of the yet to be determined effects of hypercapnic acidosis.

A concern regarding the safety of the ventilation trials conducted in patients with ARDS has recently been raised. In a review of the controlled trials of mechanical ventilation in ARDS, Eichacker and associates presented the argument that 12 mL/kg was potentially excessive, and that the use of this tidal volume as the reference intervention was inappropriate, placing patients in the control arm at risk.[117] The authors argued that there should have been a control group that better reflected "conventional" treatment. What tidal volume this control group would have actually been managed with is speculative. The reader is referred to an excellent review of the controversy and its consequences by Steinbrook.[118] The implications for this issue for the design and conduct of subsequent trials remain to be seen, but at present the ARDSNet strategy for ventilation of ARDS patients should be viewed as the standard.

In addition to lung overdistention, VILI also incorporates the concept that underdistention of alveolar units can also lead to injury. At present there are only two clinical trials that have evaluated the effects of an "open lung" approach to patients with ARDS. The first study by Amato and colleagues examined the effect of a multifaceted strategy that (1) minimized tidal volume, (2) recruited alveoli through a sustained inflation, (3) used a level of PEEP above the closing pressure of the lung, and (4) utilized a pressure-volume curve to define the optimum lung volume and PEEP.[119] Consequently the specific effects of maintaining alveolar patency cannot be determined from this trial. Nonetheless, using this

strategy they demonstrated an impressive reduction in mortality. However, the major criticism of this study is that the control group was significantly disadvantaged by a protocol that allowed for significant overventilation, and that the observed results were not due to a benefit in the treatment arm, but rather a detrimental outcome in the control group.

In order to make specific recommendations about the optimum strategy, the relative effects of tidal volume reduction, alveolar recruitment, and level of PEEP need to be determined. To this end two multicenter trials are evaluating the effect of lung recruitment and high PEEP on outcome in ARDS. The ARDS Network has reported the results of their trial (ALVEOLI trial) that was closed after enrolling 550 patients, citing a finding of futility in the trial being able to determine a treatment effect during an interim analysis.[124] In an ongoing Canadian trial over 800 patients will be randomized to either low tidal volumes (identical to the ARDSNet low stretch trial) or a low tidal volume with an open lung approach. The open lung approach will utilize both periodic sustained inflations to 40 cm H_2O continuous positive airway pressure for 40 seconds and high levels of PEEP (up to 20 cm H_2O). It is hoped that this strategy will ensure both alveolar recruitment and maintenance of alveolar patency, respectively. Preliminary evidence suggests that this strategy may lead to a significant improvement in oxygenation in a subset of patients with early ARDS and no impairment in chest wall mechanics.[120] Whether this physiologic improvement and attendant reduction in atelectasis will lead to an improvement in survival has yet to be proven.

High-frequency oscillation (HFO) may accomplish many of the goals of a lung-protective strategy. It utilizes small tidal volume excursions at a high mean airway pressure. Consequently lung overdistention may be prevented and alveolar patency may be maintained. In a study of HFO in 70 pediatric patients with ARDS, Arnold and associates reported an improvement in oxygenation and requirement for supplemental oxygen at 30 days in the HFO group.[121] However there was no difference in duration of mechanical ventilation or survival. These observed improvements in physiologic parameters were also found in a study by Derdak and coworkers.[122] In a multicenter randomized controlled trial of HFO compared to what was at that time a conventional ventilatory strategy, in 148 adults with ARDS they found no difference in survival or duration of mechanical ventilation.

However the oxygenation was better in the HFO group during the study. These reports suggest that HFO is at least as safe as conventional mechanical ventilation, and may be associated with a more rapid improvement in oxygenation. However, both trials were hampered by the fact that the control group likely did not represent the current standard of care, namely tidal volumes of 6 mL/kg PBW. It remains to be seen if HFO is any more efficacious than a strategy that restricts tidal volume (with or without a strategy to maintain alveolar patency).

Even in the face of overwhelming experimental evidence and convincing results of a large controlled study, one of the major challenges faced by intensivists seems to be implementing these recommendations in practice. Two studies have demonstrated that compliance with the ARDS Network tidal volume goals are poor, even in those centers that participated in the original trial. Clearly education and protocolization of care will need to occur to allow best evidence to be translated into clinical practice.[3,116]

ARDS continues to be a common component of multisystem organ dysfunction and primary lung injury. Unfortunately, no pharmacologic intervention has proven to be efficacious in reducing mortality in patients with ARDS. An improved understanding of ARDS and the notion that prior ventilator strategies may have been injurious has led to rethinking how these patients should be supported.

Summary

In addition to theoretical concerns and experimental data in animals, evidence is evolving that our traditional goals of ventilation need to be modified to incorporate a lung-protective strategy (see Table 12-1). The low-lung-volume ARDSNet trial demonstrated a reduction in mortality with the implementation of a lung-protective strategy. However, it is a matter of perspective as to whether the intervention produced benefit, or simply that harm was avoided. Given the complex nature of ARDS, it is likely that a multifaceted strategy that incorporates several principles of VILI will need to be adopted. Limiting tidal volume may only be a component of a lung-protective strategy. Support is evolving for attempting to recruit alveoli and for the use of liberal PEEP. Future research on the effects of mechanical ventilation on regional and distal cellular signaling, apoptosis, and distal organ injury need to be explored further, incorporating recent advances in genomic and proteomic methods.[123]

References

1. Slutsky AS: Mechanical ventilation. American College of Chest Physicians' Consensus Conference. *Chest* 104:1833, 1993.
2. The Acute Respiratory Distress Syndrome Network: Ventilation with lower tidal volumes as compared with traditional tidal volumes for acute lung injury and the acute respiratory distress syndrome. *N Engl J Med* 342:1301, 2000.
3. Weinert C R, Gross CR, Marinelli WA: Impact of randomized trial results on acute lung injury ventilator therapy in teaching hospitals. *Am J Respir Crit Care Med* 5:5, 2003.
4. Gattinoni L, Bombino M, Pelosi P, et al: Lung structure and function in different stages of severe adult respiratory distress syndrome. *JAMA* 271:1772, 1994.
5. Maunder RJ, Pierson DJ, Hudson LD: Subcutaneous and mediastinal emphysema. Pathophysiology, diagnosis, and management. *Arch Intern Med* 144:1447, 1984.
6. Pelosi P, D'Andrea L, Vitale G, et al: Vertical gradient of regional lung inflation in adult respiratory distress syndrome. *Am J Respir Crit Care Med* 149:8, 1994.
7. Mead J, Takishima T, Leith D: Stress distribution in lungs: a model of pulmonary elasticity. *J Appl Physiol* 28:596, 1970.
8. Gattinoni L, Pesenti A, Avalli L, et al: Pressure-volume curve of total respiratory system in acute respiratory failure. Computerized tomographic study. *Am Rev Respir Dis* 136:730, 1987.
9. Marcy TW: Barotrauma: detection, recognition, and management. *Chest* 104:578, 1993.
10. Macklin MT, Macklin CC: Malignant interstitial emphysema of the lungs and mediastinum as an important occult complication in many respiratory diseases and other conditions: an interpretation of the clinical literature in the light of laboratory experiments. *Medicine* 23:281, 1944.
11. Gammon BR, Shin MS, Buchalter SE: Pulmonary barotrauma in mechanical ventilation. Patterns and risk factors. *Chest* 102:568, 1992.
12. Gammon RB, Shin MS, Groves RH Jr, et al: Clinical risk factors for pulmonary barotrauma: A multivariate analysis. *Am J Respir Crit Care Med* 152:1235, 1995.
13. Williams TJ, Tuxen DV, Scheinkestel CD, et al: Risk factors for morbidity in mechanically ventilated patients with acute severe asthma. *Am Rev Respir Dis* 146:607, 1992.
14. Petersen GW, Baier H: Incidence of pulmonary barotrauma in a medical ICU. *Crit Care Med* 11:67, 1983.
15. Eisner MD, Thompson BT, Schoenfeld D, et al, and the Acute Respiratory Distress Syndrome Network: Airway pressures and early barotrauma in patients with acute lung injury and acute respiratory distress syndrome. *Am J Respir Crit Care Med* 165:978, 2002.
16. Woodring J H: Pulmonary interstitial emphysema in the adult respiratory distress syndrome. *Crit Care Med* 13:786, 1985.
17. Broccard AF, Hotchkiss JR, Kuwayama N, et al: Consequences of vascular flow on lung injury induced by mechanical ventilation. *Am J Respir Crit Care Med* 157:1935, 1998.
18. Goldstein I, Bughalo MT, Marquette CH, et al: Mechanical ventilation-induced air-space enlargement during experimental pneumonia in piglets. *Am J Respir Crit Care Med* 163:958, 2001.
19. Nuckton TJ, Alonso JA, Kallet RH, et al: Pulmonary dead-space fraction as a risk factor for death in the acute respiratory distress syndrome. *N Engl J Med* 346:1281, 2002.
20. Slavin G, Nunn JF, Crow J, Dore CJ: Bronchiolectasis—a complication of artificial ventilation. *Br Med J (Clin Res Ed)* 285:931, 1982.
21. Sladen A, Laver MB, Pontoppidan H: Pulmonary complications and water retention in prolonged mechanical ventilation. *N Engl J Med* 279:448, 1968.
22. Webb HH, Tierney DF: Experimental pulmonary edema due to intermittent positive pressure ventilation with high inflation pressures. Protection by positive end-expiratory pressure. *Am Rev Respir Dis* 110:556, 1974.
23. Bouhuys A: Physiology and musical instruments. *Nature* 221:1199, 1969.
24. Roupie E, Dambrosio M, Servillo G, et al: Titration of tidal volume and induced hypercapnia in acute respiratory distress syndrome. *Am J Respir Crit Care Med* 152:121, 1995.
25. Hernandez LA, Peevy KJ, Moise AA, Parker JC: Chest wall restriction limits high airway pressure-induced lung injury in young rabbits. *J Appl Physiol* 66:2364, 1989.
26. Dreyfuss D, Saumon G: Role of tidal volume, FRC, and end-inspiratory volume in the development of pulmonary edema following mechanical ventilation. *Am Rev Respir Dis* 148:1194, 1993.

27. Meade MO, Cook DJ: The aetiology, consequences and prevention of barotrauma, a critical review of the literature. *Clin Intensive Care* 6:166, 1995.

28. Fu Z, Costello ML, Tsukimoto K, et al: High lung volume increases stress failure in pulmonary capillaries. *J Appl Physiol* 73:123, 1992.

29. Egan E: Lung inflation, lung solute permeability, and alveolar edema. *J Appl Physiol* 53:121, 1982.

30. Adkins KW, Hernandez LA, Coker PJ, et al: Age affects susceptibility to pulmonary barotrauma in rabbits. *Crit Care Med* 19:390, 1991.

31. Dreyfuss D, Soler P, Basset G, Saumon G: High inflation pressure pulmonary edema: respective effects of high airway pressure, high tidal volume and positive expiratory pressure. *Am Rev Respir Dis* 137:1159, 1988.

32. Hernandez LA, Coker PJ, May S, et al: Mechanical ventilation increases microvascular permeability in oleic-injured lungs. *J Appl Physiol* 69:2057, 1990.

33. Peevy KJ, Hernandez LA, Moise AA, Parker JC: Barotrauma and microvascular injury in lungs of nonadult rabbits: effect of ventilation pattern. *Crit Care Med* 18:634, 1990.

34. Corbridge TC, Wood LDH, Crawford GP, et al: Adverse effects of large tidal volume and low PEEP in canine acid aspiration. *Am Rev Respir Dis* 142:311, 1990.

35. Ranieri VM, Eissa NT, Corbeil C, et al: Effects of positive end-expiratory pressure on alveolar recruitment and gas exchange in patients with the adult respiratory distress syndrome. *Am Rev Respir Dis* 144:544, 1991.

36. Pestana D, Hernandez-Gancedo C, Royo C, et al: Adjusting positive end-expiratory pressure and tidal volume in acute respiratory distress syndrome according to the pressure-volume curve. *Acta Anaesthesiol Scand* 47:326, 2003.

37. Veldhuizen RA, Welk B, Harbottle R, et al: Mechanical ventilation of isolated rat lungs changes the structure and biophysical properties of surfactant. *J Appl Physiol* 92:1169, 2002.

38. Faridy EE: Effect of ventilation on movement of surfactant in airways. *Respir Physiol* 27:323, 1976.

39. Cereda M, Foti G, Musch G, et al: Positive end-expiratory pressure prevents the loss of respiratory compliance during low tidal volume ventilation in acute lung injury patients. *Chest* 109:480, 1996.

40. Marini JJ: Tidal volume, PEEP and barotrauma. An open and shut case? *Chest* 109:302, 1996.

41. Muscedere JG, Mullen JBM, Gan K, Slutsky AS: Tidal ventilation at low airway pressures can augment lung injury. *Am J Respir Crit Care Med* 149:1327, 1994.

42. Argiras EP, Blakeley CR, Dunnill MS, et al: High PEEP decreases hyaline membrane formation in surfactant deficient lungs. *Br J Anaesth* 59:1278, 1987.

43. Paré PD, Warriner B, Baile EM, Hogg JC: Redistribution of pulmonary extravascular water with positive end-expiratory pressure in canine pulmonary edema. *Am Rev Respir Dis* 127:590, 1983.

44. Duggan M, McCaul CL, McNamara PJ, et al: Atelectasis causes vascular leak and lethal right ventricular failure in uninjured rat lungs. *Am J Respir Crit Care Med* 27:27, 2003.

45. Tremblay LN, Slutsky AS: Ventilator-induced injury: from barotrauma to biotrauma. *Proc Assoc Am Physicians* 110:482, 1998.

46. Uhlig S: Ventilation-induced lung injury and mechanotransduction: stretching it too far? *Am J Physiol Lung Cell Mol Physiol* 282:L892, 2002.

47. Tremblay L, Valenza F, Ribeiro SP, et al: Injurious ventilatory strategies increase cytokines and c-fos m-RNA expression in an isolated rat lung model. *J Clin Invest* 99:944, 1997.

48. Held H-D, Boettcher S, Hamann L, Uhlig S: Ventilation-induced chemokine and cytokine release is associated with activation of nuclear factor-κB and is blocked by steroids. *Am J Respir Crit Care Med* 163:711, 2001.

49. Jobe AH, Kramer BW, Moss TJ, et al: Decreased indicators of lung injury with continuous positive expiratory pressure in preterm lambs. *Pediatr Res* 52:387, 2002.

50. Tremblay LN, Miatto D, Hamid Q, et al: Injurious ventilation induces widespread pulmonary epithelial expression of tumor necrosis factor-alpha and interleukin-6 messenger RNA. *Crit Care Med* 30:1693, 2002.

51. Naik AS, Kallapur SG, Bachurski CJ, et al: Effects of ventilation with different positive end-expiratory pressures on cytokine expression in the preterm lamb lung. *Am J Respir Crit Care Med* 164:494, 2001.

52. Veldhuizen RA, Slutsky AS, Joseph M, McCaig L: Effects of mechanical ventilation of isolated mouse lungs on surfactant and inflammatory cytokines. *Eur Respir J* 17:488, 2001.

53. Ranieri VM, Suter PM, Tortorella C, et al: Effect of mechanical ventilation on inflammatory mediators in patients with acute respiratory distress syndrome: a randomized controlled trial. *JAMA* 282:54, 1999.

54. Valenza F, Ribeiro SP, Slutsky AS: High volume-low pressure mechanical ventilation up-regulates IL-1ß production in an ex vivo lung model. *Am J Respir Crit Care Med* 151:A552, 1995.

55. Pugin J, Dunn I, Jolliet P, et al: Activation of human macrophages by mechanical ventilation in vitro. *Am J Physiol* 275(6 Pt 1):L1040, 1998.

56. Slutsky AS: Lung injury caused by mechanical ventilation. *Chest* 116(1 Suppl):9S, 1999.

57. Liu M, Tremblay L, Cassivi SD, et al: Alterations of nitric oxide synthase expression and activity during rat lung transplantation. *Am J Physiol Lung Cell Mol Physiol* 278:L1071, 2000.

58. Mourgeon E, Xu J, Tanswell AK, et al: Mechanical strain-induced posttranscriptional regulation of fibronectin production in fetal lung cells. *Am J Physiol* 277(1 Pt 1):L142, 1999.

59. Imanaka H, Shimaoka M, Matsuura N, et al: Ventilator-induced lung injury is associated with neutrophil infiltration, macrophage activation, and TGF-beta 1 mRNA upregulation in rat lungs. *Anesth Analg* 92:428, 2001.

60. Zhang H, Downey GP, Suter PM, et al: Conventional mechanical ventilation is associated with bronchoalveolar lavage-induced activation of polymorphonuclear leukocytes: a possible mechanism to explain the systemic consequences of ventilator-induced lung injury in patients with ARDS. *Anesthesiology* 97:1426, 2002.

61. Bhattacharya S, Sen N, Yiming MT, et al: High tidal volume ventilation induces proinflammatory signaling in rat lung endothelium. *Am J Respir Cell Mol Biol* 28:218, 2003.

62. Andonegui G, Bonder CS, Green F, et al: Endothelium-derived toll-like receptor-4 is the key molecule in LPS-induced neutrophil sequestration into lungs. *J Clin Invest* 111:1011, 2003.

63. Al-Jamal R, Ludwig MS: Changes in proteoglycans and lung tissue mechanics during excessive mechanical ventilation in rats. *Am J Physiol Lung Cell Mol Physiol* 281:L1078, 2001.

64. Mascarenhas MM, Day RM, Ochoa CD, et al: Low molecular weight hyaluronan from stretched lung enhances IL-8 expression. *Am J Respir Cell Mol Biol* 8:8, 2003.

65. Foda HD, Rollo EE, Drews M, et al: Ventilator-induced lung injury upregulates and activates gelatinases and EMMPRIN: Attenuation by the synthetic matrix metalloproteinase inhibitor, Prinomastat (AG3340). *Am J Respir Cell Mol Biol* 25:717, 2001.

66. Ohta N, Shimaoka M, Imanaka H, et al: Glucocorticoid suppresses neutrophil activation in ventilator-induced lung injury. *Crit Care Med* 29:1012, 2001.

67. Ribeiro SP, Rhee K, Tremblay L, et al: Heat stress attenuates ventilator-induced lung dysfunction in an ex vivo rat lung model. *Am J Respir Crit Care Med* 163:1451, 2001.

68. Meduri GU, Belenchia JM, Estes RJ, et al: Fibroproliferative phase of ARDS. Clinical findings and effects of corticosteroids. *Chest* 100:943, 1991.

69. Meduri GU, Headley S, Kohler G, et al: Persistent elevation of inflammatory cytokines predicts a poor outcome in ARDS. Plasma

IL-1 and IL-6 levels are consistent and efficient predictors of outcome over time. *Chest* 107:1062, 1995.

70. Meduri UG, Eltorky M, Winer-Muram HT: The fibroproliferative phase of late adult respiratory distress syndrome. *Semin Repir Infect* 10:154, 1995.

71. Meduri GU, Headley AS, Golden E, et al: Effect of prolonged methylprednisolone therapy in unresolving acute respiratory distress syndrome: A randomized controlled trial [see comments]. *JAMA* 280:159, 1998.

72. Montgomery BA, Stager MA, Carrico CJ, Hudson LD: Causes of mortality in patients with the adult respiratory distress syndrome. *Am Rev Respir Dis* 132:485, 1985.

73. Doyle RL, Szaflarski N, Modin GW, et al: Identification of patients with acute lung injury. Predictors of mortality. *Am Rev Respir Crit Care Med* 152:1818, 1995.

74. Parker JC, Hernandez LA, Longenecker GL, et al: Lung edema caused by high peak inspiratory pressures in dogs. Role of increased microvascular filtration pressure and permeability. *Am Rev Respir Dis* 142:321, 1990.

75. Parker JC, Hernandez LA, Peevy KJ: Mechanisms of ventilator-induced lung injury. *Crit Care Med* 21:131, 1993.

76. Dreyfuss D, Saumon G: Ventilator-induced lung injury, in Tobin MJ, (ed): *Principles and Practice of Mechanical Ventilation*, 1st ed. New York, McGraw-Hill, 1994, p 793.

77. Albert RK, Lakshminarayan WK, Butler J: Lung inflation can cause pulmonary edema in zone I of in situ dog lungs. *J Appl Physiol* 49:815, 1980.

78. Smith JC, Mitzner W: Analysis of pulmonary vascular interdependence in excised dog lobes. *J Appl Physiol* 48:450, 1980.

79. Parker JC, Townsley MI, Rippe B, et al: Increased microvascular permeability in dog lungs due to high peak airway pressures. *J Appl Physiol* 57:1809, 1984.

80. Dreyfuss D, Soler P, Saumon G: Spontaneous resolution of pulmonary edema caused by short periods of cyclic overinflation. *J Appl Physiol* 72:2081, 1992.

81. Lesur O, Hermans C, Chalifour JF, et al: Mechanical ventilation-induced pneumoprotein CC-16 vascular transfer in rats: effect of KGF pretreatment. *Am J Physiol Lung Cell Mol Physiol* 284:L410, 2003.

82. Murphy DB, Cregg N, Tremblay L, et al: Adverse ventilatory strategy causes pulmonary-to-systemic translocation of endotoxin. *Am J Respir Crit Care Med* 162:27, 2000.

83. Savel RH, Yao EC, Gropper MA: Protective effects of low tidal volume ventilation in a rabbit model of Pseudomonas aeruginosa-induced acute lung injury. *Crit Care Med* 29:392, 2001.

84. Nahum A, Hoyt J, Schmitz L, et al: Effect of mechanical ventilation strategy on dissemination of intratracheally instilled *Escherichia coli* in dogs. *Crit Care Med* 25:1733, 1997.

85. Choi WI, Quinn DA, Park KM, et al: Systemic microvascular leak in an in vivo rat model of ventilator-induced lung injury. *Am J Respir Crit Care Med* 27:27, 2003.

86. Imai Y, Parodo J, Kajikawa O, et al: Injurious mechanical ventilation and end-organ epithelial cell apoptosis and organ dysfunction in an experimental model of acute respiratory distress syndrome. *JAMA* 289:2104, 2003.

87. Albertine KH, Soulier MF, Wang Z, et al: Fas and fas ligand are up-regulated in pulmonary edema fluid and lung tissue of patients with acute lung injury and the acute respiratory distress syndrome. *Am J Pathol* 161:1783, 2002.

88. Matute-Bello G, Liles WC, Steinberg KP, et al: Soluble Fas ligand induces epithelial cell apoptosis in humans with acute lung injury (ARDS). *J Immunol* 163:2217, 1999.

89. Imai Y, Parodo J, Kajikawa O, et al: Injurious mechanical ventilation and end-organ epithelial cell apoptosis and organ dysfunction in an experimental model of acute respiratory distress syndrome. *JAMA* 289:2104, 2003.

90. Brower RG: Mechanical ventilation in acute lung injury and ARDS. Tidal volume reduction. *Crit Care Clin* 18:1, 2002.

91. Crotti S, Mascheroni D, Caironi P, et al: Recruitment and derecruitment during acute respiratory failure: a clinical study. *Am J Respir Crit Care Med* 164:131, 2001.

92. Pelosi P, Goldner M, McKibben A, et al: Recruitment and derecruitment during acute respiratory failure: An experimental study. *Am J Respir Crit Care Med* 164:122, 2001.

93. Hickling KG: Best compliance during a decremental, but not incremental, positive end-expiratory pressure trial is related to open-lung positive end-expiratory pressure: A mathematical model of acute respiratory distress syndrome lungs. *Am J Respir Crit Care Med* 163:69, 2001.

94. Holzapfel L, Robert D, Perrin F, et al: Static pressure-volume curves and effect of positive end-expiratory pressure on gas exchange in adult respiratory distress syndrome. *Crit Care Med* 11:591, 1983.

95. Darioli R, Perret C: Mechanical controlled hypoventilation in status asthmaticus. *Am Rev Respir Dis* 129:385, 1984.

96. Menitove SM, Goldring RM: Combined ventilator and bicarbonate strategy in the management of status asthmaticus. *Am J Med* 74:898, 1983.

97. Hickling KG, Henderson SJ, Jackson R: Low mortality rate associated with low volume pressure limited ventilation with permissive hypercapnia in severe adult respiratory distress syndrome. *Intensive Care Med* 16:372, 1990.

98. Hickling KG, Walsh J, Henderson S, Jackson R: Low mortality rate in adult respiratory distress syndrome using low-volume, pressure-limited ventilation with permissive hypercapnia: A prospective study. *Crit Care Med* 22:1568, 1994.

99. Feihl F, Perret C: Permissive hypercapnia. How permissive should we be ? *Am J Respir Crit Care Med* 150:1722, 1994.

100. Laffey JG, Kavanagh BP: Carbon dioxide and the critically ill—too little of a good thing? *Lancet* 354:1283, 1999.

101. Walley K, Lewis TH, Wood LDH: Acute respiratory acidosis decreases left ventricular contractility but increases cardiac output in dogs. *Circ Res* 67:628, 1990.

102. Puybasset L, Stewart T, Rouby JJ, et al: Inhaled nitric oxide reverses the increase in pulmonary vascular resistance induced by permissive hypercapnia in patients with acute respiratory distress syndrome. *Anesthesiology* 80:1254, 1994.

103. Kavanagh B: Normocapnia vs. hypercapnia. *Minerva Anestesiol* 68:346, 2002.

104. Hori M, Kitakaze M, Sato H, et al: Staged reperfusion attenuates myocardial stunning in dogs. Role of transient acidosis during early reperfusion. *Circulation* 84:2135, 1991.

105. Nomura F, Aoki M, Forbess JM, Mayer JE Jr: Effects of hypercarbic acidotic reperfusion on recovery of myocardial function after cardioplegic ischemia in neonatal lambs. *Circulation* 90(5 Pt 2):II321, 1994.

106. Kitakaze M, Weisfeldt ML, Marban E: Acidosis during early reperfusion prevents myocardial stunning in perfused ferret hearts. *J Clin Invest* 82:920, 1988.

107. Laffey JG, Engelberts D, Kavanagh BP: Buffering hypercapnic acidosis worsens acute lung injury. *Am J Respir Crit Care Med* 161:141, 2000.

108. Laffey JG, Tanaka M, Engelberts D, et al: Therapeutic hypercapnia reduces pulmonary and systemic injury following in vivo lung reperfusion. *Am J Respir Crit Care Med* 162:2287, 2000.

109. Broccard AF, Hotchkiss JR, Vannay C, et al: Protective effects of hypercapnic acidosis on ventilator-induced lung injury. *Am J Respir Crit Care Med* 164:802, 2001.

110. Shibata K, Cregg N, Engelberts D, et al: Hypercapnic acidosis may attenuate acute lung injury by inhibition of endogenous xanthine oxidase. *Am J Respir Crit Care Med* 158(5 Pt 1):1578, 1998.

111. Sonett J, Baker LS, His C, et al: Sodium bicarbonate versus Carbicarb in canine myocardial hypercarbic acidosis. *J Crit Care* 8:1, 1993.

112. Brochard L, Roudot-Thoraval F, Roupie E, et al: Tidal volume reduction for prevention of ventilator-induced lung injury in acute respiratory distress syndrome. The Multicenter Trial Group on Tidal Volume Reduction in ARDS. *Am J Respir Crit Care Med* 158:1831, 1998.

113. Brower RG, Shanholtz CB, Fessler HE, et al: Prospective, randomized, controlled clinical trial comparing traditional versus reduced tidal volume ventilation in acute respiratory distress syndrome patients. *Crit Care Med* 27:1492, 1999.

114. Stewart TE, Meade MO, Cook DJ, et al: Evaluation of a ventilation strategy to prevent barotrauma in patients at high risk for acute respiratory distress syndrome. Pressure- and Volume-Limited Ventilation Strategy Group. *N Engl J Med* 338:355, 1998.

115. Eisner MD, Thompson T, Hudson LD, et al: Efficacy of low tidal volume ventilation in patients with different clinical risk factors for acute lung injury and the acute respiratory distress syndrome. *Am J Respir Crit Care Med* 164:231, 2001.

116. Brower RG, Rubenfeld GD: Lung-protective ventilation strategies in acute lung injury. *Crit Care Med* 31(4 Suppl):S312, 2003.

117. Eichacker PQ, Gerstenberger EP, Banks SM, et al: Meta-analysis of acute lung injury and acute respiratory distress syndrome trials testing low tidal volumes. *Am J Respir Crit Care Med* 166:1510, 2002.

118. Steinbrook R: How best to ventilate? Trial design and patient safety in studies of the acute respiratory distress syndrome. *N Engl J Med* 3481393, 2003.

119. Amato MB, Barbas CS, Medeiros DM, et al: Effect of a protective-ventilation strategy on mortality in the acute respiratory distress syndrome. *N Engl J Med* 338:347, 1998.

120. Grasso S, Mascia L, Del Turco M, et al: Effects of recruiting maneuvers in patients with acute respiratory distress syndrome ventilated with protective ventilatory strategy. *Anesthesiology* 96:795, 2002.

121. Arnold JH, Hanson JH, Toro-Figuero LO, et al: Prospective, randomized comparison of high-frequency oscillatory ventilation and conventional mechanical ventilation in pediatric respiratory failure. *Crit Care Med* 22:1530, 1994.

122. Derdak S, Mehta S, Stewart TE, et al: High-frequency oscillatory ventilation for acute respiratory distress syndrome in adults: a randomized, controlled trial. *Am J Respir Crit Care Med* 166:801, 2002.

123. Matthay MA, Zimmerman GA, Esmon C, et al: Future research directions in acute lung injury: Summary of a National Heart, Lung, and Blood Institute Working Group. *Am J Respir Crit Care Med* 167:1027, 2003.

124. http://www.ardsnet.org/ards04.php

125. Sinclair SE, Kregenow DA, Lamm WJ, et al: Hypercapnic Acidosis is protective in an in vivo model of ventilator-induced lung injury. *Am J Respir Crit Care Med* 166:403, 2002.

Chapter 38

ACUTE LUNG INJURY AND THE ACUTE RESPIRATORY DISTRESS SYNDROME

JASON D. CHRISTIE
PAUL N. LANKEN

KEY POINTS

- *Acute lung injury (ALI) and its more severe form, the acute respiratory distress syndrome (ARDS), are common causes of acute hypoxemic respiratory failure (AHRF).*

- *Both ALI and ARDS are characterized by hypoxemia that is resistant to oxygen therapy; this is due to widespread alveolar filling or collapse.*

- *Initial therapy for all patients with ALI and ARDS should be supplemental oxygen in the highest concentration available; failure to achieve 95% arterial saturation or greater confirms the presence of a large right-to-left shunt.*

- *Most patients with ALI and ARDS require early intubation because their hypoxemic respiratory failure is typically severe and may be prolonged.*

- *If a patient with severe hypoxemia as indicated by arterial blood gas analysis has a clear chest radiograph, consider a possible error (e.g., incorrect fractional inspired oxygen [$F_{I_{O_2}}$] or arterial oxygen tension [Pa_{O_2}]); in such situations, also consider the possibility of other types of right-to-left shunts (e.g., intracardiac shunts or pulmonary arteriovenous malformations) or the continued perfusion of an unventilated or poorly ventilated lung (e.g., due to acute mucous plugging of one main bronchus).*

- *The acute phase of ALI and ARDS is characterized by an exudative alveolar flooding due to pulmonary capillary leak and by extensive alveolar collapse due to loss of normal surfactant activity; while interventions directed at modulating inflammatory or other pathways of lung injury or restoring surfactant function hold theoretical promise, at present no specific pharmacologic therapy has been shown to improve outcomes; in this phase one provides mechanical ventilation and other supportive care while identifying and treating the precipitating cause or causes of ALI or ARDS.*

- *Ventilator management of patients with ALI and ARDS should use a strategy with low tidal volumes and limits to end-inspiratory pressure (i.e., plateau pressures [Pplat]), to reduce the risk of ventilator-induced lung injury (VILI); such a strategy gives higher priority to the goal of decreasing the risk of VILI by limiting end-inspiratory volume and pressure than the traditional goal of keeping arterial carbon dioxide tension (P_{CO_2}) and pH in the normal range.*

- *The target for oxygenation should be a Pa_{O_2} between 55 and 80 mm Hg (88% to 95% saturation); one should achieve this by adjusting $F_{I_{O_2}}$ and positive end-expiratory pressure (PEEP) with the goal of decreasing $F_{I_{O_2}}$ to 0.5 to 0.6 (or less),*

concentrations that are less concerning for pulmonary oxygen toxicity.

- *In general, the ventilatory strategy should use a tidal volume of 6 mL/kg of predicted body weight (PBW) with a Pplat target that does not exceed 30 cm H_2O; if Pplat exceeds 30 cm H_2O with a 6 mL/kg PBW tidal volume, the latter should be decreased to 5 mL/kg PBW; if Pplat still exceeds 30 cm H_2O, tidal volume should be further decreased to 4 mL/kg PBW.*

- *When changing to low tidal volume ventilation, one should increase the respiratory rate (RR) up to 35/min to maintain minute ventilation; the target for ventilation should be a pH of 7.30 to 7.45; if the pH is between 7.15 and 7.29, one may correct the respiratory acidosis by giving intravenous sodium bicarbonate ($NaHCO_3$) (if RR is 35/min and arterial carbon dioxide tension [Pa_{CO_2}] is <25 mm Hg); if the pH remains <7.15 with RR of 35/min and $NaHCO_3$ is considered or given, one can increase the tidal volume in 1–mL/kg PBW increments until pH exceeds 7.15 (i.e., the Pplat target may be exceeded).*

- *During assisted ventilation, use sedation to synchronize the patient's respiratory efforts with the ventilator and to decrease oxygen consumption ($\dot{V}_{O_2}$); one may also need to induce muscle paralysis by use of neuromuscular blocking agents, which despite their clinical utility, likely increase the risk of diffuse weakness in survivors.*

- *Despite the lack of results of a randomized clinical trial (RCT) to support its use, some clinicians favor a "dry" fluid management strategy to reduce edemagenesis and the duration of assisted ventilation; however, this approach generally lowers cardiac output and risks worsening or inducing nonpulmonary organ dysfunction.*

- *If one uses a "dry" fluid management strategy, one should be guided by daily and cumulative net intake and output volumes and laboratory indices of hypovolemia (blood urea nitrogen [BUN]:creatinine ratio and serum total bicarbonate) while monitoring for adequate urine output (>0.5 mL/kg PBW/h), effective circulation (by physical signs, or measurements of cardiac index or venous co-oximetry or both), adequate perfusing pressure (i.e., mean arterial pressure [MAP] ≥60 mm Hg), and electrolyte abnormalities (serum sodium and potassium).*

- *Caution! Although this strategy is supported by observational studies, no prospective RCT to date has established whether the "dry" fluid management strategy improves outcomes compared to a "non-dry" strategy; nor has the efficacy or safety of using a pulmonary artery or central venous catheter for this purpose been established.*

- *Late-phase or fibroproliferative-phase ARDS (corresponding to persistent ARDS of 1 week duration or more) is characterized by subacute inflammation, proliferation of alveolar lining cells and interstitial cells, and varying degrees of fibrosis.*

- *In severe late-phase ARDS, a prolonged course of high-dose methylprednisolone sodium succinate (MPSS) can improve gas exchange and mechanics in some patients; however, use of MPSS increases the risk of diffuse weakness that may be prolonged; preliminary results from one RCT found that MPSS administration when added to a low-tidal-volume ventilation strategy that limited Pplat as described above did not significantly improve mortality at 60 days (or ICU or hospital lengths of stay) compared with ventilation using a low tidal volume and limited plateau pressure strategy alone.*

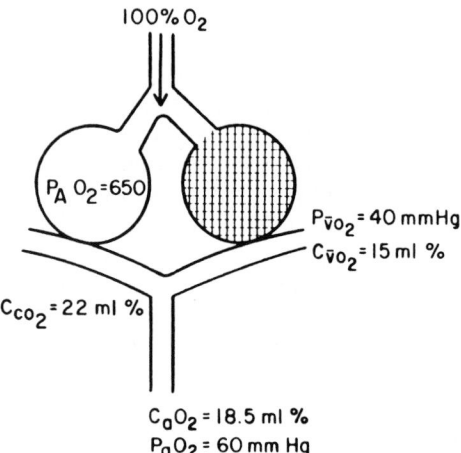

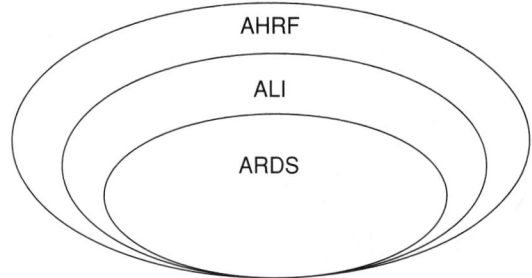

FIGURE 38-2 Schematic representation of the relationships among acute hypoxemic respiratory failure (AHRF), acute lung injury (ALI) and the acute respiratory distress syndrome (ARDS). Note that ALI is a more severe subgroup of AHRF and that ARDS is a more severe form of ALI.

FIGURE 38-1 Diagram of a two-compartment model of lung perfusion and ventilation demonstrating the basis for failure of oxygenation in ALI and ARDS. When large portions of the lung are nonventilated owing to alveolar collapse or flooding (*hatched area*), blood flow to these units with mixed venous P_{O_2} ($P\bar{v}_{O_2}$) of 40 mm Hg and content of 15 vol% is effectively shunted through the lungs without being resaturated. Thus despite a high concentration of supplemental oxygen (100% in this example) and a high alveolar P_{O_2} in ventilated units, these blood flows mix in accord with their oxygen contents (i.e., the resulting left atrial blood has an oxygen content that is the weighted mean of the oxygen content of the shunted and non-shunted blood). In this example of a 50% shunt, the left atrial and systemic arteries have an arterial P_{O_2} of 60 mm Hg. Ca_{O_2}, arterial oxygen content; Cc_{O_2}, capillary oxygen content; $C\bar{v}_{O_2}$, mixed venous oxygen content; P_A, alveolar pressure; Pa_{O_2}, arterial oxygen pressure; $P\bar{v}_{O_2}$, partial pressure of oxygen in the mixed venous blood.

Severe arterial hypoxemia that is resistant to supplemental oxygen is a common reason for admission to the ICU. This form of respiratory failure, termed *acute hypoxemic respiratory failure* (AHRF), arises from widespread flooding or collapse of alveoli. As a result, a substantial fraction of mixed venous blood traverses nonventilated alveoli (i.e., alveoli with ventilation-perfusion ratio of 0). This in turn results in a large right-to-left intrapulmonary shunt (Fig. 38-1). In addition to its adverse effects on oxygenation, fluid that accumulates in alveoli and interstitial tissues increases lung stiffness, which decreases lung compliance. This imposes a larger mechanical load on the patient's respiratory system, resulting in an increased elastic work of breathing. Without treatment with supplementary oxygen and assisted ventilation, the gas exchange derangement and abnormal lung mechanics can result in progressive hypoxemia, respiratory muscle fatigue, and eventual respiratory arrest and death.

This chapter describes two notable forms of AHRF: *acute lung injury* (ALI) and its more severe subgroup, *the acute respiratory distress syndrome* (ARDS) (Fig. 38-2). ALI and ARDS affect an estimated 50,000 to 150,000 patients each year in the United States alone.[1,2] Despite recent advances in ventilatory management and improvements in nonrespiratory supportive ICU care, the mortality rate remains high (e.g., ~25% to over 50%, depending on the characteristics of the population studied and the ventilatory strategy utilized).[3–9]

The overall goal of this chapter is to provide a comprehensive and updated clinical approach to ALI and ARDS that

is grounded in current concepts of pathogenesis and pathophysiology. Objectives include: (1) to present the definitions, epidemiology, and precipitating causes of ALI and ARDS; (2) to describe the pathogenesis and pathophysiology of ALI and ARDS; (3) to describe the differential diagnosis of ALI and ARDS and clinical approaches to distinguish among various causes of acute hypoxemic respiratory failure; (4) to review the current status of treatment for ALI and ARDS and their precipitating causes; and (5) to provide current recommendations for ventilatory management of ALI and ARDS. The last objective includes a detailed description of the low-tidal-volume ventilatory strategy used by the ARDS Clinical Trials Network (ARDSNet) investigators in the clinical trials sponsored by the National Heart, Lung and Blood Institute (NHLBI) of the National Institutes of Health (NIH).[3,4]

Description and Definitions of ALI and ARDS

ARDS was initially described in 1967 by Ashbaugh and coauthors as a syndrome characterized by the acute onset of dyspnea, severe hypoxemia, diffuse lung infiltrates, and decreased compliance of the respiratory system.[10] Following this initial report, different authors utilized varying definitions that incorporated the elements of acute timing of onset, hypoxemia, radiographic infiltrates, and absence of overt clinical congestive heart failure.[11–15] In 1988, Murray and coauthors proposed using a Lung Injury Score (LIS), in part to take into account the effects of respiratory system compliance and the pressures delivered using the mechanical ventilator.[14] The LIS combined elements of severity of chest radiograph infiltrates, hypoxemia, respiratory system compliance, and amount of administered positive end-expiratory pressure (PEEP) on the mechanical ventilator.[14]

AMERICAN EUROPEAN CONSENSUS CONFERENCE DEFINITIONS

In 1994, the first American European Consensus Conference (AECC) published these consensus-derived definitions of ALI and ARDS: acute onset, bilateral pulmonary infiltrates on chest radiograph consistent with pulmonary edema, poor systemic oxygenation, and the absence of evidence of left atrial hypertension (Table 38-1).[16] The ratio of arterial oxygen tension (Pa_{O_2}) to the fraction of inspired oxygen (F_{IO_2}), Pa_{O_2}:F_{IO_2},

TABLE 38-1 American European Consensus Conference Criteria for Acute Lung Injury (ALI) and the Acute Respiratory Distress Syndrome (ARDS)

Clinical Variable	Criteria for ALI	Criteria for ARDS
Onset	Acute	Acute
Hypoxemia	$Pa_{O_2}/F_{I_{O_2}} \leq 300$ mm Hg	$Pa_{O_2}/F_{I_{O_2}} \leq 200$ mm Hg
Chest radiograph	Bilateral infiltrates consistent with pulmonary edema	Bilateral infiltrates consistent with pulmonary edema
Noncardiac cause	No clinical evidence of left atrial hypertension **or,** if measured, pulmonary artery occlusion pressure ≤ 18 mm Hg	No clinical evidence of left atrial hypertension **or,** if measured, pulmonary artery occlusion pressure ≤ 18 mm Hg

SOURCE: Reproduced with permission from Bernard et al.[16]

was chosen to reflect the degree of hypoxemia even when measured at different $F_{I_{O_2}}$.[17] The syndrome is called ALI when this ratio is ≤ 300 and ARDS when ≤ 200. The AECC coined the term *acute lung injury* in order to identify patients who are early in the course of their ARDS and those who may have a form of AHRF that is milder than ARDS. The AECC definitions of ALI and ARDS were intentionally quite broad in order to encompass different types of AHRF occurring in a wide variety of settings. Most patients with ALI progress to ARDS, prompting some to use the use the term "ALI/ARDS" to describe all patients with a $Pa_{O_2}:F_{I_{O_2}}$ ratio ≤ 300 who also meet the other AECC criteria (see Table 38-1).

Several clinical trials have used these standardized definitions of ALI and ARDS to specify the trial's inclusion criteria for their study populations.[3,4,8] Using the AECC definition of ALI and ARDS in these and other clinical trials contributes to the comparability of their study populations and facilitates generalizability of their results. For example, in order for clinicians to extrapolate the results of a trial to their own patients, they must first be reasonably sure that their patients resemble those in the clinical trial. This requires that they meet the same inclusion criteria for ALI or ARDS as those used in the clinical trial. However, having the same inclusion criteria is necessary but not sufficient, since the clinician must also take into account the exclusion criteria used in the clinical trial to assess comparability.

VALIDITY AND RELIABILITY OF AECC DEFINITIONS

Despite standardization, these definitions have not been formally validated beyond their face validity. In addition, problems remain with the reliability of the various components of the definitions.[1] For example, interpretation of chest radiographs can be inaccurate and variable among different observers.[18,19] However, formal training sessions can improve this variability.[19] Likewise, the $Pa_{O_2}:F_{I_{O_2}}$ criterion also suffers from variability since it can be influenced by the level of PEEP used in mechanical ventilation and other transient factors, such as airway secretions or inadequate sedation. For example, higher PEEP generally increases Pa_{O_2} at a given $F_{I_{O_2}}$. This in turn may raise a patient's $Pa_{O_2}:F_{I_{O_2}} > 300$ so that the patient no longer meets the inclusion criteria for ALI. Conversely, in the absence of PEEP a $Pa_{O_2}:F_{I_{O_2}} < 300$ may reflect the presence of simple basilar atelectasis rather than ALI or ARDS. In such a case, adding PEEP may recruit enough atelectatic lung to raise $Pa_{O_2}:F_{I_{O_2}} > 300$, so that the patient no longer meets this criterion for ALI.[20]

Finally, exclusion of congestive heart failure (left atrial hypertension) also presents problems with reliability. Diagnostic criteria for left atrial hypertension on purely clinical grounds may be inaccurate.[1,21] Insertion of a pulmonary artery catheter for this purpose may also be inconclusive since the pulmonary artery occlusion pressure may be higher than 18 mm Hg due to intravascular volume loading (e.g., in patients with shock), rather than due to congestive heart failure.[21] Conversely, many patients with pulmonary edema due to congestive heart failure and high left atrial pressures may have normal pulmonary artery occlusion pressures by the time the catheter is inserted and measurements taken.[22]

Further refinement of the reliability and validity of definitions of ALI and ARDS are desirable goals. More reliable definitions will not only improve estimates of the public health impact of these syndromes, but also decrease misclassification errors that are especially problematic for research aimed at clarifying molecular and genetic mechanisms in ALI and ARDS.[23]

Epidemiology

INCIDENCE

Inconsistent definitions for ALI and ARDS in large databases of diagnoses for hospital admissions or complications, variations in the application of the AECC definition in different studies, and variations in different at-risk populations (such as sepsis, trauma, surgeries, and bone marrow transplants) have hampered obtaining accurate estimates of the incidence of ALI and ARDS. Recent studies have used data from the ARDSNet clinical trials, as well as regional cohort studies to arrive at estimates in the United States in the range of 25 to 65 cases per 10,000 person-years.[1,2,24] Thus the number of patients with ARDS and ALI in the U.S. each year is estimated to be between 53,000 and 140,000. If one assumes a short-term mortality of $\sim 30\%$ to 40%, the annual number of deaths in the U.S. directly attributable to ALI and ARDS is between 16,000 and 56,000. These estimates of attributable mortality are greater than from the acquired immune deficiency syndrome (AIDS), asthma, or cervical cancer.[1,2] In addition, ARDS and ALI contribute significantly to long-term mortality, morbidity, and diminished quality of life. (see Chap. 19).[25–28] In addition to these estimates in the U.S., two non-U.S. studies arrived at similar incidence rates for ARDS in Berlin[29] and Scandinavia.[29] Several useful reviews have

TABLE 38-2 Examples of Direct and Indirect Precipitating Causes of Acute Lung Injury (ALI) and the Acute Respiratory Distress Syndrome (ARDS)

Direct Precipitating Cause	Indirect Precipitating Cause[a]
Aspiration of gastric contents	Acute pancreatitis
Bacterial pneumonia (e.g., Legionnaire's disease)	Blood product transfusions with transfusion-related acute lung injury (TRALI)
Chest trauma with lung contusion	Post–cardiopulmonary bypass
Near-drowning	Primary graft failure of lung transplantation
Pneumonia due to *Pneumocystis carinii*	Severe sepsis and septic shock
Toxic inhalations (e.g., smoke inhalation, inhaled crack cocaine ["crack" lung])	Toxic ingestions (e.g., aspirin, tricyclic antidepressants)
Viral pneumonia (e.g., influenza, the severe acute respiratory syndrome [SARS])	Trauma with multiple fractures and fat-emboli syndrome

[a] In indirect or systemic mechanisms of lung injury the lung injury results from deleterious effects on the alveolar endothelium by inflammatory or other mediators delivered via the pulmonary circulation.

summarized the important public health impact of ALI and ARDS.[1,2,30]

PRECIPITATING CAUSES

ALI and ARDS can be considered to be a "final common pathway" reaction of the lung to a large variety of precipitating causes. Some authors have classified these causes as representing *direct* (pulmonary) or *indirect* (extrapulmonary or systemic) injury to the lung.[31,32] (Table 38-2). Although the methodology for applying these labels is not standardized and thus may be inconsistent between studies, this construct may have pathogenetic and pathophysiologic underpinnings since indirect causes may have different mechanisms of injury compared to direct injury to the lung.[33] Not all patients with these precipitating conditions develop ALI/ARDS. Indeed, the frequency of ALI/ARDS is quite variable. Depending on the precipitating cause, it ranges from ~10% to 40%. If patients have more than one of these precipitating causes, they are at an even higher increased risk for development of ALI or ARDS. Although most studies of the incidence of ARDS among different at-risk subgroups were performed before the AECC standardization of the definitions, they nonetheless provide broad estimates of the risk of development of ARDS in these subgroups.[11–13,34]

RISK FACTORS FOR THE DEVELOPMENT OF ALI AND ARDS

Why certain individuals with the same precipitating cause develop ALI and ARDS while others don't is not known. Some of this differential risk can be attributed to other acquired risk factors, such as chronic alcoholism.[35] In addition, certain individuals may have an inherent predisposition to developing ALI or ARDS while others may have inherent protections against ALI or ARDS. These considerations are discussed below.

ALI and ARDS arise from diverse populations. Within these populations, specific clinical variables may affect both the risk of ARDS and ultimate outcomes if ARDS develops.[34,36,37] Clinical variables and outcomes associated with an increased risk of ARDS include chronic alcohol abuse;[38] lack of diabetes;[39] hypoproteinemia;[40] age and gender;[13] severity of injury and illness as measured by injury severity score (ISS) or Acute Physiology, Age, and Chronic Health Evaluation (APACHE) score;[13] hypertransfusion of blood products;[13] and

possibly cigarette smoking.[41] The mechanistic underpinnings of these associations are the subject of ongoing research. Nonetheless, these observations highlight the influence of the heterogeneity of a diverse source population on the risks of ALI and ARDS. Human studies aimed at investigating genetic or molecular mechanisms that predispose or protect individuals from developing ALI and ARDS must take into account the effects of these population and environmental differences.

DETERMINANTS OF ARDS OUTCOME

Clinical variables with reported associations with increased mortality among patients with ALI and ARDS include advanced age, low $Pa_{O_2}:F_{IO_2}$, high plateau pressure (i.e., low compliance), extent of pulmonary infiltrates, chronic liver disease, nonpulmonary organ dysfunction, severity of illness, hypoproteinemia, and length of hospitalization prior to ARDS.[4,38,42–48] In addition, magnitude of the dead space fraction has been identified as a risk factor for mortality, possibly indicating the importance of loss of the pulmonary vascular bed in disease severity.[49]

Different precipitating causes of ALI and ARDS carry different prognoses. For example, trauma-associated ALI or ARDS has a better prognosis than other causes, even after adjustment is made for other baseline variables such as age.[48] Although response to some therapeutic interventions in ALI or ARDS varies according to direct or indirect cause of lung injury,[50,51] low-tidal-volume ventilation is equally efficacious in both of these subgroups.[52]

Despite recent advances in therapy, the mortality rates reported in clinical trials in the past decade have ranged from ~25% to more than 50%.[3–9] The lowest mortality rates have been achieved with low-tidal-volume ventilation, which also limited end-inspiratory (plateau) pressure.[3,4] Although no recent studies have explicitly examined the cause of death in nonsurvivors, previously the majority of deaths were found to be due to multiorgan failure or sepsis, while progressive respiratory failure accounted for only a small minority of deaths (e.g., ~15%).[53,54]

ALI and ARDS impact the health and lives of survivors beyond the ICU. Long-term functional, neuropsychiatric, and cognitive dysfunction following ALI and ARDS has been described (see Chap. 19). In the aggregate, these deficits represent an important aspect of the impact of ARDS and its associated morbidity on the general population.

Pathology and Pathophysiology

In cases of ALI and ARDS, it is useful to distinguish between the early phases of lung injury and subsequent events.[36,55,56] By light microscopy, the early appearance is of interstitial and alveolar edema, capillary congestion, and intra-alveolar hemorrhage with minimal evidence of cellular injury (Fig. 38-3). By electron microscopy, changes of endothelial cell swelling, widening of intercellular junctions, increased numbers of pinocytotic vesicles, and disruption and denudation of the basement membrane are prominent. Inflammatory cell infiltration of the lung interstitium may be seen (particularly in ARDS complicating sepsis or trauma) as well as neutrophil sequestration in alveolar capillaries, but it usually a subtle finding. During this early *exudative* phase of diffuse alveolar damage (DAD), pulmonary edema and its clinical effects are most pronounced (see Fig. 38-3). It is also a time when manipulations to decrease the rate of edemagenesis are most likely to have impact as discussed below.

Over the ensuing days, hyaline membrane formation in the alveolar spaces becomes prominent. Hyaline membranes contain condensed fibrin and plasma proteins. Intra-alveolar activation of the coagulation system results in the formation of the fibrin, while plasma proteins are deposited in the alveolar space as part of the inflammatory exudate that leaks across the alveolar-capillary membrane. Inflammatory cells become more numerous within the lung interstitium. As the process of DAD progresses, there is extensive necrosis of type I alveolar epithelial cells. If the patient with ALI and ARDS does not recover or die during the first week, they may have a prolonged course of illness, termed *late-phase ARDS*.

FIGURE 38-3 A schematic representation showing the time course of evolution of the acute respiratory distress syndrome (ARDS). During the early or exudative phase, the lesion is characterized by a pulmonary capillary leak with interstitial and alveolar edema and hemorrhage, followed by hyaline membrane formation. Within as short a period of time as 7 to 10 days, a proliferative phase may appear with marked interstitial and alveolar inflammation and cellular proliferation, which is followed by fibrosis and disordered healing (see text for discussion). (*Reproduced with permission from Katzenstein AA, Askin FB: Surgical Pathology of Non-Neoplastic Lung Diseases, 2nd ed. Philadelphia, Saunders, 1990.*)

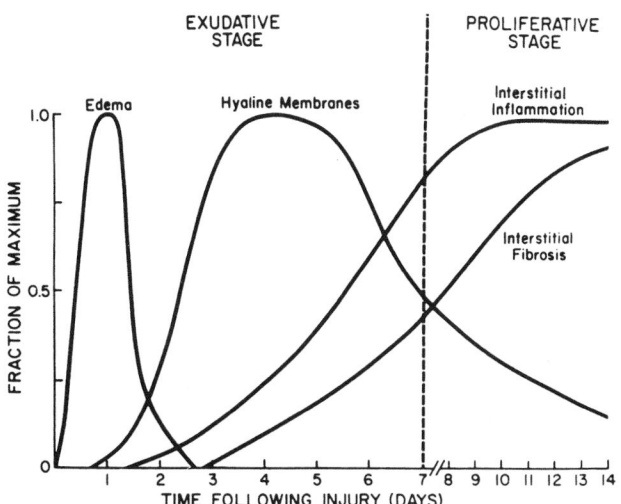

The late phase of ARDS is dominated by disordered healing. This can occur as early as 7 to 10 days after initial injury and may eventually result in extensive pulmonary fibrosis. This has been termed the *proliferative* or *fibroproliferative* phase. Type II alveolar cells proliferate along alveolar septae and the alveolar walls; fibroblasts and myofibroblasts become more numerous. Evidence of lung flooding is less prominent and may be minimal at this point. Changes in the clinical manifestations of ALI and ARDS parallel the changes in pathology. One study found that patients in late-phase ARDS typically had a large dead space fraction, a high minute ventilation requirement, progressive pulmonary hypertension, slightly improved intrapulmonary shunt that is less responsive to PEEP, and a further reduction in lung compliance.[57]

Pathogenesis

A number of closely inter-related pathophysiologic mechanisms and systems contribute to the development of ALI and ARDS (Fig. 38-4). Inflammatory cytokines, oxygen radicals, activation of coagulation and complement, platelet and immune cell activation, proteases, leukotrienes, and eicosanoids have been hypothesized to play a role in the early stages of ALI and ARDS.[33,36,37,58] In addition to ongoing inflammation and oxidation, factors specific to apoptosis, edema fluid resolution, fibrosis, and repair are likely to be important in the resolving and late phases of ALI and ARDS.[33,36,37,58,59]

INFLAMMATORY CYTOKINES AND CHEMOKINES

Cytokines are small signaling proteins that participate in host defense by binding to cell surface receptors. Many types of cells produce cytokines in response to a variety of stimuli. Cytokines teleologically must provide a net benefit in terms of contributing to host defense. However, when inflammation is overly exuberant, they have been implicated in disease states, including ALI and ARDS.[60,61]

Two of the major early proinflammatory cytokines are *tumor necrosis factor-α* (TNF-α) and *interleukin-1* (IL-1), both of whose production can be increased by hypoxia.[62] These cytokines have similar effects in initiating and propagating inflammation.[60,63–66] Their actions include: (1) recruitment, differentiation, amplification, and localization of macrophages to the lung parenchyma; (2) stimulation of other inflammatory cytokines such as interleukins-6 and -8 (IL-6 and IL-8); and (3) adherence of neutrophils to endothelium (see Fig. 38-4).[58,67–70]

In clinical studies, the most convincing evidence of the involvement of TNF-α and IL-1 in ARDS has been from direct measurement in bronchoalveolar lavage (BAL) or pulmonary edema fluid. Both fluids have consistently been reported to contain elevated levels of TNF-α and IL-1 in ARDS patients.[71–75] Furthermore, some suggest that much of the proinflammatory state of BAL in ARDS may be mediated through IL-1.[76] More recent studies suggest that an imbalance between inflammatory cytokines and their soluble receptors are an important pathogenetic mechanism in ARDS.[77]

Not only do TNF-α and IL-1 play an important role in the early pathogenesis and risk of developing ALI and ARDS,

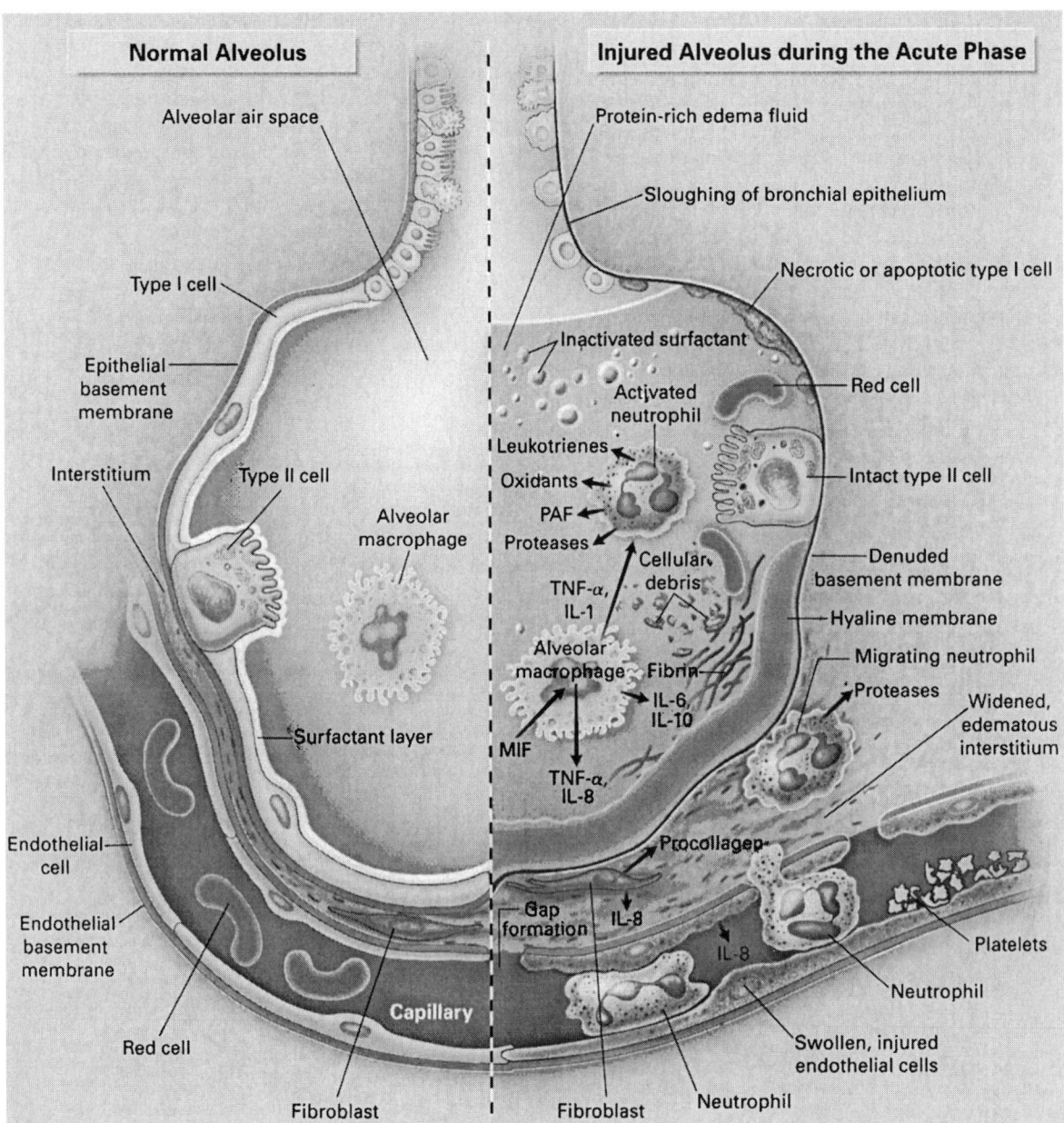

FIGURE 38-4 Schematic representation of the alveolus under normal conditions (*left-hand side*) and during development of acute lung injury (ALI) and the acute respiratory distress syndrome (ARDS) (*right-hand side*). In the acute phase of the syndrome (*right-hand side*), there is sloughing of both the bronchial and alveolar epithelial cells, with the formation of protein-rich hyaline membranes on the denuded basement membrane. Neutrophils are shown adhering to the injured capillary endothelium and marginating through the interstitium into the air space, which is filled with protein-rich edema fluid. In the air space, an alveolar macrophage is secreting cytokines such as interleukins-1, -6, -8, and -10, (IL-1, 6, 8, and 10), and tumor necrosis factor-α (TNF-α), which act locally to stimulate chemotaxis and activate neutrophils. Macrophages also secrete other cytokines, including interleukins-1, -6, and -10. Interleukin-1 can also stimulate the production of extracellular matrix by fibroblasts. Neutrophils can release oxidants, proteases, leukotrienes, and other proinflammatory molecules, such as platelet-activating factor (PAF). A number of anti-inflammatory mediators are also present in the alveolar milieu, including interleukin-1–receptor antagonist, soluble tumor necrosis factor receptor, autoantibodies against interleukin-8, and cytokines such as interleukins-10 and -11 (not shown). The influx of protein-rich edema fluid into the alveolus has led to the inactivation of surfactant. MIF denotes macrophage inhibitory factor. (*Reproduced with permission from Ware et al.[36]*)

but persistently high levels of TNF-α and IL-1 in plasma and in BAL have also been associated with an increased risk of death in patients with ALI and ARDS.[61,78]

In addition to IL-1 and TNF-α, *interleukin-6* (IL-6) has been suggested as an important mediator of lung injury. IL-6, a product of macrophages that have been stimulated by TNF-α and IL-1, has diverse functions. In mediating acute lung injury, IL-6 has traditionally been viewed as a proinflammatory cytokine. This view is based largely on the clinical observations of elevated levels in sepsis and ARDS.[79,80] However, laboratory experiments indicate that IL-6 may also have anti-inflammatory effects.[81]

Like TNF-α and IL-1, persistently elevated IL-6 levels have been associated with an increased risk of death in ARDS patients.[78] In addition, in the ARDSNet randomized clinical trial (RCT) that compared lower- and higher-tidal-volume ventilatory strategies, the lung protective treatment arm that had decreased mortality showed a significantly steeper fall in IL-6 levels over the first 72 hours compared to the higher-tidal-volume arm.[3] In a separate RCT comparing low-tidal-volume versus traditional-tidal-volume ventilation in early ARDS, the former had lower concentrations of inflammatory mediators (TNF-α, IL-1, and IL-6) in BAL fluid and plasma over the first 36 hours of the trial.[82] Thus although the exact mechanisms of IL-6 in mediating acute lung injury are uncertain, it may have an important role in clinical ALI and ARDS.

Interleukin-10 (IL-10) is a potent anti-inflammatory cytokine produced by monocytes as well as by both T and B lymphocytes. IL-10 is a potent inhibitor of proinflammatory molecules including TNF-α and IL-1.[83] Lower levels of IL-10 in blood and lung lavage fluid have been association with development of ARDS.[77,84,85] Furthermore, lower circulating levels of IL-10 have been associated with death in patients with established ARDS.[86]

Chemokines are small polypeptides that certain cells elaborate in response to a variety of proinflammatory mediators. Chemokines act locally on modulating leukocyte immune response. The most studied chemokine in ARDS is *interleukin-8* (IL-8), which has been implicated in neutrophil chemotaxis. In a variety of lung injury models, blockage of IL-8 with directed antibodies has led to attenuation of the injury.[87–89] IL-8 has also been associated with greater numbers of neutrophils in BAL fluid of patients with ARDS as well as with mortality.[61,90–92]

Given the interrelationship and overlapping regulatory mechanisms of cytokine and chemokine molecules, future studies will need to focus on cytokine and chemokine imbalances, (i.e., their interactions with antagonist molecules and soluble receptors), as well as time-dependent differences. Finally, many studies have measured cytokine concentrations, whereas given the existence of inactivating molecules, measuring biological activity may be more productive.

NEUTROPHILS AND OXIDANT STRESS

Neutrophil migration into the airspaces is evident in the early histopathology of ARDS.[93,94] BAL fluid of subjects with ARDS reveals a predominance of neutrophils.[95] Conversely, recovery is associated with resolution of neutrophilia.[96] Normally, neutrophils become apoptotic and are then removed by macrophages. Recent evidence suggests that impaired neutrophil apoptosis may be an important mechanism in early ARDS,[97] and that elevated levels of granulocyte-macrophage colony-stimulating factor (GM-CSF) may play a role in this mechanism.[98–100]

Neutrophils in the alveolar and interstitial spaces may result in lung injury due to neutrophil-mediated release of reactive oxidant species (ROS) and resulting oxidant stress. Oxidant stress refers to an imbalance between endogenously produced oxidants and endogenous antioxidants. Products of oxidant stress include superoxide, hydroxyl radicals, and peroxynitrite.[101] Although some levels of ROS may be important in normal homeostasis, ROS are highly unstable and

react quickly with surrounding proteins, DNA, and lipids, resulting in molecular damage.[101]

A widely held hypothesis is that excessive oxidant stress is a major early contributor in the pathogenesis of acute lung injury.[102–109] ROS can be generated by neutrophils (polymorphonuclear [PMN] cells),[102,104,110] or by the pulmonary endothelium.[111,112] Both PMN-mediated and endothelial generation of ROS may be important to initiation and development of lung injury.

Evidence from clinical studies supporting excess ROS in ALI and ARDS include findings of: increased hydrogen peroxide in exhaled breath of ARDS patients;[113,114] decreased levels of glutathione in lung lavage fluids of ARDS patients;[115,116] increased nitrotyrosine and chlorotyrosine in lavage fluids of ARDS patients;[117] increased lipid peroxidation products in plasma;[118,119] increased protein carbonyl levels;[120] increased plasma hypoxanthine;[121] increased levels of nitrated fibrinogen in the plasma of ALI/ARDS patients;[122] and increased serum ferritin levels in ARDS patients compared with at-risk patients.[123,124] Although some of these findings may be nonspecific for ARDS,[58] taken together, they make a strong case for the role of oxidant stress in the pathogenesis of ARDS. In addition, evidence of higher levels of oxidant stress in nonsurvivors of ARDS is illustrated by lower levels of plasma thiol groups,[125] and higher levels of hydrogen peroxide in urine of ARDS patients who are nonsurvivors.[126]

COAGULATION AND FIBRINOLYSIS

As noted above, the histopathology of the early exudative phase of ALI and ARDS is notable for diffuse alveolar fibrin deposition in the form of hyaline membranes (see Fig. 38-3).[55,56,94,127,128] In addition, a shift in the procoagulant and anticoagulant balance to favor coagulation has been demonstrated in the BAL fluid of patients with ARDS.[129–133] Furthermore, there are likely important links between the coagulation system activation and activation of the inflammatory system. For example, TNF-α and IL-1 can act synergistically to produce a procoagulant state through effects on tissue factor, thrombomodulin, and plasminogen activator inhibitor.[134–136] Given the success of intravenous activated protein C in treating sepsis (see Chap. 46),[137] as well as the observation that the mortality benefit in this trial was also evident in subjects with severe sepsis and pulmonary dysfunction as a single organ system dysfunction,[138] interventions aimed at correcting abnormalities in coagulation and fibrinolysis in ALI and ARDS are a promising future research direction.

ALVEOLAR EDEMA CLEARANCE

Considerable evidence supports the active transport of sodium and water by the pulmonary epithelium from the distal airspaces of the lung.[139] This process appears to be regulated by epithelial sodium channels predominantly on alveolar type I cells, potentially stimulated by catecholamines.[140,141] In addition, recent evidence suggests a potential role for the cystic fibrosis transmembrane conductance regulator (CFTR) in alveolar fluid transport.[142] Furthermore, the directional flow of fluid across the alveolus may be altered in conditions of hypoxia,[143,144] as well as by reactive nitrogen and oxygen species.[145]

In ALI and ARDS, the pulmonary epithelium is injured, resulting in altered fluid transport. Clinical studies in ventilated patients have illustrated impaired fluid transport in ARDS when compared with hydrostatic pulmonary edema.[36,146,147] In addition, subjects who could rapidly remove alveolar fluid had a lower hospital mortality.[147,148] Whether these findings are simply a result of disruption of the alveolar epithelium, or whether they represent a finding potentially amenable to therapy (such as with β-adrenergic receptor agonists), awaits the results of interventional clinical trials.

FIBROPROLIFERATION AND REPAIR MECHANISMS

Although there is considerable temporal overlap with the exudative and inflammatory phases (see Fig. 38-3), the late phase of ARDS is characterized by accumulation of matrix and cells in the interstitial and alveolar spaces, contributing to disruption of the alveolar architecture.[55,56] Recovery from ARDS requires resolution of this phase of the tissue injury–repair spectrum with some degree of the normal lung architecture. Clinical studies of ARDS patients indicate that the alveolus is repaired under conditions of ongoing inflammation.[61] In addition, soluble collagen precursor, type III procollagen peptide (PCP III), in the edema fluid of early ARDS can differentiate between subjects who will have longer or shorter courses of ARDS.[149] This suggests that fibroproliferation begins early in the course of lung injury. In addition to these findings with PCP III, other evidence of the prognostic significance of fibroproliferation in ARDS includes the finding that fibroblast mitogenic activity in BAL fluid is lower in survivors of ARDS than nonsurvivors.[150,151]

A complex balance of different growth factors, cytokines, and chemokines occurs in the fibroproliferative and reparative phases of acute lung injury.[58,152] A variety of animal, basic, and clinical studies have demonstrated the importance of transforming growth factor-β (TGF-β) to fibroproliferation in the lung.[153,154] A key step in fibroproliferation involves the activation of TGF-β from its latent form. This can be accomplished through interaction with a variety of mediators, including matrix metalloproteinases (MMPs), thrombospondin, plasmin, acid environments, α_2-macroglobulin, and reactive oxygen species.[153] In addition, TGF-β has extensive interactions with inflammatory cytokines, chemokines, and interferon-γ in regulating fibrosis.

Other important modulators of the remodeling process include matrix and cell surface proteoglycans and glycosaminoglycans;[155–157] matricellular proteins that affect cell adhesion;[158,159] matrix metalloproteases;[160] and the balance of coagulation and fibrinolysis (particularly through the actions of plasminogen activator inhibitor-1 [PAI-1]).[129] The interplay of these mediators with the potential for targeted therapies is the focus of current investigations.

Approach to Diagnosis of ALI and ARDS

CLINICAL PRESENTATION AND DIFFERENTIAL DIAGNOSIS

Acute hypoxemic respiratory failure has many etiologies besides ALI and ARDS (Table 38-3). However, the bedside appearance of patients with various forms of AHRF is remarkably similar. Marked tachypnea and dyspnea are invariably present. Physical examination reveals diffuse crackles in cases

TABLE 38-3 Differential Diagnosis of Acute Hypoxemic Respiratory Failure (AHRF)

- ALI or ARDS
- Acute (or "flash") cardiogenic pulmonary edema
- Bilateral aspiration pneumonia
- Lobar atelectasis of both lower lobes
- Severe unilateral lower lobe atelectasis, especially when patient is receiving vasodilators, such as intravenous nitrates, calcium channel blockers, or sodium nitroprusside, that blunt hypoxic vasoconstriction
- Acute loss of ventilation to one lung due to complete or near-complete obstruction of its main stem bronchus (e.g., due to a mucous plug or blood clot)
- Loss of ventilation to one or both lungs due to large pneumothorax/pneumothoraces
- Loss of ventilation to one or both lungs due to large pleural effusion(s)
- Diffuse alveolar hemorrhage, especially in patients post–bone marrow transplantation
- Massive pulmonary embolus
- Acute opening of a patent foramen ovale in patients with pre-existing pulmonary hypertension

ALI, acute lung injury; ARDS, acute respiratory distress syndrome.
SOURCE: Reprinted with permission from Christie JD, Schmidt G, Lanken PN: Acute respiratory distress syndrome. http://pier.acponline.org/physicians/diseases/d349/d349.html. Physicians' Information and Education Resource. Philadelphia, American College of Physicians, July 2004.

of cardiogenic pulmonary edema and focal findings of consolidation in cases of lobar pneumonia. Cardiogenic pulmonary edema may be accompanied by evidence of airflow obstruction, including wheezing and hypercapnia.[161] The presence of crackles, a radiologic appearance of high-pressure edema (see below), and hypoxemia refractory to oxygen therapy, all suggest cardiogenic pulmonary edema as the primary process. Cough and purulent sputum are hallmarks of infectious processes, while copious clear or pink-colored airway secretions result from fulminant ("flash") cardiogenic pulmonary edema.

Distressed patients with AHRF typically have initial room air arterial blood gas results with Pa_{O_2} in the 30 to 55 mm Hg range and pulse oximetry less than 85% of arterial O_2 saturation. If supplemental oxygen by mask or cannula raises arterial saturation to above 95%, a large intrapulmonary shunt is unlikely. Other causes of respiratory distress should then be considered, including airways disease, pulmonary embolus, or severe metabolic acidosis. Failure to achieve >95% saturation of arterial blood with supplemental oxygen indicates the presence of a large right-to-left shunt. The specific process should be investigated via physical examination and chest radiograph. In the rare instances that the chest radiograph is entirely clear of alveolar infiltrates, one should consider that the blood gas data are erroneous, that there is an anatomic right-to-left shunt at another site (e.g., pulmonary arteriovenous malformations or intracardiac shunt), or that there is continued perfusion of an unventilated lung due to recent complete or nearly complete occlusion of its main bronchus (but before the lung has collapsed due to absorption atelectasis) (see Table 38-3).

The differential diagnosis of ALI and ARDS (i.e., AHRF with diffuse pulmonary infiltrates consistent with pulmonary edema in the absence of a cardiac etiology) includes a variety of disorders and etiologies. Identifying the etiologies of the diffuse infiltrates is important because specific treatments exist for several of these conditions (e.g., acute eosinophilic pneumonia or diffuse alveolar hemorrhage). Table 38-4 lists the major clinical and diagnostic characteristics of these disorders.

CLINICAL SETTING

The clinical setting in which the disorder develops can provide important diagnostic information. *Cardiogenic edema* is most often accompanied by systolic left ventricular or valvular dysfunction, and the abnormal heart sounds and murmurs

TABLE 38-4 Differential Diagnosis of Acute Lung Injury (ALI) and Acute Respiratory Distress Syndrome (ARDS)

Disorder	Characteristics	Comments
Pulmonary edema due to left heart failure	History of cardiac disease, enlarged heart on chest radiograph, third heart sound (S_3)	Rapid improvement with diuresis and/or afterload reduction
Noncardiogenic pulmonary edema	History of one or more precipitating causes (see Table 38-2), crackles absent or not prominent, normal cardiac size on chest radiograph	Usual etiology for ALI and ARDS: rarely some patients with ALI or ARDS have no obvious precipitating cause
Diffuse alveolar hemorrhage (DAH)	Often associated with autoimmune diseases (e.g., vasculitis) or following bone marrow transplantation; often patients do not have bloody sputum; renal disease or other evidence of systemic vasculitis may be present; hemosiderin-laden macrophages in bronchoalveolar lavage (BAL) fluid can confirm diagnosis of DAH; may respond to apheresis, corticosteroids, or cyclophosphamide, depending on etiology	May meet diagnostic criteria for ARDS, but has different pathophysiology and management
Acute eosinophilic pneumonia	Cough, fever, pleuritic chest pain, and myalgia are often present; patients often do not have peripheral blood eosinophilia, but generally have >15% eosinophils in BAL fluid; usually responds rapidly to high-dose corticosteroid therapy	May meet diagnostic criteria for ARDS, but has different pathophysiology and management
Lupus pneumonitis	Usually associated with active lupus; may respond to high-dose corticosteroid therapy or cyclophosphamide	May meet diagnostic criteria for ARDS, but has different pathophysiology and management
Acute interstitial pneumonia (AIP)	Slower onset than ARDS (over 4–6 weeks) with progressive course; however, it may present in an advanced state, mimicking ARDS	Associated with >90% mortality; AIP includes Hamman-Rich syndrome
Pulmonary alveolar proteinosis (PAP)	Slower onset than ARDS (over 2–12 months) with progressive course; can be treated with whole lung lavage	Characteristic "crazy paving" pattern on high-resolution computed tomography scan
Bronchiolitis obliterans-organizing pneumonia (BOOP) or cryptogenic organizing pneumonia	May be precipitated by viral syndrome; slower onset than ARDS (over >2 weeks) with progressive course; however, it may present in an advanced state, mimicking ARDS; may respond to high-dose corticosteroid therapy	
Hypersensitivity pneumonitis	Typically slower onset than ARDS (over weeks) with progressive course; however it may present in an advanced state, mimicking ARDS; may respond to high-dose corticosteroid therapy and removal from offending agent	
Leukemic infiltration	May be rapid in onset during active disease states; usually leukemia is clinically apparent	
Drug-induced pulmonary edema and pneumonitis	May follow use of heroin, other opioids, overdose of aspirin, tricyclic antidepressants, or exposure to paraquat	May progress to overt ARDS
Acute major pulmonary embolus (PE)	Occurs acutely, occasionally accompanied by severe hypoxemia that may be resistant to O_2 therapy like ARDS, and by hypotension, requiring pressors, mimicking ARDS with sepsis; patients typically have risk factors for acute PE and may not have common precipitating causes of ARDS	Chest radiograph in ARDS should have bilateral infiltrates consistent with pulmonary edema; chest radiograph in acute major PE may have unilateral or no infiltrates; acute major PE needs a confirmatory study (e.g., pulmonary angiogram)
Sarcoidosis	The onset is not acute, but its clinical recognition may be; oxygenation is often impaired and the chest radiograph can be diffusely abnormal	Historical features and the frequent presence of hilar adenopathy in sarcoidosis usually eliminate confusion with ARDS
Interstitial pulmonary fibrosis	The onset is not acute, but its clinical recognition may be; oxygenation is often impaired and the chest radiograph can be diffusely abnormal	Prior chest radiographs and a history of chronic and progressive dyspnea characterize the collection of diseases causing interstitial pulmonary fibrosis

SOURCE: Reprinted with permission from Christie JD, Schmidt G, Lanken PN: Acute respiratory distress syndrome. http://pier.acponline.org/physicians/diseases/d349/d349.html. Physicians' Information and Education Resource. Philadelphia, American College of Physicians, July 2004.

associated with each should be sought. Electrocardiographic (ECG) and serum enzyme evidence of ischemia should be considered and suggest an obvious cause for cardiogenic edema. Review of intravascular volume administration often will supply information suggesting the explanation for pulmonary edema in patients with left ventricular or renal dysfunction.

ALI and ARDS commonly arise in a typical clinical context (see Table 38-2). Sepsis, pneumonia, trauma, transfusion of blood products, and acid aspiration account for the majority of cases of ALI and ARDS.[3,4,13,36] Less common causes include pancreatitis, near-drowning, leukoagglutination reactions, lung infections with viral agents or *Pneumocystis carinii*, fat embolism syndrome, and drug toxicities.[34]

CHEST RADIOGRAPH

The chest radiograph is a simple and widely available test used to assess patients with AHRF. Unfortunately, the accuracy of the routine radiograph in distinguishing hydrostatic from increased permeability edema is not high.[162,163] Criteria that have been suggested to support a diagnosis of hydrostatic edema include increased heart size, increased width of the vascular pedicle, vascular redistribution toward upper lobes, septal lines, and a centrifugal pattern of spread with a perihilar bat's-wing distribution of the edema. The lack of these findings and patchy peripheral infiltrates that extend to the lateral lung margins suggest ARDS. However, all these signs overlap, and in the best of hands this test is unlikely to yield better than a 60% to 80% accuracy of diagnosis when applied without other diagnostic tools.[162]

ECHOCARDIOGRAPHY

Echocardiography is a useful source of noninvasive information regarding cardiovascular function.[164,165] Left ventricular dilatation, regional or global wall motion abnormalities, and substantial mitral regurgitation on Doppler imaging support a diagnosis of cardiogenic edema. A heart with echocardiographically normal dimensions and function (both systolic and diastolic) in a patient with pulmonary edema suggests pulmonary vascular leakage, although prior ventricular or valvular dysfunction with intercurrent resolution of the high pulmonary vascular pressures predisposing to cardiogenic edema must be kept in mind.

RIGHT HEART CATHETERIZATION

Right heart catheterization is often performed in patients with pulmonary edema, although the benefits of this invasive procedure continue to be debated;[166–168] it has even been suggested that this technology itself contributes to a poor patient outcome.[169,170] An observational study suggested that routine right heart catheterization was harmful, with a 33% increased risk of death if used in seriously ill patients with acute hypoxemic respiratory failure.[169] In addition, several investigations have demonstrated that physician understanding of and facility with the information generated are remarkably poor.[169,171] Thus until results of the current NIH NHLBI ARDSNet clinical trial that is testing the safety and efficacy of pulmonary artery catheters versus central venous catheters in patients with ALI and ARDS are available, right heart catheterization cannot be recommended as a routine procedure in patients with ALI/ARDS.

However, it is recommended that clinicians use invasive hemodynamic methods, including right heart catheterization, to address specific questions regarding ventricular function, the adequacy of volume resuscitation, the degree of intrapulmonary shunt, and the adequacy of cardiac output and oxygen saturation of mixed venous or central venous blood. The specific pulmonary capillary wedge pressure (Ppw) that the AECC definition (see Table 38-1) used as the criterion to distinguish noncardiogenic from cardiogenic pulmonary edema (i.e., 18 mm Hg), was an arbitrary decision based on physiologic experiments, tradition, and volume resuscitation practices circa 1992. Since then, reports have indicated that some patients who originally met criteria for ALI or ARDS as listed in Table 38-1, but who have been volume loaded to increase their cardiac output, have periods when measurements of their Ppw are above 18 mm Hg.[21] In the mechanically ventilated patient with normal lung function and serum oncotic pressure, cardiogenic edema is typically associated with a Ppw of 28 mm Hg or above.[172] However, lower plasma oncotic pressure (e.g., due to hypoalbuminemia) will result in pulmonary edema at somewhat lower values of Ppw.[173] Finally, caution should be used when trying to rule in cardiogenic pulmonary edema by simply measuring the Ppw after a bout of acute pulmonary edema, since such patients often have Ppw less than 18 mm Hg by the time the catheter has been passed.[22]

BRONCHOALVEOLAR LAVAGE

Acute eosinophilic pneumonia is a rare disorder that is characterized by diffuse AHRF due to eosinophilic infiltrates in the lungs.[174–176] It is notable for its responsiveness to corticosteroid therapy. When the precipitating cause for ARDS is unclear, it is recommended to perform a bronchoalveolar lavage and measure the percentage of eosinophils in the lavage fluid.[174] Lavages can generally be done safely in many patients with ALI and ARDS except those with the lowest values of Pa_{O_2} : FI_{O_2} or hemodynamic instability.[177,178]

Likewise, a bedside bronchoscopy with BAL can be diagnostic for diffuse alveolar hemorrhage (DAH). In this case, the bronchoscopy may or may not reveal fresh blood in the trachea and major bronchi. However, BAL generally produces a bloody return, which may deepen in red color as the lavage continues. DAH occurs commonly in the first week or two post–bone marrow transplantation.[179,180] DAH also occurs in association with a variety of vasculitic disorders. These include Goodpasture's syndrome, Wegener's granulomatosis, systemic lupus erythematosus, and antiphospholipid antibody syndrome (see Chap. 104).[181–186] Finally, DAH also may result from inhalation of crack cocaine.[181] For this cause of DAH, careful history taking and sending the patient's urine for toxicology analysis for cocaine may help determine the etiology.

Approach to Treatment of Patients with ALI and ARDS

TREAT THE PRECIPITATING CAUSE OF ALI AND ARDS AND OTHER SERIOUS COMORBIDITIES

A key early step in treating patients with ALI and ARDS is to identify and treat the precipitating cause or causes of the ALI and ARDS as well as any other serious and life-threatening

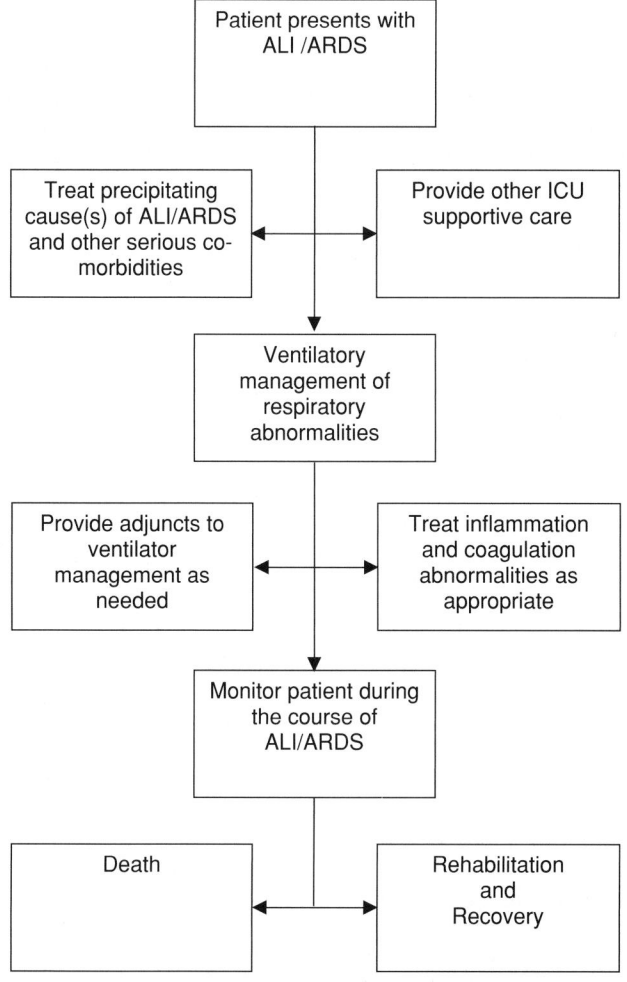

FIGURE 38-5 Schematic summary of approach to treatment of patients with ALI and ARDS. Note that the box, "Treat inflammation and coagulation abnormalities as appropriate," is currently limited to high-dose steroid therapy for late-phase ARDS (see text for details).

TABLE 38-5 Treatable Precipitating Causes of Acute Lung Injury (ALI) and Acute Respiratory Distress Syndrome (ARDS)

Infectious etiologies
Bacterial or other sepsis responsive to antimicrobial therapy
Diffuse bacterial pneumonias (e.g., *Legionella* species)
Diffuse viral pneumonias (e.g., cytomegalovirus, influenza A)
Diffuse fungal pneumonias (e.g., *Candida* and *Cryptococcus* species)
Pneumocystis carinii pneumonia
Other diffuse lung infections (e.g., miliary tuberculosis)

Noninfectious etiologies
Diffuse alveolar hemorrhage post–bone marrow transplant
Diffuse alveolar hemorrhage due to vasculitis (e.g., Goodpasture's syndrome)
Acute eosinophilic pneumonia
Lupus pneumonitis
Toxic drug reactions (e.g., aspirin)

performing early fiberoptic bronchoscopy to obtain bronchial washings for cytologic and microbiologic analyses, or in selected cases, surgical lung biopsy.

VENTILATOR MANAGEMENT OF RESPIRATORY ABNORMALITIES

MAINTAINING ADEQUATE ARTERIAL OXYGENATION

The hallmark respiratory abnormality of ALI and ARDS is hypoxemia that is resistant to oxygen therapy. This is due to the presence of a large right-to-left intrapulmonary shunt arising from fluid-filled and collapsed alveoli (see Fig. 38-1). Maintaining adequate arterial oxygenation is a goal given high priority by both traditional and more recent approaches to ventilator management, as noted below. One should use sufficient PEEP to reduce the right-to-left shunt to oxygenate the patient. By this approach, clinicians should be able to avoid prolonged exposure of such patients to potentially toxic concentrations of high inspired oxygen (e.g., F_{IO_2} of 0.7 and above).

PEEP improves arterial oxygenation, primarily by recruiting collapsed and partially fluid-filled alveoli and thereby increasing the functional residual capacity (FRC) at end-expiration.[187,188] PEEP also redistributes alveolar fluid into the interstitium,[189] which should also improve oxygenation.

NONINVASIVE VENTILATION

Assisted ventilation is generally done invasively via an endotracheal tube, but in selected cases noninvasive ventilation (NIV) may be successful[190,191] (see Chap. 33). Although NIV seems to be useful in respiratory failure in immunocompromised hosts,[190] we believe it is generally not a good choice for most patients with ALI and ARDS. This is because ARDS typically has a long course and is often associated with hemodynamic instability, coma, and multiorgan system failure (including ileus).[192]

COMPARISON OF TRADITIONAL AND CURRENT APPROACHES TO VENTILATOR MANAGEMENT
Goals and Priorities of the Traditional Approach

The traditional approach to ventilator management of patients with ALI and ARDS gave high priority to these goals: (1) to maintain arterial O_2 saturation (O_2sat) above 88% to 90% to provide for adequate tissue oxygenation while

comorbidities (Fig. 38-5). The ventilatory and other supportive management of ALI and ARDS is inadequate if not accompanied by aggressive attempts at diagnosis and treatment of the precipitating cause(s) (Table 38-2). *Because ARDS is a syndrome based on nonspecific radiographic and physiologic criteria (Table 38-1), making the diagnosis of ALI or ARDS is **not** equivalent to diagnosing the patient's underlying problem.* Not appreciating this seemingly obvious fact will delay diagnostic procedures in these patients and may delay therapy of a potentially treatable underlying disorder (Table 38-5).

For example, although appropriate supportive therapy may transiently stabilize a patient with ARDS due to sepsis from an abdominal abscess, if clinicians delay performing diagnostic tests such as abdominal CT scan or ultrasonography of the biliary tract in a timely manner, the underlying source of sepsis will go undiagnosed and the patient will eventually deteriorate. Likewise, the timely start of empiric antimicrobial therapy in patients with ALI or ARDS associated with severe sepsis or septic shock is as important as a timely diagnostic work-up (see Chaps. 45 and 46). Finally, if the precipitating cause of ALI and ARDS is unclear, one should consider

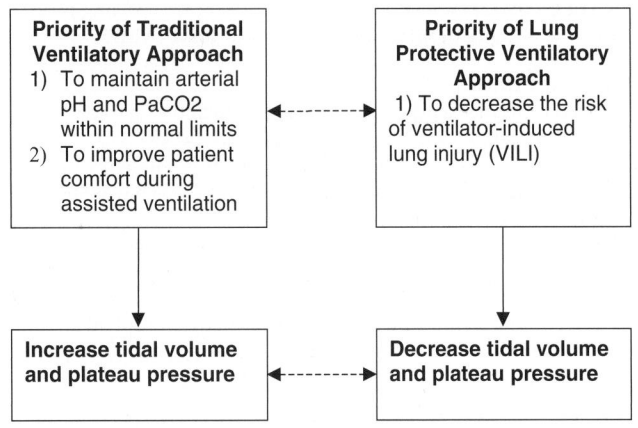

FIGURE 38-6 Schematic illustration that demonstrates how traditional and lung-protective approaches to mechanical ventilation of patients with ALI or ARDS have different priorities. The traditional approach gives higher priority to keeping arterial pH and Paco₂ normal (and possibly to keeping the patient more comfortable) than the lung-protective approach, which gives higher priority to prevention of ventilator-induced lung injury (VILI). Plateau pressure = static end-inspiratory pressure in the alveoli.

trying to minimize lung injury due to high concentrations of inspired oxygen (oxygen toxicity); (2) to provide sufficient ventilation to keep arterial pH and Pa_{CO_2} within normal limits[193] (Fig. 38-6).

To achieve the first goal, clinicians applied various levels of PEEP. This use of PEEP was first described in the initial description of ARDS by Ashbaugh and coworkers in 1967.[10] Clinicians increased levels of PEEP in order to decrease F_{IO_2} to below 70% while monitoring for adverse circulatory effects of PEEP.[194] Since arterial oxygenation was found to be determined in part by mean airway pressure, they also used relatively large tidal volumes of 10 to 15 mL/kg. These were double to triple spontaneous tidal volumes, which are of the order of 5 mL/kg. Both the use of PEEP and traditional large tidal volumes (delivered at high flow rates) generally result in relatively high peak and end-inspiratory pressures (plateau pressure [Pplat]) in patients with ALI or ARDS, whose lungs typically have decreased compliance.

To achieve the second goal, clinicians ventilated patients with ALI and ARDS with relatively large tidal volumes of 10 to 15 mL/kg at high respiratory rates if needed. The resulting high minute ventilation was needed to produce a normal alveolar ventilation. This is because patients with ALI and ARDS typically have increased physiologic dead spaces and elevated dead space:tidal volume ratios (VDS:VT) (e.g., up to 75%).[195,196] In some cases, patients were exposed to high peak and end-inspiratory pressures due to the large tidal volumes in order to maintain normal arterial blood P_{CO_2} and pH. Clinicians also used large tidal volumes and high inspiratory flow rates as a supplement to sedation to decrease patient discomfort while receiving assisted ventilation.

For example, if a patient with ARDS had a normal CO_2 production (e.g., 200 mL/min), and a normal VDS:VT of 0.3, then a minute ventilation of ~7 L/min is needed to keep the patient's Pa_{CO_2} at 40 mm Hg.[197] However, when the patient's VDS:VT increases, then additional minute ventilation is needed to keep Pa_{CO_2} at 40 mm Hg. In this example, *14 L/min* of minute ventilation is needed if the VDS:VT is 0.66, and *18 L/min* is needed if the VDS:VT is 0.75,[197] both of which occur in patients with ARDS.[195,196] For a patient with a predicted (lean) body weight (PBW) of 60 kg, one can easily achieve a minute ventilation of 18 L/min with tidal volumes of 600 to 900 mL at rates of 20 to 30 per minute.

Goals and Priorities of Lung-Protective Approach

The lung-protective approach to ventilator management has the same goal for oxygenation as the traditional approach (i.e., to maintain an arterial saturation greater than 88% to 90%). However, it gives higher priority to protection from ventilator-induced lung injury (VILI) (see Chap. 37) than to normalization of arterial P_{CO_2} and pH.[193] The lung-protective approach's goal to decrease risk of VILI often conflicts with the traditional approach's goal to provide a high minute ventilation to keep arterial pH and P_{CO_2} within normal limits (see Fig. 38-6). This conflict arises since the current lung-protective approach reduces the risk of VILI by decreasing the size of the tidal volume from the traditional 10 to 15 mL/kg body weight to tidal volumes of 4 to 6 mL/kg predicted body weight (PBW). Even with respiratory rates up to 35/min, such low tidal volumes will limit the resultant minute ventilation. This may result in a degree of permissive hypercapnia in some patients with ALI and ARDS.

For example, for a 60-kg PBW patient, a tidal volume of 6 mL/kg PBW (360 mL) with a respiratory rate of 35/min produces a minute ventilation of only 12.6 L. If one needs to reduce the tidal volume for the same 60-kg PBW patient to 4 mL/kg PBW (240 mL), in order to keep the Pplat from exceeding the threshold of 30 cm H_2O, at the same respiratory rate of 35/min it provides only 8.4 L of minute ventilation. It is likely that a patient with ARDS ventilated with tidal volumes of 4 to 6 mL/kg PBW has a VDS:VT of 0.66 or greater. This is due to the combined effects of an increased physiologic dead space in ARDS[195,196] and the fact that ventilating with a lower tidal volume ventilation decreases the denominator of the patient's VDS:VT. If the patient had a VDS:VT of 0.66, low tidal volume ventilation, which provides 8.4 to 12.6 L/min, will result in permissive hypercapnia since, as described above, 14 L/min is needed to maintain this patient's Pa_{CO_2} at 40 mm Hg. For example, for a patient with a VDS:VT of 0.66, a minute ventilation of 12.6 L/min would result in a Pa_{CO_2} of ~45 mm Hg, while 8.4 L/min of minute ventilation would result in a Pa_{CO_2} of ~65 mm Hg.[197]

Decreasing the Risk of Ventilator-Induced Lung Injury

The important change in priority of the lung protective approach of ventilator management of patients with ALI and ARDS compared to the traditional approach is the result of a remarkable confluence of two lines of scientific research that culminated in a landmark confirmatory randomized controlled clinical trial[3] (Fig. 38-7). The first line of basic research initially studied effects of mechanical forces (high pressure or high volume or both) in animal models of lung injury and then extended these observations to isolated lungs in situ or in vitro, and eventually to isolated lung cells. The second line of research involved careful clinical observations of patients with ALI and ARDS that examined the effects of systematic

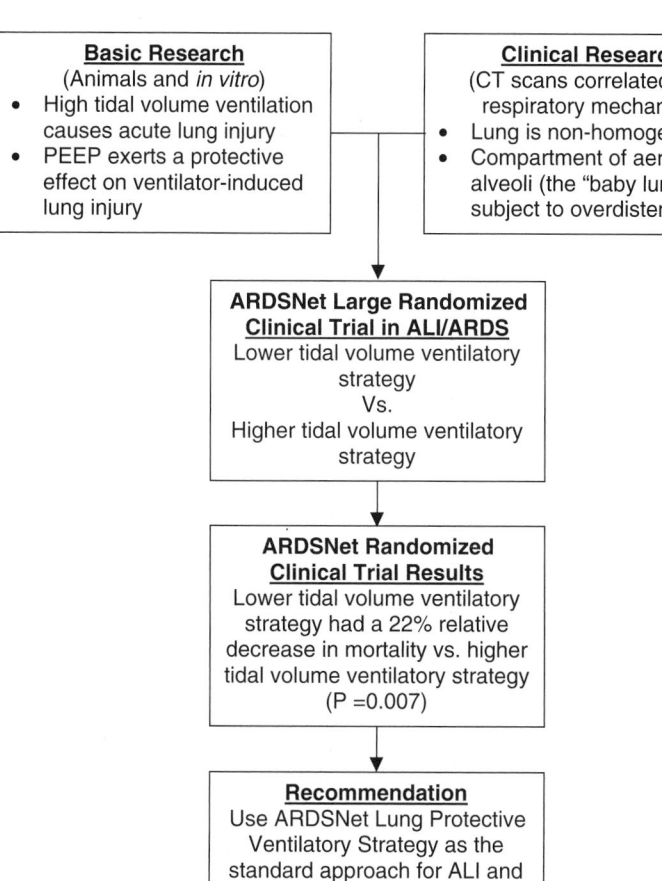

Basic Research
(Animals and *in vitro*)
- High tidal volume ventilation causes acute lung injury
- PEEP exerts a protective effect on ventilator-induced lung injury

Clinical Research
(CT scans correlated with respiratory mechanics)
- Lung is non-homogeneous
- Compartment of aerated alveoli (the "baby lung") is subject to overdistension

ARDSNet Large Randomized Clinical Trial in ALI/ARDS
Lower tidal volume ventilatory strategy
Vs.
Higher tidal volume ventilatory strategy

ARDSNet Randomized Clinical Trial Results
Lower tidal volume ventilatory strategy had a 22% relative decrease in mortality vs. higher tidal volume ventilatory strategy
(P =0.007)

Recommendation
Use ARDSNet Lung Protective Ventilatory Strategy as the standard approach for ALI and ARDS in clinical practice and in future clinical trials

FIGURE 38-7 Schematic illustration of the confluence of basic and clinical research that resulted in a large randomized clinical trial by investigators in the NHLBI ARDS Clinical Trials Network (ARDSNet).[3] This trial showed that a lower-tidal-volume ventilatory strategy was superior to a traditional-tidal-volume ventilatory strategy. As such, it confirmed that the hypothesis of ventilator-induced lung injury was important in the augmentation of the lung injury in ALI and ARDS. It also established that a lung-protective ventilatory strategy should be generally used to treat patients with ALI and ARDS. Finally, until there is new evidence to suggest otherwise, the ARDSNet lung protective protocol is recommended as the standard approach in clinical practice and future clinical trials.

changes in selected ventilatory parameters with their physiologic effects and radiographic changes.[187]

BASIC RESEARCH RELATED TO VENTILATOR-INDUCED LUNG INJURY

Although Chap. 37 provides a more comprehensive description of this research, review of some of the early reports may prove useful since it specifically relates to this chapter's recommendations for ventilating patients with ALI and ARDS. In 1974 Webb and Tierney reported that mechanical ventilation using large tidal volumes and high inflation pressures could cause a fatal lung injury (similar morphologically to ARDS) in rats with otherwise normal lungs.[198] In 1985, Dreyfuss and colleagues[199] reproduced these experiments and carefully studied the changes that occurred within the lung. They observed that the injury that occurred was morphologically and pathophysiologically similar to ARDS and hypothesized that mechanical ventilation with large tidal volumes or high inflation pressures might exacerbate or perpetuate the lung injury in patients suffering from ARDS. Two major questions were raised by this early work: Did high inflation pressures or large tidal volume excursions cause the lung injury? Did positive end-expiratory pressure (PEEP) worsen or attenuate this injury?

Dreyfuss and associates[200] then designed a set of experiments to answer these questions. They studied animals with normal lungs subjected only to varied protocols of mechanical ventilation. Some were ventilated with high pressures and large tidal volumes. Others had chest banding to limit chest wall and lung excursion during ventilation at high airway pressures. Another group was subjected to negative-pressure ventilation to assess the effect of large tidal volume excursions in the absence of high airway pressures. PEEP (10 cm H_2O) was applied to the lungs of some animals undergoing high-pressure/large-tidal-volume ventilation. Finally, control animals were ventilated using parameters typical of conventional ventilation. These investigators found that large tidal volumes were associated with lung injury, but that high inflation pressure in the absence of large tidal volume excursion was not. Surprisingly, PEEP had the effect of limiting the injury that occurred in animals ventilated with large tidal volumes and high pressures. The application of PEEP not only preserved gas exchange, but also prevented the morphologic progression of the lesion caused by this pattern of ventilation. These observations have been verified in larger animals.[201–204] (see Chap. 37 for more details).

A summary of these and subsequent animal experiments indicated that: (1) high-tidal-volume ventilation results in a lung injury morphologically similar to ARDS in humans, (2) PEEP is protective to some degree against this injury, (3) high-tidal-volume ventilation also can result in multiorgan system failure in otherwise healthy animals,[205,206] and (4) high-tidal-volume ventilation results in the release of inflammatory cells and proinflammatory cytokines.[207,208]

Clinical Research Utilizing Lung Imaging

The second parallel line of research, noted above, studied patients with ARDS by use of CT scans (see Fig. 38-7). The initial observations indicated that despite a homogeneous "white-out" pattern of diffuse pulmonary edema infiltrates on chest radiographs of patients with ALI and ARDS, the CT scans of the same patients often proved the infiltrates to have remarkable heterogeneity.[188,209] Based on strata of Hounsfield units to define different densities, the lung in ARDS could be partitioned into various compartments: nonaerated, poorly aerated, and normally aerated.[187] Moreover, these compartments could be tracked before and after PEEP was added or subtracted and before and after tidal volumes of different sizes were delivered to the lung.

The end result was a reconceptualization of the mechanical changes in the ARDS lung.[187] The traditional interpretation was that the stiffness of lungs in ARDS (e.g., low static compliances of 20 to 40 mL/cm H_2O) represented many alveoli with similarly low specific compliances (i.e., essentially a single compartment in terms of its mechanical properties). Instead, studies using the CT scans and their pathophysiologic correlations indicated that a more accurate picture is that the lung in ARDS is multicompartmental and that there is a small part of the ARDS lung that has relatively normal compliance. Gattinoni and coworkers coined the term "baby lung" when referring to this compartment and its vulnerability to overdistension.[187] In this revised conception of the acutely injured lung, some alveoli are normally compliant and vulnerable to overdistension while others are flooded or collapsed. The loss of functional alveoli necessitates that the tidal volume be distributed to far fewer aerated alveoli than in a healthy lung. Indeed, the apparent stiffness of the lungs of ARDS patients is regarded as the result of a small fraction of the lung containing relatively normal alveoli that becomes stiff as those alveoli reach their limits of distension, rather than due to generalized parenchymal "stiffness."

Based on the consistent results from the animal and in vitro studies referred to above and the insights provided by the results of the CT scans, it was hypothesized that traditional tidal volumes (e.g., 10 to 15 mL/kg) caused overdistension of alveoli in the lungs of patients with ALI and ARDS. This in turn not only resulted in exacerbation and perpetuation of their lung injury, but also, through the possible release of proinflammatory cytokines and other mechanisms, possibly contributed to the development and worsening of multiorgan system dysfunction and failure.

Intersection of Basic and Clinical Research

The intersection of these two lines of research, one basic and one clinical, resulted in two hypotheses of how patients with ALI and ARDS should be ventilated (see Fig. 38-7). First, the end-inspiratory lung volume should be limited to avoid alveolar overdistension (so-called "volutrauma") and second, sufficient PEEP should be applied so as to prevent cycles of end-expiratory derecruitment followed by inspiratory recruitment (Chap. 37 discusses the basis for both of these ventilatory recommendations in detail).

The next step was to test these hypotheses in prospective randomized controlled clinical trials (RCT) (see Fig. 38-7). Four large multicenter RCTs were conducted (Table 38-6). Three RCTs tested lower- vs. higher-tidal-volume strategies.[3,8,9] The fourth RCT tested a multifactorial lung-protective strategy (including lower tidal volume, higher PEEP based on static pressure-volume curves of the respiratory system, and recruitment maneuvers) against conventional ventilation.[7]

The strategies tested were based on interpretations of the static pressure-volume (P-V) curve of the respiratory system in ARDS (Fig. 38-8). The curve in Fig. 38-8 has a lower inflection point (LIP) and an upper inflection point (UIP). One of the RCTs used such curves, which were obtained by use of a super-syringe on paralyzed patients, to set PEEP above the LIP in the group receiving the lung protective strategy,[7] but examination of the schematized curve in Fig. 38-8 can be useful for understanding the strategies for trying to prevent VILI used in all four of the RCTs.

It was hypothesized that the LIP indicated the point at which most of the collapsed or partially fluid-filled alveoli in the lung became recruited.[210,211] At pressures higher than the LIP these recruited alveoli exhibited near-normal specific compliance. It was also hypothesized that the UIP represented the point above which the ventilated alveoli in the lung were overdistended, with a resulting low specific compliance of aerated but overdistended alveoli. Based on such P-V curves, it was suggested that PEEP above LIP should prevent the recruitment-derecruitment cycles of alveoli, and

TABLE 38-6 Phase III Randomized Controlled Clinical Trials Using Lung-Protective Strategies

Authors	Year Published (Years of Enrollment)	Number of Subjects Enrolled	Mortality in Lower-Tidal Volume Group	Mortality in Higher-Tidal-volume Group	*p* Value
Amato et al[7]	1998 (1990–1995)	53	38%[a] (45%)[b]	71%[a] (71%)[b]	<0.0001 (0.37)
Brochard et al[8]	1998 (1994–1996)	116	46.5%[c]	37.9%[c]	0.39
Stewart et al[9]	1998 (1995–1996)	120	50.0%[d]	47%[d]	0.72
ARDSnet[3e]	2000 (1996–1999)	861	31.0%[f]	39.8%[f]	0.007

[a] Mortality at 28 days.
[b] As of hospital discharge.
[c] Mortality at 60 days.
[d] Mortality at hospital discharge (up to ~100 days in hospital).
[e] NHLBI Acute Respiratory Distress Syndrome Clinical Trials Network.
[f] Mortality before discharge to home without assisted ventilation or as of 180 days, whichever occurred first.

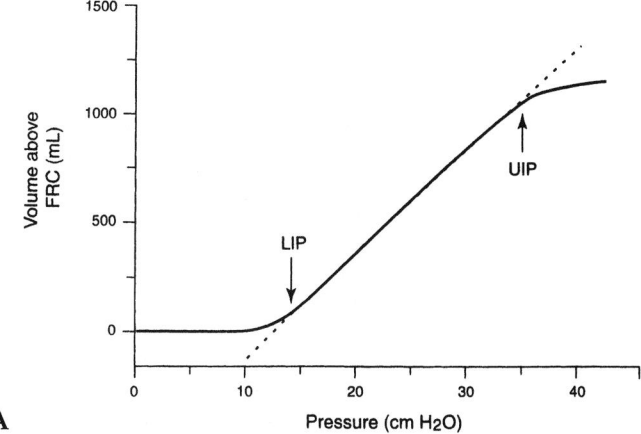

A

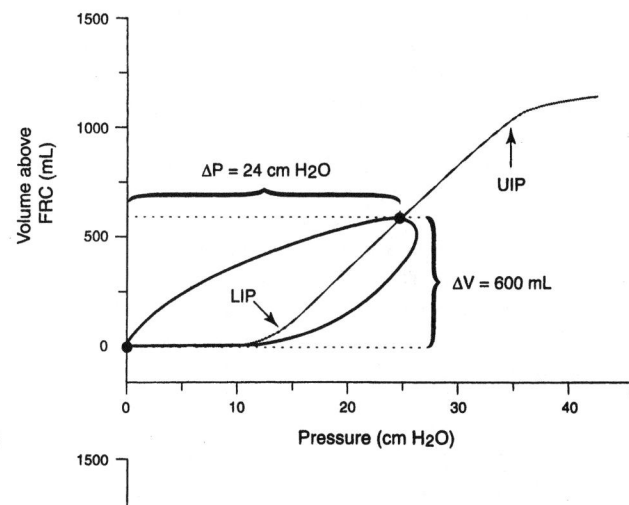

B

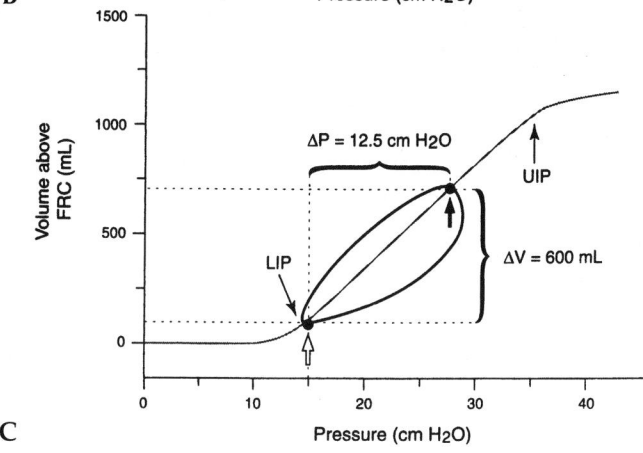

C

FIGURE 38-8 *A.* Schematic inspiratory static pressure-volume (P-V) curve of the respiratory system (lung and chest wall combined) in ARDS with a lower inflection point (LIP) at ~14 cm H_2O and an upper inflection point (UIP) at ~35 cm H_2O. The abscissa is recoil pressure of the respiratory system and the ordinate is lung volume above functional residual capacity (FRC). *B.* Same static P-V as in *A,* plus a dynamic P-V curve of 600 mL tidal volume starting at PEEP = 0, which is below the LIP. This tidal volume results in a plateau pressure of 25 cm H_2O, which is below the UIP. Static compliance (Cstat = $\Delta V/\Delta P$ = 600 mL/25 cm H_2O) is 24 mL/cm H_2O. *C.* PEEP of 15 cm H_2O has moved the starting point for the 600 mL tidal volume up the static P-V curve to a new FRC (*open arrow*), which is just above the LIP. The tidal volume results in a plateau pressure of 27.5 cm H_2O (*closed arrow*), which is well *below* the UIP. Cstat ($\Delta V/\Delta P$ = 600 mL/12.5 cm H_2O) is increased to 48 mL/cm H_2O, compared to *B. D.* Dynamic P-V curve of a 1000 mL tidal volume, starting at 14 cm H_2O PEEP, results in a plateau pressure of 38 cm H_2O (*closed arrow*). Note the decrease in Cstat ($\Delta V/\Delta P$ = 1000 mL/24 cm H_2O = 41.7 mL/cm H_2O) compared to Cstat derived from the tidal volume of 600 mL in *C.* The 1000 mL tidal volume's plateau pressure exceeds the UIP, which implies overdistension and is believed to put the lung at risk for ventilator-induced lung injury (see text). (*Reproduced with permission from Lanken PN: Acute respiratory distress syndrome, in Lanken PN, Hanson CW III, Manaker S (eds): The Intensive Care Unit Manual.* Philadelphia, WB Saunders, 2001, p 824.)

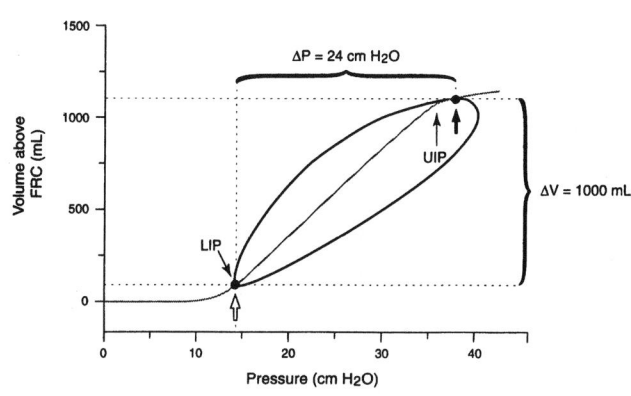

D

as such prevent the lung injury resulting from these cycles ("atelectrauma" [see Chap. 37]). Based on this interpretation, tidal volumes that resulted in end-inspiratory (plateau pressures) below the UIP should decrease alveolar overdistension and thus prevent VILI from this cause.

However, despite the attractiveness of this interpretation of the static pressure-volume curve, subsequent reports indicate that the situation is more complex and that recruitment of alveoli in experimental models and in patients with ALI and ARDS extends beyond the pressure at the LIP and continues over a wide range of airway pressures up to 45 cm H_2O.[212–214]

NHLBI ARDS Clinical Trials Network Low-Tidal-Volume Ventilatory Strategy Clinical Trial

The NHLBI ARDS Clinical Trials Network conducted the landmark RCT that investigated the use of lung-protective ventilation in patients with ALI and ARDS[3] This ARDSNet RCT compared a ventilator strategy with lower tidal volumes designed to limit stretch of the lungs during mechanical ventilation with a strategy that utilized traditional larger tidal volumes. The randomized clinical trial enrolled 861 patients at multiple centers. Briefly, one study arm received a tidal volume of 6 mL/kg PBW if the Pplat did not exceed 30 cm H_2O, and tidal volumes of 4 or 5 mL/kg PBW if Pplat did exceed 30 cm H_2O (see Table 38-9 for complete details of the protocol of this arm). The other arm received tidal volumes of 12 mL/kg PBW if the Pplat did not exceed 50 cm H_2O, and tidal volumes as low as 4 mL/kg PBW if the Pplat did exceed 50 cm H_2O. There was a 9% absolute mortality reduction (22% relative mortality reduction) in the group receiving the lower-tidal-volume ventilation strategy (see Table 38-6). This corresponds to a number needed to treat of ~11 patients in order to prevent one death. Importantly, plasma levels of IL-6 were lower among the 6-mL/kg group, as were the number of organ-failure-free days, indicating that the lower tidal volume strategy was associated with a faster clearance of IL-6, a

proinflammatory cytokine, from the plasma, and less organ dysfunction.

This ARDSNet RCT differed from two prior, smaller studies that showed no apparent benefit to the lower-tidal-volume strategies[8,9] (see Table 38-6; Table 38-7). These differences may have been due to chance alone since the earlier studies were of limited sample size, with an associated lack of statistical power to detect this degree of difference in mortality. Other possible reasons for these differences include the fact that the ARDSNet RCT used smaller tidal volumes in the low-tidal-volume group than the others (see Table 38-7). In addition, the protocols differed in how they dealt with respiratory acidosis due to lower tidal volumes and permissive hypercapnia. Related to respiratory acidosis, the ARDSNet RCT protocol required increases in ventilator rate as the tidal volume was initially decreased, or if the pH fell below normal limits. In addition, bicarbonate infusions were allowed. In the other two earlier RCTs, similar respiratory rate increases were not mandated. Possibly as a result of these differences in protocols, there were smaller differences in Pa_{CO_2} and arterial pH between study groups in the ARDSNet RCT compared to the other two RCTs (see Table 38-7).

Although the ARDSNet RCT was subsequently criticized for its design in relying on strict ventilator protocols for the higher-tidal-volume group,[215–217] the ARDSnet lower-tidal-volume ventilatory strategy has become accepted as the standard for ventilator management of ALI-ARDS patients. This is based both on the results of the ARDSnet RCT, but also on the plethora of basic and clinical studies, as described above and in Chap. 37, relating to ventilator-induced lung injury that support its hypothetical mode of efficacy.

Using Higher Levels of PEEP to Decrease the Risk of VILI

There is controversy about whether higher-than-traditional levels of PEEP can decrease the risk of ventilator-induced lung injury in patients with ALI and ARDS. In addition, if

TABLE 38-7 Comparison of Pa_{CO_2}, Arterial pH, and Tidal Volume in Phase III Randomized Controlled Clinical Trials Using Lung-Protective Strategies

Authors	Group	Tidal Volume[a] on Study Day 1 (mL/kg)	Pa_{CO_2} (mm Hg)	Arterial pH
Amato et al[7]	Lower tidal volume	~6 mL/kg	55.0 ± 1.2[b]	7.25 ± 0.01[b]
Amato et al[7]	Higher tidal volume	~12 mL/kg	33.2 ± 1.7[b]	7.40 ± 0.01[b]
Brochard et al[8]	Lower tidal volume	7.1 ± 1.3	59.5 ± 15.0[c]	N/A
Brochard et al[8]	Higher tidal volume	10.3 ± 1.7	41.3 ± 7.6[c]	N/A
Stewart et al[9]	Lower tidal volume	7.0 ± 0.7	54.4 ± 18.8[d] (28–116)	7.29[d] (6.99–7.49)
Stewart et al[9]	Higher tidal volume	10.7 ± 1.4	45.7 ± 9.8[d] (29–72)	7.34[d] (7.08–7.51)
ARDSNet[3e]	Lower tidal volume	6.2 ± 0.9	40 ± 10[c]	7.38 ± 0.08[c]
ARDSNet.[3]	Higher tidal volume	11.8 ± 0.8	$35. \pm 8$[c]	7.41 ± 0.07[c]

Values are given as mean ± standard deviation unless otherwise indicated; values in parentheses are the range.
[a] Tidal volumes are given as milliliters per kilogram of body weight, but each study used a different method for calculating body weight: Amato and coworkers used actual body weight, but expressed the results only as milliliters.[7] Brochard and associates used "actual weight minus the estimated weight gain due to water and salt retention."[8] Stewart[337] and the ARDSNet researchers[3] used body weight predicted by two different equations.[193]
[b] Values over the first 36 hours of the study.
[c] Values of Pa_{CO_2} on Study Day 1.
[d] Maximal value of Pa_{CO_2} during the study; the corresponding arterial pH is the value at the time of the maximal Pa_{CO_2}.
[e] NHLBI Acute Respiratory Distress Syndrome Clinical Trials Network.

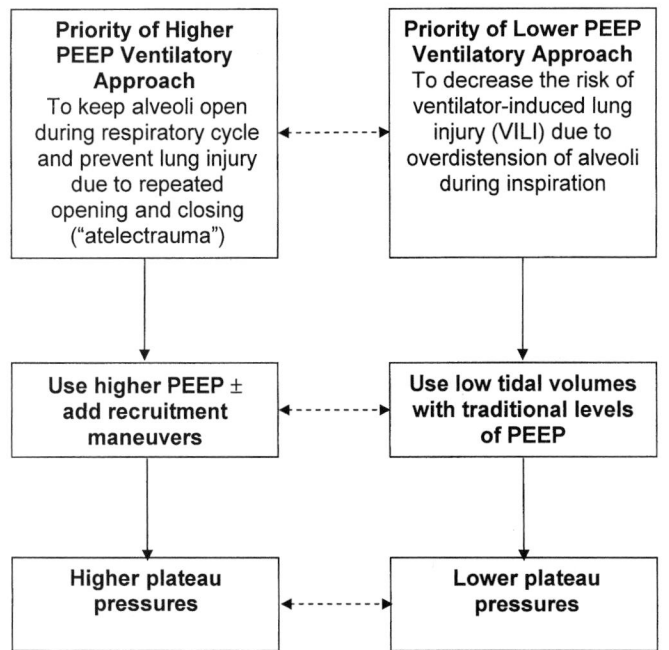

FIGURE 38-9 Schematic diagram illustrating the conflicting priorities of higher- and lower-PEEP ventilator approaches and their hypothetical associated effects. Studies that use a higher PEEP approach may combine the higher PEEP with recruitment maneuvers, which are sustained inflations (e.g., 35 to 40 cm H_2O of continuous positive airway pressure for 30 seconds or more[4,7]). For a given low tidal volume, using a higher PEEP will result in a higher plateau (end-inspiratory) pressure than using a lower PEEP. Hypothetically, this higher plateau pressure, which represents the static end-inspiratory distending pressure in open alveoli, may increase the risk of ventilator-induced lung injury due to overdistension (see text and Chap. 17 for details).

higher PEEP is effective against VILI, the question of what level of PEEP should be used clinically remains. When the pressure-volume relationship is measured in patients with ARDS, the lower inflection point (LIP) (see Fig. 38-8) is in the range of 8 to 15 cm H_2O.[7] In an earlier CT study of patients with ARDS,[211,218] the amount of reopening-collapsing tissue became insignificant only when PEEP reached 20 cm H_2O (although the greatest reduction was seen between 10 and 15 cm H_2O of PEEP).

However, as noted above, more recent animal and human studies have shown that the LIP is not the originally hypothesized simple threshold above which no further recruitment occurs. Instead, recruitment continues from below the LIP to inflation pressures of 45 cm H_2O.[212,213] In other words, there is a broad "inflection zone" from 0 to 45 cm H_2O over which there is progressive recruitment with progressively higher PEEP. The implication of these findings is that preventing cycles of recruitment and derecruitment in most of the alveoli necessitates that many open alveoli will be overdistended. Hence, prevention of injury to alveoli from cycles of recruitment-derecruitment will increase the risk of VILI from overdistension (see Figure 38-9).

Clinical Studies of Higher PEEP Ventilator Strategies
Proponents of a high-PEEP strategy (also called "open lung" strategy) were encouraged by a relatively small but statistically significant RCT performed by Amato and colleagues and published in 1998[7] (see Table 38-6). As noted above, in this RCT the group of subjects with ARDS in the "open lung" arm were treated by a combination of three interventions: (1) a low-tidal-volume ventilatory strategy, (2) higher-than-traditional levels of PEEP as dictated by the patient's LIP as described below, and (3) recruitment maneuvers. The control group of subjects was treated by a conventional ventilatory strategy for the participating ICUs, which did not include any of the three interventions of the open lung group and was not protocolized. In this study, the higher level of PEEP was determined by using a super-syringe to derive a static pressure-

volume curve on paralyzed subjects at the start of the study. From inspection of the static pressure-volume curve, the LIP (see Fig. 38-8) was identified and the PEEP was set at 2 cm H_2O above the LIP. If a sharp LIP could not be determined on the pressure-volume curve, then the PEEP was set empirically at 16 cm H_2O.[7]

Although this study found that the group receiving the open lung approach had significantly lower mortality than the group receiving conventional ventilation (see Table 38-6), it was unclear which intervention or combination of interventions was responsible for the observed improvement. Was the lower mortality due to the low-tidal-volume ventilatory strategy, the higher-than-traditional levels of PEEP, or the recruitment maneuvers, or a combination of two or all three?

To try to answer these questions, which had also been raised in an earlier report by Amato and colleagues,[219] the NHLBI ARDSNet investigators decided to study one intervention at a time in separate RCTs. As noted above, the first ARDSNet RCT compared a lower-tidal-volume ventilatory strategy to a strategy using traditional tidal volumes.[3] This RCT found a significant decrease in mortality in the group treated with the lower-tidal-volume ventilatory strategy (see Table 38-6). After completion of this RCT, the ARDSNet investigators conducted a second RCT ("ALVEOLI") to try to answer the question: When used in addition to the lower-tidal-volume strategy of ventilation, do higher PEEP levels improve survival?

The results of the ALVEOLI study[4] are presented in Table 38-8. In summary, ALVEOLI found that mortality rates were similar in those treated with higher and traditional levels of PEEP despite significant increases in Pa_{O_2} : FI_{O_2}. The higher-PEEP group had a higher mean plateau pressure despite a lower mean tidal volume (see Table 38-8). Although hypothetical, it is possible that the benefits of the higher PEEP in reducing the acute lung injury due to shear stress created by recruitment-derecruitment were negated by its adverse effects, such as worsening lung injury by overdistension (see Figure 38-9).

TABLE 38-8 ARDSNet[a] Clinical Trial of Lower versus Higher Levels of PEEP in Patients with Acute Lung Injury (ALI) or Acute Respiratory Distress Syndrome (ARDS)

Group	Number of Subjects Enrolled	PEEP[b] (cm H_2O)	Pa_{O_2}:$F_{I_{O_2}}$ Ratio[c]	Plateau Pressure[c] (cm H_2O)	Tidal Volume[c] (mL/kg Predicted Body Weight)	Mortality[d] (95% CI[f])	Adjusted Mortality[e] (95% CI[f])
Lower PEEP	273	8.3 ± 3.2	169 ± 69	24 ± 6	6.1 ± 1.1	24.9% (19.8–30.0%)	27.5% (23.0–31.9%)
Higher PEEP	276	13.2 ± 3.5	206 ± 76	26 ± 7	5.8 ± 1.0	27.5% (22.3–32.8%)	25.1% (20.7–29.5%)
p value		<0.001	<0.01	<0.05	<0.05	0.48	0.47

[a] NHLBI Acute Respiratory Distress Syndrome Clinical Trials Network.
[b] Means ($\pm$ SD) over the first 4 days after randomization.
[c] Means ($\pm$ SD) on Study Day 3.
[d] Mortality before discharge to home without assisted ventilation or as of 60 days, whichever occurred first.
[e] Mortality adjusted for imbalances in baseline variables by multivariable modeling.[4]
[f] 95% Confidence interval.
SOURCE: Data from ARDSnet.[4]

RECOMMENDED CORE VENTILATOR MANAGEMENT

As the core ventilator management in ALI and ARDS, we recommend that clinicians use the lower-tidal-volume ventilatory strategy ("ARDSnet lung-protective strategy") that the ARDSNet investigators showed to be superior to traditional tidal volume strategy (Table 38-9). Because this strategy that used traditional levels of PEEP was shown to yield similar outcomes compared to using higher PEEP levels[4] (see Table 38-8), we also recommend using the same combinations of PEEP and $F_{I_{O_2}}$ that were an integral part of the ventilator protocol for the lower-tidal-volume strategy (see Table 38-9). Clinicians should be cautious in utilizing this protocol strictly for patients with ALI and ARDS who have conditions for which respiratory acidosis due to permissive hypercapnia are contraindicated (Tables 38-10 and 38-11).

In addition to this core ventilator management, some clinicians use various interventions as adjuncts (Table 38-12). Finally, clinicians may choose to use alternative ventilatory strategies whose efficacy is unproven (e.g., salvage therapies for patients in dire clinical circumstances) (Table 38-13).

Adjuncts to Core Ventilator Management

Clinicians may use one or more interventions as adjuncts to "customize" the recommended core ventilator management to try to improve pulmonary physiology and otherwise benefit individual patients (see Table 38-13). Most of these adjuncts hold the possibility of benefit based on extrapolation from animal or clinical research that generally uses physiologic end points as suggestions of efficacy. However, it is inaccurate to extrapolate from an improvement in physiologic outcomes to efficacy in terms of clinically meaningful outcomes (e.g., survival or days of mechanical ventilation). For example, in the first ARDSNet RCT, the lower-tidal-volume group had better survival than the higher-tidal-volume group, despite having lower mean values for Pa_{O_2}: $F_{I_{O_2}}$.[3] Furthermore, the safety of these adjuncts is generally uncertain. Clinicians who want to use high-level evidence to guide care of patients with ALI and ARDS should be warned that to date, all of the following adjuncts fall short of that level of scientific evidence.

RESTRICTIVE ("DRY") FLUID MANAGEMENT The optimal fluid management in patients with ALI and ARDS remains uncertain. The rationale for restricting fluids in ALI and ARDS

suggests that if edemagenesis could be diminished early after the lung injury, the duration of potentially dangerous ventilator, PEEP, and oxygen therapy could be reduced and outcome conceivably improved. In this regard it is interesting that most patients with ARDS do not die during the early phase of disease as a consequence of severe hypoxemia, but rather over days to weeks, frequently with evidence of hypermetabolism, nosocomial infection, and multiple organ system failure.[53,54] On the other hand, some have argued that maximizing oxygen delivery (so-called "supercharging") to peripheral tissues is a necessary strategy in critically ill patients such as those with sepsis and ARDS, and advocate approaches such as volume loading to achieve this goal.[220,221] This latter position has fallen out of favor because the oxygen extraction defect purported to exist in patients with sepsis and ARDS now seems to have been artifactual, or at least not clinically relevant.[222,223] Moreover, controlled clinical trials of such goal-oriented hemodynamic therapy showed no improvement in survival[224] or worse survival.[225] In patients with ALI and ARDS, the consequence of an approach of maximizing oxygen delivery could be escalating requirements for mechanical ventilation, oxygen, and PEEP. To the extent that intensity and duration of supportive therapy are major determinants of complications and organ dysfunctions, the net result could be detrimental. Fluid management strategies in ALI and ARDS are currently the focus of an ongoing ARDSNet investigation (the Fluids and Catheter Treatment Trial, or FACTT). FACTT also is comparing use of central venous catheters to pulmonary artery catheters to guide fluid management. Until the results of this study are known, we favor an approach that aims for a cautious reduction in central venous pressure (CVP) or pulmonary artery wedge pressure (Ppw) while maintaining adequate circulation early in the course of ARDS as a strategy to minimize edemagenesis and to avoid adverse effects of its treatment. Although this approach is controversial, its justification derives from both animal experiments[226–233] and clinical data (see below).

Several retrospective or noninterventional studies have reported data showing a correlation between survival and net diuresis or reduction in Ppw.[234–236] Prospective data collection also has demonstrated that titration of therapy to minimize extravascular lung water in patients with ARDS results in decreased ventilator and ICU days.[237] Until a prospective,

TABLE 38-9 NIH NHLBI ARDS Network Low-Tidal-Volume Ventilation Strategy

Part I. Ventilator set-up and adjustment

1. Calculate ideal body weight (IBW).[a]
2. Use assist/control mode and set initial tidal volume (TV) to 8 mL/kg IBW (if baseline TV >8 mL/kg).
3. Reduce TV by 1-mL/kg intervals every 2 hours until TV = 6 mL/kg IBW.
4. Set initial rate to approximate baseline minute ventilation (but not >35 bpm).
5. Adjust TV and respiratory rate (RR) to achieve pH and plateau pressure (Pplat) goals listed below.
6. Set the inspiratory flow rate above patient demand (usually >80 L/min); adjust flow rate to achieve goal of inspiratory : expiratory ratio of 1:1.0–1.3

Part II. Oxygenation goal: Pa_{O_2} = 55–80 mm Hg or Sp_{O_2} = 88–95%

1. Use these incremental $F_{I_{O_2}}$-PEEP combinations to achieve oxygenation goal:

$F_{I_{O_2}}$	0.3	0.4	0.4	0.5	0.5	0.6	0.7	0.7
PEEP	5	5	8	8	10	10	10	12
$F_{I_{O_2}}$	0.7	0.8	0.9	0.9	0.9	1.0	1.0	1.0
PEEP	14	14	14	16	18	20	22	24

Part III. Plateau Pressure (Pplat) Goal: = 30 cm H_2O

1. Check Pplat (use 0.5-s inspiratory pause), Sp_{O_2}, total RR, TV, and arterial blood gases (ABG) (if available) at least every 4 hours and after each change in PEEP or TV.
2. If Pplat >30 cm H_2O, decrease TV by 1-mL/kg steps (minimum 4 mL/kg IBW).
3. If Pplat <25 cm H_2O and TV <6mL/kg, increase TV by 1 mL/kg until Pplat >25 cm H_2O or TV = 6 mL/kg.
4. If Pplat <30 cm H_2O and breath stacking occurs, one may increase TV in 1-mL/kg IBW increments (to a maximum of 8 mL/kg) as long as Pplat<30 cm H_2O.

Part IV. pH Goal: 7.30–7.45
Acidosis management: pH <7.30

1. If pH = 7.15 −7.30, increase RR until pH >7.30 or Pa_{CO_2} <25 mm Hg (Maximum RR = 35); if RR = 35 and Pa_{CO_2} <25 mm Hg, may give $NaHCO_3$.
2. If pH <7.15 and $NaHCO_3$ considered or infused, TV may be increased in 1-mL/kg steps until pH >7.15 (Pplat goal may be exceeded).

Alkalosis management: pH >7.45: Decrease RR if possible.

[a] Male IBW = 50 + 2.3 [height (inches) − 60]; female IBW = 45.5 + 2.3 [height (inches) − 60]. Sp_{O_2}, oxygen saturation by pulse oximetry, ABG, arterial blood gas.
From the NIH NHLBI ARDS Network (complete protocol is available at www.ardsnet.org).
SOURCE: Reproduced with permission from Lanken PN: Acute respiratory distress syndrome, in Lanken PN, Hanson CW III, Manaker S (eds): *The Intensive Care Unit Manual*. Philadelphia, WB Saunders, 2001, p. 828.

randomized trial of a strategy of conservative fluid management in ALI and ARDS patients provides evidence regarding efficacy and safety, the circulatory management of these patients can be described as a therapeutic dilemma.[238,239] On the one hand, judicious volume reduction may improve lung function. In the extreme, however, hypoperfusion and other organ failure could occur.

In order to reduce Ppw safely in patients with ALI and ARDS, the clinician's attention should be focused on the parameters of organ function that should be followed in all critically ill patients (e.g., mental status, urine output and concentration, circulatory adequacy, and metabolic evidence of anaerobic metabolism). *This should not be misinterpreted as trading reduced pulmonary edema for a hypoperfused state.* Rather, the aim of this approach is to find the lowest Ppw or CVP compatible with *adequate* functioning of the circulatory system. Preload can be reduced in part by meticulous attention to limit all extraneous fluid administration. Furosemide is often used to achieve diuresis and net negative fluid balance. However, this may confound interpretation of renal function as an indicator of the adequacy of perfusion. In selected patients, particularly those with manifest systolic dysfunction, dobutamine can be used to maintain perfusion at a reduced Ppw.

Interpreting right heart catheterization data during mechanical ventilation with PEEP can be challenging.[240] The usual measurement made at right heart catheterization is the Ppw. Measurements of Ppw may fail to reflect left ventricular filling pressure for a number of reasons. First, if alveolar pressure is greater than left atrial pressure at the site of measurement (West zone 1 or 2), then the downstream pressure is not measured, and the right heart catheter reflects alveolar pressure. Existence of zone 1 or 2 conditions can be inferred from the excursion of the pulmonary arterial and wedge pressure waveforms during positive pressure ventilation.[241] *This possibility must be considered if one attempts preload reduction in patients with ARDS requiring high PEEP levels.*

Second, it is often difficult to identify end-inspiration in many patients with ALI or ARDS. This is especially problematic if patients are spontaneously breathing while receiving assisted ventilation. To improve accuracy in making routine measurements of Ppw as well as CVP, it is recommended that the airway pressure be transduced and its transducer's output be printed simultaneously with the pressure tracing.

TABLE 38-10 Effects of Permissive Hypercapnia and Respiratory Acidosis

Hemodynamic effects

Activation of sympathetic nervous system and catechol secretion, normally resulting in increased heart rate and stroke volume with peripheral vasodilatation

Impaired myocardial contractility and worse congestive heart failure

Coronary vasodilation and potential for vasodilation-induced steal resulting in less blood flow to ischemic myocardium

Pulmonary arteriolar vasoconstriction, potentiating hypoxic pulmonary vasoconstriction

Rightward shift of the oxygen dissociation curve with potential for less loading of O_2 at the alveolar level and arterial desaturation

Effects on the central nervous system

Increased cerebral blood flow due to arterial hypertension and cerebral vasodilatation (vasodilatation may be lost in areas subject to trauma or ischemia)

Cerebral vasodilation and potential vasodilation-induced steal resulting in less blood flow to ischemic regions of the brain

Increases intracranial pressure

SOURCE: Reproduced with permission from Feihl.[247]

The transduced airway pressure tracing clearly identifies the start of inspiration by the start of its positive deflection in patients who are not assisting the ventilator. Likewise the airway pressure tracing also easily identifies the start of an assisted breath by the occurrence of the associated negative pressure deflection. This simple change can significantly decrease interobserver variability.[242]

Some have suggested that the nadir in Ppw after an airway disconnect might better reflect left ventricular filling pressure.[243,244] This approach may be dangerous and is not recommended since even relatively short discontinuation of PEEP can have adverse effects on oxygenation that may take hours to recover.

PERMISSIVE HYPERCAPNIA Traditionally physicians have attempted to ventilate patients to a normal arterial P_{CO_2} (see Fig. 38-6). In patients with severe lung disease, however, this arbitrary goal has a mechanical cost: the probable amplification of lung injury (i.e., VILI). Increasing evidence points to the safety and efficacy of allowing the arterial P_{CO_2} to rise

TABLE 38-11 Contraindications to Permissive Hypercapnia and Respiratory Acidosis

Increased intracranial pressure from any cause (trauma, mass lesion, malignant hypertension)

Acute cerebrovascular disorders (e.g., stroke)

Acute or chronic myocardial ischemia

Severe pulmonary hypertension

Right ventricular failure

Uncorrected severe metabolic acidosis

Sickle-cell anemia

Tricyclic antidepressant overdose

Patients taking β-blockers

Pregnancy (potential for decreased fetal blood flow due to vasodilatation-induced steal syndrome; in addition, shift to the right of the oxygen dissociation curve may decrease maternal-fetal oxygen gradient)

TABLE 38-12 Adjuncts to Low-Tidal-Volume Ventilation for Treatment of Acute Lung Injury (ALI) and Acute Respiratory Distress Syndrome (ARDS)

Restrictive ("dry") fluid management strategy

Increasing cardiac output and/or oxygen delivery to supranormal levels

Permissive hypercapnia

Prone positioning

Recruitment maneuvers

above 40 mm Hg when used in combination with a ventilatory strategy that uses low tidal volumes and low plateau pressures. When patients with ALI and ARDS are ventilated with volume- and pressure-limited ventilation as described above, the mean Pa_{CO_2} may rise modestly (into the low 40s mm Hg) or higher (into the mid-to-high 50s mm Hg) with corresponding falls in arterial pH (see Table 38-7). Occasional patients may have a Pa_{CO_2} above 100 mm Hg[245,246] (see Table 38-7).

Respiratory acidosis has many physiologic effects, including cellular metabolic dysfunction, depression of myocardial contractility, coronary vasodilation, systemic vasodilation, pulmonary vasoconstriction, enhanced hypoxic pulmonary vasoconstriction, cerebral vasodilation, increased intracranial pressure, and renal vasoconstriction, among others[247,248] (see Table 38-10). Yet even very high levels of P_{CO_2} seem remarkably well tolerated by adequately sedated patients. Perhaps this is related to highly efficient and rapidly acting cellular compensatory mechanisms that tend to defend intracellular pH. Because respiratory acidosis raises intracranial pressure, permissive hypercapnia should not be used in patients with cerebral edema, trauma, or space-occupying lesions. This and other contraindications are listed in Table 38-11.

PRONE POSITIONING Multiple studies have shown that about two-thirds of patients with ARDS exhibit improved oxygenation with prone positioning ("proned").[249–252] Hypotheses offered to explain the improvement in oxygenation include (1) increased FRC, (2) change in regional diaphragm motion, (3) redistribution of perfusion, and (4) better clearance of secretions.[253] FRC has been shown to be increased in the prone position in intubated, mechanically-ventilated patients without lung injury who are undergoing general anesthesia for surgery.[254] Animal models of ventilation-perfusion distribution have suggested that gravity has far less influence on the distribution of perfusion in the prone position, and that the distribution of blood flow to regions of the lung is relatively unaffected by the change from the supine to the prone position.[255] This, coupled with the observation that turning to the prone position is associated with a migration

TABLE 38-13 Salvage Interventions for Patients with Severe Hypoxemia in Acute Respiratory Distress Syndrome (ARDS)

Tracheal gas insufflation (TGI)

Pressure-controlled inverted ratio ventilation (PC-IRV)

Extracorporeal membrane oxygenation (ECMO)

High-frequency oscillatory ventilation (HFOV)

Inhaled nitric oxide (NO) or inhaled prostacyclin (epoprostenol)

Corticosteroids

of the edema fluid to the dependent portions of the lung (as demonstrated by CT scan), has suggested to some investigators that ventilation-perfusion relationships might be favorably altered by the prone position.[256] In patients managed in the prone position, special attention is necessary to prevent pressure necrosis of the nose, face, and ears, and to ensure maintenance and patency of the endotracheal tube. Pressure on the eye could lead to retinal ischemia, especially in hypotensive patients. Some patients experience cardiac arrhythmias or hemodynamic instability on being turned.

These considerations led to a large clinical trial performed by Gattinoni and colleagues.[252] In this study, subjects were placed in the prone position for six or more hours daily for 10 days. The results, published in 2001, revealed that although oxygenation was transiently improved, prone positioning offered no survival advantage over routine supine positioning.[252] Further post-hoc analyses indicated that a patient's response to prone positioning may have prognostic value. Patients whose Pa_{CO_2} *fell* by 1 mm Hg or more when placed in the prone position had a lower mortality rate than those whose Pa_{CO_2} didn't fall or rose (mortality of 35.1% vs. mortality of 52.2%).[257]

Prone positioning may have a role in the future, when combined with lower tidal volume ventilation, such as the ARDSNet protocol (see Table 38-9), ventilator sighs,[258] or when employed using a different treatment protocol. Clinicians may reserve use of prone positioning as salvage therapy for severe hypoxemia, but they should understand that there are no controlled studies that support its efficacy in this circumstance, even in those patients whose oxygenation improves (see below). Finally, although some advocate the routine use of prone positioning as part of a multifactorial lung protective strategy,[259] no controlled clinical trials support such routine use, especially given its potential adverse effects listed above.

RECRUITMENT MANEUVERS   Recruitment maneuvers evolved from traditional "sighs," which are extra-large breaths of the order of two or three normal-sized tidal volume breaths. Sighs normally occur 4 to 10 times per hour and increase the surfactant's surface-tension-lowering properties, thus stabilizing small alveoli and resisting atelectasis.

Recruitment maneuvers were part of the "open lung" strategy in the clinical trial of low tidal volume ventilation by Amato et al[7] (see Tables 38-6 and 38-7). In the Amato trial, recruitment maneuvers consisted of application of continuous positive airway pressure (CPAP) of 35 to 40 cm H_2O for 30-second periods. Others have advocated longer periods at the same or higher airway pressures.[259] The justification for recruitment maneuvers is to "recruit" or open totally or partially collapsed alveoli, which then would be kept inflated during expiration by a high level of PEEP.[259]

Evidence is lacking that recruitment maneuvers alone improve clinically significant outcomes such as mortality or ventilator-free days. Most studies of recruitment maneuvers have used physiologic end points, such as improvement in oxygenation. The ARDSNet studied recruitment maneuvers as a substudy of 96 subjects in the higher-PEEP group in the ALVEOLI study[260] (see Table 38-8). There were no clinically relevant improvements in arterial saturation, but complications occurred, such as transient hypotension and slight drops in arterial saturation during the recruitment maneuver. Other studies have shown more consistent improvement in oxygenation after recruitment maneuvers if relatively low levels of PEEP were being used,[261-263] if larger tidal volumes were used,[264] or if the patients are paralyzed.[265]

Given the lack of controlled clinical trials that demonstrate efficacy in clinically relevant end points and the potential adverse effects, we don't recommend routine use of recruitment maneuvers. Furthermore, because they exceed the threshold of 30 cm H_2O used in the ARDSnet clinical trial that showed improved survival, and the lack of studies that demonstrate improved outcomes,[266-268] we don't recommend routine use of "sighs" either.

SALVAGE INTERVENTIONS   When treating subjects with severe ARDS, some clinicians may try unproven interventions if the patient is deteriorating with severe hypoxemia (e.g., Pa_{O_2} less than 45 to 50 mm Hg) or needing an F_{IO_2} of 0.9 or more to maintain Pa_{O_2} above 55 mm Hg. These may be referred to as "salvage" interventions. These clinicians justify their use of these interventions on two grounds: (1) the dire condition of the patient, and (2) a hope of clinical efficacy. The latter is based on results from basic science studies suggesting a reasonable rationale, from their use in animal models, and from clinical usage that showed improvements in certain physiologic parameters (e.g., Pa_{O_2}: F_{IO_2}).

Despite the failure to improve survival in phase III clinical trials of patients with ALI/ARDS who were not necessarily in such dire straits, these clinicians may feel ethically obligated through the "Rule of Rescue[269]" to provide an intervention that may help as long as the risk is acceptable. Because of expense, lack of proven efficacy, and potential for harm, we do not advocate routine use of any of these "salvage interventions." Rather, we support a management strategy guided by evidence and including active observation of critically ill patients with ARDS. We urge those who advocate for their use to conduct clinical trials in the targeted population of patients with severe ARDS to assess their safety and efficacy.

Nonetheless, when there are severe problems with oxygenation in an otherwise salvageable patient, some clinicians will want to utilize certain adjunctive therapies. *It is important to realize that these therapies should not distract caregivers from the fundamentals of good critical care*, including nutrition, aspiration precautions, hygiene and prevention of nosocomial infections, appropriate sedation practices, and careful vigilance for complications of critical care.

TRACHEAL GAS INSUFFLATION   Tracheal gas insufflation (TGI), involves introducing fresh gas near the carina through a modified endotracheal tube. This added flow washes CO_2-rich gas out of the trachea (and, through turbulence, out of smaller airways as well), reducing anatomic dead space.[270] The Pa_{CO_2}-reducing effect of TGI is lessened by acute lung injury, but this is partially counterbalanced by the higher Pa_{CO_2} values used during permissive hypercapnia.[271] In patients with ARDS, TGI with 100% humidified oxygen, delivered throughout the respiratory cycle at a flow of 4 L/min, successfully lowered P_{CO_2} from 108 to 84 mm Hg.[272] Potential risks of TGI include tracheal erosion, oxygen toxicity related to the unknown F_{IO_2}, hemodynamic compromise or barotrauma due to the occult presence of auto-PEEP, and a larger tidal volume than the ventilator is set to deliver (i.e., potentially increasing the risk of VILI).

INHALED NITRIC OXIDE AND INHALED PROSTACYCLIN (EPOPROSTENOL) Since Roissant and colleagues published their initial experience using inhaled nitric oxide as a therapy for ARDS, there has been a rapid expansion of interest and literature in this field.[273-278] Given via inhalation, NO has several potentially salutary effects in ARDS. It selectively vasodilates pulmonary capillaries and arterioles that subserve *ventilated* alveoli, diverting blood flow to these alveoli (and away from areas of shunting). The vasodilating effect, signaled by a fall in pulmonary artery pressure and pulmonary vascular resistance, appears maximal at very low concentrations (0.1 ppm) in patients with ARDS.[277] The beneficial effects on oxygenation take place at somewhat higher inspired concentrations of NO (1 to 10 ppm).[277] The rapid inactivation of NO via hemoglobin binding prevents unwanted systemic hemodynamic side effects, but also mandates the continuous delivery of gas to the ventilator circuit. Thus, if continuous delivery of NO is interrupted (e.g., during patient transport or due to supply exhaustion), precipitous and life-threatening hypoxemia and right-sided heart failure may occur.[279] A recent large clinical trial compared the use of NO to placebo in subjects with ALI not due to sepsis, with no other organ failures.[280] The trial showed no benefit in survival with use of NO despite some patients having a transient improvement in oxygenation. Trials in other subgroups of ALI may be the focus of future investigations, but there is no consensus evidence for routine use of NO in ALI.

Even as a salvage intervention, inhaled NO is unattractive since there is a reasonable alternative available at much less expense. Whereas the cost of inhaled NO for 1 day is in the thousands of dollars, the daily cost of inhaled prostacyclin (epoprostenol) is in the hundreds of dollars. Inhaled prostacyclin, although less well studied, appears to provide the same degree of improvement in oxygenation in a majority of patients with ALI and ARDS at much less expense.[281-284]

CORTICOSTEROIDS Although it is commonly accepted that steroids have little or no role to play in treating the early acute phase of ARDS,[285,286] their role in later phases remains controversial. A number of anecdotal reports and small series have suggested that high-dose corticosteroids may be of some benefit during the proliferative phase of ARDS.[287-289] The rationale behind this therapy is that much of the scarring that occurs during this phase of the illness is a consequence of unattentuated inflammation that can cause severe damage to the affected alveoli.[290] There is an obvious risk, however, of immunosuppressing already debilitated patients who are still in an environment in which they are exposed to multiple resistant organisms (and frequently have multiple indwelling appliances), as well as a potential risk for long-term neuromuscular sequelae. The NHLBI ARDSNet recently completed a double-blind RCT (Late Steroid Rescue Study or LaSRS) designed to evaluate the benefits and risks of this therapy in 180 patients with ARDS lasting 7 to 21 days. The ARDSNet presented preliminary results at the 2004 International Meeting of the American Thoracic Society. These indicated that there was no difference in 60-day mortality, or ICU or hospital length of stay between those treated with high-dose methylprednisolone and those treated with placebo.[291] In addition, investigators reported more adverse events related to weakness in the steroid-treated group than in the placebo-treated group. Pending publication of the final results of this study, the routine use of steroids, specifically for late-phase ARDS, cannot be advocated on firm scientific grounds.

PRESSURE-CONTROL VENTILATION AND INVERSE-RATIO VENTILATION Pressure-control ventilation (PCV) is favored by some clinicians because it limits the maximal peak airway pressure. It also limits static end-inspiratory or alveolar pressure. However, some intensivists and respiratory care providers may not appreciate what that limit is. For example, if a patient with ARDS is being ventilated with PCV with an inspiratory pressure of 30 cm H_2O and PEEP of 10 cm H_2O, then the total end-inspiratory pressure is the sum of 30 cm H_2O plus 10 cm H_2O, or 40 cm H_2O (Fig. 38-10). Some clinicians may mistakenly believe that the alveoli are being exposed to only 30 cm H_2O, and thus do not decrease the inspiratory pressure such that the end-inspiratory pressure does not exceed 30 cm H_2O, the threshold used in the pivotal ARDSNet study.[3]

Although one could possibly mimic the tidal volumes and end-inspiratory pressures that were used in the ARDSnet low-tidal-volume ventilatory strategy (see Table 38-9), it would be challenging. It is possible that the low tidal volume per se in the ARDSnet trial was a factor in decreasing the mortality, apart from the benefits of keeping the plateau pressures limited to 30 cm H_2O or less.

Inverse ratio ventilation (IRV) entails the use of prolonged inspiratory times (inspiratory:expiratory ratio >1) with either a volume-cycled or pressure-cycled mode of mechanical ventilation (see Fig. 38-10). A subset of patients with hypoxia refractory to conventional modes of mechanical ventilation responded to IRV.[292,293] Unfortunately, there is no way to prospectively identify which patients will respond to IRV. The exact mechanisms by which IRV improves gas exchange in some patients with ARDS remain obscure, but are believed to involve both alveolar recruitment at lower airway pressures and more optimal distribution of ventilation.[294,295] Although it is tempting to attribute the beneficial effect of IRV to intrinsic PEEP, anecdotal reports have excluded intrinsic PEEP or gas trapping as the mechanism by which gas exchange improves in at least some patients.[295] An important caution when using this mode is that both auto-PEEP and the higher mean alveolar pressure typical of IRV tend to reduce cardiac output. In one study that examined PCV with or without IRV, cardiac output fell with IRV so that systemic oxygen delivery actually worsened.[296] Some investigators have noted a very gradual (over several hours) but progressive tendency for oxygenation to improve following a change to IRV.[297] This phenomenon has led some to suggest that a subset of lung units may be recruitable only through the combined effects of prolonged inspiration and time. Further studies are needed to shed light on this interesting aspect of IRV.

Inverse ratio pressure-control ventilation has been employed as part of the open lung strategy for ventilating patients with ARDS, with specific attention to keeping the tidal volume at or less than 6 mL/kg and limiting the driving (inspiratory) pressure.[7] The role of volume-control IRV remains poorly defined, and it is best regarded as a salvage therapy for patients with hypoxia refractory to more conventional approaches. Whichever approach is used, the intensivist should monitor auto-PEEP regularly, since the shortened expiratory times of IRV predispose to this effect.

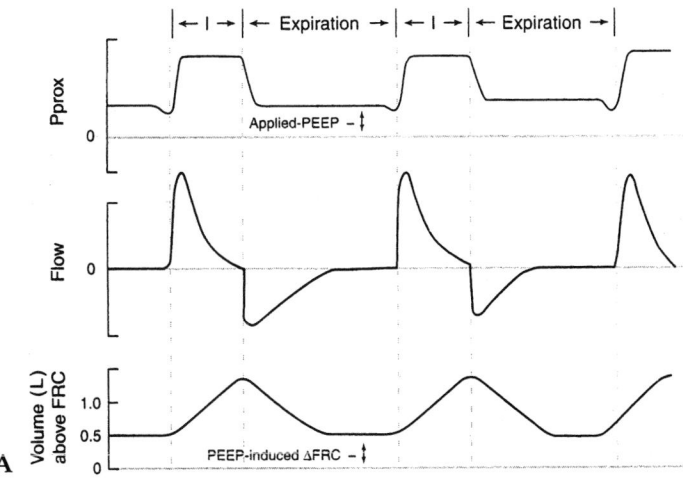

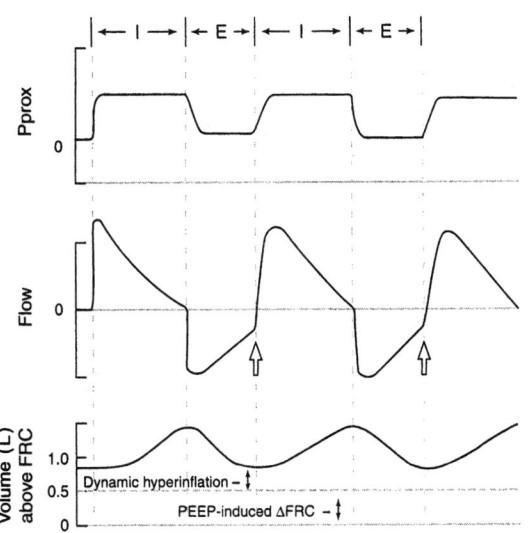

FIGURE 38-10 Schematic pressure, flow, and volume waveforms during pressure control ventilation (PCV) with applied PEEP. A. The inspiratory-to-expiratory (I:E) time is about 1:2. The pressure waveform resembles pressure support mode with the patient triggering each breath, but with a marked decelerating flow pattern. The applied PEEP increases the functional residual capacity (FRC) by about 500 mL (PEEP-induced ΔFRC). B. In pressure-controlled inverse ratio ventilation (PC-IRV), the I:E time is "reversed," with I>E. Because of this, the next breath starts before expiratory flow has returned to zero (open arrows), resulting in auto-PEEP and dynamic hyperinflation of about 300 mL. The latter is in addition to the increased FRC due to the applied PEEP (PEEP-induced ΔFRC). The patient is not initiating any breaths. E, expiration; I, inspiration; PEEP, positive end-expiratory pressure; Pprox, pressure at the proximal end of the endotracheal tube. *(Reproduced with permission from Lanken PN: Acute respiratory distress syndrome, in Lanken PN, Hanson CW III, Manaker S (eds):* **The Intensive Care Unit Manual.** *Philadelphia, WB Saunders, 2001, p 829.)*

Clinicians have also used other modalities of ventilation that depend on computerized ventilators, none of which have been compared to current low-tidal-volume strategies in RCTs (see Chap. 32).

HIGH-FREQUENCY OSCILLATORY VENTILATION If excessive lung excursion during tidal volume breathing is associated with injury to the lung, then it seems reasonable that ventilation with very small tidal volumes at high frequencies would be associated with the least possible ventilator-induced lung injury and potentially with improved outcome. Although the FDA has approved a ventilator for adults that provides high-frequency oscillatory ventilation (HFOV), its role in clinical practice remains unclear.[298] A study of HFOV[299] published in 2002 demonstrated a trend towards decreased mortality compared to conventional mechanical ventilation. However, the conventional ventilation was not based on a low-tidal-volume strategy such as ARDSNet (see Table 38-9). Because the mean airway pressure ($\pm$ SD) was higher in the group of patients treated with HFOV than the conventionally-treated group (e.g., 29 ± 6 cm H_2O vs. 23 ± 6 cm H_2O during the first 24 hours), caution must be raised about the possibility of VILI due to the high distending pressures. Until a RCT is

done comparing HFOV to the ARDSNet protocol, clinicians will not have evidence to guide them about when or if to employ HFOV.

High-frequency jet ventilation is different from HFOV. High-frequency jet ventilation typically employs tidal volumes of 1 to 5 mL/kg (or higher) and respiratory rates of 60 to 300 breaths per minute. Multiple trials of high-frequency ventilation have failed to demonstrate any benefit compared with conventional mechanical ventilation.[300-302] Nor has high-frequency jet ventilation has been associated with either improved oxygenation, reduced barotrauma, or decreased days of mechanical ventilation. On the basis of these negative results and the potential promise of HFOV, we recommend avoiding the use of high-frequency jet ventilation, even as a salvage intervention.

EXTRACORPOREAL MEMBRANE OXYGENATION AND EXTRACORPOREAL CO_2 REMOVAL The use of extracorporeal gas exchange, such as extracorporeal membrane oxygenation (ECMO) or extracorporeal CO_2 removal ($ECCO_2R$), to adequately oxygenate and ventilate the patient while allowing the lung to remain at rest was viewed as an attractive strategy for the management of patients with acute lung injury.

However, this promise has not been supported by clinical outcome studies. The earliest large-scale attempt to use ECMO in patients with severe ARDS in the 1970s demonstrated no survival benefit to its use, although it did generate a large database and a great deal of insight into patients with this problem.[303] Unfortunately, enrollment criteria in this study were such that the mortality among all patients entered into it was certain to be high (e.g., ~90% in both groups). Hence it was unlikely that any difference would be demonstrated between groups. Some believe that more careful patient selection, earlier randomization of patients, and better technology might have demonstrated a benefit to ECMO. A second wave of studies using ECMO or ECCO$_2$R was reported throughout the 1980s.[304–306] A number of techniques have been described, including venovenous ECMO, to assist in the elimination of carbon dioxide. However, the most recent report of ECMO in adult patients with ARDS also failed to demonstrate any survival benefit.[307] Despite these results, some specialized centers have continued to offer ECMO to adults with severe ARDS, based on their opinion that it is a relatively safe life-saving salvage intervention.[308]

Experimental (Non-FDA Approved) Interventions

PARTIAL LIQUID VENTILATION Partial liquid ventilation using perfluorocarbons instilled into the trachea of adults and children with the respiratory distress syndrome has been described.[309–312] Preliminary results from adult usage[313] and the more extensive experience in pediatric patients suggest that this mode of therapy may be both safe and efficacious in improving gas exchange. Partial liquid ventilation may allow oxygenation in patients who might otherwise be quite difficult to oxygenate with conventional modes of ventilation, in part because the perfluorocarbon is able to recruit dependent alveoli (by virtue of the hydraulic column) that PEEP is not. A practical problem is that perflubron is radiodense, making the lungs appear white, so it is impossible to use chest radiographs to detect infection or to follow the progress of healing. Currently, perfluorocarbons are available only as experimental agents.

EXOGENOUS SURFACTANT It has long been known from both animal models and human studies that surfactant levels are decreased or that the ratios of the surfactants are abnormal in humans and animals with ARDS.[314,315] Intensivists caring for adults have been encouraged by the dramatic results of surfactant therapy in infants with the respiratory distress syndrome (RDS) of prematurity. Surfactant therapy of RDS improves gas exchange and lung mechanics, decreases the requirement for CPAP, and lessens barotrauma.[316–318] Anzueto and associates[6] reported the first large prospective RCT of surfactant in ARDS. Their results were disappointing: There was no benefit associated with the exogenous surfactant delivered by inhalation. Because there were concerns about the appropriate dose, alternative modes of delivery, timing of therapy, and the precise surfactant formulation studied, investigators did not view this study as definitive evidence against the use of exogenous surfactant. Since then a number of RCTs, large and small, have been carried out and more are underway. Results so far have been mixed.[319–323] Large phase III trials with different surfactant preparations are underway. Like perflubron, currently exogenous surfactant for adults is available only as an experimental agent.

Supportive Care and Monitoring Patients with ALI and ARDS

SUPPORTIVE THERAPY Current management of ARDS does not benefit from proven pharmacologic interventions to limit acute lung injury or restore physiologic function. The largest strides in the recent management of ARDS have come from therapies aimed at the delivery of mechanical ventilation.[3] While it is possible that further explication of the mechanisms of lung injury will provide new avenues for pharmacologic intervention, at present, management of these patients relies on application of proven mechanical ventilation strategies, combined with meticulous supportive therapy. Appropriate management includes timely diagnosis and treatment of underlying diseases, nosocomial infections, and other problems. Indeed, even if new pharmacologic agents become available, the same supportive therapy will be necessary to maintain a viable patient to benefit from treatment. For a detailed description of elements of supportive care, please refer to the relevant other chapters in this text.

Reducing PEEP, even for short periods of time, is often associated with alveolar derecruitment and hence rapid arterial hemoglobin desaturation. Thus once endotracheal tube suctioning has been accomplished for diagnostic purposes, nursing and respiratory therapy staff should be instructed to keep airway disconnections to a minimum or to use an in-line suctioning system that maintains sterility and positive pressure, usually via the suctioning catheter residing in a sterile sheath and entering the endotracheal tube via a tight-sealing diaphragm. These suctioning systems generally are effective for lesser levels of PEEP (<15 cm H_2O) but often leak if higher levels are attempted.

MONITORING Patients with ARDS, by virtue of their serious gas exchange (and sometimes hemodynamic) impairment, combined with the effects of therapy (sedation, therapeutic paralysis, and PEEP), are at risk of sudden and life-threatening deterioration. Changes in intrapulmonary shunt, oxygen consumption, and systemic perfusion are frequent, making arterial saturation and oxygen delivery volatile. Accordingly, careful monitoring for hypoxemia and the adequacy of oxygen delivery is advisable. Continuous pulse oximetry is generally reliable (barring gross hypoperfusion) and should be used routinely. In addition, frequent sampling of arterial blood gases is advisable throughout the first day of management, as well as following major interventions or changes in clinical appearance of the patient.

Monitoring the patient's airway, ventilator function, and the ventilator-patient interface are equally important, as is assessment for liberation from assisted ventilation, and if needed, weaning (see Chap. 44).

Finally, hemodynamic monitoring, including use of a pulmonary artery catheter, has been discussed earlier in this chapter (see Chap. 13).

Long-term Sequelae of ARDS

Over the past two decades, as treatment for ARDS has decreased hospital mortality,[324] clinicians and clinical investigators have become more interested in the long-term health problems of ARDS survivors. Pulmonary function is usually mildly impaired after hospital discharge from ARDS and improves slightly over the next year.[325,326] Thus survivors with worsening dyspnea may have another superimposed respiratory lesion, such as tracheal stenosis, and should be evaluated as such. Despite their young age, ARDS survivors score well below the reference standards and other critical care controls on quality-of-life measures,[27,326–329] and many have evidence of cognitive dysfunction,[330] posttraumatic stress disorder,[328] and physical debilitation,[25] many months after hospital discharge. The long-term sequelae of critical illness and ARDS are an active area of ongoing research, covered in detail in Chap. 19.

Conclusion

Standardization of the criteria that define ALI and ARDS has aided in identification of specific at-risk groups. This in turn has spurred further research into the underlying reasons why certain risk groups (such as alcoholics[331,332]) are at greater risk for ALI. A recent NHLBI consensus statement summarized the important directions for future research, including functional response to injury and interaction between biochemical pathways and different cell types.[23] The completion of the human genome project has led to characterization of many of the genes encoding mediators of lung injury.[333] The effect of variation in these genes on predisposition to ALI in at-risk groups, such as sepsis, pneumonia, and trauma, may help to identify subgroups whose genotypes place them at unusually high risk or low risk for developing ALI and ARDS. Identifying these putative enabling and protective polymorphisms for developing ALI will provide hypotheses for interventions for prevention and for treatment of patients with ALI and ARDS in the future.

However, while waiting for those new genetically tailored therapies, much can be done in the present. The landmark ARDSNet low-tidal-volume ventilation strategy trial proved that ventilator therapy can be protocolized to reduce ventilator-induced lung injury.[3] Arguably this simple and inexpensive strategy can save thousands of lives of ALI and ARDS patients if widely accepted and utilized. Unfortunately, studies since the publication of the ARDSnet study in 2000 have indicated that that there are challenges to the widespread and timely acceptance and implementation of this low-tidal-volume strategy.[334–336] Thus the present challenges include not only improving on this therapy, but also overcoming the obstacles so that clinicians can consistently make a diagnosis of ALI and ARDS early, and then begin appropriate ventilatory support.

References

1. Neff M, Rubenfeld G: Clinical epidemiology of acute lung injury. *Semin Respir Crit Care Med* 22:237, 2001.
2. Rubenfeld GD: Epidemiology of acute lung injury. *Crit Care Med* 31:S276, 2003.
3. ARDSnet Investigators. Ventilation with lower tidal volumes as compared with traditional tidal volumes for acute lung injury and the acute respiratory distress syndrome. *N Engl J Med* 342:1301, 2000.
4. The National Heart, Lung, and Blood Institute ARDS Clinical Trials Network: Higher versus lower positive end-expiratory pressures in patients with the acute respiratory distress syndrome. *N Engl J Med* 351:327, 2004.
5. Derdak S, Mehta S, Stewart TE, et al: Multicenter oscillatory ventilation for acute respiratory distress syndrome trial study

I. High-frequency oscillatory ventilation for acute respiratory distress syndrome in adults: a randomized, controlled trial [see comment]. *Am J Respir Crit Care Med* 166:801, 2002.
6. Anzueto A, Baughman RP, Guntupalli KK, et al: Aerosolized surfactant in adults with sepsis induced acute respiratory distress syndrome. *N Engl J Med* 334:1417, 1996.
7. Amato MB, Barbas CS, Medeiros DM, et al: Effect of a protective-ventilation strategy on mortality in the acute respiratory distress syndrome. *N Engl J Med* 338:347, 1998.
8. Brochard L, Roudot-Thoraval F, Roupie E, et al: Tidal volume reduction for prevention of ventilator-induced lung injury in acute respiratory distress syndrome. The Multicenter Trial Group on Tidal Volume Reduction in ARDS. *Am J Respir Crit Care Med* 158:1831, 1998.
9. Stewart TE, Meade MO, Cook DJ, et al: Evaluation of a ventilation strategy to prevent barotrauma in patients at high risk for acute respiratory distress syndrome. Pressure- and Volume-Limited Ventilation Strategy Group. *N Engl J Med* 338:355, 1998.
10. Ashbaugh DG, Bigelow DB, Petty TL, Levine BE: Acute respiratory distress in adults. *Lancet* 2:319, 1967.
11. Fowler AA, Hamman RF, Good JT, et al: Adult respiratory distress syndrome: risk with common predispositions. *Ann Intern Med* 98:593, 1983.
12. Pepe PE, Potkin RT, Reus DH, et al: Clinical predictors of the adult respiratory distress syndrome. *Am J Surg* 144:124, 1982.
13. Hudson LD, Milberg JA, Anardi D, Maunder RJ: Clinical risks for development of the acute respiratory distress syndrome. *Am J Respir Crit Care Med* 151:293, 1995.
14. Murray JF, Matthay MA, Luce JM, Flick MR: An expanded definition of the adult respiratory distress syndrome. *Am Rev Respir Dis* 138:720, 1988.
15. Sloane PJ, Gee MH, Gottlieb JE, et al: A multicenter registry of patients with acute respiratory distress syndrome. *Am Rev Respir Dis* 146:419, 1992.
16. Bernard GR, Reines HD, Brigham KL, et al: The American European consensus conference on ARDS: definitions, mechanisms, relevant outcomes and clinical trials coordination. *Am J Resp Crit Care Med* 149:818, 1994.
17. Gilbert R, Keighley JF: The arterial-alveolar oxygen tension ratio. An index of gas exchange applicable to varying inspired oxygen concentrations. *Am Rev Respir Dis* 109:142, 1974.
18. Rubenfeld GD, Caldwell ES, Granton J, et al: Interobserver variability in applying a radiographic definition of ARDS. *Chest* 116:1347, 1999.
19. Meade MO, Cook RJ, Guyatt GH, et al: Interobserver variation in interpreting chest radiographs for the diagnosis of acute respiratory distress syndrome. *Am J Resp Crit Care Med* 161:85, 2000.
20. Ferguson ND, Kacmarek RM, Chiche JD, et al: Screening of ARDS patients using standardized ventilator settings: influence on enrollment in a clinical trial. *Intensive Care Med* 30:1111, 2004.
21. Ferguson ND, Meade MO, Hallett DC, Stewart TE: High values of the pulmonary artery wedge pressure in patients with acute lung injury and acute respiratory distress syndrome. *Intensive Care Med* 28:1073, 2002.
22. Bindels AJ, van der Hoeven JG, Meinders AE: Pulmonary artery wedge pressure and extravascular lung water in patients with acute cardiogenic pulmonary edema requiring mechanical ventilation. *Am J Cardiol* 84:1158, 1999.
23. Matthay MA, Zimmerman GA, Esmon C, et al: Future research directions in acute lung injury: summary of a National Heart, Lung, and Blood Institute working group. *Am J Respir Crit Care Med* 167:1027, 2003.
24. Goss CH, Brower RG, Hudson LD, Rubenfeld GD: Incidence of acute lung injury in the United States [comment]. *Crit Care Med* 31:1607, 2003.
25. Herridge MS, Cheung AM, Tansey CM, et al: Canadian Critical Care Trials G. One-year outcomes in survivors of the acute

respiratory distress syndrome [comment]. *N Engl J Med* 348:683, 2003.

26. Angus DC, Musthafa AA, Clermont G, et al: Quality-adjusted survival in the first year after the acute respiratory distress syndrome. *Am J Respir Crit Care Med* 163:1389, 2001.

27. Davidson T, Caldwell E, Curtis J, et al: Reduced quality of life in survivors of acute respiratory distress syndrome compared with critically ill control patients. *JAMA* 281:354, 1999.

28. Davidson T, Rubenfeld G, Caldwell E, et al: The effect of acute respiratory distress syndrome on long-term survival. *Am J Respir Crit Care Med* 160:1838, 1999.

29. Lewandowski K, Metz J, Deutschmann C, et al: Incidence, severity, and mortality of acute respiratory failure in Berlin, Germany. *Am J Respir Crit Care Med* 151:1121, 1995.

30. Neff MJ: The epidemiology and definition of the acute respiratory distress syndrome. *Respir Care Clin North Am* 9:273, 2003.

31. Gattinoni L, Pelosi P, Suter PM, et al: Acute respiratory distress syndrome caused by pulmonary and extrapulmonary disease. Different syndromes? *Am J Respir Crit Care Med* 158:3, 1998.

32. Pelosi P, Gattinoni L: Acute respiratory distress syndrome of pulmonary and extra-pulmonary origin: fancy or reality? *Intensive Care Med* 27:457, 2001.

33. Gunther A, Walmrath D, Grimminger F, Seeger W: Pathophysiology of acute lung injury. *Semin Respir Crit Care Med* 22:247, 2001.

34. Steinberg KP, Hudson LD: Acute lung injury and acute respiratory distress syndrome. The clinical syndrome. *Clin Chest Med* 21:401, 2000.

35. Moss M, Parsons PE, Steinberg KP, et al: Chronic alcohol abuse is associated with an increased incidence of acute respiratory distress syndrome and severity of multiple organ dysfunction in patients with septic shock. *Crit Care Med* 31:869, 2003.

36. Ware LB, Matthay MA: The acute respiratory distress syndrome. *N Engl J Med* 342:1334, 2000.

37. Parsons P: Mediators and mechanisms of acute lung injury. *Clin Chest Med* 21:467, 2000.

38. Moss M, Bucher B, Moore FA: The role of chronic alcohol abuse in the development of acute respiratory distress syndrome in adults. *JAMA* 275:50, 1996.

39. Moss M, Guidot DM, Steinberg KP, et al: Diabetic patients have a decreased incidence of acute respiratory distress syndrome. *Crit Care Med* 28:2187, 2000.

40. Mangialardi RJ, Martin GS, Bernard GR, et al: Hypoproteinemia predicts acute respiratory distress syndrome development, weight gain, and death in patients with sepsis. Ibuprofen in Sepsis Study Group. *Crit Care Med* 28:3137, 2000.

41. Iribarren C, Jacobs DR Jr, Sidney S, et al: Cigarette smoking, alcohol consumption, and risk of ARDS: a 15-year cohort study in a managed care setting. *Chest* 117:163, 2000.

42. Moss M, Mannino DM: Race and gender differences in acute respiratory distress syndrome in the United States: an analysis of multiple-cause mortality data (1979–1996). *Crit Care Med* 30:1679, 2002.

43. Suchyta MR, Clemmer TP, Elliott CG, et al: Increased mortality of older patients with acute respiratory distress syndrome. *Chest* 111: 1334, 1997.

44. Doyle RL, Szaflarski N, Modin GW, et al: Identification of patients with acute lung injury. Predictors of mortality. *Am J Respir Crit Care Med* 152:1818, 1995.

45. Monchi M, Bellenfant F, Cariou A, et al: Early predictive factors of survival in the acute respiratory distress syndrome. A multivariate analysis. *Am J Respir Crit Care Med* 158:1076, 1998.

46. Luhr OR, Antonsen K, Karlsson M, et al: Incidence and mortality after acute respiratory failure and acute respiratory distress syndrome in Sweden, Denmark, and Iceland. The ARF Study Group. *Am J Respir Crit Care Med* 159:1849, 1999.

47. Zilberger MD, Epstein SK: Acute lung injury in the medical ICU: comorbid conditions, age, etiology, and hospital outcome. *Am J Respir Crit Care Med* 157:1159, 1998.

48. Lanken PN, Ancukiewicz M, Christie JD, et al: Baseline risk factors for mortality in 902 subjects with acute lung injury (ALI)/acute respiratory distress syndrome (ARDS). *Am J Respir Crit Care Med* 169:A18, 2004.

49. Nuckton TJ, Alonso JA, Kallet RH, et al: Pulmonary dead-space fraction as a risk factor for death in the acute respiratory distress syndrome. *N Engl J Med* 346:1281, 2002.

50. Pelosi P, Gattinoni L: Acute respiratory distress syndrome of pulmonary and extra-pulmonary origin: fancy or reality? *Intensive Care Med* 27:457, 2001.

51. Gattinoni L, Pelosi P, Suter PM: Acute respiratory distress syndrome caused by pulmonary and extrapulmonary disease. Different syndromes? *Am J Respir Crit Care Med* 158:3, 1998.

52. Eisner MD, Thompson T, Hudson LD, et al: Efficacy of low tidal volume ventilation in patients with different clinical risk factors for acute lung injury and the acute respiratory distress syndrome. *Am J Respir Crit Care Med* 164:231, 2001.

53. Montgomery AB, Stager MA, Carrico CJ, et al: Causes of mortality in patients with the adult respiratory distress syndrome. *Am J Respir Crit Care Med* 132:485, 1985.

54. Bell RC, Coalson JJ, Smith JD, et al: Multiple organ system failure and infection in adult respiratory distress syndrome. *Ann Intern Med* 99:293, 1983.

55. Tomashefski JF: Pulmonary pathology of acute respiratory distress syndrome. *Clin Chest Med* 21:435, 2000.

56. Tomashefski JF Jr: Pulmonary pathology of the acute respiratory distress syndrome. Diffuse alveolar damage, in Ma M (ed): *Acute Respiratory Distress Syndrome*. New York, Marcel Dekker, 2003, p 75.

57. Meduri GU, Belenchia JM, Estes RJ, et al: Fibroproliferative phase of ARDS: Clinical findings and effects of corticosteroids. *Chest* 100:943, 1991.

58. Pittet JF, Mackersie RC, Martin TR, Matthay MA: Biological markers of acute lung injury: prognostic and pathogenetic significance. *Am J Respir Crit Care Med* 155:1187, 1997.

59. Clark JG, Milberg JA, Steinberg KP, Hudson LD: Type III procollagen peptide in the adult respiratory distress syndrome. Association of increased peptide levels in bronchoalveolar lavage fluid with increased risk for death [see comments]. *Ann Intern Med* 122:17, 1995.

60. Tracey KJ, Lowry SF, Cerami A: Cachetin/TNF-alpha in septic shock and septic adult respiratory distress syndrome. *Am Rev Respir Dis* 138:1377, 1988.

61. Goodman RB, Strieter RM, Martin DP, et al: Inflammatory cytokines in patients with persistence of the acute respiratory distress syndrome. *Am J Respir Crit Care Med* 154:602, 1996.

62. Ghezzi P, Dinarello CA, Bianchi M, et al: Hypoxia increases production of interleukin-1 and tumor necrosis factor by human mononuclear cells. *Cytokine* 3:189, 1991.

63. Dinarello CA: Biology of interleukin 1. *FASEB J* 2:108, 1988.

64. Li XY, Donaldson K, Brown D, MacNee W: The role of tumor necrosis factor in increased airspace epithelial permeability in acute lung inflammation. *Am J Respir Cell Mol Biol* 13:185, 1995.

65. Tracey KJ, Fong Y, Hesse DG, et al: Anti-cachectin/TNF monoclonal antibodies prevent septic shock during lethal bacteraemia. *Nature* 330:662, 1987.

66. Beutler B, Cerami A: Cachectin: more than a tumor necrosis factor. *N Engl J Med* 316:380, 1987.

67. Gamble JR, Harlan JM, Klebonoff SJ, Vados MA: Stimulation of the adherence of neutrophils to umbilical vein endothelium by human recombinant tumor necrosis factor. *Proc Natl Acad Sci U S A* 82:8667, 1985.

68. Pohlman TH, Stanness KA, Beatty PG, et al: An endothelial cell surface factor(s) induced in vitro by lipopolysaccharide, interleukin 1, and tumor necrosis factor-alpha increases neutrophil adherence by a CDw18-dependent mechanism. *J Immunol* 136:4548, 1986.

69. Bevilacqua MP, Pober JS, Wheeler ME, et al: Interleukin-1 activation of vascular endothelium. Effects on procoagulant activity and leukocyte adhesion. *Am J Pathol* 121:394, 1985.
70. Bevilacqua MP, Pober JS, Wheeler ME, et al: Interleukin 1 acts on cultured human vascular endothelium to increase the adhesion of polymorphonuclear leukocytes, monocytes, and related leukocyte cell lines. *J Clin Invest* 76:2003, 1985.
71. Bauer TT, Monton C, Torres A, et al: Comparison of systemic cytokine levels in patients with acute respiratory distress syndrome, severe pneumonia, and controls. *Thorax* 55:46, 2000.
72. Parsons PE, Moore FA, Moore EE, et al: Studies on the role of tumor necrosis factor in adult respiratory distress syndrome. *Am Rev Respir Dis* 146:694, 1992.
73. Hyers TM, Tricomi SM, Dettenmeier PA, Fowler AA: Tumor necrosis factor levels in serum and bronchoalveolar lavage fluid of patients with the adult respiratory distress syndrome. *Am Rev Respir Dis* 144:268, 1991.
74. Millar AB, Foley NM, Singer M, et al: Tumour necrosis factor in bronchopulmonary secretions of patients with adult respiratory distress syndrome. *Lancet* 2:712, 1989.
75. Suter PM, Suter S, Girardin E, et al: High bronchoalveolar levels of tumor necrosis factor and its inhibitors, interleukin-1, interferon, and elastase, in patients with adult respiratory distress syndrome after trauma, shock, or sepsis. *Am Rev Respir Dis* 145:1016, 1992.
76. Pugin J, Ricou B, Steinberg KP, et al: Proinflammatory activity in bronchoalveolar lavage fluids from patients with ARDS, a prominent role for interleukin-1. *Am J Respir Crit Care Med* 153:1850, 1996.
77. Park WY, Goodman RB, Steinberg KP, et al: Cytokine balance in the lungs of patients with acute respiratory distress syndrome. *Am J Respir Crit Care Med* 164:1896, 2001.
78. Meduri GU, Headley S, Kohler G, et al: Persistent elevation of inflammatory cytokines predicts a poor outcome in ARDS. Plasma IL-1 beta and IL-6 levels are consistent and efficient predictors of outcome over time. *Chest* 107:1062, 1995.
79. Schutte H, Lohmeyer J, Rosseau S, et al: Bronchoalveolar and systemic cytokine profiles in patients with ARDS, severe pneumonia and cardiogenic pulmonary oedema. *Eur Respir J* 9:1858, 1996.
80. Martin TR: Lung cytokines and ARDS: Roger S. Mitchell Lecture. *Chest* 116:2S, 1999.
81. Xing Z, Gauldie J, Cox G, et al: IL-6 is an antiinflammatory cytokine required for controlling local or systemic inflammatory responses. *J Clin Invest* 101:311, 1998.
82. Ranieri VM, Suter PM, Tortorella C, et al: Effect of mechanical ventilation on inflammatory mediators in patients with acute respiratory distress syndrome: A Randomized Controlled Trial. *JAMA* 282:54, 1999.
83. Moore KW, de Waal Malefyt R, Coffman RL, O'Garra A: Interleukin-10 and the interleukin-10 receptor. *Annu Rev Immunol* 19:683, 2001.
84. Armstrong L, Millar AB: Relative production of tumour necrosis factor alpha and interleukin 10 in adult respiratory distress syndrome. *Thorax* 52:442, 1997.
85. Parsons PE, Moss M, Vannice JL, et al: Circulating IL-1ra and IL-10 levels are increased but do not predict the development of acute respiratory distress syndrome in at-risk patients. *Am J Respir Crit Care Med* 155:1469, 1997.
86. Donnelly SC, Strieter RM, Reid PT, et al: The association between mortality rates and decreased concentrations of interleukin-10 and interleukin-1 receptor antagonist in the lung fluids of patients with the adult respiratory distress syndrome. *Ann Intern Med* 125:191, 1996.
87. Sekido N, Mukaida N, Harada A, et al: Prevention of lung reperfusion injury in rabbits by a monoclonal antibody against interleukin-8. *Nature* 365:654, 1993.
88. Yokoi K, Mukaida N, Harada A, et al: Prevention of endotoxemia-induced acute respiratory distress syndrome-like lung injury in rabbits by a monoclonal antibody to IL-8. *Lab Invest* 76:375, 1997.
89. Matsumoto T, Yokoi K, Mukaida N, et al: Pivotal role of interleukin-8 in the acute respiratory distress syndrome and cerebral reperfusion injury. *J Leukoc Biol* 62:581, 1997.
90. Torre D, Zeroli C, Giola M, et al: Levels of interleukin-8 in patients with adult respiratory distress syndrome. *J Infect Dis* 167:505, 1993.
91. Villard J, Dayer-Pastore F, Hamacher J, et al: GRO alpha and interleukin-8 in *Pneumocystis carinii* or bacterial pneumonia and adult respiratory distress syndrome. *Am J Respir Crit Care Med* 152:1549, 1995.
92. Miller EJ, Cohen AB, Nagao S, et al: Elevated levels of NAP-1/interleukin-8 are present in the airspaces of patients with the adult respiratory distress syndrome and are associated with increased mortality. *Am Rev Respir Dis* 146:427, 1992.
93. Abraham E: Neutrophils and acute lung injury. *Crit Care Med* 31:S195, 2003.
94. Bachofen M, Weibel ER: Structural alterations of lung parenchyma in the adult respiratory distress syndrome. *Clin Chest Med* 3:35, 1982.
95. Steinberg KP, Milberg JA, Martin TR, et al: Evolution of bronchoalveolar cell populations in the adult respiratory distress syndrome. *Am J Respir Crit Care Med* 150:113, 1994.
96. Baughman RP, Gunther KL, Rashkin MC, et al: Changes in the inflammatory response of the lung during acute respiratory distress syndrome: prognostic indicators. *Am J Respir Crit Care Med* 154:76, 1996.
97. Matute-Bello G, Liles WC, Radella F 2nd, et al: Neutrophil apoptosis in the acute respiratory distress syndrome. *Am J Respir Crit Care Med* 156:1969, 1997.
98. Matute-Bello G, Liles WC, Radella F 2nd, et al: Modulation of neutrophil apoptosis by granulocyte colony-stimulating factor and granulocyte/macrophage colony-stimulating factor during the course of acute respiratory distress syndrome [see comment]. *Crit Care Med* 28:253, 2000.
99. Lesur O, Kokis A, Hermans C, et al: Interleukin-2 involvement in early acute respiratory distress syndrome: relationship with polymorphonuclear neutrophil apoptosis and patient survival. *Crit Care Med* 28:3814, 2000.
100. Goodman ER, Stricker P, Velavicius M, et al: Role of granulocyte-macrophage colony-stimulating factor and its receptor in the genesis of acute respiratory distress syndrome through an effect on neutrophil apoptosis. *Arch Surg* 134:1049, 1999.
101. Beckman JS, Koppenol WH: Nitric oxide, superoxide, and peroxynitrite: the good, the bad, and ugly. *Am J Physiol* 271:C1424, 1996.
102. Weiss SJ: Tissue destruction by neutrophils. *N Engl J Med* 320:365, 1989.
103. Buhl R, Meyer A, Vogelmeier C: Oxidant-protease interaction in the lung. Prospects for antioxidant therapy. *Chest* 1996.110:267S–272S.
104. Gadek JE, Pacht ER: The interdependence of lung antioxidants and antiprotease defense in ARDS. *Chest* 110:273S, 1996.
105. Eiserich JP, Hristova M, Cross CE, et al: Formation of nitric oxide-derived inflammatory oxidants by myeloperoxidase in neutrophils. *Nature* 391:393, 1998.
106. Gutteridge JM, Quinlan GJ, Mumby S, et al: Primary plasma antioxidants in adult respiratory distress syndrome patients: changes in iron-oxidizing, iron-binding, and free radical-scavenging proteins. *J Lab Clin Med* 124:263, 1994.
107. Kooy NW, Royall JA, Ye YZ, et al: Evidence for in vivo peroxynitrite production in human acute lung injury. *Am J Respir Crit Care Med* 151:1250, 1995.
108. Ischiropoulos H, al-Mehdi AB: Peroxynitrite-mediated oxidative protein modifications. *FEBS Lett* 364:279, 1995.

109. Ischiropoulos H, al-Mehdi AB, Fisher AB: Reactive species in ischemic rat lung injury: contribution of peroxynitrite. *Am J Physiol* 269:L158, 1995.

110. Zimmerman GA, Renzetti AD, Hill HR: Functional and metabolic activity of granulocytes from patients with the adult respiratory distress syndrome: evidence for activated neutrophils in the pulmonary circulation. *Am Rev Resp Dis* 127:290, 1983.

111. Fisher AB, Dodia C, Tan Z, et al: Oxygen-dependent lipid peroxidation during lung ischemia. *J Clin Invest* 88:674, 1991.

112. Fisher PW, Huang YC, Kennedy TP: PO2-dependent hydroxyl radical production during ischemia-reperfusion lung injury. *Am J Physiol* 265:L279, 1993.

113. Baldwin SR, Simon RH, Grum CM: Oxidant activity in expired breath of patients with adult respiratory distress syndrome. *Lancet* 1:11, 1986.

114. Sznajder JI, Fraiman A, Hall JB, et al: Increased hydrogen peroxide in the expired breath of patients with acute hypoxemic respiratory failure. *Chest* 96:606, 1989.

115. Pacht ER, Timerman AP, Lykens MG, Merola AJ: Deficiency of alveolar fluid glutathione in patients with sepsis and the adult respiratory distress syndrome. *Chest* 100:1397, 1991.

116. Bunnell E, Pacht ER: Oxidized glutathione is increased in the alveolar fluid of patients with the adult respiratory distress syndrome. *Am Rev Respir Dis* 148:1174, 1993.

117. Lamb NJ, Gutteridge JM, Baker C, et al: Oxidative damage to proteins of bronchoalveolar lavage fluid in patients with acute respiratory distress syndrome: evidence for neutrophil-mediated hydroxylation, nitration, and chlorination. *Crit Care Med* 27:1738, 1999.

118. Richard C, Lemonnier F, Thibault M, et al: Vitamin E deficiency and lipoperoxidation during adult respiratory distress syndrome. *Crit Care Med* 18:4, 1990.

119. Quinlan GJ, Evans TW, Gutteridge JM: 4-hydroxy-2-nonenal levels increase in the plasma of patients with adult respiratory distress syndrome as linoleic acid appears to fall. *Free Radic Res* 21:95, 1994.

120. Quinlan GJ, Evans TW, Gutteridge JM: Oxidative damage to plasma proteins in adult respiratory distress syndrome. *Free Radic Res* 20:289, 1994.

121. Quinlan GJ, Lamb NJ, Tilley R, et al: Plasma hypoxanthine levels in ARDS: implications for oxidative stress, morbidity, and mortality. *Am J Respir Crit Care Med* 155:479, 1997.

122. Gole MD, Souza JM, Choi I, et al: Plasma proteins modified by tyrosine nitration in acute respiratory distress syndrome. *Am J Physiol Lung Cell Mol Physiol* 278:L961, 2000.

123. Connelly KG, Moss M, Parsons PE, et al: Serum ferritin as a predictor of the acute respiratory distress syndrome. *Am J Respir Crit Care Med* 155:21, 1997.

124. Sharkey RA, Donnelly SC, Connelly KG, et al: Initial serum ferritin levels in patients with multiple trauma and the subsequent development of acute respiratory distress syndrome. *Am J Respir Crit Care Med* 159:1506, 1999.

125. Quinlan GJ, Evans TW, Gutteridge JM: Linoleic acid and protein thiol changes suggestive of oxidative damage in the plasma of patients with adult respiratory distress syndrome. *Free Radic Res* 20:299, 1994.

126. Mathru M, Rooney MW, Dries DJ, et al: Urine hydrogen peroxide during adult respiratory distress syndrome in patients with and without sepsis. *Chest* 105:232, 1994.

127. McDonald JA: The yin and yang of fibrin in the airways [comment]. *N Engl J Med* 322:929, 1990.

128. Idell S: Extravascular coagulation and fibrin deposition in acute lung injury. *New Horiz* 2:566, 1994.

129. Abraham E: Coagulation abnormalities in acute lung injury and sepsis. *Am J Respir Cell Mol Biol* 22:401, 2000.

130. Fuchs-Buder T, de Moerloose P, Ricou B, et al: Time course of procoagulant activity and D dimer in bronchoalveolar fluid of patients at risk for or with acute respiratory distress syndrome. *Am J Respir Crit Care Med* 1:163, 1996.

131. Idell S, James KK, Levin EG, et al: Local abnormalities in coagulation and fibrinolytic pathways predispose to alveolar fibrin deposition in the adult respiratory distress syndrome. *J Clin Invest* 84:695, 1989.

132. Idell S: Coagulation, fibrinolysis, and fibrin deposition in acute lung injury. *Crit Care Med* 31:S213, 2003.

133. Idell S, Gonzalez K, Bradford H, et al: Procoagulant activity in bronchoalveolar lavage in the adult respiratory distress syndrome. Contribution of tissue factor associated with factor VII. *Am Rev Respir Dis* 136:1466, 1987.

134. Bevilacqua MP, Pober JS, Majeau GR, et al: Recombinant tumor necrosis factor induces procoagulant activity in cultured human vascular endothelium: characterization and comparison with the actions of interleukin 1. *Proc Natl Acad Sci U S A* 83:4533, 1986.

135. Clouse LH, Comp PC: The regulation of hemostasis: the protein C system. [review]. *N Engl J Med* 314:1298, 1986.

136. Esmon CT: The regulation of natural anticoagulant pathways. *Science* 235:1348, 1987.

137. Bernard GR, Vincent JL, Laterre PF, et al: Recombinant human protein C Worldwide Evaluation in Severe Sepsis (PROWESS) study group. Efficacy and safety of recombinant human activated protein C for severe sepsis [comment]. *N Engl J Med* 344:699, 2001.

138. Ely EW, Laterre PF, Angus DC, et al: Drotrecogin alfa (activated) administration across clinically important subgroups of patients with severe sepsis [see comment]. *Crit Care Med* 31:12, 2003.

139. Matthay MA, Folkesson HG, Clerici C: Lung epithelial fluid transport and the resolution of pulmonary edema [review]. *Physiol Rev* 82:569, 2002.

140. Sakuma T, Okaniwa G, Nakada T, et al: Alveolar fluid clearance in the resected human lung [see comment]. *Am J Respir Crit Care Med* 150:305, 1994.

141. Sakuma T, Folkesson HG, Suzuki S, et al: Beta-adrenergic agonist stimulated alveolar fluid clearance in ex vivo human and rat lungs. *Am J Respir Crit Care Med* 155:506, 1997.

142. Fang X, Fukuda N, Barbry P, et al: Novel role for CFTR in fluid absorption from the distal airspaces of the lung. *J Gen Physiol* 119:199, 2002.

143. Suzuki S, Noda M, Sugita M, et al: Impairment of transalveolar fluid transport and lung Na(+)-K(+)-ATPase function by hypoxia in rats. *J Appl Physiol* 87:962, 1999.

144. Vivona ML, Matthay M, Chabaud MB, et al: Hypoxia reduces alveolar epithelial sodium and fluid transport in rats: reversal by beta-adrenergic agonist treatment. *Am J Respir Cell Mol Biol* 25:554, 2001.

145. Hu P, Ischiropoulos H, Beckman JS, Matalon S: Peroxynitrite inhibition of oxygen consumption and sodium transport in alveolar type II cells. *Am J Physiol* 266:L628, 1994.

146. Verghese GM, Ware LB, Matthay BA, Matthay MA: Alveolar epithelial fluid transport and the resolution of clinically severe hydrostatic pulmonary edema. *J Appl Physiol* 87:1301, 1999.

147. Ware LB, Matthay MA: Alveolar fluid clearance is impaired in the majority of patients with acute lung injury and the acute respiratory distress syndrome [see comment]. *Am J Respir Crit Care Med* 163:1376, 2001.

148. Matthay MA, Wiener-Kronish JP: Intact epithelial barrier function is critical for the resolution of alveolar edema in humans [see comment]. *Am Rev Respir Dis* 142:1250, 1990.

149. Clark JG, Milberg JA, Steinberg KP, Hudson LD: Type III procollagen peptide in the adult respiratory distress syndrome. Association of increased peptide levels in bronchoalveolar lavage fluid with increased risk for death [see comments]. *Ann Intern Med* 122:17, 1995.

150. Marshall RP, Bellingan G, Webb S, et al: Fibroproliferation occurs early in the acute respiratory distress syndrome and impacts on outcome. *Am J Respir Crit Care Med* 162:1783, 2000.

151. Clark JG, Milberg JA, Steinberg KP, Hudson LD: Elevated lavage levels of N-terminal peptide of type III procollagen are associated with increased fatality in adult respiratory distress syndrome. *Chest* 3:126S, 1994.

152. Toews GB: Cellular alterations in fibroproliferative lung disease [Review]. *Chest* 116:112S, 1999.

153. Zhu HJ, Burgess AW: Regulation of transforming growth factor-beta signaling. [Review]. *Mol Cell Biol Res Commun* 4:321, 2001.

154. Madtes DK, Rubenfeld G, Klima LD, et al: Elevated transforming growth factor-alpha levels in bronchoalveolar lavage fluid of patients with acute respiratory distress syndrome. *Am J Respir Crit Care Med* 158:424, 1998.

155. Woods A: Syndecans: transmembrane modulators of adhesion and matrix assembly. *J Clin Invest* 107:935, 2001.

156. Bensadoun ES, Burke AK, Hogg JC, Roberts CR: Proteoglycan deposition in pulmonary fibrosis. *Am J Respir Crit Care Med* 154:1819, 1996.

157. Savani RC, Hou G, Liu P, et al: A role for hyaluronan in macrophage accumulation and collagen deposition after bleomycin-induced lung injury. *Am J Respir Cell Mol Biol* 23:475, 2000.

158. Bornstein P: Thrombospondins as matricellular modulators of cell function. *J Clin Invest* 107:929, 2001.

159. Murphy-Ullrich JE: The de-adhesive activity of matricellular proteins: is intermediate cell adhesion an adaptive state?[see comment] [Review] [36 refs]. *J Clin Invest* 107:785, 2001.

160. Shapiro SD, Senior RM: Matrix metalloproteinases. Matrix degradation and more. *Am J Respir Cell Mol Biol* 20:1100, 1999.

161. Aberman A FM: The metabolic and respiratory acidosis of acute pulmonary edema. *Ann Intern Med* 76:173, 1972.

162. Aberle DR, Brown K: Radiologic considerations in the adult respiratory distress syndrome. *Clin Chest Med* 11:737, 1990.

163. Aberle DR, Wiener-Kronish, J, Webb WR, et al: Hydrostatic versus increased permeability pulmonary edema: Diagnosis based on radiographic criteria in critically ill patients. *Radiology* 168:73, 1988.

164. Kaul S, Stratienko SA, Pollock SG, et al: Value of two-dimensional echocardiography for determining the basis of hemodynamic compromise in critically ill patients: A prospective study. *J Am Soc Echocardiol* 7:598, 1994.

165. Foster E, Schiller NB: Transesophageal echocardiography in the critical care patient. *Cardiol Clin* 11:489, 1993.

166. Fein AM, Goldberg SK, Walkenstein MD, et al: Is pulmonary artery catheterization necessary for the diagnosis of pulmonary edema? *Am J Respir Crit Care Med* 129:1006, 1984.

167. Matthay MA, Chatterjee K: Bedside catheterization of the pulmonary artery: Risks compared with benefits. *Ann Intern Med* 109:826, 1988.

168. Dalen JE, Bone RC: Is it time to pull the pulmonary artery catheter? *JAMA* 276:916, 1996.

169. Connors AF, Speroff T, Dawson NV, et al: The effectiveness of right heart catheterization in the initial care of critically ill patients. *JAMA* 276:889, 1996.

170. Robin ED: The cult of the Swan-Ganz catheter: Overuse and abuse of pulmonary flow catheters. *Ann Intern Med* 103:445, 1985.

171. Iberti TJ, Fischer EP, Leibowitz AB, et al: A multicenter study of physicians' knowledge of the pulmonary artery catheter. *JAMA* 264:2928, 1990.

172. McHugh TJ, Forrester JS, Adler L, et al: Pulmonary vascular congestion in acute myocardial infarction: hemodynamic and radiologic correlations. *Ann Intern Med* 76:29–33, 1972.

173. Sibbald WJ, Cunningham DR, Chin DN: Non-cardiac or cardiac pulmonary edema? A practical approach to clinical differentiation in critically ill patients. *Chest* 84:452, 1983.

174. Hogan TF, Riley RS, Thomas JG: Rapid diagnosis of acute eosinophilic pneumonia (AEP) in a patient with respiratory failure using bronchoalveolar lavage (BAL) with calcofluor white (CW) staining. *J Clin Lab Anal* 11:202, 1997.

175. Pope-Harman AL, Davis WB, Allen ED, et al: Acute eosinophilic pneumonia. A summary of 15 cases and review of the literature. *Medicine* 75:334, 1996.

176. Allen JN, Davis WB: Eosinophilic lung diseases. *Am J Respir Crit Care Med* 150:1423, 1994.

177. Steinberg KP, Mitchell DR, Maunder RJ, et al: Safety of bronchoalveolar lavage in patients with adult respiratory distress syndrome. *Am Rev Respir Dis* 148:556, 1993.

178. Trouillet JL, Guiguet M, Gibert C, et al: Fiberoptic bronchoscopy in ventilated patients. Evaluation of cardiopulmonary risk under midazolam sedation. *Chest* 97:927, 1990.

179. Yen KT, Lee AS, Krowka MJ, Burger CD: Pulmonary complications in bone marrow transplantation: a practical approach to diagnosis and treatment. *Clin Chest Med* 25:189, 2004.

180. Afessa B, Tefferi A, Litzow MR, et al: Diffuse alveolar hemorrhage in hematopoietic stem cell transplant recipients. *Am J Respir Crit Care Med* 166:641, 2002.

181. Schwarz MI, Fontenot AP, Afessa B, et al: Drug-induced diffuse alveolar hemorrhage syndromes and vasculitis. *Clin Chest Med* 25:133, 2004.

182. Bar J, Ehrenfeld M, Rozenman J, et al: Pulmonary-renal syndrome in systemic sclerosis. *Semin Arthritis Rheum* 30:403, 2001.

183. Lee JG, Joo KW, Chung WK, et al: Diffuse alveolar hemorrhage in lupus nephritis. *Clin Nephrol* 55:282, 2001.

184. Specks U: Diffuse alveolar hemorrhage syndromes. *Curr Opin Rheumatol* 13:12, 2001.

185. Franks TJ, Koss MN: Pulmonary capillaritis. *Curr Opin Pulm Med* 6:430, 2000.

186. Green RJ, Ruoss SJ, Kraft SA, et al: Pulmonary capillaritis and alveolar hemorrhage. Update on diagnosis and management. *Chest* 110:1305, 1996.

187. Gattinoni L, Caironi P, Pelosi P, Goodman LR: What has computed tomography taught us about the acute respiratory distress syndrome? [Review] *Am J Respir Crit Care Med* 164:1701, 2001.

188. Gattinoni L, Pesenti A, Bombino M, et al: Relationships between lung computed tomographic density, gas exchange and PEEP in acute respiratory failure. *Anesthesiology* 69:824, 1988.

189. Pare PD, Warriner B, Baile EM, Hogg JC: Redistribution of pulmonary extravascular water with positive end-expiratory pressure in canine pulmonary edema. *Am J Respir Crit Care Med* 127:590, 1983.

190. Hilbert G, Gruson D, Vargas F, et al: Noninvasive ventilation in immunosuppressed patients with pulmonary infiltrates, fever, and acute respiratory failure. *N Engl J Med* 344:481, 2001.

191. Antonelli M, Conti G, Rocco M, et al: A comparison of noninvasive positive-pressure ventilation and conventional mechanical ventilation in patients with acute respiratory failure. *N Engl J Med* 339:429, 1998.

192. Antonelli M, Conti G, Moro ML, et al: Predictors of failure of noninvasive positive pressure ventilation in patients with acute hypoxemic respiratory failure: a multi-center study. *Intensive Care Med* 1718:28, 2001.

193. Brower RG: Mechanical ventilation in acute lung injury and ARDS. *Crit Care Clin* 18:1, 2002.

194. Suter PM, Fairley B, Isenberg MD: Optimum end-expiratory airway pressure in patients with acute pulmonary failure. *N Engl J Med* 292:284, 1975.

195. Dantzker DR, Brook CJ, Dehart P, et al: Ventilation-perfusion distributions in the adult respiratory distress syndrome. *Am Rev Respir Dis* 120:1039, 1979.

196. Lemaire F, Harf A, Teisseire BP: Oxygen exchange across the acutely injured lung, in Zapol WM, Falke KJ (eds): *Acute Respiratory Failure*. New York, Marcel Dekker, 1985, p 521.

197. Selecky PA, Wasserman K, Klein M, Ziment I: A graphic approach to assessing interrelationships among minute ventilation, arterial carbon dioxide tension, and ratio of physiologic dead space to tidal volume in patients on respirators. *Am Rev Respir Dis* 117:181, 1978.

198. Webb HH, Tierney DF: Experimental pulmonary edema due to intermittent positive pressure ventilation with high inflation pressures: Protection by positive end-expiratory pressure. *Am Rev Respir Dis* 110:556, 1974.

199. Dreyfuss D, Basset G, Soler P, Saumon G: Intermittent positive-pressure hyperventilation with high inflation pressures produces pulmonary microvascular injury in rats. *Am Rev Respir Dis* 132:880, 1985.

200. Dreyfuss D, Soler P, Basset G, Saumon G: High inflation pressure pulmonary edema. Respective effects of high airway pressure, high tidal volume, and positive end-expiratory pressure. *Am Rev Respir Dis* 137:1159, 1988.

201. Kolobow T, Moretti MP, Fumagalli R, et al: Severe impairment in lung function induced by high peak airway pressure during mechanical ventilation. An experimental study. *Am Rev Respir Dis* 135:312, 1987.

202. Hernandez LA, Peevy KJ, Moise AA, et al: Chest wall restrictions limit high airway pressure induced lung injury in young rabbits. *J Appl Physiol* 66:2364, 1989.

203. Carlton DP, Cummings JJ, Scheerer RG, et al: Lung overexpansion increases pulmonary microvascular protein permeability in young lambs. *J Appl Physiol* 69:557, 1990.

204. Corbridge TC, Wood LD, Crawford GP, et al: Adverse effects of large tidal volume and low PEEP in canine acid aspiration. *Am J Respir Crit Care Med* 142:311, 1990.

205. Mandava S, Kolobow T, Vitale G, et al: Lethal systemic capillary leak syndrome associated with severe ventilator-induced lung injury: an experimental study. *Crit Care Med* 31:885, 2003.

206. Imai Y, Parodo J, Kajikawa O, et al: Injurious mechanical ventilation and end-organ epithelial cell apoptosis and organ dysfunction in an experimental model of acute respiratory distress syndrome [see comment]. *JAMA* 289:2104, 2003.

207. Tremblay LN, Miatto D, Hamid Q, et al: Injurious ventilation induces widespread pulmonary epithelial expression of tumor necrosis factor-alpha and interleukin-6 messenger RNA [see comment]. *Crit Care Med* 30:1693, 2002.

208. Zhang H, Downey GP, Suter PM, et al: Conventional mechanical ventilation is associated with bronchoalveolar lavage-induced activation of polymorphonuclear leukocytes: a possible mechanism to explain the systemic consequences of ventilator-induced lung injury in patients with ARDS. *Anesthesiology* 97:1426, 2002.

209. Maunder RJ, Shuman WP, McHugh JW, et al: Preservation of normal lung regions in the adult respiratory distress syndrome. *JAMA* 255:2463, 1986.

210. Roupie E, Dambrosio M, Servillo G, et al: Titration of tidal volume and induced hypercapnea in acute respiratory distress syndrome. *Am J Respir Crit Care Med* 152:121, 1995.

211. Holzapfel L, Robert D, Perrin F, et al: Static pressure-volume curves and effect of positive end-expiratory pressure on gas exchange in adult respiratory distress syndrome. *Crit Care Med* 11:591, 1983.

212. Crotti S, Mascheroni D, Caironi P, et al: Recruitment and derecruitment during acute respiratory failure: a clinical study. *Am J Respir Crit Care Med* 164:131, 2001.

213. Pelosi P, Goldner M, Mckibben A, et al: Recruitment and derecruitment during acute respiratory failure. An experimental study. *Am J Respir Crit Care Med* 164:122, 2001.

214. Hickling KG: Best compliance during a decremental, but not incremental, positive end-expiratory pressure trial is related to open-lung positive end-expiratory pressure: a mathematical model of acute respiratory distress syndrome lungs. *Am J Respir Crit Care Med* 163:69, 2001.

215. Eichacker PQ, Gerstenberger EP, Banks SM, et al: Meta-analysis of acute lung injury and acute respiratory distress syndrome trials testing low tidal volumes [see comment]. *Am J Respir Crit Care Med* 166:1510, 2002.

216. Steinbrook R: How best to ventilate? Trial design and patient safety in studies of the acute respiratory distress syndrome [comment]. *N Engl J Med* 348:1393, 2003.

217. Steinbrook R: Trial design and patient safety—the debate continues [comment]. *N Engl J Med* 349:629, 2003.

218. Gattinoni L PP, Crotti S, et al: Effects of positive end-expiratory pressure on regional distribution of tidal volume and recruitment in adult respiratory distress syndrome. *Am J Respir Crit Care Med* 151:1807, 1995.

219. Amato MB, Barbas CS, Medeiros DM, et al: Beneficial effects of the "open lung approach" with low distending pressures in acute respiratory distress syndrome. *Am J Respir Crit Care Med* 152:1835, 1995.

220. Shoemaker WC: Goal-oriented hemodynamic therapy. *N Engl J Med* 334:799, 1996.

221. Boyd O, Grounds RM, Bennett ED: A randomized clinical trial of the effect of deliberate perioperative increase of oxygen delivery on mortality in high-risk surgical patients. *JAMA* 270:2699, 1993.

222. Ronco JJ, Fenwick JC, Tweeddale MG, et al: Identification of the critical oxygen delivery for anaerobic metabolism in critically ill septic and nonseptic humans. *JAMA* 270:1724, 1993.

223. Ronco JJ, Phang PT, Walley KR, et al: Oxygen consumption is independent of changes in oxygen delivery in severe adult respiratory distress syndrome. *Am J Respir Crit Care Med* 143:1267, 1991.

224. Gattinoni L, Brazzi L, Pelosi P, et al: The SvO2 Collaborative Group. A trial of goal-oriented hemodynamic therapy in critically ill patients. *N Engl J Med* 333:1025, 1995.

225. Hayes MA, Timmins AC, Yau E, et al: Elevation of systemic oxygen delivery in the treatment of critically ill patients. *N Engl J Med* 330:1717, 1994.

226. Prewitt RM, McCarthy J, Wood LDH: Treatment of acute low pressure edema in dogs: Relative effects of hydrostatic and oncotic pressure, nitroprusside, and positive end expiratory pressure. *J Clin Invest* 67:409, 1981.

227. Long GR, Breen PH, Mayers I, Wood LD: Treatment of canine aspiration pneumonitis: Fluid volume reduction vs. fluid volume expansion. *J Appl Physiol* 65:1736, 1988.

228. Sznajder JI, Zucker AR, Wood LD, Long GR: Effects of plasmapheresis and hemofiltration on acid aspiration pulmonary edema. *Am J Respir Crit Care Med* 134:222, 1986.

229. Gottlieb SS, Wood LD, Hansen DE, Long GR: The effect of nitroprusside on pulmonary edema, oxygen exchange, and blood flow in hydrochloric acid aspiration. *Anesthesiology* 67:47, 1987.

230. Zucker AR, Becker CJ, Berger S, et al: Pathophysiology of treatment of canine kerosene pulmonary injury: The effects of plasmapheresis and positive end-expiratory pressure on canine kerosene pulmonary injury. *J Crit Care* 4:184, 1989.

231. Oppenheimer L, Wood LD, Prewitt RM: Acute effects of nitroprusside in patients with hypoxemic respiratory failure. *Surg Forum* 32:306, 1981.

232. Zucker AR, Wood LD, Curet-Scott M, et al: Partial lung bypass reduces kerosene lung injury in dogs. *J Crit Care* 6:29, 1991.

233. Wood LD: Acute effects of nitroprusside in patients with hypoxemic respiratory failure. *Am J Cardiol* 47:963, 1981.

234. Mitchel JP, Schuller D, Calandrino FS, et al: Improved outcome based on fluid management in critically ill patients requiring pulmonary artery catheterization. *Am J Respir Crit Care Med* 145:990, 1992.

235. Simmons RS, Berdine GG, Seidenfeld JJ, et al: Fluid balance and the adult respiratory distress syndrome. *Am J Respir Crit Care Med* 135:924, 1987.

236. Humphrey H, Hall J, Sznajder I, et al: Improved survival in ARDS patients associated with a reduction in pulmonary capillary wedge pressure. *Chest* 97:1176, 1990.

237. Eisenberg PR, Hansbrough JR, Anderson D, Schuster DP: A prospective study of lung water measurements during patient management in an intensive care unit. *Am J Respir Crit Care Med* 136:662, 1987.

238. Hyers TM: ARDS: The therapeutic dilemma. *Chest* 97:1025, 1990.

239. Hudson LD: Fluid management strategy in acute lung injury. *Am J Respir Crit Care Med* 145:988, 1992.

240. O'Quinn R, Marini JJ. Pulmonary artery occlusion pressure: Clinical physiology, measurement, and interpretation. *Am J Respir Crit Care Med* 128:319, 1983.

241. Teboul JL, Besbes M, Andrivet P, et al: A bedside index assessing the reliability of pulmonary artery occlusion pressure measurements during mechanical ventilation with positive end-expiratory pressure. *J Crit Care* 7:22, 1992.

242. Rizvi K, de Boisblanc B, Dhillon G, Arroliga A, the NIH/NHLBI ARDS Network. Effect of airway pressure display on inter-observer variability in assessment of vascular pressure in the ARDSnet Fluids and Catheters Treatment Trial (FACTT). *Am J Respir Crit Care Med* 167:A617, 2003.

243. Pinsky M, Vincent JL, De Smet JM: Estimating left ventricular filling pressure during positive end-expiratory pressure in humans. *Am J Respir Crit Care Med* 143:25, 1991.

244. Carter RS, Snyder JV, Pinsky MR: LV filling pressure during PEEP measured by nadir wedge pressure after airway disconnection. *Am J Physiol* 249:H770, 1985.

245. Hickling KG, Henderson S, Jackson R: Low mortality associated with low volume pressure limited ventilation with permissive hypercapnea in severe adult respiratory distress syndrome. *Intensive Care Med* 16:372, 1990.

246. Hickling KG, Walsh J, Henderson S, Jackson R: Low mortality rate in adult respiratory distress syndrome using low-volume, pressure-limited ventilation with permissive hypercapnea: A prospective study. *Crit Care Med* 22:1568, 1994.

247. Feihl F, Perret C: Permissive hypercapnia: How permissive should we be? *Am J Respir Crit Care Med* 150:1722, 1994.

248. Tuxen DV: Permissive hypercapnic ventilation. *Am J Respir Crit Care Med* 150:870, 1994.

249. Langer M, Mascheroni D, Marcolin R, Gattinoni L: The prone position in ARDS patients: A clinical study. *Chest* 94:103, 1988.

250. Pappert D, Rossaint R, Slama K, et al: Influence of positioning on ventilation-perfusion relationships in severe adult respiratory distress syndrome. *Chest* 106:1511, 1994.

251. Douglas W, Rehder K, Beynen RM, et al: Improved oxygenation in patients with acute respiratory failure. *Am J Respir Crit Care Med* 115:559, 1977.

252. Gattinoni L, Tognoni G, Pesenti A, et al: Effect of prone positioning on the survival of patients with acute respiratory failure. *N Engl J Med* 345:568, 2001.

253. Lamm WJ, Graham MM, Albert RK: Mechanism by which the prone position improves oxygenation in acute lung injury. *Am J Respir Crit Care Med* 150:184, 1994.

254. Pelosi P, Croci M, Calappi E, et al: The prone positioning during general anesthesia minimally affects respiratory mechanics while improving functional residual capacity and increasing oxygen tension. *Anesth Analg* 80:955, 1995.

255. Glenny RW, Lamm WJ, Albert RK, Robertson HT: Gravity is a minor determinant of pulmonary blood flow distribution. *J Appl Physiol* 71:620, 1991.

256. Gattinoni L, Pelosi P, Vitale G, et al: Body position changes redistribute lung computed-tomography density in patients with acute respiratory failure. *Anesthesiology* 74:15, 1991.

257. Gattinoni L, Vagginelli F, Carlesso E, et al: Prone-Supine Study G. Decrease in PaCO2 with prone position is predictive of improved outcome in acute respiratory distress syndrome [see comment]. *Crit Care Med* 31:2727, 2003.

258. Pelosi P, Bottino N, Chiumello D, et al: Sigh in supine and prone position during acute respiratory distress syndrome. *Am J Respir Crit Care Med* 167:521, 2003.

259. Marini JJ, Gattinoni L: Ventilatory management of acute respiratory distress syndrome: a consensus of two. *Crit Care Med* 32:250, 2004.

260. The ARDS Clinical Trials Network NHLBI, National Institutes of Health. Effects of recruitment maneuvers in patients with acute lung injury and acute respiratory distress syndrome ventilated with high positive end-expiratory pressure. *Crit Care Med* 31:2592, 2003.

261. Foti G, Cereda M, Sparacino ME, et al: Effects of periodic lung recruitment maneuvers on gas exchange and respiratory mechanics in mechanically ventilated acute respiratory distress syndrome (ARDS) patients [see comment]. *Intensive Care Med* 26:501, 2000.

262. Van der Kloot, Thomas E, Blanch L, et al: Recruitment maneuvers in three experimental models of acute lung injury. Effect on lung volume and gas exchange. *Am J Respir Crit Care Med* 161:1485, 2000.

263. Villagra A, Ochagavia A, Vatua S, et al: Recruitment maneuvers during lung protective ventilation in acute respiratory distress syndrome. *Am J Respir Crit Care Med* 165:165, 2002.

264. Richard J-C, Maggiore SM, Jonson B, et al: Influence of tidal volume on alveolar recruitment. Respective role of PEEP and a recruitment maneuver. *Am J Respir Crit Care Med* 163:1609, 2001.

265. Lim CM, Koh Y, Park W, et al: Mechanistic scheme and effect of "extended sigh" as a recruitment maneuver in patients with acute respiratory distress syndrome: a preliminary study. *Crit Care Med* 29:1255, 2001.

266. Pelosi P, Bottino N, Chiumello D, et al: Sigh in supine and prone position during acute respiratory distress syndrome. *Am J Respir Crit Care Med* 167:521, 2003.

267. Pelosi P, Cadringher P, Bottino N, et al: Sigh in acute respiratory distress syndrome. *Am J Respir Crit Care Med* 159:872, 1999.

268. Patroniti N, Foti G, Cortinovis B, et al: Sigh improves gas exchange and lung volume in patients with acute respiratory distress syndrome undergoing pressure support ventilation [see comment]. *Anesthesiology* 96:788, 2002.

269. Hadorn DC: Setting health care priorities in Oregon. Cost-effectiveness meets the rule of rescue [see comment]. *JAMA* 265:2218, 1991.

270. Carter C, Adams AB, Stone M, et al: Tracheal gas insufflation during late exhalation efficiently reduces PaCO(2) in experimental acute lung injury. *Intensive Care Med* 28:504, 2002.

271. Nahum A, Shapiro RS, Ravenscraft SA, et al: Efficacy of expiratory tracheal gas insufflation in a canine model of lung injury. *Am J Respir Crit Care Med* 152:489, 1995.

272. Belghith M, Fierobe L, Brunet F, et al: Is tracheal gas insufflation an alternative to extrapulmonary gas exchangers in severe ARDS? *Chest* 107:1416, 1995.

273. Roissant R, Falke KJ, Lopez F, et al: Inhaled nitric oxide for the adult respiratory distress syndrome. *N Engl J Med* 328:399, 1993.

274. Rossaint R, Gerlach H, Schmidt-Ruhnke H, et al: Efficacy of inhaled nitric oxide in patients with severe ARDS. *Chest* 107:1107, 1995.

275. Bigatello LM, Hurford WE, Kacmarek RM, et al: Prolonged inhalation of low concentrations of nitric oxide in patients with severe adult respiratory distress syndrome. *Anesthesiology* 80:761, 1994.

276. Puybasset L, Stewart T, Rouby JJ, et al: Inhaled nitric oxide reverses the increase in pulmonary vascular resistance induced by permissive hypercapnea in patients with adult respiratory distress syndrome. *Anesthesiology* 80:1254, 1994.

277. Lowson SM, Rich GF, McArdle PA, et al: The response to varying concentrations of inhaled nitric oxide in patients with acute respiratory distress syndrome. *Anesth Analg* 82:574, 1996.

278. Benzing A, Brautigam P, Geiger K, et al: Inhaled nitric oxide reduces pulmonary transvascular albumin flux in patients with acute lung injury. *Anesthesiology* 83:113, 1996.

279. Lavoie A, Hall JB, Olson DM, Wylam ME: Life-threatening effects of discontinuing inhaled nitric oxide in severe respiratory failure. *Am J Respir Crit Care Med* 1996.153:1985.

280. Taylor RW, Zimmerman JL, Dellinger RP, et al: Low-dose inhaled nitric oxide in patients with acute lung injury: a randomized controlled trial. *JAMA* 291:1603, 2004.

281. Reily DJ, Tollok E, Mallitz K, et al: Successful aeromedical transport using inhaled prostacyclin for a patient with life-threatening hypoxemia. *Chest* 125:1579, 2004.

282. Dahlem P, van Aalderen WM, de Neef M, et al: Randomized controlled trial of aerosolized prostacyclin therapy in children with acute lung injury [see comment]. *Crit Care Med* 32:1055, 2004.

283. Siobal MS, Kallet RH, Pittet JF, et al: Description and evaluation of a delivery system for aerosolized prostacyclin. *Respiratory Care.* 48:742, 2003.

284. Lowson SM: Inhaled alternatives to nitric oxide [see comment]. *Anesthesiology* 96:1504, 2002.

285. Bernard GR, Luce JM, Sprung CL, et al: High-dose corticosteroids in patients with adult respiratory distress syndrome. *N Engl J Med* 317:1565, 1987.

286. Bone RC, Fisher CJ Jr, Clemmer TP, et al: Ineffectiveness of high-dose methylprednisolone in preventing parenchymal lung injury and improving mortality in patients with septic shock. *Chest* 92:1032, 1987.

287. Meduri GU, Chinn AJ, Leeper KV, et al: Corticosteroid rescue treatment of progressive fibroproliferation in late ARDS. Patterns of response and predictors of outcome. *Chest* 105:1516, 1994.

288. Hooper RG, Kearl RA: Established ARDS treated with a sustained course of adrenocortical steroids. *Chest* 97:138, 1990.

289. Ashbaugh DG, Maier RV: Idiopathic pulmonary fibrosis in adult respiratory distress syndrome: Diagnosis and treatment. *Arch Surg* 120:530, 1985.

290. Meduri GU, Tolley EA, Chrousos GP, Stentz F: Prolonged methylprednisolone treatment suppresses systemic inflammation in patients with unresolving acute respiratory distress syndrome: evidence for inadequate endogenous glucocorticoid secretion and inflammation-induced immune cell resistance to glucocorticoids. *Am J Respir Crit Care Med* 165:983, 2002.

291. Hudson L: Preliminary results from the NHLBI ARDS Clinical Trials Network's LaSRS trial. Presented at International Meeting of the American Thoracic Society. Orlando, FL. 2004.

292. Tharratt RS, Allen RP, Albertson TE: Pressure controlled inverse ratio ventilation in severe adult respiratory failure. *Chest* 94:755, 1988.

293. Cole AG, Weller SF, Sykes MK: Inverse ratio ventilation compared with PEEP in adult respiratory failure. *Intensive Care Med* 10:227, 1984.

294. Gurevitch MJ, Van Dyke J, Young ES, Jackson K: Improved oxygenation and lower peak airway pressure in severe adult respiratory distress syndrome: Treatment with inverse ratio ventilation. *Chest* 89:211, 1986.

295. Manthous CA, Schmidt GA. IRV in ARDS: Improved oxygenation without autoPEEP. *Chest* 103:953, 1992.

296. Mercat A, Graini L, Teboul JL, et al: Cardiorespiratory effects of pressure-controlled ventilation with and without inverse ratio in the adult respiratory distress syndrome. *Chest* 104:871, 1993.

297. Sydow M, Burchardi H, Ephraim E, et al: Long term effects of two different ventilatory modes on oxygenation in acute lung injury: Comparison of airway pressure release ventilation and volume-controlled inverse ratio ventilation. *Am J Respir Crit Care Med* 149:1550, 1994.

298. Derdak S: High-frequency oscillatory ventilation for acute respiratory distress syndrome in adult patients. *Crit Care Med* 31:S317, 2003.

299. Derdak S, Mehta S, Stewart TE, et al: Multicenter Oscillatory Ventilation For Acute Respiratory Distress Syndrome Trial Study I. High-frequency oscillatory ventilation for acute respiratory distress syndrome in adults: A randomized, controlled trial [see comment]. *Am J Respir Crit Care Med* 166:801, 2002.

300. Holzapfel L, Robert D, Perrin F, et al: Comparison of high frequency jet ventilation to conventional ventilation in adults with respiratory distress syndrome. *Intensive Care Med* 13:100, 1987.

301. Carlon GC, Howland WS, Ray C, et al: High frequency jet ventilation: A prospective randomized evaluation. *Chest* 84:551, 1983.

302. Schuster DP, Klain M, Snyder JV: Comparison of high frequency jet ventilation to conventional ventilation during severe acute respiratory failure in humans. *Crit Care Med* 10:625, 1982.

303. Zobel G, Kuttnig-Haim M, Decar D, et al: Extracorporeal membrane oxygenation in severe acute respiratory failure. *JAMA* 242:2193, 1979.

304. Egan TM, Duffin J, Glynn MF, et al: Ten-year experience with extracorporeal membrane oxygenation for severe respiratory failure. *Chest* 94:681, 1988.

305. Snider MT Campbell DB, Kofke WA, et al: Venovenous perfusion of adults and children with severe acute respiratory distress syndrome. *ASAIO* 34:1014, 1988.

306. Gattinoni L, Pesenti A, Mascheroni D, et al: Low-frequency positive-pressure ventilation with extracorporeal CO2 removal in severe acute respiratory failure. *JAMA* 256:881, 1986.

307. Morris AH, Wallace CJ, Menlove RL, et al: Randomized clinical trial of pressure controlled inverse ratio ventilation and extracorporeal CO2 removal for adult respiratory distress syndrome. *Am J Respir Crit Care Med* 149:295, 1994.

308. Anderson H 3rd, Steimle C, Shapiro M, et al: Extracorporeal life support for adult cardiorespiratory failure. *Surgery* 114:161, 1993.

309. Hirschl RB, Pranikoff T, Wise C, et al: Initial experience with partial liquid ventilation in adult patients with the acute respiratory distress syndrome. *JAMA* 275:383, 1996.

310. Spitzer AR, Lipsky CL: Partial liquid ventilation with Perflubron in premature infants with severe respiratory distress syndrome. *Clin Pediatr* 36:181, 1997.

311. Pranikoff T, Gauger PG, Hirschl RB: Partial liquid ventilation in newborn patients with congenital diaphragmatic hernia. *J Pediatr Surg* 31:613, 1996.

312. Leach CL, Greenspan JS, Rubenstein SD, et al: Partial liquid ventilation with perflubron in premature infants with severe respiratory distress syndrome: The LiquiVent Study Group. *N Engl J Med* 335:761, 1996.

313. Hirschl RB, Croce M, Gore D, et al: Prospective, randomized, controlled pilot study of partial liquid ventilation in adult acute respiratory distress syndrome. *Am J Respir Crit Care Med* 165:781, 2002.

314. Hallman M, Spragg R, Harrell JH, et al: Evidence of lung surfactant abnormality in respiratory failure. *J Clin Invest* 70:673, 1982.

315. Lewis JF, Jobe AH: Surfactant and the adult respiratory distress syndrome. *Am Rev Resp Dis* 147:218, 1993.

316. Jobe A, Ikegami M: Surfactant for the treatment of respiratory distress syndrome. *Am J Respir Crit Care Med* 136:1256, 1987.

317. Merritt TA, Hallman M, Bloom BT, et al: Prophylactic treatment of very premature infants with human surfactant. *N Engl J Med* 315:785, 1986.

318. Horbar JD, Soll RF, Sutherland JM, et al: A multicenter, randomized, placebo-controlled trial of surfactant therapy for respiratory distress syndrome. *N Engl J Med* 320:959, 1989.

319. Spragg RG, Lewis JF, Wurst W, et al: Treatment of acute respiratory distress syndrome with recombinant surfactant protein C surfactant. *Am J Respir Crit Care Med* 167:1562, 2003.

320. Spragg RG, Rathgeb F, Hafner D, et al: Intratracheal instillation of rSP-C surfactant improves oxygenation in patients with ARDS (Abstract). *Am J Respir Crit Care Med* 165:A22, 2002.

321. Seeger W, Hafner D, Lewis JF, et al: Treatment with rSP-C surfactant reduces mortality in ARDS due to primary pulmonary events (Abstract). *Am J Respir Crit Care Med* 165:A219, 2002.

322. Gregory TJ, Steinberg KP, Spragg R, et al: Bovine surfactant therapy for patients with acute respiratory distress syndrome. *Am J Respir Crit Care Med* 155:1309, 1997.

323. Spragg RG, Lewis JF, Walmrath H-D, Johannigman J, et al: Effect of recombinant surfactant protein C-based surfactant on the acute respiratory distress syndrome. *N Engl J Med* 351:884, 2004.

324. Milberg JA, Davis DR, Steinberg KP, Hudson LD: Improved survival of patients with acute respiratory distress syndrome (ARDS). *JAMA* 273:306, 1995.

325. McHugh L, Milberg J, Whitcomb M, et al: Recovery of function in survivors of the acute respiratory distress syndrome. *Am J Respir Crit Care Med* 150:90, 1994.

326. Orme J Jr, Romney JS, Hopkins RO, et al: Pulmonary function and health-related quality of life in survivors of acute respiratory distress syndrome. *Am J Respir Crit Care Med* 167:690, 2003.

327. Weinert CR, Gross CR, Kangas JR, et al: Health-related quality of life after acute lung injury. *Am J Respir Crit Care Med* 156:1120, 1997.

328. Schelling G, Stoll C, Haller M, et al: Health-related quality of life and posttraumatic stress disorder in survivors of the acute respiratory distress syndrome. *Crit Care Med* 26:651, 1998.

329. Angus DC, Musthafa AA, Clermont G: Quality-adjusted survival in the first year after the acute respiratory distress syndrome. *Am J Respir Crit Care Med* 163:1389, 2001.

330. Hopkins R, Weaver L, Pope D, et al: Neuropsychological sequelae and impaired health status in survivors of severe acute respiratory distress syndrome. *Am J Respir Crit Care Med* 160:50, 1999.

331. Moss M, Parsons PE, Steinberg KP, et al: Chronic alcohol abuse is associated with an increased incidence of acute respiratory distress syndrome and severity of multiple organ dysfunction in patients with septic shock. *Crit Care Med* 31:869, 2003.

332. Moss M, Burnham EL: Chronic alcohol abuse, acute respiratory distress syndrome, and multiple organ dysfunction. *Crit Care Med* 31:S207, 2003.

333. Collins FS, Green ED, Guttmacher AE, Guyer MS: A vision for the future of genomics research. *Nature* 422:835, 2003.

334. Rubenfeld GD, Cooper C, Carter G, et al: Barriers to providing lung-protective ventilation to patients with acute lung injury. *Crit Care Med* 32:1289, 2004.

335. Young MP, Manning HL, Wilson DL, et al: Ventilation of patients with acute lung injury and acute respiratory distress syndrome: has new evidence changed clinical practice? [see comment]. *Crit Care Med* 32:1260, 2004.

336. Weinert CR, Gross CR, Marinelli WA: Impact of randomized trial results on acute lung injury ventilator therapy in teaching hospitals [see comment]. *Am J Respir Crit Care Med* 167:1304, 2003.

337. Stewart TE: Effective ventilation strategies for acute respiratory distress syndrome. *Can Respir J* 10:171, 2003.

Chapter 39 _____

ACUTE-ON-CHRONIC RESPIRATORY FAILURE

IVOR S. DOUGLAS
GREGORY A. SCHMIDT
JESSE B. HALL

KEY POINTS

- *Acute-on-chronic respiratory failure (ACRF) occurs when relatively minor, although often multiple, insults cause acute deterioration in a patient with chronic respiratory insufficiency.*

- *ACRF is usually seen in patients known to have severe chronic obstructive pulmonary disease (COPD), but occasionally it manifests as cryptic respiratory failure or postoperative ventilator dependence in a patient with no known lung disease.*

- *The wide variety of causes of ACRF may be compartmentalized into causes of incremental load, diminished neuromuscular competence, or depressed drive, superimposed on a limited ventilatory reserve.*

- *Intrinsic positive end-expiratory pressure (PEEPi) is a central contributor to the excess work of breathing in patients with ACRF.*

- *The most important therapeutic interventions are administration of oxygen, bronchodilators, and corticosteroids, and noninvasive positive pressure ventilation (NIPPV).*

- *NIPPV can be used in most patients to avoid intubation and has been shown to improve survival.*

- *The decision to intubate a patient with ACRF benefits from clinical judgment and a bedside presence. Hypotension and severe alkalemia commonly complicate the immediate periintubation course, but they are usually avoidable.*

- *Ventilator settings should mimic the patient's breathing pattern, with a relatively rapid rate (e.g., 20/min) and small tidal volume (e.g., 450 mL); some positive end-expiratory pressure (e.g., 5 cm H_2O) should be added.*

- *Prevention of complications such as gastrointestinal hemorrhage, venous thrombosis, and nosocomial infection is a crucial component of the care plan.*

- *The key to liberating the patient from the ventilator is to increase neuromuscular competence while reducing respiratory system load.*

- *In selected patients, extubation to NIPPV despite failed spontaneous breathing trials reduces ventilator and ICU days and further improves survival.*

In the past three decades, mortality from chronic obstructive pulmonary disease (COPD) has risen dramatically, making COPD the fourth leading cause of death in 2000.[1] Compared with people with normal lung function, subjects with severe COPD (forced expiratory volume in 1 second [FEV_1] <50% predicted) followed for 22 years as part of the National Health and Nutrition Examination Survey (NHANES I) had a 2.7-fold increased risk of death (95% CI 2.1 to 3.5) in an adjusted analysis.[2] This trend is apparent in men and women,

more prominent in black Americans, and clearly related to cigarette smoking. For the first time, in 2000 more women than men died of COPD in the U.S.[1] Admissions to ICUs for exacerbations of COPD account for a substantial portion of bed-days,[3] since these patients often require prolonged ventilatory support. In surgical ICUs, COPD is an important problem as well, since it is one of the more common reasons for a prolonged postoperative recovery. An approach to this disease is an essential component of the intensivist's armamentarium.

This chapter describes the pathophysiology and management of patients with chronic pulmonary disease (most with COPD) who require intensive care for decompensation of their normally precariously balanced ventilatory state. This acute deterioration superimposed on stable disease is termed acute-on-chronic respiratory failure (ACRF). Patients may present to the ICU with worsening dyspnea, deteriorating mental status, or respiratory arrest. Especially when there is a preexisting diagnosis of lung disease, the diagnosis of ACRF can be made easily. However, it is important to remember that not all patients with severe COPD will have been so identified. In many patients with respiratory distress, congestive heart failure or pulmonary thromboembolism is considered first; making a correct diagnosis of ACRF requires a high index of suspicion. On occasion the disease is even more occult, for example in a postoperative patient who fails extubation and then is noted to have hyperinflation on the chest radiograph. Since optimal therapy depends on accurate diagnosis, underlying COPD should be part of the differential diagnosis for most patients with dyspnea or inability to sustain unassisted ventilation.

A severe exacerbation of COPD is characterized by a sustained worsening from the stable state that is acute in onset and requires hospitalization.[4] The typical symptoms are dyspnea that has been worsening over days, often with increased cough and sputum production. Physical examination typically demonstrates respiratory distress, accessory muscle use, a prolonged expiratory time, recruitment of expiratory muscles, and wheezing. As discussed below, the absence of respiratory distress is not necessarily reassuring and when associated with somnolence is a grave and ominous sign of impending respiratory arrest. The chest radiograph is usually abnormal, reflecting the chronic lung disease, but only in 15% to 20% of cases reveals a finding (eg, pneumonia, pneumothorax, pulmonary infarction, or pulmonary edema) that results in a change of management.[5] Sometimes there are indicators of acute infection, such as purulent sputum, fever, leukocytosis, and a new radiographic infiltrate. Typical initial arterial blood gas values on room air show a partial oxygen pressure (P_{O_2}) of 35 to 45 mm Hg and a partial arterial carbon dioxide pressure (Pa_{CO_2}) of 60 to 70 mm Hg. Comparison with values obtained when the patient is stable can be useful, as many patients have compensated metabolic acidosis with chronically elevated Pa_{CO_2} at baseline. Electrocardiography (ECG) may show signs of right atrial enlargement or right ventricular hypertrophy and strain. P-wave amplitude >1.5 mm is universal in patients with acute exacerbation of COPD (but not necessarily ACRF), although classic P pulmonale (P-wave amplitude in leads II, III, and/or aVF >2.5 mm) is uncommon. Resolution of the exacerbation is associated with an amplitude reduction of approximately 0.8 mm.[6] Thus serial ECGs may be useful in assessing response to therapy.

Although the short-term risk of death is high for ACRF, the prognosis for patients with ACRF is not uniformly poor despite severe underlying pulmonary impairment. In a prospective analysis of 250 admissions (180 patients) to an ICU for acute respiratory failure complicating COPD, hospital mortality was 21% and was strongly associated with the development of extrapulmonary organ failures.[7] One-year survival following ACRF ranges from 22% to 72%.[8,9] Some patients will return to an acceptable quality of life, and some even go back to work. In a cohort of 1016 patients admitted with a COPD exacerbation and a Pa_{CO_2} >50 mm Hg, 1-year survival was 47%, but only 26% of the patients rated their quality of life as good or better when surveyed at 6 months.[3] Other than the underlying cause of chronic respiratory failure, predictors of poor survival include premorbid functional status, baseline dyspnea, lower body mass index,[3] older age,[3] lower ratio of oxygen pressure to fraction of inspired oxygen $(P_{O_2}:F_{I_{O_2}})$[3], history of congestive heart failure, presence of serious comorbid disease,[10] development of extrapulmonary organ failures,[7] serum albumin level,[3,11] cor pulmonale,[3] and requirement for >72 hours of ventilation,[10] but these indicators are not refined enough to allow accurate prognostication for individual patients.

Critical care resource utilization and costs for ACRF and COPD are substantial. Ely and coworkers calculated that respiratory care costs were almost twice as much for patients with COPD compared with non-COPD–related respiratory failure ($2422 [$1157 to $6100] vs. $1580 [$738 to $3322]) respectively; $p = 0.01$, 1996 dollars), despite similar ICU lengths of stay and mechanical ventilation days.[12]

Ideally, patients followed in the clinic with known severe COPD will be encouraged to discuss with their physicians their wishes regarding intensive care before acute deterioration. Unfortunately this is only occasionally accomplished. It is our approach to fully support patients with ACRF who believe their quality of life is acceptable, especially since most will be successfully managed with noninvasive ventilation, and most of those intubated will eventually be successfully liberated from the ventilator and survive to hospital discharge.[8,13] On the other hand, when mechanical ventilation seems excessive to the patient or physician, defining the goals of care as the provision of comfort and relief from dyspnea and pain is appropriate. We urge clinicians caring for COPD patients with compensated respiratory failure to address advance directives and desire for life-sustaining therapies during routine ambulatory clinic appointments when informed and deliberate decision making can be shared by the patient and their loved ones.

Pathophysiology

Alveolar ventilation is maintained by the central nervous system, which acts through nerves and the respiratory muscles to drive the respiratory pump. The three subsets of ventilatory failure are loss of adequate drive, impaired neuromuscular competence, and excessive respiratory load. This concept is elucidated in Fig. 39-1. The central nervous system drives the inspiratory muscles via the spinal cord and phrenic and intercostal nerves. Inspiratory muscle contraction lowers pleural pressure, thereby inflating the lungs. The pressure generated by the inspiratory muscles (neuromuscular competence) must be sufficient to overcome the elastance of the lungs and chest wall (elastic load), as well as the flow resistance of the airways (resistive load). Spontaneous ventilation can be sustained only as long as the inspiratory muscles are able to maintain adequate pressure generation.[14]

Relatively few patients develop ventilatory failure from loss of drive. Most often this occurs in the setting of drug or alcohol overdose or physician-directed sedation. Typically these patients present little challenge, requiring only supportive care until the drug can be reversed or metabolized. One exception is the group of patients with undiagnosed sleep-disordered breathing. Although sleep-disordered breathing is no more common in people with mild COPD than in healthy controls,[15] many patients with chronic respiratory failure have a significant component of central apnea with nocturnal desaturation. Specific therapy directed at relief of their sleep disorder, including nocturnal bilevel pressure support

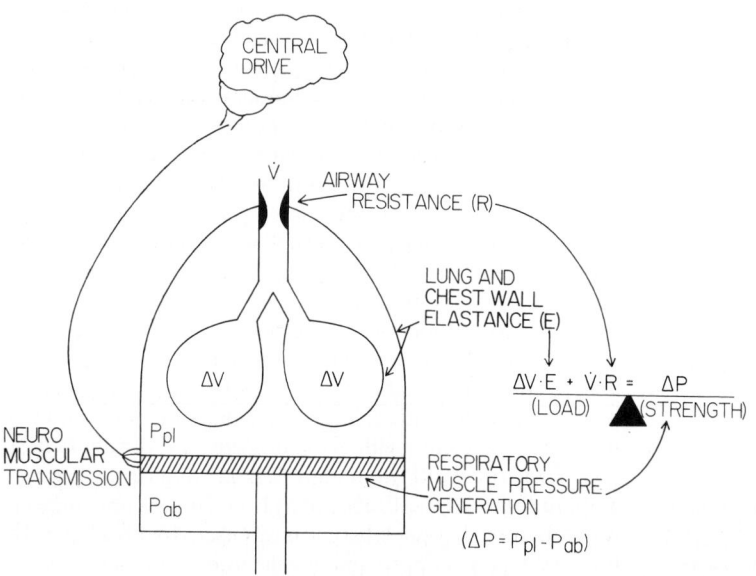

FIGURE 39-1 A drawing of the key elements of the respiratory system. The drive to breathe derives from CNS regulators of respiratory pattern. Neural afferents are the path for signals causing respiratory muscle contraction. Diaphragm contraction generates a pleural pressure (Ppl) and is opposed by any increased abdominal pressure (Pab). The Ppl generated must overcome the resistive (R) and elastic (E) forces acting on the respiratory system in producing a given minute ventilation ($\dot{V}E$). (*Reproduced with permission from Schmidt et al.[81]*)

and supplemental oxygen, may be required. Far more common and difficult are patients who have adequate drive but have inadequate neuromuscular function, excessive load, or both.

A useful approach to understanding the pathophysiology of ACRF is that inspiratory muscle fatigue is a primary determinant.[16] A muscle is fatigued when it can no longer develop the degree of tension possible before fatigue, no matter what the degree of stimulation, yet the muscle recovers with rest. Skeletal muscles fatigue when their rate of energy consumption exceeds the energy supplied by blood flow.[17] Similarly, for the respiratory muscles, endurance time during inspiratory resistive loading is closely tied to the oxygen cost of breathing ($\dot{V}_{O_2resp}$).[18] The primary determinants of $\dot{V}_{O_2resp}$ are the time-tension index, work rate, and lung volume.[19] Several experiments in humans indicate that the intensity required of the contracting respiratory muscles, as well as their strength, is a crucial factor in determining fatigue.[20] In contrast to patients with ACRF, patients with stable, moderately severe COPD do not demonstrate low frequency diaphragmatic fatigue after maximal exercise effort when measured with a nonvolitional magnetic coil–induced twitch,[21,22] despite excessive muscle loading manifest by significant slowing of the respiratory muscle maximal relaxation rate after a volitional sniff maneuver.[23] This would suggest that the superimposition of infection, heart failure, or other precipitants potentiates muscle fatigue. Once fatigue of the respiratory muscles is established, neuromuscular competence is unable to sustain the mechanical load imposed on the respiratory system, and ventilatory failure ensues. The intensivist must therefore address both the precipitant and resultant respiratory muscle fatigue for treatment to be successful.

In health, neuromuscular function far exceeds that necessary to sustain ventilation against the normally small load. Dramatic increments in load (as in status asthmaticus) or decrements in strength (as in the Guillain-Barré syndrome) are required to cause hypoventilation. In patients with COPD, however, the respiratory system load as judged by the $\dot{V}_{O_2resp}$ is elevated to 17% to 46% of the total body volume of oxygen utilization ($\dot{V}_{O_2}$), owing to abnormal airway resistance and increased elastance.[24] The increase in airway resistance is caused by bronchospasm, airway inflammation, and physical obstruction by mucus and scarring.

The most significant contributor to the elastic load is dynamic hyperinflation. Airflow obstruction, compounded by decreased elastic recoil in patients with emphysema, leads to prolongation of expiration. When the rate of alveolar emptying is slowed, expiration cannot be completed before the ensuing inspiration. Rather than reaching the normal static equilibrium of lung and chest wall recoil at functional residual capacity (FRC) at the end of each breath, the respiratory system empties incompletely. Expiration terminates at this higher, dynamically determined FRC. At end expiration, there remains a positive elastic recoil pressure, which is called intrinsic positive end-expiratory pressure (PEEPi). Accordingly, alveolar pressure remains positive with respect to end-expiratory pressure at the airway opening, such that a greater effort must be generated by the inspiratory muscles on the subsequent breath. This adds a threshold load to spontaneous inspiration, and in mechanically ventilated patients makes triggering of assisted breaths more difficult.[25] Determinants

of the magnitude of PEEPi include the degree of expiratory obstruction (including both patient and ventilator), elastic recoil, minute ventilation, and expiratory time (and therefore the respiratory rate, inspiratory flow rate, and inspiratory flow profile). PEEPi of about 10 cm H_2O is present in most, if not all, COPD patients with acute ventilatory failure,[26,27] and PEEPi can be measured in many ambulatory outpatients as well.[28] As discussed more fully below, counterbalancing this PEEPi with external positive end-expiratory pressure (PEEP) provides a means by which to lower the work of breathing (or the work of triggering). The impact of PEEPi on the work of breathing is illustrated in Fig. 39-2.

At the same time that the respiratory system load is elevated, the inspiratory muscles are poorly able to tolerate it. The hyperexpansion that occurs during COPD forces the inspiratory muscles to operate in a disadvantageous portion of their force-length relationship. Diaphragm strength (measured by sniff esophageal pressure) in patients with severe but stable COPD is only two-thirds that of normal individuals, virtually all of this ascribable to the diaphragm position rather than to inherent muscle weakness.[29] Still, patients presenting with ACRF may have not only worsening hyperinflation but also other conditions (e.g., protein-calorie malnutrition[30] or steroid myopathy[31]) that cause intrinsic muscle weakness. Even when patients with severe COPD are in a state of compensation, the increased load and diminished neuromuscular competence are precariously balanced. Only minor additional decrements in strength or increments in load are sufficient to precipitate inspiratory muscle fatigue and respiratory failure. It is this incremental deterioration in the balance of neuromuscular competence and respiratory system load that defines ACRF. Its many potential contributors are enumerated in Fig. 39-3.

ADDITIONAL CAUSES OF DECREASED NEUROMUSCULAR COMPETENCE

DEPRESSED DRIVE

In the usual patient who is dyspneic, tachypneic, diaphoretic, and using accessory muscles of respiration, impairment of drive is clearly not the cause of ACRF. When drive has been assessed in this setting it is greatly elevated,[32] as it is in most patients who fail to be weaned from mechanical ventilation.[33] Nevertheless, there are patients in whom new central nervous system (CNS) insults or drug effects contribute to respiratory failure. Even small doses of sedatives or narcotics may cause respiratory failure when superimposed on chronic ventilatory insufficiency; a careful history is essential to exclude this possibility. Occult hypothyroidism is not rare in the elderly, particularly in women. Thyroid function testing should be part of the routine screening of patients with ventilatory failure attributed to decreased drive.

It has been proposed that central depression of drive contributes to the terminal stages of respiratory failure, regardless of the precipitating factor. According to this "central wisdom" hypothesis, overworked respiratory muscles reach a threshold of loading at which point muscle injury results in the elaboration of inhibitory signals, which feedback to the CNS to reduce drive, thereby protecting the muscles from fatigue.[34–36] The relevance of this mechanism to respiratory failure remains to be demonstrated.

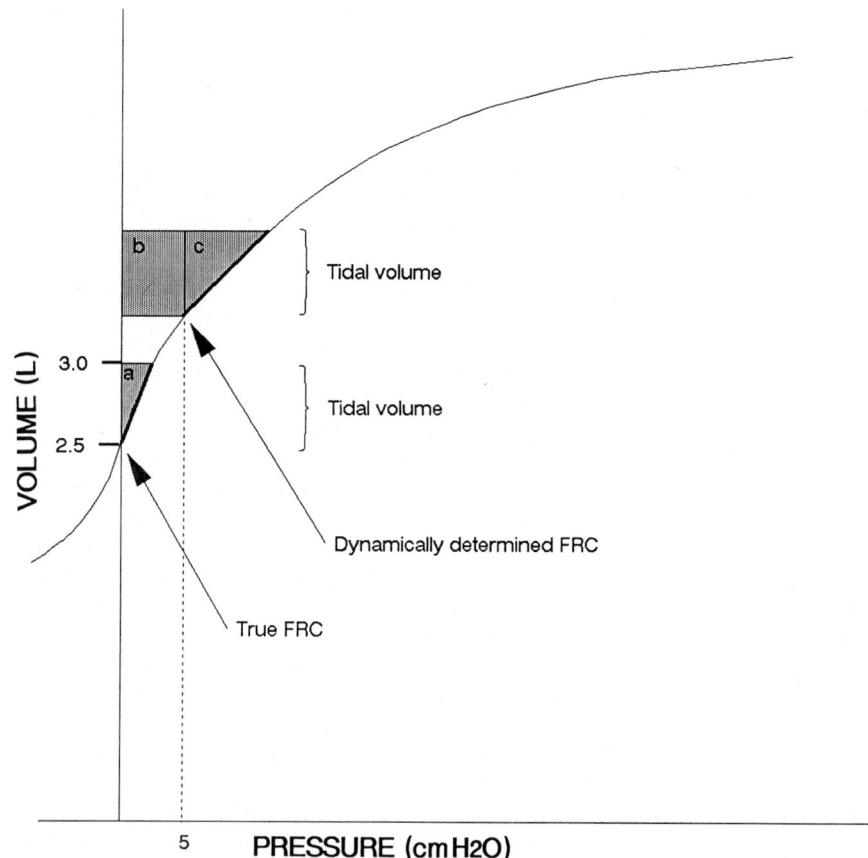

FIGURE 39-2 The effects of PEEPi on work of breathing. A volume-pressure curve for the respiratory system is shown. Under normal conditions, alveolar pressure is atmospheric at end expiration (shown as True FRC). As transpulmonary pressure is generated by the respiratory muscles, there is a tidal volume (VT) change (here from 2.5 to 3.0 L, a VT of 0.5 L). The pressure-volume product or the external work is shown by shaded area *a*. With gas trapping due to airflow obstruction, FRC can become dynamically determined. In this example, the end-expiratory pressure (PEEPi) is 5 cm H_2O, which raises the end-expired lung volume. Now, for the same VT generation, the respiratory muscles must overcome the positive alveolar pressure (PEEPi) before flow occurs, and the work of breathing is increased accordingly ($b + c$). In addition, the VT change can occur on a flatter portion of the volume-pressure curve, resulting in yet another increment in elastic load. The addition of continuous positive airway pressure (CPAP) in an amount to counterbalance the PEEPi has the ability to reduce the work of breathing from $b + c$ to *c* only.

FIGURE 39-3 The balance between the load on the respiratory system and the strength of the system determines progression to and resolution of ACRF.

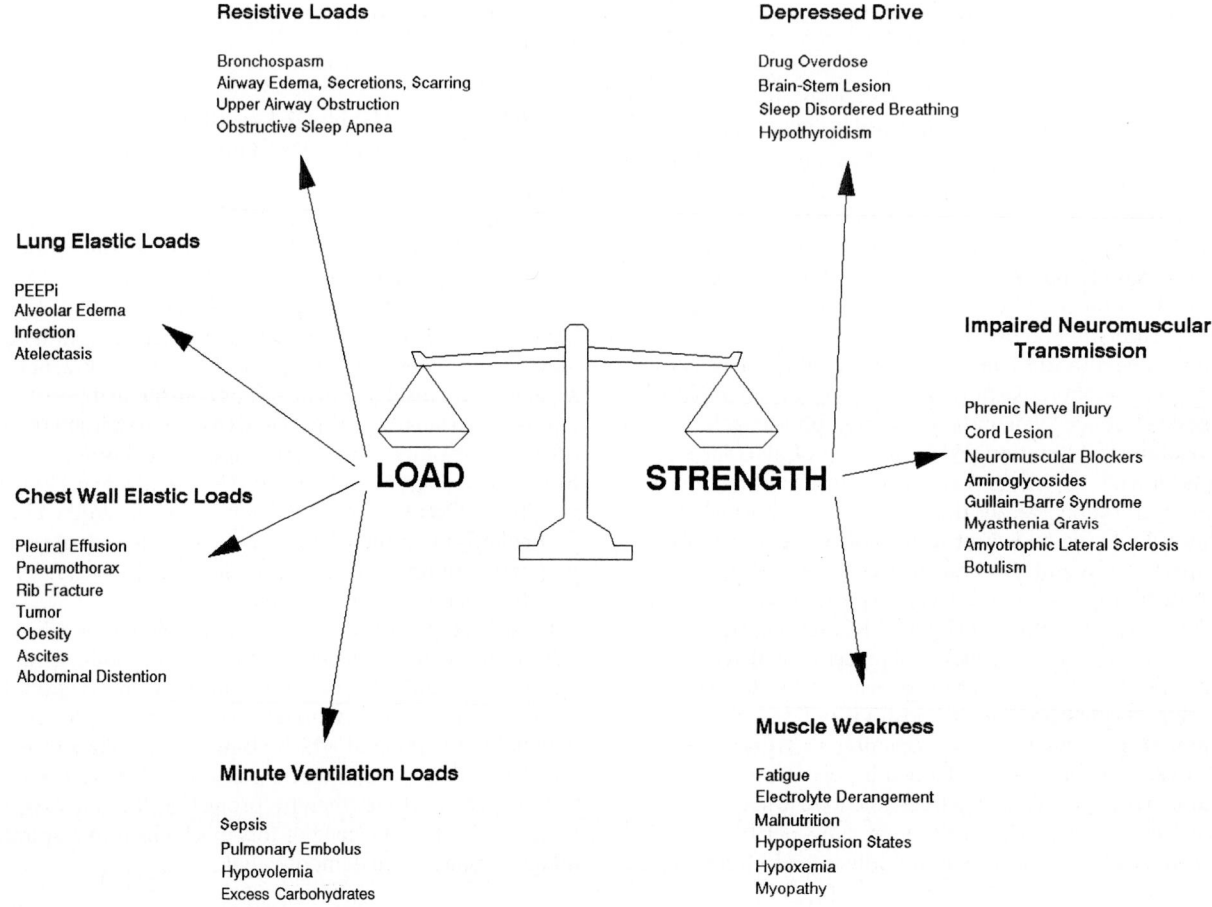

Resistive Loads

Bronchospasm
Airway Edema, Secretions, Scarring
Upper Airway Obstruction
Obstructive Sleep Apnea

Depressed Drive

Drug Overdose
Brain-Stem Lesion
Sleep Disordered Breathing
Hypothyroidism

Lung Elastic Loads

PEEPi
Alveolar Edema
Infection
Atelectasis

Impaired Neuromuscular Transmission

Phrenic Nerve Injury
Cord Lesion
Neuromuscular Blockers
Aminoglycosides
Guillain-Barre Syndrome
Myasthenia Gravis
Amyotrophic Lateral Sclerosis
Botulism

Chest Wall Elastic Loads

Pleural Effusion
Pneumothorax
Rib Fracture
Tumor
Obesity
Ascites
Abdominal Distention

Minute Ventilation Loads

Sepsis
Pulmonary Embolus
Hypovolemia
Excess Carbohydrates

Muscle Weakness

Fatigue
Electrolyte Derangement
Malnutrition
Hypoperfusion States
Hypoxemia
Myopathy

FAILED NEUROMUSCULAR TRANSMISSION

In order to effect adequate ventilation, the CNS must transmit drive to the working muscles via the spinal cord and peripheral nerves. Therefore causes of neuromuscular failure such as spinal cord lesions, primary neurologic diseases, and neuromuscular blocking drugs, may produce ACRF. Aminoglycosides[37] and procainamide[38] act as mild neuromuscular blockers, a feature unimportant in the great majority of patients, but relevant in those with neuromuscular diseases such as myasthenia gravis. The clinical setting may be a clue to one of the unusual causes, such as phrenic nerve injury following cardiopulmonary bypass. This occult lesion may be induced by direct trauma to the nerve, or more indirectly by cold cardioplegia.

MUSCLE WEAKNESS

The most important causes of decreased neuromuscular competence fall into the category of muscle weakness. In patients with COPD, respiratory muscle changes represent a balance between factors capable of impairing respiratory muscle function and metabolic adaptation of the diaphragm (Table 39-1).

Changes in chest wall geometry and diaphragm position are particularly important and adversely affect the muscles of inspiration (diaphragm and intercostal muscles) and expiration (abdominal muscles). The inspiratory muscles are poorly able to tolerate the maximal loading that occurs in emphysema. Hyperexpansion forces them to operate on a disadvantageous portion of their force-length curve. The piston-like displacement of the diaphragm is compromised and expansion of the lower thoracic cage is disturbed. In addition, a flattened diaphragm generates less transmural pressure for a given tension than the normally curved one, as described above. Electrolyte disturbances such as hypokalemia, hypophosphatemia,[39] and hypomagnesemia[40] may potentiate muscle weakness. Disturbances of the myofibrillar contractile unit have been demonstrated in humans[41] and in animal models of loaded resistive breathing that simulates ACRF. Disturbances of the sarcomere length/tension relationship, activation of proteolytic enzymes such as calpain that can degrade actin and intercellular adhesions,[42] oxidative stress, and elaboration of proinflammatory cytokines have also been proposed to play a role.[43]

Hypophosphatemia may be exacerbated by many of the drugs used to treat ventilatory failure, such as methylxanthines, β-adrenergic agonists, corticosteroids, and diuretics, accounting for its striking prevalence in COPD patients (about 20%).[44] Malnutrition, which is present in 40% to 50% of hospitalized patients with emphysema,[45] has been suggested to be associated with respiratory muscle weakness,[44] yet one study demonstrated that diaphragmatic strength was comparable between stable COPD patients with reduced body mass index (BMI; 17.3 kg/m^2) and those with normal BMI.[46] Short-term refeeding can improve indices of respiratory muscle function[30] and immune response.

Myopathy due to corticosteroids may also contribute.[31,47] Rarely, other myopathies such as an adult variant of acid maltase deficiency or mitochondrial myopathy may cause cryptic respiratory failure due to muscle weakness. Cellular and molecular adaptations of the respiratory musculature differ between the diaphragm and the intercostal muscles. The diaphragmatic myocytes adopt an "aerobic" type I phenotype with prolonged loading (see Table 39-1). By contrast the intercostal muscles undergo relatively greater glycolytic adaptation to chronic loading.[48]

TABLE 39-1 Factors Impairing Respiratory Muscle Structure/Function and Mechanisms of Chronic Adaptation In Patients at Risk for Acute-on-Chronic Respiratory Failure

Respiratory Muscle Change	Impairment	Adaptation
Thoracoabdominal geometric changes	Changes in chest wall geometry and diaphragm position resulting from hyperinflation	Structural remodeling changes in the diaphragm and accessory muscles of respiration
Respiratory muscle sarcomeric changes	Deleterious shortening of diaphragm sarcomere length disturbs intrinsic sarcomeric length-tension relationship	Transformation of myosin isoforms from fast to slow phenotype
	Disorganization of contractile myofibrils (Z-band streaming and filament misalignment)	Increase in proportion and cross-sectional area of type I fibers, and decreased type II fibers
		Increases in mitochondrial volume density and oxidative capacity
Cytosolic protein changes	Local activation of proteases (e.g., calpain) cause respiratory muscle proteolysis	New contractile protein and protease inhibitor synthesis
Oxidant/antioxidant mediator changes	Generation of reactive oxygen species from respiratory muscles and inflammatory cells overwhelm endogenous antioxidants (e.g., catalase, superoxide dismutase), resulting in respiratory muscle injury	Increased inducible antioxidant acitivity
Nutritional, pharmacologic, and aging changes	Malnutrition, steroids, and aging can impair respiratory muscles by reduction in type II muscle fibers (atrophy); glycogen, high-energy phosphate and ketone accumulation	
Inflammatory changes	Deleterious effects of infection/inflammation on skeletal muscle and systemic organ function	

SOURCE: Modified with permission from Orozco-Levi.[48]

As discussed above, muscle fatigue is the reversible loss of force generation despite adequate neural stimulation. Fatigue is itself a cause of muscle weakness and can be short-lasting (high-frequency fatigue), or long-lasting (low-frequency fatigue) which can persist for days to weeks. To the extent that fatigue is central to the development of respiratory failure, it may be caused by an inadequate supply of nutrients, excess generation of metabolites such as lactate or hydrogen ion, or depletion of muscle glycogen. Evidence to support the importance of blood supply in the genesis of fatigue comes from studies of respiratory failure in animals with hemorrhagic, cardiogenic, or septic shock.[49,50] In these animals, fatigue is hastened by circulatory insufficiency. The magnitude of blood flow to the respiratory muscles seems to be important beyond aerobic needs, as demonstrated by experiments in which flow was manipulated independently of oxygen delivery.[51] Hypoperfusion states, hypoxemia, and severe anemia have the potential to contribute to muscle fatigue and thereby hasten respiratory failure. Although fatigue is likely to contribute to the precipitation of an ACRF event, systematic evaluation has failed to demonstrate that low-frequency fatigue contributes to prolonged mechanical ventilation and failure to liberate. For example, none of 17 "weaning-failure" patients developed objective fatigue (transdiaphragmatic pressure changes with phrenic nerve stimulation), despite three quarters of patients having a diaphragmatic tension-time index (TTdi) greater than 0.15—a level associated with diaphragmatic fatigue by several other investigators.[52]

ADDITIONAL CAUSES OF INCREASED LOAD

INCREASED RESISTIVE LOAD

In patients with COPD, the respiratory system load is chronically elevated owing to abnormal airway resistance and increased elastance. The increase in airway resistance is caused by bronchospasm, airway inflammation, and physical obstruction by mucus and scarring. One common cause of increased flow resistance, and the one most amenable to pharmacologic intervention, is bronchospasm. The disease course in most patients with COPD includes an asthmatic component, and bronchial hyperreactivity to provocation may be as common in COPD as in asthma.[53] Exacerbations of bronchospasm increase resistive workload, precipitating ACRF. Superimposed heart failure may also cause increased airway resistance, mimicking asthma ("cardiac asthma"). Upper airway obstruction is much less common, but since these patients frequently have a history of prior intubation, tracheal stenosis should be considered. Finally, sleep-disordered breathing, which commonly coexists with COPD, may need to be excluded. Especially once the patient is intubated, clues to this underlying cause of dynamic upper airway obstruction (e.g., snoring) may be impossible to discern. In the proper setting (an obese, hypersomnolent patient), this possibility should be vigorously pursued. The endotracheal tube (ETT) itself presents a significant resistive workload, especially when a small size (<7.5 mm internal diameter) is chosen.[54] The angulation and length of the tube and the presence of secretions also affect flow resistance. Additionally, ventilator circuit heat and moisture exchangers (HME filters) impose significantly greater dead space and tube resistance than heated humidifiers in ventilated ACRF patients.[55] Automatic tube compensation (ATC) algorithms available on some modern ventilators are designed to maintain airway pressure by continuously calculating pressure drop across the ETT during inspiration and to decrease airway pressure during expiration to maintain constant alveolar pressure. However, ATC may be insufficient to compensate fully for the imposed resistive load of the ETT.[56]

INCREASED LUNG ELASTIC LOAD

Contributors to lung stiffness include pulmonary edema (cardiogenic and noncardiogenic), pneumonia, interstitial fibrosis or inflammation, tumor, and atelectasis. As noted above, bronchospasm not only causes increased flow resistance, but simultaneously worsens the elastic load by augmenting PEEPi.

INCREASED CHEST WALL ELASTIC LOAD

The chest wall includes the thorax, diaphragm, and abdomen. Therefore obesity, rib fracture, pneumothorax, pleural effusion, ascites, chest wall abnormalities, and abdominal distention (see Chap. 42) contribute to the work of breathing. These factors are particularly relevant in the postoperative setting.

MINUTE VENTILATION LOADS

Dividing the work of breathing into resistive and static components is a useful way of analyzing the effort of each breath. However, even if the work of each breath remains constant, an increase in respiratory rate increases the load. Increased minute ventilation ($\dot{V}E$) requirements can be divided into those due to excess carbon dioxide production ($\dot{V}_{CO2}$) and those from worsened dead space. The first category includes excessive caloric intake, fever, agitation, muscular exertion (including shivering and respiratory distress), and hypermetabolism due to injury or infection. New dead space may be caused by pulmonary embolism, hypovolemia, PEEP (including PEEPi), or shallower breathing (which raises the dead space fraction, V_{DS}/V_T). Partitioning of the lung mechanics into resistive and static components in the intubated COPD patient may be inaccurate if the end-inspiratory pause maneuver is too short and if there is a rapid spontaneous respiratory rate.[57]

MULTIFACTORIAL RESPIRATORY FAILURE

In order to analyze respiratory failure in a way that facilitates management, it is important to dissect the very complex real-life patient into simple components of deranged neuromuscular competence and load. However, the patient with ACRF due to isolated rib fracture or hypokalemia is uncommon. More often numerous contributors to both decreased strength and increased load are implicated. For example, a patient admitted with pneumonia and worsening bronchospasm may also have hypophosphatemia, heart failure, and malnutrition. Aspiration at the time of intubation, abdominal distention related to attempts to feed enterally, and overzealous parenteral nutrition complete the picture of multifactorial ACRF. Although the situation in such a patient may seem overwhelmingly complex, we caution against a "shotgun" approach to evaluation and management of patients with multifactorial respiratory failure. Despite the temptation to provide all possible interventions for these very ill patients, a systematic approach to each component of respiratory failure leads logically to a plan for treatment.

Approach to the Patient

Failure to aggressively treat mild to moderate acute exacerbations of COPD prior to the development of ACRF and other organ failure is associated with an increased risk of emergency hospitalization and delayed recovery.[58] The unequivocal role of noninvasive positive pressure mechanical ventilation (NIPPV) justifies its position as the cornerstone in the therapeutic approach to critically ill patients with ACRF (see Chap. 33). We consider NIPPV to be the "bookends" in the therapeutic library of therapy for ACRF, providing firm support on either end of an exacerbation of ACRF. This approach is discussed below, but it incorporates early initiation of NIPPV to avoid mechanical ventilation (MV) and improve survival, and later use of this tool for early liberation from MV. We describe below three phases of management of the ACRF patient: early ACRF, late ACRF requiring intubation for MV, and liberation from the ventilator.

PHASE 1: EARLY ACUTE-ON-CHRONIC RESPIRATORY FAILURE

The goals of management in the patient not yet intubated are to avoid MV whenever possible and to recognize progressive respiratory failure when it is not. The proven efficacy of NIPPV, that its use can avert mechanical ventilation in about 75% of patients with ACRF, is one of the most important developments in the management of these patients, because it buys time for the physician to treat precipitants of ACRF and for the patient to improve.

Current guidelines recommend NIPPV as definitive and first-line therapy for COPD-related ACRF.[59,60] Most centers use a face or nasal mask and pressure-support ventilation, although helmet interfaces, poncho wraps, and other ventilator modes can support NIPPV. A tight-fitting mask allows substantial ventilatory assistance yet provides for brief periods off the ventilator during which patients can speak, inhale nebulized medications, expectorate, and swallow liquids. NIPPV has been systematically evaluated in several large studies. The outcomes from these studies have been synthesized in a Cochrane meta-analysis of 14 randomized controlled studies of NIPPV versus usual medical care (UMC) that enrolled a total of 758 patients with ACRF.[61] Age ranged from 63 to 76 years, admission pH was 7.26 to 7.34, admission partial pressure of arterial carbon dioxide (Pa_{CO_2}) was 57 to 87 mm Hg, admission Pa_{O_2} was 39 to 73 mm Hg, and the FEV_1 ranged from 0.68 to 1.03 L. The eight largest studies enrolled 40 or more patients. The combined analysis demonstrated that: treatment failure was less likely with NIPPV than UMC (RR 0.48; 95% CI 0.37, 0.63) with a number needed to treat (NNT) of 5 (95% CI 4, 6), and mortality was reduced by 48% (RR for death 0.52; 95% CI 0.35, 0.76; NNT 10; 95% CI 7, 20). Notably, the mortality reduction was evident regardless of whether ACRF was treated in an ICU or in a general ward. Additionally, there was a 60% reduction in requirement for intubation with NIPPV, and rapid improvements in respiratory rate, Pa_{CO_2} and pH. Hospital length of stay (LOS) was reduced by 3.24 days, although the trend to reduced ICU LOS (4.71 fewer days) did not reach significance.[61] Interestingly, the improvement in Pa_{O_2} was heterogeneous between studies and was not significantly different at 1 hour after initiation of treatment. The finding of another meta-analysis revealed essentially similar findings for survival and clinical improvement, but subgroup analysis suggested that the benefit was limited to patients with severe but not mild ACRF. This hypothesis has not been tested in a prospective stratified fashion.[62]

NIPPV has been used for prolonged periods (more than 1 week) and has been shown to relieve symptoms, reduce respiratory rate, increase tidal volume, improve gas exchange,[63] and to lessen the amplitude of both the diaphragmatic electromyogram and the transdiaphragmatic pressure.[64] Complications of the mask have been minor and few;[61] local skin breakdown has been attributed to the tight-fitting mask, but can be avoided by applying a patch of wound care dressing. Only a few patients cannot tolerate face or nasal masks, and some of these patients respond to judicious and carefully monitored use of anxiolytics. Aspiration of gastric contents has only rarely been noted in these patients, even when a nasogastric tube is not routinely placed; however, impaired mentation probably increases this risk.

Careful patient selection is essential for successful NIPPV in ACRF and is summarized in Table 39-2.[65] Although a nasal mask is objectively as effective and well tolerated as a full face mask,[66] we typically begin therapy with a full face mask held lightly against the face. Positive pressure of 5 to 8 cm H_2O is delivered using a pressure limited mode on a noninvasive ventilator until the patient is able to tolerate the mask comfortably and synchronize with the ventilator.[67] After applying head straps, we aim to achieve an expiratory positive pressure of 2 to 5 cm H_2O (to counterbalance PEEPi) and an inspiratory positive pressure of 15 to 18 cm H_2O (equivalently, 2 to 5 cm H_2O PEEP with 13 to 16 cm H_2O pressure support) to assist alveolar ventilation. Higher pressures can sometimes be used, but they tend to be limited by air leak or mask discomfort. The PEEP component of NIPPV is important[68] and does not usually cause incremental hyperinflation.[69] Indeed, continuous positive airway pressure (CPAP) alone (without ventilatory assistance) reduces the work of breathing, improves gas exchange, leads to subjective benefit, and sometimes can avert intubation[70–72] when applied to patients with ACRF. When PEEP was added to pressure-support ventilation in ventilated patients with COPD, inspiratory effort fell another 17%, and patient-ventilator synchrony improved.[45]

TABLE 39-2 Selection Criteria for Noninvasive Positive Pressure Ventilation (NIPPV) for Acute-on-Chronic Respiratory Failure

Appropriate diagnosis with potential reversibility
Establish need for ventilatory assistance:
    Moderate to severe respiratory distress
    Tachypnea
    Use of accessory muscles or abdominal paradox
    Blood gas derangement
    pH <7.35, Pa_{CO_2} >45 mm Hg, or P_{O_2}:F_{IO_2} ratio <200
Exclude patients with contraindications to NIPPV:
    Respiratory arrest
    Medically unstable
    Unable to protect airway
    Excessive secretions
    Uncooperative or agitated
    Unable to fit mask
    Recent upper airway or gastrointestinal surgery

F_{IO_2}, fraction of inspired oxygen; Pa_{CO_2}, partial pressure of arterial carbon dioxide; P_{O_2}, oxygen pressure.
SOURCE: Reproduced with permission from Liesching et al.[65]

NIPPV is not uniformly successful in patients with ACRF.[73] Essential to successful patient-NIPPV synchrony are trigger settings for inspiration, pressurization rates (rapid pressurization reduces diaphragm work but results in increased leakage), and inspiratory-to-expiratory cycling (mask leaks can result in delayed cycling). These aspects are reviewed in detail in Chap. 33. A salutary response is typically evident within 10 minutes of beginning NIPPV, as indicated by a falling respiratory rate and heart rate as well as by the patient's subjective assessment. Occasional patients feel claustrophobic and may show objective worsening with NIPPV. Although we occasionally use pharmacologic anxiolytic therapy with success, this course has obvious attendant risks and should only be undertaken with appropriate safeguards.

A risk of NIPPV that is not often discussed is its potential to lull the physician-nurse-respiratory therapist team into a sense of comfort while the patient continues to worsen. In these patients, time spent trying NIPPV may potentially lead to a later, more urgent intubation in a more exhausted patient with significantly greater tissue hypoxia.

Avoiding intubation and conventional mechanical ventilation nearly always depends on discerning the cause of ACRF and reversing it. Thus while NIPPV is initiated, each of the potential causes enumerated in Fig. 39-3 should be reviewed in light of the clinical presentation. On occasion, impending respiratory failure can be averted by a specific intervention targeted to one precipitant, such as rib fracture (intercostal nerve block) or pulmonary edema (diuresis or afterload reduction). More often, several contributors are identified, such as worsened bronchospasm, electrolyte derangement, and infection, and treatment must be broad-based. The treatments of many of these precipitants are discussed elsewhere in this text; here, the use of oxygen and drugs will be discussed.

OXYGEN

One of the most pervasive myths surrounding the treatment of ACRF is that these patients rely on hypoxic drive to breathe. Physicians are often hesitant to supply oxygen, fearing that patients will stop breathing, necessitating intubation. Since these patients are typically hypoxemic on presentation (P_{O_2} is usually about 30 to 40 mm Hg), failure to supply adequate oxygen is a potentially devastating treatment error. Unrelieved hypoxemia in the face of acidemia, fatiguing respiratory muscles, and an often failing right ventricle risks arrhythmia, myocardial infarction, cerebral injury, renal failure, and respiratory arrest.

In several studies performed over the past decade, patients with COPD have been convincingly shown to nearly maintain $\dot{V}_E$ despite treatment with even 100% oxygen,[74,75] and to augment their drive in response to hypercarbia.[76] When oxygen is given, the P_{CO_2} typically rises, but this effect is attributed largely to worsened matching of ventilation and perfusion and the Haldane effect, not to hypoventilation. In one series, patients with ACRF had a mean initial P_{O_2} of 38 mm Hg and P_{CO_2} of 65 mm Hg.[17] They were then placed on 100% oxygen, which caused a rise in the mean P_{O_2} to 225 mm Hg, while the mean P_{CO_2} plateaued at 88 mm Hg. $\dot{V}_E$ fell by a small amount, and drive remained supranormal. Three further studies have confirmed that worsened respiratory acidosis is modest and manageable in ACRF patients receiving O_2 therapy titrated to a functional oxygen saturation (Sp_{O_2})

of 90%.[77–79] Our point is not to claim that hypoxic drive in patients with ACRF does not exist—it clearly does[80]—but to emphasize that oxygen should nevertheless be given. High concentrations of inspired oxygen are not usually necessary in ACRF, unless pneumonia or pulmonary edema is present, since hypoxemia is due largely to ventilation-perfusion ($\dot{V}/\dot{Q}$) mismatching, not to shunting. Nevertheless, we believe that the risks of oxygen therapy have been greatly overstated,[81] often leading physicians to withhold a potentially life-saving therapy. The goal of oxygen therapy is to maintain 90% saturation of an adequate amount of circulating hemoglobin. This goal can usually be attained with a face mask at 30% to 35% or a nasal cannula at 3 to 5 L/min. A rise in P_{CO_2} is likely, but that in itself is of little importance. Patients may progress to respiratory failure despite oxygen therapy, but not because of it. For this reason, careful serial assessments by the ICU team of the physician, nurse, and respiratory therapist are essential.

PHARMACOTHERAPY

Bronchodilators are an essential part of the early management of these patients (Table 39-3). While much of the airflow obstruction of COPD is irreversible, most patients have some reversible component.[82,83] In stable COPD, combinations of a β-agonist and ipratropium have been demonstrated to be superior to either drug alone.[84] However, in a meta-analysis of four randomized studies, combination therapy for acute exacerbations of COPD does not result in greater short-term bronchodilation compared with either albuterol or ipratropium alone.[85] Despite these data, current practice continues to support combination therapy if airflow obstruction persists despite maximal doses of β-agonists or if treatment-limiting tachycardia is experienced. Respiratory stimulants would be predicted not to work in this setting, since drive is already supranormal. Indeed, doxapram and similar drugs are now rarely used since their toxicity is substantial and their efficacy minimal,[86,87] particularly when compared with NIPPV.[88] We believe there is no role for these drugs. Similarly there is no evidence to support routine use of mucolytic agents or chest percussion.

TABLE 39-3 Bronchodilator Therapy in Acute-on-Chronic Respiratory Failure

β-Agonists
  Albuterol or metaproterenol by MDI (three to six puffs every
  30 to 60 min)
  or
  Albuterol or metaproterenol by nebulizer (0.5 mL albuterol or
  0.3 mL metaproterenol in 2.5 mL normal saline solution every
  2 h)
Ipratropium
  Three to ten puffs every 2 to 6 h by MDI
  Consider high doses (400 μg every 2 to 6 h) in intubated patients
Aminophylline
  Loading dose is 5 mg/kg
  Maintenance dose is approximately 0.5 mg/(kg·h)
  Must be titrated against serum levels
Corticosteroids
  Methylprednisolone, 0.5 to 1 mg/kg every 6 h
  Assess ongoing need after 72 h

MDI, metered-dose inhaler.

Beta-Agonists

Inhaled β_2-selective agents (albuterol, bitolterol, terbutaline, or metaproterenol) should be given by metered-dose inhaler (MDI), unless patient distress makes that impractical, since this route seems to be equally efficacious in nonventilated patients.[5] Administration may be facilitated by the use of a chamber device. Higher doses than usual can be given, such as 4 to 10 (or more) puffs every 20 to 60 minutes, although there is no clear benefit from frequent doses. A hand-held nebulizer (0.5 mL albuterol or 0.3 mL metaproterenol mixed with 2.5 mL saline solution) may be useful in patients who cannot use an MDI reliably, but otherwise this route confers no additional efficacy. Parenteral agents (e.g., epinephrine 0.3 mL subcutaneously) and their accompanying toxicity can nearly always be avoided. The longer-acting β_2-agonist formoterol (but not salmeterol) has a fast onset of action and has been demonstrated to provide equally effective bronchodilation in mild COPD exacerbations when administered in high doses.[89] However, because of concerns about activity as a partial receptor antagonist, significant additional cost, and therapeutic equivalence, we do not recommend long-acting inhaled β_2-agonist agonists for ACRF.

Ipratropium

The anticholinergic agent ipratropium bromide is as effective as metaproterenol in the treatment of ACRF,[85,90] and may even be better in stable COPD. An additional advantage of this drug is that compared to metaproterenol, its use is associated with a small rise in Pa_{O_2} rather than the small decline usually seen with β-agonists. The addition of ipratropium to a regimen containing inhaled β-agonists yields incremental benefit in patients with stable COPD,[84] but as discussed above, does not result in improved bronchodilation in acute exacerbations. The usual dose of ipratropium in ACRF is three puffs every 30 to 60 minutes. Much higher doses (400 μg) have been shown to be optimal in stable patients with COPD, but this question has not been examined in ACRF.[91]

Tiotropium

Tiotropium, a recently released long-acting inhaled anticholinergic, has demonstrated great promise in patients with stable COPD by reducing symptoms, the decline in FEV_1, and frequency of exacerbations. Preliminary evidence of its potential efficacy in patients with acute exacerbations was suggested by a randomized prospective study conducted by a Veterans Administration collaborative involving 1829 men with severe COPD (FEV_1 1 L, 36% predicted) at risk for exacerbations.[92] Significantly fewer patients treated with once-daily tiotropium experienced exacerbations (27.9% vs. 32.3%; $p = 0.037$) that were associated with 26% fewer hospital days ($p = 0.001$). To date, however, there is no published experience with tiotropium as a specific therapy for ACRF.

Phosphodiesterase Inhibitors

AMINOPHYLLINE   Aminophylline is a mildly effective nonselective phosphodiesterase (PDE) inhibitor in patients with COPD. In addition to its actions as a bronchodilator, aminophylline has salutary effects on the diaphragm in experimental settings. These include inotropy and resistance to fatigue seen in patients on this agent, although the clinical relevance of these findings has yet to be demonstrated, and recent studies have challenged the underpinnings of these clinical trials.[93] Whether aminophylline should be given to patients with ACRF is controversial, and recent trends show it falling out of favor. A controlled trial in patients hospitalized for an acute exacerbation of COPD failed to show any benefit of aminophylline when added to a standard regimen of β-agonists and corticosteroids.[94] On the other hand, theophylline causes demonstrable (although generally minor) physiologic improvement in stable COPD patients, even when superimposed on a regimen of a β-agonist[83] or on a combination of a high-dose inhaled β-agonist plus ipratropium.[95] Meta-analysis of four randomized controlled trials including 169 patients demonstrated no improvement in bronchodilation or hospital LOS in patients with acute exacerbations. However, not all patients had severe ACRF.[96] Toxicity of these drugs is substantial, including arrhythmogenesis and CNS effects. In the meta-analysis, there were fivefold greater odds of gastrointestinal symptoms occurring in theophylline-treated patients.[96] Daily serum level measurement is necessary for safe use, especially in light of the significant interactions with other drugs. Even when serum levels are considered to be therapeutic, aminophylline may have important toxicity. In a multivariate analysis of 100 patients receiving theophylline, drug level was the most important predictor of arrhythmia,[97] ahead of age and gender. Both atrial and ventricular arrhythmias were seen and correlated with theophylline level. In the group with therapeutic levels 48% had arrhythmias. Particularly worrisome was the finding of multifocal atrial tachycardia in patients on theophylline, including those with nontoxic levels. Two of six patients with this rhythm disturbance died suddenly during hospitalization, without antecedent ventricular ectopy.

Consistent with guidelines from expert panels,[59,98] we rarely use intravenous aminophylline, and then only as an adjunct to other, more effective management (standard bronchodilators and steroids). Aminophylline is initiated as a loading dose of 5 mg/kg infused over 30 minutes, then continued as an intravenous infusion at a rate of 0.5 mg/kg per hour. In patients who are already taking an oral methylxanthine, intravenous loading and maintenance dosing should be guided by serum levels. Given the minor efficacy of the drug and its substantial toxicity, it is difficult to justify empirical partial loading doses.

Selective Phosphodiesterase Inhibitors

Selective inhibitors of type IV PDE (such as cilomilast) are likely to have a major impact on the management of patients with stable COPD with recent studies (unpublished at the time of this writing) demonstrating modest improvements in lung function compared to placebo and a significant reduction in acute exacerbations. However, as for many newer therapies, PDE-IV inhibitors have not been evaluated in the treatment of COPD exacerbations. Additionally, a single dose of cilomilast appears to confer no additional bronchodilatory effect in stable COPD patients who respond to albuterol or ipratropium.[82]

Corticosteroids

Patients with ACRF given methylprednisolone 0.5 mg/kg every 6 hours, in addition to standard bronchodilators, show greater improvement in spirometric values than patients who do not receive this drug.[99] This benefit is demonstrable at least as early as 12 hours, and in some studies of patients with asthma possibly after 1 hour. In another study of patients with ACRF, 0.8 mg/kg of prednisolone given intravenously reduced the inspiratory resistance and PEEPi when measured at 90 minutes.[100] A meta-analysis that included 537 patients in 7 randomized controlled studies yielded an aggregate beneficial effect of steroid treatment that translated into an early FEV_1 improvement of 120 mL (95% CI; 5 mL to 190 mL) compared with controls, an effect that persisted for 3 to 5 days.[101] Although there was no survival benefit derived from the addition of steroids, treatment failure and hospital LOS were significantly reduced. Although there is significant debate about the optimal dose and duration of steroids,[5] current guidelines recommend methylprednisolone 0.5 to 1 mg/kg every 6 hours. Since these drugs have important detrimental effects on metabolic, muscular, and immune function, their continued use should be re-evaluated after the first 72 hours with a transition to oral therapy when tolerated. Although no effect of corticosteroids on respiratory muscle function can be shown in the short term (<2 weeks[102]), they do contribute to muscle weakness in the long term.[31] No additional benefit is derived from prolonging steroid therapy beyond 2 weeks. A possible alternative may be to use high doses of the nebulized steroid budesonide (2 mg every 6 hours), which may be as effective as an oral steroid regimen in patients with a COPD exacerbation.[103] Notably, hyperglycemia was less common in the budesonide-treated patients. However, this approach is significantly more expensive.

Antibiotics
Bacterial bronchitis is a common precipitant of ACRF. Nevertheless the efficacy of antibiotics is controversial. Since benefit has been demonstrated in several studies and a trend towards benefit in some others,[5] an inexpensive oral broad-spectrum antibiotic (e.g., ampicillin, doxycycline, or trimethoprim-sulfamethoxazole) should be provided in the absence of clinical features of pneumonia. Community-acquired pneumonia should be treated with a cephalosporin-macrolide combination or a high-dose single-agent fluoroquinolone.

Anabolic Steroids
Inflammation is not limited to the lungs during an acute exacerbation of COPD. Peripheral and diaphragmatic skeletal muscle weakness is pronounced during ACRF and is associated with markers of systemic inflammation such interleukin-6 and interleukin-8.[104] A combination of anabolic steroids (nandrolone decanoate 25 to 50 mg IM every 2 weeks) and caloric supplementation (420 kcal/d supplement) raised the mouth pressure during a maximal static inspiratory maneuver in patients with clinically stable COPD.[105] Similarly, COPD patients treated with oxandrolone experienced a significant increase in lean body mass.[106] However, this effect may only be clinically useful in patients receiving long-term oral steroids.[107] We are aware of no trials showing clinically important benefits in patients with ACRF.

ARRHYTHMIAS
Arrhythmias are common in the setting of respiratory failure. Fortunately, they are rarely a serious problem, but they can serve to distract the physician from more important issues, may limit the dose of bronchodilating drugs, and sometimes are significant in themselves. The most common rhythms are sinus tachycardia, atrial fibrillation, atrial flutter, multifocal atrial tachycardia, and ventricular premature beats. β-Agonists, macrolides, and electrolyte disturbances can cause transmural dispersion of repolarization abnormalities such as QT prolongation, T-wave alternans, and P-wave dispersion as precursors to serious arrhythmias. It can be difficult to judge the contributions of hypoxemia, cor pulmonale, metabolic derangements, underlying coronary artery disease, and drug toxicity to arrhythmogenesis. Treatment should focus on rectifying the underlying respiratory failure, since doing so usually has a beneficial impact on arrhythmias. Hypoxemia and electrolyte abnormalities should be corrected as a first priority. Monitoring should be initiated, and if arrhythmias continue despite correction of apparent exacerbating factors, myocardial ischemia should be excluded. Atrial fibrillation can be controlled with a calcium channel blocker or digoxin (see Chap. 24). β-Blockers should generally be avoided for fear of worsening lung function, although short-acting selective drugs have occasionally been used with success. Multifocal atrial tachycardia often responds to verapamil, sometimes with restoration of sinus rhythm,[108] and there appears to be a role for parenteral magnesium as well (see Chap. 24).

RECOGNIZING IMPENDING RESPIRATORY FAILURE
Despite aggressive attempts to find and reverse the causes of ACRF, some patients will progress to frank respiratory failure. The decision to intubate requires clinical judgment and is best assessed by a physician present at the bedside (Table 39-4). Assessment of respiratory failure based solely on results of arterial blood gas studies is fraught with error. Certainly a rising Pa_{CO_2} in a patient with progressively worsening symptoms and signs of distress should be interpreted as heralding respiratory arrest. However, the absolute level of the Pa_{CO_2}, isolated from other clinical data, may be less useful. We have taken care of a small number of patients in whom the Pa_{CO_2} rose to 150 mm Hg while the patients were alert and conversing, and mechanical ventilation did not become necessary. On the other hand, many patients with ACRF will progress to respiratory arrest long before progressive hypercarbia is clearly documented. Patients who have had an unsuccessful attempt at stabilization with NIPPV are at particular risk for underappreciated clinical instability. Those patients may have very little tissue oxygen reserve, low effective circulating volume, and are at substantial risk of cardiopulmonary arrest if transition to intubation is delayed. Respiratory arrest may be complicated

---

TABLE 39-4 Assessment of the Need for Intubation in Acute-on-Chronic Respiratory Failure

1. This judgment must be made by the physician at the bedside.
2. Predictors of frank ventilatory failure:
   Respiratory rates that remain >36/min despite NIPPV
   Worsening tachycardia
   Continued use of all accessory muscles
   Mental status deterioration
   Patient's subjective sense of exhaustion
3. Arterial blood gas studies are of limited use in making this judgment, usually merely confirming clinical assessment.
4. Concomitant hemodynamic instability or inability to protect the airway may mandate intubation.

NIPPV, noninvasive positive pressure ventilation.

by aspiration or cardiovascular instability, compromising future efforts to return the patient to spontaneous breathing. Indeed, the survival of patients who are allowed to progress to respiratory arrest is significantly lower than that of patients ventilated for acute deterioration of COPD who are intubated electively prior to arrest. The goal at this stage of management is to intubate the patient electively once mechanical ventilation becomes unavoidable. In some cases this will require foregoing NIPPV and opting for immediate airway intubation for mechanical ventilation to avoid respiratory arrest.

Useful bedside parameters of impending respiratory arrest include respiratory rate, mentation, pattern of breathing, and the patient's own assessment. The patient may be able to tell the physician whether improvement is occurring or not; the degree of dyspnea over time is a useful guide to the likelihood of success without intubation. Most patients with ACRF are tachypneic, reflecting their excessive drive. A rate that remains above 35 to 40 breaths/min, or a rate that continues to rise despite therapy and NIPPV is predictive of respiratory failure. Deterioration of mentation commonly precedes respiratory arrest. Patients become confused, less able to converse, then poorly rousable. Thoracoabdominal paradox and respiratory alternans are rarely seen and are probably not useful signs.

PHASE 2: LATE ACUTE-ON-CHRONIC RESPIRATORY FAILURE REQUIRING INTUBATION

This phase consists of the immediate peri-intubation management and the first few days of mechanical ventilation. In many respects, treatment begun in the preintubation phase (bronchodilator administration in particular) is continued, but several additional concerns become relevant. Care consists of stabilizing the patient on the ventilator, ensuring rest of the patient and respiratory muscles, improving neuromuscular competence, reducing load, and giving prophylaxis against complications, while optimizing definitive therapy for any precipitant such as infection. Optimal treatment at this time is likely to facilitate eventual liberation from mechanical ventilation.

PERI-INTUBATION RISKS

There are two common pitfalls in the immediate postintubation period: life-threatening alkalosis and hypotension. Both are related to overzealous ventilation, and both are avoidable by taking the patient's own ventilatory pattern prior to intubation into consideration. Hypotension is a consequence of escalating PEEPi following intubation. The degree of dynamic hyperinflation is proportional to $\dot{V}_E$. PEEPi has the same deleterious consequences on venous return as externally applied PEEP and can cause serious hypoperfusion. This can be particularly prominent in patients with ineffective circulating volumes (preload) and concomitant right heart dysfunction when vasodilatory and sympatholytic sedatives are used for intubation. The key to avoiding this pitfall is to prevent excessive ventilation, particularly during bag-valve-mask preoxygenation before intubation attempts. When hypotension occurs, the circulation can usually be promptly restored by simply ceasing ventilation for 30 seconds, then reinstituting ventilation along with measures to reduce PEEPi and restore circulating volume. It is also our practice in patients without

decompensated left heart failure to administer a fluid bolus immediately prior to sedation for intubation.

Most patients with ACRF have a minute ventilation of 10 L/min or less and breathe at tidal volumes of about 300 mL. Physicians commonly choose ventilator settings with a higher tidal volume and a correspondingly lower ratio of dead space to tidal volume. In addition, a minute ventilation higher than 10 L/min often is employed, particularly during the first few minutes of manual-assisted ventilation. Finally, as the work of breathing is assumed by the ventilator, $\dot{V}_{CO_2}$ drops by as much as 20%. All of these factors join to dramatically lower the patient's Pa_{CO_2} once assisted ventilation begins. Since preexisting compensatory metabolic alkalosis is the rule, life-threatening alkalemia (pH >7.7) can easily be achieved. This scenario can be avoided by simply aiming for a more reasonable minute ventilation, approximating the patient's own pattern of breathing. Typical initial ventilator settings are described below. There is no need to attempt to normalize pH, a maneuver that merely serves to waste the bicarbonate that has been so vigorously conserved during the evolution of respiratory failure.

We generally recommend head-up intubation with a large-diameter endotracheal tube, not laryngeal mask. Depolarizing muscle relaxants should be avoided and if necessary, short-acting nondepolarizing agents such as rocuronium or cisatracurium should be considered.

INITIAL VENTILATOR SETTINGS

We generally initiate ventilation using the assist-control mode, since one of the goals in this phase is to rest the loaded respiratory muscles (see Chap. 36). Tidal volumes of about 5 to 7 mL/kg are used (about 350 to 500 mL) with a respiratory rate of 20 to 24 breaths/min. As discussed above, PEEPi presents an inspiratory threshold load to the patient with ACRF. The patient must generate enough force to counterbalance PEEPi before the breathing effort results in any inspiratory flow and before it can trigger the ventilator. This difficulty cannot be sidestepped by lowering the triggering sensitivity on the ventilator or by using flow triggering. Applying external PEEP that is roughly equal to the PEEPi does reduce the work of breathing (and triggering) by a significant amount, as depicted in Fig. 39-2.[68,109] In some patients, externally applied PEEP causes additional hyperinflation, with detrimental hemodynamic effects and a potentially increased risk of barotrauma.[110,111] However, most patients with ACRF demonstrate flow limitation so that external PEEP (in amounts up to about 85% of the PEEPi) has no significant impact on the expiratory flow-volume relationship, lung volume, or hemodynamics.[112,113] Strategies to shorten ventilator inflation time are not generally helpful unless inspiratory flow is inordinately low (we typically use 60 L/min), although PEEPi can be reduced modestly.[114]

ENSURING REST AND RECOVERY

Following intubation, most patients are exhausted and will sleep for the first day and experience significant diuresis. Little or no sedation is typically necessary, although close monitoring for delirium and alcohol or substance withdrawal may be required. The respiratory muscles will require 48 to 72 hours for full recovery, so that resumption of breathing efforts before that point is counterproductive and is likely to lead to recurrence of respiratory muscle fatigue.[115] However, as discussed below this does not preclude extubation to NIPPV if there is convincing evidence that extrapulmonary organ dysfunction has stabilized and cognitive function has improved. We continue to encourage rest by maintaining ventilation, adding sedation and antidelirium agents when necessary. Rest can be achieved using any mode of ventilation, including bilevel NIPPV, as long as settings are chosen that minimize patient effort. It is important to emphasize that having the patient connected to a ventilator is no guarantee that the patient is relieved of the work of breathing. Even when the ventilator is set at a very sensitive trigger point, the presence of PEEPi causes the patient to have to make a substantial inspiratory effort to get a breath, even on volume assist-control mode. For example, with a triggered sensitivity of 1 cm H_2O and PEEPi of 10 cm H_2O, the patient must lower his airway pressure by 11 cm H_2O to trigger a breath. It is incumbent on the physician to ensure that the patient is in fact rested. We evaluate inspiratory muscle activation, synchrony, and the presence of PEEPi by palpating the epigastric area during the respiratory cycle[116] while monitoring the pressure-time and flow-time waveforms on the mechanical ventilator. When optimal ventilatory rest is achieved, respiratory muscle strength usually improves demonstrably over the first few days.

IMPROVING NEUROMUSCULAR COMPETENCE

Each of the factors discussed in phase 1 (and shown in Fig. 39-3) that contribute to depressed neuromuscular competence should be reviewed daily in the ventilated patient. In this phase the importance of nutrition must be recognized. Malnutrition is a common comorbidity of advanced COPD[117] and may contribute to respiratory muscle dysfunction as well as to immune suppression. In a randomized trial of standard feeding versus supplementation (1000 kcal above usual), malnourished inpatients with COPD were shown to develop greater respiratory muscle endurance and strength in only 16 days when given extra calories.[30] However, excessive refeeding should be avoided since unnecessarily high levels of carbon dioxide production ($\dot{V}_{CO_2}$) may result. Harris-Benedict predictions of resting energy expenditure provide a reasonable estimate in stable COPD patients;[117] however, detailed nutritional information including indirect calorimetry may be helpful to guide nutritional management in ACRF (see Chap. 11). When caloric requirements have been assessed, it is usually advisable to supply a large fraction (50% or more) of total calories in the form of lipids, to minimize the respiratory quotient (RQ) and hence $\dot{V}_{CO_2}$. Especially with refeeding, hypophosphatemia commonly develops while the patient is in the ICU, and serum phosphate content should be assessed on a daily basis.

Once the respiratory muscles are rested, a program of exercise should be initiated in conjunction with daily evaluations of readiness for liberation from mechanical ventilation. The goal is to encourage muscle power, tone, and coordination by allowing the patient to assume nonfatiguing respirations, possibly in combination with inspiratory resistive training. This can be achieved by progressively lowering the triggered sensitivity on assist-control, lowering the inspiratory pressure on pressure-support, or through graded T-piece sprints. After a period of work, the patient is returned to full rest to facilitate sleep at night. As strength improves, the amount of exercise can be increased in stepwise fashion until the breathing can be sustained and the patient passes a trial of spontaneous breathing.

During this phase, meticulous attention should be paid to harm reduction and risk avoidance. Prevention and early recognition of venous thromboembolism, gastrointestinal stress ulceration, ventilator-associated pneumonia, integument breakdown (including nasal bridge integrity in NIPPV patients), corneal desiccation, drug side effects, drug-drug interactions, substance withdrawal, and delirium are recommended.

DECREASING LOAD

Efforts to decrease load should continue. Once the patient is ventilated, it becomes possible to apportion the load into resistive and elastic components (see Chap. 36). These determinations may provide insight into the precipitants of respiratory failure and serve to guide therapy. For example, if the resistive load and PEEPi are minimal, but the elastic load is excessive, there is little to be gained from more aggressive use of bronchodilators. Rather, the source of the elastic load (lung, chest wall, or abdomen; see Fig. 39-3) should be determined and corrected.

It is important to continue treatment with bronchodilators, but whether MDIs and nebulizers are equally effective is controversial.[60,118] On the one hand, in a study of drug deposition in ventilated patients, a MDI (plus a holding chamber) was more efficient than a nebulizer.[119] In another trial of ventilated patients, MDIs were completely ineffective, despite a cumulative dose in 1 hour of 100 puffs.[120] The magnitude and duration of effectiveness of medications given via an MDI and a nebulizer appear to be similar.[118] There may be substantial differences related to the method of administration or to the specific equipment used to deliver the drug. We recommend that these drugs be given to effect, whether by MDI or nebulizer. If MDIs are used, the usual number of puffs should be doubled as a starting point to compensate for the reduced delivery of drug to the patient, and the dose increased as needed until bronchodilation is achieved (as assessed by determining respiratory mechanics).

Other contributors to increased load, such as congestive heart failure, pulmonary embolization, and respiratory infection, may be easier to discern once the patient is mechanically ventilated, and they should be sought during this phase. Congestive heart failure can usually be excluded by the physical examination and chest radiograph, although pulmonary edema may have an atypical appearance in patients with advanced emphysema. Only occasionally is the additional information from pulmonary artery catheterization useful. Pulmonary embolism (PE) is much more difficult to exclude. The incidence of PE as a precipitant of ACRF is unknown. The reported frequency of deep venous thrombosis ranges from 9% to 45%.[17,121] Large pulmonary emboli are much less common, although the incidence of smaller emboli may not be. Nevertheless, PE is commonly found at autopsy. In patients with ACRF, pulmonary hypertension is virtually universal and diagnosis of PE is difficult. Ventilation-perfusion lung scanning nearly always gives abnormal results, and computed tomographic angiography has been incompletely evaluated in patients with underlying structural lung disease (see Chap. 27). Noninvasive leg studies have been challenged in this setting as well. Capnography has been suggested as a method for excluding PE in patients with ACRF.[122]

PHASE 3: LIBERATION FROM THE VENTILATOR

The fundamental principle that guides management in this phase is that successful liberation from the ventilator requires that the premorbid compensated relationship between neuromuscular competence and load be re-established. Therefore a strategy for successfully discontinuing mechanical ventilation emphasizes increasing the strength and decreasing the load, while avoiding sedatives that may impair drive. We use a nurse- or respiratory therapist–led protocol that emphasizes daily testing of readiness for spontaneous breathing, targeted sedation strategies with daily sedation withdrawal, formal spontaneous breathing trials, and triggers for liberation including early extubation to NIPPV as discussed below and reviewed in further detail in Chap. 44. This approach has been demonstrated to be particularly effective in achieving successful ventilator liberation.[123] However, similar results may be achieved in well-staffed, well-organized closed-management ICUs where decisions to liberate are directed by expert intensivists.[124] Therapy may be highly focused, by measures such as repleting inorganic phosphate, relieving a pneumothorax, addressing neuropsychiatric components including delirium, or managing right heart syndrome. More often a broad assault on many potential precipitants, namely bronchospasm, infection, electrolyte derangement, and fatigue, is used. In either case, when load has been reduced and neuromuscular competence promoted, the patient will be able to breathe free of assistance. On the other hand, if a compensated balance of strength and load cannot be restored, attempts at spontaneous breathing will be futile. A corollary is that the specifics of ventilator management, such as the mode chosen or the device used, are less important.[125,126] Only the patient's improving physiology determines the ability to maintain ventilation as determined by the patient's ability to tolerate short periods of unassisted breathing (spontaneous breathing trial). This point has been confirmed by recent trials of weaning methods, which have shown that frequent T-piece trials are superior to intermittent mandatory ventilation (and in some cases, also to pressure-support ventilation), probably because they more readily demonstrate to the physician that the ventilator is no longer necessary.[123,126–128] This issue is more fully elaborated in Chap. 44.

Respiratory parameters (negative inspiratory force [NIF], peak pressure [Ppk], plateau pressure [Pplat], and PEEPi; see Chaps. 32 and 36) have historically been used to evaluate the progress of the patient and resolution of the load-strength imbalance. However, the poor individual performance characteristics of these maneuvers make them unreliable for predicting sustained spontaneous breathing and successful liberation.[129] However, by daily integrating respiratory parameters of load-strength balance with other validated parameters such as the frequency:tidal volume ratio, the readiness for a spontaneous breathing trial can be determined. Additionally, the impact of therapeutic maneuvers can be assessed by serially evaluating respiratory parameters. For example, while PEEPi remains at 10 cm H_2O, there is little point in trying to make the patient breathe without assistance. Indeed, in such a circumstance efforts should be directed to attempting to reduce the work of breathing.[130] On the other hand, when PEEPi has resolved and strength is adequate (usually when the NIF >30 cm H_2O), mechanical ventilation is no longer necessary and the patient should be able to tolerate at least 30 minutes of spontaneous minimally-assisted breathing.

When discontinuation of mechanical ventilation is imminent, it is useful to anticipate the respiratory pattern that the patient will soon assume. We have been impressed that patients ventilated at supraphysiologic tidal volumes, such as 800 to 1000 mL, experience respiratory distress and agitation when they resume their usual pattern of 30 breaths/min at a tidal volume of 300 mL. By choosing a pattern of mechanical ventilation that more closely approximates spontaneous respiration (e.g., assist-control mode, tidal volume of 420 mL, and a rate of 20 breaths/minute), the transition from the ventilator is smoothed.

For patients that fail to re-establish load-strength balance within 72 hours of initiating therapy, there is a significant prospect of prolonged mechanical ventilation, tracheostomy, and complications that increase the attributable morbidity and mortality. A significant shift in approach involves elective extubation to NIPPV for patients who consistently fail spontaneous breathing trials after 48 to 72 hours. In a randomized controlled trial of NIPPV versus continued intubation and ventilation in 50 ACRF patients failing a T-piece trial at 24 to 36 hours of initial ventilation via an endotracheal tube, NIPPV reduced the period of mechanical ventilation (16.6 ± 11.8 days vs. 10.2 ± 6.8 days; $p = 0.021$), ICU days (24.0 ± 13.7 days vs. 15.1 ± 5.4 days; $p = 0.005$), the incidence of nosocomial pneumonia, and mortality at 60 days (8% NIPPV vs. 28% of those on invasive ventilation; $p = 0.009$), while increasing approximately fourfold the number of patients liberated from ventilation at day 21.[131] These findings have been confirmed by others randomizing patients (75% of whom had ACRF) after three failed daily T-piece trials.[132] In a meta-analysis of five studies involving 171 patients, extubation to NIPPV translated into an aggregate relative risk reduction of 0.41 [95% CI 0.22 to 0.76].[133] NIPPV is likely to tide the patient over the additional days until the balance of neuromuscular competence and respiratory system load is re-established.

Even with appropriate institution of rest on the ventilator, rapid application of the algorithms given above or correction of abnormalities of neuromuscular competence and load, and progressive exercise of the patient, some patients require protracted periods of ventilator support. Indeed, with the wider use of NIPPV and the avoidance of intubation in all but the most severely impaired patients, it may be the case that in the future ICUs will encounter truly difficult-to-wean patients. The principles elaborated above still apply to this group, with a few additional comments. After approximately 7 days of ventilator dependence, we typically assess the patient for tracheostomy (see Chap. 35). If it appears that liberation from mechanical ventilation may succeed within another week, tracheostomy is usually not performed, and efforts continue to extubate the patient. If we judge that the course will be protracted, we prefer bedside percutaneous tracheostomy for purposes of patient comfort, communication, and avoidance of complications associated with translaryngeal intubation. If progress to liberation is likely to be very slow after the first couple of weeks, many ICUs will consider transferring the stable patient to a long-term acute care facility with dedicated expertise in pulmonary rehabilitation and liberation from mechanical ventilation. Despite the overall poor prognosis for such compromised patients, these facilities have demonstrated superior expertise in liberating a significant proportion even after long periods of ventilation for ACRF.[134] Optimal results are achieved when a protocolized multidisciplinary care pathway involves specialist respiratory care, rehabilitation, nutrition, and physical therapy departments.

Following extubation, careful serial assessments are in order. Deterioration in the hours just following extubation suggests upper airway edema. In the uncomplicated patient, the respiratory rate falls slightly through the first day, most often into the mid-twenties to low thirties. Efforts to build strength and reduce load should continue in order to protect the gains that have been made. Once the patient is stable off the ventilator, a prompt transfer to the more benign setting of the general ward should be encouraged.

Recurrence of respiratory failure is an ominous but not infrequent complication for which efforts to stave off intubation may prove fruitless and potentially harmful. When 221 patients with recurrent respiratory failure within 48 hours of initial ventilator liberation (only 12% had COPD) were randomized to either NIPPV or usual care, equal numbers progressed to intubation (48%), but the ICU mortality rate at an interim analysis was 25% in the NIPPV vs. 14% in the usual care arm (RR 1.78; 95% CI 1.03 to 3.20; $p = 0.048$).[135]

For many patients, liberation from prolonged mechanical ventilation is associated with a decision to change the goals of care from "treatment-for-cure" to "treatment-for-comfort." Decisions to withhold and withdraw life-sustaining therapy entail extensive involvement of the patient, as well as their care providers, ICU staff, chaplaincy, hospital ethics, and social work support. Pertinent to the terminal care of the ACRF patient are meticulous attention to palliation of terminal dyspnea, pain, and delirium. This subject is covered in Chap. 17.

References

1. Mannino DM, Homa DM, Akinbami LJ, et al: Chronic obstructive pulmonary disease surveillance—United States, 1971–2000. *Morb Mortal Wkly Rep Surveill Summ* 51:1, 2002.
2. Mannino DM, Buist AS, Petty TL, et al: Lung function and mortality in the United States: data from the First National Health and Nutrition Examination Survey follow up study. *Thorax* 58:388, 2003.
3. Connors AF Jr., Dawson NV, Thomas C, et al: Outcomes following acute exacerbation of severe chronic obstructive lung disease. The SUPPORT investigators (Study to Understand Prognoses and Preferences for Outcomes and Risks of Treatments). *Am J Respir Crit Care Med* 154:959, 1996.
4. Rodriguez-Roisin R: Toward a consensus definition for COPD exacerbations. *Chest* 117(5 Suppl 2):398S, 2000.
5. McCrory DC, Brown C, Gelfand SE, Bach PB: Management of acute exacerbations of COPD: a summary and appraisal of published evidence. *Chest* 119:1190, 2001.
6. Asad N, Johnson VM, Spodick DH: Acute right atrial strain: regression in normal as well as abnormal P-wave amplitudes with treatment of obstructive pulmonary disease. *Chest* 124:560, 2003.
7. Afessa B, Morales IJ, Scanlon PD, Peters SG: Prognostic factors, clinical course, and hospital outcome of patients with chronic obstructive pulmonary disease admitted to an intensive care unit for acute respiratory failure. *Crit Care Med* 30:1610, 2002.
8. Breen D, Churches T, Hawker F, Torzillo PJ: Acute respiratory failure secondary to chronic obstructive pulmonary disease treated in the intensive care unit: a long term follow up study. *Thorax* 57:29, 2002.
9. Sukumalchantra Y, Dinakara P, Williams MH Jr.: Prognosis of patients with chronic obstructive pulmonary disease after hospitalization for acute ventilatory failure: a three-year follow-up study. *Am Rev Respir Dis* 93:215, 1966.
10. Nevins ML, Epstein SK: Predictors of outcome for patients with COPD requiring invasive mechanical ventilation. *Chest* 119:1840, 2001.
11. Menzies R, Gibbons W, Goldberg P: Determinants of weaning and survival among patients with COPD who require mechanical ventilation for acute respiratory failure. *Chest* 95:398, 1989.
12. Ely EW, Baker AM, Evans GW, Haponik EF: The distribution of costs of care in mechanically ventilated patients with chronic obstructive pulmonary disease. *Crit Care Med* 28:408, 2000.
13. Claessens MT, Lynn J, Zhong Z, et al: Dying with lung cancer or chronic obstructive pulmonary disease: insights from SUPPORT. Study to Understand Prognoses and Preferences for Outcomes and Risks of Treatments. *J Am Geriatr Soc* 48(5 Suppl):S146, 2000.
14. Grassino A, Macklem PT: Respiratory muscle fatigue and ventilatory failure. *Annu Rev Med* 35:625, 1984.
15. Sanders MH, Newman AB, Haggerty CL, et al: Sleep and sleep-disordered breathing in adults with predominantly mild obstructive airway disease. *Am J Respir Crit Care Med* 167:7, 2003.
16. Zakynthinos SG, Vassilakopoulos T, Roussos C: The load of inspiratory muscles in patients needing mechanical ventilation. *Am J Respir Crit Care Med* 152(4 Pt 1):1248, 1995.
17. Derenne JP, Fleury B, Pariente R: Acute respiratory failure of chronic obstructive pulmonary disease. *Am Rev Respir Dis* 138:1006, 1988.
18. McCool FD, Tzelepis GE, Leith DE, Hoppin FG, Jr.: Oxygen cost of breathing during fatiguing inspiratory resistive loads. *J Appl Physiol* 66:2045, 1989.
19. Mador MJ, Acevedo FA: Effect of inspiratory muscle fatigue on breathing pattern during inspiratory resistive loading. *J Appl Physiol* 70:1627, 1991.
20. Roussos C, Fixley M, Gross D, Macklem PT: Fatigue of inspiratory muscles and their synergic behavior. *J Appl Physiol* 46:897, 1979.
21. Mador MJ, Kufel TJ, Pineda LA, Sharma GK: Diaphragmatic fatigue and high-intensity exercise in patients with chronic obstructive pulmonary disease. *Am J Respir Crit Care Med* 161:118, 2000.
22. Polkey MI, Kyroussis D, Keilty SE, et al: Exhaustive treadmill exercise does not reduce twitch transdiaphragmatic pressure in patients with COPD. *Am J Respir Crit Care Med* 152:959, 1995.
23. Kyroussis D, Polkey MI, Keilty SE, et al: Exhaustive exercise slows inspiratory muscle relaxation rate in chronic obstructive pulmonary disease. *Am J Respir Crit Care Med* 153:787, 1996.
24. Jounieaux V, Mayeux I: Oxygen cost of breathing in patients with emphysema or chronic bronchitis in acute respiratory failure. *Am J Respir Crit Care Med* 152(6 Pt 1):2181, 1995.
25. Smith TC, Marini JJ: Impact of PEEP on lung mechanics and work of breathing in severe airflow obstruction. *J Appl Physiol* 65:1488, 1988.
26. Murciano D, Aubier M, Bussi S, et al: Comparison of esophageal, tracheal, and mouth occlusion pressure in patients with chronic obstructive pulmonary disease during acute respiratory failure. *Am Rev Respir Dis* 126:837, 1982.
27. Broseghini C, Brandolese R, Poggi R, et al: Respiratory mechanics during the first day of mechanical ventilation in patients

with pulmonary edema and chronic airway obstruction. *Am Rev Respir Dis* 138:355, 1988.

28. Aldrich TK, Hendler JM, Vizioli LD, et al: Intrinsic positive end-expiratory pressure in ambulatory patients with airways obstruction. *Am Rev Respir Dis* 147:845, 1993.

29. Polkey MI, Kyroussis D, Hamnegard CH, et al: Diaphragm strength in chronic obstructive pulmonary disease. *Am J Respir Crit Care Med* 154:1310, 1996.

30. Whittaker JS, Ryan CF, Buckley PA, Road JD: The effects of refeeding on peripheral and respiratory muscle function in malnourished chronic obstructive pulmonary disease patients. *Am Rev Respir Dis* 142:283, 1990.

31. Decramer M, Lacquet LM, Fagard R, Rogiers P: Corticosteroids contribute to muscle weakness in chronic airflow obstruction. *Am J Respir Crit Care Med* 150:11, 1994.

32. Aubier M, Murciano D, Fournier M, et al: Central respiratory drive in acute respiratory failure of patients with chronic obstructive pulmonary disease. *Am Rev Respir Dis* 122:191, 1980.

33. Montgomery AB, Holle RH, Neagley SR, et al: Prediction of successful ventilator weaning using airway occlusion pressure and hypercapnic challenge. *Chest* 91:496, 1987.

34. Respiratory Muscle Fatigue Workshop Group: NHLBI Workshop summary. Respiratory muscle fatigue. Report of the Respiratory Muscle Fatigue Workshop Group. *Am Rev Respir Dis* 142:474, 1990.

35. Yanos J, Keamy MF 3rd, Leisk L, et al: The mechanism of respiratory arrest in inspiratory loading and hypoxemia. *Am Rev Respir Dis* 141(4 Pt 1):933, 1990.

36. Roussos C, Koutsoukou A: Respiratory failure. *Eur Respir J* 47(Suppl):3s, 2003.

37. Pittinger C, Adamson R: Antibiotic blockade of neuromuscular function. *Annu Rev Pharmacol* 12:169, 1972.

38. Miller B, Skupin A, Rubenfire M, Bigman O: Respiratory failure produced by severe procainamide intoxication in a patient with preexisting peripheral neuropathy caused by amiodarone. *Chest* 94:663, 1988.

39. Aubier M, Murciano D, Lecocguic Y, et al: Effect of hypophosphatemia on diaphragmatic contractility in patients with acute respiratory failure. *N Engl J Med* 313:420, 1985.

40. Dhingra S, Solven F, Wilson A, McCarthy DS: Hypomagnesemia and respiratory muscle power. *Am Rev Respir Dis* 129:497, 1984.

41. Orozco-Levi M, Lloreta J, Minguella J, et al: Injury of the human diaphragm associated with exertion and chronic obstructive pulmonary disease. *Am J Respir Crit Care Med* 164:1734, 2001.

42. Reid WD, Belcastro AN: Time course of diaphragm injury and calpain activity during resistive loading. *Am J Respir Crit Care Med* 162:1801, 2000.

43. Vassilakopoulos T, Divangahi M, Rallis G, et al: Differential cytokine gene expression in the diaphragm in response to strenuous resistive breathing. *Am J Respir Crit Care Med* 170:154, 2004.

44. Fiaccadori E, Coffrini E, Ronda N, et al: Hypophosphatemia in course of chronic obstructive pulmonary disease. Prevalence, mechanisms, and relationships with skeletal muscle phosphorus content. *Chest* 97:857, 1990.

45. Openbrier DR, Irwin MM, Rogers RM, et al: Nutritional status and lung function in patients with emphysema and chronic bronchitis. *Chest* 83:17, 1983.

46. Hamnegard CH, Bake B, Moxham J, Polkey MI: Does undernutrition contribute to diaphragm weakness in patients with severe COPD? *Clin Nutr* 21:239, 2002.

47. Decramer M, de Bock V, Dom R: Functional and histologic picture of steroid-induced myopathy in chronic obstructive pulmonary disease. *Am J Respir Crit Care Med* 153(6 Pt 1):1958, 1996.

48. Orozco-Levi M: Structure and function of the respiratory muscles in patients with COPD: impairment or adaptation? *Eur Respir J* 46(Suppl):41s, 2003.

49. Aubier M, Trippenbach T, Roussos C: Respiratory muscle fatigue during cardiogenic shock. *J Appl Physiol* 51:499, 1981.

50. Hussain SN, Graham R, Rutledge F, Roussos C: Respiratory muscle energetics during endotoxic shock in dogs. *J Appl Physiol* 60:486, 1986.

51. Ward ME, Magder SA, Hussain SN: Oxygen delivery-independent effect of blood flow on diaphragm fatigue. *Am Rev Respir Dis* 145:1058, 1992.

52. Laghi F, Cattapan SE, Jubran A, et al: Is weaning failure caused by low-frequency fatigue of the diaphragm? *Am J Respir Crit Care Med* 167:120, 2003.

53. Grootendorst DC, Gauw SA, Baan R, et al: Does a single dose of the phosphodiesterase 4 inhibitor, cilomilast (15 mg), induce bronchodilation in patients with chronic obstructive pulmonary disease? *Pulm Pharmacol Ther* 16:115, 2003.

54. Wright PE, Marini JJ, Bernard GR: In vitro versus in vivo comparison of endotracheal tube airflow resistance. *Am Rev Respir Dis* 140:10, 1989.

55. Girault C, Breton L, Richard JC, et al: Mechanical effects of airway humidification devices in difficult to wean patients. *Crit Care Med* 31:1306, 2003.

56. Fujino Y, Uchiyama A, Mashimo T, Nishimura M: Spontaneously breathing lung model comparison of work of breathing between automatic tube compensation and pressure support. *Respir Care* 48:38, 2003.

57. Barberis L, Manno E, Guerin C: Effect of end-inspiratory pause duration on plateau pressure in mechanically ventilated patients. *Intensive Care Med* 29:130, 2003.

58. Wilkinson TMA, Donaldson GC, Hurst JR, et al: Early therapy improves outcomes of exacerbations of chronic obstructive pulmonary disease. *Am J Respir Crit Care Med* 169:1298, 2004.

59. National Collaborating Centre for Chronic Conditions: National clinical guideline on management of chronic obstructive pulmonary disease in adults in primary and secondary care. *Thorax* 59(Suppl 1):1, 2004.

60. Newhouse MT, Fuller HD: Rose is a rose is a rose? Aerosol therapy in ventilated patients: nebulizers versus metered dose inhalers—a continuing controversy. *Am Rev Respir Dis* 148(6 Pt 1):1444, 1993.

61. Ram FS, Picot J, Lightowler J, Wedzicha JA: Non-invasive positive pressure ventilation for treatment of respiratory failure due to exacerbations of chronic obstructive pulmonary disease. *Cochrane Database Syst Rev* 1:CD004104, 2004.

62. Keenan SP, Sinuff T, Cook DJ, Hill NS: Which patients with acute exacerbation of chronic obstructive pulmonary disease benefit from noninvasive positive-pressure ventilation? A systematic review of the literature. *Ann Intern Med* 138:861, 2003.

63. Kramer N, Meyer TJ, Meharg J, et al: Randomized, prospective trial of noninvasive positive pressure ventilation in acute respiratory failure. *Am J Respir Crit Care Med* 151:1799, 1995.

64. Brochard L, Isabey D, Piquet J, et al: Reversal of acute exacerbations of chronic obstructive lung disease by inspiratory assistance with a face mask. *N Engl J Med* 323:1523, 1990.

65. Liesching T, Kwok H, Hill NS: Acute applications of noninvasive positive pressure ventilation. *Chest* 124:699, 2003.

66. Anton A, Tarrega J, Giner J, et al: Acute physiologic effects of nasal and full-face masks during noninvasive positive-pressure ventilation in patients with acute exacerbations of chronic obstructive pulmonary disease. *Respir Care* 48:922, 2003.

67. Hill NS: Noninvasive ventilation for chronic obstructive pulmonary disease. *Respir Care* 49:72, 2004; discussion 87.

68. Appendini L, Purro A, Patessio A, et al: Partitioning of inspiratory muscle workload and pressure assistance in ventilator-dependent COPD patients. *Am J Respir Crit Care Med* 154:1301, 1996.

69. Appendini L, Purro A, Gudjonsdottir M, et al: Physiologic response of ventilator-dependent patients with chronic obstructive pulmonary disease to proportional assist ventilation and

continuous positive airway pressure. *Am J Respir Crit Care Med* 159(5 Pt 1):1510, 1999.

70. Appendini L, Patessio A, Zanaboni S, et al: Physiologic effects of positive end-expiratory pressure and mask pressure support during exacerbations of chronic obstructive pulmonary disease. *Am J Respir Crit Care Med* 149:1069, 1994.

71. de Lucas P, Tarancon C, Puente L, et al: Nasal continuous positive airway pressure in patients with COPD in acute respiratory failure. A study of the immediate effects. *Chest* 104:1694, 1993.

72. Miro AM, Shivaram U, Hertig I: Continuous positive airway pressure in COPD patients in acute hypercapnic respiratory failure. *Chest* 103:266, 1993.

73. Nava S, Ceriana P: Causes of failure of noninvasive mechanical ventilation. *Respir Care* 49:295, 2004.

74. Aubier M, Murciano D, Milic-Emili J, et al: Effects of the administration of O_2 on ventilation and blood gases in patients with chronic obstructive pulmonary disease during acute respiratory failure. *Am Rev Respir Dis* 122:747, 1980.

75. Sassoon CS, Hassell KT, Mahutte CK: Hyperoxic-induced hypercapnia in stable chronic obstructive pulmonary disease. *Am Rev Respir Dis* 135:907, 1987.

76. Erbland ML, Ebert RV, Snow SL: Interaction of hypoxia and hypercapnia on respiratory drive in patients with COPD. *Chest* 97:1289, 1990.

77. Gomersall CD, Joynt GM, Freebairn RC, et al: Oxygen therapy for hypercapnic patients with chronic obstructive pulmonary disease and acute respiratory failure: a randomized, controlled pilot study. *Crit Care Med* 30:113, 2002.

78. Agusti AG, Carrera M, Barbe F, et al: Oxygen therapy during exacerbations of chronic obstructive pulmonary disease. *Eur Respir J* 14:934, 1999.

79. Moloney ED, Kiely JL, McNicholas WT: Controlled oxygen therapy and carbon dioxide retention during exacerbations of chronic obstructive pulmonary disease. *Lancet* 357:526, 2001.

80. Dunn WF, Nelson SB, Hubmayr RD: Oxygen-induced hypercarbia in obstructive pulmonary disease. *Am Rev Respir Dis* 144(3 Pt 1):526, 1991.

81. Schmidt GA, Hall JB: Oxygen therapy and hypoxic drive to breathe: Is there danger in the patient with COPD? *Intensive Crit Care Dig* 8:124, 1989.

82. Grootendorst DC, Rabe KF: Mechanisms of bronchial hyperreactivity in asthma and chronic obstructive pulmonary disease. *Proc Am Thorac Soc* 1:77, 2004.

83. Thomas P, Pugsley JA, Stewart JH: Theophylline and salbutamol improve pulmonary function in patients with irreversible chronic obstructive pulmonary disease. *Chest* 101:160, 1992.

84. Petty TL: The combination of ipratropium and albuterol is more effective than either agent alone. *Chest* 107(5 Suppl):183S, 1995.

85. McCrory DC, Brown CD: Anti-cholinergic bronchodilators versus beta2-sympathomimetic agents for acute exacerbations of chronic obstructive pulmonary disease. *Cochrane Database Syst Rev* 4:CD003900, 2002.

86. Pourriat JL, Baud M, Lamberto C, et al: Effects of doxapram on hypercapnic response during weaning from mechanical ventilation in COPD patients. *Chest* 101:1639, 1992.

87. Greenstone M, Lasserson TJ: Doxapram for ventilatory failure due to exacerbations of chronic obstructive pulmonary disease. *Cochrane Database Syst Rev* 1:CD000223, 2003.

88. Angus RM, Ahmed AA, Fenwick LJ, Peacock AJ: Comparison of the acute effects on gas exchange of nasal ventilation and doxapram in exacerbations of chronic obstructive pulmonary disease. *Thorax* 51:1048, 1996.

89. Cazzola M, D'Amato M, Califano C, et al: Formoterol as dry powder oral inhalation compared with salbutamol metered-dose inhaler in acute exacerbations of chronic obstructive pulmonary disease. *Clin Therapeutics* 24:595, 2004.

90. Karpel JP, Pesin J, Greenberg D, Gentry E: A comparison of the effects of ipratropium bromide and metaproterenol sulfate in acute exacerbations of COPD. *Chest* 98:835, 1990.

91. Gross NJ, Petty TL, Friedman M, et al: Dose response to ipratropium as a nebulized solution in patients with chronic obstructive pulmonary disease. A three-center study. *Am Rev Respir Dis* 139:1188, 1989.

92. Niewoehner D, Rice K, Cote C, et al: Reduced COPD exacerbations and associated health care utilization with once-daily tiotropium (TIO) in the VA medical system. Presented at the 100th International Conference of the American Thoracic Society. *Am J Respir Crit Care Med* 2004, Abstract [A84; in press].

93. Levy RD, Nava S, Gibbons L, Bellemare F: Aminophylline and human diaphragm strength in vivo. *J Appl Physiol* 68:2591, 1990.

94. Rice KL, Leatherman JW, Duane PG, et al: Aminophylline for acute exacerbations of chronic obstructive pulmonary disease. A controlled trial. *Ann Intern Med* 107:305, 1987.

95. Nishimura K, Koyama H, Ikeda A, et al: The additive effect of theophylline on a high-dose combination of inhaled salbutamol and ipratropium bromide in stable COPD. *Chest* 107:718, 1995.

96. Barr RG, Rowe BH, Camargo CA: Methylxanthines for exacerbations of chronic obstructive pulmonary disease. *Cochrane Database Syst Rev* 2:CD002168, 2003.

97. Bittar G, Friedman HS: The arrhythmogenicity of theophylline. A multivariate analysis of clinical determinants. *Chest* 99:1415, 1991.

98. NHLBI/WHO Workshop Report: Global Initiative for Chronic Obstructive Lung Disease. Global Strategy for the Diagnosis, Management and Prevention of Chronic Obstructive Pulmonary Disease. Available at GOLD website (www.goldcopd.com). Accessed June 07, 2004.

99. Albert RK, Martin TR, Lewis SW: Controlled clinical trial of methylprednisolone in patients with chronic bronchitis and acute respiratory insufficiency. *Ann Intern Med* 92:753, 1980.

100. Rubini F, Rampulla C, Nava S: Acute effect of corticosteroids on respiratory mechanics in mechanically ventilated patients with chronic airflow obstruction and acute respiratory failure. *Am J Respir Crit Care Med* 149(2 Pt 1):306, 1994.

101. Wood-Baker R, Walters EH, Gibson P: Oral corticosteroids for acute exacerbations of chronic obstructive pulmonary disease. *Cochrane Database Syst Rev* 2:CD001288, 2001.

102. Wang YM, Zintel T, Vasquez A, Gallagher CG: Corticosteroid therapy and respiratory muscle function in humans. *Am Rev Respir Dis* 144:108, 1991.

103. Maltais F, Ostinelli J, Bourbeau J, et al: Comparison of nebulized budesonide and oral prednisolone with placebo in the treatment of acute exacerbations of chronic obstructive pulmonary disease: a randomized controlled trial. *Am J Respir Crit Care Med* 165:698, 2002.

104. Spruit MA, Gosselink R, Troosters T, et al: Muscle force during an acute exacerbation in hospitalised patients with COPD and its relationship with CXCL8 and IGF-I. *Thorax* 58:752, 2003.

105. Schols AM, Soeters PB, Mostert R, et al: Physiologic effects of nutritional support and anabolic steroids in patients with chronic obstructive pulmonary disease. A placebo-controlled randomized trial. *Am J Respir Crit Care Med* 152(4 Pt 1):1268, 1995.

106. Yeh SS, DeGuzman B, Kramer T: Reversal of COPD-associated weight loss using the anabolic agent oxandrolone. *Chest* 122:421, 2002.

107. Creutzberg EC, Wouters EF, Mostert R, et al: A role for anabolic steroids in the rehabilitation of patients with COPD? A double-blind, placebo-controlled, randomized trial. *Chest* 124:1733, 2003.

108. Salerno DM, Anderson B, Sharkey PJ, Iber C: Intravenous verapamil for treatment of multifocal atrial tachycardia with and without calcium pretreatment. *Ann Intern Med* 107:623, 1987.

109. Petrof BJ, Legare M, Goldberg P, et al: Continuous positive airway pressure reduces work of breathing and dyspnea during

weaning from mechanical ventilation in severe chronic obstructive pulmonary disease. *Am Rev Respir Dis* 141:281, 1990.

110. Gay PC, Rodarte JR, Hubmayr RD: The effects of positive expiratory pressure on isovolume flow and dynamic hyperinflation in patients receiving mechanical ventilation. *Am Rev Respir Dis* 139:621, 1989.

111. Tuxen DV: Detrimental effects of positive end-expiratory pressure during controlled mechanical ventilation of patients with severe airflow obstruction. *Am Rev Respir Dis* 140:5, 1989.

112. Ranieri VM, Giuliani R, Cinnella G, et al: Physiologic effects of positive end-expiratory pressure in patients with chronic obstructive pulmonary disease during acute ventilatory failure and controlled mechanical ventilation. *Am Rev Respir Dis* 147:5, 1993.

113. Baigorri F, de Monte A, Blanch L, et al: Hemodynamic responses to external counterbalancing of auto-positive end-expiratory pressure in mechanically ventilated patients with chronic obstructive pulmonary disease. *Crit Care Med* 22:1782, 1994.

114. Laghi F, Segal J, Choe WK, Tobin MJ: Effect of imposed inflation time on respiratory frequency and hyperinflation in patients with chronic obstructive pulmonary disease. *Am J Respir Crit Care Med* 163:1365, 2001.

115. Braun NMT, Faulkner J, Hughes RL: When should respiratory muscles be exercised? *Chest* 84:76, 1983.

116. Kress JP, O'Connor MF, Schmidt GA: Clinical examination reliably detects intrinsic positive end-expiratory pressure in critically ill, mechanically ventilated patients. *Am J Respir Crit Care Med* 159:290, 1999.

117. Tang NL, Chung ML, Elia M, et al: Total daily energy expenditure in wasted chronic obstructive pulmonary disease patients. *Eur J Clin Nutr* 56:282, 2002.

118. Duarte AG, Momii K, Bidani A: Bronchodilator therapy with metered-dose inhaler and spacer versus nebulizer in mechanically ventilated patients: comparison of magnitude and duration of response. *Respir Care* 45:817, 2000.

119. Fuller HD, Dolovich MB, Posmituck G, et al: Pressurized aerosol versus jet aerosol delivery to mechanically ventilated patients. Comparison of dose to the lungs. *Am Rev Respir Dis* 141:440, 1990.

120. Manthous CA, Hall JB, Schmidt GA, Wood LD: Metered-dose inhaler versus nebulized albuterol in mechanically ventilated patients. *Am Rev Respir Dis* 148(6 Pt 1):1567, 1993.

121. Erelel M, Cuhadaroglu C, Ece T, Arseven O: The frequency of deep venous thrombosis and pulmonary embolus in acute exacerbation of chronic obstructive pulmonary disease. *Respir Med* 96:515, 2002.

122. Chopin C, Fesard P, Mangalaboyi J, et al: Use of capnography in diagnosis of pulmonary embolism during acute respiratory failure of chronic obstructive pulmonary disease. *Crit Care Med* 18:353, 1990.

123. Ely EW, Baker AM, Dunagan DP, et al: Effect on the duration of mechanical ventilation of identifying patients capable of breathing spontaneously. *N Engl J Med* 335:1864, 1996.

124. Krishnan JA, Moore D, Robeson C, et al: A prospective, controlled trial of a protocol-based strategy to discontinue mechanical ventilation. *Am J Respir Crit Care Med* 169:673, 2004.

125. Schmidt GA, Hall JB: Acute on chronic respiratory failure. Assessment and management of patients with COPD in the emergency setting. *JAMA* 261:3444, 1989.

126. Vitacca M, Vianello A, Colombo D, et al: Comparison of two methods for weaning patients with chronic obstructive pulmonary disease requiring mechanical ventilation for more than 15 days. *Am J Respir Crit Care Med* 164:225, 2001.

127. Esteban A, Frutos F, Tobin MJ, et al: A comparison of four methods of weaning patients from mechanical ventilation. Spanish Lung Failure Collaborative Group. *N Engl J Med* 332:345, 1995.

128. Brochard L, Rauss A, Benito S, et al: Comparison of three methods of gradual withdrawal from ventilatory support during weaning from mechanical ventilation. *Am J Respir Crit Care Med* 150:896, 1994.

129. Conti G, Montini L, Pennisi MA, et al: A prospective, blinded evaluation of indexes proposed to predict weaning from mechanical ventilation. *Intensive Care Med* 30:830, 2004.

130. Marini JJ: Strategies to minimize breathing effort during mechanical ventilation. *Crit Care Clin* 6:635, 1990.

131. Nava S, Ambrosino N, Clini E, et al: Noninvasive mechanical ventilation in the weaning of patients with respiratory failure due to chronic obstructive pulmonary disease. A randomized, controlled trial. *Ann Intern Med* 128:721, 1998.

132. Ferrer M, Esquinas A, Arancibia F, et al: Noninvasive ventilation during persistent weaning failure: A randomized controlled trial. *Am J Respir Crit Care Med* 168:70, 2003.

133. Burns KE, Adhikari NK, Meade MO: Noninvasive positive pressure ventilation as a weaning strategy for intubated adults with respiratory failure. *Cochrane Database Syst Rev* 4:CD004127, 2003.

134. Schonhofer B, Euteneuer S, Nava S, et al: Survival of mechanically ventilated patients admitted to a specialised weaning centre. *Intensive Care Med* 28:908, 2002.

135. Esteban A, Frutos-Vivar F, Ferguson ND, et al: Noninvasive positive-pressure ventilation for respiratory failure after extubation. *N Engl J Med* 350:2452, 2004.

Chapter 40 _____
STATUS ASTHMATICUS
THOMAS CORBRIDGE
JESSE B. HALL

KEY POINTS

- *Severe asthma exacerbation is defined by several, but not necessarily all, of the following features: dyspnea at rest, upright positioning, inability to speak in phrases or sentences, respiratory rate >30 breaths per minute (bpm), use of accessory muscles of respiration, pulse >120 beats/min, pulsus paradoxus >25 mm Hg, peak expiratory flow rate <50% predicted or personal best, hypoxemia, and eucapnia or hypercapnia.*

- *Altered mental status, paradoxical respirations, bradycardia, a quiet chest, and absence of pulsus paradoxus from respiratory muscle fatigue identify imminent respiratory arrest.*

- *Airway wall inflammation, bronchospasm, and intraluminal mucus cause progressive airflow obstruction. Fewer patients develop sudden-onset asthma from a more pure form of bronchospasm.*

- *Severe exacerbations and death can occur in patients with mild asthma.*

- *Airflow obstruction causes ventilation-perfusion inequality, lung hyperinflation, and increased work of breathing.*

- *Oxygen, β agonists, and systemic corticosteroids are first-line treatments. Agents of debated efficacy include ipratropium bromide, magnesium sulfate, leukotriene modifiers, theophylline, inhaled steroids, and heliox.*

- *Noninvasive ventilation is potentially useful in hypercapneic patients not requiring intubation.*

- *Postintubation hyperinflation decreases preload to the right ventricle and may cause barotrauma, hypotension, or cardiac arrest. A ventilator strategy that lowers lung volume decreases complications.*

- *Treating airflow obstruction and prolonging expiratory time decreases lung hyperinflation. Expiratory time is prolonged on the ventilator by lowering minute ventilation (even at the cost of hypercapnia) and increasing inspiratory flow rate.*

- *Deep sedation allows for safe and effective mechanical ventilation in most intubated patients. Paralysis increases the risk of myopathy.*

- *Patient education, environmental control, and pharmacotherapy are crucial to prevent exacerbations and death.*

Asthma is characterized by wheezing, dyspnea, cough, hyperreactive airways, and reversible airflow obstruction.[1–3] In the vast majority of cases, the disease is managed uneventfully in the ambulatory setting. However, severe attacks and death can occur regardless of severity classification, and in some cases there is little warning before a terminal event.[4] Deaths often occur outside the hospital; patients who have not arrested prior to emergency department (ED) arrival generally have a good prognosis.[5] Underestimation of severity, a gap in communication between health care provider and patient, airway inflammation (even in mild disease), and failure to

use inhaled corticosteroids all contribute to asthma morbidity and mortality.[6–10]

Severe asthma exacerbation is defined by several, but not necessarily all, of the following features: dyspnea at rest, upright positioning, inability to speak in phrases or sentences, respiratory rate >30 bpm, use of accessory muscles of respiration, pulse >120/min, pulsus paradoxus >25 mm Hg, peak expiratory flow rate <50% predicted or personal best, hypoxemia, and eucapnia or hypercapnia.[1] Altered mental status, paradoxical respirations, bradycardia, a quiet chest, and absence of pulsus paradoxus from respiratory muscle fatigue identify imminent respiratory arrest.[1]

The objectives of this chapter are to review the pathophysiology of severe asthma exacerbations, discuss clinical assessment and differential diagnosis, assess pharmacologic treatment, and provide a ventilatory strategy for intubated patients. It is perhaps in this last area of acute severe asthma management that intensivists have made their greatest strides over the last two decades, with indirect evidence suggesting that current strategies decrease morbidity and mortality. In the final analysis, however, the greatest gains will come from optimal outpatient management and prevention of attacks.

Pathophysiology

Exacerbations often evolve over hours to days before patients seek medical help.[11,12] There is thus a window of opportunity to treat inflammation through initiation or escalation of corticosteroids. Indeed, the "best treatment of status asthmaticus is to treat it three days before it occurs [with corticosteroids]."[13] Instead, too many patients rely on increasing doses of inhaled β agonists, eventually to no avail.

One consequence of airway inflammation is plugging of large and small airways with tenacious mucus. This can be quite striking at postmortem analysis.[14] Mucus plugs consist of sloughed epithelial cells, eosinophils, fibrin, and other serum components that leak readily through the denuded airway epithelium. In a smaller subset of patients, an unexpected exacerbation, termed sudden-onset asthma, results from a more pure form of smooth muscle–mediated bronchospasm. Sudden-onset asthma can be lethal, but it can also improve rapidly with bronchodilators.[15,16] Compared to attacks of slower tempo, there are more submucosal neutrophils and fewer airway secretions.[17,18] Triggers of sudden attacks include use of nonsteroidal anti-inflammatory agents and β-blockers in susceptible patients, allergen or irritant exposure, exercise, stress, sulfites, and inhalation of crack cocaine or heroin.[19–22] Respiratory tract infection is not a usual trigger; commonly no cause is found.[23]

ABNORMALITIES OF GAS EXCHANGE

Airway obstruction causes ventilation-to-perfusion (V/Q) mismatch. Intrapulmonary shunting is trivial, so modest enrichment of oxygen (1 to 3 L/min by nasal cannula) generally corrects hypoxemia.[24] Refractory hypoxemia is rare and suggests additional pathology: pneumonia, aspiration, acute lobar atelectasis, or barotrauma. There is a rough correlation between airflow obstruction as measured by the forced expiratory volume in 1 second (FEV_1) or peak expiratory flow rate (PEFR) and hypoxemia.[25,26] However, there is no cutoff value that accurately predicts hypoxemia. In recovering patients, multiple inert gas elimination technique (MIGET) analysis demonstrates that airflow rates commonly improve before partial pressure of arterial oxygen (Pa_{O_2}) and V/Q inequality.[27] One explanation for this is that spirometry tracks large-airway function and indices of gas exchange reflect the function of smaller peripheral airways.[27,28]

Supplemental oxygen improves oxygen delivery to respiratory muscles, reverses hypoxic pulmonary vasoconstriction, and bronchodilates airways. It further protects from β-agonist–induced hypoxemia resulting from pulmonary vasodilation and increased blood flow to low V/Q units.[29,30]

Increases in dead space are expected when regions of hyperinflated lung limit blood flow to create West's zone 1 conditions (where alveolar pressure exceeds pulmonary capillary pressure).[27] However, MIGET analysis demonstrates only small areas of high V/Q and slightly increased dead space in acute asthma.[24,30]

Respiratory alkalosis is a feature of mild acute asthma. If present long enough, there is compensatory renal bicarbonate wasting that may subsequently manifest as a normal anion-gap metabolic acidosis (posthypocapneic metabolic acidosis). As the severity of airflow obstruction increases, the partial pressure of arterial carbon dioxide ($PaCO_2$) generally increases due to inadequate alveolar ventilation (reflecting a decrease in minute ventilation as the patient nears respiratory arrest) and possible elevated CO_2 production from increased work of breathing. Hypercapnia usually does not occur unless the FEV_1 is less than 25% of predicted.[25] Importantly the absence of hypercapnia does not preclude a severe attack or potential for respiratory arrest.[26]

LUNG MECHANICAL ABNORMALITIES

Incomplete emptying of alveolar gas and positive end-expiratory alveolar pressure are hallmarks of expiratory airflow obstruction. In ventilated patients, end-expiratory alveolar pressure is not reflected at the airway opening if the expiratory port of the ventilator is open (which allows airway-opening pressure to approach atmospheric pressure or the level of ventilator-applied positive end-expiratory pressure [PEEP]). If the expiratory port is closed at end-expiration, central airway pressure generally equilibrates with alveolar pressure, permitting measurement of auto- or intrinsic PEEP (PEEPi). PEEPi reflects gas trapping only in relaxed patients, since expiratory muscle contraction elevates end-expired pressure. Low levels of PEEPi may underestimate the degree of lung hyperinflation. Leatherman and Ravenscraft[31] measured low levels of PEEPi in four ventilated asthmatics with significant lung hyperinflation, suggesting the presence of noncommunicating airspaces.

The pressure-volume relationship of the lung parenchyma predicts that hyperinflation correlates with decreased static compliance. However, lung compliance may be normal despite hyperinflation, suggesting a stretch-relaxation response in parenchymal tissue.[32] This state is not favorable to expiratory flow, but may protect against complications of lung hyperinflation.

CIRCULATORY EFFECTS OF SEVERE AIRWAY OBSTRUCTION

Circulatory abnormalities reflect a state of cardiac tamponade resulting from dynamic hyperinflation (DHI) and pleural pressure changes associated with breathing against obstructed airways. During expiration, high intrathoracic pressures decrease right-sided preload. Vigorous inspiration augments right ventricular filling and shifts the intraventricular septum leftward to cause a conformational change in the left ventricle (LV), diastolic dysfunction, and incomplete LV filling. Additionally, large negative pleural pressures directly impair LV emptying.[33,34] Rarely diastolic dysfunction and increased LV afterload cause pulmonary edema. Finally, lung hyperinflation increases RV afterload and may cause transient pulmonary hypertension.[35] The net effect of these cyclical events is to accentuate the normal inspiratory reduction in stroke volume, a phenomenon termed *pulsus paradoxus* (PP). Pulsus paradoxus is a valuable marker of asthma severity;[36] however, the absence of a widened PP does not ensure a mild attack.[37] The PP falls in improving patients, but also in the fatiguing asthmatic who is unable to generate large changes in pleural pressure.

PROGRESSION TO VENTILATORY FAILURE

Several pathophysiologic mechanisms appear to be responsible for ventilatory failure in acute asthma. PEEPi is a threshold pressure that must be overcome before inspiratory flow occurs, increasing inspiratory work of breathing. Airway resistance is increased, and if lung compliance is low, greater transpulmonary pressure is required. Work of breathing can overwhelm the fatiguing respiratory muscles to cause ventilatory failure, even in young and otherwise healthy individuals.

These mechanical loads are imposed on a diaphragm that is placed in a disadvantageous position by hyperinflation and at a time when circulatory abnormalities may result in hypoperfusion. Respiratory acidosis further decreases diaphragm force generation.[38] Lactic acidosis is a marker of severity rather than a cause of diaphragm dysfunction per se.[38–40]

Clinical Presentation, Differential Diagnosis, and Assessment of Severity

Multifactorial analysis including the history, physical examination, measures of airflow obstruction, response to therapy, arterial blood gases, and chest radiography is important to assess disease severity and risk for deterioration. Such analysis is necessary because no single clinical measurement predicts outcome reliably.[41]

MEDICAL HISTORY

Characteristics of prior exacerbations that predict a fatal or near fatal episode include intubation, hypercapnia, barotrauma, hospitalization despite corticosteroids, psychiatric illness, and medical noncompliance.[42,43] Prior intubation is the greatest single predictor of subsequent asthma death.[44] Substance abuse, alcohol ingestion, and excessive, long-term use of β agonists are also associated with increased risk of death.[45,46] Pharmacogenetic studies have suggested an association between polymorphisms of β adrenoreceptors, the severity of asthma, and its response to therapy.[47] Survivors of near-fatal asthma may also have diminished ventilatory drive in the face of hypoxemic or mechanical stimuli (i.e., poor perceivers of airflow obstruction).[48] Other concerning features include symptoms of long duration (which suggests a substantial component of airway wall inflammation and slow recovery), late arrival for care, fatigue, altered mental status, and sleep deprivation. Deterioration despite optimal treatment, including the concurrent use of oral steroids, identifies patients who are unlikely to improve quickly.

"All that wheezes is not asthma" is an appropriate clinical aphorism to consider. In most cases, the history and examination identify conditions that are confused for or complicate acute asthma. The absence of a history of asthma should alert the physician to other diagnoses (although asthma can first occur at any age). A history of smoking suggests chronic obstructive pulmonary disease (COPD), which may be associated with fixed airflow obstruction, pulmonary hypertension, and chronic respiratory acidosis. Cardiac asthma refers to the airway hyperreactivity that occurs in congestive heart failure.[49] Heart failure is generally discernible by examination, but the distinction between LV dysfunction and airway obstruction can be difficult. As discussed above, severe airflow obstruction is a rare cause of pulmonary edema, and bronchodilators may improve airflow obstruction in LV failure.[50] Foreign body aspiration must be considered in children and in adults with an abnormal swallow, a history of altered mental status, or recent dental work. Upper airway obstruction from granulation tissue, tumor, laryngeal edema, or vocal cord dysfunction may be confused for acute asthma. In classic extrathoracic obstruction, there is flattening of the inspiratory portion of the flow-volume loop and poor response to asthma medication. Fiberoptic laryngoscopy can confirm laryngeal obstruction. For patients with tracheal stenosis (e.g., from prior intubation), CT imaging and fiberoptic bronchoscopy establishes the diagnosis. Important clues to focal obstruction include localized wheeze, and rarely, asymmetric hyperinflation on the chest radiograph.[51] Pneumonia complicating asthma is unusual but should be considered when there is fever, purulent sputum, localizing signs, and refractory hypoxemia. Purulent sputum in asthma contains an abundance of eosinophils and not polymorphonuclear leukocytes. In large series of patients with pulmonary embolus, wheezing was not a reported sign. However, this association has been described anecdotally.[52] If dyspnea is out of proportion to measures of airflow obstruction, this diagnosis should be considered.

PHYSICAL EXAMINATION

The general appearance of the patient (i.e., posture, pattern of speech, positioning, and level of alertness) allows for quick assessment of status, response to therapy, and need for intubation. Adults who assume the upright position have a higher heart rate (HR), respiratory rate (RR), and PP and a significantly lower Pa_{O_2} and PEFR than patients who are able to lie supine.[53] Diaphoresis is associated with an even lower PEFR. Accessory muscle use and PP indicate severe airflow obstruction; the absence of either finding does not rule out severe obstruction.[37]

Examination of the head and neck should focus on identifying barotrauma and upper airway obstruction. Tracheal deviation, asymmetric breath sounds, a "mediastinal crunch," and subcutaneous emphysema suggest pneumomediastinum or pneumothorax. Rarely, atelectasis from a central mucus plug causes tracheal deviation. The mouth and neck should be inspected for mass lesions or signs of previous surgery. The lip and tongue should be inspected for angioedema.

Wheezing correlates poorly with the degree of airflow limitation.[54] A silent chest suggests insufficient airflow for wheezes to occur, and in general, wheezes that emerge in a previously silent chest signal clinical improvement. Localized wheezing or crackles should prompt consideration of atelectasis, pneumonia, pneumothorax, endobronchial lesions, or foreign body.

Asthmatics are generally tachycardic on presentation.[55] Bradycardia is an ominous sign of impending arrest. The usual rhythm is sinus tachycardia. Supraventricular and ventricular arrhythmias are not uncommon, particularly in older patients.[56]

Clinical signs of right-sided and left-sided heart failure suggest primary cardiac disease. Yet, acute asthma alone can cause examination and electrocardiographic findings of right-sided heart strain and pulmonary edema which resolve within hours of response to therapy.[55,57] Jugular venous distention also occurs when DHI or tension pneumothorax limit venous return to the right heart. Myocardial ischemia should be considered in older patients with coronary artery disease. Asthma may cause myocardial oxygen supply/demand imbalance if large drops in intrathoracic pressure increase LV afterload and decrease coronary blood flow.[58] β Agonists, theophylline, and hypoxemia may further disrupt this balance.

MEASUREMENT OF AIRFLOW OBSTRUCTION

The degree of airflow obstruction is determined by measuring PEFR or FEV_1. A PEFR or FEV_1 <50% of predicted or the patient's personal best characterizes severe exacerbation.[1] Objective measures are necessary because physician estimates are often wrong.[59] In most cases it is easier to measure PEFR than FEV_1, but neither is easy to obtain in critical patients. In these patients it is wise to defer measurements, since they may worsen bronchospasm[60] and rarely precipitate respiratory arrest.[61] In most cases, however, peak flow determinations are safe.

Measurement of the change in PEFR or FEV_1 is a good way to assess and follow patients. Several studies have demonstrated that failure of initial therapy to improve expiratory flow after 30 minutes predicts a refractory course and need for hospitalization or continued treatment in an ED.[41,62–64] Changes in PEFR before 30 minutes of treatment have elapsed do not predict clinical outcome.[65]

ARTERIAL BLOOD GASES

When FEV_1 is less than 50% predicted or of the patient's personal best, an arterial blood gas should be considered. In early (mild) acute asthma, mild hypoxemia and respiratory alkalosis are common. Hypercapnia indicates severe disease and impending respiratory failure, but not necessarily the need for intubation.[66] Importantly, hypercapnia is not always present in cases of severe obstruction and impending respiratory arrest.[67]

Metabolic acidosis with a normal anion gap occurs when there is bicarbonate wasting in response to respiratory alkalosis. An elevated anion gap suggests excess serum lactate, possibly secondary to increased work of breathing, tissue hypoxia, intracellular alkalosis, or decreased lactate clearance by the liver. Lactic acidosis correlates with the severity of airflow obstruction, is more common in men, and occurs more frequently when β agonists are administered parenterally.[68,39]

Serial blood gases are usually not necessary to determine clinical course. Physical examinations and peak flows allow for valid judgements in most cases. Patients who deteriorate on clinical grounds with impending respiratory failure should be intubated regardless of Pa_{CO_2}. Conversely, improving patients should not be intubated despite hypercapnia. Serial blood gases are helpful in intubated patients to guide ventilator management.

RADIOGRAPHIC STUDIES

Chest radiography plays little role in the assessment or management of patients with acute asthma. Even in hospitalized patients, radiographic findings influence treatment in 1% to 5% of cases.[69–72] In one study[72] that reported major radiographic abnormalities in 34% of cases (which the authors felt impacted management), the majority of findings were classified as focal parenchymal opacities or increased interstitial markings, common indicators of atelectasis in asthma. Chest radiography is indicated when there are localizing signs, barotrauma is suspected, or it is not clear that asthma is the cause of respiratory distress. In mechanically ventilated patients, chest radiography further identifies endotracheal tube position.

ADMISSION CRITERIA

Patients demonstrating a good response to initial therapy in the ED may be discharged home with close follow-up. There should be significant improvement in breathlessness, improved air movement on physical examination, and a FEV$_1$ or PEFR $\geq$70% of predicted or personal best.[1] Observation for 60 minutes after the last β-agonist dose helps ensure stability prior to discharge. Written medication instructions and an action plan to be followed in the event of worsening symptoms should be provided. In general, patients should be discharged on oral corticosteroids. We advise initiation and/or continuation of inhaled corticosteroids by proper technique in the ED. Follow-up appointments are essential.

Patients with severe airflow obstruction demonstrating a poor response to therapy (e.g., <10% increase in PEFR) or patients who deteriorate despite therapy should be admitted to an ICU. Other indications for ICU admission include respiratory arrest, altered mental status, arrhythmias, myocardial ischemia or infarction, and need for frequent inhaler treatments.

An incomplete response to treatment is defined as the persistence of wheezing or dyspnea and a PEFR or FEV$_1$ between 50% and 70% of predicted.[1] Patients in this group require ongoing treatment either in the ED or medical ward. In general, we treat for up to 6 hours in the ED before deciding on disposition. This length of time allows for assessment of the initial response to steroids, and for those who are discharged home decreases the risk of relapse and return to the ED.[37] If the patient has demonstrated a good response to treatment over that period of time and close follow-up can be established, discharge home is appropriate. Discharged patients not optimally treated prior to the ED have better outcomes if they receive a course of oral steroids.[73] Patients who continue to have an incomplete response should be admitted to a medical ward. Admission is also recommended when there is a harmful home environment or when noncompliance favors directly observed therapy.

Therapy Prior to Intubation

PHARMACOTHERAPY

BETA AGONISTS

Asthmatic smooth muscle has increased shortening capacity and increased velocity of shortening[74] that mandate treatment in the setting of an acute attack. Use of a β agonist by inhalation is preferred and should begin immediately regardless of prior use (Table 40-1).[75] Large and frequent doses are needed in acute asthma because the dose-response curve and duration of action are adversely affected by airway narrowing. Fortunately, high doses are generally well tolerated. In one study, albuterol delivered by metered dose inhaler (MDI) and spacer to a total dose of 1600 μg over 90 minutes did not increase cardiovascular morbidity in well-oxygenated patients with acute asthma.[76]

Albuterol is preferred over metaproterenol because of its greater β_2 selectivity and longer duration of action.[77,78] Some clinicians prefer metaproterenol or isoetharine for initial therapy, despite the tendency of these drugs to increase side effects, because of their faster onset of action.[79] Levalbuterol is the R-isomer of racemic albuterol. Preclinical data demonstrate that the S-isomer has undesirable proinflammatory effects.[80] The clinical relevance of these effects (particularly in those receiving high doses of the racemate) is under investigation. Clinical data do show that 1.25 mg levalbuterol increases FEV$_1$ to a greater extent than 2.5 mg of the racemate in stable patients with FEV$_1$ $\leq$60% of predicted.[81] In acute asthma, an open-label study of 91 patients with an FEV$_1$ of 20% to 55% of predicted, stratified into cohorts receiving 0.63 to 5 mg levalbuterol or 2.5 to 5 mg albuterol (three treatments

TABLE 40-1 Drugs Used in the Initial Treatment of Acute Severe Asthma

Albuterol: 2.5 mg by nebulization every 20 minutes or 4–6 puffs by MDI with spacer every 20 minutes; for intubated patients titrate to physiologic effect. Alternative: levalbuterol (see text)

Epinephrine: 0.3 mL of a 1:1000 solution subcutaneously every 20 minutes × 3. Terbutaline is favored in pregnancy when parenteral therapy is indicated. Use with caution in patients >age 40 and in the presence of cardiac disease

Ipratropium bromide: 0.5 mg combined with albuterol by nebulization every 20 minutes or 4–6 puffs by MDI with spacer combined with albuterol every 20 minutes

Corticosteroids: Methylprednisolone 60 mg IV every 6 hours or prednisone PO 40 mg every 6 hours

Magnesium sulfate: 2 g IV over 20 minutes, repeat in 20 minutes if clinically indicated (total 4 g unless hypomagnesemic)

Theophylline: 5 mg/kg IV over 30 minutes loading dose in patients not on theophylline, followed by 0.4 mg/kg per hour IV maintenance dose. Watch for drug interactions and disease states that alter clearance. Follow serum levels

Leukotriene modifiers: Consider montelukast 10 mg PO (the chewable formulation may have quicker onset of action)

Heliox: 80:20 or 70:30 helium:oxygen mix by tight-fitting, nonrebreathing face mask. Higher helium concentrations are needed for maximal effect in 1 hour), demonstrated faster onset of action and a greater degree of bronchodilation with levalbuterol.[82] Results from a larger multicenter study are expected in the near future.

Long-acting β agonists are not indicated in the initial treatment of acute asthma, but may be considered as add-on therapy in hospitalized patients. The addition of salmeterol to albuterol in hospitalized asthmatics is safe and improves FEV_1 after 48 hours compared with placebo.[83]

Subcutaneous administration is not indicated unless the patient is unable to carry out inhaled therapy (such as those with an altered mental status or cardiopulmonary arrest), and is associated with greater toxicity.[84–86] Subcutaneous epinephrine, however, benefits some patients not responding to several hours of an inhaled β agonist.[87] Known cardiac disease and age >40 years are relative contraindications to parenteral therapy,[88] although older patients without recent myocardial ischemia or infarction tolerate subcutaneous epinephrine reasonably well. Intravenous infusion of β agonists is not recommended. Inhaled drug achieves greater airflow rates with lesser toxicity compared to intravenous drug.[89–92] Combinations of inhaled and intravenous treatment have not been adequately studied.

Inhaled β agonists are delivered equally well by MDI with spacer or hand-held nebulizer.[93] Even in severe obstruction, four puffs of albuterol (0.36 mg) delivered by MDI with an InspirEase is as effective as 2.5 mg of albuterol by nebulization.[94] MDIs with spacers are less expensive and able to achieve faster drug delivery times; hand-held nebulizers require fewer instructions, less supervision, and less coordination.

The recommended initial dose is albuterol 2.5 mg by nebulization; three treatments can be given in the first hour depending on clinical response and side effects. A single high-dose treatment (e.g., 7.5 mg) is no better than multiple treatments (2.5 mg every 20 minutes 3 times), and causes more side effects.[95] Depending on the study, there is either no difference in efficacy or toxicity between continuous or intermittently nebulized albuterol, or a slight benefit to continuous nebulization (at the same total dose per hour) in severe obstruction.[96–98]

There are two dose response patterns to high and cumulative doses of albuterol. Approximately two-thirds of patients respond to inhaled albuterol in a dose-dependent fashion, generally allowing discharge home from the ED.[99] In these patients 1.2 to 2.4 mg albuterol delivered by MDI and spacer or 5 to 7.5 mg by nebulizer in the first hour is effective. In the remaining one-third of patients, even in high doses, albuterol has minimal effect, presumably because of airway inflammation and mucus plugging.

IPRATROPIUM BROMIDE

Data support the addition of ipratropium bromide to albuterol in acute asthma.[100–106] Karpel and colleagues studied 384 patients randomized to nebulized albuterol 2.5 mg or albuterol 2.5 mg with ipratropium 0.5 mg at entry and at 45 minutes.[107] At 45 minutes, there were more responders in the ipratropium group; however, the median change of FEV_1 from baseline did not differ between groups, and by 90 minutes there was no difference between groups in the percentage of responders and median change in FEV_1. There was no difference in the number of patients requiring additional ED or hospital treatment. Garrett and colleagues ran-

domized 338 asthmatics to a single dose of nebulized ipratropium bromide 0.5 mg combined with salbutamol 3.0 mg, or salbutamol 3.0 mg alone.[108] Mean FEV_1 at 45 and 90 minutes was significantly higher with combined therapy. Lin and colleagues demonstrated that combination therapy resulted in greater improvement in PEFR than albuterol alone in 55 adult asthmatics.[109] O'Driscoll and colleagues also demonstrated a benefit to combination therapy, particularly in patients with PEFR <140 L/min.[110] In children, combination therapy decreases ED treatment time, albuterol dose requirements, and hospitalization rates.[106,111,112]

To the contrary, Weber and colleagues performed a prospective, randomized, double-blind, placebo-controlled trial of 67 patients receiving combination albuterol and ipratropium bromide or albuterol alone by continuous nebulization for a maximum of 3 hours.[113] Primary outcome measures were improvement in PEFR, hospital admission rates, and length of stay in the ED. All outcome measures favored combination therapy, but differences were not statistically significant. Fitzgerald and coworkers reported similar results.[114] McFadden and colleagues showed no benefit in PEFR, admission rate, or ED length of stay with combination therapy used for the first hour.[115] In children, Ducharme and Davis did not demonstrate benefit from combination therapy in their study of nearly 300 asthmatics with mild to moderate acute asthma.[116]

The above studies demonstrating modest (or no) benefit to combination therapy generally used small doses of ipratropium bromide. Few trials have studied high and cumulative doses of both ipratropium bromide and albuterol. In one such study, Rodrigo and Rodrigo conducted a double-blind, randomized, prospective trial of albuterol and ipratropium bromide (120 μg of albuterol and 21 μg of ipratropium per puff, combined in one inhaler) vs. albuterol (120 μg per puff) and placebo in 180 patients with acute asthma.[117] Four puffs were administered through an MDI with a spacer every 10 minutes for 3 hours. Combination therapy resulted in a 20.5% greater improvement in PEFR and a 48.1% greater improvement in FEV_1 compared with albuterol alone. The rate of hospitalization decreased significantly, from 39% in the albuterol with placebo group to 20% with combination therapy. Subgroup analysis showed that patients most likely to benefit from high doses of ipratropium bromide were those with FEV_1 <30% of predicted and symptoms for >24 hours prior to ED presentation.

Overall, the data suggest an advantage in maximal bronchodilation response when high doses of ipratropium bromide and albuterol are combined in the emergency treatment of asthma. Combination therapy is recommended in any patient who is extremely ill on first presentation or not responding quickly (e.g., within 30 minutes) to albuterol alone.

CORTICOSTEROIDS

Systemic corticosteroids should be administered quickly to treat the inflammatory component of acute asthma. The data are mixed regarding benefit in the first few hours. McFadden's group demonstrated no differences in physiologic or clinical variables in the first 6 hours in 38 patients receiving hydrocortisone.[118] Rodrigo and Rodrigo similarly showed that early administration of steroids did not improve spirometry in the first 6 hours.[119] However, Littenberg and Gluck demonstrated that methylprednisolone 125 mg IV on arrival decreased admission rates compared to placebo,[120] and Lin and colleagues demonstrated improved peak flows after 1 and 2 hours of solumedrol.[121] A systematic review of 12 studies for the Cochrane Review demonstrated that corticosteroids within 1 hour of arrival in the ED reduced admissions.[122] Use of early systemic steroids also reduces the number of relapses in the first 7 to 10 days and the risk of death.[123–126] In hospitalized patients, systemic steroids speed the rate of improvement.[127] Oral and intravenous routes are equally effective,[128] but oral steroids should be avoided if there is concern regarding intubation.

There is no clear dose-response relationship to steroids in acute asthma.[129,130] In one meta-analysis by Manser and colleagues, there was no difference in clinical outcomes between low-dose corticosteroids ($\leq$80 mg/d solumedrol or $\leq$400 mg/d hydrocortisone) and higher doses in the initial management of hospitalized asthmatics.[131] Haskell and colleagues demonstrated that 125 mg IV methylprednisolone every 6 hours resulted in faster improvement compared to 40 mg every 6 hours, but there was no difference in peak improvement.[132] Both doses were superior to 15 mg every 6 hours in terms of rate and absolute response. Emerman and Cydulka compared 500 mg and 100 mg of methylprednisolone and found no benefit to the higher dose.[133]

The Expert Panel from the National Institutes of Health (NIH) recommends 120 to 180 mg per day of prednisone or methylprednisolone in three or four divided doses for 48 hours, then 60 to 80 mg/d until PEFR reaches 70% predicted or personal best.[1] Prednisone is tapered at variable rates depending on a number of factors, including PEFR, the duration of high-dose therapy required to treat the acute exacerbation, and whether oral steroids had been used for maintenance therapy. Automatic tapering schedules are not recommended because patients may taper prematurely.

Recent trials have demonstrated efficacy of inhaled corticosteroids in acute asthma. In children discharged from the ED, short-term use of budesonide, starting at a high-dose and tapered over 1 week, was as effective as a tapering course of oral prednisolone.[134] Rodrigo and Rodrigo conducted a randomized, double-blind trial of the addition of flunisolide 1 mg or placebo to 400 μg salbutamol every 10 minutes for 3 hours in 94 ED subjects not receiving systemic steroids.[135] They found that PEFR and FEV$_1$ were approximately 20% higher in the flunisolide group, beginning at 90 minutes. McFadden suggests this benefit stems from steroid-induced vasoconstriction, decreasing airway wall edema, vascular congestion, and plasma exudation, and not anti-inflammatory effects.[136] Recently Rodrigo and Rodrigo demonstrated therapeutic benefit from triple drug therapy (flunisolide, albuterol, and ipratropium bromide) in high doses in patients not receiving systemic steroids.[137]

To the contrary, Guttman and colleagues found no benefit from the addition of beclomethasone 7 mg every 8 hours by MDI with spacer to nebulized salbutamol and systemic corticosteroid therapy.[138] Further study demonstrated that beclomethasone (5 mg delivered by MDI) during the initial 4 hours of ER treatment did not confer added benefit to albuterol in adults with mild to moderately severe asthma.[139]

Our view is that there is little benefit to the addition of inhaled steroids to high-dose β agonists and systemic corticosteroids in the management of acute asthma. Still, consideration should be given to the use of high-dose inhaled corticosteroids in refractory patients.

AMINOPHYLLINE

There is no benefit to adding aminophylline to inhaled β agonists in the initial treatment of acute asthma.[140] In a meta-analysis by Parameswaran and colleagues there was a trend toward higher PEFR at 12 and 24 hours, but at the cost of arrhythmias and vomiting.[141] Others have reported a delayed benefit.[142] In another recent meta-analysis in children, aminophylline was shown to improve FEV$_1$ by 6 to 8 hours and provide sustained benefit for 24 hours.[143] Nonbronchodilating properties of aminophylline may be useful in refractory cases. Anti-inflammatory effects and enhanced diaphragm function may explain one report that ED administration of aminophylline decreased hospitalizations, even when airflow rates were no different than placebo.[144]

We rarely use aminophylline in refractory patients, but generally continue its use (after confirming a nontoxic serum concentration) in patients already taking theophylline. This approach is safe if attention is paid to serum drug levels and to factors that increase levels, such as congestive heart failure, ciprofloxacin, macrolide antibiotics, and cimetidine, and if the drug is discontinued in the presence of side effects.

MAGNESIUM SULFATE

Three prospective trials failed to confirm a benefit to administering magnesium sulfate (MgSO$_4$) to asthmatics in the ED.[145–147] In 135 asthmatics randomized to 2 g MgSO$_4$ IV or placebo after 30 minutes and followed for 4 hours, admission rates and FEV$_1$ were no different between magnesium-treated patients and controls.[147] However, subgroup analysis revealed MgSO$_4$ decreased admission rates and improved FEV$_1$ in subjects with FEV$_1$ <25% of predicted. Subsequently, a placebo-controlled, double-blind, randomized trial in 248 patients with FEV$_1$ $\leq$30% showed a small but statistically significant increase in FEV$_1$ after 240 minutes in the magnesium group, but no difference in hospitalization rates.[148] Meta-analysis of 9 trials and 665 patients demonstrated nonsignificant improvements in peak flows and admission rates for all patients, but in those with severe exacerbations, MgSO$_4$ increased FEV$_1$ by nearly 10% compared to placebo, and decreased admissions.[149] Additional evidence supporting benefit in severe disease comes from an uncontrolled study of five intubated asthmatics given magnesium.[150] In this study, there was a fall in peak airway pressure (43 cm H$_2$O to 32 cm H$_2$O) after high doses of MgSO$_4$ (10 to 20 g) were administered over 1 hour. Other investigators have suggested that gender may play a role in magnesium responsiveness, since estrogen augments the bronchodilator effect of magnesium.[151] Routine use of MgSO$_4$ is not justified, but MgSO$_4$ is safe, inexpensive, and may be beneficial in severe exacerbations.

Magnesium sulfate can also be administered by inhalation. Nannini and colleagues studied the effects of MgSO$_4$ (225 mg) vs. saline as the vehicle for nebulized albuterol in a randomized, double-blind fashion.[152] At 20 minutes, patients treated with MgSO$_4$ and albuterol had a greater PEFR compared to the saline-albuterol group (134 ± 70 L/m vs. 86 ± 64 L/m). Hughes and colleagues have published similar data.[153]

LEUKOTRIENE MODIFIERS

Cysteinyl leukotrienes are elevated in asthmatic sputum compared to controls and higher in subjects studied within 48 hours of exacerbation.[154] Preliminary data demonstrating benefit to a leukotriene receptor antagonist came from a double-blind, randomized trial of two doses (20 mg and

160 mg) of zafirlukast orally versus placebo in 641 asthmatics after 30 minutes of standard treatment.[155] Zafirlukast 160 mg decreased admission rates, relapses, and treatment failures. In another double-blind, placebo-controlled study of 20 patients not receiving systemic steroids in an ED, oral montelukast 10 mg resulted in a trend toward a shorter duration of stay and higher peak flows, and fewer patients requiring aminophylline or steroids.[156] In the most compelling trial to date, Camargo and colleagues randomized 201 acute asthmatics to standard therapy plus montelukast 7 mg or 14 mg IV or placebo.[157] Montelukast improved FEV_1 over the first 20 minutes (14.8% vs. 3.6% with placebo). Benefits were seen within 10 minutes and lasted for 2 hours; both treatment doses were equivalent. Montelukast also tended to result in less β-agonist use and fewer treatment failures.

HELIOX

Heliox is a mixture of 20% oxygen and 80% helium (30%:70% and 40%:60% mixtures are also available). As the percentage of helium decreases, so does the benefit of breathing this gas blend. Concentrations of helium less than 60% are ineffective, precluding its use in significant hypoxemia. Heliox is slightly more viscous than air, but significantly less dense, resulting in a more than threefold increase in kinematic viscosity (the ratio of gas viscosity to gas density) compared to air. Theoretically, this property decreases the driving pressure required for gas flow by two mechanisms. First, for any level of turbulent flow, breathing low-density gas decreases the pressure gradient required for flow. Second, heliox decreases the Reynolds number, favoring conversion of turbulent flow to laminar flow.[158] Heliox does not treat bronchospasm or airway wall inflammation.

Heliox promptly improves dyspnea, work of breathing, and arterial blood gases in upper airway obstruction.[159] Benefits have also been reported in acute asthma. In adults treated in an ED, an 80:20 mix delivered by tight-fitting face mask increased PEFR and decreased PP, suggesting improved airway resistance and work of breathing.[160] Similar results have been published in children.[161] Other studies have failed to demonstrate benefit.[162-164] In a recent meta-analysis by Rodrigo and colleagues of four randomized trials and 288 patients, the authors concluded that the evidence does not support the use of heliox in nonintubated asthmatics in the ED.[165] However, methodologic differences between studies limit the ability to draw conclusions.

If heliox is effective, it may give time for concurrent therapies to work, and thereby avert the need for intubation in some cases. Of theoretical concern is the potential for heliox to mask worsening airflow obstruction, so there is less time (and no margin for error) to control the airway when intubation is required.

Whether heliox augments the bronchodilator effect of inhaled β agonists compared to delivery in air (presumably due to low-density gas facilitating albuterol deposition) is unclear. Data are available demonstrating benefit to heliox as a driving gas,[166] but there are also data to the contrary.[167]

ANTIBIOTICS

Because viruses trigger most infectious exacerbations of asthma and bacterial pneumonia is rare, there is likely no role for antibiotics in treating acute asthma. Antibiotics are frequently prescribed for an increase in sputum volume and purulence. However, purulence may reflect an abundance of eosinophils, not polymorphonuclear leukocytes. The importance of *Mycoplasma pneumoniae* in acute asthma is unknown. A recent study by Lieberman using paired serology demonstrated evidence for mycoplasma infection in 18% of patients hospitalized for acute asthma.[168] In their 2002 update, the Expert Panel from the NIH did not recommend the use of antibiotics in asthma exacerbation unless there was fever with purulent sputum, evidence for pneumonia, or suspected bacterial sinusitis.[169] In a separate review of the literature, Graham and associates recently selected 2 out of 128 possible studies adequate for review, concluding that the role of antibiotics is difficult to assess.[170]

NONINVASIVE POSITIVE PRESSURE VENTILATION

Noninvasive positive pressure ventilation (NPPV) by face mask is an option for patients with hypercapneic respiratory failure who do not require intubation. Continuous positive airway pressure (CPAP) helps overcome the adverse effects of PEEPi and decreases the inspiratory work of breathing.[171] Bronchial dilation also occurs during CPAP.[172] Advantages of NPPV over intubation include decreased need for sedation and paralysis, decreased incidence of nosocomial pneumonia, decreased incidence of otitis and sinusitis, and improved patient comfort.[173] Disadvantages include increased risk of aspiration when there is gastric insufflation, skin necrosis, and diminished control of ventilatory status compared with invasive ventilation. Data regarding the efficacy of NPPV in acute asthma are limited. In one study[174] of 21 acute asthmatics with a mean PEFR of 144 L/min, nasal CPAP of 5 or 7.5 cm H_2O decreased respiratory rate and dyspnea compared to placebo. In another study,[175] Meduri and colleagues reported their observational experience with NPPV during 17 episodes of acute severe asthma. NPPV was achieved using a loose-fitting full-face mask with initial settings of 0 cm H_2O CPAP and 10 cm H_2O pressure support ventilation. CPAP was increased to 3 to 5 cm H_2O and pressure support was titrated to achieve an exhaled tidal volume of ≥ 7 mL/kg and a respiratory rate of <25/min. The average duration of NPPV was 16 hours. NPPV generally improved dyspnea, HR, RR, and blood gases. Two NPPV-treated patients required intubation for worsening Pa_{CO_2}. There were no NPPV complications.

Management of the Intubated Asthmatic

INTUBATION

The goals of intubation and mechanical ventilation are to maintain oxygenation and prevent respiratory arrest. Patients who are intubated before they arrest generally do well (if ventilated appropriately); patients who are intubated after respiratory arrest and the development of anoxic brain injury do not. Approximately 40% of deaths in ventilated asthmatics are due to cerebral anoxia resulting from respiratory arrest prior to mechanical ventilation.[176]

Intubation is indicated for impending respiratory failure and cardiopulmonary arrest. Changes in posture, mental status, speech, accessory muscle use, and RR can indicate progressive ventilatory failure that does not need blood-gas or PEFR confirmation. In the final analysis, the decision to intubate rests on a clinician's estimate of the patient's ability to maintain spontaneous respiration.

Oral intubation is preferred because it allows for placement of an adequately sized endotracheal tube (e.g., 8.0 mm inside diameter [ID] for adult women, 8.0 to 9.0 mm ID for adult men) to facilitate removal of mucus and decrease airflow resistance. Nasal intubation is acceptable in an awake patient anticipated to be difficult to position and intubate (fiberoptic guidance may facilitate intubation in this setting), but is complicated by the need for a smaller endotracheal tube and the high incidence of nasal polyps and sinusitis in asthma.

POSTINTUBATION HYPOTENSION

Hypotension has been reported in 25% to 35% of patients following intubation.[176] It occurs for several reasons. First, there is loss of vascular tone due to a direct effect of sedation and loss of sympathetic activity. Second, patients may be hypovolemic from high insensible losses and decreased oral fluid intake. Third, overzealous Ambu Bag ventilation results in DHI because adequate time is not provided for exhalation. When this occurs, breath sounds diminish, BP falls, and HR rises. Manual breaths take considerable effort because the hyperinflated lung is stiff (noncompliant). A trial of hypopnea (2 to 3 breaths/min) or apnea in a preoxygenated patient deflates the lung. After 30 to 60 seconds of hypoventilation, intrathoracic pressure falls, allowing for greater preload to the right atrium; BP rises, HR falls, and breaths become easier to deliver, confirming DHI.

A trial of hypopnea or apnea is both diagnostic and therapeutic for DHI. However, hemodynamic improvement during such a trial does not exclude tension pneumothorax. Tension pneumothoraces may have been responsible for >6%

of deaths of patients who required mechanical ventilation for severe asthma.[176] Careful inspection of the chest x-ray is mandatory because the lungs may not collapse completely in the setting of DHI and widespread mucus plugging. Unilateral pneumothorax conceivably increases ventilation to the contralateral lung, increasing the risk of bilateral pneumothoraces. Given these considerations, chest tubes should not be placed until a trial of hypoventilation has failed or there is radiographic evidence of pneumothorax.

INITIAL VENTILATOR SETTINGS AND DYNAMIC HYPERINFLATION

Expiratory time, tidal volume, and severity of airway obstruction determine the level of DHI (Fig. 40-1). Minute ventilation and inspiratory flow determine expiratory time.[177,178] To avoid dangerous levels of DHI, initial minute ventilation should not exceed 115 mL/kg per minute or approximately 8 L/min in a 70-kg patient.[179] To this end, we recommend a RR between 12 and 14/min and a tidal volume between 7 and 8 mL/kg. The use of low tidal volumes avoids excessive peak lung inflation, which can occur even with low minute ventilation.

Shortening the inspiratory time by use of a high inspiratory flow rate further prolongs expiratory time. We favor a flow rate of 80 L/min, using a constant flow rate pattern. High inspiratory flows increase peak airway pressure by elevating airway resistive pressure, but peak airway pressure per se does not correlate with morbidity or mortality. Rather it is the state of lung hyperinflation that predicts outcome (see below). High inspiratory flow and high airway pressures

FIGURE 40-1 Effects of ventilator settings on airway pressures and lung volumes during normocapneic ventilation of eight paralyzed asthmatic patients. V_{EE} = lung volume at end expiration; V_{EI} = lung volume at end inspiration; Ppk = peak airway pressure; Pplat = end inspiratory plateau pressure; V_E = minute ventilation; V_I = inspiratory flow. A. As inspiratory flow

is decreased from 100 L/min to 40 L/min at the same V_E, Ppk falls, but hyperinflation increases due to dynamic gas trapping. B. Dynamic hyperinflation is reduced by low respiratory rates and high tidal volumes (as long as V_E is decreased), but high tidal volumes result in high Pplat. (*Reproduced with permission from Tuxen et al.[178]*)

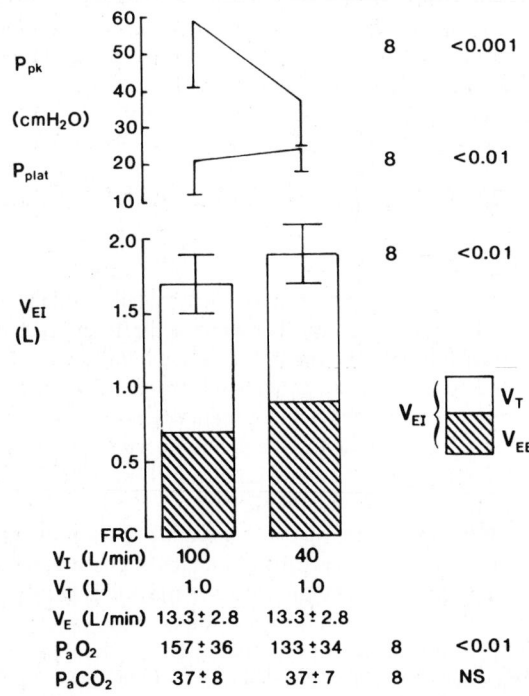

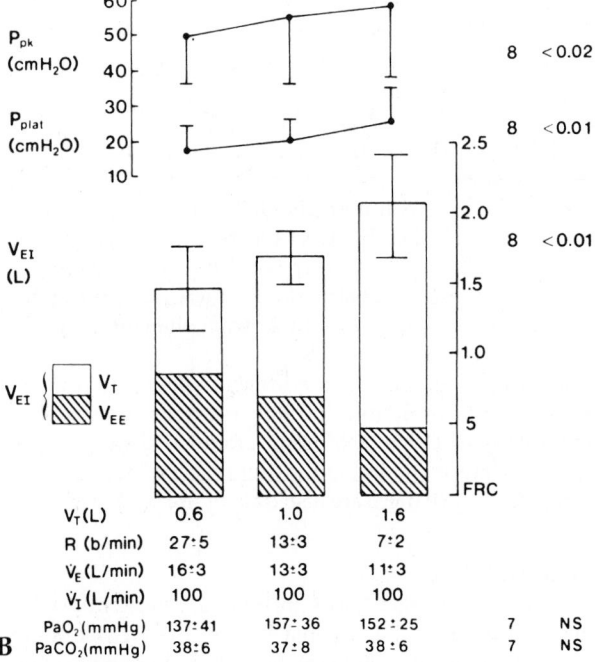

may redistribute ventilation to low-resistance lung units, risking barotrauma, but these concerns are based largely on mathematical and mechanical lung models,[180,181] and have no supporting clinical data. Another concern in spontaneously breathing patients is that high inspiratory flow rates in the assist-control mode can increase RR and thereby decrease expiratory time.[182]

There is no consensus as to which ventilator mode should be used in asthmatics. In paralyzed patients, synchronized intermittent mandatory ventilation (SIMV) and assist-controlled ventilation (ACV) are equivalent. In patients triggering the ventilator, SIMV is generally preferred because of the unproven concern that minute ventilation will be higher during ACV, since each triggered breath receives a guaranteed tidal volume.[183] However, in spontaneously breathing patients, SIMV may increase work of breathing and machine-patient dyssynchrony if set minute ventilation is low.[184] Volume-controlled ventilation (VCV) is recommended over pressure-controlled ventilation (PCV) for several reasons, including staff familiarity with its use. PCV offers the advantage of limiting peak airway pressure to a predetermined set value. However, during PCV, tidal volume is inversely related to PEEPi and minute ventilation is not guaranteed. Peak inspiratory flow rates may be extremely high in PCV (to compensate for decelerating flow) to maintain a short inspiratory time.

Ventilator-applied PEEP is not recommended in sedated and paralyzed patients because it may increase lung volume if used excessively.[185] In spontaneously breathing patients, small amounts of ventilator-applied PEEP (e.g., 5 cm H$_2$O) decrease inspiratory work of breathing by decreasing the pressure gradient required to overcome PEEPi.

ASSESSING LUNG INFLATION

Determining the level of DHI is central to risk assessment and ventilator adjustment. Numerous methods have been proposed to measure DHI. The volume at end-inspiration, termed V$_{EI}$, is determined by collecting all expired gas from the end-inspiratory volume to functional reserve capacity (FRC) during 40 to 60 seconds of apnea (Fig. 40-2). Although V$_{EI}$ may underestimate the degree of air trapping if there are very slowly emptying air spaces, V$_{EI}$ greater than 20 mL/kg correlates with barotrauma.[179] The utility of this measure is limited by the need for paralysis, and the fact that most clinicians and respiratory therapists are unfamiliar with expiratory gas collection.

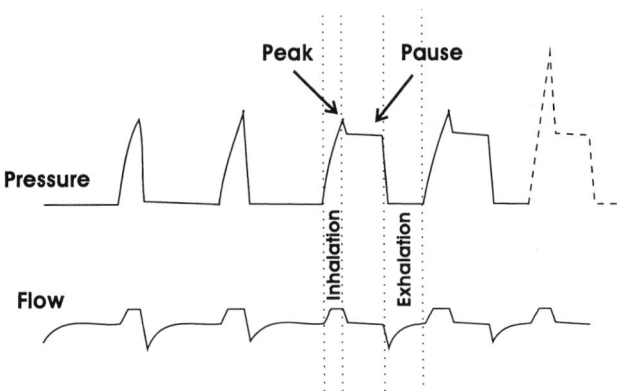

FIGURE 40-3 Simultaneous plots of flow and airway pressure in a mechanically ventilated patient. The peak-to-pause or peak-to-plateau gradient is determined by temporarily occluding inspiratory flow. End-inspiratory occlusions should be done cautiously and briefly in patients with status asthmaticus, since expiratory time may be shortened and gas trapping may worsen. Under conditions of constant inspiratory flow and absence of patient effort, the peak-plateau gradient can be used as a measure of the severity of inspiratory airway resistance, and of the efficacy of bronchodilator therapy. The dotted line indicates a high peak-pause gradient as one would see in status asthmaticus. The plateau pressure is a reflection of the respiratory system pressure change resulting from the delivery of the tidal volume, added to any level of intrinsic PEEP (PEEPi). Hence the plateau pressure is a useful marker for the degree of lung hyperinflation, and should be maintained at <30 cm H$_2$O.

Surrogate measures of DHI include the single-breath plateau pressure (Pplat) and PEEPi. Neither is perfect. Pplat is an estimate of average end-inspiratory alveolar pressures that is determined by stopping flow at end-inspiration (Fig. 40-3). PEEPi is the lowest average alveolar pressure achieved during the respiratory cycle. It is obtained by measuring airway-opening pressure during an end-expiratory hold maneuver (Fig. 40-4). In the presence of PEEPi, airway-opening pressure increases to the amount of PEEPi present. Persistence of expiratory gas flow at the beginning of inspiration (which can be detected by auscultation or monitoring of flow tracings) also demonstrates PEEPi.[186]

Accurate measurement of Pplat and PEEPi requires patient-ventilator synchrony and patient relaxation. Paralysis is generally not required. Unfortunately neither measure has been validated as a predictor of complications. Pplat is affected by the lung and surrounding structures so that variations in DHI occur at the same pressure. For example, an obese patient will have a higher Pplat than a thin patient for the same degree of DHI. Despite these limitations, experience suggests that a Pplat <30 cm H$_2$O is generally safe.

PEEPi may underestimate the severity of DHI (see above). This may occur when airway closure limits communication between the alveolus and airway opening, so that during an end-exhalation hold maneuver, airway-opening pressure does not rise. In most cases, however, PEEPi <15 cm H$_2$O is acceptable.

VENTILATOR ADJUSTMENTS

Relying on Pplat as a measure of DHI, we provide the following suggestions for ventilator adjustments. If initial settings

FIGURE 40-2 One way to measure lung hyperinflation is to collect the total exhaled volume during a period of apnea (usually 20 to 60 seconds). This volume, termed V$_{EI}$, is the volume of gas at end-inspiration above FRC, and is the sum of the tidal volume and volume at end-exhalation above FRC (V$_{EE}$). V$_{EI}$ above a threshold value of 20 mL/kg (1.4 L in an average-size adult) has been shown to predict complications of hypotension and barotrauma. (*From Tuxen et al.*[177])

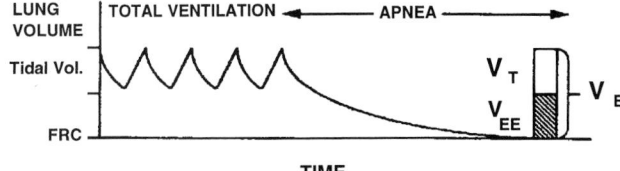

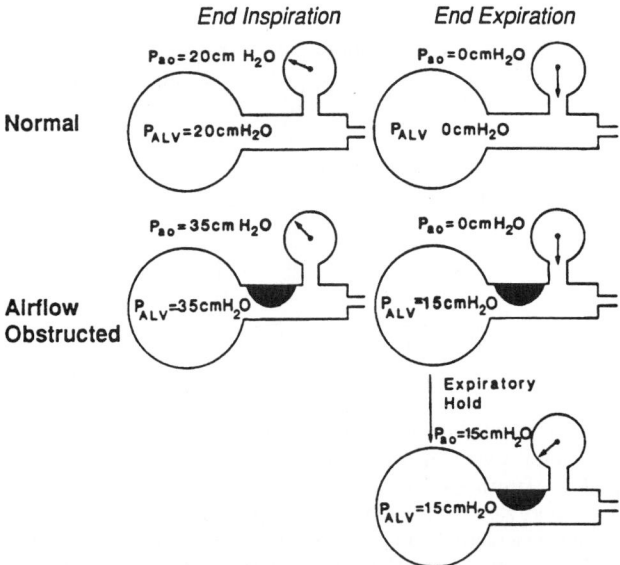

End Inspiration   *End Expiration*

Normal

$P_{ao} = 20cm\ H_2O$ $P_{ao} = 0cmH_2O$

$P_{ALV} = 20cmH_2O$ P_{ALV} $0cmH_2O$

Airflow Obstructed

$P_{ao} = 35\ cm\ H_2O$ $P_{ao} = 0cmH_2O$

$P_{ALV} = 35cmH_2O$ $P_{ALV} = 15cmH_2O$

Expiratory Hold

$P_{ao} = 15cmH_2O$

$P_{ALV} = 15cmH_2O$

FIGURE 40-4 Measurement of auto- or intrinsic PEEP (PEEPi). Under normal conditions, alveolar pressure (P_{ALV}) closely tracks pressure at the airway opening (Pao), which is reported on the ventilator manometer. At end-expiration, P_{ALV} falls to atmospheric pressure (0 cm H_2O) and is accurately reflected by Pao. In severe airflow obstruction, P_{ALV} may increase because of gas trapping, and at end-expiration P_{ALV} has not fallen to atmospheric pressure and does not equal Pao. If an expiratory hold maneuver is performed, Pao will rise, reflecting the degree of gas trapping.

result in Pplat >30 cm H_2O, RR is decreased until this goal is achieved, even at the cost of hypercapnia. Hypercapnia is generally well tolerated in oxygenated patients, even to Pa$_{CO_2}$ values nearing 90 mm Hg, as long as sudden changes do not occur.[187,188] Anoxic brain injury and myocardial dysfunction are contraindications to permissive hypercapnia, which may induce cerebral vasodilation, decrease myocardial contractility, and constrict the pulmonary vascular bed.[189] Lowering minute ventilation may not cause the expected rise in P$_{CO_2}$ if dead space decreases concurrently.

If hypercapnia results in a blood pH of less than 7.20 (and RR can not be increased because of the Pplat limit), we consider a slow infusion of sodium bicarbonate, although this has not been shown to improve outcome.[190] If Pplat is less than 30 cm H_2O and pH is less than 7.20, RR can be safely increased for the purpose of lowering Pa$_{CO_2}$ and elevating arterial pH until Pplat nears the threshold pressure. Commonly, patients can be ventilated to a pH >7.20 with a Pplat <30 cm H_2O.

SEDATION AND PARALYSIS
Sedation is indicated to improve comfort, safety, and patient-ventilator synchrony. This is particularly true when hypercapnia serves as a potent stimulus to respiratory drive. Some patients (such as those with sudden-onset asthma) may be ready for extubation within hours. In these patients, propofol is attractive because it can be rapidly titrated to a deep level of sedation, and there is quick reversal of sedation after discontinuation.[191] Lorazepam and midazolam are less expensive alternatives.[192] Time to awakening after discontinuation of benzodiazepines is longer and less predictable than with propofol.

In order to provide the best combination of amnesia, sedation, analgesia, and suppression of respiratory drive, we recommend the addition of a narcotic by continuous infusion to propofol or a benzodiazepine.[193] Morphine and fentanyl are the two most commonly used narcotics. Fentanyl has a quicker onset of action than morphine. Narcotics may release histamine and worsen bronchospasm if they are delivered by bolus administration. Daily interruption of sedatives avoids unwanted drug accumulation.[194]

Ketamine, an IV anesthetic with sedative, analgesic, and bronchodilating properties, is reserved for use in intubated patients with severe bronchospasm that precludes safe mechanical ventilation.[195–197] Ketamine must be used with caution because of its sympathomimetic effects and ability to cause delirium.

When safe and effective mechanical ventilation cannot be achieved by sedation alone, short-term muscle paralysis is indicated. Short- to intermediate-acting agents include atracurium, cis-atracurium, and vecuronium. Pancuronium is longer acting and less expensive, and its vagolytic effects cause tachycardia. Pancuronium and atracurium release histamine, but this is of doubtful clinical significance.[198] We prefer cis-atracurium because it is essentially free of cardiovascular effects, does not release histamine, and does not require hepatic and renal function for clearance.

Paralytics may be given intermittently by bolus or continuous IV infusion. If a continuous infusion is used, a nerve stimulator should be used or the drug should be withheld every 4 to 6 hours to avoid drug accumulation. Paralytic agents should be minimized whenever possible because of the risk of postparalytic myopathy.[199–201] In one study of 25 ventilated asthmatics, 19 (76%) patients had an increase in serum creatine kinase, and 9 (36%) had clinically detectable myopathy.[201] Elevated creatine kinase was associated with prolonged mechanical ventilation whether or not there was clinically detectable myopathy. In a retrospective cohort study of 107 episodes of asthma requiring intubation, the concurrent use of steroids and a paralytic was associated with muscle weakness in 29% of episodes; steroid treatment alone was not associated with weakness.[199] Importantly, this study demonstrated that the duration of paralysis correlated with the incidence of myopathy, which is rare when paralytics are used for less than 24 hours. Findings of a separate study confirm this correlation.[200] Most patients with postparalytic myopathy recover, but may require weeks of rehabilitation.

ADMINISTRATION OF BRONCHODILATORS DURING MECHANICAL VENTILATION

Many questions remain regarding the administration of inhaled bronchodilators to intubated patients. In one study,[202] only 2.9% of a radioactive aerosol delivered by nebulizer was deposited in the lungs of mechanically ventilated patients. Manthous and colleagues compared the efficacy of albuterol delivered by MDI via a simple inspiratory adapter (no spacer) to nebulized albuterol in intubated patients.[203] Using the peak-to-pause pressure gradient at a constant inspiratory flow to measure airway resistance, they found no effect (and no side effects) from the administration of 100 puffs (9.0 mg) of albuterol. Albuterol delivered by nebulizer to a total dose of 2.5 mg reduced the inspiratory flow-resistive pressure 18%. Increasing the nebulized dose to a total of 7.5 mg reduced airway resistance further in 8 of 10 patients, but caused side effects in half of the patients. Thus if MDIs are used during mechanical ventilation, use of a spacer on the inspiratory limb of the ventilator improves drug delivery.[204]

Regardless of whether an MDI with spacer or nebulizer is used, higher drug dosages are required and the dosage should be titrated to achieve a fall in the peak-to-pause airway pressure gradient. Nebulizers should be placed close to the ventilator, and in-line humidifiers stopped during treatments. Inspiratory flow should be reduced to approximately 40 L/min during treatments to minimize turbulence, although this strategy may worsen DHI and must be time-limited. Patient-ventilator synchrony is crucial to optimize drug delivery. The use of heliox as a driving gas may enhance the delivery of albuterol to target airways. When no measurable drop in airway resistance occurs, other causes of elevated airway resistance such as a kinked or plugged endotracheal tube should be excluded. Bronchodilator nonresponders should also be considered for a drug holiday. Data from randomized controlled trials are needed to determine the effects of bronchodilators in intubated patients, and to provide evidence for or against usual clinical recommendations for bronchodilator use.[205]

OTHER CONSIDERATIONS

Rarely, the above strategies are unable to stabilize the patient on the ventilator. In these situations other therapies are available. Halothane and enflurane are general anesthetic bronchodilators that acutely reduce Ppk and Pa_{CO_2}.[206,207] These agents cause myocardial depression, arterial vasodilation, and arrhythmias, and their benefit does not last after drug discontinuation. Heliox delivered through the ventilator circuit may decrease Ppk and Pa_{CO_2}.[208] However, safe use of heliox requires significant institutional expertise and careful planning. Flow meters (which are gas-density dependent) must be recalibrated for heliox, and a spirometer should be placed on the expiratory port of the ventilator during heliox administration to measure tidal volume. A trial of heliox use in a lung model is recommended prior to patient use.

Strategies to mobilize mucus such as chest physiotherapy or treatment with mucolytics or expectorants have not been proven effective in controlled trials. Bronchoalveolar lavage using either saline or acetylcysteine may be useful in nonintubated patients.[209–211] This procedure is theoretically risky because the bronchoscope increases expiratory airway resistance and may worsen bronchospasm and PEEPi.

EXTUBATION

Patients with sudden-onset asthma may respond quickly to bronchodilators. More often 24 to 48 hours of bronchodilator/anti-inflammatory therapy is required before patients are ready for extubation. As a general rule, we perform a spontaneous breathing trial once Pa_{CO_2} normalizes at a minute ventilation that does not cause significant DHI, airway resistive pressure is <20 cm H_2O, mental status is intact, and significant muscle weakness is not seen. Depending on clinical status, we extubate within 30 to 120 minutes (as the endotracheal tube itself may perpetuate bronchospasm). Shortly after extubation, we administer albuterol and ipratropium bromide by nebulization. Observation in the ICU is recommended for an additional 12 to 24 hours. During this period, the focus can switch to safe transfer to a medical ward and maximizing outpatient management.

References

1. National Asthma Education and Prevention Program (NAEPP): Expert Panel Report 2: Guidelines for the Diagnosis and Management of Asthma. National Heart, Lung, and Blood Institute (NHLBI), National Institutes of Health (NIH). NIH Publication No. 97-4051, April 1997.
2. Busse WW, Calhoun WF, Sedgewick JD: Mechanism of airway inflammation in asthma. *Am Rev Respir Dis* 147:S20, 1993.
3. Reed CE: New therapeutic approaches to asthma. *J Allergy Clin Immunol* 77:537, 1986.
4. Robertson CF, Rubinfeld AR, Bowes G: Pediatric asthma deaths in Victoria: The mild are at risk. *Pediatr Pulmonol* 13:95, 1992.
5. Nanini L: Morbidity and mortality, in Hall JB, Corbridge T, Rodrigo C, Rodrigo G (eds): *Acute Asthma: Assessment and Management.* New York, McGraw-Hill, 2000, p 11.
6. Asthma in America Survey: A Landmark Survey. Executive summary. Schulman, Ronca and Bucuvalas, Inc.(SRBI) 1998, p 1.
7. Van den Toorn LM, Overbeek SE, de Jongste JC, et al: Airway inflammation is present during clinical remission of atopic asthma. *Am J Respir Crit Care Med* 164:2107, 2001.
8. Laitinen LA, Laitinen A, Haahtela T: A comparative study of the effects of an inhaled corticosteroid, budesonide, and a beta 2-agonist, terbutaline, on airway inflammation in newly diagnosed asthma: a randomized, double-blind, parallel group controlled trial. *J Allergy Clin Immunol* 90:32, 1992.
9. Donahue JG, Weiss ST, Livingston JM, et al: Inhaled steroids and the risk of hospitalization for asthma. *JAMA* 277:887, 1997.
10. Suissa S, Ernst P, Benayoun S, et al: Low-dose inhaled corticosteroids and the prevention of death from asthma. *N Engl J Med* 343:332, 2000.
11. Corbridge T, Hall JB: State of the art: The assessment and management of adults with status asthmaticus. *Am J Respir Crit Care Med* 151:1296, 1995.
12. Arnold AG, Lane DJ, Zapata E: The speed of onset and severity of acute severe asthma. *Br J Dis Chest* 76:157, 1982.
13. Petty TL: Treat status asthmaticus three days before it occurs. *J Intensive Care Med* 4:135, 1989.
14. Hogg JC: The pathology of asthma. *Clin Chest Med* 5:567, 1984.
15. Wasserfallen JB, Schaller MD, Feihl F, et al: Sudden asphyxic asthma: a distinct entity? *Am Rev Respir Dis* 142:108, 1990.
16. Arnold AG, Lane DJ, Zapata E: The speed of onset and severity of acute severe asthma. *Br J Dis Chest* 76:157, 1982.
17. Sur S, Crotty TB, Kephart GM, et al: Sudden-onset fatal asthma: a distinct clinical entity with few eosinophils and relatively more neutrophils in the airway submucosa. *Am Rev Respir Dis* 148:713, 1993.
18. Ried LM: The presence or absence of bronchial mucus in fatal asthma. *J Allergy Clin Immunol* 80:415, 1987.
19. Rome LA, Lippmann ML, Dalsey WC, et al. Prevalence of cocaine use and its impact on asthma exacerbation in an urban population. *Chest* 117:1324, 2000.
20. Cygan J, Trunsky M, Corbridge T: Inhaled heroin-induced status asthmaticus. *Chest* 117:272, 2000.
21. Levenson T, Greenberger PA, Donoghue ER, Lifshultz BD: Asthma deaths confounded by substance abuse: an assessment of fatal asthma. *Chest* 110:604, 1996.
22. Krantz AJ, Hershow RC, Prachand N: Heroin insufflation as a trigger for patients with life-threatening asthma. *Chest* 123:510, 2003.
23. Rodrigo G, Rodrigo C: Rapid-onset asthma attack: a prospective cohort study about characteristics and response to emergency department treatment. *Chest* 118:1547, 2000.
24. Rodriguez-Roisin R, Ballester E, Roca J, et al: Mechanisms of hypoxemia in patients with status asthmaticus requiring mechanical ventilation. *Am Rev Respir Dis* 139:732, 1989.

25. Nowak RM, Tomlanovich MC, Sarker DD, et al: Arterial blood gases and pulmonary function testing in acute bronchial asthma: Predicting patient outcomes. *JAMA* 249:2043, 1983.

26. McFadden ER Jr, Lyons HA: Arterial-blood gas tension in asthma. *N Engl J Med* 278:1027, 1968.

27. Roca J, Ramis LI, Rodriguez-Roisin R, et al: Serial relationships between ventilation-perfusion inequality and spirometry in acute severe asthma requiring hospitalization. *Am Rev Resp Dis* 137:1055, 1988.

28. Ferrer A, Roca J, Wagner PD, et al: Airway obstruction and ventilation-perfusion relationships in acute severe asthma. *Am Rev Respir Dis* 147:579, 1993.

29. West JB: State of the art: Ventilation-perfusion relationships. *Am Rev Respir Dis* 116:919, 1977.

30. Ballester E, Reyes A, Roca J, et al: Ventilation-perfusion mismatching in acute severe asthma: effects of salbutamol and 100% oxygen. *Thorax* 44:258, 1989.

31. Leatherman JW, Ravenscraft SA: Low measured auto-positive end-expiratory pressure during mechanical ventilation of patients with severe asthma: Hidden auto-positive end-expiratory pressure. *Crit Care Med* 24:541, 1996.

32. Van der Touw T, Mudaliar Y, Nayyar V: Static pressure-volume relationship of the respiratory system and pulmonary hyperinflation in mechanically ventilated patients with acute severe asthma. *Am J Respir Crit Care Med* 153:A370, 1996.

33. Scharf S, Brown R, Tow D, et al: Cardiac effects of increased lung volume and decreased pleural pressure. *J Appl Physiol* 47:257, 1979.

34. Scharf S, Brown R, Saunders N, et al: Effects of normal and loaded spontaneous inspiration on cardiovascular function. *J Appl Physiol* 47:582, 1979.

35. Permutt S, Wise RA: Mechanical interaction of respiration and circulation, in Fishman A (ed): *Handbook of Physiology*, Vol 3. Baltimore, Williams & Wilkins, 1986, p 647.

36. Knowles G, Clark TJ: Pulsus paradoxus as a valuable sign indicating severity of asthma. *Lancet* 2:1356, 1973.

37. Kelsen SG, Kelsen DP, Fleegler BF, et al: Emergency room assessment and treatment of patients with acute asthma. *Am J Med* 64:622, 1978.

38. Yanos J, Wood LD, Davis K, et al: The effect of respiratory and lactic acidosis on diaphragm function. *Am Rev Respir Dis* 147:616, 1993.

39. O'Connell MB, Iber C: Continuous intravenous terbutaline infusions for adult patients with status asthmaticus. *Ann Allergy* 64:213, 1990.

40. Appel D, Rubenstein R, Shrager K, et al: Lactic acidosis in severe asthma. *Am J Med* 75:580, 1983.

41. Rodrigo G, Rodrigo C: Assessment of the patient with acute asthma in the emergency department: A factor analytic study. *Chest* 104:1325, 1993.

42. Greenberger PA, Patterson R: The diagnosis of potentially fatal asthma. *NER Allergy Proc* 9:147, 1988.

43. Lowenthal M, Patterson R, Greenberger PA: The application of an asthma severity index in patients with potentially fatal asthma. *Chest* 104:1329, 1996.

44. Rea HH, Scragg R, Jackson R, et al: A case-controlled study of deaths from asthma. *Thorax* 41:833, 1986.

45. Suissa S, Ernst P, Boivin JF, et al: A cohort analysis of excess mortality in asthma and the use of inhaled beta-agonists. *Am J Respir Crit Care Med* 149:604, 1994.

46. Levenson T, Greenberger PA, Donoghue ER, et al: Asthma deaths confounded by substance abuse: An assessment of fatal asthma. *Chest* 110:604, 1996.

47. Liggett SB: Polymorphisms of the beta2-adrenergic receptor and asthma. *Am J Respir Crit Care Med* 156:S156, 1997.

48. Kikuchi Y, Okabe S, Tamura G, et al: Chemosensitivity and perception of dyspnea in patients with a history of near-fatal asthma. *N Engl J Med* 330:1329, 1994.

49. Fishman AP: Cardiac asthma—a fresh look at an old wheeze. *N Engl J Med* 320:1346, 1989.

50. Cabanes LR, Weber SN, Matran R, et al: Bronchial hyperresponsiveness to methacholine in patients with impaired left ventricular function. *N Engl J Med* 320:1317, 1989.

51. Baughman RP, Loudon RC: Stridor: differentiation from wheezing or upper airway noise. *Am Rev Respir Dis* 139:1407, 1989.

52. Hall JB, Wood LDH: Management of the critically ill asthmatic patient. *Med Clin North Am* 74:779, 1990.

53. Brenner BE, Abraham E, Simon RR: Position and diaphoresis in acute asthma. *Am J Med* 74:1005, 1983.

54. Shim CS, Williams MH: Relationship of wheezing to the severity of obstruction in asthma. *Arch Intern Med* 143:890, 1983.

55. Grossman J: The occurrence of arrhythmias in hospitalized asthma patients. *J Allergy Clin Immunol* 57:310, 1976.

56. Josephson GW, Kennedy HL, MacKenzie EJ: Cardiac dysrhythmias during the treatment of acute asthma: A comparison of two treatment regimens by a double blind protocol. *Chest* 78:429, 1980.

57. Rebuck AS, Read J: Assessment and management of severe asthma. *Am J Med* 51:788, 1971.

58. Scharf S: Mechanical cardiopulmonary interactions with asthma. *Clin Rev Allergy* 3:487, 1985.

59. Shim CS, Williams MH Jr: Evaluation of the severity of asthma: patients versus physicians. *Am J Med* 68:11, 1980.

60. Lim TK, Ang SM, Rossing TH, et al: The effects of deep inhalation on maximal expiratory flow during intensive treatment of spontaneous asthmatic episodes. *Am Rev Respir Dis* 140:340, 1989.

61. Lemarchand P, Labrune S, Herer B, et al: Cardiorespiratory arrest following peak expiratory flow measurement during attack of asthma. *Chest* 100:1168, 1991.

62. Banner AS, Shah RS, Addington WW: Rapid prediction of need for hospitalization in acute asthma. *JAMA* 235:1337, 1976.

63. Fanta CH, Rossing TH, McFadden ER Jr: Emergency room treatment of asthma: Relationships among therapeutic combinations, severity of obstruction and time course of response. *Am J Med* 72:416, 1982.

64. Stein LM, Cole RP: Early administration of corticosteroids in emergency room treatment of acute asthma. *Ann Intern Med* 112:822, 1990.

65. Martin TG, Elenbaas RM, Pingleton SH: Failure of peak expiratory flow rate to predict hospital admission in acute asthma. *Ann Emerg Med* 11:466, 1982.

66. Mountain RD, Sahn S: Clinical features and outcome in patients with acute asthma presenting with hypercapnia. *Am Rev Respir Dis* 138:535, 1988.

67. McFadden ER Jr, Lyons HA: Arterial-blood gas tension in asthma. *N Engl J Med* 278:1027, 1968.

68. Mountain RD, Heffner JE, Brackett NC: Acid-base disturbances in acute asthma. *Chest* 98:651, 1990.

69. Findley LJ, Sahn SA: The value of chest roentgenograms in acute asthma in adults. *Chest* 5:535, 1980.

70. Zieverink SE, Harper AP, Holden RW, et al: Emergency room radiography of asthma: An efficacy study. *Radiology* 145:27, 1982.

71. Sherman S, Skoney JA, Ravikrishnan KP: Routine chest radiographs in exacerbations of acute obstructive pulmonary disease. *Arch Intern Med* 149:2493, 1989.

72. White CS, Cole RP, Lubetsky HW, et al: Acute asthma: admission chest radiography in hospitalized adult patients. *Chest* 100:14, 1991.

73. Feil SB, Swartz MA, Glanz K, et al: Efficacy of short-term corticosteroid therapy in outpatient treatment of acute bronchial asthma. *Am J Med* 75:259, 1983.

74. Ma X, Cheng Z, Kong H, et al: Changes in biophysical and biochemical properties of single bronchial smooth muscle cells from asthmatic subjects. *Am J Physiol Lung Cell Mol Physiol* 283:L1181, 2002.

75. Rossing TH, Fanta CH, McFadden ER: Effect of outpatient treatment of asthma with beta-agonists on the response to sympathomimetics in an emergency room. *Am J Med* 75:781, 1983.

76. Newhouse MT, Chapman KR, McCallum AL, et al: Cardiovascular safety of high doses of inhaled fenoterol and albuterol in acute severe asthma. *Chest* 110:595, 1996.

77. Gern JE, Lemanske RF: Beta-adrenergic agonist therapy. *Immunol Allergy Clin North Am* 13:839, 1993.

78. Paterson JW, Evans RJC, Prime FJ: Selectivity of bronchodilator action of salbutamol in asthmatic patients. *Br J Dis Chest* 65:21, 1971.

79. Shrestha M, Gourlay S, Robertson S, et al: Isoetharine versus albuterol for acute asthma: greater immediate effect, but more side effects. *Am J Med* 100:323, 1996.

80. Handley D: The asthma-like pharmacology and toxicology of (S)-isomers of beta agonists. *J Allergy Clin Immunol* 104:S69, 1999.

81. Nelson H, Bensch G, Pleskow WW, et al: Improved bronchodilation with levalbuterol compared with racemic albuterol in patients with asthma. *J Allergy Clin Immunol* 102:943, 1998.

82. Nowak R, Emerman CL, Schaefer K, et al: A pilot study to determine the safety and efficacy of escalating doses of levalbuterol in the treatment of acute asthma in the emergency department. *Emerg Med* 7:433, 2000.

83. Peters JI, Shelledy DC, Jones AP, et al: A randomized, placebo-controlled study to evaluate the role of salmeterol in the in-hospital management of asthma. *Chest* 118:313, 2000.

84. Fanta CH, Rossing TH, McFadden ER: Treatment of acute asthma: is combination therapy with sympathomimetics and methylxanthines indicated. *Am J Med* 80:5, 1986.

85. Uden DL, Goetz DR, Kohen DP, et al: Comparison of nebulized terbutaline and subcutaneous epinephrine in the treatment of acute asthma. *Ann Emerg Med* 14:229, 1985.

86. Becker AB, Nelson NA, Simons FER: Inhaled salbutamol (albuterol) vs injected epinephrine in the treatment of acute asthma in children. *J Pediatr* 102:465, 1983.

87. Appel D, Karpel JP, Sherman M: Epinephrine improves expiratory airflow rates in patients with asthma who do not respond to inhaled metaproterenol sulfate. *J Allergy Clin Immunol* 84:90, 1989.

88. Cydulka R, Davison R, Grammer L, et al: The use of epinephrine in the treatment of older adult asthmatics. *Ann Emerg Med* 17:322, 1990.

89. Lawford P, Jones BMJ, Milledge JS: Comparison of intravenous and nebulised salbutamol in initial treatment of severe asthma. *Br Med J* 1:84, 1978.

90. Williams SJ, Winner SJ, Clark TJH: Comparison of inhaled and intravenous terbutaline in acute severe asthma. *Thorax* 36:629, 1981.

91. Bloomfield P, Carmichael J, Petrie GR, et al: Comparison of salbutamol given intravenously and by intermittent positive-pressure breathing in life-threatening asthma. *Br Med J* 1:848, 1979.

92. Salmeron S, Brochard L, Mal H, et al: Nebulized versus intravenous albuterol in hypercapnic acute asthma: a multicenter, double-blind, randomized study. *Am J Respir Crit Care Med* 149:1466, 1994.

93. Cates CJ, Rowe BH, Bara A: Holding chambers versus nebulisers for beta-agonist treatment of acute asthma (Cochrane Review), in *The Cochrane Library*, Issue 2, 2003. Oxford, Update Software, Cochrane Review, 2/2002.

94. Idris AH, McDermott MF, Raucci JC, et al: Emergency department treatment of severe asthma: metered-dose inhaler plus holding chamber is equivalent in effectiveness to nebulizer. *Chest* 103:665, 1993.

95. Cydulka RK, McFadden ER, Sarver JH, et al: Comparison of single 7.5-mg dose treatment vs sequential multidose 2.5-mg treatments with nebulized albuterol in the treatment of acute asthma. *Chest* 122:1982, 2002.

96. Reisner C, Kotch A, Dworkin G: Continuous versus intermittent nebulization of albuterol in acute asthma: a randomized, prospective study. *Ann Allergy Asthma Immunol* 75:41, 1995.

97. Rudnitsky GS, Eberlein RS, Schoffstall JM, et al: Comparison of intermittent and continuously nebulized albuterol for treatment of asthma in an urban emergency department. *Ann Emerg Med* 22:1842, 1993.

98. Lin RY, Astiz ME, Saxon JC, et al: Continuous versus intermittent albuterol nebulization in the treatment of acute asthma. *Ann Emerg Med* 22:1847, 1993.

99. Rodrigo C, Rodrigo G: Therapeutic responsive patterns to high and cumulative doses of salbutamol in acute severe asthma. *Chest* 113:593, 1998.

100. Bryant DH: Nebulised ipratropium bromide in the treatment of acute asthma. *Chest* 88:24, 1985.

101. Bryant DH, Rogers P: Effects of ipratropium bromide nebulizer solution with and without preservatives in the treatment of acute and stable asthma. *Chest* 102:742, 1992.

102. Shuh S, Johnson DW, Callahan S, et al: Efficacy of frequent nebulized ipratropium bromide added to frequent high-dose albuterol in severe childhood asthma. *J Pediatr* 126:639, 1995.

103. Kelly HW, Murphy S: Should anticholinergics be used in acute severe asthma? *DICP Ann Pharmacother* 24:409, 1990.

104. Stoodley RG, Aaron SD, Dales RE: The role of ipratropium bromide in the emergency management of acute asthma exacerbation: a meta-analysis of randomized clinical trials. *Ann Emerg Med* 34:8, 1999.

105. Lanes SF, Garrett JE, Wentworth CE 3rd, et al: The effect of adding ipratropium bromide to salbutamol in the treatment of acute asthma: a pooled analysis of three trials. *Chest* 114:365, 1998.

106. Plotnick LHJ, Ducharme FM: Combined inhaled anticholinergics and beta2-agonists for initial treatment of acute asthma in children (Cochrane Review), in *The Cochrane Library*, Issue 2. Oxford, Update Software, 2003.

107. Karpel JP, Schacter EN, Fanta C, et al: A comparison of ipratropium and albuterol vs albuterol alone for treatment of acute asthma. *Chest* 110:611, 1996.

108. Garrett JE, Town GI, Rodwell P, Kelly AM: Nebulized salbutamol with and without ipratropium bromide in the treatment of acute asthma. *J Allerg Clin Immunol* 100:165, 1997.

109. Lin RY, Pesola GR, Bakalchuk L, et al: Superiority of ipratropium bromide plus albuterol over albuterol alone in the emergency department management of adult asthma: a randomized clinical trial. *Ann Emerg Med* 31:208, 1998.

110. O'Driscoll BR, Taylor RJ, Horsley MG, et al: Nebulised salbutamol with and without ipratropium in acute airflow obstruction. *Lancet* 1:1418, 1989.

111. Qureshi F, Pestian J, Davis P, Zaritsky A: Effect of nebulized ipratropium on hospitalization rates of children with asthma. *N Engl J Med* 339:1030, 1998.

112. Zorc JJ, Pusic MV, Ogborn CJ, et al. Ipratropium bromide added to asthma treatment in the pediatric emergency department. *Pediatrics* 103:748, 1999.

113. Weber EJ, Levitt A, Covington JK, Gambrioli E: Effect of continuously nebulized ipratropium bromide plus albuterol on emergency department length of stay and hospital admission rates in patients with acute bronchospasm. *Chest* 115:937, 1999.

114. Fitzgerald JM, Grunfeld A, Pare PD, et al, and the Canadian Combivent Study Group: The clinical efficacy of combination nebulized anticholinergic and adrenergic bronchodilators vs nebulized adrenergic bronchodilator alone in acute asthma. *Chest* 111:311, 1997.

115. McFadden ER, El Sanadi N, Strauss L, et al: The influence of parasympatholytics on the resolution of acute attacks of asthma. *Am J Med* 102:7, 1997.

116. Ducharme FM, Davis GM: Randomized controlled trial of ipratropium bromide and frequent low doses of salbutamol in the

management of mild and moderate acute pediatric asthma. *J Pediatrics* 133:479, 1998.

117. Rodrigo GJ, Rodrigo C: First-line therapy for adult patients with acute severe asthma receiving a multiple-dose protocol of ipratropium bromide plus albuterol in the emergency department. *Am J Respir Crit Care Med* 161:1862, 2000.

118. McFadden ER Jr, Kiser R, deGroot WJ, et al: A controlled study of the effects of single doses of hydrocortisone on the resolution of acute attacks of asthma. *Am J Med* 60:52, 1976.

119. Rodrigo C, Rodrigo G: Early administration of hydrocortisone in the emergency room treatment of asthma: a controlled clinical trial. *Respir Med* 88:755, 1994.

120. Littenberg B, Gluck EH: A controlled trial of methylprednisolone in the emergency treatment of acute asthma. *N Engl J Med* 314:150, 1986.

121. Lin RY, Pesola GR, Bakalchuk L, et al: Rapid improvement of peak flow in asthmatic patients treated with parenteral methylprednisolone in the emergency department: a randomized controlled study. *Ann Emerg Med* 33:487, 1999.

122. Rowe BH, Spooner CH, Ducharme FM, et al: Early emergency department treatment of acute asthma with systemic corticosteroids (Cochrane Review), in *The Cochrane Library*, Issue 3. Oxford, Update Software, 2003.

123. Rowe BH, Spooner CH, Ducharme FM, et al: Corticosteroids for preventing relapse following acute exacerbations of asthma (Cochrane Review), in *The Cochrane Library*, Issue 3. Oxford, Update Software, 2003.

124. Chapman KR, Verbeek PR, White JG, et al: Effect of a short course of prednisone in the prevention of early relapse after the emergency room treatment of acute asthma. *N Engl J Med* 324:788, 1991.

125. Rowe BH, Keller JL, Oxman AD: Effectiveness of steroid therapy in acute exacerbations of asthma: a meta-analysis. *Am J Emerg Med* 10:301, 1992.

126. Benatar SR: Fatal asthma. *N Engl J Med* 314:423, 1986.

127. Fanta C, Rossing TH, McFadden ER Jr: Glucocorticoids in acute asthma. A critical controlled trial. *Am J Med* 74:845, 1983.

128. Engel T, Dirksen A, Frolund L, et al: Methylprednisolone pulse therapy in acute severe asthma. A randomized, double-blind study. *Allergy* 45:224, 1990.

129. McFadden ER Jr: Clinical commentary: Dosages of corticosteroids in asthma. *Am Rev Respir Dis* 147:1306, 1993.

130. Bowler SD, Mitchell CA, Armstrong JG: Corticosteroids in acute severe asthma: effectiveness of low doses. *Thorax* 47:584, 1992.

131. Manser R, Reid D, Abramson M: Corticosteroids for acute severe asthma in hospitalized patients, Cochrane Review, in *The Cochrane Library*, Issue 3. Oxford, Update Software.

132. Haskell RJ, Wong BM, Hansen JE: A double-blind, randomized clinical trial of methylprednisolone in status asthmaticus. *Arch Intern Med* 143:1324, 1983.

133. Emerman CL, Cydulka RK: A randomized comparison of 100 mg vs 500 mg dose of methylprednisolone in the treatment of acute asthma. *Chest* 107:1559, 1995.

134. Volovitz B, Bentur L, Finkelstein Y, et al: Effectiveness and safety of inhaled corticosteroids in controlling acute asthma attacks in children who were treated in the emergency department: a controlled comparative study with oral prednisone. *J Allerg Clin Immunol* 102:605, 1998.

135. Rodrigo G, Rodrigo C: Inhaled flunisolide for acute severe asthma. *Am J Respir Crit Care Med* 157:698, 1998.

136. McFadden Jr ER: Inhaled glucocorticoids in acute asthma. Therapeutic breakthrough or nonspecific effect. *Am J Respir Crit Care Med* 157:677, 1998.

137. Rodrigo GJ, Rodrigo C: Triple inhaled drug protocol for the treatment of acute severe asthma. *Chest* 123:1908, 2003.

138. Guttman A, Afilalo M, Colacone A, et al: The effects of combined intravenous and inhaled steroids (beclomethasone dipropionate) for the emergency treatment of acute asthma. The Asthma ED Study Group. *Acad Emerg Med* 4:100, 1997.

139. Afilalo M, Guttman A, Colacone A, et al: Efficacy of inhaled steroids (beclomethasone dipropionate) for treatment of mild to moderately severe asthma in the emergency department: a randomized clinical trial. *Ann Emerg Med* 33:304, 1999.

140. Rodrigo C, Rodrigo G: Treatment of acute asthma: lack of therapeutic benefit and increase of the toxicity from aminophylline given in addition to high doses of salbutamol delivered by metered-dose inhaler with a spacer. *Chest* 106:1071, 1994.

141. Parameswaran K, Belda J, Rowe BH: Addition of intravenous aminophylline to beta2-agonists in adults with acute asthma (Cochrane Review), in *The Cochrane Library*, Issue 2. Oxford, Update Software, 2003.

142. Evans WV, Monie RDH, Crimmins J, et al: Aminophylline, salbutamol and combined intravenous infusions in acute severe asthma. *Br J Dis Chest* 74:385, 1980.

143. Mitra A, Bassler D, Ducharme FM: Intravenous aminophylline for acute severe asthma in children over 2 years using inhaled bronchodilators (Cochrane Review), in *The Cochrane Library*, Issue 3. Oxford, Update Software, 2003.

144. Wrenn K, Slovis CM, Murphy F, et al: Aminophylline therapy for acute bronchospastic disease in the emergency room. *Ann Intern Med* 115:241, 1991.

145. Green SM, Rothrock SG: Intravenous magnesium for acute asthma: failure to decrease emergency treatment duration or need for hospitalization. *Ann Emerg Med* 21:260, 1992.

146. Tiffany BR, Berk W, Todd IK, et al: Magnesium bolus or infusion fails to improve expiratory flow in acute asthma exacerbations. *Chest* 104:831, 1993.

147. Bloch H, Silverman R, Mancherje N, et al: Intravenous magnesium sulfate as an adjunct in the treatment of acute asthma. *Chest* 107:1576, 1995.

148. Silverman RA, Osborn H, Runge J, et al: IV magnesium sulfate in the treatment of acute severe asthma: a multicenter randomized controlled trial. *Chest* 122:489, 2002.

149. Rowe BH, Bretzlaff JA, Bourdon C, et al: Magnesium sulfate for treating exacerbations of acute asthma in the emergency department (Cochrane Review), in: *The Cochrane Library*, Issue 3. Oxford, Update Software, 2003.

150. Sydow M, Crozier TA, Zielmann S, et al: High-dose intravenous magnesium sulfate in the management of life-threatening status asthmaticus. *Intensive Care Med* 19:467, 1993.

151. Skobeloff EM, Spivey WH, McNamara RM: Estrogen alters the response of bronchial smooth muscle (abstract). *Ann Emerg Med* 21:647, 1992.

152. Nannini LJ, Pendino JC, Corna RA, et al: Magnesium sulfate as a vehicle for nebulized salbutamol in acute asthma. *Am J Med* 108:193, 2000.

153. Hughes R, Goldkorn A, Masoli M, et al: Use of isotonic nebulised magnesium sulfate as an adjunct to salbutamol in treatment of severe asthma in adults: randomised placebo-controlled trial. *Lancet* 361:2114, 2003.

154. Pavord ID, Ward R, Woltmann G, et al. Induced sputum eicosanoid concentrations in asthma. *Am J Respir Crit Care Med* 160:1905, 1999.

155. Silverman R, Miller C, Chen Y, et al: Zafirlukast reduces relapses and treatment failures after an acute asthma episode. *Chest* 116:296S, 1999.

156. Ferreira MB, Santos AS, Pregal AL, et al: Leukotriene receptor antagonists (Montelukast) in the treatment of asthma crisis: preliminary results of a double-blind placebo controlled randomized study. *Allerg Immunol (Paris)* 33:315, 2001.

157. Camargo CA Jr, Smithline HA, Malice MP, et al: A randomized controlled trial of intravenous montelukast in acute asthma. *Am J Respir Crit Care Med* 167: 528, 2003.

158. Madison JM, Irwin RS: Heliox for asthma: A trial balloon. *Chest* 107:597, 1995.

159. Curtis JL, Mahlmeister M, Fink JB, et al: Helium oxygen gas therapy: Use and availability for the emergency treatment of inoperable airway obstruction. *Chest* 90:455, 1986.

160. Manthous CA, Hall JB, Caputo ME, et al: The effect of heliox on pulsus paradoxus and peak flow in non-intubated patients with severe asthma. *Am J Respir Crit Care Med* 151:310, 1995.

161. Kudukis TM, Manthous CA, Schmidt GA, et al: Inhaled helium-oxygen revisited: effect of inhaled helium-oxygen during the treatment of status asthmaticus in children. *J Pediatrics* 130:217, 1997.

162. Verbeek PR, Chopra A: Heliox does not improve FEV1 in acute asthma patients. *J Emerg Med* 16:545, 1998.

163. Dorfman TA, Shipley ER, Burton JH, et al: Inhaled heliox does not benefit ED patients with moderate to severe asthma. *Am J Emerg Med* 18:495, 2000.

164. Carter ER, Webb CR, Moffitt DR: Evaluation of heliox in children hospitalized with acute severe asthma. A randomized crossover trial. *Chest* 109:1256, 1996.

165. Rodrigo G, Rodrigo C, Pollack C, Rowe B: Helium-oxygen mixture for nonintubated acute asthma patients (Cochrane Review), in *The Cochrane Library*, Issue 2. Oxford Update Software, 2003.

166. Kress JP, Noth I, Gehlbach BK, et al: The utility of albuterol nebulized with heliox during acute asthma exacerbation. *Am J Respir Crit Care Med* 165:1317, 2002.

167. Henderson SO, Acharya P, Kilaghbian T, et al: Use of heliox-driven nebulizer therapy in the treatment of acute asthma. *Ann Emerg Med* 33:141, 1999.

168. Lieberman D, Lieberman D, Printz S, et al: Atypical pathogen infection in adults with acute exacerbations of bronchial asthma. *Am J Respir Crit Care Med* 167:406, 2003.

169. National Asthma Education and Prevention Program: Expert Panel Report. Guidelines for the Diagnosis and Management of Asthma. Update on Selected Topics—2002. *J Allergy Clin Immunol* 110:S141, 2002.

170. Graham V, Lasserson TJ, Rowe BH: Antibiotics for acute asthma (Cochrane Review), in *The Cochrane Library*, Issue 2. Oxford, Update Software, 2003.

171. Martin JG, Shore S, Engel LA: Effect of continuous positive airway pressure on respiratory mechanics and pattern of breathing in induced asthma. *Am Rev Respir Dis* 126:812, 1982.

172. Barach AL, Swensen P: Effect of breathing gases under positive pressure on lumens of small and medium sized bronchi. *Arch Intern Med* 63:946, 1939.

173. Meduri GU, Abou-Shala N, Fox RC, et al: Noninvasive face mask mechanical ventilation in patients with acute hypercapnic respiratory failure. *Chest* 100:445, 1991.

174. Shivaram U, Miro AM, Cash ME, et al: Cardiopulmonary responses to continuous positive airway pressure in acute asthma. *J Crit Care* 8:87, 1993.

175. Meduri GU, Cook TR, Turner RE, et al: Noninvasive positive pressure ventilation in status asthmaticus. *Chest* 110:767, 1996.

176. Tuxen D: Mechanical ventilation in asthma, in Evans T, Hinds C (eds): *Recent Advances in Critical Care*, 4th ed. London: Churchill Livingstone, 1996, p 165.

177. Tuxen DV, Williams TJ, Scheinkestel CD, et al: Use of a measurement of pulmonary hyperinflation to control the level of mechanical ventilation in patients with acute severe asthma. *Am Rev Respir Dis* 146:1136, 1992.

178. Tuxen DV, Lane S: The effects of ventilatory pattern on hyperinflation, airway pressures, and circulation in mechanical ventilation of patients with severe air-flow obstruction. *Am Rev Respir Dis* 136:872, 1987.

179. Williams TJ, Tuxen DV, Scheinkestel CD, et al: Risk factors for morbidity in mechanically ventilated patients with acute severe asthma. *Am Rev Respir Dis* 146:607, 1992.

180. Otis A, McKerrow C, Bartlett R, et al: Mechanical factors in distribution of pulmonary ventilation. *J Appl Physiol* 8:427, 1956.

181. Bates J, Rossi A, Milic-Emili J: Analysis of the behavior of the respiratory system with constant inspiratory flow. *J Appl Physiol* 58:1840, 1985.

182. Corne S, Gillespie D, Roberts D, Younes M: Effect of inspiratory flow rate on respiratory rate in intubated patients. *Am J Respir Crit Care* 156:304, 1997.

183. Marini JJ, Capps JS, Culver BH: The inspiratory work of breathing during assisted mechanical ventilation. *Chest* 87:612, 1985.

184. Tobin MJ: Advances in mechanical ventilation. *N Engl J Med* 344:1986, 2001.

185. Tuxen DV: Detrimental effects of positive end-expiratory pressure during controlled mechanical ventilation of patients with severe airflow obstruction. *Am Rev Respir Dis* 140:5, 1989.

186. Kress JP, O'Connor MF, Schmidt GA: Clinical examination reliably detects intrinsic positive end-expiratory pressure in critically ill, mechanically ventilated patients. *Am J Respir Crit Care Med* 159: 290, 1999.

187. Feihl F, Perret C: State of the art: Permissive hypercapnia: how permissive should we be? *Am J Respir Crit Care Med* 150:1722, 1994.

188. Darioli R, Perret C: Mechanical controlled hypoventilation in status asthmaticus. *Am Rev Respir Dis* 129:385, 1984.

189. Tuxen DV: Permissive hypercapnic ventilation. *Am J Respir Crit Care Med* 150:870, 1994.

190. Cooper DJ, Calles JB, Scheinkestel CD, Tuxen DV: Does bicarbonate improve cardiac or respiratory function during respiratory acidosis and acute severe asthma—a prospective randomized study. *Am Rev Respir Dis* 147:614A, 1993.

191. Kress JP, O'Connor MF, Pohlman AS, et al: Sedation of critically ill patients during mechanical ventilation: a comparison of propofol and midazolam. *Am J Respir Crit Care Med* 153:1012, 1996.

192. Pohlman A, Simpson K, Hall J: Continuous intravenous infusions of lorazepam vs. midazolam for sedation during mechanical ventilatory support: a prospective, randomized study. *Crit Care Med* 22:1241, 1994.

193. Murray MJ, DeRuyter ML, Harrison BA: Opioids and benzodiazepines. *Crit Care Clin* 4:849, 1995.

194. Kress JP, Pohlman A, O'Connor MF, Hall JB: Daily interruption of sedative infusions in critically ill patients undergoing mechanical ventilation. *N Engl J Med* 342:1471, 2000.

195. Corseen G, Gutierrez J, Reves JG, et al: Ketamine in the anaesthetic management of asthmatic patients. *Anesth-Analg* 51:588, 1972.

196. Sarma VJ: Use of ketamine in acute severe asthma. *Acta Anaesthesiol Scand* 36:106, 1992.

197. Rock MJ, Reyes de la Rocha S, L'Hommedieu ET: Use of ketamine in asthmatic children to treat respiratory failure refractory to conventional therapy. *Crit Care Med* 14:514, 1986.

198. Caldwell JE, Lau M, Fisher DM: Atracurium versus vecuronium in asthmatic patients. A blinded, randomized comparison of adverse events. *Anesthesiology* 83:986, 1995.

199. Leatherman JW, Fluegel WL, David WS, et al: Muscle weakness in mechanically ventilated patients with severe asthma. *Am J Respir Crit Care Med* 153:1686, 1996.

200. Behbehani NA, Al-Mane F, D'yachkova Y, et al: Myopathy following mechanical ventilation for acute severe asthma: the role of muscle relaxants and corticosteroids. *Chest* 115:1627, 1999.

201. Douglass JA, Tuxen D, Horne M, et al: Myopathy in severe asthma. *Am Rev Respir Dis* 146:517, 1992.

202. MacIntyre NR, Silver RM, Miller CW, et al: Aerosol delivery in intubated, mechanically ventilated patients. *Crit Care Med* 13:81, 1985.

203. Manthous CA, Hall JB, Schmidt GA, et al: Metered-dose inhaler versus nebulized albuterol in mechanically ventilated patients. *Am Rev Respir Dis* 148:1567, 1993.

204. Manthous CA, Hall JB: Update on using therapeutic aerosols in mechanically ventilated patients. *J Crit Illness* 11:457, 1996.

205. Jones A, Peters J, Camargo C, et al: Inhaled beta-agonists for asthma in mechanically ventilated patients (Cochrane Review), in *The Cochrane Library*, Issue 3. Oxford, Update Software, 2003.

206. Saulnier FF, Durocher AV, Deturck RA, et al: Respiratory and hemodynamic effects of halothane in status asthmaticus. *Intensive Care Med* 16:104, 1990.

207. Echeverria M, Gelb AW, Wexler HR, et al: Enflurane and halothane in status asthmaticus. *Chest* 89:153, 1986.

208. Gluck EH, Onorato DJ, Castriotta R: Helium-oxygen mixtures in intubated patients with status asthmaticus and respiratory acidosis. *Chest* 98:693, 1990.

209. Smith DL, Deshazo RD: Bronchoalveolar lavage in asthma. State of the art. *Am Rev Respir Dis* 148:523, 1993.

210. Millman M, Millman FM, Goldstein IM, et al: Use of acetyl-cysteine in bronchial asthma—another look. *Ann Allergy* 54:294, 1985.

211. Lang DM, Simon RA, Mathison DA, et al: Safety and possible efficacy of fiberoptic bronchoscopy with lavage in the management of refractory asthma with mucous impaction. *Ann Allergy* 67:324, 1991.

Chapter 41
MASSIVE HEMOPTYSIS
RICHARD K. ALBERT

KEY POINTS
- *Assure adequate oxygenation.*
- *Look for and correct coagulation abnormalities.*
- *For localized bleeding, bronchoscopy and/or computed tomography scanning can generally establish the region of the lung from which the bleeding is coming.*
- *Kidney or lung biopsy may be needed to establish the cause of diffuse bleeding.*
- *Treatment depends on cause, but bronchial arterial embolization should generally be considered prior to surgery.*

Hemoptysis is defined as coughing of blood, and can be caused by numerous diseases and conditions (Table 41-1). Most series indicate that bronchiectasis is the most common cause, but the prevalence of any specific causal entity is a function of the time frame studied (with tuberculosis being more common in older series), and the nature of the population encountered (e.g., bronchiectasis in patients with cystic fibrosis, cancer in older smokers).

Most patients with hemoptysis do not require intensive care. Those who do generally have either such rapid rates of bleeding that they are hemodynamically unstable, or they have life-threatening hypoxemia as a result of diffuse parenchymal hemorrhage or extensive aspiration of blood that originates from a localized source.

"Massive" hemoptysis has been variably defined as production of more than 300 to 600 mL of blood in 12 to 24 hours, depending on the study. Although this connotation is perhaps important from a descriptive standpoint, the distinction has little clinical utility, as it is difficult for patients to accurately quantify the volume of blood they are producing, and the volume of hemoptysis may vary considerably from hour to hour (or even from minute to minute). In addition, some patients with diffuse pulmonary hemorrhage can present with life-threatening hypoxemia and diffuse parenchymal infiltrates, meeting all the criteria for the acute respiratory distress syndrome (ARDS), yet have no hemoptysis. Although any of the conditions listed in Table 41-1 may cause hemoptysis, those more commonly associated with massive hemoptysis are bronchiectasis, mycetoma, tuberculosis, bronchogenic carcinoma, lung abscess, and vascular-bronchial fistulas. A recent study of 29 patients from Singapore found that 62% had bronchiectasis, 13% had mycetomas, 10% had tuberculosis, 6% had tumors, and 3% had a pulmonary hemorrhage syndrome.[1]

Older reviews of hemoptysis comment that bleeding from the nose, pharynx, or even the gastrointestinal system may present with what was thought to be hemoptysis. The point has been made that blood coming from the lungs is usually bright red and has an alkaline pH, whereas that from the stomach will be dark and acidic. Clinically, the distinction is only rarely difficult.

Stabilization

Attention should initially be directed at assuring adequate ventilation and perfusion as with any patient requiring intensive care. The most common cause of death in patients with hemoptysis is asphyxia from aspirated blood. Clearance of blood from the airway may be facilitated by utilizing the Trendelenburg position. If the site of bleeding is known, right or left lateral decubitus positioning may serve to protect the opposite lung.

Some patients (particularly those with diffuse parenchymal hemorrhage) may require intubation and mechanical ventilation. While intubation generally facilitates removal of blood from the lower airway, the tube may become obstructed by coagulated blood with a resultant limitation in ventilation. In extreme circumstances the mainstem bronchus of the non-bleeding lung can be intubated in an attempt to protect the other lung. Alternatively, many reports describe placing occluding catheters in the mainstem bronchus of the bleeding lung. In the setting of extensive bleeding, however, intubation and/or precise placement of endotracheal tubes may be extremely difficult because of the inability to visualize the airway.

Small doses of codeine or morphine may be used to blunt the cough reflex and perhaps slow the rate of bleeding, but agents that depress the sensorium must be used cautiously as they may also increase the risk of aspiration.

Initial Evaluation

Bleeding disorders should be sought; in the appropriate setting the patient should be screened for conditions associated with pulmonary hemorrhage syndromes, and attempts made to determine the site of bleeding. The nose and mouth should be carefully inspected to exclude an upper airway source of bleeding. Rhinoscopy and/or laryngoscopy may at times be useful. A history consistent with rheumatic fever might lead to the suspicion of mitral stenosis, which is readily diagnosed by echocardiography.

Coagulation screening should include a platelet count, a prothrombin time, and a partial thromboplastin time. If patients have had substantial bleeding for a prolonged period of time, a fibrinogen level should also be determined.

Blood should be sent for urea nitrogen and creatinine, a urinalysis should be obtained, and if clinical indications point to diffuse parenchymal hemorrhage, serology should be sent to screen for connective tissue disease and vasculitis (e.g., antinuclear antibodies, rheumatoid factor, complement levels, cryoglobulins, the anti–glomerular basement antibody causing Goodpasture syndrome, anti-phospholipid antibodies, and the antinuclear cytoplasmic antibody that is seen in Wegener granulomatosis and pauci-immune vasculitis) (see Table 41-1).

DETERMINING THE SITE OF BLEEDING

The chest x-ray will identify the region of bleeding in approximately 60% of patients. Fiberoptic or rigid bronchoscopy can be used to determine the site of bleeding, as can CT imaging. In most instances the site may be investigated electively after the patient stabilizes and the rate of bleeding slows. However,

TABLE 41-1 Causes of Hemoptysis and Pulmonary Hemorrhage

Localized bleeding
  Infections
    Bronchitis
    Bacterial pneumonia (particularly *Streptococcus pneumoniae* and *Klebsiella*)
    Tuberculosis (particularly in the setting of cavitary disease)
    Fungal infections (particularly mycetomas from *Aspergillus* or *Candida*)
    Bronchiectasis (e.g., cystic fibrosis or immune deficiencies)
    Lung abscess
    Leptospirosis
  Tumors
    Bronchogenic (i.e., squamous cell)
    Necrotizing parenchymal cancer (usually adenocarcinoma)
    Bronchial adenoma
  Cardiovascular problems
    Mitral stenosis
  Pulmonary vascular problems
    Pulmonary arteriovenous malformations (e.g., Rendu-Osler-Weber syndrome)
    Pulmonary embolus with infarction
    Behçet syndrome
    Pulmonary artery catheterization with pulmonary arterial rupture
  Trauma
  Others
    Broncholithiasis
    Sarcoidosis (usually from cavitary lesions with mycetoma)
    Ankylosing spondylitis

Diffuse bleeding
  Drug- and chemical-induced
    Anticoagulants
    D-penicillamine (rare, seen with prior treatment of Wilson disease)
    Trimellitic anhydride (encountered during manufacturing of plastics, paint, and epoxy resins)
    Cocaine
    Propylthiouracil
    Amiodarone
    Phenytoin
  Blood dyscrasias
    Thrombotic thrombocytopenic purpura
    Hemophilia
    Leukemia
    Thrombocytopenia
    Uremia
    Antiphospholipid antibody syndrome
  Pulmonary-renal syndrome
    Goodpasture syndrome (anti–glomerular basement membrane antibody disease)
    Wegener granulomatosis
    Pauci-immune vasculitis
  Vasculitis
    Pulmonary capillaritis (with or without a connective tissue disease, pauci-immune vasculitis, lung transplant rejection, propylthiouracil, or the retinoic acid syndrome)
    Polyarteritis
    Churg-Strauss syndrome
    Henoch-Schönlein purpura
    Necrotizing vasculitis
    Connective tissue diseases (i.e., systemic lupus erythematosus, rheumatoid arthritis, mixed connective tissue disease, or rarely scleroderma)
    Pulmonary veno-occlusive disease
  Hemosiderosis

TABLE 41-2 Comparative Utility of Chest X-Ray, Fiberoptic Bronchoscopy, and Chest Computed Tomography

Diagnostic Modality	SITE OF BLEEDING		CAUSE OF BLEEDING	
	N	%	N	%
Chest x-ray	37	46	28	35[a]
Fiberoptic bronchoscopy	58	73	6	7
Chest CT	56	70	62	77

[a] Footnote?
SOURCE: Reproduced with permission from Revel et al.[2]

in selected patients (e.g., trauma), immediate surgical intervention may be needed. In others, especially those with rapid rates of ongoing bleeding, the choice of diagnostic evaluation may be more difficult. A recent study of 29 consecutive patients admitted to intensive care with more than 300 mL/d of hemoptysis found that fiberoptic bronchoscopy localized the bleeding in 90% of cases.[1]

Fiberoptic bronchoscopy may demonstrate a specific endobronchial lesion, or may at least indicate a specific lung lobe or segment from which the bleeding is coming. However, with rapid rates of bleeding, visualization through a fiberoptic scope is likely to be suboptimal because of an inability to clear blood from the airway. Rigid bronchoscopy allows for better suctioning, but is more invasive and only the central airways can be inspected. Nonetheless, when the rate of bleeding precludes accurate assessment of the airway anatomy by fiberoptic bronchoscopy, there should be no delay in moving to rigid bronchoscopy.

A retrospective study of 80 patients with "large or massive" hemoptysis compared the utility of chest x-rays, fiberoptic bronchoscopy, and chest computed tomography (CT).[2] The results indicated that chest CT was superior in determining the cause of bleeding, and suggested that it should become the first-line procedure (Table 41-2). A recent study of 40 consecutive patients assessed the accuracy of CT angiography for determining whether patients with massive hemoptysis (i.e., 300 to 600 mL/d) had a systemic artery as the source of the bleeding.[3] Using conventional angiography as the gold standard, CT angiography had an 80% sensitivity, an 84% specificity, and an 84% positive predictive value. More than 3 mm of pleural thickening in a region located adjacent to a parenchymal abnormality, and contrast-enhancing vascular structures in the extrapleural fat correlated with the presence of a nonbronchial systemic arterial supply.[3]

Patients with diffuse alveolar hemorrhage more commonly have diffuse rather than localized infiltrates on their chest x-rays or CT scans, but diffuse infiltrates may also result from localized bleeding if the blood is extensively aspirated. The diagnosis of diffuse alveolar hemorrhage is suggested by finding blood in bronchoalveolar lavage fluid.

Treatment

GENERAL MEASURES

The platelet count should be maintained above 50,000 mm^3 in an actively bleeding patient. Immune platelet destruction may be treated with intravenous gamma globulin prior to platelet transfusion. The platelet dysfunction associated with uremia may be treated with dialysis or by administration of cryoprecipitate and desmopressin (DDAVP). DDAVP has also recently been shown to be remarkably effective in stopping the massive hemoptysis associated with leptospirosis,[4] and may, along with cryoprecipitate, be useful in treating patients with von Willebrand disease and hemophilia A.

The prothrombin time and partial thromboplastin time should be corrected to near normal. Deficiencies are treated with vitamin K, or for a more rapid effect, with large volumes of fresh frozen plasma.

SPECIFIC INTERVENTIONS

A number of treatment modalities may be used to treat life-threatening hemoptysis. These include endobronchial ablation of specific lesions, bronchial arterial embolization, external beam irradiation, and surgical resection.

Endobronchial ablation is generally reserved for tumors affecting the larger airways as a form of palliative therapy for patients with unresectable disease. External beam irradiation has been used successfully in a few patients with massive hemoptysis resulting from mycetomas[5] and can also be used for patients with unresectable neoplasms if the rate of bleeding is sufficiently slow that the course of treatment can be completed.

Bronchial arterial embolization is the treatment of choice for most patients with life-threatening hemoptysis resulting from a localized parenchymal lesion. Recent studies indicate that the hemoptysis is controlled in as many as 85% of patients up to 1 month following the procedure, although recurrence is seen in approximately 15% of patients within the first 30 days.[6]

SURGICAL VERSUS MEDICAL MANAGEMENT

When hemoptysis occurs in the setting of diffuse disease (e.g., cystic fibrosis, extensive pulmonary tuberculosis, or other forms of bronchiectasis), surgery is precluded. For patients with localized disease the decision about when to operate continues to be based on clinical judgement and individual patient assessment, as there are no randomized trials comparing the outcomes achieved with surgery versus repeated embolization. The major indications for surgery are: **1.** recurrence of bleeding after bronchial arterial embolization, **2.** inability to perform the embolization because of anatomic problems, and **3.** multiple bleeding vessels seen on angiography.[7] Accordingly, with the possible exception of endobronchial carcinomas that require ablation, bronchial arterial embolization should generally be the initial treatment of choice for patients with localized disease who can be sufficiently stabilized to attempt the procedure.

DIFFUSE ALVEOLAR HEMORRHAGE

Diffuse alveolar hemorrhage (DAH) occurs in conjunction with, and may be the initial manifestation of, numerous diseases, conditions, and effects of medications (see Table 41-1). Up to one-third of patients with DAH will *not* have hemoptysis, but many will have other systemic manifestations of a systemic disease (e.g., rash, myalgias, arthralgias, or conjunctivitis). Chest x-rays generally show diffuse infiltrates, but localized disease may also be seen. DAH occurs in up to 10% of patients with Wegener granulomatosis, and up to 33% of patients with microscopic polyangiitis (all of whom will have evidence of glomerulonephritis). DAH is also seen in approximately 5% of patients with systemic lupus erythematosus, and rarely in conjunction with polymyositis, rheumatoid arthritis, and mixed connective tissue disease. Most patients with Goodpasture syndrome (which is caused by an antibody to the type 4 collagen found in the basement membranes of alveolar walls and glomeruli) present with DAH and glomerulonephritis, but up to 10% may have only DAH.

DIAGNOSIS

Establishing a diagnosis of DAH is not difficult when patients present with hemoptysis, diffuse pulmonary infiltrates, a falling hematocrit, and other manifestations of systemic disease. However, in those without hemoptysis or diffuse infiltrates the diagnosis becomes much more difficult. Bronchoalveolar lavage showing progressively more blood with serial aspirations may be considered diagnostic, but DAH must be suspected before this procedure is considered. When DAH is diagnosed, a kidney biopsy or an open or thoracoscopic lung biopsy is frequently recommended to allow differentiation among the various types of vasculitis, and to definitively either diagnose or exclude Goodpasture syndrome, as patients with vasculitis are treated with high doses of systemic corticosteroids and with cyclophosphamide, whereas those with Goodpasture should receive plasmapheresis.

Unfortunately, despite treatment, over half of patients with DAH resulting from a systemic vasculitis or a collagen vascular disease require mechanical ventilation, and the mortality ranges from 25% in patients with Wegener granulomatosis to 50% in patients with lupus. The 5-year survival rate for these conditions is also reduced.

References

1. Ong T-H, Eng P: Massive hemoptysis requiring intensive care. *Intensive Care Med* 29:317, 2003.
2. Revel MP, Fournier LS, Hennebicque AS, et al: Can CT replace bronchoscopy in the detection of the site and cause of bleeding in patients with large or massive hemoptysis? *Am J Roentgenol* 179:1217, 2002.
3. Yoon W, Kim TH, Kim JK, et al: Massive hemoptysis: prediction of nonbronchial systemic arterial supply with chest CT. *Radiology* 227:232, 2003.
4. Pea L, Roda L, Boussaud V, Lonjon B: Desmopressin therapy for massive hemoptysis associated with severe leptospirosis. *Am J Respir Crit Care Med* 167:726, 2003.
5. Falkson C, Sur R, Pacella J: External beam radiotherapy: A treatment option for massive haemoptysis caused by mycetoma. *Clin Oncol (R Coll Radiol)* 14:233, 2002.
6. Swanson KL, Johnson CM, Prakash UB, et al: Bronchial artery embolization: experience with 54 patients. *Chest* 121:789, 2002.
7. Endo S, Otani S, Saito N, et al: Management of massive hemoptysis in a thoracic surgical unit. *Eur J Cardiothoracic Surg* 23:467, 2003.

Chapter 42

RESTRICTIVE DISEASE OF THE RESPIRATORY SYSTEM AND THE ABDOMINAL COMPARTMENT SYNDROME

THOMAS CORBRIDGE
LAWRENCE D.H. WOOD

KEY POINTS

- *Scoliotic curves greater than 100 ° may cause dyspnea; curves greater than 120° are associated with alveolar hypoventilation and cor pulmonale.*

- *Most patients with chest wall deformity survive their first episode of acute respiratory failure. Common precipitants include upper and lower respiratory tract infections and congestive heart failure.*

- *Biphasic positive airway pressure may be effective in patients with acute hypercapnic respiratory failure.*

- *Low tidal volumes and high respiratory rates likely minimize the risk of barotrauma during mechanical ventilation; however, gradual institution of anti-atelectasis measures may improve gas exchange and static compliance.*

- *Nocturnal hypoxemia is common and may contribute to cardiovascular deterioration; routine polysomnography is recommended.*

- *Strategies for management of patients with chronic ventilatory failure include daytime intermittent positive pressure ventilation, nocturnal noninvasive ventilation, and ventilation through tracheostomy.*

- *Abdominal compartment syndrome (ACS) is caused by an acute increase in intra-abdominal pressure resulting from a number of surgical and medical conditions.*

- *By elevating the diaphragm and decreasing respiratory system compliance, ACS causes a restrictive defect. However, ACS affects a number of other organs and may cause multiorgan system failure.*

- *Diagnosis relies on measurement of intra-abdominal bladder pressure and identification of organ dysfunction.*

- *The abdomen should be decompressed before critical organ dysfunction develops.*

- *Failure to recognize and treat ACS portends a poor prognosis.*

- *Acute deterioration in respiratory status can occur from disease progression or a number of other infectious and noninfectious processes.*

- *Patients with idiopathic pulmonary fibrosis admitted to the ICU with acute respiratory failure have an extremely poor prognosis.*

- *If mechanical ventilation is deemed appropriate, the use of low tidal volumes and high respiratory rates during mechanical*

- *ventilation likely minimizes ventilator-induced lung injury.*

- *Idiopathic pulmonary fibrosis is typically refractory to drug treatment.*

- *Lung transplantation is a viable option in selected patients with end-stage fibrosis.*

Thoracic cage deformity and pulmonary fibrosis both result in a restrictive limitation to breathing. Although relatively rare in the context of pulmonary intensive care, these disorders present unique challenges that complicate ICU management. More commonly a tense and distended abdomen decreases thoracic volume and respiratory system compliance. In this chapter, we describe the pathophysiologic derangements in cardiopulmonary function associated with these disorders and how they affect management during acute illness. A primary goal of this chapter is to offer a strategy for cardiovascular management and mechanical ventilation that minimizes the risk of ventilator-induced complications and maximizes the chance for early, successful extubation.

Patients with Thoracic Cage Deformity

Although a number of disorders can deform and restrict the movement of the respiratory system (Table 42-1), kyphoscoliosis (KS) is the prototypical cause of severe thoracic deformity. Kyphoscoliosis is the combination of kyphosis (posterior deformity of the spine) and scoliosis (lateral deformity of the spine). It is far more common than isolated cases of kyphosis or scoliosis, placing as many as 200,000 people in the United States at risk of developing respiratory failure.[1] Most cases are idiopathic and begin in childhood. Other cases result from congenital defects, poliomyelitis, thoracoplasty, syringomyelia, vertebral and spinal cord tumors, and tuberculosis.

The pathophysiologic consequences of KS correlate with the degree of spinal curvature, but there is considerable variability.[1,2] Patients with severe deformity can lead long and relatively symptom-free lives,[3] while patients with lesser degrees of curvature may develop ventilatory failure and cor pulmonale at a relatively young age. The reason for this variability is not clear, although sleep-disordered breathing appears to contribute to clinical deterioration in some cases.[4,5]

The combination of a moderate kyphotic deformity and a moderate scoliotic deformity is functionally equivalent to a severe deformity of either alone.[2] Of the two, however, scoliosis produces greater physiologic derangements. In KS, scoliotic curves less than 70° (Fig. 42-1) rarely cause problems, while angles greater than 70° increase the risk of respiratory failure.[1] The earlier in life this angle is achieved, the greater the risk of eventually developing respiratory failure because curvature increases by an average of 15° over 20 years from an initial angle of 70°.[6,7] Angles greater than 100° can cause dyspnea. Angles ≥120° can result in alveolar hypoventilation and cor pulmonale.[1]

In order to decrease respiratory effort, patients with severe deformity take rapid and shallow breaths. Examination of the chest reveals decreased excursion and crackles or coarse wheezes from atelectasis or failure to clear secretions. Cardiac examination may demonstrate a loud P_2, right ventricular

TABLE 42-1 Selected Diseases of the Chest Wall

Pectus excavatum
Pectus carinatum
Poland syndrome
Kyphoscoliosis
Thoracoplasty
Fibrothorax
Chest wall tumors

heave, or jugular venous distention, indicating the presence of pulmonary hypertension.[2]

RESPIRATORY MECHANICS

Kyphoscoliosis reduces total lung capacity (TLC) and functional residual capacity (FRC) (Fig. 42-2). Residual volume (RV) may be normal or decreased to a lesser extent than FRC. Vital capacity (VC), inspiratory capacity (IC = TLC − FRC), and expiratory reserve volume (ERV = FRC − RV) are all decreased. Interestingly, in adolescents pulmonary function is only weakly related to the angle of scoliosis. In these patients, VC is also influenced by the degree of thoracic kyphosis, location of the curve, and number of vertebral bodies involved.[8] Furthermore, spinal column rotation, respiratory muscle strength, and duration of the curve are not clearly

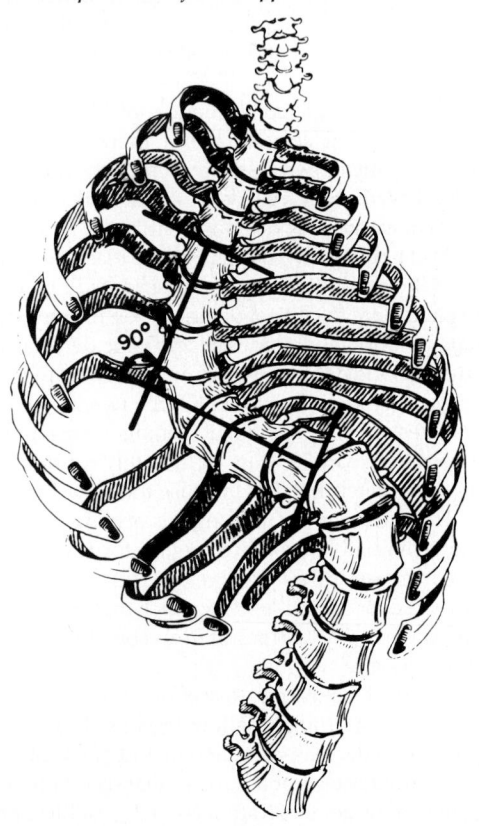

FIGURE 42-1 Determination of the scoliotic angle by the Cobb method. The scoliotic deformity consists of a primary initiating curve and a secondary compensatory curve. The scoliotic angle is commonly determined by the intersection of lines estimating the position of the upper and lower components of the primary curve. (*Reprinted with permission from Grippi et al.[13]*)

related to pulmonary function in these patients.[8] Decreasing chest wall compliance with age increases the risk of developing ventilatory failure.[9]

Patients with fibrothorax or thoracoplasty have similar abnormalities.[1] By contrast, obesity mainly reduces FRC and ERV without much change in RV, VC, or TLC. In patients with ankylosing spondylitis, ERV and IC excursions are restricted around a normal FRC, such that RV increases and TLC decreases to reduce VC, a pattern similar to that seen in neuromuscular diseases of the chest wall.

In each of these disorders, it is the chest wall that limits the excursion of the respiratory system; the lungs and respiratory muscles are affected secondarily and to a lesser degree. In health, TLC is largely determined by the pressure-volume (P-V) curve of the lung, but in KS the P-V curve of the noncompliant chest wall dominates, lowering TLC and FRC while RV is relatively spared (Fig. 42-3). Note that the P-V curve of the respiratory system is shifted downward and to the right, requiring patients to generate large efforts to take in little air. Normal lung compliance and respiratory muscle strength are assumed in Fig. 42-3, although reductions in both contribute to low lung volumes in selected patients. Indeed in four patients with severe KS requiring mechanical ventilation for acute respiratory failure, both lung and chest wall compliance was decreased.[10] Decreased lung compliance may occur as a result of infection, edema, atelectasis, or abnormalities in alveolar surface tension and may respond to intermittent positive-pressure ventilation (see below).[11]

Inspiratory muscle dysfunction occurs when the deformed thorax places inspiratory muscles at a mechanical disadvantage or there is respiratory muscle fatigue.[12] When KS is a manifestation of neuromuscular disease (e.g., postpolio syndrome), inspiratory muscles may be affected directly by the neuromuscular disease.

GAS EXCHANGE

Significant daytime hypoxemia rarely occurs until the development of daytime hypercapnia.[1] However, nocturnal hypercapnia with hypoxemia occurs early, particularly during rapid eye movement (REM) sleep, and may underlie cardiovascular deterioration in some patients.[4,5]

The alveolar-arterial gradient [$(A-a)_{O_2}$] is usually ≤25 mm Hg, even in late stages of KS.[1] This modest increase in $(A-a)_{O_2}$ results primarily from ventilation-perfusion ($\dot{V}/\dot{Q}$) inequality caused by atelectasis or underventilation of one hemithorax. $\dot{V}/\dot{Q}$ inequality further contributes to a low diffusing capacity, as does the failure of the vascular bed to grow normally in a distorted chest.

Alveolar hypoventilation results in part from an increase in the dead space to tidal volume ratio (V_{DS}/V_T). This ratio is increased because V_T is reduced in hypercapnic patients, whereas anatomic and alveolar dead space are usually normal.[1] Minute ventilation is often normal but maintained by higher respiratory rates. The use of small V_T minimizes the work of breathing and is a sign of inspiratory muscle dysfunction.[12,13] As inspiratory muscle strength falls, the partial pressure of arterial carbon dioxide (Pa_{CO_2}) rises and further affects diaphragm function.[11,14]

Ventilatory response to high concentrations of inspired CO_2 is normal in normocapnic patients with KS. However, in hypercapnic patients, the response is blunted by buffering of

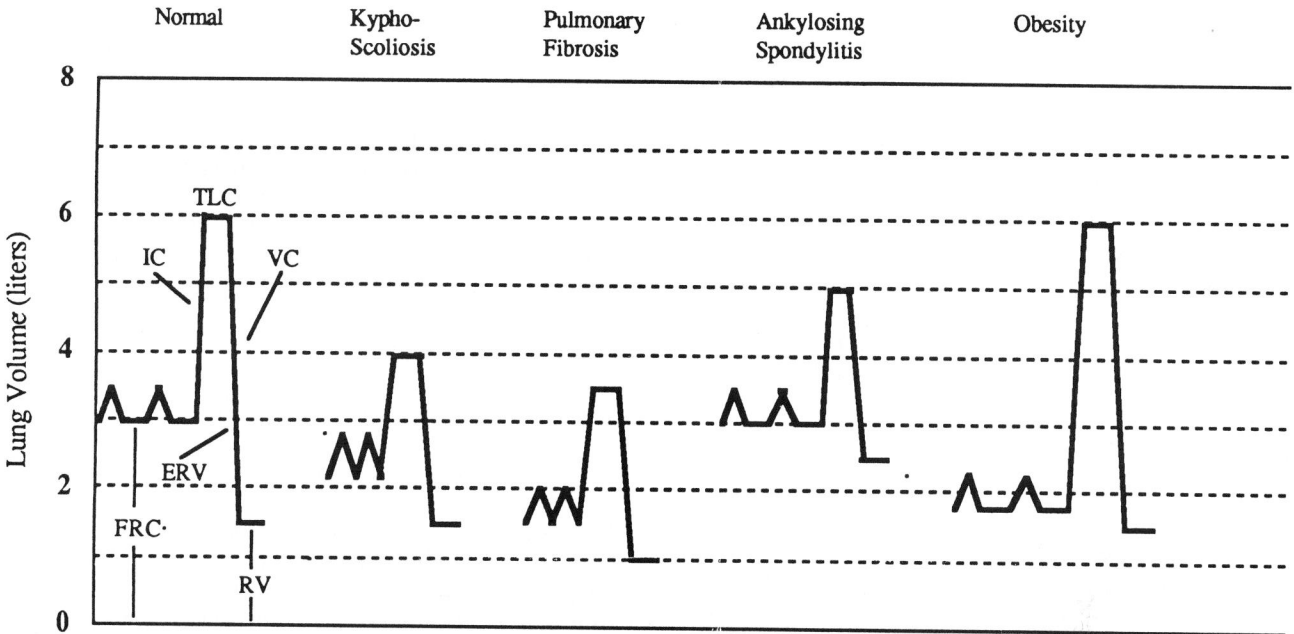

FIGURE 42-2 Schematic drawing of the abnormalities of lung volumes in common restrictive diseases. By contrast with normal subdivisions (*left trace*) of plethysmographic gas volumes (TLC, FRC, and RV) and spirometric volumes (IC, VC, and ERV), kyphoscoliosis and pulmonary fibrosis reduce VC and TLC by restricting IC, with lesser reductions in FRC (*traces 2 and 3*).

Ankylosing spondylitis (like neuromuscular diseases of the chest wall) limits IC and ERV excursions around a normal FRC, so TLC is reduced and RV is increased, causing a large decrease in VC (*panel 4*). Obesity greatly reduces FRC to eliminate ERV without much change in TLC or RV, so VC is normal and IC is increased (*panel 5*).

the signal by elevated cerebrospinal fluid bicarbonate, or by a derangement in the central drive to breathe.[13]

EFFECTS ON THE PULMONARY CIRCULATION

A further consequence of severe KS is pulmonary hypertension and cor pulmonale. Left untreated, patients with cor pulmonale typically die within 1 year.[2] Initially, pulmonary hypertension occurs only with exercise, but over time it occurs at rest as well. Pulmonary hypertension is usually caused by increased pulmonary vascular resistance (PVR) and not ele-

vated left atrial pressure.[1] Thus there is an increased gradient between the pulmonary artery diastolic pressure and the pulmonary capillary wedge pressure. Identifying and treating reversible conditions such as pulmonary embolism, hypoxemia, and sleep-disordered breathing lowers pulmonary artery pressure and delays the onset of right ventricular failure.[15–17] However, there also may be irreversible changes associated with proliferation of the media in smaller, precapillary pulmonary vessels.[2] The mechanism by which this occurs is not known, but blood flow through vessels narrowed by low lung volumes, blood flow through fewer vessels, and the

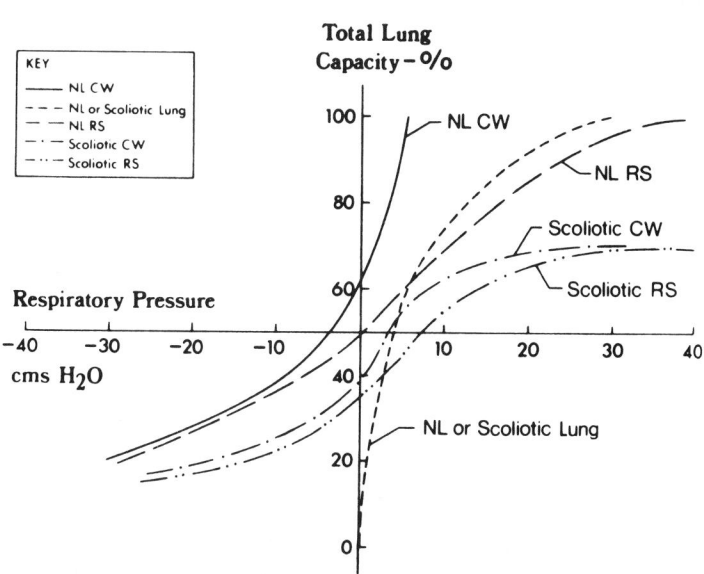

FIGURE 42-3 Pressure-volume curves of the chest wall, lung, and respiratory system in scoliosis. The P-V curve is shifted downward and to the right, requiring patients to generate large transpulmonary pressures for small amounts of air. CW = chest wall; NL = normal lung; RS = respiratory system. (*Reprinted with permission from Bergofsky.[1]*)

vascular effects of chronic hypoxia and hypercapnia are likely important. Kinking of larger vessels as they travel through deformed lung may further increase pulmonary artery pressures in some cases.[1]

Acute Cardiopulmonary Failure

OUTCOME

In 20 patients with mean deformity of 113° in acute respiratory failure (ARF) for the first time, admission blood gases showed severe arterial hypoxemia (partial pressure of arterial oxygen [Pa_{O_2}] of 35 ± 7 mm Hg), acute-on-chronic hypercapnia (Pa_{CO_2} of 63 ± 9 mm Hg), and mild arterial acidemia (pH of 7.34 ± 0.08).[18] Cor pulmonale was present in 60% of patients. Seven (35%) patients required intubation and mechanical ventilation, while the remaining patients were managed successfully without mechanical ventilation in an age when noninvasive positive-pressure ventilation (NPPV) was not routinely available. There were no statistical differences in admission blood gases, cause of respiratory failure, age, or degree of spinal curvature between patients who required mechanical ventilation and those who did not. Outcome was surprisingly good. All patients survived their initial episode of ARF and subsequently experienced 2.4 episodes of ARF each during the follow-up period (median of 6 years). Median survival after the first episode of ARF was 9 years. On discharge, mean Pa_{O_2} was 63 mm Hg and mean Pa_{CO_2} was 55 mm Hg. This study demonstrates the utility of aggressive treatment of ARF, even in cases of severe deformity.

ETIOLOGY

ARF is usually precipitated by pneumonia, upper respiratory tract infection, or congestive heart failure.[18] Triggers are often minor and may remain obscure, but even trivial insults can precipitate ARF when respiratory muscle reserve is decreased and work of breathing is increased. Because chest wall deformity theoretically affects the swallowing mechanism, aspiration should be considered in the differential diagnosis of ARF. Risk factors for clotting (pulmonary hypertension and decreased mobility) mandate consideration of pulmonary embolism, particularly when the cause of deterioration is obscure. Finally, identifying and treating airflow obstruction can help restore the delicate balance between strength and respiratory system load. Limited data suggest that airway resistance is increased in mechanically ventilated patients with KS ($\sim$20 cm H_2O/L per second) and refractory to bronchodilators.[10] Bronchoscopic examination of patients with bronchodilator-unresponsive increases in airway resistance may reveal torsion and narrowing of central airways.[19]

OXYGEN THERAPY

A primary goal is to correct hypoxemia. This is best accomplished by increasing the fraction of inspired oxygen until an oxygen saturation of 90% to 92% is achieved. Adequate saturation by pulse oximetry should be confirmed by subsequent blood gas analysis, which also helps establish the acid-base status. If adequate oxygenation cannot be achieved with face-mask oxygen, biphasic positive airway pressure (BIPAP) should be initiated unless there are indications for intubation (see below).

Hypoxemia, in addition to its many adverse effects, causes pulmonary vasoconstriction and may precipitate right ventricular failure in patients with pre-existing right heart disease (see Chap. 26). Its causes include alveolar hypoventilation, $\dot{V}/\dot{Q}$ inequality, and intrapulmonary shunt. Right-to-left intracardiac shunts have also been reported in the setting of thoracic deformity.[20] Low mixed venous P_{O_2} ($P\bar{v}_{O_2}$), a frequent finding in patients with pulmonary hypertension and low cardiac output, further lowers arterial oxygenation when there is $\dot{V}/\dot{Q}$ inequality.

HEMODYNAMIC MANAGEMENT

Evaluation of shock in patients with KS is similar to that described elsewhere in this text. When sepsis causes shock, patients with KS and pulmonary hypertension may not mount the usual hyperdynamic response. Hypotensive patients not responding to an initial aggressive volume challenge should be considered for right heart catheterization and/or bedside echocardiography to further direct therapy. Mechanical ventilation is indicated for nearly all patients with persistent shock, in part to redirect blood flow from the diaphragm, which can be as much as 25% of the cardiac output. Mechanical ventilation and sedation decrease oxygen consumption (and thus supplemental oxygen requirement) and lactic acid generation.

When right ventricular failure causes shock, a vicious cycle ensues. As the right ventricle fails, cardiac output and systemic blood pressure fall, limiting perfusion to the right ventricle from the aortic root. Right ventricular end-diastolic volume increases and shifts the interventricular septum to the left, decreasing left ventricular compliance, and further reducing cardiac output and blood pressure. Ensuring an adequate circulating volume and correcting hypoxemia to reduce pulmonary vasoconstriction are the first goals of therapy. Increasing systemic blood pressure and thus perfusion pressure to the right ventricle with norepinephrine may be helpful.[21]

To exclude venous thromboembolism we routinely perform lower extremity Doppler exams; however, roughly 50% of patients with acute pulmonary embolism have negative lower extremity Doppler exams. Serially negative Doppler exams provide an added sense of security, as does a negative D-dimer. Chest computed tomography (CT) with pulmonary embolism protocol is preferable to ventilation-perfusion imaging in chest wall deformity, and may provide additional clues regarding the etiology of respiratory failure. In select cases, pulmonary angiography is required to establish a firm diagnosis. In the absence of venous thromboembolism, preventive therapy with unfractionated heparin or low molecular weight heparin is indicated.

NONINVASIVE VENTILATION

Decreased pulmonary compliance lowers lung volume, which in turn limits cough efficiency and mucus clearance.[22] To improve compliance and treat atelectasis, short periods (15 to 20 minutes) of intermittent positive-pressure ventilation (IPPV) delivered by mouthpiece 4 to 6 times daily using inflation pressures between 20 and 30 cm H_2O have been recommended.[11] IPPV increases lung compliance by 70% for up to 3 hours in acutely ill patients, suggesting that IPPV lowers surface tension by altering the surfactant lining layer.[11]

Alternatively, a volume-preset, time-cycled device may be used.[23]

In patients with acute ventilatory failure, NPPV by full face mask or nasal mask should be considered first-line therapy (see Chap. 33). Advantages of NPPV over invasive ventilation include decreased need for sedation and paralysis, decreased incidence of nosocomial pneumonia, decreased incidence of otitis and sinusitis, and improved patient comfort. Disadvantages include increased risk of aspiration and skin necrosis, and less control of the patient's ventilatory status compared with invasive ventilation.[24]

Although nocturnal NPPV is firmly established in the management of KS patients with chronic respiratory failure,[25,26] there are limited data regarding its efficacy in acutely ill patients.[27–29] In one report of the use of noninvasive ventilation in 164 patients with heterogeneous forms of ARF, only five patients had restrictive lung disease.[30] All five patients improved on noninvasive ventilation, although one subsequently required intubation. Noninvasive ventilation was also helpful in four patients with KS and ARF failing conventional medical therapy.[31]

Following the guidelines of Meduri and colleagues,[30] we initiate NPPV using a loose-fitting full face mask. We start with 0 cm H_2O continuous positive airway pressure (CPAP) and 10 cm H_2O pressure support, and increase CPAP to 3 to 5 cm H_2O and pressure support to the level required to achieve an exhaled tidal volume ≥ 7 mL/kg and a respiratory rate ≤ 25/min.

Noninvasive negative pressure ventilators are not feasible in most acute situations because they generally require patients to lie flat and coordinate their breaths with the ventilator. Difficulties with fit and applying the device adequately to the distorted chest wall further complicate their use. Still, negative pressure ventilators have averted intubation in rare cases,[18] and have been used successfully in the long-term management of patients with KS.[32]

INTUBATION AND MECHANICAL VENTILATION

Intubation is indicated for cardiopulmonary arrest, impending arrest, refractory hypoxemia, mental status changes, and shock. Intubation can be difficult because of spinal curvature and tracheal distortion, and because patients with small lung volumes desaturate quickly. Assessment of the upper airway with fiberoptic bronchoscopy may be useful in some cases. During the peri-intubation period, a fraction of inspired oxygen ($F_{I_{O_2}}$) of 1.0 is desirable, although it should be decreased to nontoxic levels if possible once the patient has been stabilized on the ventilator. Decreasing O_2 consumption with sedatives, use of positive end-expiratory pressure (PEEP), and increasing $P\bar{v}_{O_2}$ are strategies that allow for nontoxic $F_{I_{O_2}}$ in most patients. Positional maneuvers, such as placing the patient in the lateral decubitus position, may improve oxygenation in patients with asymmetric chest walls, but care must be taken to secure the airway.

Ventilatory failure results from an imbalance between respiratory muscle strength and respiratory system load. Thus identifying and correcting reversible elements of this imbalance is fundamental to restoring the ability to breathe. While this occurs, patients should be ventilated to baseline values of Pa_{CO_2} to avoid alkalemia and bicarbonate wasting.

Respiratory muscle fatigue is treated with 48 to 72 hours of complete rest on the ventilator, with early nutritional supplementation and correction of metabolic irregularities. To rest, patients must be comfortable, quiet, and synchronized with the ventilator. If the patient is not synchronized, work of breathing remains high despite ventilator settings that appear to supply most of the minute ventilation.

In patients with bronchospasm and an increase in the peak-to-plateau gradient, we add inhaled bronchodilators and consider systemic steroids. With attention to delivery technique, bronchodilator responsiveness is assessed by measuring airway resistance 15 to 30 minutes after a treatment. Bronchoscopy may be indicated in nonresponders to exclude bronchial torsion that may benefit from placement of an endobronchial stent.[19] Theophylline titrated to a serum level of 10 μg/mL may increase respiratory muscle strength, help clear secretions, and decrease airway resistance without significant toxicity.

Although there are no controlled trials to help guide ventilator management in patients with thoracic deformity, we suggest small tidal volumes (6 to 7 mL/kg) and high respiratory rates (20 to 30/min) to minimize the hemodynamic effects of positive-pressure ventilation and the risk of barotrauma. We maintain plateau pressures <30 cm H_2O to avoid overdistention beyond physiologic TLC and hyperinflation-induced lung injury (pneumothorax, pneumomediastinum, interstitial emphysema, and volutrauma). One consequence of small tidal volume ventilation is reduced alveolar ventilation and hypercapnia. Fortunately, hypercapnia is generally well tolerated as long as Pa_{CO_2} does not exceed 90 mm Hg and acute increases in Pa_{CO_2} are avoided. Associated low values of arterial pH are generally well tolerated. Hypercapnia does cause cerebral vasodilation, cerebral edema, decreased myocardial contractility, vasodilation with a hyperdynamic circulation, and pulmonary vasoconstriction. Accordingly, it should be avoided in patients with raised intracranial pressure (as might occur in the setting of anoxic brain injury after arrest) and severely depressed myocardial function. The use of small tidal volumes demands added attention to lung volume recruitment and prevention of atelectasis. To this end, we initially apply 5 cm H_2O of PEEP to prevent alveolar closure at end-expiration, and gradually increase tidal volume when atelectasis is suspected, keeping plateau pressure <30 cm H_2O.

In refractory hypoxemia a trial of increasing PEEP (in an attempt to achieve 90% saturation of the arterial blood with a $F_{I_{O_2}}$ ≤ 0.6) helps clarify the pathophysiology. To avoid overdistention at end-inspiration, tidal volume should be decreased during PEEP titration. Since the chest wall is stiff in KS, high alveolar pressures increase pleural pressure more than in diseases characterized by stiff lungs, thereby further decreasing venous return to the right atrium and reducing cardiac output. PEEP may also increase pulmonary vascular resistance and worsen right-to-left intracardiac shunt.

The approach to liberation from mechanical ventilation is similar to that described elsewhere in this text. We favor early determination of respiratory muscle strength as assessed by the maximum negative inspiratory force (NIF), and of respiratory system load as determined by the resistive and static pressures generated during positive pressure ventilation. Inadequate strength for a given load manifests as a rapid shallow breathing pattern, which generates a high frequency:tidal volume ratio. A slower and deeper pattern is achieved when strength increases and/or load decreases. Respiratory muscle strength is improved by correction of shock, anemia, acidosis, electrolyte abnormalities, and with the institution of nutrition, and a nonfatiguing graded program of respiratory muscle exercise. Treating pulmonary edema, atelectasis, pneumonia, and airflow obstruction decreases load. When time of extubation is near, ventilation with tidal volumes that mimic the patient's spontaneous tidal volume allows for a smoother transition to spontaneous breathing. In borderline cases, NPPV can be used to facilitate return to spontaneous breathing and reduce ICU length of stay.[33] Tracheostomy may be required in more difficult cases and may be technically difficult in patients with cervical spine curvature and a distorted airway.

LONG-TERM MANAGEMENT

Primary considerations for long-term management include the use of home oxygen therapy and nocturnal NPPV. Patients with moderate to severe KS may demonstrate significant oxygen desaturation on exercise that is prevented by ambulatory oxygen therapy.[34] Derangements in breathing pattern and oxygen desaturation during sleep should be excluded with polysomnography once the patient is stable. A broad spectrum of abnormalities, including central and obstructive sleep apnea, has been identified that may contribute to chronic hypoxemia, cor pulmonale, and early death. Chronic ventilatory failure is an indication for noninvasive nocturnal ventilatory support, which can improve daytime blood gases, sleep pattern, and respiratory muscle strength.[35] Other useful strategies include daytime IPPV (25 cm H_2O for several minutes, 4 to 6 times daily), negative-pressure ventilation, and nighttime mechanical ventilation through a tracheostomy. The role of orthopedic surgery in adolescents is debated and beyond the scope of this chapter.

We recommend serial assessments of right ventricular function and pulmonary artery pressure by echocardiography. The presence of pulmonary hypertension gives added importance to oxygen therapy and mandates exclusion of other treatable causes such as pulmonary embolism.

Abdominal Compartment Syndrome

DEFINITION AND ETIOLOGY

Abdominal compartment syndrome (ACS) is characterized by critical organ dysfunction within and beyond the abdomen resulting from increased intra-abdominal pressure.[36–38] Importantly, the critical value for intra-abdominal hypertension that defines ACS varies from patient to patient, and is dependent on abdominal wall compliance and tissue perfusion pressure.[39] Studies have suggested that an intra-abdominal pressure >25 mm Hg is associated with the development of ACS; other reports have demonstrated that pressures as low as 10 mm Hg can lead to organ dysfunction in select cases.[40,41] Conditions that increase abdominal wall compliance (e.g., prior pregnancy, obesity, and cirrhosis) appear to be protective, while inflexible surgical closures or scars increase risk.[42,43] Given these considerations, the use of a strict cutoff value for intra-abdominal hypertension to define ACS is not recommended. Rather a combination of elevated intra-

TABLE 42-2 Selected Conditions Associated with Abdominal Compartment Syndrome

Abdominal trauma
Burns
Liver transplantation
Pancreatitis
Bowel obstruction
Peritonitis
Intraperitoneal hemorrhage
Tense ascites

abdominal pressure and the presence of organ dysfunction is required for proper diagnosis (see below).

A number of surgical and nonsurgical conditions have been associated with intra-abdominal hypertension. Particularly at risk is the trauma patient requiring large-volume resuscitation and emergent abdominal surgery. Use of temporary closure techniques as an alternative to tight surgical closure increases abdominal wall compliance and minimizes intra-abdominal pressure in patients at risk.[44] Other conditions associated with ACS are included in Table 42-2.

CARDIOPULMONARY EFFECTS

Cephalad displacement of the diaphragm results in mechanical compression, atelectasis, $\dot{V}/\dot{Q}$ inequality, decreased respiratory system compliance, and increased work of breathing.[45] These effects are associated with a fast and shallow respiratory pattern, hypoxemia, and hypercapnia. In mechanically ventilated patients peak and plateau pressures are elevated, leading to a common recommendation to lower tidal volume until plateau pressure is <30 cm H_2O.

Elevation of the diaphragm also reduces ventricular compliance and contractility; by reducing inferior vena caval blood flow, ACS decreases cardiac preload to further drop cardiac output.[46] Hypovolemia further aggravates this physiology, whereas hypervolemia is protective as intra-abdominal pressure increases.[47,48] Despite decreased venous return, pulmonary capillary wedge pressure does not always fall; however, intravascular pressure in this setting does not adequately reflect transmural pressure or intravascular volume.

GASTROINTESTINAL, RENAL, AND CENTRAL NERVOUS SYSTEM EFFECTS

Intra-abdominal hypertension decreases mesenteric arterial flow, an effect that is amplified by decreased cardiac output, hemorrhage, and hypovolemia.[49] Direct compression of mesenteric veins increases venous pressure, promoting visceral edema and further increases in intra-abdominal pressure that decrease gut perfusion.[50] The final event is bowel wall ischemia and translocation of bacteria through a disrupted mucosal barrier that may be central to multiorgan system failure.[51]

Increased venous resistance is also central to the rise in renal venous pressure and renal failure in ACS.[52] As intra-abdominal pressure increases, urine output falls with oliguria potentially developing at an intra-abdominal pressure of 15 mm Hg and anuria at 30 mm Hg.[53]

There is an association between abdominal compartment syndrome and raised intracranial pressure, likely mediated by the effects of intra-abdominal pressure on central venous pressure.[54] A critical situation occurs when systemic hypotension and increased intracranial pressure combine to decrease cerebral perfusion pressure.

DIAGNOSIS

The diagnosis of ACS should be considered in any patient with a tense or distended abdomen who also has hemodynamic instability, a falling urine output, mental status changes, or progressive lactic acidosis. Failure to recognize that intra-abdominal hypertension can occur in the absence of abdominal distension or that multiorgan failure is a manifestation of ACS can lead to a missed diagnosis. The importance of early detection is emphasized because mortality rates in established ACS are generally >50%.[55]

Although there are clues to ACS on abdominal CT imaging, definitive diagnosis requires measurement of intra-abdominal pressure.[56] The usual approach is to use intra-abdominal bladder pressure (IABP) as a surrogate measure of intra-abdominal pressure, based on extensive data that indicate that the two are strongly correlated.[57] The technique relies on measurements taken directly from a Foley catheter with a pressure-transducer zeroed to the level of the pubic symphysis.[57] Accurate measurements rely on ready transmission of intra-abdominal pressure to the bladder, and the bladder not adding its own effects to pressure measurements. Thus there is potential for inaccuracy when the bladder is diseased or when there is critical pathology in the vicinity of the bladder. In general, ACS is not likely when IABP is <10 mm Hg, but should be considered when the pressure is >25 mm Hg. As mentioned, however, strict cutoff values for IABP are neither sensitive nor specific enough to establish ACS, requiring concurrent assessment of organ dysfunction at any level of intra-abdominal pressure.[55]

TREATMENT

Abdominal compartment syndrome resulting from tense ascites is an indication for immediate paracentesis. Pre- and postparacentesis measurements of IABP, urine output, hemodynamics, and airway pressures help confirm ACS and demonstrate the benefit of therapeutic intervention. In most other cases of ACS, prompt surgical decompression is indicated. Determining the appropriate timing for surgical intervention is challenging and may require serial measurement of IABP and assessment of organ function. It is vital to intervene before the development of critical organ dysfunction. To aid in the determination of timing of surgery, some surgeons assess abdominal perfusion pressure (APP = MAP − IABP). An APP <50 mm Hg is associated with a poor outcome and the need for quick intervention.[58] While the operating room is prepared, volume resuscitation and low tidal volume ventilation are useful temporizing measures.

Pulmonary Fibrosis

When normal air spaces and blood vessels are replaced by fibrotic tissue, the lungs become small and stiff. In some disease processes there may be adjacent areas of inflammation amenable to immunosuppressive therapy. However, it is generally well accepted that fibrosis without inflammation is unresponsive to current pharmacologic treatment.

A number of acute and chronic disorders of known and unknown etiology are associated with pulmonary fibrosis. These include idiopathic pulmonary fibrosis (IPF), which is highlighted in this chapter.

As the name implies, IPF is a disease of unknown etiology, characterized by the histologic appearance of usual interstitial pneumonia.[59,60] It most often presents insidiously in patients >50 years old and is progressive regardless of therapy. The hallmarks of IPF are dyspnea and cough. Initially dyspnea occurs only with exercise, but even limited dyspnea can bring about a sedentary lifestyle that further adds to functional disability. As dyspnea progresses, patients develop a rapid and shallow breathing pattern, often maintaining higher-than-normal levels of minute ventilation.[61] Constitutional symptoms include fatigue, malaise, and weight loss; symptoms of sleep-disordered breathing may occur.

Auscultation of the chest frequently reveals dry, "velcro-like" crackles heard loudest at the bases of the lungs; in the late stages of the disease, cardiac examination may reveal signs of pulmonary hypertension. Clubbing of the fingers and toes commonly occurs in IPF (and asbestosis) and rarely in other interstitial lung diseases.

LABORATORY ABNORMALITIES

Hypoxemia that worsens with exercise or sleep and respiratory alkalosis are common in IPF. The development of hypercapnia is an ominous sign of imminent death. Despite hypoxemia, polycythemia is rare.[62] Elevations of sedimentation rate, serum immunoglobulins, antinuclear antibodies, and rheumatoid factor can occur; an increase in angiotensin-converting enzyme or antineutrophil cytoplasmic antibodies suggests a different diagnosis.[59]

The radiographic distribution of infiltrates often suggests the underlying disorder. Peripheral reticular opacities most prominent at the bases and low lung volumes are classic in IPF. Traction bronchiectasis occurs when fibrotic lung tissue tethers open adjacent airways. Ground-glass opacifications are either absent or minimal.[59] Subpleural honeycombing at bases of both lungs is characteristic of IPF.[59]

Other causes of lower lobe–predominant infiltrates include fibrosis associated with connective tissue disorders, asbestosis, and chronic aspiration. Upper lobe–predominant lesions include sarcoidosis, tuberculosis, fungal infections, silicosis, allergic bronchopulmonary aspergillosis, eosinophilic granuloma, ankylosing spondylitis, berylliosis, cystic fibrosis, and hypersensitivity pneumonitis. If hilar adenopathy is present, sarcoidosis, tuberculosis, histoplasmosis, malignancy, and berylliosis should be considered. Pleural effusion suggests lymphangioleiomyomatosis, connective tissue disorder, asbestosis, or drug-induced lung disease. Extensive parenchymal cysts occur in eosinophilic granuloma or lymphangioleiomyomatosis. These conditions can result in diffuse infiltrates with normal or increased lung volumes, as can a mixed process of emphysema and IPF.

RESPIRATORY MECHANICS

In end-stage pulmonary fibrosis, pulmonary function tests typically show reduced TLC, VC, and IC (see Fig. 42-2). FRC and RV are also reduced, though usually to a lesser extent

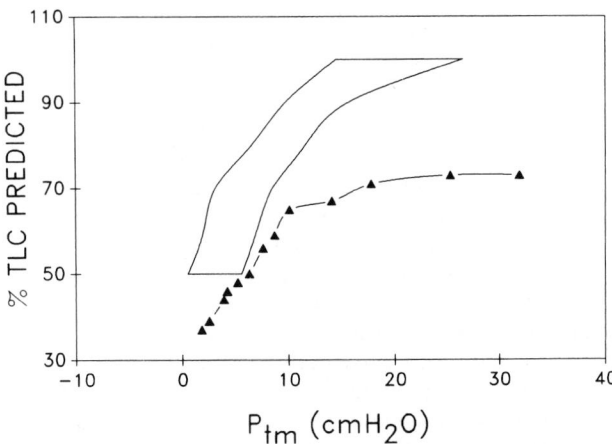

FIGURE 42-4 Pressure-volume curve of the lung in a 48-year-old man with sarcoidosis. The P-V curve is shifted downward and to the right of the normal range, such that increased elastic recoil of the lung limits TLC despite a large maximum transpulmonary pressure. This requires patients to generate prohibitively large negative pleural pressures to inspire minimal amounts of air.

than TLC or VC. Rarely, RV is normal when there is early airway closure or decreased elastic recoil pressure at low lung volumes.[63] Both the forced vital capacity (FVC) and the forced expiratory volume in 1 second (FEV_1) are decreased, but FEV_1/FVC is increased; in this instance, high expiratory flow rates relative to volume reflect increased elastic recoil pressure. Airway resistance is usually normal or low, although reversible and irreversible obstructive defects do occur.

Since chest wall compliance and respiratory muscles are normal in most patients with pulmonary fibrosis,[64] lung volumes are affected by changes in the pressure-volume relationship of the noncompliant lung (Fig. 42-4).[64] The P-V curve is shifted downward and to the right, such that increased elastic recoil of the lung limits TLC despite a very large transpulmonary pressure. This requires patients to generate large negative pleural pressures during inspiration, and is the reason why patients prefer a fast and shallow respiratory pattern. Smaller tidal volumes are an adaptive response to minimize work of breathing, which can be five to six times normal.[65]

GAS EXCHANGE

Exercise-induced hypoxemia and a low single-breath diffusing capacity (DLCO) are hallmarks of early disease. Indeed they may occur before dyspnea or radiographic changes.[63] With time, arterial hypoxemia and a widened $(A-a)_{O_2}$ are found at rest. In 20% of patients, arterial hypoxemia is worse when they are in the upright position and is improved on recumbency.[62] This paradoxical pattern is also seen with patent foramen ovale, intrapulmonary arteriovenous malformation, and hepatopulmonary syndrome. Arterial saturation also falls significantly in many patients during REM sleep.[66] Sleep-related desaturation is due to the exaggerated effects of normal nocturnal hypoventilation and $\dot{V}/\dot{Q}$ variance, or to abnormal alveolar hypoventilation from respiratory muscle dysfunction or obstructive sleep apnea.

The importance of an anatomic barrier to the diffusion of oxygen (secondary to a thickened, fibrotic interstitium) has been debated. In eight patients with varying types of intersti-

tial lung disease, multiple inert gas analysis $\dot{V}/\dot{Q}$ inequality was the principal defect; diffusion limitation contributed to none of the $(A-a)_{O_2}$ at rest and only 19% of the $(A-a)_{O_2}$ during exercise.[67] However, in 15 patients with IPF also studied by multiple inert gas elimination, 19% of the $(A-a)_{O_2}$ at rest and 40% of the $(A-a)_{O_2}$ during exercise was attributed to diffusion limitation.[68] $\dot{V}/\dot{Q}$ inequality remained the principal defect, contributing to 81% of the $(A-a)_{O_2}$ at rest, and a combination of low $P\bar{v}_{O_2}$ from an inadequate cardiac output, diffusion limitation, and high $\dot{V}/\dot{Q}$ variance accounted for the widening of the $(A-a)_{O_2}$ during exercise. Intrapulmonary shunt was small, averaging 2% of cardiac output at rest and 3% during exercise.

The dead space:tidal volume ratio (VDS/VT) may exceed 0.4 (normal = <0.3) in end-stage fibrosis.[69] This reflects an increase in the volume of alveolar dead space and a decrease in tidal volume. When VDS/VT is high, greater minute ventilation is required to maintain alveolar ventilation and a normal Pa_{CO_2}. Patients may surpass these heightened requirements to achieve respiratory alkalosis, perhaps in response to greater afferent stimuli from the fibrotic lung.[61] The development of hypercapnia is an ominous sign of imminent death.

EFFECTS ON THE PULMONARY CIRCULATION

Pulmonary hypertension and cor pulmonale are common in patients with end-stage pulmonary fibrosis, correlating with a DLCO <45% predicted and a VC <50% predicted.[70] Pulmonary hypertension occurs when blood vessels are altered by the fibrotic process, microthrombi, or hypoxic pulmonary vasoconstriction. Since polycythemia and high cardiac output are rare in IPF, they rarely contribute to pulmonary hypertension. Supplemental oxygen may alleviate hypoxic pulmonary vasoconstriction, but pulmonary hypertension resulting from destroyed and distorted vasculature is likely irreversible. Pulmonary hypertension has been associated with redistribution of pulmonary blood flow to the upper lobes,[62] a pattern that rarely normalizes after corticosteroids.[69] Because pulmonary vascular resistance is high, the gradient between the pulmonary artery diastolic pressure and the pulmonary capillary wedge pressure is wide.

ACUTE CARDIOPULMONARY FAILURE

Whether acute deterioration is reversible depends on the severity of pulmonary fibrosis, the extent of comorbidities, the nature and severity of the acute insult, and whether the acute insult accelerates the underlying disease process.

OUTCOME

ICU management including the use of mechanical ventilation may be appropriate for select patients with pulmonary fibrosis: (1) patients with early/mild disease, particularly in absence of a firm diagnosis, (2) patients with previously mild disease who present with an acute, seemingly reversible insult, (3) patients who have experienced adverse effects of therapy (e.g., drug-induced lung disease), (4) patients who may undergo imminent lung transplant, and (5) patients with pulmonary fibrosis associated with connective tissue disease or vasculitis with ground-glass opacifications or consolidation that may represent a treatable form of pneumonitis or alveolar hemorrhage. Appropriately excluded from this practice are patients with progressive, end-stage disease in whom outcome is invariably poor. In these cases, a prospective discussion and decision not to initiate resuscitative efforts should precede the anticipated terminal event.

The results of several recent studies demonstrate the grim prognosis of patients with IPF admitted to the ICU for acute respiratory failure. Blivet and colleagues described the course of 15 patients admitted to the ICU with IPF and respiratory failure.[71] Twelve patients required intubation either at the time of admission or after failure of noninvasive ventilation; three patients received only noninvasive ventilation. Eleven patients died either from respiratory failure or septic shock; four patients were discharged alive from the ICU, but two died shortly thereafter. Stern and colleagues reported their experience in 23 patients with IPF requiring intubation for acute respiratory failure.[72] With the exception of one patient who received a single-lung transplant 6 hours after initiating mechanical ventilation, all patients died while receiving mechanical ventilation. Fumeaux and colleagues similarly reported 100% mortality in 14 consecutive patients with IPF admitted to the ICU for mechanical ventilation after a mean of 7.6 days.[73] Finally, in the study by Saydain and colleagues of 38 patients with IPF admitted to the ICU mainly for respiratory failure, ICU mortality was 43% and hospital mortality was 61%.[74] However, 92% of hospital survivors died a median of 2 months after discharge.

DETECTING REVERSIBLE FEATURES

Although clinical deterioration may reflect disease progression, the differential diagnosis of an acute change in status is quite broad (Table 42-3).[59] In our experience it is often difficult to distinguish disease progression from respiratory tract infection. Frequently the cause of acute respiratory failure is not identified.[72] Acute deterioration stemming from IPF progression is essentially an untreatable condition (see above).

Pneumonia in IPF generally results from community-acquired bacteria; opportunistic infection is rare despite the widespread use of immunosuppressive agents.[70] However, *Pneumocystis carinii* pneumonia should be considered in immunosuppressed patients, particularly when ground-glass infiltrates are identified on CT imaging. Mycobacterial infection should also be considered. The incidence of tuberculosis is increased in patients with chronic interstitial lung disease, particularly in those with silicosis;[75] atypical mycobacterial superinfection may also underlie clinical deterioration in some cases. When fibrosis is associated with connective tissue disease or vasculitis, an acute deterioration may represent pneumonitis, bronchiolitis obliterans-organizing pneumonia, or alveolar hemorrhage. Patients with diffuse alveolar opacifications not responsive to antibiotics or diuresis should be considered for bronchoalveolar lavage or lung biopsy in selected cases to confirm the diagnosis.

When pneumothorax causes acute deterioration, re-expansion is countered by low parenchymal compliance occasionally requiring high levels of negative pleural pressure for prolonged periods of time.

Clinical deterioration may represent acute right or left heart failure. Right ventricular ischemia or pulmonary embolism may provoke right ventricular failure. Left-sided failure is difficult to establish without echocardiography or hemodynamic measurements because bibasilar crackles are invariably present and jugular venous distention may reflect isolated right ventricular failure.

If deterioration occurs over a period of weeks to months, progressive fibrosis, bronchogenic carcinoma, steroid myopathy, drug toxicity, cor pulmonale, and left ventricular failure should be considered.

OXYGEN THERAPY

Identification and correction of arterial hypoxemia are vital to the initial evaluation. We recommend titration of supplemental oxygen until 90% saturation is achieved. It is not unusual for patients with fibrosis to require higher flow rates than patients with chronic obstructive pulmonary disease or asthma. Hypoxemia, in addition to its many other adverse effects, causes hypoxic pulmonary vasoconstriction and may precipitate right ventricular failure in patients with pre-existing pulmonary hypertension.

CARDIOVASCULAR MANAGEMENT

Evaluation of shock in patients with pulmonary fibrosis is similar to that described elsewhere in this text (see Chaps. 20 and 21). Hypotension with cool and clammy extremities and a narrow pulse pressure suggests an inadequate cardiac output from hypovolemia, left ventricular failure, cor pulmonale, pericardial effusion, or valvular heart disease. Hypotension with a warm and bounding circulation and a wide pulse pressure suggests sepsis; however, patients with pulmonary hypertension may be unable to mount a hyperdynamic response to peripheral vasodilation. Adrenal insufficiency contributing to shock should be excluded, particularly when corticosteroids have been used for therapy.

VENTILATOR MANAGEMENT

When deemed appropriate, intubation is indicated for cardiopulmonary arrest, refractory hypoxemia, progressive ventilatory failure, mental status changes, and shock. Once the decision to intubate has been made, the goals are to achieve adequate arterial oxygen saturation and avoid ventilator-induced lung injury. Although there are no controlled trials to guide specific recommendations, we advocate an approach to mechanical ventilation that is similar to that recommended in the acute respiratory distress syndrome.[76] To avoid excessive tidal volume excursions and alveolar overinflation, we use tidal volumes in the range of 6 to 7 mL/kg combined with respiratory rates of 20 to 30 breaths/min when ventilating patients with pulmonary fibrosis. The goal is to maintain airway plateau pressures below 30 cm H_2O in an attempt to avoid overdistention beyond physiologic TLC and

TABLE 42-3 Selected Causes of Deterioration in Patients with Pulmonary Fibrosis

Progression of the underlying disease
Pneumonia
Pulmonary embolism
Left ventricular failure
Cor pulmonale
Aspiration
Bronchospasm
Pneumothorax
Bronchogenic carcinoma

hyperinflation-induced lung injury. A consequence of small tidal volume ventilation is reduced alveolar ventilation and hypercapnia. Hypercapnia can be reduced for a given minute ventilation by decreasing CO_2 production (i.e., treating fever and agitation and avoiding excessive caloric intake), repleting intravascular volume, and avoiding excessive PEEP to decrease V_{DS}/V_T. Still, in order to achieve desired airway pressures, hypercapnia is unavoidable in many cases. In patients with chronic ventilatory failure, we further desire a minute ventilation that maintains Pa_{CO_2} greater than or equal to baseline to avoid alkalemia and bicarbonate wasting.

The use of PEEP avoids tidal collapse of alveoli at low lung volumes and may help recruit fluid-filled and atelectatic lung units. We generally start with 5 cm H_2O PEEP and increase in an attempt to achieve 90% saturation of the arterial blood with a F_{IO_2} of 0.6 or less. Though F_{IO_2} of 1.0 is desirable in the peri-intubation period, it should be decreased as quickly as possible (to no greater than 0.6) to avoid oxygen toxicity. The use of sedatives and muscle relaxants to decrease oxygen consumption, PEEP, and increasing $P\bar{v}_{O_2}$ allows for nontoxic F_{IO_2} in many cases.

High alveolar pressures compress alveolar vessels, diverting blood flow from ventilated units and increasing dead space. Increasing V_{DS}/V_T from 0.4 to 0.6 requires an increase in minute ventilation of 50% to maintain a constant Pa_{CO_2}.[77] Increasing minute ventilation, however, increases alveolar pressure and V_{DS}/V_T further, creating a vicious cycle if minute ventilation is continually increased in a misguided attempt to lower Pa_{CO_2}. High alveolar and pleural pressures also increase right atrial pressure and thereby decrease venous return to the right atrium, cardiac output, $P\bar{v}_{O_2}$, and blood pressure. Additionally, diversion of blood flow using high alveolar pressure increases flow to nonventilated units, as in pneumonic consolidation.

LONG-TERM MANAGEMENT OF IDIOPATHIC PULMONARY FIBROSIS

Because no drug therapy has clearly been demonstrated to benefit patients with IPF, long-term management is largely supportive.[60] We suggest referral to a regional center of expertise for consideration of enrollment in a clinical trial or evaluation for lung transplantation. The poor outcomes in patients with IPF admitted to the ICU underscores the importance of advance directives.

References

1. Bergofsky EH: Respiratory failure in disorders of the thoracic cage. *Am Rev Respir Dis* 119:643, 1979.
2. Bergofsky EH, Turino GM, Fishman AP: Cardiorespiratory failure in kyphoscoliosis. *Medicine* 38:263, 1959.
3. Rom WN, Miller A: Unexpected longevity in patients with severe kyphoscoliosis. *Thorax* 33:106, 1978.
4. Mezon BL, West P, Israels J, et al: Sleep breathing abnormalities in kyphoscoliosis. *Am Rev Respir Dis* 122:617, 1980.
5. Guilleminault C, Kurland G, Winkle R, et al: Severe kyphoscoliosis, breathing, and sleep. *Chest* 79:626, 1982.
6. Caro CG, DuBois AB: Pulmonary function in kyphoscoliosis. *Thorax* 16:282, 1961.
7. Collins DK, Ponseti IV: Long term follow-up of patients with idiopathic kyphoscoliosis not treated surgically. *J Bone Joint Surg* 51A:425, 1969.
8. Kearon C, Viviani GR, Kirkley A, et al: Factors determining pulmonary function in adolescent idiopathic thoracic scoliosis. *Am Rev Respir Dis* 148:288, 1993.
9. Jones RS, Kennedy JD, Hasham F, et al: Mechanical inefficiency of the thoracic cage in scoliosis. *Thorax* 36:456, 1981.
10. Conti G, Rocco M, Antonelli M, et al: Respiratory system mechanics in the early phase of acute respiratory failure due to severe kyphoscoliosis. *Intensive Care Med* 23:539, 1997.
11. Sinha R, Bergofsky EH: Prolonged alteration of lung mechanics in kyphoscoliosis by positive pressure hyperinflation. *Am Rev Respir Dis* 106:47, 1972.
12. Lisboa C, Moreno R, Fava M, et al: Inspiratory muscle function in patients with severe kyphoscoliosis. *Am Rev Respir Dis* 132:48, 1985.
13. Grippi MA, Fishman AP: Respiratory failure in structural and neuromuscular disorders involving the chest bellows, in Fishman AP (ed): *Pulmonary Diseases and Disorders*, 2nd ed. New York, McGraw-Hill, 1988, p 2299.
14. Keamy MF III, Yanos J, Davis K, et al: Canine diaphragm contractility is depressed by respiratory but not lactic acidosis. *Am Rev Respir Dis* 137:386, 1988 (abstract).
15. Hoeppner VH, Cockcroft DW, Dosman JA, et al: Nighttime ventilation improves respiratory failure in secondary kyphoscoliosis. *Am Rev Respir Dis* 129:240, 1984.
16. Simonds AK, Carroll N, Branthwaite MA: Kyphoscoliosis as a cause of cardio-respiratory failure—pitfalls of diagnosis. *Respir Med* 83:149, 1989.
17. Schlenker E, Feldmeyer F, Hoster M, Ruhle KH: Effect of noninvasive ventilation on pulmonary artery pressure in patients with severe kyphoscoliosis. *Med Klin* 92(Suppl 1):40, 1997.
18. Libby DM, Briscoe WA, Boyce B, et al: Acute respiratory failure in scoliosis and kyphosis. Prolonged survival and treatment. *Am J Med* 73:532, 1982.
19. Al-Kattan K, Simonds A, Chung KF, Kaplan DK: Kyphoscoliosis and bronchial torsion. *Chest* 111:1134, 1997.
20. Herry I, Iung B, Piechaud JY, et al: Cardiac cause of hypoxaemia in a kyphoscoliotic patient. *Eur Respir J* 14:1433, 1999.
21. Molloy WD, Lee KY, Girling L, et al: Treatment of shock in a canine model of pulmonary embolism. *Am Rev Respir Dis* 130:870, 1984.
22. Azarian R, Lofaso F, Zerah F, et al: Assessment of respiratory compliance in awake subjects using pressure support. *Eur Resp J* 6:552, 1993.
23. Simonds AK, Parker RA, Branthwaite MA: The effect of intermittent positive-pressure hyperinflation in restrictive chest wall disease. *Respiration* 55:136, 1989.
24. Meduri GU, Abou-Shala N, Fox RC, et al: Noninvasive face mask mechanical ventilation in patients with acute hypercapnic respiratory failure. *Chest* 100:445, 1991.
25. Masa JF, Celli B, Riesco JA, et al: The obesity hypoventilation syndrome can be treated with noninvasive mechanical ventilation. *Chest* 119:1102, 2001.
26. Gonzalez C, Ferris G, Diaz J, et al: Kyphoscoliosis ventilatory-insufficiency: Effects of long-term intermittent positive-pressure ventilation. *Chest* 124:857, 2003.
27. Leger P, Bedicam JM, Cornette A, et al: Nasal intermittent positive pressure ventilation. *Chest* 105:100, 1994.
28. Hill NS, Eveloff SE, Carlisle CC, et al: Efficacy of nocturnal nasal ventilation in patients with restrictive thoracic disease. *Am Rev Respir Dis* 145:365, 1992.
29. Simonds AK, Elliott MW: Outcome of domiciliary nasal intermittent positive pressure ventilation in restrictive and obstructive disorders. *Thorax* 50:604, 1995.
30. Meduri GU, Turner RE, Abou-Shala N, et al: Noninvasive positive pressure ventilation via face mask: First-line intervention in patients with acute hypercapnic and hypoxemic respiratory failure. *Chest* 109:179, 1996.

31. Finlay G, Concannon D, McDonnell TJ: Treatment of respiratory failure due to kyphoscoliosis with nasal intermittent positive pressure ventilation (NIPPV). *Irish J Med Sci* 164:28, 1995.

32. Jackson M, Kinnear W, King M, et al: The effects of five years of nocturnal cuirass-assisted ventilation in chest wall disease. *Eur Respir J* 6:630, 1993.

33. Udwadia ZF, Santis GK, Steven MH, et al: Nasal ventilation to facilitate weaning in patients with chronic respiratory insufficiency. *Thorax* 47:715, 1992.

34. Jones DJ, Paul EA, Bell JH: Ambulatory oxygen therapy in stable kyphoscoliosis. *Eur Respir J* 8:819, 1995.

35. Ellis ER, Grunstein RR, Chan S, et al: Noninvasive ventilatory support during sleep improves respiratory failure in kyphoscoliosis. *Chest* 94:811, 1988.

36. Bailey J, Shapiro M: Abdominal compartment syndrome. *Crit Care* 4:23, 2000.

37. Ivatury RR, Sugarman HJ: Abdominal compartment syndrome: A century later, isn't it time to pay attention? *Crit Care Med* 28:2137, 2000.

38. McNelis J, Marini CP, Simms HH: Abdominal compartment syndrome: clinical manifestations and predictive factors. *Curr Opin Crit Care* 9:133, 2003.

39. Cheatham ML, White MW, Sagraves SG, et al: Abdominal perfusion pressure: a superior parameter in the assessment of intra-abdominal hypertension. *J Trauma* 49:621, 2000.

40. Schein M, Ivatury R: Intra-abdominal hypertension and the abdominal compartment syndrome. *Br J Surg* 85:1027, 1998.

41. Ivatury RR, Diebel L, Porter JM, Simon RJ: Intra-abdominal hypertension and the abdominal compartment syndrome. *Surg Clin North Am* 77:783, 1997.

42. Sugerman HJ, DeMaria EJ, Felton WL, Nakatsuka M: Increased intra-abdominal pressure and cardiac filling pressures in obesity-associated pseudotumor cerebri. *Neurology* 49:507, 1997.

43. Hobson KG, Young KM, Ciraulo A, et al: Release of abdominal compartment syndrome improves survival in patients with burn injury. *J Trauma* 53:1129, 2002.

44. Mayberry JC, Goldman RK, Mullins RJ, et al: Surveyed opinion of American trauma surgeons on the prevention of abdominal compartment syndrome. *J Trauma* 47:509, 1999.

45. Obeid F, Saba A, Fath J, Guslits B: Increases in intra-abdominal pressure affect pulmonary compliance. *Arch Surg* 130:544, 1995.

46. Cullen DJ, Coyle JP, Teplick R, Long MC: Cardiovascular, pulmonary and renal effects of massively increased intra-abdominal pressure in critically ill patients. *Crit Care Med* 17:118, 1989.

47. Kashtan J, Green JF, Parsons EQ, Holcroft JW: Hemodynamic effect of increased intraabdominal pressure. *J Surg Res* 30:249, 1981.

48. Ridings PC, Bloomfield GL, Blocher CCR, Sugerman HJ: Cardiopulmonary effects of raised intra-abdominal pressure before and after intravascular volume expansion. *J Trauma* 39:1071, 1995.

49. Friedlander MH, Simon RJ, Ivatury R, DiRaimo R: Effect of hemorrhage on superior mesenteric artery flow during increased intra-abdominal pressures. *J Trauma* 45:433, 1994.

50. Diebel LN, Wilson RF, Dulchavsky SA, Saxe J: Effect of intra-abdominal pressure on hepatic arterial, portal venous and hepatic microcirculatory blood flow. *J Trauma* 33:279, 1992.

51. Diebel LN, Dulchavsky SA, Brown WJ: Splanchnic ischemia and bacterial translocation in the abdominal compartment syndrome. *J Trauma* 43:852, 1997.

52. Doty JM, Saggi BH, Sugerman HJ, Blocher CR: Effect of increased renal venous pressure on renal function. *J Trauma* 47:1000, 1999.

53. Richards WO, Scovill W, Shin B, Reed W: Acute renal failure associated with increased intra-abdominal pressure. *Ann Surg* 197:183, 1983.

54. Citero G, Vascotto E, Villa F, Celotti S: Induced abdominal compartment syndrome increases intracranial pressure in neurotrauma patients: a prospective study. *Crit Care Med* 29:1466, 2001.

55. Burch JM, Moore EE, Moore FA, Franciose R: The abdominal compartment syndrome. *Surg Clin North Am* 76:833, 1996.

56. Pickhardt PJ, Shimony JS, Heiken JP, Buchman TG: The abdominal compartment syndrome: CT findings. *Am J Roentgenol* 173:575, 1999.

57. Fusco MA, Martin RS, Chang MC: Estimation of intra-abdominal pressure by bladder pressure measurement: validity and methodology. *J Trauma* 50:297, 2001.

58. Cheatham ML, White MW, Sagraves SG, Johnson JL: Abdominal perfusion pressure: a superior parameter in the assessment of intra-abdominal hypertension. *J Trauma* 49:621, 2000.

59. American Thoracic Society: Idiopathic pulmonary fibrosis: diagnosis and treatment. International consensus statement. American Thoracic Society and the European Respiratory Society. *Am J Respir Crit Care Med* 161:646, 2000.

60. Gross TJ, Hunninghake GW: Idiopathic pulmonary fibrosis. *N Engl J Med* 345:517, 2001.

61. Lourenco RV, Turino GM, Davidson LAG, et al: The regulation of ventilation in diffuse pulmonary fibrosis. *Am J Med* 38:199, 1965.

62. Crystal RG, Fulmer JD, Roberts WC, et al: Idiopathic pulmonary fibrosis: Clinical, histologic, radiographic, scintigraphic, cytologic and biochemical aspects. *Ann Intern Med* 85:769, 1976.

63. Kern JA, Fishman AP: End-stage fibrotic lung disease: Treatment and prognosis, in Fishman AP (ed): *Pulmonary Diseases and Disorders*, 2nd ed. New York, McGraw-Hill, 1988, p 2237.

64. De Troyer A, Yernault JC: Inspiratory muscle force in normal subjects and patients with interstitial lung disease. *Thorax* 35:92, 1980.

65. West JR, Alexander JK: Studies on respiratory mechanics and the work of breathing in pulmonary fibrosis. *Am J Med* 27:529, 1959.

66. Bye PTP, Issa F, Berthon-Jones M, et al: Studies on oxygenation during sleep on patients with interstitial lung disease. *Am Rev Respir Dis* 129:27, 1984.

67. Wagner PD, Dantzker DR, Dueck R, et al: Distribution of ventilation-perfusion ratios in patients with interstitial lung disease. *Chest* 69(Suppl):256, 1976.

68. Agusti AGN, Roca J, Gea J, et al: Mechanisms of gas exchange impairment in idiopathic pulmonary fibrosis. *Am Rev Respir Dis* 143:219, 1991.

69. McCarthy D, Cherniak RM: Regional ventilation-perfusion and hypoxia in cryptogenic fibrosing alveolitis. *Am Rev Respir Dis* 107:200, 1973.

70. Panos RJ, Mortenson RL, Niccoli SA, et al: Clinical deterioration in patients with idiopathic pulmonary fibrosis: causes and assessment. *Am J Med* 88:396, 1990.

71. Blivet S, Philit F, Sab JM, et al: Outcome of patients with idiopathic pulmonary fibrosis admitted to the ICU for respiratory failure. *Chest* 120:209, 2001.

72. Stern J-B, Mal H, Groussand O, et al: Prognosis of patients with advanced idiopathic fibrosis requiring mechanical ventilation for acute respiratory failure. *Chest* 120:213, 2001.

73. Fumeaux T, Rothmeier C, Jolliet P: Outcome of mechanical ventilation for acute respiratory failure in patients with pulmonary fibrosis. *Intensive Care Med* 27:1868, 2001.

74. Saydain G, Islam A, Afessa B, et al: Outcome of patients with idiopathic fibrosis admitted to the intensive care unit. *Am J Respir Crit Care Med* 166:839, 2002.

75. Sachor Y, Schindler D, Siegal A, et al: Increased incidence of pulmonary tuberculosis in patients with chronic interstitial lung disease. *Thorax* 44:151, 1989.

76. The Acute Respiratory Distress Network: Ventilation with lower tidal volumes as compared with traditional volumes for acute lung injury and the acute respiratory distress syndrome. *N Engl J Med* 342:1301, 2000.

77. Snyder JV, Froese A: Respirator lung, in Snyder JV, Pinsky MR (eds): *Oxygen Transport in the Critically Ill*. Chicago, Year Book Medical, 1987, p 358.

Chapter 43 _____

VENTILATOR-ASSOCIATED PNEUMONIA

JEAN CHASTRE
JEAN-YVES FAGON

KEY POINTS

- *The risk of nosocomial pneumonia is considerably higher in the subset of ICU patients treated with mechanical ventilation, with an incremental risk of about 1% per day of ventilation.*

- *Ventilator-associated pneumonia (VAP) is associated with mortality in excess of that caused by the underlying disease alone, particularly in case of infection due to high-risk pathogens, such as Pseudomonas aeruginosa and Acinetobacter spp. and when initial antibiotic therapy is inappropriate.*

- *The predominant organisms responsible for infection are Staphylococcus aureus, P. aeruginosa, and Enterobacteriaceae, but etiologic agents differ widely according to the population of hospital patients, duration of hospital stay, and prior antimicrobial therapy.*

- *Although appropriate antibiotics may improve survival in patients with VAP, use of empirical broad-spectrum antibiotics in patients without infection is potentially harmful, facilitating colonization and superinfection with multiresistant microorganisms. Any strategy designed to evaluate patients suspected of having developed VAP therefore should be able to withhold antimicrobial treatment in patients without pneumonia.*

- *Because even a few doses of a new antimicrobial agent can negate results of microbiologic cultures, pulmonary secretions in patients suspected of having developed VAP always should be obtained before new antibiotics are administered.*

- *Bronchoscopic techniques, when performed before introduction of new antibiotics, enable physicians to identify most patients who need immediate treatment and help to select optimal therapy in a manner that is safe and well tolerated.*

- *Empirical treatment of patients with VAP should be selected based on available epidemiologic characteristics, information provided by direct examination of pulmonary secretions, intrinsic antibacterial activities of antimicrobial agents, and their pharmacokinetic characteristics.*

- *Once the microbiologic data become available, antimicrobial therapy should be re-evaluated in order to avoid prolonged use of a broader spectrum of antibiotic therapy than is justified by the available information. For many patients, including those with late-onset infection, the culture data will not show the presence of highly resistant pathogens, and in these individuals, therapy can be narrowed or even reduced to a single agent in light of the susceptibility pattern of the causative pathogens without risking inappropriate treatment.*

- *Some very simple, no-cost measures, such as judicious use and prompt removal of a useless nasogastric tube, removal of ventilator tubing condensates with minimal exposure to patients,*

placement of ventilated patients in a semirecumbent position, prevention of sinusitis, and use of sucralfate instead of H_2 blockers, may have an impact on the frequency of VAP.

Ventilator-associated pneumonia (VAP) remains a major cause of mortality and morbidity despite the introduction of potent broad-spectrum antimicrobial agents, major advances in the management of ventilator-dependent patients admitted to ICUs, and the use of preventive measures, including the routine use of effective procedures to disinfect respiratory equipment. Rates of pneumonia are considerably higher among patients hospitalized in ICUs compared with those in hospital wards, and the risk of pneumonia is increased three- to tenfold for the intubated patient on mechanical ventilation (MV).[1–10] In contrast to infections of more frequently involved organs (e.g., urinary tract and skin), for which mortality is low, ranging from 1% to 4%, the mortality rate for VAP, defined as pneumonia occurring more than 48 hours after endotracheal intubation and initiation of MV, ranges from 24% to 50% and can reach 76% in some specific settings or when lung infection is caused by high-risk pathogens.[8–18] Because several studies have shown that appropriate antimicrobial treatment of patients with VAP significantly improves outcome, more rapid identification of infected patients and accurate selection of antimicrobial agents represent important clinical goals.[12,19,20] However, consensus on appropriate diagnostic, therapeutic, and preventive strategies for VAP has yet to be reached.

Epidemiology

Accurate data on the epidemiology of VAP are limited by the lack of standardized criteria for its diagnosis. Conceptually, VAP is defined as an inflammation of the lung parenchyma caused by infectious agents not present or incubating at the time MV was started. Despite the clarity of this conception, the past three decades have witnessed the appearance of numerous operational definitions, none of which is universally accepted. Even definitions based on histopathologic findings at autopsy may fail to find consensus or provide certainty. Pneumonia in focal areas of a lobe may be missed, microbiologic studies may be negative despite the presence of inflammation in the lung, and pathologists may disagree on the findings.[21–24] The absence of a "gold standard" continues to fuel controversy about the adequacy and relevance of many studies in this field. Prolonged (>48 hours) MV is the most important factor associated with nosocomial pneumonia. However, VAP may occur within the first 48 hours following intubation. Since the seminal study by Langer and colleagues,[25] it is usual to distinguish early-onset VAP, which occurs during the first 4 days of MV, from late-onset VAP, which develops 5 days or more after initiation of MV. Not only are the causative pathogens commonly different, but the disease also is usually less severe and the prognosis better in early-onset than late-onset VAP.[26,27]

INCIDENCE

The majority of studies have reported incidence rates of nosocomial pneumonia in general ICU populations varying between 8% and 20%. These rates are much higher than the mean annual incidence of nosocomial lower respiratory tract

TABLE 43-1 Incidence and Crude Mortality Rates of VAP

First Author, Ref.	Year of Publication	No. of Patients	Incidence (%)	Diagnostic Criteria	Mortality Rate (%)
ICU patients					
Salata, 33	1987	51	41	Clinical, autopsy	76
Craven, 13	1986	233	21	Clinical	55
Langer, 6	1989	724	23	Clinical	44
Fagon, 9	1989	567	9	PSB	71
Kerver, 34	1987	39	67	Clinical	30
Driks, 35	1987	130	18	Clinical	56
Torres, 12	1990	322	24	Clinical, PSB	33
Baker, 36	1996	514	5	PSB/BAL	24
Kollef, 37	1993	277	16	Clinical	37
Fagon, 38	1996	1118	28	PSB/BAL	53
Timsit, 39	1996	387	15	PSB/BAL	57
Cook, 29	1998	1014	18	Clinical, PSB/BAL	24
Tejada Artigas, 40	2001	103	22	PSB	44
ARDS patients					
Sutherland, 31	1995	105	15	PSB/BAL	38
Declaux, 15	1997	30	60	PTC/BAL	63
Chastre, 14	1998	56	55	PSB/BAL	78
Meduri, 32	1998	94	43	PSB/BAL	52
Markowicz, 16	2000	134	37	PSB/BAL	57

NOTE: PSB = protected specimen brush; BAL = bronchoalveolar lavage; PTC = plugged telescoping catheter.

infection of approximately 0.6 episodes per 100 hospitalizations recorded by the National Nosocomial Infection Study (NNIS), which included all patients regardless of their location in the hospital.[28]

The risk of pneumonia seems to be considerably higher in the subset of ICU patients treated with mechanical ventilation. Cross and Roup[5] have published specific data on overall rates of nosocomial pneumonia in relation to the use of respiratory devices. Pneumonia rates in patients with an endotracheal tube and mechanical ventilation were increased 10-fold over patients with no respiratory therapy devices. Similarly, in the Study on the Efficacy of Nosocomial Infection Control (SENIC), the pneumonia rate was 21-fold higher for patients treated with continuous ventilatory support than for patients not receiving mechanical ventilation.[28]

The VAP rates reported in the more recent studies evaluating homogeneous groups of patients receiving mechanical ventilation are shown in Table 43-1. In their prospective investigation on pneumonia in 23 Italian ICUs that included 724 critically ill patients who had received prolonged (>24 hour) ventilatory assistance since admission, Langer and colleagues[6] found a mean rate of nosocomial pneumonia of 23%; the incidence rose from 5% in patients receiving 1 day of respiratory assistance to 68.8% in patients mechanically ventilated for more than 30 days. Using quantitative culture of specimens obtained with a protected specimen brush (PSB) during fiberoptic bronchoscopy (FOB) to define pneumonia in 567 ventilated patients, Fagon and colleagues[9] reported a nosocomial pneumonia rate of 9%. Using an actuarial method, the cumulative risk of pneumonia in this context was estimated to be 6.5% at 10 days and 19% at 20 days after the onset of MV. Furthermore, the incremental risk of pneumonia was virtually constant throughout the entire ventilation period, with a mean rate of about 1% per day. In contrast, Cook and colleagues[29] demonstrated in a large series of 1014

mechanically ventilated patients that although the cumulative risk for developing VAP increased over time, the daily hazard rate decreased after day 5. The risk per day was evaluated at 3% on day 5, 2% on day 10, and 1% on day 15. Independent predictors of VAP retained by multivariable analysis were a primary admitting diagnosis of burns (risk ratio [RR] = 5.1; 95% confidence interval [CI] = 1.5–17.0), trauma (RR = 5.0; 95% CI = 1.9–13.1), central nervous system (CNS) disease (RR = 3.4; 95% CI = 1.3–8.8), respiratory disease (RR = 2.8; 95% CI = 1.1–7.5), cardiac disease (RR = 2.7; 95% CI = 1.1–7.0), MV during the previous 24 hours (RR = 2.3; 95% CI = 1.1–4.7), witnessed aspiration (RR = 3.2; 95% CI = 1.6–6.5), and paralytic agents (RR = 1.6; 95% CI = 1.1–2.4). Exposure to antibiotics conferred protection (RR = 0.4; 95% CI = 0.3–0.5), but this effect was attenuated over time. Thus the daily risk for developing VAP is highly dependent on the population being studied as well as on many other factors, particularly the number of patients in the given population who received antibiotics immediately after their admission to the ICU.

VAP is thought to be a common complication of the acute respiratory distress syndrome (ARDS) (see Table 43-1). Most clinical studies have found that pulmonary infection affects between 34% and more than 70% of patients with ARDS, often leading to the development of sepsis, multiple-organ failure, and death. When the lungs of patients who died of ARDS were examined histologically at autopsy, pneumonia could be demonstrated in as many as 73%.[10,30] The diagnosis of pulmonary infection in patients with ARDS, however, is often difficult. Several studies have clearly demonstrated the inability of physicians to accurately diagnose nosocomial pneumonia in this setting based on clinical criteria alone.[30] Using PSB and/or bronchoalveolar lavage (BAL) techniques at predetermined times from days 3 to 21 after the onset of the syndrome in a series of 105 patients with ARDS, Sutherland

and colleagues[31] concluded that VAP indeed may occur far less frequently than expected in this group of patients. Only 16 (15.2%) of their 105 patients met the quantitative criteria for pneumonia (PSB > 10^3 colony-forming units [cfu]/mL or BAL > 10^4 cfu/mL), and no correlations were found between total colony counts in BAL fluid or PSB cultures and severity of ARDS, as judged by Pa_{O_2}/Fi_{O_2} ratios, days on MV, static lung compliance, and/or survival. Unfortunately, these results are probably not of general value because most patients included in the study were lavaged while receiving antibiotics and at predetermined times during the course of ARDS rather than at the time of clinically suspected infection. According to four other studies, the VAP rate was higher in ARDS patients than in other mechanically ventilated patients.[14–16,32] In one study on 56 ARDS patients, PSB and BAL were used to define pneumonia, and the VAP rate was 55%,[14] whereas it was only 28% for 187 non-ARDS patients diagnosed with the same criteria during the same period. It was specified that early-onset VAP (occurring before day 7) was relatively rare in ARDS patients: only 10% of the first VAP episodes, as opposed to 40% of non-ARDS patients. These observations were confirmed in 30 ARDS patients for whom repeated quantitative culture results of specimens obtained with a plugged catheter were available and in 94 ARDS patients with suspected VAP who underwent 172 bronchoscopies, with VAP rates of 60% (incidence density = 4.2/100 ventilator-days) and 43%, respectively.[15,32] In another prospective multicentric study, VAP was confirmed bacteriologically in 49 (37%) of 134 ARDS patients versus 23% of ventilated non-ARDS patients ($p < 0.002$).[16]

MORTALITY, MORBIDITY, AND COST

Crude ICU mortality rates of 24% to 76% have been reported for VAP at a variety of institutions[6,9,12,13,29,33–41] (see Table 43-1). ICU ventilated patients with VAP appear to have a two- to tenfold higher risk of death compared with patients without pneumonia. In 1974, fatality rates of 50% for ICU patients with pneumonia versus 4% for patients without pneumonia were reported.[42] The results of several studies conducted between 1986 and 2001 have confirmed this observation. Despite variations among studies that partly reflect the populations considered, overall mortality rates for patients with or without VAP were, respectively, 55% versus 25%,[13] 71% versus 28%,[9] 33% versus 19%,[12] 38% versus 9%,[37] and 44% versus 19%.[40] These rates correspond to increased risk ratios of mortality of VAP patients of 2.2, 2.5, 1.7, 4.4, and 2.3, respectively.

Although these statistics indicate that VAP is a severe disease, previous studies have not demonstrated clearly that pneumonia is indeed responsible for the higher mortality rate of these patients. Two independent factors make it difficult to assign responsibility unambiguously. The first is, once again, the difficulty in establishing a firm diagnosis, i.e., to clearly identify patients with VAP; thus the widely diverging VAP mortality rates reported may reflect not only differences in the populations studied but also differences in the diagnostic criteria used. Second, numerous studies have demonstrated that severe underlying illness predisposes ICU patients to the development of pneumonia, and their mortality rates are, consequently, high.[3,4,8,37,43–45] Therefore, it is difficult to de-

termine whether such patients would have survived if VAP had not occurred.

The prognosis for aerobic gram-negative bacilli (GNB) VAP is considerably worse than that for infection with gram-positive pathogens when these organisms are fully susceptible to antibiotics. Death rates associated with *Pseudomonas* pneumonia are particularly high, ranging from 70% to more than 80% in several studies.[9,42,46–50] According to one study, mortality associated with *Pseudomonas* or *Acinetobacter* pneumonia was 87% compared with 55% for pneumonias due to other organisms.[9] Similarly, Kollef and colleagues[51] demonstrated that patients with VAP due to high-risk pathogens (*Pseudomonas aeruginosa*, *Acinetobacter* spp., and *Stenotrophomonas maltophilia*) had a significantly higher hospital mortality rate (65%) than patients with late-onset VAP due to other microbes (31%) or patients without late-onset pneumonia (37%). Concerning gram-positive pathogens, in a study comparing VAP due to methicillin-resistant *Staphylococcus aureus* (MRSA) or methicillin-sensitive *S. aureus* (MSSA), mortality was found to be directly attributable to pneumonia for 86% of the former cases versus 12% of the latter, with a relative risk of death equal to 20.7 for MRSA pneumonia.[52]

Multivariate analyses conducted to evaluate the independent role played by VAP in inducing death failed to identify VAP as a variable independently associated with mortality in two studies.[13,37] In contrast, the EPIC study's stepwise logistic regression analyses demonstrated that ICU-acquired pneumonia increased the risk of death with an odds ratio of 1.91 (95% CI = 1.6–2.3) independently of clinical sepsis and bloodstream infection.[3] Another study based on 1978 ICU patients including 1118 patients on MV demonstrated that in addition to the severity of illness, the presence of dysfunctional organ(s); stratification according to the McCabe and Jackson criteria of underlying disease as fatal, ultimately fatal, or not fatal; and nosocomial bacteremia and nosocomial pneumonia independently contributed to the deaths of ventilated patients.[38] Using the Cox model in a series of 387 patients, it was demonstrated that patients with clinically suspected pneumonia had an increased risk of mortality; however, confirmation of the diagnosis with invasive techniques added no prognostic information (respective RR = 2.1 and 1.7).[39]

Case-control studies have been used to assess mortality attributable to nosocomial pneumonia, i.e., the difference between the mortality rates observed for case patients (patients with pneumonia) and control subjects (patients without pneumonia). The results of matched cohort studies evaluating mortality and relative risk attributable to nosocomial pneumonia are given in Table 43-2.[36,50,53–57] Of these seven studies, five concluded that VAP was associated with a significant attributable mortality. For example, it was reported that the mortality rate attributable to VAP exceeded 25%, corresponding to a relative risk of death of 2.0 (with respective values of 40% and 2.5 for cases of pneumonia caused by *Pseudomonas* or *Acinetobacter* spp.).[50] These results were supported by those of other authors, who reported that the risk of mortality was almost three times higher in patients with pneumonia (RR = 2.95; 95% CI = 1.73–5.03) than those without, with a major impact being observed for patients with intermediate-grade severity.[58]

A recent clinical investigation to determine whether VAP is an independent risk factor for death matched 108 nonsurvivors with 108 survivors for their underlying diseases, age,

TABLE 43-2 Mortality Rates and Risk Ratios for Death Attributable to Nosocomial Pneumonia in Matched Case-Control Studies

First Author, Ref.	Diagnostic Criteria	Type of Patient	No. of Cases	CRUDE MORTALITY		Attributable Mortality (%)	Risk Ratio	p Value
				Cases (%)	Controls (%)			
Craig, 53	Clinical	ICU	54	20.4	5.6	14.8	3.6	<0.01
Fagon, 50	PSB + BAL	Ventilated	48	54.2	27.1	27.1	2.0	<0.01
Cunnion, 54	Clinical	Surgical	20	55.0	5.0	50.0	23.2	<0.002
		ICU	20	55.0	7.5	47.5	15.1	<0.002
Baker, 36	PSB/BAL	Medical	62	24.0	24.0	0	1	NS
Papazian, 55	PSB	ICU	85	40.0	38.8	1.2	1.3	NS
Heyland, 56	PSB/BAL	Trauma	177	23.7	17.9	5.8	1.3	NS
Bercault, 57	PSB	Ventilated	135	41.0	14.0	27.0	2.7*	0.03

admission date, severity of illness, and duration of MV[59]; 39 patients in each group developed VAP. This finding contrasts with those of other investigations, which identified the occurrence of VAP as an independent determinant of hospital mortality. Other factors beyond the simple development of VAP, such as the severity of the disease or the responsible pathogens, may be more important determinants of outcome for patients in whom VAP as well as other nosocomial infections develop. Indeed, it may well be that VAP increases mortality only in the subset of patients with intermediate severity[58] and/or in patients with VAP caused by high-risk pathogens, as indicated earlier.[9,51,52] It is probable that several case-control studies were confounded by the fact that patients with very low severity and early-onset pneumonia due to organisms such as *Haemophilus influenzae* or *Streptococcus pneumoniae* have excellent prognoses with or without VAP, whereas very ill patients with late-onset VAP occurring while they are in a quasi-terminal state would die anyway.

It is impossible to accurately evaluate the morbidity and excess costs associated with nosocomial pneumonia. However, with respect to morbidity measures, the prolonged hospital stay as a direct consequence of pneumonia has been estimated in several studies. Jimenez and colleagues[45] demonstrated that nosocomial pneumonia extended the duration of MV from 10 to 32 days, and Craig and Connelly[53] found that pneumonia lengthened the ICU stay threefold. Fagon and colleagues[50] observed that the median length of stay in the ICU for the patients who developed VAP was 21 days versus a median of 15 days for controls ($p < 0.02$). Recently, Baker and colleagues[36] reported mean durations of MV, ICU stay, and hospital stay of 12.0, 20.5, and 43.0 days in trauma patients with pneumonia compared with 8.0, 15.0, and 34.0, respectively, in their matched controls ($p < 0.001$). Similarly, Cunnion and colleagues[54] demonstrated that the mean hospital stay after admission to the ICU was greater for cases of nosocomial pneumonia in surgical ICU patients (30.0 days versus 22.3 days in controls) and in medical and respiratory ICU patients (40.9 days versus 23.1 days in controls).

These prolonged hospitalizations underscore the considerable financial burden imposed by the development of nosocomial pneumonia. For Baker and colleagues,[36] the extra hospital charges related to nosocomial pneumonia occurring in trauma patients were evaluated to be $40,000.

ETIOLOGIC AGENTS

Microorganisms responsible for VAP may differ according to the population of ICU patients, the durations of hospital and ICU stays, and the specific diagnostic method(s) used. The high rate of respiratory infections due to GNB in this setting has been documented repeatedly.[9,12,17,60–64] Several studies have reported that more than 60% of VAPs are caused by aerobic GNB. More recently, however, some investigators have reported that gram-positive bacteria have become increasingly common in this setting, with *S. aureus* being the predominant gram-positive isolate. For example, *S. aureus* was responsible for most episodes of nosocomial pneumonia in the EPIC study, accounting for 31% of the 836 cases with identified responsible pathogens.[64] The data from 24 investigations conducted on ventilated patients, for whom bacteriologic studies were restricted to uncontaminated specimens, confirmed those results: GNB represented 58% of recovered organisms[9,12,14,16–19,32,36,39,65–78] (Table 43-3). The predominant GNB were *P. aeruginosa* and *Acinetobacter* spp., followed by *Proteus* spp., *Escherichia coli*, *Klebsiella* spp., and *H. influenzae*. A relatively high rate of gram-positive pneumonias also was reported in those studies, with *S. aureus* involved in 20% of the cases.

The high rate of polymicrobial infection in VAP has been emphasized repeatedly. In a study on 172 episodes of bacteremic nosocomial pneumonia, 13% of lung infections were caused by multiple pathogens.[46] Similarly, when the PSB technique was used to identify the causative agents in 52

TABLE 43-3 Etiology of VAP as Documented by Bronchoscopic Techniques in 24 Studies for a Total of 1689 Episodes and 2490 Pathogens

Pathogen	Frequency (%)
Pseudomonas aeruginosa	24.4
Acinetobacter spp.	7.9
Stenotrophomonas maltophilia	1.7
Enterobacteriaceae[a]	14.1
Haemophilus spp.	9.8
Staphylococcus aureus[b]	20.4
Streptococcus spp.	8.0
Streptococcus pneumoniae	4.1
Coagulase-negative staphylococci	1.4
Neisseria spp.	2.6
Anaerobes	0.9
Fungi	0.9
Others (<1% each)[c]	3.8

[a] Distribution when specified: *Klebsiella* spp., 15.6%; *Escherichia coli*, 24.1%; *Proteus* spp., 22.3%; *Enterobacter* spp., 18.8%; *Serratia* spp., 12.1%; *Citrobacter* spp., 5.0%; *Hafnia alvei*, 2.1%.
[b] Distribution when specified: MRSA, 55.7%; MSSA, 44.3%.
[c] Including *Corynebacterium* spp., *Moraxella* spp., and *Enterococcus* spp.

consecutive cases of VAP, a 40% polymicrobial infection rate was found,[9] a value similar to that observed in another study conducted at the same time on a comparable population of ventilated patients.[63]

Underlying diseases may predispose patients to infection with specific organisms. Patients with chronic obstructive pulmonary disease (COPD) are, for example, at increased risk for *H. influenzae, Moraxella catarrhalis,* or *S. pneumoniae* infections; cystic fibrosis increases the risk of *P. aeruginosa* and/or *S. aureus* infections, whereas trauma and neurologic patients are at increased risk for *S. aureus* infections.[26,36,52,79] Furthermore, the causative agent for pneumonia differs among ICU surgical populations,[80] with 18% of the nosocomial pneumonias being due to *Haemophilus* or pneumococci, particularly in trauma patients but not in patients with malignancy, transplantation, or abdominal or cardiovascular surgery.

Despite somewhat different definitions of early-onset pneumonia, varying from less than 3 to less than 7 days,[26,77] high rates of *H. influenzae, S. pneumoniae,* MSSA, or susceptible Enterobacteriaceae were constantly found in early-onset VAP, whereas *P. aeruginosa, Acinetobacter* spp., MRSA, and multiresistant GNB were significantly more frequent in late-onset VAP.[26,76,77] This different distribution pattern of etiologic agents between early- and late-onset VAP is also linked to the frequent administration of prior antimicrobial therapy in many patients with late-onset VAP. In a prospective study that included 129 episodes of nosocomial pneumonia documented by PSB specimens, the distributions of responsible pathogens were compared according to whether or not the patients had received antimicrobial therapy before pneumonia onset.[17] The most striking finding was that the rate of pneumonia caused by gram-positive cocci or *H. influenzae* was significantly lower ($p < 0.05$) in patients who had received antibiotics, whereas the rate of pneumonia caused by *P. aeruginosa* was significantly higher ($p < 0.01$). A stepwise logistic regression analysis retained only prior antibiotic use (odds ratio [OR] = 9.2; $p < 0.0001$) as significantly influencing the risk of death from pneumonia.[17] Very similar results were obtained when multivariate analysis was used to determine risk factors for VAP caused by potentially drug-resistant bacteria such as MRSA, *P. aeruginosa, A. baumannii,* and/or *S. maltophilia* in 135 consecutive episodes of VAP.[77] Only three variables remained significant: duration of MV before VAP onset ≥ 7 days (OR = 6.0), prior antibiotic use (OR = 13.5), and prior use of broad-spectrum drugs (third-generation cephalosporin, fluoroquinolone, and/or imipenem) (OR = 4.1).[77] Not all studies, however, have confirmed this distribution pattern. For example, one recent study found that the most common pathogens associated with early-onset VAP were *P. aeruginosa* (25%), MRSA (18%), and *Enterobacter* spp. (10%), with similar pathogens being associated with late-onset VAP.[81] Their finding may be due in part to the prior hospitalization and use of antibiotics in many patients developing early-onset VAP before their transfer to the ICU.

The incidence of multiresistant pathogens is also closely linked to local factors and varies widely from one institution to another. Consequently, each ICU has to collect meticulous epidemiologic data continuously. With these aims, variations of VAP etiology among three Spanish ICUs were analyzed[76] and compared with data collected in Paris.[77] The authors concluded that VAP pathogens varied widely among these four

treatment centers, with marked differences in all the microorganisms isolated from VAP episodes in Spanish centers as compared with the French site. Clinicians clearly must be aware of the common microorganisms associated with both early- and late-onset VAP in their own hospitals in order to avoid the administration of initial inadequate antimicrobial therapy.

Legionella spp.[82,83] anaerobes,[67] fungi,[84] viruses,[85] and even *Pneumocystis carinii* should be mentioned as potential causative agents but are not considered to be common in the context of pneumonia acquired during MV. However, several of these causative agents may be more common and potentially underreported because of difficulties involved with the diagnostic techniques used to identify them, including anaerobic bacteria and viruses.[67,85] In a study conducted to determine the frequency of anaerobes in 130 patients with a first episode of bacteriologically documented VAP with special precautions taken to preserve anaerobic conditions during PSB transport and microbiologic procedures,[67] anaerobes were involved in 23% of the total number of episodes, and the main strains isolated were *Prevotella melaninogenica* (36%), *Fusobacterium nucleatum* (17%), and *Veillonella paravula* (12%). The probability of recovering anaerobic bacteria was particularly high in orotracheally intubated patients and patients in whom pneumonia occurred during the 5 days after ICU admission. However, in a study conducted among 143 patients who developed 185 episodes of suspected VAP and 25 patients with aspiration pneumonia, only 1 anaerobic organism (*V. paravula*) was isolated from 1 patient with aspiration pneumonia, and none from patients with VAP.[66] Thus, examining currently available data, the clinical significance of anaerobes in the pathogenesis and outcome of VAP remains unclear, except as etiologic agents in patients with necrotizing pneumonitis, lung abscess, or pleuropulmonary infections. Anaerobic infection and coverage with antibiotics, such as clindamycin or metronidazole, probably also should be considered for patients with Gram-stained respiratory secretions documenting numerous extra- and intracellular microorganisms in the absence of positive cultures for aerobic pathogens.

Isolation of fungi, most frequently *Candida* species, at significant concentrations poses interpretative problems. Invasive disease has been reported in VAP, but more frequently, yeasts are isolated from respiratory tract specimens in the apparent absence of disease. One prospective study examined the relevance of isolating *Candida* spp. from 25 nonneutropenic patients who had been mechanically ventilated for at least 72 hours.[84] Just after death, multiple culture and biopsy specimens were obtained with bronchoscopic techniques. Although 10 patients had at least one biopsy specimen positive for *Candida* spp., only 2 had evidence of invasive pneumonia, as demonstrated by histologic examination. Many of the endotracheal aspirates, PSB specimens, and BAL specimens also yielded positive cultures for *Candida* spp., sometimes in high concentrations, but they did not contribute to diagnosing invasive disease. Based on these data, the use of the commonly available respiratory sampling methods (bronchoscopic or nonbronchoscopic) in mechanically ventilated patients appears insufficient for the diagnosis of *Candida* pneumonia. At present, the only sure method to establish that *Candida* is the primary lung pathogen is to demonstrate yeast or pseudohyphae in a lung biopsy. However, the significance of *Candida* isolation from the respiratory samples of mechanically

TABLE 43-4 Independent Factors for VAP Identified by Multivariate Analysis in Selected Studies

Host Factors	Intervention Factors	Other
Serum albumin <2.2 g/dL	H₂ blockers ± antacids	Season
Age ≥60 years	Paralytic agents, continuous intravenous	
ARDS	sedation	
COPD, pulmonary disease	>4 units of blood products	
Coma or impaired consciousness	Intracranial pressure monitoring	
Burns, trauma	MV >2 days	
Organ failure	Positive end-expiratory pressure	
Severity of illness	Frequent ventilator circuit changes	
Large-volume gastric aspiration	Reintubation	
Gastric colonization and pH	Nasogastric tube	
Upper respiratory tract colonization	Supine head position	
Sinusitis	Transport out of the ICU	
	Prior antibiotic or no antibiotic therapy	

ventilated patients merits being investigated in greater depth.[86]

Predisposing Factors

A number of factors have been suspected or identified to increase the risk of pneumonia in the ICU, including those identified in the subset of mechanically ventilated patients; these factors are listed in Table 43-4. The data indicated specific high-risk populations (patients with COPD and ARDS, patients undergoing MV for more than 3 days, those requiring intracranial pressure monitoring, those with coma or impaired consciousness, and more generally, those with severe underlying medical conditions as evaluated by a high APACHE II or APACHE III score or the presence of organ failure) and specific treatment modalities or therapeutic intervention (use of H₂ blockers or antacids; previous antibiotics; use of drugs that are markers for severe underlying disease such as dopamine, dobutamine, or barbiturate therapy; reintubation; and frequent changes of ventilator circuits, bronchoscopy, or nasogastric tube) as being independently associated with nosocomial pneumonia.

SURGERY

Postoperative patients are at increased risk for pneumonia. In a study reported in 1981 by Garibaldi and colleagues,[44] the incidence of pneumonia during the postoperative period was 17.2%. In this study, the authors stated that development of pneumonia was closely associated with preoperative markers of the severity of the underlying disease, such as low serum albumin concentration and a high score on the American Society of Anesthesiologists (ASA) preanesthesia physical status classification. A history of smoking, longer preoperative stays, longer surgical procedures, and thoracic or upper abdominal operative sites also were significant risk factors for postoperative pneumonia. In their study comparing adult critical care populations, Cunnion and colleagues[54] demonstrated that surgical ICU patients were found to have consistently higher rates of nosocomial pneumonia than medical ICU patients with a risk ratio of 2.2. Multiple logistic regressions were performed to determine independent predictors for nosocomial pneumonia in the two groups; in SICU patients, mechanical ventilation (>2 days)

and APACHE II score were identified by the model; in MICU patients, only mechanical ventilation (<2 days) remained significant. The relative importance of the surgical procedure itself versus intubation, prophylactic antibiotics, and/or other variables therefore remains to be clearly elucidated in surgical patients.

ANTIMICROBIAL AGENTS

The use of antibiotics in the hospital setting has been associated with an increased risk of nosocomial pneumonia and selection of resistant pathogens.[17,37,49,64,77,79,87–89] In a cohort study of 320 patients, prior antibiotic administration was identified by logistic regression analysis to be one of the four variables independently associated with VAP along with organ failure, age greater than 60 years, and the patient's head positioning (i.e., flat on the back or supine versus head and thorax raised 30 to 40 degrees or semirecumbent).[37] However, other investigators found that antibiotic administration during the first 8 days was associated with a lower risk of early-onset VAP.[90,91] For example, Sirvent and colleagues[92] showed that a single dose of a first-generation cephalosporin given prophylactically was associated with a lower rate of early-onset VAP in patients with structural coma. Moreover, multiple logistic regression analysis of risk factors for VAP in 358 medical ICU patients identified the absence of antimicrobial therapy as one of the factors independently associated with VAP onset.[75] The same result was obtained for a particular subset of 250 patients with very early onset VAP, occurring within 48 hours of intubation, that was investigated to identify potential risk factors for developing VAP.[93] Multivariate analysis selected cardiopulmonary resuscitation (OR = 5.13) and continuous sedation (OR = 4.40) as significant risk factors for pneumonia, whereas antibiotic use (OR = 0.29) had a protective effect. Finally, the results of the multicenter Canadian study on the incidence of and risk factors for VAP indicated that antibiotic treatment conferred protection against VAP.[29] This apparent protective effect of antibiotics disappears after 2 to 3 weeks, suggesting that a higher risk of VAP cannot be excluded beyond this point. Thus risk factors for VAP change over time, thereby explaining why they differ from one series to another.

In contrast, prolonged antibiotic administration to ICU patients for primary infection is thought to favor selection and subsequent colonization with resistant pathogens responsible for superinfections.[9,77,87,94-96] According to our data on 567 ventilated patients, those who had received antimicrobial therapy within the 15 days preceding lung infection were not at higher risk for development of VAP,[9] but 65% of the lung infections that occurred in patients who had received broad-spectrum antimicrobial drugs versus only 19% of those developing in patients who had not received antibiotics were caused by *Pseudomonas* or *Acinetobacter* spp. In a 1988 investigation on mechanically ventilated baboons treated with a variety of regimens of intravenous and topical antibiotics or no antibiotics at all,[94] polymicrobial pneumonia occurred in almost all untreated animals. However, baboons that had received prophylactic topical polymycin had only a slightly lower incidence of pneumonia, and the prevalence of drug-resistant microorganisms in the tracheal secretions was very high: 60% and 78% after 4 and 8 days of MV, respectively. Therefore, strong arguments suggest that the prophylactic use of antibiotics in the ICU increases the risk of superinfection with multiresistant pathogens while only delaying the occurrence of nosocomial infection.

STRESS ULCER PROPHYLAXIS

According to meta-analyses of the efficacy of stress-ulcer prophylaxis in ICU patients, respiratory tract infections were significantly less frequent in patients treated with sucralfate than in those receiving antacids or H_2 blockers.[97-106] However, this conclusion was not fully confirmed in a very large, multicenter, randomized, blinded, placebo-controlled trial that compared sucralfate suspension (1 g every 6 hours) with the H_2-receptor antagonist ranitidine (50 mg every 8 hours) for the prevention of upper gastrointestinal bleeding in 1200 patients who required MV.[107] Clinically relevant gastrointestinal bleeding developed in 10 of the 596 (1.7%) patients receiving ranitidine as compared with 23 of the 604 (3.8%) patients receiving sucralfate (RR = 0.44; 95% CI = 0.21−0.92; p = 0.02). In the ranitidine group, 114 of 596 (19.1%) patients had VAP, as diagnosed by an adjudication committee using a modified version of the Centers for Disease Control and Prevention (CDC) criteria, versus 98 of 604 (16.2%) in the sucralfate group (RR = 1.18; 95% CI = 0.92−1.51; p = 0.19). Thus, although pneumonia rates were similar for the two groups, the relative risks suggest a trend toward a lower pneumonia rate for patients receiving sucralfate. Furthermore, VAP occurred significantly less frequently in patients receiving sucralfate when the diagnosis of pneumonia was based on Memphis VAP Consensus Conference criteria (if there was radiographic evidence of abscess and a positive needle aspirate or histologic proof of pneumonia at biopsy or autopsy) (p = 0.03).[107]

Sucralfate appears to have a small protective effect against VAP because stress-ulcer prophylactic medications that raise the gastric pH might themselves increase the incidence of pneumonia. This contention is supported by direct comparisons of trials of H_2-receptor antagonists versus no prophylaxis, which showed a trend toward higher pneumonia rates among the patients receiving H_2-receptor antagonists (OR = 1.25; 95% CI = 0.78−2.00).[105] Furthermore, the comparative effects of sucralfate and no prophylaxis are unclear. Among 226 patients enrolled in two randomized trials, those receiving sucralfate tended to develop pneumonia more frequently

than those given no prophylaxis (OR = 2.11; 95% CI = 0.82−5.44).[108,109]

ENDOTRACHEAL TUBE—REINTUBATION

The presence of an endotracheal tube by itself circumvents host defenses, causes local trauma and inflammation, and increases the probability of aspirating nosocomial pathogens from the oropharynx around the cuff. Sottile and colleagues[110] studied 25 endotracheal tubes by scanning electron microscopy and found that 96% had partial bacterial colonization and 84% were completely covered by bacteria in a biofilm or glycocalyx. The authors suggested that aggregates of bacteria in biofilm dislodged during suctioning may not be killed by antibiotics or cleared effectively by host immune defenses. Clearly, the type of endotracheal tube also may influence the incidence of aspiration. With low-volume, high-pressure endotracheal cuffs, an incidence of 56% was reported, which decreased to 20% with the advent of high-volume, low-pressure cuffs. In addition to the presence of endotracheal tubes, reintubation is per se a risk factor for nosocomial pneumonia, as indicated by Torres and colleagues.[111] This result is probably related to an increased risk of aspiration of colonized oropharyngeal secretions into the lower airways in patients with glottic dysfunction and/or impaired consciousness after several days of intubation. Another explanation is direct aspiration of gastric contents into the lower airways, particularly when a nasogastric tube is kept in place after extubation.

TRACHEOSTOMY

The role of early tracheostomy in VAP prevention remains controversial, with only a few studies that examined this issue.[112-119] While some studies found a reduction in the rate of VAP in patients with early tracheostomy,[115,116,118] others could not demonstrate any benefit.[112] For example, in a randomized, prospective multicenter trial on 112 patients who were thought to need prolonged MV, there were no differences, at least until day 14, among ICU length of stay, pneumonia rate, and mortality between the 53 patients who underwent early (days 3 to 5) tracheostomy and the 59 who were managed using translaryngeal intubation.[112] The major problem that doomed that study was the overwhelming physician bias, which led to limited patient entry and premature arrest of the study. In the absence of any meaningful data, practice patterns are influenced and guided by strong assumptions and quasi-religious dogma. Until a properly constructed randomized trial is performed to define the timing and utility of tracheostomy in the ICU, its true impact on decreasing VAP will remain merely speculative.[120]

NASOGASTRIC TUBE, ENTERAL FEEDING, AND PATIENT POSITION

Nearly all patients receiving mechanical ventilation have a nasogastric tube inserted to manage gastric and enteral secretions, prevent gastric distention, or provide nutritional support. The nasogastric tube is not widely considered to be a potential risk factor for pneumonia, but it may increase oropharyngeal colonization, cause stagnation of oropharyngeal secretions, and increase reflux and the risk of aspiration. Using multivariate analysis, Joshi and colleagues[43] identified the presence of a nasogastric tube as one of the three independent risk factors for nosocomial pneumonia in a series of 203 patients admitted to the ICU for 72 hours or more.

Early initiation of enteral feeding generally is regarded as beneficial in critically ill patients, but it may increase the risk of gastric colonization, gastroesophageal reflux, aspiration, and pneumonia. Pingleton and colleagues[121] evaluated simultaneous daily gastric, tracheal, and oropharyngeal cultures in 18 ventilator-dependent patients not receiving antacids or H_2 antagonists. After starting enteral feeding, the number of gram-negative isolates increased significantly, and 5 patients (28%) had gram-negative rods that were first recovered in the stomach and subsequently identified in the trachea.

Maintaining mechanically ventilated patients with a nasogastric tube in place in the supine position is also a risk factor for aspiration of gastric contents into the lower airways. Torres and colleagues[122] injected radioactive material via a nasogastric tube directly into the stomachs of 19 mechanically ventilated patients and found that mean radioactive counts in endobronchial secretions were higher in a time-dependent fashion in samples obtained while patients were in the supine position than in those obtained while patients were in the semirecumbent position. The same microorganisms were isolated from stomach, pharynx, and endobronchial samples in 32% of the specimens taken while patients were semirecumbent and in 68% of those taken while patients were in the supine position. These results suggest that placing mechanically ventilated patients in the semirecumbent position is a simple and effective means to minimize aspiration of gastric contents into lower airways and hence constitutes a recommendable, no-cost prophylactic measure for those who can tolerate this position. Such experimental results were confirmed indirectly by Kollef,[37] who demonstrated that supine patient head positioning during the first 24 hours of mechanical ventilation was an independent risk factor for acquiring VAP.

RESPIRATORY EQUIPMENT

Respiratory equipment itself may act as a source of bacteria responsible for nosocomial pneumonia. In past years, the major risk of infection was associated with contaminated reservoir nebulizers designed to deliver small-sized particles suspended in the effluent gas. These observations led to current trends in respiratory therapy toward the use of cascade humidifiers, which do not generate microaerosols. Nevertheless, respiratory equipment continues to provide a source of bacterial contamination. For example, medication nebulizers inserted into the inspiratory-phase tube of the mechanical ventilator circuit may produce bacterial aerosols after a single use.

Mechanical ventilators with humidifying cascades often have high levels of tubing colonization and condensate formation that also may be risk factors for pneumonia. The rate of condensate formation in the ventilator circuit is linked to the temperature difference between the inspiratory-phase gas and the ambient temperature and may be as high as 20 to 40 mL/h.[123] Craven and colleagues[124] examined condensate colonization in 20 circuits and found a median level of 2.0×10^5 organisms/mL, and 73% of the 52 gram-negative isolates present in the patient's sputum were isolated subsequently from condensate. Since most of the tubing colonization was derived from the patient secretions, the high-

est bacterial counts were present near the endotracheal tube. Simple procedures such as turning the patient or raising the bed rail may accidently wash contaminated condensate directly into the patient's tracheobronchial tree. Inoculation of large amounts of fluid with high bacterial concentrations is an excellent way of overwhelming pulmonary defense mechanisms and producing pneumonia. Heating ventilator tubing markedly reduces the rate of condensate formation, but heated circuits often are nondisposable and are expensive. To date, no scientific evidence confirms that heated circuits reduce the incidence of VAP. In-line devices with one-way valves to collect condensate are probably the easiest way to handle this problem. They should be positioned correctly into disposable circuits and emptied regularly.

SINUSITIS

While many studies have compared the risk of nosocomial sinusitis as a function of the intubation method used and the associated risk of VAP,[125-141] only a few were powered adequately to give a clear answer. In one study on 300 patients who required MV for at least 7 days and were randomly assigned to undergo nasotracheal or orotracheal intubation, computed tomographic (CT) evidence of sinusitis was observed slightly more frequently in the nasal than oral endotracheal group ($p = 0.08$), but this difference disappeared when only bacteriologically confirmed sinusitis was considered.[137] The rate of infectious maxillary sinusitis and its clinical relevance also were studied prospectively in 162 consecutive critically ill patients who had been intubated and mechanically ventilated for 1 hour to 12 days before enrollment.[135] All had a paranasal CT scan within 48 hours of admission that was used to divide them into three groups (no, moderate, or severe sinusitis) according to the radiologic appearance of the maxillary sinuses. Patients who had no sinusitis at admission ($n = 40$) were randomized to receive endotracheal and gastric tubes via the nasal or oral route, and based on radiologic images, respective sinusitis rates were 96% and 23% ($p < 0.03$), yet, no differences in the rates of infectious sinusitis were documented according to the intubation route. However, VAP was more common in patients with infectious sinusitis, with 67% of them developing lung infection in the days following the diagnosis of sinusitis.[135] Therefore, whereas it seems clear that infectious sinusitis is a risk factor for VAP, no studies have yet been able to demonstrate definitively that orotracheal intubation decreases the infectious sinusitis rate compared with nasotracheal intubation, and thus no firm recommendations on the best route of intubation to prevent VAP can be advanced.

INTRAHOSPITAL PATIENT TRANSPORT

A prospective cohort study conducted on 531 mechanically ventilated patients evaluated the impact of transporting the patient out of the ICU to other sites within the hospital.[142] Results showed that 52% of the patients had to be moved at least once for a total of 993 transports and that 24% of the transported patients developed VAP compared with 4% of the patients confined to the ICU ($p < 0.001$). Multiple logistic regression analysis confirmed that transport out of the ICU was independently associated with VAP (OR $= 3.8$; $p < 0.001$).

Diagnosis

BACKGROUND AND DESCRIPTION

The diagnosis of VAP usually is based on three components: systemic signs of infection, new or worsening infiltrates seen on the chest roentgenogram, and bacteriologic evidence of pulmonary parenchymal infection.[30] The systemic signs of infection, such as fever, tachycardia, and leukocytosis, are nonspecific findings and can be caused by any condition that releases cytokines.[143] In trauma and other surgical patients, fever and leukocytosis should prompt the physician to suspect infection, but during the early posttraumatic or postoperative period (i.e., during the first 72 hours), these findings usually are not conclusive. However, later, fever and leukocytosis are more likely to be caused by infection, but even then, other events associated with an inflammatory response (e.g., devascularized tissue, open wounds, pulmonary edema, and/or infarction) can be responsible for these findings.

Although the plain (usually portable) chest roentgenogram remains an important component in the evaluation of hospitalized patients with suspected pneumonia, it is most helpful when it is normal and rules out pneumonia. When infiltrates are evident, the particular pattern is of limited value for differentiating among cardiogenic pulmonary edema, noncardiogenic pulmonary edema, pulmonary contusion, atelectasis (or collapse), and pneumonia. Because atelectasis is common in ICU patients, the contribution of repeating the chest x-ray after vigorous pulmonary physiotherapy was emphasized to differentiate infiltrates caused by atelectasis from those due to infection.[144] Few studies have examined the accuracy of the portable chest radiograph in the ICU.[30,145–150] In a review of 24 patients with autopsy-proven pneumonia who were receiving MV, no single radiographic sign had a diagnostic accuracy of more than 68%.[145] The presence of air bronchograms was the only sign that corresponded well to pneumonia, correctly predicting 64% of pneumonias in the entire group. When the group was divided into patients with and without ARDS, however, a significant difference was noted. The presence of air bronchograms or alveolar opacities in patients without ARDS correlated with pneumonia, whereas no such correlation was found for patients with ARDS. A number of causes other than pneumonia can explain asymmetric consolidation in patients with ARDS, e.g., atelectasis, emphysema, pulmonary edema, and thromboembolic disease. Marked asymmetry of radiographic abnormalities also has been reported in patients with uncomplicated ARDS.[151]

Microscopic evaluation and nonquantitative culture of tracheal secretions and/or expectorated sputum also frequently are inconclusive for patients clinically suspected of having pneumonia because the upper respiratory tract of most ICU patients is colonized with potential pulmonary pathogens whether or not parenchymal pulmonary infection is present.[63,89,152–154] Based on specimens obtained simultaneously from the deep trachea and lung for culture from 48 patients with respiratory failure undergoing open-lung biopsy, culture results agreed for only 40% of these paired samples.[155] For patients with histologically documented pneumonia, endotracheal aspirate sensitivity was 82%, but its specificity was only 27%.

Ideally, any diagnostic strategy intended to be used in patients suspected clinically of having developed VAP should be able to reach the three following objectives: (1) to accurately identify patients with true pulmonary infection and, in case of infection, to isolate the causative microorganisms (in order to initiate immediate appropriate antimicrobial treatment and then to optimize therapy based on susceptibility patterns), (2) to identify patients with extrapulmonary sites of infection, and (3) to withhold and/or withdraw antibiotics in patients without infection.

Two diagnostic algorithms can be used in case of VAP suspicion. One option is to treat every patient suspected clinically of having a pulmonary infection with new antibiotics, even when the likelihood of infection is low, arguing that several studies showed that immediate initiation of appropriate antibiotics was associated with reduced mortality.[19,156–158] In this option, the selection of appropriate empirical therapy is based on risk factors and local resistance patterns and involves qualitative testing to identify possible pathogens, antimicrobial therapy being adjusted according to culture results or clinical response (Fig. 43-1). This "clinical" approach has two potential advantages: First, no specialized microbiologic techniques are requested, and second, the risk of missing a patient who needs antimicrobial treatment is minimal, at least when all suspected patients are treated with new antibiotics. However, such a strategy leads to overestimation of the incidence of VAP because tracheobronchial colonization and noninfectious processes mimicking it are included. Qualitative endotracheal aspirate cultures contribute indisputably to the diagnosis of VAP only when they are completely negative for a patient with no modification of prior antimicrobial treatment. In such a case, the negative-predictive value is very high, and the probability of the patient having pneumonia is close to null.[24]

Concern about the inaccuracy of clinical approaches to VAP recognition had led numerous investigators to postulate that "specialized" diagnostic methods, including quantitative cultures of endotracheal aspirates or specimens obtained with bronchoscopic or nonbronchoscopic techniques such as BAL and/or PSB, could improve identification of patients with true VAP and facilitate decisions about whether or not to treat and thus clinical outcome.[19,27,74,159,160] Using such a strategy, the decision algorithm is similar to the one described in Figure 43-1, except that therapeutic decisions are taken based on results of direct examination of distal pulmonary samples and results of quantitative cultures (Fig. 43-2).

SUMMARY OF THE EVIDENCE

Other than decision-analysis studies[161,162] and one retrospective study,[163] only four trials have so far assessed the impact of a diagnostic strategy on antibiotic use and outcome of patients suspected of having VAP using a randomized scheme.[72–74,164] No differences in mortality and morbidity were found when either invasive (PSB and/or BAL) or noninvasive (quantitative endotracheal aspirate cultures) techniques were used to diagnose VAP in three Spanish randomized studies.[72,73,164] However, those studies were based on relatively few patients (51, 76, and 88, respectively), and antibiotics were continued in all patients despite negative cultures, thereby neutralizing one of the potential advantages of any diagnostic test in patients clinically suspected of having VAP. Concerning the latter, several prospective studies have concluded that antibiotics indeed can be stopped in patients with negative

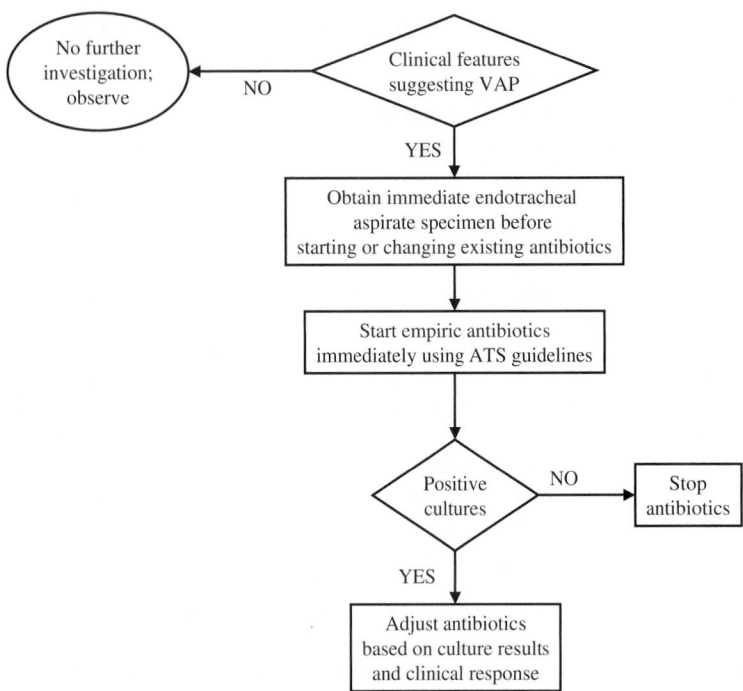

FIGURE 43-1 Diagnostic and therapeutic strategy applied to patients with a clinical suspicion of VAP managed according to the "clinical" strategy. ATS, American Thoracic Society.

quantitative cultures with no adverse effects on the recurrence of VAP and mortality.[19,70,163,165,166] One of the first studies to clearly demonstrate a benefit in favor of invasive techniques was a prospective, randomized trial that compared the two strategies in 413 patients suspected of having VAP.[74] Compared with patients managed clinically, those receiving invasive management had a lower mortality rate on day 14 (16% and 25%; $p = 0.02$) and lower mean sepsis-related organ failure assessment scores on days 3 and 7 ($p = 0.04$). At 28 days, the invasive-management group had significantly more antibiotic-free days (11 ± 9 versus 7 ± 7; $p < 0.001$), and only multivariate analysis showed a significant difference in mortality (hazards ratio [HR] = 1.54; 95% CI = 1.10–2.16; $p = 0.01$).[74] Thus implementation of bronchoscopic techniques for the diagnosis of VAP may reduce antibiotic use and improve patient outcome.

Because VAP in the ICU has substantial attributable mortality, there is justification, albeit unwarranted at times, to use antibiotics for patients with pulmonary infiltrates despite a low likelihood of infection. A recent randomized study proposed to minimize excessive use of antibacterial agents but still allow clinicians flexibility in managing patients with a perceived treatable infection.[167] Patients with a clinical pulmonary infection score (CPIS) of 6 or less (implying low likelihood of pneumonia) were randomized to receive either standard therapy (choice and duration of antibiotics at the discretion of physicians) or ciprofloxacin monotherapy with re-evaluation on day 3; ciprofloxacin was discontinued when CPIS remained 6 or less. Antibiotics were continued beyond 3 days for 90% (38 of 42) of the patients receiving standard therapy compared with 28% (11 of 39) in the ciprofloxacin group ($p = 0.0001$). Mortality and length of ICU stay did not differ despite the shorter duration ($p = 0.0001$) and lower cost ($p = 0.003$) of antimicrobial therapy in the monotherapy than in the standard-therapy arm. Antimicrobial resistance, superinfections, or both developed in 15% of the patients in

the ciprofloxacin versus 35% of the patients in the standard-therapy group ($p = 0.017$). Such an approach thus may lead to significantly lower antimicrobial therapy costs, antimicrobial resistance, and superinfections without adversely affecting the length of stay or mortality and merits prospective analysis in a large study sample. However, it should be emphasized that this strategy was tested in relatively few patients ($n = 81$) and that only 42% of patients included in the study did not require MV. Thus it remains to be precisely determined whether this strategy can perform as well when it is applied to mechanically ventilated patients.

Operating characteristics of nonbronchoscopic techniques for diagnosing VAP are probably very similar to those based on bronchoscopy, with only small differences in their sensitivities, specificities, positive predictive values, and likelihood ratios.[168] Therefore, the choice of procedure(s) eventually may depend on the preferences and experiences of individual physicians and the patient's underlying disease(s). Despite broad clinical experience with the PSB and BAL techniques, it remains, nonetheless, unclear which one should be used in clinical practice. Most investigators prefer to use BAL rather than PSB to diagnose bacterial pneumonia because BAL (1) has a slightly higher sensitivity to identify VAP-causative microorganisms, (2) enables better selection of an empirical antimicrobial treatment before culture results are available, (3) is less dangerous for many critically ill patients, (4) is less costly, and (5) may provide useful clues for the diagnosis of other types of infections.[27] However, it must be acknowledged that a very small return on BAL may contain only diluted material from the bronchial rather than alveolar level and thus give rise to false-negative results, particularly for patients with very severe COPD. In these patients, the diagnostic value of BAL techniques is greatly diminished, and the PSB technique should be preferred.[169]

Cultures of pulmonary secretions for diagnostic purposes after initiation of new antibiotic therapy in patients suspected

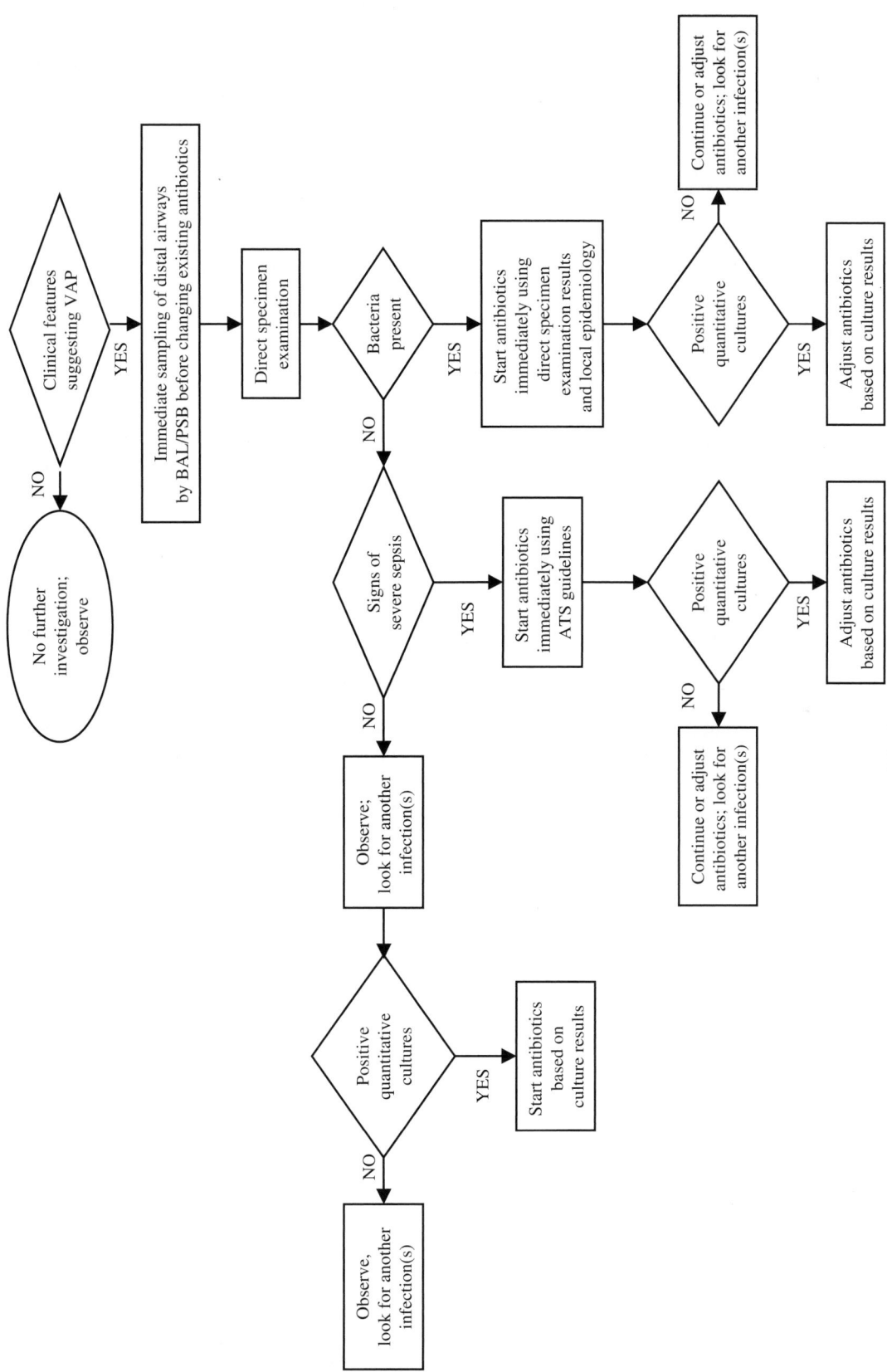

FIGURE 43-2 Diagnostic and therapeutic strategy applied to patients with a clinical suspicion of VAP managed according to the "invasive" strategy. ATS, American Thoracic Society.

of having developed VAP clearly can lead to a high number of false-negative results regardless of the way in which these secretions are obtained. Using a lower threshold to define a positive quantitative result in such a setting may be inaccurate because follow-up cultures can be completely negative in at least 40% of true cases of VAP.[65,170,171] Pulmonary secretions therefore need to be obtained before new antibiotics are administered, as is the case for all microbiologic samples.

CONCLUSIONS AND RECOMMENDATIONS

Available evidence suggests that reliance on clinical signs and endotracheal aspirate culture results leads to overdiagnosis of VAP. When performed before introduction of new antibiotics, the use of quantitative culture techiques after having obtained PSB and/or BAL specimens from the lung of patients with signs suggestive of VAP allows definition of a therapeutic strategy that is superior to that based exclusively on clinical evaluation, minimizing the use of unnecessary antibiotics with no adverse effects on patient outcome (see Fig. 43-2). In patients with clinical evidence of severe sepsis or patients with a very high pretest probability of the disease, the initiation of antibiotic therapy should not be delayed, and patients should be treated immediately with broad-spectrum antibiotics, even when no bacteria are detected using microscopic examination of pulmonary secretions. Although the true impact of this decision tree on patient outcome remains controversial, being able to withhold antimicrobial treatment from some patients without infection may constitute a distinct advantage in the long term by minimizing the emergence of resistant microorganisms in the ICU and redirecting the search for another (the true) infection site.

When quantitative culture techniques are not available to physicians treating patients clinically suspected of having VAP, we recommend following a clinical strategy, emphasizing that antimicrobial treatment should be re-evaluated on day 3, when susceptibility patterns of the microorganism(s) considered to be causative are available, in order to select treatment with a narrower spectrum or even to stop antimicrobial therapy if the clinical outcome is barely compatible with a diagnosis of pneumonia.[167]

Treatment

EVALUATION OF CURRENT ANTIMICROBIAL STRATEGIES

Despite many advances in antimicrobial therapy, successful treatment of patients with nosocomial pneumonia remains a difficult and complex undertaking. No consensus has been reached concerning issues as basic as the optimal antimicrobial regimen for therapy or duration of treatment. Although some investigators have recommended two-drug parenteral therapy for most cases, recent data have demonstrated the efficacy of newer β-lactam antibiotics as monotherapy for some patients. Similarly, the efficacy of endotracheal or aerosolized antibiotics as either the sole or adjunctive therapy for gram-negative pneumonia remains controversial. In fact, to date, evaluation of various antimicrobial strategies for the treatment of bacterial pneumonia in mechanically ventilated patients has been difficult for several reasons.

First, as indicated earlier, obtaining a definitive diagnosis of pneumonia in critically ill patients is far from easy. Although clinically distinguishing between bacterial colonization of the tracheobronchial tree and true nosocomial pneumonia is difficult, nearly all previous therapeutic investigations have relied solely on clinical diagnostic criteria and therefore probably have included patients who did not have pneumonia. Second, most of these studies used cultures of tracheal secretions as the major source of samples for microbiologic analysis despite the fact that the upper respiratory tract of most ventilated patients usually is colonized with multiple potential pathogens. Finally, the lack of an adequate technique to directly sample the infection site in the lung has hampered study of both the ability or inability of antibiotics to eradicate the causative pathogens from the lower respiratory tract and therefore the ability to predict their bacteriologic efficacy.

Recently, Montravers and colleagues[65] evaluated the bacteriologic and clinical efficacy of antimicrobial therapies selected on the basis of the etiologic microorganisms identified by cultures of PSB samples obtained during bronchoscopy for the treatment of nosocomial bacterial pneumonia in 76 patients receiving MV. Using follow-up PSB sample culture to assess the infection site in the lung directly, their results demonstrated that the administration of an antimicrobial therapy combining, in most cases, two effective agents was able to sterilize or contain the lower respiratory tract infection after only 3 days of treatment in 67 (88%) of the patients included in the study. The only two bacteriologic failures were observed in patients who did not receive adequate treatment because of errors in the selection of antimicrobial drugs. Early superinfection caused by bacteria resistant to the initial antibiotics was, however, documented in 7 (9%) patients, emphasizing the need to monitor carefully the impact of treatment on the initial microbial flora for optimal management of such patients when the clinical response is suboptimal. Furthermore, results of cultures of follow-up PSB samples were well correlated with the clinical outcome noted during the 15-day observation period, making this test a good prognostic indicator in patients with nosocomial bacterial pneumonia. Whereas the percentage of patients with clinical improvement was 96% and 82% in those with sterilized or persistent low-grade infection, respectively, it was only 44% in those with persistent high-grade infection.[65] Using such techniques to sample the infection site in the lung directly therefore may provide a more rigorous evaluation of different antimicrobial strategies.

FACTORS CONTRIBUTING TO SELECTION OF INITIAL TREATMENT

The important prognostic role played by the adequacy of the initial empirical antimicrobial therapy was analyzed by several investigators and is summarized in Table 43-5.[19,73,158,164,172–174] Factors to be considered for the optimal selection of initial antibiotic therapy include (1) putative causative pathogens and their patterns of antibiotic susceptibilities, based on the clinical setting and previous epidemiologic studies, (2) data obtained by surveillance cultures in the same patient, (3) information given by direct microscopic examination of pulmonary secretions, and (4) intrinsic antibacterial activities of antimicrobial agents and their pharmacokinetic characteristics.

TABLE 43-5 Mortality Rates According to Initial Empirical Antibiotic Therapy

| | CRUDE MORTALITY RATES OF PATIENTS RECEIVING | | |
First Author, Ref.	Inadequate Antibiotic Therapy	Adequate Antibiotic Therapy	p Value
Luna, 172	92.2% ($n = 34$)	37.5% ($n = 15$)	<0.001
Alvarez-Lerma, 158	34.9% ($n = 146$)	32.5% ($n = 284$)	NS
Rello, 19	63.0% ($n = 27$)	41.5% ($n = 58$)	0.06
Kollef, 173	60.8% ($n = 51$)	26.6% ($n = 79$)	0.001
Sanchez-Nieto, 164	42.9% ($n = 14$)	25.0% ($n = 24$)	NS
Ruiz, 73	50.0% ($n = 18$)	39.3% ($n = 28$)	NS
Dupont, 174	60.7% ($n = 56$)	47.3% ($n = 55$)	NS

CLINICAL SETTING

Underlying diseases and specific risk factors may predispose patients to infection with specific organisms, as well as some intrinsic factors linked to each hospital or ICU.[26] Therefore, selection of initial antimicrobial therapy needs to be tailored to each institution's local patterns of antimicrobial resistance.[76] Patients with COPD, for example, are at increased risk of *H. influenzae* infection, whereas cystic fibrosis would increase the risk of *P. aeruginosa* and *S. aureus* infection. On the other hand, trauma and neurosurgical patients are at increased risk of *S. aureus* infection. Based on the results of a French prospective study in which the responsible microorganisms for infection in 135 consecutive episodes of VAP observed in the ICU were documented using bronchoscopic specimens, the distribution of infecting pathogens was influenced markedly by prior duration of MV and prior antibiotic use.[77] While early-onset pneumonias in patients who had not received prior antimicrobial treatment were caused mainly by susceptible Enterobacteriaceae, *Haemophilus* spp., MSSA, or *S. pneumoniae*, early-onset pneumonias in patients who had received prior antibiotics commonly were caused by nonfermenting GNB such as *P. aeruginosa*, in addition to streptococci and *Haemophilus* spp. On the other hand, late-onset pneumonias that occurred without antibiotics during the 15 days preceding the onset of infection largely were caused by streptococci, MSSA, or Enterobacteriaceae; however, some of these GNBs were class I cephalosporinase producers, which may require treatment with a new cephalosporin, such as cefepime or cefpirome, for optimal therapy. Late-onset pneumonias in patients having recently received antibiotics were caused by multiresistant pathogens such as *P. aeruginosa*, *A. baumannii*, or MRSA in more than 40% of cases. Taking these epidemiologic characteristics into account allowed the authors to devise a rational decision tree for selecting initial treatment in this setting that prevents resorting to broad-spectrum drug coverage in all patients (Table 43-6). A computerized decision-support program linked to computer-based patient records can facilitate the dissemination of such information to physicians for immediate use in therapy decision making and improve the quality of care.[175]

ROUTINE SURVEILLANCE CULTURE RESULTS

Several investigators have recommended routine surveillance cultures of ICU patients because they may be predictive of patients who are at high risk of invasive disease, and furthermore, should invasive disease develop, empirical therapy can be selected based on the predominant pathogens identified in these cultures.[15] However, the accuracy of this approach for selecting initial antimicrobial treatment for ICU patients requiring new antibiotics for VAP has not yet been established. This hypothesis was retested recently in a prospective study conducted on 125 patients who required MV for more than 48 hours and for whom strict bronchoscopic criteria were applied to diagnose pneumonia and identify the causative pathogens.[176] Although a large number of various prior microbiologic specimen culture results (mean = 45 ± 43 per episode) were obtained before FOB for each VAP episode, only 73 (33%) of the 220 VAP-causative microorganisms were isolated by these routine analyses and their susceptibility patterns available to guide initial antimicrobial treatment. When the analysis focused on VAP episodes for which prior (within 72 hours) respiratory secretion culture results were available, hypothesizing that this microbiologic information might be particularly useful for identifying the responsible organisms in the case of subsequent pneumonia, results were better but still disappointing because all causative pathogens were recovered for less than 60% of them. Such a strategy also may increase the workload of the microbiology laboratory considerably without having any positive impact on patient management.

Colonization with potentially drug-resistant pathogens, such as MRSA or extended-spectrum β-lactamase-producing strains of *Klebsiella pneumoniae* or other Enterobacteriaceae, is associated with an increased risk of infection caused by the corresponding microorganism. These results were confirmed

TABLE 43-6 Recommended Initial Antimicrobial Therapy in Patients with VAP

Early-onset VAP, no prior antibiotics:
  Nonpseudomonal third-generation cephalosporin *or*
  β-Lactam–β-lactamase inhibitor combination
Early-onset VAP, prior antibiotics; or late-onset VAP, no prior antibiotics:
  Aminoglycoside or ciprofloxacin
  Plus one of the following:
    Ceftazidime
    Cefepime
    Cefoperazone
    Piperacillin-tazobactam
    Ticarcillin-clavulanic acid
Late-onset VAP, prior antibiotics:
  Aminoglycoside or ciprofloxacin
  Plus piperacillin-tazobactam or imipenem
  Plus vancomycin

in the study by Hayon and colleagues,[176] with positive predictive values of recovering such a microorganism from a specimen of 62%, 52%, or 24% for VAP caused by MRSA, *P. aeruginosa*, or *A. baumannii*, respectively. However, because the sensitivity of prior microbiologic culture results for identifying bacteria causing VAP do not exceed 70%, selection of initial antimicrobial therapy for patients with VAP hardly can be based only on these results, especially for deciding to use (or not) vancomycin and/or a broad-spectrum β-lactam, which are effective against *P. aeruginosa* and/or *A. baumannii*. However, when one of the three microorganisms (or any pathogen) is isolated from respiratory secretions within 72 hours of VAP, it probably should be covered by the antimicrobial regimen selected, even though predictive values do not exceed 50% to 60%.

INFORMATION GIVEN BY DIRECT EXAMINATION OF PULMONARY SECRETIONS

Direct microscopy of pulmonary secretions is extremely important not only to identify patients with true VAP but also to select appropriate treatment, especially when BAL specimens are used to prepare cytocentrifuged Gram-stained smears. In patients with pneumonia, the morphology and Gram staining of bacteria are closely correlated with the results of bacterial cultures, enabling early formulation of a specific antimicrobial regimen before the culture results are available. In a study of 94 mechanically ventilated patients with suspected VAP who underwent FOB with BAL and PSB, direct BAL fluid examination results were available within 2 hours, BAL and PSB culture results were available after 24 hours, and antibiotic susceptibility was available after 48 hours.[71] At each step in the strategy, the senior physician and the resident in charge of the patient were asked their diagnoses and their therapeutic

plans based on the available data. Using a threshold of 1% infected cells, direct BAL examination discriminated well between patients with and without VAP (sensitivity 94%, specificity 92%, area under the receiver operating characteristic curve 0.95). In contrast, the senior clinical judgment before FOB was correct for only 71% of the patients compared with the definitive diagnosis and final antibiotic susceptibility test results. In addition, the therapeutic prediction was correct for 65% using clinical judgment (15 untreated patients, 3 ineffective treatments, and 15 unnecessary treatments), 66% using airway visualization (14 untreated VAP patients, 4 ineffective treatments, and 14 unnecessary treatments), and 88% using direct BAL examination results (1 untreated patient, 6 ineffective treatments, and 4 unnecessary treatments). Therefore, a strategy based on bronchoscopy and direct examination of BAL fluid may lead to more rapid and appropriate treatment of VAP than a strategy based only on clinical evaluation.

INTRINSIC ANTIBACTERIAL ACTIVITIES OF ANTIMICROBIAL AGENTS

Intrinsic antibacterial activities of antimicrobial agents used for the treatment of nosocomial pneumonia, based on frequently reported pathogens associated with this type of infection, are indicated in Table 43-7. Effective antibiotic treatment of bacterial pneumonia depends on adequate delivery of antibacterial agents to the infection site, and therefore, scrupulous attention must be given to optimal doses, route of administration, and pharmacodynamic characteristics of each agent used to treat this infection. Owing to major methodologic problems, published data concerning the penetration of most antibiotics into the lung probably should be viewed with caution, and only general trends concerning concentrations

TABLE 43-7 Intrinsic Antibacterial Activities of Antimicrobial Agents Used for Treatment of Nosocomial Pneumonia

	"Sensitive" GNB[a]	"Resistant" GNB[b]	ESBL Producer GNB[c]	*P. aeruginosa*	*A. baumannii*	Gram-Positive Cocci[d]
Carboxypenicillins	+[e]	+	−	++	+	+/−
Ureidopenicillins β-Lactams + β-lactamase inhibitor (BLI)	++	+	−	++	+/−	+
Ticarcillin-clavulanic acid	++	+[f]	+[g]	++	+/−	++
Piperacillin-tazobactam	++	+[f]	+[g]	++	+/−	++
β-Lactam-sulbactam	++	+[f]	+[g]	++	+[h]	++
Third-generation cephalosporin						
Cefotaxime-ceftriaxone	++	+[i]	−	−	−	++
Cefoperazone	++	+[i]	−	++	−	+
Ceftazidime	++	+[i]	−	++	−	+
Cefepime-cefpirome	++	++[j]	−	+	−	++
Carbapenems	++	++	++	++[i]	++	++
Monobactams	++	+	−	++	−	−
Ciprofloxacin	++	++[i]	−	++[i]	+/−	++[k]

[a] *E. coli, K. pneumoniae, P. mirabilis, H. influenzae,* and *M. catarrhalis.*
[b] *Enterobacter* spp., *Citrobacter* spp., *M. morgannii,* Indole+ *Proteus* spp., and *Serratia* spp.
[c] Extended-spectrum betalactamases (ESBL)-producer gram-negative bacilli.
[d] Except methicillin-resistant *S. aureus* and enterococci.
[e] Except *K. pneumoniae* which is naturally resistant to ticarcillin.
[f] BLIs exhibit no activity against cephalosporinases.
[g] Clinical experience with these agents for treatment of nosocomial pneumonia is limited.
[h] Sulbactam exhibits intrinsic anti-*Acinetobacter* activity.
[i] Initial resistance or emergence of resistant organisms during treatment are possible.
[j] These agents exhibit a better activity against cephalosporinase-producing strains.
[k] Except methicillin-resistant *S. aureus,* enterococci, and *S. pneumoniae.*

achievable at the infected site in lung tissue can be derived from those studies.[177]

For penicillins and cephalosporins, the bronchial secretion-to-serum-drug-concentration ratios range between 0.05 and 0.25. Fluoroquinolones have better penetration characteristics, and bronchial secretion concentrations are between 0.8 and 2 times those in serum. Aminoglycosides and tetracyclines have ratios of 0.2 to 0.6. Host-related as well as drug-related factors may, however, influence the penetration of antimicrobial drugs across the blood-bronchus and alveolar-capillary barriers. Thus, for those drugs, such as the β-lactams and the glycopeptides, which do not cross membranes readily, penetration may increase in the presence of inflammation because of enhanced membrane permeability.[178]

Several published reports have demonstrated a relationship among serum concentrations of β-lactams or other antibiotics, the in vitro minimal inhibitory concentration (MIC) of the infecting organism, and the rate of bacterial eradication from respiratory secretions in patients with lung infection, thereby emphasizing that clinical and bacteriologic outcomes can be improved by optimizing the therapeutic regimen according to pharmacokinetic properties of the agent(s) selected for treatment.[179–182] Most investigators distinguish between antimicrobial agents that kill by a concentration-dependent mechanism (e.g., aminoglycosides and fluoroquinolones) and those that kill by a time-dependent mechanism (e.g., β-lactams and vancomycin).

Development of a priori dosing algorithms based on MIC, patient creatinine clearance and weight, and a clinician-specified pharmacokinetic-pharmacodynamic variable, such as the 24-hour area under the concentration-time curve divided by the MIC (AUIC), therefore may be a valid way to improve treatment of these patients, leading to a more precise approach than current guidelines for optimal use of antimicrobial agents.

DE-ESCALATION

Once the microbiologic data become available, it is necessary to de-escalate therapy to avoid prolonged use of a broader spectrum of antibiotic therapy than is justified by the available information.[183] For many patients, including those with late-onset infection, the culture data will not show the presence of highly resistant pathogens, and in these individuals, therapy can be narrowed or even reduced to a single agent in light of the susceptibility pattern of the causative pathogens without risking inappropriate treatment. While a de-escalating approach to antibiotic therapy (i.e., culture-guided treatment) may not help individual patients, it could benefit the ICU as a whole by reducing the selection pressure for resistance. Every possible effort therefore should be made to obtain, before new antibiotics are administered, reliable pulmonary specimens for direct microscope examination and cultures from each patient clinically suspected of having developed VAP.

MONOTHERAPY VERSUS COMBINATION THERAPY

Several studies have examined the use of a single antibiotic, e.g., a third-generation cephalosporin, imipenem-cilastatin, or a fluoroquinolone, to treat VAP.[27,184] In general, monotherapy has proven to be a useful alternative to combination therapy, with the same success rate and no more superinfections or colonizations by multiresistant pathogens.[185] Because

these studies included nonhomogeneous populations of patients with different types of infections, and given the potential inaccuracy of using only clinical criteria to diagnose lung infection, further trials are needed to clarify all these uncertainties. Furthermore, for patients with severe infection due to *P. aeruginosa* or other multiresistant bacteria, such as *Klebsiella* spp. or *Acinetobacter* spp., combining an antipseudomonal β-lactam with an aminoglycoside or ciprofloxacin is likely to obtain a much better outcome than monotherapy, as shown previously. In a prospective clinical study of 200 patients with *P. aeruginosa* bacteremia, mortality rates for patients with pneumonia receiving monotherapy or combination therapy as the initial empirical treatment were 88% (7 of 8 patients) and 35% (7 of 20 patients), respectively ($p = 0.03$).[186] Similarly, for the subgroup of 55 patients who experienced hypotension within 72 hours prior to or on the day of the positive blood culture in a prospective observational study on 230 *Klebsiella* bacteremias, the mortality rate was significantly lower for patients who received combination therapy (24%) than for those given monotherapy (50%).[187] It should be noted, however, that the β-lactam agents used in these studies were older agents with less potent activity than the advanced cephalosporins or carbapenems available today.

Based on these data, it is probably safer to use a β-lactam antibiotic in combination with an aminoglycoside or a quinolone for patients with severe VAP, at least for the first days of therapy while culture results of pulmonary secretions are pending. It may be that monodrug therapies for nosocomial pneumonia would best be reserved for infections in which *P. aeruginosa* or other multiresistant microorganisms, such as *Klebsiella, Enterobacter, Citrobacter, Serratia,* or *Acinetobacter* spp. have been excluded as the etiologic agents.

DURATION OF ANTIMICROBIAL THERAPY

The optimal antimicrobial regimen and duration of therapy for patients who develop pneumonia have not been established. Most experts recommend that the duration be adapted to the severity of the disease, the time to clinical response, and the microorganism(s) responsible.[26] A "long" treatment, i.e., a minimum of 14 to 21 days, is prescribed for the following situations: multilobular involvement, malnutrition, cavitation, gram-negative necrotizing pneumonia, and isolation of *P. aeruginosa* or *Acinetobacter* spp., which correspond to the majority of pulmonary infections occurring in patients requiring mechanical ventilation. This duration is essentially justified by the high theoretical risk of relapse, especially in case of infection caused with *P. aeruginosa,* which is particularly difficult to eradicate from the respiratory tract.[188] Thus, at present, a short-term regimen is rarely prescribed in patients who develop VAP, despite the potential major advantages it could have in terms of bacterial ecology and the prevention of emergence of multiresistant bacteria. Lowering the amount of antibiotics administered to patients hospitalized in ICUs is indeed a primary objective of every strategy aimed at reducing the emergence and dissemination of such bacteria.[189]

Prevention

Because VAP has been associated with increased morbidity, longer hospital stays, increased health care costs, and higher mortality rates, prevention of this infection is a major challenge for intensive care medicine. A number of preventive strategies have been tested, and a number of recommendations have been published.[120,190–194] However, evaluation of the impact of such interventions is a complex issue. Three methodologic difficulties make the measurement of potential efficacy of prevention strategies for VAP of limited value: (1) the difficulty of obtaining an accurate diagnosis of VAP (in fact, only patients who develop true VAP are likely to benefit from preventive measures), (2) the difficulty of precisely determining the impact of prophylactic measures on the overall mortality of a general ICU population (i.e., to identify preventable deaths directly attributable to VAP among all deaths occurring in a population of ventilated ICU patients), and (3) the difficulty of assessing the consequences of a preventive measure on a potentially pathogenic mechanism—a surrogate outcome (e.g., to determine the exact role played by prevention or reduction or modulation of tracheal colonization in modifying the development of VAP).

CONVENTIONAL INFECTION CONTROL APPROACHES

These measures should be the first step taken in any prevention program.[195] The design of the ICU has a direct effect on the potential for nosocomial infections. Adequate space and lighting, proper functioning of ventilation systems, and adequate facilities for hand washing lead to lower infection rates.[196] However, it should be kept in mind that physical upgrading of the environment does not per se reduce the infection rate unless personnel attitude and practices are improved. In any ICU, one of the most important factors is probably the team that staffs it: the number, quality, and motivation of its medical, nursing, and ancillary members. The team should include a sufficient number of nurses to avoid having them move from one patient to another and to avoid working under constant pressure.[197] The importance of personal cleanliness (education and awareness programs) and attention to aseptic procedures (simple barrier isolation methods based on the use of disposable gowns and nonsterile gloves) must be emphasized at every possible opportunity. It is clear that careful monitoring, decontamination, and compliance with the usage guidelines of respiratory equipment decrease the incidence of nosocomial pneumonia.[198] In any case, hand washing or hand rubbing with alcohol-based solutions remains uncontested as the most important infection control practice.[197,199]

A bacterial monitoring policy facilitates the early recognition of colonization and infection and has been associated with statistically significant reductions in nosocomial infection rates.[200] The focal point for infection control activities in the ICU is a surveillance system designed to establish and maintain a database that describes endemic rates of nosocomial infection. Awareness of the endemic rates enables recognition of the onset of an epidemic when infection rates rise above a calculated threshold.

Preventing infection by modifying host risk has focused on treatment of underlying diseases and complications and control of antibiotic use. Adoption of an antibiotic policy restricting the prescription of broad-spectrum agents and useless antibiotics is of major importance.[201] Simple, safe, inexpensive, logical, but unproven measures, including the use of physiotherapy,[202] the judicious use and prompt removal

of nasogastric tubes,[43] and removal of tubing condensate, may have tremendous impact on the frequency of nosocomial pneumonia in mechanically ventilated patients.[124]

SPECIFIC PROPHYLAXIS AGAINST VAP

Since invasive MV is a risk factor for VAP, strategies that reduce its duration may reduce its incidence. Optimization of weaning protocols is a first way to reduce the duration of exposure to risk.[203,204] Noninvasive ventilation is an alternative approach to the use of artificial airways to avoid infectious complications and injury of the trachea in patients with acute respiratory failure. Many observations and studies, unfortunately small and not blinded, suggest that patients who tolerate noninvasive ventilation have a lower incidence of pneumonia than those intubated tracheally, whatever the possible explanations: noninvasive ventilation itself or differences in disease severity, in the distribution of risk factors for VAP, or in the duration of exposure to each of the two ventilation methods.[205–208] However, although seven randomized trials have compared noninvasive ventilation with conventional MV for prevention of pneumonia, only one could demonstrate a statistically significant benefit in favor of noninvasive ventilation.[204,209–214]

Apart from these protocols aiming at reducing the duration of mechanical ventilation, seven prophylactic approaches have been studied: semirecumbent positioning, oscillating and rotating beds, continuous or intermittent aspiration of subglottic secretions, ventilator circuits management, methods of enteral feeding, stress ulcer prophylaxis, and antibiotic use, including selective digestive decontamination.

SEMIRECUMBENT POSITIONING
Supine patient positioning has been shown to be independently associated with the development of VAP.[37] Placing ventilated patients in a semirecumbent position to minimize reflux and aspiration of gastric contents is a simple measure, although some practical problems can occur in unstable patients. Three trials have evaluated the potential efficacy of semirecumbent positioning,[122,215,216] but only one measured the incidence of VAP.[215] This trial, which included 86 intubated and mechanically ventilated patients, was stopped after the planned interim analysis because the frequency and risk of VAP were significantly lower for the semirecumbent group. These findings were confirmed indirectly by demonstration that the head position of the supine patient during the first 24 hours of MV was an independent risk factor for acquiring VAP.[215] No adverse effects were observed in patients assigned to semirecumbent positioning.

Semirecumbent positioning is a low-cost, low-risk preventive approach that merits being considered in all ventilated patients, whenever feasible.

OSCILLATING AND ROTATING BEDS
Immobility in critically ill patients treated with MV results in atelectasis and impaired secretions drainage and potentially predisposes to pulmonary complications, including VAP. Oscillating and rotating beds may help in preventing pneumonia.[217–224] Six randomized trials, including mostly surgical and trauma patients, ventilated or not, summarized in a meta-analysis by Choi and Nelson[225] have compared continuous lateral rotational therapy with standard beds for

the prevention of nosocomial pneumonia. The meta-analysis found a statistically significant reduction in the risk for pneumonia, principally concerning early-onset (<5 days) pneumonia, and a decreased duration of ICU stay. However, five of these studies were limited to surgical patients or those with neurologic impairment. The sixth study, which included primarily medical patients, found no significant benefit.[219] A recent randomized, controlled trial of medical and surgical patients not included in the meta-analysis also found no benefit to oscillating beds.[226] Some adverse events have been described with these beds, including disconnection of catheters or pressure ulceration; in addition, nursing care potentially is complicated with oscillating beds. Despite the cost of such beds, cost-benefit analyses performed in those studies seem favorable, mainly due to the shorter duration of the ICU stay.

Although oscillating or rotating beds have no apparent benefit in general populations of medical patients, there is reasonably good evidence that this practice may be effective in surgical patients or patients with neurologic problems. Use of these beds in these select patient populations therefore should be considered.

ASPIRATION OF SUBGLOTTIC SECRETIONS

Continuous or intermittent aspiration of oropharyngeal secretions has been proposed to avoid chronic aspiration of secretions through the tracheal cuff of intubated patients. Aspiration of subglottic secretions requires the use of a specially designed endotracheal tube with a separate lumen that opens into the subglottic region. Three randomized, controlled trials have studied aspiration of subglottic secretions for the prevention of VAP.[227–229] Mahul and colleagues[227] found that pneumonia was significantly less frequent in patients with endotracheal tubes having a separate dorsal lumen for hourly suctioning of stagnant secretions above the cuff than in others and that VAP development was delayed. Similarly, in a 3-year prospective, randomized, controlled study, Valles and colleagues[228] documented a lower VAP rate when continuous subglottic aspiration was performed. However, this difference was fully explained by the VAP occurring during the first week, whereas late-onset pneumonias were more frequent in the aspiration group. Furthermore, detailed microbiologic analysis demonstrated that this reduction concerned only pneumonia due to *H. influenzae* or gram-positive cocci. The incidence of VAP due to *P. aeruginosa* or Enterobacteriaceae did not differ between the two groups.[228] Kollef and colleagues[229] performed a randomized trial on 343 post–cardiac surgery patients to compare continuous subglottic aspiration and standard postoperative medical care. Although those authors found similar rates of VAP in both groups, VAP episodes occurred significantly later in patients receiving subglottic aspiration than in those treated conventionally. No difference in mortality rates was observed in these three studies. Whereas no adverse events were reported with aspiration of subglottic secretions in the three studies just reported, experimental data have suggested the possibility of tracheal damage in sheeps intubated with this type of tube.[230]

Aspiration of subglottic secretions is a promising strategy for the prevention of early-onset VAP but cannot be recommended for general use because of the mixed results in the literature. Further study of this approach is warranted.

VENTILATOR CIRCUIT MANAGEMENT

Decreased frequency of ventilator circuit changes, replacement of heated humidifiers by heat and moisture exchangers, decreased frequency of heat and moisture exchanger changes, and closed suctioning systems all have been tested for preventing VAP. Four randomized trials of decreased frequency of ventilator circuit changes have been published[231–234] comparing changes every 2 days, 7 days, and no scheduled change and did not find any significant differences in the rate of VAP, as summarized in a recent meta-analysis.[235] One meta-analysis summarized the results of five randomized, controlled trials that compared the effects of heated humidifiers and heat and moisture exchangers on the risk of VAP.[194] Only one out of these five studies found a significant reduction of VAP rate with the use of heat and moisture exchangers.[236] The efficacy of both humidification strategies seems comparable; however, two studies reported increased rates of endotracheal tube occlusion with the use of heat and moisture exchangers.[194] Another potential caveat of these devices includes an increased resistive load resulting in difficulties in the ventilation and weaning process of patients with severe ARDS.[237] Finally, one study evaluated the impact of less frequent changes (daily versus every 5 days) of heat and moisture exchangers on the development of VAP.[238] No differences in the VAP rates were observed.

A policy of no circuit changes or infrequent circuit changes is simple to implement, does not lead to increased development of VAP, and costs less than frequent, regular circuit changes. Such a policy should be considered in all mechanically ventilated patients. The favorable impact of the use of heat and moisture exchangers on the risk of VAP has to be confirmed before being recommended for general use.

To avoid hypoxia, hypotension, and contamination of suction catheters entering the tracheal tube, investigators have examined closed suctioning systems.[239–241] While some found a nonsignificantly lower prevalence rate of VAP for patients managed with the closed system compared with those with the open system,[241] others not only failed to show a statistically significant protective effect of the closed system on the incidence of VAP but also observed an increased frequency of endotracheal colonization associated with the closed device.[239] At the present time, use of theses devices cannot be recommended for preventing VAP.

METHODS OF ENTERAL FEEDING

Nearly all patients receiving mechanical ventilation have a nasogastric tube inserted to manage gastric and enteral secretions, prevent gastric distention, or provide nutritional support. The nasogastric tube may increase the risk for gastroesophageal reflux, aspiration, and VAP.[43] Four randomized, controlled trials have evaluated various methods of enteral feeding aimed at preventing VAP: postpyloric or jejunal feeding (versus gastric feeding), the use of motility agents (metoclopramide versus placebo), acidification of feeding (with addition of hydrochloric acid), and intermittent (versus continuous) feeding.[242–245] These studies did not find differences in the incidence of VAP and/or mortality rates. Potentially serious adverse effects have been observed in patients receiving acidified feeding (gastrointestinal bleeding) or intermittent enteral feeding (increased gastric volume and lower volumes of feeding). Thus, to date, methods of enteral feeding aimed to reduce the incidence of VAP cannot be recommended for routine use.

STRESS ULCER PROPHYLAXIS

Gastric colonization by potentially pathogenic organisms has been shown to increase with decreasing gastric acidity.[246] Thus medications that decrease gastric acidity (antacids, H_2 blockers) may increase organism counts and increase the risk for VAP. In contrast, medications that do not affect gastric acidity, such as sucralfate, may not increase this risk.

Seven meta-analyses of more than 20 randomized trials have evaluated the risk for VAP associated with the methods used to prevent gastrointestinal bleeding in critically ill patients.[97,98,100,105,106,247,248] Four of these seven meta-analyses reported a significant reduction in VAP incidence with sucralfate therapy compared with H_2 blockers[97,100,106] and three a statistically significant mortality benefit.[98,100,105]

However, the relationships between prophylaxis of stress ulcer and prophylaxis of VAP are complex: (1) VAP is a possible indirect consequence of the use of drugs that raise the stomach pH, (2) gastrointestinal bleeding is a serious complication in critically ill patients at high risk for stress ulcer (e.g., patients with coagulopathy or the need for prolonged mechanical ventilation) but is extremely rare in patients at low to moderate risk, (3) the largest randomized trial comparing ranitidine with sucralfate showed that ranitidine was superior in preventing gastrointestinal bleeding and did not increase the risk of VAP,[107] and (4) the risk of VAP is unknown when accurate methods of enteral feeding or other preventive measures are used in combination with stress ulcer prophylaxis.

Clinicians must weigh the potential benefit of sucralfate (with potentially less VAP and more gastrointestinal bleeding) versus H_2 blockers (with potentially more VAP and less gastrointestinal bleeding) and probably limit stress ulcer prophylaxis to high-risk patients.

SELECTIVE DIGESTIVE DECONTAMINATION

There is theoretical interest in using topical antibiotics to sterilize the oropharynx and stomach in mechanically ventilated patients, with the goal of reducing the incidence of VAP.[249] Several groups have used topical prophylactic antibiotics for selective decontamination of the oropharynx and digestive tract (SDD) in patients at high risk for nosocomial pneumonia. The SDD regimen usually includes a short course of systemic antibiotic therapy, such as cefotaxime, trimethoprim, or a fluoroquinolone, and nonabsorbable local antibiotic prophylaxis consisting of a combination of an aminoglycoside, polymyxin B, and amphotericin.[249] Since the original studies published by Stoutenbeck and colleagues[250,251] in 1984, which demonstrated a decrease of the overall infection rate in patients receiving the SDD regimen, more than 40 randomized, controlled trials and 7 meta-analyses have been published.[91,252–258] All seven meta-analyses reported a significant reduction in the risk of VAP, and four reported a significant reduction in mortality.[91,254,255,257] No mortality benefit occurred with topical prophylaxis alone.[91,252,254,257] However, a clear consensus as to the effectiveness of SDD has not been established owing to limitations and methodologic deficiencies of the studies analyzed.[104,259] Furthermore, the

impact of SDD on the emergence of resistant organisms is currently unknown but potentially important.[260,261]

Conclusions drawn based on meta-analyses of SDD studies may be summarized as follows: (1) SDD reduces the incidence of VAP and, when a combined topical and systemic regimen is used, may reduce mortality, (2) an inverse relationship has been described between methodologic quality of the studies and benefit, questioning the overall value of results reported in the meta-analyses, (3) the long-term effects of SDD on emergence of resistance and risk of superinfections currently are unknown, and finally, (4) the impact of SDD on the duration of MV, ICU stay, and hospital stay appears to be limited. Thus, at present, this approach cannot be recommended for overall populations of ICU patients treated with MV, although SDD may be effective for specific populations, particularly surgical or trauma patients.

Early attempts at systemic prophylaxis with parenteral antibiotics alone against pneumonia clearly were unsuccessful.[262,263] In contrast, recent studies showed that a short-course antibiotic regimen in patients with structural coma or severe burns was an effective prophylactic strategy to decrease the VAP rate.[92] The influence of rotating of antibiotics (generally associated with restrictive use) in the ICU on VAP prevalence was investigated recently by comparing successive periods during which one antibiotic was used in place of another for the empirical treatment of suspected gram-negative bacterial infections. Some investigators found that VAP occurred significantly less frequently during the after period compared with the before period.[264–266]

References

1. Chastre J, Fagon JY: Pneumonia in the ventilator-dependent patient, in Tobin MJ (ed): *Principles and Practice of Mechanical Ventilation.* New York, McGraw-Hill, 1994, p 857.

2. Haley RW, Hooton TM, Culver DH, et al: Nosocomial infections in U.S. hospitals, 1975–1976: Estimated frequency by selected characteristics of patients. *Am J Med* 70:947, 1981.

3. Vincent JL, Bihari DJ, Suter PM, et al: The prevalence of nosocomial infection in intensive care units in Europe: Results of the European Prevalence of Infection in Intensive Care (EPIC) Study. EPIC International Advisory Committee (see comments). *JAMA* 274:639, 1995.

4. Chevret S, Hemmer M, Carlet J, Langer M: Incidence and risk factors of pneumonia acquired in intensive care units: Results from a multicenter prospective study on 996 patients. European Cooperative Group on Nosocomial Pneumonia. *Intensive Care Med* 19:256, 1993.

5. Cross AS, Roup B: Role of respiratory assistance devices in endemic nosocomial pneumonia. *Am J Med* 70:681, 1981.

6. Langer M, Mosconi P, Cigada M, Mandelli M: Long-term respiratory support and risk of pneumonia in critically ill patients. Intensive Care Unit Group of Infection Control. *Am Rev Respir Dis* 140:302, 1989.

7. Craven DE, Steger KA: Nosocomial pneumonia in mechanically ventilated adult patients: Epidemiology and prevention in 1996. *Semin Respir Infect* 11:32, 1996.

8. Celis R, Torres A, Gatell JM, et al: Nosocomial pneumonia: A multivariate analysis of risk and prognosis. *Chest* 93:318, 1988.

9. Fagon JY, Chastre J, Domart Y, et al: Nosocomial pneumonia in patients receiving continuous mechanical ventilation: Prospective analysis of 52 episodes with use of a protected specimen

brush and quantitative culture techniques. *Am Rev Respir Dis* 139:877, 1989.

10. Bell RC, Coalson JJ, Smith JD, Johanson WG: Multiple organ system failure and infection in adult respiratory distress syndrome. *Ann Intern Med* 99:293, 1983.

11. Pennington JE: Nosocomial respiratory infection, in Mandell GL, Douglas RG Jr, Bennet JE (eds): *Principles and Practice of Infectious Diseases.* New York, Churchill Livingstone, 1990, p 2199.

12. Torres A, Aznar R, Gatell JM, et al: Incidence, risk, and prognosis factors of nosocomial pneumonia in mechanically ventilated patients. *Am Rev Respir Dis* 142:523, 1990.

13. Craven DE, Kunches LM, Kilinsky V, et al: Risk factors for pneumonia and fatality in patients receiving continuous mechanical ventilation. *Am Rev Respir Dis* 133:792, 1986.

14. Chastre J, Trouillet JL, Vuagnat A, et al: Nosocomial pneumonia in patients with acute respiratory distress syndrome. *Am J Respir Crit Care Med* 157:1165, 1998.

15. Delclaux C, Roupie E, Blot F, et al: Lower respiratory tract colonization and infection during severe acute respiratory distress syndrome: Incidence and diagnosis. *Am J Respir Crit Care Med* 156:1092, 1997.

16. Markowicz P, Wolff M, Djedaini K, et al: Multicenter prospective study of ventilator-associated pneumonia during acute respiratory distress syndrome: Incidence, prognosis, and risk factors. ARDS Study Group. *Am J Respir Crit Care Med* 161:1942, 2000.

17. Rello J, Ausina V, Ricart M, et al: Impact of previous antimicrobial therapy on the etiology and outcome of ventilator-associated pneumonia (see comments). *Chest* 104:1230, 1993.

18. Rello J, Rue M, Jubert P, et al: Survival in patients with nosocomial pneumonia: Impact of the severity of illness and the etiologic agent. *Crit Care Med* 25:1862, 1997.

19. Rello J, Gallego M, Mariscal D, et al: The value of routine microbial investigation in ventilator-associated pneumonia. *Am J Respir Crit Care Med* 156:196, 1997.

20. Kollef MH, Sherman G, Ward S, Fraser VJ: Inadequate antimicrobial treatment of infections: A risk factor for hospital mortality among critically ill patients. *Chest* 115:462, 1999.

21. Corley DE, Kirtland SH, Winterbauer RH, et al: Reproducibility of the histologic diagnosis of pneumonia among a panel of four pathologists: Analysis of a gold standard. *Chest* 112:458, 1997.

22. Marquette CH, Copin MC, Wallet F, et al: Diagnostic tests for pneumonia in ventilated patients: Prospective evaluation of diagnostic accuracy using histology as a diagnostic gold standard. *Am J Respir Crit Care Med* 151:1878, 1995.

23. Rouby JJ, Martin De Lassale E, Poete P, et al: Nosocomial bronchopneumonia in the critically ill: Histologic and bacteriologic aspects (see comments). *Am Rev Respir Dis* 146:1059, 1992.

24. Kirtland SH, Corley DE, Winterbauer RH, et al: The diagnosis of ventilator-associated pneumonia: A comparison of histologic, microbiologic, and clinical criteria. *Chest* 112:445, 1997.

25. Langer M, Cigada M, Mandelli M, et al: Early onset pneumonia: A multicenter study in intensive care units. *Intensive Care Med* 13:342, 1987.

26. Hospital-acquired pneumonia in adults: Diagnosis, assessment of severity, initial antimicrobial therapy, and preventive strategies. A consensus statement, American Thoracic Society, November 1995. *Am J Respir Crit Care Med* 153:1711, 1996.

27. Chastre J, Fagon JY: Ventilator-associated pneumonia. *Am J Respir Crit Care Med* 165:867, 2002.

28. National Nosocomial Infections Surveillance (NNIS) System report: Data summary from January 1990–May 1999, issued June 1999. *J Infect Control* 27:520, 1999.

29. Cook DJ, Walter SD, Cook RJ, et al: Incidence of and risk factors for ventilator-associated pneumonia in critically ill patients (see comments). *Ann Intern Med* 129:433, 1998.

30. Andrews CP, Coalson JJ, Smith JD, Johanson WG: Diagnosis of nosocomial bacterial pneumonia in acute, diffuse lung injury. *Chest* 80:254, 1981.

31. Sutherland KR, Steinberg KP, Maunder RJ, et al: Pulmonary infection during the acute respiratory distress syndrome. *Am J Respir Crit Care Med* 152:550, 1995.

32. Meduri GU, Reddy RC, Stanley T, El-Zeky F: Pneumonia in acute respiratory distress syndrome: A prospective evaluation of bilateral bronchoscopic sampling. *Am J Respir Crit Care Med* 158:870, 1998.

33. Salata RA, Lederman MM, Shlaes DM, et al: Diagnosis of nosocomial pneumonia in intubated, intensive care unit patients. *Am Rev Respir Dis* 135:426, 1987.

34. Kerver AJ, Rommes JH, Mevissen-Verhage EA, et al: Colonization and infection in surgical intensive care patients: A prospective study. *Intensive Care Med* 13:347, 1987.

35. Driks MR, Craven DE, Celli BR, et al: Nosocomial pneumonia in intubated patients given sucralfate as compared with antacids or histamine type 2 blockers: The role of gastric colonization. *N Engl J Med* 317:1376, 1987.

36. Baker AM, Meredith JW, Haponik EF: Pneumonia in intubated trauma patients: Microbiology and outcomes. *Am J Respir Crit Care Med* 153:343, 1996.

37. Kollef MH: Ventilator-associated pneumonia: A multivariate analysis. *JAMA* 270:1965, 1993.

38. Fagon JY, Chastre J, Vuagnat A, et al: Nosocomial pneumonia and mortality among patients in intensive care units. *JAMA* 275:866, 1996.

39. Timsit JF, Chevret S, Valcke J, et al: Mortality of nosocomial pneumonia in ventilated patients: Influence of diagnostic tools. *Am J Respir Crit Care Med* 154:116, 1996.

40. Tejada Artigas A, Bello Dronda S, Chacon Valles E, et al: Risk factors for nosocomial pneumonia in critically ill trauma patients. *Crit Care Med* 29:304, 2001.

41. Rodriguez de Castro F, Sole-Violan J, Aranda Leon A, et al: Do quantitative cultures of protected brush specimens modify the initial empirical therapy in ventilated patients with suspected pneumonia? *Eur Respir J* 9:37, 1996.

42. Stevens RM, Teres D, Skillman JJ, Feingold DS: Pneumonia in an intensive care unit: A 30-month experience. *Arch Intern Med* 134:106, 1974.

43. Joshi N, Localio AR, Hamory BH: A predictive risk index for nosocomial pneumonia in the intensive care unit. *Am J Med* 93:135, 1992.

44. Garibaldi RA, Britt MR, Coleman ML, et al: Risk factors for post-operative pneumonia. *Am J Med* 70:677, 1981.

45. Jimenez P, Torres A, Rodriguez-Roisin R, et al: Incidence and etiology of pneumonia acquired during mechanical ventilation. *Crit Care Med* 17:882, 1989.

46. Bryan CS, Reynolds KL: Bacteremic nosocomial pneumonia: Analysis of 172 episodes from a single metropolitan area. *Am Rev Respir Dis* 129:668, 1984.

47. Tillotson JR, Lerner AM: Characteristics of nonbacteremic *Pseudomonas* pneumonia. *Ann Intern Med* 68:295, 1968.

48. Tillotson JR, Lerner AM: Characteristics of pneumonias caused by *Bacillus proteus. Ann Intern Med* 68:287, 1968.

49. Tillotson JR, Finland M: Secondary pulmonary infections following antibiotic therapy for primary bacterial pneumonia. *Antimicrob Agents Chemother* 8:326, 1968.

50. Fagon JY, Chastre J, Hance AJ, et al: Nosocomial pneumonia in ventilated patients: A cohort study evaluating attributable mortality and hospital stay. *Am J Med* 94:281, 1993.

51. Kollef MH, Silver P, Murphy DM, Trovillion E: The effect of late-onset ventilator-associated pneumonia in determining patient mortality. *Chest* 108:1655, 1995.

52. Rello J, Torres A, Ricart M, et al: Ventilator-associated pneumonia by *Staphylococcus aureus:* Comparison of methicillin-resistant

and methicillin-sensitive episodes. *Am J Respir Crit Care Med* 150:1545, 1994.

53. Craig CP, Connelly S: Effect of intensive care unit nosocomial pneumonia on duration of stay and mortality. *Am J Infect Control* 12:233, 1984.

54. Cunnion KM, Weber DJ, Broadhead WE, et al: Risk factors for nosocomial pneumonia: Comparing adult critical-care populations. *Am J Respir Crit Care Med* 153:158, 1996.

55. Papazian L, Bregeon F, Thirion X, et al: Effect of ventilator-associated pneumonia on mortality and morbidity. *Am J Respir Crit Care Med* 154:91, 1996.

56. Heyland DK, Cook DJ, Griffith L, et al: The attributable morbidity and mortality of ventilator-associated pneumonia in the critically ill patient. The Canadian Critical Trials Group. *Am J Respir Crit Care Med* 159:1249, 1999.

57. Bercault N, Boulain T: Mortality associated with ventilator-associated pneumonia in an adult intensive care unit: A prospective 135 matched-paired cohort study. *Crit Care Med* (in press).

58. Bueno-Cavanillas A, Delgado-Rodriguez M, Lopez-Luque A, et al: Influence of nosocomial infection on mortality rate in an intensive care unit. *Crit Care Med* 22:55, 1994.

59. Bregeon F, Ciais V, Carret V, et al: Is ventilator-associated pneumonia an independent risk factor for death? *Anesthesiology* 94:554, 2001.

60. Horan TC, Culver DH, Gaynes RP, et al: Nosocomial infections in surgical patients in the United States, January 1986–June 1992. National Nosocomial Infections Surveillance (NNIS) System. *Infect Control Hosp Epidemiol* 14:73, 1993.

61. LaForce FM: Hospital-acquired gram-negative rod pneumonias: An overview. *Am J Med* 70:664, 1981.

62. Levison ME, Kaye D: Pneumonia caused by gram-negative bacilli: An overview. *Rev Infect Dis* 7(suppl 4):S656, 1985.

63. Torres A, Puig de la Bellacasa J, Xaubet A, et al: Diagnostic value of quantitative cultures of bronchoalveolar lavage and telescoping plugged catheters in mechanically ventilated patients with bacterial pneumonia. *Am Rev Respir Dis* 140:306, 1989.

64. Spencer RC: Predominant pathogens found in the European Prevalence of Infection in Intensive Care Study. *Eur J Clin Microbiol Infect Dis* 15:281, 1996.

65. Montravers P, Fagon JY, Chastre J, et al: Follow-up protected specimen brushes to assess treatment in nosocomial pneumonia. *Am Rev Respir Dis* 147:38, 1993.

66. Marik PE, Careau P: The role of anaerobes in patients with ventilator-associated pneumonia and aspiration pneumonia: A prospective study (see comments). *Chest* 115:178, 1999.

67. Dore P, Robert R, Grollier G, et al: Incidence of anaerobes in ventilator-associated pneumonia with use of a protected specimen brush. *Am J Respir Crit Care Med* 153:1292, 1996.

68. Rello J, Valles J, Jubert P, et al: Lower respiratory tract infections following cardiac arrest and cardiopulmonary resuscitation. *Clin Infect Dis* 21:310, 1995.

69. Rello J, Ausina V, Castella J, et al: Nosocomial respiratory tract infections in multiple trauma patients: Influence of level of consciousness with implications for therapy. *Chest* 102:525, 1992.

70. Croce MA, Fabian TC, Schurr MJ, et al: Using bronchoalveolar lavage to distinguish nosocomial pneumonia from systemic inflammatory response syndrome: A prospective analysis. *J Trauma* 39:1134, 1995; discussion 1139.

71. Timsit JF, Cheval C, Gachot B, et al: Usefulness of a strategy based on bronchoscopy with direct examination of bronchoalveolar lavage fluid in the initial antibiotic therapy of suspected ventilator-associated pneumonia. *Intensive Care Med* 27:640, 2001.

72. Sole Violan J, Fernandez JA, Benitez AB, et al: Impact of quantitative invasive diagnostic techniques in the management and outcome of mechanically ventilated patients with suspected pneumonia (see comments). *Crit Care Med* 28:2737, 2000.

73. Ruiz M, Torres A, Ewig S, et al: Noninvasive versus invasive microbial investigation in ventilator-associated pneumonia: Evaluation of outcome. *Am J Respir Crit Care Med* 162:119, 2000.

74. Fagon JY, Chastre J, Wolff M, et al: Invasive and noninvasive strategies for management of suspected ventilator-associated pneumonia: A randomized trial. *Ann Intern Med* 132:621, 2000.

75. George DL, Falk PS, Wunderink RG, et al: Epidemiology of ventilator-acquired pneumonia based on protected bronchoscopic sampling. *Am J Respir Crit Care Med* 158:1839, 1998.

76. Rello J, Sa-Borges M, Correa H, et al: Variations in etiology of ventilator-associated pneumonia across four treatment sites: Implications for antimicrobial prescribing practices. *Am J Respir Crit Care Med* 160:608, 1999.

77. Trouillet JL, Chastre J, Vuagnat A, et al: Ventilator-associated pneumonia caused by potentially drug-resistant bacteria. *Am J Respir Crit Care Med* 157:531, 1998.

78. Leal-Noval SR, Marquez-Vacaro JA, Garcia-Curiel A, et al: Nosocomial pneumonia in patients undergoing heart surgery. *Crit Care Med* 28:935, 2000.

79. Antonelli M, Moro ML, Capelli O, et al: Risk factors for early onset pneumonia in trauma patients. *Chest* 105:224, 1994.

80. Singh N, Falestiny MN, Rogers P, et al: Pulmonary infiltrates in the surgical ICU: Prospective assessment of predictors of etiology and mortality. *Chest* 114:1129, 1998.

81. Ibrahim EH, Ward S, Sherman G, Kollef MH: A comparative analysis of patients with early-onset vs late-onset nosocomial pneumonia in the ICU setting. *Chest* 117:1434, 2000.

82. Kirby BD, Snyder KM, Meyer RD, Finegold SM: Legionnaires' disease: Report of sixty-five nosocomially acquired cases of review of the literature. *Medicine* 59:188, 1980.

83. Girod JC, Reichman RC, Winn WC, et al: Pneumonic and nonpneumonic forms of legionellosis: The result of a common-source exposure to *Legionella pneumophila*. *Arch Intern Med* 142:545, 1982.

84. el-Ebiary M, Torres A, Fabregas N, et al: Significance of the isolation of *Candida* species from respiratory samples in critically ill, non-neutropenic patients: An immediate postmortem histologic study. *Am J Respir Crit Care Med* 156:583, 1997.

85. Papazian L, Fraisse A, Garbe L, et al: Cytomegalovirus: An unexpected cause of ventilator-associated pneumonia. *Anesthesiology* 84:280, 1996.

86. Rello J, Esandi ME, Diaz E, et al: The role of *Candida* sp isolated from bronchoscopic samples in nonneutropenic patients. *Chest* 114:146, 1998.

87. Rello J, Ausina V, Ricart M, et al: Risk factors for infection by *Pseudomonas aeruginosa* in patients with ventilator-associated pneumonia. *Intensive Care Med* 20:193, 1994.

88. Jarvis WR, Edwards JR, Culver DH, et al: Nosocomial infection rates in adult and pediatric intensive care units in the United States. National Nosocomial Infections Surveillance System. *Am J Med* 91:185S, 1991.

89. Johanson WG, Pierce AK, Sanford JP, Thomas GD: Nosocomial respiratory infections with gram-negative bacilli: The significance of colonization of the respiratory tract. *Ann Intern Med* 77:701, 1972.

90. Rello J, Torres A: Microbial causes of ventilator-associated pneumonia. *Semin Respir Infect* 11:24, 1996.

91. D'Amico R, Pifferi S, Leonetti C, et al: Effectiveness of antibiotic prophylaxis in critically ill adult patients: Systematic review of randomised controlled trials. *Br Med J* 316:1275, 1998.

92. Sirvent JM, Torres A, El-Ebiary M, et al: Protective effect of intravenously administered cefuroxime against nosocomial pneumonia in patients with structural coma. *Am J Respir Crit Care Med* 155:1729, 1997.

93. Rello J, Diaz E, Roque M, Valles J: Risk factors for developing pneumonia within 48 hours of intubation. *Am J Respir Crit Care Med* 159:1742, 1999.

94. Johanson WG, Seidenfeld JJ, de los Santos R, et al: Prevention of nosocomial pneumonia using topical and parenteral antimicrobial agents. *Am Rev Respir Dis* 137:265, 1988.

95. Feeley TW, Du Moulin GC, Hedley-Whyte J, et al: Aerosol polymyxin and pneumonia in seriously ill patients. *N Engl J Med* 293:471, 1975.

96. de Man P, Verhoeven BA, Verbrugh HA, et al: An antibiotic policy to prevent emergence of resistant bacilli (see comments). *Lancet* 355:973, 2000.

97. Tryba M: Sucralfate versus antacids or H$_2$-antagonists for stress ulcer prophylaxis: A meta-analysis on efficacy and pneumonia rate. *Crit Care Med* 19:942, 1991.

98. Tryba M: Prophylaxis of stress ulcer bleeding: A meta-analysis. *J Clin Gastroenterol* 13(suppl 2):S44, 1991.

99. Tryba M: Stress ulcer prophylaxis and gastric alkalinization: Death of a myth? *Intensive Care Med* 18:1, 1992.

100. Tryba M, Cook DJ: Gastric alkalinization, pneumonia, and systemic infections: The controversy. *Scand J Gastroenterol Suppl* 210:53, 1995.

101. Tryba M, Cook D: Current guidelines on stress ulcer prophylaxis. *Drugs* 54:581, 1997.

102. Tryba M: Research on stress ulcer prophylaxis: Wrong questions, wrong answers? *Crit Care Med* 27:16, 1999.

103. Cook DJ, Witt LG, Cook RJ, Guyatt GH: Stress ulcer prophylaxis in the critically ill: A meta-analysis. *Am J Med* 91:519, 1991.

104. Craven DE, Steger KA: Ventilator-associated bacterial pneumonia: Challenges in diagnosis, treatment, and prevention. *New Horizons* 6:S30, 1998.

105. Cook DJ, Reeve BK, Guyatt GH, et al: Stress ulcer prophylaxis in critically ill patients: Resolving discordant meta-analyses. *JAMA* 275:308, 1996.

106. Messori A, Trippoli S, Vaiani M, et al: Bleeding and pneumonia in intensive care patients given ranitidine and sucralfate for prevention of stress ulcer: Meta-analysis of randomised controlled trials (in process citation). *Br Med J* 321:1103, 2000.

107. Cook D, Guyatt G, Marshall J, et al: A comparison of sucralfate and ranitidine for the prevention of upper gastrointestinal bleeding in patients requiring mechanical ventilation. Canadian Critical Care Trials Group (see comments). *N Engl J Med* 338:791, 1998.

108. Ben-Menachem T, Fogel R, Patel RV, et al: Prophylaxis for stress-related gastric hemorrhage in the medical intensive care unit: A randomized, controlled, single-blind study. *Ann Intern Med* 121:568, 1994.

109. Eddleston JM, Pearson RC, Holland J, et al: Prospective endoscopic study of stress erosions and ulcers in critically ill adult patients treated with either sucralfate or placebo. *Crit Care Med* 22:1949, 1994.

110. Sottile FD, Marrie TJ, Prough DS, et al: Nosocomial pulmonary infection: Possible etiologic significance of bacterial adhesion to endotracheal tubes. *Crit Care Med* 14:265, 1986.

111. Torres A, Gatell JM, Aznar E, et al: Re-intubation increases the risk of nosocomial pneumonia in patients needing mechanical ventilation. *Am J Respir Crit Care Med* 152:137, 1995.

112. Sugerman HJ, Wolfe L, Pasquale MD, et al: Multicenter, randomized, prospective trial of early tracheostomy. *J Trauma* 43:741, 1997.

113. Kluger Y, Paul DB, Lucke J, et al: Early tracheostomy in trauma patients. *Eur J Emerg Med* 3:95, 1996.

114. D'Amelio LF, Hammond JS, Spain DA, Sutyak JP: Tracheostomy and percutaneous endoscopic gastrostomy in the management of the head-injured trauma patient. *Am Surg* 60:180, 1994.

115. Lesnik I, Rappaport W, Fulginiti J, Witzke D: The role of early tracheostomy in blunt, multiple organ trauma. *Am Surg* 58:346, 1992.

116. Rodriguez JL, Steinberg SM, Luchetti FA, et al: Early tracheostomy for primary airway management in the surgical critical care setting. *Surgery* 108:655, 1990.

117. Armstrong PA, McCarthy MC, Peoples JB: Reduced use of resources by early tracheostomy in ventilator-dependent patients with blunt trauma. *Surgery* 124:763, 1998; discussion 766.

118. Brook AD, Sherman G, Malen J, Kollef MH: Early versus late tracheostomy in patients who require prolonged mechanical ventilation. *Am J Crit Care* 9:352, 2000.

119. Stocchetti N, Parma A, Songa V, et al: Early translaryngeal tracheostomy in patients with severe brain damage. *Intensive Care Med* 26:1101, 2000.

120. Livingston DH: Prevention of ventilator-associated pneumonia. *Am J Surg* 179:12S, 2000.

121. Pingleton SK, Hinthorn DR, Liu C: Enteral nutrition in patients receiving mechanical ventilation: Multiple sources of tracheal colonization include the stomach. *Am J Med* 80:827, 1986.

122. Torres A, Serra-Batlles J, Ros E, et al: Pulmonary aspiration of gastric contents in patients receiving mechanical ventilation: The effect of body position. *Ann Intern Med* 116:540, 1992.

123. Craven DE, Lichtenberg DA, Goularte TA, et al: Contaminated medication nebulizers in mechanical ventilator circuits: Source of bacterial aerosols. *Am J Med* 77:834, 1984.

124. Craven DE, Goularte TA, Make BJ: Contaminated condensate in mechanical ventilator circuits: A risk factor for nosocomial pneumonia? *Am Rev Respir Dis* 129:625, 1984.

125. Vandenbussche T, De Moor S, Bachert C, Van Cauwenberge P: Value of antral puncture in the intensive care patient with fever of unknown origin. *Laryngoscope* 110:1702, 2000.

126. Le Moal G, Lemerre D, Grollier G, et al: Nosocomial sinusitis with isolation of anaerobic bacteria in ICU patients. *Intensive Care Med* 25:1066, 1999.

127. Geiss HK: Nosocomial sinusitis. *Intensive Care Med* 25:1037, 1999.

128. Holzapfel L, Chastang C, Demingeon G, et al: A randomized study assessing the systematic search for maxillary sinusitis in nasotracheally mechanically ventilated patients: Influence of nosocomial maxillary sinusitis on the occurrence of ventilator-associated pneumonia. *Am J Respir Crit Care Med* 159:695, 1999.

129. Westergren V, Lundblad L, Hellquist HB, Forsum U: Ventilator-associated sinusitis: A review. *Clin Infect Dis* 27:851, 1998.

130. George DL, Falk PS, Umberto Meduri G, et al: Nosocomial sinusitis in patients in the medical intensive care unit: A prospective epidemiological study. *Clin Infect Dis* 27:463, 1998.

131. Talmor M, Li P, Barie PS: Acute paranasal sinusitis in critically ill patients: Guidelines for prevention, diagnosis, and treatment. *Clin Infect Dis* 25:1441, 1997.

132. Bert F, Lambert-Zechovsky N: Sinusitis in mechanically ventilated patients and its role in the pathogenesis of nosocomial pneumonia. *Eur J Clin Microbiol Infect Dis* 15:533, 1996.

133. Bert F, Lambert-Zechovsky N: Microbiology of nosocomial sinusitis in intensive care unit patients. *J Infect* 31:5, 1995.

134. Spapen H, Deron P, Hamels K, et al: Nosocomial pansinusitis in orotracheally intubated critically ill patients. *Acta Otorhinolaryngol Belg* 49:251, 1995.

135. Rouby JJ, Laurent P, Gosnach M, et al: Risk factors and clinical relevance of nosocomial maxillary sinusitis in the critically ill (see comments). *Am J Respir Crit Care Med* 150:776, 1994.

136. Heffner JE: Nosocomial sinusitis: Den of multiresistant thieves? *Am J Respir Crit Care Med* 150:608, 1994.

137. Holzapfel L, Chevret S, Madinier G, et al: Influence of long-term oro- or nasotracheal intubation on nosocomial maxillary sinusitis and pneumonia: Results of a prospective, randomized, clinical trial. *Crit Care Med* 21:1132, 1993.

138. Bach A, Boehrer H, Schmidt H, Geiss HK: Nosocomial sinusitis in ventilated patients: Nasotracheal versus orotracheal intubation. *Anaesthesia* 47:335, 1992.

139. Salord F, Gaussorgues P, Marti-Flich J, et al: Nosocomial maxillary sinusitis during mechanical ventilation: A prospective comparison of orotracheal versus the nasotracheal route for intubation. *Intensive Care Med* 16:390, 1990.

140. Guerin JM, Meyer P, Barbotin-Larrieu F, Habib Y: Nosocomial bacteremia and sinusitis in nasotracheally intubated patients in intensive care. *Rev Infect Dis* 10:1226, 1988.

141. Deutschman CS, Wilton P, Sinow J, et al: Paranasal sinusitis associated with nasotracheal intubation: A frequently unrecognized and treatable source of sepsis. *Crit Care Med* 14:111, 1986.

142. Kollef MH, Von Harz B, Prentice D, et al: Patient transport from intensive care increases the risk of developing ventilator-associated pneumonia. *Chest* 112:765, 1997.

143. Ayala A, Perrin MM, Meldrum DR, et al: Hemorrhage induces an increase in serum TNF which is not associated with elevated levels of endotoxin. *Cytokine* 2:170, 1990.

144. Wunderink RG: Radiologic diagnosis of ventilator-associated pneumonia. *Chest* 117:188S, 2000.

145. Wunderink RG, Woldenberg LS, Zeiss J, et al: The radiologic diagnosis of autopsy-proven ventilator-associated pneumonia. *Chest* 101:458, 1992.

146. Meduri GU, Mauldin GL, Wunderink RG, et al: Causes of fever and pulmonary densities in patients with clinical manifestations of ventilator-associated pneumonia. *Chest* 106:221, 1994.

147. Winer-Muram HT, Jennings SG, Wunderink RG, et al: Ventilator-associated *Pseudomonas aeruginosa* pneumonia: Radiographic findings. *Radiology* 195:247, 1995.

148. Winer-Muram HT, Rubin SA, Ellis JV, et al: Pneumonia and ARDS in patients receiving mechanical ventilation: Diagnostic accuracy of chest radiography. *Radiology* 188:479, 1993.

149. Lefcoe MS, Fox GA, Leasa DJ, et al: Accuracy of portable chest radiography in the critical care setting: Diagnosis of pneumonia based on quantitative cultures obtained from protected brush catheter. *Chest* 105:885, 1994.

150. Torres A, el-Ebiary M, Padro L, et al: Validation of different techniques for the diagnosis of ventilator-associated pneumonia: Comparison with immediate postmortem pulmonary biopsy. *Am J Respir Crit Care Med* 149:324, 1994.

151. Meduri GU, Belenchia JM, Estes RJ, et al: Fibroproliferative phase of ARDS: Clinical findings and effects of corticosteroids (see comments). *Chest* 100:943, 1991.

152. Villers D, Derriennic M, Raffi F, et al: Reliability of the bronchoscopic protected catheter brush in intubated and ventilated patients. *Chest* 88:527, 1985.

153. Lambert RS, Vereen LE, George RB: Comparison of tracheal aspirates and protected brush catheter specimens for identifying pathogenic bacteria in mechanically ventilated patients. *Am J Med Sci* 297:377, 1989.

154. Baselski V: Microbiologic diagnosis of ventilator-associated pneumonia. *Infect Dis Clin North Am* 7:331, 1993.

155. Hill JD, Ratliff JL, Parrott JC, et al: Pulmonary pathology in acute respiratory insufficiency: Lung biopsy as a diagnostic tool. *J Thorac Cardiovasc Surg* 71:64, 1976.

156. Kollef MH: Inadequate antimicrobial treatment: An important determinant of outcome for hospitalized patients. *Clin Infect Dis* 31(suppl 4):S131, 2000.

157. Kollef MH, Ward S: The influence of mini-BAL cultures on patient outcomes: Implications for the antibiotic management of ventilator-associated pneumonia. *Chest* 113:412, 1998.

158. Alvarez-Lerma F: Modification of empiric antibiotic treatment in patients with pneumonia acquired in the intensive care unit. ICU-Acquired Pneumonia Study Group. *Intensive Care Med* 22:387, 1996.

159. Croce MA, Fabian TC, Waddle-Smith L, et al: Utility of Gram's stain and efficacy of quantitative cultures for posttraumatic pneumonia: A prospective study. *Ann Surg* 227:743, 1998; discussion 751.

160. Bonten MJ, Bergmans DC, Stobberingh EE, et al: Implementation of bronchoscopic techniques in the diagnosis of ventilator-associated pneumonia to reduce antibiotic use. *Am J Respir Crit Care Med* 156:1820, 1997.

161. Baker AM, Bowton DL, Haponik EF: Decision making in nosocomial pneumonia: An analytic approach to the interpretation of quantitative bronchoscopic cultures. *Chest* 107:85, 1995.

162. Sterling TR, Ho EJ, Brehm WT, Kirkpatrick MB: Diagnosis and treatment of ventilator-associated pneumonia—impact on survival: A decision analysis. *Chest* 110:1025, 1996.

163. Heyland DK, Cook DJ, Marshall J, et al: The clinical utility of invasive diagnostic techniques in the setting of ventilator-associated pneumonia. Canadian Critical Care Trials Group. *Chest* 115:1076, 1999.

164. Sanchez-Nieto JM, Torres A, Garcia-Cordoba F, et al: Impact of invasive and noninvasive quantitative culture sampling on outcome of ventilator-associated pneumonia: A pilot study (see comments) *Am J Respir Crit Care Med* 157:371, 1998; published erratum appears in *Am J Respir Crit Care Med* 157:1005, 1998.

165. Fagon JY, Chastre J, Hance AJ, et al: Detection of nosocomial lung infection in ventilated patients: Use of a protected specimen brush and quantitative culture techniques in 147 patients. *Am Rev Respir Dis* 138:110, 1988.

166. Dreyfuss D, Mier L, Le Bourdelles G, et al: Clinical significance of borderline quantitative protected brush specimen culture results. *Am Rev Respir Dis* 147:946, 1993.

167. Singh N, Rogers P, Atwood CW, et al: Short-course empiric antibiotic therapy for patients with pulmonary infiltrates in the intensive care unit: A proposed solution for indiscriminate antibiotic prescription. *Am J Respir Crit Care Med* 162:505, 2000.

168. Campbell GD: Blinded invasive diagnostic procedures in ventilator-associated pneumonia. *Chest* 117:207S, 2000.

169. Baselski VS, Wunderink RG: Bronchoscopic diagnosis of pneumonia. *Clin Microbiol Rev* 7:533, 1994.

170. Prats E, Dorca J, Pujol M, et al: Effects of antibiotics on protected specimen brush sampling in ventilator-associated pneumonia. *Eur Respir J* 19:944, 2002.

171. Souweine B, Veber B, Bedos JP, et al: Diagnostic accuracy of protected specimen brush and bronchoalveolar lavage in nosocomial pneumonia: Impact of previous antimicrobial treatments (see comments). *Crit Care Med* 26:236, 1998.

172. Luna CM, Vujacich P, Niederman MS, et al: Impact of BAL data on the therapy and outcome of ventilator-associated pneumonia. *Chest* 111:676, 1997.

173. Kollef MH, Bock KR, Richards RD, Hearns ML: The safety and diagnostic accuracy of minibronchoalveolar lavage in patients with suspected ventilator-associated pneumonia (see comments). *Ann Intern Med* 122:743, 1995.

174. Dupont H, Mentec H, Sollet JP, Bleichner G: Impact of appropriateness of initial antibiotic therapy on the outcome of ventilator-associated pneumonia. *Intensive Care Med* 27:355, 2001.

175. Pestotnik SL, Classen DC, Evans RS, Burke JP: Implementing antibiotic practice guidelines through computer-assisted decision support: Clinical and financial outcomes. *Ann Intern Med* 124:884, 1996.

176. Hayon J, Figliolini C, Combes A, et al: Role of serial routine microbiologic culture results in the initial management of ventilator-associated pneumonia. *Am J Respir Crit Care Med* 165:41, 2002.

177. Baldwin DR, Honeybourne D, Wise R: Pulmonary disposition of antimicrobial agents: In vivo observations and clinical relevance. *Antimicrob Agents Chemother* 36:1176, 1992.

178. Lamer C, de Beco V, Soler P, et al: Analysis of vancomycin entry into pulmonary lining fluid by bronchoalveolar lavage in critically ill patients. *Antimicrob Agents Chemother* 37:281, 1993.

179. Forrest A, Nix DE, Ballow CH, et al: Pharmacodynamics of intravenous ciprofloxacin in seriously ill patients. *Antimicrob Agents Chemother* 37:1073, 1993.

180. Kashuba AD, Nafziger AN, Drusano GL, Bertino JS Jr: Optimizing aminoglycoside therapy for nosocomial pneumonia caused by gram-negative bacteria. *Antimicrob Agents Chemother* 43:623, 1999.

181. Schentag JJ: Antimicrobial action and pharmacokinetics/pharmacodynamics: The use of AUIC to improve efficacy and avoid resistance (in process citation). *J Chemother* 11:426, 1999.

182. Moise PA, Forrest A, Bhavnani SM, et al: Area under the inhibitory curve and a pneumonia scoring system for predicting outcomes of vancomycin therapy for respiratory infections by *Staphylococcus aureus*. *Am J Health Syst Pharm* 57:S4, 2000.

183. Hoffken G, Niederman MS: Nosocomial pneumonia: The importance of a de-escalating strategy for antibiotic treatment of pneumonia in the ICU. *Chest* 122:2183, 2002.

184. Fink MP, Snydman DR, Niederman MS, et al: Treatment of severe pneumonia in hospitalized patients: Results of a multicenter, randomized, double-blind trial comparing intravenous ciprofloxacin with imipenem-cilastatin. The Severe Pneumonia Study Group (see comments). *Antimicrob Agents Chemother* 38:547, 1994.

185. Cometta A, Baumgartner JD, Lew D, et al: Prospective randomized comparison of imipenem monotherapy with imipenem plus netilmicin for treatment of severe infections in nonneutropenic patients. *Antimicrob Agents Chemother* 38:1309, 1994.

186. Hilf M, Yu VL, Sharp J, et al: Antibiotic therapy for *Pseudomonas aeruginosa* bacteremia: Outcome correlations in a prospective study of 200 patients (see comments). *Am J Med* 87:540, 1989.

187. Korvick JA, Bryan CS, Farber B, et al: Prospective observational study of *Klebsiella* bacteremia in 230 patients: Outcome for antibiotic combinations versus monotherapy. *Antimicrob Agents Chemother* 36:2639, 1992.

188. Rello J, Mariscal D, March F, et al Recurrent *Pseudomonas aeruginosa* pneumonia in ventilated patients: Relapse or reinfection? *Am J Respir Crit Care Med* 157:912, 1998.

189. Kollef MH, Fraser VJ: Antibiotic resistance in the intensive care unit. *Ann Intern Med* 134:298, 2001.

190. Kollef MH: The prevention of ventilator-associated pneumonia (see comments). *N Engl J Med* 340:627, 1999.

191. Bassin AS, Niederman MS: Prevention of ventilator-associated pneumonia: An attainable goal? *Clin Chest Med* 16:195, 1995.

192. Guidelines for prevention of nosocomial pneumonia. Centers for Disease Control and Prevention. *MMWR* 46:1, 1997.

193. Cook D, De Jonghe B, Brochard L, Brun-Buisson C: Influence of airway management on ventilator-associated pneumonia: Evidence from randomized trials. *JAMA* 279:781, 1998; published erratum appears in *JAMA* 281:2089, 1999.

194. Collard HR, Saint S, Matthay MA: Prevention of ventilator-associated pneumonia: An evidence-based systematic review. *Ann Intern Med* 138:494, 2003.

195. Flaherty JP, Weinstein RA: Infection control and pneumonia prophylaxis strategies in the intensive care unit. *Semin Respir Infect* 5:191, 1990.

196. du Moulin G: Minimizing the potential for nosocomial pneumonia: Architectural, engineering, and environmental considerations for the intensive care unit. *Eur J Clin Microbiol Infect Dis* 8:69, 1989.

197. Pittet D, Mourouga P, Perneger TV: Compliance with handwashing in a teaching hospital infection control program. *Ann Intern Med* 130:126, 1999.

198. Craven DE, De Rosa FG, Thornton D: Nosocomial pneumonia: Emerging concepts in diagnosis, management, and prophylaxis. *Curr Opin Crit Care* 8:421, 2002.

199. Girou E, Loyeau S, Legrand P, et al: Efficacy of handrubbing with alcohol based solution versus standard handwashing with antiseptic soap: Randomised clinical trial. *Br Med J* 325:362, 2002.

200. Haley RW, Culver DH, White JW, et al: The efficacy of infection surveillance and control programs in preventing nosocomial infections in US hospitals. *Am J Epidemiol* 121:182, 1985.

201. Gruson D, Hilbert G, Vargas F, et al: Rotation and restricted use of antibiotics in a medical intensive care unit: Impact on the incidence of ventilator-associated pneumonia caused by antibiotic-resistant gram-negative bacteria. *Am J Respir Crit Care Med* 162:837, 2000.

202. Ntoumenopoulos G, Presneill JJ, McElholum M, Cade JF: Chest physiotherapy for the prevention of ventilator-associated pneumonia. *Intensive Care Med* 28:850, 2002.

203. Kollef MH, Shapiro SD, Silver P, et al: A randomized, controlled trial of protocol-directed versus physician-directed weaning from mechanical ventilation. *Crit Care Med* 25:567, 1997.

204. Nava S, Ambrosino N, Clini E, et al: Noninvasive mechanical ventilation in the weaning of patients with respiratory failure due to chronic obstructive pulmonary disease: A randomized, controlled trial. *Ann Intern Med* 128:721, 1998.

205. Girou E, Schortgen F, Delclaux C, et al: Association of noninvasive ventilation with nosocomial infections and survival in critically ill patients (in process citation). *JAMA* 284:2361, 2000.

206. Kagramanov V, Lyman A: Noninvasive ventilation and nosocomial infection. *JAMA* 285:881, 2001.

207. Carlucci A, Richard JC, Wysocki M, et al: Noninvasive versus conventional mechanical ventilation: An epidemiologic survey. *Am J Respir Crit Care Med* 163:874, 2001.

208. Nourdine K, Combes P, Carton MJ, et al: Does noninvasive ventilation reduce the ICU nosocomial infection risk? A prospective clinical survey. *Intensive Care Med* 25:567, 1999.

209. Brochard L, Mancebo J, Wysocki M, et al: Noninvasive ventilation for acute exacerbations of chronic obstructive pulmonary disease. *N Engl J Med* 333:817, 1995.

210. Confalonieri M, Potena A, Carbone G, et al: Acute respiratory failure in patients with severe community-acquired pneumonia: A prospective, randomized evaluation of noninvasive ventilation. *Am J Respir Crit Care Med* 160:1585, 1999.

211. Wood KA, Lewis L, Von Harz B, Kollef MH: The use of noninvasive positive pressure ventilation in the emergency department: Results of a randomized clinical trial. *Chest* 113:1339, 1998.

212. Antonelli M, Conti G, Rocco M, et al: A comparison of noninvasive positive-pressure ventilation and conventional mechanical ventilation in patients with acute respiratory failure. *N Engl J Med* 339:429, 1998.

213. Antonelli M, Conti G: Noninvasive positive pressure ventilation as treatment for acute respiratory failure in critically ill patients. *Crit Care* 4:15, 2000.

214. Kramer N, Meyer TJ, Meharg J, et al: Randomized, prospective trial of noninvasive positive pressure ventilation in acute respiratory failure. *Am J Respir Crit Care Med* 151:1799, 1995.

215. Drakulovic MB, Torres A, Bauer TT, et al: Supine body position as a risk factor for nosocomial pneumonia in mechanically ventilated patients: A randomised trial (in process citation). *Lancet* 354:1851, 1999.

216. Orozco-Levi M, Torres A, Ferrer M, et al: Semirecumbent position protects from pulmonary aspiration but not completely from gastroesophageal reflux in mechanically ventilated patients. *Am J Respir Crit Care Med* 152:1387, 1995.

217. Kelley RE, Vibulsresth S, Bell L, Duncan RC: Evaluation of kinetic therapy in the prevention of complications of prolonged bed rest secondary to stroke. *Stroke* 18:638, 1987.

218. deBoisblanc BP, Castro M, Everret B, et al: Effect of air-supported, continuous, postural oscillation on the risk of early ICU pneumonia in nontraumatic critical illness. *Chest* 103:1543, 1993.

219. Summer WR, Curry P, Haponik EF, et al: Continuous mechanical turning of intensive care patients shortens length of stay in some diagnostic-related groups. *J Crit Care* 4:45, 1989.

220. Whiteman K, Nachtmann L, Kramer D, et al: Effects of continuous lateral rotation therapy on pulmonary complications in liver transplant patients. *Am J Crit Care* 4:133, 1995.

221. Fink MP, Helsmoortel CM, Stein KL, et al: The efficacy of an oscillating bed in the prevention of lower respiratory tract infection in critically ill victims of blunt trauma: A prospective study. *Chest* 97:132, 1990.

222. Gentilello L, Thompson DA, Tonnesen AS, et al: Effect of a rotating bed on the incidence of pulmonary complications in critically ill patients. *Crit Care Med* 16:783, 1988.

223. Sahn SA: Continuous lateral rotational therapy and nosocomial pneumonia. *Chest* 99:1263, 1991.

224. O'Donohue WJ Jr: Prevention and treatment of postoperative atelectasis: Can it and will it be adequately studied? *Chest* 87:1, 1985.

225. Choi SC, Nelson LD: Kinetic therapy in critically ill patients: Combined results based on meta-analysis. *J Crit Care* 7:57, 1992.

226. Traver GA, Tyler ML, Hudson LD, et al: Continuous oscillation: outcome in critically ill patients. *J Crit Care* 10:97, 1995.

227. Mahul P, Auboyer C, Jospe R, et al: Prevention of nosocomial pneumonia in intubated patients: Respective role of mechanical subglottic secretions drainage and stress ulcer prophylaxis. *Intensive Care Med* 18:20, 1992.

228. Valles J, Artigas A, Rello J, et al: Continuous aspiration of subglottic secretions in preventing ventilator-associated pneumonia. *Ann Intern Med* 122:179, 1995.

229. Kollef MH, Skubas NJ, Sundt TM: A randomized clinical trial of continuous aspiration of subglottic secretions in cardiac surgery patients (see comments). *Chest* 116:1339, 1999.

230. Berra L, Panigada M, De Marchi L, et al: New approaches for the prevention of airway infection in ventilated patients: Lessons learned from laboratory animal studies at the National Institutes of Health. *Minerva Anestesiol* 69:342, 2003.

231. Kollef MH, Shapiro SD, Fraser VJ, et al: Mechanical ventilation with or without 7-day circuit changes: A randomized controlled trial (see comments). *Ann Intern Med* 123:168, 1995.

232. Dreyfuss D, Djedaini K, Weber P, et al: Prospective study of nosocomial pneumonia and of patient and circuit colonization during mechanical ventilation with circuit changes every 48 hours versus no change. *Am Rev Respir Dis* 143:738, 1991.

233. Long MN, Wickstrom G, Grimes A, et al: Prospective, randomized study of ventilator-associated pneumonia in patients with one versus three ventilator circuit changes per week. *Infect Control Hosp Epidemiol* 17:14, 1996.

234. Mermel LA, Eveloff S, Short K, et al: The risk of pneumonia associated with the use of heated wire versus conventional ventilator circuits: A prospective trial. 4th Annual Meeting of the Society for Hospital Epidemiology of America, New Orleans, 1994.

235. Stamm AM: Ventilator-associated pneumonia and frequency of circuit changes. *Am J Infect Control* 26:71, 1998.

236. Kirton OC, DeHaven B, Morgan J, et al: A prospective, randomized comparison of an in-line heat moisture exchange filter and heated wire humidifiers: Rates of ventilator-associated early-onset (community-acquired) or late-onset (hospital-acquired) pneumonia and incidence of endotracheal tube occlusion. *Chest* 112:1055, 1997.

237. Le Bourdelles G, Mier L, Fiquet B, et al: Comparison of the effects of heat and moisture exchangers and heated humidifiers on ventilation and gas exchange during weaning trials from mechanical ventilation. *Chest* 110:1294, 1996.

238. Davis K Jr, Evans SL, Campbell RS, et al: Prolonged use of heat and moisture exchangers does not affect device efficiency or frequency rate of nosocomial pneumonia (see comments). *Crit Care Med* 28:1412, 2000.

239. Deppe SA, Kelly JW, Thoi LL, et al: Incidence of colonization, nosocomial pneumonia, and mortality in critically ill patients using a Trach Care closed-suction system versus an open-suction system: Prospective, randomized study. *Crit Care Med* 18:1389, 1990.

240. Johnson KL, Kearney PA, Johnson SB, et al: Closed versus open endotracheal suctioning: Costs and physiologic consequences. *Crit Care Med* 22:658, 1994.

241. Combes P, Fauvage B, Oleyer C: Nosocomial pneumonia in mechanically ventilated patients: A prospective, randomised evaluation of the Stericath closed suctioning system. *Intensive Care Med* 26:878, 2000.

242. Bonten MJ, Gaillard CA, van der Hulst R, et al: Intermittent enteral feeding: The influence on respiratory and digestive tract colonization in mechanically ventilated intensive-care-unit patients (see comments). *Am J Respir Crit Care Med* 154:394, 1996.

243. Heyland DK, Cook DJ, Schoenfeld PS, et al: The effect of acidified enteral feeds on gastric colonization in critically ill patients: Results of a multicenter randomized trial. Canadian Critical Care Trials Group. *Crit Care Med* 27:2399, 1999.

244. Yavagal DR, Karnad DR, Oak JL: Metoclopramide for preventing pneumonia in critically ill patients receiving enteral tube feeding: A randomized, controlled trial. *Crit Care Med* 28:1408, 2000.

245. Kearns PJ, Chin D, Mueller L, et al: The incidence of ventilator-associated pneumonia and success in nutrient delivery with gastric versus small intestinal feeding: A randomized clinical trial (in process citation). *Crit Care Med* 28:1742, 2000.

246. Donowitz LG, Page MC, Mileur BL, Guenthner SH: Alteration of normal gastric flora in critical care patients receiving antacid and cimetidine therapy. *Infect Control* 7:23, 1986.

247. Cook DJ: Stress ulcer prophylaxis: Gastrointestinal bleeding and nosocomial pneumonia. Best evidence synthesis. *Scand J Gastroenterol Suppl* 210:48, 1995.

248. Cook DJ, Laine LA, Guyatt GH, Raffin TA: Nosocomial pneumonia and the role of gastric pH: A meta-analysis. *Chest* 100:7, 1991.

249. van Saene HK, Stoutenbeek CC, Stoller JK: Selective decontamination of the digestive tract in the intensive care unit: Current status and future prospects. *Crit Care Med* 20:691, 1992.

250. Stoutenbeek CP, van Saene HK, Miranda DR, et al: The prevention of superinfection in multiple trauma patients. *J Antimicrob Chemother* 14(suppl B):203, 1984.

251. Stoutenbeek CP, van Saene HK, Miranda DR, Zandstra DF: The effect of selective decontamination of the digestive tract on colonisation and infection rate in multiple trauma patients. *Intensive Care Med* 10:185, 1984.

252. Meta-analysis of randomised controlled trials of selective decontamination of the digestive tract. Selective Decontamination of the Digestive Tract Trialists' Collaborative Group. *Br Med J* 307:525, 1993.

253. Kollef MH: The role of selective digestive tract decontamination on mortality and respiratory tract infections: A meta-analysis. *Chest* 105:1101, 1994.

254. Heyland DK, Cook DJ, Jaeschke R, et al: Selective decontamination of the digestive tract: An overview. *Chest* 105:1221, 1994.

255. Hurley JC: Prophylaxis with enteral antibiotics in ventilated patients: Selective decontamination or selective cross-infection? *Antimicrob Agents Chemother* 39:941, 1995.

256. Vandenbroucke-Grauls CM, Vandenbroucke JP: Effect of selective decontamination of the digestive tract on respiratory tract infections and mortality in the intensive care unit. *Lancet* 338:859, 1991.

257. Nathens AB, Marshall JC: Selective decontamination of the digestive tract in surgical patients: A systematic review of the evidence (see comments). *Arch Surg* 134:170, 1999.

258. Liberati A, D'Amico R, Pifferi S, Telaro E: Antibiotic prophylaxis in intensive care units: Meta-analyses versus clinical practice. *Intensive Care Med* 26:S38, 2000.

259. Bonten MJ, Kullberg BJ, van Dalen R, et al: Selective digestive decontamination in patients in intensive care. The Dutch Working Group on Antibiotic Policy. *J Antimicrob Chemother* 46:351, 2000.

260. Ebner W, Kropec-Hubner A, Daschner FD: Bacterial resistance and overgrowth due to selective decontamination of the digestive tract. *Eur J Clin Microbiol Infect Dis* 19:243, 2000.

261. Bartlett JG: Selective decontamination of the digestive tract and its effect on antimicrobial resistance. *Crit Care Med* 23:613, 1995.

262. Mandelli M, Mosconi P, Langer M, Cigada M: Prevention of pneumonia in an intensive care unit: A randomized multicenter clinical trial. Intensive Care Unit Group of Infection Control. *Crit Care Med* 17:501, 1989.

263. Petersdorf RG, Merchant RK: A study of antibiotic prophylaxis in patients with acute heart failure. *N Engl J Med* 260:565, 1959.

264. Kollef MH, Vlasnik J, Sharpless L, et al: Scheduled change of antibiotic classes: A strategy to decrease the incidence of ventilator-associated pneumonia (see comments). *Am J Respir Crit Care Med* 156:1040, 1997.

265. Gruson D, Hilbert G, Vargas F, et al: Strategy of antibiotic rotation: Long-term effect on incidence and susceptibilities of gram-negative bacilli responsible for ventilator-associated pneumonia. *Crit Care Med* 31:1908, 2003.

266. Raymond DP, Pelletier SJ, Crabtree TD, et al: Impact of a rotating empiric antibiotic schedule on infectious mortality in an intensive care unit. *Crit Care Med* 29:1101, 2001.

Chapter 44
LIBERATION FROM MECHANICAL VENTILATION

CONSTANTINE A. MANTHOUS
GREGORY A. SCHMIDT
JESSE B. HALL

KEY POINTS

- *Patients are candidates for liberation from mechanical ventilation when gas exchange or circulatory disturbances that precipitated respiratory failure have been reversed.*

- *More than half of all critically ill patients can be liberated successfully from mechanical ventilation after a brief trial of spontaneous breathing on the first day that reversal of precipitating factors is recognized. Gradual reduction of mechanical support, termed* weaning, *frequently is unnecessary and can prolong the duration of mechanical ventilation.*

- *Once a patient has been liberated from the ventilator, extubation should follow if mechanisms of airway maintenance (e.g., cough, gag, and swallow) are sufficient to protect the airway from secretions. Whether to extubate is a decision that follows successful liberation from the ventilator.*

- *In patients who fail their first trial of spontaneous breathing, attention should turn to defining and treating the pathophysiologic processes underlying failure.*

- *Weaning regimens that use ventilator modes with the goal of improving respiratory muscle endurance have not been proved to expedite liberation, but data from animal models suggest that "exercise" may be beneficial. Approaches attempting to exercise the respiratory muscles should not substitute for daily interrogation of readiness for spontaneous breathing.*

- *One weaning regimen, the gradual reduction of intermittent mandatory breaths, prolongs patients' time on mechanical ventilation.*

- *Liberation from mechanical ventilation is achieved most expeditiously if patients with a stable circulation (not on pressors or with evolving myocardial infarction) and adequate oxygenation are given a trial of spontaneous breathing (T piece or pressure support ≤ 7 cm H_2O) each day. Patients remain on ventilators unnecessarily when clinicians do not put this simple plan in place.*

- *Patients who have had most correctable factors addressed and remain marginal with regard to ventilatory capacity in most circumstances should undergo a trial extubation rather than remain intubated for protracted periods. Noninvasive positive-pressure ventilation is extremely useful in these patients to transition them to fully spontaneous breathing following extubation.*

Respiratory failure occurs when the lungs and respiratory pump fail to exchange oxygen and carbon dioxide adequately (see Chap. 31). Hypoxemic (type 1) respiratory failure usually results from flooding or collapse of the distal airspaces leading to intrapulmonary shunt and inadequate arterial oxygenation despite generous concentrations of inspired oxygen (see Chap. 38). Hypercapnic (type 2) respiratory failure results from inability to sustain sufficient alveolar ventilation to eliminate the CO_2 produced from aerobic metabolism. Perioperative respiratory failure, a special case of types 1 and 2, results when postoperative pain and recumbency result in atelectasis and hypoxemia or when medications to alleviate pain reduce respiratory drive, leading to hypercapnia. Shock-related respiratory failure is another special case in which the underperfused respiratory muscles are unable to compensate for the acidosis resulting from inadequate global tissue perfusion. Mechanical ventilation substitutes for the respiratory pump until these disturbances have been reversed adequately to allow resumption of spontaneous breathing and gas exchange.

Institution of positive-pressure ventilation can be lifesaving for the disorders just described but is also associated with many complications (Table 44-1), and if this form of life support is extended beyond the point at which it is absolutely necessary, it may result in unnecessary morbidity and mortality for the patient. Most studies have demonstrated that earlier withdrawal of mechanical ventilatory support, when feasible, is associated with better outcomes for the patient. We will discuss the cardiopulmonary effects of positive-pressure ventilation and then outline principles and approaches to the withdrawal of mechanical ventilation in a way to achieve this milestone of critical care management at the earliest possible time and in the safest possible fashion.

Cardiopulmonary Effects of Positive-Pressure Ventilation and Its Cessation

PULMONARY EFFECTS

Positive-pressure ventilation (PPV) is the most common mode of mechanical ventilation used in critically ill patients. PPV can deliver an inspiratory volume or pressure to the lungs and can provide positive end-expiratory pressure (PEEP). PEEP reduces the likelihood of end-expiratory alveolar collapse, thus preserving functional residual capacity.[1,2] When used properly, PPV and PEEP can achieve and maintain alveolar recruitment and improve oxygenation. Excessive PPV or PEEP levels also can have adverse effects on gas exchange by reducing cardiac output or by increasing physiologic dead space.[2,3]

The discontinuation of mechanical ventilation increases the propensity for atelectasis, especially in patients with respiratory muscle weakness, restrictive physiology (e.g., obesity), or respiratory depression. In patients with lung injury, surfactant depletion and ultrastructural lung changes increase the likelihood of alveolar collapse (see Chap. 38). Thus cessation of PPV or PEEP may lead to atelectasis and hypoxemia (Table 44-2). In addition, the transition to spontaneous ventilation frequently is associated with increased venous return, which can precipitate pulmonary edema and hypoxemia. Finally, for patients with unrepaired imbalance between respiratory system load and neuromuscular competence, discontinuation of mechanical ventilation will precipitate

TABLE 44-1 Complications Associated with Endotracheal Intubation and Mechanical Ventilation

COMPLICATIONS RELATED TO THE ENDOTRACHEAL TUBE
Endotracheal tube malfunction—mucus plug, cuff leak
Endotracheal tube malposition
Self-extubation
Nasal or oral necrosis
Pneumonia
Laryngeal edema
Tracheal erosion
Sinusitis

COMPLICATIONS RELATED TO THE VENTILATOR
Alveolar hypoventilation/hyperventilation
Atelectasis
Hypotension
Pneumothorax
Diffuse alveolar damage

EFFECTS ON OTHER ORGAN SYSTEMS
Gastrointestinal hypomotility
Pneumoperitoneum
Stress gastropathy and gastrointestinal hemorrhage
Arrhythmias
Salt and water retention
Malnutrition

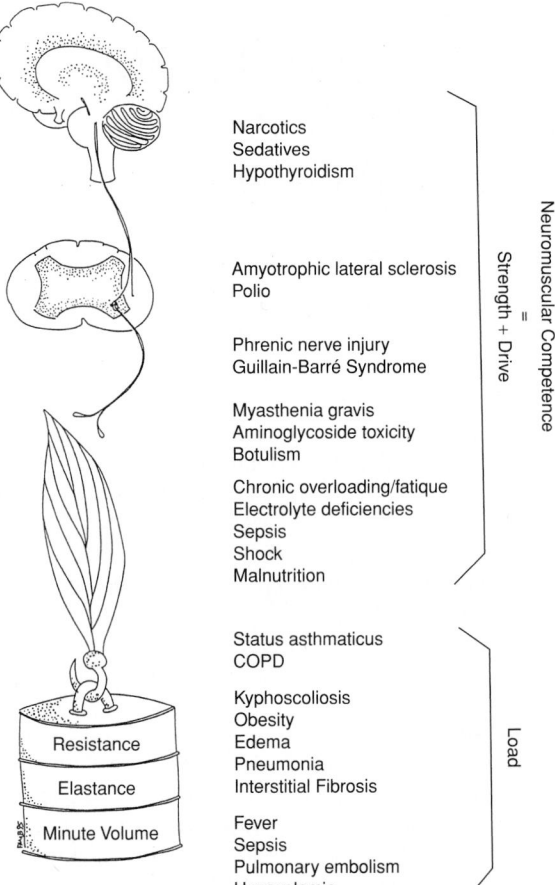

FIGURE 44-1 The neuromuscular circuit. This diagram summarizes the components of neuromuscular competence and respiratory muscle load and illustrates processes that can affect the strength-load balance leading to ventilatory failure. *(Reproduced with permission from Manthous CA, Siegel M: Ventilatory failure, in Matthay et al (eds): Pulmonary and Critical Care Yearbook, vol 3. St. Louis, Mosby, 1996, Chap 2.)*

the symptoms and signs of recurrent ventilatory failure (Fig. 44-1).

CARDIOVASCULAR EFFECTS

The principal circulatory effects of PPV and PEEP are to reduce biventricular preload[4–9] and left ventricular afterload.[4,10–13] PPV and PEEP also may increase right ventricular afterload by increasing lung volumes.[14] When patients begin to breathe spontaneously, intrathoracic pressures that were positive on inspiration during PPV and PEEP become negative. Accordingly, the transition from PPV and PEEP to

TABLE 44-2 Pathogenesis of Hypoxemia and Hypercapnia with Cessation of Mechanical Ventilation

FACTORS CONTRIBUTING TO HYPOXEMIA
Pulmonary edema due to mobilization of peripheral edema
Atelectasis due to recumbency, old age, obesity, residual sedatives, surfactant depletion
    (in patients with diffuse alveolar damage)
Hypoventilation
Withdrawal of PEEP
Increased $\dot{V}_{O_2}$ due to the work of breathing
Congestive heart failure precipitated by increased work of breathing

FACTORS CONTRIBUTING TO HYPERCAPNIA
Hypercapnia due to strength-load imbalance = ventilatory failure (see Table 44-3)
    Reduced respiratory muscle strength
        Sepsis, malnutrition, electrolyte derangements, prolonged mechanical ventilation,
            dyssynchronous mechanical ventilation, corticosteroids, postparalytic syndrome
    Increased respiratory muscle loads
        Resistance—bronchospasm, excessive secretions, endotracheal tube
        Elastance—pulmonary edema, dynamic hyperinflation, obesity
        Minute volume—hypermetabolism, increased dead space, fever, overfeeding
Other hypercapnia—does not necessarily signal ventilatory failure
    Compensation for metabolic alkalosis
    Acute return to premorbid P_{CO_2} after iatrogenic hyperventilation
    Hyperoxic hypercapnia (in chronic hypercapnic respiratory failure patients)
    Residual sedatives/narcotics

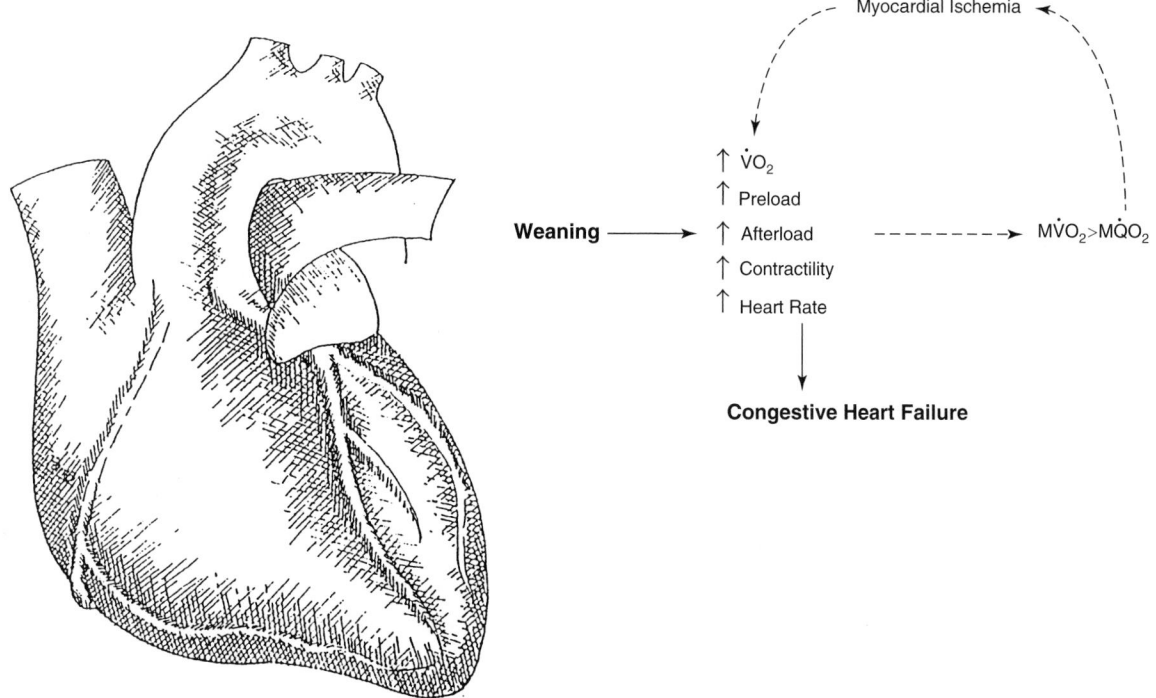

FIGURE 44-2 Pathophysiologic mechanisms of weaning-related ischemia and congestive heart failure. $\dot{V}O_2$, global oxygen consumption; $M\dot{V}O_2$, myocardial oxygen consumption; $M\dot{Q}O_2$, myocardial oxygen supply.

unassisted breathing causes acute increases in venous return and left ventricular afterload. In patients with normal hearts, these circulatory changes usually are well tolerated. However, in patients with left ventricular dysfunction, augmentation of venous return and increased left ventricular afterload increase left heart transmural pressures substantially. In addition, increased cardiac loads during weaning may precipitate ischemia in patients with coronary artery disease. Thus the transition from PPV to spontaneous breathing is accompanied by multiple events that can contribute to left ventricular failure and cardiogenic pulmonary edema (Fig. 44-2).

Expediting Liberation from Mechanical Ventilation

In order to minimize the duration of ventilator dependence, the clinician must:

1. Identify the pathogenesis of respiratory failure in each patient and institute appropriate treatment based on this pathophysiology.
2. Prevent iatrogenic complications associated with mechanical ventilation.
3. Detect when the patient is ready to breathe without the machine.

Since mechanical ventilation has numerous risks, including infection and barotrauma[15–17] (see Table 44-1), it is appropriate to work aggressively to repair the "broken" patient and determine each day whether the patient still requires the ventilator. In this section we delineate the physiologic changes that occur during and the impact of underlying diseases on the transition to spontaneous breathing. We highlight

methods used to expedite readying the patient for liberation and to identify patients who are appropriate candidates for liberation from mechanical ventilation. We also describe an approach to patients who do not succeed rapidly at being liberated from mechanical ventilation.

ITEM 1: FIX THE PATIENT

Although it may seem intuitive that an organized systematic approach aimed at remedying the pathogenesis of disease should expedite liberation from mechanical ventilation, only recently has a study examined the efficacy of such an approach. Smyrnios and colleagues[18] examined the utility of a combined protocol to identify and repair pathophysiology that binds patients to ventilators *and* recognize readiness to breathe spontaneously. This approach resulted in a substantial reduction in ventilator days and costs and expedited patient throughput. However, it is not possible to determine the degree to which the specific systematic approach of fixing the patient versus the liberation protocol contributed to the observed improvements. While from this study or the available literature it is not possible to determine the relative importance of each of these arms of treatment of respiratory failure, it is certain that both are crucial. Accordingly, from the very first day a patient requires intubation, it is worthwhile to define the mechanisms causing the need for initiation of mechanical ventilation. This can be approached through the following questions:

1. Did the patient need the ventilator, an artificial airway, or both? A significant number of patients are intubated for airway incompetence in the absence of significant hypoxemia or causes of hypercapneic respiratory failure. Disorders leading to an incompetent airway include primary neurologic diseases that attenuate airway protective reflexes

or primary mechanical airway problems such as airway obstruction or insufficient cough to expectorate secretions.

2. If the patient needed the ventilator, was the mechanism of respiratory failure acute hypoxemia, hypercapnia (ventilatory failure), or a combination of these abnormalities? This is usually apparent from the clinical presentation combined with data obtained shortly after intubation. Patients whose initial presentation is poor oxygenation despite high concentrations of inspired oxygen (i.e., 100% facemask) most often have shunt physiology with atelectasis and/or alveolar flooding with blood, pus, or edema. Patients with acute hypercapnia can be separated into two categories: those with diminished drive to breathe (e.g., narcotic/sedative overdose) manifesting as a relatively comfortable patient with diminished level of consciousness and no respiratory distress *or* those who are uncomfortable and tachypneic, suggesting an imbalance between respiratory muscle strength and endurance and the load on the respiratory system. Some patients present with elements of both elevated work of breathing *and* hypoxemia, such as a patient with pneumonia with both a large intrapulmonary shunt producing hypoxemia and the consolidated lung increasing lung elastance and the work of breathing.

Hypotheses regarding pathogenesis can be confirmed shortly after intubation by evaluation of the chest radiograph and by using the mechanical ventilator as a pulmonary function machine. Lobar atelectasis usually is seen as an abnormal opacity, but subsegmental atelectasis can cause a shunt that is not obvious on a chest radiograph. Atelectasis often improves with PPV unless caused by airway obstruction. Patients with hypoxemia requiring high F_{IO_2} and PEEP levels and lung opacities generally have alveolar flooding processes. Other clinical data are then used to confirm the mechanism of flooding. Appropriate history, purulent endotracheal secretions, and leukocytosis point to pneumonia. A dropping hematocrit with or without bloody endotracheal secretions suggests alveolar hemorrhage. Four-quadrant, relatively homogeneous airspace filling on chest radiograph suggests pulmonary edema (in the absence of hemorrhage), and attention turns to determining whether left ventricular dysfunction and/or hypervolemia are responsible or if capillary leak has resulted in hypoxemia (i.e., acute lung injury, acute respiratory distress syndrome). Clinicians should define the pathophysiology and treat underlying causes as appropriate.

In patients with hypercapnic respiratory failure, attention turns to examination of the elements of neuromuscular capacity and respiratory load. Although *primary* respiratory "pump" failure occurs occasionally (requiring one to consider a series of neurologic disorders, including CNS depression, polio or ALS, Guillain-Barré syndrome, phrenic nerve dysfunction, myasthenia gravis, and muscle dysfunction due to electrolyte deficiencies, medications, or sepsis; see Fig. 44-1), most commonly hypercapnic failure results from overloading of the neuromuscular apparatus. The three respiratory muscle loads are

1. *Flow-resistive pressure cost of breathing.* This is a function of the magnitude of flow and the resistance of the conducting airways, where Pr = flow × resistance. When the patient is on the ventilator and flow is delivered in a constant (square-wave) regime, Pr = (peak airway pressure – plateau airway pressure)/flow. If measured with a constant flow of 60 L/min (1 L/s), Pr = peak – plateau pressure yields resistance in centimeters of water per liter per second. These are the units used in the pulmonary function laboratory; since a 6- to 8-mm endotracheal tube and ventilator tubing contribute 5 to 10 cm H_2O/L per second and normal airway resistance is less than 5 cm H_2O/L per second, total resistance that is greater than 10 to 15 cm H_2O/L per second after the patient is intubated is abnormal. Removal of airway secretions and administration of bronchodilators and, if required, corticosteroids are used to treat elevated airway resistance related to airway disease. Left-sided heart dysfunction also may contribute to increased airway resistance (cardiac asthma) and should be considered in patients with known or suspected cardiac disease.

2. *Elastic pressure cost of breathing.* This refers to the pressure required to expand the lung and chest wall from functional residual capacity to a given tidal volume; Pel = Ers × V_T, where Ers = elastance of the respiratory system and V_T = tidal volume. The elastic (plateau) pressure can be measured on the ventilator with an inspiratory pause of 0.5 to 1.0 second. The inverse of the elastance—the compliance—can be computed as V_T/plateau pressure – PEEP, normal being 50 mL/cm H_2O. If compliance is decreased (elastance increased), one must determine whether the lung or chest wall is responsible. Chest wall noncompliance, which arises from conditions such as abdominal distention, obesity, and kyphoscoliosis, is usually readily apparent by clinical examination. Lung noncompliance usually is associated with lung infiltrates, large pleural effusions, or dynamic hyperinflation (due to increased airway resistance and/or hyperventilation).

3. *Minute volume.* This is not a *mechanical* load of breathing, but insofar as a higher minute volume requires more resistive and elastic pressure work of breathing (more breaths per minute), a higher minute volume loads the neuromuscular apparatus. Since minute volume equals alveolar ventilation plus dead space, any process that increases these will increase minute volume requirements. Alveolar ventilation can be increased by excess CO_2 production, such as occurs in sepsis/systemic inflammatory responses and overfeeding, or by inefficient elimination (high dead space), such as occurs in late-stage acute respiratory distress syndrome (ARDS), chronic obstructive pulmonary disease (COPD), and pulmonary embolism.

After stabilizing patients on a ventilator, the three loads are measured easily, and if they are elevated, they likely contributed to respiratory muscle failure and hypercapnia. If they are completely normal, one reconsiders the possibility of either diminished drive to breathe or a cause of neuromuscular weakness that includes the respiratory muscles.

Hypercapnic respiratory failure occurs clinically in one of three ways: acute, chronic, and acute on chronic. In *acute hypercapnic respiratory failure,* a sudden mismatch of respiratory load to neuromuscular competence places the patient in acute respiratory failure over minutes to hours. There is an abrupt increase in Pa_{CO_2} with no metabolic correction and a blood pH consistent with an acute respiratory acidosis. In *chronic hypercapnic respiratory failure*, the mismatch of respiratory load to neuromuscular competence has been long-standing and usually gradual in evolution—over days to weeks or even years. Pa_{CO_2} elevation exists, but metabolic correction is near complete. Typically, pH is 7.30 to 7.36. These patients are particularly vulnerable to acute increments of load or decrements of capacity, termed *acute-on-chronic hypercapnic respiratory failure.* The respiratory muscles are unable to respond to the new insult, and Pa_{CO_2} rises too fast for immediate renal compensation. pH is usually less than 7.30, Pa_{CO_2} is much greater than 40 mm Hg, and bicarbonate is elevated (>24 mEq/L), the "footprint of chronicity." In such cases, clinicians should seek to understand the pathogenesis of the chronic component and to define which loads and/or decrements of capacity have contributed to the acute component.

ITEM 2: PREVENT IATROGENIC COMPLICATIONS OF MECHANICAL VENTILATION

Although not emphasized in most discussions of weaning from mechanical ventilation, strategies that avoid further lung injury during mechanical support are extremely important to returning the patient to spontaneous breathing. *Ventilator-induced lung injury* (VILI) (see Chap. 37) refers to a number of mechanisms by which lung injury can occur in patients with acute lung injury and ARDS.[17] Patients with severe airflow obstruction are at risk for dynamic hyperinflation and adverse consequences such as hypotension and diminished venous return[20] (see Chap. 40). In both cases, ventilation with plateau airway pressures of less than 30 to 35 cm H_2O appears to be associated with improved outcomes. Some patients with excessive chest wall stiffness (e.g., severe obesity) may require higher plateau airway pressures to maintain alveolar recruitment, but we seldom use tidal volumes that yield plateau airway pressures in excess of 35 cm H_2O. A common misconception is that the peak airway pressure is the primary marker for risk of lung injury—indeed, this is an alarm parameter usually followed during mechanical ventilation. Very high peak airway pressures are well tolerated by the patient if plateau (i.e., end-inspiratory) alveolar pressures are maintained at less than 35 cm H_2O, a circumstance encountered commonly in patients with status asthmaticus undergoing mechanical ventilation (see Chap. 40).

Aspiration should be prevented by maintaining the head of the bed of all ventilated patients at 30 degrees unless contraindicated.[21] Ventilated patients usually are sedentary and therefore at risk of deep venous thrombosis, justifying universal prophylaxis with subcutaneous heparin or pneumatic compression boots.[22] Gastric mucosal protection also should be provided for ventilated patients.[23] Proton pump inhibitors, H_2 receptor blockers, carafate, and antacids have been used to protect the stomach. Whether continuous feeding of the gut, which usually neutralizes pH, obviates the need for prophylaxis remains unclear. Ventilated patients often require sedatives and narcotics to maintain their comfort and synchrony with the ventilator. However, these medications have a cost. If overused, they delay patients' return to consciousness and full respiratory drive, thereby prolonging the duration of mechanical ventilation. One method of reducing the amount of sedative is to titrate ventilator volumes/flows/rates/modes to patient comfort before resorting to large doses of sedatives and narcotics. When these medications are used, they should be used on an "as needed" basis,[24] or when a continuous infusion is used, a period of daily awakening should be encouraged.[25]

ITEM 3: RECOGNIZE READINESS—THE LOGISTICS OF LIBERATION

Weaning implies gradual, rather than rapid, withdrawal of ventilatory assistance. This word suggests that the mechanism for separating the patient and the ventilator successfully resides in the machine next to the patient rather than in the patient himself or herself. The remainder of this chapter will emphasize a very simple truism that "many patients do not require repetitive measurements or involved plans for discontinuation of mechanical ventilation—if intercurrent problems causing respiratory muscle weakness or abnormal lung mechanics have not arisen, the most easily effected plan for discontinuation of mechanical ventilation is to wheel the machine out of the room."[26] Thus *liberation* more accurately describes the process by which most patients are freed from the ventilator. In patients who cannot breathe independently, liberation will be possible only after the patient is treated and recovers.

Weaning Parameters

Historically, weaning parameters have been used to *predict* patients' ability to breathe without the ventilator. However, despite decades of research, no weaning parameter has predictive accuracy sufficient to be used exclusively to make liberation decisions.[27,28] Moreover, it seems wasted effort to spend time trying to predict whether a patient can breathe without the ventilator when the question can be answered directly with a trial of spontaneous breathing. Accordingly, we do not use weaning parameters routinely to make liberation decisions. In the last edition of this book we dedicated a great deal of space to discussing weaning parameters. Now we provide instead references to demonstrate why clinicians simply should perform spontaneous breathing trials (SBTs) in most of their patients to determine their candidacy for extubation.[29–46]

To consider a patient for an SBT, he or she should be stable hemodynamically, without evidence of myocardial ischemia and, preferably, not excessively tachycardic. Oxygenation must be adequate,[47] and the Pa_{O_2}/F_{IO_2} should be greater than 120 (i.e., $Pa_{O_2} > 60$ mm Hg on a concentration of oxygen less than or equal to 50%) at nominal levels of PEEP (PEEP $\leq$ 5.0 cm H_2O). If these two criteria are met, then attention turns to determining whether the patient can ventilate and oxygenate *without* the machine (Fig. 44-3).

Can the Patient Breathe without the Ventilator?

PREPARATION

Sedatives and narcotics should be discontinued several hours before a breathing trial to reduce the likelihood of inadequate drive to breathe. Indeed, while several studies have

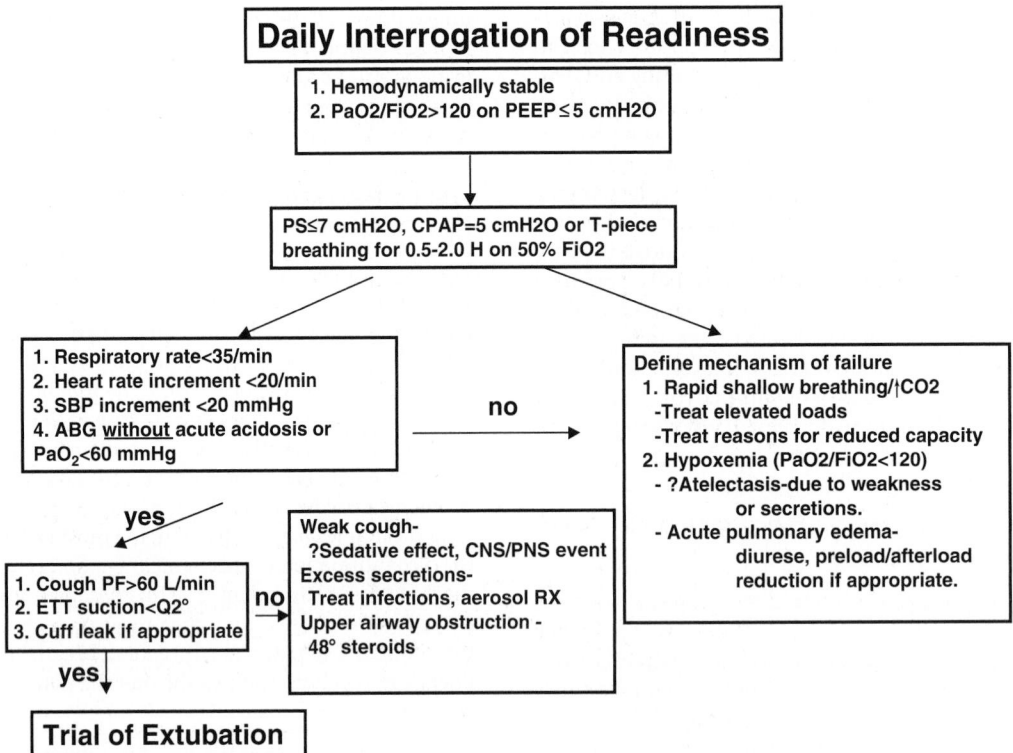

FIGURE 44-3 A simple bedside algorithm for liberating patients from mechanical ventilation and performing a trial of extubation.

indicated that protocol-driven approaches to weaning have identified patients earlier for extubation than routine care by clinicians on a day-to-day basis, other investigations protocolizing a daily interruption of sedatives have been associated with a decreased time of mechanical ventilation and diminished time in the ICU.[25] It is likely that these are two tightly linked ICU activities—sedation and mechanical ventilatory support—and that clinicians are not extremely adept at identifying prospectively when patients do not need one or the other. A simple approach to this problem is to discontinue sedatives frequently and, in those patients awakening in a stable condition, to perform an SBT.

VENTILATOR MODE AND DURATION OF THE SBT

Pressure support, continuous positive airway pressure (CPAP), and T-piece trials are the most common methods used to test readiness for liberation from mechanical ventilation. The choice of whether to use pressure support or to allow the patient to breathe without inspiratory assistance through the endotracheal tube remains a point of physician style. Some data suggest that the endotracheal tube can increase resistive load significantly,[48] which theoretically could contribute to failure. Consequently, many investigators have suggested that a pressure support of 5 to 8 cm H_2O can be used to counter this tube-related load. Recent studies have suggested, however, that pressure support intended to overcome tube resistance unloads the respiratory muscles compared with extubated breathing. These data suggest that T-piece breathing most closely approximates the work of unassisted breathing after extubation.[49,50] Nonetheless, one study suggested that the rate of extubation failure following successful trials of

pressure support equal to 8 cm H_2O was not greater than following successful T-piece trials.[51] Another study found similar rates of successful extubation following trials of pressure support of 7 cm H_2O versus T piece.[52]

The first SBT need be only 30 minutes[53] because extending the trial longer does not enhance the clinician's ability to assess the patient's readiness for extubation. The proper duration of subsequent SBTs in those who fail has not been studied (30 to 120 minutes generally are used). Thus the available data suggest that patients should be considered for a trial of extubation after a successful trial (30 to 120 minutes) of either T piece, CPAP, or pressure support of 5 to 8 cm H_2O.

THE PATIENT WHO FAILS INITIAL SBTs

Failure of an SBT is most often a clinical diagnosis. The clinical signs of failure include rapid-shallow breathing, tachycardia (>110 beats per minute), hypertension (increment of more than 20 mm Hg), mental status changes, and subjective distress. These signs result from (1) decrements in gas exchange, (2) cardiovascular events, and/or (3) other (noncardiopulmonary) issues. When a patient fails an SBT, clinicians frequently focus on specific ventilator regimes aimed at improving respiratory muscle function. Although some studies in animal models have suggested that respiratory muscle exercise may be helpful,[54] to date no study has suggested that the ventilator can be used to expedite the recovery from respiratory failure. If "exercise" is attempted, all attempts should be made to avoid exhausting the patient (generally accomplished if respiratory rates stay below 30/min). However, instead of concentrating on the ventilator, the clinician should turn attention to treatable factors underlying the patient's respiratory failure (Table 44-3). Some traditional weaning parameters are helpful in making this determination. For example, a markedly reduced maximum negative inspired pressure suggests respiratory muscle weakness. An elevated rapid-shallow breathing index (the respiratory rate per minute divided by the tidal volume in liters) suggests imbalance of respiratory muscle load and capacity. Reasons for abnormalities then can be examined by systematic diagnostic and therapeutic interventions.

ANALYZING FAILURE OF AN SBT

Acute hypercapnia during weaning frequently results from an imbalance between respiratory pump capacity and load. Normal individuals who are subjected to resistance loading exhibit rapid-shallow breathing as a sign of impending respiratory failure.[55,56] When the patient is clearly failing an SBT, it should be discontinued (even before a blood gas analysis demonstrates gas exchange abnormalities) because patients who are "weaned" to exhaustion frequently take several days to recover adequately to resume trials.

Many factors may reduce respiratory muscle strength or increase respiratory muscle loads in critically ill patients. In patients who fail due to strength-load imbalance, we quantify neuromuscular function and the three elements of respiratory muscle load (resistance, elastance, and minute volume; see above) each day so as to define/treat reversible elements. Critical illness frequently is associated with a catabolic state, malnutrition, and electrolyte deficiencies that can contribute to respiratory muscle weakness. Some patients recovering from severe illness develop a polyneuropathy[57-60] that has been hypothesized to contribute to reduced respiratory pump function and prolonged need for mechanical ventilation.[58,59] Sepsis occurs frequently in critically ill patients and is a relatively common reason for weaning failure. Numerous studies suggest that sepsis has a negative impact on respiratory muscle function,[61-65] and this effect is mediated by cytokines.[63,64] In addition, treatments that are used commonly in critically ill patients, such as administration of corticosteroids[66-68] and neuromuscular blockers,[69-71] also negatively affect respiratory muscle function. Mechanical ventilation itself may contribute to disuse atrophy of the respiratory muscles, thus contributing to the pathogenesis of prolonged ventilator dependence.[54,72] Bronchospasm and increased airway secretions frequently contribute to resistive loading of the respiratory muscles. Elevated airway resistance greater than 15 cm H_2O/L per second frequently can be reversed by removing excessive airway secretions[73] or treating with aerosolized bronchodilators.[74] If resistance remains greater than 15 cm H_2O/L per second despite bronchodilators in a patient who repeatedly fails to wean, a therapeutic trial of corticosteroids may be helpful.

Finally, numerous factors contribute to increased respiratory system elastance, ranging from acute lung injury to abdominal distention. Pulmonary edema and pneumonia are common reversible causes of increased lung elastance. Occult PEEP also increases elastic load[75] and can contribute to respiratory muscle fatigue by increasing the work of assisted[76] and unassisted breathing. Increased minute volumes associated with lung injury, hypermetabolic states of critical illness (e.g., sepsis), pulmonary embolism, and overfeeding could contribute to dynamic hyperinflation during the recovery process, thus increasing mechanical loads on the recovering respiratory muscles.

Acute hypercapnia does not necessarily connote weaning failure. In three relatively common situations, hypercapnia during an SBT trial is not accompanied by physiologic decompensation and does not signal ventilatory failure. First, occasional patients with chronic hypercapnia are hyperventilated iatrogenically to a normal P_{CO_2}, and over the course of days in the ICU, the bicarbonate concentration also decreases to normal. When these patients resume spontaneous breathing, their P_{CO_2} rises to their baseline level, leading to an acute respiratory acidosis. The clinician must decipher whether the acute acidosis is arising from strength-load imbalance, in which case the patient usually shows other signs of failure, or from preceding iatrogenic hyperventilation. Similarly, when some patients with chronic hypercapnic respiratory failure are given a high fraction of inspired oxygen, they acutely retain CO_2 in the absence of strength-load imbalance.[77-79] Reduction in the supplemental oxygen to yield a saturation of 90% to 92% may reverse this iatrogenic cause of hypercapnia. Finally, some patients who have primary metabolic alkalosis will have compensatory hypoventilation and hypercapnia.

Hypoxemia (Pa_{O_2} <60 mm Hg or saturation less than 90% on 50% inspired oxygen) can occur during weaning for several reasons. Old age, obesity, and recumbency predispose to a lower functional residual capacity (FRC), which can contribute to atelectasis and subsequent hypoxemia during the transition to unassisted breathing. Thus patients should be sitting at greater than a 30-degree angle during spontaneous breathing. Respiratory muscle weakness and sedatives or narcotics may lead to shallow breathing and atelectasis. Lung injury, a common complication of critical illness, is associated with surfactant depletion and an increased propensity for atelectasis during the withdrawal of positive-pressure ventilation. Thus many pulmonary factors can contribute to hypoxemia during SBTs. Hypoxemia also can result from cardiovascular changes during weaning.

The transition to unassisted breathing is associated with centralization of blood and increased left heart afterload, which may predispose patients with baseline left ventricular dysfunction to develop cardiogenic pulmonary edema.[6-15] SBTs also may increase the level of circulating catechols,[80] which could induce increases in heart rate, blood pressure, and arrhythmias. Tachycardia during weaning frequently is a sign of inadequate cardiopulmonary reserve and subsequent weaning failure. Moreover, in patients with coronary artery disease, if mechanical loads and catechol-induced changes are sufficient, weaning can trigger cardiac ischemia that could contribute to the clinical signs of weaning failure[81-84] (see Fig. 44-2). In a study of 93 medical patients being weaned from mechanical ventilation, ST-segment changes were noted in 6% of all patients and in 10% of those with a preceding history of coronary artery disease. Moreover, weaning-related ischemia tended to increase the risk of weaning failure.[84]

In patients who are clinically hypervolemic or who have left ventricular dysfunction, pre-emptive diuresis and nitrate therapy can be helpful in attenuating acute increases in preload during SBTs. Continuous monitoring of ST segments and treatment with additional nitrates also may be helpful in patients who experience ischemia during weaning.[84]

OTHER REASONS FOR SBT FAILURE

Even though most weaning failures are of cardiopulmonary etiology, other exogenous factors also may contribute to failure.

VENTILATOR AND CIRCUIT ELEMENTS

The ventilator and its circuitry can contribute to weaning failure by two mechanisms: (1) by increasing respiratory loads enough during an SBT to fatigue the respiratory muscles and (2) by imposing significant respiratory muscle work during "rest" periods. The resistance of the endotracheal tube increases with time, and this increase occasionally can be of sufficient magnitude to impede weaning. The ventilator circuit provides increased dead space and in some modes (for older ventilators) can require excessive work to trigger a "sticky" demand valve. Some studies suggest that flow triggering may reduce the ventilator-imposed work of breathing compared with pressure-triggered modalities.[85,86] Thus the ventilator circuit can load[87,88] and covertly fatigue the respiratory muscles when patients are presumed to be "resting," as well as when they are weaning. Patient-ventilator synchrony during "rest" periods reduces the likelihood that the ventilator is contributing to weaning failure.[87,89,90] Irregular pressure-volume curves or frequent, large esophageal or intravascular pressure fluctuations during assisted ventilation may help to identify patients who are working hard on the ventilator.[91] Empirical manipulation of inspiratory flow rates, waveforms, and triggering mechanisms may aid in improving patient-ventilator synchrony.[86] Finally, in patients with obstructive lung disease, intrinsic PEEP may increase significantly the work required to trigger ventilator-supported breaths (so-called trigger asynchrony). In selected patients, addition of applied PEEP to nearly match intrinsic PEEP can reduce this ventilator-induced load.[76]

PSYCHOLOGICAL AND HOUSEKEEPING ISSUES

Subjective distress, including anxious appearance and sweating, are nonspecific signs of weaning failure. Anxiety during breathing trials may manifest as rapid-shallow breathing, tachycardia, and hypertension that are interpreted as weaning failure by caregivers. Bedside personnel should explain the weaning process; so-called verbal anesthesia is effective in some patients. The use of sedatives to treat anxiety must be undertaken with caution because most of these drugs also depress respiratory function. Haloperidol or very low doses of benzodiazepines can be used to facilitate comfort in these exceptional patients. However, subjective distress most frequently signals that the cardiopulmonary system requires additional repair before resuming unassisted breathing.

The effect of re-establishing patient day-night cycles remains to be well studied.[92–94] In patients who fail initial trials of breathing, we are careful to ensure sleep at night and wakefulness, if not exercise, during the day.

LIBERATION STRATEGIES

Many intensivists have reasoned that by reducing ventilatory support gradually, the respiratory muscles exercise at subfatiguing loads, leading to gradual improvement in function. Some studies have suggested that respiratory exercises (repetitions of low-load resistive breathing) can lead to successful extubation in patients who have failed previously.[95] However,

there are as yet no studies proving that respiratory muscle training, through the use of graded withdrawal of ventilatory support, hastens the recovery to unassisted breathing.

Two recent studies have assessed the role of "weaning" strategies in expediting *liberation of the subset of those who fail initial SBTs*. Brochard and colleagues[51] studied 456 medical-surgical patients being considered for weaning, of whom 347 (76%) were extubated successfully on the first day of weaning. One hundred and nine patients who failed an initial SBT were randomized to be weaned by one of three strategies: (1) T-piece trials of increasing length until 2 hours could be tolerated, (2) intermittent mandatory ventilation with attempted reductions of 2 to 4 breaths per minute twice a day until 4 breaths per minute could be tolerated, and (3) pressure-support ventilation (PSV) with attempted reductions of 2 to 4 cm H_2O twice a day until 8 cm H_2O could be tolerated. Patients randomized to the three strategies were similar with regard to disease severity and duration of ventilation before weaning. Patients assigned to T-piece were placed on assist control overnight, whereas synchronized intermittent mandatory ventilation (SIMV) patients remained on an unspecified SIMV rate, and PSV patients remained at an unspecified level of pressure support. There was no difference in the duration of weaning between the T-piece and SIMV groups, but PSV led to significantly shorter weaning compared with the combined T-piece and SIMV cohorts. Interestingly, PSV and T-piece were not compared directly. These authors concluded that "the outcome of weaning from mechanical ventilation was influenced by the ventilatory strategy chosen, and the use of PSV resulted in significant improvement compared with other strictly defined weaning protocols using T-piece or SIMV."

Esteban and colleagues[96] performed a similar study of 546 medical-surgical patients, 416 (76%) of whom were extubated successfully on their first day of weaning. The 130 patients who failed were randomized to undergo weaning by (1) once-a-day T-piece trial, (2) two or more T-piece or CPAP trials each day as tolerated, (3) PSV with attempts at reduction of 2 to 4 cm H_2O at least twice a day, and (4) SIMV with attempts at reducing 2 to 4 breaths per minute at least twice a day. Patients assigned to the four groups were similar with regard to demographic characteristics, acuity of illness, and a number of cardiopulmonary variables. Duration of ventilation before weaning was shorter in the SIMV group than in other groups. The mode of ventilation at night was not specified. The weaning success rate was significantly better with once-daily T-piece trials than for PSV and SIMV. Twice-daily T-piece trials were not significantly better, and PSV was not superior to SIMV. The median duration of weaning was 5 days for SIMV, 4 days for PSV, and 3 days for the T-piece regimens. These authors concluded that "a once-daily trial of spontaneous breathing led to extubation about three times more quickly than intermittent mandatory ventilation and about twice as quickly as pressure-support ventilation."

The statistical methods used in these studies warrant some comment. The first study[51] asserts the superiority of pressure-support weaning to T-piece but does not compare these directly. The second study[96] presents "adjusted" rates of successful weaning—the nature of the adjustments and their impact on the results are unclear because raw data were not presented. However, several important conclusions can be drawn from these relatively large studies. First, and most important, most patients can be extubated successfully on the first day that physicians recognize readiness after a brief trial (30 to 120 minutes) of breathing through a T-piece. *Weaning is not necessary for most patients.* Second, both studies suggest that in patients who have failed an initial T-piece trial, SIMV weaning prolongs the duration of mechanical ventilation. These conclusions depend on the precise algorithms used in the studies—it is possible that if a more "aggressive" SIMV algorithm were used, no difference would be noted. However, if one considers the results of these studies together, *choices of ventilator mode do not appear to have a major impact in speeding the recovery to unassisted breathing.* Clinicians frequently use SIMV or PSV as the initial approach before attempting a T-piece trial. Since most patients are extubated successfully after a brief T-piece trial, such an approach is likely to prolong mechanical ventilation for many patients. PSV weaning may be equivalent to T-piece weaning in carefully controlled protocols. However, in our experience, in busy ICUs, respiratory therapists and nurses frequently are unable to "keep up" with the demands of such protocols—so pressure-support withdrawal protocols have the risk of prolonging ventilation unless followed strictly.

Extubation

There is an important distinction between liberation from mechanical ventilation and extubation. Once a patient has been liberated, i.e., has passed the SBT, he or she does not need the ventilator. The endotracheal tube, aside from providing the avenue for PPV, allows removal of secretions for patients whose airway protective mechanisms have been altered by disease. Accordingly, after a patient has performed a successful trial of unassisted breathing (is liberated from the ventilator), the physician must determine whether the patient still needs the artificial airway.

One consideration is whether the patient has an upper airway lesion that would collapse to a critically small size after extubation. Patients at risk of this problem include those who were initially intubated for upper airway stenosis and stridor and those who have had a traumatic or prolonged intubation.[97] A number of studies have suggested that the ability to breathe around a deflated endotracheal tube cuff[98–100] or a cuff leak of greater than 110 mL during volume-cycled ventilation[100] reduces the likelihood of postextubation failure. However, lack of a cuff leak does not absolutely predict extubation failure.

The patient's mental status, airway protective mechanisms, ability to cough, and amount of secretions are also determinants of extubation outcome. Patients with cough peak flows of 60 L/min or less are five times as likely to fail a trial of extubation (TOE) compared with those with cough peak flows of more than 60 L/min. Those who cannot cough and wet a white card placed 1 to 2 cm from the end of the open endotracheal tube are three times as likely to fail a TOE. Those who require endotracheal suctioning more than every 2 hours are also at increased risk of extubation failure.[47,101] Thus, in general, we are disinclined to extubate patients if they have excessive or tenacious secretions and a weak cough or are not cooperative enough to aid in their own pulmonary toilet (deep breathing and expectoration of secretions). Patients with severe cerebral vascular accidents (CVAs) frequently present with this constellation. It remains unclear as to whether early elective tracheostomy to prevent aspiration and aid in pulmonary toilet is superior to a trial of extubation. When the cause of impaired airway protection is thought to be reversible, treating and attempting a TOE at a later time are reasonable. Recent data suggest that swallowing is abnormal in more than 30% of patients following extubation.[102] Accordingly, all patients, especially those with altered mentation or CVA, should be observed carefully after extubation, and formal swallowing assessment is advisable for many patients.

Postextubation stridor arising from upper airway edema is fairly common after extubation. Pulmonary edema can develop in some of these patients[103] because large negative intrathoracic pressures during inspiration can increase left ventricular afterload dramatically.[11] Nebulized racemic epinephrine and parenteral corticosteroids have been used for the treatment of airway edema but have not been studied systematically. Heliox or mask CPAP may be used to reduce upper airway resistance temporarily in selected patients who do not require immediate reintubation.[104]

Noninvasive face-mask positive-pressure ventilation (NIPPV) may prevent the need for reintubation in selected patients who appear to be failing immediately after extubation.[105–107] One study prospectively randomized 39 patients with COPD and normal sensorium who had failed a T-piece trial to pressure-support weaning or extubation to NIPPV. Patients assigned to NIPPV were more likely to be liberated from mechanical ventilation and succeeded 5 days sooner than those who were weaned using pressure support.[107] In a multicenter trial of 221 patients failing extubation (only 10% having COPD), NIV was ineffective in preventing reintubation and did not reduce mortality.[107a] Thus NIPPV remains unproved for extubation failure, but may be useful in cooperative patients who appear to be failing extubation and who do not require immediate reintubation for impending respiratory arrest.

Deep-breathing exercises and incentive spirometry after extubation may help to prevent atelectasis in at-risk patients. Intermittent positive-pressure breathing treatments may be helpful to reduce atelectasis in patients who have not recovered adequately to cough and deep breathe. Continuous ST-segment monitoring can identify some patients with myocardial ischemia; early recognition and treatment may reduce the likelihood of recurrent respiratory failure. There are few data to support these suggestions, but common sense may not require prospective validation.

Breaking the Rules

Most experienced clinicians have treated patients whose SBTs suggested that they would fail but who were liberated and extubated successfully nonetheless. When the numbers look bad but the patient looks good or there is concern that the presence of the endotracheal tube is responsible for weaning failure, it is reasonable to perform a careful TOE. The following are among the clinical situations that could prompt consideration for a TOE in such patients:

1. When an endotracheal tube has been in place for more than 7 days. Endotracheal tube resistance increases with time and can contribute to failed SBTs.

2. When the patient experiences repeated episodes of bronchospasm on awakening from sedation. The endotracheal tube can cause reflex bronchospasm in some individuals.

3. When patients become overwhelmingly anxious when awakened to breathe through the endotracheal tube and the amount of sedative required to make them comfortable causes hypoventilation. We are particularly careful to ensure that cardiopulmonary reasons for failure have been reversed in these patients.

4. When patients with restrictive chest wall disease (e.g., obesity) repeatedly desaturate every time PEEP is decreased to less than 10 cm H_2O. Some obese patients require more than 5 cm H_2O to prevent atelectasis while intubated yet maintain adequate oxygenation when extubated.

5. When patients with severe restrictive or obstructive lung disease breathe rapidly and shallowly (a rapid-shallow breathing index or frequency/V_T > 125 breaths per minute per liter). For some end-stage patients, rapid-shallow breathing is their chronic baseline.

In these relatively rare situations, extubation should *not* be performed casually. We consider breaking the rules outlined in this chapter only after numerous failed trials of unassisted breathing and after treating reversible causes of failure. The clinical risks associated with failure and reintubation must be weighed against those of continued mechanical ventilation. We extubate these unusual patients with personnel who are skilled at endotracheal intubation nearby, should reintubation be required. In addition, we ensure ready access to NIPPV, which may avert the need for reintubation in carefully selected patients.

A Practical Approach

At many institutions, patients remain bound to ventilators for longer than necessary because clinicians either do not obtain weaning parameters in a timely manner or are hesitant to extubate even when parameters and breathing trials are favorable. Mechanical ventilation can cause complications.[15–17] Conversely, there is a small risk associated with extubation failure. The relative risks of each vary from patient to patient and from institution to institution. A simple approach can minimize both risks. Each day the clinician should ask: *Can my patient be liberated from the ventilator?* The use of interdisciplinary weaning teams[108–110] or respiratory therapist–driven protocols may expedite successful liberation by actively addressing this question each day.

Ely and colleagues studied 300 mechanically ventilated adult medical patients, of whom 149 were prospectively randomized to receive algorithm-guided *attention* to weaning, and the remaining 151 received "routine" care.[110] All patients were assessed daily to delineate recovery to adequate oxygenation (Pa_{O_2}/Fi_{O_2} > 200 on PEEP $\leq$ 5 cm H_2O), hemodynamic stability, and a frequency/V_T of 105 breaths per minute per liter or less (measured on CPAP). When all these criteria were met, a note was left in the charts of patients assigned to the treatment group suggesting that they were ready for liberation. Overall, patients whose care was guided by these criteria were liberated 1.5 days more rapidly than patients in the control group. The median weaning time after satisfaction of the criteria was 2 days shorter in the treatment group.

TABLE 44-3 Reversible Factors Contributing to Ventilatory Failure—Daily Correction of Reversible Contributors to Ventilatory Failure Expedites Patient Recovery

Reduce Respiratory Load	Improve Respiratory Strength
Resistance	Replace K^+, Mg^{2+}, PO_4^{2-} to normal
Inhaled bronchodilators	Treat sepsis
Corticosteroids	Nutritional support without
Removal of excess airway secretions	overfeeding (aim to achieve a normal prealbumin)
Treatment of upper airway obstructions	Consider stopping aminoglycosides
	Rule out:
Elastance	Neurologic disease/occult seizures
Treat pneumonia	Hypothyroidism
Treat pulmonary edema	Oversedation
Reduce dynamic hyperinflation	Critical illness myopathy/ polyneuropathy
Drain large pleural effusions	
Evacuate pneumothoraces	
Treat ileus	
Minute volume	
Detect intrinsic PEEP	
Bronchodilators	
Antipyretics	
Treat sepsis	
Therapy for pulmonary embolism	
Maintain least PEEP possible	
Correct metabolic acidoses	
Resuscitate shock	
Prevent hypovolemia	
Avoid overfeeding	

This reduction in ventilator days translated to a trend toward reduced ICU length of stay and a significant reduction (by $5000) in ICU costs of care. Interestingly, median weaning time from satisfaction of the screening criteria was 1 day in the treatment group, suggesting that further reductions could have been realized if the gentle "reminder" led to a prompt trial of unassisted breathing. Other studies[47] have suggested that the oxygenation criteria used in this study may be conservative (e.g., $Pa_{O_2} \geq$ 80 mm Hg on 40% oxygen). In addition, roughly 50% of patients with a frequency/V_T of 100 to 125 breaths per minute per liter can be extubated successfully.[32] Thus additional reductions in duration of mechanical ventilation can potentially be achieved using a more aggressive algorithm (Fig. 44-3). Note also that these results cannot necessarily be generalized to all institutions because "routine care" (the control group in this study) likely varies considerably among hospitals. However, this study strongly suggests that many patients are inappropriately retained on mechanical ventilators. Other studies have applied very different algorithms to achieve significant reductions in duration of ventilation.[18,111] However, they all have one thing in common: They substitute a program of daily systematic scrutiny of readiness for breathing for the individual variation occurring in unstructured care systems. Whether achieved by protocol or by individual clinician perseverance, we believe that patients can be liberated from mechanical ventilation more expeditiously if they are screened on a daily basis for this potential event.

Our approach can be summarized as follows: If the patient is hemodynamically stable, awake, and triggering the ventilator with a $Pa_{O_2}/F_{I_{O_2}}$ greater than 120 on PEEP of 5.0 cm H_2O or less, we perform an SBT. Alternatively, patients can be screened with a 1-2-minute T-piece trial using the frequency/VT to guide whether to lengthen the trial (as in the Ely and colleagues study).[110] We prefer pressure support at a low level or T piece on 50% oxygen for 30 minutes (60 minutes after a first-day failure). If the patient remains comfortable, with an oxygen saturation greater than 90% and without tachycardia or hypertension, and the breathing rate remains less than 35/min at 30 minutes, we will obtain an arterial blood gas and consider a TOE using independent judgments to gauge the patient's ability to do without the endotracheal tube itself (see above). For patients who fail an initial SBT, we aggressively assess the pathogenesis of their failure and perform daily trials of either T piece or pressure support of less than 7 cm H_2O until the patients can tolerate a greater than 30-minute trial of unassisted breathing and then proceed to liberation from the ventilator and assessment for extubation.

References

1. Annest SJ, Gottlieb M, Paloski WH, et al: Detrimental effects of removing end-expiratory pressure prior to endotracheal extubation. *Ann Surg* 191:539, 1980.
2. Larsson A, Gilbert JT, Bunegin L, et al: Pulmonary effects of body position, PEEP and surfactant depletion in dogs. *Acta Anaesthesiol Scand* 36:38, 1992.
3. Nieman GF, Paskanik AM, Bredenberg CE: Effect of positive end-expiratory pressure on alveolar capillary perfusion. *J Thorac Cardiovasc Surg* 95:712, 1988.
4. Luce JM: The cardiovascular effects of mechanical ventilation and positive end-expiratory pressure. *JAMA* 252:807, 1984.
5. Scharf SM: Ventilatory support in cardiac failure, in Kvetan V, Dantzker DR (eds): *The Critically Ill Cardiac Patient.* Philadelphia, Lippincott-Raven, 1966, p 29.
6. Prewitt RM, Wood LDH: Effect of positive end-expiratory pressure on ventricular function in dogs. *Am J Physiol* 236:H534, 1979.
7. Fewell JE, Abendschein DR, Carlson CJ, et al: Continuous positive-pressure ventilation decreases right and left ventricular end-diastolic volumes in the dog. *Circ Res* 46:125, 1980.
8. Marini JJ, Culver BH, Butler J, et al: Effect of positive end-expiratory pressure on canine ventricular function curves. *J Appl Physiol* 51:1367, 1981.
9. Fessler HE, Brower RG, Wise RA, Permutt S: Effects of positive end-expiratory pressure on the gradient for venous return. *Am Rev Respir Dis* 143:19, 1991.
10. Pinsky MR, Summer WR, Wise RA, et al: Augmentation of cardiac function by elevation of intrathoracic pressure. *J Appl Physiol* 54:950, 1983.
11. Buda AJ, Pinsky MR, Ingels NB, et al: Effect of intrathoracic pressure on left ventricular performance. *N Engl J Med* 301:453, 1979.
12. Bradley TD, Holloway RM, McLaughlin PR, et al: Cardiac output responses to continuous positive airway pressure in congestive heart failure. *Am Rev Respir Dis* 145:377, 1992.
13. Naughton MT, Rahman A, Hara K, et al: Effect of continuous positive airway pressure on intrathoracic and left ventricular transmural pressures in patients with congestive heart failure. *Circulation* 91:1725, 1995.
14. Roos A, Thomas LJ, Nagel EL, Prommas DC: Pulmonary vascular resistance as determined by lung inflation and vascular pressures. *J Appl Physiol* 16:77, 1961.
15. Zwillich CW, Pierson DJ, Creagh CE, et al: Complications of assisted ventilation: A prospective study of 354 consecutive episodes. *Am J Med* 57:161, 1974.
16. Pingleton SK: Complications of acute respiratory failure. *Am Rev Respir Dis* 137:1463, 1988.
17. Mutlu GM, Factor P: Complications of mechanical ventilation. *Respir Care Clin* 6:213, 2000.
18. Smyrnios NA, Connolly A, Wilson MM, et al: Effects of a multifaceted, multidisciplinary, hospital-wide quality improvement program on weaning from mechanical ventilation. *Crit Care Med* 30:1224, 2002.
19. ARDSnet investigators: Ventilation with lower tidal volumes as compared with traditional tidal volumes for acute lung injury and the acute respiratory distress syndrome. The Acute Respiratory Distress Syndrome Network. *N Engl J Med* 342:1301, 2000.
20. Corbridge TC, Hall JB: The assessment and management of adults with status asthmaticus. *Am J Respir Crit Care Med* 151:1296, 1995.
21. Drakulovic MB, Torres A, Bauer TT, et al: Supine body position as a risk factor for nosocomial pneumonia in mechanically ventilated patients: A randomised trial. *Lancet* 354:1851, 1999.
22. Attia J, Ray JG, Cook DJ, et al: Deep vein thrombosis in critically ill adults. *Arch Intern Med* 161:1268, 2001.
23. Cook D, Guyatt G, Marshall J, et al: A comparison of sucralfate and ranitidine for the prevention of upper gastrointestinal bleeding in patients requiring mechanical ventilation. *N Engl J Med* 338:791, 1998.
24. Kollef MH, Levy NT, Ahrens TS, et al: The use of continuous IV sedation is associated with prolongation of mechanical ventilation. *Chest* 114:541, 1998.
25. Kress JP, Pohlman AS, O'Connor MF, Hall JB: Daily interruption of sedative infusions in critically ill patients undergoing mechanical ventilation. *N Engl J Med* 342:1471, 2000.
26. Hall JB, Wood LDH: Liberation of the patient from mechanical ventilation. *JAMA* 257:1621, 1987.
27. Epstein SK: Weaning parameters. *Respir Care Clin North Am* 6:253, 2000.
28. MacIntyre NR, Cook DJ, Ely EW Jr, et al: Evidence-based guidelines for weaning and discontinuing ventilatory support: A collective task force facilitated by the American College of Chest Physicians, the American Association for Respiratory Care, and the American College of Critical Care Medicine. *Chest* 120(suppl):375S, 2001.
29. Sahn SA, Lakshminarayan S: Bedside criteria for discontinuation of mechanical ventilation. *Chest* 63:1002, 1973.
30. Tahvanainen J, Salmenpera M, Nikki P: Extubation criteria after weaning from intermittent mandatory ventilation and continuous positive airway pressure. *Crit Care Med* 11:702, 1983.
31. Yang KL, Tobin MJ: A prospective study of indexes predicting the outcome of trials of weaning from mechanical ventilation. *N Engl J Med* 324:1445, 1991.
32. Chatila W, Jacob B, Guanglione D, Manthous CA: The unassisted respiratory rate:tidal volume ratio accurately predicts weaning outcome. *Am J Med* 101:61, 1996.
33. Jacob B, Chatila W, Manthous CA: The unassisted respiratory rate:tidal volume ratio accurately predicts weaning outcome in post-operative patients. *Crit Care Med* 25:253, 1996.
34. Herrera M, Blasco J, Venegas J, et al: Mouth occlusion pressure ($P_{0.1}$) in acute respiratory failure. *Intensive Care Med* 11:134, 1985.
35. Sassoon CSH, Te TT, Mahutte CK, Light RW: Airway occlusion pressure: An important indicator for successful weaning in patients with chronic obstructive pulmonary disease. *Am Rev Respir Dis* 135:107, 1987.
36. Montgomery AB, Holle RHO, Neagley SR, et al: Prediction of successful ventilatory weaning using airway occlusion pressure and hypercapnic challenge. *Chest* 91:496, 1987.

37. Milbern SM, Downs JB, Jumper LC, et al: Evaluation of criteria for discontinuing mechanical ventilation support. *Arch Surg* 113:1441, 1978.

38. Nishimura M, Taenaka N, Takeqawa J: Oxygen cost of breathing and inspiratory work of ventilator as weaning monitor in critically ill. *Crit Care Med* 12:258, 1984.

39. Kemper M, Weissman C, Askanazi J, et al: Metabolic and respiratory changes during weaning from mechanical ventilation. *Chest* 92:979, 1987.

40. Hubmayr RD, Loosbrock LM, Gillespie DJ, Rodarte JR: Oxygen uptake during weaning from mechanical ventilation. *Chest* 94:1148, 1988.

41. Mohsenifar Z, Hay A, Hay J, et al: Gastric intramucosal pH as a predictor of success or failure in weaning from mechanical ventilation. *Ann Intern Med* 119:794, 1993.

42. Tobin MJ, Perez W, Guenther SM, et al: The pattern of breathing during successful and unsuccessful trials of weaning from mechanical ventilation. *Am Rev Respir Dis* 134:1111, 1986.

43. Lee KH, Hui KP, Chan TB, et al: Rapid shallow breathing (frequency-tidal volume ratio) did not predict extubation outcome. *Chest* 105:540, 1994.

44. Epstein SK: Evaluation of the rapid shallow breathing index in the clinical setting. *Am J Respir Crit Care Med* 152:545, 1995.

45. Epstein SK, Ciubotaru RL: Influence of gender and endotracheal tube size on preextubation breathing pattern. *Am J Respir Crit Care Med* 154:1647, 1996.

46. Gluck EH, Corigan L: Predicting eventual success or failure to wean in patients receiving long-term ventilation. *Chest* 110:1018, 1996.

47. Khamiees M, Raju P, DeGirolamo A, et al: Predictors of extubation outcome in patients who have successfully completed a spontaneous breathing trial. *Chest* 120:1262, 2001.

48. Wright PE, Marini JJ, Bernard GR: In vitro versus in vivo comparison of endotracheal tube airflow resistance. *Am Rev Respir Dis* 140:10, 1989.

49. Swinamer DL, Fedoruk LM, Jones RL, et al: Energy expenditure associated with CPAP and T-piece spontaneous ventilatory trials. *Chest* 96:867, 1989.

50. Ishaaya AM, Nathan SD, Belman MJ: Work of breathing after extubation. *Chest* 107:204, 1995.

51. Brochard L, Rauss A, Benito S, et al: Comparison of three methods of gradual withdrawal from ventilatory support during weaning from mechanical ventilation. *Am J Respir Crit Care Med* 150:896, 1994.

52. Esteban A, Alia I, Gordo F, et al: Extubation outcome after spontaneous breathing trials with T-tube or pressure support ventilation. The Spanish Lung Failure Collaborative Group. *Am J Respir Crit Care Med* 156:459, 1997.

53. Esteban A, Alia I, Tobin MJ, et al: Effect of spontaneous breathing trial duration on outcome of attempts to discontinue mechanical ventilation. Spanish Lung Failure Collaborative Group. *Am J Respir Crit Care Med* 159:512, 1999.

54. Sassoon CS, Caiozzo VJ, Manka A, Sieck GC: Altered diaphragm contractile properties with controlled mechanical ventilation. *J Appl Physiol* 92:2585, 2002.

55. Eastwood PR, Hillman DR, Finucane KE: Ventilatory responses to inspiratory threshold loading and role of muscle fatigue in task failure. *J Appl Physiol* 76:185, 1994.

56. Robicsek A, Kruger J, Rucker, et al: Rapid shallow breathing is a natural response to maximal ventilatory effort. *Am J Respir Crit Care Med* 153:A611, 1996.

57. Hund EF, Fogel W, Krieger D, et al: Critical illness polyneuropathy: Clinical findings and outcomes of a frequent cause of neuromuscular weaning failure. *Crit Care Med* 24:1328, 1996.

58. Coronel B, Mercatello A, Couturier JC, et al: Polyneuropathy: Potential cause of difficult weaning. *Crit Care Med* 18:486, 1990.

59. Wijdicks EFM, Litchy WJ, Harrison BA, Gracey DR: The clinical spectrum of critical illness polyneuropathy. *Mayo Clin Proc* 69:955, 1994.

60. Witt NJ, Zochodne DW, Bolton CF, et al: Peripheral nerve function in sepsis and multiple organ failure. *Chest* 99:176, 1991.

61. Mier-Jedrzejowick A, Brophy C, Green M: Respiratory muscle weakness during upper respiratory tract infections. *Am Rev Respir Dis* 138:5, 1988.

62. Boczkowski J, Dureuil B, Branger C, et al: Effects of sepsis on diaphragmatic function in rats. *Am Rev Respir Dis* 138:260, 1988.

63. Wilcox P, Osborne S, Bressler B: Monocyte inflammatory mediators impair in vitro hamster diaphragm contractility. *Am Rev Respir Dis* 146:462, 1992.

64. Wilcox P, Milliken C, Bressler B: High-dose tumor necrosis factor α produces an impairment of hamster diaphragm contractility: Attenuation with a prostaglandin inhibitor. *Am J Respir Crit Care Med* 153:1611, 1996.

65. Amoateng-Adjepong Y, Jacob B, Ahmad M, Manthous CA: The effect of sepsis on breathing pattern and weaning outcomes in patients recovering from respiratory failure. *Chest* 112:472, 1997.

66. Decramer M, Stas KJ: Corticosteroid-induced myopathy involving respiratory muscles in patients with COPD and asthma. *Am Rev Respir Dis* 146:800, 1992.

67. Weiner P, Azgad Y, Weiner M: The effect of corticosteroids on inspiratory muscle performance in humans. *Chest* 104:1788, 1993.

68. Decramer M, Lacquet LM, Fagard R, et al: Corticosteroids contribute to muscle weakness in chronic airflow obstruction. *Am J Respir Crit Care Med* 150:11, 1994.

69. Segredo V, Caldwell JE, Matthay MA, et al: Persistent paralysis in critically ill patients after long-term administration of vecuronium. *N Engl J Med* 327:524, 1992.

70. Shapiro JM, Condos R, Cole RP: Myopathy of status asthmaticus: Relation to neuromuscular blockade and corticosteroid administration. *J Intensive Care Med* 8:144, 1993.

71. Hansen-Flaschen J, Cowen J, Raps EC: Neuromuscular blockade in the intensive care unit: More than we bargained for. *Am Rev Respir Dis* 147:234, 1993.

72. Anzueto A, Tobin MJ, Moore G, et al: Effect of prolonged mechanical ventilation on diaphragmatic function: A preliminary study of a baboon model. *Am Rev Respir Dis* 135:A201, 1987.

73. Chatila W, Hall JB, Manthous CA: The effect of pulmonary secretions on respiratory mechanics in intubated patients. *Respir Care* 40:1048, 1995.

74. Manthous CA, Chatila W, Schmidt GA, Hall JB: Treatment of bronchospasm by metered dose inhaler albuterol in mechanically ventilated patients. *Chest* 107:210, 1995.

75. Similowski T, Yan S, Gauthier AP, et al: Contractile properties of the human diaphragm during chronic hyperinflation. *N Engl J Med* 325:917, 1991.

76. Petrof BJ, Legare M, Goldberg P, et al: Continuous positive airway pressure reduces work of breathing and dyspnea during weaning from mechanical ventilation in severe chronic obstructive pulmonary disease. *Am Rev Respir Dis* 141:281, 1990.

77. Sassoon CSH, Hassell KT, Mahutte CK: Hyperoxic-induced hypercapnia in stable chronic obstructive pulmonary disease. *Am Rev Respir Dis* 135:907, 1987.

78. Aubier M, Murciano D, Fournier M, et al: Effects of the administration of O_2 on ventilation and blood gases in patients with chronic obstructive pulmonary disease during acute respiratory failure. *Am Rev Respir Dis* 122:747, 1980.

79. Dunn WF, Nelson SB, Hubmayr RD: Oxygen-induced hypercarbia in obstructive pulmonary disease. *Am Rev Respir Dis* 144:526, 1991.

80. LeMaire F, Teboul J, Cinotti L, et al: Acute left ventricular dysfunction during unsuccessful weaning from mechanical ventilation. *Anesthesiology* 69:171, 1988.

81. Hurford WE, Lynch KE, Strauss HW, et al: Myocardial perfusion as assessed by thallium-201 scintigraphy during the discontinuation of mechanical ventilation in ventilator-dependent patients. *Anesthesiology* 74:1007, 1991.

82. Hurford WE, Favorito F: Association of myocardial ischemia with failure to wean from mechanical ventilation. *Crit Care Med* 23:1475, 1995.

83. Abalos A, Leibowitz AB, Distefano D, et al: Myocardial ischemia during the weaning period. *Am J Crit Care* 3:32, 1992.

84. Chatila W, Jacob B, Adjepong Y, et al: Cardiac ischemia during weaning from mechanical ventilation. *Chest* 109:1577, 1996.

85. Polese G, Massara A, Poggi R, et al: Flow-triggering reduces inspiratory effort during weaning from mechanical ventilation. *Intensive Care Med* 21:682, 1995.

86. Sassoon CS, DelRosario N, Fei R, et al: Influence of pressure- and flow-triggered synchronous intermittent ventilation on inspiratory muscle work. *Crit Care Med* 22:1933, 1994.

87. Marini JJ, Rodriguez RM, Lamb V: The inspiratory workload of patient-initiated mechanical ventilation. *Am Rev Respir Dis* 134: 902, 1986.

88. Marini JJ, Crapps JS, Culver BH: The inspiratory work of breathing during assisted mechanical ventilation. *Chest* 87:612, 1985.

89. Ward ME, Corbeil C, Gibbons W, et al: Optimization of inspiratory muscle relaxation during mechanical ventilation. *Am Rev Respir Dis* 69:29, 1988.

90. Slutsky AS, Brochard L, Dellinger P, et al: ACCP Consensus Conference: Mechanical ventilation. *Chest* 104:1833, 1993.

91. Imsand C, Feihl F, Perret C, Fitting JW: Regulation of inspiratory neuromuscular output during synchronized intermittent mechanical ventilation. *Anesthesiology* 80:13, 1994.

92. Cooper KR, Phillips BA: Effect of short-term sleep loss on breathing. *J Appl Physiol* 53:855, 1982.

93. DeKeyser F: Psychoneuroimmunology in critically ill patients. *AACN Clin Issues* 14:25, 2003.

94. Parthasarathy S, Tobin MJ: Effect of ventilator mode on sleep quality in critically ill patients. *Am J Respir Crit Care Med* 166:1423, 2002.

95. Aldrich TK, Karpel JP, Uhrlass RM, et al: Weaning from mechanical ventilation: Adjunctive use of inspiratory muscle resistive training. *Crit Care Med* 17:143, 1989.

96. Esteban A, Frutos F, Tobin MJ, et al: A comparison of four methods of weaning patients from mechanical ventilation. *N Engl J Med* 332:345, 1995.

97. Darmon JY, Rauss A, Dreyfuss D, et al: Evaluation of risk factors for laryngeal edema after tracheal extubation in adults and its prevention by dexamethasone: A placebo-controlled, double-blind, multicenter study. *Anesthesiology* 77:245, 1992.

98. Fisher MM, Raper RF: The "cuff leak" test for extubation. *Anaesthesia* 47:10, 1992.

99. Marik PE: The cuff-leak test as a predictor of postextubation stridor: A prospective study. *Respir Care* 41:509, 1996.

100. Miller RL, Cole RP: Association between reduced cuff leak volume and postextubation stridor. *Chest* 110:1035, 1996.

101. Coplin, WM, Pierson, DJ, Cooley, KD, et al: Implications of extubation delay in brain-injured patients meeting standard weaning criteria. *Am J Respir Crit Care Med* 161:1530, 2000.

102. Tolep K, Getch CL, Criner GJ: Swallowing dysfunction in patients receiving prolonged mechanical ventilation. *Chest* 109:167, 1996.

103. Willms D, Sure D: Pulmonary edema due to upper airway obstruction in adults. *Chest* 94:1090, 1988.

104. Boorstein JM, Boorstein SM, Humphries GN, Johnston CC: Using helium-oxygen mixtures in the emergency management of upper airway obstruction. *Ann Emerg Med* 18:688, 1989.

105. Wysocki M, Tric L, Wolff MA, et al: Noninvasive pressure support ventilation in patients with acute respiratory failure. *Chest* 107:761, 1995.

106. Udwadia ZF, Santis GK, Steven MH, Simonds AK: Nasal ventilation to facilitate weaning in patients with chronic respiratory insufficiency. *Thorax* 47:715, 1992.

107. Nava S, Bruschi C, Orlando A, et al: Noninvasive mechanical ventilation (NINMV) facilitates the weaning from traditional mechanical ventilation (MV) in severe COPD. *Am J Respir Crit Care Med* 153:A763, 1996.

107a. Esteban A, Frutos-Vivar F, Ferguson ND, et al: Noninvasive positive-pressure ventilation for respiratory failure after extubation. *N Engl J Med* 350:2452, 2004.

108. Anton WR, Wilhelm P, Jordan T: Reduction of length of time on mechanical ventilation by use of a multidisciplinary weaning protocol. *Respir Care* 37:1279, 1992.

109. Cohen IL, Bari N, Strosberg MA, et al: Reduction of duration and cost of mechanical ventilation in an intensive care unit by use of a ventilatory management team. *Crit Care Med* 19:1278, 1991.

110. Ely EW, Baker AM, Dunagan DP, et al: Effect of the duration of mechanical ventilation of identifying patients capable of breathing spontaneously. *N Engl J Med* 335:1864, 1996.

111. Kollef MH, Shapiro SD, Silver P, et al: A randomized, controlled trial of protocol-directed versus physician-directed weaning from mechanical ventilation. *Crit Care Med* 25:567, 1997.

112. Tanios M, Nevins ML, Hendra KP, et al: The use of weaning parameters prolongs mechanical ventilation time. *Chest* 120:190S, 2001.

PART V
INFECTIOUS DISORDERS

Chapter 45 _____

PRINCIPLES OF ANTIMICROBIAL THERAPY AND THE CLINICAL PHARMACOLOGY OF ANTIMICROBIAL DRUGS

FRED Y. AOKI

KEY POINTS

- *Rational antibiotic use requires the most specific diagnosis that can be made, knowledge of commonly used antimicrobial agents, and appropriate monitoring of therapy.*
- *Antimicrobial prophylaxis against bacterial infections is indicated in selected patients undergoing surgical procedures and in those with cardiac valvular disease.*
- *When suspected infection threatens life or major organ function, antimicrobial therapy should be directed at all infectious possibilities of more than trivial probability until the results of definitive investigations are available.*
- *Knowledge of the clinical pharmacology of antibiotics commonly prescribed in the intensive care unit is essential for the intensivist.*

Antimicrobial Use in Critically Ill Patients

The importance of antimicrobial drugs in the management of patients admitted to the intensive care unit (ICU) is beyond question. The prevention and treatment of infections in ICU patients pose formidable challenges despite advances in our understanding of the pathophysiology of specific infections, the availability of more rapid, sensitive, and specific diagnostic tests, and an array of potent antimicrobial agents.

PROPHYLAXIS OF INFECTIOUS DISEASES IN ICU PATIENTS

The efficacy of short-term systemic antibacterial administration to prevent operative site infections after surgery is well established. Effective prophylaxis requires that the antibacterial agent inhibit specific pathogenic agents that cause the infection and be present at therapeutic concentrations in the operative site at the time the incision is made. It is imperative that surgical wound prophylaxis be prescribed, when appropriate, in the management of ICU patients. Recommended drugs, doses, and duration of prophylaxis for some specific surgical procedures are listed in Table 45-1.[1]

Unlike perioperative antimicrobial prophylaxis for the prevention of wound infection, the efficacy of antibiotics to prevent bacterial endocarditis has not been established by controlled trials. Nevertheless, to prevent bacterial endocarditis, it is recommended that patients with valvulopathy (congenital or acquired) or prosthetic valves (bioprosthetic and homograft valves) be given antimicrobial prophylaxis.[2] Table 45-2 lists the cardiac conditions for which endocarditis prophylaxis is recommended, Table 45-3 presents the surgical procedures for which antibacterial prophylaxis is recommended, and Table 45-4 lists the recommended injectable drugs and doses, all of which were adapted with permission from Dajani and associates.[3]

In contrast, the usefulness of antimicrobial agents to prevent infections other than endocarditis and infections related to surgery remains limited or controversial. Two general approaches have been evaluated. In one, antibiotics are applied to sterile sites or clean skin wounds to prevent local infection; in the other, antibiotics are used to selectively eradicate the potentially pathogenic bacteria of the gastrointestinal tract and simultaneously preserve the anaerobic "nonpathogenic" flora. The former approach includes endotracheal administration of nonabsorbable antibacterial drugs, such as the aminoglycosides, instillation of antibiotics into the urinary bladder, and the covering of wounds by creams mixed with antibacterial agents. With the exception of topical use of sulfonamide creams in the management of burned patients, these methods have been associated with inconsistent prophylactic effects and a high incidence of relapse, resistance, and superinfection that renders this strategy unacceptable.

The second approach is referred to as *selective decontamination of the digestive tract* (SDD).[4] The strategy of SDD is based on the hypothesis that eradication of selected components of the bacterial and fungal flora of the oropharyngeal or gastrointestinal tract can decrease the risk of infection and maintain the natural defense of these mucosal surfaces conferred by the anaerobic flora. SDD studies include various systematic antimicrobial agents plus oral administration of nonabsorbable agents such as polymyxin E, tobramycin, plus amphotericin B, but other regimens use only nonadsorbable drugs. The antibiotics are administered for the entire duration of the critical illness; in this respect, SDD differs from short-term perioperative surgical prophylaxis. The technique has received intensive investigative attention over the past decade and evidence that SDD is effective in decreasing ICU mortality but the relative importance of antibiotic resistance varies among institutions so that SDD cannot be recommended for routine use.[5]

THERAPY OF INFECTIOUS DISEASES IN ICU PATIENTS

Rational antibiotic use requires a systematic approach to the assessment of suspected infection, knowledge of commonly used agents, and appropriate selection and monitoring of drugs.

Regardless of whether infection is suspected in an ICU patient because of the development of florid symptoms and signs of inflammation (rubor, calor, dolor, tumor, or functio laesa) or of subtle deterioration in the level of consciousness or gas exchange, the same thorough, systematic evaluation is recommended: The first question to be addressed is whether infection can be reasonably inferred to be present. Does the history show systemic or local symptoms of inflammation?

TABLE 45-1 Recommended Antibiotic Prophylaxis for Some Commonly Performed Surgical Procedures

Surgical Procedure	Recommended Prophylactic Regimen[a]
Gynecologic surgery	
Cesarean section	Cefazolin (1 g IV) after clamping the cord and 6 and 12 h later
	Prophylaxis is not indicated in uncomplicated elective procedures
	Uterine irrigation with antibiotics may be comparable to systemic therapy; if irrigating antibiotics are used, 2 g cefoxitin in 1 L normal saline is effective; in patients with β-lactam allergy, metronidazole (500 mg IV) after cord clamping is effective
Orthopedic surgery	
Open reduction of fracture or insertion of hardware[b]	Cefazolin (1 g IV) preoperatively and q 6 h (3 doses). Complex (open) fractures are considered contaminated and cefazolin therapy (1 g q 8 h for 10 d beginning at admission) is indicated
Laminectomy and spinal fusion	Prophylactic antimicrobials have not proved to be beneficial
Amputation of lower limb	Cefoxitin (2 g IV) preoperatively and q 6 h (4 doses)
General surgery	
Cholecystectomy	Cefazolin (2 g IV) preoperatively in "high-risk" patients, i.e., >60 y, previous biliary surgery, history of acute symptoms, or jaundice
	In patients with β-lactam allergy, gentamicin (80 mg IV) preoperatively and q 8 h (3 doses) is effective.
Colon surgery	Neomycin and erythromycin base, 1 g of each orally at 1, 2, and 11 PM on the day before surgery
	For emergency colon surgery or situations precluding preoperative oral prophylaxis, cefoxitin (2 g IV) preoperatively and q 4 h (3 doses) is effective
	In patients with β-lactam allergy, metronidazole (500 mg IV) and gentamicin (1.7 mg/kg IV) preoperatively and q 8 h postoperatively (3 doses) are effective
Primary appendectomy	Cefoxitin (2 g IV) preoperatively and q 6 h (3 doses) in nonperforated appendixes; in perforated appendixes, therapy is continued for 3–5 d
	Although combined aerobic and anaerobic coverage appears to be preferable, in patients with β-lactam allergy, metronidazole (500 mg IV) preoperatively is effective; with perforated appendixes, this is continued q 8 h (IV or oral administration) for 3–5 d
Gastric resection	Cefazolin (1 g) preoperatively in "high-risk" patients only, i.e., bleeding gastric or duodenal ulcer, obstructive duodenal ulcer, gastric ulcer, gastric cancer, or morbid obesity (prophylaxis is not indicated for cases of chronic uncomplicated duodenal ulcers)
	In patients with β-lactam allergy, 1 preoperative IV dose of gentamicin (120 mg) and clindamycin (600 mg) may be effective, but data are limited
Surgery for penetrating abdominal trauma	Cefoxitin (2 g IV) on admission to the hospital
	For patients with intestinal perforation, 2 g cefoxitin IV q 6 h for 2–5 d is effective
Surgery on nose, mouth, and pharynx	
Major head, neck, and oral surgery	In major surgical procedures involving an incision through oral or pharyngeal mucosa, a combination of gentamicin (1.7 mg/kg) and clindamycin (300 mg IV) preoperatively and q 8 h (2 doses) is recommended; cefazolin and third-generation cephalosporins also have demonstrated effectiveness when given over 24 h perioperatively
Rhinoplasty and repair of nose	Prophylactic antimicrobials have not proved to be effective
Cardiothoracic and vascular surgery	
Median sternotomy, coronary artery bypass grafting, and valve surgery	Cefazolin (1 g IV) preoperatively and q 6 h for 48 h
	In patients with β-lactam allergy, vancomycin (15 mg/kg IV) preoperatively, after initiation of bypass (10 mg/kg), and q 8 h postoperatively for 48 h may be effective
Pacemaker insertion	Cefazolin (1 g) as above; in patients with β-lactam allergy, no prophylaxis may be a reasonable alternative, given the low incidence of infection
Thoracic surgery procedure including lobectomy and pneumonectomy	Cefazolin (1 g) preoperatively and q 6 h postoperatively for 24 h; the optimal duration of postoperative prophylaxis has not been established
	In penetrating thoracic trauma and in the placement of chest tubes in trauma management, prophylactic antibiotics have not been effective
Peripheral vascular surgery	Cefazolin (1 g) preoperatively and q 6 h postoperatively for 24 h
	The usefulness of antibiotic prophylaxis in carotid artery surgery has not been established, but cefazolin should be used as described above when infection rates increase
Vascular surgery that involves the abdominal aorta or a groin incision	Cefazolin (1–2 g IV) preoperatively and q 4–8 h for the duration of the procedure[b]

TABLE 45-1 (Continued)

Surgical Procedure	Recommended Prophylactic Regimen[a]
Neurosurgical procedures	
Cerebrospinal fluid shunting procedures	Antibiotic prophylaxis is not indicated in institutions with low infection rates (<10%) Trimethoprim (160 mg) plus sulfamethoxazole (800 mg) IV preoperatively and q 12 h (3 doses) may be beneficial in institutions with high infection rates (>20%)
Craniotomy	For high-risk procedures (e.g., re-exploration and microsurgery), clindamycin (300 mg IV) preoperatively and q 4 h has been effective, as has vancomycin (1 g IV) plus gentamicin (80 IM) preoperatively

[a] Unless otherwise noted, the preoperative dose of intravenous antibiotic should be administered at about the time of the operative incision. Preoperative intramuscular antibiotic should be administered 30 minutes to 1 hour before the incision.
[b] From reference 2.
ABBREVIATIONS: IM, intramuscularly; IV, intravenously.
SOURCE: Reproduced with permission from Kaiser.[1]

Are signs of inflammation present? Can other causes of inflammation such as tissue injury due to drugs, immunologic diseases, and physical agents (thermal energy or electromagnetic irradiation) be excluded? Is there laboratory evidence of inflammation—visible pus or polymorphonuclear leukocytes in microscopic examinations of body fluids?

The second question for the intensivist is: What is the infectious disease that is occurring? Is this meningitis, pneumonitis, intraabdominal sepsis, intravascular, catheter-related bacteremia, or some other process? This question must be answered as specifically as possible, because an accurate diagnosis will logically lead to collection of the appropriate specimens for microbiologic testing before antibiotic therapy is initiated, and an appropriate working conclusion about the probable etiologic agents involved.

An outline of the investigation of particular infections is beyond the scope of this chapter and is detailed elsewhere in the text. Contemporary intensivists have access to a wide range of noninvasive radiologic imaging techniques that have been invaluable in confirming the diagnosis of deep visceral infections and assisting in their repeated evaluation during treatment. Occasionally, however, the patient will be too ill to tolerate the most appropriate diagnostic evaluation. This may limit the accuracy of the initial assessment, but the initiation of antimicrobial therapy must not be delayed. It is axiomatic in the critically ill patient that initial antimicrobial therapy be directed at all infectious possibilities of more than trivial probability until the results of definitive investigations are available.

TABLE 45-2 Endocarditis Prophylaxis Recommendations: Cardiac Conditions

Prophylaxis Recommended

Prosthetic cardiac valves, including bioprosthetic and homograft valves
Previous bacterial endocarditis, even in the absence of heart disease
Most congenital cardiac malformations
Rheumatic and other acquired valvular dysfunction, even after valvular surgery
Hypertrophic cardiomyopathy
Mitral valve prolapse with valvular regurgitation

Prophylaxis not recommended

Isolated secundum atrial septal defect
Surgical repair without residua beyond 6 months of secundum atrial septal defect, ventricular septal defect, or patent ductus arteriosus
Previous coronary artery bypass graft surgery
Mitral valve prolapse without valvular regurgitation
Physiologic, functional, or innocent heart murmurs
Previous Kawasaki disease without valvular dysfunction
Previous rheumatic fever without valvular dysfunction
Cardiac pacemakers and implanted defibrillators

SOURCE: Reproduced with permission from Dajani et al.[3] Copyright 1990 American Medical Association.

TABLE 45-3 Endocarditis Prophylactic Recommendations: Surgical Procedures

Prophylaxis Recommended (clinically important risk of bacteremia)

Tonsillectomy and/or adenoidectomy
Surgical operations that involve intestinal or respiratory mucosa
Bronchoscopy with a rigid bronchoscope
Sclerotherapy for esophageal varices
Esophageal dilation
Gallbladder surgery
Cystoscopy
Urethral dilation
Urethral catheterization if urinary tract infection is present
Urinary tract surgery if urinary tract infection is present[a]
Prostatic surgery
Incision and drainage of infected tissue[a]
Vaginal hysterectomy
Vaginal delivery in the presence of infection[a]

Prophylaxis not recommended (risk of bacteremia considered to be negligible)[b]

Tympanostomy tube insertion
Endotracheal intubation
Bronchoscopy with a flexible bronchoscope, with or without biopsy
Cardiac catheterization
Endoscopy with or without gastrointestinal biopsy
Cesarean section
In the absence of infection for urethral catheterization, dilation and curettage, uncomplicated vaginal delivery, therapeutic abortion, sterilization procedures, or insertion or removal of intrauterine devices

[a] In addition to prophylactic regimen for genitourinary procedures, antibiotic therapy should be directed against the most likely bacterial pathogen.
[b] In patients who have prosthetic heart valves, history of endocarditis, or surgically constructed systemic-pulmonary shunts or conduits, physicians may choose to administer prophylactic antibiotics even for low-risk procedures that involve the lower respiratory, genitourinary, or gastrointestinal tracts.

SOURCE: Reproduced with permission from Dajani et al.[3] Copyright 1990 American Medical Association.

TABLE 45-4 Endocarditis Prophylaxis Regimens

Drug	Dosing Regimen
	Oral and Upper Respiratory Tract Procedures
Ampicillin	IV or IM administration of ampicillin, 2.0 g, 30 min before procedure; then IV or IM administration of ampicillin, 1.0 g, or oral administration of amoxicillin, 1.5 g, 6 h after initial dose
	For patients allergic to ampicillin, amoxicillin, or penicillin
Clindamycin	IV administration of 300 mg 30 min before procedure and IV or oral administration of 150 mg 6 h after initial dose
	For patients considered high risk and not candidates for standard regimen
Ampicillin, gentamicin, and amoxicillin	IV or IM administration of ampicillin, 2.0 g, plus gentamicin, 1.5 mg/kg (not to exceed 80 mg), 30 min before procedure; followed by amoxicillin, 1.5 g, orally 6 h after initial dose; alternatively, the parenteral regimen may be repeated 8 h after initial dose
	For high-risk patients allergic to ampicillin, amoxicillin, or penicillin
Vancomycin	IV administration of 1.0 g over 1 h, starting 1 h before procedure; no repeated dose necessary
	Genitourinary and Gastrointestinal Procedures
	Standard regimen
Ampicillin, gentamicin, and amoxicillin	IV or IM administration of ampicillin, 2.0 g, plus gentamicin, 1.5 mg/kg (not to exceed 80 mg), 30 min before procedure; followed by amoxicillin, 1.5 g, orally 6 h after initial dose; alternatively, the parenteral regimen may be repeated once 8 h after initial dose
	For patients allergic to ampicillin, amoxicillin, or penicillin
Vancomycin and gentamicin	IV administration of vancomycin, 1.0 g, over 1 h plus IV or IM administration of gentamicin, 1.5 mg/kg (not to exceed 80 mg), 1 h before procedure; may be repeated once 8 h after initial dose
	Alternative regimen for low-risk patients
Amoxicillin	3.0 g orally 1 h before procedure, then 1.5 g 6 h after initial dose

ABBREVIATIONS: IM, intramuscular; IV, intravenous.
SOURCE: Reproduced with permission from Dajani et al.[3] Copyright 1990 American Medical Association.

Ideally, the choice of antibiotic agent(s) for the treatment of a specific infectious disease in a given host in the ICU should be based on unequivocal results from rigorous, controlled clinical trials. With a few exceptions, such data do not exist. Therefore, the selection of the proper antimicrobial agent depends on careful consideration of the known or likely susceptibility patterns of the putative pathogen in this specific type of patient at this particular institution, the natural history of the infection, and the spectrum of agents likely or known to be effective for treatment of this type of infection. The two former areas are reviewed in other sections of this book and are not elaborated on here. This chapter emphasizes the importance of knowledge of the clinical pharmacology of antibiotics as one critical element in the rational use of drugs for treatment of infectious disease in the ICU patient.

The selection of the proper drug is essential to minimize toxicity and maximize efficacy. The following key steps relative to knowledge of the antimicrobial agents in humans should be systematically considered in the selection process. These steps are essential to the rational use of any drug.

A. *Individualize* the treatment by considering the following in choosing drugs and designing dosage regimens.
  1. Processes that alter the pharmacokinetics of the drug
    a. Physiologic
      - Extremes of age
      - Pregnancy
      - Barriers to drug penetration (e.g., blood-brain barrier, intraocular fluid)
    b. Disease induced
      - Barriers to drug penetration (avascular abscess wall, infarcts, burn eschar, wet gangrene, etc.)
      - Changes in drug clearance because of hepatic, renal, or other disease (e.g., enhanced aminoglycoside clearance in burned patients, penicillins in cystic fibrosis patients)
    c. Drugs administered concurrently
      - Chemical interaction (e.g., penicillins inactivate aminoglycosides in azotemic plasma)
      - Enhanced metabolism
      - Competitive inhibition of renal or metabolic clearance in the kidney or liver
      - Displacement of highly bound drug from plasma protein
  2. Processes that alter the pharmacodynamics of the drug
    a. Allergy to the drug
    b. Other (e.g., reduced seizure threshold)
B. *Select* and *monitor* therapeutic end points.
  1. Clinical symptoms and signs of infection
  2. Laboratory measures of
    a. Efficacy (e.g., leukocyte concentration, erythrocyte sedimentation rate, serial imaging results such as brain abscess shrinkage on serial computed tomographic scans)
    b. Toxicity (e.g., creatinine concentration and urinalysis in patients receiving aminoglycosides)
  3. Microbiologic (e.g., serial cultures, serum bactericidal titers)
  4. Pharmacologic—serum concentrations of drugs

Selecting the proper antimicrobial agent, skillfully individualizing the dose regimen, and choosing the appropriate parameters to monitor for beneficial and adverse effects of drugs are closely related to knowledge of the pharmacologic effects of antimicrobial agents in humans. The remainder of this chapter reviews these aspects of many classes of antimicrobial agent from the intensivist's perspective.

Antibacterial Agents

This section reviews selected aspects of commonly used groups of antimicrobial agents likely to be prescribed by intensivists, with an emphasis on the clinical pharmacology of the drugs rather than on their molecular pharmacology and mechanisms of action.

PENICILLINS

MECHANISM OF ACTION   The penicillins are natural and semisynthetic compounds that have in common a thiazolidine ring connected to a β-lactam ring to which is attached a side chain of variable composition. The composition of the side chain affects the antibacterial spectrum of the molecule. The integrity of the β-lactam ring is essential for the antibacterial activity of the penicillins. Hence, its enzymatic hydrolysis by β-lactamases is the most important mechanism of bacterial resistance to penicillins.

Penicillins are generally bactericidal. The antibacterial effect of penicillins involves binding to penicillin binding proteins (PBPs), which are peptidases in the cell wall of susceptible bacteria.[6] The types of PBPs found in different bacterial species vary. High activity of penicillins against susceptible bacteria correlates with high affinity binding to certain PBPs, especially PBPs 1, 2, and 4. Modifications in the penicillin side chain of some semisynthetic penicillins have enhanced their antibacterial activity against gram-negative bacteria by increasing their ability to pass through the lipopolysaccharide outer layer to reach PBP ligands in the peptidoglycan layer and, less importantly, by increasing their resistance to β-lactamase, which these organisms all contain in small amounts in the periplasmic space between the inner and outer membranes.

Penicillin binding to PBPs inhibits peptidoglycan assembly and cross-linking. Cell death is usually the result of activation of endogenous autolysins (peptidoglycan hydrolases), which cause structural defects, resulting in cell lysis. Occasionally, stable round forms develop that continue to grow for several generations before lysis ultimately occurs.[7] Hence, although different penicillins, carbapenems, and cephalosporins may have different molecular sites of action, combining two or more of these agents to achieve additive or synergistic antibacterial effects is of unproven value.

The antibacterial effect of the penicillins when susceptible organisms are exposed to intermittent doses of the drugs is determined by composite events occurring during three periods: the time during which the antibacterial drug exerts its maximal effect, the time during which the drug is present at concentrations that have a definite but lesser bactericidal effect, and the period after which concentrations have decreased to levels that are not bactericidal but during which some bacteria continue to die at a faster rate than the surviving cells can multiply (now known as the period of the *postantibiotic effect* [PAE]).[8]

Bacterial killing during exposure to penicillins in vitro occurs most rapidly when exposure occurs during the logarithmic phase of bacterial growth. The killing effect of penicillins during this phase shows little dependence on concentration in excess of minimal inhibitory levels. The PAE of the penicillins usually lasts 1 to 3 hours against gram-positive coccal bacteria and 1 hour against susceptible *Enterobacteriaceae* and other enteric gram-negative bacteria. The duration of the PAE is more closely related to the duration of exposure to inhibitory concentrations of penicillin than to concentration per se. Beyond these facts, the relation between penicillin concentration and bacterial killing is complex even in vitro and more so in patients in whom host factors contribute to the antibacterial effect. It has been difficult to use these observations to optimize the way we give penicillins to patients—by intermittent administration or continuous infusion.[9] Morever, because the concentrations at the site of infection cannot be predicted, it is conventional to administer penicillins in relatively large doses at frequent intervals, or else continuously, to ensure the maximal antibacterial effect.[10] The effectiveness of this strategy depends more on the duration that penicillin concentrations exceed the inhibitory level than on the absolute concentration of drug. Extremely high peak concentrations may only increase the frequency of concentration-related adverse effects of penicillins (see below).

MECHANISMS OF RESISTANCE   Enzymatic hydrolysis of the β-lactam bond by β-lactamase is the most important mechanism of bacterial resistance to penicillins. Many gram-negative bacteria are inherently insusceptible to penicillins because the penicillins cannot diffuse through the lipopolysaccharide layer to interact with PBPs. In other bacteria, mutations in genes encoding PBPs may yield altered transpeptidases that no longer bind penicillins. Mutant streptococci have been described in which exposure to penicillins triggers synthesis of inhibitors of autolysins.

CLASSIFICATION   The penicillins can be divided into five classes based on their clinically most important antibacterial activity, notwithstanding substantial degrees of overlap demonstrable in vitro.

Natural Penicillins
Penicillin G, the prototypical member of this group, is the drug of choice for infections caused by susceptible streptococci, staphylococci, *Clostridia* and *Neisseria* species, and oral anaerobes including *Bacteroides melaninogenicus.*

Aminopenicillins
Ampicillin is the only member of this group, which includes amoxicillin and bacampicillin among others, that can be administered parenterally. It is the drug of initial choice for the treatment of community-acquired meningitis in adults, in addition to a third-generation cephalosporin and, when combined with an aminoglycoside, for the therapy of subacute bacterial endocarditis in individuals with native valves and pyelonephritis suspected to be or caused by *E. faecalis.* Although ampicillin was widely used for treatment for *Haemophilus influenzae* infections, 19% to 24% of *H. influenzae* type B bacteria causing respiratory infection in adults are now resistant to ampicillin, usually by virtue of producing β-lactamase.[11] Accordingly, in the seriously ill patients in whom *H. influenzae* is a potential pathogen, it is prudent to use a drug other than ampicillin until the organism can be shown to lack β-lactamase by in vitro testing.

Penicillinase-Resistant Penicillins

These penicillins, such as cloxacillin and nafcillin, are the antibacterial drugs of choice for therapy of *Staphylococcus aureus* infection suspected or known to be susceptible (collectively referred to as methicillin-sensitive *S. aureus* [MSSA].

Antipseudomonal Penicillins

Ticarcillin has been superseded by the extended-spectrum penicillins (see below) for treatment of patients with suspected or proven infection caused by *Pseudomonas aeruginosa*. The activity of ticarcillin against *Proteus vulgaris*, *Proteus rettgeri*, and *Morganella morganii* exceeds that of ampicillin, but against other enteric aerobic gram-negative bacilli its potency is similar to that of ampicillin and inferior to the extended-spectrum penicillins. In addition, ticarcillin and carbenicillin may interfere more with platelet function, an undesirable side effect in critically ill patients with thrombocytopenia or other potential causes of hemorrhage (e.g., stress ulcers). Because development of resistance during therapy can be a problem, ticarcillin is generally used with an aminoglycoside when *P. aeruginosa* sepsis is suspected or diagnosed.

Extended-Spectrum Penicillins

Piperacillin and mezlocillin inhibit *P. aeruginosa* in a manner similar to the antipseudomonal penicillins but also have considerably more clinically useful activity against a number of other enteric gram-negative aerobic and anaerobic organisms. Mezlocillin is more active than ticarcillin against most *Enterobacteriaceae*, but many strains are resistant through production of β-lactamase. Mezlocillin is active against oropharyngeal gram-negative anaerobic bacilli, but *Bacteroides fragilis* group organisms are not uniformly susceptible. Mezlocillin is highly active against *H. influenzae*, meningococci and gonococci, *Streptococci* (including *S. faecalis*), and penicillin-sensitive *S. aureus* strains. Because of its greater potency against *P. aeruginosa* in vitro, piperacillin is the antipseudomonal penicillin of choice.

Combining piperacillin with the β-lacatamase inhibitor tazobactam (or ticarcillin with clavulanate) extends the spectrum of piperacillin to include a number of β-lactamase–producing bacteria, including *S. aureus*, and some gram-negative bacilli such as *Serratia* species, *Acinetobacter* species, and *B. fragilis*. Thus, piperacillin/tazobactam and ticarcillin/clavulanate have utility in the ICU as broad-spectrum antibiotics in patients in whom *P. aeruginosa* is also a significant concern as an etiologic agent (see section on β-lactamases).

CLINICAL PHARMACOLOGY The absorption of orally administered penicillins is sufficiently variable among even ambulatory patients that, for this reason alone, these drugs are administered only intravenously in the critically ill patient. The range of doses of some penicillins recommended for adult patients with moderate to severe infection, with normal or impaired renal function, and dialysis-dependent kidney disease are presented in Table 45-5.

In the circulation, penicillins are bound to plasma proteins, chiefly albumin, to different degrees, ranging from 18% for ampicillin to 96% for dicloxacillin. This affects the apparent volume of distribution (AVD), the theoretical calculated volume in which a drug must be uniformly distributed if present at the concentration measured in plasma[12] expressed as liters per kg of body weight. The AVD of penicillins is approximately inversely related to the degree of protein binding, ranging from 9% of body weight for dicloxacillin to 41% for ampicillin. Although protein-bound antibiotic is not pharmacologically active,[12a] serum protein binding of penicillins has not proved to be clinically important because the binding is loose and rapidly reversible in vivo, and the doses used in clinical practice greatly exceed the capacity of the plasma proteins to bind drug. The clinical relevance of coadministering

TABLE 45-5 Recommended Intravenous Doses of Selected Penicillins for Adult Patients with Moderate to Severe Infection and Normal or Impaired Renal Function or Undergoing Dialysis

	CREATININE CLEARANCE (mL/min)				DOSE WITH END-STAGE RENAL FAILURE	
	>60	40–49	10–39	<10	Peritoneal Dialysis	Hemodialysis
Natural						
Penicillin G	1–3 million U q 4 h	Up to 2 million U q 4 h	Up to 1 million U q 4 h	Up to 1 million U q 8 h	As for creatinine clearance <10 mL/min	500,000 U q 6 h during dialysis
Amino						
Ampicillin	1–3 g q 6 h	No change	No change	1–3 g q 12 h	As for creatinine clearance <10 mL/min	0.5 g q 6 h
Penicillinase resistant						
Cloxacillin	1.5–3 g q 6 h	No change	No change	1–2 g q 12 h	?	?
Nafcillin	1.5–3 g q 6 h	No change	No change	No change	No change	No change
Antipseudomonal						
Ticarcillin	2–3 g q 3 h	No change	3 g initial dose, then 2 g q 8 h	3 g initial dose, then 2 g q 12 h	As for creatinine clearance <10 mL/min	3 g after dialysis, then 2 g q 12 h
Extended spectrum						
Piperacillin	2–4 g q 4–6 h	No change	2–4 g q 8 h	4 g q 12 h	2 g after dialysis, then 2 g q 12 h	2–4 g after dialysis, then 4 g q 12 h
Mezlocillin	3–4 g q 6 h	5 g q 12 h	5 g q 24 h	5 g q 48 h	3 g q 12 h	Normal doses

drugs that compete for the same albumin binding sites as penicillins is unclear but unlikely, with an interaction due to altered protein becoming likely only when binding exceeds 90%.[13]

Penicillins are largely eliminated from the body as unchanged drug by renal proximal tubular secretion and glomerular filtration, but some metabolic transformation occurs and can compensate for diminished renal clearance of some penicillins. For example, in anuric patients, the plasma elimination half-life ($t_{1/2}$) of penicillin G is increased from 0.5 to 10.0 hours, and doses must be reduced to obviate dose-related toxic effects (see below). However, the serum elimination $t_{1/2}$ of cloxacillin increases only threefold, to 1.5 hours, and no dose reduction is required.

Probenecid, an organic acid like the penicillins, competitively inhibits renal tubular secretion of penicillins. Coadministration results in an array of pharmacokinetic effects including increased plasma concentrations (double in the case of penicillin G), higher concentrations in the cerebrospinal fluid (CSF) because of inhibition of penicillin secretion from CSF into blood by the choroid plexus, and higher free drug concentrations in plasma because of displacement from albumin. The magnitude of these effects is greatest for those penicillins primarily eliminated by renal proximal tubular secretion.

Various other organic acids also compete with penicillins for secretion by renal tubular cells and produce probenecid-like effects on penicillin disposition. These acids include aspirin, phenylbutazone, sulfonamides, indomethacin, thiazide diuretics, furosemide, and ethacrynic acid. The clinical importance of concurrent administration of these drugs on the antibacterial effects of penicillin is not known but is unlikely to be significant.

ADVERSE DRUG REACTIONS   Adverse drug reactions (ADRs) include all unwanted effects of drugs. They are classified into those that are immunologically mediated (hypersensitivity or allergic reactions) and those that are dose or concentration related. For antibiotics, the latter class also includes all unwanted or undesired complications arising from perturbations in the normal microbiologic flora (e.g., pseudomembranous colitis and yeast vaginitis) and from superinfections caused by agents resistant to the antibiotics being administered to the patient. A third class comprises ADRs for which the mechanism is not understood. This includes anaphylactoid reactions (similar clinically to anaphylaxis but without a demonstrated immunologic basis) and idiosyncratic effects. ADRs to penicillins mostly are of the first two classes. Although they may rarely be fatal (1 per 100,000 cases treated), hypersensitivity reactions are much more important than dose-related penicillin ADR in the ICU, because such intolerance precludes the use of this useful class of drugs. Allergic reactions to penicillins are not uncommon.[14] The overall incidence in different studies ranges from 0.7% to 10.0%. In order of decreasing frequency, hypersensitivity reactions to penicillins include urticaria, fever, bronchospasm, vasculitis, serum sickness, exfoliative dermatitis, and anaphylaxis. Hypersensitivity reactions may be induced by any member of this group, and cross-reactions must be anticipated. Anaphylaxis has been reported more commonly with penicillin G than with other members of the penicillin group, but this probably reflects the frequency of its use. Anaphylaxis and accelerated urticarial reactions, rash, and serum sickness are triggered

by immunobinding of penicillin antigens to immunoglobulin (Ig) E, IgM, and IgG antibodies, respectively.[15] Atopic individuals are not more prone to have allergic reactions to penicillins. Approximately 75% of persons without medical exposure to penicillins have IgM antibody to penicilloyl, the most important penicillin antigen produced by breakage of the β-lactam ring. It acts as a hapten by covalently binding to plasma proteins. The formation of two other antigens, penicilloic acid and penicillanic acid, are increased by high and low pH, respectively. Together, penicilloic and penicillanic acids are known as major determinants because 95% of tissue-bound penicillin is in the form of penicilloyl and penicillanic acid conjugates with body proteins. IgG and IgM antibodies to these moieties occur in most patients treated with penicillins, but the allergic reactions that occasionally result are generally limited to skin rash rather than accelerated, systemic reactions. The term *penicillin minor determinants*, however, refers to benzylpenicillin itself, sodium benzyl penicilloate, and penilloate. IgE-mediated reactions to minor determinants are responsible for most anaphylactic reactions due to penicillins.

Interstitial nephritis associated with methicillin may be a delayed-type hypersensitivity reaction in which the drug induces autoimmunity to renal tubular basement membranes. This unusual immunologically mediated ADR is most commonly seen in patients treated with methicillin for extended periods in large doses, but it has been reported after therapy with most other penicillins and some cephalosporins.

The most important aspect of management of patients with hypersensitivity to penicillins is avoidance. A reliable story of anaphylaxis or an accelerated reaction to any member of this group of drugs (or a cephalosporin or carbapenem) is an absolute contraindication to their use. A history of any other form of hypersensitivity reaction should be given appropriate weight in the therapeutic decision-making process and, in particular, should be balanced against the fact that, perhaps, apart from the treatment of syphilis in the pregnant woman, there are no infectious diseases for which penicillins are absolutely the only effective antibacterial available. If it is decided to administer penicillins to a person with a history of a hypersensitivity reaction, skin testing is advised to identify those with severe hypersensitivity. Testing should be done with major and minor determinant mixtures.[16,17] The reagents themselves appear safe: 1% of patients with a history of penicillin allergy developed reactions to the skin test reagents, mostly urticaria. Negative results of skin testing with both preparations have a high negative predictive value in individuals despite a history of penicillin allergy. Ninety-seven percent to 99% did not experience any reaction on administration of penicillin. However, two (22%) of nine patients with positive skin tests to major or minor determinant mixture given penicillin experienced reactions compatible with IgE-mediated or accelerated penicillin allergy, indicating the positive predictive value of such testing.

Even if no reaction to a skin test reagent is observed, it is prudent to administer the first dose with epinephrine and resuscitation equipment at hand and to inject only a fraction of the initial dose. If none occurs after 15 to 30 min, the remainder of the initial dose may be administered. If a reaction occurs during skin testing, penicillin should, in general, be avoided, although in selected cases consultation with a clinical immunologist to effect desensitization may be appropriate.

Rashes caused by ampicillin should be distinguished from those caused by other penicillins. The rashes occur in 7% to 8% of patients, an incidence three times greater than with all other penicillins, and are not considered to be immunologically mediated. Certain patients are more prone to experience ampicillin-induced skin reactions: females, hyperuricemic patients receiving allopurinol, individuals with acute mononucleosis caused by Epstein-Barr virus (EBV) or cytomegalovirus (CMV), and those with lymphocytic leukemia, reticulosarcoma, and other lymphomas. The rashes typically are morbilliform, appear 4 to 5 days after initiation of therapy, are not accompanied by other signs of allergy, and usually subside during continued therapy. Skin testing with ampicillin and major and minor penicillin determinants will be negative. Such rashes should not be considered a contraindication to subsequent therapy with one of the other penicillins.

A few adverse reactions to penicillins are neither immunologically mediated nor dose related. Neutropenia occurs in about 15% of patients treated with methicillin and somewhat less commonly with other penicillins. Neutropenia generally occurs 10 to 20 days after initiation of therapy and resolves rapidly on discontinuation of therapy. Reversible thrombocytopenia and bone marrow suppression have also been described in patients receiving penicillins. Hypokalemia has been described in up to 81% of patients without significant renal dysfunction who were treated with methicillin or carbenicillin. The mechanism of this ADR is unclear. Although these two penicillins likely behave like a nonabsorbable anion in the distal renal tubule, increasing passive potassium urinary excretion, some have proposed that the hypokalemia may instead be caused by an intracellular shift of potassium because of a membrane-altering effect.

Four dose-related side effects of the penicillins are uncommon but may be clinically important. First, undesirable augmentation of body sodium or potassium content can occur in patients with salt and water overload (e.g., congestive heart failure or renal failure) who are treated with large doses of penicillins because the penicillins are formulated for injection as salts of one of these cations (Table 45-6).

Second, penicillins may cause neurotoxic effects including seizures. This is related to an innate pharmacologic effect of the molecule and, hence, to the concentration of drug in the body. Penicillin G is the most inherently epileptogenic of the group. Seizures usually will be seen only in patients with impaired renal function given large doses. Impairment of the blood-brain barrier due to meningeal inflammation, uremia, and cardiopulmonary bypass may contribute to the effect, as may hyponatremia or concomitant probenecid therapy that

blocks penicillin excretion from the CSF. Neurotoxicity will progress from muscular irritability with choreiform, involuntary twitching, or myoclonic jerking to a depressed level of consciousness and, ultimately, seizures, unless penicillin administration is halted. Penicillin concentrations in lumbar sac CSF in excess of 5 mg/L have been associated with seizures,[18] but the critical concentration in the CSF contiguous with cortical neurons has not been described. This toxic effect of penicillins will resolve with discontinuation of therapy and elimination of penicillin. Unfortunately, in those most predisposed to this ADR (patients with severe renal failure),[19] penicillin clearance will be slower than in those with normal renal function.

A third dose-related side effect of penicillins is impaired platelet aggregation that may lead to clinically important bleeding. Ticarcillin is the most potent in this regard, although piperacillin, mezlocillin, and penicillin G can induce this defect.[20] The effect is caused by a concentration-dependent blocking of receptor sites on platelet membranes, thereby interfering with adenosine-induced aggregation. The defect may persist for up to 12 days after drug discontinuation, suggesting an effect on megakaryocytes and circulating platelets. Impaired platelet aggregation can be avoided by limiting dose size and avoiding these agents in patients with conditions predisposing to hemorrhage, such as thrombocytopenia or severe hepatic dysfunction.

A fourth category of ADR caused by penicillin is that related to suppression of endogenous bacterial flora. The most important example is *Clostridium difficile* toxin-induced pseudomembranous colitis or diarrhea. As a group, the penicillins (and cephalosporins) rank close behind clindamycin as the most common antibacterials causing this undesirable and potentially life-threatening complication.

CEPHALOSPORINS

The cephalosporins resemble the penicillins structurally and in their mode of action, versatility, and general lack of toxicity. They possess a β-lactam structure in which the thiazolidine ring characteristic of penicillins is replaced by a six-member dihydrothiazine ring. Modification in the side chains at the 3 and 7 positions of the nucleus has yielded molecules with different pharmacokinetic and pharmacodynamic characteristics, respectively.[21] Side chain modifications at position 7 alter and extend the spectrum of antibacterial activity but, in some cases, also cause unusual adverse pharmacologic effects such as inhibition of vitamin K–dependent hepatocyte synthesis of clotting factors II, VII, IX, and X and induction of reactions to disulfiram (Antabuse) in individuals ingesting or being treated with alcohol concurrently.

The potency of third-generation cephalosporins against a wide range of clinically important bacteria and a general lack of serious toxicity have led to an emerging consensus that certain members of this group are drugs of first choice for a number of severe bacterial infections, especially nosocomial ones, including meningitis, pneumonitis, bacteremia, and urinary tract infections.[22] This is particularly true for infection caused by increasingly resistant organisms and for initial, empirical therapy in the ICU setting. The first- and second-generation cephalosporins, however, are not drugs of first choice for any acute life-threatening infectious disease that might be seen in ICU patients, although they continue to be important first-line

TABLE 45-6 Cation Content of Some Penicillins

	Sodium Content
Penicillin G[a]	2 mEq/million units
Ampicillin	2.6 mEq/g
Cloxacillin	2.3 mEq/g
Nafcillin	2.9 mEq/g
Ticarcillin	5.9 mEq/g
Piperacillin	2.0 mEq/g
Mezlocillin	1.9 mEq/g

[a] Potassium penicillin G has a sodium content of 1.7 mEq/million units.

drugs for a variety of less severe infections such as cellulitis and community-acquired pneumonia.

MECHANISM OF ACTION The mechanism of action of the cephalosporins is identical to that of the penicillins and involves binding to, and inactivation of, PBPs in the inner aspect of the cell wall of susceptible bacteria.

MECHANISM OF RESISTANCE Resistance to cephalosporin antibiotics is also mediated by mechanisms that confer resistance to penicillins. Cephalosporins may not penetrate through the lipopolysaccharide cell wall to the site of the PBPs. The cephalosporin may be inactivated by β-lactamase. Substantial evidence indicates that exposure to some third-generation cephalosporins may induce synthesis of large amounts of β-lactamase with high affinity for the cephalosporins. As a result, the antibiotic is avidly bound by the enzyme and unable to interact with PBPs.[23] This is hypothesized to be the mechanism of resistance observed in *Enterobacter, Serratia, Citrobacter,* and *Pseudomonas* species exposed to third-generation cephalosporins.

CLASSIFICATION Cephalosporins are arbitrarily classified as belonging to one of three generations. This classification is based solely on the spectrum of antibacterial activity. None of the cephalosporins is useful for infections caused by *Streptococcus faecalis* or methicillin-resistant *Staphylococcus epidermidis* and *S. aureus* (MRSA). However, cephalosporins are useful antibacterials for treatment of a wide range of infections and for surgical prophylaxis (Table 45-1).

The *first-generation cephalosporins* are potent inhibitors of aerobic gram-positive cocci such as *S. aureus* and *S. pneumoniae*, with moderate activity against a limited number of aerobic gram-negative bacilli including *Escherichia coli, Klebsiella pneumoniae,* and indole-negative proteus. They are active against some anaerobic gram-positive and gram-negative oropharyngeal organisms, as is penicillin G, but are not consistently effective against *B. fragilis* group and other fecal anaerobic organisms. Cefazolin is the prototypical agent of this group, which contains the most active cephalosporins against susceptible aerobic gram-positive cocci.

The *second-generation cephalosporins* as a group exhibit enhanced potency against *E. coli, K. pneumoniae,* and indole-negative proteus, compared with first-generation agents. Individual members of this class have clinically important antibacterial activity against β-lactamase–producing *H. influenzae* (cefamandole, cefuroxime, and cefotetan), *B. fragilis* group organisms (cefoxitin, cefotetan), *Neisseria meningitidis* and *N. gonorrhoeae,* and some species of enteric gram-negative bacilli. However, activity against the last group of organisms is sufficiently variable so that it is more appropriate to initially prescribe a third-generation cephalosporin, aminoglycoside, or perhaps fluoroquinolone. The extended spectrum of some of these second-generation agents has made them drugs of importance, albeit not first choice, in some serious infections: mixed aerobic and anaerobic pulmonary, gastrointestinal, genital tract, and skin and soft tissue infections, such as aspiration pneumonia, intra-abdominal and pelvic peritonitis, pelvic inflammatory disease, and diabetic foot infection (cefoxitin), respectively. For pneumonia caused by an exacerbation of chronic bronchitis, cefuroxime is commonly prescribed.

The *third-generation cephalosporins* are particularly noteworthy for their potency against aerobic gram-negative bacilli, which they inhibit in concentrations 10 to 100 times less than required for aminoglycosides. These cephalosporins inhibit a wide range of this group of bacteria that are resistant to first- and second-generation cephalosporins, extended-spectrum penicillins, and aminoglycosides. The lack of inherent toxicity of third-generation cephalosporins is another advantage in treating ICU patients with multisystem dysfunction, especially renal failure. Two of the third-generation cephalosporins, cefoperazone and, particularly, ceftazidime, have clinically useful activity against most strains of *P. aeruginosa,* although susceptibility may differ substantially across institutions. Third-generation cephalosporins are not more resistant to penicillinase produced by *S. aureus,* nor are they more active against this organism than are the penicillinase-resistant penicillins or first-generation cephalosporins, which are preferred for therapy of such infections.

Recommended intravenous doses of selected cephalosporins for adult patients with moderate to severe infection and normal or impaired renal function or undergoing dialysis are presented in Table 45-7.

CLINICAL PHARMACOLOGY Like the penicillins, the cephalosporins are variably bound to plasma proteins; the range is 15% (cephalexin) to 84% (cefazolin) with AVDs of 0.10 (cefoxitin) to 0.30 (cefuroxime) L/kg. These characteristics are independent of the generation to which the agent belongs. They differ from the penicillin group pharmacokinetically:

1. Hepatic biotransformation is a significant route of elimination for some members of this group. Moreover, cefotaxime hepatic biotransformation yields metabolites with antibacterial activity that contribute to the overall antibacterial effect, although their precise contribution is unclear.
2. Some have prolonged plasma $t_{1/2}$ in patients with normal renal function. For example, the extended plasma $t_{1/2}$ of 8 hours for ceftriaxone has made once- to twice-daily dosing feasible without a loss in efficacy.
3. The third-generation drugs readily cross the blood-brain barrier. Therefore, unlike the first- and second-generation cephalosporins, the third-generation ones predictably attain therapeutic concentrations in the CSF and are efficacious for treatment of meningitis. However, therapeutic concentrations of cephalosporins are attained in the vitreous and aqueous humors of the eye only by sub-Tenon or intraocular injection or topical administration of antibiotic, respectively.

Probenecid inhibits renal proximal tubule secretion of cephalosporins just as for penicillins. Moderate to severe renal dysfunction necessitates reduction in the doses of some of the cephalosporins (see Table 45-7). Hemodialysis or peritoneal dialysis may remove sufficient drug (see Table 45-7) to necessitate additional postdialysis doses. Only cefoperazone doses must be reduced in patients with moderate to severe hepatic dysfunction.

ADVERSE DRUG REACTIONS Hypersensitivity reactions to the cephalosporins qualitatively similar to those produced

TABLE 45-7 Recommended Intravenous Doses of Selected Cephalosporins for Adult Patients with Moderate to Severe Infection and Normal or Impaired Renal Function or Undergoing Dialysis

	CREATININE CLEARANCE (mL/min)				DOSE WITH END-STAGE RENAL FAILURE	
	>60	40–59	10–39	<10	Peritoneal Dialysis	Hemodialysis
First generation						
Cefazolin	0.5–2 g q 8 h	0.5 g initially, then 0.5–2 g q 12 h	0.5 g initially, then 0.25–1 g q 24 h	0.5 g initially, then 0.1–0.5 g q 24 h	As for creatinine clearance <10 mL/min	As for creatinine clearance <10 mL/min plus 0.25 g after dialysis
Second generation						
Cefuroxime	0.75–1.5 g q 8 h	No change	0.75–1.5 g q 12 h	0.75 g q 24 h	0.75 g q 24 h	0.75 g after each dialysis and each 24 h
Cefoxitin	1–2 g q 6–8 h	Same dose at interval of 8–12 h	Same dose at interval of 12–24 h	Same dose at interval of 24–36 h	As for creatinine clearance <10 mL/min	1–2 g after each dialysis and each 72 h
Third generation						
Ceftriaxone	1–4 g q 24 h	No change	No change	No change	No change	1 g q 24 h
Cefotaxime	0.5–2 g q 4–8 h	No change	0.5–2 g q 12–24 h	0.5–2 g q 24 h	As for creatinine clearance <10 mL/min	As for creatinine clearance <10 mL/min plus 0.5–2 g after each dialysis
Ceftazidime	0.5–2 g q 8 h	0.5–1.5 g q 12 h	0.5–1.5 g q 24 h	0.5–1 g q 48 h	0.5 g q 24 h	0.25–0.5 g q 24 h plus 0.5–1 g after dialysis
Cefoperazone	0.5–2 g q 6–12 h	No change	No change	No change	No change	No change

by penicillins are the most common adverse effects.[15] They are no more common with any single cephalosporin or generation of cephalosporins and likely are related to the shared bicyclic nuclear structure. However, cephalosporins lose both their ring structures when exposed to β-lactamases, in contrast to penicillin degradation. Thus, molecules unique to cephalosporins that may function as haptens are generated. This probably accounts for the lack of predictable cross-allergenicity between penicillins and cephalosporins. Haptenic activity of acyl side chains at position 7 of the β-lactam ring further complicates the predicting of reactions induced by cephalosporins in individuals with a history of penicillin intolerance. Cross-reactions do occur in penicillin-sensitive patients treated with cephalosporins.[24] However, the frequency of such cross-reactions is minimally, if at all, increased in patients with penicillin allergy. Nevertheless, a history of penicillin allergy of the immediate or accelerated type precludes use of cephalosporins. No established testing methods identify cephalosporin allergy.

Dose-related side effects of cephalosporins are generally less marked than those induced by penicillins. The likelihood of cation overloading even with large doses of cephalosporins is small. Although they are mostly sodium salts containing up to 3.6 mEq Na^1/g (Ceftriaxone), the total sodium load administered even with very large doses is unlikely to be clinically important except in rare patients with severe sodium and water overload. The epileptogenic potential of the cephalosporins is less than that of the penicillins. All cephalosporins in high concentration except cephaloridine are similar to penicillins in interfering with platelet aggregation.

Modifications induced by altering the side chain on the dihydrothiazine ring at position 3 have yielded cephalosporins with unusual pharmacologic side effects: cefamandole, cefoperazone, cefotetan, and moxalactam have a methyltetrazolethiol side chain that provokes a disulfiram-like reaction in patients ingesting or receiving ethanol. Inhibition of hepatic aldehyde dehydrogenase with accumulation of acetaldehyde during metabolism of alcohol is the presumed mechanism. These four agents may also predispose the patient to bleeding because of interference with synthesis of vitamin K–dependent clotting factors[25] in addition to their inhibition of platelet aggregation. Bleeding may only occur in patients whose oral intake of vitamin K and synthesis of endogenous vitamin K by colonic flora are impaired concomitantly. As a consequence, cefamandole, cefoperazone, and moxalactam are no longer widely used.

Superinfections are surprisingly uncommon given the wide antibacterial spectrum of third-generation cephalosporins, with occurrences from 1% of cefotaxime recipients up to 3% to 5% for cefoperazone-treated patients.[26] Superinfections in patients treated with moxalactam have been observed to frequently be caused by *S. faecalis*. Otherwise, superinfection caused by resistant aerobic enteric gram-negative bacilli, *Clostridia* species, and yeast has been the most common.

Adverse effects of cephalosporins on the kidney are rare with two exceptions: cephaloridine in doses of 4 to 6 g/d causes acute tubular necrosis, and cephalothin appears to enhance the nephrotoxic effect (but not vestibular or cochlear toxic effects) of gentamicin and tobramycin.

OTHER β-LACTAM DRUGS

Carbapenems and monobactams are two new classes of β-lactam antibiotics of importance to intensivists (Table 45-8).

TABLE 45-8 Recommended Intravenous Doses of Selected Carbapenems, Monobactams, and Combinations of a β-Lactam Antibiotic with a β-Lactam Inhibitor for Adult Patients with Moderate to Severe Infection and Normal or Impaired Renal Function or Requiring Dialysis

	CREATININE CLEARANCE (mL/min)				DOSE WITH END-STAGE RENAL FAILURE	
	>60	40–59	10–39	<10	Peritoneal Dialysis	Hemodialysis
Carbapenem						
Imipenem	0.25–1 g q 6 h	No change	0.5 q 8–12 h	0.25 g q 12 h	0.25 g q 12 h	As for creatinine clearance <10 mL/min plus 0.5 g after dialysis
Meropenem	1 g q 8 h	No change	0.5 g q 12 h	0.5 g q 24 h	0.5 g q 24 h	As for creatinine clearance <10 mL/min plus dose after dialysis
Ertapenem	1.0 g q 24 h	1.0 g q 24 h	0.5 g q 24 h	0.5 g q 24 h	?	0.5 g q 24 h; if dosed <6 h before dialysis, give 150 mg after dialysis
Monobactam						
Aztreonam	1–2 g q 6–12 h	0.75–1.5 g q 6–12 h	0.5–1 g q 6–12 h	0.25–0.5 g q 6–12 h	?	?
β-Lactamase inhibitor plus β-lactam antibiotic						
Ticarcillin clavulanate	3 g/0.1 g q 3–6 h	3 g/0.1 g q 6 h	3 g/0.1 g q 12 h	2.0 g/0.1 g q 24 h	3 g/0.1 g q 2 h	2 g/0.1 g q 24 h plus 3 g/0.1 g after dialysis
Piperacillin/tazobactam	3 g/0.375 g q 6 h	No change	3 g/0.375 g q 8 h	3 g/0.375 g q 12 h	?	As for creatinine clearance <10 ml/min plus 0.75 g/.094 g after dialysis

ª Use the 3 g/10.1 g combination for kidney infection.

CARBAPENEMS

Carbapenems possess novel stereochemical characteristics that distinguish them from the other bicyclic β-lactams, the penicillins, and cephalosporins. Imipenem, meropenem, and ertapenem are currently licensed carbapenems.

Imipenem and meropenem have the widest spectrum of any β-lactam antibiotic studied to date. They are potent inhibitors of nearly all common bacterial pathogens, including those resistant to aminoglycosides and newer cephalosporins, in concentrations as low as, or lower than, any other β-lactams. Imipenem binds primarily to PBP-2 and is not hydrolyzed by most β-lactamases, penicillinases, or cephalosporinases. The wide spectrum of activity appears to be related to the ability of this relatively compact β-lactam molecule to diffuse readily through porin channels of gram-negative enteric bacilli, in addition to the β-lactamase resistance conferred on the molecule by the unusual transconformation related to the hydroxyethyl side chain. Tolerance is not observed when bacteria are exposed to imipenem (i.e., there is no major discrepancy between inhibitory and bactericidal concentrations), and, unique among β-lactams, imipenem exerts a marked PAE on gram-positive and gram-negative bacteria. Imipenem inhibits gram-positive cocci other than *E. faecium* and MRSA, most *Enterobacteriaceae*, and gram-negative bacilli including *P. aeruginosa* but excluding most *Pseudomonas cepacia* and *S. maltophilia* strains, and all oral and most fecal anaerobic bacteria. There is no cross-resistance between imipenem and other β-lactams.

Meropenem differs from imipenem in possessing slightly greater activity against gram-negative bacteria due to more rapid penetration through the cell wall. Thus, it inhibits some *P. aeruginosa* strains resistant to imipenem.[27]

Ertapenem has a narrower spectrum of activity than does imipenem or meropenem. It is more similar to meropenem than to imipenem against *Enterbacteriaceae* including most anaerobes. However, unlike imipenem and meropenem, it possesses no activity against *P. aeruginosa* or *Acinetobacter* species.[28]

The place of the carbapenems in the therapy of infection in ICU patients continues to evolve. Clinical experience suggests that meropenem and imipenem are therapeutically equivalent.[29] For treatment of lower respiratory tract infection in patients in the ICU, meropenem is more effective than ceftazidime.[30] Ertapenem has been demonstrated to be comparable to piperacillin/tazobactam in patients with intra-abdominal, skin and skin structure, and pelvic infections;[31] its efficacy compared with imipenem and meropenem has not been described. For treatment of patients with meningitis, meropenem is the carbapenem of choice (imipenem use is associated with a significant risk of seizures and ertapenem has not been studied in patients with meningitis).

Overall, imipenem and meropenem are appropriate as monotherapy for treatment of serious nosocomial and community-acquired infections due to aerobic and/or anaerobic bacteria. Ertapenem may be as efficacious, but data are not available to support that conclusion and ertapenem should not be administered where *P. aeruginosa* is a probable or proven cause of infection. In general, they are appropriate for indications such as those for which extended-spectrum cephalosporins would be used. As monotherapy, they are probably as effective as clindamycin combined with an aminoglycoside for treatment of seriously ill patients with intra-abdominal infections.[32] Imipenem and meropenem should not be used as monotherapy of *P. aeruginosa* infections because of the risk of resistance, and ertapenem should not be used at all. The greatest value of the carbapenems may be that their broad spectrum permits their use conveniently in place of multiple-drug regimens for polymicrobial infections, with an attendant reduction in the risk of adverse reactions. Recommended intravenous doses of the carbapenems for adult patients with moderate to severe infections and variable renal function are listed in Table 45-8.

CLINICAL PHARMACOLOGY The carbapenems are not absorbed after oral administration and therefore are available only in parenteral formulations. Imipenem and meropenem are only 2% to 20% protein bound, whereas ertapenem is highly bound. They penetrate into a wide variety of tissues and brain cells but poorly into other cells. These characteristics make them unsuitable for treatment of infections caused by bacteria that are primarily intracellular pathogens and may account in part for the epileptogenic potential of imipenem in particular.

The carbapenems are eliminated from plasma by a first-order process primarily by glomerular filtration, with a mean $t_{1/2}$ of 1 hour for imipenem and meropenem; the $t_{1/2}$ for ertapenem is 4 hours, due in part to its high protein binding. Renal tubular secretion is minimal.

Renal handling of filtered carbapenems differs markedly. Imipenem is remarkably stable to bacterial β-lactamase but its β-lactam ring structure is susceptible to metabolic degradation in humans, primarily by peptidases in the brush border of renal tubular epithelial cells. Inhibition of these enzymes (by cilastatin, see below) increases urinary recovery of undegraded imipenem from 7% to 38% up to 70% to 85%. Meropenem and ertapenem are not degraded by renal tubular peptidase and, unlike imipenem, therefore are formulated without cilastatin.

Like cephaloridine, imipenem is toxic to proximal renal tubule epithelial cells. The toxic moiety appears to be a hydrolysis product, the formation of which can be safely blocked by coadministration of cilastatin, which inhibits the catalytic effect of dehydropeptidase I in the brush border and completely eliminates renal tubular damage without affecting the plasma $t_{1/2}$ of imipenem. A ratio of 1:1 for imipenem to cilastatin is optimal, and imipenem is marketed in this fixed combination.[33]

ADVERSE DRUG REACTIONS The carbapenems are generally well tolerated, like other β-lactams. Major adverse effects such as diarrhea, superinfection, or pseudomembranous colitis are infrequent. Allergic reactions, including rashes and drug fever, occur in 2% to 3% of subjects, and cross-allergenicity to penicillins has been observed. The relatively high incidence of seizures, 0.2% in series of patients treated with imipenem,[34] is unique among β-lactam antibiotics and also not seen with meropenem or ertapenem. Pre-existing central nervous system (CNS) disease, advanced age, and renal insufficiency predispose patients to this serious but reversible side effect.

Seizures ought to be preventable by appropriate dose reductions in patients with renal disease, a maneuver of particular importance in patients with CNS disease.

MONOBACTAMS

Aztreonam is the first marketed member of a new completely synthetic class of monocyclic β-lactam antibiotics called *monobactams*. Aztreonam has no clinically important activity against gram-positive or anaerobic bacteria because of failure to bind to PBPs of these organisms. Aztreonam binds primarily to PBP 3 in *Enterbacteriaceae*, *P. aeruginosa*, and other gram-negative aerobic bacteria and, hence, has a bactericidal effect; its narrow spectrum of activity most resembles that of the aminoglycosides. When combined with other β-lactam antibiotics to treat gram-negative aerobic bacterial infections, the net effect is unpredictable. Aztreonam is more predictably synergistic, or at least additive, with aminoglycosides.[35] Lack of susceptibility is caused by failure of aztreonam to cross the outer cell wall and failure to bind to PBPs. Aztreonam is stable in the presence of a wide variety of β lactamases,[36] so inactivation by this process is less important as a mechanism of bacterial resistance than for other β-lactam antibacterial agents.

The exact niche of aztreonam in the treatment of gram-negative aerobic bacterial infections in ICU patients is unclear at present. The most logical, albeit rare, circumstance for which it could be used would be in treating patients with significant allergy to β-lactam antibiotics (see below) in whom its combination with another agent, such as an aminoglycoside to obtain a synergistic or additive effect, is deemed necessary. Aztreonam also may be used alone in such patients if an aminoglycoside is considered contraindicated, but its relative utility compared with aminoglycosides and other alternatives such as fluoroquinolones and trimethoprim-sulfamethoxazole (TMP-SMX) has not been evaluated in controlled trials.

CLINICAL PHARMACOLOGY Aztreonam is poorly absorbed after enteral administration because of intragastric hydrolysis and, hence, must be administered intramuscularly or intravenously. After such injection, aztreonam distributes widely and achieves therapeutic concentrations in all body tissues and fluids except perhaps the vitreous humor. Metabolism has a minimal effect on aztreonam clearance. Aztreonam is eliminated primarily by renal filtration and tubular secretion, but some excretion in bile into the gut occurs.[37] Elimination is a first-order process with a plasma $t_{1/2}$ of 1.7 hours that is inversely related to glomerular filtration rate and increases to 6 hours in anephric patients. The usual dose, 1 to 2 g every 6 to 12 hours (maximum, 8 g/d), should be reduced in patients with renal insufficiency. The drug is removed by hemodialysis and peritoneal dialysis, but alternative schedules for such patients (see Table 45-8) have not been established.

ADVERSE DRUG REACTIONS Aztreonam shares the general safety profile of other β-lactam antibiotics. Up to 7% of patients experience rash, diarrhea, nausea, or vomiting, and isolated elevations of serum transaminase concentrations. Aztreonam is unique among β-lactams in being weakly immunogenic and not cross-allergenic with other penicillins or cephalosporins.[15] Aztreonam has been administered safely to penicillin-allergic patients, including those with positive skin test results. This unique property appears to result from the fact that aztreonam lacks the allergenic bicyclic nuclear structure of penicillins, cephalosporins, and carbapenem β-lactam antibiotics.

β-LACTAMASE INHIBITORS

Clavulanate, sulbactam, and tazobactam are β-lactam compounds that possess weak, insignificant antibacterial activity but are clinically useful because they extend the spectrum of activity of many β-lactam antibiotics by inhibiting β-lactamases. The three compounds differ in their potency and the range of lactamases they inhibit.[38] Tazobactam inhibits a wider range of plasmid- and chromosome-encoded lactamases than clavulanate and sulbactam. This fact and the greater intrinsic antibacterial effect of piperacillin in comparison with ticarcillin or amoxicillin/ampicillin account for the wider antibacterial spectrum and greater potency of piperacillin-tazobactam than the other two combinations of drugs. Thus, although injectable formulations of ampicillin-sulbactam and ticarcillin-clavulanate exist, piperacillin-tazobactam has largely supplanted the other two compounds. Moreover, the combination of tazobactam with piperacillin makes the combination an effective inhibitor of MSSA, thereby converting piperacillin into a broad-spectrum antimicrobial with attendant added utility for ICU patients.

The efficacy and safety of piperacillin-tazobactam compared with standard therapy has been demonstrated in controlled trials of patients with intra-abdominal infection, postpartum endometritis or pelvic inflammatory disease, community-acquired pneumonia, and skin and skin-structure infections.[39,40] The usual dose is 3 g piperacillin with 375 mg tazobactam every 6 hours, but for patients seriously ill with proven or suspected *Pseudomonas* species infection, 4 g plus 500 mg for every 4 hours with another drug is recommended. Studies suggest that piperacillin-tazobactam combined with amikacin is more efficacious (61% efficacy) than ceftazidime with amikacin (54%) for treatment for febrile episodes in neutropenic cancer patients.[41]

The value of piperacillin-tazobactam compared with piperacillin alone for treatment of serious infection caused by *Pseudomonas* species is unclear[39] because most lactamase-mediated resistance of *Pseudomonas* species is a result of the production of inhibitor-insusceptible enzymes. Therefore, for the treatment of serious *Pseudomonas* infections, Sanders and Sanders recommend piperacillin-tazobactam (4 g/0.5 g) every 4 hours with an additional agent such as an aminoglycoside.[39]

CLINICAL PHARMACOLOGY Clavulanate, sulbactam, and tazobactam share many clinical pharmacologic characteristics common to β-lactam antibiotics. Only the characteristics of tazobactam combined with piperacillin are discussed here; the characteristics of amoxicillin-clavulanate,[42] ampicillin-sulbactam,[43] and ticarcillin-clavulanate[44] have been reviewed elsewhere.

When piperacillin and tazobactam are administered together in a ratio of 8:1, the pharmacokinetic activities of piperacillin are unaffected. However, the pharmacokinetic characteristics of tazobactam are significantly affected, largely owing to competitive inhibition of renal proximal tubular secretion of tazobactam by the much larger quantity of piperacillin. When the peak plasma concentration of tazobactam was increased by about 30% and the plasma $t_{1/2}$ by about 100% from a mean of 0.45 to 0.94 hours, renal clearance was reduced approximately 25%.[45]

Piperacillin and tazobactam are eliminated primarily into urine by glomerular filtration and tubular secretion. Less than 1% of piperacillin and no tazobactam are secreted into bile. In patients with renal impairment, the renal clearances of piperacillin and tazobactam are proportionately reduced. Dose reductions are recommended for patients with creatinine clearances lower than 40 mL/min (see Table 45-8). Hemodialysis removes approximately 35% of piperacillin-tazobactam and peritoneal dialysis removes approximately 20% of piperacillin-tazobactam. Hence, the supplementary doses recommended after the two types of dialysis are different (see Table 45-8).

In patients with hepatic cirrhosis, the elimination $t_{1/2}$ of piperacillin and tazobactam increases by about 20%, but no dose reductions are recommended in such patients.

ADVERSE DRUG REACTIONS Adverse effects of piperacillin-tazobactam have been generally mild to moderate in severity.[34] Gastrointestinal complaints, mostly diarrhea, were noted in 4.6% of patients, but with a range from 0% to 32%; skin rash occurred in 0% to 12% of subjects. In their review, Sanders and Sanders concluded that, overall, the rates and character of adverse reactions are comparable to, or less than, those reported for piperacillin alone, ticarcillin-clavulanate, ampicillin-sulbactam, and imipenem-cilastin.[39]

AMINOGLYCOSIDE ANTIBIOTICS

One or more of the aminoglycoside antibiotics (streptomycin, kanamycin, gentamicin, tobramycin, netilmicin, amikacin, and neomycin) has been a mainstay of our antibacterial armamentarium since the discovery of streptomycin in 1943. Streptomycin currently is limited to use in the combination therapy of tuberculosis and for treatment of *Francisella*, *Yersinia pestis* infection, and brucellosis. Neomycin is too toxic for systemic use but is still administered orally for the treatment of portosystemic encephalopathy (see Chaps. 83 and 84). The remaining agents—kanamycin, gentamicin, tobramycin, netilmicin, and amikacin—are first-line drugs for the treatment of serious infection caused by *Enterobacteriaceae* and *Pseudomonas* and *Serratia* species. The importance of these bacterial species as causes of nosocomial infection has progressively increased in the antibacterial era, and the importance of the aminoglycosides has increased in parallel. Kanamycin utility has been limited by widespread resistance among many *Enterobacteriaceae* and innate inefficacy against *P. aeruginosa*. Gentamicin, tobramycin, amikacin, and netilmicin share similar spectra of activity with the following caveats. Tobramycin is twice as potent as gentamicin or netilmicin in inhibiting *P. aeruginosa* in vitro, although the clinical relevance of this superiority is not clear. Netilmicin is the most potent inhibitor of *S. epidermidis*. Amikacin is the most resistant to aminoglycoside-inactivating enzymes. As a result, many enteric bacilli resistant to kanamycin, gentamicin, and netilmicin remain susceptible to amikacin.

Unfortunately, the utility of these agents in the therapy of patients with significant infection in the ICU has been limited by their inherent toxic effects on the proximal tubule epithelial cells of the kidney and the hair cells of the cochlea, saccule, and utricle and by the emergence of resistance.

MECHANISMS OF ACTION   The aminoglycosides are rapidly bactericidal in contrast to β-lactam antibacterial drugs, which cause bacterial cell death only after a lag period.[9] Although their mode of action has been extensively studied,[46] the precise mechanism(s) of their lethal effect remains unclear. It is generally accepted that aminoglycosides interfere with bacterial protein synthesis by binding to the 30S subunit of bacterial ribosomes, resulting in misreading of mRNA codons and synthesis of faulty bacterial proteins, but the resulting alterations in protein molecules are not considered sufficient by themselves to cause cell death. Aminoglycoside uptake by bacteria depends in part on energy derived from aerobic metabolism. Thus, all of these agents are inactive under anaerobic conditions. In vitro, aminoglycosides cause bacterial cell death in a concentration-dependent manner,[47] and this effect is little affected by inoculum size.[48] This pharmacologic effect underlies, in part, the attractiveness of once-daily aminoglycoside dosing to attain greater efficacy (and less toxicity) than is achieved with multiple doses each day. Moreover, these agents consistently produce a concentration- and time-dependent PAE on gram-positive and gram-negative aerobic bacteria.[49] The PAE persists longer (usually longer than 3 hours) for gram-negative aerobic bacilli than for gram-positive aerobic bacteria (usually less than 2 hours). The mechanism of the PAE of aminoglycosides is likely related to the time required for organisms to resynthesize proteins essential for replication.

MECHANISMS OF RESISTANCE   Aminoglycoside resistance of aerobic organisms is mediated primarily by aminoglycoside-inactivating enzymes.[50] Less commonly, ribosomal mutation and diminished permeability of bacterial cells to aminoglycoside molecules account for resistance. Different enzymes may acetylate, adenylate, or phosphorylate aminoglycosides and, by these changes, preclude binding of the drug to ribosomes. The aminoglycosides differ considerably in their susceptibility to enzymatic modification. For example, gentamicin is susceptible to modification by at least five different enzymes elaborated by gram-negative bacilli, but amikacin is susceptible only to an acetyltransferase found in some *P. aeruginosa* and *Acinetobacter* species strains. The genes encoding aminoglycoside-modifying enzymes are most commonly acquired on plasmids. This usually occurs in the setting of heavy and widespread use of these agents (antibiotic selection pressure).[50] As a result, gentamicin resistance emerging under antibiotic selection pressure in institutions is more common than resistance of bacteria to amikacin; resistance of bacteria to tobramycin, netilmicin, and kanamycin is of intermediate prevalence. Although aminoglycoside resistance is to some extent a function of use, this association is not entirely predictable because other factors are probably involved.[52]

CLINICAL PHARMACOLOGY   The aminoglycosides are polycations whose polarity is responsible in part for many of their shared clinical pharmacokinetic characteristics. They are poorly absorbed after oral administration, have an AVD that is mathematically similar to the extracellular fluid volume, are excluded from the normal subarachnoid space, vitreous

humor, and prostatic fluid, and are eliminated almost exclusively by the kidney.[53]

After intramuscular administration, the aminoglycosides are rapidly and completely absorbed. Their AVD is equal to 25% to 30% of ideal body weight. The AVD is approximately 25% less in obese than in nonobese individuals and approximately 20% greater in patients with protein-calorie malnutrition. This information must be used to calculate the initial dose, which is a function of the desired plasma concentration multiplied by the AVD. For gentamicin, tobramycin, and netilmicin, the minimal inhibitory concentration (MIC) of most susceptible aerobic enteric gram-negative bacilli is 2 to 4 mg/L, and toxicity has been shown to increase at peak concentrations in excess of 10 mg/L. It is therefore conventional to prescribe an initial dose to attain a serum concentration (Cs) of 7 mg/L, which for a 70-kg adult would be 7 mg/kg $\times$ 70 kg $\times$ 0.25, or approximately 120 mg. For kanamycin and amikacin, for which desired Cs values are 25 to 30 mg/L, the initial dose, similarly calculated, would be 500 mg.

Aminoglycosides are actively concentrated in the endolymph of the cochlea, saccule, and utricle and in epithelial cells of the proximal renal tubule, a fact important in the production of aminoglycoside toxicity[54] (see below). Less than 1% of an injected dose appears in the feces and none in saliva.

Aminoglycosides are eliminated exclusively by glomerular filtration. An inverse relation exists between plasma $t_{1/2}$ and creatinine clearance as a measure of glomerular filtration rate. At creatinine clearance rates of 100 mL/min, the plasma $t_{1/2}$ averages 2 hours.[55] As the creatinine clearance declines, the plasma $t_{1/2}$ increases. In the presence of renal disease, it is possible to prescribe maintenance doses by repeating the initial dose at intervals equal to three times the estimated $t_{1/2}$ of the drug. However, it has been found to be more practical to maintain the interval at the conventional 8 or 12 hours but to reduce the dose administered proportionate to renal function (e.g., if estimated remaining renal function is 50% of normal, one can administer 50% of the dose at 8-hour intervals[51]); such a dose regimen will result in a lower peak plasma aminoglycoside concentration but in trough plasma concentrations comparable to those achieved by maintaining the dose (milligrams per kilogram) constant and increasing the dose interval. The efficacy and safety of these two approaches has not been compared in patients with renal insufficiency. Maderazo and colleagues confirmed the utility of the following formulas for adjusting the dosing regimen for aminoglycosides (and other drugs eliminated almost wholly by glomerular filtration).[56]

A. To reduce the dose and maintain the same interval as in a person with normal renal function, use this formula:

$$\text{reduced dose} = \frac{\text{creatine clearance}}{100} \times n, \text{ and}$$

B. To maintain the dose but decrease the dose frequency, use this formula:

$$\text{new dose interval} = \frac{100}{\text{creatine clearance}} \times u$$

where the creatinine clearance (milliliters per minute) is calculated from the formula of Cockcroft and Gault[57] and n represents dose (milligrams) and u represents the dose interval (hours) in a person with normal renal function.

If possible, it is preferable to use antibiotics other than aminoglycosides in patients with significant renal insufficiency. If aminoglycosides must be used, serum aminoglycoside measurements should be used to maximize efficacy and minimize toxicity (see below). The importance of serum aminoglycoside measurements is greater when renal function is fluctuating or when disease or other drugs may be affecting aminoglycoside disposition. For example, in burned and febrile patients, aminoglycoside pharmacokinetic characteristics are altered, and larger doses will be required. In patients with renal failure given aminoglycosides and penicillins in large doses, aminoglycosides are inactivated. The rate and extent of the inactivation depend on the concentration of the penicillin. Kanamycin, gentamicin, and tobramycin are most susceptible to inactivation in this manner, and amikacin the least with netilmicin of intermediate susceptibility.

The concentration in plasma (Cp)-versus-time curve after intravenous administration of an aminoglycoside dose is affected by the pre-existing Cp, the dose administered, and the method of administration (intramuscular or intravenous injection, bolus, or infusion and the rate of infusion). These variables particularly affect the time and magnitude of peak Cp. Trough Cp is less affected by these factors. This variability has made it more difficult to define the relation between post-dose aminoglycoside concentration and therapeutic effect than that between trough Cp and toxic effects. Although incontrovertible data do not exist, some data demonstrate that Cp measured 60 minutes after intramuscular or 15 minutes after an intravenous infusion of the aminoglycoside is related to efficacy. For gentamicin, a post-dose Cp of 8 mg/L or larger is associated with a better outcome than lower Cp in patients being treated for gram-negative aerobic bacillary pneumonia, whereas concentrations of at least 5 mg/L are associated with a better outcome in patients being treated for non-pneumonia, non-CNS, gram-negative aerobic bacillary infections.[58] It is assumed that the same relation holds for netilmicin and tobramycin. For amikacin and kanamycin, post-dose Cp values of 20 to 40 mg/L are desirable.

A direct relation between predose or trough aminoglycosides Cp and toxicity was first demonstrated in 1950 for streptomycin.[59] Trough Cp higher than 3 mg/L during once-daily intramuscular administration of streptomycin for therapy of tuberculosis was associated with an increased risk of dizziness, presumably owing to vestibulotoxicity. Old age was also a factor. At other times Cp values were much more variable, and often higher, but did not correlate with this toxic effect. Subsequent studies have suggested an increased risk of gentamicin nephrotoxicity, demonstrated by a rise in serum creatinine concentration, when trough gentamicin Cp exceeds 2 mg/L.[60] This interpretation is supported by studies in animals.

Compelling in vitro and correlative in vivo data provide strong support for the current practice of administering aminoglycosides intermittently rather than by constant infusion to optimize efficacy and minimize toxicity. Extrapolating further, some have argued for once-daily dosing in individuals with normal renal function.[49] These expectations are based on in vitro observations including a concentration-dependent aminoglycoside antibacterial effect over a wide range of concentrations beginning at the MIC and extending beyond tolerable serum concentrations in patients, and concentration-dependent PAE. Moreover, these observations have been supported by studies in animals with experimental infection and provide the rationale for dosing to achieve high aminoglycoside concentrations in plasma and at the site of infection. However, clinical trials comparing conventional multiple-daily doses with once-daily administration of aminoglycosides have demonstrated little or no advantage of this practice over traditional 8- or 12-hour administration in terms of efficacy or safety.[61,62] It may only be more convenient than dosing two or three times daily.

The methodologically best-designed controlled trials included almost exclusively immunocompetent adults with normal renal function; a few had mildly impaired renal function (serum creatinine <300 mmol/L).[63] Controversy exists concerning virtually all other aspects of the practice. This includes the question of whether it is appropriate to prescribe aminoglycosides once daily to infected patients with neutropenia, sepsis syndrome, and moderate to severe renal insufficiency.[64] Additional subgroups for whom few or no data are available to support once-daily aminoglycoside use include pediatric patients and patients with severe burns, endocarditis, pregnancy, or ascites. Moreover, uncertainty exists about optimal dose size[65] and the rationale for, and specifics of, serum aminoglycoside concentration measurement for monitoring.[66] Despite these limitations of the available data, as early as 1993, 19% of a random sample of 336 acute care hospitals in the United States reported that aminoglycosides were being prescribed once daily in their institutions, albeit with the anticipated variability in practice expected given the incomplete database.[67]

Until definitive data become available to guide the practice of once-daily administration of aminoglycosides, the following guidelines are recommended:

1. Restrict the practice to the prescription of netilmicin, gentamicin, tobramycin, and amikacin.
2. Once-daily administration is acceptable to treat adult patients with normal or mildly impaired renal function (serum creatinine <300 mmol/L or estimated creatinine clearance >30 mL/min). Patients should not be pregnant; endocarditis, neutropenia, severe burns, or sepsis and moderate or severe renal impairment are relative contraindications.
3. Doses: netilmicin 6 mg/kg; gentamicin and tobramycin 4 mg/kg; and amikacin 15 mg/kg.
4. Infuse the drug over 60 min, preferably by a pump, to permit interpretation of the peak serum concentration result as described by Moore and colleagues.[68]
5. Measure aminoglycoside Cp:
   A. To enhance efficacy, measure the Cp 60 minutes after the end of the infusion "peak."[68] If the peak Cp is below 5 mg/L for netilmicin, gentamicin, or tobramycin, increase the dose proportionately (e.g., if Cp = 4 mg/L, increase the dose by at least 20%).
   B. To minimize toxicity, measure the Cp just before the dose. If the Cp is above 2 mg/L for netilmicin, gentamicin, or tobramycin or above 10 mg/L for amikacin, reduce the dose proportionately.

6. Measure aminoglycoside Cp at the peak and trough every 3 days if renal function (serum creatinine concentration) is stable and more frequently if it is not.

ADVERSE DRUG REACTIONS All aminoglycosides share three dose-related, largely reversible toxic effects, although quantitative differences exist among members of this family. These are neuromuscular paralysis, nephrotoxicity, and cochleovestibular toxicity. The mechanisms of the unwanted effects are not well characterized, but an interaction of the cationic aminoglycoside molecule with calcium, magnesium, and membrane phospholipids[69] may be common to all. These effects of aminoglycosides are a result of their inherent pharmacologic properties occurring at doses close to those required for treatment. As such, the effects are not likely completely avoidable.

Neuromuscular paralysis of clinical consequence is likely to be seen only in patients receiving neuromuscular blocking drugs or with diseases such as botulism or myasthenia gravis. Aminoglycoside-induced skeletal muscle paralysis involves inhibition of acetylcholine release and blockage of acetylcholine receptors. The postsynaptic inhibitory effect is directly related to high concentrations of aminoglycoside at the neuromuscular end plate as seen when the antibiotic is injected rapidly as a bolus or when large quantities of aminoglycoside are administered and absorbed (e.g., by injection in the pleural or peritoneal cavity). The effect can be avoided by slow intravenous administration over 30 to 60 minutes or intramuscular injection and mitigated by calcium injection.

Aminoglycoside nephrotoxicity spans a wide spectrum, ranging from asymptomatic increased urinary excretion of renal tubular epithelial cell brush border enzymes to renal failure necessitating dialysis. In between is diminished creatinine clearance demonstrated by elevated serum creatinine concentration. Enzymuria is almost universally demonstrable in patients receiving therapeutic doses of aminoglycosides, whereas oliguric renal failure is rare. Elevated serum creatinine concentration is observed in 5% to 25% of treated patients.

The nephrotoxic effect is associated with accumulation of aminoglycoside in renal proximal tubule epithelial cells with resultant cell damage and, possibly, inhibition of synthesis of vasodilatory prostaglandins resulting in renal afferent arteriolar vasoconstriction and diminished glomerular filtration. Renal injury manifest as elevations in serum creatinine concentration usually occurs several days after initiation of therapy and is largely reversible because of epithelial cell regeneration. Animal and clinical studies have indicated that neomycin is the most nephrotoxic and amikacin the least nephrotoxic of currently used aminoglycosides. Gentamicin is more nephrotoxic than tobramycin.[70]

The nephrotoxic effect of aminoglycosides in animal studies is related directly to the height of the trough serum aminoglycoside concentration and the area under the serum concentration-time curve, which in turn are the important determinants of aminoglycoside uptake and sequestration in proximal tubule epithelial cells. This leads to the recommendation that trough serum aminoglycoside concentrations should be as low as possible.[61] For gentamicin, levels below 3 mg/L at trough are recommended.[62] Intuitively, the same level would seem to be appropriate for tobramycin and netilmicin, which have similar pharmacokinetic proper-

ties and antibacterial potency to gentamicin. The appropriate trough Cp for amikacin is 5 to 10 mg/L.

Additional risk factors for nephrotoxicity include older age, female sex, concomitant liver disease, hypotension, and concomitant drug therapy with cephalothin, cisplatin, amphotericin B, and cyclosporine.

Ototoxic effects of aminoglycosides include hearing loss caused by cochlear injury and vertigo caused by vestibular damage. Neither has been as well studied as nephrotoxicity because of difficulties in assessing cochlear and vestibular functions in critically ill patients. Nevertheless, available data suggest that all the injected aminoglycosides can cause both types of injury. Tobramycin is more ototoxic than netilmicin.[71]

The incidence of clinically detectable hearing loss ranges from 0.5% to 5.0% and that of vestibular dysfunction causing vertigo or nystagmus ranges from 0.4% to 4.0%. Auditory toxicity is caused by selective destruction of the outer hair cells of the organ of Corti, especially at the basal turn, with subsequent retrograde degeneration of the associated fibers of the auditory nerve. The vestibular toxicity is caused by similar injury to hair cells of the ampullae cristae. Because these are highly differentiated cells that do not regenerate if destroyed, ototoxicity is irreversible. Animal and some clinical data suggest that ototoxic effects are related to selective concentration and trapping of the cation aminoglycoside molecules in the perilymph and endolymph of the cochlea and vestibular apparatus and this in turn to high trough serum aminoglycoside concentrations,[59,72] although other data show no relation.[73] Renal insufficiency is the most important risk factor,[73] but dose is important in patients with normal renal function; duration of therapy and older age are of variable pertinence. Concomitant ethacrynic acid, but not furosemide therapy, increases the risk of ototoxicity.

Other adverse effects of aminoglycosides are uncommon. These include pseudomembranous colitis due to *C. difficile* toxin and hypersensitivity reactions such as rash, fever, Stevens-Johnson syndrome, and delirium.

Although dose-related toxic effects of aminoglycosides may be unavoidable despite assiduous attention to dose selection plus monitoring of serum concentrations, the small risk of toxic effects that are generally reversible should not engender use of small, potentially inefficacious doses of these drugs in critically ill ICU patients.

POLYMYXINS B AND E (COLISTIN)

The polymyxins are a group of basic polypeptide antibiotics that inhibit only aerobic gram-negative bacteria. Their antimicrobial action is mediated by binding to phospholipids in the cytoplasmic membrane, with disruption of membrane permeability, macromolecular and ion disequilibria, and cell lysis. Intrinsic resistance is caused in part by inability of the drug to gain access to the cytoplasmic membrane; acquired resistance is rarely observed. The potency and spectrum of activity of polymyxin are similar to those of the aminoglycosides. However, because of more marked nephrotoxicity, only polymyxins B and E (colistin) are used clinically. Polymyxin B continues to be used in topical or oral formulations from which it cannot be absorbed. Thus, polymyxin B has been administered orally to suppress aerobic gram-negative bacterial intestinal flora in immunocompromised patients. Polymyxin E (colistin) alone, or combined with another antibiotic, has a limited role as a parenteral agent for the treatment of infection caused by multiply resistant, nosocomial pathogens for which no alternative agents are available. Polymyxin E has been administered with rifampicin to treat multiresistant nosocomial *S. marcesens* infection[74] and with cotrimoxazole, to treat *P. cepacia* and *S. marcescens* infections.[75,76] It is unaffected by enzymes that degrade β-lactam and aminoglycoside antibiotics.

CLINICAL PHARMACOLOGY Like aminoglycosides, polymyxins are eliminated unchanged by glomerular filtration. The plasma elimination $t_{1/2}$ of colistin is 1.6 to 3.0 hours. No reliable data exist on the relation between serum concentrations and therapeutic or toxic effects. Accordingly, when polymyxin E is administered parenterally, avoidance of drug toxicity depends solely on clinical evaluation, urinalysis, and measurement of changes in glomerular filtration rate. In the critically ill ICU patient, the confounding effect of concurrent changes owing to disease and other drugs makes this more difficult than usual.

The usual dose of polymyxin E is 2.5 to 5.0 mg/kg per day as two or four divided intramuscular or intravenous doses or a continuous intravenous infusion at a rate of 5 to 6 mg/h. Polymyxin E accumulates in patients with renal failure so that the total daily dose should be reduced:

Creatine Clearance (mL/min)	Dose
>20	Standard dose
5–19	25.0% of standard dose every 12 h
<5 and hemodialysis and peritoneal dialysis	15% of standard dose every 12 h

ADVERSE DRUG REACTIONS Adverse reactions after topical or oral administration are uncommon, although nausea, vomiting, and diarrhea are caused by administration of large doses ($\geq$600 mg) by mouth. After parenteral administration, side effects are similar to those caused by aminoglycosides. Reversible dizziness, paresthesias especially affecting the face, incoordination caused by vestibulotoxicity and proteinuria, microscopic hematuria, and progressive azotemia or acute tubular necrosis may occur. Respiratory paralysis owing to neuromuscular blockade occurs rarely; unlike that owing to aminoglycosides, respiratory paralysis cannot be reversed by neostigmine.

A recent report described the nephrotoxicity of polymyxin B in 80 patients with nosocomial multidrug-resistant gram-negative bacterial infections.[77] Mortality rate was 20%; the organism was cleared in 88% of patients. Nephrotoxicity, defined as a doubling in serum creatinine occurred in 14% of patients, all of whom had normal baseline creatinine levels. Older age was the only predictor of nephrotoxicity; neither total dose nor duration of polymyxin B therapy was a significant predictive factor. This study is encouraging in demonstrating that this drug, which is often active against multidrug-resistant gram-negative nosocomial bacteria, can be used, if necessary, with a reasonable therapeutic-to-toxic index.

GLYCOPEPTIDE ANTIBIOTICS

Vancomycin and teicoplanin are structurally and functionally related members of the glycopeptide family of antibacterial drugs.

VANCOMYCIN

The antibacterial activity of vancomycin is essentially restricted to gram-positive bacteria. It is the drug of first choice for initial therapy of MRSA and *S. epidermidis* infection.[22] It is a significant alternative agent for treatment of enterococcal infection as ampicillin resistance continues to increase. *Staphylococcus aureus*, *S. epidermidis*, streptococci, and *Corynebacterium* and *Clostridium* species are almost uniformly sensitive to vancomycin. However, strains of vancomycin-resistant *S. aureus* (MIC >32 mg/L) are being reported.[78] Fortunately, their prevalence has not yet significantly compromised the utility of vancomycin as initial therapy for infections suspected to be caused by these organisms. In combination with gentamicin or tobramycin, vancomycin synergically inhibits *S. aureus* strains, including those resistant to methicillin and nearly all strains of *S. faecalis*. A major crisis in antimicrobial therapeutics is looming with the emergence of vancomycin-resistant enterococci (VRE), which are often resistant to all other available antibiotics.

MECHANISMS OF ACTION AND RESISTANCE Vancomycin is bactericidal by inhibiting an early stage in the formation of the peptidoglycan of the cell wall. Resistance to it, at least in enterococci, is associated with synthesis of a plasmid-encoded ligase that results in synthesis of cell wall precursors that will not bind vancomycin but can still be cross-linked by enterococcal transpeptidases to form a normal cell wall. Concern is increasing that this vancomycin resistance may be transferred to MRSA, because this can be effected readily in vitro. This appears to have occurred in a case of vancomycin-resistant *S. aureus*[78] in which vancomycin resistance was mediated by acquisition of the *Van A* gene.

CLINICAL PHARMACOLOGY Vancomycin is poorly absorbed after oral administration. For systemic therapy, it must be injected intravenously because intramuscular injection causes marked discomfort and possibly tissue necrosis. It is 30% to 55% protein bound and distributes widely into inflamed tissues and spaces in effective concentrations, including the subarachnoid space in patients with meningitis and the peritoneal cavity in patients with renal failure and peritonitis complicating chronic peritoneal dialysis. The AVD is approximately 40% of total body weight. It may be 50% less on average in morbidly obese patients, but the implication of this for dose calculation is unclear. The drug is eliminated primarily unchanged by glomerular filtration. The plasma elimination $t_{1/2}$ varies widely, with a range of 3 to 13 hours (average, 6 hours) even in patients with normal renal function. Plasma $t_{1/2}$ is prolonged with renal insufficiency and may be as long as 17 days in anuric patients. In patients with liver disease without concomitant renal dysfunction, plasma $t_{1/2}$ is also increased and has been reported to be as long as 37 hours. This observation and the incomplete recovery of injected vancomycin in urine collections from healthy volunteers indicate that vancomycin is partly eliminated by a nonrenal, presumably hepatic, route.

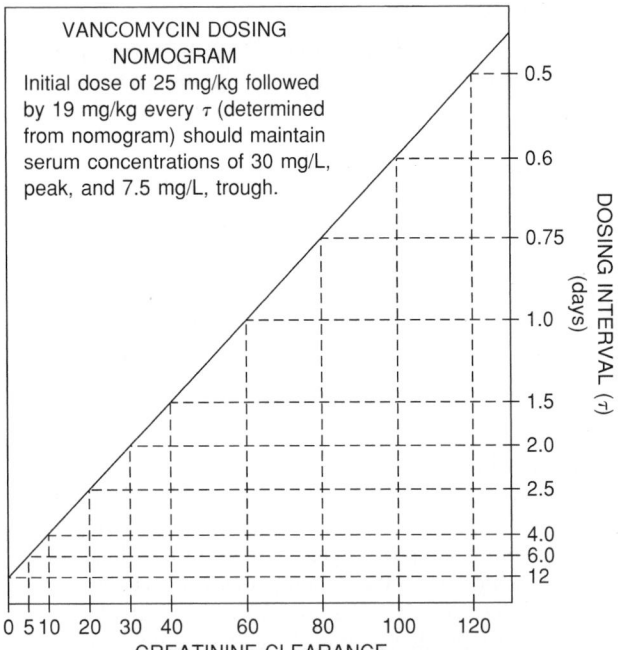

FIGURE 45-1 Dosage nomogram for vancomycin in patients with various degrees of renal function. The creatinine clearance can be estimated by a formula using the patient's age, sex, and serum creatinine as follows. In males, creatinine clearance (mL/min) = {wt(kg) [140 − age (years)]}/0.81 [serum creatinine (mL/L)]. In females, multiply the above value by 0.85. (*Reproduced, with permission, from Matzke GR, et al.[79]*)

Vancomycin Cp is directly proportional to dose. The Cp 2 hours after infusion of 0.5, 1.0, and 2.0 g in adult volunteers averages 2 to 10, 25, and 45 mg/L, respectively. The mean Cp 6 hours after infusion of 0.5 g is 6 mg/L and that 12 hours after infusion of 1.0 g is 5 mg/L.

The usual adult dose of vancomycin is 6.5 to 8.0 mg/kg administered every 6 hours or 15 mg/kg every 12 hours, given in a relatively dilute solution infused over 60 min. More rapid infusion is frequently associated with the occurrence of the *red-man syndrome*, an important adverse reaction (see below). In adults with impaired renal function, dose reductions are recommended to avoid ototoxic and, purportedly, nephrotoxic side effects (see below). One nomogram that permits calculation of the appropriate dose interval is shown in Fig. 45-1.[79]

In patients with fluctuating renal function and those with clinically important liver disease, dose intervals should be based on vancomycin concentrations in serum after the usual initial dose. Although the data demonstrating a relation between vancomycin Cp and beneficial or toxic effects are not robust[80] and lack consensus in some countries,[81] avoiding maximum concentrations of 30 mg/L is conventional after the distribution phase is complete (30 minutes after the end of infusion) to obviate ototoxicity and perhaps the red-man syndrome, as is avoiding trough concentrations above 10 mg/L, to minimize nephrotoxicity. However, in patients with gram-positive bacteremia receiving vancomycin alone, peak serum vancomycin above 20 mg/L and trough concentrations above 10 mg/L were associated with an "improved outcome."[82] If a

continuous infusion of vancomycin is administered, the target Cp should be 15 mg/L.

In functionally anephric patients who are being dialyzed, 1 g vancomycin infused weekly yields maximum Cp values of 40 to 50 mg/L that are usually well tolerated and remain therapeutic after 7 days (Cp 5 to 7 mg/L). Thus, once-weekly vancomycin infusions are a practical and convenient method for treating serious infection in patients requiring dialysis. Hemodialysis does not remove significant amounts of vancomycin so that no supplemental doses need be administered after completion of dialysis.

Vancomycin administered by mouth is effective for therapy of pseudomembranous colitis.[83] It is considered the drug of choice for severe cases, whereas metronidazole is no less effective for mild to moderately severe disease.[84] The recommended dose is 125 mg administered four times per day; the maximum dose is 500 mg administered four times per day. In patients with adynamic ileus, the optimal therapy for pseudomembranous colitis is unknown. Some experts recommend vancomycin administration intravenously and by nasogastric tube. When cholestyramine is administered by mouth for treatment of pseudomembranous colitis, coadministration of vancomycin should be avoided because it will be inactivated by binding to the resin. In patients with severe pseudomembranous colitis and moderate to severe renal dysfunction treated with vancomycin by mouth, vancomycin Cp values have been reported to reach peak concentrations as high as 13 mg/L depending on the dose given.[85] It was estimated that only an average of 4.0% of oral doses were absorbed and that the accumulation of vancomycin in serum was primarily a function of concurrent renal insufficiency in those patients. Monitoring of vancomycin Cp values has been recommended if such therapy is prolonged (>28 days) or involves higher than conventional doses (>2 g/d).

Vancomycin administered intraperitoneally in dialysis fluid is the preferred mode for treatment of gram-positive coccal peritonitis complicating peritoneal dialysis. This choice is predicated on the knowledge that peritonitis in such patients is a superficial and localized infection of the serosal surface of the peritoneum. Absence of fever in 80% to 90% of milder cases and the rarity of bacteremia support this view. Vancomycin moves readily bidirectionally across the inflamed peritoneal lining into the blood stream, and vice versa. Accordingly, the Cp ultimately attained approaches that in the peritoneal fluid. One vancomycin treatment schedule for peritonitis begins with a dose of 1 g in the initial dialysate, followed by 50-mg maintenance doses in subsequent exchanges. On such therapy, mean vancomycin Cp rises to 9 mg/L at 5 hours and averages 6 to 9 mg/L during subsequent dwell periods. In patients with severe peritonitis, it is not certain that concomitant intravenous therapy alters the outcome, but vancomycin may be administered by both routes. In such patients, the need for frequent measurement of vancomycin Cp to avoid excessively high levels becomes more acute.

ADVERSE DRUG REACTIONS The red man syndrome is the most important immediate adverse effect of vancomycin infusion. It appears to be caused by histamine release. The reaction may begin within minutes of starting the infusion or shortly after its completion and definitely occurs more commonly with rapid infusions. In general, tingling and flushing of the neck, face, and thorax develop during the course of a rapid infusion, sometimes with progression to hypotension and shock. The flushed appearance usually resolves over several hours. Antihistamines can prevent vancomycin-induced hypotension in humans,[86] but the value of antihistamines for treating hypotension after the onset of the reaction is unclear. Nevertheless, treatment with fluid administration, antihistamines, and steroids has been advocated for severe reactions. Many, but not all, occurrences of the syndrome can be prevented by following the manufacturer's strong recommendation that vancomycin be infused over at least 60 min. A maximum rate of administration of 10 mg/min may further reduce the risk of hypotension, as demonstrated in a study in volunteers.[87]

A maculopapular rash (sometimes accompanied by pruritus, fever, and rigors), not dissimilar to the cutaneous flushing seen as a component of the red man syndrome, may occur in up to 3% of patients treated with vancomycin. This adverse effect appears to be an allergic reaction, so intensivists may have to decide whether to risk readministration of the antibiotic in such patients. In those in whom the reaction is part of a typical red man syndrome, continued therapy with cautious, slower administration has been advocated; however, if allergy is diagnosed, use of alternative agents is more prudent.

Ototoxicity owing to vancomycin does not appear to be common, but definitive data are lacking.[88] In one prospective study, reversible tinnitus and dizziness occurred in 2 of 34 patients.[89] However, tinnitus may herald high-frequency hearing loss and deafness that will progress despite discontinuation of vancomycin therapy. Ototoxicity is probably caused by injury to the hair cells of the cochlea, a toxic effect identical to that caused by aminoglycoside antibiotics. It is therefore not surprising that vancomycin ototoxicity is more likely when aminoglycosides are administered concomitantly. Ototoxicity is also more frequent in elderly patients and those with renal failure. It is associated with peak vancomycin Cp above 80 mg/L but is infrequent if drug is administered so the peak and trough Cp values are below 30 mg/L and below 10 mg/L, respectively.

The nephrotoxic potential of vancomycin administered alone or in combination with an aminoglycoside is not clear despite several careful prospective observational studies. Nephrotoxicity demonstrated by a rise in creatinine Cp values has been reported in 5% to 75% of patients treated with vancomycin alone and in 0% to 22% of patients treated with vancomycin plus an aminoglycoside. In one study, trough vancomycin Cp values above 30 mg/L were associated with nephrotoxicity,[80] but others could not identify such an association.[80] Renal dysfunction developing during vancomycin therapy is usually mild and reversible, but as many as 9% of patients may have persisting evidence of diminished renal function.[89]

Even though the nephrotoxicity of vancomycin and the relevance of monitoring serum vancomycin concentration are debated, until the issue is clarified serum creatinine levels should be monitored in patients being treated with vancomycin and doses should be adjusted to obtain peak and trough Cp values below 30 mg/L and below 10 mg/L, respectively. Combination therapy with an aminoglycoside plus vancomycin requires even more careful attention to these measures.[90]

TEICOPLANIN

Teicoplanin is, like vancomycin, a glycopeptide antibiotic. It is produced by *Actinoplanes teichomyceticus* and is formulated as a complex mixture of six closely related molecules.[91]

Teicoplanin, like vancomycin, inhibits a wide range of gram-positive aerobic and anaerobic bacteria ranging from MRSA to *Clostridia* species. It is indicated for treatment of infections caused by susceptible gram-positive bacteria including MRSA and VRE. In the ICU, it probably represents an alternative to vancomycin. Administered orally, teicoplanin may be an alternative to metronidazole or vancomycin for the treatment of *C. difficile* toxin diarrhea and colitis.

The usual dose is 400 mg infused intravenously over 30 minutes or by intramuscular injection (unlike vancomycin) once daily or as often as every 12 hours for treatment of more severe infection.

MECHANISM OF ACTION Teicoplanin is bactericidal like vancomycin, presumably through its inhibition of peptidoglycan synthesis and, hence, the cell wall of daughter cells. It binds to the alanine residue of the terminal portion of the muramyl pentapeptide, resulting in inhibition of the transglycosylation reaction and cell wall biosynthesis.

Compared with vancomycin, it contains more fatty acid chains that, it is hypothesized, facilitate penetration through the bacterial cell wall and result in greater potency and a longer biological $t_{1/2}$. These fatty acids also may account for its solubility at pH 7.4, which permits good local tolerance and rapid absorption after intramuscular injection.

MECHANISM OF RESISTANCE Some bacteria are inherently insensitive to glycopeptide antibiotics; these include *Leuconostic*, *Pediococcus*, *Lactobacillus*, and *Erysipelothrix* species. Of greater clinical importance are strains that are differentially inhibited by teicoplanin and vancomycin. *Enterococcus faecalis* and *E. faecium* strains expressing the *Van A* gene exhibit high-level resistance to both drugs. Resistance is transferable by conjugation and inducible by the glycopeptides. *Enterococcus faecium* strains with the Van B phenotype exhibit susceptibility to teicoplanin but moderate resistance to vancomycin. Differential susceptibility of *S. epidermidis* or *S. haemolyticus* to the two glycopeptides has been observed. In vitro selection of stepwise resistance to teicoplanin has been observed in coagulase-negative staphylococci and *S. aureus* strains with heterogeneous patterns of β-lactam susceptibility.

Overall, these data suggest that teicoplanin may be an alternative to vancomycin for some vancomycin-resistant infections.

CLINICAL PHARMACOLOGY Absorption after intramuscular injection is equivalent in extent to intravenous injection. The AVD is 0.8 to 1.62 L/kg body weight. The drug does not penetrate into the CSF. Elimination from plasma is almost wholly by renal mechanisms; only 3% of teicoplanin is metabolized. The elimination $t_{1/2}$ is 155 to 168 hours.

Renal and total body clearance correlate with creatinine clearance, and doses must be reduced in patients with impaired renal function. Dose reductions are recommended to begin after the fourth day of treatment. For patients with creatinine clearance 40 to 60 ml/min, maintenance doses should be halved by administering one-half the dose daily or the usual dose every 2 days. For those with creatinine clearance slower than 40 mL/min and in patients on hemodialysis (teicoplanin is not removed by dialysis), the maintenance dose should be one-third the usual dose by administering one-third the usual dose daily or the full dose every 3 days.

For treatment of peritonitis due to susceptible patients on continuous ambulatory peritoneal dialysis (CAPD), a loading dose of 400 mg intravenously or intramuscularly should be accompanied by addition of teicoplanin to yield 20 mg/mL in the dialysate for the first week and then 20 mg/mL on alternate days in the second week and then in each bag in the third week.

ADVERSE DRUG REACTIONS Teicoplanin is generally well tolerated. In a large trial in Europe, 10.3% of 3377 patients treated with teicoplanin had an adverse reaction: allergic-type reactions in 2.6%, local intolerance in 1.7%, fever in 6.8%, and ototoxicity in 0.3%. Abnormal liver and renal function tests developed in 1.7% and 0.6% of patients, respectively.

Anaphylactoid reactions to vancomycin, described as "red man syndrome," have seldom been reported in patients treated with teicoplanin. The extent of cross-allergenicity to teicoplanin in patients allergic to vancomycin is uncertain, but some reactions have been reported.

Nephrotoxicity due to teicoplanin appears to be very uncommon, including a lesser propensity than with vancomycin to increase creatinine concentration when administered with an aminoglycoside.

Overall, based on a lesser likelihood than vancomycin of causing nephrotoxicity when coadministered with an aminoglycoside and greater ease of administration intravenously or intramuscularly once daily, with probable equal efficacy, teicoplanin may be a preferred alternative to vancomycin for initial broad-spectrum therapy of nosocomial infection, especially when the prevalence of MRSA and VRE is of any concern. Conversely, the lack of availability of a serum teicoplanin assay and knowledge of levels associated with safety and efficacy makes it more complicated to administer teicoplanin than vancomycin. More data from head-to-head comparative trials are needed.

SULFONAMIDES

The discovery of the antibacterial action of sulfonamides in the 1930s and the administration of these agents systemically to prevent and cure bacterial infections represented a revolutionary breakthrough in medicine and opened the chemotherapeutic era. When first introduced for general use, this group of antibiotics was effective against a wide range of infections caused by aerobic gram-positive and gram-negative bacteria, actinomycetes (*Nocardia* and *Actinomyces*), protozoa (*Pneumocystis carinii, Toxoplasma gondii,* and malarial parasites), and *Chlamydia trachomatis*. Since that time, their usefulness has declined markedly because of a number of factors: the advent of a wide range of alternative agents, the frequent emergence of resistance to sulfonamides in many formerly susceptible microorganisms, an awareness of the frequency and severity of ADR caused by some sulfonamides, and the relative unavailability of parenteral formulations.

CLASSIFICATION Sulfonamides may be classified as follows:

1. *Sulfonamides rapidly absorbed and eliminated after oral administration.* Sulfisoxazole is the prototypical agent; sulfamethoxazole and sulfadiazine are other widely used members of this class.
2. *Poor absorption of orally administered sulfonamide.* Sulfasalazine is used to treat ulcerative colitis and Crohn's disease. About 20% of an oral dose is absorbed in the small intestine, a small portion (~10%) of which is excreted into urine, and the rest is secreted in bile and enters the enterohepatic circulation.[92] This portion plus unabsorbed drug passes into the colon, where it is split into two metabolites, sulfapyridine and 5-aminosalicylic acid, which accounts for the therapeutic effect of sulfasalazine in inflammatory bowel disease.
3. *Sulfonamides for topical use.* Sulfacetamide is approximately 90 times more soluble in aqueous solution than is sulfadiazine at neutral pH and is nonirritating to the eye. It is formulated as 30% and 10% ophthalmic solutions and a 10% ointment. Ocular fluids and tissues are thus exposed to high concentrations of antibiotic during topical ophthalmic application. However, topical ophthalmic use is associated with a risk of sensitization, and this consideration plus the insensitivity of most nosocomial bacteria to sulfonamides limit the usefulness of sulfacetamide for treatment of bacterial conjunctivitis and keratitis.

   Two sulfonamides have an established place in the ICU for the topical therapy of patients with second- and third-degree burns. Silver sulfadiazine is relatively insoluble. It reacts with chloride and protein components of tissue exudate to form silver chloride, silver protein complexes, and sodium sulfadiazine. The relative contributions of each of these products to the potent inhibitory effect of silver sulfadiazine on the growth of a broad spectrum of microorganisms is unclear, but inhibition of growth of bacteria, including some species resistant to sulfonamides and fungi,[93] is observed. This suggests that inhibition other than by interference with folate synthesis (see below) contributes to the antibiotic effect.

   Mafenide is a sulfonamide marketed as 8.5% cream. Like silver sulfadiazine, it is effective for the prevention of colonization of burns by a large variety of gram-negative and gram-positive bacteria, including some anaerobes. However, *Candida* species are not inhibited as they are by silver sulfadiazine. Mafenide is rapidly absorbed and converted to a nontoxic metabolite, *p*-carboxy-benzene-sulfonamide, which is excreted in urine. Unlike all other sulfonamides, mafenide is active in the presence of blood, pus, and serum.
4. *Long-acting sulfonamides.* Sulfadoxine has a singularly long $t_{1/2}$ of 7 to 9 days. This has made it an attractive choice for malaria prophylaxis in combination with pyrimethamine (Fansidar) for the prevention and treatment of illness owing to chloroquine-resistant strains of *Plasmodium falciparum*. It has no uses as an antibacterial agent.

MECHANISM OF ACTION Sulfonamides are structural analogues of para-aminobenzoic acid. They exert a bacteriostatic effect by competitively inhibiting dihydropteroate synthetase. This enzyme catalyzes the synthesis of dihydropteroic acid, the immediate precursor of folic acid, from para-aminobenzoic acid. Folic acid is required for 1-carbon transfer reactions for purine synthesis. Most bacterial cells are impermeable to folic acid, in contrast to mammalian cells. These facts concerning the mechanism of action of sulfonamides on susceptible cells account for the selective toxicity of sulfonamides for bacterial but not for mammalian cells, the mechanism of bacterial resistance to sulfonamides, inhibition of sulfonamide action in sites of tissue necrosis, and, as will be discussed later, synergistic inhibition of some bacteria by combination with dihydrofolate reductase inhibitors such as trimethoprim (TMP) or pyrimethamine.

Because mammalian cells are permeable to folic acid, sulfonamides do not cause dose-related or concentration-related adverse effects on cellular metabolism in humans. Side effects are predominantly idiosyncratic or allergic (see below).

MECHANISMS OF RESISTANCE   Acquired bacterial resistance to sulfonamides arises by random mutation and selection or by transfer of resistance by plasmids. Such resistance is a stable characteristic whose cumulative prevalence currently limits the use of sulfonamides as initial therapy to a few infections such as brucellosis and nocardiosis. Sulfonamide resistance may be mediated by an alteration in the affinity of dihydrofolate reductase for sulfonamide, use of alternative pathways for purine and pyrimidine synthesis, and compensatory overproduction of the natural substrate, para-aminobenzoic acid. Acquired resistance to silver sulfadiazine cream in burn units has been reported and necessitated use of alternative therapy such as silver nitrate and chlorhexidine cream.[94]

CLINICAL PHARMACOLOGY   Most orally administered sulfonamides are rapidly absorbed from the stomach and small intestine, but the efficiency of this process in acutely ill patients has not been described. Absorbed sulfonamides bind to serum proteins, in particular albumin, from 20% to more than 90% and affect disposition. High protein binding of sulfadoxine (97%) accounts in part for its long disappearance $t_{1/2}$ from plasma. High protein binding of other sulfonamides administered to neonates can contribute to the development of kernicterus. This is hypothesized to be due to displacement of bilirubin from albumin binding sites, although this is disputed.[95] The lipid-soluble sulfonamides diffuse readily into inflamed and noninflamed tissues and body fluids including pleural, peritoneal, and ocular fluids, and the CSF. They readily cross the placenta and enter the fetal circulation in sufficient concentration to exert antibacterial and toxic effects.

A varying proportion of sulfonamide is acetylated in the liver or inactivated by other metabolic pathways. The rate of acetylation is genetically determined, and slow acetylators are more likely to experience certain side effects than are rapid acetylators (see below). Unchanged non–protein-bound sulfonamides and metabolites are excreted mainly by glomerular filtration into urine. Different agents are reabsorbed to different degrees in the renal tubules. In the case of sulfadoxine, resorption is so extensive and efficient that this contributes to its long $t_{1/2}$ of 7 to 9 days.

The pH of the urine influences urinary excretion of sulfonamides because they are weak acids. Thus, their clearance is enhanced in the presence of alkaline urine. In general, however, sufficient free drug reaches the urine to make sulfonamides effective agents for therapy of urinary tract infections caused by susceptible organisms. In patients with significant renal insufficiency, too little sulfonamide reaches the urine to be effective. Doses must be reduced if they are used to treat nonrenal or nonurinary infection. In burned patients with renal failure, mafenide should be used with caution (see below).

ADVERSE DRUG REACTIONS   Overall, sulfonamides cause ADR in about 5% of recipients. The types and severity of ADR are quite varied. They are due largely to allergy and only occasionally to direct dose-related toxic effects.

The best understood dose-related toxic effects include renal colic, urethral pain, hematuria and obstruction due to crystalluria, and hemolysis in patients (and fetuses) with glucose-6-phosphate dehydrogenase deficient erythrocytes. Pseudocyanosis owing to methemoglobinemia or sulfhemoglobinemia was seen with earlier sulfonamide formulations; it is rarely seen now. Mafenide causes a unique dose-related toxic effect. Mafenide and its metabolite inhibit carbonic anhydrase, which results in a metabolic acidosis usually compensated for by hyperventilation. In patients with significant renal dysfunction, high concentrations of mafenide and its metabolite will accumulate and exaggerate this effect. The absorption of silver from silver sulfadiazine and its deposition in different organs has recently been identified as a possible cause of ocular injury and of leucopenia and renal, hepatic, and neurologic toxicities.[96,97]

The slow acetylator phenotype is associated with severe, delayed hypersensitivity reactions to sulfonamides in patients with[98] and without[99] the human immunodeficiency virus. These reactions occur much less commonly than do typical exanthematous or urticarial rashes caused by sulfonamides, which resolve rapidly on discontinuation of therapy. The reactions occur late in the course of sulfonamide therapy and are typically heralded by the onset of high fever followed by development of a skin rash such as erythema multiforme. Patients with the slow acetylator phenotype are postulated to have more parent sulfonamide available for oxidative metabolism to intermediates that have been shown to mediate those adverse reactions.[100] The slow acetylator phenotype is also associated with the common side effects of sulfasalazine therapy: nausea, vomiting, anorexia, and headache are related to serum sulfapyridine concentrations above 20 mg/L,[92] which are more commonly observed in slow acetylators given the standard dose of sulfasalazine.

Sulfonamides may also cause ADR because of interactions with other drugs being administered concurrently. Sulfadiazine, sulfamethizole, and sulfaphenazole may impair hepatic metabolism of phenytoin and warfarin. Cotrimoxazole may cause an exaggerated hypoprothrombinemic effect in patients taking warfarin if their warfarin dose requirements are high and the plasma albumin level is low (see below).

Allergic and idiosyncratic reactions to sulfonamides are relatively common, occasionally may be severe, and rarely are fatal. Skin rashes are fairly frequent, usually occur after treatment of approximately 1 week, and may be maculopapular or urticarial. Erythema nodosum, erythema multiforme, and, rarely, Stevens-Johnson syndrome may occur. The risk of developing Stevens-Johnson syndrome is increased by prior sulfonamide therapy (because of the risk of sensitization) and administration of long-acting sulfonamides. Cross-allergy between sulfonamides makes it unwise to administer another agent from this group. Moreover, cross-allergy with other non-antibacterial sulfonamide drugs may occur: diuretics (acetazolamide, thiazides, bumetanide, and furosemide), oral sulfonylurea hypoglycemic agents, and antithyroid drugs (propylthiouracil). There is no skin test for sulfonamide allergy.

Idiosyncratic reactions include acute agranulocytosis. This rare reaction may be reversible on cessation of administration. However, leukopenia is seen in as many as 3% to 5% of burned patients treated with silver sulfadiazine, usually within 2 to 4 days of initiation of therapy. It is usually self-limiting even with continued use of the drug. Fatal aplastic anemia has been described with sulfonamides but less commonly than with chloramphenicol; megaloblastic anemia responsive to folic acid in patients with inflammatory bowel disease treated with sulfasalazine and thrombocytopenia has been reported.

Hepatotoxicity is a rare idiosyncratic hypersensitivity reaction to sulfasalazine administration. The toxic effect appears to be caused by sulfapyridine, the major absorbed metabolite of sulfasalazine breakdown by colonic bacteria. That this reaction is a result of hypersensitivity is suggested by additional features such as rash, lymphadenopathy, arthralgia, and eosinophilia often observed concurrently 2 to 4 weeks after initiation of therapy.

Drug interactions involving sulfonamides may cause ADR because of interference with hepatic metabolism of the concomitantly administered drug by sulfonamide and displacement of drug from plasma protein by highly bound sulfonamides. For example, tolbutamide, phenytoin, and warfarin metabolism is inhibited by usual therapeutic doses of sulfaphenazole, sulfadiazine, and sulfamethizole. Sulfamethoxazole may displace warfarin from plasma albumin and predispose the patient to an exaggerated anticoagulant effect (however, interference with hepatic metabolism of warfarin is more important).

TRIMETHOPRIM COMBINED WITH SULFAMETHOXAZOLE

TMP is marketed commercially alone and in combination with SMX in oral and parenteral formulations in a fixed ratio of 1:5. Due to its greater lipid solubility, TMP distributes more rapidly and widely than the sulfonamide, yielding a plasma TMP:SMX ratio of approximately 1:20 throughout the dose interval, the optimal ratio for in vitro synergistic antibacterial effects. This ratio is maintained relatively constant because the two agents have similar elimination $t_{1/2}$ values of about 10 hours in persons with normal renal function.

MECHANISM OF ACTION   TMP inhibits dihydrofolate reductase of bacteria about 50,000 times more efficiently than that of mammalian cells. It interferes with purine synthesis in the same pathway that sulfonamides act. The combination, therefore, produces synergistic inhibition of replication in certain bacteria.

TMP is more active than sulfonamide against many bacterial species except *Nocardia*, *Neisseria*, and *Brucella* species. The net inhibitory effect of the combination of TMP-SMX against bacteria is not consistently predictable. However, a synergistic effect is likely when a bacterium is sensitive to both agents. Moreover, when synergy is demonstrable in vitro, the net antibacterial effect may be bactericidal, although the component agents alone are only bacteriostatic.

The clinical advantage of prescribing TMP-SMX together to achieve a synergistic therapeutic effect or to minimize the emergence of resistant isolates during therapy is not well supported by clinical studies. For example, in urinary tract infection, the activity of TMP greatly exceeds that of SMX, and the potential synergy expected is not observed.[101] Resistance to TMP is increased by TMP use, but its administration with SMX has not been shown to substantially decrease this occurrence.[102]

TMP enhances the antibacterial activity of antibiotics other than sulfonamides. It enhances the inhibitory effect of rifampin against *H. influenzae* and *Brucella* species. In combination with carbenicillin and rifampicin, TMP is often synergistic against *S. maltophilia*, a frequently multiply-resistant nosocomial pathogen.[103] The potential utility of these combination therapies in critically ill patients with resistant infections should not be overlooked, but appropriate in vitro testing will be necessary to permit confident administration of these combinations.

MECHANISMS OF RESISTANCE   Resistance to TMP is most commonly associated with acquisition of a plasmid that codes for an altered dihydrofolate reductase enzyme. Some species have acquired resistance as a result of the selection of mutants that do not use the tetrahydrofolate pathway to synthesize thymidine. It is not uncommon for 30% to 40% of aerobic gram-negative enteric bacteria in hospitals to be resistant to TMP and, usually, also SMX.

CLINICAL PHARMACOLOGY   TMP is a lipid-soluble, weak base. Its AVD, 1.8 L/kg body weight, greatly exceeds that of SMX, 0.24 L/kg body weight. It diffuses freely into most tissues and body fluids and concentrates in prostatic and vaginal fluids, which are more acidic than plasma. TMP is eliminated primarily by glomerular filtration as unchanged drug, with a small amount eliminated with bile. Approximately 10% of drug in the urine is inactive metabolites formed in the liver. The elimination $t_{1/2}$ of TMP from plasma is approximately 10 hours in patients with normal renal function but increases with diminished renal function. In severe renal failure, the serum $t_{1/2}$ of SMX is increased slightly more than that of TMP, to ranges of 22 to 50 hours and 14 to 46 hours, respectively. This is attributable to the more efficient clearance of TMP than of SMX by nonrenal mechanisms.

The usual adult doses for those with normal renal function are 160 to 240 mg of TMP and 800 to 1200 mg of SMX infused intravenously every 6, 8, or 12 hours, depending on the severity of the infection. The dose should be diluted to minimize phlebitis: each 5-mL ampule (TMP 80 mg and SMX 400 mg) should be diluted in a minimum of 75 mL of 5% dextrose, 0.15 M NaCl, or Ringer solution. Extravasation causes local irritation and inflammation. In patients with renal dysfunction, a modified dose is advised: for patients with creatinine clearance faster than 25 mL/min, there is no reduction in the standard dose; for those with creatinine clearance of 15 to 24 mL/min, one-half the usual dose is given; for those with creatinine clearance slower than 15 mL/min, use is not recommended.

For *P. carinii* infection, it has been recommended that TMP-SMX doses should be adjusted to achieve TMP concentrations 1.5 to 2 hours after administration of 3 to 10 mg/L (or SMX concentrations of 100 to 150 mg/L).[104] These concentrations are usually achieved with oral or intravenous doses of TMP and SMX of 20 and 100 mg/kg per day in three to four divided doses, respectively, using the fixed-dose formulation of TMP with SMX. However, in one trial, only 32% of SMX levels were in the desired range after dose adjustments.[104] Thus, although no beneficial clinical effect on the therapeutic outcome or side effects was observed, this trial was not able to answer the question of whether sustained maintenance of SMX levels in the target range would be beneficial.

ADVERSE DRUG REACTIONS   In many cases, it is difficult to separate side effects caused by the components of TMP-SMX. TMP causes fewer reactions than the combination, but it is not known whether the combination causes a "synergistic" increase in adverse effects.

Although interference with folic acid metabolism and, hence, erythropoiesis can be demonstrated with high TMP concentrations in normal human bone marrow cells cultured in vitro, concentrations observed during therapy in humans do not attain these levels and do not produce such impairment, and this is corroborated by clinical experience. However, in individuals with pre-existing megaloblastic anemia, TMP can aggravate neutropenia and thrombocytopenia and interfere with the therapeutic response to vitamin B_{12} or folic acid. Therefore, the drug is relatively contraindicated in patients with megaloblastic anemia or in those who may be predisposed to it: pregnant women, patients on anticonvulsant drugs (phenytoin, primidone, or barbiturates), and those with macrocytic erythrocytes. For these individuals, regular blood cell counts are advised if prolonged therapy is prescribed.

Combination TMP-SMX may cause an apparent dose-related impairment of renal function in renal transplant patients or individuals with pre-existing renal insufficiency, especially if inappropriately high doses of TMP-SMX are used. TMP-SMX should be prescribed cautiously to such patients. TMP-SMX administration may cause a temporary rise in serum creatinine concentration not due to a reduction in glomerular filtration rate. This has been attributed to TMP competitive inhibition of creatinine secretion by the renal tubular cation transport system.

Gastrointestinal reactions are the most common side effects of oral TMP-SMX therapy: 3% of recipients experience nausea, vomiting, and anorexia and approximately 0.5% experience diarrhea. *Clostridium difficile* toxin-induced diarrhea and pseudomembranous colitis have been reported in patients treated with these agents.

Skin rashes occur in 1.6% to 8% of patients treated with TMP-SMX. Most of these are probably caused by the sulfonamide, but TMP occasionally causes rashes when administered alone. The rashes usually present as morbilliform eruptions and less frequently as urticarial or vasculitic processes.

QUINOLONES

The quinolone antibiotics comprise three relatively distinct generations of drugs.[105,106] The first-generation quinolones, nalidixic acid, oxolinic acid, and cinoxacin, achieve effective concentrations only in urine, thus limiting their usefulness to the oral therapy of uncomplicated urinary tract infection and, hence, are not discussed further. The second-generation quinolones are 4-fluorinated analogues of nalidixic acid: nor-

floxacin, ciprofloxacin, pefloxacin, ofloxacin, and enoxacin. They have enhanced potency against enteric bacteria compared with the first-generation agents but have inconsistent inhibitory activity against gram-positive cocci including streptococci of groups A, B, C, and G, *S. pneumoniae*, viridans group *streptococci*, *Streptococci*, or *E. faecalis*. Ciprofloxacin is distinguished by its potency against *P. aeruginosa*, for which it is the most useful fluoroquinolone for systemic therapy, although, for *P. aeruginosa* urine infection, some of the other members of this group achieve therapeutic concentrations in urine. All members of this group, apart from norfloxacin, exhibit sufficient oral bioavailability to make them useful to treat systemic infection. Only 26% to 32% of a norfloxacin dose is recovered in the urine over 24 hours compared with 75% to 95% for the other agents.

A third generation of fluoroquinolones consists of levofloxacin, moxifloxacin, and gatifloxacin. This group is characterized by clinically useful antibacterial activity against *Chlamydia*, *Legionella*, and *Mycoplasma* species and by streptococcal and staphylococcal pathogens and, hence, is also referred to as respiratory fluoroquinolones; they possess variable activity against *E. faecalis*. They inhibit penicillin-sensitive and penicillin-resistant pneumococci. Moxifloxacin and gatifloxacin are the only fluoroquinolones that inhibit *B. fragilis* species.

In the ICU setting, ciprofloxacin is particularly useful as therapy for systemic *P. aeruginosa* infection. All the second- and third-generation fluoroquinolones are effective for most enteric bacterial infections, especially as less toxic alternatives to aminoglycosides, as are third-generation cephalosporins, carbapenems, and extended-spectrum β-lactams. The respiratory quinolones are alternatives to the macrolide agents for treatment of atypical pneumonia caused by *Chlamydia*, *Mycoplasma*, and *Legionella* species. Thus, the third-generation fluoroquinolones can be administered as broad-spectrum agents for nosocomial infection and for a wide range of community-acquired respiratory and genitourinary infections.

MECHANISMS OF ACTION   The quinolones exert a bactericidal effect by selectively inhibiting two type II DNA topoisomerase enzymes, DNA gyrase and topoisomerase IV, but not the analogous cellular enzyme, topoisomerase; both normally cut segments of replicating bacterial DNA strands to prevent tangling.

MECHANISMS OF RESISTANCE   Resistance among gram-negative enteric bacteria including *P. aeruginosa* and *S. aureus*, although varying in prevalence in different countries, has emerged since widespread use of ciprofloxacin began in 1984.[107] Such strains are usually completely cross-resistant to other quinolones. Resistance arises due to chromosomal mutations in the DNA gyrase and topoisomerase IV and, to a lesser extent, to reduced drug accumulation in the bacterial cell due to active efflux of the agents by antibiotic efflux pumps.[108]

CLINICAL PHARMACOLOGY   The oral bioavailability of the fluoroquinolones, apart from norfloxacin, exceeds 75%; however, for the ill patient in the ICU, intravenous administration is recommended. Ciprofloxacin, levofloxacin, and gatifloxacin are formulated for intravenous and oral administrations, and the plasma $t_{1/2}$ values in patients with normal renal function are 4.0, 6.0, and 8.4 hours, respectively; therefore, for levofloxacin and gatifloxacin, once-daily dosing is adequate. The usual doses are 400 mg every 12 hours and 500 and 400 mg once daily, respectively. Renal elimination accounts for 60%, 95%, and 90% of the drug clearance, so $t_{1/2}$ is not unexpectedly inversely related to creatinine clearance. When creatinine clearance declines to 50 mL/min, doses should be halved. Hemodialysis patients should receive 50% of the standard dose supplemented by 200 mg every 12 hours, no extra doses, and 200 mg every 24 hours after dialysis for the three drugs, respectively.

Dose reductions are generally unnecessary for healthy elderly patients or patients with mild to moderately severe hepatic disease (Child-Pugh class B).

ADVERSE DRUG EFFECTS Quinolones and fluorinated quinolones are generally well tolerated. Gastrointestinal symptoms including nausea, anorexia, vomiting, and diarrhea occur in fewer than 5% of patients. First- and second-generation quinolones on the market cause neurologic symptoms whose pathogenesis is unclear. Dizziness and headache are the most common, being reported in 2% of patients. Giddiness, excitation or depression, visual disturbances, lethargy, agitation, somnolence, syncope, and, rarely, convulsions and acute psychosis have been reported with the first-generation quinolones and norfloxacin but not with ciprofloxacin. These effects may be more common in patients given larger doses in the presence of renal dysfunction. Some quinolones interfere with the inhibitory neurotransmitter γ-aminobutyric acid, but no clear relation exists between this characteristic of the quinolones and their propensity to cause neurotoxic symptoms. Nevertheless, the quinolones should be used with caution in patients with CNS disease or renal impairment.

Hypersensitivity reactions are uncommon; urticarial rash with eosinophilia has been reported in 0.5% to 1.0% of patients.

Rare side effects observed with nalidixic acid that may occur with second-generation quinolones include intracranial hypertension, lactic acidosis, and hemolytic anemia.

Quinolones interfere with cartilage formation in young animals and are therefore relatively contraindicated in prepubertal patients. In addition, fluoroquinolones appear to double the risk of tendinopathy compared with other antibiotics.[109] This appears to be a class effect, although pefloxacin is the most commonly associated agent (up to 68% of cases). Achilles tendon rupture is the most common and dramatic manifestation and can manifest after only 1 to 2 days of fluoroquinolone therapy. The mechanism is unknown, and the pathology is nonspecific. Concomitant renal dysfunction may predispose the patient to this adverse effect.

Drug interactions include enhancement of warfarin activity because of displacement from albumin by nalidixic acid, elevated plasma theophylline concentrations caused by impairment of metabolism by ciprofloxacin, and increased risk of CNS toxic effects in patients given nonsteroidal anti-inflammatory drugs and ciprofloxacin concurrently.

Fluoroquinolones as a class effect can increase QTc intervals. QTc prolongation can result in *torsade de pointes*, which can lead to ventricular fibrillation and sudden death. Thus, ciprofloxacin, levofloxacin, and gatifloxacin should not be given in excess of recommended doses and should be avoided in patients with known QTc prolongation and hypokalemia and those receiving class Ia (e.g., quinidine and procainamide) or class III (e.g., amiodarone, sotalol) antiarrhythmic drugs. These fluoroquinolones also should be given with caution concurrently with other drugs that prolong QTc intervals including cisapride, erythromycin, cotrimoxazole, astemizole, terfenadine, haloperidol, phenothiazine, tricyclic antidepressants, and vasopressin.[106]

Anaphylactoid reactions reported after administration of ciprofloxacin, pefloxacin, and norfloxacin may be another adverse class effect of the fluoroquinolones.[110] Hypotension, shock, asthma, laryngeal edema and urticaria, and angioedema have been reported as manifestations of these reactions. Having the acquired immunodeficiency syndrome (AIDS) may predispose to the reaction. It has been reported within 5 minutes after a first dose in individuals previously unexposed to fluoroquinolones. Although life-threatening, no deaths have been reported. The exact incidence is not known, but the adverse reaction is one with which intensivists need to be aware.

Hypoglycemia has been reported in diabetic patients receiving insulin or glyburide plus fluoroquinolone, so their coadministration must be undertaken with care.

METRONIDAZOLE

Metronidazole is one of a group of 5-nitroimidazoles, including tinidazole, nimorazole, carnidazole, and sulnidazole, that possesses a broad spectrum of antiprotozoal and antibacterial activities. Only metronidazole is available in North America. The following comments pertain to metronidazole only and its antibacterial action.

The clinically important antibacterial activity of metronidazole is restricted to obligate anaerobic bacteria. In vitro, metronidazole is a potent bactericidal antimicrobial against anaerobic gram-negative and gram-positive organisms. More than 99% of 341 blood culture isolates of *B. fragilis* from U.S. patients collected from 1987 to 1999 were susceptible to metronidazole, whereas 22% were not susceptible to clindamycin. Thus, metronidazole continues to be a potentially, uniformly efficacious, antimicrobial agent for initial treatment of *B. fragilis* infection before susceptibility test results can be available.[111] Resistant anaerobic organisms include *Proprionobacterium* species, many strains of *Bifidobacterium*, *Actinomyces*, and *Arachnia*. *Lactobacillus* species and aerobic and microaerophilic streptococci are also resistant.

Oral metronidazole is the drug of choice for *C. difficile* toxin-associated diarrhea and colitis.[84] When administered with penicillin, metronidazole is the drug of choice for the treatment of brain abscess complicating paranasal sinusitis, caused primarily by aerobic streptococci, in particular *Streptococcus milleri*, together with β-lactamase–producing *Bacteroides* species. Metronidazole is used similarly in the combined therapy of temporal lobe brain abscesses of otitic origin commonly caused by anaerobic bacteria, in particular *B. fragilis* and aerobic enteric bacilli. Metronidazole combined with an aminoglycoside is efficacious therapy for mixed aerobic and anaerobic bacterial infections of the peritoneal cavity and female genital tract. In general, this combination is not different in efficacy from clindamycin, ticarcillin, cefoxitin, or chloramphenicol combined with the aminoglycoside.[32]

Advantages arise from differences in the frequency, nature, and severity of adverse effects.

MECHANISM OF ACTION   Metronidazole is rapidly bactericidal by an immediate inhibition of DNA synthesis, but the mechanism of this action has not been fully elucidated.

MECHANISM OF RESISTANCE   Acquired resistance to metronidazole occurs extremely rarely.[111] Isolated reports have documented resistance to metronidazole associated with clinical failure in B. fragilis strains. Resistance appeared to be related to a decreased rate of metronidazole uptake and to an insufficiently low intracellular redox potential to reduce metronidazole to its active form.

CLINICAL PHARMACOLOGY   The clinical pharmacology of metronidazole and its two principal metabolites has been studied extensively.[112] It can be administered intravenously, orally, and rectally as a suppository to treat bacterial infection. The absolute bioavailability of orally administered metronidazole approaches 100%. After intravenous administration of 500 mg over 20 min, the mean metronidazole Cp 30 minutes after the completion of infusion was 27 mg/L and the trough concentration was 16 mg/L.[112] After rectal administration of a 500-mg suppository, mean peak Cs after about 3 hours was 19 mg/L, with the level remaining at approximately 10 mg/L over the next 8 hours.[113] These data suggest that rectal administration may be effective in those who cannot take the drug orally. The drug diffuses widely throughout the body: concentrations in saliva and breast milk are comparable to those in the serum; CSF concentrations in normal volunteers average 43% of the simultaneous Cp and are therapeutic; urine concentrations range from 76 to 115 mg/L after a 500-mg dose. Only about 14% of an oral dose of metronidazole is excreted in the feces, but concentrations attained in feces are much greater than the MIC of metronidazole for C. difficile, which is 4 mg/L or lower.

Metronidazole undergoes extensive metabolism, probably in the liver, to two oxidation products, an "alcohol" metabolite and a "hydroxy" metabolite.[112] The latter is produced in larger amounts, can be readily detected in the plasma of patients with normal renal function, and accumulates in the plasma of those with renal insufficiency. The metabolites possess 5% and 30%, respectively, of the antibacterial activity of the parent compound, so that they probably contribute in part to the therapeutic effect of metronidazole, particularly in patients with renal failure. Of 500 mg of metronidazole administered intravenously to healthy volunteers, 44% was recovered in the urine, consisting of parent drug (8%) and the hydroxy (24%) and alcohol (12%) metabolites. The mean plasma t$_{1/2}$ of metronidazole is 8.5 hours.

In patients with renal insufficiency, metabolites accumulate, but the parent compound does not. It is conventional not to reduce the dose of metronidazole for such patients, including those undergoing peritoneal dialysis or hemodialysis. Severe hepatic disease would be expected to reduce the metabolism of metronidazole, but its disposition in such patients and a need for dose reduction have not been described.

Interactions of metronidazole have been described in adults ingesting phenytoin and barbiturates, which induce its metabolism. Phenobarbital decreased the plasma t$_{1/2}$ of metronidazole to 3.5 hours.

ADVERSE DRUG EFFECTS   In experimental nonhuman systems, metronidazole is teratogenic, mutagenic, and carcinogenic. Comparable effects have not been demonstrated in humans, but avoiding its use during the period of organogenesis in the first trimester of pregnancy is considered prudent. Metronidazole is generally well tolerated. Gastrointestinal side effects occur occasionally. These include a metallic taste, furred tongue, and nausea. Paradoxically, two confirmed reports of pseudomembranous colitis have been described in patients receiving only metronidazole. In one, this side effect appeared to be caused by a metronidazole-resistant strain of C. difficile,[114] but in the other, the organism was susceptible. Transient reversible leukopenia occurs infrequently, but it is the most common hematologic side effect. Peripheral sensory neuropathy has been described in patients receiving large doses for prolonged periods. The cause is not known. One child developed seizures during metronidazole therapy that ultimately resolved completely.

Interactions of metronidazole with a few other drugs are well documented; it can produce an Antabuse-like reaction after alcohol ingestion. This is probably caused by inhibition of hepatic alcohol metabolism resulting in accumulation of acetaldehyde, which causes the adverse symptoms. Metronidazole augments the hypoprothrombinemic effect of warfarin sodium (Coumadin) owing to a stereoselective inhibition of the S(2)-moiety (levo warfarin).

MACROLIDES, LINCOSAMIDES, AND KETOLIDES

ERYTHROMYCIN, CLARITHROMYCIN, AZITHROMYCIN, CLINDAMYCIN, LINCOMYCIN, AND TELITHROMYCIN

These six antibiotics are considered together because they share similar mechanisms of action and resistance spectra of antibacterial activity, and clinical pharmacologic properties. Structurally, they comprise three groups, macrolides (erythromycin, clarithromycin, and azithromycin), lincosamides (lincomycin and clindamycin), and ketolides (telithromycin).

Erythromycin

Erythromycin is produced by Streptomyces erythreus. It is a member of the macrolide group of antibacterial compounds, which also includes spiramycin (used in Europe to treat T. gondii infection), azithromycin, and clarithromycin.

Erythromycin base is poorly soluble in water, has a pKa of 8.8, and is rapidly inactivated by gastric acid. Many alternative oral formulations have therefore been developed to enhance oral bioavailability over that of the base. Two water-soluble salts, erythromycin-gluceptate and erythromycin-lactobionate, have been developed for intravenous administration. In ICU patients, only the intravenous formulation can ensure adequate systemic delivery of drug, so this discussion does not include the characteristics of the oral products.

In vitro, erythromycin has a broad spectrum of antimicrobial activity that includes bacteria (including chlamydia), mycoplasma, spirochetes (Treponema pallidum), Ureaplasma, and some strains of rickettsias. Its useful antibacterial activity includes gram-positive organisms (S. aureus, S. pyogenes, S. pneumoniae, and viridans group streptococci, Cornyebacterium diphtheriae, Clostridium perfringens, and Listeria monocytogenes). Unfortunately, increased use of macrolides over a long duration has resulted in the emergence of substantial levels of resistance to macrolides in *S. pneumoniae*. Macrolide resistance increased from 13% to 23%, from 9% to 11%, from 15% to 25%, and from 34% to 41%, between 1997 and 1999 in the United States, Canada, Europe, and the Asia-Pacific region, respectively.[115] Some gram-negative organisms (*B. pertussis*, *H. influenzae*, *N. gonorrhoeae*, *N. meningitidis*, and *B. catarrhalis*), *Legionella pneumophila*, *Mycoplasma pneumoniae*, *Ureaplasma urealyticum*, and *C. trachomatis* are susceptible.

Clinically, erythromycin is used to treat *M. pneumoniae* and *L. pneumophila* infections. It is the alternative drug of choice for *C. trachomatis* infection of pregnant women and children who cannot be treated with tetracycline and for *C. diphtheriae* infection in penicillin-allergic patients. Although formerly used as the alternative to penicillin in allergic patients with *T. pallidum*, *M. catarrhalis*, and *L. monocytogenes* infections, erythromycin use in these infections has been largely superseded by other agents.

MECHANISM OF ACTION Erythromycin and the other macrolide antibiotics inhibit bacterial growth by interfering with protein synthesis. Erythromycin binds specifically to the 50S subunit of the ribosome. The precise molecular mechanism is not known but is hypothesized to interfere with the translocation reaction. This reaction, catalyzed by the enzyme translocase, involves the movement of the growing peptide chain, with its tRNA, from the acceptor to the donor site on the ribosome. Erythromycin is thought to bind to the donor site and thereby interfere with translocation of the peptide chain from the acceptor to the donor site. In humans, erythromycin is likely only bacteriostatic.

MECHANISM OF RESISTANCE Gram-negative enteric bacilli are uniformly resistant to erythromycin. This is probably a result of the inability of the drug to penetrate the cell wall to reach the ribosomal site of action. In certain other resistant bacteria, a plasmid-mediated mutational change in the 50S subunit, resulting in methylation of the tRNA erythromycin receptor, precludes erythromycin binding. Two other plasmid-mediated mechanisms confer erythromycin resistance: diminished permeability of the cell envelope of gram-positive bacteria as occurs with *S. epidermidis* and production of an esterase that hydrolyzes erythromycin in some *Enterobacteriaceae*.

Overall, the prevalence of erythromycin resistance among important pathogens such as *S. pneumoniae* currently limits the utility of these agents as first-line antimicrobials for some serious infections such as community-acquired pneumonia.

CLINICAL PHARMACOLOGY Therapeutic concentrations are attained in all sites except the brain and subarachnoid space. Although inflammation enhances erythromycin penetration into brain tissue and CSF, this effect is unpredictable, and erythromycin is thus relatively contraindicated for therapy of brain abscess and meningitis. Disappearance from plasma is first order with $t_{1/2}$ of 1.6 hours. Approximately 15% of an injected dose appears as unchanged drug in the urine; high concentrations of drug are observed in bile, but the overall contribution of this route of drug clearance to erythromycin elimination is not known. A large proportion of injected erythromycin cannot be accounted for by drug in urine or bile, so extensive biotransformation, probably in the liver, is hypothesized.

The normal plasma $t_{1/2}$ of 1.6 hours is prolonged to 4.8 to 5.8 hours in anuric patients. In patients with alcoholic liver disease and ascites, plasma $t_{1/2}$ was increased to an average of 1.6 hours as opposed to 1.3 hours in concurrently studied healthy controls.[116] In both groups, no dose reduction was necessary in view of the low risk of dose-related ADR. In patients with more severe liver disease, dose reduction would appear prudent. However, no explicit guidelines for such patients have been proposed or validated.

ADVERSE DRUG EFFECTS Erythromycin is one of the safest antibacterial agents in clinical use, but tolerance is limited by the frequent occurrence of irritating side effects. First, abdominal cramps, dyspepsia, nausea, vomiting, and diarrhea occur, which result, in part, from a direct smooth muscle–stimulating effect of erythromycin.[117] They are observed after oral and intravenous administrations. Although the smooth muscle–stimulating effect can be inhibited in vitro by the antimuscarinic agent atropine, this strategy has not been studied in humans. Second, intravenous administration predictably causes phlebitis, which can be ameliorated only partly by slow infusion of drug diluted in large volumes of intravenous fluid.

Tinnitus and reversible severe deafness occur after large intravenous doses of erythromycin.[118] Old age, renal failure, and hepatic insufficiency appear to predispose to this unusual adverse effect. The mechanism of this reaction is not known. Pseudomembranous colitis has been reported. Hypersensitivity reactions such as skin rash, fever, and eosinophilia are rare.

Cholestatic jaundice caused by erythromycin estolate (and rarely by the stearate) appears to be specifically related to the propionyl ester linkage of the 29 position so that cross-sensitivity is said not to occur.[119] Thus, a history of cholestatic jaundice during therapy with oral erythromycin estolate is not an absolute contraindication to intravenous therapy with erythromycin gluceptate or lactobionate.

In some individuals, erythromycin can inhibit elimination of astemizole, terfenadine, methylprednisolone, theophylline, carbamazepine, warfarin, and cyclosporine, with significant clinical consequences.

Clarithromycin and Azithromycin

Clarithromycin and azithromycin are recently approved analogues of erythromycin.[120,121] They differ in several respects, but few of these differences are clinically important, particularly for the intensivist.

In vitro, both drugs differ qualitatively from erythromycin in their potent inhibitory effect on *Mycobacterium avium* intracellulare. They differ quantitatively from erythromycin in being up to 10-fold more potent against *C. trachomatis*, *H. pylori*, *M. catarrhalis*, *N. gonorrhoeae*, and *H. ducreyi*.

Bacteria resistant to erythromycin are cross-resistant to clarithromycin and azithromycin.

CLINICAL PHARMACOLOGY Only azithromycin is available in a parenteral formulation. Clarithromycin and azithromycin are well absorbed after oral administration, although bioavailability has not been assessed in critically ill patients. Their good oral bioavailability is attributable in part to the changes in the lactone ring that prevent acid degradation. Reduced acid degradation, moreover, decreases the formation of ketal products that have prokinetic effects on the gastrointestinal smooth muscle, thereby decreasing the frequency of adverse gastrointestinal effects of clarithromycin and azithromycin compared with erythromycin (see Adverse Effects, below). Clarithromycin undergoes first-pass hepatic metabolism, with 20% of an oral dose being converted to a 14-hydroxymetabolite that possesses antibacterial properties similar to those of the parent molecule. Like erythromycin, these two newer macrolides have a low degree of ionization at physiologic pH and are lipid soluble, so they distribute extensively in body fluids and tissues. The AVD of clarithromycin is 2 to 3 L/kg versus 0.6 L/kg for erythromycin. Azithromycin is distributed even more widely, with an AVD of 23 L/kg.

Clarithromycin is primarily eliminated by hepatic oxidation and hydrolysis. Metabolism is characterized by a disproportionate 13-fold increase in clearance when the dose is increased from 150 to 1200 mg. Elimination $t_{1/2}$ increases from 4.4 to 11.3 hours over the same dose range. Unchanged clarithromycin increases from 18% to 30% of the dose over the 250- to 1200-mg dose range. Doses should be reduced by one-half when creatinine clearance is less than 30 mL/min; dose adjustments in the presence of hepatic disease are likely necessary but as yet remain undefined.

Azithromycin kinetic characteristics are distinguished by low Cp values and a prolonged elimination $t_{1/2}$ that reflects extensive tissue sequestration. The liposomal phospholipid complex of azithromycin is mainly excreted unchanged in the feces, with a polyphasic serum $t_{1/2}$ of 10 to 57 hours, depending on the dose and the sampling intervals. Azithromycin doses need not be adjusted in the elderly or in the presence of mild renal or mild to moderate hepatic impairment.

Clarithromycin, unlike erythromycin or azithromycin, is embryolethal and has induced congenital anomalies (cardiovascular) in preclinical studies. Its use in pregnant patients is relatively contraindicated because of uncertainty about the relevance of these data to humans.

Azithromycin appears less likely than clarithromycin or erythromycin to interact with drugs that are metabolized by hepatic cytochrome P450 enzymes. Elevated theophylline, carbamazepine, and terfenadine plasma concentrations have been demonstrated during concurrent administration of clarithromycin. These have not been observed during concomitant administration with azithromycin, but careful observation during combined therapy is recommended by the manufacturer.

The following agents interact adversely with erythromycin and warrant prudence during coadministration with clarithromycin and azithromycin: cyclosporin, valproic acid, and phenytoin.

ADVERSE DRUG EFFECTS Like erythromycin, clarithromycin and azithromycin are well tolerated. Overall, side effects are observed in 20% to 10% of recipients of clarithromycin and azithromycin, respectively; 80% to 90% of these adverse symptoms are mild to moderate in severity. Gastrointestinal side effects are the most common adverse symptoms with both drugs but occur half as often as with erythromycin. Like erythromycin, azithromycin administration has been associated with transient deafness.[122]

A uniquely prolonged adverse effect observed with azithromycin is noteworthy: rare patients have developed serious allergic reactions including angioedema and anaphy-laxis. Despite successful initial symptomatic therapy, allergic symptoms reappeared when therapy was discontinued, even without further azithromycin exposure, presumably owing to the slow clearance of azithromycin from the body. Thus, intensivists should be aware of the possible risk of protracted serious allergic reactions even after discontinuation of azithromycin therapy.

In summary, clarithromycin and azithromycin are new macrolide antibiotics that broaden the therapeutic spectrum of this class of drugs and decrease the incidence of gastrointestinal side effects but may not offer any solution to the problem observed with the prototype, erythromycin, of adverse interactions with other drugs given concomitantly.[123] The usual dose of clarithromycin for serious infection is 250 to 500 mg twice daily. A loading dose of 500 mg azithromycin is recommended, followed by 250 mg once daily; for single-dose therapy of C. trachomatis infection, a 1-g dose is administered.

Clindamycin and Lincomycin

Lincomycin was marketed only for oral administration. Chemical modification of lincomycin led to the development of clindamycin, which is superior in activity to lincomycin and is available for oral administration as the hydrochloride salt and for intravenous injection as the phosphate ester. This characteristic has led to the exclusive use of clindamycin in critically ill patients. Accordingly, only clindamycin is reviewed here.

In vitro, the antibacterial spectrum of clindamycin exceeds that of erythromycin as follows: resistance of S. aureus to clindamycin tends to be less common than to erythromycin, but resistance levels can range from 5% to 20% depending on the region. Many of these clindamycin-resistant S. aureus strains are also resistant to multiple other antibiotics, including methicillin. Clindamycin is much more potent than erythromycin against species of the B. fragilis group, although up to 22% of B. fragilis strains[111] and up to 15% of Bacteroides vulgatus strains are relatively resistant to clindamycin. Nevertheless, this degree of activity against enteric gram-negative anaerobic bacilli is exceeded only by metronidazole. Clostridium difficile strains are resistant, but other species such as Clostridium welchii and Clostridium tetani are sensitive. Mycoplasma pneumoniae, H. influenzae, and N. meningitidis are resistant.

Clindamycin in combination with an aminoglycoside is arguably the antibiotic of first choice for the therapy of serious mixed aerobic and anaerobic enteric bacterial infection of the abdomen and pelvis.[32] A meta-analysis has suggested that the dose of 900 mg every 8 hours may be more efficacious than 600 mg every 8 hours for treatment of intra-abdominal infection (although results of treating female pelvic infection with either dose are similar).[125] In similar infections of the soft tissues and skin of the feet of diabetic patients, this combination is also highly efficacious. Clindamycin alone is superior to penicillin as a single agent for treatment of serious anaerobic lung infection,[124] but their combined use for treatment of such infections is currently recommended. Clindamycin is also considered to be as effective as penicillins for the therapy of non-endocarditis infections caused by S. aureus, S. pyogenes, and S. pneumoniae and as effective as a single injection of benzathine penicillin in eradicating C. diphtheriae from the nasopharynx of asymptomatic carriers. Clindamycin is an acceptable alternative to penicillin for treatment of cervicofacial actinomycosis. Incidentally, clindamycin and quinine sulfate are effective for treatment of *Falciparum malaria* infection.

In summary, clindamycin is a valuable alternative to penicillin in patients who are allergic to the β-lactam agents and is a first-line agent, when combined with an aminoglycoside, for intra-abdominal and pelvic infections, and with penicillin, for mixed anaerobic and aerobic lung infection.

MECHANISM OF ACTION The mechanism of action of clindamycin is identical to that of erythromycin, and both are bacteriostatic.

MECHANISM OF RESISTANCE Resistance is caused by modification of the ribosomal target of clindamycin. Clindamycin-resistant *S. aureus* strains are usually resistant to erythromycin. Clindamycin resistance in *B. fragilis* group organisms is caused by at least two different mechanisms, one of which is plasmid mediated.

CLINICAL PHARMACOLOGY After intravenous injection, clindamycin distribution is analogous to that of erythromycin. Clindamycin does not predictably attain therapeutic concentrations in the fluids of the eye, the cavity or wall of brain abscess, or the CSF even in patients with meningitis. High concentrations are demonstrable in bone, but the relevance of this observation to treatment of osteomyelitis is not clear. High concentrations are attained in polymorphonuclear leukocytes, which may contribute to enhanced killing of phagocytosed bacteria.

The elimination of clindamycin is incompletely understood but probably similar to that of lincomycin, which has been more extensively documented. After intravenous injection, approximately 30% appears in urine and 5% to 15% in feces as unchanged drug and metabolites (N-dimethyl clindamycin, clindamycin sulfoxide, and others). The remainder is hypothesized to be metabolized to inactive compounds. The mean plasma $t_{1/2}$ is normally 3 hours. Severe renal failure is associated with a doubling of peak Cp, and, on this basis, halving of the usual dose is recommended. Neither hemodialysis nor peritoneal dialysis enhances its clearance from plasma. The effect of liver disease on the clinical pharmacokinetics of clindamycin is not clear; increases in plasma $t_{1/2}$ from 40% to 500% have been described. It would seem reasonable to reduce clindamycin doses in patients with severe liver disease, but no clear guidelines have been tested or validated. The usual dose for adults with moderate to severe infection is 900 to 2400 mg/d in two or three divided equal intravenous doses.[125]

ADVERSE DRUG EFFECTS Intravenous clindamycin commonly causes local phlebitis, which can be reduced by slow infusion of dilute solutions. The manufacturer recommends dilution to a concentration of 12 mg/L or lower and infusion longer than 10 minutes (preferably >25 min).

The most important adverse effect of clindamycin administration is diarrhea. This occurs in 2% to 20% of patients treated intravenously or by mouth and varies in severity. Clindamycin is the most common antibiotic cause of diarrhea. The precise pathogenesis of diarrhea associated with clindamycin is not known. However, in that subgroup of patients in whom diarrhea and, in florid cases, pseudomembranous colitis is associated with production of enterotoxin by *C. difficile* in the

colon, a direct toxic effect on the colonic mucosa is responsible. Continuation of clindamycin will intensify the severity of the colitis. When clindamycin cannot be discontinued, concomitant oral administration of metronidazole or vancomycin may permit safe continuation of the clindamycin.

Hypersensitivity reactions caused by clindamycin occur occasionally. In one study, rash occurred in 10% of patients. Drug fever and eosinophilia have also been reported.

It is worth reiterating that no cross-allergenicity exists between clindamycin and penicillin.

Unlike erythromycin, clindamycin does not cause clinically important interactions with other drugs.

Telithromycin

Telithromycin is the first ketolide antibiotic to be licensed. Ketolides are analogues of the macrolide class, molecularly modified specifically to inhibit respiratory tract bacterial pathogens that have acquired resistance to the macrolide agents.[126]

In vitro, the spectrum of activity of telithromycin is comparable to that of other macrolides except it is a potent inhibitor of *S. pneumoniae* and *S. pyogenes* strains that are resistant to macrolides by virtue of the *erm* B–resistance genotype. It does not inhibit erythromycin-resistant *S. aureus* strains.

It is available only for oral administration. The usual dose is 800 mg once daily. Clinical trials comparing telithromycin with conventional treatments for community-acquired pneumonia and exacerbations of chronic obstructive airway disease and acute sinusitis have generally demonstrated comparable efficacy and good tolerance. Limited data suggest very good efficacy in patients with macrolide-resistant *S. pneumoniae* infection. Based on the limited published data, the availability of other antibiotics to treat macrolide-resistant *S. pneumoniae* infection, and the lack of a parenteral formulation, a role for telithromycin in the ICU remains undefined.

MECHANISM OF ACTION Like erythromycin from which it is synthesized, telithromycin is bacteriostatic by inhibiting protein synthesis by binding near the peptidyl transfer site on the bacterial 50S ribosomal subunit.

MECHANISM OF RESISTANCE Resistance to macrolides is mediated most commonly by *mef*-encoded efflux and *erm* A- and B-encoded methylation of 23srRNA. Bacterial strains possessing *mef* and *erm* A genotypes are susceptible to telithromycin (see above). In vitro and in vivo experiments have demonstrated that streptococci exposed to ketolides are less likely to develop such resistance genotypes than are those exposed to macrolides.

CLINICAL PHARMACOLOGY The oral bioavailability is approximately 60% under controlled conditions in healthy volunteers; fractional absorption in ill ICU patients is not known and may be less. Telithromycin distributes widely throughout the body; of note is active transport into polymorphonuclear cells, which may contribute to its clinical efficacy in infections caused by intracellular pathogens such as *Chlamydia*. Approximately 70% of a telithromycin dose is metabolized (33% presystemic and 37% systemic) primarily by cytochrome P450, specifically CYP 3A4, hepatic enzymes. Elimination is a first-order process with $t_{1/2}$ of 9.5 hours, mediated by hepatic biotransformation and biliary and renal excretion.

The doses should be halved in patients with severe renal insufficiency. No dose adjustment is recommended in the presence of mild, moderate, or severe hepatic impairment.

ADVERSE DRUG EFFECTS Available data suggest that telithromycin is well tolerated, with a tolerance profile similar to those of clarithromycin and azithromycin. Gastrointestinal symptoms were the most common adverse symptoms (diarrhea in 13%, nausea in 8%, and vomiting in 2%). Most (69%) of these symptoms were mild in severity.

Less common (0.4%) but more severe side effects included hepatitis, pseudomembranous colitis, and erythema multiforme.

Laboratory abnormality, specifically elevated liver enzymes in comparative trials, occurred with similar frequency in groups treated with other conventional antibiotics. Fewer than 1.0% of telithromycin recipients had elevated liver enzymes.

Telithromycin may prolong the QT interval when large doses are administered (see below).

Drug interactions due to competitive metabolism of telithromycin by CYP 3A4 and other drugs administered concurrently have demonstrated inhibition of simvastatin, cisapride, itraconazole, ketoconazole, and theophylline. No interaction with concomitant warfarin has been demonstrated.

STREPTOGRAMINS

Quinupristin and dalfopristin are streptogramin antibacterial drugs recently licensed for the treatment of vancomycin-resistant *E. faecium* infection and complicated skin and skin-structure infection caused by *S. pyogenes* and MSSA. The drugs are formulated as a 30:70 mixture for intravenous injection. The standard dose is 7.5 mg/kg infused over 60 minutes every 8 to 12 hours in 5% dextrose in water; it is incompatible with saline.[127]

MECHANISM OF ACTION Quinupristin and dalfopristin inhibit susceptible gram-positive bacteria including *E. faecium*, MSSA, MRSA, *S. pyogenes*, and *S. pneumoniae* by binding to the 50S ribosome. The two streptogramins produce a synergistic effect. Against *Staphylococcus*, including MRSA, quinupristin and dalfopristin are bactericidal; against *E. faecium*, the effect is generally bacteriostatic. The locus of ribosomal binding is near to, but different from that of, the macrolides.

A prolonged PAE of 9 to 10 hours from *S. aureus* and *S. pneumoniae* permits dosing every 8 or 12 hours despite a short elimination $t_{1/2}$.

MECHANISM OF RESISTANCE The macrolide antibiotics, lincosamide, and streptogramin antimicrobial agents have a common mechanism of action so that shared resistance is common. However, quinupristin and dalfopristin bind to a proximate but different locus on the 70S ribosome, so that cross-resistance with the aforementioned agent is uncommon as is resistance to quinupristin or dalfopristin.

CLINICAL PHARMACOLOGY Only a parenteral formulation is available. Dose and peak plasma concentrations are linearly related over the dose range of 1.4 to 29.4 mg/kg, suggesting indirectly that the apparent volume of distribution is constant. The mean plasma $t_{1/2}$ is similar for both drugs and ranges from 30 to 50 min. Protein bindings range from 11% to 26% for dalfopristin and from 55% to 78% for quinupristin.

Quinupristin and dalfopristin are eliminated primarily (about 75%) by hepatic biotransformation, followed by secretion into the bile and elimination in feces; 15% to 20% is eliminated as metabolite into urine.

Plasma concentrations are significantly increased in patients with hepatic insufficiency (Child-Pugh classes A and B). Dose reduction in such patients is appropriate, but precise regimens have not been formulated or validated.

Severe renal dysfunction (creatinine clearance 6 to 28 mL/min) did not significantly alter quinupristin and dalfopristin kinetics.

Pharmacokinetic studies in elderly (69 to 74 years) adults or obese patients did not yield clinically important differences from values in healthy male volunteers.

Quinupristin and dalfopristin inhibit CYP 3A4 and, at doses in excess of 10 mg/kg, prolong QT intervals. Thus, this combination must be given with care to patients receiving other drugs primarily metabolized by the CYP 3A4 P450 isozyme and with a narrow therapeutic window, particularly those that can prolong the QT interval (cisapride, lidocaine, quinidine, and disopyramide), and other drugs such as cyclosporine and tacrolimus, some antiretroviral drugs (delavirdine, neviapine, indinavir, and ritonavir), antineoplastic agents (vinca alkaloids, docetaxel, and paclitaxel), benzodiazepines (midazolam and diazepam), calcium channel blockers (dihydropyrines, verapamil, and diltiazem), antiepileptics (carbamazepine), and cholesterol-lowering drugs (statins).

ADVERSE DRUG EFFECTS Local pain and inflammation with edema and phlebitis are common during quinupristin or dalfopristin intravenous infusion, being observed in almost 50% of treated patients. Arthralgia, myalgia, and/or nausea resulted in treatment discontinuation in 22% of 90 treated patients with MRSA infection.

The major adverse effect of quinupristin and dalfopristin is phlebitis. This may be ameliorated by increasing the volume of the diluent, slowing the infusion rate even more, and delivering the drugs through a central venous catheter rather than a peripheral one.

Conjugated hyperbilirubinemia has been reported in 9% of treated patients, possibly related to competition for hepatocyte biliary secretion.

OXAZOLIDINONE

Linezolid is a synthetic, recently licensed member of a new class of antibiotics, the oxazolidinones.[128] It has a unique mechanism of action on susceptible bacterial ribosomes that differs from that of the macrolides, aminoglycosides, streptogramins, and lincosamides, making cross-resistance unlikely.

Linezolid is indicated for a wide range of gram-positive coccal infections in adult patients: VRE *faecium* infection; nosocomial pneumonia caused by MSSA, MRSA, and *S. pneumoniae* (penicillin-susceptible strains only); complicated skin and skin-structure infection due to MSSA, MRSA, *S. pyogenes*, or *S. agalactiae*; and uncomplicated skin and soft tissue infection caused by MSSA or *S. pyogenes*; and community-acquired pneumonia (CAP) due to penicillin-susceptible *S. pneumoniae* or MSSA.

Linezolid is formulated as oral tablets or for intravenous injection. The usual adult dose is 600 mg every 12 hours (400 mg every 12 hours for uncomplicated skin infection).

MECHANISM OF ACTION The precise molecular mechanism of action is not known, but linezolid inhibits bacterial protein synthesis. It is hypothesized to do so by interfering with the interaction of tRNA with the 50S ribosomal subunit during the initiation phase.

MECHANISM OF RESISTANCE Resistance of *S. aureus* and *S. epidermidis*, including methicillin-resistant strains, has been difficult to induce during serial passage in vitro in the presence of linezolid. A few *E. faecium* clinical isolates resistant to linezolid have been observed in a compassionate-use treatment program.[129]

CLINICAL PHARMACOLOGY Linezolid is 100% orally bioavailable in volunteers, but it is not known whether the same completeness of absorption can be confidently expected in critically ill patients; for such patients, intravenous administration is preferable. It is metabolized principally by oxidation to a biologically inactive form and excreted in urine as metabolites (70%) and unchanged drug (30%). The plasma $t_{1/2}$ is 4.6 to 5.4 hours.

Pharmacokinetic studies in volunteers with different degrees of renal dysfunction have indicated that linezolid doses need not be adjusted in persons with creatinine clearance faster than 10 mL/min. However, hemodialysis removes 38% of a dose, so the drug should be given after a hemodialysis treatment or an additional 200-mg dose can be given at the end of dialysis.

Linezolid pharmacokinetic characteristics in subjects with mild to moderate hepatic dysfunction did not differ from those in controls.

ADVERSE DRUG REACTIONS Linezolid can cause two unusual, clinically important adverse effects, myelosuppression and drug–drug interactions with adrenergic and serotonergic drugs.

Linezolid causes dose- and time-dependent myelosuppressions in 2% to 10% of patients at therapeutic doses; most commonly, thrombocytopenia is observed. The effect appears to be generally reversible on discontinuation of therapy; no irreversible blood dyscrasias have been reported. Complete blood counts at weekly intervals are recommended during therapy to facilitate early detection of this adverse effect.

Linezolid is a mild, reversible, competitive inhibitor of monoamine oxidase; therefore, in patients in the ICU, concomitant administration of linezolid with indirectly acting adrenergic or dopaminergic drugs including serotonin reuptake inhibitors may cause exaggerated sympathomimetic effects and occasionally signs and symptoms of the serotonin syndrome (e.g., hyperpyrexia and cognitive dysfunction). This adverse effect was expected but not observed in controlled clinical trials of linezolid in part because patients treated concurrently with dopaminergic and adrenergic drugs were excluded and because the monoamine oxidase inhibitory effect of linezolid is a relatively weak one.

In comparative clinical trials, linezolid was more likely than control comparator antibiotics to cause diarrhea (8.3% vs. 6.3% for comparators), nausea (6.2% vs. 4.6%), vomiting (3.7%

vs. 2.0%), and insomnia (2.5% vs. 1.7%). Linezolid caused thrombopenia in 2.4% of recipients of linezolid versus 1.5% in recipients of comparative antibiotics. Bleeding effects were not observed in those randomized trials but were observed during open-label compassionate use.

Overall, in the ICU, linezolid may become a valuable niche agent with particular utility for treatment of infection caused by nosocomial drug-resistant pathogens such as MRSA and VRE *faecium*.

Antiviral Drugs

Community-acquired and nosocomial viral infections may cause acute organ dysfunction or failure that necessitates admission of adult patients to the ICU or may complicate their management. A moderate number of different drugs are currently available that specifically and selectively inhibit virus replication and have an established role in the management of selected, serious, acute infections caused by DNA and RNA viruses in immunocompetent and immunocompromised hosts. The following agents are discussed in more detail: acyclovir, valacyclovir, famciclovir, foscarnet, ganciclovir, amantadine, rimantadine, zanamivir, oseltamivir, ribavirin, and some of the 16 currently licensed HIV-1 inhibitor drugs.

All these agents are virustatic only, which partly explains their limited value or failure in patients with defective immune responses.

VIDARABINE

Vidarabine (ara-A) was the first antiviral drug administered parenterally to humans whose efficacy was demonstrated unequivocally in a controlled trial (in patients with *Herpes simplex virus* [HSV] encephalitis).[130]

Ara-A has been approved for the treatment of HSV-1 encephalitis. Controlled trials have demonstrated that it is efficacious for the therapy of otherwise healthy neonates with HSV infection (mostly HSV-2) and immunocompromised patients with chickenpox, mucocutaneous HSV infection, and localized herpes zoster with a duration shorter than 72 hours. Acyclovir has replaced it for these indications, owing to greater ease of administration and better tolerance.[131] Ara-A is no longer marketed and is not further discussed.

ACYCLOVIR

Acyclovir is a synthetic, acyclic, purine nucleoside analogue of guanine in which the deoxyribose moiety has been replaced by a hydroxy-ethoxy-methyl substituent. In vitro, acyclovir inhibits HSV-1 and HSV-2 equally in concentrations 10 to 100 times less than are required with ara-A. Varicella zoster virus (VSV) is 10 times less sensitive than HSV, and the susceptibility of VZV to ara-A and acyclovir is similar. EBV is 10 to 20 times less sensitive than VZV, and CMV is 10 times less sensitive than EBV, to acyclovir.

Acyclovir is approved for the treatment of initial and recurrent mucocutaneous HSV infections in immunocompromised children and adults and for initial episodes of genital herpes in the normal host. It is the drug of choice for treatment of HSV encephalitis[131] and perinatal HSV infection.[131a] In neonates, it is no more effective than ara-A, but it is more acceptable because it can be administered in smaller volumes of intravenous fluid. It is also the drug of choice for the treatment of chickenpox[132] in normal and immunocompromised hosts and for recurrent VZV skin infections[133] in immunocompromised patients. In these patients, acyclovir accelerates resolution of the cutaneous eruption and prevents cutaneous and visceral dissemination. Acyclovir efficacy for other serious, non-neurologic HSV infections such as esophagitis and hepatitis in normal and immunodeficient hosts has been suggested in case reports.

CMV infections do not respond in a predictable manner to acyclovir because of the relative insusceptibility of CMV to acyclovir and the host immunodeficiency commonly present. To treat CMV infection, ganciclovir is currently recommended (see below). However, therapeutic and limited antiviral effects with acyclovir treatment were observed in renal transplant recipients with CMV pneumonia, enteritis, hepatitis, nephritis, and retinitis,[134] bone marrow transplant recipients with CMV pneumonitis,[135] and children with congenital CMV infection.

Infectious mononucleosis in normal hosts is favorably affected by acyclovir,[136] but steroids are more likely to be useful to treat oropharyngeal airway obstruction owing to lymphatic hyperplasia and hypertrophy. The usefulness of intravenous acyclovir to treat life-threatening EBV complications such as hepatitis or polyclonal B-cell lymphoproliferative disease in immunodeficient individuals (X-linked lymphoproliferative syndrome, renal transplantation, severe combined immunodeficiency, and ataxia telangiectasia) is unclear, although some favorable effects have been observed.

Herpesvirus simiae, also called *herpes B virus*, commonly causes infection in Old World monkeys. In rare instances, infection has been transmitted to monkey handlers and laboratory workers manipulating simian tissue. Infection usually results in severe, fatal encephalomyelitis. If an animal handler is scratched or bitten by a monkey suspected or known to be carrying B virus, an experimental study has suggested that intravenous, but not topical, acyclovir can prevent infection.[137] Its value in patients with established neurologic infection is less clear, but its use would seem reasonable.[138]

MECHANISM OF ACTION Acyclovir inhibits HSV with low toxicity for uninfected host cells. Its therapeutic:toxic ratio in vitro is 30 to 300:1. Acyclovir acts as a prodrug that diffuses freely into and out of host cells. In HSV-infected cells, viral thymidine kinase phosphorylates acyclovir to a monophosphate nucleotide. This conversion selectively traps the drug and contributes to its lack of toxicity for uninfected cells. Cellular enzymes convert the monophosphate form to di- and triphosphate nucleotides. Acyclovir triphosphate mediates the antiviral effect by inhibiting viral DNA polymerase and by inserting into DNA, precluding further addition of bases to the DNA strand, a process known as *chain termination.*

Because EBV possesses little thymidine kinase and CMV possesses none, acyclovir lacks a similar potent inhibitory effect on these two herpesvirus strains.

MECHANISM OF RESISTANCE Strains of HSV relatively resistant to acyclovir exist in nature and may comprise up to 10% of HSV viruses.[139] In addition, acyclovir-resistant strains of HSV and VZV may be selected in vitro and in patients during therapy. In patients, acyclovir inefficacy associated with emergence of resistant strains is almost exclusively observed in immunocompromised hosts.[139] Acyclovir-resistant strains

of HSV and VZV remain susceptible to ara-A and foscarnet in vitro, and these agents have been reported to be effective when acyclovir is not.[140]

Acyclovir resistance in HSV and VZV is mediated by genetic alterations that result in production of thymidine kinase–defective mutants (mostly) and DNA polymerase-insusceptible mutants (less commonly).[141]

CLINICAL PHARMACOLOGY[142] Acyclovir is available in topical, oral, and intravenous formulations. Although it is freely soluble in water, solutions have a high pH of 9 to 11, so it is not recommended for intramuscular or subcutaneous injection because it causes tissue inflammation and pain. After intravenous injection, concentrations in CSF and aqueous humor are 35% to 50% of those in the plasma. Binding to plasma proteins is relatively low (9% to 22%), so adverse interactions owing to displacement by other drugs have not been described.

The elimination $t_{1/2}$ of acyclovir from plasma is directly related to renal function because acyclovir is eliminated by glomerular filtration and renal tubular secretion. The latter mechanism is dominant as demonstrated by a mean acyclovir clearance rate that is four to six times greater than the creatinine clearance rate and by elevated C_p and prolonged $t_{1/2}$ values in patients given probenecid concurrently. The plasma elimination $t_{1/2}$ ranges from 2.5 hours in adults with normal renal function to 18 hours in those who are anuric. Nonrenal elimination of acyclovir contributes minimally to acyclovir clearance except in the presence of severe renal insufficiency. Up to 14% of a dose is eliminated as a glucuronide metabolite in urine, and less than 2% appears in feces.

Mean acyclovir plasma $t_{1/2}$ during hemodialysis is approximately 5 hours, which reflects removal of about 50% of drug during 6 hours of dialysis.

The usual doses of acyclovir are 5 mg/kg for patients with mucocutaneous HSV infection and 10 mg/kg for patients with HSV encephalitis or VZV infection. The dose is repeated at intervals inversely related to creatinine clearance:

Creatine Clearance (mL/min)	Dose Interval (h)
>50	8
25–50	12
10–25	24
0–10	24–48

Hemodialysis patients should be given a standard initial dose that is repeated every 48 hours and after each dialysis.

ADVERSE DRUG REACTIONS Acyclovir is relatively free of serious toxicity. Crystalluria with renal tubular obstruction and elevated serum creatinine concentration can be avoided by not exceeding the recommended doses and by not administering a dose in less than 60 min. Phlebitis can be avoided by infusing acyclovir in concentrations below 10 mg/mL. Tissue inflammation will develop if drug extravasates during infusion.

Neurotoxic symptoms of lethargy, agitation, tremor, disorientation, or transient paraesthesias have been observed in bone marrow transplant recipients during prolonged intravenous acyclovir therapy.[143] These symptoms resolved on withdrawal of therapy, but their relation to acyclovir dose, duration of therapy, or plasma or CSF concentrations remains unknown. Psychiatric side effects including hallucinations and depression have been observed in patients with renal failure given doses in excess of those currently recommended, suggesting a dose-related effect. Delirium has been reported as a side effect of acyclovir in a hemodialysis patient receiving appropriately reduced doses,[144] and coma has been reported, beginning 24 to 48 hours after development of peak acyclovir serum concentration after a severe overdose.[145] Based on pharmacokinetic calculations, a loading oral dose of 400 mg followed by 200 mg twice daily with a supplemental oral dose of 400 mg has been proposed for oral doses to minimize neurotoxicity.[146] However, the utility of these calculated doses has not been validated prospectively.

Serious neurotoxic effects of acyclovir are likely to occur primarily in individuals with renal insufficiency in whom these effects can largely be avoided by careful attention to dose, frequency, and rate of administration; it has been suggested that the adverse effects can be treated by hemodialysis.[146]

VALACYCLOVIR AND FAMCICLOVIR

Valacyclovir is the ester oral prodrug of acyclovir.[147] Esterification increases oral bioavailability of acyclovir approximately twofold, from 15% to 30% to 55%. Famciclovir is a well-absorbed (77% oral bioavailability) analogue of acyclovir.[148]

Neither of these oral agents offers any unique advantage over intravenous acyclovir for treatment of ICU patients and they are not discussed further.

GANCICLOVIR[149]

Ganciclovir is a synthetic, acyclic, nucleoside analogue of guanine that differs from acyclovir in possessing a hydroxymethyl group on the ribose remnant. This modest structural alteration nevertheless profoundly affects its antiviral potency and its cellular toxicity. Compared with acyclovir, ganciclovir in vitro is on average three times less potent against HSV-1 and HSV-2, 10 times less potent against VZV, similarly potent against EBV, and 10 to 100 times more potent against CMV (0.2 to 2.8 mg/L is inhibitory). Ganciclovir concentrations of approximately 0.6 mg/L are toxic to human bone marrow progenitor cells compared with concentrations in excess of 20 mg/L for acyclovir. The clinically important feature of ganciclovir is its antiviral effect against CMV, but its therapeutic:toxic ratio is 1 or less.

In addition to its low therapeutic:toxic ratio, ganciclovir is mutagenic, teratogenic, and carcinogenic in laboratory animals. Accordingly, its use is limited to patients with serious CMV infections, almost all of whom are immunoincompetent owing to iatrogenic factors, such as immunosuppressive drug therapy in transplant recipients, or disease, such as HIV infection. Controlled clinical trials have demonstrated ganciclovir efficacy for treatment of CMV retinitis in HIV-infected individuals.[150] Less substantive data suggest that ganciclovir produces improvement in 65% of HIV-infected patients with CMV enteritis, esophagitis, wasting illness, and, possibly, pneumonitis.[151] Ganciclovir for 3 weeks is effective to suppress CMV-emia in allogeneic bone marrow recipients.[152] However, controlled trials in bone marrow transplant recipients with CMV pneumonitis have demonstrated that ganciclovir is inefficacious when administered

alone or in combination with corticosteroids but decreases mortality rate when administered with CMV hyperimmune globulin.[153]

Intravitreal ganciclovir appears to be effective for treatment of CMV retinitis in HIV-infected patients and to obviate the toxicity observed with intravenous therapy.

MECHANISMS OF ACTION   Ganciclovir inhibits viral DNA replication after intracellular conversion to the triphosphate nucleotide form. Phosphorylation is catalyzed by the virus-encoded enzyme UL97. Ganciclovir triphosphate acts like acyclovir triphosphate in selectively inhibiting viral DNA polymerase; its incorporation into viral DNA causes a slowing of DNA chain elongation and ultimately effects chain termination of the viral DNA strand. However, because it possesses two hydroxyl groups on the acyclic side chain, ganciclovir can be incorporated into host and viral DNA without abruptly interfering with chain elongation the way acyclovir triphosphate does.

MECHANISM OF RESISTANCE   Ganciclovir-resistant CMV strains have been selected during serial passage of virus in the laboratory in the presence of the drug. Resistance associated with failure of ganciclovir therapy has been reported in immunocompromised patients. Foscarnet was effective in two such patients. Resistance was associated with reduced intracellular accumulation of ganciclovir in infected cells mediated by one or more specific point mutations in the UL97 gene.[154] The presence of the mutation can be demonstrated by direct sequencing of CMV DNA in the patient's plasma.

CLINICAL PHARMACOLOGY   Oral and intravenous formulations of ganciclovir are available. There are two oral formulations, ganciclovir in capsules, which is 3% to 6% bioavailable, and valganciclovir in tablets, a prodrug that increases systemic ganciclovir availability to 61% of injected drug.[155] Valganciclovir increases ganciclovir oral bioavailability 10-fold, likely due to recognition of valganciclovir as a substrate by intestinal peptide transporters.

Oral ganciclovir capsules in large doses (3000 mg/d) deliver sufficient ganciclovir systemically to maintain CMV suppression achieved initially by intravenous drug. Thus, it is efficacious for suppressing CMV retinitis in HIV patients. Oral valganciclovir will replace oral ganciclovir capsules because of its more favorable bioavailability. It also likely will be a stepdown alternative to intravenous ganciclovir, which remains the recommended mode of administration for ill patients.

Ganciclovir diffuses readily into lungs, liver, aqueous and vitreous humors, and CSF. Elimination from plasma is by a first-order process with a $t_{1/2}$ of 2.5 to 3.6 hours that is inversely related to creatinine clearance. Ganciclovir is excreted into urine as unaltered drug.

The recommended dose of intravenous ganciclovir for adults with normal renal function is 5 mg/kg infused intravenously over 1 hour every 12 hours. Oral valganciclovir, 900 mg in a single dose, yields a serum area under the plasma-concentration versus time curve (AUC) of 0 to 24 hours similar to that observed after a single ganciclovir intravenous infusion of 5 mg/kg (41.7 vs. 48.2 mg/L per hour). For patients with impaired renal function, the dose or interval for intravenous ganciclovir scheduling should be adjusted as follows:

Creatine Clearance (mL/min)	Ganciclovir Dose (mg/kg)	Dose Interval (h)
>80	5.0	12
59–79	2.5	12
25–49	2.5	12
<25	1.25	24

Hemodialysis for 4 hours removes an average of 53% of the body load of ganciclovir; one-half (2.5 mg/kg body weight) the standard dose should be administered after each dialysis.

ADVERSE DRUG REACTIONS Primarily because of incorporation in replicating host DNA, ganciclovir causes significant toxic effects in rapidly proliferating tissues and organs. Thus, in laboratory animals, ganciclovir causes hematopoietic, gonadal, and gastrointestinal toxicities.

In humans, hematopoietic toxicity has been the most common adverse side effect observed. Neutropenia and thrombocytopenia have been observed in 40% and 20%, respectively, of HIV-infected patients, and anemia has been noted less frequently. Concomitant administration of zidovudine and ganciclovir increases the frequency of neutropenia. Neutropenia and thrombocytopenia are almost always promptly reversible when ganciclovir is discontinued. In up to 15% of patients, ganciclovir, similar to the antiviral nucleosides acyclovir and ara-A, causes CNS toxicity, with manifestations ranging from headaches to behavioral changes, psychosis, convulsions, and coma. The mechanism is not known. Ganciclovir CNS toxicity may be difficult to differentiate from CNS dysfunction owing to concurrent disease and other drug therapy in seriously ill patients.

Oral ganciclovir capsules, oral valganciclovir, and intravenous ganciclovir in clinically equivalent doses caused diarrhea in 13%, 42%, and 7%, respectively, of patients; nausea in 7%, 28%, and 13%, respectively; anemia in 7%, 25%, and 14%, respectively; and leucopenia in 22%, 36%, and 25%, respectively.

FOSCARNET[156]

Foscarnet (trisodium phosphonoformate hexahydrate) is a relatively insoluble (aqueous solubility 5% [wt/wt]) antiviral drug. In vitro, foscarnet inhibits several DNA and RNA viruses at concentrations from 6 to 120 mg/L, but cellular cytotoxicity is observed at concentrations of 150 to 300 mg/L, yielding toxic:therapeutic ratios ranging from 1 to 7:1.

Intravenous foscarnet is licensed only for treatment of CMV retinitis in AIDS patients. However, studies have suggested that foscarnet may have value for a wider range of CMV infections (pneumonitis and encephalitis) in immunocompromised patients (HIV-infected patients and renal and bone marrow transplant recipients). Foscarnet is effective for therapy of acyclovir-resistant HSV or VZV and ganciclovir-resistant CMV infections. Six patients with fulminant hepatitis caused by hepatitis B or concomitant Delta virus infection survived in association with intravenous foscarnet therapy. Although the number of patients studied was small and historical controls were used to analyze therapeutic benefit, fos-

carnet may have a role in fulminant hepatitis B infection because no other specific treatment for this infection is currently available.

Foscarnet is the drug of choice for the treatment of CMV infections in individuals unable to tolerate ganciclovir, for patients with acyclovir-resistant HSV and VZV infection, and for those with ganciclovir-resistant CMV infections.

MECHANISM OF ACTION Foscarnet is an analogue of pyrophosphate, a metabolite of nucleic acid synthesis. Foscarnet acts by inhibiting DNA and RNA polymerases, including HIV reverse transcriptase. Foscarnet inhibits DNA polymerase activity noncompetitively by binding at the pyrophosphate binding site.

MECHANISMS OF RESISTANCE Naturally occurring foscarnet-resistant HSV strains seem uncommon (1 of 41 HSV isolates in one study). Foscarnet-resistant mutants of HSV-1 and HSV-2 and non-HIV retroviruses can be cultivated in in vitro experimental systems. These mutants possess DNA polymerase resistant to foscarnet. However, resistance development has not been observed during foscarnet therapy of experimental HSV infection in laboratory animals or during clinical trials in patients with HSV or CMV infection.

Resistance appears to be mediated by a mutation in the foscarnet binding site on the DNA polymerase. Some, but not all, of these foscarnet-resistant strains exhibit diminished susceptibility to nucleoside analogues such as ara-A, suggesting that the mutational alteration affected a binding site on the enzyme common to both drugs. In addition, an acyclovir-resistant HSV-1 strain with intact thymidine kinase but mutated DNA polymerase exhibited increased sensitivity to foscarnet and ara-A, suggesting that a change in the acyclovir triphosphate binding site affects the interaction of foscarnet and the ara-A triphosphate metabolite with the polymerase.

CLINICAL PHARMACOLOGY[156] Foscarnet oral bioavailability is low, with only 12% to 22% of oral doses being absorbed. The combination of poor oral bioavailability and the large doses required (100 to 200 mg/kg per day) even when foscarnet is given intravenously make oral therapy impractical. Intravenous regimens used to treat CMV infections consist of an initial dose of 20 mg/kg over 30 minutes followed by continuous infusion of 230 mg/kg per day or 60 mg/kg three times per day to achieve a target C_p of 45 to 135 mg/L. Infusion requires several hours because the maximum concentration of drug recommended for intravenous administration is 2000 mg/L. Steady-state plasma foscarnet concentrations range from 40 to 400 mg/L (mean, 100) with a peak C_p of approximately 150 mg/L.

After intravenous administration, the drug disappears from plasma in a tri-exponential manner, with $t_{1/2}$ values of 0.5, 3, and 18 hours. The long terminal $t_{1/2}$ probably reflects the slow release of foscarnet from bone. The kinetic AVD is about 0.6 to 0.7 L/kg. Plasma protein binding is 17%. CSF concentrations average 43% (range, 13% to 68%) of simultaneous C_p. Penetration into the retina seems sufficient to inhibit CMV replication and ameliorate retinitis. Knowledge of foscarnet distribution in humans is otherwise incomplete. In animals, foscarnet, being a phosphate analogue, is incorporated into the mineral matrix of bone. Foscarnet does not undergo metabolic transformation. It is eliminated unchanged into the urine. Renal clearance averages 130 to 175 mL/min per 1.73 m^2 of surface area, suggesting that renal tubular secretion and glomerular filtration contribute to foscarnet elimination.

The kinetic characteristics of foscarnet in patients undergoing dialysis require further study. Available data indicate that the Cp of foscarnet declines rapidly during hemodialysis. This is consistent with the knowledge that foscarnet is a small molecule (molecular weight, 300 kd) that is minimally protein bound. Tissue binding of foscarnet likely will preclude extensive removal by dialysis. This facet of foscarnet disposition and its implications for dosing require further study. However, one recommendation suggests reducing the foscarnet dose by 30 mg/kg per day for each 20 mmol/L increase in creatinine concentration above 70 mmol/L.[157]

ADVERSE DRUG EFFECTS Although foscarnet commonly causes biochemical evidence of toxicity (anemia, leukopenia, thrombocytopenia, and elevation in serum creatinine, etc.), symptomatic toxicity is uncommon. Hallucinations and a flapping tremor, temporally directly related to foscarnet therapy, were associated with a relatively high Cp of 449 mg/L for foscarnet and disappeared when foscarnet was discontinued; these were therefore considered to represent direct toxic effects of the drug.

Anemia without alterations in white blood cell count or platelet concentration and mild elevations in the serum creatinine level occurs in 15% to 50% of patients, but the contributions of concurrent other drugs (e.g., cyclosporine) and underlying disease have been difficult to exclude. Hypercalcemia occurs in about 20% of patients and abnormal transaminase in 5% to 10%. Local phlebitis is uncommon. Adverse interactions of foscarnet with other drugs have not been described.

AMANTADINE

Amantadine is a synthetic, tricyclic, basic amine antiviral agent with antimicrobial utility limited to the prevention and treatment of *influenza A virus* infection.

In vitro, amantadine inhibits influenza A viruses in low concentrations of 0.2 to 0.4 mg/L. This effect has been uniformly demonstrable against all three major pandemic strains of influenza A virus and their subtypes.

Amantadine is approved for the prevention and treatment of influenza A virus infection. It has been demonstrated to be efficacious in preventing nosocomial influenza A infection in patients in acute general hospital wards, and it should be similarly effective in ICU patients, although no data exist on this issue.[158] Treatment of otherwise healthy, young adults with uncomplicated influenza illness accelerates resolution of systemic symptoms and some respiratory tract symptoms by 50% and hastens the resolution of increased peripheral airways resistance that is presumably related to inflammatory narrowing of small and medium bronchioles. In addition, treatment decreases the frequency and duration of virus shedding. Unfortunately, no data demonstrate that similar beneficial effects can be achieved by amantadine therapy in ICU patients with influenza A infection complicating severe obstructive airways disease or other severe underlying parenchymal lung disease, or with primary influenza A pneumonia in the absence of pre-existing lung disease.

For outbreak control, amantadine should be administered to all patients if epidemic influenza A infection is suspected or documented in the institution. When amantadine is used for outbreak control, it should be administered to all patients regardless of whether they received influenza vaccine recently and to unvaccinated staff. All unimmunized staff and patients given prophylactic amantadine should be offered immunization with the current vaccine simultaneously if the epidemic strain(s) is identical to, or closely related to, the vaccine strain(s). Amantadine prophylaxis should be continued until the outbreak is over, that is, until an interval equivalent to two incubation periods, 48 and 72 hours, after the period of communicability of the last case in the institution (about 5 to 6 days after onset) has passed.

MECHANISM OF ACTION Amantadine inhibits replication of influenza A virus by interfering with uncoating of the virus and release of the RNA genome in lysosomes. This effect requires that drug be present continuously in the extracellular milieu. Thus, the prophylactic or therapeutic effect is rapidly lost as drug is excreted from the body after discontinuation of drug administration.

MECHANISM OF RESISTANCE Susceptibility to the antiviral effect of amantadine is influenced by the virion M2 protein in the influenza virion envelope. Even single changes of amino acid in M2 decrease susceptibility to amantadine. Resistance to amantadine is readily selected for in vitro, during passage in mice experimentally infected with influenza A virus, and during amantadine treatment in patients. More studies are required to define the precise clinical relevance of these observations.

CLINICAL PHARMACOLOGY[159] Amantadine is highly water soluble with a pKa of 11. Its utility in the ICU setting is limited by its availability only in enteral forms as capsules of 100 mg or a syrup containing 10 mg/mL. Although data from studies in experimentally infected mice and patients with severe natural infection suggest that inhalation of amantadine as an aerosol may be more effective for influenza therapy than administration enterally, no formulation suitable for aerosol administration is available. For healthy adults 65 years of age, the recommended amantadine dose is 200 mg/d; for those older than 65 years, the dose is 100 mg/d.

In healthy adults including the elderly, amantadine is slowly (time to peak Cp, 6 to 12 hours after ingestion) but virtually completely absorbed, but no data have confirmed that similar results occur in acutely ill ICU patients. It is widely distributed with a mean AVD of 6.6L/kg that probably decreases with advanced age. As expected, there are two consequences of this pharmacokinetic characteristic. First, Cp values are low, averaging 0.5 to 0.8 mg/L at peak and 0.3 mg/L at trough at steady state, in young, healthy adults ingesting 200 mg/d and elderly men with normal creatinine Cp ingesting 100 mg/d. Second, negligible amounts are removed by hemodialysis. Amantadine is found in highest concentration in the brain, liver, lung, and kidneys in treated animals; a similar localization in humans may explain the propensity of this drug to cause CNS side effects (and, in part, ameliorate symptoms of Parkinson disease). Nasal mucus concentrations of amantadine only approximate concurrent Cp. This may explain the superiority of administration of amantadine as an aerosol for therapy of influenza A in experimentally infected mice and volunteers because aerosol administration of amantadine resulted in a mean nasal washing fluid (and presumably mucus and respiratory epithelial cell) concentration of 66,658 mg/L after long-term oral ingestion of 200 mg/d and 30,300 to 111,300 mg/L after inhalation of aerosol generated from a reservoir containing 10 g/L amantadine in volunteers.

Elimination is a first-order process, with a plasma $t_{1/2}$ averaging 14 hours in healthy, young adults and 28 hours in healthy, elderly men (and, presumably, women). Renal clearance exceeds creatinine clearance by approximately three times, implying significant renal tubular secretion of amantadine in addition to elimination by glomerular filtration. The plasma $t_{1/2}$ is inversely related to creatinine clearance, and this fact led to the following recommendation for dose modification in patients with stable renal dysfunction:

Creatine Clearance (mL/min per 1.73 m² surface area)	Amantadine Dosage
>80	200 mg/d
60–80	200–100 mg on alternate days
40–60	100 mg/d
30–40	200 mg twice weekly
20–30	100 mg thrice weekly
10–20	200–100 mg at alternate weeks

In patients on hemodialysis, a single 200-mg loading dose should be sufficient. The plasma $t_{1/2}$ of amantadine may be as long as 30 days in such individuals.

ADVERSE DRUG REACTIONS Amantadine is generally well tolerated. Mild, amphetamine-like adverse symptoms occur in 1% to 10% of young adults, manifesting as insomnia, difficulty concentrating, nightmares, jitteriness, and depression. These symptoms are rapidly reversible on discontinuation of drug administration. Rarely, severe neurotoxic adverse symptoms ranging from seizures (in those with underlying convulsive disorders), psychosis, to convulsions occur. These generally occur in patients given excessive doses or with renal insufficiency. Amantadine Cp values are usually above 1 mg/L in these individuals.

Isolated instances of congestive heart failure, vision loss, and urinary retention have been reported. Livedo reticularis and peripheral edema during chronic therapy have been described.

Anticholinergic and antihistamine drugs may increase adverse effects caused by amantadine. A diuretic containing triamterene and hydrochlorothiazide was associated with neurotoxicity and increased amantadine Cp owing to reduced renal clearance. Because amantadine is a cationic drug, its renal tubular secretion would be expected to be decreased by concurrent administration of other basic drugs such as quinidine, nicotine, and trimethoprim. The possibility of such concomitant therapy increasing the frequency or severity of amantadine side effects requires further study.

RIMANTADINE

Rimantadine, a methylated analogue of amantadine, is approved in the United States as an oral agent for prophylaxis of influenza A infection in children and adults and for the treatment of influenza A infection in adults. Rimantadine thus may be used to prevent infection in ICU patients and personnel during an outbreak. Rimantadine was better tolerated than amantadine in a comparative trial in young adults but no more efficacious than amantadine at the same dose, 200 mg/d. An experimental formulation of rimantadine was administered as aerosol to volunteers with influenza A infection. Aerosolized rimantadine caused mild nasal irritation but was as effective as a small oral dose (150 mg/d) of rimantadine and more effective than placebo. The value of such treatment in intubated, ventilated patients with severe influenzal illness in the ICU has not been described. No injectable formulation is available.

MECHANISMS OF ACTION AND RESISTANCE See mechanism of action of amantadine (above). Rimantadine is more potent in vitro than amantadine, with 50% inhibitory concentrations being two to eight times less than for amantadine; the clinical importance of this difference is uncertain.

MECHANISM OF RESISTANCE Resistance emerges as readily during therapy with rimantadine as during therapy with amantadine, being demonstrable in 30% of recipients after 2 to 3 days of treatment. The mechanism of rimantadine resistance is identical to that for amantadine resistance. Cross-resistance is complete.

CLINICAL PHARMACOLOGY[160] Rimantadine is available only as tablets or syrup for oral administration. Some clinical pharmacokinetic characteristics of rimantadine differ substantially from those of amantadine. Rimantadine is absorbed as well and completely (>90%) as amantadine. The AVD is similar to that of amantadine, about 10 L/kg. Greater than 75% of a rimantadine dose is metabolized compared with less than 10% of an amantadine dose. Rimantadine undergoes hydroxylation, conjugation, and glucuronidation. A 2-OH metabolite has 10% the activity of the parent compound; the others are devoid of antiviral activity. The metabolites are eliminated into urine. Rimantadine clearance, averaging 350 mL/min, is not affected by age in otherwise healthy adults. The elimination serum $t_{1/2}$ of rimantadine averages 25 to 37 hours, approximately twice as long as that of amantadine. The recommended dose for healthy adults younger than 65 years is 200 mg/d. Based on the incomplete pharmacokinetic data, a reduced dose of 100 mg/d is recommended for prophylaxis and treatment of adults with severe renal dysfunction (creatinine clearance < 10 mL/min) or hepatic dysfunction and of elderly nursing home patients. In patients with mild or moderate renal insufficiency, the standard dose should be administered and patients closely observed for adverse reactions. In patients with end-stage renal failure, mean elimination $t_{1/2}$ is 44 hours. A 50% reduction in dose is recommended. Rimantadine is not removed by hemodialysis. In patients with mild or moderate liver disease (no ascites, normal albumin, total bilirubin <46 mmol), rimantadine kinetics were not different from those in normal subjects.

ADVERSE DRUG REACTIONS Comparative trials have demonstrated that rimantadine, like amantadine, is generally well tolerated. It causes a lower incidence of adverse symptoms than does amantadine, and, unlike that drug, it causes predominantly gastrointestinal ADR (nausea, anorexia, dry mouth, abdominal pain, and diarrhea). Rimantadine enters the brain, but CNS toxic symptoms are less commonly seen with it than with amantadine.

No clinically important interactions of rimantadine with other drugs have been reported.

There are no trials comparing the efficacy or safety of amantadine or rimantadine used to treat patients in the ICU, but the differences in pharmacokinetic characteristics are important to note in selecting one or the other in patients with severe renal or hepatic insufficiency.

ZANAMIVIR AND OSELTAMIVIR

These drugs have recently been approved for the prevention and treatment of influenza A and B infections.[161,162] Zanamivir is administered as an orally inhaled powder, whereas oseltamivir is administered as oral capsules; no intravenous formulations are available commercially, although intravenous zanamivir was well tolerated and effective in preventing experimental influenza A infection in volunteers.

These agents differ from the M2 ion channel inhibitors, amantadine and rimantadine, in three characteristics. First, zanamivir and oseltamivir inhibit influenza A and B viruses, whereas the M2 ion channel inhibitors only inhibit influenza A strains. Second, these agents do not cause dose-related side effects of consequence (oseltamivir causes mild nausea and/or vomiting after initial doses in 10% to 15% of subjects vs. 5% to 8% of placebo recipients and zanamivir rarely causes bronchospasm in those with underlying obstructive airways disease). Third, these agents do not seem to share the propensity of amantadine and rimantadine to engender the emergence of drug-resistant virus. Amantadine- and rimantadine-resistant influenza A viruses would be expected to be susceptible to zanamivir and oseltamivir.

Zanamivir and oseltamivir are effective for the prevention of influenza A and B, and the treatment of uncomplicated influenzal illness. Neither drug appears more efficacious than the other or more efficacious than amantadine or rimantadine. No available data demonstrate that either of these agents is effective for treatment of established primary influenza pneumonia.

MECHANISM OF ACTION Zanamivir and oseltamivir inhibit influenza virus replication by inhibiting the virus-encoded enzyme neuraminidase, which is essential for release of daughter virions from infected cells. Human neuraminidase is 10^6 to 10^7 times less susceptible to inhibition by these drugs.[163]

MECHANISM OF RESISTANCE Resistance evolves in two steps. Initially, mutational changes in the viral hemagglutinin enzymatic pocket result in diminished affinity of the hemagglutinin for sialic acid, resulting in decreased dependency on the neuraminidase for virus elution. Such viruses would be less susceptible to the inhibitory effect of these drugs. Subsequently, resistance arises due to mutations in the enzymatic pocket of the neuraminidase itself, which impairs the ability of the drugs to interfere with the neuraminidase-mediated catalytic function.

CLINICAL PHARMACOLOGY Orally inhaled zanamivir is administered in a dose of two puffs (10 mg) once (for prophylaxis) or twice (for treatment) each day. The recommended dose of oseltamivir is 75 mg once or twice a day for prevention or treatment of influenza, respectively. From 4% to 17%

of a zanamivir dose is absorbed, mostly through the lungs. Oseltamivir is 80% orally bioavailable, although this has not been confirmed in seriously ill patients in the ICU.

Both drugs exhibit low levels of protein binding (<5%). Inhaled zanamivir distributes through the upper and lower airways, whereas oseltamivir distributes throughout the body, with an AVD equivalent to about 36% of total body weight; the anatomic correlate is not known.

Both drugs are eliminated from the body largely unchanged by glomerular filtration and by renal tubular secretion by a first-order process, with a serum $t_{1/2}$ of 1.8 hours in persons with normal renal function. Renal clearance is decreased by renal dysfunction and dose reductions by half are recommended for oseltamivir in patients with creatinine clearance slower than 30 mL/min. Systemic exposure to zanamivir after oral inhalation is so low and the tolerance of zanamivir sufficiently high that dose reduction of zanamivir is not needed in patients with renal dysfunction.

DRUG INTERACTIONS In both cases, low protein binding and systemic clearance as unchanged drug without significant metabolism suggest that drug interactions due to alterations in binding or competitive inhibition of metabolism will not affect other drugs administered concurrently. Animal studies and limited human studies have confirmed these predictions. Oseltamivir, which is secreted by a renal tubular anionic transporter, might interfere with the renal secretion of other anionic drugs such as probenecid. A clinical study confirmed that such an interaction could occur; probenecid clearance was reduced 50%.

ADVERSE DRUG REACTIONS Zanamivir rarely can cause worsening of airway obstruction in patients with severe or decompensated chronic pulmonary or airway disease or asthma, and the manufacturer recommends against its use in these patients.

Oseltamivir causes nausea and/or vomiting, usually after only the initial dose, in 5% to 10% of oseltamivir recipients in excess of rates in concurrent placebo recipients. No serious or fatal drug-related adverse events have been observed in oseltamivir recipients.

In conclusion, these two new anti-influenza drugs have substantial advantages over amantadine and rimantadine as agents for preventing and treating influenza A and B infections in the ICU. Unfortunately and of primary concern, no studies have demonstrated their efficacy for treating patients with influenza pneumonia.

RIBAVIRIN

Ribavirin is a synthetic analogue of guanosine. In vitro, it inhibits the replication of a wide range of RNA and DNA viruses. Clinically, its value in the management of ICU patients is limited to the treatment of individuals with influenza A or B or respiratory syncytial virus respiratory tract infection with aerosolized drug and the intravenous therapy of patients with Lassa fever, an enzootic infection of rodents in West Africa that may be imported in returning travelers and be transmitted from patients to health care workers.

In clinical trials, ribavirin has been efficacious when administered as an aerosol to children and adults with respiratory syncytial virus infection and otherwise healthy adults with uncomplicated influenza A or B virus infection. Intravenous ribavirin decreases mortality rate in patients with Lassa fever and it is likely effective, although incompletely studied, for some other viral hemorrhagic fevers.[164] A rigorous evaluation failed to demonstrate any beneficial effect of intravenous plus intracerebroventricular ribavirin in an adult with symptomatic rabies encephalomyelopathy. An uncontrolled study suggested efficacy when given intravenously to three patients with severe lower respiratory tract infection with influenza or parainfluenza viruses.[165] The utility of ribavirin for therapy of alphavirus encephalitides caused by Eastern, Western, or Venezuelan equine encephalitis viruses that are susceptible in vitro has not been reported.

Recently, ribavirin combined with pegylated interferon α_{2b} has been licensed for the treatment of chronic hepatitis C infection. The recommended dose is 200 mg, or five capsules per day for patients weighing less than 75 kg or six capsules per day for those weighing more than 75 kg, plus 3 million U interferon α_{2b} injected subcutaneously three times per week, for 24 to 48 weeks.

MECHANISM OF ACTION The precise molecular basis of the antiviral effects of ribavirin is not known. Multiple mechanisms probably are involved with differences between RNA and DNA viruses and virus-specific differences within each of these two groups.

Within cells, ribavirin behaves in part like an adenosine analogue, being phosphorylated to its mono-, di-, and triphosphate nucleotide forms by cellular adenosine kinase. Ribavirin-5′-phosphate seems to be the principal metabolite mediating the antiviral effect of ribavirin on influenza replication by inhibition of cellular inosine monophosphate dehydrogenase resulting in guanosine depletion and inhibition of viral RNA synthesis. This antiviral effect can be reversed by exogenous guanosine. However, ribavirin-5′-triphosphate also selectively inhibits influenza RNA polymerase, suggesting another locus for the antiviral effect of ribavirin on influenza replication. The multiple modes of action of ribavirin may account for the absence of reports of ribavirin resistance in clinical isolates.

CLINICAL PHARMACOLOGY Ribavirin is a water-soluble agent that has been administered to patients by aerosol, mouth, and intravenous injection.

For aerosol administration to patients with viral pulmonary infection, the drug has been prepared as a solution containing 20 g/L, which must be aerosolized in a special generator to yield particles of about 1.4 μm in diameter that will reach terminal airways and alveoli. Oral ribavirin is approximately 45% bioavailable due to substantial first-pass metabolism. Intravenous administration yields Cp values of 17 and 24 mg/L after doses of 500 and 1000 mg, respectively. These are approximately 10-fold higher than after comparable oral doses. Ribavirin distributes widely throughout the body. It accumulates within erythrocytes owing to trapping by phosphorylation. CSF concentrations average 50% to 65% of concurrent plasma levels. The drug undergoes extensive hepatic biotransformation as demonstrated by recovery of only 24% of an intravenous dose as unchanged drug in urine. Elimination from plasma is a triphasic process, with $t_{1/2}$ values of 0.2, 2, and 36 hours. Attainment of plateau concentrations in plasma will take 1 to 2 weeks.

The effect of concomitant hepatic or renal disease or other drugs on ribavirin disposition remains largely unstudied.

ADVERSE DRUG REACTIONS After administration by aerosol, ribavirin is generally well tolerated except for mild conjunctival irritation. Wheezing and cough have been observed in patients with asthma or mild chronic obstructive airway disease. These adverse effects were reversible by discontinuation of aerosol therapy or administration of aerosolized β agonist.[166] When administered to intubated patients by mechanical ventilator, ribavirin aerosol droplets deposit on the tubing and hoses, absorb water owing to their hygroscopic nature, and thereby interfere with efficient ventilation. The use of in-line filters, modified circuitry, and careful attention to pressure build-up can minimize deleterious effects on pulmonary gas exchange.

Ribavirin given intravenously for Lassa fever therapy only caused reversible anemia, which did not require transfusion, as a side effect.

Chronic oral ribavirin therapy causes CNS and gastrointestinal complaints including headache, lethargy, fatigue, insomnia, and anorexia. A dose-dependent macrocytic hemolytic anemia with a contribution from myelosuppression in those receiving larger doses commonly occurs. During treatment of chronic active hepatitis C infection, 10% of patients developed hemolysis resulting in hemoglobin levels below 10 g/dL.

Adverse interactions of ribavirin with other drugs or diseases have not been described.

In view of possible ribavirin teratogenic and embryotoxic effects in humans, like those observed in small laboratory animals, pregnant members of the nursing staff are advised to avoid protracted exposure to ribavirin aerosol.

NUCLEOSIDE REVERSE TRANSCRIPTASE INHIBITORS

Nucleoside reverse transcriptase inhibitors (NRTIs) are antiretroviral inhibitors comprising seven agents that are analogues of purines and pyrimidines used in the transcription of the HIV genome. The drugs require intracellular activation to a triphosphate nucleotide form, which is the active antiviral molecule. That is, they are in effect prodrugs. All NRTIs share a dual mechanism of action, namely as competitive inhibitors of reverse transcriptase (RT) and as chain terminators of HIV-DNA elongation, when they are incorporated into the elongating chain in place of the natural nucleotide. Mutation in the RT gene leads to viruses that are variably cross-resistant to other NRTIs. Genotypic resistance testing is needed to determine which NRTI will inhibit resistant mutants.

Collectively, NRTIs have a relatively short plasma $t_{1/2}$ of one to several hours but their intracellular half-life is longer, at least 3 hours, thereby permitting their administration one to three times per day. As a class, they have low affinity for hepatic cytochrome P450 drug-metabolizing enzymes, so they do not cause important adverse drug interactions by this mechanism. In contrast, NRTIs as a class cause depletion of mitochondrial DNA by inhibiting human DNA polymerase γ and, hence, replication of mitochondrial DNA.[167] As a result, mitochondrial DNA is depleted and drug toxicity occurs. Adverse reactions due at least in part to mitochondrial toxicity include hepatic steatosis, skeletal muscle and cardiac myopathies, peripheral neuropathy, and pancreatitis. Asymptomatic elevated serum lactate levels and fatal lactic acidosis also have been described as probable additional manifestations of NRTI mitochondrial toxicity. Mitochondrial toxicity is reversible on discontinuation of NRTI therapy.

All NRTI drugs are approved for use in combination therapy even though there are robust data supporting the use of azidothymidine (AZT) alone for peripartum prophylaxis to prevent transmission of HIV to the neonate.

These drugs competitively inhibit the use of different purines or pyrimidines by HIV RT. They also differ in the nature of the adverse reactions they cause.

The NRTIs and their analogous natural nucleosides are:

Azidothymidine (AZT)	Thymidine
Lamivudine (3TC)	Cytidine
Didanosine (ddI)	Adenosine
Stavudine (d4T)	Thymidine
Zalcitabine (ddC)	Cytidine
Abacavir	Guanosine
Tenofovir	Adenosine

The following discussion aims to highlight noteworthy, clinically important aspects of these drugs because they might cause morbidity necessitating ICU admission or cause significant iatrogenic disease when administered to ICU patients.

ZIDOVUDINE

CLINICAL PHARMACOLOGY[168] From 63% to 95% (mean, 90%) of an oral dose of AZT is absorbed. However, because of first-pass metabolism, the average oral bioavailability is 65% (range, 52% to 75%).[169] Absorption is rapid, with peak Cp appearing within 30 to 90 minutes after ingestion. The effect of gastrointestinal disease, including HIV enteropathy, on AZT absorption has not been described. The drug distributes widely throughout the body. Concentrations in CSF average 15% to 64% of concurrent Cp. Hepatic glucuronidation yields an inactive, nontoxic metabolite. The plasma elimination $t_{1/2}$ of AZT is approximately 1 hour. AZT and its glucuronide metabolite are eliminated primarily through the kidneys, contributing 14% and 74%, respectively, to urinary recovery. Renal elimination is by glomerular filtration and renal tubular secretion. Probenecid interferes with glucuronidation of AZT and inhibits renal excretion of the nontoxic glucuronide. In anuric patients, the plasma $t_{1/2}$ of AZT increased to only 1.4 hours compared with 1 hour for controls with normal renal function. However, the plasma $t_{1/2}$ of the principal metabolite (glucuronyl AZT) increased from 1 to 8 hours, with as yet incompletely understood clinical consequences. Hemodialysis has a negligible effect on AZT removal but accelerates clearance of the metabolite. Thus, AZT dose need not be adjusted for patients with renal disease, including those undergoing dialysis.

The effect of hepatic disease on AZT disposition has not been described. AZT accumulation to levels higher than that seen in subjects with normal liver function would be expected. Until more data permit development of validated dose schedules for patients with hepatic disease, one might try the following strategies for minimizing dose-related toxicity: use of smaller doses (e.g., 300 mg/d) and frequent assessment of reticulocytes, hemoglobin, and neutrophil concentrations,

because these appear to be the most sensitive to toxic effects caused by AZT. Measuring Cp of AZT has no established place in this setting and is impractical.

ADVERSE DRUG REACTIONS In adults with HIV disease, AZT ADRs were more common in those with more advanced HIV disease and in those receiving larger doses.[170] In all placebo-controlled studies, anemia and granulocytopenia were the most common ADRs observed: Anemia (hemoglobin <75 g/L) was observed in 9% and 5% of volunteers with asymptomatic and advanced HIV disease, respectively, treated with placebo and 1% (500 mg/d) or 6% (1500 mg/d) up to 29% (1500 mg/d) in AZT recipients in the two respective groups. Similarly, granulocytopenia (<750 cells/mm^3, or <0.75 × 10^9/L) was observed in 2% and 10% of subjects in the two groups treated with placebo and 2% (500 mg/d) or 6% (1500 mg/d) up to 47% (1500 mg/d) in the two groups, respectively, treated with AZT. These hematologic toxic effects generally appeared after 4 to 6 weeks of therapy and reversed with reduction of AZT doses or temporary discontinuation.

Other reactions intensivists may see include severe headache (42% of AZT recipients and 37% of placebo-treated subjects), nausea (46% to 61% and 18% to 41%, respectively, in severe and asymptomatic HIV infection), vomiting (25% and 13%, respectively), insomnia (5% of AZT recipients and 1% of placebo-treated subjects), and myalgia (8% and 2%, respectively).

Considering the number of drugs administered concomitantly to HIV-infected patients receiving AZT, a paucity of clinically important interactions has been described. Ganciclovir and AZT produce additive suppression of myeloid precursors with granulocytopenia, acetaminophen may inhibit AZT metabolism and increase its Cp, and dapsone plus AZT increases the risk of anemia. Ribavirin antagonizes the anti-HIV effect of AZT by inhibiting its phosphorylation to AZT phosphate.

LAMIVUDINE

Lamivudine (3TC), a dideoxy analogue of cytidine, is a potent, selective inhibitor of HIV-1 and HIV-2 replications in vitro.

CLINICAL PHARMACOLOGY[171] Absolute oral bioavailability is 85%. The Cp rises linearly over the dose range of 0.25 to 20 mg/kg (usual oral dose is 150 mg twice daily or ~2 mg/kg per dose). Mean elimination $t_{1/2}$ is 2 to 4 hours. Mean ratio of CSF to serum in HIV-infected patients without clinical CNS disease is 0.06, similar to, or better than, that for ddC and ddI (0.0 to 0.2) but less than that for AZT (0.25 to 0.75). Metabolism of 3TC is a minor route of elimination. The majority of 3TC is eliminated unchanged in urine. 3TC clearance is markedly affected by renal functional impairment, with mean $t_{1/2}$ values of 11.5, 14.1, and 20.7 hours in subjects with normal renal function, moderate renal impairment (creatinine clearance 10 to 40 mL/min), and severe dysfunction (creatinine clearance <10 mL/min), respectively. TMP decreases 3TC renal elimination, causing a 40% increase in 3TC Cp, probably by interfering with renal tubular secretion. This is not clinically important because 3TC has no dose-related toxic effects. 3TC dose reduction is recommended in patients with renal insufficiency; the dose should be halved for those with creatinine clearance of 30 to 49 mL/min; for patients with creatinine clearance of 15 to 29 mL/min, an initial dose of 150 mg followed by 100 mg/d is recommended; for patients with creatinine clearance of 5 to 14 mL/min, a 150-mg initial dose followed by 50 mg/d is recommended; for patients with creatinine clearance lower than 5 mL/min, a 50-mg initial dose is recommended followed by 25 mg/d. Dose adjustments for patients on dialysis are not available.

ADVERSE DRUG REACTIONS   3TC causes no dose-related adverse effects. Unlike the other marketed nucleoside RT inhibitors (AZT, d4T, ddC, and ddI), 3TC is noteworthy for causing few ADRs. The exception is a risk of pancreatitis in pediatric patients treated with 3TC combined with AZT. In one trial in which adult subjects ingested AZT 600 mg/d, 3TC 600 mg/d, or 3TC 300 or 600 mg/d plus AZT 600 mg/d, the 3TC groups reported no more adverse effects than the AZT-only group.

DIDANOSINE

CLINICAL PHARMACOLOGY[171,172]   Didanosine (ddI) was initially licensed in 1991 in the United States. It is rapidly degraded at acid pH, so oral formulations contain buffers to decrease gastric pH and facilitate absorption as chewable or water-dispersible tablets administered twice daily.

Oral bioavailability has ranged from 20% to 40%, likely due to variations in gastric degradation by acid, motility, and transit time. As of 2002, a convenient new enteric-coated tablet has been licensed that provides oral bioavailability equivalent to the buffered tablets without the need to chew them or disperse them in water before ingestion. More recently, it has been demonstrated that tenofovir administered concurrently increases ddI oral bioavailability in 44% to 60% of subjects.

Didanosine undergoes extensive intracellular metabolism in the purine pool, resulting in formation of hypoxanthine and uric acid. From 35% to 60% of a dose is recovered unchanged in urine.

In patients weighing more than 60 kg with renal impairment, doses should be reduced: for creatinine clearance of 30 to 59 mL/min, the daily dose should be 200 mg; for creatinine clearance lower than 29 mL/min, the daily dose should be 125 mg. For patients on dialysis, the daily dose should be administered after dialysis. There is no need to give supplementary doses after dialysis because ddI is not dialyzable.

In patients with hepatic impairment, the risk of ddI toxicity may be increased but no specific recommendations for reducing doses are available.

ADVERSE DRUG REACTIONS   Important serious adverse drug reactions include diarrhea, pancreatitis, peripheral neuropathy, lactic acid with hepatic steatosis, fulminant hepatic necrosis, and retinal depigmentation and vision loss. The risk of pancreatitis is 1% to 10%.

Allopurinol given concurrently appears to increase ddI AUC fourfold and thereby increases the risk of pancreatitis. Coadministration of ddI and allopurinol is not recommended.

Didanosine does not interact with other HIV-inhibitor drugs.

STAVUDINE

CLINICAL PHARMACOLOGY[173]   Only an oral capsule formulation of stavudine (d4T) is currently available. Oral bioavailability is 82% to 99%, but absorption in critically ill patients in the ICU is not known. AVD is 47.3 to 70 L in adults. Peak CSF concentrations are 16% to 72% of the concurrent plasma concentration. Plasma elimination $t_{1/2}$ is 1.6 hours in HIV-infected patients, but the intracellular $t_{1/2}$ is 3.5 hours, thus permitting twice-daily dosing.

About 40% of a dose is eliminated unchanged into urine. Renal clearance of d4T is about twice the creatinine clearance, indicating that net tubular secretion and glomerular filtration contribute to its renal elimination. Nonrenal clearance is hypothesized to involve intracellular metabolism and entry of metabolites into the pyrimidine pool. Less than 1% enters the bile.

Twice-daily doses are recommended to be reduced in adults with renal impairment: with creatinine clearance faster than 50 mL/min, doses are 40 mg twice daily for patients weighing at least 60 kg and 30 mg twice daily for those weighing less than 60 kg; with creatinine clearance of 26 to 50 mL/min, doses are 20 and 15 mg twice daily, respectively, for the two weight groups; with creatinine clearance of 10 to 25 mL/min, doses are 20 and 15 mg once daily, respectively, for the two weight groups.

No adjustment for patients with stable hepatic impairment is recommended.

ADVERSE DRUG REACTIONS   Peripheral neuropathy is the most important ADR. It has occurred in 15% to 24% of patients in controlled trials, is dose related, requires drug discontinuation or reduction, and is generally reversible.

Elevated levels of lactic acid of long duration due to mitochondrial toxicity associated with NRTI have been observed particularly during therapy with d4T. Symptoms include fatigue, shortness of breath, weight loss, and lipid abnormalities.[174] This syndrome is distinct from rare, potentially fatal lactic acidosis seen during NRTI therapy.

ZALCITABINE

CLINICAL PHARMACOLOGY[175]   Oral bioavailability of zalcitabine (ddC) in adults is approximately 85%. AVD is 0.6 L/kg. Plasma $t_{1/2}$ is 1.5 hours (range, 1.1 to 1.8 hours), and elimination is a first-order process. Urinary excretion of unchanged drug is the principal route of elimination, accounting for 62% to 75% of a dose. Approximately 10% of a dose is excreted unchanged in feces.

Renal clearance is decreased in the presence of renal dysfunction, suggesting a need for dose reduction in such patients. Doses of ddC should be reduced from 0.75 mg three times daily to 0.75 mg twice daily in adult patients with creatinine clearance of 10 to 40 mL/min and 0.75 mg once daily in those with creatinine clearance lower than 10 mL/min.

Apart from 25% reduced bioavailability when given with aluminum and magnesium hydroxide, no important drug interaction has been described.

ADVERSE DRUG REACTIONS   Peripheral neuropathy occurs with a frequency up to 12%, pancreatitis in 1%, and ulcerative stomatitis in 0.2%. Anemia and neutropenia occurred in 6% to 8% of ddC recipients versus 6% to 9% of ddI recipients in one study.

The peripheral neuropathy is dose related and generally reversible with discontinuation of treatment.

TENOFOVIR

Tenofovir disoproxil fumarate is an acyclic nucleotide analogue of adenosine monophosphate that acts as an HIV RT inhibitor.[176,177]

MECHANISM OF ACTION Unlike NRTIs such as AZT, tenofovir only undergoes two catalytic steps to convert it to its active antiviral molecule, tenofovir. Tenofovir inhibits RT and causes DNA chain termination on being incorporated into the elongating chain.

CLINICAL PHARMACOLOGY Only an oral formulation is available. A high-fat meal increases oral bioavailability from 25% to 39%; tenofovir $t_{1/2}$ in HIV patients averages 12 hours. Elimination is a first-order process. Drug is eliminated largely (75% of a dose) unchanged into urine. Renal clearance exceeds creatinine clearance, suggesting that glomerular filtration and tubular secretion contribute to tenofovir renal elimination.

As expected, renal impairment decreases tenofovir clearance. In the United States, tenofovir is relatively contraindicated in patients with moderate renal impairment (creatinine clearance <60 mL/min). In Europe, it is considered relatively contraindicated for patients with severe renal dysfunction (creatinine clearance not specified).

Tenofovir is efficiently removed by dialysis; median extraction is 54%. It can be inferred that one-half the dose should be administered after dialysis, but the validity of this inference has not been examined. Tenofovir is relatively contraindicated in patients with creatinine clearance lower than 60 mL/min.

Like the NRTIs, tenofovir is not metabolized by cytochrome P450 isozymes, so no interactions with drugs biotransformed by the isozyme are expected.

The most important drug interaction is a 28% to 44% increase in ddI AUC during concurrent administration. Tenofovir AUC is not affected. The effect is believed to be due to enhanced ddI bioavailability, although the molecular mechanism is unclear.

ADVERSE DRUG REACTIONS Tenofovir is generally well tolerated. Adverse symptoms are primarily gastrointestinal, but placebo-controlled trials showed few differences between treatments in the incidence of adverse symptoms: nausea 11% and 10%, diarrhea 9% and 8%, and vomiting 5% and 2% in tenofovir recipients and placebo recipients, respectively, and abdominal pain 3% in both groups. Severe biochemical abnormalities were similarly not different between the tenofovir and placebo groups.

Postmarketing studies have described pancreatitis, lactic acidosis, and several other ADRs during tenofovir therapy.

Overall, tenofovir appears to be a potent, useful addition to the NRTI group of antiretroviral drugs due to its potency and tolerability.

ABACAVIR

CLINICAL PHARMACOLOGY[178] Absolute oral bioavailability at 83% is excellent. Abacavir kinetics are nonlinear at doses smaller than 600 mg/d; however, because the recommended doses exceed this level, nonindependence of kinetics at smaller doses may not be clinically important.

Abacavir undergoes extensive hepatic metabolism, with less than 2% of a dose appearing in urine as parent drug.

Metabolism in the liver yields two principal metabolites that are biologically inactive. They are eliminated (83%) into the urine. Plasma $t_{1/2}$ is shorter than 2 hours, whereas intracellular $t_{1/2}$ of the antiviral metabolite is 3.3 hours, thereby supporting administration two or three times daily.

Abacavir does not undergo substantial metabolism by cytochrome P450 enzymes and no important interactions with other retroviral inhibitors or other drugs have been described.

ADVERSE DRUG REACTIONS Hypersensitivity reactions occur in 4% (range, 0% to 7%) of patients given this agent. Manifestations include respiratory symptoms (pharyngitis, dyspnea, or cough), gastrointestinal complaints (nausea, vomiting, diarrhea, or abdominal pain), and skin rash. The reactions usually occur in the first 6 weeks after initiation of therapy (median, 11 days) and can appear within hours of reintroduction of abacavir in patients who interrupted therapy after an uneventful initial course of treatment. The cause is not known, but the scenario fits with the generalized propensity of HIV patients to develop hypersensitivity reactions to sulfonamides and fluoroquinolones. This reaction may be fatal, so abacavir is absolutely contraindicated in a patient diagnosed with a hypersensitivity reaction to it.

Overall, abacavir is a useful NRTI for combination therapy. Intensivists restarting abacavir in patients in the ICU must be aware of the small but definite risk of the hypersensitivity reaction.

NON-NUCLEOSIDE REVERSE TRANSCRIPTASE INHIBITORS

Three non-nucleoside RT inhibitor (NNRTI) drugs are currently marketed: delavirdine, nevirapine, and efavirenz. All NNRTI, unlike NRTI, agents act directly to inhibit RT. They do not require intracellular phosphorylation, as do NRTIs, to generate antiviral molecules. The NNRTIs bind at a hydrophobic site close to the RT catalytic site and cause conformational change in the enzyme, whereas NRTIs bind to the catalytic site. The NNRTIs are noncompetitive inhibitors of RT, whereas NRTIs are competitive inhibitors. NNRTIs also inhibit HIV replication by inactivating RT, whereas NRTIs cause chain termination as their second antiviral mechanism of action.

NNRTIs differ structurally, so cross-allergenicity does not occur. Nonetheless, rash is a common adverse effect of all currently licensed members of the class and represents the major adverse effect of the NNRTI drugs. Most cases are mild and not life-threatening. Although the mechanism of rash is not known, "... most experts do not recommend use of any NNRTI in a patient who has had a severe hypersensitivity reaction to one of the drugs."[179,180]

All NNRTIs are approved for treatment of HIV infection in combination with other HIV-inhibitor drugs. Although nevirapine monotherapy was reported to be more effective than AZT to prevent HIV transmission from infected pregnant women to their neonates, it is not approved for that indication. A mutation in the RT gene at amino acid 103 can cause 20-fold decreased susceptibility to all NNRTIs.

From the point of view of their clinical pharmacology, they demonstrate different capacities to interact with a host of other compounds catabolized by hepatic cytochrome P450 isozymes and cause clinically important interactions. As a class, all NNRTIs are cleared primarily by the hepatic cytochrome P450 isozyme CYP 3A4, although other isozymes may contribute (efavirenz is also cleared by CYP 2B6 and delavirdine, possibly by CYP 2D6). Concomitant administration of other drugs has resulted in a range of interactions extending from asymptomatic reduction in clearance (demonstrated as increased AUC) to fatal adverse effects. Accordingly, caution always must be exercised in co-prescribing other drugs cleared by the liver and in some cases should be avoided. The following drugs are contraindicated in patients receiving delavirdine or efavirenz:

Drug Class	Agent	Potentially Fatal ADR
Gastrointestinal prokinetic	Cisapride	Cardiac arrhythmia
Antiarrhythmic	Amiodarone, quinidine	Cardiac arrhythmia
Sedative-hypnotic	Midazolam, triazolam	Prolonged sedation and respiratory depression
Neuroleptic	Pimozide	Cardiac arrhythmia
Ergot alkaloid derivatives	Dihydroergotamine, ergonovine, methylergonovine	Peripheral vasospasm and ischemic, injury
Antihistamine	Astemizole, terfenadine	Cardiac arrhythmia

The clearance of many other drugs that are also metabolized by hepatic CYP 3A4 and other isozymes may be altered during concomitant therapy with NNRTI agents. Effects of the interactions are less predictably serious than those for the agents listed above, so they are considered to be only relatively contraindicated.[180]

The following review focuses on clinical pharmacologic characteristics and adverse reactions that are deemed important for intensivists to be aware of as they consider prescribing these drugs to ICU patients.

DELAVIRDINE

CLINICAL PHARMACOLOGY[180,181] Only an oral formulation is available. Oral bioavailability is 85%. Antacids and gastric hypoacidity due to inhibition of gastric acid secretion or disease decrease oral bioavailability by approximately 50%. The AVD is about 65 L. Delavirdine is highly protein bound (~98%), mainly to albumin, so drug–drug interactions due to displacement of other highly bound drugs such as warfarin or phenytoin can occur. It is almost completely metabolized by hepatic cytochrome P450 isozymes CYP 3A (major) and CYP 2D6 (minor). Less than 5% of a dose is eliminated into urine. Half the metabolites appear in urine and half in feces, presumably with bile.

Delavirdine elimination is dose dependent and not first order as demonstrated by an increase in plasma $t_{1/2}$ from 2.4 to 4.1 hours as dose is increased from 200 to 400 mg three times daily.

Due to its extensive biotransformation by cytochrome P450 isozymes, delavirdine interacts with a wide range of drugs given concurrently because similar biotransformation is a common route of elimination for many agents.

ADVERSE DRUG REACTIONS Delavirdine is generally well tolerated in combination therapy for HIV. The most common adverse effects are skin rash (38% vs. 5% for AZT or ddI), headache (24% vs. 15%), nausea (15% vs. 5%), and pruritus (10% vs. 7%).

Skin rash is usually a pruritic erythematous maculopapular eruption that appears 7 to 15 days after initiation of therapy. Rash does not resolve more rapidly with discontinuation of delavirdine. Severe or life-threatening rash (e.g., Stevens-Johnson syndrome) has rarely been reported (1 case per 1000).

Clinical and biomedical hepatotoxicities have not been observed more frequently in delavirdine-treated patients than in recipients of control HIV treatment.

NEVIRAPINE

CLINICAL PHARMACOLOGY Nevirapine is currently available as an oral formulation, and its bioavailability exceeds 90%.[182,183] It is lipophilic and thus distributes widely. AVD is 1.4 to 1.5 L/kg body weight in adults. The ratio of CSF to plasma is 29%.

The principal route of elimination is by hepatic biotransformation followed by renal excretion. Only 3% is excreted as the parent compound in urine. Nevirapine hydroxylation and glucuronidation of metabolites are catalyzed by cytochrome P450 isozymes, primarily CYP 3A4 and CYP 2B6. The elimination $t_{1/2}$ decreases over 2 weeks due to autoinduction of metabolism: plasma $t_{1/2}$ after initial doses averages 40 hours and then 20 to 30 hours 2 weeks later. This well-described phenomenon underlies the strategy of giving 200 mg daily for 2 weeks followed thereafter by 200 mg twice daily in adults.

When administered to pregnant women to prevent neonatal HIV infection, its pharmacokinetic characteristics in women in the third trimester are not different from those in nonpregnant women. However, if initiated in labor, its kinetic characteristics are significantly altered. Systemic clearance increases on average by 30%, AVD doubles on average, AUC decreases by 15%, and $t_{1/2}$ increases by 70%. The drug readily crosses the placenta as demonstrated by high concentrations in cord blood. Breast milk concentrations average 61% of maternal blood concentrations, but the total amount of drug delivered to the baby is small if given to the woman during labor.

Nevirapine not only induces its own metabolism but also has the potential to interact with a wide range of other drugs also catabolized by CYP 3A4 and CYP 2B6 isozymes (see above).

Nevirapine pharmacokinetic features have not been described in patients with renal or hepatic impairment. However, because less than 5% of the drug is excreted into urine as the active parent compound, it is unlikely that nevirapine disposition is significantly affected by renal impairment or that dose reductions are required to minimize toxicity. Pre-existing hepatic impairment is likely to affect nevirapine clearance, so caution is recommended when nevirapine is administered to patients with moderate to severe hepatic dysfunction; no specific dose recommendations have been provided by the manufacturer.

ADVERSE DRUG REACTIONS The most common ADR is rash, observed in approximately 17% of adults, usually within 6 weeks of initiation of therapy. The rash is usually an erythematous maculopapular eruption of mild to moderate severity.

It may be treated with antihistamines or topical glucocorticoids.

In 6% of patients, the rash is severe enough to necessitate discontinuation of therapy. In 0.5%, it progresses to Stevens-Johnson syndrome.

Uncommonly (<5% of patients), nausea and elevated hepatic enzymes are observed. Although uncommon, hepatitis and fatal hepatic necrosis have been associated with nevirapine use. The manufacturer therefore recommends intensive monitoring in the first 8 to 12 weeks of nevirapine therapy to detect the earliest manifestation of severe and life-threatening skin rash or hepatitis. "Intensive" monitoring of liver function tests during this period is recommended without specification of an exact frequency. In the ICU setting, once-weekly testing seems reasonable.

EFAVIRENZ

CLINICAL PHARMACOLOGY[184] Efavirenz is administered orally once daily. Absorption increases with increasing doses from 100 to 1600 mg but not proportionately, suggesting a saturable mechanism or process. A fatty meal increases AUC by 50%. Most of a dose (16% to 61%) is eliminated in feces as unchanged drug, 14% to 34% in urine as metabolites, and less than 1% in urine as unchanged drug. The drug is 99.5% bound to human plasma protein, so interaction due to displacement of other highly bound drugs with a narrow therapeutic:toxic ratio may cause clinically significant effects (e.g., warfarin and phenytoin).

Efavirenz crosses the blood-brain barrier, but CSF concentrations are 0.26% to 1.19% of plasma levels, suggesting minimal diffusion. It is metabolized in the liver, predominantly by cytochrome P450 CYP 3A4 and 2B6 isozymes, as is the case for nevirapine. The $t_{1/2}$ is 40 to 55 hours at steady state.

Efavirenz pharmacokinetic features have not been rigorously studied in patients with renal or hepatic impairment. However, because less than 5% of efavirenz is excreted unchanged into urine, it is unlikely that renal dysfunction would cause significant accumulation of the pharmacologically active parent molecule. Conversely, efavirenz probably should be decreased in patients with significant hepatic dysfunction. However, no validated dose recommendations are available and therapeutic drug monitoring is not practicable. Caution in this circumstance is recommended.

ADVERSE DRUG REACTIONS Neurologic symptoms are the most common side effect. Headache, dizziness, insomnia, and fatigue were reported by 48% and 54% of patients receiving efavirenz plus indinavir or AZT plus 3TC, respectively. Rash was the second most common side effect, being reported by 10% and 15% of subjects receiving efavirenz plus AZT and 3TC or indinavir, respectively. Neurologic and dermatologic ADRs with efavirenz tend to be mild to moderate in severity. Rashes may respond to antihistamines and topical corticosteroids, and neurologic symptoms may be decreased by drug administration at bedtime.

PROTEASE INHIBITORS OF HIV

Six protease inhibitors of HIV have recently been licensed for combination therapy of HIV-1 infection: saquinavir, ritonavir, indinavir, amprenavir, nelfinavir, and lopinavir. These agents inhibit HIV replication by preventing cleavage of polyprotein precursors essential for synthesis of progeny virions. Protease inhibitors used in combination with other retrovirus inhibitors have produced the most marked and sustained reductions in HIV plasma concentrations observed to date. They are generally active against strains sensitive and resistant to NRTI and NNRTI, and cross-resistance is not uniform. The durability of this effect and the effectiveness of these drugs in patients measured by clinical and laboratory end points, and their efficacy in patients with advanced HIV-1 disease are substantial.

The protease inhibitor drugs, like the NNRTIs, are cleared primarily by transformation to inactive metabolites by the hepatic cytochrome P450 CYP 3AP isozyme. In addition, they may be substrates for one or more isozymes: lopinavir is also catabolized by CYP 2D6, whereas ritonavir also is a substrate for CYPs 2C9, 2C19, 2A6, 1A2, and 2E6. Not surprisingly, ritonavir interacts with a wide variety of other drugs administered concurrently. As noted for the NNRIs, the same list of drugs considered contraindicated in patients receiving one of those three agents should be considered contraindicated in patients receiving a protease inhibitor agent.

The protease inhibitor agents cause a variety of adverse effects, of which one collection of metabolic or endocrine effects appears to be a common class effect: hyperglycemia with a diabetogenic effect, adipogenic effects, hyperlipidemia and hypercholesterolemia, and spontaneous bleeding episodes.[191]

SAQUINAVIR[185]

MECHANISM OF RESISTANCE Decreased sensitivity to saquinavir does not occur readily in vitro or in treated patients. In vitro, saquinavir resistance is associated with mutations at amino acid 90 (more common; leucine to methionine) or at amino acid 48 (less common; glycine to valine). In patients treated with saquinavir alone, 45% had saquinavir-resistant phenotypes at 1 year, which did not differ from the incidence in patients treated with saquinavir plus AZT or ddC. However, the three-drug combination of saquinavir with ddC and AZT seemed to restrict emergence of resistance to AZT and saquinavir (to 22%).

Saquinavir-resistant HIV strains do not appear to be cross-resistant to indinavir or ritonavir.

CLINICAL PHARMACOLOGY Saquinavir is poorly bioavailable, with less than 1% of oral doses being absorbed under fasting conditions. Food enhances saquinavir absorption to about 30%, but only 4% reaches the systemic circulation owing to extensive first-pass metabolism. Saquinavir partitions extensively into tissues as demonstrated by an AVD of 10 L/kg body weight.

Saquinavir is extensively metabolized by the hepatic microsomal cytochrome P450 system into a number of inactive hydroxylated compounds. These are secreted into the bile and, hence, into the feces. Less than 5% is excreted into urine. Mean residence time is 7 hours. Doses need not be adjusted for patients with mild to moderate renal or hepatic insufficiency; in those with severe hepatic or renal disease, the drug should be prescribed with caution.

ADVERSE DRUG REACTIONS Saquinavir is well tolerated. Diarrhea, abdominal discomfort, nausea, and dyspepsia occur in 2% to 4% of saquinavir recipients and in 2% to 3% of recipients of saquinavir plus ddC or AZT. Nervous system side effects such as headache, dizziness, and myalgias occur with low (1% to 3%) frequency at similar rates in saquinavir recipients and recipients of saquinavir plus ddC or AZT. Adverse symptoms are generally mild. Studies have indicated that saquinavir does not alter the rate or severity of adverse effects from AZT or ddC; this finding correlates with studies finding no pharmacokinetic interactions during combination therapy.

RITONAVIR[186,187]

MECHANISM OF RESISTANCE Decreased HIV sensitivity to ritonavir appears to develop at a rate similar to that of saquinavir, although only limited data are available. Genotypically, ritonavir-resistant HIV-1 strains have changes at amino acids 54, 71, and 84. These alterations are distinct from those associated with saquinavir resistance. Clinically, waning of the antiviral effect of ritonavir monotherapy was observed beginning at 4 weeks and was inversely related to dose. In those receiving the largest dose, 600 mg twice daily, mean reductions in plasma HIV-1 RNA concentration were 15-fold at 4 weeks (maximal) and sixfold at 32 weeks. In recipients of 300 or 400 mg twice daily, mean concentrations at 32 weeks did not differ from pretreatment levels. Ritonavir potency when used alone appears to be similar to that of indinavir or AZT combined with 3TC and greater than that observed with saquinavir alone.

Ritonavir-resistant strains are not uniformly cross-resistant to indinavir and saquinavir.

CLINICAL PHARMACOLOGY Ritonavir is well absorbed and produces high concentrations in serum that exceed the minimum inhibitory concentration despite 90% serum protein binding. The serum $t_{1/2}$ is 3 to 4 hours. Elimination is primarily by hepatic metabolism.

ADVERSE DRUG REACTIONS Given alone, ritonavir caused adverse effects including nausea, vomiting, diarrhea, asthenia, and circumoral and peripheral paresthesias and altered taste in 5% to 26% of subjects compared with 1% to 6% in placebo recipients. Greater than twofold increases in serum concentrations of triglycerides, creatinine phosphokinase, and transaminases were observed in 6% to 15% of ritonavir recipients and in 1% to 7% in placebo recipients. These appear to be independent of dose, being observed in more than 85% of recipients receiving ritonavir 600 to 1200 mg/d. The mechanism of the elevated triglyceride level is not clear but does not appear to be caused by pancreatitis.

Many drugs interact with ritonavir because of metabolism by the same common pathway involving hepatic cytochrome P450 isozymes. At least 25 drugs are considered to be contraindicated in patients receiving ritonavir.[188] Ritonavir should be administered with caution and appropriate monitoring due to pharmacokinetic interactions: ritonavir causes a large increase in the AUC of the coadministered drug (AUC increase greater than three- to fourfold; 33 drugs), a moderate increase (1.5-fold to threefold increase; 39 drugs), a moderate increase or decrease (17 drugs), or a possible decrease in AUC (19 drugs).[188]

INDINAVIR SULFATE[189]

MECHANISM OF RESISTANCE Resistance to indinavir was observed in 43% of individuals receiving the recommended dose of 2.4 g/d after 24 weeks of therapy compared with 65% receiving only AZT and 18% receiving indinavir plus AZT. These initial data suggest that resistance to indinavir appears at a slightly slower rate than resistance to ritonavir during monotherapy and that combined therapy with AZT decreases the rate of emergence of indinavir resistance. Indinavir resistance is directly associated with cumulative amino acid mutations in as many as 11 RT sites.

Indinavir-resistant HIV-1 strains are cross-resistant to ritonavir and variably resistant to saquinavir.

CLINICAL PHARMACOLOGY Indinavir is readily absorbed, although large meals reduce absorption by 75% judging by reduction in AUC. Less than 10% of a dose is excreted unchanged in urine. The majority of the drug undergoes metabolism before elimination in feces and urine. The serum $t_{1/2}$ is 1.8 hours in subjects with normal renal and hepatic functions. In patients with mild to moderate hepatic insufficiency, the $t_{1/2}$ almost doubles. The effects of severe hepatic disease or renal insufficiency have not been studied. Penetration into CSF has not been described.

ADVERSE DRUG REACTIONS Indinavir is generally tolerated as well as, or better than, AZT or ritonavir. Nephrolithiasis with flank pain and hematuria occurs in 4% of patients, and asymptomatic indirect hyperbilirubinemia occurs in 10%. Other ADRs include abdominal pain (9% vs. 5% AZT alone), fatigue (4% vs. 8% AZT alone), diarrhea (5% vs. 2% AZT alone), and insomnia (3% vs. 0% AZT alone).

Phlebitis owing to the alkaline pH of the solution also has been reported.

NELFINAVIR

CLINICAL PHARMACOLOGY[190] Oral nelfinavir is 70% to 80% bioavailable when administered with food. Bioavailability is 50% to 73% less when administered in a fasting state. AVD is 2 to 7 L/kg. Plasma protein binding is high at 98%, primarily to α_1-acid glycoprotein.

Nelfinavir is metabolized in the liver by cytochrome P450 isozymes CYP 3A4, 2C9, 2C19, and 2D6. Elimination is primarily by fecal (biliary) excretion of a hydroxylated metabolite (78%); 22% of drug excreted in feces is unchanged drug, and 1% to 2% of nelfinavir is excreted in urine as unchanged drug. Plasma $t_{1/2}$ is 3.5 to 5 hours.

The pharmacokinetic characteristics of nelfinavir have not been described in patients with renal or hepatic impairment. Less than 2% of nelfinavir is excreted into urine as unchanged drug, so renal dysfunction is unlikely to significantly affect the pharmacodynamics of the active parent compound. Because the drug is primarily inactivated in the liver, caution is recommended when it is administered to patients with hepatic impairment, but the manufacturer provides no specific dose recommendations.

ADVERSE DRUG REACTIONS Nelfinavir is generally well tolerated, but ADRs were severe enough to necessitate treatment discontinuation in 1.5% to 4% of 690 subjects in controlled trials. A retrospective comparison suggested nelfinavir tolerability exceeds that of indinavir, saquinavir, or amprenavir.

Diarrhea is the commonest ADR but is generally mild to moderate in severity and usually can be controlled with drugs that decrease gastrointestinal motility (e.g., loperamide).

Diarrhea of moderate to severe intensity was reported by 20% of recipients of nelfinavir with AZT and 3TC compared with 3% in recipients of AZT and 3TC alone. A comparison of ADRs concluded that nelfinavir has better gastrointestinal tolerability than indinavir, saquinavir soft gel capsules, or ritonavir in causing only diarrhea (26% incidence) and nausea (5% incidence) but no vomiting, dyspepsia, abdominal pain, or taste perversion.[191]

AMPRENAVIR

CLINICAL PHARMACOLOGY[192,193] From 35% to 90% of an oral dose of amprenavir is absorbed. AUC increases proportionally to dose over the range of 300 to 1600 mg (the therapeutic adult dose is 1200 mg twice daily). The drug is 90% bound to plasma proteins; α_1-acid glycoprotein is the principal amprenavir binding protein. AVD is said to be 430 L in adults, suggesting sequestration in tissues outside the plasma compartment.

Elimination is by hepatic cytochrome P450 isozymes, primarily CYP 3A4. The plasma elimination $t_{1/2}$ is 7 to 11 hours, which is the longest for any of the licensed protease inhibitors. Amprenavir is excreted predominantly as metabolites into feces (75%) and urine (14%). Hence, amprenavir pharmacokinetics would not be expected to be affected by renal impairment. Clearance is decreased as the severity of cirrhosis increases (Child-Pugh score). The manufacturer recommends caution in the use of amprenavir in such patients, without recommending specific dose reductions.

ADVERSE DRUG REACTIONS The most common adverse reactions observed in two controlled trials involving 358 patients who received highly active antiretroviral therapy (HAART) including amprenavir were nausea (15%), diarrhea (14%), rash (11%), and vomiting (5%). In a controlled trial in which all subjects received AZT plus 3TC with amprenavir or its placebo, the incidence of all the aforementioned complaints was 20% to 100% less in the placebo recipients. Grade 3 or 4 increases in alanine aminotransferase and/or aspartate aminotransferase and neutropenia also were more common in amprenavir than placebo recipients (5% vs. 3% and 5% vs. 0%, respectively).

LOPINAVIR

CLINICAL PHARMACOLOGY[194,195] Lopinavir is marketed as a soft gel capsule containing 133.3 mg lopinavir and 33.3 mg ritonavir. The absolute bioavailability of lopinavir-ritonavir has not been established. Compared with ingestion in a fasting state, administration of lopinavir-ritonavir capsules with a moderately fat meal (23% to 25% fat) or high fat meal (56% fat) increased lopinavir AUC by 48% or 97%, respectively.

Lopinavir is 98% to 99% protein bound in human plasma, more to α_1-acid glycoprotein than to albumin. AVD has not been described.

Lopinavir is catabolized by hepatic cytochrome P450 isozymes, primarily CYP 3A4. This process yields metabolites with relatively little antimicrobial activity. Ritonavir is a potent inhibitor of CYP 3A4, which inhibits lopinavir metabolism and thereby increases lopinavir AUC. A study using isotope-labeled lopinavir reported that 89% of the plasma radioactivity after a single oral dose of isotope-labeled lopinavir with unlabeled ritonavir (400/100 mg) was parent lopinavir compound. The AUC of lopinavir (100 to 800 mg) increases greater than 100-fold when coadministered with ritonavir 50 to 200 mg. Lopinavir plasma $t_{1/2}$ was 5.8 hours at steady state during treatment with lopinavir-ritonavir 400 and 100 mg twice daily. After a single dose of the same mixture, 10% and 83% of isotope-labeled lopinavir was recovered in urine and feces, respectively, over 8 days. Unchanged lopinavir accounted for about 2% and 20% of drug in urine and feces, respectively.

Lopinavir pharmacokinetics have not been studied in patients with renal impairment, but no or perhaps trivial effect of renal insufficiency is anticipated.

Lopinavir-ritonavir disposition has not been studied in patients with hepatic impairment, but decreased clearance of both would be expected. In such patients the manufacturer recommends caution in the administration of lopinavir-ritonavir but has provided no specific dose guidelines.

Other drug interactions due to lopinavir and/or ritonavir inhibition on CYP 3A4 are to be expected during concurrent therapy. A list of drugs that could be affected has been published.[188]

ADVERSE DRUG REACTIONS In controlled trials involving 612 patients receiving HAART and including lopinavir-ritonavir or nelfinavir, the drug was generally well tolerated. ADRs necessitated discontinuation of lopinavir-ritonavir in 3% of patients in the groups treated with lopinavir-ritonavir and nelfinavir.

The most common ADR in lopinavir-ritonavir recipients was diarrhea (14%), which occurred with the same frequency in recipients receiving nelfinavir, d4T, and 3TC. In lopinavir-ritonavir recipients given therapy for another 48 weeks, diarrhea was reported by 24% of patients. Grade 3 or 4 increases in alanine aminotransferase and/or aspartate aminotransferase were observed in fewer than 1% of lopinavir-ritonavir recipients compared with 2% to 2.5% of subjects receiving nelfinavir, d4T, and 3TC. The rates of neutropenia at 24 weeks were 0.6% and 1.6% in the two groups, respectively.

Antifungals

Despite its inherent toxicity and the continuing development of new, potent, better tolerated imidazole antifungal drugs, amphotericin B administered alone or in combination with another antifungal agent remains the standard therapy for serious systemic mycoses. Although the arbitrary distinction between antifungal drugs used exclusively for topical therapy of superficial infection or for treatment of mycotic infections of viscera (deep mycoses) is becoming blurred with the development of the newer imidazoles, this discussion is limited to those agents that are licensed for therapy for deep mycoses:[196] amphotericin B, 5-fluorocytosine, some of the imidazoles (ketoconazole), structurally related N-substituted triazoles (fluconazole, itraconazole, and voriconazole), and an echinocandin (caspofungin).

AMPHOTERICIN B[197]

Amphotericin B is an antifungal antibiotic produced by *Streptomyces nodosus*. It exhibits amphoteric behavior, forming relatively soluble salts in basic or acid aqueous media, but is extremely insoluble in aqueous solutions at physiologic pH. Accordingly, for clinical use, amphotericin B is formulated for intravenous administration as a colloidal suspension by using the bile salt deoxycholate and sodium phosphate buffer. Recently, interest was focused on the formulation of amphotericin B with lipids to decrease its toxic effects.[198] Three lipid-associated amphotericin B preparations are currently on the market.[199] AmBisome is a true liposomal suspension consisting of vesicles comprising a phospholipid bilayer stabilized with cholesterol resulting in an intravesicular hydrophilic and external hydrophobic environment. The amphipathic character of amphotericin B makes it ideal for entrapment in those liposomes. Abelcet consists of a suspension of 1600- to 11,000-nm ribbon-like bilayers in which the amphotericin B is trapped. Amphocil consists of a colloidal dispersion of amphotericin embedded in 120- to 140-nm disks of cholesteryl sulfate.

In vitro susceptibility testing of fungi and yeasts, as with viruses, remains an inexact science. Although improvements are being made in all facets of standardization of techniques and interpretation,[200] published data from different laboratories are difficult to compare. Notwithstanding this fact, there is general agreement that an inverse relation exists between concentrations of antifungal agents required to inhibit growth in vitro and their therapeutic efficacy. The following yeasts and fungi have MIC values below 1 mg/L to amphotericin B and are considered highly sensitive to this drug: *Cryptococcus neoformans, Blastomyces dermatitidis, Histoplasma capsulatum, Coccidioides immitis, Sporotrichum schenckii, Candida albicans, Paracoccidiodes brasiliensis*, and the zygomycoses (*Mucor, Rhizopus, Absidia*, and *Cunninghamella*). *Aspergillus* species are usually sensitive. The causative agents of chromomycosis (*Phialophora* species and *Cladosporidium carrionii*) are usually resistant to amphotericin B alone but can be effectively inhibited by amphotericin B in combination with 5-fluorocytosine. *Prototheca* species, which cause chronic persistent granulomatous skin and visceral infections, are usually sensitive to amphotericin B.

Combining amphotericin B with certain antibacterial drugs such as rifampicin and tetracycline in vitro yields additive or synergistic antifungal effects, owing to enhanced penetration of the fungal cell by these two inhibitors of protein synthesis, because of enhanced permeability caused by amphotericin B. However, data from studies of animals with experimental fungal infections do not suggest a consistent, predictable, additive or synergistic effect of the combinations sufficient to warrant their use in patients.

Studies of amphotericin B combined with other selected antifungal agents in vitro, in animals with experimental fungal infections and some patients, have demonstrated effects that are at least additive. Amphotericin B with 5-fluorocytosine is at least additive in vitro and in animals with experimental candida and cryptococcal infections. This has permitted the use of smaller doses of amphotericin B with lesser attendant toxicity in patients with cryptococcal meningitis and perhaps candidal meningitis and arthritis. In a murine model of systemic aspergillosis, these two drugs produced better results than either agent administered alone, and some clinicians recommend their combined use in patients with serious aspergillus infection, especially with significant immunosuppression.

Results have been conflicting when amphotericin B is combined with imidazole antifungal drugs. Indifference, synergy, and antagonism have been observed in studies in vitro and in vivo in animals with experimental mycoses. In view of the unpredictable effects of combining imidazoles and amphotericin, intensivists should be careful about the use of combined therapy in ICU patients.

Specific recommendations for the treatment of deep mycoses are found in Chaps. 46, 49, and 50. Amphotericin B alone is the drug of choice for some *C. albicans* infections (esophagitis, peritonitis complicating peritoneal dialysis, fungemia, and endophthalmitis), coccidioidomycosis (progressive pulmonary infection and meningitis), histoplasmosis, zygomycoses, and sporotrichosis (systemic, articular, or pulmonary). Amphotericin B combined with 5-fluorocytosine is recommended for therapy of cryptococcal meningitis or disseminated infection especially in the immunocompromised host, systemic candidiasis except as noted above, *Candida* (formerly *Torulopsis*) *glabrata* endocarditis, invasive aspergillosis, and chromomycosis.

To date, no unambiguous proof of consistently enhanced efficacy of any lipid-associated amphotericin B formulations compared with the standard colloidal suspension in desoxycholate solution has been reported. Overall, at this time, it appears that lipid-associated amphotericin B formulations require larger doses to achieve comparable therapeutic benefits and cause fewer of the significant adverse effects of colloidal amphotericin B, namely hypokalemia, nephrotoxicity, and infusion-related reactions.

MECHANISM OF ACTION The antifungal action of amphotericin B is complex and largely dependent on its interaction with sterols, primarily ergosterol, in the cytoplasmic membrane of sensitive fungi. The drug appears to form channels or pores that lead to leakage of essential metabolites and, eventually, lysis of the cell. In low concentrations, the effect is reversible and the result is inhibition of fungal cell growth. However, at higher concentrations, the effect is irreversible; hence, the drug is fungicidal.

Amphotericin B potentiates the antifungal effect of 5-fluorocytosine and other agents by enhancing their entry into fungal cells.

MECHANISM OF RESISTANCE[201] Natural and acquired resistances to amphotericin B during therapy with clinical failure have been considered to be uncommon and not a clinical problem. However, in one survey, 7% of 747 strains of *C. albicans, Candida tropicalis*, and *C. glabrata* were resistant to amphotericin B. Resistance was observed only in isolates obtained from oncology patients. These data suggest, contrary to general opinions, that resistance may not be uncommon and that selection pressure from extensive amphotericin B use in granulocytopenic oncology patients may contribute to resistance development. It is postulated that a major reason that *C. albicans* resistance to amphotericin B antibiotics is uncommon is because it lacks a haploid sexual stage in its life cycle. Thus, the frequency of mutational events that will alter the specific locus where amphotericin B acts will be low. This would also explain the higher frequency of resistance observed with *C. glabrata*, which is haploid.

CLINICAL PHARMACOLOGY Absorption of amphotericin B after oral administration is negligible. Amphotericin B may be administered intravenously, intrathecally, intra-articularly, instilled into the infected urinary bladder, and in dilute solution into the peritoneal cavity of patients with fungal peritonitis.

After intravenous infusion, the drug dissociates from deoxycholate in the blood, binds extensively (90%) to plasma proteins (mostly β lipoprotein), and distributes widely throughout the body but not into CSF or the vitreous humor. Even in patients with cryptococcal meningitis, amphotericin B concentrations in CSF were less than 10% of serum values. The AVD is 4 L/kg but with wide variation. This is consistent with the observed, extensive binding of biologically active amphotericin B in tissues, particularly to sterols in hepatocytes and erythrocytes, in which the concentration is up to 30 times greater than in plasma. The Cp of amphotericin B declines in a biexponential manner after intravenous infusion. There is an initial phase of rapid decline, with $t_{1/2}$ of 24 to 48 hours and a slow terminal phase of 15 days. Kinetically, this biphasic pattern is consistent with amphotericin B infusion into a central compartment and its equilibration rapidly into two peripheral compartments. The rapid decline in plasma amphotericin B represents equilibration into the former, and the phase of slow decline represents the slow release of amphotericin B back into the central compartment from which it was eliminated.

Approximately 2% to 5% of a dose is recovered as unchanged drug in the urine. From 16% to 94% (median, 33%) of injected doses can be recovered unchanged by extraction of tissues. The remainder is assumed to be metabolized, but data are not available on this aspect of its disposition. Blood levels are unaffected by hepatic or renal failure. Dose modifications are not required in patients with renal failure to compensate for any effect of oliguria on amphotericin B disposition, but doses may be decreased to mitigate further nephrotoxic effects of the drug. Hemodialysis does not enhance amphotericin B clearance, so such patients do not require alterations in the standard dose. At steady state, plasma amphotericin B concentrations after infusion of 0.5 mg/kg are 1.0 to 1.5 mg/L, with reduction to 0.5 to 1.0 mg/L 24 hours later. Hyperlipidemic and dyslipidemic states, such as occur in animals with uncontrolled experimental diabetes, alter the distribution of amphotericin B, with reduced liver and kidney concentrations, diminished nephrotoxicity, and reduced clearance, associated paradoxically with a fourfold increase in apparent volume of distribution. The clinical implications of such altered disposition of amphotericin B remain to be elucidated.

The disposition of amphotericin B administered other than intravenously has not been extensively studied. Limited data on the decline in amphotericin B concentrations in CSF after instillation of drug into the lumbar sac or cerebral ventricle have been published. Intrathecally administered amphotericin B (0.3 mg) produces peak concentrations of 0.6 to 0.8 mg/L, which decline to 0.2 to 0.3 mg/L after 24 hours. Amphotericin B injected into a cerebral ventricle (0.5 mg) yielded mean ventricular CSF concentrations of 1.7, 0.27, and 0.16 mg/L at 4, 24, and 48 hours, respectively, after injection. For treatment of yeast peritonitis in renal failure patients undergoing chronic dialysis, amphotericin B is diluted to yield a final dialysate concentration of 1 mg/L. Between dialysis sessions, 25 mg amphotericin B is instilled in 250 mL 5% dextrose in water solution, with 25 mg hydrocortisone every 48 hours. With this regimen, peritoneal fluid predose concentration increased from 1.6 to 2.2 mg/L, and concentrations 4 hours after instillation increased from 2.5 to 3.6 mg/L. Concurrent serum amphotericin B concentrations were 15% to 33% as high. These data suggest amphotericin B is sequestered in the peritoneal cavity because the diluent solution is absorbed and that little diffuses into serum.

The clinical pharmacokinetic features of liposome-encapsulated amphotericin B also have not been well studied. In mice and rabbits, liposomal amphotericin B distribution was primarily to organs rich in reticuloendothelial cells, including liver, spleen, and bone marrow. A pharmacokinetic study in mice reported a reduced area under the serum concentration-time curve for liposomal compound compared with colloidal amphotericin B. It was suggested that liposomal amphotericin B is sequestered in tissues until the vesicles are removed from the circulation by phagocytic cells in the liver and other organs.

ADVERSE DRUG REACTIONS   The inherent toxicity of amphotericin B is demonstrated by a high frequency of adverse effects whether the drug is administered intravenously or by any other route. This propensity to cause side effects is compounded by the need, in most patients, for prolonged therapy.

Some patients may tolerate full intravenous doses of amphotericin B without difficulty, but immediate and long-term side effects frequently necessitate dose reductions or interruptions in therapy. Acute intolerance manifested by fever, chills, malaise, muscle and joint pain, nausea, vomiting, and hypotension often begins within 1 to 2 hours after initiation of therapy and lasts 2 to 4 hours. The observation that liposomal encapsulation of amphotericin B decreases production of proinflammatory cytokines by phagocytic cells is consistent with the lesser propensity of lipid-associated amphotericin B to cause infusion-related toxicity. Antipyretic, antiemetic, and antihistaminic drugs may provide some symptomatic relief, but controlled trials have provided little support for these practices.

Therapy should be initiated with a test dose of 1 mg in 20 mL 5% dextrose in water infused over 20 to 30 min, followed by a dose of 0.3 mg/kg infused over 2 to 3 hours. Thereafter, to minimize infusion-associated adverse effects, the dose should be gradually increased, if the acuity and severity of the illness permits, to the usual dose of 0.5 mg/kg per day. The maximum recommended dose is 1.5 mg/d. However, there is no proof from controlled trials that this regimen decreases infusion-related adverse effects, at least one of which was observed in 71% of patients in one large survey.[202] No more effective in preventing infusion-related toxicity was intravenous administration of amphotericin B in 4 hours versus 1 hour, although toxic reactions occurred sooner with the latter (at approximately 2 to 3 hours vs. 1 to 2 hours, respectively).[203]

Some prophylactic measures have been demonstrated to be efficacious in controlled trials:

1. Ibuprofen, 10 mg/kg, a potent inhibitor of prostaglandin synthesis, administered orally 30 minutes before initiation of amphotericin B infusion decreased the frequency of chilling from 87% to 49% in placebo recipients.[204]
2. Hydrocortisone, 25 mg, injected directly into the intravenous tubing at the start of amphotericin B therapy decreased the frequency of fever and chills from 78% to 56% in placebo recipients. However, the severity of chills and

the level of fever was not less in the hydrocortisone-treated group. Hydrocortisone 50 mg was possibly more effective than 25 mg (reactions decreased from 36% to 22%). Hydrocortisone 50 mg was not different from pretreatment with 900 mg aspirin plus 50 mg diphenhydramine.[205]

3. Meperidine in an average intravenous dose of 45 mg (range, 25 to 60 mg) stopped shaking chills induced by amphotericin B in 11 minutes, whereas interruption of amphotericin B resulted in cessation of the reaction spontaneously in an average of 38 minutes (range, 8 to 95 minutes).[206]

4. In experiments in dogs and patients, pretreatment by infusion of 0.15 M NaCl aqueous solution decreased the nephrotoxic effect of amphotericin B. Administration of 1 L physiologic saline before administration of the daily dose of amphotericin B, where the patient's condition permits, was recommended.[207]

Nephrotoxicity is the most important adverse effect of amphotericin B therapy. Creatinine clearance decreases by about 40% soon after commencing therapy in all patients and usually stabilizes at 20% to 60% of normal thereafter during continued treatment. The appearance of red and white blood cells, albumin, and casts in the urine usually accompanies the decrease in glomerular filtration rate. Thus, no nonnephrotoxic therapeutic dose of amphotericin B exists. However, evidence indicates that the severity of the renal injury is increased by larger doses, so the manufacturer recommends an absolute limit of 1.5 mg/kg per day. The nephrotoxic effect of amphotericin B appears related to induction of renal vasoconstriction and cortical ischemia. In some patients, amphotericin B causes a syndrome similar to renal tubular acidosis with its attendant risk of nephrocalcinosis and renal failure. Early recognition and alkali therapy may help avert or minimize irreversible renal injury. In about 25% of patients being treated with amphotericin B, hypokalemia and mild to moderate hypomagnesemia from renal potassium and magnesium wasting, respectively, occur and require careful monitoring and replacement.

Amphotericin B administration can be made more convenient by giving 2 days' total dose on alternate days, provided the dose to be infused is less than 1.5 mg/kg. This strategy does not affect efficacy if the alternative dose is twice the daily dose and does not decrease the nephrotoxic ADR. Animal studies demonstrating that intravenous mannitol could attenuate amphotericin B nephrotoxicity were not borne out in a controlled study in patients. Other nephrotoxic drugs such as the aminoglycosides and cyclosporine can add to the adverse effect of amphotericin B on the kidney and should be avoided.

If the patient's serum creatinine level increases from the normal range to 170 mmol/L or higher, amphotericin B should be stopped until the creatinine concentration decreases below that level. However, the severity of the fungal infection may necessitate continuing therapy at a smaller dose despite evidence of mild to moderate renal dysfunction. This appears acceptable because the renal dysfunction usually resolves after completion of a full course treatment unless the total dose exceeds 4 to 5 g.

A reversible normochronic, normocytic anemia occurs in most patients during amphotericin B therapy; the hematocrit frequently declines to stable levels of 22% to 35%. Anemia appears to be due to a suppressive effect of amphotericin B on erythropoietin production. Leukopenia and thrombocytopenia are rarely observed.

Hepatic dysfunction is rare; anaphylaxis and hypersensitivity rashes are uncommon.

Extravasated drug may cause cellulitis. Whether this is caused by the polyene drug or the deoxycholate is unclear. A similar reaction probably accounts for the arachnoiditis commonly observed with intrathecal injection. This chemical meningitis can cause nerve palsies, manifest as difficulty in voiding, impaired vision, paraplegia, and convulsions.

An adverse interaction of amphotericin B with leukocyte transfusion, causing acute dyspnea, hypoxemia, and interstitial infiltrates has been described by one group but challenged by others. However, since amphotericin B can cause polymorphonuclear leukocytes to aggregate in vitro, such an adverse interaction is biologically plausible.

Liposomal amphotericin B has been demonstrated in animals with experimental fungal infections and small numbers of patients[208] to have a better therapeutic index than the colloidal formulation available commercially. Both acute infusion-related and chronic renal toxicity side effects were less frequent and severe and liposomal amphotericin B appeared to be effective in patients unresponsive to colloidal amphotericin B. This has been hypothesized to be due to specific, selective delivery of amphotericin B to fungal cells, often in the reticuloendothelial system. However, absence of data from controlled trials comparing results of therapy with liposomal and standard amphotericin B precludes conclusions about the advantages of the liposomal formulation.

CASPOFUNGIN

Caspofungin is the first marketed member of a new class of antifungals, the glucan synthesis inhibitors or echinocandins.[209]

It is approved for the treatment of invasive candidiasis, most commonly fungemic infection, esophageal candidiasis, and invasive aspergillosis in individuals who are refractory to or intolerant of other therapies. Caspofungin is as good as, or superior to, amphotericin B and fluconazole in controlled clinical trials. The usual dose is 50 mg/d infused over 60 minutes. A 70-mg loading dose is administered initially. Treatment is continued to the point of clinical and/or mycologic cure.

MECHANISM OF ACTION   Caspofungin inhibits the synthesis of $\beta(1,3)$-D-glucan, an essential component of the cell wall of many filamentous fungi and yeast. $\beta(1,3)$-D-glucan is not a component of mammalian cells, so the drug has specificity limited to fungal cells, with a resultant paucity of adverse effects on the patient's tissues.

MECHANISM OF RESISTANCE   Resistance to caspofungin is not readily induced in the laboratory. The prevalence of resistance in various clinical isolates has not been described. Experience with treatment of patients with invasive candidiasis or aspergillus continues to accumulate. However, as of July 2003, drug resistance in such patients has not been reported.

CLINICAL PHARMACOLOGY   Only an injectable formulation is available. Caspofungin distributes slowly and widely. It is hydrolyzed and N-acetylated in the liver: 41% of the drug is recovered as metabolites in urine and 34% is recovered in feces.

Mild hepatic insufficiency (Child-Pugh score 5 to 6) does not necessitate any dose reduction. For patients with moderately severe hepatic insufficiency (Child-Pugh score 7 to 9), 35 mg/d is recommended.

Caspofungin clearance was decreased 30% to 50% in patients with moderate to severe renal insufficiency. However, no dose reduction is required for patients with renal insufficiency, including end-stage renal impairment.

In patients on hemodialysis, caspofungin kinetic features are not affected, so no supplementary doses are required after dialysis.

ADVERSE DRUG REACTIONS Caspofungin is generally very well tolerated, as would be expected given its specificity for fungal cell metabolism.

A possible histamine-mediated adverse reaction with rash, facial swelling, itch, and bronchospasm has been reported. Anaphylaxis has been reported during caspofungin infusion.

Drug-related adverse reactions occurred much less frequently (28.9%) in caspofungin recipients than in patients receiving amphotericin B (58.4%). Infusion-related toxicity (chills and fever) also was much less common (20.2% vs. 48.8%) in patients treated with amphotericin B.

Caspofungin does not inhibit cytochrome P450 enzymes, making adverse interactions due to competitive inhibition or induction unlikely.

Overall, caspofungin will be a substantial improvement over amphotericin B for treatment of deep mycoses, if results from wider clinical use mirror results from comparative controlled trials.

5-FLUOROCYTOSINE

5-Fluorocytosine is a fluorinated analogue of cytosine. It is an oral, narrow-spectrum, synthetic antifungal drug usually used in combination with amphotericin B.[210]

In vitro, 5-fluorocytosine inhibits *C. neoformans*, *Candida* species such as *C. krusei*, *C. tropicalis*, and *C. parapsilosis*, *T. glabrata*, and the agents of chromomycosis. The MICs of susceptible fungi are usually 6.25 mg/L or less; resistant species have MICs greater than 25 mg/L. *Aspergillus* species are generally moderately to strongly resistant. Other causes of deep mycoses such as *B. dermatitidis* and *H. capsulatum* are resistant to 5-fluorocytosine in vitro and clinically.

Clinically, 5-fluorocytosine has a beneficial effect against cryptococcosis, candidiasis, and chromomycosis. However, as a single agent, it is the drug of choice only for the latter disease because its efficacy in the former two is inferior to that of amphotericin B, largely because of the rapid emergence of drug resistance.

MECHANISM OF ACTION 5-Fluorocytosine inhibits growth of susceptible fungi by at least two mechanisms. It is taken up by susceptible cells and rapidly converted by cytosine deaminase to 5-fluorouridine triphosphate, which is then incorporated in place of uracil into replicating fungal RNA, causing mistranslation and cessation of growth. Another metabolite of 5-fluorocytosine, 5-fluoro-deoxyuridine monophosphate, interferes with thymidylate synthesis and thereby inhibits DNA synthesis. The synergistic effect of 5-fluorocytosine with am-

photericin B against some fungi results from enhanced penetration of 5-fluorocytosine because of alteration of cell membrane permeability caused by the amphotericin B.

MECHANISM OF RESISTANCE Naturally occurring resistance to 5-fluorocytosine is not uncommon. With *C. neoformans*, it is of the order of 1% to 2%. Resistance among *Candida* species is more variable, being demonstrable in 1% to 37% of isolates.

5-Fluorocytosine–resistant strains of *Candida* species and *C. neoformans* can be readily induced in vitro by serial passage in the presence of increasing concentrations of the drug. Such secondary resistance also has been demonstrated in patients with cryptococcal, candidal, and torulopsis infections being treated with this agent. In one study, two-thirds of isolates recovered from patients being treated with 5-fluorocytosine were resistant.

Resistance is associated with loss of the membrane permease that transports cytosine (and 5-fluorocytosine) into the cell, with diminished activity of cytosine deaminase or uridine monophosphate pyrophosphorylase that catalyzes conversion to 5-fluorodeoxyuridine. In most *C. albicans* strains resistant to 5-fluorocytosine, resistance results from a deficiency of uridine monophosphate pyrophosphorylase. The loss of the enzyme does not alter the pathogenicity of the resistant strains.

CLINICAL PHARMACOLOGY Only an oral formulation is available. In healthy volunteers, greater than 90% of an oral dose is absorbed, but absorption in critically ill ICU patients may be markedly less. Protein binding in plasma is negligible. 5-Fluorocytosine distributes widely throughout all organs and fluids. Concentrations in CSF are 71% to 85% of concomitant serum levels and those in the aqueous humor, 10 to 40 mg/L, which in one study was 20% of concomitant serum concentrations. The AVD approximates that of total body water. Elimination is a first-order process directly related to creatinine clearance and, by inference, glomerular filtration. The plasma $t_{1/2}$ is 3 to 6 hours in normal individuals and inversely related to creatinine clearance. In functionally anephric patients, plasma $t_{1/2}$ approaches 85 hours. A small amount of drug in the body is converted to 5-fluorouracil. This is hypothesized to be a result of conversion of drug in the bowel by bacteria. This metabolite may account for the hematologic and gut toxicities of 5-fluorocytosine.

The recommended daily dose is 50 to 150 mg/kg administered in four equal portions. In view of the unpredictable effects of altered gastrointestinal absorption and fluctuating renal function on 5-fluorocytosine kinetics in ICU patients, 5-fluorocytosine Cp values should be measured frequently to permit dose adjustments to maintain levels in the effective and nontoxic range. Effective Cp values range from 35 to 70 mg/L; Cp values higher than 100 mg/L are associated with an increased risk of toxicity.

The effect of urinary acidification and alkalinization on 5-fluorocytosine in humans has not been described; in other species, prolongation and shortening, respectively, of the plasma $t_{1/2}$ of 5-fluorocytosine have been observed. The effect of fluctuating pH in critically ill patients would further reinforce the need to monitor Cp values in ICU patients.

5-Fluorocytosine is cleared by dialysis; after hemodialysis, a supplemental dose of 37.5 mg/kg is recommended. Patients with creatinine Cp values higher than 150 mmol/L usually require dose reduction. The following reduced doses should be administered every 6 hours: with creatinine clearance of 40 to 49 mL/min, the dose is 27.5 mg/kg; with creatinine clearance to 20 to 29 mL/min, the dose is 18.5 mg/kg; and with creatinine clearance slower than 10 mL/min, the dose is 9.5 mg/kg.

Abnormal liver function appears neither to alter 5-fluorocytosine disposition nor to necessitate dose adjustments.

ADVERSE DRUG REACTIONS 5-Fluorocytosine causes myelosuppression and enterocolitis. The myelosuppressive effect is mediated by direct cytotoxic effects of 5-fluorocytosine on granulocyte and erythroid progenitor cells, as demonstrated in culture systems ex vivo. However, 5-fluorouracil may contribute to the hematologic toxicity of 5-fluorocytosine. The risk of these side effects correlates with 5-fluorocytosine Cp values above 100 mg/L.

Hematologic side effects of 5-fluorocytosine occur more commonly in patients with diseases such as leukemia or drug or radiation therapy that has affected marrow reserves. In extreme instances, fatal bone marrow aplasia has been reported. More commonly observed are leukopenia and thrombocytopenia, which are reversible if 5-fluorocytosine can be removed rapidly. Accordingly, in anephric patients with 5-fluorocytosine Cs values of 100 to 150 mg/L in whom elimination will be prolonged, dialysis to remove drug may be warranted.

Gastrointestinal side effects (nausea and diarrhea) are uncommon. More severe symptoms, including vomiting, abdominal pain, and copious diarrhea warrant careful re-evaluation because they may reflect acute mucositis, resembling acute ulcerative colitis.

Hypersensitive rashes are rare. In 5% of patients, hepatotoxicity, as demonstrated by mild elevations of transaminase Cp values, occurs. These patients should be monitored closely and 5-fluorocytosine Cp values measured because the hepatotoxic effect may be related to dose and concentration.

IMIDAZOLES AND TRIAZOLES

Imidazoles and the structurally related N-substituted triazoles are considered together because they share similar broad spectra of antifungal activity and the same mechanism of action. Their potency and high therapeutic indexes suggest that they may ultimately displace amphotericin B as the standard therapy for many serious fungal infections.[211]

Ketoconazole is the prototypical imidazole for therapy of deep mycoses. It is of limited value because it is available only as an oral formulation with erratic bioavailability and it interferes with steroidogenesis and the metabolism of other drugs administered concurrently by inhibition of cytochrome P450.

N-substitution of the imidazole ring has given rise to a second generation of derivatives called *triazoles* that have an antifungal spectrum similar to that of ketoconazole but less effect on steroid metabolism. This discussion describes two triazoles that are licensed for use, fluconazole and itraconazole.

KETOCONAZOLE[212]
Ketoconazole is a weak dibasic synthetic compound soluble in aqueous solution only at a pH below 3. As a consequence,

sufficient gastric acid is a prerequisite for adequate dissolution and absorption of this compound, a requirement commonly absent in ICU patients being treated with antacids of H_2-blocking drugs to prevent stress-induced gastric bleeding. Thus, although ketoconazole is currently the drug of choice to treat some uncomplicated deep mycoses in immunocompetent patients who are not gravely ill, it has a limited role in the therapy of fungal infections in ICU patients.

In vitro, ketoconazole is a potent inhibitor of a wide variety of fungi. Although MIC results from such studies do not correlate uniformly with susceptibility in humans, especially for some *C. albicans* strains, the following organisms are susceptible in vitro and in vivo: *Candida* species including *C. krusei*, *C. tropicalis*, *C. albicans*, *C. parapsilosis*, and *C. glabrata*; *Sporothrix schenckii*; *B. dermatitidis*; *C. immitis*; *H. capsulatum*; and *P. brasiliensis*. *Pseudallescheria boydii*, *C. neoformans*, *Aspergillus* species, and the agents of mucormycosis are variably susceptible to ketoconazole in vitro. Ketoconazole is not uniformly effective in infections caused by these agents.

Data are conflicting on the effects of ketoconazole combined with amphotericin B in vitro, and currently no evidence indicates a beneficial effect when these agents are combined.

Ketoconazole is the current drug of choice for treatment of mild to moderately severe nonmeningeal blastomycosis, histoplasmosis, coccidioidomycosis, pseudallescheriasis, and paracoccidioidomycosis in immunocompetent patients. Ketoconazole is also the drug of choice for therapy of oral and esophageal candidiasis and chronic mucocutaneous candidiasis.

MECHANISMS OF ACTION The molecular mechanisms of the antimycotic action of all imidazoles, including ketoconazole, are complex, with no single primary target responsible for all observed effects. However, at least two mechanisms of action have been described. At low concentrations, ketoconazole and the other imidazole agents exert a fungistatic effect on susceptible fungi. They inhibit 14-demethylation of lanosterol by binding to the cytochrome P450 enzyme C14 demethylase. This results in accumulation of 14-methylsterols and decreased concentrations of ergosterol, which is essential for normal fungal cytoplasmic membrane synthesis. At high concentrations in vitro, which probably can not be attained in human tissues, imidazoles are fungicidal to susceptible fungi. This effect is owing to direct cell membrane damage with leakage of essential components from the cells, an effect similar to that caused by amphotericin B.

MECHANISM OF RESISTANCE Acquired resistance to ketoconazole is increasingly being reported in *C. albicans* during chronic therapy in AIDS patients. Diminished susceptibility of some *C. albicans* strains isolated during chronic suppressive therapy in children with chronic mucocutaneous candidiasis has also been reported. Resistant strains are not uniformly resistant to other imidazole or triazole antifungal drugs. Resistance development in other susceptible fungi has been reported rarely. Resistance is associated with diminished uptake of ketoconazole at the cytoplasmic membrane.

CLINICAL PHARMACOLOGY After oral administration, in the presence of sufficient hydrochloric acid, ketoconazole is transformed into the hydrochloride salt, which is absorbed rapidly. Peak Cp after administration of 200 to 800 mg increases as a function of dose, but the disproportionate prolongation of the time to maximal Cp at doses of 800 mg suggests saturation of enzymes responsible for presystemic elimination of ketoconazole. In dogs, the absolute bioavailability of oral ketoconazole was 50% to 57% compared with intravenous doses, but a comparable study has not been described in humans. Food does not affect the absorption of ketoconazole. If H_2-blocking drugs or antacids must be administered to patients receiving ketoconazole, the drugs or antacids should be given 2 hours after the antifungal agent. However, given the prolonged inhibition of gastric HCl secretion produced by H_2 blockers administered orally or intravenously, it is speculative whether this strategy will permit ketoconazole to be adequately absorbed.

After absorption into the circulation, ketoconazole is more than 95% bound to plasma proteins. Its Cp declines biexponentially. The mean $t_{1/2}$ of ketoconazole in the initial distribution phase is 1 to 2 hours. The mean elimination phase $t_{1/2}$ was dose dependent after single oral doses of 100, 200, or 400 mg, with times of 6.5, 8.1, and 9.6 hours, respectively. Ketoconazole, a lipophilic drug, distributes widely, with an average AVD of approximately 2.4 L/kg. Ketoconazole is detectable in almost all fluids and tissues, although CSF concentrations are low, consistent with the drug's inefficacy in fungal meningitis.

The major route of elimination of ketoconazole involves hepatic biotransformation and excretion via the biliary tract. The major metabolic pathways involve oxidation and degradation of the imidazole ring, O-dealkylation, and aromatic hydroxylation to inactive metabolite. Clearance of ketoconazole declines out of proportion to doses beyond the range of 200 to 800 mg, suggesting that ketoconazole undergoes first-pass metabolism.

Ketoconazole kinetic features are not affected by renal insufficiency, but, as expected, significant hepatic insufficiency affects its elimination. Strategies for adjusting ketoconazole doses in patients with liver disease have not been described.

ADVERSE DRUG REACTIONS Ketoconazole at small doses is a drug of comparatively low toxicity; at larger doses, significant side effects are observed. The usual dose is 200 mg once or twice daily, but doses of 800 mg/d have been used, albeit with a higher frequency of side effects.

The most common adverse effects are dose-dependent anorexia, nausea, and vomiting, which occur in about 20% of patients receiving 400 mg/d. Administration with food may improve tolerance without affecting bioavailability.

Hepatitis demonstrated by asymptomatic elevation of serum transaminases affects a small percentage of patients, with return to normal without interruption of therapy. More severe, occasionally fatal, hepatitis occurs in about 1 in 12,000 recipients. This appears to be an idiosyncratic, unpredictable reaction, although pre-existing liver disease may be a risk factor. Therefore, liver function should be assessed before initiation of ketoconazole therapy, and the potential benefits of pretreatment should be weighed carefully against the risk of further liver damage.

Ketoconazole at doses of 800 mg/d or larger significantly interferes with normal steroid metabolism. Testosterone synthesis is blocked with the possibility of gynecomastia, diminished libido, oligospermia, and hair loss; in women, menometrorrhagia has been observed, although the mechanism is not clear; cortisol secretion and the response to adrenocorticotropin may be suppressed. All these effects are reversible by stopping ketoconazole therapy or reducing the dose.

Interactions with other drugs are clinically important. Administration of ketoconazole with cyclosporine and the nonsedating antihistamines, terfenadine and astemizole, result in increased cyclosporine and antihistamine concentrations with an attendant risk of nephrotoxicity and cardiac dysrhythmias, respectively, because of interference with hepatic drug metabolism. Rifampin coadministration decreases serum ketoconazole levels, presumably by induction of cytochrome P450 metabolism of the antifungal drug.

Ketoconazole is not thought to potentiate the anticoagulant action of warfarin, as does miconazole, another imidazole drug, but this is debated. It seems prudent to monitor the prothrombin time frequently in patients receiving ketoconazole and warfarin until the data are more clear.

ITRACONAZOLE

Itraconazole is a triazole antifungal drug that differs from ketoconazole in several respects. It is more potent in vitro than ketoconazole and more lipophilic; therefore, it possesses significantly different clinical pharmacokinetic properties. However, the place of itraconazole in the armamentarium of antifungal drugs for therapy of deep mycoses appears similar to that of ketoconazole except that there is evidence to suggest it may also be useful to treat sporotrichosis and invasive aspergillosis.[196]

The mechanism of action of itraconazole is identical to that of ketoconazole. Primary and secondary resistances to itraconazole have undefined prevalence and clinical importance at this time.

CLINICAL PHARMACOLOGY[213] The clinical pharmacokinetic characteristics of itraconazole differ significantly from those of ketoconazole. Itraconazole is a weak base that is highly ionized and poorly absorbed at the pH of gastric juice. It is insoluble in water, and this has largely precluded the development of an injectable formulation. The absolute bioavailability of itraconazole is approximately 50% in dogs; the comparable kinetic parameter in humans is not known. The usual adult dose is 200 to 400 mg/d. Ingestion of itraconazole with food doubles its absorption, so it should be taken immediately after a meal to ensure optimal oral bioavailability. As with ketoconazole, oral bioavailability appears to be enhanced at larger doses (>500 mg). This augmented oral bioavailability at larger doses likely results from transient saturation of metabolic processes in the liver. Plasma protein binding of itraconazole is 99%, mainly to albumin. Itraconazole distributes widely and, as is characteristic of lipophilic drugs, possesses a large AVD, which is 20 times greater than that of ketoconazole, and reflects extensive tissue sequestration. However, itraconazole has negligible CSF penetration.

The metabolic fate of itraconazole has been studied in detail only in laboratory animals. However, its metabolic fate in humans is expected to be comparable to that in animals. Itraconazole undergoes extensive biotransformation, presumably in the liver. More than 30 metabolites have been identified, none of which has antifungal activity. About 54% of an oral dose is secreted through the bile into the feces and 35% into urine primarily as inactive metabolites. The mean elimination $t_{1/2}$ from plasma ranges from 13 to 18 hours. Peak Cp of itraconazole attains steady state after about 2 weeks and averages 0.4 to 0.6 mg/L. In uremic patients with creatinine clearance slower than 12 mL/min who are not yet on maintenance hemodialysis and in volunteers with cirrhosis, itraconazole kinetics were not different from those in normal volunteers. Thus, dose alterations are not recommended for such patients.

Despite the high level of protein binding of itraconazole and its displacement from albumin by other drugs with similar high-level affinity, the clinical relevance of such interactions remains uncertain.

ADVERSE DRUG REACTIONS Like ketoconazole, itraconazole is reasonably well tolerated; 10% to 15% of patients experience nausea or vomiting, but the intensity does not usually require interruption of therapy. Unlike ketoconazole, itraconazole appears to neither cause hepatitis nor alter steroidogenesis.

No significant effect of itraconazole on the metabolism of warfarin has been reported. Concomitant itraconazole therapy reduces cyclosporine dose requirement by about 50%. Concurrent administration with terfenadine and astemizole inhibits their metabolism and increases the risk of cardiac dysrhythmias. Interaction with a single dose of rifampin, a potent inducer of hepatic drug-metabolizing enzymes, causes an initial inhibition of itraconazole metabolism followed by increased clearance (metabolism). The net effect of chronic dosing is hard to predict based on these limited data.

FLUCONAZOLE

Fluconazole is a novel, low-molecular-weight antifungal with two azole rings.[214,215] Its development provides intensivists with a potent, injectable, broad-spectrum antifungal of the imidazole and triazole class that is unique pharmacokinetically in penetrating readily into CSF across even uninflamed meninges and in being eliminated primarily as unchanged drug directly into the urine to yield high bioactive antifungal activity therein.

In vitro, the spectrum of action of fluconazole is comparable to that of ketoconazole, as is the scope of resistance (becoming more common) and its basis (diminished uptake by fungal cell membranes). It is efficacious in animal models of several deep fungal infections in normal and immunocompromised hosts. However, at this time, its relative usefulness compared with amphotericin B for serious visceral fungal infections is being evaluated.

Clinically, in addition to being injectable, fluconazole has two potential advantages over ketoconazole, which mirror the distinctive kinetic properties of fluconazole. First, fluconazole may be valuable for treatment and long-term suppression of fungal meningitis in immunocompetent and immunosuppressed patients such as those with AIDS; second, it may be effective for treatment of fungal urinary tract infection. Fluconazole shows great promise as a potent, safe agent for the treatment of fungal meningitis.[196] Its potential for management of this and other deep mycoses alone and in combination with amphotericin B remains to be elucidated in controlled trials.

CLINICAL PHARMACOLOGY Fluconazole is highly soluble in water; injectable and oral formulations are available. The usual daily adult dose in patients with normal renal function ranges from 100 to 400 mg. Peak Cp values average 4 to 8 mg/L after repetitive doses of 100 mg/d.

After oral administration, greater than 90% is absorbed, although whether this occurs in seriously ill ICU patients is unclear. Oral bioavailability is not affected by food or gastric pH. Fluconazole is 15% bound to plasma protein, so adverse interactions with other drugs because of displacement from plasma proteins are unlikely to be observed. CSF concentrations average 50% (range, 74% to 89%) of concurrent Cp in patients with normal and inflamed meninges. Elimination is primarily by glomerular filtration into urine as unchanged drug, so high, therapeutic antifungal concentrations are attained. The plasma $t_{1/2}$ in adults with normal renal function is approximately 30 hours, making once-daily dosing appropriate. In adults with creatinine clearance slower than 10 mL/min, fluconazole plasma $t_{1/2}$ is 48 hours, so a 50% reduction in dose is recommended. Hemodialysis for 3 hours decreases fluconazole Cp by 48%. A supplemental dose of 200 mg after dialysis is recommended. Fluconazole added to peritoneal fluid is almost completely bioavailable to the systemic circulation. Fluconazole administered orally yields peritoneal fluid concentrations 60% of corresponding Cp values. For patients requiring fluconazole and receiving peritoneal dialysis, dose reduction by 50% is recommended. *Candida* species peritonitis also can be treated by adding fluconazole 150 mg into the peritoneal dialysate every 2 days. The effect of dialysis or severe hepatic disease on fluconazole disposition and the details of associated dose adjustments needed in such patients remain to be defined.

ADVERSE DRUG REACTIONS Initial studies suggest that fluconazole shares the same safety profile as itraconazole: Gastrointestinal upset is the most common side effect. Transient elevations in serum transaminases have been described. No interference with steroid hormone synthesis has been observed.

Fluconazole administered concurrently with other drugs can affect their metabolism. Addition of fluconazole causes Cp values of terfenadine, astemizole, phenytoin, sulfonylureas, warfarin, and cyclosporine to increase, presumably by interference with their hepatic metabolism by the cytochrome P450 oxidation system.

It is expected that renal dysfunction will reduce fluconazole clearance and cause total body content and fluconazole Cp to rise if doses are not reduced. Although the clinical importance of these increased fluconazole Cp values has not yet been demonstrated, reducing fluconazole doses as renal function declines would seem prudent.

VORICONAZOLE

Voriconazole is a broad-spectrum triazole antifungal agent derived from fluconazole.[216,217] It is approved for the treatment of invasive aspergillosis in the United States and Europe for treatment of serious infections caused by *Fusarium*, *Scedosporium*, and azole-resistant *Candida* species.

In addition to caspofungin, the availability of voriconazole presents intensivists with an alternative to amphotericin B for treating patients with invasive aspergillosis and off-label uses for other serious fungal infections.

Recommended doses are 6 mg/kg intravenously 12 hours apart for two doses, followed by 4 mg/kg every 12 hours; patients may be switched to 100 mg ($\leq$40 kg body weight) or 200 mg (>40 kg) orally every 12 hours.

MECHANISM OF ACTION   Like all azole antifungals, voriconazole inhibits 14-α-sterol demethylase, an enzyme involved in synthesis of sterols for the fungal cell membrane and wall. The effect is fungistatic. Voriconazole is as or more potent an inhibitor of *Aspergillus* species and other fungi than is itraconazole, fluconazole, or amphotericin B, although the exact clinical relevance of in vitro susceptibility tests for fungi remains uncertain.

MECHANISM OF RESISTANCE   Voriconazole resistance has been observed in isolates recovered from HIV-infected pediatric patients with oropharyngeal candidiasis previously treated with azole antifungal drugs. This suggests that some cross-resistance between voriconazole and other azole antifungals is observed. However, voriconazole has been observed to inhibit fluconazole-resistant *C. albicans* from HIV patients with fluconazole-resistant esophageal candidiasis.

CLINICAL PHARMACOLOGY   Oral and intravenous formulations are available. Oral bioavailability is 96% and is not affected by gastric pH. AVD is 4.6 L/kg body weight, implying wide distribution.

Voriconazole is eliminated from serum by hepatic metabolism by cytochrome P450 isoforms 2C19, 2C9, and 3A4. Less than 2% of a dose can be recovered unchanged in urine. Due to saturable metabolism, its kinetic features are nonlinear. However, at recommended doses, serum $t_{1/2}$ is approximately 6 hours.

Clearance is decreased by 50% in patients with moderate hepatic impairment (Child-Pugh class B). It has been suggested that the loading dose for such patients can be the same as in patients with normal hepatic function, but maintenance doses should be halved. Pharmacokinetic data on voriconazole in patients with severe hepatic impairment (Child-Pugh class C) are not available, and no specific validated dose recommendations are available for such individuals.

Renal impairment, including severe dysfunction, does not alter voriconazole kinetics. Although the carrier, cyclodextrin, may accumulate in such patients, it probably will not cause adverse effects.

ADVERSE DRUG REACTIONS   Voriconazole is generally well tolerated, particularly in comparison with amphotericin B. However, it causes disturbances of vision (8% to 44% incidence), rash (5% to 6% incidence), and elevated liver function tests in about 10% of patients. In addition, because of its metabolism by hepatic CYP 3A4, a principal drug metabolizing enzyme, it has the potential to cause significant drug interactions during concurrent administration with a host of other drugs.

Vision changes consist of altered visual perception, blurring, color vision alterations, and photophobia. They were generally transient and did not necessitate interruption of treatment in published trials.

Skin rashes include Stevens-Johnson syndrome, toxic epidermal necrolysis, and erythema multiforme, although most rashes were only mild to moderate in severity.

Voriconazole markedly increases systemic exposure of concurrent warfarin, cyclosporine, phenytoin, omeprazole, sirolimus, and tacrolimus. It is predicted to increase systemic exposure of concurrent terfenadine, astemizole, cisapride, pimozide, or quinidine and potentially prolong QT intervals and cause dysrhythmias.

Concomitant treatment with nevirapine, rifampicin, rifabutin, or phenytoin decreases systemic exposure to voriconazole. Coadministration of voriconazole with erythromycin, delavirdine, and ritonavir increase voriconazole levels.

Clearly, voriconazole has the potential to cause significant drug interactions in patients, and vigilance will be required to anticipate and deal with adverse reactions arising from its use.

References

1. Kaiser AB: Antimicrobial prophylaxis in surgery. *N Engl J Med* 315:1129, 1986.
2. Antimicrobial prophylaxis in surgery. *Med Lett Drugs Ther* 37:79, 1995.
3. Dajani AS, Bisno AL, Chung KJ, et al: Prevention of bacterial endocarditis. Recommendations of the American Heart Association. *JAMA* 264:2919, 1990.
4. Van Saene HKF, Stoutenbeeck CP, Zandstra DF: Concept of selective decontamination of the digestive tract in the critically ill, in Van Saene HKF, Stoutenbeeck CP, Lawin P, Ledingham IMcA (eds): *Update in Intensive Care and Emergency Medicine.* Berlin, Springer-Verlag, 1989, p 88.
5. Vincent JL: Selective digestive decontamination: For everyone, everywhere? *Lancet* 362:1006, 2003.
6. Tomasz A: Penicillin-binding proteins in bacteria. *Ann Intern Med* 96:502, 1982.
7. Curtis NAC, Orr D, Ross GW, Boulton MG: Affinities of penicillins and cephalosporins for the penicillin-binding proteins of *Escherichia coli* K-12 and their antibacterial activity. *Antimicrob Agents Chemother* 16:533, 1979.
8. Craig WA, Vogelmann B: The postantibiotic effect. *Ann Intern Med* 106:900, 1987.
9. Turnidge JD: The pharmacodynamics of beta-lactams. *Clin Infect Dis* 27:10, 1998.
10. Drusano GL: Role of pharmacokinetics in the outcome of infections. *Antimicrob Agents Chemother* 32:289, 1988.
11. Zhanel GG, Palatnic L, Nichol KA, et al: Antimicrobial resistance in *Haemophilus influenzae* and *Moraxella catarrhalis* respiratory tract isolates: Results of the Canadian Respiratory Organism Susceptibility Study, 1997–2002. *Antimicrob Agents Chemother* 47:1875, 2003.
12. Gibaldi M, Perrier D: Apparent volumes of distribution, in *Pharmacokinetics.* New York, Marcel Dekker, 1975, p 175.
13. Barza M, Cuchural G: General principles of antibiotic tissue penetration. *J Antimicrob Chemother* 15(suppl A):59, 1985.
14. Isbister T: Penicillin allergy: A review of the immunological and clinical aspects. *Med J Austral* 1:1067, 1971.
15. Saxon A, Beall GN, Rohr AS, Adelman DC: Immediate hypersensitivity reactions to beta-lactam antibiotics. *Ann Intern Med* 107:204, 1987.
16. Sogn DD, Evans R, Shepherd GM, et al: Results of the National Institute of Allergy and Infectious Diseases Collaborative Clinical Testing trial to test the predictive value of skin testing with major and minor penicillin derivatives in hospitalized adults. *Arch Intern Med* 152:1025, 1992.

17. Gadde J, Spence M, Wheeler B, et al: Clinical experience with penicillin skin testing in a large inner-city STD clinic. *JAMA* 270:2456, 1993.

18. Smith H, Lerner PI, Weinstein L: Neurotoxicity and "massive" intravenous therapy with penicillin. *Arch Intern Med* 120:47, 1967.

19. Bloomer HA, Barton LJ, Maddock RJ Jr: Penicillin-induced encephalopathy in uremic patients. *JAMA* 200:121, 1967.

20. Editorial: Antimicrobials and hemostasis. *Lancet* I:510, 1983.

21. Petri WA Jr: Antimicrobial agents: Penicillins, cephalosporins, and other beta-lactam antibiotics, in Hardman JG, Limbird LL (eds): *The Pharmacological Basis of Therapeutics.* New York, McGraw-Hill, 2001, p 1189.

22. The choice of antibacterial drugs. *Med Lett Drugs Ther* 43:69, 2001.

23. Sanders CC, Sanders WE Jr: Microbial resistance to newer generation *b*-lactam antibiotics: Clinical and laboratory implications. *J Infect Dis* 151:399, 1985.

24. Anne S, Reisman RE: Risk of administering cephalosporin antibiotics to patients with histories of penicillin allergy. *Ann Allergy Asthma Immunol* 74:167, 1995.

25. Shevchuk YM, Conly JM: Antibiotic-associated hypoprothrombinemia: A review of prospective studies, 1966–1988. *Rev Infect Dis* 12:1109, 1990.

26. Neu HC: Third-generation cephalosporins: Safety profiles after 10 years of clinical use. *J Clin Pharmacol* 30:396, 1990.

27. Satabe S, Yoshihara E, Nakac T: Diffusion of beta-lactam through liposome membranes reconstituted from purified outer membranes of *Pseudomonas aeruginosa*. *Antimicrob Agents Chemother* 34:685, 1990.

28. Livermore DM, Oakton KJ, Carter MW, et al: Activity of ertapenem (MK-0826) versus *Enterbacteriaceae* with potent beta-lactamases. *Antimicrob Agents Chemother* 45:2831, 2001.

29. Colardyn F, Faulkner KL: Intravenous meropenem versus imipenem/cilastatin in the treatment of serious bacterial infections in hospitalized patients. Meropenem Serious Infection Study Group. *Antimicrob Agents Chemother* 38:523, 1996.

30. Hurst M, Lam HM: Meropenem. A review of its use in patients in intensive care. *Drugs* 59:653, 2000.

31. Ertapenem (Invanz)—A new parenteral carbapenem. *Med Lett Drugs Ther* 44:25, 2002.

32. McClean KL, Sheehan GJ, Harding GKM: Intraabdominal infection: A review. *Clin Infect Dis* 19:100, 1994.

33. Norrby SR: Imipenem/cilastatin: Rationale for a fixed combination. *Rev Infect Dis* 7(suppl 3):S447, 1985.

34. Calandra GB, Brown KR, Grad LC, et al: Review of adverse experiences and tolerability in the first 2,516 patients treated with imipenem/cilastatin. *Am J Med* 78(suppl 6A):73, 1985.

35. Aronoff SC, Klinger JD: *In vitro* activities of aztreonam, piperacillin and ticarcillin combined with amikacin against amikacin-resistant *Pseudomonas aeruginosa* and *P. cepacia* isolates from children with cystic fibrosis. *Antimicrob Agents Chemother* 25:279, 1984.

36. Sykes RB, Bonner DP, Bush K, Georgopapadakou NH: Aztreonam (Sq 26, 776) a synthetic monobactam specifically active against aerobic Gram-negative bacteria. *Antimicrob Agents Chemother* 32:85, 1982.

37. Swabb EA: Review of the clinical pharmacology of the monobactam antibiotic aztreonam. *Am J Med* 78(2A):11, 1985.

38. Livermore DM: Determinants of the activity of beta-lactam inhibitor combinations. *J Antimicrob Chemother* 31(suppl A):9, 1993.

39. Sanders WE Jr, Sanders CC: Piperacillin/tazobactam: A critical review of the evolving literature. *Clin Infect Dis* 22:107, 1996.

40. Offenstadt G, Vassal T, Lesage D, et al: Piperacillin/tazobactam treatment of serious infections in an intensive care unit. *Complications Surg* 12(suppl A):65, 1993.

41. Cometta A, Zinner S, DeBock R, et al: Piperacillin-tazobactam plus amikacin versus ceftazidime plus amikacin as empiric therapy for fever in granulocytopenia patients with cancer. *Antimicrob Agents Chemother* 39:445, 1995.

42. Brogden RN, Carmine A, Heel RC, et al: Amoxicillin/clavulanic acid: a review of its antibacterial activity, pharmacokinetics and therapeutic use. *Drugs* 22:337, 1985.

43. Benson JM, Nahata MC: Sulbactam/ampicillin, a new beta-lactamase/beta-lactam antibiotic combination. *Drug Intell Clin Pharm* 22:534, 1988.

44. Leigh DA, Phillips I, Wise R (eds): Timentin-ticarcillin plus clavulanic acid, a laboratory and clinical perspective. *J Antimicrob Chemother* 17(suppl C):1, 1986.

45. Sörgel F, Kinzig M: The chemistry, pharmacokinetics and tissue distribution of piperacillin/tazobactam. *J Antimicrob Chemother* 31(suppl A):39, 1993.

46. Bryan LE, Kwan S: Role of ribosomal binding, membrane potential, and electron transport in bacterial uptake of streptomycin and gentamicin. *Antimicrob Agents Chemother* 23:835, 1983.

47. Vogelman B, Craig W: Kinetics of antimicrobial activity. *J Pediatr* 5:835, 1986.

48. Davis BD: Mechanism of the bactericidal action of aminoglycosides. *Microbiol Rev* 57:341, 1987.

49. Craig WA, Gudmundsson S: Postantibiotic effect, in Lorian V (ed): *Antibiotics in Laboratory Medicine,* 3rd ed. Baltimore, Williams & Wilkins, 1991, p 403.

50. Davis BD: Resistance to aminoglycosides: Mechanisms and frequency. *Rev Infect Dis* 4(suppl 2):261, 1983.

51. Kapusnik JE, Hackbarth CJ, Chambers HT, et al: Single, large, daily dosing versus intermittent dosing of tobramycin for treating experimental Pseudomonas pneumonia. *J Infect Dis* 158:7, 1988

52. Price KE, Kresel PA, Farchione LA, et al: Epidemiological studies of aminoglycoside resistance in the USA. *J Antimicrob Chemother* 8(suppl A):89, 1981.

53. Pechere J-C, Dugal R: Clinical pharmacokinetics of aminoglycoside antibiotics. *Clin Pharmacokinet* 4:170, 1979.

54. Dulon M, Aran J-M, Zajic G, Schacht J: Comparative uptake of gentamicin, netilmicin and amikacin in the guinea pig cochlea and vestibule. *Antimicrob Agents Chemother* 30:96, 1986.

55. Cutler RE, Gyselynck A-M, Fleet WP, Forrey AW: Correlation of serum creatinine concentration and gentamicin half-life. *JAMA* 219:1037, 1972.

56. Maderazo EG, Sun H, Jay GH: Simplification of antibiotic dose adjustments in renal insufficiency: The DREM system. *Lancet* 340:767, 1992.

57. Cockroft DW, Gault MH: Prediction of creatinine clearance from serum creatinine. *Nephron* 16:31, 1976.

58. Noone P, Parsons TMC, Pattison JR, et al: Experience in monitoring gentamicin therapy during treatment of serious Gram-negative sepsis. *Br Med J* I:477, 1974.

59. Line DH, Poole GW, Waterworth PM: Serum streptomycin levels and dizziness. *Tubercle* 51:76, 950.

60. Dahlgren JG, Anderson ET, Hewitt WL: Gentamicin blood levels: A guide to nephrotoxicity. *Antimicrob Agents Chemother* 8:58, 1975.

61. Hatala R, Dinh T, Cook DJ: Once-daily aminoglycoside dosing in immunocompetent adults: A meta-analysis. *Ann Intern Med* 124:717, 1996.

62. Ferriols-Lisart R, Alos-Alminana M: Effectiveness and safety of once-daily aminoglycosides: A meta-analysis. *Am J Health Syst Pharm* 53:1141, 1996.

63. Prins JM, Büller HR, Kuijper EJ, et al: Once versus thrice daily gentamicin in patients with serious infections. *Lancet* 341:335, 1993.

64. Hustinx WNM, Hoepelman IM: Aminoglycoside dosage regimens. Is once a day enough? *Clin Pharmacokinet* 25:427, 1993.

65. Denaro C: Once daily dosing of aminoglycosides (letter). *Aust N Z J Med* 24:731, 1994.

66. Prins JM, Weverling GH, de Blok K, et al: Validation and nephrotoxicity of a simplified once-daily aminoglycoside dosing schedule and guidelines for monitoring therapy. *Antimicrob Agents Chemother* 41:2494, 1996.

67. Schumock GT, Raber SR, Crawford SY, et al: National survey of once-daily dosing of aminoglycoside antibiotics. *Pharmacotherapy* 15:201, 1995.

68. Moore RD, Smith CR, Lietman PS: The association of aminoglycoside plasma levels with mortality in patients with Gram-negative bacteremia. *J Infect Dis* 149:443, 1984.

69. Weiner ND, Schact J: Biochemical model of aminoglycoside-induced hearing loss, in Lerner SA, Matz GJ, Hawkins JE Jr (eds): *Aminoglycoside Toxicity.* Boston, Little, Brown, 1981, p 113.

70. Smith CR, Lipsky JJ, Laskin OL, et al: Double-blind comparison of the nephrotoxicity and auditory toxicity of gentamicin and tobramycin. *N Engl J Med* 302:1106, 1980.

71. Lerner AM, Reyes MP, Cone LA, et al: Randomized, controlled trial of the comparative efficacy, auditory toxicity and nephrotoxicity of tobramycin and netilmicin. *Lancet* 1:1123, 1983.

72. Nordstrom L, Banck G, Belfrage S, et al: Prospective study of the ototoxicity of gentamicin. *Acta Path Microbiol Scand B* 81(suppl 241):58, 1973.

73. Jackson GG, Arcieri G: Ototoxicity of gentamicin in man: A survey and controlled analysis of clinical experience in the United States. *J Infect Dis* 124(suppl):S130, 1971.

74. Traub WH, Kleber I: In vitro additive effect of polymyxin B and rifampin against *Serratia marcescens. Antimicrob Agents Chemother* 7:874, 1975.

75. Noriega ER, Rubinstein E, Simberkoff MS, Rahal JJ Jr: Subacute and acute endocarditis due to *Pseudomonas cepacia* in heroin addicts. *Am J Med* 59:29, 1975.

76. Thomas FE Jr, Leonard JM, Alfred RH: Sulfamethoxazole-trimethoprim-polymyxin therapy of serious multiple drug-resistant serratia infections. *Antimicrob Agents Chemother* 9:201, 1976.

77. Ouderkirk JP, Nord JA, Turett GS, et al: Polymyxin B nephrotoxicity and efficacy against nosocomial infections caused by multiresistant gram-negative bacteria. *Antimicrob Agents Chemother* 47:2659, 2003.

78. Chang S, Sievert DM, Hageman JC, et al: Infection with vancomycin-resistant *Staphylococcus aureus* containing the *van*A resistant gene. *N Engl J Med* 348:1342, 2003.

79. Matzke GR, McGory RW, Halstenson CE, Keane WF: Pharmacokinetics of vancomycin in patients with various degrees of renal function. *Antimicrob Agents Chemother* 25:433, 1984.

80. Cantu TG, Yamanaka-Yuen NR, Lietman PS: Serum vancomycin concentrations: Reappraisal of their clinical value. *Clin Infect Dis* 18:533, 1994.

81. Tobin CM: Vancomycin therapeutic drug monitoring: Is there a consensus view? The results of a UK National External Quality Assessment Scheme (UK NEQAS) for Antibiotic Assays Questionnaire. *J Antimicrob Chemother* 50:713, 2002.

82. Zimmerman AE, Katona BG, Plaisance KI: Association of vancomycin serum concentrations with outcomes in patients with Gram-positive bacteremia. *Pharmacotherapy* 15:85, 1995.

83. Keighley MRB, Burdon DW, Arabi Y, et al: Randomized controlled trial of vancomycin for pseudomembranous colitis and postoperative diarrhea. *Br Med J* 2:1667, 1978.

84. Teasley DG, Gerding DN, Olson MM, et al: Prospective randomized trial of metronidazole versus vancomycin for *Clostridium difficile*–associated diarrhoea and colitis. *Lancet* 2:1043, 1983.

85. Matzke GR, Halstenson CE, Olson PL, et al: Systemic absorption of oral vancomycin in patients with renal insufficiency and antibiotic associated colitis. *Am J Kidney Dis* 9:422, 1987.

86. Sahai J, Healy DP, Garris R, et al: Influence of antihistamine pre-treatment on vancomycin-induced red-man-syndrome. *J Infect Dis* 160:876, 1989.

87. Newfield P, Roizen MF: Hazards of rapid administration of vancomycin. *Ann Intern Med* 91:581, 1979.

88. Farber BF, Moellering RC Jr: Retrospective study of the toxicity of preparations of vancomycin from 1974 to 1981. *Antimicrob Agents Chemother* 23:138, 1970.

89. Mellor JA, Kingdom J, Cafferkey M, Keane CT: Vancomycin toxicity: A prospective study. *J Antimicrob Chemother* 15:773, 1985.

90. Chow AW, Azar RM: Glycopeptides and nephrotoxicity. *Intens Care Med* 20(suppl 4):S23, 1994.

91. Brogden RN, Peters DH: Teicoplanin. *Drugs* 47:823, 1994.

92. Peppercorn MA: Sulfasalazine: Pharmacology, clinical use, toxicity and related new drug development. *Ann Intern Med* 101:377, 1984.

93. Speck WT, Rosenkranz HS: Activity of silver sulfadiazine against dermatophytes. *Lancet* 2:895, 1974.

94. Lowbury EJL, Babb JR, Bridges K, Jackson DM: Topical chemoprophylaxis with silver sulfadiazine and silver nitrate chlorhexidine creams: Emergence of sulfonamide-resistant Gram-negative bacilli. *Br Med J* 1:493, 1976.

95. Baskin CG, Law S, Wenger NK: Sulfadiazine rheumatic fever prophylaxis during pregnancy: Does it increase the risk of kernicterus in the newborn? *Cardiology* 65:222, 1980.

96. Wan AT, Canyers RA, Coombs CJ, et al: Determination of silver in blood, urine and tissues of volunteers and burn patients. *Clin Chem* 37:1683, 1991.

97. Fuller FW, Parrish M, Nance FC: A review of the dosimetry of 1% silver sulfadiazine in burn wound treatment. *J Burn Care Rehabil* 5:213, 1994.

98. Carr A, Gross AS, Hoskins JM, et al: Acetylator phenotype and cutaneous hypersensitivity to trimethoprim-sulfamethoxazole in HIV-infected patients. *AIDS* 8:333, 1994.

99. Rieder MJ, Shear NH, Kanee A, et al: Prominence of slow acetylator phenotype among patients with sulfonamide hypersensitivity reactions. *Clin Pharmacol Ther* 49:13, 1991.

100. Rieder MJ, Utrecht J, Shear NH, et al: Diagnosis of sulfonamide hypersensitivity reactions by in vitro "rechallenge" with hydroxylamine metabolite. *Ann Intern Med* 110:286, 1989.

101. Lacey RW: Do sulfonamide-trimethoprim combinations select less resistance to trimethoprim than the use of thimethoprim alone? *J Med Microbiol* 15:403, 1982.

102. Huovinen P, Mattila T, Kiminki O, et al: Emergence of trimethoprim resistance in fecal flora. *Antimicrob Agents Chemother* 28:354, 1985.

103. Yu VL, Felegie TP, Yee RB, et al: Synergistic interaction *in vitro* with use of three antibiotics simultaneously against *Pseudomonas maltophilia. J Infect Dis* 142:602, 1980.

104. Joos B, Blaser J, Opravil M, et al: Monitoring of co-trimoxazole concentrations in serum during treatment of *Pneumocytis carinii* pneumonia. *Antimicrob Agents Chemother* 39:2661, 1995.

105. Schentag JJ, Scully BE. Quinolones, in Yu VL, Merigan TC Jr, Barriere SL (eds): *Antimicrobial Therapy & Vaccines.* Baltimore, Williams & Wilkins, 1999, p 875.

106. Zhanel GG, Ennis K, Vercaigne L et al: A critical review of the fluoroquinolones. Focus on respiratory tract infections. *Drugs* 62:13, 2002.

107. Kresken M, Hafner D, Mittermayer H, et al: Prevalence of fluoroquinolone resistance in Europe. *Infection* 22(suppl 2): S90, 1994.

108. Poole K: Efflux-mediated resistance to fluoroquinolones in Gram-negative bacteria. *Antimicrob Agents Chemother* 44:2233, 2000.

109. Khaliq Y, Zhanel GG. Fluroquinolone-associated tendinopathy: A critical review of the literature. *Clin Inf Dis* 36:1404, 2003.

110. Davis H, McGoodwin E, Reed TG: Anaphylactoid reactions reported after treatment with ciprofloxacin. *Ann Intern Med* 111:1041, 1989.

111. Aldridge KE: Bacteremia due to *Bacteroides fragilis* group: distribution of species, beta-lactamase production and antimicrobial susceptibility patterns. *Antimicrob Agents Chemother* 47:148, 2003.

112. Houghton GW, Smith J, Thorne PS, Templeton R: The pharmacokinetics of oral and intravenous metronidazole in man. *J Antimicrob Chemother* 5:621, 1979.

113. Ioannides L, Somogyi A, Spicer J, et al: Rectal administration of metronidazole provides therapeutic plasma levels in postoperative patients. *N Engl J Med* 305:1569, 1987.

114. Saginur R, Hawley CR, Bartlett JG: Colitis associated with metronidazole therapy. *J Infect Dis* 141:772, 1980.

115. Hoban D, Doern V, Fluit AC, et al: Worldwide prevalence of antimicrobial resistance in *Streptococcus pneumoniae, Haemophilus influenzae,* and *Moraxella catarrhalis* in the SENTRY Antimicrobial Surveillance Program, 1997–1999. *Clin Infect Dis* 32(suppl 2):581, 2001.

116. Krobath PD, Brown A, Lyon JA, et al: Pharmacokinetics of single-dose erythromycin in normal and alcohol liver disease subjects. *Antimicrob Agents Chemother* 21:135, 1982.

117. Sarna SK, Soergel KH, Koch TR, et al: Gastrointestinal motor effects of erythromycin in humans. *Gastroenterology* 101:1488, 1991.

118. Van Marion WF, Van der Meer JWM, Kalff MW, Schnicht SM: Ototoxicity of erythromycin. *Lancet* 2:214, 1978.

119. Tolman KG, Sannella JJ, Freston JW: Chemical structure of erythromycin and hepatotoxicity. *Ann Intern Med* 81:58, 1974.

120. Piscitelli SC, Danzinger LH, Rodvold KA, et al: Clarithromycin and azithromycin: New macrolide antibiotics. *Clin Pharmacol* 11:137, 1992.

121. Garey KW, Amsden GW: Intravenous azithromycin. *Ann Pharmacother* 33:218, 1999.

122. Bizjak ED, Haug III MT, Schilz RJ, et al: Intravenous azithromycin-induced ototoxicity. *Pharmacotherapy* 19:345, 1999.

123. Amsden GW: Erythromycin, clarithromycin and azithromycin: Are the differences real. *Clin Ther* 18:56, 1996.

124. Levinson ME, Mangura CT, Lorber B, et al: Clindamycin compared with penicillin for the treatment of anaerobic lung abscess. *Ann Intern Med* 98:466, 1983.

125. Rovers JP, Ilersich AL, Einarson TR: Meta-analysis of parenteral clindamycin dosing regimens. *Ann Pharmacother* 29:852, 1995.

126. Zhanel GG, Walters M, Noreddin A, et al: The ketolides. A critical review. *Drugs* 62:1771, 2002.

127. Cada DJ, Baker DE, Levien T: Quinupristin/dalfopristin. *Hosp Pharm* 23:77, 2000.

128. Perry CM, Jarvis B: Linezolid. A review of its use in the management of serious gram-positive infections. *Drugs* 61:525, 2001.

129. Mutnick AH, Enne V, Janes RN: Linezolid resistance since 2001: SENTRY antimicrobial surveillance program. *Ann Pharmacother* 37:769, 2003.

130. Whitley RJ, Soong S-J, Dolin R, et al: Adenine arabinoside therapy of biopsy-proved herpes simplex encephalitis: National Institute of Allergy and Infectious Diseases Collaborative Antiviral Study. *N Engl J Med* 297:289, 1977.

131. Whitley RJ, Alford CA Jr, Hirsch MS, et al, and the NIAID Collaborative Antiviral Study Group: Vidarabine versus acyclovir therapy in herpes simplex encephalitis. *N Engl J Med* 314:144, 1986.

131a. Whitley R, Arvin A, Prober C, et al: A controlled trial comparing vidarabine with acyclovir in neonatal herpes simplex virus infection. Infectious Diseases Collaborative Antiviral Study Group. *N Engl J Med* 324:444, 1991.

132. Prober CG, Kirk LE, Keeney RE: Acyclovir therapy of chickenpox in immunosuppressed children—A collaborative study. *J Pediatr* 101:622, 1982.

133. Shepp DH, Dandliker PS, Meyers JD: Treatment of varicella-zoster virus infection in severely immunocompromised patients. A randomized comparison of acyclovir and vidarabine. *N Engl J Med* 314:208, 1986.

134. Balfour HH Jr, Bean B, Mitchell CD, et al: Acyclovir in immunocompromised patients with cytomegalovirus disease. A controlled trial at one institution. *Am J Med* 73:241, 1982.

135. Wade JC, Hintz M, McGuffin RW, et al: Treatment of cytomegalovirus pneumonia with high-dose acyclovir. *Am J Med* 73:249, 1982.

136. Andersson J, Skoldenberg B, Ernberg I, et al: Acyclovir treatment in primary Epstein-Barr virus infection. A double-blind, placebo-controlled study. *Scand J Infect Dis* (suppl)47:107, 1985.

137. Boulton EA, Thornton B, Bauer DJ, Bye A: Successful treatment of experimental B virus (*Herpesvirus simiae*) infection with acyclovir. *Br Med J* 280:681, 1980.

138. Artenstein AW, Hicks CB, Goodwin BS Jr, Hilliard JK: Human infection with B virus following a needlestick injury. *Rev Infect Dis* 13:288, 1991.

139. Dekker C, Ellis MN, McClaren C, et al: Virus resistance in clinical practice. *J Antimicrob Chemother* 12(suppl B):137, 1983.

140. Birch CJ, Tachedjian G, Goherty RR, et al: Altered sensitivity to antiviral drugs of herpes simplex virus isolates from a patient with the acquired immunodeficiency syndrome. *J Infect Dis* 162:731, 1990.

141. Coen DM: General aspects of virus drug resistance with special reference to herpes simplex virus. *J Antimicrob Chemother* 18(suppl B):1, 1986.

142. Acyclovir pharmacokinetics and tolerance in man, in King DH, Galasso G (eds): *Proceedings of a Symposium on Acyclovir.* 1982, p 165.

143. Wade JC, Meyers JD: Neurologic symptoms associated with parenteral acyclovir treatment after marrow transplantation. *Ann Intern Med* 98:921, 1983.

144. Revankar SG, Applegate AL, Markovitz DM: Delirium associated with acyclovir treatment in a patient with renal failure. *Clin Infect Dis* 21:435, 1995.

145. Haefeli WE, Schoenenberger RA, Weiss P, et al: Acyclovir-induced neurotoxicity: Concentration-side effect relationship in acyclovir overdose. *Am J Med* 94:212, 1993.

146. Almond MK, Fan S, Dhillon S, et al: Avoiding acyclovir neurotoxicity in patients with chronic renal failure undergoing hemodialysis. *Nephron* 69:428, 1995.

147. Perry CM, Faulds D: Valaciclovir. A review of its antiviral activity, pharmacokinetic properties and therapeutic efficacy in herpesvirus infections. *Drugs* 52:754, 1996.

148. Perry CM, Wagstaff AJ: Famciclovir: A review of its pharmacological properties and therapeutic efficacy in herpesvirus infections. *Drugs* 50:396, 1995.

149. Faulds D, Heel RC: Ganciclovir: a review of its antiviral activity, pharmacokinetic properties and therapeutic efficacy in cytomegalovirus infections. *Drugs* 39:596, 1990.

150. Masur H, Whitcup SM, Cartwright C, et al: Advances in the management of AIDS-related cytomegalovirus retinitis. *Ann Intern Med* 125:126, 1996.

151. Jacobson MA, Mills J: Serious cytomegalovirus disease in the acquired immunodeficiency syndrome (AIDS). *Ann Intern Med* 108:585, 1988.

152. Singhal S, Mehta J, Powles R, et al: Three weeks of ganciclovir for cytomegaloviremia after allogenic bone marrow transplantation. *Bone Marrow Transplant* 15:777, 1995.

153. Zaia JA: Prevention and treatment of cytomegalovirus pneumonia in transplant recipients. *Clin Infect Dis* 17(suppl 2):S392, 1993.

154. Wolf DG, Smith IL, Lee DJ, et al: Mutations in human cytomegalovirus UL97 gene confer clinical resistance to ganciclovir and can be detected directly in patient plasma. *J Clin Invest* 95:257, 1995.

155. Curran M, Noble S: Valganciclovir. *Drugs* 61:1145, 2001.

156. Chrisp P, Clissold SP: Foscarnet. A review of its antiviral activity, pharmacokinetic properties and therapeutic use in immunocompromised patients with cytomegalovirus retinitis. *Drugs* 41:1, 1991.

157. Walmsley SL, Chew E, Read SE, et al: Treatment of cytomegalovirus retinitis with trisodium phosphonoformate hexahydrate (Foscarnet). *J Infect Dis* 157:569, 1988.

158. O'Donoghue JM, Ray CG, Terry DW Jr, Beaty HN: Prevention of nosocomial influenza infection with amantadine. *Am J Epidemiol* 97:276, 1973.

159. Aoki FY, Sitar DS: Amantadine hydrochloride. *Clin Pharmacokinet* 14:35, 1988.

160. Wintermeyer SM, Nahata MC: Rimantadine: A clinical perspective. *Ann Pharmacother* 29:299, 1995.

161. Doucette K, Aoki FY: Oseltamivir: a clinical and pharmacological perspective. *Expert Opin Pharmacother* 2:1, 2001.

162. Cheer SM, Wagstaff AJ: Zanamivir. An update of its use in influenza. *Drugs* 62:71, 2002.

163. Von Itzstein M, Wu W-Y, Kok GB, et al: Rational design of potent sialadase-based inhibitors of influenza virus replication. *Nature* 363:418, 1993.

164. McCormick JB, King IJ, Webb PA, et al: Lassa fever: Effective therapy with ribavirin. *N Engl J Med* 314:20, 1986.

165. Hayden FG, Sable CA, Connor JD, et al: Intravenous ribavirin by constant infusion for serious influenza and parainfluenza infection. *Antiviral Ther* 1:51, 1996.

166. Light RB, Aoki FY, Serrette C: Tolerance of ribavirin aerosol inhaled by normal volunteers and patients with asthma or chronic obstructive airways disease, in Smith RA, Knight V, Smith JAD (eds): *Clinical Applications of Ribavirin*. Orlando, Academic Press, 1984, p 97.

167. Lewis W, Dalakas MC: Mitochondrial toxicity of antiretroviral drugs. *Nat Med* 1:417, 1995.

168. Wilde M, Langtry MD: Zidovudine. An update on its pharmacodynamic and pharmacokinetic properties, and therapeutic efficacy. *Drugs* 46:515, 1993.

169. Acosta EP, Page LM, Fletcher CV: Clinical pharmacokinetics of zidovudine. An update. *Clin Pharmacokinet* 30:251, 1996.

170. Rachlis A, Fanning MM: Zidovudine toxicity. Clinical features and management. *Drug Saf* 8:312, 1993.

171. Perry CM, Faulds D: Lamivudine. A review of its antiviral activity, pharmacokinetic properties and therapeutic efficacy in the management of HIV infection. *Drugs* 53:657, 1997.

172. Perry CM, Noble S: Didanosine. An updated review of its use in HIV infection. *Drugs* 58:1099, 1999.

173. Hurst M, Noble S: Stavudine. An update on its use in the treatment of HIV infection. *Drugs* 58:919, 1999.

174. John M, Moore CB, James JR, et al: Chronic hyperlactatemia in HIV-infected patients taking antiretroviral therapy. *AIDS* 15:717, 2001.

175. Adkins JC, Peters DH, Faulds D: Zalcitabine. An update of its pharmacodynamic and pharmacokinetic properties and clinical efficacy in the management of HIV infection. *Drugs* 53:1654, 1997.

176. Chapman TM, McGavin JK, Noble S: Tenofovir disoproxil fumarate. *Drugs* 63:1597, 2003.

177. Grim SA, Romanelli F: Tenofovir disoproxil fumarate. *Ann Pharmacother* 37:849, 2003.

178. Hervey PS, Perry CM: Abacavir. A review of its clinical potential in patients with HIV infection. *Drugs* 60:447, 2000.

179. Anonymous: American hospital formulary service, in McEvoy GK (ed). American Society of Health-System Pharmacists, 2003, p 604.

180. Piscitelli SC, Gallicano KD: Interactions among drugs for HIV and opportunistic infections. *N Engl J Med* 3344:984, 2001.

181. Scott LJ, Perry CM: Delavirdine. A review of its use in HIV infection. *Drugs* 60:1411, 2000.

182. Mirochnick M, Clarke DF, Dorenbaum A: Nevirapine: Pharmacokinetic considerations in children and pregnant women. *Drugs* 39:281, 2000

183. Murphy RL, Montaner J: Nevirapine: A review of its development, pharmacological profile and potential for use. *Exp Opin Invest Drugs* 5:1183, 1996.

184. Adkins JC, Noble S: Efavirenz. *Drugs* 56:1055, 1998.

185. Figgit DP, Plosker GL: Saquinavir soft gel capsule: An updated review of its use in the management of HIV infection. *Drugs* 60:481, 2000.

186. Hse A, Grannemon R, Bertz RJ: Ritonavir. Clinical pharmacokinetics and interactions with other anit-HIV agents. *Clin Pharmacokinet* 35:275, 1998.

187. Lea AP, Faulds D: Ritonavir. *Drugs* 52:541, 1996.

188. Repchinsky C (ed): *Compendium of Pharmaceuticals & Specialties*. Ottawa: Canadian Pharmacists Association, 2004, p 1358.

189. Plosker GL, Noble S: Indinavir: A review of its use in the management of HIV infection. *Drugs* 58:1165, 1999.

190. Bardsley-Elliot A, Plosker GL: Nelfinavir: An update on its use in HIV infection. *Drugs* 59:581, 2000.

191. Moyle GJ, Gazzard BG: A risk benefit assessment of HIV protease inhibitors. *Drug Saf* 20:299, 1999.

192. Noble S, Goa KL: Amprenavir: A review of its clinical potential in patients with HIV infection. *Drugs* 60:1383, 2000.

193. Sadler BM, Stain DS: Clinical pharmacoology and pharmacokinetics of amprenavir. *Ann Pharmacother* 36:102, 2000.

194. Hurst M, Fauld D: Lopinavir. *Drugs* 60:1371, 2000.

195. Mangum EM, Graham KK: Lopinavir-ritonavir: A new protease inhibitor. *Pharmacother* 21:1352, 2001.

196. Lyman CA, Walsh TJ: Systemically administered antifungal agents. A review of their clinical pharmacology and therapeutic applications. *Drugs* 44:9, 1992.

197. Gallis HA, Drew RH, Pickard WW: Amphotericin B. 30 Years of clinical experience. *Rev Infect Dis* 12:308, 1990.

198. Schmidt H-J: New methods of delivery of amphotericin B. *Clin Infect Dis* 17(suppl 2):S501, 1993.

199. Singh RM, Perdue BE: Amphotericin B: A class review. *Formulary* 33:424, 1998.

200. Pfaller MA, Bale M, Buschelman B, et al: Quality control guidelines for National Committee for Clinical Laboratory. Standards recommended for broth macrodilution testing of amphotericin B, fluconazole and flucytosine. *J Clin Microbiol* 33:1104, 1995.

201. Balkin MM, Leidich SD, Mukherju PK, et al: Mechanisms of fungal resistance: an overview. *Drugs* 62:1025, 2002.

202. Grasela TH Jr, Goodwin SD, Walawander MK, et al: Prospective surveillance of intravenous amphotericin B use patterns. *Pharmacotherapy* 10:341, 1990.

203. Oldfield EC III, Garst PD, Hostettler C, et al: Randomized, double-blind trial of 1- versus 4-hour amphotericin B infusion durations. *Antimicrob Agents Chemother* 34:1402, 1990.

204. Gigliotti F, Shenep JL, Lott L, Thornton D: Induction of prostaglandin synthesis as the mechanism responsible for the chills and fever produced by infusing amphotericin. *Br J Infect Dis* 156:784, 1987.

205. Tynes BS, Utz JP, Bennett JE, Alling DW: Reducing amphotericin B reactions. A double-blind study. *Am Rev Respir Dis* 87:264, 1963.

206. Burks LC, Aisner J, Fortner CL, Wiernik PH: Meperidine for the treatment of shaking, chills and fever. *Arch Intern Med* 140:483, 1980.

207. Branch RA: Prevention of amphotericin B-induced renal impairment. *Arch Intern Med* 148:2389, 1988.

208. Rapp RP, Gubbins PO, Evans ME: Amphotericin B lipid complex. *Pharmacotherapy* 31:1174, 1997.

209. Keating G, Jarvis B: Caspofungin. *Drugs* 61:1121, 2001.

210. Bennett JE: Flucytosine. *Ann Intern Med* 86:319, 1977.

211. Como JA, Dismukes WE: Oral azole drugs as systemic antifungal therapy. *N Engl J Med* 330:263, 1994.

212. Lyman CA, Walsh TJ: Systematically administered antifungal agents. A review of their clinical pharmacology and therapeutic applications. *N Engl J Med* 330:263, 1994.

213. Heykants J, Michiels M, Meuldermans W, et al: The pharmacokinetics of itraconazole in animals and man: An overview, in Fromtling RA (ed): *Recent Trends in the Discovery, Development and Evaluation of Antifungal Agents.* Barcelona, JR Prous Science Publishers, 1987, p 223.

214. Zervos M, Meunier F. Fluconazole (Diflucan). A review. *Int J Antimicrob Agents* 54:269, 1993.

215. Goa KL, Barradell LB: Fluconazole. An update on its pharmacodynamic and pharmacokinetic properties and therapeutic uses in major superficial and systemic mycoses in immunocompromised patients. *Drugs* 50:558, 1995.

216. Ghannoum MA, Kuhn DM: Voriconazole—Better chances for patients with invasive mycoses. *Eur J Med Res* 7:242, 2002.

217. Muijsers RBR, Goa KL, Scott LJ: Voriconazole in the treatment of invasive aspergillosis. *Drugs* 62:2655, 2002.

SEPSIS WITH ACUTE ORGAN DYSFUNCTION

E. WESLEY ELY
RICHERT E. GOYETTE

KEY POINTS

- *Sepsis is the combination of a known or suspected infection and an accompanying systemic inflammatory response.*

- *Severe sepsis is sepsis with acute dysfunction of one or more organ systems; septic shock is a subset of severe sepsis.*

- *Severe sepsis is common, frequently fatal, and expensive. More than 750,000 cases occur annually in the United States.*

- *Effective management of patients with severe sepsis requires early identification, cardiopulmonary support, antibiotics, source control, and general supportive care.*

- *The prognosis of the patient with severe sepsis is related to the number of dysfunctional organs.*

- *Cardiopulmonary support consists of early and aggressive fluid resuscitation, maintenance of mean arterial pressure at 65 mm Hg or higher, and measures to maximize and maintain tissue oxygenation; judging the adequacy of tissue oxygenation is informed by measurement of the mixed venous oxygen saturation, and supportive therapy is most effective and beneficial when provided in the first hours of presentation.*

- *Patients should receive early intravenous empirical antibiotics directed at all possible sources of infection. Appropriate antibiotics decrease the mortality rate by 10% to 15% in patients with severe sepsis.*

- *Source control can be surgical or nonsurgical and is intended to remove or lessen the burden from the primary focus of infection.*

- *Despite appropriate antibiotics, source control, and organ support, the mortality rate in patients with severe sepsis remains at 28% to 50%.*

- *Specific antisepsis interventions have recently been introduced that target multiple pathophysiologic aspects of the sepsis cascade and can improve outcomes.*

- *To maximize outcomes, supportive measures must be introduced to ensure proper nutrition; maintain fluid, glucose, and electrolyte homeostasis; promote tissue oxygenation; and prevent complications.*

Sepsis with acute organ dysfunction (severe sepsis) is common and frequently fatal and represents a significant health care burden. The incidence and associated mortality and morbidity rates of severe sepsis are commonly underestimated. This is a function of a number of factors. Severe sepsis is not generally reported as a primary diagnosis. For example, although steps are underway to address this issue, the most recent edition of the *International Classification of Diseases, Ninth Revision, Clinical Modification* lacks a diagnostic code for severe sepsis. Instead, severe sepsis is often coded as a complication of another disorder (e.g., cancer or pneumonia). Several recent publications have evaluated the epidemiology of

severe sepsis in the United States.[1,2] They have estimated that the annual incidence of severe sepsis in the United States is in the range of 240 to 300 cases per 100,000 population. Further, in 2003, there were approximately 750,000 cases of sepsis in the United States. In Europe, the incidence of severe sepsis exceeds 200,000 annually.[3] Reported mortality rates in patients with severe sepsis range from 28% to 50% or higher.[1,4] Thus, in the United States and Europe, at least 700 to 1300 patients die daily from severe sepsis. Patients with severe sepsis account for annual health care expenditures in excess of $16 billion in the United States and £5.2 billion in Europe.[1,3]

The incidence of severe sepsis peaks in children younger than 12 months, remains low until midlife, and then progressively increases.[1] In a study by Angus et al[1] of the patients who developed severe sepsis, nearly 66% were older than 65 years. This population also accounted for more than 75% of the overall health care costs of the disease. The incidence of severe sepsis is anticipated to increase approximately 1.5% per year until at least 2050.[1] This increase is due to a number of factors, including age shifts in the population, prevalence of more critically ill patients (e.g., transplant recipients), and increases in the numbers of invasive diagnostic procedures and monitoring techniques. This predicted increase has significant implications for the critical care community because it has been estimated that by 2020 there will be a 22% shortfall of available intensivists' hours to meet this demand.[5]

Definitions

In 1992, members of the American College of Chest Physicians (ACCP) and the Society of Critical Care Medicine (SCCM) developed a set of consensus definitions for sepsis and related disorders (Table 46-1).[6] The consensus committee believed that standardized terminology would improve the ability of clinicians to make an early diagnosis of sepsis, provide for more reliable reporting of the incidence and severity of sepsis, and facilitate early therapeutic interventions. In addition, they hoped that acceptance of the definitions would help to standardize research protocols and improve the dissemination and application of clinical information from subsequent studies. The consensus committee acknowledged that the clinical presentation of sepsis spanned a continuum of severity; however, they recognized certain common phases and provided specific definitions for them (Fig. 46-1). Sepsis was defined as the presence of at least two of the four systemic inflammatory response syndrome (SIRS) criteria developing in response to a documented or suspected infection. Severe sepsis was sepsis plus acute organ dysfunction (Table 46-2). Although these definitions have provided an important framework, they have been criticized as being too sensitive and not providing enough information for clinicians attempting to make a diagnosis.[7] In addition, the definitions lack a clear pathologic basis and fail to incorporate the hemostatic component of severe sepsis.[6]

However, the ACCP/SCCM definitions have endured the test of time. For example, the critical importance of organ dysfunction and outcomes first emphasized by the conferees was recently reaffirmed by a study of risk factors for hospital mortality rate in 3608 intensive care unit (ICU) patients included in the European Sepsis Study (Fig. 46-2).[8] In December 2001, representatives from the SCCM, the ACCP, the

TABLE 46-1 American College of Chest Physicians/Society of Critical Care Medicine Consensus Criteria for Sepsis and Related Disorders

Infection	Microbial phenomenon characterized by an inflammatory response to the presence of microorganisms or the invasion of normally sterile host tissue by those organisms
Bacteremia	The presence of viable bacteria in the blood
SIRS	SIRS represents the systemic response to several clinical insults; it is manifested by at least two of the following: (1) temperature >38°C or <36°C; (2) heart rate >90 beats/minute; (3) respiratory rate >20 breaths/minute or partial pressure of CO_2 <32 mm Hg; and (4) white blood cell count >12,000/μL, <4000 μL, or >10% immature (band) forms
Sepsis	Systemic response to infection, manifested by two or more SIRS criteria developing as the result of infection
Severe sepsis	Sepsis associated with acute organ dysfunction, hypoperfusion, or hypotension; hypoperfusion and perfusion abnormalities may include, but are not limited to, lactic acidosis, oliguria, or acute alterations in mental status (see Table 46-2)
Septic shock	Sepsis-induced hypotension despite fluid resuscitation in addition to the presence of perfusion abnormalities that may include, but are not limited to, lactic acidosis; oliguria, or an acute alteration in mental status; patients receiving inotropic or vasopressor agents may not be hypotensive at the time that perfusion abnormalities are measured
Sepsis-induced hypotension	Systolic blood pressure <90 mm Hg or a reduction ≥40 mm Hg from baseline without other causes for hypotension
Multiple organ dysfunction syndrome	Presence of altered organ function in an acutely ill patient such that homeostasis cannot be maintained without intervention

ABBREVIATION: SIRS, systemic inflammatory response syndrome.
SOURCE: Printed with permission from Bone et al.[6]

European Society of Intensive Care Medicine, the American Thoracic Society, and the Surgical Infection Society met to revisit the definitions of sepsis and related disorders.[9] After an intensive review, the group concluded that there was no evidence that would justify altering the definitions first proposed by the ACCP/SCCM. As part of the discussion, however, they expanded the lists of signs and symptoms of sepsis that are reflected by experience gained at the bedside that prompts a clinician to say that the patient "looks septic." Among these criteria, they included additional general (e.g., altered mental status, significant edema or positive fluid balance, or hyperglycemia), inflammatory (increased C-reactive protein [CRP] or pro-calcitonin [PCT]), hemodynamic (O_2

saturation in venous blood >70%, cardiac index >3.5 L/min per square meter), organ dysfunction (coagulation abnormalities, ileus, or hyperbilirubinemia), and tissue perfusion (decreased capillary refill or mottling) abnormalities. They also emphasized the need for a precise method to characterize and stage patients with sepsis. Creation and validation of such a system would bring an increased degree of precision to clinical trials and facilitate the ability of clinicians to more fully characterize the disease and to select appropriate therapies. As a subject for debate, they proposed the Predisposition, Insult/Infection, Response, Organ Dysfunction (PIRO) model, a staging process that uses concepts from the Tumor Nodes Metastases (TNM) system of clinical oncology.

Pathogenesis

The pathogenesis of the septic response involves interaction of the host with a microbial invader. The outcome of the process depends on the capability of the immune system, endothelium and hemostatic mechanisms to contain and then eliminate the process, and the ability of the patient to restore homeostasis over time.

MICROBIAL FACTORS

Microbes possess several factors that facilitate their growth in a normally sterile environment (Fig. 46-3). These include properties of their capsule or envelope, cell wall, and metabolic factors such as the production of exotoxins. Some such factors are cited by way of example.

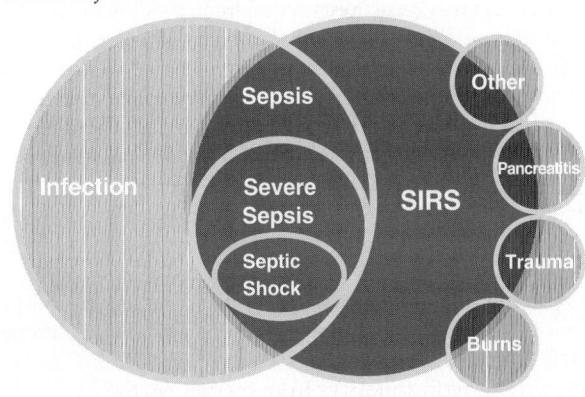

FIGURE 46-1 Relation among systemic inflammatory response syndrome (SIRS), sepsis, and severe sepsis. (*Reproduced with permission from Bone et al.[6]*)

TABLE 46-2 Clinical Manifestations of Acute Organ Dysfunction

Cardiovascular system	Arterial systolic blood pressure ≤90 mm Hg or MAP ≤70 mm Hg for ≥1 h despite adequate fluid resuscitation, adequate intravascular volume status, or the use of vasopressors in an attempt to maintain a systolic blood pressure ≥90 mm Hg or MAP ≥65 mm Hg; tachycardia; arrhythmias; cardiac arrest
Respiratory system	Ratio of Pa_{O_2} to $F_{I_{O_2}}$ ≤250 in the presence of other dysfunctional organs or systems or ≤200 if the lung is the only dysfunctional organ; Pa_{O_2} <70 mm Hg; Sa_{O_2} <90%; tachypnea; mechanical ventilator dependence with or without PEEP
Renal	Urine output <0.5 mL/kg of body weight per hour for 1 h despite adequate fluid resuscitation; acute elevation of serum creatinine; oliguria; anuria; requirement for renal replacement therapy
Hematologic	Platelet count <80,000/μL or decreased by 50% in the preceding 3 d; leukocytosis/leukopenia; increased prothrombin time; elevated partial thromboplastin time; decreased protein C; increased D-dimer; impaired leukocyte function
Gastrointestinal	Elevated pancreatic enzymes (amylase, lipase), decreased gastric pHi; ileus; gastrointentinal bleeding or perforation; intestinal ischemia; acalculous cholecystitis, acute pancreatitis; intolerance of enteral nutrition
Hepatic	Hyperbilirubinemia; elevated aminotransferases; increased LDH; elevated alkaline phosphatase; hypoalbuminemia; elevated prothrombin time; jaundice; asterixis
Neurologic	Delirium; altered consciousness; impaired mentation; confusion; psychosis; abnormal bispectral EEG
Metabolic/endocrine	pH <7.30 or a base deficit ≥5.0 mmol/L in association with a plasma lactate level >1.5 times the upper limit of the normal value; hyperglycemia; hypertriglyceridemia; hypoalbuminemia

ABBREVIATIONS: EEG, electroencephalogram; $F_{I_{O_2}}$, fraction inspired O_2; LDH, lactate dehydrogenase; MAP, mean arterial pressure; Pa_{O_2}, arterial partial pressure of O_2; PEEP, positive end-expiratory pressure; Sa_{O_2}, arterial oxygen saturation.

SOURCES: Printed with permission from: Balk RA: Pathogenesis and management of multiple organ dysfunction or failure in severe sepsis and septic shock. *Crit Care Clin* 16:337, 2000; Balk RA, Ely EW, Goyette RE: *The Sepsis Handbook.* Nashville, TN: National Initiative in Sepsis Education, Vanderbilt University Medical Center, 2001; Bernard GR, Vincent J-L, Laterre P-F, et al: Efficacy and safety of recombinant human activated protein C for severe sepsis. *N Engl J Med* 344:699, 2001.

Pili of strains of *Escherichia coli* can enable the coliform bacillus to adhere to Tamm-Horsfall protein coating the epithelium of the lower urinary tract or P-blood group antigens expressed on the epithelium of the renal pelvis. Capsular polysaccharides of certain strains of *Streptococcus pneumoniae* render the organism resistant to phagocytosis. The cell wall of gram-negative bacteria consists of an inner phospholipid bilayer with embedded transport proteins and an outer layer composed of lipoproteins, lipopolysaccharides (LPS), outer membrane proteins, and capsular polysaccharides. Bacterial LPS is generally considered to be the principal element in the initiation of the septic response in patients with severe

gram-negative infections. Whereas components of the cell wall of gram-positive bacteria may be able to elicit some of the effects of endotoxin, much of the pathogenicity of gram-positive organisms is the result of exotoxins. Some of these exotoxins can function as superantigens: chemical substances that simultaneously bind to common sequences on the major histocompatibility complex and the T-cell receptor. Superantigen binding and T-cell activation can produce a flood of cytokines and is independent of the antigenic specificity normally required for activation of various T-cell clones and the need for costimulatory molecules. Streptococcal and staphylococcal pyrogenic exotoxins acting as superantigens are believed to play a critical role in the pathogenesis of toxic shock syndrome. Hyaluronidase secreted by some bacteria can facilitate their spread along tissue planes.

HOST FACTORS

The host has a spectrum of mechanisms that supports its ability to resist the invasive properties of some microorganisms (Table 46-3). The epithelium is the first line of defense against

FIGURE 46-2 Organ dysfunction as a major outcome parameter. This graph is from a study by Alberti et al on the relation among mortality, systemic inflammatory response syndrome (SIRS), infection, organ dysfunction, and shock. Observe that the mortality curves are virtually identical for infection and infection with SIRS (sepsis). The increase in mortality rate is related to the presence of sepsis with organ dysfunction (severe sepsis, septic shock). Risk of death increased from sepsis to severe sepsis (hazard ratio = 1.53, $p < 0.0001$) and septic shock (hazard ratio = 2.64, $p < 0.0001$). (Adapted with premission from Alberti et al.[8])

FIGURE 46-3 Pathogenic microbial factors.

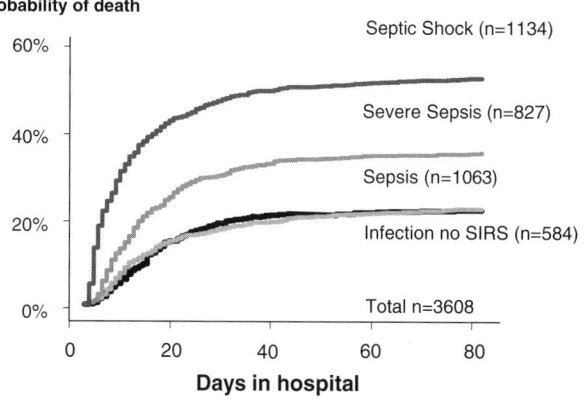

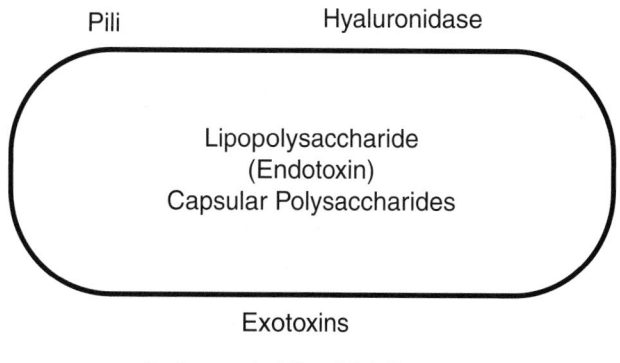

TABLE 46-3 Host Factors That Have Been Established to Contribute to an Increased Risk for Sepsis

Break in membrane integrity (surgery, toxic injury to epithelium)
Age (very young, elderly)
Gender (men > women)
Race (nonwhite > white)
Genetic polymorphisms (e.g., tumor necrosis factor promoter gene, toll-like receptors)
Comorbidities (e.g., diabetes mellitus, immunosuppression)

infection. It not only provides a mechanical barrier but also contributes other protective functions in a site-specific fashion (e.g., mucociliary flow in the respiratory tract and gastric pH). The immune status of the host is a function of inherited and acquired components. Genetic polymorphisms can be responsible for dissimilar responses to infection. For example, polymorphisms in *toll-like receptors* (TLRs) may govern an individual's response to endotoxin, whereas variants in the promoter region of the tumor necrosis factor (TNF) gene can help determine the risk for sepsis after trauma.[10] Age, disease, exposures, and interventions are acquired risk factors for sepsis. Young children and the elderly have an increased incidence of sepsis. Various morbidities can increase the risk of sepsis. Patients with diabetes mellitus are at increased risk of infection for a variety of reasons. Hyperglycemia appears to facilitate colonization and growth of organisms such as *Staphylococcus aureus* and *Candida* species. In addition, they have a variety of defects in cell-mediated immunity and phagocytosis. Genetic and acquired factors often interact to determine susceptibility to disease. For example, patients positive for the human immunodeficiency virus (HIV) who are heterozygous for a deletion in the gene for the macrophage CCR5 receptor or in the promoter region of the gene have slow progression of HIV disease compared with patients with the wild-type genotype.

INNATE IMMUNE SYSTEM

The human immune system is composed of adaptive and innate components. The adaptive elements are specialized B and T cells. Each of these cells has a structurally unique B- or T-cell antigen receptor that is generated randomly (i.e., not genomically encoded). When a lymphocyte bearing a useful receptor encounters a pathogen, it is selected for clonal expansion. Although adaptive immunity contributes significantly to the overall immune response and provides protection against future encounters with the organism, generation of a significant primary humoral or cellular immune response takes days to weeks, time that is unavailable to a patient with severe sepsis. Unlike the adaptive immune system, elements of the innate immune system can respond instantly to a challenge. This property helps explain the overwhelming systemic inflammatory response generated in patients with severe sepsis. Therefore, we focus the remainder of this section on innate immunity.

CELLULAR COMPONENTS OF INNATE IMMUNITY

In humans, cellular effectors of innate immunity are monocytes/macrophages, neutrophils, natural killer cells, and platelets. The monocyte/macrophage is the human analogue of the amebocyte, an innate immune cell present in invertebrates. Monocytes originate in the bone marrow and then transit the peripheral blood to lodge in tissues as macrophages, Kupffer cells, and other reticuloendothelial elements. Pathogen-associated molecular pattern receptors comprise a key component of the innate immune system.[11] Unlike the antigen receptors of B and T cells, these receptors are encoded in the germline, are functionally divided into three classes (secreted, endocytic, and signaling), and trigger an immediate effector function. Secreted pathogen-associated molecular pattern identification is discussed in the section on fluid-phase elements of innate immunity (below). Endocytic pattern recognition receptors such as the macrophage mannose or scavenger receptor recognize highly conserved molecular components of microbial cell walls and mediate their phagocytosis by monocytes/macrophages. Signaling receptors on monocytes/macrophages identify microbial molecular patterns and activate signal transduction pathways that upregulate a spectrum of immune response genes responsible for a variety of cellular functions, including cytokine release.

The *toll* gene, a transmembrane signaling protein present in organisms as primitive as the fruit fly, is believed to be very important to humans in the septic state. Humans possess at least 10 *toll* gene homologues known as TLRs. The TLR genes code for cell membrane molecular pattern receptors that play an integral role in the generation of local and systemic inflammatory responses. Natural ligands of the various TLRs include LPS (TLR4), peptidoglycan (TLR2), and flagellin (TLR5). The role of TLR proteins can be illustrated by the response of the innate immune system to LPS. LPS is an outer leaflet compound molecule that is unique to gram-negative bacteria; after infusion into humans, LPS reproduces many of the features of sepsis, including activation of the coagulation and complement systems.[12,13] After entering the plasma, LPS is recognized, bound, and transported to innate immune effector cells by LPS-binding protein. The cell membrane CD14 receptor on monocytes and neutrophils accepts the LPS from LPS-binding protein and forms a trimeric complex with TLR4 and MD-2, another membrane protein. Once formed, the complex activates a signal transduction pathway that phosphorylates IκB. As a result, IκB undergoes degradation and releases bound nuclear factor κB. The latter then migrates into the nucleus, where it induces transcription of a wide variety of immune- and inflammatory-response genes.[11] Transcription of these genes is responsible for the upregulation of tissue factor (TF) on monocytes/macrophages and endothelium and for the cytokine cascade that creates many of the elements of SIRS in patients exposed to LPS. These key elements of the inflammatory response are therefore linked to the coagulation cascade, with these two responses combining to form the major facets of the pathophysiologic derangements in septic humans. Surfactant appears to play an important role in maintaining innate immunity within the lung. This may be due to the protein's ability to block LPS signaling by inhibiting mitogen-activated protein and IκB kinases of alveolar macrophages.[14]

TF is responsible for initiating coagulation through the previously named *extrinsic pathway*, now called the *TF pathway*. TF is expressed constitutively on a limited number of cells and can be induced in a wide variety of cells after exposure to endotoxin or cytokines. Cells normally expressing TF include extravascular monocytes/macrophages and fibroblasts.[15] Sequestered from circulating factor VIIa, these cells are poised to activate coagulation immediately after disruption of a blood vessel wall. TF expression can be upregulated in a variety of other cells that do not express the cell membrane protein constitutively. As a result, after exposure to TNFα, CRP, CD40 ligand, or other substances, TF expression can be identified on subsets of cells including circulating monocytes, vascular smooth muscle cells, a subset of endothelial cells, and possibly alveolar epithelial cells.[16] During acute inflammation, activation of the cytokine cascade is followed by rapid upregulation of TF on monocytes and a shift of components of the hemostatic system from an antithrombotic to a prothrombotic state. Circulating TF antigen and microparticles shed from inflammatory cells and platelets contribute to the process.

FLUID-PHASE ELEMENTS: CYTOKINES AND COMPLEMENT

Once monocytes/macrophages have been activated, there is a response by fluid-phase elements. These include cytokines and activated components of the complement system. TNFα is a central cytokine in this process. Once released, it functions in an autocrine, paracrine, and endocrine fashion in a positive feedback loop to stimulate additional TNFα production and production of other cytokines. Other proinflammatory cytokines are released, including interleukin (IL)–1, IL-2, IL-6, IL-8, IL-10, platelet activating factor (PAF), and interferon γ. The cytokine cascade produces a vast array of biological effects recognized as the systemic inflammatory reaction.

However, as sepsis persists, there may be a shift in the cytokine profile from an inflammatory to a predominantly anti-inflammatory one.[17] Loss of T cells, B cells, and follicular dendritic cells through apoptosis may contribute to the immunosuppression through two processes: loss of immunocytes and the direct immunosuppressive effect of apoptotic cells.[18,19] As the anti-inflammatory reaction progresses, the septic patient may become anergic. Although it may be helpful to think that the response of the immune system to a septic insult progresses in discrete and identifiable stages, this may not be true. Some have proposed that, distant from the original source or inflammatory focus, the body's reaction is predominantly anti-inflammatory from the onset.[20] The complex nature of this process may partly explain why clinical trials of various biologic response modifiers such as TNFα antagonists have not improved overall survival rate and have even been detrimental in some cases.

Plasma components of the complement system circulate in an inactive state and develop enzymatic activity only after proteolysis or a conformational change. The system works by depositing components of complement on foreign substances or organisms requiring opsonization and by promoting inflammation. Complement can be activated through three pathways: (1) classic pathway, (2) alternate pathway, and (3) mannan-binding lectin pathway. The classic pathway is activated by immunoglobulin (Ig) M or IgG antibodies bound to a particular pathogen or by CRP released during the acute phase reaction. The classic pathway serves as a link between the complement and hemostatic systems. Components generated during activity of the classic pathway increase the exposure of phosphatidylserine on endothelial cell surfaces.[21] This action provides the phospholipid that is essential for various phases of clot formation. Activation of the alternate pathway results when complement binds directly to pathogen-associated molecular patterns on the surfaces of bacteria or fungi. Mannan-binding lectin is an example of a secreted pathogen-associated molecular pattern receptor. It is synthesized in the liver and secreted into the plasma during the acute-phase reaction. It binds to carbohydrate structures common to gram-positive and gram-negative bacteria, yeasts, and some viruses and parasites. Once binding occurs, mannan-binding lectin-associated proteases are activated and help to destroy the organism. After complement activation, some of the molecular elements of the system are cleaved, thus producing fragments with biological activity. For example, N-terminal proteolysis of C3, C4, and C5 release small peptides (e.g., C5a) that bind to G protein–coupled receptors on a variety of cells to produce chemotaxis, increase vascular permeability, and so forth. It has been proposed that C5a in excess can paralyze neutrophil function.[22] In an experimental model, antibody-mediated neutralization of excess C5a protected animals against septic death.[22]

ENDOTHELIAL CELL DYSFUNCTION

With approximately 10^{11} endothelial cells and a surface area estimated to exceed 1000 m^2, the endothelium surpasses the skin as the largest organ in the body.[23,24] The great majority of the endothelium is located in the microvasculature; in that region, the endothelial surface area per unit of blood volume is 2000 to 3000 times greater than in the larger blood vessels.[25] The endothelium serves as the interface between inflammation and coagulation.[26] Situated at the junction of the flowing blood and extracellular space, the endothelium influences a variety of inflammatory and hemostatic processes (e.g., cell-trafficking, vasoregulation, thrombosis, and antithrombosis) and plays a key role in the inflammatory, prothrombotic, and impaired fibrinolytic components of sepsis.[27]

Endothelial dysfunction is a key element in the pathogenesis of severe sepsis. This may be secondary to the effects of endotoxin or proinflammatory cytokines on endothelial cells. For example, a single injection of endotoxin in rabbits produces desquamation of approximately 25% of the aortic endothelial surface area within 5 days.[28] Alternatively, organisms such as *Rickettsiae* can directly infect endothelial cells. Severe endothelial injury can produce a microvascular coagulopathy and acute organ dysfunction.[29] Importantly, however, endothelial cells are differentially regulated in space and time. That is, the endothelium of the lung may respond differently to a septic insult than similar cells in the spleen.[30] The phenotype of endothelial cells also changes over time. For example, an endothelial cell population with an antithrombotic phenotype may transiently switch to predominantly prothrombotic activity for some period after exposure to TNFα.

Thrombomodulin (TM), intercellular adhesion molecule 1, E-selectin, and von Willebrand factor (VWF) are normal membrane-bound and intracellular endothelial cell components. Therefore, elevated circulating levels of the soluble forms of these proteins are markers of endothelial dysfunction and injury.[31] In children with septic shock, soluble TM (sTM) levels are increased, and the levels correlate with survival status and the extent of organ dysfunction.[32] Immunohistochemical studies of skin biopsy samples from patients with meningococcal septicemia have demonstrated decreased stainable TM and endothelial cell protein C receptor (EPCR).[33] This appears to result from a combination of shedding of cell surface TM and EPCR plus downregulation of endothelial cell synthesis and/or expression of these essential molecules. These changes suggest that many patients with sepsis may have insufficient TM and EPCR to convert protein C (PC) to activated PC (APC), although this is not universally true.[34] In a population of patients with sepsis, plasma levels of VWF, intercellular adhesion molecule 1, and sE-selectin were significantly increased within 8 hours of the development of the acute respiratory distress syndrome (ARDS).[35] Damaged endothelium and activated leukocytes and platelets also release microparticles with procoagulant properties (e.g., microparticle-associated TF).[36]

Apoptosis differs from necrosis because it is a highly regulated physiologic process that plays an important role in cell physiology. Apoptosis can be identified through morphologic and molecular techniques. Cytokines and inflammatory cells can damage the endothelium and induce apoptosis.[24] In patients with severe sepsis, the apoptotic process also changes in space and time. That is, the apoptotic process may not occur uniformly, in all organs, at the same time, or with all types of infections.[19,37] This may help to explain the commonality of ARDS in patients with severe sepsis. Endothelial cell apoptosis may produce abnormalities in cell trafficking, vasoregulation, and antithrombosis/thrombosis that may contribute to the pathogenesis of septic manifestations, such as multiple organ dysfunction, impaired microvascular blood flow, and inability of the body to restore homeostasis.

Pathophysiology

CARDIOVASCULAR SYSTEM

Severe sepsis is accompanied by significant alterations in cardiovascular physiology. Sepsis-induced hypotension is multifactorial in origin. Contributory factors include redistribution of blood flow, impaired metabolic autoregulation, release of vasoactive mediators, third-spacing of fluids, dehydration, increased insensible fluid losses, vomiting, diarrhea, etc. Early in the process, systemic vascular resistance may be high and cardiac output ($\dot{Q}_T$) may be decreased. However, the SVR typically decreases and $\dot{Q}_T$ increases, thus producing a hyperdynamic circulatory state.

MYOCARDIUM

Reversible myocardial dysfunction of variable severity may occur in as many as 40% of patients with severe sepsis.[38] Myocardial depression often occurs in survivors very early in the septic process, progresses over the first 3 days, and then resolves after 7 to 10 days.[39] Dysfunction may be systolic, diastolic, left ventricular, or biventricular. Potential explanations include myocardial injury mediated by cytokines such as TNF, release of noncytokine mediators such as prostanoids and nitric oxide (NO), catecholamine-induced myofibrillar damage, and myocardial ischemia with reperfusion injury.[40] An aggregate of clinical studies suggests that a circulating myocardial depressant factor, not global myocardial ischemia, is a major contributor to myocardial dysfunction in patients with severe sepsis. In a study of coronary hemodynamics in patients with severe sepsis and septic shock, Dhainaut et al reported that coronary blood flow and net myocardial lactate consumption are increased in this disorder.[41]

Cardiovascular dysfunction may also manifest as ventricular dilation, abnormalities of wall motion, increased levels of cardiac troponin, and electrocardiographic changes. The explanation for the paradoxical association of a hyperdynamic circulation and myocardial dysfunction involves an interaction of compensatory mechanisms that may maintain $\dot{Q}_T$ in the face of impaired myocardial contractility. Fluid resuscitation raises the mean systemic pressure while sepsis acts on the systemic vessels to reduce the resistance to venous return. These factors combine to maintain venous return (i.e., cardiac output) in the face of pump dysfunction (see chapters 20 and 21). It is important to note that, by the time initial resuscitation measures are conducted, most patients with severe sepsis will exhibit high-output hypotension; when this circulatory abnormality is encountered in the critically ill, sepsis should be considered to be present if it has not already been contemplated.

The introduction of pulmonary artery catheters with thermodilution $\dot{Q}_T$ capacity and portable radionuclide cineangiographic techniques has allowed a greater understanding of cardiovascular physiology and outcomes in patients with severe sepsis. Parker et al reported that patients who survived severe sepsis experienced an acute decrease in left ventricular EF that was accompanied by left ventricular dilatation, pathophysiologic abnormalities that resolved over a 7- to 10-day period.[42] This was associated with a negative correlation between EF and left ventricular end-diastolic volume index.[43] Conversely, nonsurvivors did not undergo left ventricular dilation, had preserved EF, exhibited a lower SVR, and had a positive relation between EF and left ventricular end-diastolic volume index. There are several potential explanations for this apparently paradoxical phenomenon. The lower SVR in nonsurvivors may allow them to maintain their $\dot{Q}_T$ without the need for ventricular dilation. Alternatively, the endothelial damage and microvascular dysfunction may be more severe in nonsurvivors; this could lead to a significant microcapillary leak, severe interstitial edema of the myocardium, and impaired cardiac compliance. The inability of the heart to dilate may be a surrogate for significant multiorgan dysfunction and inability of the host to respond to the multiple alterations associated with severe sepsis.

VASCULAR SYSTEM

Vasoconstriction is the physiologic response to low blood pressure (BP) in patients with hemorrhagic or cardiogenic shock. In contrast, shock in patients with severe sepsis is vasodilatory in nature. That is, their peripheral blood vessels not only dilate but all too often fail to show an adequate physiologic or pharmacologic contractile response to vasopressors. Severe sepsis is the most common cause of vasodilatory shock.[44] However, vasodilatory shock is also a component of disorders with impaired tissue oxygenation, such as carbon monoxide intoxication, and can serve as a final common pathway of any form of profound and long-lasting shock. At the vascular level, the pathophysiology of shock in patients with severe sepsis involves three major mechanisms: (1) activation of adenosine triphosphate–sensitive potassium (K_{ATP}) channels in vascular smooth muscle cells, (2) synthesis of increased amounts of NO through induction of the inducible form of NO synthase (iNOS), and (3) vasopressin deficiency.[44]

VASCULAR SMOOTH MUSCLE CELL MEMBRANE HYPERPOLARIZATION IN VASODILATORY SHOCK

When the membrane potential of vascular smooth muscle cells is within the physiologic range of −30 to −60 mV, vasopressors such as norepinephrine and angiotensin II open voltage-gated calcium channels and allow calcium to enter cells; through a complex process involving calmodulin, myosin phosphorylation, and myosin ATPase, cytosolic hypercalcemia produces muscle contraction. Under conditions of tissue hypoxia or increased tissue metabolic activity, lactic acidosis activates the K_{ATP} channels. The resultant entry of potassium into the cell hyperpolarizes the vascular cell membrane, closes the calcium channels, decreases intracellular calcium concentrations, relaxes smooth muscle, and dilates the blood vessels. In patients with severe sepsis, elevated circulating levels of atrial natriuretic peptide, calcitonin gene-related peptide, NO, and adenosine can also open K_{ATP} channels and contribute to membrane hyperpolarization.[45–47]

ROLE OF NITRIC OXIDE IN VASODILATORY SHOCK

NO is a potent endogenous vasodilator. In patients with severe sepsis and shock, cytokines upregulate iNOS in a number of cells including vascular smooth muscle and endothelium.[48] NO then presumably exerts its vasodilatory activity through activation of myosin light-chain phosphatase and perhaps by activating vascular smooth muscle cell potassium channels such as the calcium-sensitive channel. The latter would then augment the K_{ATP}-induced hyperpolarization of the membrane of vascular smooth muscle cells.

ROLE OF VASOPRESSIN DEFICIENCY IN VASODILATORY SHOCK

In addition to its role in water conservation, vasopressin secreted under baroreceptor control constricts vascular smooth muscle. During the initial phases of shock in patients with severe sepsis, vasopressin helps to maintain arterial BP. However, over time, neurohypophyseal stores of the hormone become depleted, and plasma vasopressin concentrations decline.[44] Administration of vasopressin in doses large enough to produce plasma concentrations comparable to those seen in acute hypotension will raise arterial BP by 25 to 50 mm Hg.[49] This marked hypersensitivity to exogenous vasopressin in patients with vasodilatory shock appears to result from a number of factors, including: (1) availability of receptors for occupancy by the exogenous hormone, (2) autonomic dysfunction, (3) ability of vasopressin to potentiate the activity of high levels of circulating endogenous catecholamines, (4) direct and indirect blunting of the contributions of NO to vasodilation, and (5) inactivation of K_{ATP} channels with restoration of vascular smooth muscle cell membrane potential toward normal. The role of vasopressin in inhibiting the effects of NO and blocking vascular K_{ATP} channels has been used clinically in patients with severe sepsis and shock who are refractory to other maneuvers to raise mean arterial BP (MAP). The efficacy of vasopressin in septic shock is currently being evaluated within the context of a multicenter, randomized controlled trial in Canada.

RESPIRATORY SYSTEM

Approximately 40% of cases of acute lung injury (ALI) are ascribed to sepsis (see Chap. 38).[50] Presumably, this is a consequence of the organ's large microvascular surface area. In patients with severe sepsis of extrapulmonary origin, ALI initially occurs through an indirect process; however, as the disease progresses, secondary pneumonia, mechanical ventilation, and its associated complications may contribute to ALI and, through direct and indirect mechanisms, produce ARDS.

SYSTEMIC COMPONENTS OF ACUTE LUNG INJURY

The alveoli and pulmonary capillary bed are separated by two layers of cells: pneumocytes (types I and II) and endothelial cells. In patients with severe sepsis, ALI appears to begin with endothelial injury from circulating bacterial products plus cytokines released into the circulation during the initial stages of SIRS. Endotoxin has been shown to be a potent proinflammatory molecule that can induce a variety of endothelial cell inflammatory responses and produce endothelial cell dysfunction or apoptosis.[51] Under the influence of IL-1, TNFα, components of complement and other endogenous mediators, the endothelial phenotype is altered. Activated endothelial cells become prothrombotic, upregulate adhesion molecules, and secrete different inflammatory mediators including chemoattractants.[24] Neutrophilic leukocytes attracted to the pulmonary microvasculature become adherent and activated and migrate from the capillary lumen into the alveolar space, a process accompanied by the release of different oxidants, proteases, leukotrienes, and inflammatory mediators such as PAF. In response to alveolar wall damage, pulmonary macrophages also secrete cytokines that amplify the process. Damage to endothelium and the easily injured type I pneumocytes allows flooding of alveoli by proteinaceous edema fluid. Injury to type II pneumocytes decreases the production and turnover of surfactant, whereas the protein-rich alveolar fluid inactivates it.[52,53] All of these factors contribute to the dyspnea, tachypnea, pulmonary infiltrates, and decreased ratio of arterial partial pressure of O_2 (Pa_{O_2}) to fractional inspired O_2 (Fi_{O_2}) of ALI.

The coagulopathy of sepsis is also seen at the individual organ level and can contribute to the development and progression of ALI. Compared with controls, the bronchoalveolar lavage fluid of patients with ARDS showed significant increases in the concentrations of TF and activated coagulation factor VII ($p < 0.001$).[54] Activation of the TF pathway of coagulation in the presence of large amounts of fibrinogen-rich intra-alveolar exudate can lead to extravascular fibrin deposition, hyaline membrane formation, inflammation, and pulmonary dysfunction.[55] With the passage of time, this exudative stage can be replaced by proliferative and fibrotic changes that can lead to pulmonary fibrosis. Deposition and persistence of alveolar fibrin are potentiated by depression of pulmonary fibrinolytic activity.[56] The fibrinolytic defect is largely the consequence of local amplification of plasminogen activator inhibitor 1 coupled with inhibition of urokinase plasminogen activator and downregulation of its receptor.[57] Failure of urokinase plasminogen activator to bind to urokinase plasminogen activator receptor on pneumocytes and alveolar macrophages can impair the remodeling that is an essential element of recovery from ALI and ARDS. At autopsy, patients with ARDS also showed a predictable gamut of vascular changes that mirror those within the pulmonary parenchyma.[55] For example, postmortem angiograms of patients with ARDS demonstrated the presence of serial vascular alterations that included thrombotic, fibroproliferative, and obliterative changes. The clinical significance of these lesions is signified by the development of pulmonary hypertension in patients with severe ARDS.

MECHANICAL VENTILATION AND ACUTE LUNG INJURY

Mechanical ventilation is a common supportive measure in patients with severe sepsis who develop respiratory failure. In addition to its many life-saving benefits, mechanical ventilation is potentially harmful to patients with severe sepsis and other types of critical illness (see Chaps. 37 and 43). The presence of an endotracheal tube bypasses normal airway defenses. When combined with impaired host defenses and malnutrition, patients with severe sepsis from an extrapulmonary source are at risk of a ventilator-associated pneumonia (VAP). In the absence of pre-existing disease, pneumonia may be the primary cause of ALI and ARDS. Further, high concentrations of inspired oxygen can damage alveolar membranes and worsen ALI. Moreover, barotrauma can mechanically stress alveolar and capillary walls, and shear forces generated during intratidal opening and closing of pulmonary units can damage lung tissue.[58] In addition to regional effects, barotrauma can induce release of cytokines into the pulmonary parenchyma and systemic circulation. These cytokines can contribute to the development of the multiple organ dysfunction syndrome (MODS) in mechanically ventilated patients with severe sepsis.[59] As an example of how dysfunctional organs may interact in the septic patient, it is thought that ALI (and mechanical ventilation) may contribute to dysfunction of other organs; through its effects on splanchnic blood flow, neurohumoral systems and proinflammatory cytokines, mechanical ventilation has the potential to adversely affect the gastrointestinal (GI) tract and predispose the patient to GI complications.[60] In the Acute Respiratory Distress Syndrome Network (ARDSNet) Lower Tidal Volume Study, patients ventilated with the lower tidal volumes (6 mL/kg ideal body weight) had lower levels of IL-6, more days without organ failure, and improved survival rate.[61] The complicated therapeutic considerations regarding mechanical ventilatory support in ALI are discussed later in this chapter.

GASTROINTESTINAL SYSTEM

With the decrease in the effective arterial blood volume, hypoperfusion of the gut becomes an important pathophysiologic component of severe sepsis. Early in the process, experimental evidence indicates that autoregulation of the microcirculatory blood flow is largely intact.[62] Before adequate fluid resuscitation, this regulatory process diverts blood from the muscularis mucosa to the more metabolically active mucosa. Redistribution of blood flow within the gut may preserve the mucosal barrier protection and prevent bacterial translocation. However, this redistribution of blood flow may not always be sufficient to meet mucosal oxygen demand. During this time, the intracellular PH of the gut decreases and lactate levels in the portal venous blood rise. Experiments have indicated that mesenteric lymph, rather than portal blood, may be the avenue that disseminates cytokines, endotoxin and other bacterial products, and microorganisms from the compromised gut to other parts of the body. In separate experiments, Magnotti, Sambol, and their associates showed that gut-derived mesenteric lymph, not portal blood, increases endothelial cell permeability and promotes lung injury after hemorrhagic shock and that ligation of the mesenteric lymphatic duct provides long-term organ protection.[63,64] However, Alverdy et al cautioned that experimental demonstra-

tions of alterations in the permeability of the gut mucosa to substances such as labeled dextran do not indicate a cause-and-effect relation between the "leaky mucosa" and gut-derived sepsis or multiorgan failure.[65] Instead, the two processes may be unrelated, and gut-derived sepsis may be a manifestation of nosocomial pathogens that express "potent virulence traits while competing for scarce resources in the hostile environment of the intestinal tract of a critically ill patient." Whatever the mechanism of gut-derived sepsis, experimental evidence has shown that early enteral feeding protects against bacterial translocation.[66] Whether or not such effects of enteral feeding are beneficial to overall patient outcomes is the point of ongoing study.

HEPATOBILIARY TRACT

The liver plays multiple key roles in patients with severe sepsis.[67] As previously described with regard to the lungs, the liver is a source and a target of inflammatory mediators. Its central role in the pathophysiology of severe sepsis is a function of the organ's blood flow and its cellular composition. In the postabsorptive state, the liver receives approximately 25% of $\dot{Q}_T$. Decreased perfusion is the most important event initiating hepatic dysfunction in the first hours after a septic insult.[68]

The three most important cellular elements participating in the liver's response to severe sepsis are Kupffer cells, hepatocytes, and endothelial cells. Although described separately, the liver's reaction to severe sepsis represents a collective and interactive response of all three cellular elements. The central role of the endothelium in sepsis pathogenesis has been discussed in detail above.

KUPFFER CELLS

Kupffer cells are the fixed macrophages of the liver. They represent approximately 70% of the organ's total macrophage pool. They clear the portal blood of endotoxin, bacteria, cytokines, toxins, and activated coagulation factors. Once primed, Kupffer cells secrete a variety of cytokines, including TNFα, IL-1, IL-6, IL-8, IL-12, IL-18, granulocyte colony-stimulating factor (GCSF), and granulocyte-macrophage colony-stimulating factor (GM-CSF). In a paracrine fashion, Kupffer cells modulate the response of adjacent hepatocytes to inflammatory signals through synthesis and release of acute-phase proteins and other mediators.

HEPATOCYTES

Hepatocytes play an integral role in the body's response to severe sepsis.[67] They bear receptors for endotoxin, vasoactive substances, various inflammatory mediators, and a number of cytokines. As a result of metabolic alterations during sepsis, hepatocytes re-prioritize their metabolism toward gluconeogenesis, amino acid uptake, and protein synthesis. Alterations in protein synthesis, however, are nonuniform, with levels of albumin, PC and antithrombin (AT) decreasing and concentrations of a variety of acute-phase proteins increasing. The latter include α_1-antitrypsin (α_1AT), ceruloplasmin, α_2-macroglobulin (α_2MG), CRP, fibrinogen, C4-binding protein, and thrombin-activated fibrinolysis inhibitor (TAFI). Antiproteinases such as α_1AT neutralize elastase and other proteases released by leukocytes. Ceruloplasmin and α_2MG serve a scavenger function by inactivating superoxides, hydroxyl radicals, and cytokines such as IL-6. Because many of the aforementioned proteins are involved in the hemostatic response to sepsis, they are discussed in the following section. As the septic process evolves, patients may develop a secondary hepatocellular dysfunction. This is a consequence of hepatocellular inflammation that results from the local release of inflammatory mediators and damage to the hepatic parenchyma by activated neutrophils within the hepatic sinusoids.

BLOOD AND BONE MARROW

Although dispersed in space, the blood and bone marrow comprise an organ system equal in importance to any other. During severe sepsis, the hematologic system attempts to restore homeostasis by eliminating the pathogen and isolating the infected focus. In patients with a localized infection, this process functions to the complete benefit of the host. However, in patients with severe sepsis, an exuberant response of the hematologic system can have detrimental effects. Elements of the hematologic system can be divided into cellular and fluid components.

Although the cellular elements originate in the marrow, the response of the bone marrow to sepsis is reflected in the peripheral blood. Fluid-phase elements of the hematologic system consist of various coagulation proteins. Changes in the hematologic system in patients with severe sepsis are the result of the influences of cytokines and hematopoietic growth factors, such as GM-CSF.

CELLULAR RESPONSE TO SEPSIS

Cellular elements of the peripheral blood involved in patients with severe sepsis include red blood cells, leukocytes, and platelets.[69] During the initial stages of severe sepsis, the hematocrit (HCT) reflects the opposing effects of third spacing of fluids and results of aggressive fluid resuscitation. Over time, the HCT decreases due to changes in the erythron, the red blood cell component of the hematologic system. Although an infection by a hemolytic organism such as *Clostridium perfringens* can acutely lower the HCT, the principal change in the mass of the erythron is due to a block in the reticuloendothelial transfer of iron to erythroid progenitors, erythroid hypoplasia, and a shortened survival of red blood cells. Changes in iron metabolism sequester this essential element from species of microorganisms that require iron as a growth factor. The white blood cell count may be high, normal, or low in patients with severe sepsis. The initial leukocytosis results from recruitment of neutrophils from the marginating pool and release of the more mature granulocytic elements from the bone marrow. As the process continues, the white cells show a "left shift" as less mature granulocytic elements enter the blood. This is associated with morphologic changes such as toxic granulation, Döhle bodies, and toxic vacuolation. Leukopenia may result from migration of large numbers of granulocytes into the infected focus or failure of the bone marrow to meet the demand; leukopenia resulting from infection itself is a sign of poor prognosis. Severe sepsis is usually accompanied by a variable degree of thrombocytopenia. Thrombocytopenia is a sign of dysfunction of the hematologic system and is due to platelet adhesion and aggregation throughout the microvasculature.

FLUID-PHASE RESPONSE TO SEPSIS

Severe sepsis is a prothrombotic state. This is the result of ongoing coagulation and impaired fibrinolysis. In response to acute inflammation, hepatic synthesis of the natural anticoagulants PC and AT decreases. At the same time, other elements of the PC system are compromised. Increased synthesis and release of α_1 AT and α_2 MG inhibit PC, whereas elevated levels of C4-binding protein bind protein S and prevent it from serving as a cofactor for activation of PC. In combination with the effects of microbial elements and cytokines, release of CRP by the liver upregulates the expression of TF on various cells. Increased production and release of fibrinogen and TAFI also contribute to the ongoing coagulopathy: the former by providing extra substrate for clotting, and the latter by inhibiting clot dissolution. The ongoing coagulopathy of sepsis is marked by a variable degree of thrombocytopenia; increased levels of D-dimer, a fibrin split product; and an elevation in the ratio of thrombin-antithrombin (TAT) to plasmin-antiplasmin (PAP). The TAT/PAP ratios are higher in patients with severe sepsis than in those who have sepsis without acute organ dysfunction.[21] This rise in TAT/PAP may precede the development of organ dysfunction, suggesting that enhanced coagulation and depressed fibrinolysis have a cause-and-effect relationship with the development of the MODS.

KIDNEY

Different factors present during an episode of severe sepsis have the potential to damage the kidneys. These include systemic hypotension or redistribution of blood flow, renal vasoconstriction, the effects of endotoxin and cytokines on the endothelium of the renal vasculature, and activation of inflammatory cells by LPS and inflammatory mediators.[70] In patients with severe sepsis, systemic vasodilation decreases the effective arterial blood volume. As the blood volume decreases, intrarenal vasoconstriction helps to maintain glomerular blood flow. Substances are released locally that promote intrarenal vasoconstriction in patients with severe sepsis and decreased effective arterial blood volume. They include endothelin, thromboxane A_2, and leukotrienes.[71] Eventually, however, compensatory mechanisms fail, the glomerular filtration rate decreases, prerenal azotemia develops, and acute tubular necrosis can develop. Endothelial injury from proinflammatory mediators, contents of neutrophilic granules, and components of complement can impair autoregulation of renal blood flow and may lead to microvascular thrombosis. Because the hypoperfused kidney is sensitive to nephrotoxic agents that are commonly administered in severe sepsis, these patients may be predisposed to the development of acute renal failure. For example, nonsteroidal anti-inflammatory drugs used to treat fever can inhibit the production of prostaglandins by the afferent arterioles and impair the ability of the kidney to regulate its blood flow. In the patient with severe sepsis and decreased blood volume, this may be enough to precipitate acute tubular necrosis.

NERVOUS SYSTEM

Patients with severe sepsis have abnormalities of their central, autonomic, and peripheral nervous systems.

ABNORMALITIES OF THE CENTRAL NERVOUS SYSTEM
Septic encephalopathy is common in patients with severe sepsis. In a prospective study of 69 patients with sepsis, Young et al reported that 71% exhibited mild to marked abnormalities of cerebral function.[72] The diagnosis of septic encephalopathy in a patient with severe sepsis requires evidence of extracranial infection plus impaired cerebral function. In patients without previous neurologic disease, septic encephalopathy is characterized by symmetrical neurologic findings without the asterixis, tremor, and multifocal myoclonus observed in subjects with metabolic encephalopathies of hepatic, renal, or endocrine origin.[73]

Delirium is perhaps the most costly and prevalent form of septic encephalopathy. This form of organ dysfunction has been shown to occur in more than 80% of all mechanically ventilated patients and is an independent predictor of poor outcomes.[74] Delirium can now be diagnosed by bedside techniques in 1 to 2 minutes with a high degree of accuracy and reliability by using the Confusion Assessment Method for the ICU (CAM-ICU).

The etiology of disordered function of the central nervous system in patients with severe sepsis is multifactorial. It includes abnormalities in the blood-brain barrier, alterations in cerebral blood flow, abnormal cellular physiology, and changes in the composition of neurotransmitters in the reticular activating system. In contrast to hemorrhagic shock, in which there is no change, the blood-brain barrier is disrupted in patients with septic shock.[75,76] This appears to be secondary to effects of circulating cytokines on cerebral endothelial cells. Accumulated perivascular edema fluid may impede the diffusion of oxygen and metabolic substrates, with a resultant decrease in cerebral oxygen consumption. The latter can occur despite an increase in cerebral blood flow and may also reflect the presence of mitochondrial dysfunction.[77] Although severe sepsis is vasodilatory in nature, defects in the blood-brain barrier in some patients can allow vasopressors with α_1-adrenergic activity to constrict cerebral vessels in patients with this disease.[78] Glial and neuronal defects are also present in patients with severe sepsis. Damage to astrocytes can further impair the blood-brain barrier, disrupt the autoregulation of cerebral blood flow, disturb the transfer of metabolic substrates to adjacent neurons, and increase the susceptibility of neural elements to toxic oxygen radicals. Elevated concentrations of the breakdown products of aromatic amino acids in the brain tissue of patients with septic encephalopathy may disrupt central noradrenergic pathways.[73]

ROLE OF THE AUTONOMIC NERVOUS SYSTEM
In an experimental model of sepsis, the parasympathetic nervous system plays an important role in the body's response to sepsis. Stimulation of afferent vagal nerve fibers produces the release of corticotropin-releasing hormone (CRH), adrenocorticotropic hormone (ACTH), and cortisol.[79] Subdiaphragmatic vagotomy blocks cortisol release in this situation. Stimulation of the vagus nerve prevents the onset of shock in a mouse model of endotoxemia.[80] The febrile response to IL-1 can be attenuated by experimental vagotomy.[81]

ROLE OF THE PERIPHERAL NERVOUS SYSTEM
AND SKELETAL MUSCLES
Abnormalities of the peripheral nervous system and neuromuscular units are a major cause of morbidity in patients with severe sepsis (see Chap. 66). Two major types of defects can be identified. The primary manifestation in this arena in survivors of severe sepsis and other types of prolonged serious disorders is electromyographic abnormalities. In a study by Fletcher et al, 95% of patients with prolonged critical illness had electromyographic changes indicative of chronic partial denervation, changes that were found up to 5 years after discharge from an ICU in more than 90% of patients who were in the unit for 28 days or longer.[82] Another manifestation is myoneuropathy, a critical illness present in almost 66% of patients. Clinical manifestations can be sensory or motor. The exact etiology of this process is unknown; however, it appears to result from a combination of factors including cytokines, impaired blood flow in the vasa nervosum, extended neuromuscular blockade, immobility, compression, and disuse.[83]

Diagnosis of Sepsis

After immediate stabilization, efforts should be directed toward determining the nature of the infection and identifying the presence of organ dysfunction. Special attention should be directed toward any predisposing condition such as trauma, surgery, organ transplantation, or immunosuppression (e.g., HIV infection, chemotherapy, and malignancy). Steps that define the nature of the infection and assess the degree of organ dysfunction include a complete history and physical examination, laboratory testing including selected microbiology procedures, and medical imaging studies.

CLINICAL EVALUATION

Vital signs are routinely recorded and monitored, although the frequency and method of monitoring depend on the severity of the process. As a general rule, patients can be considered febrile when they have a temperature of at least 38.0°C (100.4°F) or hypothermic with a temperature no higher than 35°C (95°F). Although the presence of fever is most accurately evaluated by assessing core temperature with a bladder or intravascular thermistor, electronic probes in body orifices (e.g., ear) are acceptable in appropriate patients. Notably, temperature must be assessed in a fashion that does not facilitate the transfer of nosocomial pathogens. Importantly, fewer than 50% of febrile episodes are infectious in origin, and almost 50% of septic patients are normothermic or hypothermic.[84] Variables related to fever may help in the differential diagnosis. Temperatures higher than 41.1°C are most probably noninfectious (e.g., drug fever or thyroid storm). Fever with a relative bradycardia and a rash may be drug induced or indicate *Salmonella typhi* or *S. paratyphi* infection. Vital signs can also provide a wealth of information about the patient's prognosis. In a study of community-acquired pneumonia (CAP), a temperature below 35°C or 40°C or higher, a pulse 125 beats/min or faster, a respiratory rate of at least 30 breaths/min, and a systolic BP lower than 90 mm Hg were independently associated with increased mortality rate.[85]

Altered mental status of the patient is an important clue to the presence of organ dysfunction. Delirium is an acute disorder of attention and cognition. It develops in 60% of older hospitalized patients and in more than 80% of mechanically ventilated patients.[76,86] Delirium may be hyperactive (agitated) or hypoactive. Whereas health care workers commonly recognize the former, hypoactive delirium is commonly missed. The presence of delirium is often an important early indication of sepsis, and it can be very hazardous and prolonged in the elderly. Delirium is associated with prolonged hospital stays, institutionalization, and death. Photophobia, nuchal rigidity, papilledema, or cranial nerve palsies should direct attention to a focus of infection, such as meningitis, within the central nervous system. Orbital pain, periorbital erythema, proptosis, or unilateral rhinorrhea may be seen in a patient with bacterial or fungal sinusitis. Although this may be the presenting illness in an immunocompromised patient, it can also be a secondary infection resulting from the obstruction of sinus ostia by nasotracheal or nasogastric tubes. Fetid breath may be detected in some patients with anaerobic oropharyngeal or pulmonary infections. Oral candidiasis may be a clue to fungal septicemia, although it is more commonly a local phenomenon. Immunosuppressed and neutropenic patients may be unable to produce purulent sputum or other exudates and may be unable to vigorously cough. Tachypnea may be the only sign of pneumonia. Careful auscultation of the lung fields may detect localized rales (crackles). Patients with lower lobe pneumonia may sometimes complain of upper abdominal pain. Associated hypoactive bowel sounds in these patients may be mistakenly ascribed to an intra-abdominal focus of infection. Tenderness over the right upper quadrant may indicate the presence of a hepatic or subphrenic abscess or acalculous cholecystitis. Abdominal tenderness and hypoactive bowel sounds may be the only evidence of a localized intra-abdominal infection or peritonitis. Pain or tenderness (direct and/or rebound) localized to the right or left lower quadrant may be evidence of appendicitis or a ruptured sigmoid diverticulum, respectively. Right lower quadrant pain in a neutropenic patient (often leukemic) may indicate the presence of typhlitis, an inflammation of the cecum that may require altered medical management or surgery.

The skin should be carefully examined. Livedo reticularis and poor capillary refill are a signs of impaired cutaneous perfusion and are associated with a poor prognosis in patients with severe sepsis. In neutropenic patients, the nail folds, axillae, perianal region, and groin provide ready entry for systemic pathogens. In this subset of patients, pain and erythema may be more reliable clues to infection than the leukocyte count. The dressings around any implanted device should be removed, and the area should be carefully inspected for purulent discharge, erythema, increased warmth, pain, and crepitus. Patients with vascular catheters also should be carefully checked for evidence of vascular compromise or embolic events originating from an infected device. Sudden hypotension after access of a vascular access device or line is a clue to the presence of an infected line. Operative wound infections are the second most common type of hospital-acquired infection. All surgical dressings should be removed to allow adequate inspection of operative sites. Patients with recent GI or gynecologic surgery, diabetes mellitus, or peripheral vascular disease are at risk for invasive polymicrobial infections such as necrotizing fasciitis or synergistic gangrene. Clues to the diagnosis include swelling around the wound, rapidly advancing border, crepitus, blisters, necrosis, or the radiographic appearance of gas within the soft tissues.

MEDICAL IMAGING STUDIES

Although universally obtained in critically ill patients, technical limitations of plain radiographs from portable machines render them of limited value in characterizing the nature of the infection in patients with severe sepsis. For example, in the critically ill population with pneumonia, portable chest radiographs have a diagnostic accuracy of 0.5, a sensitivity of 0.6, and a specificity of only 0.28.[87] Notably, chest radiographs may be essentially normal if the films are taken within the first 24 hours after the onset of symptoms or if the patient is neutropenic. Importantly, portable supine chest radiographs may be of value for other diagnostic purposes, such as estimating the patient's intravascular volume status or the nature of pulmonary edema by using the vascular pedicle width (especially when other invasive procedures are not planned).[88] Therefore, imaging studies should be selected based on the presumed nature of the infection, the clinician's need for other data related to the patient's overall clinical status, and the advantages and disadvantages of various approaches.

Plain films and ultrasound have limited utility in establishing the diagnosis of sinusitis. Therefore, a clinical diagnosis of septic sinusitis should be evaluated by computed tomographic (CT) scans of the paranasal sinuses. Although the presence of air or fluid levels is abnormal, the diagnosis is not established without recovery of infected material by sinus puncture, aspirate, and culture. A flat plate of the abdomen may demonstrate the presence of an ileus, a potential explanation for bacteremia in a patient without localizing findings. Abdominal radiographs may also show evidence of a perforated viscus or an intra-abdominal abscess. Ultrasonography of the gallbladder may demonstrate evidence of calculus or acalculous cholecystitis or of biliary tract obstruction in a patient with biliary sepsis. Ultrasound or CT studies of the abdomen may demonstrate localized fluid collections, abscesses, ureteral dilation or a perinephric abscess.

MICROBIOLOGY

All potential infected foci should be cultured in patients with severe sepsis. For example, the presence of pleural fluid adjacent to an infiltrate on a chest radiograph may provide valuable diagnostic information regarding the cause of a patient's severe sepsis. However, in 20% to 30% of patients, a definite site of infection cannot be identified.[89] The search for the responsible pathogen should include all measures necessary to establish the site and nature of infection, including direct examination and culture of material from the lower respiratory tract, fine-needle aspirates, and cultures of infected lines. The blood is also an appropriate material to culture. However, 70% of patients with sepsis will not have organisms recovered from the blood.[89] Material obtained for culture should be immediately gram stained. Cultures should also be supplemented with appropriate immunologic procedures such as detection of microbial antigens in body fluids and immunostaining. In patients with intra-abdominal infections, wound infections, and lung abscesses, the material should also be cultured anaerobically.

LABORATORY MARKERS OF SEPSIS

Several biochemical markers have been used to identify the patient with systemic activation of the cytokine cascade. None of the markers are currently widely used to diagnose sepsis, although some clinicians have argued that they should be incorporated into the entry criteria for patients in clinical trials of severe sepsis. Elevated levels of IL-6, IL-1, IL-8, TNFα, and monocyte chemotactic proteins 1 and 2 are present in septic patients and often correlate with the severity of the disease. Levels of IL-6 are increased in most patients with sepsis and have been shown to correlate with prognosis, but IL-6 is not used in clinical practice for diagnosis or prognostication.[90] Although the level of IL-6 may be able to differentiate cases of infectious from noninfectious SIRS, no correlation has been established between the concentration of IL-6 and outcomes.

CRP is an acute-phase reactant synthesized in the liver. After exposure to IL-1, IL-6, or TNFα, CRP levels increase. Levels of CRP have been used for years as a diagnostic marker of systemic inflammation. Whereas levels are normally low, they rise rapidly in patients with sepsis, paralleling the course of infection.[91] The complement system is activated in patients with sepsis; this may be mediated in part through CRP. Interactions of the complement system with microorganisms generate increased amounts of C3a and terminal components of the cascade. Elevated levels of C3a have been found to be one of the single and most sensitive and specific laboratory markers that can differentiate between sepsis and noninfectious causes of SIRS.[90]

PCT is derived from the preprohormone, pre-PCT. Although PCT levels are elevated in patients with sepsis, little is known about its source and function. Interestingly, calcitonin levels are normal in this population. In a porcine model of polymicrobial sepsis, immunoneutralization of calcitonin precursors was found to attenuate the adverse physiologic response to the infection.[92] For diagnostic purposes in critically ill patients, PCT levels have a better predictive value for sepsis than do IL-6 or CRP. When PCT concentration was combined with levels of C3a in a "sepsis score," the combination had a sensitivity of 91% and a specificity of 80% for sepsis versus noninflammatory SIRS.[90] As a prognostic marker, PCT levels have been shown to correlate with mortality rate, although the clinical utility of this prognostic marker remains uncertain at this time.[93–95]

Management

Severe sepsis is a medical emergency. The first priority should be to assess and address abnormalities in the "A,B,Cs": airway, breathing, and circulation. In many instances, the clinical assessment of tissue perfusion and response to therapy can be aided by monitoring devices and laboratory measurements (Table 46-4). Once immediate stabilization has been accomplished, the source of the infection should be established and controlled, and specific antimicrobial agents should be administered. After stabilization, source control, initiation of appropriate antimicrobial agents, and further support for dysfunctional organs, disease-specific interventions should be considered. The Surviving Sepsis Campaign is a collaborative effort by the SCCM, European Society of Intensive Care Medicine, and the International Sepsis Forum. The group's primary aim is to decrease the relative mortality rate of sepsis by 25% over a 5-year period. To reach this objective, the group has a number of goals. One of these is to improve the therapy of patients with severe sepsis. To achieve this, they reviewed published literature and achieved consensus on a number of management issues for patients with severe sepsis. These are described in the published Surviving Sepsis Campaign Practice Guidelines and listed in Table 46-5 and Figure 46-6.

TABLE 46-4 Clinical, Hemodynamic, and Ventilatory Goals for the Treatment of Patients with Severe Sepsis

Clinical goals
   Alert and oriented
   Normal skin color, warmth, perfusion and capillary refill
   Able to breathe spontaneously
   Vasopressor free
Hemodynamic goals
   Adequate perfusion pressure (MAP > 65 mm Hg)
   Cardiac index ≥ 2.5 L/min per square meter
   Urinary output ≥ 1.0 mL/kg per hour
   Lowest filling pressure and vasoactive drug dose necessary to achieve the above
Ventilatory goals
   PF ratio ≥ 300
   Sa_{O_2} >88%
   FI_{O_2} <0.4 to 0.5
   PEEP ≤ 5 cm H_2O
   RR: $V_T \leq 105$ breaths/min per liter

ABBREVIATIONS: FI_{O_2}, fraction inspired O_2; MAP, mean arterial pressure; PEEP, positive end-expiratory pressure; PF, partial pressure of O_2 to fraction inspired O_2; RR, respiratory rate; Sa_{O_2}, arterial oxygen saturation; V_T, tidal volume.

Initial Resuscitation

The initial therapeutic intervention in patients with severe sepsis is to reverse organ hypoperfusion. Patients with severe sepsis often have a relative intravascular hypovolemia. As a consequence, initial therapy often consists of the rapid administration of large amounts of fluids.

FLUID RESUSCITATION

Large amounts of fluids may be required to restore tissue perfusion and oxygen delivery. In some instances, correction of large fluid deficits may require at least 6 to 10 L of crystalloids.[96] Fluid resuscitation is often titrated by the responses of clinical end points of heart rate, BP, and urine output.[97] Appropriate amounts of fluid will improve the cardiac index by 25% to 40%. In approximately 50% of patients with severe sepsis who present with hypotension, fluid resuscitation alone will normalize BP and restore hemodynamic stability. Hemodynamic monitoring should be considered for patients who do not respond rapidly to the initial fluid challenge and those with a history of coronary heart disease.

CHOICE OF FLUIDS

There has been an ongoing debate as to whether fluid resuscitation is best accomplished with crystalloids or colloids. Choi et al conducted an evaluation of randomized clinical trials of crystalloids versus colloids in adult patients requiring fluid resuscitation.[98] They reported that there were no apparent differences in the incidences of pulmonary edema, mortality rate, or length of stay in patients who received crystalloid or colloid fluid resuscitation. In contrast, Schierhout et al compared crystalloid with colloid resuscitation in 26 clinical trials using stringent selection criteria.[99] They reported that resuscitation with colloids was accompanied by an increased absolute risk of mortality of 4% (95% confidence interval = 0% to 8%). Because colloids were not associated with improved survival rate and are significantly more expensive

TABLE 46-5 Synopsis of Major Surviving Sepsis Campaign Practice Guidelines

Intervention	Guidelines/Recommendations
Initial resuscitation	1. Resuscitate within 60 min to achieve MAP ≥65 mm Hg, urine output ≥0.5 mL/kg per hour, and CVP of 8–12 mm Hg (12–15 mm Hg in mechanically ventilated patients) 2. Packed red blood cells or dobutamine to achieve Scv_{O_2} ≥70%
Fluids	1. Crystalloids or colloids 2. Packed red blood cells to achieve a target Hb of 7–9 g/dL
Source control and antibiotics	1. The site of infection should be rapidly identified and appropriate source control measures instituted 2. When the specific infecting organism is unknown, empiric antibiotics should be administered within the first hour of treatment
Mechanical ventilation	1. 6 mL/kg tidal volume (ideal body weight) for patients with ALI/ARDS 2. Avoid increased V_T plus increased PP, maintain end-expiratory PP <30 cm H_2O 3. PEEP should be used to avoid oxygen toxicity in patients treated with high $F_{I_{O_2}}$ 4. Consider prone positioning in patients with dangerous $F_{I_{O_2}}$ levels
Drotrecogin alfa (activated)	1. Indicated for patients at high risk of death 2. No absolute contraindication 3. Administer as soon as possible after "high-risk of death" identified
Steroids	1. Indicated for patients with vasodepressor-dependent shock despite fluids 2. Administer 200–300 mg/d × 7 d by continuous intravenous infusion or in divided doses at 6-h intervals 3. The following steroid-related issues remain unresolved: ACTH stimulation test, weaning, mineralocorticoids, need to discontinue after resolution of shock
Glycemia control	1. Maintain blood glucose <150 mg/dL with insulin and glucose[a] 2. Monitor glucose concentrations at the bedside
Sedation	1. Intermittent as required 2. Continuous with daily interruption

[a] The Surviving Sepsis Campaign group expressed concerns that an initial recommendation for strict glycemic management (80 to 110 mg/dL) might be so stringent that it would not be adopted.
ABBREVIATIONS: ACTH, corticotropin; ALI, acute lung injury; ARDS; acute respiratory distress syndrome; CVP, central venous pressure; $F_{I_{O_2}}$, fraction inspired O_2; Hb, hemoglobin; MAP, mean arterial pressure; PP, plateau pressure; Scv_{O_2}, O_2 saturation of blood in the superior vena cava or right atrium; VT, tidal volume.
Extracted from Dellinger RP, et al: Surviving Sepsis Campaign guidelines for management of severe sepsis and septic shock. *Crit Care Med* 32:858, 2004.

than crystalloids, they concluded that the evidence does not support the continued use of colloids for volume replacement in the critically ill. The crystalloid versus colloid controversy continues.[100] However, in the presence of normal oncotic pressure, most patients are managed with crystalloids; patients requiring osmotic support can also be treated with colloids such as 25% albumin.[100]

Pyruvate is a potent antioxidant and free radical scavenger.[101] Although it is unstable in aqueous solution, its ethyl derivative has greater stability. Ringer ethyl pyruvate has been evaluated in different preclinical models and has been shown to improve survival rate and decrease inflammatory markers in acute endotoxemia, acute bacterial peritonitis, hemorrhagic shock, and mesenteric ischemia/reperfusion injury.[102] There is some basic science and clinical evidence that suggests that infusions of small amounts of hypertonic saline may have some future role in the resuscitation of patients with severe sepsis. In 1980, Velasco et al reported that administration of a hypertonic solution of 7.5% saline had

beneficial effects in a canine model of hemorrhagic shock.[103] Experimental studies in models of severe sepsis confirmed beneficial effects similar to those originally reported. Small clinical studies have also reported beneficial effects on cardiac indices, SVR, and oxygen transport.[104,105] Although it was initially proposed that the beneficial effect of this intervention was on cardiac preload, increasing evidence suggests that its effects extend far beyond the osmotic properties of hypertonic saline. Hypertonic saline also appears to improve myocardial contractility, reduce endothelial and interstitial edema, improve microcirculatory blood flow, and exert immunomodulatory activity.[106] Its effects on endothelial cell function and microvascular blood flow are particularly interesting in light of the growing evidence of endothelial cell dysfunction in patients with severe sepsis. Endothelial cell edema can serve as a surrogate for endothelial injury and potential dysfunction. Edema of the endothelial cells occurs in the initial phases of hypovolemia. Small infusions of hypertonic saline can reduce endothelial volume by approximately 20%, increase tissue perfusion, and improve cellular function.[107] Microcirculatory blood flow is also improved because the hypertonic fluid produces hemodilution and decreased blood viscosity.

Patients with severe sepsis very often have dramatic decreases in hemoglobin (Hb) levels. This is secondary to a number of factors including hemodilution and impaired erythropoiesis. Further, fluid resuscitation may decrease Hb levels by up to 1 to 3 g/dL.[97] This degree of anemia is tolerated by most patients because the resultant decrease in blood viscosity reduces afterload and improves venous return. Potential benefits of transfusion in this population include an increase in arterial oxygen content and an improvement in systemic oxygen availability. However, transfusions of packed red blood cells have several potentially detrimental effects. These include rheologic changes that decrease red blood cell deformability and increase blood viscosity, immunosuppression, disease transmission, risk of nonhemolytic transfusion reactions, and the fact that oxygen delivery is not immediately restored after transfusion because the infused red blood cells must restore their depleted 2,3-diphosphoglycerate levels to improve oxygen release.

Hebert et al conducted a multicenter, controlled trial of restrictive versus liberal transfusion strategies in a population of critically ill patients.[108] They enrolled 838 euvolemic, critically ill patients who had Hb concentrations below 9.0 g/dL within 72 hours of admission to the ICU. Patients were then randomized to a restrictive transfusion strategy in which Hb concentrations were maintained within the range of 7.0 to 9.0 g/dL and transfusions were administered only if the Hb dropped below 7.0 g/dL or to a strategy in which Hb levels were maintained in the range of 10.0 to 12.0 g/dL and transfusions were given if the Hb dropped below 10.0 g/dL. Even though the overall 30-day mortality rate was similar in the two groups, patients who were less severely ill as stratified by a score no higher than 20 on the Second Acute Physiology and Chronic Health Evaluation (APACHE II) and patients who were younger than 55 years had a significantly lower in-hospital mortality rate (22.2% versus 28.1%; $p = 0.05$). This benefit did not extend to patients with acute coronary syndromes. However, Rivers et al recently released the results of a clinical trial of early goal-directed therapy (EGDT) that suggest that there may be some benefit of Hb concentrations of 10 g/dL or greater, at least as part of a strategy of early resuscitation of patients with severe sepsis and septic shock.[109] Although these results are discussed below, they emphasize the importance of proper tissue oxygenation.

At this time, the optimal Hb level for patients with severe sepsis is unclear. The default transfusion threshold currently used by many ICUs is a conservative one of 7.0 g/dL, unless patients are elderly and have a history of myocardial infarction, in which case a more liberal threshold of 10 g/dL is supported by an 80,000-patient observational study by Wu et al.[110]

CARDIORESPIRATORY SUPPORT

VASOPRESSORS

Patients who remain hypotensive despite aggressive fluid resuscitation are candidates for pressor support; however, vasopressors should not be considered in lieu of adequate fluid resuscitation. BPs determined by a cuff are often inaccurate, and an arterial cannula is usually inserted to monitor intra-arterial BP in patients receiving vasopressor therapy. Many agents with different pharmacodynamic properties are available to treat the hypotensive patient with severe sepsis (Table 46-6). Patients receiving pressor support should be monitored to ensure that treatment restores perfusion to vital organs without compromising stroke volume. Surrogates of improved peripheral perfusion and splanchnic blood flow include an increase in MAP (≥65 mm Hg is often used), warming of the extremities, and resolution of cutaneous mottling and impaired capillary refill. Increased urinary output and improved mentation are other good surrogates of adequate systemic perfusion. Goals should be a urine output greater than 0.5 mL/kg per hour and an alert and oriented cognitive status.

One of the obstacles to determine the "best" pressor in patients with severe sepsis is the lack of large-scale, randomized controlled trials. Most studies of various pressor agents have been observational in nature. Norepinephrine appears to be the preferred agent for initial BP support in patients

TABLE 46-6 Vasoactive Drugs: Usual Hemodynamic Effects[a]

Drug	Dose	Paop	Q_T	BP	SVR	Comments
Norepinephrine	2–30 μg/min	↑	↑	↑↑	↑↑	Usual first-line drug; more potent than dopamine
Vasopressin	0.01–0.04 U/min	↔	↔	↑	↑	Caution advised pending large clinical trials; occasionally effective when catecholamines fail
Dobutamine	2–20 μg/kg/min	↓	↑	↓ or ↑	↓	Most useful when Q_T is low, typically due to cardiac dysfunction. Can cause hypotension, especially when hypovolemia is present
Phenylephrine	2–10 μg/kg/min	↑	↓	↑↑	↑↑	Increase in BP purely by peripheral vasoconstriction will reduce Q_T; best used when Q_T is elevated
Dopamine	2–20 μg/kg/min	↑	↑	↑	↔↑	Not effective in renal protection
Epinephrine	5–30 μg/min	↑↔	↑↑	↑↑	↑	Effects and indications similar to norepinephrine, but more often worsens lactic acidosis

[a]Dose of all agents is generally titrated upward from the lower range until a clinically desired hemodynamic effect is achieved.

ABBREVIATIONS: BP, blood pressure; Paop, pulmonary artery occlusion pressure; Q_T, cardiac output; SVR, systemic vascular resistance.

with severe sepsis who remain hypotensive despite an adequate fluid challenge. Because of its pure α-adrenergic activity, phenylephrine may be useful in patients with coronary heart disease who may be at risk for tachycardia or arrhythmias from agents with β-agonist properties. Meadows et al evaluated the effects of norepinephrine on reversal of shock in 10 patients with severe sepsis.[111] Patients with severe sepsis who remained hypotensive and oliguric despite expansion of their plasma volume to a target Paop and infusions of increasing doses of dopamine and dobutamine were then treated with norepinephrine monotherapy. After discontinuation of dopamine and dobutamine, an infusion of norepinephrine significantly elevated the MAP, reversed the hypotension, and increased the SVR, left ventricular stroke work index, and urinary output without significantly affecting heart rate. In a separate study, Martin et al evaluated the effect of norepinephrine on the outcome of patients with septic shock.[112] These investigators evaluated the effects of various independent variables that might affect outcome in an observational cohort of 97 adult patients with severe sepsis. Patients who received norepinephrine as a component of their hemodynamic support had a significantly lower hospital mortality rate than did those treated with large-dose dopamine and/or epinephrine (62% versus 82%; 95% confidence interval = 0.68, range = 0.54 to 0.87; $p < 0.001$). Further support for the use of norepinephrine as the pressor of choice was provided by Di Giantomasso et al.[113] They evaluated the effects of norepinephrine on vital organ blood flow in a sheep model. They concluded that norepinephrine infusion does not induce ischemia in vital organs in normal mammalian circulation. In addition, infusion of norepinephrine significantly increases coronary and renal blood flow, with associated improvements in urine output and serum creatinine.

Over a short period, tachyphylaxis may appear as vascular smooth muscle becomes resistant to the effects of norepinephrine and other catecholamines. Vasopressin is involved in cardiovascular homeostasis. Normally, it plays only a minor role in BP control. However, in hypotensive patients, vasopressin released under baroreflex receptor control stimulates vascular smooth muscle and helps restore BP. During the initial phases of severe sepsis-induced hypotension, high levels of vasopressin contribute to the effects of endogenous catecholamines in attempting to restore BP. However, as shock worsens, plasma concentrations of vasopressin decline significantly and become inappropriately low for the patient's MAP, presumably because neurohypophyseal stores of the hormone are depleted in the face of constant baroreceptor stimulation. In support of this hypothesis, Landry et al demonstrated by immunohistochemistry in a canine model that, after 1 hour of hemorrhagic shock, the stainable hormone was essentially absent in tissue from the animal's neurohypophysis.[44] In patients with severe sepsis and other forms of vasodilatory shock, administration of vasopressin to produce concentrations similar to those identified during acute episodes of hypotension increases arterial BP by 25 to 50 mm Hg. It has been postulated that the marked sensitivity of BP to vasopressin in this situation is multifactorial in origin: (1) in patients with severe sepsis and established hypotension, plasma levels of vasopressin are low and its receptors on vascular smooth muscle are unoccupied; (2) patients with severe sepsis may have dysfunction of the sympathetic nervous system and be more responsive to noncatecholamine

pressor agents; (3) plasma concentrations of norepinephrine are markedly elevated in patients with vasodilatory shock, and vasopressin potentiates the effects of the catecholamine; (4) vasopressin directly activates K_{ATP} channels in vascular smooth muscle, and; (5) vasopressin directly and indirectly inhibits the vasodilatory activity of NO.[44] Studies have supported the role of vasopressin in this situation. Landry et al reported that an infusion of 0.04 U/min of vasopressin in 10 hypotensive patients with severe sepsis increased arterial BP from a mean of 92/52 mm Hg to 146/66 mm Hg.[114] Importantly, however, withdrawal of vasopressin resulted in hypotension in six patients in whom it was the only pressor. In a blinded study of 24 patients with septic shock, Patel et al compared the effects of norepinephrine and vasopressin.[115] Doses of vasopressin and norepinephrine, starting at 0.01 U/min and 2 μg/min, respectively, were titrated to maintain a clinically acceptable MAP. Treatment with vasopressin produced an important catecholamine-sparing activity ($p < 0.001$), and its use was accompanied by a larger volume of urine output and an improved creatinine clearance ($p < 0.05$). Although these preliminary observations require a large-scale randomized trial to confirm the beneficial effects of vasopressin in patients with vasodilatory shock, critical care specialists are commonly treating patients with severe sepsis who are refractory to catecholamines with vasopressin.

INOTROPIC AGENTS

Patients with severe sepsis have a normal to low BP, elevated cardiac index, and decreased SVR. However, myocardial depression is common.[97] It is characterized by a decreased EF, ventricular dilation, impaired contractile response to volume loading, and a low ratio of peak systolic pressure to end-systolic volume. In patients who are unable to maintain an adequate cardiac index, MAP, mixed venous oxygen content, and/or urine output, an inotropic agent such as dobutamine may be useful.[109] However, because inotropic agents can produce clinically significant tachycardia in patients who have not been adequately resuscitated with fluid, it is important to ensure that the dobutamine candidate has adequate or increased intravascular volume. In addition, the increased myocardial oxygen consumption in patients treated with an inotrope can produce angina or an acute coronary syndrome.

OXYGEN AND MECHANICAL VENTILATION

Sepsis places significant stress on the respiratory system. At presentation, most patients are tachypneic and hypoxemic. These clinical manifestations result from a combination of factors including increased oxygen requirements, decreased pulmonary compliance, increased airway resistance, and impaired efficiency of the respiratory and other muscles.[89] Approximately 88% of patients with severe sepsis will require ventilatory support, generally for 5 to 10 days. Therefore, the patient's arterial oxygen saturation (Sa_{O_2}) and/or the Pa_{O_2} should be evaluated and steps taken to maintain the Sa_{O_2} at 88% or greater by increasing the amount of $F_{I_{O_2}}$ or improving respiratory physiology with institution and adjustments of mechanical ventilation. Prone positioning has the potential to improve oxygenation in critically ill patients with severe sepsis. Position-related changes in respiratory physiology are a function of changes in end-expiratory lung volume, ventilation-perfusion matching, and chest wall mechanics. However, although the maneuver improves oxygenation,

Gattinoni et al were unable to demonstrate an advantage with respect to mortality rate of ARDS patients when using a protocol of prone positioning for 6 hours/day over 10 days.[116] The disconnect between improved oxygenation and mortality rate in this study may be a function of several trial design considerations, including statistical power, low severity of illness of many of the enrolled patients, and the duration of prone positioning employed.[117]

Most patients with severe sepsis will require an F_{IO_2} greater than 50%. Although high-flow oxygen through a face mask can provide an F_{IO_2} in the 70% range, in general, patients with severe sepsis requiring high levels of oxygen supplementation should be treated with positive pressure ventilation. Importantly, the clinician should be proactive and recognize the signs of impending respiratory failure, so that patients can be intubated early and receive respiratory support before they aspirate, develop hypoxemic encephalopathy, or develop a potentially fatal arrhythmia. During intubation and immediately thereafter, the patient should receive an F_{IO_2} in the 95% to 100% range to maximize Sa_{O_2}. However, to avoid potential oxygen toxicity through the formation of free radicals and other mechanisms, the F_{IO_2} should be tapered to no greater than 50% as soon as possible, and Sa_{O_2} should be maintained above 88%.

Oxygen delivery (Q_{O_2}) is a function of $\dot{Q}T$, Hb level, and Sa_{O_2} ($Q_{O_2} = 10 \times \dot{Q}T \times [1.34\ Hb \times Sa_{O_2} + 0.003 \times Pa_{O_2}]$). If filling pressures are low, the $\dot{Q}T$ can be raised by fluids; alternatively, patients who do not respond to fluids and have normal or elevated filling pressures may benefit from an inotrope. Although it is important that Q_{O_2} be adequate, the therapy required to achieve supranormal Q_{O_2} may be injurious in some patients.[118] In a prospective randomized study of 109 critically ill patients, Hayes et al attempted to maximize D_{O_2} by volume expansion.[119] Patients failing volume expansion alone were randomized to a control group or a treatment group. The intervention group was treated with intravenous dobutamine (5 to 200 μg/kg per minute). All nine patients who responded to volume replacement alone survived to leave the hospital. The predicted risk of death for the remaining 100 patients was 34%. However, the in-hospital mortality rate was lower in the control group (34%) than in the supranormal Q_{O_2} (54%) group, suggesting that the aggressive efforts to increase tissue Q_{O_2} were detrimental.

One reasonable ventilatory strategy in patients requiring mechanical ventilation is to employ assist-control ventilation to provide 75% to 100% of the minute ventilation. Positive end-expiratory pressure can be employed to reduce the risk of ventilator-induced injury and reduce the F_{IO_2} required to maintain the Sa_{O_2} at 88% or greater. The results of the ARDSNet Tidal Volume Study indicated that a lung protective strategy using tidal volumes of 6 mL/kg (versus 12 mL/kg) can significantly improve outcomes in patients with ALI or ARDS.[61] Patients who were randomized to the lower tidal volume had a significantly lower mortality rate (31.0% versus 39.8%; $p = 0.007$), more days without a ventilator (12 versus 10; $p = 0.007$), more days without organ failure (15 versus 12; $p = 0.006$), and lower levels of the proinflammatory cytokine, IL-6. It is important that every effort be made to reduce mechanical ventilation settings to detect readiness for extubation from the ventilator. The spontaneous breathing trial is the best indicator of the patient's ability to breathe without mechanical support.[120] Ely et al reported that a spontaneous breathing trial protocol using respiratory therapists and nurses

significantly reduced the number of days that patients spent on a ventilator (1 versus 3; $p < 0.001$), decreased the complication rate by half, and cut the costs of ICU care by more than $5000 per patient.[121,122]

IMPORTANCE OF EARLY GOAL-DIRECTED THERAPY

Rivers et al conducted a randomized, nonblinded trial of standard therapy versus early goal-directed therapy (EGDT) in patients with SIRS criteria and systolic BP no higher than 90 mm Hg and who were unresponsive to 20–30 mL/kg of crystalloid or had a lactate concentration of 4 mmol/L or greater.[109] Patients were randomized into two groups and treated by protocol. Hemodynamic goals were identical in the two groups: central venous pressure between 8 and 12 mm Hg, vasopressors for a systolic BP of 90 mm Hg or lower, urinary output maintained at 0.5 mL/kg per hour or greater, and a MAP established at 65 mm Hg or higher. Patients in the group randomized to EGDT also received an oximetric central venous catheter capable of measuring the saturation of blood in the superior vena cava or right atrium (Scv_{O_2}) and were treated early in the emergency department according to protocol for at least 6 hours before they were transferred to the first available inpatient bed. If the Scv_{O_2} of patients in the EGDT group was less than 70%, they received transfusions of packed red blood cells until their HCT was at least 30%. If the Scv_{O_2} was still less than 70%, patients were treated with dobutamine up to a dose of 20 μg/kg per minute. If necessary, mechanical ventilation and sedation were employed to raise Scv_{O_2} to the goal concentration, and interventions were directed at lowering oxygen consumption and, hence, raising the saturation of blood returning to the right heart.

Patients treated with EGDT received approximately 1.5 L of additional fluid during the first 6 hours (5000 versus 3500 mL); they also received significantly more transfusions of packed red blood cells (PRBCs; 64.1% versus 18.5%; $p < 0.001$). Vasopressor support was not significantly different in the two groups during the first 6 hours; however, the EGDT group received significantly fewer vasopressors after 7 hours than did the standard group ($p = 0.03$). Whereas fewer than 1% of the standard therapy group received an inotrope, dobutamine was administered to approximately 14% of the EGDT group. Early EGDT significantly affected outcomes. Patients treated in the EGDT arm of the protocol had a significant benefit in mortality rate at 28 days (30.5% versus 46.5%; $p = 0.009$) and at 60 days (44.3% versus 56.9%; $p = 0.03$). The number needed to treat (NNT) to prevent one death with EGDT was six to eight patients. The results of this study indicated the importance of early identification of patients with severe sepsis at high risk for cardiovascular collapse and implementation of measures designed to restore equilibrium between oxygen demand and supply. The specific features of the protocol that contributed to the benefit with respect to mortality rate (e.g., the relatively large quantity of PRBCs and dobutamine used in the intervention group and the titration of Scv_{O_2} using oximetric central venous catheters) require further study.

INFECTION MANAGEMENT

Infection management consists of source control and the administration of anti-infectives that cover the spectrum of microbial organisms suggested by the patient's initial presentation. Importantly, appropriate cultures should be obtained; in some cases, this is accomplished during the process of source control (e.g., removal of an infected intravascular device).

SOURCE CONTROL

The term *source control* has replaced *surgical intervention* to describe measures to control the source of infection. This change in terminology is intended to highlight the fact that interventions falling into this category are not limited to surgery. Source control can be divided into three broad categories: (1) drainage of an abscess, (2) débridement of devitalized and infected tissue, and (3) removal of foreign bodies colonized by pathogens and diversion, repair, or excision of an infected focus in a hollow viscus.[123] Attention directed to source control should be included in the initial management of all patients with severe sepsis. Whereas septic foci resulting from a ruptured appendix or a perforated duodenal ulcer may be obvious, other presentations may be subtle. For example, a patient with CAP who remains septic may have an associated empyema. The timing of source control measures must take the patient's clinical condition into account. For example, removal of an infected central line should be performed immediately. Alternatively, transferring an unstable patient to the medical imaging suite, where monitoring may not be as intense, for percutaneous drainage might be best deferred until resuscitative measures have restored cardiopulmonary homeostasis. In other instances, surgical intervention should be early in aggressive disease processes in which early intervention clearly leads to improved outcomes such as necrotizing fasciitis.

ANTI-INFECTIVE THERAPY

Several general principles govern antibiotic therapy of the patient with severe sepsis (Table 46-7). Antibiotic therapy is delayed in approximately 10% of cases, a situation responsible for a mortality rate that can be 10% to 15% higher than that in patients treated early.[124,125] Iregui et al evaluated the basis and consequences of delayed appropriate antibiotic therapy in a study of 107 consecutive patients with VAP.[126] In 75.8% of

TABLE 46-7 Principles of Anti-infective Therapy of the Patient with Severe Sepsis

Obtain cultures of suspected sources of infection
Promptly administer parenteral antibiotics
Antibiotic selection(s) should be based on the following:
    Most probable diagnosis and suspected pathogens
    Site of acquisition (ie, community or nosocomial)
    Results of Gram stain
    History of prior antimicrobial treatment
    Known resistance patterns in the community or institution
    Tissue penetration of drug
    Comorbidities
    Patient's hepatic and renal function
    History of allergy to antibiotics
    Potential toxicity
    Risk of influencing resistance
Initial therapy should be broad spectrum and progressively
    narrowed as microbiological data become available
Patients should be monitored closely for
    Evidence of a response
    Development of drug toxicity
    Selection of antibiotic-resistance strains
    Appearance of a superinfection

patients, delays of 24 hours or longer were due to the simple failure to write the order for antibiotics after the diagnosis was made. Microbial resistance could explain only 18.2% of the cases in which therapy was classified as inappropriate. The initial delay of appropriate antibiotic therapy was associated with a significant 41.1% increase in hospital mortality rate from VAP ($p < 0.01$). Kreger et al evaluated the epidemiology and response to therapy in 612 patients with gram-negative bacteremia.[127] They reported that appropriate antibiotic therapy reduced the frequency at which shock developed by approximately 50%. In addition, even after shock had developed, appropriate antibiotic therapy significantly decreased mortality rates. As essential as antimicrobial therapy is, the mortality rate of patients with severe sepsis treated with appropriate antibiotics remains unacceptably high. Pittet et al analyzed bedside predictors of mortality rate in 176 ICU patients with bacteremic sepsis and found that appropriate antibiotic therapy reduced mortality rate by 11%.[124] Nevertheless, in-hospital mortality rate remained at an unacceptable 43%. Kollef et al reported even stronger evidence for the importance of appropriate antibiotic therapy.[128] The infection-related mortality rate for patients receiving inadequate antimicrobial therapy was significantly greater than that seen in patients treated appropriately (42.0% versus 17.7%; $p < 0.001$). Analysis of their data in a logistic regression model indicated that inadequate antimicrobial therapy of infection is the most important independent determinant of hospital mortality rate in critically ill patients admitted to a medical or surgical ICU. Table 46-8 lists some general guidelines for the selection of initial antibiotics for patients with severe sepsis.

PNEUMONIA

Major potential pathogens in patients with serious CAP include *S. pneumoniae*, *Haemophilus influenzae*, and *Legionella* species (see Chap. 51). Initial therapy can be an extended-spectrum cephalosporin or a β-lactam/β-lactamase inhibitor combination plus a macrolide (azithromycin, clarithromycin, or erythromycin) or an antipseudomonal fluoroquinolone (ciprofloxacin, levofloxacin, or gatifloxacin) alone. If there are concerns about infection by a strain of drug-resistant *S. pneumoniae*, the β-lactam should be cefotaxime or ceftriaxone. Notably, some researchers have advised against fluoroquinolone monotherapy in this situation because most therapeutic trials studying these drugs excluded seriously ill patients.[129] For patients with structural disease of the lung (e.g., bronchiectasis), an antipseudomonal regimen would be an excellent one. If aspiration is suspected, treatment should be clindamycin, metronidazole, or a β-lactam/β-lactamase inhibitor combination, with or without fluoroquinolone. Patients allergic to β-lactams can be treated with a fluoroquinolone with or without the addition of clindamycin. The most probable organisms in a patient with nosocomial pneumonia are *S. aureus* and aerobic gram-negative rods. A possible initial therapy for these patients might be an antipseudomonal β-lactam (cefepime, imipenem/cilastatin, meropenem, or piperacillin/tazobactam) plus an intravenous antipseudomonal fluoroquinolone such as ciprofloxacin.

INTRA-ABDOMINAL INFECTIONS

In serious community-acquired intra-abdominal infections, the major pathogens are most likely to be *E. coli*, *Klebsiella pneumoniae*, and *Bacteroides fragilis* (see Chap. 89). Initial treatment in the ICU to cover these organisms may

TABLE 46-8 Empirical Antibiotics for Initial Treatment of Adults with Severe Sepsis

Suspected Source of Sepsis	Reasonable Initial Antimicrobial Regimen	Alternative Agents
Primary bacteremia (no source evident): normal host	Third-generation cephalosporin Cefotaxime 2 g IV q 6 h *or* Ceftriaxone 2 g IV q 12 h *or* Ceftizoxime 2 g IV q 8 h	Nafcillin and gentamicin, piperacillin/tazobactam, imipenem
Primary bacteremia (no source evident): IV drug user	Ceftazidime 2 g IV q 8 h and nafcillin 2 g IV q 4 h	Piperacillin/tazobactam or imipenem and gentamicin
Febrile neutropenia	Monotherapy: cefepime 2 g IV/IM q 8–12 h Duotherapy: piperacillin 3 g IV q 4 h plus gentamicin 1.5 mg/kg IV q 8 h Vancomycin indicated: add cefepime ± aminoglycoside	Ceftazidime or cefepime plus nafcillin, imipenem or cefepime plus gentamicin
Bacterial meningitis	Ceftriaxone 2 g IV/IM q 12–24 h; if patient >50 y, add ampicillin 3 g IV q 4–6 h	Gram-positive cocci: vancomycin plus broad-spectrum cephalosporin Gram-negative cocci; penicillin G Gram-positive bacilli: ampicillin (or penicillin) plus an aminoglycoside Gram-negative bacilli: broad-spectrum cephalosporin plus aminoglycoside
Cellulitis/erysipelas/fasciitis	Limb-threatening: ciprofloxacin 400 mg IV q 12 h plus clindamycin 900 mg IV q 8 h Life-threatening: imipenem/cilastin 1 g IV q 6–8 h	Vancomycin, metronidazole, aminoglycoside
Community-acquired acute bacterial pneumonia	Third-generation cephalosporin in combination with a fluoroquinolone or a macrolide	Piperacilin/tazobactam plus a fluoroquinolone or a macrolide
Hospital-acquired acute bacterial pneumonia/ventilator-associated pneumonia	Ceftazidime 2 g IV q 8 h and gentamicin 1.5 mg/kg IV q 8 h ± macrolide	Ciprofloxacin ± vancomycin
Mixed aerobic/anaerobic infections Intra-abdominal infections Mediastinitis Fulminant aspiration pneumonia Necrotizing cellulitis and fasciitis Septic abortion, endometritis	Third-generation cephalosporin and clindamycin 900 mg IV q 8 h; *or* Metronidazole 500 mg IV q 8 h plus ampicillin 2 g IV q 4 h plus gentamicin 1.5 mg/kg IV q 8 h	Imipenem or piperacillin/tazobactam plus gentamicin, cefoxitin plus gentamicin, clindamycin plus co-trimoxazole
Urinary tract infection	Gentamicin 1.5 mg/kg IV q 8 h ± ampicillin 2 g IV q 4 h	Third-generation cephalosporin ± gentamicin

ABBREVIATIONS: IM, intramuscularly; IV, intravenously, q, every.

consist of imipenem/cilastatin, ampicillin/sulbactam, or piperacillin/tazobactam with or without an aminoglycoside. The spectrum of potential pathogens increases in patients with nosocomial intra-abdominal infections to include aerobic gram-negative rods, including those that might produce an extended-spectrum β-lactamase, other anaerobes, and *Candida* species.

SKIN AND SOFT TISSUE

In patients with severe sepsis from community-acquired skin and soft tissue infections, the most common pathogens are group A streptococci, *S. aureus*, *Clostridium* species, polymicrobial organisms, various enteric gram-negative rods, and *Pseudomonas aeruginosa* (see Chap. 55). The risk that the infecting organism will be a gram-negative rod increases in patients who are neutropenic. In these patients, initial treatment in the ICU might consist of vancomycin with imipenem/cilastatin or piperacillin/tazobactam. The most probable pathogens in patients with serious nosocomial skin and soft tissue infections are *S. aureus* (including methicillin-resistant *S. aureus*)

and aerobic gram-negative rods. A reasonable initial antibiotic regimen in these patients might consist of vancomycin plus cefepime. Patients with vancomycin-resistant organisms can be treated with the streptogramin combination, quinupristin/dalfopristin or the first oxazolidinone, linezolid. If microbiological studies demonstrate that a *Staphylococcal* strain is not resistant to methicillin, nafcillin should be administered instead of vancomycin because of its comparatively superior efficacy and to prevent the emergence of vancomycin-resistant strains. This allows vancomycin to be reserved for infections resistant to other agents.

In patients presenting with severe sepsis from a cutaneous or soft tissue infection with diabetes mellitus, peripheral vascular disease or neutropenia, or a history of recent GI or gynecologic surgery, the index of suspicion should be high for potentially fatal necrotizing fasciitis. These infections are usually polymicrobial and are produced by a combination of anaerobic organisms and aerobic gram-negative rods. This disorder has a high mortality rate unless treated aggressively. Percutaneous aspirates or biopsies should be obtained, gram stained, and cultured aerobically and anaerobically. If crepitation is detected or radiographs show gas in the deep tissues, the wound and surrounding tissues should be immediately débrided surgically.

UROSEPSIS

The most probable organisms in patients with severe community-acquired urosepsis are *E. coli, Klebsiella* species, *Enterobacter* species, and *Proteus* species (see Chap. 56). Reasonable antibiotic selections for urosepsis include a parenteral fluoroquinolone, an aminoglycoside with or without ampicillin, or an extended-spectrum cephalosporin with or without an aminoglycoside. If a gram stain of the urine demonstrates the presence of gram-positive cocci, a rational choice for initial therapy would be ampicillin/sulbactam with or without an aminoglycoside to cover enterococci. A reasonable initial antibiotic combination in patients presenting with this diagnosis would be ciprofloxacin with or without an aminoglycoside. Although bacteriuria or candiduria is common in catheterized patients in the ICU, an indwelling catheter is uncommonly the cause of urosepsis. Nosocomial urosepsis is most common in patients with a urinary tract obstruction or those who have recently undergone instrumentation of the lower urinary tract. Likely pathogens in patients with serious nosocomial urosepsis are aerobic gram-negative rods and enterococci. Unless the prevalence of vancomycin-resistant enterococci is high in the institution, a reasonable initial choice of antibiotics would be vancomycin plus cefepime.

MENINGITIS

The most probable organisms in patients with serious community-acquired meningitis are *S. pneumoniae, Neisseria meningitidis, Listeria monocytogenes, E. coli,* and *H. influenzae.* Initial treatment of meningitis should be guided by results of the cerebrospinal fluid examination, including examination of a gram stain of an ultracentrifuged specimen of cerebrospinal fluid, plus tests for antigens of *S. pneumoniae,* type B *H. influenzae,* and *N. meningitidis* in patients with purulent meningitis (see Chap. 52). Without a probable pathogen from initial microbiological studies of the cerebrospinal fluid, a reasonable initial treatment regimen for adults 18 to 50 years old would be a broad-spectrum cephalosporin. For patients older than 50 years or those with impaired cell-mediated immunity, ampicillin plus ceftazidime would be appropriate. Organisms that should be suspected in cases of nosocomial meningitis are *Pseudomonas aeruginosa, E. coli, Klebsiella* species, and *Staphylococcal* species. A reasonable initial treatment in these cases would consist of cefepime or meropenem plus vancomycin.

LINE SEPSIS

Readily accessible, stable vascular access is a routine requirement in critically ill patients and chemotherapy recipients. The most common pathogens in patients with an infected line are coagulase-negative staphylococci, *S. aureus,* aerobic gram-negative bacilli, and *Candida albicans*[130] (see Chap. 50). Infections of these devices are a major cause of morbidity and mortality in the United States. In a meta-analysis of 2573 cases of line sepsis, Byers et al reported an overall case fatality rate of 14%.[131] Of the various pathogens, *S. aureus* and *S. epidermidis* had the highest and lowest attributable mortality rates, respectively.

Management varies by the type of catheter. In most cases, infected, non-tunneled catheters should be removed and replaced. The decision to replace a tunneled catheter or implanted device is based on documentation that the device is infected, the type of pathogen, and the presence of complications such as septic thrombosis, metastatic infection, or tunnel infection. Until the susceptibility is known, staphylococcal strains should be treated with vancomycin. If the isolate is susceptible to β-lactams, a semi-synthetic penicillin such as nafcillin should be used. Patients who are allergic to penicillin and lack a history of anaphylaxis or angioedema can be treated with a first-generation cephalosporin such as cefazolin; 90% of patients treated in this fashion will not have an allergic response.[130] Empirical antibiotic therapy for patients with gram-negative line sepsis should include drugs active against *P. aeruginosa.* Patients with severe sepsis due to systemic candidiasis have several options, including amphotericin B, fluconazole, voriconazole, and caspofungin. Often patients at high risk of *Candida* species infection and no positive cultures will be treated with presumptive therapy if they are doing poorly on a well-chosen antibiotic regimen.

Specific Antisepsis Interventions

Despite early institution of appropriate antibiotics and organ support measures, 28% to 50% or more of patients with severe sepsis die. This has stimulated basic scientists and clinical investigators to seek and develop unique compounds that can serve as specific antisepsis interventions (Table 46-9). As with any new intervention, however, an evidence-based approach should be taken to ascertain whether the data, in aggregate, are sufficient to change clinical practice.[132] The analysis should include the quality of the evidence, magnitude of treatment effect, precision of treatment effect, magnitude of hazards, cost-benefit analysis, and various intangibles.

The magnitude of treatment effect can be expressed as absolute risk reduction (ARR), relative risk reduction, or NNT. The NNT represents the number of patients who must be treated with a specific intervention to prevent one adverse outcome or to attain one additional benefit. Clinicians can use the NNT, calculated as the reciprocal of the ARR, or 1/ARR, as a tool to guide them in reaching rational therapeutic decisions. Although there are few large-scale, randomized, placebo-controlled trials of specific antisepsis interventions to use as comparators, information from a large database of interventional trials in clinical cardiology has provided measures of the NNT in various medically accepted interventions. Thrombolytic therapy, for example, provides a survival benefit for patients with acute myocardial infarction. An analysis of nine randomized, placebo-controlled trials, each with 1000 patients or more with suspected acute myocardial infarction, demonstrated that thrombolytic therapy saved one life for every 55 patients treated (NNT = 55).[133] In the Thrombolysis in Myocardial Infarction 11B trial of patients with unstable angina pectoris or non–Q-wave myocardial infarction, enoxaparin prevented one composite end point (death, nonfatal myocardial infarction, or severe recurrent ischemia requiring urgent revascularization), compared with unfractionated heparin, for every 40 patients treated (NNT = 40).[134] Clinicians can use the NNT as a yardstick to make a relative comparison among the various interventions described below.

TABLE 46-9 Past, Present, and Potential Future Antisepsis Interventions

Specific Intervention	Established	Probable	Undetermined	Probably Negative	Negative
Source control	×				
Antibiotics	×				
Organ support	×				
Drotrecogin alfa (activated)	×				
Replacement dose steroids		×			
Tifacogin				×	
Antithrombin				×	
Heparin			×		
Inhibitor of activated coagulation factor VII			×		
Soluble thrombomodulin			×		
Anti–tumor necrosis factor			×		
Vagus nerve stimulation			×		
Poly(adenosine 5'-diphosphate-ribose) synthase inhibition			×		
Anti-C5a			×		
Interleukin 1 receptor antagonist					×
Prostaglandin inhibitors					×
Anti-endotoxin					×
Bacterial permeability increasing protein					×
Anti–interleukin 1					×
Nitric oxide antagonists					×
Platelet activating factor acetyl-hydrolase				×	
Bradykinin receptor antagonists					×

ACTIVATED PROTEIN C

PC is a vitamin K–dependent protein that circulates in the blood as an inactive precursor. Conversion of PC to APC requires thrombin and TM. Once thrombin is bound to endothelial cell TM, the serine protease undergoes a conformational alteration that shifts the substrate specificity of thrombin from fibrinogen to PC. Activation of PC is accelerated by the presence of the EPCR in concert with its plasma cofactor, protein S. APC modulates endothelial cell function, an effect whose phenotypic manifestations include antithrombotic, profibrinolytic, and anti-inflammatory properties.[135] Physiologically, APC limits coagulation and restores endogenous fibrinolytic activity by (1) inactivating coagulation factors Va and VIIIa, (2) inhibiting release of plasminogen activator inhibitor 1, and (3) downregulating activation of TAFI by thrombin. The anti-inflammatory activity of APC results from downregulation of thrombin-induced inflammation, modulation of nuclear factor κB activity, and inhibition of TNFα and macrophage migration inhibitory factor production in monocytes.[136,137] Experimentally, APC also blocked the accumulation of leukocytes at inflammatory foci by inhibiting the ability of leukocytes to bind to endothelial cell selectins.[138] In another experimental model, the activated molecule also blocked p53-mediated endothelial cell apoptosis, an effect that contributes to its neuroprotective activity in ischemic human brain tissue and may help explain its antisepsis activity.[139] In a baboon model, an infusion of *E. coli* at a concentration of 4.0×10^{10} organisms/kg produced septic shock, decreased concentrations of PC, fibrinogen, and platelets, and induced death within 24 to 36 hours.[140] These outcomes can be prevented when plasma-derived APC is added to the *E. coli* infusion. If activation of PC is prevented by preinfusion administration of antibody to PC, shock develops more rapidly, the coagulopathy is worse, and the animals die more quickly. Im-

portantly, the levels of endogenous PC in the experimental animals remained within normal limits during the experiment. These preclinical data suggested that APC had the potential to protect against the morbidity and mortality of severe sepsis.

Low levels of PC are present in more than 85% of patients with severe sepsis.[141] Levels of endogenous PC decrease before the appearance of the clinical signs and symptoms of sepsis with acute organ dysfunction. In a population of cancer patients with chemotherapy-induced neutropenia, Mesters et al determined that the concentrations of PC decreased 16 hours before a diagnosis of severe sepsis could be made.[142] In a review of published experimental and clinical studies, Yan et al reported that the lower levels of PC in patients with sepsis occurred in the absence of appreciable conversion to APC. The safety and efficacy of a range of doses of drotrecogin alfa (activated), a recombinant form of human APC, were tested by Bernard et al in a double-blind, randomized, placebo-controlled, multicenter, dose-ranging (sequential), phase II clinical trial of 139 adult patients with severe sepsis.[141] The investigators demonstrated that the drug was safe and well tolerated and that it produced a significant dose-dependent reduction in D-dimer and IL-6, markers of coagulopathy and inflammation, respectively. Because the endothelium is the largest organ in the body and a component of all other organ systems, the ability of infused recombinant human APC to protect endothelial cells may explain the drug's ability to improve outcomes in patients with MODS.

In the phase III randomized, double-blind, placebo-controlled, multicenter, international Protein C Worldwide Evaluation in Severe Sepsis (PROWESS) trial of 1690 patients, treatment with drotrecogin alfa (activated) produced significant relative and absolute reductions of 19.4% and 6.1%, respectively, in the risk of death ($p = 0.005$).[143] The NNT with drotrecogin alfa (activated) to save a life in the PROWESS trial was 16. Patients treated with the drug showed a trend

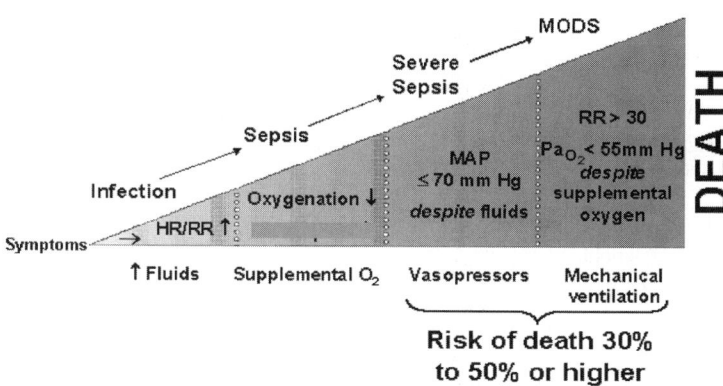

FIGURE 46-4 Sepsis continuum: identifying patients at high risk of death. HR, heart rate; MAP, mean arterial pressure; MODS, multiple organ dysfunction syndrome; Pa_{O_2}, arterial partial pressure of O_2; RR, respiratory rate. *(Reproduced with permission from the National Initiative in Sepsis Education.)*

toward a higher incidence of serious bleeding (3.5% versus 2.0%; $p = 0.06$). In patients at higher risk of death, as stratified by APACHE II scores, the ARR of death was 13% and the NNT was eight. In addition, the benefits of drotrecogin alfa (activated) persisted after discharge. In a cross-sectional observational study of the PROWESS cohort followed for up to 3.6 years, Angus et al reported that patients who were treated with the drug had an increased median survival of 9 months compared with placebo; these persistent benefits were greatest in patients with the most severe disease.[144] In those who have a reasonable life expectancy if they survive the episode, targeting drotrecogin alfa (activated) to the most severely ill patients with severe sepsis has been found to be cost effective according to societal standards.[144,145] Drotrecogin alfa (activated) therapy has recently been approved for inclusion in the hospital prospective payment system and for reimbursement under Section 533 of the Medicare Benefits Improvement and Protection Act of 2000.

IDENTIFYING CANDIDATES FOR DROTRECOGIN ALFA (ACTIVATED) THERAPY

As the first approved therapy specifically for patients with severe sepsis, drotrecogin alfa (activated) has been subjected to intensive evaluations to help determine the ideal candidates and to assess the drug's risk:benefit profile. Drotrecogin alfa (activated) is currently indicated for patients with severe sepsis at high risk of death who are felt to be candidates for aggressive care and lack contraindications for anticoagulation (Fig. 46-4).

In the PROWESS trial, mortality rates in nearly all of the prospectively defined subgroups were lower in the group that received drotrecogin alfa (activated) than in the group that received placebo infusion. However, analysis of the data from the PROWESS trial showed that the greater the baseline predicted risk of death (e.g., APACHE II score ≥ 25 or sepsis-induced organ dysfunction in two or more vital systems), the greater the ARR in mortality rate.[146] At this time, patients with the greatest likelihood of benefit are those who fulfill the following three criteria: (1) severe sepsis with vasopressor dependence and/or requiring mechanical ventilation; (2) no active bleeding, platelet count above $30,000/\mu L$, and international normalized ratio (INR) below 3.0, and no identifiable risks of central nervous system bleeding; and (3) the patient/family and medical team approve of an aggressive approach to management of sepsis in the patient, with a reasonable baseline quality of life to return to after the patient's

stay in the ICU. A useful treatment algorithm is provided in Figure 46-5.

Vasopressor dependence can be defined as a systolic BP of 90 mm Hg or lower or a MAP 70 mm Hg or lower despite aggressive fluid resuscitation to maintain adequate intravascular volume status. In the PROWESS trial, the mortality rate of patients treated with conventional therapy with an APACHE II score of 25 or higher was 25%. In this same group, the mortality rate of vasopressor-dependent patients was 32%. As a consequence, vasodepressor dependence is used by some as a surrogate for APACHE II scores of at least 25 (i.e., high risk of death). In the PROWESS trial, patients treated with drotrecogin alfa (activated) had significantly higher MAP by day 5 ($p = 0.01$) and were able to achieve a MAP above 70 mm Hg without vasopressor support over days 1 through 7 more rapidly compared with controls ($p = 0.01$).[147] Likewise, patients with severe sepsis and significantly impaired oxygenation (e.g., respiratory rate > 30 breaths/min, Pa_{O_2} < 55 mm Hg) are at high risk of death. In the PROWESS trial, treatment with drotrecogin alfa (activated) resulted in significantly improved oxygenation by day 7 ($p = 0.01$) and enabled recipients to achieve Pa_{O_2}/F_{IO_2} ratios greater than 400 without ventilator support significantly faster over days 1 through 7 ($p = 0.009$).

In the PROWESS trial, the rate of serious bleeding events attributable to drotrecogin alfa (activated) during drug infusion

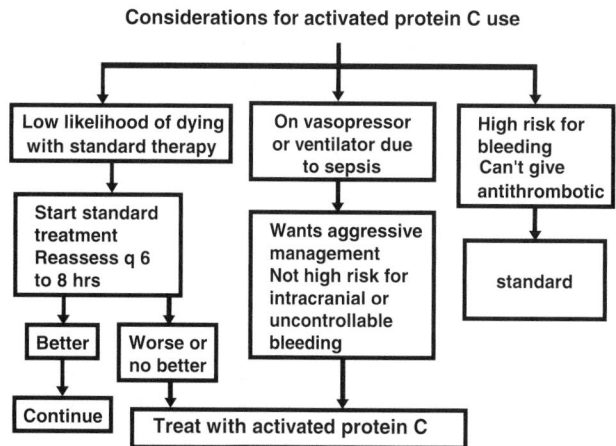

FIGURE 46-5 Algorithm for activated protein C use. *(Adapted with permission from Lawson WE, Ely EW: Managing severe sepsis with activated protein C: Reaping the benefits requires careful patient selection. J Respir Dis 24:384, 2003.)*

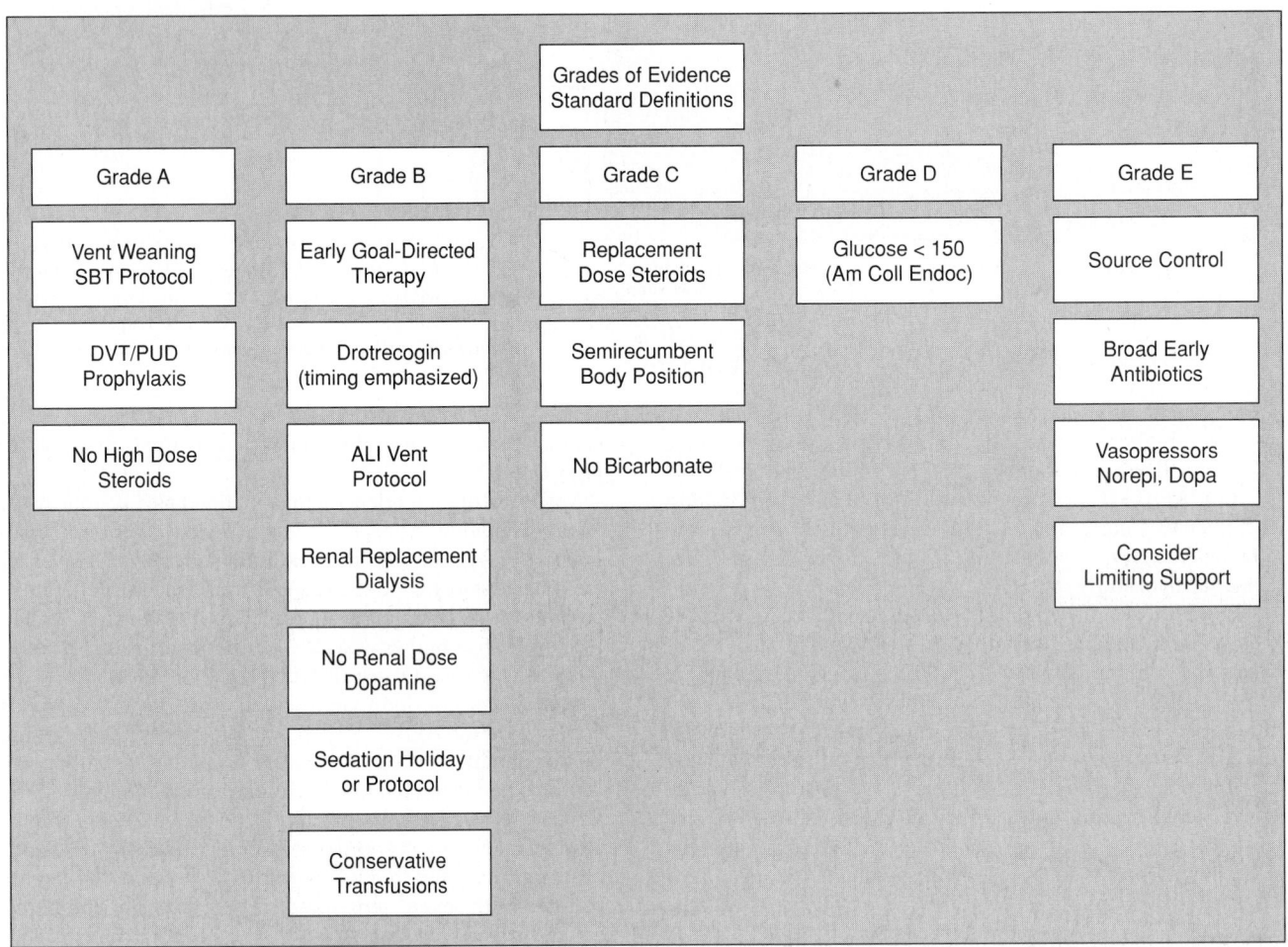

FIGURE 46-6 Surviving sepsis guidelines by grade of recommendation. From Dellinger RP, et al: Surviving Sepsis Campaign guidelines for management of severe sepsis and septic shock. *Crit Care Med* **32:858, 2004.**

was 1.5%. Most serious bleeding events in the population treated with drotrecogin alfa (activated) occurred in patients with predisposing factors such as GI ulceration, traumatic injury of a blood vessel or a highly vascular organ, or markedly abnormal tests of coagulation. Notably, the presence of material in a nasogastric aspirate that tests positive for heme (e.g., guaiac test) in the absence of overt bleeding should not be considered a contraindication to treatment with drotrecogin alfa (activated). Drotrecogin alfa (activated) therapy should be used with caution in patients with markedly abnormal hemostasis (e.g., platelet count <30,000/μL). An INR above 3.0 is also used as a relative guide; in patients with INRs above this level, the benefits must be carefully weighed against the risks. The potential for intracranial hemorrhage (ICH) represents the most important complication warranting screening. In a review of approximately 3000 patients, the ICH rate was 0.5%; in an ongoing open-label study, the incidence was 0.2%. This incidence should be viewed from the perspective of the placebo rate of ICH in other large-scale, randomized clinical trials of patients with severe sepsis. For example, in the trial of large-dose AT III in severe sepsis, the incidence of ICH in the control arm was 0.4%.[148]

In elderly patients, the cost:benefit ratio for drotrecogin alfa (activated) depends on the patient's potential to have a reasonable quality of life after recovery from the episode of severe sepsis. In general, age should not be used to stratify patients for potential life-saving interventions such as drotrecogin alfa (activated) therapy. In the Study to Understand Prognoses and Preferences for Outcomes and Risks of Treatments (SUPPORT), life support measures such as mechanical ventilation were withheld more often in patients older than 70 years, even after adjusting for severity of illness.[149] However, analysis of the ARDSNet data indicates that, despite a decreasing survival rate with advancing age, 50% of patients 80 years and older survived an episode of ARDS.[150] In the PROWESS trial, the ARR of drotrecogin alfa (activated) in patients 75 years and older was 15%, and the NNT to save a life was six to seven patients.[151] Importantly, this benefit was not accompanied by an increase in the risk of bleeding compared with that of the younger cohort. Although the pivotal study was conducted in a broad range of patients with severe sepsis, the data clearly showed that drotrecogin alfa (activated) produces the greater absolute benefit in those patients with high risk of death. Because a mortality benefit was not demonstrated in PROWESS for patients with a lower severity of illness (using APACHE II scores) and potential for harm could exist in those not likely to benefit, these low-risk patients are currently being evaluated in an 11,000-patient randomized controlled trial.

Several trial design issues have been raised and answered about PROWESS that may have limited its early adoption.[152] These include concerns regarding mid-trial changes to the study protocol and drug preparation, high acquisition costs, and bleeding.[153] The U.S. Food and Drug Administration (FDA) and the principal investigators of the trial have addressed these issues with firm conclusions: (1) large-scale clinical trials are routinely amended, and analysis of PROWESS by the FDA does not support the belief that changes in the protocol or drug were responsible for the outcomes; and (2) the greatest benefits of drotrecogin alfa (activated) are in the most severely ill patients.[154,155] In acknowledging the benefits seen in the most severely ill, the FDA indication specifies that the drug should be prescribed to patients with severe sepsis at high risk of death. In addition, the FDA requested that the manufacturer provide additional clinical trial data on the use of drotrecogin alfa (activated) in patients with severe sepsis at lower risk of death; trials in such low-risk patients are ongoing.

ADMINISTRATION AND MONITORING OF DROTRECOGIN ALFA (ACTIVATED)

Once a decision has been made to treat a patient with drotrecogin alfa (activated), the infusion should be started immediately. Although there was no indication from the clinical trials to indicate that watchful waiting is harmful within the 48-hour window after the development of sepsis-induced organ failure, it would seem prudent to treat a patient with severe sepsis at high risk of death earlier rather than later. This is supported by analysis of data from the ENHANCE trial. Patients treated with Drotrecogin alfa (activated) within the first twenty-four hours had a lower 28-day mortality by degree of organ dysfunction before treatment ($P = 0.014$) and by time to treatment stratified by APACHE II quartile. Patients treated within the first twenty-four hours also had significantly fewer days on the ventilator and lower ICU and hospital lengths of stay ($P < 0.004$). Treatment consists of an infusion of 24 μg/kg per hour of drotrecogin alfa (activated) for a total infusion duration of 96 hours. The dosage is based on the patient's actual body weight rather than ideal body weight. There is no need to monitor the infusion with tests of hemostasis or levels of PC or APC. In the event of clinically significant bleeding, the infusion should be stopped immediately. Drotrecogin alfa (activated) is rapidly cleared by plasma proteases, including PC inhibitor and α_1 antitrypsin: 80% is eliminated within 13 minutes and 98% is cleared within 2 hours. If the nature and severity of bleeding has been clarified and appropriate actions have been successfully taken, the drug infusion may be resumed for the remainder of the total 96-hour duration as long as the management team feels that treatment with an antithrombotic is now safe.

The increased rate of bleeding in patients treated with drotrecogin alfa (activated) is usually related to procedure and predominantly develops during the time of drug infusion. Because of its short half-life, there is no significant residual drug effect if the infusion is temporarily interrupted 2 hours before any surgical procedure. The decision as to when to restart the infusion should be based on the nature of the procedure and assessment of the patient.[156] For minor procedures such as tracheostomy or change or placement of an arterial line or a femoral venous catheter, the drotrecogin alfa (activated) infusion can be restarted immediately thereafter

if there is no sign of bleeding. In the absence of bleeding or complications, the drug infusion can be restarted 2 hours after procedures such as placement of a Swan-Ganz catheter or placement of a chest tube. The 2-hour postprocedure interval before the infusion is resumed is also reasonable for patients undergoing lumbar puncture, percutaneous drainage, nephrostomy, or sinus puncture. In the absence of bleeding, the infusion can be restarted after 12 hours in patients undergoing major surgical procedures or removal of an epidural catheter. Once the infusion is restarted, the drug should be administered so that the patient continues to receive the calculated amount for the full 96-hour duration. No attempt should be made to accelerate or "catch-up" and bolus infusions are contraindicated.

Investigational Natural Anticoagulants

Hemostatic abnormalities are common in patients with severe sepsis.[157] In addition to APC, the body has a number of other natural antithrombotics that have the potential to improve outcomes in patients with severe sepsis. These include AT, TF pathway inhibitor (TFPI), and endothelial cell glycosaminoglycans.

ANTITHROMBIN

AT III is a serine protease that is a slow, progressive inhibitor of thrombin and factor Xa; binding of heparin to a lysine site on the AT protein produces a conformational change in the molecule that converts it to a rapid inactivator of thrombin and factors Xa, IXa, XIa, and XIIa.[158] Experimentally, AT III supplementation has been shown to decrease inflammatory changes associated with severe sepsis.[159] Based on experimental and early clinical studies, Warren et al evaluated the safety and efficacy of AT III in a double-blind, placebo-controlled, multicenter study of 2314 adult patients with severe sepsis.[148] At 28 days, overall mortality rates were 38.9% in the treated group and 38.7% in the placebo group ($p = 0.94$). Study subjects who received AT III had a relative risk of bleeding greater than 1.7. Studies of this natural antithrombotic for the treatment of severe sepsis have been discontinued.

TISSUE FACTOR PATHWAY INHIBITOR

TFPI is a Kunitz-type inhibitor; after binding and inactivating factor Xa, TFPI then inhibits factor VIIa within the factor VIIa/TF complex.[160] Circulating TFPI has been shown to modulate the activity of the extrinsic pathway. Experimentally, TFPI inhibits LPS-induced pulmonary edema and tissue damage.[161] These features suggest that recombinant human (rh) TFPI (tifacogin) therapy might decrease the coagulopathy and inflammatory changes of severe sepsis in a fashion similar to that of rhAPC. Because the proposed benefits of tifacogin would be anticipated to be through stabilization of coagulation, trials of the drug have focused on patients with a mild coagulopathy (INR $\geq$ 1.2). Although a phase II trial showed a trend toward reduction in the 28-day all-cause mortality rate in the rhTFPI group compared with placebo, the phase III OPTIMIST (Optimized Phase III Tifacogin in Multicenter International Sepsis Trial) study failed to show a mortality benefit.[162,163] Overall mortality rate at 28 days in the group treated with tifacogin ($n = 880$) was 34.2% versus 33.9% in the placebo group ($n = 874$), a difference that did not reach statistical significance ($p = 0.88$). In addition, there was an increase in serious adverse events for bleeding in the treatment group; this difference was irrespective of the patients' INR. A second phase III study of TFPI is now being conducted to determine if a higher dose of the drug will produce a survival advantage.

GLYCOSAMINOGLYCANS

Endothelial cells have important anticoagulant systems, including the heparan sulfate-AT system. Heparan sulfate is an endothelial cell glycosaminoglycan similar in structure and pharmacodynamic properties to heparin. By interacting with endothelial cell surface heparan sulfate, endogenous AT III stimulates prostacyclin generation and inhibits cytokine and TF production in endothelial cells and monocytes.[164] It may also be involved in the AT III–associated desensitization of leukocyte chemoattractant receptors. Ahmed et al demonstrated that heparin also possesses clinically significant anti-inflammatory properties that are independent of AT III.[165] They showed that inhaled enoxaparin can produce a dose-dependent, statistically significant inhibition of exercise-induced bronchoconstriction independent of the drug's anti–factor Xa activity. In a hypothesis-generating exercise, Davidson et al reported that their analysis of the PROWESS and AT III trials suggests that administration of small-dose heparin to enrollees in the two trials is associated with a 45% (95% confidence interval = 1.18 to 1.78; $p < 0.001$) improvement in the odds for survival among the placebo recipients compared with those who did not receive heparin.[166] Similar observations have been made about a heparin effect in the trials of other natural anticoagulants. In the AT trial, mortality rate was lower in the placebo group who received heparin.[148] In the OPTIMIST trial, mortality rate was lower in patients receiving placebo and heparin than in those who did not.[163] Heparin's potential anti-inflammatory and antileukoadhesive properties were investigated in a human endotoxemia model by Derhaschnig et al.[167] They showed that, although the drug displayed little effect on cytokine production and endothelial cell activation in endotoxemia, it downregulated expression of L-selectin and produced lymphocytopenia. As intriguing as these observations are, experimental studies in a sepsis model reported that heparin does not prevent ALI produced by smoke inhalation.[168] Thus, the clinical relevance of heparin's anti-inflammatory properties is unclear and requires further studies.

OTHER AGENTS

Several experimental approaches are underway to investigate other hemostasis-related agents for the treatment of patients with severe sepsis. They include soluble TM (sTM), an inhibitor of activated coagulation factor VII (rhFVIIa), and PAF inhibitor. TM is an endothelial cell protein that alters thrombin's substrate specificity from fibrinogen to PC, thereby converting PC to APC. Studies have indicated that endotoxin and proinflammatory cytokines such as TNFα decrease endothelial cell TM expression. This may be a consequence of downregulation of TM expression, increased degradation of the protein, or some combination thereof. When coupled with a glycosaminoglycan moiety, a soluble form of TM can block

the fibrin formation and cell activation, convert PC to APC, and promote thrombin inhibition by AT III and heparin cofactor II.[169] These properties suggest that sTM might be useful in sepsis. In an experimental model, rh-sTM blocked endotoxin-induced disseminated intravascular coagulation (DIC) and pulmonary vascular injury.[170,171] Although rh-sTM has been shown to be safe in normal human volunteers, no clinical trials have been published describing its efficacy in patients with severe sepsis.[172]

Upregulation of TF on monocytes and perhaps endothelial cells is a significant element in the evolution of severe sepsis. Although clinical trials of TFPI failed to demonstrate a survival benefit, the extrinsic pathway of coagulation remains an attractive target. Active site-inhibited rhFVIIa can act as a competitive inhibitor of factor VIIa generated during activation of coagulation. Welty-Wolf et al and Carraway et al demonstrated in a primate model that rhFVIIa can prevent sepsis-induced pulmonary and renal dysfunction and attenuate organ damage in established sepsis.[173,174] However, Jilma et al reported that, although rhFVIIa was an effective inhibitor of TF-induced thrombin generation, it did not alter endotoxin-induced changes in fibrinolysis, cytokine release, or markers of endothelial cell or platelet activation.[175] Studies of this drug are ongoing.

During the systemic inflammatory response to infection, phospholipase A$_2$ is released. This enzyme catalyzes conversion of cell membrane phospholipids to PAF and arachidonic acid. It has been hypothesized that a phospholipase A$_2$ inhibitor administered within the first 18 hours of sepsis-induced organ failure may improve survival rate. However, a recent multicenter, double-blind, placebo-controlled trial of 14-kd group IIA secretory phospholipase A$_2$ inhibitor failed to provide evidence that this approach offers a survival benefit.[176]

PAF acts as a signaling molecule that can trigger and amplify inflammatory and coagulation signals.[177] Levels of PAF are increased in patients with severe sepsis and there is evidence that PAF signaling is defective. Human recombinant PAF-acetyl-hydrolase inhibits monocyte/macrophage and neutrophil activation in response to inflammation. In patients at risk for multiple organ dysfunction syndrome, rhPAF-acetyl-hydrolase was safe and improved organ scores.[178] However, a phase II clinical trial failed to demonstrate benefits of this drug compared with placebo on survival rate, hemodynamic status, respiratory function, or organ failure scores.[179]

The results of these studies raise an interesting issue: with the demonstrated efficacy of drotrecogin alfa (activated) and preclinical data that support the use of other natural antithrombotics in patients with severe sepsis, why have the results of the clinical studies of these compounds been so disappointing? The answers to these questions are unknown but several possibilities exist. Recombinant human APC has multiple mechanisms of action that may be additive to its antithrombotic properties. These include several anti-inflammatory, profibrinolytic, and endothelial cell survival properties. Other issues may be related to trial design. In the trials of AT III and TFPI, the lack of overall benefit may have been related to the dose, the ability of thromboprophylactic doses of heparin to block the drug's anti-inflammatory effect, or the concept. For example, the continuous infusion of AT III may have been insufficient to maintain supraphysiologic levels of AT III in severely septic patients. Because AT III must bind to endothelial cell and neutrophil glycosaminoglycans to promote local anticoagulant and anti-inflammatory activities, prophylactic heparin administered to some patients may have prevented the infused drug from significantly binding to its target on endothelial cells.

Replacement-Dose Steroids (see Chap. 79)

Cortisol is the predominant glucocorticoid secreted by the adrenal cortex. During acute illness, cortisol production increases as much as sixfold, an increase that is roughly proportional to the severity of the illness.[180] Increased cortisol levels in acutely ill patients are a result of a combination of increased production of CRH and ACTH plus a reduction in the degree of cortisol-mediated feedback inhibition. Other factors that may contribute to the adrenal cortical stress response include loss of the normal diurnal secretory pattern, increased levels of free cortisol resulting from a combination of a decrease in the levels of cortisol-binding globulin and cleavage of cortisol-binding globulin by neutrophil elastase, plus inflammatory cytokine-mediated alterations in peripheral cortisol metabolism and changes in the affinity of cellular glucocorticoid receptors for their ligand.

There are several potential mechanisms of action that suggest that glucocorticoid therapy might be beneficial in patients with severe sepsis: (1) correction of a state of relative adrenal insufficiency, (2) inhibition of the synthesis of iNOS, (3) improved hemodynamics secondary to restoration of the sensitivity of vascular catecholamine receptors, and (4) liberation of bound IκB-a with decreased transcription of inflammatory cytokines and increased synthesis and release of the receptor antagonist for IL-1.[181,182]

Megadose steroid therapy for patients with severe sepsis was abandoned in the late 1980s when it failed to improve mortality rate.[183] However, in 1998, Bollaert et al reported the results of a prospective, randomized, double-blind, placebo-controlled study of small doses of hydrocortisone (100 mg intravenously, three times daily for 5 days) on hemodynamics and survival.[184] After 28 days, patients treated with glucocorticoids demonstrated a significant ability to reverse the hemodynamic alterations of shock ($p = 0.005$) and had a 31% reduction in mortality rate (32% versus 63%; 95% confidence interval = 1% to 61%; $p = 0.091$). Because there was no correlation between the outcomes and the results of a short corticotropin test, the investigators commented that the results do not appear to be related to the presence of adrenal cortical insufficiency. However, in 2000, Annane et al described a three-level prognostic classification for septic shock based on cortisol levels and response to a short corticotropin stimulation test.[185]

In a follow-up placebo-controlled, randomized, double-blind, parallel-group trial, Annane et al reported the effect of hydrocortisone and fludrocortisone on mortality rate in 300 medical and surgical patients with severe sepsis.[186] Other eligibility criteria included mechanical ventilation, hypotension unresponsive to fluids, and dysfunction of other organ systems characteristic of severe sepsis. Patients who fulfilled the usual criteria for septic shock were enrolled after undergoing a short ACTH stimulation test. Steroid therapy consisted of 200 mg of hydrocortisone (50 mg at 6-hour intervals) and a single 50-μg dose of fludrocortisone daily for 7 days. In patients characterized on the basis of the short ACTH stimulation test as having relative adrenal insufficiency (i.e., nonresponders), steroid therapy significantly decreased mortality rate and the duration of vasopressor therapy. Steroid treatment of the nonresponder population produced 16% and 10% relative and absolute reductions, respectively, in the risk of 28-day mortality ($p = 0.04$). Further, steroid treatment of this subpopulation improved hemodynamics and enabled the investigators to wean patients from vasopressors 3 days earlier than placebo-treated controls. The contribution of the administered mineralocorticoid to the outcomes is unclear. Adverse events potentially associated with steroids such as superinfection, GI bleeding, and psychiatric disorders did not increase in the treatment group.

IDENTIFYING CANDIDATES FOR LOW-DOSE STEROID THERAPY

As opposed to absolute adrenal insufficiency, which is relatively uncommon in patients with severe sepsis, evidence of inadequate adrenal reserves is common. Annane et al reported that evidence of an inability of the adrenal cortex to respond to ACTH-releasing hormone (nonresponders) was present in approximately 66% of patients with severe sepsis in their study.[186] This observation coupled with the results of the study and the ready availability of glucocorticoids and mineralocorticoids provide preliminary support for low-dose steroids in appropriate patients with severe sepsis. Notably, however, steroids did not provide uniform benefits in all subgroups: in patients with normal adrenal function (i.e., responders to ACTH stimulation), administration of low doses of hydrocortisone plus fludrocortisone was associated with increased mortality rate (61% versus 53%; $p = $ not significant). Although the results were not statistically significant, when combined with previous studies indicating that steroids can have adverse effects in patients with severe sepsis, the possibility was raised that steroid therapy may be detrimental to patients in this population with adequate adrenal reserve.[187] Because the number of patients in this study was small and demonstrated interesting results, an ongoing large European trial is evaluating this intervention.

ADMINISTRATION AND MONITORING OF LOW-DOSE STEROID THERAPY

In patients with severe sepsis at high risk of death, it is reasonable to administer combination glucocorticoid/mineralocorticoid therapy with the 7-day protocol described by Annane et al.[186] Therapy should begin immediately after a short ACTH stimulation test (ACTH 250 μg [one vial of Cosyntropin] intravenously or intramuscularly with a serum cortisol level 45 to 60 minutes later). Once the results become available, steroids can be discontinued in patients whose baseline serum cortisol is increased by 10 μg/dL or greater (i.e., responders). Nonresponders, patients with a change in their serum cortisol levels of 9 μg/dL or less, can continue to receive low-dose steroids for the full 7-day period. The significance of the level of serum total cholesterol in patients with sepsis is unclear since values fall with the development of critical illness-associated hypoproteinemia. Serum free cholesterol may more accurately reflect adrenal function. Consequently, some patients may be selected for low-dose steroid therapy unnecessarily. There is no evidence that steroids and drotrecogin alfa (activated) are competitive therapies. Patients in the PROWESS trial received the best therapy as determined by their treating physicians; in many cases, this included steroids plus drotrecogin alfa (activated) or placebo. In an editorial accompanying the low-dose steroid trial, Abraham et al pointed out that more than 50% of the patients with inadequate adrenal reserve died despite treatment.[187] They emphasized that this observation underscores the need for additional therapies that can reverse organ dysfunction and improve outcomes in this population.

Other Investigational Approaches

TUMOR NECROSIS FACTOR ANTAGONISTS

TNFα is thought to play a major role in the pathogenesis of the clinical manifestations of patients with severe sepsis. Evidence supporting the cytokine's central role in the process includes: (1) experimentally, TNFα levels increase after an endotoxin or a bacterial challenge; (2) increased levels of TNFα can be demonstrated in preclinical models and patients with sepsis; (3) presence of increased levels in patients with the disease and persistent high concentrations are associated with nonsurvival; (4) TNFα challenge simulates manifestations of sepsis and can lead to organ dysfunction; and (5) neutralization of TNFα frequently leads to a decrease in sepsis-associated symptoms and increases survival rate in experimental models.[188] Compounds designed to test the efficacy of TNF antagonists can be divided into two broad groups: (1) monoclonal antibodies against human TNFα (e.g., afelimomab, CDP571) and (2) soluble TNFα receptors (e.g., p55-IgG). Studies of these compounds have indicated that they may produce small survival benefits in some subgroups of patients with severe sepsis.[188,189] Future studies of these agents require methods to better indicate patients who might benefit from the drugs and multimodal therapy that also includes TNFα neutralization.

OTHER POTENTIAL STRATEGIES

The autonomic nervous system plays a major role in the pathophysiology of severe sepsis. Studies have shown that electrical stimulation of the vagus nerve attenuates the release of TNF and other cytokines in response to endotoxin and can prevent the development of shock.[80] At a molecular level, strategies to neutralize macrophage migration, block apoptosis, or inhibit the activity of poly(adenosine 5'-diphosphate-ribose) synthase can also provide protection against the effects of severe sepsis.[190–192] Activation of the classic or alternate pathway of complement generates C5 convertase. This enzyme converts C5 to C5a and C5b. In the presence of C6, C7, and C8, C5b forms the membrane attack complex responsible for complement's lytic activity. In contrast, C5a is a proinflammatory peptide also known as anaphylatoxin. Antibodies to the C5a peptide decrease bacteremia, inhibit apoptosis, and improve survival in experimental models of sepsis.[193–195]

General Supportive Measures

NUTRITIONAL SUPPORT AND GLYCEMIC CONTROL

IMPORTANCE OF ADEQUATE NUTRITION
Severe sepsis is a catabolic state. Metabolic changes associated with the disease include rapid breakdown of proteins, carbohydrates, and lipids, protein diversion, negative nitrogen balance, hyperglycemia with insulin resistance, and altered blood flow to key metabolic sites. As with any other critically ill population, patients with severe sepsis require adequate nutritional support to correct any previous nutritional deficiencies, maintain organ system structure and function, compensate for anticipated or existent inadequate self-feeding, improve wound healing, promote immune function, decrease susceptibility to superinfection, and increase survival rate (see Chap. 11).

Energy needs can be calculated by determining the patient's basal energy expenditure from the patient's weight, height, and age inserted into the Harris-Benedict equation.[196] The weight inserted into the equation should be based on clinical evaluation. Although it is reasonable to use the ideal body weight for obese patients, the pre-illness weight can be used for those patients whose weight has been stable before hospital admission. In most instances, the basal energy expenditure will be approximately 25 to 30 kcal/kg per day; however, due to the catabolic nature of severe sepsis, which seems to reach its maximum during the second week, the basal energy expenditure may be multiplied by a stress factor of 0.5 to 2.5.[197,198] The normal protein requirements for a well-nourished individual are 0.6 to 1.0 g/kg per day.[199] In contrast, patients with severe sepsis may require up to 2.0 g/kg per day. Glutamine and arginine supplementation may improve outcomes.[200,201] Glucose should consist of 30% to 70% of the total nonprotein calories to maintain blood glucose within an acceptable range (see below). Lipids should comprise 15% to 30% of nonprotein calories. The ω-6 polyunsaturated fatty acid content of nutritional support for a septic patient should be decreased while maintaining a level that will prevent a deficiency of essential fatty acids. The ω-3 fatty acids are important for cell membrane integrity, receptor expression and function, and activation and signal transduction. Enteral preparations supplemented with these important lipids are available.

ENTERAL VERSUS PARENTERAL NUTRITION
Enteral nutrition offers several advantages including lower cost, preservation of the GI mucosal barrier, buffering of gastric acid, preservation of enteral hormone secretion, provision of unique nutrients, decreased incidence of infections, improved wound healing, and avoidance of parenteral nutritional catheters and their complications.[202] Immunomodulatory enteral preparations that are supplemented with arginine, nucleotides, and fish oil have been shown to improve outcomes in critically ill patients, although much work is needed in this area.[203,204] For septic patients who cannot tolerate enteral nutrition because of an ileus or other complications, parenteral nutrition is a consideration. Heyland et al conducted a meta-analysis of 26 randomized clinical trials of 2211 patients that compared morbidity and mortality rates in patients receiving enteral or total parenteral nutrition.[205] The mortality rate of critically ill patients was higher among those receiving TPN (RR, 1.78; 95% CI, 1.11–2.85). Notably, the

hypothesis that parenteral nutrition is superior to no nutrition during the acute episode has not been rigorously tested.

MANAGEMENT OF BLOOD GLUCOSE LEVELS

Stress-induced hyperglycemia (>200 mg/dL) is common in patients with severe sepsis. If doubt exists, it can be differentiated from chronic diabetic hyperglycemia by an assay of HbA_{1c} concentrations, values that will be within the normal range in a previously healthy patient. The etiology of this metabolic derangement in patients with severe sepsis is insulin resistance coupled with increased gluconeogenesis, abnormalities that can be compounded by excessive parenteral nutritional support. Insulin resistance is multifactorial in origin and can result from a combination of endotoxin, elevated levels of cytokines such as $TNF\alpha$, IL-1, and increased circulating concentrations of epinephrine, glucocorticoids, and growth hormone. The effects of cytokines and hormones on blood glucose levels result primarily from the development of insulin resistance in skeletal muscles.[206,207] Despite hyperglycemia, the liver is also resistant to the effects of insulin and is driven to gluconeogenesis by counterregulatory hormones such as glucagon, epinephrine, and growth hormone. An associated cause that may be overlooked in a critically ill patient is provision of excess parenteral glucose. Rosmarin et al reported that nondiabetic patients who received total parenteral nutrition in which dextrose was infused at rates greater than 4 mg/kg per minute had a 50% chance of developing hyperglycemia.[208]

The deleterious effects of hyperglycemia in patients with severe sepsis have been considered to be predominantly related to concerns about an increased risk of infection.[209] Although it is not completely clear whether secondary infections in critically ill patients with hyperglycemia is directly due to the elevated glucose or is another manifestation of latent or overt diabetes mellitus, evidence suggests that hyperglycemia directly impairs immune function.[210,211] Prolonged elevation of blood glucose may potentiate the coagulopathy of severe sepsis. Rao et al demonstrated that prolonged hyperglycemia activates the TF pathway of blood coagulation.[212] Activation of the extrinsic pathway of coagulation was independent of insulin levels, hypertriglyceridemia, and hyperosmolality. This was presumably due to activation of monocytes and/or endothelial cells, upregulation of TF expression, and enhanced conversion of factor VII to VIIa.[213]

Good glycemic control requires regular monitoring of the blood glucose and attention to parenteral nutrition and insulin therapy. However, the target blood glucose level has been unclear. For example, long-term outcomes are improved in patients with diabetes who have had a myocardial infarction if their blood glucose level is maintained at a level below 215 mg/dL or 11.9 mmol/L.[214,215] Recently, van den Berghe et al reported the results of a prospective, randomized controlled trial of more than 1500 mechanically ventilated surgical ICU patients treated with intensive versus conventional insulin therapy.[216] They reported that patients who were randomly assigned to intensive insulin therapy (target blood glucose = 80 to 110 mg/dL, or 4.4 to 6.1 mmol/L) or standard care (target blood glucose = 180 to 200 mg/dL, or 10 to 11.1 mmol/L) had significantly different outcomes. Tight glucose control produced the following advantages: (1) decreased overall ICU mortality rate (4.6% versus 8.0%); (2) decreased ICU mortality rate in patients admitted longer than 5 days

(10.6% versus 20.2%; $p = 0.005$); and (3) lower in-hospital mortality rate (7.2% versus 10.9%). Other benefits included a 46% relative reduction in bloodstream infections, a 41% decrease in the need for renal replacement therapy (RRT), a 50% decrease in the median number of red blood cell transfusions, and a 44% reduction in the incidence of critical-illness polyneuropathy. More than 97% of the patients in the tight-control group received intravenous insulin, compared with 33% in the control group. Episodes of hypoglycemia (glucose < 40 mg/dL, or 2.2 mmol/L) were more common in the intensive-control group (5.0% versus 0.7%); however, these episodes were not accompanied by hemodynamic instability or seizures. Although these findings need to be confirmed, they suggest that patients with severe sepsis should receive intensive insulin therapy to maintain their blood glucose levels between 80 and 110 mg/dL (4.4–6.1 mmol/L). Realistically, accomplishing tight glycemic control is often difficult. Many internists have adopted protocols that have adjusted glucose in the range of 100 to 140 mg/dL (5.6–7.8 mmol/L). A point of interest deserving future research is whether or not the benefits of this approach are due primarily to the lower glucose area under the curve or result from glucose-independent effects of insulin.[217] Recently, Finney et al evaluated the relation between glucose control and mortality rate in 523 critically ill patients.[218] They reported a positive association between increased insulin administration and death, independent of prevailing glucose level. They suggested that it is the control of glucose rather than absolute levels of exogenous insulin administered for glucose management that accounts for the mortality benefits of glycemic control. Further, regression analysis of their data suggests that the mortality benefit occurs at blood glucose levels below 145 mg/dL. If these data are supported by others, less stringent glycemic management may provide many of the benefits without intense resource utilization.

RENAL REPLACEMENT THERAPY

Transient oliguria is common in patients with severe sepsis and vasodilatory hypotension or shock. Notably, anuria is rare, and fewer than 5% of patients with severe sepsis develop acute renal failure requiring RRT.[89] Importantly, when it occurs, acute renal failure and its associated metabolic derangements increase the risk for potentially fatal extrarenal complications.[219,220] Therefore, steps should be taken to preserve renal function in the setting of severe sepsis. Important measures include adequate volume replacement, monitoring drug dosage and avoiding nephrotoxins, and excluding lower urinary tract obstruction as the cause for oliguria or anuria. There is no evidence that low-dose dopamine administered by continuous intravenous infusion can protect against renal dysfunction in the critically ill population.[221] If potential nephrotoxins such as aminoglycosides must be used, the dosage should be adjusted for the patient's degree of renal impairment, and drug levels should be monitored. In a patient with severe sepsis and acute renal failure, renal replacement therapy should be considered early in the disease course. In addition to providing renal replacement, continuous renal replacement therapy (CRRT) has become a part of the overall management of the critically ill.

In the ICU, peritoneal dialysis and conventional forms of hemodialysis have been superseded by various forms of

CRRT (see Chap. 75).[222] CRRT is better tolerated than other renal replacement therapies because solutes and fluids are removed in a slower fashion. The choice of a CRRT modality is based on a number of factors, including access to the equipment, experience of the staff, the degree of hemodynamic stability, vascular access, and whether the primary need is for fluid and/or solute removal. Detailed explanations of these interventions are beyond the scope of this chapter and are discussed elsewhere in the textbook.

In addition to removal of metabolic wastes, other indications for CRRT in patients with severe sepsis include establishing hemodynamic stability and providing more precise fluid and electrolyte control. Although cytokines can be found in the dialysate or ultrafiltrate of patients undergoing renal replacement, there is no evidence that cytokine removal by CRRT improves outcomes. CRRT can help to improve outcomes in patients with severe sepsis and ARDS. This potential benefit may be primarily the effect of extravascular lung water. However, the procedure can also be used to stabilize the pH of the blood in patients treated with permissive hypercapnia. Whereas benefits of CRRT are known, until recently the "dose" of CRRT has been unclear. Schiffl et al conducted a prospective study in 160 patients with acute renal failure to compare the effect of intensive (daily) HD with conventional (alternate-day) HD on mortality rate.[223] They found that daily HD reduces mortality rate without increasing hemodynamically induced morbidity compared with the alternate-day approach. Patients treated with intensive HD had better control of uremia, fewer hypotensive episodes during the procedure, and more rapid resolution of acute renal failure (mean $\pm$ SD $= 9 \pm 2$ days versus 16 ± 6 days; $p = 0.001$) than did those undergoing conventional HD. In an intention-to-treat analysis, the mortality rates were 28% for intensive HD and 46% for alternate-day dialysis ($p = 0.01$). In a multiple regression analysis, conventional (versus daily) HD was an independent risk factor for death. Currently, large-scale, multicenter trials are evaluating the effects of CRRT on survival rate in critically ill patients.

THROMBOPROPHYLAXIS

Patients with severe sepsis have at least one risk factor that places them at increased risk for venous thromboembolism (VTE). In addition to immobilization, they may have risk factors such as advanced age, recent trauma or surgery, respiratory failure, or the presence of a central venous access device. Serial scans with radiolabeled fibrinogen or ultrasonograms have indicated that approximately 30% of critically ill patients have evidence of VTE.[224,225] Importantly, VTE can occur even in patients receiving pharmacologic thromboprophylaxis. Thrombi are most common in the lower extremities, and most pulmonary emboli arise from veins in that region. The incidence of embolic events increases as the thrombus extends proximally to the popliteal fossae. Thrombi can also occur in the veins of the upper extremities; the presence of cancer or a central venous catheter increases the risk of VTE originating in this region.

All patients with severe sepsis should be assessed for VTE risk factors, and, in the absence of contraindications, they should receive pharmacologic thromboprophylaxis. Treatment can be with low-dose unfractionated heparin (UFH), adjusted-dose UFH, or low-molecular-weight heparin (LMWH). The most widely employed regimen is 5000 U of UFH administered subcutaneously, twice daily. Although LMWHs are more expensive, they offer several advantages over UFH. These include improved pharmacokinetics and negligible effects on standard tests of coagulation. The thromboprophylactic dose of a specific LMWH should be the one recommended by the manufacturer. In a meta-analysis, LMWH was demonstrated to provide at least equivalent prophylactic activity as UFH for the prevention of postoperative VTEs and was shown to be associated with less bleeding.[226] Fondaparinux is a chemically synthesized anticoagulant that possesses the critical pentasaccharide sequence responsible for the anti–factor Xa of UFH and LMWH. Its acquisition cost should be balanced with a safety and efficacy profile that is superior to LMWH for the reduction of VTE events demonstrated in patients undergoing major orthopedic surgery.[227,228] Treatment with thromboprophylactic doses of UFH or LMWH is not contraindicated during or after a 96-hour infusion of drotrecogin alfa (activated). The incidence of serious bleeding events in those who received drotrecogin alfa (activated) alone and in those who were also treated with heparin was similar (3.7% versus 3.5%).[143] In patients with severe sepsis who are judged to be at high risk of serious bleeding or who are actively bleeding, mechanical prophylaxis with graduated compression stockings or intermittent pneumatic compression devices can be employed. However, the efficacy of these devices is significantly less than that of available antithrombotic drugs. Therefore, once the bleeding risk has decreased, pharmacologic thromboprophylaxis can be started or resumed.

STRESS ULCER PROPHYLAXIS

Patients with severe sepsis have an increased risk for GI bleeding. The incidence of GI bleeding is proportional to the number of risk factors, including prolonged mechanical ventilation, coagulopathy, head injury, solid organ transplant, burns, severe sepsis, and a history of peptic ulcer disease.[229] In a prospective study of 174 patients admitted to a medical ICU, Schuster et al reported that overt or occult GI bleeding developed in 14%.[230] Risk factors for bleeding were mechanical ventilation for longer than 48 hours and/or the presence of a coagulopathy. Patients who developed GI bleeding had a higher mortality rate (64% versus 9%), longer duration of ICU stay (median $= 14.2$ days versus 4.2 days), increased risk for mechanical ventilation (84% versus 26%), and a requirement for extended duration of mechanical ventilation (9.5 versus 4.2 days) compared with those who did not bleed. The risk of bleeding can be reduced by strategies that decrease acid secretion (H_2 blockers), buffer the acid (antacids), or protect the gastric mucosal barrier (sucralfate). In a study of 1200 mechanically ventilated patients, Cook et al compared the efficacy of sucralfate and ranitidine for the prevention of GI bleeding in this population.[231] They reported that administration of ranitidine was significantly more effective than sucralfate in reducing the rate of clinically significant GI bleeding. The incidences of clinically important GI bleeding were 1.7% in patients treated with the H_2 blocker and 3.8% in those receiving mucosal protection ($p = 0.02$). The NNT to prevent one clinically significant bleed with ranitidine over sucralfate was 48.

Nevertheless, it has been hypothesized that mucosal protective strategies such as sucralfate might be superior to H$_2$ blockers for raising gastric pH above 4.0 because gastric acidity would prevent proliferation of bacteria in the stomach. That is, the raised pH with H$_2$ blockers might result in an increased risk of nosocomial pneumonia from reflux of bacteria colonizing the stomach into the respiratory tract. However, there is little evidence to support this hypothesis. Prod'hom et al randomized 244 intubated patients to GI bleeding prophylaxis with ranitidine (150 mg as a continuous infusion), sucralfate (1 g every 4 hours), or antacids (20 mL of aluminum and magnesium hydroxide every 2 hours).[232] Although the incidence of early onset pneumonia was not significantly different among the three groups, among 213 patients observed longer than 4 days, late onset pneumonia was less common in the mucosal protective group than in those treated with antacid or ranitidine (5%, 16%, and 21%, respectively; $p = 0.022$). However, there are several problems with this hypothesis, and the studies by Cook et al found no significant differences in the rates of VAP among those treated with sucralfate or ranitidine.[231] Therefore, in patients with severe sepsis, stress ulcer prophylaxis with ranitidine or the newer available intravenous proton pump inhibitors may decrease the incidence of serious GI bleeding without a convincing increase in cases of VAP.

SEPSIS COAGULOPATHY

In patients with severe sepsis, coagulation is activated and fibrinolysis is suppressed. A sepsis-associated coagulopathy is a sign of dysfunction of the hematologic organ system. In the Ibuprofen in Sepsis Trial, a coagulopathy with elevated levels of D-dimer and decreased levels of PC was almost universal in patients with severe sepsis.[233] The coagulopathy in patients with this disease is linked to endothelial cell dysfunction and fibrin deposition, pathologic processes that contribute to multiple organ system dysfunction and death. Thrombocytopenia, prolongation of the prothrombin time and/or the activated partial thromboplastin time, or any combination thereof are uncommon in patients with severe sepsis. Although there is no single clinical manifestation or laboratory value that is diagnostic of DIC, the following changes are reasonably consistent with the diagnosis: (1) presence of a disorder such as severe sepsis that is known to be linked with DIC, (2) musculocutaneous bleeding and dysfunction of one or more organ systems, and (3) ongoing consumption of coagulation factors. The first two criteria are detected by clinical examination; the last criterion can be recognized by thrombocytopenia and prolongation of one or more global tests of coagulation. Taylor et al proposed a scoring system for the diagnosis of DIC.[234] It uses the characteristics described above to provide a DIC score; values of at least 5 are characteristic of DIC.

In the absence of bleeding, patients with severe sepsis-associated coagulopathy can simply be monitored. In most instances, once the infection is controlled, the abnormal laboratory parameters return toward normal. In patients who are bleeding despite active treatment of the infection, a careful examination should be conducted to rule out a discrete and correctable anatomic lesion (e.g., peptic ulcer) as the cause of the bleed. If bleeding is from multiple sites, treatment is generally broken down into three general areas: (1) platelets and coagulation factor replacement, (2) antithrombotics, and (3) fibrinolysis inhibitors. Replacement of platelets and coagulation factors is generally the first step. Platelet transfusions are often used to maintain the platelet count above 20,000/μL, although the risk of spontaneous bleeding in the absence of anticoagulants occurs at platelet counts lower than 10,000/μL. Importantly, to avoid the risk of intracranial hemorrhage in patients who are to receive drotrecogin alfa (activated), platelet counts should be above 30,000/μL. In patients with severe sepsis, platelet turnover is accelerated; therefore, patients receiving platelets should be monitored with regular platelet counts. Although some patients are transfused with platelets to maintain the threshold, drotrecogin alfa (activated) is not usually given to patients who require multiple platelet transfusions or who have bleeding diathesis due to DIC. Coagulation factors can be replaced with cryoprecipitate or fresh frozen plasma. Each unit of these products has the equivalent of 1 U of fresh whole blood. Cryoprecipitate contains fibrinogen, factor VIII, factor XIII, VWF, and fibronectin. Each bag of cryoprecipitate has approximately 250 mg of fibrinogen and 100 U of factors VIII and XIII in a volume of approximately 10 mL. One unit of fresh frozen plasma contains all hemostatic proteins and albumin, globulins, and electrolytes in 1 U of fresh whole blood. It consists of approximately 225 mL of plasma. Cryoprecipitate may be administered to maintain the fibrinogen level above 100 mg/dL and the level of coagulation factors above 0.5 U/mL. Notably, platelets, cryoprecipitate, and fresh frozen plasma can transmit blood-borne infectious agents.

Low-dose heparin has been used in the past to interrupt the vicious cycle of coagulation, thrombosis, and factor depletion in patients with DIC. However, despite 20 years of calls for such studies, its efficacy has not been demonstrated in large-scale randomized clinical trials.[235] Aoki et al reported that low-dose rhAPC corrected the clinical and laboratory abnormalities in patients with DIC more effectively than UFH.[236] The 28-day all-cause mortality rates in patients treated with APC and heparin were 20.4% and 40%, respectively ($p < 0.05$). In addition, patients treated with APC had significantly less bleeding ($p = 0.009$). Joyce et al performed a retrospective subgroup analysis to determine the effect of drotrecogin alfa (activated) on patients with severe sepsis and DIC.[237] Treatment with drotrecogin alfa (activated) produced a 42% reduction in the relative risk of death compared with placebo (95% confidence interval = 58 to 19). Fibrinolytic inhibitors are not recommended in patients with severe sepsis and DIC because they may convert a hemorrhagic DIC to a thrombotic DIC. These agents are recommended only for patients with primary or excessive secondary fibrinolysis.

TEMPERATURE MANAGEMENT

An abnormality in temperature (i.e., $\leq 36°C$ or $\geq 38°C$) is one of the four SIRS criteria and a manifestation of sepsis that will resolve once the infection is controlled. In most instances, mild hypothermia does not need to be actively corrected; however, hypothermia that leads to shivering can increase tissue oxygen requirements and usually can be managed by covering the patient with a blanket. If the patient is to receive large amounts of refrigerated blood, significant hypothermia can be prevented by the use of an in-line blood warmer. For every 1°C above 37°C, fever increases basal oxygen consumption 13%. In most instances, mild fever requires no treatment. However, fever in patients can aggravate pre-existing cardiac or pulmonary disease and worsen behavioral changes in patients with organic brain disease. Measures to lower core temperatures are prudent in patients with temperatures above 40°C to 41°C (104°F to 105.8°F). Steps taken in this situation can include antipyretics such as acetaminophen and measures such as a cooling blanket or tepid water sponging. Notably, however, cooling measures may induce shivering with its undesirable metabolic effects. Therefore, to prevent shivering, the patient can be treated with parenteral meperidine (25 to 50 mg). Muscle relaxants such as pancuronium or vecuronium may be required on rare occasions to control shivering and rigors in adequately sedated and mechanically ventilated patients who are hyperpyrexic.

Prognostic Assessment

In the past two decades, several scoring systems have been developed to identify and describe patient populations in the ICU. These scoring systems also have been useful for ensuring comparability in clinical trial populations. These outcome prediction models and organ dysfunction scores are discussed in detail in Chapter 6. Therefore, we confine our discussion specifically to points relevant to prognostic assessment in patients with severe sepsis. These models can be subdivided into two broad categories: outcome prediction models and organ dysfunction scoring systems.

OUTCOME PREDICTION MODELS (SEE CHAP. 6)

General outcome prediction models include the APACHE, Mortality Probability Model (MPM), and the Second Simplified Acute Physiology Score (SAPS). The APACHE score has become the most commonly used survival prediction model in the critical care unit. APACHE II is a simplified version with a point score derived from initial values of 12 physiologic measurements, age, and previous health status. The APACHE III model was developed in 1991. It is complex, requires software to determine values, and is proprietary; therefore, most investigators have continued to use APACHE II. The MPM consists of two scores: MPM_0, the admission model with 15 variables, and, MPM_{24}, the 24-hour model that uses five of the admission variables and eight additional variables. The SAPS II uses 12 physiologic variables, age, type of admission, and three variables related to the nature of the underlying disease. When attempting to apply outcome prediction models at the bedside, three caveats should be kept in mind. (1) Outcome prediction models are incorporated into clinical trials of severe sepsis interventions to predict and evaluate mortality rate for cohorts of patients; at this time, it is inappropriate to use them to predict outcome or determine therapy for individual septic patients. (2) For the sake of comparability, the models must be used as originally validated. For example, the APACHE II model is validated for the use at the time of admission or within the first 24 hours. However, to obtain consistency in clinical trials, the APACHE II score is often computed from the worst values in the first 24 hours before *randomization*, not during the first 24 hours after admission. Because many of the physiologic variables used to compute the APACHE II score can be corrected within the first 24 hours in a patient with severe sepsis (e.g., pH,

electrolytes), this trial design practice limits comparison to the original APACHE database. (3) There are other inherent limitations of outcome prediction models. For example, they are cumbersome to use outside a clinical trial setting, imprecise diagnoses can invalidate the results, they are poor discriminators, and they have lead-time bias.[238,239] Lead-time bias is reflected by the fact that the admission source predicts hospital mortality rate independent of APACHE II. For example, a septic patient who is admitted to the ICU from an inpatient floor has a higher probability of death than one who is admitted from the emergency department.[240]

ORGAN DYSFUNCTION SCORING SYSTEMS

The risk of death in patients with severe sepsis is a function of the number of dysfunctional organs. Organ dysfunction scoring systems supply a tool to characterize the severity of illness in patients with sepsis. Commonly used organ dysfunction scoring systems in patients with severe sepsis include the Sequential Organ Failure Assessment (SOFA), the Multiple Organ Dysfunction Score, the Logistic Organ Dysfunction System, and the Brussels Score. Vincent et al used the SOFA Score to assess the incidence of organ dysfunction in critically ill patients.[241] They reported that mortality rates were lowest in patients without organ dysfunction (9%) and that rates increased progressively in patients with dysfunction in one (22%), two (38%), three (69%), and four or more organs (83%; $p < 0.00001$). Using logistic regression analysis of the results of a simple Multiple System Organ Failure Score, Hebert et al reported that the type of dysfunctional organ system was also linked to mortality rate.[242] The odds ratios for covariates most predictive of mortality rate by organ system were hematologic (odds ratio = 6.2), neurologic (odds ratio = 4.4), hepatic (odds ratio = 3.4), and cardiovascular (odds ratio = 2.6). However, like the outcome prediction models, there are caveats when attempting to employ organ dysfunction scores for the management of individual patients with severe sepsis. (1) The nature of the score is a morbidity, not a mortality, score. (2) Organ dysfunction is an analog parameter that varies from mild laboratory abnormalities to overt organ failure. (3) The degree of organ dysfunction is not static; instead, it changes over time. For example, the platelet count can change considerably over time. Therefore, trends are sometimes more important than absolute values. (4) Because the degree of organ dysfunction must be evaluated over time, by different individuals, and in a variety of community and academic settings, any variables employed in organ dysfunction scores should be objective, routinely measured, and easy to assess.

Acknowledgments

The authors thank George H. Karam, MD, Paul Garvey Manship Professor of Medicine, Louisiana State University School of Medicine, New Orleans for his thoughtful review of the infectious disease and antibiotic issues in this chapter.

References

1. Angus DC, Linde-Zwirble WT, Lidicker J, et al: Epidemiology of severe sepsis in the United States: Analysis of incidence, outcome, and associated costs of care. *Crit Care Med* 29:1303, 2001.

2. Martin GS, Mannino DM, Eaton S, Moss M: The epidemiology of sepsis in the United States from 1979 through 2000. *N Engl J Med* 348:1546, 2003.

3. Davies AGC, Hutton J, et al: Severe sepsis—A European estimate of the burden of disease in the ICU. Paper presented at the European Society of Intensive Care Medicine Meeting, 2001.

4. Zeni F, Freeman B, Natanson C: Antiinflammatory therapies to treat sepsis and septic shock: A reassessment (editorial). *Crit Care Med* 25:1095, 1997.

5. Angus DC, Kelley MA, Schmitz RJ, et al: Caring for the critically ill patient. Current and projected workforce requirements for care of the critically ill and patients with pulmonary disease: Can we meet the requirements of an aging population? *JAMA* 284:2762, 2000.

6. Bone RC, Balk RA, Cerra FB, et al: Definitions for sepsis and organ failure and guidelines for the use of innovative therapies in sepsis. The ACCP/SCCM Consensus Conference Committee. American College of Chest Physicians/Society of Critical Care Medicine. *Chest* 101:1644, 1992.

7. Vincent JL: Dear SIRS, I'm sorry to say that I don't like you. *Crit Care Med* 25:372, 1997.

8. Alberti C, Brun-Buisson C, Goodman SV, et al: Influence of systemic inflammatory response syndrome and sepsis on outcome of critically ill infected patients. *Am J Respir Crit Care Med* 168:77, 2003.

9. Levy MM, Fink MP, Marshall JC, et al: 2001 SCCM/ESICM/ACCP/ATS/SIS International Sepsis Definitions Conference. *Crit Care Med* 31:1250, 2003.

10. O'Keefe GE, Hybki DL, Munford RS: The G→A single nucleotide polymorphism at the −308 position in the tumor necrosis factor-alpha promoter increases the risk for severe sepsis after trauma. *J Trauma* 52:817, 2002.

11. Medzhitov R, Janeway C Jr: Innate immunity. *N Engl J Med* 343:338, 2000.

12. Suffredini AF, Fromm RE, Parker MM, et al: The cardiovascular response of normal humans to the administration of endotoxin. *N Engl J Med* 321:280, 1989.

13. Tapper H, Herwald H: Modulation of hemostatic mechanisms in bacterial infectious diseases. *Blood* 96:2329, 2000.

14. Raychaudhuri B, Abraham S, Bonfield TL, et al: Surfactant blocks lipopolysaccharide signaling by inhibiting both mitogen-activated protein and IkappaB kinases in human alveolar macrophages. *Am J Respir Cell Mol Biol* 30:228, 2004.

15. Doshi SN, Marmur JD: Evolving role of tissue factor and its pathway inhibitor. *Crit Care Med* 30(suppl):S241, 2002.

16. Marshall BC, Brown BR, Rothstein MA, et al: Alveolar epithelial cells express both plasminogen activator and tissue factor. Potential role in repair of lung injury. *Chest* 99(suppl):25S, 1991.

17. Hotchkiss RS, Karl IE: The pathophysiology and treatment of sepsis. *N Engl J Med* 348:138, 2003.

18. Hotchkiss RS, Tinsley KW, Swanson PE, et al: Sepsis-induced apoptosis causes progressive profound depletion of B and CD4+ T lymphocytes in humans. *J Immunol* 166:6952, 2001.

19. Hotchkiss RS, Tinsley KW, Swanson PE, et al: Depletion of dendritic cells, but not macrophages, in patients with sepsis. *J Immunol* 168:2493, 2002.

20. Mumford RS, Pugin J: Normal responses to inury prevent systemic inflammation and can be immunosuppressive. *Am J Respir Crit Care Med* 163:361, 2001.

21. Vervloet MG, Thijs LG, Hack CE: Derangements of coagulation and fibrinolysis in critically ill patients with sepsis and septic shock. *Semin Thromb Hemost* 24:33, 1998.

22. Riedemann NC, Guo RF, Neff TA, et al: Increased C5a receptor expression in sepsis. *J Clin Invest* 110:101, 2002.

23. Sporn LA, Huber P: Endothelial cell biology, in Coleman RWH, Marder VJ, et al (eds): *Hemostasis and Thrombosis*, 4th ed. Philadelphia, Lippincott Williams & Wilkins, 2001.

24. Hack CE, Zeerleder S: The endothelium in sepsis: Source of and a target for inflammation. *Crit Care Med* 29(suppl):S21, 2001.

25. Esmon CT: The normal role of Activated Protein C in maintaining homeostasis and its relevance to critical illness. *Crit Care* 5(suppl 2):S7, 2001.

26. Levi M, ten Cate H, van der Poll T: Endothelium: Interface between coagulation and inflammation. *Crit Care Med* 30(suppl):S220, 2002.

27. Gross PL, Aird WC: The endothelium and thrombosis. *Semin Thromb Hemost* 26:463, 2000.

28. Leclerc J, Pu Q, Corseaux D, et al: A single endotoxin injection in the rabbit causes prolonged blood vessel dysfunction and a procoagulant state. *Crit Care Med* 28:3672, 2000.

29. Vincent JL: Microvascular endothelial dysfunction: a renewed appreciation of sepsis pathophysiology. *Crit Care* 5(suppl 2):S1, 2001.

30. Aird WC: Endothelial cell heterogeneity. *Crit Care Med* 31(suppl):S221, 2003.

31. Reinhart K, Bayer O, Brunkhorst F, Meisner M: Markers of endothelial damage in organ dysfunction and sepsis. *Crit Care Med* 30(suppl):S302, 2002.

32. Krafte-Jacobs B, Brilli R: Increased circulating thrombomodulin in children with septic shock. *Crit Care Med* 26:933, 1998.

33. Faust SN, Levin M, Harrison OB, et al: Dysfunction of endothelial protein C activation in severe meningococcal sepsis. *N Engl J Med* 345:408, 2001.

34. de Kleijn ED, de Groot R, Hack CE, et al: Activation of protein C following infusion of protein C concentrate in children with severe meningococcal sepsis and purpura fulminans: A randomized, double-blinded, placebo-controlled, dose-finding study. *Crit Care Med* 31:1839, 2003.

35. Moss M, Gillespie MK, Ackerson L, et al: Endothelial cell activity varies in patients at risk for the adult respiratory distress syndrome. *Crit Care Med* 24:1782, 1996.

36. Combes V, Simon AC, Grau GE, et al: In vitro generation of endothelial microparticles and possible prothrombotic activity in patients with lupus anticoagulant. *J Clin Invest* 104:93, 1999.

37. Hotchkiss RS, Tinsley KW, Swanson PE, Karl IE: Endothelial cell apoptosis in sepsis. *Crit Care Med* 30(suppl):S225, 2002.

38. Fernandes CJ Jr, Akamine N, Knobel E: Cardiac troponin: A new serum marker of myocardial injury in sepsis. *Intensive Care Med* 25:1165, 1999.

39. Kumar A, Haery C, Parrillo JE: Myocardial dysfunction in septic shock. *Crit Care Clin* 16:251, 2000.

40. Ruiz Bailen M: Reversible myocardial dysfunction in critically ill, noncardiac patients: A review. *Crit Care Med* 30:1280, 2002.

41. Dhainaut JF, Huyghebaert MF, Monsallier JF, et al: Coronary hemodynamics and myocardial metabolism of lactate, free fatty acids, glucose, and ketones in patients with septic shock. *Circulation* 75:533, 1987.

42. Parker MM, Shelhamer JH, Bacharach SL, et al: Profound but reversible myocardial depression in patients with septic shock. *Ann Intern Med* 100:483, 1984.

43. Parker MM, Shelhamer JH, Natanson C, et al: Responses of left ventricular function in survivors and nonsurvivors of septic shock. *J Crit Care* 4:19, 1989.

44. Landry DW, Oliver JA: The pathogenesis of vasodilatory shock. *N Engl J Med* 345:588, 2001.

45. Schneider F, Lutun P, Couchot A, Bilbault P, Tempe JD. Plasma cyclic guanosine 3′-5′ monophosphate concentrations and low vascular resistance in human septic shock. *Intensive Care Med* 19:99, 1993.

46. Arnalich F, Hernanz A, Jimenez M, et al: Relationship between circulating levels of calcitonin gene-related peptide, nitric oxide metabolites and hemodynamic changes in human septic shock. *Regul Pept* 65:115, 1996.

47. Martin C, Leone M, Viviand X, et al: High adenosine plasma concentration as a prognostic index for outcome in patients with septic shock. *Crit Care Med* 28:3198, 2000.

48. Taylor BS, Geller DA: Molecular regulation of the human inducible nitric oxide synthase (iNOS) gene. *Shock* 13:413, 2000.

49. Zerbe RL, Henry DP, Robertson GL: Vasopressin response to orthostatic hypotension. Etiologic and clinical implications. *Am J Med* 74:265, 1983.

50. Martin GS, Bernard GR: Airway and lung in sepsis. *Intensive Care Med* 27(suppl 1):S63, 2001.

51. Bannerman DD, Goldblum SE: Mechanisms of bacterial lipopolysaccharide-induced endothelial apoptosis. *Am J Physiol Lung Cell Mol Physiol* 284:L899, 2003.

52. Banna P, Marcello MF, Murabito R, et al: Ultrastructural changes of the pulmonary parenchyma after experimentally induced endotoxic shock in dogs with and without drug protection. *Respiration* 47:177, 1985.

53. Whitsett JA, Weaver TE: Hydrophobic surfactant proteins in lung function and disease. *N Engl J Med* 347:2141, 2002.

54. Idell S, James KK, Levin EG, et al: Local abnormalities in coagulation and fibrinolytic pathways predispose to alveolar fibrin deposition in the adult respiratory distress syndrome. *J Clin Invest* 84:695, 1989.

55. Tomashefski JF Jr: Pulmonary pathology of the adult respiratory distress syndrome. *Clin Chest Med* 11:593, 1990.

56. Idell S: Coagulation, fibrinolysis, and fibrin deposition in acute lung injury. *Crit Care Med* 31(suppl):S213, 2003.

57. Idell S: Endothelium and disordered fibrin turnover in the injured lung: Newly recognized pathways. *Crit Care Med* 30(suppl):S274, 2002.

58. Gattinoni L, Vagginelli F, Chiumello D, et al: Physiologic rationale for ventilator setting in acute lung injury/acute respiratory distress syndrome patients. *Crit Care Med* 31(suppl):S300, 2003.

59. Gattinoni L, Pelosi P, Suter PM, et al: Acute respiratory distress syndrome caused by pulmonary and extrapulmonary disease. Different syndromes? *Am J Respir Crit Care Med* 158:3, 1998.

60. Mutlu GM, Mutlu EA, Factor P: GI complications in patients receiving mechanical ventilation. *Chest* 119:1222, 2001.

61. Acute Respiratory Distress Syndrome Network: Ventilation with lower tidal volumes as compared with traditional tidal volumes for acute lung injury and the acute respiratory distress syndrome. *N Engl J Med* 342:1301, 2000.

62. Hiltebrand LB, Krejci V, tenHoevel ME, et al: Redistribution of microcirculatory blood flow within the intestinal wall during sepsis and general anesthesia. *Anesthesiology* 98:658, 2003.

63. Magnotti LJ, Upperman JS, Xu DZ, et al: Gut-derived mesenteric lymph but not portal blood increases endothelial cell permeability and promotes lung injury after hemorrhagic shock. *Ann Surg* 228:518, 1998.

64. Sambol JT, Xu DZ, Adams CA, et al: Mesenteric lymph duct ligation provides long term protection against hemorrhagic shock-induced lung injury. *Shock* 14:416, 2000.

65. Alverdy JC, Laughlin RS, Wu L: Influence of the critically ill state on host-pathogen interactions within the intestine: Gut-derived sepsis redefined. *Crit Care Med* 31:598, 2003.

66. Gianotti L, Nelson JL, Alexander JW, et al: Post injury hypermetabolic response and magnitude of translocation: Prevention by early enteral nutrition. *Nutrition* 10:225, 1994.

67. Dhainaut JF, Marin N, Mignon A, Vinsonneau C: Hepatic response to sepsis: Interaction between coagulation and inflammatory processes. *Crit Care Med* 29(suppl):S42, 2001.

68. Szabo G, Romics L Jr, Frendl G: Liver in sepsis and systemic inflammatory response syndrome. *Clin Liver Dis* 6:1045, 2002.

69. Goyette RE: *Hematology: A Comprehensive Guide to the Diagnosis and Treatment of Blood Disorders*. Los Angeles, PMIC, 1997.

70. Abernethy VE, Lieberthal W: Acute renal failure in the critically ill patient. *Crit Care Clin* 18:203, 2002.

71. Khan RZ, Badr KF: Endotoxin and renal function: Perspectives to the understanding of septic acute renal failure and toxic shock. *Nephrol Dial Transplant* 14:814, 1999.

72. Young GB, Bolton CF, Austin TW, et al: The encephalopathy associated with septic illness. *Clin Invest Med* 13:297, 1990.

73. Papadopoulos MC, Davies DC, Moss RF, et al: Pathophysiology of septic encephalopathy: A review. *Crit Care Med* 28:3019, 2000.

74. Ely EW, Margolin R, Francis J, et al: Evaluation of delirium in critically ill patients: Validation of the Confusion Assessment Method for the Intensive Care Unit (CAM-ICU). *Crit Care Med* 29:1370, 2001.

75. Corday E, Williams JH Jr: Effect of shock and of vasopressor drugs on the regional circulation of the brain, heart, kidney and liver. *Am J Med* 29:228, 1960.

76. Ely EW, Siegel M.D., Inouye SK: Delirium in the intensive care unit: An under-recognized symptom of organ dysfunction. *Semin Respir Crit Care Med* 22:115, 2001.

77. Bowton DL, Bertels NH, Prough DS, Stump DA: Cerebral blood flow is reduced in patients with sepsis syndrome. *Crit Care Med* 17:399, 1989.

78. Breslow MJ, Miller CF, Parker SD, et al: Effect of vasopressors on organ blood flow during endotoxin shock in pigs. *Am J Physiol* 252(2 pt 2):H291, 1987.

79. Gaykema RP, Dijkstra I, Tilders FJ: Subdiaphragmatic vagotomy suppresses endotoxin-induced activation of hypothalamic corticotropin-releasing hormone neurons and ACTH secretion. *Endocrinology* 136:4717, 1995.

80. Borovikova LV, Ivanova S, Zhang M, et al: Vagus nerve stimulation attenuates the systemic inflammatory response to endotoxin. *Nature* 405:458, 2000.

81. Fleshner M, Goehler LE, Schwartz BA, et al: Thermogenic and corticosterone responses to intravenous cytokines (IL-1beta and TNF-alpha) are attenuated by subdiaphragmatic vagotomy. *J Neuroimmunol* 86:134, 1998.

82. Fletcher SN, Kennedy DD, Ghosh IR, et al: Persistent neuromuscular and neurophysiologic abnormalities in long-term survivors of prolonged critical illness. *Crit Care Med* 31:1012, 2003.

83. Marinelli WA, Leatherman JW: Neuromuscular disorders in the intensive care unit. *Crit Care Clin* 18:915, 2002.

84. Rizoli SB, Marshall JC: Saturday night fever: Finding and controlling the source of sepsis in critical illness. *Lancet Infect Dis* 2:137, 2002.

85. Fine MJ, Auble TE, Yealy DM, et al: A prediction rule to identify low-risk patients with community-acquired pneumonia. *N Engl J Med* 336:243, 1997.

86. Ely EW, Gautam S, Margolin R, et al: The impact of delirium in the intensive care unit on hospital length of stay. *Intensive Care Med* 27:1892, 2001.

87. Lefcoe MS, Fox GA, Leasa DJ, et al: Accuracy of portable chest radiography in the critical care setting. Diagnosis of pneumonia based on quantitative cultures obtained from protected brush catheter. *Chest* 105:885, 1994.

88. Ely EW, Haponik EF: Using the chest radiograph to determine intravascular volume status: The role of vascular pedicle width. *Chest* 121:942, 2002.

89. Wheeler AP, Bernard GR: Treating patients with severe sepsis. *N Engl J Med* 340:207, 1999.

90. Selberg O, Hecker H, Martin M, et al: Discrimination of sepsis and systemic inflammatory response syndrome by determination of circulating plasma concentrations of procalcitonin, protein complement 3a, and interleukin-6. *Crit Care Med* 28:2793, 2000.

91. Luzzani A, Polati E, Dorizzi R, et al: Comparison of procalcitonin and C-reactive protein as markers of sepsis. *Crit Care Med* 31:1737, 2003.

92. Wagner KE, Martinez JM, Vath SD, et al: Early immunoneutralization of calcitonin precursors attenuates the adverse physiologic response to sepsis in pigs. *Crit Care Med* 30:2313, 2002.

93. Pettila V, Hynninen M, Takkunen O, et al: Predictive value of procalcitonin and interleukin 6 in critically ill patients with suspected sepsis. *Intensive Care Med* 28:1220, 2002.

94. Wanner GA, Keel M, Steckholzer U, et al: Relationship between procalcitonin plasma levels and severity of injury, sepsis, organ failure, and mortality in injured patients. *Crit Care Med* 28:950, 2000.

95. Van der Kaay DC, De Kleijn ED, De Rijke YB, et al: Procalcitonin as a prognostic marker in meningococcal disease. *Intensive Care Med* 28:1606, 2002.

96. Rackow EC, Falk JL, Fein IA, et al: Fluid resuscitation in circulatory shock: a comparison of the cardiorespiratory effects of albumin, hetastarch, and saline solutions in patients with hypovolemic and septic shock. *Crit Care Med* 11:839, 1983.

97. Task Force of the American College of Critical Care Medicine, Society of Critical Care Medicine: Practice parameters for hemodynamic support of sepsis in adult patients in sepsis. *Crit Care Med* 27:639, 1999.

98. Choi PT, Yip G, Quinonez LG, Cook DJ: Crystalloids vs. colloids in fluid resuscitation: A systematic review. *Crit Care Med* 27:200, 1999.

99. Schierhout G, Roberts I: Fluid resuscitation with colloid or crystalloid solutions in critically ill patients: A systematic review of randomised trials. *BMJ* 316:961, 1998.

100. Wilkes MM, Navickis RJ: Patient survival after human albumin administration. A meta-analysis of randomized, controlled trials. *Ann Intern Med* 135:149, 2001.

101. Fink MP: Ethyl pyruvate: A novel anti-inflammatory agent. *Crit Care Med* 31(suppl):S51, 2003.

102. Fink MP: Ringer's ethyl pyruvate solution: A novel resuscitation fluid for the treatment of hemorrhagic shock and sepsis. *J Trauma* 54(suppl):S141, 2003.

103. Velasco IT, Pontieri V, Rocha e Silva M Jr, Lopes OU: Hyperosmotic NaCl and severe hemorrhagic shock. *Am J Physiol* 239:H664, 1980.

104. Hannemann L, Reinhart K, Korell R, et al: Hypertonic saline in stabilized hyperdynamic sepsis. *Shock* 5:130, 1996.

105. Oliveria E, Weingrtner R, Oliveria ES, et al: Hemodynamic effects of a hypertonic saline solution in sepsis (abstract). *Shock* 6, 1996.

106. Oliveira RP, Velasco I, Soriano F, Friedman G: Clinical review: Hypertonic saline resuscitation in sepsis. *Crit Care* 6:418, 2002.

107. Corso CO, Okamoto S, Leiderer R, Messmer K: Resuscitation with hypertonic saline dextran reduces endothelial cell swelling and improves hepatic microvascular perfusion and function after hemorrhagic shock. *J Surg Res* 80:210, 1998.

108. Hebert PC, Wells G, Blajchman MA, et al: A multicenter, randomized, controlled clinical trial of transfusion requirements in critical care. Transfusion Requirements in Critical Care Investigators, Canadian Critical Care Trials Group. *N Engl J Med* 340:409, 1999.

109. Rivers E, Nguyen B, Havstad S, et al: Early goal-directed therapy in the treatment of severe sepsis and septic shock. *N Engl J Med* 345:1368, 2001.

110. Wu WC, Rathore SS, Wang Y, et al: Blood transfusion in elderly patients with acute myocardial infarction. *N Engl J Med* 345:1230, 2001.

111. Meadows D, Edwards JD, Wilkins RG, Nightingale P: Reversal of intractable septic shock with norepinephrine therapy. *Crit Care Med* 16:663, 1988.

112. Martin C, Viviand X, Leone M, Thirion X: Effect of norepinephrine on the outcome of septic shock. *Crit Care Med* 28:2758, 2000.

113. Di Giantomasso D, May CN, Bellomo R: Norepinephrine and vital organ blood flow. *Intensive Care Med* 28:1804, 2002.

114. Landry DW, Levin HR, Gallant EM, et al: Vasopressin deficiency contributes to the vasodilation of septic shock. *Circulation* 95:1122, 1997.

115. Patel BM, Chittock DR, Russell JA, Walley KR: Beneficial effects of short-term vasopressin infusion during severe septic shock. *Anesthesiology* 96:576, 2002.

116. Gattinoni L, Tognoni G, Pesenti A, et al: Effect of prone positioning on the survival of patients with acute respiratory failure. *N Engl J Med* 345:568, 2001.

117. Slutsky AS: The acute respiratory distress syndrome, mechanical ventilation, and the prone position. *N Engl J Med* 345:610, 2001.

118. Gattinoni L, Brazzi L, Pelosi P, et al: A trial of goal-oriented hemodynamic therapy in critically ill patients. SvO2 Collaborative Group. *N Engl J Med* 333:1025, 1995.

119. Hayes MA, Timmins AC, Yau EH, et al: Elevation of systemic oxygen delivery in the treatment of critically ill patients. *N Engl J Med* 330:1717, 1994.

120. MacIntyre NR, Cook DJ, Ely EW Jr, et al: Evidence-based guidelines for weaning and discontinuing ventilatory support: A collective task force facilitated by the American College of Chest Physicians; the American Association for Respiratory Care; and the American College of Critical Care Medicine. *Chest* 120(suppl):375S, 2001.

121. Ely EW, Baker AM, Dunagan DP, et al: Effect on the duration of mechanical ventilation of identifying patients capable of breathing spontaneously. *N Engl J Med* 335:1864, 1996.

122. Ely EW, Meade MO, Haponik EF, et al: Mechanical ventilator weaning protocols driven by nonphysician health-care professionals: Evidence-based clinical practice guidelines. *Chest* 120(suppl):454S, 2001.

123. Jimenez MF, Marshall JC: Source control in the management of sepsis. *Intensive Care Med* 27(suppl 1):S49, 2001.

124. Pittet D, Thievent B, Wenzel RP, et al: Bedside prediction of mortality from bacteremic sepsis. A dynamic analysis of ICU patients. *Am J Respir Crit Care Med* 153:684, 1996.

125. Opal SM, Fisher CJ Jr, Dhainaut JF, et al: Confirmatory interleukin-1 receptor antagonist trial in severe sepsis: A phase III, randomized, double-blind, placebo-controlled, multicenter trial. The Interleukin-1 Receptor Antagonist Sepsis Investigator Group. *Crit Care Med* 25:1115, 1997.

126. Iregui M, Ward S, Sherman G, et al: Clinical importance of delays in the initiation of appropriate antibiotic treatment for ventilator-associated pneumonia. *Chest* 122:262, 2002.

127. Kreger BE, Craven DE, McCabe WR: Gram-negative bacteremia. IV. Re-evaluation of clinical features and treatment in 612 patients. *Am J Med* 68:344, 1980.

128. Kollef MH, Sherman G, Ward S, Fraser VJ: Inadequate antimicrobial treatment of infections: A risk factor for hospital mortality among critically ill patients. *Chest* 115:462, 1999.

129. Bartlett JG, Dowell SF, Mandell LA, et al: Practice guidelines for the management of community-acquired pneumonia in adults. Infectious Diseases Society of America. *Clin Infect Dis* 31:347, 2000.

130. Mermel LA, Farr BM, Sherertz RJ, et al: Guidelines for the management of intravascular catheter-related infections. *Clin Infect Dis* 32:1249, 2001.

131. Byers K, Adal K, Anglim A, et al: Case fatality rate for catheter-related blood stream infections (CRBSI): A meta-analysis (abstract 43). Paper presented at: Proceedings of the 5th Annual Meeting of the Society for Hospital Epidemiology of America, 1995.

132. Giroir BP: An evidence-based aproach for the evaluation of new therapies for severe sepsis: Analysis of the PROWESS trial, in Balk RA (ed): *Advances in the Diagnosis and Management of the Patient with Severe Sepsis.* London, Royal Society of Medicine Press, 2002.

133. Group FTTFC: Indications for fibrinolytic therapy in suspected acute myocardial infarction: Collaborative overview of early mortality and major morbidity results from all randomized trials of more than 1000 patients. *Lancet* 343:311, 1994.

134. Antman EM, McCabe CH, Gurfinkel EP, et al: Enoxaparin prevents death and cardiac ischemic events in unstable angina/non–Q-wave myocardial infarction. Results of the thrombolysis in myocardial infarction (TIMI) 11B trial. *Circulation* 100:1593, 1999.

135. Yan SB, Dhainaut JF: Activated protein C versus protein C in severe sepsis. *Crit Care Med* 29(suppl):S69, 2001.

136. Joyce DE, Grinnell BW: Recombinant human activated protein C attenuates the inflammatory response in endothelium and monocytes by modulating nuclear factor-kappaB. *Crit Care Med* 30(suppl):S288, 2002.

137. Schmidt-Supprian M, Murphy C, While B, et al: Activated protein C inhibits tumor necrosis factor and macrophage migration inhibitory factor production in monocytes. *Eur Cytokine Netw* 11:407, 2000.

138. Grinnell BW, Hermann RB, Yan SB: Human protein C inhibits selectin-mediated cell adhesion: Role of unique fucosylated oligosaccharide. *Glycobiology* 4:221, 1994.

139. Cheng T, Liu D, Griffin JH, et al: Activated protein C blocks p53-mediated apoptosis in ischemic human brain endothelium and is neuroprotective. *Nat Med* 9:338, 2003.

140. Taylor FB Jr, Chang A, Esmon CT, et al: Protein C prevents the coagulopathic and lethal effects of *Escherichia coli* infusion in the baboon. *J Clin Invest* 79:918, 1987.

141. Bernard GR, Ely EW, Wright TJ, et al: Safety and dose relationship of recombinant human activated protein C for coagulopathy in severe sepsis. *Crit Care Med* 29:2051, 2001.

142. Mesters RM, Helterbrand J, Utterback BG, et al: Prognostic value of protein C concentrations in neutropenic patients at high risk of severe septic complications. *Crit Care Med* 28:2209, 2000.

143. Bernard GR, Vincent JL, Laterre PF, et al: Efficacy and safety of recombinant human activated protein C for severe sepsis. *N Engl J Med* 344:699, 2001.

144. Angus DC, Linde-Zwirble WT, Clermont G, et al: Cost-effectiveness of drotrecogin alfa (activated) in the treatment of severe sepsis. *Crit Care Med* 31:1, 2003.

145. Manns BJ, Lee H, Doig CJ, et al: An economic evaluation of activated protein C treatment for severe sepsis. *N Engl J Med* 347:993, 2002.

146. Ely EW, Laterre PF, Angus DC, et al: Drotrecogin alfa (activated) administration across clinically important subgroups of patients with severe sepsis. *Crit Care Med* 31:12, 2003.

147. Vincent JL, Angus DC, Artigas A, et al: Effects of drotrecogin alfa (activated) on organ dysfunction in the PROWESS trial. *Crit Care Med* 31:834, 2003.

148. Warren BL, Eid A, Singer P, et al: Caring for the critically ill patient. High-dose antithrombin III in severe sepsis: A randomized controlled trial. *JAMA* 286:1869, 2001.

149. Hamel MB, Davis RB, Teno JM, et al: Older age, aggressiveness of care, and survival for seriously ill, hospitalized adults. SUPPORT Investigators. Study to Understand Prognoses and Preferences for Outcomes and Risks of Treatments. *Ann Intern Med* 131:721, 1999.

150. Ely EW, Wheeler AP, Thompson BT, et al: Recovery rate and prognosis in older persons who develop acute lung injury and the acute respiratory distress syndrome. *Ann Intern Med* 136:25, 2002.

151. Ely EW, Angus DC, Williams MD, et al: Drotrecogin alfa (activated) treatment of older patients with severe sepsis. *Clin Infect Dis* 37:187, 2003.

152. Warren HS, Suffredini AF, Eichacker PQ, Munford RS: Risks and benefits of activated protein C treatment for severe sepsis. *N Engl J Med* 347:1027, 2002.

153. Angus DC, Crowther MA: Unraveling severe sepsis: Why did OPTIMIST fail and what's next? *JAMA* 290:256, 2003.

154. Siegel JP: Assessing the use of activated protein C in the treatment of severe sepsis. *N Engl J Med* 347:1030, 2002.

155. Ely EW, Bernard GR, Vincent JL: Activated protein C for severe sepsis. *N Engl J Med* 347:1035, 2002.

156. Laterre PF, Heiselman D: Management of patients with severe sepsis, treated by drotrecogin alfa (activated). *Am J Surg* 184(suppl):S39, 2002.

157. Balk RA, Goyette RE: Multiple organ dysfunction syndrome in patients with severe sepsis: more than just inflammation, in Balk RA (ed): *Advances in the Diagnosis and Management of the Patient with Severe Sepsis.* London, Royal Society of Medicine Press, 2002.

158. Hirsh J, Warkentin TE, Shaughnessy SG, et al: Heparin and low-molecular-weight heparin: Mechanisms of action, pharmacokinetics, dosing, monitoring, efficacy, and safety. *Chest* 119(suppl):64S, 2001.

159. Inthorn D, Hoffmann JN, Hartl WH, et al: Effect of antithrombin III supplementation on inflammatory response in patients with severe sepsis. *Shock* 10:90, 1998.

160. Golino P, Ragni M, Cimmino G, Forte L: Role of tissue factor pathway inhibitor in the regulation of tissue factor-dependent blood coagulation. *Cardiovasc Drug Rev* 20:67, 2002.

161. Enkhbaatar P, Okajima K, Murakami K, et al: Recombinant tissue factor pathway inhibitor reduces lipopolysaccharide-induced pulmonary vascular injury by inhibiting leukocyte activation. *Am J Respir Crit Care Med* 162:1752, 2000.

162. Abraham E, Reinhart K, Svoboda P, et al: Assessment of the safety of recombinant tissue factor pathway inhibitor in patients with severe sepsis: A multicenter, randomized, placebo-controlled, single-blind, dose escalation study. *Crit Care Med* 29:2081, 2001.

163. Abraham E, Reinhart K, Opal S, et al: Efficacy and safety of tifacogin (recombinant tissue factor pathway inhibitor) in severe sepsis: A randomized controlled trial. *JAMA* 290:238, 2003.

164. Wiedermann CJ, Romisch J: The anti-inflammatory actions of antithrombin—A review. *Acta Med Austriaca* 29:89, 2002.

165. Ahmed T, Gonzalez BJ, Danta I: Prevention of exercise-induced bronchoconstriction by inhaled low-molecular-weight heparin. *Am J Respir Crit Care Med* 160:576, 1999.

166. Davidson BL, Geerts WH, Lensing AW: Low-dose heparin for severe sepsis. *N Engl J Med* 347:1036, 2002.

167. Derhaschnig U, Pernerstorfer T, Knechtelsdorfer M, et al: Evaluation of antiinflammatory and antiadhesive effects of heparins in human endotoxemia. *Crit Care Med* 31:1108, 2003.

168. Murakami K, Enkhbaatar P, Shimoda K, et al: High-dose heparin fails to improve acute lung injury following smoke inhalation in sheep. *Clin Sci (Lond)* 104:349, 2003.

169. Dhainaut JF, Yan SB, Cariou A, Mira JP: Soluble thrombomodulin, plasma-derived unactivated protein C, and recombinant human activated protein C in sepsis. *Crit Care Med* 30(suppl):S318, 2002.

170. Gonda Y, Hirata S, Saitoh K, et al: Antithrombotic effect of recombinant human soluble thrombomodulin on endotoxin-induced disseminated intravascular coagulation in rats. *Thromb Res* 71:325, 1993.

171. Uchiba M, Okajima K, Murakami K, et al: Recombinant human soluble thrombomodulin reduces endotoxin-induced pulmonary vascular injury via protein C activation in rats. *Thromb Haemost* 74:1265, 1995.

172. Nakashima M, Kanamaru M, Umemura K, Tsuruta K: Pharmacokinetics and safety of a novel recombinant soluble human thrombomodulin, ART-123, in healthy male volunteers. *J Clin Pharmacol* 38:40, 1998.

173. Welty-Wolf KE, Carraway MS, Miller DL, et al: Coagulation blockade prevents sepsis-induced respiratory and renal failure in baboons. *Am J Respir Crit Care Med* 164(10 pt 1):1988, 2001.

174. Carraway MS, Welty-Wolf KE, Miller DL, et al: Blockade of tissue factor: treatment for organ injury in established sepsis. *Am J Respir Crit Care Med* 167:1200, 2003.

175. Jilma B, Marsik C, Mayr F, et al: Pharmacodynamics of active site-inhibited factor VIIa in endotoxin-induced coagulation in humans. *Clin Pharmacol Ther* 72:403, 2002.

176. Abraham E, Naum C, Bandi V, et al: Efficacy and safety of LY315920Na/S-5920, a selective inhibitor of 14-kDa group IIA secretory phospholipase A2, in patients with suspected sepsis and organ failure. *Crit Care Med* 31:718, 2003.

177. Zimmerman GA, McIntyre TM, Prescott SM, Stafforini DM: The platelet-activating factor signaling system and its regulators in syndromes of inflammation and thrombosis. *Crit Care Med* 30(suppl):S294, 2002.

178. Pribbler J, Yu A, Peterman G: Evaluations of the safety, pharmacokinetics, and clinical pharmacology of recombinant human platelet activating factor acetyl hydrolase (rPAF-AH) in healthy subjects and critically ill patients. Paper presented at the 6th International Congress on PAF and Related Lipid Mediators, New Orleans, 1998.

179. Vincent JL, Spapen H, Bakker J, et al: Phase II multicenter clinical study of the platelet-activating factor receptor antagonist BB-882 in the treatment of sepsis. *Crit Care Med* 28:638, 2000.

180. Cooper MS, Stewart PM: Corticosteroid insufficiency in acutely ill patients. *N Engl J Med* 348:727, 2003.

181. Carlet J: From mega to more reasonable doses of corticosteroids: A decade to recreate hope. *Crit Care Med* 27:672, 1999.

182. van Leeuwen HJ, van der Bruggen T, van Asbeck BS, Boereboom FT: Effect of corticosteroids on nuclear factor-kappaB activation and hemodynamics in late septic shock. *Crit Care Med* 29:1074, 2001.

183. Cronin L, Cook DJ, Carlet J, et al: Corticosteroid treatment for sepsis: A critical appraisal and meta-analysis of the literature. *Crit Care Med* 23:1430, 1995.

184. Bollaert PE, Charpentier C, Levy B, et al: Reversal of late septic shock with supraphysiologic doses of hydrocortisone. *Crit Care Med* 26:645, 1998.

185. Annane D, Sebille V, Troche G, et al: A 3-level prognostic classification in septic shock based on cortisol levels and cortisol response to corticotropin. *JAMA* 283:1038, 2000.

186. Annane D, Sebille V, Charpentier C, et al: Effect of treatment with low doses of hydrocortisone and fludrocortisone on mortality in patients with septic shock. *JAMA* 288:862, 2002.

187. Abraham E, Evans T: Corticosteroids and septic shock. *JAMA* 288:886, 2002.

188. Reinhart K, Karzai W: Anti-tumor necrosis factor therapy in sepsis: Update on clinical trials and lessons learned. *Crit Care Med* 29(suppl):S121, 2002.

189. Reinhart K, Menges T, Gardlund B, et al: Randomized, placebo-controlled trial of the anti-tumor necrosis factor antibody fragment afelimomab in hyperinflammatory response during severe sepsis: The RAMSES Study. *Crit Care Med* 29:765, 2001.

190. Calandra T, Echtenacher B, Roy DL, et al: Protection from septic shock by neutralization of macrophage migration inhibitory factor. *Nat Med* 6:164, 2000.

191. Soriano FG, Liaudet L, Szabo E, et al: Resistance to acute septic peritonitis in poly(ADP-ribose) polymerase-1-deficient mice. *Shock* 17:286, 2002.

192. Goldfarb RD, Marton A, Szabo E, et al: Protective effect of a novel, potent inhibitor of poly(adenosine 5'-diphosphate-ribose) synthetase in a porcine model of severe bacterial sepsis. *Crit Care Med* 30:974, 2002.

193. Czermak BJ, Sarma V, Pierson CL, et al: Protective effects of C5a blockade in sepsis. *Nat Med* 5:788, 1999.

194. Guo RF, Huber-Lang M, Wang X, et al: Protective effects of anti-C5a in sepsis-induced thymocyte apoptosis. *J Clin Invest* 106:1271, 2000.

195. Huber-Lang MS, Sarma JV, McGuire SR, et al: Protective effects of anti-C5a peptide antibodies in experimental sepsis. *FASEB J* 15:568, 2001.

196. Harris JA, Benedict FG: *Biometric Study of Basal Metabolism in Man.* Publication 279. Washington, DC, Carnegie Institute of Washington, 1919.

197. Perez J, Dellinger RP: Other supportive therapies in sepsis. *Intensive Care Med* 27(suppl 1):S116, 2001.

198. Uehara M, Plank LD, Hill GL: Components of energy expenditure in patients with severe sepsis and major trauma: A basis for clinical care. *Crit Care Med* 27:1295, 1999.

199. Ackerman MH, Evans NJ, Ecklund MM: Systemic inflammatory response syndrome, sepsis, and nutritional support. *Crit Care Nurs Clin North Am* 6:321, 1994.

200. Novak F, Heyland DK, Avenell A, et al: Glutamine supplementation in serious illness: A systematic review of the evidence. *Crit Care Med* 30:2022, 2002.

201. Barbul A: Arginine: Biochemistry, physiology, and therapeutic implications. *JPEN* 10:227, 1986.

202. Heyland DK: Nutritional support in the critically ill patients. A critical review of the evidence. *Crit Care Clin* 14:423, 1998.

203. Atkinson S, Sieffert E, Bihari D: A prospective, randomized, double-blind, controlled clinical trial of enteral immunonutrition in the critically ill. Guy's Hospital Intensive Care Group. *Crit Care Med* 26:1164, 1998.

204. Gadek JE, DeMichele SJ, Karlstad MD, et al: Effect of enteral feeding with eicosapentaenoic acid, gamma-linolenic acid, and antioxidants in patients with acute respiratory distress syndrome. Enteral Nutrition in ARDS Study Group. *Crit Care Med* 27:1409, 1999.

205. Heyland DK, MacDonald S, Keefe L, Drover JW: Total parenteral nutrition in the critically ill patient: A meta-analysis. *JAMA* 280:2013, 1998.

206. Fan J, Li YH, Wojnar MM, Lang CH: Endotoxin-induced alterations in insulin-stimulated phosphorylation of insulin receptor, IRS-1, and MAP kinase in skeletal muscle. *Shock* 6:164, 1996.

207. Youd JM, Rattigan S, Clark MG: Acute impairment of insulin-mediated capillary recruitment and glucose uptake in rat skeletal muscle in vivo by TNF-alpha. *Diabetes* 49:1904, 2000.

208. Rosmarin DK, Wardlaw GM, Mirtallo J: Hyperglycemia associated with high, continuous infusion rates of total parenteral nutrition dextrose. *Nutr Clin Pract* 11:151, 1996.

209. Fietsam R Jr, Bassett J, Glover JL: Complications of coronary artery surgery in diabetic patients. *Am Surg* 57:551, 1991.

210. Khaodhiar L, McCowen K, Bistrian B: Perioperative hyperglycemia, infection or risk? *Curr Opin Clin Nutr Metab Care* 2:79, 1999.

211. Kwoun MO, Ling PR, Lydon E, et al: Immunologic effects of acute hyperglycemia in nondiabetic rats. *JPEN* 21:91, 1997.

212. Rao AK, Chouhan V, Chen X, et al: Activation of the tissue factor pathway of blood coagulation during prolonged hyperglycemia in young healthy men. *Diabetes* 48:1156, 1999.

213. Boeri D, Almus FE, Maiello M, et al: Modification of tissue-factor mRNA and protein response to thrombin and interleukin 1 by high glucose in cultured human endothelial cells. *Diabetes* 38:212, 1989.

214. Malmberg K, Norhammar A, Wedel H, Ryden L: Glycometabolic state at admission: Important risk marker of mortality in conventionally treated patients with diabetes mellitus and acute myocardial infarction: long-term results from the Diabetes and Insulin-Glucose Infusion in Acute Myocardial Infarction (DIGAMI) study. *Circulation* 99:2626, 1999.

215. Malmberg K: Prospective randomised study of intensive insulin treatment on long term survival after acute myocardial infarction in patients with diabetes mellitus. DIGAMI (Diabetes Mellitus, Insulin Glucose Infusion in Acute Myocardial Infarction) Study Group. *BMJ* 314:1512, 1997.

216. van den Berghe G, Wouters P, Weekers F, et al: Intensive insulin therapy in the critically ill patients. *N Engl J Med* 345:1359, 2001.

217. Van den Berghe G, Wouters PJ, Bouillon R, et al: Outcome benefit of intensive insulin therapy in the critically ill: Insulin dose versus glycemic control. *Crit Care Med* 31:359, 2003.

218. Finney SJ, Zekveld C, Elia A, Evans TW: Glucose control and mortality in critically ill patients. *JAMA* 290:2041, 2003.

219. Levy EM, Viscoli CM, Horwitz RI: The effect of acute renal failure on mortality. A cohort analysis. *JAMA* 275:1489, 1996.

220. Chertow GM, Levy EM, Hammermeister KE, et al: Independent association between acute renal failure and mortality following cardiac surgery. *Am J Med* 104:343, 1998.

221. Bellomo R, Chapman M, Finfer S, et al: Low-dose dopamine in patients with early renal dysfunction: A placebo-controlled randomised trial. Australian and New Zealand Intensive Care Society (ANZICS) Clinical Trials Group. *Lancet* 356:2139, 2000.

222. Meyer MM: Renal replacement therapies. *Crit Care Clin* 16:29, 2000.

223. Schiffl H, Lang SM, Fischer R: Daily hemodialysis and the outcome of acute renal failure. *N Engl J Med* 346:305, 2002.

224. Cade JF: High risk of the critically ill for venous thromboembolism. *Crit Care Med* 10:448, 1982.

225. Hirsch DR, Ingenito EP, Goldhaber SZ: Prevalence of deep venous thrombosis among patients in medical intensive care. *JAMA* 274:335, 1995.

226. Jorgensen LN, Wille-Jorgensen P, Hauch O: Prophylaxis of postoperative thromboembolism with low molecular weight heparins. *Br J Surg* 80:689, 1993.

227. Bauer KA, Eriksson BI, Lassen MR, Turpie AG: Fondaparinux compared with enoxaparin for the prevention of venous thromboembolism after elective major knee surgery. *N Engl J Med* 345:1305, 2001.

228. Eriksson BI, Bauer KA, Lassen MR, Turpie AG: Fondaparinux compared with enoxaparin for the prevention of venous thromboembolism after hip-fracture surgery. *N Engl J Med* 345:1298, 2001.

229. Cook DJ, Fuller HD, Guyatt GH, et al: Risk factors for gastrointestinal bleeding in critically ill patients. Canadian Critical Care Trials Group. *N Engl J Med* 330:377, 1994.

230. Schuster DP, Rowley H, Feinstein S, et al: Prospective evaluation of the risk of upper gastrointestinal bleeding after admission to a medical intensive care unit. *Am J Med* 76:623, 1984.

231. Cook D, Guyatt G, Marshall J, et al: A comparison of sucralfate and ranitidine for the prevention of upper gastrointestinal bleeding in patients requiring mechanical ventilation. Canadian Critical Care Trials Group. *N Engl J Med* 338:791, 1998.

232. Prod'hom G, Leuenberger P, Koerfer J, et al: Nosocomial pneumonia in mechanically ventilated patients receiving antacid, ranitidine, or sucralfate as prophylaxis for stress ulcer. A randomized controlled trial. *Ann Intern Med* 120:653, 1994.

233. Yan SB, Helterbrand JD, Hartman DL, et al: Low levels of protein C are associated with poor outcome in severe sepsis. *Chest* 120:915, 2001.

234. Taylor FB Jr, Toh CH, Hoots WK, et al: Towards definition, clinical and laboratory criteria, and a scoring system for disseminated intravascular coagulation. *Thromb Haemost* 86:1327, 2001.

235. Feinstein DI: Diagnosis and management of disseminated intravascular coagulation: The role of heparin therapy. *Blood* 60:284, 1982.

236. Aoki N, Matsuda T, Saito H, et al: A comparative double-blind randomized trial of activated protein C and unfractionated heparin in the treatment of disseminated intravascular coagulation. *Int J Hematol* 75:540, 2002.

237. Joyce D, Yan B, Basson BR, et al: Disseminated intravascular coagulation in severe sepsis patients treated with recombinant human activated protein C (abstract). *Blood* 98:445a, 2001.

238. Lemeshow S, Klar J, Teres D: Outcome prediction for individual intensive care patients: Useful, misused, or abused? *Intensive Care Med* 21:770, 1995.

239. Cowen JS, Kelley MA: Errors and bias in using predictive scoring systems. *Crit Care Clin* 10:53, 1994.

240. Escarce JJ, Kelley MA: Admission source to the medical intensive care unit predicts hospital death independent of APACHE II score. *JAMA* 264:2389, 1990.

241. Vincent JL, de Mendonca A, Cantraine F, et al: Use of the SOFA score to assess the incidence of organ dysfunction/failure in intensive care units: results of a multicenter, prospective study. Working group on "sepsis-related problems" of the European Society of Intensive Care Medicine. *Crit Care Med* 26:1793, 1998.

242. Hebert PC, Drummond AJ, Singer J, et al: A simple multiple system organ failure scoring system predicts mortality of patients who have sepsis syndrome. *Chest* 104:230, 1993.

Chapter 47 _____

APPROACH TO INFECTION IN PATIENTS RECEIVING CYTOTOXIC CHEMOTHERAPY FOR MALIGNANCY

E.J. BOW

KEY POINTS

- *Risk of infection increases as the circulating absolute neutrophil count (ANC) declines below 1.0×10^9/L. The greatest risk of bacteremic infection occurs when the ANC is $<0.1 \times 10^9$/L.*

- *Cytotoxic therapy for remission-induction therapy for acute myeloid leukemia or conditioning therapy for bone marrow transplantation (high-risk patients) is associated with periods when the ANC is $<0.1 \times 10^9$/L for 14 to 21 days. The time to marrow recovery (ANC $> 0.5 \times 10^9$/L) can vary from 21 to 42 days.*

- *Intermittent administration of cytotoxic therapy for solid tissue malignancies or lymphoreticular malignancies (low-risk patients) is often associated with a neutrophil nadir at 10 to 14 days from beginning treatment and with periods of neutropenia (ANC $< 0.5 \times 10^9$/L) of less than 5 to 7 days. This pattern of neutrophil recovery influences the natural history of febrile neutropenic episodes.*

- *Febrile episodes during neutropenia are defined by an oral temperature of $38.3°C$ ($101°F$) or more in the absence of other noninfectious causes of fever such as administration of blood products or pyrogenic drugs (e.g., cytotoxic therapy or amphotericin B), the underlying disease, thromboembolic or thrombophlebitic events, or hemorrhagic events.*

- *A single neutropenic episode may be characterized by one or more febrile episodes, of which one or more may represent infections.*

- *Body sites most often associated with infection in the neutropenic patient are those associated with integumental surfaces (skin, upper and lower respiratory tract, and upper and lower gastrointestinal tract).*

- *Antibacterial prophylaxis with oral agents such as cotrimoxazole, norfloxacin, or ciprofloxacin can reduce the frequency of febrile episodes and bacteremic events in patients with protracted neutropenia.*

- *Patients undergoing remission-induction for acute myeloid leukemia or bone marrow transplantation with a history of herpetic stomatitis or who are IgG seropositive for herpes simplex virus (HSV) are at risk for severe herpetic mucositis. Such patients should be given acyclovir prophylaxis.*

- *Empiric antimicrobial therapy for suspected infection in the febrile neutropenic patient usually is composed of a broad-spectrum antibacterial regimen of an anti-pseudomonal penicillin or carbapenem administered as a single agent*

(monotherapy). Aminoglycoside-based combinations do not add to the efficacy of the single agent, but do add toxicity.

- *Neutropenic patients responding to empiric antibacterial therapy generally require at least 5 days for the response to be observed in half the cases. Patients remaining febrile at 5 days should be systematically re-evaluated, while consideration of modification of the antimicrobial regimen can be made at day 7 or 8 unless clinical deterioration is evident. Glycopeptides administered as second-line empiric therapy for persistent fever after 3 to 5 days do not influence time to defervescence or febrile episode-related mortality.*

Critical care physicians are often called on to provide metabolic, hemodynamic, and respiratory support for patients with various inherited or acquired defects in host defense that render them susceptible to potentially lethal infections. Patients with single host defense system defects, such as those with inherited immune deficiency syndromes such as congenital agammaglobulinemia, are susceptible to particular encapsulated respiratory pathogens such as *Streptococcus pneumoniae* that require the presence of opsonizing antibody for clearance. In contrast, cancer patients undergoing potentially curative high-intensity myeloablative cytotoxic therapy acquire defects in multiple host defense systems that lead to increased susceptibility to different groups of pathogens normally contained and controlled by the absent or damaged systems. Four broad categories of defects in host defense are clinically relevant: disruption of the integrity of the integumental surfaces, quantitative neutrophilic phagocyte defects, diminished B lymphocyte (humoral) function, and diminished T lymphocyte system function. A working knowledge of the sources of failure in these host defense systems is particularly important for predicting the types of offending pathogens likely to be involved in the kind of life-threatening infections requiring the services of the critical care team. This, in turn, provides a basis for a rational approach to the choice of antimicrobial therapy. This chapter reviews the approach to managing suspected or proven infection in patients with multiple defects in host defense systems, with a particular emphasis on patients undergoing active myelosuppressive cytotoxic therapy, since this represents the largest group of immunocompromised patients who will require critical care services. Infections in patients with the acquired immunodeficiency syndrome (AIDS) are discussed in Chap. 48, and infections in those with organ or bone marrow transplantation are discussed in Chaps. 73 and 90; the problem of lung infiltrates in immunocompromised patients is covered in Chap. 51.

Hematologists and oncologists have long recognized the existence of the direct relationship between dose and response in cancer therapy. Over the last 10 to 15 years, the supportive care strategies for cancer patients undergoing remission-induction or salvage therapy have improved sufficiently to permit the extension of dosing to the very limits of toxicity and beyond. For many malignant diseases this has translated into significantly higher response rates and disease-free survival. Cure is now a goal that can be adopted realistically for many more patients with these diseases.

Despite these encouraging results, newer dose-intensive therapeutic approaches render patients highly susceptible to life-threatening infection, which in itself or in association with tumor-related end-organ damage may be accompanied by multisystem failure. Whereas some investigators have suggested that admission of cancer patients to the ICU is costly and ultimately futile,[1-4] others have challenged this assumption.[3,5-7] The outcome for cancer patients admitted to an ICU is directly related to the degree of end-organ damage rather than to the status of the underlying malignancy.[6,8,9] The rates of mortality are highest (80% to 100%) when cancer patients admitted to intensive care units (ICUs) have serious damage to three or more organ systems,[8,9] or those who develop respiratory failure and require mechanical ventilation.[6,7,10-13] Further need for critical care services beyond 14 days has been associated with a 100% hospital mortality rate in a number of studies.[8,9] Some factors are additive for ICU-related mortality. For example, a German study reported a mortality rate of 55% in patients with persistent severe neutropenia, 72% for neutropenic cancer patients requiring mechanical ventilation, and 90% for neutropenic cancer patients with invasive fungal infection who require mechanical ventilation.[7] The critical care consultant must give careful consideration to these factors to estimate the probability that a critically ill febrile neutropenic patient will survive the episode long enough for the antineoplastic treatments to have their desired effect.

Deficits in Host Defenses Related to Cancer Chemotherapy

MYELOSUPPRESSION AND NEUTROPENIA

The absolute number of circulating segmented neutrophils (ANC) represents the most important single parameter predictive of the risk for life-threatening infection.[14] An ANC of 1.5 to 8.0 $\times$ 10^9/L can be considered normal for adults. As the ANC declines below 1.0 $\times$ 10^9/L the risk of infection increases, with greatest risk for bacteremic infection at neutrophil counts below 0.1 $\times$ 10^9/L. Figure 47-1 illustrates the relationship between the neutrophil count and infection for a series of patients undergoing remission-induction therapy for acute leukemia.

The ANC is calculated by multiplying the proportion of white blood cells (WBCs) that are segmented neutrophils on a Romanovsky-stained blood smear by the total number of WBCs in a specified volume of blood measured in an automated blood cell counter. Since neutropenic patients with acute leukemia undergoing cytotoxic therapy frequently have total WBC counts of <0.5 $\times$ 10^9/L, neutrophils may be difficult to detect on a manually reviewed stained smear; accordingly, the range of error for the procedure increases dramatically. Further, automated blood cell counters may give misleading results when abnormal cells such as leukemic blasts of similar size as segmented neutrophils are present in the circulation. This should dissuade the clinician from relying too heavily on a single ANC to judge the risk of infection. Rather, the clinical relevance of the ANC lies in the recognition of the range associated with a specific infection risk.

The pattern of change of the ANC also has a significant independent influence on infection risk. In one study, 29% of the bacteremic episodes occurred as the neutrophil count was falling but before the ANC fell below 0.5 $\times$ 10^9/L.[15] Therefore, with a falling neutrophil count, multiple observations over time are necessary to establish a pattern for the neutrophil profile and to estimate the relative infection risk. Survival of an infection during severe neutropenia is also intimately linked to marrow recovery and recovery of the circulating neutrophil count.[16,17] The poorest outcomes for the infectious episodes occur among patients in whom the ANC continues to decline or fails to increase.[18,19]

The duration of severe neutropenia (ANC < 0.5 $\times$ 10^9/L) is also related directly to infection risk. For example, bacteremic infections occur 3.5 times and 5.4 times more often when neutropenia lasts 6 to 15 days and >15 days, respectively.[20] The duration of neutropenia is related to the degree of hemopoietic stem cell damage caused by the underlying disease

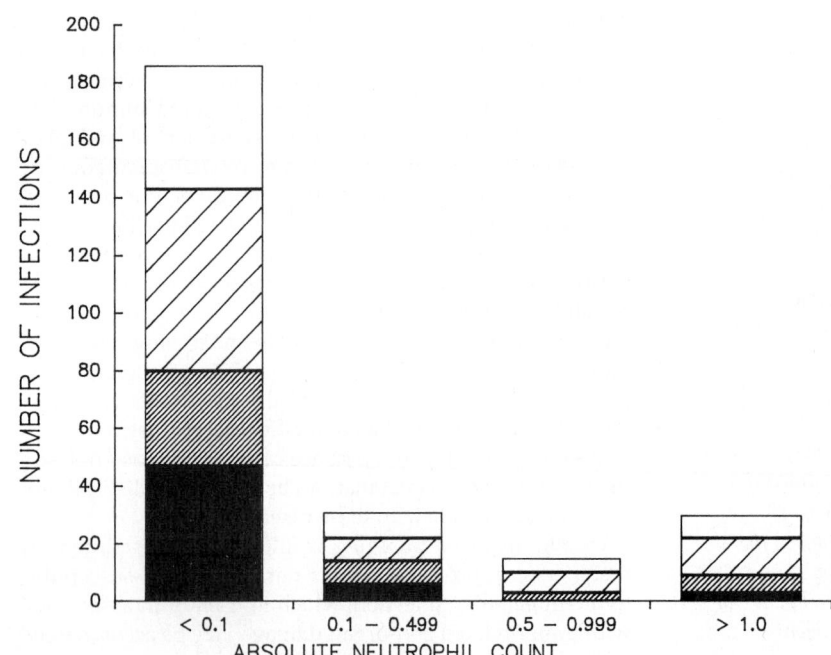

FIGURE 47-1 The relationship between the ANC and occurrence of infection in 98 patients undergoing remission-induction therapy for acute myeloid leukemia (AML). The proportions of the infections classified as possible infection, clinical infections, nonbacteremic microbiologically documented infection, and bacteremic infection are shown. The greatest risk for infection occurs when the ANC is <0.1 $\times$ 10^9/L. Possible infections, open bars; clinical infections, open crosshatch bars; nonbacteremic microbiologically documented infections, close crosshatch bars; bacteremia, black bars.

process and by myelosuppressive regimens. Following stem cell suppression, the peripheral neutrophil count falls at a rate inversely proportional to the size of the circulating and marginated peripheral neutrophil pools and the size of the marrow storage pool of mature segmented neutrophils. Marrow recovery follows the recruitment of committed stem cells that are the precursors of granulocytic, monocytic, erythroid, and megakaryocytic cell lines from the resting pluripotential stem cell pool. These hemopoietic stem cells must be able to proliferate to increase their numbers and then differentiate to provide the functional effector cell populations.

Patients receiving pulse doses of chemotherapy for solid tissue malignancies or lymphoreticular malignancies sustain only temporary damage to the hemopoietic stem cell pool. The expected circulating neutrophil nadir generally occurs between days 10 and 14. Although the neutrophil nadirs may be <0.5 × 10^9/L, the duration of neutropenia is rarely longer than 5 to 7 days (median = 3 to 5 days). For example, a patient receiving cyclophosphamide, doxorubicin (hydroxy-daunomycin), vincristine (Oncovin), and prednisone (CHOP) beginning on day 1 of a 21-day cycle of treatment for an intermediate- to high-grade non-Hodgkin's lymphoma might develop a febrile episode on day 12 in association with an ANC of 0.1 × 10^9/L. The patient's neutrophil count would be expected to have reached its nadir, and a rise in circulating neutrophils would be predicted to occur between days 15 and 21. The likelihood that this prediction is correct is increased if a relative monocytosis is observed on the differential WBC count. The recovery of peripheral blood monocytes precedes that of circulating neutrophils in chemotherapy-induced aplasia and often heralds the recovery of the ANC.

In general, the more dose-intensive myelosuppressive regimens are associated with more hemopoietic stem cell damage and longer durations of neutropenia. Standard remission-induction regimens for acute myeloid leukemia (AML) are composed of anthracycline drugs such as daunorubicin administered in intravenous doses of 30 to 60 mg/m^2 daily over 3 days, and an antimetabolite, cytarabine, administered as an intravenous bolus or as a continuous infusion at doses of 100 to 200 mg/m^2 daily over 5 to 7 days. These regimens predictably produce periods of profound myelosuppression, in which a median of 24 days passes until the circulating neutrophil count rises above 0.5 × 10^9/L.[21] If more than one cycle of therapy is required to achieve a complete remission, then the median time until marrow recovery may be prolonged by as long as 6 weeks. This additional period of myelosuppression is associated with a significant increase in infectious morbidity.[21,22]

More intensive regimens using high-dose cytarabine (HDA RAC) in doses 15 to 30 times that for standard induction regimens have been successful for salvage therapy of relapsed or resistant leukemia, for initial remission-induction therapy, and for postremission consolidation therapy for acute leukemia.[21] The median time until neutrophil recovery (>0.5 × 10^9/L) following administration of HDARAC (3.0 g/m^2 infused over 1 hour every 12 hours for 12 consecutive doses) is 25 to 30 days. Surprisingly, this period of myelosuppression is not substantially longer than for standard induction regimens. However, the period of risk for infection can be significantly longer (e.g., extending the time to neutrophil recovery to 40 to 60 days) for heavily pretreated patients, in whom there may be more prolonged direct

effects of cytotoxic therapy on the marrow stem cell pool or the marrow microenvironment.

OTHER IMMUNOSUPPRESSIVE EFFECTS OF CYTOTOXIC THERAPY

The remission-induction regimens commonly used for acute leukemia have important immunosuppressive effects in addition to the myelosuppressive effects discussed above. Anthracyclines and similar agents (e.g., doxorubicin, daunorubicin, idarubicin, epirubicin, amacrine, mitoxantrone, and rubidazone), antimetabolites (e.g., cytarabine, methotrexate, thioguanine, and mercaptopurine), and alkylating agents (e.g., cyclophosphamide, ifosfamide, melphalan, busulfan, and platinum analogues) have profound suppressive effects on the numbers of circulating T and B lymphoid cells that parallel the acquired functional defects in cell-mediated and humoral immune mechanisms. At the clinical level, the consequences of these effects are reflected by an increased susceptibility to pathogens normally controlled by these mechanisms. The ultimate impact on immune responsiveness appears to depend on the schedule of administration.

T-LYMPHOCYTE FUNCTION
Indications from in vitro testing of lymphoid cell responsiveness to mitogen-induced blastogenesis suggest that T-cell function may be moderately depressed in patients with acute leukemia. Among patients undergoing remission-induction therapy for acute leukemia, decreased cell-mediated immune responsiveness can be detected for up to 6 months following chemotherapy-induced remission.[23,24] Immune function has been observed in some patients to decline once again as a herald to relapse.[23]

The clinical consequences of T-cell dysfunction vary with the underlying disease and the cytotoxic regimen. For example, *Pneumocystis carinii* infection is an uncommon phenomenon among adult patients undergoing remission-induction for AML, but relatively common among children undergoing consolidation and maintenance-phase chemotherapy for acute lymphoblastic leukemia (ALL).[25] An intermediate degree of risk for pneumocystosis appears to be present in those undergoing bone marrow allografting or autografting. The immunosuppressive potential of the conditioning regimens for bone marrow transplantation (BMT) appears to be greater than that associated with AML induction regimens. Accordingly, most centers managing these patients recommend administering primary prophylaxis for *P. carinii* in BMT recipients or patients with ALL. These infections rarely occur during the primary period of myelosuppressive therapy–induced neutropenia.

B-LYMPHOCYTE FUNCTION
Modern cytotoxic therapy for acute leukemia appears to have a more profound effect on humoral immune competence than on T-lymphocyte function. Serum immunoglobulin concentrations and the efficiency of new antigen-induced immunoglobulin synthesis have been observed to decline following institution of remission-induction therapy, reaching a nadir at approximately 5 weeks. It has been difficult to separate the effects of the underlying malignant disease from the effects of the cytotoxic therapy. There does not appear to be a prognostically useful parameter of T- or B-cell function

that predicts infection risk in neutropenic patients that is analogous to the predictive value of the ANC for pyogenic bacterial or fungal infection. However, presence of hypogammaglobulinemia may help identify increased risk of infection by encapsulated bacteria.

INTEGUMENTAL BARRIERS

Integumental barriers are among the most important and most often damaged defense systems for cancer patients. These barriers include the epithelial surfaces of the skin, the upper and lower respiratory tract, the upper and lower gastrointestinal (GI) tract, and the mucosal surfaces lining the genitourinary tract. In critically ill patients, the barrier function of these surfaces also may be compromised by procedures such as percutaneous intravenous catheterization, endotracheal intubation, endoscopic procedures, nasogastric intubation, and indwelling urinary catheterization (Table 47-1).

Integumental damage secondary to cytotoxic therapy has become more prevalent as the dose intensity of the remission-induction regimens has increased.[26] The epithelial surfaces of the GI tract appear to be at greatest risk. The antiproliferative effect of therapy prevents cell recruitment into mucosal areas denuded by erosion or by cellular attrition, resulting in the appearance of superficial erosion and ulceration. The absorptive capacity of the GI mucosa also may be impaired significantly among recipients of regimens such as HDARAC, and both anatomic mucosal disruption and absorptive dysfunction appear to temporally parallel that of the neutrophil profile.

A high proportion of patients receiving cytoreductive therapy also experience painful, often debilitating inflammatory lesions within the oral cavity.[27] The tissues of the periodontium, gingival surfaces, oral mucosa, and mucosal surfaces of the upper and lower bowel are affected.[26] Cytotoxic regimens affect the developing basal epithelial cells of the oral mucosa in a manner that parallels the effect on the marrow system cell pool and the intestinal mucosal surface.[28] Mucosal atrophy, cytolysis, and denudation of the mucosal surface result in the painful foci of local ulceration typically observed 4 to 7 days after the administration of the cytotoxic agents and which usually resolve spontaneously between days 14 and 21.[27,29]

Cytotoxic therapy–induced intestinal mucosal damage has been described in three stages.[28] The first stage of initial injury begins during the first week of cytotoxic therapy and is characterized by replacement of the normal crypts and mucus-secreting goblet cells by atypical undifferentiated cells. The second stage represents progressive mucosal injury that occurs during the second and third weeks. This stage is characterized histologically by cellular necrosis, lack of mitotic activity, and focal loss of villous surfaces, and clinically by abdominal pain, diarrhea, electrolyte loss, and invasive infection. The third stage of cellular regeneration occurs after the third week and is characterized by resumption of mitotic activity and cellular proliferation in the crypts with subsequent repopulation of the denuded surfaces by differentiated cells.

The maximum cytotoxic therapy–induced intestinal epithelial damage occurs in the second week between days 10 and 14.[30–32] This corresponds to the median time of onset of bacteremic infection on day 14 due to the microorganisms that normally colonize these surfaces.[33] To a limited extent, the type of pathogens recovered in bacteremic infections can be predicted from the pool of microorganisms colonizing damaged mucosal surfaces. Oral mucosal ulceration, particularly that involving periodontal tissues, is often associated with viridans group streptococcal bacteremia.[34,35] Colonic mucosal damage is more likely to be associated with aerobic gram-negative bacillary infection with *Escherichia coli*, *Klebsiella* species, *Pseudomonas aeruginosa*, or opportunistic yeasts when these pathogens are colonizing the lower GI tract.[33]

Mucositis not only predisposes patients to invasive infection, but also imposes a significant cost with respect to the resources needed to manage the consequences of mucositis.[36,37] Recent cost estimates suggest that an episode of severe mucositis may cost an average of $7985 (U.S. dollars; USD) (year 2002) per patient (95% CI $6164 to $9806).[37] Neutropenia with or without infection is estimated to cost an average of $9316 USD (year 2002) per inpatient (95% CI $8522 to $10,110). In times of fiscal restraint, these complications have great significance for institutions charged with the responsibility for managing cancer patients.

INFECTIONS AND PATHOGENS

In a review of bloodstream infections occurring in patients with hematologic malignancies over a 14-year period in a tertiary cancer center in Sweden, gram-negative bacilli accounted for 45% and gram-positive organisms accounted for 55%.[38] Coagulase-negative staphylococci accounted for 17.5%; *Escherichia coli* for 16.3%; viridans group streptococci for 12.7% (with *S. mitis* being the most common in 50 of 178 isolates); *Klebsiella* and *Enterobacter* spp. for 12.7%; *Staphylococcus aureus* for 8.9%; *Enterococcus* spp. for 7.3%; and *Pseudomonas aeruginosa* for 5.5%.[38] Of note in this experience was the rising incidence of enterococcal bloodstream infections due to penicillin-resistant *E. faecium* and the high 30-day mortality (24%) compared to other gram-positive 30-day mortality rates (~15%).[38]

The infections documented among febrile neutropenic patients have been classified as microbiologically documented with the identification of a pathogen and a focus of infection; as clinically documented with the identification of a clinical focus of infection without isolation of a putative pathogen; and as an unexplained fever wherein neither a

---

TABLE 47-1 Integumental Defects

Damage to mucosal surfaces
  Endotracheal tube
  Nasogastric tube
  Cytotoxic agent–induced damage to gastrointestinal and
    respiratory epithelial barriers
  Endoscopic diagnostic procedures
Damage to skin and supporting structures
  IV catheters
    Peripheral IV lines
    Indwelling central venous catheters
  Indwelling urinary catheters
  Biopsy sites
    Bone marrow
    Lymph nodes
    Skin

clinical focus nor a pathogen are identified.[39] Among febrile neutropenic cancer patients not receiving fluoroquinolone chemoprophylaxis managed during the early 1990s, Cornelissen and colleagues reported that microbiologically-documented infections were observed in 33% of patients, with gram-negative infections comprising 18%, gram-positive infections in 9%, and mixed gram-negative and gram-positive infections in 6%.[40] Forty-two percent of patients had clinically documented infections and the remaining 24% had unexplained fevers. Among a similar group of patients who had received ciprofloxacin chemoprophylaxis, there were no gram-negative infections. Gram-positive infections were observed in 38% of patients, clinically-documented infections in 47% of patients, and unexplained fevers in only 15%.

A more recent study wherein the investigators identified all potential clinical foci of infections reported the GI tract as the focus of infection in 41% of patients with the oropharynx accounting for 70%, the esophagus 3%, clinical neutropenic enterocolitis 17%, and perirectal soft tissue infection 10%.[41] Other foci included the respiratory tract in 10%, urinary tract in 6%, and skin and soft tissue in 10%. Of the skin foci, indwelling central venous catheter sites accounted for 59%, folliculitis for 6%, and cellulitis for 35%.[41] Unexplained fevers accounted for only 10% of cases and microbiologically-documented bloodstream infections were seen in 23% of patients, of which gram-negative bacillemia accounted for 37%, coagulase-negative staphylococcemia 19%, streptococcemia 27%, and other gram-positive microorganisms in 16%.[41] These observations illustrate that with clinical diligence, clinical foci of infection may be identified in the majority of febrile neutropenic patients receiving cytotoxic therapy.

Approach to Fever Associated with Neutropenia

Fever is the hallmark of infection for most patients during periods of prolonged severe neutropenia. The definition of what constitutes a febrile episode due to suspected infection in a neutropenic patient has varied greatly in different studies.[18–20,34,41–52] The International Antimicrobial Therapy Cooperative Group (IATCG) of the European Organization for Research and Treatment of Cancer (EORTC),[20,47,48] the Intercontinental Antimicrobial Study Group,[50] and others[49] have used an oral temperature of >38°C (100.8°F) sustained over a 12-hour period or a single oral temperature of >38.5°C as the criterion for infection-related fever. The recently published German guidelines define an unexplained fever by a single oral temperature of >38.3°C or >38.0°C lasting over an hour or measured twice within 12 hours.[53] The National Cancer Institute of Canada Clinical Trials Group also has used a single oral temperature of >39°C together with chills or rigors instead of a single temperature of >38.5°C.[18,54] In order to avoid the administration of antimicrobial therapy to patients with noninfectious causes of fever, a qualifier often has been added to these definitions stipulating that other causes of noninfectious fever should be excluded. Such causes include blood products, pyrogenic drugs such as amphotericin B, thrombophlebitis, or hematoma. The Infectious Diseases Society of America (IDSA) has suggested that a single oral temperature of >38.3°C (101°F) in the absence of other obvious environmental causes would be a reasonably safe

working definition for an infection-related fever in neutropenic patients.[55]

The extent to which characteristics of the febrile episode predict a bacteremic event has been somewhat variable in different studies; however, most agree that initial oral temperatures of >39°C (102.2°F), shaking chills, clinical shock, initial ANC of <0.1 × 10⁹/L, and initial platelet count of <10 × 10⁹/L are to some degree predictive of gram-negative bacteremia.[15,20,42,56] Viscoli and associates[20] demonstrated an 8.4-fold increase in risk for bacteremic infection in neutropenic patients with initial temperatures of >39°C (102.2°F). The duration of fever prior to evaluation, however, does not appear to influence the risk of gram-negative bacteremia.[15]

The risk of developing a febrile neutropenic episode during each cycle of outpatient cancer chemotherapy for solid tissue malignancies or lymphoreticular malignancies is generally low.[57] However, this risk increases with the number of cycles administered and with the dose intensity of the regimen selected.[58] In a study of patients with lymphoma from the M.D. Anderson Cancer Center, the cumulative incidence of febrile neutropenic episodes increased from 12% among recipients of cyclophosphamide, vincristine (Oncovin), and prednisone (COP) to 27% among patients receiving a related regimen where doxorubicin (hydroxydaunomycin) was substituted for the cyclophosphamide (HOP) and 46% among recipients of cyclophosphamide, doxorubicin, vincristine (Oncovin), and prednisone (CHOP).[59] In recent studies, the incidence of infection among CHOP recipients has been lower, approximately 15% of all cycles.[60] Similarly to the findings of the study by Feld and Bodey,[59] the addition of cytotoxic agents to a chemotherapy regimen has the effect of increasing the likelihood of myelosuppression. For example, the addition of paclitaxel or docetaxel to carboplatin for the treatment of gynecologic malignancies increased the incidence of severe neutropenia (ANC < 0.5 × 10⁹/L) from <1% to 7% and 73%, respectively.[61] However, the addition of irinotecan to carboplatin and paclitaxel increased the incidence of severe neutropenia from 7% to 61%, but did not enhance the odds of developing a febrile neutropenic episode (odds ratio 3.56, 95% CI 0.71 to 17.94).[61] The median incidence of febrile neutropenic episodes in patients with small-cell lung cancer is reported as 35% for recipients of cyclophosphamide, doxorubicin, and etoposide (CAE) compared with 18% for recipients of a less myelosuppressive regimen containing cyclophosphamide, doxorubicin (Adriamycin), and vincristine (CAV).[62] In addition to the factor of neutropenia, the propensity of a given regimen to induce mucosal damage resulting in mucositis correlates directly with the incidence of febrile neutropenic episodes. The severity of mucositis is directly related to the incidence of febrile events, the duration of hospitalization, the costs of medical care, and treatment-related mortality.[36]

In contrast, febrile neutropenic episodes occur in 70% to 90% of patients receiving intensive cytotoxic therapy for acute leukemia and bone marrow transplantation.[54,63] This difference is due to the more prolonged cytotoxic therapy-induced myelosuppression and greater intestinal epithelial damage in these patients.[32]

Prolonged neutropenic periods may be punctuated by one or more febrile episodes, and a single febrile neutropenic episode may represent more than one infectious process. For example, a febrile neutropenic episode associated with a viridans group streptococcal bacteremia may not be seen to defervesce promptly despite the administration of appropriate antibacterial therapy and despite the documentation of a microbiologic cure on the basis of subsequent sterile blood cultures. This phenomenon of a persistent febrile state may occur in association with the concomitant administration of pyrogenic blood products, the presence of a coexisting infection such as a herpes simplex virus (HSV) mucositis, or a possible fungal superinfection. It is frequently impossible to distinguish clinically the boundaries defining separate sequential infectious processes by the pattern of fever unless a clear pattern of defervescence is seen between one infection and the next. This is particularly frustrating for clinicians managing febrile neutropenic patients without a defined clinical focus of infection or a defined pathogen.

DIAGNOSIS

Most febrile neutropenic episodes are assumed to represent infection. The diagnosis of a febrile state in a neutropenic patient requires a complete but directed clinical history and physical examination designed to identify potentially infected foci for which those patients are at special risk.

Important historical facts may be obtained from the patient, from significant others, and from the patient's medical record. The physician must verify that the patient is neutropenic, the degree of neutropenia, and when the patient is a recipient of cytotoxic therapy, the day of the chemotherapy cycle. The latter is determined relative to the first day of the last cycle of chemotherapy, or in the case of BMT recipients, the day of the BMT.

To avoid omitting the consideration of other noninfectious causes of fever in neutropenic patients, the clinical evaluation should include questions pertaining to the temporal association of the febrile episode to the administration of blood products, to a history of fever associated with the underlying disease, to the administration of chemotherapeutic agents or amphotericin B, to the presence of thrombophlebitis, and to the possible association of the febrile episode with thromboembolic or hemorrhagic events. For example, in a series of neutropenic patients undergoing remission-induction therapy for acute leukemia,[17] 26 of 72 (36%) febrile episodes were due to noninfectious causes (blood products in 33%, underlying disease or cytotoxic drugs in 15%, and unexplained causes in 47%). However, the majority of these patients had further febrile episodes for which a diagnosis of infection could not be excluded confidently.

The physical signs of inflammation and infection are influenced by the ANC. The incidence and magnitude of localizing findings such as exudate, fluctuance, ulceration, or fissure formation are reduced in a direct relationship to the ANC.[64] Other localizing findings, such as erythema and focal tenderness, appear to remain as useful and reliable signs of infection regardless of the ANC.

The body systems most often involved with infection in neutropenic patients are those associated with integumental surfaces (i.e., the upper and lower respiratory tracts, the upper and lower GI tracts, and the skin).[42,64,65] Table 47-2 lists the pertinent historical and physical clues to be sought in the clinical evaluation of a febrile neutropenic patient.

Examination of the head and neck area should include eyegrounds, the external auditory canals and tympanic membranes, the anterior nasal mucosa, the vermilion border of the lips, and the mucosal surfaces of the oropharynx. The eyeground examination should look for retinal hemorrhages as evidence of a bleeding diathesis and retinal exudates (often described as "cotton wool" exudates) that would suggest endophthalmitis associated with disseminated candidiasis. Examination of the external auditory canals and tympanic membranes for erythema or vesicular lesions can implicate this as a focus for infection by respiratory pathogens or herpes viruses. The anterior nasal mucosal surfaces should be examined for ulcerated lesions that might suggest the presence of a local filamentous fungal infection such as that due to *Aspergillus* species. The skin of the external nares should be examined for vesicular or crusted lesions that would suggest HSV infection. Nasal stuffiness and tenderness over the maxillary sinuses suggests that sinusitis is the infectious problem.

The oropharyngeal examination consists of inspection of the dentition, gingival surfaces, mucosal surfaces of the cheeks, hard and soft palate, tongue surfaces, and posterior pharyngeal wall. The presence of decaying teeth and gingival hyperemia implicates those sites as possible sources of bacteremic infection. The presence of shallow, painful mucosal ulcers on an erythematous base suggests herpes mucositis. Progression of this kind of lesion with local tissue necrosis can suggest a polymicrobic infection due to oropharyngeal anaerobic bacteria (e.g., *Fusobacterium nucleatum, Bacteroides melaninogenicus,* and peptostreptococci), particularly if cultures for HSV are negative or if such lesions develop during prophylactic or therapeutic administration of acyclovir. Oral thrush or pseudomembranous pharyngitis evolves from an overgrowth of opportunistic yeasts such as *Candida* species. These lesions are characterized by a thick creamy pseudomembrane consisting of masses of fungi existing in both the yeast and the mycelial phases. The distribution may be patchy, confluent, or discrete. The pseudomembrane is frequently closely adherent to the underlying mucosal surface such that attempts at removal reveal an erythematous or hemorrhagic base. The diagnosis is suspected by the clinical appearance and confirmed by the demonstration of the pathogen in culture and by the microscopic appearance of budding yeasts and pseudohyphae on a Gram's stain or potassium hydroxide preparation.

Chest examination should emphasize evaluation of the lower respiratory tract and central venous catheter sites. The typical signs of pulmonary consolidation may be muted or absent in neutropenic patients; however, localized crepitation on auscultation often precedes the appearance of pulmonary infiltrates radiologically, and thus often represents the earliest clue (and often the only clue) to a developing pneumonia in a neutropenic patient. Purulent sputum is similarly reduced in incidence and amount. Therefore the symptoms of the neutropenic patient with a developing pneumonia may manifest only as febrile illness associated with an increased respiratory rate and a few localized crepitations, with or without an associated cough or radiologic changes.[66] The clinician must search for additional differential diagnostic clues such as the origin of the suspected pneumonia (community- or hospital-acquired), the tempo of the illness, the association of the illness with other potentially noninfectious factors such as pulmonary edema, exposure to certain chemotherapeutic agents associated with lung injury (bleomycin, busulfan, or cytarabine), radiation therapy, pulmonary thromboemboli,

TABLE 47-2 Clinical Evaluation of the Febrile Neutropenic Patient

Body System	FINDINGS TO BE SOUGHT	
	Historical	Physical

Eye	Blurring of vision
	Double vision
	Loss of vision
	Pain
		Scleral abnormalities
		  Icterus
		  Hemorrhage
		  Local swelling
		Conjunctival abnormalities
		  Focal erythema
		  Petechiae
		Retina
		  Hemorrhage
		  "Cotton wool"exudates
		    (e.g., candidal
		    endophthalmitis)

Skin	Skin rash
	Pruritus (focal or diffuse)
	History of drug reactions
	Focal pain/swelling
	
	IV catheter site(s)
		Central venous catheters
		  Insertion site erythema/pain
		  Tunnel site erythema/pain
		  Exit site
		    erythema/pain/exudate
		Peripheral IV catheters
		  Focal tenderness
		  Focal erythema
		  Exudate at the insertion site
		Skin rash
		  Papular/macular/vesicular
		  Ulceration
		  Focal areas of necrosis
		    (e.g., ecthyma gangrenosum)
		  Distribution

Upper respiratory	Painful ear Nasal stuffiness Sinus tenderness Epistaxis	External auditory canals Thympanic membrane erythema
Lower respiratory	Cough Increased respiratory secretions Dyspnea Hemoptysis Chest pain	Tachypnea Tachycardia Hyperpnea Localized crepitations Consolidation

Upper
  gastrointestinal
	Odynophagia
	Dysphagia
	History of denture use
	History of herpes stomatitis
		Gingival bleeding
		Pseudomembranous exudate
		  over buccal and gingival
		  surfaces and tongue
		Mucosal erythema
		Mucosal ulceration
		Focal pain
		Preexisting periodontitis

Lower
  gastrointestinal
	Abdominal pain
	Constipation
	Diarrhea ± bleeding
	Perianal pain with
	  defecation
	
	Jaundice
		Focal abdominal pain
		  Right upper quadrant
		    (e.g., biliary tree)
		  Right lower quadrant
		    (e.g., cecum/ascending
		    colon)
		  Left lower quadrant
		    (e.g., diverticular disease)
		Perianal abnormalities
		  Focal tenderness
		  Focal/diffuse erythema
		  Fissures
		  Ulcerations
		  Hemorrhoidal tissues

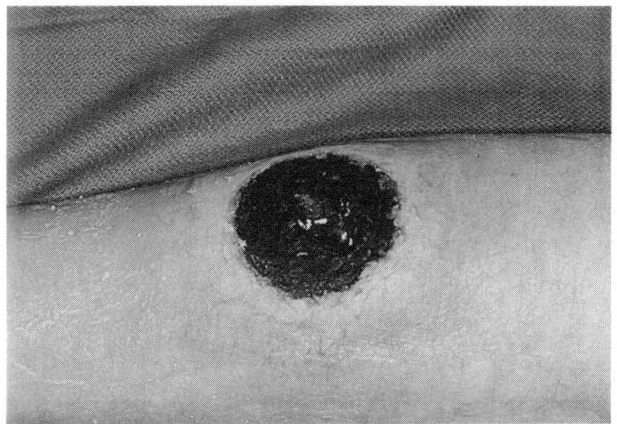

A

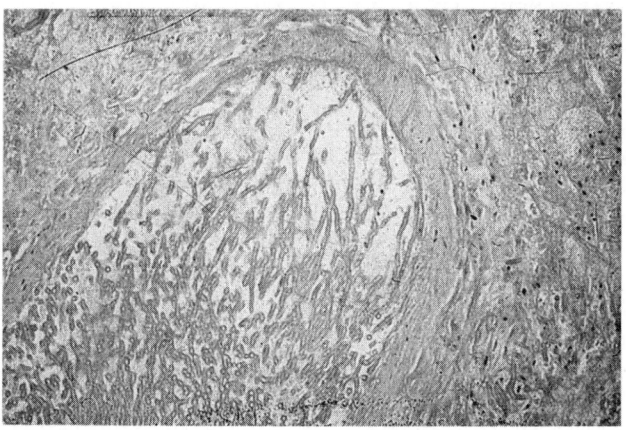

B

FIGURE 47-2 *A.* Necrotic ulcerated skin lesion in a 53-year-old man on day 15 of remission-induction therapy for acute myeloid leukemia (AML). This lesion was caused by skin infarction secondary to angioinvasive infection due to Aspergillus flavus.

B. Periodic acid–Schiff stain of a biopsy from this lesion demonstrates the invasion of broad, acutely branching septate hyphae into blood vessels.

pulmonary hemorrhage, or hyperleukocytosis. The physical assessment of the chest can do little to differentiate infectious or noninfectious causes of pulmonary findings, but it can help identify the lower respiratory tract as the potential infected focus.

The symptoms and signs of an intra-abdominal infection may be obvious or muted, focal or diffuse. The most important finding is focal tenderness.[64] For example, tenderness in the right lower quadrant might suggest neutropenic enterocolitis (typhlitis); right upper quadrant tenderness might suggest a biliary tract focus or hepatomegaly; epigastric pain suggests an upper GI focus; and left lower quadrant tenderness suggests colitis or diverticular disease. It is important to examine the perianal tissues for signs of excoriation, local erythema, swelling, tenderness, fissure formation, or hemorrhoidal tissues, since this area is frequently the site of major life-threatening infection in neutropenic patients. Digital examination of the rectum is not recommended in neutropenic patients because of the additional risk of tissue damage, bleeding, and infection. However, a light perianal digital examination can be informative about focal areas of cellulitis without increasing the risk of bacteremic infection.

The examination of the skin should consist of a thorough search for focal areas of pain, swelling, or erythema, especially in association with indwelling vascular access devices. Particular attention should be paid to the venous insertion, tunnel, and exit sites associated with central venous catheters. In contrast, nonspecific local pocket tenderness may be the only clue to infection associated with the totally implantable venous access port-reservoir systems.

Skin rashes are a common phenomenon among neutropenic patients. The differential diagnosis must include both infectious and noninfectious causes. Among the former group are focal ulcerative and necrotic lesions caused by metastatic pyogenic bacterial infection such as that associated with bacteremic *P. aeruginosa* or *Staphylococcus aureus* (infections causing ecthyma gangrenosum), or by disseminated angioinvasive filamentous fungi such as that due to *Aspergillus* species, *Pseudallescheria boydii* (formerly called *Allescheria boydii*; the conidial [asexual] state is *Scedosporium apiospermum*), or *Fusarium* species (Fig. 47-2). Pustular erythematous

lesions diffusely distributed over the skin surface suggest the possibility of disseminated fungal infection such as that caused by *Candida tropicalis*. Vesicular skin lesions suggest the possibility of infection due to HSV or herpes zoster virus.

The list of possible noninfectious causes of skin rash is long. The three most important considerations are hemorrhagic petechial or ecchymotic rashes associated with profound thrombocytopenia; hypersensitivity rashes associated with specific drugs such as β-lactam antibacterial drugs, allopurinol, or trimethoprim-sulfamethoxazole (TMP-SMX); and specific chemotherapy regimen–related rash syndromes (e.g., the exfoliative palmar/plantar syndrome associated with high-dose cytarabine; Fig. 47-3). These skin rash syndromes may coexist simultaneously. For example, experience has shown that patients undergoing remission-induction therapy with high-dose cytarabine for AML may develop hemorrhagic petechial rashes due to thrombocytopenia, palmar/plantar erythema, and edema due to cytarabine; macular penicillin-related hypersensitivity rash; and hemorrhagic cutaneous infarcts secondary to angioinvasive bacteremic or fungemic infection, all simultaneously. Only careful attention to the pertinent details of history and thorough laboratory

FIGURE 47-3 Palmar/plantar desquamation occurring on day 9 of treatment in a patient receiving high-dose cytarabine.

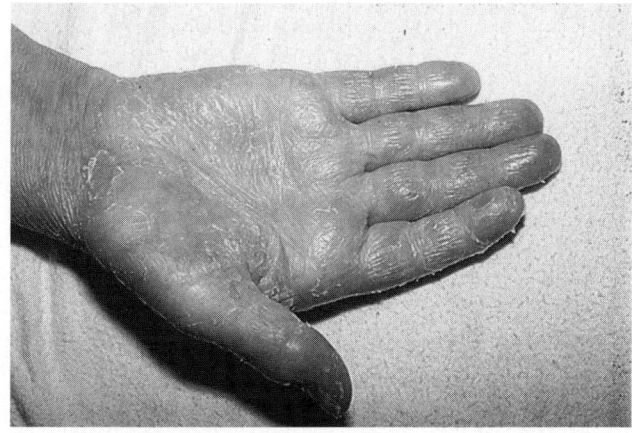

investigations can increase the likelihood that the correct diagnosis and therapeutic decisions will be made.

Once the relevant historical details and physical findings are established, the complete evaluation of the febrile neutropenic patient should include a series of laboratory and radiologic investigations designed to complement the clinical examination. Specimens of body fluids such as blood, urine, cerebrospinal fluid, and lower respiratory secretions should be submitted to the clinical microbiology laboratory for culture and antimicrobial susceptibility testing where appropriate. At least two sets of blood cultures should be obtained, at least one of which should be taken from a peripheral venous site. Furthermore, it has been recommended that for patients with multilumen indwelling central venous catheters, each lumen of the catheter should be sampled in addition to blood from the peripheral venous site.[55]

The basic radiologic investigation is the chest radiograph (posteroanterior and lateral views). When suggested by clinical clues, sinus radiographs are useful for detecting sinus opacification or fluid levels. Panoramic x-ray radiographs can be helpful for evaluating periodontal infection. High-resolution computed tomographic (HRCT) examinations of the lungs has a high yield of abnormalities in febrile neutropenic patients despite normal or nondiagnostic chest radiographs.[67,68] In one study, 60% of febrile neutropenic patients with normal chest radiographs had a pulmonary infiltrate demonstrable on the chest HRCT.[67] Computed tomography (CT) of the abdomen or hepatic ultrasonography is valuable for assessing the significance of abnormalities in cholestatic enzymes (γ-glutamyltransferase [GGT] and alkaline phosphatase). This is particularly important if the possibility of hepatosplenic candidiasis exists. Abdominal pain and tenderness with diarrhea in a persistently febrile neutropenic patient suggests the possibility of neutropenic enterocolitis. Abdominal CT examination looking for evidence of bowel wall thickening, pneumatosis, wall nodularity, mucosal enhancement, bowel dilation, ascites, and mesenteric stranding is very useful in making the diagnosis.[69]

Tissue obtained by biopsy of infected sites can be important in the diagnostic evaluation. Biopsied material should be submitted to the clinical microbiology laboratory for culture and to the pathology laboratory for histopathologic or etiologic evaluation. It is relatively common for pathogens to be observed histopathologically in infected tissue specimens without recovery of the organism by culture. Such is the case in the syndrome of hepatosplenic candidiasis, where budding yeasts and pseudohyphae observed in liver biopsy specimens frequently fail to grow in microbiologic cultures. Skin biopsies are often helpful to distinguish drug-related lesions from those caused by specific pathogenic microorganisms. Although ideally desirable for a complete evaluation, tissue biopsies of suspect sites in neutropenic thrombocytopenic patients carry the additional risks of further infection and bleeding. In addition to skin, the body sites most often considered for biopsy are esophagus (to differentiate mucositis secondary to fungi, pyogenic microorganisms, herpes viruses, or chemotherapeutic agents), liver (to evaluate hepatic lesions due to fungi, herpes viruses, pyogenic bacteria, and drug-related or disease-related hepatic damage), and lung (to evaluate the etiology of progressive infiltrates). Institutions caring for these patients should have a protocol for specimen collection and handling developed in consultation with the appropriate laboratories, the operating theaters, and surgical services.

RISK ASSESSMENT

Neutropenia-related febrile episodes are heterogeneous with respect to the cause of neutropenia, the duration of neutropenia, the risks of developing fever, the cause of fever, and the cause of infection. Furthermore, patients differ in their response to treatment and in the risks of complications, including those which are serious and life threatening. Accordingly, the practice standard has been to hospitalize all febrile neutropenic patients for assessment, administration of empiric broad-spectrum intravenous antimicrobial therapy,[55] and monitoring for and management of complications. Such complications include management of hemodynamic instability and hypotension; respiratory insufficiency requiring oxygen administration; control of pain, nausea, vomiting, and dehydration; investigation and management of confusion, delirium, and altered mental status; hemorrhage requiring blood product transfusion; cardiac dysrhythmia requiring monitoring; changes in metabolic function requiring intervention; and death.

Investigators from the Dana-Farber Cancer Institute[70] examined the natural history of febrile neutropenic patients to identify patients at risk for complications due to the neutropenia, the infection, the underlying cancer, and other comorbid conditions. Concurrent comorbidity included hypotension (defined by a systolic blood pressure of <90 mm Hg), altered mental status, respiratory failure (defined by a partial pressure of arterial oxygen of <60 mm Hg), uncontrolled bleeding, severe thrombocytopenia (defined by a platelet count of $<40 \times 10^9$/L), inadequate outpatient fluid intake or pain control, suspected spinal cord compression, symptomatic hypercalcemia, the need for hospitalization for induction therapy, serious localized infections, acute abdomen, new deep venous thrombosis, syncope, bowel obstruction, and poor performance status (Karnofsky performance status of <50%). Medical complications included hypotension, respiratory failure, new cardiac dysrhythmia or electrocardiographic changes, altered mental status, new focal neurologic abnormalities, hemorrhage requiring >3 units of packed red blood cell transfusion within 24 hours, congestive heart failure, emergency surgery, acute abdomen, pulmonary thromboembolism, acute renal failure, and diabetic ketoacidosis. Based on these comorbidities and complications, febrile neutropenic patients could be classified into three groups at high risk for complications and one low-risk group. Group 1 (39% of the total) was comprised of hospitalized patients usually with hematologic malignancies or hemopoietic stem cell transplant. Complication and morbidity rates were 34% and 23%, respectively. Group 2 (8% of the total) was comprised of outpatients with concurrent comorbidity and had complication and mortality rates of 55% and 14%, respectively. Group 3 (10% of the total) was comprised of outpatients with as yet uncontrolled or progressive cancer and had complication and mortality rates of 31% and 15%, respectively. Group 4 (the low-risk group, 43% of the total) was comprised of outpatients with controlled or responding cancer and no comorbid processes. This group had a complication rate of 2% and no deaths. These observations were prospectively validated in follow-up studies.[70,71] These results suggest that high-risk patients with characteristics corresponding to groups 1 to 3 should be admitted and managed as inpatients with careful monitoring for serious complications, whereas low-risk patients corresponding to group 4 can be managed safely and effectively on an outpatient basis.[71-79]

The Multinational Association for Supportive Care in Cancer developed a scoring system to identify low-risk patients for serious medical complications that would require admission to the hospital.[26,80] Identifying factors included absence of symptoms, hypotension, airflow obstruction, hematologic malignancy, invasive fungal infection, or dehydration. Furthermore, status as an outpatient at the onset of the febrile neutropenic episode and age <60 years were also identifying factors. A score of >21 of a possible 26 identified low-risk patients with a positive predictive value of 91%, specificity of 68%, and sensitivity of 71%. This system has been offered as a strategy for identifying patients eligible for studies of more cost-effective, safe, outpatient-based management strategies.

EMPIRIC ANTIMICROBIAL THERAPY

The empiric initial therapy for suspected infection in febrile neutropenic patients is based on three assumptions:

1. The majority of infections are due to bacteria.[81]
2. The principal pathogens are aerobic gram-negative bacilli (*E. coli, Klebsiella pneumoniae,* and *P. aeruginosa*).[42,81]

3. Inappropriate therapy for aerobic gram-negative bacillemia is associated with high mortality with a median survival of less than 72 hours.[82]

Accordingly, the antibiotic regimens that have been recommended for empiric first-line therapy of first fever in neutropenic cancer patients are designed to have excellent activity against these pathogens. With the recognition of various factors favoring infection by gram-positive organisms,[83] the addition of agents with an improved spectrum of activity against these pathogens when appropriate also has been recommended.[84]

Empiric antibacterial therapies may be administered either as combination regimens or as single-agent regimens (monotherapy) (Tables 47-3 and 47-4). Combination regimens include β-lactam agents combined together[18,85,86] (double β-lactam regimens), combined with aminoglycosides,[42-44,47,49,50,87] or combined with fluoroquinolones.[41,88] Single-agent regimens consist of β-lactam agents[48-50,52,89-92] with or without β-lactamase inhibitors (tazobactam, clavulanic acid, or sulbactam) or fluoroquinolones.[93-95] Monotherapy with aminoglycosides is not recommended.[55]

β-Lactam antibacterial agents may be categorized as extended-spectrum antipseudomonal penicillins (e.g., carbenicillin, ticarcillin with or without clavulanic acid, piperacillin with or without tazobactam, azlocillin, or mezlocillin), third- or fourth-generation antipseudomonal cephalosporins

TABLE 47-3 Antimicrobial Therapy Used for Therapy in Febrile Neutropenic Patients

β-Lactam antibiotics	
Ticarcillin ± clavulanic acid	
Piperacillin ± tazobactam	200–300 mg/kg per day IV
Azlocillin	4–6 divided doses daily
Mezlocillin	3 g q4–6h IV
Cefoperazone	2 g q12h IV
Ceftriaxone	2 g q24h IV
Ceftazidime	2 g q8h IV
Imipenem/cilastatin	500 mg q6h IV
Meropenem	1 g q8h IV
Aminoglycosides	
Gentamicin	1.5–2 mg/kg q8h IV
Netilmicin	1.5–2.0 mg/kg q8h IV
Tobramyicn	1.5–2 mg/kg q8h IV
Amikacin	7.5 mg/kg q12h IV
Fluoroquinolones	
Ciprofloxacin	400 mg q12h IV
	500–750 mg q12h PO
Ofloxacin	400 mg q12h PO
Perfloxacin	400 mg q12h PO
Enoxacin	400 mg q12h PO
Other agents	
Vancomycin	1.0 g q12h IV or 30 mg/kg per 24 h
Metronidazole	500 mg q8h IV/PO
Erythromycin	0.5–1.0 g q6h IV
TMP-SMX	10–20 mg/50–100 mg/kg per day in 4 divided doses
Acyclovir	250–500 mg/m^2 q8h IV
Ganciclovir	5 mg/kg q8-12 h IV
Amphotericin B	0.5–1.5 mg/kg per day IV
Amphotericin B lipid complex	5 mg/kg per day IV
5-Fluorocytosine	150 mg/kg per day PO in 4 divided doses
Fluconazole	200–400 mg IV/PO qd
Itraconazole	200–400 mg PO qd

TMP-SMX, trimethoprim-sulfamethoxazole.

TABLE 47-4 Considerations Governing the Choice of Empiric Antibacterial Regimen

β-Lactam	High-risk neutropenia
+	Risk of *P. aeruginosa* infection
Fluoroquinolone or	Nosocomial infection
aminoglycoside	Prolonged severe neutropenia
Monotherapy	Patients with renal impairment
	Recipients of other nephrotoxic agents
	High-risk neutropenia
Oral therapy	Short-term neutropenia
	Low-risk neutropenia
Other agents	
Vancomycin	Suspect coagulase-negative staphylococcal infection
	Suspect vascular catheter infection
	Skin or soft tissue infection
Metronidazole	Suspect intra-abdominal infection
	Necrotizing gingivitis
	Severe oral mucositis
	Suspect perianal infection

(e.g., moxalactam, ceftriaxone, ceftazidime, cefoperazone with or without sulbactam, cefpirome, or cefepime), or as carbapenems (e.g., imipenem-cilastatin, meropenem, or ertapenem). The addition of β-lactamase inhibitors to the broad-spectrum antipseudomonal penicillins, ticarcillin and piperacillin, enhances their spectrum of activity against β-lactamase–producing bacteria and their roles in the management of the febrile neutropenic patient.[47,51,96–115]

In a recent review of physician prescribing behavior for 214 febrile neutropenic patients in Canadian centers, initial empiric therapy with a single agent was administered in 42% of cases in which a third-generation cephalosporin such as ceftazidime was used in 32%, a carbapenem in 2.3%, and a fluoroquinolone in 0.9%.[116] Combination therapy was administered in 58% of cases in which an antipseudomonal penicillin plus an aminoglycoside was given in 29% of cases, an antipseudomonal cephalosporin plus an aminoglycoside in 15%, and an antipseudomonal β-lactam plus a glycopeptide in 11%.[116] Vancomycin was part of the initial empiric antibacterial therapy in 15% of cases. First modification with second-line therapy for persistent fever was administered in 87% of the 214 cases after a median of 5 days. Systemic empiric amphotericin B was administered for persistent fever in 48% of the 214 febrile neutropenic episodes after a median of 9 days. Previous studies have demonstrated that glycopeptides are employed as empiric second-line therapy in 40% to 50% of cases in which extended-spectrum cephalosporins are administered as first-line empiric therapy.[48,51,97–100,117–128]

THE ROLE OF AMINOGLYCOSIDES IN TREATMENT OF FEBRILE NEUTROPENIC PATIENTS

Aminoglycosides were part of the standard combination empiric antibacterial therapy for the management of febrile neutropenic patients from the early 1970s to the 1990s. The combination of an aminoglycoside with an antipseudomonal β-lactam antibacterial agent was designed to have a broad spectrum of antibacterial activity, achieve bactericidal serum concentrations, exert a synergistic antibacterial effect, and prevent emergence of resistance. Such combinations have been recommended in published guidelines by the Infectious

Diseases Society of America (IDSA),[55] the National Comprehensive Cancer Network,[129] and the Infectious Diseases Working Party of the German Society of Hematology and Oncology,[53] but not the Spanish guidelines, however.[130] The aminoglycoside antibiotics having proven roles for use with β-lactam antibiotics in neutropenic patients include gentamicin, netilmicin, tobramycin, and amikacin. The choice of aminoglycoside must be based on local institutional bacterial susceptibility patterns, the availability of a mechanism for serum aminoglycoside concentration monitoring, and drug cost.

A recent large randomized controlled trial from the University of Perugia, Italy, compared piperacillin-tazobactam to piperacillin-tazobactam plus amikacin.[51] The primary outcome was defervescence of all signs and symptoms of infection without modification of the initial antibacterial regimen. Response was observed in 179 of 364 (49%) monotherapy recipients and in 196 of 369 (53%) combination recipients ($p = 0.2$). The response rates in single-pathogen gram-positive bacteremias were low (27% and 32 %, respectively) because of the high proportion of coagulase-negative staphylococcal bacteremias (response rates 17% and 18%, respectively; $p = 0.8$). In contrast, the response rates for streptococcal and enterococcal bacteremias between the two groups were significantly higher (60% and 71%, respectively, $p = 0.7$). The response rates for single gram-negative bacteremias were also similar (36% and 34%, respectively; $p = 0.9$). The aminoglycoside failed to enhance the response rates in any circumstance. Studies such as this question the therapeutic value of combination antibacterial therapy with an aminoglycoside.

Two systematic reviews of the literature have examined the safety and efficacy of β-lactam plus aminoglycoside combinations in febrile neutropenic patients.[131,132] Furno and associates reviewed 4795 heterogeneously treated febrile neutropenic episodes entered into 29 randomized controlled clinical trials comparing monotherapy (ceftazidime, 9 trials; cefepime, 2 trials; cefoperazone, 1 trial; imipenem-cilastatin, 9 trials; meropenem, 4 trials; ciprofloxacin, 2 trials; and ofloxacin, 2 trials) and aminoglycoside-based combination therapy. The pooled odds ratios for overall treatment failure and for treatment failure in bloodstream infections were 0.88 (95% CI, 0.78 to 0.99) and 0.70 (95% CI 0.54 to 0.92), respectively, demonstrating fewer failures in the monotherapy groups.[131] Paul and colleagues examined 7807 febrile neutropenic patients entered into 47 randomized controlled trials comparing β-lactam monotherapy to β-lactam plus aminoglycoside combination therapy. The main outcome was overall mortality. While there was no significant difference in overall mortality (relative risk 0.85; 95% CI 0.72 to 1.02), there were fewer failures among β-lactam monotherapy recipients (relative risk 0.92; 95% CI 0.85 to 0.99).[132] Monotherapy recipients also experienced fewer adverse events overall (relative risk 0.85; 95% CI 0.73 to 1.00) and less nephrotoxicity (relative risk 0.42; 95% CI 0.32 to 0.56).[132] On the basis of these analyses, β-lactam plus aminoglycoside combinations offer no advantages over broad-spectrum β-lactam monotherapy. Rather they present significant disadvantages with respect to toxicity and costs related to drug monitoring and administration. Based on these observations and considerations, investigators are now recommending that the standard of care for initial therapy of febrile neutropenic cancer patients should be with a broad-spectrum β-lactam agent as monotherapy.[132]

FLUOROQUINOLONES IN THE TREATMENT OF FEBRILE NEUTROPENIC PATIENTS

The fluoroquinolones evaluated in studies of the empiric treatment of febrile neutropenic patients include ciprofloxacin,[41,133] perfloxacin,[134] ofloxacin,[73,74] levofloxacin,[135] and clinifloxacin.[94,95] These agents have the advantage of availability in both oral and intravenous formulations, which can facilitate intravenous-to-oral conv- ersion.[133,136,137]

The studies of empiric fluoroquinolones as first-line therapy for febrile neutropenic patients have largely targeted those patients at lower risk for medical complications.[129] Ciprofloxacin as well as other agents such as clindamycin, aztreonam, or amoxicillin have been the most completely studied.[72,73,75–78,108,135,138–142] The administration of ciprofloxacin 750 mg orally and amoxicillin-clavulanate 625 mg orally both every 8 hours was well tolerated and as effective as intravenous ceftriaxone plus amikacin[138] or ceftazidime[139] administered on an inpatient basis. Similar results have been reported for trials comparing oral ciprofloxacin-based regimens and intravenous regimens on an outpatient basis.[72,73,75–78,108,135,138–142] These strategies appear to be safe and effective for low-risk patients. The National Comprehensive Cancer Network Clinical Practice Guidelines in Oncology have included as an alternative regimen for initial empiric antibacterial therapy of higher-risk febrile neutropenic cancer patients the use of ciprofloxacin plus an antipseudomonal penicillin.[129] One large trial compared piperacillin plus ciprofloxacin and piperacillin plus tobramycin in a group of intermediate- to high-risk febrile neutropenic cancer patients.[41] Success rates (i.e., defervescence with initial regimen modification) were similar, 27% and 22% for the piperacillin-ciprofloxacin and piperacillin-tobramycin groups, respectively; however, times-to-defervescence were faster among the piperacillin-ciprofloxacin recipients, 5 days versus 6 days ($p = 0.005$).

Reports of fluoroquinolone resistance among aerobic gram-negative bacilli associated with bloodstream infections in neutropenic cancer patients began to emerge in the early 1990s.[143–145] The incidence of fluoroquinolone-resistant *Escherichia coli* (FREC) bacteremia among patients treated on the EORTC-IATCG clinical trials from 1983 to 1993 increased from zero during the period from 1983 to 1990 to 28% during the period from 1991 to 1993.[143] Of note, the incidence of resistance among strains of *Pseudomonas aeruginosa* and *Klebsiella pneumoniae* remained largely unchanged at less than 10%.[143] This has been more of a problem among cancer patients treated in institutions with high prevalence rates for gram-negative bacillary fluoroquinolone resistance (>10%) despite community-related resistance prevalences of less than 1%.[146] Carratala and colleagues reported in 1995 a 37% incidence of fluoroquinolone resistance in 35 of 230 neutropenic cancer patients previously treated with norfloxacin.[145]

Fluoroquinolone resistance among community-derived gram-negative bacilli, and FREC in particular, has emerged in parallel with the increased prescribing of these products in the community.[147–149] There is a significant correlation between the incidence of ciprofloxacin-resistant *Escherichia coli* bloodstream infection and the increased community and hospital use of fluoroquinolones ($r = 0.974$, $p = 0.005$ and $r = 0.975$, $p = 0.005$, respectively).[147] Among those who had not heretofore received fluoroquinolone therapy, Garau and colleagues reported the prevalence of FREC in the stools of adults and children in the Province of Barcelona, Spain,

to be 24% and 26%, respectively.[149] These investigators also observed a very high prevalence of FREC in the stools of pigs (45%) and poultry (90%) and argued that the increased prevalence of human carriage of FREC may be linked to the high prevalence in animal-based food products. The increased use of fluoroquinolones in animal feeds and in humans is believed to play a role in the selection for FREC. In an environment with a high (15%) prevalence of fluoroquinolone resistance among gram-negative bacilli, cancer patients receiving ciprofloxacin antibacterial chemoprophylaxis while undergoing high-dose chemotherapy with stem cell rescue became colonized with FREC in one third of cases,[150] a phenomenon that increases the likelihood of FREC bloodstream infections in such patients.[151]

In addition, inappropriate use of fluoroquinolones is common. A recent case-control study of fluoroquinolone use in emergency departments in Philadelphia demonstrated inappropriate prescription of these agents in 81% of cases.[152] Lastly, gram-negative bacilli that are co-resistant to fluoroquinolones and other antibacterials such as aminoglycosides, cefotaxime, ampicillin, amoxicillin-clavulanate and trimethoprim-sulfamethoxazole are more frequently being reported.[149,153] Thus overuse and inappropriate use of fluoroquinolones in the community is common and is strongly linked to resistance, and ultimately will reduce the likelihood that this class of agents will be useful in a variety of patient populations, including neutropenic cancer patients, who require critical care services.[143,145] It is incumbent upon prescription writers of empiric antibacterial therapy to have some understanding of the prevalence of gram-negative bacillary resistance in the institution and the community.

DOUBLE BETA-LACTAM COMBINATIONS

Regimens consisting of an antipseudomonal broad-spectrum β-lactam plus an extended-spectrum third-generation cephalosporin are relatively safe and effective alternatives to regimens of a β-lactam plus an aminoglycoside,[18,85,86] but they are costly and do not offer any advantages over those of broad-spectrum β-lactam monotherapies. Cost, hypokalemia, selection of bacterial resistance, and antagonism have been cited as potential disadvantages, although these regimens may have an occasional role in the setting of preexisting renal insufficiency, in which the patient is receiving concomitant nephrotoxic agents such as cyclosporine or cisplatin-containing chemotherapeutic regimens, or where gram-positive organisms such as viridans streptococci are suspected.[18,54] The availability of effective β-lactam and fluoroquinolone or β-lactam monotherapy-based regimens has largely rendered double β-lactam regimens obsolete. Of note, these combinations appear in the National Comprehensive Cancer Network guidelines.[129]

EXTENDED-SPECTRUM CEPHALOSPORINS

The intrinsic activity of many of the third- and fourth-generation cephalosporins such as ceftriaxone, cefoperazone, ceftazidime, or cefepime against aerobic gram-negative bacilli is high. These agents have been used effectively as single agents for empiric treatment of suspected infection.[42–45,47–50,87,92,154] Empiric monotherapy has been shown to be effective in both low- and high-risk febrile neutropenic patient populations and in those in whom the expected duration of severe neutropenia (ANC $< 0.5 \times 10^9/L$) is either longer or shorter than 7 days. The experience to date suggests that single-agent empiric regimens will require modification, usually by the addition of other antimicrobials, in one third to one half of patients with neutropenic periods in excess of 1 week.[48–50,87] There is a lower likelihood that modifications will be necessary for patients with short-term (<1 week) neutropenia.

A meta-analysis examining the efficacy of ceftazidime monotherapy compared to standard combination therapy for the empiric treatment of febrile neutropenic patients failed to demonstrate a difference with respect to the odds of overall treatment failure and failure in bloodstream infections (odds ratio 1.27; 95% CI 0.79 to 2.03 in 1077 patient episodes; and OR 0.72, 95% CI 0.33 to 1.58 in 248 patient episodes, respectively).[92] Another meta-analysis[154] compared the efficacy of ceftriaxone with (7 trials) or without (1 trial) an aminoglycoside and ceftazidime with (6 trials) or without (1 trial) an aminoglycoside or azlocillin plus an aminoglycoside (1 trial). The pooled odds ratio for overall treatment failure in the eight trials was 1.04 (95% CI 0.84 to 1.29), demonstrating no differences in the comparison for this outcome. There was also no difference in overall mortality (OR 0.84; 95% CI 0.57 to 1.24). These analyses demonstrate that empiric antibacterial therapy of febrile neutropenic patients with oncedaily ceftriaxone is as effective as thrice daily ceftazidime. This has important implications for potential outpatient oncedaily intravenous therapy.

CARBAPENEMS FOR TREATMENT OF FEBRILE NEUTROPENIC PATIENTS

Both imipenem-cilastatin and meropenem have been studied widely as empiric therapy in febrile neutropenic patients. A meta-analysis examined the efficacy of imipenem-cilastatin compared to a β-lactam plus aminoglycoside combinations (11 trials) and to β-lactam monotherapy (ceftazidime, 4 trials; cefoperazone-sulbactam, 1 trial), or β-lactam plus glycopeptide (ceftazidime, 3 trials) or double β-lactam therapy (cefoperazone-mezlocillin, 1 trial; cefoperazone-piperacillin, 1 trial). There were fewer treatment failures among imipenem-cilastatin recipients compared to β-lactam plus aminoglycoside combinations (OR 0.77; 95% CI 0.61 to 0.98) or to non–aminoglycoside-containing regimens (OR 0.67; 95% CI 0.54 to 0.84).[91] These analyses support the superiority of imipenem-cilastatin over control arms largely based on thirdgeneration cephalosporins.

Another meta-analysis comparing carbapenem monotherapy to β-lactam plus aminoglycoside combination therapy demonstrated fewer treatment failures among the carbapenem recipients (OR 0.80; 95% CI 0.66 to 0.96, Peto fixed effects model),[131] in contrast to antipseudomonal cephalosporin monotherapy (OR 0.92; 95% CI 0.77 to 1.10, Peto fixed effects model). A similar analysis of the published clinical trials of meropenem monotherapy compared to ceftazidime-based regimens with or without an aminoglycoside demonstrated greater response rates among meropenem recipients (OR 1.28; 95% CI 1.08 to 1.51).[155] These systematic observations suggest the inferiority of third-generation cephalosporin monotherapy regimens compared to the carbapenem monotherapy.

PIPERACILLIN-TAZOBACTAM FOR THE TREATMENT OF FEBRILE NEUTROPENIC PATIENTS

Piperacillin-tazobactam plus amikacin therapy was successful in 210 of 342 (61%) febrile neutropenic patients studied by the European Organisation for the Research and Treatment of Cancer, compared to 196 of 364 (54%) patients receiving cef-

tazidime plus amikacin ($p = 0.05$).[47] Furthermore, the timeto-defervescence was shorter among piperacillin-tazobactam recipients ($p = 0.01$), and the frequency with which the initial regimen was modified by the addition of a glycopeptide was lower (24% versus 35%; $p = 0.002$) in that study. Another large Italian trial examined the role of the aminoglycoside amikacin, when combined with piperacillin-tazobactam.[51] The response rates overall between the two groups were similar regardless of the classification of the febrile neutropenic episode as bacteremic, clinically documented, or unexplained fever. Clearly, the aminoglycoside offered no advantage over the piperacillin-tazobactam monotherapy. Piperacillin-tazobactam monotherapy has been studied compared to extended-spectrum cephalosporins with or without aminoglycosides.[96–100] Overall unmodified success rates were significantly higher among piperacillin-tazobactam recipients (OR 1.39; 95% CI 1.08 to 1.79).[100] Furthermore, the frequency of second-line therapy with glycopeptides was significantly lower among piperacillin-tazobactam recipients (OR 0.77; 95% CI 0.60 to 0.99).[100] These observations demonstrate the superiority of initial piperacillin-tazobactam monotherapy over extended-spectrum cephalosporins with or without aminoglycosides. Furthermore, the need to modify the initial antibacterial regimen by the addition of a glycopeptide such as vancomycin or teicoplanin for persistent fever is also significantly less than for the cephalosporin-based comparator groups. This has important implications with respect to cost, drug-related toxicities, and for selection for resistant microorganisms such as vancomycin-resistant *Enterococcus* spp.

THE ROLE OF GLYCOPEPTIDES AS FIRST-LINE AND SECOND-LINE THERAPY IN FEBRILE NEUTROPENIC PATIENTS

There has been a significant increase in the proportion of the microbiologically documented infections observed in neutropenic patients that are due to gram-positive bacteria. Two decades ago approximately 70% of bacteremic isolates were gram-negative bacilli, whereas more recently approximately 60% to 70% are gram-positive cocci.[41,83] Previously published clinical trials of ceftazidime-based empiric antibacterial therapy observed more fatal gram-positive superinfections than expected.[156] A subsequent small study demonstrated that the addition of vancomycin to ceftazidime therapy reduced the superinfection rate from 24% to zero and the infection-related mortality rate by 91% (OR 0.07; 95% CI 0.01 to 0.63).[157] Such observations have led investigators to advocate the inclusion of glycopeptides vancomycin or teicoplanin as part of the first-line empiric antibacterial therapy in febrile neutropenic patients. In contrast, two further studies from the National Cancer Institute suggested that the vancomycin therapy may be safely delayed without increased morbidity or mortality.[49,158] In order to examine this question further, the European Organization for Treatment and Research in Cancer and the National Cancer Institute of Canada Clinical Trials Group conducted a large randomized trial comparing empiric therapy with ceftazidime plus amikacin (CA) and ceftazidime plus amikacin plus vancomycin (CAV).[45] The overall response rate among the 377 CAV recipients was 288 (76%), whereas the response rate for 370 CA recipients was 232 (63%; $p < 0.001$), the difference largely due to differential response rates for gram-positive bloodstream infections among CAV recipients. Despite the apparent superiority of the CAV arm, persistently febrile CA patients at day +3 received vancomycin, resulting in no differences in overall success rates or mortality.

Treatment failures were due to lack of prompt response and to persistent fever observed at a time very early after the initiation of the allocated regimen rather than objective indicators of failure such as persistence of resistant pathogens or progression at foci of infection. Patients receiving CA were more likely to receive vancomycin with persistence of fever at day +3 than recipients of the CAV regimen.[159] Since the median time to defervescence among high-risk febrile neutropenic patients is day 5 (range = day +3 to day +7),[41,47,48,50,128] many patients were considered failures unnecessarily because of regimen modification before they would have had a chance to defervesce. The physician compulsion to modify the initial antibacterial regimen for reasons of persistent fever at day +3 is driven in part by previously published protocols[49] reinforced by previously published guidelines.[160]

Three other trials[161–163] examining the role of initial glycopeptide therapy in febrile neutropenic cancer patients came to similar conclusions as for the EORTC/NCIC trial;[45] that is, the inclusion of glycopeptides as initial therapy in febrile neutropenic patients results in modest improvements in response rates, particularly in the circumstances of gram-positive bacteremia, but has no impact on overall survival of the neutropenic episode. Accordingly, it is recommended in the recent American, German and Spanish guidelines that glycopeptides not be used as part of the initial empiric antibacterial regimen for the treatment of fever in neutropenic cancer patients unless there is evidence of gram-positive infection.[53,55,130,164]

The above trials demonstrated that among patients with persistent fever due to gram-positive infection at day +3 vancomycin could be added to the regimen at that time with no excess morbidity or mortality.[45,49,158,163] Accordingly, second-line glycopeptide-based empiric antibacterial therapy for persistent fever has become quite common. As noted above, almost half of cases enrolled in clinical trials have a glycopeptide administered for these reasons.[48,51,97–100,117–128] The efficacy of empiric second-line glycopeptide therapy has been studied in two randomized controlled trials.[101,165] Both studies failed to demonstrate a significant treatment effect with regard to defervescence or overall mortality (OR 1.05; 95% CI 0.66 to 1.67 and OR 0.80; 95% CI 0.33 to 1.90, respectively) compared to placebo.[166] The results of these two trials together with the small published meta-analysis confirm that in stable, persistently febrile, neutropenic patients, empiric second-line glycopeptide therapy after 48 to 96 hours is unnecessary.[166] Furthermore, the initial antibacterial therapy can be safely extended in such patients unmodified for an additional 72 to 96 hours for a total of 4 to 8 days.

The use of glycopeptide antibiotics as part of the initial first-line regimen should be reserved for patients at highest risk for serious gram-positive infection.[55,129] Such circumstances include clinical catheter-related infection, infection in patients receiving fluoroquinolone-based antibacterial chemoprophylaxis associated with severe mucositis predisposing patients to viridans group streptococcal bloodstream infections,[34,35,167] infection in the setting of colonization by methicillin-resistant *Staphylococcus aureus* (MRSA), a bloodstream isolate characterized as gram-positive cocci in groups and clusters (suggesting *Staphylococcus* spp. and the likelihood of a methicillin-resistant coagulase-negative *Staphylococcus*), and the setting of hypotension or septic shock syndrome without an identified pathogen. The caveat is that the glycopeptide antibiotic should be discontinued in 2 to 3 days if a resistant gram-positive infection has not been identified.

THE ROLE OF HEMATOPOIETIC GROWTH FACTORS IN THE MANAGEMENT OF FEBRILE NEUTROPENIC PATIENTS

The inclusion of hematopoietic growth factors (HGF), granulocyte and granulocyte-macrophage colony-stimulating factors (G-CSF; GM-CSF) in strategies for the prevention and management of febrile neutropenic patients remains unsettled.[168] Berghmans and colleagues published a systematic review of the literature with a meta-analysis to critically examine the evidence for or against use of these products in the treatment of febrile neutropenic episodes.[169] Eleven studies encompassing 1218 febrile neutropenic episodes published between 1990 and 1998 were considered in the analysis. Although six trials reported treatment effects for the primary outcome analyzed (mortality), overall there was no effect on mortality (relative risk 0.71; 95% CI 0.44 to 1.15). Furthermore, there were no differences when analysis was conducted by HGF and G-CSF versus GM-CSF. The impact of HGF on length of hospitalization was decreased in four trials, unaffected in four trials, and not reported in three trials. Only three of six trials reporting on the impact of HGF on duration of antibacterial therapy demonstrated a reduction in this outcome. In nine trials in which the impact of HGF on the duration of fever was reported, no treatment effects were observed in seven trials, fever reduction was observed in one trial, and no analysis was provided in one other. The studies included in this analysis were flawed by the failure to control for important variables, including the duration and intensity of neutropenia, type of cytotoxic therapy, and type of malignancy. On the basis of this review, Berghmans and colleagues could not recommend routine use of HGF in the treatment of febrile neutropenic episodes.[169]

The guidelines of the American Society of Clinical Oncology do not recommend their use as adjunctive therapy for neutropenic patients who are febrile and have suspected infection.[170] However, less than half of specialists follow these guidelines, given that usage appears to be influenced more by reimbursement than evidence.[171–173]

HGF have been evaluated in other non-neutropenic patient populations including patients with community-acquired pneumonia, human immunodeficiency virus–infected patients, neonatal sepsis, diabetic foot ulcer infections, acute hepatic failure or cirrhosis, in orthotopic liver transplantation, and in the critical care unit. While there appears to be some promising results in some subgroups of patients, HGF have no proven clinical benefit in non-neutropenic critically ill patients with regard to morbidity or mortality.[174]

THE ROLE OF SECOND-LINE THERAPY FOR PERSISTENT FEVER IN NEUTROPENIC PATIENTS

Patients with fever persisting beyond 72 hours on broad-spectrum antibiotic therapy should be re-evaluated carefully.[55,129] Table 47-5 lists several of the possible explanations for this. A nonbacterial etiology for the febrile episode should be considered. The various noninfectious causes have been discussed already. Factors such as localized tenderness,

TABLE 47-5 Differential Diagnosis of Fever >72 Hours Despite Broad-Spectrum Antibacterial Therapy

Fever is due to a nonbacterial process
   Viral infection (HSV, CMV)
   Fungal infection (candidiasis, invasive aspergillosis)
   Noninfectious fever (blood products, drugs, etc.)
Bacterial infection is resistant to the antibiotic regimen
Second or subsequent infection has developed
Bacterial infection is not responding because of inadequate antibiotic
   serum/tissue levels
Infection is associated with an undrained focus (e.g., abscess or
   prosthetic material [IV catheters])

CMV, cytomegalovirus; HSV, herpes simplex virus.

change in sensorium, hyperventilation, hypotension, progressive renal insufficiency, and acidosis suggest an infectious cause. The re-evaluation should occur between day 3 and day 5 and include a thorough examination to identify a focus. Cultures of blood (one set from each lumen of the central venous catheter and one set from a peripheral vein), urine, and other potentially infected sites should be submitted to the clinical microbiology laboratory. Repeat chest radiography or diagnostic imaging studies such as ultrasonography or high-resolution computed tomographic studies may be performed when abnormalities suggest a specific organ as a potential site for infection. When re-evaluation fails to identify the etiology of the persistent fever, the clinician may elect either to continue the initial empiric antibacterial regimen if the patient's condition shows no clinical change or deterioration, or to modify the empiric regimen appropriate to the findings of the re-evaluation (Table 47-6).

Persistently febrile severely neutropenic patients despite administration of at least 3 to 5 days of broad-spectrum antibacterial therapy are at risk of having an invasive fungal infection as the cause for the ongoing fever.[55] Such patients are candidates for empiric antifungal therapy with amphotericin B deoxycholate,[175,176] a lipid formulation of amphotericin B,[177] an echinocandin, or with an extended-spectrum azole.[178,179] The two randomized clinical trials upon which the practice of empiric antifungal therapy was based failed to demonstrate a treatment effect with respect to defervescence compared to an untreated control group (OR 0.13; 95% CI 0.01 to

1.26 for the study by Pizzo and colleagues[175] and OR 0.14; 95% CI 0.02 to 1.23 for the EORTC study[176]).

While it is widely felt that the majority of persistent fevers in the setting of severe neutropenia do not represent invasive fungal infections, approximately 20% may be related to invasive fungal infection with an attendant high mortality rate sufficient to compel physicians to administer empiric antifungal therapy. Such strategies may be considered in patients persistently febrile after 7 days of broad-spectrum antibacterial therapy. Patients should undergo a second workup for persistent fever to investigate the possibility of invasive fungal infection which includes blood cultures from peripheral and indwelling central venous access sites and sensitive HRCT images of the chest.[67,68] In 60% of persistently febrile neutropenic patients with normal or nondiagnostic chest roentgenograms the HRCT scan of the chest demonstrated a pulmonary infiltrate.[67] Such procedures can permit the earlier diagnosis and management of invasive mold infections involving the lungs by approximately 1 week.[180]

Surveillance cultures for detecting potential fungal pathogens have had some limited usefulness for predicting fungal infection. The recovery of filamentous fungi (e.g., *Aspergillus* species) in a nasopharyngeal surveillance culture in the clinical setting of a persistently febrile, profoundly neutropenic patient receiving broad-spectrum antibiotics and who develops new focal pulmonary infiltrates are to some extent predictive of *Aspergillus* pneumonia.[181] The recovery of *Candida albicans* from oropharyngeal, rectal, or urine surveillance cultures has had a positive predictive value of 10% to 15% for systematic candidiasis. The recovery of other non-albicans *Candida* species such as *Candida tropicalis*, particularly from multiple sites, has had a positive predictive value of >70% for systemic infection. In contrast, the failure to recover *Candida* species in surveillance cultures has been associated with a negative predictive value of >90% for invasive disease from *C. albicans* or *C. tropicalis*.[182] This experience suggests that clinicians cannot use surveillance cultures to predict the presence of a candidal infection (except perhaps for *C. tropicalis*). However, the clinician may be reassured by negative surveillance cultures that are properly obtained and processed, that antifungal therapy may not be indicated.[55]

TABLE 47-6 Considerations for Regimen Modification: Day 5

Progressive necrotizing mucositis/gingivitis	Anaerobic coverage (metronidazole)
Progressive ulcerating mucositis/gingivitis	Antiviral therapy (acyclovir)
Dysphagia	Antifungal (± antiviral) therapy if pseudomembranous pharyngitis
Cellulitis or inflammatory changes at venous access sites	Antistaphylococcal therapy (vancomycin)
Interstitial pulmonary infiltrates	TMP-SMX ± erythromycin Consider bronchoalveolar lavage
Focal pulmonary infiltrates	Observe if ANC is recovering Consider lung biopsy Empiric amphotericin B
Abdominal foci	*Typhlitis* Diverticulitis Anaerobic disease coverage Perirectal focus

ANC, absolute neutrophil count; TMP-SMX, trimethoprim-sulfamethoxazole.

Surrogate molecular markers of yeasts and molds are showing promise in the diagnosis of invasive fungal infection. Galactomannan is a component of the cell wall of *Aspergillus* spp., certain dematiaceous fungi such as *Alternaria* spp., and some *Penicillium* spp.,[183–185] and has been used to aid in the diagnosis of invasive aspergillosis.[180,186] A enzyme-linked immunosorbent serum assay which uses a rat monoclonal antibody EB-A2 that targets the D-galactofuranoside side chains of the *Aspergillus* spp. galactomannan[187] has been developed for the diagnosis of invasive aspergillosis.[188] The antibody may cross react with galactomannan-like materials from other molds such as *Penicillium* spp., *Paecilomyces* spp., and *Alternaria* spp.,[189] or from foods that are exposed to molds originating from the soil during growth or harvesting, such as rice, pasta, cereals, and vegetables,[190] and even milk[191] consumed by premature infants.[192] Translocation of dietary antigens into the blood of healthy adults is well documented.[193] The antibody also cross-reacts with *Bifidobacterium* spp. lipoteichoic acid, an organism that heavily colonizes the gut of neonates and infants.[194] Translocation of *Bifidobacterium* spp. has occurred in the setting of reduced integrity of the intestinal mucosal barrier.[195] The clinical setting of severe mucositis or intestinal graft-versus-host disease with intestinal mucosal damage may be circumstances in which false-positive serum galactomannan tests may be expected. In addition, false-positive serum tests have been reported in association with administration of certain antibiotics such as piperacillin-tazobactam or amoxicillin derived from cross-reacting species of mold such as *Penicillium* spp.[190,196–198] This has implications for clinicians using this test to investigate the possibility of invasive aspergillosis while administering drugs like piperacillin-tazobactam for the treatment of infection.

DURATION OF ANTIBACTERIAL THERAPY

In general, the IDSA recommendations for duration of the antibacterial regimen encompass the period until neutrophil recovery (ANC > 0.5×10^9/L for at least two consecutive days), all signs and symptoms of infections have resolved, and the temperature has remained normal for 48 hours or more.[55] For patients with prolonged severe neutropenia who have defervesced and for whom no focus of infection appears to be ongoing, the antibiotic regimen may be discontinued after 2 weeks provided the patient remains under careful observation. Some investigators have advocated substituting a fluoroquinolone-based antibacterial chemoprophylaxis regimen for the systemic antibacterial regimen under these circumstances.[199] The response assessment definitions used in clinical trials of antibacterial therapy have often included a stipulation that the patient must remain afebrile for 4 to 5 days in addition to resolution of other signs and symptoms of infection in order for a response to be valid. This seems prudent and consistent with the natural history of these episodes. While the time until response to empiric antibacterial therapy varies with the underlying causes of neutropenia,[17,50,200] the median time to response (defervescence) for high-risk patients is 5 to 7 days[41,45,47,50,87,88,100] and 2 to 4 days for low-risk patients.[138,139] If the antibacterial regimen is to be administered for an additional 4 to 5 days by the above criteria, then high-risk patients and low-risk patients would be expected to have received a 9- to 12-day and 6- to 9-day course of antibacterial therapy, respectively.

Specific Infection Syndromes in Patients Undergoing Cytotoxic Chemotherapy

Infections occur at a limited number of body sites in febrile neutropenic patients and usually involve the microorganisms colonizing those sites.[129] The three systems most commonly involved are the gastrointestinal (GI) tract (oropharynx, gingiva and teeth, esophagus, gut, and perirectal tissues), the respiratory system (sinuses, middle ear, nasopharynx, tracheobronchial tree, and pulmonary parenchyma), and the skin (including biopsy sites and sites of vascular access such as indwelling central venous catheter exit sites, tunnel sites, or insertion sites).

OROPHARYNGEAL MUCOSAL AND ESOPHAGEAL INFECTIONS

The natural history of oral mucositis is influenced by the cytotoxic therapy–induced neutropenia,[34] which plays a permissive role in the clinical expression of acute-on-chronic periodontal infections.[201] This process usually reaches its maximum intensity at the time of neutropenic nadir, approximately days 10 to 14.[27,29–31] At this time, polymicrobial infection becomes superimposed on the chemotherapy-induced mucositis. This in turn extends the morbidity into the third and fourth weeks following the commencement of chemotherapy. Although oropharyngeal bacterial flora (viridans group streptococci, anaerobic gram-negative bacilli, and anaerobic gram-positive cocci) probably contribute to disease in most cases of simple mucositis, in several studies fungi (e.g., *C. albicans*) have played important pathogenic roles in up to 60% of the oral infections among patients with acute leukemia.[202] In addition, reactivated latent HSV infections of the oral cavity have been reported in 50% to 90% of seropositive patients undergoing remission-induction therapy or BMT with a median onset between 7 and 11 days.[203,204] Acute exacerbations of preexisting, asymptomatic, chronic periodontitis occurred in 59% of one series of adult patients undergoing remission-induction therapy for acute leukemia.[201] These infections typically occurred when the ANC was <0.13×10^9/L. The severity and duration of chemotherapy-associated mucositis correlate to some degree with the extent of preexisting dental plaque and periodontal disease.[205]

CLINICAL APPROACH

Herpetic infections of the oropharynx and esophagus may be anticipated in patients with a history of herpetic stomatitis or in those known to possess IgG antibodies to HSV, indicating infection in the past. Although the typical discrete vesicular lesions on an erythematous base may be observed in neutropenic patients, herpetic infections also may manifest as areas of painful ulceration over a diffusely erythematous base. Such lesions must be distinguished from a typical presentation of oropharyngeal candidiasis or cytotoxic therapy–induced mucositis. Pseudomembranous pharyngitis suggests yeast infection. A thorough examination of the gingival and periodontal tissues for focal areas of pain, erythema, swelling, and bleeding can suggest the periodontium as a potential focus of infection (particularly as a source of bacteremic infection) by viridans streptococci and oropharyngeal gram-negative anaerobic bacilli.[206]

Laboratory aids include virus culture techniques, direct fungal stains, direct electron microscopic examination for virus particles, cytologic examination of cellular material from the base of the ulcer (e.g., Tzanck preparation for the detection of multinucleated giant cells and intranuclear inclusions), or direct herpes simplex antigen detection techniques. The material from a specific lesion should be submitted to the clinical microbiology laboratory for culture and for direct examination. Routine Gram's stain can be helpful in demonstrating the presence of budding yeasts and pseudohyphae suggestive of *Candida* species. A potassium hydroxide mount (to digest extraneous unwanted cellular material) also can provide a clue to this diagnosis by demonstrating the presence of these structures.

MANAGEMENT

The morbidity associated with oropharyngeal or esophageal mucositis can be life threatening, particularly when local pain interferes with an adequate nutritional intake. Pain control becomes a high priority. A topical anesthetic such as lidocaine in a 2% water-soluble gel or 5% water-insoluble ointment has been used widely with inconsistent success. Continuous intravenous morphine infusions have been successful for symptom control among BMT recipients with cytotoxic therapy–induced mucositis or acute oral graft-versus-host disease. Herpetic mucositis involving the oropharynx or esophagus should be treated with acyclovir. Intravenous acyclovir ($250 \, mg/m^2$ q8h) may be administered for severe cases until oral administration (200 mg q4h) can be tolerated for a total course of 7 days. Pseudomembranous candidiasis involving the oropharynx or esophagus may be treated with various approaches. Topical therapy with oral nystatin suspension (2 to 30 million units daily in four divided doses) remains a popular first-line approach. Many physicians prefer to prescribe orally absorbed azole antifungal agents such as ketoconazole (200 to 600 mg daily) or fluconazole (50 to 400 mg daily). It is important to remember that the efficacy of ketoconazole may be compromised by concomitant use of antacid therapy or in the setting of gastric achlorhydria. Invasive candidal esophagitis should be treated with intravenous amphotericin B to a cumulative dose of 500 to 1500 mg (approximately 5 to 15 mg/kg), while oropharyngeal candidiasis has been treated successfully with cumulative doses of about 500 mg (5 mg/kg). Necrotizing polymicrobial anaerobic mucositis responds well to metronidazole (500 mg PO or IV q8h).[129]

Evidence is accumulating that much of the extra morbidity caused by these infections superimposed on chemotherapy-induced mucositis can be reduced significantly by the prophylactic use of antiviral agents such as acyclovir among HSV-seropositive individuals,[207] antiseptics such as chlorhexidine,[208] and antifungal agents such as oral azoles.[209] Further work is required to determine the optimal dose schedules and routes of administration for these agents.

ENTERIC INFECTIONS

Invasive enteric bacterial infections of the gut due to *Salmonella* or *Shigella* species are relatively uncommon in neutropenic patients. Two clinical entities, however, must be considered in febrile neutropenic patients with abdominal pain and diarrhea: toxigenic enterocolitis due to the toxin elaborated from an overgrowth of Clostridium difficile and neutropenic enterocolitis (typhlitis).

CLOSTRIDIUM DIFFICILE–ASSOCIATED DIARRHEA

Clostridium difficile–associated diarrhea (CDAD) is not a rare problem among neutropenic patients receiving broad-spectrum antibiotic therapy, particularly those who are recipients of antibacterial agents that have high biliary excretion rates and are active against intestinal anaerobic bacteria. Approximately 5% to 10% of high-dose chemotherapy recipients have been reported with this complication.[210–212] This problem must be considered when such patients develop abdominal pain in association with watery diarrhea with or without blood. The differential diagnosis includes other infectious (cytomegalovirus [CMV] enterocolitis or typhlitis) and noninfectious (cytotoxic therapy–induced mucosal damage or peptic ulcer disease) causes. Protozoa and helminths are unlikely causes of this syndrome unless there is an associated history of travel to or immigration from areas where pathogens such as *Giardia lamblia* or *Strongyloides stercoralis* are endemic.

Diarrheal stools from outpatient clinics should be submitted to the clinical microbiology laboratory for bacterial culture (to rule out the remote possibilities of salmonellosis, shigellosis, and *Campylobacter* or *Yersinia* infection), examination for ova and parasites (unless this has been done earlier in the patient's course), and culture for *C. difficile* and the detection of *C. difficile* toxin. CDAD is much more common among hospitalized patients. If *C. difficile* is cultured or the toxin detected, this is sufficient to warrant therapy with either metronidazole (500 mg PO q8h for 10 days) or vancomycin (125 to 250 mg PO q6h for 10 days) without a sigmoidoscopic examination for detection of the pseudomembranous changes associated with this infection. In patients with a sufficiently typical clinical presentation, it is also reasonable to begin therapy empirically before laboratory confirmation is available.

TYPHLITIS AND NEUTROPENIC ENTEROCOLITIS

Typhlitis, also called *neutropenic enterocolitis, necrotizing enterocolitis*, or *ileocecal syndrome*, is a serious, potentially life-threatening infection of the bowel wall seen in up to 32% of patients undergoing remission-induction therapy for acute leukemia.[213–216] The pathologic process includes diffuse dilatation and edema of the bowel walls, with varying degrees of mucosal and submucosal hemorrhage and ulceration.[217] The cecum appears to be favored for the development of this syndrome, possibly related to its relatively tenuous blood supply. Bacterial invasion through an ischemic gut wall in the setting of neutropenia and cytotoxic therapy–induced mucosal surface damage is the probable pathogenesis.[213,214] The syndrome presents a spectrum of severity from mild self-limiting cecal inflammation to fulminant bowel wall necrosis with perforation. The clinical syndrome is typically characterized by a triad of diarrhea, abdominal pain, and fever in the setting of cytotoxic therapy–induced neutropenia.[217,218] Abdominal distention, nausea, vomiting, and diffuse watery or bloody diarrhea are also commonly observed. Bacteremia with enteric microorganisms (*E. coli* or *Klebsiella* species) and *Pseudomonas aeruginosa* is associated with typhlitis in up to 28% of cases.[213] Clinical examination usually reveals a diffusely tender abdomen; however, localization to the right lower or upper quadrant is not uncommon.

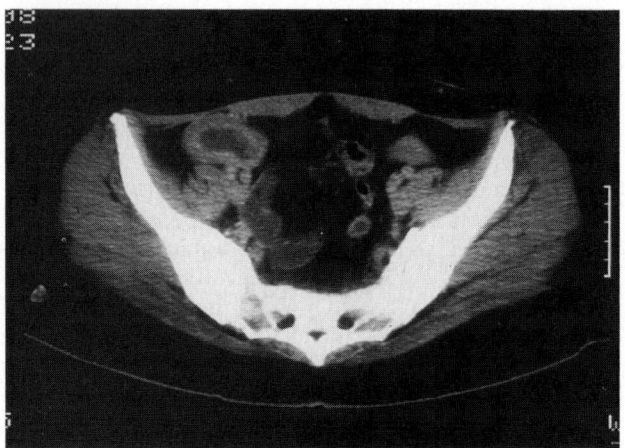

FIGURE 47-4 CT scan of the abdomen of a woman receiving high-dose cytarabine for acute leukemia who complained of severe right lower quadrant pain. The wall of the cecum is thickened and edematous consistent with typhlitis.

Ultrasonographic[219] or CT imaging of the abdomen frequently demonstrates thickening and edema of the colonic walls with or without inflammatory changes in the surrounding pericolic tissues (Fig. 47-4). Gas in the intestinal wall (pneumatosis) or an inflammatory phlegmon also may be seen in approximately 20% of cases.[69] CDAD is associated with the greatest degree of bowel wall thickening.[69] There appears to be a correlation between the thickness of the bowel wall, presumably reflecting the degree of inflammation, and mortality. Cartoni and colleagues, using ultrasonographic examinations, noted mortality rates of 60% among those with mural thickness of more than 10 millimeters.[219] Mural thickness also correlated with prolonged duration of symptoms of more than a week compared to patients without thickening (mean duration of symptoms was 7.9 vs. 3.8 days).[219]

Neutropenic enterocolitis is associated with significant impairment in the functional integrity of the gut mucosal surface. Malabsorption of D-xylose has been shown to precede clinical neutropenic enterocolitis by at least a week.[32] This intestinal mucosal damage increases the risk for translocation of bacteria and opportunistic fungi that colonize the intestinal lumen. For example, *Candida* mannoprotein antigen associated with intestinal colonizing *Candida* spp. may be detected in patients with neutropenic enterocolitis.[220] Translocation of colonizing yeast in the setting of cytotoxic therapy–induced neutropenic enterocolitis is part of the pathogenesis of invasive candidiasis with portal fungemia and subsequent hepatosplenic fungal infection.[32,221]

Management consists of early recognition, bowel rest with nasogastric decompression, intravenous fluid replacement, blood product transfusion, and broad-spectrum antibacterial agents directed against the aerobic, microaerophilic, and anaerobic enteric microflora (e.g., piperacillin-tazobactam, imipenem-cilastatin, and meropenem plus an agent effective against obligate anaerobic bacteria such as metronidazole). Although surgical consultation early in the evolution of the syndrome is recommended so that all potential management strategies can be planned before an intra-abdominal catastrophe occurs, medical management is recommended for the majority of patients who do not have evidence of a major intra-abdominal catastrophe. Surgical intervention

with right hemicolectomy or local resection of necrotic segments of bowel with anastomosis or diverting ileostomy or colostomy should only be considered in the setting of cecal perforation, massive uncontrollable GI bleeding, uncontrollable sepsis, complete bowel obstruction, or pneumatosis cystoides intestinalis.[215] With optimal management, the mortality rate has declined from over 50% to less than 20%.[217,218] The optimal outcome for these patients appears to require a high index of suspicion for the syndrome, aggressive supportive care, and marrow recovery. It is important to recognize the high risk of recurrence (up to two-thirds of cases) with subsequent cycles of cytotoxic therapy.[214]

PERIRECTAL INFECTIONS

Infections of the perirectal tissues may be life threatening in neutropenic patients. The majority of cancer patients with this complication have received cytotoxic therapy for leukemia or lymphoreticular malignancy within the preceding month and are severely neutropenic (ANC $< 0.5 \times 10^9$/L) at the time of presentation.[222] Although the presence of neutropenia may preclude the development of frank suppuration, perirectal infection must be suspected if there is focal tenderness, perirectal induration, or erythema with or without fluctuance or tissue necrosis.[64] Although some cases may be associated with a preexisting pathologic process such as an anal fissure or thrombosed hemorrhoidal tissues, most patients present no obvious predisposing factor. Conceivably, small abrasions or tears in the rectal mucosa may be the primary event allowing tissue invasion by the microflora colonizing the rectum, anus, and perineum. The etiology of these infections is polymicrobial.[223,224] The most common microorganisms associated with perirectal infections are enteric gram-negative bacilli (e.g., *E. coli*, *Klebsiella* spp., or *Enterobacter* spp.), *P. aeruginosa*, obligately anaerobic gram-negative bacilli (e.g., *Bacteroides* spp.), enterococci, and peptostreptococci. Recurrent episodes of infection are frequent (up to 26% of episodes in one series) among patients recovering from one perirectal infection and receiving subsequent cycles of cytotoxic therapy.[222]

The optimal approach to management is controversial. In general, neutropenic patients should be managed medically unless local care, systemic antimicrobials, and blood product support fail to contain the infection, or if an obvious inflammatory collection must be surgically drained. The likelihood of success of medical management is increased if the antimicrobial regimen contains agents effective in severe intra-abdominal sepsis,[225] and should include a single agent such as piperacillin-tazobactam or a carbapenem, imipenem-cilastatin or meropenem, or a combination regimen including an agent effective against anaerobic bacteria (e.g., clindamycin or metronidazole) and either a cephalosporin or a fluoroquinolone. Furthermore, vancomycin may be added if despite these antimicrobials the cellulitis appears to progress. The therapeutic role of antimicrobial agents active against *Enterococcus* spp. remains difficult to evaluate since the role of these bacterial species in the pathogenesis of these infections is controversial. Cephalosporins are inactive against *Enterococcus* spp. and the carbapenem-related susceptibility profiles tend to mirror that of ampicillin and therefore are less reliable.[226] Enterococcal colonization must be differentiated from infection. Furthermore, the rising incidence of vancomycin-resistant *Enterococcus* species argues to minimize the use of vancomycin for suspected but unproven enterococcal infection.[129] Recent observations with regard to the emergence of vancomycin-resistant *Enterococcus* species following piperacillin-based antibacterial therapy[227] are of concern given the frequency of use of this agent in the treatment of bacterial infections in cancer patients.

INVASIVE FUNGAL INFECTIONS

OPPORTUNISTIC YEAST INFECTIONS

This group of opportunistic unicellular fungal organisms of the form-class Blastomycetes and form-family Cryptococcaceae includes six genera: *Cryptococcus* (e.g., *C. neoformans*, the agent of cryptococcal meningitis), *Malassezia* (e.g., *M. furfur*, the agent of pityriasis versicolor), *Rodotorula* (e.g., *R. rubra*, an agent causing pulmonary and systemic infections), *Candida* (e.g., *C. albicans*, the most common cause of candidiasis), *Trichosporon* (e.g., *T. beigelii*, the agent of white piedra and systemic infections in compromised hosts), and *Torulopsis* (e.g., *T. glabrata*, now reclassified under the genus *Candida*). *C. albicans*, *C. tropicalis*, *C. glabrata*, and *Trichosporon* species are part of the normal microflora of the mouth, colon, and vagina. Consequently, it is not surprising to find these agents involved in the pathogenesis of infections among immunocompromised patients with damaged mucosal and integumental surfaces. This has been recently reviewed.[228]

Invasive candidiasis encompasses deep infections of various organ sites with *Candida* species.[229,230] *C. albicans* is the most commonly observed; however, *C. tropicalis*, *C. glabrata*, *C. parapsilosis*, *C. krusei*, and *C. guilliermondii* are causal agents of infection in neutropenic patients as well. When multiple organ sites are involved, the term *disseminated candidiasis* may be more appropriate. The most common forms of invasive candidiasis encountered in neutropenic patients are candidemia with or without associated central venous catheter infection, chronic systemic candidiasis (hepatosplenic candidiasis), endophthalmitis, hematogenously spread skin infection, and renal candidiasis. The pathogenesis is the invasion of damaged integumentary surfaces by colonizing yeasts during severe immunosuppression and myelosuppression.

Candidemia without evidence of metastatic infection is frequently associated with indwelling central venous catheters. Such patients should have the catheter removed and should receive antifungal therapy[229,231] with intravenous amphotericin B deoxycholate 0.6 to 1.0 mg/kg per day to a total dose of 500 to 1000 mg, or with intravenous or oral fluconazole 400 to 800 mg daily, or intravenous caspofungin 70 mg on day 1 followed by 50 mg daily.[232] Patients with evidence of dissemination to other organs should be treated with amphotericin B deoxycholate or a lipid-based formulation of amphotericin B to total doses of 30 to 60 mg/kg (2 to 4 g for a 70-kg patient). The overall response rates for amphotericin B in candidemia have been as high as 70% in teaching hospitals.[233] Patients with CNS involvement probably also should receive 5-flucytosine (5-FC). Imidazoles such as ketoconazole or miconazole are not recommended under these circumstances. The role of the newer triazoles fluconazole and itraconazole in the treatment of invasive candidiasis in neutropenic patients appears promising.[230]

Two randomized trials in non-neutropenic surgical and ICU patients with invasive candidiasis have demonstrated equivalency of fluconazole and amphotericin B.[234,235] One retrospective, matched-cohort study[236] and one randomized controlled study comparing fluconazole and amphotericin B in a mixture of neutropenic and non-neutropenic cancer patients with invasive candidiasis also have demonstrated similar response rates of 64% to 73%.[236,237]

The combination of a triazole and a polyene antifungal may be potentially antagonistic given that both classes act on the fungal cell membrane.[238,239] Azoles interfere with the 14-demethylation of lanosterol in the synthetic pathway of ergosterol, the predominant sterol in the fungal cell membrane to which polyene antifungal agents such as amphotericin B bind to produce their fungicidal effects. Clinical reports have suggested that sequential treatment with lipophilic azoles such as itraconazole followed by amphotericin B may be deleterious.[240] This effect may not be as prominent with the more lipophobic azoles such as fluconazole, with less accumulation of the agent in the lipid-rich environment of the cell membrane. A recent randomized blinded placebo-controlled trial from the National Institutes of Allergy and Infectious Disease Mycoses Study Group compared the safety and efficacy of fluconazole with or without amphotericin B for the treatment of candidemia in severely ill non-neutropenic patients with high Acute Physiology and Chronic Health Evaluation (APACHE) II scores.[241] The response rates were somewhat higher in the combination group (60 of 107, 56% vs. 77 of 112, 69%; $p = 0.043$) and no evidence of antagonism was observed. The odds of treatment failure were increased by high APACHE II scores (OR 1.09; 95% CI 1.03 to 1.14), and decreased if *C. parapsilosis* was the etiology of the bloodstream infection.[241]

Most episodes of candidemia are caused by *C. albicans*;[230] however, there is an increasing incidence of non-albicans candidemia.[242–245] In a multicenter prospective, observational study of candidemia in 427 consecutive patients from four tertiary care hospitals,[242] *C. albicans* accounted for 52% of the bloodstream isolates overall. However, over the course of the 3.5-year study, the proportion of all bloodstream isolates that were non-albicans candidal species increased from 40% to 53%. Risk factors for candidemia due to *C. albicans* included no prior use of antifungal therapy, solid organ transplant recipient, and having a wound as portal of entry. The single most important risk factor for *C. tropicalis* fungemia was neutropenia. Prognostic factors for *C. glabrata* fungemia included prior use of amphotericin B, hemodialysis, and an abdominal portal of entry; for *C. krusei* fungemia, prior use of fluconazole, and neutropenia; and for *C. parapsilosis*, prior use of fluconazole. Breakthrough candidemia occurred in 13% of patients receiving an antifungal agent for prophylaxis or empiric therapy. Under these circumstances, the candidemias were due to non-albicans species that were resistant to fluconazole. These observations have important implications for neutropenic patients in whom agents such as fluconazole are being used more widely for prophylaxis[246,247] and therapy.[236,237,241,248]

Chronic systemic candidiasis, also referred to as granulomatous hepatitis, focal hepatic candidiasis, or hepatosplenic candidiasis, has emerged as a significant problem among recipients of high-dose cytotoxic therapy.[230,249–253] The typical clinical presentation is a patient who has received high-dose cytarabine, followed by a febrile illness that persists despite broad-spectrum antimicrobial therapy and recovery of the circulating neutrophil count. There may be associated right upper quadrant tenderness, hepatomegaly,

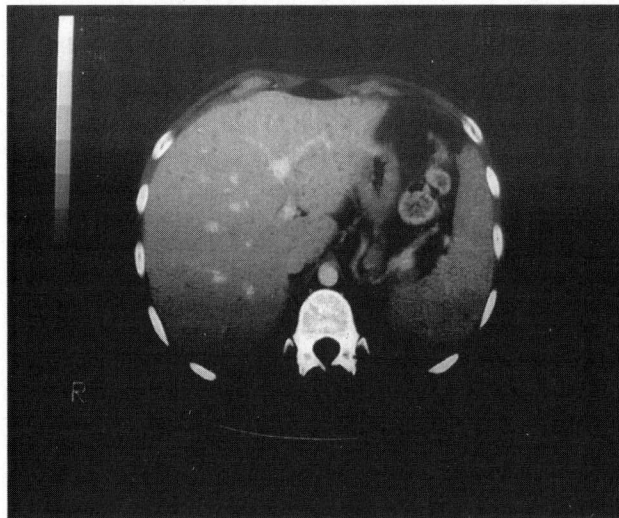

FIGURE 47-5 CT scan of the abdomen in a 22-year-old male recipient of high-dose cytarabine for relapsed high-grade non-Hodgkin's lymphoma. Multiple areas of decreased attenuation are noted in the hepatic and splenic parenchyma consistent with hepatosplenic candidiasis.

splenomegaly, and elevated serum alkaline phosphatase and γ-glutamyltransferase levels. The diagnosis may be established by imaging studies of the abdomen using ultrasonography or CT showing multiple abscesses in the liver and splenic parenchyma (Fig. 47-5). Where possible, a tissue biopsy should be considered for histopathologic and microbiologic confirmation. Biopsy of these lesions demonstrates the presence of necrotizing granulomata, frequently (but not uniformly) containing budding yeasts and pseudohyphal elements consistent with Candida species. Liver biopsy specimens should be submitted in a dry, sterile container to the clinical microbiology laboratory and processed for pyogenic bacteria, mycobacteria, viruses, and fungi. Specimens for histopathologic evaluation may be submitted to the pathology laboratory in fixative and processed for staining with hematoxylin and eosin, with periodic acid-Schiff (PAS), with an acid-fast stain, and with methenamine silver. Multiple sections through the paraffin-embedded tissue fragments may be necessary to detect the pathogens. Open liver biopsy is the most reliable means of definitively establishing the diagnosis. The pathogen is often not grown despite appropriate culture of the tissue specimen. The determination of a correct diagnosis becomes an important factor contributing to the planning of potentially curative postremission therapeutic strategies.

About half the patients respond to systemic amphotericin B (1.0 to 1.5 mg/kg per day) with or without 5-FC (100 mg/kg per day) in cumulative amphotericin B doses as high as 9 g. However, even in those who respond, the difficulty with diagnosis and the requirement for prolonged antifungal therapy frequently result in failure to complete planned postremission therapeutic regimens for the underlying malignancies, leading to shortened disease-free survival.[221] The toxicities of prolonged systemic amphotericin B (anemia, renal insufficiency, hypokalemia, fever, chills, and nausea) and 5-FC (myelosuppression) are also limiting. More recently, experience with the newer triazole antifungal agent fluconazole has suggested that this may be a useful approach for patients unable to tolerate or failing amphotericin B–containing regimens.[230]

Amphotericin B toxicity is often a limiting factor in therapy. Acute infusional toxicities occur in approximately 70% of patients during the first 7 days of therapy,[254] and include fever (51%), chills (28%), nausea (18%), and headache (9%). Prophylactic use of diphenhydramine, acetaminophen, and corticosteroids (alone or in combination) has been no more effective than no prophylaxis in preventing these infusional toxicities.[254] Meperidine (0.2 to 0.5 mg/kg) may ameliorate the rigors. Hydrocortisone has not been shown to be effective, and as a sterol itself, may compete with fungal cell membrane ergosterol for the binding of amphotericin B.[255] Metabolic toxicities including potassium and magnesium wastage or elevated serum creatinine occur in more than 80% of patients.[256] Approximately one third of amphotericin B deoxycholate recipients can be expected to experience a doubling of the serum creatinine from pretreatment levels.[177]

The newer lipid-based formulations of amphotericin B have been developed to reduce the amphotericin B–related toxicities and to permit the administration of larger doses.[230] These agents include liposomal amphotericin B, amphotericin B colloidal dispersion, and amphotericin B lipid complex (ABLC). At least one randomized controlled trial comparing ABLC (5 mg/kg per day) with conventional amphotericin B (0.6 mg/kg per day) in patients with invasive candidiasis has shown similar results with respect to efficacy and infusional toxicities, but with reduced nephrotoxicity in ABLC recipients.[257] Lipid-based formulations of amphotericin B have been studied in clinical trials of empiric antifungal therapy.[177,179]

The optimal dosing protocol for amphotericin B for empiric therapy in the setting of persistent fever unresponsive to broad-spectrum antibacterial therapy in neutropenic patients has never been established. A daily dose of at least 0.5 mg/kg amphotericin B until marrow recovery has been recommended.[258] Medoff suggested a total cumulative amphotericin B dose of 5 to 20 mg/kg given over 3 to 6 weeks for candidemia.[259] The recommended doses for invasive candidiasis have ranged from 0.5 to 1.0 mg/kg per day to cumulative doses of 2 to 4 g.[260] For a 70-kg patient receiving 0.5 mg/kg per day, this amount would require between 2 and 4 months to administer. It is unknown whether the efficacy of amphotericin B therapy is correlated with total cumulative dose or with duration of therapy.

The IDSA has suggested that patients with prolonged neutropenia who are persistently febrile despite 4 to 7 days of broad-spectrum antibacterial therapy are candidates for empiric antifungal therapy with amphotericin B.[55] This recommendation is based on two previously published trials.[175,176] The incidence of empiric amphotericin B use is significantly higher compared with the incidence of documented invasive fungal disease in neutropenic patients with acute leukemia (36% to 69% vs. 3% to 11%, respectively).[261–264] In BMT recipients, empiric amphotericin B use is also significantly higher than the incidence of invasive fungal infection (38% to 82% vs. 3% to 28%, respectively).[265–268] These differences are likely related to the difficulties in diagnosing invasive fungal infection in these patients. At least one randomized controlled clinical trial[248] compared fluconazole (6 mg/kg per day up to 400 mg/d) and amphotericin B (0.8 mg/kg per day), and demonstrated similar efficacy but with less drug-related toxicity in the fluconazole recipients compared with amphotericin B recipients (32% vs. 82%, respectively). These results are consistent with those in neutropenic and non-neutropenic patients with invasive candidiasis.[234–237,241]

The echinocandins, a class of antifungal agents that inhibit the activity of 1, 3-β glucan synthase at a critical step in fungal cell wall synthesis, are fungicidal against species of *Candida*. Among patients with candidemia, caspofungin recipients have responded only marginally better than conventional amphotericin B deoxycholate recipients, 73% vs. 62%, respectively.[269] However, caspofungin was associated with fewer adverse events such as nephrotoxicity. Among the small number of neutropenic patients enrolled into that study, the response rates were 3 of 8 (38%) for amphotericin B deoxycholate recipients and 6 of 8 (75%) among caspofungin recipients (OR 5.0; 95% CI 0.42 to 42.3). Based on these observations and those from the fluconazole trials, the National Comprehensive Cancer Network Clinical Practice guidelines in Oncology recommend the use of either caspofungin 70 mg intravenously as a loading dose followed by 50 mg intravenously daily, or fluconazole 400 to 800 mg daily in adults with invasive candidiasis instead of conventional amphotericin B deoxycholate on the basis of equivalence of efficacy and superior safety profiles.[129] Furthermore, caspofungin or a lipid formulation of amphotericin B may be recommended for clinically unstable patients with candidemia due to *C. krusei* or *C. glabrata*.

The duration of antifungal therapy for fungemic patients should be at least 14 days following the last positive blood culture and resolution of signs and symptoms of fungal infection in neutropenic and non-neutropenic adult patients.[232] The duration for patients with hepatosplenic fungal infections is a period of 3 to 6 months along with resolution of signs and symptoms of infection or calcification of radiologically detectable lesions. The duration for oropharyngeal candidiasis should be 7 to 14 days after clinical improvement and 7 to 21 days for esophageal candidiasis.[232]

The IDSA guidelines recommend the removal of all indwelling vascular access catheters in candidemic patients.[232] The purpose of this recommendation is to reduce the risk for metastatic visceral infections and excess mortality.[270] Earlier studies suggested that catheter removal at diagnosis of candidemic episodes reduced the duration of candidemia[271] and mortality.[270] More recent studies among candidemic patients receiving either caspofungin or amphotericin B deoxycholate with or without central venous catheters left in situ failed to confirm those earlier observations with regard to response rates and to duration of candidemia.[269]

OPPORTUNISTIC FILAMENTOUS FUNGAL INFECTIONS

Opportunistic filamentous fungal infections are frequently life threatening complications among neutropenic patients undergoing remission-induction treatment for acute leukemia or hemopoietic stem cell transplantation. These infections are most often caused by *Aspergillus* species, and more often by fumigatus *Aspergillus* spp. as compared to nonfumigatus *Aspergillus* spp., including *A. flavus*, *A. niger*, and *A. terreus*, *Fusarium* spp., the dematiaceous fungi (black molds), or the Zygomycetes (e.g., *Absidia* spp., *Rhizopus* spp., *Rhizo- mucor* spp., *Mucor* spp. or *Cunninghamella* spp.).[228] They produce similar clinical syndromes in compromised hosts, including necrotizing nasal mucosal infection, sinusitis, endophthalmitis, cerebral parenchymal infection, pulmonary parenchymal infection, cutaneous infection, typhlitis,

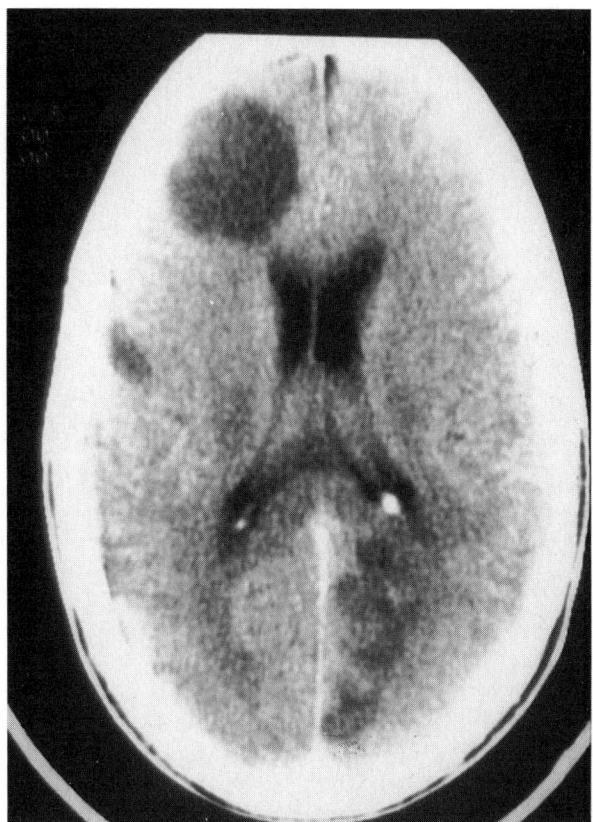

FIGURE 47-6 CT scan of the brain shows an intracerebral infarct in a 27-year-old man being treated for acute myeloid leukemia (AML) complicated by disseminated aspergillosis.

hepatosplenic abscesses, osteomyelitis, and intravascular infections.[272]

Infections by these molds are characterized by blood vessel invasion resulting in thrombosis and blood vessel obstruction, which in turn cause ischemia and infarction of the distal tissues.[273–276] This is the mechanism for the clinical manifestations such as pulmonary cavitary disease, hemoptysis, cutaneous infarcts (see Fig. 47-2), stroke-like syndromes due to intracranial infection (Fig. 47-6), and parenchymal hepatic infarction (Fig. 47-7). Infection occurs following the germination of inhaled conidia on the respiratory epithelium with the production of invasive hyphae.[275]

Characterization of these infections is important in determining prognosis and outcome of antifungal therapy. The National Institute of Allergy and Infectious Diseases Mycoses Study Group (NIAID/MSG) of the National Institutes of Health and the European Organization for the Treatment and Research of Cancer/Invasive Fungal Infections Cooperative Group (EORTC/IFICG) have developed an international consensus of diagnostic criteria for invasive fungal infections (IFI).[277] These infections are classified into three levels of probability as proven, probable, or possible, based on the robustness of the evidence supporting the diagnosis. A recent study from Spain conducted among patients undergoing peripheral blood stem cell transplants who developed IFI reported that mortality rates were related to the classification of the IFI as possible (mortality 20%), probable (mortality 57%), or proven (mortality 80%).[278] Ascioglu and colleagues caution, however, that these criteria were developed in the context of clinical

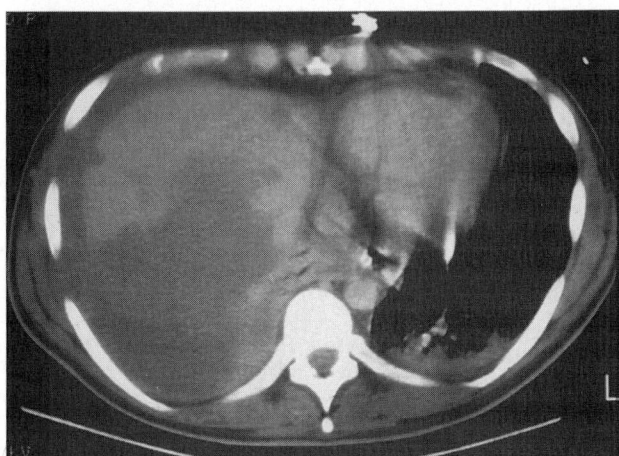

FIGURE 47-7 CT scan of the abdomen in a patient with acute myeloid leukemia (AML) shows massive hepatic infarction secondary to disseminated aspergillosis.

trials rather than for clinical application.[277] The clinical applicability is limited by false-negative observations wherein patients classified as only probable IFI may ultimately have widespread IFI at postmortem examination.[279] These observations underscore the need for more sensitive and predictive tests. However, despite the limitations of diagnostic technology, it seems prudent to use these criteria as guidelines for determining the robustness of the clinical diagnosis and the need to proceed to more invasive diagnostic procedures or for epidemiologic research.[280]

Molds are ubiquitous in the environment[183,273] and present in a wide variety of natural and synthetic materials such as soil,[274] decaying vegetation,[274] fireproofing materials,[281] water,[282] and air.[283] *Aspergillus* species frequently have been detected in the air of hospital rooms, and in particular, in circumstances associated with construction and renovation.[284,285] The management of leukemia and BMT patients in specialized self-contained hospital nursing units outfitted with high-efficiency particulate air filtration (HEPA) has reduced the incidence of invasive aspergillosis,[286] and overall mortality rates, particularly among hemopoietic stem cell transplant recipients.[287] Guidelines are available for planning infection control strategies to contain the excess risk of invasive mold infections among high-risk patients managed in environments where hospital maintenance and renovation projects are underway.[288–290] HEPA-filtered nursing units have lower concentrations of airborne fungal conidia than their non–HEPA-filtered counterparts.[291]

Invasive aspergillosis in leukemia and hemopoietic stem cell transplant patients has been reported to have extremely high mortality rates almost regardless of treatment.[292] The risk of this infection increases with the duration of neutropenia to a plateau of 70% to 80% at 5 weeks.[293] Marrow recovery represents the single most important factor relating to survival of invasive fungal infection in neutropenic patients.[294]

The clinical findings relate to the infected organ site. Fever is almost invariably present. Evidence of tissue ischemia and infarction may provide clues to the diagnosis. The most common presentation is that of focal pulmonary infiltrates in a persistently febrile, severely neutropenic patient unresponsive to broad-spectrum antibacterial therapy. Some investiga-

tors have suggested that nasal cultures positive for *Aspergillus* species in this setting can be highly predictive (∼90%) of invasive aspergillosis.[181] Positive cultures from other respiratory specimens such as sputum, bronchial brushings, or bronchoalveolar lavage fluid also can be predictive of invasive aspergillosis in high-risk patients;[230,295] however, these relationships have not been universally accepted. Based on multivariate analysis of patients with acute leukemia, a number of factors predictive of invasive opportunistic fungal disease have been identified by different investigators.[293,296–298] In each of these studies the duration of severe neutropenia was the most important independent variable. Other related variables were the duration of cytotoxic therapy (which gives rise to prolonged neutropenia), the duration of neutropenia associated with antibacterial therapy, and colonization by fungi at surveillance culture sites.

The definitive diagnosis of invasive aspergillosis usually requires microscopic and microbiologic examination of tissue biopsied from sites of infection.[273] The demonstration of septate hyphae branching at acute angles in methenamine silver stained or periodic acid-Schiff–stained tissue sections suggests the diagnosis; however, these morphologic characteristics in stained tissue sections are also shared by species of *Fusarium* and *Scedosporium*.[273] Microbiologic identification in culture is required to confirm the diagnosis. This is important because organisms such as *Fusarium* spp., *S. apiospermum*, and *S. prolificans* are not susceptible to amphotericin B. Where available, immunodiagnostic techniques may increase the positive predictive value of the classic microscopic appearance of these organisms in tissue sections.[299]

In leukemia patients the reported mortality rates from invasive pulmonary aspergillosis have had a wide range (between 13% and 100%), whereas in BMT patients the mortality rate approaches 100%.[292] Marrow recovery represents the single most important determinant of survival.[294] Aspergillosis can develop and progress despite the concomitant administration of amphotericin B at daily doses of 0.5 mg/kg.[300] Improved responses and survival rates for leukemia patients have been reported with the use of high-dose amphotericin B (1.0 to 1.5 mg/kg per day in contrast to a more standard dose of 0.5 to 0.7 mg/kg per day) without serious or permanent renal damage.[300] Anecdotal reports and studies in animal models support the use of 5-FC with amphotericin B.[239,292] Doses of 5-FC of 100 to 150 mg/kg per day in four divided doses orally usually result in serum levels of 50 to 100 mg/L. There is an increased risk of excess myelosuppression with serum levels above these values. Since 5-FC is excreted predominantly in the urine and concomitant amphotericin B therapy is almost always associated with a significant decline in renal function, regular monitoring of 5-FC levels and appropriate adjustment of dose to maintain levels in this range are mandatory.

Caspofungin has recently been approved in the United States for the treatment of invasive aspergillosis in patients refractory or intolerant of polyene-based therapy.[301] The initial experience in such patients demonstrated response rates of 50% in invasive pulmonary aspergillosis, 23% in disseminated aspergillosis, and 26% in neutropenic patients. Among patients receiving caspofungin for empiric therapy of suspected fungal infection in neutropenic patients and in whom invasive aspergillosis ultimately was determined to be the cause of the persistent fever, the response rate was 42% compared to only 8% among liposomal amphotericin B recipients.[302]

Amphotericin B lipid complex (ABLC) has been widely used in patients with invasive fungal infections refractory to or intolerant of conventional amphotericin B deoxycholate. In a review of 556 such patients receiving ABLC on an emergency drug release program, the response rate among 130 patients with invasive aspergillosis was 42%.[303] A 47% response rate was reported in an historic control study of ABLC in 39 solid organ transplant recipients with invasive aspergillosis.[304] In a series of pediatric patients with invasive aspergillosis, a 56% response rate was reported.[305]

Amphotericin B–related nephrotoxicity impacts upon patient morbidity, mortality, and the cost of management.[306–308] The safety profiles of the lipid formulations of amphotericin B in the published literature have been consistent in demonstrating advantages of reduced amphotericin B–related nephrotoxicity.[177,307] Even among patients with elevated serum creatinine levels at the outset of ABLC therapy, the advantage persists. The elevated serum creatinine levels have been observed to fall after the first week with continued administration of the drug.[309] This reduction in elevated serum creatinine after the first week of therapy may occur even when initially normal serum creatinine levels rise within the first week of ABLC therapy.[308] This experience is useful to physicians managing severely ill patients with impaired renal function and for whom polyene-based antifungal therapy is deemed necessary.

The extended-spectrum azoles such as itraconazole, voriconazole, and posiconazole have proven useful in the management of invasive mold infections.[310–313] Voriconazole proved to be superior to conventional amphotericin B deoxycholate or other licensed antifungal therapy for the management of invasive aspergillosis in a large multinational trial.[312] The treatment effect was observed in different analyses including hemopoietic stem cell transplant recipients, neutropenic patients, patients with proven or probable invasive aspergillosis, and those with pulmonary and extrapulmonary aspergillosis.

There is a high risk of relapse (>50%) in cancer patients surviving an initial episode of invasive aspergillosis during subsequent cytotoxic treatments.[314] For this reason many investigators recommend secondary prophylaxis with antifungal agents such as itraconazole or lipid formulations of amphotericin B for patients with treated invasive aspergillosis undergoing subsequent high-dose cytotoxic therapy.[315] A combination of high-dose amphotericin B (1.0 mg/kg per day) and 5-FC (100 mg/kg per day) has been used successfully to protect leukemia patients who developed invasive pulmonary aspergillosis during initial remission-induction against reactivation of the infection during subsequent cycles of cytotoxic therapy, without delay of marrow recovery.[316–318] This seems to be a rational approach for leukemic patients, but its validity for BMT patients remains to be proven.[318] The role of combinations of amphotericin with other agents such as rifampin or the azoles remains unclear and cannot be recommended at the present time.[239]

INDWELLING VASCULAR ACCESS DEVICE INFECTIONS

Indwelling peripheral and central vascular access catheters have long been recognized as a source of sepsis for critically ill cancer patients. This subject has been reviewed recently.[231,319,320] Venous and arterial cannulas physically disrupt the integrity of the skin and blood vessels, thus providing an avenue for ingress of bacteria or fungi colonizing the skin surfaces at the site of cannula placement. Determinants of intravenous cannula infection include the type of cannula, the duration of use, the technique of skin preparation for insertion, and the use of venotoxic infusates. The most common microorganisms causing intravenous site infection are gram-positive organisms such as *Staphylococcus aureus*, the coagulase-negative staphylococci, and *Corynebacterium jeikeium*; gram-negative bacilli such as the Enterobacteriaceae, *P. aeruginosa*, *Stenotrophomonas maltophilia*, and *Acinetobacter* spp; and fungi such as *Candida* species. Erythema, swelling, exudate, and focal tenderness at a peripheral intravenous catheter site should always alert the clinician to these etiologic possibilities. Suspect catheters should be removed promptly and carefully using aseptic technique and submitted to the clinical microbiology laboratory in a sterile dry container for microbiologic evaluation.

Venous access is a major problem for patients with complex multisystem problems. The need for repeated blood sampling for monitoring and for the administration of different therapies has led to the widespread use of indwelling tunneled central venous catheters. These devices provide reliable access for venous blood sampling and administration of chemotherapy, blood products, antimicrobial agents, total parenteral nutrition, crystalloids, and vasoactive agents. Infection of these devices may occur at the exit site (the point at which the catheter exits the skin), the tunnel site (that portion of the catheter buried subcutaneously and extending from the exit site to the insertion site), and the insertion site (the site, often associated with an infraclavicular or small lateral neck incision, where the catheter is inserted into a large central vein, such as the subclavian or internal jugular vein).

Erythema, exudate, and focal tenderness at the exit site suggest, but do not prove, the presence of infection. A quantitative increase in bacterial colony counts in culture swabs from the exit site has been associated with an increased probability that central venous catheter infection is present.[321,322] *Staphylococcus epidermidis* and *C. jeikeium* are the most commonly isolated colonizing microorganisms at the exit site and represent the most common etiologic agents of catheter sepsis in cancer patients.[323,324] Catheter-related sepsis is suspected if bacteremia or fungemia is present unassociated with any other site of suspected infection. The predominant mechanism of infection appears to be bacterial migration from the exit site along the outside surface of the catheter.[320] Suspected catheter exit-site infection, with or without bacteremia, may be treated with antimicrobials without removing the line.[325] Unless exit-site surveillance cultures dictate otherwise, the empiric antibacterial therapy should include an agent such as vancomycin that is active against *S. epidermidis* and *C. jeikeium*, in addition to *S. aureus* and streptococci. Infection of the subcutaneous tunnel site is more difficult to control with antimicrobial agents alone and often requires catheter removal.[326] Catheter removal is also often recommended in the setting of bacteremia due to more highly pathogenic organisms such as *S. aureus*, *P. aeruginosa*, or *Serratia marcescens*, catheter-related fungemia, or persistent catheter-related bacteremia that has not responded to appropriate antibacterial therapy. The differential time-to-positivity (i.e., the time difference between the time that the blood culture from the peripheral site and central venous catheter site was obtained to the time the cultures became positive) of >2 hours has been used as a method for predicting catheter-related infections.[327]

Infection Prevention in the Neutropenic Host

ANTIBACTERIAL PROPHYLAXIS

Antibacterial chemoprophylaxis is used widely for preventing or modifying the etiology of bacterial infection in patients for whom the expected duration of neutropenia is longer than 7 days. Oral nonabsorbable antimicrobial regimens consisting of agents such as aminoglycosides including neomycin, gentamicin, or tobramycin, vancomycin, polymyxin B, colistin, and oral nystatin or amphotericin B have not been consistently effective for reducing the incidence of febrile neutropenic episodes, documented superficial or invasive infection, or overall mortality. In addition, they are unpalatable and costly. On the other hand, oral absorbable antibacterial regimens consisting of trimethoprim-sulfamethoxazole (TMP-SMX) or fluoroquinolones including norfloxacin, ciprofloxacin, enoxacin, ofloxacin, levofloxacin, or perfloxacin have proved useful, although investigators have cautioned that efficacy appears to be intimately linked with compliance,[328] personal hygiene, the spectrum of antimicrobial activity of the regimen,[329] the cytotoxic potential of the antineoplastic regimen, and the timing of the administration of the regimen relative to the onset of the neutropenia-related risk for bacterial infection.[17,330]

The experience with oral fluoroquinolones has shown a significant reduction in the morbidity and mortality due to infection by aerobic gram-negative bacilli compared with TMP-SMX.[17,331] The tradeoff for this appears to be an increase in the risk of infection due to gram-positive organisms such as coagulase-negative staphylococci, *Enterococcus* spp., and viridans group streptococci. The presence of a tunneled indwelling central venous catheter adds to the risk for infections due to coagulase-negative staphylococci,[332] whereas severe mucositis and periodontal disease appear to predispose to viridans streptococcal infection.[34,35,206,333] A syndrome of viridans streptococcal bacteremia has been recognized among high-dose cytarabine or BMT recipients that is often associated with pulmonary infiltrates and hypotension.[34,334,335] The pathogenesis is believed to involve severe cytotoxic therapy–induced intestinal mucosal damage in the setting of severe prolonged neutropenia and gastrointestinal luminal colonization by these organisms. Oral fluoroquinolone use tends to select for these microorganisms.[336] Of clinical importance is the inconsistent susceptibility of these organisms to penicillin G and the apparent need to modify the empiric antibacterial regimen by the addition of intravenous vancomycin to improve the likelihood of a successful outcome for the febrile neutropenic episode. Bacterial infections among TMP-SMX recipients have been due to coagulase-negative staphylococci, viridans streptococci, and TMP-SMX–resistant aerobic gram-negative bacilli such as *P. aeruginosa*.[330]

Four meta-analyses have been published examining the role of fluoroquinolone-based antibacterial chemoprophylaxis in neutropenic cancer patients.[63,167,337,338] Within each of these publications are contained multiple meta-analyses. Cruciani and colleagues examined 13 trials comprising 1155 randomized subjects comparing fluoroquinolones to TMP-SMX, nonabsorbable antimicrobials, or placebo.[63] These investigators also reported on a meta-analysis examining the efficacy of fluoroquinolones plus additional agents that augmented coverage for gram-positive microorganisms.[63,167] Rotstein and associates reported on four meta-analyses; namely, five trials with 394 randomized subjects comparing fluoroquinolones to placebo, 16 trials with 1362 randomized subjects comparing fluoroquinolones to other antibacterial agents, 3 trials with 902 randomized subjects comparing ciprofloxacin to other fluoroquinolones, and 6 trials with 922 subjects comparing fluoroquinolones plus additional gram-positive coverage to control regimens.[337] Lastly, Engels and colleagues reported two meta-analyses; first, 9 trials with 731 randomized subjects comparing fluoroquinolones and untreated controls, and second, 9 trials with 677 randomized subjects comparing fluoroquinolones to TMP-SMX.[338]

These systematic reviews were able to detect prophylactic treatment effects for the fluoroquinolones in a variety of outcomes, including microbiologically documented infection overall, gram-negative infections overall, and gram-negative bacteremia regardless of whether the controls were placebo, no treatment, or TMP-SMX. Infection-related mortality and overall mortality were not affected by fluoroquinolone prophylaxis. Reduction in the incidence of febrile episodes was demonstrable only in the 8 placebo-controlled trials (OR 0.85; 95% CI 0.75 to 0.99); however, this effect was observed only among unblinded trials and not blinded trials.[338] Treatment effects were not observed for clinically documented infections or for gram-positive infections.

The combination of fluoroquinolones with agents with additional gram-positive activity such as penicillin, macrolides, or rifampin effectively prevents gram-positive bacteremias as well.[54,339–341] A recent updated meta-analysis from the University of Padua encompassing 1202 randomized subjects in 9 trials comparing fluoroquinolones plus augmented gram-positive coverage to fluoroquinolones alone demonstrated a reduction in total bacteremic episodes (relative risk 1.54; 95% CI 1.26 to 1.88), streptococcal infections (RR 2.2; 95% CI 1.44 to 3.37), coagulase-negative staphylococcal infections (RR 1.46; 95% CI 1.04 to 2.04), and incidence of fever (RR 1.08; 95% CI 1.00 to 1.16).[167] The incidence of clinically documented infections, unexplained fever, and infection-related mortality were not affected. Gram-positive prophylaxis, however, increased the incidence of prophylaxis-related drug toxicities (RR 0.46; 95% CI 0.28 to 0.76), particularly with the use of rifampin.[167]

Based upon these observations, antibacterial chemoprophylaxis using oral fluoroquinolones under circumstances in which the prevalence of fluoroquinolone-resistant *Escherichia coli* (FREC) is low (<3% to 5%) can reliably reduce the risk for invasive gram-negative bacillary infection, and if supplemented by gram-positive agents such as rifampin, penicillin, or macrolides, can reduce the risk for invasive infections due to gram-positive microorganisms including viridans streptococci and coagulase-negative staphylococci. Fluoroquinolone-based chemoprophylaxis does not reliably reduce the incidence of febrile neutropenic episodes, neutropenic episode-related mortality, or physician-initiated systemic antimicrobial prescribing behavior.

Under the appropriate conditions, it is possible that fluoroquinolone-based antibacterial chemoprophylaxis can influence physician prescribing behavior for febrile neutropenic episodes.[342-344] A study from Duke University among autologous hemopoietic transplant recipients with ciprofloxacin prophylaxis demonstrated that febrile neutropenic episodes could be safely treated with an empiric glycopeptide-based regimen.[343] A study from the University of Manitoba, Canada, demonstrated that patients developing febrile neutropenic episodes while receiving ciprofloxacin prophylaxis during remission-induction therapy for acute myeloid leukemia could be treated safely and effectively with a vancomycin plus ceftazidime–based strategy wherein the ceftazidime was discontinued before the patient defervesced, provided the serial rectal surveillance cultures and 24- to 36-hour blood cultures revealed no evidence of aerobic gram-negative bacilli.[344] In both these studies, the oral ciprofloxacin prophylaxis regimen was continued throughout the treatment for the febrile neutropenic episode. A third study from Europe demonstrated that empiric systemic antibacterial therapy for febrile neutropenic episodes could be safely discontinued after 72 to 96 hours if the initial work-up failed to provide evidence for clinically or microbiologically documented infection and if prophylaxis was continued.[342] These observations, while provocative, have not been followed up in large randomized controlled studies.

Not all fevers in neutropenic patients represent infection; thus fever is a poor outcome for clinical trials of antibacterial prophylaxis in this patient population. Better discriminators for infection are needed before the kinds of strategies suggested by these trials can enter the domain of standard practice.[345] Although the results of antibacterial prophylaxis studies have not yet had a major influence on how physicians use empiric antibacterial therapies, there is reason to believe that they will do so in the future.[345] The prophylaxis-related decrease in documented infections has been offset by an increase in unexplained fevers.[54] It is possible that these unexplained fevers may be due to increased absorption of pyrogenic endotoxins through cytotoxic therapy–induced damage to the intestinal epithelium.[346] This consideration, if true, suggests that at least some unexplained fevers do not require continued antibacterial therapy.

ANTIFUNGAL PROPHYLAXIS

The major goals of antifungal prophylaxis strategies are to reduce the morbidity and mortality due to superficial and invasive opportunistic fungal infections, and to reduce the use of toxic expensive antifungal therapy. Prophylactic strategies should be applied with a clear understanding of the pathogenesis of the microorganisms involved.

FILAMENTOUS FUNGI

Filamentous fungi such as *Aspergillus* species, the dematiaceous fungi, *Fusarium* spp., Zygomycetes, and *Scedosporium* spp. are acquired by inhalation of spores called *conidia*. The conidia germinate on the respiratory epithelium to produce invasive hyphae. There are three possible ways to prevent this. First, patients may be managed in nursing units outfitted with HEPA filtration systems. This reduces the concentration of airborne conidia and the risk of patient exposure. Although this approach is effective for reducing the risk of filamentous

fungal infection,[286,287,347] it is expensive and has no impact for patients exposed to high concentrations of airborne conidia outside the nursing unit or for those who are already infected before entering the unit. Second, topical agents such as amphotericin B sprayed by aerosol into the nares theoretically might reduce the risk of conidial germination. One randomized study from the Institute Jules Bordet in Brussels[348] evaluated the use of intranasal amphotericin B (5 mg/mL in sterile water with a total daily dose of 10 mg in three divided doses) in 90 neutropenic episodes. There was no significant difference in the empiric use of intravenous amphotericin B (35% versus 27%); however, only 1 of 46 recipients of aerosolized amphotericin B developed suspected or proven invasive aspergillosis compared with 7 of 44 controls. Although this is encouraging, intranasal amphotericin cannot be accepted as a satisfactory alternative to air filtration until further studies are done. Inhalation of aerosolized amphotericin B has been studied as a strategy to reduce invasive aspergillosis.[349] The incidence of possible, probable, or proven invasive aspergillosis in the aerosolized amphotericin B recipients was 4% compared to 7% in untreated control subjects. Furthermore, there were no differences in overall mortality or in infection-related mortality. Third, systemic antifungal therapy might prevent the progression of hyphal growth once germination occurs. Systemic amphotericin B plus 5-FC has been used successfully to prevent reactivation of previously documented invasive pulmonary aspergillosis among leukemia patients undergoing further postremission cytotoxic therapy.[316] Since this combination may be myelotoxic as well as nephrotoxic, it may be prudent to reserve this approach for those in whom opportunistic filamentous fungal infection has been proved by microbiologic or histopathologic methods. The prophylactic role of newer approaches such as lipid formulations of amphotericin B, echinocandins including caspofungin and micafungin, or the extended-spectrum triazole antifungal agents such as itraconazole, voriconazole, or posaconazole, with greater in vitro activity against *Aspergillus* species is being studied.

Itraconazole, a lipophilic extended-spectrum azole, has been evaluated for antifungal prophylaxis in a number of trials of very heterogeneous patient populations.[350-352] A recent meta-analysis of these trials failed to identify a prophylactic benefit of itraconzole against fungal disease due to *Aspergillus* spp.[247] However, studies performed in patients at higher risk for invasive aspergillosis have been more positive.[353,354] In hemopoietic stem cell allograft recipients Winston and colleagues evaluated itraconazole administered intravenously 200 mg twice daily for 2 days, then 200 mg intravenously daily for 12 days, then 200 mg orally daily until day 100, compared to fluconazole 400 mg given intravenously daily for 14 days, then 400 mg orally until day 100.[353] There was a significant reduction in the overall incidence of proven invasive fungal infection (OR 0.37; 95% CI 0.15 to 0.88), but the protective effect on mold infection was not statistically significant (OR 0.38; 95% CI 0.11 to 1.32). A similar study from the Fred Hutchison Cancer Center was able to demonstrate a significant reduction in the overall incidence of invasive fungal infection (15% to 7%; OR 0.46; 95% CI 0.56 to 0.99) and in invasive mold infections (12% to 5%; OR 0.44; 95% CI 0.17 to 0.98).[354] Despite this promising result, treatment-related adverse events necessitating treatment withdrawal resulted in a higher overall mortality among itraconazole recipients. The study drug was discontinued for reasons of intolerance in 36% of itraconazole recipients compared to only 16% of fluconazole recipients.[354] A recent meta-analysis from the University of Bonn, Germany, critically examined the efficacy of itraconazole for antifungal prophylaxis against invasive fungal infection in 13 randomized controlled trials encompassing 3597 randomized subjects, and demonstrated reductions in the mean relative risks for invasive fungal infection overall (relative risk reduction [RRR] 40% ± 13%), invasive yeast infection (RRR 53% ± 19%), and fungal infection–related mortality (RRR 35% ± 17%) in neutropenic cancer patients.[355] The risk for invasive aspergillosis was reduced only in trials in which the cyclodextrin-based oral or intravenous formulations of itraconazole were used (OR 0.52; 95% CI 0.30 to 0.90; RRR 48% ± 21%).[355]

Echinocandin antifungal agents may also be useful for prophylaxis in high-risk patient populations. A study comparing a newer echinocandin, micafungin, to fluconazole in a heterogeneous group of autologous and allogeneic transplant recipients demonstrated a significant reduction in the use of empiric systemic antifungal therapy among the micafungin recipients (15% compared to 21%; $p = 0.018$).[356] The incidence of invasive aspergillosis was 0.2% and 1.5% in micafungin and fluconazole recipients, respectively ($p = 0.07$).

OPPORTUNISTIC YEASTS

Yeast infections, primarily *Candida* spp., colonize the patient and cause infection by invading damaged integumental surfaces. HEPA filtering plays no role in the prevention of these infections. The use of topical agents such as nystatin or amphotericin B has had a small impact on colonization profiles, but no significant impact on the incidence of invasive fungal infection or the need to use empiric systemic amphotericin B for suspected invasive fungal infection. Topical chlorhexidine mouth rinses (0.12% chlorhexidine digluconate three times daily) have been effective in reducing the morbidity of oropharyngeal candidiasis in a series of marrow allograft recipients.[208] Furthermore, a reduction in candidemia also was noted, suggesting the oropharynx as a possible source for these events. The overall value of this strategy must be evaluated in further trials in different populations at risk.

Systemic antifungal therapy for the prevention of opportunistic yeast infections is better established.[246,247,355,357] Published studies using the imidazoles ketoconazole, clotrimazole, and miconazole have demonstrated a reduction in yeast colonization, but have failed to demonstrate a consistent reduction in clinical disease or the need to use empiric systemic amphotericin B. There also has been a selection for more resistant yeasts such as *Candida krusei* and *Candida glabrata* in the surveillance cultures of azole recipients.[242] The triazole antifungal agents fluconazole and itraconazole have been shown to be effective in reducing the need for empiric antifungal therapy with amphotericin B, superficial fungal infection, proven invasive yeast infection, and fungal infection–related mortality.[247] Furthermore, these agents are effective when applied to patient populations with a high risk for invasive fungal infection (10% to 15%),[246,247] when doses of 400 mg or more daily are administered,[247,355] and when the agents are absorbed.[355]

It is recommended that antifungal prophylaxis be administered only to defined populations at highest risk for invasive fungal infection and for whom clinical trials have been able to demonstrate a treatment effect. Accordingly, the populations of patients for whom this applies include patients undergoing remission-induction or reinduction therapy for acute leukemia, patients undergoing allogeneic hemopoietic stem cell transplantation, and those undergoing autologous hemopoietic stem cell transplantation without hemopoietic growth factor support.[358,359] Furthermore, the duration of prophylaxis should be from day 1 of the cytotoxic regimen until neutrophil recovery for acute leukemia patients. For allogeneic hemopoietic stem cell transplant recipients, treatment from the first day of conditioning until day 75 to 100 is recommended.[347,360]

ANTIVIRAL PROPHYLAXIS

Reactivation of herpes simplex virus (HSV) infection is one of the most common causes of oropharyngeal and esophageal mucositis in patients undergoing remission-induction for leukemia or BMT.[361] This complication is painful and can substantially impair adequate nutritional intake and drug administration. Herpes mucositis, stomatitis, or esophagitis can be prevented largely by prophylactic use of acyclovir. Patients at risk for these infections are those with a history of previous herpetic infection. They may be reliably identified by a clear history of the typical vesicular lesions of herpetic stomatitis or by the identification of IgG antibodies against HSV in their sera. Between 60% and 80% of HSV-seropositive patients will reactivate during cytotoxic therapy. It has been recommended that patients undergoing remission-induction therapy, consolidation therapy, or salvage therapy for acute leukemia and those undergoing bone marrow allografting or autografting who are IgG-seropositive for HSV-1 are candidates for acyclovir prophylaxis.[207,362,363] Oral and intravenous routes of administration have been studied and found effective. It remains unclear whether oral administration is as effective as intravenous administration in patients receiving regimens highly toxic to intestinal mucosal surfaces, such as high-dose cytarabine or etoposide-containing regimens or BMT conditioning regimens. Acyclovir in doses of 250 mg/m² administered intravenously every 12 to 8 hours or oral acyclovir administered in doses of 200 to 400 mg four to five times daily has prevented HSV mucositis successfully.[207] Prophylaxis for 1 month or less from initiation of treatment has been associated with recurrences in 58% to 70% of patients after the acyclovir was discontinued. Accordingly, it has been recommended that prophylaxis be continued for 6 weeks from the beginning of induction or conditioning,[207] or up to 6 weeks following marrow recovery in BMT recipients. Acyclovir doses of 800 mg orally every 12 hours appear to be effective for this. Valacyclovir has been shown to be as effective as acyclovir.

References

1. Chassin MR: Costs and outcomes of medical intensive care. *Med Care* 20:165, 1982.
2. Turnbull A, Goldiner P, Silverman D, Howland W: The role of an intensive care unit in a cancer center. An analysis of 1035 critically ill patients treated for life-threatening complications (editorial). *Cancer* 37:82, 1976.
3. Schapira DV, Studnicki J, Bradham DD, et al: Intensive care, survival, and expense of treating critically ill cancer patients. *JAMA* 269:783, 1993.
4. Gelder MS: Life and death decisions in the intensive care unit. *Cancer* 76(10 Suppl):2171, 1995.

5. Chalfin DB, Carlon GC: Age and utilization of intensive care unit resources of critically ill cancer patients. *Crit Care Med* 18:694, 1990.

6. Azoulay E, Moreau D, Alberti C, et al: Predictors of short-term mortality in critically ill patients with solid malignancies. *Intensive Care Med* 26:1817, 2000.

7. Maschmeyer G, Bertschat FL, Moesta KT, et al: Outcome analysis of 189 consecutive cancer patients referred to the intensive care unit as emergencies during a 2-year period. *Eur J Cancer* 39:783, 2003.

8. Lloyd-Thomas AR, Dhaliwal HS, Lister TA, Hinds CJ: Intensive therapy for life-threatening medical complications of haematological malignancy. *Intensive Care Med* 12:317, 1986.

9. Torrecilla C, Cortes JL, Chamorro C, et al: Prognostic assessment of the acute complications of bone marrow transplantation requiring intensive therapy. *Intensive Care Med* 14:393, 1988.

10. Groeger JS, White P Jr., Nierman DM, et al: Outcome for cancer patients requiring mechanical ventilation. *J Clin Oncol* 17:991, 1999.

11. Price KJ, Thall PF, Kish SK, et al: Prognostic indicators for blood and marrow transplant patients admitted to an intensive care unit. *Am J Respir Crit Care Med* 158:876, 1998.

12. Faber-Langendoen K, Caplan AL, McGlave PB: Survival of adult bone marrow transplant patients receiving mechanical ventilation: A case for restricted use. *Bone Marrow Transplant* 12:501, 1993.

13. Tremblay LN, Hyland RH, Schouten BD, Hanly PJ: Survival of acute myelogenous leukemia patients requiring intubation/ventilatory support. *Clin Invest Med* 18:19, 1995.

14. Schimpff SC: Dilemmas and choices in infection management of the cancer patient. *Eur J Cancer Clin Oncol* 25:1351, 1989.

15. Pizzo PA, Robichaud KJ, Wesley R, Commers JR: Fever in the pediatric and young adult patient with cancer. A prospective study of 1001 episodes. *Medicine (Baltimore)* 61:153, 1982.

16. Bow EJ, Louie TJ: Changes in endogenous microflora among febrile granulocytopenic patients receiving empiric antibiotic therapy: Implications for fungal superinfection. *CMAJ* 137:397, 1987.

17. Bow EJ, Rayner E, Louie TJ: Comparison of norfloxacin with cotrimoxazole for infection prophylaxis in acute leukemia—the trade-off for reduced gram-negative sepsis. *Am J Med* 84:847, 1988.

18. Feld R, Louie TJ, Mandell L, et al: A multicenter comparative trial of tobramycin and ticarcillin vs. moxalactam and ticarcillin in febrile neutropenic patients. *Arch Intern Med* 145:1083, 1985.

19. European Organization for Research and Treatment of Cancer (EORTC) International Antimicrobial Therapy Cooperative Project Group: Ceftazidime combined with a short or long course of amikacin for empirical therapy of gram-negative bacteremia in cancer patients with granulocytopenia. *N Engl J Med* 317:1692, 1987.

20. Viscoli C, Bruzzi P, Castagnola E, et al: Factors associated with bacteraemia in febrile, granulocytopenic cancer patients. The International Antimicrobial Therapy Cooperative Group (IATCG) of the European Organization for Research and Treatment of Cancer (EORTC). *Eur J Cancer* 30A:430, 1994.

21. Bow EJ, Kilpatrick MG, Scott BA, et al: Acute myeloid leukemia in Manitoba. The consequences of standard "7 + 3" remission-induction therapy followed by high dose cytarabine postremission consolidation for myelosuppression, infectious morbidity, and outcome. *Cancer* 74:52, 1994.

22. Kurrle E, Dekker AW, Gaus W, et al: Prevention of infection in acute leukemia: A prospective randomized study on the efficacy of two different drug regimens for antimicrobial prophylaxis. *Infection* 14:226, 1986.

23. Hersh EM, Gutterman JU, Mavligit GM, et al: Serial studies of immunocompetence of patients undergoing chemotherapy for acute leukemia. *J Clin Invest* 54:401, 1974.

24. Dupuy JM, Kourilsky FM, Fradelizzi D, et al: Depression of immunologic reactivity of patients with acute leukemia. *Cancer* 27:323, 1971.

25. Walzer PD, Perl DP, Krogstad DJ, et al: *Pneumocystis carinii* pneumonia in the United States: Epidemiologic, diagnostic, and clinical features. *Natl Cancer Inst Monogr* 43:55, 1976.

26. Sonis ST, Elting LS, Keefe D, et al: Perspectives on cancer therapy-induced mucosal injury: Pathogenesis, measurement, epidemiology, and consequences for patients. *Cancer* 100 (9 Suppl): 1995, 2004.

27. Lockhart PB, Sonis ST: Relationship of oral complications to peripheral blood leukocyte and platelet counts in patients receiving cancer chemotherapy. *Oral Surg Oral Med Oral Pathol* 48:21, 1979.

28. Slavin RE, Dias MA, Saral R: Cytosine arabinoside induced gastrointestinal toxic alterations in sequential chemotherapeutic protocols: A clinical-pathologic study of 33 patients. *Cancer* 42:1747, 1978.

29. Sonis ST. Mucositis as a biological process: A new hypothesis for the development of chemotherapy-induced stomatotoxicity. *Oral Oncol* 34:39, 1998.

30. Meropol NJ, Somer RA, Gutheil J, et al: Randomized phase I trial of recombinant human keratinocyte growth factor plus chemotherapy: Potential role as mucosal protectant. *J Clin Oncol* 21:1452, 2003.

31. Wardley AM, Jayson GC, Swindell R, et al: Prospective evaluation of oral mucositis in patients receiving myeloablative conditioning regimens and haemopoietic progenitor rescue. *Br J Haematol* 110:292, 2000.

32. Bow EJ, Loewen R, Cheang MS, et al: Cytotoxic therapy-induced D-xylose malabsorption and invasive infection during remission-induction therapy for acute myeloid leukemia in adults. *J Clin Oncol* 15:2254, 1997.

33. Bow EJ, Loewen R, Cheang MS, Schacter B: Invasive fungal disease in adults undergoing remission-induction therapy for acute myeloid leukemia: The pathogenetic role of the antileukemic regimen. *Clin Infect Dis* 21:361, 1995.

34. Bochud P-Y, Eggiman P, Calandra T, et al: Bacteremia due to viridans streptococcus in neutropenic patients with cancer: Clinical spectrum and risk factors. *Clin Infect Dis* 18:25, 1994.

35. Cordonnier C, Buzyn A, Leverger G, et al: Epidemiology and risk factors for gram-positive coccal infections in neutropenia: Toward a more targeted antibiotic strategy. *Clin Infect Dis* 36:149, 2003.

36. Sonis ST, Oster G, Fuchs H, et al: Oral mucositis and the clinical and economic outcomes of hematopoietic stem-cell transplantation. *J Clin Oncol* 19:2201, 2001.

37. Elting LS, Shih YC: The economic burden of supportive care of cancer patients. *Support Care Cancer* 12:219, 2004.

38. Cherif H, Kronvall G, Bjorkholm M, Kalin M: Bacteraemia in hospitalised patients with malignant blood disorders: A retrospective study of causative agents and their resistance profiles during a 14-year period without antibacterial prophylaxis. *Hematol J* 4:420, 2003.

39. Immunocompromised Host Society: The design, analysis, and reporting of clinical trials on the empirical antibiotic management of the neutropenic patient. *J Infect Dis* 161:397, 1990.

40. Cornelissen JJ, de Graeff A, Verdonck LF, et al: Imipenem versus gentamicin combined with either cefuroxime or cephalothin as initial therapy for febrile neutropenic patients. *Antimicrob Agents Chemother* 36:801, 1992.

41. Peacock JE, Herrington DA, Wade JC, et al: Ciprofloxacin plus piperacillin compared with tobramycin plus piperacillin as empirical therapy in febrile neutropenic patients. A randomized, double-blind trial. *Ann Intern Med* 137:77, 2002.

42. European Organization for Research and Treatment of Cancer (EORTC) International Antimicrobial Therapy Cooperative Project Group: Three antibiotic regimens in the treatment of

infection in febrile granulocytopenic patients with cancer. *J Infect Dis* 137:14, 1978.

43. European Organization for Research and Treatment of Cancer (EORTC) International Antimicrobial Therapy Cooperative Project Group: Combination of amikacin and carbenicillin with or without cefazolin as empirical treatment of febrile neutropenic patients. *J Clin Oncol* 1:597, 1983.

44. Klastersky J, Glauser MP, Schimpff SC, et al: Prospective randomized comparison of three antibiotic regimens for empirical therapy of suspected bacteremic infection in febrile granulocytopenic patients. *Antimicrob Agents Chemother* 29:263, 1986.

45. European Organisation for Research and Treatment of Cancer (EORTC) IATCG, National Cancer Institute of Canada CTG: Vancomycin added to empirical combination antibiotic therapy for fever in granulocytopenic cancer patients. European Organization for Research and Treatment of Cancer (EORTC) International Antimicrobial Therapy Cooperative Group and the National Cancer Institute of Canada-Clinical Trials Group. *J Infect Dis* 163:951, 1991.

46. International Antimicrobial Therapy Cooperative Group of the European Organisation for Research and Treatment of Cancer: Efficacy and toxicity of single daily doses of amikacin and ceftriaxone versus multiple daily doses of amikacin and ceftazidime for infection in patients with cancer and granulocytopenia. The International Antimicrobial Therapy Cooperative Group of the European Organization for Research and Treatment of Cancer. *Ann Intern Med* 119(7 Pt 1):584, 1993.

47. Cometta A, Zinner S, de Bock R, et al: Piperacillin-tazobactam plus amikacin versus ceftazidime plus amikacin as empiric therapy for fever in granulocytopenic patients with cancer. The International Antimicrobial Therapy Cooperative Group of the European Organization for Research and Treatment of Cancer. *Antimicrob Agents Chemother* 39:445, 1995.

48. Cometta A, Calandra T, Gaya H, et al: Monotherapy with meropenem versus combination therapy with ceftazidime plus amikacin as empiric therapy for fever in granulocytopenic patients with cancer. The International Antimicrobial Therapy Cooperative Group of the European Organization for Research and Treatment of Cancer and the Gruppo Italiano Malattie Ematologiche dell'Adulto Infection Program. *Antimicrob Agents Chemother* 40:1108, 1996.

49. Pizzo PA, Hathorn JW, Hiemenz J, et al: A randomized trial comparing ceftazidime alone with combination antibiotic therapy in cancer patients with fever and neutropenia. *N Engl J Med* 315:552, 1986.

50. De Pauw BE, Deresinski SC, Feld R, et al: Ceftazidime compared with piperacillin and tobramycin for the empiric treatment of fever in neutropenic patients with cancer. A multicenter randomized trial. The Intercontinental Antimicrobial Study Group. *Ann Intern Med* 120:834, 1994.

51. Del Favero A, Menichetti F, Martino P, et al: A multicenter, double-blind, placebo-controlled trial comparing piperacillin-tazobactam with and without amikacin as empiric therapy for febrile neutropenia. *Clin Infect Dis* 33:1295, 2001.

52. Freifeld AG, Walsh T, Marshall D, et al: Monotherapy for fever and neutropenia in cancer patients: A randomized comparison of ceftazidime versus imipenem. *J Clin Oncol* 13:165, 1995.

53. Link H, Bohme A, Cornely OA, et al: Antimicrobial therapy of unexplained fever in neutropenic patients—guidelines of the Infectious Diseases Working Party (AGIHO) of the German Society of Hematology and Oncology (DGHO), Study Group Interventional Therapy of Unexplained Fever, Arbeitsgemeinschaft Supportivmassnahmen in der Onkologie (ASO) of the Deutsche Krebsgesellschaft (DKG-German Cancer Society). *Ann Hematol* 82(Suppl 2):S105, 2003.

54. Bow EJ, Mandell LA, Louie TJ, et al: Quinolone-based antibacterial chemoprophylaxis in neutropenic patients: Effect of augmented gram-positive activity on infectious morbidity. National

Cancer Institute of Canada Clinical Trials Group. *Ann Intern Med* 125:183, 1996.

55. Hughes WT, Armstrong D, Bodey GP, et al: 2002 Guidelines for the use of antimicrobial agents in neutropenic patients with cancer. *Clin Infect Dis* 34:730, 2002.

56. Bates DW, Cook EF, Goldman L, Lee TH: Predicting bacteremia in hospitalized patients. A prospectively validated model. *Ann Intern Med* 113:495, 1990.

57. American Society of Clinical Oncology (ASCO) Ad Hoc Colony-stimulating Factor Guideline Expert Panel: Recommendations for the use of hematopoietic colony-stimulating factors: evidence-based, clinical practice guidelines. *J Clin Oncol* 12:2471, 1994.

58. Blay JY, Chauvin F, Le Cesne A, et al: Early lymphopenia after cytotoxic chemotherapy as a risk factor for febrile neutropenia. *J Clin Oncol* 14:636, 1996.

59. Feld R, Bodey GP: Infections in patients with malignant lymphoma treated with combination chemotherapy. *Cancer* 39:1018, 1977.

60. Doorduijn JK, van der HB, van Imhoff GW, et al: CHOP compared with CHOP plus granulocyte colony-stimulating factor in elderly patients with aggressive non-Hodgkin's lymphoma. *J Clin Oncol* 21:3041, 2003.

61. Markman J, Zanotti K, Webster K, et al: Experience with the management of neutropenia in gynecologic cancer patients receiving carboplatin-based chemotherapy. *Gynecol Oncol* 92:592, 2004.

62. Nichols CR, Fox EP, Roth BJ, et al: Incidence of neutropenic fever in patients treated with standard-dose combination chemotherapy for small-cell lung cancer and the cost impact of treatment with granulocyte colony-stimulating factor. *J Clin Oncol* 12:1245, 1994.

63. Cruciani M, Rampazzo R, Malena M, et al: Prophylaxis with fluoroquinolones for bacterial infections in neutropenic patients: A meta-analysis. *Clin Infect Dis* 23:795, 1996.

64. Sickles EA, Greene WH, Wiernik PH: Clinical presentation of infection in granulocytopenic patients. *Arch Intern Med* 135:715, 1975.

65. Walsh TJ: The febrile granulocytopenic patient in the intensive care unit. *Crit Care Clin* 4:259, 1988.

66. Rubin RH, Greene R: Etiology and management of the compromised host with fever and pulmonary infiltrates, in *Clinical Approach to Infection in the Compromised Host*. New York, Plenum Press, 1988, p 131.

67. Heussel CP, Kauczor HU, Heussel GE, et al: Pneumonia in febrile neutropenic patients and in bone marrow and blood stem-cell transplant recipients: use of high-resolution computed tomography. *J Clin Oncol* 17:796, 1999.

68. Caillot D, Casasnovas O, Bernard A, et al: Improved management of invasive pulmonary aspergillosis in neutropenic patients using early thoracic computed tomographic scan and surgery. *J Clin Oncol* 15:139, 1997.

69. Kirkpatrick ID, Greenberg HM: Gastrointestinal complications in the neutropenic patient: Characterization and differentiation with abdominal CT. *Radiology* 226:668, 2003.

70. Talcott JA, Siegel RD, Finberg R, Goldman L: Risk assessment in cancer patients with fever and neutropenia: A prospective, two-center validation of a prediction rule. *J Clin Oncol* 10:316, 1992.

71. Talcott JA, Whalen A, Clark J, et al: Home antibiotic therapy for low-risk cancer patients with fever and neutropenia: A pilot study of 30 patients based on a validated prediction rule. *J Clin Oncol* 12:107, 1994.

72. Rolston KV, Rubenstein EB, Freifeld A: Early empiric antibiotic therapy for febrile neutropenia patients at low risk. *Infect Dis Clin North Am* 10:223, 1996.

73. Malik IA, Abbas Z, Karim M: Randomised comparison of oral ofloxacin alone with combination of parenteral antibiotics in neutropenic febrile patients. *Lancet* 339:1092, 1992.

74. Malik IA, Khan WA, Karim M, et al: Feasibility of outpatient management of fever in cancer patients with low-risk neutropenia: Results of a prospective randomized trial. *Am J Med* 98:224, 1995.

75. Minotti V, Gentile G, Bucaneve G, et al: Domiciliary treatment of febrile episodes in cancer patients: A prospective randomized trial comparing oral versus parenteral empirical antibiotic treatment. *Support Care Cancer* 7:134, 1999.

76. Petrilli AS, Dantas LS, Campos MC, et al: Oral ciprofloxacin vs. intravenous ceftriaxone administered in an outpatient setting for fever and neutropenia in low-risk pediatric oncology patients: Randomized prospective trial. *Med Pediatr Oncol* 34:87, 2000.

77. Mullen CA, Petropoulos D, Roberts WM, et al: Outpatient treatment of fever and neutropenia for low risk pediatric cancer patients. *Cancer* 86:126, 1999.

78. Rubenstein EB, Rolston K, Benjamin RS, et al: Outpatient treatment of febrile episodes in low-risk neutropenic patients with cancer. *Cancer* 71:3640, 1993.

79. Hidalgo M, Hornedo J, Lumbreras C, et al: Outpatient therapy with oral ofloxacin for patients with low risk neutropenia and fever. *Cancer* 85:213, 1999.

80. Klastersky J, Paesmans M, Rubenstein EB, et al: The Multinational Association for Supportive Care in Cancer risk index: A multinational scoring system for identifying low-risk febrile neutropenic cancer patients. *J Clin Oncol* 18:3038, 2000.

81. Chang HY, Rodriguez V, Narboni G, et al: Causes of death in adults with acute leukemia. *Medicine* 55:259, 1976.

82. Schimpff S, Satterlee W, Young VM, Serpick A: Empiric therapy with carbenicillin and gentamicin for febrile patients with cancer and granulocytopenia. *N Engl J Med* 284:1061, 1971.

83. Zinner SH: Changing epidemiology of infections in patients with neutropenia and cancer: Emphasis on gram-positive and resistant bacteria. *Clin Infect Dis* 29:490, 1999.

84. Feld R: Vancomycin as part of initial empirical antibiotic therapy for febrile neutropenia in patients with cancer: Pros and cons. *Clin Infect Dis* 29:503, 1999.

85. Fainstein V, Bodey GP, Bolivar R, et al: Moxalactam plus ticarcillin or tobramycin for treatment of febrile episodes in neutropenic cancer patients. *Arch Intern Med* 144:1766, 1984.

86. Jones P, Rolston K, Fainstein V, et al: Aztreonam plus vancomycin (plus amikacin vs. moxalactam plus ticarcillin for the empiric treatment of febrile episodes in neutropenic cancer patients. *Rev Infect Dis* 7(Suppl 4):S741, 1985.

87. European Organisation for Research and Treatment of Cancer (EORTC) International Antimicrobial Therapy Cooperative Project Group: Efficacy and toxicity of single daily doses of amikacin and ceftriaxone versus multiple daily doses of amikacin and ceftazidime for infection in patients with cancer and granulocytopenia. *Ann Intern Med* 119:584, 1993.

88. Flaherty JP, Waitley D, Edlin B, et al: Multicenter, randomized trial of ciprofloxacin plus azlocillin versus ceftazidime plus amikacin for empiric treatment of febrile neutropenic patients. *Am J Med* 87(5A):278S, 1989.

89. Riikonen P: Imipenem compared with ceftazidime plus vancomycin as initial therapy for fever in neutropenic children with cancer. *Pediatr Infect Dis J* 10:918, 1991.

90. Norrby SR, Vandercam B, Louie TJ, et al: Imipenem/cilastatin versus amikacin plus piperacillin in the treatment of infections in neutropenic patients: A prospective randomized multiclinic study. *Scand J Infect Dis* 52(Suppl):65, 1987.

91. Deaney NB, Tate H: A meta-analysis of clinical studies on imipenem-cilastatin for empirically treating febrile neutropenic patients. *J Antimicrob Chemother* 37:975, 1996.

92. Sanders JW, Powe NR, Moore RD: Ceftazidime monotherapy for empiric treatment of febrile neutropenic patients: A meta-analysis. *J Infect Dis* 164:907, 1991.

93. Bayston KF, Want S, Cohen J: A prospective, randomized comparison of ceftazidime and ciprofloxacin as initial empiric

94. Winston DJ, Lazarus HM, Beveridge RA, et al: Randomized, double-blind, multicenter trial comparing clinafloxacin with imipenem as empirical monotherapy for febrile granulocytopenic patients. *Clin Infect Dis* 32:381, 2001.

95. Glauser MP, Brennscheidt U, Cornely O, et al: Clinafloxacin monotherapy (CI-960) versus ceftazidime plus amikacin for empirical treatment of febrile neutropenic cancer patients. *Clin Microbiol Infect* 8:14, 2002.

96. Bohme A, Shah PM, Stille W, Hoelzer D: Piperacillin/tazobactam versus cefepime as initial empirical antimicrobial therapy in febrile neutropenic patients: A prospective randomized pilot study. *Eur J Med Res* 3:324, 1998.

97. Hess U, Bohme C, Rey K, Senn HJ: Monotherapy with piperacillin/tazobactam versus combination therapy with ceftazidime plus amikacin as an empiric therapy for fever in neutropenic cancer patients. *Support Care Cancer* 6:402, 1998.

98. Bauduer F, Cousin T, Boulat O, et al: A randomized prospective multicentre trial of cefpirome versus piperacillin-tazobactam in febrile neutropenia. *Leuk Lymphoma* 42:379, 2001.

99. Gorschluter M, Hahn C, Fixson A, et al: Piperacillin-tazobactam is more effective than ceftriaxone plus gentamicin in febrile neutropenic patients with hematological malignancies: A randomized comparison. *Support Care Cancer* 11:362, 2003.

100. Bow EJ, Noskin GA, Schwarer AP, et al: Efficacy of piperacillin/tazobactam as initial empiric therapy for febrile neutropenia in patients with hematological malignancy. *Blood* 102:281a, 2003.

101. Cometta A, Kern WV, de Bock R, et al: Vancomycin versus placebo for treating persistent fever in patients with neutropenic cancer receiving piperacillin-tazobactam monotherapy. *Clin Infect Dis* 37:382, 2003.

102. Sanz MA, Lopez J, Lahuerta JJ, et al: Cefepime plus amikacin versus piperacillin-tazobactam plus amikacin for initial antibiotic therapy in haematology patients with febrile neutropenia: Results of an open, randomized, multicentre trial. *J Antimicrob Chemother* 50:79, 2002.

103. Fleischhack G, Schmidt-Niemann M, Wulff B, et al: Piperacillin, beta-lactam inhibitor plus gentamicin as empirical therapy of a sequential regimen in febrile neutropenia of pediatric cancer patients. *Support Care Cancer* 9:372, 2001.

104. Shenep JL, Hughes WT, Roberson PK, et al: Vancomycin, ticarcillin, and amikacin compared with ticarcillin-clavulanate and amikacin in the empirical treatment of febrile, neutropenic children with cancer. *N Engl J Med* 319:1053, 1988.

105. Fanci R, Paci C, Leoni F, et al: Ticarcillin-clavulanic acid plus amikacin versus ceftazidime plus amikacin in the empirical treatment of fever in acute leukemia: A prospective randomized trial. *J Chemother* 15:253, 2003.

106. Fleming DR, Ziegler C, Baize T, et al: Cefepime versus ticarcillin and clavulanate potassium and aztreonam for febrile neutropenia therapy in high-dose chemotherapy patients. *Am J Clin Oncol* 26:285, 2003.

107. Petrilli AS, Cypriano M, Dantas LS, et al: Evaluation of ticarcillin/clavulanic acid versus ceftriaxone plus amikacin for fever and neutropenia in pediatric patients with leukemia and lymphoma. *Braz J Infect Dis* 7:111, 2003.

108. Innes HE, Smith DB, O'Reilly SM, et al: Oral antibiotics with early hospital discharge compared with in-patient intravenous antibiotics for low-risk febrile neutropenia in patients with cancer: A prospective randomised controlled single centre study. *Br J Cancer* 89:43, 2003.

109. Yu LC, Shaneyfelt T, Warrier R, Ode D: The efficacy of ticarcillin-clavulanate and gentamicin as empiric treatment for febrile neutropenic pediatric patients with cancer. *Pediatr Hematol Oncol* 11:181, 1994.

110. Marie JP, Vekhoff A, Cony-Makhoul P, et al: Piperacillin/tazobactam combination + amikacin versus ceftazidime +

amikacin in patients with neutropenia and fever. An open multi-center study. Group d'etudes dea Aplasies Febriles. *Presse Medicale* 24:397, 1995.

111. Marie JP, Marjanovic Z, Vekhoff A, et al: Piperacillin/tazobactam plus tobramycin versus ceftazidime plus tobramycin as empiric therapy for fever in severely neutropenic patients. *Support Care Cancer* 7:89, 1999.

112. Sage R, Hann I, Prentice HG, et al: A randomized trial of empirical antibiotic therapy with one of four beta-lactam antibiotics in combination with netilmicin in febrile neutropenic patients. *J Antimicrob Chemother* 22:237, 1988.

113. Bolton-Maggs PH, van Saene HK, McDowell HP, Martin J: Clinical evaluation of ticarcillin, with clavulanic acid, and gentamicin in the treatment of febrile episodes in neutropenic children. *J Antimicrob Chemother* 27:669, 1991.

114. Schaison G, Reinert P, Leverger G, Leaute JB: Timentin (ticarcillin and clavulanic acid) in combination with aminoglycosides in the treatment of febrile episodes in neutropenic children. *J Antimicrob Chemother* 17(Suppl C):177, 1986.

115. Krieger O, Bernhart M, Plohowich R, et al: Timentin in combination with tobramycin as empirical therapy in febrile neutropenic patients with haematological malignances. *J Antimicrob Chemother* 17(Suppl C):211, 1986.

116. Laverdire M, Bow EJ, Rotstein C, et al: Antimicrobial regimens prescribed by Canadian physicians for chemotherapy-induced febrile neutropenic episodes. *Can J Infect Diseases* 10:353, 1999.

117. Cordonnier C, Herbrecht R, Pico JL, et al: Cefepime/amikacin versus ceftazidime/amikacin as empirical therapy for febrile episodes in neutropenic patients: A comparative study. The French Cefepime Study Group. *Clin Infect Dis* 24:41, 1996.

118. Cornely OA, Bethe U, Seifert H, et al: A randomized monocentric trial in febrile neutropenic patients: Ceftriaxone and gentamicin vs cefepime and gentamicin. *Ann Hematol* 81:37, 2002.

119. Erman M, Akova M, Akan H, et al: Comparison of cefepime and ceftazidime in combination with amikacin in the empirical treatment of high-risk patients with febrile neutropenia: A prospective, randomized, multicenter study. *Scand J Infect Dis* 33:827, 2001.

120. Chandrasekar PH, Arnow PM: Cefepime versus ceftazidime as empiric therapy for fever in neutropenic patients with cancer. *Ann Pharmacother* 34:989, 2000.

121. Chuang YY, Hung IJ, Yang CP, et al: Cefepime versus ceftazidime as empiric monotherapy for fever and neutropenia in children with cancer. *Pediatr Infect Dis J* 21:203, 2002.

122. Meropenem Study Group of Leuven LaN: Equivalent efficacies of meropenem and ceftazidime as empirical monotherapy of febrile neutropenic patients. The Meropenem Study Group of Leuven, London and Nijmegen. *J Antimicrob Chemother* 36:185, 1995.

123. Vandercam B, Gerain J, Humblet Y, et al: Meropenem versus ceftazidime as empirical monotherapy for febrile neutropenic cancer patients. *Ann Hematol* 79:152, 2000.

124. de la Camara R, Figuera A, Sureda A, et al: Meropenem versus ceftazidime plus amikacin in the treatment of febrile episodes in neutropenic patients: A randomized study. *Haematologica* 82:668, 1997.

125. Lindblad R, Rodjer S, Adreasson B, et al: Empiric monotherapy for febrile neutropenia—a randomized study comparing meropenem with ceftazidime. *Scand J Infect Dis* 30:237, 1998.

126. Behre G, Link H, Maschmeyer G, et al: Meropenem monotherapy versus combination therapy with ceftazidime and amikacin for empirical treatment of febrile neutropenic patients. *Ann Hematol* 76:73, 1998.

127. Akova M, Akan H, Korten V, et al: Comparison of meropenem with amikacin plus ceftazidime in the empirical treatment of febrile neutropenia: A prospective randomised multicentre trial in patients without previous prophylactic antibiotics.

Meropenem Study Group of Turkey. *Int J Antimicrob Agents* 13:15, 1999.

128. Feld R, De Pauw B, Berman S, et al: Meropenem versus ceftazidime in the treatment of cancer patients with febrile neutropenia: A randomized, double-blind trial. *J Clin Oncol* 18:3690, 2000.

129. Freifeld AG, Brown AE, Elting L, et al: Fever and neutropenia. National Comprehensive Cancer Network—Clinical Practice Guidelines in Oncology Ver 1.2004, 1-64. 2004.

130. Garcia-Rodriguez JA, Gobernado M, Gomis M, et al: [Clinical guide for the evaluation and treatment of patients with neutropenia and fever.] *Rev Esp Quimioter* 14:75, 2001.

131. Furno P, Bucaneve G, Del Favero A: Monotherapy or aminoglycoside-containing combinations for empirical antibiotic treatment of febrile neutropenic patients: A meta-analysis. *Lancet Infect Dis* 2:231, 2002.132.

132. Paul M, Soares-Weiser K, Leibovici L: Beta lactam monotherapy versus beta lactam-aminoglycoside combination therapy for fever with neutropenia: Systematic review and meta-analysis. *BMJ* 326:1111, 2003.

133. Giamarellou H, Bassaris HP, Petrikkos G, et al: Monotherapy with intravenous followed by oral high-dose ciprofloxacin versus combination therapy with ceftazidime plus amikacin as initial empiric therapy for granulocytopenic patients with fever. *Antimicrob Agents Chemother* 44:3264, 2000.

134. Studena M, Hlavacova E, Helpianska L, et al: Once-daily pefloxacin + teicoplanin vs netilmicin + teicoplanin in empirical therapy for fever and neutropenia. *Drugs* 49(Suppl 2):483, 1995.

135. Cornely OA, Wicke T, Seifert H, et al: Once-daily oral levofloxacin monotherapy versus piperacillin/tazobactam three times a day: A randomized controlled multicenter trial in patients with febrile neutropenia. *Int J Hematol* 79:74, 2004.

136. Horowitz HW, Holmgren D, Seiter K: Stepdown single agent antibiotic therapy for the management of the high risk neutropenic adult with hematologic malignancies. *Leuk Lymphoma* 23:159, 1996.

137. Marra CA, Frighetto L, Quaia CB, et al: A new ciprofloxacin step-down program in the treatment of high-risk febrile neutropenia: A clinical and economic analysis. *Pharmacotherapy* 20:931, 2000.

138. Kern WV, Cometta A, de Bock R, et al: Oral versus intravenous empirical antimicrobial therapy for fever in patients with granulocytopenia who are receiving cancer chemotherapy. International Antimicrobial Therapy Cooperative Group of the European Organization for Research and Treatment of Cancer. *N Engl J Med* 341:312, 1999.

139. Freifeld A, Marchigiani D, Walsh T, et al: A double-blind comparison of empirical oral and intravenous antibiotic therapy for low-risk febrile patients with neutropenia during cancer chemotherapy. *N Engl J Med* 341:305, 1999.

140. Niho S, Ohe Y, Goto K, et al: Randomized trial of oral versus intravenous antibiotics in low-risk febrile neutropenic patients with lung cancer. *Jpn J Clin Oncol* 34:69, 2004.

141. Paganini H, Rodriguez-Brieschcke T, Zubizarreta P, et al: Oral ciprofloxacin in the management of children with cancer with lower risk febrile neutropenia. *Cancer* 91:1563, 2001.

142. Mullen CA: Ciprofloxacin in treatment of fever and neutropenia in pediatric cancer patients. *Pediatr Infect Dis J* 22:1138, 2003.

143. Cometta A, Calandra T, Bille J, Glauser MP: *Escherichia coli* resistant to fluoroquinolones in patients with cancer and neutropenia. *N Engl J Med* 330:1240, 1994.

144. Kern WV, Andriof E, Oethinger M, et al: Emergence of fluoroquinolone-resistant *Escherichia coli* at a cancer center. *Antimicrob Agents Chemother* 38:681, 1994.

145. Carratala J, Fernandez-Sevilla A, Tubau F, et al: Emergence of quinolone-resistant *Escherichia coli* bacteremia in neutropenic patients with cancer who have received prophylactic norfloxacin. *Clin Infect Dis* 20:557, 1995.

146. Zaidi Y, Hastings M, Murray J, et al: Quinolone resistance in neutropenic patients: The effect of prescribing policy in the UK and Pakistan. *Clin Lab Haematol* 23:39, 2001.

147. Pena C, Albareda JM, Pallares R, et al: Relationship between quinolone use and emergence of ciprofloxacin-resistant *Escherichia coli* in bloodstream infections. *Antimicrob Agents Chemother* 39:520, 1995.

148. Farra A, Skoog G, Wallen L, et al: Antibiotic use and *Escherichia coli* resistance trends for quinolones and cotrimoxazole in Sweden. *Scand J Infect Dis* 34:449, 2002.

149. Garau J, Xercavins M, Rodriguez-Carballeira M, et al: Emergence and dissemination of quinolone-resistant *Escherichia coli* in the community. *Antimicrob Agents Chemother* 43:2736, 1999.

150. Perea S, Hidalgo M, Arcediano A, et al: Incidence and clinical impact of fluoroquinolone-resistant *Escherichia coli* in the faecal flora of cancer patients treated with high dose chemotherapy and ciprofloxacin prophylaxis. *J Antimicrob Chemother* 44:117, 1999.

151. Gomez L, Garau J, Estrada C, et al: Ciprofloxacin prophylaxis in patients with acute leukemia and granulocytopenia in an area with a high prevalence of ciprofloxacin-resistant *Escherichia coli*. *Cancer* 97:419, 2003.

152. Lautenbach E, Larosa LA, Kasbekar N, et al: Fluoroquinolone utilization in the emergency departments of academic medical centers: Prevalence of, and risk factors for, inappropriate use. *Arch Intern Med* 163:601, 2003.

153. Lautenbach E, Strom BL, Bilker WB, et al: Epidemiological investigation of fluoroquinolone resistance in infections due to extended-spectrum beta-lactamase-producing *Escherichia coli* and *Klebsiella pneumoniae*. *Clin Infect Dis* 33:1288, 2001.

154. Furno P, Dionisi MS, Bucaneve G, et al: Ceftriaxone versus beta-lactams with antipseudomonal activity for empirical, combined antibiotic therapy in febrile neutropenia: A meta-analysis. *Support Care Cancer* 8:293, 2000.

155. Bow EJ: Meropenem as empirical monotherapy for febrile neutropenic cancer patients—a meta-analysis. Unpublished, 2004.

156. Ramphal R, Kramer BS, Rand KH, et al: Early results of a comparative trial of ceftazidime versus cephalothin, carbenicillin and gentamicin in the treatment of febrile granulocytopenic patients. *J Antimicrob Chemother* 12(Suppl A):81, 1983.

157. Kramer BS, Ramphal R, Rand KH: Randomized comparison between two ceftazidime-containing regimens and cephalothin-gentamicin-carbenicillin in febrile granulocytopenic cancer patients. *Antimicrob Agents Chemother* 30:64, 1986.

158. Rubin M, Hathorn JW, Marshall D, et al: Gram-positive infections and the use of vancomycin in 550 episodes of fever and neutropenia. *Ann Intern Med* 108:30, 1988.

159. Viscoli C: Management of infection in cancer patients. Studies of the European Organization for Research and Treatment of Cancer (EORTC) International Antimicrobial Therapy Group (IATG). *Eur J Cancer* 38(Suppl 4):S82, 2002.

160. Hughes WT, Armstrong D, Bodey GP, et al: 1997 Guidelines for the use of antimicrobial agents in neutropenic patients with unexplained fever. *Clin Infect Dis* 25:551, 1997.

161. Kelsey SM, Collins PW, Delord C, et al: A randomized study of teicoplanin plus ciprofloxacin versus gentamicin plus piperacillin for the empirical treatment of fever in neutropenic patients. *Br J Haematol* 76(Suppl 2):10, 1990.

162. Martino P, Micozzi A, Gentile G, et al: Piperacillin plus amikacin vs. piperacillin plus amikacin plus teicoplanin for empirical treatment of febrile episodes in neutropenic patients receiving quinolone prophylaxis. *Clin Infect Dis* 15:290, 1992.

163. Ramphal R, Bolger M, Oblon DJ, et al: Vancomycin is not an essential component of the initial empiric treatment regimen for febrile neutropenic patients receiving ceftazidime: A randomized prospective study. *Antimicrob Agents Chemother* 36:1062, 1992.

164. Feld R: Vancomycin as part of initial empirical antibiotic therapy for febrile neutropenia in patients with cancer: Pros and cons. *Clin Infect Dis* 29:503, 1999.

165. Erjavec Z, Vries-Hospers HG, Laseur M, et al: A prospective, randomized, double-blinded, placebo-controlled trial of empirical teicoplanin in febrile neutropenia with persistent fever after imipenem monotherapy. *J Antimicrob Chemother* 45:843, 2000.

166. Wade JC, Glasmacher A: Vancomycin does not benefit persistently febrile neutropenic people with cancer. *Cancer Treat Rev* 30:119, 2004.

167. Cruciani M, Malena M, Bosco O, et al: Reappraisal with meta-analysis of the addition of Gram-positive prophylaxis to fluoroquinolone in neutropenic patients. *J Clin Oncol* 21:4127, 2003.

168. Forrest GN, Schimpff SC, Cross A: Febrile neutropenia, colony-stimulating factors and therapy: Time for a new methodology? *Support Care Cancer* 10:177, 2002.

169. Berghmans T, Paesmans M, Lafitte JJ, et al: Therapeutic use of granulocyte and granulocyte-macrophage colony-stimulating factors in febrile neutropenic cancer patients. A systematic review of the literature with meta-analysis. *Support Care Cancer* 10:181, 2002.

170. Ozer H, Armitage JO, Bennett CL, et al: 2000 Update of recommendations for the use of hematopoietic colony-stimulating factors: Evidence-based, clinical practice guidelines. American Society of Clinical Oncology Growth Factors Expert Panel. *J Clin Oncol* 18:3558, 2000.

171. Bennett CL, Smith TJ, Weeks JC, et al: Use of hematopoietic colony-stimulating factors: The American Society of Clinical Oncology survey. The Health Services Research Committee of the American Society of Clinical Oncology. *J Clin Oncol* 14:2511, 1996.

172. Bennett CL, Bishop MR, Tallman MS, et al: The association between physician reimbursement in the US and use of hematopoietic colony stimulating factors as adjunct therapy for older patients with acute myeloid leukemia: Results from the 1997 American Society of Clinical Oncology survey. Health Services Research Committee of the American Society of Clinical Oncology. *Ann Oncol* 10:1355, 1999.

173. Swanson G, Bergstrom K, Stump E, et al: Growth factor usage patterns and outcomes in the community setting: Collection through a practice-based computerized clinical information system. *J Clin Oncol* 18:1764, 2000.

174. Azoulay E, Delclaux C: Is there a place for granulocyte colony-stimulating factor in non-neutropenic critically ill patients? *Intensive Care Med* 30:10, 2004.

175. Pizzo PA, Robichaud KJ, Gill FA, Witebsky FG: Empiric antibiotic and antifungal therapy for cancer patients with prolonged fever and granulocytopenia. *Am J Med* 72:101, 1982.

176. European Organization for Research and Treatment of Cancer (EORTC) International Antimicrobial Therapy Project Group: Empiric antifungal therapy in febrile granulocytopenic patients. EORTC International Antimicrobial Therapy Cooperative Group. *Am J Med* 86(6 Pt 1):668, 1989.

177. Walsh TJ, Finberg RW, Arndt C, et al: Liposomal amphotericin B for empirical therapy in patients with persistent fever and neutropenia. *N Engl J Med* 340:764, 1999.

178. Boogaerts M, Winston DJ, Bow EJ, et al: Intravenous and oral itraconazole versus intravenous amphotericin B deoxycholate as empirical antifungal therapy for persistent fever in neutropenic patients with cancer who are receiving broad-spectrum antibacterial therapy. A randomized, controlled trial. *Ann Intern Med* 135:412, 2001.

179. Walsh TJ, Pappas P, Winston DJ, et al: Voriconazole compared with liposomal amphotericin B for empirical antifungal therapy in patients with neutropenia and persistent fever. *N Engl J Med* 346:225, 2002.

180. Maertens J, Van Eldere J, Verhaegen J, et al: Use of circulating galactomannan screening for early diagnosis of invasive

aspergillosis in allogeneic stem cell transplant recipients. *J Infect Dis* 186:1297, 2002.

181. Aisner J, Murillo J, Schimpff SC, Steere AC: Invasive aspergillosis in acute leukemia: Correlation with nose cultures and antibiotic use. *Ann Intern Med* 90:4, 1979.

182. Sandford GR, Merz WG, Wingard JR, et al: The value of fungal surveillance cultures as predictors of systemic fungal infections. *J Infect Dis* 142:503, 1980.

183. Latge JP: *Aspergillus fumigatus* and aspergillosis. *Clin Microbiol Rev* 12:310, 1999.

184. Latge JP: The pathobiology of *Aspergillus fumigatus*. *Trends Microbiol* 9:382, 2001.

185. Kappe R, Schulze-Berge A: New cause for false-positive results with the Pastorex *Aspergillus* antigen latex agglutination test. *J Clin Microbiol* 31:2489, 1993.

186. Herbrecht R, Letscher-Bru V, Oprea C, et al: *Aspergillus* galactomannan detection in the diagnosis of invasive aspergillosis in cancer patients. *J Clin Oncol* 20:1898, 2002.

187. Stynen D, Sarfati J, Goris A, et al: Rat monoclonal antibodies against *Aspergillus* galactomannan. *Infect Immun* 60:2237, 1992.

188. Stynen D, Goris A, Sarfati J, Latge JP: A new sensitive sandwich enzyme-linked immunosorbent assay to detect galactofuran in patients with invasive aspergillosis. *J Clin Microbiol* 33:497, 1995.

189. Swanink CM, Meis JF, Rijs AJ, et al: Specificity of a sandwich enzyme-linked immunosorbent assay for detecting *Aspergillus* galactomannan. *J Clin Microbiol* 35:257, 1997.

190. Ansorg R, van den BR, Rath PM: Detection of *Aspergillus* galactomannan antigen in foods and antibiotics. *Mycoses* 40:353, 1997.

191. Gangneux JP, Lavarde D, Bretagne S, et al: Transient aspergillus antigenaemia: Think of milk. *Lancet* 359:1251, 2002.

192. Siemann M, Koch-Dorfler M, Gaude M: False-positive results in premature infants with the Platelia *Aspergillus* sandwich enzyme-linked immunosorbent assay. *Mycoses* 41:373, 1998.

193. Husby S, Jensenius JC, Svehag SE: Passage of undegraded dietary antigen into the blood of healthy adults. Quantification, estimation of size distribution, and relation of uptake to levels of specific antibodies. *Scand J Immunol* 22:83, 1985.

194. Mennink-Kersten MA, Klont RR, Warris A, et al: Bifidobacterium lipoteichoic acid and false ELISA reactivity in aspergillus antigen detection. *Lancet* 363:325, 2004.

195. Naaber P, Smidt I, Tamme K, et al: Translocation of indigenous microflora in an experimental model of sepsis. *J Med Microbiol* 49:431, 2000.

196. Sulahian A, Touratier S, Ribaud P: False positive test for aspergillus antigenemia related to concomitant administration of piperacillin and tazobactam. *N Engl J Med* 349:2366, 2003.

197. Viscoli C, Machetti M, Cappellano P, et al: False-positive galactomannan platelia *Aspergillus* test results for patients receiving piperacillin-tazobactam. *Clin Infect Dis* 38:913, 2004.

198. Adam O, Auperin A, Wilquin F, et al: Treatment with piperacillin-tazobactam and false-positive *Aspergillus* galactomannan antigen test results for patients with hematological malignancies. *Clin Infect Dis* 38:917, 2004.

199. Cornelissen JJ, Rozenberg-Arska M, Dekker AW: Discontinuation of intravenous antibiotic therapy during persistent neutropenia in patients receiving prophylaxis with oral ciprofloxacin. *Clin Infect Dis* 21:1300, 1995.

200. Rubin M, Hathorn JW, Pizzo PA: Controversies in the management of febrile neutropenic cancer patients. *Cancer Invest* 6:167, 1988.

201. Overholser CD, Peterson DE, Williams LT, Schimpff SC: Periodontal infection in patients with acute nonlymphocyte leukemia. Prevalence of acute exacerbations. *Arch Intern Med* 142:551, 1982.

202. DeGregorio MW, Lee WM, Ries CA: *Candida* infections in patients with acute leukemia: Ineffectiveness of nystatin prophylaxis and relationship between oropharyngeal and systemic candidiasis. *Cancer* 50:2780, 1982.

203. Wade JC, Newton B, McLaren C, et al: Intravenous acyclovir to treat mucocutaneous herpes simplex virus infection after marrow transplantation: A double-blind trial. *Ann Intern Med* 96:265, 1982.

204. Montgomery MT, Redding SW, LeMaistre CF: The incidence of oral herpes simplex virus infection in patients undergoing cancer chemotherapy. *Oral Surg Oral Med Oral Pathol* 61:238, 1986.

205. Lindquist SF, Hickey AJ, Drane JB: Effect of oral hygiene on stomatitis in patients receiving cancer chemotherapy. *J Prosthet Dent* 40:312, 1978.

206. Peterson DE, Minah GE, Overholser CD, et al: Microbiology of acute periodontal infection in myelosuppressed cancer patients. *J Clin Oncol* 5:1461, 1987.

207. Gold D, Corey L: Acyclovir prophylaxis for herpes simplex virus infection. *Antimicrob Agents Chemother* 31:361, 1987.

208. Ferretti GA, Ash RC, Brown AT, et al: Control of oral mucositis and candidiasis in marrow transplantation: A prospective, double-blind trial of chlorhexidine digluconate oral rinse. *Bone Marrow Transplant* 3:483, 1988.

209. Brammer KW: Management of fungal infection in neutropenic patients with fluconazole. *Haematol Blood Transfus* 33:546, 1990.

210. Tomblyn M, Gordon L, Singhal S, et al: Rarity of toxigenic *Clostridium difficile* infections after hematopoietic stem cell transplantation: Implications for symptomatic management of diarrhea. *Bone Marrow Transplant* 30:517, 2002.

211. Bilgrami S, Feingold JM, Dorsky D, et al: Incidence and outcome of *Clostridium difficile* infection following autologous peripheral blood stem cell transplantation. *Bone Marrow Transplant* 23:1039, 1999.

212. Husain A, Aptaker L, Spriggs DR, Barakat RR: Gastrointestinal toxicity and *Clostridium difficile* diarrhea in patients treated with paclitaxel-containing chemotherapy regimens. *Gynecol Oncol* 71:104, 1998.

213. Shamberger RC, Weinstein HJ, Delorey MJ, Levey RH: The medical and surgical management of typhlitis in children with acute nonlymphocytic (myelogenous) leukemia. *Cancer* 57:603, 1986.

214. Keidan RD, Fanning J, Gatenby RA, Weese JL: Recurrent typhlitis. A disease resulting from aggressive chemotherapy. *Dis Colon Rectum* 32:206, 1989.

215. Moir CR, Scudamore CH, Benny WB: Typhlitis: Selective surgical management. *Am J Surg* 151:563, 1986.

216. Kunkel JM, Rosenthal D: Management of the ileocecal syndrome. Neutropenic enterocolitis. *Dis Colon Rectum* 29:196, 1986.

217. Gomez L, Martino R, Rolston KV: Neutropenic enterocolitis: Spectrum of the disease and comparison of definite and possible cases. *Clin Infect Dis* 27:695, 1998.

218. Kasper K, Loewen R, Bow E: Neutropenic enterocolitis (NEC) in adult leukemia (AL) patients (pts) in Manitoba. *Clin Infect Dis* 23:866, 1996.

219. Cartoni C, Dragoni F, Micozzi A, et al: Neutropenic enterocolitis in patients with acute leukemia: Prognostic significance of bowel wall thickening detected by ultrasonography. *J Clin Oncol* 19:756, 2001.

220. Girmenia C, Micozzi A, Cartoni C, et al: Detection of *Candida* mannoproteinemia in patients with neutropenic enterocolitis. *Eur J Clin Microbiol Infect Dis* 18:55, 1999.

221. Bow EJ, Loewen R, Cheang MS, Schacter B: Invasive fungal disease in adults undergoing remission-induction therapy for acute myeloid leukemia: The pathogenetic role of the antileukemic regimen. *Clin Infect Dis* 21:361, 1995.

222. Glenn J, Cotton D, Wesley R, Pizzo P: Anorectal infections in patients with malignant diseases. *Rev Infect Dis* 10:42, 1988.

223. Bodey GP: Unusual presentations of infection in neutropenic patients. *Int J Antimicrob Agents* 16:93, 2000.

224. Cohen JS, Paz IB, O'Donnell MR, Ellenhorn JD: Treatment of perianal infection following bone marrow transplantation. *Dis Colon Rectum* 39:981, 1986.

225. Solomkin JS, Mazuski JE, Baron EJ, et al: Guidelines for the selection of anti-infective agents for complicated intra-abdominal infections. *Clin Infect Dis* 37:997, 2003.
226. Weinstein MP: Comparative evaluation of penicillin, ampicillin, and imipenem MICs and susceptibility breakpoints for vancomycin-susceptible and vancomycin-resistant *Enterococcus faecalis* and *Enterococcus faecium*. *J Clin Microbiol* 39:2729, 2001.
227. Stiefel U, Pultz NJ, Helfand MS, Donskey CJ: Increased susceptibility to vancomycin-resistant *Enterococcus* intestinal colonization persists after completion of anti-anaerobic antibiotic treatment in mice. *Infect Control Hosp Epidemiol* 25:373, 2004.
228. Segal BH, Bow EJ, Menichetti F: Fungal infections in nontransplant patients with hematologic malignancies. *Infect Dis Clin North Am* 16:935, vii, 2002.
229. Crislip MA, Edwards JE Jr.: Candidiasis. *Infect Dis Clin North Am* 3:103, 1989.
230. Walsh TJ, Hiemenz JW, Anaissie E: Recent progress and current problems in treatment of invasive fungal infections in neutropenic patients. *Infect Dis Clin North Am* 10:365, 1996.
231. Mermel LA, Farr BM, Sherertz RJ, et al: Guidelines for the management of intravascular catheter-related infections. *Clin Infect Dis* 32:1249, 2001.
232. Pappas PG, Rex JH, Sobel JD, et al: Guidelines for treatment of candidiasis. *Clin Infect Dis* 38:161, 2004.
233. Harvey RL, Myers JP: Nosocomial fungemia in a large community teaching hospital. *Arch Intern Med* 147:2117, 1987.
234. Kujath P, Lerch K, Kochendorfer P, Boos C: Comparative study of the efficacy of fluconazole versus amphotericin B/flucytosine in surgical patients with systemic mycoses. *Infection* 21:376, 1993.
235. Rex JH, Bennett JE, Sugar AM, et al: A randomized trial comparing fluconazole with amphotericin B for the treatment of candidemia in patients without neutropenia. Candidemia Study Group and the National Institute. *N Engl J Med* 331:1325, 1994.
236. Anaissie EJ, Vartivarian SE, Abi-Said D, et al: Fluconazole versus amphotericin B in the treatment of hematogenous candidiasis: A matched cohort study. *Am J Med* 101:170, 1996.
237. Anaissie EJ, Darouiche RO, Abi-Said D, et al: Management of invasive candidal infections: Results of a prospective, randomized, multicenter study of fluconazole versus amphotericin B and review of the literature. *Clin Infect Dis* 23:964, 1996.
238. Scheven M, Schwegler F: Antagonistic interactions between azoles and amphotericin B with yeasts depend on azole lipophilia for special test conditions in vitro. *Antimicrob Agents Chemother* 39:1779, 1995.
239. Steinbach WJ, Stevens DA, Denning DW: Combination and sequential antifungal therapy for invasive aspergillosis: Review of published in vitro and in vivo interactions and 6281 clinical cases from 1966 to 2001. *Clin Infect Dis* 37(Suppl 3):S188, 2003.
240. Schaffner A, Bohler A: Amphotericin B refractory aspergillosis after itraconazole: Evidence for significant antagonism. *Mycoses* 36:421, 1993.
241. Rex JH, Pappas PG, Karchmer AW, et al: A randomized and blinded multicenter trial of high-dose fluconazole plus placebo versus fluconazole plus amphotericin B as therapy for candidemia and its consequences in nonneutropenic subjects. *Clin Infect Dis* 36:1221, 2003.
242. Nguyen MH, Peacock JE, Jr, Morris AJ, et al: The changing face of candidemia: Emergence of non-*Candida albicans* species and antifungal resistance. *Am J Med* 100:617, 1996.
243. Pfaller MA, Jones RN, Doern GV, et al: Bloodstream infections due to *Candida* species: SENTRY antimicrobial surveillance program in North America and Latin America, 1997–1998. *Antimicrob Agents Chemother* 44:747, 2000.
244. Diekema DJ, Messer SA, Brueggemann AB, et al: Epidemiology of candidemia: 3-year results from the emerging infections and the epidemiology of Iowa organisms study. *J Clin Microbiol* 40:1298, 2002.
245. Trick WE, Fridkin SK, Edwards JR, et al: Secular trend of hospital-acquired candidemia among intensive care unit patients in the United States during 1989–1999. *Clin Infect Dis* 35:627, 2002.
246. Kanda Y, Yamamoto R, Chizuka A, et al: Prophylactic action of oral fluconazole against infection in neutropenic patients—a meta-analysis of 16 randomized, controlled trials. *Cancer* 89:1611, 2000.
247. Bow EJ, Laverdiere M, Lussier N, et al: Antifungal prophylaxis for severely neutropenic chemotherapy recipients: A meta analysis of randomized-controlled clinical trials. *Cancer* 94:3230, 2002.
248. Viscoli C, Castagnola E, Van Lint MT, et al: Fluconazole versus amphotericin B as empirical antifungal therapy of unexplained fever in granulocytopenic cancer patients: A pragmatic, multicentre, prospective and randomised clinical trial. *Eur J Cancer* 32A:814, 1996.
249. Bodey GP, Anaissie EJ: Chronic systemic candidiasis. *Eur J Clin Microbiol Infect Dis* 8:855, 1989.
250. Jones JM: Granulomatous hepatitis due to *Candida albicans* in patients with acute leukemia. *Ann Intern Med* 94(4 Pt 1):475, 1981.
251. Tashjian LS, Abramson JS, Peacock JE Jr.: Focal hepatic candidiasis: A distinct clinical variant of candidiasis in immunocompromised patients. *Rev Infect Dis* 6:689, 1984.
252. Haron E, Feld R, Tuffnell P, et al: Hepatic candidiasis: An increasing problem in immunocompromised patients. *Am J Med* 83:17, 1987.
253. Thaler M, Pastakia B, Shawker TH, et al: Hepatic candidiasis in cancer patients: The evolving picture of the syndrome. *Ann Intern Med* 108:88, 1988.
254. Goodwin SD, Cleary JD, Walawander CA, et al: Pretreatment regimens for adverse events related to infusion of amphotericin B. *Clin Infect Dis* 20:755, 1995.
255. Hoeprich PD: Clinical use of amphotericin B and derivatives: Lore, mystique, and fact. *Clin Infect Dis* 14(Suppl 1):S114, 1992.
256. Butler WT, Bennett JE, Alling DW, et al: Nephrotoxicity of amphotericin B: Early and late effects in 81 patients. *Ann Intern Med* 61:175, 1964.
257. Anaissie EJ, White M, Uzun O, et al: Amphotericin lipid complex versus amphotericin B for the treatment of hematogenous and invasive candidiasis: A prospective randomized multicenter trial. Proceedings of the 35th Interscience Conference on Antimicrobial Agents and Chemotherapy, LM21. 1995, (abstract).
258. Holleran WM, Wilbur JR, DeGregorio MW: Empiric amphotericin B therapy in patients with acute leukemia. *Rev Infect Dis* 7:619, 1985.
259. Medoff G: Controversial areas in antifungal chemotherapy: Short-course and combination therapy with amphotericin B. *Rev Infect Dis* 9:403, 1987.
260. Gallis HA, Drew RH, Pickard WW: Amphotericin B: 30 years of clinical experience. *Rev Infect Dis* 12:308, 1990.
261. Winston DJ, Chandrasekar PH, Lazarus HM, et al: Fluconazole prophylaxis of fungal infections in patients with acute leukemia. Results of a randomized placebo-controlled, double-blind, multicenter trial. *Ann Intern Med* 118:495, 1993.
262. Schaffner A, Schaffner M: Effect of prophylactic fluconazole on the frequency of fungal infections, amphotericin B use, and health care costs in patients undergoing intensive chemotherapy for hematologic neoplasias. *J Infect Dis* 172:1035, 1995.
263. O'Hanley P, Easaw J, Rugo H, Easaw S: Infectious disease management of adult leukemic patients undergoing chemotherapy: 1982 to 1986 experience at Stanford University Hospital. *Am J Med* 87:605, 1989.
264. Bow EJ, Sutherland JA, Kilpatrick MG, et al: Therapy of untreated acute myeloid leukemia in the elderly: Remission-induction using a non-cytarabine-containing regimen of mitoxantrone plus etoposide. *J Clin Oncol* 14:1345, 1996.

265. Goodman JL, Winston DJ, Greenfield RA, et al: A controlled trial of fluconazole to prevent fungal infections in patients undergoing bone marrow transplantation. *N Engl J Med* 326:845, 1992.

266. Slavin MA, Osborne B, Adams R, et al: Efficacy and safety of fluconazole prophylaxis for fungal infections after marrow transplantation—a prospective, randomized, double-blind study. *J Infect Dis* 171:1545, 1995.

267. Perfect JR, Klotman ME, Gilbert CC, et al: Prophylactic intravenous amphotericin B in neutropenic autologous bone marrow transplant recipients. *J Infect Dis* 165:891, 1992.

268. Riley DK, Pavia AT, Beatty PG, et al: The prophylactic use of low-dose amphotericin B in bone marrow transplant patients. *Am J Med* 97:509, 1994.

269. Mora-Duarte J, Betts R, Rotstein C, et al: Comparison of caspofungin and amphotericin B for invasive candidiasis. *N Engl J Med* 347:2020, 2002.

270. Anaissie EJ, Rex JH, Uzun O, Vartivarian S: Predictors of adverse outcome in cancer patients with candidemia. *Am J Med* 104:238, 1998.

271. Rex JH, Bennett JE, Sugar AM, et al: Intravascular catheter exchanges and the duration of candidemia. *Clin Infect Dis* 21:994, 1995.

272. Marr KA, Carter RA, Crippa F, et al: Epidemiology and outcome of mould infections in hematopoietic stem cell transplant recipients. *Clin Infect Dis* 34:909, 2002.

273. Denning DW: Invasive aspergillosis. *Clin Infect Dis* 26:781, 1998.

274. Latge JP: *Aspergillus fumigatus* and aspergillosis. *Clin Microbiol Rev* 12:310, 1999.

275. Latge JP: The pathobiology of *Aspergillus fumigatus*. *Trends Microbiol* 9:382, 2001.

276. Marr KA, Patterson T, Denning D: Aspergillosis. Pathogenesis, clinical manifestations, and therapy. *Infect Dis Clin North Am* 16:875, vi, 2002.

277. Ascioglu S, Rex JH, de Pauw B, et al: Defining opportunistic invasive fungal infections in immunocompromised patients with cancer and hematopoietic stem cell transplants: An international consensus. *Clin Infect Dis* 34:7, 2002.

278. Martino R, Subira M, Rovira M, et al: Invasive fungal infections after allogeneic peripheral blood stem cell transplantation: Incidence and risk factors in 395 patients. *Br J Haematol* 116:475, 2002.

279. Subira M, Martino R, Rovira M, et al: Clinical applicability of the new EORTC/MSG classification for invasive pulmonary aspergillosis in patients with hematological malignancies and autopsy-confirmed invasive aspergillosis. *Ann Hematol* 82:80, 2003.

280. Cornet M, Fleury L, Maslo C, et al: Epidemiology of invasive aspergillosis in France: A six-year multicentric survey in the Greater Paris area. *J Hosp Infect* 51:288, 2002.

281. Aisner J, Schimpff SC, Bennett JE, et al: *Aspergillus* infections in cancer patients. Association with fireproofing materials in a new hospital. *JAMA* 235:411, 1976.

282. Anaissie EJ, Stratton SL, et al: Pathogenic molds (including *Aspergillus* species) in hospital water distribution systems: A 3-year prospective study and clinical implications for patients with hematologic malignancies. *Blood* 101:2542, 2003.

283. Hay RJ, Clayton YM, Goodley JM: Fungal aerobiology: How, when and where? *J Hosp Infect* 30(Suppl):352, 1995.

284. Arnow PM, Andersen RL, Mainous PD, Smith EJ: Pulmonary aspergillosis during hospital renovation. *Am Rev Respir Dis* 118:49, 1978.

285. Cooper EE, O'Reilly MA, Guest DI, Dharmage SC: Influence of building construction work on *Aspergillus* infection in a hospital setting. *Infect Control Hosp Epidemiol* 24:472, 2003.

286. Sherertz RJ, Belani A, Kramer BS, et al: Impact of air filtration on nosocomial *Aspergillus* infections. Unique risk of bone marrow transplant recipients. *Am J Med* 83:709, 1987.

287. Passweg JR, Rowlings PA, Atkinson KA, et al: Influence of protective isolation on outcome of allogeneic bone marrow transplantation for leukemia. *Bone Marrow Transplant* 21:1231, 1998.

288. Construction-related nosocomial infections in patients in health care facilities. Decreasing the risk of *Aspergillus, Legionella* and other infections. *Can Commun Dis Rep* 27(Suppl 2):i, 2001.

289. Streifel AJ: Design and maintenance of hospital ventilation systems and prevention of airborne nosocomial infections, in Mayhall CG (ed): *Hospital Epidemiology and Infection Control*. Philadelphia, Lippincott, Williams & Wilkins, 1999, p 1211.

290. Center for Disease Control: Isolation techniques for use in hospitals, 2nd ed. U.S. Government Printing Office, 1976 (pamphlet).

291. Cornet M, Levy V, Fleury L, et al: Efficacy of prevention by high-efficiency particulate air filtration or laminar airflow against *Aspergillus* airborne contamination during hospital renovation. *Infect Control Hosp Epidemiol* 20:508, 1999.

292. Denning DW, Stevens DA: Antifungal and surgical treatment of invasive aspergillosis: Review of 2121 published cases. *Rev Infect Dis* 12:1147, 1990.

293. Gerson SL, Talbot GH, Hurwitz S, et al: Prolonged granulocytopenia: The major risk factor for invasive pulmonary aspergillosis in patients with acute leukemia. *Ann Intern Med* 100:345, 1984.

294. Albelda SM, Talbot GH, Gerson SL, et al: Pulmonary cavitation and massive hemoptysis in invasive pulmonary aspergillosis. Influence of bone marrow recovery in patients with acute leukemia. *Am Rev Respir Dis* 131:115, 1985.

295. Levitz SM: Aspergillosis. *Infect Dis Clin North Am* 3:1, 1989.

296. Schwartz RS, Mackintosh FR, Schrier SL, Greenberg PL: Multivariate analysis of factors associated with invasive fungal disease during remission induction therapy for acute myelogenous leukemia. *Cancer* 53:411, 1984.

297. Wiley JM, Smith N, Leventhal BG, et al: Invasive fungal disease in pediatric acute leukemia patients with fever and neutropenia during induction chemotherapy: A multivariate analysis of risk factors. *J Clin Oncol* 8:280, 1990.

298. Tollemar J, Ringden O, Bostrom L, et al: Variables predicting deep fungal infections in bone marrow transplant recipients. *Bone Marrow Transplant* 4:635, 1989.

299. Jensen HE, Salonen J, Ekfors TO: The use of immunohistochemistry to improve sensitivity and specificity in the diagnosis of systemic mycoses in patients with haematological malignancies. *J Pathol* 181:100, 1997.

300. Burch PA, Karp JE, Merz WG, et al: Favorable outcome of invasive aspergillosis in patients with acute leukemia. *J Clin Oncol* 5:1985, 1987.

301. Maertens J, Boogaerts M: Caspofungin in the treatment of candidosis and aspergillosis. *Int J Infect Dis* 7:94, 2003.

302. Walsh TJ, et al: A randomized, double-blind, multicenter trial of caspofungin versus liposomal amphotericin B for empirical antifungal therapy of persistently febrile neutropenic patients. 43rd International Conference on Antimicrobial Agents and Chemotherapy, Chicago, IL, 2003 (abstract).

303. Walsh TJ, Hiemenz JW, Seibel NL, et al: Amphotericin B lipid complex for invasive fungal infections: Analysis of safety and efficacy in 556 cases. *Clin Infect Dis* 26:1383, 1998.

304. Linden P, Williams P, Chan KM: Efficacy and safety of amphotericin B lipid complex injection (ABLC) in solid-organ transplant recipients with invasive fungal infections. *Clin Transplant* 14(4 Pt 1):329, 2000.

305. Walsh TJ, Seibel NL, Arndt C, et al: Amphotericin B lipid complex in pediatric patients with invasive fungal infections. *Pediatr Infect Dis J* 18:702, 1999.

306. Wingard JR, Kubilis P, Lee L, et al: Clinical significance of nephrotoxicity in patients treated with amphotericin B for suspected or proven aspergillosis. *Clin Infect Dis* 29:1402, 1999.

307. Cagnoni PJ, Walsh TJ, Prendergast MM, et al: Pharmacoeconomic analysis of liposomal amphotericin B versus conventional

amphotericin B in the empirical treatment of persistently febrile neutropenic patients. *J Clin Oncol* 18:2476, 2000.

308. Wingard JR, White MH, Anaissie E, et al: A randomized, double-blind comparative trial evaluating the safety of liposomal amphotericin B versus amphotericin B lipid complex in the empirical treatment of febrile neutropenia. *Clin Infect Dis* 31:1155, 2000.

309. Walsh TJ, Hiemenz JW, Seibel NL, et al: Amphotericin B lipid complex for invasive fungal infections: Analysis of safety and efficacy in 556 cases. *Clin Infect Dis* 26:1383, 1998.

310. Denning DW, Lee JY, Hostetler JS, et al: NIAID Mycoses Study Group Multicenter Trial of Oral Itraconazole Therapy for Invasive Aspergillosis. *Am J Med* 97:135, 1994.

311. Mellinghoff IK, Winston DJ, Mukwaya G, Schiller GJ: Treatment of *Scedosporium apiospermum* brain abscesses with posaconazole. *Clin Infect Dis* 34:1648, 2002.

312. Herbrecht R, Denning DW, Patterson TF, et al: Voriconazole versus amphotericin B for primary therapy of invasive aspergillosis. *N Engl J Med* 347:408, 2002.

313. Rubin ZA, Somani J: New options for the treatment of invasive fungal infections. *Semin Oncol* 31(2 Suppl 4):91, 2004.

314. Robertson MJ, Larson RA: Recurrent fungal pneumonias in patients with acute nonlymphocytic leukemia undergoing multiple courses of intensive chemotherapy. *Am J Med* 84:233, 1988.

315. Uzun O, Anaissie EJ: Antifungal prophylaxis in patients with hematologic malignancies: A reappraisal. *Blood* 86:2063, 1995.

316. Karp JE, Burch PA, Merz WG: An approach to intensive antileukemia therapy in patients with previous invasive aspergillosis. *Am J Med* 85:203, 1988.

317. Walsh TJ, Whitcomb PO, Revankar SG, Pizzo PA: Successful treatment of hepatosplenic candidiasis through repeated cycles of chemotherapy and neutropenia. *Cancer* 76:2357, 1995.

318. Offner F, Cordonnier C, Ljungman P, et al: Impact of previous aspergillosis on the outcome of bone marrow transplantation. *Clin Infect Dis* 26:1098, 1998.

319. Greene JN: Catheter-related complications of cancer therapy. *Infect Dis Clin North Am* 10:255, 1996.

320. O'Grady NP, Alexander M, Dellinger EP, et al: Guidelines for the prevention of intravascular catheter-related infections. Centers for Disease Control and Prevention. *Morb Mortal Wkly Rep Recomm Rep* 51(RR-10):1, 2002.

321. Conly JM, Grieves K, Peters B: A prospective, randomized study comparing transparent and dry gauze dressings for central venous catheters. *J Infect Dis* 159:310, 1989.

322. Armstrong CW, Mayhall CG, Miller KB, et al: Clinical predictors of infection of central venous catheters used for total parenteral nutrition. *Infect Control Hosp Epidemiol* 11:71, 1990.

323. Landoy Z, Rotstein C, Lucey J, Fitzpatrick J: Hickman-Broviac catheter use in cancer patients. *J Surg Oncol* 26:215, 1984.

324. Lowder JN, Lazarus HM, Herzig RH: Bacteremias and fungemias in oncologic patients with central venous catheters: Changing spectrum of infection. *Arch Intern Med* 142:1456, 1982.

325. Benezra D, Kiehn TE, Gold JW, et al: Prospective study of infections in indwelling central venous catheters using quantitative blood cultures. *Am J Med* 85:495, 1988.

326. Mermel LA, Farr BM, Sherertz RJ, et al: Guidelines for the management of intravascular catheter-related infections. *Clin Infect Dis* 32:1249, 2001.

327. Blot F, Schmidt E, Nitenberg G, et al: Earlier positivity of central-venous versus peripheral-blood cultures is highly predictive of catheter-related sepsis. *J Clin Microbiol* 36:105, 1998.

328. Pizzo PA, Robichaud KJ, Edwards BK, et al: Oral antibiotic prophylaxis in patients with cancer: A double-blind randomized placebo-controlled trial. *J Pediatr* 102:125, 1983.

329. Bow EJ, Rayner E, Scott BA, Louie TJ: Selective gut decontamination with nalidixic acid or trimethoprim-sulfamethoxazole for infection prophylaxis in neutropenic cancer patients: Relation-

ship of efficacy to antimicrobial spectrum and timing of administration. *Antimicrob Agents Chemother* 31:551, 1987.

330. Bow EJ, Louie TJ: Emerging role of quinolones in the prevention of gram-negative bacteremia in neutropenic cancer patients and in the treatment of enteric infections. *Clin Invest Med* 12:61, 1989.

331. Dekker AW, Rozenberg-Arska M, Verhoef J: Infection prophylaxis in acute leukemia: A comparison of ciprofloxacin with trimethoprim-sulfamethoxazole and colistin. *Ann Intern Med* 106:7, 1987.

332. Wade JC, Schimpff SC, Newman KA, Wiernik PH: *Staphylococcus epidermidis*: An increasing cause of infection in patients with granulocytopenia. *Ann Intern Med* 97:503, 1982.

333. Elting LS, Bodey GP, Keefe BH: Septicemia and shock syndrome due to viridans streptococci: A case-control study of predisposing factors. *Clin Infect Dis* 14:1201, 1992.

334. Weisman SJ, Scoopo FJ, Johnson GM, et al: Septicemia in pediatric oncology patients: The significance of viridans streptococcal infections. *J Clin Oncol* 8:453, 1990.

335. Marron A, Carratala J, Gonzalez-Barca E, et al: Serious complications of bacteremia caused by Viridans streptococci in neutropenic patients with cancer. *Clin Infect Dis* 31:1126, 2000.

336. Tunkel AR, Sepkowitz KA: Infections caused by viridans streptococci in patients with neutropenia. *Clin Infect Dis* 34:1524, 2002.

337. Rotstein C, Mandell L, Goldberg N: Fluoroquinolone prophylaxis for profoundly neutropenic cancer patients: A meta-analysis. *Curr Oncol* 4(Suppl 2):S2, 1997.

338. Engels EA, Lau J, Barza M: Efficacy of quinolone prophylaxis in neutropenic cancer patients: A meta-analysis. *J Clin Oncol* 16:1179, 1998.

339. Reduction of fever and streptococcal bacteremia in granulocytopenic patients with cancer. A trial of oral penicillin V or placebo combined with pefloxacin. International Antimicrobial Therapy Cooperative Group of the European Organization for Research and Treatment of Cancer. *JAMA* 272:1183, 1994.

340. Kern WV, Hay B, Kern P, et al: A randomized trial of roxithromycin in patients with acute leukemia and bone marrow transplant recipients receiving fluoroquinolone prophylaxis. *Antimicrob Agents Chemother* 38:465, 1994.

341. Tjan-Heijnen VC, Postmus PE, Ardizzoni A, et al: Reduction of chemotherapy-induced febrile leucopenia by prophylactic use of ciprofloxacin and roxithromycin in small-cell lung cancer patients: An EORTC double-blind placebo-controlled phase III study. *Ann Oncol* 12:1359, 2001.

342. de Marie S, van den Broek PJ, Willemze R, van Furth R: Strategy for antibiotic therapy in febrile neutropenic patients on selective antibiotic decontamination. *Eur J Clin Microbiol Infect Dis* 12:897, 1993.

343. Gilbert C, Meisenberg B, Vredenburgh J, et al: Sequential prophylactic oral and empiric once-daily parenteral antibiotics for neutropenia and fever after high-dose chemotherapy and autologous bone marrow support. *J Clin Oncol* 12:1005, 1994.

344. Bow EJ, Loewen R, Vaughan D: Reduced requirement for antibiotic therapy targeting gram-negative organisms in febrile, neutropenic patients with cancer who are receiving antibacterial chemoprophylaxis with oral quinolones. *Clin Infect Dis* 20:907, 1995.

345. Bow EJ, Ronald AR: Antibacterial chemoprophylaxis in neutropenic patients—where do we go from here? *Clin Infect Dis* 17:333, 1993.

346. Jackson SK, Parton J, Barnes RA, et al: Effect of IgM-enriched intravenous immunoglobulin (Pentaglobin) on endotoxaemia and anti-endotoxin antibodies in bone marrow transplantation. *Eur J Clin Invest* 23:540, 1993.

347. Cornely OA, Ullmann AJ, Karthaus M: Evidence-based assessment of primary antifungal prophylaxis in patients with hematologic malignancies. *Blood* 101:3365, 2003.

348. Meunier F: New methods for delivery of antifungal agents. *Rev Infect Dis* 11(Suppl 7):S1605, 1989.

349. Schwartz S, Behre G, Heinemann V, et al: Aerosolized amphotericin B inhalations as prophylaxis of invasive *Aspergillus* infections during prolonged neutropenia: Results of a prospective randomized multicenter trial. *Blood* 93:3654, 1999.

350. Nucci M, Biasoli I, Akiti T, et al: A double-blind, randomized, placebo-controlled trial of itraconazole capsules as antifungal prophylaxis for neutropenic patients. *Clin Infect Dis* 30:300, 2000.

351. Harousseau JL, Dekker AW, Stamatoullas-Bastard A, et al: Itraconazole oral solution for primary prophylaxis of fungal infections in patients with hematological malignancy and profound neutropenia: A randomized, double-blind, double-placebo, multicenter trial comparing itraconazole and amphotericin B. *Antimicrob Agents Chemother* 44:1887, 2000.

352. Menichetti F, Del Favero A, Martino P, et al: Itraconazole oral solution as prophylaxis for fungal infections in neutropenic patients with hematologic malignancies: A randomized, placebo-controlled, double-blind, multicenter trial. GIMEMA Infection Program. Gruppo Italiano Malattie Ematologiche dell' Adulto. *Clin Infect Dis* 28:250, 1999.

353. Winston DJ, Maziarz RT, Chandrasekar PH, et al: Intravenous and oral itraconazole versus intravenous and oral fluconazole for long-term antifungal prophylaxis in allogeneic hematopoietic stem-cell transplant recipients. A multicenter, randomized trial. *Ann Intern Med* 138:705, 2003.

354. Marr KA, Crippa F, Leisenring W, et al: Itraconazole versus fluconazole for prevention of fungal infections in patients receiving allogeneic stem cell transplants. *Blood* 103:1527, 2004.

355. Glasmacher A, Prentice A, Gorschluter M, et al: Itraconazole prevents invasive fungal infections in neutropenic patients treated for hematologic malignancies: Evidence from a meta-analysis of 3597 patients. *J Clin Oncol* 21:4615, 2003.

356. van Burik J, Ratanatharathorn V, Lipton J, et al: Randomised, double-blind trial of micafungin versus fluconazole for the prophylaxis of invasive fungal infection in patients undergoing haematopoietic stem cell transplant. Programme and Abstracts of the 42nd Interscience Conference on Antimicrobial Agents and Chemotherapy, 401 (Abst. M-1238), 27-9-2002.

357. Gotzsche PC, Johansen HK: Meta-analysis of prophylactic or empirical antifungal treatment versus placebo or no treatment in patients with cancer complicated by neutropenia. *BMJ* 314:1238, 1997.

358. Rotstein C, Bow EJ, Laverdiere M, et al: Randomized placebo-controlled trial of fluconazole prophylaxis for neutropenic cancer patients: Benefit based on purpose and intensity of cytotoxic therapy. The Canadian Fluconazole Prophylaxis Study Group. *Clin Infect Dis* 28:331, 1999.

359. Dykewicz CA: Summary of the guidelines for preventing opportunistic infections among hematopoietic stem cell transplant recipients. *Clin Infect Dis* 33:139, 2001.

360. Marr KA, Seidel K, Slavin MA, et al: Prolonged fluconazole prophylaxis is associated with persistent protection against candidiasis-related death in allogeneic marrow transplant recipients: Long-term follow-up of a randomized, placebo-controlled trial. *Blood* 96:2055, 2000.

361. Saral R, Ambinder RF, Burns WH, et al: Acyclovir prophylaxis against herpes simplex virus infection in patients with leukemia. A randomized, double-blind, placebo-controlled study. *Ann Intern Med* 99:773, 1983.

362. Sullivan KM, Dykewicz CA, Longworth DL, et al: Preventing opportunistic infections after hematopoietic stem cell transplantation: The Centers for Disease Control and Prevention, Infectious Diseases Society of America, and American Society for Blood and Marrow Transplantation Practice Guidelines and beyond. *Hematology* (Am Soc Hematol Educ Program) 392, 2001.

363. Management of herpes virus infections following transplantation. *J Antimicrob Chemother* 45:729, 2000.

Chapter 48 _____
AIDS IN THE INTENSIVE CARE UNIT
PETER PHILLIPS
JULIO S. G. MONTANER
JAMES A. RUSSELL

KEY POINTS

- *The acquired immunodeficiency syndrome (AIDS) is caused by chronic infection with the human immunodeficiency virus (HIV), which through its relentless replication causes progressive depletion of T-helper lymphocytes leading to severe cellular immunodeficiency.*

- *In the absence of treatment, after a variable period, usually years from infection, multiple opportunistic infections or neoplasms characteristic of AIDS develop. Despite substantial progress in antiretroviral therapy, cure of the disease remains elusive.*

- *HIV transmission is limited to sexual exposure (homosexual or heterosexual), exposure to blood or blood products (including transplanted organs), and perinatal exposure (transplacentally, at the time of delivery, or through lactation).*

- *HIV cannot be transmitted through casual contact. Universal precautions, however, should be implemented and enforced to minimize the risk of occupational exposure to HIV as well as other infectious agents. The rate of seroconversion following a single accidental needle stick or mucous membrane exposure appears to be well below 1%.*

- *Combination antiretroviral therapy has been shown to prolong survival as well as disease-free interval. The widespread availability of plasma viral load monitoring and increasing access to genotype resistance testing in developed countries have led to further optimization of therapy and hence further improvement in outcomes.*

- *Acute respiratory failure (ARF) secondary to* Pneumocystis carinii *pneumonia (PCP) is a frequent cause of ICU admission among HIV-infected individuals.*

- *PCP usually is diagnosed in the ICU using bronchoalveolar lavage (BAL). BAL fluid always should be processed to allow identification of* P. carinii, *fungi, common bacteria, mycobacteria, and viruses.*

- *PCP-related ARF should be treated aggressively with specific antimicrobials, adjunctive systemic corticosteroids, and oxygenation support.*

- *The mortality of PCP-related ARF has decreased substantially with the use of adjunctive systemic corticosteroids. Patients developing ARF despite corticosteroid treatment, however, continue to have a dismal prognosis.*

- *Initiation of highly active antiretroviral therapy or revision of a failing regimen should be delayed until completion of PCP therapy because of the risk of pulmonary deterioration related to PCP immune reconstitution syndrome.*

- *The issue of life support should be discussed early and reassessed frequently with HIV-infected individuals. ICU admission and life support, however, should be discouraged for patients with*

multiple life-threatening complications for which there is no effective therapy. Because the outlook of AIDS and its related diseases is changing rapidly, rigid policies regarding ICU eligibility should be strongly discouraged.

HUMAN IMMUNODEFICIENCY VIRUS INFECTION

The acquired immunodeficiency syndrome (AIDS) is caused by chronic infection with the human immunodeficiency viruses (HIV-1, HIV-2). Continuous HIV replication leads to progressive dysfunction and gradual depletion of the helper T-lymphocytes or CD4+ lymphocytes.[1,2] It is clear, however, that HIV can infect other cells, including macrophages and B-lymphocytes. Eventually, this results in the development of the otherwise unusual opportunistic infections and neoplasms characteristic of AIDS.

The total number of people infected with HIV/AIDS globally as of December 2000 has been estimated to be 58 million, of whom 21.8 million have died since the beginning of the epidemic. The number of people in the United States living with HIV or AIDS was estimated to be 920,000 and 320,000, respectively.[3]

The proportion of AIDS cases requiring either hospitalization or admission to the ICU has declined since the introduction of highly active anti-retroviral therapy (HAART) in 1996. In recent years, HIV-related hospitalizations are less often due to opportunistic diseases compared with the pre-HAART era. Since the increase in HIV infection among injection drug users, a significant proportion of hospital admissions for HIV patients now are accounted for by other complications of injection drug use (e.g., liver disease from chronic hepatitis B and C, cellulitis, endocarditis etc.).

TRANSMISSION

The most common route of transmission of HIV remains sexual intercourse. It must be emphasized that homosexual and heterosexual transmission occurs, and in both cases, bidirectional transmission is possible.[4] The second most prevalent form of transmission is through exposure to infected blood or blood products, including transplanted organs. Since the widespread adoption of HIV screening of donated blood, however, parenteral transmission of HIV is limited almost exclusively to intravenous drug use. Finally, the infection also can be transmitted perinatally. This refers to infection of offspring transplacentally, at the time of delivery, or through lactation.[5]

It is important to emphasize that HIV is not transmitted through casual contact. After a single accidental needle stick exposure to contaminated material, the rate of seroconversion is approximately 1 per 300 exposures, or 0.3 percent. This is particularly reassuring for the families and health care providers of AIDS patients. In the ICU setting, the "universal precautions" recommended for patients infected with the hepatitis B virus are sufficient to deal appropriately with HIV.[6] Nevertheless, the risk of acquiring HIV infection in the workplace is real; this issue, therefore, should not be hidden but rather discussed openly, and health care institutions should adopt exemplary policies to deal fairly and compassionately with such occurrences. A case-control study conducted by the Centers for Disease Control and Prevention (CDC) showed that zidovudine use following accidental exposure to HIV in health care workers reduced the risk of transmission by approximately 80%.[7] Consequently, the need for antiretroviral therapy immediately following accidental exposure to HIV should be evaluated on a case-by-case basis by qualified specialists. According to published guidelines, counseling and possibly combination antiretroviral therapy, depending on the details of the potential exposure, should be offered immediately to health care workers.[8]

PATHOPHYSIOLOGY

HIV preferentially infects T-lymphocytes bearing the surface marker CD4, the so-called helper T cells or T4 cells. This tropism is mediated through a specific interaction between GP160, a viral envelope glycoprotein, and the CD4 molecule itself. HIV is also capable of infecting a number of other bone-marrow-derived cells, including monocytes, macrophages, Langerhans dendritic cells, microglial cells, B-lymphocytes, and bone marrow stem cells.[9]

Once within the cell, the viral ribonucleic acid (RNA) and reverse transcriptase are released. The reverse transcriptase generates a deoxyribonucleic acid (DNA) sequence complementary to the viral RNA, which then integrates into the host cell's genome to produce new viral particles, which in turn will infect other susceptible cells. Relentless HIV replication causes T4 cell dysfunction and death, leading to severe cellular immunodeficiency.[9]

NATURAL HISTORY

Acute HIV infection is associated with retrospectively identified transient symptomatic illness in 40% to 90% of patients.[10] This is most often a nonspecific flulike illness often confused with acute infectious mononucleosis and characterized by fever (>80% to 90%), fatigue (>70% to 90%), rash (>40% to 80%), headache (32% to 70%), lymphadenopathy (40% to 70%), pharyngitis (50% to 70%), and aseptic meningitis (24%), as well as other symptoms. This usually benign and self-limited syndrome, also known as *seroconversion illness,* is believed to be an immune-complex-mediated phenomenon resulting from early antibody response to the infection by HIV. Typically, after a variable period (rarely less than 2 years) with few or no symptoms, progressive immunodeficiency develops, rendering the individual susceptible to the development of opportunistic infections, wasting, and/or neoplasms characteristic of AIDS. AIDS remains incurable despite considerable progress in antiretroviral therapy. The often-prolonged period of clinical latency is characterized by continued viral replication and decline of the immune system, as illustrated by the progressive destruction of the lymph node architecture.[11]

SURROGATE MARKERS

A number of laboratory tests have been shown to correlate with prognosis among HIV-infected individuals. These tests generally are referred to as surrogate markers of disease progression.[12] The CD4+ lymphocyte count traditionally has been the most commonly used surrogate marker. A range of 400 to 1400 cells/μL (0.40 to 1.40 $\times$ 10^9/L) is considered normal in most laboratories. The CD4 count usually is reported as a fraction and an absolute count. Although the absolute CD4 count is usually a good reflection of the degree of immun-

odeficiency in a given patient, it must be noted that under specific circumstances this may be misleading. It is therefore advisable to monitor the CD4 fraction to ensure that this is in general agreement with the absolute CD4 count. CD4 counts are used widely to guide therapeutic decisions regarding the use of antiretrovirals and preventive strategies, yet they are subject to considerable variability. CD4 counts show circadian variation, which is lowest in the morning and highest in the evening. In normal individuals, the evening CD4 cell count can be nearly double the morning nadir. Although this variation may be reduced in HIV-infected patients, specimens for CD4 counting should be collected in a standardized fashion. Other factors that may affect the count include acute infections such as common viral illnesses, certain pharmaceutical agents, stress, smoking, and exercise. The results also may be influenced by differing laboratory methodologies. Despite controlling the time of collection, HIV-infected individuals who are stable clinically will still show considerable variation in CD4 counts. Short-term CD4 count fluctuations of nearly 30% may occur that are not attributable to a change in disease status. In addition, correlation between CD4 count and clinical status can be quite different from one patient to the next. Overall, it is important to monitor the trends in CD4 counts over time to avoid placing too much emphasis on the specific number derived from a single determination. Despite these limitations, the CD4 count remains a valuable tool when attempting to establish the differential diagnoses in a given patient. For example, it would be very unusual (although still possible, particularly in the context of immune reconstitution syndromes) to have a case of PCP, *Mycobacterium avium* complex (MAC), or cytomegalovirus (CMV) disease with a CD4 count within the normal range.

Strong evidence has been generated regarding the prognostic value of viral load determinations in seroincidence and seroprevalent cohorts. In one such study, seroprevalent individuals who had high viral loads were shown to have a substantially worse prognosis with regard to survival. Whereas median survival was in excess of 10 years for individuals with a plasma viral load under 5000/mL, those with plasma viral loads over 34,000/mL had a median survival on the order of 3 years.[13] These data were confirmed by the results of virologic studies within the AIDS Clinical Trials Group Protocol 175 (ACTG 175). This study demonstrated a 10-fold increase in the rate of death and progression to AIDS or death when individuals with lower viral loads (<5000 copies/mL) were compared with those with high loads (>54,000 copies/mL). In this study, CD4 counts and viral load were shown to be independent prognostic markers at enrollment. More important, decreases in viral load with treatment between weeks 0 and 8 were shown to be statistically significantly associated with improved survival and decreased progression to AIDS within this protocol. Of note, increases in CD4 counts with treatment, during the same period, failed to demonstrate a statistical association with clinical outcomes. These data strongly support the independent contribution that viral load determinations can have in terms of monitoring prognosis and response to antiretroviral therapy. Plasma viral load determinations should be obtained in tandem with CD4 counts. However, although viral load determinations play a major role in the management of HIV-infected individuals, this marker has no demonstrated role in the ICU care of HIV-infected individuals.

ANTIRETROVIRAL TREATMENT

Combination therapy regimens have been shown to prolong survival and the disease-free interval substantially among HIV-infected individuals. More recently, a number of new drugs have been added to our therapeutic armamentarium. The currently available classes of antiretrovirals are the nucleoside or nucleotide reverse-transcriptase inhibitors (NRTIs, NtRTIs), nonnucleoside reverse-transcriptase inhibitors (NNRTIs), protease inhibitors (PIs), and fusion inhibitors. The NRTIs include zidovudine (AZT), didanosine (ddI), stavudine (D4T), lamivudine (3TC), abacavir, and tenofovir. The NNRTIs include nevirapine, delavirdine, and efavirenz. The protease inhibitors include indinavir, ritonavir, saquinavir (hard-gel [Invirase], soft-gel [Fortovase]), nelfinavir, amprenavir (and fos-amprenavir), atazanavir, tipranavir, and the coformulation of lopinavir plus ritonavir (known commercially as Kaletra). PIs are increasingly coadministered with low-dose ritonavir for the purpose of taking advantage of the drug interaction, which results in higher drug levels (pharmacologic boosting) of the coadministered PI. This applies to indinavir/ritonavir, saquinavir/ritonavir, amprenavir/ritonavir, tipranavir/ritonavir, and lopinavir/ritonavir; such combinations are considered to count only as a single drug from the antiviral perspective. Currently, triple (or quadruple) drug combinations, including two nucleosides (zidovudine or stavudine plus lamivudine or didanosine) and a PI (or boosted dual PI combination) or NNRTI are recommended to achieve a greater level of suppression of viral replication.[14] Recently, regimens containing both d4T and ddI have been associated with high rates of toxicity. Alternative NRTIs (or NtRTI) include abacavir and tenofovir, which cannot be given together due to a yet to be understood interaction that compromises their antiviral effect.

In the ICU, it is particularly important to be aware of the more prevalent adverse effects of these agents (Table 48-1). As patients are increasingly treated with multiple antiretroviral agents, often including experimental agents, it is important to remain open to the possibility of new and previously unrecognized adverse effects. Also, whenever antiretroviral therapy is discontinued, viral replication will rebound within days to weeks. Patients receiving combination therapy who develop an adverse effect or drug intolerance to one of the antiretrovirals precluding its continuation should be reviewed by an HIV specialist. Temporary interruption of one drug or part of the antiretroviral regimen in particular may seriously compromise the long-term efficacy of the regimen by promoting the development of resistance to the remaining agents in the regimen.[14] Under these circumstances, interruption of the full antiretroviral regimen is a more appropriate strategy.

It is likely that as experience with some of the newer antiretroviral agents increases, new adverse effects and toxicities will be uncovered. Also, physicians should pay particular attention to possible drug interactions in these often heavily medicated patients.[15] In particular, the profound effect of ritonavir on drug metabolism always should be kept in mind in this setting.

THE SPECTRUM OF DISEASE IN THE ICU

Although HIV-infected individuals develop many medical complications, those leading to ICU admission are few. The complications may be divided according to their relationship to the HIV infection. Causes of ICU admission unrelated to the HIV infection generally are similar to those found in non-HIV-infected individuals of comparable age and risk groups (i.e., young intravenous drug users or homosexual males in North America), and since HIV infection generally is asymptomatic early in its course, many patients with clinically unsuspected HIV infection are treated in ICUs and emergency rooms. Patients with these conditions usually respond to standard management, and their prognosis appears to be similar to that of non-HIV-infected patients who have the same condition unless there is concomitant severe immunodeficiency, in which case the prognosis tends to be determined by the severity of the immunodeficiency.

Of the causes of ICU admission related to the HIV infection, acute respiratory failure (ARF) secondary to *Pneumocystis carinii* pneumonia (PCP) is much less common than in previous years. However, it remains a problem among patients who have barriers to accessing medical care and others who are nonadherent or fail to respond to antiretrovirals and PCP prophylaxis. Various conditions, such as cerebral toxoplasmosis, bacterial pneumonia, disseminated infections (such as bacterial sepsis or mycobacterial infection), gastrointestinal bleeding, Kaposi's sarcoma, lymphoma, endocarditis, and cardiomyopathy account for other HIV-related ICU admissions. The broad differential diagnosis of opportunistic diseases should be kept in mind to avoid delays in diagnosis.[16] Less frequently, a person with AIDS may be admitted to the ICU without prior knowledge of her or his HIV status. Certainly, the presence or history of minor or major opportunistic infections, wasting, otherwise unexplained extensive herpes zoster, or persistent generalized lymphadenopathy combined with a history (or clinical evidence) of high-risk activities will necessitate consideration of HIV infection and related diseases in the differential diagnosis. Also, a number of laboratory features found commonly among HIV-infected individuals can provide the initial basis for considering HIV infection within the differential diagnosis. Among them, lymphopenia, anemia, thrombocytopenia, and hypergammaglobulinemia are the most common. It must be emphasized, however, that HIV infection should not be diagnosed unless this has been confirmed using specific serologic tests, most commonly, enzyme-linked immunosorbent assay (ELISA) and Western blot.

Respiratory Disease Complicating HIV Infection

Acute respiratory failure secondary to PCP remains a frequent cause of ICU admission among HIV-infected individuals. Despite this, the initial diagnostic workup of patients with acute pulmonary disease always should consider less frequent causes, among them fungal, bacterial, mycobacterial, and viral infections. Other infections that may mimic PCP both clinically and radiologically include various causes of "atypical" pneumonia (influenza, *Mycoplasma pneumoniae*), miliary tuberculosis, disseminated histoplasmosis, cryptococcosis, coccidioidomycosis, and acute respiratory distress syndrome (ARDS). Although severe acute respiratory syndrome (SARS) has not been reported in HIV-infected patients, its progression to diffuse pulmonary infiltrates in association with lymphopenia[17] would resemble PCP in an HIV-positive

TABLE 48-1 Main Toxicities of Licensed Antiretroviral Agents

Agent	Toxicities
Nucleoside RT Inhibitors (NRTIs)	
Zidovudine (ZDV, AZT or RETROVIR)	Bone marrow suppression: macrocytic anemia, leukopenia (these effects can be accentuated when zidovudine is combined with lamivudine). GI intolerance, headache, insomnia, rash, lactic acidosis and hepatic steatosis and myositis (with elevated CPK).
Didanosine (ddI or VIDEX)	Pancreatitis, GI intolerance, sensory peripheral neuropathy, hypertriglyceridemia, hyperuricemia, gout, lactic acidosis and hepatic steatosis.
Zalcitabine (ddC or HIVID)	Sensory peripheral neuropathy, painful mouth ulcers, pancreatitis, lactic acidosis and hepatic steatosis.
Stavudine (d4T or ZERIT)	Pancreatitis, sensory peripheral neuropathy, neuromuscular weakness (resembling Guillian-Barre), lactic acidosis and hepatic staetosis.
Lamivudine (3TC or EPIVIR)	Neutropenia, anemia, lactic acidosis and hepatic steatosis
Abacavir (ZIAGEN)	Hypersensitivity reaction may be fatal (symptoms may include fever, rash, fatigue, vomiting, abdominal pain, diarrhea, cough, shortness of breath). If hypersensitivity diagnosed, then abacavir should be stopped and never restarted.
Nucleotide RT Inhibitors (NtRTIs)	
Tenofovir disoproxil fumarate (VIREAD)	GI intolerance, renal dysfunction, lactic acidosis and hepatic steatosis.
Nonnucleoside RT Inhibitors (NNRTIs)	
Nevirapine (NVP or VIRAMUNE)	Rash, hepatitis. Drug interactions caused by induction of cytochrome P450.
Delavirdine (RESCRIPTOR)	Rash, elevated transaminase levels, headaches. Drug interactions caused by inhibition of cytochrome P450.
Efavirenz (SUSTIVA)	Rash, central nervous system symptoms (e.g. abnormal dreams, confusion, agitation, hallucinations), hepatitis, teratogenic in monkeys. Drug interactions caused by induction of cytochrome P450.
Protease inhibitors (PIs)	
Saquinavir (SQV or INVIRASE or FORTOVASE)	GI intolerance, headache, transaminase elevation, hyperglycemia, fat redistribution, lipid abnormalities, possible increased bleeding episodes in hemophilia.
Ritonavir (RTV or NORVIR)	GI intolerance, peripheral and circumoral paresthesias, headache, muscle weakness, fever and lightheadedness, liver enzyme abnormalities, elevated CK, uric acid, blood glucose, fat redistribution, lipid abnormalities. Drug interactions caused by inhibition of cytochrome P450. Possible increased bleeding episodes in hemophilia.
Indinavir (IDV or CRIXIVAN)	Nephrolithiasis, GI intolerance, benign indirect hyperbilirubinemia, headache, blurred vision, rash, alopecia, transaminase elevation, thrombocytopenia, hemolytic anemia, hyperglycemia, fat redistribution, lipid abnormalities, possible increased bleeding episodes in hemophilia.
Nelfinavir (VIRACEPT)	Diarrhea, hyperglycemia, transaminase elevation, fat redistribution, lipid abnormalities, possible increased bleeding episodes in hemophilia.
Atazanavir (REYATAZ)	hyperglycemia, transaminase elevation, fat redistribution, asymptomatic hyperbilirubinemia, QT interval prolongation, possible increased bleeding episodes in hemophilia
Tipranavir	Rash, diarrhea.
Fusion Inhibitors (FI)	
T20 (ENFURVIRTIDE)	Injection site reactions, pneumonia, eosinophilia.

patient. Among 19 AIDS patients hospitalized together with 95 SARS patients on the same floor of a hospital in the Province of Guangdong, none developed SARS, in contrast to 6 of 28 medical staff who did.[18] This has raised the questions of whether HIV-1 interferes with SARS virus replication in the same host or combination antiretroviral regimens may prevent SARS.[18] Although Kaposi's sarcoma (KS) can result in ARF, this seldom occurs in the absence of overt mucocutaneous disease. Progression to ARF in KS patients is usually a reflection of overwhelming disease.

Patients who have ARF present with varying degrees of hypoxemia, hypocapnia, and other nonspecific abnormalities related to the underlying HIV disease, as discussed earlier.[19] If available, the CD4 count can aid in the differential diagnosis because the occurrence of PCP when the CD4 count is greater than 250 cells/μL would be unusual. An elevated lactic dehydrogenase (LDH) concentration in a patient with known HIV infection and respiratory distress is typical of PCP, and the LDH level tends to correlate with the severity of the episode. Furthermore, changes in the LDH level tend to parallel the course of PCP.[23] However, an elevated LDH concentration is nonspecific because this enzyme also can be elevated in various other settings, including other pneumonias, pulmonary embolism, lymphoma, megaloblastic anemia, liver disease, shock liver, and hemolysis (commonly seen among HIV-infected patients receiving dapsone treatment or prophylaxis for PCP) or during long-term AZT therapy.

By the time ARF secondary to PCP requiring ICU admission develops, the chest radiograph usually has evolved to a diffuse alveolar pattern characteristic of ARDS. However, a careful review of previous radiographs can, at times, aid in the differential diagnosis, as shown in Table 48-2.[20,21] The clinical, laboratory, and radiologic pattern is seldom specific enough to establish the diagnosis, which should be confirmed using appropriate laboratory examinations. This is particularly important when the patient does not yet carry a diagnosis of AIDS because of the serious prognostic and therapeutic implications of this diagnosis. If sputum is available, this should be cultured for bacteria, fungi, and mycobacteria. Blood cultures also should be obtained, and in selected patients, mycobacterial and fungal blood cultures should be obtained. The key to the etiologic diagnosis relies on obtaining tracheobronchial secretions.[19] In the ICU setting, particularly in ventilated patients, bronchoscopic bronchoalveolar lavage (BAL) is the preferred approach. This should be performed by an experienced specialist. Bronchoscopy should be performed using appropriate cardiorespiratory monitoring, including pulse oximetry and an electrocardiogram (ECG).

TABLE 48-2 Major Radiologic Differential Diagnosis of Lung Involvement in AIDS

Normal chest x-ray:	PCP, CMV, MAC, MTB
Diffuse or localized interstitial pattern:	PCP, MTB, CMV, ALI/ARDS, cryptococcosis
Diffuse alveolar pattern:	PCP, viral pneumonia, cryptococcosis, cardiogenic pulmonary edema, ALI/ARDS, VALI, ventilator-associated pneumonia
Miliary pattern or reticulonodular:	MTB, histoplasmosis, coccidiodomycosis
Consolidation:	common bacteria, MTB, PCP, KS, ventilator-associated pneumonia
Nodular opacity:	PCP, common bacteria, KS, cryptococcosis
Upper lung field involvement:	PCP, MTB
Pneumothorax:	PCP, ventilator-associated barotrauma
Cavity:	Aspergillosis, PCP, bacteria, MTB
Pleural effusion:	KS, common bacteria, mycobacteria

ABBREVIATIONS: PCP, Pneumocystis carinii pneumonia; CMV, Cytomegalovirus; MAC, Mycobacterium avium complex; MTB, M. tuberculosis; KS, Kaposi's sarcoma; ALI, acute lung injury; VALI, ventilator-associated lung injury; ARDS, adult respiratory distress syndrome.

The sensitivity of BAL for *P. carinii* and other treatable pathogens commonly found in AIDS patients exceeds 95%. BAL specimens should be concentrated to increase sensitivity. Aliquots should be referred for viral, bacterial, fungal, and mycobacterial studies. *P. carinii* screening should be requested specifically because this is not performed routinely in most laboratories. Sputum induction and transbronchial biopsies, although valuable techniques in the routine evaluation of less critically ill patients, are not recommended in critically ill and ventilated patients. In the few patients for whom the initial BAL does not provide a diagnosis, a transbronchial or open lung biopsy should be considered.[20] However, the appropriateness of such intervention is best decided on a case-by-case basis after careful assessment of the general status of the patient, as well as the likelihood of diagnosing a treatable condition.

P. CARINII PNEUMONIA

P. carinii, recently reclassified as a fungus but having some properties of protozoa, is a ubiquitous organism that produces human disease throughout the world, usually in the setting of severe immunosuppression. Asymptomatic primary infection generally occurs early in life. Rarely, *P. carinii* can be found incidentally at autopsy in the absence of symptoms. It is not clear whether this represents late infection or early disease not yet manifested clinically.

PCP was the index disease that facilitated the clinical recognition of AIDS. Since then, it also has become the first major AIDS-related opportunistic infection for which development of effective therapy has led to important improvement in survival. Despite these advances, PCP remains a serious opportunistic infection among those infected with HIV, typically occurring among those who do not get tested for HIV or who have problems with access or adherence to antiretroviral and prophylactic therapies. PCP is generally a late event in the evolution of HIV infection, usually occurring when the CD4 count is below 200 cells/μL.[22] Therefore, it is recommended that all HIV-infected individuals with CD4 counts below 200 cells/μL or those who have had an episode of PCP should receive lifelong PCP prophylaxis unless immune reconstitution occurs owing to antiretroviral therapy (sustained increase in absolute CD4 count to more than 200 cells/μL for at least 3 months)[22] (Table 48-3).

CLINICAL AND RADIOLOGIC FEATURES

Dyspnea, nonproductive cough, and fever are the classic features of PCP. In critically ill patients, the physical examination usually demonstrates evidence of acute respiratory distress, with surprisingly few adventitious sounds on auscultation of the chest. Acute hypoxemic respiratory failure requiring mechanical ventilation has been reported to occur in as many as 20% of hospitalized patients.[23] Most often this occurs within the first 3 days of starting antimicrobial therapy; less frequently acute hypoxemic respiratory failure develops as a complication of diagnostic bronchoscopy and rarely as the initial presentation to the emergency room.[23]

Clinically overt PCP usually develops over a period of several days to weeks, and in this time, the radiologic picture tends to progress from a normal chest radiograph to a diffuse bilateral interstitial pattern. Varying degrees of alveolar involvement can be seen; even frank consolidation may occur, as seen in Figs. 48-1 through 48-3. A number of atypical

TABLE 48-3 Guidelines for Discontinuation of Primary and Secondary Prophylaxis for Selected Opportunistic Infections Following Antiretroviral-induced Immune Reconstitution

Opportunistic Infection	Initiate Primary Prophylaxis	Discontinue Primary Prophylaxis	Discontinue Secondary Prophylaxis
Pneumocyctis carinii Pneumonia	• CD4 < 200 cells/μL or history ororpharyngeal candidiasis	• CD4 > 200 cells/μL for ≥ 3 months	• CD4 > 200 cells/μL for ≥ 3 months
Toxoplasma encephalitis	• Toxoplasma seropositive and CD4 < 100 cells/μL	• CD4 > 200 cells/μL for ≥ 3 months	• CD4 > 200 cells/μL for ≥ 6 months‡
Mycobacterium avium Complex	• CD4 < 50 cells/μL	• CD4 > 100 cells/μL for ≥ 3 months	• CD4 > 100 cells/μL for ≥ 6 months*
Crypotcoccus neoformans	not indicated	not applicable	• CD4 > 100–200 cells/μL for ≥ 6 months¶

‡ if asymptomatic from toxoplasma encephalitis and initial therapy completed
* if asymptomatic from MAC and 12 months of MAC therapy completed
¶ if asymptomatic from cryptococcosis and initial therapy completed
SOURCE: Derived from Montaner et al.[22]

radiologic presentations have been described, including cystic changes, pneumothoraces (Fig. 48-4), nodular or masslike opacities, and even cavities.[20] Upper lung field involvement, as seen in Fig. 48-5, also has been recognized increasingly, particularly (but not exclusively) in the context of aerosol pentamidine prophylaxis. To what extent aerosol pentamidine prophylaxis is responsible for the apparent increased frequency of PCP-related pneumothoraces remains controversial.

DIAGNOSIS

As discussed earlier, given the nonspecific nature of the clinical, laboratory, and radiologic picture of PCP, diagnostic confirmation is desirable. BAL is a rapid, safe, and effective means of obtaining tracheobronchial secretions to provide an adequate diagnostic specimen. Lung biopsy is seldom required to confirm the diagnosis of PCP. As seen in Fig. 48-6 (Color Figure 48-6), the usual pathologic picture of PCP consists of a mild to moderate interstitial inflammatory reaction with predominance of lymphocytes and alveolar macrophages and the presence of a foamy alveolar exudate (as seen with hematoxylin and eosin [H&E] staining). The foamy appearance of

FIGURE 48-2 Posteroanterior chest x-ray of PCP demonstrating extensive bilateral basilar lung involvement.

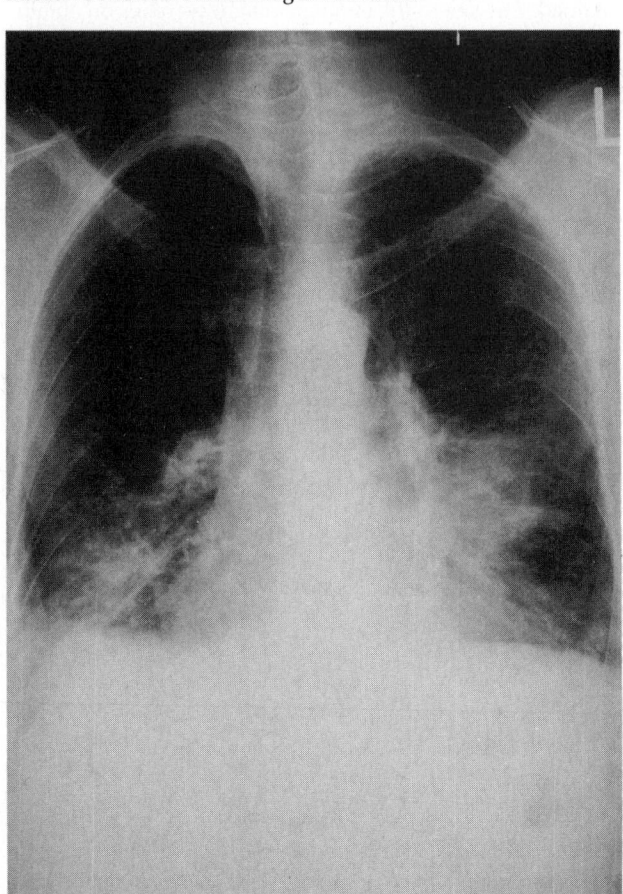

FIGURE 48-1 Posteroanterior chest x-ray of PCP patient demonstrating interstitial disease preferentially localized to the right hilum and lower lung zone.

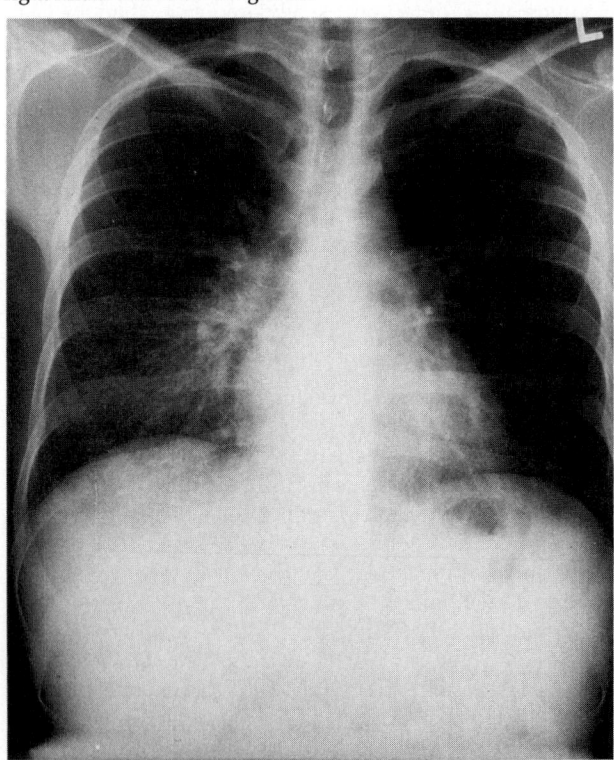

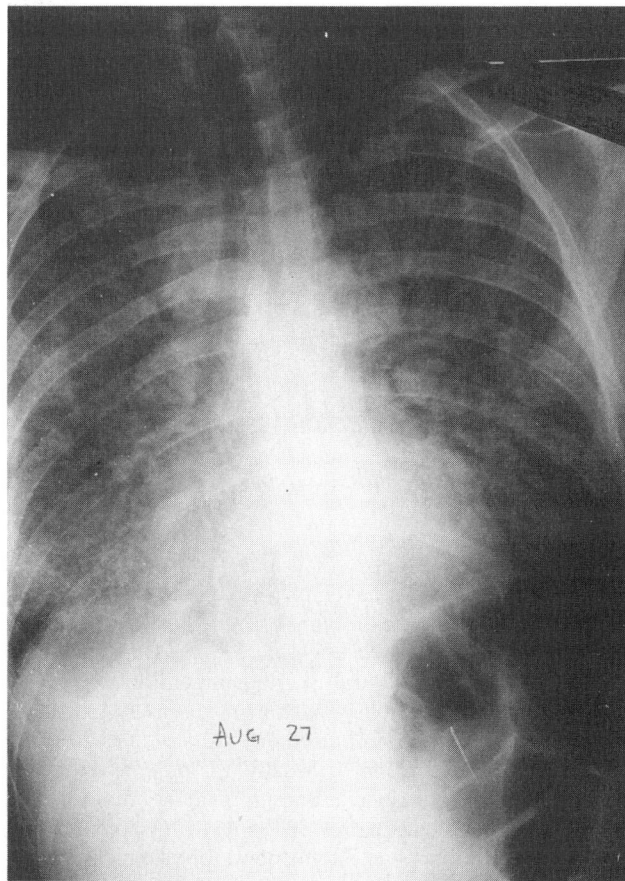

FIGURE 48-3 Anteroposterior chest x-ray demonstrating diffuse bilateral lung disease secondary to PCP in a patient with respiratory failure immediately prior to intubation. Air bronchograms can be seen throughout the lung, particularly in the upper lung fields bilaterally.

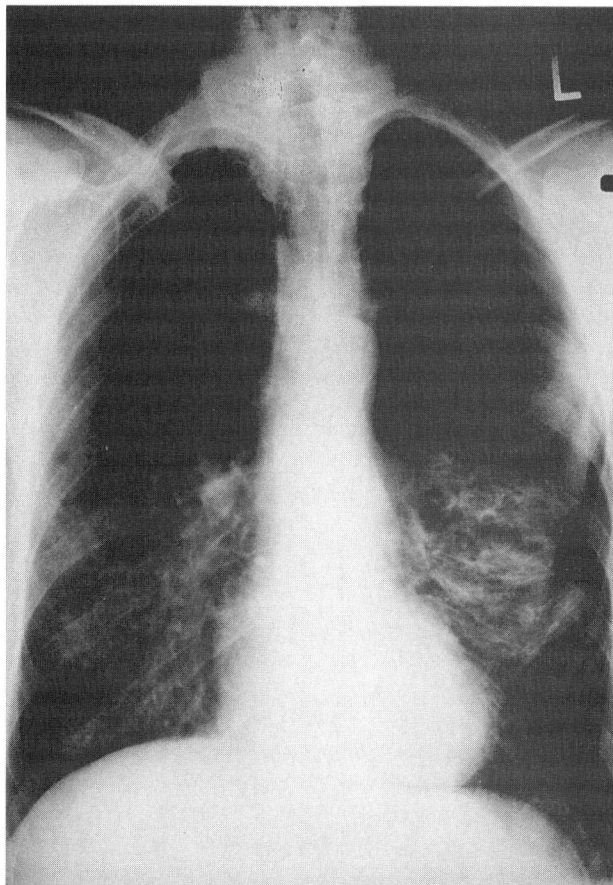

FIGURE 48-4 Posteroanterior chest x-ray of a patient with PCP who presented with a left-sided pneumothorax.

the alveolar exudate is caused by the presence of the cystic form of the organism, which is not stained with H&E but can be easily recognized using readily available special stains (Fig. 48-7 and Color Figure 48-7). As seen in Fig. 48-8 (Color Figure 48-8), BAL allows clear identification of the organism if the specimen is concentrated and stained appropriately.[19,20] The composition of the alveolar exudate has not been established conclusively. However, BAL studies suggest that this is an inflammatory exudate rich in immunoglobulins, macrophages, and suppressor cytotoxic lymphocytes.[24] Although *P. carinii* infection usually is confined to the lungs, systemic pneumocystosis (involving liver, spleen, lymph nodes, adrenals, and eyes), has been reported occasionally.[25] Polymerase chain reaction (PCR) methodology has been applied to the diagnosis of PCP using blood, sputum, and BAL but is not widely available and remains investigational.

PCP IMMUNE RECONSTITUTION SYNDROME

Immune reconstitution syndrome (IRS; also known as *immune reconstitution inflammatory syndrome*) is the clinical deterioration or "paradoxical reaction" that may develop in almost any organ system as a result of augmented immune response to preexisting clinical or subclinical infection.[26,27] Among HIV-negative patients, this phenomenon occurs occasionally during the course of chronic hepatitis B and during treatment for

borderline lepromatous leprosy (reversal reaction, Lepra type I) or tuberculosis (e.g., central nervous system tuberculomas) and is due to improvement in cell-mediated immunity.[28] A similar pathogenesis is believed to account for IRS among HIV-infected patients. IRS has been reported increasingly since the introduction of highly active antiretroviral therapy (HAART) in 1996. IRS has been described as both an unmasking of subclinical latent infection or a worsening of already documented preexisting disease. Most of the reports have been related to CMV retinitis, tuberculosis (TB), MAC, PCP, cryptococcosis, progressive multifocal leukoencephalopathy, and herpes zoster infection.

A diagnosis of IRS begins with a suspicion of clinical events occurring usually within weeks or months after initiating or revising an antiretroviral regimen. The differential diagnosis may include adverse drug effects and coexisting unrecognized infections (nosocomial or community-acquired). Some opportunistic infections show atypical features in the context of IRS, particularly MAC, CMV retinitis, and cryptococcal meningitis.[29] The diagnosis cannot be made without convincing evidence of a response to the antiretroviral regimen (e.g., ≥ 1 $\log_{10}$ reduction in HIV RNA and usually a CD4 increase). For preexisting opportunistic infections (e.g., TB), the diagnosis of IRS is one of exclusion. In contrast, MAC IRS is usually an unmasking of subclinical infection, and when the organism is recovered from a normally sterile body site, the diagnosis is established. It is important to make the

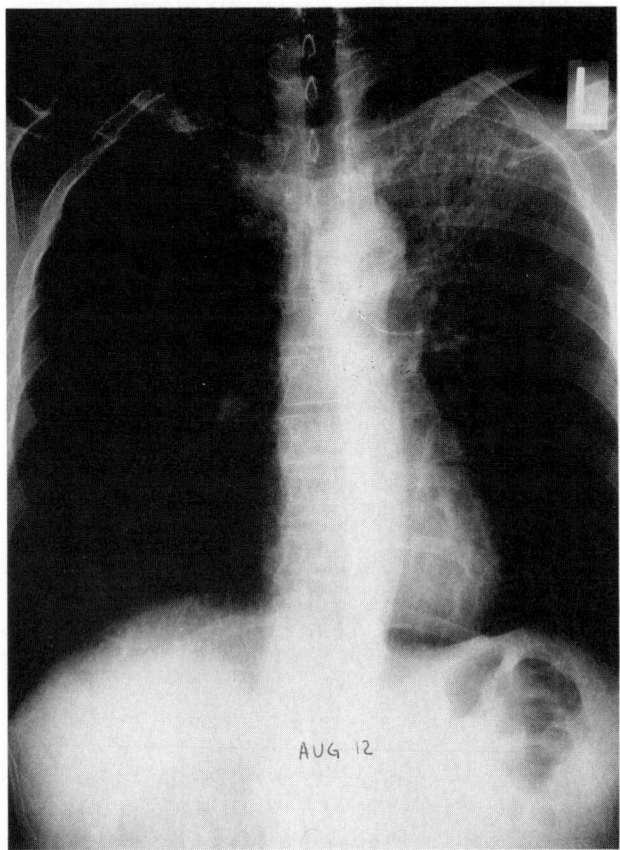

FIGURE 48-5 Posteroanterior chest x-ray of a patient with PCP who presented with bilateral upper lung disease.

diagnosis of IRS in order to avoid inappropriate therapy (e.g., chemotherapy for suspected multidrug resistant TB).

Initiation of combination antiretrovirals during therapy for PCP has been associated with a paradoxical worsening of the pulmonary infiltrates and lung function in up to 5% to 18% of patients.[30] Among the 17 patients with PCP immune reconstitution syndrome reported to date, the clinical worsening was observed 3 to 17 days after starting the antiretroviral regimen. Flow cytometry of BAL specimens in such patients may show a higher CD4/CD8 ratio than usually observed in PCP owing to an influx of CD4 cells during immune reconstitution.[31]

FIGURE 48-6 Characteristic foamy honeycomb material seen in alveolar spaces in *Pneumocystis* pneumonia (H&E stain, × 3100). (See color version of figure.)

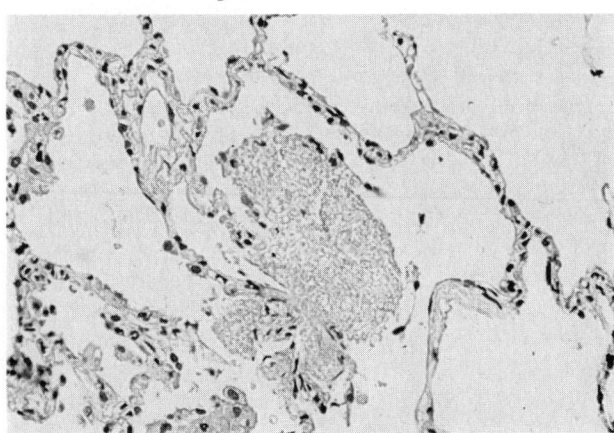

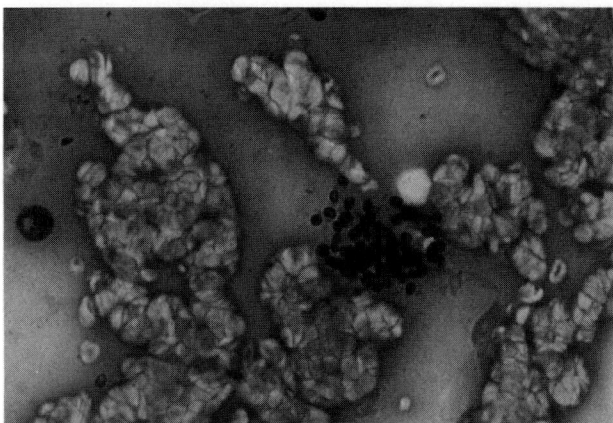

FIGURE 48-7 Cup-and-saucer–shaped *Pneumocystis* organisms seen on BAL (GMS 3 100). (See color version of figure.)

Transbronchial lung biopsy may reveal a prominent alveolar infiltrate consisting of lymphocytes, macrophages, and neutrophils with few or no demonstrable PCP organisms.[32] The diagnosis is established by endoscopy and transbronchial biopsy in order to demonstrate the above-mentioned findings and exclude other possible opportunistic diseases. Any diagnosis of IRS should be supported by evidence of a virologic (HIV viral load reduction of usually ≥ 1 $\log_{10}$) and/or immunologic (CD4 count increase) response to the antiretroviral regimen. Some patients with PCP IRS have developed respiratory failure and appeared to respond to systemic corticosteroids. The incidence of this complication may be reduced by delaying the initiation of antiretrovirals until after PCP therapy has been completed because reported cases usually have developed within the first few weeks following the dagnosis of PCP.

MANAGEMENT

Trimethoprim-sulfamethoxazole (TMP-SMX) is effective against *P. carinii*, as well as various gram-negative and gram-positive bacterial organisms. TMP-SMX is administered intravenously or orally at a dose of 15 and 75 mg/kg daily, respectively, in three divided doses for 14 to 21 days. Poor tolerance of TMP-SMX among HIV-infected patients is a significant problem, with adverse drug reactions occurring in

FIGURE 48-8 BAL specimen showing characteristic granular material found in *Pneumocystis* pneumonia infection (H&E stain, × 3100). (See color version of figure.)

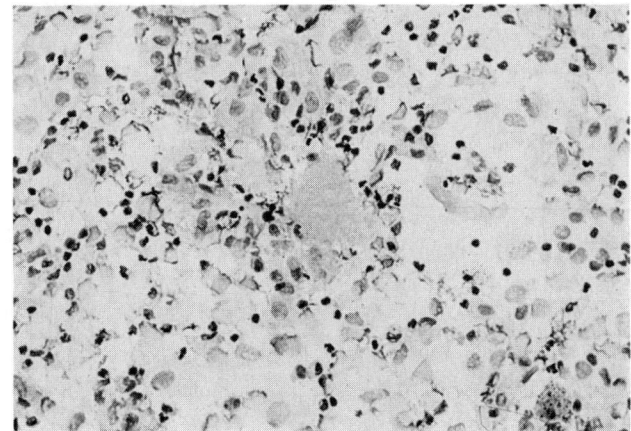

60% to 100% of patients. These include rash, fever, liver dysfunction, renal dysfunction, leukopenia, thrombocytopenia, hyponatremia, anemia, and gastrointestinal upset. Less common but at times severe are mucocutaneous reactions, occurring generally at the end of the first week of treatment. A number of reports have documented successful desensitization of TMP-SMX-allergic patients using progressively larger doses of the drug. Hypersensitivity-type reactions such as fever or rash also can be treated with diphenhydramine or corticosteroids.[33,34]

Pentamidine isethionate was used initially for the treatment of African trypanosomiasis. Since 1958, it has been known to be effective against *P. carinii*. Pentamidine usually is administered intravenously once daily at a dose of 4 mg/kg diluted in 250 mL of 5% dextrose and water for 14 to 21 days. Adverse reactions are common, occurring in up to 100% of patients in some series. Common adverse drug reactions include renal and liver dysfunction, neutropenia, thrombocytopenia, hyponatremia, rash, fever, and gastrointestinal upset. Hypotension is commonly associated with pentamidine infusion. This can be minimized by administering the drug slowly over several hours; if severe or long-lasting hypotension occurs, this should be treated supportively because it is readily reversible. Occasionally, carbohydrate metabolism abnormalities (hypo- or hyperglycemia) may develop, including insulin-dependent diabetes mellitus. Ventricular arrhythmias and pancreatitis also have been reported. Finally, observations suggest an increased risk of pancreatitis among patients receiving didanosine and systemic pentamidine concomitantly. Coadministration of these two drugs therefore is contraindicated. Owing to delayed elimination of intravenous pentamidine, ddI should not be coadministered for several weeks after stopping IV pentamidine. Because adverse reactions to pentamidine are related to its systemic concentration, and because of its poor absorption through the alveolar surface, aerosol therapy has been investigated. In a pilot study, a high cure rate with no significant systemic toxicity was achieved using 5 mg/kg daily via a nebulizer in a highly selected group of patients with mild PCP. The only reported adverse effects were cough and bronchospasm in the majority of patients; however, these adverse effects were easily prevented by premedication with a β_2-agonist bronchodilator. However, because of variable efficacy and increasing concern regarding the possibility of uneven drug distribution, early relapse, and extrapulmonary pneumocystosis, aerosol pentamidine therapy is not recommended; it should be reserved for use as a prophylactic agent only.[35–37]

Dapsone (DPS), a sulfone used for the treatment of leprosy and dermatitis herpetiformis, has been shown to be effective against *P. carinii*, particularly when DPS, 100 mg by mouth daily, is combined with trimethoprim (TMP), 320 mg by mouth q8h (or 15 mg/kg daily, divided q8h). DPS-TMP has been shown to have similar efficacy and better tolerability than TMP-SMX.[38] Adverse reactions are common, including hemolytic anemia with methemoglobinemia, thrombocytopenia, neutropenia, liver dysfunction, rash, and gastrointestinal upset, which often interferes with oral administration. The DPS-induced methemoglobinemia and hemolytic anemia are particularly severe among individuals with glucose-6-phosphate dehydrogenase deficiency. It is also important to note that the hemolytic anemia will produce an increase in LDH that should not be misinterpreted as a sign of worsening PCP.[19]

Atovaquone, a newly developed hydroxynaphthoquinone, has been shown to be a useful second-line agent for the treatment of PCP. Although slightly less effective than TMP-SMX, atovaquone has shown similar efficacy to IV pentamidine, with a very favorable safety profile. This agent is available only in an oral formulation. Furthermore, the drug is not to be used in the presence of moderate to severe diarrhea. For these reasons, atovaquone does not lend itself well to use in the critical care setting.[39]

Clindamycin-primaquine also has been shown to be effective in the treatment of PCP. This regimen usually is reserved for those who fail or are intolerant to TMP-SMX and IV pentamidine. Clindamycin is given orally or intravenously at doses of 450 to 600 mg four times daily, and primaquine is given orally at a dose of 15 to 30 mg daily.[40] Finally, trimetrexate has failed to find a place in the therapeutic armamentarium against PCP despite early favorable reports.[41]

Prospective, randomized placebo-controlled studies have demonstrated a beneficial short-term effect of adjunctive corticosteroid therapy,[42] which prevents the characteristic early deterioration in gas exchange seen in untreated patients and results in a faster resolution of the episode (as measured by respiratory rate, temperature, heart rate, Pa_{O_2}, and LDH). Adjuvant corticosteroids also have been shown to decrease mortality significantly among patients with PCP-related ARF in a prospective, placebo-controlled trial.[43] Systemic corticosteroids are recommended routinely as adjuvant therapy for moderate and severe PCP if no contraindications are present.[44] A regimen consisting of oral prednisone 40 mg twice daily for the initial 7 days followed first by 40 mg orally daily for 7 days and then by 20 mg orally daily for the final 7 days is recommended.[44] Corticosteroids should be started early in the course of the disease, and to this end, a Pa_{O_2} threshold of 70 mm Hg has been proposed.[44] It must be emphasized that adjuvant corticosteroid therapy should be continued while patients are on anti-PCP antimicrobials to avoid the rapid deterioration often seen following premature discontinuation of adjuvant corticosteroids. Adjuvant corticosteroids also may exert a similarly beneficial effect even among patients with milder forms of PCP.[45]

The initial selection of the antimicrobial agent usually occurs outside the ICU. Patients with mild to moderate PCP generally are started on dapsone-trimethoprim or TMP-SMX orally. If there is a concern regarding superimposed bacterial infection, additional antibacterial coverage should be added for community-acquired pneumonia.[46] Pentamidine generally should be reserved for in-patients with PCP and documented intolerance to TMP-SMX. If the patient is first diagnosed in the ICU, TMP-SMX intravenously generally will be the preferred antimicrobial. Corticosteroids should be started at once in any patient whose Pa_{O_2} is below 70 mm Hg while breathing room air. Response to antimicrobials generally is slow, and significant improvement usually does not occur until after 5 to 7 days.[33] With the use of adjunctive corticosteroids, however, significant improvement can be observed within the first 3 days of treatment.[42] Patients who fail to improve within the first 5 days of therapy should be reviewed thoroughly to rule out potential intercurrent infections (such as ventilator-associated pneumonia) or other complications, including pneumothorax and fluid volume overload. Evidence of *P. carinii* resistance to sulfamethoxazole has been demonstrated in patients with prior sulfonamide exposure by the presence of mutations in the gene of sulfamethaxazoles' target enzyme, dihydropteroate synthase (DHPS).[47] The results of studies that have evaluated the clinical significance of such mutations are conflicting. A retrospective Danish study suggested that DHPS mutations are predictive of mortality,[48] whereas another did not confirm this prediction.[49] Lack of improvement within 7 days of therapy generally is interpreted as a failure of treatment and therefore an indication for a trial of the alternative agent. A change in antimicrobial also would be warranted if severe adverse reactions develop despite the use of adjunctive corticosteroids. There is no evidence of increased efficacy, but there is increased toxicity when combining TMP-SMX with pentamidine. However, when switching from TMP-SMX to pentamidine, it may be advisable to administer both drugs for a few days until therapeutic levels of pentamidine can be expected in lung tissue.

PROGNOSIS

Untreated, PCP is universally fatal. With the use of appropriate antimicrobials, overall mortality of AIDS-related PCP is below 10%. However, the mortality clearly increases with the severity of the episode.[21,23,44] The expected mortality of a mild first episode of PCP, therefore, usually is negligible. In addition, young age and early diagnosis have been correlated with better outcome.[21,23,50] The mortality of ARF secondary to AIDS-related PCP appears to be changing. In the early days of the epidemic, mortality was greater than 80% in most series.[51,52] Mortality has been reduced to less than 50% with the addition of systemic corticosteroids.[23,43,44] However, if PCP-related ARF develops despite early intervention with maximal therapy, including corticosteroids and appropriate antimicrobial agents, the prognosis appears to be dismal, with a mortality greater than 90% in some series.[53]

MYCOBACTERIUM TUBERCULOSIS (MTb)

Tuberculosis occurs with varying degrees of frequency among HIV-infected individuals, reaching 20% in some series. Because the risk of developing tuberculosis is proportional to the risk of developing it prior to the acquisition of HIV, its incidence in North America is greatest among intravenous drug users, blacks, and Latin Americans. Tuberculosis usually develops within the year prior to the diagnosis of other AIDS-defining conditions. Either pulmonary or disseminated tuberculosis in an HIV-infected individual is diagnostic of AIDS according to the CDC classification of HIV disease.

The symptoms of tuberculosis in the context of HIV generally are nonspecific. This is particularly the case because "classic" tuberculosis symptoms such as fatigue, malaise, weight loss, fever, and night sweats are extremely common, even in moderately advanced stages of HIV disease. In contrast to the immunocompetent host, in the context of HIV disease, reactivating tuberculosis usually has radiologic features similar to those of primary tuberculosis, including hilar and/or mediastinal adenopathy, middle and lower lung infiltrates, pleural effusions, or a miliary pattern. Apical infiltrates or cavities are seen only in a minority of patients. As many as 9% of patients with CD4 counts of less than 200 cells/μL have a normal chest x-ray with a positive sputum culture for MTb.[54] Furthermore, PCP is diagnosed simultaneously in as many as 25% of the cases of tuberculosis. Prospective tuberculin skin testing (PPD) is useful among HIV-infected individuals because tuberculosis develops more frequently in patients

known to have a previously positive test; however, at the time of diagnosis of AIDS, at least 30% of patients are anergic. MTb usually can be diagnosed with smear and culture of sputum or BAL. Of particular note is the diagnostic yield of blood culture (2% to 12%) in some patients. Rapid diagnostic tests have been approved for the detection of *M. tuberculosis* RNA or DNA in respiratory tract specimens within 24 hours. Such tests are particularly useful in the management of selected patients who are positive or negative for an acid-fast bacilli smear, particularly for those with an intermediate pretest probability of having tuberculosis.[55] Treatment guidelines for tuberculosis have been revised recently by the American Thoracic Society (ATS) and the CDC. Tuberculosis (i.e., first-line antituberculous drug–susceptible) in HIV-infected adults should be treated with isoniazid (plus pyridoxine), rifampin, pyrazinamide, and ethambutol for the initial 2 months (initial phase) of therapy. Ethambutol and pyrazinamide are then discontinued. The continuation phase of treatment consists of isoniazid (plus pyridoxine) and rifampin for 4 more months (total 6 months). Patients who respond slowly to treatment should have the continuation phase of treatment increased to 7 months (total 9 months, or 6 months after documented culture conversion). During the continuation phase, treatment may be administered either on a daily basis or three times weekly. However, twice-weekly therapy is not recommended, particularly for those with CD4 counts of less than 100 cells/μL.[56] Numerous significant drug interactions have been identified between rifamycins and many antiretrovirals, except for NRTIs and NtRTIs. Patients with CD4 counts of less than 300 cells/μL likely will require concurrent antituberculous and antiretroviral therapy. Those with CD4 counts between 200 and 300 cells/μL should be considered for antiretroviral therapy. Rifabutin may be substituted for rifampin and has the advantage of being associated with fewer and less profound antiretroviral drug interactions.[56,57]

A high proportion of patients with multi-drug-resistant tuberculosis (MDR-TB) have been HIV-infected. MDR-TB should be suspected in patients with persistent fevers after 14 days of therapy, particularly in areas of high prevalence.[58] Persistent fevers also have been associated with extensive pulmonary or miliary disease in cases of non-MDR-TB. In contrast to previous reports, HIV-infected patients with MDR-TB had survival rates similar to those with non-MDR-TB when an early diagnosis was established and treatment was initiated with a regimen containing at least two drugs to which the isolate was susceptible in vitro.[58] Expert consultation is recommended for the management of patients with suspected or proven drug-resistant TB. Principles of therapy include the use of at least three previously unused drugs, not limiting regimens to three drugs if other active unused drugs are available (since four- to six-drug regimens appear to be more effective), using directly observed therapy (DOT), and avoiding intermittent therapy except possibly for injectable drugs after the first 2 to 3 months.[56] MTb IRS is important to consider in the differential diagnosis of any HIV+ patient who appears to worsen during the course of therapy for MTB.

M. TUBERCULOSIS IMMUNE RECONSTITUTION SYNDROME

M. tuberculosis immune reconstitution syndrome (MTb-IRS) is a paradoxical worsening of the signs and symptoms of tuberculosis during the course of antituberculous therapy.

This phenomenon was reported occasionally in the pre-AIDS era and considered to be a consequence of resolution of mycobacterial-induced suppression of cell-mediated immunity. MTb-IRS has been reported to occur in up to 36% of HIV-infected patients who initiate HAART.[59] MTb-IRS is important to consider in the differential diagnosis of any HIV+ patient who appears to worsen during the course of therapy for MTb infection. The manifestations may include fever, worsening pulmonary infiltrates, lymphadenopathy, and CNS granulomas. Case reports suggest a possible benefit of systemic corticosteroids for the management of moderate to severe IRS related to MTb and IRS related to other organisms. The diagnosis of MTb-IRS is one of exclusion, including consideration of coexisting opportunistic infections and also multi-drug-resistant MTb.

Among tuberculosis patients with advanced HIV disease (CD4 count <200 cells/μL), HAART recipients have improved 12-month survival compared with historic controls in the pre-HAART era (95% versus 85%).[60] However, problems related to polypharmacy and overlapping drug toxicities argue against the simultaneous initiation of antituberculous and antiretroviral therapy. Consequently, a more appropriate time to begin HAART may be after 4 to 8 weeks of antituberculous therapy[56]; furthermore MTb-IRS may be less likely to occur then.[61]

Mycobacterium Avium Complex (MAC) Disease

MAC disease is usually disseminated (90%) and occurs later than MTb in the course of HIV infection, typically when the CD4 lymphocyte count has fallen below 50 cells/μL. A number of nonspecific symptoms, signs, and routine laboratory abnormalities are encountered frequently in patients with MAC, including fever (87%), night sweats (78%), diarrhea (47%), weight loss (38%), anemia (hemoglobin = 8.5 g/dL; 85%), and elevated serum alkaline phosphatase levels (53%).[62] Clinical and radiologic evidence of lower respiratory tract involvement (4% to 10%) is usually absent. Occasional patients have few or no symptoms in the face of MAC bacteremia.

The diagnosis is established by isolating the organism from blood (mycobacterial blood culture, using radiometric broth or lysis-centrifugation method) or less often from tissue biopsy (e.g., bone marrow, liver) or other normally sterile body fluids. Recovery of the organism from sputum, BAL, bowel, or stool specimens may represent colonization or localized or disseminated disease. In a prospective study, multivariate analysis identified three independent predictors of mycobacteremia in patients with CD4 counts of less than 50 cells/μL: (1) fever for 30 days during the previous 3 months, (2) serum albumin concentration of less than 3.0 g/dL, and (3) hematocrit of less than 30%.[63] When applied prospectively to a validation set, the presence of at least one of the three predictors provided a sensitivity of 94%, a specificity of 42%, and a positive predictive value of 30%.

Significantly improved survival (median = 8.6 versus 5.2 months) and eradication of mycobacteremia was demonstrated with a three-drug combination of clarithromycin, ethambutol, and rifabutin (versus a four-drug regimen of ciprofloxacin, rifampin, ethambutol, and clofazimine) in a prospective, randomized trial.[64] Adverse effects of rifabutin

included uveitis, which occurred much less often at a daily dose of 300 mg (6%) compared with 600 mg (38%).[64] Results from a randomized trial of combination therapy for MAC bacteremia indicated a survival benefit for a regimen containing clarithromycin 500 mg bid compared with 1000 mg bid.[65] In a randomized trial, Chaisson and coworkers[66] reported higher mortality among patients receiving clofazimine (61%) compared with placebo (38%, $p = 0.032$) in combination with clarithromycin and ethambutol.

Rifabutin does not need to be added to clarithromycin-ethambutol for treatment of AIDS-related MAC bacteremia, as outlined below. No clinical or microbiologic benefit was associated with the addition of rifabutin (versus placebo) to a clarithromycin-ethambutol regimen in AIDS-related MAC bacteremia. Among those who responded to therapy, subsequent development of clarithromycin resistance occurred in 2% (1 of 44) and 14% (6 of 42) who received rifabutin and placebo, respectively ($p = 0.055$).[67] However, the significance of the protective effect of rifabutin on subsequent clarithromycin resistance is doubtful in the HAART era because long-term survival and subsequent MAC bacteremia relapses are related primarily to immune reconstitution rather than continued clarithromycin susceptibility of the MAC isolate.

Primary prophylaxis of MAC is indicated for patients with CD4 counts below 50 cells/μL. A randomized comparative study indicated that azithromycin 1200 mg once weekly is a more effective prophylactic than rifabutin 300 mg daily,[68] in addition to being less expensive and less problematic with respect to drug interactions. Clarithromycin is also effective for MAC prophylaxis; however, when breakthrough mycobacteremia occurs, 29% to 58% of MAC isolates are clarithromycin-resistant. MAC drug resistance has not been a problem among failures of rifabutin prophylaxis and was observed in only 11% of azithromycin failures.[68] The interest in preserving clarithromycin as an active drug for treatment of MAC bacteremia provides the rationale for restricting its use as an alternative prophylaxis drug. Primary prophylaxis for MAC bacteremia may be discontinued if there is a sustained rise in the CD4 count to more than 100 cells/μL for at least 3 months[22] (see Table 48-3).

CYTOMEGALOVIRUS (CMV) DISEASE

CMV isolation from pulmonary secretions in AIDS patients appears to have little prognostic value, even when corticosteroids are added to the treatment of PCP. Patients with confirmed PCP respond to anti-*Pneumocystis* treatment whether or not CMV is also recovered in BAL specimens.[69] However, the prominent role of CMV as a gastrointestinal or ocular pathogen among these patients is clearly recognized.

CMV pneumonitis in the context of AIDS should be diagnosed only if hypoxemia and diffuse pulmonary infiltrates coexist with evidence of CMV cytopathic effect (i.e., intranuclear and intracytoplasmic inclusions) in lung tissue and with histologic absence of other likely causes to explain the pulmonary disorder.[70] Unfortunately, CMV blood and urine cultures have poor diagnostic and predictive value in the setting of HIV disease, and the likelihood of a positive result correlates inversely with CD4 count.[71] CMV disease usually is treated with ganciclovir or foscarnet, as outlined in Table 48-4. Long-term maintenance therapy is required for CMV retinitis but may not always be needed in gastrointestinal

TABLE 48-4 Antimicrobial Therapy of Common Infections in AIDS Patients

Infection	Drug of Choice	Total Daily Dose	Dose Interval	Route	Usual Duration	Alternative Therapy
Protozoa Toxoplasmosis (*Toxoplasma gondii*)	Pyrimethamine[1]	200 mg loading dose, then 50–75 mg	Daily	PO	4–6 weeks[2]	Pyrimethamine *plus* clindamycin 600–900 mg IV[3] q6h until marked clinical improvement, then 450 mg PO q6h
	plus Sulfadiazine	4–8 g (100 mg/kg)	6 h	PO	4–6 weeks	
	Maintenance therapy: Pyrimethamine[1] *plus*	25–50 mg	Daily	PO	Indefinitely	Pyrimethamine[1] 25–50 mg/d PO *plus* clindamycin 300–450 mg PO q6h (at least 1200 mg daily)
	Sulfadiazine	2 g	6 h	PO	Indefinitely	
Cryptosporidiosis (*Cryptosporidium*)	No proven effective therapy					Azithromycin 600 mg PO daily plus Paromomycin 1 gm PO BID (optimize antiretroviral therapy)
	Restore immune function					
Giardiasis (*Giardia lamblia*)	Metronidazole	750 mg	8 h	PO	5 d	Tinidazole 2g once (not marketed in North America), or furazolidone 100 mg qid for 7–10 days, or albendazole 400 mg PO daily for 5 days
Amebiasis (symptomatic) (*Entamoeba histolytica*)	Metronidazole[4]	2.25 g	8 h	PO, IV	10 d	Tinidazole 1 gm BID for 3 days (800 mg tid for 5 days for liver abscess) (not marketed in North America), followed by a luminal agent (e.g., iodoquinol, diloxanide furoate, or paromomycin)
	followed by paromomycin	1.5 g	8 h	PO	7 d	
Isosporiasis (*Isospora belli*)	Trimethoprim-sulfamethoxazole	640 mg 3200 mg	6 h	PO, IV	10 d[5]	Pyrimethamine 50–75 mg PO daily plus folinic acid 5–10 mg PO daily for 4 weeks; or ciprofloxacin 500 mg PO BID × 7d
	Maintenance therapy: Trimethoprim, 160 mg, sulfamethoxazole, 800 mg		3 times per week	PO	Indefinitely	Pyrimethamine 25 mg PO daily *plus* folinic acid 5 mg PO daily
Pneumocystosis (*P. carinii*)	*Intravenous therapy* Trimethoprim,	15 mg/kg	6–8 h	IV	21 d	Pentamidine 4 mg/kg per day IV, (IM[6]) *or* clindamycin 600 mg q6h IV *plus* primaquine 15–30 mg daily PO
	sulfamethoxazole *Oral therapy* Trimethoprim	75 mg/kg 15 mg/kg	8 h	PO	21 d	Trimethoprim-sulfamethoxazole 2 DS tablets q8h PO; *or* clindamycin 450 mg q6h PO *plus* primaquine
	plus dapsone	100 mg	Daily	PO	21 d	15 mg (base) daily PO; or atovaquone 750 mg q12h PO with food
Candidiasis Oropharyngeal	Fluconazole	100 mg	Daily	PO/IV	7–14 d	Itraconazole 100 mg PO daily for 14 d[7] (or 100 mg BID for 7 d); or topical antifungal (nystatin or clotrimazole 3–5 times daily)

(cont.)

TABLE 48-4 (Continued)

Infection	Drug of Choice	Total Daily Dose	Dose Interval	Route	Usual Duration	Alternative Therapy
Esophageal	Fluconazole	200 mg loading dose then 100–200 mg	Daily	PO/IV	3 weeks	Itraconazole 200 mg PO daily (3 wks),[7] *or* amphotericin B 0.3–0.6 mg/kg, or caspofungin 50 mg IV daily for 7–14 d
Fluconazole-refractory mucosal candidiasis (oral, esophageal)	Itraconazole oral solution[7]	200 mg–400 mg	12 h	PO (swish and swallow)	2 weeks	Higher-dose fluconazole (400–800 mg/day), or caspofungin 50 mg IV daily *or* amphotericin B 0.3–0.6 mg/kg per day IV for 1–2 weeks
Candidemia a) Unstable	Amphotericin B	0.8–1.0 mg/kg	Daily	IV (± step down after 7d to fluconazole)	14 d after last positive blood culture	Caspofungin 70 mg 1st dose, then 50 mg IV daily; or fluconazole 400–800 mg IV daily (PO after 7 days); or Amphotericin B lipid complex (ABLC, ABELCET) 5 mg/kg per day
b) Stable	Fluconazole	400 mg	Daily	IV	14 d after last positive blood culture	Amphotericin B 0.5–1.0 mg/kg/d (total dose 0.5–1.0 gm); or caspofungin 70 mg 1st dose, then 50 mg IV daily
c) Focal invasive or disseminated candidiasis	Amphotericin B	0.7–1.0 mg/kg	Daily	IV	Until total dose 1–2 g and clinical resolution	Fluconazole 400–800 mg/d; or caspofungin 70 mg 1st dose, then 50 mg IV daily; *or* Amphotericin B lipid complex (ABLC, ABELCET) 5 mg/kg per day
	plus/minus 5-Flucytosine[8]	100 mg/kg	6 h	PO/IV		
Cryptococcal meningitis (*Cryptococcus neoformans*)	Amphotericin B	0.7–1.0 mg/kg	Daily	IV	2–3[9] weeks	Liposomal amphotericin B 3 mg/kg/d IV (Ambisome); or fluconazole 800 mg/d, plus 5-flucytosine 100 mg/kg per day (divided q6h)
	plus 5-Flucytosine *then*	100 mg/kg	6 h	PO/IV	2–3 weeks	
	Fluconazole *Maintenance therapy:*	400 mg	Daily	PO/IV	8 weeks	Itraconazole 200 mg bid PO[7]
	Fluconazole	200 mg	Daily	PO	Indefinitely	Itraconazole 200 mg bid[10]
Histoplasmosis (*Histoplasma capsulatum*)	Liposomal Amphotericin B	3 mg/kg	Daily	IV	14 d	Amphotericin B 0.5–1.0 mg/kg/d (total dose 10–15 mg/kg). For mild disease itraconazole 300 mg bid for 3 days, then 200 mg BID for 12 weeks[7]
	Maintenance therapy[11]*:* Itraconazole	400 mg[7]	BID	PO	Indefinitely	Amphotericin B, 50 mg IV once weekly
Coccidioidomycosis (*Coccidioides immitis*) a) Diffuse Pneumonia	Amphotericin B	0.7–1.0 mg/kg	Daily	IV	until clinical improvement (2–3 gm total dose), then step down to azole indefinitely	fluconazole 400–800 mg/d IV/PO; or itraconazole 200 mg IV/PO BID
b) Meningitis	Fluconazole	400–800 mg	Daily	IV/PO	Indefinite	Amphotericin B 0.5–1.0 mg/kg per day IV until total dose 1–2 g IV plus intrathecal[12] amphotericin (dose range 0.01–1.5 mg daily to once weekly); *or* itraconazole 200–300 mg bid,[7]

(cont.)

TABLE 48-4 (Continued)

Infection	Drug of Choice	Total Daily Dose	Dose Interval	Route	Usual Duration	Alternative Therapy
	Maintenance therapy: Fluconazole	400 mg	Daily	PO	Indefinitely	Itraconazole 200 mg bid[7]
Viruses						
Herpes simplex Mucocutaneous	Acyclovir	2.0 g	5 ×/d	PO	14–21 d[13]	Famciclovir 500 mg bid for 7 days; *or* valacyclovir 500–1000 mg PO BID for 7 days; or acyclovir 5 mg/kg IV q8h for 7 days
Severe or refractory mucocutaneous	Acyclovir	15 mg/kg	8 h	IV (over 1 h)	7–10 d[13]	Acyclovir 800 mg PO 5 times daily, *or* famciclovir 500 mg bid-tid PO, or foscarnet 40–60 mg/kg IV q8h (infusion over 1 h by infusion pump)[14], *or* trifluridine (topically) in a 5% ophthalmic solution; or topical cidofovir
Visceral or disseminated	Acyclovir	30 mg/kg	8 h	IV (infusion over 1 h)	10–21 d	Foscarnet 60 mg/kg IV q8h (infusion over 1 h by infusion pump)[14]
Herpes zoster Dermatomal	Famciclovir	1500 mg	8 h	PO	7 d	Valacyclovir 1000 mg tid for 7 days; or acyclovir 800 mg PO 5 times daily or 10–12 mg/kg IV (infusion over 1 h) q8h; or foscarnet 40 mg/kg IV q8h (infusion over 1 h by infusion pump)[14]
Disseminated (cutaneous or visceral) or ophthalmic zoster	Acyclovir	30–36 mg/kg	8 h	IV (infusion over 1 h)	7–14 d	Foscarnet 40–60 mg/kg IV q8h (infusion over 1 h by infusion pump)[14]
CMV cytomegalovirus)	Ganciclovir	10 mg/kg	12 h	IV	21 d	Foscarnet 90–100 mg/kg IV q12h (infusion over 2 h by pump)[14]. For non-ICU patients with CMV retinitis; valganciclovir 900 mg PO BID for 21 d
	Maintenance therapy[15] Ganciclovir	5 mg/kg	Daily	IV	Indefinite	Valganciclovir 900 mg PO daily; or foscarnet 90–120 mg/kg once daily IV (infusion over 2 h by pump) 5–7 d/week, or other options for CMV retinitis (e.g., intraocular sustained release ganciclovir implant)
Bacteria *Streptococcus pneumoniae* a) Uncomplicated pneumonia	Penicillin G	12–18 million units	4 h	IV	7–10 d	ceftriaxone, or cefotaxime or respiratory quinolone eg. levofloxacin, moxifloxacin, gatifloxacin
b) Pneumonia (decreased pneumococcus susceptibility)[16] Intermediate Resistance (penicillin MIC >0.1 and ≤1.0 μg/mL)	ceftriaxone	1–2 gm	Daily	IV	7–10 d	Cefotaxime, imipenem, respiratory quinolone (eg. Levofloxacin, moxifloxacin, gatifloxacin). (Penicillin > 10 million units/d likely adequate for pneumonia)

(cont.)

TABLE 48-4 (Continued)

Infection	Drug of Choice	Total Daily Dose	Dose Interval	Route	Usual Duration	Alternative Therapy
c) Pneumonia[16] : High-level Resistance (penicillin MIC ≥2 μg/mL)	Vancomycin	2 g	12 h	IV	7–10	Imipenem or respiratory quinolone (eg. levofloxacin, moxifloxacin, gatifloxacin) or cefotaxime or ceftriaxone (if cefotaxime and ceftriaxone MIC <2 μg/mL)
Staphylococcus aureus Pneumonia, bacteremia (uncomplicated)	Nafcillin *or* oxacillin *or* cloxacillin[17]	12 g	4 h	IV	21–28 d, 14 (if bacteremia with removable focus, no endocardi-tis)	Cefazolin 2 gm IV q8h; or if MRSA: vancomycin 15 mg/kg IV q12h
Hemophilus influenzae Pneumonia	Ceftriaxone	1–2 g	Daily	IV	10–14 d	Ampicillin 2 g IV q6h (if susceptible) *or* cefotaxime 2 g IV q8h *or* cefuroxime 1.5 g IV q8h or trimethoprim-sulfamethoxazole, or respiratory quinolone
Salmonella Bacteremia	Ciprofloxacin	800 mg	12 h	IV	2–4 weeks	Step down to ciprofloxacin 750 mg PO BID when possible. Ampicillin 2 g IV q6h for 1–4 weeks (if susceptible), then amoxicillin 500 mg tid to complete a 2–4 week course of therapy;[18] or cefotaxime; *or* ceftriaxone[18]
Listeria Meningitis	Ampicillin *plus* Gentamicin[19]	200 mg/kg 5–7 mg/kg	4 h 8 h	IV IV	6–8 weeks 2 weeks	Trimethoprim-Sulfamethoxazole (TMP-SMX) 20 mg/kg per day (based on the trimethoprim component) divided q6h plus/minus ampicillin; or meropenem
Syphilis[20] Primary, secondary, and early latent (i.e. aquired during preceding year)[21]	Benzathine penicillin G	2.4 million units	Once	IM	(some specialists recommend weekly doses × 3)	Doxycycline 100 mg PO bid for 2 weeks *or* tetracycline 500 mg PO qid for 2 weeks[22]
Late Latent[23] (acquired > 1yr before, or unknown)	Benzathine penicillin G	2.4 million units	Weekly	IM	3 weeks (3 doses)	Aqueous crystalline penicillin G 18–24 million units/d divided q4h IV for 10–14 days; or procaine penicillin G 2.4 million units IM daily *plus* probenecid 500 mg qid PO; or ceftriaxone 2g IV/IM daily for 10–14 days[23,24]
Neurosyphilis (includes meningitis or ocular syphilis)	Aqueous crystalline penicillin G	18–24 million	4 h	IV	10–14 d	Ceftriaxone 2 g IM or IV daily for 10–14 d[24,25]; *or* procaine penicillin G 2.4 million units IM daily plus probenecid 500 mg PO qid for 10–14 d[24]

(cont.)

TABLE 48-4 (Continued)

Infection	Drug of Choice	Total Daily Dose	Dose Interval	Route	Usual Duration	Alternative Therapy
Mycobacteria						
Mycobacterium tuberculosis	Isoniazid[26]	5 mg/kg (max. 300 mg)	Daily	PO	6–9 months[27]	For suspected drug resistant TB obtain expert consultation
	Plus					
	Pyridoxine (vitamin B6)	50 mg	Daily	PO	6–9 months	
	plus					
	Rifampin	10 mg/kg (maximum 600 mg)	Daily	PO, IV	6–9 months[27]	
	plus					
	Pyrazinamide	25 mg/kg	Daily	PO	2 months	
	plus					
	Ethambutol	25 mg/kg	Daily	PO	2 months	
M. avium complex (MAC)	Clarithromycin	1000 mg	12 h	PO	Indefinite	Alternatives include azithromycin 500 mg daily (instead of clarithromycin)[28] and ciprofloxacin 750 mg bid
	plus					
	Ethambutol	15 mg/kg	Daily	PO	Indefinite	
	plus/minus					
	Rifabutin	300 mg	Daily	PO	Indefinite	

ABBREVIATIONS: PO, by mouth; IV, intravenous; IM, intramuscular; d, days; q6h, every 6 h; tid, three times per day; qid, four times per day.

[1]Pyrimethamine should be used in conjunction with folinic acid (10–50 mg/d for primary therapy, 10–20 mg/d for maintenance therapy) in order to minimize hematologic toxicity (anemia, leukopenia, thrombocytopenia). AZT should be used with caution during the acute phase of treatment of toxoplasmosis.

[2]Primary therapy for toxoplasmosis should be continued until complete resolution or marked improvement has occurred clinically and radiologically (usually 4–6 weeks).

[3]Clindamycin (plus pyrimethamine) is as effective as sulfadiazine (plus pyrimethamine) for induction but less effective for maintenance therapy of cerebral toxoplasmosis.

[4]Indicated for intestinal disease and or liver abscess. Asymptomatic cyst passers may be treated with a luminal agent, e.g., paromomycin 500 mg PO tid for 7 d (alternatives: iodoquinol 650 mg tid for 20 d or diloxanide furoate 500 mg tid for 10 d). Chloroquine phosphate 600 mg base (1 g)/d for 2 d, then 300 mg base (500 mg) daily for 2–3 weeks may be used in the management of amebic liver abscess.

[5]Continue treatment for 3 more weeks with trimethoprim (160 mg)-sulfamethoxazole (800 mg) 1 DS tablet PO bid (see Pape et al[123]).

[6]Intramuscular pentamidine may be associated with sterile abscess formation. The preferred route is slow IV infusion over 2 to 4 h.

[7]Take itraconazole capsules with food or cola. However, itraconazole solution is best absorbed fasting.

[8]Consider addition of 5-flucytosine (100 mg/kg per day PO, IV in 4 divided doses) in patients with overwhelming infection or local involvement with meningitis or endophthalmitis.

[9]Patients should receive amphotericin B with 5-flucytosine (100 mg/kg per day in 4 divided doses) until significantly improved and stable (usually by 2–3 weeks), at which time treatment can be changed to fluconazole 400 mg/d PO/IV to complete a 10-week course of treatment. Itraconazole 200 mg bid PO is an alternative to fluconazole in this situation provided that drug interactions and poor absorption are not a concern.

[10]High relapse rate (24%) associated with lower dose of itraconazole 200 mg daily.

[11]Relapse rates for maintenance therapy are as follows: itraconazole, 5%; amphotericin B, 19%; fluconazole, 33%; ketoconazole, 50%.

[12]Intrathecal (IT) amphotericin B (cisternal, cervical, ventricular, or lumbar) should be started at a low dose (0.01–0.025 mg) and increased gradually as tolerated to a dose of 0.1–0.3 mg 3 times weekly. The best intrathecal route of administration is cisternal. IT amphotericin B should be given 3 times per week for 3 months then 1–2 times per week for several months. Further dosage tapering is based upon clinical course and spinal fluid parameters.

[13]Treatment should be continued until all lesions have crusted. Long-term suppressive therapy (acyclovir 200–400 mg 3–4 times daily) may be required to control frequent relapses.

[14]Saline loading may reduce foscarnet-associated nephrotoxicity.

[15]Maintenance therapy is mandatory for CMV retinitis but not always required for gastrointestinal involvement.

[16]Meningitis caused by S. pneumoniae with decreased susceptibility should be treated with vancomycin plus ceftriaxone.

[17]Vancomycin is less effective than β-lactam antibiotics against methicillin-susceptible S. aureus infections.

[18]If recurrence of bacteremia, then consider indefinite ciprofloxacin 500 mg bid or trimethoprim-sulfamethoxazole.

[19]Some specialists also recommend intrathecal gentamicin.

[20]Some specialists advise CSF examination and/or treatment with a regimen appropriate for neurosyphilis for all patients coinfected with syphilis and HIV, regardless of the clinical stage of syphilis. HIV-infected patients should have frequent follow-up and serologic testing at 1, 2, 3, 6, 9, and 12 months. Any patient without a four-fold decline in nontreponemal serology (i.e. RPR or VDRL) by 3 months for primary or secondary syphilis, or 6 months in early latent syphilis, or a four-fold rise in titer at any time should have a CSF examination and be treated with the neurosyphilis regimen unless reinfection can be established as the cause of the increased titre (see reference No. 80 Centers for Disease Control and Prevention. Sexually transmitted diseases guidelines 2002).

[21]Failed therapy and development of neurosyphilis has been reported with benzathine penicillin G (see Gordon et al[81]). CSF abnormalities are common in early syphilis in HIV patients and are of uncertain prognostic significance. Some specialists recommend CSF examination and modification of treatment accordingly.

[22]Treponemacidal antibiotics (e.g., penicillin rather than doxycycline) are preferred for syphilis in HIV-infected patients. Document penicillin allergy (history ± skin testing) and consider desensitization.

[23]HIV-infected patients who have late latent syphilis should undergo cerebrospinal fluid examination. Those patients who have a normal spinal fluid examination (including negative CSF VDRL) do not require high-dose IV penicillin therapy and should receive benzathine penicillin G 2.4 million units IM weekly for 3 doses If lumbar puncture not done to exclude asymptomatic neurosyphili (present in half of such patients), then treat with high-dose IV penicillin, or IV/IM ceftriaxone, or IM procaine penicillin G. Therapy with either benzathine penicillin G IM or ceftriaxone IV/IM is associated with serologic or clinical failures in > 20% of HIV-infected patients with latent syphilis or asymptomatic neurosyphilis.

(cont.)

TABLE 48-4 (Continued)

[24]Since the durations of these regimens are shorter than that recommended for latent syphilis, some specialists recommend benzathine penicillin 2.4 million unit IM (once) after completion of any of the 10–14 day regimens

[25]Significant failure rate in HIV-related neurosyphilis, even with high dose IV penicillin.

[26]Isoniazid: higher dose of 10 mg/kg recommended for tuberculous meningitis until clinical response observed.

[27]Antituberculous therapy should be continued for at least 6 months. Slow responders should receive 9 months of treatment, or at least 6 months after conversion to culture negative state.

[28]A possible regimen for macrolide (clarithromycin and azithromycin) resistant disseminated MAC may include: moxifloxacin, ethambutol, rifabutin, plus/minus amikacin; however optimal management depends upon antiretroviral therapy with immune reconstitution which should be the therapeutic priority.

disease. In the context of AIDS, CMV disease tends to occur at a late stage, usually when the CD4 count is less than 50 cells/μL. Mean survival with intravenous or oral ganciclovir maintenance therapy following an episode of CMV retinitis is approximately 13 months without HAART.[72]

OTHER CAUSES OF PULMONARY INFILTRATES

Bacterial pneumonias tend to occur with increased frequency among HIV-infected individuals. Community-acquired pneumonias usually are caused by *Streptococcus pneumoniae*, *Haemophilus influenzae*, *Staphylococcus aureus*, or gram-negative bacilli. *Legionella* pneumonitis, contrary to early reports, occurs infrequently among HIV-infected individuals. Clinical features of community-acquired bacterial pneumonia are indistinguishable from those described in the immunocompetent host. Chest radiographs usually demonstrate segmental or lobar consolidation. Treatment of bacterial infections is included in Table 48-4.[73,74]

Nosocomial pneumonias among HIV-infected individuals are indistinguishable from those occurring in other hospitalized patients. These are usually caused by gram-negative organisms and tend to have a high mortality despite appropriate therapy.

Ventilator-associated pneumonia (VAP) may complicate the course of HIV-infected patients who require mechanical ventilation. There is an increasing frequency of *S. aureus* (methicillin-resistant *S. aureus* [MRSA] or methicillin-sensitive *S. aureus* [MSSA]) as the cause of VAP. In addition, aerobic gram-negative bacilli remain common causes of VAP. The other diagnosis to consider in patients who have pulmonary infiltrates and who require mechanical ventilation is ventilator-associated lung injury. The details of mechanical ventilation are discussed in Chaps. 36 and 38. HIV-infected patients who have acute lung injury (diffuse bilateral infiltrates, Pa_{O_2}/FI_{O_2} <300 mm Hg, and no cardiac cause of pulmonary edema) should receive lung-protective ventilation.[75]

Fungal pneumonias are a rare cause of respiratory failure among HIV-infected individuals. Disseminated infection is often present. Aspergillosis, cryptococcosis, histoplasmosis, and coccidioidomycosis are encountered most frequently and usually are associated with advanced HIV disease. Although reported rarely in AIDS prior to 1990, invasive aspergillosis had an incidence estimated to be between 0.9% and 8.6% among patients with AIDS in the pre-HAART era.[76] Respiratory tract syndromes caused by *Aspergillus* spp. in AIDS include invasive pulmonary aspergillosis, obstructing bronchial lesions, and tracheobronchitis. The presenting symptoms frequently are cough and fever; less common complaints include dyspnea, chest pain, and hemoptysis.[76]

A common radiologic finding in AIDS-related invasive pulmonary aspergillosis is a thick-walled cavity.[77]

Candidiasis of the trachea, bronchi, or lungs, despite being recognized by the CDC as an AIDS-defining condition, is a very infrequent problem among these patients. Treatment of fungal disease is outlined in Table 48-4.[78–81]

Kaposi's sarcoma (KS) involves the lungs in up to 25% of patients with mucocutaneous KS. Clinically significant pulmonary KS without obvious mucocutaneous involvement is rare. Pulmonary KS often is indistinguishable from other HIV-related pulmonary diseases. Cough and dyspnea are common presenting features. Fever, wheezing, hoarseness, and even upper airway obstruction can occur. Sputum production usually is scant or absent. Hemoptysis, however, is relatively frequent. Chest radiograph usually shows nodular opacities of varying sizes coexisting with varying degrees of interstitial disease. Pleural and nodal involvement is also frequent. Bronchoscopic evaluation usually helps to rule out a superimposed treatable HIV-related disease in patients with pulmonary KS. It also may allow visualization of the characteristic red-violaceous lesions in the endobronchial tree. Although biopsy of these lesions at times can provide diagnostic confirmation, this is rarely required. No definitive therapy is currently available for the treatment of systemic KS, although significant improvement has been observed among some patients treated with HAART. Interferon has been used with some limited success for the treatment of early disease. Radiation therapy and chemotherapy have had some success in providing palliation. Given the poor prognosis of KS-related ARF at this time, these patients are unlikely to benefit from ICU support.[82]

Neurologic Complications in HIV-Infected Patients

Neurologic disease secondary to opportunistic infection or neoplasm may be associated with a depressed level of consciousness and occasionally precipitate ICU consultation and care. Often the neurologic disease may be a concomitant problem in patients requiring ICU care for other reasons.

The most frequently encountered neurologic syndromes in HIV-infected patients are meningitis, dementia, encephalopathy, focal neurologic deficits, myelopathy, peripheral neuropathy, and myopathy.[83,84] The various etiologic agents responsible for these syndromes, in addition to key points of clinical presentation and diagnostic evaluation, are summarized in Table 48-5. In general, most of the treatable infections complicating AIDS produce either meningitis or progressive focal neurologic deficits owing to localized inflammatory lesions in the brain, and both these syndromes

TABLE 48-5 Neurologic Complications in HIV-Infected Patients

Neurologic Syndrome	Etiologic Agents	Clinical Presentation	Diagnostic Evaluation
Meningitis	*C. neoformans*	Often headache, fever, and vomiting; sometimes confusion, seizure, meningismus, cranial nerve palsies; occasionally meningitis symptoms are minimal and presentation is fever, fungemia and/or extrameningeal lesion (e.g., skin, pneumonia).	CSF white blood count usually $< 20/\mu L$; CSF, glucose and protein often normal; cryptococcal antigen positive in CSF ($> 90\%$) and serum (99%); positive India ink smear $50\% - 90\%$; fungal cultures (blood, CSF, urine).
	Aseptic (?HIV)	Headache, meningismus, and fever (all less common in chronic cases), with/without cranial neuropathies (V, VII, VIII); may occur with seroconversion, but more common later in HIV disease.	CSF examination: mild mononuclear pleocytosis, protein elevated, glucose normal (differential diagnosis also includes syphilis and lymphomatous meningitis).
	M. tuberculosis	Usually subacute-chronic meningitis. Clinical manifestations similar to those in HIV-negative patients. Fever (89%), headache (59%), meningeal signs (65%), altered mentation (43%), focal deficits (19%), and clinical or radiologic evidence of extrameningeal tuberculosis (65%).[a]	CSF exam: lymphocytic pleocytosis, low glucose, and increased protein; smear for acid-fast-bacilli insensitive; cultures for *M. tuberculosis.* Rapid CSF diagnosis by polymerase chain reaction (PCR) appears promising,[b] but remains investigational. Detection of extrameningeal MTB facilitates early diagnosis.[a] Prior to obtaining positive CSF smears or culture, empiric therapy is indicated if clinical and spinal fluid profile are compatible with MTB.
	Coccidioides immitis	Fever, lethargy, headache, with/without meningismus, confusion (consider if travel/residence history for endemic zone, e.g., southwestern United States).	Serum tube precipitin or complement-fixing (CF) antibody titer positive in 83% of patients with AIDS-related coccidioidomycosis.[c] Any positive CSF titer of CF antibodies is usually diagnostic of meningitis. CSF profile: lymphocytic pleocytosis usually > 50 cells$/\mu L$, elevated protein, low glucose. Fungal cultures of blood and CSF.
	Bacterial (pneumococcus, meningococcus, *Listeria, H. influenzae*)	Fever, headache with/without meningeal signs, confusion, seizures. Bacterial meningitis rare in HIV-infected patients.	CSF exam: polymorphonuclear pleocytosis, high protein, low glucose, with/without positive Gram stain and/or bacterial antigens (pneumococcus, meningococcus, *H. influenzae*); bacterial cultures of blood and CSF.
Diffuse brain disease AIDS dementia complex	HIV	Usually alert, but impaired cognition (usually concentration and memory), behavior (apathy, personality change), and motor function (slowing and reduced coordination); sometimes organic psychosis or mania.	Abnormalities on neuropsychologic testing Other findings may include hyperreflexia, ataxia, release signs, leg weakness, incontinence and mutism. Nonspecific CSF abnormalities may include elevated protein, IgG, $\beta2$-microglobulin, neopterin, and positive HIV-1 p24 core antigen. CT or MRI: atrophy $\pm$ patchy or diffuse abnormalities of hemispheric white matter seen on MRI (T2-weighted).[d]
Diffuse encephalopathies	Toxic metabolic disorders (e.g., hypoxia, sepsis, drugs), CNS toxoplasmosis, CNS lymphoma, occasionally viral infection (CMV, HSV).	Impaired alertness and cognition, with/without focal neurologic deficits.	Blood chemistry to exclude metabolic causes, with/without drug levels, serology for toxoplasmosis. MRI or contrast-enhanced CT head scan: focal lesions may be seen in toxoplasmosis, lymphoma, *Herpes simplex* encephalitis.

(cont.)

TABLE 48-5 (Continued)

Neurologic Syndrome	Etiologic Agents	Clinical Presentation	Diagnostic Evaluation
Focal brain disease Toxoplasmosis	*Toxoplasma gondii*	Headache (55%), confusion (52%), fever (47%), seizures (29%), reduced level of consciousness (42%), and focal deficits (69%) usually progressing over days.	MRI or contrast-enhanced CT scan: spherical ring-enhancing lesions in cortex, thalamus, or basal ganglia, but may have atypical appearances. Toxoplasma serum serology (IgG) usually positive (84%); possible brain biopsy (see Fig. 48-9).
Lymphoma	Strong association with Epstein-Barr virus (EBV)	Confusion, lethargy, memory loss, progressive focal deficit(s), headache, seizure; more slowly progressive than toxoplasmosis. CD4 count usually < 50 cells/μL.	MRI or contrast-enhanced CT scan: usually 1–2 lesions in white matter (often periventricular), may mimic toxoplasmosis but enhancement usually weaker and homogenous; possible brain biopsy. Spinal fluid PCR for EBV DNA has sensitivity and specificity of 80–90% and almost 100%, respectively. Combined sensitivity of positive PCR for EBV DNA or increased uptake on thallium SPECT scan almost 100%.
Progressive multifocal leukoencephalopathy (PML)	JC virus (papovavirus)	Slowly progressive focal deficits (over weeks), but no systemic toxicity or reduced level of consciousness in the early stage.	MRI or contrast-enhanced CT scan: non-enhancing white matter lesions without mass effect. Definitive diagnosis requires brain biopsy. Spinal fluid PCR for JCV 60–100% sensitive depending on case definitions and methodology. Compatible clinical presentation plus positive PCR supports diagnosis; negative PCR does not exclude PML.
Neurosyphilis	*Treponema pallidum*	Focal neurologic deficits (meningovascular involvement) with prodromal symptoms for weeks–months such as headache and behavioral changes. Syphilitic meningitis may include cranial nerve palsies. Ocular syphilis (e.g., optic neuritis) often associated with CNS involvement.	Positive serum VDRL, and FTA-ABS; CSF exam: mononuclear pleocytosis, elevated protein, with/without positive VDRL; CSF profile (if VDRL negative) may be indistinguishable from CSF abnormalities caused by HIV.
Myelopathy a) Subacute, chronic (diffuse)	HIV (vacuolar), HTLV-1	Slowly progressive, painless ataxia and spasticity; bowel-bladder dysfunction occurs late; often coexistent with dementia. Usually no distinct sensory/motor level.	MRI or CT scan, with/without myelography are negative and are not indicated in typical cases (best reserved for patients with atypical findings where segmental lesions are to be excluded). Consider HTLV-1 serology.
b) Acute, subacute (transverse myelitis, segmental)	Varicella zoster, lymphoma, cytomegalovirus	More rapid onset of myelopathy than for HIV.	CT scan or MRI, myelography.
Peripheral neuropathy a) Axonal neuropathy	?HIV	Distal, mainly sensory, painful ("burning feet"), symptoms more prominent than signs.	With/without nerve conduction studies.
b) Toxic axonal neuropathy	ddI, ddC, d4T, others	As for axonal neuropathy. Neuropathy may progress for a few weeks after stopping the offending drug.	With/without nerve conduction studies.
Acute-chronic demyelinating neuropathy	?Autoimmune response to HIV	Similar to Guillain-Barré syndrome; usually occurs during the early period (CD4 >500/μL) of HIV infection, or at the time of seroconversion.	Nerve conduction studies. CSF abnormalities: elevated protein, and mild pleocytosis.
Radiculopathies	Varicella zoster virus	Herpes *zoster* dermatomal vesicular lesions.	Clinical diagnosis, with/without viral antigen detection in smears prepared from skin lesions. Tzanck smear is rapid but insensitive. Viral culture is slow for demonstration of cytopathic effect.

(cont.)

TABLE 48-5 (Continued)

Neurologic Syndrome	Etiologic Agents	Clinical Presentation	Diagnostic Evaluation
	Cytomegalovirus	Subacute and progressive ascending polyradiculopathy with sensory loss, urinary retention, and flaccid paraparesis.	CSF: polymorphonuclear pleocytosis, elevated protein, low glucose, with/without CSF culture positive for CMV; rule out bacterial and tuberculous meningitis.
Mononeuritis multiplex	Autoimmune vascular lesion in early HIV (CD4 200–500/μL). Multifocal CMV infection later in HIV disease (CD4 <200 μL)	Findings compatible with involvement of multiple distinct peripheral nerves. More severe in advanced HIV disease.	Nerve conduction studies.
Myopathy	AZT	Ranges from asymptomatic elevation of CPK to progressive myalgia, atrophy, and weakness (especially proximal leg muscles).	Consider muscle biopsy (mitochondrial abnormalities with/without inflammatory cell infiltrates) if persists after stopping AZT.
	HIV?	As for AZT-induced myopathy.	Consider muscle biopsy: myopathic changes (variable fiber size, vacuolar change and fiber destruction), with/without inflammatory infiltrates; ultrasound if localized inflammation to rule out pyomyositis.

[a] See Berenguer et al.[83]
[b] See Scarpellini et al.[84]
[c] See Fish et al.[85]
[d] See Price.[78]

usually are associated with headache. However, most of the causes of diffuse brain involvement are not associated with headache. A suggested sequence of investigations in the HIV-infected patient with headache or CNS dysfunction is outlined in Fig. 48-9. Antimicrobial therapy is outlined in Table 48-4.[85–88]

MENINGITIS

The clinical presentation of both acute and chronic meningitis is little different in the AIDS patient from that seen in the immunocompetent host; presentation includes headache, fever, and nuchal rigidity of variable duration and severity.

The most important cause of meningitis in the HIV-infected patient is *Cryptococcus neoformans*. Uncommon etiologies include *Mycobacterium tuberculosis*,[89,90] *Coccidioides immitis*,[91] *Histoplasma capsulatum*, *Treponema pallidum* (syphilis), *Listeria monocytogenes*, and the usual causative agents of bacterial meningitis (pneumococcus, meningococcus, *Haemophilus influenzae*). Antimicrobial therapy is outlined in Table 48-4. HIV-related aseptic meningitis may occur at the time of seroconversion but is more common later in the course of HIV disease, when both acute and chronic presentations have been described. The role of antiretroviral therapy for HIV-related aseptic meningitis has not been evaluated.

DIFFUSE BRAIN DISEASE (DEMENTIA AND ENCEPHALOPATHY)

AIDS dementia complex (ADC) appears to be caused by chronic HIV infection of the CNS. Patients with ADC manifest varying degrees of impaired cognition, behavior, and motor function but usually remain alert. In contrast, the diffuse encephalopathies associated with toxic and metabolic disorders, CNS toxoplasmosis, lymphoma, or viral infection (e.g., herpes simplex or CMV) usually result in impairment of cognition associated with a disturbance in the level of consciousness. Patients with ADC should be treated with combination antiretroviral therapy. There is evidence that antiretroviral therapy can both prevent and ameliorate ADC. Zidovudine (AZT) has been associated with sustained improvement in neurologic performance in up to 50% of patients.[92] The role of other antiretroviral agents in the management of ADC has not been determined; however, in a meta-analysis of clinical trials of patients switching from AZT to didanosine (ddI), there was no evidence of any increase in the incidence of ADC during ddI therapy. Despite the absence of definitive clinical trials clarifying the efficacy of HAART for the prevention or treatment of ADC, extrapolation from the monotherapy trials and anecdotal experience supports this approach. Although unproven, improved clinical response may be associated with regimens that include drugs that have good brain penetration (AZT, abacavir, stavudine, and nevirapine).

FOCAL NEUROLOGIC DISEASE

Patients presenting with focal neurologic deficits should have urgent magnetic resonance imaging (MRI) or a computed tomographic (CT) head scan with contrast material, which usually yields evidence of CNS toxoplasmosis (Fig. 48-10), lymphoma (Fig. 48-11), or progressive multifocal leukoencephalopathy (PML). Occasional cases of subacute focal brain disease may be caused by aspergillosis, cryptococcoma, tuberculoma, varicella-zoster virus infection, or herpes simplex

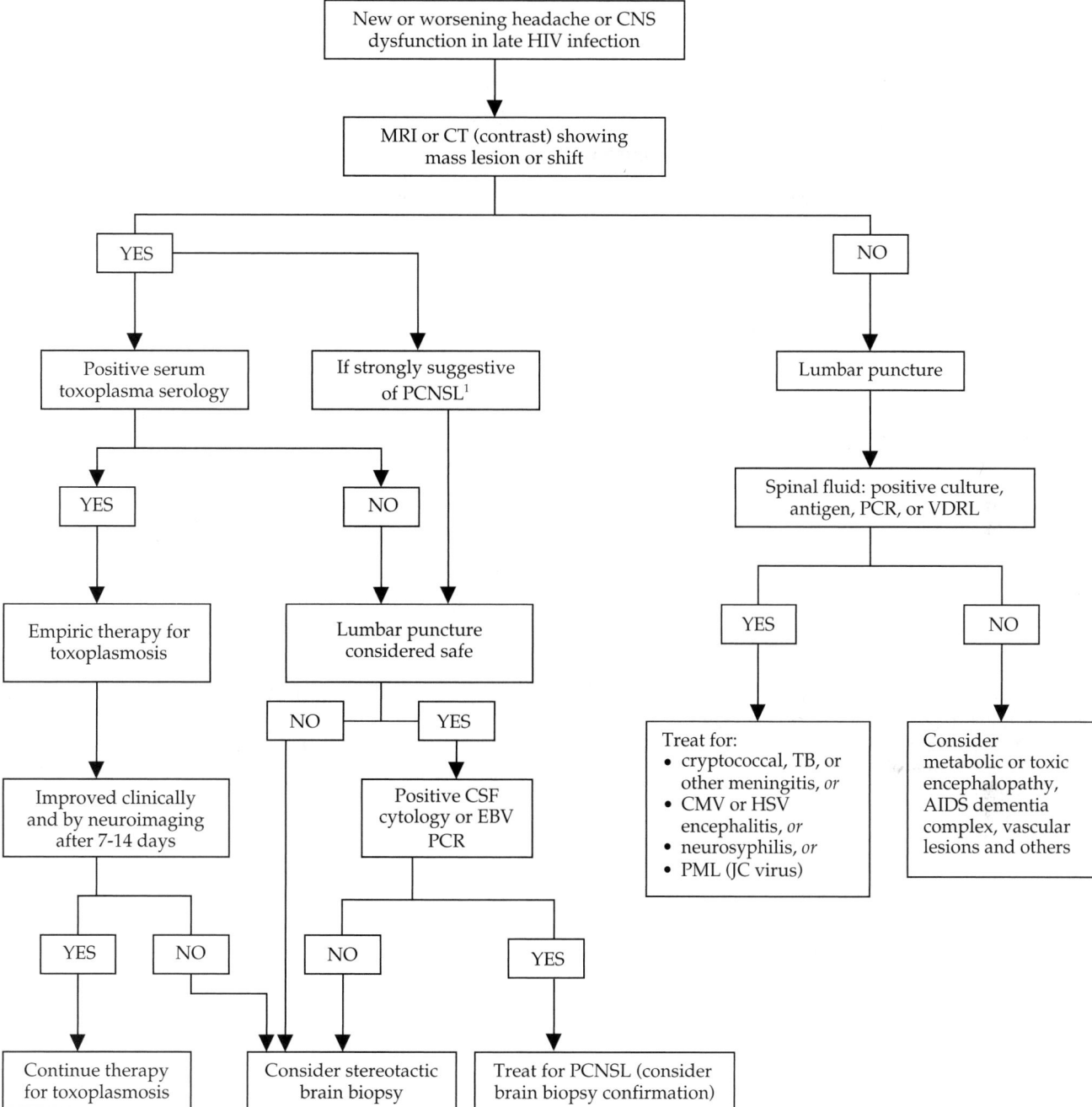

FIGURE 48-9 Approach to the HIV-infected patient with headache or CNS dysfunction.
[1]Factors which favor PCNSL include: i) negative serum serology for toxoplasma, ii) on chronic prophylaxis with TMP-SMX or dapsone, and iii) neuroimaging lesions which are periventricular, or involve deep white matter, or demonstrate diffuse (vs ring enhancement) or weak contrast enhancement.
Abbreviatons: PCNSL, primary central nervous system lymphoma; PCR, polymerase chain reaction; EBV, Epstein-Barr virus; PML, progressive multifocal leukoencephalopathy.

encephalitis. The abrupt onset of focal neurologic deficit suggests either a seizure or vascular disorder. Patients with a CT scan or MRI compatible with toxoplasmosis should be treated empirically (see Table 48-4). The diagnosis of toxoplasmosis usually is presumptive on the basis of a clinical and radiologic response to empirical therapy, without brain biopsy. Early brain biopsy should be considered for patients with mass lesion(s) who are unlikely to have toxoxplasmosis based on the combination of neuroimaging findings, toxoplasma serology, and whether the patient developed the

lesions while taking TMP-SMX or dapsone prophylaxis (see Fig. 48-9). Corticosteroids should be avoided unless there is life-threatening cerebral edema and the risk of brain herniation. Since lymphoma may respond transiently to corticosteroids, coadministration with empirical toxoplasmosis therapy may confound the assessment of response to therapy and reduce the diagnostic yield of brain biopsy. Those who are not responding to empirical therapy, particularly when associated with negative serum serology (IgG) for toxoplasmosis, should be considered for brain biopsy.[93]

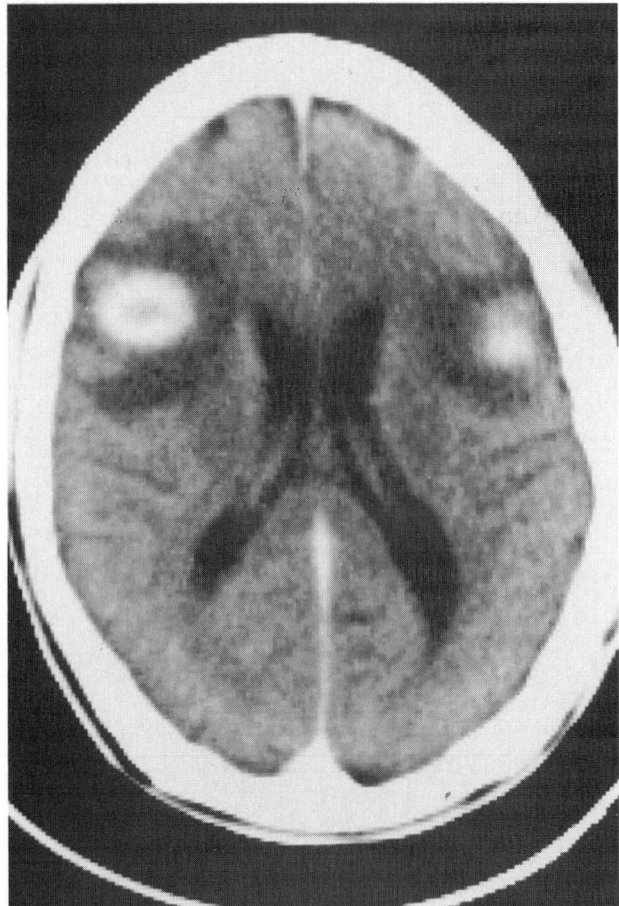

FIGURE 48-10 Double-dose delayed CT scan of the head demonstrating two lesions of cerebral toxoplasmosis. Note the ring-enhancing appearance of the right cerebral lesion.

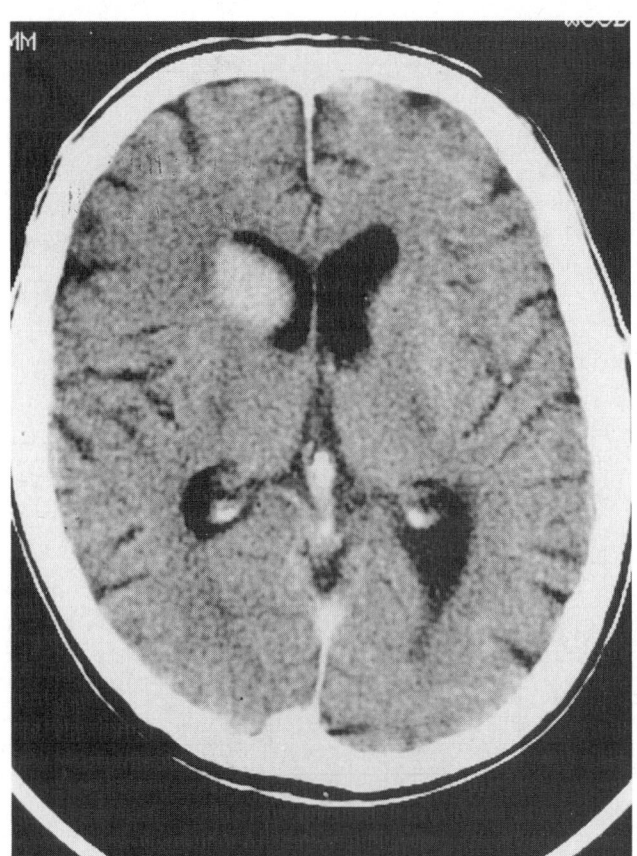

FIGURE 48-11 Double-dose delayed CT scan of the head demonstrating a lesion of cerebral lymphoma in a patient with HIV infection. Note the subependymal localization of the lesion, which is common in cerebral lymphoma.

Although less responsive to therapy, some patients with CNS lymphoma may have a significant response to radiotherapy and chemotherapy. HAART has been associated with improved clinical course and survival time in HIV-related PML for the subset of patients having relatively high CD4 counts and low spinal fluid JC viral load at the time of diagnosis.[94] JC viral load in spinal fluid usually becomes undetectable for PML patients who respond to HAART. A possible role for cidofovir in the management of PML has been suggested by observational studies.[95] Neurosyphilis is responsible only occasionally for focal neurologic deficit, but it is important to consider this treatable condition.[86]

MYELOPATHY, PERIPHERAL NEUROPATHY, AND MYOPATHY

Vacuolar myelopathy is slowly progressive and characterized by diffuse involvement of the spinal cord in HIV-infected individuals. A clinically indistinguishable presentation may be seen in human T-cell lymphotropic virus 1 (HTLV-1) infection. In contrast, a much less common form of myelopathy has a more rapid onset and is associated with segmental pathology of the spinal cord (transverse myelitis). The etiologic agents for this latter condition include lymphoma, varicella-zoster virus (VZV) infection, CMV infection, and toxoplasmosis. CMV occasionally

may cause a subacute progressive polyradiculopathy[96]; patients present with sacral sensory loss, urinary retention, and flaccid paraparesis within days to weeks. The cerebrospinal fluid (CSF) is markedly abnormal in CMV polyradiculopathy, with a polymorphonuclear pleocytosis, hypoglycorrhachia, and elevated protein. CMV may be cultured or demonstrated by PCR from the CSF, but treatment should be started empirically with ganciclovir. Herpes zoster may result in a painful radiculopathy that persists long after resolution of the dermatomal vesicular lesions. However, postherpetic neuralgia is less common in HIV-infected patients.

Peripheral neuropathy may occur at any time during the course of HIV infection. During seroconversion or the latent period (usually CD4 count >500 cells/μL), an inflammatory demyelinating neuropathy may occur with a presentation similar to that of the Guillain-Barré syndrome. This neuropathy may respond to corticosteroids, intravenous immune globulin, or plasmapheresis. Later in the course of HIV infection, an axonal neuropathy, possibly caused by HIV, results in a painful distal neuropathy that is predominantly sensory. Treatment is symptomatic with analgesics or pain-modifying agents (e.g., gabapentin, amitriptyline, or carbamazepine). A similar picture may be caused by drugs, particularly didanosine (ddI), or stavudine (d4T).

AZT has been associated with myopathy, which may present with asymptomatic elevation in the creatine kinase (CK) level or progressive myalgia and weakness, particularly in the proximal leg muscles. AZT should be discontinued in symptomatic patients, and clinical improvement and a decrease in the CK level usually occur within 2 weeks.[97] Muscle biopsy should be considered if the myopathy persists after withdrawal of AZT. If muscle biopsy shows significant inflammatory infiltrates but no opportunistic pathogens or mitochondrial changes, then an immune-mediated myopathy should be suspected. HIV-1-associated myopathy may be mediated by an immune mechanism, and some patients have responded to corticosteroids.[97]

Fungal Infections in the HIV-Infected Patient

CANDIDIASIS

Although candidiasis is the most common opportunistic fungal infection in AIDS, most such infections are limited to mucosal disease involving the oropharynx, esophagus, or vagina. Treatment therefore is aimed at control of symptoms, as outlined in Table 48-4. Deep *Candida* infections (e.g., endophthalmitis or vertebral osteomyelitis) and disseminated candidiasis are encountered rarely in the setting of HIV infection, and in such instances, the usual risk factors for invasive candidiasis often can be identified. These include granulocytopenia, immunosuppressive therapy, prolonged vascular catheterization, recent surgery (e.g., gastrointestinal, cardiac), broad-spectrum antibiotic use, and intravenous drug abuse. Management of candidemia includes removal of any potentially infected vascular catheters and careful assessment for the presence of metastatic sites of infection such as endophthalmitis. Antifungal treatment options for candidemia and other invasive forms of candidiasis include fluconazole,[80,81] amphotericin B, lipid formulations of amphotericin B, and caspofungin, as outlined in Table 48-4.

CRYPTOCOCCOSIS

Although less common now since the introduction of HAART, cryptococcosis occurred in approximately 5% to 10% of individuals at some point during the course of HIV infection in the pre-HAART era (i.e., before 1996). Cryptococcal disease in AIDS usually presents as a subacute to chronic meningitis. However, up to 9% of patients with AIDS-related cryptococcosis develop ARF, which in one series was associated with a 100% mortality rate.[98] The diagnosis of cryptococcal ARF often is not considered before death, but a serum cryptococcal antigen titer is a rapid and sensitive screening test. Predictors of ARF in AIDS-related cryptococcosis are African-American ethnicity, serum LDH concentration of more than 500 IU/L, interstitial infiltrates, and cutaneous lesions.[98] The duration of symptoms before presentation varies from a few days to several weeks. It is important to note that the diagnosis of meningitis may be overlooked because headache and other neurologic symptoms may be mild or absent. Furthermore, meningeal signs are present in only a minority of cases. Other presentations of cryptococcosis include skin lesions and unexplained fever.[99]

An elevated opening pressure at lumbar puncture is common in cryptococcal meningitis. However, the abnormalities in CSF cell count and glucose and protein concentrations may be minimal or absent despite positive results for India ink smear, fungal culture, and cryptococcal antigen. The CSF white blood cell count usually is less than 20/μL and predominantly lymphocytic. The CSF glucose concentration is usually normal but may be low. The serum cryptococcal antigen determination provides a rapid, noninvasive test that is particularly helpful in identifying the HIV-positive patient with extrapulmonary cryptococcal disease.[99] The organism may be cultured from spinal fluid, blood, urine, sputum, and skin lesions. Patients with *C. neoformans* isolated from an extraneural site should be investigated for the presence of disseminated disease, including a lumbar puncture, even in the absence of headache or neurologic symptoms.

A suggested sequence of investigations in the HIV-infected patient with headache or CNS dysfunction is outlined in Fig. 48-9. An HIV-infected patient presenting with an illness compatible with cryptococcosis whose serum cryptococcal antigen titer is positive (except if the titer is 1:8 or less, which may represent a false-positive result) should be started on antifungal therapy before completion of the investigations if there are delays involved in obtaining a CT head scan (or MRI) or contraindications to performing a lumbar puncture (e.g., mass lesion or shift on CT head scan or coagulopathy). Initial treatment of AIDS-related cryptococcal meningitis (see Table 48-4) should be initiated with amphotericin B at 0.7 mg/kg per day (plus flucytosine) rather than with fluconazole.[100,101] The role of flucytosine in the management of AIDS-related cryptococcal meningitis has been controversial, although in a recent randomized trial the addition of flucytosine to amphotericin B was associated with improved CSF sterilization at 2 weeks of treatment (confirmed by multivariate analysis) and fewer subsequent relapses. However, there was no survival benefit.[102] The best-studied alternative treatment is liposomal amphotericin B, which appears to be of equal efficacy but is better tolerated than amphotericin B.[103] Similar results were obtained with liposomal amphotericin at 3 or 6 mg/kg per day compared with conventional amphotericin B at 0.7 mg/kg per day.[103] Limited human and animal studies provide evidence of delayed CSF sterilization with amphotericin B–lipid complex (Ablecet), arguing against its use in the management of cryptococcal meningitis.[104] Investigational approaches to salvage therapy include high-dose fluconazole (800 to 1200 mg/d) plus 5-flucytosine (100 to 150 mg/kg per day divided q6h).[105] Increased intracranial pressure is common, and its documentation and management should not be overlooked.[106] Usually this entails serial lumbar punctures or placement of a CSF shunt in order to reduce intracranial pressure. After a clinical response has been obtained (usually after 2 to 3 weeks), patients should be switched to oral fluconazole at 400 mg daily in order to complete 10 weeks of therapy.[102] Thereafter, the fluconazole dosage is reduced to 200 mg daily and continued lifelong as suppressive therapy, unless the patient undergoes immune reconstitution with antiretroviral therapy (see Table 48-3).[107] An unacceptably high relapse rate has been observed during suppressive therapy with itraconazole at 200 mg daily (24%) compared with fluconazole at 200 mg daily (4%).[108] Despite its importance for initial diagnosis, the serum cryptococcal antigen titer has not been helpful in assessing either the response to initial treatment or a suspected relapse of cryptococcal meningitis.[109]

IRS (immune reconstitution syndrome) has been described in patients with cryptococcosis who subsequently receive

HAART. Presentations may include pulmonary or soft tissue lesions that often are culture-negative but demonstrate organisms consistent with cryptococcus on smear or histology.[110] Others may experience an exacerbation of cryptococcal meningitis associated with a negative CSF culture and a higher than usual CSF pleocytosis.[111] Cryptococcal meningitis also may be unmasked by HAART-induced immune reconstitution. HAART may precipitate symptomatic disease in those with latent CNS cryptococcal infection. Cryptococcal meningitis IRS exacerbation may respond to systemic corticosteroids, according to anecdotal reports. Antiretroviral therapy should be interrupted for life-threatening IRS and possibly reintroduced at a later date along with corticosteroid coadministration.

HISTOPLASMOSIS

In North America, histoplasmosis is usually restricted geographically to the endemic zone extending from Mexico and Texas up through the central United States (especially the Mississippi Valley area) and into eastern Canada. Most patients with histoplasmosis will have a history of exposure to endemic areas. Although less common at present, during the pre-HAART era (before 1996), histoplasmosis occurred in 2% to 5% of HIV-infected patients in endemic areas but in as many as 25% in certain cities. Although over 90% of cases have occurred in patients whose CD4 count was less than 100 cells/μL, histoplasmosis was the first AIDS-defining illness in half the cases.

Histoplasmosis in the context of AIDS is almost always a disseminated infection. The clinical presentation is usually that of a nonspecific febrile illness often accompanied by other features such as pulmonary infiltrates, hepatosplenomegaly, lymphadenopathy, pancytopenia, and liver enzyme elevations.[112] The spectrum of disease ranges from a nonspecific febrile illness (often with constitutional and/or respiratory symptoms) to a syndrome resembling septic shock (10% of patients) with respiratory and multiorgan failure. Chest radiographs reveal diffuse infiltrates (interstitial or reticulonodular) in approximately half the patients, but radiologic findings are normal in one-third of patients.[113] A rapid presumptive diagnosis can be obtained by demonstrating the organism in a buffy coat smear (30% sensitivity), bone marrow biopsy, or occasionally other tissues. The small intracellular yeast forms may be seen within leukocytes. The diagnosis is confirmed by fungal culture (blood, bone marrow, respiratory tract specimens, lymph node, or skin biopsy), although a positive result may take several weeks. Complement-fixation titers are negative in up to 30% of non-AIDS patients with histoplasmosis. Similarly, in AIDS patients, a negative serology for histoplasmosis does not reliably exclude the disease. However, antigen detection in serum and urine is rapid and reliable,[114] but the test is not widely available, and specimens must be sent to the reference laboratory. A helpful clue to the diagnosis of disseminated histoplasmosis is the presence of a markedly elevated serum LDH concentration (>600 IU in 73% of patient in one series),[115] which also may be seen in AIDS-related disseminated toxoplasmosis. Therapy is outlined in Table 48-4. A prospective, double-blind study in moderate to severe AIDS-related disseminated histoplasmosis demonstrated greater efficacy and significantly increased survival with liposomal amphotericin B (3 mg/kg per day) compared with conventional amphotericin B (0.7 mg/kg per day) as induction therapy.[116] Itraconazole is effective therapy for patients with mild to moderate disease.

COCCIDIOIDOMYCOSIS

The endemic zone for coccidioidomycosis in North America is limited to the southwestern United States and extends into northern Mexico. Coccidioidomycosis is an important opportunistic infection in endemic areas, occurring in 6% of HIV-infected patients in Arizona during the pre-HAART era (before 1996).[91] Most patients have a CD4 count of less than 250 cells/μL at the time of diagnosis. This infection should be considered in HIV-infected individuals who have history of exposure to endemic areas and who present with a compatible illness. Clinical features are nonspecific and may include fevers, dyspnea, focal or diffuse pulmonary infiltrates, meningitis, skin lesions, arthritis, and lymphadenopathy. Some patients have fevers and weight loss with no focal lesions.[117] The most common clinical presentations include diffuse or focal pulmonary infiltrates and meningitis. The diagnosis is made by histologic examination and fungal culture of respiratory secretions, tissue biopsies (skin or lymph node), spinal fluid, and blood. The characteristic coccidioidal spherules may be identified using lactophenol cotton blue stain, Gomori's silver methenamine stain, or Papanicolaou's stain. The CSF characteristics in coccidioidal meningitis usually include a pleocytosis of greater than 50 cells/μL that consists of predominantly lymphocytes. The CSF glucose concentration is low, and the protein concentration is elevated. Serology for coccidioidomycosis is positive in approximately 90% of HIV-related cases.[117] Positive CSF serology (complement fixation) for *C. immitis* usually indicates the presence of coccidioidal meningitis. Therapy is outlined in Table 48-4. Fluconazole represents an important advance in the therapy of coccidioidomycosis because of the efficacy and lower side-effect profile of fluconazole compared with amphotericin B. Lifelong suppressive azole therapy is required in coccidioidal meningitis.[118–120] Survival is shortest among patients with diffuse pulmonary disease.

Supportive Care for AIDS Patients in the ICU

Resuscitation and supportive care of AIDS patients in the ICU includes airway protection, noninvasive ventilation, mechanical ventilation, cardiovascular monitoring and support, gastrointestinal and nutritional management, and psychological supportive care. Airway assessment is important in patients who have a depressed level of consciousness, usually because of neurologic problems or systemic sepsis, and in patients who have acute respiratory failure. Detailed discussion of the management of acute hypoxemic respiratory failure is presented in Chap. 38. In general, patients with arterial hypoxemia require supplemental high-flow, high-concentration oxygen. If hypoxemia is refractory to supplemental oxygen, then mask continuous positive airway pressure (CPAP) of 5 to 10 cm H$_2$O may improve arterial hypoxemia and decrease respiratory rate in alert patients who are able to protect their airway.[123] Mask CPAP has been used for up to 11 days. Pneumothorax occurs infrequently, in approximately

5% of patients.[121] Mask CPAP also allows speech and therefore ongoing discussion regarding prognosis and therapeutic options. Noninvasive ventilation using BiPAP also may preclude the need for intubation and mechanical ventilation. Endotracheal intubation and mechanical ventilation are indicated in patients who require airway protection, or who do not respond to CPAP or BiPAP. Assist-control ventilation with positive end-expiratory pressure is usually necessary for PCP patients who require mechanical ventilation.

In patients who meet the criteria of acute lung injury (ALI),[75] lung-protective ventilation with a tidal volume of 6 mL/kg of ideal body weight is recommended because this decreases the mortality of ALI from 40% to 30% (ARDSnet). It is recommended to use the ARDSnet protocol, which includes titration of positive end-expiratory pressure (PEEP) and F_{IO_2} according to a simple algorithm. Use of higher PEEP generally is not recommended because of the risk of barotrauma (especially in PCP) and because a randomized, controlled trial of higher PEEP versus "usual" PEEP (ALVEOLI trial, in press at present time) found no significant improvement in mortality.

Critically ill AIDS patients may develop cardiovascular instability. Systemic arterial catheterization is appropriate for continuous arterial pressure monitoring and arterial blood gas determinations. Hypotension may be caused by hypovolemia, autonomic neuropathy, pentamidine, or septic shock. Hypovolemia may be caused by increased insensible fluid losses, diarrhea, and inadequate intake. Autonomic neuropathy occurs in some AIDS patients and appears to explain the occasionally sudden fatal hypotension and bradycardia.[122] The hypotension that may occur during infusion of pentamidine can be minimized by administering the drug slowly over 4 hours, as described earlier. Hypotension in critically ill AIDS patients may be the result of septic shock owing to bacterial sepsis (e.g., pneumococcus, *H. influenzae, Staphylococcus,* or enteric gram-negative bacilli), PCP, or other systemic fungal infection such as histoplasmosis. Patients who have PCP, similar to patients who have bacterial sepsis, have tachycardia, decreased systemic vascular resistance, increased cardiac output, and hypotension.[123] The clinical approach to management is similar to that for other critically ill patients, detailed in Chap. 46. The evaluation of adrenal insufficiency and use of corticosteroids for septic shock[124] are relevant; furthermore, patients with PCP or suspected PCP should be treated with hydrocortisone, as discussed earlier.

HIV-positive patients who have severe sepsis in the ICU may be eligible for consideration of treatment with recombinant human activated protein C (rhAPC). This treatment option is discussed in more detail in Chap. 46. A large, pivotal randomized clinical trial showed that rhAPC decreased mortality of severe sepsis from 31% to 25%.[125] RhAPC is approved for treatment of patients who have severe sepsis and who are at high risk of death (defined as an APACHE II score >25 or organ system failure involving two or more organs). End-stage disease and end-stage HIV were exclusions in the pivotal trial. However, we recommend consideration of rhAPC in HIV-positive patients admitted to the ICU who have at least an otherwise moderately good prognosis.

Enteropathy, malnutrition, and weight loss are very common gastrointestinal problems in AIDS patients. Up to 30% of AIDS patients have multiple gastrointestinal pathogens.[126]

TABLE 48-6 Causes of Common Gastrointestinal Problems in AIDS Patients

Problem	Organisms
Esophagitis	*Candida*, CMV, HSV
Gastroenteritis	*Cryptosporidium, Microsporidium, Giardia lamblia, Isospora belli, Salmonella,* MAC, CMV
Enterocolitis	*Shigella, Campylobacter, Entamoeba histolytica,* CMV, *Cryptosporidium,* MAC, *Clostridium difficile*
Sexually transmitted proctitis	*N. gonorrhea, Chlamydia trachomatis, Treponema pallidum,* HSV

ABBREVIATIONS: CMV = cytomegalovirus; HSV = herpes simplex virus; MAC = *Mycobacterium avium complex.*

The causes of common gastrointestinal problems in AIDS patients are listed in Table 48-6, and their treatment is outlined in Table 48-4. Esophagitis may be caused by *Candida,* CMV, and herpes simplex virus (HSV). *Candida* esophagitis usually presents with dysphagia, but marked odynophagia suggests either HSV or CMV esophagitis. Oropharyngeal and esophageal *Candida* infection rarely gives rise to deep visceral involvement or disseminated candidiasis. Diarrhea occurs in about 50% of AIDS patients and is caused by gastrointestinal infections, AIDS-associated enteropathy, and much less commonly, gastrointestinal neoplasms. Gastroenteritis may be secondary to *Cryptosporidium, Giardia, Isospora, Salmonella,* MAC, and CMV. *Cryptosporidium* and *Microsporidia* may cause severe diarrhea, and although specific antimicrobial therapy for cryptosporidiosis has not been proved effective, clinical and microbiologic resolution has been reported anecdotally in association with HAART-induced immune reconstitution. Enterocolitis may be the result of infection with *Shigella, Campylobacter, Entamoeba histolytica,* and CMV. Finally, sexually transmitted proctitis caused by gonorrhea, syphilis, *Chlamydia,* or HSV may produce severe rectal symptoms accompanied by frequent small-volume stools associated with blood and mucus. *Clostridium difficile* colitis also should be considered in patients treated recently with antibacterial agents. Others have diarrhea caused by AIDS-associated enteropathy,[127] which may represent an unidentified infectious cause, possibly HIV or an autoimmune disorder.

AIDS patients with esophageal symptoms and thrush may be treated empirically with fluconazole 100 to 200 mg daily. If there is no response, then esophagoscopy and biopsy should be performed. Investigation of diarrhea includes examination of stool for ova and parasites, stool culture and *C. difficile* toxin assay, and occasionally, flexible sigmoidoscopy and upper gastrointestinal endoscopy.[128] The treatment of critically ill AIDS patients who have diarrhea includes bowel rest, antimicrobial therapy for isolated pathogens[126,129] (see Table 48-4), intravenous fluid and electrolytes, symptomatic antidiarrheal therapy, and nutritional therapy. Antimotility agents should be avoided when certain enteric pathogens (e.g., *Salmonella, Shigella, E. histolytica,* and *C. difficile*) are suspected. Total parenteral nutrition may be necessary in critically ill patients who have significant diarrhea because enteral nutrition frequently exacerbates the diarrhea. Malnourished AIDS patients who are critically ill and do not have diarrhea often respond adequately to enteral nutrition supplemented as appropriate with potassium, magnesium, calcium, and phosphate.

AIDS patients, family, and friends also may suffer important emotional and psychological problems that require counseling, psychological support, and the empathy of health care workers. In many communities with a high prevalence of AIDS patients, active peer support groups may be extremely helpful. In addition, family physicians and referring specialists who have long-term care relationships with patients can provide valuable support to the critical care team.

ICU Eligibility of AIDS Patients

The two fundamental issues determining ICU eligibility in a patient with AIDS are the patient's prognosis and the patient's wishes regarding life support. Concerning prognosis, it is necessary to assess both the prognosis of the acute illness necessitating life support and the prognosis of the underlying HIV disease. Prior to the development of AIDS, the prognosis of HIV disease generally was dictated by the CD4 count and the remaining antiretroviral treatment options available. A prognostic staging system had been suggested for patients with AIDS.[130] Various clinical and laboratory abnormalities were scored, and higher scores were associated with shorter survival times. Although this information had been useful in the assessment of eligibility of AIDS patients for life support in the ICU,[131] its applicability in the setting of HAART is unclear.

As in any other critical illness, it is of utmost importance to involve the patient or those close to the patient, whenever possible, in discussions regarding the appropriateness of ICU admission and life support. Often the issue of life support has been considered previously, and the patient has already made his or her wishes known to primary physicians, friends, or relatives.[132] ICU admission and life support generally are inappropriate for patients with life-threatening complications for which there is no particularly effective therapy (e.g., high-grade lymphoma). It is reasonable, however, to offer ICU admission and life support to patients with an acceptable quality of life who have a potentially reversible acute illness.[133]

In every instance, clear goals of ICU admission should be established with the patient, family, and treating physicians. Obviously, a lucid, well-informed patient and his or her family may refuse life support. Finally, it must be emphasized that the outlook of AIDS and its related conditions has improved considerably. For this reason, rigid policies regarding ICU admission are undesirable, and detailed evaluation of each situation on a case-by-case basis is required. For patients who still have antiretroviral therapy options and in whom there is some expectation of partial immune reconstitution, there is no CD4 count that by itself would be considered justification for exclusion of the patient from admission to the ICU. It also should be noted that the initiation of HAART may be associated with clinical improvement in patients with opportunistic diseases for which there is no proven specific effective therapy (e.g., microsporidiosis, cryptosporidiosis, PML, and macrolide-resistant disseminated MAC infection).

Acknowledgment

This work was supported in part by the National Health and Research Development Programme, Health and Welfare, Ottawa, Canada, and the National Institutes of Health. We thank Kelly Hsu for assistance in preparation of the manuscript.

References

1. Ho DD, Neumann AU, Perelson AS, et al: Rapid turnover of plasma virions and CD4 lymphocytes in HIV-1 infection. *Nature* 373:123, 1995.
2. Perelson AS, Neumann AU, Markowitz M, et al: HIV-1 dynamics in vivo: Virion clearance rate, infected cell life-span, and viral generation time. *Science* 271:1582, 1996.
3. UNAIDS AIDS epidemic update, December 2000. Available at http://www.unaids.org/en/default.asp. Accessed on August 20, 2004.
4. Johnson AM, Laga M: Heterosexual transmission of HIV. *AIDS* 2:S49, 1988.
5. Anderson RM, Medley GF: Epidemiology of HIV infection and AIDS: Incubation and infection periods, survival and vertical transmission. *AIDS* 2:S57, 1988.
6. CDC: Guidelines for prevention of transmission of human immunodeficiency virus and hepatitis B virus to health-care and public-safety workers. *MMWR* 38:1, 1989.
7. Cardo DM, Culver DH, Ciesielski CA, et al: A case-control study of HIV seroconversion in health care workers after percutaneous exposure. *N Engl J Med* 337:1485, 1997.
8. Gerberding JL: Occupational exposure to HIV in health care settings. *New Engl J Med* 348:826, 2003.
9. Pantaleo G, Graziosi C, Fauci AS: New concepts in the immunopathogenesis of human immunodeficiency virus infection. *N Engl J Med* 328:327, 1993.
10. Kahn JO, Walker BD: Acute human immunodeficiency virus type-1 infection. *N Engl J Med* 339:33, 1998.
11. Pantaleo G, Graziosi C, Demarest JM, et al: HIV infection is active and progressive in lymphoid tissue during the clinically latent stage of disease. *Nature* 362:355, 1993.
12. Schechter MT, Craib KJP, Le TN, et al: Progression to AIDS and predictors of AIDS in seroprevalent and seroincident cohorts of homosexual men. *AIDS* 3:347, 1989.
13. Mellors JW, Rinaldo CR Jr, Gupta P, et al: Prognosis in HIV-1 infection predicted by the quantity of virus in plasma. *Science* 272:1167, 1996.
14. Yeni PG, Hammer SM, Carpenter CCJ, et al: Antiretroviral treatment for adult HIV infection in 2002. *JAMA* 288:222, 2002.
15. Dybul M, Fauci AS, Bartlett JG, et al: Guidelines for using antiretroviral agents among HIV-infected adults and adolescents: Recommendations of the panel on clinical practices for treatment of HIV. *MMWR* 52:1, 2002.
16. Flora GS, Modilevksy T, Antoniskis D, Barnes PF: Undiagnosed tuberculosis in patients with human immunodeficiency virus infection. *Chest* 98:1056, 1990.
17. Lee N, Hui D, Wu A, et al: A major outbreak of severe acute respiratory syndrome in Hong Kong. *N Engl J Med* 348:1986, 2003.
18. Chen XP, Li GH, Tang XP, et al: Lack of severe acute respiratory syndrome in 19 AIDS patients hospitalized together. *J AIDS* 34:242, 2003.
19. Montaner JSG, Zala C: The role of the laboratory in the diagnosis and management of AIDS-related *Pneumocystis carinii* pneumonia. *Ballieres Clin Infect Dis* 2;471, 1995.
20. Levine SJ, White DA: *Pneumocystis carinii*. *Clin Chest Med* 9:395, 1988.
21. Golden JA, Sollitto RA: The radiology of pulmonary disease. *Clin Chest Med* 9:481, 1988.
22. Masur H, Kaplan JE, Holmes KK: Guidelines for preventing opportunistic infections among HIV-infected persons—2002. *Ann Intern Med* 137:435, 2002.
23. Montaner JSG, Russell JR, Lawson LM, Ruedy J: Acute respiratory failure secondary to *Pneumocystis carinii* pneumonia in

the acquired immunodeficiency syndrome: A potential role for systemic corticosteroids. *Chest* 95:881, 1989.

24. Young KR, Rankin JA, Naegel GP, Reynolds HY: Bronchoalveolar lavage cells and proteins in patients with acquired immunodeficiency syndrome. *Ann Intern Med* 103:522, 1985.

25. Telzak EE, Cote RJ, Gold JWM, et al: Extrapulmonary *Pneumocystis carinii* infections. *Rev Infect Dis* 12:380, 1990.

26. DeSimone JA, Pomerantz RJ, Babinchak TJ: Inflammatory reactions in HIV-1-infected persons after initiation of highly active antiretroviral therapy. *Ann Intern Med* 133:447, 2000.

27. Shelburne SA, Hamill RJ, Rodriguez-Barradas MC, et al: Immune reconstitution inflammatory syndrome: Emergence of a unique syndrome during highly active antiretroviral therapy. *Medicine* 81:213, 2002.

28. Chen VCC, Yuen K, Chan W, et al: Immunorestitution disease involving the innate and adaptive response. *Clin Infect Dis* 30:882, 2000.

29. Phillips P, Kwiatkowski MB, Copland M, et al: Mycobacterial lymphadenitis associated with the initiation of combination antiretroviral therapy. *J AIDS* 20:122, 1999.

30. Dean GL, Williams DI, Churchill DR, et al: Transient clinical deterioration in HIV patients with *Pneumocystis carinii* pneumonia after starting highly active antiretroviral therapy: Another case of immune restoration inflammatory syndrome. *Am J Resp Crit Care Med* 165:1670, 2002.

31. Barry SM, Lipman MCI, Deery AR, et al: Immune reconstitution pneumonitis following *Pneumocystis carinii* pneumonia in HIV-infected subjects. *HIV Med* 3:207, 2002.

32. Wislez M, Bergot E, Antoine M, et al: Acute respiratory failure following HAART introduction in patients treated for *Pneumocystis carinii* pneumonia. *Am J Respir Crit Care Med* 164:847, 2001.

33. Wharton BM, Coleman DL, Wofsy CB, et al: Prospective, randomized trial of trimethoprim-sulfamethoxazole versus pentamidine for *Pneumocystis carinii* pneumonia in the acquired immunodeficiency syndrome. *Ann Intern Med* 105:37, 1986.

34. Gordin FM, Simon GL, Wofsy CB, Mills J: Adverse reactions to trimethoprim-sulfamethoxazole in patients with acquired immunodeficiency syndrome. *Ann Intern Med* 100:495, 1984.

35. Leoung GS, Feigal DW, Montgomery AB, et al: Aerosolized pentamidine for prophylaxis against *Pneumocystis carinii* pneumonia. The San Francisco Community Prophylaxis Trial. *N Engl J Med* 323:769, 1990.

36. Montaner JSG, Lawson LM, Gervais A, et al: Aerosol pentamidine for the secondary prophylaxis of AIDS-related *Pneumocystis carinii* pneumonia: A placebo-controlled study. *Ann Intern Med* 114:948, 1991.

37. Armstrong G, Bernard E: Aerosol pentamidine. *Ann Intern Med* 109:852, 1988.

38. Medina I, Mills J, Leoung G, et al: Oral therapy for *Pneumocystis carinii* pneumonia in the acquired immunodeficiency syndrome: A controlled trial of trimethoprim-sulfamethoxazole versus trimethoprim-dapsone. *N Engl J Med* 323:776, 1990.

39. Hughes W, Leoung G, Kramer F, et al: Comparison of Atovaquone (566C80) with trimethoprim-sulfamethoxazole to treat *Pneumocystis carinii* pneumonia in patients with AIDS. *N Engl J Med* 328:1521, 1993.

40. Toma E, Fournier S, Dumont M, et al: Clindamycin/primaquine versus trimethoprim-sulfamethoxazole as primary therapy for *Pneumocystis carinii* pneumonia in AIDS: A randomized, double-blind pilot trial. *Clin Infect Dis* 17:178, 1993.

41. Allegra CJ, Chabner BA, Tauzon CV, et al: Trimetrexate for the treatment of *Pneumocystis carinii* pneumonia in patients with the acquired immunodeficiency syndrome. *N Engl J Med* 317:978, 1987.

42. Montaner JSG, Lawson LM, Levitt N, et al: Corticosteroids prevent early deterioration in patients with moderately severe AIDS-related *Pneumocystis carinii* pneumonia and the acquired immunodeficiency syndrome (AIDS). *Ann Intern Med* 113:15, 1990.

43. Gagnon S, Boota AM, Fischl MA, et al: Corticosteroids as adjunctive therapy for severe *Pneumocystis carinii* pneumonia in the acquired immunodeficiency syndrome: A double-blind placebo-controlled study. *N Engl J Med* 323:1444, 1990.

44. Consensus statement on the use of corticosteroids as adjunctive therapy for *Pneumocystis* pneumonia in the acquired immunodeficiency syndrome. *N Engl J Med* 323:1500, 1990.

45. Guillemi S, Belzberg A, Lawson LM, et al: Adjunctive corticosteroid therapy decreases lung permeability in patients with AIDS-related *Pneumocystis carinii* pneumonia. *Can Respir J* 2:55, 1995.

46. Bartlett JG, Dowell SF, Mandell LA, et al: Practice guidelines for the management of community-acquired pneumonia in adults. *Clin Infect Dis* 31:347, 2000.

47. Mei Q, Gurunathan S, Masur H, et al: Failure of co-trimoxazole in *Pneumocystis carinii* infection and the mutations in dihydropteroate synthase gene. *Lancet* 351:1631, 1998.

48. Helweg-Larsen J, Benfield TL, Eugen-Olsen J, et al: Effects of mutations in *Pneumocystis carinii* dihydropteroate synthase gene on outcome of AIDS-associated *P. carinii* pneumonia. *Lancet* 354:1318, 1999.

49. Navin TR, Beard CB, Huang L, et al: Effects of mutations in *Pneumocystis carinii* dihydropteroate synthase gene on outcome of *P. carinii* pneumonia in patients with HIV-1: A prospective study. *Lancet* 358:545, 2001.

50. El-Sadr W, Simberkoff MS: Survival and prognostic factors in severe *Pneumocystis carinii* pneumonia requiring mechanical ventilation. *Am Rev Respir Dis* 137:1264, 1988.

51. Wachter MW, Luce JM, Turner J, et al: Intensive care of patients with the acquired immunodeficiency syndrome: Outcome and changing patterns of utilization. *Am Rev Respir Dis* 134:891, 1986.

52. Steinbrook R, Lo B, Moulton J, et al: Preferences of homosexual men with AIDS for life-sustaining treatment. *N Engl J Med* 314:457, 1986.

53. Quieffen J, Ronco JJ, Russell JA, et al: Worsening survival of mechanically ventilated acute respiratory failure secondary to AIDS-related PCP. *Clin Invest Med* B21:123, 1990.

54. Perlman DC, El-Sadr WM, Nelson ET, et al: Variation of chest radiographic patterns in pulmonary tuberculosis by degree of human immunodeficiency virus–related immunosuppression. *Clin Infect Dis* 25:242, 1997.

55. Havlir D. Barnes PF. Tuberculosis in patients with human immunodeficiency virus infection. *N Engl J Med* 340:367, 1999.

56. American Thoracic Society/Centers for Disease Control and Prevention/Infectious Diseases Society of America: Treatment of tuberculosis. *Am J Respir Crit Care Med* 167:603, 2003.

57. Bloch AB, Cauthen GM, Onorato IM, et al: Nationwide survey of drug-resistant tuberculosis in the United States. *JAMA* 271:665, 1994.

58. Salomon N, Perlman DC, Friedmann P, et al: Predictors and outcome of multidrug-resistant tuberculosis. *Clin Infect Dis* 21:1245, 1995.

59. Narita M, Ashkin D, Hollender ES, et al: Paradoxical worsening of tuberculosis following antiretroviral therapy in patients with AIDS. *Am J Respir Crit Care Med* 158:157, 1998.

60. Burman W, Benator D, Vernon A, et al: Use of antiretroviral therapy during treatment of active tuberculosis with a rifabutin-based regimen. Conference on Retroviruses and Opportunistic Infections, Boston, 2003, abstract 136.

61. Navas E, Martin-Davila P, Moreno L, et al: Paradoxical reactions of tuberculosis in patients with the acquired immunodeficiency syndrome who are treated with highly active antiretroviral therapy. *Arch Intern Med* 162:97, 2002.

62. Benson CA, Ellner JJ: *Mycobacterium avium* complex infection and AIDS: Advances in theory and practice. *Clin Infect Dis* 17:7, 1993.

63. Chin DP, Reingold AL, Horsburg CR, et al: Predicting *Mycobacterium avium* complex bacteremia in patients infected with human immunodeficiency virus: A prospectively validated model. *Clin Infect Dis* 19:668, 1994.

64. Shafran SD, Singer J, Zarowny DP, et al: Rifabutin, ethambutol and clarithromycin versus rifampin, ethambutol, clofazimine and ciprofloxacin for *Mycobacterium avium* complex bacteremia in AIDS patients: A prospective, randomized, multicenter, comparative trial (CTN 010). *N Engl J Med* 335:377, 1996.

65. Cohn DL, Fisher EJ, Peng GT, et al: A prospective, randomized trial of four three-drug regimens in the treatment of disseminated *Mycobacterium avium* complex disease in AIDS patients: Excess mortality associated with high-dose clarithromycin. *Clin Infect Dis* 29:125, 1999.

66. Chaisson RE, Keiser P, Pierce M, et al: Clarithromycin and ethambutol with or without clofazimine for the treatment of bacteremic *Mycobacterium avium* complex disease in patients with HIV infection. *AIDS* 11:311, 1997.

67. Gordin FM, Sullam PM, Shafran SD, et al: A randomized, placebo-controlled study of rifabutin added to a regimen of clarithromycin and ethambutol for treatment of disseminated infection with *Mycobacterium avium* complex. *Clin Infect Dis* 28:1080, 1999.

68. Havlir DV, Dube MP, Sattler FR, et al: Prophylaxis against disseminated *Mycobacterium avium* complex with weekly azithromycin, daily rifabutin, or both. *N Engl J Med* 335:392, 1996.

69. Bozzette SA, Arcia J, Bartok AE, et al: Impact of *Pneumocystis carinii* and cytomegalovirus on the course and outcome of atypical pneumonia in patients with advanced human immunodeficiency virus. *J Infect Dis* 165:93, 1992.

70. Jacobson MA, Mills J: Cytomegalovirus infection. *Clin Chest Med* 9:443, 1988.

71. Zurlo JJ, O'Niell D, Polis MA, et al: Lack of clinical utility of cytomegalovirus blood and urine cultures in patients with HIV infection. *Ann Intern Med* 118:12, 1993.

72. Drew WL, Ives D, Lalezari JP, et al: Oral ganciclovir as maintenance treatment for cytomegalovirus retinitis in patients with AIDS. *N Engl J Med* 333:615, 1995.

73. Friedland IR, McCracken GH Jr: Management of infections caused by antibiotic-resistant streptococcus pneumoniae. *N Engl J Med* 331:377, 1994.

74. Levine DP, Fromm BS, Reddy BR: Slow response to vancomycin or vancomycin plus rifampin in methicillin-resistant staphylococcus aureus endocarditis. *Ann Intern Med* 114:674, 1991.

75. The Acute Respiratory Distress Syndrome Network: Ventilation with lower tidal volumes as compared with traditional tidal volumes for acute lung injury and the acute respiratory distress syndrome. *N Engl J Med* 342:1301, 2000.

76. Khoo SH, Denning DW: Invasive aspergillosis in patients with AIDS. *Clin Infect Dis* 19(suppl 1):S41, 1994.

77. Staples CA, Kang EY, Wright JL, et al: Invasive pulmonary aspergillosis in AIDS: Radiographic, CT, and pathologic findings. *Radiology* 196:409, 1995.

78. Laine L, Dretler RH, Conteas CN, et al: Fluconazole compared with ketoconazole for the treatment of *Candida* esophagitis in AIDS: A randomized trial. *Ann Intern Med* 117:655, 1992.

79. Phillips P, Zemcov J, Mahmood W, et al: Itraconazole cyclodextrin solution for fluconazole-refractory orpharyngeal candidiasis in AIDS: Correlation of clinical response with in vitro susceptibility. *AIDS* 10:1369, 1996.

80. Rex JH, Bennett JE, Sugar AM, et al: A randomized trial comparing fluconazole with amphotericin B for the treatment of candidemia in patients without neutropenia. Candidemia Study Group and the National Institute. *N Engl J Med* 331:1325, 1994.

81. Phillips P, Shafran S, Garber G, et al: Multicentre randomized trial of fluconazole versus amphotericin B for treatment of candidemia in non-neutropenic patients. *Eur J Clin Microbiol Infect Dis* 16:337, 1997.

82. Ognibene FP, Shelhamer JH: Kaposi's sarcoma. *Clin Chest Med* 9:459, 1988.

83. McArthur JC: Neurologic manifestations of AIDS. *Medicine* 66:407, 1987.

84. Price RW: Neurologic disease, in Dolin R, Masur H, Saag M (eds): *AIDS Therapy,* 2d ed. New York, Churchill Livingstone, 2003, p 737.

85. Dannemann B, McCutchan A, Israelski D, et al: Treatment of toxoplasmic encephalitis in patients with AIDS: A randomized trial comparing pyrimethamine plus clindamycin to pyrimethamine plus sulfadiazine. *Ann Intern Med* 116:33, 1992.

86. Centers for Diseases Control and Prevention: Sexually transmitted diseases treatment guidelines—2002. *MMWR* 51:1, 2002.

87. Gordon SM, Eaton ME, Goerge R, et al: The response of symptomatic neurosyphilis to high-dose intravenous penicillin G in patients with human immunodeficiency virus infection. *N Engl J Med* 331:1469, 1994.

88. Hook EW: Management of syphilis in human immunodeficiency virus-infected patients. *Am J Med* 93:477, 1992.

89. Berenguer J, Moreno S, Labuna F, et al: Tuberculous meningitis in patients infected with the human immunodeficiency virus. *N Engl J Med* 326:668, 1992.

90. Scarpellini P, Racca S, Cinque P, et al: Nested polymerase chain reaction for diagnosis and monitoring treatment response in AIDS patients with tuberculous meningitis. *AIDS* 9:895, 1995.

91. Fish DG, Ampel NM, Galgiani JN, et al: Coccidioidomycoasis during human immunodeficiency virus infection: A review of 77 patients. *Medicine* 59:384, 1990.

92. Sidtis JJ, Constantine G, Price RW, et al: Zidovudine treatment of the AIDS dementia complex: Results of a placebo-controlled trial. *Ann Neurol* 33:343, 1993.

93. Murray HW, Katlama C: Toxoplasmosis, in Dolin R, Masur H, Saag M (eds): *AIDS Therapy,* 2d ed. New York, Churchill Livingstone, 2003, p 419.

94. Taoufik Y, Delfraissy J-F, Gasnault J: Highly active antiretroviral therapy does not improve survival of patients with high JC virus load in the cerebrospinal fluid at progressive multifocal leukoencephalopathy diagnosis. *AIDS* 14:758, 2000.

95. De Luca A, Giancola ML, Ammasari A, et al: Cidofovir added to HAART improves virologic and clinical outcome in AIDS-associated progressive multifocal leukoencephalopathy. *AIDS* 14:F117, 2000.

96. Miller RG, Storey JR, Greco CM: Ganciclovir in the treatment of progressive AIDS-related polyradiculopathy. *Neurology* 40:596, 1990.

97. Till M, MacDonell KB: Myopathy with human immunodeficiency virus type 1 (HIV-1) infection: HIV-1 or zidovudine. *Ann Intern Med* 113:492, 1990.

98. Visnegarwala F, Graviss EA, Lacke CE, et al: Acute respiratory failure associated with cryptococcosis in patients with AIDS: Analysis of predictive factors. *Clin Infect Dis* 27:1231, 1998.

99. Chuck SL, Sande MA: Infections with *Cryptococcus neoformans* in acquired immunodeficiency syndrome. *N Engl J Med* 321:794, 1989.

100. Larsen RA, Leal MAE, Chan LS: Fluconazole compared with amphotericin B plus flucytosine for cryptococcal meningitis in AIDS: A randomized trial. *Ann Intern Med* 113:183, 1990.

101. Saag MS, Powderly WG, Cloud GA, et al: Comparison of amphotericin B with fluconazole in the treatment of acute AIDS-associates cryptococcal meningitis. *N Engl J Med* 326:83, 1992.

102. van der Horst C, Saag MS, Cloud GA, et al: Treatment of cryptococcal meningitis associated with the acquired immunodeficiency syndrome. *N Engl J Med* 337:15, 1997.

103. Hamill RJ, Sobel J, El-Sadr W, et al: Randomized double-blind trial of AmBisome [liposomal amphotericin B] and amphotericin B in acute cryptococcal meningitis in AIDS patients. ICAAC Meeting, San Francisco, 1999, abstract 1161.

104. Sharkey PK, Graybill JR, Johnson ES, et al: Amphotericin B lipid complex compared with amphotericin B in the treatment of cryptococcal meningitis in patients with AIDS. *Clin Infect Dis* 22:315, 1996.

105. Milefchik E, Leal M, Haubrich R, et al: A phase II dose escalation trial of high dose fluconazole with and without flucytosine for AIDS associated cryptococcal meningitis. Fourth Conference on Retroviruses and Opportunistic Infections, Washington, January 1997, abstract 5.

106. Graybill JR, Sobel J, Saag M, et al: Diagnosis and management of increased intracranial pressure in patients with AIDS and cryptococcal menigitis. *Clin Infect Dis* 30:47, 2000.

107. Vibhagool A, Sungkanuparph S, Mootsikapun P, et al: Discontinuation of secondary prophylaxis for cryptococcal meningitis in human immunodeficiency virus–infected patients treated with highly active antiretroviral therapy: A prospective, multicenter, randomized study. *Clin Infect Dis* 36:1329, 2003.

108. Saag MS, Cloud GC, Graybill JR, et al: Comparison of fluconazole versus itraconazole as maintenance therapy of AIDS-associated cryptococcal meningitis. Thirty-Fifth Interscience Conference on Antimicrobial Agents and Chemotherapy, San Francisco, September 17–20, 1995, abstract I218, p 244.

109. Powderly WG, Cloud GA, Dismukes WE, Saag MS.: Measurement of cryptococcal antigen in serum and cerebrospinal fluid: Value in the management of AIDS-associated cryptococcal meningtitis. *Clin Infect Dis* 18:789, 1994.

110. Jenny-Avital ER, Abadi M: Immune reconstitution cryptococcosis after initiation of successful highly active antiretroviral therapy. *Clin Infect Dis* 35:e128033, 2002.

111. Woods, ML, MacGinley R, Eisen DP, Allworth AM: HIV combination therapy: Partial immune restitution unmasking latent cryptococcal infection. *AIDS* 12:1491, 1998.

112. Wheat LJ, Connoly-Stringfield PA, Baker RL, et al: Dissemnated histoplasmosis in the acquired immunodeficiency syndrome: Clinical findings, diagnosis and treatment, and review of the literature. *Medicine* 69:361, 1990.

113. Sarosi GA, Johnson PC: Disseminated histoplasmosis in patients infected with human immunodeficiency virus. *Clin Infect Dis* 14(suppl 1):S60, 1992.

114. Wheat J, Kohler RB, Tewari RP: Diagnosis of disseminated histoplasmosis by detection of *Histoplasma capsulatum* antigen in serum and urine specimens. *N Engl J Med* 314:83, 1986.

115. Corcoran GR, Al-Abdely H, Flanders CD, et al: Markedly elevated serum lactate dehydrogenase levels are a clue to the diagnosis of disseminated histoplasmsosis in patients with AIDS. *Clin Infect Dis* 24:942, 1997.

116. Johnson PC, Wheat LJ, Cloud GA, et al: Safety and efficacy of liposomal amphotericin B compared with conventional amphotericin B for induction therapy of histoplasmosis in patients with AIDS. *Ann Intern Med* 137:135, 2002.

117. Galgiani JN, Ampel NM: Coccidioidomycosis in human immunodeficiency virus–infected patients. *J Infect Dis* 162:1165, 1990.

118. Galgiani JN, Catazaro A, Cloud GA, et al: Fluconazole therapy for coccidioidal meningitis. *Ann Intern Med* 119:28, 1993.

119. Tucker RM, Denning DW, Dupont B, Stevens DA: Itraconazole therapy for chronic coccidioidal meningitis. *Ann Intern Med* 112:108, 1990.

120. Dewsnup DH, Galgiani JN, Graybill R, et al: Is it ever safe to stop azole therapy for coccidioides immitis meningitis? *Ann Intern Med* 124:305, 1996.

121. Greg RW, Friedman BC, Williams JF, et al: Continuous positive airway pressure by face mask in *Pneumocystis carinii* pneumonia. *Crit Care Med* 18:21, 1990.

122. Craddock C, Pasvol G, Bull R, et al: Cardiorespiratory arrest and autonomic neuropathy in AIDS. *Lancet* 2:16, 1987.

123. Ronco JJ, Montaner JSG, Fenwick JC, et al: Pathologic dependence of oxygen delivery in acute respiratory failure secondary to AIDS-related *Pneumocystis carinii* pneumonia. *Chest* 98:1463, 1990.

124. Annane D, Sébille V, Charpentier C, et al: Effect of treatment with low doses of hydrocortisone and fludrocortisone on mortality in patients with septic shock. *JAMA* 288:862, 2002.

125. Bernard GR, Vincent J, Laterre P, et al, for the Recombinant Human Activated Protein C Worldwide Evaluation in Severe Sepsis [PROWESS] Study Group: Efficacy and safety of recombinant human activated protein C for severe sepsis. *N Engl J Med* 344;699, 2001.

126. Smith PD, Quinn TC, Strober W, et al: Gastrointestinal infections in AIDS. *Ann Intern Med* 116:63, 1992.

127. Bartlett JG, Belitsos PC, Sears CL: AIDS enteropathy. *Clin Infect Dis* 15:726, 1992.

128. Johanson JR, Sonnenberg A: Efficient management of diarrhea in the acquired immunodeficiency syndrome (AIDS). *Ann Intern Med* 112:942, 1990.

129. Pape JW, Verdier RI, Johnson WD Jr: Treatment and prophylaxis of *Isospora belli* infection in patients with the acquired immunodeficiency syndrome. *N Engl J Med* 320:1044, 1989.

130. Justice AC, Feinstein AR, Wells CK: A new prognostic staging system for the acquired immunodeficiency syndrome. *N Engl J Med* 320:1288, 1989.

131. Wachter RM, Luce JM, Lo B, Raffin TA: Ethics in cardiopulmonary medicine: Life-sustaining treatment for patients with AIDS. *Chest* 95:647, 1989.

132. Smedira NG, Evans BH, Grais LS, et al: Withholding and withdrawal of life support from the critically ill. *N Engl J Med* 322:309, 1990.

133. Bone RC, Rackow EC, Weg JC, and members of the ACCP/SCCM Consensus Panel: Ethical and moral guidelines for the initiation, continuation, and withdrawal of intensive care. *Chest* 94:949, 1990.

Chapter 49 _____

ENDOCARDITIS AND OTHER INTRAVASCULAR INFECTIONS

JAMES M. SIZEMORE, JR.
C. GLENN COBBS
MARK B. CARR

KEY POINTS

- *The possibility of intravascular infection should be considered in all critically ill patients with bacteremia or fungemia of uncertain origin, particularly when there are known intravascular or endocardial abnormalities or intravascular devices; fever or hemodynamic instability of unclear origin; or signs of inflammation related to an indwelling intravascular device.*

- *Blood cultures are the most important diagnostic test for this group of infections because most intravascular infections will result in persistent bacteremia or fungemia.*

- *Successful therapy often requires prolonged administration of microbicidal agents plus removal of devices.*

- *Certain microbes, including staphylococci, enterococci, aerobic gram-negative bacilli, and yeasts, are especially likely to cause intravascular infectious disease.*

Patients hospitalized in ICUs may have an intravascular infectious disorder as their primary problem, as a complication of their main disorder, or as a nosocomial infection occurring during their stay. Specific populations common to the ICU, including hemodialysis patients, injection drug users, HIV-infected patients, and those with congenital heart disease, are at increased risk of intravascular infection. Furthermore, violation of anatomic barriers by indwelling intravascular devices and by surgery, as well as impairment of cellular or humoral immune function related to critical illness, contributes to invasion by a variety of microbial pathogens. Infections of intravascular foreign bodies or native vascular structures themselves are likely to be associated not only with symptoms and signs of local inflammation but also with evidence of disseminated disease due to metastatic spread of infectious agents. This chapter provides the clinician caring for patients in an ICU with an approach to the patient with suspected or proved intravascular infectious disorders. We will emphasize the underlying clinical situations that predispose to intravascular infection, the pathogenesis of the disorders, the symptoms and signs of disease, and the appropriate diagnostic procedures, particularly those that provide assistance in the choice of antimicrobial therapy and selection of ancillary medical and surgical procedures. Table 49-1 lists the intravascular infections of native vessels and those associated with intravascular devices, respectively.

Intravascular Infections in the Absence of Any Foreign Device

INFECTIVE ENDOCARDITIS ON A NATIVE VALVE

PATHOGENESIS

The pathogenesis of infective endocarditis (IE) usually involves transient bloodstream invasion by microorganisms, followed by adherence of the organism to the endocardial surface and multiplication of the microorganism within a layer of platelets and fibrin that is relatively inaccessible to host phagocytic defenses. The likelihood that a patient with or without underlying valvular heart disease may develop IE depends on the species and concentration of microorganisms in the blood, the duration of the bloodstream invasion, the presence or absence of antimicrobial agents in serum at the time of bacteremia/fungemia, and the characteristics of the endocardium. Clearly, some microorganisms are much more likely to adhere to endocardium than others. *Staphylococcus aureus*, enterococci, and other streptococci are most adherent. Enteric gram-negative bacilli and anaerobic microorganisms are less so. Since *S. aureus* is adherent and invasive, is found commonly on the skin, and causes skin infection that can result in transient bacteremia, this organism is associated with acute bacterial endocarditis, even in patients without significant underlying valvular heart disease. *Viridans*-type streptococci, which are normal flora of the upper airway, may gain access to the bloodstream from trauma to the teeth or gingiva (as in dental work) and cause IE nearly always in a patient with a significant predisposing valvular abnormality. Many distinctions between acute and subacute endocarditis are blurred. Enteric gram-negative organisms, because they are much less adherent to endocardium, cause fewer cases of endocarditis relative to the frequency of bacteremia caused by these organisms. However, gram-negative organisms that have a greater propensity to adhere to surfaces, such as *Pseudomonas aeruginosa*, and that can gain access to the circulation via contaminated intravenous injections (as in drug abusers) or infection at other body sites produce a significant proportion of cases. The most common nosocomial pathogenesis of IE in critically ill patients is from central venous catheters, with peripheral IVs and urologic instrumentation also identified as sources.[1–4]

CLINICAL AND LABORATORY FEATURES

Table 49-2 lists the most common signs and symptoms encountered in patients with native-valve IE. Table 49-3 lists the most commonly encountered laboratory abnormalities. Because most reports stress community-acquired disease, patients developing IE while hospitalized in an ICU may not manifest identical findings. Fernandez-Guerrero and colleagues[1] reported fever in 100% of patients with hospital-acquired IE. A murmur was present in only 20% of patients with vascular catheter–associated IE but was present in 75% of patients with IE following a urologic procedure. Still, fever and a heart murmur are the most common findings in IE; both are found in at least 80% of patients with community-acquired left-sided IE. The incidence is less in patients with right-sided disease only.[5]

A number of peripheral manifestations may be present in patients with IE. A number of skin lesions occur, petechiae

TABLE 49-1 Intravascular Infection of Native Vessels and Implanted Intravascular Devices

Site	Infectious Disorder	Comment
Medium and large arteries	Mycotic aneurysm	Abdominal aortic aneurysms; various sites complicating endocarditis
Intracranial	Cavernous sinus thrombosis	Follows facial cellulitis, *Staphylococcus aureus* common etiology
Heart and major vessels	Native-valve endocarditis	Usually occurs at site of prior endocardial damage
	Prosthetic-valve endocarditis	Risk of infection on mitral equals aortic valve risk
	Permanent pacemaker infection	Risks include diabetes, malignancy, corticosteroid use, bacteremia, or skin erosion over generator box
	Arterial graft infection	Increased risk if graft crosses groin; risk greatest in first year after placement
Head and neck venous structures	Postanginal sepsis	*Fusobacterium, Bacteroides* common; metastatic disease frequent
Pelvic veins	Pelvic vein thrombophlebitis	Following septic abortion, pelvic inflammatory disease in women
Portal veins	Pylephlebitis	Complication of intra-abdominal abscess; perforated appendix, peridiverticular abscess, etc.

being most common. These are 1- to 2-mm red, nonblanching macules that become darker and fade within 2 to 3 days. These are seen in less than 50% of patients but, when present, are seen most often on the conjunctiva, soft palate, and distal portions of the extremities.[6] Vascular hemorrhages in the optic fundus are referred to as *Roth spots*. Splinter hemorrhages are vascular hemorrhages occurring under the nails, and often they are difficult to distinguish from traumatic lesions. Splinter hemorrhages due to trauma are more common and are more typically an isolated finding. Osler nodes are erythematous, tender subcutaneous papules that occur on the finger pads (Fig. 49-1 and Color Figure 49-1). They are 2 to 5 mm in diameter and may be multiple. Janeway lesions are painless, erythematous macules, larger than Osler nodes, that occur on the palms and soles (Fig. 49-2 and Color Figure 49-2). It is unclear whether Osler nodes and Janeway lesions are due to septic emboli directly or to immunologic phenomena.

Systemic emboli occur in approximately 40% of patients with left-sided valvular infection. In the central nervous system (CNS), embolic occlusion of peripheral arteries results in the stroke syndrome. Emboli to the spleen and kidney often cause abdominal pain. Emboli to mesenteric arteries may cause ischemic bowel disease or frank infarction of bowel. Emboli to muscles are common but usually clinically unap-

parent. Embolic disease can occur after the institution of antibiotics; patients at increased risk for this complication include those with embolic disease prior to the institution of antibiotics, those with larger vegetations, those with mitral valve involvement, and those infected with staphylococci.[7] Drug abusers with right-sided IE frequently have evidence of septic pulmonary emboli on chest x-ray.[5]

Patients with IE also may present with heart failure due to valve malfunction, embolic myocardial infarction, myocarditis, or systemic toxicity owing to sepsis syndrome. Renal insufficiency is also a prominent sequela of untreated IE, whether occurring on a native or prosthetic valve.

Disorders of the CNS are prominent in patients with IE. Between 10% and 50% of patients with IE will develop some neurologic abnormality. Mental status changes such as confusion, delirium, and psychosis are most common. Focal neurologic symptoms and signs may be caused by an embolic stroke, a bleeding mycotic aneurysm, meningitis, or cerebral artery vasculitis. Overall, approximately 30% of patients with IE will have evidence of a focal neurologic event during their illness.

Anemia is common in patients with IE. Leukocytosis occurs in about 40% of patients. Changes in the renal sediment, particularly proteinuria and microscopic hematuria, usually are present in patients with IE. In long-standing disease, rheumatoid factor is present in about one-half of patients.

TABLE 49-2 Frequency of Symptoms and Signs at Presentation of Infective Endocarditis

Symptoms	Frequency, %	Signs	Frequency, %
Fever	85	Fever	95
Malaise	25	Murmur	85
Myalgias arthralgias	25	Petechiae	35
Headache	20	Osler's nodes	10
Back pain	25	Hemiparesis	10
Delirium	10	Coma	5

TABLE 49-3 Frequency of Various Laboratory Abnormalities in Infective Endocarditis

Laboratory Finding	Frequency, %
Anemia	80
Thrombocytopenia	20
Leukocytosis	30
Increased erythrocyte sedimentation rate	95
Hypergammaglobulinemia	25
Hematuria	40
Proteinuria	60

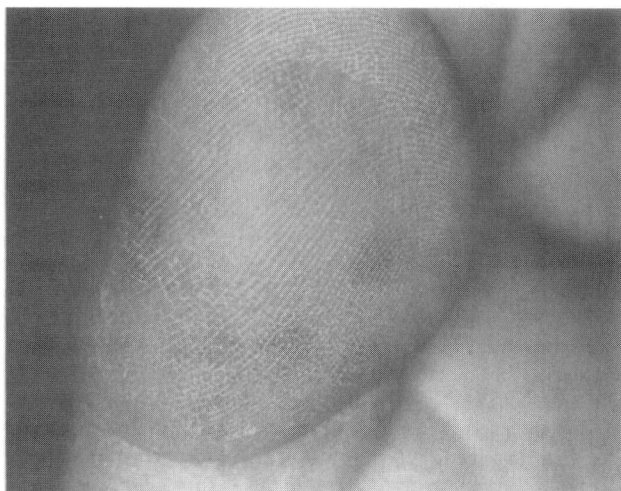

FIGURE 49-1 Subacute bacterial endocarditis: nontender, purpuric macules with irregular borders scattered on the toes (Janeway lesions). (See Color Plate 49-1.)

DIAGNOSIS

Blood cultures are the most important laboratory tests in the diagnosis of IE. The vast majority of blood cultures obtained when a patient is not receiving antimicrobial therapy will be positive. In approximately 5% to 10% of patients with presumed IE, no etiologic organism is isolated initially. The causes of culture-negative endocarditis are prior antibiotics and endocarditis due to fastidious organisms, including anaerobes, nutritionally deficient streptococci, *Coxiella burnetii, Legionella pneumophila, Chlamydia psittaci, C. pneumoniae,* members of the HACEK group, and various fungi. *HACEK* is an acronym for a group of small, fastidious, gram-negative bacilli that includes *Haemophilus* spp., *Actinobacillus actinomycetemcomitans, Cardiobacterium hominis, Eikenella corrodens,* and *Kingella kingae.*[8] Longer incubation of cultures, special culture techniques to aid in isolation of fastidious microorganisms, and use of serologic studies for *Coxiella, Bartonella,* and *Chlamydia* may aid in diagnosis. Other potentially useful laboratory techniques currently under study for intravascular infections and endocarditis include the urinary histoplasmo-

sis antigen, polymerase chain reaction (PCR) using universal bacterial (16S) and fungal (18S, 28S, and 5.8S) RNA primers,[9] and serology for lipid S, a component of the gram-positive cell wall.[10]

Echocardiography is useful in identifying vegetations or local complications of IE. Transthoracic echocardiography has around 60% sensitivity in detecting vegetations in IE. Transesophageal echocardiography (TEE) has emerged as a major tool in the diagnosis and management of native-valve endocarditis (NVE). The sensitivity of TEE in the diagnosis of NVE is 90% to 99%, with a specificity of 90%. Therefore, when NVE is likely clinically but blood cultures are sterile, a TEE may be obtained to assist in diagnosis.[11–13] A TEE also should be obtained in patients with an equivocal transthoracic echocardiogram (TTE) or those with a complicated course. One study has suggested that if the pretest probability of IE is between 4% and 60%, it is cost-effective to proceed to TEE without TTE.[15] Durack and colleagues[12] have proposed criteria for diagnosis of infective endocarditis, and they have been proved useful by other investigators.[13] Finally, intracardiac echocardiography is an emerging diagnostic tool that has been used to identify pacemaker lead vegetations even in patients whose TEE is unremarkable.[16]

MANAGEMENT

Patients encountered in the ICU with fever, cardiac murmurs, or other findings suggesting the possibility of IE always should be evaluated for the possibility of valve infection; this evaluation should include multiple blood cultures and echocardiography. While this evaluation proceeds, two central questions arise: Which clinical situations warrant empirical antimicrobial therapy, and what empirical therapy should be selected? In general, physicians managing patients with *possible* IE should initiate therapy when one of the following situations is present: (1) the patient is critically ill, (2) antimicrobial therapy appears be necessary for some other infectious disorder, (3) early valve replacement is contemplated because of valve malfunction, and (4) IE is suspected clinically and one or more blood cultures are positive for an etiologic microorganism.

In patients with undiagnosed fever or other findings suggesting IE as a diagnostic consideration but without any of these indications for immediate therapy, withholding antimicrobials is reasonable until blood cultures and the results of other investigations provide support for the diagnosis.

In centers with lower rates of methicillin-resistant *S. aureus* (MRSA), it is still reasonable to initiate therapy with IV nafcillin at 2 g every 4 hours plus IV ampicillin at 2 g every 4 hours and gentamicin. Gentamicin doses should be at lower levels (1 mg/kg q8h) because synergistic killing with β-lactam agents does not require conventional gentamicin dosage. In the many hospitals and communities where increasing rates of infection with MRSA have been identified, empirical therapy with vancomycin rather than nafcillin should be considered. However, this regimen may not be adequate for IE secondary to vancomycin-resistant enterococci (VRE), which are being reported from many centers. Newer agents, such as linezolid and quinupristin-dalfopristin (*faeceium* isolates only), may be useful alternatives if VRE are identified and other agents, especially ampicillin, are also unavailable because of resistance profiles.[14]

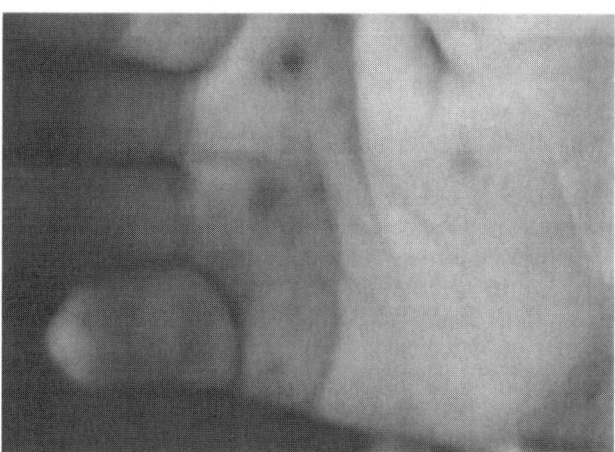

FIGURE 49-2 Osler's nodes: randomly distributed tender nodules on the palm of the hand in a patient with *Staphylococcus aureus* endocarditis. (See Color Plate 49-2.)

TABLE 49-4 Etiology and Valve Involvement in Native-Valve Endocarditis

Microorganism	Percentage
Streptococci	55
Enterococci	7
Staphylococcus aureus	25
Staphylococcus epidermidis	6
Gram-negative bacilli	6
Fungi	1
Culture negative	7
Distribution of valvular lesions:	
Aortic	35–50
Mitral	50
Tricuspid	10
Pulmonic	1

In a febrile patient without the usual risk factors for coronary artery disease admitted with acute myocardial infarction, careful consideration of a diagnosis of IE should be undertaken prior to the administration of thrombolytics because catastrophic CNS bleeds from ruptured mycotic aneurysms have been reported.[17]

In patients with an established diagnosis of IE, management entails a careful choice of antimicrobial therapy based on identification of the etiologic microorganism and ongoing consideration of surgical measures that may be necessary. Table 49-4 lists the most common etiologic microorganisms causing community-acquired NVE and the valves involved. Staphylococci, enterococci, and *Candida* are the most common microorganisms responsible for nosocomial IE.[1] Table 49-5 describes the recommended antimicrobial regimens for treatment of IE. Certain principles are followed when treating patients with IE. Parenteral antibiotics are preferred over oral agents because of more sustained antibacterial activity associated with IV antibiotics and erratic absorption associated with many oral drugs. Bactericidal agents are superior to bacteriostatic drugs. Long-term antimicrobial therapy almost always is required for cure. However, 2 weeks of antibiotics may be adequate in selected patients with uncomplicated *viridans* streptococcal IE or staphylococcal IE of the tricuspid valve.[18,19] Determination of minimal inhibitory concentrations (MICs) and minimal bactericidal concentrations (MBCs) of antimicrobial agents necessary to inhibit or kill the microorganism, respectively, are useful in choosing treatment regimens in patients with streptococcal or enterococcal infections. The serum bactericidal test (Schlicter test) is a measurement of antibacterial activity of the patient's serum, at peak and trough antimicrobial concentrations, against the patient's microorganisms. This test remains somewhat controversial. However, some investigators believe that a peak serum inhibitory concentration (SIC) of 1:8 or greater is more likely to be associated with successful treatment of IE.

Valve replacement may be life-saving in patients with IE. Indications for urgent valve replacement include severe heart failure, valvular obstruction, fungal endocarditis, ineffective antimicrobial therapy, and the presence of an unstable prosthetic device.[20] A point system to aid in evaluation of the need for surgical intervention in IE has been described.[21] The various complications that develop during IE are assigned a weighted point value according to their importance as indicators for valve replacement. A total of five or more points indicates the need for urgent surgery. Table 49-6 lists the conditions associated with need for valve replacement and their relative point ratings. Severe heart failure is considered heart failure that does not respond to maximal medical therapy (see Chaps. 22 and 23). Moderate heart failure is failure that is still present after routine but not maximal medical therapy.

PROGNOSIS

The outcome of treatment for IE is heavily influenced by the relative pathogenicity of the infecting organism, the location of the infected valve, and the presence of complications of the infection. *S. aureus* typically produces a severe and destructive endocarditis that is fatal in more than a third of patients when the infection occurs on the aortic or mitral valve. In patients with tricuspid valve endocarditis, as typically occurs in intravenous drug users, the prognosis is substantially better.[5] Recent data indicate that patients with large (>1 cm) vegetations have an increased morbidity and mortality.[22] Other factors associated with worse prognosis include mitral valve involvement, severe cardiac failure, shock, major arterial emboli, myocardial abscess formation, and associated major organ system failure. As noted earlier, several of these would constitute indications for surgical intervention.

ANTIMICROBIAL PROPHYLAXIS

Prevention of IE in susceptible individuals has been emphasized for many years because of the significant morbidity and mortality associated with the disease. Prophylactic antimicrobial therapy is based on evidence suggesting that bacteremia commonly occurs during certain procedures and that certain cardiac abnormalities place patients at an increased risk for the development of IE following bacteremia. Procedures most frequently associated with bacteremia and for which prophylaxis is recommended include dental extractions, periodontal surgery, lower gastrointestinal procedures, and genitourinary procedures. Bronchoscopy, endoscopy, and barium enemas are also associated with bacteremia but much less commonly, and none of these procedures routinely justifies antimicrobial prophylaxis. Most of the common procedures carried out in ICUs, including endotracheal intubation, urethral catheterization, and insertion of central vascular catheters percutaneously, pose little risk of bacteremia and do not require prophylaxis (except for urethral catheterization in the presence of a urinary tract infection).

Cardiac abnormalities that appear to especially predispose patients to IE following bacteremia include significant aortic and mitral valve deformity/disease, unrepaired ventricular septal defects, patent ductus arteriosus, coarctation of the aorta, prosthetic heart valves, and previously infected native valves. Patients with atrial septal defects, cardiac pacemakers, and atherosclerotic lesions are at much less risk. Mitral valve prolapse with a systolic murmur and/or redundancy of the valve seen on echocardiogram may be an indication for prophylaxis.

The specific antimicrobial agents chosen for prophylaxis depend on the specific procedure to be performed, the cardiac abnormality present, and the presence or absence of penicillin allergy (Table 49-7). In critically ill patients with underlying cardiac abnormalities who are undergoing procedures with a risk of bacteremia, a parenteral regimen usually is appropriate.

TABLE 49-5 Antimicrobial Therapy for Infective Endocarditis and Other Intravascular Infections[a]

Organism	Recommended Therapy	Penicillin-Allergic
1. Penicillin-sensitive streptococci (MIC □ 0.1)	Penicillin G 10–20 million units IV qd for 4 wks *plus* aminoglycoside[c] for first 2 wks (streptomycin 7.5 mg/kg [< or = 500 mg] IM q12h *OR* Gentamicin 1.0 mg/kg IM or IV q8h	Cefazolin 2 g IV q8h for 4 wks[b] *plus* aminoglycoside for 2 weeks Ceftriaxone 2 g IV qd for 4 wks
2. Relatively "resistant" streptococci (Penicillin MIC-0.2–0.5)	Penicillin G 20 million units/d for 4 wks plus aminoglycoside[d] for 4 wks	Cefazolin 2 g IV q8h for 4 weeks[b] *plus* aminoglycoside for 4 wks
3. Resistant streptococci and enterococci (MIC > 0.5)	Penicillin G 20–30 million units IV qd for 6 wks (ampicillin 12 g IV qd is alternative) *plus* aminoglycoside[d] for 6 wks[b]	Vancomycin 30 mg/kg qd for 6 wks[a]
4. Staphylococci (methicillin-sensitive)—in absence of prosthetic valve	Nafcillin 2.0 g IV q4h for 4–6 wks[e] or nafcillin 2 g IV q4h *or* gentamicin 1 mg/kg q8h for 2 wks[h]	Cefazolin 2 g IV q8h for 4–6 wks[b]
5. Methicillin-resistant staphylococci—in absence of prosthetic valve	Vancomycin 30 mg/kg IV per day +/− rifampin 300 mg PO q8h for 6 wks	Same
6. Staphylococci (methicillin-sensitive)	Nafcillin 2.0 g IV q4h for 6–8 wks *plus* rifampin 300 mg[f] PO q8h for 6–8 wks *plus* aminoglycoside for 2 wks	Cefazolin 2 g IV[b] q8h for 6–8 wks *plus* rifampin[f] plus aminoglycoside for 2 wks
7. Staphylococci (methicillin-resistant)—in presence of prosthetic valve	Vancomycin 30 mg/kg 24h IV for 6–8 wks, rifampin 300 mg q8h for 6–8 wks[f] *plus* aminoglycoside for 2 wks	Same
8. *Corynebacterium*	Penicillin G 20–30 million units IV qd for 6 wks *plus* aminoglycoside for 6 wks	Vancomycin 30 mg/kg qd IV for 6 wks
9. Gram-negative bacilli Enterobacteriaceae	Therapy should be directed by in vitro susceptibilities	Same
Pseudomonas	Therapy should be directed by in vitro susceptibilities, though usual regimen includes tobramycin (8 mg/kg per day) plus extended-spectrum penicillin	Same, though ceftazidime *plus* tobramycin (8 mg/kg per day) frequently used
HACEK group	Ampicillin 2.0 g IV q4h is commonly used, though therapy should be directed by in vitro susceptibilities (aminoglycoside frequently used in combination)	Third-generation cephalosporins (e.g., ceftriaxone 2g IV qd for 4 wks)
10. Rickettsia *Coxiella burnetti*	Tetracycline 500 mg PO q6h for at least 1 yr *plus* trimethoprim 480 mg plus sulfamethoxazole 2400 mg qd until there is no evidence clinically of disease or phase I antibody titer is < .1:128	Same
11. Fungal	Amphotericin B plus surgery	Same

[a] Duration of treatment given applies to native-valve infective endocarditis only.

[b] If patient sensitivity to penicillin is of the immediate hypersensitivity type, vancomycin is recommended.

[c] Aqueous crystalline penicillin G should be used alone in patients over 65 years of age or in those who have renal disease or hearing impairment.

[d] Choice of aminoglycoside should depend on in vitro susceptibilities.

[e] Addition of an aminoglycoside is optional.

[f] Use of rifampin in coagulase-negative staphylococcal infection is recommended. The value of rifampin in coagulase-positive staphylococcal infections is controversial.

[g] Vancomycin is indicated for penicillin-resistant strains; consult when treating vancomycin-resistant strains.

[h] Optional in uncomplicated right-sided IE in intravenous drug users.

MYCOTIC ANEURYSM

PATHOGENESIS AND MICROBIAL ETIOLOGY

Mycotic aneurysms are aneurysmal dilations of arteries caused by infection of the vessel wall with consequent weakening of the vessel's structure. These aneurysms occur most commonly in patients with IE and in that instance usually involve vessels of smaller caliber. The pathogenesis probably involves embolic localization of a valvular vegetation with extension of suppuration from the lumen circumferentially into the vessel wall. Another proposed mechanism is embolization of the vasa vasorum by infected material from the valve. In the absence of underlying IE, mycotic aneurysm may occur following transient bacteremia with seeding of a previously damaged site in a large artery, most commonly an

TABLE 49-6 Point System for Assessing the Need for Cardiac Surgery in Infective Endocarditis

Complication	POINT RATING[a] Native-Valve IE	POINT RATING[a] Prosthetic-Valve IE
Heart failure		
Severe	5	5
Moderate	3	5
Mild	1	2
Fungal etiology	5	5
Persistent bacteremia	5	5
Organism other than streptococci	1	2
Relapse after medical therapy	2	3
Single major embolus	2	2
Two or more emboli	4	4
Vegetations by echocardiography (2D)	1	1
Early closure of mitral valve by echocardiography (2D)	2	NA
Ruptured chordae tendineae or papillary muscle	3	NA
Heart block	3	3
Rupture of sinus of Valsalva or ventricular septum	4	4
Unstable prosthesis	NA	5
Early prosthetic valve endocarditis	NA	2
Periprosthetic leak	NA	2
Valvular obstruction	5	5

[a] Accumulation of five or more points implies need for valve replacement; NA - not applicable.
SOURCE: Adapted from Alsip and colleagues.[9]

ulcerated atherosclerotic plaque in the abdominal aorta. Mycotic aneurysms also may occur in intravenous drug abusers who both damage and contaminate the wall of a large artery by direct intra-arterial injections of drugs; mycotic aneurysms of the lower extremity, particularly the femoral artery, are most common in this population.

Endocarditis-associated mycotic aneurysms are caused by the same microorganisms causing the IE—streptococci, staphylococci, and occasionally, gram-negative enteric bacilli, the latter being more common among drug abusers. *S. aureus* and *Salmonella* spp. are the most frequent causes of mycotic aneurysms of the abdominal aorta and usually are not associated with IE.

CLINICAL FEATURES

Intracranial mycotic aneurysms are encountered most commonly in patients who already carry a diagnosis of IE. These aneurysms usually are asymptomatic unless they rupture. In that circumstance, symptoms and signs are consistent with subarachnoid or intracerebral hemorrhage, with sudden onset of severe headache, decrease in the level of consciousness, and focal neurologic signs. Mycotic aneurysms of visceral arteries have a variable presentation based on the organ involved. In the case of the small bowel, there may be colicky abdominal pain and symptoms of small-bowel obstruction. In the case of hepatic arterial aneurysms, an important differential diagnostic consideration is ascending cholangitis because of fever, right upper quadrant pain, and jaundice. Mycotic aneurysms of the external iliac artery may present with pain in the lower anterior abdomen, quadriceps wasting, diminished deep tendon reflexes, and arterial insufficiency of the ipsilateral lower extremity.[23]

Patients with mycotic aneurysms of the abdominal aorta present with pain and fever, often of weeks' or months' duration. In as many as one-third of patients with abdominal aortic aneurysms, there is extension into the lumbar or thoracic vertebrae with resulting osteomyelitis. Aortoenteric fistula may occur if an aneurysm erodes into bowel lumen. On physical examination, in addition to fever, there may be a palpable mass in the abdomen.

DIAGNOSIS

In patients with IE, clinical suspicion of a mycotic aneurysm usually arises after an episode of new neurologic symptoms in the case of intracranial aneurysms or local findings suggestive of aneurysms, as noted earlier. Clinical suspicion of a leaking intracerebral aneurysm should prompt contrast- and non–contrasted-enhanced computed tomographic (CT) examinations initially; however, an angiogram generally is necessary to exclude or confirm the diagnosis. The diagnosis of mycotic aneurysm of the abdominal aorta is also made on the basis of clinical suspicion, demonstration of bacteremia, and radiologic examination. CT scan of the abdomen may indicate a perivascular collection of fluid or actual blood in an aneurysm or pseudoaneurysm. Arteriography also may be helpful in demonstrating an aortic mycotic aneurysm, and bone films may show erosion of adjacent vertebral bodies.

MANAGEMENT

The management of mycotic aneurysm depends on the organ involved. In the case of intracranial mycotic aneurysms, there

TABLE 49-7 Endocarditis Prophylaxis

Procedure	Standard Regimen	Standard Oral Regimen for PCN-Allergic Patients	Alternative Parenteral Regimens
Dental or respiratory tract procedure	Amoxicillin 3.0 g PO 1 h before, then 1.5 g 6 h later	Erythromycin 1.0 g PO 2 h before, then 500 mg 6 h later *or* clindamycin 300 mg PO 1 h before, then 150 mg 6 h later	Ampicillin 2.0 g IV or IM 30 min before, then 1.0 g 6 h later *or* clindamycin 300 mg IV 30 min before, then 150 mg 6 h later *or* vancomycin 1.0 g IV over 1 h
Gastrointestinal or genitourinary tract procedure	Ampicillin 2.0 g IV or IM *plus* gentamicin 1.5 mg/kg of body weight IV or IM given 30 min before, repeat 8 h later		Vancomycin 1.0 g IV slowly over 1 h, *plus* gentamicin 1.5 mg/kg of body weight IV or IM, given 1 h before, repeat 8 h later

TABLE 49-8 Recommended Duration of Antimicrobial Therapy for Patients with Various Intravascular Infections

Infectious Disorder	PATIENTS WITHOUT INTRAVASCULAR FOREIGN BODIES Duration of Treatment
Cavernous sinus thrombosis	2 weeks following the resolution of all signs of the disease (usually 4 weeks)
Mycotic aneurysm	4–6 weeks; 2–4 weeks after resection of the aneurysm
Postanginal sepsis	4 weeks or 10 days following resolution of local symptoms and signs
Pelvic vein thrombophlebitis	4 weeks (consider anticoagulation)
Pylephlebitis	4–6 weeks; if associated with liver abscess, consider additional treatment until abscess is resolved

is debate regarding the most appropriate therapy. For peripheral intracranial aneurysms, clipping probably is indicated. For deep lesions, for which a surgical approach is felt to be hazardous, antimicrobial therapy alone is advisable because many aneurysms will resolve spontaneously with medical treatment. A history of bleeding, large aneurysm size, and persistence of the aneurysm following antimicrobial therapy are all factors that increase the advisability of surgery for accessible lesions. In the case of abdominal aortic aneurysms, surgical resection of the involved aorta is almost always necessary. Antimicrobial therapy for mycotic aneurysms and other intravascular infections without foreign bodies is outlined in Tables 49-5 and 49-8.

CAVERNOUS SINUS THROMBOSIS

Cavernous sinus thrombosis usually results from direct spread of bacteria from a contiguous focus of infection. Extension of bacteria may occur by several routes, including septic thrombophlebitis of the angular and ophthalmic veins from facial cellulitis, along the lateral sinus and petrosal sinuses from middle ear infections, via the pterygoid venous plexus from a peritonsillar abscess, following a dental infection from osteomyelitis of the maxilla or from a cervical abscess, and along the venous plexus surrounding the internal carotid artery from the middle ear or jugular bulb.

S. aureus is the cause of cavernous sinus thrombosis in about 60% to 70% of patients. Streptococci, anaerobes, and other aerobes account for most of the rest.[24] Patients with cavernous sinus thrombosis generally present with the early onset of external ophthalmoplegia with decreased sensation around the eye. The physical examination reveals periorbital edema and chemosis, and as the illness develops, meningismus, altered mental status, and cranial nerve palsies, especially of cranial nerves III, IV, V, and VI, become evident. Examination of the fundus often reveals striking venous congestion. The differential diagnosis of cavernous sinus thrombosis includes orbital cellulitis and rhinocerebral phycomycosis (mucormycosis). The distinction between cavernous sinus thrombosis and orbital cellulitis is sometimes difficult. Bilateral involvement and fifth nerve palsy, a fixed, dilated pupil, and signs of meningitis are all more likely in cavernous sinus thrombosis than in orbital cellulitis.

Although the diagnosis may be evident on clinical grounds alone, several imaging modalities can be useful. Ultrasound examination of the orbit can be useful in defining a periorbital abscess that may require surgical intervention. CT examination with contrast or MRI also can aid in this, will be useful in demonstrating sinusitis or underlying osteomyelitis, and may establish the diagnosis of cavernous sinus thrombosis as well. Carotid angiography and orbital venography also have been used to establish the diagnosis but are not recommended because they are unlikely to influence management. Following CT scan, a lumbar puncture is warranted, but it is usually sterile (80%)[24] with a parameningeal inflammatory pattern: pleocytosis and elevated protein without significant hypoglycorrhachia. Blood cultures are mandatory and often are positive (70%)[24]; if sinus or abscess drainage is performed, fluid should be cultured for both aerobic and anaerobic bacteria. When rhinocerebral mucormycosis is a consideration, usually in a diabetic patient with blackish nasal discharge in addition to the rest of the syndrome, surgical exploration with biopsy and histologic examination for fungi is needed to establish the diagnosis.

Successful management of cavernous sinus thrombosis depends on early, effective antimicrobial therapy. Even with the best medical and surgical therapy, the outcome is often unsatisfactory. For this reason, adjunctive therapies such as corticosteroids and anticoagulation have been tried without success, and they cannot be recommended. The regimens shown in Tables 49-5 and 49-8 can be used when a bacterial etiology has been established. Prior to bacteriologic confirmation, empirical therapy depends on the underlying infection suspected.

POSTANGINAL SEPSIS

In 1936, in an article entitled, "On Certain Septicemias Due to Anaerobic Organisms," Lemierre[25] described a group of patients with pharyngitis complicated by bacteremia due to anaerobic microorganisms. Subsequently, this disorder, usually referred to as *postanginal sepsis,* has been described frequently.[26] The pathogenesis is thought to involve bacterial invasion of the mucosa of the posterior pharynx with extension of suppurative thrombophlebitis (ST) into the internal jugular veins. Bacteremic spread of the infection is common, with lung, liver, and joints the most common sites of metastatic disease. Clinically, patients present with sore throat, chills, fever, and occasionally jaundice. On physical examination, in addition to the toxicity and fever, there may be palpable tender thrombosis of the jugular vein as well as evidence of septic arthritis, pleuropulmonary disease, or jaundice. An enhanced CT scan usually will demonstrate internal jugular vein thrombophlebitis and is useful to localize purulent collections requiring drainage. Chest radiograph may show scattered infiltrates owing to septic pulmonary emboli. *Fusobacterium necrophorum* has been isolated most commonly from blood, although *Bacteroides fragilis* and other mouth anaerobes have been reported as well.

Management includes early recognition and treatment of the disorder with effective antimicrobial therapy. Antibiotics should be directed against anaerobic bacteria, with drugs such as metronidazole, chloramphenicol, imipenem-cilastatin, or ticarcillin-clavulanic acid. Prompt surgical intervention to drain any purulent material present locally or distantly is required in addition to antibiotics.

SEPTIC PELVIC VEIN THROMBOPHLEBITIS

Pelvic vein thrombophlebitis develops most often 1 to 2 weeks after delivery or gynecologic surgical intervention or in the setting of pelvic suppuration, such as following septic abortion or post–Cesarean section endometritis. Symptoms include fever, chills, anorexia, nausea, vomiting, and abdominal pain.[27] On physical examination, there may be tenderness in the lower quadrants, and tender venous structures may be palpated in one-third of patients.[28] Eighty percent of pelvic vein thromboses complicating pregnancy and delivery occur on the right side, perhaps because of compression of the right ovarian vein at the pelvic brim by the enlarged uterus. In 5% of episodes, thrombosis is apparent only on the left, and in 14%, it is bilateral. Spread distally to femoral veins is unusual.

The most serious complication of suppurative pelvic vein thrombosis is pulmonary embolization. When this occurs, the patient presents with respiratory distress associated with pulmonary opacities that often are pleural-based. Even though the process is associated with thrombosis and bacterial suppuration in the venous lumen, bacteremia is unusual, with an overall prevalence of only 30%. Microorganisms isolated from the blood, or from the veins if surgery is carried out, include those that are normally present in the pelvis, particularly *Peptostreptococcus* spp., *Peptococcus* spp., *B. fragilis*, aerobic gram-negative bacilli such as *Escherichia coli*, *Klebsiella*, and *Enterobacter*, group A and group B β-hemolytic streptococci, and rarely, staphylococci.

The diagnosis can be difficult because the findings are similar to a wider range of other pelvic and lower abdominal inflammatory conditions. Probably the best imaging modality to support the diagnosis is contrast-enhanced CT scan; ultrasound examination also may be useful if the intravascular thrombus can be demonstrated.

Successful treatment frequently requires both antimicrobial therapy and heparinization; indeed, in the appropriate clinical context, fever that is failing to respond to apparently appropriate antimicrobials and that responds to the addition of intravenous heparin can be regarded as support for the diagnosis.[29] Complications are mainly those related to suppurative pulmonary emboli.

PYLEPHLEBITIS

Pylephlebitis is septic thrombosis of the portal vein and its branches. It is a rarely seen complication of intra-abdominal suppuration and was first described in patients with appendicitis or diverticulitis. The illness evolves in three phases. In the first phase, symptoms and signs of the original intra-abdominal disorder such as acute appendicitis or perforated diverticulum predominate. The second phase involves portal bacteremia, with resulting invasion and thrombosis of portal veins. In the third phase, abscesses form in the liver owing to proximal spread of the suppurative material. Late signs and symptoms include fever, abdominal pain, jaundice, and right upper quadrant tenderness. The liver is enlarged in one-half of patients. Laboratory studies reveal an elevated white blood cell count with increased numbers of immature granulocytes and abnormal liver function tests, particularly elevations of the alkaline phosphatase and aspartate amino-

transferase (AST) levels. Bacteremia is not a consistent finding. CT scan is especially useful in demonstrating this disorder, showing clot in the portal veins and occasionally gas in portal vein radicals in the liver. The microorganisms responsible reflect large bowel flora and include aerobic gram-negative bacilli such as *E. coli*, *Klebsiella*, and *Enterobacter*; anaerobic microorganisms such as *Peptococcus*, *Peptostreptococcus*, *B. fragilis*, and *Fusobacterium*; and gram-positive aerobic species such as staphylococci and enterococci.

Successful therapy requires surgical correction of the primary problem, as well as high-dose antibacterial therapy directed against the offending pathogens. Pyogenic liver abscesses resulting from this disorder usually are best treated with prolonged medical therapy alone, unless they are few and relatively large, in which case percutaneous drainage may be useful. Surgical drainage of multiple small abscesses is very difficult, often requires a transperitoneal approach, and is not recommended. The effectiveness of antibacterial therapy may be judged by physical examination, resolution of fever and leukocytosis, and improvement of abnormalities demonstrated by ultrasound or CT scan.

Infections of Intravascular Prosthetic Devices

PROSTHETIC VALVE ENDOCARDITIS

PATHOGENESIS AND MICROBIOLOGY

Prosthetic heart valves may become infected early following implantation or later during the life of the device. Overall, about 2% of patients with prosthetic heart valves become infected, one-third in the first few months after valve implantation and two-thirds later. In early prosthetic valve endocarditis (PVE), the presumed pathogenesis involves inoculation of the operative site at the time of surgery or the localization of microorganisms on the new device following transient bacteremia associated with indwelling lines used in the perioperative period. Factors associated with an increased risk of PVE include IE of the native valve prior to valve resection and replacement, use of a mechanical valvular device in contrast to a tissue heterograft or homograft, a history of intravenous drug abuse, male gender (possibly because of the greater likelihood of superficial cellulitis as a result of shaving prior to surgery), and longer cardiopulmonary bypass time.[30]

In late PVE, i.e., disease appearing more than 12 months after replacement, the pathogenesis more closely resembles that of native-valve disease.[31] Extension of local tissue disease via lymphatics to the bloodstream or direct inoculation of microorganisms via capillary beds, as occurs during dental work, results in transient bacteremia with localization on the prosthetic device. Nosocomial PVE is acquired most commonly via intravascular devices but may be initiated by cutaneous and other infections as well.[32]

Microorganisms most commonly responsible for PVE are listed in Table 49-9. *Staphylococcus epidermidis* is the most common cause of early PVE. *S. aureus* and gram-negative bacilli are also prominent etiologic microorganisms during this period. Other less commonly encountered microorganisms are enterococci, other streptococci, and yeast. Microorganisms found in patients with late PVE tend to be similar to those seen in native-valve disease. *Viridans* streptococci

TABLE 49-9 Etiology of Prosthetic-Valve Endocarditis

Microorganism	Early PVE, %	Late PVE, %
Staphylococci		
S. epidermidis	30	20
S. aureus	20	11
Streptococci		
Group D streptococci	5	12
Viridans streptococci	4	25
Gram-negative bacilli	20	12
Corynebacterium		
(not *C. diphtheriae*)	8	3
Fungi	10	5
Other or		
culture-negative	3	12

are common, as is *S. aureus; S. epidermidis* and gram-negative bacilli are less common. Nosocomial PVE is most commonly due to staphylococci, *epidermidis* followed by *aureus;* enterococci, gram-negative bacilli, *Candida,* and *viridans* streptococci are less common pathogens.[32]

CLINICAL FEATURES

The signs, symptoms, and clinical laboratory abnormalities seen in PVE generally are similar to those encountered in patients with NVE, except that patients with PVE have a higher prevalence of cardiac complications. Clinical evidence of these cardiac complications may include new and changing regurgitant murmurs caused by paravalvular leak from dehiscence of the valve ring, intraventricular and atrioventricular conduction defects resulting from extension of a paravalvular abscess into the interventricular septum, and muffling of prosthetic heart sounds or new stenotic murmurs related to malfunction of the valve caused by a vegetation. Fang and colleagues [31] reported on patients with nosocomial PVE having peripheral stigmata in 20%, splenomegaly in 5%, stroke in 3%, and a new or changing murmur in 31%.

DIAGNOSIS

Diagnostic difficulty arises in the immediate postoperative period when bacteremia occurs in a patient with a new prosthetic valve. In this setting, blood cultures yielding staphylococci, "diphtheroids," and yeasts are more likely to represent true prosthetic valve infection than is gram-negative bacilli bacteremia, which more likely results from indwelling venous catheter infection.

In patients with late PVE caused by staphylococci or streptococci, bacteria usually are recovered consistently from blood cultures, provided that the patient has not received prior antimicrobial therapy. Generally, three sets of blood cultures obtained over a brief period from different venipuncture sites are sufficient to identify the etiology of prosthetic valve infection. Echocardiography helps identify vegetations and local suppurative complications, as well as determine ventricular function and valvular integrity, although the metallic devices tend to result in distorted echo signals, confusing the interpretation. TEE is superior to TTE in visualizing the mitral valve; visualization of aortic valve prostheses with TEE is less clear. The reported sensitivity and specificity of TEE for detection of morphologic abnormalities are 86% and 88%, respectively.[11] Patients with neurologic symptoms associated

with PVE also should undergo a contrast-enhanced CT scan of the head to detect embolic hemorrhagic infarcts and abscesses. Since a CT scan does not reliably exclude mycotic aneurysm, cerebral angiography also may be indicated when CT findings do not explain the neurologic symptoms adequately.

MANAGEMENT

The same principles described for the treatment of NVE apply for the treatment of PVE.[33] The antimicrobial agents used in the treatment of PVE are outlined in Table 49-5. In general, initial antimicrobial therapy is chosen on the basis of identification and susceptibility tests of the infecting microorganism. When the infecting microorganism has not been identified, initial therapy should include vancomycin and gentamicin to cover the likely possibilities of *S. epidermidis, S. aureus,* and streptococci. This combination would cover most nosocomial pathogens as well; however, the choice of antibiotics also should be determined by the usual organisms encountered at the specific hospital environ. In addition, previous or current antibiotic use should be considered when choosing an empirical regimen, especially for nosocomial PVE. Ill, bacteremic patients who may have IE should be treated without delay. In addition, if heart surgery is scheduled because of valve deterioration or antimicrobial therapy is required for some other indication in a patient with suspected endocarditis, therapy should be initiated without waiting for the results of blood cultures. Relative indications for valve replacement in PVE include early PVE, nonstreptococcal late PVE, and periprosthetic leak. Patients with PVE should be treated for 6 to 8 weeks in most instances whether or not the valve is removed. If microorganisms can be cultured at the time of valve replacement, we recommend 6 to 8 additional weeks of therapy beginning at that time.

CARDIAC PACEMAKER INFECTIONS

Four major varieties of pacemakers are presently in use: transvenous and epicardial temporary pacemakers with external generators and transvenous and epicardial pacemakers of the permanent variety with implanted generator boxes. The pathogenesis and management of infections of temporary transvenous pacemakers are essentially identical to those for other percutaneous central vascular catheters and are not discussed further here (see Chap. 50). The most common complication affecting permanently implanted pacemakers is mechanical failure (failure to pace or sense correctly), but infection is the next most common. Approximately 4% of pacemakers become infected at some point after placement. Generator box infections, infection of the electrode along its subcutaneous course, and bacteremic infection of the intravascular portion of the electrode, with or without associated endocarditis, each contribute approximately one-third to the overall infection problem. Diabetes mellitus, cancer, and corticosteroid therapy all have been noted to predispose to infection of the device. Skin erosion adjacent to a generator pouch also predisposes to direct invasion of the apparatus. As with PVE, pacemaker infections can be classified as early or late; early infections occur in the first 3 to 6 months. Early infections generally can be attributed to wound contamination by skin organisms at the time of implantation, whereas late infection, particularly of the intravascular electrode, often results from transient bacteremia with adherence of organisms to the surface of the device. Particularly in the case of staphylococcal infections, adherence to the foreign material is facilitated by an exopolysaccharide glycocalyx produced by the organism. This material also forms a protective layer over the biofilm on the foreign body, contributing to impairment of the local antibacterial activity of polymorphonuclear leukocytes and reducing the effectiveness of antimicrobial therapy.

S. epidermidis and *S. aureus* are the most common microorganisms isolated from patients with generator pocket or electrode infections. In one large study of pacemaker infections, *S. epidermidis* accounted for 44% of episodes and *S. aureus*, 29%.[34] They are also the most common organisms isolated from the blood of patients with pacemaker infections in the absence of obvious generator pocket or electrode disease. Other etiologic microorganisms that have been reported include *Corynebacterium* spp., gram-negative aerobic bacilli, and occasionally, fungi.

Chills, fever, and other constitutional symptoms without another evident source constitute the usual presentation of pacemaker infection. The diagnosis is made by inspecting the generator pocket and the subcutaneous electrodes and obtaining blood cultures. Generator pocket and subcutaneous electrode infections usually evidence local inflammation without bacteremia or with transient bacteremia. Persistent bacteremia in a patient with an intravascular pacemaker suggests intravascular electrode infection or IE. Since most pacemakers are implanted in the right ventricle, the associated endocarditis is usually not accompanied by systemic embolic phenomena but may produce septic pulmonary emboli or multifocal pneumonia, as in right-sided endocarditis of other causes. TEE is more sensitive than TTE with regard to detecting pacemaker-related vegetations. As mentioned previously, intracardiac echocardiography is an emerging technology that also may prove useful in identifying pacemaker lead vegetations.[16]

There are three main considerations in developing a therapeutic plan for the management of pacemaker infection. One is the identity of the suspected or proved infecting microorganisms, second is the particular component of the apparatus that is involved, and the third is the presence or absence of bacterial infection at sites other than the pacemaker itself. Infected pacemakers must be removed when the generator box is infected, when there is persistent bacteremia, and when there is evidence of IE. A few authors have suggested that patients with permanent transvenous pacemakers that have been present for a long duration and who have bacteremia without evidence of generator box infection or IE can be tried on antibacterial therapy in the hope that the infection on the device may be cured without replacement. If treatment of pacemaker infection is attempted without removal of the device, 4 to 6 weeks of intravenous antimicrobial therapy probably is necessary as an initial trial. In the case of fungal agents or mycobacteria, a longer duration of therapy is necessary and is more likely to be unsuccessful. If the decision is made to remove the pacemaker, then the new transvenous generator should be located in a deeper pocket. Antimicrobial therapy is chosen on the basis of the microorganism isolated from the skin and subcutaneous tissue or bloodstream and is described in Tables 49-5 and 49-10. Two weeks of antimicrobial therapy after removal of the device probably is sufficient in the case of most generator pocket infections resulting from pyogenic microorganisms unless there is metastatic disease or secondary

TABLE 49-10 Recommended Duration of Antimicrobial Therapy for Infections of Intravascular Devices

Infectious Disorder	Recommended Duration of Treatment
Pacemaker infection, generator box, and/or bacteremia	2 weeks after device removed, 4–6 weeks if not removed
Ventricular assist device	No uniform recommendations at this time; prolonged antibiotics and removal of device if possible
Prosthetic heart valves replacement	6–8 weeks; if culture positive at valve, 6–8 additional weeks beginning at that time
Arterial vascular grafts	6–8 weeks

NVE, in which case the usual duration of treatment for NVE is used after the device is removed. Transvenous lead infections also require device removal and parenteral antimicrobial therapy. It is sometimes difficult to extricate the transvenous electrode tip from the right side of the heart. Tricuspid valve or ventricular wall tears have occurred. If percutaneous electrode removal is impossible, thoracotomy is required.

VENTRICULAR ASSIST DEVICE INFECTIONS

Ventricular assist devices (VADs) are becoming more common in ICU patients. VADs often serve as bridges to cardiac transplantation. Because they are an intravascular device, VADs may become colonized and serve as a site for recurrent bacteremias or fungemias. It has been estimated that 25% to 50% of VAD placements are complicated by infection.[35] VAD-associated infections often involve the pump driveline, the pocket, or both. Commonly reported etiologic organisms include *S. aureus*,[35] *S. epidermidis*,[35,36] *P. aeruginosa*,[35] and *Candida* species.[35,36] If this complication should develop, replacement is one consideration; however, others would argue that this approach will fail more often than not owing to reinfection of the subsequent device and that these patients should receive priority for transplantation. However, lack of donor organs often leaves the former as the only available option.

ARTERIAL GRAFT INFECTIONS

Arterial grafts have an infection rate that has varied between 2% and 6% in different studies,[37–39] with a mortality rate as high as 50%. The pathogenesis of graft infection is analogous to that of prosthetic valve disease, with some patients presumably developing infectious disorders of the graft owing to inoculation of microorganisms at the time of surgery and others developing infection later owing to adherence of microorganisms that have gained access to the circulation. Grafts remain susceptible to infection for a rather long period because of the slow process of pseudointima formation in the graft lumen. Overall, graft infections present a mean of 8 months after implantation, but late disease may occur as long as 7 to 10 years after graft placement.[40] Autogenous vein grafts are the least susceptible to infection. Knitted Dacron grafts appear to be more susceptible, and woven Dacron grafts have a risk of infection somewhere in between. Grafts that cross the femoral area seem to be at greatest risk for infection, possibly due to contamination by bowel flora at the time of implantation.

TABLE 49-11 Microorganisms Responsible for Infections of Implanted Intravascular Devices

Organisms	PVE[a]	Pacemaker, %	Vascular Graft, %
S. epidermidis	27	42	10
S. aureus	14	35	15
Streptococci (includes enterococci)	26	—	30
Gram-negative rods	14	—	30
Diphtheroids and gram-positive rods	7	—	3
Fungi	9	—	2
Unknown	3	23	10

[a] Prosthetic-valve endocarditis.

The microbial etiology of vascular graft infection is shown in Table 49-11. Gram-positive microorganisms, particularly *S. aureus,* are the most common cause of graft infections, particularly in the groin or popliteal area. Gram-negative enteric microorganisms such as *E. coli, Proteus,* or *Pseudomonas* are more often the cause of abdominal graft suppuration.

Graft infections generally present with variable systemic constitutional symptoms, nonspecific laboratory evidence of an inflammatory process (leukocytosis, elevated erythrocyte sedimentation rate [ESR]), and findings at the graft site that vary depending on the location of the graft. Early infections (occurring less than 4 months after graft placement) more often present as sepsis or wound infection, whereas late infections present with graft malfunction or cutaneous sinus formation. Intraluminal infection may present as fever and nonspecific constitutional complaints resulting from bacteremia. Patients with a vascular graft who have persistent bacteremia with no other known source must be approached as if they have a graft infection. Extraluminal infection may present with evidence of local graft infection with erythema, tenderness, and swelling over the graft site; with systemic inflammatory symptoms without definite localizing findings; or with graft occlusion. Rapid swelling suggests disruption of the suture line with bleeding and false aneurysm formation and frequently implies graft infection. The most common presentation of groin or leg graft site infection is a localized abscess or draining sinus. Graft thrombosis should be suspected when signs and symptoms of peripheral arterial insufficiency develop. Exteriorization of the graft secondary to breakdown of tissue overlying the graft is rare but, when present, is pathognomonic of infection.

With infection of abdominal aortic grafts, swelling of tissues surrounding the graft may produce a mass effect, sometimes with evidence of ureteral obstruction or hydronephrosis. In addition, symptoms and signs of lower extremity ischemia may occur. The development of an aortoduodenal fistula between an infected aortic graft and the duodenum is a catastrophic complication. Patients in this group present with hematemesis or circulatory collapse.

Not infrequently, a diagnosis of graft infection must be based predominantly on the clinical features noted earlier because blood cultures are negative. The most useful imaging procedure is scanning with indium- or technetium-labeled white blood cells, which can demonstrate the inflammatory process along the course of the vascular graft.[41] CT scan or MRI is perhaps preferable if soft-tissue edema resulting from infection surrounding the graft or false aneurysm formation can be demonstrated. Vascular imaging may be combined with percutaneous fine-needle aspiration of perigraft fluid that can be Gram-stained and cultured. When the graft is removed for presumed infection, the graft itself and swabs from the graft bed should be cultured for both aerobes and anaerobes and examined for fungi.

Management of an infected intravascular graft almost always requires specific antimicrobial therapy chosen on the basis of the presumed or demonstrated infecting microorganism, as well as graft removal. When antimicrobial therapy alone is attempted, graft infection usually persists. If a graft provides the only blood supply to a distal organ or extremity, then some variety of revascularization must be carried out at the time of graft removal. An example is the use of an axillofemoral graft to bypass an infected aortic bifurcation prosthesis.

Specific antimicrobial regimens and suggested duration of therapy are indicated in Tables 49-5 and 49-10.

An Approach to Patients with Fever and Suspected Intravascular Infection

Intravascular infection is usually suspected in a critically ill patient when fever or other clinical or laboratory features of sepsis are present without a satisfactory alternative explanation. Blood cultures are mandatory in all such patients as an initial step, and all permanent or temporary intravascular devices should be inspected carefully for local evidence of infection.

Patients with otherwise unexplained positive blood cultures in the presence of an intravascular device must be presumed to have an infection of the device. When the device is a temporary one, such as a peripheral intravenous line, central venous catheter, or temporary pacemaker, it should be removed. In most cases, IV antimicrobial agents appropriate for the organism should be given for 1 to 2 weeks. If pus can be expressed from the puncture site or there is persistent bacteremia, surgical exploration of the peripheral veins is indicated. Tunneled central venous catheters call for a more selective approach (see Chap. 50). When positive blood cultures are attributed to an infected permanent intravascular device, the initial clinical decision is whether the device should be removed. Indications for permanent intravascular device removal depend on the variety of the device and have been discussed previously.

Positive blood cultures in the absence of an intravascular device and without an evident infection such as cellulitis, pneumonia, urinary tract infection, cholangitis, or intra-abdominal abscess predisposing to bacteremia most commonly result from an occult abscess or an intravascular suppuration. When sufficient clinical suspicion suggests the possibility of an intravascular infection such as a mycotic aneurysm, NVE, postanginal sepsis, pelvic vein thrombophlebitis, or pylephlebitis, appropriate special diagnostic studies outlined earlier should be performed promptly, and appropriate antimicrobial therapy for the bacteremia should be initiated. In addition, when the diagnosis has been established, appropriate surgical intervention frequently is required, as noted earlier.

Another group of critically ill patients in whom intravascular infection must be considered consists of those with fever and persistently sterile blood cultures, either while receiving antimicrobial therapy or not. When antimicrobial agents are being administered for some other reason, making a diagnosis of the precise etiology of intravascular infection may be especially difficult. Even if antimicrobial therapy can be discontinued, blood cultures may still take as long as 2 weeks to become positive again. In the patient with a prosthetic heart valve, blood-culture–negative IE is a consideration. In those with permanent pacemakers or vascular grafts, infection with a fastidious organism that is difficult to detect by usual methods is also a possibility, as is infection of a part of the device that is extravascular. The approach to these infections involves blood cultures designed to detect more fastidious organisms (see above), serologic studies for infections not detected by culture, and imaging studies aimed at acquiring nonmicrobiologic support for the diagnosis of infection. An echocardiogram demonstrating a vegetation on a valve, an arteriogram showing a mycotic aneurysm, or a scan with labeled white blood cells demonstrating increased uptake around a vascular graft may be sufficient to raise the index of suspicion high enough to proceed to more definitive therapy.

Patients with fever, negative blood cultures, and temporary devices in place should be examined carefully for evidence of local inflammation at the site of the device, and if present, the device should be removed and cultured semiquantitatively: A colony count of less than 15 when the intracutaneous portion of a vascular catheter is rolled on an agar plate virtually excludes sepsis due to infection of that line, whereas higher bacterial counts provide some support for the diagnosis.[42]

A common practice in some centers involves changing the central venous line over a guidewire in the febrile patient whose central vascular catheter exit site does not look infected and who is not bacteremic; if the line tip culture is positive, then the central venous line is replaced in a sterile site. Data to support or refute this practice are not compelling; therefore, one must weigh the risk of the catheter being the source of sepsis against the risk associated with placement of a new catheter or doing without it. A more complete discussion of the problem of suspected temporary intravascular device infection is given in Chap. 50.

Finally, even in the patient with fever of unknown source, negative blood cultures, and no intravascular device in place, an intravascular infection remains an important diagnostic consideration. Mycotic aneurysms, culture-negative NVE, pelvic vein septic thrombophlebitis, and pylephlebitis are all examples. The key points in the diagnostic approach are a careful history and physical examination and consideration of the clinical context. Examples include a woman with fever without bacteremia following delivery, in whom a pelvic vein thrombophlebitis, a new or previously demonstrated pathologic heart murmur (raising the possibility of culture-negative IE), or known intravenous drug abuse suggesting the possibility of mycotic aneurysm must be considered.

References

1. Fernandez-Guerrero M, Verdejo C, Azofra J, et al: Hospital-acquired infections endocarditis not associated with cardiac surgery: An emerging problem. *Clin Infect Dis* 20:16, 1995.

2. Farmer JA, Torres G: Endocarditis. *Curr Opin Cardiol* 12:123, 1997.

3. Moreillon P, Que YA: Infective endocarditis. *Lancet* 363:139, 2004.

4. Mylonakis E, Calderwood SB: Infective endocarditis in adults. *N Engl J Med* 345:1318, 2001.

5. Hecht SR, Berger M: Right-sided endocarditis in intravenous drug users. *Ann Intern Med* 117:560, 1992.

6. Watanakunakorn C, Burkert T: Infective endocarditis at a large community teaching hospital, 1980–1990: A review of 210 episodes. *Medicine* 72:90, 1993.

7. Vilacosta I, et al: Risk of embolization after institution of antibiotic therapy for infective endocarditis. *J Am Coll Cardiol* 39:1489, 2002.

8. Berbari EF, Cockerill FR, Steckleberg JM: Infective endocarditis due to unusual or fastidious microorganisms. *Mayo Clin Proc* 72:532, 1997.

9. Millar B, et al: Molecular diagnosis of infective endocarditis. *Scand J Infect Dis* 33:673, 2001.

10. Connaughton M, et al: Rapid serodiagnosis of gram-positive bacterial endocarditis. *J Infect* 42:140, 2001.

11. Daniel WG, Mugge A: Transesophageal echocardiography. *N Engl J Med* 332:1268, 1995.

12. Durack DT, Lukes AS, Bright DK, et al: New criteria for diagnosis of infective endocarditis: Utilization of specific echocardiographic findings. *Am J Med* 96:200, 1994.

13. Jessurun C, Mesa A, Wilansky S: Utility of transesophageal echocardiography in infective endocarditis. *Tex Heart Inst J* 23:98, 1996.

14. Hunter AJ, et al: Thrombolytics in infectious endocarditis associated myocardial infarction. *J Emerg Med* 21:401, 2001.

15. Heidenreich PA, et al: Echocardiography in patients with suspected endocarditis: A cost-effective analysis. *Am J Med* 107:198, 1999.

16. Dalal A, et al: Intracardiac echocardiography in the detection of pacemaker lead endocarditis. *J Am Soc Echocardiogr* 15:1027, 2002.

17. Hunter AJ, et al: Thrombolytics in infectious endocarditis associated myocardial inferction. *J Emerg Med* 21:401, 2001.

18. Chambers HF, Miller RT, Newman MD: Right-sided *S. aureus* endocarditis in intravenous drug abusers: Two-week combination therapy. *Ann Intern Med* 109:619, 1988.

19. Roberts SA, Lang SDR, Ellis-Pegler PB: Short course treatment of penicillin-susceptible *viridans* streptococcal infective endocarditis with penicillin and gentamicin. *Infect Dis Clin Pract* 2:191, 1993.

20. Dinubile MJ: Surgery in active endocarditis. *Ann Intern Med* 96:650, 1982.

20a. DiSalvo G, et al: Echocardiography predicts embolic events in infective endocarditis. *J Am Coll Cardiol* 37:1069, 2001.

21. Alsip SG, Blackstone EH, Kirk JW, et al: Indications for cardiac surgery in patients with active infective endocarditis. *Am J Med* 78(suppl 6B):138, 1985.

22. Bayer AS: Infective endocarditis. *Clin Infect Dis* 17:313, 1993.

23. Feinsod FM, Norfleet RG, Hoehn JL: Mycotic aneurysm of the external iliac artery: A triad of clinical signs facilitating early diagnosis. *JAMA* 238:245, 1977.

24. Ebright JR, et al: Septic thrombosis of the cavernous sinuses. *Arch Intern Med* 161:2671, 2001.

25. Lemierre A: On certain septicemias due to anaerobic organisms. *Lancet* 1:701, 1936.

26. Sinave CP, Hardy GJ, Fardy PW: The Lemierre syndrome: Suppurative thrombophlebitis of the internal jugular vein secondary to oropharyngeal infection. *Medicine* 68:85, 1989.

27. Josey WF, Staggers SR: Heparin therapy in septic pelvic thrombophlebitis: A study of 46 cases. *Am J Obstet Gynecol* 120:228, 1974.

28. Munster AM: Septic thrombophlebitis: A surgical disorder. *JAMA* 230:1010, 1974.

29. Josey WE, Cook CC: Septic pelvic thrombophlebitis: Report of 17 patients treated with heparin. *Obstet Gynecol* 35:891, 1970.

30. Ivert TSA, Dismukes WE, Cobbs CG, et al: Prosthetic valve endocarditis. *Circulation* 69:223, 1984.

31. Karchmer AW, Dismukes WE, Buckley MJ, et al: Late prosthetic valve endocarditis: Clinical features influencing therapy. *Am J Med* 64:199, 1978.

32. Fang G, Keys TF, Gentry LO, et al: Prosthetic valve endocarditis resulting from nosocomial bacteremia. *Ann Intern Med* 119:560, 1993.

33. Mayer KH, Schoenbaum SC: Evaluation and management of prosthetic valve endocarditis. *Prog Cardiovasc Dis* 25:43, 1982.

34. Bluhm G: Pacemaker infections in a clinical study with special reference to prophylactic use of some isoxozolyl penicillins. *Acta Med Scand Suppl* 699:1, 1985.

35. Myers TJ, et al: Infectious complications associated with ventricular assist systems. *ASAIO J* 46:S28, 2000.

36. Holman WL, et al: Infection during circulatory support with ventricular assist devices. *Ann Thorac Surg* 68:711, 1999.

37. Wolma FJ, Derrick JR, McCoy J: Management of infected arterial grafts. *Am J Surg* 126:798, 1973.

38. Goldstone J, Moore WS: Infection in vascular prostheses: Clinical manifestations and surgical management. *Am J Surg* 128:225, 1974.

39. Ilgenfritz FM, Jordan FT: Microbiological monitoring of aortic aneurysm wall and contents during aneurysmectomy. *Arch Surg* 123:506, 1988.

40. Willwerth BM, Waldhausen JA: Infection of arterial prostheses. *Surg Gynecol Obstet* 139:446, 1974.

41. Rubin RH, Fischman AJ, Callahan RJ, et al: ^{111}In-labeled non-specific immunoglobulin scanning in the detection of focal infection. *N Engl J Med* 321:935, 1989.

42. Maki DG, Weis CE, Sarafin HW: A semiquantitative culture method for identifying intravenous-catheter-related infections. *N Engl J Med* 296:1305, 1977.

Chapter 50

INFECTIOUS COMPLICATIONS OF INTRAVASCULAR ACCESS DEVICES USED IN CRITICAL CARE

J. M. CONLY

KEY POINTS

- *Intravascular access device–associated infections may be either local or bacteremic, and the risk of developing an infection varies with the patient population, the type of device, the microbe, and the patient-microbe-device interaction.*

- *The status of all indwelling vascular access devices should be reviewed daily by the critical care team, with attention to the duration of placement, appearance of the exit site, and continued clinical indication for the intravascular device.*

- *Central venous catheters account for over 90% of all intravascular device–related bacteremias.*

- *Most intravascular device–related bacteremias are caused by endogenous skin flora at the catheter insertion site that migrate along the transcutaneous portion of the catheter with subsequent colonization of the catheter tip.*

- *Coagulase-negative staphylococci and* Staphylococcus aureus *account for just over 50% of all intravascular device–related bacteremias, followed in frequency by gram-negative bacilli and yeast.*

- *Diagnosis of intravascular device–related infection, either local or bacteremic, is best approached using a combination of clinical and laboratory criteria.*

- *Although treatment of central line infections due to coagulase-negative staphylococci may be successful without catheter removal, infections caused by* S. aureus *necessitate catheter removal.*

- *Central intravascular catheter infections are essentially preventable infections. Successful prevention entails attention to a careful needs assessment for the device, careful site selection, maximal barrier precautions and aseptic technique on insertion, insertion by the most skilled operators, rigorous catheter-site care, and interrupting the integrity of the system as little as possible.*

The use of intravascular access devices has become an integral part of modern patient care, and nowhere is this more evident than the ICU. Progress over the last two to three decades has provided an increasing array of devices other than the original peripheral and single-lumen central catheters. Included in the list of devices currently in use are multilumen central venous catheters (CVCs); tunneled CVCs such as the Hickman, Broviac, Cook, and Quinton catheters; flow-directed pulmonary artery catheters (PACs), peripherally inserted

central and midline catheters, peripheral arterial catheters, and totally implantable devices. These indwelling intravascular devices provide a route for the administration for fluids, blood products, nutritional products, and medications; allow the monitoring of hemodynamic functions; and permit bloodletting and the maintenance of emergency access. However, vascular access devices may be associated with several complications, including local and bacteremic infections related to the device, thrombosis, thrombophlebitis, and septic thrombophlebitis. Infectious complications are the most frequent and among the most serious of these complications. The magnitude of CVC-related infectious complications can be appreciated when one realizes there are an estimated 15 million days of exposure to CVCs in patients in ICUs in the United States each year.[1] Bacteremias caused by intravascular devices are associated with increased morbidity, prolonging hospitalization a mean of 7 days, and have a reported attributable mortality of up to 35% in studies that are not controlled for severity of illness.[1–4]

Epidemiology

The risk of developing device-related infection (either local or bacteremic) varies considerably with the patient population, the type of device and its intended use, the microorganisms involved, and the patient-microbe-device interaction. The risk factors for device-associated infection that have been identified for the host, the microbe, the device, and the interaction among them are listed in Table 50-1. In addition, representative incidence-density rates for device-associated bacteremias are shown in Table 50-2.

Of the many intravascular devices available, the peripheral venous catheter is by far the most commonly used. Most peripheral venous catheters currently are made of polyurethane, Teflon, or steel and are associated with a very low risk of bacteremia, with less than 1 episode of bacteremia per 500 devices.[5,6] There is little difference currently in the risk of bacteremia regardless of whether polyurethane, Teflon, or steel needles are used if the same level of asepsis is applied at the time of placement.

Peripheral arterial catheters are in widespread use in ICUs for blood pressure monitoring and for obtaining arterial samples for blood gas determination. The incidence of bacteremia related to peripheral arterial devices is about 1%,[7–9] and the rate of significant colonization ($\geq$15 colony-forming units [cfu] on semiquantitative culture) is about 5%.[7–11] Insertion by cutdown, catheterization lasting 4 days or longer, and inflammation at the catheter exit site are associated with a higher risk of significant catheter colonization.

CVCs are estimated to account for over 90% of all catheter-related bacteremias. Prospective studies of noncuffed, short-term single or multilumen catheters inserted into either internal jugular or subclavian sites have found bacteremia rates of 1% to 5% and rates of significant colonization of the catheters ($\geq$15 cfu on semiquantitative culture) ranging between 5% and 30%[12–18] depending on the use and duration of the catheter plus the patient population. Peripherally inserted central catheters (PICCs) have somewhat lower catheter-related bacteremia rates, ranging between 1% to 2%.[19] Many of the factors that may influence the risk of catheter colonization and/or catheter-related bacteremia are listed in

TABLE 50-1 Risk Factors for Catheter-Related Infection

Patient-related factors
    Age (age ≤1 year or ≥60 years)
    Loss of skin integrity (burns)
    Presence of neutropenia (absolute neutrophil count ≤1000)
    Chemotherapy and radiotherapy
    Distant focus of infection
    Severity of underlying illness
Device-related risk factors
    Type of device material (steel, polyurethane, Teflon, and silicone more resistant to bacterial adherence than polyethylene and polyvinylchloride)
    Frequency of surface irregularities
    Thrombogenecity of catheter materials (predisposes to bacterial colonization)
    Use of antibiotic or antiseptic impregnated catheters (reduces risk)
Microbe-related risk factors
    Adherence properties (adherence to fibronectin or directly to polymer materials)
    Extracellular slime substance (antiphagocytic and may potentiate pathogenecity by acting as a barrier to antimicrobial penetration)
Host-microbe–device interaction risk factors
    Type of placement (cutdown higher risk than percutaneous)
    Emergent placement (higher risk than elective placement)
    Site of placement (jugular greater risk than subclavian)
    Duration of use (longer duration increases the risk)
    Use of aseptic technique at the time of insertion (use of maximal barrier precautions—mask, sterile gown and gloves, and large drape—decreases risk)
    Dense cutaneous colonization at device entry site (higher density of bacteria per unit area increases risk)
    Dressing material (gauze dressing associated with lower risk for central lines)
    Skill of puncturist (greater operator skill decreases risk)
    Type of skin antiseptic used for insertion (chlorhexidine preparations may be associated with less risk)
    Use of topical antimicrobial ointment (may decrease risk)
    Frequency of entry into the system (greater frequency of entry represents greater risk)

Table 50-1. The presence of a distant focus of infection, bacteremia, tracheostomy, loss of skin integrity, emergent placement, internal jugular placement, absence of appropriate barrier precautions, transparent dressings, a high frequency of entry into the system, and multilumen catheters increase the risk of significant catheter colonization.[1,12–15,20–27]

The use of less stringent barrier precautions, the use of 10% povidone-iodine or 70% alcohol alone as compared with 2% chlorhexidine as an antiseptic, the use of transparent dressings (in some but not all randomized studies), duration of catheterization of 4 days or more, and heavy cutaneous insertion-site colonization all have been associated with an increased risk of catheter-related bacteremia for central catheters.[12–15,20,28–30] Antibiotic-coated and antiseptic-impregnated[31–33] CVCs reduce catheter colonization and bloodstream infection, but a recent meta-analysis suggests that the benefit is only during the first week after insertion.[34] Replacement of existing catheters over a guidewire is associated with a significantly lower rate of mechanical complications than replacement by insertion at a new site but more frequently results in infection of the newly placed catheter.[35]

PACs, which are used frequently in the management of hemodynamically unstable, critically ill patients, carry many of the same risk factors and rates of bacteremia as CVCs. Most PACs consist of a polyurethane catheter that passes through a percutaneous indwelling Teflon introducer sheath. Prospective studies have identified several risk factors associated with significant catheter colonization, including placement with less stringent barrier precautions, internal jugular vein placement, prolonged catheterization (≥4 days), and heavy microbial colonization at the catheter insertion site.[20,36,37] Exposure of a PAC to bacteremia from a distant focus of infection, catheterization for 4 days or more, and difficulty with insertion also have been found to increase the risk of bacteremia. The incidence of bacteremia from PACs is about 1%.[37]

Pathogenesis

Microorganisms can gain entry (Fig. 50-1) to the intravascular device (usually an intravascular catheter) and the intravenous delivery system in several ways to cause device- or catheter-related bacteremia, including contamination of infusate, contamination of the catheter hub–infusion tubing junction, hematogenous seeding of the catheter tip, and colonization at the cutaneous catheter exit site.

Contamination of infusate may be *intrinsic*, occurring at the manufacturing level, or *extrinsic*, occurring via the administration sets, the extension tubing, the use of outdated intravenous solutions, or a break in aseptic technique allowing faulty admixtures. The potential for proliferation of organisms in various infusate fluids after intrinsic contamination has been well documented with strains of *Klebsiella, Enterobacter,* and *Serratia.*[38,39] *Candida* species have a propensity to grow in hypertonic glucose solutions used in parenteral solutions, and the commercially available lipid emulsions support

TABLE 50-2 Representative Rates for Intravascular Device-Associated Bacteremia

Type of Device	Setting	Incidence Density Rate
Peripheral		
Short-term, infusion lock	Med/surg wards	<1/1000 catheter-days
Arterial, PICC	Med/surg ICU	2/1000 catheter-days
Central		
Non-cuffed venous	Med/surg ICU, CCU	5–7/1000 catheter-days
(single- or multilumen)	Pediatric ICU	11.4/1000 catheter-days
	Burn units	30.2/1000 catheter-days
Cuffed venous (Hickman, Broviac)	Med/surg wards	2.0/1000 catheter-days
Pulmonary arterial	Med/surg ICU	4.8/1000 catheter-days

PICC = peripherally inserted central catheter.

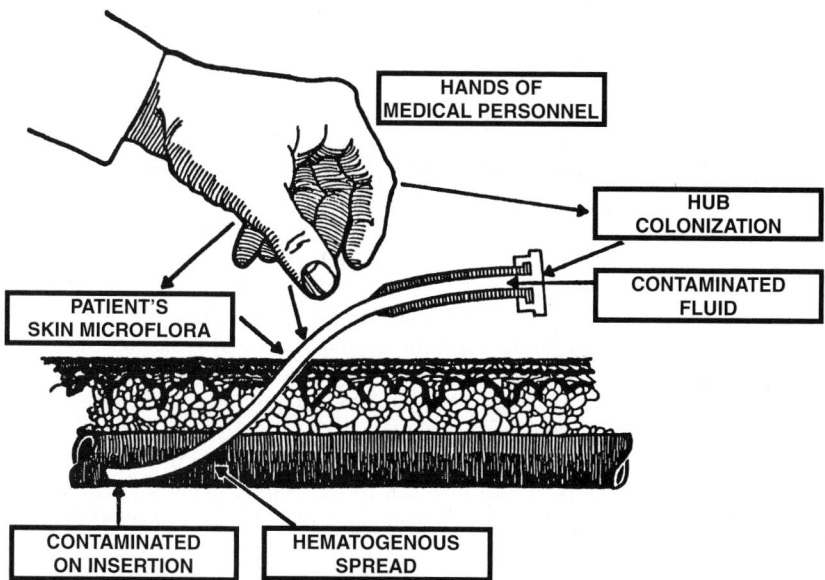

FIGURE 50-1 Potential sources for contamination of intravascular devices.

the growth of most organisms.[40] Nosocomial bacteremias secondary to contaminated infusate usually have occurred in epidemics or clusters but with improvement in manufacturing standards are now exceedingly rare. Extrinsic contamination of infusate causing central catheter–related bacteremia is also a very uncommon problem, with an estimated incidence of less than 1 per 1000 cannula-related septicemias. Most are reported in epidemics occurring as a result of the exposure to a common source of microbial contamination such as multidose vials, administration sets, or contaminated water-bath warmers. The risk of fluid becoming extrinsically contaminated is related to the duration of infusion through the administration set. Most hospitals now have policies that require replacement of the entire delivery system every 72 hours, which represents one of the most important control measures for reducing the complications of contaminated infusates. Similar to intrinsic contamination, hematogenous seeding of the catheter tip with consequent bacteremia is considered to be a rare event.

Most cannula-related bacteremias are thought to result from local endogenous microflora colonizing skin at the insertion site and/or the transcutaneous wound[29,41,42] that migrate along the subcutaneous tunnel, colonize the subcutaneous portion of the catheter, and then finally colonize the tip of the catheter. Another mechanism is colonization of the internal surface of the catheter hub, with subsequent colonization of the internal surface of the catheter and eventual colonization of the catheter tip.[43–45] This could occur as a result of obligate manipulations of the connection during tubing replacements or improper connection. After the hub has been contaminated, the microbes would be carried intraluminally, reach the catheter tip, and colonize the fibrin sheath. The origin of these microorganisms colonizing the hub is often the hands of those manipulating the hub rather than the flora of the patient's skin. This latter mechanism of catheter tip colonization is considered an important contributor to intraluminal colonization of long-term catheters.[43–45]

Studies of central line infections (short indwelling insertion times) using molecular subtyping techniques to differentiate the different strains of infecting and colonizing organisms

have demonstrated that approximately 80% of the microorganisms from distal catheter tips are concordant with organisms present on the skin at the catheter insertion site. The source of the remaining organisms was either contamination of the catheter hub, hematogenous colonization from remote sites, or unknown sources. Of episodes of catheter-related bacteremia, concordance of organisms at the catheter insertion site, the catheter tip, and the blood varied between 86% and 100%.

It also has been shown in several studies[15,20,41] that heavy colonization at the catheter insertion site is strongly associated with significant catheter colonization, which in turn is associated with catheter-related bacteremia. Using quantitative insertion-site cultures, the presence of $\geq 10^3$ cfu/mL per 25 cm^2 has been strongly associated with the presence of significant catheter colonization.

Once microorganisms gain access to the catheter tip, they act as a nidus for further colonization because of a loosely formed fibrin sheath that develops around the distal portion of the cannula. This sheath acts as a reservoir within which microorganisms can multiply and be shielded from the body's normal host defense mechanisms. The presence of grossly visible thrombus formation on the catheter tip is also highly correlated with the presence of bacterial colonization.

Microbiology

The species of the microorganism causing a bacteremia is frequently an important clue suggesting the intravascular device as the source of the bacteremia. Coagulase-negative staphylococci (mainly *Staphylococcus epidermidis*) and *Staphylococcus aureus* are the most frequently encountered organisms causing cannula-related infections. These two species account for well over 50% of all cannula-related infections. Enteric gram-negative bacilli are the next most frequent group of causative organisms, followed by yeast, especially *Candida albicans*. Other less commonly identified organisms include *Pseudomonas* species, *Corynebacterium jeikeium*, and *Malassezia furfur*.

TABLE 50-3 Frequently Encountered Microorganisms Associated with Device-Associated Bacteremia

Source	Microorganisms
Peripheral venous catheters	Coagulase-negative *Staphylococci*
	S. aureus
	Candida species
	Bacillus species
	Malassezia furfur
Peripheral arterial catheters	*Klebsiella-Enterobacter* species
	Serratia species
	Coagulase-negative *Staphylococci*
	S. aureus
Central venous and arterial catheters	Coagulase-negative *Staphylococci*
	S. aureus
	Candida species
	Corynebacterium jeikeium
	Klebsiella-Enterobacter species
	Trichophyton beiglii
	Malassezia furfur

Several studies have suggested that coagulase-negative staphylococci may have an intrinsic propensity to adhere to plastic catheters that results in a selective advantage for these organisms in causing device-associated infections.[46]

Unusual isolates such as *Enterobacter* species, *Burkholderia cepacia*, *Flavobacterium* species, and *Stenotrophomonas* and *Acinetobacter* species are uncommonly found as a cause for CVC-associated infection and should suggest the possibility of a contaminated infusion product or a common environmental reservoir.[47,48] A summary of the organisms commonly associated with device-associated bacteremia is given in Table 50-3.

Definitions and Diagnosis of Device-Related Infections

There is currently no uniform method for defining local device-related infection or device-related bacteremia. Establishing a firm diagnosis of device-related bacteremia may be very difficult. Basing the diagnosis and subsequent definition of device-related infection on clinical or laboratory criteria alone has its own intrinsic limitations. In addition, the definitions used for clinical purposes may differ from those used for surveillance.[49]

Several laboratory techniques are available to assist the diagnosis of catheter-related infection. These include qualitative culture of vascular catheters in broth, semiquantitative culture of catheters on solid media, and quantitative culture of catheters in broth, removing organisms by flushing or sonication. Qualitative culture in broth is not specific, is prone to contamination, and probably should not be done. The use of semiquantitative cultures of catheter tips or of the intracutaneous portion of the catheter or central-line sheath using the roll-plate method described by Maki and colleagues[50] defines significant colonization as 15 cfu or more. Using this laboratory definition and applying it to diagnosing catheter-related bacteremia, a specificity of 76% to 96% and a positive predictive value of 16% to 31% have been reported. Owing to its simplicity, the roll-plate method has been adopted widely in many hospital microbiology laboratories. The use

of quantitative cultures of broth, in which the catheter has been flushed or sonicated, may be more sensitive but is too time-consuming and laborious for routine use.

Quantitative blood cultures have been used as a laboratory method to assist in the diagnosis of catheter-related bacteremia when catheter removal is not possible.[51,52] Blood cultures are obtained simultaneously from the central catheter (a retrograde "drawback" culture) and from a peripheral venipuncture. A 10-fold or higher differential count from blood obtained from the central catheter is considered to be indicative of catheter-related bacteremia. The use of quantitative cultures is laborious, and concerns over contamination of drawback cultures have limited the usefulness of this technique. Recent studies have evaluated endoluminal brush sampling and differential blood culture growth rates, which may provide acceptable accuracy without requiring removal of indwelling catheters, but the accuracy of these techniques needs to be confirmed in other studies.[53–56]

Using clinical criteria alone to make a diagnosis of catheter-related infection also may be difficult. Whereas the presence of culture-positive purulent exudate at the catheter insertion site in the presence of bacteremia with the same organism would define a catheter-related bacteremia, making the diagnosis is much more difficult with bacteremia in the absence of any inflammation at the catheter insertion site. Signs of local inflammation at the catheter insertion site are present in only about 50% of the cases of catheter-related bacteremia. Several clinicoepidemiologic features are helpful in distinguishing catheter-related bacteremia from bacteremia caused by another source. These findings, which may be present alone or in combination, include the following:

1. Absence of an alternative source for bacteremia on clinical examination
2. Patient not considered at high risk for bacteremia
3. Presence of local purulence at the catheter exit site
4. Presence of *Candida* endophthalmitis in patients who are receiving total parenteral nutrition
5. A septic picture that is refractory to antimicrobial theapy
6. Bloodstream infection caused by staphylococci or *Candida* species
7. Dramatic improvement of a febrile syndrome following catheter removal
8. Clusters of bacteremia due to *Enterobacter* species for seemingly unapparent reasons (suggesting common-source contamination of IV fluids)

Many definitions for catheter-related infections have been used, but none is considered standard or uniform. However, any definition used should incorporate both clinical and laboratory criteria in an attempt to increase the utility of the definition. Examples of definitions for local and bacteremic catheter-related infections that may be used are given below. For local infections, definitions include

- Purulent discharge at the exit site, either spontaneous or expressed on palpation of the site, regardless of whether an organism is cultured from the site
- Erythema, tenderness, and/or induration (any two of the three) at the exit site with serous or serosanguineous discharge, either spontaneous or expressed on palpation, in the

presence of a positive exit-site culture (moderate to heavy growth of a single or predominant organism)

Definitions for bacteremic infection include those for *definite* infection:

- A single positive peripheral blood culture from a patient with clinical and microbiologic data disclosing no other source of the bacteremia in the presence of a semiquantitative or quantitative culture of a catheter segment (proximal or distal) from which the same organism (species, antibiogram) was isolated
- Differential quantitative blood cultures with a 10-fold or greater colony-count difference between blood cultures drawn from the catheter and simultaneously from a peripheral venous blood culture
- A single positive peripheral blood culture from a patient with isolation of the same organism (species, antibiogram) from purulent, serous, or serosanguineous discharge from the catheter exit site or along the path of a subcutaneously tunneled catheter or from the subcutaneous pocket containing a reservoir of a totally implantable device

Definitions for *probable* infection include

- Two or more positive blood cultures for the same organism (species, antibiogram) from any source (peripheral or retrograde intravascular device cultures) from a patient with clinical and microbiologic data disclosing no other source for the bacteremia except the intravascular device
- One positive blood culture for *S. aureus* or *Candida* species from any source (peripheral or retrograde intravascular device culture) in a patient with clinical and microbiologic data disclosing no other source for the bacteremia except the intravascular device
- One positive blood culture for any organism commonly associated with intravascular device–related infection (coagulase-negative staphylococci, *Bacillus* species, *Corynebacterium* species, and *M. furfur*) from any source (peripheral or retrograde culture) in an immunocompromised patient or a neutropenic patient (neutrophils <500 cells/μL) with clinical and microbiologic data disclosing no other source for the bacteremia except a *centrally* placed intravascular device

Management of Infection

The management of intravascular device–associated infections depends on several variables, including the type of infection (local or bacteremic), the microorganism(s) involved, the type of device (peripheral or central catheter, totally implanted device), and the severity of illness of the patient. A guideline was published recently that outlines these variables in detail and provides detailed recommendations for the management of intravascular catheter–related infections.[57] Local infections at the catheter insertion site may be treated with catheter removal, local care, and topical and/or systemic antimicrobial agents as appropriate. If a spreading cellulitis develops, extending along the course of the catheter, then systemic antimicrobials and catheter removal are indicated. The antimicrobials chosen should be based on microbiologic cultures obtained from the discharge present at the insertion site.

The management of bacteremic infections is more complex and depends on the microorganism, the type of device, and the clinical status of the patient. Any peripheral (venous or arterial) or noncuffed central catheters (venous or pulmonary arterial) that are being used in the short term and are suspected of being the source of a bacteremic infection in a patient with no other obvious source should be removed, the administration set changed, and the catheter tip and intracutaneous portion of the insertion sheath sent for culture. The catheter should be removed regardless of whether there is evidence of inflammation at the insertion site because over 50% of the catheter-related bacteremias occur without any evidence of local site inflammation.

An option for the management of CVC-related bacteremia due to coagulase-negative staphylococci, without removal of the catheter, is the use of systemic antimicrobials and the antibiotic-lock technique,[57] but the risk of recurrent bacteremic infection is approximately 20%.[58] Thus this option must be considered carefully on an individual basis. In general, if the indication for the central catheter remains, a new catheter should be inserted into a new site if the catheter is proved to be or is strongly suspected as the source of the infection. In the absence of inflammation or local purulence at the catheter insertion site, and when the evidence suggesting the line as the source for infection is not compelling, it is reasonable to do a guidewire catheter exchange at the same site, but the catheter that is removed should be cultured, and if it is positive, the newly inserted catheter should be removed and another catheter inserted in a different site.[35]

Device-related bacteremia that is suspected to arise from cuffed central long-term indwelling catheters (Hickman, Broviac, or Cook catheter) or totally implanted devices does not necessarily require removal of the device.[57] If there is obvious local purulence, bacteremia due to *S. aureus* or *Candida* species, a spreading tunnel-associated cellulitis, septic thrombophlebitis, tricuspid valve endocarditis, or a persisting bacteremia despite appropriate parenteral antimicrobial therapy, removal of the device is required, often with surgical dissection. Retention of a cuffed long-term central catheter with catheter-related *S. aureus* bacteremia has been associated with a higher relapse rate of bacteremia and higher sepsis-related mortality.[59] In the setting of bacteremia due to other microorganisms and in the absence of complications, a course of parenteral antimicrobial therapy with or without antibiotic-lock therapy without removal of the cuffed central catheter or implantable device may be sufficient in as many as two-thirds of cases.[57,60,61] Following treatment, these patients should be monitored carefully for recurrences of bacteremic infection.

Definitive antimicrobial therapy for device-associated bacteremia depends on appropriate identification and susceptibility testing of the infecting microorganism. Empirical therapy prior to the identification and susceptibility results will be influenced by local microbiologic patterns of line-related infection and susceptibilities. However, a combination of an IV antistaphylococcal penicillin (vancomycin if methicillin-resistant *S. aureus* is prevalent) and an aminoglycoside or a third-generation cephalosporin will provide coverage for most gram-positive and gram-negative microorganisms. Any catheter-related bacteremic infections caused by *S. aureus* should be treated for 14 days with parenteral therapy to avoid metastatic infectious complications. The optimal duration of therapy for infections caused by organisms other than

TABLE 50-4 Strategies for Prevention of Vascular Device–Related Infections

Process or System	Preventive Strategy	Rationale
Device itself	Institute careful needs assessment prior to insertion of any intravascular device.	Avoid unnecessary insertions. Use of peripheral catheter, midline, or PICC line should be considered if appropriate.
	Choose least thrombogenic material for type of device being inserted based on the needs assessment.	Polyvinylchloride > polyurethane > silicone > steel with respect to thrombogenecity and colonization with certain microorganisms.
	Consider use of antiseptic-antimicrobial bonded devices or use of subcutaneous cuffs impregnated with antimicrobial agent.	Significant reductions in catheter infection rates (50%–80%) have been found in several randomized controlled trials using chlorhexidine silver-bonded catheters, silver-impregnated cuffs, and antibiotic-coated catheters.
	Minimize the number of lumens and the number of accesses whenever possible.	This strategy is somewhat controversial, since several but not all studies have demonstrated an increased risk of catheter infection with multilumen lines. A greater number of lumens will increase the frequency of entry to the system, which is associated with a greater risk of catheter-related infection.
Device insertion	Choose site associated with least risk for local and systemic device-related infection.	Risk of local and systemic catheter-related infection is independently associated with density of flora at the catheter insertion site; femoral > jugular/subclavian > antecubital fossa.
	Use aseptic technique.	Good hand washing and use of maximal barrier precautions (masks, sterile drapes, gloves, gown) are associated with less risk of catheter-related bacteremia than minimal barrier precautions (mask, sterile gloves, small drapes).
	Insertion is done by skilled operators.	Organized, specifically trained IV teams have been associated with lower catheter infection rates, but the key ingredient is a highly skilled operator with excellent technique. Difficulty of insertion has been associated with higher local catheter-related infection rates.
	Place device in as controlled an environment as possible.	Emergency catheter insertions are associated with a higher risk of infection than elective placement.
	Use prophylactic antibiotics at time of insertion.	Prospective randomized controlled trials have shown no benefit, and prophylactic antibiotics are not generally recommended.
Catheter site care	Use cutaneous antiseptic with maximal efficacy, ease of application, and compliance with recommendations for usage.	Chlorhexidine (0.5% tincture or 2% aqueous) may offer best approach to cutaneous antisepsis considering all criteria for use. Povidone iodine, although effective, is often used improperly despite best efforts to improve compliance.
	Apply topical antiseptics/antimicrobials at the insertion site.	Clinical trials to date have shown only marginal or no benefit but may be of benefit in selected settings.
	Choose dry gauze or other permeable dressings for site care.	Transparent semipermeable dressings have been associated with both a significantly increased density of flora at the catheter insertion site and local catheter-related infection rates. Some prospective studies have demonstrated a significantly increased risk of catheter-related bacteremia.
Catheter care	Minimize the number of interruptions to the integrity of the line.	With TPN there is an increased risk of catheter-related infection with line violations. The system should be kept closed as much as possible.
Delivery system	Minimize the number of interruptions to the integrity of the delivery system.	With TPN the risk of catheter-related infections increases significantly with interruptions to the integrity of the system.
	Change administration set every 72 hours.	Changes of the administration sets at 72-hour intervals have not been shown to be associated with any increased risk of catheter-related infection compared to changes at 24-hour intervals.

PICC = peripherally inserted central catheter; TPN = total parenteral nutrition.

S. aureus is unknown, but 7 to 14 days has been suggested.[57] Catheter-related candidemia may be treated with a short course of amphotericin B (3 to 7 mg/kg total dose) or fluconazole (200 to 400 mg/day for 10 to 14 days). In the susceptible patient population most often found in the ICU, a thorough evaluation for metastatic candidal infection, including careful funduscopic examination, is necessary. The finding of persistently positive blood cultures after catheter removal and initiation of antifungal therapy or the finding of metastatic candidal lesions would necessitate more prolonged therapy.

Preventive Strategies

Attention to detail in all aspects of the placement and care of intravascular devices is necessary to minimize the risks of device-related infection. This attention to detail is particularly important in the ICU, where the use of lines is intensive and patients, by nature of their underlying illnesses, are at high risk of device-related infections. The processes to which preventive strategies may be applied may be divided conveniently into the catheter itself, the catheter insertion, catheter site care, catheter care, and the delivery system (Table 50-4). The details on which attention should be focused, as well as the accompanying rationale for the specific strategy, are presented. Detailed guidelines for the prevention of intravascular device–related infections are available from the Centers for Disease Control and Prevention.[49]

Although new scientific approaches to establishing improved techniques for catheter care are necessary and new technologic advances such as microbe-resistant materials will help to reduce the incidence of catheter-related infection, there is no substitute for meticulous care and attention to detail in care of the lines.

References

1. Mermel LA: Prevention of intravascular catheter-related infections. *Ann Intern Med* 132:391, 2000.
2. Smith RL, Meixler SM, Simberkoff MS: Excess mortality in critically ill patients with nosocomial bloodstream infections. *Chest* 100:164, 1991.
3. Digiovine B, Chenoweth C, Watts C, Higgins M: The attributable mortality and costs of primary nosocomial bloodstream infections in the intensive care unit. *Am J Respir Crit Care Med* 60:976, 1999.
4. Pittet D, Tarara D, Wenzel RP: Nosocomial bloodstream infection in critically ill patients: Excess length of stay, extra costs, and attributable mortality. *JAMA* 162:1598, 1994.
5. Craven DE, Lichtenberg A, Kunches LM, et al: A randomized study comparing a transparent polyurethane dressing to a dry gauze dressing for peripheral intravenous catheter sites. *Infect Control* 6:361, 1985.
6. Maki DG, Ringer M: Evaluation of dressing regimens for prevention of infection with peripheral intravenous catheters. *JAMA* 258:2396, 1987.
7. Thomas F, Burke JP, Parker J, et al: The risk of infection related to radial vs femoral sites for arterial catheterization. *Crit Care Med* 11:807, 1988.
8. Gardner RM, Schwartz R, Wong HC, Burke JP: Percutaneous indwelling radial-artery catheters for monitoring cardiovascular function. *N Engl J Med* 290:1227, 1974.
9. Raad I, Umphrey I, Khan A, et al: The duration of placement as a predictor of peripheral and pulmonary arterial catheter infections. *J Hosp Infect* 23:17, 1993.
10. Norwood SH, Cormier B, McMahon NG, et al: Prospective study of catheter-related infection during prolonged arterial catheterization. *Crit Care Med* 16:836, 1988.
11. Pinilla JC, Ross DF, Martin T, Crump H: Study of the incidence of intravascular catheter infection and associated septicemia in critically ill patients. *Crit Care Med* 11:21, 1983.
12. Powell C, Regan C, Fabri PJ, Ruberg RL: Evaluation of op-site catheter dressings for parenteral nutrition: A prospective, randomized study. *J Parenter Enteral Nutr* 6:43, 1982.
13. Richet H, Hubert B, Nitemberg G, et al: Prospective multicentre study of vascular-catheter-related complications and risk factors for positive central-catheter cultures in intensive care unit patients. *J Clin Microbiol* 28:2520, 1990.
14. Powell CR, Traetow MJ, Fabri PJ, et al: Op-Site dressing study: A prospective, randomized study evaluating povidone-iodine

15. Conly JM, Grieves K, Peters B: A prospective, randomized study comparing transparent and dry gauze dressings for central venous catheters. *J Infect Dis* 159:310, 1989.
16. Raad II, Hohn DC, Gilbreath BJ, et al: Prevention of central venous catheter-related infections by using maximal sterile barrier precautions during insertion. *Infect Control Hosp Epidemiol* 15:231, 1994.
17. Armstrong CW, Mayhall G, Miller KB, et al: Prospective study of catheter replacement and other risk factors for infection of hyperalimentation catheters. *J Infect Dis* 154:808, 1986.
18. Flowers RH III, Schwenzer KJ, Kopel RJ, et al: Efficacy of an attachable subcutaneous cuff for the prevention of intravascular catheter-related infection. *JAMA* 261:878, 1989.
19. Raad I, Davis S, Becker M, et al: Low infection rate and long durability of non-tunneled Silastic catheters: A safe cost-effective alternative for long-term venous access. *Arch Intern Med* 153:1791, 1993.
20. Mermel LA, McCormick RD, Springman SR, Maki DG: The pathogenesis and epidemiology of catheter-related infection with pulmonary artery Swan-Ganz catheters: A prospective study utilizing molecular subtyping. *Am J Med* 38:197S, 1991.
21. Pemberton L, Lyman B, Lauder V, et al: Sepsis from triple- vs single-lumen catheters during total parenteral nutrition in surgical or critically ill patients. *Arch Surg* 121:591, 1986.
22. Hilton E, Haslett T, Borenstein M, et al: Central catheter infections: Single vs triple-lumen catheters influence of guidelines on infection rates when used for replacement of catheters. *Am J Med* 84:667, 1988.
23. Bjornson H, Colley R, Bower R, et al: Association between microorganisms growth at the catheter insertion site and colonization of catheter in patients receiving total parenteral nutrition. *Surgery* 92:7207, 1982.
24. Pettigren R, Lang D, Haycock D, et al: Catheter-related sepsis in patients on intravenous nutrition: A prospective study of quantitative catheter cultures and guideline changes for suspected sepsis. *Br J Surg* 72:52, 1985.
25. Armstrong C, Mayhall C, Miller K, et al: Prospective study of catheter replacement and other risk factors for infection of hyperalimentation catheters. *J Infect Dis* 154:808, 1986.
26. Ryan J, Abel R, Abbott W, et al: Catheter complications in total parenteral nutrition: A prospective study of 200 consecutive patients. *New Engl Med* 290:757, 1974.
27. Michel L, McMichan J, Bachy J: Microbial colonization of indwelling central venous catheters: Statistical evaluation of potential contaminating factors. *Am J Surg* 137:745, 1979.
28. Hoffman KK, Western S, Kaiser DL, et al: Bacterial colonization and phlebitis-associated risk with transparent polyurethane film for peripheral intravenous site dressings. *Am J Infect Control* 16:101, 1988.
29. Conly J, Stein K, Peters B: The pathogenesis of catheter-related infection in central venous catheters using gauze versus transparent dressings, in Wadstrom T, Eliasson I, Holder I, Ljungh A (eds): *Pathogenesis of Wound and Biomaterial Association Infections*. London, Springer-Verlag, 1990, p 508.
30. Maki DG, Ringer M, Alvarado CJ: Prospective randomized trial of povidone-iodine, alcohol, and chlorhexidine for prevention of infection associated with central venous and arterial catheters. *Lancet* 338:339, 1991.
31. Maki DG, Stolz SM, Wheeler S, et al: Prevention of central venous catheter–related bloodstream infection by use of an antiseptic-impregnated catheter: A randomized, controlled trial. *Ann Intern Med* 127:257, 1997.
32. Raad I, Darouiche R, Dupuis J, et al: Central venous catheters coated with minocycline and rifampin for the prevention of

catheter-related colonization and bloodstream infections: A randomized, double-blind trial. *Ann Intern Med* 127:267, 1997.

33. Chaiyakunapruk N, Veenstra DL, Lipsky BA, Saint S: Chlorhexidene compared with povidone-iodine solution for vascular-site care: A meta-analysis. *Ann Intern Med* 136:792, 2002.

34. Waldner B, Pittet D, Tramer M: Prevention of bloodstream infections with central catheters treated with anti-infective agents depends on cathetere type and insertion time: Evidence from a meta–analysis. *Infect Control Hosp Epidemiol* 23:748, 2002.

35. Cobb DK, High KP, Sawyer RG, et al: A controlled trial of scheduled replacement of central venous and pulmonary-artery catheters. *N Engl J Med* 327:1062, 1992.

36. Rello J, Coll P, Net A, Prats G: Infection of pulmonary artery catheters: Epidemiologic characteristics and multivariate analysis of risk factors. *Chest* 103:132, 1993.

37. Mermel LA, Maki DG: Infectious complications of Swan-Ganz pulmonary artery catheters: Pathogenesis, epidemiology, prevention and management. *Am J Respir Crit Care Med* 149:1020, 1994.

38. Maki DG, Rhame FS, Mackel DC, Bennett JV: Nationwide epidemic of septicemia caused by contaminated intravenous products. *Am J Med* 60:471, 1976.

39. Jarvis WR, Highsmith AK: Bacterial growth and endotoxin production in lipid emulsion. *J Clin Microbiol* 19:17, 1984.

40. Plouffe JF, Brown DG, Silva J, et al: Nosocomial outbreak of *Candida parapsilosis* fungemia related to intravenous infusions. *Arch Intern Med* 137:1686, 1977.

41. Maki D, Ringer M: Evaluation of dressing regimens for prevention of infection with peripheral intravenous catheters: Gauze, a transparent polyurethane dressing, and an iodophor-transparent dressing. *JAMA* 258:2396, 1987.

42. Syndman D, Murray S, Kornfeld S, et al: Total parenteral nutrition-related infections: Prospective epidemiologic study using semiquantitative methods. *Am J Med* 73:695, 1982.

43. Sitges-Serra A, Puig P, Linares J, et al: Hub colonization as the initial step in an outbreak of catheter-related sepsis due to coagulase negative *Staphylococci* during parenteral nutrition. *J Parent Enteral Nutr* 8:668, 1984.

44. Linares J, Sitges-Serra A, Garau J, et al: Pathogenesis of catheter sepsis: A prospective study with quantitative and semiquantitative cultures of catheter hub and segments. *J Clin Microbiol* 21:357, 1985.

45. Raad II, Costerton W, Sabharwal U, Sacilowski M, Anaissie E, Bodey GP: Ultrastructural analysis of indwelling vascular catheters: a quantitative relationship between luminal colonization and duration of placement. *J Infect Dis* 168:400, 1993.

46. Peters G, Locci R, Pulverer G: Adherence and growth of coagulase-negative staphylococci on surfaces of intravenous catheters. *J Infect Dis* 146:479, 1982.

47. Bollet C, Elkouby A, Pietri P, et al: Isolation of *Enterobacter amnigenus* from a heart transplant recipient. *Eur J Clin Microbiol Infect Dis* 10:1071, 1991.

48. Henderson D, Baptiste R, Parrillo J, et al: Indolent epidemic of *Pseudomonas cepacia* bacteremia and pseudobacteremia in an intensive care unit traced to a contaminated blood gas analyzer. *Am J Med* 84:75, 1988.

49. Centers for Disease Control Prevention: Guidelines for the prevention of intravascular catheter–related infections. *MMWR* 51:1, 2002.

50. Maki D, Weise C, Sarafin H: A semiquantitative method for identifying intravenous catheter–related infection. *N Engl J Med* 296:1305, 1977.

51. Mosca R, Curtas S, Forbes B, et al: The benefits of isolator cultures in the management of suspected catheter sepsis. *Surgery* 102:718, 1987.

52. Ascher PD, Shoupe BA, Robb M, et al: Comparison of standard and quantitative blood cultures in the evaluation of children with suspected central venous line sepsis. *Diagn Microbiol Infect Dis* 15:499, 1992.

53. Kite P, Dobbins BM, Wilcox MH, et al: Evaluation of a novel endoluminal brush method for in situ diagnosis of catheter related sepsis. *J Clin Pathol* 50:278, 1997.

54. Kite P, Dobbins BM, Wilcox MH, McMahon MJ: Rapid diagnosis of central-venous-catheter-related bloodstream infection without catheter removal. *Lancet* 354:1504, 1999.

55. Seifert H, Cornely O, Seggewiss K, et al: Bloodstream infection in neutropenic cancer patients related to short-term nontunneled catheters determined by quantitative blood cultures, differential time to positivity, and molecular epidemiological typing with pulsed-field gel electrophoresis *J Clin Microbiol* 41:118, 2003.

56. Blot F, Nitenberg G, Chachaty E, et al: Diagnosis of catheter-related bacteraemia: A prospective comparison of the time to positivity of hub-blood versus peripheral-blood cultures. *Lancet* 354:1071, 1999.

57. Mermel LA, Farr BM, Sherertz RJ, et al: Guidelines for the management of intravascular catheter–related infections. *Clin Infect Dis* 32:1249, 2001.

58. Raad I, Davis S, Khan A, et al: Impact of central venous catheter removal on the recurrence of catheter-related coagulase-negative staphylococcal bacteremia. *Infect Control Hosp Epidemiol* 13:215, 1992.

59. Dugdale DA, Ramsey PG: *Staphylococcus aureus* bacteremia in patients with Hickman catheters. *Am J Med* 89:137, 1990.

60. Press OW, Ramsey PG, Larson EB, et al: Hickman catheter infections in patients with malignancies. *Medicine* 63:189, 1984.

61. Schuman ES, Winters V, Gross GF, Hayes JF: Management of Hickman catheter sepsis. *Am J Surg* 149:627, 1985.

Chapter 51 _____

PNEUMONIA
R. BRUCE LIGHT

KEY POINTS

- *Pneumonia is one of the leading causes of respiratory failure leading to admission to the intensive care unit and is by far the most common nosocomial infection in critically ill patients.*

- *Mortality rate may exceed 50% for severe community-acquired pneumonia (CAP) requiring admission to the intensive care unit and varies from 30% to 60% in nosocomial cases.*

- *The initial approach to diagnostic testing and empiric therapy is guided by the clinical presentation of the pneumonia, which can be categorized as follows: CAP, acute CAP, aspiration pneumonia/lung abscess, and chronic pneumonia; nosocomial pneumonia; and pulmonary infiltrate in immunocompromised host.*

- *Investigation of acute pneumonia should always include a blood culture and Gram stain and culture of lower respiratory tract secretions. Smear and culture for* Legionella *species and serologic testing for other atypical pathogens should be done when atypical pneumonia features are present and in otherwise undiagnosed cases of severe pneumonia.*

- *Fiberoptic bronchoscopy with quantitative bacteriology of a protected brush specimen or bronchoalveolar lavage specimen is the procedure of choice for diagnosis of acute CAP and nosocomial pneumonia that respond poorly to treatment and resist diagnosis by noninvasive means.*

- *Empiric intravenous antimicrobial therapy should be begun immediately in all critically ill patients with an acute pneumonia. Antimicrobial coverage should include all pathogens of more than trivial probability and should always include* Streptococcus pneumoniae, Staphylococcus aureus, *and* Enterobacteriaceae. *In cases of severe pneumonia of unknown cause, a fluoroquinolone should be included to cover* Legionella *species, and dual antimicrobial coverage for* Pseudomonas *species should be given to patients at special risk of carrying this organism.*

- *Empiric antimicrobial therapy initially can be withheld in less severely ill patients in whom the diagnosis of infectious pneumonia is in doubt and in patients with a chronic pneumonia presentation, pending definitive diagnosis.*

- *Pulmonary infiltrates in an immunocompromised host may be caused by any of the infectious agents affecting the normal population, by opportunistic infections, or by noninfectious processes. The required approach combines empiric therapy, selected on the basis of the particular infectious agents for which the patient is at special risk, with a timely stepwise diagnostic approach that moves from noninvasive testing to fiberoptic bronchoscopy to open lung biopsy at a rate determined by the rate of progression of the patient's undiagnosed pneumonia.*

Pneumonia remains the leading infectious cause of death in the developed world. It is also the most frequent infection leading to admission to most intensive care units (ICUs) and by far the most important nosocomial infection complicating the treatment of patients admitted to ICUs for other problems. Roughly 5% to 10% of patients hospitalized for community-acquired pneumonia (CAP) require ICU admission, with a mortality rate of 30% to 50%.[1–3] Pneumonia is also the most important nosocomial infection leading to ICU admission and a frequent complication of treatment in an ICU, occurring in 5% to 50% of patients requiring mechanical ventilation.[4] A systematic approach and an aggressive attitude toward diagnosis and treatment of pneumonia therefore are fundamental to good critical care practice.

The discussion that follows categorizes the major pneumonia syndromes as CAP, nosocomial pneumonia, and pulmonary infiltrates in the immunocompromised host. Whereas the etiologies of pneumonia in these three categories overlap to some degree, the underlying pathogeneses, etiologic differential diagnoses, and approaches to empiric antimicrobial therapy differ considerably.

Community-Acquired Pneumonia

Pneumonia in patients presenting from outside the hospital can lead to ICU admission for a variety of reasons: hypoxemic or hypercapnic respiratory failure, depressed level of consciousness caused by hypoxia or sepsis, or hypotension related to relative hypovolemia or septic shock. Although supportive management for these problems is generally similar for all types of pneumonia and the principles of circulatory and respiratory management differ little from those for shock and respiratory failure of other causes, there are major differences among the different forms of pneumonia in the approach to diagnosis and empiric antimicrobial therapy. The great majority of CAPs are caused by common bacterial pathogens such as *Streptococcus pneumoniae, Staphylococcus aureus,* and *Haemophilus influenzae.* However, in most series of pneumonia severe enough to require ICU admission, a significant minority of cases is caused by a number of less common pathogens with widely differing antimicrobial susceptibilities.[1–7] Approximate percentages for the major causes of CAP are shown in Table 51-1. The distribution of etiologies varies widely among different geographic areas.

PATHOGENESIS

Pathogenic mechanisms of pneumonia vary greatly among the different etiologic agents, depending on the relative virulence of the organism, which host defenses are most important in preventing infection with that organism, and the common route of entry of the organism into the lung. The three major routes of entry are aspiration of oropharyngeal or gastric contents into the lung, inhalation of aerosols or particles containing organisms, and hematogenous spread of organisms into the lung from another infected site.

Aspiration accounts for the vast majority of pulmonary infections, with the particular clinical syndrome being determined by the quantity of material aspirated, the nature of the bacteria in the aspirated material, and the efficiency of the host's pulmonary defense mechanisms. The upper airway of normal human beings is frequently colonized by *S. pneumoniae, H. influenzae,* and, occasionally, *S. aureus,* in addition to the normal microflora consisting of mixed aerobic and anaerobic bacteria. Colonization by enteric gram-negative

TABLE 51-1 Infectious Etiologic Agents Implicated in Severe Community-Acquired Pneumonia Requiring Intensive Care Support

Etiologic Agent	Cases Admitted (%)[a]
Acute community-acquired pneumonia	85
Streptococcus pneumoniae	40
Staphylococcus aureus	10
Enterobacteriaceae	10
Legionella pneumophila	10
Haemophilus influenzae	5
Mycoplasma pneumoniae	5
Chlamydia psittaci	2
Coxiella burnetii	1
Viral	2
Aspiration pneumonia/lung abscess	10
Chronic pneumonia syndrome	5
Mycobacterium tuberculosis	3
Endemic dimorphic fungi	2

[a] The percentage shown are approximate only, based on published studies from different geographic locations and population bases. Because these percentages represent cases requiring hospital admission and care in the intensive care unit, pneumonias that more commonly cause severe illness or that occur more commonly in patients with significant underlying disease (*S. aureus*, enteric gram-negative bacilli, *Legionella* spp., etc.) are over-represented compared with unselected community-acquired pneumonia. Also note that most published series include 20% to 50% for which no etiologic diagnosis was made and that are not included in this table.

bacilli, such as *Escherichia coli* or *Klebsiella pneumoniae*, is much less frequent, occurring in fewer than 1% of persons in the community at large, although it is more frequent in alcoholics, persons with poor oral hygiene, and the institutionalized elderly.[8,9] Even people who have normal upper airway reflexes aspirate small quantities of oropharyngeal material during sleep.[10] Normally, the organisms so aspirated are cleared by the bronchial mucociliary clearance mechanism, and any residual debris is cleared by the phagocytic cells present in alveoli and on the bronchial mucosa. However, if the aspirate contains organisms with significant potential for virulence, and if the aspiration occurs in a human host with impaired pulmonary clearance mechanisms, the organism can proliferate in the pulmonary parenchyma and cause pneumonia. Pneumonia caused by relatively high-grade pathogens such as *S. pneumoniae*, *S. aureus*, and enteric gram-negative bacilli generally occurs as an acute infection without clinically obvious major aspiration (i.e., the aspiration is subclinical) in patients with damaged or deficient host defenses. Examples include pneumonia after a viral respiratory infection (which impairs ciliary clearance mechanisms), pneumonia in alcoholics or others with intermittently depressed level of consciousness (greater opportunity for subclinical aspiration), and pneumonia in patients with impaired mucociliary clearance (chronic obstructive pulmonary disease, or chronic bronchitis) or relative immunologic impairment (diabetes mellitus, uremia, or hypogammaglobulinemia).

The normal microflora of the upper airway has limited virulence and therefore causes pulmonary infection mainly when aspiration is more florid, when the aspirated oropharyngeal material is present in greater quantity, or when there is severe local impairment of tracheobronchial clearance.

Examples of these conditions include risk factors for major aspiration, such as uncontrolled epileptic seizures or abnormal motor control of the upper airway; periodontal disease; and bronchial obstruction caused by foreign body aspiration or neoplasm. The infection produced by these relatively nonpathogenic bacteria is usually an indolent one producing a subacute, but necrotizing, pneumonia, with eventual liquefaction of pulmonary parenchyma and abscess formation.

Because the numbers of microorganisms reaching the lung usually are extremely small when the route of entry is inhalation, only organisms that are highly efficient pathogens produce infection by this mechanism. This does not include most of the common bacterial pathogens but does include most respiratory viruses, *Legionella* species, *Mycoplasma pneumoniae*, *Chlamydia* species, *Coxiella burnetii*, *Mycobacterium tuberculosis*, and most of the endemic fungal pneumonias. These pathogens are inhaled and deposited within alveoli, evading tracheobronchial mucociliary clearance. For the most part they share the ability to resist phagocytosis or to survive intracellularly within phagocytes, requiring the development of a humoral and cell-mediated immune response to limit infection.

For hematogenous spread of infection to the lung, the organisms must gain access to the venous circulation; the organisms lodge in the pulmonary microvasculature of the lung and proliferate. The pneumonia is usually diffuse or multinodular throughout both lung fields. In most cases, there is an established infection elsewhere, which is then carried to the lung, or organisms are injected directly into the bloodstream, as with intravenous drug abusers and persons given contaminated intravenous fluid infusions. The common pathogens are *S. aureus* and aerobic gram-negative bacilli such as *Pseudomonas aeruginosa*. A few rare pulmonary infections caused by very virulent organisms that gain entry directly through damaged skin are also transmitted to the lung hematogenously; such pulmonary involvement may occur in tularemia, brucellosis, and melioidosis.

PATHOPHYSIOLOGY

The proliferation of microorganisms within the pulmonary parenchyma elicits the host's full acute inflammatory response, with exudation of protein-rich fluid and influx of large numbers of phagocytic cells into alveoli and airways. The local mechanical consequences of this include impaired distribution of ventilation and a decrease in lung compliance, which contribute to increased work of breathing and the symptom of dyspnea. Ventilation/perfusion mismatch is increased somewhat, particularly in predominantly interstitial pneumonias; in most acute bacterial pneumonias, the major mechanism for arterial hypoxemia is intrapulmonary shunt caused by maintenance of pulmonary arterial blood flow to consolidated lung.[11,12] There is also evidence that metabolically active inflammatory cells within the consolidated lung consume oxygen, thus further decreasing pulmonary venous oxygen content and arterial oxygenation.[12–14]

The local inflammatory response includes activation of mononuclear phagocytic cells, which are the main source of interleukin 1, cachectin, and other cytokines that act as hormones mediating the acute-phase response. These effects result in fever, leukocytosis, and the many other metabolic changes of infection. In more severe cases, bacteremia or microbial antigenemia may activate the inflammatory response systemically, leading to frank septic shock (see Chap. 46).

CLINICAL AND RADIOGRAPHIC FEATURES

The basic features common to most forms of pneumonia include (a) the presence of a systemic inflammatory response manifest as fever, elevation of the white blood cell count, and, in severe cases, other features of the sepsis syndrome; (b) pulmonary symptoms such as cough, sputum production, or hemoptysis, dyspnea, and pleuritic chest pain (if the pleura is involved); (c) physical findings consistent with an inflammatory pulmonary parenchymal process, such as tachypnea, rales, or signs of consolidation (bronchial breathing, dullness to percussion, increased vocal fremitus over the consolidated lung region); (d) evidence of abnormal lung function, such as arterial hypoxemia and hypocapnia (in a hyperventilating, dyspneic patient) or hypercapnia (in a patient with acute-on-chronic respiratory failure); and (e) a radiographic pulmonary infiltrate consistent with pneumonia.

There are major differences in the time course, frequency, and pattern of these findings among the many forms of pneumonia caused by the multiplicity of etiologic agents. Characterizing the patient's presentation based on the clinical, epidemiologic, and radiographic features—information generally available for most patients when they are initially seen—is a useful starting point in the assessment of pneumonia. These clinical presentations include:

1. Acute CAP
2. Aspiration pneumonia
3. Chronic pneumonia

ACUTE COMMUNITY-ACQUIRED PNEUMONIA
Bacterial Pneumonia

The typical history for CAP caused by conventional bacteria, most commonly *S. pneumoniae*, is acute onset of fever, with chills or rigors, associated with dyspnea and a cough productive of purulent or bloody sputum, sometimes with pleuritic chest pain. Patients with no chronic underlying disease often report a preceding upper respiratory tract infection, but most pneumonias occur in the presence of a predisposing illness, such as alcohol abuse, chronic lung disease, chronic cardiac or renal failure, or malignancy. In more severely debilitated patients or the institutionalized elderly, a specific history may be unavailable; new or worsened confusion and tachypnea noted by attendants is often the only history in these instances.

Physical examination shows a tachypneic, apprehensive patient with tachycardia, fever, and diaphoresis. Crackles are heard over the involved lung fields on auscultation. There may be signs of pulmonary consolidation (bronchial breathing, dullness to percussion, or increased tactile fremitus).

The chest radiograph usually demonstrates airspace consolidation with a lobar or a bronchopneumonic pattern. A dense lobar infiltrate, particularly with an air bronchogram, very strongly suggests acute bacterial pneumonia (Fig. 51-1); bronchopneumonic and patchy infiltrates are less specific.

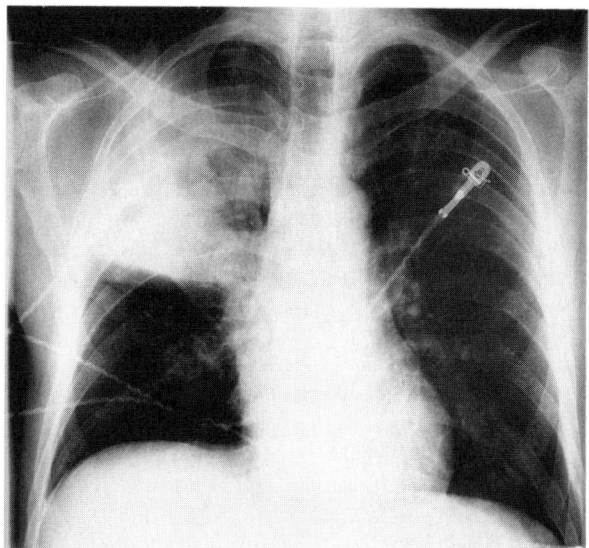

FIGURE 51-1 Dense localized infiltrate consistent with acute bacterial pneumonia. Note the air bronchogram, the downward-bulging transverse fissure, and the cavitation within the infiltrate, suggesting necrotizing infection with a mucoid organism such as *Klebsiella pneumoniae*, which proved to be the pathogen in this case.

Interstitial infiltrates virtually exclude the usual bacterial pneumonias, although diffuse reticulonodular patterns or multicentric pneumonia sometimes occur with hematogenous pneumonia (e.g., in intravenous drug abusers; Fig. 51-2).

The polymorphonuclear leukocyte count is usually elevated and shifted leftward but may be depressed in severely ill patients with shock or may even be within the normal range in debilitated or elderly patients.

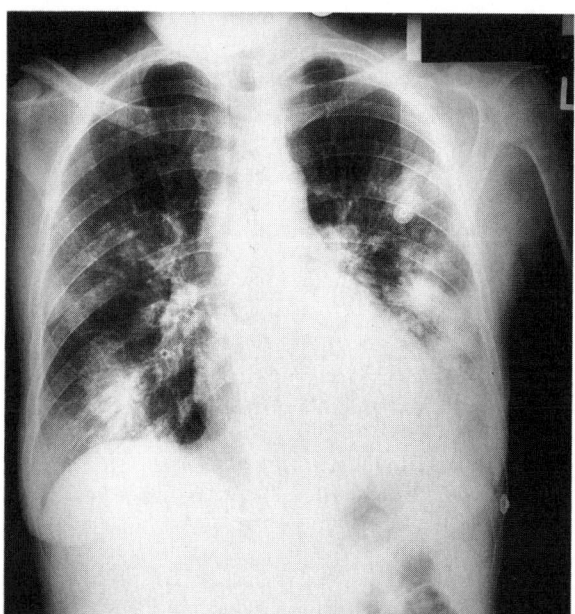

FIGURE 51-2 Multicentric hematogenous *Staphylococcus aureus* pneumonia in an intravenous drug abuser with severe cellulitis at an injection site. Note the multicentric regions of airspace consolidation.

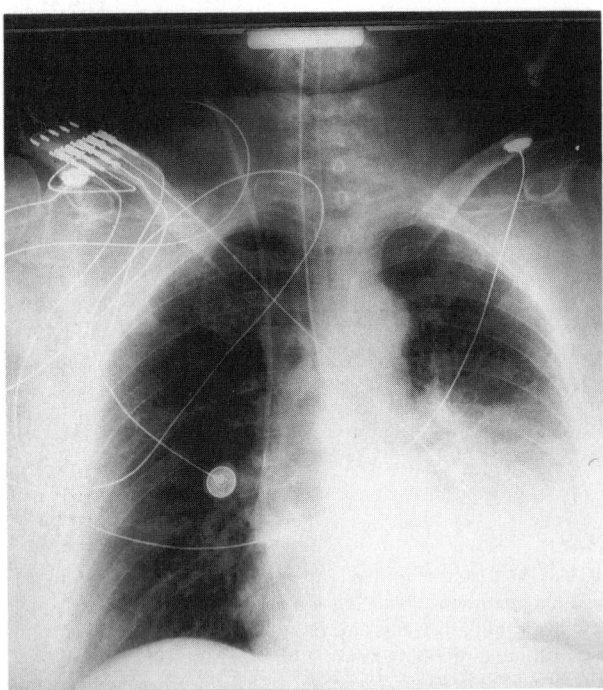

FIGURE 51-3 Ill-defined, large airspace density in the left lower lobe of a patient with community-acquired *Legionella pneumophila* pneumonia.

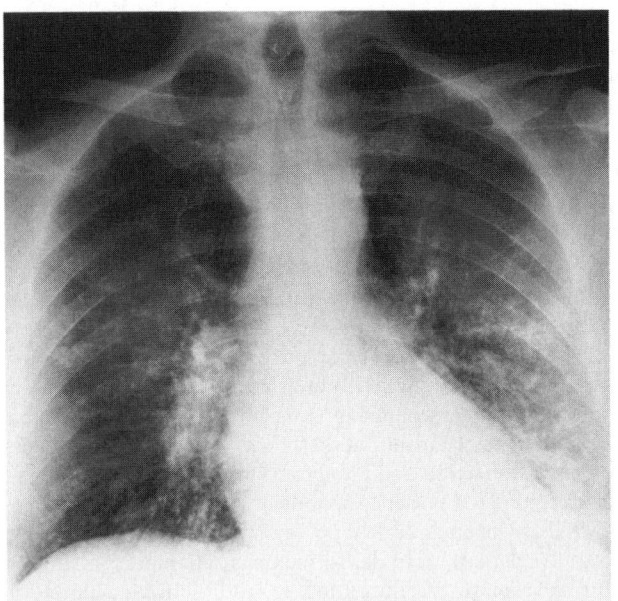

FIGURE 51-4 Diffuse interstitial and alveolar infiltrates in a patient with acute *Mycoplasma pneumoniae* pneumonia complicated by acute respiratory failure.

Legionnaire's Disease

Whereas early descriptions of community-acquired Legionnaire's disease emphasized many clinical features that set it apart from usual bacterial pneumonia,[15] we now know that Legionnaire's disease can present in ways clinically indistinguishable from disease caused by pneumococcus.[16] Clinical features that may suggest the diagnosis include dry cough, preceding diarrhea or other gastrointestinal (GI) symptoms, and encephalopathy not explained by other features of the illness. Epidemiologic clues include exposure to aerosols of *Legionella*-contaminated water in cooling towers or potable water distribution systems, underlying chronic lung disease, and immunologic impairment, particularly that caused by corticosteroid therapy. In patients requiring intensive care, the course is usually one of rapidly progressive pneumonia, sometimes with the aforementioned clinical features, or extrapulmonary involvement complicated by acute hypoxemic respiratory failure. The radiologic abnormalities are variable; most characteristic is peripheral rounded airspace consolidation with ill-defined margins (Fig. 51-3); however, patchy infiltration is also common.[17]

Mycoplasma pneumoniae *Pneumonia*

The term *atypical pneumonia* was coined to describe the pneumonia syndrome caused by *M. pneumoniae*, a pneumonia usually occurring in people in the second and third decades of life without major underlying disease predisposing to acute bacterial pneumonia. The clinical syndrome consists of a prodromal upper respiratory tract infection followed by an increasingly persistent dry cough associated with low-grade fever, frequently with extrapulmonary symptoms such as diarrhea, myalgia, arthralgia, and skin rash. In severe cases, the patient is tachypneic and cyanotic, but examination of

the chest generally shows only widespread crackles without signs of pulmonary consolidation. The pharynx may be red; bullous myringitis is occasionally present, and a rash is sometimes seen. The chest radiograph most typically shows a unilateral segmental infiltrate but may show patchy or interstitial infiltrates bilaterally. In patients requiring intensive care for respiratory failure caused by this infection, diffuse bilateral interstitial and alveolar infiltrates are usual (Fig. 51-4). Other extrapulmonary features can also lead to the need for intensive care, in particular encephalomyelitis or myocarditis (manifest more commonly as prolonged QT interval or ventricular arrhythmias than as congestive heart failure). A moderately "septic" appearance and hemodynamic assessment is usual; however, frank septic shock is not, and hypotension is more often caused by volume depletion.

In the more severe cases seen in the ICU, the polymorphonuclear leukocyte count is elevated and shifted leftward, and thrombocytopenia may be present. Hemolytic anemia may be present because of the presence of high-titer cold agglutinins, which may also produce erroneous red cell indices, or "error flags," on automated cell counters because of red cell agglutination. Moderate elevation of hepatic transaminase levels is common. Although most patients do not produce sputum, in those who do it is usually purulent grossly and on microscopic examination; organisms are conspicuously absent on Gram stain.

Chlamydia psittaci

The major epidemiologic clue to psittacosis is exposure to infected birds, often pets (budgerigars and other related species which may or may not be visibly ill) in homes or pet stores, or commercial birds, such as turkeys, which may shed the organism when killed and eviscerated in processing plants.[18] The pneumonia follows exposure by 1 to 2 weeks. High fever and a persistent dry cough are frequently associated with a variety of atypical features: myalgias, headache, GI symptoms, and occasionally a macular rash. On auscultation of the lungs, crackles over involved lung regions, without signs of pulmonary consolidation, are usual. Extrapulmonary physical findings are not infrequent: hepatomegaly, splenomegaly, pleural and pericardial friction rubs, and, in the rare case with complicating endocarditis, pathologic cardiac murmurs. In severe cases, dyspnea and hypoxia are prominent; encephalopathy, with confusion, obtundation, or even coma, may occur. The pulmonary infiltrate is generally a patchy infiltrate in all lung fields, with lower lobe predominance, but this is too variable to be a major differential point. Other routine laboratory studies are equally nonspecific, demonstrating only the usual hematologic and biochemical changes common in patients with serious infections.

Other *Chlamydia* species may also cause pneumonia (*C. pneumoniae* commonly, *C. trachomatis* rarely) but generally do not cause acute CAP sufficiently severe to require intensive care, unless the disease occurs in patients with severe underlying debility.

Q Fever Pneumonia

Coxiella burnetii is a rickettsia-like organism that is transmitted to human beings by inhalation of aerosols or suspended particulate matter from a wide variety of domestic and wild animals, including sheep, goats, cattle, domestic fowl, mice, rabbits, and parturient cats.[19] Usually the infected animal is not ill. The illness begins with fever and chills, associated with myalgia and severe diffuse headache in most cases. Some persons with Q fever have GI symptoms. Cough is usually not severe and is nonproductive; however, in cases likely to be referred for intensive care, dyspnea and hypoxemia are prominent. Peripheral segmental infiltrates or rounded opacities are the most common radiographic findings, but no radiologic pattern excludes the diagnosis. Leukocytosis, elevated hepatic transaminase levels, and electrolyte disturbances are common but not specific.

Viral Pneumonia

In adults, the major viral causes of pneumonia that produce illnesses severe enough to lead to ICU admission are influenza viruses A and B. Rarely, severe pneumonia can be caused by respiratory syncytial virus (RSV) or cytomegalovirus (CMV), especially in the debilitated elderly or the immunocompromised; by *Varicella zoster* virus in healthy adults with primary chicken pox or secondary to disseminated herpes zoster in the immunocompromised; by Epstein-Barr virus in nonimmunocompromised adults with unusually severe infectious mononucleosis; or by adenovirus in susceptible young adults in close contact (e.g., military recruits). Severe influenza occurs during epidemic periods of the year ("flu season," usually winter or early spring), particularly in nonimmunized patients who are elderly or have significant underlying disease. A "flu-like" illness, with fever, myalgia, headache, sore throat, and harsh cough with burning retrosternal chest pain, is followed by increasing dyspnea and prostration. Physical findings include pharyngitis, crackles and wheezes in all lung fields, tachypnea, and cyanosis. The chest radiograph generally shows diffuse interstitial infiltrates (Fig. 51-5) unless there is also a complicating acute bacterial pneumonia, which is a common circumstance.[20]

In autumn 2002, an apparently novel, highly contagious form of severe pneumonia appeared in southern China and

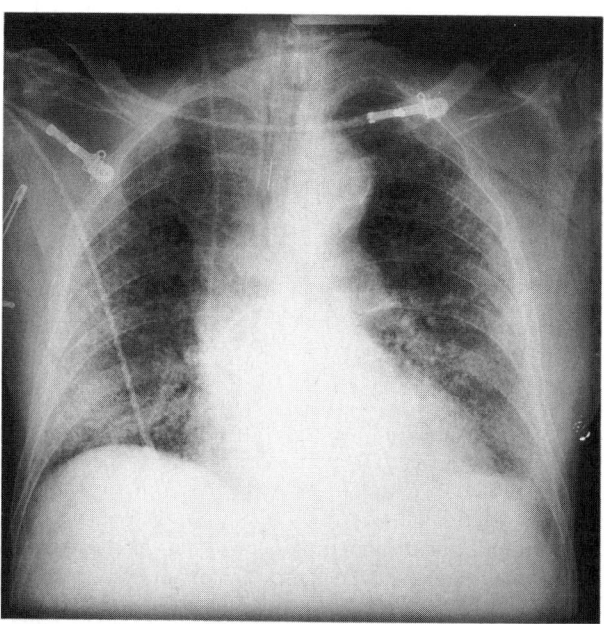

FIGURE 51-5 Diffuse interstitial infiltrates caused by influenza A pneumonia in an elderly, but otherwise well, individual.

over the ensuing months was transmitted by air travelers throughout the world, leading to multiple local outbreaks of different degrees of severity.[21] Termed *severe acute respiratory syndrome* (SARS), the illness has been shown to be caused by a coronavirus of animal origin transmitted to humans.[22] Typically, after close contact with an infected individual, there is an incubation period of 2 to 10 days followed by abrupt onset of fever with rigors.[23] Three to 5 days after the onset of fever, there follows the development of dyspnea associated with headache, malaise, and dry cough. Physical examination at this time is unremarkable except for crackles and signs of consolidation on chest examination. The white blood cell count is generally unremarkable except for moderate lymphopenia. The chest radiograph may be unremarkable in less severe cases, but in definite cases shows airspace opacities of variable (focal or patchy) distribution. In the more severe cases, pulmonary infiltrates progress over 5 to 10 days to full-blown acute respiratory distress syndrome (ARDS) radiologically and histopathologically, which requires intensive care for mechanical ventilatory support. Mortality rate worldwide has averaged about 15%, ranging from 1% to 5% in younger, previously well, people to higher than 50% in the elderly or debilitated. At the time of this writing, ongoing transmission of this infection appears to be halted; however, the potential for re-emergence of the disease clearly exists, requiring physicians to remain alert to this possibility when faced with rapidly advancing undiagnosed pneumonia in a returned traveler.

Pneumocystis carinii *Pneumonia*

Although this infection is an opportunistic pneumonia occurring only in the severely immunocompromised, the current prevalence of the human immunodeficiency virus (HIV) among people who previously were well requires the physician to consider it as a possible diagnosis in patients presenting with diffuse pneumonia even in the absence of a prior diagnosis of HIV infection. It presents as a relatively insidious illness characterized by low-grade fever, dry cough, and increasing dyspnea, usually with diffuse infiltrates on the chest radiograph (see Chap. 48). Although *Pneumocystis carinii* pneumonia (PCP) would be the immediate consideration with this presentation in a patient with known advanced HIV infection, the diagnosis is less obvious when this diagnosis has not been made, particularly when the patient is not known to be at increased risk for HIV infection (high-risk sexual activity, prior transfusion with potentially HIV-contaminated blood products, illicit intravenous drug use, or exposure to multiply-used nonsterile needles, etc.).

ASPIRATION PNEUMONIA

Frank aspiration of oropharyngeal or gastric contents can produce any of a number of different clinical presentations, depending on the amount and nature of the material aspirated.[24] Large-particle aspiration causes airway obstruction with acute asphyxia (the "cafe coronary"), atelectasis, unilateral or localized hyperinflation, or, subacutely, bacterial pneumonia or lung abscess caused by impaired mucociliary clearance in the airway obstructed by a foreign body. Small-particle or liquid aspiration usually causes a low-grade chemical pneumonitis, with a pulmonary infiltrate that clears over a few days without treatment. When the aspirated liquid is gastric acid, a more severe chemical burn is the result, with rapid exudation of fluid into the lung. Consequences can include acute hypovolemic hypotension and, if the region of damaged lung is relatively large, acute hypoxemic respiratory failure.

In most cases of witnessed pulmonary aspiration, the number and pathogenicity of aspirated bacteria are low, and no infection requiring immediate antimicrobial therapy is present. In addition, no evidence indicates that administering antimicrobials at this point decreases the risk of subsequent infective pneumonia, which, when it occurs, becomes evident 3 days to 1 week after the episode of aspiration.[24,25] A major exception to this rule is aspiration of gastric contents that have become heavily contaminated with mixed enteric organisms. This occurs in the setting of bowel obstruction with accumulation of large amounts of feculent upper GI fluid, which may be aspirated. It may also occur after upper abdominal surgery or in the presence of upper GI bleeding or paralytic ileus, particularly when there is absence of the normal low gastric pH on account of achlorhydria or treatment with antacids or histamine-blocking agents. Aspiration of feculent gastric contents can result in a fulminant necrotizing pneumonia caused by mixed aerobic and anaerobic enteric bacteria. Prompt broad-spectrum antimicrobial therapy is mandatory.

A much more common syndrome related to pulmonary aspiration is pneumonia or lung abscess caused by the predominantly anaerobic normal microflora of the mouth. Persons at particular risk are those who have a propensity toward aspiration because of a continuously or intermittently depressed level of consciousness (alcohol or drug abuse, epileptic seizures, stupor or coma of any cause), an impaired swallowing mechanism (esophageal or neurologic disease), or an impairment of tracheobronchial clearance mechanisms (endobronchial lesion or foreign body). After the aspiration episode, a low-grade pneumonia, manifest as cough, fever, and malaise, begins within a few days to 1 week. A chest radiograph at this time usually shows a patchy infiltrate, which

may be unilateral or bilateral, occurring a little more commonly in the right lung and predominantly in lung zones that would be dependent in the supine patient (posterior segments of the upper and lower lobes). If the patient does not seek medical attention at this stage, the illness evolves over 1 to 4 weeks, with a persistent fever with night sweats, malaise, anorexia, and weight loss. The onset of production of large amounts of foul-smelling, watery sputum signals the development of a lung abscess, manifest on a chest radiograph as a cavity (or multiple smaller cavities), often with an air–fluid level, surrounded by a pulmonary infiltrate (Fig. 51-6). Involvement of the pleura often results in empyema, as demonstrated by clinical examination and radiographic findings consistent with a pleural effusion related to the region of pulmonary consolidation. Most patients with this syndrome are subacutely, rather than acutely, ill, but very large empyema collections or relatively extensive pneumonia can produce respiratory failure. In particular, the onset of respiratory insufficiency caused by re-expansion pulmonary edema after drainage of large empyemas may require intensive supportive therapy.

Leukocytosis may be mild or marked; many patients are anemic, especially those with a more protracted course. Electrolyte disturbances, in particular hyponatremia, are common. A variety of biochemical abnormalities related to lengthy illness and malnutrition may be present, including hypoalbuminemia, hypophosphatemia, and hypomagnesemia. None of these is particularly valuable in categorizing the syndrome.

CHRONIC PNEUMONIA

Pneumonia in intensive care practice is predominantly an acute problem; in a significant minority of cases, however, a chronic progressive pulmonary process presents with impending or established respiratory failure or with circulatory consequences of the inflammatory process. It is critically important to recognize the presentation as subacute or chronic, because the approaches to diagnosis and empiric therapy are entirely different from those employed in patients with acute pneumonia. Because the differential diagnosis can be extremely large, including many relatively exotic infectious diseases and a number of noninfectious entities, a systematic and aggressive diagnostic approach is more rewarding than wide-spectrum empiric therapy, the initial approach generally adopted for acute pneumonias.

The usual definition of chronic pneumonia is progressive pulmonary symptoms (cough, dyspnea, and pain) for a period of 3 weeks to several months, associated with radiographic evidence of an inflammatory pulmonary parenchymal process. The patient generally appears chronically, rather than acutely, ill and is often malnourished or cachectic. Hematologic and routine biochemical testings show the usual evidence of a longstanding inflammatory process: mild leukocytosis, lymphopenia, and anemia, more often with thrombocytosis than with thrombocytopenia; hypoalbuminemia; and multiple mild electrolyte abnormalities. Depending on the cause of the process and the specific other organs involved, a wide variety of other findings may be present.

DIAGNOSIS

Pneumonia is often an obvious diagnosis, particularly when respiratory symptoms associated with a new pulmonary

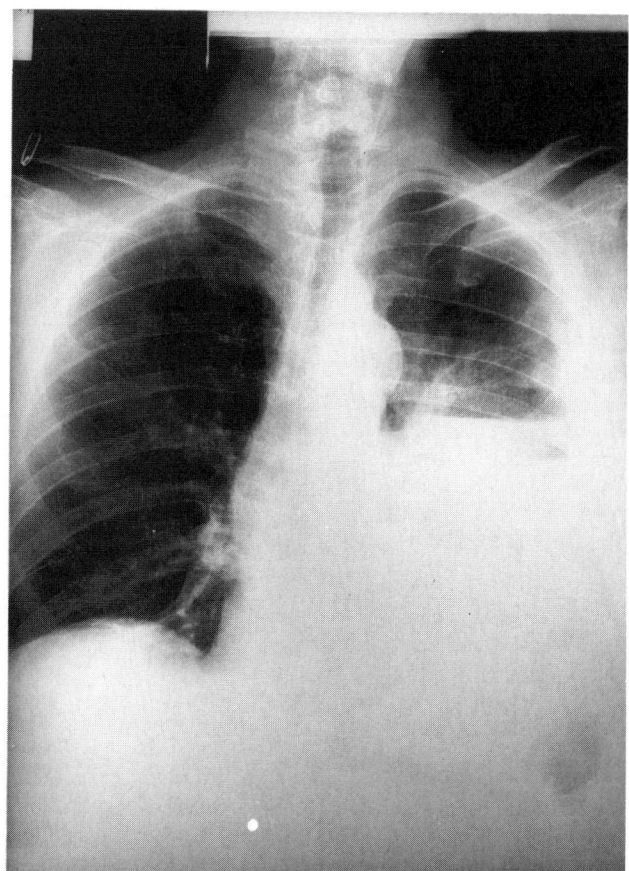

A

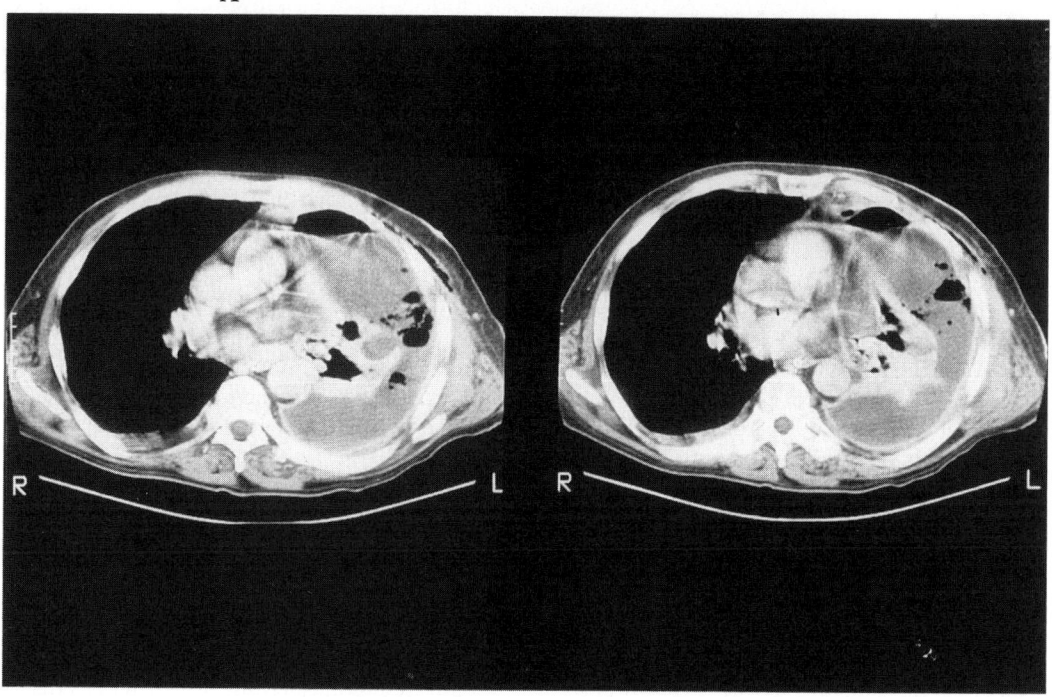

B

FIGURE 51-6 Aspiration-associated anaerobic pneumonia and empyema. A. Chest radiograph demonstrates multiple fluid levels with incompletely drained empyema fluid and underlying atelectasis or consolidation. B. Computed tomogram of the thorax shows multiple loculations of empyema fluid and, predominantly, atelectasis of the underlying lung. This patient required decortication to achieve adequate drainage and re-expansion of the lung.

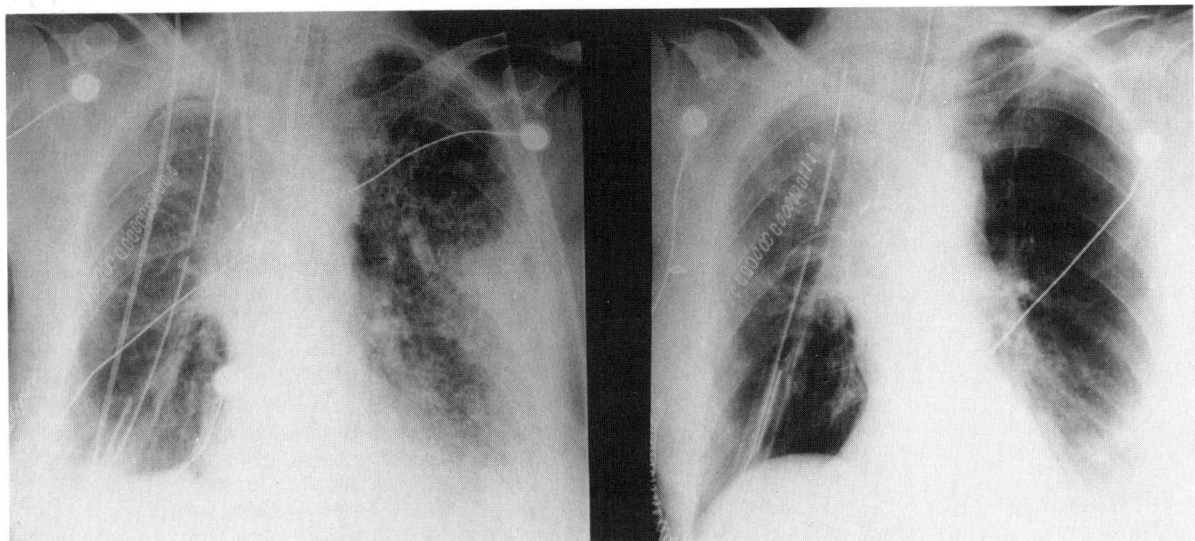

FIGURE 51-7 Example of delay of radiologic diagnosis of pneumonia attributable to volume depletion. These chest radiographs were obtained just 4 hours apart. *Right.* At the time this radiograph was obtained, the patient had severe dyspnea, crackles in the left lung, and hypoxemia requiring urgent intubation; until then she had been treated vigorously with diuretics for presumed cardiac failure, although no radiologic evidence and only equivocal clinical evidence were present. *Left.* After fluid resuscitation for hypotension (and demonstration of a low pulmonary wedge pressure), extensive pulmonary infiltrates quickly became evident in the left lung. These were attributed to acute *Escherichia coli* nosocomial pneumonia.

infiltrate and systemic signs of infection occur in a previously well patient. However, in patients with underlying lung or cardiac disease, the diagnosis may be more difficult. Increased dyspnea and cough with low-grade fever in a patient with an underlying chronic lung disease associated with long-term abnormalities on chest radiograph may be caused by pneumonia but may also represent a viral bronchitis or even an infection or inflammatory process elsewhere in the body. In a patient with known congestive cardiac failure, respiratory deterioration with a moderate leukocytosis and asymmetric radiographic findings of pulmonary edema may be due simply to heart failure, but the radiographic asymmetry may be caused by an underlying pneumonia. These less certain situations can be approached in one of two ways, depending on a clinical assessment of the relative likelihood that superimposed pneumonia is present, the severity of the illness, and the potential consequences of a wrong judgment. When pneumonia seems less likely and the patient is relatively stable, it is often reasonable to treat the underlying condition and withhold antimicrobial therapy with the expectation that the patient will improve without it. In the patient with congestive heart failure, steady clearing of the pulmonary edema, including the asymmetric region, without increasing systemic signs of infection helps to exclude the diagnosis of pneumonia; but failure of the local infiltrate to clear with diuresis, persistent productive cough, fever, and leukocytosis mandate further investigation and empiric treatment for pneumonia. In a more severely ill patient in whom it is felt that any delay in treatment for pneumonia would adversely affect outcome, it is more prudent to initiate empiric antimicrobial therapy at the outset and to stop that therapy later if the clinical course does not support the initial impression of possible pneumonia.

Cough with sputum production, fever, and leukocytosis without a convincing pulmonary infiltrate on chest radiograph is usually caused by viral bronchitis or, in the patient with chronic lung disease, an exacerbation of chronic bronchitis caused by a viral infection, or increased endobronchial bacterial microflora. However, in occasional cases, pneumonia may be present but not visible on the radiograph. This is usually caused by intravascular volume depletion delaying the appearance of the infiltrate (Fig. 51-7) or by a technically inadequate radiograph. Repeating the radiograph with a better technique or after volume resuscitation usually clarifies these situations.

When one has made a clinical diagnosis of pneumonia, the next major issues are making an etiologic diagnosis and prescribing antimicrobial therapy. These tasks can be made difficult by the fact that, although most pneumonias are caused by a small number of common pathogens, a significant minority is caused by a wide range of less common pathogens that require different approaches to investigation and treatment. The differential diagnosis also includes a large number of noninfectious causes of pulmonary infiltrates associated with an acute inflammatory response. For acute pneumonias, these include pulmonary atelectasis, chemical pneumonitis from aspiration or toxic inhalation, pulmonary infarction from pulmonary embolism, lung contusion in trauma cases, and a range of immunologically mediated acute pneumonitis syndromes. Noninfectious causes of subacute and chronic pneumonias are even more common. Many of these diagnoses can be suspected on the basis of the clinical context; in severe cases otherwise consistent with an infectious etiology, one usually should proceed with investigation and initial empiric therapy for infection until such an etiology is excluded.

The first step in the diagnostic assessment is to try to categorize the pneumonia presentation as outlined under Clinical and Radiographic Features. The diagnostic and immediate therapeutic approach to each is different: severe acute CAP mandates empiric antimicrobial therapy and investigation directed at identifying the offending organism; aspiration pneumonia or lung abscess is generally treated empirically with agents directed at the predominantly anaerobic, normal oral microflora, with investigation aimed mainly at uncovering an underlying anatomic cause for the pneumonia; and the chronic pneumonia syndrome, which has an extremely large differential diagnosis including infectious and noninfectious entities, usually does not require empiric therapy but does mandate a systematic and often invasive approach to establishing the diagnosis.

ACUTE COMMUNITY-ACQUIRED PNEUMONIA

All patients with a clinical diagnosis of pneumonia leading to ICU admission should have a blood culture, a Gram stain, and culture of lower respiratory tract secretions. If a significant pleural effusion is present it should be aspirated. In nonintubated patients, the immediately available lower respiratory tract sample is sputum, which is a mixture of materials from the lung and the upper respiratory tract and that has many well-known limitations in diagnosis: The patient may not be able to produce a good specimen; the specimen may contain potentially pathogenic organisms that come from the upper respiratory tract but are not the cause of the pneumonia; and contaminating organisms from the upper airway may overgrow the real pathogen on the culture plate and prevent its detection. Despite these problems, sputum examination remains a good place to start, mainly because in a significant minority of cases, and particularly in the most severe cases of bacterial pneumonia, the Gram stain, with subsequent confirmation by culture, can be diagnostic.

The utility of the Gram stain can be maximized by microscopic evaluation of the degree to which the sample is contaminated by upper respiratory secretions.[26] A specimen with large numbers of polymorphonuclear leukocytes, more than 25 per high-power field, and few large epithelial cells, fewer than 10 per high-power field, is reasonably likely to represent a good-quality lower respiratory tract specimen and can usefully be examined further to determine the predominant bacterial morphotype present. Those specimens with large numbers of epithelial cells and few leukocytes are mostly saliva; they are unlikely to yield useful diagnostic information and should be discarded after another and better specimen has been obtained. In a patient with a clinical presentation consistent with acute bacterial pneumonia, a microscopically acceptable specimen that contains large numbers of bacteria of a single morphotype and few bacteria of other types is strong evidence that this is the cause of the pneumonia. A fairly definitive result such as this occurs in fewer than 33% of cases; however, it occurs more commonly in the most severe cases—those with extensive pneumonia caused by *S. pneumoniae*, *S. aureus*, and enteric facultatively aerobic gram-negative bacilli—and in cases in which an endotracheal tube has been placed, which permits the collection of a less heavily contaminated lower respiratory tract specimen.

Preliminary results of blood and sputum cultures are usually available at 24 to 48 hours. Whereas a positive blood culture for a recognized pneumonia pathogen is definitive, sputum cultures must be interpreted in light of the original Gram stain of the specimen, bearing in mind that potential pathogens grown from a specimen that contained mainly upper respiratory tract material may not be the cause of the pneumonia and that, if the patient received antimicrobials before providing the specimen, susceptible pathogens such as *S. pneumoniae* might not be detected.

In most cases of acute bacterial pneumonia, the investigations described above are all that is needed. Patients with severe bacterial pneumonia leading directly to ICU admission very frequently have positive blood or respiratory secretion cultures, whereas those who are less ill at the time of hospital admission usually improve with empiric antimicrobial therapy (whether or not a positive culture is obtained). Further investigation is needed in patients whose condition deteriorates or fails to improve and in whom the initial investigation has failed to provide an etiologic diagnosis to guide changes in therapy. The first step in a newly intubated patient is to repeat the Gram stain and culture of lower respiratory tract secretions. In deteriorating nonintubated pneumonia patients, the procedure of choice is fiberoptic bronchoscopy using a protected brush to collect a specimen from the consolidated lung segment or bronchoalveolar lavage (BAL) of the region. Because many of these patients have significantly compromised respiratory function, the procedure should be performed by an experienced bronchoscopist with other personnel present to continually monitor the patient's respirations, blood pressure and pulse, and oxygenation. A pulse oximeter to monitor arterial oxygen saturation continuously is mandatory. In patients who have significant arterial hypoxemia to begin with, it is usually best to insert an endotracheal tube and provide supplemental oxygen and assisted ventilation to facilitate bronchoscopy. The specimens obtained should be Gram stained and cultured quantitatively for conventional bacteria; the finding of more than 10^5 colony-forming units/mL from a BAL specimen (or 10^3 colony-forming units/mL from a protected brush) of a recognized pathogen is diagnostic of infection.[27–29] The specimen also should be stained and cultured for *Legionella* species, mycobacteria, and fungi and, where available, cultured for viruses. In most cases, it is also wise to do cytologic examination of the specimen.

Among the major pneumonia pathogens not detectable by routine Gram stain and culture of respiratory secretions, the one with the greatest propensity to present with an illness indistinguishable from usual acute bacterial pneumonia is *Legionella pneumophila*. For this reason, some hospital laboratories in areas of high prevalence routinely culture all submitted lower respiratory tract secretions for this organism. If this culture is not done routinely, it should be ordered specifically for all patients in whom an etiologic diagnosis is not immediately evident from the Gram stain. A direct fluorescent antibody stain for *Legionella* is also available. This can be done on sputum, endobronchial aspirates, or bronchoscopy specimens, but, particularly with sputum, the sensitivity of the test is not high, and false-positive results can result from cross-reaction of the fluorescent antibody with other gram-negative species. A urinary antigen detection test for *Legionella* is available in many centers and has excellent specificity; however, particularly early in the course of the illness, the sensitivity is not sufficiently high to exclude the diagnosis.[16]

In cases of severe pneumonia that resist diagnosis, particularly when the clinical course suggests the possibility of infection with an "atypical pneumonia " pathogen, additional investigations should be ordered according to the epidemiologic features of the case. In appropriate cases, culture of respiratory secretions and stool for viruses is worthwhile. Acute and 2- to 4-week blood specimens for serologic examination will establish the diagnosis in *M. pneumoniae*, *Chlamydia* speceis, *C. burnetii*, and the major viruses causing pneumonia (influenzae A and B, adenovirus, RSV, and CMV). Single high-titer–specific antibody levels can also be used to make most of these diagnoses earlier in the clinical course. Serology is also valuable in diagnosing some rare bacterial infections, such as *Francisella tularensis* pneumonia and brucellosis. Legionnaire's disease also can be detected serologically, but, because the antibody response to the organism may be slow, convalescent blood specimens should be drawn at 2 weeks and 6 weeks.

Direct enzyme immunoassay antigen detection performed on respiratory secretions is widely available for diagnoses of influenza A and RSV and is very useful in establishing a diagnosis quickly. At the time of this writing, rapid diagnostic testing for the SARS coronavirus is still under development; the diagnosis still relies on clinical case definitions associated with investigation of the outbreak (probable case: exposure to a known case or travel to an area of local transmission, fever, respiratory symptoms, and pulmonary infiltrate on chest radiograph without an alternative diagnosis).

Suspicion of PCP, generally based on the clinical and radiographic features and history of factors placing the patient at increased risk of HIV infection, should prompt early consideration of fiberoptic bronchoscopy with BAL. Serologic testing for HIV is usually also a part of this investigation.

ASPIRATION PNEUMONIA

The approach to aspiration-associated acute bacterial pneumonia caused by the usual pyogenic aerobic organisms is the same as that for pneumonia caused by subclinical aspiration. However, most aspiration CAPs, particularly those progressing to lung abscess, are caused by organisms constituting the normal flora of the oropharynx. These are predominantly anaerobic. Culture of sputum or endotracheal aspirates will always demonstrate some of these organisms because of the inevitable contamination of these specimens with saliva, and the microbiology laboratory will report the result of aerobic cultures as containing "normal flora." Anaerobic culture of such specimens is not worthwhile because they also would demonstrate "normal flora" in virtually all patients whether or not these organisms were pathogenically important. When the clinical presentation suggests aspiration pneumonia and conventional sputum or endobronchial aspirate cultures show only "normal flora," in most cases it is reasonable to make a clinical diagnosis of pneumonia caused by mixed oropharyngeal anaerobic bacteria and to treat accordingly. In less obvious cases, in which bronchoscopy is done to establish an etiologic diagnosis, it is reasonable to perform aerobic and anaerobic cultures on protected brush or BAL specimens because they are less likely to be contaminated by saliva. Bronchoscopy at some time in the treatment course is indicated in many patients with anaerobic pneumonia or lung abscess, particularly those with no clearly increased risk of significant aspiration, to exclude a predisposing endobronchial lesion.

CHRONIC PNEUMONIA

Some of the many infectious and noninfectious diseases that may present as a chronic pneumonia are listed in Table 51-2. Patients with an undiagnosed chronic pneumonia are less common in the ICU environment because the chronicity of progressive symptoms usually leads patients to seek medical attention before intensive care is required. In those who

TABLE 51-2 Infectious and Noninfectious Etiologies of Chronic Pneumonia

Bacterial and mycobacterial infections
  Tuberculosis
  Chronic cavitary bacterial pneumonia (*Klebsiella pneumoniae*, *Pseudomonas aeruginosa*, others)
  Actinomycosis
  Nocardiosis
  Melioidosis
  Aspiration-induced anaerobic pneumonia and lung abscess
Fungal infections
  Blastomycosis
  Coccidioidomycosis
  Paracoccidioidomycosis
  Histoplasmosis
  Cryptococcosis
  Chronic necrotizing aspergillosis
Noninfectious causes
  Systemic vasculitides
  Malignancy
  Interstitial pneumonitis (fibrosing alveolitis) and other idiopathic infiltrative pulmonary diseases
  Cryptogenic organizing pneumonia
  Lymphomatoid granulomatosis
  Sarcoidosis
  Toxic exposures and drug reactions

do present in respiratory failure, there are usually extensive bilateral pulmonary infiltrates, and the radiologic pattern is sometimes helpful in suggesting the diagnosis. However, almost every "characteristic" radiologic pattern can be caused by several different disease processes.

Among infectious causes of chronic pneumonia, reactivating pulmonary fibrocaseous tuberculosis generally demonstrates characteristic upper lobe predominance, with cavities and pleural thickening and scarring, but only rarely causes significant hypoxemia, generally when spillage of infected material from tuberculous cavities into otherwise normal lung produces acute airspace inflammation termed *acute tuberculous pneumonia* (Fig. 51-8). Somewhat less rarely, miliary tuberculosis or chronic hematogenous tuberculosis usually presents with a diffuse miliary or reticulonodular pattern on a chest radiograph (Fig. 51-9), often with respiratory failure, particularly when the disease produces a systemic inflammatory response complicated by the ARDS.[30] Infections that can mimic upper lobe tuberculosis reactivation include chronic necrotizing bacterial pneumonia (usually caused by *K. pneumoniae*, occasionally by *P. aeruginosa* or *S. aureus*), melioidosis, and some fungal infections. Miliary or reticulonodular disease (with or without ARDS) causing respiratory failure also occasionally occurs with fungal pneumonias, in particular blastomycosis[31] (Fig. 51-10), malignancy, and noninfectious granulomatous diseases.

The initial step in the investigation of a patient with a chronic pneumonia is recognizing that the pace and pattern of the disease do not fit with one of the acute bacterial or atypical pneumonias. Appropriately directed, additional history taking for exposure to tuberculosis or residence in an area endemic for one of the dimorphic fungi can be obtained, and extrapulmonary symptoms or signs associated with the noninfectious diseases listed in Table 51-2 can be sought. Lower respiratory tract secretions should be sent for routine Gram stain and culture for bacteria, and several

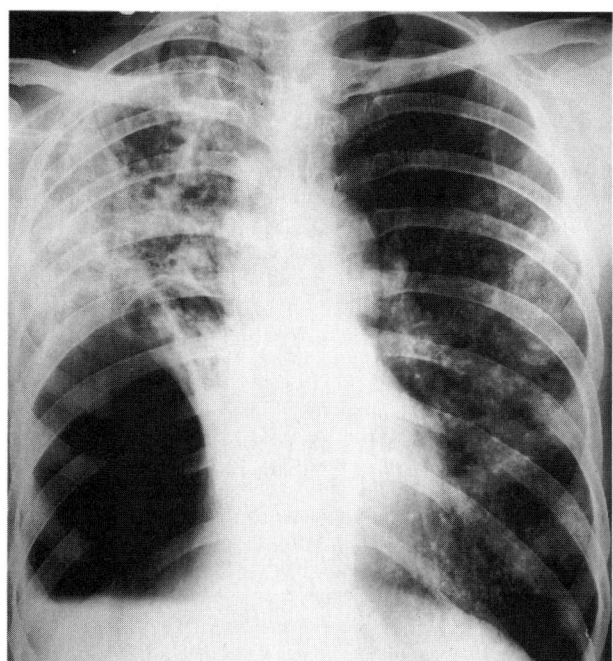

FIGURE 51-8 Tuberculous pneumonia. Fairly discrete acinar shadows are present in the left lung, remote from the confluent airspace disease on the right. (*Courtesy of Dr. Richard Long, Edmonton, Canada.*)

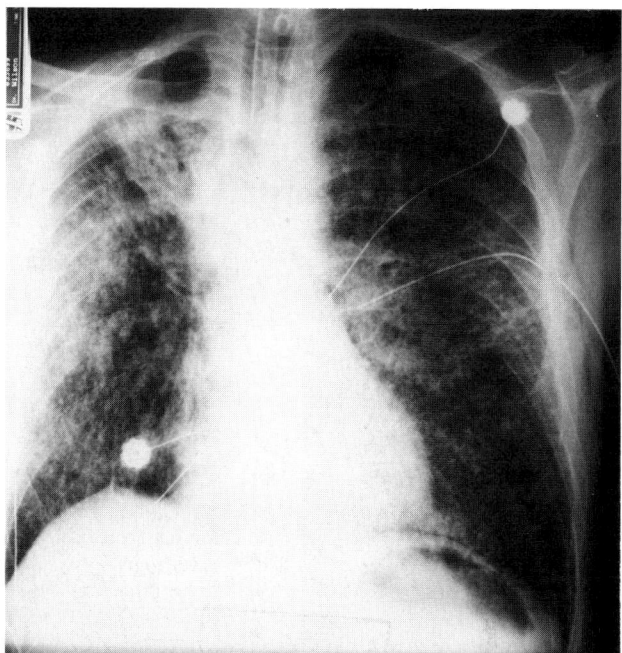

FIGURE 51-10 Severe pulmonary blastomycosis with a miliary pattern. This patient had an associated septic arthritis of the right knee caused by blastomycosis, the likely source of hematogenous dissemination to the lung.

specimens should be examined and cultured for mycobacteria and fungi. In patients who have spent time in the Far East, examination for ova and parasites should be done to exclude infection with *Paragonimus westermani*. Cytologic studies for malignancy should be done in most cases. If sputum or endobronchial secretions are used, these should be sent repeatedly (three to five specimens) to maximize yield. In patients from whom satisfactory secretions cannot be obtained, fiberoptic bronchoscopy with BAL is most satisfactory.

Other noninvasive tests for infectious agents, such as serologic testing and skin tests, which are often of some diagnostic value in less severely ill patients, are not helpful in critically ill patients. However, for some of the noninfectious diseases, in particular systemic vasculitides and other immunologically mediated diseases with pulmonary involvement, testing for the specific autoantibodies associated with these syndromes can be very useful (see Chap. 104).

Many of the causes of the chronic pneumonia syndrome also cause extrapulmonary manifestations. The nature of these associated findings is frequently of considerable help in suggesting the correct diagnosis; examples include skin or bone involvement with pulmonary blastomycosis, sinusitis with Wegener granulomatosis, lymphocytic meningitis with coccidioidomycosis or tuberculosis, granulomatous oral lesions with paracoccidioidomycosis, and glomerulonephritis with Goodpasture syndrome and other immunologically mediated systemic diseases. When other organ systems are involved, it is often less risky for a patient with significantly compromised respiratory function to undergo biopsy of the extrapulmonary site of involvement rather than of the lung.

If a diagnosis is not promptly established by the initial examination of lower respiratory tract secretions, if the clinical constellation of findings is not characteristic enough to establish a diagnosis on these grounds, and if no extrapulmonary site of involvement suitable for biopsy is present, most critically ill patients with chronic pneumonia immediately should undergo open lung biopsy. The range of potential diagnoses and risks associated with empiric therapy for most of the diagnostic entities is simply too large to attempt management without establishing a definitive diagnosis. In a patient who has reached a stage of the disease requiring intensive care,

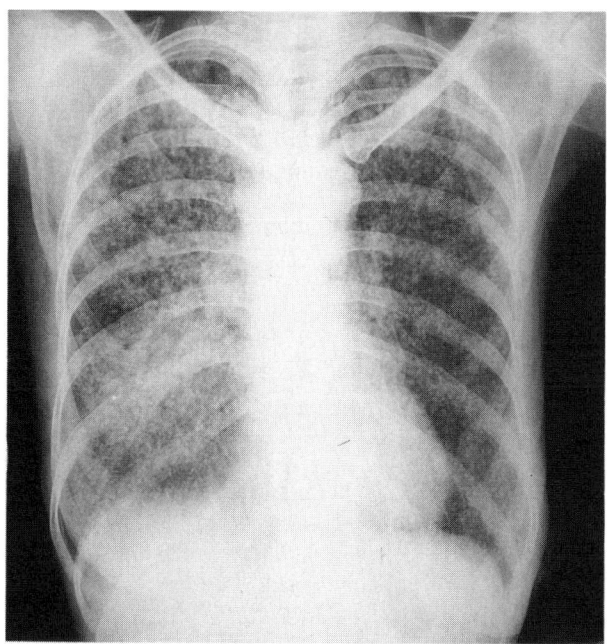

FIGURE 51-9 Miliary tuberculosis. Discrete small nodules (1 to 3 mm) are uniformly distributed throughout the lungs. (*Courtesy of Dr. Richard Long, Edmonton, Canada.*)

TABLE 51-3 Initial Antimicrobial Therapy for Acute Pneumonia of Known Etiology in Critically Ill Patients[a]

	Recommended Antimicrobial Therapy	Alternative Antimicrobial Agents
Streptococcus pneumonia and other streptococci		
Penicillin susceptible	Penicillin G 1 million U IV q 4 h	Cefazolin, clindamycin, or vancomycin
Intermediate susceptibility (MIC 0.1–1.0 μg/mL)	Penicillin G 3 million U IV q 4 h or cefotaxime 2 g IV q 8 h	Clindamycin, fluoroquinolone, vancomycin
Penicillin resistant (MIC > 2 μg/mL)	Vancomycin 1 g IV q 12 h	Linezolid, fluoroquinolone
Staphylococcus aureus		
Methicillin sensitive	Nafcillin 2 g IV q 4 h	Cefazolin, clindamycin, or vancomycin
Methicillin resistant	Vancomycin 500 mg IV q 6 h	Linezolid, cotrimoxazole (if susceptible)
Haemophilus influenzae		
β-Lactamase negative	Ampicillin 2 g IV q 6 h	Cefuroxime, cotrimoxazole
β-Lactamase positive	Cefuroxime 1.5 g IV q 8 h	Cotrimoxazole
Moraxella catarrhalis	Cefuroxime 1.5 g IV q 8 h	Cotrimoxazole
Klebsiella, Escherichia coli, etc.	Cefotaxime 2 g IV q 6 h *and* gentamicin 4.5 mg/kg q 24 h	Piperacillin/tazobactam or carbapenam *and* gentamicin, cotrimoxazole, or ciprofloxacin
Enterobacter spp.	Meropenem 500 mg IV q 8 h *and* ciprofloxacin 400 mg IV q 12 h	Cotrimoxazole
Pseudomonas aeruginosa	Ceftazidime 2 g IV q 8 h *and* tobramycin 4.5 mg/kg q 24 h	Carbapenem or anti-pseudomonal penicillin and tobramycin or ciprofloxacin
Anaerobic pneumonia/ lung abscess	Penicillin 2 million U IV q 4 h *and* metronidazole 750 mg IV q 8 h	Clindamycin, chloramphenicol
Legionella pneumophila	Ciprofloxacin 400 mg IV q 12 h ± rifampin 600 mg IV daily	Macrolide and rifampin
Mycoplasma pneumoniae	Azithromycin 500 mg IV once daily	Tetracycline, macrolide or fluoroquinolone
Chlamydia psittaci (psittacosis)	Doxycycline 100 mg IV q 12 h	Macrolide, fluoroquinolone
Coxiella burnetii (Q fever)	Doxycycline 100 mg IV q 12 h	Macrolide with rifampin
Yersinia pestis (plague)	Gentamicin 5 mg/kg IV once daily	Ciprofloxacin, doxycycline
Francisella tularensis (tularemia)	Gentamicin 5 mg/kg IV once daily	Ciprofloxacin, doxycycline
Bacillus anthracis (anthrax)	Ciprofloxacin 400 mg IV q 12 h *and* clindamycin 600 mg IV q 8 h	Doxycycline, rifampin, penicillin G (if susceptible)
Influenza A or respiratory syncytial virus (severe with respiratory failure)	Ribavirin aerosol 1 g/d over 12–18 h	
Varicella zoster	Acyclovir 10 mg/kg q 8 h	

[a] All drug dosages cited are for patients with normal renal function; dosage adjustment for renal insufficiency is required for several of the agents listed. Monitoring of blood drug levels is strongly advised for the aminoglycosides.

ABBREVIATIONS: IV, intravenously; MIC, minimum inhibitory concentration.

the necessary time for further observation of the course or attempts at empiric trials of therapy is lacking.

ANTIMICROBIAL THERAPY

ACUTE COMMUNITY-ACQUIRED PNEUMONIA

When a specific etiologic diagnosis for pneumonia has been established on the basis of the blood culture or Gram stain and culture of secretions from the respiratory tract, antimicrobial therapy directed specifically at that pathogen can be prescribed (Table 51-3). The regimens suggested in this chapter are applicable when in vitro testing demonstrates that the organism is susceptible to the listed antimicrobial agents; resistant strains would require appropriate alternative therapy. However, in most cases of pneumonia, the etiologic diagnosis is not available at the outset, and empiric therapy must be directed at the most probable microbial etiologies in the particular patient being treated. Because patients requiring intensive care are usually in a relatively precarious state that makes the consequences of undertreatment unacceptable, it is a principle of therapy in this class of patient that antimicrobial treatment should be very conservative; that is, it should

cover all etiologic possibilities except the quite remote ones. Some suggested empiric regimens are presented in Table 51-4; these are loosely congruent with, but not identical to, some recent recommendations from expert panels[1–3] that thus far have been unable to reach a consensus, mainly because definitive comparative studies of antimicrobial regimens do not exist.

For most cases of severe acute pneumonia, a third-generation cephalosporin combined with quinolone or a macrolide is appropriate because it works against most conventional bacteria likely to be acquired in the community and atypical pathogens such as *Legionella* and *Mycoplasma*. A respiratory quinolone or macrolide alone is not advised in the more severely ill ICU population because of the emergence of significant resistance to these agents in *Streptococcus pneumoniae* and some other species.

When the clinical context suggests the possibility of infection caused by *C. burnetii* or *C. psittaci*, a tetracycline such as doxycycline 100 mg intravenously (IV) every 12 hours should be included in the regimen. Rifampin 600 mg IV or orally can be added for patients with fulminant atypical pneumonia and for patients with pneumonia caused by *L. pneumophila*

TABLE 51-4 Empiric Antimicrobial Therapy for Critically Ill Patients with Acute Community-Acquired Pneumonia[a]

Clinical Setting	Recommended Antimicrobial Therapy	Alternative Agents
Acute community-acquired pneumonia (including nursing home patients and those with COPD or alcohol abuse)	Cefotaxime 2 g IV q 8 h *or* other third-generation cephalosporin	β-Lactam / β-lactamase inhibitor, carbapenem, respiratory fluoroquinolone
Legionellosis or suspected atypical pneumonia	Ciprofloxacin 400 mg IV q 12 h *or* azithromycin 500 mg IV once daily	
Anaerobic aspiration pneumonia/lung abscess	Penicillin G 2 million U IV q 4 h *and* metronidazole	Clindamycin, carbapenam, β-lactam / β-lactamase inhibitor
Severe/fulminant pneumonia	Piperacillin/tazobactam 3.375 g IV q 6 h *and* ciprofloxacin 400 mg IV q 12 h	Carbapenem or third-generation cephalosporin *and* ciprofloxacin or macrolide

[a] Dosages cited are for patients with normal renal function; dosage adjustment for renal insufficiency is required for several of these agents.
ABBREVIATIONS: COPD, chronic obstructive pulmonary disease; IV, intravenously.

or Q fever that is responding poorly to the initial treatment regimen.

ASPIRATION PNEUMONIA

Most cases of witnessed or otherwise recent aspiration of oropharyngeal or gastric contents associated with a new pulmonary infiltrate represent an acute chemical pneumonitis rather than an infection. These cases usually resolve without antimicrobial therapy, with deep breathing and coughing, or with chest physiotherapy, when required. There is no convincing evidence that early administration of antimicrobials decreases subsequent incidences of complicating bacterial pneumonia, although there is evidence that such treatment may be associated with subsequent pneumonia caused by a relatively antimicrobial-resistant organism.[24,25] Aspiration that has resulted in pneumonia, lung abscess, or empyema caused by oropharyngeal anaerobic bacteria has usually been treated, at least initially, with penicillin. However, in a critically ill patient with this syndrome, therapy should usually begin with penicillin 2 million U IV every 4 hours and metronidazole 750 mg IV every 6 hours or with clindamycin 900 mg every 8 hours. Aspiration can also be complicated by later development of aerobic acute bacterial pneumonia; in these cases, the regimens listed in Tables 51-3 and 51-4 apply. Much less commonly, aspiration can produce an acute, rapidly progressive necrotizing pneumonia. This infection usually involves anaerobes and facultatively aerobic enteric gram-negative bacilli. The clinical context is often major aspiration in a patient without gastric acid (and therefore a large gastric bacterial population) or with an accumulation of feculent material in the stomach caused by adynamic ileus, upper GI bleeding, or bowel obstruction. Treatment must include adequate coverage for anaerobes, including *Bacteroides fragilis*, and aerobic gram-negative organisms. As in other acute gram-negative pneumonias, it is unwise to rely on an aminoglycoside alone for aerobic gram-negative coverage. Acceptable initial regimens include piperacillin/tazobactam 3.375 g IV every 6 hours with gentamicin 4.5 mg/kg every 24 hours, clindamycin 900 mg IV every 8 hours with cefotaxime 2 g IV every 6 hours, and meropenem 1 g every 8 hours with gentamicin 4.5 mg/kg IV every 24 hours. Ciprofloxacin can be substituted for the aminoglycoside when toxicity is a concern.

CHRONIC PNEUMONIA

Empiric therapy is seldom indicated for patients presenting with a chronic pneumonia. The pace of the illness is generally such that a delay of hours or a few days in establishing the diagnosis is not critical, and the large differential diagnosis makes selection of empiric treatment difficult. One occasional exception to this rule is extensive pneumonitis or pulmonary hemorrhage in a patient with sufficient extrapulmonary evidence to support a clinical diagnosis of a systemic inflammatory disease such as lupus erythematosus, Goodpasture syndrome, polyarteritis, or Wegener granulomatosis (see Chap. 104).

A full discussion of specific therapies for all the infectious and noninfectious causes of chronic pneumonia is beyond the scope of this chapter; however, treatment regimens for the more common fungal pneumonias are listed in Table 51-5. Drugs used in the treatment of critical illness or respiratory failure caused by tuberculosis are listed in Table 51-6. In general, in seriously ill patients, use of four antituberculous drugs initially (isoniazid, rifampin, pyrazinamide, and streptomycin; ethambutol substituted for streptomycin, if necessary, or added if drug resistance is suspected) is recommended.[32] Addition of a corticosteroid (methylprednisolone 125 mg IV every 12 hours) can also be considered in the nonimmunocompromised patient with severe tuberculosis in an attempt to speed resolution of the exudative

TABLE 51-5 Treatment Regimens for Fungal Pneumonia Associated with Critical Illness in the Nonimmunocompromised Host

Etiologic Agent	Recommended Antimicrobial Therapy
Blastomyces dermatitidis	Amphotericin B 0.5–1.0 mg/kg IV daily to total dose of 2–2.5 g
Histoplasma capsulatum	As above
Coccidioides immitis (without CNS involvement)	Amphotericin B 0.5–0.8 mg/kg IV daily to total dose of 3–4 g
Cryptococcus neoformans	Amphotericin B 0.4–0.6 mg/kg IV daily *and* flucytosine 75–100 mg/kg daily in 4 divided doses (adjusted according to monitored blood levels)

ABBREVIATIONS: CNS, central nervous system; IV, intravenously.

TABLE 51-6 Drugs Used in the Treatment of Critical Illness due to Tuberculosis

Drug	Daily Dose	Route	Comments
Isoniazid	10 mg/kg up to 300 mg (given with pyridoxine 50 mg)	PO, IM, IV	Hepatotoxic—monitor liver enzymes
Rifampin	20 mg/kg up to 600 mg	PO, IV	Hepatotoxic—monitor liver enzymes
Pyrazinamide	30 mg/kg up to 2 g	PO	Monitor liver enzymes and serum uric acid
Streptomycin	15 mg/kg up to 1 g	IM	Nephrotoxic—monitor renal function; neurotoxic to cranial nerve VIII
Ethambutol	25 mg/kg	PO	

ABBREVIATIONS: IM, intramuscular; IV, intravenous; PO, oral.

inflammatory response, but controlled studies to support this practice are lacking.

SUPPORTIVE THERAPY

In most respects, supportive therapy for patients with pneumonia resembles that for other patients with infections requiring intensive care. The most frequent reason for a patient with pneumonia to require intensive care is respiratory failure. An approach to management of this problem is detailed in Chapter 38. Most patients have intravascular volume depletion at presentation and require some intravenous volume expansion with crystalloid solutions. However, septic pneumonia patients are also at increased risk of developing more generalized pulmonary edema, as in ARDS (see Chap. 38). Hypotension that does not respond to reasonable volume expansion is usually due to septic shock, the management of which is detailed in Chapter 46.

As in other critically ill patients, a multiplicity of metabolic, hematologic, and blood electrolyte abnormalities occur and may require correction. Especially important in the pneumonia patient is hyponatremia caused by inappropriate vasopressin secretion, leading to impaired water excretion by the kidney; this is common and makes administration of hypotonic intravenous solutions potentially hazardous.[33] The correction of metabolic alkalosis of any cause also may be important because this may be associated with an improvement in arterial oxygenation caused by improved ventilation/perfusion matching related to potentiation of regional hypoxic pulmonary vasoconstriction.[34]

Because patients with acute pulmonary infections frequently shed potentially pathogenic organisms into their immediate environment, the risk of exposure of caregivers and other patients to these pathogens must be considered. Many of the common acute respiratory pathogens causing pneumonia are normal flora of the respiratory tract (e.g., *S. pneumoniae*, *H. influenzae*, and *Moraxella catarrhalis*) and therefore require no special precautions during patient care. However, some bacterial pathogens do pose significant risk to other patients if transmitted via aerosol or on the hands or equipment of caregivers. These include *S. aureus* (especially methicillin-resistant *S. aureus*) and multiply-resistant gram-negative bacilli. When these organisms are cultured or suspected patients should be cared for in separate rooms, where possible, using appropriate infection control precautions[35] (see Chap. 4). Some viral infections also pose a risk to staff

and other patients. Examples include influenzae A and B (for which staff vaccination is highly effective), RSV, and acute *Varicella zoster*.

During the SARS outbreak of March 2002, transmission of infection to caregivers accounted for the majority of cases in some centers, with several fatalities among those infected. Most transmissions occurred by direct contact or by respiratory droplet spread from undiagnosed infected patients to staff not using personal protective precautions. When active case identification was put in place, potential cases were rapidly put in isolation, and caregivers were protected by using N95 masks, eye protection, gloves, gowns, and strict hand washing for all patient contact, transmission was quickly halted. Patients requiring ventilatory support in the ICU were particularly important vectors of infection, mainly related to droplet spread of the virus during endotracheal intubation and other respiratory care procedures. The following measures to minimize risk to staff during intubation for SARS-related respiratory failure are suggested:

1. Anticipate the need for ventilatory support to ensure that intubation occurs in a well-prepared, nonemergent controlled setting.
2. Intubation should be performed by the most skilled individual available.
3. Minimize staff in procedure room.
4. Intubate in a closed-door, well-ventilated, and preferably negative-pressurized room.
5. Minimize coughing and other droplet-generating respiratory efforts by the patient by using good preintubation sedation; consider using muscle relaxation to facilitate intubation.
6. Personnel in the room should have N95 masks checked for correct fit, face shields, gowns, and gloves.
7. Meticulous hand washing should occur after any procedure, particularly after removing protective clothing.
8. Surfaces in the procedure room should be disinfected before the area is used for another purpose.
9. Continue these infection control procedures during subsequent ICU care for respiratory failure.

Nosocomial Pneumonia

Nosocomial pneumonia differs significantly from CAP in aspects of pathogenesis and in the range of usual microbial pathogens seen.[36,37] Approaches to diagnosis are generally

TABLE 51-7 Bacterial Causes of Nosocomial Pneumonia in Patients Requiring Intensive Care

Organism	Frequency (% of Cases)[a]
Enterobacteriaceae (*Klebsiella, Escherichia coli, Enterobacter, Proteus, Acinetobacter, Serratia,* etc.)	30–50
Staphylococcus aureus	10–30
Pseudomonas aeruginosa	10–20
Streptococci (including *Streptococcus pneumoniae*)	10–15
Legionella spp.	5–15
Haemophilus influenzae	2–10
Moraxella (*Branhamella*) *catarrhalis*	2–10
Anaerobes	2–5

[a] Ranges shown are derived from several studies from different geographic areas and different patient populations. The incidence of each infection greatly depends on local circumstances.

similar to those for CAP; however, the approach to antimicrobial therapy differs considerably, reflecting the different spectrum of pathogens. In addition, because nosocomial pneumonia by definition occurs in patients already under medical care for illnesses requiring hospitalization, the possibility of preventing its occurrence exists and is an important aspect of the day-to-day care of the critically ill patient (see Chaps. 4 and 10).

PATHOGENESIS AND MICROBIOLOGY

The most common microbial causes of nosocomial pneumonia are listed in Table 51-7. This table was constructed from data gathered in a number of surveys of different patient populations, and it must be emphasized that hospital populations are not identical with respect to risk for pneumonia caused by each of these pathogens. As in CAP, the basic event leading to pneumonia is usually subclinical aspiration of oropharyngeal material, an event for which hospitalized patients are at increased risk on account of disease and medical intervention. These increased risks include depressed level of consciousness caused by head injury, metabolic disease, or sedative and anesthetic drugs, and impaired laryngeal reflexes and esophageal sphincter function caused by neurologic disease or instrumentation of the airway or esophagus. Although endotracheal intubation with a cuffed tube may prevent frank aspiration of gastric contents, it is no barrier to the minor degrees of aspiration required to transfer potential pathogens from the upper to the lower respiratory tract. The patient's ability to deal effectively with contamination of the lower respiratory tract may also be compromised. Mucociliary clearance may be impaired by damage to the tracheal mucosa by endotracheal tubes, metabolic disease, or drugs; immunologic defenses may be impaired by underlying disease or by immunosuppressive therapy.

The explanation for the nature of the common pneumonia pathogens is the pattern of colonization of the upper airway, which determines which organisms gain access to the lung when aspiration occurs. In previously well patients admitted to ICUs with acute illness that compromises airway defenses, pneumonia in the few days after admission is caused most often by organisms that are frequent colonizers of the upper airway in normal persons: *S. aureus, Streptococcus* species,

and, to a lesser extent, *H. influenzae* and *M. catarrhalis*.[38] Patients with underlying chronic lung disease are frequently colonized with these same pathogens, but nontypeable *H. influenzae* and *M. catarrhalis* are more frequent in patients with underlying lung disease than in normal persons and therefore cause early nosocomial pneumonia more frequently in these patients.[39,40] Patients who have other chronic debilitating diseases or those who have been in the hospital for a number of days are at increased risk of having upper airway colonization and subsequent pneumonia caused by enteric facultatively aerobic gram-negative bacilli such as *K. pneumoniae, E. coli,* and *Enterobacter* species, whereas patients with underlying structural lung disease, the immunosuppressed, and those who have been treated with antimicrobials or who have had a lengthy stay in an ICU are at increased risk for colonization or infection with more antimicrobial-resistant hospital-acquired pathogens such as *P. aeruginosa, Stenotrophomonas maltophilia,* or *Acinetobacter* species.[41] The source of staphylococci or *Enterobacteriaceae* causing these infections is most often the patient's own endogenous microflora; however, many of the more resistant pathogens may be transmitted to patients by contact spread from the hands of caregivers or, particularly with water-borne organisms such as *Pseudomonas* or *Acinetobacter*, by contaminated respiratory therapy equipment.

Among the pathogens in the atypical pneumonia group, only viruses and *L. pneumophila* are notable causes of nosocomial pneumonia. Influenza A and RSV are sporadically reported to cause outbreaks of pneumonia in the hospital, generally by respiratory or hand-to-hand spread from other infected individuals, and there is reason to believe that CMV can also occasionally cause pneumonia leading to respiratory failure in immunocompetent hospitalized patients; the pathogenesis of nosocomial infection in this population is unknown. In the March 2002 SARS coronavirus outbreak, much of the disease transmission was nosocomial, mainly by direct contact or droplet spread from patients with undiagnosed SARS to health care workers not using any personal protection against infection, and from them to other patients by the same mechanisms.[21] For nosocomial infection with *Legionella* species, the pathogenesis is inhalation of aerosols containing the organism. In outbreak situations, this can usually be traced to presence of the organism in hospital water supplies, with dissemination by showers and baths and the like, or to cooling tower contamination. Ground excavation near an outside air intake has also been implicated. It is likely that many hospitalized patients are exposed to *Legionella*, given its widespread presence in hospital water supplies; however, most cases continue to occur among the immunosuppressed hospitalized population, particularly those on corticosteroid treatment for prevention of organ transplant rejection. This is presumably because a patient with suppressed cell-mediated immunity has a reduced capacity to clear even small inhaled inocula of this intracellular pathogen, with which a patient with intact cell-mediated immunity can cope easily.

DIAGNOSIS

The clinical features and radiographic findings associated with nosocomial pneumonia are similar to those of CAP but may be greatly confounded by other disease processes common in hospitalized patients, particularly those in intensive care. The diagnosis is suggested by the presence of a pulmonary infiltrate consistent with pneumonia on chest radiograph, increased amount and purulence of lower respiratory tract secretions (sputum or endobronchial aspirates), deterioration in gas exchange and increased dyspnea, and an increase in temperature or leukocyte count. There are problems with the sensitivity and specificity of this clinical definition. Postmortem studies of critically ill patients with extensive lung disease of other causes have indicated that many patients have clinically unsuspected bacterial pneumonia at the time of death. However, there is evidence that, in the general ICU patient population, other processes, such as chemical pneumonitis caused by aspiration, atelectasis, and purulent tracheobronchitis, can produce many of or all the same clinical findings as pneumonia, and that pneumonia can be significantly overdiagnosed in this context.[42] In intubated, ventilated patients in particular, quantitative bacteriologic evaluation of bronchoscopic specimens of secretions from the lower respiratory tract has been advocated as a way of overcoming this problem, and this approach is discussed comprehensively in Chapter 43.

For most patients, a careful clinical assessment combined with conventional microbiologic studies for the diagnosis of nosocomial pneumonia in ward patients and in intubated ICU patients remains a reasonable first approach. Some patients have clinical presentations with such marked pyrexia, leukocytosis, deterioration in lung function, and advancing infiltrates that the diagnosis is fairly certain. It remains only to obtain the appropriate specimen to establish the etiology; in most such cases, this is sputum or endobronchial aspirates, a blood culture, and needle aspirate of pleural fluid if a significant amount is present. It is mainly in patients with less florid presentations, with marginal changes in the major diagnostic parameters and with infiltrates that could be atelectasis or pneumonia, in whom the diagnosis is substantially in doubt. In these cases, the usual best policy is to obtain endobronchial secretions for Gram stain and culture, provide chest physiotherapy and or frequent posturing of the patient and endobronchial suctioning, and withhold antimicrobial treatment initially. Over the ensuing hours to days, the result of the culture will become available; the additional information regarding the progress of the pulmonary process, the systemic inflammatory response without antimicrobial treatment, the presence and quantitation of leukocytes and bacteria on Gram stain, and the results of initial cultures will aid in making the judgment about whether an infection requiring antimicrobial treatment is present. In cases in which substantial uncertainty remains, fiberoptic bronchoscopy with a protected specimen brush or BAL with quantitative bacteriology is a reasonable next step.

MANAGEMENT

The principles of supportive management for nosocomial pneumonia are identical to those outlined for CAP. However, there are several differences in antimicrobial therapy because of the considerably different range of etiologic agents seen. Atypical pneumonia is much less common in hospitalized patients and, when it occurs, is most often caused by *Legionella* species. Bacterial pneumonias make up the vast majority of cases and are much more likely to be caused by *S. aureus* or enteric gram-negative bacilli and, in particular subgroups of patients, by relatively antimicrobial-resistant gram-negative bacilli. Suggested empiric antimicrobial regimens for hospital-acquired pneumonia are listed in Table 51-8 and those for specific proven pathogens are listed in Table 51-3.

The pathogens causing hospital-acquired pneumonia are much more likely to cause a destructive necrotizing pneumonia than are the common community-acquired pathogens and therefore are more likely to result in formation of abscesses and empyema, pneumothorax, and permanent fibrosis of involved lung regions. These pathogens also are more difficult to eradicate permanently from the lung with antimicrobial therapy. Accordingly, duration of antimicrobial therapy is generally longer, usually at least 3 weeks to as many as 6 or 8 weeks, depending on the initial response, presence of abscess cavities, and susceptibility of the organism. Treatment should always be parenteral initially and for most enteric gram-negative organisms should usually include two different agents effective against the pathogen, generally a β-lactam drug and an aminoglycoside or a quinolone. After 7 to 10 days, if a good clinical response has been observed, completion of the treatment course with an appropriate oral agent is reasonable. Oral agents considered suitable for gram-negative

TABLE 51-8 Empiric Antimicrobial Therapy for Nosocomial Pneumonia Associated with Critical Illness[a]

Clinical Setting	Recommended Antimicrobial Therapy	Alternative Antimicrobial Therapy
Acute nosocomial pneumonia (postoperative or complicating medical illness)	Cefotaxime 2 g IV q 8 h *and* gentamicin 4.5 mg/kg IV q 24 h	Co-trimoxazole IV; ciprofloxacin or ofloxacin IV ± a β-lactam
Nosocomial pneumonia with increased risk of resistant aerobic gram-negatives (i.e., prior broad-spectrum antibiotics, acute leukemia, endemic resistant organisms, etc.)	Piperacillin/tazobactam 3.375 g IV q 6 h and ciprofloxacin 400 mg IV q 12 h or gentamicin 4.5 mg/kg IV q 24 h	Carbapenem or ceftazidime *and* gentamicin or quinolone
Severe pneumonia after aspiration	Clindamycin 900 mg IV q 8 h *and* cefotaxime 2 g IV q 8 h	Clindamycin and cotrimoxazole IV, metronidazole and cefotaxime
Suspect legionellosis (endemic, organ transplant, steroid use, or undiagnosed fulminant pneumonia)	*Add* ciprofloxacin 400 mg IV q 12 h ± rifampin 600 mg IV daily to one of the above regimens	Azithromycin ± rifampin
Suspect methicillin-resistant *Staphylococcus aureus*	*Add* vancomycin 500 mg IV q 6 h	

[a] Doses cited are for patients with normal renal function; dosage adjustments for renal insufficiency are required for several of the listed agents. Monitoring of blood drug levels is strongly advised for aminoglycosides. Gentamicin is shown as the preferred aminoglycoside; however, where resistance to this agent is common, selection of an alternative aminoglycoside may be necessary.

pneumonias include cotrimoxazole, amoxicillin/clavulanic acid, cefuroxime axetil, cefixime, and, for resistant organisms such as *Pseudomonas* species, ciprofloxacin.

As in outpatients, pulmonary aspiration in hospital patients can result in a simple chemical pneumonitis or atelectasis that does not require antimicrobial therapy. Hospitalized patients are much more likely to have been receiving antimicrobial agents for other indications, agents that decrease gastric acidity, and are more likely to have conditions predisposing to development of large numbers of pathogenic bacteria in the oropharynx and the stomach (e.g., recent surgery, adynamic ileus, or tube feeding). This increases the risk of an acute necrotizing bacterial pneumonia in these patients. Accordingly, if there is evidence to support an active infectious process after presumed or witnessed aspiration, antimicrobial therapy directed at GI anaerobes and relatively resistant enteric gram-negative bacilli should be given.

Antimicrobial selection for hospital-acquired pneumonia, to a much greater extent than that for CAP, must be based on knowledge of which pathogens are prevalent in the environment in a particular hospital or even in a particular unit within the hospital, because antimicrobial resistance patterns vary greatly in different locations. The recommendations listed in the tables must therefore be used with caution and with knowledge of local conditions.

PREVENTION

The considerable morbidity rate associated with nosocomial pneumonia, particularly in critically ill patients, has led to much interest in developing methods to prevent these infections.[43,44] Prevention would clearly depend on breaking the pathogenetic chain leading from colonization of the upper respiratory and GI tracts with potential pathogens to aspiration of these colonizers into the lower respiratory tract; establishment of lower respiratory tract colonization; and then failure of the pulmonary clearance mechanisms and immune system to contain the organism, leading to invasion of the pulmonary parenchyma. Attempts to break the chain at each of the points mentioned have been tried by various investigators, with limited success.

Minimizing the potential for the transmission of relatively antimicrobial-resistant pathogens between patients clearly is the first priority. Basic measures to accomplish this include hand washing before and after patient contact by all caregivers, avoiding the sharing of bedside or respiratory therapy equipment between patients, and isolation of patients known to be infected or colonized with multiply-resistant bacterial pathogens.

Interventions to prevent upper airway and gastric colonization by enteric gram-negative bacilli have recently been tried in many centers. Based on evidence that stomach acid helps minimize such colonization and that administration of H_2 blockers or antacids for prophylaxis against upper GI bleeding increases colonization, use of sucralfate, an agent that protects the mucosa and prevents bleeding without increasing stomach pH, has been advocated, and studies from some centers have been demonstrated that its use decreases the rate of nosocomial pneumonia in intubated patients. However, others have been unable to confirm that gastric colonization is a risk for airway colonization and pneumonia or that use of sucralfate rather than antacids or histamine blockers is

protective. Although the controversy on this issue continues, it should be pointed out that sucralfate is cheap, nontoxic, and probably as effective as other agents, so if bleeding prophylaxis is used, sucralfate may be preferable to an H_2 blocker or antacid, except in patients at special risk for upper GI bleeding. Other suggested strategies to limit bacterial proliferation in the stomach and subsequent spread to the respiratory tract include using small bowel feeding tubes instead of gastric tubes, intermittent feeding to maintain gastric acidity, and acidification of feeds, but none of these has been convincingly shown to be effective.

Different prophylactic antimicrobial regimens, topical and systemic, have also been used to prevent colonization and pneumonia. These regimens have often been shown to be effective in limiting the incidence of pneumonia in ICU patients, but there continues to be concern that their use may eventually lead to an increase in the prevalence of antimicrobial resistance. Also, in most reported studies, the decreased rate of pneumonia was not associated with a decrease in mortality rate or in use of ICU resources. For these reasons, none of the currently available prophylactic antimicrobial regimens can be recommended.

Decreasing the risk of aspiration in seriously ill patients involves mainly commonsense measures. For a nonintubated patient who has difficulty in swallowing or decreased level of consciousness, nursing the patient on his or her side with the head slightly down may be helpful. Frequent and careful suctioning and mouth care are also important. In patients with endotracheal or nasogastric tubes and those with otherwise disturbed esophageal sphincter function, the upright position and sleeping with the head of the bed up reduces the risk of gastroesophageal reflux and aspiration. When the nasogastric tube is in place solely for feeding purposes, and it has been established that gastric emptying is adequate, the large-bore tube can be changed to a soft small-bore tube, which is less likely to interfere with the esophageal sphincter and is also more comfortable. In orally intubated patients, use of an orogastric tube rather than a nasogastric tube is also preferred.

For intubated patients, exemplary nursing care can have a substantial role in decreasing the risk of pneumonia. Frequent turning of patients while they are in bed and minimizing the use of deep sedation or muscle relaxants help avoid dependent secretion accumulation in the lungs. Use of oscillating beds to accomplish this has had mixed success with respect to efficacy and tolerance by patients, so their routine use is not currently recommended. Frequent gentle suctioning of the endotracheal tube and careful monitoring of endotracheal cuff seal and pressure are also likely to help minimize secretion accumulation and prevent pneumonia.[45] Good mouth care, suctioning of the oropharynx before endotracheal tube cuff deflation or before turning of the patient, no-touch sterile suctioning technique, and early detection and correction of gastroesophageal reflux problems are other measures that have yet to be studied in a systematic way with regard to infection rate; but they almost certainly account for much of the extremely wide variation in nosocomial pneumonia rates in different ICUs.

An active infection control program is also critical to minimizing nosocomial pneumonia risk.[46] Careful monitoring of infection rates and the occurrence of pathogens with a propensity for nosocomial spread is needed to detect potential reservoirs for cross-infection of patients and to guide

TABLE 51-9 The More Common Opportunistic Pulmonary Infections of the Immunocompromised Host[a]

Immunodeficiency	Predominant Pulmonary Infections	Most Frequent Clinical Settings
Humoral immunodeficiency	Pyogenic bacterial pneumonias	Hypogammaglobulinemia, chronic lymphocytic leukemia, multiple myeloma
Phagocytic cell deficiency	Bacterial pneumonia, fungal pneumonias, aspergillosis, candidemia with pulmonary involvement, cryptococcosis	Chemotherapy-induced granulocytopenia, acute myelogenous leukemia
Cell-mediated immunodeficiency	*Pneumocystis carinii* pneumonia, legionellosis, nocardiosis, CMV pneumonia, cryptococcosis, mycobacteriosis	Lymphoma or acute lymphocytic leukemia undergoing chemotherapy, high-dose corticosteroid therapy, organ transplantation, advanced HIV infection

[a] These categories are not mutually exclusive. For example, bone marrow transplant recipients develop mainly bacterial and fungal infections associated with phagocytic cell deficits early after transplantation but develop infections related to chronic suppression of cell-mediated immunity after recovery from transplantation.
ABBREVIATIONS: CMV, cytomegalovirus; HIV, human immunodeficiency virus.

institution of infection control measures. In general, an ICU with a pneumonia rate higher than approximately 10% in patients ventilated for longer than 48 hours, with a sustained increase in pneumonia rate over baseline, or with a predominance of water-borne gram-negative organisms such as *Pseudomonas* species or *Acinetobacter* species or any other single species as a cause of most cases of pneumonia, probably has a potentially correctable infection control problem.

Pulmonary Infiltrates in the Immunocompromised Host

Immunocompromised patients with fever and new pulmonary infiltrates usually come to the attention of the intensive care physician when they develop imminent or established acute respiratory failure or when a period of endotracheal intubation with mechanical ventilatory support is needed to facilitate an invasive diagnostic procedure. That both of these events occur relatively frequently says a great deal about the many special problems posed by this group of patients: The differential diagnosis of pulmonary inflammatory processes is wide, establishing a definitive diagnosis is often difficult, empiric antimicrobial therapy is often ineffective, and the patient's condition can deteriorate rapidly.

The nature of the immunologic abnormality that is present in a given case has a major bearing on the nature of the infective processes likely to be present. The major categories of immunologic abnormality include (a) deficient humoral immunity (these are patients with agammaglobulinemia and multiple myeloma or chronic lymphocytic leukemia, without intensive chemotherapy), (b) deficient phagocytic cell function or number (patients with chemotherapy-induced granulocytopenia make up the majority in this group), and (c) deficient cell-mediated immune function (includes patients on corticosteroids or other immunosuppressive drugs for the control of a variety of inflammatory diseases, control of rejection after organ transplantation, and less intensive chemotherapy for a variety of malignancies; it also includes patients with advanced HIV infection, which is discussed in

more detail in Chap. 48). Many patients have mixed immune dysfunctions, especially those on rigorous chemotherapeutic regimens for cancer. Table 51-9 lists the major pulmonary infections most strongly associated with each type of immune dysfunction.

CLINICAL FEATURES

In addition to the information regarding the nature of the immunodeficiency noted above, clues to the etiologic diagnosis may be available from details of the history and physical examination.

The timing of the onset of the illness, with respect to previous chemotherapy and duration of immunosuppression, is often very helpful. After cytotoxic chemotherapy resulting in granulocytopenia, acute bacterial infections predominate in the first 2 to 3 weeks. Subsequently, especially with illnesses occurring in the face of broad-spectrum antimicrobial therapy, opportunistic fungal infections are increasingly common. After bone marrow and other transplantation procedures, bacterial infections also predominate early, with viral and fungal infections occurring weeks to months later. In this patient population, CMV pneumonia is of particular importance, occurring with increased frequency in patients known to be seropositive for CMV; in bone marrow recipients, CMV pneumonitis is also more common in older patients, those who have received total-body irradiation, and those with severe graft-versus-host disease.[47,48] Some noninfectious causes of pulmonary infiltrates also follow a somewhat predictable time course: radiation pneumonitis usually occurs 4 to 10 weeks after treatment; pulmonary edema caused by acute toxic myocarditis after high-dose doxorubicin therapy usually occurs a few days to a few weeks after treatment, whereas cardiomyopathy from doxorubicin and daunorubicin is increasingly frequent with increasing cumulative dose; and interstitial pneumonitis caused by bleomycin is common at cumulative doses larger than 450 U, although damaging pulmonary reactions to this cytotoxic drug and to others can occur with much smaller doses.[49]

Although the pace at which the pulmonary process progresses is to some degree characteristic for each etiologic agent, this is highly variable and greatly dependent on the nature and severity of the underlying immunologic deficit. *Aspergillus* species, for example, produce an indolent localized pneumonia in patients treated with immunosuppressive drugs and corticosteroids if phagocytic cell function is relatively preserved, but in patients with severe combined immunodeficiency and in some with long-term granulocytopenia from chemotherapy for myelogenous leukemia, the illness may be fulminant.[50] *Pneumocystis carinii* causes a severe, rapidly progressive diffuse pneumonia in patients with lymphoma or leukemia but usually is an insidious illness in those with HIV. It is also worth bearing in mind that an apparent change in the pace of progression of disease may signal the presence of more than one process, for example, an acute bacterial infection superimposed on a more slowly progressive disease, such as interstitial pneumonitis.

The physical examination is only occasionally revealing in this patient group. Examination of the chest almost never adds to the radiologic assessment. However, extrapulmonary findings may be very helpful in the differential diagnosis and may provide a potential alternative site for diagnostic testing. Central nervous system involvement (meningitis or encephalitis) indicates systemic fungal infections, tuberculosis, bacteremia with metastatic foci, or disseminated viral infections and mandates computed tomography of the brain followed by lumbar puncture. Disseminated aspergillus infection, in addition to involving the lung and brain, may produce necrotizing skin lesions. *Ecthyma gangrenosum* signals bacteremia, usually with *P. aeruginosa* and usually producing a diffuse multinodular pneumonia. Staphylococcal bacteremia and pneumonia may be associated with widespread cutaneous pustules, whereas the rare case of disseminated candidiasis with pulmonary involvement may be associated with a papular rash, myalgias, or "cotton wool" exudates on funduscopic examination.

RADIOGRAPHIC FEATURES

The chest radiographic appearance of the pulmonary infiltrate can be a useful guide to a differential diagnosis but is seldom specific enough to establish the diagnosis. The most important differentiation to be made is whether the infiltrate is a localized or a diffuse process.

Diffuse infiltrates, if they are of infectious origin, imply infection with a pathogen that has reached the lung hematogenously in large numbers or has spread rapidly along the respiratory mucosa early in the course of the infection. Examples include viral infections such as CMV, which is actually a systemic infection; hematogenous bacterial pneumonia (*P. aeruginosa* most commonly); miliary or chronic hematogenous tuberculosis; and candidemia with secondary candidal pneumonitis. PCP also is typically a diffuse pneumonia (Fig. 51-11). Noninfectious processes producing diffuse infiltrates are those in which the entire lung is exposed equally to the damaging agent through the bloodstream or the lymphatics (Table 51-10). Examples include drug-associated lung injury, leukemic infiltration or lymphangitic carcinomatosis of the lung, and idiopathic interstitial pneumonitis.[51]

Localized infiltrates caused by infections are generally those in which the organism has gained access to the lung

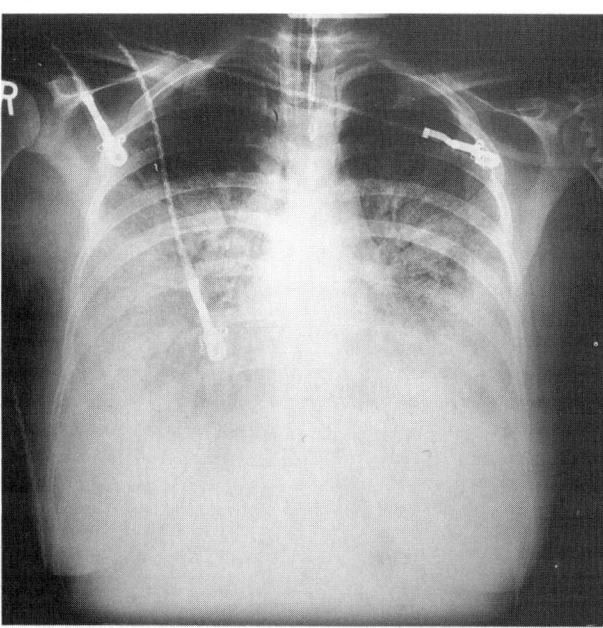

FIGURE 51-11 Severe *Pneumocystis carinii* pneumonia in a patient with acute myelogenous leukemia undergoing induction chemotherapy. Note the lower lobe and perihilar predominance of the mainly alveolar infiltrate, with areas of frank consolidation; in the right lower lobe, note an air bronchogram.

by aspiration of oropharyngeal material or by inhalation of the pathogen. Examples include most cases of acute bacterial pneumonia, including nocardial pneumonia and *L. pneumophila* pneumonia, and most cases of opportunistic fungal pneumonia, such as those caused by *Aspergillus*, *Mucor*, and *Cryptococcus* species. The appearance of the infiltrate sometimes provides a diagnostic clue. *Legionella pneumophila* often produces airspace consolidation with a peripheral, ill-defined, rounded density, often with rapid subsequent progression (see Fig. 51-4).[16] Localized infiltrates caused by *Aspergillus* usually begin as enlarging nodular infiltrates or as patchy bronchopneumonia in the granulocytopenic patient (Fig. 51-12), with the development of central necrosis, cavitation, and "air crescent" signs associated with marrow recovery.[52] Hematogenous spread of infection causing a localized infiltrate also occurs occasionally, although this most often produces multiple, locally spreading infiltrates that may not be anatomically adjacent; hematogenous bacterial infections, especially septic thromboembolia, are examples of this. The major noninfectious entities producing localized infiltrates are atelectasis, pulmonary embolism with infarction, and metastatic neoplastic disease.

APPROACH TO DIAGNOSIS AND MANAGEMENT

Diagnosis and management must be considered together, particularly for patients requiring support in an ICU. There are usually two phases to the approach. In the first phase, a presumptive diagnosis or group of potential diagnoses is formulated and empiric therapy is begun while relatively noninvasive diagnostic testing is implemented. Many patients respond to initial therapy or, if they do not, have a tenable diagnosis established on the basis of the initial investigation, leading to a revision of the initial therapeutic regimen. In the second phase, which is marked by the increasingly clear need

TABLE 51-10 Noninfectious Causes of Pulmonary Infiltrates in the Immunocompromised Host and the Clinical Settings in Which They Are Most Frequently Seen

Noninfectious Diagnosis	Clinical Settings
Diffuse pulmonary infiltrates	
Interstitial pneumonitis due to cytotoxic drug therapy	Bleomycin (>150 mg total) or not related to dose
	Reaction to bleomycin, cyclophosphamide, methotrexate, and others
Cardiogenic pulmonary edema	Pre-existing cardiac disease
	Chemotherapy with daunorubicin or doxorubicin
Lymphangitic carcinomatosis	Carcinoma poorly responsive to therapy
Leukemic infiltration of lung	Uncontrolled acute leukemia
Acute low-pressure pulmonary edema (diffuse alveolar damage)	Leukemic cell lysis after chemotherapy
	Leukoagglutination reaction after transfusion
Focal pulmonary infiltrates	
Pulmonary metastasis	Untreated or poorly responsive primary carcinoma
Atelectasis	Endobronchial lesion
	Chest wall or upper abdominal pain
	Depressed cough or respiration (narcotics)
Pulmonary infarction (pulmonary thromboembolism)	Hypercoagulable state owing to carcinoma or paraproteinemia, immobility, venous obstruction
Radiation pneumonitis	Recent (4–12 wk) radiotherapy with lung exposure

for a definitive diagnosis because of the failure of empiric therapy or the pace and severity of progression of disease, increasingly invasive diagnostic testing is performed until the diagnosis is established and definitive therapy begun. The key to appropriate management is to take great care to neither abandon the frequently correct initial diagnosis and treatment too soon (thereby subjecting many patients to the risk of an unnecessary lung biopsy) nor wait too long to proceed to a definitive diagnostic procedure (making the diagnosis too late to reverse the disease).

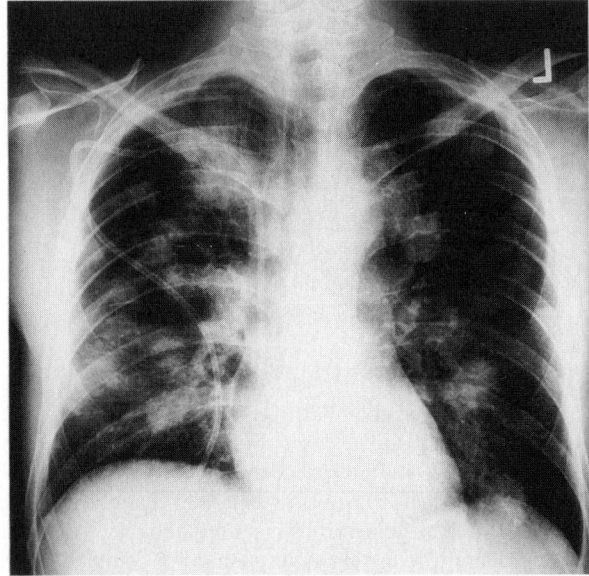

FIGURE 51-12 Pulmonary aspergillosis in a patient with acute myelogenous leukemia and protracted granulocytopenia. Note the multiple, dense, alveolar infiltrates forming large expanding nodules.

The major considerations governing the initial empiric antimicrobial approach and the selection of diagnostic procedures are (a) the underlying disease and the timing of the pulmonary process with respect to it, (b) the presence of major clues to the diagnosis from the initial clinical evaluation, (c) the radiologic pattern, and (d) the physiologic stability of the patient and the rate of progression of the disease. Patients with pulmonary infiltrates that fit a commonly seen clinical and radiologic pattern quite well and who are physiologically stable can be treated empirically pending the results of initial diagnostic testing. Those who have less certain clinical and radiologic patterns and who are unstable or getting worse quickly require prompt and definitive diagnostic testing.

Patients with diffuse infiltrates should receive intravenous wide-spectrum antimicrobials directed at hematogenous bacterial pneumonia, at least until initial culture results are available. Piperacillin/tazobactam 3.375 g IV every 6 hours and ciprofloxacin 400 mg IV every 12 hours is usually acceptable. Cotrimoxazole (20 mg/kg trimethoprim with 100 mg/kg sulfamethoxazole per day in four divided doses) may be added to cover *P. carinii* (unless the patient has been receiving cotrimoxazole prophylaxis, in which case the diagnosis is essentially excluded). Investigations include blood cultures, respiratory and stool specimens for viral culture, culture of blood for CMV, respiratory secretions for Gram stain and culture, and examination for acid-fast bacilli and fungi. In patients with predominantly cell-mediated immune impairment (lymphoma, steroid, or immunosuppressive drug therapy or organ transplant) who have not received cotrimoxazole and have negative blood cultures, PCP is the leading infectious possibility. Unlike what is seen in HIV patients with PCP, the number of organisms in the lung is not large; hence sputum examination for the organism is not useful. Early bronchoscopy with BAL or a protected specimen brush is advised.[53] The specimen obtained should be examined

TABLE 51-11 Initial Antimicrobial Therapy for Opportunistic Lung Infections in Critically Ill Immunocompromised Patients

Pulmonary Infection	Antimicrobial Regimen
Pneumocystis carinii pneumonia	Cotrimoxazole 5 mg/kg TMP and 25 mg/kg SMX IV q 6 h *or* clindamycin 600 mg IV q 8 h with primaquine 30 mg PO once daily
Nocardia asteroids, pneumonia, or abscess	Cotrimoxazole 2.5 mg/kg TMP and 12.5 mg/kg SMX IV q 6 h *or* imipenem 500 mg IV q 6 h ± amikacin 5 mg/kg IV q 8 h
Aspergillosis	Voriconazole 6 mg/kg q 12 h × 2, then 4 mg/kg IV q 12 h *or* amphotericin B 0.6–1.0 mg/kg IV q 24 h
Candida pneumonia due to associated candidemia	Amphotericin B 0.5–0.8 mg/kg IV q 24 h *or* fluconazole 400 mg IV q 24 h
CMV pneumonia	Ganciclovir 2.5 mg/kg IV q 8 h *and* CMV immunoglobulin 400–500 mg/kg on alternate days (4–10 doses)
Varicella zoster, disseminated, with pneumonia	Acyclovir 10 mg/kg IV q 8 h

ABBREVIATIONS: CMV, cytomegalovirus; IV, intravenously; PO, orally; SMX, sulfamethoxazole; TMP, trimethoprim.

for the full range of pathogens mentioned above. Cytologic examination of cells for evidence of CMV, culture of respiratory secretions, and blood for CMV will help in establishing that diagnosis. Bronchoscopic methods have excellent diagnostic yield for infectious diagnoses in this setting but are somewhat less useful in defining noninfectious etiologies for diffuse infiltrates.[54] Accordingly, for patients who are at lesser risk for PCP and CMV, for those in whom the initial investigation excludes these possibilities, and for those with rapidly progressive diffuse lung disease, open lung biopsy should be considered. Open lung biopsy remains controversial in this setting: Although a definitive diagnosis can be established in most patients and therapy can be adjusted appropriately, in severely ill patients this often does not lead to survival. Further, significant morbidity caused by the procedure is not uncommon. Nevertheless, there is evidence that in selected cases open biopsy can be very useful by offering the best chance of survival to the subset of patients with reversible disease.[55,56] In the face of progressing disease, if a biopsy is to be done, it is important to make the decision to proceed before the patient has progressed to frank respiratory failure.

The diagnosis of localized pulmonary infiltrates caused by conventional bacterial pneumonia can usually be established with sufficient certainty by blood cultures, Gram stain and culture of respiratory secretion and culture, direct fluorescent antibody staining and culture of respiratory secretions for *L. pneumophila*, and the clinical response to empiric antimicrobial therapy, usually piperacillin/tazobactam and ciprofloxacin, unless it is known that the patient is colonized with a pathogen resistant to these antimicrobials. If the diagnosis is not immediately forthcoming or the patient does not respond promptly to empiric therapy, bronchoscopy should be done and BAL or protected brush specimens sent for examination for bacteria; acid-fast bacilli; direct fluorescent antibody, and culture for *Legionella*; fungal elements; and cytologic examination. If there is no contraindication, transbronchial biopsy may increase the yield for invasive fungal infection and for malignancy. However, as many as 50% of cases of invasive fungal infections may not be detected by bronchoscopic methods and require open lung biopsy

for diagnosis. Culture of aspergilli from nasal scrapings or sputum can be helpful in this regard. Although culture of aspergilli is not indicative of disease in normal persons, in severely immunocompromised patients with granulocytopenia and acute leukemia, such positive cultures are strongly associated with invasive disease.

When the diagnosis has been established, definitive therapy is begun and other agents started empirically are discontinued unless other indications for their use remain. A discussion of the full range of therapies for noninfectious etiologies of pulmonary infiltrates is beyond the scope of this chapter; drug regimens for the major infectious causes of opportunistic pneumonia are presented in Table 51-11.

References

1. Bartlett JG, Dowell SF, Mandell LA, et al. Practice guidelines for the management of community-acquired pneumonia in adults. *Clin Infect Dis* 31:347, 2000.
2. Mandell LA, Marrie TJ, Grossman RF, et al. Canadian guidelines for the initial management of community-acquired pneumonia: an evidence-based update by the Canadian Infectious Disease Society and the Canadian Thoracic Society. *Clin Infect Dis* 31:383, 2000.
3. Neiderman MA, Mandell LA (co-chairs) for the American Thoracic Society: Guidelines for the management of adults with community-acquired pneumonia. *Am J Respir Crit Care Med* 163: 1730, 2001.
4. George DL: Epidemiology of nosocomial pneumonia in intensive care unit patients. *Clin Chest Med* 16:29, 1995.
5. Torres A, Serra-Batlles J, Ferrer A, et al: Severe community-acquired pneumonia. *Am Rev Respir Dis* 144:312, 1991.
6. British Thoracic Society: The etiology, management and outcome of severe community-acquired pneumonia in the intensive care unit. *Respir Med* 86:7, 1992.
7. Rello J, Quintana E, Ausina V et al: A three year study of severe community-acquired pneumonia with emphasis on outcome. *Chest* 103:232, 1993.
8. Mackowiak PA, Martin RM, Jones SR, Smith JW: Pharyngeal colonization by gram-negative bacilli in aspiration-prone persons. *Arch Intern Med* 138:1224, 1978.

9. Valenti WM, Trudell RG, Bently DW: Factors predisposing to oropharyngeal colonization with gram-negative bacilli in the aged. *N Engl J Med* 298:1108, 1978.

10. Huxley EJ, Viroslav J, Gray WR, Pierce AK: Pharyngeal aspiration in normal adults and patients with depressed consciousness. *Am J Med* 64:564, 1978.

11. Davidson FF, Glazier JB, Murray JF: The components of the alveolar-arterial oxygen tension difference in normal subjects and in patients with pneumonia and obstructive lung disease. *Am J Med* 52:754, 1972.

12. Light RB, Mink SN, Wood LDH: Pathophysiology of gas exchange and pulmonary perfusion in pneumococcal pneumonia in dogs. *J Appl Physiol* 50:524, 1981.

13. Light RB: Intrapulmonary oxygen consumption in experimental pneumococcal pneumonia. *J Appl Physiol* 64:2490, 1988.

14. Hensel M, Kox WJ: Increased intrapulmonary oxygen consumption in mechanically ventilated patients with pneumonia. *Am J Respir Crit Care Med* 160:137, 1999.

15. Miller AC: Early clinical differentiation between Legionnaires' disease and other sporadic pneumonias. *Ann Intern Med* 90:526, 1979.

16. Stout JE, Yu VL: Legionellosis. *N Eng J Med* 337:682, 1997.

17. Dietrich PA, Johnson RD, Fairbank JT, Walke JS: The chest radiograph in Legionnaires' disease. *Radiology* 127:577, 1978.

18. Verweij PE, Meis JF, Eijk R, et al Severe human psittacosis requiring artificial ventilation: Case report and review. *Clin Infect Dis* 20:440, 1995.

19. Marrie TJ: *Coxiella burnetii* pneumonia. *Eur Respir J* 4:713, 2003.

20. Oliveira EC, Marik PE, Colice G. Influenza pneumonia: A descriptive study. *Chest* 19:1717, 2001.

21. Consensus document on the epidemiology of Severe Acute Respiratory Distress Syndrome (SARS). World Health Organization, 2003. Available at: www.who.int/csr/sars/WHOconsensus.pdf

22. Holmes KV: SARS coronavirus: A new challenge for prevention and therapy. *J Clin Invest* 111:1605, 2003.

23. Booth CM, Matukas LM, Tomlinson GA, et al. Clinical features and short-term outcomes of 144 patients with SARS in the greater Toronto area. *JAMA* 289:2801, 2003.

24. Wynne JW, Modell JH: Respiratory aspiration of stomach contents. *Ann Intern Med* 87:466, 1977.

25. Bynum LJ, Pierce AK: Pulmonary aspiration of gastric contents. *Am Rev Respir Dis* 114:1129, 1976.

26. Murray PR, Washington JA: Microscopic and bacteriologic analysis of expectorated sputum. *Mayo Clin Proc* 50:339, 1975.

27. Thorpe J, Baugham R, Frame PT, et al: Bronchoalveolar lavage for diagnosing acute bacterial pneumonia. *J Infect Dis* 155:855, 1987.

28. Khan FW, Jones JM: Diagnosing bacterial respiratory infections by bronchoalveolar lavage. *J Infect Dis* 155:862, 1987.

29. Jimenez P, Saldias F, Meneses M, et al: Diagnostic fiberoptic bronchoscopy in patients with community-acquired pneumonia. Comparison between bronchoalveolar lavage and telescoping plugged catheter cultures. *Chest* 103:1023, 1993.

30. Penner C, Roberts D, Kunimoto D, et al: Tuberculosis as a primary cause of respiratory failure requiring mechanical ventilation. *Am J Resp Crit Care Med* 151:867, 1995.

31. Meyer KC, McManus EJ, Maki DG: Overwhelming pulmonary blastomycosis associated with the adult respiratory distress syndrome. *N Engl J Med* 329:1231, 1993.

32. Blumberg HM, Burman WJ, Chaisson RE, et al: American Thoracic Society/Centers for Disease Control and Prevention/Infectious Diseases Society of America: Treatment of tuberculosis. *Am J Respir Crit Care Med* 167:602, 2003.

33. Dreyfuss D, Leviel F, Paillard M, et al: Acute infectious pneumonia is accompanied by a latent vasopressin-dependent impairment of renal water excretion. *Am Rev Respir Dis* 138:583, 1988.

34. Brimioulle S, Kahn RJ: Effects of metabolic alkalosis on pulmonary gas exchange. *Am Rev Respir Dis* 141:1185, 1990.

35. Centers for Disease Control and Prevention: Guidelines for prevention of nosocomial pneumonia. *MMWR Recomm Rep* 46:1, 1997.

36. American Thoracic Society: Hospital-acquired pneumonia in adults: Diagnosis, assessment of severity, initial antimicrobial therapy, and preventive strategies. A consensus statement. *Am J Respir Crit Care Med* 153:1711, 1995.

37. Craven DE, Steger KA: Hospital-acquired pneumonia: perspectives for the healthcare epidemiologist. *Infect Control Hosp Epidemiol* 18:783, 1997.

38. Baker AM, Meredith JW, Haponik EF: Pneumonia in intubated trauma patients: Microbiology and outcomes. *Am J Respir Crit Care Med* 153:343, 1996.

39. Murphy TF: Respiratory infections caused by non-typable *Haemophilus influenzae. Curr Opin Infect Dis* 6:129, 2003.

40. Hager H, Verghese A, Alvarez S, Berk SL: Branhamella catarrhalis respiratory infections. *Rev Infect Dis* 9:1140, 1987.

41. Maloney SA, Jarvis WR: Epidemic nosocomial pneumonia in the intensive care unit. *Clin Chest Med* 16:209, 1995.

42. Fagon JY, Chastre J, Hance AJ, et al: Detection of nosocomial lung infection in ventilated patients: Use of a protected specimen brush and quantitative culture techniques in 147 patients. *Am Rev Respir Dis* 138:110, 1988.

43. Kollef MH: The prevention of ventilator-associated pneumonia. *N Eng J Med* 340:627, 1999.

44. Collard HR, Saint S, Matthay MA: Prevention of ventilator-associated pneumonia: An evidence-based systematic approach. *Ann Intern Med* 138:494, 2003.

45. Rello J, Sonora R, Jubert P, et al: Pneumonia in intubated patients: Role of respiratory airway care. *Am J Respir Crit Care Med* 154:111, 1996.

46. Haley RW, Culver DH, White JW, et al: The efficacy of infection surveillance and control programs in preventing nosocomial infections in US hospitals. *Am J Epidemiol* 121:182, 1985.

47. Winston DJ, Ho WG, Champlin RE: Cytomegalovirus infections after allogeneic bone marrow transplantation. *Rev Infect Dis* 12(suppl 7):S776, 1990.

48. Konoplev S, Champlin RE, Giralt S, et al: Cytomegalovirus pneumonia in adult autologous blood and bone marrow recipients. *Bone Marrow Transplant* 27:877, 2001.

49. Cooper JAD, White DA, Matthay RA: Drug-induced pulmonary disease. Part 1: Cytotoxic drugs. *Am Rev Respir Dis* 133:321, 1986.

50. Soubani AO, Chandrasekar PH: The clinical spectrum of pulmonary aspergillosis. *Chest* 121:1988, 2002.

51. Crawford SW: Noninfectious lung disease in the immunocompromised host. *Respiration* 65:385, 1999.

52. Albelda SM, Talbot GH, Gerson SL, et al: Pulmonary cavitation and massive hemoptysis in invasive pulmonary aspergillosis. *Am Rev Respir Dis* 131:115, 1985.

53. Williams DE, Yungbluth M, Adams G, Glassroth J: The role of fiberoptic bronchoscopy in the evaluation of immunocompromised hosts with diffuse pulmonary infiltrates. *Am Rev Respir Dis* 131:880, 1985.

54. Rano A, Jiminez CA, Angrill J, et al: Pulmonary infiltrates in non-HIV immunocompromised patients: A diagnostic approach using non-invasive and bronchoscopic procedures. *Thorax* 56:379, 2001.

55. Kramer MR, Berkman N, Mintz B, et al: The role of open lung biopsy in the management and outcome of patients with diffuse lung disease. *Ann Thorac Surg* 65:198, 1998.

56. White DA, Wong PW, Downey R: The utility of open lung biopsy in patients with hematologic malignancies. *Am J Respir Crit Care Med* 161:723, 2000.

Chapter 52 ⎯⎯⎯⎯⎯⎯⎯⎯⎯⎯⎯⎯

BACTERIAL INFECTIONS OF THE CENTRAL NERVOUS SYSTEM

ALLAN R. TUNKEL
W. MICHAEL SCHELD

KEY POINTS

- *More than 80% of adults with bacterial meningitis present clinically with fever, headache, meningismus, and signs of cerebral dysfunction; elderly patients, however, may present with insidious disease manifested only by lethargy or obtundation, variable signs of meningeal irritation, and no fever.*

- *Occasionally, a patient with acute bacterial meningitis has a low cerebrospinal fluid (CSF) white cell count despite high bacterial concentrations in CSF; therefore, a Gram stain and culture should be performed on every CSF specimen, even if the cell count is normal.*

- *Neuroimaging techniques have little role in the diagnosis of acute bacterial meningitis. However, computed tomography (CT) should be performed before lumbar puncture when a space-occupying lesion of the central nervous system (CNS) is suspected. Clinical features at baseline associated with an abnormal CT image (in patients with suspected meningitis) are age of at least 60 years, immunocompromise, a history of CNS disease, a history of seizure within 1 week before presentation, and specific neurologic abnormalities.*

- *Empirical antimicrobial therapy, based on the patient's age and underlying disease status, should be initiated as soon as possible in patients with presumed bacterial meningitis; therapy should never be delayed while diagnostic tests such as CT are awaited.*

- *Adjunctive dexamethasone therapy has been shown to decrease the morbidity rate in infants and children with acute* Haemophilus influenzae *type b meningitis and, if commenced with or before antimicrobial therapy, is also beneficial for pneumococcal meningitis in childhood. A recent study has associated adjunctive dexamethasone with decreased morbidity and mortality rates in adults with pneumococcal meningitis when administered before the first dose of antimicrobial therapy.*

- *Only about 50% of patients with brain abscess present with the classic triad of fever, headache, and focal neurologic deficit; the clinical presentation of brain abscess in immunosuppressed patients may be masked by the diminished inflammatory response.*

- *The diagnosis of brain abscess has been revolutionized by the development of CT; magnetic resonance imaging may offer advantages over CT in the early detection of cerebritis, cerebral edema, and satellite lesions.*

- *Aspiration of brain abscess under stereotaxic CT guidance is useful for microbiologic diagnosis, drainage, and relief of increased intracranial pressure.*

- *A short course of corticosteroids may be useful in patients with brain abscess who have deteriorating neurologic status and increased intracranial pressure.*

- *Cranial subdural empyema should be suspected in patients with headache, vomiting, fever, change in mental status, and rapid progression of focal neurologic signs.*

- *Spinal epidural abscess may develop acutely or chronically, with symptoms and signs of focal vertebral pain, nerve root pain, motor or sensory defects, and paralysis; the transition to paralysis may be rapid, indicating the need for emergent evaluation, diagnosis, and treatment.*

- *Surgical therapy is essential for the management of subdural empyema because antibiotics do not reliably sterilize these lesions.*

- *Rapid surgical decompression should be performed in patients with spinal epidural abscess who have increasing neurologic deficit, persistent severe pain, or increasing temperature or peripheral white blood cell count.*

- *Lateral gaze palsy may be an early clue to the diagnosis of cavernous sinus thrombosis because the abducens nerve is the only cranial nerve traversing the interior of the cavernous sinus.*

- *The noninvasive diagnostic procedure of choice for suppurative intracranial thrombophlebitis is magnetic resonance imaging, which can differentiate between thrombus and normally flowing blood.*

Bacterial infections of the central nervous system (CNS) are frequently devastating. The brain possesses several defense mechanisms (e.g., intact cranium and blood-brain barrier) to prevent entry of bacterial species; but once microorganisms have gained entry to the CNS, host defense mechanisms are inadequate to control the infection. Antimicrobial therapy is limited by the poor penetration of many agents into the CNS and by the ability of antibiotics to induce inflammation in the CNS via their bacteriolytic action, thereby contributing to brain damage. We review meningitis, brain abscess, subdural empyema, epidural abscess, and intracranial thrombophlebitis, with an emphasis on recent developments in diagnosis and therapy as they pertain to the care of the critically ill patient.

Meningitis

EPIDEMIOLOGY AND ETIOLOGY

The rates of morbidity and mortality from bacterial meningitis remain unacceptably high despite the availability of effective antimicrobial therapy. In a surveillance study of all cases of bacterial meningitis in 27 states of the United States from 1978 to 1982, the overall annual attack rate of bacterial meningitis was approximately 3.0 cases per 100,000 population, although there was variability according to geographic area, sex, and race;[1] incidences for the various meningeal pathogens are listed in Table 52-1. Bacterial meningitis is also a significant problem in hospitalized patients. In a review of 493 episodes of bacterial meningitis in adults 16 years or older from the Massachusetts General Hospital from 1962 through 1988, 40% of cases were nosocomial in origin, and these episodes carried a high mortality rate (35% for single episodes of nosocomial meningitis).[2] With the introduction of *Haemophilus influenzae* type b conjugate vaccines in the

TABLE 52-1 Etiology of Bacterial Meningitis in the United States

Organism	PERCENT OF TOTAL	
	1978–1981	1995
Haemophilus influenzae	48	7
Neisseria meningitidis	20	25
Streptococcus pneumoniae	13	47
Streptococcus agalactiae	3	12
Listeria monocytogenes	2	8
Other[a]	8	—
Unknown	6	—

[a] Includes *Escherichia coli,* other Enterobacteriaceae, staphylococci, *Pseudomonas* species, and other streptococcal and *Haemophilus* species.
SOURCE: Adapted from Schlech et al[1] and Shuchat et al.[4]

United States and elsewhere, dramatic declines in the incidence of invasive *H. influenzae* type b disease have been reported; these conjugate vaccines have been licensed for routine use in all children beginning at age 2 months.[3] In a study that evaluated the epidemiology of bacterial meningitis in the United States during 1995 in laboratories serving all the acute care hospitals in 22 counties in four states (Georgia, Tennessee, Maryland, and California),[4] the incidence of bacterial meningitis decreased dramatically as a result of the vaccine-related decline in meningitis caused by *H. influenzae* type b (see Table 52-1).

Before the development of effective vaccines against it, *H. influenzae* type b was isolated in almost half of all cases of bacterial meningitis in the United States, but this microorganism currently accounts for only 7% of cases. About 40% to 60% of cases were seen in children ages 2 months to 6 years; of these, 90% were due to capsular type b strains. Disease is most likely initiated after nasopharyngeal acquisition of a virulent organism with subsequent systemic invasion. *Haemophilus influenzae* is unusual after age 6 years; isolation of the organism in this older group should suggest the possible presence of certain predisposing factors, including sinusitis, otitis media, epiglottitis, pneumonia, head trauma with a cerebrospinal fluid (CSF) leak, diabetes mellitus, alcoholism, splenectomy or asplenic states, and immune deficiency (e.g., hypogammaglobulinemia).[5]

Meningitis due to *Neisseria meningitidis* is most often found in children and young adults and may occur in epidemics. Nasopharyngeal carriage of virulent organisms accounts for initiation of infection.[6] The incidence of meningococcal serogroup C disease has been increasing in North America, with several recent outbreaks reported in the United States and Canada.[7,8] Infection is more likely in persons who have deficiencies in the terminal complement components (C5, C6, C7, C8, and perhaps C9), the so-called membrane attack complex; the incidence of neisserial infections is more than 8000-fold greater in this group than among other persons.[9]

Pneumococcal meningitis is observed most frequently in adults (>30 years) and is often associated with distant foci of infection, such as pneumonia, otitis media, mastoiditis, sinusitis, and endocarditis; this organism currently accounts for 47% of cases of bacterial meningitis in the United States.[4] Serious pneumococcal infections may be observed in persons with predisposing conditions, such as splenectomy or asplenic states, multiple myeloma, hypogammaglobulinemia, and alcoholism. *Streptococcus pneumoniae* is the most common

meningeal isolate in head trauma patients who have basilar skull fracture with subsequent CSF leakage.[10]

Listeria monocytogenes accounts for only about 8% of all cases of bacterial meningitis but carries a high mortality rate.[4] Infection with *Listeria* is more likely in neonates, the elderly, alcoholics, cancer patients, and immunosuppressed adults (e.g., renal transplant patients).[11,12] *Listeria* meningitis is found infrequently in patients with human immunodeficiency virus infection,[13] despite its increased incidence in patients with deficiencies in cell-mediated immunity. However, up to 30% of adults and 54% of children and young adults with listeriosis have no apparent underlying condition. Listeriosis has been associated with several food-borne outbreaks involving contaminated cole slaw, milk, cheese, and processed meats.

Meningitis due to aerobic gram-negative bacilli is observed in specific clinical situations.[14] *Escherichia coli* is isolated in 30% to 50% of infants younger than 2 months with bacterial meningitis. *Klebsiella* species, *E. coli,* and *Pseudomonas aeruginosa* may be isolated in patients who have had head trauma or neurosurgical procedures, in the elderly, in immunosuppressed patients, and in patients with gram-negative septicemia. Despite the low frequency of meningitis due to this group of organisms, the mortality rates are very high (~84% with *P. aeruginosa,* until recently).

Specific clinical situations also predispose to the development of meningitis due to staphylococcal species.[15] *Staphylococcus epidermidis* is the most common cause of meningitis in persons with CSF shunts. Meningitis due to *Staphylococcus aureus* is frequently found (when compared with other pathogens) soon after neurosurgery. Underlying diseases among persons with no prior CNS disease who develop *S. aureus* meningitis include diabetes mellitus, alcoholism, chronic renal failure requiring hemodialysis, and malignancies. Conditions that increase *S. aureus* nasal carriage rates (e.g., injection drug abuse, insulin-requiring diabetes, and hemodialysis) may also predispose to staphylococcal infection of the CNS.

Group B streptococcus (*Streptococcus agalactiae*) is a common cause of meningitis in neonates.[16] The risk of transmission from the mother to her infant is increased when the inoculum of organisms and number of sites of maternal colonization are large; horizontal transmission has also been documented from the hands of nursery personnel to the infant. Risk factors for group B streptococcal meningitis in adults include age older than 60 years, diabetes mellitus, parturient status in women, cardiac disease, collagen vascular disease, malignancy, alcoholism, hepatic failure, renal failure, and corticosteroid therapy.[17–19] No underlying illnesses were found in 43% of patients in one review.[18]

CLINICAL PRESENTATION

The classic clinical presentation in adults with bacterial meningitis includes fever, headache, meningismus, and signs of cerebral dysfunction;[20] these symptoms and signs are found in more than 80% of cases. Also seen are nausea, vomiting, rigors, profuse sweating, weakness, and myalgias. The meningismus may be subtle or marked or accompanied (rarely) by the Kernig and/or Brudzinski sign. The Kernig sign is elicited by flexing the thigh on the abdomen with the knee flexed; the leg is then passively extended, and, if there is meningeal inflammation, the patient resists leg extension.

The Brudzinski sign is present when passive flexion of the neck leads to flexion of the hips and knees. However, these signs are elicited in fewer than 20% of cases of bacterial meningitis in adults. Cerebral dysfunction is manifested by confusion, delirium, or a declining level of consciousness ranging from lethargy to coma. Cranial nerve palsies (especially involving cranial nerves III, IV, VI, and VII) and focal cerebral signs are uncommon (10% to 20% of cases). Seizures occur in about 30% of all cases. Papilledema is rare (<5%) and should suggest an alternate diagnosis, such as an intracranial mass lesion. Late in the disease, patients may develop signs of increased intracranial pressure, including coma, hypertension, bradycardia, and third-nerve palsy; these findings are ominous prognostic signs.

Certain symptoms and signs may suggest an etiologic diagnosis in patients with bacterial meningitis.[20] Persons with meningococcemia present with a prominent rash, principally on the extremities (~50% of cases). Early in the disease course, the rash may be erythematous and macular, but it quickly evolves into a petechial phase, with further coalescence into a purpuric form. The rash often matures rapidly, with new petechial lesions appearing during the physical examination. A petechial, purpuric, or ecchymotic rash may also be seen in other forms of meningitis (i.e., those due to echovirus type 9, *Acinetobacter* species, *S. aureus*, and, rarely, *S. pneumoniae* or *H. influenzae*), in Rocky Mountain spotted fever or *S. aureus* endocarditis, and in overwhelming sepsis (due to *S. pneumoniae* or *H. influenzae*) in splenectomized patients. An additional suppurative focus of infection (e.g., otitis media, sinusitis, or pneumonia) is present in 30% of patients with pneumococcal or *H. influenzae* meningitis but is rarely found in meningococcal meningitis. Meningitis due to *S. pneumoniae* is relatively likely after head trauma in persons who have basilar skull fractures in which a dural fistula is produced between the subarachnoid space and the nasal cavity, paranasal sinuses, or middle ear.[10] These persons commonly present with rhinorrhea or otorrhea due to a CSF leak; a persistent defect is a common explanation for recurrent bacterial meningitis.

Certain subgroups of patients may not manifest the classic signs and symptoms of bacterial meningitis. Usually in a neonate there is no meningismus or fever, and the only clinical clues to meningitis are listlessness, high-pitched crying, fretfulness, refusal to feed, or irritability. Elderly patients, especially those with underlying conditions such as diabetes mellitus or cardiopulmonary disease, may present with insidious disease manifested only by lethargy or obtundation, variable signs of meningeal irritation, and no fever. In this subgroup, altered mental status should not be ascribed to other causes until bacterial meningitis has been excluded by CSF examination. A patient after neurosurgery or a patient who has undergone head trauma also presents a unique clinical situation because these patients already have many of the symptoms and signs of meningitis from their underlying disease processes.[10] One must have a low threshold for CSF examination in these patients should they develop any clinical deterioration.

DIAGNOSIS

The diagnosis of bacterial meningitis rests on the CSF examination.[20] The opening pressure is elevated in virtually all cases; values above 600 mm H_2O suggest cerebral edema, the presence of intracranial suppurative foci, or communicating hydrocephalus. The fluid may be cloudy or turbid if the white blood cell count is elevated (>200/μL). If the lumbar puncture is traumatic, the CSF may appear bloody initially, but it should clear as flow continues. Xanthochromia, a pale-pink to yellow-orange color of the supernatant of centrifuged CSF, is found in patients with subarachnoid hemorrhage, usually within 2 hours after hemorrhage.

The CSF white cell count is usually elevated in untreated bacterial meningitis, ranging from 100 to at least 10,000 per microliter, with a predominance of neutrophils. About 10% of patients present with a lymphocytic predominance (>50%) in CSF. Some patients have a very low CSF white cell count (0 to 20/μL) despite high bacterial concentrations in CSF; these patients have a poor prognosis. Therefore, a Gram stain and culture should be performed on all CSF specimens, even those with a normal cell count. A CSF glucose concentration of less than 40 mg/dL is found in about 60% of patients with bacterial meningitis, and a CSF:serum glucose ratio of less than 0.31 is observed in 70% of cases. The CSF glucose level must always be compared with a simultaneous serum glucose concentration. The CSF protein concentration is elevated in virtually all cases of bacterial meningitis, presumably because of disruption of the blood-brain barrier.

CSF examination by Gram stain permits a rapid, accurate identification in 60% to 90% of cases of bacterial meningitis; the likelihood of detecting the organism by Gram stain correlates with the specific bacterial pathogen and the concentration of bacteria in CSF. False-positive findings may occur as a result of contamination in the collection of tubes or during staining. Cultures of CSF are positive in 70% to 80% of cases. These percentages may be lower in patients who have received prior antimicrobial therapy.

Several rapid diagnostic tests have been developed to aid in the diagnosis of bacterial meningitis.[21] Tests using staphylococcal coagglutination or latex agglutination are rapid and sensitive, although many of the kits do not include tests for group B meningococcus, and other kits probably are poor detectors of this antigen because of the limited immunogenicity of group B meningococcal polysaccharide. Performance of one of these rapid diagnostic tests (preferably latex agglutination) should be considered on all CSF specimens from patients in whom bacterial meningitis is suspected when the Gram stain is negative. Recently, the routine use of CSF bacterial antigen tests for the etiologic diagnosis of bacterial meningitis has been questioned; positive results have not modified therapy and false-positive and false-negative results may occur. Measurement of serum C-reactive protein or pro-calcitonin may also be useful in discriminating between bacterial and viral meningitis because elevated serum concentrations of these proteins have been observed in patients with acute meningitis.[22] In patients with acute meningitis in whom the CSF Gram stain is negative, serum concentrations of C-reactive protein or pro-calcitonin that are normal or below the limit of detection have a high negative predictive value in the diagnosis of bacterial meningitis. Polymerase chain reaction has been used to amplify DNA from patients with meningococcal meningitis; it showed a sensitivity and specificity of 91% in one study.[23] Further refinements in polymerase chain reaction may render it useful in the diagnosis of bacterial meningitis when the CSF Gram stain and cultures are negative.

Neuroimaging techniques have little role in the diagnosis of acute bacterial meningitis, except to rule out the presence of other pathologic conditions or to identify a parameningeal source of infection. However, computed tomography (CT) or magnetic resonance imaging (MRI) may be useful in patients who have a persisting fever several days after initiation of antimicrobial therapy, prolonged obtundation or coma, new or recurrent seizure activity, signs of increased intracranial pressure, or focal neurologic deficits. MRI is better than CT for evaluation of subdural effusions, cortical infarctions, and cerebritis, although it is more difficult to obtain an MRI in a critically ill patient, which limits its usefulness in many patients with meningitis.

TREATMENT

ANTIMICROBIAL THERAPY

The initial approach to the patient with suspected bacterial meningitis is to perform a lumbar puncture to determine whether the CSF findings are consistent with that diagnosis.[20,24] Patients should receive empirical antimicrobial therapy based on their age and underlying disease status, if no etiologic agent is identified by Gram stain or rapid diagnostic tests. In patients with a focal neurologic examination, CT should be performed immediately to exclude an intracranial mass lesion because lumbar puncture is relatively contraindicated in that setting. However, obtaining a CT scan generally entails some delay, so empirical antimicrobial therapy should be started immediately, before the CT scan and lumbar puncture are done and after obtaining blood cultures, because of the high mortality rate in patients with bacterial meningitis in whom antimicrobial therapy is delayed. Although many clinicians routinely perform CT before lumbar puncture, this is probably not necessary in most patients. In a recent retrospective study of 301 adults with suspected meningitis,[25] the clinical features at baseline that were associated with an abnormal finding on CT of the head were an age of at least 60 years, immunocompromise, a history of CNS disease, a history of seizure within 1 week before presentation, and the following neurologic abnormalities: an abnormal level of consciousness, an inability to answer two consecutive questions correctly or to follow two consecutive commands, gaze palsy, abnormal visual fields, facial palsy, arm drift, leg drift, and abnormal language. These results need to be validated but are a reasonable guide in determining which patients require CT before lumbar puncture.

Our choices for empirical antibiotic therapy in patients with presumed bacterial meningitis, based on age, are presented in Table 52-2.[20,24] For neonates younger than 1 month, the most likely infecting organisms are *E. coli*, *S. agalactiae*, and *L. monocytogenes*; for those ages 1 to 23 months, infection may be due to *S. pneumoniae*, *N. meningitidis*, *S. agalactiae*, *E. coli*, or *H. influenzae*. From age 2 to 50 years, most cases of meningitis are due to *N. meningitidis* and *S. pneumoniae*. In older adults (≥50 years), the meningococcus and the pneumococcus are possible causes, as are *L. monocytogenes* and gram-negative bacilli. For all patients in whom *S. pneumoniae* is a possible causative pathogen, vancomycin should be added to empirical therapeutic regimens because highly penicillin- or cephalosporin-resistant strains of *S. pneumoniae* may be likely (see below). One other situation deserves comment: In patients after neurosurgery or patients with CSF shunts or foreign bodies, likely infecting organisms include staphylococci (*S. epidermidis* or *S. aureus*), diphtheroids, and gram-negative bacilli (including *P. aeruginosa*). Antimicrobial therapy in these situations should consist of vancomycin plus ceftazidime or cefepime pending culture results.

Once an infecting microorganism has been isolated, antimicrobial therapy can be modified for optimal treatment.[20,24] Our antibiotics of choice are listed in Table 52-3. Dosages for adults are listed in Table 52-4. For bacterial meningitis due to *S. pneumoniae* or *N. meningitidis*, penicillin G and ampicillin are equally efficacious. However, although in past years pneumococci remained uniformly susceptible to penicillin (minimal inhibitory concentration ≤ 0.06 μg/mL), worldwide reports have now documented relatively and highly resistant strains of pneumococci, with minimal inhibitory concentrations of 0.1 to 1.0 μg/mL and at least 2 μg/mL, respectively. In view of these recent trends, and because sufficient CSF concentrations of penicillin are difficult to achieve with standard high parenteral doses (initial CSF concentrations of ~1 μg/mL), penicillin can never be recommended as empirical antimicrobial therapy when *S. pneumoniae* is considered a likely infecting pathogen. Further, susceptibility testing must be performed on all CSF isolates. For relatively resistant strains, a third-generation cephalosporin (e.g., cefotaxime or ceftriaxone) should be used; for highly resistant strains, vancomycin in combination with a third-generation cephalosporin is the antimicrobial regimen of choice. Vancomycin used alone may not be optimal therapy for patients with pneumococcal meningitis. In one report of 11 consecutive patients with culture-proven pneumococcal meningitis caused by relatively penicillin-resistant strains,[26] four patients experienced a therapeutic failure with vancomycin, necessitating a change in therapy. These data indicate the need

TABLE 52-2 Empirical Therapy of Purulent Meningitis

Age	Standard Therapy	Alternative Therapies
<1 mo	Ampicillin plus cefotaxime	Ampicillin plus an aminoglycoside[b]
1–23 mo	Vancomycin plus a third-generation cephalosporin[a]	Vancomycin plus ampicillin plus chloramphenicol
2–50 y	Vancomycin plus a third-generation cephalosporin[a]	Meropenem
>50 y	Vancomycin plus ampicillin plus a third-generation cephalosporin[a]	Vancomycin plus ampicillin plus aztreonam; vancomycin plus trimethoprim-sulfamethoxazole; meropenem

[a]Cefotaxime or ceftriaxone.
[b]Gentamicin, tobramycin, or amikacin.

TABLE 52-3 Antimicrobial Therapy of Bacterial Meningitis

Organism	Antibiotic of Choice
Streptococcus pneumoniae	
Penicillin MIC < 0.1 μg/mL	Penicillin G or ampicillin
Penicillin MIC 0.1–1.0 μg/mL	Third-generation cephalosporin[a]
Penicillin MIC $\geq$ 2.0 μg/mL	Vancomycin plus a third-generation cephalosporin[a]
Neisseria meningitidis	Penicillin G or ampicillin; or a third-generation cephalosporin[a]
Haemophilus influenzae	
β-Lactamase–negative	Ampicillin
β-Lactamase–positive	Third-generation cephalosporin[a]
Enterobacteriaceae	Third-generation cephalosporin[a]
Pseudomonas aeruginosa	Ceftazidime or cefepime[b]
Streptococcus agalactiae	Penicillin G or ampicillin[b]
Listeria monocytogenes	Ampicillin or penicillin G[b]
Staphylococcus aureus	
Methicillin sensitive	Nafcillin or oxacillin
Methicillin resistant	Vancomycin
Staphylococcus epidermidis	Vancomycin[c]

[a] Cefotaxime or ceftriaxone.
[b] Addition of an aminoglycoside should be considered.
[c] Addition of rifampin may be indicated.
ABBREVIATION: MIC, minimal inhibitory concentration.

for careful monitoring, perhaps even including measurement of CSF vancomycin concentrations, in adult patients who are receiving vancomycin alone for pneumococcal meningitis. We recommend the combination of vancomycin plus a third-generation cephalosporin (cefotaxime or ceftriaxone) for documented pneumococcal meningitis pending results of susceptibility testing. Some investigators have recommended the addition of rifampin (if the organism is susceptible) to

TABLE 52-4 Recommended Doses of Antibiotics for Intracranial Infections in Adults with Normal Renal Function

Antibiotic	Total Daily Dose in Adults (Dosing Interval)
Amikacin	15 mg/kg (q 8 h)
Ampicillin	12 g (q 4 h)
Aztreonam	6–8 g (q 6–8 h)
Cefepime	6 g (q 8 h)
Cefotaxime	8–12 g (q 4–6 h)
Ceftazidime	6 g (q 8 h)
Ceftriaxone	4 g[a] (q 12–24 h)
Chloramphenicol	4–6 g[b] (q 6 h)
Ciprofloxacin	800–1200 mg (q 8–12 h)
Gentamicin, tobramycin	5 mg/kg (q 8 h)
Meropenem	6 g (q 8 h)
Metronidazole	30 mg/kg (q 6 h)
Nafcillin, oxacillin	9–12 g (q 4 h)
Penicillin G	24 million U (q 4 h)
Rifampin[c]	600 mg (q 24 h)
Trimethoprim-sulfamethoxazole	10–20 mg/kg[d] (q 6–12 h)
Vancomycin	2–3 g (q 8–12 h)

[a] Actual dose studied was 50 mg/kg every 12 hours.
[b] Higher dose recommended for pneumococcal meningitis.
[c] Oral administration.
[d] Dosage based on trimethoprim component.

vancomycin for the treatment of meningitis caused by highly resistant pneumococcal strains,[27] although there are no firm data to support this. Meropenem, a carbapenem antimicrobial agent, yields microbiologic and clinical outcomes similar to those of cefotaxime or ceftriaxone in the treatment of patients with bacterial meningitis.[28] The newer fluoroquinolones (e.g., moxifloxacin, gatifloxacin) have in vitro activity against resistant pneumococci and have shown activity in experimental animal models of resistant pneumococcal meningitis but should not be used as first-line therapy in patients with bacterial meningitis, pending results of ongoing clinical trials. Trovafloxacin was recently shown to be therapeutically equivalent to ceftriaxone with or without vancomycin for the treatment of pediatric bacterial meningitis,[29] although this agent is no longer used because of concerns of liver toxicity.

Meningococcal strains that are relatively resistant to penicillin have also been reported from several areas (in particular Spain); however, most patients harboring these strains have recovered with standard penicillin therapy, so their clinical significance is unclear. In the United States, approximately 3% of meningococcal strains have shown intermediate resistance to penicillin.[30] Some authorities would treat meningococcal meningitis with a third-generation cephalosporin (cefotaxime or ceftriaxone) pending results of in vitro susceptibility testing.

Treatment of *H. influenzae* type b meningitis has been hampered by the emergence of β-lactamase–producing strains of the organism, which accounted for approximately 25% to 33% of all isolates in the United States.[1] Chloramphenicol resistance also has been reported in the United States (<1% of isolates) and Spain ($\geq$50% of isolates). In addition, a study found chloramphenicol to be bacteriologically and clinically inferior to certain β-lactam antibiotics (ampicillin, ceftriaxone, and cefotaxime) in childhood bacterial meningitis, and most of these cases were due to *H. influenzae* type b.[20] From these findings and those of other studies, the third-generation cephalosporins (e.g., cefotaxime and ceftriaxone) seem to be at least as effective as ampicillin plus chloramphenicol for therapy of *H. influenzae* meningitis. Cefuroxime, a second-generation cephalosporin, has also been evaluated for therapy of *H. influenzae* meningitis. Although initial studies documented an efficacy for this drug similar to that of ampicillin plus chloramphenicol, recent case reports have documented delayed CSF sterilization and the development of epiglottitis in patients receiving cefuroxime for meningitis. In addition, a prospective randomized study of ceftriaxone versus cefuroxime for the treatment of childhood bacterial meningitis documented the superiority of ceftriaxone; patients receiving this drug had milder hearing impairment and more rapid CSF sterilization than did those receiving cefuroxime.[31] We currently recommend a third-generation cephalosporin for empirical therapy when *H. influenzae* is considered a likely infecting pathogen.

The treatment of bacterial meningitis in adults that is caused by gram-negative enteric bacilli has been revolutionized by the third-generation cephalosporins,[20] with cure rates of 78% to 94%. Ceftazidime or cefepime is also active against *P. aeruginosa* meningitis; ceftazidime, alone or in combination with an aminoglycoside, resulted in cure of 19 of 24 patients with *Pseudomonas* meningitis in one report. Intrathecal or intraventricular aminoglycoside therapy should be considered if there is no response to systemic therapy, although this therapy is now rarely needed. The fluoroquinolones (e.g., ciprofloxacin or pefloxacin) have been used in some patients with gram-negative bacillary meningitis, but at this time they can be considered only for patients with meningitis due to multidrug-resistant gram-negative bacilli or for patients in whom conventional therapy has failed.

The third-generation cephalosporins are inactive against meningitis caused by *L. monocytogenes*, an important meningeal pathogen; this is a major drawback of these agents. Therapy in this situation should consist of ampicillin or penicillin G; addition of an aminoglycoside should be considered in documented infection, at least for the first several days of treatment.[12,20] Alternatively, trimethoprim-sulfamethoxazole can be used. Patients with *S. aureus* meningitis should be treated with nafcillin or oxacillin; vancomycin should be reserved for patients allergic to penicillin and patients with disease caused by methicillin-resistant organisms.[15] Infection with *S. epidermidis*, the most likely isolate in a patient with a CSF shunt, should be treated with vancomycin, with rifampin added if the patient fails to improve. Shunt removal is often essential to optimize therapy.

The durations of therapy for bacterial meningitis should be 10 to 14 days for most causes of non-meningococcal meningitis and 3 weeks for meningitis due to gram-negative enteric bacilli.[20,32] Seven days of therapy appear adequate for meningococcal meningitis; several reports have suggested that 7 days of therapy is effective also for *H. influenzae* meningitis. Patients with *S. agalactiae* meningitis should be treated for 14 to 21 days, and patients with meningitis caused by *L. monocytogenes* should be treated for at least 21 days. However, therapy must be individualized; on the basis of clinical response, some patients may require longer courses of treatment.

ADJUNCTIVE THERAPY

Despite the availability of effective antimicrobial therapy, the morbidity and mortality rates of bacterial meningitis remain unacceptably high. Recent studies have focused on the pathogenesis and pathophysiology of bacterial meningitis, in the hope of developing innovative strategies for adjunctive treatment.[20,24] Recent work in experimental animal models of meningitis has suggested a potentially useful role for anti-inflammatory agents (e.g., corticosteroids and nonsteroidal anti-inflammatory agents) in decreasing the inflammatory response in the subarachnoid space, which may be responsible for the development of neurologic sequelae. Adjunctive dexamethasone therapy has been evaluated over the past decade in a number of published trials, mostly in infants and children with *H. influenzae* type b meningitis.[20,24] A meta-analysis of clinical studies published from 1988 to 1996 confirmed the benefit of adjunctive dexamethasone (0.15 mg/kg every 6 hours for 2 to 4 days) in infants and children with *H. influenzae* type b meningitis and, if commenced with or before parenteral antimicrobial therapy, suggested benefit for pneumococcal meningitis in childhood.[33] Administration of dexamethasone before or with initiation of antimicrobial therapy is recommended for optimal attenuation of the subarachnoid space inflammatory response; patients must be carefully monitored for the possibility of gastrointestinal hemorrhage. In a recently published prospective, randomized, double-blind trial in adults with bacterial meningitis, adjunctive treatment with dexamethasone was associated with a reduction in the proportion of patients who had unfavorable outcome and in the proportion of patients who died; the benefits were most striking in the subset of patients with pneumococcal meningitis.[34] The use of adjunctive dexamethasone, however, is of particular concern in patients with pneumococcal meningitis caused by highly penicillin- or cephalosporin-resistant strains who are treated with vancomycin because a diminished inflammatory response may significantly decrease CSF vancomycin penetration and delay CSF sterilization, perhaps leading to a worse outcome. In the study cited above, only 72% of the 108 CSF cultures that were positive for *S. pneumoniae* were submitted for susceptibility testing, and all were susceptible to penicillin. However, based on the results of this trial and the apparent absence of serious adverse outcomes in the patients who received dexamethasone, routine use of adjunctive dexamethasone is warranted in most adults with pneumococcal meningitis.[35] In patients with meningitis caused by pneumococcal strains resistant to penicillin and/or cephalosporins, careful observation and follow-up are critical to determine whether dexamethasone therapy is associated with an adverse outcome. When dexamethasone is used, the timing of administration is crucial. Administration of dexamethasone before or concomitant with the first dose of antimicrobial therapy is recommended for optimal attenuation of the subarachnoid space inflammatory response. Dexamethasone is not recommended in patients who have already received antimicrobial therapy. If the meningitis is found not to be caused by *S. pneumoniae* in adults, dexamethasone therapy should be discontinued.

Other adjunctive therapies may be useful in critically ill patients with bacterial meningitis.[20] Patients who are stuporous or comatose (precluding assessment of worsening neurologic function) and who show signs of increased intracranial pressure (e.g., altered level of consciousness; dilated, poorly reactive or nonreactive pupils; and ocular movement disorders) may benefit from the insertion of an intracranial pressure monitoring device. Increased intracranial pressure can be lowered by elevating the head of the bed to 30 degrees to maximize venous drainage with minimal compromise of cerebral perfusion, by the use of hyperosmolar agents, and by hyperventilation. However, the routine use of hyperventilation (to maintain the partial arterial pressure of CO_2 between 27 and 30 mm Hg) has been questioned in patients with bacterial meningitis. Infants and children with bacterial meningitis and normal initial CT scans can be treated with hyperventilation to decrease elevated intracranial pressure because it is unlikely that cerebral blood flow will be decreased to ischemic thresholds. However, in children in whom CT shows cerebral edema, cerebral blood flow is likely to be normal or decreased, so hyperventilation might decrease intracranial pressure at the expense of cerebral blood flow, possibly reducing flow to ischemic thresholds. The use of hyperosmolar agents (e.g., mannitol, glycerol) may be useful in reducing increased intracranial pressure in patients with bacterial meningitis. In one recent study in infants and children with bacterial meningitis, oral glycerol appeared to help prevent neurologic sequelae,[36] although further studies are needed before adjunctive glycerol can be routinely recommended. A detailed discussion of the management of raised intracranial pressure is found in Chap. 65. Seizures must be treated promptly to avoid status epilepticus, which might lead to anoxic brain injury (see Chap. 64). Another important adjunctive measure in patients with bacterial meningitis is fluid restriction to combat hyponatremia caused by excess secretion of antidiuretic hormone, although this measure is not appropriate in the presence of shock or dehydration because hypotension may predispose the patient to cerebral ischemia. Many patients, particularly children, with bacterial meningitis are hyponatremic (serum sodium level < 135 mEq/L) at presentation; the degree and duration of hyponatremia may contribute to neurologic sequelae. The management of hyponatremia is discussed in greater depth in Chap. 76.

PREVENTION

A final point concerns chemoprophylaxis of contacts of meningitis cases, which is indicated for contacts of patients with *N. meningitidis* or *H. influenzae* type b meningitis.[20] For meningococcal meningitis, chemoprophylaxis usually is administered only to intimate contacts (e.g., household contacts, day-care contacts, nursery school contacts, contacts who eat or sleep in the same dwelling, and close contacts such as in a military barracks or boarding school); it is not indicated for other groups (e.g., office coworkers or classmates) unless there has been intimate contact. However, one study has suggested that school-aged children may be at increased risk of secondary infection when classrooms are crowded and/or when contact during lunch or recess is frequent. Prophylaxis is not necessary for medical personnel caring for cases unless there has been intimate contact (e.g., mouth-to-mouth resuscitation, or those who perform endotracheal intubation or endotracheal tube management). All contacts (children and adults) of a patient with *H. influenzae* meningitis should receive chemoprophylaxis if exposure has occurred in a household or day-care center containing children 4 years or younger (other than the index case), provided that the exposure to *H. influenzae* type b was in the week before presentation. The recommended drug of choice for chemoprophylaxis, for contacts of patients with either type of meningitis, is rifampin. For contacts of patients with *H. influenzae* meningitis, rifampin at a daily dose of 20 mg/kg (not exceeding 600 mg) for 4 consecutive days is most effective. For contacts of meningococcal cases, one rifampin dose of 10 mg/kg (not exceeding 600 mg) twice a day for 2 days is effective. One dose of ciprofloxacin (500 or 750 mg) may also be effective for eradicating nasopharyngeal carriage of meningococci; ciprofloxacin is not recommended in pregnant women or in persons younger than 18 years because of concerns of cartilage damage. Ciprofloxacin may well supplant rifampin for chemoprophylaxis in adults. On one study, ceftriaxone (250 mg intramuscularly in adults or 125 mg in children) was shown to eliminate the meningococcal serogroup A carrier state in 97% of patients for up to 2 weeks and is probably the safest alternative for meningococcal chemoprophylaxis in pregnant women. Azithromycin (500 mg orally once) was also shown to be as effective as a four-dose regimen of rifampin in the eradication of meningococci from the nasopharynx.[37]

Brain Abscess

EPIDEMIOLOGY AND ETIOLOGY

Brain abscess is one of the most serious complications of head and neck infections. Even in the antibiotic era, mortality from brain abscess was not appreciably different from that in the era before antibiotics (about 40% to 60%) until the past decade, when mortality decreased to between 5% and 10%.[38] This improvement is likely due to recent developments in diagnosis and treatment, which are discussed below. There is a large geographic variability in the incidence of brain abscess, with approximately 4 to 10 cases seen annually on active neurosurgical services in developed countries.

Bacteria can reach the brain by several different mechanisms. The factors predisposing to brain abscess and the etiologic agents in each circumstance are presented in Table 52-5.[38-40] The most common pathogenic mechanism of brain abscess formation is spread from a contiguous focus of infection, most often in the middle ear, mastoid air cells, or paranasal sinuses. Early studies associated 40% of brain abscesses with otitis media, but this number has been decreasing in recent years. However, if antibiotic therapy of otitis is neglected, there is an increased risk of intracranial complications. Brain abscess secondary to otitis media is bimodally distributed, with peaks in children (acute otitis media) and in persons older than 40 years (chronic otitis media). Most cases of brain abscess due to otitis media occur in the temporal lobe and cerebellum. The etiologic agents in brain abscess secondary to otitis media include a broad range of bacterial species, including streptococci, *Bacteroides fragilis*, and members of the *Enterobacteriaceae*.

TABLE 52-5 Predisposing Conditions and Microbiology in Brain Abscess

Predisposing Condition	Usual Bacterial Isolates
Otitis media or mastoiditis	Streptococci (anaerobic or aerobic), *Bacteroides* sp., *Enterobacteriaceae*
Sinusitis (frontoethmoidal or sphenoidal)	Streptococci, *Bacteroides* sp., *Enterobacteriaceae*, *Staphylococcus aureus*, *Haemophilus* sp.
Dental sepsis	Mixed *Fusobacterium*, *Bacteroides*, and *Streptococcus* sp.
Penetrating trauma or postneurosurgical state	*Staphylococcus aureus*, streptococci, *Enterobacteriaceae*, *Clostridium* sp.
Congenital heart disease	Streptococci, *Haemophilus* sp.
Lung abscess, empyema, bronchiectasis	*Fusobacterium*, *Actinomyces*, and *Bacteroides* sp. *Nocardia asteroides*; streptococci
Bacterial endocarditis	*Staphylococcus aureus*, streptococci
Immunosuppressed host	*Nocardia*, Enterobacteriaceae

SOURCE: Adapted from Tunkel et al.[38]

Paranasal sinusitis continues to be an important condition predisposing to brain abscess, most commonly in persons ages 10 to 30 years. The frontal lobe is the predominant abscess site; when brain abscess complicates sphenoid sinusitis, the temporal lobe or sella turcica is usually involved.[38–40] Streptococci are the predominant bacterial species involved in brain abscess secondary to sinusitis, although anaerobes, *S. aureus,* and gram-negative bacilli have been isolated.

Dental infections are a less common source of brain abscess; infections of molar teeth seem most often to be the cause. The frontal lobe is usually involved, but temporal lobe extension has also been described.

A second mechanism of brain abscess formation is hematogenous dissemination to the brain from a distant focus of infection. These abscesses are usually multiple and multiloculated, and they have a higher mortality rate than do abscesses that arise secondary to contiguous foci of infection.[38–40] The most common sources in adults are chronic pyogenic lung diseases, especially lung abscess, bronchiectasis, empyema, and cystic fibrosis. Anaerobes (*Fusobacterium* and *Bacteroides* species) and streptococci are likely infecting pathogens in this situation, as are *Nocardia* and *Actinomyces* species. Brain abscess may also occur hematogenously from wound and skin infections, osteomyelitis, pelvic infection, cholecystitis, and other intra-abdominal infections. Another predisposing factor leading to hematogenously acquired brain abscess is cyanotic congenital heart disease (accounting for 5% to 10% of all brain abscess cases, with higher percentages in some pediatric series), most commonly due to tetralogy of Fallot and transposition of the great vessels.[41] Brain abscess is rare during bacterial endocarditis (<5% of cases in most series), despite the presence of persistent bacteremia.[42] Hereditary hemorrhagic telangiectasia is a predisposing factor almost always observed in patients with co-existing pulmonary arteriovenous malformations; perhaps it allows septic emboli to cross the pulmonary circulation without capillary filtration. Brain abscesses have also developed after esophageal dilatation and sclerosing therapy for esophageal varices.

Trauma is a third pathogenic mechanism in the development of brain abscess, whether secondary to an open cranial fracture with dural breach, to neurosurgery, or (especially in children) to a foreign body injury.[38–40] The incidence of brain abscess formation after head trauma ranges from 3% to 17% in military populations, where it is usually secondary to retained bone fragments or contamination of initially "sterile" missile sites with bacteria from skin, clothes, and the environment. Predisposing traumatic conditions in the civilian population include compound depressed skull fractures, dog bites, rooster pecking, and, especially in children, injury from lawn darts and pencil tips. Likely infective microorganisms after trauma include staphylococci, streptococci, gram-negative bacilli, and anaerobes.

Brain abscess is cryptogenic in about 20% of patients. Many of these cases are secondary to unrecognized dental foci of infection. In this subgroup of patients, broad antimicrobial therapy is indicated pending culture results (see section on Treatment, below).

Overall, the most commonly isolated bacterial species in brain abscess are streptococci (aerobic, anaerobic, and microaerophilic), which are present in 60% to 70% of cases.[38–40] These bacteria (especially the *Streptococcus milleri* group) normally reside in the oral cavity, appendix, and female genital tract and have a proclivity for abscess formation. *Staphylococcus aureus,* which was isolated in 25% to 30% of cases in the era before antibiotics, currently accounts for 10% to 15% of isolates, although the frequency of isolation of *S. aureus* is increased in certain clinical situations (e.g., cranial trauma and endocarditis). Attention to proper culture techniques has increased the rate of isolation of anaerobes, with *Bacteroides* species isolated in 20% to 40% of cases, often in mixed culture. Enteric gram-negative bacilli (*Proteus* species, *E. coli, Klebsiella* species, and *Pseudomonas* species) are isolated in 23% to 33% of patients. Other bacterial species occur less commonly (<1% of cases) and include *H. influenzae, S. pneumoniae, L. monocytogenes,* and *Nocardia asteroides* (*Nocardia* is more often isolated in patients with T-lymphocyte or mononuclear phagocyte defects). Nocardial brain abscesses have increased in incidence with the increasing numbers of immunosuppressed patients, although up to 48% of patients with nocardiosis have no underlying conditions. Brain abscesses due to *Actinomyces* species are commonly associated with pulmonary and odontogenic infections.

CLINICAL PRESENTATION

The clinical course of brain abscess may be indolent or fulminant; 75% of patients have symptoms for less than 2 weeks. Most of the clinical manifestations are due to the presence of space-occupying lesions within the brain.[38–40] The most common symptom is headache, present in more than 70% of patients. The headache is usually moderate to severe and hemicranial, but it may be generalized. Other findings include nausea and vomiting (~50% of cases), nuchal rigidity (~25%), and papilledema (~25%). Mental status changes ranging from lethargy to coma occur in the majority of cases. Seizures, usually generalized, occur in 25% to 35% of patients. Fever appears in only 45% to 50% of cases; afebrile patients tend to be older and to have a longer duration of illness and a higher mortality rate. Only about 50% of patients present with the classic triad of fever, headache, and focal neurologic deficit. Patients with frontal lobe abscess often present with headache, drowsiness, inattention, and deterioration in mental status; the most common focal neurologic signs are hemiparesis, with unilateral motor signs, and a motor speech disorder. The clinical presentation of cerebellar abscess may include ataxia, nystagmus, vomiting, and dysmetria. Persons with abscess of the temporal lobe may present with ipsilateral headache and aphasia, if the lesion is in the dominant hemisphere. A visual field defect (e.g., an upper homonymous quadrantanopia) may be the only presenting sign of a temporal lobe abscess. Persons with brain stem abscesses usually present with facial weakness, fever, headache, hemiparesis, dysphagia, and vomiting. Clues to the site of origin of the infection should also be sought; these include otorrhea, orbital cellulitis, purulent nasal discharge, dental sepsis, and postoperative or posttraumatic cranial infection; such findings occur in about 60% of cases. It is important to note that the clinical presentation of brain abscess in immunosuppressed patients may be masked by the diminished inflammatory response.

DIAGNOSIS

The diagnosis of brain abscess has been revolutionized by CT, which not only is an excellent means to examine the brain parenchyma but also is superior to standard radiologic procedures for examination of the paranasal sinuses, mastoid cells, and middle ear.[38–40] The sensitivity of CT is 95% to 99% for brain abscess; it also yields information concerning the extent of surrounding edema, the presence or absence of a midline shift, the presence of hydrocephalus, and the possibility of imminent ventricular rupture. The characteristic appearance of brain abscess on CT is a hypodense center with a uniform peripheral ring enhancement after the injection of contrast material; this is surrounded by a variable hypodense area of brain edema. A similar appearance is seen with neoplasms, granulomas, cerebral infarction, or resolving hematoma. Contrast enhancement of the ependymal lining suggests ventriculitis. Other CT findings include nodular enhancement and areas of low attenuation without enhancement; the latter finding is observed during the early stage of cerebritis, before abscess formation; as the abscess progresses, contrast enhancement is observed. In later stages, as the abscess becomes encapsulated, contrast no longer differentiates the lucent center, and the CT appearance is similar to that in the early stage of cerebritis. The use of delayed films may be helpful because the presence of contrast material in the center of the lesion suggests cerebritis. The absence of contrast material likely indicates a well-encapsulated lesion. This difference is important therapeutically because cerebritis may respond to medical therapy alone, whereas most encapsulated lesions require surgical intervention. CT is also useful for following the course of brain abscess, although, after aspiration, improvement in the CT appearance may not be seen for up to 5 weeks or longer. Complete resolution may take 4 to 5 months.

Scintigraphy with ^{111}In-labeled leukocytes has also been evaluated in the diagnosis of brain abscess.[43] Radiolabeled leukocytes migrate to, and accumulate in, an area of active inflammation, thereby differentiating brain abscess from other cerebral mass lesions, although false-positive scans can be observed in necrotic tumors and false-negative scans in patients receiving corticosteroids. This modality is most useful as a complement to CT.

MRI has an important role in the diagnosis of brain abscess, for which it has several advantages over CT.[38] MRI is more effective for the early detection of cerebritis. Also, in cases of cerebral edema, MRI shows a stronger contrast between an edematous and a normal brain and more clearly shows the spread of inflammation into the ventricles and subarachnoid space. MRI also permits earlier detection of satellite lesions. T1-weighted images characteristically demonstrate a peripheral zone of mild hypointensity (representative of edema formation) related to adjacent brain, which surrounds a central zone of more marked hypointensity (indicative of the necrotic center of the abscess); these two regions are separated by a capsule that appears as a discrete rim, which is isointense to mildly hyperintense. On T2-weighted images, there is an area of marked hyperintensity in the zone of edema when compared with adjacent brain, whereas the central core is isointense to hyperintense compared with gray matter; the capsule appears as a well-defined hypointense rim at the margin of the abscess. Contrast-enhanced MRI, using the paramagnetic agent gadolinium diethylenetriamine penta-acetic acid, has the advantage of clearly differentiating the central abscess, the surrounding contrast-enhancing rim, and the cerebral edema surrounding the abscess. MRI is the current diagnostic procedure of choice for detection of brain abscess, although it is not always feasible in critically ill patients.

A major advance in the use of CT is the availability of stereotaxic CT-guided aspiration of the abscess to facilitate bacteriologic diagnosis. However, aspiration during the early cerebritis stage may be complicated by hemorrhage. At the time of aspiration, a specimen should be sent for Gram stain (and other special stains, e.g., Ziehl-Nielsen, modified acid-fast, and silver stains, when appropriate), routine culture, and anaerobic culture. The use of this modality in the treatment of brain abscess is discussed under Surgical Therapy in the section on Treatment.

Lumbar puncture is contraindicated in patients with suspected or proven brain abscess because of the risk of life-threatening cerebral herniation after removal of CSF. When lumbar puncture is performed, the CSF profile is nonspecific, with a predominantly mononuclear pleocytosis and an elevated protein concentration. Hypoglycorrhachia is present in only 25% of cases, and fewer than 10% of CSF cultures are positive. Microorganisms usually are not demonstrated on Gram stain, unless the abscess has ruptured into the subarachnoid space or there is accompanying meningitis.

TREATMENT

ANTIMICROBIAL THERAPY

Perhaps related to the alteration of the blood-brain barrier in the area of the brain abscess, there is increased penetration of normally excluded antibiotics into the brain. However, this increased penetration into the brain does not predict penetration into cerebral abscesses. Brain abscess concentrations of antibiotics have been measured, and several generalizations can be made:[38] (a) metronidazole can be expected to achieve inhibitory levels for sensitive anaerobic microorganisms; (b) chloramphenicol concentrations in the brain are likely to be high relative to serum; and (c) concentrations of various penicillins and cephalosporins in brain tissue and abscess are usually poor, although when given in large parenteral doses, these agents achieve therapeutic concentrations for sensitive microorganisms.

When a diagnosis of brain abscess is made, whether presumptively on the basis of radiologic studies or through aspiration of the abscess, antimicrobial therapy should be initiated. Aspiration may provide an etiologic diagnosis on Gram stain examination, but when aspiration is impractical or delayed, we recommend empirical therapy based on the likely etiologic agent, if a predisposing condition can be identified (Table 52-6).[38] Because of the high rate of isolation of streptococci (particularly the *S. milleri* group) from brain abscesses of various etiologies (see Table 52-5), high-dose penicillin G (20 to 24 million U/day) or another drug that is active against this organism (e.g., a third-generation cephalosporin, either cefotaxime or ceftriaxone) should be included in the initial therapeutic regimen. Penicillin is also active against most anaerobic species, with the notable exception of *B. fragilis*, which is isolated in a high percentage (20% to 40%) of brain abscess cases. When *B. fragilis* is suspected, we recommend the addition of metronidazole (7.5 mg/kg every 6 hours). The advantages of metronidazole over other agents include its bactericidal activity against *B. fragilis* (the others are frequently bacteriostatic for this organism) and the high concentrations it attains in brain abscess pus, even with concomitant corticosteroid administration. In addition, one retrospective review has suggested that metronidazole may improve mortality rates in patients with brain abscess.[44] In cases in which *S. aureus* is a likely infecting pathogen (e.g., cranial trauma or prior neurosurgery), nafcillin should be used.

TABLE 52-6 Empirical Antimicrobial Therapy for Brain Abscess

Predisposing Condition	Antimicrobial Regimen
Otitis media or mastoiditis	Metronidazole plus a third-generation cephalosporin[a]
Sinusitis	Vancomycin plus metronidazole plus a third-generation cephalosporin[a]
Dental sepsis	Penicillin plus metronidazole
Cranial trauma or postneurosurgical state	Vancomycin plus a third-generation cephalosporin[a]
Congenital heart disease	Third-generation cephalosporin[a]
Unknown	Vancomycin plus metronidazole plus a third-generation cephalosporin[a]

[a] Cefotaxime or ceftriaxone; ceftazidime or cefepime is used if *Pseudomonas aeruginosa* is suspected.

Vancomycin, which penetrates into brain abscess fluid,[45] is reserved for patients who are allergic to penicillin or in whom methicillin-resistant organisms are likely or have been isolated. The penetration of clindamycin, erythromycin, and the first-generation cephalosporins into brain abscesses is usually inadequate to achieve therapeutic concentrations, thus precluding their use in this setting. For empirical therapy when members of the *Enterobacteriaceae* are suspected (e.g., in cases of abscess of otitic origin), a third-generation cephalosporin or trimethoprim-sulfamethoxazole should be used.

One regimen that has theoretical advantages and covers a broad range of possible infecting bacterial pathogens is metronidazole, vancomycin, and a third-generation cephalosporin (cefotaxime or ceftriaxone; see Table 52-6). In addition to activity against gram-negative bacilli, these third-generation cephalosporins have excellent antistreptococcal activity and possess antistaphylococcal action. However, it is important to note that there are no clinical trials comparing this regimen with traditional penicillin-containing formulas. If *P. aeruginosa* is a likely infecting pathogen, ceftazidime or cefepime is the agent of choice. However, if ceftazidime is the third-generation cephalosporin used in empirical therapy of brain abscess, the regimen must also include penicillin G to treat a possible streptococcal infection because ceftazidime has unreliable activity against gram-positive organisms.

Once an infecting pathogen is isolated, antimicrobial therapy can be modified (Table 52-7).[38] Antimicrobial therapy

with large-dose intravenous antibiotics should be continued for 6 to 8 weeks and is often followed by oral antibiotic therapy for 2 to 6 months, if an appropriate agent is available. A shorter course (3 to 4 weeks) may be adequate for patients undergoing excision of the abscess. Surgical therapy (see below) is often required for treatment of brain abscess, although certain subgroups of patients can be managed without surgery.[46,47] These include patients with medical conditions that increase the risks from surgery, patients with multiple abscesses or an abscess in a deep or dominant location, patients with coexisting meningitis or ependymitis, patients in whom antimicrobial therapy results in early abscess reduction and clinical improvement, and patients with an abscess smaller than approximately 3 cm.

SURGICAL THERAPY
Most patients require surgical management for optimal treatment of brain abscess. The two procedures judged equivalent by outcome are aspiration of the abscess after burr hole placement and complete excision after craniotomy.[38,48,49] Drainage and marsupialization are rarely used. The choice of procedure must be individualized for each patient. Aspiration may be performed using stereotaxic CT guidance, which affords the surgeon rapid, accurate, and safe access to virtually any intracranial point. Aspiration can also be used for swift relief of increased intracranial pressure. Incomplete drainage of multiloculated lesions is a major disadvantage of aspiration;

TABLE 52-7 Antimicrobial Therapy for Brain Abscess

Organism	Standard Therapy	Alternative Therapies
Streptococcus milleri and other streptococci	Penicillin G	Third-generation cephalosporin,[a] vancomycin
Bacteroides fragilis	Metronidazole	Chloramphenicol, clindamycin
Fusobacterium sp., *Actinomyces*	Penicillin G	Metronidazole, chloramphenicol, clindamycin
Staphylococcus aureus	Nafcillin	Vancomycin[c]
Enterobacteriaceae	Third-generation cephalosporin[a]	Aztreonam,[b] trimethoprim-sulfamethoxazole, fluoroquinolone, meropenem
Haemophilus sp.	Third-generation cephalosporin[a]	Aztreonam,[b] trimethoprim-sulfamethoxazole
Nocardia asteroides	Trimethoprim-sulfamethoxazole	Minocycline, third-generation cephalosporin,[a] imipenem (all[b])

[a] Cefotaxime or ceftriaxone.
[b] Limited data available for use of these agents; firm recommendations are not possible at this time.
[c] Use vancomycin if methicillin-resistant S. *aureus* is isolated.

these lesions frequently require excision. Other risks of aspiration are that it may allow the abscess to rupture into the ventricle, and that pus may leak into the subarachnoid space, resulting in ventriculitis or meningitis.

Complete excision after craniotomy is most often employed in patients in a stable neurologic condition. Surgery is also indicated for abscesses exhibiting gas on radiologic evaluation and for posterior fossa abscesses. In patients with worsening neurologic deficits, including deteriorating consciousness or signs of increased intracranial pressure, surgery should be performed emergently. Excision is contraindicated in the early stages, before a capsule is formed. All brain abscesses larger than 2.5 cm in diameter should be aspirated or excised for optimal management.[50]

ADJUNCTIVE THERAPY

Intracranial pressure monitoring has become important in the intensive care management of brain abscess patients who have cerebral edema (see Chap. 65). The use of these monitoring devices has diminished the likelihood of transtentorial herniation, brain stem compression, and further injury from cerebral ischemia.

Corticosteroids have been used as one method to manage increased intracranial pressure, although their use remains controversial.[38] These agents may retard the encapsulation process, reduce antibiotic entry into the CNS, increase necrosis, and alter the appearance of ring enhancement on CT as inflammation subsides, thereby obscuring information from sequential studies. Steroids (at a dexamethasone dose for adults of 4 to 6 mg every 6 hours) are most useful in the patient with deteriorating neurologic status and increased intracranial pressure, for whom steroids may prove lifesaving. When used to treat cerebral edema, steroids should be used for the shortest time possible and withdrawn when the mass effect no longer poses a significant danger to the patient. The management of increased intracranial pressure is discussed in Chap. 65.

Subdural Empyema and Epidural Abscess

EPIDEMIOLOGY AND ETIOLOGY

The term *subdural empyema* refers to a collection of pus in the space between the dura and arachnoid. This process accounts for about 20% of all localized intracranial infections.[51–53] The disease was essentially lethal before the advent of antimicrobial therapy; with current methods of diagnosis and treatment, mortality rates are 10% to 20%. The most common pre-

disposing conditions are otorhinologic infections, especially infection of the paranasal sinuses, which are affected in 50% to 80% of cases.[51,52,54] The pathogenesis involves spread of infection to the subdural space through valveless emissary veins in association with thrombophlebitis or by extension of an osteomyelitis of the skull with accompanying epidural abscess. The mastoid cells and middle ear are the source in 10% to 20% of patients, especially in geographic areas where many cases of otitis media are not treated promptly with antibiotics. Other predisposing conditions include skull trauma, neurosurgical procedures, and infection of a pre-existing subdural hematoma. The infection is metastatic in a minority of cases (~5%), principally from the pulmonary system. In infants, meningitis is an important predisposing condition for the development of subdural empyema, which occurs in about 2% of infants with bacterial meningitis. Different bacterial species have been isolated from cranial subdural empyemas[53–55] (Table 52-8), including streptococci (35% to 40% of cases), staphylococci (~15%), aerobic gram-negative bacilli (~3%), and anaerobes (33% to 100%, when careful culturing is performed); these organisms constitute the microbial flora that are frequently isolated from patients with chronic sinusitis and cranial abscesses.

Spinal subdural empyema is a rare condition occurring secondary to metastatic infection from a distant site.[56] *Staphylococcus aureus* is the most frequent isolate, whereas streptococci are found less frequently.

The term *epidural abscess* refers to a localized infection between the dura mater and the overlying skull or vertebral column. Cranial epidural abscess can cross the cranial dura along emissary veins, so subdural empyema often is also present. Therefore, the etiology, pathogenesis, and bacteriology of intracranial epidural abscess are usually identical to those described for subdural empyema (see above), with the initial focus of infection in the middle ear, paranasal sinuses, or mastoid cells.

In contrast, spinal epidural abscess usually follows hematogenous dissemination from foci elsewhere in the body to the epidural space or, by extension, from vertebral osteomyelitis.[57,58] Hematogenous spread occurs in 25% to 50% of cases, secondary to infections of the skin (furuncles, cellulitis, or infected acne), urinary tract infections, periodontal abscesses, pharyngitis, pneumonia, or mastoiditis. Mild blunt spinal trauma may provide a devitalized site susceptible to transient bacteremia. Infection of the epidural space has also been reported after penetrating injuries, extension of decubitus ulcers or paraspinal abscesses, back surgery, lumbar puncture, and epidural anesthesia. Bacteremia may be an

TABLE 52-8 Bacteriology of Cranial Subdural Empyema and Spinal Epidural Abscess

Organism	Cranial Subdural Empyema (%)	Spinal Epidural Abscess (%)
Staphylococci (including *S. aureus* and *S. epidermidis*)	15	65
Streptococci (aerobic, anaerobic, and microaerophilic)	36	8
Aerobic gram-negative bacilli	3	17
Other anaerobes	18	2
Other	8	2
Unknown	20	6

SOURCE: Data summarized from Kaufman et al,[53] Yoshikawa et al,[55] Danner and Hartman,[58] and Koppel et al.[59]

important predisposing factor because the incidence of spinal epidural abscess is increased in patients who use injection drugs[59] or have intravenous catheters. The infecting microorganism in the vast majority of cases is *S. aureus* (50% to 95% in various series; see Table 52-8). Other isolates include aerobic and anaerobic streptococci (~8% of cases) and gram-negative aerobic bacilli (~18%), especially *E. coli* and *P. aeruginosa*.

CLINICAL PRESENTATION

Persons with subdural empyema can present in a rapidly progressive, life-threatening clinical condition.[51–53] Symptoms and signs relate to the presence of increased intracranial pressure, meningeal irritation, or focal cortical inflammation. In addition, 60% to 90% of patients have evidence of the antecedent infection (e.g., sinusitis or otitis). Headache, initially localized to the infected sinus or ear is a prominent complaint and can become generalized as the infection progresses. Vomiting is common as intracranial pressure increases. Early in the infection, about 50% of patients have altered mental status, which can progress to obtundation if the patient is not treated. Fever with a temperature above 39°C is present in most cases. Focal neurologic signs appear in 24 to 48 hours and progress rapidly, with eventual involvement of the entire cerebral hemisphere. Hemiparesis and hemiplegia are the most common focal signs, although ocular palsies, dysphasia, homonymous hemianopsia, dilated pupils, and cerebellar signs have been observed. Seizures (focal or generalized) are observed in more than 50% of cases. Signs of meningeal irritation (e.g., meningismus) are found in approximately 80% of patients, although fewer have Kernig or Brudzinski sign. If the patient remains untreated, neurologic deterioration occurs rapidly, with signs of increased intracranial pressure and cerebral herniation. Papilledema develops in fewer than 50% of patients. This fulminant picture may not be seen in patients with subdural empyema after cranial surgery or trauma, in patients who have received prior antimicrobial therapy, in patients with infected subdural hematomas, or in patients with infections metastatic to the subdural space.

Spinal subdural empyema usually manifests as radicular pain and symptoms of spinal cord compression, which may occur at multiple levels.[56] Clinically, this lesion is difficult to distinguish from a spinal epidural abscess (see the section on Diagnosis, below).

The onset of symptoms in cranial epidural abscess may be insidious and overshadowed by the primary focus of infection (e.g., sinusitis or otitis media).[51] Headache is a usual complaint, but the patient may otherwise feel well unless the clinical course is complicated (e.g., by development of subdural empyema or involvement of deeper intracranial structures). Because the dura is closely opposed to the inner surface of the cranium, the abscess usually enlarges too slowly to produce sudden major neurologic deficits (in contrast to subdural empyema) unless there is deeper intracranial extension. However, there may eventually be development of focal neurologic signs and focal or generalized seizures. In the absence of treatment, papilledema and other signs of increased intracranial pressure develop as the abscess enlarges. An epidural abscess near the petrous bone may present as Gradenigo syndrome, characterized by involvement of cranial nerves V and VI, with unilateral facial pain and weakness of the lateral rectus muscle.[50]

Spinal epidural abscess may develop within hours to days (after hematogenous seeding) or may grow slowly over months (associated more often with vertebral osteomyelitis).[57–61] Most abscesses pass through the following stages: focal vertebral pain; root pain; defects of motor, sensory, or sphincter function; and paralysis. Pain is the most consistent symptom and is accompanied by local tenderness at the affected level in more than 90% of cases. Subsequently, radicular pain develops; it is followed by progression to weakness and paralysis. Fever occurs in most patients during the course of the illness. Headache and neck stiffness may also occur. Respiratory function may be impaired if the cervical spinal cord is involved. The usually irreversible manifestations of cord involvement include muscle weakness, sensory deficits, and disturbances of sphincter control. At this juncture there may be rapid transition to paralysis (usually within 24 hours from onset of weakness), indicating the need for emergent evaluation, diagnosis, and treatment.

DIAGNOSIS

Subdural empyema should be suspected in any patient with meningeal signs and a focal neurologic deficit. Lumbar puncture is contraindicated in this setting because of the risk of cerebral herniation. When lumbar puncture is performed, CSF findings are nonspecific and include elevated opening pressure, moderate neutrophilic pleocytosis, and an increased protein concentration. Unless the course is complicated by bacterial meningitis, CSF Gram stain and cultures are negative. Skull radiographs may demonstrate evidence of concurrent sinusitis or osteomyelitis.

The diagnostic procedures are CT with contrast enhancement or MRI.[51,62] The typical CT appearance is a crescentic or elliptical area of hypodensity below the cranial vault or adjacent to the falx cerebri. Loculations may also be seen. Depending on the extent of disease, there is often an associated mass effect with displacement of midline structures. After the administration of contrast material, a fine, intense line of enhancement can be seen between the subdural collection and the cerebral cortex. However, false-negative CT scans do occur. MRI provides greater clarity of morphologic detail and may detect empyema not clearly seen on CT; it is of particular value in identifying subdural empyemas located at the base of the brain, along the falx cerebri, or in the posterior fossa. On the basis of signal intensity, MRI can differentiate extra-axial empyemas from most sterile effusions and chronic hematomas. Based on these findings, MRI is considered the modality of choice for the diagnosis of subdural empyema. CT and MRI are also useful for demonstrating sinusitis and otitis, although CT is better than MRI at imaging bone and should be used in cases of penetrating injury or osteomyelitis. MRI is the diagnostic procedure of choice for spinal subdural empyema because it more accurately defines the extent of the lesion than does CT.[60,61]

CT and MRI are also the diagnostic procedures of choice for cranial epidural abscess because both demonstrate a superficial, circumscribed area of diminished density.[51] The possibility of adjacent subdural empyema or other intracranial involvement can also be assessed. MRI or CT should be performed in cases of suspected spinal epidural abscess. MRI is recommended as the diagnostic procedure of choice because it can visualize the spinal cord and epidural space in sagittal and transverse sections and can identify accompanying osteomyelitis, intramedullary spinal cord lesions, and joint space infection; the response to therapy also can be assessed readily with this technique.

TREATMENT

The therapy of subdural empyema and epidural abscess optimally requires a combined medical and surgical approach. Surgical therapy is essential for three reasons: because antibiotics do not reliably sterilize these lesions without concurrent drainage; because cultures of purulent material guide antimicrobial therapy; and because surgical decompression is useful in controlling increased intracranial pressure.

ANTIMICROBIAL THERAPY

Once purulent material is aspirated, antimicrobial therapy should be initiated; it should be based on a Gram stain and on the site of primary infection[51,63] (Table 52-9). For suspected *S. aureus*, nafcillin (1.5 to 2.0 g every 4 hours) should be used, with vancomycin (1.0 g every 12 hours) reserved for patients allergic to penicillin and for cases where methicillin-resistant organisms are suspected. Metronidazole (15 mg/kg loading dose and then 7.5 mg/kg every 6 to 8 hours) is used when anaerobes (e.g., *B. fragilis*) are suspected. For aerobic gram-negative bacilli, a third-generation cephalosporin (cefotaxime or ceftriaxone) should be used, with ceftazidime or cefepime reserved for cases in which *P. aeruginosa* is likely. Parenteral antibiotics should be continued for 3 to 6 weeks, depending on the patient's clinical response. Longer periods of intravenous therapy (and perhaps oral therapy) may be required if an associated osteomyelitis is present.

Presumptive antimicrobial therapy for spinal epidural abscess must include a first-line antistaphylococcal agent (nafcillin or vancomycin); coverage for gram-negative organisms should be included for any patient with a history of a spinal procedure or of injection drug abuse.[58,60] In addition, pending culture results, empirical antimicrobial therapy in patients who have undergone a spinal procedure should include vancomycin for presumed involvement by *S. epidermidis*.

SURGICAL THERAPY

The optimal surgical approach for subdural empyema is controversial, and there are several unanswered questions with regard to management.[51] First, should drainage be performed by craniotomy or via burr holes? Previous studies have documented a lower mortality rate in patients undergoing craniotomy, although it may be that a larger percentage of gravely ill patients were treated with burr holes because of the greater surgical risk. Burr hole therapy may be more efficacious in the early stages of subdural empyema, when the pus is liquid, because thickening occurs as the disease progresses, making aspiration more difficult. If burr holes are to be placed, they should be multiple to allow extensive irrigation. However, craniotomy may be essential for posterior fossa subdural empyema, and it is also needed in 10% to 20% of patients initially treated with trephination. Thus, burr hole drainage, even with catheter irrigation, may not adequately drain the empyema. When craniotomy is performed, wide exposure should be afforded to allow adequate exploration of all areas where subdural pus is suspected. Second, should antibiotics be instilled locally to irrigate the subdural space? Although antibiotic irrigation has become common, there are no data on the potential benefits of this practice. Third, should drains, or catheters, be left in the subdural space? This decision is best made by the neurosurgeon intraoperatively; however, with drains in place, the risk of nosocomial superinfection must be kept in mind. Further, surgical correction of the antecedent otorhinologic infection may also be necessary. In patients with spinal epidural abscess, laminectomy with decompression and drainage may need to be performed as a surgical emergency to minimize the likelihood of permanent neurologic sequelae. However, in a literature review of 38 patients with spinal epidural abscess treated with antimicrobial therapy alone, 23 recovered, two died, one worsened, and the rest remained the same or improved.[64] However, there have been no prospective, randomized trials comparing the efficacy of antimicrobial agents plus surgery with antimicrobial therapy

TABLE 52-9 Empirical Antibiotic Therapy for Subdural Empyema, Epidural Abscess, and Septic Intracranial Thrombophlebitis

Condition	Site of Primary Infection	Antibiotics
Cranial subdural empyema, cranial epidural abscess, or septic intracranial thrombophlebitis	Paranasal sinusitis, otitis media, or mastoiditis	Vancomycin plus metronidazole plus a third-generation cephalosporin[a]
	Cranial surgery	Vancomycin plus a third-generation cephalosporin[a]
	Hematogenous from distant and/or unknown site	Vancomycin plus metronidazole plus a third-generation cephalosporin[a]
Spinal epidural abscess or spinal subdural empyema	Extension of osteomyelitis or paravertebral infection	Vancomycin plus a third-generation cephalosporin[a]
Spinal epidural abscess	Hematogenous spread	Vancomycin plus a third-generation cephalosporin[a]
Spinal subdural empyema	Hematogenous spread	Vancomycin

[a] Cefotaxime or ceftriaxone should be used. If *Pseudomonas aeruginosa* is suspected, ceftazidime or cefepime is indicated instead.
SOURCE: Modified from Bleck and Greenlee.[63]

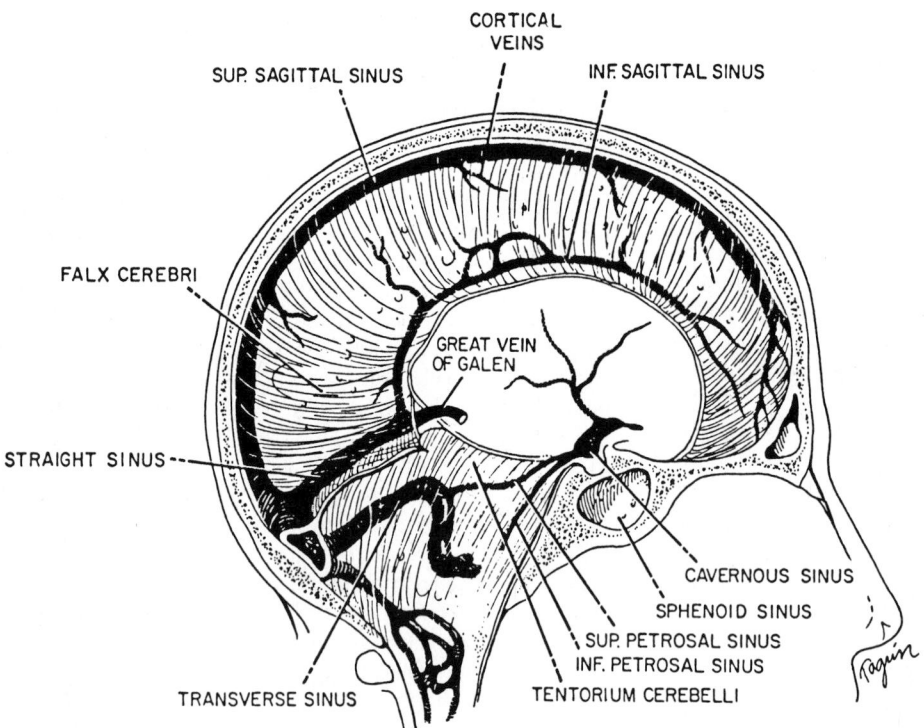

FIGURE 52-1 Lateral cross section of the skull, demonstrating the major dural venous sinuses. Note that the cavernous sinus is close to the sphenoid air sinus and that the anterior segment of the superior sagittal sinus is near the frontal air sinus. (*Reproduced with permission from Southwick et al.[66]*)

alone. Rapid surgical decompression should be performed in patients with increasing neurologic deficit, persistent severe pain, or increasing temperature or peripheral white blood cell count.[65]

ADJUNCTIVE THERAPY

Patients may also require various adjunctive measures to control increased intracranial pressure. Preoperative use of mannitol, hyperventilation, and/or dexamethasone may be effective in controlling intracranial pressure before surgical decompression. However, corticosteroids should be tapered rapidly after surgical therapy because of the increased risk of secondary infection. We believe a short course of corticosteroids is appropriate in cases in which surgical intervention is delayed or contraindicated. Anticonvulsants should be used in patients with seizures.

Suppurative Intracranial Thrombophlebitis

EPIDEMIOLOGY AND ETIOLOGY

Septic intracranial thrombophlebitis involves venous thrombosis and suppuration. It may begin within veins and venous sinuses or may follow infection of the paranasal sinuses, middle ear, mastoid, face, or oropharynx, and it may involve additional vessels by propagation or discontinuous spread. Septic thrombophlebitis may also occur in association with epidural abscess, subdural empyema, or bacterial meningitis. Occasionally, there is metastatic spread from distant sites of infection. Conditions that increase blood viscosity or coagulability, such as dehydration, polycythemia, pregnancy, oral contraceptive use, sickle cell disease, malignancy, and trauma, increase the likelihood of thrombosis.

The antecedent conditions that predispose to the development of intracranial venous sinus thrombosis depend on the close proximity of various structures to the dural venous sinuses[66,67] (Fig. 52-1). The usual predisposing conditions for cavernous sinus thrombosis are paranasal sinusitis (especially frontal, ethmoidal, or sphenoidal) and infection of the face or mouth. Likely infecting bacterial pathogens depend on the initial source: staphylococci, streptococci, gram-negative bacilli, and anaerobes, if the antecedent condition is sinusitis, and predominantly *S. aureus* in the case of facial infections. Otitis media and mastoiditis are infections associated with lateral sinus thrombosis and infection of the superior and inferior petrosal sinuses. Infections of the face, scalp, subdural space, and epidural space and meningitis are associated with suppurative thrombophlebitis of the superior sagittal sinus. The likely infecting microorganisms depend on the associated primary condition (see Table 52-5).

In cavernous sinus thrombosis, *S. aureus* is the most important infecting microorganism, having been isolated in more than 66% of cases. This relates to the importance of this organism in infections of the face and scalp and in acute sphenoid sinusitis. Less common isolates include streptococci (isolated in about 17% of cases), pneumococci and gram-negative bacilli (5% each), and *Bacteroides* species (2%).

CLINICAL PRESENTATION

The clinical manifestations of suppurative cortical thrombophlebitis depend on the location of involvement. With involvement of the cortical venous system, the appearance of neurologic deficits depends on the adequacy of collateral venous drainage.[68] Persons with inadequate collateral flow present with impairment of consciousness, focal or generalized seizures, symptoms of increased intracranial pressure, and focal neurologic signs (e.g., hemiparesis). Aphasia is common if the dominant cerebral hemisphere is involved.

The findings in dural venous sinus thrombosis also depend on location.[66,67] In cavernous sinus thrombosis, the most common complaints are periorbital swelling (73% of cases) and headache (52%). Headache is more common if the antecedent condition is sinusitis rather than a facial infection. Other symptoms include drowsiness, diplopia, eye tearing, photophobia, and ptosis. Fever is present in more than 90% of patients. Other common signs are proptosis, chemosis, periorbital edema, and weakness of the extraocular muscles (due to involvement of cranial nerves III, IV, and VI). Because the abducens nerve is the only cranial nerve traversing the interior of the cavernous sinus, lateral gaze palsy may be an early neurologic finding. Papilledema or venous engorgement and a change in mental status are observed in 65% and 55% of patients, respectively. Meningismus is present in about 40% of cases, usually secondary to retrograde spread of the thrombophlebitis. About 25% of patients have dilated or sluggishly reactive pupils, decreased visual acuity (frequently progressing to blindness), and dysfunction of cranial nerve V. As the infection spreads to the opposite cavernous sinus through the intercavernous sinuses, findings are duplicated in the opposite eye. Persons with septic cavernous sinus thrombosis may present with acute or chronic illness.[67] In the acute presentation (generally secondary to facial infection), the time between primary infection and cavernous sinus thrombosis is short (<1 week), and the patient presents in a significantly toxic state, with rapid development of the symptoms and signs described above; there is also rapid progression to bilateral eye signs. In contrast, there is a more indolent form of cavernous sinus thrombosis, usually secondary to dental infection, otitis media, or paranasal sinusitis. In these patients, the orbital manifestations are often unimpressive, and involvement of the contralateral eye is a late and inconsistent finding.

Patients with septic lateral sinus thrombosis complain predominantly of headache (>80% of cases); earache, vomiting, and vertigo also may occur because otitis media is a common predisposing condition.[66,68] Fever and abnormal ear findings are observed in most patients (79% and 98%, respectively), and there may be seventh nerve palsy, facial pain and altered facial sensation, papilledema, and mild nuchal rigidity. Thrombosis of the superior sagittal sinus produces an abnormal mental status, motor deficits, nuchal rigidity, and papilledema. Seizures occur in more than 50% of these patients. Patients with sinusitis as a predisposing condition tend to have a subacute onset of symptoms. Involvement of the inferior petrosal sinus may produce ipsilateral facial pain and lateral rectus muscle weakness (Gradenigo syndrome).

DIAGNOSIS

The noninvasive diagnostic procedure of choice for suppurative intracranial thrombophlebitis is MRI.[69] This technique visualizes blood vessels and differentiates between thrombus and normally flowing blood. It can also demonstrate the evolution and resolution of the entire veno-occlusive process. CT, with and without use of intravenous contrast material, also permits diagnosis of venous sinus thrombosis,[67] although it is considerably less sensitive and reliable than MRI. CT usually visualizes unilateral or bilateral multiple irregular filling defects in the enhancing cavernous sinus, with or without

orbital inflammatory change. An additional benefit of MRI and CT is the ability to fully evaluate the paranasal sinuses and to provide information concerning subdural and epidural infection, cerebral infarction, cerebritis, hemorrhage, and cerebral edema.

Other laboratory studies are usually nonspecific.[66,67] Lumbar puncture demonstrates a mild pleocytosis (mononuclear, neutrophilic, or mixed) and an elevated protein concentration (consistent with a parameningeal focus of infection), although, in septic thrombosis of the superior sagittal sinus, there may be findings consistent with frank meningitis; often the causative organism is isolated on CSF culture. Blood cultures may be positive, especially in patients with a rapidly progressive course. Chest radiographs may show evidence of septic pulmonary emboli after propagation of thrombus into the inferior petrosal sinus and jugular vein. Sinus radiographs may document involvement of the paranasal sinuses, although conventional radiographs are inferior to MRI and CT in the detection of sphenoid sinusitis.

TREATMENT

ANTIMICROBIAL THERAPY

Appropriate antimicrobial therapy of septic intracranial thrombophlebitis depends on the antecedent clinical condition. The likely organisms are similar to those observed in cranial subdural empyema and epidural abscess; empirical antibiotic therapy should be directed toward those organisms[68] (see Table 52-9). If the antecedent condition is paranasal sinusitis, empirical therapy should be directed toward grampositive organisms (staphylococci and streptococci), aerobic gram-negative bacilli, and anaerobes. In cavernous sinus thrombosis, an antistaphylococcal agent should always be included (because of the high incidence of *S. aureus* isolates) in the empirical therapeutic regimen pending culture results. Nafcillin should be used, with vancomycin reserved for penicillin-allergic patients and cases in which methicillin-resistant organisms are suspected.

SURGICAL THERAPY

Surgical intervention may be required for optimal therapy. Surgical drainage of infected sinuses is necessary when antimicrobial therapy alone is ineffective. This is especially important in patients with cavernous sinus thrombosis secondary to sphenoid sinusitis; some investigators have recommended operative intervention for patients who develop cavernous venous thrombosis as a complication of sinusitis. Internal jugular vein ligation has been used for lateral sinus vein thrombosis, and thrombectomy has also been used in some situations, but the efficacy of these procedures is poorly defined. Surgical therapy may also be required for other infections (e.g., dental abscess).

ADJUNCTIVE THERAPY

The use of anticoagulants (e.g., heparin) is controversial, although there is literature to support their use in prevention of the spread of thrombus from the cavernous sinus to other dural venous sinuses and cerebral veins.[66] Recent evidence has indicated that anticoagulation (in combination with antibiotics) decreases mortality rate and is most beneficial early in the treatment of cavernous sinus thrombosis to reduce the morbidity rate among survivors.[70] However, the hazards of intracranial hemorrhage (bleeding from sites of cortical venous infarction or from sites on the intracavernous walls of the carotid artery) must be recognized. In the absence of specific contraindications, anticoagulation is most likely to be useful early in the course of cavernous sinus thrombosis.

References

1. Schlech WF, Ward JI, Band JD, et al: Bacterial meningitis in the United States, 1978 through 1981. The national bacterial meningitis surveillance study. *JAMA* 253:1749, 1985.

2. Durand ML, Calderwood SB, Weber DJ, et al: Acute bacterial meningitis in adults. A review of 493 episodes. *N Engl J Med* 328:21, 1993.

3. Murphy TV, White KE, Pastor P, et al: Declining incidence of *Haemophilus influenzae* type b disease since the introduction of vaccination. *JAMA* 269:246, 1993.

4. Schuchat A, Robinson K, Wenger JD, et al: Bacterial meningitis in the United States in 1995. *N Engl J Med* 337:970, 1997.

5. Spagnuolo PT, Ellner JJ, Lerner PI, et al: *Haemophilus influenzae* meningitis: The spectrum of disease in adults. *Medicine* 61:74, 1982.

6. McGee ZA, Stephens DS, Hoffman LH, et al: Mechanisms of mucosal invasion by pathogenic *Neisseria*. *Rev Infect Dis* 5:S708, 1983.

7. Jackson LA, Schuchat A, Reeves MW, et al: Serogroup C meningococcal outbreaks in the United States: An emerging threat. *JAMA* 273:383, 1995.

8. Whalen CM, Hockin JC, Ryan A, et al: The changing epidemiology of invasive meningococcal disease in Canada, 1985 through 1992. *JAMA* 273:390, 1995.

9. Ross SC, Densen P: Complement deficiency states and infection: Epidemiology, pathogenesis and consequences of neisserial and other infections in an immune deficiency. *Medicine* 63:243, 1984.

10. Kaufman BA, Tunkel AR, Pryor J, et al: Meningitis in the neurosurgical patient. *Infect Dis Clin North Am* 4:677, 1990.

11. Gellin BG, Broome CV: Listeriosis. *JAMA* 261:1313, 1989.

12. Lorber B: Listeriosis. *Clin Infect Dis* 24:1, 1997.

13. Decker CF, Simon GL, DiGioia RA, et al: *Listeria monocytogenes* infections in patients with AIDS: Report of five cases and review. *Rev Infect Dis* 13:413, 1991.

14. Cherubin CE, Marr JS, Sierra MF, Becker S: *Listeria* and gram-negative bacillary meningitis in New York City, 1972–1979. Frequent causes of meningitis in adults. *Am J Med* 71:199, 1981.

15. Schlesinger LS, Ross SC, Schaberg DR: *Staphylococcus aureus* meningitis: A broad-based epidemiologic study. *Medicine* 66:148, 1987.

16. Saez-Llorens X, McCracken GH Jr: Bacterial meningitis in neonates and children. *Infect Dis Clin North Am* 4:623, 1990.

17. Farley MM, Harvey RC, Stull T, et al: A population-based assessment of invasive disease due to group B streptococci in nonpregnant adults. *N Engl J Med* 328:1807, 1993.

18. Dunne DW, Quagliarello V: Group B streptococcal meningitis in adults. *Medicine* 72:1, 1993.

19. Domingo P, Barquet N, Alvarez M, et al: Group B streptococcal meningitis in adults: Report of twelve cases and review. *Clin Infect Dis* 25:1180, 1997.

20. Tunkel AR, Scheld WM: Acute meningitis, in Mandell GL, Bennett JE, Dolin R (eds): *Mandell, Douglas and Bennett's Principles and Practice of Infectious Diseases*, 5th ed. Philadelphia, Churchill-Livingstone, 2000, p 959.

21. Gray LD, Fedorko DP: Laboratory diagnosis of bacterial meningitis. *Clin Microbiol Rev* 5:130, 1992.

22. Nathan BR, Scheld WM: The potential roles of C-reactive protein and procalcitonin in the serum and cerebrospinal fluid in the diagnosis of bacterial meningitis, in Remington JS, Swartz MN (eds): *Current Clinical Topics in Infectious Diseases*, vol 22. Oxford, Blackwell Science, 2002, p 155.

23. Ni H, Knight AL, Cartwright K, et al: Polymerase chain reaction for diagnosis of meningococcal meningitis. *Lancet* 340:1432, 1992.

24. Tunkel AR, Scheld WM: Acute bacterial meningitis. *Lancet* 346:1675, 1995.

25. Hasbun R, Abrahams J, Jekel J, Quagliarello VJ: Computed tomography of the head before lumbar puncture in adults with suspected meningitis. *N Engl J Med* 345:1727, 2001.

26. Viladrich PF, Gudiol F, Linares J, et al: Evaluation of vancomyin for therapy of adult pneumococcal meningitis. *Antimicrob Agents Chemother* 35:2467, 1991.

27. Kaplan SL, Mason EO: Management of infections due to antibiotic-resistant *Streptococcus pneumoniae*. *Clin Microbiol Rev* 11:628, 1998.

28. Odio CM, Puig JR, Feris JM, et al: Prospective, randomized, investigator-blinded study of the efficacy of meropenem vs. cefotaxime therapy in bacterial meningitis in children. *Pediatr Infect Dis J* 18:581, 1999.

29. Saez-Llorens X, McCoig C, Feris JM, et al: Quinolone treatment for pediatric bacterial meningitis: A comparative study of trovafloxacin and ceftriaxone with or without vancomycin. *Pediatr Infect Dis J* 21:14, 2002.

30. Rosenstein NE, Stocker SA, Popovic T, et al: Antimicrobial resistance of *Neisseria meningitidis* in the United States, 1997. *Clin Infect Dis* 30:212, 2000.

31. Schaad UB, Suter S, Gianella-Borradori A, et al: A comparison of ceftriaxone and cefuroxime for the treatment of bacterial meningitis in children. *N Engl J Med* 322:141, 1990.

32. Radetsky M: Duration of treatment in bacterial meningitis: A historical inquiry. *Pediatr Infect Dis J* 9:2, 1990.

33. McIntyre PB, Berkey CS, King SM, et al: Dexamethasone as adjunctive therapy in bacterial meningitis: A meta-analysis of randomized clinical trials since 1988. *JAMA* 278:925, 1997.

34. de Gans J, van de Beek D: Dexamethasone in adults with bacterial meningitis. *N Engl J Med* 347:1549, 2002.

35. Tunkel AR, Scheld WM: Corticosteroids for everyone with meningitis? *N Engl J Med* 347:1613, 2002.

36. Kilpi T, Peltola H, Jauhiainen T, et al: Oral glycerol and intravenous dexamethasone in preventing neurologic and audiologic sequelae of childhood bacterial menigitis. *Pediatr Infect Dis J* 14:270, 1995.

37. Girgis N, Sultan Y, Frenck RW Jr, et al: Azithromycin compared with rifampin for eradication of nasopharyngeal colonization by Neisseria meningitidis. *Pediatr Infect Dis J* 17:816, 1998.

38. Tunkel AR, Wispelwey B, Scheld WM: Brain abscess, in Mandell GR, Bennett JE, Dolin R (eds): *Mandell, Douglas and Bennett's Principles and Practice of Infectious Diseases*, 5th ed. Philadephia, Churchill Livingstone, 2000, p 1016.

39. Mathisen GE, Johnson JP: Brain abscess. *Clin Infect Dis* 25:763, 1997.

40. Heilpern KL, Lorber B: Focal intracranial infections. *Infect Dis Clin North Am* 10:879, 1996.

41. Saez-Llorens XJ, Umaña MA, Odio CM, et al: Brain abscess in infants and children. *Pediatr Infect Dis J* 8:449, 1989.

42. Tunkel AR, Kaye D: Neurologic complication of infective endocarditis. *Neurol Clin* 11:419, 1993.

43. Rehncrona S, Brismar J, Holtas S: Diagnosis of brain abscesses with indium-111 labeled leukocytes. *Neurosurgery* 16:23, 1985.

44. Alderson D, Strong AJ, Ingham MR, Selkon JB: Fifteen year review of the mortality of brain abscess. *Neurosurgery* 8:1, 1981.

45. Levy RM, Gutin PH, Baskin DS, Pons VG: Vancomycin penetration of a brain abscess: Case report and review of the literature. *Neurosurgery* 18:632, 1986.

46. Boom WH, Tuazon CU: Successful treatment of multiple brain abscesses with antibiotics alone. *Rev Infect Dis* 7:189, 1985.

47. Carpenter JL: Brain stem abscesses: Cure with medical therapy, case report, and review. *Clin Infect Dis* 18:219, 1994.

48. Stephanov S: Surgical treatment of brain abscess. *Neurosurgery* 22:724, 1988.

49. Mampalam TJ, Rosenblum ML: Trends in the management of bacterial brain abscesses: A review of 102 cases over 17 years. *Neurosurgery* 23:451, 1988.

50. Mamelak AN, Mampalam TJ, Obana WG, et al: Improved management of multiple brain abscesses: A combined medical and surgical approach. *Neurosurgery* 36:76, 1995.

51. Silverberg AL, DiNubile MJ: Subdural empyema and cranial epidural abscess. *Med Clin North Am* 69:361, 1985.

52. Coonrod JD, Dans PE: Subdural empyema. *Am J Med* 53:85, 1972.

53. Kaufman DM, Miller MH, Steigbigel NH: Subdural empyema: Analysis of 17 recent cases and review of the literature. *Medicine* 54:485, 1975.

54. Kaufman DM, Litman N, Miller MH: Sinusitis-induced subdural empyema. *Neurology* 33:123, 1983.

55. Yoshikawa TT, Chow AW, Guze LB: Role of anaerobic bacteria in subdural empyema. Report of four cases and review of 327 cases from the English literature. *Am J Med* 58:99, 1975.

56. Dacey RG, Winn HR, Jane JA, Butler AB: Spinal subdural empyema: Report of two cases. *Neurosurgery* 3:400, 1978.

57. Baker AS, Ojemann RG, Swartz MN, Richardson EP Jr: Spinal epidural abscess. *N Engl J Med* 293:463, 1975.

58. Danner RL, Hartman BJ: Update of spinal epidural abscess: 35 Cases and review of the literature. *Rev Infect Dis* 9:265, 1987.

59. Koppel BS, Tuchman AJ, Mangiardi JR, et al: Epidural spinal infection in intravenous drug abusers. *Arch Neurol* 45:1331, 1988.

60. Bleck TP, Greenlee JE: Epidural abscess, in Mandell GL, Bennett JE, Dolin R (eds): *Mandell, Douglas and Bennett's Principles and Practice of Infectious Diseases,* 5th ed. Philadephia, Churchill Livingstone, 2000, p 1031.

61. Lasker BR, Harter DH: Cervical epidural abscess. *Neurology* 37:1747, 1987.

62. Weingarten K, Zimmerman RD, Becker RD, et al: Subdural and epidural empyemas: MR imaging. *AJR* 152:615, 1989.

63. Bleck TP, Greenlee JE: Subdural empyema, in Mandell GL, Bennett JE, Dolin R (eds): *Mandell, Douglas and Bennett's Principles and Practice of Infectious Diseases,* 5th ed. Philadelphia, Churchill Livingstone, 2000, p 1028.

64. Wheeler D, Keiser P, Rigamonti D, et al: Medical management of spinal epidural abscess: Case report and review. *Clin Infect Dis* 15:22, 1992.

65. Baker AS, Ojemann RG, Baker RA: To decompress or not to decompress—Spinal epidural abscess. *Clin Infect Dis* 15:28, 1992.

66. Southwick FS, Richardson EP Jr, Swartz MN: Septic thrombosis of the dural venous sinuses. *Medicine* 65:82, 1985.

67. DiNubile MJ: Septic thrombosis of the cavernous sinuses. *Arch Neurol* 45:567, 1988.

68. Bleck TP, Greenlee JE: Suppurative intracranial phlebitis, in Mandell GL, Bennett JE, Dolin R (eds): *Mandell, Douglas and Bennett's Principles and Practice of Infectious Diseases,* 5th ed. Philadelphia, Churchill Livingstone, 2000, p 1034.

69. Macchi PJ, Grossman RI, Gomori JM, et al: High field MR imaging of cerebral venous thrombosis. *J Comput Assist Tomogr* 10:10, 1986.

70. Levine SR, Twyman RE, Gilman S: The role of anticoagulation in cavernous sinus thrombosis. *Neurology* 38:517, 1988.

Chapter 53
ENCEPHALOMYELITIS

JOHN C. GALBRAITH
ROBERT VERITY
D. LORNE TYRRELL

KEY POINTS

- *Herpes simplex virus (HSV) is the most common cause of fatal sporadic encephalitis. Early recognition and early treatment with acyclovir significantly improve outcome.*

- *A diagnosis of encephalomyelitis should be suspected in patients with fever, headache, behavioral changes, unexplained focal neurologic signs, seizures, or altered mental status without an obvious alternative explanation.*

- *Focal neurologic abnormalities are demonstrable either clinically or with neurodiagnostic evaluation in 90% of cases of HSV encephalitis (HSVE).*

- *If focal neurologic signs are present, computed tomography or magnetic resonance imaging should be performed before lumbar puncture. Diagnostic imaging is helpful in ruling out other treatable causes of altered mental status and also may identify patients with increased intracranial pressure in whom lumbar puncture may be dangerous.*

- *Unless contraindicated, an early lumbar puncture should be performed. This measure is especially important to rule out bacterial meningitis.*

- *The cerebrospinal fluid (CSF) is almost always abnormal in encephalomyelitis, usually demonstrating increased leukocytes, generally between 10 and 500 cells per microliter. The CSF glucose value is usually normal, and the protein content is usually normal or slightly elevated. Although a completely normal CSF does not rule out encephalomyelitis, it should heighten suspicion for a toxic or metabolic encephalopathy.*

- *Treatment with acyclovir must be commenced early when HSVE is suspected clinically. Polymerase chain reaction detection of HSV in CSF is the gold standard for the diagnosis of HSVE. However, a negative result on polymerase chain reaction does not always exclude HSVE and does not, by itself, provide justification for the termination of acyclovir treatment.*

- *Arboviruses are the most common cause of encephalitis worldwide. Their frequency varies dramatically, depending mainly on the season and geographic locale. West Nile virus has recently emerged as an important cause of encephalitis in North America.*

- *Although viruses are the most common cause of encephalomyelitis, nonviral causes should be carefully ruled out because they are often readily treatable.*

- *The threat of bioterrorism has increased the likelihood that unusual organisms may be etiologic agents.*

- *Intensive supportive care is indicated in patients with encephalitis because these patients may make remarkable recoveries even after prolonged unconsciousness.*

Encephalitis and *myelitis* refer to inflammation of the brain and spinal cord, respectively. These processes may occur together, often with meningeal involvement; hence, the terms *meningoencephalitis* and *meningoencephalomyelitis*. Encephalomyelitis may result from direct invasion of a microorganism into the central nervous system (CNS) or from an autoimmune process that results in demyelination; the latter process is often triggered by a recent vaccination or infection. Up to 20% of all encephalitides result from autoimmune reactions; they have been variously termed *postinfectious, parainfectious* (when they occur simultaneously with an infection), and *postvaccinial* (when they occur after a vaccination). Regardless of the pathogenesis, the clinical manifestations and differential diagnosis of these processes overlap to such a degree that they may be considered together.

Approach to the Patient with Suspected Encephalomyelitis

There are a multiplicity of etiologies for encephalomyelitis[1] (Table 53-1). Unfortunately, most patients do not present with symptoms and signs pathognomonic of a certain cause, but rather with nonspecific problems of fever, headache, and behavioral changes or altered mental status. Therefore, one must have a clear approach in the workup of such patients. This should begin with a careful history and physical examination. The clinical features alone are not generally sufficient to establish an etiologic diagnosis, but they do influence the likelihood of some diagnoses. For instance, age can be a factor because neonates are the group at highest risk for meningoencephalitis from herpes simplex virus type 2 (HSV-2). Enteroviruses and bacterial infections, including infections with group B streptococcus and *Listeria monocytogenes*, should also be considered in the differential diagnosis of progressive encephalopathy in neonates. At the other end of the age spectrum, *Varicella zoster* virus (VZV) is a leading cause of encephalitis in the elderly.

The setting of disease may provide helpful clues. Arbovirus encephalitis depends more or less on the season, locale, degree of insect exposure, and current prevalence of disease in a given community. Most outbreaks of eastern equine encephalitis are preceded by enzootics of disease in local horses and pheasants. West Nile virus infections are heralded by outbreaks and deaths among birds. Epidemics of St. Louis encephalitis are often preceded by serologic changes in chickens. Tick exposure in specific geographic areas should heighten the suspicion for Lyme disease, Rocky Mountain spotted fever, or ehrlichiosis. Similarly, exposure to certain animals may be suggestive of rabies or leptospirosis.

The progression of disease often suggests certain causes. Encephalitis developing 1 to 2 weeks after immunization or a viral syndrome is more likely postinfectious, whereas an acute fulminant course is more in keeping with herpes simplex virus encephalitis (HSVE) or eastern equine encephalitis. A slowly progressive neurologic disease is more characteristic of Creutzfeldt-Jakob disease, variant Creutzfeldt-Jakob disease, subacute sclerosing panencephalitis (SSPE), or encephalopathy due to acquired immunodeficiency syndrome (AIDS). A chronic or fluctuating course suggests mycobacterial or fungal infections, although mucormycosis may progress very rapidly. The diagnosis of CNS tuberculosis is difficult and requires a high index of suspicion.

TABLE 53-1 Causes of Encephalomyelitis[a]

Viral	Nonviral
Herpetoviridae	Bacterial meningitis, brain abscess
Herpes simplex virus	Parameningeal infection
Varicella zoster virus	Infective endocarditis
Cytomegalovirus	*Mycobacterium*
Epstein-Barr virus	*Listeria*
Human herpesvirus type 6	*Anthrax*
Herpes B virus	Brucellosis
Togaviridae	*Mycoplasma*
Alphaviruses	*Coxiella burnetii*
Eastern equine encephalitis virus	*Rickettsia*
Western equine encephalitis virus	*Borrelia*
Venezuelan equine encephalitis virus	*Leptospira*
Flaviviridae	*Treponema pallidum*
St. Louis encephalitis virus	*Cryptococcus*
Murray Valley encephalitis virus	*Nocardia*
Japanese B encephalitis virus	*Actinomycosis*
Dengue fever virus	*Coccidioides*
West Nile Virus	Mucormycosis
Tick-borne complex	*Histoplasma*
Bunyaviridae	*Toxoplasma*
California (La Crosse) encephalitis virus	*Plasmodium falciparum*
Picornaviridae	*Trypanosoma*
Echovirus	*Acanthamoeba*
Coxsackievirus	*Naegleria*
Poliovirus	Connective tissue diseases, vasculitis
Hepatitis A virus	
Arenaviridae	
Lymphocytic choriomeningitis virus	
Lassa fever virus	
Rhabdoviridae	
Rabies virus	
Retroviridae	
Human immunodeficiency virus	
Human T-cell lymphotropic virus (myelitis)	
Paramyxoviridae	
Measles virus	
Mumps virus	
Nipah virus	
Myxoviridae	
Influenza virus	
Rubivirus	
Rubella virus	
Adenoviridae	
Adenovirus	
Filoviridae	
Marburg virus	
Ebola virus	

[a]Conditions that may resemble encephalitis include tumor, toxic or metabolic encephalopathy, intracranial hemorrhage or hematoma, and cerebrovascular disease.

A subacute neurologic process with certain associated systemic symptoms may suggest immunologic disorders (e.g., systemic lupus erythematosus or sarcoidosis) or a neoplastic disease such as lymphoma, leukemia, and breast or lung carcinoma.

The immune status of the patient is also important when considering the various etiologic possibilities. Patients who are immunocompromised frequently develop unusual forms of encephalitis. Hypogammaglobulinemic patients may develop chronic encephalitis with enteroviruses. Rhinocerebral mucormycosis most often occurs in diabetics with ketoacidosis and in neutropenic leukemics who have been on broad-spectrum antibiotics. Toxoplasmosis is the most common cause of encephalitis in AIDS patients. Other causes of encephalitis in AIDS include cytomegalovirus (CMV) and other herpesviruses, fungi (especially *Cryptococcus*), *Mycobacterium,* and uncommon pathogens such as *Nocardia, Listeria, Acanthamoeba,* and papovavirus.

Physical examination lends little to the diagnostic approach except in cases in which a characteristic rash is present, as in varicella, measles, Lyme disease, or Rocky Mountain spotted fever. A cutaneous eschar may aid in the diagnosis of anthrax. Evidence of disease outside the CNS can suggest certain causes. For example, most patients with CNS disease associated with *Mycoplasma pneumoniae* have antecedent or concurrent respiratory tract infection. Pulmonary symptoms may accompany lymphocytic choriomeningitis or legionella infections. A thorough neurologic examination is important because the presence of focal neurologic signs heightens the likelihood of treatable infectious causes and mandates the commencement of empirical antimicrobial therapy. Although it is noteworthy that encephalitis caused by HSV is associated with focal neurologic findings in the vast majority of patients, these findings are nonspecific. Even when present in patients with fever, they could represent other CNS diseases, such as parameningeal infection, subdural empyema, brain abscess, cerebral malaria, hemorrhage, vascular disease, or tumor.

The presence of focal neurologic abnormalities clearly mandates urgent diagnostic imaging with computed tomography (CT) or magnetic resonance imaging (MRI). Although the sensitivity of these techniques is limited in diagnosing encephalitis, they are essential and invaluable in ruling out other CNS processes that could be confused clinically with encephalitis and that require a different specific therapy. In addition, CT or MRI can identify patients with increased intracranial pressure (ICP) in whom lumbar puncture is contraindicated.

A lumbar puncture is an important step in the diagnostic evaluation of encephalitis and should be performed early unless there is a specific contraindication. It is especially important to rule out bacterial meningitis. If there is concern about increased ICP and possible herniation, a cisternal puncture should be considered. Cerebrospinal fluid (CSF) should be sent for cell count, chemistry, viral studies (including polymerase chain reaction [PCR] for HSV and other viruses), and stains and culture for fungi and bacteria (including mycobacteria). Completely normal findings on lumbar puncture significantly decrease the likelihood of encephalitis and raise the possibility of toxic or metabolic encephalopathy. Reye syndrome must be distinguished from encephalitis. This syndrome has been associated with several viral infections, especially influenza and VZV, together with salicylate use. It occurs most often in children who are usually afebrile but have altered mental status and hepatomegaly. CSF protein and cell counts are normal, but the blood ammonia level is almost always elevated. Other clues to the diagnosis of Reye syndrome include elevated liver enzyme levels in serum and hypoglycemia. Patients with normal CSF examinations should be monitored carefully; if the index of suspicion for encephalitis remains high, further neurodiagnostic evaluation, including a second lumbar puncture, should be considered. Further evaluation of patients with encephalitis includes an electroencephalogram (EEG) and CT or MRI. Ancillary studies, such as serology, should be performed depending on the specific characteristics of each case. If no specific diagnosis is established, then brain biopsy should be considered. In patients with suspected HSVE, it is important to commence empirical treatment early with acyclovir. Ongoing surveillance for alternative diagnoses must be maintained.

AIDS patients are unique. The approach to management in these patients requires a complete neurodiagnostic assessment and serologic testing for *Toxoplasma*. If the encephalitis is compatible with toxoplasmosis, then empirical treatment with pyrimethamine and sulfadiazine is begun. Clinical and radiographic improvements are expected to occur within 10 days of the start of therapy. However, if there is evidence of disease progression, then brain biopsy for definitive diagno-

sis should be performed. At least one pathogen is occasionally isolated in AIDS patients with CNS disease. There are other possibilities to consider in the patient who is infected with human immunodeficiency virus (HIV) and presents with CNS mass lesions, including CNS lymphoma and progressive multifocal leukoencephalopathy (see Chap. 48).

Myelitis

The diagnostic and therapeutic approach to myelitis without encephalitis is somewhat different. Polio should be suspected in cases in which there is a history of recent immunization or contact with a recently immunized individual. The pattern of myelitis caused by poliovirus and other enteroviruses is primarily lower motor neuron disease; characteristically, there is an asymmetric flaccid paralysis with preserved sensation and bladder function. The diagnosis is established by isolation of virus from stools, the throat, or the CSF, in addition to serologic confirmation. It is noteworthy that Japanese virus encephalitis and West Nile virus infection can also produce a polio-like myelitis.

Patients with transverse myelitis usually present with limb weakness and a sensory level with loss of bowel and bladder control. This syndrome may result from a variety of infectious diseases; however, in most cases, there is no identifiable cause. It is important to exclude the potentially treatable causes, such as tuberculosis, syphilis, herpes zoster, schistosomiasis, and HIV infection. The numerous parainfectious etiologies of transverse myelitis include measles, mumps, rubella, influenza, and *M. pneumoniae* infection, and the management of these causes is strictly supportive. Regardless of the exact etiology, early neurodiagnostic evaluation with myelography and CT or MRI is important to rule out spinal cord compression, epidural abscess, or hemorrhage.

A syndrome known as *tropical spastic paraparesis* is associated with human T-lymphotropic virus type I infection. Tropical spastic paraparesis is characterized by spastic paraparesis or paraplegia with pyramidal signs, occasional mild distal sensory loss, and occasional sphincter incontinence. Human T-lymphotropic virus type I is endemic in certain geographic regions, including Africa, southern Japan, and the Caribbean basin.

Herpes Simplex Virus Encephalitis

EPIDEMIOLOGY AND PATHOGENESIS

HSVE is the most common fatal nonepidemic encephalitis. It accounts for 5% to 10% of all reported cases of encephalitis.[2] The exact incidence is unknown, but the disease has been estimated to have an incidence of 1 in 250,000 population per year.[3] It is seen in all age groups, in both sexes, and in all seasons.[4] The patient is seldom immunocompromised, and one cannot predict who is at risk for HSVE. HSVE is particularly important because it has a very high mortality rate if untreated, whereas early therapy with acyclovir significantly improves the outcome.[5]

A temporal lobe syndrome is the most common clinical presentation for HSVE, but atypical presentations may occur, with involvement of parietal or frontal lobes. The predilection of the disease for the frontal or temporal lobes has led to

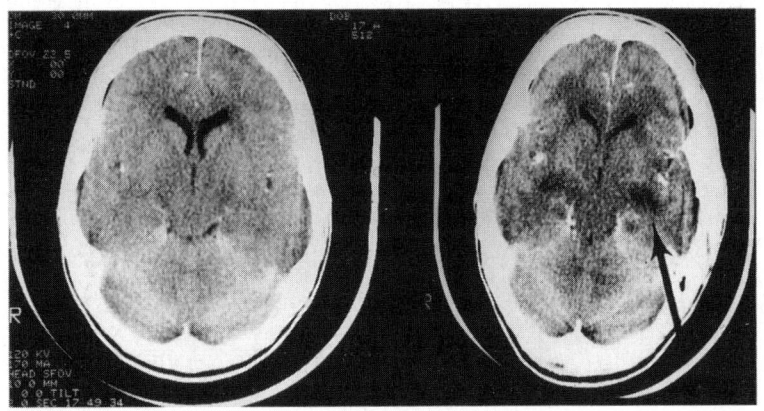

FIGURE 53-1 Computed tomographic scan of the head in a patient with herpes simplex virus encephalitis demonstrating bilateral hippocampal hypodensities. Involvement of the temporal lobes is classic for herpes simplex virus encephalitis.

the speculation that HSVE results from the retrograde spread of infection from the nasopharynx along the olfactory pathway to the basal portion of the frontal and temporal lobes. Alternatively, latent virus in the trigeminal ganglia may become activated and may reach the CNS along a neurotropic route.[6] Either of these pathogenetic mechanisms may explain why HSV-1 more commonly causes adult encephalitis than HSV-2. Serologic evaluation indicates that approximately 70% of HSVE is due to reactivation of latent HSV, whereas approximately 30% is due to primary infection. The median age for patients developing primary HSVE is 15 years, whereas the median age for recurrent infection is 50 years.[5]

CLINICAL AND LABORATORY FEATURES

There are no pathognomonic clinical symptoms or signs of HSVE that distinguish it from encephalitis of other etiologies. The clinical presentation may be abrupt or insidious. There may be an influenza-like prodrome. Clinical findings include fever (90%), headache (81%), alteration of consciousness (97%), personality changes (85%), dysphasia (76%), autonomic dysfunction (60%), ataxia (40%), hemiparesis (38%), seizures (38%), cranial nerve defects (32%), visual field loss (14%), and papilledema (14%). Eighty-five percent of patients have clinical findings indicative of focal neurologic disease.[4]

Adult HSVE may occur in the presence or absence of mucocutaneous HSV lesions. Although a history of recurrent HSV lesions was obtained in 22% of patients with HSVE, this history was also found with equal frequency in patients with encephalitis of other etiologies.[4]

Examination of the CSF shows an abnormality in 90% to 97% of cases.[4,7] Usually there is a lymphocytic predominance with 10 to 500 leukocytes per microliter, although early in the course of illness, polymorphonuclear cells (PMNs) may predominate. Red blood cells are present in 75% to 80% of samples, indicating the hemorrhagic nature of this encephalitis. The glucose level is generally normal, and the protein content is only moderately elevated. Viral cultures are almost always negative. PCR analysis to detect HSV DNA in CSF is the gold standard for the diagnosis of HSVE,[8] especially in the early phase of the disease. It has a sensitivity of 96% and a specificity of 99%.[9] Later in the course of the disease, intrathecal antibody detection may be used to confirm the diagnosis, although this is seldom used in practice.[10] When the index of suspicion remains high for HSVE even though PCR has not produced a positive result, a full course of acyclovir is recommended.[11]

Neurodiagnostic tests, such as EEG, brain scan, CT, and MRI, are useful in confirming and localizing the CNS lesion. EEG has been shown to be more sensitive than brain scan or CT early in the course of HSVE.[4] In 80% to 90% of cases, the initial EEG is abnormal, with predominantly spiked and slow wave patterns localized to the area of the brain involved. Paroxysmal lateral epileptiform discharges are characteristic of HSVE but are neither pathognomonic nor common.[12] Sodium pertechnetate ^{99}Tc brain scans are abnormal in only about 50% of cases of HSVE and demonstrate radionuclide uptake in the involved area of the brain. Similarly, CT scans are abnormal early in the course of illness in only about 50% of cases of HSVE. Abnormalities include localized edema, low-density lesions, mass effect, contrast enhancement, and hemorrhage (Fig. 53-1).[4] MRI may be the most sensitive neurodiagnostic test and has excellent delineation of the temporobasal lobe of the brain[13] (Fig. 53-2). MRI is more specific than the EEG and has been advocated by some as the preferred imaging test in the evaluation of suspected HSVE,[14–16] although single-photon emission CT has shown abnormalities in the temporo occipital area of two HSVE patients with normal MRI.[17]

DIAGNOSIS AND MANAGEMENT

For optimal patient care, acyclovir treatment must be commenced early when HSVE is clinically suspected. The diagnosis can be confirmed subsequently by PCR detection of HSV DNA in the CSF. Although PCR detection is an extremely useful technique, false-positive and false-negative results have been reported.[10,18,19] Brain biopsy should be considered in very select circumstances, when the diagnosis remains uncertain despite all available investigations, and particularly when the patient is deteriorating clinically despite empirical therapy. When the diagnosis is not established, it is important to continue diagnostic investigations to rule out other disorders that mimic HSVE, such as bacterial abscess, tuberculosis, cryptococcosis, toxoplasmosis, rickettsial infections, anthrax, and neoplastic or vascular diseases. If a brain biopsy specimen is taken, the pathology and microbiology laboratories should be notified. Specimens should be submitted for the detection and culture of bacteria (including mycobacteria), viruses, and fungi and for histopathology.[20,21]

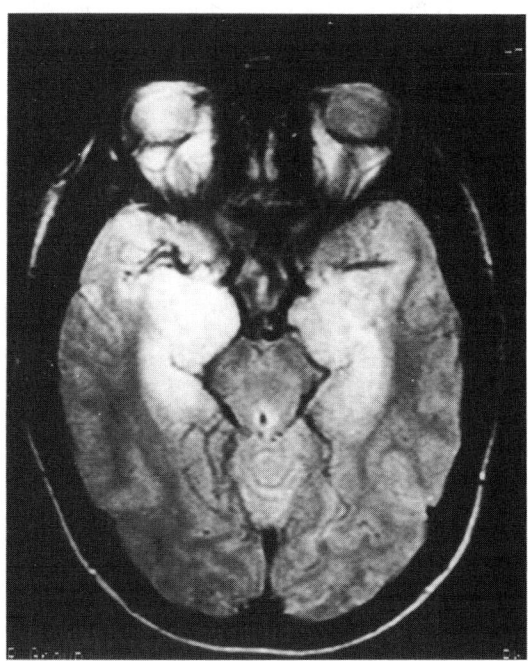

FIGURE 53-2 T2-weighted magnetic resonance image of the head demonstrating increased signal intensity involving the medial aspects of the temporal lobes in the region of the hippocampus. Increased signal intensity is present bilaterally but is more marked on the right side than on the left. These findings are highly suggestive for herpes simplex virus encephalitis.

The recommended treatment of HSVE is acyclovir at a dose of 10 mg/kg every 8 hours for 10 to 14 days.[22] Relapse of HSVE has been described after successful treatment and may necessitate a second course of therapy.[23,24] In most cases, the relapses occurred within 2 weeks of completing antiviral therapy. The precise etiology and the frequency of relapses remain unclear, although it appears to be more common in children than in adults.

The toxicity of acyclovir is minimal. Uncommonly, precipitation of crystals in renal tubules can occur in poorly hydrated patients. This is manifested by a rise in serum creatinine and blood urea levels, which can be reversed by increased hydration, dosage adjustment, or discontinuation of therapy. Patients at a higher risk of nephrotoxicity include those with pre-existing renal disease and those concurrently receiving nephrotoxic drugs. The dosage of acyclovir should be adjusted in patients with renal failure[25] (Table 53-2).

TABLE 53-2 Dose of Intravenous Acyclovir for Herpes Simplex and Varicella-Zoster Encephalitis According to Renal Function

Creatinine Clearance (mL/min per 1.7 m^2)	Dose Schedule
>50	10 mg/kg q 8 h
25–50	10 mg/kg q 12 h
10–25	10 mg/kg q 24 h
0–10	5 mg/kg q 24 h
Hemodialysis (3 times/wk)	5 mg/kg q 24 h
Postdialysis	6.0 mg/kg after dialysis

SOURCE: Adapted with permission from Deeter and Khanderia.[25]

Patients who receive acyclovir for suspected HSVE should also receive broad-spectrum antibiotics, such as cloxacillin, cefotaxime, and metronidazole, for the first 48 to 72 hours until CSF and other cultures for bacteria are reported negative.

The precise factors that determine the therapeutic response are unknown. Patients who are younger than 30 years and present with a Glasgow coma score higher than 10 have the best outcome.[5] Patients who present with a Glasgow coma score below 6, irrespective of age, have a very poor prognosis. Other markers of poor outcome include bilateral abnormalities on the EEG and the presence of identifiable lesions on the original CT scan.

Long-term complications of HSVE infection are common and include residual dysphasias, paresis, paresthesias, behavioral changes, and a Korsakoff-like amnesia. Even with acyclovir treatment, the mortality rate is 28%, and only 38% of patients recover with little or no residuum.[5,26]

Herpes Simplex Virus Type 2

HSV-2 as a cause of encephalitis is seen primarily, although not exclusively, in neonates. In adults it is more frequently seen as a cause of aseptic meningitis concurrent with primary genital infection.

Neonatal infection occurs with the frequency of 26 per 100,000 deliveries, and, although infection may be localized to the skin, it is more often disseminated.[27] Infection is acquired by passage of infants through the birth canal of infected mothers, especially mothers with primary infection. It is recommended that all women in labor be examined for genital HSV-like lesions and, if lesions are present (and if the membranes are intact), that a cesarean section be performed.[28] Unfortunately, most neonatal exposure to HSV results from excretion of virus by asymptomatic mothers at delivery. Asymptomatic shedding in pregnant women has been documented to be not infrequent. One can neither predict nor prevent these exposures. Because HSV-2 causes 90% of primary genital herpes and 99% of recurrent infections, neonatal HSV infections are usually caused by HSV-2. HSV-2 causes more morbidity than HSV-1 in neonatal encephalitis.[29] Approximately 50% of neonates with encephalitis are premature, and clinical illness typically begins 1 to 3 weeks after birth. Although CNS disease can occur in isolation, more commonly there is evidence of diffuse disease with accompanying skin lesions, hepatitis, pneumonitis, or disseminated intravascular coagulation.[6]

The diagnosis should be suspected in any infant who becomes encephalopathic during the first weeks of life. Skin vesicles are, if present, the easiest source of viral isolation and confirmation of diagnosis, but up to 20% of newborns with HSV infection never have skin involvement.[30] These infants often excrete virus from peripheral sites in the absence of skin lesions; hence, conjunctival, throat, and CSF specimens should be submitted for viral studies. As with HSV-1, PCR testing for HSV-2 DNA in CSF is important to confirm the diagnosis. Further diagnostic evaluation may include EEG, brain scan, CT, ultrasonography, and MRI, alone or in combination, depending on the circumstances. Early empirical treatment with acyclovir is important in decreasing mortality and morbidity rates. Without treatment, the mortality rate is

50% to 85% and the morbidity rate is 100%. A new larger-dose regimen of acyclovir at 20 mg/kg every 8 hours for 21 days is the current recommended dose for neonatal HSVE.[31] With this larger-dose treatment, the mortality rate has decreased to 5% in neonates and about 40% of survivors develop normally.

Varicella Zoster Virus

Primary VZV infection (chickenpox) is only rarely complicated by encephalitis, aseptic meningitis, transverse myelitis, or Guillain-Barré syndrome. There are two forms of encephalitis with primary VZV.[32,33] The cerebellar form is seen in children and occurs with a frequency of 1 per 1000 cases of chickenpox. It is characterized by ataxia, nystagmus, headache, nausea, vomiting, and nuchal rigidity. This illness is usually self-limited, lasting 2 to 4 weeks, and most children have a complete recovery. The mortality rate is only 0.5%.[34] A more severe form of encephalitis occurs mostly in adults and infants, with an incidence of one to two episodes per 10,000 cases of VZV. It most often begins about 1 week after the varicella rash and is manifested by altered sensorium, seizures, and focal neurologic signs; it has a mortality rate of 5% to 10%.[33]

After chickenpox ends, the virus becomes latent, but it may reactivate later in the form of shingles (herpes zoster). Viral invasion of the CNS is not uncommon with zoster, occurring in 35% of patients in one study.[35] However, CNS complications of zoster such as meningoencephalitis or myelitis are rare. Zoster encephalitis may take the form of a stroke. This is more commonly observed in the elderly and can occur weeks to months after an episode of herpes zoster, typically involving the first division of the trigeminal nerve. It is thought that VZV directly invades cerebral arteries by extension along intracranial branches of the trigeminal nerve. Diagnosis is usually supported by angiography. The mortality rate is 20% to 25%, and there is a strong probability of permanent neurologic sequelae.[33]

Chronic zoster encephalitis is seen almost exclusively in immunocompromised patients, especially those with AIDS. The presentation is subacute, with headache, fever, mental status changes, seizures, and focal neurologic signs. The onset may occur months after the zoster rash, making the diagnosis more difficult. The clinical course is often progressive deterioration and death.[33]

A fulminant necrotizing zoster encephalitis with concomitant lymphoma related to Epstein-Barr virus (EBV) and CMV ventriculitis in an AIDS patient has been reported.[36] This highlights the potential for simultaneous infection with multiple pathogens in immunodeficient patients.

The diagnosis of VZV encephalitis may be suspected on the basis of the characteristic lesions of varicella or zoster. The virus may be identified from vesicular scrapings on immunofluorescence, electron microscopy, or culture.[27] The virus grows slowly, usually requiring 2 to 3 weeks for a positive culture. Serologic recognition of the presence of specific immunoglobulin M (IgM) may be useful for diagnosing primary chickenpox. It has been noted that primary varicella encephalitis and zoster encephalitis can occur in the absence of any rash.[37,38] As with HSVE, PCR analysis of CSF VZV DNA and VZV antibody may be used to confirm the diagnosis.[39] Intravenous acyclovir is the drug of choice for

VZV encephalitis, at doses of 10 mg/kg every 8 hours. In one study, foscarnet was added and a favorable outcome was reported in one patient with zoster encephalitis who was not responding to acyclovir alone.[40]

Cytomegalovirus

CMV encephalitis (CMVE) is not uncommon in immunocompromised patients.[41,42] The presentation is typically subacute, with lethargy, confusion, cranial nerve palsies, and coma being prominent clinical features. A large majority of these patients has AIDS, and most have a history of another CMV disease, especially retinitis. CSF viral cultures are typically negative. PCR detection for the presence of CMV DNA in CSF has a sensitivity of 79% and a specificity of 95%.[42] Unfortunately, it does not always correlate with histologic evidence of encephalitis in immunocompromised patients.[43] A high level of CMV DNA in the CSF may be an indicator of significant CMV encephalitis. MRI is more sensitive than CT and characteristically demonstrates periventricular enhancement. The diagnosis is especially challenging in AIDS patients because the clinical presentation is widely variable and because there may be coexisting processes including HIV encephalopathy, toxoplasmic encephalitis, CNS lymphoma, or coinfection with HSV or VZV.[41,42]

CMVE is rare in immunocompetent individuals but has been reported.[42,44] Patients tend to be relatively young, 20 to 64 years. The pathogenesis is unclear. The typical clinical picture is similar to that of HSVE, with severe headache, fever, and focal neurologic signs. CSF examination shows a mild pleocytosis, and the EEG may be markedly abnormal. Differentiation from HSVE requires specific virologic studies. In contrast to AIDS patients, in whom progressive deterioration is the rule, immunocompetent patients with CMVE usually recover but may have long-term sequelae.

Ganciclovir, a nucleoside analogue, is the accepted antiviral agent of choice for CMV.[25,42] The standard dose is 5.0 mg/kg intravenously every 12 hours, given for 2 to 3 weeks. Dosage must be adjusted in patients with renal dysfunction. Possible adverse effects include granulocytopenia, thrombocytopenia, anemia, and elevated serum concentrations of bilirubin, alkaline phosphatase, and creatinine. In AIDS patients adding foscarnet to ganciclovir may be more efficacious.[45]

Epstein-Barr Virus

Neurologic complications occur in fewer than 1% of cases of mononucleosis but are the leading cause of death in infections with EBV.[6] CNS manifestations can include aseptic meningitis, Guillain-Barré syndrome, Bell palsy, transverse myelitis, or encephalitis.[27]

EBV encephalitis typically is acute in onset and may be diffuse or focal, with abnormalities localized usually to the cerebellum or temporal lobe. The diagnosis may be readily evident if the encephalitis occurs in the setting of fever, pharyngitis, lymphadenopathy, and positive EBV serology. CSF changes usually demonstrate a mononuclear pleocytosis with fewer than 200 cells per microliter. Atypical lymphocytes may be seen in the CSF. The protein content may be normal or mildly elevated, and the glucose level is usually normal.[27] PCR detection of EBV DNA is a reliable method of diagnosing EBV encephalitis or myelitis.[46] Although EBV encephalitis may be severe, it is usually self-limited, and almost all survivors recover without sequelae. Successful treatment with intravenous ganciclovir has been reported in immunocompromised patients with EBV encephalitis.[47,48]

Arboviruses

Arboviruses are a group of enveloped RNA viruses that are transmitted by insects. There are numerous viruses in this group that are known to cause encephalitis; together, they are the most common cause of encephalitis worldwide.[6] The relative predominance of the different arboviruses depends on the geographic locale, season, and weather conditions (Table 53-3). In temperate climates, infections tend to be seasonal, occurring mainly in the summer when arthropod populations are high. Human beings are incidental hosts and do not play a part in the natural history of the arboviruses that cause encephalitis. Asymptomatic and mild infections are most common. Serologic evidence indicates that the proportion of infections manifested as disease depends on the specific virus and on the age of the host. In eastern equine encephalitis, 1 in 10 to 40 infections results in encephalitis, whereas in Murray Valley encephalitis, only 1 in 1000 infections results in encephalitis. For West Nile virus, approximately 1 in 150 infections result in meningoencephalitis.[49,50] Historically, California serogroup encephalitis was the most frequently reported arbovirus infection in the United States; the number of cases reported has remained relatively constant since the 1970s. In 1994 a case of Powassan encephalitis was reported in Massachusetts. This tick-borne flavivirus illness occurs infrequently, with only 24 confirmed cases having been reported in North America between 1958 and 1994.[51] More recently, West Nile virus has arrived on the North American

continent, and annual cases of West Nile virus meningoencephalitis may surpass those of California serogroup encephalitis.

The pathogenesis of arbovirus encephalitis is believed to begin with an initial viremia followed by localization in the CNS. The virus likely crosses the blood-brain barrier by infected cells that migrate through the blood vessels of the brain. Once within the CNS, the virus may replicate in neurons or glial elements.

The clinical features of the different arbovirus encephalitides are presented in Table 53-4. In general, arbovirus encephalitides follow the typical pattern of acute onset of fever, headache, and meningismus, with progression to an alteration in mental status. Examination of the CSF usually shows fewer than 500 leukocytes per microliter; most leukocytes are mononuclear, although early on there may be a PMN predominance. The protein content is usually normal or slightly elevated. The glucose level is characteristically normal. Virus isolation is rare; hence, distinguishing among the different viruses requires careful consideration of epidemiologic and clinical variables in addition to serology.[52-56] There is an enzyme immunoassay that detects virus-specific IgM antibodies in blood or CSF of patients with suspected Japanese B encephalitis.[57] Similarly, the diagnosis of West Nile virus encephalitis can be established by the presence of IgM antibody in blood or CSF.[50] Molecular assays are also rapidly becoming more available.

At present, there is no proven antiviral therapy for arboviral encephalitis. In vitro activity of interferon α against West Nile virus and other flaviviruses has been demonstrated. Open clinical trials using interferon α for patients with St. Louis encephalitis and Japanese encephalitis have produced promising results. During an Israeli outbreak of West Nile virus infection in 2000, large-dose ribavirin was given without detectable benefit. Immunoglobulin from patients previously

TABLE 53-3 Epidemiology of the Major Arboviruses

Disease	Virus	Vector	Reservoir	Geographic Location	Approximate Number of U.S. Cases/Year
Eastern equine encephalitis	Togavirus (alphavirus)	Mosquito	Birds	North, Central, and South America (especially Atlantic and Gulf states)	0–12
Western equine encephalitis	Togavirus (alphavirus)	Mosquito	Birds	North, Central, and South America (in U.S. in regions west of the Mississippi; in Canada in prairie provinces)	3–50
Venezuelan equine encephalitis	Togavirus (alphavirus)	Mosquito	Horses	Florida, Texas, Central, and South America	0–5
St. Louis encephalitis	Flavivirus	Mosquito	Birds (especially chickens)	North, Central, and South America	20–2500
West Nile meningoencephalitis	Flavivirus	Mosquito	Birds (especially Corvidae family)	North and Central America, Africa, parts of Asia and southern Europe	20–2500
Japanese B encephalitis	Flavivirus	Mosquito	Pigs and birds	Asia (especially southern and eastern Asia)	0
Murray Valley encephalitis	Flavivirus	Mosquito	Birds	Australia, New Guinea	0
California (La Crosse) encephalitis	Bunyavirus	Mosquito	Rodents	Midwestern U.S.	50–200

TABLE 53-4 Clinical Aspects of Arbovirus Infection

Disease	Clinical Features	Morbidity and Mortality Rates in Patients Who Develop Encephalitis
EEE	Mainly affects children and the elderly Abrupt onset with fulminant course Seizures are common; diffuse signs	50–75% mortality rate; 30% of survivors have severe sequelae: mental retardation, behavior changes, seizures, and paralysis
Western equine encephalitis	Mainly affects infants and the elderly Subclinical infections are common Similar to EEE but milder (except in infants)	3–7% mortality rate; fewer sequelae than with EEE
Venezuelan equine encephalitis	Many subclinical infections <4% develop encephalitis Myalgias are prominent	10–20% mortality rate
St. Louis encephalitis	<1% infected people develop encephalitis Most severe in elderly May have tremor, seizures, paresis, syndrome of inappropriate antidiuretic hormone, urinary symptoms	5–15% mortality rate; mortality rate increase with age; neurasthenia may be a persistent problem
Japanese B encephalitis	Most common arbovirus worldwide Mainly among children <2% of infected develop encephalitis A vaccine is available	10–50% mortality rate, especially among children; up to 70% of survivors have neuropsychiatric sequelae
Murray Valley encephalitis	Patients frequently present in coma Rapid disease progression in infants	20–50% mortality rate; 40–100% of survivors have neurologic sequelae
California (La Crosse) Encephalitis	Mainly affects boys (ages 3–10 y) Fulminant onset with seizures Rapid recovery after 2–5 d	<2% mortality rate; up to 15% have behavioral problems or recurrent seizures
West Nile meningoencephalitis	Incubation period 2–14 d 1 in 150 people infected develop encephalitis More severe in the elderly 1–7 d febrile prodrome May have polio-like flaccid paralysis	4–14% mortality rate for patients admitted to the hospital; higher in the elderly

ABBREVIATIONS: EEE, eastern equine encephalitis.

infected with West Nile virus has been given to some patients and is being considered for clinical trials.[50] The mortality and morbidity rates depend on the specific arbovirus and the age and health of the patient.

Enteroviruses

Enteroviruses are very common causes of meningitis but cause only a small proportion of cases of encephalitis. They rank behind arboviruses, HSV, and lymphocytic choriomeningitis virus as causes of encephalitis that proved to be viral in the United States. Enteroviruses are distributed worldwide, and infections are most prevalent in the summer and autumn months in the temperate climates. At least 50% to 80% of nonpolio enteroviral infections are completely asymptomatic.[58] When encephalitis develops, the signs and symptoms may vary, from lethargy, drowsiness, and personality changes to seizures, paresis, and coma. The clinical findings suggest generalized involvement in most cases, but focal abnormalities, including partial motor seizures, hemichorea, and acute cerebellar ataxia, have been reported. Enteroviral encephalitis can mimic HSVE, and distinguishing CNS enteroviral infection from other bacterial and viral causes of encephalitis can be clinically difficult.

CSF examination typically shows 10 to 500 leukocytes per microliter, with a lymphocytic predominance, although neutrophils may predominate early in infection. The CSF protein content is normal or slightly elevated, and the glucose level is normal. In the past, the diagnosis was established by culture of virus from the CSF. However, CSF viral cultures were often negative, and the diagnosis had to be inferred from isolation of virus from non-neurologic sites, such as throat washings or feces. More recently, PCR detection of enterovirus RNA in CSF has become the optimal method for confirming the diagnosis.[59]

The course of illness is generally benign, and treatment is supportive. However, neonates may develop a severe illness culminating in death, and infants younger than 1 year often have persistent neurologic sequelae. In addition, patients with antibody deficiencies may have severe infection. A syndrome of chronic enteroviral meningoencephalitis occurs in agammaglobulinemia.[60] Most of these patients present with a dermatomyositis-like syndrome and many have hepatitis. The course is prolonged, and clinical manifestations may vary and fluctuate. Neurologic manifestations include headaches, seizures, lethargy or coma, weakness, and ataxia. In this syndrome the mortality rate is high. The administration of specific neutralizing antibody has been shown to be effective.[60,61] A case of chronic enteroviral meningoencephalitis also has been reported associated with HIV.[62] Pleconaril may be used to treat patients with serious enteroviral infections. Pleconaril is given orally at a dose of 200 to 400 mg three times daily, although the appropriate dosing has not been clearly established.[62,63] A recent report on two cases of chronic enteroviral meningoencephalitis suggested that perfusion single-photon emission tomographic scans are useful for clinically monitoring treatment.[62]

Poliovirus is a neurotropic enterovirus, but owing to the widespread use of polio vaccines, the incidence of poliovirus infection has dramatically declined. Poliomyelitis still occurs in patients who have not received the vaccine and in underdeveloped countries. Rarely, paralytic polio develops in association with the use of the live vaccine. Currently, this is a very rare event, given that inactivated poliovirus vaccine has largely replaced oral poliovirus vaccine. Paralysis occurs in 0.1% of all poliovirus infections. In adults, poliomyelitis often begins with muscle pain, particularly involving the neck or lumbar region. This pain may be relieved by motion. Subsequently, there is progression to weakness and paralysis, usually over 2 to 3 days. A characteristic feature of the paralysis of poliomyelitis is its asymmetric distribution. Another key point to note in the clinical diagnosis of poliomyelitis is that sensation is usually preserved. If sensory loss is present, then an alternate diagnosis should be considered. Poliomyelitis very rarely takes the form of encephalitis.[64] When poliovirus encephalitis does occur, it is seen principally in infants. It is manifested primarily by disturbances in consciousness. In addition, seizures and spastic paralysis may be seen. The illness is not distinguishable clinically from encephalitis due to many other viruses. The diagnosis is established when virus is isolated from the CSF. Unfortunately, it is rare to isolate poliovirus from these patients. Most often, throat and stool cultures should be taken, in addition to acute and convalescent sera. PCR technology promises to aid in the confirmation of the diagnosis.[59]

Enterovirus 71 is a picornavirus that can cause an epidemic paralytic disease indistinguishable from poliomyelitis. Like other enteroviruses, it may cause hand-foot-mouth disease. Paralysis may be accompanied by encephalitis or cranial nerve involvement. The diagnosis is established when enterovirus 71 is isolated from vesicle fluid, feces, oropharyngeal sections, urine, or CSF. The treatment is supportive. The mortality rate is 29.5% in patients with paralytic disease but increases to as high as 65% in patients with bulbar disease.[65]

Lymphocytic Choriomeningitis Virus

Lymphocytic choriomeningitis virus is an arenavirus that is endemic in mice and can be transmitted to human beings.[66] Lymphocytic choriomeningitis virus infection may occur worldwide but has been demonstrated only in Europe and the Americas. Human infection is most commonly seen in young adults, although persons of all ages may be affected. Most cases occur in the autumn. The exact mode of transmission is not known but may be related to aerosols, direct contact with rodents, or rodent bites. The incubation period is usually from 5 to 10 days. The illness typically has an influenza-like prodrome followed later by a severe headache. A few patients develop a clinical picture of encephalomyelitis, with confusion, psychosis, paraplegia, or disturbances of cranial, sensory, or autonomic nerve function. Other occasional complications include orchitis, myopericarditis, arthritis, and alopecia. Laboratory findings show a leukopenia and thrombocytopenia. The CSF typically shows several hundred lymphocytes per microliter, with a normal to elevated protein level and a normal to reduced glucose content. Infection is usually diagnosed by a fourfold rise in antibodies or isolation of virus.[27] The treatment is supportive, and rarely is the illness fatal.

Rabies Virus

Rabies virus is usually transmitted to human beings by the bite of an infected mammal, although infection by the respiratory route can occur. In countries where domestic anima rabies is well controlled, most disease is associated with infection from wild animals. Human disease is rare in the United States, with only 36 cases being reported to the Centers for Disease Control and Prevention from 1980 to 1996.[67] In countries where domestic animal rabies has not been controlled, human rabies remains a significant problem. In 1996, 33,209 cases of human rabies were reported to the World Health Organization, but, because this reporting is voluntary, it underestimates the actual number of cases.[68] The incubation period is usually 20 to 90 days, although in reported cases it has varied from 4 days to 19 years. During the incubation period, the patient is well. A prodrome of 2 to 10 days, which may include paresthesia at the bite site, is followed by evidence of CNS infection, which may include agitation, hydrophobia, bizarre behavior, or delirium. About 20% of patients present with a paralytic form. The mental status gradually deteriorates, with disorientation, stupor, and coma.[68,69] The case fatality rate is virtually 100%. No tests are currently available to diagnose rabies infection before the onset of clinical disease. A diagnosis of rabies should be suspected even in the absence of a definitive history of an animal bite because this may be missing in some cases. Diagnosis can be established rapidly by using immunofluorescent procedures to detect viral antigens on biopsy of the skin of the posterior neck. Other methods for diagnosis before death include detecting antibodies to rabies virus in serum or CSF from patients with a long clinical course and virus isolation or nucleic acid detection in saliva.[70] Rabies is a disease that is much easier to prevent than cure. However, cases have occurred even in patients receiving optimal prophylaxis. Patients should be isolated because rabies virus may be present in saliva, tears, urine, CSF, and other body fluids or tissues.

Treatment is supportive, but the outcome is dismal. High-dose passive rabies immunoglobulin has been used in some cases, with no clear benefit.[71] Although no single therapeutic agent is effective, a combination of therapies such as rabies vaccine, rabies immunoglobulin, monoclonal antibodies, ribavirin, interferon α, and ketamine may be considered.[72]

Two survivors in a review of 38 human rabies cases in the United States received rabies vaccine before the onset of their illness and intensive supportive care after the onset of illness.[69]

Human Immunodeficiency Virus

HIV is a neurotropic pathogen that may cause CNS disease varying from aseptic meningitis to encephalitis resulting in dementia and death (see Chap. 48 for more details). Postmortem studies of patients dying of HIV-related complications have suggested that CNS infection is always present, even when it is not clinically apparent. The diagnosis should be suspected in patients with encephalitis who have risk factors for or clinical evidence of HIV infection. Serology is used to confirm HIV infection, but there are no good means at present of antemortem diagnosis of CNS disease. Measurement of CSF levels of HIV RNA might prove to be a useful monitor of CNS infection.[73]

Measles

Measles is an acute infection caused by a paramyxovirus. This virus is highly contagious and causes infections with a worldwide distribution. It remains a significant problem, especially in unimmunized children and adults. Acute postinfectious measles encephalomyelitis is the most common neurologic complication of measles. Although it is rare in children younger than 2 years, it complicates approximately 1 of 1000 measles infections in older children.[74] It probably has an autoimmune pathogenesis.[75] The illness is of abrupt onset and typically begins 1 week after the onset of the rash. However, it has been reported to have occurred before the onset of the rash or weeks after. The illness is manifest by recurrence of fever, seizures, motor abnormalities, and a depressed level of consciousness. The abrupt onset of the encephalomyelitis in the setting of the typical exanthem is a characteristic feature that helps to differentiate postinfectious encephalomyelitis from other forms of viral encephalitis that have a more gradual onset. The CSF is normal in approximately 33% of patients. Neither viral RNA nor measles-specific antibody is present in the CSF. However, antibodies to myelin basic protein are present in the CSF. Up to 50% of patients with measles have detectable EEG abnormalities.[76] MRI is a sensitive modality.[77] Treatment is supportive; the mortality rate is 10% to 20%, and most survivors have neurologic sequelae.[74]

A less common complication of measles infection is SSPE, which occurs in about 1 in 300,000 cases. SSPE occurs months to years after measles, most often in children. Although the exact pathogenesis is unknown, it appears that persistent infection results from defective viral production of membrane or envelope proteins, which allow the virus to escape immunosurveillance.[78] The onset is insidious, with subtle personality changes and declining intellectual performance. The disease is progressive, with mental deterioration followed by convulsive and motor signs and invariably coma and death.[79] The most useful laboratory findings in SSPE include an abnormal EEG with the typical pattern consisting of well-defined periodic bursts of high-voltage activity with an interval of 3 to 5 seconds between bursts and increased levels of γ globulin and measles antibody in CSF or detection of viral RNA.[80–82] Biopsy is not considered necessary for the diagnosis because the clinical findings combined with the finding of measles antibody or viral RNA in the CSF are sufficient to establish the diagnosis in almost all cases. There is no well-established effective treatment for this condition; however, isoprinosine (inosiplex) has been reported to produce remission for longer than 2 years in 5 of 15 patients in one study.[83] Other reports have described mixed benefits.[84–86] Combination therapy with interferon α, ribavirin, and inosiplex has been described in one case report.[87]

Subacute measle encephalitis (SME) is a third form of measles encephalitis. SME occurs mainly in immunosuppressed children in whom it acts like an opportunistic infection. Measles virus RNA can be detected in the brain of SME patients, and it follows a rapidly progressive course. More recently, one case report documented SME in an immunocompetent adult.[88]

Mumps

Meningitis occurs in 15% of mumps cases, although CSF abnormalities may occur in up to 50%. Meningitis is a common benign condition, to be distinguished from encephalitis, which is rare and more serious. Encephalitis occurs in approximately 1 in 6000 cases of mumps.[89] There is bimodal distribution of illness: an early-onset illness that coincides with parotitis and represents damage to neurons directly due to viral invasion, and a more common late-onset illness that develops 7 to 10 days after the onset of parotitis and is a postinfectious demyelinating process.

The clinical features are diffuse encephalitis with fever, marked change in level of consciousness, seizures, paresis, aphasia, and involuntary movements. The CSF examination shows the typical picture of viral meningoencephalitis, with a lymphocytic pleocytosis and a normal or slightly elevated CSF protein level. However, there may be a PMN cell predominance and hypoglycorrhachia. No rapid procedures are available for diagnosing mumps.[24,65] Virus may be isolated from CSF on tissue culture. Serology may be used to confirm the diagnosis. Encephalitis may occur secondary to mumps in the absence of parotitis. The treatment is supportive, and sequelae of psychomotor retardation and convulsive disorders have been reported. The mortality rate is 1.4%.[66] Other neurologic syndromes rarely associated with mumps include deafness, cerebellar ataxia, facial palsy, transverse myelitis, ascending polyradiculitis, and a poliomyelitis-like syndrome.

Nipah Virus

A paramyxovirus, Nipah virus, was identified as the etiologic agent of an outbreak of severe encephalitis in Malaysia and Singapore that occurred among people who had close contact exposure to pigs.[90] Nipah virus is closely related to another zoonotic paramyxovirus, Hendra virus, which infects horses and rarely humans. Both viruses have the ability to infect a broad range of species. After an incubation period of 10 days, patients present with nonspecific symptoms such as fever, headache, myalgia, sore throat, and altered mental state.[91,92] Other clinical features may include segmental myoclonus, areflexia, hypertension, and tachycardia. The mortality rate reported from the outbreak in Malaysia was 41%.[92] An open-label trial of ribavirin for treatment has suggested some benefit.[93]

Rubella

Encephalitis is a rare postinfectious complication of rubella. It occurs with a frequency of approximately 1 in 3000 to 1 in 24,000 rubella patients.[94] It occurs more frequently in adults than in children.[95] The symptoms are similar to but milder than those seen with measles. Diagnosis maybe established on the basis of serology or on the detection of anti–rubella virus IgM in the CSF. The treatment is supportive. The case fatality rate has been found to vary between 0% and 30%.[94] A rubella SSPE-like syndrome occurs mainly in young adults, as opposed to measles-associated SSPE, which tends to occur in children.

Mycoplasma Pneumoniae

Mycoplasma pneumoniae is a frequent cause of upper and lower respiratory tract infections in otherwise healthy people. Approximately 1 in 1000 patients with *M. pneumoniae* respiratory disease develop complicating CNS disease.[96] The pathogenesis of the CNS disease is unclear; however, it has been postulated that the disease may result from direct invasion by the organism, a neurotoxin elaborated by the organism, or an autoimmune reaction precipitated by the *Mycoplasma* infection.[96,97] Multiple patterns of CNS involvement associated with *M. pneumoniae* have been reported. These include meningitis, encephalitis, psychosis, cerebellar ataxia, hemiplegia, transverse myelitis, and polyradiculitis.[98] The encephalitis may be focal, mimicking HSVE, or nonfocal. Most patients have antecedent respiratory symptoms. In encephalitis, the CSF usually shows a lymphocytic predominance combined with a moderate elevation of the protein content and a normal glucose level. *Mycoplasma pneumoniae* genomic material has been identified in cases of encephalitis related to mycoplasmal disease by using PCR techniques after CSF was collected early in the disease process.[99] *Mycoplasma pneumoniae* has rarely been identified histologically or recovered from biopsy specimens. In the absence of PCR, the diagnosis can be established by serology. The treatment is mainly supportive, and no controlled prospective trials have evaluated the role of antibiotics. However, intravenous tetracycline would seem to be an appropriate agent. The mortality rate was 5% in one series and 23% had severe sequelae.[96]

Rocky Mountain Spotted Fever

Encephalitis may occur as a complication of Rocky Mountain spotted fever. This disease is caused by *Rickettsia rickettsii* and is transmitted by the bite of an infected tick. It is seen most frequently in the eastern United States, especially in younger people. The illness is characterized by the sudden onset of fever, malaise, headache, chills, and conjunctival injection. This is followed 2 to 3 days later by a maculopapular rash that appears first on the wrist and ankles and then rapidly spreads to the rest of the body, including the palms and soles. The rash is often petechial or may become confluent and hemorrhagic. Routine laboratory tests for rapid diagnosis early in the illness are not readily available. A fourfold rise in antibody titer between acute- and convalescent-phase sera is considered diagnostic. PCR detection has been reported, but its clinical usefulness has not been established.[100] Doxycycline or other tetracycline is considered by many to be the agent of choice, but chloramphenicol is preferred in pregnant patients.[101] Unfortunately, neurologic involvement with this disease is associated with a bad prognosis. Of 37 patients followed for 1 to 8 years after acute Rocky Mountain spotted fever, 21 had residual neurologic abnormalities.[102]

Bacillus Anthracis

Since the events of September 11, 2001 and the months following in the United States, anthrax meningoencephalitis (AME) has moved up the differential diagnostic list of meningoencephalitis because of the possibility of a bioterrorist act. Patients with AME present with fever, headache, nausea, vomiting, meningeal signs, and altered mentation associated with symptoms and signs related to the source of infection.[103] The three main sources of infection are cutaneous, inhalational, and gastrointestinal. The CSF studies typically show findings of hemorrhagic meningitis. Gram-stained smears of CSF may show large gram-positive bacilli suggestive of *Bacillus anthracis*. The organism will subsequently grow on CSF culture. PCR testing may be used to rapidly detect anthrax DNA in CSF.[104] Blood cultures are positive in approximately 70% of cases. Chest radiographs are usually abnormal in those with inhalational anthrax, with findings including pleural effusion, hilar adenopathy, widened mediastinum, infiltrates, and soft tissue edema. CT or MRI of the head in these patients may show focal intracerebral hemorrhage, subarachnoid hemorrhage, intraventricular hemorrhage, diffuse cerebral edema, or prominent leptomeningeal enhancement.

The prognosis for AME is not good, with 75% of patients dead within 24 hours of presentation. Survival rate is at most 15%, but there have been no reported cases in the world literature of survival after AME associated with inhalational anthrax. The Centers for Disease Control and Prevention have indicated that ciprofloxacin or doxycycline should be included as essential components of initial treatment for anthrax from any portal of entry. Rifampin plus vancomycin would be reasonable to add given the concern of possible antibiotic resistance in bioengineered strains.[103] Antianthrax serum and/or steroids have been recommended for consideration as adjunct agents in AME.

Brucella

Brucella, like anthrax, is a potential bioterrorism threat. Symptoms of brucella are nonspecific and include fever, sweats, malaise, anorexia, headache, and back pain. Brucellosis may involve any organ or system. Invasion of the CNS occurs in fewer than 5% of cases. Complications in the nervous system include meningitis most frequently, and encephalitis, myelitis-radiculoneuronitis, brain abscess, epidural abscess, demyelinating syndromes, and meningovascular syndromes. CSF shows a lymphocytic pleocytosis, elevated protein, and low to normal glucose levels. The diagnosis of brucellosis is generally made by recovering brucella from blood culture. CNS disease can be confirmed by culturing brucella from CSF, but cultures are positive in only about 25%. The diagnosis also can be established by detecting antibodies in the CSF. Doxycycline with trimethoprim-sulfamethoxazole and rifampin has been used to successfully treat neurobrucellosis. When the CNS is involved with brucella, therapy is often continued for 6 to 9 months.[105]

Cat Scratch Disease

Bartonella (formerly *Rochalimaea*) *henselae* has been shown to be the cause of cat scratch disease. Case reports of a variety of

CNS manifestations have been reported in cases of cat scratch disease, including encephalitis, myelitis, radiculitis, and cerebellar ataxia.[106] PCR has been used in a number of reports to identify *B. henselae* in tissue; however, such testing currently is not widely available.[107] The initial therapy of choice for these infections is doxycycline or erythromycin.[108]

Lyme Disease

Lyme disease is the most common vector-borne infection in North America and Europe. It is a multisystem disease that results from infection with the spirochete *Borrelia burgdorferi* transmitted by a tick bite.[109] Neurologic involvement occurs in 15% to 25% of patients, usually occurring weeks to months after infection. The typical pattern is fluctuating symptoms of meningitis with superimposed cranial or peripheral radiculoneuropathies. Acute or chronic encephalomyelitis may also occur. In patients with CNS involvement, the CSF may show a lymphocytic pleocytosis with elevated protein levels. Unfortunately, a test that uniformly indicates active infection in the CNS is lacking. The diagnosis has traditionally been made when patients with a clinically compatible illness are demonstrated to have positive serology. With the advent of PCR techniques, the difficult diagnosis of Lyme neuroborreliosis may be more firmly established in suspected cases.[110] In patients who have Lyme disease with neurologic abnormalities, the recommended treatment is ceftriaxone 2 g daily for 2 to 4 weeks.

Leptospirosis

Leptospirosis is a multisystem disease that may involve the CNS.[111] It is caused by spirochetes of the genus *Leptospira* and is a zoonosis of worldwide distribution. Humans become infected by direct or indirect contact with infected animals or by recreational exposure, especially in South Atlantic, Gulf, and Pacific coastal states in the United States (especially, in Hawaii). Subclinical infection occurs commonly. Clinical infection is commonly mild and anicteric; however, there is a severe icteric form. Leptospirosis is typically a biphasic illness, beginning with a septicemic phase characterized by an abrupt onset of fever, headache, myalgias, and nausea and vomiting. This persists for 4 to 7 days and is followed by a second or immune phase when fever is usually low grade or absent. The headache during this stage is characteristically intense and may be accompanied by mild delirium. Common physical findings include muscle tenderness, conjunctival suffusion, adenopathy, hepatosplenomegaly, and rashes. Examination of the CSF demonstrates a mild mononuclear pleocytosis with a normal or slightly elevated protein level. In this milder form of leptospirosis, focal neurologic signs and evidence of encephalitis are uncommon.

In icteric leptospirosis, the illness is more severe and is characterized by impaired renal and hepatic function, hemorrhage, myocarditis, and severe alterations in consciousness. The definitive diagnosis requires isolation of the organism or seroconversion. With the use of specialized media, the organisms may be isolated from the blood or CSF during the first 10 days of the illness or from the urine during the second week. PCR, where available, may be helpful in the detection of *Leptospira*.[112] Treatment consists of intravenous penicillin and general supportive therapy to manage the life-threatening complications of renal failure, hypotension, and hemorrhage. The mortality rate in the more severe cases is between 5% and 10%.[111]

Cryptococcus Neoformans

Cryptococcosis is a systemic infection caused by the ubiquitous yeast-like fungus *Cryptococcus neoformans*. Infection most frequently occurs in patients who are immunocompromised, especially those with AIDS. Infection tends to localize to the CNS. Onset may be abrupt in patients receiving corticosteroid therapy or those receiving treatment for lymphoreticular malignancies, but most frequently it is insidious, with mild and nonspecific complaints such as headache, irritability, somnolence, and clumsiness. Often there are behavioral changes. On physical examination, the patient is frequently afebrile with minimal or no nuchal rigidity. Papilledema is noted in about 33% of cases, and cranial nerve palsies are seen in about 20%.[113] CSF examination may show an elevated opening pressure with elevated protein content, decreased glucose level, and small numbers of leukocytes. It should be emphasized that in AIDS patients there are minimal or no abnormalities of the CSF, but cryptococci grow in culture. In 50% of patients with cryptococcal meningoencephalitis, the organism may be identified in India ink smears of CSF. Latex agglutination detects antigen in CSF, but positive tests must be confirmed by cultures before a definite diagnosis of cryptococcosis can be made. The recommended treatment is amphotericin B at a dose of 0.7 mg/kg body weight daily intravenously for 2 weeks followed by fluconazole 400 mg daily for at least 10 weeks.[114] Eradication of infection seldom, if ever, occurs in AIDS patients. Even after a 6-week course of amphotericin, the relapse rate was 50% to 60%.[115] It is therefore currently recommended that AIDS patients receive fluconazole, 200 to 400 mg daily, indefinitely after initial therapy with amphotericin.[113,116] The benefits of larger doses of fluconazole have yet to be determined. Even in immunocompetent hosts, the mortality rate in treated cryptococcal meningoencephalitis is approximately 25% to 30%.[113,117]

Toxoplasmosis

Toxoplasma gondii is the causative agent in toxoplasmosis. It is an obligate intracellular protozoan parasite that infects virtually all mammalian species and has a worldwide distribution. Toxoplasmic encephalitis historically was a relatively rare disease seen sporadically in immunocompromised patients, in particular those with malignancies of the reticuloendothelial system and organ transplant recipients. However, this disease has risen to prominence in association with AIDS. It is now recognized as the most common cause of intracerebral mass lesions in AIDS patients.[118] It is believed that toxoplasmic encephalitis results from reactivation of chronic latent infection. Clinically, the CNS manifestations of toxoplasmosis are nonspecific and highly variable. They may take the form of cerebral mass lesions, meningoencephalitis, or diffuse encephalitis. Focal abnormalities are common and include focal seizures, hemiparesis, hemiplegia, cerebellar tremor, cranial nerve palsies, personality changes, and severe headache. Generalized abnormalities may also occur, including weakness, myoclonus, confusion, lethargy, and coma. Immunocompromised patients with toxoplasmosis have predominantly CNS manifestations; however, extraneural manifestations of the disease include chorioretinitis, pneumonitis, myocarditis, orchitis, and peritonitis.[108]

CSF examination of patients with toxoplasmic encephalitis generally shows an elevated protein content with a mononuclear pleocytosis of up to several hundred cells per microliter. The glucose level is normal or slightly depressed. However, results of CSF analysis may be completely normal. CT of the brain in AIDS patients with cerebral toxoplasmosis visualizes abnormalities in more than 90% of patients.[119,120] Most commonly, the lesions are in the region of the basal ganglia, midbrain, or brain stem and are rounded and hypodense with peripheral "ring" enhancement, but they may show diffuse or no contrast enhancement. Lesions may be single or multiple, with multiple lesions being more specific for toxoplasmosis. MRI is reportedly more sensitive than CT.[121]

The diagnostic serologic changes associated with toxoplasmosis infection in immunocompetent individuals are seldom seen in AIDS patients with toxoplasmic encephalitis. Moreover, although negative toxoplasmosis serology in AIDS patients reduces the likelihood of toxoplasmosis infection, there are several reports of false-negative tests.[122,123] Local antibody production to *T. gondii* in the CSF is specific but lacks sensitivity and therefore is of limited diagnostic usefulness. PCR has been used to amplify parts of the *T. gondii* genome and appears promising for diagnosis.[124] Larger studies are required to characterize the role of PCR, especially in light of the current recommendations for empirical therapy.

In AIDS patients with suspected toxoplasmic encephalitis, it is desirable to have a confirmed diagnosis because similar lesions may be due to tuberculosis, other bacteria, fungi, or lymphoma. Hence, AIDS patients who have encephalitis that is clinically and radiographically compatible with toxoplasmosis are usually given a therapeutic trial with pyrimethamine and sulfadiazine. Biopsy is reserved for patients who fail to respond to therapy or whose neurologic status is rapidly deteriorating. Clinical and radiographic responses to therapy should be seen within 10 days of starting therapy. The standard treatment regimen is pyrimethamine (a 200-mg oral loading dose followed by 50 to 75 mg/day orally), folinic acid (10 to 20 mg/day orally or intravenously), and sulfadiazine (1 to 1.5 g orally every 6 hours).[125] This therapy is continued for at least 6 weeks. In AIDS patients, discontinuation of therapy has been associated frequently with relapse of toxoplasmic encephalitis, and maintenance therapy should be continued indefinitely. Toxoplasmosis occasionally progresses to death even with appropriate therapy.

Acanthamoeba

Granulomatous amebic encephalitis (GAE) is caused *by Acanthamoeba castellani, Acanthamoeba culbertsoni, Acanthamoeba astronyxis, Acanthamoeba palestinensis,* and *Balamuthia mandrillaris.* These are free-living amebae that have been isolated from soil, water, and air from diverse geographic locations. GAE is a subacute opportunistic infection that spreads hematogenously from pulmonary or skin lesions to the CNS. It occurs predominantly in debilitated or immunosuppressed

individuals. Typically these patients present with mental status abnormalities, seizures, fever, headache, and hemiparesis. They may also demonstrate meningismus, visual disturbances, or ataxia. The diagnosis is frequently made postmortem. Brain biopsy is the only way to make the diagnosis antemortem. Little is known about the treatment of GAE; however, it has been recognized that the diamidine derivatives (pentamidine) have the greatest activity against *Acanthamoeba.*[126]

Naegleria

Naegleria fowleri is another free-living ameba that causes primary amebic meningoencephalitis (PAM). This ameba has been isolated from soil, river, and lake water and is especially prominent in warmer thermally polluted freshwater lakes. PAM appears primarily in healthy children and young adults who have a history of recent swimming in warm fresh water. The illness is characterized by abrupt onset of fever, nausea and vomiting, headache, and meningismus. The encephalitis is fulminant and in most patients progresses to coma and death. CSF examination typically shows a neutrophilic pleocytosis, elevated protein level, and normal or reduced glucose value. Gram stain shows pus cells but no bacteria. However, if a wet mount is made of the CSF, motile trophozoites of *N. fowleri* may be seen. Molecular methods to rapidly and specifically diagnose *Naegleria* infections are a recent development. Only six patients are known to have survived PAM. Their treatment included large-dose systemic and intrathecal amphotericin B. Passive immunotherapy with anti-*Naegleria* immune serum or an anti-*Naegleria* monoclonal antibody may in the future prove to be useful adjunctive therapy.[126]

Supportive Therapy in the Intensive Care Unit

Intensive supportive care is indicated in patients with encephalitis because these patients may make remarkable recoveries even after prolonged periods of unconsciousness.

The usual first principles of establishing and maintaining airway patency, oxygenation, and adequate ventilation in patients with disordered CNS function should be applied. A poor gag reflex and ineffective cough are markers of the need for airway protection. Special care must be taken in the intubation of patients with suspected encephalomyelitis to prevent potentially catastrophic increases in ICP. Intubation should be performed early in an elective fashion by an experienced person. Hypotension is also dangerous for patients with increased ICP and, if present, should be treated with intravenous fluids and appropriate inotropic support.

Strict monitoring of fluid, electrolyte, and glucose balance is necessary because of the possibility of hypothalamic involvement in the encephalitic process. Moreover, depending on the specific etiologic agent of encephalitis, there may be concurrent dysfunction of other organ systems compromising the patient's normal mechanisms of autoregulation and homeostasis. Nutrition must be maintained, preferably with enteral alimentation, but parenteral nutritional support may be necessary. Routine skin and eye care should not be neglected.

Although controversial, ICP monitoring is advocated by some for adults with severe encephalitis. Treatment of increased ICP has been required in up to 75% of patients in some series.[5] Major rises in ICP may lead to further neurologic compromise or death. Elevated ICP has been associated with a poor prognosis.[127] Therapy for raised ICP includes optimizing head position, hyperventilation to maintain a partial pressure of CO_2 of 25 or 30 mm Hg, osmotic agents such as mannitol (100 g in 500 mL of 5% dextrose in water) infused intravenously over 10 to 20 minutes every 4 to 6 hours, as needed, in an effort to keep the ICP below 20 mm Hg (see Chap. 65).

Seizures are also a recognized complication of encephalitis and are best managed by phenytoin at a loading dose of 15 to 18 mg/kg. This should be infused at a rate not exceeding 50 mg/min in a glucose-free solution to prevent precipitation. Transient hypotension and heart block can occur during intravenous phenytoin administration, so blood pressure and electrocardiographic monitoring are required. A therapeutic plasma level of 10 to 20 mg/mL is usually achieved with a daily maintenance dose of phenytoin of 300 to 500 mg (4 to 8 mg/kg). This dose may be given intravenously or orally. The half-life of phenytoin is long (36 hours); therefore, a steady state is not achieved until 5 to 7 days have elapsed.

If seizures persist despite loading with phenytoin, then phenobarbital may need to be added (see Chap. 64). One should not assume that the seizures are secondary to the encephalitis until other treatable precipitating causes, such as structural or metabolic abnormalities, have been ruled out. Complications of prolonged seizures may include cerebral edema, aspiration, rhabdomyolysis, myoglobinuria, hyperthermia, and hypoxia. These should be treated as they arise. Extreme hyperthermia may develop secondary to the encephalitis itself and be an aggravating cause of seizures. It should be controlled by appropriate cooling measures. Medical and nursing staffs frequently ask questions about contagiousness. Except for a very few causes of encephalomyelitis, there is very little risk of disease transmission. Enteric precautions should be exercised when caring for patients with suspected enteroviral (including polio viral) infection. Isolation precautions against respiratory secretions should be taken in patients with suspected tuberculosis, rabies, measles, mumps, or lymphocytic choriomeningitis virus infection. Viral hemorrhagic fevers require strict isolation. Secretions from lesions of patients with VZV are potentially infectious, and appropriate precautions should be used. Standard precautions, including masks, gowns, gloves, and eye protection, should be worn by all personnel participating in acute resuscitation, especially those involved in endotracheal intubation.

References

1. Griffin DE: Encephalitis, myelitis and neuritis, in Mandell GL, Bennett JE, Dolin R (eds): *Mandell, Douglas and Bennett's Principles and Practice of Infectious Diseases*, 5th ed. Philadelphia, Churchill Livingstone, 2000, p 1009.
2. Whitley RJ: Viral encepalitis. *N Engl J Med* 323:242, 1990.
3. Whitley RJ: Herpes simplex virus infections of the central nervous system. *Am J Med* 85(S2A):61, 1988.
4. Whitley RJ, Soong S-J, Linneman C Jr, et al: Herpes simplex encephalitis. *JAMA* 247:317, 1982.
5. Whitley RJ, Alford CA, Hirsch MS, et al: Vidarabine versus acyclovir therapy in herpes simplex encephalitis. *N Engl J Med* 31:144, 1986.
6. Ho DD, Hirsch MS: Acute viral encephalitis. *Med Clin North Am* 69:415, 1985.
7. Koskiniemi M, Vaheri A, Taskinen E: Cerebrospinal fluid alterations in herpes simplex virus encephalitis. *Rev Infect Dis* 6:608, 1984.
8. Lakeman FD, Whitley, RJ, et al: Diagnosis of herpes encephalitis: Application of polymerase chain reaction to cerebral spinal fluid from brain-biopsied patients and correlation with disease. *J Infect Dis* 171:857, 1995.
9. Tebas P, Nease RF, Storch GA: Use of the polymerase chain reaction in the diagnosis of herpes simplex encephalitis:a decision analysis model. *Am J Med* 105:287, 1998.
10. Sauerbrei A, Eichhorn G, Hottenrott G, Wutzler P: Virological diagnosis of herpes simplex encephalitis. *J Clin Virol* 17:31, 2000.
11. Puchhammer-Stockl E, Heinz FX, Kundi M, et al: Evaluation of the polymerase chain reaction for diagnosis of herpes simplex encephalitis. *J Clin Microbiol* 31:146, 1993.
12. Ch'ien LT, Boehm RM, Robinson H, et al: Characteristic early electroencephalographic changes in herpes simplex encephalitis. *Arch Neurol* 34:361, 1977.
13. Schroth G, Gawehn J, Thron A, et al: Early diagnosis of herpes simplex encephalitis by MRI. *Neurology* 37:179, 1987.
14. Demaerel P, et al: MRI of herpes encephalitis. *Neuroradiology* 34:490, 1992.
15. Schroth G: Reply to letter. *Neurology* 38:335, 1988.
16. Domingues RB, Fink MC, Tsanaclis AM, et al: Diagnosis of herpes simplex encephalitis by magnetic resonance imaging and polymerase chain reaction assay of cerebrospinal fluid. *J Neurol Sci* 157:148, 1998.
17. Hasegawa Y, Morishita M, Ikeda T, Suzumura A: Early diagnosis of herpes simplex virus encephalitis by single photon emission computed tomography in patients with normal MRI. *Rinsho Shinkeigaku* 36:475, 1996.
18. Landry M: False positive polymerase chain reaction results in the diagnosis of herpes simplex encephalitis. *J Infect Dis* 172:1641, 1995.
19. Akhan SC, Coskunkan F, Mutlu S, et al: A probable case of herpes simplex encephalitis despite negative PCR findings. *Infection* 29:359, 2001.
20. Whitley RJ, Cobbs CG, Alford CA, et al: Diseases that mimic herpes simplex encephalitis. *JAMA* 262:234, 1989.
21. Morawitz RB, Whitley RJ, Murphy DM: Experience with brain biopsy for suspected herpes encephalitis: A review of 40 consecutive cases. *Neurosurgery* 12:654, 1983.
22. Sköldenberg B, Forsgren M, Alestig K, et al: Acyclovir versus vidarabine in herpes simplex encephalitis. *Lancet* 2:707, 1984.
23. Ito Y, Kimura H, Yabuta Y, et al: Exacerbation of herpes simplex encephalitis after successful treatment with acyclovir. *Clin Infect Dis* 30:185, 2000.
24. Yamada S, Kameyama T, Nagaya S, et al: Relapsing herpes simplex encephalitis: Pathological confirmation of viral reactivation. *J Neurol Neurosurg Psychiatry* 74:262, 2003.
25. Deeter RG, Khanderia U: Recent advances in antiviral therapy. *Clin Pharmacokinet* 5:961, 1986.
26. McGrath N, Anderson NE, Croxson MC, Powell KF: Herpes simplex encephalitis treated with acyclovir: Diagnosis and long term outcome. *J Neurol Neurosurg Psychiatry* 63:321, 1997.
27. Chonmaitree T, Baldwin CD, Lucia HL: Role of the virology laboratory in diagnosis and management of patients with central nervous system disease, in Morello JA (ed): *Clinical Microbiology Reviews*. Chicago, American Society of Microbiology, 1989, p 1.
28. Prober CG, Hensleigh PA, Boucher FD, et al: Use of routine viral cultures at delivery to identify nenoates exposed to herpes simplex virus. *N Engl J Med* 318:887, 1988.

29. Corey L, Stone ET, Whitley RJ, et al: Difference between herpes simplex type I and type II neonatal encephalitis in neurological outcome. *Lancet* 1:1, 1988.

30. Whitley RJ, Nahmias AJ, Visintine AM, et al: The natural history of herpes simplex virus infection of mother and newborn. *Pediatrics* 66:489, 1980.

31. Whitley RJ, Gnann JW: Viral encephalitis: Familiar infections and emerging pathogens. *Lancet* 359:507, 2002.

32. Straus SE, Ostrove JM, Enchauspé G, et al: Varicella-zoster virus infections. *Ann Intern Med* 108:221, 1988.

33. Gnann JW: Varicella-zoster virus: atypical presentations and unusual complications. *J Infect Dis* 186:S91, 2002.

34. Barnes DW, Whitley RJ: CNS diseases associated with varicella zoster virus and herpes simplex virus infection: Pathogenesis and current therapy. *Neurol Clin* 4:265, 1986.

35. Haanpaa M, Dastidar MD, Weinberg MD, et al: CSF and MRI findings in patients with acute herpes zoster. *Neurology* 51:1405, 1998.

36. Nebuloni M, Vago L, Boldorini R, et al: VZV fulminant necrotizing encephalitis with concomitant EBV-related lymphoma and CMV ventriculitis: Report of an AIDS case. *J Neurovirol* 4:457, 1998.

37. Koskiniemi M, Piiparinen H, Rantalaiho T, et al: Acute central nervous system complications in varicella zoster virus infections. *J Clin Virol* 25:293, 2002.

38. Hausler M, Schaade L, Kemeny S, et al: Encephalitis related to primary varicella-zoster virus infection in immunocompetent children. *J Neurol Sci* 195:111, 2002.

39. Puchhammer-Stockyl E, Popow-Kraupp T, Heinz FX, et al: Detection of varicella-zoster virus DNA by polymerase chain reaction in the cerebrospinal fluid of patients suffering from neurologic complications associated with chicken pox or herpes zoster. *J Clin Microbiol* 29:1513, 1991.

40. Tauro S, Toh V, Osman H, Mahendra P: Varicella zoster meningoencephalitis following treatment for dermatomal zoster in an alloBMT patient. *Bone Marrow Transplant* 26:795, 2000.

41. Morgello S, Cho ES, Nielsen S, et al: Cytomegalovirus encephalitis in patients with acquired immunodeficiency syndrome. *Hum Pathol* 18:289, 1987.

42. Arribas JR, Storch GA, Clifford DB, Tselis AC: Cytomegalovirus encephalitis. *Ann Intern Med* 125:577, 1996.

43. Tyler KL: Polymerase chain reaction and the diagnosis of viral central nervous system disease. *Ann Neurol* 36:809, 1994.

44. Siegman-Igra Y, Michaeli D, Doron A, et al: Cytomegalovirus encephalitis in a noncompromised host. *Isr J Med Sci* 20:163, 1984.

45. Redington JJ, Tyler KL: Viral infections of the nervous system, 2002. *Arch Neurol* 59:712, 2002.

46. Langren M, Kyllerman M, Bergstrom T, et al: Diagnosis of Epstein-Barr-virus–induced central nervous system infections by DNA amplification from cerebrospinal fluid. *Ann Neurol* 35:631, 1994.

47. Garamendi I, Montejo M, Cancelo L, et al: Encephalitis caused by Epstein-Barr virus in a renal transplant recipient. *Clin Infect Dis* 34:287, 2002.

48. Dellemijn PLI, Branderburg A, Niesters HGM, et al: Successful treatment with ganciclovir of presumed Epstein-Barr meningoencephalitis following bone marrow transplant. *Bone Marrow Transplant* 16:311, 1995.

49. Petersen LR, Marfin AA: West Nile virus: A primer for the clinician. *Ann Intern Med* 137:173, 2002.

50. Solomon T, Ooi MH, Beasley DWC, et al: West Nile encephalitis. *BMJ* 326:865, 2003.

51. Centers for Disease Control: Arboviral disease—United States 1994. *MMWR* 44:641, 1995.

52. Kaplan MH: Central nervous system infections. *Curr Opin Infect Dis* 2:287, 1989.

53. Tsai TF: Flaviviruses, in Mandell GL, Bennett JE, Dolin R (eds): *Mandell, Douglas and Bennett's Principles and Practice of Infectious Diseases*, 5th ed. Philadephia, Churchill Livingstone, 2000, p 1714.

54. Monath TP: Alphaviruses, in Mandell GL, Bennett JE, Dolin R (eds): *Mandell, Douglas and Bennett's Principles and Practice of Infectious Diseases*, 5th ed. Philadelphia, Churchill Livingstone, 2000, p 1703.

55. Peters CJ: California encephalitis, hantavirus pulmonary syndrome and bunyavirid hemorrhagic fevers, in Mandell GL, Bennett JE, Dolin R (eds): *Mandell, Douglas and Bennett's Principles and Practice of Infectious Diseases*, 5th ed. Philadelphia, Churchill Livingstone, 2000, p 1849.

56. Centers for Disease Control: Provisional Surveillance Summary of the West Nile Virus Epidermic—United States, January–November 2002. *MMWR* 51:1129, 2002.

57. Burke DS, Nisalak A, Ussevy MA, et al: Kinetics of IgM and IgG responses to Japanese encephalitis virus in human serum and cerebrospinal fluid. *J Infect Dis* 151:1093, 1985.

58. Modlin JF: Introduction to Picornaviridae, in Mandell GL, Bennett JE, Dolin R (eds): *Mandell, Douglas and Bennett's Principles and Practice of Infectious Diseases*, 5th ed. Philadelphia, Churchill Livingstone, 2000, p 1888.

59. Rotbart HA: Enteroviral infections of the central nervous system. *Clin Infect Dis* 20:971, 1995.

60. McKinney RG, Keitz SL, Wilfert CM: Chronic enteroviral meningoencephalitis in agammaglobulinemic patients. *Rev Infect Dis* 9:334, 1987.

61. Kondoh H, Kobayashi K, Sugio Y, Hayashi T: Successful treatment of echovirus meningoencephalitis in sex-linked agammaglobulinaemia by intrathecal and intravenous injection of high titre gammaglobulin. *Eur J Pediatr* 146:610, 1987.

62. Tormey VJ, Buscombe JR, Johnson MA, et al: SPECT Scans for monitoring response to pleconaril therapy in chronic enteroviral meningoencephalitis. *J Infect* 46:138, 2003.

63. Rotbart HA, Webster AD: Treatment of potentially life-threatening enterovirus infections with pleconaril. *Clin Infect Dis* 32: 228, 2001.

64. Modlin JF: Poliovirus, in Mandell GL, Bennett JE, Dolin R (eds): *Mandell, Douglas and Bennett's Principles and Practice of Infectious Diseases*, 5th ed. Philadelphia, Churchill Livingstone, 2000, p 1895.

65. Modlin JF: Coxsackie, echovirus and newer enteroviruses, in Mandell GL, Bennett JE, Dolin R (eds): *Mandell, Douglas and Bennett's Principles and Practice of Infectious Diseases*, 5th ed. Philadelphia, Churchill Livingstone, 2000, p 1888.

66. Peters CJ: Lymphocytic choriomeningitis virus, Lassa virus and the South American hemorrhagic fevers, in Mandell GL, Bennett JE, Dolin R (eds): *Mandell, Douglas and Bennett's Principles and Practice of Infectious Diseases*, 5th ed. Philadelphia, Churchill Livingstone, 2000, p 1855.

67. Noah DL, Drenzek CL, Smith JS, et al: Epidemiology of human rabies in the United States, 1980–1996. *Ann Intern Med* 128:922, 1998.

68. Bleck TP, Rupprecht CE: Rabies virus, in Mandell GL, Bennett JE, Dolin R (eds): *Mandell, Douglas and Bennett's Principles and Practice of Infectious Diseases*, 5th ed. Philadelphia, Churchill Livingstone, 2000, p 1811.

69. Anderson LJ, Nicholson KG, Tauxe RV, Winkler WG: Human rabies in the United States, 1960 to 1979: Epidemiology, diagnosis and prevention. *Ann Intern Med* 100:728, 1984.

70. Plotkin SA: Rabies. *Clin Infect Dis* 30:4, 2000.

71. Fishbein DB, Robinson LE: Rabies. *N Engl J Med* 329:1632, 1993.

72. Jackson AC, Warrell MJ, Rupprecht CE, et al: Management of rabies in humans. *Clin Infect Dis* 36:60, 2003.

73. Gisslen M, Hagberg L: Antiretroviral treatment of central nervous system HIV-1 infection: A review. *HIV Med* 2:97, 2001.

74. Johnson RT, Griffin DE, Hirsch RL, et al: Measles encephalomyelitis—Clinical and immunologic studies. *N Engl J Med* 310:137, 1984.

75. Moench TR, Griffen DE, Obriecht CR, et al: Acute measles in patients with and without neurologic involvement: distribution of measles virus antigen and RNA. *J Infect Dis* 158:433, 1988.

76. Gibbs FA, Gibbs EL, Carpenter PR, et al: Electroencephalographic changes in uncomplicated childhood diseases. *JAMA* 171:1050, 1959.

77. Lee KY, Cho WH, Kim SH, et al: Acute encephalitis associated with measles: MRI features. *Neuroradiology* 45:100, 2003.

78. Dhib-Jalbut S, McFortand HF, Mingidie ES, et al: Humoral and cellular immune responses to matrix protein of measles virus in subacute sclerosing panencephalitis. *J Virol* 62:2483, 1988.

79. Jabbour JT, Garad JH, Lemmi H, et al: Subacute sclerosing panencephilitis. A multidisciplinary study of eight cases. *JAMA* 207:2248, 1969.

80. Sever JL: Persistent measles infection of the central nervous system: Subacute sclerosing panencephalitis. *Rev Infect Dis* 4:467, 1983.

81. Sever JL, Krebs H, Ley A, et al: Diagnosis of subacute panencephalitis. The value and availability of measles antibody determinations. *JAMA* 228:604, 1974.

82. Nakayama T: The detection of measles virus genome directly from clinical samples by reverse transcriptase–polymerase chain reaction and genetic variability. *Virus Res* 35:1, 1995.

83. Huttenlocher PR, Mattson RH: Isoprinosine in subacute sclerosing panencephalitis. *Neurology* 29:763, 1979.

84. Jones CE, Dyken PR, Huttenlocher PR, et al: Inosiplex therapy in subacute sclerosing panencephalitis. *Lancet* 1:1034, 1982.

85. DuRant RH, Dyken PR: The effect of inosiplex on the survival of subacute sclerosing panencephalitis. *Neurology* 33:1053, 1983.

86. Noetzel MJ, Dodson WE: Progressive CT abnormalities despite clinical improvement in SSPE treated with inosiplex. *Ann Neurol* 13:457, 1983.

87. Solomon T, Hart CA, Vinjamuri S, et al: Treatment of subacute sclerosing panencephalitis with interferon-alpha, ribavirin and inosiplex. *J Child Neurol* 17:703, 2002.

88. Croxson MC, Anderson NE, Vaughan AA, et al: Subacute measles encephalitis in an immunocompetent adult. *J Clin Neurosci* 9:600, 2002.

89. Baum SG, Litman N: Mumps virus, in Mandell GL, Bennett JE, Dolin R (eds): *Mandell, Douglas and Bennett's Principles and Practice of Infectious Diseases*, 5th ed. Philadelphia, Churchill Livingstone, 2000, p 1776.

90. Chua KB, Bellini WJ, Rota PA, et al: Nipah virus: A recently emergent deadly paramyxovirus. *Science* 288:1432, 2000.

91. Goh KJ, Tan CT, Chew NK, et al: Clinical features of Nipah virus encephalitis among pig farmers in Malaysia. *N Engl J Med* 342:1229, 2000.

92. Chong H-T, Kunjapan SR, Thayaparan T, et al: Nipah encephalitis outbreak in Malaysia, clinical features in patients from Seremban. *Can J Neurol Sci* 29: 83, 2002.

93. Chong H-T, Kamarulzaman A, Tan C-T, et al: Treatment of acute Nipah encephalitis with ribavirin. *Ann Neurol* 49:810, 2001.

94. Lau KK, Lai ST, Lai JY, et al: Acute encephalitis complicating rubella. *Hong Kong Med J* 4:325, 1998.

95. Heggie, AD, Robbins FC: Natural rubella acquired after birth. *Am J Dis Child* 118:12, 1969.

96. Koskiniemi M: CNS manifestations associated with *Mycoplasma pneumonae* infections: Summary of cases at the University of Helsinki and review. *Cli Infect Dis* 17(suppl 1):S52, 1993.

97. Lerer RJ, Kalavsky SM: Central nervous system disease associated with *Mycoplasma pneumoniae* infection: Report of five cases and review of the literature. *Pediatrics* 52:658, 1973.

98. Westenfelder GO, Akey DT, Corwin SJ, Vick NA: Acute transverse myelitis due to *Mycoplasma pneumoniae* infection. *Arch Neurol* 38:317, 1981.

99. Narita M, Itakura O, Matsuzono Y, Togashi T: Analysis of mycoplasmal central nervous system involvement by polymerase chain reaction. *Pediatr Infect Dis J* 14:236, 1995.

100. Sexton DJ: The use of a polymerase chain reaction as a diagnostic test for Rocky Mountain spotted fever. *Am J Trop Med Hyg* 50:59 1994.

101. Walker DH, Raoult D: *Rickettsia rickettsii* and other spotted fever group rickettsiae, in Mandell GL, Bennett JE, Dolin R (eds): *Mandell, Douglas and Bennett's Principles and Practice of Infectious Diseases*, 5th ed. Philadelphia, Churchill Livingstone, 2000, p 2035.

102. Rosenblum MJ, Masland RL, Harrell TG: Residual effect of rickettsial disease on the central nervous system. *Arch Intern Med* 90:444, 1952.

103. Lanksa, DJ: Anthrax meningoencephalitis. *Neurology* 59:327, 2002.

104. Meyer, MA: Neurologic Complications of Anthrax. *Arch Neurol* 60:483, 2003.

105. Young EJ: Brucella species, in Mandell GL, Bennett JE, Dolin R (eds): *Mandell, Douglas and Bennett's Principles and Practice of Infectious Diseases*, 5th ed. Philadelphia, Churchill Livingstone, 2000, p 2386.

106. Marra C: Neurologic complications of *Bartonella henselae* infection. *Curr Opin Neurol* 8:164, 1995.

107. Anderson B, Sims k, Regnery R, et al: Detection of *Rochalimaea henselae* DNA in specimens from cat-scratch disease patients by PCR. *J Clin Microbiol* 32:942, 1994.

108. Luccy D, Dolan MJ, Moss CW, et al: Relapsing illness due to *Rochalimaea henselae* in immunocompetent hosts: Implication for therapy and new epidemiologic associations. *Clin Infect Dis* 14:683, 1992.

109. Steere AC: Lyme disease. *N Engl J Med* 321:586, 1989.

110. Nocton JJ, Bloom BJ, Rutledge BJ, et al: Detection of *Borrelia burgdorferi* DNS by polymerase chain reaction in cerebrospinal fluid in lyme neuroborreliosis. *J Infect Dis* 174:623, 1996.

111. Farr RW: Leptospirosis. *Clin Infect Dis* 21:1, 1995.

112. Merien F, Amouriaux P, Perolat P, et al: Polymerase chain reaction for detection of *Leptospira* spp. in clinical samples. *J Clin Microbiol* 30:2219, 1992.

113. Diamond RD: *Cryptococcus neoformans*, in Mandell GL, Bennett JE, Dolin R (eds): *Mandell, Douglas and Bennett's Principles and Practice of Infectious Diseases*, 5th ed. Philadelphia, Churchill Livingstone, 2000, p 2707.

114. van der Horst CM, Saag MS, Cloud MA, et al: Treatment of cryptococcal meningitis associated with the acquired immunodeficiency syndrome. National Institute of Allergy and Infectious Diseases Mycosis Study Group and AIDS Clinical Trials Group. *N Engl J Med* 337:15, 1997.

115. Zuger A: Cryptococcal disease in patients with the acquired immunodeficiency syndrome. Diagnostic features and outcome of treatment. *Ann Intern Med* 49:234, 1986.

116. Robinson PA, et al: Fluconazole for life-threatening fungal infections in patients who cannot be treated with conventional antifungal agents. *Rev Infect Dis* 12(suppl 3):S349, 1990.

117. Diamond RD, Bennett JE: Prognostic factors in cryptococcal meningitis. A study of 111 cases. *Ann Intern Med* 80:176, 1974.

118. Luft JL, Remington JS: Toxoplasmic encephalitis. *J Infect Dis* 157:1, 1988.

119. Post MJD, Kursunoglu SJ, Hensley GT, et al: Cranial CT in acquired immunodeficiency syndrome: Spectrum of diseases and optimal contrast enhancement technique. *AJR* 145:929, 1985.

120. Levy RM, Rosenbloom S, Perrett LV: Neuroradiologic findings in AIDS: A review of 200 cases. *AJR* 147:977, 1986.

121. Ramsey RG, Gerenia GK: CNS complications of AIDS: CT and MR findings. *AJR* 151:449, 1988.

122. Wanke C, Tuazon C, Kovacs A, et al: Toxoplasma encephalitis in patients with acquired immune deficiency syndrome: Diagnosis and response to therapy. *Am J Trop Med Hyg* 36:509, 1987.

123. Gotzsche PC, Bygbjerg IC, Olesen B, et al: Yield of diagnostic tests for opportunistic infections in AIDS: A survey of 33 patients. *Scand J Infect Dis* 20:396, 1988.

124. Ostergaard L, Nielsen AK, Black FT: DNA amplification on cerebrospinal fluid for diagnosis of cerebral toxoplasmosis among HIV positive patients with signs or symptoms of neurologic disease. *Scand J Infect Dis* 25:227, 1993.

125. Montoya JG, Remington JS: *Toxoplasma gondii*, in Mandell GL, Bennett JE, Dolin R (eds): *Mandell, Douglas and Bennett's Principles and Practice of Infectious Diseases*, 5th ed. Philadelphia, Churchill Livingstone, 2000, p 2858.

126. Singh U, Petri WA: Free-living amebas, in Mandell GL, Bennett JE, Dolin R (eds): *Mandell, Douglas and Bennett's Principles and Practice of Infectious Diseases*, 5th ed. Philadelphia, Churchill Livingstone, 2000, p 2811.

127. Barnett GH, Ropper AH, Romeo J: Intracranial pressure and outcome in adult encephalitis. *J Neurosurg* 68:585, 1988.

Chapter 54

LIFE-THREATENING INFECTIONS OF THE HEAD, NECK, AND UPPER RESPIRATORY TRACT

ANTHONY W. CHOW

KEY POINTS

- *A thorough knowledge of the fascial relations and the potential anatomic routes of infection is a prerequisite to optimal management of deep neck infections.*

- *The microbial etiology of deep infections of the head and neck is complex and typically polymicrobial. Anaerobes generally outnumber aerobes by a factor of 10:1.*

- *The development of marked asymmetry in the course of a submandibular space infection should be viewed with great concern because it may be indicative of extension to the lateral pharyngeal space.*

- *In immunocompromised patients, the classic manifestations of infection, such as edema and fluctuance at the local site and features of systemic toxicity, may be absent.*

- *Penicillin with metronidazole is the antibiotic regimen of choice for odontogenic deep neck infections, but immunocompromised patients require a broader spectrum against organisms such as* Staphylococcus aureus *and enteric gram-negative rods.*

- *Chronic sinusitis, otitis, and mastoiditis are the most important causes of parameningeal infection and intracranial suppuration. Computed tomography is the single neuroimaging technique proved to be the most useful for the diagnosis of these conditions.*

Life-threatening infections of the head, neck, and upper respiratory tract have become less common in the postantibiotic era. As a consequence, many physicians are unfamiliar with these conditions. Further, with widespread use of antibiotics and profound immunosuppression in some patients, the classic manifestations of these infections are often altered. Features of systemic toxicity, such as chills and fever, and local signs, such as edema and fluctuance, may be absent. Thus, physicians unfamiliar with these entities may underestimate their extent and severity. The situation is made more serious by the fact that these infections often have a rapid onset and may progress to fatal complications. In this chapter, the key clinical manifestations of several life-threatening infections of the head, neck, and upper respiratory tract are highlighted, and the critically important anatomic relations that underlie their diagnosis and management are emphasized.

General Anatomic Considerations

Life-threatening infections of the head, neck, and upper respiratory tract most commonly originate from suppurative complications of dental, oropharyngeal, or otorhinolaryngeal infections. From these sites, infection may extend along natural fascial planes into deep cervical spaces or vascular compartments (Fig. 54-1).[1] The deep cervical fascia ranges from loose areolar connective tissue to dense fibrous bands. It invests muscles and organs, thus forming planes and spaces. Notably, these fascial planes separate and connect distant areas, thereby limiting and directing the spread of infection. These infections may be fatal by local airway occlusion or by direct extension to vital structures such as the mediastinum or carotid sheath. Otorhinocerebral infections may cause intracranial suppuration such as cerebral or epidural abscess, subdural empyema, and cavernous or cortical venous sinus thrombosis (Fig. 54-2).[2] A thorough knowledge of the fascial relations and the potential anatomic routes of infection is a prerequisite to understanding the etiology, manifestations, and complications of deep neck infections. Such knowledge will not only provide valuable information on the nature and extent of infection but also suggest the optimum surgical approach for effective drainage.

Microbial Etiology and Pathogenesis

The microbial etiology of deep infections of the head and neck is complex and typically polymicrobial. As a rule, it reflects the autochthonous microflora of the contiguous mucosal surfaces from which the infection originated. Owing to their close anatomic relation, the resident flora of the oral cavity, the upper respiratory tract, and certain parts of the ears and eyes share many common organisms (Fig. 54-3).[3] Anaerobes generally outnumber aerobes at all sites by a factor of 10:1.[4] Although less is known about the pathogenic potential of individual species, it is clear that as a group these organisms are structural opportunists and invade deep tissues when normal mucosal barriers are broken (e.g., during pharyngitis, odontogenic infections, or direct trauma). Invasiveness is often enhanced by synergistic interactions of multiple species, aerobic and anaerobic. Moreover, certain species or combinations may be more invasive or more resistant to therapy than others.

Bacteria most commonly isolated from deep space infections include *Bacteroides, Peptostreptococcus, Veillonella, Actinomyces, Fusobacterium,* and microaerophilic streptococci. Most are sensitive in vitro to penicillin G, but more species are now resistant.[5] Although anaerobes are likely to be involved in most head and neck infections, a small but significant proportion of cases in immunocompromised patients will also involve other pathogens such as *Staphylococcus aureus* and facultative gram-negative rods, including *Pseudomonas aeruginosa.*

Clinical Syndromes

CERVICAL FASCIAL SPACE INFECTIONS

Deep fascial space infections of the head and neck are most frequently odontogenic in origin (Fig. 54-4).[1,6,7] The potential pathways of extension of these infections from one space to another are illustrated in Fig. 54-5.[8] Cervical fascial space infections considered to be life-threatening include those of the submandibular space, the lateral pharyngeal space, and

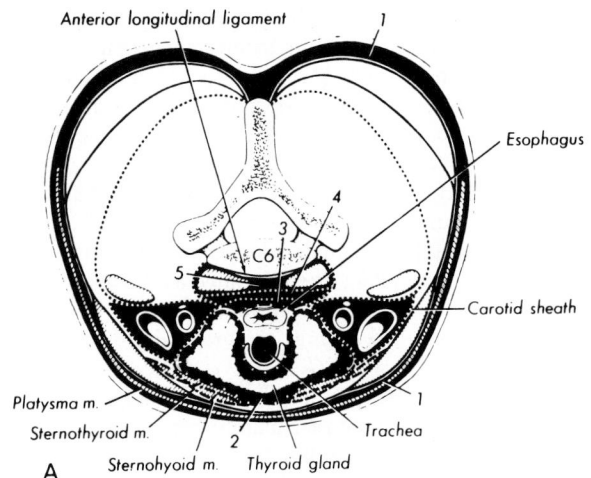

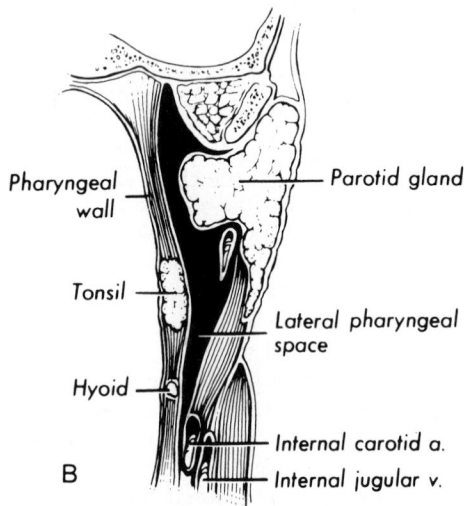

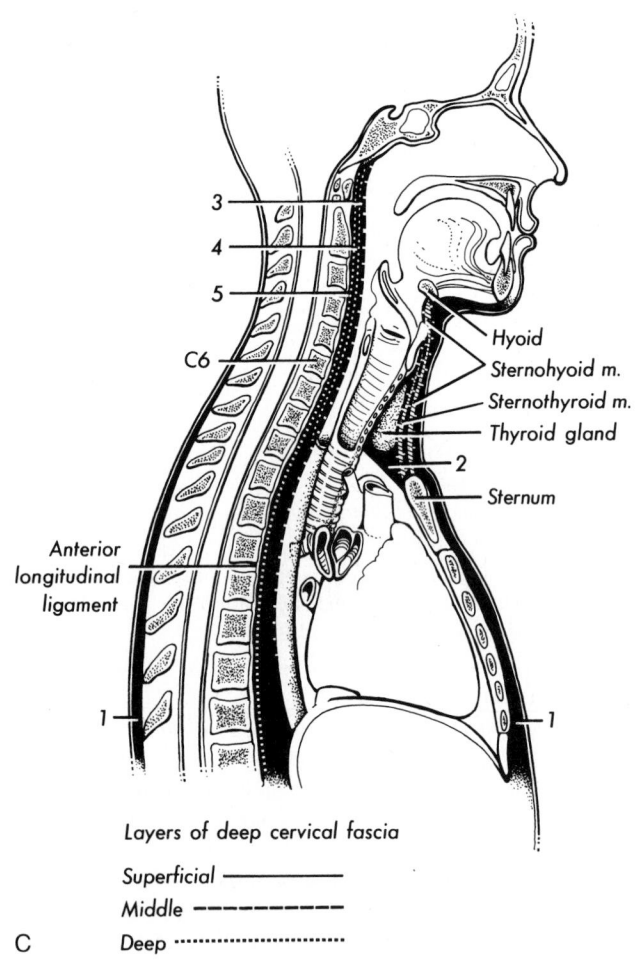

Layers of deep cervical fascia

Superficial ————————
Middle ------------
Deep ·················

FIGURE 54-1 Relation of lateral pharyngeal, retropharyngeal, and prevertebral spaces to the posterior and anterior layers of deep cervical fascia: *1,* superficial space; *2* pretracheal space; *3,* retropharyngeal space; *1,* "danger" space; *1,* prevertebral space. *A.* Cross section of the neck at the level of thyroid isthmus. *B.* Coronal section in the suprahyoid region of the neck. *C.* midsagittal section of the head and neck. *(Reproduced with permission from Chow.[1])*

the retropharyngeal, "danger," and prevertebral spaces. Their salient clinical features are presented in Table 54-1.[9] The approach to radiographic and microbiologic diagnoses is discussed toward the end of this chapter. Recommended antimicrobial regimens for initial empirical therapy are presented in Table 54-2.[7]

SUBMANDIBULAR SPACE INFECTIONS

The prototypical infection of this space is known as Ludwig angina. In 1836, von Ludwig described five patients with "gangrenous induration of the connective tissues of the neck which advances to involve the tissues that cover the small muscles between the larynx and the floor of the mouth." The infection is characteristically an aggressive, rapidly spreading "woody" or brawny cellulitis involving the submandibular space. Although the submandibular space is divided by the mylohyoid muscle into the sublingual space above and the submylohyoid space below (Fig. 54-6), it can be considered a

single unit owing to a direct communication around the posterior aspect of the mylohyoid muscle. Ludwig angina most commonly follows infection of the second or third mandibular molar teeth (70% to 85% of cases). The submylohyoid space is initially involved because the roots of these teeth are located below the attachments of the mylohyoid muscle to the mandible (see Fig. 54-4). Also, because the lingual aspects of periodontal bone around these teeth are thinner, medial spread of infection is facilitated. Infection extends contiguously (rather than by the lymphatics, which would limit the infection to one side) to involve the sublingual and thus the entire submandibular space in a symmetrical manner. Less commonly, an identical process initially involving the sublingual space arises from infection of the premolars and other teeth or from trauma to the floor of the mouth. Once established, infection can evolve rapidly. The tongue may enlarge to two or three times its normal size and distend posteriorly into the hypopharynx, superiorly against the palate, and anteriorly out of the mouth. Immediate posterior extension

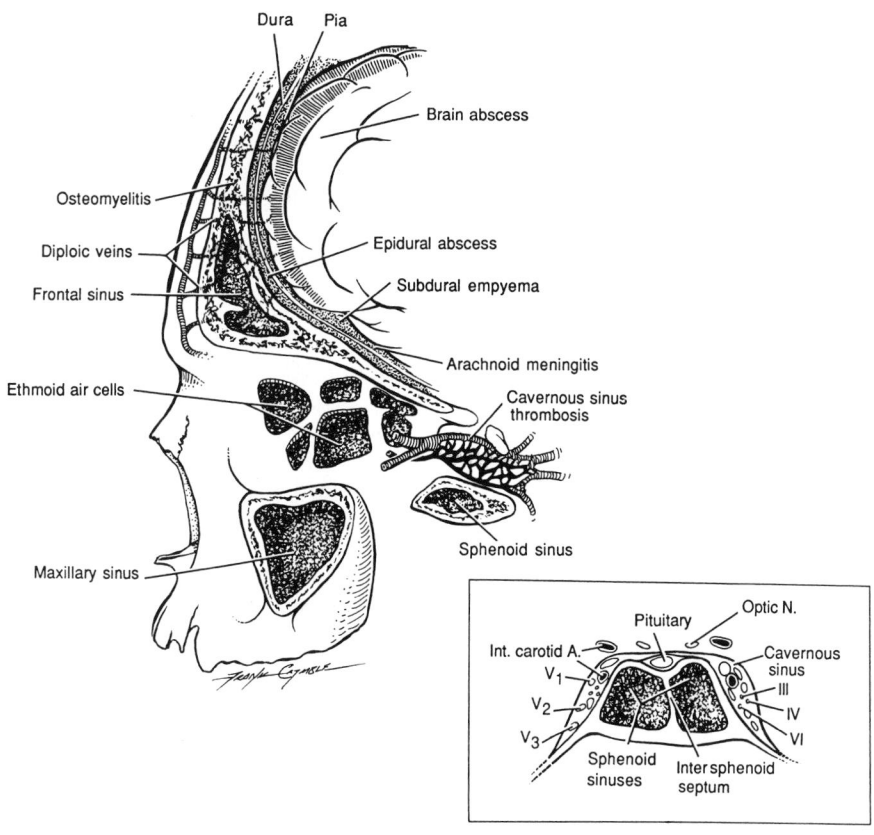

FIGURE 54-2 Major routes for intracranial extension of infection directly or through the vascular supply. The coronal section demonstrates the structures adjoining the sphenoid sinus. *(Reproduced with permission from Chow.[2])*

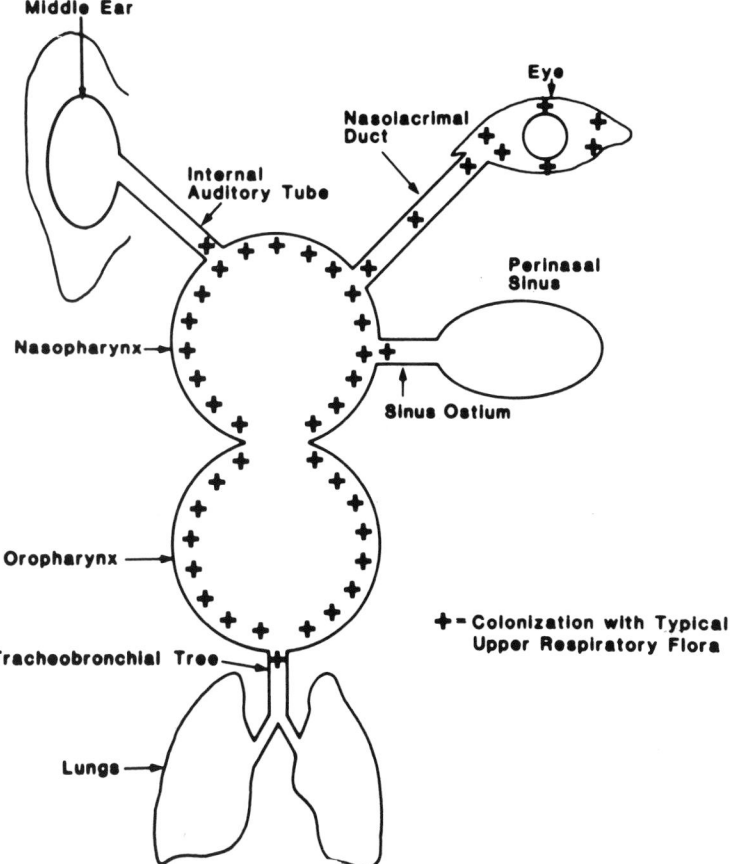

FIGURE 54-3 Diagram of the anatomic relations of head and neck structures and distribution of the indigenous flora. *(Reproduced with permission from Todd.[3])*

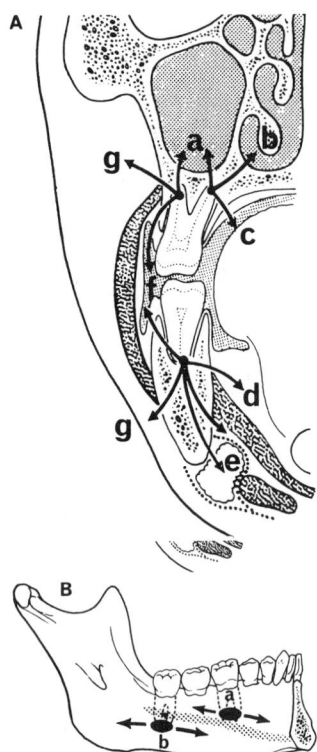

FIGURE 54-4 Routes of spread of odontogenic infections.
A. Coronal section at first molar teeth: *a*, maxillary antrum;
b, nasal cavity; *c*, palatal plate; *d*, sublingual space (above
mylohyoid muscle); *e*, submylohyoid space; *f*, intraoral
presentation with infection spreading through the buccal plates
inside the attachment of the buccinator muscle; *g*, extraoral
presentation to buccal space with infection spreading through the
buccal plates outside the attachment of the buccinator muscle.
B. Lingual aspect of the mandible: *a*, tooth apices above the
mylohyoid muscle with spread of infection into sublingual space;
b, tooth apices below the mylohyoid muscle with spread of
infection into submylohyoid space. *(Reproduced with permission
from Chow.[30])*

of the process directly involves the epiglottis (see Fig. 54-6).
There exists a little-regarded dangerous connection between
the submandibular and lateral pharyngeal spaces known as
the *buccopharyngeal gap*. This gap is created by the styloglos-
sus muscle as it leaves the tongue and passes between the
middle and superior constrictor muscles to attach on the styloid process. Thus, cellulitis of the submandibular space may
spread directly into the lateral pharyngeal space and thereby
to the retropharyngeal space and mediastinum (see Fig. 54-6).

Clinically, the patient is febrile and complains of mouth
pain, stiff neck, drooling, and dysphagia, leaning forward
to maximize the airway diameter. A tender, symmetrical,
and indurated swelling, sometimes with palpable crepitus,
is present in the submandibular area. The mouth is held open
by lingual swelling. Respirations are usually difficult, and
stridor and cyanosis are considered ominous signs. Radiographic views of the teeth may indicate the source of infection, and lateral views of the neck will demonstrate the degree
of soft tissue swelling around the airway and possibly submandibular gas. The development of significant asymmetry
of the submandibular area should be viewed with great concern because it may be indicative of extension to the lateral

pharyngeal space. Well-timed surgical drainage decreases the
risk of spread to this space and subsequently to the superior
mediastinum.[10]

The therapy of Ludwig angina has undergone a number of
modifications since its initial description.[11] Although maintenance of an adequate airway is the primary concern and
may necessitate urgent tracheostomy, most cases can be managed initially by close observation and intravenous antibiotics. If cellulitis and swelling continue to advance rapidly or
if dyspnea occurs, artificial airway control should be gained
immediately, before stridor, cyanosis, and asphyxia require
that it be done under emergency conditions. There is general agreement that blind oral or nasotracheal intubation is
traumatic and unsafe in advanced Ludwig angina because
of the potential for induction of severe laryngospasm. A recommended approach is to use a flexible fiberoptic scope to
assess the airway and to aid in inserting an endotracheal tube.
Tracheostomy is still the most widely recommended means
of airway control, although cricothyroidotomy is advocated
by some experts because of a lower complication rate.

Penicillin G with metronidazole or a similar regimen directed at the mixed aerobic and anaerobic flora of the mouth
(see Table 54-2) is the antibiotic regimen of choice, but immunocompromised patients require a broader spectrum of
antibiotic coverage to include organisms such as facultative
gram-negative rods and *S. aureus*. Early surgical decompression, much advocated in the era before antibiotics, is unlikely
to locate pus and at best may only moderately improve the
airway. Pus collections develop relatively late (they are not
usually present in the first 24 to 36 hours) and are sometimes
difficult to detect clinically. If the patient is not responding adequately to antibiotics alone after this initial period or if fluctuance is detectable, needle aspiration or a more formal incision and drainage procedure under general anesthetic should
be performed. Preferably, this should be done with a cuffed
tracheostomy in place. In addition, the infected teeth implicated in the sepsis should be extracted.

With the combined use of systemic antibiotics and aggressive surgical intervention, the mortality rate for Ludwig
angina has declined dramatically from more than 50% before
the antibiotic era to 0% to 4% currently.

LATERAL PHARYNGEAL SPACE INFECTIONS

Lateral pharyngeal space infections are potentially life-
threatening because of involvement of vital structures within
the carotid sheath and a tendency to bacteremic dissemination. Anatomically, the lateral pharyngeal space (also known
as the *pharyngomaxillary space*) is shaped like an inverted cone
in the lateral neck, with its base at the skull and its apex
at the hyoid bone. Its medial wall is continuous with the
carotid sheath, and anteriorly it lies between the superior pharyngeal constrictor muscle medially and the internal pterygoid muscle, mandibular ramus, and parotid gland laterally
(Fig. 54-7). It is divided into an anterior (prestyloid or
muscular) compartment and a posterior (retrostyloid or
neurovascular) compartment by the styloid process and its
attached muscles, the stylomandibular ligament, and the insertion of these structures into the hyoid bone. The anterior
compartment contains no vital structures, but only fat, lymph
nodes, connective tissue, and muscle. It is the compartment
most closely related to the tonsillar fossa and the internal

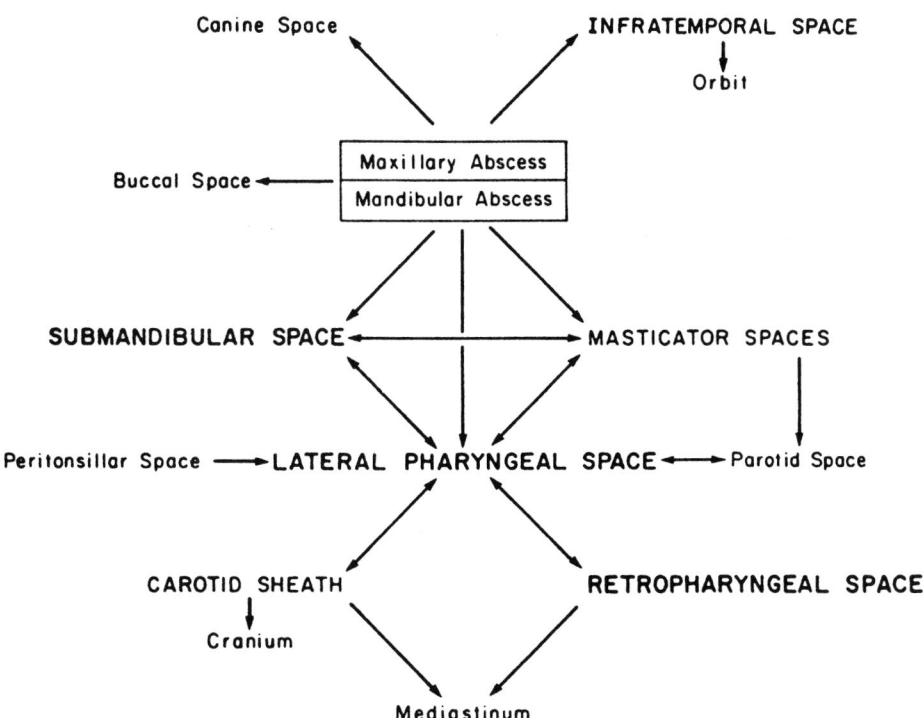

FIGURE 54-5 Potential pathways of extension in deep fascial space infections. *(Reproduced with permission from Blomquist and Bayer.[8])*

pterygoid muscle. The posterior compartment contains the ninth to twelfth cranial nerves, the carotid sheath and its contents, and the cervical sympathetic trunk. Infections of the lateral pharyngeal space may arise from sources throughout the neck. Dental infections are the most common source, followed by peritonsillar abscess (postanginal sepsis) and rarely parotitis, otitis, or mastoiditis (Bezold abscess).

Infection of the anterior compartment is often suppurative. Because most patients are already compromised by infection elsewhere, diagnosis of lateral pharyngeal involvement is often delayed. The cardinal clinical features, in order of importance, are (a) trismus, (b) induration and swelling below the angle of the mandible, (c) systemic toxicity with fever and rigors, and (d) medial bulging of the pharyngeal wall. Although not prominent, dyspnea can occur. Suppuration may advance quickly to other spaces, particularly to the retropharyngeal space and the mediastinum, or may spread to involve

the posterior compartment of the lateral pharyngeal space. In these cases, timely surgical incision and drainage are of utmost importance.

Postanginal sepsis can involve the anterior or the posterior compartment, but because lymphatic drainage is the most important mechanism of spread, it most often involves the carotid sheath alone. A history of sore throat, although usually present on admission, is not invariable; it may only be mild or unilateral, and there may be a latent period of up to 3 weeks before manifestations of deep infection develop. The patient presents in a toxic condition or insidiously with a fever of undetermined origin. Trismus is absent, and signs of local suppuration may be subtle clinically because of the tight connective tissue around and within the carotid sheath. This barrier confines the infection and may limit it to only the internal jugular vein. Dyspnea may be prominent as edema and swelling may descend directly to involve the epiglottis

TABLE 54-1 Comparative Clinical Features of Deep Fascial Space Infections

Space	Pain	Trismus	Swelling	Dysphagia	Dyspnea
Submandibular	Present	Minimal	Mouth floor; submylohyoid	Present if bilateral involvement	Present if bilateral involvement
Lateral pharyngeal					
Anterior	Severe	Prominent	Anterior lateral pharynx; angle of jaw	Present	Occasional
Posterior	Minimal	Minimal	Posterior lateral pharynx (hidden)	Present	Severe
Retropharyngeal (and danger)	Present	Minimal	Posterior pharynx	Present	Present
Masticator					
Masseteric and pterygoid	Present	Prominent	May not be seen	Absent	Absent
Temporal	Present	None	Face, orbit	Absent	Absent
Buccal	Minimal	Minimal	Cheek	Absent	Absent
Parotid	Severe	None	Angle of jaw	Absent	Absent

SOURCE: Produced with permission from Megran et al.[9]

TABLE 54-2 Usual Causative Organisms and Initial Empirical Antimicrobial Regimens for Life-Threatening Infections of the Head, Neck, and Upper Respiratory Tract

Infection	Usual Causative Organisms	ANTIMICROBIAL REGIMENS	
		Normal Host	Compromised Host
Cervical fascial space infections including Ludwig angina	Viridans and other streptococci, *Peptostreptococcus* spp., *Bacteroides* spp., and other oral anaerobes	Penicillin G 2–4 MU IV q 4–6 h, *plus* metronidazole 0.5 g IV q 6 h; *or* Ampicillin-sulbactam 2 g IV q 4 h; *or* Clindamycin 600 mg IV q 6 h; *or* Doxycycline 200 mg IV q 12 h; *or* Cefoxitin 1–2 g IV q 6 h; *or* Cefotetan 2 g IV q 12 h	Cefotaxime 2 g IV q 6 h; *or* Ceftizoxime 4 g IV q 8 h; *or* Piperacillin 3 g IV q 4 h; *or* Imipenem 500 mg IV q 6 h; *or* Meropenem 1 g IV q 8 h; *or* Gatifloxacin 200 mg IV q 24 h
Lateral pharyngeal *or* retropharyngeal space infections			
Odontogenic	Viridans and other streptococci, *Staphylococcus* spp., *Peptostreptococcus* spp., *Bacteroides* spp., and other oral anaerobes	Penicillin G 2–4 MU IV q 4–6 h, *plus* metronidazole 0.5 g IV q 6 h; *or* Ampicillin-sulbactam 2 g IV q 4 h; *or* Clindamycin 600 mg IV q 6 h	Cefotaxime 2 g IV q 6 h; *or* Ceftizoxime 4 g IV q 8 h; *or* Piperacillin 3 g IV q 4 h; *or* Imipenem 500 mg IV q 6 h; *or* Gatifloxacin 400 mg IV q 24 h
Rhinogenic	*Streptococcus pneumoniae, Haemophilus influenzae,* viridans and other streptococci, *Bacteroides* spp., *Peptostreptococcus* spp., and other oral anaerobes	Penicillin G 2–4 MU IV q 4–6 h; *or* Ciprofloxacin 0.2 g q 12 h, *plus* metronidazole 0.5 g IV q 6 h; *or* Clindamycin 600 mg IV q 6 h; *or* Gatifloxacin 400 mg IV q 24 h	Same as for odontogenic space infections
Otogenic	Same as for rhinogenic space infections	Same as for rhinogenic space infections	Same as for odontogenic space infections
Peritonsillar abscess (Quinsy)	Group A streptococcus (*S. pyogenes*), *Fusobacterium* spp., *Peptostreptococcus* spp., and other oral anaerobes	Penicillin G 2–4 MU IV q 4–6 h, *plus* metronidazole 0.5 g IV q 6 h; *or* Ampicillin-sulbactam 2 g IV q 4 h; *or* Clindamycin 600 mg IV q 6 h; *or* Cefoxitin 1–2 g IV q 6 h	Cefotaxime 2 g IV q 6 h; *or* Ceftizoxime 3 g IV q 8 h; *or* Piperacillin 3 g IV q 4 h
Suppurative parotitis	*Staphylococcus aureus,* viridans and other streptococci, *Bacteroides* spp., *Peptostreptococcus* spp., and other oral anaerobes	Nafcillin 1.5 g IV q 4–6 h *plus* metronidazole 0.5 g IV q 6 h; *or* Clindamycin 600 mg IV q 6 h	Vancomycin 0.5 g IV q 6 h *plus* cefotaxime 2 g IV q 6 h; *or* Ceftizoxime 3 g IV q 8 h; *or* Pipenacillin 3 g IV q 4 h
Extension of osteomyelitis from prevertebral space infection	*Staphylococcus aureus,* facultative gram-negative bacilli	Nafcillin 1.5 g IV q 4–6 h, *plus* tobramycin 2 mg/kg q 8 h; *or* Ciprofloxacin 0.2 g q 12 h	Vancomycin 0.5 g IV q 6 h, *plus* cefotaxime 2 g IV q 6 h; *or* Ceftizoxime 4 g IV q 8 h; *or* Imipenim 500 mg IV q 6 h
Pott's puffy tumor (frontal osteitis)	Same as for rhinogenic space infections	Same as for rhinogenic space infections	Same as for odontogenic space infections
Malignant otitis media and petrous osteitis	*Pseudomonas aeruginosa*	Ciprofloxacin 200 mg IV q 12 h; *or* Tobramycin 2 mg/kg q 8 h *plus* ceftazidime 2 g IV q 6 h; *or* Piperacillin 3 g IV q 4 h; *or* Imipenem 1 g IV q 6 h	Ciprofloxacin 200 mg IV q 12 h; *or* Tobramycin 2 mg/kg q 8 h *plus* ceftazidime 2 g IV q 6 h; *or* Piperacillin 3 g IV q 4 h; *or* Imipenem 1 g IV q 6 h

ABBREVIATIONS: IV, intravenous; MU, million units; q, every.

and larynx. Swelling of the pharyngeal wall, if present, will be behind the palatopharyngeal arch and is easily missed.

Suppurative jugular thrombophlebitis (Lemierre syndrome) is the most common vascular complication of lateral pharyngeal space infection.[12] An indurated swelling a few centimeters long may be palpable behind the sternocleidomastoid muscle or may be found more deeply behind the palatopharyngeal arch. Trismus is minimal and may be absent. Vocal cord paralysis or other neurologic signs representing lower cranial nerve involvement may be present. These signs are frequently missed unless specifically sought (they were detected in only 20% of cases antemortem in one series),

and they may be transient. The patient may thus present as having an obscure septicemia (50% of cases). Metastatic abscesses are common, characteristically involving the lungs, bones, and joints or other sites. There may be retrograde spread of infection with cerebral abscess or meningitis. A diagnosis of right-side bacterial endocarditis may be considered. In common with other anaerobic septicemias, hepatic enlargement, tenderness, abnormal liver function tests, and even frank jaundice may be present, which may misdirect investigations and further delay diagnosis.[13] Positive gallium or white-cell–labeled indium uptake in the neck is a useful diagnostic aid in these cases. Computed tomography (CT)

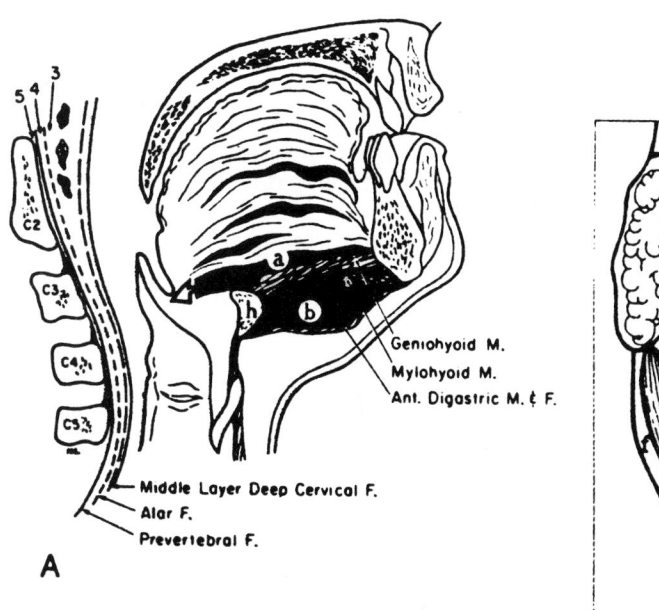

FIGURE 54-6 Anatomic relations in Ludwig angina. Sagittal (*A*) and oblique (*B*) sections of the head and neck: *a*, sublingual space; *b*, submylohyoid space; *c*, lateral pharyngeal space; *d*,

parotid gland; *f*, masticator space; *g*, peritonsillar space; *h*, hyoid bone; *3*, retropharyngeal space; *4*, danger space; *5*, prevertebral space. (*Reproduced with permission from Blomquist and Bayer.*[8])

of the neck visualizes edema within the lateral pharyngeal space and the presence of thrombus in the internal jugular vein (Fig. 54-8). Thrombosis of the jugular vein can also be demonstrated by magnetic resonance angiography. Rarely, the carotid artery is involved, leading to an arteritis and to the formation and eventual rupture of an aneurysm. This complication is usually heralded by several minor bleeds before a major hemorrhage occurs and signals the need for urgent surgical intervention. Such bleeding may involve the oral cavity, nose, or ear or appear as ecchymosis in the neck and surrounding tissues. An ipsilateral Horner syndrome and otherwise unexplained ninth to twelfth cranial nerve palsies are additional premonitory syndromes of carotid sheath involvement.

Treatment of lateral pharyngeal space infection initially depends on whether local suppuration is present, but often this is difficult to determine. CT, careful needle aspiration, or more definitive incision and drainage may be required. Most cases of postanginal sepsis with suppurative jugular thrombophlebitis can be managed medically without the need for ligation or surgical resection of the infected vein. Prolonged courses of intravenous antibiotics (3 to 6 weeks) will be required. Because anaerobic bacteremia caused by *Bacteroides* species or *Fusobacterium necrophorum* is frequently present[14] and penicillin resistance among these organisms is increasingly recognized, therapy generally requires addition of metronidazole, clindamycin, or β-lactamase–stable cephalosporins. Fever may be slow to resolve, even in cases

FIGURE 54-7 Cross sections of the lateral pharyngeal space: *P*, parotid gland; *T*, tonsil; *M*, mandible; *3*, retropharyngeal space; *4*, danger space; *5*, prevertebral space. *Inset.* Anterior and posterior

compartments of the lateral pharyngeal space. (*Reproduced with permission from Blomquist and Bayer.*[8])

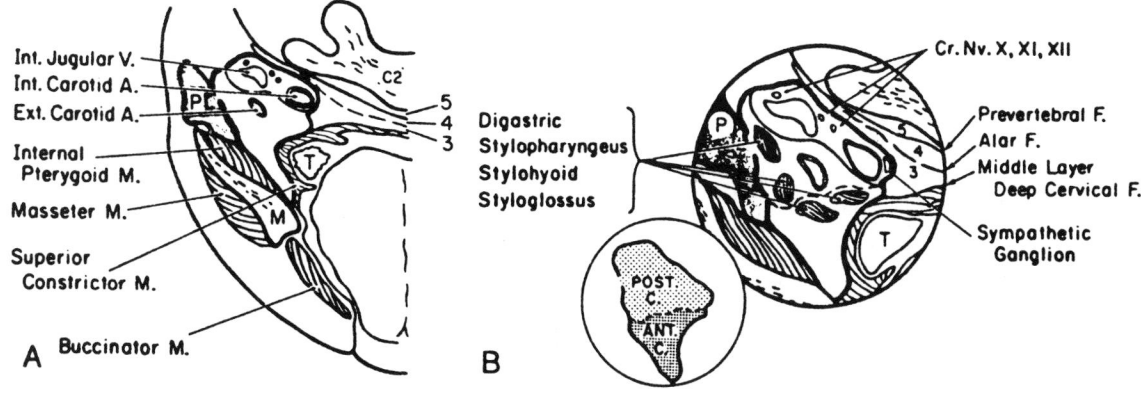

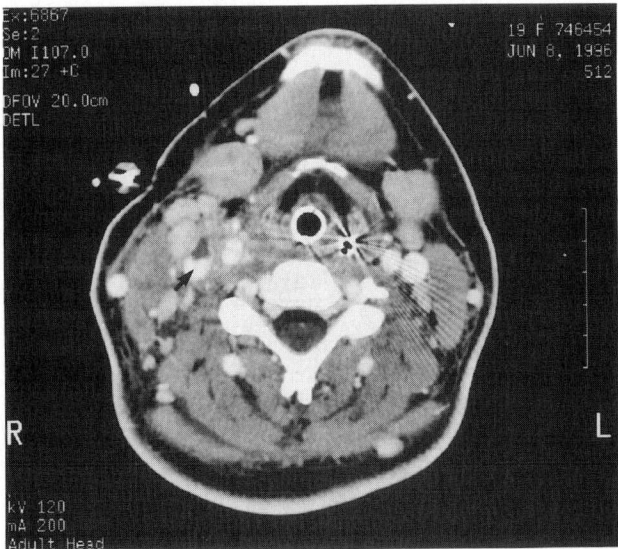

FIGURE 54-8 Computed tomographic scan of the neck in a patient with lateral pharyngeal space infection secondary to a peritonsillar infection. *Arrow* indicates a partial thrombus in the right internal jugular vein.

successfully treated, particularly if there is metastatic involvement. Anticoagulants have sometimes been used in this setting, but their efficacy is unconfirmed. Surgical ligation of the internal jugular vein, the only available therapeutic option before antibiotics, is currently required only in the rare patient who fails to respond to antibiotic therapy alone. When there is impending or frank rupture of the carotid artery, the artery must be ligated immediately, with special attention given to the airway and to restoration of blood volume. Predictably, morbidity (e.g., stroke) and mortality rates are high (20% to 40%). In all such cases, early surgical intervention is the key to a successful outcome.

INFECTIONS OF THE RETROPHARYNGEAL, "DANGER," AND PREVERTEBRAL SPACES

The retropharyngeal, "danger," and prevertebral spaces lie between the deep cervical fascia surrounding the pharynx and esophagus anteriorly and the vertebral spine posteriorly (see Fig. 54-1). The retropharyngeal space is bound anteriorly by the constrictor muscles of the neck and their fascia and posteriorly by the alar layer of the deep cervical fascia, extending from the base of the skull to the level of the superior mediastinum, where the two fascial layers fuse. The "danger" space is interposed between the retropharyngeal space anteriorly and the prevertebral space posteriorly. It extends from the base of the skull and descends freely through the entire posterior mediastinum to the diaphragm. The prevertebral space is bound by the prevertebral fascia, which originates posteriorly on the spinous processes and encircles the splenius, erector spinae, and semispinalis muscles. Before completing its circle anterior to the vertebral bodies, it fuses to the transverse processes. At this point it is split into two layers: the more anterior alar fascia and the prevertebral fascia. The prevertebral space extends from the base of the skull to the coccyx, thus allowing infectious spread as far down as the psoas muscle sheath.

Retropharyngeal abscesses are among the most serious of deep space infections because infection can extend directly into the anterior or posterior portions of the superior mediastinum or into the entire length of the posterior mediastinum through the danger space (see Fig. 54-1).

Retropharyngeal infections may occur in children and adults. In young children, infection usually reaches this space through lymphatic channels, most commonly as complications of suppurative adenitis after infections of the upper respiratory tract. The onset may be insidious, with little more than fever, irritability, drooling, or possibly nuchal rigidity. More acute symptoms include dysphagia and dyspnea. The latter may be due to a local mass effect or to laryngeal edema. In general, there is little pain, but the neck may be held rigidly and tilted to the unaffected side. Definite bulging of the posterior pharyngeal wall is usually seen but may need careful palpation to be appreciated. The main dangers are severe laryngeal edema with airway obstruction and abscess rupture with consequent aspiration pneumonia or asphyxia. Many cases will respond to antibiotic therapy alone if treatment precedes the development of frank suppuration.

In adults, infection may reach the retropharyngeal space from local or distant sites. The former usually results from penetrating trauma (e.g., from chicken bones or after instrumentation); in such cases, the presence of a sore throat or difficulty in swallowing or breathing may be the first indications of infection. More distant sources include odontogenic sepsis and peritonsillar abscess (now a rare cause). Infection from these sources often may obscure the diagnosis because of associated trismus, which makes direct examination of the posterior pharyngeal wall difficult. In this setting, CT and radiographic views of the lateral neck are especially helpful and may demonstrate cervical lordosis with swelling and gas collections in the retropharyngeal space, which causes anterior displacement of the larynx and trachea. Radiographs may also help to differentiate this infection from prevertebral space sepsis arising from cervical osteomyelitis. Once a diagnosis is made, surgical exploration and wide drainage should be carried out without delay.

Acute necrotizing mediastinitis is the most feared complication of retropharyngeal space infections.[15] The onset is rapid and is characterized by (a) widespread necrotizing process extending the length of the posterior mediastinum and occasionally into the retroperitoneal space, (b) rupture of mediastinal abscess into the pleural cavity with empyema or development of loculations, and (c) pleural or pericardial effusions, frequently with tamponade. Aspiration pneumonia is also a significant problem (50% of cases) and may be secondary to impairment of swallowing or spontaneous rupture of the abscess into the airway. As might be expected, the mortality rate in adults is high (25%), even when appropriate antibiotics are administered. Early diagnosis and timely débridement are the mainstays of successful treatment. Mediastinal drainage may be attained by the cervical mediastinal or the transthoracic approach. Although the cervical approach may be effective in early mediastinitis, thoracotomy is generally indicated once the necrotizing process has entered the danger space. In patients who are recovering, it is important to restrict all oral intake until the swallowing impairment, which may have a prolonged course, has resolved completely.

SUPPURATIVE PAROTITIS

Acute bacterial parotitis is a specific clinical entity primarily affecting the elderly, malnourished, dehydrated, or postoperative patient.[16] Ductal (Stensen) obstruction secondary to sialolithiasis appears to be a major predisposing condition. Other predisposing factors include sialogogic drugs and trauma. Clinically, there is sudden onset of firm, erythematous swelling of the pre- and postauricular areas extending to the angle of the mandible. This is associated with exquisite local pain and tenderness but not trismus. Systemic findings of high fevers, chills, and marked toxicity are generally present. Septicemic spread may lead to osteomyelitis of the adjacent facial bones. Staphylococci have been the predominant isolates, and empirical antibiotic therapy should include an antistaphylococcal agent. Early surgical drainage and decompression of the gland are generally required because spontaneous drainage is uncommon. Because of its close relation to the posterior aspect of the lateral pharyngeal space, progression of infection into the parotid space may lead to massive swelling of the neck with respiratory obstruction and has the added potential risk of direct extension into the danger and visceral spaces and, hence, to the posterior mediastinum (see Fig. 54-1).

PERITONSILLAR ABSCESS AND PHARYNGEAL DIPHTHERIA

PERITONSILLAR ABSCESS

This condition, also known as *quinsy*, is a suppurative complication of acute tonsillitis involving the peritonsillar space. The latter consists of loose areolar tissue overlying the tonsil surrounded by the superior pharyngeal constrictor muscle and the anterior and posterior tonsillar pillars. Peritonsillar abscesses may affect patients of all ages but are most common among young adults 15 to 30 years old. The patient appears ill, with fever, sore throat, dysphagia, trismus, pooling of saliva, and a muffled voice. The abscess is usually unilateral, with associated cervical lymphadenitis. Examination of the pharynx in the majority of cases shows swelling of the anterior pillar and the soft palate and, less commonly, the middle portion or lower pole of the tonsil. Initially, needle drainage in the Trendelenburg position should be attempted, and the patient should be closely monitored and managed with intravenous antibiotics alone. Failure to obtain pus is an indication for surgical incision and more formal exploration. Delays increase the risk of spontaneous rupture. Aspiration of purulent material is the main hazard, particularly in the sleeping patient. More serious complications include (a) airway obstruction, especially with bilateral disease or when laryngeal edema develops; and (b) lateral dissection (usually from infections of the middle or lower portions of the tonsil) through the superior pharyngeal constrictor muscle to involve the lateral pharyngeal space (see Fig. 54-6B). Continued signs of sepsis after drainage of the peritonsillar space usually indicate coexisting, undrained lateral pharyngeal space infection. Fatalities associated with peritonsillar abscess (>50% before antibiotics) were due largely to this complication.

Ideally, antibiotics should be tailored according to the results of cultures of aspirated pus, but these are infrequently performed. Also, results are unlikely to be helpful unless specimens are collected without oropharyngeal contamination and are transported in appropriate media. Group A β-hemolytic streptococci (often as part of a mixed flora containing anaerobes) are most commonly isolated. Occasionally other β-hemolytic streptococci, *Haemophilus influenzae*, *S. aureus*, or anaerobes alone are cultured. Penicillin G is effective therapy in most cases. Bilateral tonsillectomy should be performed once the patient has recovered to avoid recurrences. Interim antibiotic prophylaxis should be considered in high-risk cases.

PHARYNGEAL DIPHTHERIA

Widespread immunization has substantially reduced infections caused by toxigenic strains of *Corynebacterium diphtheriae*. Nevertheless, local outbreaks of infection continue to occur sporadically, where reservoirs of infections (e.g., nasopharyngeal carriage) and suboptimal levels of immunization exist. All age groups, irrespective of immunization status, may develop diphtheria, but most cases usually occur in children and young adolescents. Those previously immunized are more likely to have milder or asymptomatic infections. Tonsillitis is the commonest manifestation, but any site in the upper airway can be infected. Nasopharyngeal involvement usually occurs by contiguous spread from the tonsils. In these patients, local symptoms of sore throat and dysphagia frequently follow a prodrome of fever, malaise, headache, nausea, and vomiting. Even though infection is limited to the mucosal epithelium (toxin absorption is responsible for systemic complications), the tonsils, uvula, and pharynx may swell considerably, sometimes sufficiently to suggest the presence of a peritonsillar or retropharyngeal collection. Further, a brawny nonpitting edema or "bull neck" may develop secondary to reactive cervical lymphadenopathy. With nasopharyngeal infection, cervical lymphadenopathy may be marked. Diphtheria is known for the formation of a tenacious membrane, but this is not an invariable finding and may be confined to the tonsillar mucosa. It may be produced by other infections, but the typical membrane of diphtheria quickly becomes discolored and necrotic (Fig. 54-9).[17] Bleeding may occur after attempts to remove it and is sometimes severe. Airway obstruction by membrane and local swelling may complicate severe tonsillar and nasopharyngeal infection but is more likely when the larynx is primarily involved. Urgent tracheostomy may then be required; if this measure fails to bypass the obstruction, bronchoscopy to remove any membrane present in the lower airways should be considered.

Circulating toxin is responsible for the neurologic and cardiac manifestations of diphtheria (peripheral neuropathy and myocarditis). These manifestations develop after a latent period of 1 to 2 weeks or longer and are influenced by the rate of toxin production (increased by more available iron) and absorption (greater in the nasopharynx). Gravis, intermedius, and mitis variants of *C. diphtheriae* are similarly toxigenic, and their distinction is of primarily epidemiologic importance. Of the neurologic complications, palatal, ocular, and ciliary paralysis are the earliest to develop and may be followed by motor or sensory changes in the limbs; but these symptoms are reversible. Myocarditis may develop acutely or insidiously, with a gradually rising serum aspartic transaminase level. Manifestations include shock, heart failure, arrhythmias, and various conduction disturbances. The prognosis

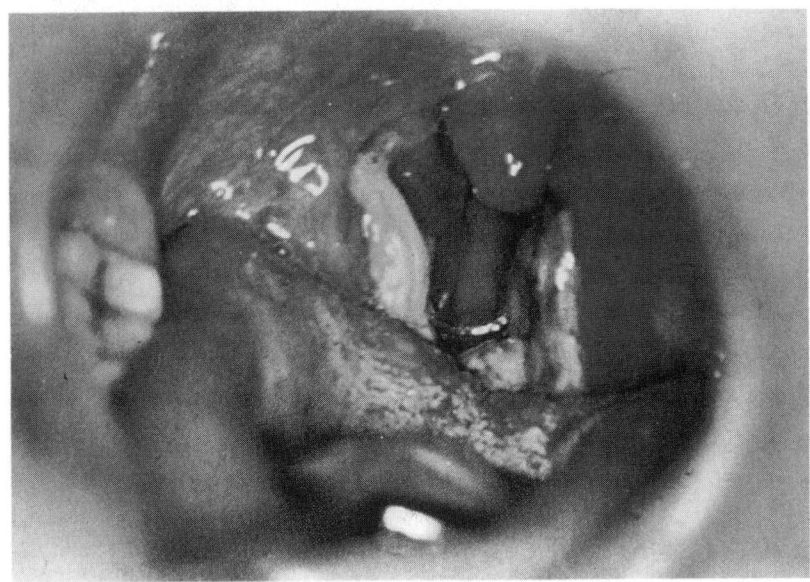

FIGURE 54-9 Tonsillar diphtheria with characteristic grayish green membrane overlying the right tonsil. (*Reproduced with permission from Whiting and Chow.*[17])

for cardiac disease is guarded, but complete recovery is the rule for those who survive.

For immediate treatment, equine diphtheria antitoxin should be given whenever clinical evidence of diphtheria exists because early administration decreases the risk of myocarditis. The dose depends on the site and severity of the infection. Testing for hypersensitivity to horse protein (and desensitization, if necessary) of all patients is mandatory. Diagnostic confirmation requires culturing *C. diphtheriae*, which must then be shown to be toxigenic. Although uncommon, toxigenic strains of *C. ulcerans* can also cause classic symptoms of laryngeal and cutaneous diphtheria.[18] These organisms are sensitive to several antibiotics, including penicillin G and erythromycin, which are equally effective and are used for treating clinical cases, carriers, and contacts.

ACUTE EPIGLOTTITIS AND LARYNGOTRACHEOBRONCHITIS

ACUTE EPIGLOTTITIS

Acute epiglottitis is an infection that produces predominantly nonsuppurative inflammatory edema involving the supraglottic structures and the epiglottis. Once caused mainly by *H. influenzae*, widespread use of vaccination against this organism in children has greatly reduced its prevalence, so that other bacteria, such as *Streptococcus pneumoniae*, *S. aureus*, *Haemophilus parainfluenzae*, and oral anaerobes, are increasingly implicated. In addition, because of vaccination, the occurrence of the disease in children has fallen dramatically; in most centers, most current cases seen are in adults.[19]

In older children and adults, the chief initial complaint is a sore throat and later odynophagia, but in younger children the physician has to rely on clinical findings alone. Typically, the triad of fever, stridor, and drooling is present. The patient tends to sit up and remain quiet, often leaning forward to facilitate breathing. The voice is muffled rather than hoarse. Inspiration tends to draw down the epiglottis and further obstruct the airway, so respirations are deliberately slow rather than rapid. Cyanosis, pallor, and bradycardia are late signs

of severe airway obstruction that signal the urgent need to establish an artificial airway.

Once the diagnosis is suspected, confirmation depends on the condition of the patient, with the knowledge that this can change rapidly and unexpectedly, particularly in younger children in whom, because of the relatively small size of the supraglottic larynx, even small degrees of swelling can rapidly lead to complete airway obstruction. Particularly in adults who appear not to be in great distress, frequently only antimicrobial therapy and close observation in an intensive care unit without endotracheal intubation are required.[19] However, in a significant minority of adults (20%) and in most children (70%), respiratory distress, worsening stridor, or inability to easily clear secretions will mandate placement of an artificial airway.[20] Whether the patient is managed expectantly or by intubation, it is worth emphasizing that the personnel involved should be highly experienced with all aspects of difficult airway management because even with close monitoring there can be abrupt changes in the clinical course. If intubation is indicated, it should be done by direct visualization and in the operating room, preferably by a skilled anesthetist. Equipment and personnel necessary for emergency tracheostomy and a bronchoscope should be immediately available. Attempts to visualize the cherry-red epiglottis by direct laryngoscopy in an awake patient in the absence of these precautions for immediate intubation are discouraged because acute airway obstruction can be precipitated by dislodging a mucus plug or causing the patient to gag. Radiographic views of the lateral neck usually show an enlarged epiglottis with edematous supraglottic structures and ballooning of the hypopharynx (Fig. 54-10).[21] However, when the clinical signs point toward the diagnosis of epiglottitis with a significant compromise of the airway, radiologic investigation should not precede airway management.

Additional laboratory data may indicate a moderate leukocytosis with a left shift and positive cultures of blood and epiglottis. A concurrent pneumonia is demonstrated on chest radiographs in about 25% of cases. Antibiotic treatment may be initiated with ampicillin-sulbactam or a *β*-lactamase–resistant cephalosporin such as cefuroxime, cefotaxime, or

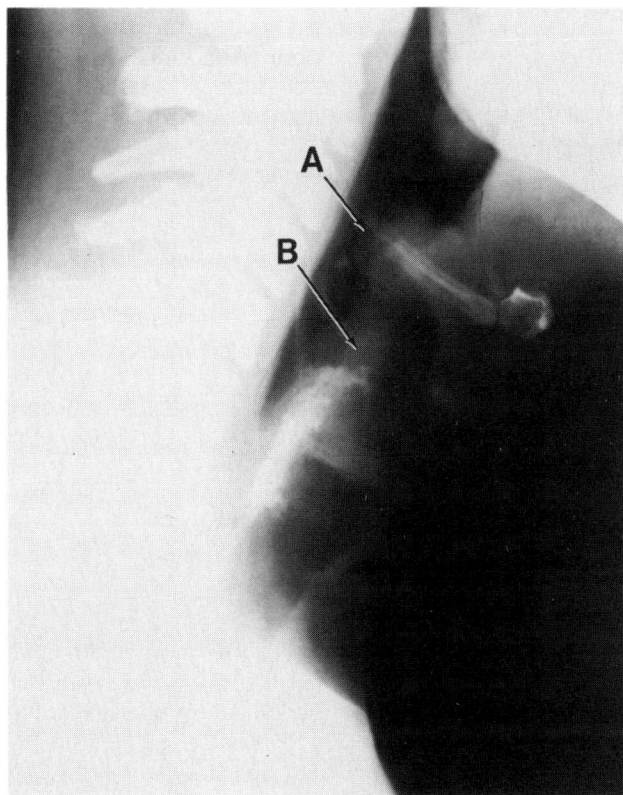

FIGURE 54-10 Lateral view of the neck in an adult with acute epiglottitis, showing soft tissue swelling of the epiglottis (*A*) and aryepiglottic folds (*B*). (*Reproduced with permission from Chow et al.[21]*)

ceftriaxone. Culture and sensitivity results will dictate the ultimate choice of antibiotic, which should be continued for 7 to 10 days. When *H. influenzae* infection is demonstrated, rifampin prophylaxis should be provided for all household contacts when the household contains contacts younger than 4 years.

LARYNGOTRACHEOBRONCHITIS (CROUP)

Laryngotracheobronchitis primarily affects young children after a viral upper respiratory infection caused by influenza, parainfluenza, respiratory syncytial virus, adenovirus, and occasionally *Mycoplasma pneumoniae*.[22] Inflammation results in edematous swelling of the conus elasticus with narrowing of the infraglottic structures. Laryngotracheobronchitis follows a more gradual course than does bacterial epiglottitis and may be self-limiting or progress to respiratory obstruction. Clinical findings include a "brassy" or "barking" nonproductive cough associated with different degrees of inspiratory stridor, hoarseness, and respiratory distress. Respirations are noisy, often accompanied by chest wall retractions and inspiratory and expiratory wheezing. Nasal discharge and pharyngeal injection are common, but the epiglottis and supraglottic structures appear normal. Fever and malaise are present as part of the upper respiratory viral syndrome. A lateral radiograph of the neck can be helpful by showing the characteristic infraglottic narrowing. Management is similar to that for supraglottic laryngitis, including humidification, hydration, oxygen administration, and antibiotic therapy for secondary bacterial infection. Use of sedatives and narcotics,

which suppress the cough reflex, is to be avoided.[23] The role of steroids remains unclear.[23] Occasionally, an artificial airway is required for 2 to 5 days or longer. Extubation is sometimes difficult because of additional edema secondary to the endotracheal tube. It seems reasonable that a tracheostomy rather than reintubation should then be considered when the patient fails extubation.

PERICRANIAL INFECTIONS AND INTRACRANIAL SUPPURATION

SINUSITIS, OTITIS, AND MASTOIDITIS

Fortunately, suppurative and life-threatening complications of acute and chronic sinusitis have become relatively infrequent in the postantibiotic era. However, because of the unique pericranial location of these airspaces and the rich vascular supply in this region, contiguous spread of infection may extend intracranially through the diploic veins and result in serious complications such as meningitis, brain abscess, subdural or epidural empyema, osteomyelitis of the skull, and cavernous and other cortical venous sinus thrombosis.[24] The clinical spectrum of such complications may be quite varied (Table 54-3). Because the roof of the frontal and ethmoidal sinuses forms the anterior cranial fossa, infection in either sinus may produce a frontal epidural abscess, subdural empyema, or a frontal lobe brain abscess (see Fig. 54-2). Frontal sinusitis may also result in thrombosis of the superior sagittal sinus, which arises in the roof of the frontal air sinuses. Extension of infection anteriorly into bone can lead to "Pott's puffy tumor of the forehead," whereas an orbital extension may lead to periorbital cellulitis. The ethmoidal sinuses are separated from the orbital cavity by a paper-thin orbital plate. Perforation of the plate allows direct spread of infection into the retro-orbital space. Ethmoidal sinusitis can also spread to the superior sagittal vein or the cavernous venous sinus (see Fig. 54-2). The sphenoid sinus occupies the body of the sphenoid bone in close proximity to the pituitary gland above, the optic nerve and optic chiasma in front, and the internal carotids, the cavernous sinuses, and the temporal lobes of the brain on each side (see Fig. 54-2). Thus, sphenoid sinusitis can spread locally to cause cavernous sinus thrombosis, meningitis, temporal lobe abscess, and orbital fissure syndromes.[7,25] The superior orbital fissure syndrome, characterized by orbital pain, exophthalmos, and ophthalmoplegia, is due to involvement of the abducens, oculomotor, and trochlear nerves and the ophthalmic division of the trigeminal nerve as they pass through the orbital fissure.[24] Extension of infection from the maxillary sinus into the adjacent structures may result in osteomyelitis of the facial bones, including prolapse of the orbital antral wall with retro-orbital cellulitis, proptosis, and ophthalmoplegia. Direct intracranial extension from the maxillary sinus is rare, except in rhinocerebral mucormycosis and other types of invasive fungal sinusitis. Infections of the middle ear or mastoid within the petrous bone may extend into the middle fossa to involve the temporal lobe or into the posterior fossa to involve the cerebellum or brain stem. The skull overlying the dura of the cerebrum is covered extracranially by the galea aponeurotica. Pericranial infections due to head trauma or to a craniotomy may result in a subgaleal abscess and cranial osteomyelitis, with possible retrograde spread through the emissary veins to the epidural, subdural, and subarachnoid spaces.

TABLE 54-3 The Clinical Spectrum and Investigation of Intracranial Complications

Complication	Clinical Signs	Cerebrospinal Fluid	COMPUTED TOMOGRAPHY	
			Plain	With Contrast
Meningitis	Headache, fever (++), stiff neck, lethargy (++), rapid course	High PMN and protein levels; low glucose level	Normal	Diffusely enhanced
Osteomyelitis	Pott's puffy tumor (±)	Normal	Bony defect	Bony defect
Epidural abscess or mucocele	Headache (±), fever (±)	Normal	Lucent area	Biconvex capsule
Subdural empyema	Headache (±), convulsions (±), hemiplegia (±), rapid course (±)	High PMN and protein levels; normal glucose level	Lucent area	Crescent-shaped enhancement
Cerebral abscess	Convulsions (+), headache (+), personality change (+)	Lymphocytosis; normal glucose level	Lucency with mass effect	Capsule
Venous sinus thrombosis (cavernous)	"Picket-fence" fever (++), rapid course (++), orbital edema (++), ocular palsies (++)	Normal or high PMN count	Nonspecific	Enhancing lesion

ABBREVIATIONS: (++) characteristically seen; (+) frequently seen; (±) may or may not be seen; PMN, polymorphonuclear leukocyte.

Sinusitis occurring after prolonged endotracheal intubation is a recognized complication among critically ill patients. The incidence of this infection likely exceeds 15% in patients intubated longer than 5 days and is probably more frequent with nasal than with endotracheal and gastric tubes.[26,27] One study pointed to the difficulties in assessing sinusitis associated with intubation.[26] In this evaluation of 162 adult patients with intubation longer than 7 days, only 25% exhibited entirely normal maxillary sinuses at the time of an initial CT scan within 48 hours of admission. Some degree of mucosal thickening or an air–fluid level was present in most patients, suggesting that subsequent imaging studies must be interpreted in light of a high incidence of baseline abnormalities in patients admitted with respiratory failure. Nonetheless, when culture-positive sinusitis did develop, aggressive diagnosis and treatment appeared beneficial, and there was an association between sinusitis and bronchopneumonia. Interestingly, use of oral intubation was associated with a lower incidence of maxillary sinusitis than of nasal intubation.

Whether the use of soft feeding tubes or the Sengstaken-Blakemore tube carries a similar risk is currently unknown. This event is probably secondary to local trauma and edema within the intubated nasal cavity and is further promoted by limited head mobility, resulting in impaired drainage of the sinuses through the natural ostia. In contrast to community-acquired sinusitis, nosocomial sinusitis in the critically ill is often clinically silent, except for unexplained fever and leukocytosis. Purulent rhinorrhea and opacification or air–fluid levels on sinus roentgenograms or CT scans may suggest the diagnosis. The sequelae of unrecognized infection can be catastrophic, with intracranial extension and fulminant sepsis. A large percentage of cases of nosocomial sinusitis is polymicrobial (42% in one series), and most patients may be receiving broad-spectrum antibiotics at the time of diagnosis. The use of antral puncture for drainage and specimen collection for Gram stain and culture is strongly recommended. Antimicrobial therapy should be guided by Gram stain of the aspirate and culture results. Broad-spectrum coverage of *S. aureus* and enteric gram-negative bacilli is generally required.

RHINOCEREBRAL MUCORMYCOSIS AND MALIGNANT OTITIS EXTERNA

Rhinocerebral mucormycosis is a progressive and destructive infection of the paranasal sinuses caused by fungi of the family Mucoraceae: *Absidia*, *Mucor*, *Rhizomucor*, and *Rhizopus*.[28,29] It occurs primarily in debilitated patients with uncontrolled diabetes and ketoacidosis, in profoundly dehydrated children, and in neutropenic patients receiving cytotoxic therapy. The infection begins in the nose or nasopharynx and spreads through the sinuses into the orbit or central nervous system. It may extend through the cribriform plate to involve the meninges and the adjacent frontal lobe and cranial nerves, or it may extend through the nasolacrimal duct to involve the orbit, producing panophthalmitis. These fungi have a predilection for the walls of arteries, and infection spreads by this route, causing thrombosis and tissue infarction. The internal carotid artery or its major branches may be involved, as may the cavernous sinus. Clinically, black necrotic lesions may be found on the nasal mucous membranes or the soft palate. When orbital involvement is seen, there is proptosis, ophthalmoplegia, blindness, chemosis, and corneal anesthesia. Extension into the cranial cavity is manifested by headache, meningismus, trigeminal or facial cranial nerve palsy, seizures, and other focal neurologic signs. Progressive obtundation is seen, culminating in coma. The diagnosis is confirmed by the presence of broad, nonseptate hyphae in biopsy specimens and a positive culture. Treatment requires aggressive surgical débridement and systemic amphotericin B. With early diagnosis, control of the underlying condition, and appropriate antimicrobial therapy, long-term survival has been reported in 85% of cases.

Malignant otitis externa is a progressive and necrotizing infection of the external ear caused by *P. aeruginosa*, with spread through the cartilaginous and bony canal to the base of the skull. Affected patients are usually debilitated and often have poorly controlled diabetes mellitus. The infection is associated with severe otalgia, hearing loss, purulent discharge, edema, and granulation tissue or "polyp" in the cartilaginous portion of the external ear canal. Three stages of progression are recognized clinically: (a) locally invasive disease,

(b) disease associated with facial palsy, and (c) disease associated with multiple cranial nerve palsies. In the latter stages, infection may involve the infratemporal fossa by extension into the temporal or occipital bone. Prolonged medical therapy in conjunction with local débridement of granulation tissue and infected cartilage is effective in the majority of patients. In patients with more extensive disease involving the base of the skull and multiple cranial nerve palsies, therapy is not as successful, and up to 20 months of antimicrobial treatment may be required to achieve eradication of infection without relapse.

INTRACRANIAL SUPPURATION

These dreaded complications, which most commonly arise from chronic sinusitis, mastoiditis, or deep fascial space infections,[30] are only briefly reviewed here. Readers are referred to Chap. 52 for a more comprehensive description of these entities.

BRAIN ABSCESS

Most brain abscesses occur in association with three identifiable clinical settings (a) a contiguous focus of infection, particularly sinusitis, otitis, or mastoiditis; (b) cranial trauma or trauma after craniotomy; and (c) hematogenous spread from an extracranial focus of infection, especially the lung and heart valves. Otogenic (e.g., temporal lobe or cerebellum) and sinusitis-related (e.g., frontal lobe) brain abscesses account for approximately 50% of all pericranial sources of infection.[31] Hematogenous brain abscesses are frequently multiple and located in the distribution of the middle cerebral artery (i.e., in the posterior frontal or parietal lobes). The clinical presentations of brain abscesses are quite variable and appear to be influenced primarily by the anatomic location of the abscesses; their proximity to the ventricles, cisterns, or dural sinuses; and major alterations in the intracranial pressure dynamics secondary to the mass effect. Thus, a pontine abscess may bulge posteriorly and block the aqueduct of Sylvius acutely to cause obstructive hydrocephalus. An occipital lobe abscess could rupture or leak into the ventricular system, causing ventriculitis, or it could involve the transverse sinus and cause septic thrombophlebitis or a subdural empyema. Four distinctive clinical presentations of a brain abscess can be recognized, based on the unique pathophysiologic events implicated: (a) rapid focal mass expansion, (b) intracranial hypertension, (c) diffuse brain destruction, and (d) focal neurologic deficit. In the last category, the temporal progression of infection is so slow that it is often misdiagnosed as a neoplasm. Fever is present in only 45% to 50% of patients; therefore, absence of fever should not be used to exclude the diagnosis of brain abscess.

SUBDURAL EMPYEMA AND CRANIAL EPIDURAL ABSCESS

Intracranial subdural empyema in the adult usually results from a suppurative infection of the paranasal sinuses, mastoid, or middle ear. An acute flare-up with local pain and increase in purulent nasal or aural discharge and onset of generalized headache and high fevers are the first indications of intracranial spread. They are followed within days by focal neurologic findings such as unilateral motor seizures, hemi-

plegia, hemianesthesia, or aphasia, and signs of increased intracranial pressure with progressive lethargy and coma. The neck is stiff, but cerebrospinal fluid examination is more consistent with an aseptic meningitis syndrome. In infants and young children, however, an intracranial subdural empyema is almost invariably a complication of bacterial meningitis. Early signs such as irritability, poor feeding, or increased head size are nonspecific, but hemiparesis, convulsions, stupor, and coma may rapidly ensue. *Streptococcus pneumoniae*, *Streptococcus agalactiae*, and *H. influenzae* are the most common causes.

Cranial epidural abscess is usually associated with an infection after craniotomy or a cranial osteomyelitis secondary to chronic sinusitis or middle ear infection. The onset of symptoms may be insidious and overshadowed by the localized inflammatory process. Focal neurologic findings are less common than in subdural empyema. Rarely, a fifth and sixth cranial nerve palsy may develop in association with infections of the petrous portion of the temporal bone (Gradenigo syndrome).

SEPTIC INTRACRANIAL THROMBOPHLEBITIS AND MYCOTIC ANEURYSM

Septic intracranial thrombophlebitis most frequently follows infection of the paranasal sinuses, middle ear, mastoid, or oropharynx. If collateral venous drainage is adequate, septic venous thrombosis may produce only transient neurologic findings or may be silent. If the thrombus outstrips collateral flow, progressive neurologic deficits will result, with impairment of consciousness, focal or generalized seizures, and increased intracranial pressure. The clinical findings differ with the location of cortical veins or dural sinuses involved. Cavernous sinus thrombosis is characterized by abrupt onset with diplopia, photophobia, orbital edema, and progressive exophthalmos. Involvement of cranial nerves III, IV, V, and VI produces ophthalmoplegia, a midposition fixed pupil, loss of the corneal reflex, and diminished sensation over the upper face. Obstruction of venous return from the retina results in papilledema, retinal hemorrhage, and visual loss. Contrast-enhanced CT (Fig. 54-11) and magnetic resonance imaging (MRI) are the imaging modalities of choice. Treatment requires early recognition, high-dose intravenous antibiotics, and surgical decompression of the underlying predisposing infection. Anticoagulation and steroids are not indicated. Mortality remains high, approximately 15% to 30%. Thrombosis of the superior sagittal sinus produces bilateral leg weakness and may cause communicating hydrocephalus. Occlusion of the lateral sinus produces pain over the ear and mastoid and may cause edema over the mastoid (Griesinger sign). Involvement of cranial nerves V and VI produces ipsilateral facial pain and lateral rectus weakness (Gradenigo syndrome). Intracranial mycotic aneurysm usually results from septic embolization as a complication of bacterial endocarditis. This produces infection and necrosis in the arterial wall, which leads to dilation and possible rupture. Mycotic aneurysms can be multiple and are usually found on distal branches of the middle or anterior cerebral arteries. The early clinical manifestations are similar to those of cerebral emboli and infarction. The weakened vessel may be seen to progressively grow on serial angiograms. Because the clinical course

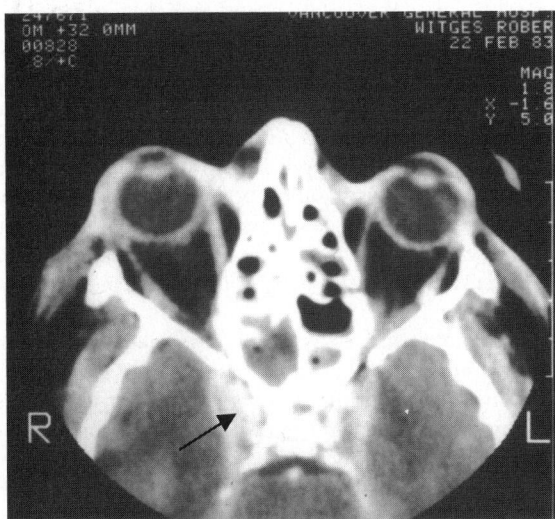

FIGURE 54-11 Computed tomographic scan of the head in a patient with cavernous sinus thrombosis secondary to sphenoid sinusitis. *Arrow* indicates thrombus in the right cavernous sinus.

of a mycotic aneurysm is quite variable and the risk of rupture with catastrophic cerebral hemorrhage cannot be predicted even after successful therapy of the underlying endocarditis, early surgical intervention is advised.

Diagnostic Considerations

MICROBIOLOGIC TECHNIQUES

It is imperative that clinical specimens for the diagnosis of deep head and neck infections be obtained without contamination by the resident oronasopharyngeal flora. This is best accomplished using a needle and syringe for aspiration of loculated pus through an extraoral approach. After the skin is cleaned, pus is aspirated into the syringe. All air is carefully expressed, and the needle tip is inserted into a rubber stopper. This allows the exclusion of air, and the specimen can then be transported directly to the laboratory. This method of specimen collection is superior to using swabs. If a swab is used, it should be saturated with purulent material and inserted into a commercially available transport tube specifically designed to transport swabs under anaerobic conditions. An additional swab should be taken for Gram staining. The Gram stain is particularly useful in the assessment of head and neck infections because a polymicrobial flora is generally present, and anaerobic bacteria may require 48 hours or longer for growth. The microscopic morphology of some of the bacteria may be characteristic enough to suggest a provisional diagnosis and, ultimately, therapy. Infected tissues obtained intraoperatively are also suitable for anaerobic and aerobic processing, provided that care is taken to prevent contamination by the normal resident flora.

IMAGING TECHNIQUES

CT and MRI are particularly useful for localization of deep fascial space infections of the head and neck.[7,32] Because CT can localize a process and define its extent, in particular invasion into the cranial vault, mediastinum, or the bone, it is an invaluable tool for guiding needle aspiration or open

drainage. A lateral radiograph of the neck may demonstrate compression or deviation of the tracheal air column or the presence of gas within necrotic soft tissues. The soft tissues of the posterior wall of the hypopharynx are approximately 5 mm deep, less than one-third the diameter of the fourth cervical vertebra (C4). The retropharyngeal soft tissues should be approximately two-thirds the width of C4, and the retrotracheal space should be slightly smaller. A lateral radiograph of the cervical spine or a CT can determine whether the soft tissue swelling or abscess originated from the retropharyngeal space or the prevertebral space. The former suggests an odontogenic or oropharyngeal source, whereas the latter likely suggests involvement of the cervical spine.

CT is the single neuroimaging technique that has been most helpful for the diagnosis of intracranial infections such as brain abscess, subdural empyema, and epidural abscess. The typical CT finding in brain abscess is an area of decreased attenuation that is surrounded by a ring of enhancement after injection of contrast. CT also detects cerebral edema, hydrocephalus, an associated mass effect, and the presence of extracranial infection. In subdural empyema, CT presents inward displacement of cerebral substance due to an extracerebral mass. In epidural abscess, CT demonstrates a thick and circumscribed area of diminished density associated with extracerebral displacement and contiguous cranial osteomyelitis. Radionuclide brain scans and cerebral angiography remain useful as complementary procedures for the localization of certain central nervous system infections, in particular posterior fossa lesions and demonstration of mycotic aneurysms. MRI appears to be more sensitive than CT in the detection of suppurative intracranial infections. It is particularly useful for the detection and characterization of the early stages of cerebritis or epidural abscess. MRI is also useful for imaging vascular lesions, such as jugular thombophlebitis.[33] It remains to be seen whether newer techniques such as positron emission tomography will improve the diagnostic yield in early pericranial or intracranial infections.

Technetium bone scanning, used in combination with gallium- or indium-labeled white blood cells, is particularly useful for the diagnosis of cranial or cervical osteomyelitis. MRI is more sensitive than CT and probably more accurate than bone scan in detecting bone involvement.[34,35] T2-weighted images may identify and localize areas of pus for drainage or aspiration. Gadolinium enhancement is important to accurately define the soft tissue component.

Therapeutic Considerations

Although resuscitation and surgical measures are of primary importance in the initial management of these life-threatening infections, appropriate antibiotics are essential for a successful outcome. Empirical antimicrobial regimens for head and neck and upper respiratory tract infections are presented in Table 54-2. Recommendations for intracranial suppurative complications are discussed in Chap. 52. Maximum doses of systemic antimicrobials should be administered to optimize penetration of bone and the blood-brain barrier. Therapy should be continued for 2 to 3 weeks. Intracranial and vascular or bone infections may require at least 6 to 8 weeks of intravenous antibiotics. Where anaerobes are implicated, penicillin G, usually in combination with metronidazole to deal with penicillin-resistant anaerobes, is the antibiotic regimen of first choice. Clindamycin is useful as an alternative in the penicillin-allergic patient and has the advantage of more effective coverage against β-lactamase–producing anaerobes. Chloramphenicol is rarely used because of its propensity for myelotoxicity. Metronidazole lacks activity against gram-positive anaerobic cocci such as *Peptostreptococcus* and facultative organisms such as streptococci and *S. aureus*, which precludes its use as monotherapy for head and neck infections. For immunocompromised and critically ill patients, broad-spectrum coverage for aerobic gram-negative rods, *S. aureus*, and anaerobes (e.g., with cefotaxime, ceftizoxime, piperacillin-tazobactam, or imipenem) is indicated (see Table 54-2). The final selection of antimicrobial therapy should be guided by culture results and susceptibility data.

Although considerable advances have been made in our understanding of these life-threatening oropharyngeal and otorhinolaryngeal infections, vigilance in terms of diagnosis and management is required to avoid the high mortality rate associated with this important group of conditions.

References

1. Chow AW: Infections of the oral cavity, neck and head, in Mandell GL, Bennett JE, Dolin R (eds): *Principles and Practice of Infectious Diseases.* New York, Churchill Livingstone, 1995, p 593.
2. Chow AW: Infections of the sinuses and parameningeal structures, in Gorbach SL, Bartlett JG, Blacklow NR (eds): *Infectious Diseases.* Philadelphia, WB Saunders, 1998, p 517.
3. Todd JK: Bacteriology and clinical relevance of nasopharyngeal and oropharyngeal cultures. *Pediatr Infect Dis* 3:159, 1984.
4. Brook I: Anaerobic bacteria in upper respiratory tract and other head and neck infections. *Ann Otol Rhinol Laryngol* 111:430, 2002.
5. Brook I: Antibiotic resistance of oral anaerobic bacteria and their effect on the management of upper respiratory tract and head and neck infections. *Semin Respir Infect* 17:195, 2002.
6. Chow AW: Life-threatening infections of the head, neck, and upper respiratory tract, in Hall JB, Schmidt GA, Wood LDH (eds): *Principles of Critical Care.* New York, McGraw-Hill, 1998, p 887.
7. Chow AW: Head and neck infections, in Baddour L, Gorbach SL (eds): *Therapy of Infectious Diseases.* Philadelphia, Saunders, 2003, p 25.
8. Blomquist IK, Bayer AS: Life-threatening deep fascial space infections of the head and neck. *Infect Dis Clin North Am* 2:237, 1988.
9. Megran DW, Scheifele DW, Chow AW: Odontogenic infections. *Pediatr Infect Dis* 3:257, 1984.
10. Barakate MS, Jensen MJ, Hemli JM, et al: Ludwig's angina: Report of a case and review of management issues. *Ann Otol Rhinol Laryngol* 110:453, 2001.
11. Busch RF: Ludwig angina: early aggressive therapy. *Arch Otolaryngol Head Neck Surg* 125:1283, 1999.
12. Hagelskjaer KL, Prag J: Human necrobacillosis, with emphasis on Lemierre's syndrome. *Clin Infect Dis* 31:524, 2000.
13. Sinave CP, Hardy GJ, Fardy PW: The Lemierre syndrome—Suppurative thrombophlebitis of the internal jugular vein secondary to oropharyngeal infection. *Medicine (Baltimore)* 68:85, 1989.
14. Armstrong AW, Spooner K, Sanders JW: Lemierre's syndrome. *Curr Infect Dis Rep* 2:168, 2000.
15. Takao M, Ido M, Hamaguchi K, et al: Descending necrotizing mediastinitis secondary to retropharyngeal abscess. *Eur Respir J* 7:1716, 1994.
16. Fattahi TT, Lyu PE, Van Sickels JE: Management of acute suppurative parotitis. *J Oral Maxillofac Surg* 60:446, 2002.
17. Whiting JL, Chow AW: Life-threatening infections of the mouth and throat. *J Crit Illness* 2:36, 1987.
18. von Hunolstein C, Alfarone G, Scopetti F, et al: Molecular epidemiology and characteristics of *Corynebacterium diphtheriae* and *Corynebacterium ulcerans* strains isolated in Italy during the 1990s. *J Med Microbiol* 52:181, 2003.
19. Frantz TD, Rasgon BM, Quesenberry CP Jr: Acute epiglottitis in adults. Analysis of 129 cases. *JAMA* 272:1358, 1994.
20. Solomon P, Weisbrod M, Irish JC, et al: Adult epiglottis: the Toronto Hospital experience. *J Otolaryngol* 27:332, 1998.
21. Chow AW, Bushkell LL, Yoshikawa TT, et al: Case report. *Haemophilus* parainfluenzae epiglottitis with meningitis and bacteremia in an adult. *Am J Med Sci* 267:365, 1974.
22. Malhotra A, Krilov LR: Viral croup. *Pediatr Rev* 22:5, 2001.
23. Stannard W, O'Callaghan C: Management of croup. *Paediatr Drugs* 4:231, 2002.
24. Chow AW: Acute sinusitis: current status of etiologies, diagnosis, and treatment. *Curr Clin Topics Infect Dis* 21:31, 2001.
25. Lew D, Southwick FS, Montgomery WW, et al: Sphenoid sinusitis. A review of 30 cases. *N Engl J Med* 309:1149, 1983.
26. Rouby JJ, Laurent P, Gosnach MCE, et al: Risk factors and clinical relevance of nosocomial maxillary sinusitis in the critically ill. *Am J Resp Crit Care Med* 150:776, 1994.
27. Holzapfel L, Chevret S, Madinier G, et al: Influence of long-term oro- or nasotracheal intubation on nosocomial maxillary sinusitis and pneumonia: Results of a prospective, randomized, clinical trial. *Crit Care Med* 21:1132, 1993.
28. deShazo RD: Fungal sinusitis. *Am J Med Sci* 316:39, 1998.
29. Gonzalez CE, Rinaldi MG, Sugar AM: Zygomycosis. *Infect Dis Clin North Am* 16:895, 2002.
30. Chow AW: Life-threatening infections of the head and neck. *Clin Infect Dis* 14:991, 1992.
31. Yoshikawa TT, Quinn W: The aching head—Intracranial suppuration due to head and neck infections. *Infect Dis Clin North Am* 2:265, 1988.
32. Salit IE: Diagnostic approaches to head and neck infections. *Infect Dis Clin North Am* 2:35, 1988.
33. Latchaw RE, Hirsch WL Jr, Yock DH Jr: Imaging of intracranial infection. *Neurosurg Clin North Am* 3:303, 1992.
34. Santiago RC, Gimenez CR, McCarthy K: Imaging of osteomyelitis and musculoskeletal soft tissue infections: Current concepts. *Rheum Dis Clin North Am* 29:89, 2003.
35. Kattapuram TM, Treat ME, Kattapuram SV: Magnetic resonance imaging of bone and soft tissue infections. *Curr Clin Topics Infect Dis* 21:190, 2001.

Chapter 55

SOFT TISSUE INFECTIONS

JOHN CONLY

KEY POINTS

- *Soft tissue infections characterized by extensive necrosis of subcutaneous tissue, fascia, or muscle are uncommon, but they require prompt recognition and urgent surgical treatment.*

- *The classic hallmarks of virulent soft tissue infections are extensive involvement of the subcutaneous tissues and a relative paucity of cutaneous involvement until late in the course of the infection.*

- *Rapidly spreading soft tissue infections present acutely with severe systemic toxicity.*

- *Successful management of these critically ill patients depends on prompt diagnosis by clinical and radiologic means.*

- *The principles of management include fluid resuscitation, hemodynamic stabilization, a broad-spectrum antimicrobial regimen, and early surgical intervention.*

- *Prompt surgery, in which a definitive diagnosis is reached and all necrotic tissue is débrided, should be considered the mainstay of treatment.*

- *The mortality rate is highest when the diagnosis is delayed or initial surgical treatment is limited.*

Classification of Soft Tissue Infections

In severe soft tissue infections, the initial cutaneous presentation often belies the relentless progression of subcutaneous tissue necrosis and dissection that lies beneath a normal-appearing skin. Successful management of these soft tissue infections depends on early recognition followed by appropriate investigations to establish a specific diagnosis. A clear understanding of a classification of these entities is required, but, unfortunately, the published literature in this area is confusing because of a lack of uniformity in descriptive terminology and the use of different classification schemes. The confusion is compounded by the fact that certain clinical entities may involve one or more anatomic planes within the subcutaneous tissue, and one or more bacterial species may be responsible for the same or different clinical entities. Although classification schemes based on microbial etiology may be the most complete, they offer little to the clinical diagnostic process necessary to expedite appropriate management.[1] To place a useful clinicoanatomic classification into perspective, a review of the basic anatomy and microbial ecology of the skin and subcutaneous tissues is necessary.

BASIC ANATOMY AND MICROBIAL ECOLOGY OF THE SKIN AND SOFT TISSUES

The skin consists of an outer layer, the *epidermis,* and an inner layer, the *dermis,* which resides on a fibrous connective tissue layer, the *superficial fascia.* Beneath this layer, the avascular *deep fascia* overlies and separates muscle groups and acts as a mechanical barrier against the spread of infections from superficial layers to the muscle compartments. Between the superficial and deep fascia lies the *fascial cleft,* which is mainly composed of adipose tissue and contains the superficial nerves, arteries, veins, and lymphatics that supply the skin and adipose tissue.

Normally, the skin has a resident and a transient flora. The resident flora includes *Corynebacterium* species, coagulase-negative staphylococci, and *Micrococcus* species. *Staphylococcus aureus* is not considered part of the resident flora, but colonization rates of 10% to 30% in the anterior nares, axillae, groins, and perineum are not uncommon. Gram-negative bacilli are not considered part of the normal resident flora, although they are occasionally found in the moist intertriginous areas, such as the toe webs, groin, and perineum. The transient flora is made up of bacteria that are collected from extraneous sources and colonize the cutaneous surface for only a short period (hours to days). These organisms are highly variable but often include pathogenic gram-negative bacilli such as *Escherichia coli, Proteus* species, *Pseudomonas aeruginosa,* among others.[2] Critically ill patients frequently have compromised natural defense barriers, with concomitant increases in transient flora colonization.[3]

CLINICOANATOMIC CLASSIFICATION OF SOFT TISSUE INFECTIONS

Most classification schemes for soft tissue infections are based on clinical presentation or microbiologic etiology. Figure 55-1 shows a practical approach to the classification that is based on the affected anatomic plane of the soft tissues, the most commonly encountered clinical terms, and the microbial etiology.

The *common superficial pyodermas* include erysipelas, impetigo, ecthyma, furunculosis, and carbunculosis. These entities do not extend beyond the skin or its appendages and are not discussed further.

The *cellulitides* include what is commonly referred to as *cellulitis, anaerobic (or gangrenous) cellulitis,* and the clinically distinctive variant of gangrenous cellulitis called *progressive bacterial synergistic gangrene (Meleney gangrene).* Cellulitis is an acute spreading infection of the skin extending below the superficial fascia and involving the upper half of the subcutaneous tissues. These infections do not involve the deep fascial layer. The production of gas by anaerobic organisms and the subsequent presence of soft tissue gas, either palpable or demonstrable radiographically, and the propensity to produce necrosis in the subcutaneous tissue (and eventually in the skin) are major differentiating features of anaerobic and classic cellulitis. *Progressive bacterial synergistic gangrene (Meleney gangrene)* was the original term used to describe a distinct form of cellulitis often occurring postoperatively, with necrotic ulcer formation in the center of a cellulitic area.[4]

Necrotizing fasciitis is an acute infection involving the deep fascia, subcutaneous tissue, and superficial fascia to variable degrees.[5] The muscle tissue beneath the deep fascia is unaffected. The skin may not be involved early in the course of the infection, but as the process continues the skin becomes involved. Fournier syndrome (or gangrene) is a form of necrotizing fasciitis that affects the scrotum and genitalia.[6] In this setting, because there is virtually no subcutaneous fat

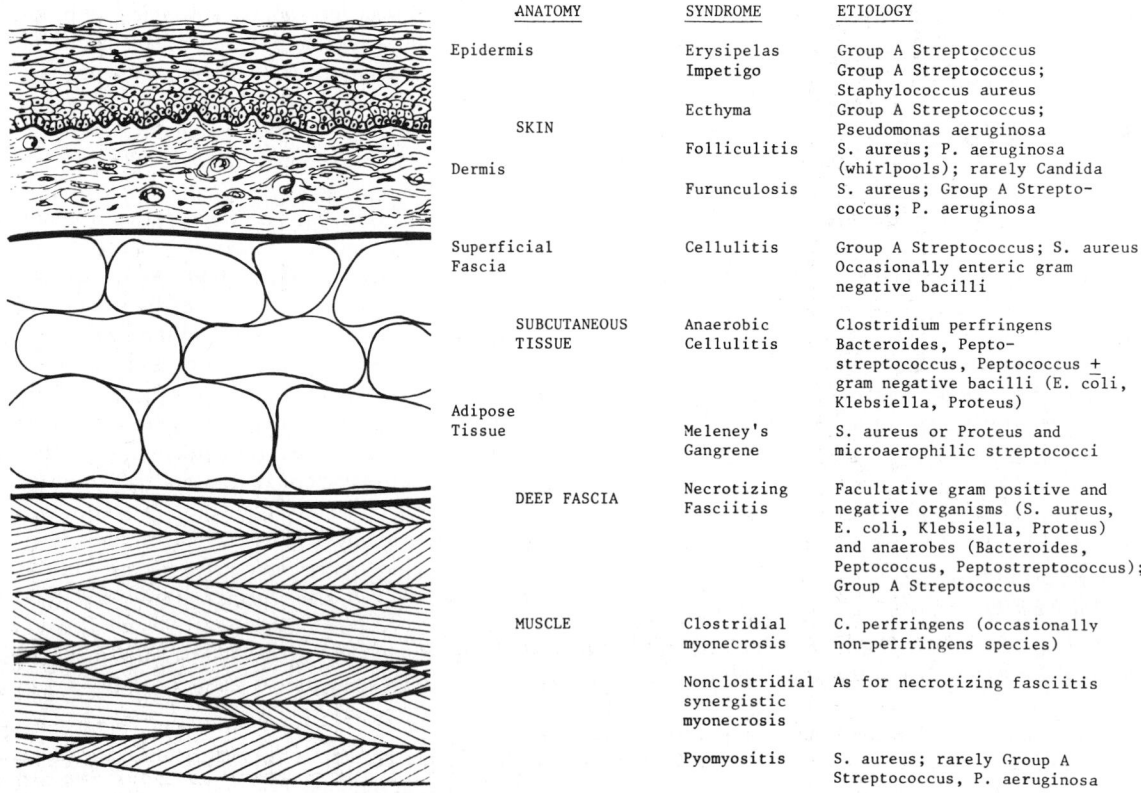

ANATOMY	SYNDROME	ETIOLOGY
Epidermis	Erysipelas	Group A Streptococcus
	Impetigo	Group A Streptococcus; Staphylococcus aureus
SKIN	Ecthyma	Group A Streptococcus; Pseudomonas aeruginosa
	Folliculitis	S. aureus; P. aeruginosa (whirlpools); rarely Candida
Dermis	Furunculosis	S. aureus; Group A Streptococcus; P. aeruginosa
Superficial Fascia	Cellulitis	Group A Streptococcus; S. aureus Occasionally enteric gram negative bacilli
SUBCUTANEOUS TISSUE	Anaerobic Cellulitis	Clostridium perfringens Bacteroides, Peptostreptococcus, Peptococcus + gram negative bacilli (E. coli, Klebsiella, Proteus)
Adipose Tissue	Meleney's Gangrene	S. aureus or Proteus and microaerophilic streptococci
DEEP FASCIA	Necrotizing Fasciitis	Facultative gram positive and negative organisms (S. aureus, E. coli, Klebsiella, Proteus) and anaerobes (Bacteroides, Peptococcus, Peptostreptococcus); Group A Streptococcus
MUSCLE	Clostridial myonecrosis	C. perfringens (occasionally non-perfringens species)
	Nonclostridial synergistic myonecrosis	As for necrotizing fasciitis
	Pyomyositis	S. aureus; rarely Group A Streptococcus, P. aeruginosa

FIGURE 55-1 Clinicoanatomic classification of soft tissue infections.

between the epidermis and dartos fascia, cutaneous gangrene readily develops.

The *myonecroses* include clostridial myonecrosis (otherwise known as *gas gangrene*), nonclostridial myonecrosis (which has also been termed *synergistic necrotizing cellulitis,* although that is a misnomer), pyomyositis, and vascular gangrene. Rapid necrosis of the muscle and subsequent necrosis of the overlying subcutaneous tissue and skin are characteristic of the myonecrotic syndromes. Pyomyositis, an exception, is a bacterial abscess localized to the muscle, usually occurring after penetrating trauma. Vascular gangrene occurs in a limb devitalized by arterial insufficiency.

Major Soft Tissue Infections

CELLULITIS

PATHOGENESIS
Cellulitis most often occurs secondary to trauma of the skin with local inoculation of microorganisms, secondary to an underlying skin lesion or a postoperative wound infection, or by contiguous spread from a suppurative infection of other soft tissues or bone. However, cellulitis may also occur in the absence of any obvious local trauma. After inoculation of microorganisms into the subcutaneous tissues and skin, an acute inflammatory response is seen in the epidermis, dermis, adipose tissue, and superficial fascia, to different degrees.

ETIOLOGY
The most common organisms causing classic cellulitis are *Streptococcus pyogenes* and *S. aureus,* with *Streptococcus pneumoniae,* other streptococci, and gram-negative bacilli encoun-

tered less frequently. Cellulitis due to gram-negative bacilli occurs primarily in immunosuppressed or granulocytopenic patients. A severe form of cellulitis may occur in individuals exposed to *Aeromonas hydrophila* in fresh water; the organism gains access through lacerations during swimming or wading. A severe and fulminant form of cellulitis that progresses rapidly to necrosis and bacteremia may be caused by *Vibrio* species, especially *Vibrio vulnificus,* acquired by exposure of a traumatic wound to salt water or raw seafood drippings.[7]

PRESENTATION
Classic cellulitis is characterized by erythema, pain, edema, and local tenderness involving an area of the skin with ill-defined borders. The area of initial cutaneous involvement expands rapidly. Occasionally there is lymphangitis and regional lymphadenopathy. Systemic manifestations include fever, malaise, and rigors. With untreated or rapidly progressive cellulitis, the process may spread to involve an entire extremity, producing severe systemic toxicity. Dehydration, mental apathy or obtundation, disseminated intravascular coagulopathy, respiratory failure, and septic shock may follow, necessitating intensive care management.

MANAGEMENT
Appropriate laboratory diagnostic studies should be performed before antimicrobial therapy is begun. Any skin abrasions or draining sites should be swabbed for immediate Gram stain and culture. The stain is examined for the presence of organisms, their morphologic appearance, and the number and types of cells. Needle aspiration after injection of 0.5 mL of nonbacteriostatic saline into the leading edge of the cellulitis may be attempted; potential pathogens have been

isolated in 10% to 38% of cases.[8,9] A combination of needle aspiration, skin biopsy, and blood cultures results in isolation of pathogens in approximately 25% of cases.[10]

For severe infections in which streptococci and staphylococci are considered possible, parenteral administration of a large-dose penicillinase-resistant penicillin (nafcillin or cloxacillin), 8 to 12 g/day in four or six divided doses, is most appropriate. Alternate agents include a first-generation cephalosporin, such as cefazolin (6 g/day in three divided doses), vancomycin (2 g/day in two divided doses), or clindamycin (1200 to 2400 mg/day in three divided doses). If the etiologic agent proves to be streptococcal, penicillin G should be substituted (6 to 12 million U/day). In the immunocompromised host or in the presence of a rapidly progressive cellulitis developing after a freshwater or saltwater injury, an aminoglycoside (gentamicin or tobramycin), 3 to 5 mg/kg in three or four divided doses or, alternatively, 5 to 7 mg/kg as a single daily dose, should also be administered.

Local care of cellulitis includes immobilization and elevation of the affected area. These measures are most appropriate when an extremity is affected. Analgesic drugs are administered as necessary. Cool compresses may help alleviate pain. The extent of the cellulitis should be outlined on the skin with an appropriate marker at the time of admission to facilitate objective daily assessments of the extent of spread. Frequent inspection of the involved area is necessary to detect any areas of crepitus or suppuration, which may require surgical drainage. Abscesses of the subcutaneous tissue are not infrequent after extensive cellulitis; judicious use of repeated needle aspiration may be necessary. Failure to achieve defervescence and a decrease in systemic toxicity within 48 to 72 hours after institution of appropriate antimicrobial therapy should arouse suspicion of suppuration or a more virulent soft tissue infection, such as necrotizing fasciitis or myonecrosis.

ANAEROBIC CELLULITIS

PATHOGENESIS

The term used for this type of cellulitis is not properly descriptive, but it persists because it is in common use. Other terms for this process include *gas abscess*, *gangrenous cellulitis*, *localized gas gangrene*, and *epifascial gangrene*. The process usually represents infection of already devitalized subcutaneous tissue without involvement of the deep fascia or underlying muscle. Microorganisms are introduced into the subcutaneous tissues from an operative or traumatic wound or from a pre-existing local infection. The subcutaneous tissues are devitalized owing to a local injury, an inadequately débrided wound, or a metabolic disturbance that compromises vascular supply (e.g., diabetes mellitus). Usually, the infectious process is not invasive but instead remains localized in the area of devitalized tissue.[11,12] Extensive gas formation and suppuration, usually limited to the area of devitalized tissue, are present.

ETIOLOGY

Anaerobic cellulitis may be clostridial or nonclostridial. *Clostridium perfringens* is the most commonly isolated clostridial species, followed by *Clostridium septicum*. Gram-negative rods, staphylococci, or streptococci are occasionally present but are not the predominant isolates. The nonclostridial form of anaerobic cellulitis is essentially the same process as

clostridial cellulitis, but has a different microbiologic etiology. Obligate anaerobes are the predominant isolates, with *Bacteroides fragilis*, *Bacteroides* species, *Peptostreptococcus*, and *Peptococcus* encountered most frequently. Other bacteria that may be present include the gram-negative enteric bacilli (*Escherichia coli* and *Klebsiella*), staphylococci, and streptococci.

PRESENTATION

The clinical pictures of clostridial and nonclostridial anaerobic cellulitis are very similar and may be discussed together. Because this infection represents the local invasion of already devitalized tissue, the process does not generally have a virulent progressive course. The onset is gradual, with mild to moderate local pain and only mild to moderate tissue swelling. Constitutional symptoms are not prominent; the relative paucity of symptoms is helpful in distinguishing this entity from myonecrotic infections. A thin, dark, malodorous discharge from the wound or inoculation site, sometimes containing fat globules, with extensive and prominent gas formation, is characteristic. A dusky erythema may be present, and there may be extensive crepitus in the involved area. Although not initially invasive beyond the area of devitalized tissue, the condition must not be considered benign. If it is inadequately managed, the infection will eventually spread and lead to a rapid and extensive undermining of the skin similar to that seen in necrotizing fasciitis, with corresponding systemic toxicity.

A distinctive variant of gangrenous cellulitis was described and named by Meleney several decades ago.[4] It has been called *progressive bacterial synergistic gangrene, postoperative progressive gangrene, Meleney gangrene*, and—if associated with burrowing necrotic tracts producing distant lesions—*Meleney ulcer*. The process usually begins postoperatively, particularly after abdominal or thoracic procedures, with a slowly developing shaggy ulcer with a gangrenous center surrounded by an inner zone of purple discoloration, which in turn is surrounded by an outer zone of erythema. Without treatment, the course is one of relentless indolent extension, but without significant systemic toxicity. Satellite lesions may occur; they represent tracts of burrowing subcutaneous infection that surface to produce a gangrenous ulcer on the skin. Pathologically, the process is usually limited to the upper third of the subcutaneous fat, but occasionally it extends down to fascia. The lesion was originally thought to be caused by a synergistic interaction between microaerophilic streptococci and *S. aureus*, but recently other microorganisms, including *Proteus* species and other gram-negative enteric bacilli, have been implicated.

MANAGEMENT

Drainage from the wound or site of local injury should be sent for immediate Gram stain and culture. A simple method for obtaining anaerobic specimens for culture is to use a needle and syringe to aseptically aspirate the crepitant area at a site removed from the wound. All air should be carefully expressed from the syringe. If a swab is used, contact with normal flora should be avoided, and a commercial anaerobic transport medium should be used. Blood cultures should also be obtained. Radiologic examination should be performed to assess the presence and extent of soft tissue gas.

Initial antimicrobial selection is guided by the Gram stain of the purulent drainage. If only large "boxcar-shaped" gram-positive bacilli are present, the causative microorganism is *Clostridium,* and moderate to large doses of parenteral penicillin G (10 to 20 million U/day in six to eight divided doses) are indicated. If multiple organisms of different morphologies are present on the Gram stain, then one may assume that the process is polymicrobial, and an empirical broad-spectrum antimicrobial regimen should be instituted. An aminoglycoside (gentamicin or tobramycin, 3 to 5 mg/kg per day in three divided doses or, alternatively, 5 to 7 mg/kg as a single daily dose) and clindamycin (1200 to 2400 mg/day in three or four divided doses), with or without penicillin G (10 to 20 million U/day in six to eight divided doses), would be appropriate. In patients with impaired or changing renal function, a third-generation cephalosporin, such as cefotaxime, ceftriaxone, or ceftazidime, can be used instead of an aminoglycoside. Alternatively, a carbapenem such as imipenem or meropenem may be used as a single agent.

The major conditions to be differentiated from anaerobic cellulitis are necrotizing fasciitis and the myonecrotic syndromes.[13] Distinguishing between clostridial myonecrosis and anaerobic cellulitis is necessary to avoid unnecessary extensive débridement. This distinction is made definitively at the time of surgery, which is mandatory to establish the diagnosis. The involved soft tissue must be laid open widely; devitalized tissue must be débrided; suppurative foci should be drained; and all involved fascial planes should be opened. The deep fascia and muscle must be carefully examined; if they are healthy, no further surgery is necessary. Further débridement may be necessary, depending on the amount of devitalized tissue present. The management of Meleney gangrene includes wide excision of the lesion plus antimicrobials as dictated by the culture results.

NECROTIZING FASCIITIS

PATHOGENESIS

Necrotizing fasciitis is an uncommon but severe infection involving the subcutaneous tissue and the deep fascia. It spreads rapidly in the fascial cleft but spares the overlying skin until the later stages. Extensive undermining of the skin is the hallmark of this infection. It affects persons of all ages but is most common in middle-age and elderly adults. However, with the resurgence of group A streptococcal infections, including soft tissue infections, the incidence of necrotizing fasciitis in previously healthy young adults has increased.[14,15] The infections may occur anywhere, but infections in the perineal region and in the extremities are most commonly reported.

The most common initiating injury leading to infection is minor trauma (~80% of reported cases); operative wounds and decubitus ulcers account for most remaining cases. The presentation is usually acute or subacute, ranging from 3 to 14 days after the injury. In some cases, particularly those associated with group A streptococcus, the onset is very sudden; the condition may progress dramatically from a tiny abrasion to septic shock, with massive subcutaneous necrosis, within 24 hours.[14,16] Many patients have underlying chronic illnesses,[17,18] with diabetes present in 20% to 50% of patients, severe arteriosclerosis in 20% to 33%, and cardiovascular or renal disease in 50%. Nutritional status is also an important consideration, with marked obesity or marked wasting noted

in many cases. With infection due to group A streptococcus, more than 50% of patients have no underlying illness and were previously in good health.

After the initial bacterial invasion, the infection spreads rapidly along fascial planes and subcutaneous fat, with ischemic tissue facilitating spread of the necrotizing process. At an early stage, histologic examination of full-thickness skin biopsies shows no abnormality. However, the subcutaneous fat and fascia show a contiguous nonspecific inflammatory reaction, with fibrinoid arteriolitis and thrombosis of vessels, and subsequent necrosis. If the condition is left untreated, the overlying skin becomes extensively necrotic because of thrombotic occlusion of the venules and arterioles supplying it.

It has been shown that traumatic surgical and vascular injuries generate areas of relative tissue anoxia, with the result that carbohydrate and protein metabolism proceed anaerobically, generating lactic acid. Buffer systems become depleted and acidosis develops, which causes lysosomal disruption and, hence, local autolysis and destruction. This environment provides an ideal milieu for anaerobic growth. Whether actual infection evolves is determined by several factors, including the means of inoculation and the size of the inoculum, altered host defense mechanisms, and the virulence of the bacteria. Altered host defenses play an important role in propagation of the infection. For example, high blood alcohol levels, steroids in large doses, and metabolic acidosis inhibit adherence of phagocytes, and patients with cirrhosis and metastatic carcinoma have poor phagocyte chemotaxis. The virulence of the bacteria is determined, to some extent, by their capacity to produce various enzymes (hemolysins, fibrinolysin, hyaluronidase, and collagenase). In addition, for *S. pyogenes,* the presence of M protein on the surface of the organism has an anticomplement effect and may function as a superantigen, leading to a massive release of potent vasoactive mediators such as tumor necrosis factor, interleukin 1, and myocardial depressant factor. The streptococcal pyrogenic exotoxins A, B, and C or other unknown antigens may also function as super-antigens and have been found to share DNA sequence homology with staphylococcal toxic shock syndrome toxin. Functioning as super-antigens, these toxins share the ability to mediate nonspecific binding to antigen-presenting macrophages and T-helper cells, leading to polyclonal activation of large numbers of these lymphocytes. The cytokine release associated with this activation is responsible for the severe toxic shock–like syndrome associated with *S. pyogenes* infections. Synergistic activity of different bacterial species has also been postulated on the basis of evidence from clinical experience and from experimental infections in animals.[19] It is commonly assumed that aerobic organisms assist the growth of anaerobes by using oxygen, diminishing redox potential, and supplying catalase. Local ischemia and reduced host defense mechanisms in the presence of virulent pathogens combine to produce a milieu that is responsible for the alarmingly rapid spread (Fig. 55-2).

ETIOLOGY

Necrotizing fasciitis may be due to a synergistic polymicrobial bacterial infection in which at least one anaerobic organism (usually a *Bacteroides, Peptostreptococcus,* or *Peptococcus* species) is isolated in combination with one or more facultative organisms (usually streptococci, *E. coli, Klebsiella*

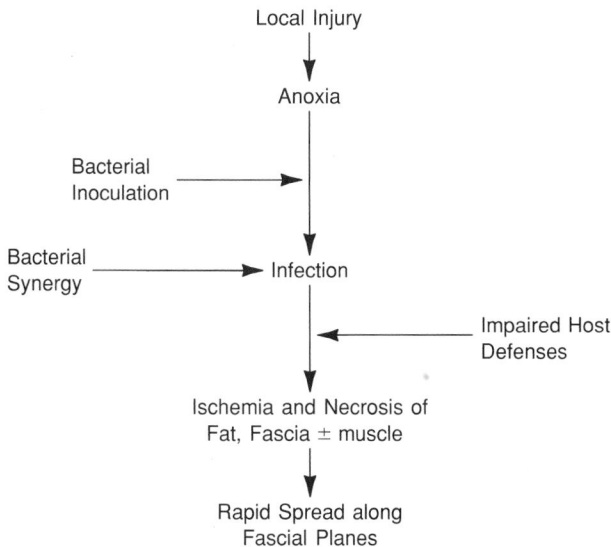

FIGURE 55-2 The pathogenic process in necrotizing fasciitis.

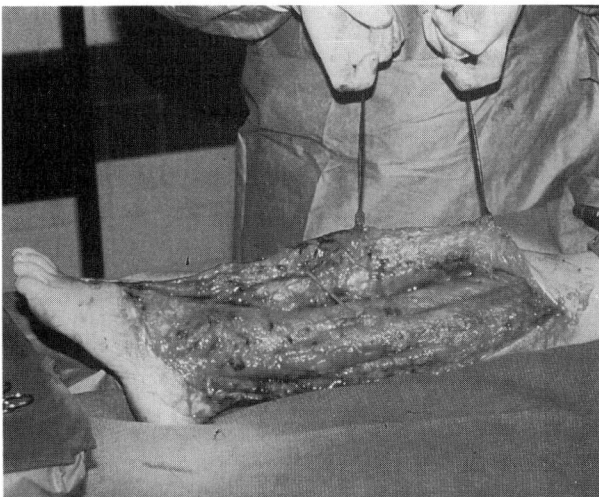

FIGURE 55-4 Postoperative appearance of the lower leg presented in Fig. 55-3 (see Color Plate 55-4). All necrotic subcutaneous tissue was excised.

or *Proteus* species, or *S. aureus*),[20] or it may be due to a single organism, usually *S. pyogenes.* In most cases of polymicrobial origin, multiple organisms are present, with an average of three or four isolates per patient. Some investigators distinguish acute group A streptococcal necrotizing fasciitis as a separate entity. *Vibrio vulnificus* and *Aeromonas hydrophila* have also been reported to cause a particularly virulent form of necrotizing fasciitis.

PRESENTATION

With necrotizing fasciitis, there is often a trivial injury followed, after several hours or days, by the onset of pain and swelling accompanied by chills and fever. The pain is progressive, relentless, and severe and is often out of proportion to the severity of the physical findings. There may be considerable pale erythema in the involved area; brown-to-bluish skin discoloration is not uncommon later in the course of the illness (Fig. 55-3 and Color Plate 55-3). If the condition is left to progress, frank cutaneous gangrene may be seen. Pain is gradually replaced by numbness or analgesia as a result of compression and destruction of cutaneous nerves. Hypesthesia of the affected area may be a useful sign of the extensive undermining that occurs. Edema is present in most patients. Crepitation is not usual, but it may be found in patients seen

FIGURE 55-3 Necrotizing fasciitis of the lower leg. Dusky erythema is present, with blistering and small patches of dermal gangrene. See Color Plate 55-3.

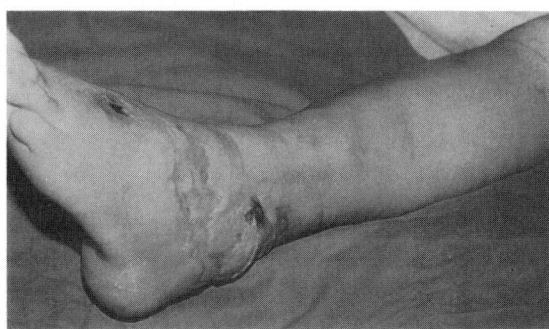

later in the course of the illness. Fluid-filled vesicles may appear in the area of erythema, often quickly followed by frank cutaneous gangrene. If an exudate is present, it may be serosanguineous and foul smelling. Systemic toxicity with disorientation is often severe. Large extracellular fluid shifts, hypotension, shock, and jaundice may follow. When these findings are present in the setting of infection due to group A streptococci, the term *streptococcal toxic shock syndrome* is used.

A significant manifestation of necrotizing fasciitis is extensive undermining of the skin (Fig. 55-4 and Color Plate 55-4) associated with necrosis of subcutaneous fat and deep fascia.[21] The undermining can be demonstrated by passing a sterile instrument along the plane just superficial to the deep fascia (Fig. 55-5); the instrument cannot be passed with ordinary cellulitis.

MANAGEMENT

Before antimicrobial therapy is started, samples for immediate Gram stain and for aerobic and anaerobic cultures should be obtained by direct needle aspiration of the involved area. Probing the lesion through an existing drainage site or through a small skin incision will reveal the characteristic undermining of skin seen in necrotizing fasciitis. The use of full-thickness skin biopsy with frozen section may aid the diagnosis.[22]

The principles of management include general supportive measures, administration of antimicrobial agents, and definitive surgery. General measures include the placement of central venous and arterial monitoring catheters, administration of intravenous fluids to correct dehydration, maintenance of adequate oxygenation, treatment of any underlying diseases (e.g., correction of ketoacidosis or congestive heart failure), and attention to the patient's nutritional needs. Total parenteral or enteral nutrition is required in the postoperative state to meet the dramatically increased nitrogen requirements associated with tissue repair, hyperthermia, sepsis, and vital organ requirements. Antibiotic selection should be guided by the initial Gram stain. In the absence of specific microbiologic data, broad-spectrum coverage should be given, including coverage for anaerobes, especially *B. fragilis.*

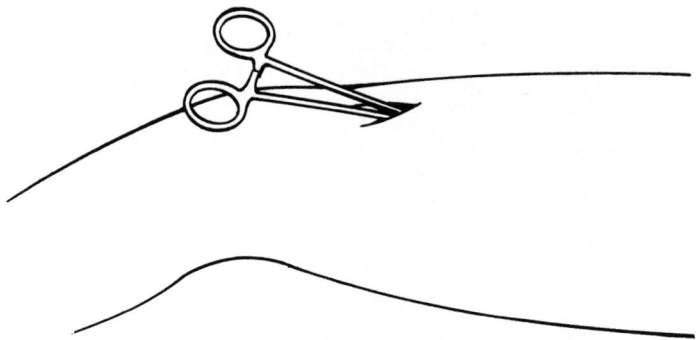

FIGURE 55-5 Necrotizing fasciitis with unopposed passage of a blunt instrument along the fascial cleft, indicating the characteristic undermining between the subcutaneous tissue and deep fascia.

An aminoglycoside (gentamicin or tobramycin), 3 to 5 mg/kg per day in three divided doses or, alternatively, 5 to 7 mg/kg as a single daily dose, plus clindamycin, 1200 to 2400 mg/day in three or four divided doses, is adequate initial therapy. If large gram-positive rods are noted, suggesting clostridia, or if group A streptococcus is suspected, penicillin G should be added (20 to 24 million U/day in divided doses). The combination of clindamycin and penicillin is considered the treatment of choice for severe soft tissue infection due to group A streptococcus. The addition of intravenous immunoglobulins, 0.4 g/kg per day for 4 to 5 days or 2 g/kg as a single dose with a repeat dose in 48 hours if the patient remains unstable, may be a useful adjunct for streptococcal toxic shock syndrome.[23–25] In penicillin-allergic patients, chloramphenicol or metronidazole is useful as an alternative anaerobic agent. In patients whose renal function is impaired or rapidly changing owing to underlying disease or acute tubular necrosis, a third-generation cephalosporin, such as cefotaxime, ceftriaxone, or ceftazidime, can be used in place of the aminoglycoside. Alternatively, a carbapenem such as imipenem or meropenem may be used as a single agent.[26]

The mainstay of management is surgical exploration, débridement, and drainage, which should be done as soon as possible. Débridement and excision of all necrotic subcutaneous adipose tissue and fascia are required. The wound should be packed open. Daily exploration under general anesthesia is indicated for truncal or perirectal infections and for all patients who remain in a toxic condition. Frequent dressing changes are performed after suitable analgesia and are continued until healthy granulation tissue appears. Careful and regular reinspection of the wound is necessary because initial débridement is seldom complete, and small foci of infection and necrotic tissue often lead to further progression. It must be emphasized that *conservative surgery leads to relapse of the process.* In the pelvic and upper thigh regions, a hip disarticulation or hemipelvectomy may be required.

Mortality rate is extremely variable, ranging from 4% to 74%. High scores on the Acute Physiology and Chronic Health Evaluation on admission, age older than 50 years, diabetes, truncal disease, and failure to achieve adequate initial débridement are associated with high mortality rates.[27]

MYONECROSIS

PATHOGENESIS

The bacterial myonecrotic syndromes involve bacterial invasion of previously undamaged healthy muscle, resulting in its rapid destruction. The process often referred to as *gas gangrene* is a fulminant, life-threatening infection for which early diagnosis and intervention are essential. Bacterial myonecrotic syndromes may be of clostridial or nonclostridial origin. Both entities have a similar pathogenesis, clinical presentation, and management.[21] Clostridial myonecrosis occurs in the setting of muscle injury and concurrent inoculation with clostridial spores from the soil or a foreign body. Although most commonly encountered in penetrating war wounds, it is seen now in the following settings: (a) trauma, especially motor vehicle or agricultural accidents involving open fractures; (b) the postoperative period, especially after bowel or biliary surgery; (c) malignancy, especially colorectal tumors; (d) arterial insufficiency in an extremity; (e) septic abortion; (f) occasionally, burn wounds; and (g) rarely, after intravascular or intramuscular injections. Although colonization of a traumatic wound by clostridia is common, the frequency of clostridial myonecrosis is only about 1%. In an animal model, the minimal dose of *C. perfringens* required to produce a fatal infection is reduced by a factor of 10^6 when the organism is injected into devitalized, as opposed to normal, muscle. Clinically, however, clostridial myonecrosis does occasionally occur even in the absence of devitalized muscle. Once the clostridia begin to proliferate, several potent exotoxins are produced that have the capacity to destroy host tissue. At least 17 toxins are produced by *C. perfringens,* including α toxin, a phospholipase that disrupts cell membranes and results in hemolysis, platelet destruction, widespread capillary damage, and myofibril destruction. The μ toxin, a hyaluronidase, facilitates tissue spread and is thought to be responsible for the massive edema associated with this condition. As the process spreads, the involved muscle undergoes rapid destruction. Early pallor, edema, and loss of elasticity give way to a discolored, noncontractile muscle, which eventually becomes friable and disintegrates. The histologic findings are of coagulation necrosis.

Myonecrosis due to organisms other than clostridia has a pathogenesis not unlike that of necrotizing fasciitis. The infection may be introduced through a break in the skin, through intravenous injection of illicit drugs,[28] a surgical wound or enterostomy, a decubitus ulcer, or a fistula. Predisposing factors include diabetes mellitus, obesity, advanced age, renal disease, and local trauma; diabetes mellitus is reported most commonly. With myonecrosis due to group A streptococci, no predisposing factors may be present. In drug addicts, infections of the extremities are more common, whereas perineal and buttock infections are more common in other populations.

When multiple microorganisms are responsible for myonecrosis, the facultative bacteria assist the growth of anaerobes by using available oxygen and destroying tissue

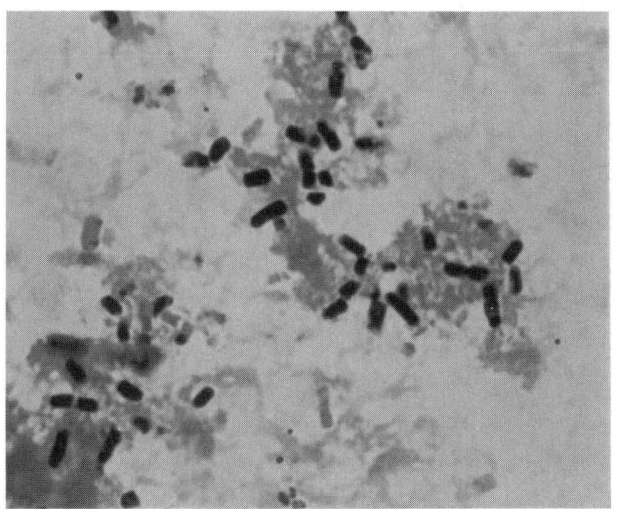

FIGURE 55-6 Gram stain of *Clostridium perfringens*. See Color Plate 55-6.

(reducing the redox potential), which promotes a favorable milieu for the proliferation of anaerobic organisms. The process often involves muscle and fascia extensively, and it may secondarily involve areas of subcutaneous tissue and skin. It should be noted that necrotizing fasciitis will ultimately involve muscle, if left to progress.

ETIOLOGY
Clostridium perfringens is the most common cause of clostridial myonecrosis, producing 80% to 95% of cases (Fig. 55-6 and Color Plate 55-6). *Clostridium novyi* and *Clostridium septicum* are responsible for 5% to 20%, with other species implicated rarely. Nonclostridial myonecrosis is usually polymicrobial, although group A streptococcus may be a single causative agent. Most commonly, a mixture of facultative bacteria (*E. coli*, *Klebsiella* species, *Enterobacter* species, *Proteus* species, and *S. aureus*) and anaerobic bacteria (*Bacteroides* species, *Peptostreptococcus* species, and *Peptococcus* species) is found, an etiology similar to that seen in necrotizing fasciitis. *Aeromonas hydrophila* has also been described as causing severe myonecrosis after penetrating muscle injury in a freshwater environment.

PRESENTATION
The incubation period of clostridial myonecrosis, from time of injury to appearance of symptoms, is usually 2 to 3 days, but it may be as brief as 6 hours. Intense pain, out of proportion to the extent of injury, is characteristic. The pain rapidly progresses in intensity and distribution. Fever is not present until later in the course. Within hours there appear signs of severe systemic toxicity: mental confusion, irritability, marked tachycardia, tachypnea, sweating, pallor, and hypotension. Delirium and stupor may supervene, although a period of intense mental alertness may occur before the onset of delirium. Renal failure, progressive hypotension and septic shock, intravascular hemolysis, and disseminated intravascular coagulopathy may ensue. Bacteremia occurs in only 10% to 15% of cases. Profound metabolic acidosis is common and can overwhelm compensatory hyperventilation, causing respiratory failure. Examination of the wound may initially show only tense edema and mild erythema. Later a spreading zone of woody edema appears, in addition to a characteristic bronzing of the skin. A thin, watery, brownish discharge with a sickly sweet odor may be present. Gas bubbles may be present in the discharge. Crepitus is usually present but is not a prominent feature. Tense blebs containing a thin serosanguineous fluid develop in the overlying skin, and areas of cutaneous necrosis appear in later stages. If an open wound is present, edematous muscle may herniate through the wound to the skin surface.

In nonclostridial myonecrosis, the process has its onset over several days. The port of entry is usually evident in the vicinity of the area of involvement. Moderate to severe pain and erythema, rather than edema, are more prominent. Progression is rapid, and systemic toxicity is severe; it may progress to shock and multisystem organ failure. Local crepitus may be present, as may a "dirty dishwater" discharge. Progression of the infection is rapid and may involve fascia and subcutaneous tissues. With infection due to group A streptococci, it is not uncommon to find myofasciitis and a toxic shock syndrome.

MANAGEMENT
Early diagnosis is critical; its importance cannot be overemphasized. Confusion about the types of gas gangrene, failure to recognize that the infection does not have the usual signs of pyogenic inflammation, and failure to recognize that clostridial infections can develop without a history of recent trauma can create diagnostic difficulties. The major considerations are other gas-forming infections of the soft tissues, including anaerobic cellulitis and necrotizing fasciitis. The severe toxemia, limited crepitus, tense edema, and characteristic bronzing of the skin are suggestive, but not definitive, evidence of clostridial myonecrosis. Similarly, areas of cutaneous necrosis in a severely toxic patient with a "dirty dishwater" discharge suggest a nonclostridial myonecrosis. Adjunctive diagnostic tools include Gram stain and radiography. A Gram stain of the discharge or of soft tissue aspirate in clostridial myonecrosis reveals large, gram-positive bacilli with blunt ends, but few or no pus cells (which are destroyed by the clostridial lecithinase). A mixed flora or gram-positive cocci (streptococci) may be seen with nonclostridial myonecrosis. Precautions should be taken to ensure that anaerobic specimens are collected appropriately and transported promptly to the laboratory. A radiograph of the involved area may visualize gas that is not palpable and will give an indication of the distribution of such gas.

The principles of management include general supportive measures, antimicrobials, and surgery. Surgical exploration is definitive and is mandatory for the mere suspicion of clostridial or nonclostridial myonecrosis. Urgent surgical intervention is the ultimate diagnostic and therapeutic maneuver, and its importance cannot be overemphasized. Bacterial myonecrosis is characterized by a darkened, "cooked" appearance of the muscle, which does not contract on stimulation and bleeds very little on incision. Excision of involved muscles—or amputation, if necessary—and decompressive fasciotomies are the mainstays of surgical treatment. Any necrotic fascia or subcutaneous tissue should be débrided. General supportive therapy includes insertion of appropriate monitoring lines, administration of isotonic crystalloid to maintain blood pressure, maintenance of adequate oxygenation, correction of severe acidosis, and maintenance of electrolyte balance. Blood should be given sparingly during the acute stages if evidence of extensive hemolysis is present. Nutritional support is necessary in these critically ill patients, especially in the postoperative period.

For clostridial myonecrosis, the antimicrobial treatment of choice is large-dose penicillin G, 20 to 24 million U/day in six to eight divided doses. The dose must be reduced appropriately if a significant degree of renal failure is present. Chloramphenicol, 1 to 2 g/day in four divided doses, or metronidazole, 1 to 2 g/day in two to four divided doses, is a good alternative in the penicillin-allergic patient. If a mixed flora is found on Gram stain, the antimicrobial regimen should include an aminoglycoside (gentamicin or tobramycin), 3 to 5 mg/kg per day in three divided doses, or 5 to 7 mg/kg per day as a single daily dose, plus clindamycin, 1200 to 2400 mg/day in three to four divided doses. If clostridia are present on Gram stain, then penicillin should also be added to the regimen because some clostridia are resistant to clindamycin.[29] If streptococcal myonecrosis or myofasciitis is suspected, the use of clindamycin plus penicillin is recommended. In addition, the use of intravenous immunoglobulin, as discussed in the previous section, may be a useful adjunct. A third-generation cephalosporin, such as cefotaxime, ceftriaxone, or ceftazidime, may be used in place of the aminoglycoside. A carbapenem such as imipenem or meropenem is a useful alternative as a single agent in nonclostridial myonecrosis.

Hyperbaric oxygen has been advocated as an adjunctive measure in patients with clostridial myonecrosis, but its role is controversial.[30] Controlled trials have not been done and are unlikely to be done because of the limited number of cases that might be seen at a given institution and ethical considerations in the randomization of critically ill patients. Evidence supporting the use of hyperbaric oxygen comes from animal experiments, case reports, and uncontrolled small series. Its role at present appears to be in the management of selected patients with extensive involvement in whom extensive surgical débridement would be so mutilating as to threaten life or limb.

References

1. Baxter CR: Surgical management of soft tissue infections. *Surg Clin North Am* 52:1483, 1972.
2. Simmons RL, Ahrenholz DM: Infections of the skin and soft tissues, in Howard RJ, Simmons RL (eds): *Surgical Infectious Diseases.* New York, Appleton-Lange, 1982, p 507.
3. Wilson MA: Skin and soft-tissue infections: Impact of resistant gram-positive bacteria. *Am J Surg* 186:35S, 2003.
4. Meleney FL: Bacterial synergism in disease processes with confirmation of synergistic bacterial etiology of certain types of progressive gangrene of the abdominal wall. *Ann Surg* 94:961, 1931.
5. Kuncir EJ, Tillou A, St. Hill CR, et al: Necrotizing soft-tissue infections. *Emerg Med Clin North Am* 21:1075, 2003.
6. Laucks SS II: Fournier's gangrene. *Surg Clin North Am* 74:1339, 1994.
7. Howard RJ, Bennett NT: Infections caused by halophilic marine vibrio bacteria. *Ann Surg* 217:525, 1993.
8. Newell PM, Norden CW: Value of needle aspiration in bacteriologic diagnosis of cellulitis in adults. *J Clin Microbiol* 26:401, 1988.
9. Kielhofner MA, Brown B, Dall L: Influence of underlying disease process on the utility of cellulitis needle aspirates. *Arch Intern Med* 148:2451, 1988.
10. Hook EW III, Hooton TM, Horton CA, et al: Microbiologic evaluation of cutaneous cellulitis in adults. *Arch Intern Med* 146:295, 1986.
11. George WL: Other infections of skin, soft tissue, and muscle, in Finegold SM, George WL (eds): *Anaerobic Infections in Humans.* San Diego, Academic Press, 1989, p 485.
12. Majeski JA, John JF Jr: Necrotizing soft tissue infections: A guide to early diagnosis and initial therapy. *South Med J* 96:900, 2003.
13. Feingold DS: The diagnosis and treatment of gangrenous and crepitant cellulitis, in Remington JS, Swartz MN (eds): *Current Clinical Topics in Infectious Diseases.* New York, McGraw-Hill, 1981, p 259.
14. Stevens D: Invasive group A *Streptococcus* infections. *Clin Infect Dis* 14:2, 1992.
15. Jallali N: Necrotizing fasciitis: Its aetiology, diagnosis and management. *J Wound Care* 12:297, 2003.
16. Davies HD, McGeer A, Schwartz B, et al: Invasive group A streptococcal infections in Ontario, Canada. *N Engl J Med* 335: 547, 1996.
17. Gozal D, Ziser A, Shupak A, et al: Necrotizing fasciitis. *Arch Surg* 121:233, 1986.
18. Green RJ, Dafoe DC, Raffin TA: Necrotizing fasciitis. *Chest* 110: 219, 1996.
19. Roberts DS: Synergistic mechanisms in certain mixed infections (editorial). *J Infect Dis* 120:720, 1969.
20. Brook I, Frazier EH: Clinical and microbiologic features of necrotizing fasciitis. *J Clin Microbiol* 33:2382, 1995.
21. Ahrenholz DH: Necrotizing soft-tissue infections. *Surg Clin North Am* 68:199, 1988.
22. Stamenkovic I, Lew DP: Early recognition of potentially fatal necrotizing fasciitis. *N Engl J Med* 310:1689, 1984.
23. Barry W, Hudgins L, Donta ST, Pesanti EL: Intravenous immunoglobulin therapy for toxic shock syndrome. *JAMA* 267:3315, 1992.
24. Kaul R, McGeer A, Norrby-Teglund A, et al: Intravenous immunoglobulin therapy for streptococcal toxic shock syndrome— A comparative observational study. *Clin Infect Dis* 28:800, 1999.
25. Crum NF, Wallace MR: Group B streptococcal necrotizing fasciitis and toxic shock-like syndrome: A case report and review of the literature. *Scand J Infect Dis* 35:878, 2003.
26. Fung HB, Chang JY, Kuczynski S: A practical guide to the treatment of complicated skin and soft tissue infections. *Drugs* 63:1459, 2003.
27. Pess ME, Howard RJ: Necrotizing fasciitis. *Surg Gynecol Obstet* 161:357, 1985.
28. Ebright JR, Pieper B: Skin and soft tissue infection in injection drug users. *Infect Dis Clin North Am* 16:697, 2002.
29. Rosenblatt JE: Antimicrobial susceptibility testing of anaerobic bacteria. *Rev Infect Dis* 6:S242, 1984.
30. Tibbles PM, Edelberg JS: Hyperbaric oxygen therapy. *N Engl J Med* 334:1642, 1996.

Chapter 56
URINARY TRACT INFECTIONS
GERARD J. SHEEHAN
BUSI MOOKA

KEY POINTS

- *All patients with severe urosepsis requiring admission to the intensive care unit should have immediate imaging of the urinary tract preferably by computed tomography with contrast because suppurative complications are common and require drainage as a priority.*

- *Percutaneous drainage can be used to drain definitively or stabilize temporarily a patient with suppurative complications.*

- *Empiric antimicrobial therapy for acute complicated urosepsis should include two agents with activity against gram-negative bacilli, such as a combination of ciprofloxacin or piperacillin/tazobactam with an aminoglycoside, until the pathogen is isolated and antimicrobial sensitivities are known.*

- *Urinary catheters are associated with a high incidence, 1% to 5% per day, of bacteriuria. Patients are also predisposed to candiduria, especially those receiving broad-spectrum antibacterial therapy.*

- *Asymptomatic bacteriuria should be treated in all patients before instrumentation of the urinary tract to avoid the development of gram-negative bacteremia.*

- *The continued usefulness of a urinary catheter needs to be reassessed on a regular basis, and removal in selected awake stable patients needs to be considered.*

- *Treatment of bacteriuria without local signs of infection should be considered only in patients with fever or sepsis after exclusion of other potential causes of infection.*

At the beginning of the 21st century, urinary tract infection (UTI) remains one of the commonest nosocomial infections, giving rise to prolonged hospitalization and additional cost. Eighty percent of nosocomial UTIs follow urinary catheterization, bacteremia arises in 1% to 3% of these, and the attributed mortality rate is then 13%.[1] Community-acquired pyelonephritis occasionally causes sepsis syndrome, especially when it arises in an obstructed urinary tract or when the host defense is compromised by poorly controlled diabetes. Urinary tract infection is thus an important initiating event for admission to the intensive care unit (ICU). Because of the almost universal insertion of urinary catheters in critically ill patients, UTI is a common sequel of intensive care and ranks in the top four of ICU-acquired infections. Bacteriuria, acquired through urinary catheterization in the ICU, constitutes a reservoir of resistant pathogens, which occasionally gives rise to epidemic spread of infection within the hospital.

Bacteriuria simply means the presence of bacteria in the urine. Significant bacteriuria implies the presence of at least 10^5 organisms per milliliter by a quantitative method. However, a count of at least 10^2 aerobic gram-negative organisms per milliliter from a woman with pyuria and symptoms of lower UTI represents true infection.[2] Low-level bacteriuria (or candiduria) of any quantity in a hospitalized, catheterized patient rapidly advances to significant bacteriuria, provided the patient is not receiving antimicrobial agents to which the organism is susceptible.[3,4] Thus, any level of bacteriuria in a catheterized ICU patient is worthy of consideration as a cause of sepsis.

Pyuria, the presence of white blood cells in urine, is commonly measured by counting the number of cells per microscopic high-power field in a centrifuged urine specimen. Using the criterion of five cells per microscopic high-powered field, pyuria, when present, is a reliable indicator of UTI, especially when cells greatly exceed this number. However, the sensitivity is not high, and the absence of such pyuria does not reliably exclude UTI. When measured with a counting chamber, using a criterion of more than 10 cells per microliter, a sensitivity of 96% is achieved for symptomatic UTIs.[5]

Acute Pyelonephritis

MICROBIOLOGY

Most (80% to 90%) of community-acquired UTIs in females are caused by *Escherichia coli*.[6] *Staphylococcus saprophyticus* is the second most common pathogen but rarely gives rise to sepsis and ICU admission. It remains fully susceptible to most antimicrobial agents used for UTI, including ampicillin and trimethoprim-sulfamethoxazole. Other Enterobacteriaceae (e.g., *Proteus* species, *Klebsiella* species, and *Enterobacter* species), *Enterococcus* species, and *Pseudomonas aeruginosa* account for only a small residual minority. In men *Escherichia coli* is also the commonest community-acquired urinary pathogen, but *Enterococcus* species and other Enterobacteriaceae are more commonly encountered.

For men and women, the spectrum of pathogens changes when UTI is acquired in the hospital environment. *Escherichia coli* (47%), *Enterococcus* species (13%), *Klebsiella* (11%), *Pseudomonas aeruginosa* (8%), *Proteus mirabilis* (5%), *Enterobacter* species (4%), and *Citrobacter* species (3%) together account for 91% of hospital-acquired bacterial UTIs, in a rank order that is consistent internationally.[7] In the ICU the spectrum shifts, with *Enterococcus* species (24%) and *Candida albicans* (21%) dominating and *E. coli* accounting for only 15%.[8] This predominance of more resistant species reflects the more widespread use of broad-spectrum antimicrobial agents and the nearly universal use of urinary catheters in ICUs.

Enterococcus species are an increasing concern as a cause of nosocomial UTI and bacteremia in the ICU. A Spanish prospective multicenter observational study of 21,979 ICU admissions between 1997 and 2001 found that 223 patients had 239 infections involving *Enterococcus* species, 14.3% of which were UTIs.[9] In ICUs the proportion of enterococci resistant to vancomycin is increasing but varies geographically. These isolates may also exhibit resistance to ampicillin and high-level aminoglycoside.[10] A retrospective study in one tertiary care center found a rate of vancomycin-resistant enterococci (VRE) bacteriuria of 23 per 10,000 admissions. Of 107 positive cultures, there were 13 symptomatic UTIs, two associated with bacteremia and one associated with death.[11] Most are *Enterococcus faecium* and are sensitive to linezolid, nitrofurantoin, and chloramphenicol.[12] Infection with VRE usually occurs in patients with significantly compromised host defenses and serious comorbidities, and this magnifies the importance of early effective antimicrobial treatment.[13]

VRE may serve as a reservoir of resistant genes for *Staphylococcus aureus*. Transfer of the VanA gene has occurred clinically, giving rise to vancomycin-resistant *S. aureus* invasive infection.[14] Isolation of *S. aureus* in a urine culture is uncommon and should always raise the possibility of seeding of the urinary tract through the bloodstream. Such patients should be reviewed for evidence of vascular cannula infections ("line sepsis"), endocarditis, osteomyelitis, and pneumonia. Multiple or single cortical renal abscesses (renal carbuncle) may be present.

Persistent or relapsing bacteriuria caused by *Proteus mirabilis* should prompt a search for a staghorn calculus. Chronic bacteriuria due to *Corynebacterium urealyticum* may be also associated with alkaline urine and renal stones. This organism is fastidious and commonly resistant to most antimicrobial agents other than vancomycin.[15]

Infection with less common nosocomial urinary pathogens may arise, sometimes in outbreaks, depending on local antimicrobial usage patterns. These include *K. pneumoniae* and *E. coli* with extended-spectrum β-lactamase resistant to cephalosporins and most other antimicrobial classes other than carbapenems[16] and *Stenotrophomonas (Xanthomonas) maltophilia*, resistant to carbapenems, cephalosporins, and aminoglycosides.[17] UTI secondary to Shiga toxin-producing *E. coli* has rarely presented with hemolytic-uremic syndrome in children and adults, sometimes accompanied by bacteremia.[18]

PATHOGENESIS

Women with recurrent UTIs often have vaginal and periurethral cells to which *E. coli* adhere more readily as compared to controls. Most *E. coli* implicated in UTIs have several virulence factors, which include diverse adhesins, siderophores, toxins, polysaccharide coatings, and other properties that assist the bacteria in avoiding or subverting host defenses, injuring or invading host cells and tissues, and stimulating a noxious inflammatory response. Thus, certain strains are "selected out" of the fecal floral that are capable of causing UTI (uropathogenic *E. coli*).[19] These various factors allow adhesion to periurethral cells, multiplication in the bladder, ascent of the ureters, and invasion of renal tissue in patients with anatomically normal urinary tracts. In contrast, those *E. coli* causing UTIs in patients with reflux nephropathy or obstruction are not specifically uropathogenic.[19]

Tamm-Horsfall protein, secreted by the loop of Henle, contains mannose residues that bind to type 1 fimbriae on *E. coli* and aggregate the organism preventing uroepithelial attachment and ascent against the urinary flow.[20] Voiding of the bladder is another important host defense mechanism. Vesicoureteric reflux frustrates this defense and allows establishment of upper UTI. The medulla and papillae of the kidney are prone to infection because of hyperosmolality and low blood flow. During pyelonephritis, an acute inflammatory exudate develops that limits infection but contributes to scarring.[19]

DIAGNOSIS

Acute pyelonephritis is a syndrome of fever with evidence of renal inflammation, such as costovertebral angle tenderness or flank pain. There are often signs of systemic toxicity and sometimes bacteremia. However, silent pyelonephritis is present in up to 33% of patients with clinical cystitis in primary care settings and may be latent for long periods. Patients with spinal cord injury are especially prone to silent, complicated, life-threatening pyelonephritis associated with urinary obstruction due to calculi and often will have fever with nonspecific abdominal discomfort, increased spasms, and autonomic dysreflexia.

Patients requiring ICU admission sometimes will have been admitted to the ward with a classic history of acute pyelonephritis. Subsequent deterioration should prompt a search for a urinary tract obstruction, such as calculus or renal papillary necrosis, or for a suppurative focus in or around the kidney (intrarenal or perinephric abscess, see below). Alternatively, such deterioration may arise if the urinary pathogen is resistant to the chosen empiric antimicrobial regimen. Features that suggest obstruction include classic renal colic, severe costovertebral angle tenderness, or a palpable kidney due to hydronephrosis.

At presentation, Gram stain of a drop of unspun urine can provide rapid, specific information. It may show gramnegative bacilli, gram-positive cocci in clumps, gram-positive cocci in chains, large gram-positive yeasts, or, much less often, a polymicrobial pattern. The stain can be valuable for distinguishing the less common etiologies (*S. aureus*, *Enterococcus* species, *Candida* species, and polymicrobial anaerobic) from the aerobic gram-negative bacilli that comprise the vast majority of pathogens.

A urine culture should always be obtained before therapy, if necessary, urinary catheterization. The culture identifies the infecting organism unless the patient has received prior antimicrobial agents or has complete obstruction or a perinephric abscess. Blood cultures also should be obtained because patients may have concomitant bacteremia. Renal function should be assessed, although acute renal failure caused directly by pyelonephritis is rare.[21] If present, it is usually due to acute tubular necrosis due to sepsis or to drug toxicity.

ANTIMICROBIAL THERAPY

A wide variety of regimens has been shown to be effective as empiric therapy of acute pyelonephritis. These include an aminoglycoside combined with ampicillin, trimethoprimsulfamethoxazole alone, third-generation cephalosporins, extended-spectrum penicillins combined with β-lactam inhibitors, carbapenems, monobactams, and quinolones. All of these are excreted through the kidneys, with the exception of moxifloxacin and gemifloxacin. The choice of the initial antimicrobial regimen for a patient with severe urosepsis hinges primarily on the absolute necessity of covering the pathogen while awaiting definitive culture and sensitivity data at 24 to 48 hours. This has become increasingly difficult with the evolution of resistance to most antimicrobial classes. An initial combination of two agents effective against aerobic gramnegative bacilli is therefore appropriate in a septic patient with UTI, with consideration given to anti-enterococcal activity and to the risk of toxicity. The prevalence of resistance to a given agent will vary geographically and evolve with time. Such rates are invariably higher for nosocomial isolates and in patients with a prior history of antimicrobial exposure. In patients with a higher risk of aminoglycoside toxicity, such as those with prior renal impairment, liver dysfunction, advanced age, shock, or oliguria, consideration should be given to a non-aminoglycoside regimen or to a limitation to a single dose to cover the first 24 hours.

Historically, a combination of an aminoglycoside and ampicillin provided cost-effective, empiric coverage against most aerobic gram-negative bacilli and enterococci. However, in many geographic locations, greater than 50% of *E. coli* and most other Enterobacteriaceae are now ampicillin resistant. The addition of a β-lactamase inhibitor, such as clavulanic acid or sulbactam, eliminates the resistance in many cases. Similarly, resistance rates in uropathogens to trimethoprim-sulfamethoxazole are growing, with an excess of 20% of isolates resistant in many areas in North America and even higher rates in Latin America and Europe.[7] A combination of a quinolone with an aminoglycoside offers initial double coverage against aerobic gram-negative bacilli but will not reliably cover enterococci because an increasing proportion has become quinolone resistant. Alternatively, piperacillin-tazobactam or ticarcillin-clavulanic acid will cover most aerobic-gram negative bacilli and enterococcal species. An aminoglycoside also can be added for double coverage until sensitivity data emerge. A third-generation cephalosporin will be active against most gram-negative bacilli but will have no activity against enterococci.

Once the organism is isolated and identified, then the antimicrobial regimen should be promptly adjusted to a single agent with the least toxicity and cost. Once fever has resolved and the patient can tolerate oral agents, an oral regimen can be started. Acute pyelonephritis requires 10 to 14 days of antimicrobial therapy. Cell wall synthesis inhibitors, such as the β-lactams, may have a higher relapse rate after completion of therapy. The hypertonic renal medulla may allow residual bacteria to survive as L forms (cell wall–deficient protoplasts).[22,23] Trimethoprim alone, trimethoprim-sulfamethoxazole, or a quinolone is preferred as oral therapy.

The optimal treatment for VRE is not known and should be chosen in consultation with an infectious diseases physician. Case reports of success and failure of treatment of difficult infections due to VRE have been published, in addition to noncomparative series with large numbers of patients. Treatment options include chloramphenicol (which may not be suitable for UTI because it is not excreted in the urine), tetracycline, high-dose ampicillin or ampicillin-sulbactam, and nitrofurantoin (for lower UTI). Newer agents (linezolid and quinupristin-dalfopristin) have been approved, and additional agents are likely to emerge in the next few years.[10]

IMAGING

Contrast-enhanced computed tomography (CT) is currently the initial study of choice for most patients with urosepsis. For patients in whom renal calculi may be present, the study should also include noncontrast images through the kidneys. CT scanning more accurately defines the anatomy of the renal parenchyma than ultrasound and gives a clear cross-sectional view of the surrounding anatomy. Helical scanning technology has greatly increased the quality and usefulness of the information CT provides. CT scan can more readily distinguish complications of upper UTI such as cortical abscess, acute focal bacterial nephritis (AFBN), and perinephric abscess. Accurate placement of percutaneous drains into suppurative collections may require CT scanning to delineate all structures precisely.[24,25]

Ultrasound can be technically inadequate because of obesity, overlying bowel gas, subcutaneous emphysema, wounds, or dressings. Although it has the advantage of being portable, the results depend on the skill and persistence of the operator. It will reliably diagnose most causes of obstruction and perinephric collections. Ultrasound may be chosen as the initial investigation for patients with severe urosepsis, when transport out of the ICU is hazardous or there are significant concerns about the risk of contrast induced nephrotoxicity. Intravenous urography currently has little or no role because helical CT scan is superior at demonstrating the collecting system and early papillary necrosis at a reversible phase and other lesions, such as tuberculosis and renal scarring due to childhood reflux nephropathy.[26]

Retrograde urography in conjunction with cystoscopy may be useful at demonstrating the anatomy of the collecting system in a nonexcreting kidney. Different adverse effects rarely result from the passage of the ureteral catheters or stents, including hemorrhage, perforation, or septicemia. However, this procedure may permit relief of obstruction by passage of a stent or manipulation of a calculus.

Acute Focal Bacterial Nephritis

Human kidneys consist of five to 11 lobes (usually eight), each of which contains a conical medullary pyramid whose apex converges into a renal papilla projecting into a calyx. Each pyramid is capped by cortical tissue to form a renal lobe and is separated from other lobes by a renal column containing the interlobar arteries and veins.[27] With the advent of CT scanning, there has been increasing recognition of AFBN.[28] This is analogous to lobar pneumonia because the abnormalities are limited to one or more renal lobes. Patients manifest the usual features of acute pyelonephritis but do not respond with defervescence within 48 hours, thereby prompting investigation for obstruction or suppurative focus. Ultrasound may be normal or may visualize a solid, hypoechoic, poorly defined mass without evidence of liquefaction. Noncontrast CT scanning is frequently normal, but with intravenous contrast enhancement, the nephrogram invariably shows one or more wedge-shaped areas of decreased density. Such lesions may be demonstrated in a significant proportion of patients with acute pyelonephritis. The differential diagnosis of AFBN includes neoplasm, evolving renal infarct, and abscess. Demonstration of enhancing tissue within the mass on delayed CT images excludes cancer and abscess. AFBN usually resolves with antimicrobial therapy, but scarring and atrophy may result. Histopathology shows intense polymorphonuclear leukocyte infiltration without liquefaction, so needle aspiration or percutaneous drainage is not indicated. *Escherichia coli* is the most common organism isolated from patients with AFBN.[28,29]

RENAL ABSCESS

AFBN may progress to suppuration, especially when associated with obstruction. The abscess may drain spontaneously into the calyxes or may rupture through the renal capsule to form a perinephric abscess. The usual pathogens are Enterobacteriaceae (*E. coli*, *K. pneumoniae*, and *Proteus* species). These organisms, which arise by the ascending route, are now commoner than cortical abscess arising from hematogenous spread. The latter was the commonest form of renal suppurative infection before the antibiotic era and usually resulted from *S. aureus*. Patients at high risk for staphylococcal septicemia, such as intravenous drug users, may present with renal cortical abscess, with or without other features of invasive staphylococcal infection, such as right-side endocarditis or multiple lung abscesses.

The clinical features of either form of renal abscess can be initially subtle. The patient often has chills, fever, and back or abdominal pain. Costovertebral angle tenderness, a flank mass, or involuntary guarding of the upper lumbar and paraspinal muscles may suggest the diagnosis. Prominent abdominal features such as nausea, vomiting, and abdominal guarding may suggest another intra-abdominal cause.

Ultrasound usually demonstrates an ovoid mass of decreased attenuation within the parenchyma. This may initially mimic AFBN, a cyst, or a tumor. Dependent echoes changing with position represent shifting debris within the abscess cavity. Gas within the abscess can be present. Definitive characterization of fluid within the mass is done by demonstration of enhanced transmission of the beam through the mass and refraction of the beam at the fluid–solid interface. The presence of debris within a cyst or an abscess is a strong indication of infection. CT shows a distinctly marginated low-attenuation (0 to 20 Hounsfield units) mass that fails to enhance. Sharp demarcation is demonstrated between the mass and the surrounding normally enhancing renal tissue. There may be a surrounding rim of increased enhancement (the ring sign). CT is more sensitive than ultrasound for small lesions (<2 cm in diameter) and for gas. Because hemorrhage within a cyst or necrotic debris within a tumor occasionally can mimic an abscess, confirmation by aspiration or nuclear medicine scanning is desirable. Alternatively, serial scanning until resolution while the patient is receiving antimicrobial therapy may suffice.

The classic therapy of intrarenal abscess is incision and drainage with a nephrectomy, if necessary, for larger abscesses. It is now clear that a trial of intravenous antimicrobial therapy will succeed in most patients once microbial etiology is established by urine, blood, or aspirate culture. Close monitoring of the response, including disappearance of fever and leukocytosis and diminution of size as assessed by ultrasound or CT, is necessary. Percutaneous drainage using ultrasound or CT guidance is another alternative to surgery and should be tried as initial therapy when the abscess cavity is large.[30]

EMPHYSEMATOUS PYELONEPHRITIS

Emphysematous pyelonephritis is a fulminant disorder, historically associated with a mortality rate of 80%. The patient typically presents acutely with features of pyelonephritis and severe sepsis with or without multiorgan failure. Gas formation occurs in the renal parenchyma and surrounding tissues due to mixed acid fermentation of glucose by Enterobacteriaceae, which forms hydrogen and carbon dioxide. Most patients have uncontrolled diabetes mellitus and some have obstruction of the urinary tract. *Escherichia coli* accounts for the majority of pathogens, with most of the rest being due to *Klebsiella* species.[31] Strict anaerobes have not been reported, but optimal anaerobic isolation techniques may not have been applied in all studies. Pathology demonstrates extensive necrotizing pyelonephritis with abscess formation and pap-

illary necrosis. Poor perfusion is present in most cases due to infarction, vascular thrombosis, arteriosclerosis, and/or glomerulosclerosis.[31]

Plain radiographs may show diffuse mottling of the parenchyma as an early sign. More advanced cases show extensive bubbles in the parenchyma and a gas crescent surrounding the kidney within the perinephric space. Ultrasound and CT are much more sensitive than plain films at detecting gas. CT identifies the gas clearly and unambiguously. Ultrasound identifies gas by the artifacts produced. Artifacts include an intense band of echoes distant to the gas and "dirty shadowing" distally with poorly defined margins and many echoes. This must be distinguished from the shadows associated with calculi, which produce "clean shadows" with sharply defined margins.[24]

Case reports published before 1982 associated surgical intervention within 48 hours and antimicrobial therapy with improved outcome. Although relief of obstruction was sometimes sufficient, nephrectomy was frequently necessary. The possible involvement of the contralateral kidney was a concern. More recent reports have suggested that a combination of antimicrobial agents, ICU support, including tight control of hyperglycemia, and percutaneous drainage guided by modern imaging techniques is successful in most cases, with nephrectomy reserved for a minority (18% mortality rate in a series of 46 cases).[31]

PERINEPHRIC ABSCESS, PYONEPHROSIS, AND PYOCYSTIS

The perinephric space, containing the kidney, renal fat pad, and adrenal gland, is conical and opens inferiorly to the pelvis. In most cases, it communicates to the contralateral perinephric space anterior to the aorta and inferior vena cava. Bridging septae exist within it, which act as lamellar barriers against the spread of infection or hematoma. Multiple loculations may arise, causing difficulty with percutaneous drainage.[32]

Most cases of perinephric abscess occur secondary to pyelonephritis caused by Enterobacteriaceae (*E. coli*, *K. pneumoniae*, and *Proteus* species). However, a minority is bacteremic in origin due to *S. aureus* or pyogenic streptococci. Polymicrobial infection involving anaerobic bacteria also occurs. There have been rare reports of perinephric abscess due to *Candida* and *Aspergillus* species. Many patients have associated renal obstruction or diabetes mellitus. Perinephric abscess is usually confined by the renal fascia, but additional spread to adjacent structures and spaces can occur.

Initial descriptions of perinephric abscess emphasized its insidious nature, delay in diagnosis, and 50% mortality rate.[33] Most patients have fever and chills. Other features may include weight loss, nausea, vomiting, dysuria, flank pain, abdominal pain, pleuritic chest pain, and pain in the thigh or groin. Symptoms usually last at least 2 weeks and sometimes persist for months.[34] The patient may present for investigation of fever of unknown origin. Other patients are given an initial diagnosis of acute pyelonephritis. Flank mass or renal tenderness will be present in most patients.

With the ready availability of ultrasound and CT, the diagnosis is now made sooner. Ultrasound demonstrates fluid that may contain debris or gas. CT shows loculated collections with decreased attenuation (0 to 20 Hounsfield units). The abscess wall may show increased attenuation after intravenous injection of contrast material. Thickening of the renal fascia (Gerota fascia) and unilateral enlargement of the kidney or psoas muscle may also be seen. The diagnosis can be confirmed by ultrasound-guided aspiration of pus. Most patients can be treated by a combination of antimicrobial agents and percutaneous drainage. Empiric antimicrobial therapy should be directed at mixed anaerobes and *S. aureus*, in addition to the usual aerobic gram-negative bacilli.[24,30,34]

Pyonephrosis arises when infection develops proximal to an obstructed hydronephrotic kidney. Unilateral loss of renal function is present, as is infection of the renal parenchyma. Occasionally gas may form; if so, the prognosis is much better than with emphysematous pyelonephritis. The clinical presentation is similar to perinephric abscess and may be insidious. Initial investigations should include a plain abdominal radiograph to look for calculi. Ultrasound will show a distended upper urinary tract. Specific features of pyonephrosis that allow distinction from simple hydronephrosis include sedimented echoes and dispersed internal echoes within the dilated collecting system. These findings are present in a minority of patients with pyonephrosis.[35] In a septic patient with hydronephrosis, direct aspiration is indicated. CT is more sensitive for detecting radiolucent calculi and will establish whether there is accompanying infection in the tissues around the kidney. Once the diagnosis is made, a nephrostomy tube should be inserted, which usually suffices to drain the infection.

Pyocystis (pus in the urinary bladder) with or without gas-forming organisms can present with sepsis, lower urinary tract signs, and pneumaturia. Patients with chronic oliguria on dialysis or those who have had diversion of urine away from the bladder (e.g., ileal conduit) are especially predisposed. Antimicrobial therapy and bladder irrigations may be sufficient therapy, but necrosis of the bladder wall as demonstrated by gas in the muscular layers on CT will require surgical resection.[36,37]

INFECTED CYSTS

Dependent debris can be demonstrated in a renal cyst by ultrasound or CT and suggests infection. However, absence of such a finding does not exclude a pyocyst. Aspiration of cyst fluid for Gram stain and culture establishes the diagnosis. Assessment is much more problematic in polycystic renal disease. Pyocysts may arise from ascending infection or by hematogenous seeding. In the presence of uremia, systemic responses to infection, such as fever and leukocytosis, are often blunted. Infected cysts may manifest as persistent sepsis unresponsive to intravenous antimicrobial agents. Ultrasound or CT frequently fails to distinguish an infected cyst from the rest of the polycystic kidney. Delineation of the infected cyst as the cause may require white blood cell scanning, magnetic resonance imaging, or positron emission tomography,[38,39] followed by percutaneous drainage of the particular cyst. Alternatively, unilateral nephrectomy can be carried out with preservation of the uninfected kidney. A trial of antimicrobial therapy should be carried out first if the patient is stable. Lipophilic agents, such as trimethoprim-sulfamethoxazole, ciprofloxacin or ofloxacin, are more likely to succeed. Lipophobic agents such as

β-lactams and aminoglycosides penetrate cysts poorly, if at all.[40]

URINARY TRACT INFECTION DUE TO *CANDIDA*

By microscopic examination, *Candida* species are readily recognized as gram-positive, ovoid, unicellular forms and grow readily on routine culture systems. Quantitative methods are commonly applied in urine; 10^4 colony-forming units per milliliter, especially when associated with pyuria, should be regarded as indicating at least infection of the bladder and possibly the upper tract.

Disseminated invasive candidiasis may originate in the urinary tract or secondarily seed it. Widespread microabscesses often form in the kidney and in other parenchymal organs. The skin, bones, spleen, eyes, liver, endocardium, myocardium, and central nervous system are typical sites of seeding, but the kidneys are almost universally involved. Renal failure may develop from bilateral renal infection. Neutropenia, loss of mucous membrane integrity due to chemotherapy, burns, steroid use, diabetes mellitus, total parenteral nutrition, and upper gastrointestinal tract surgery predispose to invasive candidiasis. Overgrowth on superficial tissues such as skin, mucous membranes, and the gastrointestinal tract frequently precedes invasion and is often associated with prolonged broad-spectrum antibacterial therapy. Although there may be extensive tissue involvement, direct proof of such deep candida infection is frequently lacking. Blood cultures are positive in only 50% of cases.[41]

Primary infection of the kidneys by *Candida* is generally associated with an indwelling urinary catheter, broad-spectrum antibacterial agents, and an obstructed urinary tract. Candiduria confined to the bladder is usually present for a variable period before renal infection. Persistent candiduria should be assumed to reflect renal infection if the patient has any of the predispositions listed above, is receiving broad-spectrum antibacterial therapy, and continues to have features of sepsis such as fever or leukocytosis. A search should be made for specific features of disseminated candidiasis such as white "cotton wool" exudates in the retina and nodular skin lesions. Unilateral or bilateral hydronephrosis should raise suspicion of a fungus ball. Microscopic examination of the urinary sediment may show *Candida* casts.[42] A careful evaluation of these clinical and laboratory data should allow selection of those patients who require early empiric antifungal therapy.

Renal or disseminated infection requires systemic amphotericin B therapy with its attendant toxicities or fluconazole.[43] Outcome is superior if intravenous catheters are removed on or before the first day of therapy.[41] Amphotericin B carries a significant risk of nephrotoxicity; fluconazole is not active against many non-*Albicans* species. However fluconazole may overcome such resistance in the urine by its high urinary levels.[44] To date, there are no clinical trials validating the efficacy of other agents, such as the less nephrotoxic lipid formulations of amphotericin B, 5-flucytosine, voriconazole, and caspofungin in the treatment of ascending *Candida* pyelonephritis or renal candidiasis. Concern has been raised that the structure of lipid formulations of amphotericin B could impair their urinary excretion. Caspofungin and voriconazole are metabolized through the liver with little urinary excretion. 5-Flucytosine is excreted in high concentration in urine, but resistance can develop rapidly when used alone.

Hydronephrosis due to a fungus ball should be relieved by a percutaneous nephrostomy tube. Irrigation of the ureter with an amphotericin B solution is effective in some cases. Lack of response radiologically should prompt surgical excision.

A more commonly encountered situation is that of the stable ICU patient who has persistent candiduria. For many individuals, this is a benign condition, which resolves spontaneously or after withdrawal of the urinary catheter. Asymptomatic patients with candiduria should receive treatment if they have undergone transplantation, are neutropenic, or are about to undergo invasive urologic procedures. Amphotericin B washouts, although effective, have been largely abandoned because they are labor intensive and require the continuation of a catheter.[44,45]

PROSTATIC INFECTIONS

Acute bacterial prostatitis rarely causes sepsis requiring ICU admission. It presents with high fever and urgency, frequency, dysuria, difficulty voiding or acute retention of urine, with suprapubic or perineal pain.[46] Rectal examination demonstrates a tender and swollen prostate. Gram-negative bacilli are the most frequent pathogens, and *E. faecalis* may also be responsible.

Because of the intense inflammatory response in acute bacterial prostatitis, most antimicrobial agents cross the prostatic epithelium effectively. Rarely, a patient with acute prostatitis may develop chronic infection, so we recommend continuing with an oral antimicrobial agent that penetrates the prostatic acini well, such as trimethoprim alone, trimethoprim-sulfamethoxazole, ciprofloxacin, or ofloxacin, for a total of 6 weeks in an attempt to eradicate the organisms from the prostate. Prostatic abscess, if present, can be confirmed by transrectal ultrasonography or CT. Transurethral resection of the prostate and unroofing or perineal aspiration of pus guided by transrectal ultrasonography usually provide adequate drainage.[46]

CATHETER-ASSOCIATED BACTERIURIA

Before the 1960s, urinary catheters had "open" drainage systems, with a significant bacteriuria prevalence of 95% within 4 days of continuous use. The principal route of acquisition was intraluminal. The widespread introduction of closed urinary drainage systems has significantly reduced these high rates to 10% to 27% in various studies. The prevalence of catheter-associated bacteriuria is time-dependent. One percent of patients will acquire bacteriuria from single "in-out" catheterizations.[47] The per-day risk of developing bacteriuria has varied from 1% to 5%, with lower figures reported in the ICU setting, but with a higher prevalence of resistant pathogens.[8,48,49] Other factors associated with a higher prevalence of catheter-associated bacteriuria include advancing age and female sex.[8] Systemic antimicrobial agents initially protect against catheter-associated bacteriuria. Subsequently, organisms manifesting extensive antimicrobial resistance become prevalent, such as enterococci, coagulase-negative staphylococci, *Candida* species, and *Pseudomonas* species. Disconnections of the collecting tube–catheter junction are associated with a two- to threefold increase in

bacteriuria. Samples should always be taken by aspiration of urine through the distal catheter or collection port, after local disinfection.

Ascent of bacteria to the bladder occurs predominantly outside the lumen when a closed drainage system is used. The space between the catheter and the urethral mucous membrane is filled by a variable amount of fluid, mucus, and inflammatory exudate. This is static and lacks inhibitory factors against bacterial proliferation. A progressive multiplication of organisms originating from the meatus occurs, which accounts for the time-dependent acquisition and for the higher rates associated with the female urethra.[50]

In a small minority of patients, the organism originates from the collecting bag and ascends intraluminally. Contamination of the collecting bag can occur in association with disconnections of the distal catheter or during emptying of the bag near the drainage port. Organisms have been carried on the hands of personnel or in the collecting urinal from one source patient to the collecting bags of others. Thus, intraluminal spread is the mechanism associated with most epidemics of catheter-associated bacteriuria.[51]

Catheterization of the bladder is unavoidable in most patients in the ICU. Indications include the monitoring of urine output in patients with shock, hemodynamic instability, or polyuric renal failure and the relief of lower urinary tract obstruction. Catheterization should not be used routinely, to avoid incontinence and contamination of the perineal skin. The almost universal use of urinary catheters in most ICUs can be reduced by early withdrawal of catheters in selected patients. These include alert and stable patients who can maintain continence, patients with anuric renal failure for whom once-a-day catheterization will suffice, and male patients with an intact voiding mechanism who can be managed with condom drainage.[1] Intermittent catheterization can be used in stable patients with neurogenic bladders and in some patients with disturbed consciousness. The necessity for the catheter should be frequently questioned and a trial of removal attempted when feasible. Once in place, there is no need for regular scheduled replacements of the catheter, which can be left indefinitely provided it is functioning well and there are no encrustations.[52] Bacteremia can arise with instrumentation, including passage of a new urinary catheter. Bacteriuria should be treated in a catheterized patient before instrumentation of the urinary tract. Catheter-associated bacteriuria is generally asymptomatic. Treatment is sometimes justified to relieve symptoms of cystitis, especially in the patient in whom removal of the catheter is imminent. Short-course treatments will work well once the catheter has been removed.[53]

Studies of recent technical innovations to reduce catheter-associated bacteriuria have shown equivocal results. These include urinary catheters impregnated with nitrofurazone or minocycline and rifampin or coated with a silver alloy-hydrogel. Conflicting opinions exist concerning their efficacy and cost effectiveness. We do not recommend them at this time.[49,54]

References

1. Warren JW: Urethral catheters, condom catheters, and nosocomial urinary tract infections. *Infect Control Hosp Epidemiol* 17:212, 1996.

2. Stamm WE, Counts GW, Running KR, et al: Diagnosis of coliform infection in acutely dysuric women. *N Engl J Med* 307:463, 1982.

3. Stark RP, Maki DG: Bacteriuria in the catheterized patient. *N Engl J Med* 311:560, 1984.

4. Bonten MJ, Weinstein RA: The role of colonization in the pathogenesis of nosocomial infections. *Infect Control Hosp Epidemiol* 17:193, 1996.

5. Stamm WE: Measurement of pyuria and its relation to bacteriuria. *Am J Med* 75:53, Suppl. 183.

6. Gupta K, Scholes D, Stamm WE: Increasing prevalence of antimicrobial resistance among uropathogens causing acute uncomplicated cystitis in women. *JAMA* 281:736-8 1999.

7. Gordon KA, Jones RN: SENTRY participant groups (Europe, Latin America, North America). Susceptibility patterns of orally administered antimicrobials among urinary tract infection pathogens from hospitalized patients in North America: Comparison report to Europe and Latin America. Results from the SENTRY Antimicrobial Surveillance Program (2000). *Diagn Microbiol Infect Dis* 45:295, 2003.

8. Laupland KB, Zygun DA, Davies HD, et al: Incidence and risk factors for acquiring nosocomial urinary tract infection in the critically ill. *J Crit Care* 17:50, 2002.

9. Alvarez Lerma F, Palomar M, Insausti J, et al: Enterococcal infections in critically ill patients admitted to ICU. *Med Clin (Barc)* 121:281, 2003.

10. Murray BE: Vancomycin-resistant enterococcal infections. *N Engl J Med* 342:710,2000.

11. Wong AH, Wenzel RP, Edmond MB: Epidemiology of bacteriuria caused by vancomycin-resistant enterococci, a retrospective study. *Am J Infect Control* 28 277, 2000.

12. Zhanel GG, Laing NM, Nichol KA, et al: Antibiotic activity against urinary tract infection (UTI) isolates of vancomycin-resistant enterococci (VRE): Results from the 2002 North American Vancomycin Resistant Enterococci Susceptibility Study (NAVRESS). *J Antimicrob Chemother* 52:382, 2003.

13. Vergis EN, Hayden MK, Chow JW, et al: Determinants of vancomycin resistance and mortality rates in enterococcal bacteremia. A prospective multicenter study. *Ann Intern Med* 135;484,2001.

14. Chang S, Sievert D, Hageman JC, et al: Infection with vancomycin-resistant *Staphylococcus aureus* containing the VanA resistance gene. *N Engl J Med* 348:1342, 2003.

15. Fernandez-Natal I, Guerra J, Alcoba M, et al: Bacteremia caused by multiply resistant *Corynebacterium urealyticum*: Six case reports and review. *Eur J Clin Microbiol Infect Dis* 20:514, 2001.

16. Ho PL, Chan WM, Tsang KW, et al: Bacteremia caused by *Escherichia coli* producing extended-spectrum beta-lactamase: a case-control study of risk factors and outcomes. *Scand J Infect Dis* 34:567, 2002.

17. Vartivarian SE, Papadakis KA, Anaissie EJ: *Stenotrophomonas (Xanthomonas) maltophilia* urinary tract infection. A disease that is usually severe and complicated. *Arch Intern Med* 156:433, 1996.

18. Chiurchiu C, Firrincieli A, Santostefano M, et al: Adult nondiarrhea hemolytic-uremic syndrome associated with Shiga toxin *Escherichia coli* O157:H7 bacteremia and urinary tract infection. *Am J Kidney Dis* 41:E4, 2003

19. Johnson JR: Microbial virulence determinants and the pathogenesis of urinary tract infection. *Infect Dis Clin North Am* 17:261, 2003.

20. Pak J, Pu Y, Zhang ZT, et al: Tamm-Horsfall protein binds to type 1 fimbriated *Escherichia coli* and prevents *E. coli* from binding to uroplakin Ia and Ib receptors. *J Biol Chem* 276:9924, 2001.

21. Jones SR: Acute renal failure in adults with uncomplicated pyelonephritis: Case reports and review. *Clin Infect Dis* 14:243, 1992.

22. Stamm WE, McKevitt M, Counts GW: Acute renal infection in women: Treatment with trimethoprim-sulfamethoxazole or ampicillin for two or six weeks. *Ann Intern Med* 106:341, 1987.

23. Preiksaitis JK, Thompson L, Harding GKM, et al: A comparison of the efficacy of nalidixic acid and cephalexin in bacteriuric women and their effect on fecal and periurethral carriage of Enterobacteriaceae. *J Infect Dis* 143:603, 1981.

24. Kaplan DM, Rosenfield AT, Smith RC: Advances in the imaging of renal infection. Helical CT and modern coordinated imaging. *Infect Dis Clin North Am* 11:681, 1997.

25. Baumgarten DA, Baumgartner BR: Imaging and radiologic management of upper urinary tract infections. *Urol Clin North Am* 24:545, 1997.

26. Lang EK, Macchia RJ, Thomas R, et al: Detection of medullary and papillary necrosis at an early stage by multiphasic helical computerized tomography. *Br J Urol* 170:94, 2003.

27. Williams PL, Warwick R, Dyson M, Bannister LH: The urogenital system, in Williams PL, Warwick R, Dyson M, Bannister LH (eds): *Gray's Anatomy*, 37th ed. Norwich, Churchill Livingstone, 1989, p 1396.

28. Huang JJ, Sung J-M, Chen K-W, et al: Acute bacterial nephritis: A clinico-radiologic correlation based on computed tomography. *Am J Med* 93:289, 1992.

29. Meyrier A, Condamin MC, Fernet M, et al: Frequency of development of early cortical scarring in acute primary pyelonephritis. *Kidney Int* 35:696, 1989.

30. Dembry LM, Andriole VT: Renal and perirenal abscesses. *Infect Dis Clin North Am* 11:663, 1997.

31. Huang JJ, Tseng CC: Emphysematous pyelonephritis: clinicoradiological classification, management, prognosis, and pathogenesis. *Arch Intern Med* 160:797, 2000.

32. Thornton FJ, Kandiah SS, Monkhouse WS, et al: Helical CT evaluation of the perirenal space and its boundaries: A cadaveric study. *Radiology* 218:659, 2001.

33. Thorley JD, Jones SR, Sanford JP: Perinephric abscess. *Medicine (Baltimore)* 53:441, 1974.

34. Sheinfeld J, Erturk E, Spataro RF, et al: Perinephric abscess: Current concepts. *J Urol* 137:191, 1987.

35. Vehmas T, Paivansalo M, Taavitsainen M, et al: Ultrasound in renal pyogenic infection. *Acta Radiol* 29:675, 1988.

36. Lees JA, Falk RM, Stone WJ, et al: Pyocystis, pyonephrosis and perinephric abscess in end stage renal disease. *J Urol* 134:716, 1985.

37. Kato H, Hosaka K, Kobayashi S, et al: Fate of tetraplegic patients managed by ileal conduit for urinary control: Long-term followup. *Int J Urol* 9:253, 2002.

38. Chicoskie C, Chaoui A, Kuligowska E, et al: MRI isolation of infected renal cyst in autosomal dominant polycystic kidney disease. *Clin Imaging* 25:114, 2001.

39. Bleeker-Rovers CP, Sevaux RG, Van Hamersvelt HW, et al: Diagnosis of renal and hepatic cyst infections by 18-F-fluorodeoxyglucose positron emission tomography in autosomal dominant polycystic kidney disease. *Am J Kidney Dis* 41:E18, 2003.

40. Sklar AH, Caruana RJ, Lammers JE, et al: Renal infections in autosomal dominant polycystic kidney disease. *Am J Kidney Dis* 10:81, 1987.

41. Eggimann P, Garbino J, Pittet D: Epidemiology of *Candida* species infections in critically ill non-immunosuppressed patients. *Lancet Infect Dis* 3:685,2003.

42. Gregory MC, Schumann GB, Schumann JL, et al: The clinical significance of candidal casts. *Am J Kidney Dis* 4:179, 1984.

43. Rex JH, Bennett JE, Sugar AM, et al: A randomised trial comparing fluconazole with amphotericin B for the treatment of candidemia without neutropenia. *N Engl J Med* 332:1100, 1994.

44. Lundstrom T, Sobel J: Nosocomial candiduria: A review. *Clin Infect Dis* 32:1602, 2001.

45. Rex JH, Walsh TJ, Sobel JD, et al: Practice guidelines for the treatment of candidiasis. *Clin Infect Dis* 30:662, 2000.

46. Liu KH, Lee HC, Chuang YC, et al: Prostatic abscess in southern Taiwan: another invasive infection caused predominantly by *Klebsiella pneumoniae*. *J Microbiol Immunol Infect* 36:31, 2003.

47. Kass EH: Asymptomatic infections of the urinary tract. *Trans Assoc Am Phys* 69:56, 1956.

48. Merle V, Germain JM, Bugel H, et al: Nosocomial urinary tract infections in urologic patients: Assessment of a prospective surveillance program including 10,000 patients. *Eur Urol* 41:483, 2002.

49. Tambyah PA, Knasinski V, Maki DG: The direct costs of nosocomial catheter-associated urinary tract infection in the era of managed care. *Infect Control Hosp Epidemiol* 23:27, 2002.

50. Garibaldi RA, Burke JP, Britt MR, et al: Meatal colonization and catheter-associated bacteriuria. *N Engl J Med* 303:316, 1980.

51. Marrie TJ, Major H, Gurwith M, et al: Prolonged outbreak of nosocomial urinary tract infection with a single strain of Pseudomonas aeruginosa. *Can Med Assoc J* 119:593, 1978.

52. Kunin CM: Care of the urinary catheter, in Kunin CM (ed): *Detection, Prevention and Management of Urinary Tract Infections*, 3d ed. Philadelphia, Lea and Febiger, 1987, p 153.

53. Harding GKM, Nicolle LE, Ronald AR, et al: How long should catheter-acquired urinary tract infection in women be treated? *Ann Intern Med* 114:713, 1991.

54. Niel-Weise BS, Arend SM, van den Broek PJ: Is there evidence for recommending silver-coated urinary catheters in guidelines? *J Hosp Infect* 52:81, 2002.

Chapter 57

GASTROINTESTINAL INFECTIONS

STEPHEN G. WEBER

KEY POINTS

- *In addition to immunologic mechanisms, physical (motility), chemical (gastric acidity), and microbiologic (normal colonizing flora) factors normally protect the gastrointestinal tract against infection.*

- *Esophagitis, most commonly caused by* Candida albicans *or herpes simplex virus, may be underrecognized among patients in the intensive care unit.*

- *Infection with* Helicobacter pylori *may play a role in the pathogenesis of gastric stress ulceration among critically ill patients.*

- *The epidemiology and microbiology of diarrheal illness is significantly different among patients in the critical care unit than is observed in the community setting. Most infectious diarrhea is hospital-acquired and is usually attributable to* Clostridium difficile.

- *A systematic approach to the critically ill patient with diarrhea includes consideration of pathogens that cause noninflammatory, inflammatory, and hemorrhagic diarrhea. Thorough history taking supplements laboratory data in the diagnosis of these patients.*

- C. difficile *infection is the single most common cause of gastrointestinal infection among patients in the intensive care unit. The spectrum of disease induced by* C. difficile *infection is broad. Timely diagnosis and treatment is critical both for the management of the infected patient and to prevent the spread of infection through the unit.*

While rarely severe enough to warrant admission to the ICU, gastrointestinal infections account for substantial morbidity and mortality among critically ill patients. Because of severe comorbid disease, impaired immune defenses, and the invasive interventions to which they are subjected, patients in the ICU are especially susceptible to hospital-acquired GI infection. Nevertheless, despite the frequency with which these infections occur, the morbidity and mortality that they cause, and the costs they incur, GI infections can go undetected and untreated in the ICU. While trying to manage patients with deteriorating cardiac function, marginal ventilatory performance, and life-threatening metabolic abnormalities, clini-

cians in the ICU may fail to recognize the important early signs of GI infection.

Any discussion of GI infections among critically ill patients must begin with a consideration of the host defenses that normally protect the alimentary tract. As such, the first section of this chapter is devoted to a description of the unique non-immunologic mechanisms normally active in the GI tract. Particular consideration is given to the means by which these defenses may be compromised in patients in the ICU. Following this introduction, the clinical manifestations of infection affecting each segment of the GI tract are discussed (Table 57-1). In addition to describing the microbiology associated with each syndrome, a rational diagnostic and therapeutic approach is offered, based on the most up-to-date experience reported in the medical literature. The chapter concludes with an expanded discussion of the unique clinical challenges presented by the patient in the ICU with *Clostridium difficile* infection.

Host Defenses

MOTILITY

GI motility, in addition to its central role in normal digestion, is one of the principal host defenses against infection. By continuously flushing the lumen of the GI tract, normal motility prevents the accumulation of infectious organisms and the virulent toxins associated with disease. When bacteria are permitted to collect and reproduce unchecked, such as in blind bowel loops rendered devoid of normal motility by surgical interventions, infection can ensue. Patients in the ICU are routinely exposed to interventions that can have the effect of impairing gut motility, rendering the patient vulnerable to infection. For example, while narcotics can provide appropriate and necessary analgesia for the critically ill patient, these agents have the side effect of inhibiting gut motility.

GASTRIC ACIDITY

Gastric acidity provides a unique chemical barrier to the establishment of upper GI colonization and infection. In the highly acidic environment of the stomach, few pathogens are able to survive, much less thrive. However, the gastric pH of patients in the ICU is often much higher, providing an environment that is more hospitable to bacteria. More importantly, ingested microbes can pass into the lower GI tract. Once again, pharmacologic interventions are primarily responsible for this disruption of normal protective physiology. The attenuation of gastric acidity is deliberate—an effort to lessen the likelihood of stress-induced gastritis and resultant GI hemorrhage. Medications such as histamine (H_2)-receptor blockers and proton pump inhibitors are

TABLE 57-1 Clinical Manifestations of Infection of Different Segments of the Gastrointestinal Tract

Site	Normal Host Defense	Clinical Syndrome	Typical Pathogens
Esophagus	Motility, acidity	Esophagitis	*Candida* species, herpes simplex virus, cytomegalovirus
Stomach	Acidity, motility	Gastritis	*Helicobacter pylori*
Small and large intestine	Normal flora, motility	Infectious diarrhea	*Clostridium difficile, Escherichia coli, Salmonella,* and *Shigella* species

commonly employed for this practice in both medical and surgical ICUs.

NORMAL COLONIZING FLORA

While not intuitively obvious as a component of host defense against infection, the normal colonizing flora of the GI tract provides as much protection as any physical or chemical barrier. Together, the host and normal GI flora comprise a delicate and varied ecology into which the introduction of new and potentially virulent flora is not favored. The bacteria that populate the GI tract are varied, depending on the anatomic segment under consideration. The mouth normally contains a mixed population of gram-positive, gram-negative, and anaerobic bacteria. In the esophagus, the population is less diverse. As already noted, the acidic environment of the stomach is distinctly inhospitable to the establishment of bacterial colonization. However, one organism, discussed in detail later, has been found to be of profound clinical relevance. Because of its ability to survive in the stomach, *Helicobacter pylori* plays a critical role in the pathogenesis of peptic ulcer disease. In contrast to the case of the stomach, the lower GI tract plays host to substantial microbiologic diversity. An enormous range of gram-negative, gram-positive, and anaerobic flora populates the intestines, especially the colon. Specific constituents include enterococci and *Bacteroides* species, as well as members of the family Enterobacteriaceae.

Disturbance of the dynamic between host and bacterial colonizers, such as occurs after exposure to broad-spectrum antimicrobials, predisposes patients to GI infection, most notably colitis caused by *Clostridium difficile*. While this association is well recognized, the factors that govern this phenomenon are still not well understood. It is not known if the normal flora compete with infecting pathogens for nutrients or substrates, occupy limited mucosal binding sites, or somehow otherwise alter the microenvironment in a way that reduces the likelihood of colonization. Regardless of the actual mechanism, an interesting therapeutic corollary can be inferred from the relationship between the normal host and GI colonizers. Deliberate intestinal colonization with so-called probiotics such as *Saccharomyces cerevisiae* may offer a means by which to preclude the onset of nosocomial infection or to attenuate the effects of these infections once established.[1]

Esophagitis

The esophagus may be easily overlooked as a site of infection in patients hospitalized in the ICU. These patients may be unable to verbalize or otherwise express to caregivers the subjective complaints that indicate the presence of infection. To make matters worse, mechanical instrumentation commonly employed in the ICU, including endotracheal, nasogastric, and orogastric tubes, may limit the clinician's ability to thoroughly examine the patient for signs of upper GI infection. Moreover, even when characteristic physical findings of infection are visualized, they may be incorrectly ascribed to mechanical irritation or inflammation associated with such tools. When the opportunity to diagnose upper GI infection is missed, directed therapy may be withheld and infection allowed to proceed unchecked.

CLINICAL PRESENTATION

Nearly 20% of ICU patients who underwent upper endoscopy in one study were incidentally noted to have esophagitis.[2] These patients typically experience dysphagia with or without odynophagia. The pain of esophagitis is described as retrosternal and is typically exacerbated by the recumbent position. In the alert, awake, and communicative patient, these hallmark complaints are easily called to the attention of caregivers. However, as was already noted, the intubated and sedated patient in the ICU may not be able to express these complaints. Fever is an unreliable clinical finding in the patient with esophagitis. Regardless of the causative organism, fewer than one third of all patients with esophagitis will experience an elevation in temperature.[3]

MICROBIOLOGY

Among hospitalized patients, esophagitis is most often caused by *Candida albicans*. While *C. albicans* remains the yeast species most frequently associated with esophagitis, an increasing proportion of cases have been linked to non-*albicans Candida* species, including *C. tropicalis*, *C. parapsilosis*, *C. krusei* and *C. glabrata*.[4] This changing epidemiology has been attributed to the increasingly common use of empiric and prophylactic therapy with triazole antifungal agents such as fluconazole, to which many non-*albicans Candida* species are resistant. This epidemiologic phenomenon needs to be incorporated into the approach to therapy for such patients.

Herpes simplex virus (HSV) is another frequent cause of esophagitis and is the most common serious viral infection of the upper GI tract among patients in the ICU. For the most part, HSV type 1 is more likely to cause esophagitis than is HSV 2, which is more typically associated with genital infections. Less frequently, other viruses, including cytomegalovirus (CMV) can cause esophageal ulceration. For patients with CMV disease, lesions may extend throughout the length of the GI tract.

DIAGNOSIS

Thorough physical examination is not only essential to the diagnosis of esophagitis, but may offer preliminary clues as to the causative pathogen. Both yeast and viral pathogens infecting the esophagus can produce telltale lesions in the oral cavity, where they will be easily detected on routine physical examination. Although present in fewer than one third of all patients with HSV esophagitis, oral or labial herpetic ulcers should not be missed in the physical examination of the critically ill patient with unexplained fever.[5] Similarly, an adherent white coating to the lateral aspects of the tongue, which when scraped away reveals patches of inflammation, should point to *Candida albicans* as the cause of a suspected case of esophagitis. Despite the utility of such findings, it is equally important to recognize that esophagitis most often occurs in the absence of such clues. Nevertheless, to miss these clinical findings, when present, is to miss a critical opportunity for early diagnosis and intervention.

Upper GI endoscopy can be a useful tool to confirm the pathologic and microbiologic diagnosis of esophagitis. Unfortunately, even when visualized through the endoscope, the lesions of *Candida* and HSV esophagitis may appear quite similar. Even the large shallow ulcers typical of CMV esophagitis may be mimicked by *Candida* or HSV. Because of this lack of discriminatory power, it is advisable to proceed to confirmatory biopsy. Brush specimens alone can be inadequate, especially as *Candida* species can be isolated as colonizers of the upper GI tract in up to 20% of normal individuals.[6] Once obtained, tissue should be sent for viral and fungal culture as well as for histopathologic examination to confirm tissue invasion.

THERAPY

Under most circumstances, directed therapy for esophagitis should be withheld until the causative organism has been identified. However, for critically ill patients with suspected esophagitis in whom endoscopy is not practical and microbiologic diagnosis is impossible, it is reasonable to treat empirically for *C. albicans*, based on the prevalence of this entity in this population. For esophagitis when *C. albicans* is known or suspected to be the cause, the most effective treatment is fluconazole given intravenously at a dose of 100 to 200 mg per day for 14 to 21 days. For those infected with *Candida* species resistant to fluconazole, or for patients with persistent infection despite first-line therapy, amphotericin B can be used as salvage therapy. The role of newer antifungal agents, including voriconazole and the echinocandins has not yet been fully clarified.

For HSV esophagitis, the antiviral agent with which there is the most clinical and published experience is acyclovir. Most patients in the ICU will require parenteral therapy—5 mg/kg intravenously every 8 hours for 7 to 14 days. If the virus is resistant to acyclovir, intravenous foscarnet can be substituted.

Gastritis

While the stomach is not typically considered an important site of infection among hospitalized patients, the potential association between *Helicobacter pylori* infection and gastric stress ulceration suggests another means by which GI pathogens may take a toll among critically ill patients. The etiologic relationship between the presence of *Helicobacter pylori* and ulcerative disease of the upper GI tract, and particularly the duodenum and stomach, has been established. Importantly, treatment of *H. pylori* infection with combinations of antimicrobial agents and inhibitors of gastric acidity will eradicate *H. pylori* infection, and in so doing promote the resolution of peptic ulcer disease.[7] Antibiotics employed for this purpose are active against *H. pylori* and include macrolides and β-lactam agents. Acid suppressive agents given concurrently include sucralfate, H_2-receptor blockers, and proton pump inhibitors.

Given these findings and a growing clinical experience with this strategy, it is not surprising that a link between *H. pylori* infection and the stress-induced gastritis that affects patients in the ICU has been proposed. Thus far, the results have been generally inconclusive. In a prospective, single-institution study of patients admitted to a medical/surgical ICU, half of all patients admitted were positive for *H. pylori* by urea breath test. After adjusting for other risk factors, *H. pylori* infection was the only clinical factor significantly associated with major mucosal injury. The organism was detected in 80% of such patients.[8] However, the same investigators observed that the prevalence of *H. pylori* infection among ICU patients declined to 8% by the third day of admission, and to 0% by 1 week, owing to intercurrent antibiotic exposure.[9]

Diarrhea

Diarrhea, the principal manifestation of intestinal infection among the critically ill, affects approximately one third of all patients admitted to the ICU.[10] Patients in the ICU with diarrhea are especially vulnerable to the clinical sequelae of infection. For the critically ill patient, the dehydration that frequently accompanies severe diarrhea strains a circulatory capacity already limited by impaired cardiac contractility and septic hemodynamics. Such individuals are at high risk for further systemic deterioration, often culminating in multisystem organ failure. In addition to life-threatening volume loss, diarrhea in the critically ill patient can precipitate metabolic derangements including electrolyte imbalances and acidosis, further exacerbating the potential for cardiac rhythm irritability. Finally, uncontrolled diarrhea in a severely ill immobile patient can predispose to compromise of the protective barrier of the skin. As such, the patient is rendered vulnerable to further infectious complications. Considering these dire clinical consequences, the prompt detection, microbiologic diagnosis, and therapy of diarrhea must be a high priority for clinicians in the ICU.

The epidemiology of diarrheal illness among patients in the ICU is substantially different from that seen among less severely ill patients in the community. Such differences render most of the schemes used to classify diarrhea in other settings less applicable to the evaluation of the critically ill patient. Infectious diarrhea acquired in the outpatient setting is rarely sufficiently severe to warrant admission to the ICU. Therefore, infectious diarrhea among patients in the ICU is most often acquired in the hospital. As a result, the spectrum of clinical disease and associated pathogens for the patient in the ICU tends to be less diverse than that encountered in the community. In fact, the majority of all cases of infectious diarrhea diagnosed in the ICU can be attributed to a single pathogen, *Clostridium difficile*. For many of these patients, the differential diagnosis consists largely of noninfectious entities, such as diarrhea induced by hyperosmolar enteral feeding solutions.[11] Norwalk-like viruses, one of the most common causes of endemic and epidemic diarrhea in the outpatient setting, are rarely identified as the cause of diarrhea in critically ill patients. Similarly, while outbreaks of food-borne gastroenteritis have been reported among hospitalized patients,[12] in the absence of an identified cluster, the work-up of the ICU patient with diarrhea usually need not include consideration of these pathogens.

It is in recognition of the rarity with which the clinician in the ICU will encounter diarrhea that is not hospital-acquired that a review of these less familiar presentations is warranted. While the distinctions between these syndromes are somewhat arbitrary, and there is considerable overlap between them, it is imperative that the clinician caring for critically ill patients at least be able to recognize these syndromes. In the sections that follow, inflammatory, noninflammatory, and hemorrhagic diarrheas are considered separately. Each is discussed with respect to the most common

TABLE 57-2 Features of Noninflammatory, Inflammatory, and Hemorrhagic Diarrhea

	Noninflammatory	Inflammatory	Hemorrhagic
Clinical presentation	Large volumes of watery stool; signs and symptoms of dehydration	Dysentery; small quantities of blood and mucus, often accompanied by fever	Grossly bloody bowel movements
Laboratory findings	Fecal leukocyte studies negative; acidosis; azotemia	Fecal leukocyte studies positive	Anemia; azotemia in the setting of hemolytic uremic syndrome (HUS)
Typical pathogens	*Vibrio cholerae*, enterotoxigenic *Escherichia coli*	*Shigella* species, *Salmonella* species, *Campylobacter jejuni*	*E. coli* type O157:H7
Pathophysiology	Toxin-mediated secretory diarrhea	Compromise of the intestinal epithelium with varying degrees of bacterial invasion	Poorly understood
Approach to therapy	Rehydration and antimicrobial therapy	Antimicrobial therapy if severely ill or immunocompromised	Supportive therapy; antimicrobials may increase the risk of HUS

clinical presentations and pathogens that could be expected in the ICU (Table 57-2). A general approach to the diagnosis and treatment of diarrhea among patients in the ICU follows. The chapter concludes with an in-depth discussion of diarrhea caused by *C. difficile*—an organism whose central role as a cause of diarrhea among patients in the ICU has already been discussed.

NONINFLAMMATORY DIARRHEA

In general, the noninflammatory diarrheal syndromes are characterized by the production of large volumes of watery stool devoid of gross blood or inflammatory cells. By definition, stool examination for fecal leukocytes in such patients will be negative. The typical presentation and pathophysiology of noninflammatory diarrhea is best exemplified by infection with *Vibrio cholerae*. While this gram-negative bacillus is the most prevalent cause of dehydrating diarrhea throughout the world, it is rarely encountered as a pathogen causing serious disease in the developed world. That said, the metabolic sequelae of cholera are capable of generating systemic illness sufficiently severe as to require ICU admission in a returning traveler.

While the diarrhea experienced by the patient infected with *V. cholerae* is characteristic of the other noninflammatory diarrheal infections, the severity of disease is unique to cholera. Diarrhea is voluminous, and patients can lose more than 1 liter of fluid *every hour*. Affected patients are at high risk for life-threatening dehydration. Vital signs will reveal tachycardia and hypotension. The metabolic abnormalities can precipitate severe acidosis. To compensate, the patient may become tachypneic. Skin evaluation in these individuals reveals decreased turgor. The mucous membranes, including conjunctivae, appear dry. In extreme cases, the patient's eyes will appear sunken, producing a characteristic facies. If fluids are not replaced promptly and in sufficient quantity, the infection will be fatal.

The diarrhea of cholera is secretory in nature. Having established itself in the lumen of the bowel, *V. cholerae* releases an extracellular protein that binds to the membrane of intestinal epithelial cells. The enterotoxin induces an increase in intracellular cyclic adenosine monophosphate (cAMP). The high concentration of cAMP induces an increase in chloride secretion and a decrease in sodium absorption, producing the massive fluid and electrolyte loss characteristic of cholera.[13]

While *V. cholerae* is the prototypical pathogen associated with noninflammatory diarrhea, an array of other organisms

can produce the same syndrome. While the diarrhea induced by these other pathogens tends to be less severe than that of cholera, the greater frequency with which these organisms cause infection in the developed world makes them more likely to be encountered as a cause of diarrhea in this setting. Most important among these are the so-called enterotoxigenic strains of *Escherichia coli*. These isolates produce an extracellular toxin, a component of which is similar to that produced by *V. cholerae*. The end result is comparable—profuse watery diarrhea that challenges patient and clinician to maintain adequate hydration.

INFLAMMATORY DIARRHEA

Spanning a broad spectrum of clinical severity, inflammatory diarrhea is strictly defined by the presence of fecal leukocytes when the stool from affected patients is examined microscopically. In terms of pathophysiology, these infections are characterized by compromise of the integrity of the intestinal epithelium. Depending on the causative organism, there may be varying degrees of bacterial invasion. As a result of this process, inflammatory cells, including both neutrophils and lymphocytes, are recruited to the affected area, where some are shed into the intestinal lumen.

In the most extreme cases, inflammatory diarrhea causes the clinical syndrome commonly referred to as dysentery. The patient with dysentery presents with semisolid or liquid bowel movements that are not as voluminous as those seen with noninflammatory diarrhea. In fact, some patients report very scant production of fecal matter. For them, bowel movements are characterized by small quantities of gross blood and mucus. Fever is often present, but is usually not exceedingly high. Patients with dysentery may experience severe cramping abdominal pain or tenesmus—pain with the passage of bowel movements. Because of the limited ability of critically ill patients to report such complaints, clinicians should be alert for the presence of the unique stool characteristics that identify the patient with dysentery and inflammatory diarrhea.

A number of pathogens have been described in association with the clinical manifestations of inflammatory diarrhea, but the classical description of the syndrome is associated with infection with *Shigella* species, particularly *S. dysenteriae*. As was true for cholera and other noninflammatory diarrheas, this association once again points to a shared pathophysiology. Pathogenic *Shigella* species elaborate an exotoxin (Shiga toxin) that acts by inhibiting protein synthesis, damaging the intestinal mucosa. Analogous shiga-like toxins have been detected in association with other bacterial species linked to inflammatory diarrhea, including both enteroinvasive and enterohemorrhagic strains of *E. coli*.

Like *Shigella*, the other bacterial species commonly identified in cases of inflammatory diarrhea are generally acquired through fecal oral transmission, often in the setting of food-borne outbreaks. In the United States, the most common such pathogens are members of the *Salmonella* species. Outbreaks of food-borne salmonellosis, while most commonly linked to undercooked poultry and dairy products, have even been reported in the context of a deliberate release associated with an episode of domestic bioterrorism.[14] Other important pathogens identified in association with inflammatory diarrhea include *E. coli* and *Campylobacter jejuni*.

HEMORRHAGIC DIARRHEA

Patients with hemorrhagic diarrhea, characterized by the presence of frank blood, are increasingly being seen in the setting of the ICU. In addition to the hemodynamic and metabolic complications that characterize other inflammatory diarrheas, patients with hemorrhagic diarrhea have been found to be predisposed to systemic illness that can warrant admission to critical care. Strains of *E. coli* belonging to serogroup O157:H7 have been epidemiologically linked to the development of the hemolytic uremic syndrome.[15] While the mechanism linking infection and this syndrome is not yet well understood, the resultant deposition of fibrin thrombi in the renal glomeruli can induce sufficient anemia, thrombocytopenia, and azotemia as to be life threatening. The hemolytic uremic syndrome typically follows the onset of diarrhea by about 1 week. While many of these patients will require intensive supportive therapy, including blood transfusion and hemodialysis, for most the condition is reversible. Of particular concern to clinicians caring for these patients is the observation that antimicrobial treatment may contribute to the emergence of this syndrome.[16]

EVALUATION OF THE CRITICALLY ILL PATIENT WITH DIARRHEA

The foremost consideration in the evaluation of the critically ill patient with diarrhea is the prompt recognition of infection with *C. difficile*. In the setting of prior exposure to antimicrobials or antineoplastic therapy, diarrhea can be presumptively attributed to *C. difficile* infection until proven otherwise. Identification of these patients is critical not only for the initiation of directed therapy, but to ensure that adequate infection control procedures are followed to limit the spread of infection to other vulnerable patients in the ICU. A comprehensive approach to the diagnosis of *C. difficile* is provided at the end of this chapter.

Whether or not *C. difficile* infection can be excluded, the evaluation of diarrhea in the ICU must progress in a systematic fashion with respect to the microbiology of the most likely infecting organism (Table 57-3). The initial assessment of these patients should include an accurate history of both the course of diarrhea and the presence of any precipitating factors that might suggest a causative organism. The patient, or for the uncommunicative patient a family member or friend, should be queried about the timing of onset of diarrhea, the progression of symptoms, associated systemic

TABLE 57-3 Diagnostic Approach to the Patient with Infectious Diarrhea

History
    Timing and rapidity of onset
    Associated signs and symptoms (fever)
    Nature and quantity of bowel movements
    Prior antibiotics or chemotherapy
Physical examination
    Hemodynamic compromise (tachycardia or hypotension)
    Signs of dehydration (orthostasis, skin tenting)
    Rectal examination for gross or occult bleeding
Laboratory
    Stool for fecal leukocytes
    Immunoassay for *C. difficile* toxins A and B
    Stool culture (especially in the setting of outbreak or community acquisition)
    Stool for ova and parasites (if travel-related)
    Endoscopy (reserve for persistent cases in which other tests are not revealing)

complaints such as fever or chills, and the nature and quantity of bowel movements (with particular emphasis on the presence or absence of bloody stools). Additional essential data includes information about recent travel, unusual dietary intake, and the presence of similar symptoms among companions with whom the patient has shared a meal. Of course, a history of prior antibiotic therapy or cancer chemotherapy will be needed to distinguish individuals at risk for *C. difficile* colitis. By the end of this process, the clinician should be able to characterize the diarrhea as acute or chronic, community- or hospital-acquired, and severe or mild. The last finding is of particular importance in that supportive therapy to alleviate severe dehydration should not be withheld pending further laboratory and microbiologic evaluation.

Given the emphasis placed on distinguishing inflammatory from noninflammatory diarrhea, it will come as no surprise that the initial laboratory work-up of the critically ill patient with diarrhea should include an objective measure of inflammation. Testing for fecal leukocytes offers a reliable means by which to do so. The test is performed by mixing a drop of stool with methylene blue on a slide, followed by examination under a microscope. Testing for stool occult blood has been suggested as another useful tool to identify patients in the ICU with inflammatory diarrhea. Unfortunately, testing for occult blood, even in the presence of a new fever in a critically ill patient, may be of little use in discriminating inflammatory infectious diarrhea from other common, noninfectious causes of bloody bowel movements among such patients, including stress-induced gastric ulceration and ischemic colitis.

In the setting of noninflammatory diarrhea, epidemiologic data must be interpreted to assess the likelihood of infection with *V. cholerae*. For a traveler returning from an endemic area presenting with signs and symptoms consistent with cholera, direct stool examination under darkfield or phase contrast microscopy can reveal the linear motility characteristic of *V. cholerae*. The organism will also grow on nonselective bacteriologic media, but the preferred method is culture on thiosulfate-citrate-bile salts-sucrose agar. If infection with enterotoxigenic *E. coli* is suspected, an assay to detect toxin is available from reference laboratories.

Especially in a patient with community-acquired diarrhea, the identification of fecal leukocytes on direct observation

TABLE 57-4 Recommended Antimicrobial Regimens for Patients Hospitalized with Bacterial Diarrhea

Pathogen	Recommended Treatment Regimen	Notes
Campylobacter jejuni	Azithromycin or ciprofloxacin	Fluoroquinolone resistance increasing in some regions
Clostridium difficile	Metronidazole	Vancomycin is not preferred because of risk of precipitating resistance; avoid antimotility agents
Escherichia coli O157:H7	No antimicrobial therapy advised	Antimicobials may increase the risk of hemolytic uremic syndrome
Salmonella species	Ciprofloxacin	Treat only if symptoms are severe or patient is immunocompromised
Shigella species	Ciprofloxacin	
Traveler's diarrhea	Fluoroquinolone	Use of antimotility agents is appropriate
Vibrio cholerae	Ciprofloxacin	Rehydration is cornerstone of therapy
Yersinia enterocolitica	Ciprofloxacin	

should warrant a search for bacterial pathogens that cause inflammatory diarrhea, including *E. coli*, *C. jejuni*, *Salmonella*, and *Shigella* species.[17] Stool culture can be particularly useful in distinguishing the bacterial pathogens that are commonly associated with these food-borne gastroenteritides. Selective media, such as MacConkey, desoxycholate, and salmonella-shigella agars, are employed in the microbiology lab to enhance the ability to detect these pathogens. It is useful to identify particular epidemiologic concerns to the microbiology lab so that the appropriate media can be employed.

The examination of stool for the presence of ova and parasites is of limited utility among patients in the ICU. First and foremost, the clinical syndromes caused by infection with these organisms tend not to be so serious as to require admission to the ICU. Moreover, the incidence of parasitic infections in ICU patients is so low as to make the positive predictive value of the stool ova and parasite examination vanishingly small. In this context, even a positive finding on stool ova and parasite exam is more likely to represent a false-positive than it is to represent actual infection. Many clinical laboratories have gone so far as to not accept stool ova and parasite specimens from patients who have been hospitalized for 48 to 72 hours.

The role of endoscopy in the evaluation of infectious diarrhea is limited. While biopsy may detect the presence of specific pathogens such as *Entamoeba histolytica*, the relatively low incidence of these infections in this population makes this the diagnostic procedure of last resort. Lower GI endoscopy will not help to discriminate or diagnose infection with common bacterial pathogens such as *E. coli* or *C. jejuni*. As discussed later, sigmoidoscopy and colonoscopy can be helpful in the detection and diagnosis of colitis caused by *C. difficile* infection.

TREATMENT

The foremost objective in the care of the patient with infectious diarrhea is to restore the patient to a normal fluid and electrolyte balance as rapidly as possible. While oral rehydration solutions, such as that recommended by the World Health Organization, have proven safe and effective in settings in which intravenous therapy is either impractical or unavailable, most patients with diarrhea in the ICU will require parenteral replenishment. Effective regimens include

lactated Ringer solution and normal saline with electrolyte supplementation. The use of large volumes of 5% dextrose and water for these patients may precipitate dangerous hyponatremia. No matter the regimen selected, serum chemistry analyses should be performed frequently to ensure adequacy of electrolyte replacement.

In general, empirical antimicrobial therapy for infectious diarrhea not associated with *C. difficile* should be avoided. Indiscriminant antibiotic use for this indication exposes the patient to needless toxicity, may precipitate the emergence of resistant organisms as a cause of systemic infection, can worsen the course of some infection (as in the case of *E. coli* serotype O157:H7), and might predispose the patient to prolonged carriage with the offending pathogen.[18] However, once a specific pathogen has been identified, therapy can be directed by documented susceptibility information—or at least trends among known or suspected pathogens. Pathogen-specific recommendations are listed in Table 57-4.

Clostridium Difficile Infection

As was already noted, *Clostridium difficile* is the single most common cause of infectious diarrhea among all hospitalized patients, including those in the ICU. When patients receiving antibiotics during hospitalization are considered, the incidence of *C. difficile* colitis approaches 10%.[19] It is estimated that fully one quarter of diarrheal episodes among hospitalized patients may be attributable to *C. difficile* infection.[20] Hospital costs for patients who acquire *C. difficile* diarrhea are more than 50% higher than for those without infection, and an episode of *C. difficile* colitis prolongs the average length of stay for infected patients by nearly 4 days.[21] Of greater concern, the incidence of *C. difficile* colitis appears to be increasing.[22]

CLINICAL PRESENTATION

The clinical presentation of patients with *C. difficile* can be quite diverse. In addition to asymptomatic carriage, some patients may report only a minimal increase in the frequency or liquidity of bowel movements. Such individuals, while at low risk of complication from infection, if not identified and appropriately isolated from other patients, represent an important reservoir for the spread of *C. difficile* within the ICU. At the other extreme, patients may experience severe clinical deterioration as a result infection with *C. difficile.* The bowel movements of the patient with *C. difficile* infection may be watery and voluminous, such as is seen in noninflammatory diarrheas. Other patients with *C. difficile* infection experience a clinical syndrome more consistent with that of the inflammatory gastroenteritides, occasionally even reporting gross blood in the stool. Fever is present in about half of patients. Leukocytosis, sometimes profound, is often a reliable indicator of the onset of *C. difficile* colitis.

In extreme cases, patients infected with *C. difficile* present with the complication of toxic megacolon. Such patients may or may not experience diarrhea. Abdominal radiography in these cases reveals grossly dilated colonic loops without evidence of mechanical obstruction. The patients frequently demonstrate end-organ dysfunction as is typical for the sepsis syndrome. The diagnosis of toxic megacolon carries with it a high degree of mortality. Colonic perforation can result if the infection is not treated promptly.

MICROBIOLOGY

C. difficile is an obligate anaerobic gram-positive bacillus whose virulence is attributed to the production of extracellular toxins. *C. difficile* can be identified as part of the normal flora in patients without overt diarrheal disease. In these individuals, toxin-negative strains of *C. difficile* are likely no more than harmless commensal organisms. In fact, there are data suggesting that progression to diarrhea occurs early after acquisition of *C. difficile* or not at all.[23] To produce diarrhea and other manifestations of clinical disease, infecting strains of *C. difficile* must produce extracellular toxins. Together, toxin A (enterotoxin) and toxin B (cytotoxin) cause epithelial cell necrosis through the disruption of the actin cytoskeleton.[24] Recently, strains of toxin A–negative, toxin B–positive *C. difficile* have been described in association with outbreaks of hospital-acquired disease.[25]

DIAGNOSIS

The spectrum of clinical disease associated with *C. difficile* infection makes diagnosis solely on the basis of clinical observations impractical. That said, experienced clinicians often point to what they consider to be a typical picture of *C. difficile* diarrhea, including foul-smelling stool that is greasy and green in color. Unfortunately, such observations are of limited value. On the other hand, readily available historical data, when accurately obtained, can be far more informative in leading the clinician to an accurate diagnosis.

While once closely linked to exposure to clindamycin or other agents from the lincosamide class, *C. difficile* colitis has since been observed to occur after therapy with nearly every antimicrobial agent available to clinicians, including metronidazole.[26] Because of their widespread use and broad spectrum of activity, there appears to be an especially close association between *C. difficile* diarrhea and prior therapy with the cephalosporin class of β-lactam agents.[26] While there may be an association between the anaerobic activity of an antibiotic and its likelihood of precipitating *C. difficile* diarrhea, the specific mechanisms and implications of this relationship remain to be explored. The observed association between some antineoplastic chemotherapy agents and *C. dif-*

ficile infection similarly challenges our understanding of the pathophysiology of these infections.

The onset of diarrhea due to *C. difficile* infection most commonly occurs in close relation to antibiotic administration. Twenty-five percent of cases present while dosing is ongoing.[27] However, both the published literature and clinical experience reveal episodes of *C. difficile* colitis that occur within 48 hours of the initiation of antibiotic therapy, and others that develop months after exposure. In addition to the pharmacologic agents already mentioned, a number of factors are thought to predispose patients to *C. difficile* colitis, including advanced age, increased severity of illness, and impaired GI motility.[28] In one study, the odds ratio for *C. difficile* infection among patients with the most severe underlying disease was 17.6.[19] Each of these factors is commonly encountered among patients in the ICU, rendering them especially susceptible to infection.

While a patient's clinical history might suggest *C. difficile* infection, accurate diagnosis depends on the prudent use of objective laboratory assays. Attempts to culture *C. difficile* from the stool have proven clinically unreliable and have little utility in the evaluation of the hospitalized patient with diarrhea. The results of fecal leukocyte testing in the setting of *C. difficile* infection are similarly unreliable as an aid to diagnosis. The accurate identification of *C. difficile* colitis depends on the detection of the characteristic toxins produced by the organism. Previously, the gold standard for diagnosis was the cytotoxic assay. With this study, diluted stool is added to monolayers of cultured cells. Observation of a cytopathic effect that is neutralized by antibody against the toxins is more than 95% sensitive and specific for the identification of toxigenic *C. difficile*.[29] Because of the labor and expertise required to perform this assay, most labs now rely on immunoassays for the direct detection of *C. difficile* toxins. Newer immunoassays capable of detecting both toxin A and B are more sensitive than earlier versions that detected only the enterotoxin.

Endoscopy can be helpful in the diagnosis of *C. difficile* colitis, but its widespread application for this purpose is limited. The characteristic finding of pseudomembranes comprised of necrotic epithelial tissue and inflammatory cells all but confirms the diagnosis of *C. difficile* colitis in the appropriate clinical setting. However, this finding is not always encountered, even in severe episodes of *C. difficile* colitis. Moreover, to perform colonoscopy or even flexible sigmoidoscopy in the setting of *C. difficile* infection is to expose the patient to the risk of unnecessary trauma that could result in the accidental perforation of an already inflamed and friable GI tract.

TREATMENT

Whenever feasible, the first and most important step in the treatment of the patient with *C. difficile* colitis is the discontinuation of the pharmacologic agent that precipitated the infection. In most cases, this means that ongoing antimicrobial therapy for other indications should be withdrawn as soon as it is safe to do so. This is a particular challenge when dealing with the critically ill patient. Broad-spectrum antimicrobial therapy, even when given empirically, is essential to the survival of the septic patients commonly encountered in this setting. For them, the discontinuation of therapy is not advisable, and an agent with activity against *C. difficile* (discussed below) must instead be added to the antimicrobial regimen.

The most appropriate antimicrobial strategy to treat *C. difficile* colitis can be the source of some controversy and confusion for even experienced caregivers in the ICU. Both metronidazole and vancomycin, when administered orally, have been shown to be effective in the treatment of *C. difficile* colitis. While many clinicians persist in the belief that vancomycin is superior to metronidazole for the treatment of *C. difficile*, the available literature does not yet support this position. Several clinical trials have pointed to the equivalence of vancomycin and metronidazole therapy.[30] However, it is worth noting that the percentage of isolates of *C. difficile* that are resistant in vitro to metronidazole may be increasing, but remains less than 10%.[31] The clinical implications of this observation have yet to be sorted out.

Reduction in the overall use of vancomycin, and specifically in the setting of initial treatment of *C. difficile* colitis, has been recommended by the Centers for Disease Control and Prevention as a means by which to stem the emergence of resistant bacteria.[32] Vancomycin-resistant enterococci are familiar to ICU physicians as a frequent cause of serious hospital-acquired infections. Strains of *Staphylococcus aureus* resistant to vancomycin have also been reported recently.[33]

For patients with *C. difficile* colitis who can tolerate oral therapy, treatment should be initiated with metronidazole, 500 mg every 8 hours. While many clinicians elect to treat for longer periods, the duration of metronidazole therapy necessary to treat *C. difficile* need not extend beyond 10 to 14 days. For patients who cannot tolerate metronidazole, vancomycin is an effective alternative, but should not be used as first-line therapy for the reasons previously outlined.

When oral therapy is not feasible, when given intravenously, metronidazole achieves adequate intraluminal concentrations to eradicate *C. difficile* colitis.[34] The recommended dosage is 500 mg every 8 hours. Intravenous vancomycin should never be used to treat *C. difficile* infection. After parenteral vancomycin administration, drug levels within the intestinal lumen are not sufficient to guarantee eradication. The role of vancomycin in treating *C. difficile* infection in the critically ill patient instead focuses on intraluminal therapy. When administered via a rectal tube or in the form of an enema, vancomycin can serve as a useful adjunct to intravenous metronidazole for the severely ill patient. Such methods are particularly useful in the setting of toxic megacolon caused by *C. difficile*, when GI motility has all but halted, and reliable delivery of drug administered orally or by a feeding tube cannot be assumed. However, caution is advised when employing these techniques. The GI mucosa is exceedingly friable in the setting of *C. difficile* infection, particularly when toxic megacolon has evolved. Such patients are at high risk for GI perforation. When the patient is critically ill as a consequence of *C. difficile* colitis (rather than critically ill and also having *C. difficile* colitis), combined therapy (500–750) mg IV every 6–8 h plus vancomycin 500 mg enterally every 6 h) has been advised.[35]

Retreatment of patients with either recurrent *C. difficile* colitis or those who fail to respond to initial metronidazole therapy is controversial and bears special attention. Clinicians should avoid the practice of routine laboratory testing to detect *C. difficile* toxin at the end of a course of therapy in an effort to confirm clearance. Infected patients may continue to shed detectable toxin after therapy is complete. Some individuals may do so intermittently for years. In these cases, additional therapy is not warranted. However, when diarrhea continues despite initial therapy or recurs soon thereafter, additional treatment is advised. In these circumstances, a switch to vancomycin or a more prolonged course of metronidazole has been advocated. However, in most cases, simple retreatment with metronidazole appears to be just as efficacious.

References

1. Bengmark S: Gut microbial ecology in critical illness: Is there a role for prebiotics, probiotics, and synbiotics? *Curr Opin Crit Care* 8:145, 2002.
2. Plaisier PW, van Buuren HR, Bruining HA: Upper gastrointestinal endoscopy at four intensive care units in one hospital: Frequency and indication. *Eur J Gastroenterol Hepatol* 10:997, 1998.
3. Baehr PH, McDonald GB: Esophageal infections: Risk factors, presentation, diagnosis, and treatment. *Gastroenterology* 106:509, 1994.
4. Wingard JR, Merz WG, Rinaldi MG, et al: Increase in *Candida krusei* infection among patients with bone marrow transplantation and neutropenia treated prophylactically with fluconazole. *N Engl J Med* 325:1274, 1991.
5. Galbraith JC, Shafran SD: Herpes simplex esophagitis in the immunocompetent patient: Report of four cases and review. *Clin Infect Dis* 14:894, 1992.
6. Andersen LI, Frederiksen HJ, Appleyard M: Prevalence of esophageal *Candida* colonization in a Danish population: Special reference to esophageal symptoms, benign esophageal disorders, and pulmonary disease. *J Infect Dis* 165:389, 1992.
7. Hopkins RJ, Girardi LS, Turney EA: Relationship between *Helicobacter pylori* eradication and reduced duodenal and gastric ulcer recurrence: a review. *Gastroenterology* 110:1244, 1996.
8. van der Voort PH, van der Hulst RW, Zandstra DF, et al: Prevalence of *Helicobacter pylori* infection in stress-induced gastric mucosal injury. *Intensive Care Med* 27:68, 2001.
9. van der Voort PH, van der Hulst RW, Zandstra DF, et al: Suppression of *Helicobacter pylori* infection during intensive care stay: Related to stress ulcer bleeding incidence? *J Crit Care* 16:182, 2001.
10. Ringel AF, Jameson GL, Foster ES: Diarrhea in the intensive care patient. *Crit Care Clin* 11:465, 1995.
11. Caines C, Gill MV, Cunha BA: Non-*Clostridium difficile* nosocomial diarrhea in the intensive care unit. *Heart Lung* 26:83, 1997.
12. Spearing NM, Jensen A, McCall BJ, et al: Direct costs associated with a nosocomial outbreak of *Salmonella* infection: An ounce of prevention is worth a pound of cure. *Am J Infect Control* 28:54, 2000.
13. Holmgren J: Actions of cholera toxin and the prevention and treatment of cholera. *Nature* 292:413, 1981.
14. Torok TJ, Tauxe RV, Wise RP, et al: A large community outbreak of salmonellosis caused by intentional contamination of restaurant salad bars. *JAMA* 278:389, 1997.
15. Slutsker L, Ries AA, Greene KD, et al: *Escherichia coli* O157:H7 diarrhea in the United States: Clinical and epidemiologic features. *Ann Intern Med* 126:505, 1997.
16. Wong CS, Jelacic S, Habeeb RL, et al: The risk of the hemolytic-uremic syndrome after antibiotic treatment of *Escherichia coli* O157:H7 infections. *N Engl J Med* 342:1930, 2000.
17. Guerrant RL, Shields DS, Thorson SM, et al: Evaluation and diagnosis of acute infectious diarrhea. *Am J Med* 78:91, 1985.
18. Gregg CR, Nassar NN: Infectious enteritis. *Curr Treat Options Gastroenterol* 2:119, 1999.
19. Kyne L, Sougioultzis S, McFarland LV, Kelly CP: Underlying disease severity as a major risk factor for nosocomial *Clostridium difficile* diarrhea. *Infect Control Hosp Epidemiol* 23:653, 2002.
20. Vasa CV, Glatt AE: Effectiveness and appropriateness of empiric metronidazole for *Clostridium difficile*-associated diarrhea. *Am J Gastroenterol* 98:354, 2003.

21. Kyne L, Hamel MB, Polavaram R, Kelly CP: Health care costs and mortality associated with nosocomial diarrhea due to *Clostridium difficile*. *Clin Infect Dis* 34:346, 2002.

22. Dallal RM, Harbrecht BG, Boujoukas AJ, et al: Fulminant *Clostridium difficile*: An underappreciated and increasing cause of death and complications. *Ann Surg* 235:363, 2002.

23. Samore MH, DeGirolami PC, Tlucko A, et al: *Clostridium difficile* colonization and diarrhea at a tertiary care hospital. *Clin Infect Dis* 18:181, 1994.

24. Poxton IR, McCoubrey J, Blair G: The pathogenicity of *Clostridium difficile*. *Clin Microbiol Infect* 7:421, 2001.

25. Alfa MJ, Kabani A, Lyerly D, et al: Characterization of a toxin A-negative, toxin B-positive strain of *Clostridium difficile* responsible for a nosocomial outbreak of *Clostridium difficile*-associated diarrhea. *J Clin Microbiol* 38:2706, 2000.

26. Thomas C, Stevenson M, Riley TV: Antibiotics and hospital-acquired *Clostridium difficile*-associated diarrhoea: A systematic review. *J Antimicrob Chemother* 51:1339, 2003.

27. Tabibian N: Diarrhea in critically ill patients. *Am Fam Physician* 40:135, 1989.

28. Brown E, Talbot GH, Axelrod P, et al: Risk factors for *Clostridium difficile* toxin-associated diarrhea. *Infect Control Hosp Epidemiol* 11:283, 1990.

29. George WL, Rolfe RD, Harding GK, et al: *Clostridium difficile* and cytotoxin in feces of patients with antimicrobial agent-associated pseudomembranous colitis. *Infection* 10:205, 1982.

30. Teasley DG, Gerding DN, Olson MM, et al: Prospective randomised trial of metronidazole versus vancomycin for *Clostridium difficile*-associated diarrhoea and colitis. *Lancet* 2:1043, 1983.

31. Pelaez T, Alcala L, Alonso R, et al: Reassessment of *Clostridium difficile* susceptibility to metronidazole and vancomycin. *Antimicrob Agents Chemother* 46:1647, 2002.

32. Recommendations for preventing the spread of vancomycin resistance. Hospital Infection Control Practices Advisory Committee (HICPAC). *Infect Control Hosp Epidemiol* 16:105, 1995.

33. Chang S, Sievert DM, Hageman JC, et al: Infection with vancomycin-resistant *Staphylococcus aureus* containing the vanA resistance gene. *N Engl J Med* 348:1342, 2003.

34. Friedenberg F, Fernandez A, Kaul V, et al: Intravenous metronidazole for the treatment of *Clostridium difficile* colitis. *Dis Colon Rectum* 44:1176, 2001.

35. Fekety R: Guidelines for the diagnosis and management of *Clostridium difficile*-associated diarrhea and colitis. American College of Gastroenterology, Practice Parameters Committee. *Am J Gastroenterol* 92:739, 1997.

SEVERE MALARIA
DAVID A. WARRELL

KEY POINTS

- *Consider the diagnosis of malaria in any acutely febrile patient with a history of recent travel to a malarious area or who might have been infected through blood transfusion, needlestick, or other nosocomial parenteral exposure.*

- *Transfer severely ill patients to an ICU and make a rapid clinical assessment, including spot measurement of blood glucose.*

- *If the diagnosis of severe falciparum malaria is proved or suspected, initiate antimalarial chemotherapy using optimal doses of an appropriate agent (licensed quinine or quinidine or an artemisinin derivative such as artesunate on a named-patient basis) administered intravenously, using a loading dose. Monitor the clinical and parasitologic responses.*

- *Prevent, or detect early and treat, the numerous complications (especially generalized convulsions, hypoglycemia, hyperpyrexia, and secondary bacterial infections).*

- *Ensure correct fluid, electrolyte, and acid-base balance. Control fluid replacement to prevent circulatory overload and pulmonary edema. Anticipate renal and respiratory failure.*

- *Expert nursing care of the unconscious patient is essential.*

- *Avoid the use of potentially harmful ancillary treatments of unproven benefit, such as corticosteroids, heparin, and epinephrine.*

Malarial Parasites and Life Cycles

Malaria is a mosquito-borne protozoal infection caused in humans by four species of *Plasmodium: P. falciparum, P. vivax, P. malariae,* or *P. ovale.*[1] Only *P. falciparum* causes life-threatening malaria, but other species can cause severe illness in debilitated individuals. *Plasmodium* sporozoites, inoculated by female *Anopheles* mosquitoes during their blood meal, invade hepatocytes where they mature into schizonts, and after 6 to 16 days rupture to release merozoites into the bloodstream. In the cases of *P. vivax* and *P. ovale,* some sporozoites remain dormant in the liver for months or years in the form of hypnozoites, and can give rise to relapsing infections months or even years later. *Plasmodium falciparum* and *P. malariae* may persist as inapparent low-grade parasitemias to cause symptomatic recrudescences. However, these species do not persist in the liver. The erythrocytic cycle consists of invasion, development from rings to mature pigmented multinucleated schizonts, and rupture with release of 4 to 32 merozoites, depending on the species. These invade erythrocytes to produce repeated cycles of infection, or develop into male and female gametocytes. Merozoites cannot reinvade the liver from the blood. Erythrocytes containing mature trophozoites and schizonts of *P. falciparum* are sequestered in the tissues. Gametocytes taken up by mosquitoes complete a sexual cycle producing sporozoites which are injected with the mosquito's saliva during a blood meal. The usual intervals between the mosquito bite and the appearance of parasitemia are 10 days for *P. falciparum,* 8 to 13 days for *P. vivax,* 9 to 14 days for *P. ovale,* and 15 to 16 days for *P. malariae.* Minimal intervals between the bite and first symptom (incubation period) are a few days longer.

EPIDEMIOLOGY

Malaria is endemic throughout tropical countries except in Pacific Islands east of Vanuatu (Fig. 58-1). *P. falciparum* is the most common cause of malaria in Africa, Haiti, some parts of South America, Southeast Asia, and New Guinea, but is now absent from Europe. *Plasmodium vivax* has been the dominant species in most parts of the Indian subcontinent where there is now a resurgence of *P. falciparum;* it is replaced by *P. ovale* in West Africa, but occurs with varying frequency throughout other parts of the malaria endemic area. *P. malariae* infections are widespread but usually infrequent.

Children who grow up in endemic areas eventually acquire, through frequent infections, immunity to symptoms and severe malaria.[1] In these regions, severe disease is confined to infants and young children. This immunity lapses in those who move outside the endemic area for several years. Thus Asian or African immigrants living in Europe or North America may become susceptible to symptomatic malaria by the time they return home on vacation. Outside the endemic areas, autochthonous malaria may occur in those living around international airports or in immigrant communities. Malaria can be transmitted by transfusion of blood products and bone marrow, by transplanted organs and contaminated needles (for example, among intravenous and subcutaneous drug abusers), and transplacentally (congenital malaria). Nosocomial outbreaks have followed contamination of intravenous lines and contrast medium, and administration of drugs.

GENETICS

So far, eighteen human genetic polymorphisms have been associated with resistance to malaria.[2] These include thalassemias, hemoglobins S, E, and C, South East Asian ovalocytosis, glucose-6-phosphate dehydrogenase (G6PD) deficiency, interferon-α and -γ receptors, toll-like receptor 4, and for vivax malaria, the Duffy blood group. The highest frequencies of these resistance genes occur in intensely malarious areas.

GENERAL PATHOPHYSIOLOGY

Symptoms and pathologic changes are attributable to the asexual erythrocytic cycle and to secondary activation of macrophages and the immune system. A malarial toxin, released at schizont rupture, stimulates macrophages to release interleukin-1, tumor necrosis factor-α (TNF-α), and other cytokines. Cytoadherence to the wall of venules by erythrocytes containing mature trophozoites and schizonts plays an important role in producing organ and tissue dysfunction. The molecular basis of cytoadherence is the binding of malarial antigens expressed on the erythrocyte surface (notably the diverse and variable adhesive antigens, PfEMP$_1$) to endothelial receptors such as intracellular adhesion molecule-1 (ICAM-1), vascular cell adhesion molecule (VCAM), E-selectin, chondroitin-4-sulfate and hyaluronic acid (on placental villi),

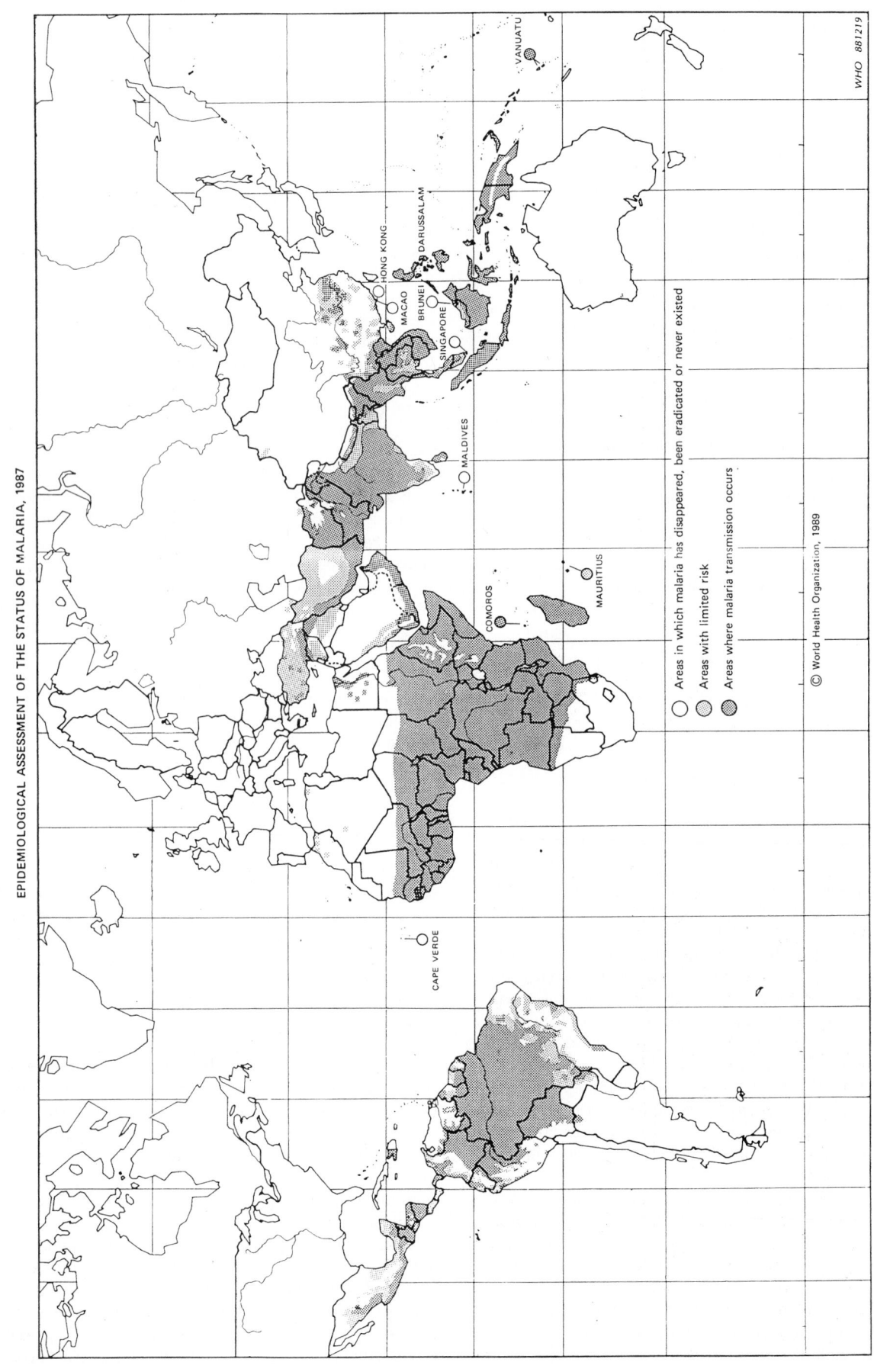

EPIDEMIOLOGICAL ASSESSMENT OF THE STATUS OF MALARIA, 1987

VANUATU

HONG KONG
BRUNEI DARUSSALAM
MACAO
SINGAPORE

MALDIVES

MAURITIUS

COMOROS

CAPE VERDE

○ Areas in which malaria has disappeared, been eradicated or never existed

Areas with limited risk

Areas where malaria transmission occurs

© World Health Organization, 1989

WHO 88.1219

FIGURE 58-1 Distribution of malaria in the world.

TABLE 58-1 Severe Manifestations of Falciparum Malaria in Adults and Children

Clinical Manifestations	Laboratory Findings
Prostration	Severe anemia (hemoglobin <5 g/dL or hematocrit <15%)
Impaired consciousness (cerebral malaria)	Hypoglycemia (blood glucose <2.2 mmol/L *or* 40 mg/dL)
Respiratory distress (acidotic breathing)	Acidosis (plasma bicarbonate <15 mmol/L or base excess >−10)
Multiple convulsions	Hyperlactatemia (>5 mmol/L)
Circulatory collapse	Hyperparasitemia
Pulmonary edema	Renal impairment
Abnormal bleeding	
Jaundice	
Hemoglobinuria	

SOURCE: Reproduced with permission from World Health Organization.[9]

membrane glycoprotein CD36, or the multifunctional adhesive glycoprotein thrombospondin.[1] Sequestration of parasitized erythrocytes is most marked in brain, kidney, gut, placenta, skeletal muscle, liver, bone marrow, and retina.[2–4] The resulting stagnation of blood flow causes hypoxia and anaerobic glycolysis with increased lactic acid production.[5]

PATHOPHYSIOLOGY OF SPECIFIC ORGAN AND TISSUE DYSFUNCTIONS

Anemia results principally from hemolysis of parasitized erythrocytes and perhaps some immune hemolysis. Enhanced splenic removal of nonparasitized erythrocytes and dyserythropoiesis may contribute. *Intravascular hemolysis* and *hemoglobinuria* in patients with inherited erythrocytic enzyme defects such as G6PD deficiency is commonly associated with the use of oxidant antimalarial drugs such as primaquine and chloroquine. Classic *blackwater fever* has been attributed to quinine-related immune hemolysis, but the evidence is inconclusive. *Thrombocytopenia* results from splenic sequestration or immune destruction; there is no evidence of reduced marrow production. There is evidence of *disseminated intravascular coagulation* (DIC) in about 15% of severe cases. Neurologic symptoms (*cerebral malaria*) are attributable to sequestration of parasitized erythrocytes in venules with some inflammatory change, especially in children. Plasma concentrations of TNF-α correlate directly with severity and incidence of neurologic sequelae.[6] In human cerebral malaria, permeability of the blood-cerebrospinal fluid barrier is only mildly deranged. Cerebral edema does not explain coma. *Acute pulmonary edema* may be precipitated by fluid overload, but is more commonly associated with normal or low pulmonary artery wedge pressures and resembles acute respiratory distress syndrome. Leukocyte sequestration in the pulmonary capillaries resembles experimental "endotoxin lung." *Hypoglycemia* may result from quinine- or quinidine-induced hyperinsulinemia or from inhibition of hepatic gluconeogenesis by TNF-α, in association with appropriately low plasma insulin levels. *Renal* and *hepatic dysfunction* result from vasoconstriction and vascular obstruction by sequestered parasitized erythrocytes.[1,7] *Shock* (*algid malaria*) is frequently associated with secondary gram-negative rod septicemia, but may also arise in patients with acute pulmonary edema, dehydration, lactic acidosis, hypoglycemia, and hemorrhagic shock following gastrointestinal hemorrhage or splenic rupture.

CLINICAL FEATURES

FALCIPARUM MALARIA

The shortest interval between the infecting mosquito bite and the first symptom is 7 days. This fact may be useful in excluding the diagnosis of malaria in patients who fall ill too soon after entering a malarial endemic region. More than 80% of patients with imported falciparum malaria become ill within 1 month of leaving the endemic area, whereas only a few percent present between 3 and 12 months or longer after leaving. None of the symptoms of malaria is specific. The illness may start with headache, a fever, a chill, tiredness, or lethargy. Backache, myalgias, postural syncope, prostration, vomiting, and diarrhea are common. Physical signs include anemia, jaundice, and tender hepatosplenomegaly. An absence of focal symptoms, lymphadenopathy, and rash (other than herpes labialis) help distinguish malaria from some other fevers. The classical tertian or subtertian fever (a fever spike every 36 or 48 hours) is rarely seen, and even the classic "paroxysm" (chill, hot phase, and diaphoresis) is uncommon.[1,8]

Life-threatening falciparum malaria is defined by the presence of any of the features listed in Table 58-1.[9] There are age and geographic variations in the frequency of these different features. In most parts of the world, cerebral malaria is the most familiar manifestation of severe malaria in adults, but jaundice is more common in Vietnam and Papua New Guinea, and in African children acidotic breathing is more common.[1,9]

Cerebral malaria[10,11] should be considered in any acutely febrile patient, possibly exposed to *P. falciparum* infection, whose level of consciousness is impaired. A typical history would be that after a few days of febrile symptoms, coma developed insidiously or suddenly with a generalized convulsion. An immediate trial of antimalarial chemotherapy is warranted in such patients even if parasitemia is not evident in the peripheral blood smear. A strict definition of cerebral malaria (essential for comparative clinical trials) demands unrousable coma (Glasgow Coma Scale score ≤11), the demonstration of asexual *P. falciparum* parasitemia, and the exclusion of other causes of coma, especially of bacterial meningitis and locally prevalent viral encephalitides.[9,12]

Other clinical features of cerebral malaria include seizures (which may be subclinical in children),[13] dysconjugate gaze, forcible jaw closure and tooth grinding (bruxism), signs of a symmetrical upper motor neuron lesion (with extensor plantar responses and absent superficial reflexes), and abnormal extensor or flexor posturing (decerebrate/decorticate rigidity). Retinal hemorrhages, and the less frequent exudates and papilledema, carry a severe prognosis. Survivors recover consciousness within a few days and are usually free of neurologic sequelae (but see discussion of children below). Psychiatric manifestations (brief reactive psychosis), involuntary (extrapyramidal) movements, and focal convulsions without loss of consciousness are seen but are uncommon. Delayed and reversible postmalaria ataxia has been described, especially in South Asia, but is not usually associated with cerebral malaria or severe disease.[1,10]

Renal functional impairment of some degree occurs in about a third of adult patients with severe falciparum malaria.[14] Acute tubular necrosis develops in a minority. Acute renal failure is a feature of classic blackwater fever.

Acute pulmonary edema is often fatal. It is associated with hyperparasitemia, renal failure, lactic acidosis, use of excessive parenteral fluid replacement, and parturition. It has been rarely reported in vivax and ovale malarias (see below).[15]

Hypoglycemia is increasingly recognized. Symptoms of hypoglycemia may be confused with those of malaria itself, and so hypoglycemia must be specifically excluded in all patients with impaired consciousness, abnormal posturing, convulsions, shock, tachypnea, and in pregnant women in whom there is evidence of fetal distress. Hypoglycemia commonly develops as a complication of treatment with cinchona alkaloids (quinine and quinidine), which induce hyperinsulinemia, even in convalescence, particularly in pregnant women who may be asymptomatic, and in adults and children with hyperparasitemia and other features of severe disease.

Shock (algid malaria) may complicate severe malaria itself or be a result of simple dehydration or acute hemorrhage, but in many patients there is superimposed gram-negative septicemia. Cardiac arrhythmias and myocardial failure are extremely rare.

Bleeding, coagulopathy, and DIC are found in about 15% of nonimmune travelers with severe falciparum malaria. Thrombocytopenia is common in both falciparum and vivax malarias; its degree is not related to prognosis.

Acidosis, usually resulting from lactic acid accumulation, presents with rapid deep respirations in severely ill patients.

Massive intravascular hemolysis and hemoglobinuria in patients with normal erythrocyte enzymes has been termed "blackwater fever." This puzzling syndrome is associated with intermittent use of quinine, mild or absent parasitemia, fever, loin pain, vomiting, diarrhea, polyuria followed by oliguria and passage of black urine, tender hepatosplenomegaly, profound anemia, and deep jaundice.

Hepatic dysfunction is manifested by deep jaundice with a major component of conjugated bilirubin, prolonged prothrombin time, increased concentrations of serum aminotransferases (rarely more than 3 to 5 times greater than normal), and a low or falling serum albumin.

Severe falciparum malaria in children[1,16,17] is found in endemic regions of the tropics, where children under the age of 5 years are the most vulnerable. The history may be very short with less than 24 hours between the first feverish symptom and loss of consciousness. Generalized and subclinical convulsions are common.[13] There is evidence of raised intracranial pressure (cerebrospinal fluid

[CSF] opening pressure at lumbar puncture is elevated), brain swelling (confirmed by computed tomography [CT] or magnetic resonance imaging [MRI]), and in some cases neurologic signs suggesting cerebral and brain stem herniation.[17] A syndrome of metabolic acidosis, respiratory distress, and profound anemia carries a particularly bad prognosis.[16] Jaundice, renal failure, hemostatic abnormalities, and pulmonary edema are much less common than in adults, but hypoglycemia is very common. The incidence of persistent neurologic sequelae after childhood cerebral malaria may exceed 10%.

The mortality of severe falciparum malaria ranges from 10% to 50%. In a recent report of imported cases of malaria managed in a European ICU, the mortality was 11%.[18] However, in adults, impaired consciousness alone, without evidence of other organ or tissue dysfunctions, carries a good prognosis.[12,18]

OTHER MALARIAS

Initial febrile and influenza-like symptoms associated with other *Plasmodium* species are as unpleasant as in falciparum malaria. The fever in untreated vivax and ovale malarias has a tertian periodicity (fever spike every 48 hours), and in *P. malariae* infection has quartan periodicity (every 72 hours). Vivax and ovale malarias may relapse 8 years or longer after the initial infection, and malarial infection may recrudesce for 50 years or more.

If, in a patient whose blood film shows only parasites of *P. vivax*, *P. ovale*, or *P. malariae*, there are clinical features of severe disease, inapparent mixed infection with *P. falciparum* should be suspected and the patient treated accordingly. Rapid antigen detection tests specific for *P. falciparum* can be useful in this situation (see below). However, *Plasmodium vivax* and *P. ovale* malarias can cause increased pulmonary capillary permeability, and on rare occasions, even clinically apparent pulmonary edema.[15] Fatal splenic rupture has been described in vivax, and some debilitated children or adults have died of severe anemia. *P. malariae* malaria may prove severe or even fatal in immunocompromised patients who acquire the infection by transfusion. *P. malariae* infection is an important cause of nephrotic syndrome, especially in Africa.

IMPACT OF OTHER CONDITIONS ON DISEASE SEVERITY

Malaria is more severe in pregnant women, especially in the third trimester, and even women with acquired malarial immunity become newly vulnerable to severe disease during their first pregnancy. Splenic dysfunction predisposes to severe disease with high parasitemia with schizonts, and other mature forms may be present in the peripheral blood smear. An interaction between human immunodeficiency virus (HIV) immunosuppression and malaria has so far been demonstrated only in pregnant women, who show higher parasitemias, and in their babies, who suffer higher perinatal mortality. Although sickle cell trait partially protects against falciparum (but not ovale) malaria, malaria may be disastrous in children with sickle cell disease.

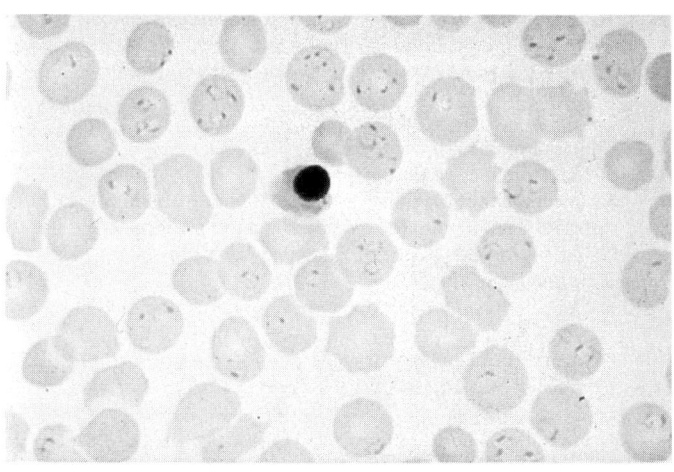

FIGURE 58-2 *Plasmodium falciparum* **hyperparasitemia in a thin blood film from a patient with cerebral malaria.** (*Copyright D.A. Warrell.*) **(See Color Plate 58-2.)**

INVESTIGATIONS

In a case of suspected malaria, the most urgent investigation is confirmation of diagnosis by microscopy or rapid antigen detection (see below). Other useful laboratory tests include a full blood count to detect anemia, thrombocytopenia (also common in vivax malaria), and neutrophil leukocytosis (of prognostic significance); examination of a thin blood film to detect malarial pigment in leukocytes (see below); measurement of plasma electrolytes (hyponatremia, hypophosphatemia, and hypocalcemia are reported); blood urea, creatinine, creatine kinase (for evidence of rhabdomyolysis), bilirubin, albumin, aminotransferases, lactate dehydrogenase and other serum enzymes (evidence of hepatic dysfunction); blood glucose; arterial blood gases, pH, bicarbonate and lactate (of prognostic significance); rapid urine testing for blood, hemoglobin, and myoglobin, and microscopy (sediment typical of acute glomerulonephritis); and, in cases of cerebral malaria, lumbar puncture and examination of CSF to exclude a bacterial, viral, fungal, or protozoal meningoencephalitis.[1]

The chest radiograph may show pulmonary edema or an incidental pneumonia or, if clear, supports the diagnosis of "acidotic breathing" in a hyperventilating patient. Electrocardiography (ECG) may confirm an arrhythmia or conduction defect attributable to quinine or quinidine. Abdominal ultrasound may show hepatosplenomegaly or evidence of splenic rupture. Electroencephalography may reveal subclinical seizure activity.[13]

BRAIN IMAGING

CT and MRI scans have been reported in patients with cerebral[19,20] and noncerebral malaria.[21] Abnormalities include diffuse cerebral edema, focal hemorrhagic and nonhemorrhagic infarcts in various parts of the brain, subarachnoid hemorrhage, areas of hypoattenuation, and symmetrical infarction of the thalamus and cerebellum in adults who died of cerebral malaria.[21] Not all those with cerebral malaria showed evidence of cerebral edema, and the prognosis was better in patients with normal scans.

DIAGNOSIS

DIFFERENTIAL DIAGNOSIS

Malaria must be included in the differential diagnosis of any acutely ill, febrile patient with an appropriate travel history.

Exposure can occur during a brief stopover in a malarious area, even if the ultimate destination was malaria-free. Routes of infection other than mosquito bites must be considered, such as blood transfusions and needlestick injuries and other nosocomial parenteral exposures to blood products. A diagnosis of malaria is more likely if the patient took no precautions against mosquito bites and no antimalarial chemoprophylaxis (or took the drugs irregularly or stopped them prematurely). The differential diagnosis of malaria includes other acute infections that cause chills and rigors, especially those that do not cause focal signs or symptoms (e.g., influenza, enteric fevers, or brucellosis); jaundice (e.g., viral hepatitis, leptospirosis, and relapsing fevers); hemorrhage (e.g., viral hemorrhagic fevers or hepatic failure); hyperpyrexia (e.g., heatstroke, neuroleptic malignant syndrome, malignant hyperthermia, or thyroid storm), gastrointestinal symptoms (e.g., gastroenteritis, traveler's diarrhea, or salmonellosis); and encephalopathy (e.g., viral, bacterial, fungal, or protozoal encephalitides, heat stroke, or metabolic coma).

LABORATORY DIAGNOSIS

Rapid antigen detection tests employing monoclonal antibodies to *P. falciparum* histidine-rich protein 2 and lactate dehydrogenase have proved to be sensitive and specific screening tests.

Microscopic diagnosis, which remains the gold standard, is achieved by examining conventional hematologic thin blood smears and thick films (a simple concentration method), preferably made at the bedside using blood straight from the patient that has not been stored with anticoagulant. Wright, Field, Leishman, and Giemsa stains are suitable (Fig. 58-2 and Color Plate 58-2). Parasites should be counted in relation to erythrocytes or leukocytes in the same field, and the parasite concentration (per microliter) calculated from total erythrocyte or leukocyte counts. Blood examinations should be repeated at least every 12 hours, as parasitemia may fluctuate. Blood sampling need not be timed to coincide with a fever spike or paroxysm. There is no advantage in using venous or arterial blood instead of blood obtained by finger prick. Blood smears should be examined at 12-hour intervals (minimum) after starting treatment until parasitemia has disappeared for at least 24 hours. Malaria parasites may not be seen or recognized in travelers who are taking antimalarial drugs prophylactically. For this reason, such drugs should be stopped immediately, in the interest of making a diagnosis. Peripheral parasitemia may sometimes be undetectable in patients subsequently found (at autopsy) to have parasitized erythrocytes sequestered in their brains, and so a therapeutic trial of antimalarial drugs should be considered if there is clinical suspicion of severe malaria. The presence of gametocytes indicates recovery from infection; their morphology distinguishes falciparum from other malarias. Malarial pigment may be found in circulating leukocytes; its density is of prognostic value.

MANAGEMENT OF SEVERE MALARIA

Severe malaria is nearly always the result of *P. falciparum* infection. Because the disease can evolve rapidly, with sudden clinical deterioration and successive involvement of many vital organs and tissues, severe falciparum malaria is a medical emergency that should ideally be managed in an ICU.

INITIAL CLINICAL ASSESSMENT AND MANAGEMENT
The clinical history, taken from the patient or accompanying friends and relatives, should include precise details (times and places) of travel to the tropics, preventive methods, recent antimalarial therapy or prophylaxis, and previous attacks of malaria. A history of ominous events such as convulsions, drowsiness, diminishing urine output, black urine, and psychosis should be elicited. It is important to know whether a female patient is pregnant. In severely ill patients, a rapid initial examination should be carried out to exclude other diagnoses (e.g., meningitis) and to detect life-threatening complications such as pulmonary edema, renal failure, shock, and hypoglycemia. In patients with malarial parasitemia, the physician must keep an open mind about other disease processes, especially in residents of the malarious zone in whom parasitemia may be irrelevant to their current illness. Initial investigations must include a parasite count (which is of prognostic importance), hematocrit, full blood count, and measurement of electrolytes, blood urea, and creatinine (Table 58-2). Frequent measurement of the blood glucose concentration is most important. It can be checked rapidly and repeatedly at the bedside using one of the many commercially available methods. The blood should be cultured. In patients with respiratory distress, arterial pH, blood gas tensions, bicarbonate, and lactic acid concentrations should be measured. In patients with impaired consciousness and other neurologic signs, lumbar puncture is important to exclude treatable meningoencephalitides. The usual precautions should be observed before carrying out a lumbar puncture: search for clinical evidence of raised intracranial pressure, lateralizing neurologic signs, and signs of imminent coning, local skin sepsis, etc. If there is any doubt, a CT or nuclear magnetic resonance (NMR) scan should be performed first. Lumbar puncture is safe in *adult* patients with cerebral malaria. However, African children may show progressive signs of cerebral compression and raised intracranial pressure, and some authorities recommend delaying lumbar puncture for 24 hours and giving presumptive antimicrobial treatment against bacterial meningitis.[17] In cerebral malaria the CSF is usually normal. However, a mild lym-

TABLE 58-2 Initial Management of Patients with Severe Malaria

1. Clear and maintain airway.
2. Position semiprone or on side.
3. Weigh the patient, calculate drug dosage.
4. Start antimalarial chemotherapy.
5. Make rapid clinical assessment.
6. Take blood for diagnostic smear, monitoring of blood sugar (rapid "stix" method), hematocrit, and other laboratory tests.
7. Exclude or treat hypoglycemia.
8. Assess state of hydration.
9. Consider need for additional drugs (antimicrobials, vitamin K, etc).
10. Measure and monitor urine output. If necessary, insert urethral catheter. Measure urine specific gravity and sodium concentration.
11. Plan first 8 hours of intravenous fluids, including diluent for antimalarial drug, glucose therapy, and blood transfusion.
12. Consider inserting central venous pressure or pulmonary artery catheter to monitor fluid replacement.
13. If rectal temperature exceeds 39°C, remove patient's clothes, tepid sponge, fan, use hypothermia mattress, and consider antipyretic (acetaminophen).
14. Do lumbar puncture to exclude meningitis. Consider other infections.

phocyte pleocytosis (up to about 15 cells/μL) and mildly raised total protein concentration are found occasionally. Low or undetectable CSF glucose concentration indicates hypoglycemia. CSF opening pressure was normal in 80% of Thai adults with cerebral malaria, but was elevated in Kenyan children.[17]

ANTIMALARIAL CHEMOTHERAPY
In patients with proven or suspected severe falciparum malaria, appropriate parenteral chemotherapy (usually with licensed quinine or quinidine) must be started immediately. Artemisinin derivatives such as artesunate, artemether (which has proved as effective as quinine in the treatment of cerebral and severe falciparum malaria),[22] or arteether, may be available for treatment on a named-patient basis. Delay in diagnosis and treatment and the use of inappropriate antimalarial drugs account for most cases of fatal imported malaria.

In severely ill patients, chloroquine-resistant *P. falciparum* infection should be assumed. Recommended parenteral regimens for treatment of severe malaria are summarized in Table 58-3.

Cinchona Alkaloids (Quinine and Quinidine)
Quinine remains effective in the treatment of severe falciparum malaria. In the United States quinidine[23] is supplied by the Centers for Disease Control and Prevention in Atlanta, Georgia, whose 24-hour malaria hotline telephone number is (404) 332-4555. Quinine and quinidine should never be given by intravenous push or bolus injection, but should be administered by slow, controlled-rate intravenous infusion using an intravenous drip with a metered chamber or an infusion pump. Unless the patient has been given quinine, quinidine, or mefloquine within the previous 12 hours, an initial loading dose should be used so that therapeutic blood concentrations can be achieved rapidly.[23–25]

TABLE 58-3 Severe Falciparum Malaria: Antimalarial Chemotherapy

1. *Quinine*: 7 mg dihydrochloride *salt*/kg (loading dose) IV by infusion pump over 30 minutes followed immediately by 10 mg *salt*/kg (maintenance dose) diluted in 10 mL/kg isotonic fluid by IV infusion over 4 hours, repeated every 8–12 hours until the patient can swallow,[c] then quinine tablets,[b] approx. 10 mg salt/kg every 8 hours to complete 7 days of treatment.[25]

or

2. *Quinine*: 20 mg dihydrochloride *salt*/kg (loading dose)[a] by IV infusion over 4 hours, then 10 mg *salt*/kg over 4 hours, every 8–12 hours until patient can swallow,[c] then quinine tablets,[b] to complete 7 days of treatment.[24]

or

3. *Quinidine*: 15 mg *base*/kg (equivalent to 20 mg/kg of quinidine gluconate) (loading dose)[a] by IV infusion over 4 hours, then 7.5 mg *base*/kg over 4 hours, every 8–12 hours until patient can swallow,[c] then quinine tablets[b] to complete 7 days of treatment.[23]

or

4. *Artesunate:* (reconstitute with 5% bicarbonate immediately before injection) 2.4 mg/kg (loading dose) by IV (bolus) or IM injection, followed by 1.2 mg/kg daily as a single dose for a minimum of 3 days or until patient can take oral therapy or another effective antimalarial.[1]

or

5. *Artemether*: 3.2 mg/kg (loading dose) by IM injection, followed by 1.6 mg/kg daily for a minimum of 3 days or until patient can take oral treatment or another effective antimalarial.[1]

---

[a] Quinine/quinidine loading dose should not be used if patient received either drug or mefloquine within the preceding 12 hours.
[b] For infections acquired in areas of quinine resistance (e.g., Thailand) add an oral course of tetracycline 250 mg, 4 times a day *or* doxycycline 200 mg a day every day for 7 days except in children under 8 years of age and pregnant women, or clindamycin 10 mg/kg twice daily for 3–7 days.
[c] In patients requiring more than 48 hours of parenteral therapy reduce the maintenance dose to one half to two thirds (i.e., quinine *salt* 5–7 mg/kg or quinidine *base* 3.75–5 mg every 8–12 hours).

The initial dose should not be reduced in pregnant women[26] or in patients with renal and hepatic dysfunction, but the maintenance dose should be reduced after 48 hours of parenteral treatment, unless the patient can continue treatment by the oral route. The dose should also be reduced if at any stage the plasma concentration exceeds 15 mg/L (45 mmol/L). In patients treated with quinidine, the ECG should be monitored for QTc prolongation, and blood pressure measured every 30 minutes during the initial loading dose infusion.[23]

TOXICITY OF CINCHONA ALKALOIDS Plasma concentrations of cinchona alkaloids above about 5 mg/L are associated with cinchonism: giddiness, tinnitus, high-tone deafness, tremors, blurred vision, nausea, and vomiting. Concentrations above 20 mg/L may cause blindness, deafness, hypotension, ECG abnormalities, and central nervous system depression. However, most patients with malaria are more tolerant of high plasma concentrations than uninfected patients who take overdoses of these drugs, due to binding of quinine by acute phase reactive proteins, especially α_1-acid glycoprotein. Quinidine more than quinine causes prolongation of the QTc interval and QRS complex, but this is rarely associated with dysrhythmia or hypotension unless the drugs are given too rapidly. The most frequent important side effect of quinine and quinidine is hypoglycemia, which may occur at any stage of treatment and may cause recurrent neurologic symptoms in patients who appear to have recovered from cerebral malaria. Normal therapeutic doses can be used safely even in the third trimester of pregnancy.[26] In these patients it is important to assess uterine activity and fetal heart rate before starting quinine, to avoid confusing the effects of malaria and high fever per se from those of the drug.[26] In severe quinine toxicity (following oral or parenteral administration), quinine elimination can be increased by oral or nasogastric administration of activated charcoal.[27]

Artemisinin Derivatives (Artesunate, Artemether, and Arteether)

These compounds are convenient to administer, rapidly clear parasitemia, and have proved safe in clinical use. Large comparative studies have demonstrated that they reduce case fatality of cerebral and severe falciparum malaria at least as effectively as quinine.[22] They are particularly valuable where quinine resistance is emerging and in patients with recurrent quinine-induced hypoglycemia.

Artesunate, a water soluble preparation for intravenous injection, is inherently unstable in aqueous solution, but can be made up with 5% bicarbonate immediately before use. Artemether is an oily suspension for intramuscular injection which is licensed for use in a number of countries (but not the United States, Canada, or the United Kingdom). Arteether, a virtually identical compound, is being prepared for registration in the United States. Artemether and arteether have proved to be neurotoxic and fetotoxic in animals, but these effects have never been observed in tens of thousands of human patients monitored during and after treatment with these drugs.

SUPPORTIVE CARE OF PATIENTS WITH SEVERE FALCIPARUM MALARIA

HYPERPYREXIA

Hyperpyrexia can cause febrile convulsions in children, fetal distress in pregnant women, and when sustained at core temperatures above 40°C, irreversible neurologic damage. Core temperature should be monitored, and when necessary the patient should be tepid-sponged and fanned, placed on a hypothermia mattress, or given an antipyretic (e.g., acetaminophen).

CEREBRAL MALARIA
Generalized or covert seizures are common, especially in children. These must be controlled rapidly with appropriate anticonvulsants such as diazepam. Single-dose phenobarbital prophylaxis effectively reduces the incidence of generalized convulsions in adult and childhood cerebral malaria, but in a large randomized, placebo-controlled trial in African children, excess mortality was associated with this treatment, and thus it is not recommended.[28] Cerebral edema does not require treatment in adult patients with cerebral malaria. However, in African children with cerebral malaria, intracranial pressure is commonly raised, and in those who are deteriorating, intravenous infusion of mannitol 1 g/kg over 20 minutes should be considered.[17] Most of the ancillary treatments for cerebral malaria advocated in the past, including dexamethasone, have proved ineffective and potentially dangerous.[12,29,30]

ANEMIA
Anemia is an inevitable consequence of severe malaria. If transfusion becomes necessary, packed red blood cells should be used while the patient is carefully monitored for evidence of incipient pulmonary edema. Diuretics, such as intravenous furosemide, may be required to reduce the risk of fluid overload. Children with profound malarial anemia may present in shock with tachycardia and tachypnea. Hypovolemia and metabolic (lactic) acidosis are usually the main problems requiring urgent correction. Blood transfusion may have little permanent effect in raising the hematocrit of patients with severe malaria because of the greatly reduced survival of even nonparasitized erythrocytes.[31]

HYPOGLYCEMIA
The possibility of hypoglycemia in patients with severe or deteriorating symptoms must constantly be borne in mind. Frequent monitoring of the blood glucose is essential. Intravenous 50% dextrose (25 to 50 mL) should be tried if hypoglycemia is suspected or proved.

METABOLIC (LACTIC) ACIDOSIS
Metabolic (lactic) acidosis results from impaired tissue perfusion caused by hypovolemia and microvascular obstruction, reduced hepatic clearance of lactate, and in patients with a large parasite burden, from the parasites' lactic acid production. Tissue perfusion and oxygenation should be improved by correcting hypovolemia, clearing the airway, increasing the inspired oxygen concentration, and providing mechanical ventilatory support if necessary. The treatment of gram-negative bacteremia, a frequently associated complication, should be considered as well. Use of epinephrine as a pressor agent may increase lactic acidosis, an effect not seen with dopamine.[32]

DISSEMINATED INTRAVASCULAR COAGULATION
Severe DIC with spontaneous bleeding and fibrin deposition in the lungs and other tissues is occasionally seen (for treatment of DIC see Chap. 69).

DISTURBANCES OF FLUID AND ELECTROLYTE BALANCE
Patients with severe falciparum malaria are commonly dehydrated and hypovolemic on admission to the hospital as a result of decreased fluid intake, increased insensible losses through sweating and hyperventilation during febrile episodes, gastrointestinal fluid losses (vomiting and diarrhea), and sometimes during the diuretic phase of recovery from acute renal failure. These patients require parenteral fluid replacement, but this must be carefully controlled or else the increases in pulmonary capillary permeability may lead to acute and catastrophic pulmonary edema. A central venous or pulmonary artery catheter should be inserted. For correction of hyponatremia, hypocalcemia, hypophosphatemia, and hyper- or hypokalemia, see Chap. 76.

PULMONARY EDEMA
This may be associated with high central venous and pulmonary wedge pressures (caused by volume overload and/or anemia), or with low pressures as in acute respiratory distress syndrome from other causes. Mechanical ventilation may be required.[18] See Chaps. 36 and 38 for a discussion of the management of these complications.

RENAL FAILURE
Oliguria may be prerenal—caused by volume depletion—or attributable to direct renal injury.[14] If dialysis is indicated (see Chap. 75), hemofiltration has proved more effective than peritoneal dialysis.[18,33]

HEMOGLOBINURIA AND BLACKWATER FEVER
Intravascular hemolysis may be associated with acute renal failure. To protect the kidney from "pigment nephropathy," hypovolemia and acidosis must be corrected. Mannitol diuresis is recommended by some nephrologists. Packed red blood cells should be transfused to maintain the hematocrit above 20%. Despite the unproven suspicion that quinine may be responsible for the massive intravascular hemolysis of blackwater fever, treatment with cinchona alkaloids should not be stopped unless an alternative drug such as an artemisinin derivative is available.

HYPERPARASITEMIA
Mortality generally increases with parasitemia, exceeding 50% at parasitemias above 500,000/μL. It has been suggested that exchange transfusion, by reducing the burden of parasitemia more rapidly than chemotherapy alone, might reduce mortality, although the introduction of artemisinin derivatives that clear parasitemia very rapidly may weaken the argument for this intervention. Other theoretical advantages of exchange transfusion include the removal of harmful metabolites, toxins, and mediators, and the replenishment of normal red blood cells, platelets, clotting factors, and other depleted blood constituents. However, these potential advantages must be weighed against potential dangers, such as electrolyte disturbances (hypocalcemia and hyperkalemia), cardiovascular complications, line infections, and contamination of transfused blood with blood-borne pathogens, notably HIV, human T-lymphocyte virus-1, hepatitis viruses, and protozoa. In more than 200 reported cases, red blood cell exchange achieved rapid reduction in parasitemia, which in some cases was accompanied by evidence of clinical

COLOR PLATES

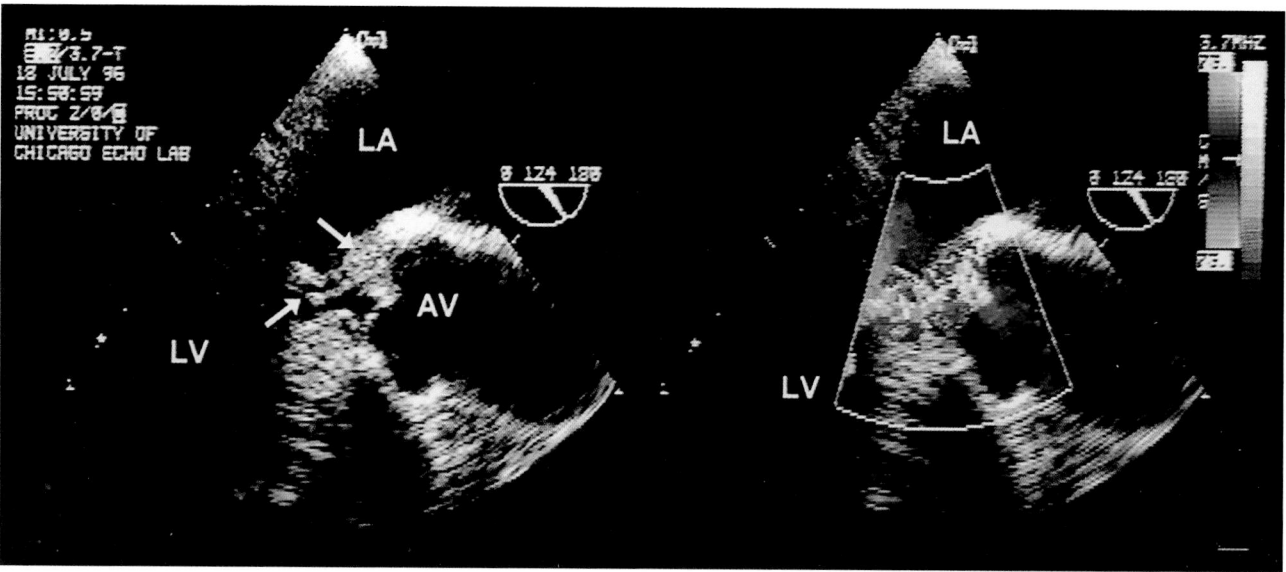

▲ PLATE 29-6 Acute aortic insufficiency secondary to endocarditis. Transesophageal echocardiogram showing a large mobile vegetation (*arrows*) extending from the aortic valve (AV) into the left ventricle (LV). Doppler echocardiography reveals significant regurgitation from the aorta into the LV. LA, left atrium.

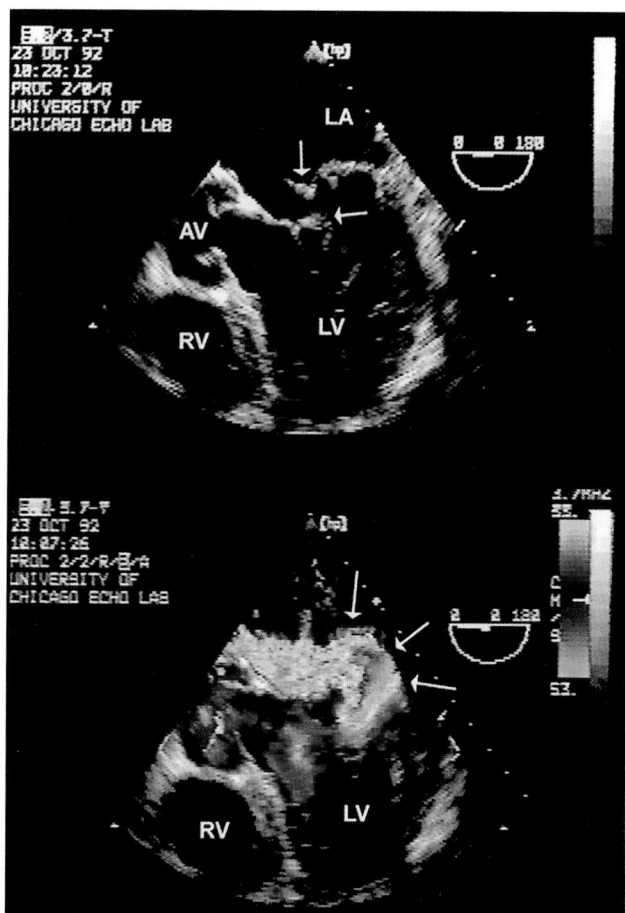

◄ PLATE 29-9 Mitral regurgitation secondary to endocarditis and a flail posterior mitral valve leaflet. Transesophageal echocardiogram showing thickened mitral valve leaflets with vegetations (*arrows*). The posterior leaflet has prolapsed from the left ventricle (LV) into the left atrium (LA). The second panel depicts severe mitral regurgitation by Doppler echocardiography (*arrows*). AV, aortic valve; RV, right ventricle.

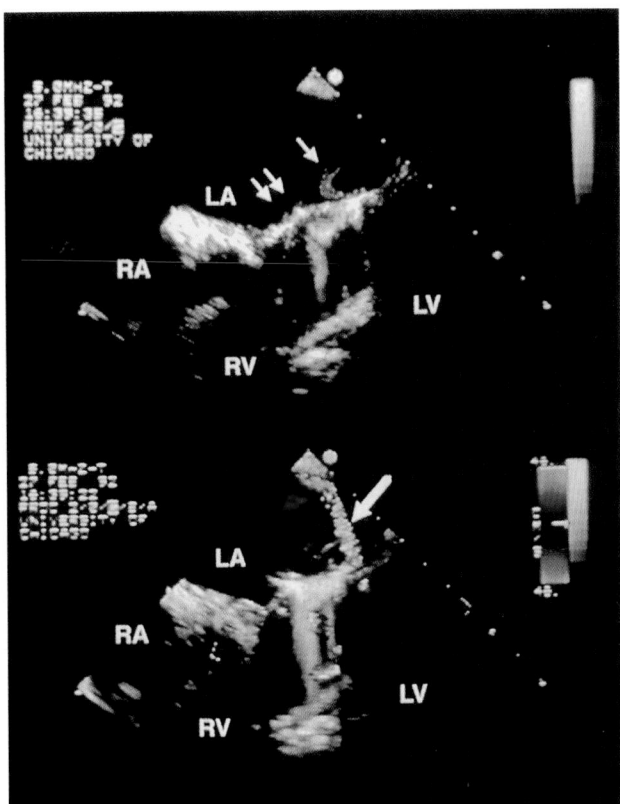

◄ PLATE 29-10 Endocarditis involving a St. Jude Medical mechanical valve in the mitral position. Transesophageal echocardiogram showing vegetations on the left atrial (LA) side of the mechanical valve (*small arrows*). Doppler echocardiography reveals perivalvular mitral regurgitation (*large arrow*). LV, left ventricle; RV, right ventricle; RA, right atrium.

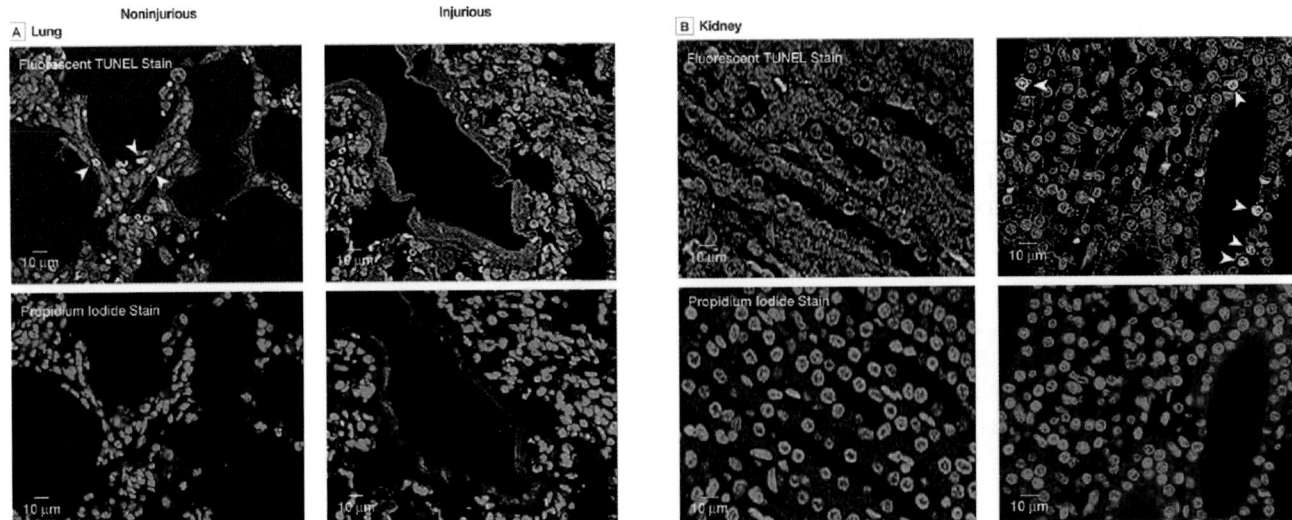

▲ PLATE 37-4 There was greater apoptosis of renal tubular epithelial cells in the group that received injurious mechanical ventilation compared to the group that received the noninjurious strategy, as evidenced by the greater number of TUNEL-positive cells (*arrowheads*) in the injurious group. Terminal deoxynucleotidyltransferase-mediated dUTP nick end-labeling (TUNEL) staining identifies the apoptotic cell, and propidium iodide staining identifies nuclei and helps ensure that noncellular background staining is not inadvertently identified as a TUNEL-positive cell (original magnification × 400). (*Reproduced with permission from Imai et al.*[89])

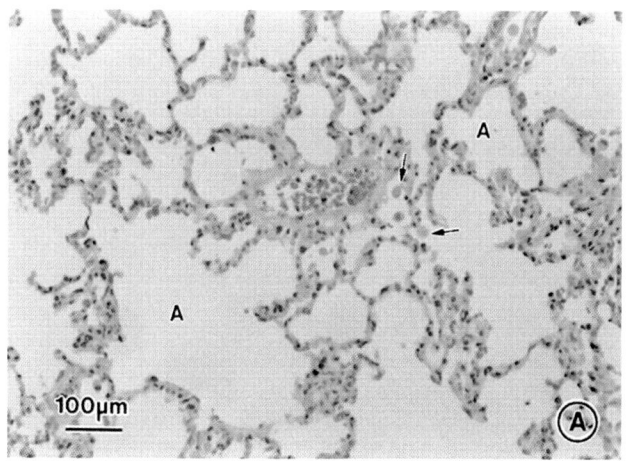

A

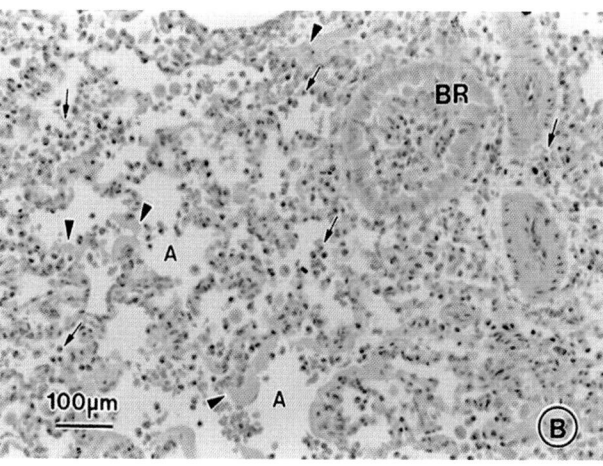

B

▲ PLATE 37-5 A representative micrograph of lung tissue from a hypercapnic animal. The alveoli are free of edema and cellular infiltrate (*A*), normal parenchymal architecture is maintained, and only a small number of macrophages are present in the alveoli (*arrow*). *B*. A comparable micrograph from the eucapnic group. There is marked cellular infiltration in the interstitium and alveoli (*arrows*), which also fills the lumen of a bronchiole (BR). Alveolar and interstitial edema, as well as hyaline membrane formation (*arrowheads*) are also present (hematoxylin and eosin stained; 120× magnification; scale indicates 100 m). (*Reproduced with permission from Sinclair et al.*[???])

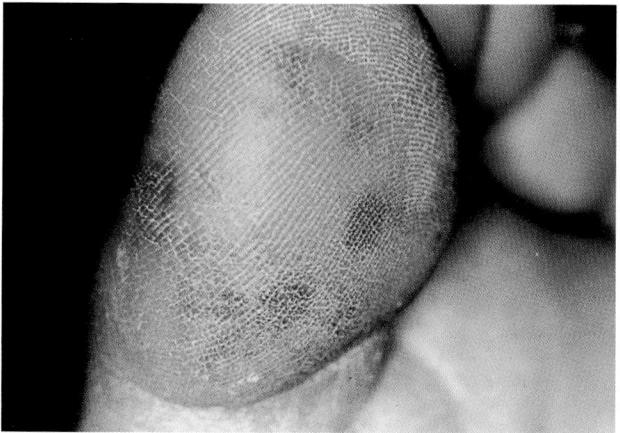

▲ PLATE 49-1 / PLATE 107-13 Subacute bacterial endocarditis: nontender, pupuric macules with irregular borders scattered on the toes (Janeway lesions). (NOTE: same as color plate 107-14)

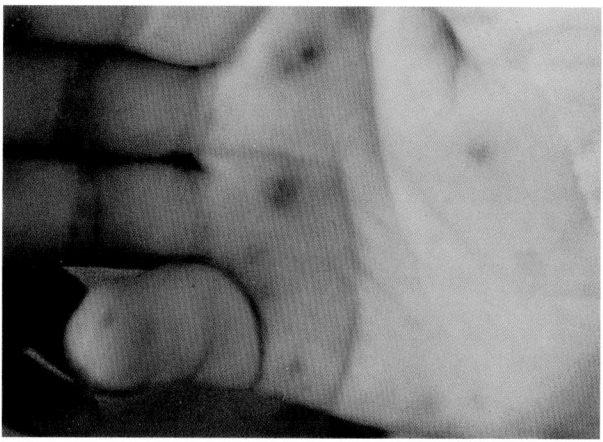

▲ PLATE 49-2 Osler's nodes: randomly distributed tender nodules on th palm of the hand in a patient with *Staphylococcus aureus* endocarditis.

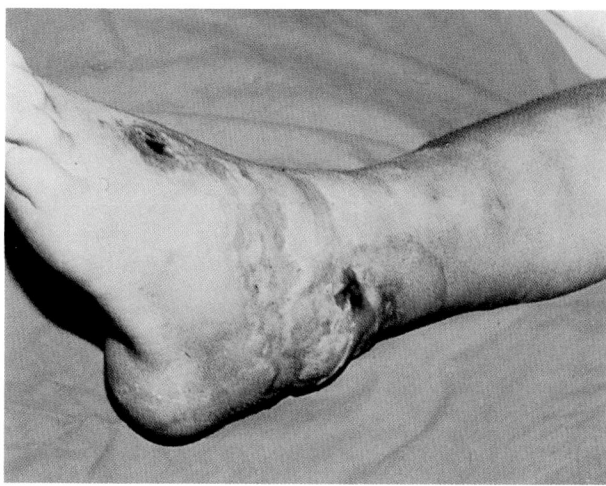

◄ PLATE 55-3 Necrotizing fasciitis of the lower leg. Dusky erythema is present, with blistering and small patches of dermal gangrene.

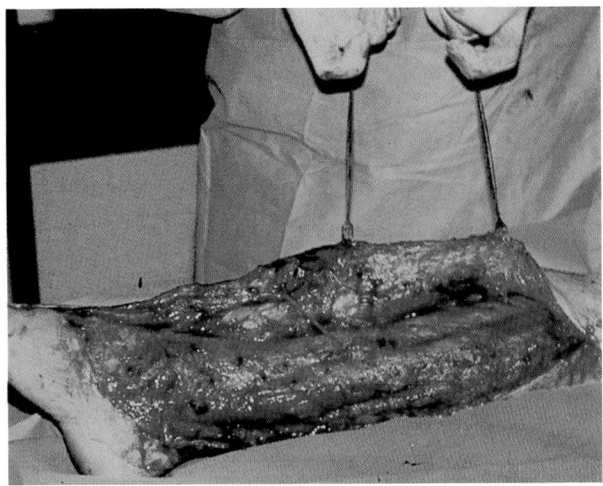

◀ PLATE 55-4 Postoperative appearance of the lower leg presented in Fig. 55-3. All necrotic subcutaneous tissue was excised.

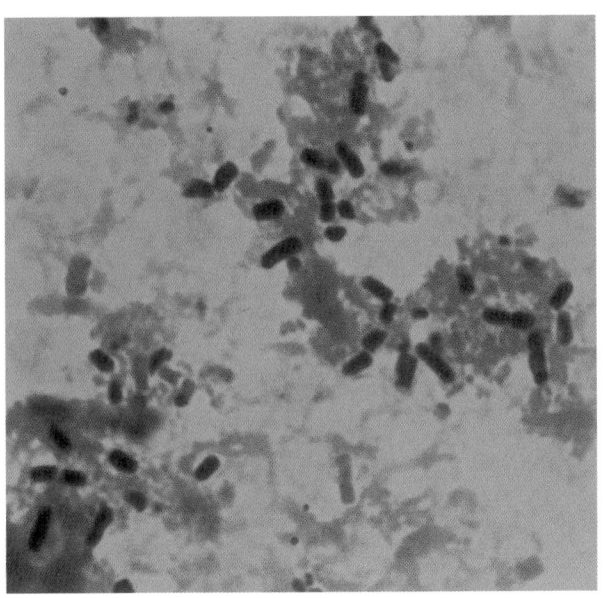

◀ PLATE 55-6 Gram stain of *Clostridium perfringens.*

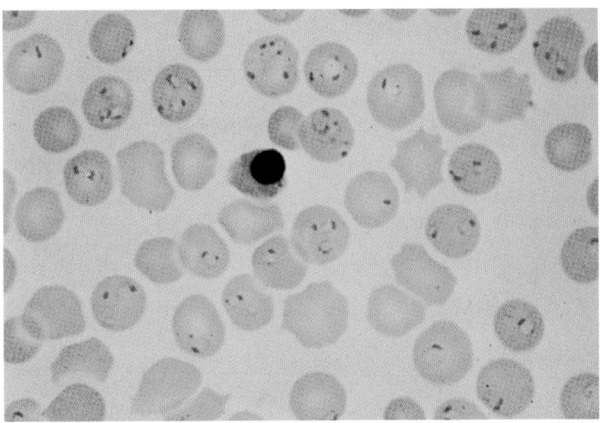

▲ PLATE 58-2 *Plasmodium falciparum* hyperparasitemia in a thin blood film from a patient with cerebral malaria. (*Copyright D.A. Warrell.*)

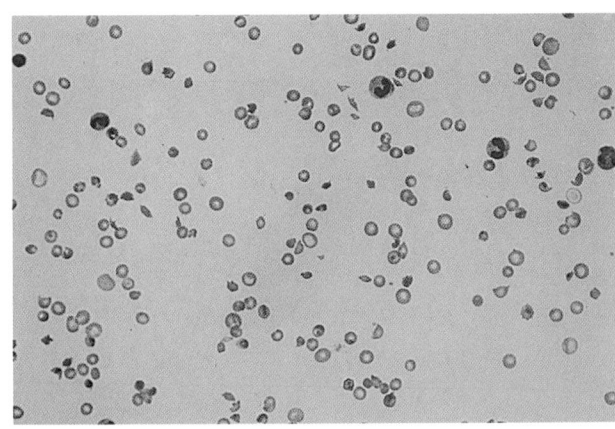

▲ PLATE 70-1 Admission (hospital day 1) peripheral blood smear (Wright-Giemsa stain) showing characteristic RBC morphology of microangiopathic hemolytic anemia (×350).

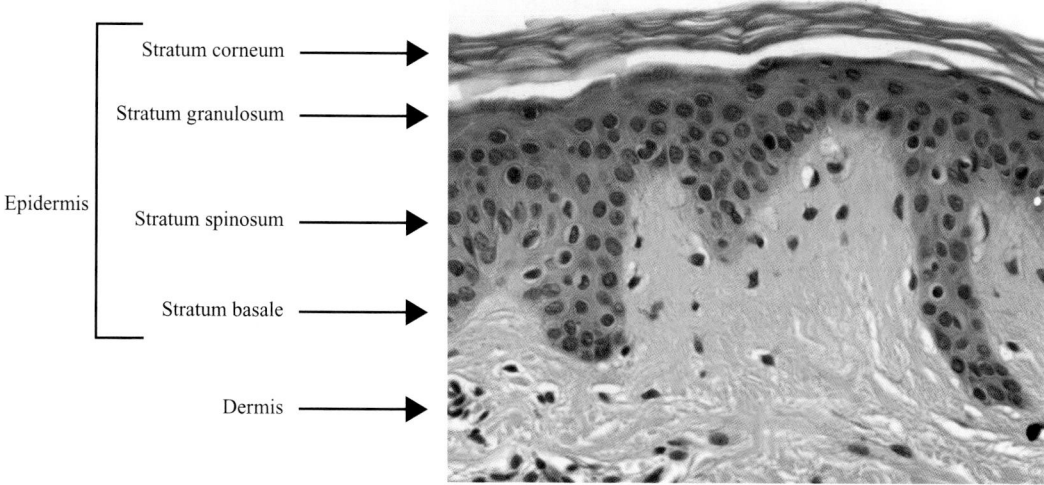

Epidermis
- Stratum corneum →
- Stratum granulosum →
- Stratum spinosum →
- Stratum basale →

Dermis →

◄ PLATE 107-1
Structure of normal
skin.

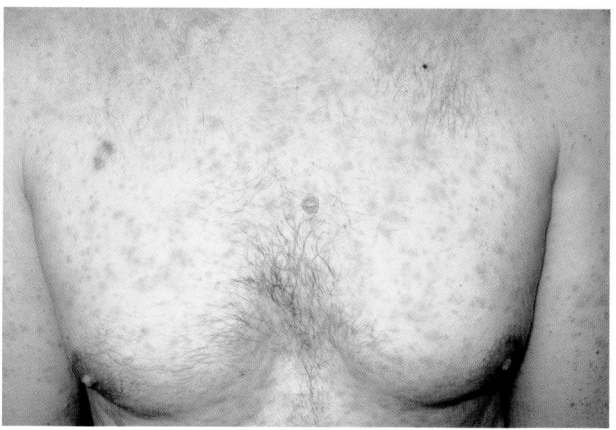

▲ PLATE 107-2 Maculopapular or morbilliform eruption. This is
the most common presentation of a cutaneous adverse drug
reaction. (*Collection of Dr. Mario Lacouture.*)

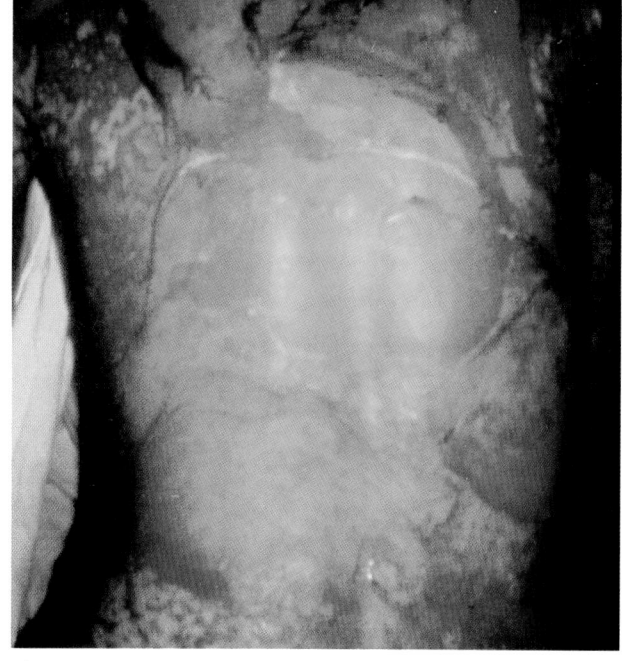

▲ PLATE 107-5 Toxic epidermal necrolysis: >30% of the body
surface area involved. Necrotic epidermis sloughs, revealing
moist, bright red dermis. (*Courtesy Dr. Iris K. Aronson collection.*)

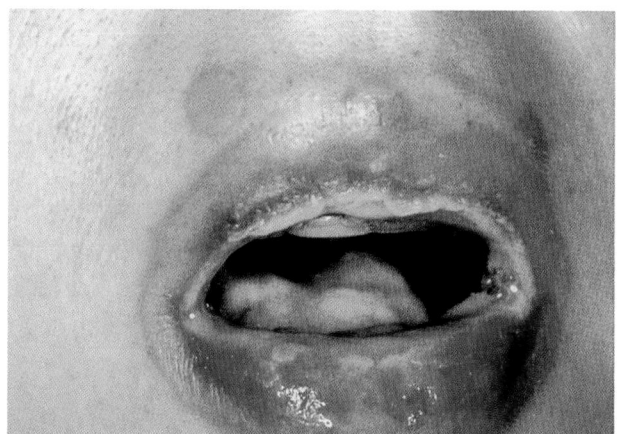

▲ PLATE 107-4 Stevens-Johnson syndrome/toxic epidermal
necrolysis. Erosive involvement of lips and oral mucosa.
(*Courtesy Dr. Iris K Aronson collection.*)

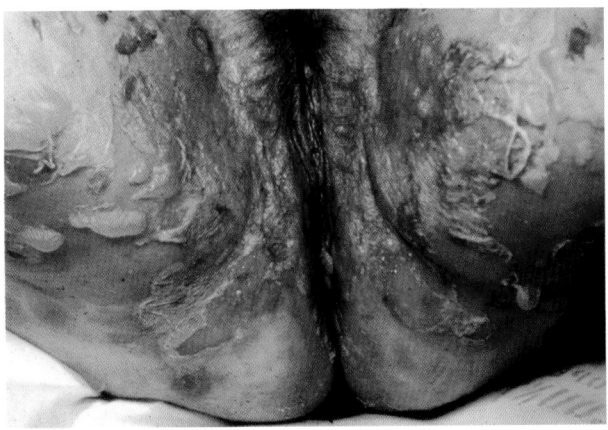

▲ PLATE 107-6 Pemphigus vulgaris. Flaccid, superficial bullae which rupture easily leaving superficial erosions. (*Courtesy Dr. Anne Laumann collection.*)

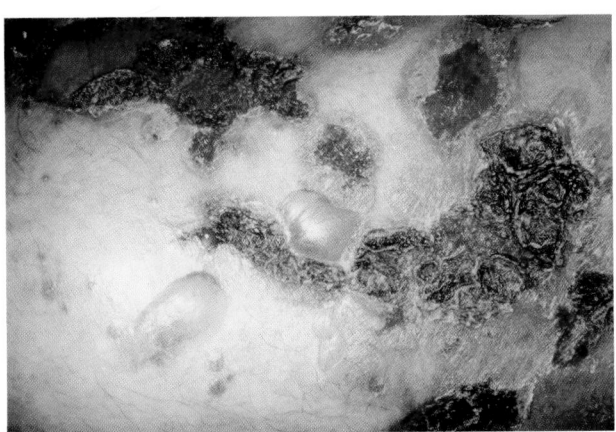

▲ PLATE 107-7 Bullous pemphigoid. Tense bullae arising on an erythematous plaque. (*Courtesy Dr. Anne Laumann collection.*)

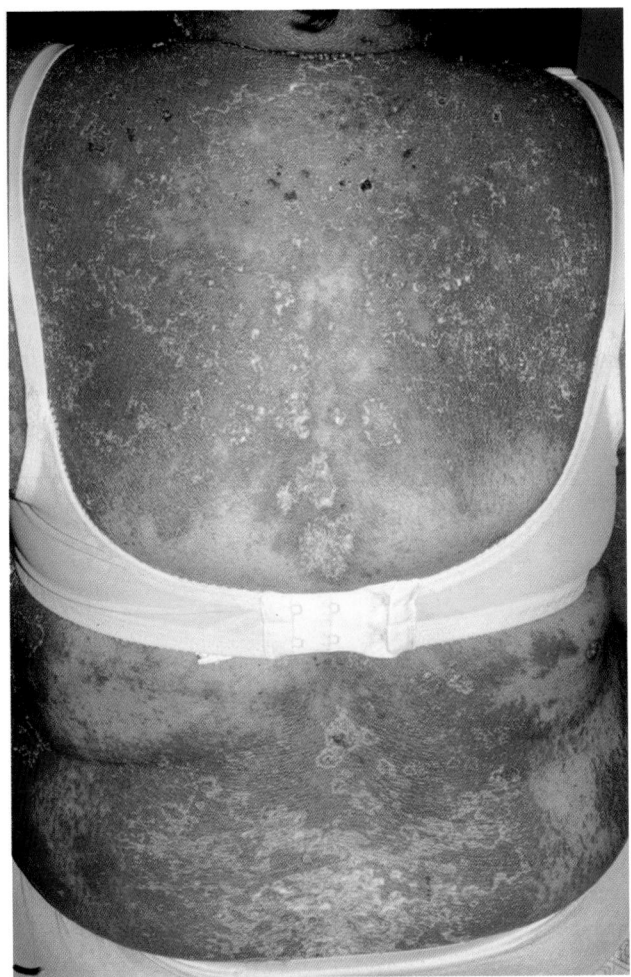

▲ PLATE 107-8 Erythroderma. Generalized erythema, edema, and scaling. (*Courtesy Dr. Anne Laumann collection.*)

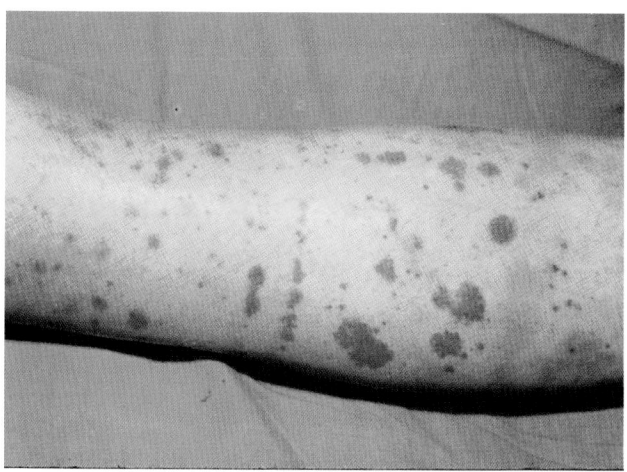

▲ PLATE 107-10 Palpable purpura (leukocytoclastic vasculitis). Erythematous to violaceous plaques on the lower extremity, which do not blanch with pressure. (*Courtesy Dr. Denise Rubenstein collection.*)

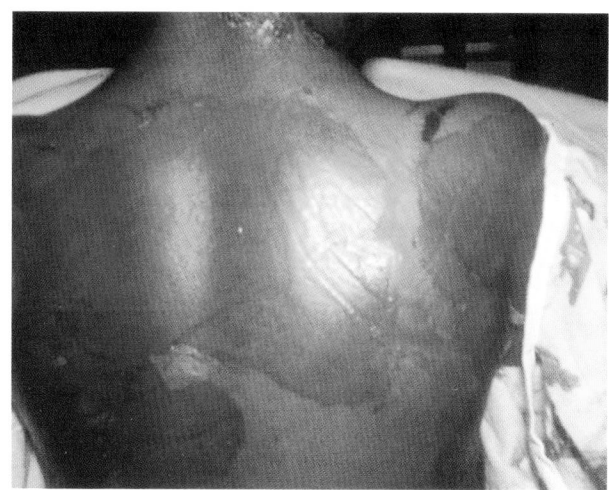

▲ PLATE 107-11 Staphylococcal scalded skin syndrome. Superficial desquamation of non-necrotic epidermis. (*Courtesy Dr. Denise Rubenstein collection.*)

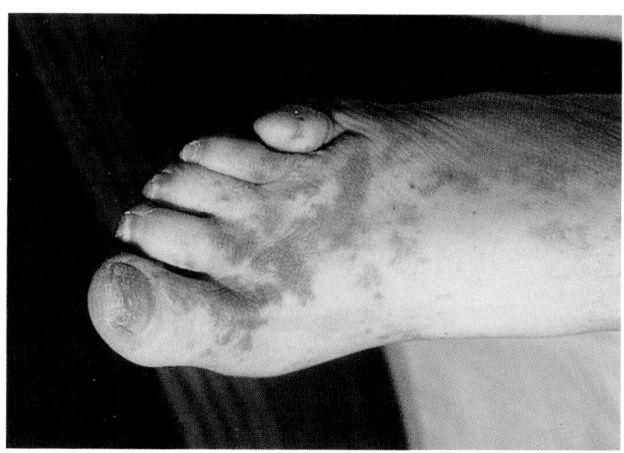

▲ PLATE 107-12 Meningococcemia. Pupuric lesions with irregularly angulated borders.

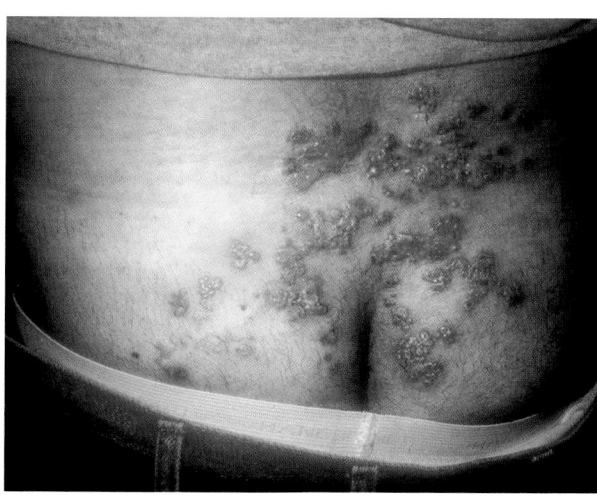

◄ PLATE 107-14 Severe recurrent herpes simplex infection associated with systemic steroid administration. Grouped vesicles and pustules on an erythematous base. (*Courtesy Dr. Anne Laumann collection.*)

improvement.[34] Exchange transfusion should be considered for nonimmune travelers who are severely ill, who have deteriorated on optimal chemotherapy, or who have parasite densities above 10% of circulating erythrocytes.[1]

RUPTURED SPLEEN

This life-threatening complication may occur in vivax or falciparum malaria. It must be suspected and excluded in patients who develop abdominal pain and shock. Ultrasound is useful for detecting free blood in the peritoneum and a tear in the splenic capsule. Invasive techniques such as needle aspiration of the peritoneal cavity, laparoscopy, or laparotomy may be required.

References

1. Warrell DA, Gilles HM (eds): *Essential Malariology*, 4th ed. London, Arnold, 2002, p 1.
2. Aucan C, Walley AJ, Hennig BJ, et al: Interferon-alpha receptor-1 (IFNAR1) variants are associated with protection against cerebral malaria in The Gambia. *Genes Immun* 4:275, 2003.
3. MacPherson GG, Warrell MJ, White NJ, et al: Human cerebral malaria: A quantitative ultrastructural analysis of parasitized erythrocyte sequestration. *Am J Pathol* 119:385, 1985.
4. Turner GDH: Cerebral malaria. *Brain Pathol* 7:569, 1997.
5. Warrell DA, White NJ, Veall N, et al: Cerebral anaerobic glycolysis and reduced cerebral oxygen transport in human cerebral malaria. *Lancet* 2:534, 1988.
6. Clark IA, Cowden WB: The pathophysiology of falciparum malaria. *Pharmacol Ther* 99:221, 2003.
7. Molyneux ME, Looareesuwan S, Menzies IS, et al: Reduced hepatic blood flow and intestinal malabsorption in severe falciparum malaria. *Am J Trop Med Hyg* 40:470, 1989.
8. Bradley DJ, Warrell DA: Malaria, in Warrell DA, Cox TM, Firth J, Benz E (eds): *Oxford Textbook of Medicine*, 4th ed. Oxford, Oxford University Press, 2003, p 721.
9. World Health Organization: Severe falciparum malaria. *Trans R Soc Trop Med Hyg* 94(Suppl 1): 1, 2000.
10. Warrell DA: Cerebral malaria, in Shakir RA, Newman PK, Poser CM (eds): *Tropical Neurology*. London, Saunders, 1996, p 213.
11. Warrell DA: Cerebral malaria, in Scheld WM, Whitley RJ, Marra CM (eds): *Infections of the Central Nervous System*, 3rd ed. Philadelphia, Lippincott Williams & Wilkins, 2004, p 735.
12. Warrell DA, Looareesuwan S, Warrell MJ, et al: Dexamethasone proves deleterious in cerebral malaria. A double-blind trial in 100 comatose patients. *N Engl J Med* 306:313, 1982.
13. Crawley J, Smith S, Muthininji P, et al: Electroencephalographic and clinical features of cerebral malaria. *Arch Dis Child* 84:247, 2001.
14. Trang TTM, Phu NH, Vinh H, et al: Acute renal failure in patients with severe falciparum malaria. *Clin Infect Dis* 15:874, 1992.
15. Anstey NM, Jacups SP, Cain T, et al: Pulmonary manifestations of uncomplicated falciparum and vivax malaria: Cough, small airways obstruction, impaired gas transfer, and increased pulmonary phagocytic activity. *J Infect Dis* 185:1326, 2002.
16. Marsh K, Forster D, Waruiru C, et al: Indicators of life-threatening malaria in African children. *N Engl J Med* 332:1399, 1995.
17. Newton CRJC, Crawley J, Sowumni A, et al: Raised intracranial pressure in Africans with cerebral malaria. *Arch Dis Child* 76:219, 1997.
18. Bruneel F, Hocqueloux L, Alberti C, et al: The clinical spectrum of severe imported falciparum malaria in the intensive care unit. *Am J Respir Crit Care Med* 167:684, 2003.
19. Looareesuwan S, Warrell DA, White NJ, et al: Do patients with cerebral malaria have cerebral oedema? A computed tomography study. *Lancet* 1:434, 1983.
20. Looareesuwan S, Wilairatana P, Krishna S, et al: Magnetic resonance imaging of the brain in patients with cerebral malaria. *Clin Infect Dis* 21:300, 1995.
21. Patankar TF, Karnad DP, Shetty PG, et al: Adult cerebral malaria: Prognostic importance of imaging findings and correlation with postmortem findings. *Radiology* 224:811, 2002.
22. Artemether-Quinine Meta-analysis Study Group: A meta-analysis using individual patient data of trials comparing artemether with quinine in the treatment of severe falciparum malaria. *Trans R Soc Trop Med Hyg* 95:1, 2001.
23. Phillips RE, Warrell DA, White NJ, et al: Intravenous quinidine for the treatment of severe falciparum malaria. Clinical and pharmacokinetic studies. *N Engl J Med* 312:1273, 1985.
24. White NJ, Looareesuwan S, Warrell DA, et al: Quinine loading dose in cerebral malaria. *Am J Trop Med Hyg* 32:1, 1983.
25. Davis TME, Supanaronond W, Pukrittayakamee S, et al: A safe and effective consecutive-infusion regimen for rapid quinine loading in severe falciparum malaria. *J Infect Dis* 161:1305, 1990.
26. Looareesuwan S, Phillips RE, White NJ, et al: Quinine and severe falciparum malaria in late pregnancy. *Lancet* 2:4, 1985.
27. Prescott LF, Hamilton AR, Heyworth R: Treatment of quinine overdosage with repeated oral charcoal. *Br J Clin Pharmacol* 27:95, 1989.
28. Crawley J, Waruiru C, Mithwani S, et al: Effect of phenobarbital on seizure frequency and mortality in childhood cerebral malaria: A randomised, controlled intervention study. *Lancet* 355:701, 2000.
29. Hoffman SL, Rustama D, Punjabi NH, et al: High-dose dexamethasone in quinine-treated patients with cerebral malaria: A double-blind placebo-controlled trial. *J Infect Dis* 158:325, 1988.
30. Warrell DA: Management of severe malaria. *Parassitologia* 41:287, 1999.
31. Looareesuwan S, Merry AH, Phillips RE, et al: Reduced erythrocyte survival following clearance of malarial parasitaemia in Thai patients. *Br J Haematol* 67:473, 1987.
32. Day NPJ, Phu NH, Bethell DP, et al: The effects of dopamine and adrenaline infusions on acid-base balance and systemic haemodynamics in severe infection. *Lancet* 348:219, 1996.
33. Phu NH, Hien TT, Mai NT, et al: Hemofiltration and peritoneal dialysis in infection-associated acute renal failure in Vietnam. *N Engl J Med* 347:895, 2002.
34. Riddle MS, Jackson JL, Sanders JW, Blazes DL: Exchange transfusion as an adjunct therapy in severe *Plasmodium falciparum* malaria: a meta-analysis. *Clin Infect Dis* 34:1192, 2002.

Chapter 59 _____

TETANUS
PERRY GRAY

KEY POINTS

- *Tetanus is a toxin-mediated disease caused by* Clostridium tetani *and characterized by trismus, dysphagia, and localized muscle rigidity near a site of injury, often progressing to severe generalized muscular spasms complicated by respiratory failure and cardiovascular instability.*

- *The diagnosis of tetanus is made on clinical grounds alone. A clinical diagnosis of presumed tetanus is sufficient to initiate treatment.*

- *Patients with tetanus should be managed in an ICU. In severe cases, the first priority is control of the airway to ensure adequate ventilation and correction of hypotension related to hypovolemia and/or autonomic instability.*

- *Antitoxin therapy with human tetanus immune globulin is given intramuscularly (3000 to 6000 IU) as early as possible. In cases that have not yet progressed to generalized spasms, 250 IU given intrathecally by lumbar puncture may be of benefit.*

- *Treatment to limit continued production and absorption of toxin includes surgical débridement of the site of injury and antimicrobial therapy with intravenous metronidazole.*

- *Traditionally muscle rigidity and spasms have been treated with high-dose benzodiazepines and narcotics. However, intravenous magnesium therapy should also be considered.*

- *Cardiovascular instability due to autonomic dysfunction is managed by ensuring normovolemia and using benzodiazepine, narcotic, and/or magnesium sulfate infusions when needed.*

- *Supportive measures include early provision of nutrition, correction of electrolyte disturbances, subcutaneous heparin administration for prophylaxis of deep venous thrombosis, and prompt antimicrobial therapy for nosocomial infection.*

- *With meticulous management of the manifestations of this disease and careful attention to prevention of its major complications, complete recovery is possible in most cases.*

Tetanus is one of the best examples of a disease for which modern intensive care can offer a truly major improvement in long-term useful survival. Often a disease of otherwise healthy active people, the fully developed form is frequently rapidly fatal unless the patient is supported through a lengthy period of painful muscle spasms complicated by respiratory failure, cardiovascular instability, and increased risk of pulmonary embolism and nosocomial infection. However, if all these problems are meticulously managed, complete recovery can be expected. In developed countries, this disease is likely to remain an uncommon but challenging problem that demands an alert and aggressive approach to initial diagnosis and management, coupled with careful attention to supportive care and avoidance of complications over a period of weeks to months to achieve the eventual excellent outcome possible in most cases.

Pathogenesis

Although tetanus is primarily a disease of underdeveloped countries, there are approximately 36 to 48 cases per year reported in the United States.[1] The male:female ratio is approximately 3:2, representing a greater incidence of tetanus-prone wounds in males. Because preformed circulating antibody to tetanospasmin can completely prevent development of the disease, tetanus occurs primarily in nonimmunized or inadequately immunized patients, particularly the poor and elderly.[1,2] However, in rare instances tetanus has developed in patients who had received their primary series, as well as proper booster doses of toxoid,[3,4] so a history of proper immunization does not exclude the diagnosis of tetanus.

The disease is caused by *Clostridium tetani*, an anaerobic bacterium that exists in both vegetative and sporulated forms and has been isolated from soil, feces of humans and animals, dust, wounds, intact skin, catgut, and talcum powder. During unfavorable conditions the organism exists in the sporulated form, which can remain viable for several months. It is resistant to boiling and antiseptics but is killed by autoclaving at 121°C for 15 minutes. *Clostridium tetani* is not locally invasive and does not provoke an inflammatory response, and inoculation of spores into viable tissue does not produce tetanus. However, tissue necrosis, foreign bodies, or concurrent anaerobic or facultative anaerobic infections lower the normal oxidation-reduction potential of the tissue, which allows conversion to the vegetative form with subsequent toxin formation. The toxins produced include tetanolysin, which is capable of causing local damage to viable tissue, thereby optimizing conditions for bacterial multiplication, and production of tetanospasmin, which is a potent neurotoxin responsible for the clinical disease state.[5] Toxin formed in a skin wound enters the underlying muscle and may spread to adjacent muscles. It then accumulates in the nerve endings of motor fibers. Retrograde transport of the toxin then occurs via intra-axonal and periaxonal pathways from nerve endings to the ventral horns of the spinal cord or motor nuclei of the cranial nerves. If toxin is produced in larger amounts, it also accumulates in the lymphatic system of the invaded muscle, enters the bloodstream via the thoracic duct, and is disseminated throughout the body. Toxin passing from blood to skeletal muscle then accumulates in the nerve endings of the motor fibers and proceeds to the ventral horns (or cranial nuclei), or is taken up by the lymphatic system and recirculated in the blood. The rate of accumulation of toxin in the ventral horns of the spinal cord depends on the length of the neural pathway and the activity of the muscles involved.[6] Since jaw muscles and spinal postural muscles have short neural pathways to the ventral horns and are continually active in the awake human, this is the likely explanation for trismus and neck stiffness early in the course of the illness.

In the anterior horn or cranial nerve nuclei the toxin accumulates in the presynaptic apparatus, impairing spontaneous secretion and evoked release of the inhibitory neurotransmitter γ-aminobutyric acid (GABA) and glycine.[1,5] Because inhibitory synapses are more sensitive to the effects of tetanus toxin than excitatory synapses, impaired inhibition of motoneurons and interneurons results in enhanced excitation and muscular rigidity. Disruption of the inhibitory interneurons within the propriospinal connections results in enhanced excitation such that stimulation from the periphery, such as light touch or visual or auditory stimuli from the reticular formation, can result in the generalized spasms seen in tetanus.

The effect of tetanus toxin on the neuromuscular junction is presynaptic inhibition of acetylcholine release, which can result in paralysis of muscles. Paralysis is less frequent and usually localized to areas of high toxin concentration because the neuromuscular junction is not as sensitive to tetanus toxin as the inhibitory neurons.

Autonomic dysfunction occurs later in the course of the disease because of the longer neuronal path. Sympathetic and parasympathetic overactivity has been attributed to impaired inhibition.[5]

Classification

There are three clinical forms of tetanus: generalized, local, and cephalic. Generalized tetanus is the most common form and is characterized by diffuse muscle rigidity. Localized tetanus is characterized by rigidity of a group of muscles in close proximity to the site of injury. Cephalic tetanus, which is a variant of local tetanus, is defined as trismus plus paralysis of one or more cranial nerves.[7] *Both local and cephalic tetanus may progress to generalized tetanus*, the latter occurring in approximately 65% of cases.

Clinical and Laboratory Manifestations

The most common means by which *C. tetani* enters the human host is through lacerations, especially if associated with tissue necrosis or foreign body. Tetanus can also follow burns or animal bites, septic abortion complicated by gangrene of the uterus, and rarely after otherwise uncomplicated abdominal surgery.[8] Untreated middle ear infections account for up to 30% of the cases of tetanus in India.[9] Intravenous drug users can develop tetanus associated with skin infections caused by use of inadequately sterilized needles.[10] However, in 15% to 25% of cases a portal of entry cannot be determined (cryptogenic tetanus).[3,9,10]

The interval between injury and onset of clinical symptoms is usually from 3 days to 3 weeks, but occasionally is as long as several months. Cephalic tetanus after scalp or facial injury tends to occur earlier with an incubation period of 1 day to 2 weeks.[7] In general, the shorter the incubation period, the more severe the disease. However, a long incubation does not guarantee a mild attack.

Muscular rigidity is the most prominent early symptom of tetanus. Rigidity of the masseter muscle (trismus) results in difficulty with opening the mouth and chewing. Rigidity of the facial muscles gives the characteristic smile of tetanus (risus sardonicus). Opisthotonos is caused by rigidity of the vertebral muscles and antigravity muscles. Abdominal muscle rigidity may simulate peritonitis. Nuchal rigidity may simulate meningitis. In the Edmondson and Flowers series of 100 patients,[3] trismus and dysphagia (described as sore throat) were the presenting symptoms in 75 cases and neck and back stiffness in 14 cases. However, in 88 cases, it was possible to demonstrate trismus on initial physical examination. In cephalic tetanus cranial nerve palsies may precede trismus.[3,11]

The *period of onset* of the disease is defined as the interval between the first symptom and the first generalized muscular spasm. A shorter period of onset is usually predictive of a severe attack.

Spasms are initially tonic, followed first by high-frequency and then low-frequency clonic activity. In very severe tetanus, spasms may occur so frequently that status epilepticus may be suspected, and may be forceful enough to cause fractures of long bones and of the spine. Spasm-induced damage to muscles can also result in rhabdomyolysis complicated by acute renal failure.[12] Spasms may be initiated by touch, noise, lights, and swallowing, even in the sleeping patient. Spasms severe enough to require treatment may persist for up to 6 weeks.

In addition to being extremely painful, spasms can produce a variety of significant secondary effects. Apnea occurs when spasms involve the respiratory muscles or larynx. Paralysis of skeletal muscles may occur following periods of sustained spasms due to presynaptic inhibition of acetylcholine release at the neuromuscular junction. Similarly, paralysis of urinary bladder musculature together with spasm of perineal muscles have been implicated in causing acute urinary retention. In pregnancy, spasms can cause abortion or miscarriage, although the fetus is not directly affected, since the toxin does not cross the placenta. Inadequately treated spasms can also produce fever, although secondary infection and direct and indirect actions of toxin on hypothalamic temperature regulation are often implicated.

The autonomic nervous system dysfunction of severe tetanus usually occurs 1 to 2 weeks after the onset of the disease but may occur earlier.[13] Manifestations of impaired sympathetic inhibition include tachycardia, labile hypertension alternating with hypotension, peripheral vasoconstriction, fever, and profuse sweating. Overactivity of the parasympathetic nervous system causes increased bronchial and salivary gland secretions, bradycardia, and sinus arrest.[14]

A complete blood count will usually show a leukocytosis with a left shift, and less frequently, a lymphocytosis. Examination of urine may reveal proteinuria and leukocytes thought to result from accumulation of tetanus toxin in the kidneys.[9] Other nonspecific laboratory abnormalities include elevation of serum transaminases, increased catecholamine levels in serum and urine, and decreased serum cholinesterase level. Creatine phosphokinase (CPK) is usually normal initially but generally rises with the onset of muscular spasms. Idoko and colleagues reported elevated cerebrospinal fluid (CSF) protein levels in 26 of 34 (76.5%) patients with tetanus.[15] The elevation of CSF protein appeared to correlate with disease severity. Nineteen patients with severe disease (10 ultimately fatal) had significantly higher CSF protein values (mean = 1582 mg/L) than mild cases (mean = 400 mg/L).

Complications of tetanus are numerous and frequent. The need for long-term endotracheal intubation and ventilatory support coupled with increased risk of aspiration may result in bacterial pneumonia. Other nosocomial infections also occur, as many patients require a long-term stay in an ICU. These may include infections of vascular access catheters, catheter-related urosepsis, and infected decubitus ulcers. Protracted immobilization places the patient at risk for deep venous thrombosis and pulmonary thromboembolism, which is commonly reported as a cause of death.

TABLE 59-1 Differential Diagnosis of Tetanus: Clinical Features

	Tetanus	Strychnine	Neuroleptics	SMS[a]	Rabies	Meningitis
Trismus	+	+	+	+	−	−
Nuchal rigidity	+	+	+	+	−	+
Risus sardonicus	+	+	−	−	−	−
Opisthotonus	+	+	+	−	+	−
Muscle rigidity (continuous)	+	+	+	−	−	−
Muscle rigidity (intermittent)	−	−	−	+	+	−
Encephalopathy	−	−	−	−	+	+
Rapid course	−	+	+	−	−	−

[a] Stiff-man syndrome.

Diagnosis

The diagnosis of tetanus is based on clinical manifestations rather than laboratory tests. Tissue cultures are positive in less than 50% of patients.[16] Since the organism is noninvasive, blood cultures are of little value except in diagnosing secondary infection. The major clinical features on which the diagnosis of tetanus is based are listed in Table 59-1 along with the features of other conditions with which it can be confused. Symptoms of strychnine poisoning usually begin 5 to 60 minutes after ingestion and resolve after 6 hours, although the hyperreflexia, stiffness, and muscle pains may last 3 to 7 days. The rapid course distinguishes strychnine poisoning and acute dystonic reactions from tetanus. Stiff-man syndrome is characterized by initially intermittent followed by continuous spasms of limb and trunk muscles that disappear during sleep. Trismus, facial palsy, nuchal rigidity, and continuous muscle rigidity are not seen in rabies. Cutaneous hyperesthesia is quite marked in rabies, as are disturbances in mentation, and both are absent in tetanus. Isolated paralysis of the facial nerve may be due to Bell palsy or an early manifestation of cephalic tetanus.[9] Patients with meningitis have nuchal rigidity but not trismus. However, examination of CSF is mandatory if the diagnosis is uncertain. Determination of serum calcium will rule out hypocalcemic tetany. Unlike trismus owing to these processes, tetanic trismus becomes more pronounced as the jaw is forced open.[9] Isolated trismus may be due to subluxation or arthritis of the temporomandibular joint or any inflammatory process involving teeth, mouth, tonsils, or pharynx.

Treatment

Patients with a presumptive diagnosis of tetanus should be admitted to an ICU.[3,16] Since the period of onset of the disease ranges from less than 1 to 12 days, even patients with mild tetanus (trismus, dysphagia, and localized rigidity) should be observed in an ICU for at least 1 week (2 weeks if no resolution of symptoms is noted). Patients with incubation periods of greater than 20 days who have only localized rigidity can be safely discharged to the ward after a few days of observation provided no progression of the disease has occurred.

The principles of initial treatment of tetanus consist of airway management, sedation, treatment of the portal of entry, antitoxin therapy, administration of appropriate antibiotics, and general supportive measures.[3,5,9,16] Drugs commonly used in the management of tetanus are listed in Table 59-2 together with their indications and usual doses.

Appropriate management of the airway is the first priority. Patients with trismus and localized rigidity with no evidence of respiratory compromise do not require prophylactic endotracheal intubation. Patients with diffuse rigidity, especially if unresponsive to benzodiazepine therapy, should be intubated, even in the absence of respiratory compromise. Intubation should be performed in all patients who have already had a generalized spasm or in any patient with evidence of respiratory compromise, including patients with severe dysphagia who are in danger of aspiration. The preferred route (nasotracheal vs. orotracheal) and method (awake vs. anesthetized) of intubation depends on the clinical situation. Ideally an anesthesiologist should perform intubation. An

TABLE 59-2 Drugs Used in Medical Management of Tetanus

Medication	Indication	Dose (Usual)
HTIG[a]	Local or cephalic tetanus	250 IU intrathecal
HTIG[a]	Generalized tetanus	3000–6000 IU intramuscular
Metronidazole	Toxin production (given in all cases)	500 mg IV/PO q6h
Midazolam	Spasms, sedation, and cardiovascular instability	0.3–30.0 mg/h IV (mean = 9.0 mg/h)
Magnesium sulfate	Spasms and cardiovascular instability	70–80 mg/kg IV load then 1–3 g IV q1h
Vecuronium	Neuromuscular blockade for severe muscle spasms	3–4 mg/h IV
Dantrolene	Rigidity and spasms	0.5–1.0 mg/kg IV q4–6h
Clonidine	Cardiovascular instability	300 μg q8h via nasogastric tube

[a] Human tetanus immune globulin.

emergency cricothyrotomy tray should be at the bedside prior to attempted intubation. If paralysis is required to facilitate intubation, a nondepolarizing agent should be used, since depolarizing neuromuscular blocking agents (e.g., succinylcholine) may cause hyperkalemia and cardiac arrest in patients withbreak tetanus.[17]

The classical approach for patients with muscular rigidity is sedation with intravenous benzodiazepines and narcotics. The doses should be titrated to reduce rigidity and provide adequate analgesia, respectively. Intubation, ventilation, sedation, and neuromuscular blockers[3,9,16,18] are the conventional therapies for tetanic spasms. However, in the early 1990s case reports suggested that neuromuscular blockade and ventilation could be avoided by using dantrolene and sedation.[19,20] More recently Attygalle and Rodrigo published their experience with 40 patients using intravenous magnesium as a first-line therapy for rigidity, spasms, and control of autonomic dysfunction.[21] In 95% of patients, control of spasms and muscle rigidity was achieved with serum magnesium levels of 2.0 to 4.0 mmol/L. The authors published their specific treatment protocol and stressed the importance of early tracheostomy for tracheal toilet. If neuromuscular blockade is required, pancuronium,[9] atracurium,[22] and vecuronium[18] have been reported as being safe and effective. Vecuronium has no cardiovascular side effects, which may be advantageous in treating patients with autonomic dysfunction.[18]

Aggressive surgical treatment of tetanus-producing wounds results in improved survival. The wound should be excised with a 2-cm margin.[23] If gangrene is present, the extremity should be amputated at least one uninvolved joint proximal to the wound.[23] The decision to perform a hysterectomy on a patient who develops tetanus following induced abortion or in the postpartum period should be based on the presence of associated invasive bacterial sepsis, gangrene of the uterus, or uterine injury. Tetanus is not itself an indication for hysterectomy.[9]

Several studies comparing mortality rates of patients with tetanus treated with and without antitoxin have produced conflicting results. However, the importance of answering this question has been markedly reduced by the availability of human tetanus immune globulin (HTIG), which has no serious adverse effects. It is now generally agreed that patients with tetanus should be treated with antitoxin as soon as possible.[1,5,16] However, controversy persists regarding the preferred route and dosage of antitoxin. There is evidence that in patients who have not yet progressed to generalized rigidity and spasms or those with very mild disease, intrathecal HTIG may reduce length of stay, prevent generalization, and in one study reduced mortality.[24,25] Conversely, once generalization has occurred, the administration of intrathecal HTIG has failed to improve survival. Intramuscular doses of HTIG ranging from 3000 to 6000 IU have been suggested.[5,16] It is important to administer antitoxin prior to débridement because the toxin may be introduced into the bloodstream during manipulation.[16]

Antibiotics are generally given both to treat infection at the injury site and to eliminate continued toxin production. Metronidazole 500 mg intravenously every 6 hours for 10 days is the antibiotic of first choice for *C. tetani*.[26] Penicillin G, tetracycline, erythromycin, clindamycin, and chloramphenicol are also effective.[5,26] Penicillin is a GABA antagonist.

Given the pathophysiology of tetanus, the use of GABA antagonists is concerning.

General supportive measures include establishing intravenous access to maintain adequate fluid and electrolyte balance. A Foley catheter should be inserted in all but the mildest cases to prevent urinary retention. Appropriate prophylaxis for stress ulcers is indicated. Ideally, intubated patients should be fed using the nasojejunal route to minimize the possibility of aspiration. Energy expenditure in patients with severe tetanus receiving appropriate sedation are within 10.5% of predicted basal metabolic rates using the Harris-Benedict equation.[27] Subcutaneous heparin is given to prevent deep venous thrombosis. Physiotherapy prevents contractures in patients treated with neuromuscular blockers.

Arterial and pulmonary artery catheterization may be useful to manage the autonomic dysfunction of severe tetanus. In the absence of cardiac disease the cardiac index tends to be elevated. Rapid changes in systemic vascular resistance are responsible for fluctuations in blood pressure.[5] The pulmonary capillary wedge pressure and central venous pressure are usually normal, but may be low in patients with severe spasms and diaphoresis, which have led to hypovolemia. It is important to ensure that hypovolemia is promptly corrected, since this will substantially increase the potential for immediately life-threatening hypotension in the presence of the autonomic instability. Core body temperature should be monitored and hyperpyrexia (core temperature greater than 41°C) avoided owing to the increased risk of sudden death.[28] Treatment of cardiovascular instability consists of deep sedation, which if unsuccessful is followed by high-dose magnesium sulfate infusions.[29–31] Continuous benzodiazepine intravenous infusion should be tried initially, followed by continuous narcotic infusion if required. Successful control of autonomic dysfunction has been achieved using a bolus (5.0 µg/kg IV) plus a continuous infusion (4.0 to 6.0 µg/kg per hour IV) of fentanyl when a benzodiazepine alone was insufficient.[30] Patients unresponsive to deep sedation have been successfully treated with intravenous magnesium sulfate. A loading dose of 70 mg/kg IV over 5 minutes is followed by a continuous infusion titrated to maintain serum magnesium levels between 2.5 and 4.0 mmol/L.[29] This usually requires infusion rates of 1 to 3 g/h. Serum calcium and magnesium levels should be measured every 4 hours.[31] Calcium supplements may be required to maintain serum calcium levels above 6.8 mg/dL (1.7 mmol/L).[29] Any magnesium-induced cardiac arrhythmias should also be treated with IV calcium and the infusion rate of magnesium should be reduced. There is conflicting opinion regarding the ability to reduce sedation and/or analgesic medications in patients who respond to intravenous magnesium therapy.[29,31] Autonomic dysfunction unresponsive or incompletely responsive to magnesium may respond to clonidine.[32,33] Continuous epidural infusion of bupivacaine and sufentanil was retrospectively evaluated in 11 patients with severe tetanus and autonomic dysfunction.[34] In two patients the epidural alone was ineffective, therefore morphine, muscle relaxation, and phenobarbitone or chlorpromazine were added. One patient developed an epidural abscess requiring a laminectomy with surgical drainage. The authors discuss in detail the risks of placing epidural catheters in patients with tetanus and suggest a caution for advocates of intrathecal therapy. In the past, β-blockers have been used. However, there is now evidence that their use is associated with a significant risk of death due to cardiac arrest,[14,35–37] and they are no longer recommended.

Prognosis

With modern intensive care management, mortality ranges from 10% to 15% overall and is no longer influenced by age.[5,38] In areas where such care is not available, mortality rates of between 25% and 50% are usual.[1,3,5,39] The general quality of critical care support is likely a key determinant of prognosis. In a recent study tracking mortality from severe tetanus in Brazil over two decades, mortality fell from 36.5% in the early time frame to 18.0% in the later period, likely related to general advances in ICU management.[40]

Finally, it is important to remember that recovery from tetanus does not guarantee natural immunity.[1] Patients should begin their primary immunization series prior to leaving the hospital; indeed, since passive immunization with HTIG does not interfere with successful active immunization, the series can begin even before the patient leaves the ICU.

References

1. Hsu SS, Grouleau G: Tetanus in the emergency department: A current review. *J Emerg Med* 20:357, 2001.
2. Gergen PJ, McQuillan GM, Kiely M, et al: A population-based serologic survey of immunity to tetanus in the United States. *N Engl J Med* 332:761, 1995.
3. Edmondson RS, Flowers MW: Intensive care in tetanus: Management, complications and mortality. *Br Med J* 1:1401, 1979.
4. Shimoni Z, Dobrousin A, Cohen J: Tetanus in an immunised patient. *BMJ* 319:1049, 1999.
5. Cook TM, Protheroe RT, Handel JM: Tetanus: A review of the literature. *Br J Anaesth* 87:477, 2001.
6. Kaeser HE, Saner A: The effect of tetanus toxin on neuromuscular transmission. *Eur Neurol* 3:193, 1970.
7. Jagoda A, Riggio S, Burguieres T: Cephalic tetanus: A case report and review of the literature. *Am J Emerg Med* 6:128, 1988.
8. Lennard TWJ, Gunn A, Sellers J, Stoddart JC: Tetanus after elective cholecystectomy and exploration of the common bile duct. *Lancet* 1:1466 (Letter), 1984.
9. Veronesi R (ed): *Tetanus, Important New Concepts.* Amsterdam: Excerpta Medica, 1981, p 1.
10. Cherubin CE: Epidemiology of tetanus in narcotic addicts. *NY State J Med* 70:267, 1970.
11. Schon F, O'Dowd L, White J, Begg N: Tetanus: Delay in diagnosis in England and Wales. *J Neurol-Neurosurg-Psychiatr* 57:1006, 1994.
12. Raman GV, Lee HA: Tetanus and renal failure. *Br J Clin Pract* 38:275, 1984.
13. Kerr JH, Corbett JL, Prys-Roberts C, et al: Involvement of the sympathetic nervous system in tetanus. Studies on 82 cases. *Lancet* 2:236, 1968.
14. Wright DK, Lalloo UG, Nayiager S, Govender P: Autonomic nervous system dysfunction in severe tetanus: Current perspectives. *Crit Care Med* 17:371, 1989.
15. Idoko JA, Amiobonomo AE, Anjorin FI: Cerebrospinal fluid changes in tetanus: raised proteins and immunoglobulins in patients with severe disease. *Trans R Soc Trop Med Hyg* 84:593, 1990.
16. Alfrey D, Rauscher LA: Tetanus: A review. *Crit Care Med* 7:176, 1979.
17. Azar I: The response of patients with neuromuscular disorders to muscle relaxants. *Anesthesiology* 61:173, 1984.
18. Powles AB, Ganta R: Use of vecuronium in the management of tetanus. *Anaesthesia* 40:879, 1985.
19. Sternlo JE, Andersen LW: Early treatment of mild tetanus with dantrolene. *Intensive Care Med* 16:345, 1990.
20. Checketts MR, White RJ: Avoidance of intermittent positive pressure ventilation in tetanus with dantrolene therapy. *Anaesthesia* 48:969, 1993.
21. Attygalle D, Rodrigo N: Magnesium as first line therapy in the management of tetanus: A prospective study of 40 patients. *Anaesthesia* 57:811, 2002.
22. Peat SJ, Potter DR, Hunter JM: The prolonged use of atracurium in a patient with tetanus. *Anaesthesia* 43:962, 1988.
23. Percy AS, Kukora JS: The continuing problem of tetanus. *Surg Gynecol Obstet* 160:307, 1985.
24. Agarwal M, Thomas K, Peter JV: A randomized double-blind sham-controlled study of intrathecal human anti-tetanus immunoglobulin in the management of tetanus. *Nat Med J India* 11:209, 1998.
25. Gupta PS, Kapoor R, Goyal S, et al: Intrathecal human tetanus immunoglobulin in early tetanus. *Lancet* 2:439, 1980.
26. Ahmadsyah I, Salim A: Treatment of tetanus: An open study to compare the efficacy of procaine penicillin and metronidazole. *Br Med J* 291:648, 1985.
27. Linton DM, Wells Y, Potgieter PD: Metabolic requirements in tetanus. *Crit Care Med* 20:950, 1992.
28. Udwadia FE, Udwadia ZF, Lall A: Autonomous dysfunction in severe tetanus. *Intensive Care Med* 16:520, 1990.
29. James MFM, Manson EDM: The use of magnesium sulphate infusions in the management of very severe tetanus. *Intensive Care Med* 11:5, 1985.
30. Moughabghab AV, Prevost G, Socolovsky C: Fentanyl therapy controls autonomic hyperactivity in tetanus. *Br J Clin Pract* 50:477, 1996.
31. Lipman J, James MFM, Erskine J, et al: Autonomic dysfunction in severe tetanus: Magnesium sulfate as an adjunct to deep sedation. *Crit Care Med* 15:987, 1987.
32. Sutton DN, Tremlett MR, Woodcock TE: Management of autonomic dysfunction in severe tetanus: The use of magnesium sulphate and clonidine. *Intensive Care Med* 16:75, 1990.
33. Gregorakos L, Kerezoudi E, Dimopoulos G: Management of blood pressure instability in severe tetanus: The use of clonidine. *Intensive Care Med* 23:893, 1997.
34. Bhagwanjee S, Bosenberg A, Muckart D: Management of sympathetic overactivity in tetanus with epidural bupivacaine and sufentanil: Experience with 11 patients. *Crit Care Med* 27:1721, 1999.
35. Wesley AG, Hariparsad D, Pather M, Rocke DA: Labetalol in tetanus. *Anaesthesia* 38:243, 1983.
36. Buchanan N, Smit L, Cane RD, De Andrade M: Sympathetic overactivity in tetanus fatality associated with propranolol. *Br Med J* 22:254, 1978.
37. Dundee JW, Morrow WFK: Labetalol in severe tetanus. *Br Med J* 1:1121, 1979.
38. Jolliet P, Magnenat J-L, Kobel T, Chevrolet J-C: Aggressive intensive care treatment of very elderly patients with tetanus is justified. *Chest* 97:702, 1990.
39. Udwadia FE, Lall A, Udwadia ZF, et al: Tetanus and its complications: Intensive care and management experience in 150 Indian patients. *Epidemiol Infect* 99:675, 1987.
40. Brauner JS, Rios Vieira SR, Bleck TP: Changes in severe accidental tetanus mortality in the ICU during two decades in Brazil. *Intensive Care Med* 28:930, 2002.

Chapter 60 _____

VIRAL HEMORRHAGIC FEVERS

SUSAN P. FISHER-HOCH

KEY POINTS

- *Viral hemorrhagic fevers (VHFs) are seen worldwide as either locally endemic disease or as imported cases in travelers.*

- *Travelers may be the source of epidemics in countries far from the source.*

- *Clinical presentation may be a flu-like syndrome, but may also be abrupt, with fever associated with generalized myalgia and headache. Severe cases progress to respiratory and gastrointestinal symptoms followed by systemic "capillary leak" causing pulmonary edema, shock, and bleeding from mucosal surfaces.*

- *Clinical diagnosis hinges on a history of potential exposure within the preceding few days up to a maximum of 4 weeks. The exposure may be to rodents, ticks, or fresh animal or human blood, or patients, usually in remote rural areas where these diseases are endemic.*

- *Management is mainly supportive, but effective antiviral therapy is available for some fevers. The critical issues are respiratory support, replacement of blood components as needed, and support of the circulation (using vasopressor drugs if necessary) while avoiding large infusions of intravenous fluids, which worsen pulmonary edema.*

- *Ribavirin is effective for several VHF infections, and when indicated should be given intravenously and as soon as possible.*

- *Prevention of transmission of infection is effected by providing routine isolation of suspect cases in a single room, preferably one with negative pressure, and use of standard universal precautions for exposure to contact with blood or body fluids, including gloves, gowns, and other barrier nursing procedures, and careful disinfection of exposed surfaces. With appropriate barrier precautions the risk of nosocomial transmission is minimal.*

- *With prompt and appropriate supportive therapy, many patients with these infections can make a rapid and complete recovery without significant sequelae.*

Overview of the Viral Hemorrhagic Fevers

Viral hemorrhagic fevers (VHFs) are endemic on every continent with the possible exception of Australia. The diseases are characterized by acute onset with high fever, and in some cases, high mortality. The bleeding by which they are known is a complication only of severe disease, but the underlying pathology is of widespread leakage from the capillaries, with prominent pulmonary edema. The clinical syndrome is mainly caused by endothelial cell dysfunction, not by tissue necrosis. Death usually results from hypovolemic shock with or without acute respiratory distress syndrome (ARDS). In survivors, recovery is rapid and usually complete.

The diseases are caused by many different enveloped RNA viruses. Almost all are zoonoses, and infection of humans is accidental, usually the consequence of intrusion of a human into the ecologic niche of the virus. The viruses belong to four major families: bunyaviridae, arenaviridae, filoviridae, and flaviviridae. The bunyaviruses include hantaviruses and Crimean Congo hemorrhagic fever (CCHF), a member of the genus *Nairovirus*. CCHF is spread by ticks, and occurs widely across Africa, Southeastern Europe, the Middle East, and Asia. Hantaviruses are found throughout the world as natural silent infections of a number of rodents. A New World hantavirus in North and South America is a pathogen of deer mice and related species, and causes the hantavirus pulmonary syndrome (HPS). Arenaviruses are also natural infections of rodents, the most important being Lassa virus, which is confined to West Africa, and the South American hemorrhagic fever viruses belonging to a complex of New World rodent viruses, four of which at present are known to cause VHF. The filoviruses are a unique family of filamentous viruses that includes Ebola and Marburg. African filoviruses have high mortality, but Asian filoviruses seen in monkeys from the Philippines do not appear to be pathogenic for humans. The flaviviridae include yellow fever virus and dengue virus, both spread by mosquitoes. Other viruses may cause hemorrhagic fever, such as Kyasanur Forest disease and Omsk hemorrhagic fever, but these are confined to very local areas and will not be discussed in detail.

EPIDEMIOLOGY

The zoonotic character of these infections means that they are primarily rural diseases in developing communities in areas with poor medical facilities, and they often go undiagnosed. Clinical reports and trials are scant, and data are limited. Essentially, VHFs are diseases of the poor. However, with increasing mobility of populations, and the migration and enrichment of individuals from poor communities who may revisit their villages for family events, infected patients can and do appear almost anywhere in the world. Missionaries and medical staff working in remote areas are also at risk and more likely than locals to reach tertiary care facilities, and thus to be diagnosed. Peace keepers and other aid workers are particularly at risk and several have been infected with Lassa fever in Sierra Leone and a few have died. Epidemics of VHFs such as yellow fever may be devastating, and there can be thousands of cases of this mosquito-borne disease. Some viruses, particularly filoviruses, have only emerged in small epidemics; however their very high mortality has given them prominence disproportionate to the number of patients. Recently Ebola outbreaks in equatorial Africa, specifically Gabon and the Republic of Congo, are associated with a massive epizootic in great apes whose populations are threatened now with extinction due to a combination of Ebola virus, logging, and hunting for bush meat. This epizootic is fueling epidemics in rural communities in the adjoining areas.

HISTORY AND CLINICAL DIAGNOSIS

The most critical element in the clinical diagnosis is a thorough history covering the incubation period, a maximum of 4 weeks prior to onset of fever. The element that alerts the physician to a viral hemorrhagic fever (and usually indicates which one it is likely to be) is the contact the patient might have had with known ecologic niches or patients who may have one of these infections (Table 60-1). Questions must include a thorough travel history; information on any possible contact with ticks, fresh animal blood, rodent urine or blood, wild animals, and mosquitoes and other insects; recent camping in exotic areas; possibly entry into bat caves; and attendance at ceremonial funerals. All of these factors can be significant, especially in remote areas. A medical care provider or other worker who might have had contact with blood from a primary case is also cause for alert.

An essential element is a short history of fever, often high and of abrupt onset. However, some patients present with a flu-like syndrome, which is of course difficult to differentiate. Severe body pains and headache are prominent and may be excruciating. Other features may be severe sore throat, nausea and vomiting, petechiae, oozing from the gums, and bradycardia. Proteinuria is frequent. Total peripheral white counts are usually unhelpful, but differential counts usually show lymphopenia and neutrophilia, which may be marked, and may actually mislead one into thinking it is caused by a bacterial infection. Thrombocytopenia is common, and platelet function is impaired. Partial thromboplastin times may be prolonged, but prothrombin times are relatively spared. Disseminated intravascular coagulation (DIC) is not a feature of VHF except as a complication of the terminal phase. As disease progresses, hypovolemic shock, pulmonary edema, and frank bleeding ensue. Serum glutamate oxaloacetate transaminase (SGOT; aspartate aminotransferase) is usually raised, and VHFs distinguish themselves from viral hepatitis because the SGOT is disproportionately high compared with the serum glutamate pyruvate transaminase (SGPT; alanine aminotransferase). Ratios of SGOT:SGPT may be as high as 11:1, and the level of the SGOT also reflects prognosis. Patients are rarely jaundiced, and the bilirubin is usually normal, the exception being yellow fever as its name suggests. The central nervous system (CNS) is relatively spared, but encephalopathy and neurologic sequelae such as ataxia and deafness occur. Isolated ocular sequelae in Ebola including blindness have been reported, as has a syndrome of polyserositis following Lassa fever.[1,2]

LABORATORY DIAGNOSIS

Care must be taken in collection, handling, and transport of specimens, and consultation with the laboratory is essential. Gloves must be worn at all times and the specimens clearly labeled as hazardous. Blood samples should be drawn, preferably into a vacuum tube system. Specimens for transport should be transferred to a leakproof plastic container and double wrapped in further leakproof containers for shipping to a suitable reference laboratory. Sera may be safely handled for immunologic tests by inactivation by heating to 60°C for 30 minutes.

The most rapid and accurate method of diagnosis is by reverse transcriptase polymerase chain reaction (RT-PCR). This technique is reliable and safe to perform directly on serum or tissues. However, availability of the assay specific for a particular virus may not be locally available and specimens need to be directed rapidly to a competent laboratory. The chemical reagents used in RT-PCR will reliably inactivate virus, so the technique also has advantages in safety, provided the initial steps are performed with care. In some circumstances antigen detection techniques in blood and tissues are available using enzyme-linked immunosorbent assay (ELISA) methodology, but once again these are usually only available in reference laboratories. Laboratory diagnosis is also by isolation of virus from serum, but this usually requires a high level of laboratory biocontainment, and takes time, often a week or more. Demonstration of a fourfold rise in antibody titer, or high-titer IgG antibody with virus-specific IgM antibody in association with compatible clinical disease is also diagnostic, but the more rapid VHFs, particularly Ebola and CCHF, evolve so quickly that patients may never develop antibody before death. Antibody detection techniques include immunofluorescence assay (IFA) and ELISA, and are increasingly being produced using recombinant antigens, thus avoiding the use of infectious agents in their preparation.

MANAGEMENT

VHFs in survivors are self-limiting diseases, so providing the acute crisis can be managed, recovery is rapid and usually complete, though convalescence may be prolonged.[3,4] Some viruses are highly treatable using the antiviral agent ribavirin, provided therapy is instituted as early as possible in the disease course (Table 60-2). Therapy with immune plasma has also been advocated, but with the exception of Argentine hemorrhagic fever, it has not been shown to have efficacy.

The main challenge is careful management of fluid balance. Patients will often present with high hematocrit due to capillary leakage aggravated by dehydration. Despite this, pulmonary edema is a real risk, and patients should be infused with caution. Blood and platelet replacement may be necessary. Full intensive care support may be required including mechanical ventilation, monitoring of central venous pressure, and dialysis. Seizures and arrhythmias will need to be controlled. DIC is not generally a major feature, and heparin is contraindicated. Exchange transfusion and use of steroids are controversial and cannot be recommended at this time. Early accurate diagnosis and good intensive care support are the most important underlying principles for the physician.

Patients with VHF do not travel well, since their cardiovascular system is often unstable, and even the moderate trauma of travel can induce bleeding or hypotension. For this reason moving a patient should be avoided whenever possible.[5] Moving the patient also increases the risk and the number of people exposed and thus the risk of secondary infections.

PREVENTION OF SPREAD

The fearsome reputation of some of these viruses, such as Ebola, Lassa, and CCHF, comes from their ability to spread to medical staff and patients in facilities where inadequate barrier nursing and other practices lead to blood-to-blood contact with the virus, such as needlestick injuries, blood spills on unprotected damaged skin, or mouth-to-mouth resuscitation. In some countries, reuse of needles and syringes has produced nosocomial and community outbreaks.[6] There are also reports of outbreaks in surgical teams who unwisely performed laparotomy on infected patients.[7] In these circumstances mortality has been high.

TABLE 60-1 Guide to Viral Hemorrhagic Fevers by Continent and Potential Exposures

RECENT TRAVEL IN CENTRAL OR SOUTH AMERICA

Exposure	Clinical Syndrome	Virus	Therapy in Addition to Routine Support of Organ Function	Prevention
Rodents	Fever with insidious onset; sore throat, myalgia; dyspnea with ARDS; bleeding, thrombocytopenia; elevated SGOT and bilirubin; seizures, obtundation, and coma	South American hemorrhagic fever viruses (Argentinian, Junin, Machupot, Sabia, Guanarito)	Immune plasma (AHF only) Ribavirin; likely that most viruses respond, but no clinical trial data are available	Oral ribavirin for high risk exposures; Vaccinate for AHF; Avoid rodent contact
Mosquitoes	Fever, bleeding, and thrombocytopenia; jaundice with raised SGOT, SGPT, and bilirubin; ARDS; wasting	Yellow fever	None	Vaccinate; Prevent mosquito bites
Mosquitoes	Fever and myalgia; thrombocytopenia, with petechiae; ARDS; shock	Dengue	None	Prevent mosquito bites
Rodents	Sudden onset of fever and myalgias; shock; prominent ARDS	Hantavirus pulmonary syndrome	Consider ribavirin	Avoid rodent contact

RECENT TRAVEL IN RURAL AFRICA

Exposure	Clinical Syndrome	Virus	Therapy	Prevention
Rodents; infected patients	Insidious onset of fever, sore throat, and myalgia; bleeding with moderate thrombocytopenia; ARDS; elevated SGOT, SGPT, and bilirubin; proteinuria; seizures and coma	Lassa fever	Ribavirin	Oral ribavirin for high-risk exposure Strict barrier nursing Avoid rodent contact
Infected patients; sick or dead monkeys Bush meat ?Unknown	Sudden onset with fever, sore throat, myalgia; severe bleeding with thrombocytopenia and elevated APTT; elevated SGOT, SGPT and bilirubin; proteinuria; effusions; ARDS	Ebola/Marburg	None	Strict barrier nursing
Mosquitoes	Bleeding and thrombocytopenia; jaundice with raised SGOT, SGPT, and bilirubin; ARDS; wasting	Yellow fever	None	Vaccinate; prevent mosquito bites
Ticks; blood from infected patients	Sudden onset of fever and myalgias; severe bleeding and ecchymoses with thrombocytopenia and elevated APTT; elevated SGOT; proteinuria	Crimean-Congo hemorrhagic fever	Ribavirin	Oral ribavirin for high-risk exposure Avoid tick contact Strict barrier nursing

RECENT TRAVEL IN RURAL EUROPE AND RURAL AND URBAN ASIA

Exposure	Clinical Syndrome	Virus	Therapy	Prevention
Rodents	Insidious onset; thrombocytopenia; proteinuria and oliguria to anuria; shock; ARDS	Hemorrhagic fever with renal syndrome; nephropathia epidemica	Ribavirin	Avoid rodent contact

(continued)

TABLE 60-1 Guide to Viral Hemorrhagic Fevers by Continent and Potential Exposures (Continued)

		RECENT TRAVEL IN RURAL EUROPE AND RURAL AND URBAN ASIA		
Exposure	Clinical Syndrome	Virus	Therapy	Prevention
Ticks; infected patients	Sudden onset with fever and myalgia; severe bleeding and ecchymoses with thrombocytopenia and elevated APTT; elevated SGOT; proteinuria	Crimean-Congo hemorrhagic fever	Ribavirin	Oral ribavirin for high-risk exposures Avoid tick contact Strict barrier nursing
Mosquitoes	Fever and myalgia; petechiae and thrombocytopenia; shock; ARDS	Dengue	None	Prevent mosquito bites

Clinical syndromes overlap considerably, particularly early in disease, so the detailed travel history is critical. This table is intended as a general guide for the clinician and advice from experts should be sought immediately if any of these diagnoses are under consideration. Note that medical personnel and possibly family members may have not traveled themselves, but may have been in contact with sick travelers.
ABBREVIATIONS: AHF, Argentine hemorrhagic fever; APTT, activated partial thromboplastin time; ARDS, acute respiratory distress syndrome; SGOT, aspartate aminotransferase; SGPT, alanine aminotransferase.

The key to prevention of transmission both in endemic and nonendemic areas has consistently been good hospital and laboratory practice, with strict isolation of febrile patients at risk of VHF and rigorous use of gloves and disinfection.[8] A small number of designated personnel should undertake direct care and be kept fully informed about the nature of the virus and the precautions to be taken.

Intensive care and full life support should not be denied. Essential surgery should be performed with meticulous attention to avoiding accidental inoculation of blood or fluids. Pregnant patients are a major challenge. They often present with absent fetal movements, and maternal survival in Lassa fever and probably other hemorrhagic fevers has been shown to depend on aggressive obstetric intervention to evacuate the uterus.[9]

Aerosol spread in hospitals has not been documented; indeed there is much published evidence that this is not a major hazard. Past recommendations for isolation of patients in a plastic isolator have long given way to simple strict barrier nursing. Indeed, the risk to personnel is about equal to that of human immunodeficiency virus (HIV) transmission, and the practices now universally adopted for HIV nursing and medical care are quite adequate to prevent transmission of VHFs, provided they are fully implemented and observed. This practice presents no excess risk to hospital personnel and allows substantially better care to be given to the patient.

The major factor in nosocomial transmission is unawareness of the possibility of VHF by a health care provider who is also inattentive to the requirements of effective barrier nursing. Many outbreaks in developing countries have been due to lack of hygiene and to unwise surgery on febrile patients. Once the diagnosis has been entertained and appropriate precautions instituted, the risk of nosocomial transmission is very small.

High risk of infection is associated with direct percutaneous or mucosal contact with blood or body fluids. Postexposure prophylaxis with ribavirin for CCHF and for arenaviruses should be offered to contacts with high-risk exposures. People with medium- or low-risk contact histories (includes most unprotected contact with blood or body fluids, and casual or social contact) may safely be observed for development of persistent high fever for 3 weeks from the last date of contact. The practice of following up airline passengers and other low-risk

TABLE 60-2 Ribavirin Therapy for Viral Hemorrhagic Fevers

Intravenous regimen:	Ribavirin 2 g IV loading dose, then 1 g IV every 6 h for 4 days, infused over at least 20 min; then 0.5 g every 8 h for 6 more days
Oral regimen:	Ribavirin 2 g loading dose, then 4 g/d in four divided doses every 6 hours; then 2 g/d in four divided doses for 6 days
Potential side effects:	Hemolysis

RESPONCE TO RIBAVIRIN THERAPY		
Highly Effective	May Have Some Efficacy	No Efficacy
Lassa fever South American hemorrhagic fevers Crimean Congo hemorrhagic fever	Hantavirus pulmonary syndrome Hemorrhagic fever with renal syndrome	Ebola and Marburg viruses Yellow fever Rift Valley fever Dengue hemorrhagic fever

exposures has been discontinued. Low-risk contacts (entered the room) do not need to be placed under surveillance.

The 1988 Centers for Disease Control and Prevention (CDC) Guidelines for the Management of Patients with VHFs recommends routine patient isolation in a single room, preferably but not necessarily with negative air pressure gradient from the hallway through an anteroom to the patient room.[3] Staff education; use of gloves, gowns, and masks; and rigorous disinfection are mandatory. The recommendations issued for patient management and handling of clinical specimens from acquired immunodeficiency virus (AIDS) patients are adequate for containment of VHFs.

Lassa and Ebola viruses in particular are robust and withstand drying. However, all the viruses can be inactivated by heat (60°C), detergents, chlorine, formalin, and ultraviolet (UV) radiation (sunlight). All the hemorrhagic fever viruses have envelopes that are disrupted by detergents and soaps, rendering them inactive. Though detergents cannot be recommended for disinfection, it is useful to remember that their liberal use will greatly reduce the number of infectious particles. Disinfection can be accomplished by washing with 0.5% phenol in detergent (e.g., Lysol), 0.5% hypochlorite solution, formaldehyde, glutaraldehyde, or paracetic acid. Care should be taken to ensure solutions are freshly and correctly made up and time allowed for disinfectant to work on spills.

Finally a problem of VHFs, particularly viruses such as Ebola, is the fear and press attention they receive. A single case can be quite traumatic for an institution unless the situation is carefully handled. A measured and informed approach from a collaborative team of doctors, nurses, administrators, and others is needed. Careful education of all medical staff, emphasizing the real risks and the way to avoid them, allaying unnecessary fears, and avoiding panic will result in appropriate management of the patient and avoid secondary infections. Press attention can be quite disruptive and is best managed by the sharing of accurate and regular information.

Bunyaviruses

Bunyaviruses are a large family of spherical (85 to 100 nm) negative-sense RNA viruses found in animals and insects. Crimean Congo hemorrhagic fever (CCHF) virus is a member of the tick-borne *Nairovirus* genus of this family, and the hantaviruses, which are rodent-borne, form their own genus.

CRIMEAN CONGO HEMORRHAGIC FEVER

CCHF is a tick-borne viral disease initially described in the USSR in the 1930s, and the virus was isolated in the Belgian Congo in the 1950s. The virus is now known to occur from Eastern Europe through Asia, the Middle East, and in all of Africa and the People's Republic of China (PRC), where the disease is known as *Xinjiang fever*.[4,10–13] Humans are infected from ticks or by handling blood or secretions from infected people or domestic animals. Because of the high mortality of infection with CCHF virus, the virus is classified as Biosafety Level 4 (BSL4).

CCHF virus infects at least 24 species of ixodid (hard) ticks, particularly *Hyalomma* species, which serve as both reservoir

and vector of this agent. CCHF infection of humans has emerged as a sporadic but important disease, particularly in arid livestock farming areas. Seasonality depends on local climatic conditions, with peaks corresponding to maximum periods of tick infestation.[14,15] A wide range of wild and domestic animals and birds may be infected.

The illness:infection ratio of CCHF virus ranges from 1:5 in the southern USSR to more than 50% of infected persons in South Africa, and mortality varies from 5% to 10% in the southern USSR to 35% in South Africa; rates of 35% to 50% or higher are possible in nosocomial outbreaks. Mild or inapparent infection appears to be the rule for most mammalian species, with the exception of humans.

The high risk of nosocomial outbreaks was first recognized in 1976, when a laparotomy was performed on a patient in Pakistan with abdominal pain, hematemesis, and melena. Eleven secondary cases in hospital staff resulted in three deaths, including a surgeon and an operating theater attendant.[7] Since then, similar nosocomial outbreaks have been reported in many countries from South Africa through countries of the former Yugoslavia, Iran, Dubai, Afghanistan, China, and Russia.[10–13,16–20] In hospital outbreaks heavy blood contamination or needlestick injury is frequently recorded.[16]

CLINICAL AND LABORATORY FEATURES

The incubation period of CCHF is only about 2 to 9 days.[21] There is a rapid, dramatic onset with severe headache, high fever, chills, and excruciating myalgia strongly localized to the lower back and joints. There is often epigastric pain. Conjunctivitis and a mild flushing of the face and chest, pharyngeal hyperemia, and petechiae on the palate are frequent. Bradycardia is typical, and diarrhea occasional.

Within 3 to 5 days after onset, signs of hemorrhagic diathesis may develop with bleeding from the gums, epistaxis, hematuria, and bloody diarrhea. Petechiae and purpura are frequent. Massive hematemesis, melena, extensive bloody effusions, bleeding from virtually every orifice and from venipuncture sites, and hypovolemic shock precede death with development of sometimes spectacular ecchymoses. Despite the high fever, bradycardia is typical, with tachypnea due to pulmonary edema.

Liver function tests may show mild to marked hepatocellular dysfunction, sometimes accompanied by renal failure. SGOT may be markedly raised, but SGPT elevation is usually minimal. There is no evidence of myocardial involvement. There is no objective evidence of direct CNS infection. Intracranial bleeding is a possibility. Changes in affect and mood, including aggressive behavior, are a feature of the convalescent phase.

Severe thrombocytopenia is invariable, frequently with counts below 20,000/μL. Prothrombin times (PTTs) and activated partial thromboplastin times (APTT) may be prolonged but usually not severely so. Platelet counts of less than 20,000/μL, PTT >60 seconds, SGOT >200 IU/L, and SGPT >150 IU/L are associated with a risk of death of more than 90% in untreated patients. Leukopenia may be profound with an early predominance of polymorphonuclear cells, giving way to a marked relative and absolute lymphopenia after 7 to 10 days. Some patients have a relative neutrophilia. During convalescence there may be lymphocytosis with atypical forms.

DIAGNOSIS

Diagnosis is most rapidly made by RT-PCR. Though there is some genetic diversity, sufficient conserved sequences may be targeted for broad specificity. Virus may also be isolated from blood of acutely ill patients, but viremia is early and of short duration, and the virus is labile, so that specimens have to be carefully taken and preserved for transportation. Antigen detection systems are also available using recombinant antigens.[11,12] Virus-specific antibodies appear 7 to 10 days after infection and neutralizing antibodies after day 14 to 16, but since the incubation period is very short, often only 3 to 4 days, acute diagnosis by antibody detection is not reliable.[22]

SPECIFIC TREATMENT

CCHF virus is sensitive to the antiviral ribavirin in vitro and in vivo in concentrations as low as 5 μg/mL, and the CDC recommends the empirical use of the intravenous preparation for treatment of CCHF infections.[3] Ribavirin has shown to be effective in vivo.[16]

Oral ribavirin has been used for postexposure prophylaxis for CCHF infection, but its efficacy has not been formally examined. Though intravenous ribavirin is the treatment of choice, oral therapy may be used if it is the only form available, since ribavirin is well absorbed from the gastrointestinal tract and would be expected to attain adequate levels in the blood. There is presently no role for immune plasma in the treatment of CCHF infection.

PREVENTION

Avoidance of tick bite using repellents applied to skin or soaked into clothing are methods of choice. Slaughter of potentially viremic animals is hazardous. Care of infected patients should avoid blood contact and high-risk procedures such as mouth-to-mouth resuscitation. The combination of epigastric pain and hematemesis has sometimes led an unwary surgeon to perform laparotomy.[16] Generalized oozing results in large blood losses and inevitably difficulty in achieving hemostasis. The patient does not survive, and the surgeon and operating attendants themselves have a high risk of fatal infection.

HANTAVIRUSES

Hemorrhagic fever with renal syndrome (HFRS) loosely describes a complex of diseases in which fever and acute renal failure are associated with bleeding, first reported from Manchuria and from Scandinavia during the 1930s. Until the early 1990s the diseases and the viruses that cause them were thought to belong exclusively to the Old World. In 1993 hantavirus pulmonary syndrome (HPS) was identified in an outbreak in the United States,[23] and since then patients and infected rodents have been found from Canada to Argentina. Both disease syndromes are now known to be caused by related viruses collectively called hantaviruses, which are members of the bunyaviridae.[24,25]

EPIDEMIOLOGY

Hantaviruses are all natural parasites of a wide variety of rodents, in which they persist for life without apparent disease. The rodents are infected at or around birth, and excrete large amounts of virus in urine, probably for life. The virus groups are determined primarily by the rodent host species, which govern geographic distribution of diseases they cause. Thus among the Old World hantaviruses, particularly in Siberia, mainland China, and Korea, the most common rodent host is the Manchurian striped field mouse, *Apodemus agrarius*. This mouse carries the Hantaan virus strain, which is the cause of the most severe clinical manifestation, HFRS. Throughout Europe, a less pathogenic group of hantaviruses, Puumala virus and related strains, cause nephropathia epidemica (NE). These viruses are endemic in the red bank vole, *Clethrionomys glareolus*. In the Balkans, Belgrade virus isolated from the yellow-neck mouse, *Apodemus flavicollis*, causes severe HFRS and is more closely related to Hantaan virus. In urban centers in the Far East and in rural areas in China, yet another strain, Seoul virus, with intermediate pathology, is endemic in house rats. Transmission appears to be from direct contact with rodent urine, but aerosol dispersal in heavily rodent urine–contaminated dust is also reported. Human disease occurs in agricultural areas with high human and rodent population densities, during military campaigns or exercises, in crowded urban housing, or in laboratories housing infected rodents. Person-to-person contact has not been reported, and these viruses do not cause nosocomial outbreaks.[26] All ages and both sexes may be affected.

Until the early 1990s, HFRS was thought to be exclusively an Old World disease. In 1993, however, a pulmonary disease emerged in the United States that was found to be associated with hantavirus infection (hantavirus pulmonary syndrome; HPS), without a significant renal component.[23] This virus, named the Sin Nombre virus, infects deer mice mainly in the southwestern United States. Risk of infection is related to exposure to infected rodent populations. By 1999, 277 cases had been reported from 31 states.[27] Canada had also reported 32 cases, but it was South America that rapidly emerged as bearing the greatest burden, with over 500 reported cases in Argentina, Uruguay, Chile, Paraguay, and Bolivia. Two more related South American viruses were identified, Andes and Laguna Negra viruses, and a number of rodents of the sigmodontine and oligoryzomys species appear to be the natural hosts. The ecology of these viruses and rodents appears to be as complex as in the Old World. On both continents the viruses persist in its chosen rodent species despite robust immune responses, probably because they are able to continuously produce quasispecies, thereby escaping immune surveillance. Such viruses probably coevolved with their rodent hosts over as long as 9 million years.

CLINICAL AND LABORATORY FEATURES

Hantaviruses are distinguished from most other hemorrhagic fever viruses by their longer incubation period of 2 to 3 weeks; for the Sin Nombre virus it is 9 to 33 days.[28] The underlying pathology of both HPS and HFRS appears to be induction of cytokines in lung or renal tissue, and there is in fact overlap between the two syndromes,[27] the difference being the predominant target tissue. The Old World hantaviruses induce a brief period of acute renal impairment, which may be as severe as anuria, requiring dialysis. However, this is usually self-limiting and of short duration. In HRFS vascular impairment and thrombocytopenia may result in bleeding that is usually minor, and the "leaky capillary syndrome," which manifests variably as shock, renal failure, and in severe cases, ARDS. Renal involvement is seen in some HPS patients, but HPS pathology is centered on the lungs, and the ensuing severe respiratory distress carries a higher mortality than HFRS, earlier thought to be about 50%, but now recorded as being on the order of 27%. Though HPS mortality in South America appears to be higher than in North America, it appears that the illness:infection ratio is lower in South America. Mortality from HRFS is about 5% to 15%, with survival often depending on experience in fluid management, and death in NE patients is rarely recorded. In all these syndromes, raised hematocrit on admission to hospital probably reflects hemoconcentration due to leaking capillaries as in other hemorrhagic fevers, and thrombocytopenia, left shift in white cell counts, and hypoxia are characteristic, with the difference in HPS being that bleeding does not appear to be a problem. Pulmonary edema, which may be aggravated by injudicious IV fluids, can coexist with profound hypovolemic shock. Pathologic lesions are compatible with endothelial dysfunction and leakage, since no evidence of endothelial damage is seen. Viral antigen is seen in lung tissue of patients with HPS, and local production of cytokines is involved in the pathology.[24,29] Recovery in survivors is rapid, and sequelae are not reported. Antibody has been found in up to 40% of some populations in South America, demonstrating that a large number of infected people have asymptomatic infection or mild disease, but in the north it is difficult to find antibody-positive people with no history of the disease.[27] There is no nonhuman primate model for hantavirus infection in which to study these processes in more detail, but recently infection of cynomolgus macaques with the most virulent strain, Andes virus, has been established.[30]

In Asia and Europe, HFRS and NE are distinct clinical entities, very familiar to physicians working in endemic areas, who normally have little difficulty in making an accurate clinical diagnosis. HFRS was first described in the literature in Eastern Siberia in 1912, and NE in Scandinavia in the 1930s. During the Second World War Japanese investigators conducted some ethically highly controversial studies in prisoners in China. Throughout the twentieth century the disease was a well recognized hazard of war, particularly with soldiers bivouacking in the open or in trenches, and NE may have been one of the causes of "trench fever" in the First World War. There were probably about 30,000 cases in American troops during the Korean War.

HRFS is classically described to exhibit five stages. First is the febrile stage, during which the patient will have headache, malaise, and muscle pains. Petechiae are found not only on the soft palate and under the axillae, but also on the face, neck, upper hips, and thighs. Flushing and edema are marked around the eyes. The liver may occasionally be palpable, and abdominal and renal tenderness are most common. Platelet counts are reduced and may be very low. White cell counts are variable, but in some severe cases, marked transient neutrophilia can lead to confusion with bacterial infection. Proteinuria is invariable. After 2 to 4 days the patient either recovers spontaneously or progresses to the shock phase. This period of low blood pressure is followed within 24 hours by the oliguric or anuric phase. Within a further 24 hours or so most patients enter the diuretic phase. Finally the convalescent phase leads to full recovery with no well-documented sequelae. Although bleeding is uncommon, when it occurs it is usually in the convalescent phase and hemorrhage may be difficult to control, and death may result from intracranial bleeding. There are no clinical and laboratory data to suggest bleeding is due to hepatic failure and consumption coagulopathy is only recorded in terminal disease.

LABORATORY DIAGNOSIS

RT-PCR on blood is the most reliable method of diagnosis for all the hantaviruses. Quantitative RT-PCR is available (qPCR), with the ability to measure as few as 10^3 copies per reaction.[27] The viruses are difficult to culture, and it appears that many virions and viral antigens are bound in immune complexes in the blood, increasing the difficulty of isolation. In any event, viremia is an early event, so for success specimens must be taken early. The disease may be immunologically mediated, occurring mostly after disappearance of the virus. Laboratory diagnosis of hantavirus infections can also be made by demonstration of a rise in specific antibodies or demonstration of virus-specific IgM. Over 90% of patients have hantavirus-specific IgM and IgG antibody when first seen. Antibodies persist for up to 3 decades and generally react to highest titer with homologous antigens. Neutralizing antibody can be detected.

SPECIFIC TREATMENT

Intravenous ribavirin may be useful in HFRS if given on or before the fourth day of disease, in doses similar to those used for Lassa fever.[31] Early treatment is essential. Ribavirin has similarly been recommended for patients with HPS,[32] but some adverse effects were noted (principally anemia) and efficacy was not demonstrated (see Table 60-2). Further studies are needed. For both of these syndromes the focus in supportive management of the patient is on careful fluid balance. Intravenous fluids given during the febrile and shock phases may leak into the extravascular space, aggravating edema, particularly during the period of shock and oliguria. Judicious use of vasopressor drugs for severe hypotension is preferred. When pulmonary edema leads to severe dyspnea and impending acute respiratory failure, intubation and mechanical ventilatory support are mandatory. Diuretics are relatively ineffective in HFRS, but peritoneal dialysis or hemodialysis may be life-saving. With these supportive measures and careful fluid management, most patients have the potential to make a spontaneous and complete recovery.

PREVENTION

The variety and ubiquity of rodent carriers and their success in many ecologic settings make the reduction of hantaviral infections by rodent control virtually impossible. Improvement of housing, particularly food storage, will help prevent those cases caused by rodent invasion of houses. However, a large number of infections occur in rural settings associated with agriculture and forestry. Education of populations to avoid direct contact with rodents in these circumstances may only have marginal effect because the virus may be made airborne by agricultural practices. Some vaccines have undergone preliminary trials in China and North and South Korea with encouraging results, but none has undergone the safety and clinical trials necessary for licensing in any country.

Arenaviruses

Rodents experience silent, lifelong infection with arenaviruses, with persistent viruria, and are the primary source of contamination of the environment. Five arenaviruses cause hemorrhagic fevers: Lassa in West Africa, and Junin, Machupo, Guanarito, and Sabia in South America, causing

Argentine, Bolivian, Venezuelan, and Brazilian hemorrhagic fevers, respectively. These viruses occupy circumscribed, sometimes remote ecologic niches, intrusion into which determines human infection. The viruses infect primarily through skin cuts and scratches and possibly the mucosae, contaminated with rodent urine, although there is evidence with Argentine hemorrhagic fever that dust generated by agricultural implements and laden with infected rodent urine may infect by aerosol. In endemic foci, the number of infected people may be very high. Human-to-human spread through blood contact is reported for Lassa fever both in community and hospital settings but is apparently rare with the other pathogenic arenaviruses.

Arenaviruses are enveloped, pleomorphic, membrane viruses containing two segments of single-stranded RNA, tightly associated with a nucleocapsid protein. The small RNA strand encodes the glycoprotein precursor and the nucleoprotein. Lassa and the South American hemorrhagic fever viruses are categorized as BSL4 laboratory agents. Disease may be severe and hemorrhagic, but with Lassa fever at least, mild or asymptomatic infection is also common.

LASSA FEVER

EPIDEMIOLOGY

Lassa fever is confined to West Africa, where it is responsible for up to 16% of all adult medical admissions and about 30% of adult deaths on medical wards.[33] It has been estimated that more than 100,000 infections with Lassa virus may occur each year, with several thousand deaths. All age groups and both sexes are affected. In endemic areas, illness:infection ratios range from 9% to 26%, and the proportion of febrile illness associated with seroconversion is between 5% and 14%. Five to eight percent of infected people may be hospitalized, of whom 17% will die if untreated. However, the fatality among all infections (hospitalized and nonhospitalized) is of the order of 2%.[34]

Person-to-person spread of Lassa virus occurs within homes as well as in hospitals. Hospital outbreaks are associated with inadequate disinfection and direct contact with infected blood and contaminated needles. Increasing and indiscriminate use of needles for intravenous therapy, or intramuscular injections in West African hospitals along with inadequate needle and syringe sterilization has led to large-scale epidemics. These epidemics can be devastating, resulting in the deaths not only of patients but also medical staff, surgeons, nurses, and other scarce personnel.[6,35]

Lassa fever is an increasing threat. It now affects communities in West Africa outside of its already broad area of rural endemicity. Indeed, urban Lassa fever in West Africa has been occurring with increasing frequency. In early 2000 hospital epidemics in large towns were again being seen in Nigeria, the most populous country in Africa. Since 1990, severe social disruption from conflicts and terror campaigns in Sierra Leone and Liberia have resulted in displacement of up to two million people—25% of the population of the area—with a substantial increase in the already large number of Lassa fever cases and deaths.[36]

Lassa fever is the exotic hemorrhagic fever most likely to occur in developed countries due to infection in returning travelers. This is because of the prevalence of disease in the endemic areas, and the relatively long incubation period (up

to 3 weeks). In the year 2000 at least four cases were imported into Europe.[37] All died, due in great part to delay in diagnosis, and therefore delay in instituting antiviral therapy. Increased cases in non-West Africans in 2000 has been seen as a result of United Nations peacekeeping efforts in Sierra Leone, where the rebels' stronghold is the center of the Lassa fever endemic area. One of the fatal cases in expatriates was an Englishman who had been working to disarm the rebel soldiers in the diamond mining area of Eastern Sierra Leone.[38]

The only known reservoir is *Mastomys natalensis*, one of the most commonly occurring rodents in Africa. Direct contact between virus-contaminated articles and surfaces and cuts and scratches on bare hands and feet may be the most important and consistent mode of transmission. The sporadic pattern of human infection in the household does not suggest aerosol transmission. Nosocomial spread in hospitals was and continues to be associated with inadequate disinfection and direct contact with infected blood and contaminated needles. Ill advised surgery performed on infected patients has resulted in infection and death among medical staff. Increasing and indiscriminant use of routine intravenous therapy in West African hospitals along with inadequate needle and syringe care has led to large-scale epidemics. Nevertheless, where simple but rigorous barrier nursing techniques have been applied, Lassa virus infection does not spread.[8] In a study in London, none of 173 unprotected hospital contacts of a severely ill Lassa fever patient were infected.[39]

CLINICAL AND LABORATORY FEATURES

Following an incubation period of 7 to 18 days, Lassa fever begins insidiously, with fever, weakness, malaise, severe headache—usually frontal—and a very painful sore throat.[15] More than 50% of patients then develop joint and lumbar pain, and 60% or more develop a nonproductive cough. Many also develop severe retrosternal chest pain, and about half will have nausea with vomiting or diarrhea and abdominal pain. On physical examination respiratory rate, temperature, and pulse rate are elevated, and blood pressure may be low. There is no characteristic skin rash in Lassa fever, and petechiae and ecchymoses are not seen. About one third of patients will have conjunctivitis. More than two thirds have pharyngitis, half with exudates, diffusely inflamed and swollen posterior pharynx and tonsils, but few if any ulcers or petechiae. The abdomen is tender in 50% of patients. Neurologic signs in the early stages are limited to a fine tremor, most marked in the lips and tongue.[40]

Up to one-third of hospitalized Lassa fever patients progress to a prostrating illness 6 to 8 days after onset, usually with persistent vomiting and diarrhea. Patients are often dehydrated with elevated hematocrit. Proteinuria occurs in two thirds of patients. About half of Lassa fever patients will have diffuse abdominal tenderness but no localizing signs or loss of bowel sounds. The severe retrosternal or epigastric pain seen in many patients may result from pleural or pericardial involvement. Bleeding is seen in only 15% to 20% of patients, limited primarily to the mucosal surfaces or occasionally conjunctival hemorrhages or gastrointestinal or vaginal bleeding. Severe pulmonary edema and acute respiratory distress syndrome is common in fatal cases, with gross head and neck edema, pharyngeal stridor, and hypovolemic shock.

Over 70% of patients may have abnormal electrocardiograms including nonspecific ST-segment and T-wave abnormalities, ST-segment elevation, generalized low-voltage complexes, and changes reflecting electrolyte disturbance, but none of these correlate with clinical or other measures of disease severity or outcome, and they are unassociated with clinical manifestations of myocarditis.[41] Neurologic signs are infrequent but carry a poor prognosis, progressing from confusion to severe encephalopathy with or without general seizures, but without focal signs. Cerebrospinal fluid is usually normal, but with a few lymphocytes, and low titers of virus relative to serum. Pneumonitis and pleural and pericardial rubs develop in early convalescence in about 20% of hospitalized patients, occasionally in association with congestive cardiac failure.

Although the mean white blood cell count in Lassa fever on admission to hospital is often normal, there may be early lymphopenia and later relative or absolute neutrophilia, as high as 30,000/μL. Thrombocytopenia is only moderate, and petechiae are uncommon. Endothelial and platelet dysfunction (despite adequate numbers of circulating platelets) are characteristic of severe disease,[42] and the capillary leak syndrome results in ARDS, as with most hemorrhagic fever viruses.

A serum aspartate aminotransferase (SGOT) level of >150 U/L is associated with a case fatality rate of 50%, and there is a correlation between an increasing level and a higher risk of fatal outcome.[34] Alanine aminotransferase (SGPT) is only marginally raised, and the ratio of SGOT to SGPT in natural infections and in experimentally infected primates is as high as 11:1. Prothrombin times and glucose and bilirubin levels are near normal, excluding biochemical hepatic failure, suggesting that some of the SGOT may be nonhepatic in origin.

Nearly 30% of patients with Lassa fever infection suffer an acute loss of hearing in one or both ears, not associated with severity of the disease.[43] About half show a near or complete recovery by 3 to 4 months after onset, but the remainder have persistent significant sensorineural deafness, which after about a year will be permanent. Many patients also exhibit cerebellar signs during convalescence, particularly tremors and ataxia, but these usually resolve with time. Infrequent complications are uveitis, pericarditis, orchitis, pleural effusion, ascites, and acute adrenal insufficiency.[44] Renal and hepatic failure are not seen.

Lassa fever may be a common cause of maternal mortality in many areas of West Africa, with case fatality about 20%.[9] Fetal loss is as much as 87%, and does not seem to vary by trimester. Lassa virus is known to be present in the breast milk of infected mothers, and neonates are therefore at risk of congenital, intrapartum, and puerperal infection with Lassa virus. Lassa fever is common in children, but may be difficult to diagnose because manifestations are so general. In very young babies marked edema has been reported. In older children the disease may manifest as diarrhea or as pneumonia or simply as an unexplained prolonged fever.

DIAGNOSIS
RT-PCR is the most rapid and accurate method for acute diagnosis and has been shown to be more sensitive even than virus isolation.[45] Virus may persist in serum into the convalescence phase and coexist with antibody, and virus has been detected in urine as many as 60 days after onset.[40] By the sixth day of Lassa illness antibodies are found in about 50% of patients. Virus is easily isolated from serum or tissues in cell culture, but this should be performed in BSL4 laboratory facilities. Virus has also been isolated from breast milk, spinal fluid, pleural and pericardial transudate, placenta, and from autopsy material, and may be recovered intermittently for 1 to 2 months in urine. Neutralizing antibodies to Lassa virus are absent in the serum of patients at the beginning of convalescence, and in most people they are never detectable.

Viral protein may be detected by monoclonal antibodies in tissue imprints (usually liver) on a microscope slide or using ELISA techniques. Efforts to detect antigen in conjunctival scrapings, buffy coat preparations, cells from pharyngeal aspirates, and urinary sediment have not been successful.

SPECIFIC TREATMENT
Ribavirin is effective in treating acute Lassa fever and should be given as early as possible.[40,46] A five- to tenfold decrease in the case fatality ratio was demonstrated in patients treated with ribavirin compared with untreated patients when therapy was given within the first 6 days of illness. Treatment later in disease is effective, but less so.

PREVENTION
Avoidance of contact with rodent urine and with blood and tissues from infected rodents is an obvious precaution in the field. In the hospital, spread of Lassa virus is by blood-to-blood contact and can be prevented by simple barrier precautions.[8] The importance of awareness by medical teams of the possibility of Lassa fever in patients in or from endemic areas cannot be overemphasized.[47] Complete support should not be denied because of the suspected diagnosis. Carefully conducted intensive care or surgery by informed and trained personnel using maximum precautions (double gloves, educated staff, limited theater personnel) does not carry major risks.

SOUTH AMERICAN HEMORRHAGIC FEVER VIRUSES

The New World arenaviruses causing human disease are Junin (Argentine hemorrhagic fever; AHF), Machupo (Bolivian hemorrhagic fever, BHF), Guanarito (Venezuelan hemorrhagic fever; VHF), and Sabia (Brazilian hemorrhagic fever). All are endemic in geographically limited areas, but new, related viruses may emerge in other yet unstudied areas. The major rodent hosts are *Calomys* species, and the viruses are related to numerous other nonpathogenic arenaviruses from South American rodents ("Tacaribe complex").

Argentine hemorrhagic fever was first recognized in the 1950s in the fertile farmland of northwestern Buenos Aires Province in Argentina, and Junin virus was first isolated in 1958. By 1990 about 21,000 cases had been reported over 30 years, but with the recent introduction of a live attenuated vaccine, this disease has diminished. Before the introduction of the vaccine, the disease was seasonal with peaks each May. The major routes of virus transmission to humans is probably through virus-infected dust and grain products, possibly from mechanical harvesters. There is no recorded person-to-person spread.

CLINICAL AND LABORATORY FEATURES
The South American hemorrhagic fevers are similar in presentation, although Guanarito may more closely resemble

Lassa fever.[48] After an incubation period of about 12 days there is insidious onset of malaise, high fever, severe myalgia, anorexia, lumbar pain, epigastric pain and abdominal tenderness, conjunctivitis, and retro-orbital pain, often with photophobia and constipation. Nausea and vomiting frequently occur after 2 or 3 days of illness. There is no lymphadenopathy or splenomegaly, sore throat or cough, but there is marked erythema of the face, neck, and thorax and conjunctivitis. Petechiae may be observed in the axillae by the fourth or fifth days of the illness. There may be a pharyngeal enanthem, but pharyngitis is uncommon. Relative bradycardia is often observed.

The second stage of illness begins with epistaxis, hematemesis, or acute neurologic disease. In contrast to the relative infrequency of bleeding in Lassa fever, the South American diseases are associated with hemorrhagic manifestations in nearly half of the patients, manifest as gingival hemorrhages, epistaxis, metrorrhagia, petechiae, ecchymoses, purpura, melena, or hematuria. Hypotensive shock, hypothermia, and pulmonary edema precede death. Renal failure has been reported. There is some electrocardiographic evidence of myocarditis. Fifty percent of AHF and BHF patients also have neurologic symptoms during the second stage of illness, such as tremors of the hands and tongue, progressing in some patients to delirium, oculogyrus, and strabismus. Meningeal signs and cerebrospinal fluid abnormalities are rare.

A low white blood cell count, under $1000/\mu$L, and a platelet count under $10,000/\mu$L are invariable. Bleeding and clot retraction times are concomitantly prolonged, although DIC is apparently not a significant feature. Proteinuria is common, and microscopic hematuria also occurs. Liver and renal function tests are only mildly abnormal. Mortality is about 16% in laboratory-confirmed hospitalized patients with untreated AHF. There are no estimates of overall mortality from population-based surveys.

A late neurologic syndrome has been described in AHF, consisting mainly of cerebellar signs, and associated with high-titer antiserum used in treatment in about 10% of cases.[49] The syndrome begins between 4 and 6 weeks after onset of acute illness and lasts less than a week. It is characterized by fever, headache, ataxia, and intention tremors, and a mild cerebrospinal fluid pleocytosis with anti-Junin virus antibody in the CSF. Most patients recover within 3 months. Mild permanent damage to acoustic centers has been detected. AHF is also reported to be severe in pregnancy, but no formal studies are available, and women are less frequently affected.

Despite the different degrees of bleeding, there are sufficient similarities between the course of disease in AHF, BHF, and Lassa fever to speculate that they share similar pathophysiologic pathways. Organ function, other than the endothelial system, appears to remain intact, and the critical period of shock is brief, lasting only 24 to 48 hours. Hepatitis is mild, and renal function is also well maintained. Bleeding is more pronounced with AHF and BHF than Lassa fever, but it is not the cause of shock and death. Capillary leakage is significant, with loss of protein and intravascular volume being much more pronounced than loss of red cells.

In marked contrast to Lassa fever, the antibody response to Junin virus is effective in clearing virus during acute disease and may also be sufficient to protect against infection. Neutralizing antibody may be detectable at the time the patient begins to recover from the acute illness, and the therapeutic efficacy of immune plasma in patients with Junin infection is directly associated with the titer of neutralizing antibody in the plasma given.

DIAGNOSIS

RT-PCR is the most rapid and accurate method of acute diagnosis. The IFA may be positive by the end of the second week of illness. Neutralizing and complement-fixing antibody to Junin are usually detectable 3 to 4 weeks after onset. IgM is more difficult to read by IFA, and an ELISA system may be preferred. Virus may also be cultured from serum, but this should be performed in Biosafety Level 4 conditions.

SPECIFIC TREATMENT

In contrast to Lassa fever, convalescent-phase plasma has been shown to be highly successful in Argentine hemorrhagic fever, reducing the mortality from 16% to 1% in patients treated in the first 8 days of illness.[49] Efficacy is directly related to the concentration of neutralizing antibodies. Late initiation of therapy is less successful. Availability of appropriately screened plasma may be a problem. Ribavirin may also be effective in treating South American hemorrhagic fever.

PREVENTION

The human-rodent encounter resulting in AHF occurs during the crop harvests, and there are no means of controlling feral rodents. A successful live attenuated vaccine, Candid 1, for AHF has now undergone phase III studies, and is in use in the endemic area of Argentina, where it has almost eliminated the disease. The vaccine has proved safe in large-scale trials, and has a protective efficacy of 84%.[50]

Filoviruses

Human infections with filoviruses are exceedingly rare, but their occurrence has invariably been dramatic and mysterious.[51] The first appearance was in Marburg in 1967. There were 7 deaths among 32 infected laboratory technicians, medical personnel, animal care personnel, and relatives. Primary cases had been exposed to tissues and blood from African green monkeys imported into Germany and Yugoslavia from Uganda. A unique virus was isolated from these with a strange looped and branched filamentous form, hence named *filovirus.* In 1976 and 1979, epidemics of a hemorrhagic disease with very high mortality in northern Zaire and in southern Sudan were found to result from two strains of a related yet distinct filovirus, named Ebola virus after a river in Zaire.

At first thought related to rhabdoviruses, it has become clear that these viruses form a family of their own, now designated *filoviridae.* Nucleotide sequence analyses now place the family in the order mononegavirales, which also includes the paramyxoviridae (e.g., respiratory syncytial virus) and rhabdoviridae (such as rabies). Filoviruses are among the largest known viruses, with highly variable length (up to 14,000 nm), but uniform 80-nm diameter, with a helical nucleocapsid, consisting of a central axis 20 to 30 nm in diameter. The virions contain a single negative-strand RNA genome.

EPIDEMIOLOGY

Since the 1967 Marburg outbreak, there have been three further, isolated, primary human Marburg infections (and only two secondary cases), all in adventurous expatriates in remote parts of Africa. In the late 1990s, epidemics in eastern Congo (formerly Zaire) were traced to miners entering disused, partially flooded gold mines. These outbreaks may be ongoing, but the civil disturbances in the area have made it impossible to get accurate information. Between 1976 and 1979 three separate major outbreaks of Ebola occurred in northern Zaire and the southern Sudan.[52,53] In each instance, early index cases were rapidly followed by dissemination, mainly in hospitals and clinics, where reuse of needles for injection and exposure of staff to blood were strongly implicated in transmission. Case mortality ranged from 53% to 88%.

Ebola disappeared after 1979, only to re-emerge in 1994 in Kikwit, Zaire, again amplified in a hospital. The outbreak involved some 315 confirmed cases, among whom 244 died (77% fatality).[54,55] The virus from the Kikwit outbreak is apparently identical to the 1976 Zaire strain of Ebola. In 1994 a Swiss animal researcher reported 30 deaths in monkeys due to Ebola in the Ivorial rainforest bordering Liberia, and in 1996, 27 cases were reported from Gabon with 18 deaths (67% fatality) in humans. In this last outbreak, 12 of the fatalities had had direct contact with the blood of a dead chimpanzee.[56]

Person-to-person spread has been the major mode of transmission in epidemics. Contact with patients ill with Ebola is the most important factor in determining risk of illness. Other risk factors associated with human-to-human transmission are infection from contaminated materials such as needles, contact with blood or secretions, preparation of a body for burial, or occasionally, sexual contact. Close contact with blood or tissues of infected monkeys is also important.[56] The virus enters through mucous membranes or skin lesions, and outbreaks have been abruptly terminated when blood transmission was interrupted.[57] Relatively frequent epidemics of Ebola Zaire in Gabon and the Congo, Ebola Sudan in Uganda, and Marburg in eastern Congo have been reported, and several outbreaks of Ebola Zaire are ongoing, and apparently closely linked to a major epizootic in great apes. This Ebola epizootic, combined with hunting and loss of habitat, is now thought to threaten chimpanzees and gorillas in the area with extinction.[58]

CLINICAL AND LABORATORY FEATURES

The incubation period is 3 to 12 days, 3 to 7 days for needle transmission, and 6 to 12 days for person-to-person spread. The illness:infection ratio for Marburg and Ebola viruses approaches unity, since few if any asymptomatic infections have ever been observed.

The disease caused by the African filoviruses is dramatic.[52,53,59,60] Onset is abrupt with fever, severe headache (usually periorbital and frontal), myalgia, arthralgia, conjunctivitis, and extreme malaise. Sore throat is a common symptom, often associated with severe swelling and dysphagia, but no exudative pharyngitis. A papular, eventually desquamating rash may occur in some patients, especially on the trunk and back; a morbilliform rash has been observed on white skin. Gastrointestinal symptoms develop in most patients on the second or third day of illness with abdominal pain, cramping, diarrhea, and vomiting. Jaundice is not a feature of Marburg or Ebola disease. Persistence of vomiting and the onset of any signs of mucosal bleeding carry a high risk of fatal outcome. Bleeding begins about the fifth day of illness and is most commonly from the mucous membranes, gastrointestinal tract, gingiva, nasopharynx, and vagina. The most profound physiologic alteration is shock (manifested by hypotension, effusions, and facial edema), which is invariably fatal. Severe, acute fluid loss often with frank bleeding into the tissue and into the gut results in dehydration, and electrolyte and acid-base imbalance. Infection in pregnancy results in high maternal fatality and virtually 100% fetal death. CNS involvement has led to hemiplegia and disorientation and sometimes frank psychosis. Even in convalescence patients show prolonged weakness and severe weight loss, and in a few survivors serious but reversible personality changes are recorded, namely confusion, anxiety, and aggressive behavior.

Thrombocytopenia is invariable, but bleeding is not usually of sufficient volume to account for the shock, nor is it associated with solid evidence of DIC in the small number of animals or humans studied so far. Platelet dysfunction has also been described in experimentally infected nonhuman primates. Profound lymphopenia early in disease is accompanied by marked neutrophilia. Laboratory evidence of moderate DIC appears only in the terminal stages. Liver enzymes (SGOT and SGPT) are raised, but the rise in SGOT is disproportionately higher than SGPT, as in Marburg disease.

At autopsy there is widespread hemorrhagic diathesis into body cavities, membranes, and soft tissue, with focal necrosis in liver, lymph nodes, ovaries, and testis. Most prominent are eosinophilic inclusion bodies in hepatocytes (Councilmanlike), without significant inflammatory response.

Very little is understood about the immunology of Ebola virus infections except for the observation, made many years ago, that neutralizing antibodies are difficult to demonstrate in both humans and primates, and that like many zoonotic viruses, notably Lassa virus and now the severe acute respiratory syndrome (SARS) human coronavirus, Ebola virus appears to be able to circulate in humans in the presence of detectable antibody and to show varying ability to persist at least for short periods following acute infection. Nevertheless protection must be achieved, since reactivation disease should have been observed by now, were it occurring. Studies using specimens from patients in Gabon have shown that the innate immune system plays a very important role in disease.[61] Evidence from these studies and from animal studies suggest that the proinflammatory response is a central figure both in pathogenesis of severe disease and in protection from disease, in that an early, orderly innate immune response was observed in infected individuals who never developed disease.[62] Conversely primate studies have shown that infection of monocuclear phagocytes is critical, and that these trigger a cascade of cytokines/chemokines and oxygen free radicals, and that it is this process, not direct viral replication destroying critical cells, which lead to the manifestations of disease. These manifestations are associated with massive intravascular apoptosis.[61,63]

DIAGNOSIS

RT-PCR is the method of choice for acute diagnosis of Ebola hemorrhagic fever.[64] Extreme care should be taken in both drawing and handling blood specimens, since virus titer may be extremely high, and the virus is stable for long periods even at room temperature. High- or rising-titer filovirus-specific IgG is diagnostic, as is the presence of IgM by ELISA or IFA. Patients may die, however, before developing detectable antibodies. Virus may be isolated and identified within 2 to 3 days if suitable facilities are available. An antigen detection ELISA system is also used, but is less sensitive than RT-PCR.[64] Antigen may also be detected in biopsies, including skin.[65] Unexplained, nonspecific reactions in antibody assays (sometimes up to 15% of sera), particularly with IFA, have plagued serologic studies.

SPECIFIC TREATMENT

Patients will require full intensive care support, including mechanical ventilation, along with blood, plasma, or platelet replacement. Provided strict barrier precautions are observed, intensive care should not be denied and may be life saving. Every effort is justified, since the crisis is short-lived, and complete recovery can be expected in most survivors.

No antiviral therapy (including convalescent plasma, ribavirin, or related compounds) has been shown to be effective against either Marburg or Ebola virus infection in patients or in experimentally infected nonhuman primates. Suitably screened and stored human plasma is in any event unavailable. Human interferon is ineffective in vitro.

Flaviviruses

Flaviviruses are positive-strand RNA viruses, spread by mosquitoes. Yellow fever and dengue virus cause hemorrhagic disease. Dengue is the only exclusively human VHF.[66]

YELLOW FEVER

EPIDEMIOLOGY

Since it was first described in 1498, yellow fever has been a recognized scourge of West Africa, and subsequent to colonization and the slave trade, the West Indies, and Central and South America. Outbreaks in the Americas in the nineteenth century were reported as far north as Hartford, Connecticut, and frequent devastating epidemics were familiar to the southern United States. Mosquito eradication programs successfully controlled epidemics from the beginning of the twentieth century, and with the introduction of an effective vaccine in the 1930s, yellow fever became a preventable disease. Nevertheless it continues to circulate in West and Central Africa, and in the interior of South America. Large epidemics are regularly seen in Africa, particularly Nigeria and the Cameroon, in areas where for political or economic reasons vaccine coverage is low.[67]

Yellow fever virus is transmitted to humans by mosquito bite; the principal vector is *Aedes aegypti*, but other *Aedes* species are also capable of transmission. Two epidemiologic forms are recognized, sylvatic and urban. In the sylvatic cycle the virus circulates from monkey to monkey via mosquitoes, with humans occasionally being infected peripherally. Several species of monkey are involved, but in general, South American nonhuman primates are much more susceptible to disease than Old World primates, and they mostly die from the infection. In the urban form of the disease, the virus

is maintained by transmission from humans to humans by mosquito. Direct person-to-person spread has not been reported. Distribution in Africa and South America generally follows that of the equatorial rain forests. For reasons that are unclear, Asia has been spared this virus. Nevertheless, globally the disease affects more than 200,000 persons a year in endemic areas and is a significant risk to unvaccinated travelers.[68]

CLINICAL AND LABORATORY FEATURES

Though the disease has been well described in the past, there are no recent data concerning either clinical disease or pathogenesis,[66,68] relegating this fulminating disease to the neglected diseases of the poor of the developing world. The incubation period is usually 3 to 6 days. Clinical presentation varies from a nonspecific low-grade febrile disease to a fulminant hepatitis with renal failure and hemorrhage, which is usually fatal. Onset is abrupt with fever and chills, intense headache, generalized myalgia, nausea, and vomiting. High fever continues for about 3 days, with conjunctival injection, edema and hyperemia of the face and neck, and occasionally a macular or scarlatiniform rash. Then epistaxis and gum bleeding may develop, and there will be proteinuria. Some patients then deteriorate to the "yellow" phase, with jaundice, hemorrhages, violent epigastric pains, and vomiting that may become black from altered blood, the "vomito negro" from which they rarely recover. The renal syndrome progresses from oliguria to anuria. Hypotension and shock appear late. Electrocardiographic changes consist of increase in PR and QT intervals, with bradycardia accompanying high fever. Terminal phases are characterized by agitation, delirium, and convulsions, leading to coma and death. Mortality as high as 50% has been recorded in urban outbreaks in Nigeria.[67] When recovery occurs, it is complete, without sequelae.

There is generalized leukopenia and thrombocytopenia. Liver function tests show high SGOT and SGPT, but as in other VHFs, SGOT is disproportionately high. Unlike other VHFs, however, bilirubin rises rapidly and continues to be high in convalescence. Elevated bilirubin and serum aminotransferase levels reflect the severity of illness, and as in Lassa fever, are of prognostic value. In fatal cases hepatic failure contributes to the hypoglycemia and metabolic encephalopathy. Virus may be recovered from the liver, and it is likely that direct viral injury accounts for most of the observations. There is marked albuminuria and oliguria, and in severe cases renal failure may be observed. Metabolic acidosis is an important component of the terminal stages of this disease.

Bleeding is common, often with upper gastrointestinal hemorrhage. Thrombocytopenia is prominent, and prolongation of the prothrombin time, APTT, and clotting time are reported along with reduced levels of clotting factors, particularly those derived from the liver. Disseminated intravascular coagulation may be an important component of the terminal stages and may be associated with the severe hepatic injury. Unlike some other flaviviruses (e.g., West Nile virus) direct involvement of the central nervous system by this virus probably does not occur; however, metabolic encephalopathy results in agitation, mania, delirium, convulsions, and coma. There are no focal neurologic signs.

Yellow fever is by far the most hepatotropic of the VHF viruses. Histology shows the characteristic Councilman bodies, consisting of eosinophilic degeneration in mesolobular or midzonal regions. Generally the liver shows coagulative necrosis with some sparing about the centrilobular veins and portal vessels.

DIAGNOSIS

RT-PCR is the method of choice. Diagnosis is made by isolation of the virus from blood, but the virus is labile and culture may be difficult, requiring suckling mouse inoculation. Though person-to-person spread is not a feature of this disease, care should nevertheless be taken that specimens are handled by persons vaccinated against yellow fever. Serologic data are more difficult to interpret than in other VHFs because of the notorious cross-reactivity of flaviviruses, particularly in persons from endemic areas who may have encountered many of the myriad of related viruses that abound. "Original antigenic sin" is a major feature of all flavivirus infections, since infected people tend to have highest antibody titers to whichever virus was their first exposure, regardless of the virus causing their current or most recent infection. Specific IgM assays using modern ELISA techniques may be helpful, but again in patients from endemic areas pre-existing flavivirus antibody may yield confusing results. For all these reasons diagnosis of yellow fever outside the setting of a known epidemic may be difficult, and RT-PCR performed on specimens (blood or tissue) early in infection is the surest means to identify the virus. Antigen detection techniques using ELISA have also been developed, but await full evaluation.

SPECIFIC TREATMENT

Management is supportive. Yellow fever virus is not susceptible to ribavirin or to any other known antiviral agent.

PREVENTION

Prevention is by vaccination with the 17D strain of yellow fever virus, one of the oldest and most successful vaccines. This is a live attenuated vaccine. A single shot apparently provides lifelong protection, although WHO recommends validity for 10 years. The current preparation has been one of the safest vaccines in existence, with millions of doses having been given over more than 50 years. Recently there have been isolated reports of actual yellow fever–like disease following vaccination. Nevertheless, the long history of safety of the 17D strain now makes it an important candidate for insertion of other genes, particularly other flavivirus genes such as dengue and hepatitis C. Mosquito control is the ultimate control method, resulting in near complete eradication of disease, as was demonstrated in Brazil and the southern United States. However, the recent resurgence of yellow fever in Brazil that accompanied the reintroduction of *Aedes aegypti* to many areas of that country is a warning that eradication is a mirage given a zoonotic focus of the virus, and that constant surveillance is essential.

Yellow fever is one of four notifiable diseases in the international health regulations of WHO. Notification of suspected as well as confirmed cases is mandatory.

DENGUE HEMORRHAGIC FEVER

Dengue virus infection is frequently asymptomatic or a mild febrile illness. However, dengue hemorrhagic fever (DHF) usually occurs in children less than 15 years of age and in some circumstances in adults. There are four dengue virus serotypes, and DHF is apparently due to infection with a second serotype, though in outbreaks due to newly introduced virus in nonimmune populations, fulminant hemorrhagic disease may be seen in young adults. It is hypothesized that the replication of the second infecting serotype is enhanced by pre-existing antibody at suboptimal levels, but this remains controversial.[66]

The epidemiology of dengue is recent, dating back to the Second World War. Whether it was the disruption of this war which allowed the virus to spread, or more likely the rapid and explosive population increases and development of large urban areas and megacities is unclear. However, the end result is clear: dengue is endemic in the cities and the countryside of Southeast Asia and has spread widely east and south to Africa and even threatens Australia.[69] Deterioration of urban environments with crowding and mosquito infestation also favors the virus. Reintroduction of dengue has now been documented in Central and South America including Brazil, Ecuador, Bolivia, Peru, Venezuela, and many Caribbean islands. It has also been reintroduced into the Pacific. Epidemics are reported each year from Central and South America, and cases are now seen in south Texas. The potential for further spread is great, particularly in the southern United States and more widely in South America. The disease must be considered in febrile travelers from all the affected areas, which now includes most of the tropical regions of the world and many subtropical regions. Unlike yellow fever, the natural history is a cycle involving only mosquito and human, the main vector for its spread is humans, but still it has proved difficult to control given the ubiquity of both mosquito and human hosts.

Large epidemics occur, often annually in all endemic areas. In areas where the virus has been recently reintroduced the most severe disease may be in adults, but in Southeast Asia, DHF is a disease of young children, thousands of whom are affected annually. Epidemics tend to occur in the hot rainy season. The vector is *Aedes aegypti,* but *Aedes albopictus* has also been implicated. *Aedes* prefer to breed in clean cool water, and in Southeast Asia are abundant in drinking water pots kept in the shade. Intercontinental trade in used tires containing moisture was thought to be responsible for the recent introduction of *Aedes albopictus* in the United States, but no disease or indeed presence of virus has been demonstrated in association with these tires.

CLINICAL AND LABORATORY FEATURES

The incubation period is 2 to 10 days. Onset is abrupt, with fever, severe headache, and a combination of myalgia, backache, photophobia, and retro-orbital pain, accompanied by anorexia and vomiting. Most patients then recover uneventfully, but some may progress to dengue hemorrhagic fever or dengue shock syndrome (DSS). These conditions are characterized by low platelet counts, petechiae, and hypovolemic shock. This is normally of short duration and self-limiting, but a few patients may deteriorate and die with pulmonary edema or intracranial bleeding. Patients may also have marginally raised liver function tests, with SGOT levels higher than SGPT levels.

The cardinal signs of dengue hemorrhagic fever are shock, with narrow pulse pressure and petechiae. Hepatic involvement is variable. There is often severe thrombocytopenia and marked intravascular volume depletion with edema as in HFRS. During the acute phase there is lymphopenia. Serous effusions are common. These are transudates with high albumin content. Endothelial cell biopsies show swelling of endothelial cells, with enlarged endothelial gaps in some sections, but no necrosis of cells themselves. Indeed since most patients recover promptly, responding to careful fluid management, it must be assumed that the increased permeability is the result of some acute metabolic or biochemical dysfunction.

The pathogenesis of DHF has been the subject of much debate. Various studies have reported complement consumption, activation of the plasma kinin system, circulating immune complexes, leukopenia, depression of T-cell function, increased natural killer cell activity, or interferon-γ production by dengue-stimulated T lymphoctyes. It has been suggested that an initial infection with one type of dengue virus, followed by a second infection with another serotype, induces an immune response resulting in enhancement of virus entry into monocytic cells where it replicates. This observation, which has been under consideration for decades, still remains controversial.

DIAGNOSIS

Serologic diagnosis is difficult to interpret, again because of cross-reactions with pre-existing flavivirus antibodies, particularly in endemic areas. The RT-PCR detecting dengue virus RNA in serum or white cells is likely to be the most practical approach where it is available and affordable. IgM assays may be useful in identifying acute infection. Identification of the specific virus type is difficult by antibody or antigen detection methods, and may require virus isolation. However, this information is principally of importance for epidemiologic evaluation of epidemic and endemic behavior of the viruses.

SPECIFIC TREATMENT

Management of DHF and DSS is supportive. Dengue virus is not susceptible to ribavirin or to any other antiviral agent.

References

1. Hirabayashi Y, Oka S, Goto H, et al: An imported case of Lassa fever with late appearance of polyserositis. *J Infect Dis* 158:872, 1998.
2. Kibadi K, Mupapa K, Kuvula K, et al: Late ophthalmologic manifestations in survivors of the 1995 Ebola virus epidemic in Kikwit, Democratic Republic of the Congo. *J Infect Dis* 179(Suppl 1):S13-4, 1999.
3. Centers for Disease Control and Prevention: Management of patients with suspected viral hemorrhagic fever. *Morb Mortal Wkly Rep* 37:S1, 1988.
4. Chen HX, Qiu FX, Dong BJ, et al: Epidemiological studies on hemorrhagic fever with renal syndrome in China. *J Infect Dis* 154:394, 1986.
5. Management of patients with suspected viral hemorrhagic fever. *Morb Mortal Wkly Rep* 37(Suppl 3):1–16, 1988.
6. Fisher Hoch SP, Tomori O, Nasidi A, et al: Review of cases of nosocomial Lassa fever in Nigeria: The high price of poor medical practice. *BMJ* 311:857, 1995.
7. Burney MI, Ghafoor A, Saleen M, et al: Nosocomial outbreak of viral hemorrhagic fever caused by Crimean Hemorrhagic fever-Congo virus in Pakistan, January 1976. *Am J Trop Med Hyg* 29:941, 1980.
8. Fisher Hoch SP, Price ME, Craven RB, et al: Safe intensive-care management of a severe case of Lassa fever with simple barrier nursing techniques. *Lancet* 2:1227, 1985.
9. Price ME, Fisher Hoch SP, Craven RB, McCormick JB: A prospective study of maternal and fetal outcome in acute Lassa fever infection during pregnancy. *BMJ* 297:584, 1988.
10. Morikawa S, Qing T, Xinqin Z, et al: Genetic diversity of the mRNA segment among Crimean-Congo hemorrhagic fever virus isolates in China. *Virology* 296:159, 2002.
11. Yashina L, Petrova I, Seregin S, V et al: Genetic variability of Crimean-Congo haemorrhagic fever virus in Russia and Central Asia. *J Gen Virol* 84(Pt 5):1199, 2003.
12. Dunster L, Dunster M, Ofula V, et al: First documentation of human Crimean-Congo hemorrhagic fever, Kenya. *Emerg Infect Dis* 8:1005, 2002.
13. Papa A, Bozovi B, Pavlidou V, et al: Genetic detection and isolation of crimean-congo hemorrhagic fever virus, Kosovo, Yugoslavia. *Emerg Infect Dis* 8:852, 2002.
14. Chapman LE, Wilson ML, Hall DB, et al: Risk factors for Crimean-Congo hemorrhagic fever in rural northern Senegal. *J Infect Dis* 164:686, 1991.
15. Fisher Hoch SP, McCormick JB, Swanepoel R, et al: Risk of human infections with Crimean-Congo hemorrhagic fever virus in a South African rural community. *Am J Trop Med Hyg* 47:337, 1992.
16. Fisher Hoch SP, Khan JA, Rehman S, et al: Crimean Congo-haemorrhagic fever treated with oral ribavirin. *Lancet* 346:472, 1995.
17. Khan AS, Maupin GO, Rollin PE, et al: An outbreak of Crimean-Congo hemorrhagic fever in the United Arab Emirates, 1994–1995. *Am J Trop Med Hyg* 57:519, 1997.
18. Papa A, Bino S, Llagami A, et al: Crimean-Congo hemorrhagic fever in Albania, 2001. *Eur J Clin Microbiol Infect Dis* 21:603, 2002.
19. Scrimgeour EM, Zaki A, Mehta FR, et al: Crimean-Congo haemorrhagic fever in Oman. *Trans R Soc Trop Med Hyg* 90:290, 1996.
20. Taverne J: Tick-borne haemorrhagic fever in Iran. *Trends Parasitol* 18:344, 2002.
21. Swanepoel R, Leham P, Abbott JC, et al: Epidemiology, diagnosis, clinical pathology and treatment of Crimean Congo hemorrhagic fever (CCHF) in South Africa. Proceedings and Abstracts of the VIIth International Congress of Virology, Berlin, 1990. Abstract
22. Saijo M, Qing T, Niikura M, et al: Recombinant nucleoprotein-based enzyme-linked immunosorbent assay for detection of immunoglobulin G antibodies to Crimean-Congo hemorrhagic fever virus. *J Clin Microbiol* 40:1587, 2002.
23. Duchin JS, Koster FT, Peters CJ, et al: Hantavirus pulmonary syndrome: a clinical description of 17 patients with a newly recognized disease. The Hantavirus Study Group [see comments]. *N Engl J Med* 330:949, 1994.
24. Khan A, Khan AS: Hantaviruses: a tale of two hemispheres. *Panminerva Med* 45:43, 2003.
25. Jonsson CB, Schmaljohn CS: Replication of hantaviruses. *Curr Top Microbiol Immunol* 256:15, 2001.
26. Vitek CR, Breiman RF, Ksiazek TG, et al: Evidence against person-to-person transmission of hantavirus to health care workers. *Clin Infect Dis* 22:824, 1996.
27. Khan AS, Young JC: Hantavirus pulmonary syndrome: At the crossroads. *Curr Opin Infect Dis* 14:205, 2001.
28. Young JC, Hansen GR, Graves TK, et al: The incubation period of hantavirus pulmonary syndrome. *Am J Trop Med Hyg* 62:714, 2000.
29. Mori M, Rothman AL, Kurane I, et al: High levels of cytokine-producing cells in the lung tissues of patients with fatal hantavirus pulmonary syndrome. *J Infect Dis* 179:295, 1999.
30. McElroy AK, Bray M, Reed DS, Schmaljohn CS: Andes virus infection of cynomolgus macaques. *J Infect Dis* 186:1706, 2002.
31. Huggins JW, Hsiang CM, Cosgriff TM, et al: Prospective, double-blind, concurrent, placebo-controlled clinical trial of intravenous ribavirin therapy of hemorrhagic fever with renal syndrome. *J Infect Dis* 164:1119, 1991.

32. Chapman LE, Mertz GJ, Peters CJ, et al: Intravenous ribavirin for hantavirus pulmonary syndrome: Safety and tolerance during 1 year of open-label experience. Ribavirin Study Group. *Antivir Ther* 4:211, 1999.

33. McCormick JB, Webb PA, Krebs JW, et al: A prospective study of the epidemiology and ecology of Lassa fever. *J Infect Dis* 155:437, 1987.

34. McCormick JB, King IJ, Webb PA, et al: A case-control study of the clinical diagnosis and course of Lassa fever. *J Infect Dis* 155:445, 1987.

35. Monath TP, Mertens PE, Patton R, et al: A hospital epidemic of Lassa fever in Zorzor, Liberia, March-April 1972. *Am J Trop Med Hyg* 22:773, 1973.

36. Allan R, Ladbury R, Skinner K, Mardel S: Emergence of epidemic Lassa fever during civil conflict in Sierra Leone. International Conference on Emerging Infectious Diseases [P21.16], 134. 1998. Abstract.

37. Lassa fever, imported case, Netherlands [news]. *Wkly Epidemiol Rec* 75:256, 2000.

38. Lassa fever imported to England. *Commun Dis Rep CDR Wkly* 10:99, 2000.

39. Cooper CB, Gransden WR, Webster M, et al: A case of Lassa fever: experience at St Thomas's Hospital. *Br Med J Clin Res Ed* 285:1003, 1982.

40. Johnson KM, McCormick JB, Webb PA, et al: Clinical virology of Lassa fever in hospitalized patients. *J Infect Dis* 155:456, 1987.

41. Cummins D, Bennett D, Fisher Hoch SP, et al: Electrocardiographic abnormalities in patients with Lassa fever. *J Trop Med Hyg* 92:350, 1989.

42. Cummins D, Fisher Hoch SP, Walshe KJ, et al: A plasma inhibitor of platelet aggregation in patients with Lassa fever. *Br J Haematol* 72:543, 1989.

43. Cummins D, McCormick JB, Bennett D, et al: Acute sensorineural deafness in Lassa fever [see comments]. *JAMA* 264:2093, 1990.

44. Cummins D, Bennett D, Fisher Hoch SP, et al: Lassa fever encephalopathy: Clinical and laboratory findings. *J Trop Med Hyg* 95:197, 1992.

45. Trappier SG, Conaty AL, Farrar BB, et al: Evaluation of the polymerase chain reaction for diagnosis of Lassa virus infection. *Am J Trop Med Hyg* 49:214, 1993.

46. McCormick JB, King IJ, Webb PA, et al: Lassa fever. Effective therapy with ribavirin. *N Engl J Med* 314:20, 1986.

47. Holmes GP, McCormick JB, Trock SC, et al: Lassa fever in the United States. Investigation of a case and new guidelines for management [see comments]. *N Engl J Med* 323:1120, 1990.

48. Maiztegui JI: Clinical and epidemiological patterns of Argentine haemorrhagic fever. *Bull World Health Organ* 52:567, 1975.

49. Enria DA, Briggiler AM, Fernandez NJ, et al: Importance of dose of neutralising antibodies in treatment of Argentine haemorrhagic fever with immune plasma. *Lancet* 2:255, 1984.

50. Maiztegui JI, McKee KT Jr, Barrera Oro JG, et al: Protective efficacy of a live attenuated vaccine against Argentine hemorrhagic fever. AHF Study Group. *J Infect Dis* 177:277, 1998.

51. Fisher-Hoch SP, McCormick JB: Filoviruses, in Zuckerman AJ (ed): *Principles and Practices of Clinical Virology.* Chichester, John Wiley and Sons, (in press).

52. Ebola haemorrhagic fever in Zaire, 1976. *Bull World Health Organ* 56:271, 1978.

53. Ebola haemorrhagic fever in Sudan, 1976. Report of a WHO/International Study Team. *Bull World Health Organ* 56:247, 1978.

54. Khan AS, Tshioko FK, Heymann DL, et al: The reemergence of Ebola hemorrhagic fever, Democratic Republic of the Congo, 1995. Commission de Lutte contre les Epidemies a Kikwit. *J Infect Dis* 179(Suppl 1):S76, 1999.

55. Bwaka MA, Bonnet MJ, Calain P, et al: Ebola hemorrhagic fever in Kikwit, Democratic Republic of the Congo: Clinical observations in 103 patients. *J Infect Dis* 179(Suppl 1):S1, 1999.

56. Georges AJ, Leroy EM, Renaut AA, et al: Ebola hemorrhagic fever outbreaks in Gabon, 1994–1997: Epidemiologic and health control issues. *J Infect Dis* 179(Suppl 1):S65, 1999.

57. Muyembe-Tamfum JJ, Kipasa M, Kiyungu C, Colebunders R: Ebola outbreak in Kikwit, Democratic Republic of the Congo: Discovery and control measures. *J Infect Dis* 179(Suppl 1):S259, 1999.

58. Kaiser J: Conservation biology. Ebola, hunting push ape populations to the brink. *Science* 300:232, 2003.

59. Ndambi R, Akamituna P, Bonnet MJ, et al: Epidemiologic and clinical aspects of the Ebola virus epidemic in Mosango, Democratic Republic of the Congo, 1995. *J Infect Dis* 179(Suppl 1):S8, 1999.

60. Rowe AK, Bertolli J, Khan AS, et al: Clinical, virologic, and immunologic follow-up of convalescent Ebola hemorrhagic fever patients and their household contacts, Kikwit, Democratic Republic of the Congo. Commission de Lutte contre les Epidemies a Kikwit. *J Infect Dis* 179(Suppl 1):S28, 1999.

61. Baize S, Leroy EM, Georges-Courbot MC, et al: Defective humoral responses and extensive intravascular apoptosis are associated with fatal outcome in Ebola virus-infected patients. *Nat Med* 5:423, 1999.

62. Leroy EM, Baize S, Volchkov VE, et al: Human asymptomatic Ebola infection and strong inflammatory response. *Lancet* 355:2210, 2000.

63. Hensley LE, Young HA, Jahrling PB, Geisbert TW: Proinflammatory response during Ebola virus infection of primate models: possible involvement of the tumor necrosis factor receptor superfamily. *Immunol Lett* 80:169, 2002.

64. Leroy EM, Baize S, Lu CY, et al: Diagnosis of Ebola haemorrhagic fever by RT-PCR in an epidemic setting. *J Med Virol* 60:463, 2000.

65. Zaki SR, Shieh WJ, Greer PW, et al: A novel immunohistochemical assay for the detection of Ebola virus in skin: Implications for diagnosis, spread, and surveillance of Ebola hemorrhagic fever. Commission de Lutte contre les Epidemies a Kikwit. *J Infect Dis* 179(Suppl 1):S36, 1999.

66. Monath TP, Heinz FX: Flaviviruses, in Fields BN, Knipe DM, Howley PM (eds): *Fields' Virology.* Philadelphia, Lippincott-Raven, 1996, p 961.

67. De Cock KM, Monath TP, Nasidi A, et al: Epidemic yellow fever in eastern Nigeria, 1986. *Lancet* 1:630, 1988.

68. Monath TP: Yellow fever: An update. *Lancet Infect Dis* 1:11, 2001.

69. Innis BL: Dengue and dengue hemorrhagic fever, in Porterfield JS (ed):. *Exotic Viral Infections.* London, Chapman and Hall, 1995, p 103.

Chapter 61

BIOWARFARE AGENTS

MANOJ KARWA
RAGHU S. LOGANATHAN
VLADIMIR KVETAN

KEY POINTS

- *Unlike other mass casualty events, mass exposure to a biological agent is unlikely to be realized until cases start presenting and a high degree of suspicion is needed to realize this.*
- *Specific knowledge of the various types of agents is required to help in the diagnosis and management.*
- *Victims of class A agents such as plague, anthrax, botulinum toxin, smallpox, and viral hemorrhagic fever are likely to be critically ill and in need of the expertise of intensivists.*
- *Preparedness for a mass casualty event is key in dealing with effective care of patients in the hospital setting, containment of spread of particularly virulent organisms, and controlling public hysteria.*

Since the terrorist attacks of September 11, 2001, and the distribution of mail containing anthrax spores that led to seven deaths in the U.S., the threat of a large-scale bioterrorist attack has become very real.[1] A recent report by the Monterey Institute for International Studies found a total of 121 biocrimes were committed since 1960, with a reported sharp rise since 1995.[2] Reports of biological agent stockpiles and their weaponization by Iraq and the former Soviet Union, as well as the use of various biological agents by cult organizations such as the Rajneesh cult, Aum Shinrikyo, and Minnesota Patriots make the possibility of their use by a rogue nation or nonmilitary organization a very real one.

Attack of a civilian target would cause a large number of casualties, panic, and civil disruption. There would be a rapid overwhelming of public health facilities and capabilities.[3–5] It is highly likely that many if not the majority of patients would need some degree of critical care such as a ventilator or hemodynamic support. Thus the critical care physician's role could be a central one that depends on specific knowledge of the various agents, and preattack preparedness, the two cornerstones in dealing with such a catastrophe. The main objectives of this chapter are to provide a concise review of individual agents likely to be used in a bioterrorist attack, and focus on key issues related to the intensivist in preparing to deal with such an event.

The Centers for Disease Control and Prevention's strategic planning workgroup categorizes biological warfare agents into groups A, B, and C, based on capability to cause illness or death, stability of the agent, ease of delivery, ease of mass production, person-to-person transmissibility, potential for creating public fear and civil disruption, and the ability of the public health systems to deal with such an attack.[6] Category A agents would have the greatest impact on public health and its infrastructure. Category B agents would have less impact on the public health and its infrastructure. Category C agents are least likely to impact on the public health and include various emerging infectious agents.[6,7] This list is not definitive and serves only as a guideline for preparation for a bioterrorist attack (Table 61-1).

Recognition of a bioterrorist attack would require prompt identification based on typical clinical syndromes, since awaiting laboratory confirmation of these otherwise rare illnesses might be delayed. Certain epidemiologic features peculiar to a bioterrorist attack help distinguish it from a natural outbreak of disease as outlined in Table 61-2.[8,9]

Because of the greater absorption surface area of the alveolar bed, a biological weapon is more likely to be delivered via an aerosol spray or a cloud. This would require an agent to be aerosolized into droplets or particle sizes of 1 to 5 μm in diameter in order to reach and be absorbed via the alveolar bed. Particles >5 to 10 μm would be filtered out by or deposited into the upper respiratory tract. However, many viruses like influenza, viral hemorrhagic fevers, and smallpox can be infective at these sites.[10–12] Aerosol delivery of an agent would also give rise to unusual presentations of diseases such as inhalational anthrax and pneumonic plague.

A bioterrorist attack through the contamination of food and water is less likely for several reasons. Most category A agents are not transmitted via food and water, while category B agents that can be transmitted by these routes usually cause short-term vomiting and diarrhea with a relatively quick recovery. Current water treatment methods effectively kill many biological agents and contaminating a water or food supply effectively would require large amounts of toxin and bacteria in order to overcome any dilution factor. Furthermore, boiling water and cooking food destroys most agents. A recent study warns of the United States' vulnerability to such an attack based on very centralized food processing methods and distribution of the foods over large areas. Likely agents are botulinum toxin, *Salmonella, Shigella, Escherichia coli,* and *Vibrio cholerae.*[13]

Contact with intact skin with any of these agents is unlikely to result in disease. However, if the skin integrity is compromised, the potential for disease exists. Current studies suggest that thorough washing with soap and water is sufficient to overcome even this threat.

Anthrax

Bacillus anthracis is a gram-positive spore-forming bacterium. It is an encapsulated, nonmotile, and nonhemolytic organism, and usually grows within 6 to 24 hours on conventional culture media. The vegetative form is incapable of surviving outside of a warm-blooded host, and colony counts are undetectable in water after 24 hours. As a biological weapon it is likely to be delivered as an aerosol. Clinically this would produce inhalational anthrax, the deadliest and rarest form of the disease.[14] The cutaneous form is not considered lethal with current antibiotic regimens, and the gastrointestinal form is exceedingly rare with essentially no cases having been reported in the U.S.[15,16]

Inhalational anthrax occurs after spores are ingested by alveolar macrophages and transported via regional lymphatics to mediastinal lymph nodes. Germination takes place in 2 to 5 days, but can be delayed as much as 60 days, after which disease rapidly occurs.[1,16,17] The major virulence factors are the antiphagocytic capsule and three toxin components (lethal factor, edema factor, and protective antigen).[18] The

TABLE 61-1 Categorization of Potential Biological Agents

Biological Agent	Disease
Category A	
Variola major	Smallpox
Bacillus anthracis	Anthrax
Yersinia pestis	Plague
Clostridium botulinum (botulinum toxin)	Botulism
Francisella tularensis	Tularemia
Filoviruses and arenaviruses (e.g., Ebola virus, Lassa virus)	Viral hemorrhagic fevers
Category B	
Coxiella burnetii	Q fever
Brucella spp.	Brucellosis
Burkholderia mallei	Glanders
Burkholderia pseudomallei	Melioidosis
Alphaviruses (VEE, EEE, WEE)	Encephalitis
Rickettsia prowazekii	Typhus fever
Toxins (e.g., ricin, staphylococcal enterotoxin B)	Toxic syndromes
Chlamydia psittaci	Psittacosis
Food safety threats (e.g., *Salmonella* spp., *Escherichia coli* O157:H7)	
Water safety threats (e.g., *Vibrio cholerae*, *Cryptosporidium parvum*)	
Category C	
Emerging threat agents (e.g., Nipah virus, hantavirus)	

ABBREVIATIONS: EEE, eastern equine encephalomyelitis; VEE, Venezuelan equine encephalomyelitis; WEE, western equine encephalomyelitis.
SOURCE: Reproduced with permission from Rotz et al.[6]

three toxins cause edema, hemorrhage, and necrosis, producing a thoracic lymphadenitis and hemorrhagic mediastinitis. Death can occur despite antibiotic administration if toxin levels have reached a critical threshold.

Clinically anthrax presents as a biphasic illness. The first stage is characterized by nonspecific symptoms of fever, chills, weakness, headache, vomiting, abdominal pain, dyspnea, cough, and chest pain, lasting for hours up to a few days.[1,16,19] This may be followed by a short period of apparent recovery. The second stage is characterized by sudden resurgence of fever, shortness of breath, profound sweating that drenches the patient, and shock. Hypocalcemia, hypoglycemia, hyperkalemia, depression of the respiratory centers, and terminal acidosis are some of the biochemical and physiologic signs that develop in severe infections.[20,21] Delirium, meningismus, obtundation, seizures, and coma secondary to hemorrhagic meningitis occur in up to 50% of

TABLE 61-2 Distinguishing Features of a Biological Attack

A rapid rise and fall of the epidemic curve over a short period of time (a few hours to days)

Instead of the peaks and troughs seen in natural outbreaks, there may be a steady rise in cases

A disproportionate number of people seeking care for similar symptoms

Large numbers of patients arriving from the same geographical area

Large numbers of rapidly fatal cases

A lower attack rate in people who were indoors compared to those who were outdoors

Appearance of an uncommon disease that has bioterrorism potential (e.g., anthrax, plague, tularemia, botulism)

Increased numbers of sick or dead animals

A large number of cases within 48–72 hours of an attack suggests a bacterial agent, while those presenting within a few hours suggests a toxic agent

cases.[14,22,23] Involvement of the gut is also a common feature of advanced disease and thought to be secondary to hematogenous spread (different from primary gastrointestinal anthrax) presenting as abdominal pain (33%), and can lead to necrotizing enteritis of the bowel.[1,22,100] In a series of 11 cases in the U.S., there was a 33% incidence of supraventricular arrhythmias and one case that had fatal pericardial effusion.[1] Severe infection leads to hypotension and cyanosis progressing rapidly to death.[1,19,24,25] The lag period between initial exposure and the onset of symptoms seems to be inversely proportional to mortality.[16]

Diagnosis of inhalational anthrax clinically requires a high degree of suspicion given that the symptoms on initial presentation can easily be confused with a seasonal viral syndrome. Presenting symptoms and routine laboratory tests are nonspecific, and the only clue prior to development of fulminant disease may be a widened mediastinum on chest x-ray[25,27,100] (Fig. 61-1). Autopsies of victims from the Sverdlovsk incident failed to reveal any diffuse bronchopneumonic process; however, 11 of the 42 autopsies did show a necrotizing lung lesion similar to a Ghon complex.[22] The recent series of cases in the U.S. suggest a parenchymal process is likely to be more common than previously thought.[1] Small pleural effusions that rapidly progress to a large size appears to be a consistent finding and may correlate with the progression of the disease. Thoracentesis yields a hemorrhagic fluid with relatively few WBC, and is positive for the bacteria by Gram stain and culture.[1] Noncontrast computed tomography (CT) scan of the chest is extremely helpful in determining the extent of mediastinal adenopathy and edema[25] (Fig. 61-2). Given the rapidity at which death can occur, a delay in administration of antibiotics greatly decreases chances of survival.[1,25,27,28]

Meningeal signs develop in 50% of cases, with contrast CT scan of the brain revealing diffuse leptomeningeal enhancement, with intracerebral and subarachnoid hemorrhages.[23]

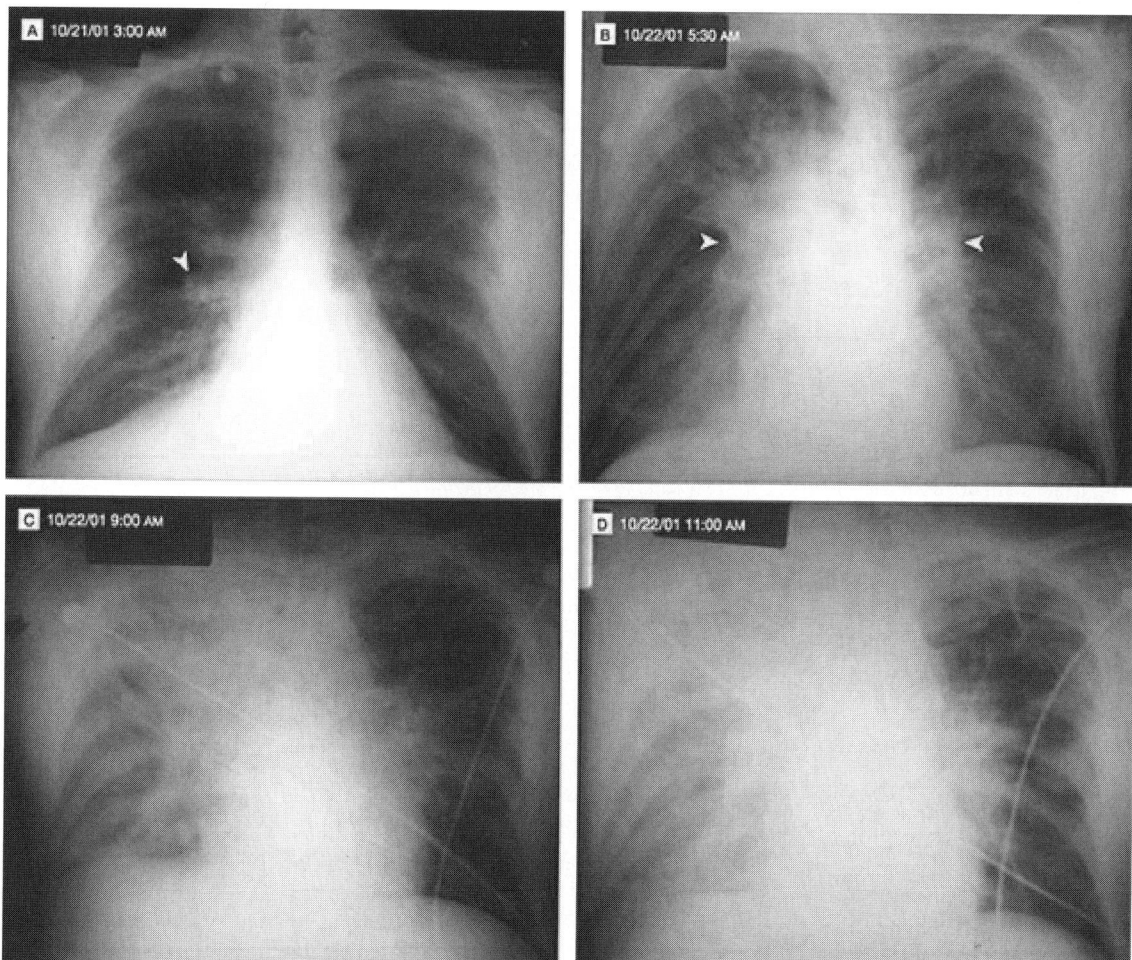

FIGURE 61-1 *A.* In this case of inhalation anthrax, initially only a subtle bilateral hilar prominence (*arrowhead*) and right perihilar infiltrate was noted, but subsequent images (*B, C,* and *D*) revealed a progressively widened mediastinum (*B, arrowheads*) and marked perihilar infiltrates, peribronchial cuffing, and air bronchograms. (*Reprinted with permission from Borio et al.[100]*)

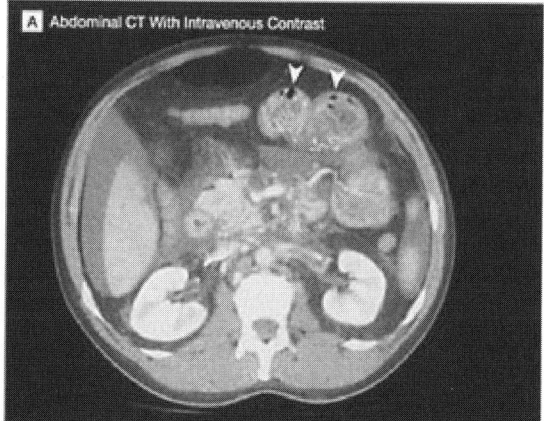
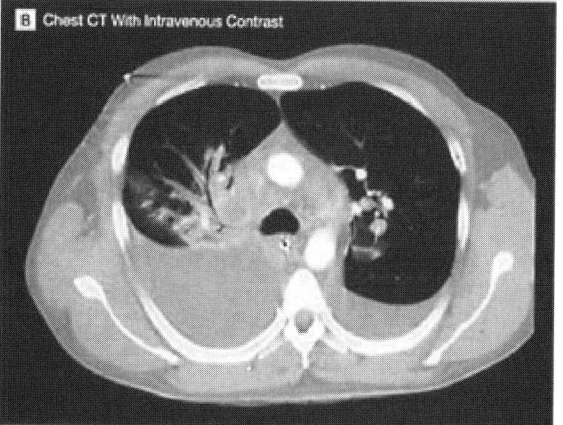

FIGURE 61-2 Abdominal and chest CT images of a patient with inhalation anthrax. *A.* Abdominal CT scan with intravenous contrast showing moderate amount of ascites, small-bowel wall edema, and intramural pneumatosis (*arrowheads*) consistent with a necrotizing enteritis. Other CT windows showed air within the hepatic branches of the portal venous system. *B.* Chest CT scan with intravenous contrast showing large bilateral perihilar infiltrates, perihilar lymphadenopathy, and widened mediastinum. Other CT windows showed high-attenuation mediastinal lymphadenopathy and blood in the mediastinum, consistent with hemorrhagic lymphadenopathy and hemorrhagic mediastinitis. (*Reprinted with permission from Borio et al.[100]*)

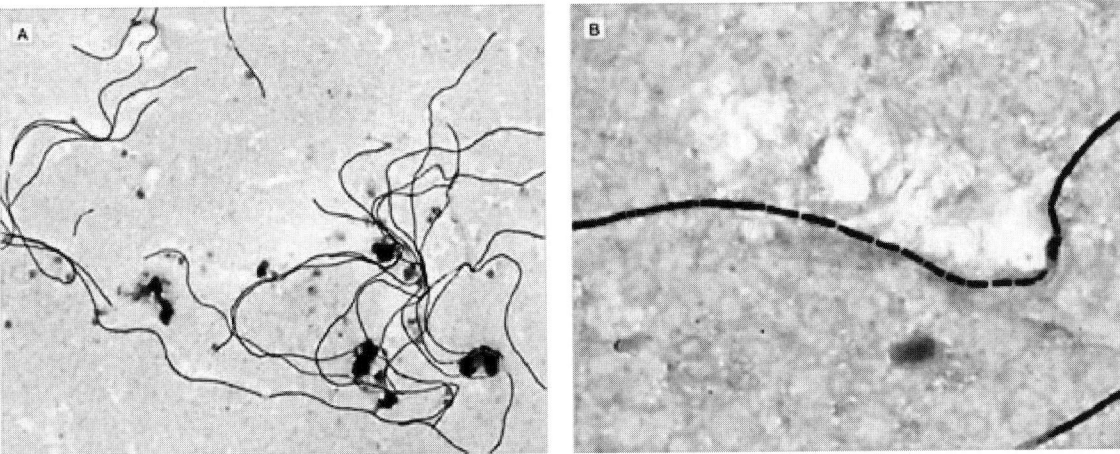

FIGURE 61-3 Gram stain of anthrax in blood in culture media. *(Reprinted with permission from Borio et al.[100])*

Cerebrospinal fluid (CSF) is usually bloody and gram-positive. Gram stains of sputum are typically negative, while those of blood and pleural fluid are more likely to be positive (Fig. 61-3). Blood cultures are almost always positive within 24 hours; however, laboratories may presumptively assume a contamination of specimens with *Bacillus cereus*.[29] Thus microbiology labs need to be notified of the suspicion, so they may use selective media to isolate anthrax.[30] Confirmatory testing such as growth on special nutrient agars, susceptibility to lysis by gamma phage, direct fluorescence antibody staining, nucleic acid signatures, and enzyme-linked immunosorbent assay (ELISA) for protective and capsule antigens are performed at level B and C laboratories of the Laboratory Response Network (LRN) for Bioterrorism, CDC, or the United States Army Medical Research Institute of Infectious Diseases (USAMRIID).[14,32] Serological testing of acute and convalescent serum is useful only retrospectively.

Postexposure prophylaxis for adults (including pregnant women and the immunosuppressed) is initially with ciprofloxacin 500 mg orally every 12 hours or doxycycline 100 mg every 12 hours. If the strain is susceptible, then amoxicillin 500 mg orally every 8 hours or the above dose of doxycycline can be taken. These regimens should be taken for 60 days owing to the unpredictable latency of inhalational anthrax.[14,33] An aluminum hydroxide adsorbed, licensed vaccine made of noninfectious sterile culture filtrate from attenuated B. anthracis is available, and evidence shows it to protect against aerosol challenge. However, currently it is not recommended for postexposure prophylaxis in either health care workers or the public. However should it become available, it would be used at 0, 2, and 4 weeks postexposure.[32]

Treatment of patients with inhalational anthrax that has progressed to its fulminant stage warrants close observation in a monitored setting. Surveillance of serum chemistries, oxygen saturation, and EKG are all warranted. Chest tube placement for moderately large pleural effusions is necessary as they can increase rapidly and worsen respiratory distress.[1] Patients with meningeal involvement may require steroids, phenytoin, and benzodiazepines to control edema and seizures. They may also need mechanical ventilation for airway protection. The additional support of mechanical ventilation and vasopressors are ominous signs.

Current CDC recommendations for empiric treatment of inhalational anthrax in adults (including pregnant women and immunosuppressed) are ciprofloxacin 400 mg intravenously every 12 hours or doxycycline 100 mg intravenously every 12 hours. These should be given with another one or two additional antibiotics that have in vitro activity against anthrax (rifampin, penicillin, ampicillin, vancomycin, imipenem, clindamycin, chloramphenicol, or clarithromycin).[33,34] If the strain of the organism is susceptible, then 4 million units of penicillin G intravenously every 4 hours can be used.[14,33] High-dose intravenous penicillin may provide better CNS penetration in cases associated with meningitis. Recent survivors of inhalational anthrax were treated with a combination of ciprofloxacin (based on official recommendations), rifampin (for increased gram-positive coverage and for its intracellular mechanism of action), and clindamycin (for its ability to prevent expression of toxin).[25] It is important to note that *B. anthracis* isolates produce cephalosporinase, making treatment with cephalosporins such as ceftriaxone useless.

As person-to-person transmission does not occur, patients can be cared for under standard precautions. However, it should be remembered that in an act of suspected bioterrorism one would not immediately know whether patients are affected with anthrax or a more transmissible agent such as plague, which warrants respiratory isolation precautions as well (Table 61-3). Patients with cutaneous anthrax should be cared for under contact isolation. Specimens should be handled under Biosafety Level (BSL) 2 precautions.[31] Decontamination of individuals exposed to the initial aerosol attack is not necessary, and washing with soap and water is sufficient to eliminate any secondary aerosolization. For contaminated hospital areas, bleach solutions and 0.5% hypochlorite solution are adequate for decontamination.[14,31]

Of the 77 cases of anthrax in the Sverdlovsk incident, only 11 patients survived. There was a reported hospital stay of 1 to 2 days for those who died and 3 weeks for those who survived. There are no details of the medical therapy that they had received but some of the survivors did need mechanical ventilation.[16] Prior to 1978, inhalational anthrax in the U.S. had a mortality of 80% to 90%.[19] However, the more recent experience in the U.S. showed a 40% mortality, and this may

TABLE 61-3 Differential for a Large Number of Persons Presenting with Febrile Illness and Respiratory Symptoms

Agent	Time to Onset	Chest X-Ray	Fatality	Onset to Respiratory Failure	Person-to-Person Infection	Complications	Diagnosis	Treatment
Anthrax[14,25,26] (inhalational)	1–6 days	Mediastinal widening; pleural effusions	90%	1–3 days	None; use standard precautions	Meningitis	Blood culture, Gram stain, ELISA for serology and antigen	Ciprofloxacin or doxycycline; addition of rifampin likely useful
Plague[35,42–44] (pneumonic)	2–3 days	Bilateral infiltrates; may have pleural effusions	90%	Within 1 day	High; use respiratory isolation	Early hemoptysis	Gram/Wayson stain, cultures, Fl Ag assay by ELISA, fluorescent Ab for F1 AG	Streptomycin or gentamicin or ciprofloxacin or doxycycline
Tularemia[53,55,58,61]	2–10 days	Bilateral infiltrates > hilar adenopathy > pleural effusions	30% w/o therapy; <5% with therapy	Low incidence	None; use standard precautions	Regional adenopathy in ulcer glandular type; sepsis/shock in typhoidal type	Cultures usually not revealing; fluorescent Ab, ELISA, and PCR	Streptomycin gentamicin, ciprofloxacin, or doxycycline
Legionella	2–10 days	Variable, bilateral subsegmental infiltrates, or consolidation	15%	Variable incidence	None; use standard precautions	Sepsis, ARDS	Urine Ag assay	Azithromycin or a fluoroquinolone; for severe cases add rifampin
Influenza	1–2 days	Variable bilateral interstitial or alveolar infiltrates	10–25% in those with underlying diseases	Variable incidence	High; use standard precautions	ARDS; secondary bacterial pneumonia	Immunofluorescence Ab staining, ELISA, tissue culture	Amantidine or oseltamivir or rimantidine; supportive care
Staphylococcal Enterotoxin B[24,94] (SEB)	3–12 hours	No abnormalities	<1%	None reported	None; use standard precautions	Gastrointestinal anorexia	Ag ELISA, Ab ELISA	Supportive, antiemetics, oxygen support
Ricin[96] (inhalation)	18–24 hours	Likely bilateral infiltrates/ARDS	High	Likely within 30 hours	None; use standard precautions	Hemoptysis likely; gastrointestinal bleeding and hepatic necrosis if ingested	ELISA for Ag, ELISA for Ab	Supportive; activated charcoal if ingested

ABBREVIATIONS: ARDS, acute respiratory distress syndrome; ELISA, enzyme-linked immunosorbent assay; PCR, polymerase chain reaction.

959

be due to early recognition, better antibiotics, and modern intensive care units.[1]

Plague

Yesinia pestis is a nonmotile, gram-negative bipolar coccobacillus that is the causative agent of plague. Recently, the organism has been used as the hypothetical biological weapon in the TOPOFF scenario,[4] theoretically causing thousands of casualties and widespread disruption of the public health system.[14,35] The most likely route of delivery during an attack would be via aerosol.

Human plague occurs worldwide and is endemic to the southwestern U.S., with an average of 10 cases reported each year.[36] Its natural reservoirs are urban and rural rodents. The transmission vector is the oriental rat flea (*Xenopsylla cheopis*). Humans become accidental hosts after being infected by an infected flea's bite. Humans very rarely are responsible for its propagation, except when they have the pneumonic form of the disease.[37]

Humans contract plague from the bite of an infected flea, inhalation of respiratory secretions of animals or humans with pneumonic forms of plague, or direct handling of infected animal tissues.[37] The former is the most common route, while the latter two are very rare in nature and usually give rise to the pneumonic form of disease. In the U.S. there were 390 cases of plague reported between 1947 and 1996. Of these 84% was bubonic, 13% septicemic, and 2% pneumonic. Fatality rates were 14%, 22%, and 57% respectively.[38]

Y. pestis has a number of virulence factors including V and W antigens, lipopolysaccharide endotoxin, capsular envelope (antiphagocytic fraction I antigen), coagulase, and fibrinolysin. Bacteria inoculated into the skin by an infected flea become phagocytosed by mononuclear cells. They multiply intracellularly, eventually lysing the cells, after which they become resistant to further phagocytosis. Bacteria are transported via lymphatics to the regional lymph nodes causing inflammation and hemorrhagic necrosis, and subsequently give rise to the typical bubo.[37,39]

The incubation period for bubonic plague is 2 to 8 days. It presents with sudden onset of fever, chills, weakness, and headache. Within a few hours to a day patients notice the bubo, which is characterized by its sudden onset, absence of overlying skin lesions, marked surrounding edema, and extreme pain that limits the motion of the region. Buboes can occur in the inguinal, axillary, or cervical nodes, and can present as an 1 to 10 cm firm, extremely tender, nonfluctuant mass.[35,37,40,41] Subsequently patients deteriorate rapidly over 2 to 4 days, having high fever, tachycardia, malaise, headache, vomiting, chills, alterations in mental status, prostration, and chest pain, eventually progressing to vasodilation and septic shock. During this time patients may have signs of disseminated intravascular coagulation (DIC), with acral purpura that may progress to gangrene. Hematogenous spread can give rise to complications such as plague pneumonia (5% to 15%), meningitis, hepatic and splenic abscesses, and endophthalmitis. Patients ultimately manifest signs of multiorgan failure and acute respiratory distress syndrome (ARDS).[37,39,41–45] A minority present with the septicemic phase of disease (primary septicemic plague without bubo formation). A distinguishing clinical feature is severe abdominal pain. Patients in this group present earlier, are more likely to be elderly, are more toxic in appearance, and are hospitalized sooner than patients with bubonic plague. Despite this they have a higher mortality, likely related to the delay in the diagnosis.[45]

Primary pneumonic plague occurs by inhalation of aerosolized bacteria from patients who have lung involvement secondary to fulminant bubonic plague, or animals (cats) with secondary plague pneumonia.[46] This is the most fatal form of the disease and its incubation time is 1 to 3 days. It manifests suddenly with fever, chills, headache, body pains, weakness, and chest discomfort.[38,47] As the disease progresses there is an increase in cough and sputum production, as well as increasing chest pain, hemoptysis, and hypoxia, progressing rapidly to frank respiratory failure. The presence of hemoptysis should alert the clinician to the possibility of primary pneumonic plague, since it is less likely to present in inhalational anthrax (see Table 61-3). Death usually occurs within 18 to 24 hours after the onset of symptoms. Pulmonary complications include localized necrosis, cavitation, pleural effusion, and ARDS.[16,18,32,41] In addition the course is complicated by endotoxemia and septic shock.

Patients with primary pneumonic plague have an infectious pneumonitis at the onset of the disease. These patients are capable of a vigorous and highly infectious cough, and are not usually debilitated like patients with bubonic disease. Secondary plague pneumonia on the other hand, is usually a result of hematogenous spread of the disease to the lungs. Usually the patient is ill for several days, debilitated, and unable to cough vigorously, making them less infectious. However, pneumonic plague (primary or secondary) should always be considered extremely infectious.[40,43]

Routine blood tests are nonspecific. Bacteremia initially is transient, and single blood cultures at presentation are only 27% positive. Blood, sputum, bubo aspirates, and CSF Gram stains can reveal gram-negative bipolar coccobacilli, while the Wayson stain shows light blue bacilli with dark blue polar bodies on a pink background (Fig. 61-4). Automated culture detection systems may present a delay or even misidentify the organism. Thus a high level clinical suspicion of the disease should prompt immediate notification of the lab. State level B or national level C (CDC or USAMRIID) laboratories should be notified through the LRN. Direct fluorescence staining for fraction 1 (F1) envelope antigen, phage lyses of cultures, or

FIGURE 61-4 Peripheral blood smear from a patient with septicemic plague. *(Reprinted with permission from Inglesby et al.[35])*

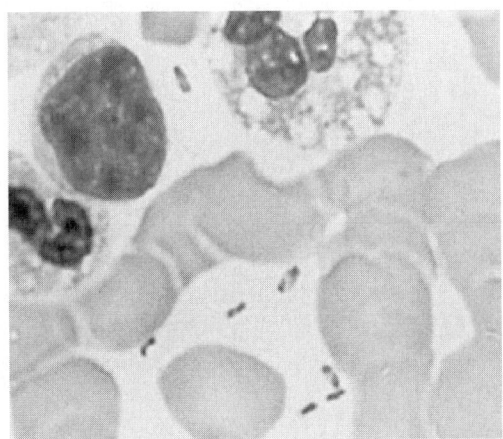

polymerase chain reaction (PCR) assay should confirm identification. Acute and convalescent serum titers for antibody to F1 antigen are retrospectively diagnostic.[31,35,37,39] Chest radiographs in cases of bubonic plague may show small transient unilateral infiltrates. However, nodular or bilateral alveolar infiltrates in these patients is strongly associated with a more fulminant and fatal course. Primary pneumonic forms of plague are associated with bilateral alveolar and nodular infiltrates, with over half of them having pleural effusions. Cavitary lesions have also been noted to occur.[42,43,44,46]

Treatment requires the prompt administration of antibiotics, especially in the septicemic and pneumonic forms. As the bacteria is capable of inducing an endotoxemia leading to DIC, septic shock, ARDS, and multiorgan failure, close observation of the patient and early resuscitative measures are warranted at the earliest sign of progression toward a more fulminant course. These patients require aggressive volume resuscitation, and may need mechanical ventilation as well as vasopressor support.[47,48]

Based on the Working Group on Civilian Biodefense's recommendations for pneumonic plague, first-line therapy is with streptomycin 1 g IV or IM twice a day, or gentamicin 0.5 mg/kg IM or IV twice daily. Alternate therapies are doxycycline 100 mg IV twice daily, ciprofloxacin 400 mg IV twice daily, or chloramphenicol 25 mg/kg IV four times daily. Therapy should be implemented in anyone exposed with a temperature >38.5°C or a new cough.[35]

In the setting of mass casualties where public health facilities may be overwhelmed, first-line therapy recommendations for postexposure prophylaxis in adults include doxycycline 100 mg orally twice daily, or ciprofloxacin 400 mg orally twice daily. Alternatively, chloramphenicol 25 mg/kg can be used. The reader is referred to the CDC article for dosing in children and pregnant women.[35] Currently no recommendations exist for vaccination of public or health care providers in the postexposure setting.[35,40,49]

Patients with pneumonic forms of plague should be kept under respiratory droplet isolation protocols (Table 61-4) until they have received at least 48 hours of appropriate antibiotic therapy or shown improvement. Persons who have been exposed who refuse to take antibiotic prophylaxis but are not symptomatic do not require isolation, but need to be watched and treated at the first sign of cough or fever. The use of standard disposable surgical masks is recommended. Microbiology lab personnel should be aware of the potential of getting infected from handling samples during high-risk lab procedures, and BSL 3 precautions should be observed during such times.[31,35,39]

Tularemia

Tularemia is caused by a gram-negative, facultative intracellular bacterium, *Francisella tularensis*. It is a zoonotic disease of small mammals and is transmitted by arthropod vectors (primarily ticks). There are two biovars of *F. tularensis*. Biovar tularensis or type A is more common in the south-central and western U.S., and is highly virulent to rabbits and humans. Biovar palearctica or type B is more common in Eurasia and less virulent to humans. The bacteria can survive for long periods in soil, water, and animal carcasses. Organisms infect humans by direct contact with mucous membranes, broken skin, ingestion, or inhalation.[50] Hunters, animal handlers, and laboratory personnel working with the bacteria are at greater risk for developing disease. Only 10 to 50 organisms are needed to cause infection in humans, via contact, inoculation, or inhalation.[51] Theoretically, a biological attack with tularemia would be with an aerosolized form. From the site of entry, bacteria are ingested by macrophages and transported to regional lymph nodes where they multiply and disseminate. At the site of the entry, a predominantly cell-mediated inflammatory reaction causes necrosis and granuloma formation. Granulomas are also formed at other target organs after dissemination.[50,52]

The incubation period is 3 to 5 days. Patients present with abrupt onset of fever, chills, headache, coryza, malaise, and weakness. A temperature-pulse deficit is noted in 42% of patients. Patients may complain of cough and chest discomfort without having signs of pneumonia. Patients may have varying degrees of sore throat, abdominal pain, arthralgias, and myalgias. If untreated, anorexia, continued weight loss, and debility occur over a period of weeks to months.[50,51,53] Clinically the disease may present as either ulceroglandular (which includes glandular, oculoglandular, and pharyngeal), or pneumonic (typhoidal) forms.

Ulceroglandular tularemia accounts for about 85% of natural cases, presenting as a cutaneous ulcer at the inoculation site within a few days of the onset of symptoms. The tender ulcer usually measures 0.4 to 3 cm in diameter, has raised edges, and is associated with regional lymphadenopathy. Affected lymph nodes are also tender, and can become fluctuant and suppurate. A minority present with the glandular form and no signs of skin involvement.[50,52,54] The oculoglandular and pharyngeal forms refer to the primary sites of inoculation, and are associated with intense inflammation, edema, hemorrhage, and granulomatous disease of the inoculation site, as well as regional lymphadenopathy. Of interest is that the pharyngeal form of the disease is frequently associated with pneumonia.[53]

Typhoidal tularemia refers to illness without lymphadenopathy or signs of a portal of entry. It occurs in 15% of natural cases. It is likely that this is actually a primary pneumonic form of the disease, acquired by inhalation of the organism. Onset is more abrupt, and patients are more toxic, with pronounced gastrointestinal symptoms such as abdominal pain, prostration, and watery diarrhea. Respiratory complaints and pneumonia are associated with 80% of cases. Pharyngitis, pleuritic chest pain, cough with minimal sputum production, and bronchiolitis are common, while hemoptysis is uncommon.[50,53-55] However, unlike both primary pneumonic plague and inhalational anthrax, the disease does not usually rapidly deteriorate to respiratory failure and death (see Table 61-3).

Both forms of tularemia are capable of causing pneumonia, ARDS, and septic shock, with the need for mechanical ventilation and vasopressor support, although only a handful of such cases exist in the postantibiotic literature.[56] Interestingly, those that did had ulceroglandular forms of the disease. Mortality is 35% in pneumonic forms of the disease without therapy. With appropriate antibiotics fatalities would be <5%. However, potential for widespread disability would be great.[24,57]

Initial laboratory tests are nonspecific. Moderate leukocytosis, elevations in lactate dehydrogenase, serum transaminases, and alkaline phosphatase are common. CSF may show a small elevation in protein, low glucose, and minimal

TABLE 61-4 Isolation Guidelines For Bioterrorism Agents

Patient Management
Nagative Pressure Rooms are:
IMPORTANT PHONE NUMBERS:
Infectious Diseases .....-.....
Infection Control .....-.....
ER ....-.........
USAMRIID 301-619-2833
CDC Emergency Response
Office 770-422-7100

	BACTERIAL AGENTS	Anthrax	Brucellosis	Cholera	Glanders	Bubonic Plague	Pneumonic Plague	Tularemia	Q Fever	VIRUSES	Smallpox	Venez. Equine Encephalitis	Viral Encephalitis	Viral Hemmorrhagic Fever	BIOTOXINS	Botulism	Ricin	T-2 Mycotoxins	Staph. Enterotoxin B
Isolation Precautions																			
Standard precautions for all aspects of patient care		X	X	X	X	X	X	X	X		X	X	X	X		X	X	X	X
Contact precautions (gown & gloves; wash hands after each patient encounter)				X^c	X^a	X^a					X			X				X^a	
Airborne precautions (negative pressure room & N95 masks for all individuals entering the room)											X			X^b					
Droplet precautions (surgical mask)							X							X^b					
Patient Placement																			
No restrictions		X	X	X	X			X	X			X	X			X	X	X	X
Cohort 'like' patients when private room unavailable				X^c	X^a	X	X				X			X				X^a	
Private room				X^c	X^a	X^a	X				X			X				X^a	
Negative pressure											X			X^b					
Door closed at all times											X			X^b					
Patient Transport																			
No restrictions		X	X	X	X	X		X	X			X	X			X	X	X	X
Limit movement to essential medical purposes only				X^c	X^a	X^a	X				X			X				X^a	
Place mask on patient to minimize dispersal of droplets							X				X			X^b					
Cleaning and Disinfection																			
Routine cleaning of rooms with hospital approved disinfectant		X	X	X	X	X	X	X	X		X	X	X			X	X	X	
Disinfect surfaces with 10% bleach solution or phenolic disinfectant														X					
Dedicated equipment (disinfect prior to leaving room)				X^c	X^a	X^a					X			X				X^a	
Linen management as with all other patients		X	X	X	X	X	X	X	X		X	X	X	X		X	X	X	X
Linens autoclaved before laundering in hot water with bleach added											X								
Post-mortem Care																			
Follow principles of standard precautions		X	X	X	X	X	X	X	X		X	X	X	X		X	X	X	X
Droplet precautions (surgical mask)							X												
Contact precautions (gown & gloves)				X^a	X^a						X			X				X^a	
Avoid autopsy or use airborne precautions & HEPA filter							X				X			X^b					
Routine terminal cleaning of rooms with hospital approved disinfectant		X	X	X	X	X	X	X	X		X	X	X			X	X	X	X
Disinfect surfaces with 10% bleach solution or phenolic disinfectant														X					
Mimimal handling of body; seal body in leak-proof material														X					
Cremate body whenever possible											X								
Discontinuation of Isolation																			
48 hrs of appropriate antibiotic and clinical improvement							X												
Until all scabs separate											X								
Until skin decontamination completed (1 hr contact time)																		X	
Duration of illness				X^c	X^a	X^a								X					

STANDARD PRECAUTIONS – Standard Precautions prevent direct contact with all body fluids (including blood), secretions, excretions, non-intact skin (including rashes), and mucous membranes. Standard Precautions routinely practiced by health care providers include: splash/spray, and gowns to protect skin and clothing during procedures.

^{a} Contact precautions needed only if the patient has skin involvement (bubonic plague: draining bubo) or until decontamination of skin is complete (T-2 Mycotoxins).

^{b} A surgical mask and eye protection should be worn if you come within 3 feet of patient. Airborne precautions are needed if patient has cough, vomiting, diarrhea, or hemorrhage.

^{c} Contact precautions needed only if the patient is diapered or incontinent.

SOURCE: Reprinted with permission from the St. Louis University School of Public Health's Center for the Study of Bioterrorism and Emerging Infections. Available at http://www.bioterrorism.slu.edu/anthrax/key_ref/Isolation.pdf. Accessed December 2004.

increases in white blood cells (WBCs).[50,53] Typically blood cultures are negative, owing to poor growth on standard media and a low index of suspicion, and historically there is usually a delay of several days before identification. However, organisms have been recovered from blood, ulcers, conjunctival exudates, sputum, gastric washings, and pharyngeal exudates.[53,58,61] Direct microscopic examination using fluorescent labeled antibodies provides a means of rapid diagnosis.[50] Antigen detection, PCR, and ELISA are also used, and these methods are available at state and national reference labs through the LRN. Manipulation of cultures is a well-known hazard to laboratory personnel, and should only be done under BSL 3 containment. A fourfold increase in serum antibody is also diagnostic, but of retrospective importance.[31,61]

In a large series of inhalation-acquired tularemia 50% of the patients had chest x-ray abnormalities; 40% had infiltrates described as 2- to 8-cm oval-shaped lesions with indistinct borders, mostly in the juxtahilar position; 21% had unilateral hilar adenopathy always associated with other x-ray abnormalities; and 11% had pleural effusions.[58] Pneumonia can occur in ulceroglandular disease, especially with the pharyngeal form. Interstitial patterns, cavitary lesions, bronchopleural fistulae, and frank ARDS have been reported on chest radiographs.[59] Pleural fluid analysis shows a serosanguineous exudate with a lymphocytic predominance. Increased adenosine deaminase, lysozyme, and β_2-microglobulin occur similarly to tuberculous effusions.[53,55,60]

Isolation of proven cases is not required since human-to-human transmission does not occur (see Table 61-4). Standard precautions should be applied to care of patients with draining lesions or pneumonia. Decontamination of soiled linen and equipment can be done with heat and standard disinfectants.

The Working Group on Civilian Biodefense's first-line therapy recommendations for treatment of adults in a contained casualty setting is streptomycin 1 g IM twice daily or gentamicin 5 mg/kg IM or IV once daily, for 10 days. Alternative therapies are doxycycline 100 mg IV twice daily for 14 to 21 days, chloramphenicol 15 mg/kg IV four times daily for 14 to 21 days, or ciprofloxacin 400 mg IV twice daily for 10 days. Of note, in the 1950s a fully virulent streptomycin-resistant strain was developed that could potentially be used in a bioterrorist attack. Fortunately the strain was sensitive to gentamicin. Since gentamicin has broader gram-negative coverage and is more readily available, it may be a more attractive first-line agent, especially if the diagnosis of tularemia is considered but in doubt.[61]

In a mass casualty setting where hospital resources are overwhelmed, adults can be treated with doxycycline 100 mg orally or ciprofloxacin 500 mg orally, twice daily for 14 days. Recovery from the illness is usually within 5 to 7 days. Currently vaccination is only recommended for microbiology laboratory workers handling cultures.[53,57,61]

Botulinum

Clostridium botulinum is a ubiquitous spore-forming anaerobic bacillus that produces a group of seven potent neurotoxins (types A through G). Botulism is the clinical syndrome produced by these toxins, and naturally occurs in three forms:

food-borne, intestinal, and wound. Sporadic outbreaks of botulism occur throughout the U.S. due to contamination of food sources.[62] No water-borne cases have ever been reported.[63,64]

All cases of botulism occur secondary to absorption of toxin from gut, lung, or wounds into the bloodstream. Toxin is not absorbed through intact skin. Once absorbed it is carried to the peripheral neuromuscular junctions, where it binds irreversibly. The toxin is made of two polypeptide subunits (light and heavy chains). Toxin is endocytosed into the nerve terminus by virtue of its heavy chain. Subsequently, the light chain cleaves various components of the synaptic fusion complex, preventing release of acetylcholine into the synaptic cleft. This causes presynaptic inhibition of neuromuscular transmission, affecting cholinergic, muscarinic, and nicotinic receptors. Recovery may take weeks or months and is dependent on regeneration of new motor axons to reinnervate muscle.[65,66]

Botulinum toxin is likely to be used as an aerosol agent in a bioterrorist attack. Aside from the general epidemiologic clues to a bioterrorist attack, identification of toxin types C, D, F, and G should arouse suspicion, since types A, B, and E are the most common forms found in the U.S.[63] Botulinum toxin is the most potent toxic agent (per weight) known. Toxin A given in doses of 0.09 to 0.15 μg IV or IM, 0.7 to 0.9 μg inhaled, or 70 μg orally is enough to kill a 70-kg human. The toxin itself is colorless, odorless, and a relatively large protein (150,000-da). It quickly denatures under environmental conditions: 12 hours in air, 3 hours in sunlight, several minutes with heat >100° C, and 20 minutes at 0.4% mg/mL free available chlorine in water.[67]

The incubation period for food-borne botulism can vary from hours to days, but typically is between 12 and 72 hours, similar to that of the inhalational form.[59,63] The rapidity of the onset of symptoms varies with the dose of the toxin, but most often is acute. Patients present initially with cranial nerve palsies and prominent bulbar signs of blurred vision, mydriasis, ptosis, diplopia, dysphonia, dysarthria, and dysphagia. A progressive symmetric descending flaccid muscle paralysis follows, the rapidity of which is also variable. It is important to note that the patient remains conscious throughout this time and is not febrile. Patients may also manifest with anticholinergic signs and postural hypotension. Nausea and vomiting may occur as nonspecific sequelae of an ileus.[62,65,68] The upper airway may collapse due to weakness of oropharyngeal musculature, and handling of secretions may be problematic if the gag reflex is absent. Later the diaphragm is involved and respiratory failure ensues. Progression to hypercapnic and secondary hypoxic respiratory failure has been noted to occur within 24 hours in severe food-borne botulism.[63,65,68,69]

The diagnosis of botulism in the scenario of a bioterrorist attack should be made on the basis of its clinical and epidemiologic features mentioned above. This is because the definitive diagnosis can be delayed for days. The differential diagnosis for isolated cases includes stroke syndromes, intoxication, Guillain-Barré (Miller-Fischer variant), myasthenia gravis, and tick paralysis. However, for multiple cases presenting within a short period of time, the differential would be organophosphate and nerve agent poisoning (Table 61-5).

Routine laboratory tests, CSF examination, and brain imaging are unremarkable. Electromyography (EMG) studies show normal nerve conduction velocity, normal sensory function, and decreased amplitude of action potentials in affected

TABLE 61-5 Differential Diagnosis of a Large Number of Afebrile People Presenting with Paralysis

	Nerve Agent/Organophosphate Toxicity	Botulinum Toxin[2]
Mechanism of action	Inhibits acetylcholinesterase	Inhibits presynaptic acetylcholine neurotransmission
Routes of acquiring	Inhalation and dermal	Inhalation, ingestion, and contamination of wounds; not dermally active
Onset to action	Minutes to hours	12 hours to several days
Central nervous system effects	Agitation, confusion, delirium, seizures, coma	Patients remain conscious but anxious
Motor system (nicotinic receptors)	Muscle fasciculations, pain, progressive weakness to rigid paralysis	Bulbar palsy (dysarthria, dysphonia, dysphagia, diplopia), progressive descending flaccid muscle paralysis
Autonomic system (muscarinic receptors)	Salivation, lacrimation, urinary incontinence, diarrhea, vomiting	Dry mouth, variable degree of gastrointestinal symptoms
Respiratory signs	Variable bronchoconstriction, rapid progression to respiratory failure within minutes	Comparatively slower progression to respiratory failure
Ocular signs	Progressive miosis	Mydriasis, early ptosis, 4th and 6th cranial nerve palsy
Cardiovascular	Bradyarrhythmias > tachycardia	None
Electromyography	Normal nerve conduction, decreased amplitude at low rates of repetitive nerve stimulation	Normal nerve conduction, increased amplitude at high rates of repetitive stimulation
Diagnosis	Blood butyrocholinesterase and erythrocyte-cholinesterase levels	Mouse neutralization bioassay, specific toxin typing
Decontamination	Only for dermal agents, charcoal and sorptive resins, do not wipe (blot only)	None needed if inhalational. If ingested give activated charcoal
Therapy	Atropine, pralidoxime. anticonvulsants, antiarrhythmics, ventilator support	Trivalent or heptavalent antitoxin, anxiolytics, ventilatory support
Recovery	Hours to a few days	Weeks to months in severe cases

muscle groups. An incremental increase in amplitude after repetitive 30- to 50-Hz stimulation helps distinguish botulism from Guillain-Barré syndrome and myasthenia gravis, but not Eaton-Lambert syndrome. The edrophonium test can be transiently positive.[70]

Ventilatory failure should be watched for by following vital capacity and carbon dioxide tension on arterial blood gases. Patients without gag reflex are at high risk for aspiration and may need endotracheal intubation. In one large series of patients many had significant hypoxia without significant hypercapnia.[69] The time to mechanical ventilation was up to 5 days after the onset of symptoms, and was required for an average of 97 days. Aspiration pneumonia was presumed to occur in 29% of patients, all of whom received mechanical ventilation. Patients generally regained respiratory muscle strength later than in other muscle groups. Death from sepsis and shock were related to aspiration or ventilator-associated pneumonia.[69]

Definitive diagnosis of botulism is by mouse neutralization (bioassay), where type-specific antitoxin is used to protect mice against toxin in a patient's serum. Serum should be obtained prior to administration of antitoxin, as it may interfere with the assay. Results may take up to 2 days. Gastric, stool, and vomitus samples can also be used.[63] Samples should be handled under BLS 2 conditions at a level B lab.[31]

The mainstays of therapy are administration of antitoxin, ventilatory assistance, and supportive care. Patients presenting with food-borne botulism should be given activated charcoal and then antitoxin when available. Currently an equine botulinum antitoxin that provides passive immunity against types A, B, and E toxins is available from the CDC through state and local health departments. Prompt administration limits the severity of disease, but does not reverse existing paralysis. An investigational heptavalent antitoxin against types A through G is available in the U.S. Army for other toxin types. Unlike organophosphate poisoning, atropine is not indicated and would possibly exacerbate symptoms.[67]

Patients unable to handle oropharyngeal secretions should be placed in reverse Trendelenburg position with frequent pulmonary and oropharyngeal toilet to avoid aspiration. Patients with clinical signs of respiratory failure require mechanical ventilation. It is important to recognize that patients remain conscious throughout and may require sedation to relieve anxiety. Aminoglycosides, clindamycin, and steroids should be avoided, as they may worsen muscle atrophy and exacerbate neuromuscular blockade and myopathy.[72,73]

Postexposure prophylaxis with antitoxin is currently neither recommended nor practical. Exposed persons who are not symptomatic should be watched closely and given antitoxin if symptoms develop. Vaccination against botulinum toxin using a multivalent toxoid is advocated only for military personnel and laboratory workers who may be at great risk.[74] Decontamination is not required, as the agent is not dermally active. However, the possible use of a nerve agent should be considered in a scenario with many patients presenting with muscular weakness, and dealt with appropriately with decontamination (see Table 61-5).

Smallpox

Smallpox vaccination ceased in 1980, after the disease was declared eradicated by the WHO.[75] This has left a civilian population under the age of 30 totally susceptible. If the virus were ever intentionally released, its properties like high person-to-person transmission, viability outside its human host, and high fatality rate would cause colossal damage.[76]

Smallpox is caused by the variola virus of the orthopoxvirus family. Smallpox is highly infectious and person-to-person spread occurs by inhalation of expectorated respiratory droplet nuclei and by direct contact of the mucous membranes. Fomites such as contaminated linen of infected patients have also been responsible for spread. The incubation period is 12 to 14 days. Following deposition on the upper airway mucosa, the virus is transported to regional lymph nodes and then other lymphoid tissues. The virus then spreads systemically and localizes in small vessels of the dermis and oropharyngeal mucosa. This prodromal phase lasts for 3 days, and is marked by high fever, rigors, malaise, vomiting, headache, and backache.[77]

The clinical manifestations of smallpox are of five types. The classic or ordinary type accounted for 90% of cases with a fatality rate of 30%. Modified type occurred in 25% of unvaccinated and 2% of vaccinated cases with rare fatalities. Flat type occurred in 7% of cases and was characterized by slow evolution of flat, soft focal skin lesions and severe systemic toxicity. It had a fatality rate of 95% and 33% in the unvaccinated and vaccinated, respectively. Hemorrhagic type was almost uniformly fatal, occurring in 3%, and was characterized by diffuse hemorrhagic manifestations and rapid progression to death even before any skin lesions could be discerned. Variola sine eruptione was seen in vaccinated persons and was characterized by a 48-hour period of febrile illness. Unfortunately the various types cannot be distinguished until they start to manifest.[77]

The classical type of disease begins acutely with prodromal symptoms, followed by an enanthema of the tongue, mouth, and oropharynx. The next day a discrete centrifugal rash, characterized by 2- to 3-mm reddish macules begins on the face, hands, and forearms. These lesions progress to become papules and then vesicles of 3 to 5 mm in size, and spread centrally to cover the whole body by the fourth to seventh day. By the eighth day pustules of 4 to 6 mm are formed. Over the next 5 to 8 days, the pustules become larger and have a central depression (umbilicated). Later they become flattened and more confluent. During this phase of rash another fever spike occurs. By the thirteenth day the lesions start to crust and over the ensuing week start to scab and separate, leaving depressed depigmented lesions. The rash is typically more peripherally distributed and homogeneous in stage when compared to the rash of chickenpox.[77,78] Secondary infections of the rashes were reportedly not common. Complications of the disease included panophthalmitis and secondary infection causing blindness in 1%, arthritis in 2% of children, and encephalitis in 1%. Bronchitis was occasionally reported; however, pneumonia was rare.[76,77]

Death from the classic type of disease was reported to be most common during the second week. The fatality rate in the classic type seems directly related to the degree of confluence among the lesions. This may have direct bearing on the degree of fluid sequestration and protein loss during the vesicular and pustular stage. Renal failure, electrolyte imbalance, protein loss, and metabolic derangements were reportedly similar to those of burn victims and likely accounted for the majority of the morbidity of shock, infection, and death.[77,79]

The two most dreaded forms of the disease are the hemorrhagic and flat types. Hemorrhagic type has a predilection for pregnant women. There was no difference in incidence between vaccinated and unvaccinated individuals. It was characterized by a shorter more severe prodromal phase and marked prostration. Diffuse hemorrhagic lesions (likely due to DIC) occurred in all mucous membranes and skin, leading to sloughing of these surfaces. Pulmonary edema and hemoptysis were common. Patients were reportedly conscious until the very end and death often occurred within a week.[77] Flat type disease was rare in vaccinated individuals. The prodromal fever was present throughout the eruptive phase of the disease, and patients were extremely toxic in appearance. Mucous membrane sloughing was also characteristic.

It is likely that the vast majority of practicing clinicians would not be able to recognize smallpox in its early stages, by which time it would already be too late to prevent its spread. The differential diagnosis of the disease is quite vast, but the most common misdiagnosis would be that of chickenpox. Chickenpox has a less pronounced prodromal illness, a more centripetal rash, asynchronous evolution of the rash, quicker scab formation (1 week), and a fatality rate of <1%. Other illnesses that can be confused with smallpox are monkeypox, various cutaneous drug reactions, atypical measles, and molluscum contagiosum. Cases of hemorrhagic and flat type smallpox would be difficult to diagnose clinically, and would likely be misdiagnosed as severe meningococcemia, DIC from other diseases, Stevens-Johnson syndrome, or a filovirus hemorrhagic fever.[80]

Notification of local, state, and national public health authorities is of the utmost importance, as the diagnosis of smallpox is an international public health emergency. Specimens should be sent to state and national health authorities using the LRN, under BSL 4 precautions. Information regarding handling of specimens is detailed on the CDC website: http://www.bt.cdc.gov/agent/smallpox/responseplan/#guided.

Demonstration of the characteristic brick-shaped virus under electron microscopy is confirmatory for an orthopoxvirus, and aggregations of variola virus particles called Guarnieri bodies can be found under light microscopy. However, none of these tests are capable of discriminating variola from other orthopoxviruses. Definitive diagnosis is by isolation of the virus on chorioallantoic membrane culture and further testing with PCR.[80,81]

In a recent report, it was estimated that if as few as 10 persons were initially infected by a covert biological attack with smallpox, within 1 year as many as 224,000 persons would be infected if the disease went unchecked. Furthermore, a combination of quarantine (25% removal of cases from society daily) and a mass vaccination program (reducing the number of transmissions by 33%), would lead to halting of an epidemic within 1 year, and the cumulative number of cases would be 4200. In order for this scenario to be feasible it was estimated that over 9 million doses of vaccine would be necessary.[82]

Strict airborne and contact isolation in a negative pressure room is of primary importance in dealing with a case of smallpox. However, this is only feasible in a small, contained outbreak. In a massive outbreak separate hospitals would need to be designated for those with complications or more severe forms of the disease. More likely, people would have to be quarantined within their homes for routine supportive care. Patients requiring admission to the hospital in a scenario like this would likely be critically ill. Keeping pace with fluid losses, electrolyte imbalances, and nutritional needs would be a major goal of therapy in these patients. This is especially true for patients with more confluent rashes, as well as flat type and hemorrhagic type variants of the disease. Meticulous skin care should be performed. Early placement of central venous access and invasive hemodynamic monitoring catheters may be warranted in severe cases as progressive distortion of the superficial anatomy occurs.[77,79] Patients with the flat and hemorrhagic types would be most likely to need some degree of mechanical ventilatory support, as the incidence of pulmonary edema is higher. In addition they would likely need transfusion therapy for complications related to DIC.

Currently there is no definitive treatment of the disease. Cidofovir (currently FDA approved for treatment of cytomegalovirus retinitis) is reportedly useful in preventing monkeypox and vaccinia in animals. It may have roles in postexposure prophylaxis and treatment of vaccinia vaccination complications. This drug would possibly be made available in a smallpox epidemic.[81]

Vaccination is done with reconstituted lyophilized vaccinia. It is applied with a bifurcated needle via 15 punctures at right angles into the skin overlying the deltoid without drawing blood. Successful vaccination is confirmed by the appearance of a characteristic Jennerian pustule after a week, and this provides immunity for up to 10 years, and 20 years with revaccination. The vaccinee must understand that there is viable vaccinia virus in the lesion from the moment the papule forms (2 to 5 days after vaccination) until the scab dislodges (on days 14 to 21). The lesions should be covered as there is a risk of transmission to an unvaccinated individual ("contact vaccinia").[101]

A three phase smallpox vaccination program was recently put forth by the U.S. government, under which medical and health care personnel are offered smallpox vaccination on a voluntary basis. The plan also calls for the creation of smallpox vaccination teams comprised of health care workers and public health officials in each state. These teams will assist in epidemiologic investigation and vaccination efforts during the first 7 to 10 days of an outbreak. Vaccination within 4 days of exposure will provide some protection from getting disease and will decrease mortality.[102] Vaccination of patients with suspected smallpox should also be considered for fear of misdiagnosis.[81] Recently it has been established that an increase in the dilution of the vaccine from 1:5 to 1:10 establishes immunity, and this practice could substantially boost the availability of the vaccine to the public.[83]

Contraindications for vaccination include immunosuppression, human immunodeficiency virus (HIV) infection, history of exfoliative dermatologic conditions, and pregnancy. Complications of vaccination in order of frequency are infection, generalized vaccinia (usually self-limited), eczema vacciniatum, postvaccinial encephalitis (with 10% significant neurologic morbidity), and vaccinia gangrenosa (occurs in immunosuppressed individuals and has a high fatality rate). Vaccinia immune globulin (VIG) is indicated for eczema vacciniatum, and vaccinia gangrenosa.[76,77,84]

Viral Hemorrhagic Fever

Viral hemorrhagic fever (VHF) is caused by a diverse group of RNA viruses that are transmitted to humans from their natural animal and arthropod reservoirs. They produce clinical syndromes characterized by fever, myalgias, prostration, increased vascular permeability, disturbances in regional circulation, and bleeding. Several of the hemorrhagic fevers (Marburg, Ebola, Lassa, Junin, and Machupo viruses) have been weaponized and experimented with for aerosol infectivity by the former Soviet Union, Russia, and the U.S. Experimental infection of animals via aerosol is highly effective. However, aerosol infection of humans has never been documented, except in the case of hantavirus. However, these agents are highly infective by direct contact with needles, fluids, and tissues of infected persons.[85] Important human pathogens are:

- Arenaviruses: Lassa, Junin, and Machupo viruses that cause Lassa fever, Argentinean, and Bolivian hemorrhagic fevers, respectively.
- Bunyaviruses: Rift Valley fever (RVF) virus and Crimean-Congo hemorrhagic fever (CCHF) viruses cause RVF and CCHF. Hantaviruses cause hemorrhagic fever renal syndrome (HFRS) and hantavirus pulmonary syndrome (HPS).
- Filoviruses: Marburg and Ebola viruses.
- Flaviviruses: Dengue fever, Kyasanur forest disease, and Omsk hemorrhagic fever.

VHF viruses target vascular endothelium, causing microvascular damage and derangement in vascular permeability. Common presenting complaints are fever, myalgias, and prostration. On examination patients may have conjunctival injection, mild hypotension, flushing, and petechial hemorrhages. Bleeding is variable and generally not life threatening, but it is an index of severity. Progression to shock and generalized bleeding from the mucous membranes is often accompanied by neurological, hematopoietic, or pulmonary involvement. Hepatic involvement is common; however, jaundice and frank hepatic failure is seen in a small percentage patients with RVF, CCHF, Marburg, and Ebola hemorrhagic fevers, and yellow fever. Death is secondary to increased vascular permeability, intravascular volume loss, and multiorgan failure.[86] The Working Group on Civilian Biodefense has concluded that CCHF and HFRS are unlikely to be employed as biowarfare agents, because they are technically difficult to produce in large quantities. Dengue is also an unlikely agent as it is not transmissible by aerosol, and only rarely causes VHF.

Each virus has unique features that set it apart clinically. Lassa fever is endemic in West Africa, and has a high mortality in children and pregnant women. Hemorrhagic and neurologic complications are not pronounced and occur only in the severely ill. Case-fatality rates in hospitalized patients average 15% to 25%.[87] In survivors deafness is a frequent sequela. In contrast, the South American arenaviruses (Argentine and Bolivian hemorrhagic fevers) have prominent neurologic and hemorrhagic manifestations.

RVF is endemic in sub-Saharan Africa. Frank hemorrhagic disease is seen in a minority of patients. Retro-orbital pain and blindness from retinitis occurs in 10%. In 1% of patients, fulminant disease with hemorrhage, jaundice, and hepatitis develops, with a 50% fatality rate. Fatal encephalitis occurs in <1%.[88] Marburg and Ebola viruses produce prominent maculopapular rashes and DIC is a major component in their pathogenesis. Both are characterized by pronounced bleeding. Forty-one percent of patients manifest bleeding from puncture sites and mucous membranes; however, this form of bleeding does not distinguish nonsurvivors from survivors. Pulmonary involvement is uncommon and death usually results from multiorgan system failure and cardiovascular collapse.[89,90] Fatality rates for Ebola and Marburg hemorrhagic fevers are 80% and 25%, respectively.[86]

Routine laboratory tests in patients with VHFs are nonspecific, but the presence of early thrombocytopenia and coagulation abnormalities should arouse suspicion. Definitive diagnosis of VHF is done by isolation in cell culture or immunohistochemical staining of formalin-fixed tissues. These techniques should only be attempted under BSL 4 conditions at the CDC or USAMRIID. In the field, viral identification can safely be done following chemical inactivation with ELISA to detect viral antigen as well as IgM and IgG antibodies. Reverse transcriptase PCR has also been successfully applied to field diagnosis.[86]

Medical management for VHF is largely supportive. Patients should be handled as gently as possible as they are especially prone to bleeding. Aspirin and other antiplatelet drugs should be avoided. Immunosuppression with steroids or other agents is contraindicated. Uncontrolled clinical observations support the transfusion of red cells for severe hemorrhage and platelet and clotting factors for DIC. Hemodialysis is of particular help in treatment of HFRS. Mechanical ventilation may be necessary. Treatment of hypotension and shock is often difficult and the use of invasive hemodynamic monitoring techniques may help to guide therapy. Limited experience has shown that rapid infusion of fluids may quickly worsen pulmonary edema because of increased vascular permeability. Fluids are best administered carefully using crystalloids first, and later with the addition of colloids.[86,91] In cases of HPS the use of inotropes may be warranted.[92]

The only specific antiviral therapy available for VHF is ribavirin, a nonimmunosuppressive nucleoside analogue with broad antiviral properties. It has been shown to reduce mortality in Lassa fever and shows promise with the treatment of other arena- and bunyaviruses. Passive immunotherapy has been used successfully in Argentine hemorrhagic fever and shows promise in Bolivian hemorrhagic fever. However, passive immunization is contraindicated in HFRS since an active immune response is already evolving in most patients who are diagnosed. Currently the only licensed vaccine is for yellow fever and is mandatory for all travelers to endemic areas.[86]

Isolation of suspected VHF cases is essential as secondary infections of close contacts and medical personnel are well documented. Until the definitive diagnosis has been made, patients with suspected VHF should be isolated in a single room with an adjoining anteroom serving as an entrance. Negative pressure rooms and strict respiratory precautions may be more appropriate in confirmed severe end-stage disease where the viral load is maximal (see Table 61-4). These precautions may not be possible in the case of large outbreaks. However, it is essential to enforce stringent barrier nursing, with the use of mask, glove, gown, and needle precautions, along with hazard labeling of all laboratory specimens. Patient access should be restricted and the incineration or autoclaving of all contaminated materials including linens is mandatory. Decontamination of areas can likely be carried out by detergents, bleach, and hypochlorite solutions, as these viruses have lipid envelopes making them susceptible.[85]

Category B Agents

Discussion of all the possible biological weapons is beyond the scope of this chapter. However, *Coxiella burnetii* (Q fever), staphylococcal enterotoxin B (SEB toxin), viral equine encephalitides, and ricin toxin deserve attention, as they have been weaponized. Furthermore they can all present as an upper respiratory viral illness, making differentiation of biological attack from a natural viral epidemic difficult (see Table 61-3).

Q fever is a zoonotic disease of herded animals. Humans acquire it via inhalation. It is extremely infectious, requiring as few as 10 organisms to produce disease. The incubation time is 2 to 14 days. Patients present with signs and symptoms of a seasonal viral syndrome that can be prolonged in two thirds for up to 2 weeks. The most frequent physical finding is rales on chest exam. Chest x-rays are abnormal in 50% to 60% of cases, most often showing consolidation, but effusions also occur. Routine blood tests commonly show elevations of liver transaminases and alkaline phosphatase up to three times normal. Fatalities are extremely rare; however, the disease is incapacitating. Treatment and prophylaxis is with doxycycline or tetracycline.[93]

SEB is a heat-stable pyrogenic toxin produced by *Staphylococcus aureus*. This toxin can be mass produced and is stable as an aerosol. When inhaled it binds to the MHC class II molecules that stimulate T cells with a massive release of cytokines including interferon-γ, interleukin-6, and tumor necrosis factor (TNF)-α. Within 3 to 12 hours of exposure high fever (up to 106°F), myalgias, nonproductive cough, chest tightness, dyspnea, headache, and vomiting develop. Conjunctival signs are notably absent. On chest examination, rales are the prominent finding. Chest x-ray typically is normal, but can show interstitial pulmonary edema. Postural hypotension as well as profound vasodilatory shock can occur. Patients usually progress rapidly to a relatively stable level of disease, but can be incapacitated for weeks. Lethality is low. Diagnosis is clinical, but serum detection of the toxin is possible with ELISA. Therapy is currently limited to supportive care.[24,94]

The viral equine encephalitides include Venezuelan, eastern, and western viruses (VEE, EEE, and WEE) of the alphavirus family. Humans are accidental hosts, acquiring the virus via a mosquito vector. However, they are highly infectious by aerosol and readily grow in cell cultures. All three of the viruses are capable of killing with varying degrees of neurologic involvement. EEE is most virulent with 50% to 70% mortality, WEE follows with <10% mortality, and VEE has <1% mortality. A febrile prodrome of 1 to 5 days marks replication in bone marrow and lymphoid tissue resulting in lymphopenia. Subsequently high viremia seeds the brain and spinal cord. Central nervous system symptoms and signs include menigismus, hyper- or hypoactive reflexes, and spastic paralysis that can progress to death. Loss of airway protection and status epilepticus may require mechanical ventilation and ICU management. CSF shows elevated protein and 50 to 2000 WBCs/mL with lymphocyte predominance. Definitive diagnosis relies on viral culture of serum or CSF, or antibody detection from serum by ELISA. Therapy is limited to supportive treatment. A live-attenuated vaccine for VEE is available, along with inactivated vaccines for VEE, WEE, and EEE. These vaccines are available under investigational new drug

(IND) release status from the US government but are only 50–85% effective for <1 year.[95]

Ricin toxin is an extract of castor beans. It is highly lethal via ingestion, injection, and inhalation. At the cellular level it kills through the inhibition of protein synthesis. Its clinical features are route-specific. Studies in primates show that within several hours of inhalation a severe diffuse acute tracheobronchitis manifests, followed by fibrin purulent pneumonia with diffuse severe alveolar flooding, peribronchovascular edema, and mediastinal lymphadenitis. Respiratory failure and ARDS are likely to occur within 30 hours. Distinguishing an attack with ricin from either anthrax or pneumonic plague would be extremely difficult. Diagnosis would be largely clinical, but antigen ELISA of nasal swabs should be done within 24 hours. Treatment would be largely supportive, though vaccination with a toxoid in animals is very effective and in development by the U.S. Army.[96]

Role of Critical Care in Bioterrorism

The scenario of a biological weapons attack poses several unique challenges for the intensivist. Although most external disasters will occur with some degree of warning, biological agent exposure is an exception. Here the diagnosis is more likely to be made within a hospital, perhaps a few days after the environmental release.[97] Patients are more likely to seek medical care at the most convenient medical facility instead of responders going to the patients.[98,99] Unlike natural disasters or conventional wars, victims in a biological attack are likely be a more homogenous population. Potentially enormous numbers of ill and exposed patients presenting with the same level of severity will rapidly overwhelm the health care system, its infrastructure, and supplies. Issues of supplies and distribution of medical resources would be a major problem, as already predicted in the TOPOFF exercise.[4] Applying conventional mass disaster triaging schemes may therefore not be possible to a such homogeneously affected population. It is thus important to consider these unique features related to biological agent attacks in both preparation and acute disaster management.

The need for the critical care personnel to be involved in the planning process cannot be overstated. The intensivist will become a key figure in governing the flow of patient traffic, making triage decisions, and allocating ICU resources for patients in the ER, OR, recovery room, and the rest of the hospital. Intensivists should understand capabilities, resources, and limitations of various governmental and nongovernmental disaster-related agencies, as well as consider their hospital's location and community resources in anticipating a likely disaster scenario.[97]

Although the full details of a hospital's preparedness plan are beyond the scope of this chapter, certain key issues deserve attention in coping with such a disaster. Readers are referred to the CDC web site for preparation and planning for a bioterrorist attack at http://www.bt.cdc.gov/planning/index. asp, as well as individual state health department guidelines for preparedness, and their own hospital's disaster management plans.

1. Define the area to be covered during a disaster scenario. Intensivists should familiarize themselves with their hospital disaster plan, and know their responsibilities relative to other departments in the plan.
2. Identification and assignment of key personnel in the hospital, emergency response personnel, state and local authorities, and key members of the community.
3. Assessment of hospital infrastructure, supplies at hand, and manpower for a given situation. This would also include knowing the vendor lists to meet sudden demand for supplies and knowledge of the absolute limits of the hospital resources (inventory of ventilators, oxygen tanks, intravenous catheters, isolation capabilities of the hospital, etc).
4. Establishing secure lines of communication internally via a central command post or incident center, as well as externally with the LRN, National Pharmaceutical Stockpile (NPS), and local, state, and federal authorities. Successful interaction with these agencies will likely define the successful management of a disaster response (Table 61-6).
5. Defining portals of entry to the hospital and creating safe arrival and triage areas, in addition to decontamination areas.
6. Establishing algorithms for triage from the ED and clinics, as well as criteria for ICU admission. As surge capacity nears, the risks and benefits of treating existing patients in the hospital and carrying out elective surgeries needs to be weighed. Knowledge of alternative beds and transfer agreements with nearby ICUs would be crucial in this regard.
7. Early efforts must be made to contain the agent. This can be achieved by education of staff and public, early efforts to identify the agent through the LRN, reporting of the agent to the local, state, and federal health authorities, early intervention and treatment of the disease, and early implementation of appropriate infection control measures (Tables 61-6 and 61-7).
8. Ensuring the safety of workers. This includes issues of isolation precautions, evaluation of the potential for spread among other patients and staff once the agent has been confirmed, postexposure prophylaxis, and vaccination. Staff exhaustion and posttraumatic stress disorder should be anticipated, and dealt with by scheduling adequate rest periods, appropriate use of volunteer staff, and a program of critical incident stress management.
9. Carrying out drills and mock events for continual assessment of flaws in organization and execution of the plan.

Summary

A bioterrorist attack of any kind has the potential to overwhelm a community and indeed an entire nation. A high degree of suspicion and prompt recognition of an event will be required in order to contain it. The likelihood of exposed patients to require hospitalization and specifically critical care is high, and specific knowledge of the possible agents and estimating the needs of a health care facility and community will be the cornerstones in disaster preparedness for a biological attack. Aside from the delivery of critical care to the patient in the ICU, the intensivist will be involved in making triage decisions (which automatically dictates how other non-ICU beds are used and managed), managing resources related to the ICU, and coordinating a multidisciplinary effort in caring for the exposed.

TABLE 61-6 Biosafety Precautions

Biosafety Level	Agents	Practices	Safety Equipment (Primary Barriers)	Facilities (Secondary Barriers)
1	Not known to cause disease in healthy adults	Standard microbiological practices	None required	Open bench-top sink required
2	Associated with human disease; hazard from autoinoculation, ingestion, mucous membrane exposure	BSL-1 practice plus: a) Limited access; b) Biohazard warning signs; c) Sharps precautions; d) Biosafety manual defining any needed waste decontamination or medical surveillance policies	Primary barriers; Class I or II BSCs or other physical containment devices used for all manipulations of agents that cause splashes or aerosols of infectious materials; PPEs: laboratory coats, gloves, face protection as needed.	BSL-1 plus: autoclave available
3	Indigenous or exotic agents with potential for aerosol transmission; disease may have serious or lethal consequences	BSL-2 practice plus: a) Controlled access; b) Decontamination of all waste; c) Decontamination of lab clothing before laundering; d) Baseline serum	Primary barriers; Class I or II BCSs or other physical containment devices used for all manipulations of agents; PPEs: protective lab clothing, gloves, respiratory protection as needed	BSL-2 plus: a) Physical separation from access corridors; b) Self-closing, double-door access; c) Exhausted air not recirculated; d) Negative airflow into laboratory
4	Dangerous/exotic agents that pose high risk of life-threatening disease, aerosol-transmitted lab infections, or related agents with unknown risk of transmission	BSL-3 practices plus: a) Clothing change before entering; b) Shower on exit; c) All material decontaminated on exit from facility	Primary barriers: All procedures conducted in Class III BSCs or Class I or II BSCs in combination with full-body, air-supplied, positive-pressure personnel suit.	BSL-3 plus: a) Separate building or isolated zone; b) Dedicated supply/exhaust, vacuum, and decon systems

ABBREVIATIONS: BSC, biosafety cabinets; PPE, personal protective equipment.

TABLE 61-7 Internet Resources

Government and Environmental Resources	Address
CDC weibsite for bioterrorism	http://www.bt.cdc.gov/
National Disaster Management System	http://ndms.dhhs.gov/index.html
Environmental Protection Agency	http://www.epa.gov
National Response Team	http:www.nrt.org/
Federal Emergency Management Agency	http://www.fema.gov/
Federal Bureau of Investigation	http://www.fbi.gov/
State Department Counter-Terrorism Coordinator	http://www.state.gov/www/global/terrorism/index.html
U.S. Army Medical Research Institute of Infectious Disease (USAMRIID)	http://www.usamriid.army.mil/
Department of Defense Global Emerging Infections	http://www.geis.ha.osd.mil/

Useful Professional Organizations	Address
Association for Professionals in Infection Control and Epidemiology (APIC)	http://www.apic.org/
American Public Health Association	http://www.apha.org/
National Association of EMS Physicians	http://www.naemsp.org/
American College of Emergency Physicians	http://www.acep.org/
American Society for Microbiology (ASM)	http://www.asmusa.org/

Institutions	Address
Johns Hopkins Center for Civilian Biodefense Studies	http://www.hopkins-biodefense.org/
Saint Louis School of Public Health/Center for the Study of Bioterrorism and Emerging Infections	http://bioterrorism.slu.edu/
Center for Nonproliferation Studies/Monterey Institute for International Studies	http://www.cns.miis.edu/

Chemical & Biological Hotline	1-800-424-8802 (Emergency Only)

Acknowledgments

This chapter is adapted from a previous publication: Karwa M, Bronzert P, Kvetan V: Bioterrorism and critical care. *Crit Care Clin* 19:279, 2003. Reproduced with permission from Elsevier.

References

1. Jernigan JA, Stephens DS, Ashford DA, et al: Bioterrorism related inhalational anthrax: The first 10 cases reported in the United States. *Emerg Infect Dis* 7:933, 2001.
2. Tucker JB: Historical trends related to bioterrorism: An empirical analysis. *Emerg Infect Dis* 5:498, 1999.
3. Health Aspects of Chemical and Biological Weapons: Report of a WHO Group of Consultants. Geneva, World Health Organization, 1970, pp 72, 99.
4. Inglesby TV, Grossman R, O'Toole T: A plague on your city: Observations from TOPOFF. *Clin Infect Dis* 32:436, 2001.
5. O'Toole T: Smallpox: An attack scenario. *Emerg Infect Dis* 5:540, 1999.
6. Rotz LD, Khan AS, Lillibridge SR, et al: Public health assessment of potential biological terrorism agents. *Emerging Infect Dis* 8:225, 2002.
7. Khan AS, Sage MJ: The Centers for Disease Control's Strategic Planning Workgroup, Biological and chemical terrorism: Strategic plan for preparedness and response. *Morb Mortal Wkly Rep* 49(RR-4):1, 2000.
8. Departments of the Army, the Navy, and the Air Force. Washington, FM 8-9, NATO Handbook on the Medical Aspects of NBC Defensive Operations AmedP-6; Part II Biological, 1996; http://www.fas.org/nuke/guide/usa/doctrine/dod/fn8-9/toc.htm, Accessed November 7, 2001.
9. English JF, Cundiff MY, Malone JD, et al: APIC Bioterrorism Task Force & CDC Hospital Infections Program Bioterrorism Working Group, Bioterrorism readiness plan: A template for healthcare facilities. April 1999. http://www.apic.org/educ/readinow.cfm. Accessed January 3, 2002.
10. Birerzvige A: Inhalation Hazard from Reaerosolized Biological Agents: a Review [report No. CRDEC-TR-413]. Aberdeen Proving Ground, MD: Chemical Research Development and Engineering Center, 1992.
11. Chinn KSK: Aerosol Penetration of Chemical Protective Overgarment [report No. DPG/JCP-94/005]. Dugway, UT: Joint Contact Point Directorate, U.S. Army Dugway Proving Ground, 1994.
12. Morrow PE, Yu CP: Models of Aerosol Behavior in Airways. Aerosols in Medicine: Principles, Diagnosis and Therapy. New York, Elsevier Science Publishers (Biomedical Division), 1985, p 149.
13. Sobel J, Khan AS, Swerdlow DL: Threat of a biological terrorist attack on the US food supply: The CDC perspective. *Lancet* 359:874, 2002.
14. Inglesby TV, Henderson DA, Bartlett JG, et al: Anthrax as a biological weapon: Medical and public health management. *JAMA* 281:1735, 1999.
15. Dixon TC, Meselson M, Guillemin J, et al: Anthrax. *N Engl J Med* 341:815, 1999.
16. Meselson M, Guillemin J, Hugh-Jones M, et al: The Sverdlosk anthrax outbreak of 1979. *Science* 266:1202, 1994.
17. Friedlander A, Welkos SL, Pitt ML, et al: Postexposure prophylaxis against experimental inhalation anthrax, *J Infect Dis* 167:1239, 1993.
18. Brossier F, Mock M: Toxins of *Bacillus anthracis*. *Toxicon* 39:1747, 2001.
19. Brachman PS: Inhalation anthrax. *Ann NY Acad Sci* 353:83, 1980.
20. Dahlgren CM, Buchanan LM, Decker HM, et al: *Bacillus anthracis* aerosols in goat hair processing mills. *Am J Hyg* 72:24, 1960.
21. Walker JS, Lincoln RE, Klein F: Pathophysiological and biochemical changes in anthrax. *Fed Proc* 26:1539, 1967.
22. Amramova FA, Grinberg LM, Yampolskaya O, et al: Pathology of inhalational anthrax in 42 cases from the Sverdlovsk outbreak in 1979. *Proc Natl Acad Sci USA* 90:2291, 1993.
23. Kim HJ, Jun WB, Lee SH, et al: CT and MRI findings of anthrax meningoencephalitis: Report of two cases and review of the literature. *Am Soc Neuroradiol* 22:1303, 2001.
24. Franz DR, Jahrling PB, Friedlander A, et al: Clinical recognition and management of patients exposed to biological warfare agents. *JAMA* 278:399, 1997.
25. Mayer TA, Matcha SB, Murphy C: Clinical presentation of inhalational anthrax following bioterrorism exposure: Report of 2 surviving patients. *JAMA* 286:2549, 2001.
26. Vessal K, Yeganehdoust J, Dutz W, Kohout E: Radiologic changes in inhalation anthrax. *Clin Radiol* 26:471, 1975.
27. Barnes JM: Penicillin and B anthracis. *J Pathol Bacteriol* 194:113, 1947.
28. Lincoln RE, Klein F, Walker JS, et al: Successful treatment of monkeys for septicemic anthrax, in *Antimicrobial Agents and Chemotherapy—1964*. Washington, American Society for Microbiology, 1965, p 759.
29. Penn C, Klotz SA: Anthrax, in Gorbach SL, Bartlett JG, Blacklow NR (eds): *Infectious Diseases*. Philadelphia, WB Saunders, 1998, p 1575.
30. Knisely RF: Selective medium for *Bacillus anthracis*. *J Bacteriol* 92:784, 1966.
31. Miller JM: Agents of bioterrorism: Preparing for bioterrorism at the community health care level. *Infect Dis Clin* 15:1127, 2001.
32. Swartz MN: Recognition and management of anthrax—an update. *N Engl J Med* 345:1621, 2001.
33. CDC guidelines for state health departments on how to handle anthrax and other biological agent threats (revised Oct. 14, 2001). Atlanta, Centers for Disease Control and Prevention. http://www.bt.cdc.gov. Accessed October 26, 2001.
34. Update: Investigation of bioterrorism-related anthrax and interim guidelines for exposure management and antimicrobial therapy, October 2001. *Morb Mortal Wkly Rep* 50:909, 2001. http://www.cdc.gov/mmwr/preview/mmwrhtml/mm5042a1.htm. Accessed February 16, 2002.
35. Inglesby TV, Dennis DT, Henderson DA, et al: Plague as a biological weapon: Medical and public health management. *JAMA* 283:2281, 2000.
36. Centers for Disease Control and Prevention: Human plague—United States, 1993–1994. *Morb Mortal Wkly Rep* 43:242, 1994.
37. Butler T: *Yesinia* species (including plague), in Mandell GL, Bennett JE, Dolin R (eds): *Principles and Practice of Infectious Diseases*. New York, Churchill Livingstone, 1995, p 2070.
38. Centers for Disease Control and Prevention: Fatal human plague. *Morb Mortal Wkly Rep* 278:380, 1997.
39. Freidlander AM, McGovern TW: Plague, in Sidell FR, Takafuji ET, Franz DR (eds): Part I: *Medical Aspects of Chemical and Biological Warfare* (Textbook of Military Medicine). Office of the Surgeon General, Department of the Army, United States of America, 1997, p 479.
40. Dennis DT, Gage K, Gratz N, et al: Plague Manual: Epidemiology, Distribution, Surveillance and Control. World Health Organization, Communicable Disease Surveillance and Response, 1999. http://www.who.int/emc_documents/plague/whocdscsredc992c.html.
41. Reyn CF, Weber NS, Tempest B, et al: Epidemiologic and clinical features of an outbreak of bubonic plague in New Mexico. *J Infect Dis* 136:489, 1977.
42. Dennis JA, Mettler FA, Mann JM: Radiographic manifestations of plague in New Mexico, 1975–1980. *Radiology* 139:561, 1981.

43. Dennis JC, Vernalo JR, Lombardi LJ, et al: Plague pneumonia: Disease caused by *Yesinia pestis. Semin Respir Med* 12:12, 1997.

44. Florman AL, Spencer RR, Sheward S: Multiple lung cavities in a 12 year old girl with bubonic plague, sepsis, and secondary pneumonia. *Am J Med* 80:1191, 1986.

45. Hull H, Montes JM, Mann JM: Septicemic plague in New Mexico. *J Infect Dis* 155:113, 1987.

46. Werner SB, Weidmer CE, Nelson BC, et al: Primary plague pneumonia contracted from a domestic cat in South Lake Tahoe, California. *JAMA* 251:929, 1984.

47. Centers for Disease Control and Prevention: Pneumonic plague—Arizona. *Morb Mortal Wkly Rep* 41:737, 1992.

48. Meyer K: Pneumonic plague. *Bacteriol Rev* 25:249, 1961.

49. Centers for Disease Control and Prevention: Prevention of plague: Recommendations of the Advisory Committee on Immunization Practices. *Morb Mortal Wkly Rep* 45:RR-14, 1996.

50. Cross JT, Penn RL: *Francisella tularensis* tularemia, in Mandell GL, et al (eds): *Principles and Practice of Infectious Diseases.* Philadelphia, Churchill Livingstone, 2000, p 2393.

51. Saslaw S, Eigelsbach HT, Prior JA, et al: Tularemia vaccine study. II: Respiratory challenge. *Arch Intern Med* 107:134, 1961.

52. Geyer SJ, Burkey A, Chandler FW: Tularemia, in Connor DH (ed): *Pathology of Infectious Diseases.* Stamford, CT, Appleton & Lange, 1997, p 869.

53. Evans ME, Gregory DW, Schaffner W, McGee ZA: Tularemia: a 30-year experience with 88 cases. *Medicine* 64:251, 1985.

54. Freidlander AM, Evans ME: Tularemia, in Sidell FR, Takafuji ET, Franz DR (eds): Part I: *Medical Aspects of Chemical and Biological Warfare* (Textbook of Military Medicine). Office of the Surgeon General, Department of the Army, United States of America, 1997, p 503.

55. Cunha BA, Gill V: Tularemia pneumonia. *Semin Respir Infect* 12:61, 1997.

56. Sunderrajan EV, Hutton J, Marienfeld D: Adult respiratory distress syndrome secondary to tularemia pneumonia. *Arch Intern Med* 145:1435, 1985.

57. Tularemia, in Kortepeter M, Christopher G, Cieslak T, et al (eds): *USAMRIID's Medical Management of Biological Casualties Handbook,* 4th ed. Ft. Detrick, MD, 2001, p 37. http://www.usamriid.army.mil/education/bluebook.html. Accessed February 18, 2002.

58. Overholt EL, Tigert WD, Kadull PJ, et al: An analysis of forty two cases of laboratory acquired tularemia. *Am J Med* 30:785, 1961.

59. Franz DR, Pitt LM, Clayton MA, et al: Efficacy of prophylactic and therapeutic administration of antitoxin for inhalation botulism, in DasGupta BR (ed): *Botulinum and Tetanus Neurotoxins: Neurotransmission and Biomedical Aspects.* New York, Plenum Press, 1993, p 473.

60. Pettersson T, Nyberg P, Nordstrom D, et al: Similar pleural fluid in pleuropulmonary tularemia and tuberculous pleurisy. *Chest* 109:572, 1996.

61. Dennis DT, Inglesby TV, Henderson DA: Tularemia as a biological weapon: Medical and public health management. *JAMA* 285:2763, 2001.

62. Shapiro RL, Hatheway C, Swerdlow DL: Botulism in the United States: a clinical and epidemiologic review. *Ann Intern Med* 129:221, 1998.

63. Centers for Disease Control and Prevention: *Botulism in the United States 1899–1996: Handbook for Epidemiologists, Clinicians, and Laboratory Workers.* Atlanta, CDC, 1998. http://www.cdc.gov/ncdod/dbmd/diseaseinfo/botulism.pdf. Accessed March 5, 2002.

64. Gangarosa EJ, Donadio JA, Armstrong RW, et al: Botulism in the United States, 1899–1969. *Am J Epidemiol* 93:93, 1971.

65. Mann JM, Martin S, Hoffman R, Marrazzo S: Patient recovery from type A botulism: Morbidity assessment following a large outbreak. *Am J Public Health* 71:266, 1981.

66. Montecucco C (ed): Clostridial neurotoxins: The molecular pathogenesis of tetanus and botulism. *Curr Top Microbiol Immunol* 195:1, 1995.

67. Botulinum toxins, in Middlebrook JL, Franz DR (EDS): *USAMRIID's Medical Management of Biological Casualties Handbook,* 4th ed. Ft. Detrick, MD, 2001, p 63. http://www.usamriid.army.mil/education/bluebook.html. Accessed March 5, 2002.

68. Hughes JM, Blumenthal JR, Merson MH, et al: Clinical features of types A and B food-borne botulism. *Ann Intern Med* 95:442, 1981.

69. Nowara WWS, Samet JM, Rosario PA: Early and late pulmonary complications of botulism. *Arch Intern Med* 143:451, 1983.

70. Cherington M: Clinical spectrum of botulism. *Muscle Nerve* 21:701, 1998.

71. Khajehdehi P: Toxemic shock, hematuria, hypokalemia, and hypoproteinemia in a case of cutaneous anthrax. *Mt Sinai J Med* 68:213, 2001.

72. Santos JI, Swensen P, Glasgow LA: Potentiation of *Clostridium botulinum* toxin by aminoglycoside antibiotics: Clinical and laboratory observations. *Pediatrics* 68:50, 1981.

73. Schulze J, Toepfer M, Schroff KC, et al: Clindamycin and nicotinic neuromuscular transmission. *Lancet* 354:1792, 1999.

74. Arnon SS, Schecter R, Inglesby TV: Botulinum toxin as a biological weapon: Medical and public health management. *JAMA* 285:1059, 2001.

75. World Health Organization: The Global Eradication of Smallpox: Final Report of the Global Commission for the Certification of Smallpox Eradication. Geneva, World Health Organization, 1980, p 5. Available at http://whqlibdoc.who.int/publications/a41438.pdf. Accessed February 2002.

76. Mcclain DJ: Smallpox, in Sidell FR, Takafuji ET, Franz DR (eds): Part I: *Medical Aspects of Chemical and Biological Warfare* (Textbook of Military Medicine). Office of the Surgeon General, Department of the Army, United States of America, 1997, p 539.

77. Fenner F, Henderson DA, Arita I, et al: Smallpox and its eradication. Geneva, World Health Organization, 1988, p 1460.

78. Breman JG, Henderson DA: Diagnosis and management of smallpox. *N Engl J Med* 346:1300, 2002.

79. Koplan JP, Foster SO: Smallpox: Clinical types, causes of death, and treatment. *J Infect Dis* 140:440, 1979.

80. Esposito JJ, Massung RF: Poxvirus infections in humans, in Murray PR, Tenover F, Baron EJ (eds): *Clinical Microbiology.* Washington, American Society of Microbiology, 1995, p 1131.

81. Henderson DA, Inglesby TV, Bartlett JG, et al: Smallpox as a biological weapon: Medical and public health management. *JAMA* 281:2127, 1999.

82. Meltzer MI, Damon I, LeDuc JW, et al: Modeling potential responses to smallpox as a bioterrorist weapon. *Emerg Infect Dis* 7:959, 2001.

83. Frey SE, Couch RB, Tacket CO, et al: Clinical responses to undiluted and diluted smallpox vaccine. *N Engl J Med* 346:1265, 2002.

84. Centers for Disease Control: Vaccinia (smallpox) vaccine recommendations of the Advisory Committee on Immunization Practices (ACIP), 2001. *Morb Mortal Wkly Rep* 50(RR-10):1, 2001.

85. Centers of Disease Control: Notice to readers update: Management of patients with suspected viral hemorrhagic fever—United States. *Morb Mortal Wkly Rep* 44:475, 1995.

86. Jahrling PB: Viral hemorrhagic fevers, in Sidell FR, Takafuji ET, Franz DR (eds): Part I: *Medical Aspects of Chemical and Biological Warfare* (Textbook of Military Medicine). Office of the Surgeon General, Department of the Army, United States of America, 1997, p 591.

87. McCormick JB, King IJ, Webb PA, et al: A case-control study of the clinical diagnosis and course of Lassa fever. *J Infect Dis* 155:445, 1987.

88. Peters CJ: Arenaviridae and bunyaviridae, in Mandell GL, Bennett JE, Dolin R (eds): *Principles and Practice of Infectious Diseases.* New York, Churchill Livingstone, 1995, p 1856.

89. Bwaka MA, Bonnet MJ, Calain P, et al: Ebola hemorrhagic fever in Kikwit, Democratic Republic of the Congo: Clinical observations in 103 patients. *J Infect Dis* 179(Suppl 1):S1, 1999.

90. Heyman DL, Barakamfitye D, Szczeniowski M, et al: Ebola hemorrhagic fever: Lessons learned from Kikwit, Democratic Republic of the Congo. *J Infect Dis* 179(Suppl 1):S283, 1999.

91. Soni A, Chugh K, Sachdev A, et al: Management of dengue in ICU. *Indian J Pediatr* 68:1051, 2001.

92. Hallin G, Simpson S, Cromwell R, et al: Cardiopulmonary manifestations of hantavirus pulmonary syndrome. *Crit Care Med* 24:252, 1996.

93. Q fever, in Middlebrook JL, Franz DR (EDS): *USAMRIID's Medical Management of Biological Casualties Handbook*, 4th ed. Ft. Detrick, MD, 2001, p 33. http://www.usamriid.army.mil/education/bluebook.html. Accessed March 5, 2002.

94. Ulrich RG, Sheldon S, Taylor T, et al: Staphylococcal enterotoxin B and related pyrogenic toxins, in Sidell FR, Takafuji ET, Franz DR (eds): Part I: *Medical Aspects of Chemical and Biological Warfare* (Textbook of Military Medicine). Office of the Surgeon General, Department of the Army, United States of America, 1997, p 621.

95. Smith JF, Davis KY, Hart MK, et al: Viral encephalitides, in Sidell FR, Takafuji ET, Franz DR (eds): Part I: *Medical Aspects of Chemical and Biological Warfare* (Textbook of Military Medicine). Office of the Surgeon General, Department of the Army, United States of America, 1997, p 561.

96. Wilhelmsen C, Pitt L: Lesions of acute inhaled lethal ricin intoxication in rhesus monkeys. *Vet Pathol* 30:482, 1993.

97. Roccaforte JD, Cushman JG: Disaster preparation and management for the intensive care unit. *Curr Opin Crit Care* 8:607, 2002.

98. Joint Commission on Accreditation of Healthcare Organizations: Emergency management in the new millennium. 21:2, 2001. Available at http://www.jcrinc.com/docviewer.aspx. Accessed August 2002.

99. Simon R, Teperman S: The World Trade Center Attack. Lessons for disaster management. *Crit Care* 5:318, 2001.

100. Borio L, Frank D, Mani V, et al. Death due to bioterrorism-related inhalational anthrax: Report of 2 patients. *JAMA* 286:2554, 2001.

101. Downie A, Dumbell K: Survival of variola virus in dried exudates and crusts in small pox patients. *Lancet* 1:550, 1947.

102. Bartlett J, Borio L, Radonovich L, et al: Small pox vaccination in 2003: Key information for clinicians. *Clin Infect Dis* 36:883, 2003.

PART VI

NEUROLOGIC DISORDERS

Chapter 62 _____
DELIRIUM IN THE INTENSIVE CARE UNIT
E. WESLEY ELY

KEY POINTS
- *Delirium may be considered to be present when there is an acute or fluctuating change in mental status and inattention coupled to disordered thinking or an altered level of consciousness.*
- *Delirium is extraordinarily common among patient populations in the intensive care unit (ICU) and is under-recognized by care providers, in part related to a previous lack of tools to assess this phenomenon.*
- *Hypoactive or mixed forms of delirium are more common than pure hyperactive delirium.*
- *The Confusion Assessment Method for the ICU is a well-validated tool to provide simple and reproducible assessment of delirium at the bedside.*
- *The risk factors for delirium may be divided into host factors, the acute illness, and environmental or iatrogenic factors.*
- *Because age and pre-existing mental impairment are powerful risk factors for delirium, it is likely to be encountered with increasing frequency in the ICU in the future.*
- *Because administration of psychoactive drugs, including sedatives and analgesics, is an important risk factor for delirium, this represents a fruitful area for modification of practice to reduce the incidence of delirium in ICU patients.*
- *Delirium is independently associated with increased morbidity, cost of care, and mortality rate, even after adjusting for severity of illness, age, coma, and other relevant covariates.*

Patients in the intensive care unit (ICU) who experience delirium are exhibiting an under-recognized form of *organ dysfunction*. Delirium is extremely common in ICU patients due to factors such as comorbidity, critical illness, and iatrogenesis. This neurologic complication can be extremely hazardous in hospitalized older persons and is associated with death, prolonged hospital stays, and institutionalization. Neurologic dysfunction compromises patients' ability to be removed from mechanical ventilation or achieve full recovery and independence. Unfortunately, health care providers in the ICU are unaware of delirium in many circumstances, especially those in which the patient's delirium is manifesting predominantly as the hypoactive (quiet) subtype as opposed to the hyperactive (agitated) subtype. In the past few years, research on ICU delirium has demonstrated the importance of this problem in critically ill patients in addition to methods for routinely monitoring delirium at the bedside. This chapter reviews the definition and salient features of delirium, its primary risk factors, validated methods for bedside delirium assessment, pharmacologic agents associated with the development of delirium, and pharmacologic and non-pharmacologic strategies for delirium management.

Historically, two words were used to describe confused patients. One was the Roman word *delirium*, which referred to an agitated and confused person (think of hyperactive delirium). The other was from the Greek word *lethargus*, which was used to describe a quietly confused person (think of hypoactive delirium). ICU patients commonly demonstrate both subtypes as they progress through different stages of their illness and therapy. In either case, the patient's brain is not functioning normally. It therefore makes sense that the original derivation of delirium comes from the Latin word *deliria*, which literally means to "be out of your furrow." For greater clarity and to avoid misuse of terms such as *dementia* and *delirium*, Table 62-1 lists basic definitions of some common cognitive syndromes.

Health care professionals in the ICU have traditionally used inadequate monitoring devices to detect dysfunction in arguably the most important organ of all, the brain. Delirium, an acute central nervous system (CNS) dysfunction resulting from any number of common insults that ICU patients experience, has largely been overlooked in critical care research until the past few years. Recent discussions of encephalopathy and organ dysfunction secondary to sepsis have not mentioned delirium as one of the clinical manifestations of CNS dysfunction.[1,2]

The ICU literature often refers to delirium as *ICU psychosis*,[3–8] which represents a potentially dangerous misnomer. The development of delirium often goes unnoticed in the ICU because we think of it as "part of the scenery" or an expected and inconsequential outcome of mechanical ventilation and other therapies. A series of investigations has recently been conducted that provide validated means of detecting delirium by nonpsychiatrists (e.g., internists, nurses, or respiratory therapists). The CNS monitoring instruments and observations from these investigations are leading to a change in the culture and practice in the ICU in which health care providers more closely follow patients for the development of delirium and modify their care to help prevent this potentially disastrous complication. The most recent clinical practice guidelines from the Society of Critical Care Medicine (SCCM)[9] have recommended routine (daily) monitoring of delirium in all mechanically ventilated patients, which is discussed later in this chapter.

Pathophysiology and Etiology of Delirium

Delirium is thought to be related to imbalances in the synthesis, release, and inactivation of neurotransmitters that modulate the control of cognitive function, behavior, and mood.[8,10] Three of the neurotransmitter systems involved in the pathophysiology of delirium are dopamine, γ-aminobutyric acid, and acetylcholine.[11,12] Whereas dopamine increases excitability of neurons, γ-aminobutyric acid and acetylcholine decrease neuronal excitability.[11] An imbalance of one or more of these neurotransmitters results in neuronal instability and unpredictable neurotransmission. In general, an excess of dopamine and depletion of acetylcholine are two major physiologic problems felt to be central to delirium. In addition to these neurotransmitter systems, others are thought to be involved in the development of delirium, such as serotonin imbalance, endorphin hyperfunction, and increased central noradrenergic activity.[10,12]

TABLE 62-1 Highlights Regarding Cognitive Syndromes

Confusion	A characteristic occurring in delirium, resulting in an altered state of consciousness, and characterized by deficits in attention, memory, visual-constructional ability, and executive functions (also defined as reduced mental clarity, coherence, comprehension, and reasoning).
	Think: Disturbed orientation with respect to person, place, and time.
Delirium	A disturbance of consciousness characterized by an *acute* onset and fluctuating course of impaired cognitive functioning, so that a patient's ability to receive, process, store, and recall information is strikingly impaired. Delirium develops over a short period (hours to days), is usually reversible, and is a direct consequence of a medical condition, substance intoxication or withdrawal, use of a medication, toxin exposure, or a combination of these factors.
	Think: Rapid onset, clouded consciousness (bewildered/confused), often worse at night, fluctuating.
Dementia	Development of a state of generalized cognitive deficits in which there is a deterioration of previously acquired intellectual abilities usually developing over weeks and months. The deficits include memory impairment and at least one of the following: aphasia, apraxia, agnosia, or a disturbance in executive functioning. The cognitive deficits must be sufficiently severe to cause impairment in occupational or social functioning, and they may be progressive, static, or reversible depending on the pathology and the availability of effective treatment.
	Think: Gradual onset, intellectual impairment, memory disturbance, personality/mood change, no clouding of consciousness.
Psychosis	A major mental disorder characterized by hallucinations, delusions, or the inability to distinguish reality from fantasy, which lead to an inability to maintain interpersonal relations and to compromised daily functioning.
	Think: Hallucinations/delusions, impaired reality testing, inappropriate mood and impulse control, no clouding of consciousness.

SOURCE: Reprinted with permission from Ely EW, et al: Delirium in the intensive care unit: An unrecognized syndrome of organ dysfunction. *Semin Respir Crit Care Med* 22:115, 2001.

Several causal factors lead to neurotransmitter imbalance, including reduction in cerebral metabolism, primary intracranial disease, systemic illness, secondary infection of the brain, exogenous toxic agents, withdrawal from substances of abuse such as alcohol or sedative-hypnotic agents, hypoxemia, metabolic disturbances, and the administration of psychoactive medications such as benzodiazepines and narcotics.[12,13] Cognitive neuroscience and psychopharmacology are active areas of research that may advance our understanding and treatment of delirium.

"Confusion" Regarding Delirium Terminology

There are more than 25 terms in the literature used to refer to delirium, such as "subacute befuddlement" and "toxic confusional state." Others simply refer to delirium as confusion or neurological impairment. The neurologic literature tends to use the terms *delirium* to refer exclusively to the hyperactive subtype[14] and *encephalopathy* to refer to hypoactive delirium. These subtypes are discussed in the next section of this chapter. *ICU psychosis* is a potentially dangerous misnomer that refers to delirious patients who demonstrate increased psychomotor activity and hallucinations (i.e., hyperactive delirium).[3–8]

Occurrence of Delirium in the ICU and Its Subtypes

The prevalence of delirium in ICU cohort studies has been reported as 20%,[15] 70%,[16] and 80%,[17] depending on the characteristics of the patient population and the instrument used. Its incidence is likely to increase in future years as older persons more frequently receive ICU care. Two events that are frequently linked during older patients' ICU course are the need for mechanical ventilation and the development of profound and possibly persistent cognitive impairment.[18]

Almost every patient in the ICU receives narcotics or benzodiazepines at some point during their stay, yet physicians rarely modify the quantity or dosing intervals of these drugs based on patients' age. Patients on mechanical ventilation are frequently sedated to the point of stupor or coma to improve oxygenation, alleviate agitation, and prevent them from removing support devices. However, age is only rarely factored into complex decisions concerning how to dose these potent medications or when to remove sedatives and liberate patients from mechanical ventilation. The result is that it is now commonplace in the ICU to find that most elderly patients receiving mechanical ventilation are in a drug-induced state of "suspended animation."[19]

The subtypes of delirium based upon motor activity are hypoactive, hyperactive, and mixed. Peterson et al recently reported on delirium subtypes from a cohort of 613 ventilated and nonventilated ICU patients in whom delirium was monitored for more than 20,000 observations.[20] These investigators found that, among patients who developed delirium, pure hyperactive delirium was rare (<5%), whereas hypoactive and mixed types of delirium were the predominant subtypes (~45% each). Interestingly, the hypoactive subtype was significantly more common in older than in young patients. The risk factors for and clinical implications of these subtypes are the subject of ongoing investigations.

The period surrounding cessation of sedation represents a typical scenario in the ICU setting in which delirium may be easily recognized or completely missed by clinicians. Patients emerging from the effects of sedation may do so peacefully or in a combative manner. At one extreme are the "peaceful" patients who are often erroneously assumed to be thinking clearly. Delirium in this context is referred to as *hypoactive delirium* and is characterized by decreased mental and physical activities and inattention.[6] Such mental status changes could lead to adverse outcomes such as reintubation, which itself has been shown to increase 10-fold the risk of nosocomial pneumonia and death. In addition, hypoactive delirium is associated with aspiration, pulmonary embolism, decubitus ulcers, and other complications related to immobility.

At the other extreme are agitated or combative patients (i.e., hyperactive delirium) who are at risk not only for self-extubation and subsequent reintubation but also for pulling out central venous access and even falling out of bed. These patients are most often given larger doses of sedatives that commit them to at least another day of mechanical ventilation. This places patients at risk for being left in a cognitively impaired state and on mechanical ventilation unnecessarily.[21] Because of this difficult cycle, it is important for health care professionals to avoid overuse of psychoactive medications and to develop better methods of assessing cognitive function, especially during the transition from drug-induced or metabolic coma to wakefulness.

Missing the Diagnosis of Delirium

The "quiet," or hypoactive, delirium is frequently overlooked by physicians and nurses.[22–25] Delirium remains unrecognized by the clinician in as many as 66% to 84% of patients experiencing this complication,[26,27] and it may be attributed incorrectly to dementia, depression, or just an "expected" occurrence in the critically ill, elderly patient.[26] Many clinicians expect delirium to present with agitation or hallucinations, features that are not required for the diagnosis. Other reasons for the lack of recognition of delirium include infrequent cognitive assessments and the fluctuating nature of delirium. The very development of delirium has been associated with fewer interactions and less time spent by nurses and physicians in direct patient care.[28,29]

Geriatric ICU Concerns and Pre-existing Cognitive Impairment

It is estimated that the cost of care for those older than 65 years will increase 10-fold over the next three decades.[30] These data have been used to argue for limiting ICU care provided to the elderly to conserve resources.[31–33] However, a recent report from Angus et al. documented that nearly 60% of all ICU days were incurred by patients older than 65 years.[34] In fact, adults younger than 65 had 37 ICU days per year per 1000 person-years versus 240 for those older than 75 years. The incidence of acute respiratory failure requiring mechanical ventilation rises 10-fold from the age of 55 to 85,[35] resulting in larger numbers of elderly patients treated in ICUs.[36]

Because of these age-related demographics and the relation between pre-existing cognitive impairment and development of delirium, clinicians are likely to discover an increased burden of delirium among hospitalized patients across the country.[37,38] Advanced age and cognitive decline have been found to lead to decreases in the level of interactions and potentially life-saving therapeutic interventions from clinicians and caregivers.[39,40] Nevertheless, more and more elderly patients are being admitted to the ICU,[41] and certainly this will include older patients with pre-existing cognitive impairment ranging from mild to overt dementia. In a cohort investigation, Pisani et al studied the effect of pre-existing cognitive impairment (mostly mild) on ICU outcomes and found that those with and without cognitive impairment had similar outcomes in terms of length of stay in the ICU and the hospital and mortality rate.[42] However, the persistence of delirium

symptoms in such patients could strongly affect discharge rates to nursing homes after hospitalization.[24,26]

Prognostic Significance of Delirium

Reports have associated CNS organ dysfunction with complications of mechanical ventilation, including aspiration, nosocomial pneumonia, reintubation, and self-extubation.[43–47] Moreover, in mechanically ventilated neurosurgical patients, the strongest predictor of failed extubation was found to be an abnormal Glasgow Coma Score.[48] In medical ICU patients, Salam et al found important interactions between cognitive dysfunction and the likelihood of failed extubation.[49] CNS "failure" is an important predictor of outcome from sepsis.[2]

In non-ICU populations, the development of delirium in the hospital is associated with an in-hospital mortality rate of 25% to 33%, prolonged hospital stay, and three times the likelihood of discharge to a nursing home.[18,24,50] In a three-site study of medical non-ICU patients, delirium was found to be an independent predictor of the combined outcome of death or nursing home placement.[51] Francis and Kapoor found that the 2-year mortality rate in patients having experienced delirium was 39% versus 23% in controls,[52] but multivariate analysis showed that this was largely explained by baseline cognitive and functional statuses. Perhaps the most convincing report of the independent association between delirium and mortality rate among non-ICU patients was published by McCusker et al,[53] which showed an adjusted hazard of dying of 2.11 associated with the development of delirium. This mortality rate increase has since been shown to be independent of dementia status.[54]

Among ICU patients, there is current evidence that delirium is a predictor of mortality at 6 months following the ICU stay (Fig. 62-1).[55] The development of delirium was associated with a threefold increase in risk of death after controlling for pre-existing comorbidities, severity of illness, coma, and the use of sedative and analgesic medications. These data also showed that delirium is not simply a transition state from coma to normal because delirium occurred just as often among those who never developed coma as among those who did and persisted in 11% of patients at the time of hospital discharge. Further, three recent prospective studies have associated delirium with an increased risk for dementia over 2 to 3 years.[56–58] In light of these findings, future studies should determine whether or not prevention or treatment of delirium changes clinical outcomes, including mortality rate, length of stay, cost of care, and long-term neuropsychological outcomes among survivors of critical illness.

Costs Associated with Delirium in the ICU Patient

Delirium complicates the hospital stay of more than 2 to 3 million elderly patients per year in the United States, involving more than 17.5 million inpatient days and accounting for more than $4 billion in Medicare expenditures.[59] In the only study to date reporting on costs associated with delirium in the ICU, Milbrandt et al found that median ICU and hospital costs were significantly higher for those with at least one episode of delirium versus those with no delirium

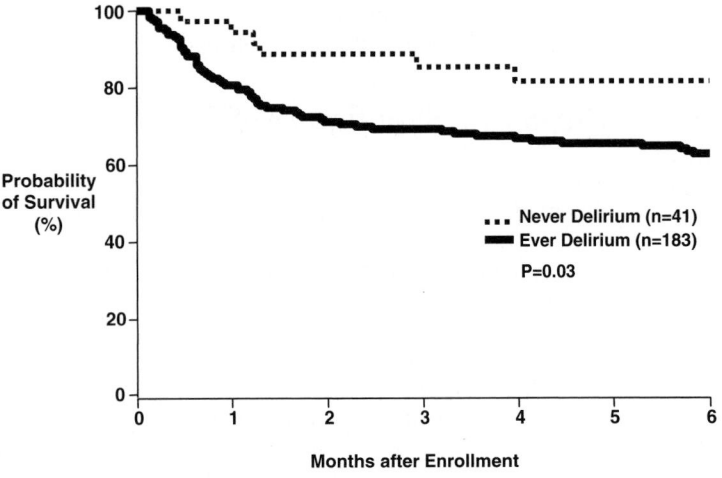

A

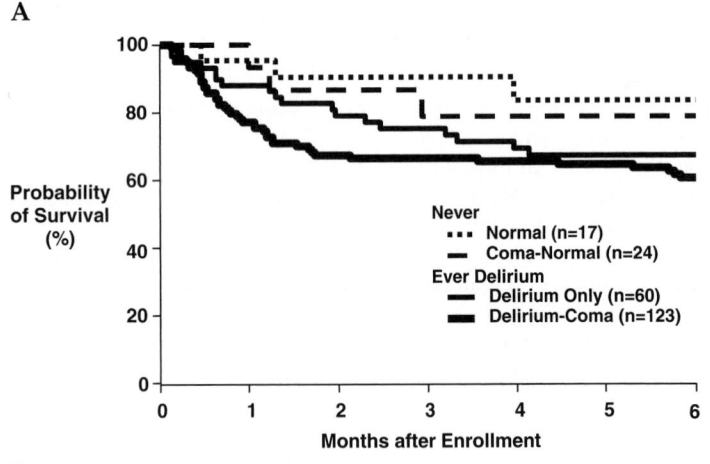

B

FIGURE 62-1 Kaplan-Meier plots show the relation between delirium and 6-month survival rate. *A.* Never-delirium versus ever-delirium groups (according to whether or not the patient ever developed delirium in the intensive care unit). *B.* Clinical severity (subdividing the never- and ever-delirium groups to better understand the phenomenology of delirium). The never-delirium group, composed of those who were always normal and those who were comatose and then normal (e.g., deeply sedated and then normal when drugs were stopped) had higher survival rates than the ever-delirium group, which was composed of those with delirium only and delirium and coma.

(Fig. 62-2).[60] Even after controlling for important potentially confounding variables, such as baseline comorbidities and severity of illness, delirium was associated with a 40% relative increase in ICU and total hospital costs. In addition, the data demonstrated a "dose-response" in which cumulative delirium severity was associated with incrementally higher cost.

The associated annual cost of ICU delirium may be enormous. In the study by Milbrandt et al,[60] delirium occurred in 82% of mechanically ventilated patients and was associated with an incremental increase in ICU cost of more than $9000 per patient. In the United States, there are approximately 880,000 to 2,760,000 ICU admissions annually for respiratory failure requiring mechanical ventilation. Therefore,

the estimated number of cases of ICU delirium may range from 721,600 to 2,263,200 per year, with an associated increase in health care costs ranging from $6.5 billion to $20.4 billion. Even if the incidence of delirium from a less severely ill ICU cohort occurred in only 19% of patients,[61] the estimated annual costs would be in the range of $1.5 billion to $4.7 billion. Because some of the additional cost associated with delirium could be attributable to unmeasured differences between patient groups, these estimates represent the upper limit of the cost attributable to ICU delirium. However, even if only 20% of the difference in costs between patients with and without delirium were due to delirium, this would be a significant public health concern, with $300 million to $4 billion in annual attributable costs.

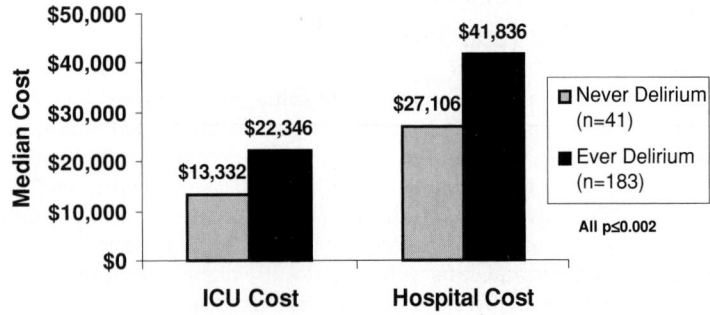

FIGURE 62-2 Median intensive care unit (ICU) and hospital costs per patient. This histogram shows cost according to clinical categorization of ever-delirium versus never-delirium. Delirium was significantly associated with increased ICU and hospital cost.

Risk Factors for Delirium

Only a few studies of ICU patients have studied risk factors for delirium, although many investigations over the past decade, by using a variety of non-ICU cohorts, have identified numerous risk factors for the development of delirium.[50] Patients who are highly vulnerable to delirium may develop the disorder after only minor physiologic stressors, whereas those with low baseline vulnerability require a greater insult to become delirious.[62] It is possible to stratify patients into risk groups depending on the number of risk factors present.[26,62-64] Three or more risk factors increase the likelihood of developing delirium to approximately 60% or higher, and it is a rare patient in the ICU who would not be in the high-risk group. Most ICU patients have more than 10 risk factors for delirium.[17,65]

In practical terms, the risk factors can be divided into three categories: (1) host factors, (2) the acute illness, and (3) iatrogenic or environmental factors (Table 62-2).[4,18,23,26,61,63,64,66-68] Issues that are ripe for study in terms of prevention or intervention have been indicated. In the only ICU cohort risk factor study published to date,[61] factors related to medical history included hypertension and smoking (thereby raising one's awareness of the risks of relative underperfusion of the brain or nicotine withdrawal). During the ICU stay, a dose-dependent risk was found for patients having been treated with opiates.

Psychoactive medications are the leading iatrogenic risk factors for delirium.[24,61,62,69,70] Benzodiazepines, narcotics, and other psychoactive drugs are associated with a 3 to 11 times increased relative risk,[24] and the number and rate of adding psychoactive medications increase the risk of delirium by 4 to 10 times.[24] By coupling these data to knowledge regarding the extreme variability in the pharmacokinetics of sedatives and analgesics according to age, ethnicity, drug metabolizing ability and other factors,[71-74] perhaps the most promising delirium interventions could be centered on delivery patterns of these medications.

Combining Sedation and Delirium Assessments at the Bedside

The SCCM guidelines suggest that all critically ill patients be simultaneously monitored for level of sedation and for delirium.[9] Bedside critical care nurses and the rest of the ICU team need to use data obtained from well-validated, reliable, objective, but brief assessment tools to monitor for both components of consciousness (arousal level and content of consciousness).[75] Neurologic monitoring in the ICU can be streamlined by using a two-step approach to sedation and delirium.

The first step in the neurologic assessment of an ICU patient is to assess that patient's level of consciousness or sedation with an objective sedation assessment. The recommended standard of care is to use objective assessment scales to avoid oversedation and to promote earlier liberation from mechanical ventilation.[9,76-80] Sedation scales help provide a common language for the multidisciplinary team to use when discussing goals and treatments for patients.[80-82] Whereas the Ramsay Scale[83] has been the most widely used instrument for decades in clinical practice and the published literature,[84] other recently developed instruments such as the Sedation-Agitation Scale[85] and Richmond Agitation Sedation Scale[86,87] have been better validated and are being widely implemented.[17,88] Chapter 14 includes a thorough discussion of how to approach sedation in the ICU, but it is appropriate to emphasize the importance of using these instruments to guide patient-targeted or goal-directed sedation. The concept of using sedation scales over time within patients was addressed in the second Richmond Agitation Sedation Scale validation study,[87] in which emphasis was placed on the fact that potent psychoactive medications should not be given without a specific agreed-on target level of effect.

The second step for assessing the brain's function in critically ill ICU patients builds on the level of arousal assessment and involves the delirium assessment. All patients who are responsive to verbal stimuli should be assessed for delirium. The first delirium assessment tools designed specifically for nonverbal, intubated ICU patients were published in 2001.[15,17,89] One of these instruments is the Intensive Care Delirium Screening Checklist,[15] which is used as a screening instrument due to its high sensitivity (99%) and moderate specificity (64%). The other is the Confusion Assessment Method for the ICU (CAM-ICU),[17,89] which has a sensitivity and specificity of approximately 95% and very high interrater reliability ($\kappa = 0.96$). The CAM-ICU was designed to be a serial assessment tool for use by bedside clinicians (nurses or physicians). Thus, it is easy to use, takes only 1 minute on

TABLE 62-2 Risk Factors for Delirium[a]

Host Factors	Acute Illness[a]	Iatrogenic or Environmental
Elderly	Severe sepsis[a]	Sedative and analgesic use[a]
Underlying comorbidities (e.g., heart, liver, or renal failure, diabetes, hypertension)	Acute respiratory distress syndrome[a]	Immobilization (e.g., restraints or catheters)[a]
Pre-existing cognitive impairment or dementia	Multiple organ dysfunction syndrome	Total parenteral nutrition[a]
Hearing or vision impairment[a]	Drug overdose or illicit drugs	Sleep deprivation[a]
Neurologic disease (stroke or seizure)	Acquisition of nosocomial infection[a]	Malnutrition[a]
Alcoholism and smoking[a]	Metabolic disturbance[a]	Anemia (phlebotomy)[a]

[a]Potentially modifiable factors through specific interventions or avoidance.

average to complete, and requires minimal training. Delirium assessment using the CAM-ICU incorporates four key features that comprise delirium as defined by the *Diagnostic and Statistical Manual of Mental Disorders, Fourth Edition* (American Psychiatric Association). These features are (1) change in mental status from baseline or fluctuating course of mental status, (2) inattention, (3) disorganized thinking, and (4) altered level of consciousness. Delirium is present when features 1 and 2 plus features 3 or 4 are present (Fig. 62-3 and Table 62-3). The CAM-ICU has been translated into many languages, and numerous aspects of neurologic monitoring are discussed and available for download from an educational Web site (www.icudelirium.org).

Strategies for Optimal Management of ICU Delirium

PRIMARY PREVENTION AND NONPHARMACOLOGIC APPROACHES

In a trial of 852 general medical patients older than 70 years,[90] strategies for primary prevention of delirium resulted in a 40% reduction in the odds of developing delirium (15% in controls versus 9.9% in the intervention patients). The protocol focused on optimization of risk factors with the following

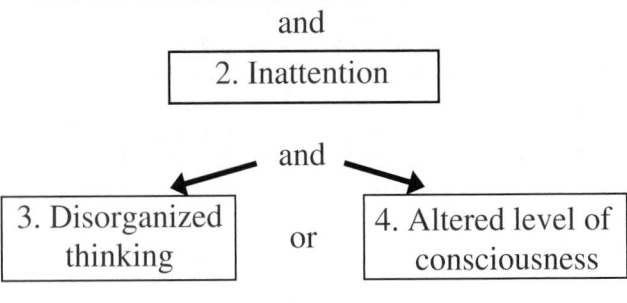

FIGURE 62-3 Definition of delirium according to the Confusion Assessment Method for the Intensive Care Unit. *(Adapted with permission from the American Psychiatric Association, Diagnostic and Statistical Manual of Mental Disorders, Fourth Edition.)*

methods: repeated reorientation of the patient by trained volunteers and nurses, provision of cognitively stimulating activities for the patient three times per day, a nonpharmacologic sleep protocol to enhance normalization of sleep and wake cycles, early mobilization activities and range of motion

TABLE 62-3 Features and Descriptions of the CAM-ICU

	Absent	Present
1. Acute onset or fluctuating course	Absent	Present
A. Is there evidence of an acute change in mental status from the baseline?		
or		
B. Did the (abnormal) behavior fluctuate (i.e., tend to come and go) during the past 24 h or increase and decrease in severity as demonstrated by fluctuation on a sedation scale (e.g., RASS), GCS, or previous delirium assessment?		
2. Inattention	Absent	Present
Did the patient have difficulty focusing attention as demonstrated by scores <8 on the auditory or visual component of the Attention Screening Examination? (Instructions on next page.)		
3. Disorganized thinking	Absent	Present
Is there evidence of disorganized or incoherent thinking as indicated by incorrect answers to ≥2 of the 4 questions and/or inability to follow the commands?		
Questions (alternative sets A and B)		

Set A	Set B
1. Will a stone float on water?	1. Will a leaf float on water?
2. Are there fish in the sea?	2. Are there elephants in the sea?
3. Does 1 lb weigh more than 2 lb?	3. Does 2 lb weigh more than 1 lb?
4. Can you use a hammer to pound a nail?	4. Can you use a hammer to cut wood?

   Other
     1. Are you having any unclear thinking?
     2. Hold up this many fingers. (Examiner holds 2 fingers in front of the patient.)
     3. Now do the same thing with the other hand. (Examiner does not repeat the gesture.)

	Absent	Present
4. Altered level of consciousness	Absent	Present
Is the patient's level of consciousness anything other than alert, such as vigilant, lethargic, or stupor (e.g., RASS other than "0" at time of assessment)?		

Alert	Spontaneously fully aware of environment and interacts appropriately
Vigilant	Hyperalert
Lethargic	Drowsy but easily aroused, unaware of some elements in the environment, or not spontaneously interacting appropriately with the interviewer; becomes fully aware and appropriately interactive when prodded minimally
Stupor	Becomes incompletely aware when prodded strongly; can be aroused only by vigorous and repeated stimuli, and as soon as the stimulus ceases, stuporous subject lapse back into the unresponsive state

	Yes	No
Overall CAM-ICU (features 1 and 2 plus feature 3 or 4)	Yes	No

ABBREVIATIONS: CAM-ICU, Confusion Assessment Method of the Intensive Care Unit; GCS, Glasgow Coma Scale; RASS, Richmond Agitation Sedation Scale.

exercises, timely removal of catheters and physical restraints, institution of the use of eyeglasses and magnifying lenses, hearing aids and earwax disimpaction, and early correction of dehydration. Unfortunately, this intervention did not show sustained benefit when the patients were followed to 6 months.[91] Other recent studies of delirium prevention reproduced success only in subgroups such as those without underlying dementia[92] or not at all.[93]

However, this study of primary prevention did not focus on critically ill patients and excluded mechanically ventilated patients. Because ICU studies using the CAM-ICU have documented delirium rates of 70% to 80%, one might view the "room for improvement" in delirium management as far greater for critically ill patients than for general medical patients. Although primary prevention of delirium is preferred, some degree of delirium is inevitable in the ICU. In these cases, the basic tenets of patient management such as restoring sleep/wake cycles, timely removal of catheters, early mobilization, use of a scheduled pain management protocol, minimization of unnecessary noise or stimuli, and frequent reorientation should be applied liberally. Family involvement can be very helpful in reorienting and soothing delirious patients. It is important to teach family members about the fluctuating course of delirium and how they can detect delirium. Preventive and management strategies for delirium in the ICU represent an important area for future investigation.

PHARMACOLOGIC THERAPY

Medications should be used only after giving adequate attention to correction of modifiable contributing factors (e.g., sleep disturbance and restraints) as discussed above and presented in Table 62-2. It is important to recognize that delirium may be a manifestation of an acute, life-threatening problem that requires immediate attention (e.g., hypoxia, hypercarbia, hypoglycemia, metabolic derangements, or shock). After addressing such concerns, delirious patients should be considered for pharmacologic management. Even though the agents used to treat delirium are intended to improve cognition, they all have psychoactive effects that may further cloud the sensorium and promote a longer overall duration of cognitive impairment. Therefore, until outcomes data confirm the beneficial effects of treatment, these drugs should be used judiciously in the smallest possible dose and for the shortest time necessary, a practice *infrequently* adhered to in most ICUs. Some patients will prove refractory to all "cocktail" approaches to sedation and delirium therapy, and these patients should be considered for a trial of complete cessation of all psychoactive drugs.

Benzodiazepines, which are used most commonly in the ICU for sedation, are not recommended for the management of delirium because of the likelihood of oversedation, exacerbation of confusion, and respiratory suppression. However, they remain the drugs of choice for the treatment of delirium tremens (and other withdrawal syndromes) and seizures. The amnestic qualities of benzodiazepines make these agents especially useful when noxious or unpleasant procedures are required. However, it is likely that residual accumulation of these drugs may lead to prolonged delirium long after the drugs have been discontinued. In certain populations, in particular elderly patients with underlying dementia, benzodiazepines may lead to increased confusion and agitation. In

such cases, one may try to take advantage of the sedative effects of haloperidol in lieu of continued benzodiazepines. Preliminary results from a prospective, randomized, but unblinded trial of sedation in postoperative cardiac surgical patients showed that those treated with dexmedetomidine, as opposed to propofol or midazolam, were less likely to develop delirium.[94] This work must be confirmed on a larger scale with documented improved outcomes before modifying standard sedation practices.

There are currently no drugs approved by the U.S. Food and Drug Administration for the treatment of delirium. The SCCM guidelines recommend haloperidol as the drug of choice, although it is acknowledged that this is based on sparse outcomes data from nonrandomized case series and anecdotal reports (i.e., level C data).[9,95–103] Nevertheless, haloperidol is a butyrophenone "typical" antipsychotic, which is the most widely used neuroleptic agent for delirium.[104] It does not suppress the respiratory drive and works as a dopamine receptor antagonist by blocking the D_2 receptor, which results in treatment of positive symptomatology (hallucinations, unstructured thought patterns, etc.) and produces a variable sedative effect.[105]

In the non-ICU setting, the recommended starting dose of haloperidol is 0.5 to 1.0 mg orally or parenterally, with repeated doses every 20 to 30 minutes until the desired effect is achieved. In the ICU setting, a recommended starting dose is 5 mg every 12 hours (intravenously or orally), with maximal effective doses usually in the neighborhood of 20 mg/day. This dose range is usually adequate to achieve the "theoretically optimal" 60% D_2 receptor blockade[106–108] and avoid complete D_2 receptor saturation associated with the adverse effects cited below. Because of the urgency of the situation in many ICU patients, due to the potential for inadvertent removal of central lines, endotracheal tubes, or even aortic balloon pumps, much larger doses of haloperidol are often used. Unfortunately, there are few data from formal pharmacologic investigations to guide dosage recommendations in the ICU. Once calm, the patient can usually be managed with much smaller maintenance doses of haloperidol.

Neither haloperidol nor similar agents (i.e., droperidol and chlorpromazine) have been extensively studied in the ICU.[9] Newer "atypical" antipsychotic agents (e.g., risperidone, ziprasidone, quetiapine, and olanzapine) may also prove helpful for delirium.[9,109] The rationale behind the use of atypical antipsychotics over haloperidol (especially in hypoactive/mixed subtypes of delirium) is theoretical and centers on the fact that they affect not only dopamine but also other potentially key neurotransmitters such as serotonin, acetylcholine, and norepinephrine. Adequately powered randomized controlled trials of these agents are not available.

Adverse effects of typical and atypical antipsychotics include hypotension, acute dystonias, extrapyramidal effects, laryngeal spasm, malignant hyperthermia, glucose and lipid dysregulation, and anticholinergic effects such as dry mouth, constipation, and urinary retention. Perhaps the most immediately life-threatening adverse effect of antipsychotics is *torsades de pointes*,[110,111] and these agents should not be given to patients with prolonged QT intervals unless thought to be absolutely necessary. Patents who receive substantial quantities of typical or atypical antipsychotics or coadministered arrhythmogenic drugs should be monitored closely with electrocardiography. Having mentioned these potential difficulties, antipsychotics (most experience having been accrued with haloperidol) are usually well tolerated from the hemodynamic and respiratory standpoints.

Summary of Key Points on ICU Delirium

Critically ill patients are at great risk for the development of delirium in the ICU. However, this form of brain dysfunction is grossly under-recognized and undertreated. Delirium is mistakenly thought to be a transient and expected outcome in the ICU and of little consequence (i.e., part of the "ICU psychosis"). It is now recognized that delirium is one of the most frequent complications experienced in the ICU; even after adjusting for covariates such as age, sex, race, and severity of illness, delirium is an independent risk factor for prolonged length of stay and higher 6-month mortality rates. In addition, many ICU survivors demonstrate persistent cognitive deficits at follow-up testing months to years later. It is essential for health care professionals to be able to recognize delirium readily at the bedside. The CAM-ICU is a valid, reliable, quick, and easy-to-use serial assessment tool for monitoring delirium in ventilated and nonventilated ICU patients. Delirium is a multifactorial problem for ICU patients that demands an interdisciplinary approach for assessment, management, and treatment. Critical care nurses and physicians should assume a position of leadership in the ICU with regard to delirium monitoring because they are the best-suited members of the ICU team to successfully implement this essential component of patient management, which is now recommended by the SCCM clinical practice guidelines. Although ongoing trials may elucidate the optimal ways to treat delirium, standard pharmacologic and nonpharmacologic management strategies have been reviewed.

Acknowledgments

Dr. Ely is the Associate Director of Research for the VA Tennessee Valley Geriatric Research and Education Clinical Center. He is a recipient of the Paul Beeson Faculty Scholar Award from the Alliance for Aging Research and a recipient of a K23 from the National Institute of Health (grant AG01023-01A1).

References

1. Papadopoulos MC, Davies DC, Moss RF, et al: Pathophysiology of septic encephalopathy: A review. *Crit Care Med* 28:3019, 2000.
2. Russell JA, Singer J, Bernard G, et al: Changing pattern of organ dysfunction in early human sepsis is related to mortality. *Crit Care Med* 28:3405, 2000.
3. Granberg A, Engberg B, Lundberg D: Intensive care syndrome: A literature review. *Intensive Crit Care Nurs* 12:173, 1996.
4. Wilson LM: Intensive care delirium: The effect of outside deprivation in a windowless unit. *Arch Intern Med* 130:22, 1972.
5. Geary SM: Intensive care unit psychosis revisited: Understanding and managing delirium in the critical care setting. *Crit Care Nurs* 17:51, 1994.
6. Meagher DJ, Hanlon DO, Mahony EO, et al: Relationship between symptoms and motoric subtype of delirium. *J Neuropsychiatry Clin Neurosci* 12:51, 2000.
7. McGuire BE, Basten CJ, Ryan CJ, Gallagher J: Intensive care unit syndrome: A dangerous misnomer. *Arch Intern Med* 160:906, 2000.
8. Justic M: Does "ICU psychosis" really exist? *Crit Care Nurs* 20:28, 2000.
9. Jacobi J, Fraser GL, Coursin DB, et al: Clinical practice guidelines for the sustained use of sedatives and analgesics in the critically ill adult. *Crit Care Med* 30:119, 2002.
10. Meagher DJ, Trzepacz PT: Motoric subtypes of delirium. *Semin Clin Neuropsychiatry* 5:75, 2000.
11. Webb JM, Carlton EF, Geeham DM: Delirium in the intensive care unit: Are we helping the patient? *Crit Care Nurs Q* 22(4):47, 2000.
12. Crippen D: Treatment of agitation and its comorbidities in the intensive care unit, in Hill NS, Levy MM (eds): *Ventilator Management Strategies for Critical Care.* New York, Marcel Dekker, 2001, p 243.
13. Lipowski ZJ: Delirium in the elderly patient. *N Engl J Med* 320:578, 1989.
14. Wijdicks EFM: *Neurologic Complications of Critical Illness.* New York, Oxford University Press, 2002.
15. Bergeron N, Dubois MJ, Dumont M, e al: Intensive Care Delirium Screening Checklist: evaluation of a new screening tool. *Intensive Care Med* 27:859, 2001.
16. McNicoll L, Pisani MA, Zhang Y, et al: Delirium in the intensive care unit: occurrence and clinical course in older patients. *J Am Geriatr Soc* 51:591, 2003.
17. Ely EW, Inouye SK, Bernard GR, et al: Delirium in mechanically ventilated patients: Validity and reliability of the confusion assessment method for the intensive care unit (CAM-ICU). *JAMA* 286:2703, 2001.
18. Levkoff SE, Evans DA, Liptzin B, et al: Delirium: The occurrence and persistence of symptoms among elderly hospitalized patients. *Arch Intern Med* 152:334, 1992.
19. Heffner JE: A wake-up call in the intensive care unit. *N Engl J Med* 342:1520, 2000.
20. Peterson JF, Truman BL, Shintani A, et al: The prevalence of hypoactive, hyperactive, and mixed type delirium in medical ICU patients. *J Am Geriatr Soc* 51:S174, 2003.
21. Kollef MH, Levy NT, Ahrens T, et al: The use of continuous IV sedation is associated with prolongation of mechanical ventilation. *Chest* 114:541, 1999.
22. Francis J: Delirium in older patients. *J Am Geriatr Soc* 40:829, 1992.
23. Francis J, Kapoor WN: Delirium in hospitalized elderly. *J Gen Intern Med* 5:65, 1990.
24. Inouye SK, Schlesinger MJ, Lyndon TJ: Delirium: A symptom of how hospital care is failing older persons and a window to improve quality of hospital care. *Am J Med* 106:565, 1999.
25. Inouye SK, Foreman MD, Mion LC, et al: Nurses' recognition of delirium and its symptoms. *Arch Intern Med* 161:2467, 2001.
26. Francis J, Martin D, Kapoor WN: A prospective study of delirium in hospitalized elderly. *JAMA* 263:1097, 1990.
27. Inouye SK: The dilemma of delirium: Clinical and research controversies regarding diagnosis and evaluation of delirium in hospitalized elderly medical patients. *Am J Med* 97:278, 1994.
28. Armstrong-Esther CA, Browne KD: The influence of elderly patients' mental impairment on nurse-patient interaction. *J Adv Nurs* 11(4):379, 1986.
29. Wray NP, Friedland JA, Ashton CM, et al: Characteristics of house staff work rounds on two academic general medicine services. *J Med Educ* 61:893, 1986.
30. Hobbs F, Damon BL, Taeuber CM: *Sixty-Five Plus in the United States.* Washington, DC, US Department of Commerce, Economics, and Statistics Administration, Bureau of the Census, 1996.
31. Sage WM, Hurst CR, Silverman JF, Bortz WM: Intensive care for the elderly: Outcome of elective and nonelective admissions. *J Am Geriatr Soc* 35:312, 1987.

32. Baltussen R, Leidl R, Ament A: The impact of age on cost-effectiveness ratios and its control in decision making. *Health Econ* 5(3):227, 1996.

33. Shaw AB: Age as a basis for healthcare rationing. Support for ageist policies. *Drugs Aging* 9(6):403, 1996.

34. Angus DC, Kelly MA, Schmitz RJ, et al: Current and projected workforce requirements for care of the critically ill and patients with pulmonary disease: Can we meet the requirements of an aging population? *JAMA* 284:2762, 2000.

35. Behrendt CE: Acute respiratory failure in the United States: Incidence and 31-day survival. *Chest* 118:1100, 2000.

36. Chelluri L, Grenvik A, Silverstein M: Intensive care for critically ill elderly: Mortality, costs, and quality of life. Review of the literature. *Arch Intern Med* 155:1013, 1995.

37. O'Keeffe S, Lavan J: The prognostic significance of delirium in older hospital patients. *J Am Geriatr Soc* 45:174, 1997.

38. Ely EW: Optimizing outcomes for older patients treated in the intensive care unit. *Intensive Care Med* 29:2112, 2003.

39. Hamel MB, Philips RS, Teno JM, et al: Seriously ill hospitalized adults: do we spend less on older patients? *J Am Geriatr Soc* 44:1043, 1996.

40. Hamel MB, Teno JM, Goldman L, et al: Patient age and decisions to withhold life-sustaining treatments from seriously ill, hospitalized adults. *Ann Intern Med* 130:116, 1999.

41. Jakob SM, Rothen HU: Intensive care 1980–1995: Change in patient characteristics, nursing workload and outcome. *Intensive Care Med* 23:1165, 1997.

42. Pisani MA, Redlich C, Ely EW, et al: Favorable ICU outcomes in older patients with preexisting cognitive impairment. *Am J Resp Crit Care Med* 167:A252, 2003.

43. Epstein SK, Ciubotaru RL, Wong JB: Effect of failed extubation on the outcome of mechanical ventilation. *Chest* 112:186, 1997.

44. Epstein SK, Ciubotaru RL: Independent effects of etiology of failure and time to reintubation on outcome for patients failing extubation. *Am J Respir Crit Care Med* 158:489, 1998.

45. Vallverdu I, Calaf N, Subirana M, et al: Clinical characteristics, respiratory functional parameters, and outcome of a two-hour T-piece trial of patients weaning from mechanical ventilation. *Am J Respir Crit Care Med* 158:1855, 1999.

46. Torres A, Gatell JM, Aznar E: Re-intubation increases the risk of nosocomial pneumonia in patients needing mechanical ventilation. *Am J Respir Crit Care Med* 152:137, 1995.

47. Esteban A, Alia I, Gordo F, et al: Extubation outcome after spontaneous breathing trials with T-tube or pressure support ventilation. *Am J Respir Crit Care Med* 156:459, 1997.

48. Namen AM, Ely EW, Tatter S, et al: Predictors of successful extubation in neurosurgical patients. *Am J Respir Crit Care Med* 163:658, 2001.

49. Salam A, Tilluckdharry L, Amoateng-Adjepong Y, Manthous CA: Neurologic status, cough, secretions and extubation outcomes. *Intensive Care Med* 30:1334, 2004.

50. American Psychiatric Association: Practice guideline for the treatment of patients with delirium. *Am J Psychiatry* 156(suppl):1, 1999.

51. Inouye SK, Rushing JT, Foreman MD, et al: Does delirium contribute to poor hospital outcomes? A three-site epidemiologic study. *J Gen Intern Med* 13:234, 1998.

52. Francis J, Kapoor WN: Prognosis after hospital discharge of older medical patients with delirium. *J Am Geriatr Soc* 40:601, 1992.

53. McCusker J, Cole M, Abrahamowicz M, et al: Delirium predicts 12 month mortality. *Arch Intern Med* 162:457, 2002.

54. Fick DM, Agostini JV, Inouye SK: Delirium superimposed on dementia: A systematic review. *J Am Geriatr Soc* 50:1723, 2002.

55. Ely EW, Shintani A, Truman B, et al: Delirium as a predictor of mortality in mechanically ventilated patients in the intensive care unit. *JAMA* 291:1753, 2004.

56. Rockwood K, Cosway S, Carver D: The risk of dementia and death after delirium. *Age Ageing* 28:551, 1999.

57. Rahkonen T, Luukkainen-Markkula R, Paanilla S, Sulkava R: Delirium episode as a sign of undetected dementia among community dwelling subjects: A 2 year follow up study. *J Neurol Neurosurg Psychiatry* 69:519, 2000.

58. McCusker J, Cole M, Dendukuri N, et al: Delirium in older medical inpatients and subsequent cognitive and functional status: A prospective study. *Can Med Assoc J* 165:575, 2001.

59. *Statistical Abstract of the United States.* Washington, DC, Bureau of the Census, 1996.

60. Milbrandt E, Deppen S, Harrison P, et al: Costs associated with delirium in mechanically ventilated patients. *Crit Care Med* 32:955, 2004.

61. Dubois MJ, Bergeron N, Dumont M, et al: Delirium in an intensive care unit: A study of risk factors. *Intensive Care Med* 27:1297, 2001.

62. Inouye SK, Charpentier PA: Precipitating factors for delirium in hospitalized elderly persons: Predictive model and interrelationship with baseline vulnerability. *JAMA* 275:852, 1996.

63. Inouye SK, Viscoli C, Horwitz RI, et al: A predictive model for delirium in hospitalized elderly medical patients based on admission characteristics. *Ann Intern Med* 119:474, 1993.

64. Marcantonio ER, Goldman L, Mangione CM, et al: A clinical prediction rule for delirium after elective noncardiac surgery. *JAMA* 271:134, 1994.

65. Ely EW, Gautam S, Margolin R, et al: The impact of delirium in the intensive care unit on hospital length of stay. *Intensive Care Med* 27:1892, 2001.

66. Williams-Russo P, Urquhart BL, Sharrock NE, Charlson ME: Post-operative delirium: Predictors and prognosis in elderly orthopedic patients. *J Am Geriatr Soc* 40:759, 1992.

67. Marcantonio ER, Juarez G, Goldman L, et al: The relationship of postoperative delirium with psychoactive medications. *JAMA* 272:1518, 1994.

68. Lynch EP, Lazor MA, Gellis JE, et al: The impact of postoperative pain on the development of postoperative delirium. *Anesth Analg* 86:781, 1998.

69. Fish DN: Treatment of delirium in the critically ill patient. *Clin Pharmacokinet* 10:456, 1991.

70. Francis J: Drug-induced delirium. *CNS Drugs* 5:103, 1996.

71. Zhou HH, Sheller JR, Nu H, et al: Ethnic differences in response to morphine. *Clin Pharmacol Therap* 1993; 54:507.

72. Salzman C (ed): *Clinical Geriatric Psychopharmacology,* 3rd ed. Baltimore, Williams & Wilkins, 1998, p 58.

73. Tateishi T, Wood AJJ, Guengerich FP, Wood M: Biotransformation of tritiated fentanyl in human liver microsomes. *Biochem Pharmacol* 50:1921, 1995.

74. Yun C, Wood M, Wood AJJ, Guengerich FP: Identification of the pharmacogenetic determinants of alfentanil metabolism: cytochrome P-450 3A4: An explanation of the variable elimination clearance. *Anesthesiology* 77:467, 1992.

75. Plum F, Posner J: *The Diagnosis of Stupor and Coma,* 3rd ed. Philadelphia, FA Davis, 1980.

76. Brook AD, Ahrens TS, Schaiff R, et al: Effect of a nursing implemented sedation protocol on the duration of mechanical ventilation. *Crit Care Med* 27:2609, 1999.

77. Kress JP, Pohlman AS, O'Connor MF, Hall JB: Daily interruption of sedative infusions in critically ill patients undergoing mechanical ventilation. *N Engl J Med* 342:1471, 2000.

78. MacIntyre NR, Cook DJ, Ely EW, et al: Evidence-based guidelines for weaning and discontinuing ventilatory support. *Chest* 120:375S, 2001.

79. Ely EW, Meade M, Haponik EF, et al: Mechanical ventilator weaning protocols driven by non-physician health care professionals: evidence based clinical practice guidelines. *Chest* 120:454S, 2001.

80. Mascia MF, Koch M, Medicis JJ: Pharmacoeconomic impact of rational use guidelines on the provision of analgesia, sedation, and neuromuscular blockade in critical care. *Crit Care Med* 28:2300, 2000.

81. Bair N, Bobek MB, Hoffman-Hogg L, et al: Introduction of sedative, analgesic, and neuromuscular blocking agent guidelines in a medical intensive care unit: Physician and nurse adherence. *Crit Care Med* 28:707, 2000.

82. Slomka J, Hoffman-Hogg L, Mion LC, et al: Influence of clinicians' values and perceptions on use of clinical practice guidelines for sedation and neuromuscular blockade in patients receiving mechanical ventilation. *Am J Crit Care* 9:412, 2000.

83. Ramsay M, Savege TM, Simpson ER, Goodwin R: Controlled sedation with alphaxalone-alphadolone. *Br Med J* 2:656, 1974.

84. Ostermann ME, Keenan SP, Seiferling RA, Sibbald W: Sedation in the intensive care unit. *JAMA* 283:1451, 2000.

85. Riker R, Picard JT, Fraser G: Prospective evaluation of the sedation-agitation scale for adult critically ill patients. *Crit Care Med* 27:1325, 1999.

86. Sessler CN, Gosnell M, Grap MJ, et al: The Richmond Agitation-Sedation Scale: Validity and reliability in adult intensive care patients. *Am J Respir Crit Care Med* 166:1338, 2002.

87. Ely EW, Truman B, Shintani A, et al: Monitoring sedation status over time in ICU patients: The reliability and validity of the Richmond Agitation Sedation Scale (RASS). *JAMA* 289:2983, 2003.

88. Ely EW, Gautam S, May L, et al: A comparison of different sedation scales in the ICU and validation of the Richmond Agitation Sedation Scale (RASS). *Am J Respir Crit Care Med* 163:A954, 2001.

89. Ely EW, Margolin R, Francis J, et al: Evaluation of delirium in critically ill patients: validation of the confusion assessment method for the intensive care unit (CAM-ICU). *Crit Care Med* 29:1370, 2001.

90. Inouye SK, Bogardus ST, Charpentier PA, et al: A multicomponent intervention to prevent delirium in hospitalized older patients. *N Engl J Med* 340:669, 1999.

91. Bogardus ST, Desai MM, Williams CS, et al: The effects of a targeted multicomponent delirium intervention of postdischarge outcomes for hospitalized older adults. *Am J Med* 114:383, 2003.

92. Marcantonio ER, Flacker JM, Wright RJ, Resnick NM: Reducing delirium after hip fracture: A randomized trial. *J Am Geriatr Soc* 49:516, 2001.

93. Cole MG, McCusker J, Bellavance F, et al: Systematic detection and multidisciplinary care of delirium in older medical inpatients: A randomized trial. *Can Med Assoc J* 167:753, 2002.

94. Maldonado JR, Wysong A, van der Starre PJ: Post-operative sedation and the incidence of ICU delirium in cardiac surgery patients. *Crit Care Med* 2004 (in press).

95. Tesar GE, Murray GB, Cassem NH: Use of high-dose intravenous haloperidol in the treatment of agitated cardiac patients. *J Clin Psychopharmacol* 5(6):344, 1985.

96. Hassan E, Fontaine DK, Nearman HS: Therapeutic considerations in the management of agitated and delirious critically ill patients. *Pharmacotherapy* 18:113, 1998.

97. Seneff MG, Mathews RA: Use of haloperidol infusions to control delirium in critically ill adults. *Ann Pharmacother* 29:690, 1995.

98. Levenson JL: High-dose intravenous haloperidol for agitated delirium following lung transplantation. *Psychosomatics* 36:66, 1995.

99. Adams F: Emergency intravenous sedation of the delirious, medically ill patient. *J Clin Psychiatry* 49(suppl):22, 1988.

100. Brown RL, Henke A, Greenhalgh DG, Warden GD: The use of haloperidol in the agitated, critically ill pediatric patient with burns. *J Burn Care Rehabil* 17:34, 1996.

101. Wise TN, Mann LS, Jani N, et al: Haloperidol prescribing practices in the general hospital. *Gen Hosp Psychiatry* 11:368, 1989.

102. Adams F, Fernandez F, Andersson BS: Emergency pharmacotherapy of delirium in the critically ill cancer patient. *Psychosomatics* 27(suppl):33, 1986.

103. Lawrence KR, Nasraway SA: Conduction disturbances associated with administration of butyrophenone antipsychotics in the critically ill: A review of literature. *Pharmacotherapy* 17:531, 1997.

104. Ely EW, Stephens RK, Jackson JC, et al: Current opinions regarding the importance, diagnosis, and management of delirium in the intensive care unit: A survey of 912 healthcare professionals. *Crit Care Med* 31:106, 2003.

105. Kapur S, Seeman P: Antipsychotic agents differ in how fast they come off the dopamine D2 receptors. Implications for atypical antipsychotic action. *J Psychiatry Neurosci* 25:161, 2000.

106. Kapur S, Remington G, Jones C, et al: High levels of dopamine d2 receptor occupancy with low-dose haloperidol treatment: A PET study. *Am J Psychiatry* 153:948, 1996.

107. Stone CK, Garver DL, Griffith J, et al: Further evidence of a dose-response threshold for haloperidol in psychosis. *Am J Psychiatry* 152:1210, 1995.

108. Wolkin A, Brodie JD, Barouche F, et al: Dopamine receptor occupancy and plasma haloperidol levels. *Arch Gen Psychiatry* 46:482, 1989.

109. Skrobik Y, Bergeron N, Dumont M, Gottfried SB: Olanzapine vs. haloperidol: treating delirium in a critical care setting. *Intensive Care Med* 30:444, 2004.

110. Riker R, Fraser G, Cox P: Continuous infusion of haloperidol controls agitation in critically ill patients. *Crit Care Med* 22:433, 1994.

111. Sharma ND, Rosman H, Padhi ID, Tisdale JE: Torsades de pointes associated with intravenous haloperidol in critically ill patients. *Am J Cardiol* 81:238, 1998.

Chapter 63 _____

CEREBROVASCULAR DISEASE

VENKATESH AIYAGARI
WILLIAM J. POWERS
MICHAEL N. DIRINGER

KEY POINTS

- *Nonarteriosclerotic causes of stroke occur more commonly in patients admitted to the ICU and should be carefully sought by appropriate diagnostic tests.*
- *In patients with acute ischemic stroke, reduction of systemic blood pressure may carry a risk of producing further neurologic deterioration.*
- *Intravenous tissue plasminogen activator improves outcome in carefully selected patients with acute ischemic stroke when treatment is instituted within 3 hours of onset.*
- *Clinical trials of anticoagulation with heparin or heparin-like drugs in patients with acute cerebral ischemia or infarction have shown no benefit. If other indications for acute anticoagulation are present, these drugs may be given safely.*
- *Emergency neurosurgical intervention should be strongly considered in patients with cerebellar infarction or hemorrhage and consequent brain stem compression.*
- *Early surgical clipping or coiling of ruptured aneurysms removes the risk of rebleeding and facilitates the effective management of delayed vasospasm and hydrocephalus.*

Etiology

Cerebrovascular diseases can be divided into three categories: cerebral ischemia and infarction, intracerebral hemorrhage, and subarachnoid hemorrhage.

Cerebral ischemia and infarction are caused by processes that reduce cerebral blood flow. Reductions in whole brain blood flow due to systemic hypotension or increased intracranial pressure (ICP) may produce infarction in the distal territories or border zones of the major cerebral arteries. More prolonged global reductions cause diffuse hemispheric damage without localizing findings, or at its most severe produce brain death. Prolonged regional reductions can lead to focal brain infarctions. Local arterial vascular disease accounts for approximately 65% to 70% of all ischemic strokes. In most cases, arterial disease serves as a nidus for local thrombus formation with or without subsequent distal embolization. Focal arterial stenosis in combination with systemic hypotension is a rare cause of focal brain infarction. Atherosclerosis is the most common cause of local disease in the large arteries supplying the brain. Disease of smaller penetrating arteries may cause small deep (lacunar) infarcts; it is unclear how often these lacunar infarcts are caused by atherosclerosis, some other arteriosclerotic process of small vessels, or by small emboli arising from more proximal sources. While emboli arising from the heart cause approximately 30% of all cerebral infarcts in a general population, they assume more importance

in ICU patients.[1] Atrial fibrillation is the most common cause. Atherosclerotic emboli following heart surgery, infective endocarditis, nonbacterial thrombotic endocarditis, and ventricular mural thrombus secondary to acute myocardial infarction or cardiomyopathy should all be considered in appropriate circumstances. Rarer causes of cerebral infarction must also be considered in the ICU. These include dissections of the carotid or vertebral artery after direct neck trauma, "whiplash" injuries or forced hyperextension during endotracheal intubation, intracranial arterial or venous thrombosis secondary to meningeal or parameningeal infections, and paradoxical embolization from venous thrombosis via a patent foramen ovale.[1]

Hemorrhages into the basal ganglia, thalamus, and cerebellum in middle-aged patients with long-standing hypertension are the most common type of intracerebral hemorrhage. In hypertensive patients with hemispheric lobar hemorrhages and patients without hypertension, other causes should be sought, such as arteriovenous malformations or saccular aneurysms.[2] Amyloid angiopathy becomes increasingly important in patients in the seventh, eighth, and ninth decades; these hemorrhages usually occur in the subcortical hemispheric white matter and may be multiple. Hemorrhage due to anticoagulant and thrombolytic drugs can affect any part of the brain. Rarer causes of intracerebral hemorrhage occurring in patients with other systemic diseases include thrombocytopenia, hemophilia, and disseminated intravascular coagulation (DIC).

Nontraumatic spontaneous subarachnoid hemorrhage (SAH) is almost always due to ruptured saccular aneurysms. Aneurysms may also rupture into the brain parenchyma, producing intracerebral hemorrhage as well. Saccular aneurysms are most commonly located on the large arteries at the base of the brain. Both congenital and acquired factors appear to play a role in the development of aneurysms. Acquired contributing factors include atherosclerosis, hypertension, and hemodynamic stress. In patients with infective endocarditis, mycotic aneurysms of more distal arteries may form and sometimes rupture. Other causes of SAH include ruptured arteriovenous malformations (cerebral and spinal) and fistulae, cocaine abuse, pituitary apoplexy, and intracranial arterial dissection.[3] In some cases, particularly SAH ventral to the midbrain, the cause cannot be determined.

Clinical and Laboratory Diagnosis

The initial diagnostic evaluation of the patient with suspected stroke serves (1) to determine whether neurologic symptoms are due to cerebrovascular disease or to some other condition, such as peripheral nerve injury, intracranial infection, tumor, subdural hematoma, multiple sclerosis, epilepsy, or hypoglycemia; and (2) to distinguish among different types of cerebrovascular disease that require different treatments. The clinical history and examination remain the cornerstone of this process. Cerebrovascular disease typically produces focal brain dysfunction of sudden onset in a single location. The primary exception to this is aneurysmal SAH, which usually presents as a sudden onset of severe headache, with or without nausea, vomiting, or loss of consciousness. In some cases, a less severe aneurysmal hemorrhage may present as a headache of moderate intensity, neck pain, and nonspecific symptoms. A high index of suspicion is needed in order to avoid missing the diagnosis of SAH. Focal brain dysfunction may not always include an obvious hemiparesis. Neurologic deficits such as neglect, agnosia, aphasia, visual field defects, or amnesia may be the only manifestations of brain infarction or hemorrhage. The clinical distinction between cerebral infarction and intracerebral hemorrhage is unreliable. Both produce sudden focal deficits. Large hemorrhages may produce vomiting or unconsciousness, but so may infarcts in the vertebrobasilar circulation. Multiple small brain infarcts may produce impaired consciousness with minimal or no focal neurologic deficits, thus mimicking metabolic or toxic encephalopathy. The initial neurologic examination provides information about the location of the brain dysfunction and provides a baseline for monitoring the subsequent clinical course. A thorough medical evaluation is necessary to detect systemic diseases that may be the cause of the cerebrovascular problem. Careful examination of the heart is imperative to detect conditions that might predispose to embolization, particularly atrial fibrillation, recent myocardial infarction, and more rarely, infective endocarditis.

X-ray computed tomography (CT) is the diagnostic neuroimaging test of choice for patients with acute stoke. It is rapid and can be performed easily on acutely ill patients. Acute intracerebral hemorrhage is easily identified by noncontrast CT. Intravenous contrast administration increases the sensitivity for detecting diseases that may mimic stroke, such as tumor, chronic subdural hematoma, and abscess. Cerebral infarction may not be demonstrated by CT for several days. If the infarct is small enough, it may never be apparent. Magnetic resonance diffusion weighted imaging is more sensitive than CT for lesion detection in the early period following ischemic infarction. Due to its superior resolution, magnetic resonance imaging (MRI) is also superior for detecting small infarcts (especially those in the posterior fossa) at any time. However, MRI is more cumbersome to perform in acutely ill patients because of longer imaging times, the need for special nonferromagnetic life support equipment, and the necessity of putting the entire body in the scanner. Demonstration of cerebral infarction by neuroimaging is rarely necessary, since the diagnosis can be made reliably by the clinical presentation together with a negative CT scan to exclude hemorrhage and other conditions. Cerebral infarction is most commonly misdiagnosed when there is no clear history of an abrupt onset.

Diagnosis of border zone infarction due to systemic arterial hypotension is almost entirely dependent on the pattern of infarction shown by CT or MRI. Border zone infarctions are often asymmetrical and patchy; rarely is the entire border zone territory between the middle cerebral artery and posterior or anterior cerebral artery involved. Furthermore, the actual location of the border zone varies from person to person.[4] When more than one area of acute infarction has occurred and all infarcted areas are within the border zones, systemic hypotension should be considered as a cause of infarction.

MRI has no advantage over CT in the demonstration of acute intracerebral hemorrhage, but it does have superior sensitivity for detecting subacute or chronic hemorrhage. Noncontrast CT has a sensitivity of >90% for detecting SAH when performed within 24 hours of hemorrhage. There is no role for standard MRI in the initial diagnosis of acute SAH since it is difficult to perform in an acutely ill agitated patient and it does not increase the likelihood of detecting SAH.

In the patient who is awake and alert with acute focal brain dysfunction in whom noncerebrovascular causes can be excluded, the immediate distinction between cerebral infarction and cerebral hemorrhage may not be necessary if no emergent treatment of the stroke is planned. In certain situations, however, differentiation between infarction and hemorrhage may be critical. Patients with ischemic stroke whose time of onset can be determined to be less than 3 hours earlier and whose other medical problems do not preclude thrombolytic therapy, will benefit from treatment with intravenous tissue plasminogen activator (t-PA).[5] In this circumstance, emergency CT to exclude cerebral hemorrhage is imperative, or t-PA cannot safely be given (see the section on treatment below). In the patient with decreased consciousness and a new focal neurologic deficit, emergency CT may be critically important in identifying an intracranial mass lesion that requires emergency neurosurgical intervention.

Except in patients with cerebral venous thrombosis, hematologic evaluation of patients with ischemic stroke is rarely of value. Antiphospholipid antibodies are found in a high percentage of patients with arterial stroke, but they confer neither a worse prognosis nor is there a benefit of long-term anticoagulation.[6] Acquired or hereditary hypercoagulable disorders have not been clearly linked to arterial ischemic stroke, whereas they are clearly of etiologic importance in cerebral venous thrombosis. In patients with intracranial hemorrhage, especially in the ICU, acquired hemorrhagic diatheses (e.g., anticoagulant or thrombolytic drugs, DIC, thrombocytopenia) should always be considered and should be sought by appropriate laboratory testing when clinical suspicion indicates.

Lumbar puncture with cerebrospinal fluid (CSF) examination can be an extremely important test in the evaluation of the patient with apparent stroke, especially in patients with acquired immune deficiency syndrome (AIDS) or when there is infection elsewhere. Meningitis may cause stroke by producing thrombosis of arteries or cortical veins. CSF pleocytosis is common following septic embolism from infective endocarditis and can serve as a valuable clue to its presence. Lumbar puncture is the most sensitive test for detection of SAH; it should be reserved for cases in which there is a strong clinical suspicion and a negative CT scan, or when CT is not available or feasible. CSF xanthochromia can help differentiate SAH from traumatic lumbar puncture. In most patients, conditions that cause increased ICP can be excluded by a careful history and neurologic examination; lumbar puncture can then be performed safely at the bedside without a prior neuroimaging study.

Electrocardiographic monitoring detects previously unsuspected atrial fibrillation in 2% of patients with acute cerebral ischemia.[7,8] This information is clinically useful, since the superiority of oral anticoagulation over aspirin for secondary stroke prevention in this circumstance has been demonstrated.[9] Transthoracic echocardiography can provide evidence of poor left ventricular function, and rarely left ventricular thrombi. In patients without clinical cardiac disease (no previous history or signs or symptoms of cardiac disease, no electrocardiographic [ECG] abnormalities, and normal cardiac silhouette on chest x-ray), significant left ventricular dysfunction is vanishingly rare. Transesophageal echocardiography has made it possible to identify atherosclerosis of the ascending aorta hitherto detectable only by cardiac catheterization, surgery, or autopsy. Large aortic arch lesions are associated with an increased risk of stroke. The most common lesion detected by echocardiography in patients with stroke who have no other evidence of heart disease is patent foramen ovale with or without atrial septal aneurysm. Although echocardiography can detect these lesions in patients with ischemic stroke, the treatment implications are problematic (see below). ECG abnormalities are extremely common in patients with SAH. However, the clinical relevance of these abnormalities is questionable since they often do not correlate with echocardiographic abnormalities, histopathologic abnormalities, or serum markers of cardiac injury. Approximately 20% of patients with SAH have elevated serum troponin-I levels. Patients with elevated troponin-I levels should undergo echocardiography, as elevated troponin-I levels have been shown to be 100% sensitive and 86% specific for the detection of left ventricular dysfunction by echocardiography.[10]

Cerebral arteriography provides high-resolution images of both extracranial and intracranial vessels, which may occasionally be useful in the identification of causes of cerebral infarction, such as arterial dissection or vasculitis. Magnetic resonance arteriography (MRA), although widely used, is not reliable and can overestimate the degree of stenosis, sometimes even portraying normal vessels as abnormal. In addition, MRA lacks the high resolution of conventional arteriography and cannot be used to exclude small aneurysms or abnormalities in distal arterial branches. In contrast, magnetic resonance venography has supplanted conventional catheter arteriography for the detection of sagittal and lateral sinus venous thrombosis. In hypertensive patients with lobar intracerebral hemorrhage and in nonhypertensive patients with intracerebral hemorrhage in any location, arteriography may demonstrate vascular malformations or aneurysms.[2] Cerebral arteriography plays an important role in the evaluation of the patient with SAH by confirming the existence of an aneurysm and providing the necessary information to plan a surgical approach. If a CT scan demonstrates SAH, a four-vessel angiogram should be performed as soon as possible. A complete study is necessary to look for multiple aneurysms. If arteriography does not reveal a cause for SAH, it should be repeated in 1 to 2 weeks. CT angiography is sometimes used to provide detailed three-dimensional reconstruction of the aneurysm and surrounding vessels to allow precise interventional planning.

Doppler ultrasound of the carotid arteries is useful to prevent subsequent stroke in screening for severe carotid stenosis at the cervical bifurcation in patients who are candidates for carotid endarterectomy. It is important to remember that the reliability of this technique varies from center to center, and that it is insensitive to stenosis above the carotid bifurcation. Patients with transient ischemic attacks (TIAs) who are good surgical candidates should be evaluated immediately since the risk of stroke following TIA can be as high as 1 in 20 within the first 2 days.[11] On the other hand, in patients with a completed stroke, there is usually no urgency in obtaining this information since carotid endarterectomy does not play a role in the management of acute stroke. Transcranial Doppler (TCD) studies can detect stenosis of intracranial vessels, but the value of this information in management

decisions remains to be demonstrated.[12] TCD can also detect increases in flow velocity in most patients with arteriographic vasospasm of the middle cerebral artery following SAH (see below). The value of regional cerebral blood flow measurements with positron emission tomography (PET), single photon emission computed tomography (SPECT), stable xenon CT, or MRI in the diagnosis and treatment of patients with cerebrovascular disease remains to be demonstrated. Since the diagnosis of cerebral infarction can be made reliably by means of the clinical picture and a CT scan, it is rarely if ever necessary to demonstrate a defect on a cerebral blood flow study. Furthermore other conditions also may produce focal regional reductions of cerebral blood flow. Cerebral blood flow measurement as an adjunct in deciding the appropriate therapeutic intervention in patients with stroke has not been shown to result in improved outcome. The combination of diffusion weighted imaging (DWI) and perfusion weighted imaging (PWI) in patients with acute ischemic stroke often reveals a central area of restricted diffusion surrounded by a larger area of low perfusion. The diffusion abnormality increases with time. These observations have led to the hypothesis that the area of perfusion-diffusion mismatch indicates tissue destined for infarction that may be salvaged by thrombolytic therapy. This hypothesis remains unproven. Clinical trials are currently under way to determine if treatment decisions based on DWI-PWI magnetic resonance scans lead to better patient outcome.

Treatment

ATHEROTHROMBOTIC INFARCTION

Immediate supportive care of the patient with atherothrombotic infarction requires attention to the patient's airway, breathing, and circulation. Although most patients have preserved pharyngeal reflexes, those with brain stem infarction or depressed consciousness may require intubation for airway protection. Coexisting heart and lung disease is common in patients with atherothrombotic stroke. Respiratory and cardiac function should be assessed fully, and appropriate interventions should be performed to maintain perfusion and oxygenation. The use of supplemental inspired oxygen is rational only if the arterial oxygen content of the blood is decreased. At the time of hospital admission, some patients may have mild intravascular volume depletion. In addition to normal maintenance requirements, careful fluid supplementation may be required. The composition of the intravenous fluid (normal saline solution, one-half normal saline solution, or 5% glucose) makes no difference as long as serum electrolyte and glucose concentrations remain normal. Care should be taken to avoid hypo-osmolarity, which potentially could exacerbate brain edema.

Systemic arterial hypertension is common following acute ischemic stroke. In most cases, blood pressure returns to baseline levels without treatment in a few days. It remains controversial what treatment is appropriate. During the period following acute cerebral infarction, the normal mechanism of cerebral autoregulation of blood flow in response to changes in cerebral perfusion pressure is impaired. Any reduction in systemic blood pressure may cause a decrease in cerebral blood flow, causing further damage in marginally perfused areas adjacent to the infarct. There are no known hazards to the brain from this spontaneous transient elevation in systemic blood pressure. When systemic hypertension causes organ damage elsewhere (e.g., myocardial ischemia, congestive heart failure, or dissecting aortic aneurysm), careful and judicious lowering of the blood pressure with constant monitoring of neurologic status is indicated. Unfortunately, there are insufficient data to permit designation of any target blood pressure levels as either safe or effective.[13]

The NINDS t-PA Stroke Trial demonstrated that intravenously administered t-PA improves outcome in carefully selected patients with acute ischemic stroke when instituted within 3 hours of onset.[5] Inclusion and exclusion criteria used in this trial are listed in Table 63-1. Owing to the strictness of these criteria, less than 5% of patients initially screened were enrolled. Patients received 0.9 mg/kg (90 mg maximum) of alteplase, 10% given as an initial bolus over 1 minute, followed by a continuous intravenous infusion of the remainder over 60 minutes. The infusion was discontinued if intracranial hemorrhage was suspected. All patients were admitted to a neurology special care area or ICU. Anticoagulant or antiplatelet drugs were not allowed for 24 hours. Blood pressure was monitored every 15 minutes for 2 hours, every 30 minutes for 6 hours, and then every 60 minutes for 16 hours. Blood pressure was kept below 185/110 mm Hg with labetalol or sodium nitroprusside. Symptomatic cerebral hemorrhage occurred more commonly in the group treated with t-PA (6%) than in the control group (<1%). Even taking into account the increased risk of intracerebral hemorrhage, there was no difference in mortality, and more t-PA–treated patients demonstrated an excellent neurologic outcome at 3 months by each of four separate outcome scales.

The use of intravenous t-PA in acute ischemic stroke has been questioned because proof of its efficacy is based only on a single well-conducted trial. Retrospective analysis of small subgroups of patients enrolled <3 hours postevent in other trials have provided supporting evidence, and there are no data to indicate that patients who meet the eligibility criteria for the NINDS trial do not benefit.[14,15] Therefore at this time, t-PA can be recommended for patients who meet the strict inclusion and exclusion criteria of the NINDS trial.[16] The diagnosis of ischemic stroke in this situation rests on clinical evidence; it should be made by a physician experienced in the evaluation of acute neurologic problems to avoid unnecessary administration of an expensive and dangerous drug to patients who will not benefit. If the time of stroke onset cannot accurately be established to be less than 3 hours, t-PA should not be given. For patients who awaken from sleep with a stroke, the time of onset must be taken to be the last time they were awake and known to be in their premorbid state, not the time of awakening. CT signs of early infarction should prompt careful reconsideration of the time of onset, as they rarely occur within 3 hours of onset, but they are not a contraindication to treatment.[17] Facilities must be available for closely monitoring blood pressure and maintaining it below 185/110 mm Hg. Recommended treatment of symptomatic intracerebral hemorrhage following t-PA includes cryoprecipitate and platelet transfusion.[18] In spite of this treatment, mortality at 3 months was 75% in the NINDS trial.[19]

The value of any thrombolytic agent delivered after 3 hours either intravenously or directly by an intra-arterial catheter is not supported by current data.[16] A single trial of intra-arterial pro-urokinase in patients with middle cerebral artery stem

TABLE 63-1 Inclusion and Exclusion Criteria from the NINDS t-PA Stroke Trial

Inclusion criteria
1. Age 18 through 80 years.
2. Clinical diagnosis of ischemic stroke causing a measurable neurologic deficit, defined as impairment of language, motor function, cognition, and/or gaze or vision, or neglect. Ischemic stroke is defined as an event characterized by the sudden onset of an acute focal neurologic deficit presumed to be due to cerebral ischemia after computed tomography (CT) has excluded hemorrhage.
3. Time of onset well established to be less than 180 minutes before treatment would begin.
4. Prior to treatment, the following must be known or obtained: complete blood cell count, platelet count, prothrombin time (if the patient has a history of oral anticoagulant therapy in the week prior to treatment initiation), partial thromboplastin time (if the patient has received heparin within 48 hours of treatment initiation), blood glucose, and CT scan (noncontrast).

Exclusion criteria
1. Minor stroke symptoms or major symptoms that are improving rapidly.
2. Evidence of intracranial hemorrhage on CT scan.
3. Clinical presentation that suggests subarachnoid hemorrhage even if initial CT scan is normal.
4. Female patient who is lactating or known or suspected to be pregnant.
5. Platelet count less than 100,000/μL; prothrombin time greater than 15 seconds; heparin has been given within 48 hours and partial thromboplastin time is greater than the upper limit of normal for laboratory; anticoagulants currently being given.
6. Major surgery or serious trauma, excluding head trauma, in the previous 14 days, or head trauma within the previous 3 months.
7. History of gastrointestinal or urinary tract hemorrhage in the previous 21 days.
8. Arterial puncture at a noncompressible site or a lumbar puncture within the previous 7 days.
9. On repeated measurement, systolic blood pressure >185 mm Hg or diastolic blood pressure >110 mm Hg at the time treatment is to begin, or patient requires aggressive treatment to reduce blood pressure to within these limits.
10. Patient has had a stroke in the previous 3 months or has ever had an intracranial hemorrhage considered to put the patient at an increased risk for intracranial hemorrhage.
11. Serious medical illness likely to interfere with this trial.
12. Abnormal blood glucose (<50 or >400 mg/dL).
13. Clinical presentation consistent with acute myocardial infarction or suggesting post–myocardial infarction pericarditis.
14. Patient cannot, in the judgment of the investigator, be followed for 3 months.
15. Seizure occurred at onset of stroke.

occlusion showing a barely statistically significant benefit was not sufficient proof for the drug to be approved for use in the United States.[20] The use of MRI (DWI, PWI, or MRA) or CT (CT angiography or perfusion studies) to identify patients beyond the 3 hour window who might benefit from thrombolytic therapy is the subject of active investigation, but lacks evidence to demonstrate that patient outcome is improved. Owing to its poor safety profile, streptokinase cannot be used as a substitute for t-PA.

Two large studies have shown that 160 or 300 mg/d of aspirin begun within 48 hours of the onset of ischemic stroke results in a net decrease in further stroke or death of 9/1000.[21] Data from several randomized controlled trials have shown that anticoagulation with heparin, low-molecular-weight heparins, or heparinoids in patients with acute ischemic stroke provides no net short- or long-term benefit in general or in any subgroup.[22,23] Ticlopidine, clopidogrel, and the combination of low-dose aspirin and extended-release dipyridamole (Aggrenox) all have been demonstrated to be modestly effective in the long-term prevention of recurrent ischemic stroke, but there are no data regarding their value during the acute period.[24]

Many drugs aimed at ameliorating ischemic neuronal damage in patients with acute stroke are currently undergoing clinical trials. Physicians treating patients with acute ischemic stroke should be aware of the results of these trials on an ongoing basis.

Cerebral edema is the major cause of early mortality following cerebral infarction; no treatment has been shown by randomized controlled trials to be effective in improving outcome. Mannitol and hyperventilation can temporarily reduce intracranial pressure. They may be of value to the patient with brain stem compression from an edematous cerebellar infarct for whom craniotomy and removal of the edematous tissue may be life-saving. Both hypothermia and hemicraniectomy are sometimes used to treat massive edema from hemispheric infarction. The value of these treatments is unproven, and the proper selection of patients is problematic.[16]

No clinical evidence or pathophysiologic rationale supports routine restriction to bed of patients with acute brain infarction. Prolonged bed rest carries an increased risk of iliofemoral venous thrombosis, pulmonary embolism, and pneumonia. Patients should be out of bed and walking as soon as possible after a stroke. Occasionally, orthostatic hypotension with worsening of neurologic deficits will occur. In these cases, a more gradual program of ambulation should be instituted. In hemiplegic patients, subcutaneous heparin should be administered to prevent iliofemoral venous thrombosis. Alternating pressure antithrombotic stockings may provide benefit as well. In the case of pulmonary embolism or deep venous thrombosis, full anticoagulation with heparin or heparin-like drugs may be instituted without risk to the brain. Fever may occur due to infection or other systemic causes. Central fevers due to hypothalamic disease are an exceedingly uncommon event and the search for other causes should be vigorously pursued. Animal studies have shown that even minor elevations in temperature of a few degrees poststroke can lead to worse brain damage. Maintaining normothermia through the use of antipyretics and cooling blankets makes good sense but is of unproven value. Trials of induced hypothermia with both external and internal cooling are now underway. It is important to remember that dysphagia occurs commonly, even with unilateral hemispheric lesions. Before oral feeding is instituted, each patient's ability to swallow should be carefully checked. Incontinence is also common following acute stroke. Careful attention must be given to the prevention of decubitus ulcers in bedridden patients.

CARDIOEMBOLIC INFARCTION

The basic supportive care of the patient with cardioembolic brain infarction is the same as for atherothrombotic infarction. Intravenous t-PA instituted within 3 hours is effective in selected patients with nonhemorrhagic cardioembolic stroke as well.[5] Patients with ischemic stroke and a cardioembolic source, including atrial fibrillation, do not benefit from acute anticoagulation.[25–27]

OTHER CAUSES OF CEREBRAL INFARCTION

In general, the principles of general care discussed above are applicable to patients with other causes of cerebral infarction. Specific causes may require specific definitive treatments, such as exchange transfusions for cerebral infarction due to sickle cell anemia. The major therapeutic question that arises in dealing with these unusual causes is whether acute anticoagulation will be of benefit. In most cases, this is unknown. Cerebral venous thrombosis can present a particularly difficult situation because of the presence of hemorrhage. Two small controlled trials have demonstrated that anticoagulation improves outcome even in patients with hemorrhagic infarction, although many of those enrolled did not receive anticoagulation within the first few days.[28]

Patent foramen ovale (PFO) is detected more commonly in patients with ischemic stroke than in nonstroke controls and is often the only abnormality found. Based on this finding, it is often concluded that the cause of stroke is paradoxical embolization from deep venous thrombosis. However, in contrast to pulmonary embolization, it is unusual to find a deep venous source in these patients. The risk of recurrent stroke is low and anticoagulation with warfarin does not reduce the risk of long-term recurrence.[29,30] Studies of acute anticoagulation are not available. Acute anticoagulation of spontaneous or traumatic dissections of the carotid or vertebral arteries is often recommended. Data to support this approach are derived only from small nonrandomized, nonblinded studies, and even these data are weak.[31]

INTRACEREBRAL HEMORRHAGE

Supportive care of patients with primary intracerebral hemorrhage (ICH) requires attention to the same basic factors as for patients with cerebral infarction. Any underlying coagulopathy should be corrected as rapidly as possible. Prophylaxis for deep venous thrombosis with low-dose subcutaneous heparin may be instituted safely on the second day after the hemorrhage.[32] Seizures are more common with lobar ICH compared to basal ganglia hemorrhage. While seizures in the acute setting warrant treatment with anticonvulsants, antiepileptic medication should be discontinued after 1 month if seizures do not recur. Prophylactic antiepileptic medications are not recommended.[33]

Systemic blood pressure is often elevated acutely, sometimes to very high levels. Whether acute treatment of hypertension following ICH is beneficial remains to be determined.[13] In patients with small to medium sized hematomas, reductions in blood pressure down to a mean arterial pressure (MAP) of 110 mm Hg or about 20% of the admission MAP do not affect cerebral blood flow in the brain as a whole or in the region around the clot. If ICP is elevated due to large hematomas or hydrocephalus, this lower limit of autoregulation may be shifted to a higher value. Calcium channel blockers and β-blockers have an equivalent minimal effect on CBF within the autoregulatory range of MAP; ganglionic blockers may have a more profound effect on cerebral blood flow.[34] In patients with increased ICP, the use of systemic antihypertensive agents that cause intracranial vasodilation (e.g., sodium nitroprusside) may further increase ICP. If the ICH is large enough to increase ICP, cerebral perfusion pressure will be reduced, making the rationale for lowering systemic blood pressure problematic. Although rebleeding is now known to occur in up to one third of patients within the first 24 hours, there is no relationship to early arterial hypertension.[13]

The value of ICP monitoring and treatment remains unknown. Corticosteroids do not reduce morbidity and mortality due to edema.[33] Ventriculostomy is of unknown value. In our experience, patients with ventricular enlargement due to intraventricular blood do not appear to benefit from ventriculostomy.[35] Mannitol and hyperventilation can be used effectively to reduce ICP temporarily. This tactic is particularly useful if a definitive surgical intervention is planned.

The primary goal of surgery is to alleviate the effects of the hematoma acting as an intracranial mass lesion, not to reverse the effects of local tissue destruction. Thus surgery has no role in the treatment of small hemorrhages. The value of surgery is best accepted for cerebellar hemorrhages resulting in brain stem compression, although no data other than anecdotal reports are available. Ideally such surgical intervention should be undertaken before brain stem damage occurs. Patients with small cerebellar hematomas (<2 cm) may do well without surgical intervention, or simply with ventricular drainage for hydrocephalus. Those with larger cerebellar hematomas usually undergo surgical evacuation, although no prospectively validated criteria for the necessity and the timing of cerebellar hematoma evacuation are available. Patients with large, deep hematomas arising from the basal ganglia or thalamus do not benefit from surgical intervention. Those with more superficial hematomas and signs of increased ICP may show improvement after surgical evacuation.[35] Intracerebral hematomas due to arteriovenous malformations or ruptured aneurysms require special consideration and careful angiographic studies prior to any surgical approach.

SUBARACHNOID HEMORRHAGE DUE TO RUPTURED INTRACRANIAL ANEURYSM

Aneurysmal SAH remains a devastating neurologic problem, with up to 25% of patients dying within 24 hours with or without medical attention. Of those patients that survive, more than half are left with neurologic deficits as a result of the initial hemorrhage or delayed complications. SAH presents the intensivist with a unique and challenging series of management issues. SAH usually presents as an acute neurologic event which triggers a predictable series of processes that lead to delayed central nervous system and systemic complications. Patients who are minimally affected by the initial hemorrhage can, over the course of hours to weeks, deteriorate due to rebleeding, hydrocephalus, or delayed ischemic deficits caused by vasospasm. Management can be complicated by spontaneous volume contraction, cardiac dysfunction, electrolyte abnormalities, infections, and a catabolic state. The treatment team should include neurosurgeons, radiologists, anesthesiologists, intensivists, and nurses experienced in the management of SAH patients. Because of the complicated nature of their surgical and medical management, SAH patients are best cared for in centers that specialize in this care.

The management of patients following rupture of intracranial aneurysms has changed significantly over the past decades. The calcium channel blocker nimodipine is now routinely used to reduce the impact of vasospasm. Attempts at early obliteration of the ruptured aneurysm with surgical clipping or endovascular placement of detachable coils within the aneurysm have become routine. Hypertensive therapy is now the cornerstone of the management of vasospasm with adjunctive endovascular treatment employed in selected cases. Several new interventions to prevent or to reduce injury from vasospasm are currently under investigation.[36]

INITIAL STABILIZATION AND EVALUATION

Initial evaluation should assess airway, breathing, circulation, and neurologic function. Patients with a diminished level of consciousness often have impaired airway reflexes. In general, patients with a Glasgow Coma Scale score of 8 or less should be intubated. This should be performed under controlled conditions by experienced personnel. Premedication with short-acting agents such as thiopental or etomidate should be used to prevent elevations in blood pressure (BP) with tracheal stimulation so the risk of rebleeding can be minimized.

As soon as the patient is stabilized, a complete neurologic examination, CT, and if indicated, lumbar puncture should be performed. Patients are graded on the basis of clinical and radiographic criteria. The two common clinical grading scales are the Hunt-Hess scale and the World Federation of Neurological Surgeons scale (Table 63-2). The Fisher grade is based on the amount of blood visible on CT scan.[37] These scales predict the likelihood of vasospasm and death.

Routine management of SAH patients usually includes anticonvulsants, steroids, and prophylaxis against deep vein thrombosis (DVT). Anticonvulsants are frequently used in patients with SAH. However, the majority of seizures in these patients occur prior to presentation, and the efficacy of anticonvulsants in preventing subsequent seizures is not conclusively established.[38] Steroids are thought to reduce meningeal irritation and headache and to make the brain less swollen at surgery; however, there are no clear data on their effectiveness. DVT is common in SAH patients, and pneumatic compression stockings are preferred to heparin for prophylaxis because of the risk of intracranial bleeding. Patients require close neurologic and cardiopulmonary monitoring to detect the early complications of hypertension, rebleeding, acute hydrocephalus, pulmonary edema, cardiac arrhythmias, and left ventricular dysfunction.

Routine treatments to reduce the impact of vasospasm include preventing volume contraction and administering nimodipine. Patients should be hydrated with 3 to 5 L of isotonic saline per day. Indicators of volume status should be monitored closely (fluid balance, weight, and in selected cases, central venous pressure or pulmonary capillary wedge pressure) and fluids adjusted accordingly. Several large, prospective, placebo-controlled studies have demonstrated that nimodipine reduces the incidence and severity of delayed ischemic deficits and improves outcome in SAH.[39] It remains uncertain whether this drug acts by causing vasodilation or by exerting direct neuroprotective effects. The recommended dose is 60 mg every 4 hours for 21 days from the time of hemorrhage.

TABLE 63-2 The Hunt-Hess, the World Federation of Neurologic Surgeons, and the Fisher Scales

HUNT-HESS SCALE

Grade	Criteria
I	Asymptomatic or mild headache
II	Moderate to severe headache, nuchal rigidity, with or without cranial nerve deficits
III	Confusion, lethargy, or mild focal symptoms
IV	Stupor and/or hemiparesis
V	Comatose and/or extensor posturing

WORLD FEDERATION OF NEUROLOGIC SURGEONS SCALE

Grade	Glasgow Coma Scale Score	Motor Deficits
I	15	Absent
II	14–13	Absent
III	14–13	Present
IV	12–7	Present or absent
V	6–3	Present or absent

FISHER SCALE (BASED ON INITIAL CT APPEARANCE AND QUANTIFICATION OF SUBARACHNOID BLOOD)

1. No subarachnoid hemorrhage on computed tomography
2. Broad diffusion of subarachnoid blood, no clots and no layers of blood greater than 1 mm thick
3. Either localized blood clots in the subarachnoid space or layers of blood greater than 1 mm thick
4. Intraventricular and intracerebral blood present, in absence of significant subarachnoid blood

At this dose, nimodipine can sometimes reduce systemic BP, an effect that is undesirable in patients with vasospasm (see below). This effect can be ameliorated by increasing fluid administration and by altering the dose to 30 mg every 2 hours, but pharmacologic blood pressure support is necessary in some patients.

EARLY COMPLICATIONS

Hypertension

Elevated BP often initially accompanies acute SAH. Several factors may contribute to increased BP, including headache, elevated ICP in patients with hydrocephalus, increased sympathetic nervous system activity, and pre-existing hypertension. The rationale for treating hypertension is to reduce the risk of aneurysmal rebleeding. There are few compelling reasons not to treat the elevated BP before the onset of vasospasm. As definitive data on optimal BP are lacking, it seems prudent to take the patient's usual BP as a target. When the patient's usual BP is not known, it is probably better to overtreat than to undertreat. There is one important exception—comatose patients in whom CT shows marked hydrocephalus. In such cases BP should be treated very cautiously until the ICP is known, to avoid causing a critical reduction in cerebral perfusion pressure. In patients who present several days after hemorrhage and are at risk for vasospasm, the appropriate management of hypertension is less clear. The benefit of preventing rebleeding must be weighed against the risk of worsening neurologic symptoms by lowering blood pressure in the presence of vasospasm.

The first step in treating elevated BP is to administer analgesics such as morphine or fentanyl. Patients are routinely given nimodipine to prevent vasospasm, and it alone may be adequate to control BP. Otherwise, short-acting agents are preferred, since BP may be labile. Labetalol administered in intermittent intravenous boluses is frequently used, since it appears to have little effect on ICP and is easily titrated. Other useful agents include intravenous hydralazine and enalapril. Sodium nitroprusside is usually avoided because of its tendency to increase ICP and thus reduce the cerebral perfusion pressure. Intravenous nicardipine is becoming more popular in the management of SAH patients.

Rebleeding

Rebleeding is most common in the first 24 hours after the initial hemorrhage. The cumulative risk after 1 week is ~20%, and the risk remains elevated for several weeks.[40] About one half of patients who rebleed die. Measures employed in the hope of preventing rebleeding include avoidance of hypertension, cough, the Valsalva maneuver, and excessive stimulation. Treatment may involve the administration of antitussives, stool softeners, and sedatives when indicated. Antifibrinolytic medications can reduce the risk of rebleeding, but do so at the cost of an increased incidence of hydrocephalus and vasospasm. With the increasingly wide use of early surgery, the use of antifibrinolytics has largely been abandoned.

The timing of surgical obliteration of the aneurysm has changed considerably. Up to the 1970s, surgery was routinely delayed because of reluctance to operate on an edematous brain. Several factors have resulted in a shift to early surgery (days 1 to 3) for patients who have a grade of I to III on the Hunt-Hess scale. These include improved surgical techniques, better results with early surgery in North America,[41] and the necessity that the aneurysm be clipped before hypertensive therapy for vasospasm is administered. The timing of surgery in poor-grade patients (Hunt-Hess grades IV or V) remains controversial, but early surgery is routinely performed in some centers.[42]

In recent years, endovascular techniques for the occlusion of intracranial aneurysms have become possible, allowing craniotomy to be avoided. Electrolytically detachable coils can be placed directly in the aneurysm, where they induce thrombosis. This technique is currently considered appropriate treatment for patients with an aneurysm unsuitable for surgical clipping and those considered to be at high risk for craniotomy.[43] In a recent multicenter randomized trial, 20% of all assessed patients had a ruptured aneurysm that was considered to be amenable to treatment with either surgical clipping or endovascular coiling. Among this subgroup of patients (predominantly of good clinical grade with small ruptured aneurysms of the anterior circulation) the risk of death or dependency at 1 year was significantly lower with endovascular coiling.[44] The long-term risk of rebleeding with this technique and the need for repeated procedures are still under investigation.

Acute Hydrocephalus

Acute hydrocephalus can develop very quickly after SAH. It is most common in patients with intraventricular blood, but can occur in the absence of this factor. The hallmark of symptomatic hydrocephalus is a diminished level of consciousness, sometimes accompanied by downward deviation of the eyes and poorly reactive pupils. The diagnostic evaluation can be complicated if the patient has received sedative drugs; it is important that analgesics be administered in doses that provide adequate relief from pain, but not excessive sedation. If sedatives are required for agitated patients, judicious administration of short-acting agents is prudent.

Hydrocephalus can be diagnosed reliably with CT and treated effectively with external ventricular drainage. Since less than half of patients with CT evidence of hydrocephalus will deteriorate clinically, ventriculostomy is usually reserved for patients with a diminished level of consciousness.

Cardiac Complications

Cardiac arrhythmias and electrocardiographic abnormalities are common in the first 24 to 48 hours after SAH. Most arrhythmias are benign. More serious arrhythmias include supraventricular and rarely ventricular tachycardia and are associated with hypokalemia.

A significant number of patients have ventricular dysfunction, which can manifest as pulmonary edema or hypotension. Increased serum levels of troponin-I and Swan-Ganz catheter recordings showing elevated pulmonary artery occlusion pressure and decreased cardiac output can serve as surrogate markers of left ventricular dysfunction and should prompt the physician to order definitive tests such as echocardiography or radionuclide ventriculography. Electrocardiographic abnormalities do not always correlate with ventricular dysfunction. Subendocardial myocardial lesions (myofibrillar degeneration and contraction-band necrosis) are seen in patients dying from SAH. These lesions are thought to be due to high levels of circulating catecholamines and/or to cardiac nerve hyperactivity and not to reflect coronary insufficiency. Cardiac pump failure is often transient, hence this condition has been called "stunned myocardium." Though catecholamines have been implicated in the pathogenesis, patients have been successfully treated with inotropes such as dobutamine.[45]

Pulmonary Complications

Pulmonary complications are seen in almost one fourth of all patients with SAH.[46,47] They include pneumonia (arising from acute or subacute aspiration, commonly with nosocomial organisms), cardiogenic pulmonary edema, neurogenic pulmonary edema, and pulmonary embolism. Neurogenic pulmonary edema is thought to be secondary to massive catecholamine release leading to systemic vasoconstriction and a relative shift of the intravascular volume to the pulmonary vasculature. Other possibilities include direct endothelial damage mediated by the sympathetic system and transient cardiac dysfunction. Management of severe pulmonary edema usually involves positive pressure ventilation and diuretics; however, diuretics may not be appropriate for neurogenic pulmonary edema if there is relative intravascular volume depletion.[45] A pulmonary artery catheter often helps guide therapy in such cases.

POSTOPERATIVE MANAGEMENT

Knowledge of the intraoperative surgical and anesthetic course facilitates the postoperative care of SAH patients. Large doses of mannitol may have been administered to shrink the brain and facilitate retraction. This measure can re-

sult in postoperative hypovolemia. If temporary clipping of cerebral vessels is required, hypothermia and/or large doses of barbiturates may be employed. These maneuvers may delay emergence from anesthesia and add to the systemic complications of hypothermia. The decision to extubate a postoperative patient must take these factors into consideration. If the aneurysm is successfully clipped, many practitioners will accept higher blood pressures in the postoperative period in anticipation of vasospasm (see below).

HYPONATREMIA AND INTRAVASCULAR VOLUME CONTRACTION

A total of 30% to 50% of SAH patients develop intravascular volume contraction and a negative sodium balance (referred to as *cerebral salt wasting*) when given volumes of fluids intended to meet maintenance needs. Low intravascular volume is associated with symptomatic vasospasm. Hyponatremia develops in 10% to 34% of patients following SAH. Administration of large volumes (5 to 8 L per day) of isotonic saline prevents hypovolemia, but patients may still develop hyponatremia. The degree of hyponatremia appears to be related to the tonicity rather than the volume of fluids administered.[48] Thus administration of large volumes of isotonic saline and restriction of *free water* are usually effective at limiting hyponatremia and preventing hypovolemia. In SAH patients with hyponatremia, the volume of fluids should never be restricted; instead only free water intake should be limited.

VASOSPASM

The term *vasospasm* was originally used to refer to segmental or diffuse narrowing of large conducting cerebral vessels. Recently, this term has taken on multiple meanings. It may refer to angiographic findings, to increased transcranial Doppler velocities, or to delayed ischemic deficits. Angiographic and transcranial Doppler vasospasm occurs in 60% to 80% of patients, whereas clinical vasospasm (or delayed ischemic deficit) occurs in 20% to 40% of patients.

The pathogenesis of vasospasm is complex. Sustained exposure of vessels to extraluminal oxyhemoglobin appears to play an important role in initiating vasospasm. In animal models of vasospasm, vessels demonstrate enhanced responses to vasoconstrictors, as well as structural changes that physically reduce luminal diameter. These changes develop in a delayed fashion after exposure to subarachnoid blood and are self-limited. In addition to changes in the large conducting cerebral vessels that traverse the subarachnoid space, small-vessel reactivity may be impaired as well.[49]

Monitoring for Vasospasm

Serial neurologic assessments are essential in monitoring for vasospasm. These must be performed frequently by physicians and nurses well versed in neurologic examination and the recognition of subtle deficits. The patients with the highest incidence of vasospasm are those with Hunt-Hess grades III through V and Fisher grade 3. These patients are often monitored in the ICU or another special care area during the period of highest risk for onset of vasospasm (days 5 to 10). Clinically vasospasm presents as a decline in the global level of function or a focal neurologic deficit. Patients may initially appear "less bright" and then become progressively less alert and finally comatose. The focal deficits mimic those seen in ischemic stroke. Middle cerebral artery vasospasm can produce hemiparesis, and if left-sided, aphasia. Anterior cerebral artery vasospasm often manifests as abulia or lower extremity weakness. The focal deficits wax and wane and therefore are not reported by all observers. The symptoms are exacerbated by hypovolemia or hypotension.

Transcranial Doppler ultrasonography detects changes in the blood flow velocity in the proximal portion of the major cerebral vessels. Very high flow velocities (>200 cm/s) in the middle cerebral and intracranial carotid arteries are closely correlated with angiographic vasospasm, while low flow velocities (<120 cm/s) suggest a low likelihood of vasospasm.[50] Patients with rapidly rising velocities are considered to be at highest risk for developing clinical vasospasm. Transcranial Doppler has several limitations. High flow velocities can be due to increased blood flow rather than narrowing of the blood vessel. Distal segments of the major arteries cannot be evaluated. The technique is also operator dependent and adequate "acoustic windows" are required. Therefore, transcranial Doppler velocities should not be used in isolation as an indication for the initiation of aggressive treatments—the clinical course must be considered as well. Angiography may be used to confirm the clinical diagnosis of vasospasm and for endovascular treatment (see below), but it has a limited role in monitoring for vasospasm.

Treatment of Vasospasm

HEMODYNAMIC AUGMENTATION Hemodynamic augmentation for the treatment of vasospasm has been referred to as *hemodilution hypervolemic hypertensive therapy* ("triple H therapy") or as *hypervolemic hypertensive therapy* (HHT). The pathophysiologic rationale is based on the high rate of spontaneous hypovolemia, the association of hypovolemia with delayed ischemic deficits, and the loss of autoregulation of cerebral blood flow in this population.

Most centers continue aggressive hydration during the period of vasospasm risk. Some will increase the rate of fluid administration if transcranial Doppler velocities are rising. The indication for starting aggressive hemodynamic augmentation is usually the onset of clinical symptoms of delayed ischemic deficit. Early descriptions of this therapy emphasized the role of volume expansion, as many of these patients had not been aggressively hydrated before the onset of symptoms. However, if intravascular volume has been maintained before the onset of symptoms, further volume expansion may not be helpful.[51] The optimal intravascular volume is unknown, and achieving cardiac filling pressures that optimize cardiac output has been advocated.

When symptoms persist despite optimal intravascular volume, vasoactive drugs are administered, usually to raise mean arterial pressure (MAP). In most cases, patients will be monitored with an arterial line and a pulmonary artery catheter. The most commonly used agents are dopamine and phenylephrine. Caution must be employed when using dopamine alone, because of a high incidence of tachyarrhythmias. When dopamine is combined with phenylephrine, this is less of a problem. It is best to monitor MAP rather than systolic pressure, because MAP more accurately reflects cerebral perfusion pressure. MAP also varies less than systolic BP with the use of different techniques for measuring blood pressure.

When therapy is initiated, the MAP should be raised to 15% to 20% above baseline rather than to an arbitrary value. If after

1 to 2 hours the delayed ischemic deficit has not resolved, the MAP should be raised further. The MAP is increased progressively until the neurologic deficit is completely resolved or the risk of systemic toxicity becomes unacceptable. Some patients may require a MAP of 150 to 160 mm Hg to completely reverse the neurologic symptoms. Often extremely high doses of vasopressors are required to produce the degree of hypertension desired. The neurologic status should be re-evaluated several times a day to determine MAP goals. Recently, the use of dobutamine to augment cardiac output has been proposed as an alternative to raising blood pressure. Both approaches are reported to produce neurologic improvement. It has not yet been determined whether the optimal therapy is to enhance cardiac output, MAP, or both.

Once instituted, the therapy is generally continued for 3 to 4 days before attempts are made to wean the patient from it. Weaning should be done gradually, with very close monitoring of neurologic status. If the initial attempt at weaning is unsuccessful, a second attempt should be made after 1 to 2 days. The patient usually is weaned from vasoactive drugs first, aggressive hydration being continued for several more days.

Hemodynamic augmentation is not without complications. Early reports indicated high rates of fluid overload, heart failure, and myocardial ischemia. A more recent study indicated that this therapy is safe when administered in a closely monitored setting, even in patients with pre-existing cardiac disease.[52] Cardiovascular monitoring should include continuous display of the electrocardiogram, peripheral oxygen saturation, MAP, and frequent measurements of pulmonary capillary wedge pressure and cardiac output. In patients with a history of ischemic heart disease, daily electrocardiograms and cardiac enzyme measurements may be helpful. Close monitoring of potassium, magnesium, and phosphate levels is important because of large losses in the urine.

ENDOVASCULAR THERAPIES: PERCUTANEOUS TRANSLUMINAL ANGIOPLASTY AND PAPAVERINE Balloon angioplasty can be used to dilate proximal segments of intracranial vessels, but it is not well suited for use in the distal vasculature. The dilatation achieved appears to be long-lasting. Complications that have been reported include artery rupture and displacement of aneurysm clips. In most cases there is clearcut angiographic improvement, but the clinical efficacy of angioplasty has not been clearly established.[36]

Papaverine is a potent vasodilator that has been used in superselective intra-arterial infusions as an adjunct to angioplasty. The vasodilator effects of papaverine persist for less than 2 hours.[53] Radiographic improvement is usually evident, but the clinical effect is less clear. Complications of papaverine treatment are increased intracranial pressure, tachycardia, arrhythmias, and transient neurologic deficits. These therapies are usually reserved for patients who do not tolerate or do not respond to hemodynamic augmentation.

OTHER POTENTIAL THERAPIES Prevention rather than treatment of the consequences of vasospasm would significantly reduce the morbidity, mortality, and cost of SAH. Intracisternal instillation of thrombolytic agents has been employed in an attempt to dissolve clots around the circle of Willis and thereby decrease vasospasm. A multicenter, randomized, blinded, placebo-controlled study found trends towards reduction of angiographic vasospasm, reduced delayed neurologic worsening, lower 14-day mortality, and improved 3-month outcome that did not achieve statistical significance in patients treated with intracisternal t-PA. Patients with thick subarachnoid clots had a significant reduction in the incidence of severe vasospasm with intracisternal t-PA.[54]

The degradation of blood deposited during an SAH involves the conversion of oxyhemoglobin to methemoglobin, which releases an activated form of oxygen that catalyzes free radical reactions, including lipid peroxide formation. The 21-aminosteroid, tirilazad mesylate, a potent scavenger of oxygen free radicals, inhibits lipid peroxidation and reduces vasospasm in animal models. A European-Australian multicenter study showed that tirilazad was associated with better outcomes compared to control patients, but this was not confirmed in a subsequent North American study.[55,56] In a multicenter, randomized, double-blind, placebo-controlled trial, nicaraven, a hydroxyl radical scavenger, significantly reduced the incidence of severe vasospasm and poor outcome at 1 month but not at 3 months.[57] Ebselen, another lipid peroxidation inhibitor, did not lower the incidence of symptomatic vasospasm in a controlled study.[58] Other potential therapies being studied include cyclosporine A, high-dose methylprednisolone, serine protease inhibitors, thromboxane A_2 inhibitors, endothelin-1 receptor antagonists, nitric oxide donors, potassium channel activators, and delivery systems capable of slow subarachnoid release of papaverine and calcitonin gene-related peptide.[36]

References

1. Levine SR: Acute cerebral ischemia in a critical care unit. A review of diagnosis and management. *Arch Intern Med* 149:90, 1989.
2. Zhu XL, Chan MS, Poon WS: Spontaneous intracranial hemorrhage: which patients need diagnostic cerebral angiography? A prospective study of 206 cases and review of the literature. *Stroke* 28:1406, 1997.
3. van Gijn J, Rinkel GJ: Subarachnoid haemorrhage: Diagnosis, causes and management. *Brain* 124(Pt 2):249, 2001.
4. van der ZA, Hillen B, Tulleken CA, et al: Variability of the territories of the major cerebral arteries. *J Neurosurg* 77:927, 1992.
5. The National Institute of Neurological Disorders and Stroke rt-PA Stroke Study Group. Tissue plasminogen activator for acute ischemic stroke. *N Engl J Med* 333:1581, 1995.
6. Levine SR, Brey RL, Tilley BC, et al: Antiphospholipid antibodies and subsequent thrombo-occlusive events in patients with ischemic stroke. *JAMA* 291:576, 2004.
7. Koudstaal PJ, van Gijn J, Klootwijk AP, et al: Holter monitoring in patients with transient and focal ischemic attacks of the brain. *Stroke* 17:192, 1986.
8. Rem JA, Hachinski VC, Boughner DR, Barnett HJ: Value of cardiac monitoring and echocardiography in TIA and stroke patients. *Stroke* 16:950, 1985.
9. EAFT (European Atrial Fibrillation Trial) Study Group: Secondary prevention in non-rheumatic atrial fibrillation after transient ischaemic attack or minor stroke. *Lancet* 342:1255, 1993.
10. Deibert E, Barzilai B, Braverman AC, et al: Clinical significance of elevated troponin I levels in patients with nontraumatic subarachnoid hemorrhage. *J Neurosurg* 98:741, 2003.
11. Johnston SC, Gress DR, Browner WS, Sidney S: Short-term prognosis after emergency department diagnosis of TIA. *JAMA* 284:2901, 2000.
12. Benesch CG, Chimowitz MI: Best treatment for intracranial arterial stenosis? 50 years of uncertainty. The WASID Investigators. *Neurology* 55:465, 2000.
13. International Society of Hypertension Writing Group: International Society of Hypertension (ISH): Statement on the Management of Blood Pressure in Acute Stroke. *J Hypertens* 21:665, 2003.
14. Lenzer J, Warlow C, Saver JL, et al: Alteplase for stroke: money and optimistic claims buttress the "brain attack" campaign. *BMJ* 324:723, 2002.
15. The NINDS t-PA Stroke Study Group: Generalized efficacy of t-PA for acute stroke. Subgroup analysis of the NINDS t-PA Stroke Trial. *Stroke* 28:2119, 1997.
16. Adams HP Jr, Adams RJ, Brott T, et al: Guidelines for the early management of patients with ischemic stroke: A scientific statement from the Stroke Council of the American Stroke Association. *Stroke* 34:1056, 2003.
17. Patel SC, Levine SR, Tilley BC, et al: Lack of clinical significance of early ischemic changes on computed tomography in acute stroke. *JAMA* 286:2830, 2001.
18. Adams HP Jr, Brott TG, Furlan AJ, et al: Guidelines for Thrombolytic Therapy for Acute Stroke: A Supplement to the Guidelines for the Management of Patients with Acute Ischemic Stroke. A statement for healthcare professionals from a Special Writing Group of the Stroke Council, American Heart Association. *Stroke* 27:1711, 1996.
19. The NINDS t-PA Stroke Study Group: Intracerebral hemorrhage after intravenous t-PA therapy for ischemic stroke. *Stroke* 28:2109, 1997.
20. Furlan A, Higashida R, Wechsler L, et al: Intra-arterial prourokinase for acute ischemic stroke. The PROACT II study: A randomized controlled trial. Prolyse in Acute Cerebral Thromboembolism. *JAMA* 282:2003, 1999.
21. Chen ZM, Sandercock P, Pan HC, et al: Indications for early aspirin use in acute ischemic stroke: A combined analysis of 40,000 randomized patients from the Chinese acute stroke trial and the international stroke trial. On behalf of the CAST and IST collaborative groups. *Stroke* 31:1240, 2000.
22. Bath PM, Lindenstrom E, Boysen G, et al: Tinzaparin in acute ischaemic stroke (TAIST): A randomised aspirin-controlled trial. *Lancet* 358:702, 2001.
23. Swanson RA: Intravenous heparin for acute stroke: What can we learn from the megatrials? *Neurology* 52:1746, 1999.
24. Antithrombotic Trialists' Collaboration: Collaborative meta-analysis of randomised trials of antiplatelet therapy for prevention of death, myocardial infarction, and stroke in high risk patients. *BMJ* 324:71, 2002.
25. Berge E, Abdelnoor M, Nakstad PH, Sandset PM: Low-molecular-weight heparin versus aspirin in patients with acute ischaemic stroke and atrial fibrillation: A double-blind randomised study. HAEST Study Group. Heparin in Acute Embolic Stroke Trial. *Lancet* 355:1205, 2000.
26. International Stroke Trial Collaborative Group: The International Stroke Trial (IST): A randomised trial of aspirin, subcutaneous heparin, both, or neither among 19435 patients with acute ischaemic stroke. *Lancet* 349:1569, 1997.
27. The Publications Committee for the Trial of ORG 10172 in Acute Stroke Treatment (TOAST) Investigators: Low molecular weight heparinoid, ORG 10172 (danaparoid), and outcome after acute ischemic stroke: a randomized controlled trial. *JAMA* 279:1265, 1998.
28. Stam J, de Bruijn S, deVeber G: Anticoagulation for cerebral sinus thrombosis. *Stroke* 34:1054, 2003.
29. Homma S, Sacco RL, Di Tullio MR, et al: Effect of medical treatment in stroke patients with patent foramen ovale: patent foramen ovale in Cryptogenic Stroke Study. *Circulation* 105:2625, 2002.
30. Mas JL, Arquizan C, Lamy C, et al: Recurrent cerebrovascular events associated with patent foramen ovale, atrial septal aneurysm, or both. *N Engl J Med* 345:1740, 2001.

31. Lyrer P, Engeleter S: Antithrombotic drugs for carotid artery dissection (Cochrane Review), in *The Cochrane Library*, Issue 2, 2003. Oxford, Update Software.

32. Boeer A, Voth E, Henze T, Prange HW: Early heparin therapy in patients with spontaneous intracerebral haemorrhage. *J Neurol Neurosurg Psychiatry* 54:466, 1991.

33. Acharya AB, Powers WJ: Intracerebral Hemorrhage, 2003. Nashville, TN, EBM Solutions. EBM Solutions Guidelines for Health Care Providers and Consumers [online database].

34. Powers WJ, Zazulia AR, Videen TO, et al: Autoregulation of cerebral blood flow surrounding acute (6 to 22 hours) intracerebral hemorrhage. *Neurology* 57:18, 2001.

35. Adams RE, Diringer MN: Response to external ventricular drainage in spontaneous intracerebral hemorrhage with hydrocephalus. *Neurology* 50:519, 1998.

36. Treggiari-Venzi MM, Suter PM, Romand JA: Review of medical prevention of vasospasm after aneurysmal subarachnoid hemorrhage: A problem of neurointensive care. *Neurosurgery* 48:249, 2001.

37. Fisher CM, Kistler JP, Davis JM: Relation of cerebral vasospasm to subarachnoid hemorrhage visualized by computerized tomographic scanning. *Neurosurgery* 6:1, 1980.

38. Rhoney DH, Tipps LB, Murry KR, et al: Anticonvulsant prophylaxis and timing of seizures after aneurysmal subarachnoid hemorrhage. *Neurology* 55:258, 2000.

39. Rinkel GJ, Feigin VL, Algra A, et al: Calcium antagonists for aneurysmal subarachnoid haemorrhage (Cochrane Review), in *The Cochrane Library*, Issue 2, 2003. Oxford, Update Software.

40. Weir B, MacDonald L: Cerebral vasospasm. *Clin Neurosurg* 40:40, 1993.

41. Haley EC Jr, Kassell NF, Torner JC: The International Cooperative Study on the Timing of Aneurysm Surgery. The North American experience. *Stroke* 23:205, 1992.

42. de Gans K, Nieuwkamp DJ, Rinkel GJ, Algra A: Timing of aneurysm surgery in subarachnoid hemorrhage: a systematic review of the literature. *Neurosurgery* 50:336, 2002.

43. Brilstra EH, Rinkel GJE, van der Graaf Y, et al: Treatment of intracranial aneurysms by embolization with coils: A systematic review. *Stroke* 30:470, 1999.

44. Molyneux A, Kerr R, Stratton I, et al: International Subarachnoid Aneurysm Trial (ISAT) of neurosurgical clipping versus endovascular coiling in 2143 patients with ruptured intracranial aneurysms: a randomised trial. *Lancet* 360:1267, 2002.

45. Macmillan CS, Grant IS, Andrews PJ: Pulmonary and cardiac sequelae of subarachnoid haemorrhage: time for active management? *Intensive Care Med* 28:1012, 2002.

46. Friedman JA, Pichelmann MA, Piepgras DG, et al: Pulmonary complications of aneurysmal subarachnoid hemorrhage. *Neurosurgery* 52:1025, 2003.

47. Solenski NJ, Haley EC Jr, Kassell NF, et al: Medical complications of aneurysmal subarachnoid hemorrhage: A report of the multicenter, cooperative aneurysm study. Participants of the Multicenter Cooperative Aneurysm Study. *Crit Care Med* 23:1007, 1995.

48. Diringer MN: Neuroendocrine regulation of sodium and volume following subarachnoid hemorrhage. *Clin Neuropharmacol* 18:114, 1995.

49. Dietrich HH, Dacey RG Jr: Molecular keys to the problems of cerebral vasospasm. *Neurosurgery* 46:517, 2000.

50. Vora YY, Suarez-Almazor M, Steinke DE, et al: Role of transcranial Doppler monitoring in the diagnosis of cerebral vasospasm after subarachnoid hemorrhage. *Neurosurgery* 44:1237, 1999.

51. Lennihan L, Mayer SA, Fink ME, et al: Effect of hypervolemic therapy on cerebral blood flow after subarachnoid hemorrhage : A randomized controlled trial. *Stroke* 31:383, 2000.

52. Miller JA, Dacey RG Jr, Diringer MN: Safety of hypertensive hypervolemic therapy with phenylephrine in the treatment of delayed ischemic deficits after subarachnoid hemorrhage. *Stroke* 26:2260, 1995.

53. Milburn JM, Moran CJ, Cross DT III, et al: Effect of intraarterial papaverine on cerebral circulation time. *Am J Neuroradiol* 18:1081, 1997.

54. Findlay JM, Kassell NF, Weir BK, et al: A randomized trial of intraoperative, intracisternal tissue plasminogen activator for the prevention of vasospasm. *Neurosurgery* 37:168, 1995.

55. Haley EC Jr, Kassell NF, Alves WM, et al: Phase II trial of tirilazad in aneurysmal subarachnoid hemorrhage. A report of the Cooperative Aneurysm Study. *J Neurosurg* 82:786, 1995.

56. Haley EC Jr, Kassell NF, Apperson-Hansen C, et al: A randomized, double-blind, vehicle-controlled trial of tirilazad mesylate in patients with aneurysmal subarachnoid hemorrhage: A cooperative study in North America. *J Neurosurg* 86:467, 1997.

57. Asano T, Takakura K, Sano K, et al: Effects of a hydroxyl radical scavenger on delayed ischemic neurological deficits following aneurysmal subarachnoid hemorrhage: results of a multicenter, placebo-controlled double-blind trial. *J Neurosurg* 84:792, 1996.

58. Saito I, Asano T, Sano K, et al: Neuroprotective effect of an antioxidant, ebselen, in patients with delayed neurological deficits after aneurysmal subarachnoid hemorrhage. *Neurosurgery* 42:269, 1998.

Chapter 64

SEIZURES IN THE INTENSIVE CARE UNIT

SARICE L. BASSIN
NATHAN B. FOUNTAIN
THOMAS P. BLECK

KEY POINTS

- *Seizures are a relatively common occurrence in the intensive care unit, but may be difficult to recognize.*
- *Seizures that persist longer than 5 to 7 minutes should be treated to prevent progression to status epilepticus.*
- *Three major factors determine outcome in status epilepticus: type of seizure, cause, and duration.*
- *Electroencephalographic (EEG) monitoring to titrate therapy should be implemented in seizing patients who do not awaken promptly after institution of antiepileptics, even if tonic-clonic motor activity resolves.*
- *Lorazepam is a preferred agent for initial treatment, followed by consideration of additional agents for long-term management or to "break" status epilepticus.*
- *Patients with refractory status epilepticus require intubation, mechanical ventilation, and aggressive treatment with antiepileptics titrated to the EEG.*
- *The underlying cause of the seizure disorder must be sought in tandem with treatment of the seizure disorder itself.*

Seizures are a relatively common occurrence in the ICU, complicating the course of about 3% of adult intensive care unit patients admitted for nonneurologic conditions.[1] Status epilepticus (SE) may be the primary indication for admission, or it may occur in any ICU patient during a critical illness.

A seizure may be the first indication of a central nervous system (CNS) complication or the result of overwhelming systemic disease. Seizures in the setting of critical illness are often difficult to recognize and require a complex diagnostic and management strategy. Delay in recognition and treatment of seizures is associated with increased mortality;[2] thus the rapid diagnosis of this disorder is mandatory.

Status epilepticus refers to a protracted seizure episode or multiple frequent seizures lasting 30 minutes or longer. Although conventional definitions of SE have used this time window, clinicians should recognize that most seizures will terminate spontaneously within a few minutes.[3] Recent data suggest that only half of seizure episodes lasting 10 to 29 minutes will stop spontaneously.[4] Therefore seizures that persist longer than 5 to 7 minutes should be treated to prevent progression to SE.[5]

Epidemiology

Limited data are available on the epidemiology of seizures in the ICU. A 10-year retrospective study of all ICU patients with seizures at the Mayo Clinic revealed that 7 patients had seizures per 1000 ICU admissions.[5] Our 2-year prospective study of medical ICU patients identified 35 with seizures per 1000 admissions.[1] The incidence of generalized convulsive SE (GCSE) in the United States is estimated to be up to 195,000 episodes per year,[6] but it is unknown how many of these patients require care in an ICU. The incidence of SE in the elderly is almost twice that of the general population.[7] Eight percent of hospitalized comatose patients in a recent series were found to be in electrographic status epilepticus.[8] Seizures are probably even more frequent in the pediatric ICU, as children in the first year of life have the highest incidence of SE of any age group studied.[5]

Table 64-1 summarizes the most common causes of SE in adults and children in the community. An analysis of 204 cases of SE in Virginia revealed that the primary etiology in children was infection with fever, followed by remote symptomatic

TABLE 64-1 Causes of Status Epilepticus Presenting from the Community

ADULTS		CHILDREN	
Prior Seizures	No Prior Seizures	Prior Seizures	No Prior Seizures
Common causes			
Subtherapeutic anticonvulsant	Ethanol-related	Subtherapeutic anticonvulsant	Febrile seizures
Ethanol-related	Drug toxicity	Intractable epilepsy	CNS infection
Intractable epilepsy	CNS infection		Head trauma
	Head trauma		
	CNS tumor		
Less common causes			
CNS infection	Metabolic aberration	Anoxic brain injury	CNS infection
Metabolic aberration	Stroke	Head trauma	Intractable epilepsy
Drug toxicity		Metabolic aberration	Metabolic aberration
Stroke			
CNS tumor			
Head trauma			

CNS, central nervous system.

SOURCE: Adapted with permission from Bleck TP, Dunatov CJ: Seizures in critically ill patients, in Shoemaker WC, Ayres SM, Grenvik A, Holbrook PR (eds): *Textbook of Critical Care*, 4th ed. Philadelphia, WB Saunders, 2000, p 1846.

epilepsy, and subtherapeutic levels of anticonvulsant drugs. In adults, cerebrovascular disease and low antiepileptic drug levels were the most prevalent causes.[5] A recent study from Brazil found anticonvulsant noncompliance to be the main cause of SE in patients with a prior history of epilepsy, and CNS infection, stroke, and metabolic disturbances predominated in the group without previous seizures.[9] A prospective study of neurologic complications in medical ICU patients determined that two thirds of patients had a vascular, infectious, or neoplastic explanation for their seizures;[1] metabolic and toxic etiologies are common in the ICU as well. A review of 100 cases of nonconvulsive SE (NCSE) demonstrated that 14% were due to acute neurologic events, 28% due to acute systemic causes, and 31% due to epilepsy, with the remainder due to multiple causes or a cryptogenic etiology.[10]

A prospective study of neurologic complications in medical ICU patients showed that having one seizure in the ICU doubled mortality.[1] Up to 61% of patients developing SE during hospitalization die.[11] SE in and of itself confers a mortality rate of 26% to adults older than 16 years and 38% to those 60 years and older.[5] Multiple reports corroborate an especially poor outcome in the elderly.[8,12] The mortality rate of SE in children is 3% in the general population and 6% in the ICU.[13]

Three major factors determine outcome in SE: the type of SE, the cause, and the duration. Myoclonic SE following an anoxic episode carries a very poor prognosis for survival. Complex partial SE (CPSE) can produce limbic system damage, usually manifested as a memory disturbance. The mortality of patients with NCSE has been reported between 18%[9] and 57%,[14] and correlates with the underlying etiology, severity of impairment of mental status, and the development of acute complications (especially respiratory failure and infection). Causes associated with increased mortality included anoxia, intracranial hemorrhage, tumor, infection, and trauma. SE in the setting of acute ischemic stroke has a very high mortality, approaching 35%.[15] Prolonged seizure duration is a negative prognostic factor.[16] A study of 253 adult SE patients showed a greater than tenfold increase in mortality rate associated with seizures lasting ≥ 60 minutes compared with those lasting 30 to 59 minutes.[17]

Classification

The International League Against Epilepsy's (ILAE) classification of seizures is generally accepted. The system allows classification on the basis of clinical criteria without inferring cause. Knowledge of interictal or ictal electroencephalographic (EEG) findings is not necessary to classify seizures except for absence seizures, which are not likely to be a problem in the ICU. The classification system divides seizures into two types: *partial*, which have a focal or localized onset, and *generalized*, in which the cortex of both cerebral hemispheres is involved simultaneously at onset. Partial seizures can further be categorized as *simple*, in which consciousness remains intact throughout the event, or *complex*, in which consciousness is disrupted or altered (but not lost), often resulting in amnesia for the event. Seizures that start locally and then spread to involve the entire cortex are termed *secondary generalized*. Generalized seizures are of two types: *convulsive*, in which tonic, clonic, or myoclonic movements are prominent, and *nonconvulsive*, in which a patient has an al-

tered level of consciousness with or without very subtle motor manifestations.

The clinical manifestation of partial seizures varies with the location of their onset. Motor seizures are usually due to a lesion in the contralateral frontal lobe. Deviation of eyes and head toward the irritative focus is often seen at the onset of seizure activity and is termed *versive* movement. Careful observation of the direction of this initial movement provides important diagnostic information regarding the location of brain pathology. Muscle contractions may be localized to a small region, such as the face or fingers, or be more extensive, involving the entire hemibody. Movements are usually tonic or clonic, but dystonic posturing is also common. Sensory seizures can be primarily auditory, somatosensory, visual, or consist of vague visceral sensations. Patients with complex partial seizures may demonstrate any combination of the above symptoms and have associated motor automatisms, such as lip smacking or swallowing.

Generalized convulsive seizures are usually of the tonic-clonic type. During the tonic phase, initial extension of the trunk is followed by extension of the arms, legs, neck, and back. The respiratory muscles may be involved in the tonic spasm, resulting in cyanosis and decreased oxygen saturation if the tonic phase is long enough, although this is rare. The clonic phase follows and is manifest by repetitive muscle contractions. Fixed and dilated pupils, tachycardia, and hypertension are well described during tonic-clonic seizures. Incontinence usually follows termination of the seizure. The frequency of the clonus eventually wanes and respiration commences when the seizure stops. Patients may initially be deeply comatose but should begin to regain consciousness within 15 to 20 minutes.

Status epilepticus refers to prolonged or serial seizures without interictal resumption of baseline mental status. *Refractory SE* refers to SE that is resistant to treatment with first-line measures and requires more aggressive therapy. Further description of specific treatment modalities will be reviewed below. *Epilepsia partialis continua* is a special type of focal motor epilepsy that consists of near constant muscle contractions of a specific muscle group. These movements can last for months or years without generalizing.

There are theoretically as many different types of SE as there are seizures, since SE is a prolonged seizure. However, SE cannot be classified in exactly the same manner as individual seizures, because seizures are discrete time-limited events with symptomatology restricted to the brief duration of their occurrence. SE, on the other hand, can evolve over time and therefore can have a symptomatology that may encompass more than one seizure type. Furthermore, NCSE can have similar signs and symptoms with different EEG signatures and etiologies. The simplest classification divides SE into generalized convulsive SE and nonconvulsive SE, depending on whether convulsive movements are present. Since NCSE includes everything that is not convulsive, it describes a wide variety of clinical entities and scenarios.

The conventional method of subcategorizing NCSE is to divide it into absence SE and complex partial SE. This works well for patients with a previous history of epilepsy. In this context, absence SE denotes confusion, typically mild, in a patient with generalized, approximately 3-Hz spike-wave discharges on EEG and a history of generalized epilepsy. Complex partial SE denotes confusion, typically waxing and waning, or recurrent complex partial seizures associated with focal seizures in a patient with focal epilepsy. As defined herein, both types of NCSE imply that the encephalopathy is due to seizure activity. Historically, NCSE was labeled "absence" type if generalized EEG changes were found and "complex partial" if focal EEG changes were found, regardless of whether a history of epilepsy was present.

Many patients with NCSE do not have a history of epilepsy and do not fit into the conventional categorization elaborated above. For example, in a retrospective study of NCSE, we did not find any association between EEG findings and mortality,[9] emphasizing that this categorization is not very useful. This is particularly a problem in ICU patients in whom there are typically numerous factors contributing to encephalopathy. This nosologic uncertainty has given rise to several terms to describe NCSE arising in the ICU, including ICU status, subtle generalized convulsive status epilepticus, EEG status, and status in the critically ill. An important aspect of ICU status is that encephalopathy often has other causes in addition to the seizure activity.

NCSE is of particular importance to the intensivist when it occurs as a sequela of inadequately treated GCSE. After prolonged generalized convulsions, visible motor activity may stop, but the electrochemical seizure continues. Patients who do not start to awaken after 20 minutes should be assumed to have entered NCSE. NCSE following GCSE is a dangerous problem because the destructive effects of SE continue even without obvious motor activity. NCSE in this setting demands emergent treatment guided by electroencephalographic monitoring to prevent further cerebral damage since there are no clear clinical criteria to indicate whether therapy is effective.

NCSE can occur as a late stage of convulsive SE from any etiology, or as an initial form of SE from another cause. Failure to recognize NCSE is common in patients presenting with nonspecific neurobehavioral abnormalities, such as delirium, lethargy, bizarre behavior, cataplexy or mutism.[18] A high level of suspicion for this disorder should be maintained in patients with unexplained alteration in level of consciousness or cognition who are admitted to the ICU.

Two special circumstances with which the intensivist should be familiar are myoclonus and febrile seizures. Brief, shock-like, involuntary muscle contractions constitute myoclonus. Myoclonic jerks are arrhythmic, of variable amplitude, and involve both small and large muscles. In patients with postanoxic coma, myoclonus may be continuous or evoked by stimuli such a noise or touch. While this disorder has been associated with epileptiform discharges in the EEG,[19] not all episodes of myoclonus are epileptic; an EEG can clarify whether it is epileptic in individual cases. Postanoxic myoclonus also occurs in patients who have regained consciousness (the Lance-Adams syndrome); in this setting the myoclonus is probably of cerebellar origin and is not a seizure. Febrile seizures are specific to young children and are usually generalized motor convulsions that occur in association with fever, typically as the temperature is rising. These seizures should not be confused with those that transpire in the setting of fever secondary to infection of the nervous system. Febrile seizures are usually brief, but can be prolonged and recurrent, prompting admission to an ICU.

Clinical judgment is required to classify seizures in the ICU. Patients in whom consciousness has already been altered by drugs, hypotension, sepsis, or intracranial pathology may be difficult to classify using only the ILAE classification because it depends heavily on whether the seizure activity has altered consciousness. However, focal seizure activity on EEG or focal neurologic deficits often helps determine whether the seizure is focal or generalized in onset. The ILAE continues to work towards revising and updating the current classification system. The goal is a multi-axis diagnostic scheme that incorporates anatomic, etiologic, therapeutic, and prognostic implications. For the most recent information regarding this ongoing project, refer to www.epilepsy.org.[20]

Pathogenesis and Pathophysiology

The systemic and cerebral pathophysiology of GCSE can be divided into early and late phases.[21] The early phase of systemic manifestations results from an adrenergic surge and excessive muscle activity.[22] The adrenergic surge causes tachycardia, hypertension, and hyperglycemia. These are augmented by extreme muscle activity that causes hyperthermia and acidosis and can lead to muscle breakdown, rhabdomyolysis, and secondary acute renal failure. This stage is generally well compensated by homeostatic mechanisms so that the excessive demands are met with increased supply or other compensatory mechanisms.

Most facets of GCSE begin to slow down late in GCSE, so only a rare patient continues to have continuous convulsive motor activity for more than an hour. Cessation of continuous motor activity would seem to be a beneficial turn of events, but this is actually coincident with a sharp increase in mortality and in complications. Although systemic factors such as heart rate and blood pressure normalize, they may be inadequate to meet increased demands of intermittent convulsions or electrographic seizure activity, even in the absence of convulsions. Thus mortality increases dramatically for SE lasting longer than an hour.[16] Death may result from a number of causes, but in a prospective study of cardiovascular changes during GCSE 58% of patients had potentially fatal arrhythmias.[23] Patients with atherosclerotic cardiovascular risk factors may have a gradual deterioration in hemodynamic parameters as their cardiovascular reserve is expended, while other patients decline acutely, presumably from arrhythmias.[24]

SE may cause neuronal injury in surviving patients. Some neuronal injury is caused by systemic factors; for example, hyperthermia causes cerebellar neuronal injury. However, neuronal injury continues during electrographic SE, even without motor manifestations or when physiologic parameters are held in the normal range. This is illustrated most clearly in experimental GCSE. Neuronal injury is prominent in the hippocampus and temporal lobe in primates with experimental GCSE. The injury persisted even when muscle activity was eliminated by paralysis, and pulse, blood pressure, temperature, and oxygenation were kept normal.

Neuronal injury during SE is due in part to the excitotoxic effects of glutamate-mediated neuronal seizure activity.[20] Glutamate is the most common excitatory neurotransmitter in the brain. It mediates transfer of information between neurons under normal conditions via several receptors. However, glutamate excessively activates the N-methyl-D-aspartate (NMDA) subtype of receptor in the robust conditions of SE. NMDA receptors have a limited normal function, but during

SE they cause very prolonged depolarization of neurons. This results in intracellular accumulation of calcium and other cellular changes that result in both immediate and delayed cell death.[20]

There are two important clinical implications of the pathophysiology of SE. First, neuronal injury continues during electrical SE even after control of motor manifestations. Therefore it is imperative to exclude ongoing seizure activity if patients are pharmacologically paralyzed after GCSE or do not awaken soon after motor activity stops. These circumstances require EEG monitoring to exclude ongoing seizure activity. Second, pharmacologic treatment is aimed at augmenting inhibition, via drugs that act on γ-aminobutyric acid (GABA), such as barbiturates and benzodiazepines. There will probably also be a role for NMDA antagonists. Ketamine is the only currently available NMDA antagonist, but others are likely to be helpful in the future.

Clinical Manifestations

Three problems complicate seizure recognition in the ICU: (1) occurrence of complex partial or nonconvulsive seizures in the setting of depressed consciousness, (2) masking of seizures by pharmacologically-induced paralysis or sedation, and (3) misinterpretation of other abnormal movements as seizures. ICU patients often have decreased levels of consciousness in the absence of seizures that are ascribable to the underlying disease and its complications.[25] An encephalopathic patient may be unable to appreciate or report symptoms of seizure. Fluctuations in mental status are frequently subtle and may go unrecognized by staff. A decline in baseline alertness may reflect a seizure; an EEG may be required to confirm that one has occurred.

Patients receiving neuromuscular junction blocking agents do not manifest the motor signs of seizures. Patients with refractory intracranial hypertension, severe pulmonary disease, or other critical illnesses may be both paralyzed and sedated, making identification of seizures particularly challenging. Tachycardia and hypertension are signs of seizure that can be misinterpreted as evidence of inadequate sedation. Continuous EEG monitoring is warranted in this population if seizures are suspected.

Patients with metabolic disturbances, anoxia, and other types of nervous system injury may demonstrate abnormal movements that can be confused with seizure. Asterixis, or flapping tremor, is a brief arrhythmic loss of tone that can appear in the setting of hepatic encephalopathy, hypercarbia, drug intoxication, or CNS pathology.[26] Myoclonus in postanoxic coma has been reported in the presence[18] and absence[27] of epileptiform discharges. Therefore EEG is absolutely indicated in this setting to evaluate for ongoing seizures. Action myoclonus in a patient recovering from hypoxic encephalopathy is evoked during movements directed at a target, such as an examiner's finger. It is frequently associated with cerebellar ataxia and postural lapses, which when combined with myoclonus can severely impair ambulation. Myoclonus associated with etomidate is described,[28] but whether it is cortically mediated remains unclear. Brain-injured patients may suffer from so-called "hypothalamic seizures." Tetanus patients do not lose consciousness during their spasms, and describe excruciating pain associated with the sustained whole-body contractions. Psychiatric disturbances in the ICU occasionally resemble complex partial seizures. If doubt about the nature of abnormal movements persists, an EEG should be performed.

Diagnostic Approach

The initial approach to seizure management is the same as that for any other acute medical problem: airway, breathing, and circulation. As described above, generalized convulsive status epilepticus often causes apnea and/or poor oxygen saturation. Hypertension and tachycardia may be marked. However, respiratory and hemodynamic dysfunction is transient, and with seizure termination rapidly returns to normal. Padded tongue blades or similar items should not be placed inside the mouth; they are more likely to obstruct the airway than to preserve it. Medication to treat tachycardia and hypertension before the seizure activity stops is not warranted.

When a patient has a seizure, one has a natural tendency to try to stop the event. This leads to both diagnostic confusion and iatrogenic complications. Beyond protecting the patient from harm, very little can be done rapidly to influence the course of the seizure. The seizures of most patients stop before any medication can reach the brain in an effective concentration. Observation is the most important activity to perform when a patient has a single seizure. This is the time to collect evidence of a partial onset in order to implicate structural brain disease. The postictal examination is similarly valuable; language, motor, sensory, or reflex abnormalities after an apparently generalized seizure are evidence of focal pathology.

Seizures in ICU patients have many potential causes that must be investigated. Drugs are a major cause of seizures in critically ill patients, especially in the setting of renal or hepatic dysfunction. Theophylline can provoke seizures or SE if it has been rapidly loaded or if high concentrations of the drug occur; however, these complications can also arise with normal serum drug levels.[10] Imipenem-cilastatin[29] and fluoroquinolones[30] have the potential to lower the seizure threshold, particularly in patients with impaired renal function. Accumulation of a metabolite of meperidine, normeperidine, causes seizures, even in patients with normal renal function. Sevoflurane, a volatile anesthetic agent, also causes electrographic and clinical seizures without a history of epilepsy or CNS pathology.[31]

Recreational drugs are frequently-overlooked offenders in patients presenting to the ICU. Acute cocaine or methamphetamine intoxication is characterized by a state of hypersympathetic activity followed by seizures.[32] Ethanol withdrawal is a common cause of seizures between 6 and 96 hours after the patient's last drink, but concomitant causes must not be overlooked. Narcotic withdrawal may produce seizures in the critically ill[5] and in newborns of opioid-dependent mothers.[33] Both bupropion hydrochloride[34] and tricyclic antidepressants are associated with seizure in overdose and occasionally at therapeutic doses. In the absence of other clear causes for seizure, a complete toxicology screen should be performed upon admission.

Serum glucose, electrolyte concentrations, and serum osmolality should also be measured. Nonketotic hyperglycemia can precipitate both focal and generalized seizures;[35,36] epilepsia partialis continua was the most common type seen in a recent series.[37] Seizure activity may infrequently be the first presenting sign of diabetes mellitus. Both severe, rapidly developing hyponatremia and hypoglycemia can cause seizures. The patient's blood glucose concentration should be measured immediately upon presentation, and dextrose and thiamine administered if hypoglycemia is present. Hypocalcemia rarely causes seizures beyond the neonatal period; identifying even moderate hypocalcemia must *not* signal the end of the diagnostic work-up. Hypomagnesemia has an equally unwarranted reputation as the cause of seizures in malnourished alcoholic patients.

The physical examination should emphasize assessment for both global and focal abnormalities of the CNS. Evidence of cardiovascular disease or systemic infection should be sought and the skin and fundi examined closely. Particular attention should be given to the funduscopic examination of infants presenting from the community with seizures, as retinal hemorrhages may be the only evidence of brain trauma induced by child abuse (the "shaken baby syndrome").

New-onset seizures almost always warrant brain imaging. Considering the large number of critically ill patients with neurologic pathology as a primary or contributing cause for seizures, acute brain processes must be ruled out. Computed tomography (CT) scanning is a rapid modality with which the trained clinician can detect acute blood, swelling, large tumors or abscesses, and subacute or remote ischemic strokes. With current technology, there are exceptionally few patients who cannot undergo CT scanning. Magnetic resonance imaging (MRI) is particularly helpful in detecting evidence of acute ischemic stroke, encephalitis, small tumors, subdural empyemas, and cerebral edema. Most cardiac pacemakers are a contraindication to MRI, but many other medical devices, such as inferior vena cava filters, intracranial pressure monitors, and cerebral aneurysm clips, are now manufactured using MRI-compatible material. Patients with altered mental status who need cerebrospinal fluid analysis require imaging of the brain first, to rule out a mass, swelling, or other cause of impending brain herniation. When CNS infection is suspected, empiric antibiotic treatment should be started while imaging studies are being obtained.

In contrast to the patient with a single or a few seizures, the SE patient requires simultaneous diagnostic and therapeutic efforts. Although 30 minutes of continuous or recurrent seizure activity usually defines SE, one should not stand by waiting for this period to pass to start treatment. Since most seizures in critically ill patients stop within 2 to 3 minutes, it is reasonable to start treatment after 5 minutes of continuous seizure activity or after the second or third seizure occurs without recovery between the spells.

THE ELECTROENCEPHALOGRAM

Treatment for recognized SE should not be delayed to obtain an EEG, but such recognition is not always straightforward. A prospective evaluation of 164 patients demonstrated that nearly half manifested persistent electrographic seizures in the 24 hours after clinical control of convulsive SE, and 14% went into electrographic status epilepticus.[38] Subclinical seizures have been observed during aggressive treatment for SE, even in patients treated with high-dose barbiturates to produce a burst-suppression pattern on EEG. These data suggest that EEG monitoring after control of convulsive SE can be essential in directing the course of treatment. Emergent EEG is necessary to exclude NCSE in those patients who do not begin to awaken soon after visible seizure activity has stopped. Patients who develop refractory SE or receive neuromuscular junction blockade require continuous EEG monitoring, since ongoing seizure activity can cause neuronal injury via excitotoxic mechanisms as outlined above.

A variety of findings may be present in the EEG, depending on the seizure type, duration, and level of pharmacologic intervention. Prospective data indicate that EEG patterns may also be helpful in determining prognosis. One study found that the presence of burst-suppression, post-SE ictal discharges, and periodic lateralized epileptiform discharges during the initial 24 hours after control of SE were statistically significantly correlated with mortality and poor outcome.[39] Burst-suppression secondary to pharmacologic coma for treatment of SE must be differentiated from burst-suppression due to widespread cortical injury, or that seen as the last stage of the EEG evolution of SE. The availability of continuous paperless electroencephalographic monitoring allows for detection of seizure activity over a long period.

Management Approach

ISOLATED SEIZURES

Not all patients who have seizures require anticonvulsant therapy. Making the decision to administer anticonvulsants to a hospitalized patient who experiences one or a few seizures mandates consideration of a provisional cause, estimation of the likelihood of recurrence, and recognition of the utility and limitations of anticonvulsants. For example, seizures due to ethanol or other hypnosedative withdrawal do not need chronic treatment, but short-term therapy with benzodiazepines for repeated or prolonged seizures may be warranted (Table 64-2). Seizures caused by metabolic disturbances such as hyponatremia are often refractory to conventional anticonvulsant medications such as phenytoin, and are best treated with correction of the underlying disorder (benzodiazepines may be useful for seizure suppression if needed while the metabolic problem is being corrected). Seizures related to nonketotic hyperglycemia respond best to correction of hyperglycemia with insulin and rehydration.[36]

A patient with CNS disease who has even one seizure should receive anticonvulsant therapy because the risk of seizure recurrence is very high. However, this treatment should be reviewed before discharge. Initiating this treatment after the first *unprovoked* seizure may help delay the appearance of subsequent seizures,[40] but probably does not influence whether epilepsy subsequently develops.[41] Prophylactic therapy in patients at high risk for seizure, especially if his or her condition would be seriously complicated by a convulsion, is not unreasonable. Patients with traumatic brain injury, intracerebral hemorrhages, and subarachnoid hemorrhages are frequently placed on anticonvulsants immediately upon admission, although no prospective randomized trials have proven a positive effect on outcome.

In the ICU setting, phenytoin is often the first drug selected due to ease of administration and rapid assessment of blood levels. While the efficacy of phenytoin in the control of seizures is well established, several inherent properties of the drug limit its tolerability. In order to improve aqueous

TABLE 64-2 Drugs for the Treatment of Acute Convulsive Status Epilepticus

Drug	Dose	Rate	Advantages	Disadvantages
Diazepam	0.15 mg/kg	IV push	Quick onset of action	Respiratory depression
Fosphenytoin	20 mg/kg	<150 mg/min	Easy transition to chronic administration	Delay to onset of action; prolonged loading time; hypotension
Lorazepam	0.1 mg/kg	IV push diluted 1:1	Quick onset of action; may prevent early recurrence	Respiratory depression
Midazolam	0.2 mg/kg	IV/IM push	Can be given IM; quick onset of action	Respiratory depression
Phenobarbital	10–20 mg/kg	50–100 mg/min	Readily available	Prolonged loading time; hypotension
Phenytoin	20 mg/kg	<50 mg/min	Readily available	Prolonged loading time; cardiac arrhythmias; necrosis if extravasation occurs; hypotension; incompatiable with dextrose-containing solutions
Valproate	25 mg/kg	12–200 mg/min diluted 2:1	Appears safe in children	Not well studied in status epilepticus

solubility, phenytoin is suspended in a highly alkaline solution that is comprised of 40% propylene glycol.[42] The propylene glycol vehicle has been linked to hypotension and cardiac arrhythmias during phenytoin infusion; however, phenytoin itself may be partly responsible for hemodynamic instability. The caustic pH of the parenteral formulation can cause injection site reactions that can range from burning at the IV site to necrosis in the event of extravasation.

The phenytoin prodrug, fosphenytoin, is water soluble; therefore the parenteral formulation is more neutral than that of phenytoin and contains no organic solvents. Cardiovascular side effects were initially thought to be less common with fosphenytoin, but subsequent experience suggests that hypotension and arrhythmias may follow its infusion. Pain at the infusion site is significantly less common with fosphenytoin than with phenytoin.[43] In patients without IV access, fosphenytoin can be safely administered intramuscularly. IM doses of fosphenytoin are well tolerated, require no cardiac monitoring, and are completely absorbed. Fosphenytoin is rapidly converted to phenytoin in vivo and free phenytoin levels after fosphenytoin administration are not markedly different compared to phenytoin, although the time to reach the peak level after IM administration is several hours.

A 20 mg/kg loading dose of phenytoin brings most patients to the desired concentration of 20 μg/mL (corresponding to an unbound or free concentration of 2 μg/mL). Fosphenytoin is dosed by phenytoin-equivalent units (PE); therefore no dosage adjustments are needed when converting patients from phenytoin to fosphenytoin. Fosphenytoin can be administered via intravenous infusion at rates of up to 150 mg PE/min, compared with a maximum rate of 50 mg/min for phenytoin. Both of these drug infusions should be started at a lower rate and increased as tolerated. When loading doses of fosphenytoin are given IM, two divided doses of 10 mg/kg each are recommended. After fosphenytoin administration, phenytoin concentrations should not be measured until the biologic conversion to phenytoin is complete and the drug has equilibrated throughout the body, about 2 hours after an intravenous infusion or 4 hours after an intramuscular injection of fosphenytoin. Phenytoin is approximately 90% protein bound in normal hosts, but the unbound fraction is the active component. Patients with renal or hepatic dysfunction or those taking drugs that compete for protein binding may benefit from measuring the free (unbound) serum phenytoin concentration before increasing phenytoin doses due to apparently subtherapeutic total phenytoin concentrations.

The maintenance dose for phenytoin is typically in the range of 5 to 7 mg/kg per day, but is highly variable because of individual differences in metabolism and interactions with other drugs metabolized via the cytochrome P450 system. Maintenance doses can be given either enterally or parenterally. Maintenance doses of IV or enteral liquid suspension phenytoin must be given in twice-daily divided doses since their half-life is less than 24 hours. Extended-release capsules can be given once a day. However, patients often do not tolerate more than 300 or 400 mg of phenytoin enterally in any one dose secondary to nausea. Therefore patients requiring more than this amount in capsules should usually receive divided doses.

Hypersensitivity is the major adverse effect of concern to the intensivist. This may manifest itself solely as fever, but commonly includes rash, eosinophilia, and elevated liver enzymes. Adverse reactions to phenytoin and other anticonvulsants have been reviewed elsewhere.[44]

Phenobarbital remains a useful anticonvulsant for those intolerant to phenytoin or those who have persistent seizures after *adequate* phenytoin administration. The loading IV dose is 15 to 20 mg/kg, and the target serum concentration is 20 to 40 μg/mL. The serum concentration may be altered by hepatic and renal dysfunction. Furthermore, phenobarbital can also induce P450-related metabolism, thereby affecting the metabolism of other drugs that undergo hepatic clearance. Since the usual clearance half-life of phenobarbital is about 96 hours, maintenance doses of this agent should be given once a day. A steady-state level takes about 3 weeks to become established. Sedation is the major adverse effect; allergy to the drug occurs rarely.

Carbamazepine is rarely initiated in the ICU because it is not available in parenteral form and absorption from the gastrointestinal tract is relatively slow. Carbamazepine has significant interactions with many drugs that are used in hospitalized patients, such as corticosteroids, theophylline, warfarin, and cimetidine. Adjusting blood levels of carbamazepine in the setting of polypharmacy can be unpredictable. Carbamazepine and the newer anticonvulsant oxcarbazepine can both cause hyponatremia with chronic use, probably due to a combination of the syndrome of inappropriate secretion of antidiuretic hormone (SIADH) and salt-wasting nephropathy.

STATUS EPILEPTICUS

Status epilepticus is a medical emergency. While proper diagnosis of the cause is critical, the most important initial goal is to expeditiously stop the clinical and electrographic seizures. The likelihood of successfully treating SE is inversely related to the duration of seizures; the longer seizures last, the more difficult they are to terminate. Aggressive and rapid management of status epilepticus is essential to limit further neurologic and systemic complications.

The conventional agents used for first-line treatment of SE are the benzodiazepines (especially lorazepam, diazepam, and midazolam), phenytoin, and phenobarbital. The Veterans Affairs Status Epilepticus Cooperative Study Group trial compared four regimens for the initial treatment of GCSE and demonstrated that lorazepam was more efficacious than phenytoin, and easier to use than phenobarbital or phenytoin plus diazepam.[45] Lorazepam has been our agent of first choice for terminating SE for many years and remains so with support from this study.

The major advantage of lorazepam over diazepam is its longer duration of action, thereby limiting seizure recurrence. Lorazepam has traditionally been given in 2-mg doses repeated at 5-minute intervals if seizures do not terminate. Since this is often an inadequate dose and valuable time passes before definitive treatment is instituted, we recommend instead a single IV dose of 0.1 mg/kg of lorazepam. If lorazepam is not available, a single IV dose of 0.15 mg/kg of diazepam is an alternative. However, another agent such as phenytoin or phenobarbital should be started immediately, as the duration of action of diazepam against SE is only about 20 minutes. In the event that IV access is unattainable, 0.2 mg/kg of midazolam administered IM will be rapidly and reliably absorbed. The use of midazolam in refractory SE will be discussed below. All benzodiazepines carry a risk of hypotension and respiratory depression. However, these are also sequelae of prolonged or inadequately treated SE. The intensivist should be prepared to intubate or use vasopressors if necessary.

Phenytoin is an effective anti-SE agent; however, the constraint on the rate of intravenous administration is of concern when treating SE. Fosphenytoin may be a better drug for use in SE since it can be loaded up to three times faster, although its 7-minute conversion half-life means that the serum phenytoin level does not reach its target much faster. Phenytoin has a long duration of action when an adequate dose is given (a 20-mg/kg dose produces a serum level above 20 mg/mL for 24 hours). Adding an additional 5 mg/kg if the initial load fails to stop SE may be useful. Intramuscular injection of fosphenytoin in SE patients may be supported by the known pharmacokinetics of this route, but it should not be considered to be acceptable therapy for SE and should be reserved for only those rare circumstances in which IV access cannot be obtained.

Phenobarbital in the management of acute SE is not routinely recommended, except when phenytoin is contraindicated. However, the Veterans Affairs study showed no difference in efficacy between lorazepam and phenobarbital as first-line agents in SE, but phenobarbital took longer to administer.[45] Furthermore, in the patients that did not respond to lorazepam or phenytoin, the response rate to phenobarbital was only 2.1% (unpublished data). We therefore recommend pursuing a more definitive treatment strategy for patients who have entered refractory SE (RSE).

REFRACTORY STATUS EPILEPTICUS

Patients in RSE require doses of medication that are highly likely to cause significant respiratory suppression and hypotension. Therefore mechanical ventilation is necessary, and invasive hemodynamic monitoring is frequently required. Concomitant continuous EEG monitoring is also mandatory to confirm treatment success and monitor depth of sedation. The traditional goal of therapy is burst-suppression pattern on EEG for 12 to 24 hours prior to any attempts to wean medication. Since the available data suggest that successful treatment and improved outcome probably required seizure suppression regardless of background EEG activity,[46] we recommend cessation of electrographic seizures as the goal instead.

High-dose barbiturates, most commonly pentobarbital, are extremely useful in RSE, but side effects can be severe and may limit use (Table 64-3). Hypotension can be refractory to initial resuscitative efforts, and the patient may benefit

TABLE 64-3 Drugs for the Treatment of Refractory Status Epilepticus

Drug	IV Loading Dose	Maintenance Dose	Advantages	Disadvantages
Ketamine	4–5 mg/kg over 2–4 min	1–5 mg/kg per h	Unlikely to cause hemodynamic instability	Not well studied for status epilepticus
Midazolam	0.2 mg/kg IV bolus	0.05–2 mg/kg per h	Fast onset of action	Tachyphylaxis
Pentobarbital	5–12 mg/kg at 50 mg/min	1–10 mg/kg per h	Readily available	Hypotension; immune suppression
Propofol	1–2 mg/kg IV bolus	1–15 mg/kg per h	Easy to adjust	High lipid and calorie content; "propofol infusion syndrome" (metabolic acidosis, and on occasion rhabdomyolysis, with doses greater than 5 mg/kg per h)
Thiopental sodium	75–125 mg IV bolus	1–5 mg/kg per h	Fast onset of action	Can have prolonged effects after extended infusions due to absorption into adipose tissue

from pulmonary artery catheterization to plan fluid and vasopressor management. Pulmonary infection is common due to prolonged intubation and impaired function of both respiratory cilia and leukocytes. The intensivist must be vigilant in monitoring for infection since barbiturate-induced poikilothermia may mask fever. Despite these side effects, barbiturate anesthesia should not be rapidly discontinued if it is successful in terminating refractory SE. Continuing therapy for at least 48 hours, gradual tapering of the infusion dose, and the administration of phenobarbital during the drug taper are recommended.[47] Pentobarbital is loaded at 5 to 12 mg/kg followed by an infusion of 1 to 10 mg/kg per hour. As an alternative, thiopental sodium may be given in 75- to 125-mg IV boluses followed by infusion rates of 1 to 5 mg/kg per hour. Both medications rapidly redistribute into adipose tissue; recovery of consciousness usually takes much longer after thiopental infusions than after pentobarbital. Elimination times can be greatly increased in obese patients after prolonged infusions.

Midazolam is a water-soluble benzodiazepine that has demonstrated high efficacy in refractory SE in adults and children.[48–50] Midazolam is loaded at 0.2 mg/kg followed by continuous infusion of 0.05 to 2.0 mg/kg per hour. Respiratory depression may be encountered less frequently than with other hypnosedatives, but should be anticipated. Since most patients with RSE are already intubated, concern for respiratory effects should not limit use. Clinically significant hypotension is rare even at the very high doses that are often required to address tachyphylaxis.[51] Sedation is quickly reversed after short-term infusions are discontinued. However, terminal half-lives of three to eight times normal have been reported with extended administration.[52] In addition, prolonged elimination times have been associated with critical illness and hepatorenal dysfunction.

Propofol is an intravenous anesthetic agent that acts primarily on the GABA$_A$ receptor. Case reports documenting its efficacy in RSE are abundant, but studies examining direct comparisons with other agents have had mixed results.[53–55] An initial bolus of 1 to 2 mg/kg should be followed with a maintenance infusion at 1 to 15 mg/kg per hour. Propofol is fast acting, highly lipid soluble, and has little propensity to accumulate even with prolonged infusions.[47] Because of its rapid clearance, propofol should not be abruptly discontinued, but instead tapered gradually. Respiratory depression and hypotension are extremely common, especially after the initial bolus. Nutritional support must be adjusted in the setting of propofol infusion due to the high lipid and calorie content of the solution. Acidosis and rhabdomyolysis have been reported in both adults[56] and children.[57] Careful monitoring of creatine kinase and blood pH are prudent.

Alternative regimens with reported success in the termination of RSE include isoflurane, intravenous valproate, ketamine, and topiramate. Further studies are indicated to elucidate the role of these agents in the treatment of seizure emergencies.

Once SE is addressed, one must manage the major systemic complications of SE. Patients with GCSE should be screened for rhabdomyolysis with urine myoglobin and serum creatinine kinase (CK) determination. If myoglobinuria is present or if the CK concentration is more than 10 times the upper limit of normal, rehydration and urinary alkalinization should be instituted.[58] Prolonged or severe hyperthermia should be aggressively treated with cooling blankets, ice packs, or other cooling modalities.

SPECIAL CONSIDERATIONS FOR CHILDREN

Treatment of seizures or SE in critically ill children generally parallels that for adults. Intravenous access is often more difficult to achieve in children. Lorazepam and diazepam can both be administered by the rectal route (usually 0.5 mg/kg *per rectum* for both agents) and midazolam (0.2 mg/kg) via the IM, nasal, or buccal routes. Lorazepam is probably the first-line drug of choice for terminating SE in children as for adults. One study of 86 children presenting with seizure found that those who received lorazepam had a higher incidence of termination of seizure activity and less frequent respiratory depression than those treated with diazepam.[59] Midazolam administered by continuous infusion appears effective in RSE in children.[60–62] Although all eight patients in one study were mechanically ventilated, none demonstrated cardiovascular instability despite midazolam doses resulting in burst-suppression.[59]

As with adults, rapid control of SE in children achieved with benzodiazepines should be followed by administration of a longer-acting agent such as phenytoin (20 mg/kg IV), fosphenytoin (20 mg PE/kg IV), or phenobarbital (10 to 20 mg/kg IV).[63] The rate of conversion of fosphenytoin to phenytoin is probably the same in children as in adults. Intramuscular injection of fosphenytoin may be particularly advantageous for prevention of recurrent seizures in children without IV access. The use of IV fosphenytoin over IV phenytoin is prudent in infants and neonates, whose small limbs are at especially high risk of extensive necrosis and amputation in the event of a phenytoin extravasation.

Intravenous valproate appears to be safe and effective in children;[64] however, more data are needed to fully evaluate its use in pediatric SE.

References

1. Bleck TP, Smith MC, Pierre-Louis JC, et al: Neurologic complications of critical medical illnesses. *Crit Care Med* 21:98, 1993.
2. Young GB, Jordan KG, Doig GS: An assessment of nonconvulsive seizures in the intensive care unit using continuous EEG monitoring: an investigation of variables associated with mortality. *Neurology* 47:83, 1996.
3. Lowenstein DH, Bleck T, Macdonald RL: It's time to revise the definition of status epilepticus. *Epilepsia* 40:120, 1999.
4. DeLorenzo RJ, Garnett LK, Towne AR, et al: Comparison of status epilepticus with prolonged seizure episode lasting 10 to 29 minutes. *Epilepsia* 40:164, 1999.
5. Wijdicks EFM, Sharbrough FW: New-onset seizures in critically ill patients. *Neurology* 43:1042, 1993.
6. DeLorenzo RJ, Hauser WA, Towne AR, et al: A prospective population-based epidemiologic study of status epilepticus in Richmond, Virginia. *Neurology* 46:1029, 1996.
7. Waterhouse EJ, DeLorenzo RJ: Status epilepticus in older patients: epidemiology and treatment options. *Drugs Aging* 18:133, 2001.
8. Towne AR, Waterhourse EJ, Boggs JN, et al: Prevalence of nonconvulsive status epilepticus in comatose patients. *Neurology* 54:340, 2000.
9. Garzon E, Fernandes RMF, Sakamoto AC: Analysis of clinical characteristics and risk factors for mortality in human status epilepticus. *Seizure* 12:337, 2003.

10. Shneker BF, Fountain NB: Assessment of acute morbidity and mortality in nonconvulsive status epilepticus. *Neurology* 61:1066, 2003.

11. Delanty N, French JA, Labar DR, et al: Status epilepticus arising de novo in hospitalized patients: an analysis of 41 patients. *Seizure* 10:116, 2001.

12. Hui AC, Joynt GM, Li H, et al: Status epilepticus in Hong Kong Chinese: aetiology, outcome and predictors of death and morbidity. *Seizure* 12:478, 2003.

13. Lacroix J, Deal C, Gauthier M, et al: Admissions to a pediatric intensive care unit for status epilepticus: A 10-year experience. *Crit Care Med* 22:827, 1994.

14. Young GB, Jordan KG, Doig GS: An assessment of nonconvulsive seizures in the intensive care unit using continuous EEG monitoring: an investigation of variables associated with mortality. *Neurology* 47:83, 1996.

15. Waterhouse EJ, Vaughan JK, Barnes TY, et al: Synergistic effect of status epilepticus and ischemic brain injury and mortality. *Epilepsy Res* 29:175, 1998.

16. Aminoff MJ, Simon RP: Status epilepticus: causes, clinical features and consequences in 98 patients. *Am J Med* 69:657, 1980.

17. Towne AR, Pellock JM, Ko D, et al: Determinants of mortality in status epilepticus. *Epilepsia* 35:27, 1994.

18. Kaplan PW: Nonconvulsive status epilepticus in the emergency room. *Epilepsia* 37:643, 1996.

19. Van Cott AC, Blatt I, Brenner RP: Stimulus-sensitive seizures in postanoxic coma. *Epilepsia* 37:868, 1996.

20. http://www.epilepsy.org. Retrieved January 24, 2004.

21. Fountain NB, Lothman EW: Pathophysiology of status epilepticus. *J Clin Neurophysiol* 12:326, 1995.

22. Simon RP, Aminoff MJ, Benowitz NL: Changes in plasma catecholamines after tonic-clonic seizures. *Neurology* 34:255, 1984.

23. Boggs JG, Painter JA, DeLorenzo RJ: Analysis of electrocardiographic changes in status epilepticus. *Epilepsy Res* 14:87, 1993.

24. Boggs JG, Marmarou A, Agnew JP, et al: Hemodynamic monitoring prior to and at the time of death in status epilepticus. *Epilepsy Res* 31:199, 1998.

25. Bleck TP: Why isn't this patient awake? *J Intensive Care Med* 8:155, 1993.

26. Gokula RM, Khasnis A: Asterixis. *J Postgrad Med* 49:272, 2003.

27. Kanemoto K, Ozawa K: A case of post-anoxic encephalopathy with initial massive myoclonic status followed by alternating Jacksonian seizures. *Seizure* 9:352, 2000.

28. Van Keulen SG, Burton JH: Myoclonus associated with etomidate for ED procedural sedation and analgesia. *Am J Emerg Med* 21:556, 2003.

29. Campise M: Neurological complication during imipenem/cilastatin therapy in uraemic patients. *Nephrol Dial Transplant* 13:1895, 1998.

30. Kushner JM, Peckman JH, Snyder CR: Seizures associated with fluoroquinolones. *Ann Pharmacother* 35:1194, 2001.

31. Jaaskelainen SK, Kaisti K, Suni L, et al: Sevoflurane is epileptogenic in healthy subjects at surgical levels of anesthesia. *Neurology* 61:1073, 2003.

32. Klein C, Balash Y, Pollak L, et al: Body packer: cocaine intoxication, causing death, masked by concomitant administration of major tranquilizers. *Eur J Neurol* 7:555, 2000.

33. So YT. Effects of drug abuse on the nervous system, in Bradley WG, Daroff RB, Fenichel GM, Marsden CD (eds): *Neurology in Clinical Practice*, 3rd ed. Boston, Butterworth Heinemann, 2000, p 1521.

34. Balit CR, Lynch CN, Isbister GK: Bupropion poisoning: A case series. *Med J Aust* 20:61, 2003.

35. Morres CA, Dire DJ: Movement disorders as a manifestation of nonketotic hyperglycemia. *J Emerg Med* 7:359, 1989.

36. Hennis A, Corbin D, Fraser H: Focal seizures and non-ketotic hyperglycemia. *J Neurol Neurosurg Psychiatry* 55:195, 1992.

37. Tiamkao S, Pratipanawatr T, Tiamkao S, et al: Seizures in nonketotic hyperglycaemia. *Seizure* 12:409, 2003.

38. DeLorenzo RJ, Waterhouse EJ, Towne AR, et al: Persistent nonconvulsive status epilepticus after the control of convulsive status epilepticus. *Epilepsia* 39:833, 1998.

39. Jaitly R, Sgro JA, Towne AR, et al: Prognostic value of EEG monitoring after status epilepticus: a prospective adult study. *J Clin Neurophysiol* 14:326, 1997.

40. First Seizure Trial Group: Randomized clinical trial of the efficacy of antiepileptic drugs in reducing the risk of relapse after a first unprovoked tonic-clonic seizure. *Neurology* 43:478, 1993.

41. Musicco M, Beghi E, Solari A, et al: Treatment of first tonic-clonic seizure does not improve the prognosis of epilepsy. First Seizure Trial Group (FIRST Group). *Neurology* 49:991, 1997.

42. DeToledo JC, Ramsay RE: Fosphenytoin and phenytoin in patients with status epilepticus. *Drug Saf* 22:459, 2000.

43. Knapp LE, Kugler AR: Clinical experience with fosphenytoin in adults: Pharmacokinetics, safety, and efficacy. *J Child Neurol* 13:S15, 1998.

44. Smith MC, Bleck TP: Toxicity of anticonvulsants, in Klawans HL, Goetz CG, Tanner CM (eds): *Textbook of Clinical Neuropharmacology*, 2nd ed. New York, Raven Press, 1992, p 45.

45. Treiman DM, Meyers PD, Walton NY, et al: A comparison of four treatments for generalized convulsive status epilepticus. Veterans Affairs Status Epilepticus Cooperative Study Group. *N Engl J Med* 339:792, 1998.

46. Krishnamurthy KB, Drislane FW: Depth of EEG suppression and outcome in barbiturate anesthetic treatment for refractory status epilepticus. *Epilepsia* 40:759, 1999.

47. Krishnamurthy KB, Drislane FW: Relapse and survival after barbiturate anesthetic treatment of refractory status epilepticus. *Epilepsia* 37:863, 1996.

48. Kumar A, Bleck TP: Intravenous midazolam for the treatment of refractory status epilepticus. *Crit Care Med* 20:483, 1992.

49. Igartua J, Silver P, Maytal J, et al: Midazolam coma for refractory status epilepticus in children. *Crit Care Med* 27:1982, 1999.

50. Hanley DF, Pozo M: Treatment of status epilepticus with midazolam in the critical care setting. *Int J Clin Pract* 54:30, 2000.

51. Shafer A: Complications of sedation with midazolam in the intensive care unit and a comparison with other sedative regimens. *Crit Care Med* 26:947, 1998.

52. Naritoku D, Sinha S: Prolongation of midazolam half-life after sustained infusion for status epilepticus. *Neurology* 54:1366, 2000.

53. Stecker MM, Kramer TH, Raps ED, et al: Treatment of refractory status epilepticus with propofol: clinical and pharmacokinetic findings. *Epilepsia* 39:18, 1998.

54. Prasad A, Worrall BB, Bertram EH, Bleck TP: Propofol and midazolam in the treatment of refractory status epilepticus. *Epilepsia* 42:380, 2001.

55. Niermeijer JM, Uiterwaal CS, Van Donselaar CA: Propofol in status epilepticus: little evidence, many dangers? *J Neurol* 250:1237, 2003.

56. Kumar M, Khaled KA, Urrutia VC, et al: Irreversible acidosis and death after prolonged propofol infusion use in two adult patients: propofol infusion syndrome in adults revisited. Abstracts presented at Neurocritical Care Society Meeting, February 2004, San Diego, CA.

57. Hanna JP, Ramundo ML: Rhabdomyolysis and hypoxia associated with prolonged propofol infusion in children. *Neurology* 50:301, 1998.

58. Bleck TP: Management approaches to prolonged seizures and status epilepticus. *Epilepsia* 40:S59, 1999.

59. Appleton R, Sweeney A, Choonara I, et al: Lorazepam versus diazepam in the acute treatment of epileptic seizures and status epilepticus. *Dev Med Child Neurol* 37:682, 1995.

60. Rivera R, Segnini M, Baltodano A, et al: Midazolam in the treatment of status epilepticus in children. *Crit Care Med* 21:991, 1993.

61. Sheth RD, Buckely DJ, Gutierrez AR, et al: Midazolam in the treatment of refractory neonatal seizures. *Clin Neuropharmacol* 19:165, 1996.

62. Igartua J, Silver P, Maytal J, et al: Midazolam coma for refractory status epilepticus in children. *Crit Care Med* 27:1982, 1999.

63. Segeleon JE, Haun SE: Status epilepticus in children. *Pediatr Ann* 25:380, 1996.

64. Yu KT, Mills S, Thompson N, et al: Safety and efficacy of intravenous valproate in pediatric status epilepticus and acute repetitive seizures. *Epilepsia* 44:724, 2003.

Chapter 65

INTRACRANIAL PRESSURE: MONITORING AND MANAGEMENT

JEFFREY I. FRANK
AXEL J. ROSENGART

KEY POINTS

- *Intracranial hypertension is the final common pathway of morbidity and mortality for diverse neurologic problems, and its proper treatment requires the timely application of the available therapeutic alternatives when the clinical situation and prognosis warrant and justify treatment.*

- *Anticipating patients at risk for brain swelling is important and allows the development of a strategic plan to limit its severity and facilitate early intervention when possible.*

- *The initial therapeutic focus for intracranial pressure reduction should be the control of factors that can aggravate intracranial hypertension, such as inappropriate head and body position, elevated body temperature, inadequate treatment of pain and agitation, elevated airway pressures, blood pressure fluctuations, seizures, and administration of hypotonic fluids.*

- *The appropriate conventional medical therapies should be selected based on the details of each specific case. It should be clear that brain tissue displacement (BTD) and intracranial hypertension are not synonymous, and the treatment of each of them can be different. Surgical removal of an intracranial mass lesion or expansion of the intracranial compartment should be considered in patients with severe BTD and/or evolving intracranial hypertension.*

- *In the end, the treatment of intracranial hypertension is heuristic, challenging the managing physician's thorough understanding of the cause of the problem and his or her ability to define the human aspects that relate to determining the appropriate level of care for individual patients. In addition, successful management depends on a partnership with nurses founded on comprehensive communication to assist with the accurate translation of the defined care priorities.*

Intracranial hypertension can be the result of a primary central nervous system process, or it can result as a complication of a concurrent systemic illness. Independent of the specific etiology, it is an important and potentially disabling and deadly complication. While it often has important prognostic implications, its successful management can protect the brain from secondary injury and improve outcome. The management of intracranial hypertension is frequently approached in an overly simplistic manner with the sequential application of various intracranial pressure (ICP)–lowering strategies in a cookbook fashion. However, such a simplistic approach to intracranial hypertension can be perilous and potentially aggravate the problem.

The management of intracranial hypertension is best tailored to each specific situation. This chapter will introduce the basic principles that should be considered when arriving at an individualized strategic management plan for a patient with brain swelling and/or intracranial hypertension. While some of these concepts and treatment strategies are discussed in Chap. 93 in the context of head injury, we will present a more global view on the management of brain swelling and intracranial hypertension

Cerebral Hemodynamic Considerations

INTRACRANIAL PRESSURE

When it is monitored, the ICP tracing is a ballistic waveform much like the systemic arterial pressure (Fig. 65-1). However, it has a narrow "pulse pressure" and is expressed, by convention, as its mean. The normal mean ICP is generally between 5 and 10 mm Hg, and it will fluctuate at times to higher levels depending on many physiologic factors.

In normal adults, the skull is a rigid container and contains brain parenchyma, fluid (interstitial and cerebrospinal), and blood (arterial and venous). The expansion of any of these compartments or the addition of a space-occupying process can lead to ICP elevation. Table 65-1 lists some of the most common causes of brain swelling. The extent of the ICP elevation depends on many factors, most importantly the patient's intracranial compliance.

INTRACRANIAL COMPLIANCE

Figure 65-2 shows the intracranial pressure-volume curve that diagrammatically describes the dynamic of intracranial compliance. When a process that adds volume to the intracranial cavity evolves, cerebrospinal fluid (CSF) from the hemispheric convexities, basal cisterns, and ventricles (except in hydrocephalus) is passively displaced into the contiguous spinal subarachnoid space. As a result, the ICP only modestly increases during the early stages of the process (A). However, once CSF cannot be passively displaced any further, the ICP rises more sharply as the space-occupying process continues to evolve (B). This relationship between added volume to the intracranial cavity and its matched rise in ICP is referred to as the intracranial compliance. There is decreasing intracranial compliance as the intracranial hemodynamic relationship shifts to the right along the intracranial pressure-volume curve.

The concepts of the intracranial pressure-volume relationships and intracranial compliance can be applied when evaluating brain imaging studies to estimate the likelihood of intracranial hypertension in a patient who suffers a space-occupying intracranial process. For example, Fig. 65-3 shows an axial computed tomography (CT) scan of the brain with brain swelling from a middle cerebral artery territory infarction. As there are still compressible spaces around the swollen brain (e.g., basal cisterns, ipsilateral lateral ventricle, and ipsilateral cortical sulci) on that scan, it is reasonable to expect that the ICP is not yet significantly or persistently elevated. On the other hand, the CT in Fig. 65-4 shows a more extensively swollen brain than in Fig. 65-3, with obliteration of all surrounding CSF spaces. In the example shown in Fig. 65-4 the ICP is likely markedly elevated. While estimating

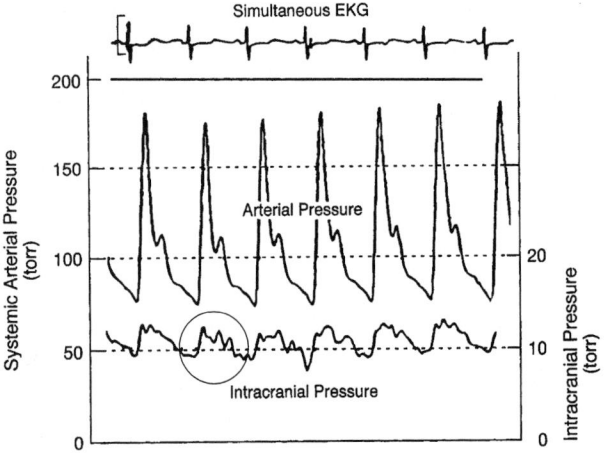

FIGURE 65-1 ICU monitor tracing demonstrating the ballistic waveform of the intracranial pressure (bottom). Note the circled ICP waveform that shows the several smaller waves that comprise it.

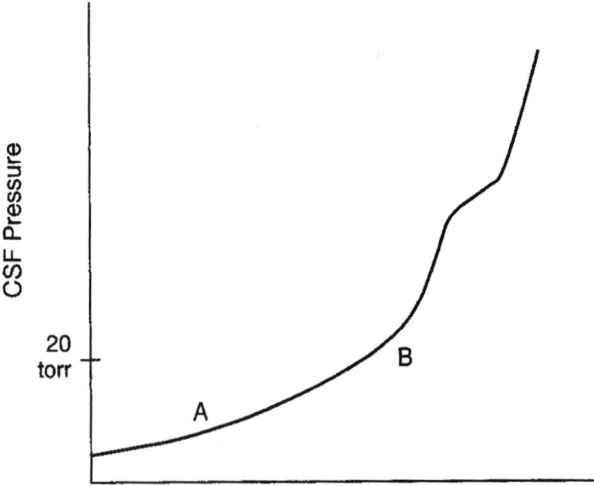

FIGURE 65-2 The intracranial pressure-volume relationship. Point A is where compliance is high. Point B indicates a state of lower intracranial compliance whereby the addition of something that takes up a certain volume will lead to a sharper rise in ICP relative to point A.

TABLE 65-1 Common Causes of Brain Swelling and Intracranial Hypertension

Cerebral abscess
Benign intracranial hypertension
Cerebral neoplasm (primary or metastatic)
Cerebral venous thrombosis
Diabetic ketoacidosis
Eclampsia
Hypertensive encephalopathy
Encephalitis
Fulminant hepatic failure
Hydrocephalus
Cerebral infarction
Meningitis
Reye's syndrome
Head trauma

the likelihood of intracranial hypertension by CT scan appearance is imperfect, it can provide some practically useful direction in management when the clinician is making decisions about whether to begin invasive ICP monitoring or considering other therapeutic maneuvers such as surgical decompression.

CEREBRAL BLOOD FLOW AND CEREBRAL PERFUSION PRESSURE

Alterations in cerebral blood flow (CBF), either too much or too little, can disturb the brain homeostatic mechanisms and lead to cerebral injury. A relatively constant supply of blood to the brain is ensured by cerebral autoregulation, a physiologic phenomenon that allows maintenance of a constant CBF over a wide range of arterial blood pressures. Figure 65-5 graphically depicts this relationship for normotensive patients. In chronic hypertensives, the autoregulatory thresholds are shifted to the right. Relative blood pressure lowering within an autoregulatory range leads to cerebral vasodilation and an increase in cerebral blood volume. Conversely, relative blood pressure elevation within an autoregulatory range leads to cerebral vasoconstriction and a decrease in cerebral blood volume. Such alterations in cerebral blood volume can importantly affect the ICP. In fact, CBF is a critical

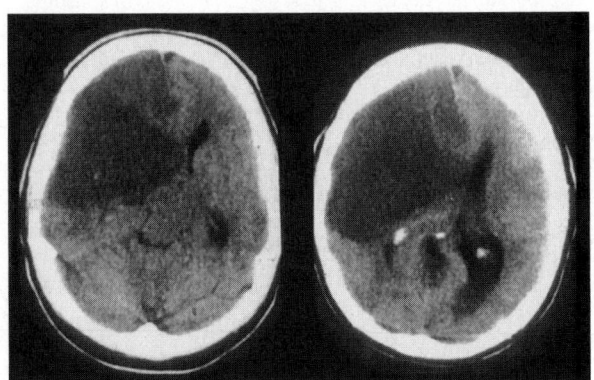

FIGURE 65-4 An unenhanced CT of the brain 96 hours after a right middle cerebral artery territory infarction. There is severe compression of all CSF spaces, an evolving more recent right anterior cerebral artery infarction from right to left subfalcine herniation. This patient has poor intracranial compliance relative to figure 65-3.

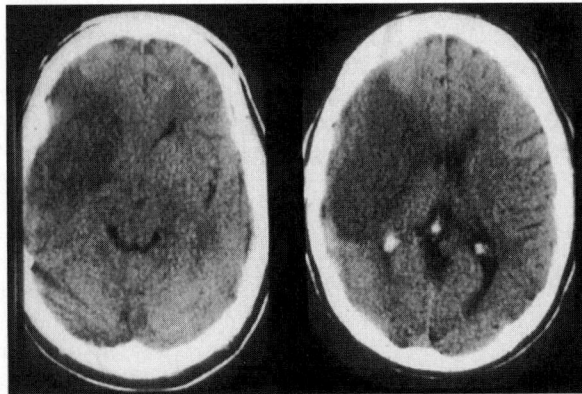

FIGURE 65-3 An unenhanced CT of the brain showing a 48-hour old right middle cerebral artery territory infarction. There are still compressible CSF spaces defining that this patient has better intracranial compliance relative to that in figure 65-4.

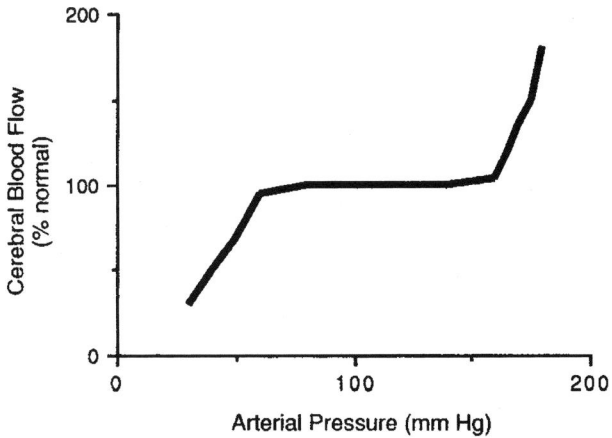

FIGURE 65-5 Cerebral autoregulatory curve demonstrating a constant cerebral blood flow over a range of blood pressures.

between ICP and blood pressure. By definition, the CPP refers to the difference between the mean arterial pressure (MAP) and the cerebral venous pressure. Since the cerebral venous pressure is approximated by the ICP in most cases, the generally accepted CPP equation is:

$$CPP = MAP - ICP$$

This equation emphasizes the important point that the primary mechanism of cerebral injury from intracranial hypertension is cerebral ischemia from compromised cerebral perfusion. Notably, CBF is not a direct correlate of CPP, since autoregulation allows the CBF to remain constant in normotensive patients once the CPP exceeds approximately 40 mm Hg in previously normotensive patients.

The physiologic relationship between blood pressure, CBF, and CPP are less predictable in damaged brain regions where autoregulation is impaired. In brain regions without intact autoregulation, relative blood pressure lowering or elevation, even within a normal range, can lead to regional cerebral ischemia or hyperemia, respectively. Table 65-2 lists several important factors that influence CBF and ICP. Control or manipulation of these factors constitutes the basis for much of the medical management of raised ICP.

In most situations, it is best to maintain CPP in the 60 to 80 mm Hg range in euthermic patients, but the target CPP

determinant of ICP, and its reduction is a major final common pathway for cerebral injury from raised ICP. A practical understanding of these concepts is critical to developing a rational therapeutic plan for patients with intracranial hypertension.

The concept of cerebral perfusion pressure (CPP) is an important guide to management of the dynamic interplay

TABLE 65-2 Factors That Influence Cerebral Blood Flow and Intracranial Pressure

Factor	Cerebral Blood Flow	Intracranial Pressure	Effect	Clinical Commentary
Raised intracranial pressure	↓	NA	—	Cerebral injury occurs through ischemia
Cerebral hyperemia	NA	↑	—	Most relevant in pediatric head injury
Hyperventilation	↓	↓	Vasoconstriction	Tromethamine may prolong effect
Hypoventilation	↑	↑	Vasodilatation	Common with posterior fossa pathology
Hypotension	+/−	↑	Vasodilatation	Early diagnosis and treatment imperative
Hypovolemia	+/−	↑	Vasodilatation	Maintain euvolemia
Acidosis	↑	↑	Vasodilation	
Alkalosis	↓	↓	Vasoconstriction	
Hyperthermia	↑	↑	Vasodilation	Linear increase in cerebral blood flow 6% per degree C.
Hypothermia	↓	↓	Vasoconstriction	May have therapeutic value
Hypoxia	↑	↑	Vasodilatation	Significant at P_{AO_2} <50mm Hg
Increased intrathoracic pressure	↓	↑	Cerebral venous outflow attenuation	Occurs with Valsalva maneuver
Pain/arousal	↑	↑	Vasodilatation	Avoid noxious stimuli and treat with analgesics
Volatile anesthetics	↑	↑	Vasodilatation	Alert anesthesia staff to intracranial pressure concerns
Seizures	↑	↑	Increased metabolism and Valsalva	Maintain low threshold for prophylaxis
Positive end-expiratory	↑	↑	Increased thoracic pressure	Variable effect on intracranial pressure

NA, not applicable.

TABLE 65-3 Classification of Cerebral Edema

Type	Location	Site	Blood-Brain Barrier	Probable Mechanism
Vasogenic	Extracellular	White	Disrupted	Increased vascular permeability
Cytotoxic	Intracellular	White or gray	Intact	Cellular failure
Ischemic	Intra- and extracellular	White and gray	Disrupted	Anoxia
Hydrostatic	Extracellular	White and gray	Disrupted	Increased blood pressure
Hydrocephalic	Extracellular	White	Intact	Impaired CSF outflow or absorption
Osmotic	Intra- and extracellular	White and gray	Intact	Relative plasma hypo-osmolality

CSF, cerebrospinal fluid; gray, gray matter, white, white matter.

must be adjusted based on the priorities dictated by each particular clinical situation. For example, when brain hyperemia is one of the causes of brain swelling, maintaining CPP at a lower level can be an important therapeutic strategy. On the other hand, maintaining CPP on the generous side can provide a useful margin of "reserve" when there are plateaus in ICP that can suddenly and unpredictably challenge brain perfusion. Furthermore, higher CPP should be tolerated in circumstances in which blood pressure augmentation is used in selected patients as a treatment strategy for raised ICP based on its ability to cause autoregulatory reflex vasoconstriction, reduced cerebral blood volume, and ICP lowering.

PLATEAU WAVES

One of the most feared and devastating complications of patients with intracranial hypertension and poor intracranial compliance are plateau waves (PW). PW are acute elevations in ICP, at times in the range of 50 to 100 mm Hg, in patients with reduced intracranial compliance. They can last from several minutes to more protracted durations in extreme cases. Resolution of a PW is often as abrupt as its occurrence. While there are many causes of PW, one important mechanism is generalized cerebral vasodilation from an autoregulatory response to a decrement in systemic blood pressure.[1] Other causes include processes that can cause an increase in CBF and/or cerebral blood volume, many of which are listed in Table 65-2. Independent of their mechanism, PW can be disabling or deadly. Since compromised CPP can play a role in the occurrence of the most severe PW, relative blood pressure lowering should be avoided and/or rapidly treated. Similarly, during a PW, maneuvers that accentuate CPP such as blood pressure augmentation will abort the process in many circumstances. Even if blood pressure augmentation does not abort the process, it can prevent cerebral ischemia until other treatment modalities can successfully lower the ICP.

Cerebral Edema, Mass Effect, and Brain Tissue Displacement

CEREBRAL EDEMA

Cerebral edema is defined as an increase in brain water content. The more classic categorization of cerebral edema by etiology differentiates that caused by cellular injury (cytotoxic edema) vs. breakdown of the blood-brain barrier (vasogenic

edema).[3] Hydrocephalic edema, ischemic edema (a combination of cytotoxic and vasogenic edema), osmotic edema, and hydrostatic edema have also been characterized as distinct entities by some authors based on their mechanisms and the location of the edema fluid.[3–5] Table 65-3 lists various categories of cerebral edema along with some of their distinguishing characteristics.

Vasogenic edema is comprised of a plasma-derived protein-rich exudate due to an alteration in the blood-brain barrier. It occurs in both gray and white matter, but it tends to predominate within the white matter. Vasogenic edema occurs in variable degrees with brain tumors, abscesses, traumatic brain injury, meningitis, infarction, and hemorrhage. Corticosteroids are useful in reducing vasogenic edema, and their effect is most profound when vasogenic is the main edema etiology, as with brain tumors, and to a lesser degree abscesses.[6] Osmotic agents (see below) have no beneficial effect on the formation or extent of vasogenic edema.[3]

Cytotoxic edema is characterized as an intracellular swelling of neurons, glia, and endothelial cells with an accompanying reduction in the extracellular space. It occurs without a disruption in the blood-brain barrier and is likely due to cellular energy depletion. This results in the failure of the adenosine triphosphate–dependent sodium pump, with resultant accumulation of sodium and water within the cells.[2,3] It occurs in both gray and white matter. Hypoperfusion injuries are most classically associated with cytotoxic edema. They have also been described with Reye's syndrome, diabetic ketoacidosis, and water intoxication. Corticosteroids have no benefit in limiting cytotoxic edema, and osmotic agents have only limited benefit in reducing brain water from cytotoxic edema due to concurrent disruption in autoregulation with most of the processes that cause this form of swelling.[3]

Ischemic edema begins as a cytotoxic edema, and is followed to variable degrees by vasogenic edema.[4] When severe ischemia occurs and is followed by reperfusion, edema formation is biphasic: cells initially take up water and sodium from the extracellular space, but there is no net increase in brain water because there is no blood flow to serve as a source of water. Hours to days after the ischemic insult, the blood-brain barrier becomes disrupted, resulting in increased permeability and rapid accumulation of vasogenic edema. There is no therapy of demonstrated benefit for this process, and steroids have not been shown to be helpful, even though one aspect of this form of edema is vasogenic.[7]

Hydrocephalic edema is defined as an increase in brain fluid caused by the blockage of CSF flow pathways. It occurs in the periventricular white matter in association with hydrocephalus. In this situation the blood-brain barrier remains intact and the edema is in the extracellular space and of the same composition as CSF. Treatment consists of relieving the obstruction to CSF outflow or providing an accessory outflow pathway with a ventricular catheter or shunt.

In general, cerebral edema does not directly affect neural activity. Its main and most severe consequences are due to its mass effect and distortion of surrounding brain tissue. This can cause regional ischemia and result in the development of pressure gradients, leading to devastating brain tissue shifts.[8-10]

BRAIN TISSUE DISPLACEMENT AND HERNIATIONS

It is important to differentiate mass effect and brain tissue displacement (BTD) from intracranial hypertension. As should be apparent from Fig. 65-2, there can be a substantial amount of mass effect without an important global elevation in ICP, and the mass effect alone can cause brain damage through its regional effect on brain perfusion and/or brain tissue displacement (e.g. herniation). BTD is a distortion of brain anatomy, and depression of consciousness is one common sign associated with such distortion. However, depressed consciousness can be a late accompaniment to BTD. Autonomic changes such as increasing blood pressure and exaggeration of the respiratory sinus arrhythmia are also changes that can occur early with evolving BTD, and recognition of these signs can serve as an early warning of this life-threatening phenomenon.[11] The consequences of BTD depend on the extent and duration of the process, and its occurrence alone should not deter attempts to reverse the process.

A more thorough discussion of the clinical signs associated with the various herniation syndromes is covered in Chap. 67 but it is useful to note the relationship between horizontal brain displacement and depressed consciousness. With acute intracranial mass lesions, lateral displacement of posterior brain structures (diencephalon and brainstem) correlate with depression of consciousness. This can be practically quantified by measuring horizontal shift of the pineal gland on noncontrast CT scans. In the classic study describing this important relationship, horizontal shift of the pineal (from midline) by 0 to 3 mm correlated with alertness; 3 to 4 mm with drowsiness; 6 to 8 mm with stupor; and >8 mm with coma.[12] This has clinical applicability in determining the cause of depressed consciousness in individual patients. When the extent of horizontal shift does not readily explain a patient's level of consciousness, other potential etiologic factors should be considered.

The falx cerebri is the dural structure that sagitally divides the left and right hemispheres. The anterior cerebral arteries course inferiorly and parallel to the falx cerebri, and they supply blood flow to the anterior, inferior, and medial frontal lobes. When there is BTD anteriorly, it can lead to herniation of brain tissue under the falx cerebri, *subfalcine herniation*, thereby compressing the anterior cerebral arteries and placing their territory of supply (inferomedial frontal lobes and caudate nucleus) in jeopardy for infarction (Fig. 65-6). Furthermore, subfalcine herniation can lead to obstruction of the outflow of the lateral ventricles (foramina of Monro), leading

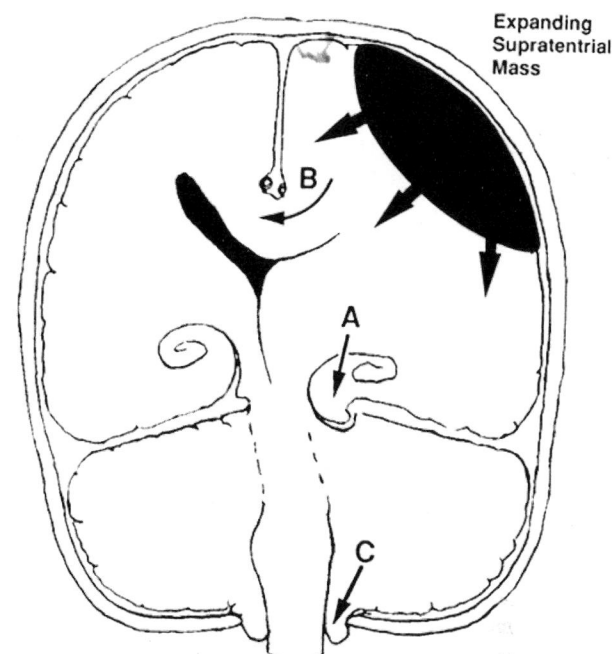

FIGURE 65-6 Shcematic representation of lateral brain tissue displacement from an expanding unilateral supratentorial mass. *A* illustrates the phenomenon of lateral transtentorial herniation. *B* illustrates the phenomenon of subfalcine herniation.

to obstructive hydrocephalus (usually contralateral to the mass lesion). Since subfalcine herniation is an anterior process, it may not lead to depressed consciousness unless it is very extreme.

The tentorium cerebelli is the dural structure that divides the supratentorial from the infratentorial space. The space between the lateral midbrain and the medial border of the tentorium cerebelli is called the tentorial incisura, and the posteromedial temporal lobe sits just above this space. When an intracranial mass or brain swelling is posterior it can cause BTD (mainly the inferomedial temporal lobe) through the tentorial incisura, called *lateral transtentorial herniation*. This can lead to compression of the posterior cerebral arteries as they course around the midbrain, placing the brain tissue they supply (occipital lobes, medial temporal lobes, and thalami) in jeopardy for infarction (see Fig. 65-6).

Central transtentorial herniation (Fig. 65-7) is most common with global processes (e.g., global ischemia/infarction, meningitis, or fulminant hepatic failure) and classically occurs as the cerebral hemispheres and basal ganglia exert downward pressure, causing BTD through the tentorial incisura bilaterally. If persistent and extreme, it results in severe brainstem compression with resultant ischemia and hemorrhage, bilateral posterior cerebral artery compression with resultant ischemia/infarction in its territory of distribution, and CSF outflow obstruction with resultant hydrocephalus.

Posterior fossa lesions produce their effects through direct pressure on the medulla, or downward displacement of the cerebellar tonsils (*cerebellar tonsillar herniation*) and lower brainstem through the foramen magnum (see Fig. 65-7). Clinically, these patients develop early depressed consciousness, autonomic disturbances, altered respiratory patterns, and signs of brainstem dysfunction. This type and location of

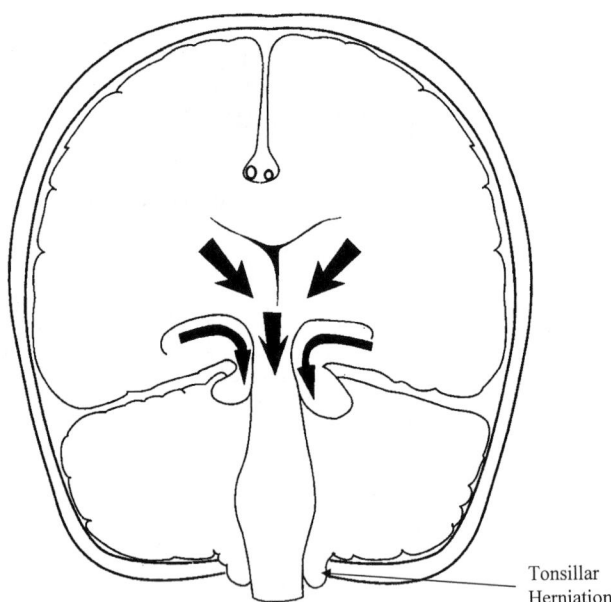

FIGURE 65-7 Schematic representation of central herniation.

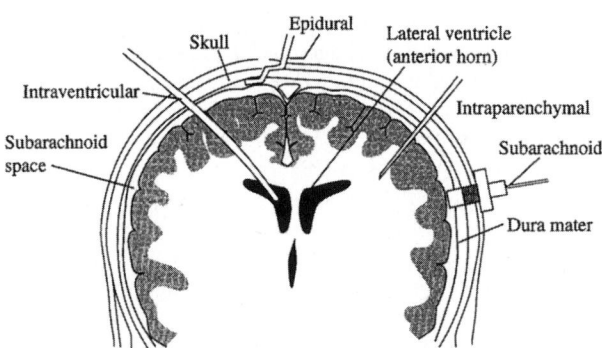

FIGURE 65-8 Various anatomic sites to monitor intracranial pressure.

BTD causes its damage by severe brainstem and upper cervical spinal cord compression, as well as obstruction of CSF outflow.

As already mentioned, BTD from regional brain swelling can occur even without important ICP elevations, and it can have devastating consequences. For an example, an acute middle cranial fossa process such as an acute temporal hematoma can cause lateral transtentorial herniation without a profound rise in ICP. As a result, successful management of BTD requires strategic consideration of its significance in individual cases. This is particularly important since the treatment for elevated ICP is not necessarily the same as it is for BTD. In fact, in certain cases ICP-directed medical treatments can accentuate BTD.

When a patient at high risk for brain swelling is encountered, a proactive approach to management should begin. This includes developing a monitoring strategy for early detection of the problem and planning the best management approach if it does occur. In at-risk patients without significant brain swelling, invasive ICP monitoring may not yet be appropriate. However, early insertion of an ICP monitor may be necessary if the risk of the problem is very high (e.g., fulminant hepatic failure), serial examination and/or imaging cannot be performed properly or readily (e.g., the intubated and/or heavily sedated patient), and/or the determination of the ICP will translate into important therapeutic changes.

Intracranial Pressure Monitors

It should be clear that the most rational and sophisticated management of intracranial hypertension should be based on continuous ICP and CPP monitoring. While active management of ICP guided by ICP monitoring has not shown a consistent benefit in outcome, it is difficult to study this well in humans for a variety of methodologic reasons. Most experienced physicians appreciate that ICP monitoring has value in properly selected patients. In particular, processes associated with life-threatening elevation of ICP, a rapidly expanding intracranial mass, or a disease in which ICP elevation is likely to be progressive and demand proactive preservation of CPP represent some generally accepted indications for monitor insertion.

ICP can be monitored from several intracranial sites (Fig. 65-8). The most commonly employed ICP monitoring devices are ventricular catheters and parenchymal monitors. Both can be readily placed at the bedside with a twist drill by neurosurgeons or experienced neurocritical care physicians. Ventricular catheters have been considered the gold standard for ICP monitoring, based on their reliability and ability to drain CSF, as an alternative for ICP control. It is the most invasive of alternatives, however, and it is associated with higher risks of infection, intracranial hemorrhage, and in our experience, seizures.

Ventricular catheters are ideally placed into a lateral ventricle. In general, right-sided (nondominant hemispheric) placement is usually preferred, since a bleeding complication from the insertion would be less likely to cause language disturbance from this location. Ventricular catheters are then connected to one of the many commercially available closed external drainage systems comprised of a drainage chamber, drainage bag, and an attached transducer. The height of the drainage chamber can be set to allow automatic drainage when the ICP rises above a designated level based on manometric concepts. A ruled measure on the drainage system facilitates accurate drainage chamber height adjustments and a stopcock system between the drainage catheter, drainage chamber, and transducer allows the physicians and nurses to choose between automatic CSF drainage and continuous ICP transduction.

One behavior we often encounter is the simultaneous transduction and recording of the ICP while the CSF chamber is set and open to automatically drain. In this situation, the ICP measure obtained is generally meaningless. For this reason, even when continuous CSF drainage to a determined level is the selected care strategy, the ICP should be transduced with the ventricular drain closed to drainage at least every 30 to 60 minutes for a 5- to 10-minute period with a recording of the ICP and CPP at the end of that time and determination if they are within the desired parameters. This is particularly important since CSF drainage to a set level does not always achieve maintenance of the ICP in the desired range. Some of the factors that limit ICP control by this method are imperfect ventricular catheter placement, collapse of the ventricle in which the catheter is placed, bubbles within the catheter or fluid column from catheter to transducer, and catheter obstruction.

Several avoidable causes of complications from ventricular drains should be mentioned. Ventricular drains should never be connected to a pressure bag. This can be a deadly error. The only connections to the ventricular catheters should be the drainage system. The drainage system should not be detached or penetrated with a needle except by individuals experienced with the management of ventricular drains. Ventricular drains should be actively closed (via the intervening stopcock apparatus) whenever a change is being made in patient position (particularly involving raising the head of the bed) or during excessive coughing or active endotracheal suctioning. Failure to do this can lead to excessive CSF drainage with dangerous consequences. In addition, ventricular catheters are structurally fragile and they can be readily broken or displaced from their placement within the cranium. All personnel moving patients with ventricular drains (or all other types of ICP monitors or intracranial drains) should be aware of their presence and reminded to take special care in the process. When transporting patients, assigning one individual to have responsibility for the head and maintenance of the monitor integrity is advisable to avoid inadvertent mishaps.

An important risk of infection is associated with their use, and its occurrence in properly handled drains is most often related to its duration of use. Catheter exchange does not have a demonstrated benefit in reducing the infection risk when prolonged external drainage is required, and the practice expands the risk of iatrogenic complications from multiple insertions. Longer subcutaneous catheter tunneling and giving prophylactic antibiotics that target common skin flora likely decrease the risk of infection.[13,14] While newer antibiotic-coated catheters promise a lower risk of infection, their use is not presently an established care standard in most medical settings. Due to the risk of infection with ventricular catheters, each day a patient has one in place should be used to maximize benefit from its placement and/or begin the process necessary to determine the best timing for its safe removal. For a patient on subcutaneous heparin or heparinoids for deep vein thrombosis prophylaxis, it is our practice to hold two doses before removing the ventricular catheter to hypothetically decrease the risk of development of hematoma during removal.

Patients with ventricular drains should have their CSF analyzed at least every other day (we do so daily) for white blood count, protein, glucose, Gram stain, and bacterial cultures. A reduction in CSF glucose to <50% of the simultaneous serum glucose is ominous for infection, particularly when accompanied by a rising CSF white blood cell count, fever, nuchal rigidity, and worsened encephalopathy. However, nuchal rigidity, fever, and worsened encephalopathy can be later findings, and their absence should not delay a real suspicion for early CSF infection. Conversely, a mild elevation in CSF white blood count alone has limited specificity since many processes that require a ventricular drain (e.g., hemorrhage) cause a delayed inflammatory response. We have observed that relative lowering of serum sodium occurs in a respectable number of patients as an early sign of evolving CSF infection in those with ventricular drains.

In general, compulsive concern about CSF infection should drive tight monitoring for its occurrence and early empiric treatment when suspected.

Parenchymal monitors offer some advantages over other systems in that they allow rapid and safe placement with accurate measurements and less risk of infection. The presently available parenchymal monitors employ either fiberoptic or strain gauge technology. Their tip can be placed anywhere within the skull, but their most common site is several millimeters into the brain parenchyma through a twist drill hole placed over the convexity. Since the maximal ICP is in the region of an intracranial mass, they are best placed ipsilateral to a mass lesion unless it is deemed unsafe based on the suspected etiology of the process.

Parenchymal monitors are often placed through and secured by a bolt screwed into the cranium after the placement of a small hole with a twist drill; avoidance of kinking is important for fiberoptic catheters since they can break if bent. The monitors based on strain gauge technology can be bent and allow a wider flexibility of placement methods and configurations relative to the fiberoptic systems. However, both technologies are widely used and the selection of monitor type is often based on institutional history and the personal experience and preferences of those who insert them. While ventricular catheters are fluid coupled systems that can be zeroed by nurses at the bedside, parenchymal monitors are zeroed prior to insertion and can only be rezeroed through removing and reinserting them. The advantages of parenchymal monitors over ventricular catheters are to some degree counterbalanced by drift in the ICP readings over time and the inability to drain CSF for ICP control.[15] While these various advantages and disadvantages are important considerations when selecting the ICP monitor type, the anatomy and physiology of the process requiring a monitor often dictate the best monitoring method.

As illustrated in Fig. 65-1, ICP monitors provide a ballistic waveform temporally associated with the systemic blood pressure. Certain characteristics about the ICP waveform can communicate important information about an evolving cerebral process, even when the ICP is not critically elevated. The ICP waveform is comprised of various smaller subwaves. The first two waves observed during systole are referred to as P1 and P2. Normally, each sequential subwave of the ICP waveform is smaller than the one before it, so P1 is usually greater than P2. However, as intracranial compliance decreases, P2 usually becomes greater than P1, even before the ICP is increased to abnormal levels. In addition, fluctuations in the baseline of the ICP waveform with breathing usually reflects a decrease in intracranial compliance, and it can occur and accentuate even before an elevation in ICP. These facts can be helpful in selected situations. For example, when a patient has fulminant hepatic failure, observation of these subtle changes in the ICP waveform can signal the evolution of brain swelling before it is clinically apparent or the ICP has increased.

As mentioned earlier in this chapter, ICP elevation can be imperfectly predicted through analysis of brain imaging studies, usually CT. When the ICP from any monitor type is either much lower or higher than expected clinically and based on imaging analysis, steps should be taken to determine the accuracy of the monitor. At times this requires rezeroing the monitor or replacement, at times even in a new position or location. Blind trust of monitoring information that is significantly contrary to clinical expectations can lead to mismanagement and avoidable complications.

Management of Intracranial Pressure

While Chap. 93 presents much about the available conventional management strategies for intracranial hypertension when it complicates traumatic brain injury, they are similar for nontraumatic etiologies. The following sections will supplement the information provided in that chapter.

CONTROLLING AGGRAVATING FACTORS

Patient positioning is an important aspect of the care of patients with intracranial hypertension. Lateral head rotation, rotating neck movements, and restrictive devices around the neck (e.g., endotracheal tube neck straps) can compromise jugular venous drainage. The head should be kept in the neutral forward position. Sometimes towel rolls placed on both sides of the head can be useful in maintaining the neutral position. Head elevation lowers ICP by enhancing CSF drainage and maximizing cerebral venous output. CSF and cerebral venous blood are maximally displaced with severe intracranial hypertension, challenging the benefits of head elevation in these patients. The logical approach is to individualize the ideal head and neck position based on clinical observation of the patient and ICP monitoring, when available. When ICP monitoring is not available, head elevations of 30° to 40° allows the most consistent reduction in ICP.[16]

Fevers should be treated aggressively because body temperature elevations increase ICP by increasing cerebral metabolism, cerebral blood flow, and cerebral edema.[17,18] Acetaminophen should be administered (assuming normal hepatic function) and a diligent search made for treatable infection. There should be a low threshold for using empiric antibiotics for the most likely source, even though centrally mediated fevers are often considered in the differential diagnosis in many of these patients. In those resistant to acetaminophen, nonsteroidal anti-inflammatory drugs (e.g., ibuprofen) should be considered when bleeding is not a primary concern. Cooling blankets can be useful, but control of shivering is necessary since it can aggravate intracranial hypertension. Newer intravascular cooling devices provide an exciting alternative to more rapidly and consistently achieve fever control in this brittle patient group.[19] Independent of the cooling method, if shivering complicates its use, it can be controlled with various medications such as meperidine, parenteral sedatives, and neuromuscular paralysis. The key point about fever control in patients with brain swelling and/or intracranial hypertension is that it is essential and requires close follow-up to assure that it is brought under control in a timely fashion.

Coughing and straining against the ventilator increases intrathoracic pressure and can reduce the venous outflow from the intracranial cavity. This can lead to elevation of the ICP. As a result, strategies to decrease these ventilator- or airway-provoked problems can be essential to the management of patients with brittle intracranial hypertension. Some of these strategies include repositioning of the endotracheal tube, inhaled nebulizations that can serve to decrease coughing, ventilator adjustments adapted to the patient's respiratory behavior, or the administration of sedation or nondepolarizing neuromuscular blockers.

Positive end-expiratory pressure (PEEP) will increase ICP only when mean airway pressures are increased, causing transmission to the mediastinum. When pulmonary compliance is reduced as occurs in acute respiratory distress syndrome or pneumonia, the effect of PEEP on ICP is attenuated. It seems fortuitous that the conditions for which higher PEEP levels are often used diminish its deleterious impact on ICP. Probably more important than the effect of PEEP on ICP is its potential effect to decrease cardiac output and blood pressure, with their deleterious impact on cerebral perfusion. In general, the presence of an ICP monitor shifts the concerns about the impact of PEEP from the theoretical to the empiric.

Frequent zealous monitoring of systemic blood pressure is a cornerstone of ICP management in patients with intracranial hypertension. Hypotension will directly cause cerebral vasodilation and increase ICP. A treatment plan should be orchestrated with pressor agents and isotonic fluids at the bedside to allow rapid intervention at the first observation of significant relative blood pressure lowering. However, when cerebral autoregulatory mechanisms are impaired, hypertension may lead to pathologic increases in regional CBF, worsened brain swelling, and aggravation of intracranial hypertension.

Pain and arousal can cause elevated ICP by increasing CBF. As a result, patients with life-threatening intracranial hypertension should generally receive sedatives and analgesics, even if their use risks clouding of the neurological exam. The present availability of short-acting sedatives and analgesics and the ready availability of neuroimaging have simplified the historical reluctance to utilize these classes of agents in the neurologically ill.

Seizures increase ICP by increasing cerebral metabolism and CBF by Valsalva. If the patient is deemed to be at risk, anticonvulsants should be administered promptly. Given the deleterious consequences of seizures and the severity of illness of these patients, drugs that can be parenterally administered with known effectiveness as monotherapy should be used (phenytoin, phenobarbital, or valproic acid). Since hypotension can accompany the administration of phenytoin and phenobarbital, close monitoring of the blood pressure is critical, with preparedness to detect any relative blood pressure lowering and promptly intervene.

MECHANICAL VENTILATION AND HYPERVENTILATION

Hyperventilation induces a rapid and effective reduction in ICP through vasoconstriction induced by hypocapnia-associated CSF alkalosis.[20] The duration of the ICP reduction is variable, but in general, the ICP returns to baseline within hours after commencing hyperventilation, due to normalization of the CSF alkalosis through compensatory adjustments in the bicarbonate buffering systems in the brain and vascular smooth muscle.

When hyperventilation is required for urgent management, it can be accomplished with an ambu mask or mechanical ventilation. Providing a 10- to 12-mL/kg tidal volume at a rate of 14 to 20 breaths/min usually achieves substantial reduction in the partial pressure of carbon dioxide (P_{CO_2}). The ideal P_{CO_2} is variable depending on the clinical situation and the individual patient's response. One of the most controversial questions is whether excessive hyperventilation can cause cerebral ischemia through extreme cerebral vasoconstriction—a phenomenon suggested by several studies in traumatic brain-injured patients.[21] The most recent work on the subject in patients with severe traumatic brain injury utilizing positron emission tomography demonstrated that hyperventilation can be safely performed (without consequent cerebral ischemia) to a P_{CO_2} of 30 mm Hg, and perhaps to <25 mm Hg in selected patients.[22] Furthermore, it has been shown that hyperoxia can improve oxygen delivery to the brain during hyperventilation.[23]

The potential benefits of hyperventilation must be balanced against some of its potential deleterious consequences, including but not limited to diminished cardiac filling pressures with resultant hypotension, decreased myocardial oxygen supply with an increase in myocardial demand, elevation in mean airway pressure leading to accentuation of intracranial hypertension, electrolyte disturbances (e.g., alkalosis, hypokalemia, and hyperchloremia), and cardiac arrhythmias.[24]

Because hyperventilation is the most rapid way to reduce ICP, it is best kept as a back-up strategy for emergent ICP elevations. A modest goal of 30 mm Hg seems safest with the present state of our knowledge, and preoxygenation may add a layer of protection that is potentially beneficial for ischemia deriving from hyperventilation. Once other ICP-lowering strategies are instituted and controlling ICP and CPP adequately, hyperventilation should be lifted. Gradual withdrawal of hyperventilation is necessary to avoid rebound elevations in ICP as the P_{CO_2} is normalized. We recommend not exceeding P_{CO_2} increases of 2 to 3 mm Hg per hour. When hyperventilation is used for a prolonged period, jugular venous oxygen saturation can be used to monitor for the feared complication of cerebral ischemia due to this maneuver. Inadvertent fluctuations in the P_{CO_2} due to variable ventilation is an important and avoidable cause of ICP plateaus. This is commonly a problem that occurs during patient transport. We recommend using transport ventilators for patients with brittle intracranial hypertension to minimize variations in P_{CO_2} during transport.

Tris(hydroxymethyl)aminomethane (THAM) is a buffer than can be used to correct acidotic states, and it can be used at times to assist in the management of patients with intracranial hypertension. The advantage of THAM is that it alkalinizes without changing plasma sodium or P_{CO_2}. THAM may have a role in limiting rebound ICP elevation during the withdrawal of hyperventilation, or prolonging the benefit of hyperventilation in some patients.[25] It is administered intravenously at a dose of 1 mL/kg per hour. Some of the complications associated with its use include local skin irritation and necrosis, hypoglycemia, and respiratory depression.

CEREBROSPINAL FLUID DRAINAGE

CSF drainage with a ventricular catheter is the primary treatment for hydrocephalus, and it can be a useful treatment strategy for intraventricular hemorrhage, through both CSF drainage and providing access for administration of intraventricular thrombolytic agents. The management of CSF drainage and ventricular catheters is discussed in the section on ICP monitoring in this chapter. While CSF drainage through lumbar puncture should generally be avoided in

patients with intracranial hypertension, it is a mainstay of treatment for patients with pseudotumor cerebri (benign intracranial hypertension).

MANNITOL

Osmotherapy is directed at increasing plasma osmolality, establishing an osmotic gradient across the relatively impermeable blood-brain barrier. This favors a net loss of brain water, thereby increasing brain compliance and decreasing ICP. In addition, mannitol, the most widely used osmotic agent, can improve cerebral perfusion through transient hypervolemia and hemodilution, leading to autoregulatory cerebral vasoconstriction, decreased cerebral blood volume, and lower ICP.[26–28] It also can increase CSF absorption.[29] However, most mechanisms of brain injury lead to disruption of the blood-brain barrier and a loss of normal autoregulation. As a result, osmotic agents are less effective in injured brain regions. This is an important consideration when strategizing management in individual patients with unilateral mass lesions and BTD.

Mannitol is typically used in a 20% solution. Its ICP-lowering effect is dose-dependent, and it appears to be maximal with a 1 g/kg dose infused over 30 minutes.[30,31]. The duration of benefit from this high-dose infusion is limited to several hours, and terminal dose-interval ICP elevations beyond the pretreatment baseline are common. Smaller doses of 0.25 to 0.5 g/kg over longer infusion periods (30 to 60 minutes) can be associated with less profound and more lasting ICP benefits within the usual 4-hour dosing interval when multidosing regimens are used. The reduction in ICP after mannitol use should be apparent within 15 minutes, and failure of a response to mannitol is considered ominous, but not hopeless, in our experience.

The goal of osmotherapy should be plasma hyperosmolality with maintenance of adequate intravascular volume. In general, the target osmolality should be in the 300 to 310 mOsm/L range with adequate maintenance intravenous fluid administration. Normal saline should be used for maintenance and replacement fluids. Hypotonic fluids are contraindicated and should be avoided because water accumulation by hyperosomolar brain can aggravate brain swelling and intracranial hypertension. The development of moderate hypernatremia should be expected and tolerated, because administration of hypotonic fluids to correct the hypernatremia is counterproductive and potentially dangerous.

Single doses of mannitol are often effective in reducing ICP and improving intracranial compliance temporarily. When single doses are used, monitoring of the plasma osmolality is unimportant. The benefit of multidosing regimens is more controversial. This is due to some experimental evidence that it can accentuate regional brain water when the blood-brain barrier is disrupted.[32–34] In addition, its disproportionate impact on uninjured brain (relative to injured brain) can potentially accentuate BTD through enhancement of regional intracranial pressure differentials.[35] Nonetheless, mannitol is an effective agent for rapidly reducing ICP in an emergency setting, and it can buy critical time to temporarily stabilize the patient while other treatment strategies are being arranged and commenced.

Rapid diuresis before administration of adequate amounts of replacement fluids can occur in some patients after receiving mannitol. This can lead to systemic hypotension, emphasizing the need for preparedness when using this treatment modality. We always have pressor agents and replacement fluids readily available at the bedside in patients with increased ICP. Other important complications include electrolyte disturbances (hypernatremia and hypokalemia), prerenal azotemia, and congestive heart failure. Sometimes, pretreatment with a dose of furosemide can circumvent some of the complications of the transient expansion of intravascular volume that occurs immediately after administration of mannitol.

HYPERTONIC SALINE

Hypertonic saline has been used with renewed enthusiasm in patients with brain swelling and intracranial hypertension.[36-39] The osmolality of 3% saline (1026 mOsm/L) is similar to that of 20% mannitol (1375 mOsm/L). The osmolality is much higher with other solutions, such as 7.5% saline (2565 mOsm/L) and 23.4% saline (8008 mOsm/L). Variable formulations of hypertonic saline have been used with different-size boluses (up to 75 mL) with occasional benefit, most recently reported in some patients with traumatic brain injury and cerebral infarction refractory to other modalities. Its use can be associated with the expected complications of hypernatremia, hypokalemia, hyperchloremia, and congestive heart failure. It is an underrecognized part of the ICP-lowering armamentarium. Its use can be a particularly well-suited treatment in patients with volume depletion or renal failure.

LOOP DIURETICS

Loop diuretics such as furosemide can reduce ICP and have been reported in selected series to reduce ICP alone or when used in conjunction with osmotic agents.[40] Diuretics exert their effect through an osmotic gradient caused by a mild diuresis, reduction in CSF formation, and reduction in brain water. They provide another alternative when mild reductions in ICP are desired. However, like osmotic agents, they can produce volume and electrolyte depletion, requiring proper treatment and surveillance for these complications.

CORTICOSTEROIDS

Corticosteroids have been shown to reduce the vasogenic edema associated with brain tumors and abscesses, but their benefit with other processes that can cause intracranial hypertension is less clear.[41] There is generally no benefit consistently demonstrated with intracerebral hemorrhage.[42-45] While it may have a theoretical advantage in certain stages of infarction-related edema, it has not been of demonstrated benefit and has been associated with worse outcomes.[46-49] Dexamethasone is the most commonly used corticosteroid for vasogenic cerebral edema, and there is a wide range of dosing alternatives. We typically use 16 to 24 mg/day of dexamethasone in two to four divided doses in extreme situations. It can be given parenterally or enterally. Higher doses can be safely used for brief periods of time with less clear benefit over more conventional dosing. Potential side effects include gastrointestinal bleeding, hyperglycemia, disturbance in nitrogen metabolism, wound breakdown and poor healing, sleep disturbances, and behavioral disturbances. The hyperglycemia is of particular concern and requires aggressive

intervention due to its increasingly recognized negative impact on outcome with most of the processes that can cause intracranial hypertension.

HYPOTHERMIA

There has been renewed interest in moderate hypothermia (32° to 34°C) as an adjunctive therapy for patients with intracranial hypertension. It can lower ICP and improve CPP in some patients, and it theoretically limits hypoperfusion brain injury due to its neuroprotective properties. However, it has not yet been demonstrated to achieve outcome benefit in scientifically valid clinical trials. In spite of the lack of scientific evidence for its benefit to date, those experienced in the management of patients with the problem have used hypothermia with success in selected patients; it is considered a useful "time-buying" trick in refractory cases.

The most classic method for hypothermia induction is with cooling blankets placed above and below the patient with the variable addition of ice-water lavage. However, newer intravascular cooling devices are increasingly available but not yet widely applied.[19] When hypothermia is used, shivering can be a complicating factor when the body temperature gets below 36°C. Since shivering can increase ICP, its occurrence should be anticipated and sedatives and/or narcotics should be rapidly administered and titrated to effect to limit its severity. Rebound intracranial hypertension is an important concern during the rewarming process.[50] When induced hypothermia is terminated, patients should be allowed to passively rewarm with close attention to slow down its pace if the patient develops a rebound increase in ICP. The most common complications of induced hypothermia include pneumonia, cardiac arrhythmia, and coagulopathy.[51]

BARBITURATE COMA

The use of barbiturate coma is an advanced treatment measure aimed at preventing patient demise from uncontrollable intracranial hypertension. While it has been used with variable degrees of success for the treatment of elevated ICP from a variety of causes, there is little evidence that it improves outcome.[52-56] In addition, it is a costly undertaking from an economic and physiologic perspective.

Some of its ICP-lowering benefit may be derived from depression of cerebral metabolism and reduction of CBF in normal areas of brain, with shunting of blood to ischemic areas. In addition, it may limit oxidative damage to lipid membranes and scavenge free radicals, reduce formation of vasogenic edema, attenuate fatty acid release, reduce intracellular calcium, and of course limit external stimuli from causing patient arousal, with the concomitant increases in CBF and cerebral blood volume.[48,54]

The induction of barbiturate coma is a weighty undertaking and demands experience to assure its safe and proper use. The agents most commonly used are thiopental and pentobarbital. Systemic hypotension, complications of prolonged immobility and mechanical ventilation, and immune suppression are the most common deleterious effects of barbiturate therapy. In addition, the need for more frequent transport and invasive line complications are other risks that should not be underestimated in their potential impact.

Pentobarbital coma requires a loading dose of 10 to 30 mg/kg. In our experience, it is best to administer the pentobarbital in small boluses of 100 to 200 mg every 10 to 20 minutes as tolerated from a blood pressure standpoint. This should be done under electroencephalographic (EEG) monitoring. While each bolus will briefly achieve either a burst-suppression pattern or a flat EEG, usually a more full loading dose is necessary to achieve a sustained effect. A continuous drip of 1 to 3 mg/kg per hour is usually necessary to maintain the desired depth of anesthesia. Optimizing depth of barbiturate therapy should be guided by EEG in these cases, usually titrating a continuous drip to achieve a burst suppression pattern in the 3 to 6 bursts/min frequency. The EEG can be monitored continuously or hourly, and ICU nurses can be taught to interpret burst-suppression frequency as part of the bedside monitoring.

In patients under prolonged barbiturate anesthesia, various strategies must be used to compensate for the loss of ability to do a neurologic examination, and can include continued evoked potential monitoring, serial imaging studies, and numerous other devices that are increasingly becoming available that can track a number of combinations of intracranial factors. The only neurologic exam that is useful in these patients is pupillary dilation, since the barbiturates usually cause bilaterally small pupils. When they become large it can be an ominous sign. However, an important phenomenon has been described in patients under pentobarbital coma: an accentuated ciliospinal reflex that manifests as pupils that are large (>6 mm) and seemingly unreactive to light, usually after a nursing maneuver such as patient turning. It can be misinterpreted as a catastrophic clinical change leading to unnecessary scans. Usually, when it occurs the pupils will react with a sustained intense light stimulus, and it spontaneously abates within minutes after it begins.[57]

As already mentioned, intensive hemodynamic monitoring is required with barbiturate coma. Since volume depletion increases the risk of hypotension from barbiturates, special attention should focus on maintaining intravascular volume with the guidance of invasive monitoring in most cases. The risk of infection and the concurrent disruption in the usual response to infection—fever—requires systematic surveillance for infection with regular cultures (at least every other day) of the endotracheal secretions, urine, and blood drawn through invasive lines.

Hypothermia is common with barbiturates, and in fact we often use barbiturates to facilitate the induction of hypothermia as a treatment modality. While permissive moderate hypothermia is recommended when using barbiturates, extreme hypothermia (<32°C) is associated with numerous complications and should be avoided.

The long half-life of pentobarbital (approximately 24 hours) allows a slow recovery, even when abruptly stopped. Shivering is common during the recovery period from barbiturate anesthesia and may require treatment with narcotics or short-acting sedatives. We prefer to use propofol for this complication. In addition, chaotic EEG patterns are common during this period and often are misinterpreted as status epilepticus.

SURGICAL PROCEDURES

Surgical procedures can be a very important part of the management of patients with intracranial mass lesions, with or without intracranial hypertension. The two primary types of procedures are removal of the primary problem (e.g.,

hematoma evacuation, neoplasm excision, etc), or creating more room to accommodate an intracranial mass and deter the deleterious effects of BTD by removing skull bone and opening the overlying dura ipsilateral to the mass through hemicraniectomy and durotomy. The application of these surgical alternatives and their timing is heuristic, based on numerous clinical factors, some of which will be discussed in the following section.

General Disease-Specific Comments

While we cannot provide an exhaustive delineation of management recommendations for all causes of intracranial hypertension, in this section we address some disease-specific recommendations for some of the causes most commonly encountered in a medical critical care setting, and not covered in other chapters of this textbook.

HYPERTENSIVE ENCEPHALOPATHY AND ECLAMPSIA

Hypertensive encephalopathy occurs when the blood pressure is elevated beyond autoregulatory thresholds. This leads to an increase in extracellular water, predominantly by hydrostatic mechanisms. In addition, there can be variable degrees of parenchymal hemorrhage, most often localized in the end-arterial border zones along the frontal and posterior parietal convexities (see Fig. 65-9). This is an important reversible cause of brain swelling in which the extent of brain swelling does not necessarily correlate with neuronal injury. Blood pressure lowering is obviously the focus of treatment

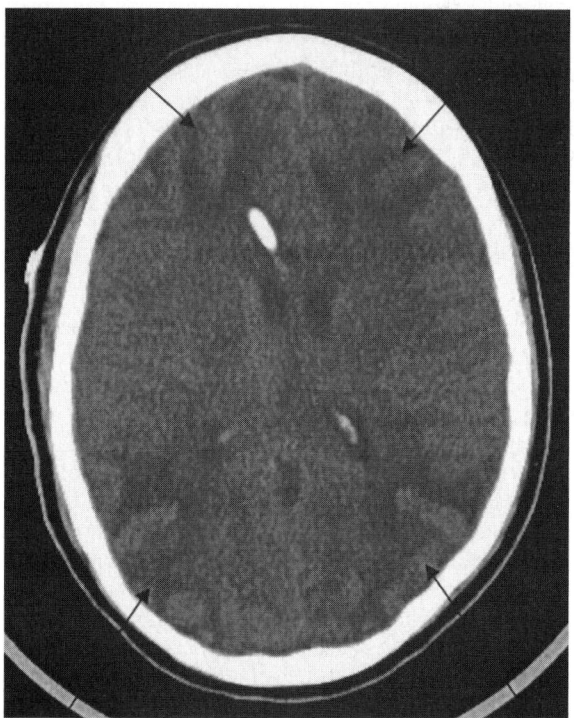

FIGURE 65-9 An unenhanced CT of the brain in a patient with the complications of hypertensive encephalopathy. The arrows are pointing to the end-arterial border zones with changes consistent with ischemic and hemorrhagic changes.

of the brain swelling with this disease. However, blood pressure lowering does not achieve immediate resolution of the cerebral edema. So, if the patient already has important intracranial hypertension and diminished intracranial compliance (an estimate guided by clinical and imaging parameters), ICP monitoring is necessary to guide the pace and degree of blood pressure lowering so as to not compromise cerebral perfusion. Any type of ICP monitor can be used, but most often global cerebral edema is associated with a loss of CSF spaces and compression of the ventricles. When that occurs, the ventricular catheters are more difficult to place, their readings are less consistently accurate, and they do not allow enough CSF removal to justify their higher risk. We find parenchymal monitors to be a more rational choice in these cases.

While the mechanism of brain swelling from eclampsia is similar but not exactly the same as hypertensive encephalopathy, the management of intracranial hypertension complicating eclampsia is generally the same. However, the management of eclampsia-associated intracranial hypertension has the added priority of urgent fetal delivery. The presence and suspected severity of intracranial hypertension should be considered when determining the method of delivery and anesthesia. Cesarean section is the preferred mode of delivery in almost all cases. Spinal anesthesia should be avoided due to the risk of precipitating central herniation with CSF drainage. General anesthesia should include close attention to the blood pressure to avoid degrees of lowering that could compromise cerebral perfusion. In general, successful management of intracranial hypertension is best guided with an ICP monitor, and easy and predominantly uncomplicated bedside placement of parenchymal monitors provides little justification for not using them.

Both hypertensive encephalopathy and eclampsia can be associated with ominous clinical presentations and imaging studies. Neither midposition unreactive pupils with extensor posturing nor CT changes suggestive of bilateral end-arterial border zone infarctions with hemorrhage should deter aggressive and optimistic management of such patients. In our experience, both scenarios can potentially lead to good outcomes when treated promptly and aggressively.

FULMINANT HEPATIC FAILURE

Cerebral edema complicates fulminant hepatic failure (FHF) in up to 50% of cases.[58] Similarly to hypertensive encephalopathy and eclampsia, the brain swelling from FHF is global and usually symmetric (Fig. 65-10). Its etiology is thought to be predominantly glial swelling from intracellular glutamine accumulation, but a variety of other mechanisms have been shown to play a variable role in its development.[59–62]

The development of brain swelling from FHF should be anticipated in all patients. Early detection of cerebral edema is imperative in order to pace its development and proactively manage its complications. However, bedside clinical evaluation does not allow its accurate detection due to the worsening hepatic encephalopathy concurrently developing in FHF patients. For example, stage IV encephalopathy patients frequently have diffuse hyperreflexia and increased motor tone with decerebrate posturing in the absence of any cerebral edema. It is not possible to differentiate uncomplicated hepatic encephalopathy from FHF-associated cerebral edema in

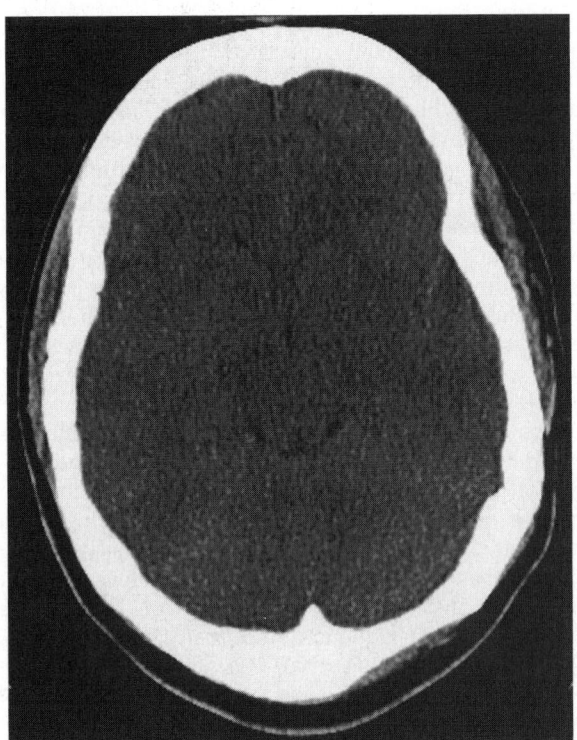

FIGURE 65-10 Unenhanced CT of the brain of a patient with cerebral edema from fulminant hepatic failure. Note the attenuation of CFS spaces and the global nature of the swelling.

patients with higher-stage encephalopathy. However, significant cerebral edema most often occurs in patients with higher-stage encephalopathy (III or IV). CT scans should be done in all patients with FHF, particularly those with stage III or IV encephalopathy, to rule out intracerebral hemorrhage and to estimate the presence and severity of cerebral edema. In our experience, patients in the early stages of cerebral edema have their CT scans misread as normal by inexperienced physicians. In addition, the presence of intracranial hypertension has been reported in FHF patients with normal CT scans.[63,64]

Once a patient drifts into the higher stages of encephalopathy with FHF, significant cerebral edema and cerebral hypoperfusion can be occurring and be undetectable in the absence of ICP monitoring. So an ICP monitor should be placed prior to stage IV encephalopathy in FHF patients. Often the frequent and severe coagulopathy observed in these patients justifiably demands thoughtful reflection on the risks and benefits of the intervention. However, in our experience, even with coagulopathy, bedside parenchymal monitors can be inserted without significant complications. We prefer to use a parenchymal monitor in the nondominant standard location. We insert it with the administration of 2 units of fresh frozen plasma (FFP) before, 1 unit of FFP during, and 2 units of FFP after the procedure. This should be carried out in collaboration with other caregivers, so invasive line insertions can be coordinated while the FFP infusions are being administered for ICP monitor insertion. Small pediatric patients require a different strategy to minimize bleeding during invasive procedures. While some neuroclinicians prefer to insert ventriculostomies in patients with potential intracranial hypertension (to allow CSF drainage as one therapeutic maneuver to treat plateaus in ICP), this modality carries a higher risk of hemorrhagic complications and the ventricles collapse (not allowing CSF drainage) in patients with consequential cerebral edema from FHF.

Once an ICP monitor is in place, management should focus on maintenance of adequate cerebral perfusion pressure. Given the likelihood of impaired autoregulation in FHF patients, extremes of blood pressure should be avoided. The patient's blood pressure should be maintained in the mid-normal range for the previously normotensive patient. In addition, normal intravascular volume should be maintained, and a state of readiness for acute response to any systemic hypotension is critical.

In patients with an elevation in ICP and poor intracranial compliance, ICP lowering may be necessary, particularly those with tenuous CPP (<60 mm Hg). Mannitol can be useful in some patients with FHF.[65,66] It should mainly be considered in nonoliguric/anuric patients without significant hypernatremia. We generally use 0.25- to 0.5-g/kg aliquots of mannitol infused over a 20 to 30 minute period. The maintenance intravenous fluid should be isotonic with serum; normal saline is a good choice, with added 5% dextrose and/or potassium, depending on the specific clinical situation.

When using osmotic agents with FHF, the patient is already in quite a hyperosmolar state, so we do not titrate the mannitol to a specific serum osmolality. Rather, it is used intermittently to achieve the desired affect of improved intracranial compliance and ICP lowering. It may lose its effectiveness after several dosings, and so other therapeutic strategies should be considered concurrently. As is typical with the use of an osmotic diuretic, volume depletion can be an important complication with resultant hypotension. Maintaining euvolemia is ideal and requires thoughtful attention to fluid balance and intermittent replacement. Administration of hypotonic fluids such as 50% dextrose without electrolytes (commonly used in FHF in some settings) should be avoided.

Most patients with FHF will develop spontaneous hyperventilation, and this can be related to an increase in circulating free fatty acids and ammonia. While the institution of hyperventilation can be beneficial in lowering ICP acutely, it has no prolonged benefit in FHF as is true with most etiologies of cerebral edema and intracranial hypertension.[67]

Induced hypothermia can be a favorable strategy for both neuroprotection and deterring the development of cerebral edema, but further research is required to clarify its preventive role in this population. A recent study supported the promising role of moderate hypothermia for lowering ICP in patients with FHF.[68] Seven consecutive FHF patients with intracranial hypertension refractory to osmotherapy and ultrafiltration were studied. Moderate hypothermia to 32° to 33°C was achieved with cooling blankets. The mean ICP before and after cooling was 45 mm Hg and 16 mm Hg, respectively. The mean CPP before and after cooling was 45 mm Hg and 70 mm Hg, respectively. The mean CBF before and after cooling was 103 mL/100 g per minute and 44 mL/100 g per minute, respectively.

We induce hypothermia in patients with refractory intracranial hypertension prior to significant cerebral hypoperfusion events. We strive for a body temperature of 32° to 34°C with the use of cooling blankets above and below the patient. Proactive strategies to allow early detection and treatment of fever should be an important part of the care plan for these patients, independent of whether hypothermia is used.

Like most other therapeutic strategies for ICP lowering in FHF, there have been few reliable clinical studies to guide the indications for and use of barbiturate therapy. It has been shown to have an impact on controlling ICP in Reye's syndrome.[69] It probably would be best considered in patients with either refractory intracranial hypertension and/or those with oliguria or anuria. One study of 13 FHF patients with acute renal failure and refractory intracranial hypertension administered thiopental slowly to a maximum of 500 mg to achieve an ICP <20 mm Hg, CPP >50 mm Hg, or until hypotension developed.[70] In each case, the ICP was reduced with the administration of anywhere between 185 and 500 mg (median = 250 mg) of thiopental over a 15-minute infusion period. In eight patients, a constant infusion was required (50 to 250 mg/h) to maintain adequate ICP and CPP. Given the small number of patients and unclearly defined end points, it is difficult to assess the true benefit of the ICP-lowering accomplishments of this strategy. However, unique to FHF, impaired barbiturate metabolism and clearance often precludes the need for a maintenance infusion after the desired effect is accomplished using a loading dose. See the section on treatment recommendations for the management of barbiturate coma elsewhere in this chapter.

GLOBAL CEREBRAL HYPOPERFUSION

The potential benefits of hypothermia on outcome in patients after cardiac arrest is beyond the scope of this chapter and is discussed in Chap. 16. However, when intracranial hypertension does occur as a result of global cerebral hypoperfusion it is a reflection of diffuse neuronal injury. As a result, when secondary intracranial hypertension occurs in this situation, it signals widespread injury and poor neurologic outcome. We strongly discourage aggressive management of this complication in these patients.

LARGE SUPRATENTORIAL HEMISPHERIC INFARCTIONS

While large supratentorial cerebral hemispheric infarctions (LHI) are not common (accounting for less than 10% of all ischemic strokes), they are among the most disabling and deadly. As a result, physicians involved with the management of these patients must be equipped with a contemporary management strategy to minimize disability and mortality in patients in whom survival is desired as the appropriate medical care focus in keeping with the patient's life philosophy. LHI defines a group of patients with disabling strokes, variable degrees of collateral circulation, and brain swelling and life-threatening deterioration from brain herniations and intracranial hypertension.

In addition to the usual priorities of general systemic care (e.g., respiratory, cardiovascular, and nutritional), and general stroke care (e.g., blood sugar control, fever management, and deep vein thrombosis prophylaxis), patients who suffer a LHI should receive thoughtful application of medical treatments and monitoring for optimizing brain perfusion (or avoiding cerebral hypoperfusion), minimizing brain swelling, and limiting brain tissue shifts. There should be early discussion with the patient, family, and surrogate regarding the patient's life priorities as they may apply to practical life-and-death decision making and procedures in the context of the disabling stroke event; a strategic monitoring plan

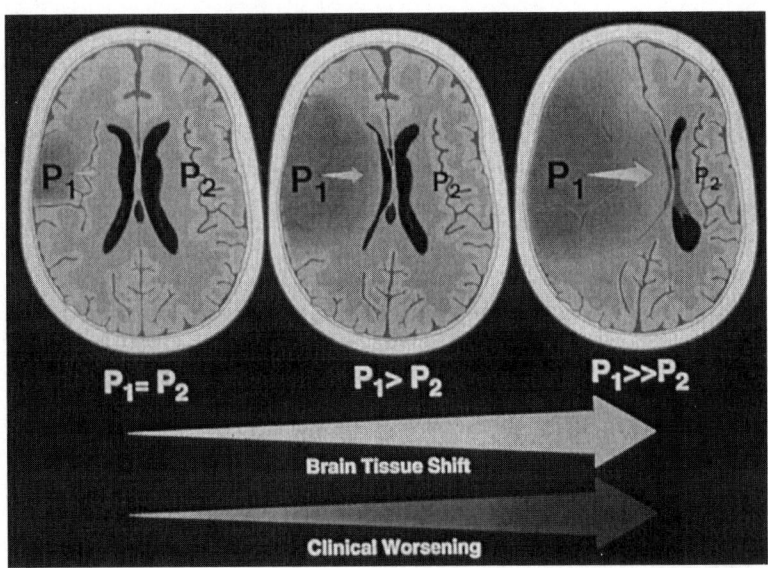

FIGURE 65-11 A schematic diagram demonstrating the concept of evolving pressure differentials with regional brain swelling from large supratentorial hemispheric infarction. Note that the clinical worsening in its early states correlates with brain tissue displacement.

for early detection of deterioration and brain swelling; and engagement of other professionals necessary for the timely application of treatments necessary in the case of significant worsening (e.g., neurosurgeons).

There have been a variety of clinical predictors studied and identified to correlate with fatal outcome from LHI. Some of these factors include high National Institutes of Health Stroke Scale scores, early drowsiness, and early nausea and vomiting.[71-75] The various identified prognostic factors are generally associated with larger infarctions, and not surprisingly, CT and magnetic resonance imaging (MRI) analyses have confirmed a correlation between infarction volume and outcome from supratentorial infarctions.[76,77] While new evolving approaches to predicting brain swelling in patients with LHI are exciting, and our wisdom on their best application will evolve over time, at this point all acute patients with LHI should be considered at risk for severe, life-threatening deterioration. This is supported by the preliminary results of the recently completed HeADDFIRST study, a prospective randomized pilot clinical trial on LHI and surgical decompression. In that study, 65% of the registered patients with at least complete MCA territory infarction (based on acute clinical and CT imaging criteria) developed life-threatening brain swelling and tissue shifts ($\geq$7 mm of anteroseptal shift or $\geq$4 mm of pineal shift from midline) within 96 hours of stroke onset.[78]

While patients with acute ischemic stroke are a heterogeneous group with variable baseline blood pressure and stroke mechanisms, those patients with LHI more likely have large-vessel narrowing or occlusion, autoregulatory dysfunction, and/or are vitally dependent on collateral circulation. At this point in our understanding, blood pressure lowering should only be done with great reluctance in patients with LHI, with clearly prioritized goals, thoughtful agent selection (to be discussed), and vigilant monitoring to avoid overtreatment. Depending on the extent of brain swelling and the degree of blood pressure lowering desired, it may be rational and appropriate to consider parenchymal ICP or CBF monitoring to avoid exacerbating regional cerebral hypoperfusion. In most cases, we recommend maintenance of the blood pressure at least in the high-normal range with LHI in order to

maintain collateral perfusion, since cerebral edema progressively challenges this vital brain-preserving source of cerebral blood flow.

It has been shown that the majority of patients who deteriorate from LHI do not have important ICP elevations or cerebral hypoperfusion as an early contributing factor to their worsening.[35] Their clinical deterioration is mainly due to BTD from evolving brain pressure differentials caused by regional cerebral edema (Fig. 65-11). Indiscriminant administration of mannitol or contralateral ventricular drain insertion and CSF drainage (the ipsilateral ventricle is usually collapsed) can lead to accentuation of the pressure differentials that drive BTD and augment the clinical worsening. However, early ICP elevation, when it does occur with LHI, stratifies the patient to higher risk of death from brain swelling, and younger patients are at higher risk for such early elevations.[35,79] It has not been shown that ICP-focused management (whether or not under the guidance of ICP monitoring) improves the outcome in LHI patients, but it has not been well-studied with appropriate standardized medical treatment protocols. In fact, some of the more widely quoted studies on LHI with aggressive ICP lowering–focused treatment strategies report some of the most dismal outcomes for this disease.[80,81]

We use ICP monitoring in young patients with LHI who already have shown evidence of significant regional brain swelling and compression of ipsilateral cerebrospinal fluid spaces. These patients have declining intracranial compliance and are at risk for ICP plateau waves. The presence of early ICP elevation in the young patient should put everyone on the alert for the escalating risk of death in that individual patient, and this can be factored into decisions regarding treatment escalation and the possible application and timing of surgical decompression. In addition, ICP monitoring in such patients may assist with strategies (positioning and medical) to improve intracranial compliance, and attempt to avoid catastrophic cerebral hypoperfusion during transport and various nursing maneuvers. When ICP monitoring is employed, we recommend using an ipsilateral (to the infarction) parenchymal monitor, since it will be the region of greatest ICP elevation. The ipsilateral placement is because the ICP will be maximal in the region of dominant brain swelling, and the ventricle ipsilateral to the infarction collapses as swelling progresses, with the various disadvantages mentioned earlier in this section.

When ICP is elevated, medical management alone carries a high mortality. However, with respect to ICP reduction, the application of conventional ICP-lowering strategies can be very helpful early in the course of management. These include: optimizing head and body positioning, avoidance of behaviors that elevate ICP in patients with poor cerebral compliance (fighting the ventilator, agitation, and seizures), tight fever control, hyperventilation, and the administration of mannitol. We rarely administer multidose regimens of mannitol in LHI patients, because its misapplication and overuse has hypothetical dangers in these patients. When ICP elevations are considered important to medically treat in patients with LHI, use of hypertonic saline can also be an effective strategy.

The theme of fluid management in patients with LHI should be avoidance of volume depletion. There is no role for dehydration as a management strategy to limit the development of brain edema. Isotonic fluids (0.9% saline) are generally recommended without clear scientific evidence for their unique advantage for patients with LHI. When patients have been exposed to hyperosomolar treatments, the use of only isotonic fluids is critical, as the hyperosmolar brain may be at risk for worsened cerebral edema when exposed to hypotonic fluids. There is some evidence of a possible benefit of albumin infusions in experimental animals with LHI from MCA occlusion, but this has not been widely applied in humans.[82,83]

The potential for surgical decompression as a method to limit infarct volume and mortality from brain swelling after stroke has been demonstrated in experimental animals and with more recently promising human work.[78,81,84–86] Unfortunately, the selection of patients for this procedure and its best timing are still unclear; the decision making for this step requires a delicate balance between the patient's medical condition, the pace and anticipated severity of clinical progression, the prognosis, premorbid patient wishes, and various ethical and psychosocial issues.

References

1. Rosner MJ, Becker DP: Origin and evolution of plateau waves. *J Neurosurg* 60:312, 1984.
2. Klatzko I: Presidential address: Neuropathological aspects of brain edema. *J Neuropathol Exp Neurol* 26:1, 1967.
3. Fishman RA: Brain edema. *N Engl J Med* 293:706, 1975.
4. Katzman R, Clasen RA, Klatzko I, et al: Brain edema in stroke. *Stroke* 8:512, 1977.
5. Manz HJ: The pathology of cerebral edema. *Human Pathol* 5:291, 1974.
6. Kaufmann AM, Cardoso ER: Aggravation of vasogenic cereberal edema by multiple dose mannitol. *J Neurosurg* 77:584, 1992.
7. Mrsulja BB, Djuricic BM, Cvejic V, et al: Biochemistry of experimental ischemic brain edema. *Adv Neurol* 28:217, 1980.
8. Hirai N, Kuchiwaki H, Misu N, et al: Study of local shifting of the brainstem in increased intracranial pressure by a supratentorial balloon. *Brain Nerve (Tokyo)* 38:371, 1986.
9. Kaufmann GE, Clark K: Continuous simultaneous monitoring of intraventricular and cervical subarachnoid cerebrospinal fluid pressure to indicate development of cerebral or tonsillar herniation. *J Neurosurg* 33:145, 1970.
10. Kuchiwaki H, Furuse M, Gonda T, et al: Mutual relations between shifting of focal brain structures and intracranial pressure, in Ishi S, Nagai H, Brock M (eds): *Intracranial Pressure V*. Berlin, Springer-Verlag, 1986, p 445.
11. Frank JI, Ropper AH, Zuniga GE: Acute intracranial lesions and respiratory sinus arrhythmia. *Arch Neurol* 49:2100, 1992.
12. Ropper AH: Lateral displacement of the brain and level of consciousness in patients with an acute hemispheral mass. *N Engl J Med* 314:953, 1986.
13. Poon WS, Ng S, Wai S: CSF antibiotic prophylaxis for neurosurgical patients with ventriculostomy: A randomized study. *Acta Neurochir Suppl (Wien)* 71:146, 1998.
14. Sundbarg G, Nordstrom CH, Soderstrom S: Complications due to prolonged ventricular fluid pressure recording. *Br J Neurosurg* 2:485, 1988.
15. Poca M, Sahuquillo J, Arribas M, et al: Fiberoptic intraparenchymal brain pressure monitoring with the Camino V420 monitor: reflections on our experience in 163 severely head injured patients. *J Neurotrauma* 19:439, 2002.
16. Durward QJ, Amacher AL, Del Maestro RF, et al: Cerebral and cardiovascular responses to changes in head elevation in patients with intracranial hypertension. *J Neurosurg* 59:938, 1983.
17. Busiga DW, Leffler CW, Pourcyrous M: Hyperthermia increases cerebral metabolic rate and blood flow in neonatal pigs. *Am J Physiol* 255:H343, 1988.
18. Clasen RA, Pandolfi S, Laiang I, et al: Experimental study of relation of fever to cerebral edema. *J Neurosurg* 41:576, 1974.
19. Diringer MN and Neurointensive Care Fever Control Trialists: Treatment of fever in the neurointensive care unit with a catheter based heat exchange system. *Crit Care Med* 32:559, 2004.
20. Muizelaar JP, Van er Poel HG, Li ZC, et al: Pial arteriole vessel diameter and CO_2 reactivity in the rabbit. *J Neurosurg* 69:923, 1988.
21. Carmona Suazo JA, Maas AI, van der Brink WA, et al: CO_2 reactivity and brain oxygen pressure monitoring in severe head injury. *Crit Care Med* 28:3268, 2000.
22. Diringer MN, Videen TO, Yundt K, et al: Regional cerebrovascular and metabolic effects of hyperventilation after severe traumatic brain injury. *J Neurosurg* 96:103, 2002.
23. Thiagarajan A, Goverdhan PD, Chari P, et al: the effects of hyperventilation and hyperoxia on cerebral oxygen saturation in patients with traumatic brain injury. *Anesth Analg* 87:850, 1998.
24. Laffey JG, Kavanagh BP: Hypocapnia. *N Engl J Med* 347:43, 2002.
25. Wolf AL, Levi L, Maramou A, et al: Effects of THAM on outcome in severe head injury: a randomized prospective trial. *J Neurosurg* 78:54, 1993.
26. Burke AM, Quest DO, Chien S, et al: The effects of mannitol on blood viscosity. *J Neurosurg* 55:550, 1981.
27. Muizelaar JP, Lutz HA III, Becker DP: Effects of mannitol on ICP and CBF and correlation with pressure autoregulation in severely head injured patients. *J Neurosurg* 61:700, 1984.
28. Muizelaar JP, Wei EP, Kontos HA, et al: Cerebral blood flow is regulated by changes in blood pressure and in blood viscosity alike. *Stroke* 17:44, 1986.
29. Ravussin P, Abou-Madi M, Archer D, et al: Changes in CSF pressure after mannitol in patients with and without elevated CSF pressure. *J Neurosurg* 69:869, 1988.
30. Node Y, Nakazawa S: Clinical study of mannitol and glycerol on raised intracranial pressure and their rebound phenomenon. *Adv Neurol* 53:359, 1990.
31. Roberts PA, Pollay M, Engles C, et al: Effect on intracranial pressure of furosemide combines with varying doses and administration rates of mannitol. *J Neurosurg* 66:440, 1987.
32. Kaufmann AM, Carduso ER: Aggravation of vasogenic cerebral edema by multiple dose mannitol. *J Neurosurg* 77:584, 1992.
33. Kofke WA: Mannitol: potential for rebound intracranial hypertension. *J Neurosurg Anesth* 5:1, 1993.
34. Rudehill A, Gordon E, Ohman G, et al: Pharmacokinetics and effects of mannitol on hemodynamics, blood, and CSF electrolytes,

and osmolality during intracranial surgery. *J Neurosurg Anesthesiol* 5:4, 1993.

35. Frank JI: Large hemispheric infarction, deterioration, and intracranial pressure. *Neurology* 45:1286, 1995.

36. Shaywitz BA, Rothstein P, Venes JL: Monitoring and management of increased ICP in Reye's syndrome: results in 29 children. *Pediatrics* 66:198, 1980.

37. Worthley LI, Cooper DJ, Jones N: Treatment of resistant intracranial hypertension with hypertonic saline. *J Neurosurg* 68:478, 1988.

38. Horn P, Munch E, Vajkoczy P, et al: Hypertonic saline solution for control of elevated intracranial pressure in patients with exhausted response to mannitol and barbiturates. *Neurol Res* 21:758, 1999.

39. Schwartz S, Georgiadis D, Aschoff A, et al: Effects of hypertonic (10%) saline in patients with raised intracranial pressure after stroke. *Stroke* 33:1166, 2002.

40. Wilkinson HA, Wepsic JG, Austin G: Diuretic synergy in the treatment of acute experimental cerebral edema. *J Neurosurg* 34:203, 1977.

41. Galicich JH, French LA: Use of dexamethasone in the treatment of cerebral edema resulting from brain tumors and brain surgery. *Am Practitioner* 12:169, 1961.

42. Duff TA, Ayeni S, Levin AB, et al: Neurosurgical management of intracerebral hemorrhage. *Neurosurgery* 9:387, 1981.

43. Shenkin HA, Zavala M: Cerebellar strokes: mortality, surgical indications, and results of ventricular drainage. *Lancet* 11:429, 1982.

44. Tellez H, Bauer R: Dexamethsaone as treatment in cerebrovascular disease. 1. a controlled study in intracerebral hemorrhage. *Stroke* 4:541, 1973.

45. Poungvarin N, Bhoopat W, Viriyavejakul A, et al: Effects of dexamethsaone in primary supratentorial intracerebral hemorrhage. *N Engl J Med* 316:1229, 1987.

46. Anderson DC, Cranford RE: Corticosteroids in ischemic stroke. *Stroke* 10:68, 1979.

47. Bauer RB, Tellez H: Dexamethsone as treatment in cerebrovascular disease. 2. a controlled study in acute cerebral infarction. *Stroke* 4:547, 1977.

48. Gaetani P, Rodriquez Y, Baena R, Marzatico F, et al: Ex vivo release of eicosanoid from human brain tissue: Its relevance in the development of brain edema. *Neurosurgery* 28:853, 1991.

49. Norris JW, Hachinski VC: Megadose steroid therapy in ischemic stroke. *Stroke* 16:150, 1985.

50. Bloch M: Cerebral effects of rewarming following prolonged hypothermia. Significance for the management of cranio-cerebral injury and acute pyrexia. *Brain* 90:769, 1967.

51. Shiozaki H, Hayakata T, Taneda M, et al: A multicenter prospective randomized controlled trial of the efficacy of mild hypothermia for severely head injured patients with low intracranial pressure. *J Neurosurg* 94:50, 2001.

52. Forbes A, Alexander GJM, O'Grady JG, et al: Thiopental infusion in the treatment of intracranial hypertension complicating fulminant hepatic failure. *Hepatology* 10:306, 1989.

53. Miller JD: Barbiturates and raised ICP. *Ann Neurol* 6:189, 1979.

54. Piatt JH, Schiff SJ: High dose barbiturate therapy in neurosurgery and intensive care. *Neurosurgery* 15:427, 1984.

55. Rockoff MA, Marshall LF, Shapiro HM: High dose barbiturate therapy in humans. a clinical review of 60 patients. *Ann Neurol* 41:26, 1984.

56. Woodcock J, Ropper AH, Kennedy SK: High dose barbiturates in non-traumatic brain swelling: ICP reduction and effect on outcome. *Stroke* 13:785, 1982.

57. Andrefsky JC, Frank JI, Chyatte D: The ciliospinal reflex in pentobarbital coma. *J Neurosurg* 90:644, 1999.

58. Gazzard BG, Portmann B, Murray-Lyon IM, et al: Causes of death in fulminant hepatic failure and relationship to quantitative histological assessment of parenchymal damage. *Q J Med* 176:615, 1976.

59. Dixit V, Chang TM: Brain edema and the blood brain barrier in galactosamine-induced fulminant hepatic failure in rats: an animal model for evaluation of liver support systems. *ASAIO Transactions* 36:21, 1990.

60. Zaki AEO, Ede RJ, Davis M, et al: Experimental studies of blood brain barrier permeability in acute hepatic failure. *Hepatology* 4:359, 1984.

61. Hirata T, Kohler RC, Brusilow SW, et al: Impaired cerebrovascular reactivity to hypocapnia during hyperammonemia is linked to glutamine synthesis. *Crit Care Med* 22:A203, 1994.

62. Traber OG, DalCanto M, Ganger D, et al: Effect of body temperature on brain edema and encephalopathy in the rat after hepatic devascularization. *Gastroenterology* 96:885, 1989.

63. Lidofsky SD, Bass NM, Prager MC, et al: Intracranial pressure monitoring and liver transplantation for fulminant hepatic failure. *Hepatology* 16:1, 1992.

64. Munoz SJ, Robinson M, Northrup B, et al: Elevated intracranial pressure and computed tomography of the brain in fulminant hepatocellular failure. *Hepatology* 13:209, 1991.

65. Canalese J, Gimson AES, Davis C, et al: Controlled trial of dexamethasone and mannitol for the cerebral edema of fulminant hepatic failure. *Gut* 23:625, 1982.

66. Hanid MA, Davies M, Mellon PJ, et al: Clinical monitoring of intracranial pressure in fulminant hepatic failure. *Gut* 21:866, 1980.

67. Ede RJ, Gimson AES, Bihari D, et al: Controlled hyperventilation in the prevention of cerebral edema in fulminant hepatic failure. *J Hepatol* 2:43, 1986.

68. Schafer DF, Shaw BW: Fulminant hepatic failure and orthotopic liver transplantation. *Semin Liver Dis* 9:189, 1989.

69. Marshall LF, Shapiro HM, Rauscher A, et al: Pentobarbital therapy for intracranial hypertension in metabolic coma: Reye's syndrome. *Crit Care Med* 6:1, 1978.

70. Forbes A, Alexander GJM, O'Grady JG: Thiopental infusion in the treatment of intracranial hypertension complicating fulminant hepatic failure. *Hepatology* 10:306, 1984.

71. Henon H, Godefroy O, Leyd D, et al: Early predictors of death and disability after acute cerebral ischemic event. *Stroke* 26:392, 1995.

72. Hanna JP, Frank JI, Furlan AJ, et al: Prediction of worsening consciousness from edema after hemispheric infarction. *J Stroke Cerebrovasc Dis* 6:25, 1996.

73. Krieger DW, Demchuk AM, Kasner SE, et al: Early clinical and radiographic predictors of fatal swelling in ischemic stroke. *Stroke* 30:287, 1999.

74. Kasner SE, Demchuk AM, Berrouschot J, et al: Predictors of fatal brain edema in massive hemispheric ischemic stroke. *Stroke* 32:2117, 2001.

75. Ropper AH, Shafran B: Brain edema after stroke: clinical syndrome and intracranial pressure. *Arch Neurol* 41:26, 1984.

76. Saver JL, Johnston KC, Homer D, et al: Infarct volume as a surrogate or auxiliary outcome measure in ischemic stroke clinical trials. *Stroke* 30:293, 1999.

77. van der Worp, Claus SP, Bar PR, et al: Reproducibility of measurements of cerebral infarct volume on CT scans. *Stroke* 32:424, 2001.

78. Frank JI, Chyatte D, Thisted R, et al: Hemicraniectomy and durotomy upon deterioration from infarction related swelling trial (HeADDFIRST): First public presentation of the preliminary findings. *Neurology* 60(5, Suppl 1):A426, 2003.

79. Kasner SE, Demchuk AM, Berrouschot J, et al: Predictors of fatal brain edema in massive hemispheric ischemic stroke. *Stroke* 32:2117, 2001.

80. Hacke W, Schwab S, Horn M, et al: Malignant middle cerebral artery territory infarction: clinical course and prognostic signs. *Arch Neurol* 53:309, 1996.

81. Rieke K, Schwab S, Krieger, et al: Decompressive surgery in space occupying cerebral hemispheric infarction. *Crit Care Med* 23:1576, 1995.

82. Schwarz S, Schwab S, Bertram M, et al: Effects of hypertonic saline hydroxyethyl starch solution and mannitol in patients with increased intracranial pressure after stroke. *Stroke* 29:1550, 1998.

83. Schwarz S, Georgiadis D, Aschoff A, Schwab S: Effects of hypertonic (10%) saline in patients with raised intracranial pressure. *Stroke* 33:136, 2002.

84. Doerfler A, Forsting M, Reith W, et al: Decompressive craniectomy in a rat model of malignant cerebral hemispheric stroke: Experimental support for an aggressive therapeutic approach. *J Neurosurg* 85:853, 1996.

85. Cho DY, Chen TS, Lee HC: Ultra-early decompressive craniectomy for malignant middle cerebral artery infarction. *Surg Neurol* 60:227, 2003.

86. Schwab S, Steiner T, Aschoff A, et al: Early hemicraniectomy in patients with complete middle cerebral artery infarction. *Stroke* 29:1888, 1998.

Chapter 66 _____
NEUROMUSCULAR DISEASES LEADING TO RESPIRATORY FAILURE

WILLIAM A. MARINELLI
JAMES W. LEATHERMAN

KEY POINTS

- *Neuromuscular disorders (NMDs) in critical care may be divided into those that precipitate admission to the ICU and those that arise during ICU management; the latter are much more common and significantly influence the pace and extent of recovery from critical illness.*

- *The maximal inspiratory pressure (MIP), maximal expiratory pressure (MEP), vital capacity (VC), and qualitative judgment of oropharyngeal function are the most important parameters to follow in patients with NMDs.*

- *An effective cough is unlikely with a MEP <40 cm H$_2$O or a VC <30 mL/kg.*

- *Sleep-related deterioration in hypoventilation and hypoxemia is common in patients with respiratory muscle impairment.*

- *Many patients with Guillain-Barré syndrome or myasthenia gravis of sufficient severity to precipitate ICU admission will benefit from treatment with plasmapheresis or intravenous immunoglobulin.*

- *Muscle biopsy is useful in the diagnosis of polymyositis, mitochondrial disease, and other myopathies, and should be considered when electrophysiologic and other testing does not offer a clear diagnosis of peripheral neuropathy or myoneural junction diseases.*

- *Critical illness myopathy and neuropathy should be considered in all patients with protracted critical illness, particularly when multisystem organ failure has been present; avoidance of paralytics, appropriate correction of the metabolic milieu, early physical therapy, and measures to shorten duration of mechanical ventilation may help ameliorate the impact of these acquired NMDs.*

Neuromuscular Disorders in Critical Care

Neuromuscular weakness may result from disorders involving the peripheral nerves, neuromuscular transmission, or skeletal muscles.[1–3] Neuromuscular disorders encountered in the critical care setting may be divided into those that result in ICU admission and those that are acquired during treatment of critical illness. In the first part of this chapter we will address neuromuscular disorders that lead to ICU admission, focusing on Guillain-Barré syndrome (GBS), myasthenia gravis (MG), and dermatomyositis/polymyositis (DM/PM), and concluding with a brief discussion of mitochondrial disease, a recently recognized metabolic myopathy. Subsequently, neuromuscular weakness that is acquired after admission to the ICU will be reviewed. However, before

discussing the various causes of neuromuscular weakness, a brief review of respiratory muscle impairment is appropriate, since respiratory failure is the most common reason that patients with a primary neuromuscular disorder are admitted to an ICU.

Although respiratory muscle impairment may occasionally develop rapidly, more often its onset is gradual. Diaphragmatic weakness may be initially manifested by orthopnea or sleep disruption due to nocturnal hypoventilation, without prominent dyspnea.[2] Because there may be a paucity of symptoms, objective testing is necessary. Maximal inspiratory pressure (MIP), maximum expiratory pressure (MEP), vital capacity (VC), and an assessment of oropharyngeal function are the most important respiratory muscle parameters to follow,[4–6] and should be measured frequently in hospitalized patients who have an evolving neuromuscular disorder, with careful attention to serial changes.[7] The most sensitive parameters of respiratory muscle strength are the MIP and MEP. Measurement of MIP and MEP requires a maximal effort at residual volume (MIP) and total lung capacity (MEP), using a bedside manometer fitted with a mouthpiece. Normal values for MIP and MEP are approximately –70 cm H$_2$O and 100 cm H$_2$O, respectively, for women, and approximately –100 cm H$_2$O and 150 cm H$_2$O, respectively, for men.[5] An effective cough is unlikely when the MEP is <40 cm H$_2$O, and there is risk of hypercapnia when the MIP is less negative than –20 cm H$_2$O. In the early stages of respiratory muscle weakness, arterial blood gas and VC measurements are commonly normal. The normal VC in adults is approximately 50 mL/kg, and elimination of secretions with coughing is impaired when the VC declines to <30 mL/kg. Serial VC measurements that decline to <15 to 20 mL/kg increase the likelihood that ventilatory assistance will be necessary.[1,8] Sleep-related deterioration in hypoventilation and hypoxemia are common in patients with respiratory muscle impairment, particularly during rapid eye movement sleep.[2] When the supine VC is <60% of the predicted value, or the MIP is less negative than –34 cm H$_2$O, sleep-disordered breathing is common.[9]

Bulbar muscle impairment may significantly increase the risk for aspiration-related respiratory failure. Unfortunately, bulbar muscle impairment is commonly unrecognized, resulting in increased risk of morbidity and mortality.[8] Intact musculature involving the mouth, pharynx, palate, tongue, and larynx are necessary for effective oropharyngeal function.[10] The assessment of oropharyngeal function is primarily based on clinical observation, and early consultation with an experienced speech pathologist is recommended to assess the patient's ability to perform the complex and coordinated action of swallowing.

Neuromuscular Disorders Leading to Intensive Care Unit Admission

Many patients who present to the ICU as a result of an underlying neuromuscular disorder will have a previously defined diagnosis. However, when a patient presents with recent onset of acute or subacute bilateral muscle weakness, a broad differential diagnosis must be considered (Table 66-1). An initial approach to differential diagnosis is based on the patient's history and a careful neurologic exam that attempts

TABLE 66-1 Causes of Acute and Subacute Bilateral Weakness

Syndrome/Level of Abnormality	Representative Disorders
Basilar artery occlusion	Embolic, thrombotic, vasculitic
Myelopathy	Cord compression (e.g., abscess, neoplasm, disc herniation, trauma)
	Transverse myelitis
Central nervous system infections	Poliomyelitis
	West Nile virus
Central nervous system toxins	Neurotoxic fish poisoning
Peripheral nerve disorders	Guillain-Barré syndrome
	Diphtheria
	Heavy metal toxicity
	Vasculitic neuropathy
Disorders of neuromuscular transmission	Myasthenia gravis
	Eaton-Lambert syndrome
	Botulism
	Tick paralysis
	Organophosphate poisoning
	Penicillamine toxicity
Myopathic disorders	Dermatomyositis/polymyositis
	Metabolic myopathy (e.g., mitochondrial disease)
	Toxic myopathy (e.g., corticosteroid injury, rhabdomyolysis)
Electrolyte disorders	Periodic paralysis
	Hypophosphatemia
	Hypokalemia

to define the principal level of abnormality (Table 66-2). Additional diagnostic tests such as nerve conduction studies and an electromyogram (EMG) are often needed to more reliably establish the underlying disorder. Although lesions involving the upper and lower motor neuron may occasionally be responsible for new-onset weakness that necessitates ICU admission, the latter is more often due to diseases that effect the peripheral nerves (e.g., GBS), neuromuscular junction (e.g., MG), or muscles (e.g., PM/DM).

GUILLAIN-BARRÉ SYNDROME

Guillain-Barré syndrome is an acute inflammatory demyelinating polyneuropathy that most often presents with ascending symmetrical weakness.[1,8,11] Weakness typically evolves over days to weeks, although a subset of patients experience a rapid decline in function over hours. Excluding trauma, GBS is the most common cause for acute flaccid paralysis in previously healthy people.[1] The ascending weakness is accompanied by depressed or absent reflexes. Sensory involvement is common, and many patients experience peripheral paresthesias as their initial symptom. In addition, an aching discomfort in the lower back and legs is common in the early phase of the syndrome. Autonomic dysfunction is common in patients with GBS, resulting in brady- or tachyarrhythmias, orthostatic hypotension, hypertension, or abnormal sweating.[8] Although bowel and bladder function are usually preserved,[12] ileus and bladder dysfunction can occur. Variants from the usual GBS presentation may be encountered, including

TABLE 66-2 Differential Diagnosis of Neuromuscular Disorders Leading to ICU Admission

Level of Abnormality	Presentation	Representative Disorders	Nerve Conduction	Electromyography
Upper motor neuron	Weakness	Cortical	Normal	Normal
	Spasticity	Subcortical		
	Hyperreflexia	Brain stem		
	Sensory/autonomic changes	Spinal cord lesions		
Lower motor neuron	Weakness	Poliomyelitis	Normal	Denervation
	Flaccidity	Post-polio syndrome		
	Hyporeflexia	Amyotrophic lateral sclerosis		
	Fasciculations			
	Bulbar changes			
	No sensory changes			
Peripheral nerve	Weakness	Guillain-Barré syndrome	Reduced	Denervation
	Flaccidity	Diphtheria		
	Hyporeflexia	Heavy metal toxicity		
	Bulbar changes	Vasculitic neuropathy		
	Sensory/autonomic changes			
Neuromuscular junction	Fluctuating weakness	Myasthenia gravis	Normal	Abnormal repetitive stimulation
	Fatigability	Eaton-Lambert		
	Normal reflexes	Botulism		
	No sensory changes	Tick paralysis		
	With or without autonomic changes	Organophosphate poisoning		
		Penicillamine		
Muscle	Weakness	Polymyositis	Normal	Small motor units
	Normal reflexes	Dermatomyositis		
	No sensory or autonomic changes	Metabolic myopathies		
	With or without pain	Muscular dystrophy		

SOURCE: Modified with permission from Luce J: Neuromuscular diseases leading to respiratory failure, in Hall JB, Schmidt GA, Wood LDH (eds): *Neuromuscular Diseases Care*, 2nd ed. New York, McGraw-Hill, 1998, p 995.

the Miller-Fischer variant, with ataxia, ophthalmoparesis, and areflexia.[1,11,13]

For unclear reasons, GBS appears to be more common in young adults and in the elderly. A preceding infectious syndrome with respiratory or gastrointestinal symptoms, usually occurring 1 to 4 weeks prior to the onset of neurologic symptoms, has been noted in approximately two thirds of patients.[1,11,14] *Campylobacter jejuni* and cytomegalovirus infections are the most commonly identified triggers for GBS.[11,14] However, a diverse and seemingly unrelated group of triggers have been identified, including infections, vaccination, general surgery, epidural anesthesia, thrombolytic agents, drugs, neoplastic disease (Hodgkin's disease), sarcoidosis, and connective tissue diseases.[1,8]

A diagnosis of GBS is based on the clinical presentation and electrodiagnostic studies compatible with a demyelinating polyneuropathy.[1,11] Elevated cerebrospinal fluid protein levels are commonly noted after the first week of symptoms and may be associated with a limited mononuclear pleocytosis (<10 cells/cm^3). Diagnoses other than GBS should be more aggressively considered if: (1) reflexes remain intact despite weakness (areflexia is present in $\sim$90% of patients when weakness is fully developed); (2) the distribution of weakness is highly asymmetric; (3) fever is present during the initial presentation; or (4) the electrodiagnostic features are not indicative of an acquired demyelinating polyneuropathy.[1] A rapidly progressive spinal lesion is the most important potentially reversible process to be excluded in a patient who presents with ascending weakness.[12]

Respiratory failure occurs at the time of initial presentation in 10% of patients, and eventually develops in up to 43% of patients during the course of their disease.[1,15] All aspects of respiratory muscle function—inspiratory strength, expiratory strength, and upper airway protection—may be impaired.[8,16] Progression to respiratory failure was predicted in one retrospective study by the presence of a VC <20 mL/kg, MIP less negative than -30 cm H_2O, and MEP <40 cm H_2O ("20/30/40 rule").[17] Inability to cough markedly increases the risk for intubation.[15] In addition, multivariate analyses have also indicated that a time from onset to admission of less than 7 days, inability to stand, and inability to lift the head or elbows are all associated with an increased risk for mechanical ventilation.[15] The risk of intubation is increased by the dysautonomia of GBS, because of an exaggeration of the hypotensive response to sedative agents, and a markedly increased risk of arrhythmias, most often bradyarrhythmias.[8,10]

Guillain-Barré syndrome is a monophasic illness with a fairly predictable natural history; at least 90% of patients reach the nadir of their neuromuscular impairment by 4 weeks.[8] Most patients recover from their illness, with two thirds experiencing mild residual deficits, and 10% to 20% of patients recovering completely.[1] The remaining 3% to 8% of patients will die as a result of pneumonia, acute respiratory distress syndrome, sepsis, pulmonary emboli, and cardiac arrest.[1,18,19] Deaths appear to be more common in the elderly, particularly in patients with pre-existing pulmonary disease.[18] In addition, the mortality and morbidity of GBS is strongly associated with the need for and duration of mechanical ventilation. The mortality rate of patients with GBS who require mechanical ventilation may be as high as 20%.[20] Mechanical ventilation for more than 2 weeks has been found to be the strongest predictor of major morbidity by multivariate

analysis, with lower respiratory tract infection being the most common complication.[21]

Treatment of GBS involves either plasmapheresis or intravenous immune globulin (IVIg). Plasma exchange was demonstrated to improve strength and reduce the incidence of respiratory failure in three multicenter trials conducted in the 1980s.[22–24] Two exchanges may be needed in patients with mild impairment, whereas four exchanges are optimal in those with more severe impairment.[25] Albumin is as effective as fresh frozen plasma as a replacement fluid during plasma exchange, and is associated with fewer adverse reactions.[26] IVIg has also been shown to be an effective therapy for GBS.[27] The mechanism by which IVIg benefits patients with GBS is not fully defined, but neutralizing neuromuscular blocking antibodies by a dose-dependent process appears likely.[28] A randomized, multicenter, international trial compared plasma exchange, IVIg, or plasma exchange followed by IVIg in 379 GBS patients who had marked weakness and whose symptoms had been present for 14 days or less.[21] There were no differences among the three treatment groups with regard to either the duration of mechanical ventilation or functional outcome 4 weeks after therapy. It was therefore concluded that IVIg and plasmapheresis are equally effective therapies, and that their combined use offered no additional benefit.[21] Because of its ease of administration and acceptable side effect profile, IVIg is often preferred. In addition, IVIg may be superior to plasmapheresis in patients with *Campylobacter jejuni* infections and antibodies to peripheral nerve gangliosides.[2,29] Screening for IgA deficiency is recommended prior to treatment with IVIg to reduce the risk of anaphylaxis during infusion. Although frequently used in the past, corticosteroids have not been shown to be beneficial in patients with GBS.[1,11,13]

MYASTHENIA GRAVIS

Myasthenia gravis is an acquired autoimmune disorder of neuromuscular junction transmission characterized by muscle weakness, progressive muscle fatigue with repetitive use, and improvement in strength after rest.[3,30] The incidence of MG is highest in younger women or older men. Generalized weakness with fatigability involving the trunk and extremity muscles is noted in approximately 85% of patients and may be the dominant complaint.[3] Ocular muscle involvement, including ptosis and diplopia, are common at presentation. Bulbar muscle impairment results in dysphonia and difficulty with chewing and swallowing. The immunopathogenesis of MG has been well defined, with identification of autoantibodies that bind to the acetylcholine receptor resulting in a significant reduction in the number of available receptors at the neuromuscular junction, thereby impairing neuromuscular transmission.[3]

Although isolated involvement of the respiratory muscles may occur, respiratory muscle impairment typically presents along with generalized muscle weakness.[31,32] Upper airway obstruction with abnormal vocal cord adduction during inspiration has also been described.[33] Lower respiratory muscle impairment is evidenced by a significant reduction in VC, MIP, and MEP. Approximately 15% to 27% of patients experience "myasthenic crises," a rapid and severe decline in respiratory muscle function that is associated with a mortality of

4% to 13%.[34–36] Multiple triggers for myasthenic crises have been identified, including infection, electrolyte abnormalities, withdrawal of anticholinesterase drugs, and the use of drugs that impair neuromuscular transmission, with infection being the most common identifiable precipitating factor. However, a trigger for the myasthenic crisis cannot be found in nearly a third of patients.[35] In a retrospective study of 73 episodes of myasthenic crises progressing to intubation, 50% of patients were extubated within 2 weeks, and the median ICU and hospital stays were 14 and 35 days, respectively.[35] Three independent predictors of prolonged intubation were identified in this study: (1) preintubation serum bicarbonate ≥30 mg/dL; (2) peak VC <25 mL/kg on day 1 to 6 postintubation; and, (3) age >50 years. Cardiac dysrhythmias are a common cause of death in patients with myasthenic crises, and continuous cardiac rhythm monitoring is strongly recommended.

In patients with a compatible clinical presentation, the diagnosis of MG centers on three principal studies: (1) a positive anticholinesterase test (rapid and transient improvement in strength after administration of edrophonium); (2) presence of acetylcholine receptor antibodies in the serum; and (3) electrophysiologic studies that are indicative of a disorder of the neuromuscular junction, with a decremental response in compound action potentials to repetitive nerve stimulation.[3] Acetylcholine receptor–binding antibodies are identified in approximately 88% to 93% of patients with generalized MG, and in approximately 71% of patients with symptoms limited to ocular muscle involvement.[37] One diagnostic strategy that has been recommended begins with an edrophonium test, followed by a repetitive nerve stimulation test and measurement of acetylcholine receptor antibodies.[3] Single-fiber EMG may be obtained if the diagnosis remains undefined.

Conditions associated with MG include thymic hyperplasia or thymoma, and autoimmune conditions such as rheumatoid arthritis, lupus, thyroiditis, and Graves disease.[3] Thyroid function testing should be obtained in all patients with MG. Thymic abnormalities are present in the majority of patients with MG, with thymic hyperplasia being most common and thymoma identified in 10% to 12% of patients.[3] The association with thymic abnormalities has led to the use of a chest computed tomographic (CT) or magnetic resonance imaging (MRI) scan as a screening tool in patients with MG.

The treatment of MG includes anticholinesterase medications to increase the concentration of acetylcholine available for receptor binding, immunosuppressive therapy, and thymectomy.[3,38,39] The first line of therapy is use of an anticholinesterase agent, most commonly pyridostigmine. Respiratory muscle function improves in approximately 50% of patients treated with anticholinesterase medications.[2,40] Muscarinic side effects include abdominal cramping with frequent defecation, increased urinary frequency, bronchospasm, bradycardia, fasciculations, increased oral secretions, and excessive lacrimation. Less commonly, these agents produce a cholinergic crisis, with increased bulbar and lower respiratory muscle weakness during the early phase of treatment. The clinical manifestations of a cholinergic crisis may overlap with those of a myasthenic crisis, making a clear distinction difficult; withholding anticholinesterase medications for 4 to 10 days may be necessary.

Most patients respond to anticholinesterase therapy, but their response is usually incomplete and symptomatic relapse during therapy is common. Unfortunately, increasing the dose of drug often leads to significant side effects.[3,38,39] Thus the majority of patients require additional therapy with immunosuppressive agents. Corticosteroid use results in a remission or marked improvement in approximately 75% of patients with MG, and these are the most commonly used agents. Azathioprine has a more delayed onset of action, usually requiring at least 3 months of therapy, thereby limiting its use as a primary agent for initial therapy. Cyclosporine reduces acetylcholine receptor antibody production, but toxicity limits its use. Cyclophosphamide has also been beneficial in patients who were refractory to other agents, but toxicity remains a significant concern.

Plasma exchange and IVIg are commonly used for intensive short-term therapy.[41,42] Plasma exchange removes acetylcholine receptor antibodies rapidly, commonly resulting in an improvement in strength within several days. Typically, 2- to 4-liter exchanges are performed two to three times per week over a 10- to 14-day period. IVIg also results in a rapid improvement in most patients. Plasma exchange should be considered as an initial intervention in patients with myasthenic crisis, with IVIg reserved for possible use after a course of plasma exchange.[38]

Thymectomy has been associated with clinical improvement and remission in patients with MG, and is generally recommended for patients with thymomas between the ages of puberty and approximately 60 years.[3,38,43] However, adequate prospective studies demonstrating a clear benefit from thymectomy are unavailable. Because postoperative decline in ventilatory function is common, thymectomy should not be performed as an emergency procedure in patients with significantly impaired ventilatory function (VC <2 L). Plasma exchange should be considered preoperatively in patients with significant ventilatory impairment.

Alternative therapeutic strategies should be considered in MG patients who are refractory to conventional therapy. For example, high-dose cyclophosphamide followed by granulocyte colony-stimulating factor therapy was reported to be effective in three patients with MG refractory to conventional immunosuppressive therapy, plasma exchange, and thymectomy.[44] In addition, lymphocyte depletion therapy with the human-mouse chimeric monoclonal antibody rituximab was associated with clinical improvement and reduction in the acetylcholine receptor antibody titer in a patient who developed MG after bone marrow transplantation.[45,46]

Disorders of neuromuscular transmission that may mimic MG include Eaton-Lambert syndrome (usually associated with small-cell carcinoma), botulism, tick paralysis, organophosphate toxicity, and a myasthenic-like syndrome induced by penicillamine.[3] Botulism results in a toxin-mediated irreversible inhibition of neuromuscular transmission, resulting in an acute symmetric descending paralysis beginning with bulbar impairment.[2,47] The early bulbar involvement of botulism may initially be confused with the Miller-Fischer variant of GBS, which predominantly involves the bulbar musculature.[1,13] Botulism is most commonly associated with food-borne and intestinal sources. Wound-related illness may also occur, especially in parenteral heroin users. Bioterroism remains a serious concern as another potential source of botulism. Tick paralysis typically affects children more than adults and is manifested by an ascending paresis or paralysis caused by a tick-borne neurotoxin.[48] A high index of clinical suspicion is critical for establishing a diagnosis of tick paralysis. Treatment of tick paralysis is centered on a careful physical exam (including scalp, ears, axilla, buttocks, perianal skin, and labia) to identify and remove all ticks and their body parts, along with close observation and supportive care. In North American tick paralysis, significant improvement in neuromuscular strength usually occurs within several hours of tick identification and removal.

DERMATOMYOSITIS AND POLYMYOSITIS

Dermatomyositis and polymyositis are idiopathic inflammatory disorders which usually present with progressive symmetrical muscle weakness over several months.[49,50] Less commonly, there is an acute presentation with rapidly evolving muscle weakness. Of the major muscle groups, the shoulder and pelvic girdle muscles are most often affected. Neck flexion muscles are weakened in up to 50% of patients, but facial muscles are usually spared. Pharyngeal muscle involvement may present with dysphonia or dysphagia. Myalgias and muscle tenderness occur in up to 50% of patients. An immune-mediated mechanism is strongly supported by the association of PM/DM with other autoimmune diseases, and by the frequent presence of autoantibodies in serum.[50]

Diagnostic criteria for PM/DM include the presence of symmetrical proximal muscle weakness, elevated skeletal muscle enzymes, and compatible findings on electromyography and skeletal muscle biopsy.[49–51] Characteristic dermatologic findings are present in dermatomyositis, including heliotropic changes of the eyelids and Gottron sign, a characteristic symmetric erythematous rash over the extensor surfaces of metacarpophalangeal, interphalangeal, elbow, and knee joints. Creatine phosphokinase (CK) elevation is the most consistent indicator of muscle inflammation. However, other muscle enzymes (aldolase, aspartate aminotransferase, alanine aminotransferase, and lactate dehydrogenase) may also be elevated. Electromyography typically reveals features of a generalized myopathic disorder, but findings may be normal in 10% to 15% of patients. Muscle biopsy is the most definitive test, demonstrating variable degrees of type I and II fiber necrosis and inflammation.

Respiratory and cardiovascular complications of DM/PM are the main concerns in the ICU.[49,52,53] Respiratory complications with DM/PM include respiratory muscle weakness, interstitial lung disease, pneumonia resulting from aspiration or immunosuppression, and drug-induced lung disease. The presence of dysphagia suggests pharyngeal muscle dysfunction, which greatly increases the risk for aspiration, the most commonly reported pulmonary complication of DM/PM. Respiratory muscle dysfunction with inspiratory and expiratory muscle involvement has been reported in up to one third of patients. Interstitial lung disease has also been identified in nearly one third of patients with DM/PM,[54] with nonspecific interstitial pneumonitis being the most common underlying histopathologic lesion.[55] Typical findings on high-resolution chest CT include reticular and ground-glass opacities in the lower lung fields, variable presence of consolidation in the lung periphery, and the absence of a fibrotic honeycomb-like appearance.[56] An analysis of 70 patients with DM/PM and diffuse interstitial lung disease found a

musculoskeletal presentation in 36%, pulmonary presentation in 30%, and a combination of musculoskeletal and pulmonary symptoms in 21%.[55] When presentation is with pulmonary disease alone, treatment with corticosteroids may suppress or obscure musculoskeletal symptoms, thereby delaying the diagnosis of DM/PM for weeks to years.[55] Cardiac features include tachyarrhythmias, conduction abnormalities, myocarditis, or heart failure with a dilated cardiomyopathy. Chronic pulmonary hypertension may result from several mechanisms, including underlying cardiomyopathy, chronic hypoxia associated with either chronic hypercapnic respiratory failure or interstitial lung disease, or the development of a primary pulmonary hypertension–like syndrome.

Most patients with DM/PM respond to corticosteroids, with normalization in muscle enzymes by 4 to 6 weeks and improvement in muscle strength within 2 to 3 months.[38,49,50] Therapy with corticosteroids is usually initiated at a dosage of 0.5 to 1.5 mg/kg prednisone, with gradual tapering after a complete response has been demonstrated. However, the clinical course of DM/PM is quite variable, ranging from a relatively indolent course to a relentlessly progressive process that is unresponsive to therapy. Symptom duration of greater than 6 months before diagnosis, severe symptoms, and the presence of dysphagia are clinical predictors of poor outcome in DM/PM.[57,58]

Alternative immunosuppressive agents, including methotrexate, azathioprine, or cyclophosphamide, should be considered in patients with poor prognostic markers or a limited response to corticosteroids.[58] These immunosuppressive agents, particularly methotrexate or azathioprine, may also be used if there is corticosteroid intolerance and for long-term maintenance therapy. Alternative therapy with IVIg, cyclosporine, tacrolimus, alkylating agents, and tumor necrosis factor inhibitors has been used for patients whose symptoms are unresponsive to standard treatment. In one study of 35 patients with PM who were refractory to therapy with prednisone and at least one additional immunosuppressive agent, significant improvement in strength was noted in 71% of patients after treatment with IVIg; all patients had a significant reduction in CK values.[59] IVIg has also been reported to be beneficial in the management of life-threatening esophageal involvement in DM/PM.[60] Pharyngeal muscle involvement in DM/PM usually responds to corticosteroid therapy. However, surgical division of the cricopharyngeal muscle may be necessary for severe cricopharyngeal achalasia that is refractory to immunosuppressive therapy. Cardiac complications are managed with appropriate pharmacologic therapy and insertion of a pacemaker-defibrillator should be considered in the event of serious conduction abnormalities or ventricular dysrhythmias.

MITOCHONDRIAL DISEASE

Mitochondrial disease may present with diverse manifestations in the critical care setting, including respiratory muscle impairment. This increasingly recognized metabolic myopathy appears to result from acquired mutations of genes coding for critical proteins in glycolysis, fatty acid oxidation, or oxidative phosphorylation.[61–63] Clues to the possible presence of this interesting disorder include unexplained dyspnea progressing to respiratory failure, sedative-related respiratory failure out of proportion to the sedative dose administered, respiratory failure with persistent unexplained lactic acidosis, prolonged paralysis following use of neuromuscular blockade, and unexplained difficulty with weaning from mechanical ventilation.[61,64,65] An elevation in the lactate:pyruvate ratio of greater than 20 is frequently present in patients with abnormalities in glycolysis. Reduction in carnitine levels may be identified in patients with a disorder in fatty acid oxidation, reflecting abnormalities in carnitine palmitoyl transferase enzymes. Muscle biopsies are usually diagnostic, demonstrating characteristic findings on light and electron microscopy. Care for patients with these unique disorders is primarily supportive, including treatment of precipitating infections and withholding sedatives and neuromuscular blockers. A diet high in carbohydrates may be of benefit in patients with abnormal carnitine palmitoyl transferase enzyme function.

Neuromuscular Disorders Acquired in the Intensive Care Unit

Acquired neuromuscular disorders have become increasingly recognized over the last two decades as a major cause of morbidity related to critical illness. Currently, acquired disorders are a much more common cause of severe generalized weakness in the ICU than are primary neuromuscular disorders.[66] Although ICU-acquired muscle weakness is usually reversible, respiratory muscle involvement may lead to prolonged mechanical ventilation and delayed weaning. Once patients are successfully extubated, they often require prolonged physical rehabilitation and may be unable to perform basic activities of daily living for weeks to months.[67] Of greater concern, recent studies have documented the persistence of significant weakness up to several years after hospital discharge, indicating that in some cases severe ICU-acquired weakness may result in permanent disability.[68–71] Without question, the medical, economic, and psychosocial costs of ICU-acquired neuromuscular weakness represent a major problem in the current practice of critical care medicine.

CAUSES OF INTENSIVE CARE UNIT–ACQUIRED WEAKNESS

Three basic causes of ICU-acquired neuromuscular weakness have been identified: (1) persistent blockade of the neuromuscular junction after discontinuing a neuromuscular blocking agent (NMBA), (2) a sensorimotor axonal polyneuropathy, and (3) an acute myopathy.[72–74] Although the clinical setting and physical examination may be of some help in elucidating the underlying cause of muscle weakness, in most cases diagnosis has been made by electrophysiologic studies, sometimes supplemented by biopsy of muscle or nerve. As will be discussed below, elucidation of the underlying cause of weakness is not always easy, and combined disorders of muscle and nerve may occur.[75]

PERSISTENT NEUROMUSCULAR JUNCTION BLOCKADE

Residual blockade of the neuromuscular junction after discontinuation of an NMBA is rarely responsible for persistent neuromuscular weakness in the ICU.[66] One possible exception is the use of vecuronium in patients with renal failure, in which case accumulation of the active metabolite

3-desacetylvecuronium may result in paralysis that is prolonged for several days.[74] If residual neuromuscular paralysis is a consideration, a repetitive nerve stimulation protocol should be performed to see if there is a progressive decrement in the compound muscle action potential (CMAP) that would indicate residual blockade at the neuromuscular junction.

CRITICAL ILLNESS POLYNEUROPATHY

In the 1980s Bolton and colleagues reported on a group of critically ill patients who developed generalized weakness after several weeks in the ICU.[72,76] Affected patients, most of whom had underlying sepsis, often underwent neurologic evaluation because of difficulty in weaning from mechanical ventilation or because of diffuse limb weakness. Distal muscles were often affected most prominently, but cranial nerves did not appear to be involved. Sensory examination was difficult to perform, but deep tendon reflexes were either reduced or absent in most cases.[72,76] Electrophysiologic evaluation with electroneurography (ENG) and EMG suggested that weakness was due to an axonal sensorimotor polyneuropathy. Key findings included a reduction in the CMAP in response to stimulation of motor nerves, often accompanied by a decrease in the sensory action potential (SAP) when sensory nerves were stimulated. The EMG revealed spontaneous fibrillations and positive sharp waves that were attributed to denervation. Survivors had improvement in their electrophysiologic studies over several months that paralleled clinical recovery. Autopsy findings included grouped fiber atrophy in muscle and axonal degeneration with loss of myelin in nerves, with distal segments most severely affected.[76] Neither muscle nor nerve showed inflammation.[76]

Numerous additional studies dealing with critical illness polyneuropathy have been published in the last 20 years, and the reported findings have been similar to those initially described, including the diffuse distribution of weakness (other than the facial muscles), frequent difficulties with weaning, and occurrence in the setting of sepsis and systemic inflammatory response syndrome (SIRS), often with multiorgan dysfunction. The pathogenetic mechanism of acquired polyneuropathy in critical illness is not understood. It has been suggested that the peripheral nervous system may be one of the many target sites for tissue damage in the setting of sepsis, and that lack of effective vascular autoregulation and increased microvascular permeability could result in neural edema and capillary occlusion, thereby damaging peripheral nerves.[72,77] As with other types of organ dysfunction in SIRS, neuronal injury may be cytokine-mediated.[77]

INTENSIVE CARE UNIT–ACQUIRED MYOPATHY (CRITICAL ILLNESS MYOPATHY)

Severe ICU-acquired myopathy was first reported 25 years ago,[78] with numerous individual case reports and case series having been published subsequently.[79–81] Myopathy most often occurred in the setting of mechanical ventilation for severe airflow obstruction, and affected individuals had typically been treated with concomitant corticosteroids and NMBAs. However, myopathy has also been documented in patients treated with corticosteroids without paralysis, and in critically ill septic patients who received neither corticosteroids nor NMBAs.[73,82–85] Some authors have attempted to subdivide the acute myopathy that develops in the ICU into a "critical illness myopathy" associated with hypercatabolic (generally septic) states, a "thick filament myopathy" related to corticosteroids and (usually) NMBAs, and a "necrotizing myopathy" characterized by prominent myonecrosis.[73] However, it is not clear that these are really distinct entities, and a recent editorial suggested the term *critical illness myopathy* be used as the sole descriptor for all instances of ICU-acquired myopathy.[86]

Like critical illness polyneuropathy, acute myopathy is usually manifested by generalized muscle weakness that becomes apparent once withdrawal of sedation allows an assessment of neuromuscular function. Although reflexes may be depressed or absent if myopathy is severe, sensation is intact. In severe cases, patients are unable to move their limbs, resulting in the commonly used descriptor "acute quadriplegic myopathy." On occasion, patients may not open their eyes in response to verbal commands, giving the impression of coma. When less severe, patients may have predominantly distal weakness, and both foot drop and wrist drop are common. In contrast to the frequent diaphragmatic involvement in critical illness polyneuropathy, asthmatic patients who develop myopathy often have relatively well-preserved inspiratory muscle function despite near-quadriplegic limb weakness.[80]

Serum creatine kinase (CK) levels may be elevated or normal, and can neither establish nor exclude an underlying myopathy as the cause of muscle weakness. The EMG reveals either normal or decreased CMAP amplitudes, depending on the degree of muscle involvement. Like critical illness polyneuropathy, needle EMG often reveals spontaneous fibrillations and positive sharp waves in resting muscle. However, with voluntary contractions there is a characteristic myopathic pattern of abundant low-amplitude, short-duration polyphasic units with early recruitment.[87] Pathologic findings in acute myopathy have been variable, with fiber atrophy and vacuolization in the absence of inflammation being the most common finding.[73] Although necrosis may be prominent, more often it is minimal or absent.[73] A key finding on electron microscopy is a selective loss of myosin, with relative sparing of actin and Z bands.[73] This pattern is very characteristic of ICU-acquired myopathy and is rarely seen in other disorders of muscle. A reduction in the myosin:actin ratio has also been documented by electrophoresis of needle aspirates of muscle, potentially offering a minimally invasive technique of diagnosing acute ICU-acquired thick filament myopathy.[88]

The underlying reason for the often near-quadriplegic muscle weakness in ICU-acquired myopathy is uncertain. Although myosin loss may interfere with normal contractility, another potential mechanism of weakness may be temporary muscle inexcitability. In a study of patients with severe ICU-acquired myopathy related to corticosteroids and NMBAs, Rich and colleagues found that they were unable to induce an action potential even when the muscle was stimulated directly.[89] Muscles later regained their ability to generate an action potential during clinical recovery.[89] In a subsequent study, inability to induce an action potential by direct muscle stimulation was also documented in a more heterogenous group of patients with ICU weakness, including a number of patients who were septic and had not received corticosteroids or NMBAs.[90] Studies in experimental animals suggest that muscle inexcitability may be due to impairment of sodium fast channels.[91]

POLYNEUROPATHY, MYOPATHY, OR "POLYNEUROMYOPATHY"

Differentiation of an axonal motor polyneuropathy and severe myopathy by EMG often rests upon the pattern of recruitment seen with voluntary muscle contraction, and inability to cooperate with the voluntary portion of the needle EMG may preclude reliable diagnosis. Marked reduction in sensory nerve amplitudes would indicate neuropathy, but tissue edema may limit the accuracy of sensory ENG, and it has been claimed that 40% to 60% of patients with critical illness polyneuropathy have normal sensory exams. Furthermore, the routine histopathologic findings in muscle biopsy specimens may be similar in myopathy and critical illness polyneuropathy. Therefore, a diagnostic dilemma is presented by patients who have a normal sensory ENG (or in whom sensory evaluation cannot be performed) and are unable to perform voluntary muscle contractions.

A recent study evaluated eight critically ill patients in whom a standard ENG/EMG and muscle histopathology could not differentiate a pure motor axonal neuropathy and a primary myopathy.[92] In all cases electron microscopy revealed a profound selective loss of myosin and normal sural nerve histology, indicating the presence of a primary myopathy rather than motor neuropathy as the cause of weakness.[92] A similar conclusion was reached when direct muscle stimulation was used to differentiate motor neuropathy and myopathy.[93] As noted earlier, muscle inexcitability has been documented in acute myopathy, but a motor neuropathy should not preclude generation of a normal CMAP in response to direct muscle stimulation. In a study of 22 consecutive patients in whom standard ENG/EMG was nondiagnostic, all but 1 patient had evidence of myopathy by direct muscle stimulation and quantitative EMG.[93] Another group has noted that with use of direct muscle stimulation they have never been able to document a single case of pure axonal motor neuropathy, and suggest that previously reported patients given the latter diagnosis almost certainly had a myopathy.[94] Direct muscle stimulation could eventually prove to be useful in the investigation of severe weakness in the ICU, because coma or deep sedation does not preclude its use.[84] It should be appreciated, however, that this technique is not as well-standardized as the routine EMG, and individual laboratories may need to establish their own normative data.

Recently, it has been suggested that some patients with ICU-acquired weakness have both an axonal polyneuropathy and myopathy. In one study muscle and nerve biopsies were performed in 24 patients with ICU-acquired weakness, all of whom had ENG/EMG evidence suggestive of polyneuropathy.[95] All but one had pathologic evidence of a myopathy and one third also had an axonal lesion. The authors concluded that polyneuropathy and myopathy often coexist. A recent prospective study of ICU-acquired paresis found that 22 patients in whom ENG/EMG could be performed uniformly had evidence of a sensorimotor axonal neuropathy, but each of the 10 patients who also underwent muscle biopsy had evidence of myopathy (type II fiber atrophy with myosinolysis).[96] This again suggested that both polyneuropathy and myopathy may coexist and together contribute to ICU-acquired weakness.

Although clarification of the underlying mechanisms of ICU-acquired weakness may be important from a research perspective, it is uncertain how it will affect individual patients in the ICU since there is no specific therapy. Indeed, it has been suggested that electrophysiologic and pathologic studies are of little practical value in the evaluation of weakness that is clearly acquired after the onset of critical illness, and that a purely clinical approach is adequate to define the presence of a critical illness weakness syndrome.[97] From a practical standpoint, the primary concern with omission of electrophysiologic studies would be missing a rare case of the Guillain-Barré syndrome, a disorder with specific therapy that may be triggered by acute nonneurologic critical illness (see above). In addition, the prognosis for recovery may be different with a pure myopathy and a severe axonal polyneuropathy (see below).

INTENSIVE CARE UNIT–ACQUIRED WEAKNESS: INCIDENCE AND RISK FACTORS

A number of studies have attempted to define the incidence of ICU-acquired weakness and the risk factors for its development. In general, two types of patient cohorts have been examined: those with status asthmaticus, and a more general ICU population in which sepsis, SIRS, and multiorgan failure were dominant.

STATUS ASTHMATICUS

Asthmatic patients who developed acute myopathy have uniformly received systemic corticosteroids while undergoing mechanical ventilation, and in the great majority of cases neuromuscular paralysis had been used to facilitate mechanical ventilation.[79–81] Two large retrospective studies found an identical 30% incidence of myopathy among mechanically ventilated asthmatic patients who had received an NMBA.[80,98] The risk of myopathy increases with the duration of paralysis. One prospective study found a striking relationship between the duration of paralysis and incidence of myopathy.[79] In a second retrospective study the mean duration of paralysis for patients who developed myopathy was 3.2 days, and 90% of patients had been paralyzed for more than 24 hours.[80] A third study also reported a mean duration of paralysis of 3 days among asthmatic patients who developed myopathy.[98] Although it was initially believed that myopathy may be related to use of steroidal NMBAs (vecuronium and pancuronium), the incidence of myopathy is similar with atracurium (a nonsteroidal NMBA) and vecuronium.[80]

These reports, as well as numerous additional publications, have suggested that mechanically ventilated patients with status asthmaticus who are treated with corticosteroids should be at minimal risk of developing acute myopathy as long as they have minimal or no exposure to NMBAs. Unfortunately, the data linking use of NMBAs with acute myopathy has been based almost entirely on retrospective analyses. In the single prospective study of myopathy in status asthmaticus, patients were uniformly paralyzed.[79] More recently, myopathy has been reported in mechanically ventilated patients with airflow obstruction who received corticosteroids and deep sedation, without paralysis.[83] Furthermore, our recent unpublished clinical experience has included a number of patients who developed severe myopathy despite minimal or no exposure to NMBAs. Therefore, while prolonged paralysis appears to increase the risk of myopathy in status asthmaticus, avoidance of NMBAs does not eliminate the risk of neuromuscular weakness.

In experimental animals a thick filament myopathy analogous to that seen in humans with status asthmaticus can be produced by combined denervation and corticosteroids, but not by either intervention alone.[99] Denervation results in a marked increase in the number of cytosolic corticosteroid receptors, but a similar effect is seen after limb immobilization by pinning and casting.[100,101] It is possible that the apparent enhancement of corticosteroid myotoxicity by prolonged paralysis in individuals with status asthmaticus is related to the induction of total muscle inactivity rather than denervation per se. This could explain the occurrence of severe myopathy in corticosteroid-treated patients who underwent deep sedation for many days.[83]

Sepsis, Systemic Inflammatory Response Syndrome, and Other Causes of Critical Illness

A number of studies have attempted to identify the incidence and risk factors for ICU-acquired weakness among populations of medical and surgical patients who had prolonged critical illness, usually as a result of sepsis and SIRS. The reported incidence of ICU-acquired weakness has varied widely due to differences in diagnostic criteria and case mix. A recent study prospectively screened 95 consecutive patients who had remained mechanically ventilated for 7 days and subsequently became sufficiently awake that they could answer simple questions.[96] Based on a complete clinical and electrophysiologic neuromuscular evaluation 1 week after awakening, clinically significant ICU-acquired paresis was diagnosed in 25% of patients.[96] Another prospective study found an incidence of 33% among patients who had been mechanically ventilated for more than 4 days.[102] When focusing on patients with sepsis and multiorgan failure, the incidence of clinically significant ICU-acquired neuromuscular disease appears to be much higher (70% to 82%).[103,104]

A variety of risk factors have been associated with risk for the development of weakness during critical illness. Sepsis is believed to be a major risk factor for ICU-acquired weakness. Although some studies found Acute Physiology and Chronic Health Evaluation (APACHE) II scores to be of no prognostic utility, a recent study found higher APACHE III score and presence of SIRS increased the risk of neuromuscular complications.[102] Duration of mechanical ventilation has also been associated with increased risk, as has the presence of multiorgan dysfunction.[96]

Despite their putative role in status asthmaticus–related myopathy, the contribution of corticosteroids and NMBAs to weakness that occurs in a mixed ICU population, in which sepsis, SIRS, and multiorgan dysfunction predominate, is uncertain.[105] Although one multicenter prospective study found corticosteroid therapy to be a strong risk factor for ICU-acquired paresis,[96] most studies have not found a relationship between corticosteroid use and ICU-acquired weakness.[105] Similarly, most studies involving mixed ICU populations have found no relationship between NMBA use and persistent muscle weakness.[95,102]

OUTCOME

The rate of recovery from ICU-acquired weakness has varied greatly in different series. When weakness occurs in the setting of severe asthma treated with corticosteroids and NMBAs, recovery may require several weeks, but near-normal muscle function is sometimes evident within 10 to 14 days after severe quadriparesis.[87] A much longer recovery time has been found in studies involving a more diverse group of critically ill patients. In the first large study of critical illness polyneuropathy, survivors recovered over 3 to 6 months.[76] A recent prospective study of ICU-acquired paresis reported a median recovery time of 21 days, and a number of patients did not achieve near-normal muscle function for 2 to 3 months.[96] Another prospective study found that all survivors had recovered by 2 to 3 months.[104]

Although earlier studies suggested that ICU-acquired weakness is nearly always reversible, more recent studies have found that long-term, perhaps permanent, disability does occur. An evaluation of 109 survivors of acute respiratory distress syndrome found significant functional limitation at 1 year that was attributed in large part to muscle wasting and weakness.[71] A second study found that one third of patients who had spent more than a month in the ICU had persistent muscle weakness 1 to 5 years after discharge.[68] An evaluation of 19 patients who had been admitted to a rehabilitation unit due to severe ICU-acquired weakness found that one-third had persistent quadriparesis 2 years after discharge.[69] Finally, 11 of 13 patients in one study had incomplete recovery by clinical and electrophysiologic criteria 1 to 2 years after ICU discharge.[70] Together, these studies suggest the disturbing possibility that some patients with severe ICU-acquired weakness may never fully recover, and that the persistent muscle weakness may have a profound impact on overall function and quality of life.

TREATMENT AND PREVENTION

There is no specific treatment for ICU-acquired muscle weakness other than physical rehabilitation. Unfortunately, it may not be possible to easily prevent this complication in patients with either severe sepsis and multiorgan failure or severe, protracted status asthmaticus that requires use of corticosteroids and either prolonged deep sedation or neuromuscular paralysis. In essence, the risk of neuromuscular weakness may be largely determined by the severity and duration of the underlying illness, whether it be sepsis syndrome or status asthmaticus. Nonetheless, to the extent that near-total muscle inactivity may contribute to myopathy, it is possible that risk of the latter might be decreased by maintaining as much muscle activity as is safely possible. A group of researchers recently found that mandated withdrawal of sedatives to determine ongoing need helped avoid oversedation and shortened the total time of mechanical ventilation, without increasing the risk of complications.[106] It is possible that periods of sedation withdrawal could decrease the incidence of myopathy by permitting increased muscle activity, avoiding oversedation, and shortening the duration of ventilatory support. Finally, one large randomized study found that tight glycemic control improved overall outcome among surgical critically ill patients, including a significant reduction in the incidence of muscle weakness,[107] suggesting an additional strategy for prevention of ICU-acquired neuromuscular weakness.

References

1. Ropper AH: The Guillain-Barré syndrome. *N Engl J Med* 326: 1130, 1992.
2. Laghi F, Tobin MJ: Disorders of the respiratory muscles. *Am J Respir Crit Care Med* 168:10, 2003.
3. Drachman DB: Myasthenia gravis. *N Engl J Med* 330:1797, 1994.
4. Rochester DF, Esau SA: Assessment of ventilatory function in patients with neuromuscular disease. *Clin Chest Med* 15:751, 1994.
5. Ward NS, Hill NS: Pulmonary function testing in neuromuscular disease. *Clin Chest Med* 22:769, 2001.
6. Tobin MJ, Brochard L, Rossi A: ATS/ERS statement on respiratory muscle testing. Assessment of respiratory muscle function in the intensive care unit. *Am J Respir Crit Care Med* 166:610, 2002.
7. Chevrolet J-C, Deléamont P: Repeated vital capacity measurements as predictive parameters for mechanical ventilation need and weaning success in the Guillain-Barré syndrome. *Am Rev Respir Dis* 144:814, 1991.
8. Fulgham JR, Wijdicks EFM: Guillain-Barré syndrome. *Crit Care Clin* 13:1, 1997.
9. Ragette R, Mellies U, Schwake C, et al: Patterns and predictors of sleep disordered breathing in primary myopathies. *Thorax* 57:724, 2002.
10. Teitelbaum JS, Borel CE: Respiratory dysfunction in Guillain-Barré syndrome. *Clin Chest Med* 15:705, 1994.
11. Hahn AF: Guillain Barré syndrome. *Lancet* 352:635, 1998.
12. Bleck TP: Treatment strategies for patients with Guillain-Barré syndrome. *Crit Care Med* 21:641, 1993.
13. Lindenbaum Y, Kissel JT, Mendell JR: Treatment approaches for Guillain-Barré syndrome and chronic inflammatory demyelinating polyradiculoneuropathy. *Neurol Clin* 19:187, 2001.
14. Jacobs BC, Rothbarth PH, van der Meché FGA, et al: The spectrum of antecedent infections in Guillain-Barré syndrome. A case-control study. *Neurology* 51:1110, 1998.
15. Sharshar T, Chevret S, Bourdain F, et al: Early predictors of mechanical ventilation in Guillain-Barré syndrome. *Crit Care Med* 31:278, 2003.
16. Hahn AF: The challenge of respiratory dysfunction in Guillain-Barré syndrome. *Arch Neurol* 58:871, 2001.
17. Lawn ND, Fletcher DD, Henderson RD, et al: Anticipating mechanical ventilation in Guillain-Barré syndrome. *Arch Neurol* 58:893, 2001.
18. Lawn ND, Wijdicks EFM: Fatal Guillain-Barré syndrome. *Neurology* 52:635, 1999.
19. Plasma Exchange/Sandoglobulin Guillain-Barré Syndrome Trial Group. Randomized trial of plasma exchange, intravenous immunoglobulin, and combined treatments in Guillain-Barré syndrome. *Lancet* 349:225, 1997.
20. Fletcher DD, Lawn ND, Wolter TD, et al: Long-term outcome in patients with Guillain-Barré syndrome requiring mechanical ventilation. *Neurology* 54:2311, 2000.
21. Henderson RD, Lawn ND, Fletcher DD, et al: The morbidity of Guillain-Barré syndrome admitted to the intensive care unit. *Neurology* 60:17, 2003.
22. The Guillain-Barré syndrome Study Group: Plasmapheresis and acute Guillain-Barré syndrome. *Neurology* 35:1096, 1985.
23. Osterman PO, Fagius J, Lundemo G, et al: Beneficial effects of plasma exchange in acute inflammatory polyradiculoneuropathy. *Lancet* 2:1296, 1984.
24. French Cooperative Group on Plasma Exchange in Guillain-Barré Syndrome: Efficiency of plasma exchange in Guillain-Barré syndrome: A role of replacement fluids. *Ann Neurol* 22:753, 1987.
25. Raphael JC, Chevret S, Auriant I, et al: Treatment of adult Guillain-Barré syndrome: Indications for plasma exchange. *Transfusion Sci* 20:53, 1999.

26. Bouget J, Chevret S, Chastang C, et al: Plasma exchange morbidity in Guillain-Barré syndrome: Results from the French prospective, double-blind, randomized, multicenter study. *Crit Care Med* 21:651, 1993.

27. van der Merché FGA, Schmitz PIM, and the Dutch Guillain-Barré Study Group: A randomized trial comparing intravenous immune globulin and plasma exchange in Guillain-Barré syndrome. *N Engl J Med* 326:1123, 1992.

28. Buchwald B, Ahangari R, Weishaupt A, et al: Intravenous immunoglobulins neutralize blocking antibodies in Guillain-Barré syndrome. *Ann Neurol* 51:673, 2002.

29. Yuki N, Ang CW, Koga M, et al: Clinical features and response to treatment in Guillain-Barré syndrome associated with antibodies to GM_{1b} ganglioside. *Ann Neurol* 47:314, 2000.

30. Younger DS, Worrall BB, Penn AS: Myasthenia gravis: Historical perspective and overview. *Neurology* 48 (Suppl 5):S1, 1997.

31. Zulueta JJ, Fanburg BL: Respiratory dysfunction in myasthenia gravis. *Clin Chest Med* 15:683, 1994.

32. Dushay KM, Zibrak JD, Jensen WA: Myasthenia gravis presenting as isolated respiratory failure. *Chest* 97:232, 1990.

33. Putman MT, Wise RA: Myasthenia gravis and upper airway obstruction. *Chest* 109:400, 1996.

34. Berrouschot J, Baumann I, Kalischewskip P, et al: Therapy of myasthenic crisis. *Crit Care Med* 25:1228, 1997.

35. Thomas CE, Mayer SA, Gungor Y, et al: Myasthenic crisis: Clinical features, mortality, complications, and risk factors for prolonged intubation. *Neurology* 48:1253, 1997.

36. Mayer SA: Intensive care of the myasthenic patient. *Neurology* 48 (Suppl 5):S70, 1997.

37. Lennon VA: Serologic profile of myasthenia gravis and distinction from the Lambert-Eaton myasthenic syndrome. *Neurology* 48 (Suppl 5):S23, 1997.

38. Younger DS, Raksdawan N: Therapy in neuromuscular disease. *Neurol Clinics* 19:205, 2001.

39. Massey JM: Treatment of acquired myasthenia gravis. *Neurology* 48 (Suppl 5):S46, 1997.

40. Keenan SP, Alexander D, Road JD, et al: Ventilatory muscle strength and endurance in myasthenia gravis. *Eur Respir J* 8:1130, 1995.

41. Gajdos P, Chevret S, Clair B, et al: Clinical trial of plasma exchange and high-dose intravenous immunoglobulin in myasthenia gravis. *Ann Neurol* 41:789, 1997.

42. Qureshi AI, Choudhry MA, Akbar MS, et al: Plasma exchange versus intravenous immunoglobulin treatment in myasthenic crisis. *Neurology* 52:629, 1999.

43. Jaretzki III A: Thymectomy for myasthenia gravis: Analysis of the controversies regarding technique and results. *Neurology* 48:(Suppl 5):S52, 1997.

44. Drachman DB, Jones RJ, Brodsky RA, et al: Treatment of refractory myasthenia: "Rebooting" with high-dose cyclophosphamide. *Ann Neurol* 53:29, 2003.

45. Zaja F, Russo D, Fuga G, et al: Rituximab for myasthenia gravis developing after bone marrow transplant. *Neurology* 55:1062, 2000.

46. Edwards JCW, Leandro MJ, Cambridge G: B-lymphocyte depletion therapy in rheumatoid arthritis and other autoimmune disorders. *Biochem Soc Trans* 30:824, 2001.

47. Arnon SS, Schechter R, Inglesby TV, et al: Botulism toxin as a biologic weapon: medical and public health management. *JAMA* 285:1059, 2001.

48. Dworkin MS, Shoemaker PC, Anderson DE: Tick paralysis: 33 human cases in Washington State, 1946–1996. *Clin Infect Dis* 29:1435, 1999.

49. Dalakas MC: Polymyositis dermatomyositis, and inclusion-body myositis. *N Engl J Med* 325:1487, 1991.

50. Wortmann RL: Inflammatory and metabolic diseases of muscle, in Klippel JH (ed): *Primer on the Rheumatic Diseases*. Atlanta, Arthritis Foundation, 2001, p 369.

51. Tymms KE, Webb J: Dermatopolymyositis and other connective tissue diseases. A review of 105 cases. *J Rheumatol* 12:1140, 1985.

52. Schwartz MI: The lung in polymyositis. *Clin Chest Med* 19:701, 1998.

53. Haupt HM, Hutchins GM: The heart and cardiac conduction system in polymyositis-dermatomyositis: A clinicopathologic study of 16 autopsied patients. *Am J Cardiol* 50:998, 1982.

54. Schnabel A, Reuter M, Biederer J, et al: Interstitial lung disease in polymyositis and dermatomyositis: Clinical course and response to treatment. *Semin Arthritis Rheum* 32:273, 2003.

55. Douglas WW, Tazelaar HD, Hartman TE, et al: Polymyositis-dermatomyositis associated interstitial lung disease. *Am J Respir Crit Care Med* 164:1182, 2001.

56. Arakawa H, Yamada H, Kurihara Y, et al: Nonspecific interstitial pneumonia associated with polymyositis and dermatomyositis. *Chest* 123:1096, 2003.

57. Fafalak RG, Peterson MGE, Kagen LJ: Strength in polymyositis and dermatomyositis: Best outcome in patients treated early. *J Rheumatol* 21:643, 1994.

58. Joffe MM, Love LA, Leff RL, et al: Drug therapy of idiopathic inflammatory myopathies: predictors of response to prednisone, azathioprine and methotrexate and a comparison of their efficacy. *Am J Med* 94:379, 1993.

59. Cherin P, Pelletier S, Teixeira A, et al: Results and long-term follow-up of intravenous immunoglobulin infusions in chronic refractory polymyositis: An open study with thirty-five adult patients. *Arthritis Rheum* 46:467, 2002.

60. Marie I, Hachulla E, Levesque H, et al: Intravenous immunoglobulins as treatment of life threatening esophageal involvement in polymyositis and dermatomyositis. *J Rheumatol* 26:2706, 1999.

61. Clay AS, Behnia M, Brown KK, et al: Mitochondrial disease. A pulmonary and critical-care medicine perspective. *Chest* 120:634, 2001.

62. Chinnery PF, Turnbull DM: Mitochondrial DNA and disease. *Lancet* 354:(Suppl 1): 17, 1999.

63. DiMauro S, Schon EA: Mitochondrial respiratory-chain diseases. *N Engl J Med* 348:2656, 2003.

64. Flaherty KR, Wald J, Weisman IM, et al: Unexplained exertional limitation. Characterization of patients with a mitochondrial myopathy. *Am J Respir Crit Care Med* 164:425, 2001.

65. Stacpoole PW: Lactic acidosis and other mitochondrial disorders. *Metabolism* 46:306, 1997.

66. Lacomis D, Petrella JT, Giuliani MJ: Causes of neuromuscular weakness in the intensive care unit: A study of ninety-two patients. *Muscle Nerve* 21:610, 1998.

67. Sliwa JA: Acute weakness syndromes in the critically ill patient. *Arch Phys Med Rehabil* 81(3 Suppl 1):S45, 2000.

68. Fletcher SN, Kennedy DD, Ghosh IR, et al: Persistent neuromuscular and neurophysiologic abnormalities in long-term survivors of prolonged critical illness. *Crit Care Med* 31:1012, 2003.

69. de Seze M, Petit H, Wiart L, et al: Critical illness polyneuropathy. A 2-year follow-up study in 19 severe cases. *Eur Neurol* 43:61, 2000.

70. Zifko U: Long-term outcome of critical illness polyneuropathy. *Muscle Nerve* 9:S49, 2000.

71. Herridge MS, Cheung AM, Tansey CM, et al, and the Canadian Critical Care Trials Group: One-year outcomes in survivors of the acute respiratory distress syndrome. *N Engl J Med* 348:683, 2003.

72. Bolton CF, Gilbert JJ, Hahn AF, Sibbald WJ: Polyneuropathy in critically ill patients. *J Neurol Neurosurg Psychiatry* 47:1223, 1984.

73. Hund E: Myopathy in critically ill patients. *Crit Care Med* 27:2544, 1999.

74. Segredo V, Caldwell JE, Matthay MA, et al: Persistent paralysis in critically ill patients after long-term administration of vecuronium. *N Engl J Med* 327:524, 1992.

75. Bednarik J, Lukas Z, Vondracek P: Critical illness polyneuromyopathy: The electrophysiological components of a complex entity. *Intensive Care Med* 29:1505, 2003.

76. Zochodne DW, Bolton CF, Wells GA, et al: Critical illness polyneuropathy. A complication of sepsis and multiple organ failure. *Brain* 110(Pt 4):819, 1987.

77. Bolton CF, Young GB, Zochodne DW: The neurological complications of sepsis. *Ann Neurol* 33:94, 1993.

78. MacFarlane I, Rosenthal F: Severe myopathy after status asthmaticus. *Lancet* 2:615, 1977.

79. Douglass J, Tuxen D, Horne M, et al: Myopathy in severe asthma. *Am Rev Respir Dis* 146:517, 1992.

80. Leatherman JW, Fluegel W, David W, et al: Muscle weakness in mechanically ventilated patients with severe asthma. *Am J Respir Crit Care Med* 153:1686, 1996.

81. Griffin D, Fairman N, Coursin D, et al: Acute myopathy during treatment of status asthmaticus with corticosteroids and steroidal muscle relaxants. *Chest* 102:510, 1992.

82. Deconinck N, Van Parijs V, Beckers-Bleukx G, Van den Bergh P: Critical illness myopathy unrelated to corticosteroids or neuromuscular blocking agents. *Neuromuscul Disord* 8(3–4):186, 1998.

83. Hanson P, Dive A, Brucher J-M, et al: Acute corticosteroid myopathy in intensive care patients. *Muscle Nerve* 20:1371, 1997.

84. Rich MM, Bird S, Raps, et al: Direct muscle stimulation in acute quadriplegic myopathy. *Muscle Nerve* 20:665, 1997.

85. Williams TJ, O'Hehir R, Czarny D, et al: Acute myopathy in severe acute asthma treated with intravenously administered corticosteroids. *Am Rev Respir Dis* 137:460, 1988.

86. Lacomis D, Zochodne DW, Bird SJ: Critical illness myopathy. *Muscle Nerve* 23:1785, 2000.

87. David WS, Roehr CL, Leatherman JW: EMG findings in acute myopathy with status asthmaticus, steroids and paralytics. Clinical and electrophysiologic correlation. *Electromyogr Clin Neurophysiol* 38:371, 1998.

88. Stibler H, Edstrom L, Ahlbeck K, et al: Electrophoretic determination of the myosin/actin ratio in the diagnosis of critical illness myopathy. *Intensive Care Med* 29:1515, 2003.

89. Rich M, Teener J, Raps E, et al: Muscle is electrically inexcitable in acute quadriplegic myopathy. *Neurology* 46:731, 1996.

90. Rich MM, Bird SJ, Raps EC, et al: Direct muscle stimulation in acute quadriplegic myopathy. *Muscle Nerve* 20:665, 1997.

91. Rich MM, Pinter MJ: Crucial role of sodium channel fast inactivation in muscle fibre inexcitability in a rat model of critical illness myopathy. *J Physiol* 547(Pt 2):555, 2003.

92. Sander HW, Golden M, Danon MJ: Quadriplegic areflexic ICU illness: selective thick filament loss and normal nerve histology. *Muscle Nerve* 26:499, 2002.

93. Trojaborg W, Weimer LH, Hays AP: Electrophysiologic studies in critical illness associated weakness: Myopathy or neuropathy—a reappraisal. *Clin Neurophysiol* 112:1586, 2001.

94. Teener JW, Rich MM, Bird SJ: Other causes of acute weakness in the intensive care unit, in Miller DH, Raps EC (eds): *Critical Care Neurology*. Blue Books of Practical Neurology Vol. 22. Boston, Butterworth-Heinemann, 1999, p 69.

95. Coakley JH, Nagendran K, Yarwood GD, et al: Patterns of neurophysiological abnormality in prolonged critical illness. *Intensive Care Med* 24:801, 1998.

96. De Jonghe B, Sharshar T, Lefaucheur JP, et al: Paresis acquired in the intensive care unit: A prospective multicenter study. *JAMA* 288:2859, 2002.

97. Morris C, Trinder J: Electrophysiology adds little to clinical signs in critical illness polyneuropathy and myopathy. *Crit Care Med* 30:2612, 2002.

98. Behbehani NA, Al-Mane F, D'yachkova Y, et al: Myopathy following mechanical ventilation for acute severe asthma: The role of muscle relaxants and corticosteroids. *Chest* 115:1627, 1999.

99. Rouleau G, Karpati G, Carpenter S, et al: Glucocorticoid excess induces preferential depletion of myosin in denervated skeletal muscle fibres. *Muscle Nerve* 10:428, 1987.

100. Dubois DC, Almon RR: A possible role for glucocorticoids in denervation atrophy. *Muscle Nerve* 4:370, 1981.

101. Dubois DC, Almon RR: Disuse atrophy of skeletal muscle is associated with an increase in number of glucocorticoid receptors. *Endocrinology* 107:1649, 1980.

102. de Letter MA, Schmitz PI, Visser LH, et al: Risk factors for the development of polyneuropathy and myopathy in critically ill patients. *Crit Care Med* 29:2281, 2001.

103. Witt NJ, Zochodne DW, Bolton CF, et al: Peripheral nerve function in sepsis and multiple organ failure. *Chest* 99:176, 1991.

104. Berek K, Margreiter J, Willeit J, et al: Polyneuropathies in critically ill patients: A prospective evaluation. *Intensive Care Med* 22:849, 1996.

105. van Mook WN, Hulsewe-Evers RP: Critical illness polyneuropathy *Curr Opin Crit Care* 8:302, 2002.

106. Kress JP, Pohlman AS, O'Connor MF, Hall JB: Daily interruption of sedative infusions in critically ill patients undergoing mechanical ventilation. *N Engl J Med* 342:1471, 2000.

107. van den Berghe G, Wouters P, Weekers F, et al: Intensive insulin therapy in the critically ill patients. *N Engl J Med* 345:1359, 2001.

Chapter 67 _____
COMA, PERSISTENT VEGETATIVE STATE, AND BRAIN DEATH

AXEL J. ROSENGART, ROBERTA L. NOVAKOVIC,
AND JEFFREY I. FRANK

KEY POINTS

- *The neuroanatomy of coma can be divided into three major categories: diffuse brain dysfunction or bithalamic injury, primary brain stem disorders, and secondary brain stem compression from supratentorial and infratentorial mass lesions.*

- *Most cases of coma are due to metabolic disorders or exogenous drug intoxication.*

- *Patient evaluation must follow an orderly sequence, beginning with vital signs, general physical examination, and neurologic examination.*

- *The most important single sign distinguishing toxic-metabolic coma from primary brain disease is the presence of pupillary light responses.*

- *The neurologic examination of the patient in coma is brief and focuses on (1) level of consciousness, (2) pupils, (3) eye movements, (4) motor responses, and (5) respiratory pattern.*

- *Computed tomographic (CT) scanning of the brain is the most valuable acute test to rule out structural causes of coma.*

- *Hypoxic-ischemic encephalopathy after cardiopulmonary arrest or shock states may be ameliorated by aggressive measures to increase cerebral blood flow after resuscitation.*

- *Serial neurologic examination over the first 72 hours is most helpful to determine the prognosis for patients with atraumatic coma; for anoxic brain injury, failure to recover pupillary responses or corneal reflexes in the first 24 hours is a poor prognostic sign.*

- *As therapies aimed at cerebral resuscitation and preservation following acute injury are developed and proved efficacious, prior guidelines for determining prognosis will require redefinition and reconfirmation.*

- *The Uniform Determination of Death Act states that "an individual who has sustained either (1) irreversible cessation of circulatory and respiratory functions, or (2) irreversible cessation of all functions of the entire brain, including the brain stem, is dead."*

- *The determination of death by brain criteria is based on clinical examination, and in most cases does not require confirmatory tests. However, the cause of coma must be known, and the cause must be sufficient to explain irreversible cessation of whole brain function.*

Normal and Impaired Consciousness: A Conceptual Approach

Consciousness is a difficult term to define, and even more complicating is the fact that many different meanings and classification systems exist for the various states of decreased level of consciousness, such as drowsiness, stupor, and coma. For practical reasons, however, in the evaluation of consciousness most clinicians give greater weight to the patient's responses and behavior than to what the patient says. Hence, consciousness can be defined in its simplest form as the patient's *awareness of self and environment* and the *responsiveness to his or her needs and external stimulation*. The level of consciousness used in clinical practice refers to the state of arousal and should be separated from the *content* of consciousness, which describes various forms of cognitive behaviors and thinking. An awake person is fully responsive (alert) to stimuli and is able to specify an awareness of self and environment.

Impaired consciousness is generally categorized by the level of responsiveness to external and internal stimuli (Table 67-1). *Drowsiness* ("lethargy") is a state of reduced physical and mental activity and a drowsy person can often not sustain wakefulness without external stimulation. It is similar in appearance to light sleep and almost always accompanied by reduced attention and concentration span and mild confusion. A *stuporous* patient requires repeated, stronger stimuli to arouse and quickly drifts back to persistent inactivity when the stimulus is withdrawn. When aroused, this patient may or may not open his or her eyes and partially respond to requests. At times restlessness and motor stereotypes are observed. *Sopor*, the Latin word for deep sleep and a term used in some European countries, denotes an intermediate state between stupor and coma. *Coma* (from the Greek *komas*, or deep sleep) is a state of unresponsiveness in which the patient is incapable of arousing to external or internal stimuli (lack of alertness). The degree of coma can vary from lighter stages (also denoted as *semicoma*) with observed changes in autonomic function or brief moaning to strong stimulation, to the deepest stage with absence of any brain stem responses (e.g., pupillary and corneal reflexes), cyclic autonomic activity, and motor tone. *Sleep* and pathologic states of consciousness undeniably share some common features; for example, the sleeping person is not aware of him- or herself and in this respect is unconscious. Of course, the important difference is that a sleeping person can be aroused to full consciousness. Furthermore, electrodiagnostic evaluation differs in the two conditions (see below) and cerebral glucose uptake does not decrease during sleep but does so in coma. For in-depth discussions of this topic the reader is referred to the major textbooks in neurology and to the seminal work by Plum and Posner.[1]

A *vegetative state* can follow coma and identifies a state in which brain stem and diencephalic (thalamic) activity is present to a degree that clinical signs of arousal are observed.[2] This condition is without meaningful mental function. The patients often show blink responses to light; intermittent eye movements (sometimes erroneously interpreted as following objects or looking at family members); stimulus-sensitive automatisms such as swallowing, bruxism, and moaning, as well as primitive motor responses and cycles of sleeping and waking. However, despite the appearance of wakefulness, the

TABLE 67-1 Clinical Levels of Altered Consciousness

Terms	Eyes	Arousability	Content
Lethargy	Closed	Arousable	Mildly impaired
Stupor	Closed	Arousable with effort	Markedly impaired
Coma	Closed	Unarousable	Not applicable
Akinetic mutism[a] (abulic state, coma vigil)	Open	Wakeful	Impaired
Locked-in syndrome[b]	Open	Wakeful	Normal

[a] Secondary to bilateral frontal/basal forebrain dysfunction.
[b] Secondary to basis pontis dysfunction.

patient's cerebral function remains severely impaired with total inattention and unawareness. If this state is long-lasting it is referred to as *persistent vegetative state* (PVS) and is used as a descriptive clinical syndrome rather than a disease-specific entity. The most common causes include cardiac arrest, head trauma, and various causes of thalamic necrosis. Vegetative states can also be seen in the terminal phase of degenerative illnesses such as Alzheimer's disease. Ambiguous terms for PVS such as apallic syndrome and neocortical death should be avoided.[3,4] *Minimal conscious state* can be diagnosed in patients displaying inconsistent behavioral evidence of awareness of the environment, but they cannot communicate and are unable to follow instructions reliably[5] (Table 67-2).

Clinical practice teaches that *consciousness* should be viewed as a continuum between different pathological conditions and not as an all-or-none phenomenon,[1] and that it is frequently difficult to identify definite signs of conscious perception of environment and self in patients with severe brain injuries. The latter limits the diagnostic certainty of remaining brain function on clinical grounds since the identification of consciousness relies purely on the deduction whether consciousness is present or absent in a particular patient.[2]

Recent data obtained in patients with PVS helps to reveal the critical brain areas involved in consciousness. Extensive loss and severe neuronal damage is causally related to loss of consciousness in patients with PVS, a finding supported by a study identifying decreased cortical radiolabeled flumazenil uptake (a benzodiazepine antagonist and neuronal marker).[6] In corroboration, several studies consistently identified decreased cerebral glucose metabolism and blood flow.[7,8] However, brain regions with the most consistent decrease in cerebral glucose consumption in patients in PVS are the polymodal association areas of the frontal, temporal, and parietal lobes[9]; interestingly, normal subjects display

higher brain metabolism during wakefulness than in sleep in similar regions.[10] Furthermore, thalamocortical disconnections can be identified using auditory and sensory external stimulations.[11]

Some carefully performed studies identified patients with PVS who activate primary and associative cortex, depending on the complexity and familiarity of the test stimuli.[12,13] It is, however, unclear whether the identified activations represent consciousness since no conclusions to the connectivity of thalamocortical brain regions and larger neuronal networks can be drawn. Similarly, brain plasticity with recovery of functional thalamocortical connections and reestablishment of neuronal networks may allow certain patients to regain consciousness after severe brain injury and PVS.[9] In recent years we have gained much insight into which brain areas seem necessary for conscious experience; however, future research should broaden our knowledge about what form of brain activity in these areas confers consciousness.

Impaired Consciousness: An Anatomic Approach

Because coma is a sleeplike state, it is not surprising to find that the neuroanatomy of coma is closely related to brain stem centers that regulate daily cycles of wakefulness and sleep: the reticular activating system (RAS). In animals the RAS lies within the center of the brain stem, extending from the midbrain into the hypothalamus and thalamus.[14,15] Electrical stimulation of this region in a sleeping animal produces arousal, and ablation causes coma. Lesions in the pathways of the brain stem reticular formation or RAS have the greatest impact on changes in consciousness.

TABLE 67-2 Characteristics of the Persistent Vegetative State (PVS) and Related Conditions

Condition	Self-Awareness	Sleep-Wake Cycles	Motor Function	Experience Suffering	EEG Activity
PVS	Absent	Intact	No purposeful movement	No	Polymorphic delta or theta, sometimes slow alpha
Coma	Absent	Absent	No purposeful movement	No	Polymorphic delta or theta
Brain death	Absent	Absent	None or only spinal reflex movements	No	Electrocerebral silence
Locked-in syndrome	Present	Intact	Quadriplegia and pseudobulbar palsy; eye movements preserved	Yes	Normal or minimally abnormal
Akinetic mutism	Present	Intact	Paucity of movement	Yes	Nonspecific slowing

SOURCE: Adapted from ref. 8 with permission.

The RAS is a loosely organized core of polysynaptic neurons reaching in the brain stem from the lower medulla through the paramedian pons to central midbrain. At the diencephalic level it includes several functionally related nuclei in the thalami (especially the medial thalamus) and cerebral projections are prominent to the inferomedial frontal lobes, but also reach almost all cerebral cortex. The essential role of the RAS is arousal and maintenance of wakefulness; injury leads to reduction or failure of arousal. As the brain stem RAS receives direct spinothalamic information, incoming sensory stimulations are not only projected to the sensory cortices, but are also needed to activate the brain stem RAS for the maintenance of consciousness. Within the brain stem and thalamus the RAS is confined to rather small anatomic areas; therefore even small lesions can severely impair arousal and consciousness. In contrast, RAS fibers are sparse and spread out as they move towards the cerebral hemispheres, hence only larger cortical lesions will lead to impaired consciousness at that level.

Lesions in the medulla and lower pons need to be quite large to induce significant coma (loss of awareness) since the RAS is rather thinned in these regions. More commonly, lesions in the *ventral pons* (such as basilar artery occlusions) lead to severe motor pathway injury sparing somatosensory and ascending RAS (arousal) systems. This state is referred to as *locked-in syndrome* or de-efferented state, as the patient has preserved consciousness. However, the patient cannot speak or respond and is unable to move cranial, trunk, or extremity muscles, but retains the ability for vertical gaze and eye blinking. In contrast, vascular occlusions of the top of the basilar artery or the posterior cerebral arteries result in injuries to the *midbrain* or *medial thalami* which lead to significant impairment of consciousness but no or only minimal focal neurologic findings.

Traumatic brain shearing injury can lead to slit-like hemorrhages and ischemia or inflammatory to necrotizing lesions of the midbrain, resulting in impaired consciousness. Cerebral masses can produce either direct or indirect (uncal or tentorial herniation) displacement and torsions of the midbrain and reduced alertness. *Akinetic mutism* refers to patients who are silent and apathetic with greatly reduced activity and no focal findings on examination. A number of pathologic lesions have been described, often associated with inferior frontal lobe damage bilaterally. Sudden injury to either or both cerebral hemispheres may produce impaired consciousness, indicating that wakefulness has no hemispheric dominance and requires some cerebral function. Bilateral, extensive acute or subacute damage to the cortex and white matter, for example due to trauma, hypoxia, or infection, impairs activation of the upper RAS, leading to impaired consciousness. Notably, even large cortical (lobar) areas can be injured and initially not affect consciousness at all until secondary injury from swelling and bleeding occurs, as evidenced by patients with penetrating wounds of the cerebral hemispheres who remain fully awake. Similarly, degenerative disorders such as Alzheimer's disease generally do not or only minimally affect the RAS since these patients remain fully awake. *Hypersomnia* refers to a condition of excessive drowsiness and sleep. It may occur in the setting of narcolepsy, hypothalamic disorders, sleep disorders, or psychiatric illness.

Several categories of consciousness-impairing mechanisms and lesions can be defined. First, one cause is an easily identifiable mass lesion compressing the upper RAS either directly or indirectly (such as tumor, abscess, meningitis, or hemorrhage); second, discrete lesions of the upper brain stem (examples are outlined above) may be the cause; and third, a larger group of patients includes those in whom suppression of the RAS is induced by metabolic derangements, toxic states, or seizures. Such functional causes of coma may be reversible by correcting the underlying metabolic derangement or removing the offending drug. "Metabolic" coma is likely the most common etiologic category resulting in impaired consciousness in medical critical care units.

The neuroanatomy of consciousness is not linked to any specific motor, sensory, or cognitive function. Coma and specific focal signs of neurologic damage may occur together or independently. Therefore, patients in coma can be divided into two major clinical categories: coma with or coma without focal neurologic signs. This simple division is often the best way to identify primary neurologic disease as the cause for coma.

Examination of the Comatose Patient: A Clinical Approach

Acute depression in level of consciousness is a critical, life-threatening emergency that requires a systematic approach for evaluation of etiology. The variety of causes of coma are myriad. Therefore, a reliable history should be obtained from family, witnesses, or medical personnel, and examination should seek representative localizing neurological and general physical findings.

HISTORICAL FEATURES

Clues can be ascertained from the onset of coma. An acute onset in a previously healthy individual may indicate a cerebral vascular etiology (i.e., subarachnoid hemorrhage, intracerebral hemorrhage, or hemispheric or brain stem stroke), generalized epileptic activity, traumatic brain injury, or drug overdose. Likewise, a subacute deterioration may point to systemic illness, evolving intracranial mass, or a degenerative infectious or paraneoplastic neurologic disorder. Moreover, the duration of a comatose state should be documented because it may have predictive value for prognosis in certain causes.

GENERAL CLINICAL FEATURES AND PROTOCOL

Frequently the etiology of acute depression in consciousness in the hospitalized patient includes sepsis, acid-base and electrolyte disorders, or hepatic, renal, or cardiac failure. Therefore careful physical examination is performed with attention to vital signs, spontaneous breathing pattern, and careful auscultation of the lungs and heart (Table 67-3). Airway patency and protective reflexes should be assessed. Emergency measures should be taken to ensure vital functions continue despite an obscure diagnosis. Furthermore, laboratory studies should be obtained to exclude metabolic and endocrine causes.

During evaluation, core body temperature is an important clue. Hypothermia can be seen in drug overdose, brain death, or acute spinal cord transection. Moreover, hyperthermia can be seen in infection; traumatic brain injury; subarachnoid,

TABLE 67-3 Useful Physical Examination Findings in Comatose Patients

Exam Focus	Specific Features	Suggested Condition
Skin	Petechiae, splinter hemorrhage	Coagulopathy; SBE
	Icteric	Hepatic encephalopathy
	Needle tracks	Drug overdose or withdrawal
	Cyanotic	CO_2 narcosis
Lymph nodes	Adenopathy	Infectious etiologies; immunocompromised hosts
Head	Contusion; postauricular ecchymosis (Battle's sign)	Trauma
	VP shunt	Hydrocephalus; shunt malfunction
Eyes	Periorbital ecchymosis (raccoon eyes)	Trauma
	Papilledema	Increased intracranial pressure
Ears	Hemotympanum	Trauma
Nose	Excessive discharge	Trauma
Neck	Stiff	Subarachnoid hemorrhage, infection
	Enlarged thyroid	Dysthyroidism
Cardiovascular	Arrhythmia, etc.	Hypoxic/iechemic encephalopathy
Abdomen	Small hard liver	Hepatic encephalopathy
Misc.	Acetone, alcohol breath	Ketoacidosis; alcohol intoxication
	Fever	Infection
	Tongue laceration; incontinence	Postictal state

SBE, subacute bacterial endocarditis; VP, ventriculoperitoneal.

intracerebral, or pontine hemorrhage; and hypothalamic dysfunction.

NEUROLOGIC EXAMINATION

The neurologic exam in a patient with depressed level of consciousness can be a valuable tool to localize the etiology. The important neurologic features include (Table 67-4): (1) respiratory pattern, (2) pupillary size and reactivity, (3) eye position and movements, (4) corneal reflexes, and (5) motor function.

Assessment of Consciousness

The determination of the level of consciousness depends on analyzing arousability and content (see Table 67-1). Initially, observe whether the patient appears asleep or wakeful with spontaneous eye opening. In a sleeping patient, quantify how much stimulation is required to arouse the patient. Attempts

TABLE 67-4 Neurologic Assessment of the Comatose Patient

Level of consciousness
  Arousability
  Content
Brain stem function
  Respiratory rate and pattern
  Blood pressure and heart rate
  Pupil size and reactivity
  Eye position and movements
    Doll's eyes maneuver
    Cold caloric testing
  Corneal reflexes
  Facial symmetry
Motor function
  Posturing
  Tone
  Spontaneous movements
  Withdrawal to noxious stimulus
  Deep tendon reflexes

should be made to elicit a behavioral response by verbal command alone. If no response is obtained, then physical stimulation should be used, first by shaking the patient. Then noxious stimulation can be applied by digital pressure to the supraorbital nerves or nailbeds of the fingers or toes. Purposeful attempts by the patient to remove the offending stimulus indicate preservation of brain stem function and intact connections to the appropriate cerebral hemisphere. Eye opening, either spontaneous or in response to stimulation, indicates preserved function of the RAS in the upper brain stem and hypothalamus. Once aroused, the patient's ability to remain wakeful and respond coherently is determined.

Lethargy (or drowsiness), stupor, and coma represent different points on a continuum of decreasing levels of consciousness. Patients in these states appear to be sleeping with eyes closed. In contrast, patients with akinetic mutism and locked-in syndrome appear to be awake with eyes opened.

The Glasgow Coma Scale (Table 67-5) is used to assign a numerical description of consciousness. The scale was devised to evaluate patients with head injury and is most reliable and reproducible in trauma patients.[16,17] Its application in nontraumatic conditions is less reliable, but it is still the most widely used clinical scale to evaluate the level of consciousness. Furthermore, it provides a reproducible tool to monitor progression.

Respiratory Control

The cerebral cortex and forebrain are important in the control of regular respiration. Patients with isolated brain injury uncomplicated by other critical medical illnesses may have characteristic breathing patterns that aid in neuroanatomic localization (Fig. 67-1). However, these patterns are not reliable in patients with multiple organ system failure who are receiving mechanical ventilation. Nevertheless, a discussion is warranted.

Cheyne-Stokes respiration is a periodic breathing pattern in which periods of hyperpnea regularly alternate with apnea

TABLE 67-5 The Glascow Coma Scale[a]

Response	Points
Eye opening	
Spontaneously	4
To speech	3
To pain	2
Never	1
Best verbal response	
Oriented	5
Confused	4
Inappropriate	3
Garbled	2
None	1
Best motor response	
Obeys commands	6
Localizes pain	5
Withdrawal	4
Abnormal flexion	3
Extension	2
None	1
	15

[a] The lower the GCS score, the more severe the head injury.

in a smooth crescendo-decrescendo pattern. This neurogenic respiratory alteration occurs with damage to the cortex and forebrain bilaterally, or secondary to cardiac or respiratory failure. It is the result of the loss of frontal lobe control over respiratory patterns with excessive dependence on blood CO_2 levels to trigger brain stem respiratory centers.

Midbrain and upper pontine lesions may cause a central neurogenic hyperventilation syndrome with persistent deep hyperventilation. It can only be diagnosed with arterial blood gas measurements, since hyperventilation also occurs secondary to hypoxemia and acidemia. Likewise, metabolic disorders, especially the early stages of hepatic coma, cause central neurogenic hyperventilation.

Lesions of the middle or lower pons are characterized by deep prolonged inspiration followed by a long pause referred to as *apneustic breathing*. Most patients with this respiratory pattern require early intubation and mechanical ventilation.

Ataxic and irregular periodic breathing occurs with lesions in the dorsomedial medulla and may be accompanied by hypersensitivity to respiratory depressants. These patterns are not compatible with sustained life.

When assessing a comatose patient, the rate and pattern of respiration should be observed. In addition, vomiting and hiccups should be noted because they may result from intrinsic brain stem pathology or transmitted pressure on the brain stem. Furthermore, spontaneous yawning may occur in comatose patients. The neurogenic networks for this complex respiratory response are integrated in the lower brain stem.

Pupillary Size and Reactivity

In one study of 346 comatose patients, the pupillary reflex was shown to be the strongest prognostic variable for awakening when compared with evoked-potential studies.[18] Pupillary size is controlled by the autonomic nervous system and is dictated by the balance between sympathetic and parasympathetic input to the pupillary dilators and constrictors, respectively. The parasympathetic efferents to the pupil originate from the Edinger-Westphal nucleus in the upper midbrain and travel with the ipsilateral third cranial nerve (oculomotor). Dysfunction within this pathway will produce unopposed sympathetic input to the pupil and relative pupillary dilation ipsilateral to the lesion. The sympathetic efferents to the pupil originate in the hypothalamus, descend through the brain stem and cervical spinal cord, and exit the upper thoracic spinal cord (T1 to T3 levels). From this point they ascend the carotid sheath and follow the vasculature to the pupil. Any disruption of the sympathetic fibers along this loop can lead to unopposed parasympathetic pupillary activity and subsequently an ipsilateral small (miotic) pupil.

A light stimulus to one eye produces constriction of the ipsilateral pupil (direct response) and contralateral pupil (consensual response), through a network of connections. Table 67-6 summarizes the pupillary changes commonly seen in coma and their significance.

Small reactive pupils may be due to a toxic-metabolic disturbance. Very small pupils (pinpoint) that react to naloxone are characteristic of narcotic overdose. Pinpoint pupils that are poorly reactive are characteristic of pontine dysfunction. Lesions rostral or caudal to the midbrain may disrupt descending sympathetics and produce small pupils.

Bilateral, widely dilated, fixed pupils are due to sympathetic overactivity from an endogenous cause (seizures or severe anoxic ischemia) or exogenous catecholamines (dopamine or norepinephrine) or atropine-like drugs.

Since the midbrain is the one location in the brain stem where parasympathetic and sympathetic pupillary fibers are adjacent, a midbrain lesion classically results in intermediate pupil size. Such pupils are seen in brain death and severe midbrain injuries.

A unilaterally dilated, unreactive pupil in a comatose patient may be caused by herniation of the ipsilateral temporal uncus through the tentorium, which compresses the ipsilateral oculomotor nerve and its parasympathetic fibers. In this

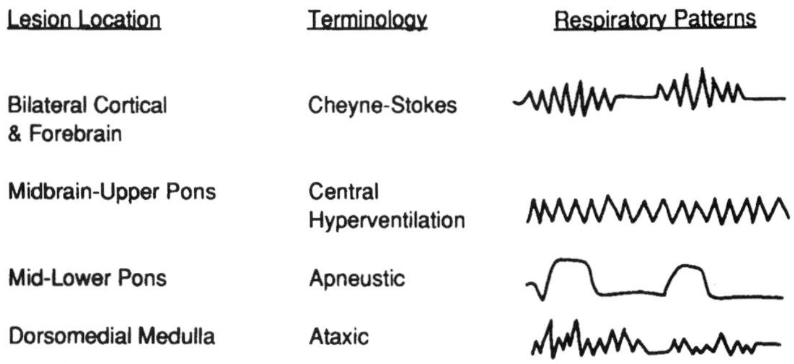

Lesion Location	Terminology	Respiratory Patterns
Bilateral Cortical & Forebrain	Cheyne-Stokes	
Midbrain-Upper Pons	Central Hyperventilation	
Mid-Lower Pons	Apneustic	
Dorsomedial Medulla	Ataxic	

FIGURE 67-1 Respiratory patterns in coma.

TABLE 67-6 Pupillary Changes in Coma

Size	Reactivity	Comments
Bilateral		
Normal or small	Normal	Toxic-metabolic disturbance
Midposition (3–5 mm)	Poor	Midbrain dysfunction; drugs (glutethimide [Doriden])
Small (pinpoint)	Poor	Pontine dysfunction; drugs (narcotics)
Large	Poor	Toxic-metabolic disturbance (anoxia); drugs (anticholinergics)
Unilateral		
Large	Unreactive	Ipsilateral midbrain pathology or compression of ipsilateral CN III: uncal herniation, posterior communicating artery aneurysm
Small	Minimal	Ipsilateral sympathetic dysfunction

setting, the large pupil is eventually accompanied by other evidence of cranial nerve (CN) III disruption (i.e., ipsilateral eye deviation inferolaterally). In the setting of head trauma, this implies an ipsilateral epidural, subdural, or intracerebral hematoma. In nontraumatic conditions, it usually occurs with large cerebral infarcts, spontaneous intracerebral hematoma, or supratentorial brain tumors.

Eye position and Movement

The eye muscles are controlled by three sets of cranial nerves, CN III, CN IV (trochlear), and CN VI (abducens), their nuclei being located in the upper midbrain, lower midbrain, and pontomedullary junction, respectively. Proper eye movement control requires a network of interconnections between these nuclei so that the eyes move conjugately. This interconnection is referred to as the medial longitudinal fasciculus (MLF), which is also integrated with the vestibular nuclei and allows

for reflex conjugate eye movement in response to positional head changes.

Figure 67-2 displays the relevant anatomy accounting for horizontal conjugate eye movements. Each frontal eye field controls gaze to the contralateral side by stimulating the contralateral pontine paramedian reticular formation (PPRF) at the pontomedullary junction. Lesions of the frontal eye fields or the PPRFs lead to conjugate eye deviation, provided that the MLF is intact. Therefore, a lesion of the right frontal eye field or left PPRF impairs leftward gaze, and thus the eyes conjugately deviate to the right. In short, the eyes turn toward the lesion with frontal eye field dysfunction and away from the lesion with PPRF dysfunction. In contrast, MLF lesions are manifested as poor adduction of the eye ipsilateral to the MLF lesion. Spontaneous "roving" eye movements in all directions in the comatose patient demonstrate integrity of a significant portion of the brain stem. If no spontaneous eye movements are observed, the intactness of the interconnections

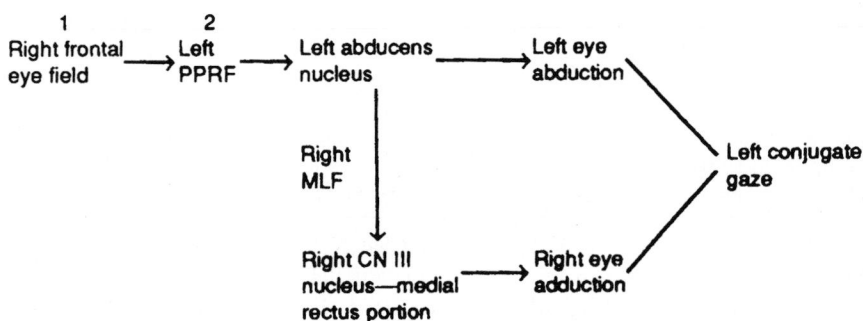

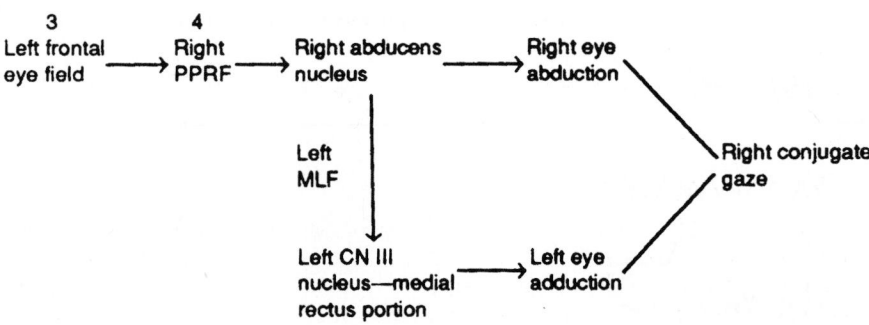

FIGURE 67-2 Schematic representation of the neurologic pathways controlling horizontal conjugate gaze. PPRF, pontine paramedian reticular formation; MLF, median longitudinal fasciculus; CN III, third cranial nerve; 1–4, sites of possible pathologic lesions (see text).

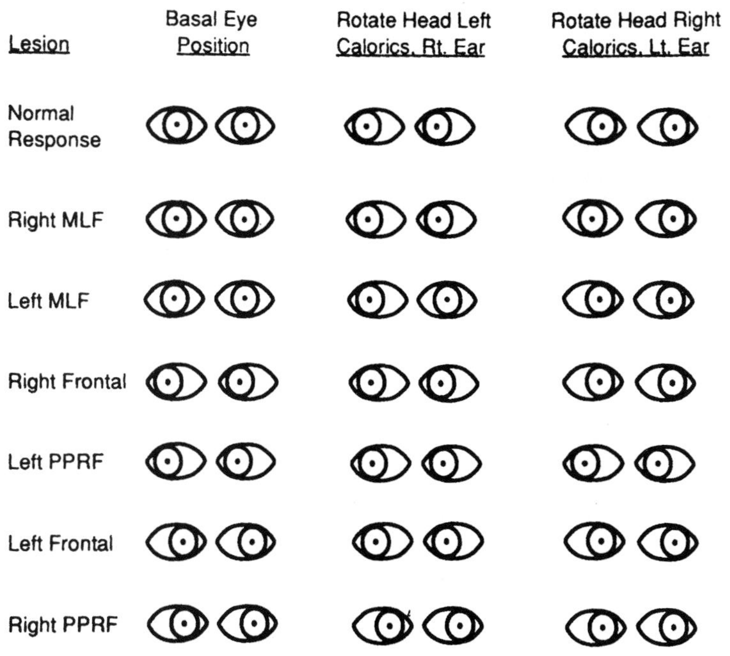

Lesion	Basal Eye Position	Rotate Head Left Calorics, Rt. Ear	Rotate Head Right Calorics, Lt. Ear
Normal Response			
Right MLF			
Left MLF			
Right Frontal			
Left PPRF			
Left Frontal			
Right PPRF			

FIGURE 67-3 Eye positions in the doll's eye maneuver and with cold caloric testing in coma. MLF, median longitudinal fasciculus; PPRF, pontine paramedian reticular formation.

responsible for eye control is in question. Since comatose patients are unable to follow commands, maneuvers that take advantage of vestibular input to ocular control must be utilized.

An oculocephalic reflex (doll's eye maneuver) is performed by rapidly rotating the head from side to side and observing the patient's eye positional changes (Fig. 67-3). The normal response in the comatose patient with intact brain stem is for the eyes to remain fixed on the same point in space. Thus when the head is turned rightward, the eyes move to the left. When the head is turned leftward, the eyes move conjugately to the right. If a comatose patient does not have normal doll's eyes, a disruption of brain stem ocular and vestibular connections may be present. Of course, in the setting of trauma, the head should not be rotated due to the possibility of cervical spine injury. In this situation or when doll's eye maneuvers are inconclusive, cold water calorics are helpful.

Oculovestibular reflexes (cold water caloric testing) depend on vestibular system stimulation by altering endolymphatic flow in the semicircular canals. The change in endolymphatic flow is achieved by instilling ice-cold water in the external auditory canal, thereby cooling the mastoid process, and in turn the semicircular canal. Prior to performing this test, the external auditory canal should be examined to confirm intactness of the tympanic membrane and remove any impacted cerumen. The head should then be elevated 30 degrees. A functional apparatus for instilling the water is a butterfly catheter (with the needle removed) connected to a syringe containing approximately 100 mL of cold water.

The responses to cold water in patients with various lesions are summarized in Fig. 67-3. In normal wakeful patients the response is horizontal nystagmus, with the slow phase toward and the fast phase away from the stimulated side and with minimal eye movement from the midline. With diminishing consciousness in patients without structural brain stem damage, the fast phase of the nystagmus disappears, and the eyes tend to deviate conjugately toward the stimulated side. Structural brain stem disease eliminates the caloric response, as does inner ear disease, deep drug coma, and anticonvulsant drug overdose. In order to ensure proper interpretation of cold water caloric testing, the opposite side should not be stimulated until 5 minutes after the initial side.

Corneal Reflex

The corneal reflex is an important protective mechanism for the cornea. it is a blinking reflex triggered when the cornea is presented with a noxious stimulus. The afferent limb is via the trigeminal nerve (CN V), and the efferent limb is via the facial nerve (CN VII). Although corneal reflexes assess brain stem function, they have limited localizing value.

Motor Function

The corticospinal tract predominantly originates from the frontal cortex and descends ipsilaterally through the corona radiata, the posterior limb of the internal capsule, and the cerebral peduncle of the midbrain and consolidates in the pyramids, the ventral swellings of the medulla. The pyramidal fibers decussate to the contralateral side at the junction of the medulla and spinal cord to form the lateral corticospinal tract.

Observation is the key to the motor examination in the comatose patient. The patient is observed for spontaneous movements or maintenance of particular postures. Lesions involving the corticospinal tract generally lead to diminished contralateral spontaneous activity. Upper midbrain or more rostral lesions may lead to decorticate posturing characterized by flexion of the contralateral arm at the elbow and hyperextension of the leg. Central midbrain and high pontine lesions, with a relatively intact brain stem inferiorly, may lead to decerebrate posturing characterized by contralateral arm and leg extension. Such posturing may also be caused by structural lesions or metabolic insults and it is often mistaken for seizure activity. The patient should be observed for the presence of tremor, myoclonus, or asterixis, because these may be associated with toxic-metabolic encephalopathies.

After observing for spontaneous movements and posturing, motor tone should be assessed by passive flexion and extension of the extremities. Tone may be increased or decreased, depending on the location of the motor system involvement. Afterward, noxious stimuli should then be applied to each limb and the supraorbital regions. Purposeful movement upon noxious stimulation suggests intactness of motor tracts to that limb, whereas decorticate or decerebrate posturing in response to noxious stimuli has the localizing significance mentioned above.

Acute corticospinal tract lesions may cause hyporeflexia because hyperreflexia may not occur for days to weeks after the injury. However, a Babinski sign, which is characterized by extension of the great toe and fanning of the other toes upon lateral plantar stimulation, may be present acutely with corticospinal tract lesions. Complete bilateral paralysis without any response to noxious stimuli usually indicates a grave prognosis. However, spinal cord injury and neuromuscular transmission blockade must be excluded because they may produce a similar state of complete paralysis.

Differential Diagnosis of Coma

Alcoholism, cerebral trauma, and cerebrovascular diseases account for a majority of comatose patients. Other major causes for admission include epilepsy, drug intoxication, diabetes, and severe infection. In the university hospital setting Plum and Posner[1] found one-quarter of comatose patients to have cerebrovascular disease, 6% were the consequence of trauma, all "mass lesions" (i.e., tumors, abscesses, hemorrhages, and infarcts) accounted for less than one-third, while subarachnoid hemorrhage, meningitis, and encephalitis accounted for another 5%. The majority of cases were the consequence of exogenous (drug overdose) and endogenous (metabolic) intoxications and hypoxia.

When the examination leads to the conclusion that the central neuraxis is affected at multiple levels or diffusely, the etiology is most likely of toxic-metabolic origin. Metabolic causes and toxic ingestions account for the largest number of patients with depressed consciousness (Table 67-7). The single most important sign distinguishing metabolic from structural coma is the presence of the pupillary light response.[19,20] In metabolic coma, confusion and stupor commonly precede symmetrical motor signs. Asterixis, myoclonus, tremor, and seizures are common. Central hyperventilation occurs frequently.

Supratentorial mass lesions causing compression or displacement of the upper brain stem (Table 67-8) usually present with focal neurologic signs that are asymmetrical. Neurologic dysfunction usually progresses in a rostral-caudal fashion, and the examination usually points to one anatomic area of the brain stem at a given point in time.

Subtentorial masses or *destructive lesions* causing coma usually are associated with brain stem dysfunction or sudden onset of coma. Brain stem signs always precede or accompany the onset of coma and always include abnormalities of eye movements. Cranial nerve palsies are usually present. Irregular respiratory patterns are common and usually appear at the onset of coma.

TABLE 67-7 Acute Metabolic-Endocrine Derangement Causing Coma

Hypoxia
  Decreased P_{O2}
  Anemia
  Cyanide poisoning
  Carbon monoxide poisoning
  Methemoglobinemia
Fluid and electrolyte disorders
  Hypo- and hyperglycemia (nonketotic hyperosmolar)
  Hypo- and hypernatremia
  Hypo- and hyperosmolality
  Acid-base disorders
  Extreme values of calcium, magnesium, phosphorus
Cofactor/vitamin deficiency
  Thiamine
  Niacin
  Pyridoxine
  Vitamin B_{12}
  Folate
Endocrine abnormalities
  Addison's disease
  Acute hypothyroidism
  Acute panhypopituitarism
Endogenous toxins
  Acute uremia
  Hyperbilirubinemia
  Hypercapnia
  Hepatic failure
Exogenous toxins and drug toxicity
  Perscribed medications
    Benzodiazepines, opiate analgesics, barbiturates, anticonvulsant, salicylates, ethanol, tricyclic antidepressants, anticholinergics, phenothiazines, lithium, monamine oxidase inhibitors, antihistamines, cimetidine, penicillins, organic phosphates
  Drugs of abuse
    Amphetamines, cocaine, lysergic acid diethylamide (LSD), paraldehyde, methanol, ethylene glycol, heavy metals
Psychiatric causes
  Lethal catatonia
  Hysterical coma
  Malingering

SELECTED CAUSES OF COMA

Metabolic derangements, cerebrovascular diseases, head trauma, and drug intoxications are reviewed in Chaps. 62, 63, 93, and 102.

Hypoxic-ischemic encephalopathy is the most common and most devastating cause of coma in most critical care units. The term is a pathologic diagnosis that refers to the effects of various degrees of global brain ischemia, sometimes complicated by hypoxemia. Cardiac arrest is the most common cause of global brain ischemia.[21–24] Each year there are 200,000 attempts at cardiac resuscitation, and only 70,000 are successful. Of the early survivors, 30% leave the hospital, but only 10% resume their former lifestyle because of permanent neurologic deficits. Other important causes of global brain ischemia include severe hypotension, cardiac failure, strangulation, cardiopulmonary bypass, status epilepticus, diffuse cerebral arteriosclerosis, increased intracranial pressure, cerebral arterial spasm, closed head trauma, and hyperviscosity.

TABLE 67-8 Focal Neurologic Lesions Causing Coma

Hemorrhage
  Subarachnoid
  Lobar
  Subdural/epidural
  Cerebellar
  Brain stem
Ischemia
  Cardiac arrest
  Shock
  Blood hyperviscosity
  Disseminated intravascular coagulation
  Hypertensive encephalopathy
  Anoxic-ischemic encephalopathy
Cerebral arterial occlusive infarction
  MCA occlusion with swelling
  Brainstem/basilar artery occlusion
  Bilateral thalamic infarcts
  Cerebellar with displacement and brain stem compression
Infection/Inflammatory
  Brain abscess
  Empyema
  Meningitis
  Systemic lupus
  Vasculitis
  Encephalitis (viral, paraneoplastic)
  Postinfectious demyelinating encephalomyelitis
Neoplasms
  Lymphoma
  Brain stem tumor
  Gliomatosis
  Multiple brain metastasis
  Cerebellar glioma
Diffuse physiologic brain dysfunction
  Generalized tonic-clonic seizures
  Porphyria
  Basilar migraine
  Idiopathic recurrent stupor
  Hypothermia and heat stroke
  Traumatic brain injury/contusions
  Osmotic demyelination syndrome
  Progressive hydrocephalus
  Leukoencephalopathy (chemotherapy or radiation)

The degree of neuronal injury in this condition depends on the degree of mismatch between metabolic demand and delivery of substrate (oxygen and glucose) to the brain.[25] For example, the brain can tolerate 45 minutes of total circulatory arrest with complete recovery if hypothermia to 18°C is induced. Conversely, a brain with metabolic activity that is eightfold above normal during status epilepticus will sustain neuronal damage after 2 hours, even with perfect maintenance of arterial oxygenation, glucose, and blood pressure.

The neurologic syndromes that follow cardiac arrest and resuscitation are diverse and depend on the duration of ischemia (time from arrest to cardiopulmonary resuscitation [CPR]), adequacy of CPR, underlying cardiovascular disease, degree of arterial atherosclerosis, adequacy of postresuscitation cerebral perfusion, and whether the patient is cooled following arrest (see Chap. 16). Patients in coma less than 12 hours after resuscitation usually make an excellent recovery. Those in coma more than 12 hours have permanent neurologic deficits due to focal or multifocal infarcts of the cere-

bral cortex in arterial border zones. They may be left with permanent amnesia, dementia, bibrachial or quadriparesis, cortical blindness, seizures, myoclonus, and ataxia.[26,27] If the coma persists for 1 week, recovery is rare, and most patients remain in a PVS due to laminar necrosis of the cerebral cortex with preservation of brain stem function.[28,29]

Early in the course of hypoxic-ischemic encephalopathy, specific neurologic signs can predict outcome with a high degree of reliability. In a study of 210 patients, the absence of pupillary responses on the first day after CPR predicted poor outcome.[30] None of 52 patients recovered, and only 3 regained consciousness. No patient who lacked corneal reflexes after the first day ever regained consciousness. After 3 days, a lack of purposeful motor responses predicted poor outcome in all patients (PVS or severe disability). Certain early signs were associated with good recovery. At 1 day, the following signs were associated with at least a 50% chance of regaining independent function: verbal responses of any type, purposeful eye movements or motor responses, normal ocular reflexes, and response to verbal commands.

The cause of hypoxic-ischemic encephalopathy is not a simple response to circulatory arrest. Evidence has accumulated that the brain can tolerate a longer period of ischemia than previously thought if certain conditions are met. After a 10-minute period of global brain ischemia, if the circulation is adequately restored, there is marked hyperemia, subsequently followed by a delayed, progressive fall in cerebral blood flow to levels considerably below prearrest values.[31] In some cases, cerebral metabolism remains high in the face of low blood flow, a situation that worsens the effects of the initial ischemia. There is experimental evidence suggesting that if cerebral blood flow can be maintained at a hyperemic level, the brain can recover.[32] It appears that some of the damage is due to a lack of adequate reperfusion after resuscitation, the no-reflow phenomenon. The mechanisms of delayed hypoperfusion and no-reflow are poorly understood but may be due to diffuse arterial spasm, calcium influx, vasoconstrictor prostaglandins, and intravascular coagulation. Even when adenosine triphosphate levels recover promptly as evidence of successful reperfusion, neurons show progressive morphologic damage, suggesting that injury may be in large part due to reperfusion rather than ischemia, per se. Persistently impaired protein synthesis following reperfusion may prevent the cell from repairing damage. In addition, apoptotic pathways appear to be activated, triggering neuronal death. In addition, other biochemical changes are initiated after ischemia that can cause delayed neuronal injury: elevation of intracellular calcium, release of neurotoxic excitatory amino acids (glutamate and aspartate), reoxygenation injury from superoxide formation, and brain lactic acidosis.[33,34]

The pathophysiology of altered cerebral blood flow and meta-bolism following CPR is complex and points to several windows of opportunity where the devastating effects of global brain ischemia may be ameliorated. Calcium channel blockers such as nimodipine, nicardipine, and lidoflazine are being investigated, experimentally and clinically, to determine if they can prevent neuronal damage following global brain ischemia and improve cerebral perfusion after resuscitation. Excitatory amino acid antagonists (MK-801) may be effective at preventing delayed neuronal injury after ischemia.[31] Free radical scavengers and excitatory amino acid antagonists have also been considered as potentially useful to improve outcome after brain injury; to date, despite some promise in animal models of central nervous system (CNS) injury, these agents have not shown benefits in clinical trials. The mechanism of benefit from induced hypothermia following anoxic brain injury is unknown, and this topic is further considered in Chap. 16.

DIAGNOSTIC PROCEDURES IN EVALUATING THE COMATOSE PATIENT

Keeping in mind the preceding differential diagnosis for states of coma, the sequence of diagnostic studies becomes clear. Rapid identification of metabolic or toxic causes of coma is determined by laboratory testing of blood, urine, gastric aspirate, and cerebrospinal fluid (CSF) (Table 67-9).

A variety of diagnostic tests are useful in evaluating comatose patients. *Computed tomographic* (CT) scanning of the head is useful in detecting changes in brain density. It is utilized mainly to detect focal brain disease, being most sensitive for diagnosing acute hemorrhage, which appears as an area of increased density. Conversely, infarction shows up as an area of lucency, subtly apparent at least several hours after onset. Neoplasms and abscesses are lucent on CT but often accumulate IV contrast material due to alterations in the blood–brain barrier. CT is the test of choice in acute trauma because it provides detailed images of bony structures of the skull base.[35] It may also show parenchymal shifts and effacements of CSF spaces, suggesting the presence of increased intracranial pressure or the presence of hydrocephalus. In addition, CT can be performed easily and rapidly in critically ill, intubated, and artificially ventilated patients.

Magnetic resonance imaging (MRI) is the most sensitive method to image the brain and define diverse pathologies. The image resolution is much better than CT, and it allows images of the central nervous system in multiple planes. MRI is particularly helpful for imaging posterior fossa structures, which often are poorly visualized on CT due to bony artifact. MRI frequently displays pathologic processes earlier than CT does, which may be critical for prompt initiation of appropriate therapy, as in herpes encephalitis.

Lumbar puncture and CSF examination are essential in the diagnosis of meningitis and encephalitis. On occasion, CSF analysis is more sensitive than CT in documenting subarachnoid hemorrhage. The major contraindication to performing a spinal tap is cerebral edema. Since processes associated with cerebral edema represent several of the etiologic considerations in the comatose patient, CT should generally be performed prior to the spinal tap in comatose patients. If it is essential to obtain CSF in states associated with intracranial masses and intracranial hypertension, ventriculostomy may be performed safely and provides an excellent tool for subsequent monitoring and treatment of intracranial hypertension.

Electroencephalography (EEG) measures brain wave activity. It is useful in detecting focal cerebral dysfunction, seizures, encephalitis, and diffuse metabolic encephalopathy, although it is nonspecific with regard to cause (i.e., uremia vs. hepatic failure).[36,37] A rare patient in coma from nonconvulsive status epilepticus will be identified by EEG.[38] It can be used as objective verification of brain death, but this application is less popular in contemporary practice.[39]

Evoked-potential studies (visual, auditory, and somatosensory) have been used extensively for assessment of brain function in comatose patients with acute brain injury, with the hope that they would provide information about prognosis.[37,39] In general, they are no more useful than the clinical examination, except for somatosensory evoked potential (SSEP). The absence of cortical waves in SSEPs performed early after onset of hypoxic-ischemic coma has a high specificity for predicting the likelihood of nonawakening. SSEPs are resistant to sedative drug intoxication and may be present in drug overdose states that cause an "isoelectric" EEG. The persistence of cortical SSEPs in comatose patients with head trauma predicts potential recovery in about one-third of patients; the absence of SSEPs predicts poor outcome in the vast majority.[37,40] Recently one study showed promising potential with more specific tests looking at the role of late auditory (N100), cognitive evoked potentials (mismatch negativity; MMN), and middle latency auditory evoked potentials (MLAEPs) for prognosis of awakening in a cohort of 346 comatose patients.[18] The strongest prognostic variable was pupillary reflex (estimated probability 79.7%), and the estimated probability rose to 87% when N100 was present, and to 89.9% when MLAEPs were present. Interestingly, when MMN was present, 88.6% of patients awakened and no patient with MMN became permanently vegetative.

In a recent small study of 34 patients with anoxic coma admitted over a 2-year period to an intensive care unit, the predictive value of combined clinical exam, SSEP, and EEG was evaluated.[41] On day 3 or thereafter, patients with extensor motor response to pain or worse and a "malignant" EEG (low amplitude, less than $50~\mu V$, delta rhythm, nonreactive; or burst-suppression; or suppression $<20~\mu V$, alpha/theta coma, nonreactive; or epileptiform discharges with burst-suppression), or those patients with flexor posturing or worse and bilaterally absent SSEPs invariably had poor outcome. However, some patients with initially malignant EEG and normal SSEPs may recover and should be supported until their prognosis becomes more definitive.

Treatment of Coma

Treatment must be instituted immediately, even when the diagnosis is uncertain, to prevent further brain damage secondary to complications. Oxygenation must be ensured, and airway protection is essential. All patients in coma should have a cuffed endotracheal tube placed quickly; the need for mechanical ventilation is determined by the degree of spontaneous breathing and the need for therapeutic hyperventilation. Trauma patients with suspected cervical spine injuries may need emergency tracheostomy to avoid extension of

---

TABLE 67-9 Emergency Laboratory Tests for Nonstructural Coma

1. Venous blood: hemoglobin, white blood count, platelets, glucose, electrolytes, calcium, blood urea nitrogen, creatinine, osmolality, coagulation studies, liver function tests, muscle enzymes, thyroid and adrenal functions, toxicology screen, blood cultures
2. Arterial blood: pH, P_{CO_2}, P_{O_2}, carboxyhemoglobin, ammonia
3. Urine: toxicology, microscopic examination
4. Gastric aspirate: toxicology
5. Cerebrospinal fluid: cell count and gram stain, protein, glucose, culture, counterimmunoelectrophoresis, viral and fungal antigens, and antibody titers

the neck during endotracheal tube placement (see Chap. 35). Subsequent ventilator adjustments are determined by arterial blood gases.

Arterial blood pressure must be maintained. Hypotension causes secondary brain ischemia. Intravascular volume replacement with blood or isotonic solutions often requires hemodynamic monitoring. The goals are to attain normal intravascular volume with normal central venous pressure, mean arterial pressure, and blood osmolality. Excessive volume replacement can aggravate intracranial hypertension, especially if hypotonic solutions are administered and serum osmolality falls. Inadequate intravascular volume will cause a fall in cardiac output and worsen brain ischemia. Inotropic and vasopressor drugs are administered as needed.

As part of the initial management of all patients with coma, glucose should be given (50 mL of 50% glucose) as soon as blood is sent to the laboratory. Although there is a theoretical risk of hyperglycemia causing brain lactic acidosis during ischemia, the risk of damage from hypoglycemic coma is much greater and requires emergency treatment. Thiamine (100 mg IM or IV) is administered with the glucose to avoid Wernicke-Korsakoff syndrome. Seizures, regardless of cause, must be stopped (see Chap. 64). Intracranial hypertension, if present, should be treated aggressively using intracranial pressure monitoring as a guideline for treatment.[35,42] Details of intracranial pressure monitoring and treatment are described in Chap. 65.

Systemic infections, especially gram-negative sepsis, can cause stupor or coma on a toxic basis and must be promptly treated. Severe acid-base disorders, while rarely responsible by themselves for coma, can worsen the overall situation by causing secondary cardiovascular and respiratory failure. Rapid correction of severe acidosis or alkalosis may be helpful.

Hyperthermia can accompany a variety of pathologic states, either infectious or secondary to hypothalamic or brain stem damage. A 1°C elevation in body temperature will increase cerebral tissue metabolic demand by 10%. Therefore, hyperthermia can itself exacerbate the harmful effects of ischemia, hypoxia, or hypoglycemia. Hyperthermia should be aggressively treated. Mild therapeutic hypothermia was first proposed as a treatment for brain trauma in the late 1950s. Hypothermia can lower ICP, alter chemical pathways that could contribute to injury, and modulate apoptosis, but the mechanism of benefit seen in animal models remains unknown. Large trials in patients with traumatic brain injury have been conflicting[43,44] while benefit seems established following out-of-hospital cardiac arrest.[45,46]

Specific antidotes may be effective in coma secondary to drug intoxication. Details of treatment for drug overdose are described in Chapter 102. Other than general measures, as outlined above, treatment depends on accurate diagnosis of cause and specific directed treatment.

Prognosis and the Persistent Vegetative State

While it is possible to describe broad prognostic likelihoods for patients with nontraumatic coma, particularly postanoxic brain injury (see above), there are no precise tools to determine which patients with coma will evolve to vegetative state.

Generally, the clinical course and long-term outcome of vegetative state depends in part on the etiology of the brain injury. A useful classification in this regard describes three broad categories: (1) acute traumatic and nontraumatic brain injuries, (2) degenerative and metabolic brain disorders, and (3) severe congenital malformations of the CNS. Recovery of consciousness from a posttraumatic PVS is unlikely after 12 months for both children and adults. For nontraumatic PVS, recovery after 3 months is exceedingly rare. Patients with degenerative disorders or congenital abnormalities are very unlikely to recover consciousness after several months of PVS. For all patients remaining in PVS, life span is substantially reduced and generally ranges from 2 to 5 years. Survival beyond 10 years is extremely unusual. Life expectancy is largely influenced by the complications accompanying chronic care of these individuals.

Patients who recover consciousness after severe head trauma are often left with marked disabilities. The overall main costs of disability from brain injury are loss of employment. Only about half of all patients with full time employment prior to the severe head injury event were able to return to full time employment,[47] most of them at lower occupational status. In a group of severely brain-injured young men, however, the re-employment rate can be significantly improved by using on-site training accompanied by a job coach, as well as continuing long-term support with use of behavioral and cognitive training strategies.[48,49]

Declaration of Death Using Neurologic Criteria

In recent years, the success rate of organ transplantation has increased dramatically, and transplantation has become standard therapy for patients with end-stage kidney, heart, and liver disease. Unfortunately, thousands of critically ill patients will not receive needed organs due to a lack of understanding of the concepts and criteria for the declaration of death. We are wasting a rare and precious resource because health professionals, as well as the public, have been misinformed about definitions and procedures necessary to declare death in the setting of massive, irreversible brain damage[50,51] (see also Chap. 91).

Although specific protocols for the determination of death vary slightly from institution to institution, guidelines in the United States were firmly established by the President's Commission in 1981 and have been uniformly accepted by the American Medical Association, American Academy of Neurology, and American Bar Association.[52–54]

The Uniform Determination of Death Act states that "an individual who has sustained either (1) irreversible cessation of circulatory and respiratory functions, or (2) irreversible cessation of all functions of the entire brain, including the brain stem, is dead. A determination of death must be made in accordance with accepted medical standards." In 1987, the state of New York adopted the preceding statement as the legal definition of death. Since that time, this definition has been widely adopted throughout North America and Europe.[55,56]

However, confusion still surrounds (1) the definition of death and (2) the criteria for determining death in a patient who has stable cardiovascular function but irreversible cessation of brain function. Part of this confusion arises from the continued use of the ambiguous term "brain death," implying that there is more than one type of death. If health professionals are confused about this concept, it is no surprise that the public remains uncertain about the terminology.

The medical and legal definitions of death are clear: brain death and cardiac death are the same. Dissenting opinions from the strict religious orthodoxy of Roman Catholicism and Orthodox Judaism persist, however, due to individual interpretations and applications of religious beliefs and laws. It is unlikely that there will ever be a unanimously accepted definition of death, due to diverse religious and ethical opinions. However, time has brought about increasing acceptance that the irreversible cessation of brain function is a mechanism of death.

The core of the clinical diagnosis of brain death is to establish unresponsiveness and brain stem areflexia. The preconditions are that (1) the cause of coma is known and (2) the cause is adequate to explain the irreversible cessation of whole brain function.[57,58] In almost all cases, cerebral circulatory arrest from intracranial hypertension is the mechanism. Confirmatory tests are appropriate in selected cases, particularly for posterior fossa processes that can cause devastating brainstem dysfunction without hemispheric injury. Careful attention to these preconditions will alert the intensivist to special circumstances that require re-evaluation and confirmatory tests. In the press for organ procurement, the cautious physician may be perceived as delaying the transplant process to ensure that the diagnosis of death is unequivocal.

The President's Commission's recommendations grew out of studies at Harvard Medical School in the 1960s and extensive collaborative studies sponsored by the National Institute of Neurological Disorders and Stroke in the years 1971 and 1972.[59,60] These clinical studies were performed before the availability of CT imaging, making the cause of coma and anatomic extent of brain damage uncertain in many cases. Therefore, the use of routine EEG became a standard part of many determination-of-death protocols. With the ability to directly visualize the extent of brain damage in comatose patients by CT, the determination of irreversibility became more precise. To this day, however, there continues to be unnecessary reliance on confirmatory laboratory tests rather than the use of objective clinical criteria. In contemporary practice, the use of transcranial Doppler to verify cerebral circulatory arrest is more relevant than EEG.

In most states in the United States and many countries around the world, clinical criteria are sufficient to diagnose brain death. Confirmatory tests are reserved for situations in which there is uncertainty regarding cause and reversibility of coma. However, there is no doubt that the diagnosis of brain death requires diagnostic respect from the physician and its proper pronouncement is best verified by physicians experienced with the diagnosis.

CLINICAL DIAGNOSIS

It is important to keep a structured approach in mind when approaching a patient with the possible diagnosis of brain death. First, imperative prerequisites that should be fulfilled prior to determination of brain death include (1) irreversible brain catastrophe which involves both the cerebral hemispheres and the brain stem; (2) core temperature >32°C; (3) no evidence of intoxication, poisoning, or the use of paralyt-

ics, anesthetics, or sedatives; and (4) no confounding medical conditions such as severe endocrine, electrolyte, and acid-base disturbances. CT scan may or may not show abnormalities consistent with brain death. For example, following cardiopulmonary arrest the CT may show abnormalities only visible to the expert and may be interpreted as normal by those who are less experienced. On the other hand, a significant and easily identifiable mass lesion seen on CT scan does not necessary imply brain death. As a rule, if the brain CT is discrepant with the clinical diagnosis of brain death, a repeat study is warranted; if the repeat CT scan remains discrepant, the search for other confounding factors should be intensified.

The examination of a potentially brain dead patient should be methodologic as well as documented in detail: Identify the lack of consciousness (coma), verify the patient's core temperature and ventilator dependency, test and describe that no movements and brain stem reflexes are present (including absence of pharyngeal and tracheal reflexes), and demonstrate the lack of spontaneous respiration to increasing arterial carbon dioxide levels (*apnea test*). The apnea test demonstrates the lack of ventilatory drive while the patient remains oxygenated; a patient fails the apnea test when an increase of arterial CO_2 to 60 mm Hg (from a baseline range of 35 to 45 mm Hg) or a 20 mm Hg increase from the pre–apnea test baseline arterial CO_2 has been documented.[61] The successful performance of an apnea test requires a specific methodology to minimize hypoxemia during testing and proactively manage hypotension to assure study completion. For these reasons, it should only be done by physicians experienced with the test. Generally, failure to adequately perform an apnea test (e.g., because of hypotension or a marked drop in oxygenation) should indicate the need for another confirmatory test.

Certain spinal movements and reflexes can be observed in brain-dead patients without casting doubt on the diagnosis. They may be especially prominent during apnea testing, and physical stimulation of the patient. They are often short-lasting and symmetric. Well-known but rather uncommon in its complete form is a brief attempt of the body to sit up to about 60° with raising of both arms (Lazarus sign). A convenient classification of spinal movements and reflexes seen in brain-dead patients[61] by body region includes but is not limited to: cervical region (tonic neck reflexes or head turning), upper extremities (flexion-withdrawal or extension pronation or flexion), trunk (opisthotonic posturing, flexion, or abdominal reflexes), and lower extremities (plantarflexion, triple flexion, or Babinski sign). Observation of any of these movements should lead to verification that they are compatible with the diagnosis of brain death (by an experienced physician) and preparation of the family of their mechanism and relevance.

CONFIRMATORY TESTING

Generally, confirmatory testing is recommended in children less than 1 year old and in situations in which adequate clinical testing cannot be performed. Lack of cerebral blood flow, that is, *cerebral circulatory arrest*, can be documented by standard arterial angiography, transcranial Doppler, or radionuclide scan, and there is some, but limited, experience with magnetic resonance imaging/angiography and CT angiography. Four-vessel cerebral angiography may be performed in clinically dead patients who have an uncertain diagnosis.[57]

Complete absence of cerebral circulation is an absolute confirmation of brain death. The major use of the technique is for rapid diagnosis of death in patients whose clinical examination is obscured by hypothermia or drug intoxication. Transcranial Doppler sonography is a noninvasive bedside technique that can measure, in a qualitative fashion, blood flow in the proximal portions of the main cerebral arteries. An ultrasonic probe is placed over the temporal bones (usually) and the direction and velocity of blood flow can be measured. A number of investigators have shown that absence or reversal of diastolic flow in the cerebral arteries can be demonstrated in patients who meet the traditional criteria for brain death;[62] the operator-dependent sensitivity ranges from 90% to 99%, and the specificity is 100%.[63] About 10% of patients cannot be insonated because of excessive skull thickness. Radioisotope brain scanning can accurately document absent brain blood flow in the cerebral hemispheres, but not in the vertebrobasilar circulation.[64] Some institutions have portable units that can be brought to the bedside in the ICU. Because this technique does not image the posterior circulation, the clinical diagnosis of brain stem areflexia becomes even more important. In situations of suspected or known drug intoxication, isotope brain scanning is not helpful, since it will not answer the question of whether brain stem areflexia is due to drug effect or irreversible damage. Xenon-enhanced CT and ^{99m}T-HMPAO single photon emission computed tomography (SPECT) are noninvasive techniques for accurately measuring brain blood flow in all arterial territories. It has been used in young children and infants with great reliability to confirm the clinical criteria of death.[65] Particularly in children it can overcome many of the problems associated with EEG and cerebral angiography. Unfortunately, the technique is only available in a referral center.

Absence of any electrical activity on a 30-minute EEG with increased sensitivity settings is consistant with brain death and has a reported sensitivity and specificity of about 90%.[66] If the cause of coma is clearly established from anatomic imaging studies of the brain, and clinical criteria are met that all brain functions are absent, EEG confirmation is not necessary.[67] Apneic coma and an isoelectric EEG in the face of normal brain imaging studies are strongly suggestive of sedative drug intoxication, and appropriate toxicology studies must be performed.

NEUROLOGIC STATES RESEMBLING BRAIN DEATH

As correct identification and verification of brain death is rather difficult and complex and misjudgment may have great negative impact, not only on the patient, but also on the family and the diagnosing medical doctor. The diagnosis should only be made by a physician with experience in careful neurologic examinations, interpretations of brain imaging studies, and skilled evaluation of confirmatory studies used to diagnose brain death. Misleading diagnoses may lead the superficial examiner to believe that the patient is brain dead, but often the history and examination together reveal details inconsistent with the diagnosis of cerebral perfusion arrest. For details, the reader is referred to current textbooks in neurology and a recent monograph by Wijdicks.[61] Examples of disorders potentially mimicking brain death include but are not limited to severe hypothermia, acute metabolic coma (e.g., endocrine and organ failure, among others); poisoning (via drugs such as antidepressants, anticonvulsants, analgesics/sedatives, and many more, or via toxins and poisons); locked-in syndrome, akinetic mutism, and possible PVS, as well as peripheral nerve disorders in which the patient may appear brain dead, but is fully awake.

Critical Care Aspects of Brain-Dead Patients

It is well known that brain injury can have immediate and delayed systemic effects on multiple organs. Hence, it is not surprising that brain-dead patients will experience significant effects on overall body function. Generally, vascular motor tone and cardiac stability and performance decreases, pulmonary edema, disseminated intravascular coagulation, and hypothermia may occur, and severe electrolyte and fluid balance disturbances are noted. Up to one-quarter of all potential donor organs are rejected because of the detrimental impact of these changes, which are commonly associated with inadequate medical management (see Chap. 91).

Since the determination of any brain dead patient as a medically suitable organ donor is only done by organ procurement organizations, all brain dead patients should be managed as potential organ donors. This requires proactive anticipatory care to avoid the expected systemic complications that can sabotage the success of organ donation once a family approves. A brief discussion of some of the more important management issues follows.

1. *Maintain hemodynamic stability*. The initial response of brain injury is massive discharge of catecholamines leading to hypertension and tachycardia and not infrequently myocardial injury. In brain death, hypotension and hypovolemia associated with electrolyte and temperature disturbances will lead to systemic vascular instability. Target hemodynamic goals in these patients could be simplified to maintain systolic blood pressure at about 100 mm Hg, heart rate <100 beats per minute, and urine output >100 mL/h. For fluid resuscitation, boluses of either 5% albumin or crystalloid infusion are recommended, the particular choice depends on the treating physician's preference and individual patient's sensitivity to low osmotic pressure–mediated tissue edema. For heart-lung donors we prefer use of colloids to reduce the risk of precipitating acute heart failure, especially in patients with brain injury–related myocardial abnormalities. Inotropic support is indicated for a volume-resuscitated patient with systolic blood pressures <100 mm Hg; principally, any vasopressor agent can be used; however, ideally use the lowest dose possible to avoid further organ impairments. We commonly initiate treatment with low-dose dopamine to stabilize cardiac function and blood pressure while dilating renal, mesenteric, and coronary vasculature. However, if myocardial contractility is already impaired, dobutamine in combination with dopamine would be an appropriate first step. Blood loss is treated with transfusions to a target hematocrit of about 30%. Consumption of blood factors and platelets due to disseminated intravascular coagulation (aggravated by massive release of brain thromboplastin) can be rapid and replacement may become increasingly difficult.

2. *Manage diabetes insipidus.* Posterior lobe pituitary injury and necrosis leading to diabetes insipidus (DI) in brain-injured and brain-dead patients is common and should be recognized immediately. Helpful clinical parameters supporting the diagnosis of DI include (1) hypotonic polyuria, identified by urine output >4 mL/kg per hour and urine specific gravity <1.005; (2) urine osmolality <300 mOsm/L; and (3) plasma osmolality >300 mOsm/L (may be confounded by the use of osmotic diuretics). Diabetes insipidus will invariably lead to dehydration, hypernatremia, and vascular collapse. Therapy is simplified by early recognition of DI and includes hypotonic fluid resuscitation on a volume-to-volume basis, and desmopressin acetate, for example, as an initial bolus of 0.3 μg IV, and then as an adjusted dose guided by clinical and laboratory parameters (e.g., titrate urine output to 2 to 3 mL/kg), given approximately every 6 hours to a total 24-hour dose ranging from 10 to 40 μg. Infusion of aqueous vasopressin can be used alternatively (start at 3 U/h); however, the infusion should be stopped prior to surgical organ recovery to diminish the dose-dependent effects on systemic vascular constriction. Recently, the addition of thyroid hormone replacement was shown to have a vasopressor-supporting effect.[68] The management of diabetes insipidus can be complex, and is best guided by those experienced with brain death management.

3. *Maintaining normothermia.* Adverse effects of hypothermia are well known and include reduction of cardiac output and peripheral vascular resistance leading to arrhythmia and hypotension, hypoxia, hyperglycemia, and coagulopathy. Brain-dead patients have lost their ability to control body temperature and are hence dependent on ambient temperature and the temperature of the infusion products they receive. For these reasons (as well as for the establishment of the diagnosis of brain death) the core temperature should be kept constantly above 36°C using conventional methods.

4. *Maintain glucose and electrolyte balance.* Hypernatremia (e.g., from untreated DI) in excess of 155 mEq/dL may lead to a higher incidence of graft loss after liver transplantation and should therefore be treated aggressively.[69] Certainly, electrolytes need to be evaluated and supplemented as needed, at least every 2 to 4 hours, especially with aggressive fluid resuscitation and treatment of DI, as hypernatremia, hypokalemia, hypocalcemia, and hypomagnesemia are common. Hypophosphatemia is frequently observed in brain-dead patients, and if untreated, may lead to hemolysis, rhabdomyolysis, and platelet dysfunction. Glucose, potassium, and ketones should also be checked regularly, as hyperglycemia due to relative insulin resistance, and use of steroid-, pressor-, and glucose-containing solutions is frequent in these patients. Often an insulin infusion is required to maintain blood glucose levels between 150 and 200 mg/dL.

The proper diagnosis and management of brain death is complex and requires expertise and respect for the diagnosis as a real mechanism of death. The need for proper diagnosis supersedes whether or not the patient will become an organ donor. However, the sensitive and thoughtful management of the patient and family can at least keep the opion of organ donation open; a decision to be finalized between organ procurement, and, usually, families. This is one situation in which proper management can potentially save several lives.

References

1. Plum F, Posner JB: *The Diagnosis of Stupor and Coma*, 3rd ed. Philadelphia, FA Davis, 1980.
2. Jennett B, Plum F: Persistent vegetative state after brain damage: A syndrome in search of a name. *Lancet* 1:734, 1972.
3. The Multi-Society Task Force on PVS: Medical aspects of the persistent vegetative state (first of two parts). *N Engl J Med* 330:1499, 1994.
4. The Multi-Society Task Force on PVS: Medical aspects of the persistent vegetative state (second of two parts). *N Engl J Med* 330:1572, 1994.
5. Giacino JT, Ashwal S, Childs N, et al: The minimally conscious state: definition and diagnostic criteria. *Neurology* 58:349, 2002.
6. Rudolf J, Sobesky J, Grond M, Heiss WD: Identification by positron emission tomography of neuronal loss in acute vegetative state. *Lancet* 355:115, 2000.
7. Levy DE, Sidtis JJ, Rottenberg DA, et al: Differences in cerebral blood flow and glucose utilization in vegetative versus locked-in patients. *Ann Neurol* 22:673, 1987.
8. Tommasino C, et al. Regional cerebral metabolism of glucose in comatose and vegetative state patients. *J Neurosurg Anesthesiol* 7:109, 1995.
9. Laureys S, Faymonville ME, Luxen A, et al: Restoration of thalamocortical connectivity after recovery from persistent vegetative state. *Lancet* 355:1790, 2000.
10. Maquet P: Functional neuroimaging of normal human sleep by positron emission tomography. *J Sleep Res* 9:207, 2000.
11. Laureys S, Faymonville MD, Peigneux P, et al: Cortical processing of noxious stimuli in the persistent vegetative state. *Neuroimage* 17:732, 2002.
12. Menon DK, Owen AM, Williams EJ, et al: Cortical processing in persistent vegetative state. *Lancet* 352:200, 1998.
13. de Jong BM, Willemsen AT, Paans AM: Regional cerebral blood flow changes related to affective speech presentation in persistent vegetative state. *Clin Neurol Neurosurg* 99:213, 1997.
14. Moruzzi G, Magoun HW: Brainstem reticular formation and activation of the EEG. *Electroencephalogr Clin Neurophysiol* 1:455, 1949.
15. Magoun HW: *The Waking Brain*, 2nd ed. Springfield, IL, Charles C Thomas, 1963.
16. Snyder BD, Hauser WA, Loewenson RB, et al: Neurologic prognosis after cardiopulmonary arrest: III. Seizure activity. *Neurology* 30:1292, 1980.
17. Pal J: The value of the Glasgow Coma Scale and Injury Severity Score in predicting outcome in multiple trauma patients with head injury. *J Trauma* 29:746, 1989.
18. Fischer C, Luaute J, Adeleine P, et al: Predictive value of sensory and cognitive evoked potentials for awakening from coma. *Neurology* 63:669, 2004.
19. Fisher CM: Some neuro-ophthalmological observations. *J Neurol Neurosurg Psychiatry* 30:383, 1967.
20. Fisher CM: The neurological examination of the comatose patient. *Acta Neurol Scand* 45(Suppl 36):1, 1969.
21. Mullie A, Buylaert W, Michem N, et al: Predictive value of Glasgow Coma Score for awakening after out-of-hospital cardiac arrest. Cerebral Resuscitation Study Group of the Belgian Society for Intensive Care. *Lancet* 1:137, 1988.
22. Bertini G, Margheri M, Giglioli C, et al: Prognostic significance of early clinical manifestations in postanoxic coma: A retrospective study of 58 patients resuscitated after prehospital cardiac arrest. *Crit Care Med* 17:627, 1989.
23. Brain Resuscitation Clinical Trial I Study Group: Randomized

clinical study of thiopental loading in comatose survivors of cardiac arrest. *N Engl J Med* 314:397, 1986.

24. Earnest MP, Yarness PR, Merrill SL, et al: Long-term survival and neurologic status after resuscitation from out-of-hospital cardiac arrest. *Neurology* 30:1298, 1980.

25. Siesjo BK: Cerebral circulation and metabolism. *J Neurosurg* 60:883, 1984.

26. Caronna JJ, Finklestein S: Neurological syndromes after cardiac arrest. *Stroke* 9:517, 1978.

27. Krumholz A, Stern BJ, Weiss HD: Outcome from coma after cardiopulmonary resuscitation: Relation to seizures and myoclonus. *Neurology* 38:401, 1988.

28. Dougherty JH, Rawlinson, DG, Levy DE, et al: Hypoxic-ischemic brain injury and the vegetative state: Clinical and neuropathologic correlation. *Neurology* 31:991, 1981.

29. Levy DE, Bates D, Caronna JJ, et al: Prognosis in nontraumatic coma. *Ann Intern Med* 94:293, 1981.

30. Levy DE, Caronna JJ, Singer BH, et al: Predicting outcome from hypoxic-ischemic coma. *JAMA* 253:1420, 1985.

31. Beckstead JE, Tweed WA, Lee J, et al: Cerebral blood flow and metabolism in man following cardiac arrest. *Stroke* 9:569, 1978.

32. Safar P: Resuscitation from clinical death: Pathophysiologic limits and therapeutic potentials. *Crit Care Med* 16:923, 1988.

33. Krause GS, White BC, Aust SD, et al: Brain cell death following ischemia and reperfusion: A proposed biochemical sequence. *Crit Care Med* 16:714, 1988.

34. Rothman SM, Olney JW: Glutamate and the pathophysiology of hypoxic-ischemic brain damage. *Ann Neurol* 19:105, 1986.

35. Fink ME: Emergency management of the head-injured patient. *Emerg Med Clin North Am* 5:783, 1987.

36. Austin EJ, Wilkus RJ, Longstreth WT: Etiology and prognosis of alpha coma. *Neurology* 38:773, 1988.

37. Ganes T, Lundar T: EEG and evoked potentials in comatose patients with severe brain damage. *Electroencephalogr Clin Neurophysiol* 69:6, 1988.

38. White SR, Hall JB, Dietrich M, Spire JP: Clinically inapparent status epilepticus as a cause of coma in the critically ill. *J Crit Care* 2:112, 1987.

39. Chatrian GE: Electrophysiologic evaluation of brain death: A critical appraisal, in Aminoff MJ (ed): *Electrodiagnosis in Clinical Neurology*, 2nd ed. New York, Churchill-Livingstone, 1986, p 669.

40. Ahmed I: Use of somatosensory evoked responses in the prediction of outcome from coma. *Clin Electroencephalogr* 19:78, 1988.

41. Chen R, Bolton CF, Young GB: Prediction of outcome in patients with anoxic coma: A clinical and electrophysiologic study. *Crit Care Med* 24:672, 1996.

42. Tasker RC, Matthew J, Helms P, et al: Monitoring in nontraumatic coma: I. Invasive intracranial measurements. *Arch Dis Child* 63:888, 1988.

43. Clifton G, Miller E, Choi SC, et al: Lack of effect of induction of hypothermia after acute brain injury. *N Engl J Med* 344:556, 2001.

44. Polderman KH, Tjong Tjin Joe R, Peerdeman SM, et al: Effects of therapeutic hypothermia on intracranial pressure and outcome in patients with severe head injury. *Intensive Care Med* 28:1563, 2002.

45. Bernard SA, Gray TW, Buist MD, et al: Treatment of comatose survivors of out-of-hospital cardiac arrest with induced hypothermia. *N Engl J Med* 346:557, 2002.

46. The Hypothermia after Cardiac Arrest Study Group: Mild therapeutic hypothermia to improve the neurologic outcome after cardiac arrest. *N Engl J Med* 346:549, 2002.

47. Stambrook M, Moore AD, Peters LC, et al: Effects of mild, moderate and severe closed head injury on long term vocational status. *Brain Injury* 4:183, 1990.

48. Wehman P, Kreutzer J, West M, et al: Employment outcome of persons following traumatic brain injury: Pre-injury, post-injury and supported employment. *Brain Injury* 3:397, 1989.

49. Wehman PH, West MD, Kregal J, et al: Return to work for persons with severe traumatic brain injury: A date-based approach to programme development. *J Head Trauma Rehabil* 10:27, 1995.

50. Bernat JL: Ethical issues in brain death and multiorgan transplantation. *Neurol Clin* 7:715, 1989.

51. O'Callahan JG, Fink C, Pitts LH, Luce JM: Withholding and withdrawing of life support from patients with severe head injury. *Crit Care Med* 23:1567, 1995.

52. Report of the Medical Consultants on the Diagnosis of Death to the President's Commission for the Study of Ethical Problems in Medicine and Biomedical and Behavioral Research: Guidelines for the determination of death. *JAMA* 246:2184, 1981.

53. Quality Standards Subcommittee of the American Academy of Neurology: Practice parameters: Assessment and management of patients in the persistent vegetative state (summary statement). *Neurology* 45:1015, 1995.

54. Wijdicks EFM: Determining brain death in adults. *Neurology* 45:1003, 1995.

55. Powner DJ: The diagnosis of brain death in the adult patient. *J Intensive Care Med* 2:181, 1987.

56. Halevy A, Brody B: Brain death: Reconciling definitions, criteria, and tests. *Ann Intern Med* 119:519, 1993.

57. Black PM: Brain death in the intensive care unit. *J Intensive Care Med* 2:177, 1987.

58. Black PM: Brain death. *N Engl J Med* 299:338, 1978.

59. Beecher HK: A definition of irreversible coma: Report of the ad hoc committee of the Harvard Medical School to examine the definition of brain death. *JAMA* 205:337, 1968.

60. NINCDS Collaborative Study: An appraisal of the criteria of cerebral death: A summary statement. *JAMA* 237:982, 1977.

61. Wijdicks EFM (ed): *Brain Death: A Clinical Guide*. Baltimore, Lippincott Williams & Wilkins, 2001.

62. Petty GW, Mohr JP, Pedley TA, et al: The role of transcranial Doppler in confirming brain death: Sensitivity, specificity, and suggestions for performance and interpretation. *Neurology* 40:300, 1990.

63. Ducrocq X, Hassler W, Moritake K, et al: Consensus opinion on diagnosis of cerebral circulatory arrest using Doppler sonography: Task Force Group on Cerebral Death of the Neurosonology Research Group of the World Federation of Neurology. *J Neurol Sci* 158:145, 1998.

64. Goodman JM, Heck LL, Moore BD: Confirmation of brain death with portable isotope angiography: A review of 204 consecutive cases. *Neurosurgery* 16:492, 1985.

65. Facco E, Zucchetta P, Munari M, et al: 99mTcHMPAO SPECT in the diagnosis of brain death. *Intensive Care Med* 24:911, 1998.

66. Buchner H, Schuchardt V: Reliability of electroencephalogram in the diagnosis of brain death. *Eur Neurol* 30:138, 1990.

67. Grigg MM, Kelly MA, Celesia GG, et al: Electroencephalographic activity after brain death. *Arch Neurol* 44:948, 1987.

68. Zuppa A, Nadkarni V, Davis L, et al: The effect of a thyroid hormone infusion on vasopressor support in critically ill children with cessation of neurologic function. *Crit Care Med* 32:2318, 2004.

69. Totsuka E, Dodson F, Urakami A, et al: Influence of high donor serum sodium levels on early postoperative graft function in human liver transplantation: effect of correction of donor hypernatremia. *Liver Transpl Surg* 5:421, 1999.

PART VII

HEMATOLOGIC AND ONCOLOGIC DISORDERS

Chapter 68

ANEMIA AND BLOOD TRANSFUSION

JUDITH A. LUCE

KEY POINTS

- *The current practice of transfusion in the ICU is conservative, reflecting a balance between the benefits and adverse consequences of transfused blood.*
- *Anemia developing in the ICU should not be attributed solely to phlebotomy; red cell loss, destruction, or underproduction should also be considered.*
- *Evaluation of the basis for anemia, beginning with analysis of the blood smear, reticulocyte count, and red cell indices, may lead to easier management of the anemia and may prove useful in overall treatment.*
- *For most critically ill patients, a transfusion target for hemoglobin of 7 to 9 g/dL is at least as safe as a higher threshold of 10 to 12 g/dL; the lower value may be superior.*
- *Transfusion is rarely associated with life-threatening complications such as transfusion-related acute lung injury, major hemolysis, or lethal infection.*
- *Erythropoietin and oxygen-carrying blood substitutes remain unproven for critically ill patients.*
- *Massively transfused patients are at risk for hypothermia and dilutional coagulopathy.*

Red blood cells are the most efficient vehicle by which oxygen is delivered to the tissues of whole organisms. The evolution of red cells and the circulatory system allowed for the development of larger, more complex organisms with higher levels of activity. Deficiency in the number and in the local delivery of red blood cells causes relative oxygen deficiency in tissues. Oxygen deficit causes metabolic insufficiency, with inadequate energy production to sustain activity, or even life. Hemoglobin, the complex molecule contained within human red blood cells, has unique properties in and of itself, allowing for the efficient uptake of oxygen in an oxygen-rich environment, and the efficient divestiture of oxygen in an oxygen-poor environment. The whole organism also has evolved to attempt to regularly recycle and reuse the important portions of the hemoglobin molecule, thus reducing the need for ongoing sources of iron. Anemia, the lack of red blood cells in normal volumes, is therefore a disorder that threatens the homeostasis of the entire organism, and when it occurs in the setting of already life-threatening illness, anemia is a potential contributor to mortality.

Blood transfusion has long been recognized as a potential remedy for blood loss, although the first efforts to transfuse blood from animals to human beings or from one human to another were marred by the lack of knowledge of the unique antigens on the surface of red blood cells and the immune response to them. Once a systematic approach to the collection, storage, cross-matching, and transfusion of blood was developed, enthusiasm for transfusion reached its peak. Tempered by the recognition of new transmissible illnesses, by the increasing limitations of the blood supply,[1] and by the awareness of the limitations of aggressive transfusion, modern critical care practice has evolved to a more conservative approach to the use of transfusion as a remedy for anemia in critically ill patients.

Anemia in the ICU

The frequency of anemia in critically ill patients has been studied in a variety of settings, all with the conclusion that it is a common problem that tends to worsen with severity of illness and duration of stay in the ICU. Up to 40% of patients admitted to the ICU in one large sequential cohort study were bleeding on admission,[2] and 40% to 50% require blood transfusion during their ICU stay.[3] By day two in the ICU, nearly 95% of patients are anemic.[4] Trauma patients are subject to higher rates of transfusion, 55%, than medical patients in one comparative study, even though these patients had lower rates of comorbid illnesses.[5]

In these studies, anemia has been defined in various ways, mostly as any deviation from the normal hemoglobin content of blood for men and women. The severity of anemia, however, may vary, and the data on the effects of anemia show that severity is an important marker of both concomitant complications and outcome. Hemodilution in laboratory animals is a relatively well tolerated phenomenon; acute hemodilution results in evidence of myocardial dysfunction and tissue ischemia demonstrable only at hemoglobin levels of 3 to 5 g/dL. Normal human volunteers also appear to tolerate hemodilution to levels of 5 g/dL.[6] However, in animal models of coronary ischemia, and in acute hemodilution in humans with coronary disease, hemoglobin levels of 7 to 10 g/dL may produce evidence of further ischemia and of depressed ventricular function.[7] Conversely, the normalization of hematocrits with transfusion and erythropoietin in patients with chronic anemia and coronary disease in one randomized trial did not result in an outcome benefit.[8]

Measurement of the effects of severe anemia in the critically ill is not straightforward. The assessment of the consequences of anemia is complicated in severely ill patients who cannot report the usual symptoms of anemia—dyspnea, fatigue, lightheadedness, angina, or claudication. The usual signs of end-organ problems due to poor oxygen delivery may also be difficult to interpret: tachycardia and tachypnea have many other causes, cardiac ischemia may be multifactorial, and physical signs of poor organ perfusion may result from a variety of other conditions.

Guidelines for the evaluation of the physiologic impact of anemia are based on what is known of the physiology of anemia. In the absence of adequate delivery of red cells over a given volume of perfused tissue, oxygen extraction rises. Thus the delivered oxygen content may remain constant, but the mixed venous oxygen content will fall compared to normal. Low mixed venous oxygen saturation, usually below 70%, is often employed as a marker of anemic physiology. Under normal circumstances, peripheral oxygen extraction is about 25%, so the ratio of oxygen saturation in mixed venous blood to that delivered ($S\bar{v}_{O_2}/Sa_{O_2}$), and the oxygen extraction ratio (Sa_{O_2} minus $S\bar{v}_{O_2}$ divided by Sa_{O_2}) all have been shown to provide indirect clues to the presence of tissue oxygen delivery problems.[9]

To make matters more complicated, there are numerous case reports of patients tolerating severe anemia in the postoperative setting in Jehovah's Witnesses, in patients with renal failure, and in situations in which matched blood could not be obtained. These reports were compiled in a formative review by Hébert and colleagues for the Canadian Guidelines on Blood Transfusion.[10] This qualitative review concluded that there was little evidence of perioperative mortality when the preoperative hemoglobin concentration was above 8 g/dL and the estimated blood loss at surgery was less than 500 mL. However, patients having the same hemoglobin level and either older age (>50 years) or greater blood loss were subject to greater mortality.[11] Hemoglobin levels below 8 g/dL are accompanied by a rise in mortality.[12]

Risk factors for adverse outcomes from anemia have been examined in a number of recent publications, and these risk factors are more prevalent in patients in the ICU.[13–15] Most of the evidence for these adverse risk factors is empiric, retrospective, and cohort based. ICU admission alone is a risk factor for poor outcome, as are advanced age and underlying cardiac, cerebrovascular, or respiratory insufficiency.[16,17] In particular, the Carson series of Jehovah's Witnesses allows for a calculation of the relative risk according to perioperative hemoglobin levels: The odds ratio for mortality in patients having a hemoglobin of 6 g/dL preoperatively is 2.5 times the risk of a nonanemic patient, but the mortality rises from 2.5- to 16-fold in the presence of cardiac disease. A retrospective review of Medicare data for patients having myocardial infarction showed that transfusion was associated with lower 30-day mortality in patients having hematocrits of 27% or lower, and with higher mortality in patients having admission hematocrits of 36% or more.[18] Perioperative transfusions after hip fracture were associated with no difference in outcome for patients with hemoglobin levels of 8 g/dL or greater. While overall severity of illness appears to be a risk factor, most of the other studies involving patients in the ICU are too small to examine the independent effects of age, cardiac and cerebrovascular disease, and degree of blood loss.

CAUSES OF ANEMIA IN THE ICU

RED CELL LOSS OR DESTRUCTION

Hemorrhage is the most common cause of anemia in the ICU; those losses arise from surgical intervention or from medical causes of bleeding, and are the sole contributor to anemia in up to 20% of anemic patients in the ICU (Table 68-1).[4] The severity of red cell loss, and the resultant need for transfusion, is also dependent on the degree of underlying illness in a particular patient, as well as the type of surgery being performed, and the exact medical cause of bleeding. Underlying conditions such as renal failure, nutritional failure, liver disease, and drug effects have been shown to increase the risk of bleeding in critically ill patients.[2]

Red cell losses attributable to phlebotomy can be considerable; when originally reported, they probably amounted to the equivalent of two units of red blood cells in an average ICU patient.[19] Phlebotomy losses are greatest in the first few days of ICU admission. Following the initial

TABLE 68-1 Causes of Anemia in the ICU

Loss of red blood cells
  Hemorrhage
    Surgery
    Nonsurgical
  Phlebotomy
  Extracorporeal circuits: hemodialysis, membrane oxygenator, hemofiltration, plasmapheresis
  Wounds and burns (until covered)
  Immune-mediated hemolysis
    Autoimmune
    Drug-induced
    Infection-related
  Nonimmune hemolysis
    Endovascular devices
    Thrombotic thrombocytopenic purpura, hemolytic-uremic syndrome
    Metabolic defects (e.g., glucose-6-phosphate dehydrogenase deficiency)
Underproduction of red blood cells
  Anemia of chronic disease
    Suppression of erythropoietin production
    ?Suppression of response to erythropoietin
    Alterations in iron metabolism and delivery
    Nutritional failure
Bone marrow suppression
  Immune
  Drugs, toxins

publications regarding the extent of red cell loss, a variety of conservation measures have been employed, including microanalytic techniques, continuous arterial sampling, the use of external oxygen monitoring, and increasing nursing precautions for blood loss at phlebotomy or other patient procedures.[20] Early closure of burns reduces red cell loss dramatically. Recently published prospective series suggest that the fraction of red cell loss attributable to "medical vampires" has been reduced to less than 20% of all calculated red cell loss.[21]

Red cell destruction also occurs in critically ill patients, although is it a less common cause of red cell loss than is blood loss. Intravascular events that cause mechanical shearing and red cell destruction include disseminated intravascular coagulation (DIC), thrombotic thrombocytopenic purpura (TTP), and endovascular devices, especially newly placed endovascular grafts and older mechanical cardiac prosthetic valves. Thermal destruction of red cells may occur in particular situations, including malfunctioning blood warmers, patients with thermal injuries and with heat exposure, but not in patients with high fever only.

Immune-mediated red cell destruction is also less common than blood loss, but often unrecognized. Autoimmune hemolytic anemia is a very rare event in a critically ill patient, but may be seen in patients with the acquired immunodeficiency syndrome (AIDS), autoimmune diseases, and lymphomas. More common is alloimmunization due to transfusion; delayed red cell hemolysis due to delayed transfusion reactions is often unrecognized and may occur in one in 4000 red cell transfusions.[22] The estimates of red cell sensitization for patients undergoing coronary bypass surgery, for example, are a risk of approximately 1% per unit of red cells transfused.

While critically ill patients are less likely to experience primary immunization to homologous red cell antigens than are either healthy volunteers or less sick patients,[23] nonetheless, prior exposures to homologous red cells may predispose to delayed transfusion reactions even though the patient is at the time quite severely compromised.

Drug-induced red cell destruction may occur by several mechanisms: glucose-6-phosphate dehydrogenase (G-6-PD) deficiency is the most common cause of metabolic hemolysis. In the presence of oxidative stress from drugs such as sulfas, primaquine, nitrofurantoin, phenazopyridine, and dapsone, G-6-PD-deficient patients may experience intravascular hemolysis, occasionally on a large scale with accompanying hyperbilirubinemia and hemoglobinuria. But other minor metabolic abnormalities, unstable hemoglobin molecules, and red cell membrane defects may also be associated with hemolysis under the stress of critical illness. More commonly, drugs bound to the red cell membrane act as antigens and stimulate an immune response or form an immune complex which then binds to the red cell surface as a by-stander site. The result is immune-mediated, usually extravascular, hemolysis and anemia. Because the antibodies only bind when the drug is present, this particular form of immune-mediated hemolysis is particularly reversible with the cessation of the drug. Other drugs such as methyldopa are capable of inducing autoantibodies; still others cause hemolysis by unknown mechanisms. Common causes of drug-induced immune hemolysis include penicillins, cephalosporins, quinine and related drugs, sulfas and sulfonylureas, and procainamide.

Another rare cause of red cell destruction in critically ill patients is sepsis due to a variety of infectious agents that can cause hemolysis. Malaria is usually recognizable by history and blood film examination. Babesiosis is a tick-borne intracellular parasite that may also be recognized on peripheral blood smear. *Bartonella bacilliformis* adheres to red cell membranes and induces their destruction in the spleen and reticuloendothelial system. Massive intravascular hemolysis may occur in patients with *Clostridium perfringens* sepsis, due to the formation by the organisms of lysolecithins and resulting red cell membrane proteolysis. Overwhelming infections with the DNA viruses Epstein-Barr, herpes, and cytomegalovirus are associated with hemolysis, probably due to immune complexes. Hemolysis has also been observed in varicella, influenza, measles, and coxsackievirus infections. Mycoplasma infections are commonly associated with the formation of cold agglutinins; occasionally these produce overt cold-mediated hemolysis. Infections with enterotoxin-inducing species of *Escherichia coli* and other enteric organisms trigger hemolytic uremic syndrome.

RED CELL UNDERPRODUCTION
The humoral response to stress and infection includes the production of a wide variety of inflammatory cytokines that have an adverse effect on red cell production, erythropoietin production and responsiveness, iron metabolism, and the reticuloendothelial system. The end result of this adaptation to stress and infection is the characteristic anemia of chronic disease (ACD). The laboratory phenomena associated with the anemia of chronic disease have all been observed in critically ill patients, and evolve rapidly at the onset of severe

illness such as sepsis and multiorgan failure.[24] The anemia of chronic disease may also be present prior to ICU admission, as it is a common manifestation of inflammatory and neoplastic disease.

Inflammatory cytokines cause suppression of marrow production of red cells. This phenomenon is seen in a wide variety of illnesses, including minor viral infections. Ordinarily it is brief in duration and produces only a small impact on red cell mass. In critical illness, however, marrow suppression is combined with other disorders of red cell synthesis to produce more profound and durable anemia. One phenomenon that has been documented in the anemia of chronic disease is shortening of red cell lifespan. There is no evidence that this is directly immune-mediated, nor that the red cells themselves are abnormal. The current theory is that the 20% to 30% reduction in lifespan is a result of exaggerated surveillance by an activated reticuloendothelial system.[25,26]

Underproduction of erythropoietin has also been documented in critically ill patients. This may be a direct consequence of hepatic or renal failure, but is more often related to suppression of production of erythropoietin and perhaps to relative refractoriness of the marrow to its effects. Serum erythropoietin levels below those expected for the degree of anemia have been demonstrated in critically ill patients.[27,28] What is more controversial is whether pharmacologic erythropoietin treatment has a significant impact on overall outcomes (see below).

Another phenomenon observed in critically ill patients and in patients with chronic disease is abnormal iron metabolism. Iron has two sources: dietary iron is absorbed in the small intestine, transferred across the epithelial cells and into the bloodstream to the carrier molecule transferrin, where it is made available to the marrow storage cells. Iron is also recycled from senescent red cells by macrophages. Transferrin and ferritin are the molecules that deliver stored iron to developing erythrocytes. In chronic illness, ferritin levels are usually normal or elevated, but iron transport via ferritin into developing erythrocytes is suppressed, probably by responses to inflammation within the macrophages themselves. Transferrin production and transfer of iron from macrophages to transferrin is also often suppressed, and serum iron and iron binding capacity levels are low as a consequence. The result is that although iron absorption is normal, iron reuse from storage is suppressed, and overall production of red cells declines.

While the suppressive effects of the anemia of chronic disease are likely to be the most important elements causing prolonged anemia in the ICU, a variety of other causes of red cell underproduction should be assessed and treated in critically ill patients. Nutritional factors are particularly important, as they lend themselves to obvious solutions. Underlying nutritional deficiency may antedate entry into the ICU, particularly in the elderly, in alcoholics, and in patients with underlying gastrointestinal or other conditions that predispose to undernutrition. Folic acid, vitamin B_{12}, micronutrients (copper, selenium, and zinc) and calorie malnutrition all may cause anemia or perpetuate it in a critically ill patient.[29] Bone marrow suppression from drugs is important in cancer patients, but should be evaluated in patients taking suppressive therapies for autoimmune diseases, and in patients on chronic nonphenothiazine antipsychotic medications and phenytoin. The presence of pancytopenia should prompt an evaluation of the peripheral blood smear for evidence of disruption of marrow architecture, and perhaps bone marrow biopsy to evaluate the anemia.

EVALUATION OF ANEMIA IN THE ICU

Patients with anemia upon admission to the ICU should have the same considerations of cause as any patient admitted to the hospital. A medical history may disclose the underlying conditions, the duration of the anemia, and prior evaluation. Patients having unknown causes or new onset of anemia upon ICU admission should be thoroughly evaluated at the onset of their stay, since the underlying cause may both prove useful in the overall treatment of the patient, and will certainly assist in the management of the anemia during the ICU stay. Patients who acquire their anemia during the ICU stay have a slightly different set of conditions to consider.

The work-up of anemic patients should begin with the evaluation of the peripheral blood smear and the reticulocyte count. Normal to low reticulocyte counts should be expected in patients sick enough to merit ICU admission, and thus a high reticulocyte count should prompt an evaluation for chronic hemolysis or other red cell destruction. Patients' mean corpuscular volume (MCV) should also be evaluated; frankly megaloblastic red cells have a limited differential diagnosis, as do frankly microcytic red blood cells. Most patients, however, will have normal red cell volumes. The evaluation of both the peripheral blood smear and the MCV are complicated by the addition of transfused red blood cells. Pancytopenia should prompt a still different set of diagnoses, including bone marrow disorders and marrow toxins.

The evaluation of hemolysis also begins with the peripheral blood smear. Red cell fragmentation and distortion, producing schistocytes and teardrop cells, are indications of intravascular events or intramedullary events that mechanically fragment red cells, and suggest the diagnosis of DIC, TTP, or marrow infiltration.

Most patients will prove to have normochromic, normocytic anemia with a low or normal reticulocyte count and no obvious alterations in red cell morphology on peripheral blood smear. Such patients are likely to have the anemia of chronic disease. This may antedate ICU admission and be due to underlying chronic illness, or may appear in the ICU as a consequence of acute illness and marrow suppression, combined with steady blood loss. Whether such a patient requires some other confirmatory test to prove the presence of ACD is controversial. For example, critically ill patients (and many other categories of chronically ill patients without renal failure) display erythropoietin levels that are below the range considered normal for their degree of anemia. However, measuring erythropoietin levels is expensive, often not readily available, and is not considered a standard for the evaluation of ACD in the ICU. Similarly, the iron transport protein ferritin should be normal or elevated in ACD, and low when ACD is accompanied by iron deficiency. However, serum iron levels themselves are often low, and transferrin levels low in ACD in the ICU. These common indices of the suppression of red cell production are in themselves only suggestive of ACD and are not widely used to make a diagnosis. Hence, the diagnosis of ACD is usually one of exclusion. The extent to which testing for other causes of anemia is undertaken depends on the clinical situation.

TRANSFUSION THERAPY IN THE ICU

INDICATIONS FOR TRANSFUSION

In spite of a long tradition of transfusion of red blood cells in critically ill patients, the precise indications for transfusion remain a source of controversy, and specific transfusion practices may vary widely among clinicians. Prior to the major randomized studies of transfusion policies, survey studies of transfusion practice showed that about half of ICU patients were receiving red cell transfusions,[30] and another showed that if the ICU stay was longer than a week, the rate of transfusion was 85%.[31] Total numbers of transfusions were high, and ICU practice was characterized by high rates of transfusions.[32]

There have been only ten randomized trials of transfusion policy in the ICU, and only one of these was large enough to draw specific, statistically significant conclusions.[33] The Canadian Critical Care Trials Group compared a liberal (target hemoglobin 10 to 12 g/dL) with a restrictive (target hemoglobin 7 to 9 g/dL) red cell transfusion policy in patients stratified for disease severity. At 30 days from randomization, the restrictive strategy was at least as good as, if not better than ($p = 0.11$) the liberal strategy, and overall hospital mortality was significantly lower for the restrictive strategy group ($p = 0.05$). For patients under 55 years of age and for patients with lower (≤ 20) Acute Physiology, Age, and Chronic Health Evaluation (APACHE) II scores, the restrictive strategy was clearly superior. In addition, liberal transfusion was not associated with shorter ICU stays, less organ failure, or shorter hospital stays; longer mechanical ventilation times and cardiac events were more frequent in the liberal strategy group. A later subgroup analysis of patients having cardiovascular disease, while small enough to have statistical doubt, suggested that for patients with severe ischemic coronary disease a more liberal transfusion strategy was probably appropriate.[34] The Canadian study has highlighted the many and complex issues involved in transfusion decision making in the ICU.

Since the publication of the Canadian study, several large reports have examined utilization of red cell transfusions in critical care units. Vincent and colleagues[3] surveyed European ICUs, and found that transfusion rates for 3534 patients were 37% during the ICU stay and 12.7% after the ICU stay. The mean pretransfusion hemoglobin level was 8.4 g/dL. Corwin and colleagues[35] studied 284 ICUs in the United States a year later and found great similarity: nearly 50% of patients received transfusions, and the mean threshold hemoglobin level was 8.6 g/dL. A single large Scottish teaching hospital reported a more parsimonious practice; the rate of transfusion was still 52% in its ICU patients, but the total volume of blood used was slightly smaller and the mean pretransfusion hemoglobin was only 7.8 g/dL.[36] All of these authors have concluded that ICU practice has not fully embraced the guidelines of the Canadian clinical trial. In contrast, eighteen hospitals in Australia and New Zealand have reported on transfusion in 1808 consecutive ICU admissions, and although the authors found a median pretransfusion hemoglobin of 8.2 g/dL, the rate of transfusion was lower, at only 19.7% of patients, 60% of whom were bleeding.[37] The "inappropriate" transfusion rate was 3%. The authors speculate that the practitioners may have been influenced by the publication of the Canadian study and their own regional survey of transfusion practices. Nonetheless, they agree that full implementation of the Canadian guidelines in their clinical setting might be controversial.

COMPONENTS AVAILABLE FROM THE BLOOD BANK
Whole Blood and Red Cell Products
Whole blood, approximately 450 to 500 mL obtained by phlebotomy, is generally stored in an acid-citrate-dextrose medium, and is most often available only for replacement during acute hemorrhage, where transfusion requirements are likely to be large. Because most donated units of blood are separated into components rather than remaining as whole blood, whole blood has become less available.

Fresh whole blood, which has been removed from donors within a few hours of its use, has not been shown to be more effective than stored whole blood, and is only very rarely available, in part because complete infection testing may take several days. Whole blood that has been stored less than 10 days does exhibit longer red cell survival than blood that has been subjected to longer storage, and there is some evidence that the red cells in whole blood have slightly longer survival than red cells that are stored as packed red blood cells. Patients who are at high risk of clinical problems from the transfusion of hemolyzed or senescent red cells may be candidates for blood that has been stored for a shorter time period. Such patients include those with anticipated difficulty clearing bilirubin, such as neonates.

Packed red blood cells (PRBCs) consist of essentially all of the red cells in a unit of whole blood, with platelets and plasma largely removed, so that the resulting cells are at a hematocrit of about 70%. Their higher viscosity may result in longer transfusion times.

Red blood cells store well when frozen, usually in glycerol. Their shelf life is vastly extended, and they can be shipped with little risk of loss. Rare donor types may be stored in one institution and made available nationwide to other blood banks. Frozen red cells are no less likely to transmit most diseases than refrigerated stored red cells. Preparation for transfusion of frozen red cells consists of careful thawing and dilution and recentrifugation in order to remove the glycerol. Opening and manipulating the stored red cells results in a short shelf life; they must be used within 24 hours in order to avoid the risk of bacterial contamination.

"Washed" red cells are produced by recentrifugation in saline solution in order to remove plasma and contaminating white blood cells. They must also be used rapidly after washing, and because of this and the cost of the washing procedure, most institutions use white blood cell filters to prevent febrile transfusion reactions prior to considering the washing procedure. Washing does permit the administration of red cell transfusions to patients with a history of major allergic responses to plasma transfusion (see below).

Irradiation of blood products renders the lymphocytes nonviable, and is used to prevent graft-versus-host disease (see below). Irradiated red cells have a normal life span, do not require expedited handling, and may perhaps be less likely to transmit viral disease.

One blood conservation strategy that is probably underused, although it is currently estimated to be the source of approximately 7.5% of all transfusions, is autologous predeposit of whole blood. Designated donor blood, which has not been shown to be safer than volunteer donor blood, comprises 1% to 2% of all transfusions. Whole blood from autologous predeposit or from designated donors is tested and stored in the same fashion as donor blood. Institutional guidelines vary with respect to the handling of autologous units that test positive for transmissible diseases. While federal regulations allow the storage and use of such units of blood, many institutions either label it with biohazard labels or do not allow its use at all in order to attempt to avoid the potential for clerical error and transfusion to another patient (see section on risks, below). Unfortunately, wastage of both autologous and designated donor blood is approximately 50%, higher than that for volunteer donor blood (about 15%). This observation suggests that overcollection may be occurring.

Red blood cells are customarily stored for 72 to 90 days; during that time they gradually become deficient in 2,3-diphosphoglycerate (2,3-DPG), and a small fraction of stored cells also gradually lyse, releasing potassium, hemoglobin, and red cell stroma into the pack. Red cell senescence is accelerated in storage, and the survival of red cells held in storage is shorter than normal. Altered conditions of storage, such as the addition of alanine, that improve red cell survival unfortunately diminish 2,3-DPG levels, and vice versa. Individual blood bank policies and practices with respect to preservation solutions vary. Usage of red cells beyond the storage limit can result in higher risks of bacterial transmission.

Heat and mechanical fragmentation both can disrupt stored red cells. Blood warmers must be checked for temperature accuracy, since exposure to temperatures over 42°C can result in significant hemolysis of red cells. Attempts to restore the 2,3-DPG levels of stored red cells are not necessary, as the cells rapidly replete when transfused. However, citrate toxicity, which results in hypocalcemia, may be seen when large volumes of blood are administered over a very short time (more than a liter in an hour or two). The intravenous administration of calcium gluconate is recommended for treatment of this problem.

Platelets, Plasma, and Other Products
Platelets do not survive refrigeration, and therefore platelets are removed from fresh whole blood and stored at 22°C under continuous agitation. They may also be obtained by pheresis of a single donor, which harvests about the same amount as five to six units of platelets. Stored platelets are viable for up to a week, and transfused platelets last up to 72 hours in normal recipients.

Platelets pheresed from a single donor may be used to reduce the risk of immunization of recipients who are repeatedly exposed to platelet transfusions. Platelets may be matched to specific platelet antigens or to human leukocyte antigen (HLA) haplotypes; both techniques may be used to successfully give platelet transfusions to recipients who have already become sensitized to random donor platelets.

Plasma may be stored whole, usually as fresh frozen whole plasma. Each unit of plasma from the blood bank is about 200 to 250 mL. Fresh frozen plasma must be thawed carefully, and thawed plasma is rarely kept in storage in blood banks. Cryoprecipitate is prepared from fresh plasma by freezing, then slow thawing to 60°F. The resulting flocculant precipitate contains factor VIII_C/von Willebrand factor (vWF), fibrinogen (about one-third of that in the unit of blood), and fibronectin. Commercial cryoprecipitate is lyophilized after the precipitate is harvested. Both of these plasma products have long shelf lives, though shorter half lives once transfused than their native counterparts. When made into cryoprecipitate, a unit of plasma yields about 80 to 100 units of factor VIII$_C$/vWF and about 200 to 300 mg of fibrinogen. Cryoprecipitate can be reconstituted in extremely small volumes, making it useful when volume overload is a concern.

Specific coagulation factors may be manufactured from pooled plasma or as recombinant DNA products. The latter are more expensive, but appear to have fewer complications, including sensitization and disease transmission. These include human recombinant factor VIII, factor IX, activated protein C, and activated factor VII.

Commercial preparations of plasma also include plasma products that are free of immunoglobulins, that consist of activated or non-activated liver-dependent clotting factors (prothrombin complex), and fibrin "glue" or fibrin sheets.

RISKS OF TRANSFUSION THERAPY
Cross-Matching and Sensitization
Red cells are cross-matched by mixing recipient serum with type-specific (ABO and Rh) donor cells at two different temperatures (major cross-match) and donor serum with recipient red cells (minor cross-match). This takes time, and only under desperate circumstances should this step be omitted. Cross-matching may be complicated by a variety of problems. Nonspecific cold agglutinins are seen in a host of medical conditions, and they cause difficulty matching at room temperature and sometimes at 37°C. Cold agglutinins are usually not associated with serious hemolytic reactions in vivo, but they make cross-matching difficult and they may mask the presence of other antibodies. The warm antibodies seen in autoimmune hemolytic anemia are usually IgG, are associated with autoimmune disease and certain malignancies, and make conventional cross-matching of red cells very difficult because they react with almost all red cells. The procedure for cross-matching in patients having warm antibodies involves eluting the warm antibodies from the patient's plasma so that a cross-match may be performed. If antibody elution is not available, the consensus is that blood banks should provide the best possible match of type-specific blood, knowing that hemolysis may be no greater than it is endogenously. Surface antigens are weakly expressed in neonates, the extremely elderly, and massively transfused patients, making cross-matching difficult. Larger volumes of blood will be needed to cross-match these patients.

In spite of cross-matching, sensitization to homologous blood transfusion occurs, and may become a clinical problem for repetitively transfused individuals, especially those who have rare blood types. The risk of sensitization to red cells is estimated at 1% per transfusion episode; in contrast, the risk of platelet sensitization is 5% to 10% per pooled random donor transfusion episode. Recipient sensitization to leukocyte antigens also occurs during red cell transfusion and may be the basis for some febrile reactions, but is otherwise usually of little clinical significance. On the other hand, the presence of leukocyte antibodies in the donor plasma, the presumed cause of transfusion-associated lung injury, can be prevented only by much more complex leukocyte typing.

Hemolytic Transfusion Reactions
Intravascular hemolysis of transfused red blood cells is caused by complement fixation and rapid intravascular destruction of ABO incompatible red cells, or by the same process in a previously sensitized patient with a high-titer antibody such as anti-Kell or antibodies to Rh system components. The syndrome that results from massive intravascular hemolysis is due to the release of red cell stroma, which causes cytokine, bradykinin, and granulocyte mediator release. Hypotension, capillary leak, and oliguria are manifestations that follow very rapidly after the onset of intense intravascular hemolysis. The most feared complications are disseminated intravascular coagulation, acute renal failure, and the acute respiratory distress syndrome (ARDS). The majority of acute hemolytic transfusion reactions are caused by clerical or nursing error, and fortunately, deaths are rare.

The treatment of hemolytic transfusion reactions is supportive. Early recognition of the syndrome and stopping the offending transfusion are critical. Recognition may be difficult during general anesthesia, and the symptoms at the bedside may also be initially confusing. The decision to stop a transfusion is often difficult unless the findings are very extreme. Most clinicians believe that supporting high urine output is important during the resuscitation of these patients, but that diuretics should be used only if the patient shows intravascular volume overload. The use of mannitol is controversial. There is no role for steroids, antihistamines, heparin, colloid, or other specific pharmacologic interventions. Treatment of the complications should be vigorous, as the majority of patients survive the event.

Delayed Transfusion Reactions
Red cell sensitization may result in an antibody response that is initially weak and does not persist. However, the patient's next exposure to that red cell antigen will arouse an anamnestic immune response, and higher titers of antibody may occur fairly rapidly after transfusion. If an extremely brisk anamnestic response produces antibodies capable of fixing complement, patients may have intravascular hemolysis of the transfused cells within a few days of transfusion. These delayed transfusion reactions usually produce jaundice, and elevated lactate dehydrogenase (LDH) and low haptoglobin levels, but may occasionally be severe and result in oliguria. If the antibody does not fix complement, extravascular hemolysis of the transfused red cells will occur. This type of delayed transfusion reaction is often subtle, but results in elevations in LDH and indirect bilirubin, occasionally the appearance of spherocytes in the peripheral blood smear, a positive direct antiglobulin (Coombs) test, and falling hemoglobin levels. Documentation of such a reaction is important so that future transfusions are more carefully screened.

Other Types of Transfusion Reactions
Febrile transfusion reactions are most often attributed to the presence of granulocytes in transfused blood, although they may also be caused by plasma factors such as exogenous immunoglobulins or rarely by bacterial pyrogens. Benign febrile transfusion reactions may be distinguished from the fever associated with intravascular hemolytic transfusion reactions by the lack of hypotension, chills, or other signs of hemolysis, and by the generally delayed onset of fever compared to hemolytic transfusion reactions. Febrile reactions are usually treated with acetaminophen or aspirin; use of these drugs and occasionally antihistamines for prophylaxis is also common. Patients who have repeated febrile reactions should receive leukocyte-filtered blood.

Urticarial transfusion reactions are thought to be caused by plasma components. One rare subset of patients with congenital IgA deficiency (about one in 650 to 900 persons) may have anaphylaxis due to plasma exposure, but in general urticarial reactions are not accompanied by a risk of anaphylaxis. Urticarial reactions are usually treated with antihistamines and may be treated prophylactically. IgA-deficient patients may be transfused with washed packed red blood cells, or failing that, with IgA-deficient red cells. Products such as platelets must be from IgA-deficient donors. Patients who have repetitive urticarial reactions in spite of prophylaxis may need to receive related-donor blood products.

Transfusion-related acute lung injury (TRALI) is an uncommon syndrome that is due to the presence of leukocyte antibodies in transfused plasma. TRALI is believed to occur in approximately one in every 5000 transfusions. Leukoagglutination and pooling of granulocytes in the recipient's lungs may occur, with release of the contents of leukocyte granules, and resulting injury to cellular membranes, endothelial surfaces, and potentially to lung parenchyma. In most cases leukoagglutination results in mild dyspnea and pulmonary infiltrates within about 6 hours of transfusion, and spontaneously resolves; occasionally more severe lung injury occurs as a result of this phenomenon and ARDS results.[38] Leukocyte filters may prevent TRALI for those patients whose lung injury is due to leukoagglutination of the donor white blood cells, but because most TRALI is due to donor antibodies to leukocytes, filters are not helpful in TRALI prevention. Transfused plasma (from any component source) may also contain antibodies that cross-react with platelets in the recipient, producing usually mild forms of posttransfusion purpura or platelet aggregation after transfusion.

Another nonspecific form of immunologic transfusion complication is mild to moderate immunosuppression consequent to transfusion. This effect of transfusion is not completely understood, but appears to be more common with cellular transfusion and may result in both desirable and undesirable effects. Mild immunosuppression may benefit organ transplant recipients and patients with autoimmune diseases; however, neonates and other already immunosuppressed hosts may be more vulnerable to infection, and cancer patients may possibly have worse outcomes postoperatively.[39]

Graft-versus-host disease (GVHD) occurs when immunocompetent lymphocytes are transfused into an immunoincompetent recipient. The lymphocytes proliferate and respond to recipient HLA antigens. The syndrome presents as fever, skin rash, and liver function abnormalities occurring 2 to 6 weeks after transfusion. Graft-versus-host disease is highly lethal in reported cases outside of the transplantation situation; it is very morbid in transplant settings as well. GVHD primarily occurs in organ transplantation, leukemia, and other severely immunosuppressed patients, but it has been reported following cardiac surgery and in neonates. GVHD has been reported only once in a patient with the acquired immunodeficiency syndrome (AIDS). The correct diagnosis is made by recognizing the syndrome and obtaining a skin biopsy. Prevention in the non–bone marrow transplant setting is to irradiate every cellular blood product before use. Treatment of active graft-versus-host disease involves further immunosuppression with cyclosporine, antithymocyte globulin, steroids, and cytotoxic drugs. Critically ill adult patients who are receiving blood transfusions from family members should have those related donor products irradiated.[40]

In order to reduce the risks of immunosuppression and GVHD, cytomegalovirus (CMV) transmission, and perhaps of alloimmunization, leukocyte reduction through the routine use of white blood cell filters has been undertaken. Several randomized trials of leukoreduced transfusions in critically ill patients have been published, but none of the trials has been large enough to demonstrate benefits unequivocally, and most are negative. However, the largest prospective study performed to date was a Canadian sequential cohort study that has shown some potential benefits to routine leukoreduction.[41] The study closely followed 6982 patients using routine practice, followed by the institution of universal leukoreduction in all blood banks and follow-up of 7804 patients' outcomes. The main outcome measure was all-cause in-hospital mortality, which was reduced during the leukoreduction period compared to the previous period (odds ratio [OR] 0.87; 95% confidence interval 0.75 to 0.99). The second outcome measure, nosocomial infections, was not changed by leukoreduction, although the frequency of fevers and the use of antibiotics were reduced. The cost effectiveness of this strategy has yet to be analyzed.

Risks of Disease Transmission

Hepatitis transmission from blood transfusion is rapidly becoming a rare event. Nucleic acid testing for hepatitis B is universal. The current estimate of the risk of hepatitis B is less than 1 in 200,000.[42] Nucleic acid–based screening tests for hepatitis C provide excellent protection. It detects more potentially infectious units of blood than the enzyme-linked immunosorbent assay (ELISA) test, and is thought to have the potential to reduce the rate of posttransfusion hepatitis to less than the current 5% nationwide.[43] Individuals who have an acute hepatitis-like illness after transfusion should be tested for hepatitis C; however, since the antibody screen is not 100% sensitive. The vast majority of individuals infected do develop antibodies within the first 6 months after transmission. Many of those people may lose their antibodies later on, hence the less-than-perfect screening test. Posttransfusion hepatitis may be caused by other as yet poorly characterized hepatitis viruses, but it is an uncommon event when donor screening by questionnaire and serology is performed.

AIDS transmission is also an unusual event. Both nucleic acid–based tests and HIV antibody tests are routinely used, and the most recent estimates of risk nationwide are less than one in two million.[44] Human T-lymphocyte virus (HTLV) I/II is also tested using ELISA antibody detection, and the total number of cases related to transmission of this virus in the U.S. is fewer than two dozen annually. Transfusion-associated HIV is more rapidly lethal than most community-acquired cases. Acute HIV infection is characterized by fever, adenopathy, and pancytopenia. For all disease testing, repetitively tested volunteer donor blood has been shown to have a higher safety profile than family donors or designated donors.

Cytomegalovirus transmission remains a clinical problem. Forty to sixty percent of adults in the U.S. are antibody-positive for CMV; most, however, are not infectious. Clinical studies have estimated transmission to occur in 3 to 12 recipients/100 units of blood transfused. Rises in antibody titers or seroconversion have been shown in up to 30% of transfused surgical patients. More than 90% of seroconverters/titer increases are asymptomatic, but in vulnerable recipients, CMV produces acute illness. Neonates, premature, or low birth weight infants are at highest risk; 13% to 37% acquire CMV, and up to one in four dies of it.[44] Bone marrow transplant recipients have a high rate of early death due to CMV pneumonitis, although most of this is thought to represent endogenous reactivation of virus replication. Other vulnerable patients include cancer patients, AIDS patients, seronegative pregnant women, and splenectomy patients. Symptomatic acute cytomegalovirus infection results in a clinical syndrome that resembles infectious mononucleosis. Treatment of cytomegalovirus disease is marginally effective; drugs used in infected patients are mostly suppressive unless remission of the immunosuppression occurs. White blood cell filters, chemoprophylaxis for seropositive patients, and use of seronegative blood products for others are important and useful strategies in the bone marrow transplant setting, and transmission is prevented in neonates by the use of seronegative donor blood products.[45]

Blood may be contaminated by bacteria at the time of collection. This is a rare event, at a rate of 0.21 per million units of red cells transfused, but it is fatal in about one third of recipients, especially if the contaminating organism is a gram-negative rod.[46] Contamination is more than twice as likely from platelets or plasma. Other blood-borne diseases that may be transmitted by transfusion include parvovirus B19, Epstein-Barr virus, human herpesvirus-8 (HHV-8), malaria, brucellosis, trypanosomiasis, syphilis, toxoplasmosis, West Nile virus, the severe acute respiratory syndrome, and possibly variant Creutzfeldt-Jakob disease (or bovine spongiform encephalopathy).

THE MASSIVELY TRANSFUSED PATIENT

Patients suffering rapid blood loss require massive transfusion, generally defined as replacement of the entire blood volume within a 24-hour period, or equaling 50% of the blood volume in 3 hours. Typical conditions leading to massive transfusion include polytrauma, peripartum hemorrhage, gastrointestinal blood loss, aortic aneurysmal rupture, and perioperative bleeding. These patients are considered separately because the large volume of blood required leads to complications not generally associated with blood transfusion, most notably a severe coagulopathy. Moreover, management may benefit from a style that relies on prevention and empiricism as well as on laboratory testing.

Coagulopathy accompanying massive transfusion is multifactorial, including contributions from direct loss, consumption, and dilution of clotting factors and platelets; hypothermia as cool fluids are infused; and shock-related hepatic dysfunction leading to impaired clearance of activated coagulation factors and their breakdown products. It is generally believed that early detection and prevention of coagulopathy is more effective than later treatment by interrupting a vicious cycle that, if not avoided, culminates in a hypothermic, acidemic patient who responds very poorly to aggressive resuscitation. Early studies implicated thrombocytopenia as being the predominant early consequence of massive transfusion, but more recent studies show that a coagulation factor deficit is the earlier derangement. Hypocalcemia can contribute to coagulopathy during truly massive transfusion (greater than 100 mL/min), but this is not often seen because citrate can be rapidly metabolized by the liver.

Initial priorities in the massively bleeding patient include achieving hemostasis when this is possible; obtaining large-bore intravenous access (number and caliber are more important than location); assessing the need for intubation and mechanical ventilation; and infusing sufficient quantities of fluid (generally normal saline). Fluid warmers should be used early in anticipation of heat losses, not only when core temperature falls to abnormal levels. Packed red blood cells should be infused rapidly, dictated by the clinical assessments of blood loss, intravascular volume, and measured hemoglobin concentration. Laboratory tests of hemoglobin, coagulation parameters, platelets, and fibrinogen are indicated, but given the delay in obtaining results and preparing and transporting blood products, cannot provide the sole basis for plasma and platelet transfusion in all patients. Instead some centers have empiric guidelines recommending transfusion of fresh frozen plasma and platelets in some proportion to the amount of blood transfused once the patient is deemed to be "massively transfused." Such a formulaic approach has not been shown to improve outcomes and is strongly discouraged by many, but others attribute their unusually good outcomes in massively bleeding patients to such protocols. The roles for cryoprecipitate, prothrombin complex concentrates, and recombinant activated factor VII remain to be determined.

Some patients transfused massively will suffer uncommon complications such as abdominal compartment syndrome (see Chap. 42); electrolyte derangements such as hypocalcemia, hyperkalemia, or hypomagnesemia (see Chap. 76); and transfusion-related acute lung injury (see Chap. 38), although this is difficult to diagnose in a patient also at risk of fluid overload and aspiration.

ALTERNATIVES TO USE OF BLOOD BANK PRODUCTS

Presurgical storage, or autologous blood donation, makes up approximately 7.5% of all transfusions, although recent studies suggest that autologous donation is underused. Generally, practice has been to have patients donate a unit every 2 to 3 weeks prior to surgery, while taking oral iron and perhaps erythropoietin. There is some evidence that more units may be predeposited with the concomitant use of erythropoietin, although the ultimate clinical impact of such use is unknown. Patients do present for surgery slightly anemic. The FDA permits the use of autologous units that are hepatitis- or HIV-infected; individual institutions may not wish to assume the risk of handling such units and may reject such autologous donors. If used, this infected donated blood should be labeled as a biohazard and handled with extreme caution.

Designated donors, usually members of a patient's family, are often requested by physicians and patients as sources of blood products, usually with the idea that designated donors are less likely to have infectious diseases. Unfortunately, the published data demonstrate that in comparison to regular volunteer donors who have been screened, designated donor blood is more likely to test positive for infectious diseases. Designated donor blood is not necessarily safer than volunteer donor banked blood.

With the availability of recombinant human erythropoietin and its success in increasing hemoglobin concentration in patients with renal failure and bone marrow failure due to HIV infection or chemotherapy, the use of erythropoietin to reduce blood transfusions in critically ill patients seemed obvious. In the past decade, six randomized studies have evaluated exogenous administration of recombinant human erythropoietin (rHuEPO) to decrease red cell transfusions in the ICU.[47] They have varied with respect to dosage regimens, the dose of concurrently administered iron, patient characteristics (trauma, medical, and surgical), and transfusion thresholds. Although the use of rHuEPO does increase hemoglobin levels compared to concurrent or historical controls, the rate at which hemoglobin rises is slow, measured over a period of weeks, not days. The largest study conducted to date using the best methodology administered weekly rHuEPO and found a 19% decrease in transfusion requirements.[48] Reduced ICU length of stay was shown in only one study of surgical/trauma patients. Reduced hospital stay after ICU discharge was found in another study of severely ill patients (APACHE II score >22), a potentially important non-ICU outcome. A variety of other outcomes were measured in these studies, but none was significantly altered by rHuEPO use. No adverse events were associated with rHuEPO use, although these studies were not designed to evaluate safety, and the target hemoglobin was higher than that used in the Canadian transfusion trial. There are to date no published cost-effectiveness analyses.

Artificial blood substitutes are still in development. Perfluorocarbon products are chemically inert polyfluorinated hydrocarbons that are insoluble in plasma, but in which oxygen is soluble. They are produced as emulsions with surfactants and added hydroxyethyl starch and they need to be stored frozen. The oxygen delivery capability of these products is good, but the use of perfluorocarbons is limited by less efficient oxygen uptake, which requires 100% inspired oxygen delivery. In addition, the total dose and carrying capacity are limited, so that at the maximum dose, the contribution to the total hematocrit by perfluorocarbon, or "fluorocrit," is very low. Finally, these drugs are short-acting, with a half-life of only about 24 hours.[49,50]

Hemoglobin conjugated to polysaccharide is available in a variety of forms, although all have drawbacks with respect to oxygen-carrying capacity, reactions, vasoconstriction, and shorter half-lives. None is currently marketed for use in critical care.

Hemodilution and intraoperative autologous transfusion are other surgical techniques used to avoid transfusion. Hemodilution lowers blood viscosity, thought to be an advantage by some. While there are no formal randomized trials of hemodilution, there are ample nonrandomized studies in cardiac bypass surgery, orthopedic surgery, and Jehovah's Witness patients to suggest that hemodilution techniques are safe and can result in saving blood transfusions.[51] Intraoperative scavenging and reuse of red cells using cell saver technology has become widespread practice in major surgeries such as cardiac and vascular procedures. It remains controversial in trauma or "dirty" operative fields, however. A large number of published nonrandomized series attest to the relative safety of most "washing" cell savers now in use, although the research methodology does not allow for unequivocal demonstration of benefit for their use.[52] One systematic review of the available trials in abdominal aortic aneurysm repair does not clearly demonstrate an advantage with respect to the use of blood products,[53] while an overall review of cell salvage use supports safety and the potential for decreasing red cell use. The use of heparin, antibiotics, filters, and other adjuncts to cell salvage is not standardized.

Additional savings in blood loss have been made with the use of continuous intra-arterial monitoring devices, laboratory microtechniques, and concerted nursing efforts in intensive care units to reduce the number and volume of phlebotomies.

References

1. Sullivan MT, McCullough J, Schreiber GB, et al: Blood collection and transfusion in the United States in 1997. *Transfusion* 42:1253, 2002.
2. Brown RB, Klar J, Teres D, et al: Prospective study of clinical bleeding in intensive care unit patients. *Crit Care Med* 16:1171, 1988.
3. Vincent JL, Baron J-F, Reinhart K, et al: Anemia and blood transfusion in critically ill patients: an epidemiological, observational study. *JAMA* 288:1499, 2002.
4. Corwin HL, Surgenor SD, Gettinger A: Transfusion practice in the critically ill. *Crit Care Med* 31(12 Suppl):S668, 2003.
5. Shapiro MJ, Gettinger A, Corwin HL, et al: Anemia and blood transfusion in trauma patients admitted to the intensive care unit. *J Trauma* 55:269, 2003.
6. Messmer K, Lewis DH, Sunder-Plassman L, et al: Acute normovolemic hemodilution: changes of central hemodynamics and microcirculatory flow in skeletal muscle. *Eur Surg Res* 4:55, 1972.
7. Leung JM, Weiskopf RB, Feiner J, et al: Electrocardiographic ST-segment changes during acute, severe, isovolemic hemodilution in humans. *Anesthesiology* 93:1004, 2000.
8. Besarab A, Bolton WK, Browne JK, et al: The effect of normal as compared with low hematocrit values in patients with cardiac disease who are receiving hemodialysis and epoetin. *N Engl J Med* 339:584, 1998.
9. Spahn DR: Perioperative transfusion triggers for red blood cells. *Vox Sang* 78(Suppl 2):163, 2000.
10. Expert Working Group: Guidelines for red blood cell and plasma transfusions for adults and children: Report of the Expert Working Group. *Can Med Assoc J* 156(Suppl 11):S1, 1997.
11. Viele MK, Weiskopf RB: What can we learn about the need for transfusion from patients who refuse blood? The experience with Jehovah's Witnesses. *Transfusion* 34:396, 1994.
12. Carson JL, Noveck H, Berlin JA, Gould SA. Mortality and morbidity in patients with very low postoperative hemoglobin levels who decline blood transfusion. *Transfusion* 42:812, 2002.
13. Cane RD: Hemoglobin: How much is enough? *Crit Care Med* 18:1046, 1990.
14. Crosby ET: Perioperative haemotherapy: I. Indications for blood component transfusion. *Can J Anesth* 39:695, 1992.
15. Welch HG, Meehan KR, Goodnough LT: Prudent strategies for elective red blood cell transfusion. *Ann Intern Med* 116:393, 1992.
16. Carson JL, Duff A, Poses RM, et al : Effects of anaemia and cardiovascular disease on surgical mortality and morbidity. *Lancet* 348:1055, 1996.
17. Hebert PC, Wells G, Tweeddale M, et al: Does transfusion practice affect mortality in critically ill patients? *Am J Respir Crit Care Med* 155:1618, 1997.
18. Wu WC, Rathmore SS, Wang Y, et al: Effectiveness of blood transfusion in elderly patients with acute myocardial infarction. *N Engl J Med* 345:1230, 2001.
19. Burnum JF: Medical vampires. *N Engl J Med* 314:1250, 1986.
20. Foulke GE, Harlow DJ: Effective measures for reducing blood loss from diagnostic laboratory tests in intensive care unit patients. *Crit Care Med* 17:11443, 1989.
21. von Ahsen N, Muller C, Serke S, et al: Important role of nondiagnostic blood loss and blunted erythropoietic response in the anemia of medical intensive care patients. *Crit Care Med* 27:2630, 1999.

22. Pineda AA, Paswell HF, Brzica SM Jr: Delayed hemolytic transfusion reaction: an immunologic hazard of blood transfusion. *Transfusion* 18:1, 1978.

23. Schmidt PJ, Leparc GF, Samia CT: Use of Rh positive blood in emergency situations. *Surg Gynecol Obstet* 167:229, 1988.

24. van de Wiel A: Anemia in critically ill patients. *Eur J Intern Med* 15:481, 2004.

25. Dinant HJ, deMaat CEM: Erythropoiesis and mean red-cell life span in normal subjects and in patients with the anemia of active rheumatoid arthritis. *Br J Haematol* 39:437, 1978.

26. Atkinson JP, Frank MM: The effect of bacillus Calmette-Guerin-induced macrophage activation on the in vivo clearance of sensitized erythrocytes. *J Clin Invest* 53:1742, 1974.

27. Rogiers P, Zhang H, Leeman M, et al: Erythropoietin response is blunted in critically ill patients. *Intensive Care Med* 23:159, 1997.

28. Elliot JM, Virankabutra T, Jones S, et al: Erythropoietin mimics the acute phase response in critical illness. *Crit Care* 7:R35, 2003.

29. Rodriguez RM, Corwin HL, Gettinger A, et al: Nutritional deficiencies and blunted erythropoietin response as causes of the anemia of critical illness. *J Crit Care* 16:36, 2001.

30. Littenberg B, Corwin HL, Gettinger A, et al: A practice guideline and decision aide for blood transfusion. *Immunohematology* 11:88, 1995.

31. Corwin HC, Parsonnet KC, Gettinger A: RBC transfusion in the ICU: is there a reason? *Chest* 108:767, 1995.

32. Groeger JS, Guntapalli KK, Strosberg M, et al. Descriptive analysis of critical care units in the United States: Patient characteristics and intensive care unit utilization. *Crit Care Med* 21:279, 1993.

33. Hebert PC, Wells G, Blajchman MA, et al: A multicenter, randomized, controlled clinical trial of transfusion requirements in critical care. *N Engl J Med* 340:409, 1999.

34. Hebert PC, Yetisir E, Martin C, et al: Is a low transfusion threshold safe in critically ill patients with cardiovascular diseases? *Crit Care Med* 29:227, 2001.

35. Corwin HL, Gettinger A, Pearl RG, et al: The CRIT study: Anemia and blood transfusion in the critically ill—Current clinical practice in the United States. *Crit Care Med* 32:39, 2004.

36. Chohan SS, McArdle F, McClelland DBL, et al: Red cell transfusion practice following the transfusion requirements in critical care (TRICC) study: Prospective observational cohort study in a large UK intensive care unit. *Vox Sanguinis* 84:211, 2003.

37. French CJ, Bellomo R, Finfer SR, et al: Appropriateness of red blood cell transfusion in Australasian intensive care practice. *Med J Aust* 177:548, 2002.

38. Looney MR, Gropper MA, Matthay MA: Transfusion-related acute lung injury: A review. *Chest* 126:249, 2004.

39. Petranyi GG, Reti M, Harsanyi V, et al: Immunologic consequences of blood transfusion and their clinical manifestations. *Int Arch Allergy Immunol* 114:303, 1997.

40. Schroeder ML: Transfusion-associated graft-versus-host disease. *Br J Haematol* 117:275, 2002.

41. Hebert PC, Fergusson D, Blajchman MA, et al: Clinical outcomes following institution of the Canadian universal leukoreduction program for red blood cell transfusions. *JAMA* 289:1941, 2003.

42. Pomper GJ, Wu YY, Snyder EL: Risks of transfusion-transmitted infections: 2003. *Curr Opin Hematol* 10:412, 2003.

43. Stramer SL, Glynn SA, Kleinman SH, et al: Detection of HIV-1 and HCV infections among antibody-negative blood donors by nucleic acid-amplification testing. *N Engl J Med* 351:760, 2004.

44. Roback JD: CMV and blood transfusions. *Rev Med Virol* 12:211, 2002.

45. Bowden RA: Transfusion-transmitted cytomegalovirus infection. *Hematol Oncol Clin North Am* 9:155, 1995.

46. Kuehnert MJ, Roth VR, Haley NR, et al. Transfusion-transmitted bacterial infection in the United States, 1998 through 2000. *Transfusion* 41:1493, 2001.

47. Pajoumand M, Erstad BL, Camamo JM: Use of epoetin alfa in critically ill patients. *Ann Pharmacother* 38:641, 2004.

48. Corwin HL, Gettinger A, Pearl RG, et al: Efficacy of recombinant human erythropoietin in critically ill patients: a randomized controlled trial. *JAMA* 288:2827, 2002.

49. Gould SA, Rosen AL, Sehgal LR, et al: Fluosol-DA as a red-cell substitute in acute anemia. *N Engl J Med* 314:1653, 1986.

50. Spahn DR, Kocian R: The place of artificial oxygen carriers in reducing allogeneic blood transfusions and augmenting tissue oxygenation. *Can J Anaesth* 50(6 Suppl):S41, 2003.

51. Gillon J, Thomas MJ, Desmond MJ: Consensus conference on autologous transfusion. Acute normovolaemic haemodilution. *Transfusion* 36:640, 1996.

52. Carless PA, Henry DA, Moxey AJ, et al: Cell salvage for minimising perioperative allogeneic blood transfusion (Cochrane Review). In: The Cochrane Library, Issue 3, 2004. Chichester, UK: John Wiley & Sons, Ltd.

53. Alvarez GG, Fergusson DA, Neilipovitz DT, et al: Cell salvage does not minimize perioperative allogeneic blood transfusion in abdominal vascular surgery: a systematic review. *Can J Anaesth* 51:425, 2004.

Chapter 69 _____

BLEEDING DISORDERS

JOSEPH M. BARON
BEVERLY W. BARON

KEY POINTS

- *Assessment of the patient with a bleeding diathesis requires careful history-taking and bedside evaluation and comprehensive baseline coagulation testing.*

- *Uncomplicated vascular injury related to trauma or surgery should be eliminated as the primary cause of bleeding before the possibility of a coagulopathy is invoked.*

- *Consideration of coagulation abnormalities should include vascular disorders, platelet problems, impairment of the fibrin generation cascade, and excessive fibrinolytic activity.*

- *Disseminated intravascular coagulation may present with either thrombotic or bleeding problems. Awareness of the possibility of this diagnosis and prompt, appropriate laboratory confirmation may improve treatment selection and outcome.*

- *Invasive procedures in critically ill patients with coagulopathies need to be performed with special caution to prevent complications. Some guidelines are presented.*

Introduction to Bedside and Laboratory Diagnosis of Coagulopathies

Accurate diagnosis of the mechanism of a bleeding disorder is based on careful history-taking and bedside evaluation of the patient, coupled with appropriate confirmatory laboratory testing.[1] Information obtainable from the patient or others about a pre-existing congenital or acquired bleeding diathesis, medications being taken, recent surgery or pregnancy, and underlying disturbed organ function (e.g., hepatic or renal insufficiency) will facilitate the diagnostic process and provide the basis for directing empirical urgent therapy should it be necessary before laboratory testing can be completed.

Careful physical examination may clarify whether observed bleeding is strictly a local problem, i.e., limited to one site and not out of proportion in severity to that expected from an observed injury or fixed lesion, or is due to a systemic bleeding diathesis, which should be suspected if multiple bleeding or bruising sites are present and cannot be accounted for by the extent or severity of known trauma. In some patients with a single mechanism of systemic coagulopathy, it may be possible to distinguish a vascular or platelet disorder, which is characterized by immediate bleeding (prolonged, continued bleeding after onset and dominant petechial/mucosal manifestations), from a problem of fibrin generation (a cascade disorder) or of fibrinolysis, which is typified by delayed bleeding (rebleeding after initial hemostasis and prominent ecchymoses or deep muscle and joint hemorrhage). Complex coagulopathies, such as disseminated intravascular coagulopathy (DIC), may have features of both categories. The presence of findings such as splenomegaly or telangiectases also may be helpful clues.

Several generalizations based on data from the history and physical examination may help in directing the workup and treatment of bleeding problems. The first consideration in the evaluation of a bleeding patient—before a coagulopathy is invoked as a contributing cause—is to exclude uncomplicated vascular injury (related to trauma or surgery) that would be amenable to surgical hemostasis techniques. Second, brisk bleeding is almost never due to spontaneous hemorrhage caused by a coagulopathy alone. Third, clinically significant bleeding often is the result of the coexistence of trauma or a potential bleeding lesion (e.g., a peptic ulcer) with a coagulopathy that may antedate the lesion or may develop while the lesion is present. Fourth, initial and follow-up laboratory screening of critically ill patients for the presence of a potential bleeding diathesis is important in predicting and preventing bleeding complications during interventions such as line placements and surgical procedures.

Systematic laboratory evaluation of the patient with a coagulopathy[2] is facilitated by consideration of the factors necessary for normal clot formation and degradation (Table 69-1). An appropriate screening laboratory survey for a hemostatic disorder in the critically ill patient would include a complete blood count including platelet count; review of a peripheral smear for the presence of schistocytes and for the evaluation of platelet number, clumping, size, and appearance; rapid screening of in vitro platelet function[3] and measurement of bleeding time (unless the platelet count is less than $50,000/\mu L$); prothrombin time (PT), activated partial thromboplastin time (PTT), thrombin time (TT), and functional fibrinogen level; and the level of fibrin degradation products (FDPs) as well as D-dimer assay. These tests should be done simultaneously rather than sequentially in the critically ill patient.

The initial response to vessel injury with formation of the platelet plug depends on normal vascular and platelet function. Defects in these components are reflected in a prolonged bleeding time. Platelet dysfunction (e.g., aspirin effect, von Willebrand's disease) may be sorted out by in vitro platelet function screening.[3] Formation of the definitive fibrin clot requires proper functioning of the clotting factor cascade (Fig. 69-1). Clotting times that are measured in vitro, such as the PT, PTT, and TT, are useful in combination for the detection of significant abnormalities in this pathway. The TT depends on the final step of the cascade (conversion of fibrinogen to fibrin) and, therefore, is sensitive for the detection of fibrinogen abnormalities and inhibitors acting at this level (e.g., heparin). The fibrin plug must be maintained for long enough to permit repair of vascular injury, or delayed or secondary bleeding may occur. Excessive fibrinolysis leading to premature clot instability and lysis is detected by FDP and D-dimer testing.

TABLE 69-1 Major Phases in the Formation, Maintenance, and Eventual Dissolution of Clot

1. Blood vessels
2. Platelets
3. Fibrin generation cascade
4. Fibrin degradation

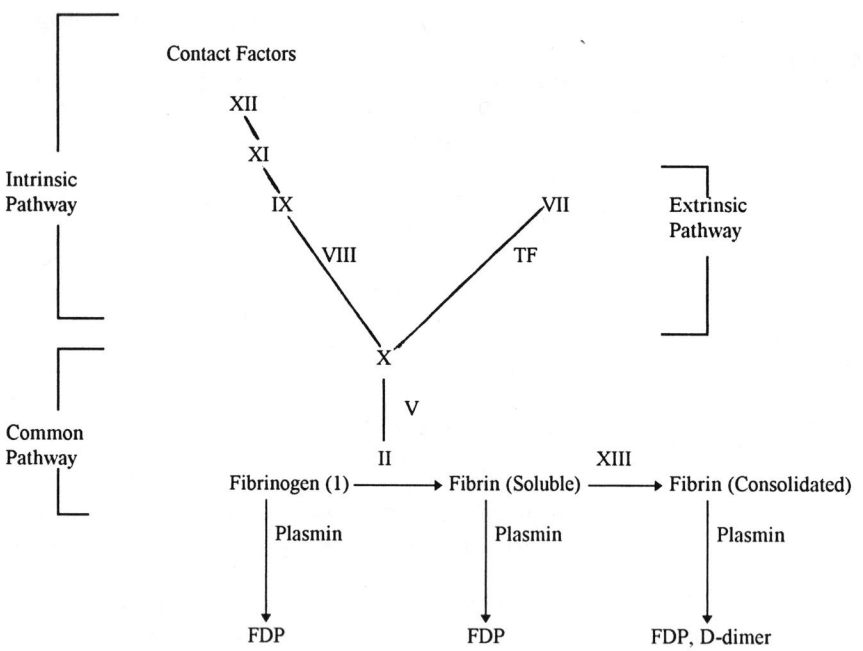

FIGURE 69-1 Fibrin generation cascade and fibrin degradation. TF = tissue factor; FDP = fibrin degradation products.

FDPs result from fibrinogenolysis and fibrinolysis, but the D-dimer is a unique product of plasmin degradation of fibrin. Thus elevated D-dimer levels imply that clotting (fibrin formation) has taken place prior to plasmin activity. Screening profiles of a number of common coagulopathies are given in Table 69-2.

Vascular Disorders

VASCULITIS[4]

Patients with vasculitis due to any of a variety of causes (e.g., drugs, infections, neoplasms, or systemic connective tissue

TABLE 69-2 Screening Coagulation Test Profiles in Selected Typical, Fully Manifest Bleeding Disorders

Disorder	Platelet No.	Bleeding Time	PT	PTT	TT	FDP Level	D-Dimer Level	Other
Vasculitis	N	I	N	N	N	N	N	Palpable purpura
Telangiectasia	N	N	N	N	N	N	N	Cutaneous and visceral lesions
Immune thrombocytopenia	D	I	N	N	N	N	N	Antiplatelet antibodies
Thrombotic thrombocytopenic purpura	D	I	N	N	N	N	N	Schistocytes, renal failure
Thrombocythemia	I	I or N	N	N	N	N	N	Large platelets
Thrombocytopathy	I, N, or D	I	N	N	N	N	N	Impaired platelet aggregation
Hypofibrinogenemia	N	N	I	I	I	N	N	Liver dysfunction
Hemophilia A	N	N	N	I	N	N	N	Low VIII:C levels
von Willebrand's disease	N	I	N	I	N	N	N	Low levels of VIII:C, and ristocetin cofactor
Vitamin K deficiency	N	N	I	I	N	N	N	
Advanced liver disease	N or D	N or I	I	I	I	I	N or I	Elevated VIII:C level, short euglobulin lysis time
Disseminated intravascular coagulation	D	I	I	I	I	I	I	Schistocytes, low fibrinogen and VIII:C levels, normal euglobulin lysis time
Heparin therapy	N	N	I	I	I	N	N	Low antithrombin III level, positive circulating anticoagulant test
Warfarin therapy	N	N	I	I	N	N	N	Negative circulating anticoagulant test
Thrombolytic therapy	N	N	I	I	I	I	I	Low fibrinogen level, short euglobulin lysis time

ABBREVIATIONS: N, normal; I, increased; D, decreased; TT, thrombin time.

diseases) may have an increased risk of bleeding complications owing to vascular fragility resulting from the inflammatory changes in vessel walls. Cutaneous rashes secondary to allergic drug reactions may have a significant vasculitic component. Vasculitis may be suspected by finding so-called palpable purpura—small hemorrhagic areas that are infiltrated and become palpable—in contrast to the typically flat purpura of thrombocytopenia.

Cutaneous vasculitis, such as that associated with drug rashes, may cause a prolonged bleeding time and may compromise the safety of even a small surgical incision through involved areas. A positive diagnosis of vasculitis may be made by a small punch biopsy of a purpuric lesion. Management consists of removing possible offending agents, treating underlying disorders (if possible), minimizing skin trauma, and administering anti-inflammatory agents such as corticosteroids, if not contraindicated by other clinical circumstances.

VASCULAR MALFORMATIONS

A variety of vascular malformations may bleed when traumatized or entered inadvertently during closed-space biopsies. Hereditary hemorrhagic telangiectasia (Osler-Weber-Rendu disease) may be associated with cutaneous, mucosal, or deep visceral malformations. Usually there is no laboratory evidence of a coagulopathy. A family history (the disorder has autosomal dominant inheritance) and careful inspection of cutaneous and mucosal sites for blanching "spiders" may suggest the diagnosis. Unfortunately, rare patients have only unsuspected deep visceral malformations, which may bleed. The disorder occasionally coexists with von Willebrand's disease or hemophilia A.

Patients with congenital cavernous hemangiomas may have a coagulopathy related to consumption of platelets and clotting factors in stagnant vascular spaces (Kasabach-Merritt syndrome).[5] There may be physical findings and laboratory features of DIC.

MICROCIRCULATORY OBSTRUCTION

Leukostasis secondary to very elevated myeloblast levels in acute nonlymphocytic leukemias may lead to small-vessel obstruction and resulting purpura.[6] Brain, lung, and skin are particularly well recognized sites of clinical importance. Similar vaso-occlusive sequelae may be seen in DIC, thrombotic thrombocytopenic purpura (TTP), heparin-induced thrombocytopenia, and fat embolism after long-bone fractures.

Platelet Disorders

THROMBOCYTOPENIAS (TABLE 69-3)

The platelet count is the result of a balance between the rate at which platelets are produced and the rate at which they are removed from the circulation. Bone marrow normally has a six- to eightfold reserve production capacity for the formed elements released into the blood, which can help to compensate for shortening of the normal platelet life span of about 10 days. Although there is no simple, readily available test for the rate of platelet production corresponding to the reticulocyte count as an indicator of new red blood cell (RBC) production, the rate of platelet production can be estimated roughly from evaluation of Wright-stained peripheral blood smears for young (large, basophilic) platelets and from particle counter estimates of mean platelet volume.

UNDERPRODUCTION STATES
Hypoplastic Marrow

Lack of platelet production, either as an isolated problem or as a factor contributing to thrombocytopenia, is suspected when decreased overall cellularity or a selective decrease in

TABLE 69-3 Thrombocytopenias in the Critically Ill

Mechanism	Selected Specific Causes
Underproduction of platelets	
Bone marrow hypoplasia/aplasia	Drugs and chemicals (cytotoxic chemotherapy, ethanol, benzene, chloramphenicol, thiazides)
	Radiation therapy
	Infections (viral hepatitis, cytomegalovirus, tuberculosis)
Ineffective bone marrow	Myelophthisic (metastatic cancers, tuberculosis)
	Megaloblastic (folic acid, B12 deficiencies)
	Primary marrow diseases (leukemia, myeloma)
Shortened platelet survival	
Immune thrombocytopenia	Drugs (rifampicin, methicillin, sulfonamides, barbiturates, diphenylhydantoin, quinidine, α-methyldopa, thiazides, furosemide, gold salts, heparin, trimethoprim-sulfamethoxazole)
	Lymphomas
	Collagen vascular diseases (systemic lupus erythematosus)
	Viral infections, including HIV-1
Intravascular consumption	DIC
	TTP
	Cardiopulmonary bypass
	Hemodialysis
Sequestration	Hypersplenism (cirrhosis, lymphoma)
Hemodilution	Massive transfusion

ABBREVIATIONS: DIC, disseminated intravascular coagulation; TTF, thrombotic thrombocytopenic purpura; HIV-1, human immunodeficiency virus type 1.

megakaryocyte number and size is found on bone marrow examination. A variety of suppressive factors may cause a generalized decrease in marrow mass or a selective decrease in megakaryocyte number. These include chemicals, both therapeutic drugs and environmental toxins; infectious agents, including bacteria, viruses, fungi, and mycobacteria; immune processes, in which the marrow may be inhibited by either a humoral or a cell-mediated mechanism; radiation injury; and idiopathic hypoplastic or aplastic marrow. Marrow hypoplasia will be evident on examination of a bone core biopsy. Care should be taken not to sample marrow that is in the port of prior radiotherapy. Hypoplasia is expected in such an area and may be misleading if interpreted as representing the status of the full marrow.

Ineffective Marrow

Ineffective marrow states are characterized by normal or increased cellularity but lack of release of precursors into the blood. Measurement of the reticulocyte response to anemia is a convenient way to monitor marrow "effectiveness" in this circumstance. A common cause of ineffective marrow function is folate deficiency causing megaloblastic hematopoiesis. The finding of hypersegmented polymorphonuclear leukocytes or ovalomacrocytes and the lack of a reticulocyte response in conjunction with thrombocytopenia should suggest this mechanism. Increased metabolic requirements, decreased folate intake in the diet, and therapy with certain chemotherapeutic agents predispose an individual to folate deficiency. Of course, vitamin B_{12} deficiency needs to be considered at the same time because of hematologic features identical to folate deficiency. Ineffective marrow function is also a feature of various myelophthisic conditions in which marrow may be replaced by tumor or granuloma or is impaired functionally by metabolic disturbances such as azotemia or hypothyroidism. A variety of inflammatory conditions may cause increased or decreased platelet counts via mechanisms not clearly defined.

SHORTENED PLATELET SURVIVAL

The survival of platelets in the blood is usually shortened in patients who are ill. Fever, bleeding, and sepsis, in general, predispose to shortened platelet survival; some specific circumstances include immune-mediated platelet removal by the reticuloendothelial system, hypersplenism, and consumptive coagulopathy. An otherwise uncomplicated shortened platelet life span can be suspected from the findings of a low circulating platelet count, normal or (usually) increased numbers of megakaryocytes on bone marrow examination, and the presence of large, basophilic platelets on a blood smear (indicative of effective marrow release of platelets).

Immune Thrombocytopenic Purpura (ITP)

Immune thrombocytopenic purpura (ITP) is confirmed by finding antiplatelet antibodies in the patient's serum or on the patient's platelets. When a drug is suspected to be the cause, these studies can be done in the presence and absence of the candidate drug in an effort to help confirm the diagnosis. Since the testing may take some time, often an empirical decision is made to stop administration of one or more suspect drugs, when possible. Immune-mediated thrombocytopenia also may be associated with such conditions as

collagen-vascular disease, lymphomas, and viral infections, including HIV-1.

The first step in therapy consists of discontinuation of any potential offending agents (e.g., quinidine, trimethoprim-sulfamethoxazole, diphenylhydantoin, thiazides). In addition, drugs that impair platelet function are contraindicated. It is often difficult to sort out a responsible drug in patients with complex medical conditions who are taking multiple medications, but in our experience, a frequent offender in the ICU setting is intravenous furosemide given repetitively. Corticosteroids may improve platelet survival by loosening the attachment of antibodies to platelets and decreasing the reticuloendothelial clearance of the antibody-coated platelets. A longer-term effect of corticosteroids is suppression of antibody production. Administration of platelets is usually of temporary benefit because their survival is shortened, presumably by mechanisms similar to those affecting the patient's platelets. Another intervention that may help to improve platelet survival is infusion of intravenous γ-globulin, 0.4 to 1 g/kg per day for 3 to 5 days.[7] This agent is thought to work by causing reticuloendothelial blockade and, possibly, because of the presence of anti-idiotypic antibodies in the preparation, by reducing the amount of antiplatelet antibody available to attach to platelets. In some patients receiving platelets, pretreatment with intravenous γ-globulin may help to prolong survival of the platelets. A benefit may not be seen for several days, and the resulting increase in platelet number, which may be life-saving and permit surgical procedures, is temporary. Subsequent repeat doses may be effective again, but cost becomes an important consideration when selecting this as an ongoing treatment.

Splenectomy may be an effective treatment for immune thrombocytopenia, but often the ICU patient is not a good candidate for the procedure, and therefore, the emphasis is more on the medical interventions just outlined. Intravenous human anti-Rh_o(D) IgG also may be effective in treating patients with immune thrombocytopenia who are Rh-positive and still have their spleen.[8] The mechanism of benefit is not fully understood, but the rationale is to coat circulating Rh-positive red cells with the anti-D antibody, thereby inducing intrasplenic sequestration of the red cells, resulting in reduced available reticuloendothelial capacity to remove antibody-coated platelets. Careful monitoring of the expected (usually limited) hemolysis is necessary. Some patients may be already significantly anemic and unable to tolerate a significant fall in RBC count. Patients who have received anti-D should receive Rh-negative red cells if transfusion is needed. Other agents, such as azathioprine, vincristine, colchicine, danazol, rituximab, mycophenolate mofetil, and cyclophosphamide, or devices (e.g., staphylococcal protein A column treatment of plasma) may be helpful, but they are usually used in subacute and chronic management situations or for individuals with persistent thrombocytopenia after splenectomy.

POSTTRANSFUSION PURPURA (PTP) Abrupt, often apparently unexplained, delayed appearance of severe thrombocytopenia may occur following blood transfusion in rare predisposed (usually P1^{A1}-negative) individuals. The life span is shortened for both P1^{A1}-positive donor platelets (to which isoantibodies have been produced) and the patient's own platelets (mechanism unclear). Infusions of intravenous γ-globulin (0.4 g/kg per day for 2 to 5 days) have been followed by good responses in patients with this potentially serious problem, regardless of the antibody implicated.[9]

THROMBOTIC THROMBOCYTOPENIC PURPURA (TTP) In TTP, intravascular clumping of platelets accounts for secondary vaso-occlusion and thrombocytopenia. Recent discoveries[10] have supported a proposed pathogenetic mechanism to explain the TTP syndrome (see Chap. 70 for an in-depth discussion of this subject).

Triggers of the acquired syndrome include infections (e.g., HIV-1), various drugs (including the antiplatelet agents ticlopidine and clopidogrel), chemotherapeutic agents (especially mitomycin), and malignancies. The important diagnostic clues are schistocytes on blood smear, a low platelet count (usually with a disproportionately low incidence of hemorrhagic symptoms), a negative direct Coombs' test in the face of laboratory evidence of hemolysis, and (usually) normal findings on coagulation studies. Evidence of vaso-occlusion by platelet hyaline agglutinates may be seen in biopsy specimens from tissues such as skin, marrow, gingiva, and kidney. Treatment with corticosteroids and plasma exchange[11] usually results in significant improvement. Also, favorable responses to intravenous vincristine, cyclophosphamide, rituximab,[12] and in otherwise refractory cases, splenectomy have been reported. Because exacerbation of the vaso-occlusive process has been noted following platelet transfusions, these should be avoided unless there is serious bleeding or an invasive procedure is mandatory.

DISSEMINATED INTRAVASCULAR COAGULATION (DIC) When thrombocytopenia is a manifestation of DIC,[13] usually other features of the process are present that permit recognition of the syndrome. Accompanying microangiopathic hemolysis, hypofibrinogenemia, elevated levels of FDPs and D-dimers, and prolonged clotting times are cardinal features. In advanced DIC, the bleeding diathesis associated with low platelet counts is compounded by qualitative platelet dysfunction owing to thrombin-induced platelet storage pool depletion, which may make platelet transfusions less effective. Schistocytes are seen less frequently in DIC than in TTP and, paradoxically, may be less evident in more advanced stages when fibrinolysis may be brisk, leading to breakdown of fibrin strands responsible for red cell shearing.

HEPARIN-INDUCED THROMBOCYTOPENIA (HIT) Bleeding is the most frequent complication of heparin therapy. An important cause of thrombocytopenia is the immune mechanism related to heparin.[14] This is of special interest in the ICU because of the almost ubiquitous exposure of patients to heparin owing to its use in access and monitoring lines and the common insertion of "heparin bonded" or "heparin coated" catheters. In addition, certain patient populations, especially those who have undergone cardiac or orthopedic surgery, appear to be at increased risk of sensitization by heparin.

It is common for patients to have a small, reversible drop in platelet count (usually within the normal range) within 1 to 2 days of the initiation of heparin therapy. This effect is thought to reflect some platelet aggregation caused by the presence of high-molecular-weight heparin species in the commercially available unfractionated heparin. The immune-mediated thrombocytopenia (seen in less than 1% of heparin-treated patients) typically appears at about 5 to 7 days after first exposure, but an anamnestic response due to persistent antibody from previous sensitization to heparin may cause thrombocytopenia to develop earlier in some patients, usually if they are within about 100 days of their initial sensitization. The clinical picture may range from no symptoms to life-threatening thrombotic events, which may be venous or arterial. Hemorrhage is less frequent, despite quite severe thrombocytopenia in some individuals. It is often necessary to make the decision about discontinuing heparin on clinical grounds.

The clinical criteria for diagnosis of HIT include an otherwise unexplained fall in platelet count below 150,000/μL or a fall of 50% or more of platelet count within the normal range. A history of any adverse reaction to heparin in the past or of necrotic changes at subcutaneous heparin injection sites should alert one to risk of serious vascular consequences on re-exposure to the drug. It is often difficult in the ICU setting to sort out mechanisms of thrombocytopenia, but a high index of suspicion is important in avoiding adverse consequences of unrecognized HIT. The "gold standard" confirmatory test (normalization of the platelet count after stopping heparin) also may be difficult to achieve because of other coexisting causes of thrombocytopenia (e.g., other drugs, sepsis).

Current notions of the pathogenesis of HIT suggest that the normally formed platelet factor 4 (PF4)–heparin complex is immunogenic in some individuals. Antibodies developed against the PF4-heparin target antigen form antigen-antibody complexes that can activate platelets after interacting with their Fc receptors. The result is intravascular obstruction by platelet clumps.

Laboratory confirmation of the presence of heparin-dependent antibodies may be helpful but is not always available in a timely fashion for decision making. In addition, false-negative tests are not infrequent. When available, various functional assays, such as heparin-induced platelet aggregation, [14C]serotonin release, and flow cytometric methods, may increase the predictability of clinically significant vaso-occlusive events beyond the detection of sensitization using enzyme-linked immunosorbent assay (ELISA) techniques for antibodies to PF4.

It is important to emphasize that the severe antibody syndrome may occur with any type of heparin (although the incidence appears to be less with low-molecular-weight heparin[15]) given via either intravenous or subcutaneous route. If the syndrome is suspected clinically, all devices and practices that expose the patient to heparin should be discontinued (including use of heparin locks, flushes of indwelling lines, and indwelling catheters that are heparin-coated).

Patients with HIT are hypercoagulable whether or not a clinically recognized vaso-occlusive event has occurred. As a result, they require immediate alternative anticoagulation. Once sensitized by unfractionated heparin (UFH), patients should not receive low-molecular-weight heparin (LMWH) as an alternative because of the high rate of cross-reactivity of antibodies to UFH with LMWH. The commonly used anticoagulants in this setting are direct thrombin inhibitors that do not cross-react with heparin-induced antibodies. Hirudin and argatroban usually are selected—the choice being made based on the patient's comorbidities (hirudin depends on renal clearance; argatroban depends on hepatic function status). Although each agent has a relatively short half-life, the lack of an antagonist for either increases the risk of bleeding complications. If patients require long-term anticoagulation with oral warfarin, it should not be started for at least 2 weeks because of reported adverse clotting problems when begun earlier in the course of HIT.

MECHANICAL SURFACE-RELATED THROMBOCYTOPENIA[16]
Variable lowering of platelet number is sometimes seen when platelets pass over or through foreign or distorted surfaces. Clinical situations of this type include cardiopulmonary bypass and the presence of intraaortic balloon pumps or pulmonary artery catheters. For cardiopulmonary bypass, at least, platelet-related bleeding during or after bypass is much more likely to be secondary to impaired platelet function (see below) than to severe depression of the platelet count.

SEQUESTRATION
Hypersplenism
Thrombocytopenia with or without anemia and neutropenia may be a feature of hypersplenism.[17] This state of increased local sequestration, usually with shortened intrasplenic survival, frequently is accompanied by increased spleen size that is detectable on physical examination or imaging studies. Bedside ultrasound is a safe noninvasive method for assessing the spleen in ICU patients.

Hypersplenism may be a chronic, stable condition antedating and then complicating a new problem (e.g., cirrhosis with splenomegaly predating acute deterioration for another reason). In addition, acute onset of hypersplenism with progressive splenic enlargement and sequestration may be a feature of such processes as splenic venous occlusion and sickle cell splenic sequestration crisis in children. It is unusual to encounter a platelet count of less than about $30,000/\mu L$ in "compensated" hypersplenism associated with cirrhosis and portal hypertension accompanied by splenomegaly. Bone marrow evaluation is expected to reveal increased megakaryocyte number and overall hypercellularity. The peripheral smear should show decreased platelet numbers but some large basophilic platelets.

In situations of progressive splenomegaly with associated thrombocytopenia (and risk of splenic rupture), splenectomy may be the only available therapy. If the splenic enlargement is secondary to leukemic or lymphomatous involvement, radiation therapy may be of some benefit in shrinking the spleen, but the effect may be temporary, and there is the risk of paradoxical thrombocytopenia or neutropenia rather than count improvement.

THROMBOCYTOSIS/THROMBOCYTHEMIA

Elevated platelet counts are seen commonly in critically ill patients because inflammation, bleeding, surgery, hemolysis, severe injury, and neoplasia are among the major causes of reactive thrombocytosis. Usually, the count is elevated to levels less than $1 \times 10^6/\mu L$, and no adverse effect is expected from such a secondary increase in qualitatively normal platelets.

In contrast, patients with elevated platelet counts secondary to myeloproliferative disorders[18] are at an increased risk of bleeding or thrombotic sequelae, especially when the platelet count exceeds $1 \times 10^6/\mu L$. The diagnosis of an underlying myeloproliferative disorder may have been established prior to the patient's presentation with a complication, or it may be suspected from associated clinical features such as splenomegaly, abnormal platelet morphology on smear, and bone marrow examination revealing panmyelosis (increase in all cell lines) as well as qualitative abnormalities in megakaryocytes, which are also markedly increased in number.

If the patient is asymptomatic, a prolonged bleeding time may portend hemorrhagic problems. No definitive laboratory tests predict impending thrombotic complications in such patients, but it appears that the risk may be increased in older persons with fixed vascular disease. It is especially important to avoid splenectomy, either intentional or inadvertent, at the time of abdominal surgery for other reasons because marked platelet elevations may cause fatal vaso-occlusive events.

Platelet levels may be reduced quickly and effectively in symptomatic thrombocythemic individuals by plateletpheresis. Treatment with anagrelide or hydroxyurea can be used to maintain normal platelet counts (the usual goal is to keep the platelet count less than $500,000/\mu L$).[18] These drugs also can help to prevent secondary rises in platelet count following surgical procedures and other factors that may precipitate reactive thrombocytosis.

THROMBOCYTOPATHY

Qualitative platelet abnormalities are encountered frequently in the ICU setting.[19] Often they contribute to other, more serious bleeding diatheses, but on occasion they present a significant problem in their own right. Exposure to external agents, such as ethanol, aspirin, and nonsteroidal anti-inflammatory drugs (NSAIDs), prior to admission is common. Other drug-induced causes of thrombocytopathy in the hospital include exposure to the parenteral NSAID ketorolac (TORADOL) and glycoprotein (GP) IIb/IIIa inhibitors (e.g., abciximab, ticlopidine, clopidogrel). The resulting prolongation of bleeding time varies in duration and severity. Once the offending agent has been removed, the bleeding problem can be overridden promptly by administration of normal platelets or, in the case of aspirin or ticlopidine, by intravenous infusion of 1-diamino-8-D-arginine vasopressin (DDAVP), if necessary. Often, unless there is significant bleeding or invasive procedures are needed, it is sufficient to wait several days and let the patient's own production of new platelets unexposed to the offending agent correct the problem.

UREMIA
A more difficult problem is the thrombocytopathy associated with uremia. A variety of interventions may be helpful temporarily. Correction of the prolonged bleeding time may be needed prior to an intended surgical intervention (e.g., renal biopsy for diagnosis). The key step is appropriate dialysis; additional benefit sometimes is noted with administration of corticosteroids, infusions of cryoprecipitate[20] (usually 10 cryopacks every 12 hours), intravenous DDAVP[21] ($0.3 \mu g/kg$), platelet transfusions, and intravenous conjugated estrogens.[22] Intravenous DDAVP, if effective in reducing the bleeding time, may be repeated at 6- to 12-hour intervals, but tachyphylaxis is expected after 1 to 2 days of this therapy. It is also important to seek and correct other coexisting coagulopathies, such as vitamin K deficiency.

MYELOPROLIFERATIVE DISORDERS

Patients with myeloproliferative disorders may have platelet dysfunction, especially when platelet counts are elevated. Usually, normalization of the platelet count results in return of the bleeding time to normal, but individuals with long-standing polycythemia vera or myeloid metaplasia, for example, may still have abnormal bleeding, especially with surgical procedures, even when all counts have been normalized.

DRUGS

Aspirin

The classic drug inhibitor of platelet function is aspirin. It causes irreversible inhibition of cyclo-oxygenase, thereby leading to impaired prostaglandin metabolism. The net effect of aspirin is the result of inhibition of production of the platelet aggregant thromboxane A_2 versus decreased synthesis of prostacyclin—the potent endothelium-derived inhibitor of platelet aggregation. In most individuals on Western diets that contain limited amounts of the omega fatty acid precursors of prostacyclin synthesis, the net result is a prolonged bleeding time. When aspirin is discontinued, the exposed platelets remain impaired, but newly synthesized platelets with normal function soon begin to contribute to normalization of the bleeding time. Usually, the effect of aspirin on bleeding time has dissipated significantly by 3 days after discontinuation.

Nonsteroidal Anti-Inflammatory Drugs (NSAIDs)

NSAIDs cause reversible inhibition of cyclo-oxygenase and, therefore, a shorter period of bleeding risk than aspirin after discontinuation.

Antibiotics

Antibiotics of the penicillin family, epitomized by carbenicillin, may cause a complex coagulopathy. In addition to disturbance of the synthesis of vitamin K by the intestinal flora, a thrombocytopathy characterized by a prolonged bleeding time is recognized. These phenomena usually are not of major clinical significance, but they may add to other coagulation defects and affect the interpretation of coagulation laboratory evaluations. When bleeding from these mechanisms is serious, platelet transfusion after discontinuation of the drug should compensate for the impaired function of platelets exposed to the drug.

DYSPROTEINEMIAS

Abnormal immunoglobulin concentrations, as seen in myeloma and Waldenstrom's macroglobulinemia, interfere with platelet function (causing prolonged bleeding times) presumably by physically "coating" platelet surfaces and thus limiting the access of clotting factors to the phospholipid surfaces of platelets, which are needed to promote key reactions in the clotting cascade. In addition, prolongation of the TT is often noted.

CARDIOPULMONARY BYPASS[16]

Acquired thrombocytopathy is regularly produced by contact of platelets with membrane surfaces in bypass circuits. In some patients this effect may add to other causes of increased bleeding risk after bypass (such as hypofibrinogenemia and inadequate heparin neutralization). Transfusion of donor platelets (if clinically urgent) is expected to normalize the bleeding time once bypass is discontinued.

THROMBIN-INDUCED STORAGE POOL DEFECT

Thrombocytopathy may contribute to the bleeding problems in DIC. During active DIC (e.g., in acute promyelocytic leukemia), an acquired platelet function defect with prolonged bleeding time may appear owing to release of granule contents by excess thrombin. This is likely to be especially troublesome when patients are thrombocytopenic as well. Control of the DIC is the key to successful correction of this problem. Infusion of donor platelets is of benefit for only limited periods because these platelets are also exposed to excess thrombin while the DIC is active.

Fibrin Generation Disorders

SAMPLE COLLECTION AND INTERPRETATION

Accurate values for clotting times, which form the basis for assessment of the integrity of the coagulation cascade, depend on collection of the correct quantity of blood relative to the amount of anticoagulant present in the sample tube; in addition, extraneous contamination by heparin must be avoided. It is important not to overfill collection tubes; rather, the vacuum should be allowed to determine the correct amount of specimen per tube, and the tube then should be inverted promptly to ensure adequate mixing with anticoagulants. Rapid delivery to the testing location decreases problems with cascade activation in the tube (which leads to prolonged clotting times). When drawing from heparinized lines, a double draw (discarding at least 10 mL initially and using the second aliquot) should prevent heparin contamination. Unexpectedly long PTTs that are not corrected by mixing the sample with an equal volume of pooled normal plasma but that are corrected by incubating the sample with heparin neutralizer powder (triethylaminoethyl cellulose) should indicate the presence of heparin contamination.

Consideration of the results of PT and PTT in combination can help to identify the site(s) of cascade deficiency (Table 69-4). Prolonged clotting times should be restudied after the patient's plasma is mixed with an equal volume of pooled normal plasma to differentiate between absence of the factors in question and inhibition of their activity by circulating inhibitors. If the clotting time is corrected by this mixing test, a deficiency is present; if the clotting time of the mix remains prolonged, an inhibitor (such as heparin or one directed against a specific clotting factor) is present.

ISOLATED FACTOR DEFICIENCIES

Isolated severe factor deficiencies may antedate and complicate the need for intensive care, as in hemophilia A or B, or may be acquired as a consequence of the critical illness, as in the case of hypofibrinogenemia secondary to DIC.

HYPOFIBRINOGENEMIA

Low functional fibrinogen levels in ICU patients most commonly result from decreased hepatic synthesis of fibrinogen or increased removal due to the action of thrombin and plasmin during DIC. Bleeding risk is increased by the anticoagulant effect of nonclottable fibrin split products in high titer. Spontaneous clinical hemorrhage from hypofibrinogenemia is not expected above a concentration of 100 mg/dL in plasma and usually is not a serious risk until levelsg of 50 mg/dL

TABLE 69-4 Use of Combined PT and PTT Results to Determine Site(s) of Fibrin Generation Cascade Defects

	PT Normal	PT Elevated
PTT Normal	Result 1	Result 2
PTT Elevated	Result 3	Result 4

Result 1: Normal results on screening tests of cascade (factor levels at least 30% to 35% of normal)
Result 2: Isolated low factor VII level—may be due to congenital deficiency or early liver disease, vitamin K deficiency, or warfarin effect
Result 3: Intrinsic pathway abnormality—low levels of factors VIII, IX, XI, or XII; typical pattern in hemophilia A and von Willebrand's disease
Result 4: Due to common pathway abnormality—factors I (fibrinogen), II, V, X— and/or combined intrinsic and extrinsic pathway defects. Seen in advanced liver disease, vitamin K deficiency, full warfarin and heparin effects, and DIC.

are reached. Fibrinogen may be replaced with fresh frozen plasma (FFP) or, more efficiently in terms of volume, with cryoprecipitate; each cryopack is expected to raise the fibrinogen level approximately 4 to 10 mg/dL in an adult. Although the plasma half-life of fibrinogen is approximately 4 days under normal circumstances, serial plasma fibrinogen level determinations will dictate the frequency of infusions (as often as every 6 to 12 hours, especially in acutely ill patients with a shortened fibrinogen half-life).

HEMOPHILIA A (FACTOR VIII DEFICIENCY)

Critical illness in a patient with hemophilia A requires careful correction of the pre-existing coagulopathy, especially when the situation is complicated by such new problems as ITP, DIC, sepsis, and hepatic or renal dysfunction. Appearance of an inhibitor to factor VIII and development of a progressive pseudotumor may further increase the complexity of management. Preparation of the severe hemophiliac for surgery consists of checking to exclude an inhibitor and then replacing with factor VIII concentrate to achieve the desired percent correction (100% equals 1 unit of factor VIII per milliliter of the patient's plasma). For major surgery, a starting level at or above 100% is desirable. Additional doses are given intraoperatively. The doses are dictated by the amount of bleeding and stat factor VIII levels. The shortened half-life of factor VIII during bleeding leads to increased requirements for replacement (both higher doses and shorter intervals between doses). To give a sample calculation: Suppose that a 70-kg patient with a hematocrit of 40% has a blood volume of 4900 mL (70 mL/kg) and a plasma volume of 2940 mL (60% of the blood volume). If the starting factor VIII level is less than 1%, approximately 3000 units of factor VIII concentrate will be needed to achieve correction to the 100% level. It is important to assess the adequacy of correction by monitoring the factor VIII level before invasive procedures and to continue support for 10 to 14 days after a major surgical procedure or hemorrhage to prevent serious delayed bleeding. Maintenance postoperative factor VIII support usually is given every 8 to 12 hours; the goal is to prevent the between-dose nadir in factor VIII plasma levels from falling below 40% to 50%. Several recombinant factor VIII products are available.

Similar considerations apply to patients with hemophilia B (Christmas disease), except that replacement is with FFP, prothrombin complex, or recombinant factor IX in severe deficiency states.

FACTOR VII DEFICIENCY

Factor VII deficiency is a much less common inherited deficiency than the preceding. It is a non–X-linked disorder with a variable severity, which in some patients presents as a severe hemophilia-like condition. Replacement with FFP or prothrombin complex is appropriate. The relatively short half-life of factor VII (4 to 7 hours) may require dosing at 6- to 8-hour intervals during major hemostatic challenges, but less frequent maintenance doses may be sufficient beyond the fourth day following some orthopedic procedures.[23]

Isolated factor VII deficiency is caused most often by vitamin K deficiency or liver disease or occurs during the initiation of warfarin anticoagulation. When factor VII deficiency cannot be corrected with vitamin K therapy, factor replacement with FFP or, when indicated, prothrombin complex can be used. Recombinant activated factor VII (rVIIa) also is available.

FACTOR XI DEFICIENCY

Factor XI deficiency is usually inherited, although in advanced liver disease a deficiency of factor XI may coexist with low levels of the other factors synthesized in liver parenchymal cells. FFP is the only currently available replacement product. For severely deficient patients with a bleeding tendency, preoperative plasma exchange may be used to establish safe hemostatic levels that can then be maintained by follow-up plasma infusions.

FACTORS II, V, AND X

These deficiencies may appear in isolation or coexist with others. Isolated factor X deficiency with significant bleeding may be seen in amyloidosis. FFP (or prothrombin complex for factors II and X) replacement therapy is indicated, if needed, but it may not readily correct an amyloid-associated factor X deficiency because of rapid clearance of the factor, which attaches to the amyloid fibrils. Splenectomy may be helpful in such instances.

FACTOR XII

Factor XII deficiency causes a prolonged PTT without a clinically significant bleeding diathesis. Some workers have suggested that, paradoxically, patients who are severely deficient in factor XII may be hypercoagulable. It is important to identify this factor deficiency both because needed invasive procedures can be done in its presence when it is an isolated abnormality and to avoid unnecessary correction of the PTT with FFP.

FACTOR XIII

Deficiency of factor XIII[24] is usually lifelong and may be associated with significant bleeding problems of the delayed type. In homozygotes there is an increased risk of fatal intracranial bleeding; spontaneous abortion also has been noted. Rarely, an acquired deficiency is seen in patients who develop an inhibitor while taking a drug such as isoniazid. The diagnosis cannot be made from the usual clotting or bleeding time tests. Rather, this deficiency must be suspected and tested for directly. Clot dissolution in $5\ M$ urea during overnight incubation indicates deficiency (<1% activity). The deficiency is readily corrected with FFP, cryoprecipitate, or a placental concentrate. Only 1% to 2% of the normal factor XIII activity is adequate for hemostasis and intact clot stability. The long half-life of this factor (8 days) permits long dosing intervals and relatively easy prophylaxis when a hemostatic challenge is anticipated.

VON WILLEBRAND'S FACTOR (VWF)[25]

Deficiency of VWF results in a bleeding disorder more akin to that associated with platelet dysfunction than to that of the hemophilias. Cardinal findings include a prolonged bleeding time and a moderately prolonged PTT with depression (usually mild) of the factor VIII coagulant (VIII:C) level. Decreased levels of ristocetin cofactor and von Willebrand's antigen also are found. Rapid screening for von Willebrand's disease using an in vitro platelet function analyzer can be helpful in diagnosis.[3] The most common variety of this disorder (type I) is characterized by a defect in secretion of normal VWF from vascular endothelial cells. Less commonly, qualitative defects in the multimeric structure of the factor (type II) or a severe deficiency in its synthesis (recessively inherited type III) is seen. Type I patients may respond to infusion of DDAVP (0.3 μg/kg IV) with a rise in VWF and other released endothelial products, some of which may have anticoagulant effects (such as prostacyclin [PGI$_2$] and tissue plasminogen activator). Usually there is a net hemostatic benefit, which is seen as an improved bleeding time over a several-hour period. Repeat doses may be given, but tachyphylaxis after 1 to 2 days precludes effective long-term therapy with DDAVP or reliance on it alone for major surgical procedures.

The Duke bleeding time was considered by some to be the best indicator of bleeding risk prior to invasive procedures, but critical review of the bleeding time[26] raises questions as to the predictability of bleeding from the result of this test in individual cases. A more extensive workup, including both functional studies (ristocetin cofactor, PTT, VIII: C, ristocetin-induced platelet aggregation) and antigenic studies (VIII-related antigen and multimer analysis), is useful in characterizing the type and potential severity of the defect. In acute situations when the diagnosis is known, measuring the VIII-related antigen level, if available, is a helpful way to monitor the patient's status and adequacy of replacement. The platelet function analyzer also may be used for rapid confirmation of improvement after treatment. The usual goal of therapy is normalization of the VWF level during active bleeding and before anticipated surgery or another invasive procedure. For severe deficiency and prolonged treatment, virucidal-treated factor VIII concentrates, which contain high levels of VWF (e.g., HUMATE P), are indicated. Monoclonal antibody–purified factor VIII concentrates are not useful because VWF is depleted from these products. DDAVP may be contraindicated in type IIB and platelet-type (or pseudo-) von Willebrand's disease—two conditions in which platelet aggregation and thrombocytopenia may ensue.

INHIBITORS[27]

Coagulation factor inhibitors may create life-threatening situations, especially in otherwise critically ill patients. The potency of the inhibitor can be determined by titration of the effect of plasma dilutions on the result of mixing the patient's plasma with pooled normal plasma (see above).

FACTOR VIII INHIBITORS

The most commonly encountered coagulation factor inhibitors are directed against factor VIII. They are seen most frequently in hemophiliac patients receiving supplementary factor replacement, but they also can occur sporadically in elderly individuals, in the postpartum period, and in persons with an autoimmune diathesis or lymphoma.[28] Factor VIII inhibition usually is measured in Bethesda units (BU); levels greater than 10 BU indicate more potent inhibitors. Testing to exclude a factor VIII inhibitor should be done before any significant invasive procedure is undertaken in a hemophiliac in order to make it possible to predict the response to factor replacement. It is also important to confirm that the expected response to factor administration has occurred before proceeding with an invasive procedure. For lesser titers, infusion of factor VIII concentrate often can override the inhibitor in the short term, although in some patients this approach will elicit a rise in the inhibitor titer. Other modes of therapy for high-titer inhibitors include bypassing the factor VIII–dependent step with prothrombin complex concentrate (PCC) or activated PCC, use of porcine factor VIII concentrates, and infusions of rVIIa. Combined immunosuppressant programs that include steroids, cytotoxic agents, plasma processing over columns that remove immunoglobulin G (IgG) and IgG-containing immune complexes,[29] and high-dose intravenous immunoglobulin are approaches to the subacute and chronic management of hemophiliacs with inhibitors. Recent favorable experience with rituximab has been noted.[30]

Inhibitors found in nonhemophiliacs tend to be more responsive to simpler immunosuppressive treatments, such as treatment with azathioprine and prednisone. There is a significant risk of bleeding in these individuals when the inhibitor is not controlled. If an underlying tumor or autoimmune disorder is present, its management may help to reduce the level of inhibitor. Surgical procedures in patients with inhibitors obviously are fraught with high risk, and meticulous hemostatic correction perioperatively is necessary. Correction needs to be maintained for at least 10 days after major procedures (as in uncomplicated hemophilia) to prevent delayed bleeding.

LUPUS ANTICOAGULANTS

The presence of the so-called lupus anticoagulant[31] is important to recognize because, although it is usually associated with a prolonged PTT, it may imply a hypercoagulable state rather than a bleeding diathesis. Rare individuals with lupus anticoagulants have a bleeding diathesis. Prolongation of the PT in addition to the PTT may be an indicator of such a case.

This phospholipid inhibitor was first identified in patients with de novo systemic lupus erythematosus (SLE), but it is known to occur also in drug-induced SLE syndromes, in individuals with other autoimmune diseases, and in otherwise normal persons. The typical laboratory result is a prolonged PTT and/or Russell's viper venom time (RVVT) with evidence of an inhibitor and interference on several of the coagulation factor assays. An abnormally steep rise in the PT with serial dilution of thromboplastin in vitro is a characteristic finding (the tissue thromboplastin inhibition [TTI] test). This latter phenomenon may be mimicked by the presence of heparin and warfarin anticoagulation; therefore, it is preferable to perform the test, if possible, before anticoagulation is begun. Absorption of the patient's plasma with platelet phospholipid in vitro may remove the inhibitor and lead to normalization of the PTT, TTI, and RVVT test results, thus enhancing the specificity of diagnosis.

Most patients with the lupus anticoagulant do not have coagulation problems, but approximately 25% have clinically important hypercoagulability. It is unclear whether empirical prophylactic long-term anticoagulation with warfarin is useful. Perioperative prophylactic dose heparinization is recommended to offset added surgical hypercoagulable risks. If thrombotic problems—typically venous (deep venous thrombosis, pulmonary emboli)—do occur, chronic anticoagulation with warfarin is recommended. Results of the PT are sometimes unpredictable in patients with lupus anticoagulants. Chromogenic factor X levels may be more reliable for monitoring the degree of warfarin effect. Increased risk for arterial clotting events also is present.

The potency of lupus anticoagulants may diminish spontaneously as a result of the discontinuation of an offending drug (e.g., procainamide, phenothiazines) or in response to immunosuppressive therapy (e.g., with prednisone).

FACTOR V INHIBITORS[32]

Some patients exposed to topical bovine thrombin used as a surgical sealant may develop an inhibitor to factor V (a contaminant of the bovine product). On occasion, there can be significant lowering of the human factor V level because of cross-reactivity. The antibodies eventually disappear in a period of weeks, but treatment with plasma and platelets (thought to be site of factor V protected from the inhibitor) may be needed in individuals who bleed significantly.

COMBINED FACTOR DEFICIENCY STATES

VITAMIN K DEFICIENCY[33]

The combination of poor dietary intake and antibiotic therapy that is so common among ICU patients predisposes them to vitamin K deficiency. Impaired absorption of fat-soluble vitamins, as in biliary obstruction, may contribute as well. Prolongation of the PT initially and then of both the PT and the PTT is characteristic. Documentation of selected reduction of the levels of factors II, IX, and X is rarely needed to make this diagnosis; usually the initial decline in factor VII in the absence of other explanations (such as liver disease or warfarin anticoagulation) is sufficient. Vitamin K supplementation may be given orally, subcutaneously, intramuscularly, or intravenously. The oral and subcutaneous routes are preferred, if feasible, to avoid a risk of hematoma or, rarely, anaphylaxis after intravenous dosing.

DYSFIBRINOGENEMIA

A qualitative abnormality of fibrinogen may or may not be associated with clinically significant hypofibrinogenemia.[34] The diagnosis is made by finding a disproportionately low functional level of fibrinogen relative to the antigenic fibrinogen level. In addition to the variety of inherited fibrinogen abnormalities associated with bleeding, clotting, and wound dehiscence problems that have been recognized, an acquired decrease in fibrinogen function is seen commonly in the presence of parenchymal liver disease[35] and hepatomas.

If it becomes clinically necessary to correct the hypofibrinogenemia, infusion of cryoprecipitate is the method of choice (see above). A functional level of 100 mg/dL or greater is the usual goal of therapy.

Fibrinolytic Disorders

DEFINITIONS AND LABORATORY TESTING METHODS

Clot strength and stability are the keys to prevention of rebleeding and consequent development of hemorrhagic infarction after initial hemostasis. The covalent cross-linking of fibrin mediated by factor XIII is important for clot strength, and carefully regulated activity of the fibrinolytic system allows eventual clot degradation once the vessel is strong enough to handle re-established flow. The details of regulation of the fibrinolytic process, including its intensity and timing, are incompletely understood.

Fibrinolytic activity is mediated by plasmin, which is derived from the inactive plasma precursor plasminogen. Plasminogen can be activated by various endogenous kinases, including tissue plasminogen activator and urokinase, as well as by exogenous agents such as streptokinase. The activity of plasmin is regulated by a series of inhibitors, the most important of which is α_2-antiplasmin. The activity of the fibrinolytic system is assessed indirectly in vitro by measurement of concentrations of substrate (fibrinogen) and plasmin-generated breakdown products of fibrinogen and fibrin (FDPs, D-dimer). Lesser degrees of fibrinolysis may be detected by measuring the level of plasmin-antiplasmin complexes.

PRIMARY FIBRINOLYSIS

It is helpful to distinguish so-called primary fibrinolysis, in which plasmin is generated from plasminogen by an activator in the plasma, from secondary fibrinolysis, in which plasmin is generated within a formed clot by an activator that is also present. Primary fibrinolysis (fibrinogenolysis) is seen in states of tissue injury such as liver disease or therapeutic administration of activators such as urokinase and streptokinase. Secondary fibrinolysis is the normal mechanism of clot degradation initiated by tissue plasminogen activator. The latter process is accelerated pathologically in DIC.

SECONDARY FIBRINOLYSIS

The in vitro tests of clot lysis, such as the euglobulin lysis time, are sensitive to generation of circulating plasmin and therefore give shortened times in primary fibrinolysis but normal times in secondary fibrinolytic states (e.g., DIC). Levels of fibrinogen and FDPs do not distinguish the two mechanisms. D-dimer is a unique degradation product of cross-linked fibrin that is not seen among the products of plasmin digestion of fibrinogen. As such, it is helpful in distinguishing fibrinogenolysis from fibrinolysis. This test is especially helpful in evaluating states of increased clot formation such as DIC. However, it must be emphasized that elevated D-dimer levels do not indicate the mechanism of clot generation. For example, high levels of D-dimer may be present during the dissolution of a hematoma, and it would be wrong to assume that DIC necessarily was the cause of the original clot.

Complex Coagulopathies

ACUTE DISSEMINATED INTRAVASCULAR COAGULATION[13]

The most important complex coagulopathy in intensive care medicine is acute DIC. DIC is essentially a state of increased propensity for clot formation; it may be triggered by a variety of stimuli related to such diverse underlying disorders as sepsis, tissue injury, and neoplasm. There may be clinical and laboratory evidence of hypercoagulability, but in acute cases, consumptive coagulopathy with hemorrhagic manifestations may predominate. The full-blown state is characterized by thrombocytopenia, prolonged clotting times, depressed circulating levels of cascade factors (especially factor VIII), and increased fibrinolysis manifested by high FDP and D-dimer levels as well as hypofibrinogenemia. There may be associated hemolysis with evidence of microangiopathic changes on blood smear (schistocytes) in some patients. Organ dysfunction secondary to vaso-occlusion or hemorrhage may be evident. DIC should be suspected when such a complex coagulopathy appears, especially if the clinical setting would predispose the patient to it.

The key step in management is treatment of the underlying condition that is responsible for the hypercoagulable state (e.g., antibiotic treatment for infection). Transfusion of blood products, including RBCs, platelets, FFP, and cryoprecipitate, if needed for the correction of severe hypofibrinogenemia, may protect the patient from hemorrhagic complications while the mechanism triggering the DIC is being eliminated. Although, in theory, blood product support may temporarily "feed the fire," often patients benefit from such treatment without requiring heparin therapy with its attendant potential complications.

In cases of purpura fulminans and massive thromboembolism, where the pace of the process is catastrophic, a trial of heparin therapy is appropriate (or drotrecogin in severe sepsis), along with blood product support, especially in patients who have potentially treatable underlying disorders that can be expected to respond reasonably promptly with appropriate specific therapy. The doses of heparin required are variable because of heparin resistance in DIC (owing to low levels of antithrombin III and elevated levels of PF4). The necessary dose may vary initially from 5 to 10 units/kg/h, given by continuous intravenous infusion up to full therapeutic levels. The criteria usually used to determine whether heparin is helpful include clinical observation of lessened bleeding and a rise in fibrinogen levels and platelet counts.

There are obvious risks to the use of heparin because of uncertainty as to the optimal dose and because the addition of an anticoagulant drug makes it difficult to interpret the results of clotting tests. Heparin therapy usually is not indicated for patients with bleeding in critical areas, such as intracranial locations. In addition, isolated antifibrinolytic therapy with agents such as ε-aminocaproic acid is contraindicated because of the risk of extensive thrombotic complications. For more chronic, low-grade DIC, subcutaneous heparin (e.g., 5000 units every 8 to 12 hours) or low-molecular-weight heparin may be helpful in preventing clinical thrombotic complications.

Laboratory parameters for following DIC include clotting times, platelet count, and fibrinogen level (assuming they are not disturbed simultaneously by an underlying process such as leukemia or liver failure). FDP levels are good markers for the detection of fibrinolysis but tend to lag as indicators of improvement.

MASSIVE TRANSFUSION

Patients who have had one to two blood volumes replaced with stored RBCs within 24 hours are subject to the development of a complex coagulopathy, the most important feature of which is thrombocytopenia owing to both dilutional and consumptive mechanisms.[36,37] In addition, there may be impaired platelet function and lowered levels of plasma factors VIII and V. Successful management of this coagulopathy depends on recognition of the developing pattern and administration of sufficient platelets and FFP to offset the effects of dilution. More serious disturbances of hemostasis appear if DIC develops as a consequence of the underlying shock and/or tissue injury (see above). There has been recent interest in use of rVIIa to help control hemorrhage and thereby reduce the need for massive transfusion.[38,39]

ANTIBIOTIC THERAPY

Use of multiple or broad-spectrum antibiotics predisposes the patient to combined coagulation defects. Vitamin K deficiency is common. Impaired platelet function manifested by prolonged bleeding time has been observed with carbenicillin[40] and related antibiotics.

LIVER DISEASE[41]

Because of the key role of the liver in clotting factor and thrombopoietin synthesis, coagulopathies are an important part of liver dysfunction. Not only are clotting times prolonged, but if there is associated hypersplenism, thrombocytopenia also may be present. Underproduction of thrombopoietin and immune thrombocytopenia secondary to hepatitis C, alcohol, and folate deficiency are also potential factors contributing to lowered platelet counts. Platelet dysfunction (usually mild) also may be present. In addition, primary fibrinolysis secondary to liver cell injury may occur, creating a picture that may mimic DIC. It is not unusual to see DIC superimposed on liver failure causing a severe complex coagulopathy. The pattern of fibrinolysis and the factor VIII:C level may be helpful for distinguishing the coagulopathy of advanced liver failure from DIC. Primary fibrinolysis (short euglobulin lysis time) and elevated factor VIII:C levels are seen in liver disease; findings of secondary-type fibrinolysis (normal euglobulin lysis time) and low factor VIII:C levels (as well as more elevated levels of D-dimer) favor DIC. Placement of shunts to drain ascites into the venous circulation may be associated with accelerated DIC and bleeding risk.

Therapy for the coagulopathy of liver disease consists of replacement of clotting factors and platelets as well as correction of vitamin K deficiency. If volume considerations permit, FFP is used first. Often it is necessary to use prothrombin complex for adequate correction prior to invasive or surgical procedures. The risks of administration of this product include enhanced coagulation and, in some instances, DIC owing to the presence of activated clotting factors in the concentrate. Prothrombin complex concentrates replace only the vitamin K–dependent factors, not all the clotting factors made in the liver. Other approaches to life-threatening hemorrhage in patients with liver failure have included use of fibrinolysis inhibitors and, more recently, rVIIa.[39]

RENAL DISEASE[41]

Uremic patients are likely to have a bleeding diathesis, which most commonly is a thrombocytopathy characterized by a prolonged bleeding time. The disease underlying the renal failure also may, of course, predispose the patient to a coagulopathy (e.g., immune thrombocytopenia due to SLE, factor X deficiency secondary to amyloid, low antithrombin III and factor IX levels in nephrotic syndrome of various causes). The thrombocytopathy becomes especially important if surgical interventions such as renal biopsy are needed. Adequate acute or subacute hemostasis usually can be achieved by using one or more of the treatments discussed earlier, but chronic protection from bleeding is more difficult to achieve. Hemostasis may be improved in uremia after treatment with recombinant human erythropoietin.[42]

DYSPROTEINEMIAS[43]

Patients with multiple myeloma or Waldenstrom's macroglobulinemia may have significant bleeding problems in addition to the thrombocytopenia that may accompany advanced disease or be a consequence of treatment. Both impaired platelet function (prolonged bleeding time) and prolonged TT secondary to interference with the conversion of fibrinogen to fibrin may be seen. The mechanism of these effects is not fully understood but is thought to involve the physical "coating" of the platelets by the paraproteins, which reduces the exposure of the phospholipid template that is needed for key steps of the cascade. Steric hindrance of the process of fibrin formation also may play a role. These adverse effects on coagulation tend to improve with a decline in paraprotein levels (owing to chemotherapy-induced decreased production and/or to removal by plasmapheresis).

Coagulation Status: Guidelines for Invasive Procedures

GENERAL CONSIDERATIONS

The following guidelines should be used in the management of patients with coagulopathies:

1. Invasive procedures should be performed only when absolutely necessary in patients who have coagulopathies or can be expected to develop them as a result of their disease or its therapy.

2. Intervention(s) should be as limited as possible, and procedures that can be performed under direct vision are preferred. Direct vision allows the operator to be sure that primary hemostasis has been achieved and facilitates follow-up for detection of delayed bleeding.

3. The clinician should be certain that the preliminary coagulation status is fully delineated so that potential bleeding risks can be anticipated accurately and the correct therapeutic agents can be available.

4. If a preparatory treatment (e.g., infusion of factor VIII concentrate) or a change in medication (e.g., discontinuation of an anticoagulant drug) is indicated, the clinician should check that the expected beneficial effect actually has occurred before the procedure is begun.

5. The timing of procedures for which supportive products will be needed should be coordinated with the providers (e.g., the blood bank or pharmacy) so that an adequate supply is available for the anticipated duration of support. One should be liberal in estimating needs so that unexpected complications can be covered.

6. The patient should be monitored carefully for both immediate and delayed bleeding to detect status changes early. Other health care personnel should be alerted to the potential for bleeding and the appropriate therapy based on previous evaluation.

7. In a patient who has been evaluated and treated for a coagulopathy, it is important to be alert to the possible effects on coagulation of changes in either medical status (e.g., the onset of sepsis) or medications. Reassessment may be necessary if the patient shows a decreasing response to therapy that was effective initially.

SPECIFIC COAGULOPATHIES

VASCULITIS

Patients with vasculitic rashes may have very long bleeding times that prohibit skin incision. Discontinuation of an offending drug and trial of corticosteroids may be useful. Administration of platelets is not indicated unless thrombocytopenia or thrombocytopathy coexists.

THROMBOCYTOPENIA

For procedures that will be performed under direct vision, such as limited biopsies or peripheral line insertions, platelet counts of 50,000 to 80,000/μL usually are adequate, depending on the extent of the planned intervention. For major surgical procedures, insertion of lines in large central vessels, or closed-space needle biopsies, initial counts in the range of 80,000 to 100,000/μL are preferred (assuming that platelet function assessed by the bleeding time is normal). Lumbar punctures usually are performed safely at platelet counts of greater than 50,000/μL.

THROMBOCYTOPATHY

Thrombocytopathic bleeding can be very difficult to manage, especially if the environment into which new platelets are transfused is deleterious to their function. Thus, in uremia, for example, multiple transfusions of normal platelets may be ineffective. Other methods of therapy discussed in earlier sections of this chapter may be helpful in this situation. The bleeding time may not be corrected significantly in some patients. The predictive value of the skin incision bleeding time in individual patients has been questioned, but it seems prudent to attempt to shorten a prolonged bleeding time, when possible, before an invasive procedure is performed.

Drug-induced thrombocytopathies may be easier to manage if the drug has a reasonably short half-life or if its inhibitory effect on platelet function is reversible (as with NSAIDs, for example). After the drug has been discontinued and its effect has dissipated, new platelets produced by the patient's marrow and (if needed for an acute intervention) transfused normal platelets will correct the prolonged bleeding time. In urgent situations, DDAVP infusions may be used to override, at least temporarily, the thrombocytopathic effects of aspirin and ticlopidine.[44]

THROMBOCYTHEMIA

Patients with myeloproliferative disorders and elevated platelet counts (usually in excess of $1 \times 10^6/\mu L$ but sometimes in the range of 0.5×10^6 to $1 \times 10^6/\mu L$) may have excessive bleeding, either spontaneously or following trauma or surgery. It is generally advisable to lower the platelet count into the normal range, but even when this goal is achieved, some patients have considerable bleeding difficulties. The bleeding time may be a helpful predictor. It is wise, when possible, to avoid or minimize invasive procedures in these individuals. Similar precautions are indicated in individuals with a bleeding diathesis due to a myelodysplastic disorder.

FIBRIN GENERATION CASCADE DEFECTS

A PT and PTT that are at least normal should be insisted on, if they are achievable, for procedures in which excess bleeding could seriously compromise the outcome (e.g., intracranial neurosurgery) or for closed-space procedures in which mechanical hemostasis is difficult to achieve or in which the extent of bleeding may not be obvious until it is significant. More precise correction of factor levels than that produced by achieving normal clotting times is indicated for such procedures in patients with known factor deficiency states, such as hemophilia A.

For procedures done under direct vision or for line placements, there may be a greater tolerance for impaired clotting times. The clotting times should not exceed 1.2 to 1.3 times the baseline value under these circumstances. In contrast to platelet-related problems, bleeding in patients with cascade deficiencies may be delayed in onset and, therefore, unexpected by uninformed medical and nursing staff. The risk of bleeding with liver biopsy, for example, may be reduced by using transjugular or laparoscopic techniques.

FIBRINOLYTIC STATES

Hyperfibrinolytic states leading to short clot survival, hypofibrinogenemia, and elevated levels of FDPs may be associated with serious bleeding during and after procedures. Intracranial bleeding, thrombotic events, and recent major surgical procedures are contraindications to the initiation of fibrinolytic therapy because of the risk of clot breakdown. If possible, invasive procedures should not be performed while the patient is in a fibrinolytic state. If bleeding occurs during fibrinolytic therapy, the usual approach is to discontinue the drug, provide blood product support (including cryoprecipitate as a source of fibrinogen, if needed), and wait until the fibrinolytic state subsides.

ANTICOAGULANT DRUG EFFECTS

Unfractionated Heparin

The heparinized patient who needs to undergo an invasive procedure usually can be managed by discontinuation of heparin approximately 6 hours beforehand. In urgent circumstances, neutralization with protamine sulfate can hasten preparation.

Low-Molecular-Weight Heparin (LMWH)

Invasive procedures, e.g., epidural anesthesia, have been complicated by bleeding in patients who stopped LMWH therapy shortly beforehand. Because of lack of a predictably effective antagonist, it is important to know the anticoagulated status of these patients before procedures are initiated. LMWH levels can be helpful in assessing residual presence of these agents and possible bleeding risk.

Warfarin

After discontinuation or tapering of warfarin therapy prior to an intended procedure, it may take 2 days or more for the PT to normalize. In emergent situations, use of FFP or prothrombin complex (if volume overload is a problem) can provide immediate correction by supplying the missing factors. Oral or intravenous vitamin K (1 to 5 mg) has its onset of effect approximately 8 to 12 hours after administration. The use of vitamin K in higher doses may lead to a subsequent state of warfarin resistance. The use of prothrombin complex may be associated with induction of a hypercoagulable state. This agent should be reserved, therefore, for urgent indications. During the period following tapering of warfarin, temporary heparinization can allow more flexible planning of interventions; heparin should be discontinued 6 hours before an invasive procedure. In patients unable to receive heparin or LMWH, warfarin can be continued throughout the perioperative period, with FFP used to override its anticoagulant effect, until it is safe to re-establish anticoagulation.

Direct Thrombin Inhibitors

Although their half-lives are short, hirudin and argatroban effects need to be monitored closely by following the PTT level once they have been discontinued to be certain that there is no lingering anticoagulation prior to an invasive procedure. Lack of an effective antagonist for either of these drugs makes rapid reversal of their effects problematic.

Drotrecogin Alfa (XIGRIS)[45]

Drotrecogin alfa is a recombinant activated protein C product with antithrombotic and profibrinolytic properties used in the management of patients with severe sepsis. Its major side effect is risk of bleeding, especially on day 1 of the 96-hour infusion period. Forty-three percent of serious bleeding events were procedure-related.[46] Coexisting thrombocytopenia of $30,000/\mu L$ or less was a frequent concomitant risk factor. It is recommended that infusion of the drug be discontinued 2 hours prior to an anticipated procedure and that the platelet count be maintained above $30,000/\mu L$. The drug variably affects the PTT and assays of intrinsic pathway factors but has little effect on the PT or assays of factors that influence the PT. If otherwise safe, it is recommended that a 12-hour period elapse after a significant procedure before cautiously restarting the infusion.

References

1. Bowie EJW, Owen CA: The clinical and laboratory diagnosis of hemorrhagic disorders, in Ratnoff OD, Forbes CD (eds): *Disorders of Hemostasis.* Orlando, FL, Grune & Stratton, 1984, p 43.

2. Thompson AR, Harker LA: *Manual of Hemostasis and Thrombosis,* 3d ed. Philadelphia, Davis, 1983, p 175 (Appendix A).

3. Ziegler S, Maca T, Alt E, et al: Monitoring of antiplatelet therapy with the PFA-100 in peripheral angioplasty patients. *Platelets* 13:493, 2002.

4. Winkelmann RK: Classification of vasculitis, in Wolff K, Winkelmann RK (eds): *Vasculitis.* London, Lloyd-Luke, 1980, p 1.

5. Kasabach HS, Merritt KK: Capillary hemangioma with extensive purpura: Report of a case. *Am J Dis Child* 259:1063, 1940.

6. McKee LC Jr, Collins RD: Intravascular leukocyte thrombi and aggregates as a cause of morbidity and mortality in leukemia. *Medicine* 53:463, 1974.

7. Bussel JB, Kimberly RP, Inman RD, et al: Intravenous gammaglobulin treatment of chronic idiopathic thrombocytopenic purpura. *Blood* 62:480, 1983.

8. Lazarus AH, Crow AR: Mechanism of action of IVIG and anti-D in ITP. *Transfusion Apheresis Sci* 28:249, 2003.

9. Ziman A, Klopper E, Pepkowitz S, et al: A second case of post-transfusion purpura caused by HPA-5a antibodies: Successful treatment with intravenous immunoglobulin. *Vox Sang* 83:165, 2002.

10. Moake JL: Thrombotic microangiopathies. *N Engl J Med* 347:589, 2002.

11. Rock GA, Shumak KH, Buskard NA, et al: Comparison of plasma exchange with plasma infusion in the treatment of thrombotic thrombocytopenic purpura. *N Engl J Med* 325:393, 1991.

12. Zheng X, Pallera AM, Goodnough LT, et al: Remission of chronic thrombotic thrombocytopenic purpura after treatment with cyclophosphamide and rituximab. *Ann Intern Med* 138:105, 2003

13. Marder VJ, Feinstein DI, Colman RW: Consumptive thrombohemorrhagic disorders, in Colman RW, Hirsh J, Marder VJ, et al (eds): *Hemostasis and Thrombosis,* 4th ed. Philadelphia, Lippincott Williams & Wilkins 2001, p 1197.

14. Hirsh J, Warkentin TE, Shaughnessy SG, et al: Heparin and low-molecular-weight heparin: Mechanisms of action, pharmacokinetics, dosing, monitoring, efficacy, and safety. *Chest* 119(suppl):64S, 2001.

15. Warkentin TE, Levine MN, Hirsh J, et al: Heparin-induced thrombocytopenia in patients treated with low-molecular-weight heparin or unfractionated heparin. *N Engl J Med* 332:1330, 1995.

16. Bick RL: Alterations of hemostasis during cardiopulmonary bypass: A comparison between membrane and bubble oxygenators. *Am J Clin Pathol* 73:300, 1980.

17. Harker LA, Finch CA: Thrombokinetics in man. *J Clin Invest* 48:963, 1969.

18. Baron BW, Mick R, Baron JM: Combined plateletpheresis and cytotoxic chemotherapy for symptomatic thrombocytosis in myeloproliferative disorders. *Cancer* 72:1209, 1993.

19. Coller BS: Disorders of platelets, in Ratnoff OD, Forbes CD (eds): *Disorders of Hemostasis.* Orlando, FL, Grune & Stratton, 1984, p 143.

20. Janson PA, Jubelier SJ, Weinstein MJ, Deykin D: Treatment of the bleeding tendency in uremia with cryoprecipitate. *N Engl J Med* 303:1318, 1980.

21. Mannucci PM, Remuzzi G, Pusineri F, et al: Deamino-8-D-arginine vasopressin shortens the bleeding time in uremia. *N Engl J Med* 308:8, 1983.

22. Livio M, Mannucci PM, Vigano CL, et al: Conjugated estrogens for the management of bleeding associated with renal failure. *N Engl J Med* 315:731, 1986.

23. Kuzel T, Green D, Stulberg SD, Baron J: Arthropathy and surgery in congenital factor VII deficiency. *Am J Med* 84:771, 1988.

24. Lorand L, Losowsky MS, Miloszewski KJM: Human factor XIII: Fibrin-stabilizing factor. *Prog Haemost Thromb* 5:245, 1980.

25. Sadler JE, Blinder M: von Willebrand's disease: Diagnosis, classification, and treatment, in Colman RW, Hirsh J, Marder VJ, Clowes AW, George JN (eds): *Hemostasis and Thrombosis,* 4th ed. Philadelphia, Lippincott Williams & Wilkins 2001, p 825.

26. Rodgers RPC, Levin J: A critical reappraisal of the bleeding time. *Semin Thromb Hemost* 16:1, 1990.

27. Shapiro SS: Acquired inhibitors to the blood coagulation factors. *Semin Thromb Hemost* 1:336, 1975.

28. Green D, Lechner K: A survey of 215 non-hemophilic patients with inhibitors to factor VIII. *Thromb Haemost* 45:200, 1981.

29. Nilsson IM, Jonsson S, Sundqvist SB, et al: A procedure for removing high titer antibodies by extracorporeal protein-A-sepharose adsorption in hemophilia: Substitution therapy and surgery in a patient with hemophilia B and antibodies. *Blood* 58:38, 1981.

30. Wiestner A, Cho HJ, Asch AS, et al. Rituximab in the treatment of acquired factor VIII inhibitors. *Blood* 100:3426, 2002.

31. Shapiro SS, Thiagarajan P: Lupus anticoagulants. *Prog Hemost Thromb* 6:263, 1982.

32. DeLoughery T: Hemorrhagic and thrombotic disorders in the intensive care setting, in Kitchens CS, Alving BM, Kessler CM (eds): *Consultative Hemostasis and Thrombosis.* Philadelphia, Saunders, 2002, p 493.

33. Olson RE: Vitamin K, in Colman RW, Hirsh J, Marder VJ, Salzman EW (eds): *Hemostasis and Thrombosis,* 2d ed. Philadelphia, Lippincott, 1987, p 846.

34. Beck EA, Charache P, Jackson D: A new inherited coagulation disorder caused by an abnormal fibrinogen (fibrinogen "Baltimore"). *Nature* 208:143, 1965.

35. Francis JL, Armstrong DJ: Acquired dysfibrinogenemia in liver disease. *J Clin Pathol* 35:667, 1982.

36. Harrigan C, Lucas CE, Ledgerwood AM, Mammen ET: Primary hemostasis after massive transfusion for injury. *Am Surg* 48:393, 1982.

37. Hewson JR, Neame PB, Kumar N, et al: Coagulopathy related to dilution and hypotension during massive transfusion. *Crit Care Med* 13:387, 1985.

38. Martinowitz U, Kenet G, Lubetske A, et al: Possible role of recombinant activated factor VII (rFVIIa) in the control of hemorrhage associated with massive trauma. *Can J Anaesth* 49:515, 2002.

39. Hedner U, Erhardtsen E: Potential role of recombinant factor VIIa as a hemostatic agent. *Clin Adv Hematol Oncol* 1:112, 2003.

40. Shattil SJ, Bennett JS, McDonough M, Turnbull J: Carbenicillin and penicillin G inhibit platelet function in vitro by impairing the interaction of agonists with the platelet surface. *J Clin Invest* 65:329, 1980.

41. Joist JH, George JN: Hemostatic Abnormalities in liver and renal disease, in Colman RW, Hirsh J, Marder VJ, Clowes AW, George JN (eds): *Hemostasis and Thrombosis,* 4th ed. Philadelphia, Lippincott Williams & Wilkins, 2001, p 995.

42. Moia M, Mannucci PM, Vizzotto L, et al: Improvement in the haemostatic defect of uraemia after treatment with recombinant human erythropoietin. *Lancet* 2:1227, 1987.

43. Furie B: Acquired coagulation disorders and dysproteinemias, in Colman RW, Hirsh J, Marder VJ, Salzman EW (eds): *Hemostasis and Thrombosis,* 2d ed. Philadelphia, Lippincott, 1987, p 841.

44. Schulman S: DDAVP—The multipotent drug in patients with co-agulopathies. *Transfusion Med Rev* 5:132, 1991.

45. Bernard GR, Vincent J-L, Laterre RF, et al: The recombinant human activated protein C worldwide evaluation in severe sepsis (PROWESS) study group: Efficacy and safety of recombinant human activated protein C for severe sepsis. *N Engl J Med* 344:699, 2001.

46. Bernard GR, Macias WL, Williams MD, et al: Safety assessment of drotrecogin alfa (activated) in the treatment of adult patients with severe sepsis. *Crit Care* 7:155, 2003.

Chapter 70

THROMBOTIC THROMBOCYTOPENIC PURPURA, HEMOLYTIC UREMIA SYNDROMES, AND THE APPROACH TO THROMBOTIC MICROANGIOPATHIES

LAWRENCE TIM GOODNOUGH

KEY POINTS

- *The thrombotic microangiopathies (TMAs) include the spectrum of thrombotic thrombocytopenic purpura (TTP) and hemolytic uremic syndromes (HUS) as well as related obstetric syndromes.*

- *The hallmarks of TMA are a microangiopathic hemolytic anemia (MAHA) and thrombocytopenia.*

- *TMA must be distinguished from other coagulopathies, such as disseminated intravascular coagulation (DIC) and collagen vascular disease with vasculitis, since therapeutic approaches differ.*

- *The clinical presentation of TTP/HUS is characterized by a pentad of findings: MAHA, thrombocytopenia, neurologic abnormalities, renal dysfunction, and fever.*

- *Plasma exchange is the therapy of choice for TTP/HUS, with adjunctive therapies including plasma infusion, corticosteroids, splenectomy, and/or immunosuppressive agents.*

- *TTP/HUS is a hematologic emergency, and patients are at risk of developing tissue anoxia, lactic acidosis, renal failure, or catastrophic central nervous system injury.*

- *Plasma exchange may be complicated by catheter accidents, air embolus, citrate toxicity, and pulmonary edema.*

Moschcowitz's original description of TTP in 1925 was based on a triad of findings: anemia (of the microangiopathic hemolytic type), thrombocytopenia, and neurologic symptoms. In 1966, 271 cases of TTP were reviewed, and the features of fever and renal impairment were added to form a clinical pentad.[1] Subsequent series have confirmed that renal involvement is common, with proteinuria, hematuria, or azotemia seen in 80% of patients with TTP.[2,3] Hemolytic uremic syndromes (MAHA, thrombocytopenia, and renal failure) are regarded as part of a spectrum of TMA, which at one end consists of TTP with predominantly neurologic findings and minimal renal abnormality, and at the other end consists of profound renal dysfunction with little or no central nervous system (CNS) pathology. The latter syndromes are more common in childhood, in the postpartum period, and following use of chemotherapeutic (mitomycin C) or immunosuppressive (cyclosporine) agents. On occasion, the evolution of renal manifestations in TTP can become indistinguishable

from HUS, so that attempts at rigid distinction are generally unrewarding.[4]

The age of onset of TTP/HUS ranges from infancy to the eighth decade, with a peak incidence in the third decade. Females are more frequently affected than males by a ratio of 2:1. Childhood HUS often presents with antecedent illness, typically gastroenteritis related to enterotoxin-producing strains of *Escherichia coli* or *Shigella*. TMA associated with pregnancy includes several syndromes with considerable overlap, making prospective differentiation difficult.[5,6] Pregnancy-induced hypertension (PIH; eclampsia and pre-eclampsia) is often associated with subtle laboratory abnormalities consistent with a degree of underlying TMA; on occasion this becomes clinically significant. When *h*ypertension, *e*levated *l*iver enzyme levels, and a *l*ow *p*latelet count occur together as a syndrome in the peripartum period, the term HELLP syndrome is applied (see Chap. 105). TTP may also be encountered in the second or third trimesters of pregnancy; unlike thrombocytopenias associated with PIH, it may not improve rapidly with termination of the pregnancy and may require further treatment. Finally, postpartum HUS is distinguished by its onset after delivery. Characterization of TMA in pregnancy is often made in the context of this clinical information.

TTP syndromes have also been described as drug-induced in patients receiving antiplatelet agents,[7,8] chemotherapeutic agents[9] (such as mitomycin C), or immunosuppressive agents (such as cyclosporine or FK 506)[10] following organ transplantation. Transplantation patient populations are growing, and these patients are likely to be encountered in the critical care environment. Transplant patients are at risk for multiple complications that may be associated with coagulopathy and cytopenia, so making the correct diagnosis is challenging. TTP/HUS has also been associated with human immunodeficiency virus (HIV) infection,[11] and more recently TTP/HUS has been identified as a complication related to antiplatelet therapy such as ticlopidine[7] and clopidogrel.[8]

TTP/HUS has also been described as a complication in patients with collagen vascular disease such as systemic lupus erythematosus (SLE).[12] Vasculitic syndromes and end-organ involvement in these patients may mimic the clinical pentad associated with the TTP syndrome, making clinical differentiation between these two syndromes problematic.

Despite the well-described association of TTP/HUS syndromes with pre-existing comorbidities or inciting agents, most cases of TTP currently present as idiopathic, community-acquired syndromes, perhaps in association with an antecedent viral syndrome. Much progress has been made in recent years regarding the pathophysiology of TTP in this setting, which is discussed below.

Clinical Presentation

The clinical presentation of TTP varies with the extent and severity of the thrombotic lesions. Neurologic findings can be nonspecific and include headache alone or with changes in mental status. Often these seemingly minor manifestations of disease are discovered by careful history-taking to have preceded more fulminant findings associated with anemia, thrombocytopenia, or renal failure. Neurologic findings may be more obvious, including seizures, obtundation, focal neurologic deficits, or coma. Altered mental status in TTP has

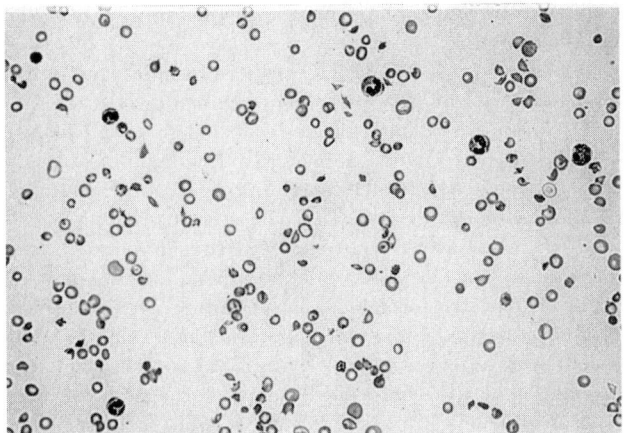

FIGURE 70-1 Admission (hospital day 1) peripheral blood smear (Wright-Giemsa stain) showing characteristic RBC morphology of microangiopathic hemolytic anemia ($\times$ 350) (see Color Plate 70-1).

also been described as secondary to nonconvulsive status epilepticus.[13] Fever is present in approximately two thirds of cases.

Although the presence or absence of renal failure may affect prognosis, the heterogeneity of patients with TMA is greater than this single clinical parameter.[4] Survival rates without (78%)[14] or with (83%)[15] acute renal failure have been reported not to be different. Thus while patients can be characterized according to their extent of neurologic or renal abnormalities, at present a clinical distinction for adult patients with TMA between TTP and HUS does not seem useful.

Laboratory findings in TTP/HUS are often striking. Thrombocytopenia may be profound, with platelet counts of <50,000/μL frequently observed. Anemia is of a microangiopathic type, and the peripheral smear is remarkable for fragmented red blood cells (RBCs), polychromatophilia, nucleated RBCs, and a markedly diminished platelet count (Fig. 70-1; Color Plate 70-1). Intravascular hemolysis frequently causes elevation of total bilirubin (predominantly the direct fraction) and lactate dehydrogenase (LDH). Urinalysis usually reveals proteinuria or hematuria; varying degrees of diminished glomerular filtration rate may be seen. Diagnosis of TTP/HUS by tissue biopsy has been advocated by some, but findings are often consistent with, but not specific for, TTP/HUS. Gingival biopsy, a previously popular test, lacks sensitivity and specificity.[16]

Pathophysiology

The earliest pathologic descriptions of TTP/HUS emphasized the presence of hyaline thrombi in the terminal arterioles and capillaries of the heart, liver, and kidneys. These hyaline deposits have subsequently been shown to consist largely of agglutinated platelets. A degree of associated fibrin deposition is regarded as a secondary phenomenon, since its presence is variable and patients with TTP do not routinely exhibit the coagulation abnormalities of DIC.

The pathogenesis of this diffuse microvascular thrombosis, while unclear,[17] is becoming better understood. The initial event is inappropriate platelet adhesion, aggregation, and

mediator release on endothelial surfaces that results in vascular occlusion, with the characteristic hyaline thrombi of platelets and fibrin. Systemic endothelial cell damage appears to be a central component of the pathogenesis of TTP/HUS,[18] particularly in patients with virutoxin-mediated HUS associated with pathogenic *E. coli* or *Shigella*.[19] Endothelial damage stimulates the release of unusually large von Willebrand factor (vWF) multimers[20] that may cause platelet agglutination and microvascular occlusions.[21] Deficiency of a vWF cleaving protease (vWFCP, or ADAMTS13) was initially reported in patients with familial or idiopathic TTP, but not in patients with HUS.[22] However, other reports found reduced vWFCP levels in HUS,[23] and in other conditions with thrombocytopenia, including DIC and idiopathic thrombocytopenic purpura (ITP),[24] and in patients with liver cirrhosis, chronic renal insufficiency, and acute inflammatory states.[25] In one report, reduced vWFCP levels were observed in other thrombocytopenic disorders, and had only moderate sensitivity (0.45) and low specificity (0.30) in patients with a clinical diagnosis of TTP/HUS.[24] In a second report using a vWVFCP cutoff level of 30%,[26] the collagen-binding assay performed with a sensitivity of 94%, specificity of 93%, and a positive predictive value of 79%. Although vWFCP activity is decreased (<30%) in a substantial proportion of patients with thrombocytopenia of various causes, a severe (<5%) deficiency is more specific for TMA commonly labeled TTP.[27]

Inhibitors (characterized as IgG antibodies) against the vWFCP have been detected in one report in two thirds of plasma samples in the acute phase from patients with TTP-HUS.[28] Another report[29] found that 79% of patients with idiopathic, community-acquired TTP/HUS have low (<5%) levels of vWFCP; of these, vWFCP inhibitor was detected in 73%. vWFCP has recently been identified as a new member of the metalloproteinase family,[30] and was subsequently cloned.[31] Levy and colleagues[32] found that vWFCP is mutated in congenital TTP, thereby proving that the protease is directly involved in protection from microangiopathy. Finally, autoantibodies to vWFCP have also been found in patients who developed ticlopidine-associated TTP.[33]

A recent report suggested that in patients with TTP and normal vWFCP activity, factor V Leiden may be an important pathophysiologic risk factor.[34] While the vWFCP deficiency may not be specific for TTP,[23] its deficiency along with the presence of vWFCP inhibitor appears to correlate with a prolonged course and multiple relapses.[29,35] It is clear that disorders of diverse causes converge on a clinical phenotype that includes TMA,[36] and laboratory evaluations based on vWFCP levels and inhibitor assays will facilitate dissection of these potentially distinct entities.

Differential Diagnosis

The differential diagnosis of the thrombotic microangiopathies includes disease processes presenting with thrombocytopenia and MAHA (Table 70-1). Most commonly, the clinician must distinguish between TTP/HUS and the DIC syndromes or distinguish TTP/HUS from a collagen vascular disease (CVD) such as systemic lupus erythematosus (SLE) with vasculitis (Table 70-2). DIC may be associated with many diseases (see Table 70-1) and results in widespread generation and deposition of intravascular fibrin in small blood vessels,

TABLE 70-1 Differential Diagnosis of Microangiopathic Hemolytic Anemia

DIC syndromes
    Purpura fulminans
    Incompatible blood transfusion reaction
    Sepsis
    Amniotic fluid embolus
    Dead fetus syndrome
    Abruptio placentae
    Massive tissue injury (trauma, burns)
    Kasabach-Merritt syndrome (cavernous hemangioma)
SLE and other vasculitic syndromes
Pregnancy-associated syndromes
    PIH
    HELLP syndrome
HUS
    Childhood-associated
    Postpartum
    Drug-induced (chemotherapy, cyclosporine, etc)
TTP

ABBREVIATIONS: DIC, disseminated intravascular coagulation; HELLP, hypertension, elevated liver enzymes, and low platelets; HUS, hemolytic uremic syndrome; PIH, pregnancy-induced hypertension; SLE, systemic lupus erythematosus; TTP, thrombotic thrombocytopenic purpura.

accompanied by a consumptive coagulopathy with clotting factor activation as a primary process. This condition is to be distinguished from TTP/HUS, in which the primary process is platelet aggregation at the vascular endothelial surface.

DISTINGUISHING THROMBOTIC THROMBOCYTOPENIC PURPURA FROM DISSEMINATED INTRAVASCULAR COAGULATION

DIC may be initiated by either endothelial injury (the intrinsic coagulation pathway) or release of tissue thromboplastin (the extrinsic coagulation pathway). Either process can cause platelets to undergo intravascular aggregation when exposed to collagen and thrombin. The clinical manifestations of DIC arise from injury related to intravascular thrombosis or from bleeding that results from consumption and depletion of clotting factors and platelets. Acute DIC syndromes usually present with bleeding and demonstrable hypo- or afibrinogenemia. In more chronic forms of DIC in which reticuloendothelial system clearance mechanisms, clotting factor production, and marrow cell production compensate

TABLE 70-2 Laboratory Findings in Thrombotic Microangiopathies and Other Disorders

Parameter	TMA	DIC	SLE
RBC fragmentation	+++	+++	+
Thrombocytopenia	+++	+++	±
PT	Normal	Prolonged	Normal
PTT	Normal	Prolonged	Normal
Fibrinogen level	Normal	Low	Normal
Level of fibrin degradation products	Low	High	Low
Complement levels	Normal	Normal	Low

ABBREVIATIONS: DIC, disseminated intravascular coagulation; PT, prothrombin time; PTT partial thromboplastin time; RBC, red blood cell; SLE, systemic lupus erythematosus; TMA, thrombotic microangiopathy.

for consumption, patients can present with thrombosis rather than hemorrhage. Typical thrombotic problems include deep vein or superficial thrombophlebitis, pulmonary embolus, cerebrovascular accidents, or nonbacterial (marantic) endocarditis.

DIC shares with TTP the features of MAHA and thrombocytopenia (see Table 70-2). In one series, the frequency of MAHA as judged by peripheral smear was 68% in patients with DIC. In the same series, thrombocytopenia (platelet count $<150,000/\mu L$) was seen in 96% of cases of DIC; however, significant thrombocytopenia (platelet count $<50,000/\mu L$) was much less common (57%).

A number of laboratory findings will help to distinguish TTP from DIC (see Table 70-2). As noted above, hypofibrinogenemia is typical of fulminant, consumptive DIC. In addition, as clotting factors are consumed, prolongation of the prothrombin time (PT) and partial thromboplastin time (PTT) is seen. Also, the systemic generation of fibrin can lead to activation of the fibrinolytic system, either by activation of plasminogen by tissue activators released from vascular endothelium or by Hageman factor–dependent activation. Fibrinolysis results in the appearance of fibrin degradation products (FDPs) in the serum that can be measured. While none one of these laboratory tests alone can distinguish TTP from DIC, in the aggregate they are sufficient to permit a specific diagnosis (see Table 70-2 and Chap. 69).

Finally, the clinical context will often help to determine if DIC is a viable explanation for the observed abnormalities. Most often, the disease or disorder that is the precipitant of DIC is apparent. Amniotic fluid embolus, retained products of conception, and abruptio placentae are obstetric complications often associated with DIC. Septicemia is the substrate for DIC in many patients encountered in the ICU. The presentation of these patients may be fulminant, as in the Waterhouse-Friderichsen syndrome (shock, bleeding diathesis, and adrenal insufficiency in association with meningococcemia), or more indolent, as in the complex postoperative patient with a "smoldering" intra-abdominal source of infection. Trauma is a well-recognized cause of DIC and fibrinolysis resulting from the exposure of tissue thromboplastins and plasminogen activators to plasma.[37] In trauma patients, unexplained bleeding during or after a surgical procedure may be the first manifestation of DIC. In the setting of head injury, as many as 70% of patients have clinical evidence of DIC.[38]

In summary, TTP/HUS can usually be distinguished readily from DIC by the clinical context and laboratory parameters. It is important to apply this principle, as all of the defining features of TTP/HUS—thrombocytopenia, MAHA, fever, neurologic dysfunction, and renal abnormality—are so common in the critically ill that a clear approach to this possible diagnosis is warranted.

APPROACH TO THE PREGNANT PATIENT

Hematologic aberrations associated with PIH (pre-eclampsia/eclampsia; see Chap. 105) include MAHA, thrombocytopenia, and alterations of the coagulation mechanism. Evidence of MAHA can be found in 2% to 15% of women with PIH, and thrombocytopenia has been reported in as many as 18% of patients. Thus a subset of patients with PIH will have two of the cardinal hematologic abnormalities of TTP/HUS.[5] It has been suggested that PIH and TTP/HUS share pathophysiologic features, specifically aberration in prostaglandin metabolism at the platelet-endothelial cell interface. In this regard it is interesting that plasma exchange has been reported to be a successful therapy in PIH. A subset of patients with PIH and thrombocytopenia may have marked elevation of liver function tests (HELLP syndrome). Right upper quadrant pain is often present and may mimic cholecystitis or peritonitis.

Postpartum HUS is characterized by predominant renal involvement; neurologic signs and fever are usually absent. It has been suggested that this syndrome is a clinical counterpart of the generalized Schwarzman reaction. It is hypothesized that bacterial endotoxins or vasoactive amines are discharged into the maternal circulation and either stimulate the coagulation cascade or initiate thrombosis by damage to the vascular endothelium.

As mentioned above, DIC syndromes accompany major complications of pregnancy. Usually these processes are associated with a catastrophic process such as amniotic fluid embolus or abruptio placentae. Less apparent and more indolent DIC may be encountered with retained products of conception.

Finally, TTP/HUS itself is encountered in pregnancy but is rare, with approximately 70 cases reported. It is likely that most pregnant patients with thrombocytopenia and MAHA are best classified as having PIH with hematologic abnormalities.[10] The key features distinguishing these patients from the group with HELLP syndrome are the emergence of disease in late pregnancy, relatively mild hematologic irregularities, and prompt resolution of thrombocytopenia, MAHA, neurologic symptoms, and liver function abnormalities following delivery. HUS begins postpartum, with a predominance of renal dysfunction. DIC differs from TTP as described above (see Table 70-2). The small remaining group of patients whose clinical presentation is best described as TTP/HUS are best managed in pregnancy with the usual treatments (see below), with expeditious delivery or termination of pregnancy.[39,40]

DISTINGUISHING THROMBOTIC THROMBOCYTOPENIC PURPURA FROM COLLAGEN VASCULAR DISEASE

An association between TTP/HUS and SLE has been reported. In one review, evidence of SLE was found in 7 of 64 cases initially diagnosed as TTP/HUS.[1] TTP/HUS has also been reported in association with other CVDs, including rheumatoid arthritis, ankylosing spondylitis, and polyarteritis nodosa. On the other hand, vasculitis in association with SLE or another CVD may mimic TTP/HUS with findings of renal failure, fever, neurologic disturbance, thrombocytopenia, and MAHA. Serum complement levels are usually low in patients with vasculitis and normal in those with TTP/HUS (see Table 70-2). Antinuclear antibodies are positive in the great majority of patients with SLE. These CVD screening tests are indicated in all patients with a tentative diagnosis of TTP/HUS. If a diagnosis of a specific CVD can be made, therapy should be directed at that disorder, rather than at the associated hematologic problems.

Therapy

TTP/HUS is a hematologic emergency. Patients will often need ICU admission because of profound anemia, shock, lactic acidosis, respiratory failure, or deteriorating neurologic function. Intubation and mechanical ventilation may be required because of ventilatory failure complicating CNS involvement or because of direct lung injury associated with pulmonary vascular involvement by TTP.[41]

PLASMA EXCHANGE

Once a diagnosis of TTP is made, plasma exchange is the therapy of choice. Since 1961, mortality for this disease has declined from >90% to <50%, likely owing to the institution of plasma exchange therapy. Some studies, however, have suggested that the overall mortality from TTP has actually increased in the United States in recent years.[3] The prognosis of TTP is improved by prompt recognition and treatment, so that emergency apheresis should be conducted in any patient diagnosed with TTP/HUS. Plasma exchange of 150% of the plasma volume is instituted (3 to 4 L for normal-sized individuals) with plasma replacement. Two intravenous sites are required for the procedure, which uses 17 gauge (draw line) and 18 gauge (return line) catheters. Ideally, plasma exchange is conducted through a double-lumen dialysis catheter. Special precautions should be taken when placing large-bore central catheters in these thrombocytopenic patients, such as ultrasound guidance or placement in a compressible vessel (jugular or femoral vein).

Potential complications of plasma exchange include those related to line placement, air embolus, citrate toxicity, pulmonary edema, and risks associated with plasma transfusion (hives, urticaria, rash, anaphylactoid reactions). In one series over a 6-year period, 54 major complications, including 3 deaths, were identified to be related to plasma exchange in 42 (28%) of 142 consecutive patients with TTP/HUS.[42] The risk of air embolus is reduced when the procedure is performed by experienced personnel. Machine safety devices include bubble traps and a bubble alarm that stops the machine when air is detected in the lines. Citrate toxicity can occur from the plasma citrate anticoagulant infused into the patient and is compounded by associated renal dysfunction. Citrate toxicity causes hypocalcemia and metabolic alkalosis and presents as oral paresthesias, numbness or tingling in the extremities, or a prolonged QT interval on the electrocardiogram. Hypocalcemia can be prevented by routinely administering 1 ampule of calcium gluconate by constant infusion per liter of plasma exchanged. An additional one half ampule may be administered if symptoms are experienced during the procedure. Periodic monitoring of ionized calcium levels is useful as well. In all cases, the relative benefits and risks of the procedure should be discussed with the patient or guardians, and informed consent obtained.

Plasma exchange should be performed daily until evidence indicates that the disease is in remission. The patient should have normal end-organ function, including normal mental status and renal function. The most sensitive indicator of response is a rising platelet count, which should be normal (>150,000/μL) for a number of days (3 to 5) before plasma exchange is discontinued. The LDH level is also a sensitive indicator of tissue hypoxia[43] and can be used to monitor the response to therapy. RBC morphology on peripheral smear [see Fig. 70-1 (Color Plate 70-1) should be examined sequentially, although improvement in cell fragmentation can lag behind clinical responses (such as improving mental status) by several days. Bone marrow reticulocyte response may not occur for 3 to 5 days, depending on the pace of presentation of the disease. The patient should be given folate (1 mg or more daily) in this setting of poor dietary intake, plasma exchange, and increased marrow requirement.

The usual course of plasma exchange lasts 5 to 14 days. Patients can be moved from the ICU when mental status has normalized and hematocrit and platelet count are increasing. The shortest treatment requirement we have observed is 3 days. Late responses in occasional patients have occurred after 14 days of therapy. Continued plasma exchange may be required for up to 4 weeks as long as the patient remains stable or is improving. Studies have suggested that under conditions of massive plasma replacement, plasma depleted of the largest multimers of von Willebrand factor (cryoprecipitate-poor plasma) might be preferable for the treatment of patients with recurrent or refractory TTP.[44] Patients have been reported to respond to this cryosupernatant fraction as replacement fluid, despite having been refractory previously to plasma replacement therapy;[45] the current standard for initial therapy, however, remains apheresis with plasma replacement.[46]

SALVAGE THERAPIES FOR PATIENTS WHO RECUR OR FAIL TO GAIN REMISSION

Early relapse rates of up to 37% have been reported in patients with TTP/HUS, and 40% of centers routinely use a tapering schedule of apheresis.[47] Occult infections have been described in association with refractory or recurrent TTP/HUS.[48]

With the emerging evidence that some fraction of patients with TTP-HUS may have an autoimmune disease, along with the recognition that sustained treatment with plasma exchange is not without risk,[42] there has been a re-examination of the potential usefulness of salvage therapies for patients with refractory TTP-HUS. Cryosupernatant plasma has been suggested to have a theoretical benefit over fresh frozen plasma (FFP) because it is depleted of vWF, and a retrospective study suggested efficacy.[45] Glucocorticoid therapy is commonly utilized in patients with TTP-HUS; despite one favorable review[49] on its value, no randomized study assessing an impact on the prognosis of TTP-HUS has been performed.[50]

Splenectomy has been reported to be of value[51–60] in patients who do not have a complete or lasting response to plasma exchange. The value of splenectomy may be due to the removal of a major site of synthesis of a pathogenic IgG.[28] In one report[51] in patients who failed exchange, 9 (70%) of 13 refractory patients treated with splenectomy survived.

ADJUNCTIVE THERAPIES

In patients with an incomplete clinical response, splenectomy should be considered. High-dose steroid therapy has been advocated by some,[61] but without convincing evidence of benefit.[50] Our current approach is to use steroids only in patients who do not respond to plasma exchange and in those with a concurrent diagnosis of collagen vascular disease. Vincristine, presumably acting as an immunosuppressant, has

also been reported to produce sustained remissions in a small series.[62]

In view of the pathophysiology of TTP/HUS, antiplatelet agents seem to be a rational addition to treatment. However, clinical trials have not shown a convincing impact of these drugs, including intravenous prostacyclin. Aspirin is difficult to give to an obtunded or comatose patient, and we discourage nasogastric tube placement for this purpose because of the risk of bleeding. Dipyridamole can be given intravenously. While larger series have shown that plasma exchange therapy coupled with antiplatelet agents results in complete remission in approximately two thirds of patients,[63] antiplatelet therapy is no longer routinely used.

Plasma infusion therapy is useful in many patients, particularly those with chronic relapsing TTP/HUS. While plasma infusion (12 U every 24 hours) can be used acutely in patients at facilities that lack apheresis capability, this therapy should not delay the institution of plasma exchange nor prevent the transfer of the patient to a fully equipped referral unit.

Platelet transfusion is relatively contraindicated in TTP, because of clinical evidence that it is associated with relapse.[64] If a diagnosis of TTP has been made, we do not recommend routine use of platelet support, except during invasive procedures. Heparin has been advocated for patients with HUS, but a randomized trial in pediatric patients failed to show benefit.[65] Supportive therapy for HUS often requires renal dialysis, and plasma exchange may be considered for patients with HUS and rapid disease progression.[40]

Therapy with rituximab, a chimeric anti-CD20 monoclonal antibody directed against B lymphocytes, along with cyclophosphamide therapy has been described to successfully treat a patient with TTP/HUS that was chronically refractory (more than 2 years) to previously administered therapies including apheresis, steroids, splenectomy, vincristine, and cyclosporine therapy.[66] This patient had a severe deficiency of vWFCP (ADAMTS13) activity and an antibody to ADAMTS13. Even during periods of clinical hematologic remission, the anti-ADAMTS13 was detectable and the ADAMTS13 levels remained low. Two courses of cyclophosphamide followed by rituximab therapy subsequently resulted in sustained clinical remission, along with disappearance of the ADAMTS13 inhibitor and detectable levels of ADAMTS activity (>17%) after more than 18 months of follow-up (see Fig. 70-2).

Prognosis

Despite a recent single-institution report of a 91% survival rate in patients with TTP,[61] a review of 52 patients treated over 10 years at our own institution revealed a 33% mortality from TTP/HUS.[51] This is in the same range as a 22% mortality rate reported in a Canadian clinical trial of plasma exchange in patients with TTP.[14] A recent review of mortality data in the United States indicated that, despite a reduction in mortality related to TTP from nearly 100% of cases before the era of plasma exchange to an approximately 70% survival rate currently, the incidence of TTP-related deaths in the United States has increased over time.[3] African-Americans and African-American females in particular, are affected disproportionately. The increased incidence of HIV infection and

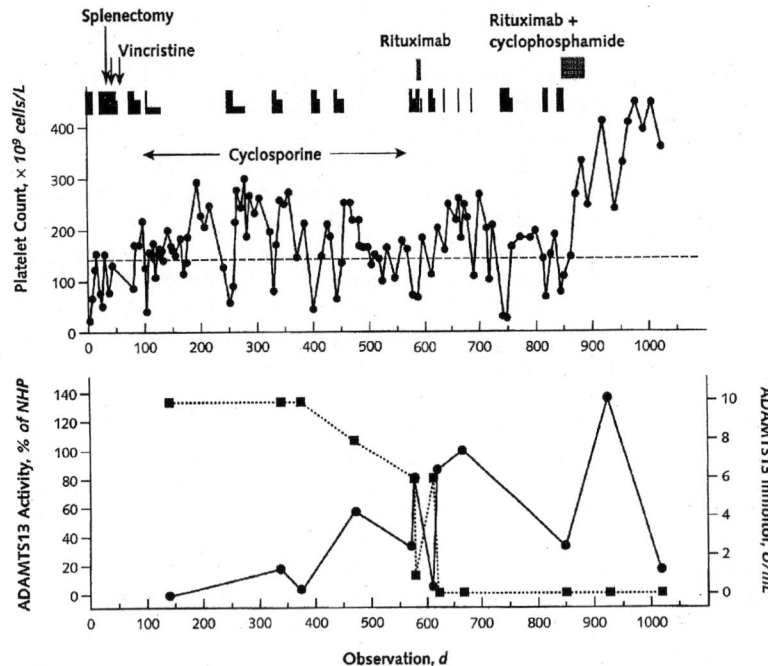

FIGURE 70-2 Platelet count (*top*) and ADAMTS13 activity (*bottom*) in a patient with TTP. Arrows indicate splenectomy and vincristine doses. Black bars indicate plasma exchange treatments; bars of full height, half height, and one third height represent treatment daily, every other day, or twice per week, respectively. The dashed line in the top panel represents the lower limit of normal platelet count (140 × 10⁹ cells/L). In the bottom panel, the solid line represents ADAMTS13 activity and the dotted line represents ADAMTS13 inhibitor. NHP, normal human plasma. (*Reprinted with permission from Zheng et al.*[66])

related disease has contributed to some of the increase in TTP mortality in recent years, but it does not completely explain most of the increase, which began before the onset of the HIV epidemic.

References

1. Amorosi EL, Ultmann J: Thrombotic thrombocytopenic purpura: Report of 16 cases and review of the literature. *Medicine* 45:139, 1966.

2. Ridolfi RL, Bell WR: Thrombotic thrombocytopenic purpura: Report of 25 cases and a review of the literature. *Medicine* 60:413, 1981.

3. Torok TJ, Holman RC, Chorba TL: Increasing mortality from thrombotic thrombocytopenic purpura in the United States. Analysis of National Mortality Data, 1968–1991. *Am J Hematol* 50:84, 1995.

4. George JN: How I treat patients with thrombotic thrombocytopenic purpura-hemolytic uremic syndrome. *Blood* 96:1223, 2000.

5. Weiner CP: Thrombotic microangiopathy in pregnancy and the postpartum period. *Semin Hematol* 24:119, 1987.

6. Ezra Y, Rose M, Eldor A: Therapy and prevention of TTP during pregnancy. *Am J Hematol* 51:1, 1996.

7. Bennett CL, Weinberg PD, Rozenberg-Ben-Dror K, et al: Thrombotic thrombocytopenic purpura associated with ticlopidine. A review of 60 cases. *Ann Intern Med* 128:541, 1998.

8. Bennett CL, Connors JM, Carwile JM, et al: Thrombotic thrombocytopenic purpura associated with clopidogrel. *N Engl J Med* 342:1773, 2000.

9. Myrgo AJ: Thrombotic microangiopathy in the cancer patient including those induced by chemotherapeutic agents. *Semin Hematol* 214:161, 1987.

10. Sarode R, McFarland JG, Flomenberg N, et al: Therapeutic plasma exchange does not appear to be effective in the management of TTP/HUS syndrome following bone marrow transplantation. *Bone Marrow Transplant* 16:271, 1995.

11. Thompson CE, Damon LE, Ries CA, Linker CA: Thrombotic microangiopathies in the 1980s: Clinical features, response to treatment, and the impact of the human immunodeficiency virus epidemic. *Blood* 80:1890, 1992.

12. Gelfand J, Truong L, Stern L, et al: Thrombotic thrombocytopenic purpura syndrome in systemic lupus erythematosus. *Am J Kid Dis* 6:154, 1985.

13. Garrett WT, Chang CW, Bleck TP: Altered mental status in TTP is secondary to nonconvulsive status epilepticus. *Ann Neurol* 40:245, 1996.

14. Rock GA, Shumak KH, Buskard NA, et al: Comparison of plasma exchange with plasma infusion in the treatment of thrombotic thrombocytopenic purpura. *N Engl J Med* 325:393, 1991.

15. Rock GA, Shamak KH, Kelton J, et al: Thrombotic thrombocytopenic purpura: outcome in 24 patients with renal impairment treated with plasma exchange. *Transfusion* 32:710, 1992.

16. Goodman A, Ramos R, Petrelli M, et al: Gingival biopsy in thrombotic thrombocytopenic purpura. *Ann Intern Med* 89:501, 1987.

17. Ruggenenti P, Remuzzi G: The pathophysiology and management of TTP. *Eur J Haematol* 56:191, 1996.

18. Dang CT, Magid MS, Weksler B, et al: Enhanced endothelial cell apoptosis in splenic tissues of patients with thrombotic thrombocytopenic purpura. *Blood* 93:1264, 1999.

19. Mead PS, Griffin PM: *Escherichia coli* O157:H7. *Lancet* 352:1207, 1998.

20. Moake JL, Rudy CK, Troll JH, et al: Unusually large plasma factor VII: von Willebrand factor multimers in chronic relapsing with thrombotic thrombocytopenic purpura. *N Engl J Med* 339:1578, 1998.

21. Moake JL, Chow TW: Increased von Willebrand factor (vWf) binding to platelets associated with impaired vWf breakdown in thrombotic thrombocytopenic purpura. *J Clin Apheresis* 13:126, 1998.

22. Furlan M, Robles R, Galbusera M, et al: Von Willebrand factor-cleaving protease in thrombotic thrombocytopenic purpura and the hemolytic uremic syndrome. *N Engl J Med* 339:1578, 1998.

23. Remuzzi G, Galbusera M, Noris M, et al: Von Willebrand factor-cleaving protease (ADAMTS13) is deficient in recurrent and familial thrombotic thrombocytopenic purpura and hemolytic uremic syndrome. *Blood* 100:778, 2002.

24. Moore JC, Hayward CPM, Warkentin TE, Kelton JG: Decreased von Willebrand factor protease activity associated with thrombocytopenic disorders. *Blood* 98:1842, 2001.

25. Mannucci PM, Canciani MT, Forza I, et al: Changes in health and disease of the metalloprotease that cleaves von Willebrand factor. *Blood* 98:2730, 2001.

26. Thimons MM, Zeigler ZR, Shadduck RK, et al: Evaluation of a new rapid collagen binding assay for von Willebrand factor (vWF) protease in thrombocytopenic disorders. *Blood* 98:34a, 2001.

27. Bianchi V, Alberio L, Furlan M, Lammie B: Von Willebrand factor-cleaving protease (ADAMTS13) in thrombocytopenic disorders: A severely deficient activity is specific for thrombotic thrombocytopenic purpura. *Blood* 100:710, 2002.

28. Tsai H-M, Lian ECY: Antibodies to von Willebrand factor-cleaving protease in acute thrombotic thrombocytopenic purpura. *N Engl J Med* 339:1585, 1998.

29. Zheng X, Kaufman R, Goodnough LT, Sadler JE: Prospective study of the effect of plasma exchange on the levels of von Willebrand factor cleaving protease and inhibitor in patients with thrombotic thrombocytopenic purpura. *Blood* 98:754a, 2001.

30. Fujikawa K, Suzuki H, McMuullen B, Chung D: Purification of human von Willebrand factor-cleaving protease and its identification as a new member of the metalloprotease family. *Blood* 98:1662, 2001.

31. Zheng X, Chung D, Takayama TK, et al: Structure of von Willebrand factor cleaving protease (ADAMTS13), a metalloprotease involved in thrombotic thrombocytopenic purpura. *J Biol Chem* 276:41059, 2001.

32. Levy GG, Nichols WC, Lian EC, et al: Mutations in a member of the ADAMTS gene family cause thrombotic thrombocytopenic purpura. *Nature* 413:488, 2001.

33. Tsai HM, Rice L, Sarode R, et al: Antibody inhibitors to von Willebrand factor (VWF) metalloproteinase and increasing binding of VWF to platelets in ticlopidine-associated TTP. *Ann Intern Med* 132:794, 2000.

34. Raife TJH, Lentz SR, Atkinson BS, et al: Factor V Leiden: A genetic risk factor for thrombotic microangiopathy in patients with normal von Willebrand factor-cleaving protease activity. *Blood* 99:437, 2002.

35. Fijnheer R, Hene RJ, Schiphorst ME, et al: Persistent inhibition of von Willebrand factor cleaving protease predicts a prolonged course and relapse in patients with thrombotic thrombocytopenic purpura. *Blood* 98:631a, 2001.

36. Zheng X, Kaufman R, Goodnough LT, et al: Effect of plasma exchange on plasma ADAMTS13 metalloprotease activity, inhibitor level, and clinical outcome in patients with idiopathic and nonidiopathic thrombotic thrombocytopenic purpura. *Blood* 103:4043, 2004.

37. Kapsch DN, Metzler M, Harrington M, et al: Fibrinolytic response to trauma. *Surgery* 95:473, 1984.

38. Miner MED, Kaufman HM, Graham SH, et al: Disseminated intravascular coagulation fibrinolytic syndrome following head injury in children: Frequency and prognostic implications. *J Pediatr* 100:687, 1982.

39. Vandekerchhove F, Noens L, Colardyn F, et al: Thrombotic thrombocytopenic purpura mimicking toxemia of pregnancy. *Am J Obstet Gynecol* 150:320, 1984.

40. Spencer CD, Crane FM, Kumar JR, Alving BM: Treatment of postpartum hemolytic uremic syndrome with plasma exchange. *JAMA* 247:2808, 1982.

41. Bone RC, Henry JE, Petterson J, Amare M: Respiratory dysfunction in thrombotic thrombocytopenic purpura. *Am J Med* 65:262, 1978.

42. McMinn JR, Thomas IA, Terrell DR, et al: Complications of plasma exchange in thrombotic thrombocytopenic purpura–hemolytic-uremic syndrome: A study of 78 additional patients. *Transfusion* 43:415, 2003.

43. Cohen JA, Brecher ME, Bandarenko N: Cellular source of serum lactate dehydrogenase elevation in patients with thrombotic thrombocytopenic purpura. *J Clin Apheresis* 13:16, 1998.

44. Byrnes JJ, Moake JL, Klug P, Perian P: Effectiveness of the cryosupernatant fraction of plasma in the treatment of refractory thrombotic thrombocytopenic purpura. *Am J Hematol* 34:169, 1990.

45. Rock G, Shumak KH, Sutton DMC, et al: Cryosupernatant as replacement fluid for plasma exchange in thrombotic thrombocytopenic purpura. *Br J Haematol* 94:383, 1996.

46. Blackall DP, Uhl L, Spitalnick SL: Cryoprecipitate-reduced plasma: rationale for use and efficacy in the treatment of thrombotic thrombocytopenic purpura. *Transfusion* 41:840, 2001.

47. Bandarenko N, Brecher ME, and the TTP Apheresis Study Group: United States Thrombotic Thrombocytopenic Purpura Apheresis Study Group. Multicenter survey and retrospective analysis of current efficacy of therapeutic plasma exchange. *J Clin Apheresis* 13:133, 1998.

48. Creager AJ, Brecher ME, Bandarenko N: Thrombotic thrombocytopenic purpura that is refractory to therapeutic plasma exchange in two patients with occult infection. *Transfusion* 38:419, 1998.

49. Rock G, Porta C, Bobbio-Pallavinci E: Thrombotic thrombocytopenic purpura treatment in year 2000. *Hematologica* 85:410, 2000.

50. Gorini M, Luliri P: Steroids: What role in TTP? *Transfus Sci* 13:73, 1992.

51. Goodnough LT, Strasburg D, Verbrugge D, Fisher C: Morbidity and mortality in adults with "idiopathic" thrombotic thrombocytopenic purpura/hemolytic uremic syndrome. *J Intensive Care* 9:167, 1994.

52. Schneider PA, Rauner AA, Linker CA, et al: The role of splenectomy in multimodality treatment of thrombotic thrombocytopenic purpura. *Ann Surg* 202:318, 1985.

53. Cuttner J: Splenectomy, steroids, and dextran 70 in thrombotic thrombocytopenic purpura. *JAMA* 227:397, 1974.

54. Reynolds PM, Jackson JM, Brine JA, Vivian AB: Thrombotic thrombocytopenic purpura—remission following splenectomy. Report of a case and review of the literature. *Am J Med* 61:439, 1976.

55. Rutkow IM: Thrombotic thrombocytopenic purpura (TTP) and splenectomy: A current appraisal. *Ann Surg* 188:701, 1978.

56. Stein SH, Aqui NA, Strobl FJ, et al: The role of splenectomy in patients with relapsed/refractory thrombotic thrombocytopenic purpura. *Blood* 98:631a, 2001.

57. Winslow GA, Nelson EW: Thrombotic thrombocytopenic purpura: Indications for and results of splenectomy. *Am J Surg* 170:558, 1995.

58. Veltman GAM, Brand A, Leeksman OC, et al: The role of splenectomy in the treatment of relapsing thrombotic thrombocytopenic purpura. *Ann Hematol* 70:231, 1995.

59. Wells AD, Majumdar G, Slater NGP, Youong AE: Role of splenectomy as a salvage procedure in thrombotic thrombocytopenic purpura. *Br J Surg* 78:1389, 1991.

60. Crowther MA, Heddle N, Hayward CPM, et al: Splenectomy done during hematologic remission to prevent relapse in patients with thrombotic thrombocytopenic purpura. *Ann Intern Med* 125:294, 1996.

61. Bell WR, Braine HG, Ness PM, Kickler TJ: Improved survival in thrombotic thrombocytopenic purpura–hemolytic uremic syndrome. *N Engl J Med* 325:398, 1991.

62. Schreeder MT, Prchal JT: Successful treatment of thrombotic thrombocytopenic purpura by vincristine. *Am J Hematol* 14:75, 1983.

63. Myers TJ: Treatment of thrombotic thrombocytopenic purpura with combined exchange plasmapheresis and antiplatelet drugs. *Semin Thromb Hemostasis* 7:37, 1981.

64. Gordon LI, Dwaan HC, Rossi EC: Deleterious effects of platelet transfusions and recovery thrombocytosis in patients with thrombotic microangiopathy. *Semin Hematol* 24:194, 1987.

65. Vitaco M, Avalos JJ, Giantantonio CA: Heparin therapy in the hemolytic-uremic syndrome. *J Pediatr* 83:271, 1973.

66. Zheng X, Pallera AM, Goodnough LT, et al: Remission of chronic thrombotic thrombocytopenic purpura after treatment with cyclophosphamide and rituximab. *Ann Intern Med* 138:105, 2003.

Chapter 71

ACUTE LEUKEMIA

RICHARD A. LARSON
MICHAEL J. HALL

KEY POINTS

- *Many patients, especially children and younger adults, can be cured of acute leukemia with the use of intensive chemotherapy and skillful supportive care.*
- *The prognosis for the leukemia patient depends on the specific type of leukemia, defined by cytogenetics and immunophenotype, its stage, prior therapy, and coexisting chronic medical problems.*
- *Infection and bleeding are due to the severe pancytopenia caused by either the leukemia itself or its myelosuppressive treatment; these problems resolve as the normal bone marrow recovers.*
- *The success of chemotherapy for acute leukemia depends not only on the drug susceptibility of the individual patient's leukemia but also on the ability of that patient to survive the toxicity of treatment.*
- *Blood transfusions should be used to maintain a hematocrit greater than 30% and a platelet count greater than 10,000/μL.*
- *Hyperleukocytosis with malignant myeloblasts must be treated as a medical emergency with leukapheresis and chemotherapy.*
- *Central nervous system (CNS) leukemia can be treated successfully with radiotherapy, intrathecal chemotherapy, and high-dose systemic chemotherapy.*
- *Tumor cell lysis, aminoglycoside antibiotics, disseminated intravascular coagulation, elevated lysozyme levels, hyperuricemia, and direct infiltration by leukemia cells can lead to acute renal failure, which is often reversible with proper care.*
- *Necrotizing enterocolitis requires aggressive medical management with antibiotics, blood transfusions, nasogastric suction, bowel rest, and maintenance of normal serum proteins and electrolytes.*
- *Hyperuricemia is proportional in severity to the leukemia tumor burden, and it responds to effective chemotherapy together with administration of fluids, bicarbonate, rasburicase, and allopurinol.*

Acute leukemia is a malignant proliferation of bone marrow or lymphoid cells that is uniformly fatal when left untreated. However, with the use of intensive chemotherapy and skillful supportive care, many patients, particularly children and younger adults, can be cured of this devastating disease. Not uncommonly, use of the medical ICU is necessary during the treatment of acute leukemia to manage either the complications of the disease itself or the complications of intensive cytotoxic therapy (Table 71-1). Such newly diagnosed patients deserve maximum aggressive supportive care in the medical ICU because most of the acute complications of leukemia resolve as a complete remission (CR) is achieved. The successful treatment of patients with acute leukemia requires a multidisciplinary approach with close collaboration among intensive care physicians, hematologic oncologists, infectious disease specialists, and the blood bank. Twenty-four-hour physician

coverage is necessary to respond to emergencies that otherwise could lead to rapid deterioration of a patient in the midst of treatment.

Appropriate decision making requires an understanding of the pathophysiology and clinical history of the leukemic disorders. The likelihood of a successful outcome from intensive care management depends in part on the specific type of leukemia and its stage; i.e., the prognosis depends on whether the patient is newly diagnosed and not yet treated or is in an advanced stage following multiple relapses. Knowledge of prior therapy aids in the evaluation of complications, especially with regard to opportunistic infections or organ dysfunction. Since accurate diagnosis and optimal initial treatment and supportive care are essential to achieving the best chance of curing acute leukemia, it is highly desirable that newly diagnosed patients be referred to regional oncology centers where appropriate expertise and resources are readily available.

This chapter briefly reviews the treatment strategy for acute leukemia and then focuses on the serious metabolic, circulatory, and infiltrative complications that most often necessitate ICU care. The far more common bleeding and infectious complications and direct drug toxicities are dealt with in Chaps. 47, 68, 69, and 74.

Differential Diagnosis

Leukemia and other cancers result from genetic alterations in somatic cells. When mutational damage alters normal growth-regulatory mechanisms in a hematopoietic stem cell, a clone of neoplastic cells may proliferate, overwhelming the normal bone marrow through a selective growth advantage, although not necessarily by more rapid growth. Cooperating mutations also affect differentiation and apoptotic pathways. Leukemia cells usually retain characteristics of their original cell lineage, allowing classification[1,2] (Table 71-2). However, because these cells are neoplastic, aberrant expression of proteins not usually manifested by normal cells in a particular hematopoietic lineage may be detected, yielding a "mixed cell" phenotype. The acute leukemias include acute myeloid (nonlymphocytic) leukemia (AML) and acute lymphoblastic leukemia (ALL), as well as the blastic transformations of chronic myelogenous leukemia (CML) and the myelodysplastic syndromes (MDS). Therapy-related AML occurs in patients following treatment with cytotoxic chemotherapy or radiotherapy for an earlier cancer or other disease.

Acute leukemia almost always causes marked abnormalities in the peripheral blood counts. Anemia may be mild, moderate, or severe, and the red blood cells may be macrocytic. Most patients will have moderate to severe thrombocytopenia. Although an elevated white blood cell count

TABLE 71-1 Complications of Leukemia Therapy and Its Treatment

- Cytopenias (anemia, leukopenia, thrombocytopenia)
- Tumor Lysis Syndrome
- Disseminated intravascular coagulation (DIC)
- Acute renal failure
- Infection
- Allergy-related reactions

TABLE 71-2 World Health Organization (WHO) Classification of Acute Leukemias and Their Clinical Features

Subtype	Type	Characteristic Features
Acute Lymphoblastic Leukemia		
	• Precursor B-cell ALL	80% of cases; t (9;22) portends a poor prognosis
	• Precursor T-cell ALL	20% of cases; 50% have a mediastinal mass
Acute Myeloid Leukemia (AML)		
	• AML with recurrent cytogenetic abnormalities	
	— t (8;21)	Neutrophil maturation
	— inv (16) or t (16;16)	Monocyte maturation; abnormal eosinophils
	— t (15; 17) (APL/M3)	Auer rods, DIC; responsive to ATRA
	— 11q23 abnormalities	Also in therapy-related leukemias
	• AML with multilineage dysplasia	Often pancytopenia, in older patients
	• AML and myelodysplastic syndromes, therapy-related	Related to prior alkylating agents, radiation, or topoisomerase II inhibitors; poor prognosis
	• AML otherwise uncatagorized	(FAB designation noted)
	—Minimal differentiation	(MO); No myeloperoxidase activity; ~5% of cases
	—Without maturation	(MI); ~10% of cases
	—With maturation	(M2); myeloid sarcomas, Auer rods; ~40% of cases
	—Myelomonocytic leukemia	(M4); Auer rods; ~25% of cases
	—Monoblastic and monocytic leukemia	(M5a/M5b); often with CNS involvement, gingival/skin infiltration; ~15% of cases
	—Erythroid leukemias	(M6); ~5% of cases
	—Megakaryoblastic leukemia	(M7); <5% of cases; often with extensive marrow fibrosis
	—Basophilic leukemia	<1% of cases
	—Panmyelosis and/or myelofibrosis	Rare; poor prognosis
	—Myeloid sarcoma	Rare; AML presenting as a solitary tumor mass
	• Acute leukemias of ambiguous lineage	~2–4% of cases; can be bilineal, biphenotypic, or undifferentiated
Chronic Myelogenous Leukemia–Blast Phase		Resembles acute leukemia; t (9;22) and/or BCR/ABL positive
	—Lymphoid blast phase	~30% of case; B-cell immunophenotype
	—Myeloid blast phase	~70% of cases; splenomegaly, fever, leukostasis, myeloid sarcomas
Burkitt Leukemia/Lymphoma		Aggressive mature B-cell neoplasm (TdT negative); high tumor burden in marrow and lymph nodes; EBV-related; *MYC* gene translocations diagnostic; high proliferative fraction

and readily recognizable circulating blast cells frequently are present, not all patients have leukocytosis. Some patients actually present with leukopenia, and malignant cells may not be observed in the peripheral blood. A careful review of a blood smear often demonstrates dysplasia in one or more cell lines. In elderly patients, AML frequently evolves from an MDS; mature granulocytes (called *pseudo-Pelger-Huet cells*) often are hypocellular with poorly condensed nuclear chromatin, and platelets may be large and may lack normal granulation. An overt or subclinical preleukemic phase may have been present for several months. The presence of greater than 20% blast cells in the marrow is the somewhat arbitrary dividing line between acute leukemia and the "preleukemic" disorder MDS.

The diagnosis and subclassification of acute leukemia rest on the interpretation of an adequate bone marrow sample. A marrow aspiration specimen, together with a bone marrow needle core biopsy from the posterior iliac crest, provides essential information. Auer rods are observed often in malignant myeloblasts. Cytochemical reactivity reveals myeloperoxidase or nonspecific esterase activity in myeloid leukemias, whereas such activity is absent in lymphoid leukemias.

Immunophenotypic analysis using flow cytometry or immunohistochemical techniques detects cell-surface antigens, whose presence supports the diagnosis. Cytogenetic analysis of bone marrow specimens provides important diagnostic and prognostic information.[3,4] Metaphase cells are karyotyped after direct preparation or short-term (24- to 48-hour) unstimulated culturing. Characteristic recurring chromosomal abnormalities include the presence of extra chromosomes, the loss of certain chromosomes, and structural rearrangements such as translocations, deletions, insertions, and inversions. Many distinct subtypes of acute leukemia can now be defined according to their characteristic morphologic, cytochemical, immunophenotypic, and cytogenetic features. These disorders have a more predictable clinical course than less well-defined leukemias, and this distinction is reflected in the current World Health Organization (WHO) classifications.[2]

Management of Acute Leukemia

The optimal chemotherapy for patients with acute leukemia has not yet been determined.[5–7] Recent clinical trials have identified different risk groups that are more or less likely to respond to standard chemotherapy programs (Table 71-3). Treatment is given in two or three phases: remission induction, consolidation, and in some cases, maintenance. The goal of *remission-induction chemotherapy* is to induce a complete remission. Any lesser response does not improve survival. *Complete remission* is defined by the absence of detectable leukemia in the bone marrow and blood, the regeneration of normal marrow elements, and the return to normal levels of all three blood cell lines for at least a month. This response reflects a reduction in the tumor cell mass by more than 3 logs (i.e., >99.9%). However, as many as 10^8 malignant cells may still persist at this point. If no postremission therapy were given, most patients with acute leukemia would relapse within 2 to 4 months. Thus *consolidation chemotherapy* (sometimes called *intensification therapy*) is directed at destroying any clonogenic leukemia cells that remain undetected after initial treatment. Consolidation therapy uses several monthly cycles (commonly one to four) of myelosuppressive chemotherapy, each sufficiently intense to produce bone marrow hypoplasia and peripheral blood pancytopenia. Various strategies using allogeneic bone marrow transplantation or high-dose chemotherapy followed by reinfusion of autologous marrow or blood stem cells collected earlier during remission are being tested as postremission consolidation treatments. Low-dose outpatient maintenance chemotherapy that does not lower the blood count has not been proved to increase the fraction of patients with AML who are cured, although 18 to 24 months of maintenance treatment seems useful for patients with ALL.

Patients who suffer a relapse of acute leukemia after completion of all therapy often can achieve a second remission with reinstitution of the original induction chemotherapy regimen. However, patients who relapse in the midst of initial treatment or while receiving maintenance therapy are less likely to achieve a second remission and rarely have long survival. Second and subsequent periods of remission usually are progressively shorter. The risks and costs of marrow/stem cell transplantation are easily justified for patients who have

TABLE 71-3 Common Chemotherapy Regimens for Acute Leukemia

AML
  Remission Induction
    Cytarabine and anthracycline* (7 days + 3 days)
    Cytarabine, Daunorubicin, and Etoposide (7+3+3 or ADE)
    High-dose cytarabine (HiDAC) and Daunorubicin
  Post-remission Consolidation
    High-dose cytarabine (HiDAC)
    Cytarabine and Daunorubicin
    Cytarabine and 6-thioguanine
    Stem-cell transplantation (autologous or allogeneic)
  Reinduction After Relapse
    High-dose cytarabine (HiDAC) and mitoxantrone
    Gemtuzumab ozogamicin (Mylotarg)
    Mitoxantrone and etoposide

APL
  Induction
    ATRA (all-trans retinoic acid) plus daunorubicin (or idarubicin) with or without cytarabine
  Consolidation
    ATRA plus daunorubicin
  Reinduction After Relapse
    Arsenic Trioxide[24]

ALL
  Induction
    Daunorubicin, vincristine, prednisone (or dexamethasone), +/− L-asparaginase +/− cyclophosphamide
  Consolidation
    High-dose cytarabine
    High-dose methotrexate
    CNS prophylaxis with intrathecal methotrexate
  Maintenance
    6-Mercaptopurine and methotrexate +/− vincristine and prednisone.

*Daunorubicin, idarubicin, or mitoxantrone have been used.

had a relapse of leukemia because otherwise disease-free survival is generally (but not always) short. Patients who are younger than 50 years of age and have a human leukocyte antigen (HLA)–identical sibling are good candidates for allogeneic transplantation. Many centers offer transplantation to selected patients up to 60 years of age. It may be possible to extend the upper age limit with the use of T-cell depletion from the donor marrow to diminish the incidence and severity of graft-versus-host disease (GVHD), as well as the introduction of less toxic "reduced intensity" stem cell transplant regimens. The use of marrow stem cells from a matched but unrelated donor is also feasible.

The success of chemotherapy for acute leukemia depends not only on the drug susceptibility of the individual patient's leukemia but also on the ability of that patient to survive the rigors of treatment. Significant advances have been made in the supportive care of patients undergoing intensive cytotoxic therapy. Prevention and early treatment of infection have been foremost. Prior to treatment, all patients should have a thorough dental evaluation and a computed tomographic (CT) scan of the sinuses to identify and eliminate potential sources for infections. Patients are placed in protective isolation in single rooms; in this way, these immunocompromised patients are protected from common infectious agents in the hospital environment. Laminar airflow rooms are not necessary for successful treatment, but patients generally are restricted from eating fresh fruits and vegetables to decrease their enteric bacterial flora. Strict attention to thorough handwashing by all medical and nursing personnel and visitors is necessary.

Infection/Sepsis

Patients with leukemia are severely immunocompromised by both their disease and their treatment. Because chemotherapy damages mucosal barriers, these patients are susceptible to infection by endogenous organisms. Most common are gram-negative enteric bacteria, gram-positive cocci, and fungi such as *Candida* and *Aspergillus* species. Patients with ALL also are susceptible to *Pneumocystis*, mycobacterial, and viral infections. Prophylactic use of oral antibiotics such as fluoroquinolones can decrease the incidence and severity of infections in leukopenic patients. Antiviral and/or antifungal prophylaxis is also employed commonly in patients with profound or prolonged leukopenia.

Standard practice dictates that broad-spectrum antibiotic therapy must be initiated promptly and empirically in a granulocytopenic patient at the time of the first fever greater than 38.5°C (101.5°F). The Infectious Disease Society of America recently published guidelines on the management of these patients.[8] Blood, urine, and sputum cultures should be obtained, but the source of infection is rarely identified in part because there is little inflammatory response in the tissues. The first priority must be to prevent septic shock. Ceftazidime or imipenem as a single agent or the combination of a semisynthetic penicillin plus an aminoglycoside is widely used, but the choice of regimen depends in part on renal function and history of allergies. High-risk patients also should be given vancomycin without delay because nosocomial gram positive organisms may be resistant to methicillin. Should initial cultures reveal a pathogen, antibiotic therapy should be adjusted for maximum bactericidal activity based on susceptibility testing in vitro.

Pulmonary infiltrates in febrile leukemia patients should be managed aggressively in an attempt to identify the etiology and treat the underlying cause (Table 71-4). In general, however, broad-spectrum treatment continues until the chemotherapy is completed and the granulocyte count recovers to near normal.

Patients with acute leukemia are characterized by bone marrow failure owing either to replacement by leukemia cells or to chemotherapy-induced hypoplasia. Red blood cell transfusions are given to maintain a hematocrit of approximately 30%. A higher hematocrit should be maintained in hypoalbuminemic patients to keep the blood volume expanded and tissues perfused. While the general practice in critically ill patients has been to restrict red blood cell transfusion until the hematocrit falls much lower than this threshold, we believe that leukemia patients are a unique population not well represented in trials of transfusion strategies. If red blood cell transfusion is, in fact, immunosuppressive, it is unlikely to have much additional impact in chemotherapy-immunosuppressed leukemic patients. Further, these patients may benefit from the additional margin of safety that a higher hematocrit provides in case of thrombocytopenia-related hemorrhage.

TABLE 71-4 Evaluation and Treatment of Pulmonary Infiltrates in Febrile Patients with Acute Leukemia

Chest radiographs—posteroanterior and lateral
Sputum specimens for Gram staining and for bacterial, fungal, and acid-fast bacillus (AFB) cultures and sensitivity testing
Broad-spectrum empirical antibiotic therapy with
   Ceftazidime (+/− vancomycin)
      or
   Imipenem (+/− vancomycin)
      or
   Ciprofloxacin + vancomycin
      or
   Piperacillin + aminoglycoside
Bronchoscopy with lavage and biopsy within the first 12–24 hours to evaluate new pulmonary infiltrates
CT-guided needle biopsy should be considered if bronchoscopy does not yield diagnostic material
After 72 hours of fever without a specific diagnosis, open lung biopsy should be considered

Bleeding is a common problem, and the risk rises as the platelet count decreases (see Chap. 69). Platelets should be transfused prophylactically to maintain a platelet count of greater than $10,000/\mu L$ to decrease the risk of spontaneous hemorrhage, such as a stroke or gastrointestinal bleeding. A higher platelet count is necessary to treat active bleeding. No salicylates or other drugs that interfere with platelet function should be given, nor should intramuscular injections be given to a thrombocytopenic patient. The use of single-donor platelets collected by apheresis will decrease the rate of alloimmunization in leukemia patients. Patients who become alloimmunized may benefit from HLA-matched platelets or antibody–cross-matched platelets to achieve adequate posttransfusion platelet counts. Blood bank techniques to remove leukocytes by filtration or centrifugation from red blood cell or platelet transfusion units may slow the rate of alloimmunization.

Granulocyte transfusions are rarely necessary for patients receiving chemotherapy for acute leukemia. The indications for their use generally are limited to severely granulocytopenic patients who remain febrile and bacteremic despite receiving antibiotics that have bactericidal activity against the particular organism in vitro. In this situation, the phagocytic activity of exogenous granulocytes can be lifesaving. One or two leukapheresis products are transfused daily for 4 to 7 days. Complications include respiratory distress from leukoagglutination, transmission of cytomegalovirus (CMV), and rapid alloimmunization. Pulmonary infiltrates may worsen as granulocytes migrate into infected lung tissues.

Over the past several years, the hematopoietic growth factors filgrastim (granulocyte colony-stimulating factor [G-CSF]) and sargramostim (granulocyte-macrophage colony-stimulating factor [GM-CSF]) have become available commercially in the United States. Pegfilgrastim (NEULASTA), a long-acting form of G-CSF also has become available recently for clinical use. They are now used routinely to support cancer patients with solid tumors or lymphoma who have received myelosuppressive chemotherapy. The American Society of Clinical Oncology has adopted guidelines for the use of colony-stimulating factors in clinical practice.[9] Colony-stimulating factors have been shown to reduce significantly the incidence of febrile neutropenia when used prophylactically in certain patients who receive intensive chemotherapy regimens. Specifically, it is recommended that patients who receive a chemotherapy program previously associated with a greater than 40% incidence of febrile neutropenia be treated prophylactically with colony-stimulating factors to reduce this risk. In addition, there is evidence that administration of colony-stimulating factors may reduce the risk of febrile neutropenia in subsequent cycles of chemotherapy for patients who had a documented occurrence in an earlier cycle. Most randomized, controlled trials have not demonstrated significant long-term clinical benefit (response rate or outcome) from using myeloid growth factors in patients with AML. However, modest benefits in decreased duration of neutropenia and hospitalization have been observed. For adults with ALL, clinical trials have demonstrated statistically significant shortening of the duration of neutropenia following remission-induction chemotherapy when G-CSF was used. The clinical benefit was greater in older patients.

The current data do not support the routine use of colony-stimulating factors as adjuncts to antibiotic therapy in febrile neutropenic patients. Nevertheless, their use along with antibiotics may be reasonable in high-risk patients. Specifically, neutropenic patients with clinical features that predict a poor outcome, such as pneumonia, documented fungal infection, or sepsis syndrome, are reasonable candidates for therapy with colony-stimulating factors.[9]

Soft Silastic right-atrial catheters (e.g., double- or triple-lumen Hickman or Groshong catheters) that tunnel under the skin and enter the innominate vein are used widely. They allow direct access to a large vein for infusion of chemotherapy agents, antibiotics, and blood transfusions and also allow painless blood sampling for laboratory monitoring. Parenteral hyperalimentation can be administered easily through these catheters, if necessary. Although a boon to both patient and physician, such chronic indwelling lines are not without hazard. They must be placed in a sterile fashion by a skilled surgeon or invasive radiologist, especially in a thrombocytopenic patient. A vigorous skin preparation preoperatively reduces the likelihood of a staphylococcal or corynebacterial subcutaneous tunnel infection or bacteremia. Although most gram-negative bacteremias can be treated successfully in a granulocytopenic patient by antibiotics alone without removing the catheter, gram-positive infections or candidal infections of the tunnel or vein may require catheter removal.

Hyperleukocytosis

A small proportion of patients with leukemia have an extraordinary elevation of circulating leukocytes. Hyperleukocytosis (>100,000 blast cells per microliter) is a true medical emergency, but the risks of circulatory complications begin to rise at counts above about 50,000/μL (Table 71-5). These patients present special problems because of the rheologic effects of leukemia blast cells in the circulation of the lung, brain, and other organs; the metabolic consequences when massive numbers of leukemia cells are destroyed simultaneously by cytotoxic drugs; and perhaps other mechanisms.[10] Although in some cases the blood viscosity is markedly increased because of the elevated leukocrit, in most cases the whole blood viscosity will not be increased above normal because hyperleukocytosis is associated most frequently with severe anemia.[11] However, red blood cell transfusions can precipitate a hyperviscosity syndrome in a patient with hyperleukocytosis and should be delayed, if possible, until the white blood cell count falls. Nevertheless, viscosity may be high in the microcirculation. The high oxygen consumption and invasiveness of leukemia cells may interact with slow flow through the capillaries to lead to hypoxemia and vascular damage.

The contribution of blood cells to the viscosity of blood is a function of the deformability of individual cells and their fractional volume. Immature leukocytes are much larger and

---

TABLE 71-5 Diagnosis and Management of Leukostasis Syndrome

Leukostasis begins to occur when the peripheral blast count rises above 50,000/μL.

Blast counts greater than 100,000/μL should be treated as a medical emergency.

The signs and symptoms of leukostasis are due to increased blood viscosity and are manifestations of decreased small vessel perfusion of end organs: mental status alterations (CNS), respiratory failure (pulmonary capillaries), renal failure (renal glomeruli), and cardiac arrhythmias (cardiac microvasculature).

Cerebral perfusion should be assessed by examination of the retinal vessels and mental status; renal perfusion should be assessed by careful measurement of urine output; perfusion of the heart and lungs should be assessed by cardiopulmonary monitoring (pulse oximetry).

Hydration should be maintained vigorously with saline infusion to decrease viscosity.

Since the viscosity of blood is a function of both the leukocrit and the hematocrit, red blood cell transfusions should be withheld until the WBC count has been reduced (unless the patient is severely anemic).

If specific chemotherapy will not be started immediately, then oral hydroxyurea should be given in a dose of 2 g every 6 hours.

A temporary large-bore catheter should be placed and leukapheresis begun as soon as possible; leukapheresis should be continued daily until the WBC count is below 100,000/μL.

Specific chemotherapy should be begun as soon as the patient is stable.

For mental status changes due to leukostasis, cranial irradiation with a single dose of 400 cGy should be considered.

Respiratory compromise with hypoxemia due to leukostasis (not infection) can be treated with 400 cGy of thoracic irradiation and supplemental oxygen.

less deformable than erythrocytes. Leukemic myeloblasts are considerably larger than lymphoblasts, which are, in turn, larger than leukemic lymphocytes. Thus the incidence of significant leukostasis is highest in CML in the blast phase, followed by AML and then ALL. In contrast, leukostasis is rare in patients with chronic lymphocytic leukemia (CLL) despite white blood cell counts as high as 500,000/μL. Similarly, well-hydrated patients with CML in the chronic phase can tolerate total white blood cell counts of 200,000/μL without difficulty because only a small fraction of the cells are blasts or promyelocytes, and most are mature granulocytes.

Leukostasis and hypoxia in the capillary beds can induce respiratory distress, cardiac arrhythmias, and central nervous system (CNS) symptoms leading to coma. Death follows rapidly unless the circulation can be restored. Emergency measures include leukapheresis to remove a large mass of tumor cells directly from the bloodstream.[10] A single efficient leukapheresis can decrease the leukocyte count by approximately 50% within 2 to 3 hours. A centrifuge technique rather than a filtration method should be used because blast cells do not adhere to glass-wool filters. Prompt use of antimetabolite drugs such as oral hydroxyurea or intravenous cytarabine can reduce cell proliferation rapidly and decrease the blast count transiently. A single dose of cranial irradiation (200 to 400 cGy) can ameliorate CNS symptoms due to leukostasis. Diffuse pulmonary infiltrates and respiratory distress also may respond to thoracic irradiation. Once the circulation through the capillaries has been restored, systemic chemotherapy should be initiated promptly. Prophylactic platelet transfusions must be given to prevent bleeding as the circulation is restored to hypoxic tissues. The invasiveness of leukemic myeloblasts may lead to injury and disruption of vascular endothelium. Lysis of these cells in situ releases proteolytic enzymes, causing further tissue damage and bleeding.

Tachypnea and pulmonary infiltrates in a patient with hyperleukocytosis can mimic pulmonary embolism or infection. Care must be taken to rule out "pseudohypoxemia," which results from the in vitro consumption of oxygen within an arterial blood-gas sample by blast cells in transit to the laboratory.[12] Such blood specimens should be transported rapidly on ice. Rarely, marked thrombocytosis can produce a similar artifact in addition to pseudohyperkalemia.

Myeloid Sarcoma

Leukemia is, from its genesis in the marrow, spleen, or thymus, a systemic disease. Malignant cells circulate through the bloodstream and lymphatics and can infiltrate the parenchyma of any tissue. ALL cells migrate preferentially to lymphoid organs such as lymph nodes, spleen, and liver, causing organomegaly. When malignant myeloblasts form a solid tumor, a granulocytic or myeloid sarcoma results. The older term *chloroma* ("green cancer") describes the greenish color that results from the myeloperoxidase reaction when a myeloid sarcoma is exposed to air. Myeloid sarcomas occur most often in patients with CML in blast phase or with myelomonocytic or monoblastic leukemia, and most commonly they involve bone and subperiosteum, lymph nodes, skin, soft tissues, and the gastrointestinal tract.[13] They most frequently cause pain but also may cause neuropathy or intestinal obstruction from their mass effect. They are quite responsive to local irradiation (1000 to 2000 cGy), but since they are a localized manifestation of a disseminated disease, systemic chemotherapy also must be used. Local therapy often is not necessary because myeloid sarcomas often shrink and disappear within a few days after chemotherapy begins.

CNS Leukemia

CNS infiltration by leukemia cells is more common in ALL than AML and is more common in children than in adults. Among patients with myeloid leukemia, the incidence of CNS involvement is greatest in children and in those with monoblastic leukemias or high circulating blast counts. Among the lymphoblastic leukemias, the risk is greatest in patients with the T-cell or mature B-cell (Burkitt) immunophenotypes.[14] When the vascular leptomeninges surrounding the brain and spinal cord are infiltrated by malignant cells, leukemia cells often (but not always) can be found in the cerebrospinal fluid (CSF) by lumbar puncture. Cranial neuropathy and spinal radiculopathy result from the impingement of an expanding mass of leukemia cells on these nerves where they traverse narrow bony foramina. In contrast, a few malignant cells in the CSF at diagnosis probably are not significant because they often disappear during the initial induction chemotherapy treatment without specific attention to the CNS.

The most frequent symptoms in patients with overt CNS leukemia are those caused by increased intracranial pressure: vomiting, headache, papilledema, and lethargy. Diplopia results from oculomotor nerve palsy, especially of the abducens nerve. Facial nerve palsies are also common. Spinal radiculopathy and the cauda equina syndrome occur more commonly in adults than in children. Mass lesions in the brain substance itself or in the spinal cord are not common, and seizures are rarely present. Meningismus is also uncommon, and its presence suggests infection or subarachnoid hemorrhage.

The diagnosis is established by finding leukemia cells in the CSF. Usually, the CSF pressure is elevated in symptomatic patients, the glucose concentration is low, and the protein concentration is moderately elevated. CT scan or magnetic resonance imaging (MRI) may demonstrate thickening or contrast enhancement of the membranes around the base of the brain or the spinal nerves. Because spinal subarachnoid hemorrhage or focal hematomas can follow lumbar puncture in thrombocytopenic patients, platelets should be transfused to counts of greater than 20,000/μL and any coagulopathy corrected before a careful lumbar puncture is done.

CNS leukemia is usually rapidly responsive to irradiation or intrathecal chemotherapy. Standard treatment for symptoms is 2400 cGy to the whole brain in 12 fractions. The posterior orbits and upper cervical spine should be included. The spinal column is rarely irradiated except in patients with symptomatic radiculopathy because of the resulting damage to the underlying bone marrow. Dexamethasone 4 mg four times per day can alleviate symptoms of increased intracranial pressure. The spinal cord is best treated with preservative-free methotrexate (12 mg/m^2 to a maximum dose of 15 mg) injected intrathecally every 3 days for at least six doses. Once the CSF is clear of malignant cells, intrathecal therapy should be administered once a month for the following year. Methotrexate can cause an inflammatory arachnoiditis with fever and nuchal rigidity. For this reason, hydrocortisone (50 mg) often is coadministered with the methotrexate. Alternative drugs for intrathecal use are cytarabine (DEPOCYTE, 50 mg), or less commonly, thio-TEPA. Slow diffusion of methotrexate out of the CSF into the systemic circulation can cause myelosuppression and gastrointestinal toxicity. This problem can be lessened by giving 5 mg leucovorin 36 hours after each dose. Leucovorin decreases methotrexate's toxic effects on normal tissues by replenishing the supply of reduced folate to cells. Too much leucovorin can interfere with subsequent doses of methotrexate. Administration of intrathecal chemotherapy via lumbar puncture has the disadvantage of not treating the ventricles at all and treating the top surface of the brain only poorly. For this reason, an Ommaya reservoir often is placed in symptomatic patients who require chronic CNS therapy to allow an intraventricular (and easier) route of administration.

Clinical trials have suggested that the CNS is a sanctuary site for leukemia cells and is poorly treated by many intravenously administered drugs. Patients can have an isolated CNS relapse even while they are in an apparent bone marrow remission. To diminish this risk in patients with ALL, all patients with lymphoblastic leukemia generally receive some prophylactic treatment of the CNS as part of their initial treatment program. Alternatives include high doses of cytarabine or methotrexate, two drugs that cross the blood-brain barrier and reach cytotoxic concentrations in the CSF even when administered intravenously. CNS prophylaxis is not commonly employed for AML.

Although uncommon, various paraneoplastic syndromes occur in patients with leukemia, such as Guillain-Barré polyneuritis and progressive multifocal leukoencephalopathy. It is not known to what extent the leukemia itself or its treatment with chemotherapy or irradiation is responsible for these disorders. High doses of cytarabine (2000 mg/m^2 for 6 to 12 doses) can cause irreversible cerebellar ataxia, especially in elderly patients and those with renal failure.

Enlargement of the Liver and Spleen

Marked leukemic infiltration of the liver and spleen is infrequent in AML and occurs principally in patients with ALL or CML in the blast phase. Signs and symptoms may mimic those of an acute hepatitis, with jaundice, tender hepatomegaly, and elevated serum transaminase levels. This problem usually resolves with effective chemotherapy, but the choice of initial chemotherapy may be restricted because many useful drugs are cleared through the liver. A biliary ultrasound examination should be performed to rule out bile duct obstruction. The spleen is rarely massively enlarged, although it may be palpable at diagnosis owing to leukemic infiltration. Vascular infarction can occur, causing painful subcapsular hematomas. A rub with respiratory variation sometimes will be heard over the left upper quadrant. Rarely, such an infarcted spleen ruptures, causing shock and signs of intraperitoneal hemorrhage. This is a surgical emergency. Splenic rupture also can occur during chemotherapy as the tumor cell mass is receding, but this event is extremely rare.

Infiltration of the Kidney

Infiltration of the kidneys is more common in ALL and monoblastic leukemias than in other types of AML. These patients present with oliguric acute renal failure. Renal ultrasound examination demonstrates homogeneous enlargement of both kidneys but no ureteral obstruction. Alternatively, enlarged retroperitoneal lymph nodes secondary to infiltration by leukemia cells can cause ureteral obstruction and renal failure without intrinsic renal disease. These signs resolve during the course of effective chemotherapy, but the inability to excrete the breakdown products of tumor cell lysis can precipitate hyperkalemia and hyperuricemia with their resulting metabolic complications (see below). One or two doses of radiation therapy (200 to 400 cGy) to include just the kidneys if they are enlarged (or the ureters as necessary) can re-establish renal excretory function prior to the use of systemic chemotherapy and thus alleviate the risk of tumor lysis syndrome.

Necrotizing Enterocolitis (Typhlitis)

Typhlitis is a necrotizing enterocolitis particularly of the terminal ileum, appendix, cecum, and right colon that occurs in granulocytopenic patients.[15] Although seen most often in young patients who have recently received intensive chemotherapy, typhlitis can occur in any granulocytopenic patient, such as those with aplastic anemia or acute leukemia not yet treated. Symptoms and signs are similar to those of inflammatory bowel disease: nausea, vomiting, abdominal pain and tenderness, profuse watery or bloody diarrhea, and fever. The intestinal mucosa is ulcerated, allowing enteric organisms to invade into and through the bowel wall. Ileus and bowel dilation result. Plasma proteins and electrolytes are lost into the bowel lumen, as occurs with toxic megacolon. Bowel perforation and peritonitis may follow. Jaundice and hepatitis are common, probably because of bacterial seeding through the portal vein.

Most patients are best managed with aggressive medical treatment: broad-spectrum antibiotics; transfusion of red blood cells, platelets, and fresh frozen plasma; maintenance of normal serum electrolyte levels (especially of potassium); and bowel rest with nasogastric suction. Narcotic analgesics and bowel paralytic agents such as LOMOTIL (diphenoxylate hydrochloride and atropine sulfate) should be avoided because they increase the risk of ileus. Granulocyte transfusions in this setting can prove lifesaving in severely neutropenic patients. With appropriate treatment of the transmural gastrointestinal infection and the recovery of granulocytes, this problem usually resolves without sequelae. Patients with clear evidence of bowel perforation require surgery with ileal diversion or bowel resection. Peritoneal lavage can establish the correct diagnosis if blood or feculent material is recovered. Although the perioperative mortality is high in such cases, the likelihood of a granulocytopenic patient surviving a disseminated peritonitis without surgery is small. Radiographic evidence of air within the bowel wall (*pneumatosis intestinalis*) does not in itself necessitate surgery, nor should a granulocytopenic patient who is otherwise doing well necessarily undergo laparotomy for intraperitoneal free air. Antibiotic-associated pseudomembranous colitis (*Clostridium difficile*), radiation enteritis, and graft-versus-host disease (GVHD) are other causes of abdominal pain and bloody diarrhea in leukemia and stem cell transplant patients.

Hyperuricemia and Tumor Lysis Syndrome

Uric acid is the product of nucleic acid catabolism, and its level is increased in diseases in which cell turnover rates are high. Uric acid is excreted largely by the kidneys through both glomerular filtration and tubular excretion. Uric acid nephropathy in leukemia may be present at diagnosis, or it may occur as a complication of therapy. Hyperuricemia may be exacerbated and uricosuria increased as a result of successful cytolytic therapy, as well as by drugs such as thiazide diuretics, probenecid, and aspirin. Hyperphosphatemia due to tumor cell lysis can cause deposition of calcium phosphate precipitates in the calyces and tubules. In acid urine, uric acid quickly supersaturates and precipitates. Uric acid has a dissociation constant of 5.4. At pH 7.0 and above, over 99% of urates are in the ionized form and thus are water-soluble. At pH 4.5, on the other hand, 80% of urate is in the form of poorly soluble uric acid, and the combined solubility of uric acid and urate falls below 8 mg/dL. In leukemia patients, therefore, the production of organic acids, together with the decreased urine formation that results from dehydration owing to anorexia or fever, frequently leads to precipitation of urates in the renal tubules and collecting system. Direct infiltration of leukemia cells into the kidneys also appears to enhance the local accumulation of uric acid. Leukemia patients with prior renal disease are more likely to develop uric acid nephropathy. Intratubular precipitation of urates leading to obstruction of urine flow is the more critical cause of nephropathy rather than renal cell injury per se.

Effective management of hyperuricemia and hyperuricosuria in leukemia patients is based on reducing the production of uric acid and at the same time promoting the solubility of uric acid in the urine. An adequate urine flow (100 mL/h) should be established by oral and intravenous hydration. The blood volume must be expanded and acidosis corrected. Acetazolamide, a carbonic anhydrase inhibitor, can be given together with sodium bicarbonate to alkalinize the urine. The optimal urine pH is 7.0 to 7.5. Allopurinol (300 mg/d) will effectively inhibit the conversion of xanthine and hypoxanthine to uric acid. Allopurinol treatment with alkalinization of the urine markedly decreases the risk of uric acid nephropathy in nearly all cases of leukemia. Rasburicase (ELITEK) (0.20 mg/kg) is a recombinant human urate oxidase that, when administered intravenously, can rapidly metabolize serum uric acid. It may be used daily for 1 to 5 days when rapid decreases in serum uric acid are needed or when a large tumor cell lysis is predicted.[16] Allopurinol should not be used in combination with rasburicase but can be restarted after the hyperuricemia resolves. Rasburicase is not recommended for patients with glucose-6-phosphate dehydrogenase (G6PD) deficiency. Once the tumor cell mass has been reduced, these measures can be discontinued safely. Allopurinol causes an allergic dermatitis in approximately 10% of patients, but this side effect usually occurs only after more than a week of treatment, allowing time for leukemia cytoreduction. Fever and the Stevens-Johnson syndrome may follow the systemic rash if allopurinol is continued.

Lysozymuria and Renal Tubular Dysfunction

Lysozyme is a small protein (molecular weight = 14,000) with an unusually high isoelectric point (pH = 11) that has a remarkable capacity to lyse the cell walls of certain bacteria. Lysozyme (also known as muramidase) is present in high concentrations in granulocytes and monocytes as well as tissue macrophages. Patients with monocytic and myelomonocytic leukemia excrete large quantities of lysozyme in the urine.[17] Lysozyme is toxic to renal tubule cells and causes tubular dysfunction. Marked hypokalemia generally has accompanied lysozymuria in patients with monoblastic and myelomonocytic leukemias. These problems resolve with effective treatment of the leukemia.

Disseminated Intravascular Coagulation

Laboratory evidence of disseminated intravascular coagulation (DIC) is almost always present at diagnosis in patients with acute promyelocytic leukemia (APL), but it can accompany any leukemia or infection where there is rapid cell lysis or tissue destruction. The pathophysiology is still controversial, but the coagulation cascade appears to be initiated by the release of intracellular thromboplastic material.[18] The syndrome is characterized by the consumption of plasma coagulation proteins and platelets, resulting in prolongation of the prothrombin time (PT), thrombin time (TT), and partial thromboplastin time (PTT), together with a decrease in fibrinogen levels and an elevation in the levels of fibrin degradation products (FDPs) and D-dimer. Oozing from venipuncture sites is common. Fibrin thrombi usually are present in the renal glomeruli, leading to moderate renal insufficiency. Aminoglycoside antibiotics should be avoided because patients with DIC are unexpectedly susceptible to renal failure despite blood level monitoring. Trauma to circulating red blood cells from fibrin strands creates schistocytes, which are apparent on the blood smear. Deep vein thrombosis and pulmonary embolism may occur. The DIC in patients with leukemia is most intense shortly after chemotherapy begins, when the destruction of leukemia cells results in the release of procoagulant-rich granules. The DIC wanes as the tumor burden declines. However, a state of low-grade DIC may persist in the setting of ongoing tumor lysis, bacteremia, or sepsis.

Management of DIC is always directed at correcting the underlying tissue destruction, whether due to leukemia, infection, a burn or crush injury, or an obstetric complication. In the meantime, the consumption of coagulation proteins through fibrin formation and its associated secondary fibrinolysis can be brought under control by administration of exogenous cryoprecipitate, platelets, and fresh frozen plasma, as well as by the use of heparin. A continuous intravenous infusion of heparin at 5 units/kg per hour is well tolerated even in thrombocytopenic patients and allows fresh frozen plasma or cryoprecipitate to be transfused safely without concern about adding substrate for renewed intravascular coagulation. Nonetheless, there are no randomized clinical trials demonstrating benefit from the use of heparin products in DIC. Subcutaneous and/or low-dose intravenous heparin should be used with great care in patients with DIC and particularly in actively bleeding patients. Cryoprecipitate infusions should be used to maintain the fibrinogen concentration at greater than 100 mg/dL. Several doses of vitamin K (10 mg/d) should be given. If the liver is functioning normally, the vitamin K–dependent factors II, VII, IX, and X, as well as antithrombin, will be repleted rapidly, thereby avoiding the need for transfusion of large volumes of fresh frozen plasma. If after 24 hours of heparin therapy the fibrinogen level has not stabilized and the FDP levels have not decreased, the heparin infusion should be increased to 10 U/kg per hour; a higher dose of heparin is rarely necessary. Lack of response to heparin may indicate a deficiency of the heparin cofactor antithrombin, which can be repleted by transfusion of fresh frozen plasma. The optimal approach to DIC in leukemia remains to be determined. It is usually possible to manage the coagulopathy associated with APL with all-*trans*-retinoic acid, intensive chemotherapy, and blood product support without the routine use of heparin.[19,20]

All-trans-Retinoic Acid and the Retinoic Acid Syndrome

All-*trans*-retinoic acid (tretinoin, ATRA) has emerged as a remarkably effective agent for inducing complete remissions in patients with acute promyelocytic leukemia (AML-M3 or APL).[21] Patients with this form of AML have a characteristic chromosomal translocation, t(15;17). The juxtaposition of the retinoic acid receptor-α (*RAR-α*) gene on chromosome 17 and the *PML* gene on chromosome 15 results in the expression of fusion gene products in the leukemia cells. The leukemic blasts undergo terminal differentiation in response to ATRA, and complete responses are achieved in the majority of patients. The best results are achieved when patients also receive cytotoxic chemotherapy concomitantly with ATRA. The success of ATRA has led to its incorporation into remission-induction regimens for all patients with APL.

ATRA has several advantages over standard induction chemotherapy: (1) Patients usually do not have an exacerbation of DIC with ATRA treatment, as can happen with chemotherapy. In fact, resolution of DIC often occurs within 24 to 48 hours. (2) Patients treated with ATRA alone do not suffer bone marrow aplasia and prolonged neutropenia, as do patients treated with chemotherapy. (3) The systemic side effects are generally less severe with ATRA than with chemotherapy.

However, ATRA does have its own unique toxicities, which must be anticipated to maximize the safety of this novel agent (Table 71-6). The two most significant toxicities of ATRA are hyperleukocytosis and the retinoic acid syndrome.[22] In contrast to patients receiving chemotherapy who undergo a rapid cytoreductive phase accompanied by increased DIC and tumor lysis syndrome, APL patients receiving ATRA sometimes exhibit a progressive leukocytosis, which may become marked. The leukocytosis occurs because ATRA causes differentiation of the leukemic blasts in the bone marrow, resulting in the accumulation of maturing forms in the peripheral blood. This is less likely to occur if early institution of concurrent cytotoxic chemotherapy (usually daunorubicin or idaru-

TABLE 71-6 Toxicities of All-*trans*-Retinoic Acid Therapy

Retinoic acid syndrome
Leukocytosis
Intracranial hypertension ("pseudotumor cerebri")
Headache
Hypertriglyceridemia
Hepatic toxicity
Congestive heart failure
Dry skin and mucous membranes; cheilosis

bicin) at full doses or hydroxyurea is used. Leukapheresis has also been used to reduce the white blood cell count in these patients.

The retinoic acid syndrome occurs in approximately 25% of patients receiving ATRA and is characterized by fever, rapidly progressive respiratory distress with diffuse pulmonary infiltrates on chest radiograph, pleural effusions, and weight gain (Table 71-7). If the syndrome is unrecognized and left untreated, progressive hypoxemia, multiorgan failure, and death frequently occur. The syndrome may occur as early as 2 days after the initiation of treatment or as late as 3 or 4 weeks. The syndrome may be more common in patients with ATRA-induced leukocytosis, but it also occurs in patients with white blood cell counts of less than 10,000/μL. Clinically, the syndrome is similar to "capillary leak" syndromes associated with certain cytokines, such as interleukin 2. This fact has led to the hypothesis that the retinoic acid syndrome may itself be cytokine-mediated. Similar symptoms may occur in chemotherapy-treated APL patients, implicating the malignant cells and not the treatment as the primary problem. Early recognition of the syndrome and prompt treatment with steroids (e.g., dexamethasone 10 mg bid for 3 days) effectively reverse the syndrome in most patients. The syndrome may be confused with an infectious complication. Thus it is important to recognize the retinoic acid syndrome promptly so that patients are not treated solely for infection, which could delay the start of corticosteroid treatment.

Another potential complication of ATRA is intracranial hypertension, or "pseudotumor cerebri." This complication is

TABLE 71-7 Clinical Features and Management of the Retinoic Acid Syndrome

The constellation of fever, respiratory distress, pulmonary infiltrates on chest radiograph, pleural effusion, and weight gain make up the retinoic acid syndrome, which occurs in 25% of APL patients treated with ATRA.

Immediate therapy should be instituted with dexamethasone, 10 mg I.V. every 12 hours for 3 days.

If there is a question of infection versus retinoic acid syndrome, then dexamethasone should be instituted together with broad-spectrum antibiotics. It is important not to delay dexamethasone treatment while the patient's response to antibiotics is assessed.

Efforts to control leukocytosis (in response to ATRA) may improve the retinoic acid syndrome.

Supportive care for pulmonary and other affected organ systems should be given until the syndrome improves.

The syndrome may recur at any point during therapy with ATRA and can be re-treated successfully with dexamethasone.

more frequent in pediatric patients receiving ATRA. Such cases of pseudotumor have been treated with lumbar puncture, corticosteroids, and narcotic analgesia.

Lactic Acidosis

Marked elevations of blood lactate or pyruvate concentrations in patients with leukemia result from an increase in the rate of lactic acid production or a decrease in the rate of pyruvic acid use or both. Whether clinical acidosis results depends in part on other metabolic and respiratory factors that influence acid-base balance. Blood lactate elevations occur more commonly in patients with acute leukemia than in those with any other neoplastic disorder.[23] Lactic acidosis also may be secondary to inadequate oxygenation of the tissues due to hyperleukocytosis, septic shock, pulmonary edema, or severe anemia. The development of lactic acidosis despite an apparently adequate supply of oxygen to the tissues sometimes reflects disseminated fungal infection with small-vessel occlusion or extensive liver necrosis. Lactic acidosis associated with massive leukemia is seen most commonly in patients with ALL and especially mature B-cell or Burkitt ALL. Experiments in vitro suggest that although malignant leukocytes exhibit little lactic acid production under aerobic conditions, they can have considerable anaerobic lactic acid production. It has been estimated that a rapidly growing mass of leukemia cells crowded into organs where the cells may be poorly oxygenated and therefore are dependent on anaerobic glycolysis for energy could produce as much as 300 to 600 mM lactic acid per hour. Any interference with hepatic blood supply or hepatic metabolism can diminish the body's ability to handle this acid load, resulting in clinical acidosis.

The successful treatment of lactic acidosis in patients with acute leukemia depends on the institution of effective antileukemia therapy. Removal of lactic acid by hemodialysis or peritoneal dialysis also may be useful.

References

1. Bennett JM, Catovsky D, Daniel MT, et al: Proposed revised criteria for the classification of acute myeloid leukemia: A report of the French-American-British Cooperative Group. *Ann Intern Med* 103:626, 1985.
2. Jaffe ES, Harris NL, Stein H, Vardiman JW (eds): *World Health Organization Classification of Tumours: Pathology and Genetics of Tumours of Hematopoietic and Lymphoid Tissues.* Lyon, France, IARC Press, 2001.
3. Le Beau MM, Larson RA: Cytogenetics and neoplasia, in Hoffman R, Benz EJ Jr, Shattil SJ, et al (eds): *Hematology: Basic Principles and Practice,* 2d ed. New York, Churchill Livingstone, 1995, p 878.
4. Byrd JC, Mrozek K, Dodge RK, et al: Cancer and Leukemia Group B (CALGB 8461): Pretreatment cytogenetic abnormalities are predictive of induction success, cumulative incidence of relapse, and overall survival in adult patients with de novo acute myeloid leukemia: Results from Cancer and Leukemia Group B (CALGB 8461). *Blood* 100:4325, 2002.
5. Larson RA: Acute leukemia, in Dale DC, Federman DD (eds): *ACP Medicine.* New York, Healtheon/WebMD, 2003, section XVI.
6. Eisenbeis CF, Larson RA: Chemotherapy of acute leukemia in adults, in Perry MC (ed): *The Chemotherapy Source Book,* 3d ed. Baltimore, Lippincott Williams & Wilkins, 2001, p 824.
7. Laport G, Larson RA: Acute lymphoblastic leukemia in adults. *Semin Oncol* 24:70, 1997.
8. Hughes WT, Armstrong D, et al: 2002 Guidelines for the use of anti-microbial agents in neutropenic patients with cancer. *Clin Infect Diseases* 34:730, 2002.
9. Ozer H, Armitage JO, et al: 2000 Update of recommendations for the use of hematopoietic colony-stimulating factors: Evidence-based, clinical practice guidelines. *J Clin Oncol* 18:3558, 2000.
10. Porcu P, Farag S, Marcucci G, et al: Leukocytoreduction in acute leukemia. *Ther Apheres* 6:15, 2002.
11. Lichtman MA, Rowe JM: Hyperleukocytic leukemias: Rheological, clinical, and therapeutic considerations. *Blood* 60:279, 1982.
12. Hess CE, Nichols AB, Hunt WB, et al: Pseudohypoxemia secondary to leukemia and thrombocytosis. *N Engl J Med* 301:361, 1979.
13. Byrd JC, Weiss RB, Arthur DC, et al: Extramedullary leukemia adversely affects hematologic complete remission rate and overall survival in patients with t(8;21) (q22;q22): Results from Cancer and Leukemia Group B 8461. *J Clin Oncol* 15:466, 1997.
14. Surapaneni UR, Cortes JE, Thomas D, et al: Central nervous system relapse in adults with acute lymphoblastic leukemia. *Cancer* 94:773, 2002.
15. Urbach DR, Rotstein OD: Typhlitis. *Can J Surgery* 42:415, 1999.
16. Navolanic PM, Pui CH, Larson RA, et al: Elitek-rasburicase: An effective means to prevent hyperuricemia associated with tumor lysis syndrome, a Meeting Report, Dallas, Texas, January 2002. *Leukemia* 17:499, 2003.
17. Muggia FM, Heinemann HO, Farhangi M, et al: Lysozymuria and renal tubular dysfunction in monocytic and myelomoncytic leukemia. *Am J Med* 47:351, 1969.
18. Menell JS, Cesarman GM, Jacovina AT, et al: Annexin II and bleeding in acute promyelocytic leukemia. *N Engl J Med* 340:994, 1999.
19. Goldberg MA, Ginsburg D, Mayer RJ, et al: Is heparin administration necessary during induction chemotherapy for patients with acute promyelocytic leukemia? *Blood* 69:187, 1987.
20. Hardaway RM, Williams CH, Vasquez Y: Disseminated intravascular coagulation in sepsis. *Semin Thromb Hemost* 27:577, 2001.
21. Lo Coco F, Diverio D, Falini B, et al: Genetic diagnosis and molecular monitoring in the management of acute promyelocytic leukemia. *Blood* 94:12, 1999.
22. Tallman, MS: Retinoic acid syndrome: A problem of the past. *Leukemia* 16:160, 2002.
23. Field M, Block JB, Levin R, et al: Significance of blood lactate elevations among patients with acute leukemias and other neoplastic proliferative disorders. *Am J Med* 40:528, 1966.
24. Soignet SL, Frankel SR, et al: United States multicenter study of arsenic trioxide in relapsed acute promyelocytic leukemia. *J Clin Oncol* 19:3852, 2001.

Chapter 72

ONCOLOGIC EMERGENCIES

ELIZABETH B. LAMONT
PHILIP C. HOFFMAN

KEY POINTS

- *Patients with malignancy are subject to life-threatening complications of the primary disease, its treatment, or coexisting medical diseases.*
- *Oncologic emergencies should be treated when they are associated with higher acute morbidity and mortality than the underlying malignancy.*
- *In patients who are terminally ill from their malignancy, restraint should be exercised in the diagnosis and management of oncologic complications.*
- *A high index of suspicion must be maintained for oncologic complications to be recognized because they often share features with other common medical illnesses.*
- *Frequent examination of critically ill patients is necessary because such patients (often intubated, bed-bound, hypotensive) are often unable to verbalize changes in their condition.*

This chapter details the epidemiology, pathophysiology, clinical presentation, diagnostic approaches, and treatment modalities of the most common oncologic emergencies. Because of the systemic nature of cancer, these emergencies often affect organ systems remote from the original cancer, making diagnosis challenging. To recognize these disorders, it is important to develop a differential diagnosis for common signs and symptoms that occur in critically ill patients (Table 72-1). Given the long natural history of many advanced cancers, the successful diagnosis and management of these emergencies may be rewarded with prolonged survival. However, when cancer patients become end stage, the same invasive diagnostic procedures and aggressive treatments may be onerous. Decisions regarding management of these patients may be best made through discussions among the patient, the primary oncologist, the family, and the treating physician.

Thoracic Syndromes

SUPERIOR VENA CAVA SYNDROME

Superior vena cava (SVC) syndrome is the clinical manifestation of SVC obstruction and occurs through external compression, thrombosis, or invasion of the vein. While previously in the realm of nonneoplastic entities such as syphilitic aortitis or histoplasmosis, SVC syndrome is now almost exclusively (>90%) secondary to malignancy.[1] The syndrome complicates 2% to 8% of primary thoracic malignancies, most frequently small cell carcinoma of the lung, followed by other lung cancer histologies, non-Hodgkin's lymphoma, and mediastinal germ cell tumors.[2–5] Studies estimate the risk of clinically evident subclavian vein thrombosis to be approximately 5%[6,7]

in cancer patients with indwelling central venous catheters, and some small percentage of these apparently evolve to SVC syndrome.[8–10]

To understand the clinical manifestations of the syndrome, an appreciation of the regional anatomy is necessary (Fig. 72-1). Because the venous drainage from the upper extremities, upper thorax, and head is obstructed, SVC syndrome presents with symptoms related to engorgement of these areas. Both the degree of SVC compromise and the extent of collateral veins determine the varied clinical presentation, which can be as mild as slight facial and upper extremity edema or as dire as intracranial swelling, seizures, hemodynamic instability, and tracheal obstruction. Table 72-2 lists the frequency of symptoms in 66 patients admitted with SVC obstruction.[1] Because of the lore of the dire symptomatologies, physicians often react to suspected SVC syndrome with panicked urgency and are tempted to initiate treatment before a pathologic diagnosis can be made. However, some argue convincingly that the SVC syndrome is rarely so urgent as to preclude timely and methodical radiologic and pathologic evaluations prior to therapy.[11]

When a patient presents with suspected SVC syndrome, the first step is to obtain an imaging study to both confirm the diagnosis and assist in treatment decisions. Of the several imaging modalities available for diagnosing the syndrome, the best study is the one that can be obtained most expediently. Magnetic resonance imaging (MRI), contrast-enhanced computed tomographic (CT) scanning, radionuclide flow study, and traditional venography are all adequate modalities, but at most centers CT scan is the most readily available. CT scan and MRI also provide information regarding possible etiologies and thus can direct the approach to a tissue diagnosis. The approach to establishing a tissue diagnosis is defined by both the patient's clinical stability and the findings on examination and radiographic studies. Table 72-3 summarizes the diagnostic yields for several tests ranging from noninvasive approaches such as sputum cytology to the maximally invasive thoracotomy. Tissue diagnoses are important because they guide treatment; specifically, they identify patients for whom SVC syndrome should be treated with combination chemotherapy rather than with local measures such as radiation therapy or percutaneous vascular procedures. Patients with known thoracic malignancies clearly do not require a further tissue diagnosis.

Treatment of SVC syndrome is divided into supportive and definitive therapy. Acutely, patients should be supported with elevation of the head of their bed and supplemental oxygen. Although dexamethasone is sometimes used, its utility has never been supported by experimental data. The definitive treatment of SVC syndrome depends on the etiology. Studies of small cell lung cancer patients with SVC syndrome reveal systemic combination chemotherapy to be more efficacious than radiation therapy, with 73% to 100% of patients experiencing symptomatic relief within 7 days.[5,12,13] Conversely, for non-small cell lung cancer and for solid tumors metastatic to the thorax, such as breast cancer, radiation therapy is the preferred treatment modality and is associated with a 56% to 70% success rate within 2 weeks.[2] Finally, in patients with non-Hodgkin's lymphoma, single-modality chemotherapy and radiation therapy appear equally efficacious, with 100% of patients experiencing relief of symptoms within 2 weeks.[3] For these patients, chemotherapy is argued to be

TABLE 72-1 Differential Diagnosis for Common Signs and Symptoms in Cancer Patients

Sign/Symptom	Differential Diagnosis
Nausea and vomiting	Hypercalcemia
	Renal failure
	Brain metastases or brain herniation
	Leptomeningeal carcinomatosis
	Gastric outlet obstruction
	Liver metastases
Abnormal mental status	Hypercalcemia
	Hyponatremia
	Renal failure
	Sepsis
	Leptomeningeal carcinomatosis
	Brain metastases or brain herniation
Hemodynamic instability	Pulmonary embolism
	Pericardial tamponade
	Pericardial constriction
	Brain herniation
	Superior vena cava syndrome
Renal failure	Hypercalcemia
	Tumor lysis syndrome; hyperuricemia
	Urinary obstruction
	Paraneoplastic changes
	Glomerulonephritis

TABLE 72-2 Presenting Symptoms and Signs of SVC Obstruction in 66 Patients

Symptoms	%	Signs	%
Face Swelling	83	Neck Vein Distention	92
Dyspnea	83	Facial Swelling	86
Cough	70	Arm Vein Distention	68
Orthopnea	64	Upper Extremity Swelling	64
Nasal Stuffiness	35	Mentation Changes	27
Hoarseness	35	Glossal Edema	24
Stridor	33	Laryngeal Edema	24
Dizziness	29	Rhinorrhea	18
Tongue Swelling	24	Stupor	14
Headache	3	Coma	6
Blackout	3	Upper Body Plethora	3
Dysphagia	1		
Epistaxis	1		

SOURCE: Lochridge, SK, Knibbe WP, Doty DB: Obstruction of the superior vena cava. *Surgery* 85:14, 1979.

the better modality because it also provides systemic therapy. Patients with recurrent or refractory symptoms may benefit from percutaneous stent placement. SVC stenting with thrombolytic therapy and/or systemic anticoagulation is associated with immediate relief of symptoms in more than 90% of patients and provides excellent palliation in most patients.[14–20] Vascular bypass surgery is a treatment modality available for similar patients, but the even higher morbidity and mortality

in such patients make it an infrequently employed therapy. Finally, for patients whose SVC syndrome is secondary to venous catheter thrombosis, thrombolytic therapy given within 5 days of the onset of symptoms is associated with a greater than 80% success rate.[21,22] For thromboses of longer duration, catheter removal in the setting of systemic anticoagulation with heparin and warfarin may be a more successful approach.

MALIGNANT PERICARDIAL DISEASE

Pericardial disease in cancer patients can result from a variety of medical conditions, including radiation, uremia, infection, and malignancy. Autopsy series have shown that malignant involvement of the pericardium complicates 5% of cancers

FIGURE 72-1 Frontal (*left*) and lateral (*right*) sections of the thorax depicting the anatomic structures adjacent to the SVC. The shaded area indicates the most common site of obstruction in SVC syndrome.

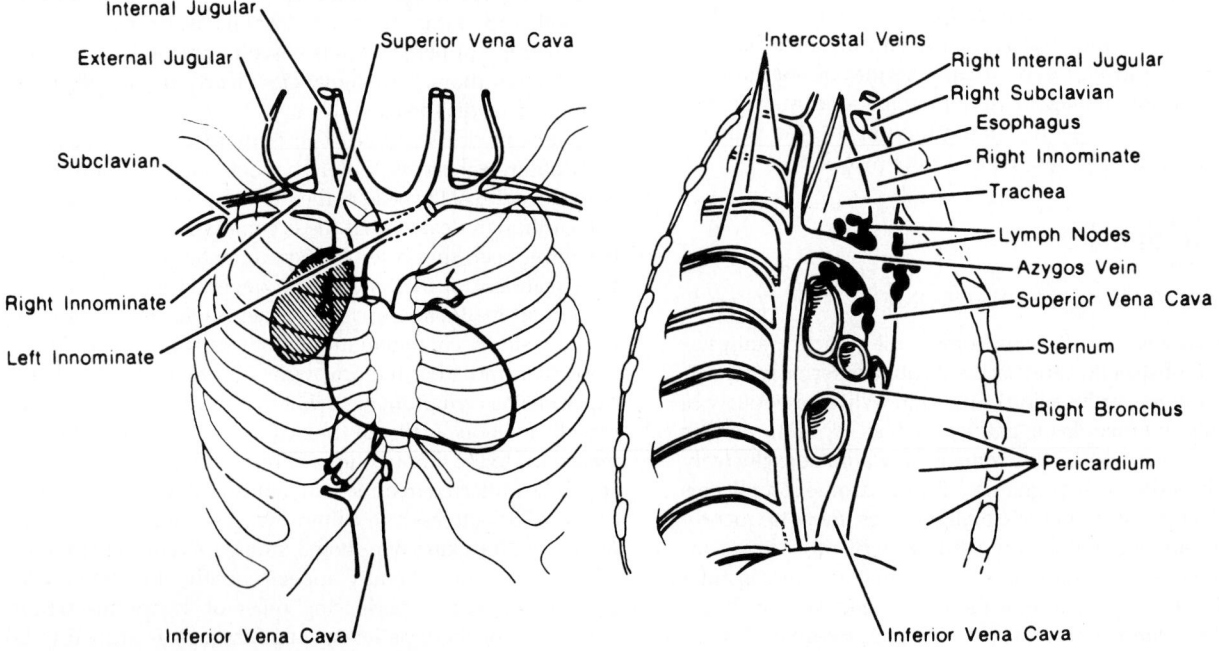

TABLE 72-3 Diagnostic Yield of Various Tests in SVC Syndrome

Test	% Positive
Thoracotomy	98
Mediastinoscopy	77
Thoracentesis	73
Lymph node biopsy	67
Bronchoscopy	90
Sputum cytology	50–90
Bone marrow biopsy	23

and is usually clinically silent.[23,24] However, the series reveal that when malignant pericardial disease is symptomatic, it is often the direct or a supporting cause of death. Thoracic tumors are the most frequent tumors to invade the pericardium directly or hematogenously, with lung cancer first, followed by lymphoma and breast cancer.[23,24]

Malignant pericardial effusion leading to tamponade can be an immediately life-threatening complication of malignant pericardial disease and should be suspected in cancer patients with new cardiopulmonary complaints (see Chap. 28). Because the right-sided cardiac chambers are compressed by surrounding fluid, signs of both right-sided heart failure and left-sided heart insufficiency result. As Table 72-4 details, the presenting symptoms reflect these circulatory disruptions and are, in decreasing order of frequency, dyspnea, cough, orthopnea, chest pain, and pedal edema.[25] Examination often reveals hypotension, tachycardia, distended jugular veins, and a paradoxical pulse of greater than 10 mm Hg. Chest radiographs reveal cardiomegaly in most and pleural effusions in approximately half of patients. However, patients with prior chest radiotherapy may not have radiographic evidence of cardiomegaly due to radiation-induced fibrosis of the pericardium. Electrocardiographic (ECG) abnormalities are protean, usually nonspecific, and commonly include sinus tachycardia and decreased voltage in the limb leads but rarely electrical alternans (i.e., alteration in the amplitude of the R wave, as shown in Fig. 72-2).[24–26] Echocardiography confirms the diagnosis by revealing effusion associated with inspiratory increase in right ventricular dimensions and right atrial and/or right ventricular collapse. Classically, right-sided heart catheterization reveals equalization of in-

traperiicardial, right atrial, right ventricular diastolic, and pulmonary capillary wedge pressures.[27] Since not all pericardial effusions in cancer patients are malignant, both the clinical setting and the results of a diagnostic pericardiocentesis or pericardial biopsy are critical to determining the etiology and therefore the correct treatment for this condition.

Management of malignant pericardial effusions can be challenging and is divided into temporizing and definitive therapies. The immediate management of a hemodynamically significant pericardial effusion is echocardiography-guided pericardiocentesis. In 97% of patients, the fluid is removed successfully, and symptoms resolve immediately.[28] Unfortunately, in approximately 50% of patients, the fluid reaccumulates, requiring subsequent pericardiocenteses. Several more definitive therapies targeted at decreasing the reaccumulation rate have been paired with pericardiocentesis, including radiation therapy, systemic chemotherapy, pericardial sclerotic therapies, and mechanical therapies. When administered following initial pericardiocentesis, these therapies have the following reaccumulation rates: radiation therapy 33%, systemic chemotherapy 30%, pericardial sclerosis with tetracycline 15% to 30%, and mechanical therapies (e.g., indwelling pericardial catheter placement, balloon pericardiotomy, thoracotomy with pericardiostomy) 0% to 15%.[29–32]

Of all the mechanical therapies, balloon pericardiotomy has the best reaccumulation profile, with 0% to 6% reaccumulation.[29–32] The procedure includes a pericardiocentesis followed by balloon catheter dilation of the pericardial needle entrance site. Typically, a balloon catheter is placed across the pericardial entrance site and inflated two to three times, each for 1 to 2 minutes for a total procedure time of 20 to 40 minutes. Side effects have been limited to asymptomatic pleural effusions in most patients.[29,30] Not only is balloon pericardiotomy more successful than other less invasive therapies, but it is also the most successful and least morbid of the other mechanical therapies, most of which require general anesthesia and thoracotomy. At centers with staff facile with this technique, patients requiring definitive management of malignant pericardial effusions should be evaluated for this therapy.

Even when fluid does not reaccumulate, cardiac function may not return to normal because of tumor infiltration of the epicardium. This causes diastolic dysfunction mimicking

TABLE 72-4 Clinical Presentation of Malignant Pericardial Effusion in 93 Patients

Symptoms	%	Signs	%
Dyspnea	91	Paradoxical Pulse (>10 mm Hg)	62
Cough	42	Elevated JVP	51
Orthopnea	32	Tachycardia (>110 beats/min)	43
Chest Pain	20	Systolic BP (<110 mmHg)	42
Peripheral Edema	17	Respiratory Rate (>20 breaths/min)	35
Nausea	12	Kussmaul's Sign	14
Impaired Level of Consciousness	5	Pericardial Friction Rub	6
Diaphoresis	4	Hepatomegaly	2
Dysphagia	3		
Hemoptysis	2		
Syncope	2		
Facial Swelling	2		

SOURCE: Maher EA, Shepherd FA, Todd TJR: Pericardial sclerosis as the primary management of malignant pericardial effusion and cardiac tamponade. *J Thorac Cardiovasc Surg* 112:637, 1996.

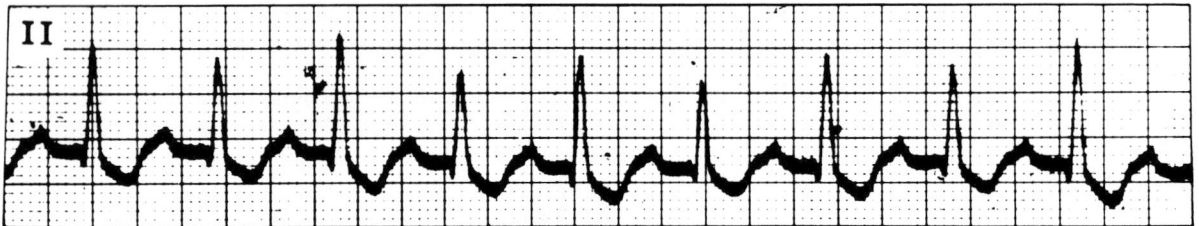

FIGURE 72-2 ECG depicting electrical alternans with variation in the amplitude of the QRS complex from beat to beat.

pericardial constriction. This combination of tamponade and cardiac restriction is termed *effusive-constrictive pericarditis* and may complicate as many as 50% of malignant effusions presenting with hemodynamic compromise. Diagnosis rests on measurement of right side of the heart and pericardial pressures both before and after draining the effusion.[33] This complication may lead to critical hemodynamic deterioration in the days following pericardiocentesis, and while some patients may benefit from pericardiectomy, most will succumb.

RADIATION-RELATED PERICARDIAL DISEASE

Three well-described pericardial syndromes that can manifest in the months to years following radiation therapy to the mediastinum are acute pericarditis with or without tamponade, pericardial effusion with or without tamponade, and pericardial constriction.[34] Such cardiac complications have been described in patients receiving radiation therapy for a variety of tumors within or adjacent to the thoracic cavity (e.g., breast cancer, Hodgkin's disease, esophageal cancer, lung cancer), and one study reported a 9% rate of pericardial effusion in patients receiving radiation therapy to esophageal tumors.[35] The authors suggest that effusions may be predictable when considering elements of radiation administration, with fraction sizes of more than 2 Gy associated with increased risk. The symptoms associated with constrictive

FIGURE 72-3 Right and left ventricular pressure recording in a patient with constrictive pericarditis. The tracing depicts equilibration of right and left ventricular diastolic pressures and the characteristic square-root sign of the diastolic waveform.

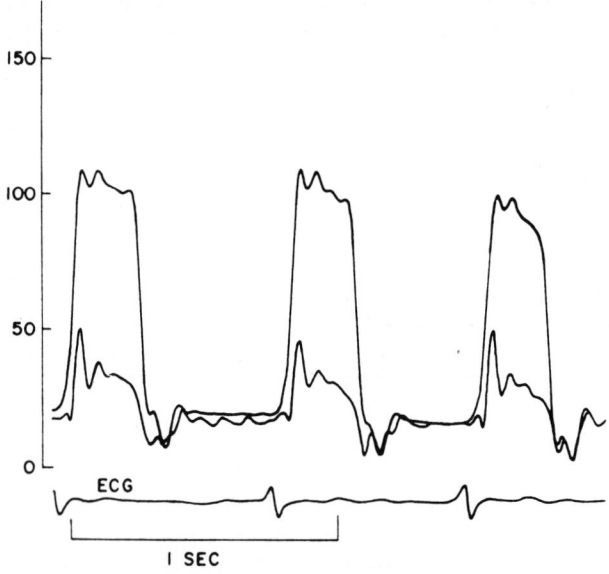

pericarditis typically develop insidiously over a period of months to years. Increasing abdominal girth and peripheral edema, along with progressive exertional dyspnea, are common complaints. As the disease progresses, symptoms suggestive of cardiac cachexia develop (e.g., weakness, dyspnea at rest, palpitations).

Patients generally have a normal or low blood pressure. Elevated venous pressure is demonstrated by jugular venous distention with a rapid *y* descent and rapid rebound. In contrast to cardiac tamponade, an inspiratory increase in jugular venous distention (Kussmaul's sign) occurs in constrictive pericarditis. The heart sounds are often distant. Hepatomegaly, pulmonary edema, and ascites are late clinical features of the syndrome. Chest radiographs show an enlarged cardiac silhouette in only slightly more than 50% of cases. Occasionally, intrapericardial calcifications are present; however, the absence of calcifications does not exclude constrictive pericarditis. ECG findings are nonspecific. Atrial fibrillation is observed in long-standing cases owing to elevated atrial pressure.

M-mode and two-dimensional echocardiography can demonstrate pericardial thickening, but most findings are nonspecific. Doppler echocardiography can demonstrate altered patterns of left ventricular filling that distinguish normal individuals from those with constrictive pericarditis. Patients with constrictive pericarditis typically have a rapid deceleration of filling velocity and a shortened filling period.

In constrictive pericarditis, cardiac catheterization will demonstrate equilibration of diastolic pressures in all four chambers. The ventricular pressure tracing will demonstrate the characteristic dip-and-plateau pattern, or square-root sign (Fig. 72-3). The early diastolic dip of ventricular pressure indicates abnormally rapid ventricular filling in constrictive pericarditis. The pulmonary artery pressure is slightly elevated, and the cardiac index is usually decreased. Angiography is able to demonstrate a thickened pericardium in most patients with constrictive pericarditis, and more recently, CT scan has been shown to effectively distinguish between restrictive myocardial disease and constrictive pericarditis by the presence of a thickened pericardium. Clinically significant pericardial effusions are managed with pericardial drainage as described earlier, and pericardial constriction is managed with cardiac surgery (e.g., pericardial stripping, pericardial resection).

Neurologic Emergencies

SPINAL CORD COMPRESSION

Malignant compression of the spinal cord complicates between 5% and 10% of all malignancies and requires emergent

TABLE 72-5 Signs and Symptoms of Epidural Spinal Cord Compression in 130 Patients

Sign/Symptom	% First Symptom	% With Symptom/Sign at Diagnosis
Pain	96	96
Weakness	2	76
Autonomic Dysfunction	0	57
Sensory Loss	0	51
Ataxia	2	3
Herpes Zoster	0	2
Flexor Spasms	0	1

SOURCE: Gilbert RW, Kim JH, Posner JB: Epidural spinal cord compression from metastatic tumor: Diagnosis and treatment. *Ann Neurol* 3:40, 1978.

initiation of therapy to stop what is often rapid and irreversible neurologic deterioration.[36] In 85% of patients, the condition results from the hematogenous spread of a previously diagnosed cancer to the vertebral body that then compresses the cord directly or causes vertebral body collapse, compressing the cord.[37] In a small number of patients (10%), the condition results from paraspinal malignancies such as lymphoma that compress neural structures traversing the foramina. The most common vertebral levels of spinal cord compression (SCC) are thoracic (70%), lumbosacral (15%), and cervical (15%), and up to 50% of patients have tumor in more than one, often noncontiguous vertebra.[37,38] Clinical series have shown that the tumors most likely to cause SCC are, in decreasing order of frequency, breast carcinoma, lung carcinoma, lymphoma, prostate carcinoma, renal cell carcinoma, and myeloma, together accounting for nearly 70% of histologies.[37]

The presenting symptoms and signs of malignant SCC in 130 patients are detailed in Table 72-5.[37] While back pain is the presenting complaint in almost all patients (96%), the pain can be either localized or radicular, and it can be challenging to distinguish SCC from benign conditions such as degenerative joint disease or disk disease. Characteristics suggestive of SCC include a history of pain worsening with Valsalva maneuver, cough, or recumbency. Subsequent examination reveals clear, objective weakness (usually bilateral and symmetric) in 87% of patients. Sensory deficits are noted in 78% and autonomic dysfunction (like urinary retention or incontinence) in 57% of patients. Patients with autonomic dysfunction at the time of diagnosis form an important poor-prognosis subgroup in which 66% lose ambulation.

After the suspicion of malignant SCC is raised by history and/or physical examination, dexamethasone should be administered (see details of dosing below), and radiologic evaluation must be obtained quickly. The absence of objective neurologic signs of SCC should not dissuade the clinician from the appropriate diagnostic evaluation. Nearly all patients (>80%) with SCC will have abnormal plain radiographs.[36,38,39] The anteroposterior (AP) view can reveal pedicle pathology such as erosion or displacement; the lateral view can reveal vertebral body pathology such as collapse; and the oblique view can reveal foramina pathology such as encroachment or enlargement. Since plain films are both highly sensitive and specific for malignant SCC, they are preferable to bone scans, which, although quite sensitive for malignant bony disease, are less sensitive for SCC.[40] An important exception to this rule occurs in lymphoma patients, 60% of whom will have no abnormalities on plain films.[41] Sub-

sequent imaging with gadolinium-enhanced MRI will both confirm the diagnosis and determine the extent of disease for radiation planning.[42,43] Of note, an MRI examination of the entire spine is often necessary, irrespective of the site of pain, because multilevel disease is often present, particularly in patients with prostate cancer and myeloma. If MRI is unavailable or contraindicated, the more invasive metrizamide myelography with or without CT scan can confirm the diagnosis.

In most cases, pretreatment neurologic function portends posttreatment function, with most ambulatory patients (approximately 80%), fewer paretic patients (<50%), and even fewer paraplegic patients (<10%) ambulatory after therapy.[37,38,40] Therapy for SCC is divided into temporizing therapy and definitive therapy. Acutely, patients should be given dexamethasone 10 mg intravenously, followed by 4 mg every 6 hours to continue until the completion of definitive therapy. The steroid will decrease cord edema and thereby transiently improve neurologic signs and symptoms in some patients. Radiation therapy and surgical decompression via laminectomy are the two definitive treatment modalities. Series examining the effect of laminectomy followed by radiation therapy compared with radiation therapy alone reveal radiation therapy alone to be equally efficacious and far less morbid than the more invasive therapy in most patients.[37–44] However, there are several instances in which surgery with radiation therapy is preferable to radiation therapy alone, including patients in whom a tissue diagnosis is needed, in whom the tumor is radio-refractory such as sarcoma or melanoma, in whom there is spinal instability requiring surgical stabilization, and in whom disease occurs in a previously irradiated field. Finally, for those patients whose SCC results from bony metastases, regular bisphosphonate therapy is an appropriate approach to decreasing the risk of subsequent skeletal complications of the malignancy. Ninety milligrams of intravenous pamidronate infused over 2 hours every 4 weeks has been found in placebo-controlled, randomized trials to reduce skeletal complications in patients with myeloma and patients with breast cancer metastatic to the bone.[45,46] Zolendronic acid, a newer bisphosphonate that can be infused more rapidly, appears to offer equivalent protection against skeletal events.[47]

CEREBRAL HERNIATION SYNDROMES

In cancer patients, cerebral herniation syndromes result from space-occupying brain tumors that increase intracranial pressure and thereby compress the brain against rigid cranial elements (see Chap. 65). Herniation can result from primary central nervous system (CNS) tumors or from those metastatic to the CNS, with lung cancer, breast cancer, melanoma, renal cell carcinoma, and lymphoma the most common.[48] With increased intracranial pressure, patients initially experience intermittent bilateral frontal or occipital headaches. The headaches often awaken patients from sleep or are present on awakening in the morning. They can be accompanied by signs of elevated intracranial pressure, such as projectile vomiting, unsteady gait, and papilledema. As intracranial pressure increases further, cerebral function decreases, leading to inattention, apathy, psychomotor retardation, and somnolence. Because the brain is compartmentalized by the falx cerebri and tentorium, increased pressure in one compartment is equalized into the other compartments through characteristic herniations. MRI may reveal the herniation, as well as the causative tumor and edema (Fig. 72-4).

Management of malignant cerebral herniation syndromes centers around decreasing intracranial pressure through several simultaneous interventions and then initiating definitive antitumor therapy. First, the patient should be loaded with dexamethasone 10 mg intravenously, followed by 4 mg every 6 hours, to mitigate cerebral edema and thereby reduce intracranial pressure. The patient then should be intubated for both airway protection and hyperventilation to a Pa_{CO_2} of roughly 30 mm Hg. Hypocapnia to this level results in cerebral vasoconstriction, which will decrease intracranial volume and thereby reduce intracranial pressure. The effect, however, is of a short duration (48 to 72 hours) because renal bicarbonate wasting will act to normalize cerebral pH and thereby normalize cerebral blood flow.[49] Finally, a loading dose of the osmotic diuretic mannitol 100 g, followed by

25 g as needed, may further reduce intracranial edema. The patient should be evaluated emergently by a radiation oncologist for more definitive therapy with cranial radiation therapy.

CARCINOMATOUS MENINGITIS

Carcinomatous meningitis results from the direct or hematogenous seeding of the meninges by tumor cells and should be suspected in cancer patients presenting with deficits in multiple areas of the neuraxis. Autopsy studies suggest that malignant involvement of the meninges is common, occurring in 8% of cancer patients. These studies reveal that patients with acute leukemias have the highest rates of leptomeningeal disease, followed by patients with non-Hodgkin's lymphoma, small cell lung cancer, and breast cancer.[48]

The diagnosis of carcinomatous meningitis is often elusive, with symptoms that can be both diffuse and localized. Diffuse symptoms result from decreased brain metabolism that is seen with malignant CNS disease, from cerebral spinal fluid (CSF) obstruction causing hydrocephalus and increased intracranial pressure, or from diffuse meningeal irritation. These patients present most frequently with headache and have signs of altered mental status on examination. Localized signs result from spinal and/or cranial nerve root invasion. In cases of spinal nerve root involvement, the most frequent presenting complaint is lower motor neuron weakness, and the most frequent examination findings are reflex asymmetry and weakness. Spinal sensory nerves also can be affected, resulting in complaints of paresthesias and findings of sensory loss. Cranial nerves damaged by tumor deposits result in cranial nerve palsies. Among those with cranial

FIGURE 72-4 *A.* Diagram depicting the brain tissue displacement that accompanies a parietal lobe tumor. *B.* Diagram showing the brain tissue displacement that accompanies a tumor in the posterior cranial fossa.

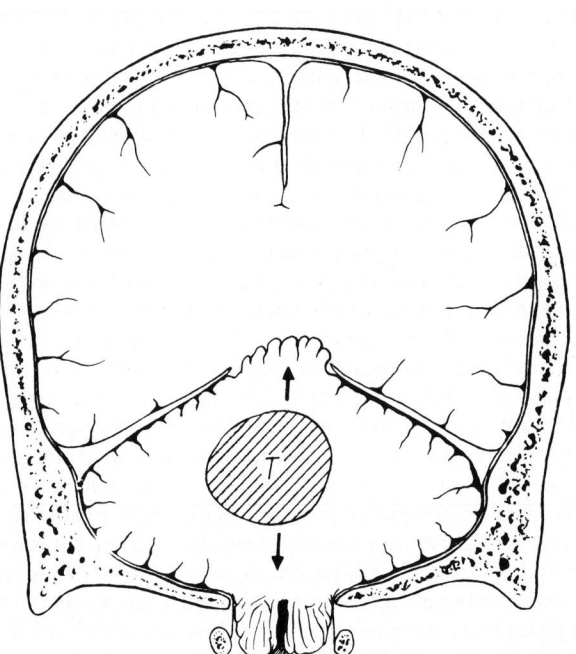

A   B

TABLE 72-6 Leptomeningeal Metastases from Solid Tumors in 90 Patients: CSF Findings

Test	% Positive on Initial LP
Protein >50 mg/dl	81
White Blood Cells >5 mcl	57
Positive Cytology	54
Opening Pressure >160 mm CSF	50
Glucose <40 mg/dl	31
Normal	3

SOURCE: Wasserstrom WR, Glass JP, Posner JB: Diagnosis and treatment of leptomeningeal metastases from solid tumors: Experience with 90 patients. *Cancer* 49:759, 1982.

nerve involvement, the most frequent presenting complaint is double vision, and the most frequent examination finding is ocular muscle paresis due to compromise of cranial nerves III, IV, and VI.[50]

Carcinomatous meningitis is diagnosed most reliably through examination of the CSF, not through neuroimaging. Once a head CT scan excludes a concomitant mass lesion that could cause herniation during lumbar puncture, the patient should undergo a lumbar puncture, followed by CSF examination. Table 72-6 details the initial CSF results of 90 patients with leptomeningeal metastases. It reveals that 97 percent of patients with carcinomatous meningitis have CSF abnormalities with the following distribution: elevated protein 81%, elevated white blood cell count 57%, positive cytology 54%, elevated opening pressure 50%, and depressed glucose 31%. The cytology yield increases to 86% if three lumbar punctures are performed.[50] MRI with gadolinium can identify leptomeningeal deposits as areas of enhancement but is positive in only 33% to 66% of cases.[51,52]

Successful treatment of carcinomatous meningitis can arrest or sometimes reverse neurologic loss, extending patient survival from weeks to months.[50] The treatment modalities are intrathecal chemotherapy and/or radiation therapy. Because the blood-brain barrier hinders the passage of systemic chemotherapeutic agents into the brain, chemotherapy must be administered intrathecally through a ventricular reservoir (e.g., Ommaya shunt) or through a lumbar puncture. Standard regimens are methotrexate 10 mg twice weekly (with systemic leucovorin to prevent bone marrow suppression), thiotepa 5 to 10 mg twice weekly, or cytarabine 90 mg twice weekly until clinical neurologic improvement occurs or until CSF cytology clears of malignant cells. The interval between doses is then increased to weekly or monthly. While acute side effects are transient nausea and vomiting, the late side effects are myelosuppression and mucositis from systemic absorption of the chemotherapeutic agent. Radiation therapy is a second treatment option for established cranial or cauda equina neuropathies and may be given either singly or in association with intrathecal chemotherapy. Focal areas of disease are irradiated rather than the entire neuraxis because the latter is associated with substantial myelosuppression. The acute side effect is transient nausea. A rare complication of concomitant methotrexate and radiation therapy is leukoencephalopathy.[50] With these therapies, approximately 50% of patients will experience either improvement or stabilization of their disease.[50] Since carcinomatous meningitis is often a late finding in the course of a patient's malignancy,

and since treatment often has limited success, the decision of whether to treat needs to be considered carefully, taking into account the patient's performance status and the state of his or her systemic cancer. It is not unusual for patients with carcinomatous meningitis to be at such a point in their illness (i.e., have widespread and refractory cancer) that the complication is managed with supportive care alone and not chemotherapy or radiation.

Metabolic Complications

LACTIC ACIDOSIS

Tumor-induced lactic acidosis is an extremely rare condition that occurs in malignancies with exceptionally high proliferative indices, such as Burkitt's lymphoma; small noncleaved, non-Burkitt's lymphoma; or acute lymphoblastic leukemia. Although the mechanism has not been established definitively, it is likely a function of tumor cell hypoxia leading to anaerobic metabolism (glycolysis) that generates lactate. Concomitant hepatic impairment by the malignancy may reduce the patient's ability to metabolize the lactate produced. The diagnosis of lactic acidosis should be suspected in cancer patients with large tumor burdens who have anion-gap acidoses and no history of toxic ingestion or clinical or laboratory evidence of diabetic ketoacidosis or uremia. Such patients usually have high levels of serum lactate dehydrogenase (LDH), indicating high tumor cell turnover. The mainstay of treatment of this condition is treatment of the malignant cause of the acidosis with urgent chemotherapy. The role of exogenous sodium bicarbonate in the management is controversial, with several animal and human studies reporting increased cellular acidosis, increased serum lactate concentration, and higher mortality in subjects treated with bicarbonate.[53–56] Although standard texts recommend supplemental bicarbonate therapy in patients with a blood pH of less than 7.1, it is not clear that this improves clinical outcome in this patient population.

TUMOR LYSIS SYNDROME

Tumor lysis syndrome is another complication of rapidly proliferating tumors. Tumor lysis syndrome is a life-threatening condition caused by the rapid release into the plasma of large quantities of cytoplasmic solutes, most notably potassium, uric acid, and inorganic phosphate, liberated by tumors with high proliferative indices (e.g., Burkitt's lymphoma) either because of rapid cell turnover or because of cell lysis by cytotoxic chemotherapy. Uric acid nephropathy may result from intrarenal precipitation of massive amounts of uric acid. Uric acid crystals in the renal collecting system obstruct urine flow, raising intrarenal pressure and thereby decreasing vascular perfusion. The end result is acute oliguric renal failure. Patients may develop lethargy, seizures, nausea, and vomiting and eventually symptoms and signs of volume overload. Laboratory evaluation typically reveals elevated potassium, uric acid, and inorganic phosphate levels and often creatinine. Urine evaluation can reveal uric acid concentrations of 150 to 200 mg/dL and both uric acid and sodium monourate crystals.[57]

The management of tumor lysis syndrome is primarily preventive, with the goal to decrease uric acid production and increase its urine solubility. Decreased production is achieved through the use of allopurinol, a xanthine oxidase inhibitor. Treatment with allopurinol should precede chemotherapy by 2 to 3 days, if possible. The initial dose of between 300 and 800 mg daily should reflect tumor burden. The dose eventually may be decreased to between 100 and 300 mg daily and should continue through the period of cytoreduction. The dose should be reduced for renal insufficiency. Increased uric acid solubility can be achieved by maximizing urine output and by making the urine alkaline through the use of sodium bicarbonate or acetazolamide.[58,59] Urinary output of 3 L/d (125 mL/h) and a urinary pH of 7 or greater often are recommended. The use of recombinant urate oxidase (rasburicase), a catalyst in the oxidation of uric acid to allantoin, in the prophylaxis or treatment of patients with hyperuricemia in the setting of leukemia and lymphoma shows promising results.[60] The drug has the advantage over allopurinol of both blocking uric acid formation and increasing its solubility and requiring administration only hours prior to chemotherapy administration. For patients in whom uric acid nephropathy develops despite these measures, hemodialysis can both acutely decrease serum uric acid and correct the volume and electrolyte effects of acute renal failure.[61]

HYPERCALCEMIA

Hypercalcemia is the most common life-threatening metabolic disorder associated with malignancy. It has been estimated that between 10% and 20% of cancer patients become hypercalcemic during the course of their disease.[62] Cancers commonly associated with hypercalcemia include both solid tumors, in particular squamous cell histologies, and hematologic malignancies, in particular multiple myeloma.

Dysregulation of bone resorption is the principal factor implicated in the hypercalcemia of malignancy, although defects in renal clearance and intestinal absorption also have been described. Current evidence suggests that this disorder is most often due to increased bone resorption secondary to diffusible factors produced in excess by cancer cells or direct malignant bone invasion. The best characterized of the diffusable factors is parathyroid hormone–related peptide (PTHrP). In cancers metastatic to bone, the bony destruction that was originally attributed to the tumor cells themselves in most cases may be secondary to high local concentrations of PTHrP resulting in osteoclast activation. Other diffusible factors also have been implicated in tumor-related osteolysis and subsequent hypercalcemia, notably tumor necrosis factor and interleukin 6 in multiple myeloma.[63,64]

The clinical manifestations of hypercalcemia of malignancy are protean and depend on both the rate of increase of serum calcium concentration and the absolute value. A slow rise to 14 mg/dL may be imperceptible, whereas a rapid elevation to 12 mg/dL could result in coma. The typical presentation is with nausea, vomiting, anorexia, fatigue, weight loss, and dehydration. Table 72-7 lists many of the common signs and symptoms. Serum calcium has diuretic properties, leading in the hypercalcemic state to volume contraction and eventually dehydration. In the setting of volume contraction, the kidney actively resorbs sodium at the distal tubule under the stimulation of antidiuretic hormone. In addition to resorbing sodium, the Na^+, K^+ pump resorbs calcium and wastes potassium. This action leads to further increases

TABLE 72-7 Symptoms and Signs of Hypercalcemia of Malignancy

Neurologic
depression, irritability, disturbed sleep
lethargy, confusion, stupor, coma
muscle weakness, hypotonia
absent deep–tendon reflexes

Cardiovascular
shortening of the QT interval
broadening of the T–wave
heart block, asystole
ventricular arrhythmias
increased sensitivity to digoxin

Gastrointestinal
anorexia, vomiting, gastric atony
constipation
acute pancreatitis

Renal
polyuria, polydipsia
dehydration
impaired glomerular filtration
nephrocalcinosis

SOURCE: Mosekilde L, Eriksen EF, Charles P: Hypercalcemia of malignancy: Pathophysiology, diagnosis and treatment. *Crit Rev Onc Hem* 11:1–27 1991.

in total body calcium and deficiency of potassium. The increased calcium, in turn, causes more volume loss, resulting in further resorption of sodium and calcium and loss of potassium. Therefore, when patients become hypercalcemic, they enter a self-perpetuating physiologic cycle of increasing hypercalcemia.

Treatment is focused on reversing the physiologic progression of hypercalcemia, as well as on attenuating the underlying pathologic process that initiated the elevation. To interrupt the physiologic progression acutely, one should rehydrate patients with intravenous fluids and correct hypokalemia. Treatment of the underlying pathology consists of both anticancer therapies and initiation of bisphosphonate therapy to attenuate release of calcium from the bone. Since the randomized trial showing pamidronate to be superior over saline alone, bisphosphonates, like pamidronate, became the cornerstone of the treatment for hypercalcemia of malignancy through their inhibition of osteoclast activity.[65] A newer bisphosphonate, zoledronic acid, has the advantage over pamidronate of both more rapid administration and more rapid resolution of hypercalcemia. A large randomized study comparing zoledronic acid with pamidronate revealed that a single 4-mg dose of zoledronic acid infused over 5 minutes was superior to a single 90-mg dose of pamidronate infused over 2 hours in normalizing serum calcium concentration within 10 days (88% versus 70%) and in the duration of response (32 versus 18 days).[66] Other therapeutic measures may be required in acute, symptomatic hypercalcemia resistant to hydration. For example, calcitonin given at the dose of 200 to 400 MRC units intramuscularly or subcutaneously every 12 hours will rapidly lower serum calcium concentration and, although its effects are short-lived, may be useful in the period before bisphosphonate therapy takes effect.

SYNDROME OF INAPPROPRIATE SECRETION OF ANTIDIURETIC HORMONE

The syndrome of inappropriate secretion of antidiuretic hormone (SIADH) was first described in the 1950s by investigators who reported the finding of hyponatremia associated with renal sodium loss and high urine osmolality in two lung cancer patients.[67] The authors correctly theorized that cancer-produced antidiuretic hormone (arginine vasopressin) was responsible for the syndrome.[68] The tumor most frequently associated with SIADH is small cell lung cancer, although many other cancers have been reported to cause the syndrome. Up to 15% of small cell lung cancer is complicated by SIADH.[69] However, as shown in Table 72-8, a host of other mechanisms can be responsible for SIADH in cancer patients, including infections, drugs, pulmonary processes, and CNS processes.

Antidiuretic hormone is normally synthesized in the posterior pituitary and functions as a critical physiologic regulator of water balance. It acts primarily on the collecting tubules of the nephron to stimulate upregulation of water channels, permitting increased free water resorption. It is controlled by a complex network of signals derived from volume and osmoreceptors in the hypothalamus, left atrium, and pulmonary veins and from circulating angiotensin II. Excessive autonomous secretion of ADH leads to excess water resorption out of proportion to sodium, resulting in progressive water intoxication and hyponatremia. The hyponatremia can lead to CNS toxicity, with headaches and fatigue ultimately progressing to confusion, seizures, coma, and death.

The mainstay of treatment of SIADH caused by tumors is therapy for the underlying malignancy. When this is not sufficient, or when the serum sodium concentration is less than 130 mEq/L, fluid restriction is the next step. For relatively mild cases, restriction of free water to 1 L/d may be adequate to correct the serum sodium concentration. Greater fluid restriction occasionally may be required, although it is difficult to accomplish, especially in the outpatient setting. Another approach is serum sodium correction with 3% saline in patients with acute (<48 hours), symptomatic hyponatremia. Care needs to be taken to avoid too rapid correction of the serum sodium concentration, however, because central pontine myelinolysis[70] and volume overload may occur because patients with SIADH are euvolemic. Specifically, the rate of change in the serum sodium concentration should not exceed 1 to 2 mEq/L per hour, and an absolute change of greater than 20 mEq/L in 24 hours should be avoided. After the serum sodium concentration reaches 120 to 125 mEq/L, therapy should be shifted to free water restriction. For chronic cases of hyponatremia, in which free water restriction is not feasible, pharmacologic therapy with demeclocycline has proven to be effective. Demeclocycline inhibits the renal effects of antidiuretic hormone and, when used in doses of 600 to 1200 mg/d, usually restores the serum sodium concentration to normal in 5 to 14 days.[71]

TABLE 72-8 Causes of SIADH

Carcinomas
  Small cell lung cancer
  Bronchial carcinoids
  Prostate
  Adrenal
  Head and neck
  Duodenal, colorectal
  Pancreas
  Esophagus
  Hodgkin's and non–Hodgkin's lymphoma

Pulmonary disorders
  Viral, bacterial pneumonias
  Abscess
  Tuberculosis

CNS
  Meningitis
  Encephalitis
  Cerebritis
  Primary or metastatic tumors
  Abscess
  Head trauma–skull fractures
  Subdural hematoma
  Subarachnoid hemorrhage
  Pain

Drugs
  Morphine
  Nicotine
  Cyclophosphamide
  Vincristine
  Alcohol
  Chlorpropramide

Urologic Emergencies

HEMORRHAGIC CYSTITIS

Hemorrhagic cystitis results from inflammation of the bladder and presents with dysuria, hematuria, and urinary frequency. In cancer patients, the condition can result from chemotherapy, radiation therapy, or viral infections. Cyclophosphamide and ifosfamide are the most frequent chemotherapeutic agents implicated in hemorrhagic cystitis and act through their metabolite acrolein to damage the bladder mucosa. While previously complicating greater than 40% of bone marrow transplants, hemorrhagic cystitis now occurs in less than 5% due to preventive management with hydration and the drug mesna.[72–76] Vigorous intravenous hydration generates a high urine output that limits bladder exposure to acrolein. Mesna is a thiol that is activated in the kidney and inactivates acrolein in the bladder. Because its half-life is shorter than that of cyclophosphamide, it must be started prior to cyclophosphamide and continued after the completion of the cyclophosphamide infusion. For patients in whom hemorrhagic cystitis develops despite these measures, emergent urologic consultation must be obtained regarding possible bladder irrigation, cystoscopy with clot extraction and fulguration, or chemical hemostasis with formalin. In refractory cases, vascular ligation or even cystectomy may be required.

Disorders of Blood Viscosity

Hyperviscosity syndrome (HVS) and leukostasis are disorders resulting from a malignant excess of blood components and requiring rapid evaluation for possible emergent apheresis, chemotherapy, and radiotherapy.

HYPERVISCOSITY SYNDROME

HVS results from high levels of serum paraprotein often elaborated by Waldenstrom's macroglobulinemia (IgM) or multiple myeloma (IgG, IgA, and very rarely light-chain disease). HVS is characterized by a clinical triad of visual changes, bleeding, and neurologic changes, with patients often presenting with blurred vision, "dizzy headache," and mucosal oozing.[77,78] The visual and neurologic symptoms result from sludging of blood through end arterioles, and the bleeding results from paraprotein-induced platelet dysfunction, clotting factor inhibition, and fibrin inhibition. Funduscopic examination can reveal tortuous vessels with a sausage-like appearance termed *fundus paraproteinaemicus*, as well as retinal hemorrhage and papilledema. The diagnosis is made by observing a serum paraprotein concentration in the setting of an elevated blood viscosity (usually >4.0 cP). Treatment is plasmapheresis to decrease the paraprotein acutely, followed by chemotherapy to decrease production of the paraprotein. Of note, some IgM paraproteins are cold-reactive, making plasmapheresis with a room-temperature cell separator problematic. These patients should undergo plasmapheresis with prewarmed equipment in a warm room.

LEUKOSTASIS

Leukostasis is a rare condition that results from an excess of the blood's cellular elements. The signs and symptoms result from end-organ ischemia, infarction, and hemorrhage due to microvascular thrombi from leukocyte aggregates. Patients may present with visual changes, confusion, and dyspnea. Evaluation may reveal mental status changes, papilledema, cardiogenic or noncardiogenic pulmonary edema, liver dysfunction, renal failure, and priapism. Blood rheology studies and clinical reports reveal the risk of leukostasis to be a complex function of white blood cell type, maturity, and number, as well as hematocrit and platelet count (see Chap. 71). Patients with acute leukemias or the accelerated phase of chronic myelogenous leukemia (CML) with blast counts greater than $50,000/\mu L$ are at a far greater risk for leukostasis than patients with chronic lymphocytic leukemia (CLL) with lymphocyte counts of even $500,000/\mu L$.[79,80] Leukemia patients who present with leukostasis should not receive blood product transfusions until their white blood cell count has been decreased substantially through leukapheresis, chemotherapy, or both because additional blood products will exacerbate their condition through increasing blood viscosity. Patients with pulmonary or CNS leukostasis may require emergent local radiation therapy to arrest organ compromise.

Acknowledgment

Financial support was provided by a grant from the National Institutes of Health (EBL, Grant No. K07 CA93892).

References

1. Lochridge SK, Knibbe WP, Doty DB: Obstruction of the superior vena cava. *Surgery* 85:14, 1979.
2. Armstrong BA, Poerez CA, Simpson JR, Hederman MA: Role of irradiation in the hemanagement of superior vena cava syndrome. *Int J Radiat Oncol Biol Phys* 13:531, 1987.
3. Perez-Soler R, McLaughlin P, Velasquez WS, et al : Clinical features and results of managment of superior vena cava syndrome secondary to lymphoma. *J Clin Oncol* 2:260, 1984.
4. Salsali M, Cliffton EE: Superior vena cava obstruction in carcinoma of the lung. *NY State J Med* 69:2875, 1969.
5. Sculier JP, Evans WK, Feld R, et al: Superior vena cava syndrome in small-cell lung cancer. *Cancer* 57:847, 1986.
6. Luciani A, Clement O, Halimi P, et al: Catheter-related upper extremity deep venous thrombosis in cancer patients: A prospective study based on Doppler ultrasound. *Radiology* 220:655, 2001.
7. Nightingale CE, Norman A, Cunningham D, et al: A prospective analysis of 949 long-term central venous access catheters for ambulatory chemotherapy in patients with gastrointestinal malignancy. *Eur J Cancer* 33:398, 1997.
8. Weber T, Huemer G, Tschernich H, et al: Catheter-induced thrombus in the superior vena cava diagnosed by transesophageal echocardiography. *Acta Anaesthesiol Scand* 42:1227, 1998.
9. Stricker PD, Manoharan A, Hanel KC: Major venous thrombosis in patients with indwelling venous access catheters. *Med J Aust* 144:601, 1986.
10. Qanadli SD, Mesurolle B, Sissakian JF, et al: Implanted central venous catheter-related acute superior vena cava syndrome: Management by metallic stent and endovascular repositioning of the catheter tip. *Eur Radiol* 10:1329, 2000.
11. Ahmann F: A reassessment of the clinical implications of the superior vena cava syndrome. *J Clin Oncol* 2:961, 1984.
12. Dombernowsky P, Hansen HH: Combination chemotherapy in the management of superior vena cava obstruction in small-cell anaplastic cancer of the lung. *Acta Med Scand* 204:513, 1978.
13. Maddox AM, Valdivieso M, Lukeman J, et al: Superior vena cava obsturction in small cell bronchogenic carcinoma. *Cancer* 52:2165, 1983.
14. Gaines PA, Belli AM, Anderson PB, et al: Superior vena caval obstruction managed by the Gianturco Z stent. *Clin Radiol* 49:202, 1994.
15. Hennequin LM, Fade O, Fays JG, et al : Superior vena cava stent placement: Results with the Wallstent endoprosthesis. *Radiology* 196:353, 1995.
16. Kishi K, Sonomura T, Mitsuzan K, et al: Self-expandable metallic stent therapy for superior vena cava syndrome: Clinical observations. *Radiology* 189:531, 1993.
17. Oudkerk M, Heystraten FM, Stoter G: Stenting in malignant vena caval obstruction. *Cancer* 71:142, 1993.
18. Shah R, Sabanathan S, Lowe RA, Mearns AJ: Stenting in malignant obstruction of superior vena cava. *J Thorac Cardiovasc Surg* 112:335, 1996.
19. Courtheoux P, Alkofer B, Al Refai M, et al: Stent placement in superior vena cava syndrome. *Ann Thorac Surg* 75:158, 2003.
20. Wilson E, Lyn E, Lynn A, et al: Radiological stenting provides effective palliation in malignant central venous obstruction. *Clin Oncol* 14:228, 2002.
21. Gray BH, Olin JW, Graor RA, et al: Safety and efficacy of thrombolytic therapy for superior vena cava syndrome. *Chest* 99:54, 1991.
22. Morales M, Comas V, Trujillo M, Dorta J: Treatment of catheter-induced thrombotic superior vena cava syndrome: A single institution's experience. *Supp Care Cancer* 8:334, 2000.
23. Skhvatsabaju LV: Secondary tumors of the heart and pericardium in neoplastic disease. *Oncology* 43:103, 1986.
24. Thurber DL, Edwards JE, Achor RW: Secondary malignant tumors of the pericardium. *Circulation* 26:228, 1962.
25. Maher EA, Shepherd FA, Todd TJR: Pericardial sclerosis as the primary management of malignant pericardial effusion and cardiac tamponade. *J Thorac Cardiovasc Surg* 112:637, 1996.
26. Laham RJ, Cohen DJ, Kuntz RE, et al: Pericardial effusion in patients with cancer: Outcome with contemporary management strategies. *Heart* 75:67, 1996.

27. Braunwald E: Pericardial disease, in Braunwald E (ed): *Heart Disease,* 3d ed. Philadelphia, Saunders, 1988, p 1492.

28. Vaitkus PT, Herrmann HC, LeWinter MM: Treatment of malignant pericardial effusion. *JAMA* 272:59, 1994.

29. Galli M, Politi A, Fausto P, et al: Percutaneous balloon pericardiotomy for malignant pericardial tamponade. *Chest* 108:1499, 1995.

30. Palacios IF, Tuzcu EM, Ziskind AA, et al: Percutaneous balloon pericardial window for patients with malignant pericardial effusion and tamponade. *Cathet Cardiovasc Diagn* 22:244, 1991.

31. Ziskind AA, Pearce AC, Lemon C, et al : Percutaneous pericardotomy for the treatment of cardiac tamponade and large pericardial effusion: Description of technique and report of the first 50 cases. *J Am Coll Cardiol* 21:1, 1993.

32. Tsang TSM, Enriquez-Sarano M, Freeman WK, et al: Consecutive 1127 therapeutic echocardiographically guided pericardiocenteses: Clinical profile, practice patterns, and outcomes spanning 21 years. *Mayo Clin Proc* 77:429, 2002.

33. Sagristà-Sauleda J, Angel J, Sànchez A, et al: Effusive-constrictive pericarditis. *N Engl J Med* 350:469, 2004.

34. Stewart JR, Fajardo LF, Gillette SM, Constine LS: Radiation injury to the heart. *Int J Radiat Oncol Biol Phys* 31:1205, 1995.

35. Martel MK, Sahijdak WM, Haken RKT, et al: Fraction size and dose parameters related to the incidence of pericardial effusions. *Int J Radiat Oncol Biol Phys* 40:155, 1998.

36. Barron KD, Hirano A, Araki S, et al: Experience with metastatic neoplasms involving the spinal cord. *Neurology* 9:91, 1959.

37. Gilbert RW, Kim JH, Posner JB: Epidural spinal cord compression from metastatic tumor: Diagnosis and treatment. *Ann Neurol* 3:40, 1978.

38. Stark RJ, Henson RA, Evans SJW: Spinal metastasis: A retrospective survey from a general hospital. *Brain* 105:189, 1982.

39. Portenoy RK, Galer BS, Salamon O, et al: Identification of epidural neoplasm: Radiography and bone scintigraphy in the symptomatic and asymptomatic spine. *Cancer* 64:2207, 1989.

40. Rodichok LD, Ruckdeschel JC, Harper GR, et al: Early detection and treatment of spinal epidural metastases: The role of myelography. *Ann Neurol* 20:696, 1986.

41. Haddad P, Thaell JF, Kiely JM, et al: Lymphoma of the spinal and extradural space. *Cancer* 38:1862, 1976.

42. Koch D, Wakhloo AK, van Velthoven V: Magnetic resonance imaging in spinal emergency. *Acta Neurochir (Wien)* 134:100, 1995.

43. Pigott KH, Baddeley H, Maher EJ: Pattern of disease in spinal cord compression on MRI scan and implications for treatment. *Clin Oncol R Coll Radiol* 6:7, 1994.

44. Young RF, Post EM, King GA: Treatment of spinal epidural metastases: Randomized prospective comparison of laminectomy and radiotherapy. *J Neurosurg* 53:741, 1980.

45. Berenson JR, Lichtenstein A, Porter L, et al for the Myeloma Aredia Study Group: Long-term pamidronate treatment of advanced multiple myeloma patients reduces skeletal events. *J Clin Oncol* 16:593, 1998.

46. Theriault RL, Lipton A, Hortobagyi GN, et al for the Protocol 19 Aredia Breast Cancer Study Group: Pamidronate reduces skeletal morbidity in women with advanced breast cancer and lytic bone lesions: A randomized, placebo-controlled trial. *J Clin Oncol* 17:846, 1999.

47. Rosen LS, Gordon D, Antonio BS, et al: Zoledronic acid versus pamidronate in the treatment of skeletal metastases in patients with breast cancer or osteolytic lesions of multiple myeloma: A phase III, double-blind, comparative trial. *Cancer J* 7:377, 2001.

48. Posner J, Chernick N: Intracranial metastases from systemic cancer. *Adv Neurol* 19:575, 1978.

49. Heffner JE, Sahn SA: Controlled hyperventilation in patients with intracranial hypertension. *Arch Intern Med* 143:765, 1983.

50. Wasserstrom WR, Glass JP, Posner JB: Diagnosis and treatment of leptomeningeal metastases from solid tumors: Experience with 90 patients. *Cancer* 49:759, 1982.

51. Sze G, Soletsky S, Bronen R, Krol G: MR imaging of the meninges with emphasis on contrast enhancement and meningeal carcinomatosis. *AJNR* 10:965, 1989.

52. Yousem DM, Patrone PM, Grossman RI: Leptomeningeal metastases: MR elevation. *J Comput Assist Tomogr* 14:255, 1990.

53. Arieff AI, Leach W, Park R, Lazarowitz VC: Systemic effects of $NaHCO_3$ in experimental lactic acidosis in dogs. *Am J Physiol* 242:F586, 1982.

54. Fields ALA, Wolman SL, Halperin ML: Chronic lactic acidosis in a patient with cancer. *Cancer* 47:2026, 1981.

55. Fraley DS, Adler S, Bruns FJ, Zett B: Stimulation of lactate production by administration of bicarbonate in a patient with a solid neoplasm and lactic acidosis. *N Engl J Med* 303:1100, 1980.

56. Park R, Arieff AI: Treatment of lactic acidosis with dichloroacetate in dogs. *J Clin Invest* 70:853, 1982.

57. Conger JD: Acute uric acid nephropathy. *Med Clin North Am* 74:859, 1990.

58. Conger JD, Falk SA: Intrarenal dynamics in the pathogenesis and prevention of acute urate nephropathy. *J Clin Invest* 59:786, 1977.

59. Kursch ED, Resnick MI: Dissolution of uric acid calculi with systemic alkalinization. *J Urol* 132:286, 1984.

60. Pui C-H, Mahmoud HH, Wiley JM, et al: Recombinant urate oxidase for the prophylaxis or treatment of hyperuricemia in patients with leukemia or lymphoma. *J Clin Oncol* 19:697, 2001.

61. Steinberg SM, Galen MA, Lazarus JM, et al: Hemodialysis for acute anuric uric acid nephropathy. *Am J Dis Child* 129:956, 1975.

62. Burt ME, Brennan MF: Incidence of hypercalcemia and malignant neoplasm. *Arch Surg* 115:704, 1980.

63. Johnson RA, Boyce BF, Mundy GR, et al: Tumors producing human tumor necrosis factor induce hypercalcemia and osteoclastic bone resorption in nude mice. *Endocrinology* 124:1424, 1989.

64. Black K, Garret IR, Mundy GR: Chinese hamster ovarian cells transfected with murine IL-6 gene causes hypercalcemia as well as cachexia, leukocytosis, thrombosis in tumor-bearing mice. *Endocrinology* 128:2657, 1991.

65. Gaculp R, Theriault R, Gill I, et al: Treatment of cancer-associated hypercalcemia. *Arch Intern Med* 154:1935, 1994.

66. Major P, Lortholary A, Hon J, et al: Zoledronic acid is superior to pamidronate in the treatment of hypercalcemia of malignancy: A pooled analysis of two randomized, controlled clinical trials. *J Clin Oncol* 19:558, 2001.

67. Schwartz WB, Bennet W, Curalop S, et al: A syndrome of renal sodium loss and hyponatremia probably resulting from inappropriate section of antidiuretic hormone. *Am J Med* 23:529, 1957.

68. Amatruda TT, Mulrow JP, Gallager JC, et al : Carcinoma of the lung with inappropriate diuresis. *N Engl J Med* 260:544, 1963.

69. Lokich JJ: The frequency and clinical biology of the ectopic hormone syndromes of small cell carcinoma. *Cancer* 50:2111, 1982.

70. Sterns R: Severe symptomatic hyponatremia: Treatment and outcome. *Ann Intern Med* 107:656, 1987.

71. Bower M, Brazil L, Coombes RC: Endocrine and metabolic complications of advanced cancer, in Doyle D, Hanks GWC, MacDonald N (eds): *Oxford Textbook of Palliative Medicine,* 2d ed. London, Oxford University Press, 1999, p 715.

72. Watson NA, Noteley RG: Urologic complications of cyclophosphamide. *Br J Urol* 45:606, 1973.

73. Antman K, Ryan L, Elias A, et al: Response to ifosfamide and mesna: 124 previously treated patients with metastatic or unresectable sarcoma. *J Clin Oncol* 7:126, 1989.

74. Williams SD, Munshi N, Einhorn LH, et al: Cyclophosphamide and ifosfamide: Role of uroprotective agents. *Cancer Invest* 8:269, 1990.

75. Andriole GL, Sandland JI, Miser JS, et al : The efficacy of mesna (2-mercaptoethane sodium sulfonate) as a uroprotectant in patients with hemorrhagic cystitis receiving further oxazaphosphorine chemotherapy. *J Clin Oncol* 5:799, 1989.

76. Shepard JD, Pringle LE, Barnett MJ, et al: Mesna versus hyperhydration for the prevention of cyclophosphamide-induced hemorrhagic cystitis in bone marrow transplantation. *J Clin Oncol* 9:2016, 1991.

77. Fahey JL, Barth WF, Solomon A: Serum hyperviscosity syndrome. *JAMA* 192:120, 1965.

78. Mehta J, Singhal S: Hyperviscosity syndrome in plasma cell dyscrasias. *Semin Thromb Hemost* 29:467, 2003.

79. Baer MR, Stein RS, Dessypris EN: Chronic lymphocytic leukemia with hyperleukocytosis: The hyperviscosity syndrome. *Cancer* 56:2865, 1985.

80. Litchman MA, Rowe JM: Hyperleukocytic leukemia: Rheologic, clinical, and therapeutic considerations. *Blood* 60(2):279, 1982.

Chapter 73

HEMATOPOIETIC STEM CELL TRANSPLANTATION AND GRAFT-VERSUS-HOST DISEASE

STEPHEN W. CRAWFORD
RODNEY J. FOLZ
KEITH M. SULLIVAN

KEY POINTS

- *The principles of and approaches to the critical care of hematopoietic stem cell transplant recipients are similar to those for other immunosuppressed hosts.*

- *Specific complications tend to occur within well-defined time periods and are influenced by the type of stem cell transplant.*

- *The primary distinguishing features of hematopoietic stem cell transplant recipients are the high prevalence of graft rejection, graft-versus-host reactions, and chemoradiotherapy-related toxicities.*

- *Acute graft-versus-host disease represents a major problem to allogeneic hematopoietic stem cell transplantation.*

- *Hepatic veno-occlusive disease is the most common lethal chemoradiotherapy-related toxicity after hematopoietic stem cell transplantation.*

- *When prophylactic treatment is used, diffuse pneumonia due to cytomegalovirus is uncommon after hematopoietic stem cell transplantation.*

- *Idiopathic pneumonia syndrome remains a major cause of mortality, and no treatment has been proved effective.*

Hematopoietic Stem Cell Transplantation

Transplantation of human marrow precursors (hematopoietic stem cell transplantation [HSCT]) has become the primary therapy for several malignant and nonmalignant diseases. HSCT serves as a "salvage" therapy for restoring marrow function after marrow-ablating doses of chemoradiotherapy have been given to eradicate malignant cells in leukemias, myelodysplastic syndromes, multiple myeloma, malignant lymphomas, and assorted solid tumors, such as breast carcinoma and neuroblastoma. HSCT also can be used to replace dysfunctional hematopoietic or lymphoreticular precursors and to correct congenital or acquired deficiencies, such as aplastic anemia, thalassemia, and congenital immune-deficiency syndromes.[1]

Antigenic differences between the marrow donor and recipient may result in graft rejection or, since the marrow graft contains immunocompetent lymphocytes, may initiate graft-versus-host (GVH) reactions. The antigenic determinants that mediate tissue graft rejection responses are primarily the human leukocyte antigens (HLAs). These are encoded by genes of the major histocompatibility complex (MHC) located on chromosome 6.

Donor marrow precursor stem cells may be obtained from several sources. Autologous hematopoietic stem cells from the marrow or peripheral blood of the patient can be used in the treatment of malignant disease if the cells are free of malignancy and were harvested before chemoradiotherapy conditioning. This type of material can be cryopreserved for an extended period prior to reinfusion. Syngeneic stem cells from an identical twin also are ideal because they are genetically indistinguishable from those of the recipient.

In many cases, HSCT is undertaken with allogeneic but phenotypically similar marrow or peripheral blood stem cells. In the best case, an HLA-identical sibling is available to serve as the donor, thus minimizing the antigenic disparity. Siblings have a 25% chance of being HLA identical. Allogeneic HSCT also may be performed using partially HLA-matched donor sources. International tissue typing banks may make it possible to identify unrelated volunteer donors who are HLA identical.

IMMUNOLOGIC ALTERATIONS

Intensive chemoradiotherapy conditioning regimens produce predictable alterations in host defenses related to granulocytopenia and ablation of humoral and cell-mediated immunity. Circulating granulocytes generally recover within the first 3 weeks after marrow infusion. Normal numbers of lymphocytes are seen within a month after HSCT, but antibody production is often delayed for 3 or more months. Host immunoglobulins may circulate for 3 months. At 1 year, serum levels of IgM and IgG are usually normal, but serum and secretory IgA levels remain low for a longer period. T-cell–dependent antigen production, response to vaccination, and skin reactivity to antigens may be delayed for months to a year. Alveolar macrophages of host origin persist for weeks to months before being replaced by donor cells (Fig. 73-1).

Patients with chronic graft-versus-host disease (GVHD) have persistently decreased cell-mediated immunity and antigen-specific antibody responses. These alterations are caused by the GVHD and are independent of immunosuppressive treatment.

Complications of Hematopoietic Stem Cell Transplantation

The morbidity and mortality of HSCT are related primarily to relapse of malignancy, conditioning-related toxicities, infection, and donor-recipient antigenic disparity (leading to graft rejection or GVHD)[2] (Table 73-1). Specific complications tend to occur within well-defined periods of immunologic alteration after intensive conditioning regimens.[3] Knowledge of these periods makes diagnostic decisions in the HSCT recipient easier than in many other immunosuppressed hosts. At major transplantation units about 40% of HSCT recipients require intensive hemodynamic monitoring or critical care procedures, such as hemodialysis or mechanical ventilation. The following section discusses the incidence and presentation of

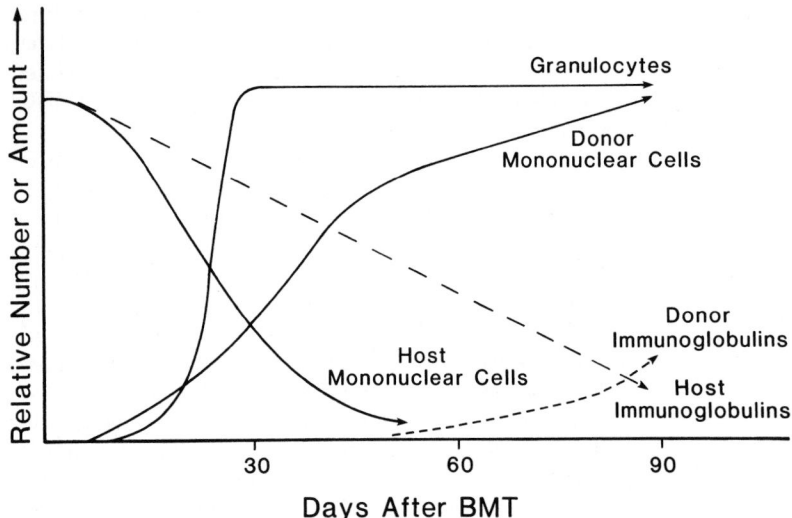

FIGURE 73-1 Alterations in host defense marrow transplantation.

complications that are of concern to the critical care provider. With the exception of the immunologic aspects, complications of HSCT are similar to those of intensive antineoplastic therapy.

COMPLICATIONS OF CYTOREDUCTIVE CHEMOTHERAPY

Infections are very common after HSCT. Bacteremia or serious bacterial infection is noted in up to 50% of HSCT recipients. Infection with *Aspergillus* species and colonization and infection with *Candida* also have become major clinical problems.[4,5] The risks for bacterial and fungal infections are related mainly to the routine use of central venous access lines (e.g., Hickman catheters), prolonged neutropenia, and immunosuppression to prevent GVHD.

TABLE 73-1 Complications after Marrow Transplantation

Rejection of marrow graft
Relapse of malignancy
Conditioning-related toxicity
  Hepatic VOD
  Oral mucositis
  Idiopathic pneumonia
  Leukoencephalopathy
  Neuropathy
  Myopericarditis
  Hepatitis
Infection
  Venous access line infection
  Bacteremia, fungemia
  Pneumonia
    Viral
    Fungal
    Bacterial
    P. carinii
GVHD
  Acute
  Chronic
Idiopathic pneumonia
Obliterative bronchiolitis

Gastrointestinal manifestations of conditioning-related toxicities are common. Desquamation of the oropharyngeal and gastrointestinal mucosa (mucositis) secondary to high-dose radiotherapy and administration of antimetabolites generally occurs within the first 3 weeks after transplantation. The mucositis and the opiate analgesics administered to temper the pain increase the risk of pulmonary aspiration and necessitate intravenous alimentation.

Although relatively uncommon, congestive cardiomyopathies and pleuropericarditis syndromes associated with preparative regimens involving cyclophosphamide and anthracycline are seen occasionally. Central nervous system (CNS) complications also may be seen with specific drug treatments. Both Guillain-Barré syndrome and peripheral neuropathies have been described after cytarabine treatment. Toxicity due to cyclosporine may cause an altered sensorium and coma. Complications of cancer therapy, such as cyclophosphamide-induced hemorrhagic cystitis, tumor lysis syndromes, and chemotherapy-related neurologic and pulmonary reactions, also may be observed.

RELAPSE AND REJECTION

Relapse of the primary malignancy and rejection of the donor marrow are fatal complications. Fortunately, immune-mediated graft rejection is relatively uncommon (<1% of patients) in recipients of HLA-identical marrow prepared with total body irradiation (TBI). Its incidence rises with increasing degree of HLA disparity and is also elevated in previously transfused patients with aplastic anemia who were not prepared with TBI. Recurrence of malignancy after transplantation is seen in approximately 20% of patients who undergo transplantation while in early-stage leukemia (i.e., in a first remission or a chronic phase) and in 50% to 70% of patients who undergo transplantation while in advanced leukemia (a relapse or blast crisis).[6] Most relapses occur with host-type cells and signal ineffective antineoplastic treatment. Extramedullary conditioning–related toxicities limit the intensity of the cytoreductive regimens that can be used. A second transplantation following repeat preparative conditioning may be successful, but mortality remains high owing to prolonged pancytopenia.

TABLE 73-2 Grading of GVHD

Grade	Degree of Organ Involvement
1	+ to ++ skin rash; no gut involvement; no liver involvement; no decrease in clinical performance
2	+ to +++ skin rash; + gut involvement or + liver involvement (or both); mild decrease in clinical performance
3	++ to +++ skin rash; ++ to +++ gut involvement or ++ to +++ liver involvement (or both); marked decrease in clinical performance
4	Similar to grade 3 but with ++ to ++++ organ involvement and extreme decrease in clinical performance

GRAFT-VERSUS-HOST DISEASE

This clinicopathologic syndrome is an immunologic reaction of donor lymphocytes to "foreign" antigens present on the surface of host cells. Transplantation (HLA) antigens are important, as are "minor" antigens not detected by current typing techniques. Overall, acute GVHD occurs in 20% to 50% of allograft recipients and in up to 80% of recipients of HLA-nonidentical grafts.[6] GVHD is categorized as acute or chronic according to time of presentation, organ involvement, and histology.

ACUTE GVHD
Incidence
Acute GVHD occurs within the first 3 months after HSCT. The reactions are seen in 20% to 50% of HLA-identical marrow recipients. The incidence increases with patient age and with the degree of HLA disparity between host and donor.

Manifestations
The histologic hallmark of acute GVHD is lymphocytic infiltration of the epidermis and gastrointestinal tract. The clinical syndrome is composed of dermatitis, enteritis, and hepatitis. The severity of GVHD is commonly determined by a grading system (Table 73-2). The grade depends on the stage of GVHD in the skin, liver, and gut (Table 73-3). Fever, diffuse macular dermatitis (often leading to bullae and desquamation), cramping abdominal pain, watery to bloody diarrhea, and jaundice with cholestasis and hepatocellular necrosis may be seen. The most dramatic presentation, in the absence of prophylactic immunosuppression occurs as early as 7 days after HSCT. This hyperacute GVHD is accompanied by exfoliative dermatitis, shock, and hyperpyrexia. Mortality increases with increasing severity of acute GVHD and often is related to associated infectious complications.

Immunology
The principal effector cells responsible for GVHD appear to be immunocompetent donor cytotoxic T-lymphocytes. These cells differentiate and proliferate in response to host histocompatibility antigens. It is likely that lymphokine production from sensitized lymphocytes recruits additional effector mononuclear cells to participate in the alloimmune response.

Although histocompatibility matching is an important first step in trying to reduce the severity of acute GVHD, this tactic alone is ineffective in preventing GVHD. Almost all recipients of unmodified allogeneic marrow develop GVHD if not given posttransplant immunosuppression. Methotrexate and cyclosporine appear to be equally effective in decreasing the incidence of acute GVHD. Their combined use gives better results than the use of either agent alone. Attempts at removing donor T-lymphocytes from the marrow inoculum have been effective in lessening GVHD, but this advantage is offset by an increase in the rates of graft rejection and recurrent leukemia.

CHRONIC GVHD
Incidence
Chronic GVHD is seen in 20% to 50% of allograft recipients. It develops more than 3 months after HSCT. While it usually occurs in patients who experienced acute GVHD, 20% to 30% of cases occur in patients without prior acute GVHD.

Manifestations
Chronic GVHD mainly involves skin, mucous membranes, and liver. The characteristic pigmentation and sclerosis of the skin, lichenoid oral plaques, esophagitis, polyserositis, and oral and ophthalmic sicca syndrome resemble the manifestations of collagen-vascular disorders. Elevated alkaline phosphatase and transaminase levels occur in 90% of patients. Chronic wasting due to anorexia is common in untreated patients. Chronic pulmonary diseases are seen in 10% to 20% of patients and are divided between diffuse pneumonias and obliterative bronchiolitis.

Mortality from chronic GVHD is related to type of onset and extent of the disease. Mortality is lower when the disease is limited to the skin and liver and when it occurs in the absence of prior acute GVHD. Death is usually caused by infection.

Immunology
Minor differences in histocompatibility antigens and deficient thymic function may play a role in the immunopathogenesis of chronic GVHD. Patients with GVHD have an increase in

TABLE 73-3 Staging of Acute GVHD

Stage	Skin	Liver	Gut
+	Maculopapular rash over <25% body surface	Bilirubin level, 2–3 mg/dL	Diarrhea of 500–1000 mL/day
++	Maculopapular rash over 25% to 50% body surface	Bilirubin level, 3–6 mg/dL	Diarrhea of 1000–1500 mL/day
+++	Generalized erythroderma	Bilirubin level, 6–15 mg/dL	Diarrhea of >1500 mL/day
++++	Desquamation and bullae	Bilirubin level, >15 mg/dL	Pain or ileus

nonspecific suppressor lymphocyte function and lack the specific suppression of cytotoxic reactivity to host alloantigens. Cytokine mediators may propagate autoimmune-like tissue injury.

Chronic immunodeficiency persists as long as the disease is active and places these patients at risk for opportunistic infection. Immunoglobulin deficiencies are common and likely are responsible for the increased incidence of fatal infections with *Streptococcus pneumoniae*.

HEPATIC VENO-OCCLUSIVE DISEASE

Liver disease is a common and complex problem after HSCT. The most serious complication is hepatic veno-occlusive disease (VOD) (Table 73-4).

Incidence

The incidence of hepatic VOD ranges from less than 2% among patients who undergo transplantation for nonmalignant conditions without TBI conditioning to 20% to 60% for those with malignancy who undergo conditioning with chemotherapy and TBI. Higher rates are seen with increasing age of marrow recipients and prior hepatitis. The mortality rate of hepatic VOD is approximately 30%. There is no known effective treatment, although there has been some recent interest in defibrotide, a novel oligodeoxyribonucleotide.[7]

Presentation

Hepatic VOD is distinguished from other liver diseases in part by the timing of presentation. Occurring within 2 weeks of HSCT, it appears earlier than hepatic manifestations of acute GVHD. Typically seen are progressive weight gain with peripheral edema, a peaking of hepatic enzyme levels within 2 weeks, jaundice, ascites, and painful hepatomegaly. Metabolic encephalopathy and renal failure consistent with the hepatorenal syndrome may occur.

Pathogenesis

The pathologic lesion is terminal hepatic venule occlusion and hemorrhage. Subendothelial thickening with edema and deposition of fibrin and clotting factors is later replaced by cellular debris and a fibrotic reaction involving terminal venules and sinusoids. Hepatocellular injury around the terminal venule is prominent.

Endothelial cell damage from high-dose chemoradiotherapy is a likely inciting event. Deposition of coagulants and microthrombosis probably lead to venular obstruction. The resulting passive congestion and ischemia cause necrosis of surrounding hepatocytes. Toxicities of antimetabolic drugs and viral hepatitis may impair cellular metabolic repair mechanisms and contribute to hepatic injury.

PNEUMONIA

Incidence and Pathogenesis

Historically, pneumonia develops in 40% to 60% of HSCT recipients; however, the rate may be substantially lower among those undergoing nonmyeloablative transplants.[8–10] Both infectious and noninfectious etiologies are seen, and the prevalence of these varies with the time after HSCT (Table 73-5).

TABLE 73-4 Gastrointestinal Disease after Marrow Transplantation

	Pretransplant	DAYS AFTER TRANSPLANTATION		
		Days 0–20	Days 20–100	Beyond Day 100
Liver disease	Viral hepatitis, leukemia, drug effect, tuberculosis	VOD, bacteremia, drug effect, fungal infection, parenteral nutrition, early GVHD	Acute GVHD, viral hepatitis, persistent VOD, fungal infection, drug effect, EBV lymphoma	Chronic GVHD, viral hepatitis (chronic), drug effect, infection (mycobacteria)
Ascites	—	VOD, peritonitis	Persistent VOD, acute GVHD, peritonitis, hepatic vein obstruction, pericarditis, pancreatitis	Chronic hepatitis (viral, chronic GVHD)
Diarrhea	Fungal infection, parasites, drug effect	Conditioning therapy, drug effect, infection, early GVHD	Acute GVHD, infection, drug effect	Persistent acute GVHD, infection, bacterial overgrowth (chronic GVHD)
Nausea/ vomiting	Bacteremia, liver disease, drug effect	Conditioning therapy, drug effect, infection, early GVHD	Infection (herpesvirus), acute GVHD, drug effect	Drug effect, chronic GVHD
Esophageal symptoms	Infection, reflux esophagitis	Esophagitis (fungal, bacterial)	Esophagitis (viral), reflux esophagitis	Chronic GVHD, reflux esophagitis
Intestinal bleeding	Peptic ulcer	Esophagitis (infections), "stress ulcers," Mallory-Weiss tears	Esophagitis (infections), "stress ulcers," GVHD, viral ulcers (mostly CMV), EBV lymphoma	Persistent acute GVHD
Abdominal pain	—	VOD, conditioning therapy enteritis	Acute GVHD, infection, drug effect (ileus), liver abscess, cholecystitis, peritonitis, pancreatitis, cystitis, herpes zoster	Persistent acute GVHD, infection

SOURCE: Adapted from McDonald et al.[33]

TABLE 73-5 Incidence of Common Etiologies for Pulmonary Infiltrates after BMT

Complications	Approximate Incidence, %
COMPLICATIONS WITHIN 100 DAYS	
Pulmonary edema syndromes	0–50
Infectious pneumonia	20–30
Bacterial	2–30
Fungal	4–13
Viral	4–10
Protozoal	<5
Idiopathic pneumonia	7–12
Pulmonary VOD	Rare
COMPLICATIONS AFTER 100 DAYS	
Bacterial bronchopneumonia	20–30
Idiopathic pneumonia	10–20
Viral pneumonia	0–10
Obliterative bronchiolitis*	2–11

*Obstructive airflow among marrow recipients with chronic GVHD

INFECTIOUS PNEUMONIA

The true incidence of bacterial bronchopneumonia is unknown but ranges from 2% (documented by open lung biopsy) to over 25% (noted at autopsy).[11] Commonly isolated bacteria can include *Pseudomonas aeruginosa, Mycobacterium avium* complex, *Enterobacter cloacae*, and *Serratia*.[12,13] The frequency of invasive fungal disease due to *Aspergillus, Zygomycetes*, and *Candida* species is increasing. *Aspergillus* infection most often involves the lung and is seen in 10% to 25% of patients with HSCT.[4,5] Both fiberoptic bronchoscopy and fine-needle aspiration may be useful in diagnosing *Aspergillus* infection.[12,14,15] Invasive *Candida* infection is also prevalent in HSCT patients, and autopsy data suggest that 50% of infected patients have pulmonary involvement.[11,16] *Zygomycetes* appears to be an emerging pathogen that has a particularly rapidly progressive course and is reported to occur in up to 1.2% of HSCT patients.[17,18]

Cytomegalovirus (CMV) pneumonia occurs primarily among HSCT recipients with previous CMV infection (documented by positive serology) or in seronegative recipients who receive stem cells from seropositive donors. Among seronegative recipients of seronegative stem cells, use of either seronegative or leukocyte-filtered blood products markedly decreases the rate of CMV infection.[19] In the absence of pre-emptive antiviral therapy, between 30 and 150 days after HSCT, 60% to 80% of diffuse pneumonias are due to CMV.[20,21] The rate of CMV pneumonia can be reduced dramatically by the administration of ganciclovir either prophylactically or at the time of first viral excretion.[22] Other herpes-group viruses, such as herpes simplex virus (HSV) and varicella-zoster virus (VZV), are seen less commonly because of the prophylactic administration of acyclovir. Likewise, *Pneumocystis carinii* pneumonia (PCP) is rare after a pretransplant course of trimethoprim-sulfamethoxazole prophylaxis. Respiratory syncytial virus (RSV) and parainfluenza virus are common causes of diffuse pneumonia during outbreaks in the community.

NONINFECTIOUS CAUSES OF PULMONARY INFILTRATES

In 20% to 30% of patients with suspected pneumonia after HSCT, no infection is demonstrated. The causes of noninfectious pulmonary disease after HSCT include pulmonary hemorrhage, edema, acute respiratory distress syndrome (ARDS), idiopathic interstitial pneumonia, and drug toxicity. Less common are thromboemboli, vasculopathy, and a leukemic/lymphoma infiltrate. Lymphangitic carcinoma also may be present. Noninfectious pneumonia is recognized to represent a spectrum of lung injuries owing to multiple causes with a common clinical presentation. These diffuse noninfectious pneumonias are now referred to collectively as the *idiopathic pneumonia syndrome*[23] (Table 73-6).

Presentation

The etiologies and severity of the lung diseases seen vary with the time after HSCT. Focal or patchy infiltrates in the first 30 days after HSCT (a period of granulocytopenia) frequently represent bacterial or fungal infection. Bacteria are an unusual cause for diffuse infiltrates. Focal radiographic lesions with a masslike appearance that develop or persist despite antibiotics are pulmonary fungal infections in most cases.[15,24] Occasionally, *Pseudomonas, Legionella,* and rarely, *Nocardia* species are identified in localized lesions.

Pulmonary edema related to excess intravascular fluid administration, cardiotoxic chemotherapy, or ARDS from chemoradiotherapy injury or sepsis, in addition to pulmonary hemorrhage (diffuse alveolar hemorrhage) due to thrombocytopenia, cause most diffuse infiltrates occurring in the first 30 days. These patients frequently suffer from multiorgan disease owing to conditioning-related toxicities or grade 2 to 4 (moderate to severe) acute GVHD. Thus pancytopenia, hepatic and renal failure, desquamating skin lesions, and mucositis complicate both evaluation and management. Within 30 days, diffuse infiltrates often are acute in onset and progress rapidly to respiratory failure. During this time, respiratory syncytial virus and parainfluenza virus are the major infectious causes of diffuse infiltrates, particularly during endemic months.[25]

Beyond 30 days, viral pneumonias, especially CMV, predominate as causes for diffuse pulmonary infiltrates in seropositive patients not receiving ganciclovir. Onset ranges from insidious to rapid progression from tachypnea to hypoxia with respiratory failure. Unfortunately, similar presentations are seen with idiopathic pneumonia or PCP. There is little to distinguish these etiologies clinically. After 30 days, the CMV pneumonia is usually milder and slower in onset. However, progression to profound respiratory failure often follows.

Late after HSCT (>100 days), diffuse pulmonary disease is most often insidious in onset. These late pneumonias occur predominantly among allogeneic marrow recipients with chronic GVHD.[26] Viral pneumonias (CMV or VZV) are seen but become less common after day 100. *Pneumocystis* infection occasionally presents in patients with chronic GVHD and inadequate trimethoprim-sulfamethoxazole prophylaxis. Late-onset noninfectious pneumonia, possibly due to late radiation- or cyclophosphamide-induced pulmonary damage, is identical in presentation clinically to other diffuse pneumonias.

TABLE 73-6 Criteria for Diagnosis of Idiopathic Pneumonia Syndrome

1. Evidence of widespread alveolar injury:
   - Multilobar infiltrates on chest radiography or computed tomography
   - Symptoms and signs of pneumonia
   - Evidence of abnormal physiology
   and
2. Absence of active lower respiratory tract infection documented by:
   - Negative bronchoalveolar lavage, lung biopsy, or autopsy with examination of stains and cultures for bacteria, fungi, and viruses, including cytomegalovirus (CMV) centrifugation culture, cytology for viral inclusions and *Pneumocystis carinii*, and immunofluorescence monoclonal antibody staining for CMV, respiratory syncytial virus, influenza virus, parainfluenza virus, and adenovirus.

OBLITERATIVE BRONCHIOLITIS

Incidence

Early estimates suggest that about 10% of allogeneic HSCT recipients develop progressive airflow obstruction usually more than 3 months after HSCT. However, more recent estimates, which use less stringent airflow obstruction parameters, indicate that the incidence may be as high as 26% overall and up to 32% incidence among patients with chronic GVHD.[27] The major risk factor is chronic GVHD, and most, but not all, patients have an obliterative bronchiolitis pattern histologically.[28] Other significant risk factors include age greater than 60 years at the time of transplant and pretransplant FEV_1/FVC ratio of less than 70%.[27] The relationship between airflow obstruction and GVHD has led to speculation that expression of class II histocompatibility antigen on bronchial epithelial cells triggers a cytotoxic lymphocyte response.

Manifestations

The diagnosis depends on demonstration of airflow obstruction by pulmonary function testing. Some HSCT recipients are asymptomatic when this alteration is detected. Typical manifestations are insidious progression of dyspnea on exertion and cough.[29,30] There may be few physical findings, and the chest radiograph may be normal. Rarely, the onset is acute, and profound wheezing is noted, particularly when symptoms are seen early after HSCT. Both viral and fungal airway infections may present similarly.

Although this disorder often is progressive and results in death because of respiratory failure, the rapidity of onset and rate of progression predict the outcome. Control of chronic GVHD with increased immunosuppression may achieve stabilization of the airway disease.

Diagnosis and Management of HSCT Complications

PRINCIPLES OF CARE

INFECTION CONTROL

Infection is a major cause of morbidity and mortality among severely immunosuppressed HSCT recipients. Prophylactic daily administration of oral trimethoprim-sulfamethoxazole for the 2 weeks prior to HSCT and twice weekly after adequate granulocyte engraftment has virtually eliminated the occurrence of PCP. Patients with sulfa allergies should undergo desensitization. Prophylaxis with either pentamidine or dapsone is associated with more failures than trimethoprim-sulfamethoxazole.[31]

Prophylactic measures have decreased the incidence of herpesvirus infections. Pretransplant serologic testing identifies previously infected recipients who are at risk for reactivation infection with CMV and HSV. Transmission of CMV infection can be avoided by providing the recipient with blood products from CMV-seronegative donors.[19] Similarly, the rate of HSV reactivation after HSCT can be reduced by prophylactic treatment with acyclovir after HSCT. Surprisingly, this treatment also decreases the incidence of CMV infection by about a third, even though acyclovir has little in vitro activity against CMV. The use of ganciclovir as prophylaxis for seropositive patients or as pre-emptive treatment at the first evidence of viral excretion or viremia significantly reduces the incidence of CMV pneumonia.[22]

GVHD PROPHYLAXIS

Morbidity and mortality increase with increasing grades of GVHD. GVHD causes direct organ damage and may lead to fatal hepatic failure, gastrointestinal bleeding, or diffuse exfoliative dermatitis. In addition, it increases the incidence of other potentially fatal complications, such as CMV enteritis, pneumonia, and bacterial and fungal infection. Virtually all allograft recipients who do not receive in vivo immunosuppressive prophylaxis develop acute GVHD. As noted earlier, prophylaxis with a combination of methotrexate and cyclosporine decreases the incidence of acute GVHD to about 25%.

SEPSIS SYNDROME

Hypotension and fever are common in marrow recipients, especially during the period of neutropenia. Whereas the basic approach to these situations is similar to that described elsewhere for other neutropenic hosts (see Chap. 47), the HSCT recipient poses several distinct problems.

Bloodstream infection is noted in up to 50% of HSCT recipients, and coagulase-negative staphylococci and *Candida* species predominate. This prevalence influences antibiotic choices and frequently prompts the empirical addition of antistaphylococcal and antifungal agents.

Systemic viral infections are seen with higher frequency after HSCT than after conventional chemotherapy. Herpesviruses, CMV in particular, almost uniformly reactivate after allogeneic HSCT in previously infected patients who develop acute GVHD, and the infection may present with a septic appearance. CMV viremia has been associated with high cardiac output and a low systemic vascular resistance (SVR), which are suggestive of the sepsis syndrome. It is unclear whether this response is due to viremia or to concomitant processes often associated with CMV infection, such as GVHD.

A diagnostic dilemma posed by sepsis syndrome is differentiation of true bacterial or fungal sepsis from acute GVHD. The cardiovascular responses to systemic cytotoxic lymphocyte activation in acute GVHD may be indistinguishable from those of endotoxemia. As with endotoxemia, acute GVHD may be associated with high levels of circulating tumor necrosis factor (TNF) and other vasoactive cytokines. In our experience, a profoundly decreased SVR and relative hypotension are seen with the acute onset of GVHD. In patients with uncompromised myocardial function, stroke volume increases, and cardiac output may exceed three times normal. These patients have fever, diffuse cutaneous hyperemia, and bounding peripheral and precordial pulses. Diffuse pulmonary infiltrates, azotemia, and altered sensorium may follow in severely ill patients.

GVHD increases the risk of infection and subsequent sepsis, and the two conditions often coexist. Allogeneic HSCT recipients with clinical sepsis therefore should be presumed to have infection. Empirical antibiotic coverage should be started and modified on the basis of culture results and local patterns of endemic infection and resistance. The assessment of potential GVHD should be made on clinical grounds and biopsy of appropriate tissues. Often the pattern of dermatitis strongly suggests acute GVHD, and biopsy may confirm this suspicion.

Confounding the evaluation and treatment of sepsis syndrome in the marrow recipient is the frequent finding of relative intravascular volume expansion. Up to 50% of HSCT recipients develop pulmonary edema within the first weeks after HSCT. This problem generally is attributable to excessive administration of crystalloid fluids. In addition to exogenous fluid administration, intravascular volume is often replete owing to fluid and sodium retention from hepatic VOD. Thus brisk volume replacement often is not necessary in these patients to maintain arterial blood pressure when SVR declines. However, blood loss, often from occult gastrointestinal sources, may complicate the volume management of the marrow recipient with sepsis.

One critical determinant of survival in such situations appears to be cardiac function. An inability to respond with an increased cardiac output is associated with high mortality. The clinical assessment of the intravascular volume necessary to provide adequate left ventricular filling is extremely difficult in these rapidly changing patients. Given the potential complexities of diagnosis and management, central hemodynamic monitoring may be useful to guide fluid and vasoactive therapy. Positive inotropic support may be provided for patients who have an inadequate stroke volume despite "normal" pulmonary artery occlusion pressures.

GVHD

Diagnosis and management of acute GVHD are crucial to success in allogeneic HSCT. These aspects of care often involve the critical care physician in collaboration with the oncologist. Acute GVHD occurs most frequently during the initial

hospitalization for HSCT. Such patients are at risk of death as a result of multisystem involvement by the GVHD and frequently require intensive care management. In addition to the acute illness associated with the onset of acute GVHD, risks of potentially fatal bacterial or fungal infection are also present.

In contrast to acute GVHD, chronic GVHD mainly represents a limitation to long-term survival. The major life-threatening problems relate to infectious complications resulting from prolonged deficits in antigen-specific antibody production, increased nonspecific suppressor lymphocyte activity, and phagocytic dysfunction. Thus acute disseminated bacterial infections and opportunistic pulmonary infections pose the greatest threats. These occur primarily in the ambulatory care setting and only later involve the critical care physician.

ACUTE GVHD

Since acute GVHD is a clinicopathologic syndrome, the presentation may only suggest the diagnosis. Dermatitis, jaundice, and enteritis may be caused by various insults, such as chemoradiotherapy, disseminated infection, or drug toxicity. Histologic confirmation of the diagnosis is made by biopsy (often repeated) of affected organs. Skin is involved most often and is biopsied; however, liver and gastrointestinal tract are also amenable to this approach. Thus invasive procedures usually are necessary to confirm the diagnosis of acute GVHD in the presence of skin, liver, or gastrointestinal tract disease. Occasionally, fever is the major manifestation, and biopsy of other organs is too risky. In this case, "blind" biopsy of skin becomes necessary for diagnosis.

However, verification of the diagnosis does not eliminate the possibility of coexisting causes of similar features, such as infection. Repeated blood cultures should be prompted by persistent fever. Nausea and vomiting should be evaluated by endoscopy to exclude viral, bacterial, or fungal infection, and diarrheal stool should be examined and stained for bacterial pathogens. Vigilant search for other etiologies should continue. Exfoliative dermatitis should be biopsied to exclude toxic epidermal necrolysis due to drug sensitivity. Liver and endoscopic gastrointestinal tract biopsies may be necessary to exclude infectious complications.

Treatment of established acute GVHD is often difficult. Current strategies use increased immunosuppression with corticosteroids (methylprednisolone, 2 mg/kg per day), antithymocyte globulin (ATG), and continued methotrexate and cyclosporine administration.[32] The survival rates for steroid-resistant GVHD are poor, and death is most often due to infection. The administration of monoclonal antibodies directed against T-lymphocytes shows promise as a method of "turning off" the disease.

Supportive care of the marrow recipient with acute GVHD assumes great importance because of the difficulties posed by treatment and the threat of fatal infectious complications. Continued surveillance for viral, bacterial, or fungal infection is mandatory. A chest x-ray is obtained at least weekly, and abnormalities are evaluated aggressively. Prophylactic broad-spectrum antibiotics should be continued for the duration of neutropenia or in the presence of fever and immunosuppressive therapy.

Adequate nutrition is vital but often poses problems in the presence of severe enteric GVHD. Malabsorption is common, and return to oral feeding often is delayed. Total parenteral nutrition (TPN) may be required for prolonged periods. Cramping and diarrhea may necessitate parenteral opiate analgesics, even at the risk of ileus.

Depression of marrow function and systemic viral infection sometimes are manifestations of severe acute GVHD. Thrombocytopenia due to decreased platelet production may be compounded by rapid turnover because of fever and bleeding. Support of hemostasis usually requires repeated transfusions of platelets. Vitamin K should be given when the prothrombin time is elevated, but it may fail to correct the problem in the presence of hepatic failure, necessitating the administration of plasma to correct the hemostatic defect. Bleeding from the gastrointestinal tract is common and may be severe. A thorough evaluation for the site(s) of severe or persistent bleeding is recommended. Often diffuse intestinal hemorrhage because of ulceration from GVHD is found at endoscopy. However, focal bleeding from infectious ulcers or peptic disease may be identified. Angiography or nuclear medicine studies may be useful, and surgical correction of localized bleeding may be successful.

HEPATIC FAILURE

Differential Diagnosis

Liver disease is common after HSCT. The etiologies are varied, and their interactions are complex (see Table 73-4). Hepatic VOD and GVHD account for the majority of cases and, in part, can be differentiated on the basis of time of presentation and biochemical patterns.[33] However, drug toxicities (of cyclosporine, antibiotics, and antimetabolites) and infections, especially viral (hepatitis B, hepatitis C, CMV, HSV, and EBV) and bacterial or fungal, also may cause liver disease. Renal impairment prevents the normal excretion of conjugated bilirubin, and continued hemolysis contributes to jaundice beyond that expected for the degree of liver disease.

Levels of hepatic transaminases rise and peak within 2 weeks of transplantation in hepatic VOD. Fluid retention and jaundice develop early in the course and may be severe. Hepatic VOD must be distinguished from passive hepatic congestion from right-sided heart failure, pancreatitis, hepatic vein thrombosis, invasive fungal disease, or septicemia with peritonitis.

Liver disease due to GVHD tends to occur after day 20 and in the presence of clinical disease in other organs. Elevations in alkaline phosphatase may peak at 20 times normal levels, much higher than seen in hepatic VOD.

Imaging modalities such as computed tomographic (CT) scanning and ultrasonography are useful in defining liver density, focal lesions, collateral circulation, and the presence of ascites. Percutaneous liver biopsy carries risks of hemorrhage in thrombocytopenic patients but may be critical in defining pathology and providing culture material in difficult cases. Transjugular approaches to the hepatic vein for liver biopsy may prove to be safer. Occasionally, paracentesis is required to exclude fungal or bacterial infection and to relieve pressure in patients with respiratory embarrassment.

Management

The management of VOD of the liver is primarily supportive and may be ineffective in preventing progressive hepatic failure. Restriction of fluid and sodium intake, along with judicious use of loop diuretics, may prevent extracellular fluid accumulation. However, ascites and edema often develop prior to overt jaundice and suggest that active sodium retention owing to renal disturbance is important. A major cause of mortality is the development of the hepatorenal syndrome. Care must be exercised to avoid compromising renal perfusion while trying to decrease ascites. Intravascular volume usually is maintained with replacement of blood products to ensure renal perfusion. However, hemodialysis may be necessary. Renal failure in these settings is often multifactorial. The administration of multiple nephrotoxic drugs appears to play a part.

Surgical shunting procedures to decompress the portal circulation are risky and have unproven benefit in this setting. Management of ascites with peritoneovenous shunt likewise poses great risks. Potential treatments to limit venule obstruction by microthrombosis may include prophylactic anticoagulation or thrombolytic therapy. This theoretical approach is certainly not without risk in the setting of prolonged thrombocytopenia. Thrombolytic therapy with recombinant tissue plasminogen activator has been successful in improving hepatic blood flow in some patients. This therapy is associated with a case-fatality rate of 10% and a response rate of 40% to 50%, and it should be used only for patients likely to die. Defibrotide, an agent with antithrombotic properties, as well as potentially beneficial endothelial effects, has been reported to be effective in some patients with hepatic VOD, particularly when given early in the course.[7]

Liver disease caused by GVHD requires intensive therapy for the GVHD. Specific interventions do not appear to be beneficial. Hepatic encephalopathy is approached as it is with any chronic liver disease (see Chap. 84). Modifications in dietary protein intake and clearing of the gastrointestinal tract with lactulose should be instituted.

PNEUMONIA

DIAGNOSTIC APPROACH

The clinical presentations of pulmonary disease after HSCT have been reviewed in this chapter and in the recent literature.[3,34] The diagnostic approach to pulmonary disease after HSCT differs from that for other categories of immunosuppressed hosts owing to the difference in prevalence of specific etiologies.

In the 30 days after HSCT, also referred to as the *preengraftment* or *neutropenic phase*, there is a low prevalence of infectious causes for diffuse pulmonary infiltrates.[8] Empirical treatment with broad-spectrum antibiotics is recommended, and diuresis and sodium restriction frequently improve the clinical status of the patient. Occasionally, pulmonary artery wedge measurement (or cardiac echocardiography) may be helpful to exclude pulmonary edema and guide therapy. Correction of bleeding disorders, including adequate platelet support, and maintenance of euvolemia may help to prevent further pulmonary hemorrhage, if present. If clinical deterioration ensues or respiratory viruses such as respiratory syncytial virus are present in the community, nasal saline irrigation and/or fiberoptic bronchoscopy with bronchoalveolar lavage (BAL) is recommended to exclude treatable pulmonary infection.[35]

More than 30 days after HSCT, most centers perform fiberoptic bronchoscopy with BAL, unless pulmonary edema is strongly suspected as the cause of diffuse pulmonary infiltrates. These specimens are processed with rapid-detection techniques for viral pathogens, especially CMV. The techniques include direct fluorescent monoclonal antibody stains and centrifugation culture (shell vial) for CMV.[21,36] High sensitivity for the detection of virus in as little as 16 hours has been reported for these tests. In addition to bacterial, fungal, and cytologic stains, a quantitative bacterial culture is performed.

Experience has shown that in the HSCT recipient, open lung biopsy for the evaluation of diffuse infiltrates is unlikely to reveal pathogens not detectable by BAL. Thoracotomy may be reserved for HSCT recipients with nondiagnostic BAL (sometimes repeated) who have high risk of undiagnosed infection, such as *P. carinii* infection, if prophylaxis was not given.

Focal pulmonary lesions are evaluated aggressively because these more likely represent bacterial or fungal infection. CT scan of the chest often reveals a masslike appearance of the lesion with a zone of attenuation highly suggestive of invasive pulmonary fungal infection. Additional lesions not appreciated on plain chest radiograph also may be seen. This finding often alters the approach to diagnosis.

The diagnostic approach to localized lesions in part depends on their radiographic appearance and location(s). Areas of bronchopneumonia usually can be approached with fiberoptic bronchoscopy and BAL. Peripheral lesions may be amenable to percutaneous needle aspiration biopsy for diagnosis; the diagnostic yield for masslike lesions is about 67%, but the negative predictive value is only 50%.[24] Thus a nondiagnostic evaluation should prompt repeat of the procedures or progression to more definitive measures. The most definitive study appears to be biopsy at thoracotomy. Complete surgical resection of pulmonary fungal infection may be both diagnostic and curative in selected patients.

TREATMENT

Bacterial Pneumonia

Fever in the HSCT recipient should be presumed to represent bacterial infection, and empirical antibiotics should be given after appropriate samples for culturing are obtained. Management is identical to that for other immunosuppressed or neutropenic hosts (see Chap. 47). HSCT recipients have a high prevalence of coagulase-negative staphylococcal infections, yet it is unclear how often these infections cause pneumonia. Late after HSCT, chronic GVHD increases the prevalence of systemic pneumococcal infections and mandates prophylactic penicillin or trimethoprim-sulfamethoxazole for the duration of active disease.

Viral Pneumonia

CMV pneumonia previously was fatal in over 85% of affected HSCT recipients. Multiple experimental treatment modalities were unsuccessful in altering the outcome. Favorable responses to combination therapy with ganciclovir and high-titer anti-CMV immunoglobulin are reported.[36–38] Various treatment regimens have been used successfully, usually initially involving administration of ganciclovir 2.5 mg/kg every 8 hours for at least 2 weeks, together with CMV immune globulin 400 to 500 mg/kg three to five times weekly for between 2 and 3 weeks. In some series, continued therapy with lower-dose ganciclovir and CMV immune globulin for

a period of several weeks after successful therapy has been suggested to avoid early relapse.

Treatment of other herpes-group viruses is with intravenous acyclovir at doses of 500 mg/m^2 every 8 hours for at least 7 days. Except for CMV, HSV, and VZV, the efficacy of therapy for other viral respiratory infections in this setting remains unproven; however, there are anecdotal reports of success with aerosolized ribavirin, in combination with intravenous immunoglobulin, as treatment for respiratory syncytial virus and parainfluenza virus pneumonias, provided treatment is started early in the disease.

Fungal Pneumonia

Aspergillus species infection is documented in up to 18% of HSCT recipients, but also seen are *Mucormycosis, Fusarium, Rhizopus,* and *Petriellidium*.[39,40] Pulmonary involvement by filamentous fungi is the rule in infected patients. Disseminated yeast infection, especially with *C. albicans,* has declined; however, approximately 50% of patients with invasive *Candida* infection have pulmonary involvement.[16] Mortality rates are as high as 88% for these infections.[5,41]

The major risk factor for invasive fungal infections is the presence of GVHD; however, the level and duration of neutropenia, patient age, total number of other infections, and corticosteroid administration play significant roles.[39,40] The frequency of *Aspergillus* infections is similar between recipients of allogeneic and autologous transplants, but these tend to occur during periods of neutropenia prior to engraftment among autologous marrow recipients and after engraftment among allogeneic marrow recipients.[42] Autologous recipients have fewer *Candida* but not *Aspergillus* infections compared with allograft recipients. Emergence of resistant species (*C. krusei* and *C. glabrata*) is increasing and has been shown to be associated with the widespread use of fluconazole.[42–44]

Among 20 patients with *Aspergillus* infection detected during life and reported by Wingard,[39] only 1 recovered. Early diagnosis and treatment, however, may improve survival rates. Favorable outcome with pulmonary filamentous fungal infection has followed treatment with amphotericin at 1 mg/kg per day to a total dose of 2 g or more.[39,45] The optimal therapy and dosing for invasive aspergillosis has not been established but likely includes amphotericin. Although most successful treatment of these pulmonary fungal infections after HSCT also has included surgical resection, the precise role of surgery is not clear. Recovery by HSCT recipients without complete surgical resection has been noted. Adjunctive therapy with granulocyte transfusions and/or granulocyte colony-stimulating factor (G-CSF) remains investigational.

Treatment for invasive *Candida* infection also is largely empirical. Amphotericin in doses of at least 0.5 mg/kg per day until clinical response occurs is employed commonly. Alternative therapeutic approaches to deep-seated fungal infections recently became available. Recent advances in amphotericin B include the development of lipid formulations. The clinical responses to these formulations are as good (or as bad, depending on your perspective) as those seen with conventional amphotericin B. The reduced toxicity profiles allow administration of significantly higher doses of amphotericin B. However, it is unclear that these higher doses lead to improved efficacy.

The most frequently used second-generation triazole antifungal agent is itraconazole. In a prospective, randomized study in patients with hematologic malignancies, response rates were better (but not statistically different) for itraconazole (47%) compared with amphotericin B (38%) when used as empirical antifungal therapy.[46] There were no differences in rates of breakthrough fungal infection or deaths. However, the amphotericin B patients experienced significantly more drug-related adverse effects. Such studies suggest that itraconazole may be a reasonable alternative to conventional amphotericin B for empirical therapy.

Voriconazole is a newer triazole antifungal with a broad spectrum of activity against most human fungal pathogens, including *Candida, Aspergillus,* and *Cryptococcus* species, filamentous fungi, and dimorphic fungi. Twice-daily dosing (both intravenously and orally) is available. Studies suggest that voriconazole may be a reasonable alternative to either conventional amphotericin B or liposomal amphotericin.[47,48]

Caspofungin acetate represents the first of a new class of antifungal drugs (echinocandins or glucan synthesis inhibitors) that inhibit the synthesis of β-(1,3)-D-glucan, an integral component of the fungal cell wall. Of note, β-(1,3)-D-glucan is not present in mammalian cells. Caspofungin is not an inhibitor of any enzyme in the cytochrome P450 (CYP) system, unlike the triazoles. The agent has in vitro and in vivo activity against *Candida* species, *Aspergillus* species, and *Histoplasma capsulatum.* Caspofungin has a very low toxicity profile. Because it has a different site and mechanism of action, there is reason to believe that it may be useful in combination with currently available antifungals, such as amphotericin or the triazoles.

Other Infections

Management of *P. carinii, Legionella* species, *Nocardia,* and other unusual infections in HSCT recipients does not differ substantially from that used elsewhere. Few data exist to suggest that the outcome of these infections after HSCT is different from that in other patient populations. Survival is more closely related to the underlying immune deficiencies, GVHD, or conditioning-related toxicities.

Idiopathic Pneumonia

No proven treatment exists for the diffuse idiopathic pneumonia syndrome after HSCT.[23] A biopsy of the lung most often reveals a histologic pattern either of diffuse alveolar damage or mononuclear interstitial infiltrate. About 60% of patients die with progressive respiratory failure, whereas in 25% the process resolves.[49] Supportive management, including assisted mechanical ventilation, is appropriate. However, the overall mortality rate in patients requiring mechanical ventilatory support approaches 95% by 6 months after the insult.[50] Treatment of ARDS-like conditions after HSCT with corticosteroids has not been evaluated in clinical trials, but it is practiced routinely in many centers. We advocate managing idiopathic pneumonia, especially if it occurs more than 100 days after HSCT, in the same manner as idiopathic pulmonary fibrosis in the nontransplant population. In the presence of active GVHD, increased immunosuppression to control that condition is also advised. Improved outcome of patients with diffuse alveolar hemorrhage has been reported with corticosteroid therapy in uncontrolled studies.

Airflow Obstruction

Obstructive airflow in the presence of chronic GVHD is managed primarily by addressing the GVHD with increased immunosuppression. This approach has been noted to halt the progression of pulmonary disease in about half the cases. Improvement in airflow has been noted in only 8% of patients. Treatment and prevention of potential coexisting infection with early and aggressive antibiotic treatment and prophylactic trimethoprim-sulfamethoxazole are encouraged. Evaluation of possible airway infection with bronchoscopy before intensifying the immunosuppression is reasonable. Most patients with chronic GVHD and airflow obstruction have hypogammaglobulinemia. It has been proposed that this deficiency contributes to the pathogenesis of the airflow obstruction by permitting recurrent sinopulmonary infection. We recommend the routine intravenous replacement of immunoglobulin for those with low class or subclass levels.

Respiratory Failure

Studies of intensive care for respiratory failure of patients with cancer and hematologic malignancies have reported low survival rates. Approximately 3% of HCST recipients receiving mechanical ventilation survived to 6 months after transplantation.[51,52] Studies of pediatric HCST recipients find the same poor prognosis as noted among adults; however, limited studies suggest an improving survival trend.[53,54] Improvement in survival rates may be seen with increased use of noninvasive ventilation and earlier intervention, as well as with less intensive radiochemotherapy regimens ("mini-allotransplantation").[3,55]

Multiple-organ failures after HSCT appear to be based on common pathophysiologic derangements and are highly fatal. Pulmonary dysfunction, CNS dysfunction, and hepatic dysfunction are all associated with significant decreases in the levels of antithrombin III and protein C and an increase in the platelet transfusion requirement.[56] Patients with these organ dysfunctions have higher levels of interleukin 6, interleukin 10, and TNF-α than patients who never develop these complications. Mortality rates for patients with these organ dysfunctions vary from 15% in patients with only one organ dysfunction to 100% in patients who have progressed to all three. Patients who develop none of these organ dysfunctions have a mortality rate that approaches zero.[56]

Studies support the idea that severe multiorgan failure with mechanical ventilation after HSCT is fatal.[51,57] Severe lung injury combined with hemodynamic instability or hepatic-renal insufficiency is a sensitive and highly specific predictor of nonsurvival in mechanically ventilated marrow transplant recipients. These overwhelmingly negative results justify a standard of care for mechanically ventilated bone marrow transplant patients that restricts prolonged intensive care. Such information should be used to counsel patients and families to the expected outcomes of such situations.

References

1. Thomas ED, Storb R, Clift RA, et al: Bone-marrow transplantation (second of two parts). *N Engl J Med* 292:895, 1975.
2. Kernan NA, Bartsch G, Ash RC, et al: Analysis of 462 transplantations from unrelated donors facilitated by the National Marrow Donor Program. *N Engl J Med* 328:593, 1993.
3. Crawford SW: Respiratory disease in bone marrow and hematopoietic stem cell transplantation, in Elias JA, Fishman JA, Grippi MA, et al (eds): *Fishman's Pulmonary Disease and Disorders.* New York: McGraw-Hill, 1998, p 2137.

4. McWhinney PH, Kibbler CC, Hamon MD, et al: Progress in the diagnosis and management of aspergillosis in bone marrow transplantation: 13 years' experience. *Clin Infect Dis* 17:397, 1993.

5. Junghanss C, Marr KA, Carter RA, et al: Incidence and outcome of bacterial and fungal infections following nonmyeloablative compared with myeloablative allogenic hematopoietic stem cell transplantation: A matched control study. *Biol Blood Marrow Transplant* 8:512, 2002.

6. Sullivan K, Storb R: Bone marrow transplantation and graft-versus-host disease, in Brend L, Sells R (eds): *Bailliere's Clinical Immunology and Allergy*. London: Bailliere Tindall, 1989. p 91.

7. Corbacioglu S, Greil J, Peters C, et al: Defibrotide in the treatment of children with veno-occlusive disease (VOD): A retrospective multicentre study demonstrates therapeutic efficacy upon early intervention. *Bone Marrow Transplant* 33:189, 2004.

8. Crawford SW, Hackman RC, Clark JG: Open lung biopsy diagnosis of diffuse pulmonary infiltrates after marrow transplantation. *Chest* 94:949, 1988.

9. Krowka MJ, Rosenow EC III, Hoagland HC: Pulmonary complications of bone marrow transplantation. *Chest* 87:237, 1985.

10. Khouri IF, Keating M, Korbling M, et al: Transplant-lite: induction of graft-versus-malignancy using fludarabine-based nonablative chemotherapy and allogeneic blood progenitor-cell transplantation as treatment for lymphoid malignancies. *J Clin Oncol* 16:2817, 1998.

11. Hackman R: Lower respiratory tract, in Sale G, Shulman H (eds): *The Pathology of Bone Marrow Transplantation*. New York: Masson. 1984, p 156.

12. Feinstein MB, Mokhtari M, Ferreiro R, et al: Fiberoptic bronchoscopy in allogeneic bone marrow transplantation: Findings in the era of serum cytomegalovirus antigen surveillance. *Chest* 120:1094, 2001.

13. Jain P, Sandur S, Meli Y, et al: Role of flexible bronchoscopy in immunocompromised patients with lung infiltrates. *Chest* 125:712, 2004.

14. Jantunen E, Piilonen A, Volin L, et al: Diagnostic aspects of invasive *Aspergillus* infections in allogeneic BMT recipients. *Bone Marrow Transplant* 25:867, 2000.

15. Jantunen E, Piilonen A, Volin L, et al: Radiologically guided fine needle lung biopsies in the evaluation of focal pulmonary lesions in allogeneic stem cell transplant recipients. *Bone Marrow Transplant* 29:353, 2002.

16. Goodrich JM, Reed EC, Mori M, et al: Clinical features and analysis of risk factors for invasive candidal infection after marrow transplantation. *J Infect Dis* 164:731, 1991.

17. Morrison VA, Haake RJ, Weisdorf DJ: Non-*Candida* fungal infections after bone marrow transplantation: Risk factors and outcome. *Am J Med* 96:497, 1994.

18. Penalver FJ, Romero R, Fores R, et al: Mucormycosis and hemopoietic transplants. *Haematologica* 83:950, 1998.

19. Bowden RA, Sayers M, Flournoy N, et al: Cytomegalovirus immune globulin and seronegative blood products to prevent primary cytomegalovirus infection after marrow transplantation. *New Engl J Med* 314:1006, 1986

20. Meyers JD, Flournoy N, Thomas ED: Nonbacterial pneumonia after allogeneic marrow transplantation: A review of ten years' experience. *Rev Infect Dis* 4:1119, 1982.

21. Crawford SW, Bowden RA, Hackman RC, et al: Rapid detection of cytomegalovirus pulmonary infection by bronchoalveolar lavage and centrifugation culture. *Ann Intern Med* 108:180, 1988.

22. Goodrich JM, Boeckh M, Bowden R: Strategies for the prevention of cytomegalovirus disease after marrow transplantation. *Clin Infect Dis* 19:287, 1994.

23. Clark JG, Hansen JA, Hertz MI, et al: NHLBI workshop summary: Idiopathic pneumonia syndrome after bone marrow transplantation. *Am Rev Respir Dis* 147:1601, 1993.

24. Crawford SW, Hackman RC, Clark JG: Biopsy diagnosis and clinical outcome of persistent focal pulmonary lesions after marrow transplantation. *Transplantation* 48:266, 1989.

25. Chakrabarti S, Avivi I, Mackinnon S, et al: Respiratory virus infections in transplant recipients after reduced-intensity conditioning with Campath-1H: High incidence but low mortality. *Br J Haematol* 119:1125, 2002.

26. Wingard JR, Santos GW, Saral R: Late-onset interstitial pneumonia following allogeneic bone marrow transplantation. *Transplantation* 39:21, 2002.

27. Chien JW, Martin PJ, Gooley TA, et al: Airflow obstruction after myeloablative allogeneic hematopoietic stem cell transplantation. *Am J Respir Crit Care Med* 168:208, 2003.

28. Chan CK, Hyland RH, Hutcheon MA, et al: Small-airways disease in recipients of allogeneic bone marrow transplants: An analysis of 11 cases and a review of the literature. *Medicine* 66:327, 1987.

29. Crawford SW, Clark JG: Bronchiolitis associated with bone marrow transplantation. *Clin Chest Med* 14:741, 1993.

30. Afessa B, Litzow MR, Tefferi A: Bronchiolitis obliterans and other late onset non-infectious pulmonary complications in hematopoietic stem cell transplantation. *Bone Marrow Transplant* 28:425, 2001.

31. Souza JP, Boeckh M, Gooley TA, et al: High rates of *Pneumocystis carinii* pneumonia in allogeneic blood and marrow transplant recipients receiving dapsone prophylaxis. *Clin Infect Dis* 29:1467, 1999.

32. Sullivan KM: Acute and chronic graft-versus-host disease in man. *Int J Cell Clon* 4(suppl 1):42, 1986.

33. McDonald GB, Shulman HM, Sullivan KM, Spencer GD: Intestinal and hepatic complications of human bone marrow transplantation, part I. *Gastroenterology* 90:460, 1986.

34. Duncker C, Dohr D, Harsdorf S, et al: Noninfectious lung complications are closely associated with chronic graft-versus-host disease: A single center study of incidence, risk factors and outcome. *Bone Marrow Transplant* 25:1263, 2000.

35. Wendt CH, Hertz MI: Respiratory syncytial virus and parainfluenza virus infections in the immunocompromised host. *Semin Respir Infect* 10:224, 1995.

36. Emanuel D, Cunningham I, Jules-Elysee K, et al: Cytomegalovirus pneumonia after bone marrow transplantation successfully treated with the combination of ganciclovir and high-dose intravenous immune globulin. *Ann Intern Med* 109:777, 1988.

37. Reed EC, Bowden RA, Dandliker PS, et al: Treatment of cytomegalovirus pneumonia with ganciclovir and intravenous cytomegalovirus immunoglobulin in patients with bone marrow transplants. *Ann Intern Med* 109:783, 1988.

38. Schmidt GM, Kovacs A, Zaia JA, et al: Ganciclovir immunoglobulin combination therapy for the treatment of human cytomegalovirus-associated interstitial pneumonia in bone marrow allograft recipients. *Transplantation* 46:905, 1988.

39. Wingard JR, Beals SU, Santos GW, et al: *Aspergillus* infections in bone marrow transplant recipients. *Bone Marrow Transplant* 2:175, 1987.

40. Martino R, Caballero MD, Canals C, et al: Reduced-intensity conditioning reduces the risk of severe infections after allogeneic peripheral blood stem cell transplantation. *Bone Marrow Transplant* 28:341, 2001.

41. Williamson EC, Millar MR, Steward CG, et al: Infections in adults undergoing unrelated donor bone marrow transplantation. *Br J Haematol* 104:560, 1999.

42. Goodman JL, Winston DJ, Greenfield RA, et al: A controlled trial of fluconazole to prevent fungal infections in patients undergoing bone marrow transplantation. *N Engl J Med* 326:845, 1992.

43. Marr KA, Seidel K, Slavin MA, et al: 2000. Prolonged fluconazole prophylaxis is associated with persistent protection against candidiasis-related death in allogeneic marrow transplant

recipients: Long-term follow-up of a randomized, placebo-controlled trial. *Blood* 96:2055, 1992.

44. Marr KA, Seidel K, White TC, Bowden RA: Candidemia in allogeneic blood and marrow transplant recipients: Evolution of risk factors after the adoption of prophylactic fluconazole. *J Infect Dis* 181:309, 2000.

45. Boutati EI, Anaissie EJ: *Fusarium*, a significant emerging pathogen in patients with hematologic malignancy: Ten years' experience at a cancer center and implications for management. *Blood* 90:999, 1997.

46. Boogaerts M, Winston DJ, Bow EJ, et al: Intravenous and oral itraconazole versus intravenous amphotericin B deoxycholate as empirical antifungal therapy for persistent fever in neutropenic patients with cancer who are receiving broad-spectrum antibacterial therapy: A randomized, controlled trial. *Ann Intern Med* 135:412, 2001.

47. Herbrecht R, Denning DW, Patterson TF, et al: Voriconazole versus amphotericin B for primary therapy of invasive aspergillosis. *N Engl J Med* 347:408, 2002.

48. Walsh TJ, Pappas P, Winston DJ, et al: Voriconazole compared with liposomal amphotericin B for empirical antifungal therapy in patients with neutropenia and persistent fever. *N Engl J Med* 346:225, 2002.

49. Kantrow SP, Hackman RC, Boeckh M, et al: Idiopathic pneumonia syndrome: Changing spectrum of lung injury after marrow transplantation. *Transplantation* 63:1079, 1997.

50. Crawford SW, Petersen FB: Long-term survival from respiratory failure after marrow transplantation for malignancy. *Am Rev Respir Dis* 145:510, 1992.

51. Faber-Langendoen K, Caplan AL, McGlave PB: Survival of adult bone marrow transplant patients receiving mechanical ventilation: A case for restricted use. *Bone Marrow Transplant* 12:501, 1993.

52. Crawford SW, Schwartz DA, Petersen FB, Clark JG: Mechanical ventilation after marrow transplantation. Risk factors and clinical outcome. *AmRev Respir Dis* 137:682, 1988.

53. Todd K, Wiley F, Landaw E, et al: Survival outcome among 54 intubated pediatric bone marrow transplant patients. *Crit Care Med* 22:171, 1994.

54. Nichols DG, Walker LK, Wingard JR, et al: Predictors of acute respiratory failure after bone marrow transplantation in children. *Crit Care Med* 22:1485, 1994.

55. Azoulay E, Alberti C, Bornstain C, et al: Improved survival in cancer patients requiring mechanical ventilatory support: Impact of noninvasive mechanical ventilatory support. *Crit Care Med* 29:519, 2001.

56. Haire WD: Multiple organ dysfunction syndrome in hematopoietic stem cell transplantation. *Crit Care Med* 30:S257, 2002.

57. Rubenfeld GD, Crawford SW: Withdrawing life support from mechanically ventilated recipients of bone marrow transplants: A case for evidence-based guidelines. *Ann Intern Med* 125:625, 1996.

Chapter 74 _____

TOXICITIES OF CHEMOTHERAPY

APURVA A. DESAI
GINI FLEMING

KEY POINTS

- *Drug toxicity is most often a diagnosis of exclusion.*
- *Dose, schedule, and drug combinations are key parameters used to determine the likelihood of drug toxicity.*
- *Not all toxicities are known, and drug regimens are modified constantly.*
- *Therapy is supportive for most chemotherapy-related toxicities.*
- *Pelvic and spinal irradiation potentiates the myelosuppressive effects of chemotherapeutic agents.*
- *Bleomycin and gemcitabine are among the causes of drug-related interstitial lung disease.*
- *Most cardiac events in cancer patients are related to pre-existing heart disease or direct invasion of the heart by cancer; nonetheless, drug toxicity must be considered, particularly when high-dose cyclophosphamide and anthracyclines have been administered.*
- *In high-dose regimens, cytosine arabinoside, ifosfamide, and methotrexate may produce dramatic central nervous system syndromes.*
- *Renal injury is often dose limiting for cisplatin.*
- *Cytokines such as interleukin-2 have a wide range of toxicities involving virtually all organ systems.*
- *Many commonly used chemotherapeutic agents and several recently introduced targeted anticancer agents are associated with hypersensitivity reactions.*
- *Thrombotic microangiopathy is associated with various chemotherapeutic agents, particularly gemcitabine and mitomycin-C.*

As more intensive anticancer regimens are being used to achieve cure, an increasing number of oncology patients are admitted to ICUs for complications of treatment. Several principles about drug-induced toxicity should be kept in mind.

Drug toxicity is often a diagnosis of exclusion. The toxic reaction to an antineoplastic drug or drugs is frequently nonspecific clinically and even pathologically. Other causes always should be considered. Infection, a tumor effect, and toxicity from other drugs such as antiemetics or antibiotics frequently are elements of the differential diagnosis.

Dose, schedule, and combination make a difference. Most antineoplastic drugs are given in combination, and drugs and radiation are often combined. The toxicities of a given combination may be more severe than the effects of the individual agents would suggest. Moreover, different drug schedules, such as a continuous infusion versus a single bolus dose, may have very different spectrums of side effects for the same agent. Formerly, the dose-limiting toxicity of most agents was myelosuppression, but the introduction of

colony-stimulating factors and the rapidly increasing use of autologous stem cell or marrow reinfusion for rescue after very-high-dose drug regimens have exposed a plethora of new toxicities.

Not all toxicities are known. New drugs and new combinations of drugs are being tried constantly and may be used widely before all toxicities are well characterized. Moreover, the diagnosis of drug reactions that are sporadic rather than dose-related is often difficult, particularly in cancer patients who have many symptoms regardless of treatment. The tables in this chapter list the most common or notorious toxicities and are not intended to be comprehensive.

Treatment is supportive. The importance of a diagnosis of treatment-related toxicity is generally that the offending agent can be stopped, and useless remedies or diagnostic procedures can be withheld. Only rarely is specific therapy indicated.

Fever and Hypersensitivity Reactions[1]

A great many commonly used antineoplastic agents can cause acute hypersensitivity reactions. These are particularly common with L-asparaginase, taxanes (paclitaxel and docetaxel), and platinum agents. None of these drugs should be administered without antianaphylaxis medications close at hand. Hypersensitivity reactions were the treatment-limiting factor in early trials of paclitaxel, and this agent is now administered routinely after premedication with corticosteroids and antihistamines, which has significantly reduced the incidence of severe reactions. For the taxanes, the reactions may be related partly to the excipients in which they are formulated. With platinum agents, the hypersensitivity often occurs in the second or third use of the regimen. Several recently approved monoclonal antibodies such as rituximab (RITUXAN) and trastuzumab (HERCEPTIN) are also associated with hypersensitivity reactions.[2,3] Most of the hypersensitivity reactions associated with antibodies can be managed by slowing the rate of infusion of the agent and by premedicating patients with corticosteroids and antihistamines.

Antitumor drugs also may cause fever in the absence of other symptoms of allergy. Bleomycin, which may cause very high fevers, is particularly notorious. Febrile reactions are also often observed with cytarabine.

Myelosuppression[4,5]

Complications of myelosuppression, including infections and bleeding, account for many therapy-related ICU admissions in cancer patients. Management of these problems is discussed elsewhere. Granulocytes (circulating half-life = 6 hours) usually are affected the earliest and most severely, followed by platelets (half-life = 5 to 7 days); red blood cells (RBCs) (half-life = 120 days) are relatively spared unless the patient has received high doses or multiple courses of chemotherapy. Bleeding and other causes of anemia must be considered before a very low hemoglobin level is attributed to antineoplastic chemotherapy alone. There is variation in which cell lines are most suppressed; the nitrosoureas and mitomycin C, for example, typically produce a late, severe thrombocytopenia. For most drugs, the granulocyte count reaches its nadir 7 to 14 days after the administration of a

TABLE 74-1 Granulocytopenia Induced by Antineoplastic Drugs

Drug	Nadir, days	Recovery, days
Most agents	7–14	21–28
Busulfan	21–28	42–56
Melphalan	21	28–40
Mitomycin C	21–28	40–55
Nitrosoureas (BCNU, CCNU)	21–28	35–60

single dose, and recovery occurs by 21 to 28 days. Some agents produce a more delayed pattern (Table 74-1). Patients who have received pelvic or spinal irradiation or who have had multiple courses of chemotherapy suffer more severe and prolonged myelosuppression. The critically ill cancer patient also may have a multitude of other causes for cytopenias, but if doubt exists as to the cause of abnormal blood counts, a bone marrow biopsy should be performed. This procedure can be performed safely on even the sickest patients and is an invaluable aid in excluding many possible diagnoses, particularly marrow infiltration by tumor. Hematopoietic growth factors, such as granulocyte colony-stimulating factor (G-CSF), may be useful in some circumstances.[6] Empirical institution of broad-spectrum antibiotic therapy based on clinical presentation can be lifesaving for febrile neutropenic patients.[7]

Mucositis and Diarrhea[4]

Like the cells in the bone marrow, cells of the gastrointestinal tract, from mouth to rectum, proliferate rapidly and therefore are particularly susceptible to damage by antineoplastic drugs. The effects of toxicity range from mild mouth sores to ulcerative stomatitis and severe bloody diarrhea. Breakdown of the mucosal barrier also contributes to morbidity and mortality by providing a portal for the entry of infectious agents, particularly in a neutropenic patient. Agents that commonly cause stomatitis or diarrhea at standard doses are listed in Table 74-2. High-dose chemotherapy regimens used in preparation for bone marrow transplantation frequently cause severe mucositis.

TREATMENT

Candida and herpesviruses commonly cause or worsen stomatitis and esophagitis. *Clostridium difficile* always should be

TABLE 74-2 Antineoplastic Drugs that Cause Stomatitis or Diarrhea

Drug	Effects
Anthracyclines	Stomatitis
Bleomycin	Stomatitis
5-Fluorouracil	Stomatitis, anal sores, diarrhea
Capecitabine	Stomatitis, diarrhea
Cytarabine	Stomatitis, diarrhea
Cyclophosphamide	Stomatitis
Dactinomycin	Stomatitis, diarrhea
Taxanes	Stomatitis
Vinca alkaloids	Stomatitis
Methotrexate	Stomatitis
Irinotecan (CPT-11)	Diarrhea
Gefitinib	Diarrhea

considered in hospitalized patients with diarrhea, particularly those receiving antibiotics, even if they also have received diarrhea-producing anticancer therapy.

Patients' mouths should be kept scrupulously clean with the use of soft swabs and saline or peroxide rinses. The discomfort caused by stomatitis may be severe. If topical anesthetics do not control the pain, systemic narcotics should be administered in ample doses. Diarrhea and stomatitis often severely compromise enteral feeding. Intravenous alimentation should be considered early.

IRINOTECAN[8]

Irinotecan (CPT-11) is an agent used frequently in the treatment of colon cancer and is somewhat unusual in having severe diarrhea in the absence of mucositis as one of its most significant side effects. Two distinct types of diarrhea have been described. The first is an early-onset diarrhea occurring during infusion of the drug or within 30 minutes of infusion. This reaction is part of an acute cholinergic response and can be controlled with atropine, 0.5 to 1.0 mg intravenously. The second type usually appears 6 to 10 days after drug administration, may be linked to a secretory process in the small intestine, and can be massive (>10 L/d). Early recognition and aggressive treatment with loperamide and octreotide can be useful in controlling this late-onset diarrhea.

Pulmonary Toxicity

A large number of antineoplastic drugs can cause pulmonary symptoms (Table 74-3). Furthermore, lungs are a common site for metastases and infections, complicating the diagnostic process in patients with advanced cancer. Pulmonary toxicity syndromes reported include acute pleuritic chest pain, hypersensitivity lung disease, and noncardiogenic pulmonary edema,[9–12] but the vast majority of cases fall into the pneumonitis/fibrosis category described below. This type of toxicity classically is associated with the "three B's": busulfan, bleomycin, and BCNU (carmustine), and for many agents, it is sporadic rather than dose related.[11] Methotrexate lung toxicity may be similar in terms of symptoms but is believed to be a form of hypersensitivity reaction.[13–15] Unlike lung toxicity associated with other antitumor agents, it also may be associated with hilar adenopathy. Some of the newly approved agents, such as all-*trans*-retinoic acid (tretinoin) and gefitinib (IRESSA) have been associated with unique pulmonary toxicities.[16–18] All-*trans*-retinoic acid (ATRA, TRETINOIN) is a derivative of vitamin A used in the treatment of acute promyelocytic leukemia (APL). It is associated with the unique *retinoic acid syndrome,* consisting of high fever, fluid retention, pulmonary infiltrates, and respiratory distress, which may occur in as many as 25% of APL patients treated with ATRA. This can be seen as soon as 2 days after beginning therapy. The syndrome has been attributed to pulmonary leukostasis but is not always associated with exceedingly high peripheral white blood cell (WBC) counts. Treatment with dexamethasone may be helpful. Gefitinib, an oral inhibitor of the epidermal growth factor receptor (EGFR) tyrosine kinase, was approved for the treatment of refractory lung cancer and has been reported to cause interstitial lung

TABLE 74-3 Antineoplastic Drugs that Have Pulmonary Toxicity

Agent	Type of Toxicity	Incidence, %	Comments
Bleomycin	Pneumonitis/fibrosis	2–40	Chest x-ray may be atypical; eosinophilia may be seen on lung biopsy; steroids felt to be useful
	Hypersensitivity pneumonitis	Rare	
	Acute chest pain	Rare	Substernal pressure or pleuritic pain; self-limited over 4–72 h
Busulfan	Pneumonitis/fibrosis	4	Insidious onset after prolonged therapy; poor prognosis
Carmustine (BCNU)	Pneumonitis/fibrosis	20–30	Toxicity is dose-related; common in pretransplantation regimens; effects may appear years after therapy has ended
Cyclophosphamide	Pneumonitis/fibrosis	<1	May potentiate toxicity of bleomycin, BCNU
High-dose cytarabine	Noncardiogenic pulmonary edema	4–20	Care is supportive, but corticosteroids are occasionally helpful; prognosis is variable
Gemcitabine	Noncardiogenic plumonary edema	1–5	Care is supportive, but corticosteroids are occasionally helpful; prognosis is variable
Methotrexate	Hypersensitivity pneumonitis	8	Prognosis is good; dramatic response to corticosteroids reported
	Acute pleuritic pain	Rare	May be associated with pleural effusion or friction rub; subsides over 3–5 days
	Noncardiogenic pulmonary edema	Rare	Few reports, most with intrathecal injection
Mitomycin C	Pneumonitis/fibrosis	3–12	High mortality reported
Procarbazine	Acute hypersensitivity		Onset within hours after drug dose; recovery rapid
Tretinoin (ATRA)	Retinoic acid syndrome	10–20	Corticosteroids suggested
Vinorelbine	Acute dyspnea	5	Readily reversible chest pain
Gefitinib	Interstitial lung disease	1–3	One-third of cases can be fatal
Trastuzumab	Organizing pneumonia	Rare	Case reports only

disease (ILD) in about 1% of the patients worldwide; approximately one-third of the reported cases have been fatal.[18] Patients often present with acute onset of dyspnea, with or without cough and low-grade fever. Prompt discontinuation of the agent with adequate supportive care is recommended when ILD is suspected. Trastuzumab also has been reported recently to cause organizing pneumonia[19]; however, details regarding the prevalence or underlying mechanisms of the toxicity are not well understood. If such pulmonary toxicity is determined eventually to be class-specific, then as an increasing number of monoclonal antibodies get approved for the treatment of cancer, such toxicities will become more common.

CLINICAL PRESENTATION

The onset of pneumonitis/fibrosis associated with the classic cytotoxic agents may occur after prolonged, continuous treatment, as is typical for busulfan; after only a few cycles of therapy, as may occur with bleomycin; or even years after therapy has ended, as can occur with BCNU. Signs and symptoms frequently are nonspecific and range from mild to life threatening. Patients invariably present with dyspnea. A dry cough, fatigue, fever, and end-expiratory rales are common but not universal features. Hemoptysis is not typical, and this finding should suggest another diagnosis. The symptoms typically appear gradually over several weeks, but acute presentations are not unusual. A patient with this disorder who is ill enough to arrive in the ICU generally will be hypoxic, with diffuse pulmonary infiltrates visible on chest x-ray, and the full spectrum of possible causes for this presentation, including infection, irradiation, cardiogenic edema, pulmonary embolus, hemorrhage, leukoagglutinin reaction, and progressive tumor, must be considered.

HISTOPATHOLOGY

The histopathology closely resembles that of idiopathic diffuse interstitial pulmonary fibrosis. There is endothelial cell swelling, necrosis of type I pneumocytes, and atypical proliferation of type II pneumocytes, with generalized fibrosis in end-stage disease. The character of the inflammatory infiltrate, when one is present, is variable; a finding of eosinophilia suggests a hypersensitivity reaction, which may be particularly responsive to corticosteroids.[14,15]

DIAGNOSTIC TESTING

The chest x-ray in drug-associated pneumonitis/fibrosis generally is normal or reveals a basilar or diffuse reticulonodular pattern, but atypical findings on chest x-ray should not rule out this diagnosis. Bleomycin is particularly notorious for occasionally producing a nodular appearance, which may mimic recurrent tumor, and methotrexate may be associated with a pleural effusion or hilar adenopathy. Pulmonary function tests reveal a reduced diffusing capacity for carbon monoxide (DL_{CO}) and, sometimes, a restrictive ventilatory defect. Since the histologic findings are not specific, even a lung biopsy may not absolutely establish the diagnosis of drug-induced toxicity, although it is usually helpful. In the case of acutely ill cancer patients with hypoxia and diffuse pulmonary infiltrates, both the choice of which patients are appropriate candidates for lung biopsy and the timing of the procedure remain controversial.[20,21]

TREATMENT

Treatment for drug-associated pneumonitis/fibrosis is supportive. The precipitating agent should be discontinued. While there are no good data establishing the efficacy of

TABLE 74-4 Antineoplastic Drugs that Have Cardiac Toxicity

Drug	Effect	Incidence, %	Comments
Anthracyclines	Acute ECG changes	Common	Almost always benign and reversible
	Acute myocarditis/ pericarditis syndrome	Rare	
	Chronic cardiomyopathy	1–2	May appear years after treatment
Cyclophosphamide	Acute hemorrhagic cardiac necrosis	Unusual	Only in very high doses
5-Fluorouracil/Capecitabine	Angina/myocardial infarction	Rare	Usually within hours of drug dose; asymptomatic ECG changes more common
Mitoxantrone	Cardiomyopathy	1–2	Drug is structurally related to anthracyclines, but incidence of cardiomyopathy is probably somewhat less; risk is <1% if cumulative dose < 120 mg/m^2
Paclitaxel	Arrhythmias	10–20	Most common is asymptomatic bradycardia
Vinca alkaloids	Angina/myocardial infarction	Rare	Scattered case reports
Trastuzumab	Cardiomyopathy	More common when combined with chemotherapy	Often managed medically

corticosteroid therapy, there are many anecdotal reports of its usefulness, and it is often given a trial. The syndrome may be reversible, particularly in mild cases, or it may be progressive even in the absence of further exposure to the drug.

BLEOMYCIN[22]

Bleomycin is a particularly frequent and well-studied cause of pneumonitis. Bleomycin is thought to cause direct injury to the pulmonary capillary endothelium and type I pneumocytes, which leads to stimulation of an inflammatory cascade. Bleomycin toxicity is sporadic rather than dose related below a threshold cumulative total dose of 450 to 500 mg; above this threshold, the incidence rises dramatically.

Attempts have been made to predict and prevent pulmonary toxicity by serially monitoring the $D_{L_{CO}}$. Stopping therapy in patients with a significant decrease in $D_{L_{CO}}$ is strongly recommended, but this practice has not been shown to alter the incidence of fatal toxicity. Many patients may present with acute decline in pulmonary function weeks to months after a normal $D_{L_{CO}}$. Age over 70 years, prior or concurrent radiation therapy to the lungs, and concurrent treatment with cyclophosphamide or methotrexate are reported to potentiate bleomycin lung toxicity. Pre-existing lung disease has not been shown to be a risk factor.

The danger posed by oxygen therapy after treatment with bleomycin is a source of some controversy in the scant literature on the subject. Some small studies have reported a high incidence of severe postoperative respiratory distress in bleomycin-treated patients, which they attributed to a high intraoperative concentration of inspired oxygen ($F_{I_{O_2}}$).[22–24] Most authors recommend limiting intra- and perioperative $F_{I_{O_2}}$ in these patients to the lowest safe concentrations.

Cardiovascular Toxicity[25]

The vast majority of cardiac events in cancer patients are related to pre-existing heart disease or to involvement of the myocardium or pericardium by tumor, not to anticancer drugs, most of which produce cardiac damage rarely and sporadically, if at all (Table 74-4). Anthracyclines are the exception. Doxorubicin and daunorubicin have very similar effects on the heart; doxorubicin is used much more commonly, and its cardiac effects have been better studied. Trastuzumab also has been reported to cause cardiac dysfunction in patients that is similar to the cardiomyopathy associated with anthracycline therapy.[26] Cardiovascular toxicity is also associated with the use of immunomodulatory agents such as interferon and interleukin-2 (IL-2), which will be addressed separately in the section describing the toxicities associated with biologic agents.

ELECTROCARDIOGRAPHIC CHANGES AND ARRHYTHMIAS

Cisplatin and other drugs may produce secondary effects through alterations in plasma potassium, calcium, and magnesium levels. Direct effects appear to be caused mainly by the anthracyclines and paclitaxel. Electrocardiographic (ECG) changes occur in up to 40% of patients during doxorubicin infusion. The most frequently noted effects are nonspecific ST-T wave changes, but premature atrial and ventricular contractions, sinus tachycardia, and decreased QRS voltage are also common; almost every conceivable type of arrhythmia has been reported. While sudden death attributed to acute anthracycline-induced arrhythmia has been reported, it is extremely rare; cardiac monitoring during drug infusion is not warranted. The ECG changes are, with the possible exception of the decreased QRS voltage, transient. They are not a reason to discontinue therapy and are not associated with the subsequent development of heart failure.

PACLITAXEL[27,28]

Paclitaxel causes asymptomatic, reversible sinus bradycardia, with heart rates ranging from 30 to 50 beats per minute, in up to 29% of patients during a 24-hour infusion. More serious bradyarrhythmias, including third-degree heart block, have been observed but are rare. Myocardial infarction and atrial and ventricular tachyarrhythmias also have been noted, but their relationship to paclitaxel therapy is uncertain.

MYOCARDIAL ISCHEMIA AND INFARCTION[29]

Anticancer drugs very rarely cause myocardial ischemia or infarction. Radiation therapy to the heart may result in accelerated atherogenesis, but this effect becomes symptomatic only years after treatment. The vinca alkaloids have been reported to precipitate myocardial infarction in a few instances, sometimes when given with bleomycin, which is known to cause Raynaud's phenomenon and other vasospastic symptoms. Up to 4% of patients treated with 5-fluorouracil (5-FU) have been reported to suffer anginal symptoms, and a greater number have transient asymptomatic ECG changes suggestive of ischemia[30]; prolonged infusions appear to cause more problems. Myocardial infarction may occur. The mechanism is unknown, but agents such as nitrates and calcium channel blockers, which reverse vasospasm, may be helpful. Capecitabine, an orally administered prodrug of 5-FU, causes many of the toxicities associated with prolonged infusion of 5-FU, including cardiac toxicities.[31]

CARDIOMYOPATHY AND PERICARDITIS

The anthracyclines and high-dose cyclophosphamide may produce fatal cardiomyopathies. Trastuzumab, which is used in the treatment of breast cancer, also has been associated with cardiomyopathy.

ANTHRACYCLINES AND TRASTUZUMAB[26,32–35]

The *myocarditis-pericarditis syndrome* consists of an acute drop in ejection fraction seen in the hours to weeks after drug administration. This reaction sometimes is associated with a pericardial effusion and may result in the sudden death of the patient from severe congestive failure. Fortunately, it is exceedingly rare.

The classic subacute presentation of cardiomyopathy, on the other hand, develops in from 1% to 10% of patients receiving 550 mg/m^2 of doxorubicin, with a steep rise in incidence in patients treated with cumulative doses greater than 600 mg/m^2. Symptoms usually appear around 30 to 60 days after what appears to have been the precipitating dose of doxorubicin, but they may be noted a year or more after the end of treatment. Patients develop tachycardia, dyspnea, cardiomegaly, and peripheral and pulmonary edema. Pathologic changes are similar to those seen in cardiomyopathy of other causes.

Total dose is the single most important risk factor for the development of doxorubicin-related cardiomyopathy. There is no cutoff dose below which cardiomyopathy never occurs. Many patients, even those with severe failure, respond well to conventional therapy, and the ejection fraction gradually may return toward normal. However, some of these patients have recurrent symptoms 5 or more years later. Less commonly, such late cardiac decompensation is seen in patients who never had subacute symptoms. There has been particular concern over anthracycline-treated survivors of childhood cancers, up to 57% of whom have abnormalities of left ventricular contractility after treatment. Adults, however, are affected by late cardiac symptoms as well, and these sequelae may occur in patients who received only moderate cumulative doses of doxorubicin. There is no specific therapy

for anthracycline-induced cardiotoxicity once it has occurred; care is supportive. Further administration of anthracycline is contraindicated.

Detailed data analyses from various clinical trials conducted with trastuzumab[26] suggest that its cardiotoxic potential is highest when it is used with other chemotherapeutic agents, especially anthraclines. Single-agent therapy with trastuzumab seems to be safer, and most patients' clinical symptoms are well controlled with congestive heart failure therapy. Ongoing clinical trials with the agent potentially will provide greater insight into the risk factors and mechanisms that lead to the cardiac dysfunction associated with this agent.

CYCLOPHOSPHAMIDE AND IFOSFAMIDE[25,36,37]

Both cyclophosphamide and ifosfamide have minimal cardiac toxicity at standard doses. However, when used at high doses, both agents can cause severe myopericarditis and arrhythmias. The major nonhematologic dose-limiting toxicity of cyclophosphamide is a severe hemorrhagic myopericarditis, which usually is seen only at doses higher than 1.5 g/m^2, as are used typically in marrow-ablative regimens. Total ifosfamide doses far in excess of 1000 mg/m^2 usually have been associated with cardiotoxicity, and these patients generally develop cardiac toxicity within 2 weeks of receiving the drug. In its most virulent form, cyclophosphamide-induced cardiotoxicity appears within 48 hours of the last drug dose. Patients die rapidly of cardiogenic shock. More typically, edema, tachycardia, and tachypnea develop 7 to 10 days after therapy, usually preceded by a decrease in QRS amplitude on the electrocardiogram. Not all patients who have a decrease in QRS amplitude will develop symptoms. However, a hemorrhagic or serosanguineous pericardial effusion develops frequently, with possible signs of tamponade. Pericardiocentesis usually does not produce any clinical improvement, possibly because of the severity of the underlying myocardial damage.

Treatment is supportive. If patients survive the acute phase, complete recovery can be expected, and there may be no residual evidence of cardiac damage even at autopsy.

Neurotoxicity[1]

Only rarely will the neurologic toxicity (Table 74-5) of an anticancer drug be severe enough to be the primary reason for admission to the ICU. Neurologic problems are common in cancer patients, but local effects of tumor produce most of them, e.g., brain or epidural metastases. The antiemetic and pain medications given to patients often include combinations of high doses of corticosteroids, narcotics, and benzodiazepines, all of which can cause dramatic neurologic changes that must be considered when symptoms developing acutely after therapy are being evaluated.

PERIPHERAL NEUROPATHY

Peripheral neuropathies are frequent side effects of some very widely used anticancer drugs. Paclitaxel and docetaxel can cause glove-stocking paresthesias and, rarely, motor dysfunction. Symptoms often improve within months after therapy is stopped. Cisplatin likewise commonly causes a peripheral neuropathy that is primarily sensory and may progress to disabling ataxia. Symptoms may continue to worsen

TABLE 74-5 Antineoplastic Drugs that Have Neurologic Toxicity

Drug	Incidence, %	Comments
ENCEPHALOPATHY		
L-Asparaginase	25–50	Ranges from drowsiness to stupor; onset usually on the day after start of therapy; generally resolves rapidly when therapy is over
High-dose busulfan	15	Acute obtundation, seizures; prophylactic anticonvulsants often used
High-dose carmustine (BCNU)	10	Severe acute or chronic encephalomyelopathy; time of onset variable; usually not reversible
High-dose cytarabine	10–20	Ranges from disorientation to coma; onset usually 5–7 days after start of therapy; prognosis variable
Fludarabine	Rare at conventional doses	Optic neuritis, altered mental status, paralysis; may appear weeks after treatment
Hexamethylmelamine	Variable	Toxicity ranges from depression to hallucinations; usually reversible when drug is withdrawn
Ifosfamide	5–30	Frequency greater with higher doses; ranges from mild somnolence to coma; onset hours after infusion, recovery usually within days; use of methylene blue might reverse or shorten the duration of toxicity
High-dose methotrexate	2–15	Onset usually 1 week after administration; most common presentation is a strokelike syndrome; usually reversible
Mitotane	40	Lethargy, somnolence, dizziness, vertigo
Pentostatin	Rare at conventional doses	Lethargy, seizures, coma
Procarbazine	10	Usually mild drowsiness or depression, rarely stupor or manic psychosis
High-dose thio-TEPA	Dose-dependent	Somnolence, seizures, coma; dose limiting extramedullary toxicity
Vincristine/vinblastine	Rare	SIADH
ACUTE CEREBELLAR SYNDROME		
High-dose cytarabine	10–20	Ranges from mild dysarthria to disabling ataxia; onset is 5–7 days after start of therapy; prognosis is variable
5-Fluorouracil	<1	Usually seen with large bolus doses; reversible in 1–6 weeks
ACUTE PARAPLEGIA		
Intrathecal administration of cytarabine, methotrexate, thio-TEPA	Rare	These are the only drugs normally given intrathecally; all cause acute reversible arachnoiditis fairly often, paralysis exceedingly rarely; paralysis may or may not be reversible
PERIPHERAL NEUROPATHIES		
Cisplatin		Dose-dependent ototoxicity; distal sensory neuropathy
Oxaliplatin	Common	Acute and chronic sensory neuropathy; reversible pharyngolaryngeal dysesthesias; cold exposure may exacerbate symptoms
Hexamethylmelamine	Variable	Peripheral paresthesias and weakness
Procarbazine	10–20	Decreased tendon reflexes, mild distal paresthesias
Paclitaxel, docetaxel	Common	Distal sensory neuropathy
Vinca alkaloids	See text	Symmetric areflexia and distal paresthesias; symmetric motor weakness starting with dorsiflexors; jaw pain; cranial nerve palsies; paralytic ileus
Thalidomide		Peripheral neuropathy

ABBREVIATION: SIADH, syndrome of inappropriate antidiuretic hormone secretion.

after treatment is completed and may persist for years. Cisplatin also can cause tinnitus and deafness and, more rarely, Lhermitte's sign (painful electric shock–like sensations elicited by neck flexion or extension), autonomic neuropathy, seizures, transient cortical blindness, and retinal injury. Acute and chronic neuropathy also has been the dose-limiting toxicity of oxaliplatin, a recently approved third-generation platinum agent.[38] Oxaliplatin causes an acute and reversible sensory neuropathy in up to 95% of patients treated with the agent and causes a more chronic sensory neuropathy in 15% to 20% of patients who have received cumulative dose in excess of 780 mg/m^2. A few patients who have received more than 1000 mg/m^2 of the agent have been described to develop Lhermittes's sign and urinary retention. Most cases of chronic peripheral neuropathies associated with oxaliplatin have been reversible. An acute and reversible syndrome of pharyngolarngeal dysesthesias has been reported to occur in 1% to 2% of patients. This toxicity often is extremely distressing to the patient owing to the overwhelming sensation of difficulty with breathing and swallowing. These symptoms frequently are triggered or exaggerated by cold exposure. Given the disturbing subjective nature of the toxicity and the fact that it is common and reversible, all patients need to be educated regarding this toxicity to avoid panic and unnecessary medical interventions.

Vinca alkaloids are tubulin poisons that disrupt microtubule function in neuronal axons. Vincristine is the most neurotoxic vinca alkaloid. The most common toxic manifestation of vincristine is a symmetric mixed sensorimotor neuropathy, which may, in severe cases, progress to quadriparesis. It is dose related and gradual in onset. Deep tendon reflexes are lost. Peripheral nerve conduction velocities are characteristically normal despite severe clinical deficits. Paresthesias and motor weakness may or may not improve gradually. No treatment is known to heal vinca-related neuropathies. Vincristine has been administered intrathecally accidentally; this is invariably fatal.

The approval of thalidomide for the treatment of multiple myeloma has increased the clinical use of the agent. Both reversible and irreversible sensory neuropathies have been well documented with the use of thalidomide in up to 60% of patients with chronic use. Nerve conduction studies indicate that the symptoms most probably result from axonal damage. The symptoms can range from mild reversible parasthesias to more severe irreversible sensory neuropathies if the agent is not withdrawn in patients with progressive peripheral neuropathy. Central nervous system manifestations are common, including sedation, dizziness, muscle incoordination, fatigue, unsteady gait, tremulousness, mood changes, confusion, and weakness.[39,40]

CRANIAL NERVE PALSIES

Various cranial nerve palsies, including vocal cord paralysis, dysphagia, optic atrophy (rare), ptosis, ophthalmoplegias, and facial nerve paralysis, are seen in up to 10% of vincristine-treated patients. Unlike the peripheral nerve findings, cranial neuropathies may be abrupt in onset and mimic a brainstem stroke. They tend to be bilateral and usually are reversible with discontinuation of the drug.

AUTONOMIC NEUROPATHY

Autonomic symptoms, including ileus, bladder atony, impotence, and orthostatic hypotension, may occur even in patients with no sign of peripheral nerve toxicity. Severe paralytic ileus presenting as an acute abdomen is not rare and can occur acutely or following long-term administration of vincristine, vinblastine, or vinorelbine. It is usually reversible over the course of several days. Nasogastric tube drainage is the only standard therapy; metoclopramide has been reported to be helpful and may be tried if there is no suspicion of mechanical obstruction.

L-ASPARAGINASE

Between 25% and 50% of patients receiving L-asparaginase on a wide variety of dosing schedules will have some evidence of cerebral dysfunction, adults more often than children. The toxicity ranges from mild depression and drowsiness to confusion, stupor, and coma. Evidence of encephalopathy often occurs on the first day after administration and usually clears rapidly after the end of therapy. The syndrome resembles hepatic encephalopathy and may or may not be associated with high ammonia levels. The electroencephalogram (EEG) in most cases shows a diffuse slowing that returns to normal when the drug is stopped. L-Asparaginase itself does not cause focal neurologic abnormalities, but thrombotic and hemorrhagic cerebrovascular accidents due to asparaginase-induced clotting abnormalities have been reported. Patients on L-asparaginase can develop exceedingly low fibrinogen levels (with elevated prothrombin time), and this can be corrected with cryoprecipitate.

CYTOSINE ARABINOSIDE[41]

Cytosine arabinoside (Ara-C, cytarabine) is not neurotoxic when used at conventional doses (100 to 200 mg/m^2). However, at high doses (e.g., 2 to 3 g/m^2 twice daily, as given for the treatment of acute leukemia), a 10% to 20% incidence of cerebellar and cerebral toxicity is observed. Larger cumulative doses and age over 55 years are associated with more frequent and more irreversible neurologic damage.

The cerebellar changes are more common and usually more severe than the cerebral ones. The onset of symptoms is usually 5 to 7 days after the start of Ara-C therapy (within 24 hours of the final dose on a typical schedule). Mild cerebellar findings may include intention tremor, dysarthria, and horizontal nystagmus; in severe cases, limb and truncal ataxia may render the patient completely unable to walk or even eat unaided. Cerebral symptoms range from mild somnolence to disorientation, memory loss, and coma. Seizures have been reported. EEGs show diffuse slowing; findings on lumbar puncture and computed tomographic (CT) scan are normal. Toxicity may abate over a few days to weeks or may be irreversible. Rarely, it is fatal. Supportive care and withdrawal of Ara-C are the only therapies. Intrathecal Ara-C has not been associated with cerebellar toxicity, although it rarely may cause a paralysis similar to that described below with intrathecal methotrexate.

METHOTREXATE[42]

Like Ara-C, methotrexate used in conventional doses is not neurotoxic. However, when used at very high doses (1 to 7 g/m^2), cytotoxic levels are achieved in the cerebrospinal fluid (CSF), and a 2% to 15% incidence of various transient central nervous system (CNS) syndromes has been reported. The time of onset ranges from several hours to several weeks after treatment, with a mean of about a week. Signs develop abruptly and often resemble a stroke, with, for example, hemiplegia and a speech disorder. Neurologic findings may fluctuate; focal or generalized seizures are common. Electrolyte levels and results of radiologic studies are normal, EEGs show a variety of abnormalities, and examination of the CSF may or may not reveal an elevated protein level. The mechanism of these neurologic reactions is unknown, and care generally is supportive. There are reports that aminophylline can reverse early neurotoxicity in children, presumably by displacement of adenosine from its receptor by aminophylline.[43] In any case, patients recover completely over several days, and symptoms may or may not recur with subsequent courses.

Intrathecal methotrexate also can cause neurologic damage. The most common symptom is an acute arachnoiditis, which resolves over 12 to 72 hours without sequelae. Rarely, the presentation is severe enough to mimic bacterial meningitis. Very rarely, an acute reaction, which may include paralysis, cranial nerve palsies, or seizures, is seen. Examination of the CSF may show increased pressure, high protein concentrations, and a reactive pleocytosis. Recovery often, but not always, is complete. A necrotizing leukoencephalopathy sometimes occurs after the combination of cranial irradiation and intrathecal methotrexate, but this is a delayed effect that usually begins insidiously months after treatment.

IFOSFAMIDE[44,45]

High-dose ifosfamide therapy is associated with encephalopathy that can present with a wide variety of symptoms ranging from subtle sensorimotor deficits to severe mental status changes and even death. Early recognition of the toxicity and discontinuation of the agent are sufficient to reverse the toxicity over a period of 24 to 48 hours in most cases. Intravenous methylene blue can be useful in reversing the neurologic deficits associated with ifosfamide encephalopathy.

Renal and Urinary Toxicity[46]

Cisplatin is the only antineoplastic drug used frequently in current oncologic practice that causes renal failure at conventional doses. Hyperuricemic nephropathy with or without a full-blown tumor lysis syndrome may occur following rapid cell lysis in sensitive cancers with large tumor volumes; it is not the effect of any particular drug and is discussed elsewhere. Uric acid levels also can be rapidly lowered by the use of rasburicase.

Cyclophosphamide and ifosfamide can cause a hemorrhagic cystitis that is difficult to manage and occasionally is fatal and is described separately in the next section. Table 74-6 lists the common renal abnormalities caused by antineoplastic drugs.

CISPLATIN[47,48]

Renal injury characterized pathologically by focal necrosis of the distal tubules and collecting ducts is a dose-limiting toxicity of cisplatin. Acute renal failure can occur. Vigorous pretreatment hydration with saline solution minimizes but does not eliminate the damage; all patients will have some decline in glomerular filtration rate with a sufficient dose. Aminoglycoside therapy and pre-existing renal dysfunction are believed to increase the incidence. The creatinine level begins to rise a few days after therapy, peaks at 3 to 14 days, and then usually declines toward pretreatment levels. Toxicity is cumulative; multiple courses and higher doses produce more severe and less reversible damage.

Cisplatin also causes a variety of electrolyte disorders. Renal magnesium wasting, not necessarily associated with azotemia, is seen in half the patients receiving cisplatin and may persist for years. Although serum magnesium levels often are strikingly low, and symptomatic muscular irritability has been reported, most patients are asymptomatic. Of particular concern in the ICU are the hypocalcemia and hypokalemia that frequently accompany the magnesium wasting and that may be refractory to treatment if serum magnesium levels are not corrected first. Aminoglycosides should be used with extreme caution. Oral magnesium therapy is of

TABLE 74-6 Antineoplastic Drugs Producing Renal and Electrolyte Abnormalities

Agent	Toxicity	Comments
Cisplatin	Magnesium, calcium, potassium, sodium wasting; renal insufficiency	—
Cyclophosphamide	Impaired free water excretion	Transient; seen with doses >50 mg/kg
Ifosfamide	Proximal tubular defect	—
High-dose methotrexate	Acute renal failure	Usually reversible
Mitomycin C	Renal failure with microangiopathic hemolytic anemia (HUS/TTP)	Common with cumulative dose >60 mg
Nitrosoureas (BCNU, CCNU, methyl-CCNU)	Progressive renal failure appearing after large cumulative doses	Decrease in renal size may be noted; effect may occur years after therapy
Streptozotocin	Renal failure, proximal renal tubular acidosis, nephrotic syndrome	Transient proteinuria is earliest manifestation

uncertain benefit; intravenous or intramuscular doses should be administered. Renal salt wasting resulting in hyponatremia and symptomatic orthostatic hypotension also has been reported.

METHOTREXATE

High doses of methotrexate (>50 mg/kg) are potentially quite toxic and normally are given in the hospital with careful hydration and urine alkalinization to promote drug excretion. Plasma methotrexate levels are measured after drug administration, and leucovorin rescue is continued until the drug concentration has fallen to a safe level. Despite these precautions, an acute azotemia believed to result from the precipitation of methotrexate crystals in the distal nephron can be seen. Methotrexate-induced renal failure is usually, although not always, reversible over the 2 to 3 weeks following drug withdrawal. However, because the kidney is the primary route of excretion for methotrexate, dangerously high drug levels will persist for some time. This situation can produce other morbidity, particularly cytopenias and mucositis. A similar situation occurs when methotrexate has been given inadvertently to a patient with a third-space fluid reservoir, such as a pleural effusion or ascites, from which the drug is released only gradually. Administration of leucovorin until plasma levels of methotrexate fall below 5×10^{-8} M is beneficial in avoiding various toxicities described earlier. Doses of leucovorin need to be increased in patients with high plasma levels of methotrexate and will not completely prevent toxicity. Methotrexate also can be dialyzed using high-flux hemodialysis membranes[49]; hence hemodialysis also could be considered for reversing acute methotrexate toxicity along with high-dose leucovorin rescue. Carboxypeptidase-G2 is an enzyme that cleaves the terminal glutamate from methotrexate and can decrease methotrexate levels rapidly in patients with renal failure.[50] Food and Drug Administration (FDA) approval for this agent is being sought, but at this time it is only available for compassionate emergent use from the National Cancer Institute.

Thrombotic and Hemorrhagic Toxicity

All myelosuppresive agents potentially can cause thrombocytopenia and resulting bleeding complications. This section will focus more on some severe and specific complications associated with cancer therapies. Hemorrhagic cystitis is a well-described complication that occurs in patients treated with cyclophosphamide and ifosfamide. Thrombotic microangiopathies also have been described with various chemotherapeutic agents and will be discussed in this section. Among the recently approved agents, thalidomide has been associated with a significant risk of thromboembolic complications. This risk is much greater when the agent is administered in combination with various chemotherapeutic agents, and clinicians administering thalidomide need to be vigilant about the potential occurrence of this complication.[39,51]

HEMORRHAGIC CYSTITIS[52,53]

Urologic complications, including bladder fibrosis, bladder cancer, and hemorrhagic cystitis, are among the most troublesome side effects of cyclophosphamide and ifosfamide.

Susceptibility to hemorrhagic cystitis is somewhat idiosyncratic, and symptoms can occur after a few small doses, but the incidence is much higher with prolonged or high-dose therapy. Excretion of the BK human polyoma virus has been associated with a greater incidence of hemorrhagic cystitis in bone marrow transplant patients. Ifosfamide, an analog of cyclophosphamide, produces even more urothelial toxicity.

PREVENTION

Local bladder irritation from acrolein, one of the metabolites of cyclophosphamide, is believed to cause the damage. Sodium-2-mercaptoethane sulfonate (mesna) can help to prevent it by providing free sulfhydryl groups, which neutralize the acrolein in the urine. Ifosfamide should not be administered without sodium-2-mercaptoethane sulfonate. Sodium-2-mercaptoethane sulfonate is not useful in treating established cystitis. Adequate prehydration with frequent voiding to decrease the length of time the acrolein is in contact with the bladder is also an important prevention measure, particularly with high single doses of cyclophosphamide. Hypotonic solutions should not be used to hydrate patients receiving high-dose cyclophosphamide therapy.

CLINICAL PRESENTATION

The acute form of hemorrhagic cystitis appears within the first few days of drug treatment. Symptoms range from minimal hematuria with mild dysuria, urgency, and frequency to massive hemorrhage requiring transfusion. The thrombocytopenia seen with high doses of cyclophosphamide aggravates the blood loss. The bleeding usually is self-limited and will stop after a median duration of a month, even in severe cases, if the patient can be supported that long.

TREATMENT

Mild episodes do not require treatment other than cessation of drug therapy. In serious cases, vigorous hydration to promote urine flow, maintenance of adequate platelet counts (50,000/μL), and constant bladder irrigation through a large-bore catheter are indicated. The catheter must be kept free of obstructing clots, which can cause renal obstruction with severe pain.

Intravesical instillation of a variety of agents has been reported to control bleeding. Formalin is the best established of these agents, but formalin administration may have significant side effects, including pain, fibrosis, and renal papillary necrosis. It must be given with the patient under anesthesia. Urinary diversion also may be useful. In intractable cases, hypogastric artery embolization may be attempted, and severe intractable cases sometimes even require cystectomy with urinary diversion.[51–53]

MICROANGIOPATHIC HEMOLYTIC ANEMIA[54–60]

Thrombotic microangiopathy has been associated with various cancers as well as cancer therapies; thus it sometimes can cause a diagnostic dilemma. Among the various cancer treatments associated with the process, mitomycin C has been associated most closely with a syndrome of renal failure with microangiopathic hemolytic anemia. However, various other agents, such as bleomycin, cisplatin, interferon, and gemcitabine, also have been associated with microangiopathy. Thrombotic thrombocytopenic purpura/hemolytic-uremic syndrome (TTP/HUS) also can be a late complication (usually occurring within 1 year) of both allogeneic and autologous bone marrow transplantation. In both settings, the symptoms resemble those of idiopathic HUS; hypertension, renal failure, and anemia predominate rather than fever and neurologic signs. Conventional plasmapheresis, which is standard therapy for sporadic TTP, does not appear to be as effective in these drug-induced disorders. The prognosis in mitomycin C–associated HUS has been reported to be very poor; staphylococcal protein A immunoadsorption may be useful. The severity of the presentation and the prognosis in transplant patients are variable. Plasma exchange with cryosupernatant, protein A immunoadsorption, intravenous immunoglobulin administration, and glucocorticoid administration are of uncertain benefit.

Hepatotoxicity[61]

Although a large number of cytoxic agents can damage the liver in a variety of ways, few of them do so regularly with any severity when used in conventional doses (Table 74-7). However, veno-occlusive disease (VOD) of the liver is a major toxicity of high-dose regimens given before transplantation.

VENO-OCCLUSIVE DISEASE OF THE LIVER[62]

VOD is seen sporadically and rarely with a number of cytotoxic drugs, particularly antimetabolites, at conventional doses. Much more important, it has an incidence of up to 20% and is a common cause of death in patients given a variety of high-dose chemotherapy regimens or chemoradiotherapy combinations prior to infusion of autologous or allogeneic marrow or stem cells. Clinically, VOD resembles Budd-Chiari syndrome. The diagnosis is based on the presence of at least two of the triad of jaundice, hepatomegaly or right upper quadrant pain, and ascites or unexplained weight gain. Hyperbilirubinemia, which generally precedes hepatomegaly and ascites by several days, usually is out of proportion to increases in transaminase concentrations.

Symptoms begin at a mean of 10 days after marrow reinfusion, whereas graft-versus-host disease, one of the major differential diagnoses in patients who have had an allogeneic transplant, more often develops after day 20. Most deaths associated with VOD occur by day 35 after transplantation, and the majority of recoveries are evident by this time. However, late-onset VOD occurs with some regimens. The pain may be acute and severe enough to suggest an abdominal catastrophe such as pancreatitis, bowel infarction, biliary obstruction, peritonitis, or pyogenic liver abscess. Drugs, such as cyclosporine, and sepsis may cause laboratory abnormalities that mimic those seen in VOD.

Pathologically, early VOD is characterized by subintimal edema and hemorrhage within small central venules and centrilobular congestion. This picture progresses to fibrous obliteration of the central venule lumina and centrilobular sinusoidal fibrosis.

Diagnosis of VOD remains largely based on the clinical picture. Percutaneous biopsy usually is contraindicated because patients generally are thrombocytopenic, may be refractory to platelet transfusions, and may have a coagulopathy caused by liver dysfunction. Transvenous liver biopsies and measurement of the hepatic venous pressure gradient (elevated in VOD) are safer but still may result in fatal hemorrhage. Ultrasound studies may show an increased mean hepatic artery resistive index or reversal of portal venous flow. However, definitive findings tend to occur late, when the disease is obvious clinically. No therapies for VOD have been evaluated in prospective, randomized fashion. Standard supportive care for liver failure is indicated (see Chap. 73 and 83).

Biologic Agents[63-68]

A number of cytokines are available for widespread use, and new ones are constantly undergoing testing. Each has a unique toxicity profile that depends on dose, schedule, and combination with other cytokines or with other anticancer

TABLE 74-7 Cytotoxic Agents that Have Hepatic Toxicity

Drug	Frequency of Toxicity	Comments
L-Asparaginase	Common	Fatty metamorphosis; decreased synthetic function; reversible
Azathioprine	Uncommon	Cholestasis/necrosis; hyperbilirubinemia; variable prognosis
High-dose cytarabine	Common	Elevated bilirubin and transaminases; reversible
Floxuridine (FUDR)	Common	Biliary sclerosis with hepatic intra-arterial infusion; chemical hepatitis
Methotrexate	Common	Cirrhosis, fibrosis, fatty metamorphosis; laboratory data may be normal; seen with prolonged daily therapy; variable prognosis
High-dose methotrexate	Common	Elevated transaminase levels, usually reversible in weeks
6-Mercaptopurine	Common	Cholestasis or necrosis; usually reversible
Mithramycin	Common	Necrosis; rarely seen with lower doses used for hypercalcemia
Nitrosoureas (BCNU, CCNU)	Occasional	Generally mild and reversible
Vincristine	Rare	May produce severe damage when combined with radiation to the liver

drugs, but they tend to share a spectrum of side effects, probably related to the "cytokine cascade," that are different from those of most chemotherapeutic agents. These include typical side effects of interferon, such as fever and myalgia, and a side effect of high-dose IL-2 treatment that consists of a sepsis-like capillary leak syndrome that can lead to hypotension and cardiovascular collapse. Attempts at fluid resuscitation may lead to pulmonary edema, and use of vasopressors may be necessary. The capillary leak syndrome, like most cytokine toxicities, resolves rapidly after discontinuation of therapy. Arrhythmias and myocardial infarction also may be seen and may result either from fluid shifts or from direct myocardial toxicity. CNS toxicity is frequent and may be related to the vascular leak phenomenon or to the function of cytokines as messenger molecules with the CNS. CNS toxicity usually is reversible, but it may persist for days after cessation of treatment.

A detailed list of the side effects of IL-2 treatment that are seen at the recommended doses for renal cancer (600,000 U/kg every 8 hours for 14 doses) is given in Table 74-8 as a prototype of cytokine toxicities.

TABLE 74-8 Toxicities of Interleukin-2

Toxicity	Comments
Febrile reaction complex	Dose-dependent fever and chills are ameliorated with antipyretics and meperidine
Cardiovascular toxicity	Capillary leak syndrome; see text. Rare cases of eosinophilic myocarditis
Central nervous system toxicity	Dose-dependent reversible somnolence, disorientation, cognitive deterioration; appears several days after beginning of a treatment course
Hematopoietic toxicity	Frequent anemia, occasional thrombocytopenia, rare neutropenia; lymphopenia with rebound lymphocytosis, dramatic eosinophilia
Gastrointestinal toxicity	Mild nausea, vomiting, diarrhea; mucositis is unusual but may be severe; profound, reversible cholestasis with hyperbilirubinemia and elevated alkaline phosphatase but normal transaminases
Infectious complications	Increase in staphylococcal bacteremia, often catheter-related
Renal toxicity	Oliguria and prerenal azotemia reversible when infusion discontinued
Cutaneous toxicity	Rash ranging from discrete nonpruritic maculopapular lesions to diffuse erythroderma with flaky exfoliation after resolution of redness
Other	Hypo- and hyperthyroidism, decrease in vitamin K–dependent coagulation factors, severe myalgias

Toxicities of Targeted Therapies[69-77]

The tremendous gains made in cancer biology in the past 10 to 15 years have led to the development of agents that inhibit specific targets such as surface receptors or intra- and extracellular proteins that are thought to play a key role in the development or progression of various malignancies, and these agents are often referred to as *targeted therapies*. Several new monoclonal antibodies and small-molecule kinase inhibitors have been approved by the FDA in the last 5 years for various therapeutic indications. With increasing use of targeted agents, a range of new clinical toxicities is being recognized and reported. Compared with various classic cytotoxic agents discussed earlier, the clinical experience with the newer targeted agents is limited; hence details regarding the prevalence and underlying pathologic mechanisms of the toxicities currently are sparse and will continue to evolve. This section describes some of the more severe adverse events that have been reported with the various targeted agents.

MONOCLONAL ANTIBODIES[26,69–71]

The past few years have seen several new humanized monoclonal antibodies approved for the management of hematologic and solid malignancies. It is anticipated that the common toxicities, such as acute infusion reactions, associated with the antibodies most likely will be similar for the different antibodies, whereas specific toxicities, such as cardiac toxicity associated with trastuzumab,[26] most likely will be related to the modulation of the targeted pathway by each specific antibody. Rituximab (RITUXAN) is a chimeric anti-CD20 antibody that is now used routinely for the treatment of various lymphoid malignancies. Recent case reports have implicated this antibody in various dermatologic and systemic toxicities.[69,70] The toxicities have ranged from mild cutaneous reactions to the much more severe Stevens-Johnson syndrome and serum sickness; the toxicities generally have resolved with discontinuation of therapy in conjunction with supportive care and steroids. The cytokines released by the targeted malignant cells, as well as the antibody itself, have been implicated as the cause of these adverse events. The specifics of the underlying pathology are poorly understood, but treating physicians should be aware of such severe toxicities because they are anticipated to become more common with increasing use of these agents. Some monoclonal antibodies that are currently in clinical use are conjugated to either a cytotoxic entity or a radioisotope.[71] The rationale behind their development is that the antibody will bring the lethal conjugated cytotoxic compounds specifically into proximity with the targeted neoplastic cells and potentially enhance the cytotoxicity of the agents. The radioisotope-labeled antibodies frequently are associated with prolonged myelosuppression.

ANTIANGIOGENIC AGENTS[72–74]

Recognition of the importance of angiogenesis in the progression and propagation of various malignancies has led to an increased emphasis on the development of agents that inhibit the complex process of angiogenesis. Although thalidomide and the monoclonal antibody bevacizumab (AVASTIN) are the only antiangiogenic agents currently approved for cancer therapy, many other agents in this class are in advanced stages of development and are anticipated to be approved in the near future. The most serious adverse events that have been described with this class of agents are bleeding, thromboses, and hypertension, and the underlying mechanisms of these toxicities are still being defined. Hence the recommendations for management or prevention of the vascular complications are also evolving. In general, for patients with the most severe complications, discontinuation of the antiangiogenic agent with the appropriate medical therapy is the most prudent approach currently. Reversible hypertension and proteinuria also have been observed routinely for various antiangiogenic therapies. Generally, both toxicities can be managed medically or can be reversed by discontinuation of the therapeutic agent.

The observation that thalidomide has modest antiangiogenic properties led to a renewed interest in its use as an anticancer agent, and the initial clinical investigation led to its approval for the treatment of multiple myeloma. Besides the well-publicized teratogenic and neurologic toxicities, it also has been associated with high rates of thromboembolic complications in several cancer clinical trials. Patients receiving thalidomide in combination with other chemotherapeutic agents seem to be the most susceptible to the thrombotic complications.[39,71] Various approaches to managing patients with these complications have been proposed from the more conservative approach of discontinuing thalidomide therapy in patients with marginal benefit from the agent to reinitiating thalidomide therapy after appropriate stable anticoagulation therapy has been established. Uniform management guidelines for such complications will emerge only after more clinical experience with this class of agents has been gained.

SMALL-MOLECULE TYROSINE KINASE INHIBITORS[75-77]

Many of the tyrosine kinase inhibitors that were thought initially to be highly specific are in some instances not as specific in their inhibitory capacity and are demonstrating activity against malignancies that they were not designed to treat initially.[75-77] Hence they are being described here as another class of cancer agents that will be used more routinely for management of different malignancies. The reader should note that the predominant toxicities of many kinase inhibitors will not always be the same and eventually will be dictated by the pathways predominantly inhibited by each agent. This section will limit the discussion only to currently FDA-approved agents.

One of the most publicized tyrosine kinase inhibitors is imatinib mesylate (GLEEVEC, STI-571).[75] Imatinib mesylate is an orally administered drug that inhibits the Bcr-Abl protein-tyrosine kinase. The Bcr-Abl fusion protein is the result of the pathognomonic 9,22 chromosome translocation that causes chronic myelogenous leukemia (CML). Imatinib mesylate treatment resulted in both hematologic and cytogenetic responses in CML patients and led to approval of the agent in United States in 2001. Subsequent studies also demonstrated that imatinib mesylate also was active against gastrointestinal stromal tumors (GISTs) that overexpress the platelet-derived growth factor receptor kinase.[75] Some of the common toxicities associated with the agent consist of mild nausea, emesis, edema, and dermatologic reactions. However, about 2% to 4% of patients have been reported to have severe fluid retention in the forms of pleural and pericardial effusions, as well as severe cutaneous reactions. The severe adverse events have been observed more commonly in patients receiving the higher doses ($\geq$600 mg/d) of the agent. Gefitinib, the epidermal growth factor receptor (EGFR) tyrosine-kinase inhibitor approved for the treatment of lung cancer, results in mild to moderately severe skin rash and diarrhea in most patients in addition to the rare but severe pulmonary toxicity discussed earlier.[18] Both toxicities are relatively easy to manage with dose reduction or supportive care when they are mild; however, in about 5% to 10% of the patients, both rash and diarrhea can be quite severe, requiring discontinuation of therapy and aggressive supportive care. Finally, as mentioned earlier in this section, oncologic therapies are anticipated to undergo some dramatic changes in the next few years with the introduction of several novel agents that differ from the traditional cytotoxic agents both in their mechanisms of action and in their typical toxicity profiles. As a result, clinicians will be challenged initially with limitations in information regarding some of the uncommon and potentially severe toxicities of the newer agents, and this will require diligence and patience while the clinical experience with such agents increases and some practice standards are established.

References

1. Weiss RB: Miscellaneous toxicities in cancer, in DeVita VT, Hellman S, Rosenberg SA (eds): *Principles and Practice of Oncology,* 6th ed. Philadelphia, Lippincott-Raven, 2001, p 2964.
2. Cersosimo RJ: Monoclonal antibodies in the treatment of cancer, part 2. *Am J Health Syst Pharm* 60:1631, 2003.
3. Weiner LM, Adams GP, Von Mehren M: Therapeutic monoclonal antibodies: General principles, in DeVita VT, Hellman S, Rosenberg SA (eds): *Principles and Practice of Oncology,* 6th ed. Philadelphia, Lippincott-Raven, 2001, p 495.
4. Fischer DS, Knobf MT, Durivage HJ: *The Cancer Chemotherapy Handbook,* 4th ed. Chicago, Mosby, 1993.
5. Gastineou DA, Hoagland HC: Hematologic effects of chemotherapy. *Semin Oncol* 19:543, 1992.
6. Griffin JD: Hematopoietic growth factors, in DeVita VT, Hellman S, Rosenberg SA (eds): *Principles and Practice of Oncology,* 6th ed. Philadelphia, Lippincott-Raven, 2001, p 2798.
7. Hughes WT, Armstrong D, Bodey GP, et al: 1997 guidelines for the use of antimicrobial agents in neutropenic patients with unexplained fever. Infectious Diseases Society of America. *Clin Infect Dis* 25:247, 1997.
8. Vanhoefer U, Harstrick A, Achterrath W, et al: Irinotecan in the treatment of colorectal cancer: Clinical overview. *J Clin Oncol* 19:1501, 2001.
9. Anderson BS, Cogan BM, Keating MJ, et al: Subacute pulmonary failure complicating therapy with high-dose Ara-C in acute leukemia. *Cancer* 56:2181, 1985.
10. Haupt HM, Hutchins GM, Moore GW: Ara-C lung: Noncardiogenic pulmonary edema complicating cytosine arabinoside therapy of leukemia. *Am J Med* 70:256, 1981.
11. Kreisman H, Wolkove N: Pulmonary toxicity of antineoplastic therapy. *Semin Oncol* 19:508, 1992.
12. Sostman HD, Matthay RA, Putman CE, et al: Methotrexate-induced pneumonitis. *Medicine* 55:371, 1976.
13. Carson CW, Cannon GW, Egger MJ, et al: Pulmonary disease during the treatment of rheumatoid arthritis with low-dose pulse methotrexate. *Semin Arthritis Rheum* 16:186, 1987.
14. White DA, Rankin JA, Stover DE, et al: Methotrexate pneumonitis: Bronchoalveolar lavage findings suggest an immunologic disorder. *Am Rev Respir Dis* 139:18, 1989.

15. White DA, Kris MG, Stover DE: Bronchoalveolar lavage populations in bleomycin-induced pulmonary toxicity. *Thorax* 42:551, 1987.

16. Frankel SR, Eardly A, Lauwerd G, et al: The "retinoic acid syndrome" in acute promyelocytic leukemia. *Ann Intern Med* 117:242, 1992.

17. Wiley JS, Firkin FC: Reduction of pulmonary toxicity by prednisolone prophylaxis during all-*trans*-retinoic acid treatment of acute promyelocytic leukemia. *Leukemia* 9:774, 1995.

18. Cohen MH, Williams GA, Sridhara R, et al: FDA drug approval summary: Gefitnib (ZD1839)(IRESSA) tablets. *Oncologist* 8:303, 2003.

19. Radzikowska E, Szczepulska E, Chabowski M, et al: Organising pnuemonia caused by trastuzumab (HERCEPTIN) therapy for breast cancer. *Eur Respir J* 21:552, 2003.

20. Cheson BD, Samlowski WE, Tang TT, Spruance SL: Value of open-lung biopsy in 87 immunocompromised patients with pulmonary infiltrates. *Cancer* 55:453, 1985.

21. Potter D, Pass HI, Brower S, et al: Prospective, randomized study of open lung biopsy versus empirical antibiotic therapy for acute pneumonitis in nonneutropenic cancer patients. *Ann Thorac Surg* 40:422, 1985.

22. Comis RL: Bleomycin pulmonary toxicity: Current status and future directions. *Semin Oncol* 19(suppl 5):64, 1992.

23. Goldiner PL, Carlon GC, Cvitkovic E, et al: Factors influencing postoperative morbidity and mortality in patients treated with bleomycin. *Br Med J* 1:1664, 1978.

24. Hulbert JC, Grossman JE, Cummings KB: Risk factors of anesthesia and surgery in bleomycin-treated patients. *J Urol* 130:163, 1983.

25. Allen A: The cardiotoxicity of chemotherapeutic drugs. *Semin Oncol* 19:529, 1992.

26. Seidman A, Hudis C, Pierri MK, et al: Cardiac dysfunction in the trastuzumab clinical trials experience. *J Clin Oncol* 20:1215, 2002.

27. Rowinsky EK, McGuire WP, Guarnieri T, et al: Cardiac disturbances during the administration of taxol. *J Clin Oncol* 9:1704, 1991.

28. Rowkinsky EK, Donehower RC: Paclitaxel (TAXOL). *N Engl J Med* 332:1004, 1995.

29. Doll DC, Ringenberg QS, Yarbro JW: Vascular toxicity associated with antineoplastic agents. *J Clin Oncol* 4:1405, 1986.

30. Rezkalla S, Kloner RA, Ensley J, et al: Continuous ambulatory ECG monitoring during fluorouracil therapy: A prospective study. *J Clin Oncol* 7:509, 1989.

31. Bertolini A, Flumano M, Fusco O, et al: Acute cardiotoxicity during capecitabine treatment: A case report. *Tumori* 87:200, 2001.

32. Schwartz RG, McKenzie WB, Alexander J, et al: Congestive heart failure and left ventricular dysfunction complicating doxorubicin therapy. *Am J Med* 82:1109, 1987.

33. Shan K, Lincoff AM, Young JB: Anthracycline-induced cardiotoxicity. *Ann Intern Med* 125:47, 1996.

34. Steinherz LJ, Steinherz PG, Tan CTC, et al: Cardiac toxicity 4 to 20 years after completing anthracycline therapy. *JAMA* 266:1672, 1991.

35. Lipshultz SE, Colan SD, Gelber RD, et al: Late cardiac effects of doxorubicin therapy for acute lymphoblastic leukemia in childhood. *N Engl J Med* 324:808, 1991.

36. Steinherz LJ, Steinherz PG: Cyclophosphamide cardiotoxicity. *Cancer Bull* 37:231, 1985.

37. Quezado ZM, Wilson WH, Cunnion RE, et al: High-dose ifosfamide is associated with severe, reversible cardiac dysfunction. *Ann Intern Med* 118:31, 1993.

38. Grothey A: Oxaliplatin-safety profile: Neurotoxicity. *Semin Oncol* 30:5, 2003.

39. Dimopoulos MA, Anagnostopoulos A, Weber D: Treatment of plasma cell dyscrasias with thalidomide and its derivatives. *J Clin Oncol* 21:4444, 2003.

40. Matthews SJ, McCoy C: Thalidomide: A review of approved and investigational uses. *Clin Ther* 25:342, 2003.

41. Baker J, Royer GL, Weiss RB: Cytarabine and neurologic toxicity. *J Clin Oncol* 9:679, 1991.

42. Jaffe N, Takaue Y, Anzai T, Robertson R: Transient neurologic disturbances induced by high-dose methotrexate treatment. *Cancer* 56:1356, 1985.

43. Bernini JC, Fort DW, Greiner JC, et al: Aminophylline for methotrexate-induced neurotoxicity. *Lancet* 345:544, 1995.

44. Kupfer A, Aeschlimann C, Cerny T: Methylene blue and the neurotoxic mechanisms of ifosfamide encephalopathy. *Eur J Clin Pharmacol* 50:249, 1996.

45. Pelgrims J, De Vos F, Van den Brande J: Methylene blue in the treatment and prevention of ifosfamide-induced encephalopathy: Report of 12 cases and a review of the literature. *Br J Cancer* 82:291, 2000.

46. Patterson WP, Reams GP: Renal toxicities of chemotherapy. *Semin Oncol* 19:521, 1992.

47. Blachley JA, Hill JB: Renal and electrolyte disturbances associated with cisplatin. *Ann Intern Med* 95:628, 1981.

48. Hutchinson FN, Perez EA, Gandara DR: Renal salt wasting in patients treated with cisplatin. *Ann Intern Med* 108:21, 1988.

49. Wall SM, Johansen MJ, Molony DA, et al: Effective clearance of methotrexate using high-flux hemodialysis membranes. *Am J Kidney Dis* 6:846, 1996.

50. Mohty M, Peyriere H, Guinet C, et al: Carboxypeptidase G2 rescue in delayed methotrexate elimination in renal failure. *Leuk Lymphoma* 3–4:441, 2000.

51. Russo P: Urologic emergencies in the cancer patient. *Semin Oncol* 20:2895, 2002.

52. Stillwell TJ, Benson RC Jr: Cyclophosphamide-induced hemorrhagic cystitis: A review of 100 patients. *Cancer* 61:451, 1988.

53. Gine E, Rovira M, Real I, et al: Successful treatment of severe hemorrhagic cystitis after hemopoietic cell transplantation by selective embolization of the vesical arteries. *Bone Marrow Transplant* 31:923, 2003.

54. Korel S, Schein PS, Smith FP, et al: Treatment of cancer-associated hemolytic uremic syndrome with staphylococcal protein A immunoperfusion. *J Clin Oncol* 4:210, 1986.

55. Lesesne JB, Rothschild N, Erickson B, et al: Cancer-associated hemolytic-uremic syndrome: Analysis of 85 cases from a national registry. *J Clin Oncol* 7:781, 1989.

56. Zeigler ZR, Shadduck RK, Nemunaitis J, et al: Bone marrow transplant–associated thrombotic microangiopathy: A case series. *Bone Marrow Transplant* 15:247, 1995.

57. Byrnes JJ, Hussein AM: Thrombotic microangiopathic syndromes after bone marrow transplantation. *Cancer Invest* 14:151, 1996.

58. Porta C, Danova M, Riccardi A: Cancer chemotherapy–related thrombotic thrombocytopenic purpura: Biological evidence of increased nitric oxide production. *Mayo Clin Proc* 6:570, 1999.

59. Walter RB, Joerger M, Pestalozzi BC: Gemcitabine-associated hemolytic-uremic syndrome. *Am J Kidney Dis* 40:E16, 2002.

60. Al-Zahrani H, Gupta V, Minden MD: Vascular events associated with alpha interferon therapy. *Leuk Lymphoma* 44:471, 2003.

61. Perry MC: Chemotherapy agents and hepatotoxicity. *Semin Oncol* 19:551, 1992.

62. Bearman SI: The syndrome of hepatic veno-occlusive disease after marrow transplantation. *Blood* 85:3005, 1995.

63. Quesada JR, Talpaz M, Rios A, et al: Clinical toxicity of interferons in cancer patients: A review. *J Clin Oncol* 4:234, 1986.

64. Deyton LR, Walker RE, Kovacs JA, et al: Reversible cardiac dysfunction associated with interferon-alpha therapy in AIDS patients with Kaposi's sarcoma. *N Engl J Med* 321:1246, 1989.

65. Rohatiner AZS, Prior P, Burton A, et al: Central nervous system toxicity of interferon. *Prog Exp Tumor Res* 29:197, 1985.

66. Lotze MT, Matory YL, Rayner AA, et al: Clinical effects and toxicity of interleukin-2 in patients with cancer. *Cancer* 58:2764, 1986.

67. Nora R, Abrams JS, Tait NS, et al: Myocardial toxic effects during recombinant interleukin-2 therapy. *J Natl Cancer Inst* 81:59, 1989.

68. DeVita T Jr, Hellman S, Rosenberg SA (eds): *Biologic Therapy of Cancer.* Philadelphia, Lippincott, 1991.

69. Dereure O, Navarro R, Rossi JF, et al: Rituximab-induced vasculitis. *Dermatology* 203:83, 2001.

70. Hellerstedt B, Ahmed A: Delayed-type hypersensitivity reaction or serum sickness after rituximab treatment. *Ann Oncol* 14:1792, 2003.

71. Bethge WA, Sandmaier BM: Targeted cancer therapy and immunosuppression using radiolabeled monoclonal antibodies. *Semin Oncol* 1:68, 2004.

72. Tonini T, Rossi F, Claudio PP: Molecular basis of angiogenesis and cancer. *Oncogene* 22:6549, 2003.

73. Kabbinavar F, Hurwitz H, Fehrenbacher L, et al: Phase II, randomized trial comparing bevacizumab plus fluorouracil (FU)/leucovorin (LV) with FU/LV alone in patients with metastatic colorectal cancer. *J Clin Oncol* 21:60, 2003.

74. Bennett CL, Schumock GT, Desai AA, et al: Thalidomide-associated deep vein thrombosis and pulmonary embolism. *Am J Med* 113:603, 2002.

75. Sawyers CL: Opportunities and challenges in the development of kinase inhibitor therapy for cancer. *Genes Dev* 24:2998, 2003.

76. Deininger MW, O'Brien SG, Ford JM, Druker BJ: Practical management of patients with chronic myeloid leukemia receiving imatinib. *J Clin Oncol* 21:1637, 2003.

77. Eisenberg BL: Imatinib mesylate: A molecularly targeted therapy for gastrointestinal stromal tumors. *Oncology* 11:1615, 2003.

PART VIII

RENAL AND METABOLIC DISORDERS

Chapter 75
ACUTE RENAL FAILURE

BHARATHI REDDY
PATRICK MURRAY

KEY POINTS

- *Prenatal azotemia and acute tubular necrosis account for the overwhelming majority of hospital-acquired acute renal failure cases, whereas acute glomerulonephritis and vasculitides are more common causes of acute renal failure developing outside the hospital.*

- *Acute renal failure occurs in at least 10% to 30% of patients admitted to an ICU and is associated with a mortality rate of about 50% despite advances in supportive care and technology.*

- *The most important diagnostic classification to be made in the evaluation of patients with acute renal failure is based on the site of the renal lesion (pre-, intra-, or postrenal).*

- *Since there are few specific therapies available in patients with established acute tubular necrosis, the major clinical focus is on prevention of ARF by identification of subjects at highest risk.*

- *All aspects of treatment of acute tubular necrosis, including renal replacement therapy, are basically supportive. The nondialytic measures of greatest importance are maintenance of nutritional, volume, and electrolyte homeostasis.*

- *Emergent renal replacement therapy is indicated in the management of acute renal failure when pulmonary edema, hyperkalemia, refractory acidosis, or symptomatic uremia develops.*

- *Prophylactic renal replacement therapy should be considered in patients with sustained anuria, persistent oliguria with progressive azotemia and glomerular filtration rate <10 mL/ min, and to prevent uncontrolled positive fluid balance.*

Acute renal failure (ARF) is defined as rapid decline (over hours to days) in glomerular filtration rate (GFR). This manifests as a rapid increase in blood urea nitrogen (BUN; azotemia) and serum creatinine, and may or may not be accompanied by a decline in urine output; specific definitions (e.g., absolute or fractional increase of serum creatinine) vary widely between studies.[1] ARF occurs in 2% to 5% of general medical-surgical admissions, but up to 10% to 30% of ICU admissions. Acute renal failure can be classified into three broad etiologic/anatomic categories: prerenal ARF, intrarenal ARF, and postrenal ARF. Prerenal ARF is caused by renal hypoperfusion with intact renal parenchyma (55% to 60% of instances of ARF). Intrarenal ARF is caused by parenchymal renal diseases (35% to 40% of instances of ARF). Postrenal ARF is caused by urinary tract obstruction (~5% of instances of ARF).[2]

Most ARF in the ICU is caused by prerenal azotemia, and the rest predominantly by renal parenchymal injury with acute tubular necrosis (ATN); the former may convert to the latter. Despite advances in critical care and dialysis technologies, the mortality of ARF requiring dialysis in critically ill patients remains 50% to 80%.[3–5] Although there is evidence that isolated ARF itself increases mortality, it is clear that

mortality of ICU ARF increases with every additional nonrenal organ failure present at the time of initiation of renal replacement therapy (RRT).[3,5] Emerging data suggest that renal ischemia-reperfusion injury and the uremic milieu actually contribute to the development of distant organ injury (increased pulmonary vascular permeability and cardiac and splanchnic organ apoptosis).[6–8] Outcome is particularly poor in septic ARF; in one study, mortality of septic ARF was 74%, compared to 45% in nonseptic cases.[9] ARF in the presence of shock (septic or cardiogenic) is an increasingly common occurrence in modern ICUs, and has driven the development of continuous renal replacement therapy (CRRT) to permit control of azotemia and fluid balance in hemodynamically unstable patients.[5,10] Although a broad differential diagnosis and therapeutic plan should be considered for every ICU patient with ARF, in most cases the approach is to reverse any element of prerenal azotemia, provide supportive care in the presence of ATN, and intervene with effective RRT when indicated, in anticipation of probable renal recovery in the event of patient survival.

Classification of Acute Renal Failure

PRERENAL ACUTE RENAL FAILURE

Prerenal azotemia is the most common cause of ARF in hospitalized patients. The main feature of prerenal ARF is the presence of intact renal parenchymal tissue and the rapid correction of GFR with restoration of renal perfusion. Uncorrected prerenal azotemia predisposes to the development of ATN. Prerenal ARF is caused by any condition leading to renal hypoperfusion, including systemic hypoperfusion with hypovolemia, cardiac failure, or vasodilatory shock, and/or regional hypoperfusion caused by renal vasoconstriction (Table 75-1; see Chap. 21).

Renal blood flow and GFR are relatively maintained during mild hypoperfusion, due to compensatory mechanisms.[11] Renal perfusion is largely preserved within a range of mean arterial pressure (MAP) between 80 to 180 mm Hg, if cardiac output is adequate. As MAP falls below 80 mm Hg there is a precipitous fall in renal blood flow and GFR.[12] There are two major mechanisms of renal blood flow autoregulation: a myogenic reflex and tubuloglomerular (TG) feedback. The myogenic reflex is mediated by stretch receptors in the afferent arterioles, which detect a decrease in perfusion pressure, leading to autoregulatory relaxation of afferent arterioles and vasodilation. TG feedback defends renal perfusion as follows: chloride concentration is continuously sensed in the tubular lumen by the macula densa, just distal to the thick ascending loop of Henle. When luminal chloride decreases (presumably reflecting decreased renal blood flow, GFR, intravascular volume, or a combination of these), a vasodilatory signal is transduced to the corresponding afferent arteriole (and vice versa if flow increases). Together these mechanisms autoregulate renal blood flow in the face of hypotension or hypertension. A third mechanism additionally helps autoregulate GFR. Increased renin secretion stimulated by hypotension/hypovolemia sensed in the afferent arteriole helps maintain GFR (but not renal blood flow) during hypotension, through the efferent arteriolar action of angiotensin II (discussed further below).

TABLE 75-1 Causes of Acute Renal Failure

Prerenal

Volume depletion: Gastrointestinal fluid loss or hemorrhage; renal losses (diuretics or glucosuria, salt-wasting nephropathy, diabetes insipidus, or adrenal insufficiency); cutaneous losses (burns, desquamation)

Volume redistribution: Peripheral vasodilation (sepsis or antihypertensives), peritonitis, burns, pancreatitis, hypoalbuminemia (nephrotic syndrome or hepatic disease)

Cardiac dysfunction: Pericardial tamponade, complications of myocardial infarction, acute or chronic valvular disease, cardiomyopathies, arrythmias

Vasodilatory shock: Sepsis, liver failure, postcardiotomy, anaphylaxis, or antihypertensives

Renal vasoconstriction: Cirrhosis, sepsis, hypercalcemia, drugs (cyclosporine, tacrolimus, nonsteroidal anti-inflammatory drugs, or pressors)

Renal

Ischemia: Trauma, surgery, sepsis, pigment nephropathy (hemolysis or rhabdomyolysis), cardiac or aortic hemorrhage

Nephrotoxic: Radiocontrast, antibiotics (aminoglycosides or amphotericin), nonsteroidal anti-inflammatory drugs, carbon tetrachloride, ethylene glycol, heavy metals (lead, mercury, arsenic, cadmium, or uranium), pesticides, fungicides, cyclosporine, or tacrolimus

Disorders of glomeruli and blood vessels: Poststreptococcal glomerulonephritis, infective endocarditis, systemic lupus erythematosus, Goodpasture's syndrome, microscopic polyarteritis, Wegener's granulomatosis, Henoch-Schönlein purpura, idiopathic rapidly progressive glomerulonephritis, polyarteritis nodosa, malignant hypertension, thrombotic microangiopathies (hemolytic uremic syndrome, thrombotic thrombocytopenic purpura, postpartum renal failure, or antiphospholipid syndrome), renal artery embolism, renal artery dissection, bilateral renal vein thrombosis, or abdominal compartment syndrome

Acute interstitial nephritis:

Allergic: Semisynthetic penicillin analogues (e.g., methicillin, ampicillin, or nafcillin), cephalosporins, rifampin, ciprofloxacin, cotrimoxazole, sulfonamides, thiazides, furosemide, allopurinol, phenytoin, tetracyclines, or warfarin

Infectious: Streptococcal, staphylococcal, leptospirosis, infectious mononucleosis, diphtheria, brucellosis, Legionnaire's disease, toxoplasmosis, or cytomegalovirus

Infiltrative: Sarcoidosis, lymphoma, leukemia

Autoimmune/alloimmune: Systemic lupus erythematosus or renal transplant rejection

Postrenal

Malignancy: Lymphoma, renal adenocarcinoma, bladder ureteral carcinoma, gynecologic cancers, prostate cancer, other pelvic tumors, or metastatic disease

Inflammatory processes: Tuberculosis, inflammatory bowel disease, retroperitoneal abscess or fibrosis, postradiation therapy

Vascular diseases: Aortic aneurysm, renal artery aneurysm

Papillary necrosis: Diabetes mellitus, sickle hemoglobinopathy, analgesic abuse, prostaglandin inhibition, or hepatic cirrhosis

Intratubular: Uric acid, calcium phosphate, Bence Jones proteins, methotrexate, acyclovir, sulfonamide antibiotics, or indinavir

Miscellaneous: Nephrolithiasis, ureteral ligation, retrograde pyelography with ureteral edema, neurogenic bladder, neuropathic ureteral dysfunction, or obstructed urinary catheter

---

Of course, in addition to local autoregulation, systemic neurohumoral influences also play a prominent role in determining the renal response to shock. Systemic hypoperfusion activates the sympathetic nervous system and renin-angiotensin-aldosterone axis. Norepinephrine and angiotensin II are systemic vasoconstrictors, and tend to increase renal blood flow by preserving renal perfusion pressure. On the other hand, both hormones are renal vasoconstrictors, though they differ in their glomerular hemodynamic effects. Angiotensin II preferentially constricts efferent arterioles, and helps preserve glomerular filtration, increasing filtration fraction (the ratio of GFR to renal plasma flow) by creating "back-pressure" to augment net filtration pressure in the glomerular capillary. Norepinephrine causes balanced afferent and efferent arteriolar constriction, similarly increasing filtration fraction in the face of decreased renal blood flow, but to a lesser extent than angiotensin II. Both angiotensin II and norepinephrine stimulate intrarenal vasodilator prostaglandin production, thus attenuating their simultaneous effect of afferent arteriolar vasoconstriction and helping preserve renal perfusion.

Drugs may unfavorably alter the glomerular hemodynamic response to renal hypoperfusion. Nonsteroidal anti-inflammatory drug (NSAIDs) administration to patients with decreased effective arterial blood volume (due to hypovolemia or congestive heart failure) or renal vasoconstriction (due to cirrhosis) leads to a decline in renal blood flow and GFR. These patients are dependent on vasodilator prostaglandins to maintain renal perfusion, so NSAIDs leave renal vasoconstrictor influences unopposed. Angiotensin-converting enzyme inhibitors (ACEIs) and angiotensin receptor blockers (ARBs) can lead to prerenal azotemia in patients who are dependent on angiotensin II for maintenance of GFR. This phenomenon is most commonly seen in patients receiving ACEIs or ARBs in the presence of hypovolemia, bilateral renal artery stenosis, or unilateral renal artery stenosis with a solitary kidney.

Prerenal azotemia also leads to avid renal tubular sodium and water reabsorption throughout the nephron. Catecholamines and angiotensin II directly increase sodium transport and reabsorption in the proximal and distal nephron. Efferent arteriolar constriction by angiotensin II and increased filtration fraction simultaneously lead to decreased peritubular capillary hydraulic pressure and increased peritubular capillary oncotic pressure. The combination of high oncotic pressure and low hydraulic pressure in peritubular capillaries increases sodium and water absorption in the proximal tubule, a process termed *glomerulotubular balance.* Angiotensin II also leads to downstream production of aldosterone, another salt-retaining influence. Severe hypovolemia/ hypotension (>10% to 15% decrease in MAP or blood volume) leads to nonosmotic vasopressin secretion, and avid water reabsorption in the collecting duct, along with systemic vasoconstriction. Finally, in hypovolemic patients decreased atrial stretch downregulates production of atrial natriuretic peptide, also favoring sodium retention (the opposite is true if renal hypoperfusion is caused by congestive heart failure). Thus the combination of glomerulotubular balance and the tubular effects of catecholamines, angiotensin II, aldosterone, and vasopressin mediate the salt and water retention which is the hallmark of prerenal azotemia. Accordingly, patients with prerenal azotemia tend to have oliguria, low urine sodium, and concentrated urine with a urine osmolality exceeding 500 mOsm/kg. Low urine sodium (and fractional excretion of sodium; see below) and increased urine osmolality (with a high urine:plasma creatinine ratio) are not seen in patients who have prerenal ARF due to renal losses (ongoing diuretic therapy, salt-wasting nephropathies, osmotic diuresis, adrenal insufficiency, and central or nephrogenic diabetes insipidus). Other common laboratory features of prerenal ARF are increased serum BUN:creatinine ratio (caused by low tubular flow and increased urea reabsorption), decreased fractional excretion of urea (see below), polycythemia/high serum albumin (hemoconcentration), mild hypercalcemia, hyperuricemia, and acid-base abnormalities (metabolic acidosis from diarrhea or shock or lactic acidosis; metabolic alkalosis from diuretics or vomiting). Hyponatremia may also be present, depending on abnormalities in water balance (see Chap. 76). The renal response to volume challenge or vasoactive drug initiation may also be used to determine the presence or absence of a reversible, "prerenal" etiology of ARF.

POSTRENAL ACUTE RENAL FAILURE

Postrenal ARF (often called obstructive uropathy) accounts for 5% of all cases of ARF, and is more common in the elderly. Unilateral obstruction is not sufficient alone to cause ARF. Renal insufficiency due to obstruction occurs only when the obstruction involves a site that affects both kidneys, or a single functioning kidney. The most common cause of postrenal obstruction is bladder neck obstruction (prostatic hypertrophy, prostate cancer, and neurogenic bladder). Postrenal obstruction is also caused by bilateral ureteral obstruction or unilateral obstruction in patients with solitary kidney (stones, clots, sloughed renal papillae, retroperitoneal fibrosis, or retroperitoneal masses). Intratubular obstruction can be caused by crystals like uric acid, calcium oxalate, calcium phosphate, acyclovir, sulfadiazine, indinavir, methotrexate, or by paraprotein (myeloma cast nephropathy). Volume expansion, sometimes with urinary alkalinization (uric acid, methotrexate, or myeloma), is the primary treatment for these causes of intratubular obstruction.

Obstruction to urine flow by increased tubular hydrostatic pressure is only partly responsible for the reduced GFR of obstructive uropathy. ARF is also caused and sustained by renal vasoconstriction that occurs in response to ureteral obstruction, mediated by thromboxanes. Obstruction should be suspected in patients with recurrent urinary tract infections, nephrolithiasis, prostate disease, or pelvic tumor. Causes of obstructive uropathy are listed in Table 75-1. These patients usually have a preceding history of obstructive symptoms followed by sudden onset of anuria or oliguria. Polyuria and nocturia due to renal concentrating defect may be seen in patients with partial or intermittent obstruction. Other features of ARF secondary to obstruction are increased BUN:creatinine

ratio, hyperkalemia, and defective urinary acidification with metabolic acidosis.

The two most important diagnostic tests when obstruction is suspected are bladder catheterization and renal ultrasonography. If urinary tract obstruction is strongly suspected, but ultrasound results are equivocal, then a "stone protocol" noninfused computed tomography (CT) scan should be performed. In some cases where false-negative ultrasound or CT scan results are suspected, cystoscopy and retrograde pyelograms may be required to definitively exclude the diagnosis of obstructive uropathy. For example, we would request retrograde pyelograms despite normal ultrasound images in a patient with anuric, hyperkalemic ARF and extensive pelvic tumor, potentially encasing the ureters and preventing dilation and hydronephrosis. Retroperitoneal fibrosis can similarly cause obstructive ARF without hydronephrosis. Early diagnosis is essential, as the extent of parenchymal damage is dependent on the duration of obstruction; complete recovery is possible up until 10 to 14 days of obstruction.

INTRINSIC ACUTE RENAL FAILURE

Intrinsic acute renal failure can be categorized anatomically, according to the site of the lesion: vascular, glomerular, or tubulointerstitial. We will discuss tubular and interstitial causes first, because they are far more common in hospitalized patients.

ACUTE TUBULAR NECROSIS

The most common cause of intrinsic ARF in hospitalized patients is acute tubular necrosis (ATN). ATN is caused by ischemia, nephrotoxins, or a combination of both, and accounts for approximately 85% to 90% of intrinsic ARF cases.[2,13] Ischemic ATN is commonly seen in patients with sepsis or severe cardiac failure, or postoperative patients, particularly after cardiac and aortic surgeries. Massive trauma or cardiac arrest are other causes of ATN. Prerenal failure can result in ischemic ATN if renal hypoperfusion is severe and not reversed by timely therapy. Although improving renal perfusion may reverse prerenal ARF (by definition), and diminish ischemic contributions to the pathogenesis of ATN, it is quite conceivable that in many cases ATN develops despite appropriate resuscitation and adequate renal perfusion. Zager has shown in an endotoxemic rat model of septic ARF that paired combinations of insults (renal cross clamp, systemic endotoxin, aminoglycoside, and temperature elevation) cause azotemia and renal pathologic findings of ATN, but these insults individually cause no renal dysfunction or injury.[13] We suspect that this synergistic injury model accurately reflects the pathogenesis of much ARF in the ICU. Positive pressure mechanical ventilation alters renal perfusion and function through a variety of mechanisms, both hemodynamic and inflammatory.[14] Other experimental data have shown that endotoxin, tumor necrosis factor, and numerous other inflammatory mediators are directly cytotoxic to renal endothelial and tubular cells.[15]

The diagnosis of ATN is usually made by clinical exclusion of alternative diagnoses such as obstruction or prerenal azotemia, and a lack of features suggestive of other intrinsic renal lesions. Characteristic urinalysis and urine chemistry findings frequently support the clinical diagnosis (see below). Ischemic ATN is usually reversible by tubular regeneration in surviving patients with previously

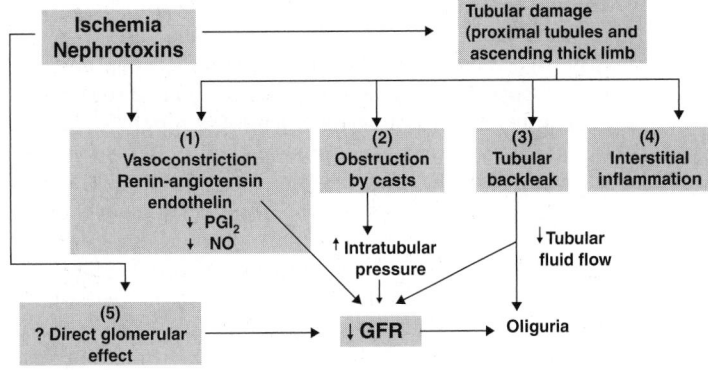

FIGURE 75-1 Pathophysiologic mechanisms of acute renal failure. Tubular damage by ischemia, nephrotoxins, or both, leads to decreased GFR by a combination of mechanisms. (1) Renal vasoconstriction via activation of tubuloglomerular feedback, and decreased vasodilator substances (PGI$_2$, prostacyclin; NO, nitric oxide) is a prominent functional mechanism of decreased GFR in ATN. (2) Backpressure from tubular obstruction by casts directly decreases GFR. (3) Backleakage of glomerular filtrate into peritubular capillaries decreases the efficiency of glomerular filtration, effectively decreasing GFR. (4) There is increasing evidence for a role of interstitial inflammation in the extension phase of ATN. (5) Direct glomerular effects (mesangial contraction, decreased filtration surface area) may also play a role in decreasing GFR in the presence of ATN. (*Reproduced with permission from Lameire et al.[21]*)

normal renal function. Failure to recover prompts consideration of a differential diagnostic list including bilateral cortical necrosis, renal atheroembolism, renal artery stenosis/thrombosis/dissection, and severe forms of other intrinsic lesions such as rapidly progressive glomerulonephritis (GN). Bilateral cortical necrosis causes irreversible renal failure and is associated with profound shock with disseminated intravascular coagulation, obstetric complications, hemolytic uremic syndrome, or snake bites.[16]

Cellular mediators that play a role in the pathogenesis of ATN include calcium, reactive oxygen species, phospholipases, proteases, adhesion molecules, and nitric oxide (NO).[17] ATN has several phases: prerenal, initiation, extension, maintenance, and repair.[18] It is not intuitive that renal tubular injury should cause decreased glomerular filtration and ARF. A decrease in glomerular ultrafiltration coefficient has been shown in several animal models of ARF, but this is a minor contributor to the observed decrement in GFR.[19,20] The pathophysiologic mechanisms that explain the reduction of GFR in ATN are hemodynamic abnormalities, tubular obstruction, and tubular backleakage of glomerular filtrate (Fig. 75-1).[21] Renal vasoconstriction is seen in ARF,[21,22] caused by activation of tubuloglomerular feedback; increased distal chloride delivery past injured tubular segments is sensed by the macula densa, causing vasoconstriction of the corresponding afferent arteriole. This reversible, functional mechanism seems to be the major cause of decreased GFR in ATN, and is in part protective. Severe hypovolemia would rapidly result if injured tubules failed to reabsorb the bulk of filtered sodium and water; thus the term "acute renal success" has been used to describe the development of decreased GFR ("acute renal failure") in the presence of tubular necrosis.[22] Furthermore, reabsorption of filtered sodium accounts for the bulk of renal oxygen consumption; continued glomerular filtration of sodium in ATN may aggravate hypoxic damage to sublethally injured tubules. The phenomenon of medullary hypoxia plays an important role in the pathogenesis of ATN. Low medullary blood flow is required for urinary concentration.[23] Reabsorption of sodium chloride by the medullary thick ascending limb of the loop of Henle (mTAL) is the major determinant of medullary oxygen consumption, resulting in a hypoxic environment under normal circumstances.[23,24] mTAL is vulnerable to ischemic injury if increased oxygen requirement is associated with decreased oxygen delivery. In addition, the inflammatory mechanisms that dominate as ATN progresses

from initiation to extension and maintenance phases of ATN result in medullary congestion and hypoperfusion.[18]

The tubular factors that are also involved in the reduction of GFR in ARF are tubular obstruction and tubular backleakage. Necrotic cell debris incorporated into casts causes obstruction of proximal and distal tubules and has been shown to play a significant role in experimental ARF.[25,26] Backleakage of tubular fluid across denuded basement membranes and injured proximal tubule cells has been demonstrated in several experimental models of ARF.[27] Subsequently it has been shown that tubular backleakage and intratubular obstruction are important factors contributing to the reduction of GFR in human ischemic ARF.[28,29]

Nephrotoxic injury is the second major cause of ATN. Nephrotoxic ATN is caused by drugs (aminoglycosides, cisplatin, amphotericin, and chemotherapy), radiocontrast agents, heme pigments (myoglobin and hemoglobin), and myeloma light chain proteins. ARF due to aminoglycosides and radiocontrast agents accounts for most cases of nephrotoxic ATN. Nephrotoxicity of cancer chemotherapy is discussed in Chap. 74; malignancy and ARF are further discussed below. Three nephrotoxic ARF syndromes will be further discussed here: aminoglycoside nephrotoxicity, radiocontrast nephropathy, and ARF caused by nonsteroidal anti-inflammatory drugs (NSAIDs).

Aminoglycoside Nephrotoxicity
Aminoglycosides like tobramicin, gentamicin, amikacin, and netilmicin are widely used for the treatment of gram-negative infections. Although they are effective antibiotics, therapy with aminoglycosides is complicated by nephrotoxicity in 10% to 20% of patients.[30] Aminoglycosides are excreted by glomerular filtration and are reabsorbed by proximal tubular cells. The mechanism of aminoglycoside-induced renal injury is not well understood. Accumulation of aminoglycosides in the proximal tubules in high concentration results in disruption of a variety of intracellular processes. Aminoglycosides are tubular toxins, and the earliest morphologic changes consist of vacuolization of proximal tubules, loss of brush border, and the presence of myeloid bodies within proximal tubule cells. Clinical evidence also attests to the tubular toxicity of aminoglycosides; maximum urine osmolality falls, and renal wasting of Mg^{2+} and K^+ ensues. The relationship between this tubule damage and reduced GFR remains unclear, although in experimental models using high doses

TABLE 75-2 Risk Factors for Aminoglycoside Nephrotoxicity

Preexisting renal disease
Advanced age
Volume depletion
Obstructive jaundice
Severe infection
Drug interactions
Cephalosporins
Vancomycin
Prostaglandin inhibitors

TABLE 75-3 Risk Factors for Radiocontrast Nephrotoxicity

Preexisting renal failure
Diabetes mellitus
Volume depletion
Previous contrast nephropathy
Multiple contrast procedures
High contrast dose (>2 mL/kg)
Congestive heart failure
Elderly patient
Multiple myeloma

of aminoglycosides, tubule obstruction and backleakage can be demonstrated. In experimental models of aminoglycoside nephrotoxicity, relatively small doses decrease glomerular permeability, while larger doses cause renal vasoconstriction. The relevance of these hemodynamic changes to human aminoglycoside nephrotoxicity is not known.

ARF generally develops 7 to 10 days after aminoglycoside therapy is started. Aminoglycoside nephrotoxicity is associated with nonoliguric ARF, due to a concentrating defect caused by tubular injury. Aminoglycoside nephrotoxicity is also accompanied by potassium and magnesium wasting. Risk factors for aminoglycoside nephrotoxicity are summarized in Table 75-2. In patients with preexisting renal insufficiency the dosing interval should be adjusted and levels monitored to minimize the risk of ototoxicity and nephrotoxicity. Once-daily dosing of aminoglycosides decreases nephrotoxicity with no apparent loss of effectiveness.[31–33] In patients with acutely deteriorating renal function who require aminoglycoside therapy, monitoring may be very difficult and require frequent reassessment. Aminoglycosides should be discontinued whenever renal dysfunction develops; increasing trough levels and decreased calculated aminoglycoside clearance may signal decreased GFR before serum creatinine increases. Recovery of renal function is expected in most cases when nephrotoxicity is recognized early and aminoglycosides held, but may be delayed for days to weeks.

Radiocontrast Nephropathy

ARF due to radiocontrast agents occurs within 24 to 48 hours of intravenous radiocontrast administration, and is termed radiocontrast nephropathy. Vasoconstriction and direct tubular toxicity due to generation of oxygen free radicals are thought to be the pathogenetic mechanisms of radiocontrast nephrotoxicity. In most cases the ARF is mild and recovery typically begins with stabilization of serum creatinine at 3 to 5 days postcontrast.[34] Renal failure is usually nonoliguric. However, in patients with preexisting severe chronic renal failure radiocontrast nephropathy may be severe, irreversible, and require chronic dialysis.

The risk of nephrotoxicity due to contrast agents varies with the type and dose of agent. Low- or iso-osmolal agents are less nephrotoxic than ionic high-osmolal agents.[35,36] The incidence of ARF due to radiocontrast agents is less than 2% in patients with normal renal function, but is inversely related to GFR in patients with chronic renal insufficiency; in high-risk patients the incidence is as high as 60%.[37] There are several important risk factors for radiocontrast nephropathy, including chronic renal insufficiency, diabetic nephropathy, severe congestive heart failure, intravascular volume depletion, high contrast dose, and multiple myeloma (Table 75-3).

Of note, the risk of radiocontrast nephropathy at any GFR level of chronic renal impairment is approximately double in diabetics compared to nondiabetics. The group at risk for radiocontrast nephropathy can be reliably identified, and a variety of prophylactic strategies have been used, several successfully.

A number of measures are used for prevention of radiocontrast nephropathy. Alternative imaging approaches (ultrasound, noninfused CT, or gadolinium-enhanced magnetic resonance angiography) are preferred to radiocontrast studies in patients with a high risk of radiocontrast nephropathy. Nonionic low-osmolal agents[35] and nonionic iso-osmolol agents[36] are less nephrotoxic, and these agents are used to decrease the incidence of ARF due to radiocontrast agents. Standard recommendations suggest that IV hydration with 0.45% saline is beneficial in reducing the incidence and severity of radiocontrast nephropathy,[38] but recently normal saline (1 mL/kg per hour for 12 hours pre- and postcontrast) was demonstrated superior for this purpose.[39] Most recently, Merten and colleagues showed that administration of an equimolar sodium bicarbonate solution was superior to normal saline for radiocontrast nephropathy prophylaxis, infused as 3 mL/kg per hour for 1 hour precontrast, then 1 mL/kg per hour for 6 hours.[40] In some studies the administration of acetylcysteine, a thiol-containing antioxidant, in combination with saline hydration has been shown to be beneficial in reducing the incidence of contrast nephropathy when administered in various oral regimens (1200 mg once or 600 mg every 12 hours before and after radiocontrast).[41–43] One successful study used intravenous acetylcysteine for radiocontrast nephropathy prophylaxis.[44] Although other studies did not show any benefit,[45,46] a recent meta-analysis of eight randomized controlled trials involving 855 patients reported that the use of acetylcysteine reduced the risk of radiocontrast by 59%.[46] However, further doubt has been cast over these inconsistent findings by emerging experimental data that suggest that the apparent efficacy of acetylcysteine in these studies may have been artifactual. Specifically, acetylcysteine causes a decrement in serum creatinine (but not cystatin C) by a GFR-independent mechanism,[47] perhaps by inhibiting creatinine phosphokinase function.[48] Nevertheless, given the available data, oral administration of acetylcysteine to patients at high risk of developing contrast nephropathy appears warranted, and should do no harm in combination with adequate volume expansion. Other approaches such as vasodilation with dopamine[49] or fenoldopam[50] failed to prevent radiocontrast nephropathy, and mannitol and furosemide appeared to increase the rate of ARF postcontrast in one study.[38] Prophylactic hemodialyis has not been shown to be beneficial in the prevention of contrast nephropathy.[51]

More recently, Marenzi and colleagues compared the effectiveness of hemofiltration with intravenous isotonic saline administration in patients with chronic renal insufficiency undergoing coronary interventions.[52] BUN and serum creatinine were measured at baseline, immediately before the procedure, and then daily for the following 3 days and at hospital discharge. In this study there was less likelihood of an increase in serum creatinine (the primary end point), less likelihood of requiring emergent hemodialysis, and less in-hospital and 1-year mortality in the hemofiltration group.[52] Adulteration of the primary end point by hemofiltration of creatinine in one arm is a fatal flaw of this study. Other flaws include an unbalanced level of care between the groups (floor vs. hemofiltration in the ICU), and more regulation of fluid balance in the hemofiltration group (and more pulmonary edema in the fluids-alone arm). Since hemofiltration is also expensive, associated with a variety of risks, and a limited resource, we do not recommend this approach to radiocontrast nephropathy prevention unless confirmed by additional prospective controlled studies.

Nonsteroidal Anti-Inflammatory Drugs and Acute Renal Failure

NSAIDs can cause hemodynamically mediated ARF. Vasodilatory prostaglandins (prostacyclin and prostaglandin E_2 [PGE_2]) are essential for the maintenance of renal blood flow and GFR in states of effective volume depletion, such as congestive heart failure, cirrhosis of the liver, nephrotic syndrome, and in states of true volume depletion.[53] Prostaglandins counterbalance the effects of vasoconstrictors such as angiotensin II and catecholamines. NSAIDs inhibit prostaglandins and thus would lead to unopposed effect of angiotensin II and catecholamines, leading to reduced GFR. Hyperkalemia may be prominent because NSAIDs impair renin secretion. Patients with chronic renal insufficiency are similarly at risk for NSAID-induced ARF, because vasodilator prostaglandins maintain hyperfiltration in remnant nephrons. Hemodynamically-mediated ARF is seen within days of taking NSAIDs in high-risk patients. Cyclooxygenase-2 (COX-2) selective drugs have the same renal effects as nonselective NSAIDs, because COX-2 is constitutively expressed and physiologically active in the kidney.[54] The second type of acute renal injury is allergic interstitial nephritis, as discussed below. Chronic NSAID use is also associated with papillary necrosis and is thought to occur in patients who are taking multiple analgesics.

ACUTE TUBULOINTERSTITIAL NEPHRITIS

ARF due to acute interstitial nephritis (AIN) is most often caused by allergic reaction to various drugs (allergic AIN), but there are also a variety of infectious (Legionnaire's disease, cytomegalovirus, and Hantavirus), autoimmune (lupus), alloimmune (renal transplant rejection), and infiltrative (sarcoidosis, leukemia, and lymphoma) disorders that can cause AIN (see Table 75-1). The most common drugs that cause allergic AIN are penicillins, cephalosporins, ciprofloxacin, rifampin, sulfonamides (furosemide, thiazide diuretics, and trimethoprim-sulfamethoxazole), cimetidine, allopurinol and NSAIDs.

Patients with AIN classically present with ARF temporally related to drug therapy or infection, associated with a triad of fever, rash, and eosinophilia.[55] Urinalysis findings include leukocyturia with eosinophiluria, leukocyte casts, and low-grade proteinuria. Although all these signs are present in the majority of patients with AIN, absence of these does not exclude the diagnosis of AIN. In particular, these findings are usually absent in NSAID-induced AIN. Proteinuria is mild to moderate except in NSAID-induced AIN, in which nephrotic syndrome caused by a minimal change lesion has been described. Tubular dysfunction (e.g., Fanconi's syndrome, distal renal tubular acidosis, or hyperkalemia) occurs in the majority of patients with AIN.

AIN is usually suspected from the history and laboratory findings. In the absence of urinary tract infection, detection of large numbers of urinary eosinophils (>5%) strongly suggests the diagnosis of drug-induced tubulointerstitial nephropathy (TIN). Hansel's stain of the urine is more sensitive than Wright's stain for the detection of urinary eosinophils.[56] The Hansel method correctly identified 10 of 11 patients with TIN, as opposed to only 2 of 11 correctly classified using Wright's stain. False-positive results with the Hansel technique are most commonly caused by rapidly progressive GN or acute prostatitis. Diagnosis can be confirmed by renal biopsy if ARF is progressive and treatment of an alternative diagnosis is considered (e.g., rapidly progressive GN), or if there is no recovery of renal function after discontinuation of the medication suspected to have caused AIN.

No therapy is recommended in patients with mild renal insufficiency, and in patients who respond after discontinuation of the offending medication. AIN is usually reversible after withdrawal of the offending agent and treatment of underlying disease; corticosteroid therapy is unproven, and generally recommended only in patients with biopsy-confirmed acute allergic interstitial nephritis who do not respond to conservative management, and have no contraindication to immunosuppression.

RAPIDLY PROGRESSIVE GLOMERULONEPHRITIS

Glomerulonephritis such as postinfectious glomerulonephritis, lupus nephritis, and Goodpasture's syndrome can cause acute or subacute renal failure (see Table 75-1). Rapidly progressive glomerulonephritis (RPGN) causing ARF is an emergency. The combination of ARF with an "active" urine sediment (heavy proteinuria, hematuria, leukocyturia, and erythrocyte/leukocyte/mixed cellular casts) should prompt urgent evaluation with renal biopsy and serologies. The underlying pathologic lesion is classically necrotizing crescentic glomerulonephritis, treated with high-dose pulse corticosteroid therapy to stabilize renal function, followed by intensive immunosuppression (with or without plasmapheresis). Causes include inflammatory disorders with immune complex deposition (lupus, postinfectious, or cryoglobulinemia), anti–glomerular basement membrane antibodies (Goodpasture's syndrome, when associated with pulmonary hemorrhage), and pauci-immune glomerulonephritis (usually with small-vessel vasculitis; see below). Associated clinical features such as pulmonary hemorrhage, sinus involvement, leukocytoclastic vasculitis, neuropathy, or other stigmata of autoimmune disease may increase the index of suspicion for this diagnosis, but it must be emphasized that a skilled urinalysis demonstrating an "active" sediment in a patient with ARF may make this diagnosis alone. In fact the presence of erythrocyte casts is pathognomonic of GN; associated with ARF, this is essentially diagnostic of RPGN.

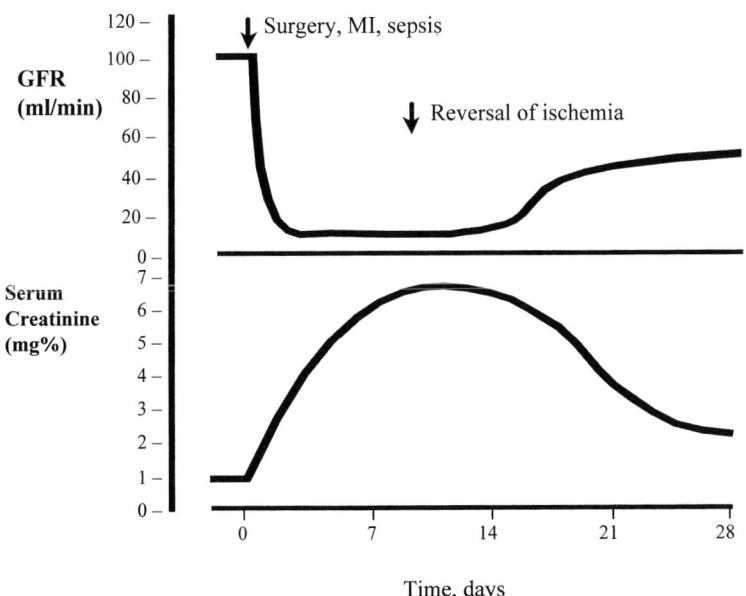

FIGURE 75-2 Dynamic relationship between serum creatinine and GFR in ARF. Moran and Myers demonstrated that elevation of serum creatinine lags significantly behind GFR decrements in ARF. In this example, an acute decrement in GFR to <10 mL/min (commonly a dialysis-requiring level) after a major ischemic insult is associated with a subsequent slow, daily rise of serum creatinine. The daily serum creatinine increment is determined by creatinine generation (muscle mass and catabolic state), volume status (volume of distribution of creatinine), and the new GFR level. Serum creatinine continues to rise until creatinine generation equals creatinine excretion at steady state. Only after a week is it fully apparent from the serum creatinine level how low the GFR is in this patient with ARF; this could have been inferred from the progressive daily serum creatinine increments, and measured by urine collection for an abbreviated creatinine clearance. *(Reproduced with permission from Star,[3] and modified with permission from Moran et al.[61])*

VASCULAR CAUSES OF ACUTE RENAL FAILURE

Vascular causes of ARF are categorized into small-vessel diseases and large-vessel diseases (see Table 75-1). Diseases involving small vessels include microscopic polyarteritis (vasculitis in polyarteritis nodosa and Kawasaki's disease involves medium-sized vessels), Wegener's granulomatosis, mixed cryoglobulinemia, and conditions that are categorized as thrombotic microangiopathies, including thrombotic thrombocytopenic purpura, hemolytic uremic syndrome, scleroderma renal crisis, malignant hypertension, and antiphospholipid antibody syndrome. Large-vessel renal vascular diseases include thromboembolic diseases and renal vein thrombosis. Atheroembolic disease should be considered in patients who develop ARF after instrumentation of the aorta, particularly in patients with known atherosclerotic disease.[57] Renal vein thrombosis is usually a complication of nephrotic syndrome, and if bilateral can cause ARF. Abdominal compartment syndrome (see Chap. 42) is present when the intra-abdominal pressure (IAP) reaches 20 to 25 cm H_2O, and unless decompressed, irreversible organ failure may result.[58] The pathogenesis of oliguria and ARF in abdominal compartment syndrome involves venous compression (decreased venous return and renal vein compression), ureteral compression with obstructive uropathy, and possibly changes in renovascular resistance and intrarenal blood flow distribution. Regardless of the underlying cause, a reduction in urine output with or without azotemia in the presence of a measured intra-abdominal pressure over 15 cm H_2O is cause for concern and should prompt intervention.

Renal Function Monitoring and Diagnostic Approach to Acute Renal Failure

MONITORING RENAL FUNCTION IN THE ICU

Attempts to develop strategies to prevent or treat ARF in the ICU have been hampered by the lack of sensitive real-time methods to monitor renal perfusion and function in the clinical setting.[59] There are no direct measures of renal perfusion in clinical use. Of the available research techniques for this purpose, para-aminohippuric acid (PAH) clearance is not a valid method to assess renal plasma flow because renal PAH extraction is impaired in critical illness, after cardiac surgery, post–renal transplantation, and in ARF.[60] Clinical indices such as plasma concentrations of urea nitrogen and creatinine, urine output, urine chemistries, and urinalysis may be assessed in combination to monitor renal perfusion and function, but alterations in these markers are insensitive, indirect, and often delayed manifestations of renal hypoperfusion and injury.[59] Although relatively insensitive, it should be recognized that progressive elevation of serum creatinine is a specific sign of decreased GFR and diagnostic of ARF. As depicted in Fig. 75-2, daily serum creatinine increments of 0.5 to 1 mg/dL (depending on muscle mass, and in the absence of rhabdomyolysis) signal severe depression of GFR.[61] In the absence of obstruction or renal hypoperfusion, this is usually diagnostic of ATN.

Direct measurement of GFR is probably the most relevant marker of renal function to monitor in the ICU, and can be used as an index of adequate systemic perfusion, a marker of organ dysfunction, a guide to medication dosing, and to determine timing of initiation of renal replacement therapy. GFR measurement methods more sensitive than monitoring serum creatinine and urea nitrogen have been validated in this population, but are not yet in widespread clinical use.[59,62] Abbreviated creatinine clearance measurements (2 to 4 hours) provide a more accurate estimate of GFR than serum creatinine alone, and are more timely than 24-hour urine collections.[63] Emerging data suggest that serial monitoring of serum cystatin C levels may provide a more sensitive index of early ARF than serum creatinine or BUN. Cystatin C is a nonglycosylated 13-kDa basic protein that is a member of the cystatin superfamily of cysteine protease inhibitors. It is produced by all nucleated cells, and its production rate is unaltered by inflammatory conditions or muscle mass; only thyroid dysfunction has been shown to alter serum levels independent of GFR in studies to date.[64–66] It undergoes purely renal excretion.

Serum cystatin C levels increase before serum creatinine levels in patients with progressive chronic kidney disease.[64,66] Emerging data suggest that plasma cystatin C levels similarly increase 1 to 2 days before serum creatinine in patients developing ARF in a variety of settings,[66] including radio-contrast nephropathy,[67] renal transplantation,[68,69] cirrhotic ARF,[70] malarial ARF,[71] and ARF in the ICU.[72,73] In the latter study of 85 critically-ill patients, Herget-Rosenthal and colleagues showed that ARF defined by elevation of cystatin C occurred 1 to 2 days before serum creatinine elevation; the area under the curve in receiver operating curve analysis was 0.82 and 0.97 on the 2 days prior to creatinine-defined ARF.[73]

In patients with azotemia and/or oliguria, traditional urine chemistry markers may provide useful information, interpreted in combination with other clinical and laboratory parameters (see below), including microscopic urinalysis.[59,74] Hopefully, more sensitive markers of early renal hypoperfusion and injury will prove clinically useful in the future.[75,76] Meanwhile, all clinically available renal function indices should be used in combination for assessment of renal perfusion and function in the ICU.

DIAGNOSTIC APPROACH TO ACUTE RENAL FAILURE

The diagnostic approach to ARF involves assignment of the cause to prerenal, renal, or postrenal categories, with further refinement of the diagnosis based on additional laboratory testing.

HISTORY AND PHYSICAL EXAMINATION IN ACUTE RENAL FAILURE

Any decrease in effective perfusion of the kidneys can result in the syndrome of prerenal ARF. This may be the result of an absolute decrease in the extracellular fluid (ECF) volume, redistribution of ECF from vascular to interstitial locations (third-spacing), or impaired delivery of blood to the kidneys such as can occur in patients with renal arterial stenosis, vasculitis, or depressed cardiac function. Third-space losses should be suspected in the presence of severe burns, pancreatitis, peritonitis, or recent abdominal surgery. Absolute decreases in the ECF volume are most common in the setting of gastrointestinal fluid losses or in patients receiving excessive doses of diuretics.

Decreases in weight, if known, can provide some information about the degree of ECF loss. However, weight changes are subject to misinterpretation if the nature of fluid loss is not taken into account (Fig. 75-3). The ability of pure water loss (which is spread out across the total-body water) to cause volume depletion is only one-third as great as an equivalent loss of isotonic fluid (all of which must come from the smaller ECF compartment). Thus the importance of changes in weight should be assessed relative to changes in serum sodium concentration.

The cardinal signs of ECF volume depletion are changes in hemodynamic parameters, jugular venous pressure, and in the skin. An orthostatic increase in pulse of 15 beats per minute or a decrease in diastolic blood pressure of 10 mm Hg can detect losses of 5% of the ECF volume. A postural increase in pulse (supine to standing) of at least 30 beats per minute is 96% specific for clinically-significant volume depletion, whereas systolic pressure may fall 20 mm Hg upon

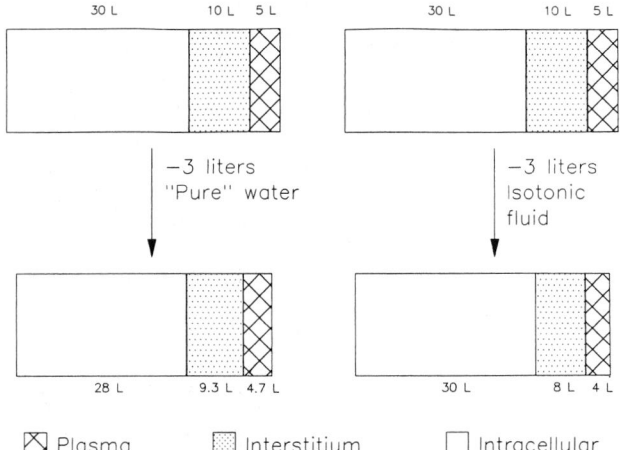

FIGURE 75-3 Effect of fluid loss on body water distribution. Because water is in osmotic equilibrium across biologic membranes, loss of 3 L of solute-free water will be spread across the total body water, resulting in a small decrease (0.3 L) in plasma volume. A similar loss of isotonic fluid, which does not obligate osmotic water movement, leads to a much greater decrease (1.0 L) in plasma volume. This is based on the assumption of 45 L of total body water, two-thirds of which is intracellular. Of the extracellular fluid, about one-third is plasma and the remainder extravascular (interstitium).

standing in 10% of normal individuals and in up to 30% of patients >age 65.[77] The inability of a patient to stand because of severe lightheadedness is a relatively specific sign of hypovolemia. In uncomplicated hypovolemia, estimated central venous pressure by examination of jugular venous pressure should be low. Skin changes that accompany volume depletion include cool, mottled extremities, dry mucous membranes and axillae, and skin tenting (particularly over the forehead and sternum, where age-related changes in skin elasticity are not as pronounced as elsewhere).

Obstruction of the urinary tract must be considered in every patient with an acute deterioration of renal function. The symptoms of acute urinary tract obstruction (severe flank pain, hematuria, and changes in urine flow) are often mistaken for urinary tract infection. Of more importance from a historical standpoint is the identification of preexisting conditions that predispose to urinary tract obstruction. Some of these are listed in Table 75-1. Physical findings suggestive of obstruction include palpably enlarged kidneys, pelvic or abdominal masses, bladder enlargement, prostatic hypertrophy, aneurysmal dilation of the aorta, and signs of inflammatory bowel disease. If oliguria or anuria develops in a critically ill patient with a Foley catheter in place, possible catheter occlusion should be assessed by sterile flushing and if necessary a catheter change.

Intrinsic ARF can be the final result of many diverse renal insults. While space limitations do not permit a thorough review of all aspects of the history and physical examination in intrinsic ARF, some points deserve comment. ARF due to therapeutic or recreational drugs (e.g., cocaine-induced rhabdomyolysis) is so common that a detailed drug history is mandatory.[78] The presence of a skin rash should suggest the possibility of a systemic vasculitis with renal involvement or acute tubulointerstitial nephritis. Palpable purpura due to leukocytoclastic vasculitis is characteristic of Henoch-Schönlein purpura. One of the pulmonary-renal syndromes should be considered if prominent thoracic complaints accompany ARF. These include, among others, Goodpasture's syndrome, Wegener's granulomatosis, microscopic polyarteritis, systemic lupus erythematosus, and Churg-Strauss syndrome.

DIAGNOSTIC TESTS IN ACUTE RENAL FAILURE

The majority of cases of ARF can be diagnosed by history and physical examination. However, in a significant minority the cause remains obscure after initial assessment, and further evaluation is necessary.

Daily urine volume must be measured in all patients with ARF. Bladder catheterization is both diagnostic and therapeutic in patients with obstruction at the level of the bladder neck or urethra. Urine volume is determined by the requirement to excrete the daily obligate solute load (electrolytes and nitrogenous wastes) in appropriately concentrated urine. Assuming maximal urine concentrating ability (1400 mOsm/kg), the minimum daily urine output required to excrete the average daily solute load is 400 mL, below which positive solute balance and azotemia develop, thus the standard definition of oliguria (<400 mL/24 hours). In terms of monitoring urine output, if urine is maximally concentrated (1400 mOsm/kg), and excretion of 10 mOsm/kg per day (700 mOsm/d in a 70-kg person) is required to avoid solute retention, this mandates urine output of 500 mL daily (21 mL/h, or 0.3 mL/kg per hour). Of course, if solute appearance increases (patient size, hypercatabolism, or hyperalimentation) or maximal urinary concentrating ability is diminished (renal dysfunction or advanced age), higher urine volumes are required to maintain adequate solute excretion. Since such conditions are more the rule than the exception, it seems more appropriate to expect solute retention at urine outputs below the more typical ICU monitoring target of 0.5 to 1 mL/kg per hour (840 to 1680 mL/d). Of course, urine output targets must be sufficient to control fluid balance as well as solute excretion, so higher urine output values may be required for patients with large obligate fluid intakes.

ARF is classified as anuric (urine output <100 mL/d), oliguric (urine output <400 mL/d), or nonoliguric (urine output >400 mL/d). Causes of ARF associated with various urine flow patterns are listed in Table 75-4. Prerenal ARF with polyuria may be seen very rarely if excessive urine losses are the cause of the prerenal state. This occurs in adrenal or mineralocorticoid deficiency states and excessive diuresis. Although occasional polyuric patients with urinary indices suggestive of prerenal ARF have been described,[79] it is believed that the majority of them in fact have polyuric ATN rather than prerenal ARF. The continued use of an indwelling bladder catheter after the cause of ARF has been determined is frequently unnecessary and merely increases the risk of nosocomial urinary tract infection. This is particularly true in the oligo-anuric patient. Intermittent bladder catheterization once or twice daily can provide useful information with a lower risk of urosepsis. An external condom-type catheter does not provide sufficient information to replace the Foley catheter in persons with ARF. Because it is also associated with an increased risk of urinary infection, it cannot be recommended in this setting.

Urinalysis is also useful in patients with ARF. The urinary specific gravity tends to be >1.020 in patients with prerenal

TABLE 75-4 Urine Flow Rates in the Diagnosis of Acute Renal Failure

Anuria (<100 mL/d)
    Complete urinary tract obstruction
    Bilateral renal arterial or venous occlusion
    Bilateral cortical necrosis
    Overwhelming acute tubular necrosis
    Severe acute glomerulonephritis
Oliguria (100–400 mL/d)
    Prerenal azotemia
    Intrinsic acute renal failure
    Tubular necrosis
    Interstitial nephritis
    Glomerulonephritis
    Partial intermittent obstruction
Polyuria nonoliguria (>400 mL/d)
    Tubular necrosis
    Interstitial nephritis
    Partial intermittent obstruction

failure. On the other hand, patients with intrinsic or postrenal ARF are generally isosthenuric, with a urine specific gravity of approximately 1.010. Substantial proteinuria (3 g/d or more) strongly suggests the possibility of a glomerular disease, with nephrotic-range proteinuria (>3.5 g per 24 hours) pathognomonic of glomerular rather than tubular disease; this may be confirmed with a "spot" urine protein:creatinine ratio (>3 suggests nephrotic-range proteinuria will be confirmed by 24-hour urine collection). Glycosuria in the absence of hyperglycemia strongly suggests proximal tubular injury with Fanconi's syndrome. A positive reaction for blood in the urine is consistent with acute glomerular or tubular injury, urinary tract infection, or nephrolithiasis. If blood is present on dipstick but not microscopically, or if the findings are disproportionate (e.g., 4+ blood on dipstick with rare erythrocytes on microscopy), a pigment nephropathy (hemoglobinuria or myoglobinuria) should be considered. The urine sediment is usually unremarkable in prerenal and postrenal azotemia, except for occasional hyaline casts. In postrenal ARF due to stones, blood and crystals can be seen. Intrinsic ARF is often associated with a characteristic (or even diagnostic) urine sediment. A careful microscopic examination frequently can distinguish between GN, AIN, ATN, and TIN. Erythrocyte casts, often accompanied by proteinuria and numerous erythrocytes and leukocytes, are pathognomonic of GN. Detection of large numbers of leukocytes, leukocyte casts, and eosinophils in uninfected urine strongly suggests the diagnosis of drug-induced AIN. ATN is suggested by findings including muddy brown granular casts, free renal tubular cells, and tubular cell casts.

Several measurements of urine composition have been suggested as ways to differentiate between prerenal azotemia and intrinsic ARF in the oliguric patient.[80] Urine electrolytes are most useful in this regard, especially the fractional excretion of sodium (FE$_{Na}$), calculated as

$$FE_{Na}(\%) = \frac{U_{Na} \times P_{Cr} \times 100}{P_{Na} \times U_{Cr}} \qquad (75\text{-}1)$$

where U$_{Na}$ and P$_{Na}$ are urine and plasma sodium concentrations, respectively, and U$_{Cr}$ and P$_{Cr}$ are urine and plasma

TABLE 75-5 Causes of Acute Renal Failure with Low Fractional Excretion of Sodium

Prerenal azotemia
Nonoliguric acute tubular necrosis
Acute glomerulonephritis
Acute obstruction (early)
Acute interstitial nephritis
Contrast nephropathy
Nontraumatic rhabdomyolysis
Uric acid nephropathy

creatinine concentrations, respectively. Values of FE_{Na} <0.01 (1%) in oliguric patients suggest avid tubular sodium reclamation and prerenal azotemia with functioning renal tubules, whereas values >.03 (3%) suggest tubular injury. The FE_{Na} is less useful in patients who are not oliguric.[81] Contrary to common belief, however, it may be useful in diuretic-treated patients. Although an elevated value may be a result of ATN or the effects of the diuretic, a low level in the face of diuretic therapy strongly suggests volume depletion and prerenal ARF. Some causes of ARF presenting with a low FE_{Na} are listed in Table 75-5. A low U_{Na} (<10 mEq/L) as an isolated measurement is often used as evidence of a prerenal state. However, this measurement depends exquisitely on the state of water balance in addition to sodium balance. It cannot be said that it is any easier to use than FE_{Na}, since an independent evaluation of water balance must be made to interpret it. Therefore it is not recommended as an isolated measurement in the routine evaluation of ARF.

Most other urinary diagnostic indices do not show any clear-cut superiority over FE_{Na} in distinguishing prerenal azotemia from ATN; however, they are independently useful in the assessment of tubular function. Recent data suggest urinary fractional excretion of urea (FE_{UN}) is superior to FE_{Na} to distinguish prerenal azotemia from ATN, particularly in diuretic-treated patients. FE_{UN} is calculated as

$$FE_{UN}(\%) = \frac{U_{UN} \times P_{Cr} \times 100}{BUN \times U_{Cr}} \quad (75\text{-}2)$$

where U_{UN} and BUN are urine and serum urea nitrogen concentrations, respectively, and U_{Cr} and P_{Cr} are urine and plasma creatinine concentrations, respectively. The normal FE_{UN} is 50% to 65%, reflecting reabsorption of approximately 50% of filtered urea in the proximal tubule; urea reabsorption is trivial in the thick ascending limb and distal convoluted tubule. Hypovolemia results in increased urea absorption, decreased urea clearance, and thus a lower FE_{UN}.[82] Loop and thiazide diuretics, which act at the thick ascending limb and distal convoluted tubule, do not interfere directly with urea reabsorption and should not alter FE_{UN}. However proximal tubule diuretics and osmotic diuresis decrease proximal reabsorption of urea and may produce an inappropriately high FE_{UN}. Carvounis and colleagues prospectively evaluated 102 hospitalized patients with ARF.[74] Patients were divided into three groups: 50 were deemed prerenal; 27 were deemed prerenal with diuretics given up to the day of consultation (details were not provided as to whether diuretics were given 1 or 23 hours prior to the urine sample); and 25 were diagnosed with ATN. Patients with AIN, GN, and obstructive nephropa-

thy were excluded. FE_{Na} was <1%, as expected, in 92% of group 1 patients, but in only 48% of the prerenal patients treated with diuretics. In contrast, 90% of the group 1 patients and 89% of those given diuretics had a FE_{UN} <35%. The ATN patients evidenced a mean FE_{UN} of 59%. A FE_{UN} <35% had 85% sensitivity, 92% specificity, 99% positive predictive value and 75% negative predictive value for a prerenal state. In this study, the urine:plasma creatinine ratio also performed better than FE_{Na} to distinguish prerenal azotemia from ATN. One other urine chemistry test may be useful in hyperuricemic patients with ARF and possible urate nephropathy (tumor lysis syndrome and hypovolemia with hyperuricemia and acid urine): urine uric acid:urine creatinine ratios >1.1 are consistent with acute urate nephropathy.[83]

Several radiographic studies are useful in the evaluation of patients with ARF. Plain films of the abdomen can assess kidney size, detect >90% of renal stones, and detect skeletal abnormalities of secondary hyperparathyroidism, which imply chronic renal insufficiency rather than ARF. In our view, the potential hazards of intravenous pyelography make this test of little benefit in the work-up of ARF. Renal ultrasound is a sensitive and specific method for detecting hydronephrosis. It is probably indicated in nearly every patient with ARF unless obstruction can be proven more quickly in another manner (e.g., by bladder catheterization in a patient with symptoms of bladder neck obstruction) or if some diagnosis other than obstruction is made with certainty early in the evaluation. If clinical suspicion of obstruction persists despite an apparently negative ultrasound, retrograde pyelography is the definitive diagnostic maneuver.[84] Computed tomography of the kidneys does not have any advantages over ultrasound and retrograde pyelography in the detection of obstruction, but may help clarify its cause. Radionuclide scans of the kidneys may be useful in the evaluation of patients with suspected vascular accidents of the kidneys.

The great majority of the time, volume status can be ascertained by history and physical examination alone. Occasionally one is presented with a patient in whom the ECF volume status cannot be determined with certainty on clinical grounds, particularly subjects with significant third-space losses. A typical example would be a patient with sepsis, hypotension, noncardiogenic pulmonary edema, anasarca, and oliguria. In this case, the clinician is often faced with the contradictory choice of using either diuretics or intravenous fluids. It is obviously inappropriate to treat a patient as if volume overload and hypovolemia were present simultaneously; in this setting, invasive hemodynamic monitoring with a central venous pressure (and central venous oxygen saturation) or a pulmonary artery catheter (and mixed venous oxygen saturation) can be an invaluable diagnostic adjunct. Complementary information may be obtained from simultaneous echocardiography.

Clinical Acute Renal Failure Syndromes

There are a number of diseases that commonly lead to ARF. In many cases of ARF in the ICU, prerenal azotemia combines with exposure to nephrotoxins (endogenous or exogenous) to cause ATN. However, the suspicion of other causes such as obstruction or specific parenchymal lesions is increased in certain patient populations.

MALIGNANCY AND ACUTE RENAL FAILURE

ARF is seen in patients with malignancy and could be caused by malignancy itself or its treatment with chemotherapeutic agents (Table 75-6). The full differential diagnosis of ARF must be considered in cancer patients, including common causes such as prerenal azotemia, drug nephrotoxicity, and obstructive uropathy, as well as rarer causes such as tumor infiltration of the kidneys and radiation nephritis. Urinary tract obstruction leading to ARF is commonly seen in patients with malignancy. Ureteral obstruction is seen in patients with abdominal and pelvic metastasis. ARF is also caused by intratubular obstruction. This is usually seen in patients with acute uric acid nephropathy as part of tumor lysis syndrome, intratubular obstruction by light chains in patients with multiple myeloma, and in patients who received high-dose methotrexate.

A variety of chemotherapeutic agents are potentially nephrotoxic, including cisplatin, nitrosoureas, and methotrexate, as discussed in Chap. 74. In addition, mitomycin is known to cause hemolytic uremic syndrome thus leading to renal failure.

If large numbers of malignant cells suddenly die, as in spontaneous necrosis or successful chemotherapy of large tumors, ARF can occur as a result of tumor lysis syndrome. This is noted most commonly in patients with germ cell tumors or hematologic malignancies because of their rapid turnover.[85] The tumor lysis syndrome is due to the toxic effects of intracellular constituents, which cause ARF, hyperkalemia, hyperphosphatemia, hypocalcemia, and hyperuricemia. The most common pathogenetic mechanism involved is acute urate nephropathy. When serum uric acid levels exceed about 20 mg/dL, the risk of ARF is high. The urinary ratio of uric acid to creatinine is >1.1.[83] Uric acid crystals may be seen in the urinary sediment. Synergistic factors in the development of the acute nephropathy include volume depletion and acidosis. The usual pathophysiology of urate nephropathy is intratubular deposition of urate crystals, causing intrarenal obstruction.[86] Less commonly, ureteral obstruction may be seen.

TABLE 75-6 Causes of Renal Dysfunction in Malignancy

Obstruction
   Ureteral
   Retroperitoneal lymphatic involvement
   Primary ureteral tumor
   Bladder neck
   Primary bladder tumor
   Prostate
Intrarenal
   Intratubular crystallization
   Light-chain proteins
Renal parenchymal invasion
   Renal cell carcinoma
   Metastases to kidneys
   Tumor infiltration (leukemias and lymphomas)
Drug effects
   Cisplatin
   Nitrosoureas
   Methotrexate
   Mithramycin
   Mitomycin
   Radiation nephritis

Once oliguria occurs, diuretics are seldom useful in restoring urine flow. Allopurinol and alkaline diuresis are effective measures when instituted prophylactically, but do not reverse established urate nephropathy.[87] Rasburicase, a recombinant form of urate oxidase, has been shown to be effective in reducing plasma uric acid levels within 4 hours after the first dose;[88] urate oxidase converts uric acid to allantoin, which is more soluble than uric acid. Severe hyperphosphatemia (levels >20 mg/dL) can be associated with tumor lysis and subsequent ARF.[89] The pathogenesis of the renal dysfunction can be either intratubular crystallization of phosphate or metastatic calcification in the renal parenchyma. It is important to make the distinction between this entity and urate nephropathy, because urinary alkalinization promotes calcium phosphate crystallization. If hyperuricemia is prevented or controlled by volume expansion, allopurinol, or uricase, it may be preferable to avoid or stop urinary alkalinization if severe hyperphosphatemia develops, to avoid hyperphosphatemia ARF and the risk of tetany (hypocalcemia combined with metabolic alkalosis). Renal replacement therapy in tumor lysis syndrome is indicated in patients in whom the resolution of ARF is unlikely, and is also indicated in patients with life-threatening electrolyte abnormalities. Normalization of uric acid and phosphorus levels is required for recovery of renal function. Hemodialysis is far more effective in the clearance of uric acid compared to peritoneal dialysis.[85] Continuous renal replacement therapies (CRRT) have been used in the management of tumor lysis syndrome. The solute clearances vary depending on the specific prescription. In these patients the uric acid and phosphorus clearances were, respectively, 45 mL/min and 47 mL/min in continuous venovenous hemodiafiltration and 39 mL/min and 40 mL/min in continuous arteriovenous hemodialysis.[90,91] These clearances were achieved with high dialysate and high replacement fluid rates. CRRT cannot correct electrolyte abnormalities as rapidly as intermittent hemodialysis, but it is a much more effective treatment for severe hyperphosphatemia, because rebound elevation of serum phosphorus postdialysis is prevented. Sequential hemodialysis to control severe evolving electrolyte abnormalities, followed by CRRT to prevent rebound may be the best approach. If RRT does not result in diuresis within a week, ureteral catheterization should be performed to exclude ureteral obstruction.

THROMBOTIC MICROANGIOPATHY AND ACUTE RENAL FAILURE

Hemolytic uremic syndrome (HUS) and the closely related entity thrombotic thrombocytopenic purpura (TTP) are characterized by renal involvement early in their course. Renal disease tends to be more fulminant in HUS than in TTP. Nearly 100% of patients with HUS have ARF at some point in their course (which is severe in at least 60%) as compared with a total incidence of renal failure of even mild severity in TTP that is <50%. Clinical features of these disorders are more thoroughly discussed in Chap. 70.

In the syndrome of disseminated intravascular coagulation (DIC), the pathologic picture is cortical necrosis. This can be prevented in some experimental models by the infusion of the angiotensin antagonist saralasin. It is unknown if activated protein C will decrease the contribution of microvascular injury and DIC to the pathogenesis of septic ARF. Numerous other causes of microangiopathic hemolytic anemia and thrombocytopenia can also cause ARF, including malignant hypertension, scleroderma renal crisis, and antiphospholipid syndrome.

PREGNANCY AND ACUTE RENAL FAILURE

The incidence of ARF complicating pregnancy has been decreasing for the past 25 years. This is attributable to improvements in prenatal care and obstetric science and fewer complications related to septic abortions. The timing of ARF in pregnancy has a bimodal distribution.[92] The early peak, which occurs during the first 20 weeks of gestation, is due to septic abortions, while the later peak (at 36 to 40 weeks) is secondary to preeclampsia and bleeding complications.

Preeclampsia and eclampsia are accompanied by decreases in GFR of 20% to 25% that are seldom clinically significant (see Chap. 105). However, in a small proportion of pregnant women, the renal dysfunction progresses to severe ARF. Women with preeclampsia are at increased risk for the development of cortical necrosis. Cortical necrosis also can occur as a complication of placental abruption (often with concealed blood loss) or prolonged intrauterine death. Although severe, irreversible renal failure may be seen, partial recovery of renal function due to patchy cortical necrosis is more common.[93] The diagnosis of complete cortical necrosis should be established by renal biopsy or arteriography to exclude patchy cortical necrosis and ATN, from either of which a degree of functional recovery is to be expected.

Coexisting ARF and fulminant hepatic failure have been described in gravid subjects. In women with acute fatty liver of pregnancy, ARF is present in over half. Although the mortality rate for both mother and fetus in this condition has been reported to be at least 70%, the prognosis may be improving because of increased recognition of less severe cases. The syndrome known by the acronym HELLP (*h*emolysis, *e*levated *l*iver enzymes, and *l*ow *p*latelets) is a variant of unusually severe preeclampsia. The great majority of these patients have evidence of hepatic dysfunction and sinusoidal congestion that may culminate in liver rupture. The mean creatinine clearance in these women is about 55 mL/min (less than half normal), while 10% have severe ARF with a creatinine clearance of <20 mL/min.

The rare but well-defined clinical entity of idiopathic postpartum ARF is characterized by the onset of ARF in the peripartum period following a previously normal pregnancy and childbirth.[94] The serum creatinine level rises rapidly within a few days to several weeks following parturition. There is often an associated consumptive coagulopathy. Other common clinical features include malignant hypertension, lethargy, seizures, and a dilated cardiomyopathy. The pathophysiology of this disorder is unknown. The outcome is poor; most patients have severe chronic renal failure, require dialysis, or die.

LIVER DISEASE AND ACUTE RENAL FAILURE

ARF frequently occurs in the setting of severe liver disease. Prerenal azotemia can be a consequence of ascitic redistribution of the ECF (or its excessive treatment with diuretics), GI fluid losses (e.g., vomiting, diarrhea, or hemorrhage), or cardiac dysfunction (e.g., alcoholic cardiomyopathy). If a

TABLE 75-7 Coexisting Renal and Liver Failure

Simultaneous liver and renal injury
Cardiovascular collapse with shock
Drugs and toxins
    Chlorinated solvents
    Heavy metals (arsenic, chromium, and copper)
    Antibiotics
    Isoniazid
    Rifampin
    Tetracyclines
    Sulfonamides
    Acetaminophen
    Mushroom poisoning (*Amanita phalloides*)
Infections
    Viral hepatitis
    Bacterial sepsis
Miscellaneous
    Reye's syndrome
    Acute fatty liver
    Systemic lupus erythematosus
    Polyarteritis nodosa
Sequential liver and renal injury
Prerenal azotemia
    Ascites
    Alcoholic cardiomyopathy
    Emesis
    Excessive diuresis
Intrinsic acute renal failure
    Cirrhotic glomerulosclerosis
    Acute tubular necrosis
    Hepatorenal syndrome
Obstructive nephropathy
    Blood clots in the collecting system
    Papillary necrosis

coagulopathy is present, blood clots in the collecting system can cause obstructive uropathy. Cirrhosis may predispose to the occurrence of papillary necrosis. Intrinsic ARF in subjects with liver disease is classified into disorders that simultaneously injure liver and kidney and those in which the renal disease is a consequence of the hepatic process (Table 75-7). The kidney is generally much more sensitive to the effects of potential nephrotoxic agents if jaundice is present. A relatively specific glomerular lesion called *cirrhotic glomerulosclerosis* has been identified and is usually asymptomatic; however, it probably predisposes to ARF of other causes. More commonly, patients with hepatitis B or C with proteinuria have membranous nephropathy or membranoproliferative (cryoglobulinemic) glomerulonephritis. Hepatitis B is also associated with polyarteritis nodosa. The most serious of coexisting hepatic and renal diseases is the hepatorenal syndrome (HRS).

HRS is difficult to distinguish from prerenal ARF in the setting of advanced liver failure; indeed, many authorities consider the two conditions to be part of a single spectrum. Perhaps the best operational definition of HRS is severe prerenal azotemia that does not respond to volume repletion. The principal functional abnormalities that have been described are renal vasospasm in the setting of peripheral vascular resistance that is abnormally low;[95] there is no "typical" structural lesion of HRS. Oliguria and a low FE_{Na} are frequent, if not universal, findings; the diagnosis of HRS should be considered untenable in their absence.

The therapy of HRS has been very disappointing.[95,96] A trial of empirical volume expansion with colloid solutions, with an end point of clear-cut increases in ascites and peripheral edema, can be used diagnostically to differentiate prerenal ARF from HRS. Attempts to modify low systemic vascular resistance have generally been unsuccessful in reversing this condition, as have attempts at selectively increasing renal perfusion. Emerging data suggest potential utility of combination treatment with midodrine and octreotide in hepatorenal syndrome;[97] vasopressin and analogues may also be useful for this indication.[96] There is little information on the use of transjugular intrahepatic portosystemic shunt in patients with HRS. Dialysis is only recommended in patients who are awaiting liver transplantation or in whom recovery of the underlying liver lesion is possible.

Paracentesis, ascitic reinfusion, and use of peritoneovenous shunts have not produced substantial improvements in patient survival in the few available controlled studies. Attempts to redistribute ascitic fluid into the vascular tree and then excrete it with various combinations of albumin, furosemide, and dopamine have not improved long-term results. Hemodialysis and related modalities have not been shown to improve survival and generally cannot be recommended except in two general settings. If there is any doubt about whether the patient may have potentially reversible ATN (such as by demonstration of a $FE_{Na} > 1\%$) or if the patient is a candidate for hepatic transplantation, all supportive measures including dialysis should be considered.

Some diseases simultaneously affect both liver and kidney. These diseases are summarized in Table 75-7.

ACUTE RENAL FAILURE IN RENAL TRANSPLANTATION

The approach to the transplant patient with ARF is no different from that in any other patient, with the exception that several unique entities must be considered. It is simplest to consider these in relation to the time since transplantation occurred. Within the first few hours or days after surgery, technical problems are the first consideration. In addition to hypovolemia and ATN, these include vascular thrombosis, ureteral stenosis, urinary leaks, and obstructive fluid collections such as hematomas or lymphoceles. Hyperacute rejection, though often apparent at the time of surgery, may not be recognized for several hours or days. Thorough diagnostic evaluation is mandatory, including renal ultrasound, confirmatory tissue typing (particularly the direct cross-match), and occasionally angiography or transplant biopsy. Surgical intervention is often required in addition to the usual supportive measures.

During the period beginning approximately a week after surgery and continuing for the next several months, drug effects, acute rejection, and infectious processes are of particular concern. It is during this time that antirejection drug dosages are at their highest levels, and as a result complications related to these drugs are most frequent. The immunosuppressive drugs cyclosporine and tacrolimus are frequent causes of dose-dependent acute nephrotoxicity, and levels should be monitored closely; thrombotic microangioipathy is a rarer

adverse effect of these calcineurin inhibitors. The clinical diagnosis of acute rejection is often difficult to make, frequently requiring histologic confirmation or empirical antirejection therapy. Although an acute rejection episode occurs in the majority of renal transplant recipients within the first year following engraftment, it is increasingly uncommon thereafter. Thus a diagnosis of acute rejection several years after transplantation is less likely as long as the patient complies with therapy.

One of the most frequent and severe infections compromising renal function in transplant recipients is cytomegalovirus (CMV), which can cause dysfunction in many organ systems, including the central nervous system, lungs, liver, and kidneys. CMV is often suspected clinically on the basis of fever, multisystem organ involvement (including ARF), and progressive leukopenia. It is more common in patients who have received intensive immunosuppression for severe or recurrent rejection episodes.

Late causes of ARF in transplant recipients include recurrence of the patient's original renal disease, de novo transplant glomerulopathy, infections, transplant artery stenosis, and urologic problems such as stricture or rejection of the ureter. In addition to renal ultrasound, transplant biopsy is often useful in defining the cause of ARF late in the course of a kidney transplant.

Prevention of Acute Renal Failure

Frequently, ARF develops in hospitalized patients in whom it is predictable and can be prevented or ameliorated. To intervene effectively, it is important to identify the patients at risk (Table 75-8). There is an additive interaction among the risk factors. Unfortunately, most attempts to modify the course of ARF are probably too late if tubular damage has already begun[4].

Although ARF may be prevented or ameliorated by judicious use and monitoring of nephrotoxic drugs, and perhaps evolving cytoprotective and anti-inflammatory therapies, the major focus in ARF prophylaxis and therapy remains optimization of renal perfusion. The primary causes of renal hypoperfusion differ between the major types of shock, and therapies vary accordingly. The role of hemodynamic monitoring and support with fluids and vasoactive drugs in the prevention of ARF in the ICU is important, but there is little high-grade evidence to guide these therapeutic choices. As discussed above, renal perfusion is optimized by using fluids and vasoactive drugs to seek an adequate perfusion pressure and cardiac output. There is generally no adequate study to

TABLE 75-8 Risk Factors for the Development of Acute Renal Failure

Preexisting chronic renal failure
Volume depletion
Diabetes mellitus
Elderly patients
Postoperative patients
Congestive heart failure
Urinary tract infection
Prior history of acute renal failure

guide the choice of specific fluid or vasoactive drug to improve renal function. It appears that colloids are not superior to crystalloids for prevention of ARF in critically ill patients. A large randomized, controlled prospective trial of albumin versus saline in almost 7000 critically ill patients found no demonstrable effect of one over the other on mortality, renal function, or the frequency of renal replacement therapy.[98] Of note, patients with cirrhosis were excluded from this trial, and limited data suggest that albumin is useful to prevent ARF in cirrhotic patients with spontaneous bacterial peritonitis,[99] or those undergoing large-volume paracentesis. As discussed above, for prevention of radiocontrast nephropathy normal saline is superior to half-normal saline,[39] and an equimolar solution of sodium bicarbonate is superior to normal saline.[40] Otherwise, despite the importance of fluid therapy in the prevention of ARF, the nature of the optimum fluid resuscitation regimen remains a disputed topic. Similarly, there are no proven advantages of any specific inotrope or vasopressor with respect to renal function. In patients with septic shock, the use of early goal-directed therapy, steroids in nonresponders to adrenocorticotropic hormone stimulation, and activated protein C may lead to a decreased incidence or severity of ARF, but there is no evidence in the literature that improved survival in the pivotal studies supporting these therapies is associated with a decreased incidence of ARF. Limited evidence suggests that tight glycemic control and lung-protective ventilation strategies may decrease the incidence of ARF in critically ill patients.[4,14]

Prevention of nephrotoxic injury is the other mainstay of ARF prevention in critically ill patients. Avoidance of potential nephrotoxins such as intravenous radiocontrast, aminoglycosides, amphotericin, and NSAIDs is prudent, when possible. Single daily dosing of aminoglycoside antibiotics is associated with a lower risk of nephrotoxicity and equivalent antimicrobial efficacy compared to multiple dosing strategies.[31–33] Drug modifications such as nonionic radiocontrast[36,37] and lipid-emulsified amphotericin B may also reduce the incidence of ATN. Aggressive diuresis must be avoided when possible, particularly in conjunction with the use of ACEIs or ARBs, and must be accompanied by careful monitoring of fluid balance and renal function. Monitoring the serum levels of potentially nephrotoxic drugs such as aminoglycosides, cyclosporine A, tacrolimus, and vancomycin is recommended, although studies proving that therapeutic drug monitoring decreases the incidence of ATN are lacking.

Numerous studies have sought to demonstrate efficacy of pharmacologic interventions for primary prevention of ARF (prophylaxis), or secondary prevention in ARF (ATN therapy to decrease dialytic requirement and improve outcome). Broadly speaking, these studies have been trials of diuretics or renal vasodilators. There have been other negative studies of agents including insulin-like growth factor and thyroxine, but these will not be further discussed here.

DIURETICS

Furosemide is a loop diuretic and vasodilator that may decrease oxygen consumption in the loop of Henle by inhibiting sodium transport, thus potentially lessening ischemic injury. By increasing urinary flow, it may also reduce intratubular obstruction and backleakage of filtrate. Based on these properties, furosemide might be expected to prevent ARF. However, there are few data to support its use. Furosemide was found to be ineffective or harmful when used to prevent ARF after cardiac surgery, and to increase the risk of ARF when given to prevent contrast nephropathy.[38,100]

Similarly, there is little evidence of benefit from diuretic therapy in established ARF. A single recent study in 100 patients with oliguric ARF after cardiac surgery suggested that a cocktail infusion of furosemide, mannitol, and dopamine improved renal function post–cardiac surgery compared to intermittent loop diuretics alone.[101] However, numerous studies in patients with established ATN have found no benefit of loop diuretics.[102–107] Their use did not accelerate renal recovery, decrease the need for dialysis, or reduce mortality. It was shown that the mortality rate of oliguric patients who responded to furosemide with a diuresis was lower than those who did not.[106–107] However, the clinical characteristics, severity of renal failure, and mortality rates were similar in patients with either spontaneous non-oliguric ARF or patients who became non-oliguric after furosemide. This implies that those patients able to respond to furosemide have less severe renal damage than nonresponders, rather than deriving any true therapeutic benefit from furosemide administration. Although administration of furosemide might facilitate improved fluid management if it induces a diuresis, a retrospective review of a recent trial in critically ill patients with ATN raised concerns of possible harm from loop diuretics in ARF. The authors found that diuretic use was associated with an increased risk of death and nonrecovery of renal function.[108] Most of the increased risk, however, was seen in those patients unresponsive to high doses of diuretics, implying they had more severe disease. Therefore, diuretics should be used with caution in critically ill patients, and iatrogenic hypovolemia and superimposed prerenal azotemia must be avoided. Diuretics should be withdrawn if there is no response, to avoid ototoxicity. Our current maximal, synergistic diuretic challenge combines furosemide 200 mg IV with chlorothiazide 500 mg IV. In patients who experience an increase in urine output, hypotension must be avoided, since kidneys with ATN are susceptible to further damage from decreases in perfusion pressure. To maintain the diuresis, a continuous infusion of drug is probably preferable to intermittent bolus administration.[109] Although there are no large randomized controlled trials, the overall evidence suggests that continuous infusion of diuretics as opposed to bolus administration is more effective and associated with less toxicity and delayed development of diuretic resistance.

Mannitol is an osmotic diuretic that can decrease cell swelling, scavenge free radicals, and cause renal vasodilatation by inducing intrarenal prostaglandin production.[110] It may be beneficial when added to organ preservation solutions during renal transplantation and may protect against ARF caused by rhabdomyolysis if given extremely early.[110–112] Otherwise, mannitol has not been shown to be useful in the prevention of ARF. In fact, mannitol may aggravate ARF due to radiocontrast agents.[38] Furthermore, mannitol may precipitate pulmonary edema if given to volume-overloaded patients who remain oliguric, can exacerbate the hyperosmolar state of azotemia, and may even cause acute renal failure ("osmotic nephrosis").[113]

RENAL VASODILATORS

ATRIAL NATRIURETIC PEPTIDE

Atrial natriuretic peptide (ANP) has been investigated in clinical trials for the treatment or prevention of ARF. ANP can lead to an increase in GFR due to arteriolar dilatation and also has a natriuretic effect. ANP improved renal function in animal studies and a phase II human ATN study.[114–115] However, larger randomized trials failed to show any benefit of ANP compared to placebo.[116–117] Hypotension was significantly more common in ANP-treated patients in these studies, and may have negated any potential benefit of renal vasodilation in these patients. Hence there is no convincing evidence to support the use of ANP in the prevention or treatment of ARF. A new, promising, but underpowered (61 patients) positive study of ANP to treat ARF immediately following cardiac surgery showed a decreased rate of postoperative renal replacement therapy compared to placebo-treated patients;[118] a larger prospective trial in this setting appears warranted.

DOPAMINE

Low-dose dopamine administration (1 to 3 μg/kg per minute) to normal individuals causes renal vasodilation and increased GFR, and acts as a proximal tubular diuretic. Due to these effects, numerous studies have used low-dose dopamine to either prevent or treat ATN in a variety of clinical settings. It has been given as prophylaxis for ARF associated with radiocontrast administration, repair of aortic aneurysms, orthotopic liver transplantation, unilateral nephrectomy, renal transplantation, and chemotherapy with interferon.[119–122] Yet despite more than 20 years of clinical experience, prevention trials with low-dose dopamine all have been small, inadequately randomized, of limited statistical power, and with end points of questionable clinical significance. Denton and associates reviewed the data on the use of renal doses of dopamine and concluded that there is no convincing data that renal-dose dopamine either prevents ARF or improves outcome in patients with established ARF.[120] Meta-analyses done by Kellum and Decker[121] and by Marik[122] similarly did not show any benefit of dopamine in the prevention or treatment of ARF. The Australian and New Zealand trial (ANZICS) studied the effects of low-dose dopamine in ICU patients with systemic inflammatory response syndrome and ARF.[123] This is a double-blind randomized study. The patients were randomly assigned to receive either dopamine at a dose of 2 μg kg^{-1} min^{-1} or placebo. The investigators found no difference in the primary outcome measure, which was the peak serum creatinine concentration during trial infusion (Fig. 75-4). The proportion of patients reaching serum creatinine values above 3.4 mg/dL and proportion of patients requiring renal replacement therapy was similar in both groups (Fig. 75-5). There was no difference in the length of ICU and hospital stay, or mortality and time to renal recovery. This study convincingly demonstrated that low-dose dopamine does not improve outcome in critically ill patients with early ARF. Furthermore, there is concern for the potential harmful effects of dopamine, even at low doses. It can trigger tachyarrhythmias and myocardial ischemia, decrease intestinal blood flow, cause digital necrosis and hypothyroidism, and suppress T-cell function.[119] It has also been shown to increase the risk of radiocontrast nephropathy when given prophylactically to patients with diabetic nephropathy.[49]

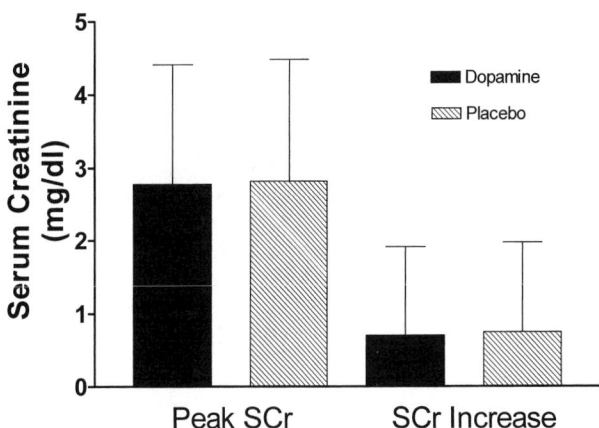

FIGURE 75-4 Primary end point of the ANZICS low-dose dopamine trial. In the ANZICS trial, there was no difference between low-dose dopamine and placebo in the primary outcome measure, which was peak serum creatinine attained during trial drug infusion. Peak urea and increments from baseline of creatinine and urea were also similar in the placebo and dopamine groups. *(This figure was produced using data from Murray.[119] Adapted from Bellomo et al.[123])*

Nondialytic Supportive Care of Acute Renal Failure

When a diagnosis of intrinsic ARF has been firmly established and potentially reversible causes have been excluded or treated, the patient is then monitored for early detection of complications. Conservative measures consist of hospital observation with attention to blood pressure, volume status, neurologic function, and evidence of hemorrhagic or infectious complications. Electrolytes (Na^+, K^+, Cl^-, HCO_3^{2-}, Ca^{2+}, and PO_4^{3-}), BUN, and creatinine should be monitored daily, although the hyperkalemic patient will require more frequent monitoring.

Fluid intake should be adjusted to replace urine and insensible losses, while Na^+ and K^+ are allowed in amounts to replace urine and GI losses. Obviously, fluid and electrolyte

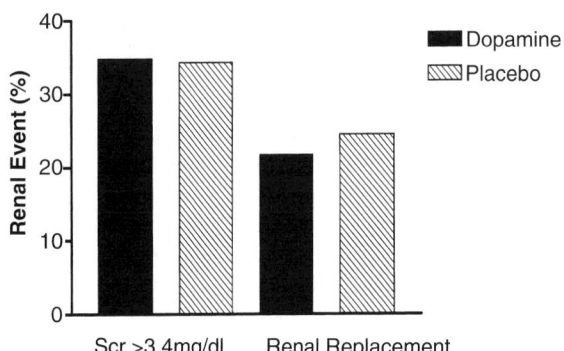

FIGURE 75-5 Secondary end points of the ANZICS low-dose dopamine trial. In the ANZICS trial, there was no significant difference between the dopamine and placebo groups in the number of patients whose serum creatinine concentration exceeded 3.4 mg/dL or who received renal replacement therapy. *(This figure was produced using data from Murray.[119] Adapted from Bellomo et al.[123])*

TABLE 75-9 Therapy of Hyperkalemia

Drug	Dose	Onset	Duration	Mechanism
Calcium gluconate	10–20 mL IV	1–5 min	0.5 h	Membrane antagonist
Sodium bicarbonate	1–2 ampules (IV 50–100 mEq)	30 min	1–4 h	Cellular shift
Glucose + insulin	500 mL $D_{10}W$ with 10 U regular insulin IV	30 min	1–4 h	Cellular shift
Sodium polystyrene sulfonate	30–50 g with sorbitol PO, or as retention enema	1–2 h	4–6 h	Increased excretion

$D_{10}W$, 10% dextrose in water.

restriction will be more severe in the oliguric patient. A small daily reduction in weight is expected in the patient with ARF, but weight loss >1 kg daily indicates severe catabolism or volume loss. On the other hand, it should be emphasized that maintenance of weight or weight gain indicates volume expansion.

Clinical trials to determine the benefit of nutritional therapy with amino acids to improve renal failure show conflicting results.[124,125] The guiding principle of nutritional management in the nondialyzed case of ARF has traditionally been slowing the accumulation of nitrogen waste products and avoiding severe electrolyte perturbations. We recommend limiting potassium and phosphorus intake to avoid severe electrolyte disturbances, but we do not limit protein intake specifically to limit production of nitrogenous waste and avoid dialysis. Whether a patient with ARF is in the period before or after initiation of renal replacement therapy, protein intake should be prescribed to provide 1.0 to 1.5 g/kg per day (higher in more catabolic patients, and in those receiving CRRT, who have additional amino acid removal). Calories can be provided in the form of simple carbohydrates such as jelly and sugar. Caloric requirements increase in proportion to the severity of the underlying illness, and intake of 3000 kcal/d or more may be necessary to blunt catabolism. Should the patient be incapable of eating due to anorexia or other reasons, a small, soft feeding tube may be inserted into the stomach and tube feeding administered by constant infusion or intermittent bolus. In general, tube feedings with lower K^+ and Na^+ concentrations are chosen. For the patient who cannot tolerate enteral feeding, total parenteral nutrition (TPN) becomes necessary. Because of the volume of fluid required for TPN, earlier institution of dialysis and ultrafiltration is often necessary. A reasonable approach is to give sufficient calories to prevent negative nitrogen balance but not to overfeed patients to the point that hepatic and platelet complications develop or that dialysis imposes additional risks.

The management of various electrolyte abnormalities often associated with ARF is described in greater detail in Chap. 76 and will only be touched on here. Administration of excessive amounts of free water is the most common cause of hyponatremia in patients with ARF. Less important causes of hyponatremia in this setting include water production from carbohydrate metabolism and water release from injured tissue. Judicious fluid management will prevent any untoward complications from hyponatremia. Hyperkalemia is the most grave of the electrolyte perturbations that may complicate ARF. The clinical consequences of hyperkalemia are largely confined to the cardiovascular and neuromuscular systems. The earliest hyperkalemic effects are manifest in the electrocardiogram (ECG). ECG changes are uniformly present above a potassium level of 8 mEq/L; below 7 mEq/L, changes may not be evident. The treatment of hyperkalemia is summarized in Table 75-9.

Disturbances of divalent ion metabolism are common in ARF. Hyperphosphatemia is an almost universal accompaniment of oliguric ARF. Control of hyperphosphatemia in the acute setting is achieved by oral administration of aluminum hydroxide gels. Short-term administration of aluminum-containing compounds to patients with renal failure does not result in aluminum intoxication. However, concurrent administration of oral citrate compounds must be avoided because citrate enhances gut absorption of aluminum and accelerates the development of aluminum intoxication.

Hypocalcemia is an expected complication of ARF but is generally of no clinical significance and does not require intervention. However, severe depression of serum Ca^{2+} may complicate rhabdomyolysis-induced ARF. Nevertheless, calcium salts are contraindicated except as part of the treatment of life-threatening hyperkalemia or if hypocalcemic tetany develops. Hypercalcemia may be observed when rhabdomyolysis-induced ARF enters the diuretic phase, and Ca^{2+} deposited in damaged muscle is released. It is usually self-limited.

Uric acid levels may rise by 1 to 2 mg/dL per day in cases of ARF not due to rhabdomyolysis, but rarely does the level exceed 15 mg/dL. This plateau is thought to result from enhanced metabolism of uric acid by gut bacteria. Extreme elevations in uric acid levels have been observed in cases of exertional rhabdomyolysis and following treatment of some lymphomas.

Metabolic acidosis occurs commonly in ARF, and in cases of trauma or sepsis the fall in plasma bicarbonate may exceed 15 mEq per 24 hours. In the catabolic patient with ARF, acid is released from metabolism of sulfur- and phosphorus-containing compounds, which contributes to a rise in the anion gap. Acidosis may be treated with sodium bicarbonate; however, the additional volume is hazardous in the patient with compromised renal function, the buffering requires increased ventilation, and adverse intracellular effects may result. Uncontrollable acidosis may mandate dialysis therapy.

Metabolic alkalosis may complicate ARF in the patient with nasogastric suction, but is a less frequent acid-base disturbance in these patients. Although nasogastric suction–induced metabolic alkalosis normally responds to saline supplementation, this maneuver is ineffective in ARF and carries the hazard of potential volume overload. Severe metabolic alkalosis in ARF may require dialysis using a reduced concentration of bicarbonate or acetate in the bath. Alternatively, 0.1 N hydrochloric acid may be administered by slow intravenous infusion. Development of metabolic alkalosis in the patient on nasogastric suction may be prevented or attenuated by use of histamine blockers such as cimetidine.

Infection continues to be a leading cause of death in the patient with ARF, and pneumonia, urinary tract infection, and wound infection are most common. Infection has been the cause of death in up to 70% of cases of ARF and has contributed to 50% of deaths occurring during the diuretic phase.[126] In several large series of ARF, the incidence of septicemia exceeds 50%, and intra-abdominal sepsis is known to be a particularly important determinant of survival. In the septic patient without an obvious source, intra-abdominal sepsis must be vigorously excluded. Imaging procedures of value for detecting an abdominal source include CT scanning and ultrasound, with CT the better of the two. The severity of infection in ARF is undiminished despite the advent of new antibiotics and other advances in general medical care. Prophylactic antibiotics are not recommended for the patient with ARF and may be harmful.

Prior to the use of antacids and histamine blockers (e.g., cimetidine and ranitidine) to prevent gastric stress ulceration in ARF, GI hemorrhage was the second leading cause of death. Now many centers report a dramatic decline in GI hemorrhage.[127] Recent advances in the therapy of uremic bleeding include use of 1-deamino-8-D-arginine vasopressin (DDAVP), cryoprecipitate, and conjugated estrogens.[128] These drugs are most useful in patients with clinically significant bleeding episodes who lack evidence of any other (nonuremic) coagulopathy. DDAVP is typically infused over 30 minutes in a dose of 0.3 μg/kg of body weight and is effective within minutes.[129] Unfortunately, because of the short duration of action of this compound (1 to 4 hours), frequent dosing may be required. The use of cryoglobulin infusions (10 units IV over 15 minutes) also may serve as a temporary expedient in patients with uremic bleeding. Conjugated estrogens (0.6 mg/kg IV daily for 5 days) have a very delayed onset of action (3 to 5 days), but the duration of the therapeutic effect can be as long as 14 days.[130]

RENAL REPLACEMENT THERAPY

In ARF, there is consensus that dialysis should be initiated if there are uremic symptoms or signs, or if volume overload, electrolyte abnormalities, or acidosis are refractory to medical management. The precise timing of RRT initiation is usually a matter of clinical judgment.[3,5] Absent the above clinical indications, hemodialysis (HD) is commonly initiated when the BUN concentration reaches 100 mg/dL, and repeated to maintain a predialysis BUN below 80 mg/dL.[5] This pattern of practice is based primarily on early experience suggesting

that uremic bleeding diathesis and hemorrhage were reduced when hemodialysis was initiated before the BUN exceeded 100 mg/dL,[5] the results of small prospective ARF studies in 1975 and 1986,[131] and extrapolation from results of the National Cooperative Dialysis Study in chronic renal failure patients. This relatively prophylactic approach is balanced against potential adverse effects of RRT, including hypotension with worsening renal ischemic acute tubular necrosis, and the renal and systemic inflammatory effects of extracorporeal membrane exposure. Although it seems prudent to start RRT aggressively in critically ill catabolic patients, studies have not shown a significant benefit of prophylactic dialysis, including a recent small study using CRRT by Bouman and colleagues.[132] It is universally accepted that emergent RRT is indicated in the management of ARF when pulmonary edema, hyperkalemia, refractory acidosis, or symptomatic uremia develops. In our opinion, initiation of RRT should also be considered in patients with sustained anuria, persistent oliguria with progressive azotemia and GFR <10 mL/min, and to control fluid balance, rather than waiting for complications of volume overload, electrolyte imbalance, or uremia to develop.

RRT modalities available include intermittent hemodialysis (IHD), peritoneal dialysis (PD), and continuous renal replacement therapy (CRRT). CRRT nomenclature includes elements denoting duration of therapy (C for continuous), vascular access (arteriovenous [AV], or venovenous [VV]), and the solute transport mechanism(s) used (diffusion [dialysis], convection [hemofiltration], or both [hemodiafiltration]). So the different modalities include continuous arteriovenous hemofiltration (CAVH), continuous venovenous hemofiltration (CVVH), continuous arteriovenous and venovenous hemodialysis (CAVHD and CVVHD), and continuous arteriovenous and venovenous hemodiafiltration (CAVHDF and CVVHDF). Solute clearance during RRT occurs either by diffusion or convection. Solute clearance during IHD and continuous dialysis therapies (CAVHD and CVVHD) occurs primarily by diffusion. Solute clearance during CVVH and CAVH is primarily by convection. In CAVHDF and CVVHDF both convective and diffusive solute transport occurs.

CRRT is thought to permit fluid and solute removal with greater hemodynamic stability than intermittent HD for two reasons. The first is the fact that fluid removal is done slowly and continuously, rather than in 1- to 4-L increments over 2- to 4-hour treatment sessions. Rapid diffusive solute clearance by intermittent HD results in loss of intravascular solutes and results in the reduction of plasma osmolality relative to surrounding tissues, which in turn causes transfer of plasma water into tissues. This leads to further depletion of extracellular volume which has been diminished by ultrafiltration.[10] So, in hemodynamically unstable patients CRRT is preferred compared to IHD, as it allows removal of excess fluid in hypotensive patients. CRRT also allows us to better manage fluid status in patients who are receiving TPN. Apart from hypovolemia and plasma hypo-osmolality, there are a variety of other causes of intradialytic hypotension (IDH) (Tables 75-10 and 75-11).[10] Although IDH is common in ICU patients, the complete differential diagnosis of this problem should be considered in every case, particularly when hypotension is profound or refractory to standard measures. Several techniques are used routinely in ICU patients

TABLE 75-10 Dialysis-Dependent Factors in Intradialytic Hypotension

Ultrafiltration
    Amount
    Rate
Autonomic reflexes
Osmolality decrease
Acetate buffer
Low dialysate calcium
Warm dialysate temperature
Membrane reaction
Air embolism

Reproduced with permission from Doshi et al.[10]

receiving IHD to improve hemodynamic stability. Intermittent isolated ultrafiltration (also called IUF) sessions, which remove fluid without diffusive solute clearance, are commonly used for acute volume removal with greater hemodynamic stability than intermittent HD. The use of higher dialysate sodium concentrations, called *sodium modeling* (e.g., beginning HD with a 160-mEq/L sodium "bath," decreasing to 140 mEq/L over 4 hours), similarly improves hemodynamic tolerance of intermittent HD, by ameliorating the tendency towards plasma hypo-osmolality. The use of cool dialysate (35.5°C) and increasing dialysate calcium concentration are among the other interventions proven to increase systemic vascular resistance and improve hemodynamic tolerance of HD; increased dialysate calcium also augments cardiac output. Numerous patients hemodynamically intolerant of isolated ultrafiltration, intermittent HD, their sequential combination, and the other modifications mentioned above, have been supported with CRRT. The capacity to alter fluid balance at will, even in hemodynamically unstable patients, is

TABLE 75-11 Dialysis-Independent Factors in Intradialytic Hypotension

Hypovolemic
    Gastrointestinal bleeding or fluid loss (emesis or diarrhea)
    Retroperitoneal bleeding
Cardiogenic
    Left ventricular dysfunction
        Systolic/diastolic
    Myocardial ischemia
    Right Ventricular dysfunction
        Pulmonary hypertension or right ventricular infarction
    Pericardial tamponade
    Valvular dysfunction
    Arrhythmias
Vasodilatory
    Sepsis
    Cirrhosis
    Adrenal insufficiency
    Antihypertensive drugs
    Anaphylaxis
    Autonomic dysfunction
Mixed
    Hypovolemia with diastolic dysfunction or vasodilation
    Vasodilation with cardiac dysfunction

Reproduced with permission from Doshi et al.[10]

in large part responsible for the attractiveness of CRRT to intensivists.

Although acute therapy of severe hyperkalemia, metabolic acidosis, or intoxications is more efficiently achieved with IHD, lesser abnormalities are corrected relatively quickly and controlled effectively with CRRT. Clinical data suggest that CRRT should be strongly considered for patients with severe hyperphosphatemia or elevated intracranial pressure (ICP), and might also be a useful component of therapy for lithium intoxication.[5] Continuous removal prevents the postdialytic rebound elevation of plasma concentration typically seen with IHD in patients with hyperphosphatemia (tumor lysis syndrome or rhabdomyolysis) or lithium intoxication.[5] In patients with cerebral edema complicating acute liver failure, intermittent machine hemofiltration, but not continuous renal replacement therapies (CAVH or CAVHD) raised ICP and decreased cerebral perfusion pressure; similar adverse effects of intermittent HD were previously demonstrated.[5] Raised ICP in this setting is due to acute solute removal and resulting plasma hypo-osmolality, causing a shift of water into the brain along with other tissues. The detrimental effect of this phenomenon on cerebral perfusion pressure may be increased by treatment-induced hypovolemia or hypotension. Despite apparent advantages over intermittent therapies in unstable patients, outcome superiority of CRRT with respect to mortality or recovery of renal function outcomes has not been demonstrated. Data from a U.S. prospective, comparative trial of intermittent HD versus CRRT in ICU ARF did not demonstrate an effect of modality on outcome.[133] In this study, Mehta and colleagues excluded patients with a mean arterial pressure below 70 mm Hg. Randomization did not balance severity of illness between groups; CRRT patients had higher severity of illness and mortality, and there was no difference in mortality between HD and CRRT groups adjusted for Acute Physiology, Age, and Chronic Health Evaluation (APACHE) II scores. Ongoing studies may determine if there is an advantage of any specific modality over others in critically ill patients.

Few RRT dosing guidelines have been established in patients with ARF, but it is clear that dialysis delivery is inadequate in the ICU, even by standards set for stable end-stage renal disease outpatients. Clearance of urea, a low-molecular-weight nitrogenous waste product, is the most commonly studied marker of adequate uremic detoxification by HD. The term Kt/V is a unitless measure of HD dose (based on urea removal): K is the urea clearance of the dialysis membrane used (in milliliters per minute), t is the duration of dialysis (in minutes), and V is the volume of distribution of urea in the patient (in milliliters). Thus, Kt/V is a measure of the volume of plasma cleared of urea during a HD session (Kt) divided by the urea distribution volume (V, assumed to be total body water: 0.5 to 0.6 L/kg), and larger Kt/V values signify greater HD dose. Kt/V measurements of delivered dialysis dose are usually calculated using the ratio of postdialysis to predialysis BUN and a nomogram. In chronic hemodialysis patients the minimum acceptable dialysis dose is a Kt/V of 1.2. Extrapolation of HD data from the chronic HD population to the ARF setting is limited by numerous poorly quantifiable variables, including effects of critical illness on urea kinetic modeling. Furthermore, Kt/V measurements extrapolated from pre- and post-BUN may be very inaccurate in ARF,

% Survival

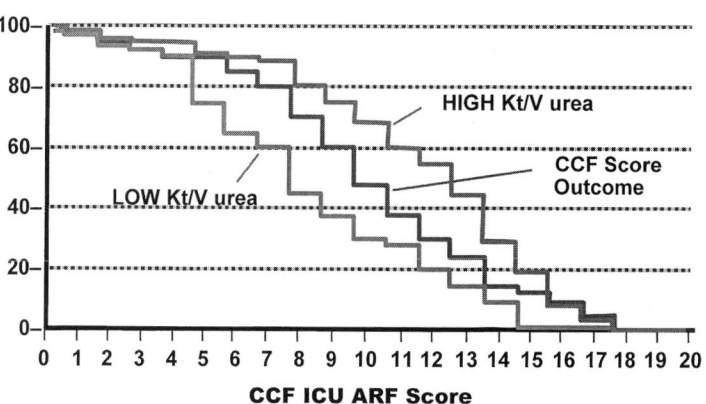

FIGURE 75-6 Relationship between RRT dose and outcome using diffusive solute clearance (hemodialysis). Paganini and colleagues demonstrated by retrospective analysis of a prospectively gathered database that delivered dialysis dose was predictive of mortality in critically ill ARF patients treated with RRT, if they had moderate-range severity of illness. Severity of illness was measured by the Cleveland Clinic Foundation ARF score (higher score predicts increased mortality). Mortality of the most and least severely ill patients was independent of dialysis dose, measured by Kt/V (see text for explanation of Kt/V). *(Reproduced with permission from Paganini et al.[135])*

because rebound postdialysis increases in BUN from tissue stores hypoperfused during IHD occurs. Furthermore, numerous patient- and technique-related factors impede effective delivery of prescribed dialysis in critically ill patients. In a prospective study which examined the prescribed and delivered dialysis dose in 40 ARF patients found that 68% of ARF treatments failed to deliver the minimum dialysis dose recommended for maintenance HD of chronic renal failure patients, and that for 49% of treatments a minimally adequate dialysis dose was not even prescribed.[134] Failure to adjust dialysis dose and/or achieve adequate dialysis delivery in larger patients was a major source of treatment failure.

In a study done by Paganini and colleagues, improved survival was seen in patients with higher Kt/V, and this survival benefit is particularly evident in patients with moderate-range severity of illness. In patients with least and most severity of illness the mortality was not affected by dialysis dose (Fig. 75-6).[135] Another study done by Schiffl and colleagues found that patients who received daily IHD had a lower mortality compared with patients who received alternate-day IHD (28% vs. 46%), and improved renal recovery.[136] In patients who received alternate-day IHD, time-averaged blood urea nitrogen level was 104 mg/dL, reflecting inadequate dialysis that is below the standard of care for most critically ill patients, so it is not surprising that their outcome was inferior to well-dialyzed patients. Nonetheless, it seems prudent to prescribe more frequent HD for ICU patients treated with intermittent dialysis, to optimize dose delivery, fluid balance, and outcome. There are also outcome data to guide CRRT dosing, provided by the landmark study of Ronco and colleagues, who conducted a large prospective study to determine the impact of hemofiltration dose on survival. In this study, patients were randomly assigned to one of three treatment doses, based on effluent volume (which is equivalent to small solute clearance by continuous hemofiltration, or by low-volume continuous hemodialysis): $20 \text{ mL h}^{-1} \text{ kg}^{-1}$ (group 1), $35 \text{ mL h}^{-1} \text{ kg}^{-1}$ (group 2), or $45 \text{ mL h}^{-1} \text{ kg}^{-1}$ (group 3). Patients assigned to group 1 had higher mortality than those in groups 2 and 3 (Fig. 75-7).[137] Based on this study, we recommend a minimum effluent volume of 35 mL/kg per hour for ICU patients with ARF treated with CRRT. Current and future studies may identify alternative markers of adequate RRT dose, such as clearance of larger molecules, or biomarkers such as leukocyte response to inflammatory stimuli.[59]

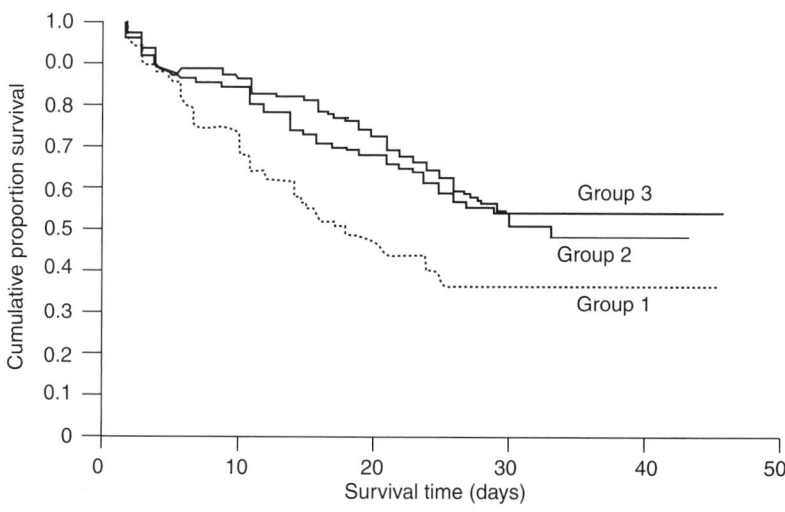

FIGURE 75-7 Relationship between RRT dose and outcome using convective solute clearance (hemofiltration). Kaplan-Meier estimation of survival curves in the three groups of ICU patients with ARF, divided based on dose delivered during CRRT: $20 \text{ mL h}^{-1} \text{ kg}^{-1}$ (group 1), $35 \text{ mL h}^{-1} \text{ kg}^{-1}$ (group 2), or $45 \text{ mL h}^{-1} \text{ kg}^{-1}$ (group 3). Survival in group 1 is significantly lower than in groups 2 and 3. Survival in groups 2 and 3 did not differ significantly. *(Reproduced with permission from Ronco et al.[137])*

References

1. Kellum JA, Levin N, Bouman C, Lameire N: Developing a consensus classification system for acute renal failure. *Curr Opin Crit Care* 8:509, 2002.

2. Hou SH, Bushinsky DA, Wish JB, et al: Hospital acquired renal insufficiency: A prospective study. *Am J Med* 74:243, 1983.

3. Star RA: Treatment of acute renal failure. *Kidney Int* 54:1817, 1998.

4. Tang I, Murray PT: Prevention of perioperative ARF: What works? *Best Pract Res Clin Anesthesiol* 18:91, 2004.

5. Murray PT, Hall JB: Renal replacement therapy for acute renal failure. *Am J Respir Crit Care Med* 162:777, 2000.

6. Kelly KJ: Distant effects of experimental renal ischemia/reperfusion injury. *J Am Soc Nephrol* 14:1549, 2003.

7. Kramer AA, Postler G, Salhab KF, et al: Renal ischemia/reperfusion leads to macrophage-mediated increase in pulmonary vascular permeability. *Kidney Int* 55:2362, 1999.

8. Rabb H, Wang Z, Nemoto T, et al: Acute renal failure leads to dysregulation of lung salt and water channels. *Kidney Int* 63:600, 2003.

9. Neveu H, Kleinknecht D, Brivet F, et al: Prognostic factors in acute renal failure due to sepsis. Results of a prospective multicentre study. *Nephrol Dial Transplant* 11:293, 1996.

10. Doshi M, Murray PT: Approach to intradialytic hypotension in ICU patients with ARF. *Artif Organs* 27:772, 2003.

11. Blantz RC: Pathophysiology of prerenal azotemia. *Kidney Int* 53:512, 1998.

12. Bersten AD, Holt AW: Vasoactive drugs and the importance of renal perfusion pressure. *New Horiz* 3:650, 1995.

13. Zager RA: Endotoxemia, renal hypoperfusion, and fever: interactive risk factors for aminoglycoside and sepsis-induced acute renal failure. *Am J Kidney Dis* 20:223, 1992.

14. Pannu N, Mehta RL: Mechanical ventilation and renal function: an area for concern? *Am J Kidney Dis* 39:616, 2002.

15. Murray PT, Wylam ME, Umans JG: Nitric oxide and septic vascular dysfunction. *Anesth Analg* 90:89, 2000.

16. Chugh KS, Jha V, Sakhuja V, Joshi K: Acute renal cortical necrosis—a study of 113 patients. *Ren Fail* 16:37, 1994.

17. Lieberthal W: Biology of acute renal failure: therapeutic implications. *Kidney Int* 52:1102, 1997.

18. Sutton TA, Fisher CJ, Molitoris BA: Microvascular endothelial injury and dysfunction during ischemic acute renal failure. *Kidney Int* 62:1539, 2002.

19. Blantz RC: The mechanisms of acute renal failure after uranyl nitrate. *J Clin Invest* 55:621, 1975.

20. Baylis C, Rennke HG, Brenner BM: Mechanism of the defect in glomerular ultrafiltration associated with gentamicin administration. *Kidney Int* 12:344, 1977.

21. Lameire N, Vanholder R: Pathophysiologic features and prevention of human and experimental acute tubular necrosis. *J Am Soc Nephrol* 12:S20, 2001.

22. Thurau K, Boylan JW: Acute renal success. The unexpected logic of oliguria in acute renal failure. *Am J Med* 61:308, 1976.

23. Brezis M, Rosen S: Hypoxia of the renal medulla—its implications for disease. *N Engl J Med* 332:647, 1995.

24. Brezis M, Agmon Y, Epstein FH: Determinants of intrarenal oxygenation. Effects of diuretics. *Am J Physiol* 267:F1059, 1994.

25. Venkatachalam MA, Bernard DB, Donohoe JF, et al: Ischemic damage and repair in the rat proximal tubule: differences among the S_1, S_2, and S_3 segments. *Kidney Int* 14:31, 1978.

26. Patel R, McKenzie JK, McQueen EG: Tamm-Horsfall urinary mucoprotein and tubular obstruction by casts in acute renal failure. *Lancet* 1:457, 1964.

27. Donohoe FJ, Venkatachalam MA, Bernard DB, et al: Tubular leakage and obstruction after renal ischemia: structure-function correlations. *Kidney Int* 13:208, 1978.

28. Myers BD, Chui F, Hilberman M, et al: Transtubular leakage of glomerular filtrate in human acute renal failure. *Am J Physiol* 237:F319, 1978.

29. Moran SM, Myers BD. Pathophysiology of protracted acute renal failure in man. *J Clin Invest* 76:1440, 1985.

30. Matzke G, Lucarotti R, Shapiro HS: Controlled comparison of gentamicin and tobramycin nephrotoxicity. *Am J Nephrol* 3:11, 1983.

31. Prins JM, Buller HR, Kuijper EJ, et al: Once versus thrice daily gentamicin in patients with serious infections. *Lancet* 341:335, 1993.

32. Hatala R, Dinh T, Cook DJ: Once-daily aminoglycoside dosing in immunocompetent adults: a meta-analysis. *Ann Intern Med* 124:717, 1996.

33. Barza M, et al: Single or multiple daily doses of aminoglycosides: a meta-analysis. *Br Med J* 312:338, 1996.

34. Rudnick MR, Berns JS, Cohen RM, et al: Contrast media-associated nephropathy. *Semin Nephrol* 17:15, 1997.

35. Rudnick MR, Goldfarb S, Wexler L, et al: Nephrotoxicity of ionic and nonionic contrast media in 1196 patients: a randomized trial. *Kidney Int* 47:254, 1995.

36. Aspelin P, Aubry P, Fransson SG, et al: Nephrotoxic effects in high-risk patients undergoing angiography. *N Engl J Med* 348:491, 2003.

37. Rudnick MR, Berns JS, Cohen RM, et al: Nephrotoxic risks of renal angiography: Contrast media associated nephrotoxicity and atheroembolism—a critical review. *Am J Kidney Dis* 24:713, 1994.

38. Solomon R, Werner C, Mann D, et al: Effects of saline, mannitol, and furosemide on acute decreases in renal function induced by radiocontrast agents. *N Engl J Med* 331:1416, 1994.

39. Mueller C, et al: Prevention of contrast media-associated nephropathy: randomized comparison of 2 hydration regimens in 1620 patients undergoing coronary angioplasty. *Arch Intern Med* 162:329, 2002.

40. Merten GJ, Burgess WP, Gray LV, et al: Prevention of contrast-induced nephropathy with sodium bicarbonate: a randomized, controlled trial. *JAMA* 291:2328, 2004.

41. Tepel M, Van Der Giet M, Schwarzfeld C, et al: Prevention of radiographic-contrast-agent-induced reduction in renal function by acetylcysteine. *N Engl J Med* 343:180, 2000.

42. Shyu KG, Cheng JJ, Kuan P: Acetylcysteine protects against acute renal damage in patients with abnormal renal function undergoing a coronary procedure. *J Am Coll Cardiol* 40:1383, 2002.

43. Kay J, Chow WH, Chan TM, et al: Acetylcysteine for prevention of acute deterioration of renal function following elective coronary angiography and intervention: a randomized controlled trial. *JAMA* 289:553, 2003.

44. Baker CSR, Wragg A, Kumar S, et al: A rapid protocol for the prevention of contrast-induced renal dysfunction: The RAPPID Study. *J Am Coll Cardiol* 41:2114, 2003.

45. Durham JD, Caputo C, Dokko J, et al: A randomized controlled trial of N-acetylcysteine to prevent contrast nephropathy in cardiac angiography. *Kidney Int* 62:2202, 2002.

46. Alonso A, et al: Prevention of radiocontrast nephropathy with N-acetylcysteine in patients with chronic kidney disease: A meta-analysis of randomized, controlled trials. *Am J Kidney Dis* 43:1, 2004.

47. Hoffmann U, Fischereder M, Kruger B, et al: The value of N-acetylcysteine in the prevention of radiocontrast agent-induced nephropathy seems questionable. *J Am Soc Nephrol* 15:407, 2004.

48. Genet S, Kale RK, Baquer NZ: Effects of free radicals on cytosolic creatine kinase activities and protection by antioxidant enzymes and sulfhydryl compounds. *Mol Cell Biochem* 210:23, 2000.

49. Weisberg LS, Kurnik PB, Kurnik BR: Risk of radiocontrast nephropathy in patients with and without diabetes mellitus. *Kidney Int* 45:259, 1994.

50. Stone GW, et al: Fenoldopam mesylate for the prevention of contrast-induced nephropathy: a randomized controlled trial. *JAMA* 290:2284, 2003.

51. Lehnert T, Keller E, Gondolf K, et al: Effect of hemodialysis after contrast media administration in patients with renal insufficiency. *Nephrol Dial Transplant* 13:358, 1998.

52. Marenzi G, Marana I, Lauri G, et al: The prevention of radiocontrast-agent-induced nephropathy by hemofiltration. *N Engl J Med* 349:1333, 2003.

53. Brater DC: Anti-inflammatory agents and renal function. *Semin Arthritis Rheum* 32(3 Suppl 1):33, 2002.

54. Breyer MD, Hao C, Qi Z: Cyclooxygenase-2 selective inhibitors and the kidney. *Curr Opin Crit Care* 7:393, 2001.

55. Linton AL, Clark WF, Driedger AA, et al: Acute interstitial nephritis due to drugs: Review of the literature with a report of nine cases. *Ann Intern Med* 93:735, 1980.

56. Nolan CR, Anger MS, Kelleher SP: Eosinophiluria: A new method of detection and definition of the clinical spectrum. *N Engl J Med* 315:1516, 1986.

57. Thadhani RI, Camargo CA Jr, Xavier RJ, et al: Atheroembolic renal failure after invasive procedures: natural history based on 52 histologically proven cases. *Medicine* 74:350, 1995.

58. McNelis J, Marini CP, Simms HH: Abdominal compartment syndrome: Clinical manifestations and predictive factors. *Curr Opin Crit Care* 9:133, 2003.

59. Murray PT, Le Gall JR, Dos Reis Miranda D, et al: Physiologic endpoints (efficacy) for acute renal failure studies. *Curr Opin Crit Care* 8:519, 2002.

60. Corrigan G, Ramaswamy D, Kwon O, et al: PAH extraction and estimation of plasma flow in human post-ischemic acute renal failure. *Am J Physiol* 277(2 Pt 2):F312, 1999.

61. Moran SM, Myers BD: Course of acute renal failure studied by a model of creatinine kinetics. *Kidney Int* 27:928, 1985.

62. Erley CM, Bader BD, Berger ED, et al: Plasma clearance of iodine contrast media as a measure of glomerular filtration rate in critically ill patients. *Crit Care Med* 29:1544, 2001.

63. Sladen RN, Endo E, Harrison T: Two-hour versus 22-hour creatinine clearance in critically ill patients. *Anesthesiology* 67:1013, 1987.

64. Newman DJ, Thakkar H, Edwards RG, et al: Serum cystatin C measured by automated immunoassay: A more sensitive marker of changes in GFR than serum creatinine. *Kidney Int* 47:312, 1995.

65. Massey D: Commentary: Clinical diagnostic use of cystatin C. *J Clin Lab Analysis* 18:55, 2004.

66. Laterza OF, Price CP, Scott MG: Cystatin C: an improved estimator of glomerular filtration rate? *Clin Chem* 48:699, 2002.

67. Rickli H, Benou K, Ammann P, et al: Time course of serial cystatin levels in comparison with serum creatinine after application of radiocontrast media. *Clin Nephrol* 61:98, 2004.

68. Christensson A, Ekberg J, Grubb A, et al: Serum cystatin C is a more sensitive and more accurate marker of glomerular filtration rate than enzymatic measurements of creatinine in renal transplantation. *Nephron Physiol* 94:19, 2003.

69. Le Bricon T, Thervet E, Benlakehal M, et al: Changes in plasma cystatin C after renal transplantation and acute rejection in adults. *Clin Chem* 45:2243, 1999.

70. Orlando R, Mussap M, Plebani M, et al: Diagnostic value of plasma cystatin C as a glomerular filtration marker in decompensated liver cirrhosis. *Clin Chem* 48:850, 2002.

71. Gunther A, Burchard GD, Slevogt H, et al: Renal dysfunction in falciparum-malaria is detected more often when assessed by serum concentration of cystatin C instead of creatinine. *Trop Med Int Health* 7:931, 2002.

72. Delanaye P, Lambermont B, Chapelle JP, et al: Plasmatic cystatin C for the estimation of glomerular filtration rate in intensive care units. *Intensive Care Med* 30:980, 2004.

73. Herget-Rosenthal S, Marggraf G, Husing G, et al: Early detection of acute renal failure by serum cystatin C. *Kidney Int* 66:1115, 2004.

74. Carvounis CP, Nisar S, Guro-Razuman S: Significance of the fractional excretion of urea in the differential diagnosis of acute renal failure. *Kidney Int* 62:2223, 2002.

75. Dagher PC, Herget-Rosenthal S, Ruehm SG, et al: Newly developed techniques to study and diagnose acute renal failure. *J Am Soc Nephrol* 14:2188, 2003.

76. Han WK, Bailly V, Abichandani R, et al: Kidney injury molecule-1 (KIM-1): A novel biomarker for human renal proximal tubule injury. *Kidney Int* 62:237, 2002.

77. McGee S, Abernethy WB 3rd, Simel DL: The rational clinical examination: Is this patient hypovolemic? *JAMA* 281:1022, 1999.

78. Koffler A, Friedler RM, Massry SG: Acute renal failure due to non-traumatic rhabdomyolysis. *Ann Intern Med* 85:23, 1976.

79. Miller PD, Krebs RA, Neal BJ, McIntyre DO: Polyuric prerenal failure. *Ann Intern Med* 140:907, 1980.

80. Miller TR, Anderson RJ, Linas SL, et al: Urinary diagnostic indices in acute renal failure: A prospective study. *Ann Intern Med* 89:47, 1978.

81. Pru C, Kjellstrand CM: The FE_{Na} test is of no prognostic value in acute renal failure. *Nephron* 36:20, 1984.

82. Goldstein MH, Lenz PR, Levitt MF: Effect of urine flow rate on urea reabsorption in man: urea as a 'tubular marker.' *J Appl Physiol* 26:594, 1969.

83. Kelton J, Kelley WH, Holmes EW: A rapid method for the diagnosis of acute uric acid nephropathy. *Arch Intern Med* 138:612, 1978.

84. Maillet PJ: Nondilated obstructive acute renal failure: Diagnostic procedures and therapeutic management. *Radiology* 160:659, 1986.

85. Davidson MB, Thakkar S, Hix JK, et al. Pathophysiology, clinical consequences, and treatment of tumor lysis syndrome. *Am J Med* 116:546, 2004.

86. Conger JD, Falk SA. Intrarenal dynamics in the pathogenesis and prevention of acute urate nephropathy. *J Clin Invest* 59:786, 1977.

87. Robinson RR, Yarger WE: Acute uric acid nephropathy (editorial). *Arch Intern Med* 137:839, 1977.

88. Goldman SC, Holcenberg JS, Finklestein JZ, et al. A randomized comparison between rasburicase and allopurinol in children with lymphoma and leukemia at high risk for tumor lysis. *Blood* 97:2998, 2001.

89. Kaplan BS, Hebert D, Morrell RE: Acute renal failure induced by hyperphosphatemia in acute lymphoblastic leukemia. *Can Med Assoc J* 124:429, 1981.

90. Agha-Razii M, Amyot SL, Pichette V, et al. Continuous venovenous hemodiafiltration for the treatment of spontaneous tumor lysis syndrome complicated by acute renal failure and severe hyperuricemia. *Clin Nephrol* 54:59, 2000.

91. Pichette V, Leblanc M, Bonnardeaux A, et al. High dialysate flow rate continuous arteriovenous hemodialysis: a new approach for the treatment of acute renal failure and tumor lysis syndrome. *Am J Kidney Dis* 23:591, 1994.

92. Chugh KS, Singhal PC, Shamra BK, et al: Acute renal failure of obstetric origin. *Obstet Gynecol* 48:642, 1976.

93. Kleinknecht D, Grunfeld JP, Gomez PC, et al: Diagnostic procedures and long-term prognosis in bilateral renal cortical necrosis. *Kidney Int* 4:390, 1973.

94. Ferris TF: Postpartum renal insufficiency. *Kidney Int* 14:383, 1978.

95. Arroyo V, Guevara M, Gines P. Hepatorenal syndrome in cirrhosis: pathogenesis and treatment. *Gastroenterology* 122:1658, 2002.

96. Cardenas A, Arroyo V: Hepatorenal syndrome. *Ann Hepatol* 2:23, 2003.

97. Angeli P, Volpin R, Gerunda G, et al. Reversal of type 1 hepatorenal syndrome with the administration of midodrine and octreotide. *Hepatology* 29:1690, 1999.

98. Finfer S, Bellomo R, Boyce N, et al: A comparison of albumin and saline for fluid resuscitation in the intensive care unit. *N Engl J Med* 350:2247, 2004.

99. Sort P, et al: Effect of intravenous albumin on renal impairment and mortality in patients with cirrhosis and spontaneous bacterial peritonitis. *N Engl J Med* 341:403, 1999.

100. Lassnigg A, et al: Lack of renoprotective effects of dopamine and furosemide during cardiac surgery. *J Am Soc Nephrol* 11:97, 2000.

101. Sirivella S, Gielchinsky I, Parsonnet V: Mannitol, furosemide, and dopamine infusion in postoperative renal failure complicating cardiac surgery. *Ann Thorac Surg* 69:501, 2000.

102. Cantarovich F, et al: High dose frusemide in established acute renal failure. *Br Med J* 4:449, 1973.

103. Minuth AN, Terrell JB Jr, Suki WN: Acute renal failure: a study of the course and prognosis of 104 patients and of the role of furosemide. *Am J Med Sci* 271:317, 1976.

104. Kleinknecht D, et al: Furosemide in acute oliguric renal failure. A controlled trial. *Nephron* 17:51, 1976.

105. Brown CB, Ogg CS, Cameron JS: High dose frusemide in acute renal failure: a controlled trial. *Clin Nephrol* 15:90, 1981.

106. Shilliday IR, Quinn KJ, Allison ME: Loop diuretics in the management of acute renal failure: A prospective, double-blind, placebo-controlled, randomized study. *Nephrol Dial Transplant* 12:2592, 1997.

107. Anderson RJ, et al: Nonoliguric acute renal failure. *N Engl J Med* 296:1134, 1977.

108. Mehta RL, et al: Diuretics, mortality, and nonrecovery of renal function in acute renal failure. *JAMA* 288:2547, 2002.

109. Martin SJ, Danziger LH: Continuous infusion of loop diuretics in the critically ill: A review of the literature. *Crit Care Med* 22:1323, 1994.

110. Schetz M: Should we use diuretics in acute renal failure? *Best Pract Res Clin Anaesthesiol* 18:75, 2004.

111. Bonventre JV, Weinberg JM: Kidney preservation ex vivo for transplantation. *Annu Rev Med* 43:523, 1992.

112. Better OS, et al: Mannitol therapy revisited (1940–1997). *Kidney Int* 52:886, 1997.

113. Visweswaran P, Massin EK, Dubose TD: Mannitol-induced acute renal failure. *J Am Soc Nephrol* 8:1028, 1997.

114. Conger JD, Falk SA, Hammond WS: Atrial natriuretic peptide and dopamine in established acute renal failure in the rat. *Kidney Int* 40:21, 1991.

115. Rahman SN, Kim GE, Mathew AS, et al: Effects of atrial natriuretic peptide in clinical acute renal failure. *Kidney Int* 45:1731, 1994.

116. Allgren RL, Marbury TC, Rahman SN, et al: Anaritide in acute tubular necrosis. Auriculin Anaritide Acute Renal Failure Study Group. *N Engl J Med* 336:828, 1997.

117. Lewis J, et al: Atrial natriuretic factor in oliguric acute renal failure. Anaritide Acute Renal Failure Study Group. *Am J Kidney Dis* 36:767, 2000.

118. Sward K, Valsson F, Odencrants P, et al: Recombinant human atrial natriuretic peptide in ischemic acute renal failure: A randomized, placebo-controlled trial. *Crit Care Med* 32:1310, 2004.

119. Murray PT: Use of dopaminergic agents for renoprotection in the ICU. Yearbook of Intensive Care and Emergency Medicine, Springer-Verlag, 2003, p 637.

120. Denton MD, Chertow GM, Brady HR. "Renal-dose" dopamine for the treatment of acute renal failure: scientific rationale, experimental studies and clinical trials. *Kidney Int* 49:4, 1996.

121. Kellum JA, Decker JM: Use of dopamine in acute renal failure: A meta-analysis. *Crit Care Med* 29:1526, 2001.

122. Marik PE: Low-dose dopamine: A systematic review. *Intensive Care Med* 28:877, 2002.

123. Bellomo R, Chapman M, Finfer S, et al: Low-dose dopamine in patients with early renal dysfunction: A placebo-controlled randomised trial. Australian and New Zealand Intensive Care Society (ANZICS) Clinical Trials Group. *Lancet* 356:2139, 2000.

124. Alvestrand A: Nutritional aspects in patients with acute renal failure/multiorgan failure. *Blood Purif* 14:109,1996.

125. Conger JD: Intervention in clinical acute renal failure: What are the data? Am J Kid Dis 26:565, 1995.

126. Montgomerie JZ, Kalmanson GM, Guze LB: Renal failure and infection. *Medicine* 47:1, 1968.

127. Remuzzi G: Bleeding in renal failure. *Lancet* 1:1205, 1988.

128. Bridges KR: Hemorrhagic complications associated with renal failure. *J Crit Illness* 4:17, 1989.

129. Mannucci PM, Remuzzi G, Pusineri F, et al: Deamino-8-D-arginine vasopressin shortens the bleeding time in uremia. *N Engl J Med* 308:8, 1983.

130. Janson PA, Kosfeld R, Marcum S. Treatment of uremic bleeding with conjugated oestrogen. *Lancet* 2:887, 1984.

131. Gillum DM, Dixon BS, Yanover MJ, et al: The role of intensive dialysis in acute renal failure. *Clin Nephrol* 25:249, 1986.

132. Bouman CS, Oudemans-Van Straaten HM, Tijssen JG, et al: Effects of early high-volume continuous venovenous hemofiltration on survival and recovery of renal function in intensive care patients with acute renal failure: a prospective, randomized trial. *Crit Care Med* 30:2205, 2002.

133. Mehta RL, McDonald B, Gabbai FB, et al: A randomized clinical trial of continuous versus intermittent dialysis for acute renal failure. *Kidney Int* 60:1154, 2001.

134. Evanson JA, Himmelfarb J, Wingard R, et al: Prescribed versus delivered dialysis in acute renal failure patients. *Am J Kidney Dis* 32:731, 1998.

135. Paganini EP, Tapolyai M, Goormastic M, et al: Establishing a dialysis therapy/patient outcome link in intensive care unit acute dialysis for patients with acute renal failure. *Am J Kidney Dis* 28:S81, 1996.

136. Schiffl H, Lang SM, Fischer R: Daily hemodialysis and the outcome of acute renal failure. *N Engl J Med* 346:305, 2002.

137. Ronco C, Bellomo R, Homel P, et al: Effects of different doses in continuous veno-venous haemofiltration on outcomes of acute renal failure: a prospective randomised trial. *Lancet* 356:26, 2000.

Chapter 76 _____

ELECTROLYTE DISORDERS IN CRITICAL CARE

JOEL MICHELS TOPF
STEVE RANKIN
PATRICK MURRAY

KEY POINTS

- *Measurement of electrolyte free water clearance is extremely useful in understanding the pathophysiology of hyponatremia and hypernatremia.*
- *Treatment of hyponatremia should be guided by the degree of symptomatology, rather than the magnitude of the hyponatremia per se.*
- *Hyperkalemia should be treated emergently if typical electrocardiographic (ECG) changes are present; hence ECG monitoring is indispensable in this setting.*
- *Hypocalcemia need only be treated urgently if it is symptomatic.*
- *Severe hypomagnesemia may have significant consequences itself, including cardiac arrhythmias and muscle weakness; lesser degrees of hypomagnesemia often accompany hypokalemia and hypocalcemia and correction of the magnesium deficit facilitates correction of the other electrolyte abnormalities.*
- *Severe hyperphosphatemia is seen in the setting of renal failure and/or massive cell lysis.*
- *Total body phosphate stores may be significantly reduced and produce organ dysfunction even in the face of normal or minimally decreased serum levels; if suspicion for a depleted state exists, treatment should be given.*

Sodium

METABOLISM

Sodium is the chief extracellular cation and is critical to regulating extracellular and intravascular volume. Total body sodium determines clinical volume status, but sodium concentration does not correlate with volume status. Both hypernatremia and hyponatremia occur in the presence of hypo-, eu-, and hypervolemia. The sodium concentration itself is the single ion that best represents serum osmolality; essentially all of the clinically relevant symptoms of dysnatremia are secondary to alterations in osmolality. Hypernatremia is largely synonymous with hyperosmolality, while hyponatremia is generally indicative of hypoosmolality.

Osmolality and tonicity are related but separate concepts. Osmolality measures all of the solutes in solution, while tonicity only includes particles that are unable to cross from the intracellular to the extracellular compartment. It is these particles which are osmotically active, and by drawing water across compartments they may alter cell volume. Sodium and potassium are the primary determinants of tonicity.

Balancing water intake and excretion is the principal means by which the body regulates sodium concentration. Water balance is maintained by thirst and antidiuretic hormone (ADH). Following a water load, osmolality falls and osmoreceptors in the hypothalamus suppress thirst and ADH release. The latter signals the kidney to produce dilute urine to clear the water load. In states of water deprivation (or a solute load) osmoreceptors detect the rise in osmolality and increase thirst and ADH.

The kidney regulates osmolality and sodium concentration by diluting or concentrating urine. Producing dilute urine allows the kidney to clear a water load, raising plasma osmolality. In order to make dilute urine, multiple criteria must be met:

1. Tubular fluid must be delivered to the diluting segment of the nephron. This can be assured in any patient with adequate effective arterial blood volume (EABV) and a normal or near normal glomerular filtration rate (GFR).
2. There must be intact sodium resorption in the diluting segments of the kidney (i.e., the thick ascending limb of the loop of Henle [TALH]) and the distal convoluted tubule. Loop and thiazide diuretics are the primary causes of inoperative diluting segments.
3. The collecting tubule must be impermeable to water. ADH increases water permeability, so the production of dilute urine requires a lack of ADH.

Concentrating urine allows the kidneys to minimize water loss and compensate for an increase in serum osmolality. In order to produce concentrated urine, the following conditions must be met:

1. A hypertonic medullary interstitium draws water from the medullary collecting ducts. The TALH creates and maintains the high concentration of the interstitium. Any factor that antagonizes the TALH (e.g., loop diuretics, hypercalcemia, or hypokalemia) will disrupt the production of concentrated urine.
2. ADH increases the permeability of the collecting tubules, allowing water to osmotically flow out of the collecting ducts into the medullary interstitium, concentrating the urine.

ANTIDIURETIC HORMONE

ADH plays a crucial role in the concentrating and diluting process. ADH, or vasopressin, is a six-peptide amino acid produced in the hypothalamus and stored in the posterior pituitary gland. Release of ADH follows increases in osmolality or dramatic drops in blood pressure or effective arterial blood volume. An increase in serum osmolality of 1% (2 mOsm/kg) will stimulate ADH, while a similar decrease inhibits release. ADH is less sensitive to changes in blood volume; a loss of 7% to 10% of blood volume is required to release ADH.[1] When osmolality suppresses and volume depletion stimulates ADH release, volume effects predominate and ADH is released. Osmolality is a more sensitive ADH stimulus, while volume is a more potent ADH stimulus. ADH is also released in response to a collection of nonosmotic, nonvolemic stimuli (Table 76-1).

TABLE 76-1 Causes of Antidiuretic Hormone (ADH) Release

Inappropriate Stimuli of ADH Release	Appropriate Stimuli of ADH Release
Pain	Hyperosmolality
Nausea	Hypovolemia
Narcotics	
Nicotine	
Clofibrate	
Vincristine	
Carbamazepine	
Ifosfamide	
Chlorpropamide	

FREE WATER CLEARANCE AND ELECTROLYTE FREE WATER CLEARANCE

The renal excretion or retention of water is central to the regulation of osmolality, so specialized concepts have been developed to model renal water handling. *Clearance* is a generic term used to quantify solute removal (x) by the kidney. Clearance is an artificial construct that represents the volume of blood that is completely cleared of a substance in a set amount of time (Equation 76-1). The clearance formula can be manipulated to calculate the clearance of free water, called the *free water clearance*. Conceptually, urine can be divided into two components: an isotonic and a free water component. The isosmotic component contains all of the excreted solute at the same concentration as that found in plasma; since the solute and water loss occur in the same proportion as found in the body, excretion of this isotonic urine does not affect osmolality. The other component is free water; this is solute-free water and excretion of this compartment raises plasma osmolality. For example: A person makes 1200 mL of urine with an osmolality of 142 mOsm/kg. This urine can be divided into 600 mL of isotonic urine (284 mOsm/kg) and 600 mL of free water. In terms of osmolality, only the 600 mL of free water needs to be considered. The loss of this 600 mL will tend to increase serum osmolality. The case is reversed with concentrated urine. A patient produces 1000 mL of urine with an osmolality of 568 mOsm/kg. This urine can be divided into 2000 mL of isotonic urine (284 mOsm/kg) and a negative 1000 mL of free water. In regards to changes in osmolality only the −1000 mL needs to be considered. The −1000 mL represents water that is added to the body and will decrease serum osmolality. Despite the patient excreting 1000 mL of urine, 1000 mL of fluid have been effectively added to the body by the production of concentrated urine. Equation 76-2 is used to calculate the free water clearance.

$$C_x = \left[\frac{U_x \times V}{P_x} \right]$$

Equation 76-1. Generic clearance formula. Using conventional units, U_x is in milligrams per deciliter of urine, V is in milliliters of urine per minute, and P_x is milligrams per deciliter of blood. After the units cancel, the equation simplifies to milliliters of blood and represents the quantity of blood that is completely cleared of the substance in 1 minute. U_x, urine concentration of x; V, urine volume over a set time period; P_x, plasma concentration of x.

$$V = C_{osm} + C_{H_2O}$$
$$C_{H_2O} = V - C_{osm}$$

$$C_{H_2O} = V - \left[\frac{U_{osm} \times V}{P_{osm}} \right]$$
$$C_{H_2O} = V \times \left[1 - \frac{U_{osm}}{P_{osm}} \right]$$

Equation 76-2. Free water clearance. The derivation of free water clearance begins with the assumption that urine volume is the sum of the solute clearance (C_{osm}) and free water clearance. From there, algebraic manipulation results in the free water clearance equation.

Free water clearance allows one to model changes in osmolality, but as described above, changes in tonicity and associated alterations in cell volume cause the clinical symptoms of dysnatremia. In order to model changes in tonicity (i.e., sodium) rather than osmolality, the free water clearance is further refined to measure electrolyte free water clearance (C_{EFW}). In electrolyte free water clearance, serum osmolality is replaced with serum sodium and urine osmolality is replaced with the sum of urine sodium and potassium (Equation 76-3). To demonstrate the utility of C_{EFW} over C_{H_2O}, consider two patients with identical urine output (800 mL) and urine and plasma osmolality (700 and 270, respectively). One has heart failure and the other has the syndrome of inappropriate secretion of antidiuretic hormone (SIADH). In both patients, the C_{H_2O} is identical at −1274. For every 800 mL of urine they produce, 1274 mL of water is added to the body. When using *electrolyte* free water the two cases look very different. In heart failure (and in all cases of decreased EABV) urine sodium is low, while in SIADH the urine sodium is elevated. Using urine sodium (U_{Na}) = 90, urine potassium (U_K) = 60, and plasma sodium (P_{Na}) = 130 for SIADH, the C_{EFW} is −123 mL. Using U_{Na} = 5, U_K = 60, and P_{Na} = 130 for congestive heart failure (CHF), the C_{EFW} is 400 mL. In the case of CHF the C_{EFW} is positive, so the kidney is appropriately excreting excess water (although it is limited by oliguria), while in SIADH the C_{EFW} is negative, so the production of urine further lowers plasma osmolality.

$$C_{EFW} = V \times \left[1 - \frac{U_{Na+} + U_K}{P_{Na}} \right]$$

Equation 76-3. Electrolyte free water clearance. This formula adapts the free water clearance formula to model changes in tonicity. C_{EFW}, free water clearance; P_{Na}, plasma sodium; U_K, urine potassium; U_{Na}, urine sodium; V, urine volume.

HYPERNATREMIA

Hypernatremia has been reported in 0.2% of hospital admissions and occurs in an additional 0.3% to 1% of patients during their hospital stay.[1a] These numbers likely underrepresent the prevelance of hypernatremia in the ICU, since studies focused on this patient population have shown that 9% of medical ICU patients had a sodium level >150 mmol/L at admission, and an additional 6% developed hypernatremia during the ICU stay.[1b] The body defends against increases in osmolality and serum sodium by increasing water intake and minimizing renal free water excretion (through the creation of a concentrated urine). Though ADH is used to minimize free water losses, drinking water alone is able to maintain a normal sodium and serum osmolality despite a total absence of ADH and the production of large amounts of dilute urine. Because the adequate ingestion of water can prevent and reverse hyperosmolality, persistent hypertonicity (and hypernatremia)

TABLE 76-2 Causes of Hypernatremia

Increased C_{EFW}[a]	Sweat and Insensible Losses	Water Loss into Cells	Increased Intake of Sodium	Central Impairment of Thirst
Central diabetes insipidus	Fever	Severe exercise	Infusions of hypertonic sodium bicarbonate	Reset osmostat
Nephrogenic diabetes insipidus	Tachypnea	Seizures	Infusions of hypertonic saline	Elderly patients
Hypercalcemia	Burns		Hypertonic dialysate	
Hypokalemia	Exercise		Overdose of salt tablets	
Recovery from acute tubular necrosis				
Postobstructive diuresis				
X-linked recessive				
Lithium				
Demeclocycline				
Osmotic diuresis				
Hyperglycemia				
Mannitol				
Urea (catabolic state, high-protein tube feedings)				
Diarrhea (osmotic)				
Lactulose				
Sorbitol				
Malabsorption				

[a] Note: Patients with increased electrolyte free water losses that are able to increase water intake will maintain eunatremia. These conditions increase the demand for water, but if that demand is met they will not cause hypernatremia.

only occurs when water ingestion is disabled, as occurs with altered mental status, lack of access to water, or inability to drink water. In a review of hypernatremia 86% of patients lacked access to free water and 94% received less than a liter of electrolyte free water.[1a] In the absence of adequate water intake hypernatremia occurs when C_{EFW} exceeds electrolyte free water intake. Causes of increased electrolyte free water clearance are listed in Table 76-2.

ETIOLOGIES
Loss of Water
Electrolyte free water clearance can exceed water intake either from enhanced renal water loss or extrarenal loss.

Renal Water Loss
Renal water losses occur when the kidney is unable to appropriately concentrate urine. This is generically referred to as diabetes insipidus (DI). Diabetes insipidus can be either central or nephrogenic. In central diabetes insipidus (CDI) there is a complete or partial lack of ADH. In nephrogenic diabetes insipidus (NDI) there is a complete or partial end-organ resistance to ADH. Patients with DI have very high C_{EFW} and present with polyuria, polydipsia, and a normal serum sodium. Hyperosmolality and hypernatremia only occur when the patient fails to drink enough water to compensate for the increased C_{EFW}. Renal water loss plays a role in 90% of hospital-acquired hypernatremia, primarily from diuretics or osmotic diuresis.[1]

Extrarenal Water Losses
The C_{EFW} equation can be modified to look at extrarenal water losses. To do this, change the urinary Na and K to the extrarenal fluid Na and K (see Equation 76-3). When the fluid Na + K is significantly less than serum Na, electrolyte free water is being lost, predisposing the patient to hypernatremia. Sweat, osmotic diarrhea, and insensible water loss all result in significant EFW loss.

Use of Hypertonic Fluids
The addition of any fluid to the body may alter osmolality. The change in osmolality is predictable using an equation that looks at the volume and electrolyte composition of both the infusate and urine. Equation 76-4 calculates the change in sodium following any combination of infusion and urine production.[2a] Figures 76-1 and 76-2 show how the change in sodium formula works to predict hypernatremia in two scenarios, one a hypertonic saline infusion and the other an increase in C_{EFW}. The change in sodium formula is a general model of sodium handling in the body and works equally well in both the etiologies and treatment of dysnatremias.

$$\Delta Na = \left\{ \frac{V_{iv} \times (Na_{iv} + K_{iv}) - V_u \times (Na_u + K_u) - \Delta V \times Na_s}{TBW + \Delta V} \right\}$$

$$\Delta Na = \left\{ \frac{0.4 \times (1000 + 0) - 0.4 \times 140}{42 + 0.4} \right\}$$

$$\Delta Na = 8.1$$

FIGURE 76-1 Change in sodium following a cardiac arrest. This patient was given 4 amps of sodium bicarbonate during a code. Each amp of bicarbonate contains 100 mL and has a concentration of 1 mmol/mL or 1000 mmol/L. The patient is anuric so the urine volume, Na, and K drop out. The patient weighs 70 kg and has 60% body water so TBW = 42. See caption to Equation 76-4 for explanation of variables.

$$\Delta Na = \left\{ \frac{V_{iv} \times (Na_{iv} + K_{iv}) - V_u \times (Na_u + K_u) - \Delta V \times Na_s}{TBW + \Delta V} \right\}$$

$$\Delta Na = \left\{ \frac{8 \times (0 + 0) - 18 \times (8 + 15) - (-14) \times 140}{42 + (-14)} \right\}$$

$$\Delta Na = 30.8$$

$$\Delta Na = \left\{ \frac{V_{iv} \times (Na_{iv} + K_{iv}) - V_u \times (Na_u + K_u) - \Delta V \times Na_s}{TBW + \Delta V} \right\}$$

Equation 76-4. Change in sodium for any combination of urine and infusate. V_{iv} is the volume of infusate and Na_{iv} is the sodium content of the infusate. Typical values are 0 for 5% dextrose in water, 77 for 0.45% normal saline, 154 for 0.9% normal saline, and 513 for 3% saline; K_{iv} is the potassium content of the infusate; V_u is the volume of urine; Na_u is the sodium content of the urine; K_u is the potassium content of the urine; ΔV is the change in total body volume ($V_{iv} - V_u$); Na_s is the current serum sodium concentration; TBW is the total body water, usually calculated by multiplying weight in kilograms by 0.7 for young men and 0.6 for women and older men.

CLINICAL SEQUELAE

The primary symptoms of hypernatremia are due to loss of cell volume (Fig. 76-3). A decrease in brain volume causes neuromuscular irritability that clinically presents as lethargy, weakness, and headache. These are nonspecific signs and can be particularly occult in the population predisposed to hypernatremia (e.g., altered mental status, dementia, and coma). As sodium rises above 158 mmol/L more severe symptoms may emerge such as seizures and coma, and death may ensue. Interestingly even relatively modest hypernatremia (Na >150 mEq/L) has been associated with increased mortality among ICU patients (RR 1.6) and general inpatients (66% hospital mortality).[1b,1c] Significant decreases in brain volume stretch cerebral bridging veins, rendering them susceptible to rupture and intracerebral hemorrhage.[2,4] Beyond cerebral effects, hypernatremia inhibits insulin release and causes insulin resistance, predisposing patients to hyperglycemia.

FIGURE 76-2 Change in sodium in a patient with central diabetes insipidus who stopped his desmopressin and is ingesting an inadequate quantity of water. The patient weighs 70 kg and has 60% body water so TBW = 42. See caption to Equation 76-4 for explanation of variables.

In response to increased serum tonicity and volume loss, cells compensate by increasing the number of intracellular osmoles. Initially cells move extracellular electrolytes into the cells, and later they transfer amino acids and other small molecules into the cell. Increased intracellular osmolality restores intracellular volume, and decreases the clinical impact of hypernatremia.

TREATMENT

The goal of treating hypernatremia is to arrest any ongoing cause of hypernatremia, and then to restore serum sodium to normal. Specific therapy should be employed to reduce ongoing water losses, such as correcting hypercalcemia-induced diuresis or administering desmopressin (DDAVP) to patients with CDI. Beyond this, correcting hypernatremia requires giving hypotonic fluid either enterally or parenterally. The enteral route is preferred, as it allows the use of electrolyte free water rather than hypotonic or dextrose-containing fluids. Though the optimum speed of correction has not been rigorously determined, studies on infants and children showed no seizures when sodium was corrected at less than 0.5 mmol/L per hour.[5] The sodium can be safely lowered by 10 mmol in the first day of therapy. Patients with acute increases in sodium (e.g., from hypertonic bicarbonate infusions) can safely be corrected at 1 mmol/L per hour.[5a] The change in serum sodium from a given amount of fluid can be calculated using Equation 76-4. An example of this is shown in Fig. 76-4.

A number of complications from the treatment of hypernatremia can occur. If the sodium is lowered too quickly cerebral edema may occur. Dextrose solutions predispose patients to hyperglycemia, which may cause an osmotic diuresis, worsening the hypernatremia. For this reason enteral fluids are preferred during treatment of hypernatremia.

HYPONATREMIA

Hyponatremia is defined as a serum sodium less than 136 mmol/L. Since serum sodium and its accompanying anions are the principal determinants of serum osmolality, hyponatremic patients are typically hypo-osmolar; however, hyponatremia may also be associated with normal or elevated osmolality. Since the primary morbidity from hyponatremia is due to decreased tonicity, hyponatremia with normal or elevated osmolality does not cause the clinical picture typically associated with hyponatremia.

Pseudohyponatremia is hyponatremia with a normal plasma osmolality. It is an artifact of two popular sodium assays, flame photometry and indirect potentiometry. Serum with elevated triglycerides, proteins (from multiple myeloma or Waldenström's macroglobulinemia, or following intravenous immunoglobulin therapy) or rarely cholesterol, has

FIGURE 76-3 Increased plasma osmolality causes a shift of water out of the intracellular compartment. Decreased cell volume impairs tissue function, particularly in the central nervous system.

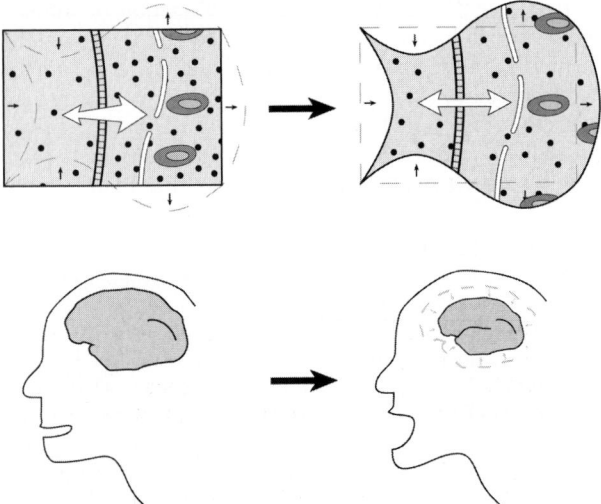

Initial Na = 168 mmol/L

$$\Delta Na = \left\{ \frac{V_{iv} \times (Na_{iv} + K_{iv}) - \Delta V \times Na_s}{TBW + \Delta V} \right\}$$

$$\Delta Na = \left\{ \frac{1 \times (0 + 0) - 1 \times 168}{42 + 1} \right\}$$

$\Delta Na = 3.9 \approx 4$

So: 6 liters free water will decrease Na by 24 to 144 mmol/L

To calculate the rate, limited to 2 mmol/L per hour :

$$\frac{24 \text{ mmol/L}}{2 \text{ mmol/L per hour}} \times 6 \text{ L} = 0.5 \text{ L/h}$$

FIGURE 76-4 Using the change in sodium formula to assist with the treatment of hypernatremia. In this example the patient is assumed to be anuric. During the treatment urine Na and K should be measured along with urine volume to better refine the estimated volume and time needed to correct the hypernatremia. See caption to Equation 76-4 for explanation of variables.

increased solute, and thus a given volume of serum contains less water. This results in a lab error due to overdilution of the sample (Fig. 76-5). Patients suspected of having pseudohyponatremia should have their sodium assessed by direct potentiometry, a technique generally employed by blood gas laboratories that is not susceptible to artifactual hyponatremia. Indirect potentiometry is used in two-thirds of clinical labs, making pseudohyponatremia a real issue.[5b] Since patients with pseudohyponatremia have normal sodium and osmolality, no specific treatment is needed.

With simultaneous hyponatremia and hyperosmolality an additional solute is contributing to the osmolality. Both glucose and mannitol can act as the additional solute. The increased extracellular osmolality draws water from the intracellular space, diluting serum sodium. The measured serum sodium falls by a predictable amount; the common cited adjustment is a decrease in sodium of 1.6 mmol/L for every 100-mg/dL increase in blood glucose.[6] However, the only empiric data that looked at this showed a more complex relationship: The adjustment of 1.6 mmol/L holds until serum glucose exceeds 400 mg/dL, at which point the sodium should fall by 4.0 mmol/L for every 100-mg/dL rise in glucose. For glucose less than 700 mg/dL, using an adjustment of 2.4 worked nearly as well as the more complex biphasic system.[7]

Hyposmotic hyponatremia, also called true hyponatremia, and in the remainder of the chapter simply called hyponatremia, occurs when electrolyte free water intake exceeds

electrolyte free water clearance (C_{EFW}). Intact kidneys are able to clear close to 20 L of electrolyte free water, so outside of exceptional water intake, hyponatremia only occurs when there is a defect in the C_{EFW}. This defect in C_{EFW} can alternatively be stated as an inability to produce an adequate volume of dilute urine. This can be due to:

- Decreased delivery of water to the diluting segments of the nephron, namely the thick ascending limb of the loop of Henle (TALH) and distal convoluted tubule (DCT). Decreased delivery of tubular fluid is due to a generalized decrease in glomerular filtration rate (GFR), as seen in renal failure, or increased proximal resorption of water, as seen with decreased EABV.
- Decreased activity in the diluting segments of the nephron due to diuretics. Loop diuretics block solute resorption in the TALH and thiazide-type diuretics block resorption in the DCT.
- ADH activity, which allows water to be resorbed in the collecting tubules, preventing C_{EFW}.

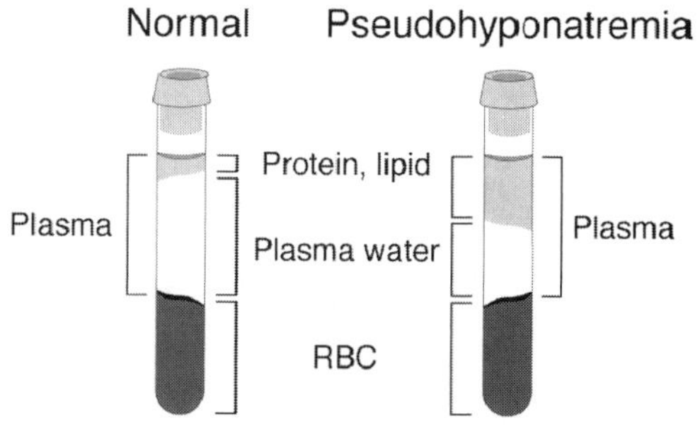

ETIOLOGIES

Hypotonic hyponatremia is traditionally broken down by clinical volume status of the patient (Table 76-3). While this may help clinically classify patients, it does not elucidate the pathophysiology of hyponatremia (e.g., CHF and vomiting both cause hyponatremia by inducing a nonosmotic release of ADH, but they are on opposite sides of the classification, as one is hypovolemic and the other hypervolemic). A pathophysiologic approach to hyponatremia categorizes the etiology based on why the patient has compromised C_{EFW}.

Decreased Delivery of Water to the Diluting Segments of the Nephron

Decreases in GFR for any reason reduce C_{EFW}. Patients with renal failure must moderate their intake of fluids or they may develop acute hyponatremia. Decreases in effective arterial blood volume can result from heart failure, cirrhosis, or volume depletion. Even in situations in which the GFR is intact, decreased EABV (due to CHF, liver failure, or nephrotic syndrome) increases resorption of fluid in the proximal tubule, reducing delivery of fluid to the diluting segments. Patients with reduced distal delivery of fluid have positive C_{EFW}, but

FIGURE 76-5 Pseudohyponatremia occurs when plasma proteins or lipids occupy an unexpectedly high volume. The decreased plasma water is overdiluted while preparing the sodium assay, so the sodium will be falsely reported as low.

Normal   Pseudohyponatremia

Plasma

Protein, lipid

Plasma water

Plasma

RBC

TABLE 76-3 Etiologies of Hyponatremia Categorized by Clinical Volume Status

Hypovolemic	Euvolemic	Hypervolemic
Diarrhea	SIADH	CHF
Vomiting	Hypothyroidism	Cirrhosis
Pancreatitis	Glucocorticoid deficiency	Nephrotic syndrome
Burns		Acute renal failure
Diuretic-induced		Chronic renal failure
Mineralocorticoid deficiency		
Salt-wasting nephropathy		
Cerebral salt wasting		

CHF, congestive heart failure; SIADH, the syndrome of inappropriate secretion of antidiuretic hormone.

the clearance is less than their intake of free water. The hyponatremia tends to be gradual in onset and of mild severity.

Decreased Activity in the Diluting Segments of the Nephron Due to Diuretics

An intact diluting segment is essential to C_{EFW}. In some patients, severe hyponatremia can follow the initiation of diuretics.[8] Diuretics promote hyponatremia by blocking at least one and possibly all three factors required to produce dilute urine:

1. Thiazide and loop diuretics both directly antagonize the production of dilute urine.
2. Diuretic-induced volume depletion reduces the delivery of water to the diluting segments of the nephron.
3. With more dramatic volume loss, diuretics stimulate a nonosmotic release of ADH, dramatically reducing C_{EFW}.

Despite the fact that thiazide-type diuretics are less potent than loop diuretics, they cause hyponatremia more frequently and hyponatremia that is more severe. The NaK2Cl channel, which is antagonized by loop diuretics, is the engine that produces the hypertonic medullary interstitium. This medullary interstitium is necessary for ADH-stimulated water resorption in the medullary collecting duct. Chronic loop diuretic use attenuates the hypertonicity of the interstitium,

so that even in the presence of ADH, little water is resorbed (Fig. 76-6).

Thiazide-induced hyponatremia is classically seen among elderly Caucasian females.[8,9] It should be noted that although these patients are classified as hypovolemic, the volume loss has repeatedly been reported as minor and subtle.[10–12] Although hyponatremia associated with diuretic use normally occurs within the first few days of therapy, hyponatremia due to chronic diuretic use may emerge in a newly sick patient.[11]

ADH Activity

The primary role of ADH is to regulate osmolality, so that it is released in response to increases in osmolality. In the presence of hypoosmolality ADH release is suppressed. However, ADH has a secondary role in maintaining perfusion, and is released in response to large decreases in blood pressure. This nonosmotic release of ADH sacrifices osmoregulation to maintain adequate perfusion. Volume depletion, heart failure, and cirrhosis are all examples in which a nonosmotic release of ADH reduces C_{EFW} and contributes to hyponatremia.

ADH may also be released without an osmotic or perfusion-related stimuli. In these cases the ADH release is considered inappropriate, as it serves no physiologic purpose. The syndrome of inappropriate secretion of ADH (SIADH) is a release of ADH despite decreased osmolality and normal EABV. Causes of SIADH are listed in Table 76-1. Among the elderly

FIGURE 76-6 In the left panel, thiazide diuretics block reabsorption in the DCT, leaving the TALH intact. ADH-induced water resorption is not dissipated. In the right panel, loop diuretics block TALH so that the medullary interstitium loses its concentration gradient. Even in the presence of ADH, little water is resorbed from the collecting tubule due to the loss of the hypertonic interstitium.

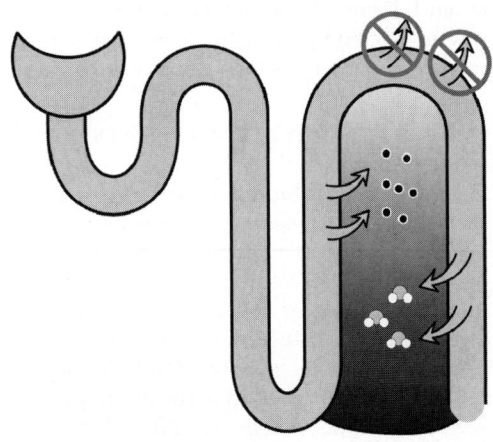
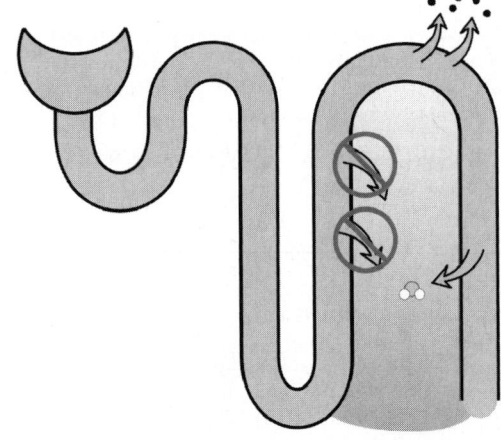

no cause of SIADH can be found in up to 10% of patients.[13] The diagnosis of SIADH requires four criteria:

1. Hypotonic (<270 mOsm/kg) hyponatremia (<135 mmol/L)
2. Inappropriately concentrated urine (>100 mOsm/kg)
3. Elevated urine sodium
4. No underlying adrenal, thyroid, pituitary, or renal disease.

UNIQUE CLINICAL SITUATIONS RESULTING IN HYPONATREMIA

Cerebral Salt Wasting

Cerebral salt wasting (CSW) is a rare clinical event that typically follows a subarachnoid hemorrhage. Patients have high urinary flow rates with elevated urine sodium, which ultimately results in severe volume deficiency and hyponatremia. The pathophysiology behind CSW has not been fully elucidated but it is likely that natriuretic proteins are released in response to the CNS injury. Atrial natriuretic peptide, brain natriuretic peptide, and an endogenous oubain-like peptide have all been proposed as possible etiologic agents. The key diagnostic dilemma is differentiating CSW from SIADH, as both can follow CNS insults and are marked by hyponatremia with elevated urine sodium. The principal differences are urine volume (in SIADH it is low, while it is high in CSW) and clinical volume status (it is normal in SIADH, while it is low in CSW). In CSW ADH release is secondary to decreased volume status, and aggressive fluid replacement is required to maintain perfusion and suppress ADH. This differentiates it from SIADH, where isotonic saline will decrease serum sodium. CSW spontaneously resolves after 2 to 3 weeks.[14]

Postoperative Hyponatremia

The postoperative period is ripe with factors that stimulate ADH: stress, positive pressure ventilation, pain, nausea, and opioids. It is not surprising that with the addition of generous quantities of IV fluids hyponatremia can occur.[15]

A unique form of postoperative hyponatremia may follow urologic or gynecologic procedures employing large amounts of hypotonic irrigants, typically 1.5% glycine.[16] The hypotonic fluid enters the systemic circulation and patients develop acute neurologic symptoms from either the rapid drop in sodium or from increased ammonia produced from the metabolism of glycine. Patients with hypotonic and neurologic symptoms should be treated for acute hyponatremia. Intact kidneys rapidly clear the irrigant so hyponatremia is only transient. Severe hyponatremia is more common following longer operations, larger resections, and high-pressure irrigation.[17]

Psychogenic Polydipsia

This disorder is most commonly seen in patients suffering from schizophrenia. They overwhelm their urinary diluting capacity by ingesting large volumes of water. Nausea and vomiting from acute hyponatremia is typical and stimulates a nonosmotic release of ADH, worsening the hyponatremia.[18] These patients demonstrate excessive diurnal weight gains, usually in excess of 10% of their body weight.

Adrenal Insufficiency

Adrenal insufficiency reliably causes hyponatremia. There are two mechanisms that cause this: hypovolemic release of ADH and corelease of ADH with adrenocorticotropic hormone (ACTH). Patients with adrenal insufficiency can be hypotensive due to either loss of cortisol, or in the case of primary adrenal insufficiency loss of aldosterone, causing a salt-wasting nephropathy resulting in hypovolemia. The hypotension and hypovolemia reduces water delivery to the diluting segments and stimulates ADH release. The second mechanism is due to enhanced ADH release in response to increased corticotropin-releasing hormone (CRH). CRH is the secretagogue of ACTH, but it also stimulates ADH release.[19,20] In primary and secondary adrenal insufficiency CRH is increased, which will cause increased ADH release, lowering C_{EFW}.

CLINICAL SEQUELAE

Symptoms seen in hyponatremia are largely neurologic and increase in severity with lower sodium and increased rate of development of the hypo-osmolar state. Symptoms are often vague and nonspecific: malaise, nausea, confusion, and lethargy. More dangerous symptoms follow: headache, obtundation, seizures, coma, and death.[10] Unusual symptoms have been reported, including hemiparesis and acute psychosis.[20a] Symptoms are largely due to cerebral edema (Fig. 76-7). With extracellular hypoosmolality the intracellular compartment becomes relatively hypertonic and water osmotically flows into cells, resulting in cell swelling and increased intracranial pressure. Following prolonged hyponatremia (24 to 72 hours) cells compensate for the chronic hyponatremia by ejecting intracellular solutes, lowering intracellular volume. With the restoration of intracellular volume in chronic hyponatremia, the condition becomes essentially asymptomatic.

Hypoxia is repeatedly reported as a common finding among patients with symptomatic hyponatremia. Some authors have attributed this to noncardiogenic pulmonary edema, though central hypoventilation may also be responsible.[20b] The average partial arterial oxygen pressure (Pa_{O_2}) of patients with symptomatic hyponatremia was 63 mm Hg and 68% of the patients in this series were ultimately

FIGURE 76-7 Decreases in extracellular osmolality cause the intracellular compartment to be relatively hypertonic. The hypertonic intracellular compartment attracts water, resulting in cellular swelling and tissue dysfunction. In the brain, cellular swelling causes cerebral edema and elevated intracranial pressure.

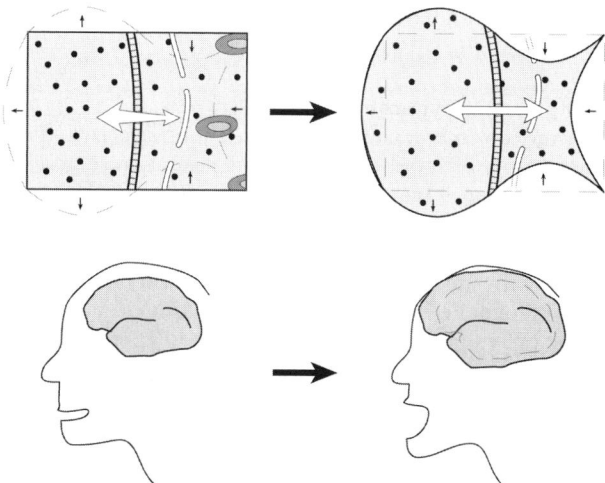

Initial Na $= 107$ mmol/L

$$\Delta Na = \left\{ \frac{V_{iv} \times (Na_{iv} + K_{iv}) - V_u \times (Na_u + K_u) - \Delta V \times Na_s}{TBW + \Delta V} \right\}$$

$$\Delta Na = \left\{ \frac{1 \times (513 + 40) - 1 \times 107}{42 + 1} \right\}$$

$$\Delta Na = 10.4$$

So : 1 liter of 3% saline will increase Na by 10 and 1.2 liters will increase it by 12, the limit for the first day of therapy.

To calculate the rate, divide 1200 mL by 24 hours :

$$\frac{1200 \text{ mL}}{24 \text{ h}} = 50 \text{ mL/h}$$

FIGURE 76-8 Using the change in sodium formula to assist with the treatment of hyponatremia. In this example the patient is assumed to be anuric. During the treatment urine Na and K should be measured along with urine volume to better refine the estimated volume and time needed to correct the hyponatremia.

intubated.[20c] Hypoxia has been shown to delay cellular compensation, resulting in persistent symptoms of acute hyponatremia despite a prolonged clinical course of over 5 days.

TREATMENT

Hyponatremia causes symptoms due to cerebral edema from the osmotic movement of water into cells. Compensation for acute hyponatremia consists of cells ejecting intracellular solutes in order to restore normal cell volume. This compensation complicates treatment decisions because rapidly restoring normal osmolality in the presence of compensated cells can cause the serum to be relatively hypertonic to the cells, resulting in the osmotic movement of water out of the cells. In the CNS this can cause a condition called central pontine myelinolysis (CPM) or osmotic demyelination syndrome (ODS) that results in severe morbidity or death. In determining the treatment plan for hyponatremia one must balance the risk of cerebral edema from the hyponatremia against the risk of ODS from treating compensated hyponatremia. Creating evidence-based guidelines is difficult because of the lack of randomized controlled trials. Recommendations are based on retrospective case series and expert opinion. The following guidelines attempt to balance the risks of these opposing outcomes.

Symptomatic Hyponatremia

In acute hyponatremia little compensation has occurred and the benefits of rapid correction and resolution of cerebral edema outweigh the risks of ODS. While acute hyponatremia has classically been defined as hyponatremia lasting less than 48 hours, a prospective (albeit not randomized) trial has shown active treatment to be superior to fluid restriction for a cohort of patients with CNS symptoms and an average duration of hyponatremia of 5.2 days (all had hyponatremia for longer than 48 hours and a gradual decrease in sodium of 0.5 mmol/L per hour). Given this, patients with symptomatic hyponatremia should be actively treated. Sodium levels should be initially raised rapidly until symptoms abate or the serum sodium has been raised by 4 to 6 mEq/L.[21] Further-

more, the sodium should be raised no more than 12 mEq/L in the first 24 hours.[22-24] The sodium concentration should be assessed frequently to maintain the permitted rate of correction. Aside from volume depletion, hypertonic saline is the best way to raise the sodium concentration to treat acute, symptomatic hyponatremia. When using hypertonic saline to correct hyponatremia Equation 76-4 allows rapid calculation of how much the serum sodium will change in response to 1 L of IV fluid. It should be noted that when using IV fluids to treat hyponatremia, potassium in the IV fluid has the same effect on serum tonicity as sodium, and needs to be added to the sodium.[25,26] Figure 76-8 gives an example of using the change in sodium formula to manage hyponatremia.

Caution should be used when estimating total body water. The common estimate of 0.7 times total body weight for men and 0.6 times total body weight for women assumes a normal hydration status and normal percentage of body fat. This calculation overestimates total body water among patients who are volume depleted or obese. Overestimating TBW leads to exceeding limits on the speed of correction and possibly increased risk of osmotic demyelinization.

In the setting of hyponatremia due to volume depletion, normal saline should be used to restore normal perfusion prior to specific therapy for hypo-osmolality. Restoring normal perfusion will remove the nonosmotic stimulus for ADH release so the kidney will increase free water clearance and auto-correct the hyponatremia. In some situations patients will correct their sodium too fast and require free water infusions to slow the rate of correction.

Asymptomatic Hyponatremia

Whereas acute symptomatic hyponatremia demands aggressive treatment to reverse cerebral edema, chronic asymptomatic hyponatremia is well tolerated and should be treated conservatively. First, any ongoing cause of the hyponatremia (e.g., water intake or diuretics) should be stopped and water restriction initiated. A spot urine sodium and potassium should be checked in order to calculate the C_{EFW}. In most cases this will be positive and can allow one to determine the degree of fluid restriction required to raise the serum sodium. However, in SIADH the C_{EFW} will be negative, which means that for every milliliter of urine the patient produces, water is added to (rather than cleared from) the body. With a negative C_{EFW} water restriction will rarely be successful at raising serum sodium. In this unique situation a loop diuretic can increase the C_{EFW} by reducing the urine sodium. A negative C_{EFW} only occurs when the urine Na plus urine K is higher than the serum Na, and loop diuretics typically reduce the urine sodium to around 70, which is sufficient to reduce the urine Na plus K to below serum Na. This will make the C_{EFW} positive and allow fluid restriction to increase the serum sodium. (Note: In patients with a positive C_{EFW}, adding a loop diuretic can have the opposite effect by increasing a low urine Na, indicative of good C_{EFW}, to around 70.)

In patients with chronic SIADH, use of the antibiotic demeclocycline acts as an ADH antagonist and so allows more liberal fluid intake. Likewise, increasing the solute load by using a high-protein diet or increased sodium and potassium intake will also allow increased daily fluid intake.

Osmotic Demyelination Syndrome

ODS is the primary complication of therapy for hyponatremia. With rapid or complete restoration of extracellular osmolality, a well adjusted intracellular environment becomes relatively hypotonic. Water then flows from the intracellular to the extracellular compartment, causing cell volume collapse. In the CNS this can cause a demyelinating lesion. Symptoms usually present within a week of the correction of the hyponatremia. Although slowly evolving neurologic symptoms similar to a pseudobulbar palsy and the "locked-in" quadriparesis are classic, findings may be more subtle. Disturbances of movement or behavior or seizures may be the presenting finding.[28] Some patients tend to be more susceptible than others. In a case-control study by Ayus and colleagues, patients with hepatic encephalopathy, hypoxia, or normalization of Na (or an increase greater than 25 mmol/L) in the first 48 hours were found to be susceptible to ODS.[27a] In the event that ODS occurs, some authors advocate relowering the sodium to 120 mEq/L by giving hypotonic fluids and DDAVP, and then allowing the sodium to slowly return to normal. However, there are no randomized trials in the literature to validate this approach, and given the devastating morbidity and mortality of ODS, an attempt to reverse the corrected sodium should be attempted in patients displaying symptoms of ODS.

Potassium

Potassium is the most common cation in the body. The ratio of the intracellular to extracellular potassium concentration is the primary determinant of the resting membrane potential (E_m). Alterations in the E_m disrupt the normal function of neural, cardiac, and muscular tissues. Normal serum potassium ranges from 3.5 to 5.2 mmol/L. The molecular weight of potassium is 39.1, so a daily potassium intake of 80 mmol is roughly equivalent to 3.1 g of potassium.

The normal physiologic handling of potassium can be viewed as a three-step process: ingestion, cellular distribution, and excretion. Irregularities at any of these steps can result in pathologic serum potassium concentrations.

METABOLISM

INTESTINAL ABSORPTION

Normal daily intake is roughly 40 to 80 mmol. Potassium is rapidly and completely absorbed by the small intestine. Net GI absorption (intake minus GI losses) is approximately 90%.[29] Lower GI secretions have high concentrations of potassium, 80 to 90 mmol/L, but due to the limited amount of stool (80 to 120 g/d), daily GI excretion of potassium is only 10 mEq.[30–32] The colonic epithelium is capable of actively excreting potassium, but this is not clinically significant. Patients with chronic renal failure have elevated stool potassium but total potassium excretion is still limited to about 12 mEq/d.[29]

CELL UPTAKE

Following absorption, potassium distributes among the intracellular and extracellular compartments. The intracellular compartment acts as the primary buffer to changes in serum potassium concentration.

The Na-K-ATPase pump, driven by a ubiquitous cell surface enzyme, moves potassium into cells while pumping sodium out of cells. The pump is stimulated by β_2-adrenergic activity, while α-adrenergic activity results in potassium efflux.[33] Insulin also stimulates the activity of this pump and is independent of its hypoglycemic activity.[34]

Extracellular pH can affect the cellular distribution of potassium. Various explanations have been proposed, including a direct effect of pH on the Na-K-ATPase, or a H^+-K^+ exchange to maintain electroneutrality. The effect of pH on potassium distribution varies depending on the nature of the acid-base disturbance. Respiratory acidosis, alkalosis, and organic acidosis all have minimal effect on potassium distribution. Inorganic acidosis can increase serum potassium, while metabolic alkalosis can lower potassium.

RENAL EXCRETION OF POTASSIUM

Renal excretion of potassium can range from 5 to 500 mEq/d.[35,36] Though 500 mmol of potassium is filtered by the glomerulus each day, essentially all of it is resorbed in the proximal tubule and loop of Henle. Any potassium that is ultimately excreted in the urine must be secreted by the distal nephron.[37] Because of this phenomenon, the study of renal potassium handling can focus exclusively on the distal nephron.

The secretion of potassium in the distal tubule is governed by two phenomena: tubular flow and aldosterone activity (Fig. 76-9). Potassium secretion by the principal cells of the collecting duct depends on a favorable electrochemical gradient. Rapid tubular flow provides a continuous supply of potassium-depleted fluid, maintaining a favorable chemical gradient. Additionally, increased tubular flow occurs with high tubular sodium delivery. Resorption of sodium by the principal cells generates a negative charge in the tubular lumen. Some of this negative charge is lost by concurrent resorption of chloride. The luminal electronegativity enhances potassium secretion. Decreased distal chloride delivery, as occurs with metabolic alkalosis, reduces chloride resorption, increasing the tubule electronegativity and enhancing potassium secretion.[38] Aldosterone is a steroid hormone produced in the zona glomerulosa of the adrenal gland. Its principal site of action is the connecting segment and collecting

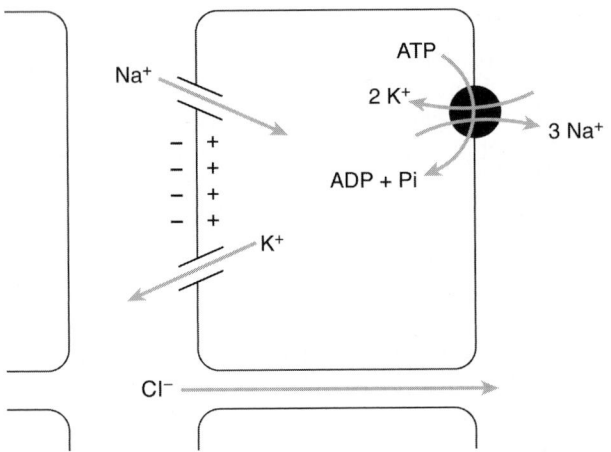

FIGURE 76-9 Potassium handling in the cortical collecting duct. The resorption of sodium creates a negatively charged tubule lumen. This charge helps drive the secretion of potassium. Chloride resorption decreases the negative charge, so increased chloride resorption decreases potassium secretion. ADP, adenosine diphosphate; ATP, adenosine triphosphate; Pi, inorganic phosphate.

tubules of the distal nephron. In the principal cells of the cortical collecting duct (CCD), aldosterone increases the resorption of sodium and hence the secretion of potassium. Aldosterone stimulates the production and activity of Na-K-ATPase, sodium channels, and potassium channels.[39] Aldosterone also has a small but measurable effect on increasing GI potassium excretion.[29] Aldosterone is secreted in response to angiotensin II and elevated serum potassium.

The fact that potassium secretion is dependent on both tubular flow and aldosterone means that renal potassium handling is independent of volume status, despite the fact that both tubular flow and aldosterone are intimately tied to volume status. With volume depletion, increased angiotensin II stimulates the release of aldosterone, which enhances potassium secretion; however, the simultaneous decrease in GFR and increased resorption by the proximal tubule decrease tubular flow, antagonizing potassium secretion. In the opposite case of volume overload, decreased aldosterone suppresses potassium secretion, but increased tubular flow enhances potassium secretion, maintaining potassium balance.

HYPOKALEMIA

Hypokalemia is defined as a serum potassium concentration below 3.5 mmol/L, and is found among 20% of the hospitalized population. However, this high frequency probably does not reflect total body potassium depletion. In a review of 70 hospitalized patients with a potassium less than 2.8 mmol/L, the potassium rose toward normal regardless if they were given potassium or not. The authors suggested that hospitalization for acute illness was associated with increased adrenergic stimulation, resulting in intracellular movement of potassium and transient hypokalemia.[40]

ETIOLOGY
See Table 76-4.

TABLE 76-4 Causes of Hypokalemia

Decreased Potassium Intake	Cellular Shift	Increased Potassium Loss
Anorexia	β-Adrenergic activity	Extrarenal losses
Malnutrition/malabsorption	Endogenous	Chronic diarrhea
Alcoholism	Albuterol	Fistulas and ostomies
Ingestion of grey clay	Dobutamine	Renal losses
	Terbutaline	Loop diuretics
	Fenoterol	Thiazide diuretics
	Insulin	Osmotic diuretics
	Alkalemia	Acetazolamide
	Periodic paralysis	Type I and II renal tubular
	Thyrotoxicosis	acidosis
	Familial	Metabolic alkalosis
	Xanthines	Bicarbonaturia (vomiting)
	Theophylline toxicity	Ketonuria
	Caffeine	Hypomagnesemia
	Barium toxicity	Carbenicillin
	Treatment of anemia	Bartter's and Gitelman's
	(rapid cell proliferation)	syndromes
		Hyperaldosteronism
		Exogenous steroids
		Adrenal adenoma
		Adrenal hyperplasia (Conn's
		syndrome)
		Syndrome of apparent
		mineralocorticoid excess
		Liddle syndrome
		Congenital adrenal hyperplasia
		Renal artery stenosis
		Renin-secreting tumor

Decreased Dietary Intake

Potassium-poor diets usually are merely contributory to hypokalemia. Even among patients with severe malnutrition due to anorexia nervosa and/or bulimia, serum potassium less than 3 mmol/L occurred in less than 2%, and in all of those patients there was enhanced potassium loss from cathartics or vomiting.[41]

Cellular Shifts

Activation of β-adrenergic receptors increases Na-K-ATPase activity. Any physiologic stress that releases epinephrine or norepinephrine can result in a transient decrease in serum potassium. Use of primarily β-adrenergic catecholamines, such as dobutamine, can cause transient hypokalemia.[42] The β-agonists used for bronchodilation or as tocolytic agents can also acutely lower potassium.

Insulin reliably stimulates Na-K-ATPase and lowers serum potassium.[34] Insulin-induced hypokalemia has been documented in the treatment of diabetic ketoacidosis, nonketotic hyperosmolar coma, and with the use of intravenous dextrose solutions.[43] Refeeding syndrome occurs among patients given a carbohydrate-rich diet or parenteral nutrition following periods of starvation. Refeeding syndrome is associated with hypokalemia and hypophosphatemia.[44]

Metabolic alkalosis is associated with the intracellular movement of potassium and increased renal potassium excretion. Increased pH results in movement of hydrogen ions from the intracellular to the extracellular compartment. Potassium shifts into cells to maintain electroneutrality. Simultaneously, increased serum bicarbonate enhances renal potassium excretion. Studies in nephrectomized dogs show a modest but measurable decrease in serum potassium of less than 0.3 mmol/L for each increase in pH of 0.1 (though these data did not account for a significant increase in serum osmolality).[45] The common association of alkalosis and hypokalemia is primarily due to enhanced renal excretion of potassium rather than a transmembrane shift.

Hypokalemic periodic paralysis is an unusual clinical entity in which transcellular shifts in potassium result in paralysis. These patients develop sudden, severe drops in serum potassium associated with skeletal muscle paralysis. Triggers include carbohydrate loads, exercise, and changes in body temperature. Acetazolamide may decrease the frequency and severity of symptoms in some families.[46] Oral potassium can be used to treat acute paralysis but patients often develop rebound hyperkalemia.[47]

Increased Potassium Loss

The cortical collecting duct is the critical site of renal potassium handling. Normally aldosterone activity and sodium delivery to the CCD are balanced so that when one is elevated the other is decreased. Excess renal potassium excretion only occurs when both aldosterone and distal sodium delivery are increased.

Most diuretics increase distal delivery of sodium and increase aldosterone, resulting in hypokalemia. Primary hyperaldosteronism causes hypertension and hypokalemia. The hypokalemia is due to the simultaneous increase in aldosterone activity and sodium delivery to the distal nephron. The increased sodium delivery is due to a spontaneous diuresis in response to the hypertension known as *aldosterone escape*. A full discussion of the causes of increased aldosterone activity is beyond the scope of this text; however, a list of causes is included in Table 76-4.

Normally, the primary anion in the tubular fluid is chloride. Various conditions can result in chloride being replaced by an unresorbable anion. Anions that are not resorbed prevent sodium from being resorbed and increase sodium and tubular fluid delivery to the distal nephron. Additionally, unresorbable anions increase tubule electronegativity, which enhances potassium secretion by the principal cells. The most common example of an unresorbable anion resulting in hypokalemia is bicarbonate. In metabolic alkalosis, increased serum bicarbonate is delivered to the distal nephron, resulting in increased renal potassium loss. Diabetic ketoacidosis increases delivery of the unresorbable anion β-hydroxybutyrate to the distal nephron.

Hypomagnesemia is associated with hypokalemia that is resistant to therapy. Decreased magnesium increases renal potassium losses and needs to be corrected prior to successful treatment of hypokalemia.[48]

Despite a high concentration of potassium in lower GI secretions, 85 to 95 mmol/L, GI potassium losses are typically modest, about 10 mEq/d.[31] Chronic diarrhea can cause hypokalemia, but the mechanism appears to be more complex than simple GI loss of potassium. In cases of experimental diarrhea, daily GI potassium loss was never higher than 24 mEq/d, a level well below average daily potassium intake.[49] In addition, studies on diarrhea show that as stool volume increases, stool potassium concentration falls, ultimately reaching a level similar to that of plasma in cases of severe cholera.[29] Explanations for the commonly seen association of diarrhea and hypokalemia include: secondary hyperaldosteronism, diminished intake of potassium, or transcellular shifts of extracellular potassium.

Gastric secretions have potassium content similar to that of plasma, 5 to 8 mmol/L. Gastric losses result in severe metabolic alkalosis and secondary hyperaldosteronism, both of which enhance *renal* potassium loss.

CLINICAL SEQUELAE

Hypokalemia is a well-known risk factor for cardiac arrhythmia. Increased ectopy with hypokalemia has been documented in ambulatory hypertensive patients, in patients undergoing coronary artery bypass grafting, and during acute myocardial infarction (AMI).[50,51] Following AMI, hypokalemia increases the risk for a number of arrhythmias; patients with hypokalemia are more than twice as likely to develop ventricular fibrillation.[52] Hypokalemia enhances the risk of digitalis toxicity and associated arrhythmias. Digitalis-induced arrhythmias may occur despite normal digitalis levels in the presence of modest hypokalemia.[53]

A drop in extracellular potassium hyperpolarizes the muscle cells, which can prevent myocyte depolarization. Clinically, this can lead to weakness, fatigue, cramping, and myalgia. Severe cases can result in paralysis. Numerous case reports of respiratory muscle weakness and respiratory failure have been reported with hypokalemia due to diabetic ketoacidosis. Severe hypokalemia can cause rhabdomyolysis. Alcoholics may be particularly prone to proximal muscle weakness due to rhabdomyolysis.[54,55]

Hypokalemia can cause polyuria due to increased thirst and by inducing a mild and reversible renal concentrating defect.[56,57] The etiology of the concentrating defect is multifactorial, but primarily represents decreased renal response to ADH.

Gastrointestinal complications are primarily related to decreased gut motility associated with hypokalemia. Serum potassium of less than 3.0 mmol/L is associated with constipation. Paralytic ileus can occur as potassium falls below 2.5 mmol/L.

Hypokalemia stimulates the proximal tubule to increase ammoniagenesis. Patients predisposed to hepatic encephalopathy can develop encephalopathy from this increased ammonia load.[58]

DIAGNOSIS

Hypokalemia is defined as a serum potassium concentration less than 3.5 mmol/L. Once hypokalemia has been established, the primary diagnostic goal is differentiating renal from extrarenal potassium loss. Urine studies are used to separate extrarenal losses, in which the kidneys are potassium avid, from renal losses, in which the kidney inappropriately wastes potassium. Three studies may be used to differentiate these states: spot urine potassium concentration, 24-hour urine potassium, and the transtubular potassium gradient (TTKG).

The spot urine is the simplest test to use. The urine potassium should be less than 20 mmol/L in the face of hypokalemia. If the spot potassium is greater than 40, renal potassium wasting should be suspected. Urine potassium of 20 to 40 mmol/L is considered nondiagnostic.[59] There are two primary problems with this test; the first is it fails to control for changes in the water content of urine. Since hypokalemia is associated with decreased ADH sensitivity, increased water content will lower the urinary potassium concentration. The second problem is that spot samples provide information for only a single moment in time. Patients with diuretic-induced hypokalemia become potassium avid after the diuretic has cleared. One study on the diagnosis of hypokalemia (mean K = 2.0 mmol/L) found spot urine potassium to have a sensitivity of 40% and specificity of 100% for excess renal potassium loss.[60]

The 24-hour urine potassium test avoids both of the above problems at the expense of increased complexity and a 24-hour delay. Patients with hypokalemia should reduce urinary potassium losses to less than 15 mEq/d. Potassium losses greater than that indicate inappropriate renal losses. The 24-hour urine provides no information on the renal potassium handling prior to the urine collection (e.g., diuretic use that is stopped prior to collection will show an appropriately potassium-avid kidney).

The transtubular potassium gradient calculates the ratio of tubular potassium to venous potassium at the end of the CCD. The CCD is responsible for potassium excretion, so increases in the TTKG indicate renal wasting of potassium, while decreases indicate renal potassium conservation (Fig. 76-10 and Equation 76-5). When serum and renal potassium handling are normal, the TTKG runs from 5 to 8.[61,59] In the face of hypokalemia, the CCD should minimize the potassium excretion, resulting in a reduced TTKG. The TTKG has been validated in patients with decreased dietary potassium, periodic paralysis, diuretic-induced hypokalemia, primary hyperaldosteronism and vomiting.[61–62]

$$TTKG = \frac{urine\,K \div \dfrac{urine\,Osm}{plasma\,Osm}}{plasma\,K}$$

Equation 76-5. The transtubular potassium gradient (TTKG). plasma Osm, plasma osmolality; urine Osm, urine osmolality.

CCD, cortical collecting duct; DCT, distal convoluted tubule; TALH, the thick ascending limb of the loop of Henle.

FIGURE 76-10 The transtubular potassium gradient measures the ratio of tubular potassium to interstitial potassium and quantifies the renal excretion of potassium. ADH, antidiuretic hormone;

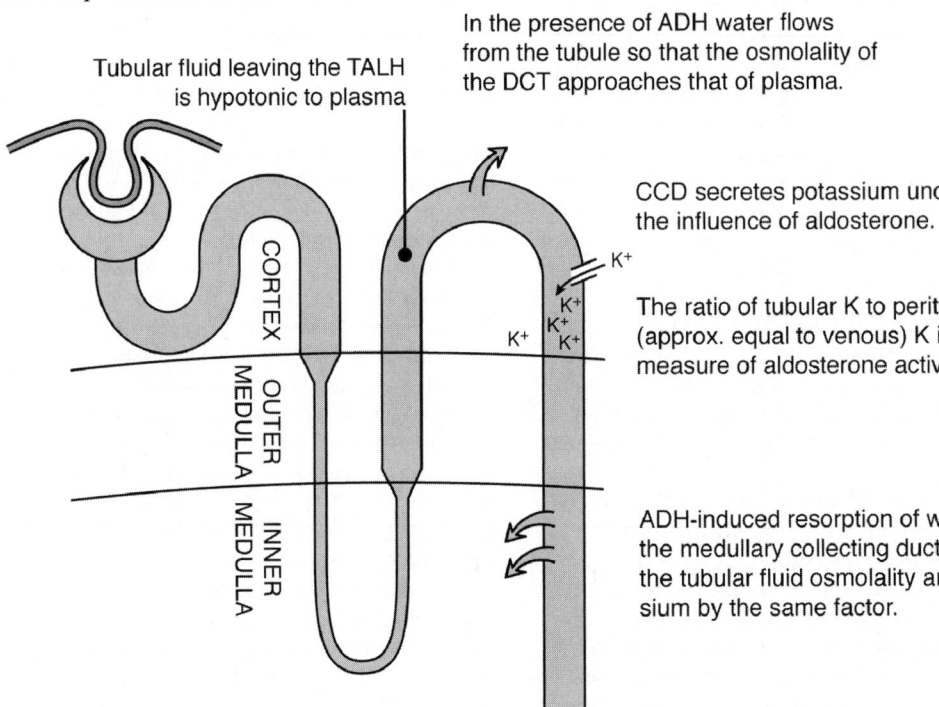

Tubular fluid leaving the TALH is hypotonic to plasma

In the presence of ADH water flows from the tubule so that the osmolality of the DCT approaches that of plasma.

CCD secretes potassium under the influence of aldosterone.

The ratio of tubular K to peritubular (approx. equal to venous) K is a measure of aldosterone activity.

ADH-induced resorption of water in the medullary collecting duct increases the tubular fluid osmolality and potassium by the same factor.

The TTKG has two assumptions that must be met prior to using this formula:[63]

1. There must be ADH activity to ensure that the osmolality of the tubular fluid approximates the osmolality of blood by the end of the cortical collecting duct. ADH activity is assured by only using the formula when urine osmolality exceeds serum osmolality.
2. There must be adequate tubular sodium to allow the cortical collecting duct to secrete potassium. The test should only be done if the urine sodium concentration is greater than 25 mmol/L.

TREATMENT

The treatment of hypokalemia can be broken down into three questions: when to treat, with which potassium salt, and with what quantity. The National Council on Potassium in Clinical Practice has published clinical practice guidelines on potassium replacement. The guidelines recommend correcting potassium in any patient with potassium below 3.0 mmol/L and select patients with serum potassium below 3.5 mmol/L. They specified the more aggressive treatment regimen for patients with hypertension, congestive heart failure, and increased risk for or history of cardiac arrhythmias or stroke.[64]

Determining the dose of potassium to correct hypokalemia is difficult because there is not a firm relationship between serum potassium and total body potassium. Balance studies have shown that potassium is disproportionately lost from the extracellular compartment rather than total body potassium (e.g., a 25% drop in serum potassium is due to less than a 25% drop in total body potassium). Sterns and colleagues analyzed the results of seven balance studies and found a linear relationship for potassium deficit and serum potassium (r = 0.893). The loss of 100 mmol of potassium lowered the serum potassium by 0.27 mmol/L, so a fall from 4 to 3 mmol/L represented a 370-mmol potassium deficit.[65] In Scribner and Burnell's review, they estimated that a drop in potassium from 4 to 3 mmol/L represented a loss of 100 to 200 mmol of potassium, and a drop in serum potassium from 3 to 2 mmol/L represented an additional 200 to 400 mmol deficit.[66] These estimates do not account for altered cellular distribution of potassium. In diabetic ketoacidosis for example, serum potassium overestimates total body potassium, while β-agonist–induced hypokalemia underestimates total body potassium. In most cases of hypokalemia due to cellular redistribution, experts advise against treatment, as the hypokalemia is transient and treatment predisposes the patient to hyperkalemia. One exception to this is symptomatic periodic paralysis in which respiratory arrest due to hypokalemia may occur, so emergent treatment is indicated. Caution should still be used, as rebound hyperkalemia is common.

The form of potassium used in repletion is most often potassium chloride. The chloride anion has some advantages over alternatives such as phosphate, bicarbonate, or citrate. The chloride anion is primarily an extracellular anion, which minimizes the movement of potassium into the cell, maximizing the change in serum potassium. Chloride also does not increase the secretion of potassium at the collecting duct. The use of alternate potassium salts should be reserved for specific clinical scenarios in which there is an indication for the anion (e.g., citrate in metabolic acidosis and phosphate in hypophosphatemia).

In patients who are asymptomatic, oral replacement is sufficient and doses from 40 to 100 mEq of KCl per day are typically sufficient to correct the hypokalemia over several days.[64] Increasing intake of potassium-rich foods is less effective than potassium chloride supplements because the anions associated with dietary potassium are primarily phosphate and citrate.

Potassium chloride can be given as a liquid, powder (often marketed as a salt substitute), or pills with multiple formulations and coatings. The bioavailability of all these formulations is identical, with greater than 70% absorption.[67] The liquid formulation has the fastest absorption and lowest patient compliance of all formulations (due to the bad taste).[68] Wax-matrix extended-release tablets are associated with gastrointestinal tract ulcers and stenotic lesions. The microencapsulated extended-release formulations have the best compliance and low rates of GI side effects.[68,64]

Parenteral potassium should be used to correct symptomatic hypokalemia or when patients are unable to take oral medications. Twenty to forty millimoles of KCl in a liter of isotonic saline or 5% dextrose is a typical solution. Both saline and dextrose solutions can cause problems. Dextrose solutions stimulate insulin release that can result in acute worsening of the hypokalemia.[43,69] The use of saline with dilute concentrations of potassium means that patients must get multiple liters of saline to correct even modest potassium deficits.

The use of concentrated potassium solutions has generated fears about the possibility of precipitating arrhythmias from local, transient hyperkalemia near the infusion site or by causing peripheral vein irritation from caustic potassium solutions. Despite these concerns, the use of concentrated potassium infusions, 200 mmol/L, at a rate of 20 mEq/h in the ICU was shown to be safe and efficacious in both a retrospective study of 495 infusions and a prospective study of 40 patients.[70,71] Twenty milliequivalents of KCl increased the serum potassium by 0.25 mmol/L 1 hour after the infusion finished. The peak rise in serum potassium, 0.48 mmol/L, was at the end of the infusion. ECG monitoring showed no change except for decreased ventricular ectopy. Potassium was infused safely through both peripheral and central sites.

Hypomagnesemia is a common cause of treatment failure. Patients who are resistant to potassium supplementation should have serum magnesium measured, and if low, repleted. Patients with diuretic-induced hypokalemia often benefit from the initiation of a potassium-sparing diuretic. Amiloride has been shown to mitigate magnesium losses associated with loop and thiazide diuretics.

Patients on amphotericin B often become hypokalemic. Both spironolactone (100 mg twice a day) and amiloride (5 mg twice a day) have been shown to increase serum potassium and decrease the use of potassium supplements in randomized prospective trials.[72,73]

In patients with recalcitrant vomiting (i.e., bulimia) and associated hypokalemia, one treatment strategy is to decrease the loss of hydrogen ions with a proton pump inhibitor or H$_2$-blocker. In one case a bulimic patient was started on lansoprazole and the patient's alkalosis and hypokalemia improved. In addition, the patient remained normokalemic for the following year despite continued vomiting.[74] Proton pump inhibitors may have a similar role in ameliorating hypokalemia associated with gastric suction.

TABLE 76-5 Causes of Hyperkalemia

Increased Potassium Intake	Cellular Shift	Decreased Potassium Excretion
Oral	β-Blockers	Decreased tubular flow
Dietary	Lack of insulin	Renal insufficiency
K supplements	Acidemia (inorganic)	Prerenal azotemia
Salt substitutes	Digitalis toxicity	Volume depletion
Ingestion of red clay	Succinylcholine	Congestive heart failure
Enteral feeding	Periodic paralysis	Cirrhosis
supplements	Hyperkalemic	NSAID use
Parenteral	Hypertonicity	Decreased stimulation of aldosterone
Medical error	Hyperglycemia	Type IV RTA (hyporeninism)
TPN	Mannitol	ACE inhibitor use
CVVH replacement	Cell destruction	Angiotensin-receptor blocker
fluid	Ischemia	Decreased synthesis of aldosterone
Peritoneal dialysis	Necrosis	Adrenal insufficiency, primary
fluid	Hemolysis	Ketoconazole
Old blood transfusions	Rhabdomyolysis	Heparin
Treatment of hypokalemia	Tumor lysis syndrome	Congenital adrenal hyperplasia
Penicillin	Chemotherapy	Decreased aldosterone activity
(K formulations)	Radiation therapy	Spironolactone
	Spontaneous	Trimethoprim
		Amiloride
		Triamterene
		Cyclosporine A
		Tacrolimus
		Type I RTA, hyperkalemic variety
		SLE, obstruction, sickle cell
		Decreased GI excretion
		Constipation in ESRD patients

ACE, angiotensin-converting enzyme; CVVH, continuous venovenous filtration; ESRD, endstage renal disease; NSAID, nonsteroidal anti-inflammatory drug; RTA, renal tubular acidosis; SLE, systemic lupus erythematosus; TPN, total parenteral nutrition.

HYPERKALEMIA

ETIOLOGIES

The ability of the kidney to excrete potassium is flexible and adaptable. If dietary ingestion of potassium is increased over a number of days, the kidney increases daily potassium excretion to match. Because of this, dietary loads of potassium do not result in hyperkalemia unless they are sudden, or paired with a defect in renal potassium handling. Likewise, conditions associated with the movement of intracellular potassium to the extracellular space are associated with only transient hyperkalemia because either the kidneys excrete or the cells reuptake the excess potassium. Decreases in the ability of the kidney to excrete potassium increase susceptibility to hyperkalemia from increased potassium intake or transcellular shifts (Table 76-5).

Increased Potassium Intake

Dietary potassium is typically in the range of 40 to 80 mEq/d. Hyperkalemia has been reported to follow the use of potassium chloride salt substitutes, even in the presence of normal renal function.[75] One teaspoon of potassium chloride contains 50 to 65 mEq of potassium. Enteral nutrition supplements may be rich sources of potassium. Ensure Plus at 100 mL/h provides 130 mEq of potassium per day.

Red blood cell transfusions can have extracellular potassium concentrations as high as 70 mmol/L.[76] The risk of hyperkalemia from transfusions rises as the age of the transfusions increases (Table 76-6). Use of "washed" packed red blood cells reduces the risk of transfusion-associated hyperkalemia.[77]

Intracellular Redistribution of Potassium

Increases in plasma osmolality, most often due to hyperglycemia, causes an osmotic movement of water from the intracellular compartment. Potassium moves out of the cell with the water. Using mannitol to increase serum osmolality from 283 to 300 mmol/kg increased potassium from 4.4 to 5.2 mmol/L.[78]

The Na-K-ATPase is critical in preventing intracellular potassium from causing hyperkalemia. Any factor that decreases the activity of this enzyme will cause potassium to leak from cells. A lack of insulin slows the Na-K-ATPase.

TABLE 76-6 Potassium Concentration in Red Blood Cell Transfusions

Age (Days)	Plasma Potassium (mmol/L)[a]	Extracellular Potassium (mmol) per 250 mL of PRBC (Hematocrit 60%)
0	1.6	0.2
7	17	1.7
14	27	2.7
35	44	4.4
42	46	4.6

PRBC, packed red blood cells.
[a] Per Murthy.[255]

In diabetic ketoacidosis hyperkalemia is typical despite total body potassium depletion, and in this setting is largely related to the hyperglycemia.

β-Blockers inhibit the Na-K-ATPase activity and are associated with a mild increase in serum potassium. Uremia reduces Na-K-ATPase activity so that renal failure patients are less able to use the intracellular compartment to buffer potassium loads. Digitalis is a Na-K-ATPase antagonist. Digitalis toxicity can cause severe hyperkalemia. Removing digitalis with binding antibodies allows rapid correction of the hyperkalemia.[79]

Inorganic acids increase serum potassium. Attempts to predict the change in potassium from changes of pH have shown tremendous variability (0.3 to 1.1 mmol/L for a decrease in pH of 0.1) and are considered unreliable.[78] Decreases in pH due to respiratory or organic acidosis have minimal effect on serum potassium.

Cell death results in release of intracellular potassium. Large-scale cell death can cause fatal hyperkalemia. Tissue necrosis and hyperkalemia can be seen with rhabdomyolysis of any etiology. Likewise, tissue ischemia can cause cell death and release large amounts of potassium. Bowel and limb ischemia are occult causes of hyperkalemia. Hemolysis causes hyperkalemia by releasing the intracellular potassium of red blood cells. Tumor destruction with chemotherapy results in release of intracellular contents. Tumor lysis syndrome is hyperphosphatemia, hyperuricemia, hyperkalemia, and hypocalcemia associated with acute renal failure. The prophylactic use of allopurinol has nearly eliminated acute renal failure, which is due to uric acid nephropathy. The syndrome most often occurs with poorly differentiated neoplasms such as Burkitt's lymphoma and acute leukemias, but it has been reported with breast cancer, medulloblastoma, and ovarian and lung cancer. In some rapidly-growing tumors, spontaneous lysis occurs prior to therapy. Hyperkalemia in tumor lysis syndrome is more common in patients with premorbid renal insufficiency.[80]

Succinylcholine is a depolarizing paralytic. It can cause hyperkalemia by two unique mechanisms. The first occurs after muscle damage from burns, trauma, or disuse (often from denervation, prolonged ICU stay, or central nervous system lesion such as stroke or Gullain-Barré syndrome). The muscle damage causes upregulation of the nicotinic acetylcholine receptors so that subsequent exposure to succinylcholine causes massive potassium efflux and hyperkalemia. The second mechanism is a drug-induced rhabdomyolysis. Nearly all of the reported cases of rhabdomyolysis occurred in patients with a preexisting myopathy, often a form of muscular dystrophy (Duchenne's or Becker's).[81]

Renal Dysfunction

Increased intake and cellular redistribution cause transient increases in potassium because the kidneys are so efficient at excreting potassium. Persistent hyperkalemia is almost always associated with a defect in renal potassium clearance. Renal potassium excretion is dependent on adequate tubular flow and adequate aldosterone activity. Besides dramatic decreases in renal function, defects in renal potassium clearance can always be traced back to one of these two problems.

Decreases in GFR from chronic renal insufficiency or prerenal azotemia reduce the flow through the distal tubule and can cause hyperkalemia. Decreases in renal function

not associated with oliguria do not typically cause hyperkalemia. Examples of this include aminoglycoside toxicity (usually associated with hypokalemia) and chronic interstitial nephritis.

Inadequate aldosterone activity can be due to pathology at any point in the aldosterone axis. Inadequate renin production causes hypoaldosteronism and subsequently type IV renal tubular acidosis (RTA). Angiotensin-converting enzyme inhibitors and angiotensin-receptor blockers prevent angiotensin II from stimulating the release of aldosterone. Since serum potassium itself can directly stimulate aldosterone release, most patients can maintain potassium homeostasis despite the loss of angiotensin II. However, patients with other defects in potassium handling (e.g., renal insufficiency or decreased insulin) can become hyperkalemic.[82]

Ketoconazole and heparin cause hyperkalemia by blocking aldosterone synthesis. Spironolactone and eplerenone act as competitive inhibitors of aldosterone. Calcineurin inhibitors cause hyperkalemia in a subset of patients, possibly by inducing tubular insensitivity to aldosterone.[83,84] Potassium-sparing diuretics such as amiloride and triamterene and the antibiotic trimethoprim all block collecting tubule sodium channels, decreasing potassium secretion.[85] Distal RTA usually causes hypokalemia; however, one subtype causes hyperkalemia due to a defect in sodium resorption at the cortical collecting duct. This is different from type IV RTA and does not respond to supplemental mineralocorticoids. This defect has been reported in chronic urinary tract obstruction, lupus, and sickle cell anemia.[86,87]

CLINICAL SEQUELAE

The potassium concentrations inside and outside of the cell are the primary determinants of the cellular resting membrane potential (E_m). Changes in the extracellular concentration can have dramatic effects on the resting membrane potential and the cell's ability to depolarize. As extracellular potassium rises, the normally negative E_m increases toward zero; this allows easier depolarization (i.e., increased excitability). However, this excitability is short-lived as chronic hyperkalemia ultimately inactivates the sodium channels critical to producing an action potential. Hyperkalemia shortens the refractory period following depolarization by facilitating faster potassium uptake.

In the myocardium, inactivated sodium channels slow conduction velocity, and high serum potassium speeds repolarization. On ECG, hyperkalemia causes widened QRS complexes (slowed conduction velocity) and shortened ST intervals with tented T waves (rapid repolarization). The slowed conduction associated with rapid repolarization predisposes the myocardium to ventricular fibrillation.

While animal models and experimental protocols document a stepwise progression of ECG changes from peaked T waves to widened QRS to disappearance of P waves, and ultimately a sinusoidal ECG, clinically patients may develop symptomatic arrhythmias without prior ECG changes.[88] Rapid increases in potassium, hyponatremia, hypocalcemia, and metabolic acidosis all increase the likelihood of arrhythmia.[89–92]

Ascending paralysis mimicking Guillain-Barré syndrome has been documented with a serum potassium of 7 mmol/L. In a review of all published cases of hyperkalemic paralysis (excluding hereditary periodic paralysis) the average

TABLE 76-7 Time Course, Expected Decrement of Potassium, and Side Effects of Each Therapy

Treatment	Dose	Onset	Duration	Magnitude	Side Effects
Calcium[a]	1 g (10 mL) of 10% calcium gluconate or calcium chloride; may repeat	Immediate (documented normalization of ECG as early as 15 s)	30–60 min		Caution/contraindicated in hypercalcemia and digoxin toxicity
Insulin and glucose[a]	10 U of regular insulin and 50 g of glucose; can omit the glucose if the patient is hyperglycemic	Significant reduction at 15 min;[a] peak action at 60 min[d]	>6 h (potassium still decreased by 0.76 mmol/L at 6 h)[e]	1 mmol/L	Hypoglycemia and hyperglycemia; hyperglycemia may increase serum potassium through solute drag
Albuterol IV[f]	0.5% mg in 100 mL of 5% dextrose solution infused over 15 min	Onset and peak action at 30 mins	6 h	1–1.5 mEq/L	Tachycardia, variable changes in BP, tremor; rise in blood glucose and insulin; rise in serum potassium in the first minute after MDI spacer use; rise averaged only 0.15 mmol/L, but 59% had a rise of at least 0.1 mmol/L and two had a rise of >0.4 mmol/L
Albuterol nebulized[g]	10–20 mg in 5 mL of normal saline inhaled over 10–15 min	5–10 min with peak action at 30–120 min	3–6 h		
Albuterol MDI with spacer[h]	1200 μg via MDI	3–5 min with potassium falling at end of study	Only one study and test ended at 60 min; K was still trending down	≥0.4 mmol/L	
Sodium bicarbonate	4-mEq/min drip for a total of 400 mEq; note: lower doses, 50–100 mEq have been shown to be ineffective	240 min;[i] note: the prolonged time for onset of hypokalemic effect	Potassium was still falling at end of 6-h study	0.6 at 4 h 0.74 mmol/L at 6 h	May precipitate tetany by decreasing ionized calcium; may antagonize cardioprotective effect of calcium

Data from these references: [a]Campieri et al,[256] [b]Allon et al,[100] [c]Allon et al,[106] [d]Lens et al,[257] [e]Mahajan et al,[110] [f]Montoliu et al,[103] [g]Montoliu et al,[102] [h]Mandelberg et al,[101] and [i]Blumberg et al.[258]

potassium was 9 mmol/L. The use of potassium-sparing diuretics was the etiology of the hyperkalemia in over half of the cases. Electromyograms showed the paralysis to be due to abnormal nerve depolarization rather than muscle pathology.[93]

DIAGNOSIS

The high intracellular potassium content results in frequent misdiagnosis of hyperkalemia. The most common cause is hemolysis following the blood draw. The lab should report this, as it is easy to detect. Increased platelets or white cells can also release potassium, especially if the specimen is allowed to clot. Thrombocytosis greater than 1,000,000 platelets or leukocytosis over 100,000 increase the likelihood of pseudohyperkalemia. Rarely, counts as low as 600,000 platelets or 70,000 leukocytes have been reported to cause the same phenomenon.[94] The other major cause of pseudohyperkalemia is fist pumping prior to phlebotomy. Forearm exercise in the presence of a tourniquet can falsely elevate potassium by 1.4 mmol/L.[95]

In the diagnosis of hyperkalemia, urine chemistries have a limited role since they are primarily useful for differentiating decreased renal excretion from increased potassium loads. Increased potassium loads, whether endogenous or exogenous, rarely are an occult cause of persistent hyperkalemia, and so the urinary chemistries nearly always point to inappropriate renal handling of potassium.

TREATMENT

The decision of when and how to treat hyperkalemia should be based on physical signs, the clinical situation, and serum potassium. Individual tolerances of hyperkalemia can vary dramatically and are influenced by pH, calcium concentration, rate of potassium rise, and underlying heart disease. Patients with rapid increases in serum potassium or hypocalcemia may have arrhythmias at serum potassium levels as low as 7 mmol/L, while newborns regularly tolerate potassium concentrations of that level. Patients with muscle weakness or ECG changes consistent with hyperkalemia should be urgently treated. Modestly elevated potassium in the absence of ECG or muscle weakness can be treated more conservatively (Table 76-7).

First-line therapy for hyperkalemia should be stopping any and all potassium sources. Total parenteral nutrition, potassium supplements, transfusions, and medications containing potassium should be stopped. Patients already on peritoneal dialysis with potassium added to the peritoneal fluid should be switched to potassium-free fluid. Patients on continuous renal replacement therapies need to have the replacement fluid potassium verified and removed.

Calcium

Calcium reverses the ECG changes seen in hyperkalemia and decreases the risk of arrhythmia. Both calcium chloride and calcium gluconate can be used, but the chloride formulation has three times the elemental calcium (0.225 mmol/mL vs. 0.68 mmol/mL of a 10% solution). Since the cardioprotective effect of calcium has been shown to be dose dependent it is presumed that the chloride salt is more effective than the gluconate.[96] The downside of calcium chloride is that it is more irritating to veins. Both compounds cause tissue necrosis if extravasated. The onset of action is immediate and duration is approximately 1 hour. If, following a dose of IV calcium, hyperkalemic ECG changes persist, the calcium should be repeated. In animal studies, calcium channel blockers ablate the cardioprotective effect of calcium.[96,97]

Calcium may be contraindicated in hyperkalemia due to digitalis toxicity.[98] Digitalis toxicity is associated with intracellular hypercalcemia. Theoretically, additional calcium can worsen the toxicity and precipitate arrhythmias. Clinical data to support this are scant. Bower and Mengle reported two cases of cardiovascular collapse and death following the administration of calcium in digitalized patients, but no information on digitalis levels, serum calcium, or potassium concentrations was provided.[99] Digitalis toxicity with hyperkalemia should be treated with digoxin FAB to rapidly remove the drug (improvement within 2 hours).

Transcellular Redistribution

The fastest method to reduce serum potassium is to induce a transcellular shift. IV insulin with glucose (to prevent hypoglycemia) will reduce potassium within 15 minutes and the lower serum levels persist for up to 6 hours.[100] This treatment can be repeated. The primary side effect is hypoglycemia.

Albuterol has been used to stimulate β_2 receptors and produce a transcellular shift of potassium. Albuterol has been shown to be effective when given IV, by nebulizer, or by metered dose inhaler with spacer.[101–103] One concern is the β-selectivity of albuterol. α-Agonists increase serum potassium. Two studies that looked at potassium immediately after administration of albuterol showed a brief increase in serum potassium.[101,104] A short-lived predominance of α activity immediately following administration of albuterol may account for the increase in serum potassium.

Combining therapies is additive but not synergistic. Combining albuterol and insulin/glucose is particularly appealing, as albuterol decreases the incidence of hypoglycemia.[105] In a well controlled trial the use of insulin and glucose with albuterol was twice as efficacious than either drug alone (1.2 mmol/L at 1 hour vs. 0.6 mmol/L).[106]

Bicarbonate has long been listed as a way to induce an intracellular potassium shift, based primarily on case reports and small trials.[107,108] Recent data have shown bicarbonate to be an ineffective agent for the treatment of hyperkalemia. Blumberg and associates found an increase in potassium of 0.2 mmol/L following bicarbonate infusions, regardless whether isotonic or hypertonic bicarbonate was used.[109] Sodium bicarbonate also was ineffective in patients with low serum bicarbonate. Additionally, increased pH lowers ionized calcium, increasing the risk of arrhythmia with hyperkalemia.

Other strategies to induce a transcellular shift include epinephrine infusions and aminophylline; however, both of these therapies are less effective than insulin and glucose.[109,110]

In patients with cardiac arrest, the ability to induce a transcellular shift is reduced.[111] This may be due to decreased blood flow to skeletal muscle and the liver, which are the primary tissues involved in cellular redistribution.[112]

Enhanced GI Clearance of Potassium

In addition to inducing a transcellular shift of potassium, patients with increases in total body potassium must get specific therapy to remove potassium from the body. Cation exchange resins can enhance intestinal potassium excretion. Sodium polystyrene (SPS) resins bind approximately 1 mEq of potassium per gram of resin. SPS maximally absorbs potassium when given orally, but enemas are effective.[113] When given at doses of 20 to 40 g, SPS resins can be effective at treating acute hyperkalemia after calcium and intracellular shift treatments have been initiated. Two recent studies have questioned the effectiveness of SPS resins, but until larger studies corroborate these findings, SPS resins remain part of the therapy for acute hyperkalemia.[114,98] SPS and sorbitol usage have rarely been associated with intestinal necrosis.[115–117]

Enhanced Renal Clearance of Potassium

In patients with decreased renal excretion of potassium, but adequate GFR, the kidneys may be used to increase potassium excretion. The best way to increase renal potassium excretion is to increase distal delivery of sodium and increase tubular flow by increasing sodium intake and using loop diuretics. Potassium-sparing diuretics should be stopped.

Dialysis

In cases of severe hyperkalemia hemodialysis is the best method to remove potassium from the body. In a study comparing various therapeutic regimens for hyperkalemia, Blumberg and colleagues found hemodialysis to be faster than insulin and glucose, with 1-hour reductions of serum potassium of 1.34 mmol/L.[109] Higher serum potassium concentrations enhance dialytic clearance of potassium. A 4-hour dialysis session with a potassium bath of 1 mmol/L can be expected to remove between 60 and 140 mmol of potassium.[118] Following dialysis the serum concentration rises significantly. Therapies that shift potassium into cells decrease the effectiveness of dialysis and increase the post-rebound serum potassium.[118] There is concern that dialyzing patients prone to cardiac arrhythmias against a low potassium dialysate may precipitate arrhythmias. In a randomized controlled trial, potassium modeling (stepwise lowering of the potassium bath during treatment) reduced premature ventricular contractions (PVCs) and PVC couplets during dialysis.[119] The use of intermittent dialysis has been successful in the face of cardiac arrest. In one case of ventricular fibrillation due to hyperkalemia, CPR provided adequate blood pressure to dialyze the patient. Cardiac function was restored after 25 minutes of dialysis.[120]

Continuous renal replacement therapy (CRRT) is also effective at reducing potassium and is better tolerated than intermittent hemodialysis in unstable patients. CRRT has been used to successfully treat hyperkalemic asystole.[121]

Other Issues in the Treatment of Hypokalemia

An important factor to consider when adopting a treatment strategy for hyperkalemia is whether the source of potassium is transient (e.g., potassium overdose) or continuous (e.g., limb or gut ischemia). In the latter situation the use of intermittent hemodialysis will provide temporary correction followed by recurrent hyperkalemia. CRRT offers a unique advantage in this situation as it prevents rebound hyperkalemia. In cases of severe hyperkalemia from a continuous potassium leak, one should consider mixed modalities: initiating intermittent hemodialysis to rapidly correct the hyperkalemia, followed by CRRT to prevent rebound hyperkalemia.

There are multiple cases in the literature of patients with remarkable neurologic recovery despite prolonged resuscitative efforts.[111,122,123] Patients with hyperkalemic cardiac arrest may have better outcomes than generally associated with

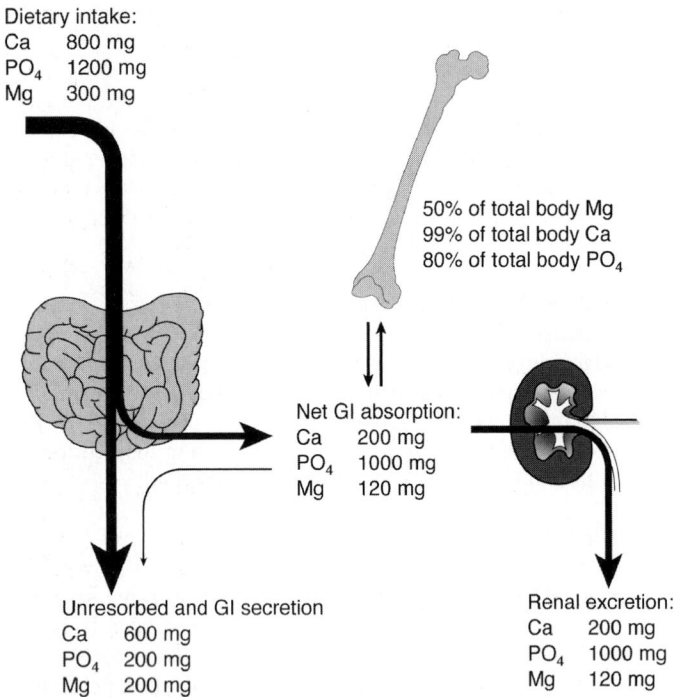

Dietary intake:
Ca   800 mg
PO₄ 1200 mg
Mg   300 mg

50% of total body Mg
99% of total body Ca
80% of total body PO₄

Net GI absorption:
Ca   200 mg
PO₄ 1000 mg
Mg   120 mg

Unresorbed and GI secretion
Ca   600 mg
PO₄ 200 mg
Mg   200 mg

Renal excretion:
Ca   200 mg
PO₄ 1000 mg
Mg   120 mg

FIGURE 76-11 Calcium, phosphorus, and magnesium have unique patterns of dietary intake, absorption, and degrees of mineralization and renal excretion. Values are typical for adult males on an American diet.

cardiac arrest and deserve aggressive and prolonged resuscitative efforts.

Calcium

Calcium is a divalent cation that regulates cellular movement, hormone release, enzyme activity, and coagulation. Calcium also plays a role in cell injury and death.[124] Ninety-nine percent of total body calcium is located in the bones and teeth. Normally, cytosolic calcium is very low, with a ratio of extracellular to intracellular ionized calcium of 10,000:1.[125]

METABOLISM
MEASURING CALCIUM
Normal serum calcium is 8.8 to 10.3 mg/dL. The molecular weight of calcium is 40; in SI units the normal range is 2.2 to 2.6 mmol/L (4.4 to 5.2 mEq/L). Forty percent of serum calcium is protein bound, primarily to albumin. An additional 10% to 15% is complexed to serum anions, such as bicarbonate, phosphate, and citrate. The remaining 45% is the physiologically active, *ionized* fraction.[126] Normal ionized calcium is 4.0 to 5.2 mg/dL (1.0 to 1.3 mmol/L). Decreases in albumin lower total serum calcium without affecting ionized calcium. Likewise, increases in albumin or globulins cause meaningless increases in total calcium, while the calcium regulatory mechanism maintains a normal ionized calcium.[127,128] Increases in pH enhance calcium binding to albumin, lowering ionized calcium; decreases in pH have the opposite effect. Free fatty acids, either from lipid infusions or endogenous lipolysis, increase calcium binding by albumin, lowering ionized calcium.[129] Despite widespread use of formulas to adjust total calcium for albumin and pH, these have been shown to be poor predictors of ionized calcium. In patients in whom total calcium is borderline or there is suspicion of disordered

protein-calcium binding, an ionized calcium level should be measured.[130,131]

CALCIUM REGULATION
Regulation of calcium balance begins with control of dietary absorption. Net calcium absorption is 100 to 200 mg per day (Fig. 76-11). Normally, people are in calcium balance and absorbed calcium is excreted in the urine. Parathyroid hormone (PTH), calcitriol, calcitonin, estrogen, and testosterone regulate calcium balance. The effects of estrogen and testosterone are complex, poorly understood, and will not be discussed here.

PTH is a peptide hormone released from the parathyroid glands in response to ionized hypocalcemia (Fig. 76-12). Elevated calcium, magnesium, and calcitriol all suppress PTH release. PTH minimizes urinary calcium excretion, stimulates the conversion of 25-hydroxyvitamin D to 1,25-dihydroxyvitamin D (calcitriol) by the kidney, and in conjunction with calcitriol, mobilizes calcium from bone.

Vitamin D is ingested or synthesized in the skin. In order for vitamin D to become metabolically active it must be hydroxylated, first in the liver, and then in the kidney, to form calcitriol. Calcitriol increases dietary absorption of both calcium and phosphorus and is active in bone metabolism. Calcitriol inhibits PTH release.

Calcitonin is a 32-amino acid peptide that decreases serum calcium.

RENAL HANDLING OF CALCIUM
Both ionized and complexed calcium, representing 55% to 60% of total calcium, are freely filtered at the glomerulus. Nearly all of this filtered calcium (98%) is resorbed by the tubules (Fig. 76-13). In the proximal tubule, calcium is resorbed with sodium. Increased proximal sodium resorption, as occurs with volume depletion, increases calcium resorption. Typically two-thirds of filtered calcium is resorbed by the proximal tubules. Calcium resorption in the TALH is

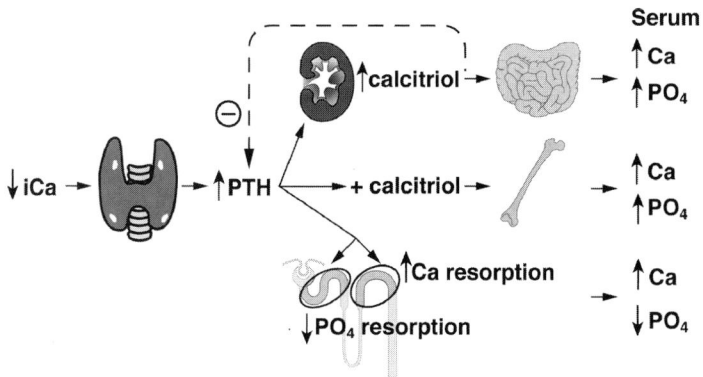

FIGURE 76-12 Decreased ionized calcium stimulates parathyroid hormone release from the parathyroid gland. PTH acts on three targets: it stimulates 1-α-hydroxylase to increase calcitriol synthesis, which increases GI calcium and PO$_4$ (phosphate) absorption (calcitriol also inhibits PTH secretion); in concert with calcitriol PTH stimulates bone resorption, releasing calcium and PO$_4$; PTH increases tubular resorption of calcium and decreases tubular resorption of phosphorus, increasing serum calcium and lowering serum phosphorus.

primarily passive, down an electrical gradient created by the Na-K-2Cl carrier and the renal outer medulla potassium (ROMK) channel (Fig. 76-14). The distal convoluted tubule (DCT) is the only area where calcium can be resorbed independent of sodium. PTH increases permeability of the paracellular tight junctions to calcium. PTH and calcitriol both stimulate calcium resorption in the DCT.

HYPOCALCEMIA

Hypocalcemia is common among ICU patients, with prevalence reported to be 20% to 88%.[131-133] Hypocalcemia is more frequent with increased severity of illness and is associated with increased mortality.[132,133]

ETIOLOGIES
Broadly speaking, hypocalcemia occurs when calcium moves out of the vascular space faster than it can be repleted by diet or the mobilization of skeletal calcium. Calcium enters the vascular space via diet or bone resorption. Calcium leaves the vascular space via renal excretion or deposition in bones and soft tissue. In addition, increased pH or chelation by an-

ions can acutely drop the ionized calcium. The etiologies of hypocalcemia are summarized in Table 76-8.

Calcium Deposition
Deposition of calcium in tissues can occur with sudden increases in phosphorus.[134] Tumor lysis syndrome releases a large amount of intracellular phosphorus that binds ionized calcium. Phosphorus overdoses from enemas (especially if mistakenly taken orally) cause hypocalcemia due to the hyperphosphatemia.[134-136] Pancreatitis results in increased serum lipase, resulting in increased free fatty acids that chelate ionized calcium. In addition, pancreatitis is associated with increased calcitonin and decreased PTH, both of which contribute to hypocalcemia.

The citrate used to preserve blood transfusions can bind calcium and causes ionized hypocalcemia. It is normally rapidly metabolized and well tolerated, despite transient decreases in calcium; 10% of patients transiently have ionized calcium levels less than 1 mmol/L.[137] Factors that inhibit citrate metabolism (liver failure, kidney failure, or hypothermia) or rapid or large transfusions predispose patients to

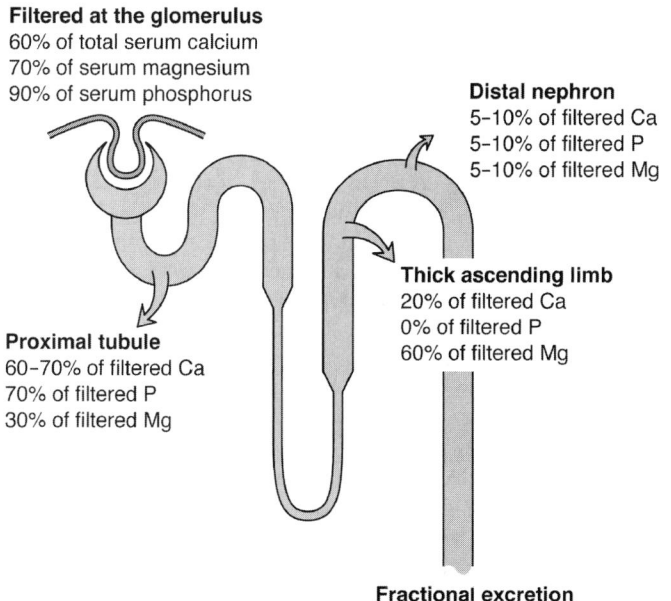

Filtered at the glomerulus
60% of total serum calcium
70% of serum magnesium
90% of serum phosphorus

Distal nephron
5–10% of filtered Ca
5–10% of filtered P
5–10% of filtered Mg

Thick ascending limb
20% of filtered Ca
0% of filtered P
60% of filtered Mg

Proximal tubule
60–70% of filtered Ca
70% of filtered P
30% of filtered Mg

Fractional excretion
Ca   1–2%
P   20%
Mg   2–4%.

FIGURE 76-13 Renal handling of calcium, phosphorus, and magnesium varies in each segment of the nephron.

TABLE 76-8 Etiologies of Hypocalcemia

Decreased Intestinal Absorption	Increased Renal Excretion	Tissue Deposition/ Serum Complexes
Vitamin D deficiency	Hypoparathyroidism	Citrate
25-D deficiency	Congenital	EDTA
Low sunlight exposure	Mutations of the calciumsensing receptor	Radiocontrast agents (gadolinium causes a pseudohypocalcemia)[d]
Liver disease	DiGeorge syndrome	Pancreatitis
Phenytoin	Pseudohypoparathyroidism	Hyperphosphatemia
Phenobarbital	Acquired	Hungry bone syndrome
Malabsorption	Surgical hypoparathyroidism	Osteoblastic metastatic lesions
Nephrotic syndrome	APECED	Breast cancer
Gastrectomy[a]	Hypermagnesemia	Pancreatic cancer
1,25 D deficiency	Hemochromatosis	Other
Renal failure	Granulomatous diseases	Pentamidine
Ketoconazole	Neoplastic infiltration	Asparaginase
Hydroxychloroquine	Amyloidosis	Doxorubicin
5-Fluorouracil	Wilson's disease	Fluoride
Leucovorin	Hyperthyroidism (thyroid crisis)[b]	
	Cimetidine[c]	

Data from these references: [a]Efstathiadou et al,[259] [b]Yamaji et al,[260] [c]Edwards et al,[261] and [d]Lin et al.[262]
APECED, autoimmune polyendocrinopathy-candidiasis-ectodermal dysplasia syndrome; EDTA ethylenediamine tetraacetic acid.

hypocalcemia. Plasmapheresis can use large amounts of citrate, predisposing patients to ionized hypocalcemia.[138]

Hypoparathyroidism

Hypoparathyroidism increases renal calcium excretion and prevents the mobilization of skeletal calcium. The most com-

FIGURE 76-14 The thick ascending limb of the loop of Henle (TALH). Calcium and magnesium are both resorbed through the paracellular space down an electrical gradient. The Na-K-2Cl carrier paired with the apical potassium channel, ROMK, generates the positive potential difference. The Na-K-2Cl carrier itself is not electrogenic because the two cations are balanced by the two chloride anions, but since potassium is recycled through the ROMK channel, the net movement of charge is one anion leaving the tubule, which generates a positive potential difference. Factors that block either the Na-K-2Cl carrier (e.g., furosemide) or the ROMK channel (e.g., hypercalcemia or magnesium depletion) increase renal excretion of calcium and magnesium. ADP, adenosine diphosphate; ATP, adenosine triphosphate; Pi, inorganic phosphate.

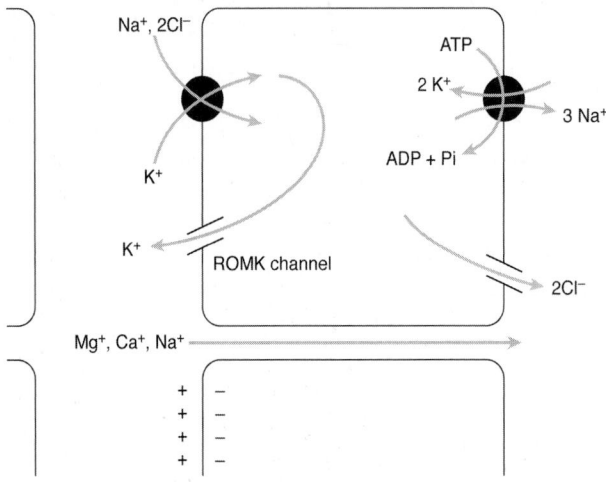

mon cause of acquired hypoparathyroidism is neck surgery. Following thyroidectomy, the parathyroid gland often stops releasing PTH. This hypoparathyroidism may be temporary or permanent. Hypoparathyroidism can follow radiation therapy, as well as autoimmune, infiltrative, and granulomatous diseases. Following parathyroidectomy for primary or tertiary hyperparathyroidism there may be widespread osteoblastic activity, resulting in hypocalcemia, hypomagnesemia, and hypokalemia. This is termed *hungry bone syndrome* and is due to the rapid mineralization of osteoid. The hypocalcemia can last for months.

Disorders of magnesium can decrease PTH activity. Modest hypomagnesemia decreases end-organ responsiveness to PTH, while more severe hypomagnesemia suppresses PTH release.[139] At high concentrations (>5 mg/dL) magnesium binds the calcium-sensing receptor on the parathyroid gland, imitating hypercalcemia, directly suppressing PTH release.

Vitamin D Deficiency

Acute hypocalcemia with vitamin D deficiency occurs because of the inability to mobilize skeletal reserves of calcium. Vitamin D deficiency is common among nursing home patients, alcoholics, and malnourished patients. Increased hepatic metabolism of vitamin D occurs in patients on phenytoin and phenobarbital. The nephrotic syndrome is commonly associated with hypocalcemia, though most of this is due to hypoalbuminemia. Ionized hypocalcemia occurs due to the loss of 25-hydroxyvitamin D and its binding protein in the urine. Decreased activation of 25-hydroxyvitamin D occurs with renal failure and hypoparathyroidism.

Critical Illness

Hypocalcemia is a pervasive disorder in the ICU. While hypocalcemia was thought to be limited to patients with sepsis, Zivin and associates have shown hypocalcemia to be common in all patients with severe illness.[133] However, despite careful assessment, a definitive etiology can be found in less than half of the patients.[132] Some authors believe that ICU-associated hypocalcemia (ICU-H) is an adaptive beneficial response to critical illness, as it may prevent intracellular hypercalcemia and associated tissue damage.[140] While not describing all patients with ICU-H, most patients have elevated levels of PTH and low levels of calcitriol.[141,142] Elevated levels of procalcitonin have also been found in ICU-H, leading some authors to wonder if this supposedly calcium-neutral precursor to calcitonin may exert a hypocalcemic effect.[142]

CLINICAL SEQUELAE

The primary manifestation of hypocalemia is neuromuscular irritability. This can range from perioral numbness and acral paresthesias to severe tetany and seizures. Seizures can occur in the absence of any other neuromuscular irritability. Grand mal, petit mal, and focal seizures have all been reported.

Tetany classically affects the upper extremities followed by the lower extremities. Patients typically demonstrate elbow extension, wrist flexion, and metacarpophalangeal flexion.[135] Tetany can cause laryngospasm or bronchospasm, resulting in respiratory failure. The classic signs of latent tetany are Trousseau's sign (carpal spasm after inflation of a blood pressure cuff on the arm and leaving it in place for 3 minutes) and Chvostek's sign (facial spasm induced by tapping on the facial nerve at the temple). The sensitivity of both is poor and the specificity of Chvostek's is particularly poor (a partial Chvostek's sign is found in 25% of eucalcemic individuals).[143] Tetany may be masked by anticonvulsant therapy.

Acute hypocalcemia can cause heart failure. Even modest hypocalcemia can precipitate heart failure and hypotension in patients with latent cardiac damage. These serious findings can precede tetany.[144] The classic electrocardiogram findings of hypocalcemia are bradycardia, prolonged QT interval, and inversion of the T wave.[138] Heart block and cardiac arrest have also been documented. The electrocardiogram is not a sensitive marker of hypocalcemia and may be normal during life-threatening hypocalcemia.

Hypotension can occur following loss of vascular tone. In one ICU study, decreased ionized calcium correlated with decreased mean arterial pressures. Digitalis acts by increasing intracellular calcium. Hypocalcemia is a cause of digitalis resistance. Patients can sometimes tolerate toxic digitalis levels with concurrent hypocalcemia. Correction of this protective hypocalcemia can precipitate arrhythmias due to digitalis toxicity.

TREATMENT
When to Treat

Unique to calcium among all electrolyte disorders is the theory that hypocalcemia may be an adaptive response to critical illness, and because of this the treatment of ICU-associated hypocalcemia (ICU-H) is controversial.[140] Care must be taken not to extrapolate this controversy to patients in whom the etiology of their hypocalcemia is understood (e.g., acute hypoparathyroidism, tumor lysis syndrome, or acute renal failure). Patients with chronic hypocalcemia and myocardial dysfunction should be given a trial of calcium supplementation. Patients with asymptomatic hypocalcemia secondary to surgical hypoparathyroidism had improved cardiac function with calcium infusions.[145] Calcium should be repleted in cases of seizures, tetany, laryngospasm, and hyperkalemia.[146] Among asymptomatic patients, the risk of significant clinical

symptoms rises as the ionized calcium falls below 3 mg/dL, and treatment is warranted in these patients.[125]

The controversy regarding the treatment of ICU-H is due to in vitro data that show intracellular calcium to be a mediator of cell injury in reperfusion and sepsis models. Abbott and colleagues looked at calcium in relation to reperfusion in isolated rat hearts and found that calcium infusion immediately following reperfusion increased mitochondrial damage and decreased cardiac function.[147] In addition, animal studies have repeatedly shown that administering calcium to hypocalcemic septic rats improves blood pressure but *increases mortality*.[148,149] The increased mortality was not reproduced in septic pigs and more recent research has questioned the appropriateness of the rat as an animal model for human sepsis.[150,151]

In critically ill hypocalcemic patients with life-threatening hypotension that is resistant to other therapies (e.g., pressors, volume resuscitation, and inotropes), a trial of IV calcium may be considered. In a study of 12 hypocalcemic patients with bacterial sepsis, seven were hypotensive despite volume resuscitation and dopamine and norepinephrine infusions. Correcting hypocalcemia restored normal blood pressure in all seven patients. Cardiac output, systemic vascular resistance, and urine output all improved following the calcium.[141] However, no studies have been done to assess whether treating ICU-H affects mortality.

It is important to note that all of the negative data on replacing calcium come from studies of sepsis in animals. The applicability to the human population with ICU-H is unclear. The multifactorial etiology of ICU-H is accepted, and it is likely that benefits of treatment vary with the etiology.

How to Treat

Patients with asymptomatic mild hypocalcemia (ionized calcium >3.2 mg/dL) can be treated with increased dietary calcium (Table 76-9). Increases of 1000 mg per day are appropriate. The 25-hydroxyvitamin D level should be checked and patients placed on vitamin D if low. In patients with renal failure, treating the hyperphosphatemia and decreased calcitriol levels will help correct the hypocalcemia.

Severe or symptomatic hypocalcemia should be treated with an infusion of 100 to 200 mg of elemental calcium. This should be given over 10 to 20 minutes to avoid cardiac toxicity. This initial infusion tends to suppress symptoms longer than it maintains a normal calcium level. In order to prevent rebound hypocalcemia a calcium infusion should be started at 0.5 to 1.5 mg elemental calcium/kg per hour (Table 76-10).

TABLE 76-9 Oral Formulations for Hypocalcemia

Agent	Elemental Calcium	How Supplied
Calcium glubionate	64 mg/g	1.8 g/5 mL
Calcium gluconate	90 mg/g	500–1000 mg tab
Calcium lactate	130 mg/g	325–650 mg tab
Calcium citrate	211 mg/g	950 mg tab
Calcium acetate	253 mg/g	667 mg tab
Calcium carbonate	400 mg/g	650–1500 mg tab
Vitamin D requirements	1 μg = 40 IU	
RDA	10 μg	400 IU
For D deficiency	40–50 μg/d	1600 IU/d

RDA, recommended daily allowance.

TABLE 76-10 Parenteral Calcium Formulations

Agent	Supplied	Elemental Ca per mL	Elemental Ca per Gram	
Calcium gluconate	1 g in 10 mL	9 mg/mL	90 mg	4.5 mEq
Calcium chloride	1 g in 10 mL	27.2 mg/mL	272 mg	13.6 mEq
Calcium gluceptate	1 g in 5 mL	18 mg/mL	90 mg	4.5 mEq

Two forms of parenteral calcium are commonly available: calcium gluconate and calcium chloride. Concerns that calcium gluconate requires hepatic metabolism have not been borne out.[152] In a randomized, double-blind trial of the two calcium salts in critically ill children, the chloride salt resulted in a higher and more consistent rise in ionized calcium levels. All of the patients receiving the chloride salt had an increase in ionized calcium versus 65% of the gluconate group.[153] Calcium chloride is caustic to veins and should be reserved for central access. Calcium gluconate can safely be infused peripherally. Both calcium compounds can cause tissue necrosis if extravasated.

Other Treatment Issues
Treatment of hypocalcemia can precipitate arrhythmias, especially in patients on digitalis. Other complications reported from treating hypocalcemia include bradycardia, pancreatitis, and vasospasm.[154]

When hypocalcemia is due to hyperphosphatemia there is concern that providing calcium could accelerate metastatic soft-tissue calcification. The degree to which this occurs is unclear. In the face of hyperphosphatemia, calcium should be limited to reversing acute toxicity (tetany, laryngospasm, and arrhythmias) and full correction of hypocalcemia should be delayed until the phosphorus is normalized.[134]

Hypomagnesemia can contribute to hypocalcemia so patients should have a magnesium level checked and repleted if low.[139] There have been reports of magnesium-responsive hypocalcemia despite normal serum magnesium levels. This is thought to be due to total body magnesium depletion despite normal serum levels (see section on the diagnosis of hypomagnesemia below for details).

The principal therapy for hypocalcemia due to citrate toxicity is metabolism of the citrate. Citrate metabolism occurs via temperature-dependent enzymes so correcting hypothermia improves hepatic metabolism. Steps to improve hypotension and hepatic blood flow should be taken. Saline loading in order to increase renal clearance may speed recovery. Be aware that saline loading will also increase renal calcium excretion. About 20% of citrate is excreted unmetabolized in the urine.

HYPERCALCEMIA

ETIOLOGIES
Hypercalcemia is a relatively common clinical finding. Hypercalcemia occurs when calcium enters the vascular compartment faster than it can be excreted. There are two mechanisms by which calcium enters the vascular space: calcitriol-mediated gut absorption and bone resorption. Likewise, there are two means by which calcium is removed from the vascular space: deposition in tissue and excretion in urine.

The most common cause of hypercalcemia is primary hyperparathyroidism, while malignancy is a distant second. Among hospitalized patients, however, this ratio is reversed, with cancer accounting for 65% of cases and hyperparathyroidism 25%. One series found milk-alkali syndrome to account for up to 12% of patients hospitalized for hypercalcemia.[155] A summary of the etiologies of hypercalcemia are listed in Table 76-11.

Increased Intake
Increased dietary intake alone rarely causes hypercalcemia because the kidney is able to increase calcium excretion dramatically. Increased intake causes hypercalcemia in patients with renal failure or in patients in whom the kidney is prevented from excreting calcium.

Milk-Alkali Syndrome
The milk-alkali syndrome (MAS) is defined by three concurrent findings: hypercalcemia, metabolic alkalosis, and renal insufficiency, and is due to the ingestion of calcium and alkali.[155] In the modern era, patients are typically women being treated for osteoporosis with calcium carbonate, which supplies both the calcium and the alkali. Historically, MAS was characterized by hyperphosphatemia due to the high phosphorus content of milk. In modern MAS, the calcium is a pharmaceutical product without phosphorus and patients tend to be hypophosphatemic, which stimulates calcitriol production, increasing calcium absorption. The hypercalcemia typically responds to stopping alkali and calcium ingestion. Additionally, saline infusions and loop diuretics are effective treatments.[155]

Endogenous Calcitriol Production
Calcitriol synthesis can be increased by chronic granulomatous disorders (e.g., tuberculosis or sarcoidosis), lymphomas, and acromegaly.[156,157] Macrophages found in granulomas convert 25-hydroxyvitamin D to calcitriol despite low PTH levels. Both Hodgkin's disease and non-Hodgkin's lymphoma can cause hypercalcemia by endogenous production of 1,25-dihydroxyvitamin D.

Increased Bone Resorption
Malignancy is the most common cause of inpatient hypercalcemia. Ten to twenty percent of patients with cancer develop hypercalcemia. The most common associated malignancies are breast cancer, lung cancer, and multiple myeloma. There are three primary mechanisms for increased bone resorption in malignancy:

1. Local osteolysis from bone metastasis
2. Tumor secretion of PTH-related peptide (PTH-rP), often called humoral hypercalcemia
3. Tumor-induced hydroxylation of 25-hydroxyvitamin D to calcitriol

PTH-rP is the most common cause of hypercalcemia of malignancy. PTH-rP is a physiologic protein that is normally

TABLE 76-11 Etiologies of Hypercalcemia

Increased Intestinal Intake	Increased Bone Resorption	Decreased Renal Excretion	Miscellaneous
Increased calcium intake	Hyperparathyroidism	Thiazide diuretics	Pheochromocytoma
Renal failure (often with vitamin D supplementation)	Primary	Familial hypocalcuric hypercalcemia	Adrenal insufficiency
Milk-alkali syndrome	Adenoma	Hyperparathyroidism	Rhabdomyolysis
Hypervitaminosis D	Hyperplasia		Theophylline toxicity
Increased intake of vitamin D or metabolites	Tertiary		Coccidioidomycosis[k]
Calcipotriol (topical treatment for psoriasis is structurally similar to 1,25-dihydroxy-vitamin D)[a]	MEN I		Pseudohypercalcemia due to thrombocytosis[l]
	MEN IIA		Human growth hormone[m]
	Lithium therapy[g]		Recovery of rhabdomyolysis-induced acute renal failure[n]
Chronic granulomatous disorders	Malignancy		
Sarcoidosis	PTH-rP (humoral hypercalcemia)		
Leprosy	Metastasis to the bones		
Tuberculosis	Breast cancer		
Berylliosis	Prostate cancer		
Histoplasmosis	Langerhans cell histiocytosis[h]		
Silicon induced granulomas[b]	Hyperthyroidism		
Disseminated candidiasis	Immobilization		
Wegener's granulomatosis[c]	Paget's disease		
Brucellosis	Estrogen and antiestrogens in metastatic breast cancer		
Talc granulomatosis[d]	Hypervitaminosis A		
Cat-scratch disease[e]	Retinoic acid		
Hodgkin's and non-Hodgkin's lymphoma[f]	PTH-rP in pregnancy and lactation[i]		
Acromegaly	Vitamin A toxicity[j]		

Data from these references: [a] Hardman et al,[263] [b] Kozeny et al,[264] [c] Bosch et al,[265] [d] Woywodt et al,[266] [e] Bosch et al,[267] [f] Seymour et al,[157] [g] Bendz et al,[268] [h] McLean et al,[269] [i] Lepre et al,[270] [j] Fishbane et al,[271] [k] Westphal,[272] [l] Howard et al,[273] [m] Knox et al,[274] and [n] Meneghini et al.[275] MEN, multiple endocrine neoplasia; PTH-rP, parathyroid-hormone–related peptide.

involved in the synthesis and development of cartilage. PTH-rP causes hypercalcemia by binding to PTH receptors. Though similar in structure to PTH, PTH-rP is not measured by PTH assays and requires a specific blood test. Hypercalcemia from PTH-rP is most common in nonmetastatic solid tumors, non-Hodgkin's lymphoma, chronic myeloid leukemia (blast phase), and adult T-cell lymphoma.

Hyperparathyroidism

Primary hyperparathyroidism is the most frequent cause of hypercalcemia. Mild hypercalcemia, hypophosphatemia, and elevated PTH are the hallmarks of this condition. Generally patients have three normal parathyroid glands with one large gland containing a functional adenoma. However, in 15% of cases there will be hyperplasia of all four glands. Parathyroid cancer accounts for less than 1% of primary hyperparathyroidism. Surgery to remove the autonomous gland is the preferred treatment, and in cases of diffuse four-gland enlargement, three and a half glands are removed. Rarely, extreme symptomatic hypercalcemia can occur with hyperparathyroidism. This is called *parathyroid crisis* and is characterized by mental status changes, severe hypercalcemia, and very high PTH levels. Surgical removal of the parathyroid tissue is indicated.

Tertiary hyperparathyroidism occurs in chronic renal failure in which chronic PTH stimuli (decreased serum calcium or decreased calcitriol) result in parathyroid glands that autonomously secrete PTH, resulting in hypercalcemia. These patients typically have four-gland hyperplasia and are resistant to medical management and require surgery.

CLINICAL SEQUELAE

Mild hypercalcemia is associated with relatively mild, nonspecific symptoms. Patients with primary hyperparathyroidism are generally asymptomatic, but may complain of weakness, fatigue, anorexia, depression, vague abdominal pain, and constipation. Gastrointestinal side effects become more severe at higher calcium levels. Hypercalcemia has been associated with increased gastrin secretion and may predispose patients to peptic ulcers. Severe hypercalcemia can cause pancreatitis.

Hypercalcemia can cause multiple forms of renal dysfunction. Long-standing hypercalcemia predisposes patients to nephrolithiasis. It also causes volume depletion by reducing sodium resorption in the TALH and decreasing the renal response to ADH. Hypercalcemia can cause acute renal failure by causing volume depletion or by vasoconstriction, reducing renal blood flow. Long-standing hypercalcemia results in irreversible renal insufficiency.

Mental status changes from mild confusion to psychosis or coma can occur in severe cases of hypercalcemia. It is clinically

TABLE 76-12 Treatment of Hypercalcemia

Drug	Dose	Onset	Effectiveness	Duration	Concerns
Saline and furosemide	Infuse saline at a rate high enough to achieve urine output of 250–300 mL/h	24–48 h	0.5–2.0 mg/dL; frequent treatment failures	3 days	Volume overload, electrolyte abnormalities
Calcitonin	4–8 IU/kg SC or IV bid–qid for 1 to 2 d	4 h	2–3 mg/dL	1–4 d	Tachyphylaxis, nausea, rash, flushing, malaise
Hemodialysis	3 h with low-calcium dialysate (0–1 mmol/L)	Significant decrease in calcium after 1 h	4–6 mg/dL in 3 h	Variable; may be repeated as needed	Cardiovascular instability from rapid decrease in calcium
Plicamycin (mithramycin)	25 μg/kg IV over 4–6 h, repeat qd	12–72 h	1–2 mg/dL per dose	2–14 d	Hepatic, renal, bone marrow toxicity; thrombocytopenia
Pamidronate[a]	Single infusion over 2, 4, or 24 h; 30 mg for Ca <12 mg/dL; 60 mg for Ca 12–13.5 mg/dL 90 mg for Ca >13.5 mg/dL	48 h with normocalcemia at 96 h	30 mg lowered Ca by 2.2 mg/dL; 60 mg lowered Ca by 3.3 mg/dL; 90 mg lowered Ca by 3.9 mg/dL	10–30 d; dosing every 2 weeks increased maintenance of normocalcemia	Limit to 30 mg in patients with renal failure; fever in 20%; hypocalcemia (asymptomatic)
Zolendronate[b]	4 mg given over 5 min; 8 mg for relapse or refractory hypercalcemia	96 h; calcium was not assessed prior to 96 h	50% remission at 4 days; 88% at 7 days	32 d for 4 mg; 43 d for 8 mg	Fever; rare (1–2%) renal insufficiency
Chloroquine[c]	250 mg bid	1–3 days	Able to normalize serum calcium in sarcoidosis	Maintenance chloroquine	Only used in patients with increased 1,25 dihydroxyvitamin D; ineffective in hypercalcemia of malignancy
Corticosteroids	Hydrocortisone 200–400 mg/d for 3–5 d	4–7 d	0.5–3 mg/dL	3–4 d	Hyperglycemia, immunosuppression, electrolyte abnormalities

Data from these references: [a] Nussbaum et al,[164] [b] Major et al,[166] and [c] Adams et al.[276]

important to note that mental status impairment can persist for days following correction of hypercalcemia.[158]

TREATMENT

The best treatment for hypercalcemia is to correct the underlying etiology. In situations in which this is not possible or specific hypocalcemic therapy is needed, the treatment should focus on the three legs of calcium physiology: calcium resorption in the kidney, calcium mobilization by the bones, and calcium absorption by the gut. A summary of therapies can be found in Table 76-12.

Calcium resorption, except in the distal convoluted tubule, is paired with sodium resorption so reducing sodium resorption will increase calcium clearance. The most effective way to do this is to infuse saline. Saline also treats the volume depletion found with hypercalcemia. Following volume repletion, loop diuretics can further reduce calcium resorption. The goal of therapy is a brisk diuresis of 250 to 300 mL/h; however, this may be difficult to achieve and poses significant risk to patients.[159] Care should be taken to monitor the patient's volume status and electrolytes. Saline and diuretics are effective short-term therapies, but significant hypercalcemia typically requires additional therapy.

Corticosteroids decrease calcium absorption at the gut and reduce extrarenal formation of calcitriol.[160] Failure of prednisone (20 to 40 mg/d) to correct the granuloma-associated hypercalcemia within 2 weeks should prompt exploration for an alternative diagnosis.[161] Chloroquine and hydroxychloroquine can block peripheral production of calcitriol and are effective treatment for sarcoid-induced hypercalcemia.[162,163] Ketoconazole has also been used in the treatment of calcitriol-induced hypercalcemia.

There are multiple pharmacologic strategies to block bone resorption. The most effective are bisphosphonates. The bisphosphonates are effective at correcting hypercalcemia of malignancy regardless of the etiology.[164] Pamidronate has achieved widespread use and has been shown to be superior in both efficacy and convenience to etidronate and clodronate.[165] Zolendronate, a newer bisphosphonate, has been shown to be superior to the maximum dose of pamidronate in two randomized controlled trials.[166] However, some have questioned the validity of these data due to the poor performance of pamidronate compared to prior trials.

Salmon calcitonin can rapidly lower serum calcium by inhibiting osteoclastic bone resorption. It also increases renal excretion of calcium. It can be given IV or SC and reduces serum calcium by 1 to 2 mg/dL within hours of administration. Unfortunately, it only works in just over half of patients with hypercalcemia of malignancy, and tachyphylaxis is common after 2 to 3 days.

Dialysis

Dialysis should be considered in patients with severe symptomatic hypercalcemia that is unresponsive to drug therapy. Low-calcium hemodialysis (dialysate calcium of 0 to 0.5 mmol/L) has repeatedly been shown to rapidly correct hypercalcemia. Calcium clearance for hemodialysis ranges from 270 to 680 mg/h. While there is a risk of rebound hypercalcemia, many patients are able to maintain normocalcemia with medical management following a single dialysis session.[167] Continuous renal replacement therapy (CRRT) has been used in cases in which rebound hypercalcemia has been a problem. CRRT can be paired with citrate regional anticoagulation, which chelates free calcium, allowing rapid and durable control of hypercalcemia.[168]

Overview

Treatment of hypercalcemia may utilize multiple modalities. Initially calcium and vitamin D preparations should be stopped. The next action should be to administer saline to restore euvolemia. In cases of endogenous calcitriol excess, steroids are an effective acute treatment and chloroquine/hydroxychloroquine or ketoconazole may be used as long-term therapies. In patients with hyperparathyroidism, surgical treatment is the definitive therapy and seldom is additional therapy required. Using bisphosphonates prior to surgery may result in severe hypocalcemia postoperatively (hungry bone syndrome). In hypercalcemia of malignancy, bisphosphonates are the standard of care, but since onset of action can be delayed up to 48 hours, calcitonin may be used as a bridge. In recalcitrant cases, saline and loop diuretics to create a brisk diuresis may be tried with careful monitoring; however, if patients are severely symptomatic, dialysis should be initiated.

Phosphorus

METABOLISM

In medicine phosphate and phosphorus are often used interchangeably, though using strict nomenclature, phosphorus refers to the element and phosphate to the PO_4^{2-} anion. Inorganic phosphorus exists as a weak acid with three protons that can dissociate: H_3PO_4, $H_2PO_4^-$, HPO_4^{2-}, and PO_4^{3-}. At a pH of 7.4 the ratio of HPO_4^{2-} to $H_2PO_4^-$ is 4:1 and the other forms are essentially nonexistent. Clinical labs report the concentration of elemental inorganic phosphorus which exists almost exclusively as phosphate (e.g., organic phospholipids and phosphorylated proteins, which represent two-thirds of all phosphorus located in the serum, are not measured in the lab assay). The normal range of phosphorus is 3 to 4.5 mg/dL. The molecular weight is 31 so the normal concentration in SI units is 1 to 1.5 mmol/L (1.7 to 2.6 mEq/L). Normal values of phosphorus vary with age (higher levels in younger people). The upper limit of normal in infants is 6.5 mg/dL and adult ranges are not found until late adolescence. The majority (80%) of phosphorus is mineralized in bone with almost all of the remainder in the intracellular

compartment. Only 0.1% of total body phosphorus is in the extracellular compartment.

RENAL HANDLING OF PHOSPHORUS

Ninety percent of serum phosphorus is filtered at the glomerulus and 75% to 99% is subsequently resorbed. Na-P co-transporters in the proximal tubule resorb 70% of the filtered phosphorus. PTH and metabolic acidosis both decrease phosphate resorption by the Na-P transporters, increasing the renal excretion of phosphorus.[169] Since phosphorus is resorbed concomitantly with sodium, any factor that decreases sodium resorption will decrease the tubular resorption of phosphorus (see Fig. 76-13).

Normal phosphorus concentrations are maintained by adjusting intestinal absorption and renal excretion. Hypophosphatemia stimulates production of calcitriol, which increases intestinal phosphorus and calcium absorption. The increased calcium suppresses PTH, and decreased PTH will increase resorption of phosphorus in the proximal tubule[170] (see Fig. 76-12).

HYPOPHOSPHATEMIA

Modest degrees of hypophosphatemia are common and of little consequence. Severe hypophosphatemia, however, is rare. In a retrospective review of 55,000 serum phosphorus measurements, persistent phosphorus levels less than 1.5 mg/dL were found in only 0.2%.[171] However, hypophosphatemia was found in 10% to 30% of patients with COPD exacerbations or those admitted to the ICU.[172,173] Because only a tiny proportion of the total body phosphorus is found in the vascular space, the serum phosphorus is not a reliable indicator of total body phosphorus. Isolated hypophosphatemia without intracellular depletion is of little consequence and is usually a transient phenomenon. Severe symptoms from hypophosphatemia are due to total body phosphorus depletion. The causes of hypophosphatemia are listed in Table 76-13.

ETIOLOGIES

Transcellular redistribution is movement of phosphorus into cells. This is usually transient, and in the face of normal total body phosphorus, harmless. However, in the face of pre-existing phosphorus depletion, this transcellular movement can provoke serious symptoms including death.[174] The most severe cases of hypophosphatemia due to transcellular distribution are found with refeeding syndrome. Starvation decreases total body phosphorus due to decreased dietary intake. Despite the phosphorus depletion, serum phosphorus typically remains normal as phosphorus leaks out of cells. With refeeding, insulin moves phosphorus into cells where it is consumed. Thirty-four percent of ICU patients experienced refeeding-associated hypophosphatemia after being NPO for as little as 48 hours.[175] Alcoholics admitted to the hospital also commonly suffer from refeeding syndrome. Alcoholics are often poorly nourished and have a renal phosphorus leak resulting in total body phosphorus depletion.

One of the most common causes of intracellular phosphorus redistribution is respiratory alkalosis.[171] The drop in the partial pressure of carbon dioxide results in intracellular alkalemia, which stimulates glycolysis, consuming phosphorus.[176] Metabolic alkalosis rarely causes

TABLE 76-13 Etiologies of Hypophosphatemia

Intracellular Shift of Phosphorus	Decreased Phosphorus Absorption	Increased Renal Excretion
Carbohydrate infusion	Dietary insufficiency	Alcoholism
Fructose	Malabsorption	Volume expansion/natriuretic
Glucose	Phosphate binders	states
Glycerol	Calcium	IV Bicarbonate
Lactate	Magnesium	Bicarbonaturia
Calcitonin	Aluminum	Glucosuria
Catecholamines	Sevelamer	Diuretics
Epinephrine	Lanthium	Acetazolamide is the most
Dopamine	Steatorrhea	phosphaturic
Terbutaline[a]	Vitamin D deficiency	Thiazides
Albuterol	Glucocorticoids	Loop diuretics[c]
Insulin[b]		Osmotic diuretics
Respiratory alkalosis	Miscellaneous	High salt diet or saline
Rapid cell proliferation	Hungry bone syndrome	infusion
Treatment of anemia	Burns	Hyperaldosteronism
CML in blast crisis	Acetaminophen overdose	SIADH
AML	Bisphosphonates	Fanconi syndrome
AMML	Gallium nitrate	Multiple myeloma
Refeeding syndrome		Aminoglycosides
Rewarming hypothermia		Heavy metal toxicity
		Chinese herbs
		Congenital
		Ifosfamide
		Cisplatin
		Cystinosis
		Wilson's disease
		Hereditary fructose
		intolerance
		Glucocorticoids
		Hyperparathyroidism
		Hypercalcemia
		Metabolic acidosis
		Paraneoplastic syndrome
		PTH-rP
		Tumor-induced osteomalacia
		Renal transplantation
		Acute malaria (falciparum)
		X-linked hypophosphatemic
		rickets (vitamin D resistant
		rickets)
		Xanthines

AML, acute myelogenous leukemia; AMML, acute myelomonocytic leukemia; CML, chronic myelogenous leukemia; PTH-rP, parathyroid-hormone–related peptide; SIADH, syndrome of inappropriate secretion of antidiuretic hormone.
Data from these references: [a] Brady et al,[178] [b] Winter et al,[191] and [c] Fiaccadori et al.[172]

hypophosphatemia because it typically fails to induce the intracellular alkalemia essential for the phenomenon.

Dietary insufficiency of phosphorus is rare, as phosphorus is ubiquitous in the diet and the body is efficient at reducing renal losses. Decreased dietary absorption can occur due to corticosteroids, either endogenous or therapeutic. Antacids that contain magnesium, calcium, or aluminum bind dietary phosphorus, preventing its absorption. Vitamin D deficiency decreases intestinal absorption of phosphorus and the lack of calcitriol increases PTH release (Fig. 76-15).

Phosphorus is primarily resorbed in the proximal tubules (see Fig. 76-13). PTH enhances phosphorus excretion. Since phosphate is resorbed in conjunction with sodium, any pro-

cess that decreases sodium resorption (volume expansion, osmotic diuretics, or glucosuria) decreases phosphorus resorption. Diuretics that act in the proximal tubules, such as osmotic diuretics and carbonic anhydrase inhibitors, have particularly potent phosphaturic effects because they block the primary site of phosphate resorption. Any process that damages the proximal tubule will increase renal excretion of phosphorus. Fanconi's syndrome is characterized by proximal tubule dysfunction and has marked phosphaturia as one of its components. Alcoholics develop a renal leak of phosphorus, which is reversible following weeks of abstinence.[177]

Hypophosphatemia also occurs during therapy for acute bronchospasm. β_2-Agonists, steroids, and IV fluids all

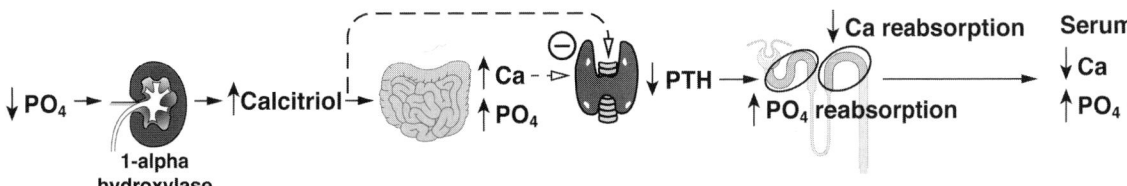

FIGURE 76-15 Decreased phosphorus directly stimulates the production of calcitriol by the kidney. Calcitriol has two principal actions: it increases gut absorption of calcium and phosphate and suppresses PTH release (the increased calcium from gut absorption also suppresses PTH release). The decreased PTH increases renal resorption of phosphorus. Increased serum phosphorus feeds back and inhibits calcitriol production.

increase renal excretion of phosphorus.[178] Since a growing body of evidence indicates that hypophosphatemia weakens muscles and impairs the ability to breathe, monitoring and replacing phosphorus in patients with obstructive pulmonary disease is prudent.[179]

CLINICAL SEQUELAE

Modest hypophosphatemia is devoid of clinical symptoms. Symptomatic hypophosphatemia generally becomes apparent as phosphorus falls below 1.0 mg/dL. Severe hypophosphatemia in the presence of intracellular phosphate depletion can result in significant cellular dysfunction. The oxygen affinity of hemoglobin is regulated by 2,3 diphosphoglycerate (2,3 DPG). Severe hypophosphatemia decreases 2,3 DPG, which increases hemoglobin's affinity for oxygen, decreasing oxygen delivery to tissues. Since phosphate is a substrate for glycolysis, intracellular phosphate depletion can slow glycolysis, decreasing ATP levels. Hypophosphatemia without intracellular phosphate depletion (i.e., transcellular redistribution) is typically benign.[180]

CNS symptoms include weakness, tremors, and paresthesias. Progressive hypophosphatemia can cause delirium, seizures, coma, and death. CNS symptoms are particularly prominent with refeeding syndrome.

Myopathy can occur due to decreased adenosine triphosphate. This can present as proximal muscle weakness, ileus, cardiomyopathy, and respiratory failure.[181] Phosphate repletion has been shown to restore cardiac contractility.[173,182] Patients with decreased total body phosphorus who undergo a superimposed intracellular shift of phosphorus resulting in severe hypophosphatemia can develop rhabdomyolysis. This classically occurs in alcoholics following hospitalization.[183] Since tissue lysis releases phosphorus, the serum phosphorus will normalize following the rhabdomyolysis.

Additionally, arrhythmias and hemolysis can occur with hypophosphatemia.[184,185]

DIAGNOSIS

A few clinical scenarios result in spurious lab results. Mannitol, multiple myeloma, and hyperbilirubinemia (>3 mg/dL) all interfere with some phosphorus assays, resulting in artifactual hypophosphatemia. Patients with very high white blood cell counts can have spurious hypophosphatemia if the specimen is allowed to clot.

Occasionally it is important to separate patients with extrarenal phosphorus losses from those with renal losses. Patients with extrarenal losses and transcellular distribution of phosphorus should have less than 100 mg (3.3 mmol) of phosphorus in a 24-hour collection. Determining the fractional re-

sorption of phosphorus ($FrPO_4$) on a spot urine can give similar information. While $FrPO_4$ normally varies from 75% to 99%, in the face of hypophosphatemia, a $FrPO_4$ less than 95% indicates renal wasting (see Equation 76-6).

$$FrPO_4 = 100 \times \left(1 - \frac{sCr \times uPO_4}{sPO_4 \times uCr} \right)$$

Equation 76-6. The fractional resorption of phosphorus ($FrPO_4$) can be used to determine if hypophosphatemia is due to abnormal renal phosphorus loss or extrarenal phosphorus loss. A $FrPO_4$ less than 95% in the face of hypophosphatemia indicates abnormal renal phosphorus wasting. sCr, serum creatinine; sPO$_4$, serum phosphorus; uCr, urine creatinine; uPO$_4$, urine phosphorus.

TREATMENT

Patients with hypophosphatemia and depletion of phosphorus should be treated. Patients with hypophosphatemia due *solely* to a transcellular shift (e.g., respiratory alkalosis) do not need repletion of phosphorus. One should be particularly aggressive about treating hypophosphatemia in patients with septic shock. Hypophosphatemia is common in sepsis and hypophosphatemia is associated with arrhythmias in this population.[184] Animal data suggest that hypophosphatemia decreases response to vasopressors.[186] Human data have shown increased left ventricular function, systolic blood pressure, and pH following normalization of phosphorus.[173,187]

Enteral Replacement

Oral replacement of phosphorus is appropriate for patients with low serum phosphorus in the absence of acute symptoms. Dietary phosphorus can be used but care should be taken not to give phosphorus with an abundance of carbohydrates, which could precipitate an intracellular shift, worsening the hypophosphatemia. In patients with refeeding syndrome and severe hypophosphatemia, in addition to supplementing phosphorus it is important to decrease the delivery of carbohydrates (use lipids and proteins as the primary source of calories). Skim milk has a safe phosphorus:carbohydrate ratio, along with potassium, calcium, and protein needed in malnourished patients (Table 76-14).

Patients should get 1000 to 4000 mg (30 to 130 mmol) of phosphorus per day divided into three or four doses. This should replace most phosphorus deficits over 7 to 10 days. Dividing the daily dose reduces diarrhea. Since it is impossible to know the exact degree of phosphorus depletion, patients should have periodic laboratory monitoring.

Parenteral Replacement

Patients with signs or symptoms consistent with hypophosphatemia should be given IV phosphorus. Various regimens

TABLE 76-14 Phosphorus Supplements

Phosphate Source	Phosphate	Sodium	Potassium
Oral formulations			
Skim cow's milk	1 mg/mL (0.032 mmol/mL)	28 mEq/L	38 mEq/L
Neutra-Phos	250 mg/pkg (8 mmol)	7.1 mEq/pkg	7.1 mEq/pkg
Fleet Phospho-Soda	150 mg/mL (5 mmol/mL)	4800 mEq/L	
Neutra-Phos K	250 mg/cap (8 mmol)		14.25 mEq/cap
K-Phos	150 mg/cap (5 mmol)		3.65 mEq/cap
K-Phos Neutral	250 mg/tab (8 mmol)	13 mEq/tab	1.1 mEq/tab
Parenteral formulations			
Potassium phosphate	93 mg/mL (3 mmol/mL)		4.4 mEq/mL
Sodium phosphate	93 mg/mL (3 mmol/mL)	4.4 mEq/mL	

recommend giving 2.5 to 5 mg/kg over 6 hours.[188] Larger and faster doses (620 mg in an hour or 25 mg/kg in 30 minutes) have been shown to be safe and effective.[173,187] Continued vigilance is important as hypophosphatemia returns in most patients. After IV therapy, patients should be continued on oral phosphates to replenish intracellular stores.

While therapy is generally safe it is not without complications. In a randomized controlled trial of phosphorus replacement in diabetic ketoacidosis, no benefit from treatment was found in terms of speed of recovery, mental status, oxygen-carrying capacity, or 2,3 DPG levels. The only significant finding was decreased ionized calcium in the phosphorus group.[189] Complications due to therapy for hypophosphatemia include hyperphosphatemia with or without associated hypocalcemia; hyperkalemia from potassium preparations; and volume overload or hypernatremia from sodium phosphorus preparations (4.4 mmol of sodium per mL is nine times the concentration of 3% saline).[190]

HYPERPHOSPHATEMIA

The kidney is responsible for excreting excess phosphorus and is so effective at this that it is able to compensate for huge increases in daily phosphate intake. Essentially the study of hyperphosphatemia can be limited to acute phosphorus loads, generalized renal failure, and specific failure in the kidney's ability to excrete phosphorus.

ETIOLOGIES

Increased Intake of Phosphorus

The ability to maintain phosphorus balance in the face of massive phosphorus loads (4000 mg/d) depends on the phosphorus load being spread over time. Sudden loads can overwhelm renal phosphate clearance, resulting in hyperphosphatemia. Phosphorus loads can be exogenous or endogenous (Table 76-15). Exogenous intake can be from diet, phosphate enemas, or parenteral sources. Fleet enemas contain 130 mg (4.15 mmol) of phosphorus per milliliter. Dietary intake of phosphorus can be enhanced by vitamin D toxicity. Calcitriol enhances gut absorption of phosphorus and the associated hypercalcemia, along with the increased calcitriol, suppresses PTH, decreasing renal phosphorus clearance.

Endogenous sources of phosphate are due to release of intracellular phosphorus from cell death or transcellular distribution. Patients who present with diabetic ketoacidosis are usually hyperphosphatemic despite decreased total body phosphorus.[191] This is due to the lack of insulin decreasing the movement of phosphorus into cells and metabolic acidosis slowing phosphorus consuming glycolysis. Tumor lysis syndrome is due to destruction of large bulky tumors with chemotherapy or radiation therapy. The tumor cells release phosphorus, potassium, and purines (metabolized to uric acid). Acute renal failure from urate nephropathy can exacerbate the electrolyte abnormalities. For more

TABLE 76-15 Etiologies of Hyperphosphatemia

Exogenous Phosphorus Intake	Endogenous Phosphorus Loads	Decreased Renal Clearance of Phosphorus
Fleet enemas	Cell death	Renal failure
Oral phosphorus overdose	Tumor lysis syndrome	Hypoparathyroidism
Parenteral phosphate	Rhabdomyolysis	Acquired
Vitamin D intoxication	Tissue infarction	Postsurgical
White phosphorus burns	Malignant hyperthermia	Hypomagnesemia
	Neuroleptic malignant syndrome	Radiation treatment
	Heat stroke	Hemochromatosis
	Transcellular movement	Congenital
	Metabolic acidosis	Pseudohypoparathyroidism
	Ketoacidosis	Hypoparathyroidism
	Lactic acidosis	DiGeorge syndrome
	Respiratory acidosis	Acromegaly
		Growth hormone therapy
		Tumoral calcinosis
		Bisphosphonates

information see the discussion in hyperkalemia section, above.

Decreased Renal Clearance of Phosphorus
Since the kidney is the primary means of excreting phosphorus, renal failure of any etiology is associated with hyperphosphatemia. The kidney maintains phosphorus balance by filtering serum phosphorus and then adjusting the fractional resorption of phosphorus via PTH. In some cases the kidneys fail to excrete phosphorus despite adequate GFR. The primary cause of this is hypoparathyroidism due to removal of the parathyroids or other neck surgery. In the former, the hypoparathyroidism is permanent, while in the latter it is usually a temporary stunning of the gland. Other causes of hypoparathyroidism are discussed under etiologies of hypocalcemia (see Table 76-8).

CLINICAL SEQUELAE
The primary clinical consequence of hyperphosphatemia is hypocalcemia and its metabolic manifestations. Increased serum phosphorus binds ionized calcium, lowering the biologically active fraction of calcium.[192]

Severe hyperphosphatemia can result in metastatic calcification in soft tissues. In rare cases this may contribute to acute renal failure or cardiac arrhythmias.[193] The risk of calcification increases as the calcium-phosphorus product (calcium times phosphorus) rises above 70 mg^2/dL^2. In patients with end-stage renal disease empiric data have shown decreased mortality in patients with a calcium-phosphorus product less than 52. In the same study isolated hyperphosphatemia also predicted increased mortality.[194]

TREATMENT
Hyperphosphatemia in patients with intact renal function is usually transient and self-correcting. Infusing saline to induce natriuresis can enhance renal clearance of phosphorus. Acetazolamide can increase renal clearance by blocking phosphate resorption in the proximal tubule.[195]

If there is decreased renal function or symptomatic hypocalcemia, dialysis is essential. Twenty to thirty millimoles of phosphorus are removed with a 4-hour dialysis session. Continuous renal replacement strategies have been shown to provide better control of hyperphosphatemia and hypocalcemia.[196]

In tumor lysis syndrome the use of sodium bicarbonate to alkalinize the urine can be detrimental. Alkalinization has been used to increase solubility of uric acid in the urine; however, urinary phosphorus solubility decreases with higher urine pH. The use of sodium bicarbonate predisposes to renal calcium deposition. In addition, raising the pH exacerbates the ionized hypocalcemia found in tumor lysis syndrome. The use of allopurinol and uricase prevent hyperuricemia, eliminating the need for alkalinization.

Phosphate binders are regularly used in patients with chronic renal failure to reduce absorption of dietary phosphorus. Though they primarily act to decrease absorption of dietary phosphorus, they have a small but measurable ability to reduce phosphorus in patients not ingesting additional phosphorus.[197] Patients with acute hyperphosphatemia should have a low-phosphorus diet and be started on phosphorus binders (i.e., magnesium, calcium, or aluminum salts, lanthanum carbonate, or sevelamer).

Magnesium

METABOLISM
Magnesium is the second most prevalent intracellular cation. It is a critical cofactor in any reaction powered by ATP, so deficiency of this ion can have dramatic effects on metabolism. Magnesium also acts as a calcium channel antagonist and plays a key role in the modulation of any activity governed by intracellular calcium (e.g., muscle contraction and insulin release).[198] The atomic weight of magnesium is 24.3. Half of total body magnesium is mineralized in bone. Almost all of the remainder is localized in the intracellular compartment with only 1% of total body magnesium in the extracellular space.[199] Normal plasma magnesium concentration is 1.8 to 2.3 mg/dL (0.75 to 0.95 mmol/L; 1.5 to 1.9 mEq/L). Magnesium exists in three states: ionized (60% of total magnesium), protein bound (30%, mostly albumin), and complexed to serum anions (10%).[200,201] Only the ionized magnesium is physiologically active; however, it is not routinely measured. Patients with low serum albumin may have low serum magnesium levels with normal ionized magnesium levels.[202]

MAGNESIUM BALANCE
Net oral magnesium intake is 100 mg (see Fig. 76-11). The kidneys are responsible for excreting this magnesium load. The bulk of magnesium resorption (60% to 70%) occurs in the thick ascending limb of the loop of Henle (TALH) (see Fig. 76-13). The resorption of magnesium in the TALH is inversely related to flow, so that any situation associated with increased tubular flow reduces magnesium resorption. Similarly, any factor that abolishes the positive luminal charge (e.g., loop diuretics or hypercalcemia) opposes magnesium resorption.

Renal resorption of magnesium varies widely to maintain magnesium homeostasis. Fractional resorption of filtered magnesium can decline to nearly zero in the presence of hypermagnesemia or reduced GFR (i.e., all of the filtered magnesium is excreted). In response to magnesium depletion or decreased intake the fractional resorption of Mg^{2+} can rise to 99.5% in order to minimize urinary losses.

HYPOMAGNESEMIA
Hypomagnesemia is common. Among ICU patients, the prevalence of hypomagnesemia ranges from 11% to 65%.[203–205] When present, hypomagnesemia is usually undetected. In a prospective study, 47% of patients undergoing clinical blood testing for electrolyte concentrations had hypomagnesemia, but physicians ordered magnesium levels in only 10% of these patients.[206]

ETIOLOGIES
Hypomagnesemia is nearly always due to increased renal or GI losses (Table 76-16). GI losses or malabsorption of magnesium occur with steatorrhea, diarrhea, and short bowel syndrome (loss of more than 75 cm of bowel).[207–209]

Renal loss of magnesium occurs most prominently in any situation in which there is increased tubular flow. Intravenous fluids or osmotic diuresis from glucosuria will increase tubular flow and magnesium wasting.[210] Loop, thiazide, and osmotic diuretics, recovery from acute tubular necrosis, and relief of urinary tract obstruction have all been documented to

TABLE 76-16 Etiologies of Hyper- and Hypomagnesemia

Hypomagnesemia	Hypermagnesemia
Extrarenal causes	*Decreased renal excretion of magnesium*
Gastrointestinal	Renal insufficiency
Diarrhea	Any etiology with a glomerular filtration rate <10 mL/min
Steatorrhea	Lithium
Congenital malabsorption	Hypocalciuria, hypercalcemia[f]
Protein calorie malnutrition	*Magnesium ingestion*
Alcoholism	Parenteral
Enteral nutrition	Dosing error
Inflammatory bowel disease[a]	Treatment of pre-eclampsia
Gastric suction	Treatment of torsades de pointes or myocardial infarction
Vomiting	Oral
Short bowel syndrome[b]	Damage to the intestinal lining may increase Mg absorption
Sprue	Mg^{2+}-containing antacids
Intestinal bypass for obesity[c]	Gaviscon [$Al(OH)_3$ and $MgCO_3$]
Chronic pancreatitis[d]	Mylanta ($CaCO_3$ and $MgCO_3$)
Skin	Milk of magnesia [$Mg(OH)_2$]
Burns	Maalox [$Al(OH)_3$ and $Mg(OH)_2$]
Toxic epidermal necrolysis	Epsom salts ($MgSO_4$)
Bone	Mg^{2+}-containing cathartics
Hungry bone syndrome	Magnesium citrate
Other	Milk of magnesia [$Mg(OH)_2$]
Pancreatitis	Magnesium-containing enemas
Renal causes	Magnesium citrate
Drugs	Aspiration
Aminoglycoside toxicity	Dead Sea near drowning
Pentamidine toxicity	*Other*
Amphotericin B toxicity	Theophylline toxicity[g]
Thiazide diuretics	
Calcineurin inhibitors	
Foscarnet	
Cisplatin	
Loop of Henle	
Loop diuretics	
Hypercalcemia	
Increased tubular flow	
Osmotic diuresis	
Diabetes types I and II	
Hyperaldosteronism[e]	
Volume expansion	
Diabetic ketoacidosis	
Tubular dysfunction	
Recovery from acute tubular necrosis	
Recovery from obstruction	
Recovery from transplantation	
Congenital renal magnesium wasting	
Bartter's syndrome (one-third of cases)	
Gittelman's syndrome (universal)	

Data from these references: [a] Galland,[277] [b] Hessov et al,[209] [c] Lipner,[278] [d] Papazachariou et al,[279] [e] Massry et al,[210] [f] Sutton et al,[211] and [g] Eshleman et al.[280]

increase magnesium loss.[211–213] Specific magnesium wasting defects can be induced by tubular toxins. Cisplatin, amphotericin B, and the aminoglycosides all cause magnesium wasting independent of any effect on GFR.[214–216] Gitelman's syndrome is a congenital syndrome characterized by hypokalemia, metabolic alkalosis, and normotension. Unlike the similar condition Bartter's syndrome, Gitelman's is often not diagnosed until early adulthood. Hypomagnesemia is a universal finding in Gitelman's, with magnesium levels typically just over 1 mg/dL.[217]

Hypomagnesemia has been reported to occur in 40% of patients with burns.[218] The decreased magnesium is due primarily to exudative skin losses.[219]

CLINICAL SEQUELAE
Hypomagnesemia is usually asymptomatic. In a retrospective review of 1576 consecutive admissions to a geriatric facility in Scotland, 169 patients with hypomagnesemia (≤1.6) showed no difference in duration of stay, survival to discharge, or 6-month survival.[220] However, a prospective study done in an

TABLE 76-17 Clinical Sequelae of Magnesium Disturbances

MAGNESIUM LEVEL			
mg/dL	mEq/L	mmol/L	Manifestation
<1.2	<1	<0.5	Tetany, seizures, arrhythmias
1.2–1.8	1.0–1.5	0.5–0.75	Neuromuscular irritability, hypocalcemia, hypokalemia
1.8–2.5	1.5–2.1	0.75–1.05	Normal magnesium level
2.5–5.0	2.1–4.2	1.05–2.1	Typically asymptomatic
5.0–7.0	4.2–5.8	2.1–2.9	Lethargy, drowsiness, flushing, nausea and vomiting, diminished deep tendon reflexes
7.0–12	5.8–10	2.9–5	Somnolence, loss of deep tendon reflexes, hypotension, electrocardiographic changes
>12	>10	>5	Complete heart block, cardiac arrest, apnea, paralysis, coma

inpatient setting showed a tremendous impact of hypomagnesemia on survival. Though there was no difference in Acute Physiology, Age, and Chronic Health Evaluation (APACHE) II scores at admission, patients with a serum magnesium level <1.5 mg/dL had a dramatically higher mortality rate than patients with normal magnesium (31% vs. 22%).[221]

Determining the clinical consequences of isolated hypomagnesemia is difficult because patients with hypomagnesemia typically also have hypokalemia, hypocalcemia, and hyponatremia. Symptoms due to hypomagnesemia become more common as serum magnesium falls below 1.2 mg/dL[222] (Table 76-17).

Neuromuscular Effects
Neuromuscular irritability is a common sign of magnesium depletion. Patients can develop Trousseau's and Chvostek's signs despite normal ionized calcium. Severe depletion can cause weakness, fatigue, vertical nystagmus, tetany, and seizures.[223] Reversible blindness due to magnesium deficiency has been reported.[224]

Metabolic Effects
Hypokalemia is commonly associated with hypomagnesemia. One series reported it to occur in 40% of patients with hypomagnesemia. The reverse is also true; 60% of patients with hypokalemia are hypomagnesemic.[206] One explanation for this phenomenon is that many of the etiologies of hypomagnesemia (diuretics, alcoholism, and diarrhea, among others) also result in hypokalemia. In addition, hypomagnesemia causes renal potassium wasting. The mechanism for potassium wasting is multifactorial. Decreased intracellular magnesium slows adenosine triphosphate (ATP) production, which decreases Na-K-ATPase activity, resulting in the loss of intracellular potassium. In the TALH and cortical collecting duct the loss of ATP increases the number of potassium channels on the apical membrane.[48] Intracellular potassium flows down its concentration gradient into the tubule and is lost in the urine.

Hypocalcemia has been reported in 12% to 50% of patients with hypomagnesemia.[220,225] Hypomagnesemia suppresses the release of PTH and causes end-organ resistance to PTH. The hypocalcemia is refractory to calcium supplementation until the magnesium deficit is corrected.[139]

Cardiovascular Effects
Hypomagnesemia has been associated with a variety of atrial and ventricular arrhythmias.[226] Zuccala and associates

prospectively studied 52 elderly patients undergoing hip surgery. He noted an association of higher rates of arrhythmias with greater perioperative drops in magnesium. The arrhythmogenic association of magnesium depletion was independent of changes in serum calcium and potassium.[227] Torsades de pointes is a unique form of ventricular tachycardia that is refractory to cardioversion, but responds to magnesium repletion. ECG findings with hypomagnesemia include flattened T waves, U waves, prolonged QT interval, and widened QRS complexes. All of these ECG effects are also found with hypokalemia, and may be secondary to changes in potassium.

Since both magnesium depletion and digitalis inhibit the Na-K-ATPase pump, it is not surprising that hypomagnesemia aggravates digitalis toxicity. In fact, hypomagnesemia was the most frequent electrolyte abnormality in a study of digitalis toxicity.[228]

DIAGNOSIS
Hypomagnesemia can be divided into extrarenal and renal causes, which can be readily distinguished by determining if the kidney is magnesium-avid or wasting magnesium. There are two ways to determine renal magnesium avidity: 24-hour urine collection and fractional excretion of magnesium. A 24-hour urine magnesium level less than 20 mg is consistent with an intact renal response to hypomagnesemia and implicates decreased intake or extrarenal losses as the cause of hypomagnesemia. A 24-hour urinary magnesium level greater than 24 mg indicates renal magnesium wasting. The fractional excretion of magnesium (FeMg) allows assessment of the renal handling of magnesium on a single urine specimen. A cutoff of 4% correctly separates patients with renal magnesium wasting (FeMg >4%) from patients with decreased magnesium absorption (FeMg <4%)[229] (Equation 76-7).

$$FeMg = 100 \times \frac{sCr \times uMg}{(0.7 \times sMg) \times uCr}$$

Equation 76-7. The fractional resorption of magnesium differentiates between magnesium-avid and magnesium-wasting states. A FeMg greater than 4% in the presence of hypomagnesemia indicates abnormal renal magnesium wasting. sCr, serum creatinine; sMg, serum magnesium; uCr, urine creatinine; uMg, urine magnesium.

Clinical sequelae of altered magnesium content are more dependent on tissue magnesium levels than blood magnesium concentration. One method to infer the tissue magnesium level in patients with normal serum magnesium is a physiologic test that measures the renal response to a magnesium load. An 800 mg infusion of magnesium is given over 8 hours, and a 24-hour urine is collected starting from the initiation of the infusion. Patients who excrete less than 560 mg (70%) are considered magnesium depleted, while those who excrete more than 640 mg (80%) are said to be magnesium replete.[230] This will only work in patients with normal renal function and normal renal magnesium handling.

TREATMENT

Patients with symptomatic hypomagnesemia should be treated with intravenous magnesium. The most common formulation is magnesium sulfate ($MgSO_4 \cdot 7H_2O$). One gram of $MgSO_4$ contains 0.1 gram of elemental magnesium. Acute symptomatic hypomagnesemia (e.g., seizures, tetany, and arrhythmias) should be treated with 2 g IV over 1 to 5 minutes. In order to restore intracellular magnesium stores the acute bolus should be followed by 8 g over 24 hours and 4 to 6 g a day for 3 or 4 days.[226,231,232]

The American College of Cardiology and the American Heart Association (AHA) recommend 1 to 2 g of magnesium sulfate as an IV bolus over 5 minutes for treatment of torsades de pointes. Because early studies demonstrated a benefit of magnesium in acute myocardial infarction (AMI) the AHA currently recommends administration of 2 g of $MgSO_4$ over 15 minutes, followed by 18 g over 24 hours for AMI in the elderly or patients for whom reperfusion therapy is contraindicated. However, the MAGIC trial failed to show any benefit (or harm) from the use of magnesium in AMI; therefore we expect the AHA to rescind any recommendations for using magnesium in AMI.[233]

Magnesium replacement should be done cautiously in patients with renal insufficiency; doses should be reduced by 50% to 75%. Patients should be monitored during infusions for decreased deep tendon reflexes and magnesium levels should be checked at regular intervals.

Oral supplementation with 360 mg of elemental magnesium per day (divided tid) was effective at treating magnesium depletion.[234] Trials at lower doses were not effective.[235] Patients with significant GI magnesium wasting who fail to raise their magnesium on one formulation of Mg^{2+} may respond to another.[236] Diarrhea frequently complicates oral magnesium repletion.

Potassium-sparing diuretics may be helpful in patients with chronic renal magnesium wasting. Amiloride and triamterene have been shown to be helpful in selected patients.[237,238]

HYPERMAGNESEMIA

Normally the kidney excretes only 2% to 4% of the filtered magnesium, but is capable of increasing fractional excretion to nearly 100% in the face of decreased GFR or increased serum magnesium levels.[211] Because of this renal reserve, hypermagnesemia is rarely seen. In a study that looked for magnesium levels greater than 6 mg/dL, only 8 cases were found among nearly 20,000 nonobstetric patients who had magnesium levels checked.[239]

ETIOLOGIES

The most common cause of hypermagnesemia is renal insufficiency. Patients with progressive renal insufficiency maintain magnesium balance by increasing the fractional excretion of magnesium (FeMg). Patients with severe renal insufficiency have a FeMg of nearly 100%, which allows preservation of magnesium balance despite severe decreases in GFR.[240]

Symptomatic hypermagnesemia (despite normal renal function) has been reported with magnesium infusions. The typical setting is the treatment of preterm labor or pre-eclampsia/eclampsia. Standard obstetric protocols (4- to 6-g load followed by 1 to 2 g/h) result in serum magnesium levels of 4 to 8 mg/dL.[241] Patients suffering accidental parenteral magnesium overdoses usually have good outcomes, despite significant short-term morbidity and magnesium levels as high as 24 mg/dL.[242,243]

Hypermagnesemia due to ingestion of magnesium is unusual in the absence of renal insufficiency. In one retrospective study of hypermagnesemia, excluding obstetric admissions all cases were due to oral intake and the average creatinine was 4.8. Oral sources of magnesium include antacids and Epsom salts.[244–246] Chronic oral ingestions of magnesium result in severe symptoms, including death. Hypermagnesemia has been repeatedly reported following the use of magnesium-containing enemas.[247–249]

CLINICAL SEQUELAE

Magnesium can block synaptic transmission of nerve impulses. Hypermagnesemia causes loss of deep tendon reflexes, and may lead to flaccid paralysis and apnea.[239,242,250,251] Neuromuscular toxicity also affects smooth muscle, resulting in ileus and urinary retention.[252] In cases of oral intoxication, the development of ileus can slow intestinal transit times, increasing absorption of magnesium.[244] Hypermagnesemia has also been reported to cause parasympathetic blockade, resulting in fixed and dilated pupils, mimicking brain stem herniation.[242] Other neurologic signs include lethargy, confusion, and coma[242,239,251] (see Table 76-17).

Cardiovascular manifestations of hypermagnesemia initially include bradycardia and hypotension.[239,244,251] Higher magnesium levels cause PR interval prolongation, increased QRS duration, and prolonged QT interval.[239] Extreme cases can result in complete heart block or cardiac arrest. One case of ventricular fibrillation has been reported with a Mg^{2+} level of 9.7 mg/dL.[243]

TREATMENT

The first principle of treatment is prevention. Patients with renal insufficiency should not be given magnesium-containing antacids or cathartics. In cases of hypermagnesemia, stopping the infusion or supply of magnesium will allow patients with intact renal function to recover.

Calcium salts can reverse hypotension and respiratory depression.[253] Patients are typically given 100 to 200 mg of elemental calcium intravenously over 5 to 10 minutes.

In patients with severe renal dysfunction, dialysis offers a way to rapidly clear magnesium. Though both peritoneal and hemodialysis can lower magnesium in an acute situation, hemodialysis is the preferred modality.[239,244,254] Continuous renal replacement therapy is also effective at lowering serum magnesium, but is slower than hemodialysis.[251]

References

1. Dunn FL, Brennan TJ, Nelson AE, Robertson GL: The role of blood osmolality and volume in regulating vasopressin secretion in the rat. *J Clin Invest* 52:3212, 1973.

1a. Palevsky PM, Bhagrath R, Greenberg A: Hypernatremia in hospitalized patients. *Ann Intern Med* 124:197, 1996.

1b. Polderman KH, Schreuder WO, Strack vSRJ, Thijs LG: Hypernatremia in the intensive care unit: An indicator of quality of care? *Crit Care Med* 27:1105, 1999.

1c. Mandal AK, Saklayen MG, Hillman NM, Markert RJ: Predictive factors for high mortality in hypernatremic patients. *Am J Emerg Med* 15:130, 1997.

2. McManus ML, Churchwell KB, Strange K: Regulation of cell volume in health and disease. *N Engl J Med* 333:1260, 1995.

2a. Barsoum NR, Levine BS: Current prescriptions for the correction of hyponatremia and hypernatremia: Are they too simple? *Nephrol Dial Transplant* 17:1176, 2002.

3. Strange K: Regulation of solute and water balance and cell volume in the central nervous system. *J Am Soc Nephrol* 3:12, 1992.

4. Moder KG, Hurley DL: Fatal hypernatremia from exogenous salt intake: Report of a case and review of the literature. *Mayo Clin Proc* 65:1587, 1990.

5. Kahn A, Brachet E, Blum D: Controlled fall in natremia and risk of seizures in hypertonic dehydration. *Intensive Care Med* 5:27, 1979.

5a. Adrogue HJ, Madias NE: Hypernatremia. *N Engl J Med* 342:1493, 2000.

5b. Bruns DE, Ladenson JH, Scott MG: Hyponatremia. *N Engl J Med* 343:886, 2000.

6. Katz MA: Hyperglycemia-induced hyponatremia—calculation of expected serum sodium depression. *N Engl J Med* 289:843, 1973.

7. Hillier TA, Abbott RD, Barrett EJ: Hyponatremia: Evaluating the correction factor for hyperglycemia. *Am J Med* 106:399, 1999.

8. Sonnenblick M, Friedlander Y, Rosin AJ: Diuretic-induced severe hyponatremia. Review and analysis of 129 reported patients. *Chest* 103:601, 1993.

9. Clark BA, Shannon RP, Rosa RM, Epstein FH: Increased susceptibility to thiazide-induced hyponatremia in the elderly. *J Am Soc Nephrol* 5:1106, 1994.

10. Adrogue HJ, Madias NE: Hyponatremia. *N Engl J Med* 342:1581, 2000.

11. Friedman E, Shadel M, Halkin H, Farfel Z: Thiazide-induced hyponatremia. Reproducibility by single dose rechallenge and an analysis of pathogenesis. *Ann Intern Med* 110:24, 1989.

12. Ashraf N, Locksley R, Arieff AI: Thiazide-induced hyponatremia associated with death or neurologic damage in outpatients. *Am J Med* 70:1163, 1981.

13. Miller M: Hyponatremia: age-related risk factors and therapy decisions. *Geriatrics* 53:32, 37, 41 passim, 1998.

14. Maesaka JK, Fishbane S: Regulation of renal urate excretion: A critical review. *Am J Kidney Dis* 32:917, 1998.

15. Arieff AI, Llach F, Massry SG: Neurological manifestations and morbidity of hyponatremia: correlation with brain water and electrolytes. *Medicine (Baltimore)* 55:121, 1976.

16. Hahn RG: Natriuresis and "dilutional" hyponatremia after infusion of glycine 1.5%. *J Clin Anesth* 13:167, 2001.

17. Sunderrajan S, Bauer JH, Vopat RL, et al: Posttransurethral prostatic resection hyponatremic syndrome: case report and review of the literature. *Am J Kidney Dis* 4:80, 1984.

18. Kawai N, Baba A, Suzuki T, Shiraishi H: Roles of arginine vasopressin and atrial natriuretic peptide in polydipsia-hyponatremia of schizophrenic patients. *Psychiatry Res* 101:39, 2001.

19. Wolfson B, Manning RW, Davis LG, et al: Co-localization of corticotropin releasing factor and vasopressin mRNA in neurones after adrenalectomy. *Nature* 315:59, 1985.

20. Kalogeras KT, Nieman LK, Friedman TC, et al: Inferior petrosal sinus sampling in healthy subjects reveals a unilateral corticotropin-releasing hormone-induced arginine vasopressin release associated with ipsilateral adrenocorticotropin secretion. *J Clin Invest* 97:2045, 1996.

20a. Ellis SJ: Severe hyponatraemia: complications and treatment. *QJM* 88:905, 1995.

20b. Gross P, Reimann D, Henschkowski J, Damian M: Treatment of severe hyponatremia: conventional and novel aspects. *J Am Soc Nephrol* 12(Suppl 17):S10, 2001.

20c. Ayus JC, Arieff AI: Chronic hyponatremic encephalopathy in postmenopausal women: association of therapies with morbidity and mortality. *JAMA* 281:2299, 1999.

21. Gross P, Reimann D, Henschkowski J, Damian M: Treatment of severe hyponatremia: conventional and novel aspects. *J Am Soc Nephrol* 12(Suppl 17):S10, 2001.

22. Berl T: Treating hyponatremia: Damned if we do and damned if we don't. *Kidney Int* 37:1006, 1990.

23. Sterns RH: Severe symptomatic hyponatremia: treatment and outcome. A study of 64 cases. *Ann Intern Med* 107:656, 1987.

24. Sterns RH, Cappuccio JD, Silver SM, Cohen EP: Neurologic sequelae after treatment of severe hyponatremia: A multicenter perspective. *J Am Soc Nephrol* 4:1522, 1994.

25. Kamel KS, Bear RA: Treatment of hyponatremia: a quantitative analysis. *Am J Kidney Dis* 21:439, 1993.

26. Rose BD: New approach to disturbances in the plasma sodium concentration. *Am J Med* 81:1033, 1986.

27. Gross P: Treatment of severe hyponatremia. *Kidney Int* 60:2417, 2001.

27a. Ayus JC, Krothapalli RK, Arieff AI: Treatment of symptomatic hyponatremia and its relation to brain damage. A prospective study. *N Engl J Med* 317:1190, 1987.

28. Lampl C, Yazdi K: Central pontine myelinolysis. *Eur Neurol* 47:3, 2002.

29. Agarwal R, Afzalpurkar R, Fordtran JS: Pathophysiology of potassium absorption and secretion by the human intestine. *Gastroenterology* 107:548, 1994.

30. Cummings JH, Bingham SA, Heaton KW, Eastwood MA: Fecal weight, colon cancer risk, and dietary intake of nonstarch polysaccharides (dietary fiber). *Gastroenterology* 103:1783, 1992.

31. Bjork JT, Soergel KH, Wood CM: The composition of "free" stool water. *Gastroenterology* 70:864, 1976.

32. Deitrick JE, Whedon GD, Shorr E: Effects of immobilization upon various metabolic and physiologic functions in normal men. *Am J Med* 4:3, 1948.

33. Williams ME, Gervino EV, Rosa RM, et al: Catecholamine modulation of rapid potassium shifts during exercise. *N Engl J Med* 312:823, 1985.

34. Zierler KL, Rabinowitz D: Effect of very small concentrations of insulin on forearm metabolism. Persistence of its action on potassium and free fatty acids without its effects on glucose. *J Clin Invest* 43:950, 1964.

35. Squires RD, Huth EJ: Experimental potassium depletion in normal human subjects. I. Relation of ionic intakes to the renal conservation of potassium. *J Clin Invest* 38:1134, 1959.

36. Rabelink TJ, Koomans HA, Hené RJ, Dorhout Mees EJ: Early and late adjustment to potassium loading in humans. *Kidney Int* 38:942, 1990.

37. Malnic G, Klose RM, Giebisch G: Micropuncture study of distal tubular potassium and sodium transport in rat nephron. *Am J Physiol* 211:529, 1966.

38. Halperin ML, Kamel KS: Potassium. *Lancet* 352:135, 1998.

39. Sanson S, Muto S, Giebisch G: Na-dependent effects of DOCA on cellular transport properties of CCDs from ADX rabbits. *Am J Physiol* 253:F753, 1987.

40. Morgan DB, Young RM: Acute transient hypokalemia: new interpretation of a common event. *Lancet* 8301:751, 1982.

41. Greenfeld D, Mickley D, Quinlan DM, Roloff P: Hypokalemia in outpatients with eating disorders [see comments]. *Am J Psychiatry* 152:60, 1995.

42. Coma-Canella I: Changes in plasma potassium during the dobutamine stress test. *Int J Cardiol* 33:55, 1991.

43. Kunin AS, Surawicz B, Sims EAH: Decrease in serum potassium concentrations and appearance of cardiac arrhythmias during

infusion of potassium with glucose in potassium-depleted patients. *N Engl J Med* 266:228, 1962.

44. Crook MA, Hally V, Panteli JV: The importance of the refeeding syndrome. *Nutrition* 17:632, 2001.

45. Swan RC, Axelrod DR, Seijs M, Pitts RF: Distribution of sodium bicarbonate infused into nephrectomized dogs. *J Clin Invest* 34:1795, 1975.

46. Johnsen T: Trial of the prophylactic effect of diazoxide in the treatment of familial periodic hypokalemia. *Acta Neurologica Scandinavica* 56:525, 1977.

47. Ko GT, Chow CC, Yeung VT, et al: Thyrotoxic periodic paralysis in a Chinese population. *QJM* 89:463, 1996.

48. Kelepouris E, Kasama R, Agus ZS: Effects of intracellular magnesium on calcium, potassium and chloride channels. *Miner Electrolyte Metab* 19:277, 1993.

49. Hammer HF, Santa Ana CA, Shiller LR, Fordtran JS: Studies of osmotic diarrhea induced in normal subjects by ingestion of polyethylene glycol and lactulose. *J Clin Invest* 84:1056, 1989.

50. Holland OB, Nixon JV, Kuhnert L: Diuretic induced ventricular ectopic activity. *Am J Med* 70:762, 1981.

51. Parks R, Boisvert D, Comunale M, et al: Preoperative serum potassium levels and perioperative outcomes in cardiac surgery patients. *JAMA* 281:2203, 1999.

52. Nordrehaug JE: Malignant arrhythmias in relation to serum potassium values in patients with an acute myocardial infarction. *Acta Med Scand* (Suppl 647):101, 1981.

53. Shapiro W: Correlative studies of serum digitalis levels and the arrhythmias of digitalis intoxication. *Am J Cardiol* 41:852, 1978.

54. Sharief MK, Robinson SF, Swash M: Hypokalaemic myopathy in alcoholism. *Neuromuscular Disord* 7:533, 1997.

55. Finsterer J, Hess B, Jarius C, et al: Malnutrition-induced hypokalemic myopathy in chronic alcoholism. *J Toxicol Clin Toxicol* 36:369, 1998.

56. Berl T, Linas SL, Aisenbrey GA, Anderson RJ: On the mechanism of polyuria in potassium depletion. The role of polydipsia. *J Clin Invest* 60:620, 1977.

57. Rubini M: Water excretion in potassium deficient man. *J Clin Invest* 40:2215, 1961.

58. Gabuzda GJ, Hall PW: Relation of potassium depletion to renal ammonium metabolism and hepatic coma. *Medicine* 45:481, 1966.

59. West ML, Marsden PA, Richardson RM, et al: New clinical approach to evaluate disorders of potassium excretion. *Miner Electrolyte Metab* 12:234, 1986.

60. Lin SH, Lin YF, Halperin ML: Hypokalaemia and paralysis. *QJM* 94:133, 2001.

61. Ethier JH, Kamel KS, Magner PO, et al: The transtubular potassium concentration in patients with hypokalemia and hyperkalemia. *Am J Kidney Dis* 15:309, 1990.

62. Joo KW, Chang SH, Lee JG, et al: Transtubular potassium concentration gradient (TTKG) and urine ammonium in differential diagnosis of hypokalemia. *J Nephrol* 13:120, 2000.

63. West ML, Bendz O, Chen CB, et al: Development of a test to evaluate the transtubular potassium concentration gradient in the cortical collecting duct in vivo. *Miner Electrolyte Metab* 12:226, 1986.

64. Cohn JN, Kowey PR, Whelton PK, Prisant LM: New guidelines for potassium replacement in clinical practice: a contemporary review by the National Council on Potassium in Clinical Practice. *Arch Intern Med* 160:2429, 2000.

65. Sterns RH, Cox M, Feig PU, Singer I: Internal potassium balance and the control of the plasma potassium concentration. *Medicine* 60:339, 1981.

66. Scribner BH, Burnell JH: Interpretation of the serum potassium concentration. *Metabolism* 5:468, 1956.

67. Skoutakis VA, Acchiardo SR, Wojciechowski NJ, et al: The comparative bioavailability of liquid, wax-matrix, and microencapsulated preparations of potassium chloride. *J Clin Pharmacol* 25:619, 1985.

68. Halpern MT, Irwin DE, Brown RE, et al: Patient adherence to prescribed potassium supplement therapy. *Clin Ther* 15:1133, 1993.

69. Agarwal A, Wingo CS: Treatment of hypokalemia [letter; comment] [erratum appears in *N Engl J Med* 340:663, 1999]. *N Engl J Med* 340:154, 1999.

70. Kruse JA, Carlson RW: Rapid correction of hypokalemia using concentrated intravenous potassium chloride infusions. *Arch Intern Med* 150:613, 1990.

71. Kruse JA, Clark VL, Carlson RW, Geheb MA: Concentrated potassium chloride infusions in critically ill patients with hypokalemia. *J Clin Pharmacol* 34:1077, 1994.

72. Ugur UA, Avcu F, Cetin T, et al: Spironolactone: is it a novel drug for the prevention of amphotericin B-related hypokalemia in cancer patients? *Eur J Clin Pharmacol* 57:771, 2002.

73. Smith SR, Galloway MJ, Reilly JT, Davies JM: Amiloride prevents amphotericin B related hypokalemia in neutropenic patients. *J Clin Pathol* 41:494, 1988.

74. Eiro M, Katoh T, Watanabe T: Use of a proton-pump inhibitor for metabolic disturbances associated with anorexia nervosa [see comments]. *N Engl J Med* 346:140, 2002.

75. Schim vdLHJ, Strack vSRJ, Thijs LG: Cardiac arrest due to oral potassium intake. *Intensive Care Med* 15:58, 1988.

76. de SM, Seghatchian MJ: Is depletion of potassium in blood before transfusion essential? *Lancet* 344:136, 1994.

77. Knichwitz G, Zahl M, Van AH, et al: Intraoperative washing of long-stored packed red blood cells by using an autotransfusion device prevents hyperkalemia. *Anesth Analg* 95:324, 2002.

78. Kurtzman NA, Gonzalez J, DeFronzo R, Giebisch G: A patient with hyperkalemia and metabolic acidosis. *Am J Kidney Dis* 15:333, 1990.

79. Carlebach M, Hasdan G, Shimoni T, Korzets Z: Vomiting, hyperkalaemia and cardiac rhythm disturbances. *Nephrol Dial Transplant* 16:169, 2001.

80. Hande KR, Garrow GC: Acute tumor lysis syndrome in patients with high-grade non-Hodgkin's lymphoma. *Am J Med* 94:133, 1993.

81. Gronert GA: Cardiac arrest after succinylcholine: Mortality greater with rhabdomyolysis than receptor upregulation. *Anesthesiology* 94:523, 2001.

82. Brater DC: Effects of nonsteroidal anti-inflammatory drugs on renal function: focus on cyclooxygenase-2-selective inhibition. *Am J Med* 107:65S, 70S, 1999.

83. Kamel KS, Ethier JH, Quaggin S, et al: Studies to determine the basis for hyperkalemia in recipients of a renal transplant who are treated with cyclosporine. *J Am Soc Nephrol* 2:1279, 1992.

84. Oishi M, Yagi T, Urushihara N, et al: A case of hyperkalemic distal renal tubular acidosis secondary to tacrolimus in living donor liver transplantation. *Transplant Proc* 32:2225, 2000.

85. Marinella MA: Trimethoprim-induced hyperkalemia: An analysis of reported cases. *Gerontology* 45:209, 1999.

86. Batlle DC, Arruda JA, Kurtzman NA: Hyperkalemic distal renal tubular acidosis associated with obstructive uropathy. *N Engl J Med* 304:373, 1981.

87. Batlle D, Itsarayoungyuen K, Arruda JA, Kurtzman NA: Hyperkalemic hyperchloremic metabolic acidosis in sickle cell hemoglobinopathies. *Am J Med* 72:188, 1982.

88. Sakemi T, Ikeda Y, Rikitake O: Tonic convulsion associated with sinus arrest due to hyperkalemia in a chronic hemodialysis patient. *Nephron* 73:370, 1996.

89. Roberts KE, Magida MG: Electrocardiographic alterations produced by an increase in plasma pH, bicarbonate and sodium as compared with those produced by an increase in potassium. *Circulation* 1:206, 1953.

90. Braun HA, Van Horne R, Bettinger JC, Bellet S: The influence of hypocalcemia induced by sodium ethylenediamine tetraacetate on the toxicity of potassium. *J Lab Clin Med* 46:544, 1955.

91. Surawicz B, Chlebus H, Mazzoleni A: Hemodynamic and electrocardiographic effects of hyperpotassemia. Differences in response to slow and rapid increases in concentration of plasma K. *Am Heart J* 73:647, 1967.

92. Surawicz B, Lepeschkin E: The electrocardiogram in hyperpotassemia. *Heart Bull* 10:66, 1961.

93. Evers S, Engelien A, Karsch V, Hund M: Secondary hyperkalaemic paralysis. *J Neurol Neurosurg Psychiatry* 64:249, 1998.

94. Howard MR, Ashwell S, Bond LR, Holbrook I: Artefactual serum hyperkalaemia and hypercalcaemia in essential thrombocythaemia. *J Clin Pathol* 53:105, 2000.

95. Don BR, Sebastian A, Cheitlin M, et al: Pseudohyperkalemia caused by fist clenching during phlebotomy. *N Engl J Med* 322:1290, 1990.

96. Bisogno JL, Langley A, Von DMM: Effect of calcium to reverse the electrocardiographic effects of hyperkalemia in the isolated rat heart: a prospective, dose-response study. *Crit Care Med* 22:697, 1994.

97. Nugent M, Tinker JH, Moyer TP: Verapamil worsens rate of development and hemodynamic effects of acute hyperkalemia in halothane-anesthetized dogs: effects of calcium therapy. *Anesthesiology* 60:435, 1984.

98. Emmett M: Non-dialytic treatment of acute hyperkalemia in the dialysis patient. *Semin Dial* 13:279, 2000.

99. Bower JO, Mengle HAK: The additive effect of calcium and digitalis. A warning and a report of two deaths. *JAMA* 106:1151, 1936.

100. Allon M, Shanklin N: Effect of bicarbonate administration on plasma potassium in dialysis patients: interactions with insulin and albuterol. *Am J Kidney Dis* 28:508, 1996.

101. Mandelberg A, Krupnik Z, Houri S, et al: Salbutamol metered-dose inhaler with spacer for hyperkalemia: how fast? How safe? *Chest* 115:617, 1999.

102. Montoliu J, Almirall J, Ponz E, et al: Treatment of hyperkalaemia in renal failure with salbutamol inhalation. *J Intern Med* 228:35, 1990.

103. Montoliu J, Lens XM, Revert L: Potassium-lowering effect of albuterol for hyperkalemia in renal failure. *Arch Intern Med* 147:713, 1987.

104. Du PWJ, Hay L, Kahler CP, et al: The dose-related hyper- and hypokalaemic effects of salbutamol and its arrhythmogenic potential. *Br J Pharmacol* 111:73, 1994.

105. Ngugi NN, McLigeyo SO, Kayima JK: Treatment of hyperkalaemia by altering the transcellular gradient in patients with renal failure: Effect of various therapeutic approaches. *East Afr Med J* 74:503, 1997.

106. Allon M, Copkney C: Albuterol and insulin for treatment of hyperkalemia in hemodialysis patients. *Kidney Int* 38:869, 1990.

107. Schwarz KC, Cohen BD, Lubash GD, Rubin AL: Severe acidosis and hyperpotassemia treated with sodium bicarbonate infusion. *Circulation* 19:215, 1959.

108. Burnell JM, Villamil MF, Uyeno BT, Scribner BH: The effect in humans of extracellular pH change on the relationship between serum potassium concentration and intracellular potassium. *J Clin Invest* 35:935, 1956.

109. Blumberg A, Weidmann P, Shaw S, Gnadinger M: Effects of various therapeutic approaches on plasma potassium and major regulating factors in terminal renal failure. *Am J Med* 85:507, 1988.

110. Mahajan SK, Mangla M, Kishore K: Comparison of aminophylline and insulin-dextrose infusions in acute therapy of hyperkalemia in end-stage renal disease patients. *J Assoc Physicians India* 49:1082, 2001.

111. Jackson MA, Lodwick R, Hutchinson SG: Hyperkalaemic cardiac arrest successfully treated with peritoneal dialysis. *BMJ* 312:1289, 1996.

112. Schummer WJ, Schummer C: Hyperkalemic cardiac arrest: the method chosen depends on the local circumstances. *Crit Care Med* 30:1674, 2002.

113. Evans BM, Hughes Jones NC, Milne MD, Yellowlees H: Ion exchange resins in the treatment of anuria. *Lancet* 265:791, 1953.

114. Gruy-Kapral C, Emmett M, Santa ACA, et al: Effect of single dose resin-cathartic therapy on serum potassium concentration in patients with end-stage renal disease. *J Am Soc Nephrol* 9:1924, 1998.

115. Wootton FT, Rhodes DF, Lee WM, Fitts CT: Colonic necrosis with Kayexalate-sorbitol enemas after renal transplantation [see comments]. *Ann Intern Med* 111:947, 1989.

116. Rashid A, Hamilton SR: Necrosis of the gastrointestinal tract in uremic patients as a result of sodium polystyrene sulfonate (Kayexalate) in sorbitol: an underrecognized condition [see comments]. *Am J Surg Pathol* 21:60, 1997.

117. Gerstman BB, Kirkman R, Platt R: Intestinal necrosis associated with postoperative orally administered sodium polystyrene sulfonate in sorbitol. *Am J Kidney Dis* 20:159, 1992.

118. Ahmed J, Weisberg L: Hyperkalemia in dialysis patients. *Semin Dial* 14:348, 2001.

119. Redaelli B, Locatelli F, Limido D, et al: Effect of a new model of hemodialysis potassium removal on the control of ventricular arrhythmias. *Kidney Int* 50:609, 1996.

120. Lin JL, Huang CC: Successful initiation of hemodialysis during cardiopulmonary resuscitation due to lethal hyperkalemia. *Crit Care Med* 18:342, 1990.

121. Torrecilla C, de la Serna JL: Hyperkalemic cardiac arrest, prolonged heart massage and simultaneous hemodialysis. *Intensive Care Med* 15:325, 1989.

122. Quick G, Bastani B: Prolonged asystolic hyperkalemic cardiac arrest with no neurologic sequelae. *Ann Emerg Med* 24:305, 1994.

123. Lin JL, Huang CC: Successful initiation of hemodialysis during cardiopulmonary resuscitation due to lethal hyperkalemia. *Crit Care Med* 18:342, 1990.

124. Marban E, Koretsune Y, Corretti M, et al: Calcium and its role in myocardial cell injury during ischemia and reperfusion. *Circulation* 80:IV17, 1989.

125. Zaloga GP: Hypocalcemia in critically ill patients. *Crit Care Med* 20:251, 1992.

126. Ladenson JH, Lewis JW, Boyd JC: Failure of total calcium corrected for protein, albumin, and pH to correctly assess free calcium status. *J Clin Endocrinol Metab* 46:986, 1978.

127. Lindgarde F, Zettervall O: Hypercalcemia and normal ionized serum calcium in a case of myelomatosis. *Ann Intern Med* 78:396, 1973.

128. Side L, Fahie-Wilson MN, Mills MJ: Hypercalcemia due to calcium binding in Waldenstrom's macroglobulinaemia. *J Clin Pathol* 48:961, 1995.

129. Zaloga G, Willey S, Tomasic P, Chernow B: Free fatty acids alter calcium binding: A cause for misinterpretation of serum calcium values and hypocalcemia in critical illness. *J Clin Endocrinol Metab* 64:1010, 1987.

130. Taylor B, Sibbald WJ, Edmonds MW, et al: Ionized hypocalcemia in critically ill patients with sepsis. *Can J Surg* 21:429, 1978.

131. Zaloga G, Chernow B, Cook D, et al: Assessment of calcium homeostasis in the critically ill surgery patient. The diagnostic pitfalls of the McLean-Hastings nomogram. *Ann Surg* 202:587, 1985.

132. Desai TK, Carlson RW, Geheb MA: Prevalence and clinical implications of hypocalcemia in acutely ill patients in a medical intensive care setting. *Am J Med* 84:209, 1988.

133. Zivin JR, Gooley T, Zager RA, Ryan MJ: Hypocalcemia: A pervasive metabolic abnormality in the critically ill. *Am J Kidney Dis* 37:689, 2001.

134. Sutters M, Gaboury CL, Bennett WM: Severe hyperphosphatemia and hypocalcemia: A dilemma in patient management. *J Am Soc Nephrol* 7:2056, 1996.

135. Edmondson S, Almquist TD: Iatrogenic hypocalcemic tetany. *Ann Emerg Med* 19:938, 1990.

136. Craig JC, Hodson EM, Martin HC: Phosphate enema poisoning in children. *Med J Aust* 160:347, 1994.

137. Howland WS, Schweizer O, Jascott D, Ragasa J: Factors influencing the ionization of calcium during major surgical procedures. *Surg Gynecol Obstet* 143:895, 1976.

138. Bashour TT, Ryan C, Kabbani SS, Crew J: Hypocalcemic acute myocardial failure secondary to rapid transfusion of citrated blood. *Am Heart J* 108:1040, 1984.

139. Hermans C, Lefebvre C, Devogelaer JP, Lambert M: Hypocalcaemia and chronic alcohol intoxication: transient hypoparathyroidism secondary to magnesium deficiency. *Clin Rheumatol* 15:193, 1996.

140. Zaloga GP: Ionized hypocalcemia during sepsis. *Crit Care Med* 28:266, 2000.

141. Zaloga GP, Chernow B: The multifactorial basis for hypocalcemia during sepsis. Studies of the parathyroid hormone-vitamin D axis. *Ann Intern Med* 107:36, 1987.

142. Lind L, Carlstedt F, Rastad J, et al: Hypocalcemia and parathyroid hormone secretion in critically ill patients. *Crit Care Med* 28:93, 2000.

143. Hofmann E: The Chvostek sign: A clinical study. *Am J Surg* 96:33, 1958.

144. Shinoda T, Aizawa T, Shirota T, et al: Exacerbation of latent heart failure by mild hypocalcemia after parathyroidectomy in a long-term hemodialysis patient. *Nephron* 60:482, 1992.

145. Wong CK, Lau CP, Cheng CH, et al: Hypocalcemic myocardial dysfunction: short- and long-term improvement with calcium replacement. *Am Heart J* 120:381, 1990.

146. Chernow B: Calcium: does it have a therapeutic role in sepsis? *Crit Care Med* 18:895, 1990.

147. Abbott AJ, Hill R, Shears L, et al: Effects of calcium chloride administration on the postischemic isolated rat heart. *Ann Thorac Surg* 51:705, 1991.

148. Zaloga G, Sager A, Black KW: Low dose calcium administration increases mortality during septic peritonitis in rats. *Circ Shock* 37:226, 1992.

149. Malcolm D, Zaloga G, Holaday J: Calcium administration increases the mortality of endotoxic shock in rats. *Crit Care Med* 17:900, 1989.

150. Carlstedt F, Eriksson M, Kiiski R, et al: Hypocalcemia during porcine endotoxemic shock: effects of calcium administration. *Crit Care Med* 28:2909, 2000.

151. Steinhorn D, Sweeney M, Layman L: Pharmacodynamic response to ionized calcium during acute sepsis. *Crit Care Med* 18:851, 1990.

152. Martin TJ, Kang Y, Robertson KM, et al: Ionization and hemodynamic effects of calcium chloride and calcium gluconate in the absence of hepatic function. *Anesthesiology* 73:62, 1990.

153. Broner CW, Stidham GL, Westenkirchner DF, Watson DC: A prospective, randomized, double-blind comparison of calcium chloride and calcium gluconate therapies for hypocalcemia in critically ill children. *J Pediatr* 117:986, 1990.

154. Jankowski S, Vincent JL: Calcium administration for cardiovascular support in critically ill patients: when is it indicated? *J Intensive Care Med* 10:91, 1995.

155. Beall DP, Scofield RH: Milk-alkali syndrome associated with calcium carbonate consumption: report of 7 patients with parathyroid hormone levels and an estimate of prevalence among patients hospitalized with hypercalcemia. *Medicine* 74:89, 1995.

156. Lemann J, Gray RW: Calcitriol, calcium, and granulomatous disease. *N Engl J Med* 311:1115, 1984.

157. Seymour JF, Gagel RF, Hagemeister FB, et al: Calcitriol production in hypercalcemic and normocalcemic patients with non-hodgkin lymphoma. *Ann Intern Med* 121:633, 1994.

158. Cardella CJ, Birkin BL, Rapoport A: Role of dialysis in the treatment of severe hypercalcemia: Report of two cases successfully treated with hemodialysis and review of the literature. *Clin Nephrol* 12:285, 1979.

159. Davidson TG: Conventional treatment of hypercalcemia of malignancy. *Am J Health System Pharm* 58:S8, 2001.

160. Seymour JF, Gagel RF: Calcitriol: The major humoral mediator of hypercalcemia in Hodgkin's disease and non-Hodgkin's lymphoma. *Blood* 82:1383, 1993.

161. Sharma OP: Vitamin D, calcium and sarcoidosis. *Chest* 109:535, 1996.

162. O'Leary TJ, Jones G, Yip A, et al: The effects of chloroquine on serum 1,25 dihydroxyvitamin D and calcium metabolism in sarcoidosis. *N Engl J Med* 315:727, 1986.

163. Adams JS, Diz MM, Sharma OP: Effective reduction in the serum 1,25-dihydroxyvitamin D and calcium concentration in sarcoidosis-associated hypercalcemia with short-course chloroquine therapy. *Ann Intern Med* 111:437, 1989.

164. Nussbaum SR, Younger J, Vandepol CJ, et al: Single-dose intravenous therapy with pamidronate for the treatment of hypercalcemia of malignancy: comparison of 30-, 60-, and 90-mg dosages. *Am J Med* 95:297, 1993.

165. Ralston SH, Patel U, Fraser WD, et al: Comparison of three intravenous bisphosphonates in cancer-associated hypercalcemia. *Lancet* 8673:1180, 1989.

166. Major P, Lortholary A, Hon J, et al: Zoledronic acid is superior to pamidronate in the treatment of hypercalcemia of malignancy: A pooled analysis of two randomized, controlled clinical trials. *J Clin Oncol* 19:558, 2001.

167. Kaiser W, Biesenbach G, Kramar R, Zazgornik J: Calcium free hemodialysis: An effective therapy in hypercalcemic crisis—report of 4 cases. *Intensive Care Med* 15:471, 1989.

168. Sramek V, Novak I, Matejovic M, et al: Continuous venovenous hemodiafiltration (CVVHDF) with citrate anticoagulation in the treatment of a patient with acute renal failure, hypercalcemia, and thrombocytopenia. *Intensive Care Med* 24:262, 1998.

169. Kempson SA, Lotscher M, Kaissling B, et al: Parathyroid hormone action on phosphate transporter mRNA and protein in rat renal proximal tubules. *Am J Physiol* 268:F784, 1995.

170. Ramirez JA, Emmett M, White MG, et al: The absorption of dietary phosphorus and calcium in hemodialysis patients. *Kidney Int* 30:753, 1986.

171. Halevy J, Bulvik S: Severe hypophosphatemia in hospitalized patients. *Arch Intern Med* 148:153, 1988.

172. Fiaccadori E, Coffrini E, Ronda N, et al: Hypophosphatemia in course of chronic obstructive pulmonary disease. Prevalence, mechanisms, and relationships with skeletal muscle phosphorus content. *Chest* 97:857, 1990.

173. Zazzo JF, Troche G, Ruel P, Maintenant J: High incidence of hypophosphatemia in surgical intensive care patients: efficacy of phosphorus therapy on myocardial function. *Intensive Care Med* 21:826, 1995.

174. Weinsier RL, Krumdieck CL: Death resulting from overzealous total parenteral nutrition: The refeeding syndrome revisited. *Am J Clin Nutr* 34:393, 1981.

175. Marik PE, Bedigian MK: Refeeding hypophosphatemia in critically ill patients in an intensive care unit. A prospective study. *Arch Surg* 131:1043, 1996.

176. Brautbar N, Leibovici H, Massry SG: On the mechanism of hypophosphatemia during acute hyperventilation: evidence for increased muscle glycolysis. *Miner Electrolyte Metab* 9:45, 1983.

177. De Marchi S, Cecchin E, Basile A, et al: Renal tubular dysfunction in chronic alcohol abuse—effects of abstinence. *N Engl J Med* 329:1927, 1993.

178. Brady HR, Ryan F, Cunningham J, et al: Hypophosphatemia complicating bronchodilator therapy for acute severe asthma. *Arch Intern Med* 149:2367, 1989.

179. Farber M, Carlone S, Palange P, et al: Effect of inorganic phosphate in hypoxemic chronic obstructive lung disease patients during exercise. *Chest* 92:310, 1987.

180. Subramanian R, Khardori R: Severe hypophosphatemia. Pathophysiologic implications, clinical presentations, and treatment. *Medicine (Baltimore)* 79:1, 2000.

181. Newman JH, Neff TA, Ziporen P: Acute respiratory failure associated with hypophosphatemia. *N Engl J Med* 296:1101, 1977.

182. O'Connor LR, Wheeler WS, Bethune JE: Effect of hypophosphatemia on myocardial performance in man. *N Engl J Med* 297:901, 1977.

183. Wada S, Nagase T, Koike Y, et al: A case of anorexia nervosa with acute renal failure induced by rhabdomyolysis; possible involvement of hypophosphatemia or phosphate depletion. *Intern Med* 31:478, 1992.

184. Schwartz A, Gurman G, Cohen G, et al: Association between hypophosphatemia and cardiac arrhythmias in the early stages of sepsis. *Eur J Intern Med* 13:434, 2002.

185. Melvin JD, Watts RG: Severe hypophosphatemia: A rare cause of intravascular hemolysis. *Am J Hematol* 69:223, 2002.

186. Saglikes Y, Massry SG, Iseki K, et al: Effect of phosphate depletion on blood pressure and vascular reactivity to norepinephrine and angiotensin II in the rat. *Am J Physiol* 248:F93, 1985.

187. Bollaert PE, Levy B, Nace L, et al: Hemodynamic and metabolic effects of rapid correction of hypophosphatemia in patients with septic shock. *Chest* 107:1698, 1995.

188. Shiber JR, Mattu A: Serum phosphate abnormalities in the emergency department. *J Emerg Med* 23:395, 2002.

189. Fisher JN, Kitabchi AE: A randomized study of phosphate therapy in the treatment of diabetic ketoacidosis. *J Clin Endocrinol Metab* 57:177, 1983.

190. Winter RJ, Harris CJ, Phillips LS, Green OC: Diabetic ketoacidosis. Induction of hypocalcemia and hypomagnesemia by phosphate therapy. *Am J Med* 67:897, 1979.

191. Kebler R, McDonald FD, Cadnapaphornchai P: Dynamic changes in serum phosphorus levels in diabetic ketoacidosis. *Am J Med* 79:571, 1985.

192. Eisenberg E: Effect of intravenous phosphate on serum strontium and calcium. *N Engl J Med* 282:889, 1970.

193. Isotalo PA, Halil A, Green M, et al: Metastatic calcification of the cardiac conduction system with heart block: an under-reported entity in chronic renal failure patients. *J Forensic Sci* 45:1335, 2000.

194. Block GA, Hulbert-Shearon TE, Levin NW, Port FK: Association of serum phosphorus and calcium x phosphate product with mortality risk in chronic hemodialysis patients: A national study. *Am J Kidney Dis* 31:607, 1998.

195. Yamaguchi T, Sugimoto T, Imai Y, et al: Successful treatment of hyperphosphatemic tumoral calcinosis with long-term acetazolamide. *Bone* 16:247S, 1995.

196. Tan HK, Bellomo R, M'Pis DA, Ronco C: Phosphatemic control during acute renal failure: intermittent hemodialysis versus continuous hemodiafiltration. *Int J Artif Organs* 24:186, 2001.

197. Schiller LR, Santa Ana CA, Sheikh MS, et al: Effect of the time of administration of calcium acetate on phosphorus binding. *N Engl J Med* 320:1110, 1989.

198. Sanders GT, Huijgen HJ, Sanders R: Magnesium in disease: A review with special emphasis on the serum ionized magnesium. *Clin Chem Lab Med* 37:1011, 1999.

199. Yu ASL: Disturbances of magnesium metabolism, in Brenner BM (ed): *The Kidney.* Philadelphia, WB Saunders, 2000, p 1055.

200. Kulpmann WR, Gerlach M: Relationship between ionized and total magnesium in serum. *Scand J Clin Lab Invest Suppl* 224:251, 1996.

201. Thienpont LM, Dewitte K, Stockl D: Serum complexed magnesium—a cautionary note on its estimation and its relevance for standardizing serum ionized magnesium. *Clin Chem* 45:154, 1999.

202. Saha H, Harmoinen A, Karvonen AL, et al: Serum ionized versus total magnesium in patients with intestinal or liver disease. *Clin Chem Lab Med* 36:715, 1998.

203. Broner CW, Stidham GL, Westenkirchner DF, Tolley EA: Hypermagnesemia and hypocalcemia as predictors of high mortality in critically ill pediatric patients. *Crit Care Med* 18:921, 1990.

204. Ryzen E, Wagers PW, Singer FR, Rude RK: Magnesium deficiency in a medical ICU population. *Crit Care Med* 13:19, 1985.

205. Hebert P, Mehta N, Wang J, et al: Functional magnesium deficiency in critically ill patients identified using a magnesium-loading test. *Crit Care Med* 25:749, 1997.

206. Whang R, Ryder KW: Frequency of hypomagnesemia and hypermagnesemia: Requested vs routine. *JAMA* 263:3063, 1990.

207. Lim P, Jacob E: Tissue magnesium level in chronic diarrhea. *J Lab Clin Invest* 80:313, 1972.

208. Nielsen JA, Thaysen EH: Acute and chronic magnesium deficiency following extensive small gut resection. *Scand J Gastroenterol* 6:663, 1971.

209. Hessov I, Hasselblad C, Fasth S, Hulten L: Magnesium deficiency after ileal resections for Crohn's disease. *Scand J Gastroenterol* 18:643, 1983.

210. Massry SG, Coburn JW, Chapman LW, Kleeman CR: The effect of long-term deoxycorticosterone acetate administration on the renal excretion of calcium and magnesium. *J Lab Clin Invest* 71:212, 1968.

211. Sutton RA, Domrongkitchaiporn S: Abnormal renal magnesium handling. *Miner Electrolyte Metab* 19:232, 1993.

212. Lim P, Jacob E: Magnesium deficiency in patients on long-term diuretic therapy for heart failure. *BMJ* 3:620-, 1972.

213. Davis BB, Preuss HG, Murdaugh HVJ: Hypomagnesemia following the diuresis of post-renal obstruction and renal transplant. *Nephron* 14:275, 1975.

214. Lam M, Adelstein DJ: Hypomagnesemia and renal magnesium wasting in patients treated with cisplatin. *Am J Kidney Dis* 8:164, 1986.

215. Barton CH, Pahl M, Vaziri ND, Cesario T: Renal magnesium wasting associated with amphotericin B therapy. *Am J Med* 77:471, 1984.

216. Green CG, Doershuk CF, Stern RC: Symptomatic hypomagnesemia in cystic fibrosis. *J Pediatr* 107:425, 1985.

217. Bettinelli A, Bianchetti MG, Borella P, et al: Genetic heterogeneity in tubular hypomagnesemia-hypokalemia with hypocalciuria (Gitelman's syndrome). *Kidney Int* 47:547, 1995.

218. Cunningham JJ, Anbar RD, Crawford JD: Hypomagnesemia: A multifactorial complication of treatment of patients with severe burn trauma. *JPEN J Parenter Enteral Nutr* 11:364, 1987.

219. Berger MM, Rothen C, Cavadini C, Chiolero RL: Exudative mineral losses after serious burns: a clue to the alterations of magnesium and phosphate metabolism. *Am J Clin Nutr* 65:1473, 1997.

220. Martin BJ, Black J, McLelland AS: Hypomagnesaemia in elderly hospital admissions: A study of clinical significance. *Q J Med* 78:177, 1991.

221. Rubeiz GJ, Thill-Baharozian M, Hardie D, Carlson RW: Association of hypomagnesemia and mortality in acutely ill medical patients. *Crit Care Med* 21:203, 1993.

222. Kingston ME, Al-Siba'i MB, Skooge WC: Clinical manifestations of hypomagnesemia. *Crit Care Med* 14:950, 1986.

223. Shils ME: Experimental human magnesium depletion. *Medicine* 48:61, 1969.

224. Al-Tweigeri T, Magliocco AM, DeCoteau JF: Cortical blindness as a manifestation of hypomagnesemia secondary to cisplatin therapy: Case report and review of literature. *Gynecol Oncol* 72:120, 1999.

225. Dickerson RN, Brown RO: Hypomagnesemia in hospitalized patients receiving nutritional support. *Heart Lung* 14:561, 1985.

226. Al-Ghamdi SM, Cameron EC, Sutton RA: Magnesium deficiency: Pathophysiologic and clinical overview. *Am J Kidney Dis* 24:737, 1994.

227. Zuccala G, Pahor M, Lattanzio F, et al: Detection of arrhythmogenic cellular magnesium depletion in hip surgery patients. *Br J Anaesth* 79:776, 1997.

228. Young IS, Goh EM, McKillop UH, et al: Magnesium status and digoxin toxicity. *Br J Clin Pharmacol* 32:717, 1991.
229. Elisaf M, Panteli K, Theodorou J, Siamopoulos KC: Fractional excretion of magnesium in normal subjects and in patients with hypomagnesemia. *Magnes Res* 10:315, 1997.
230. Gullestad L, Dolva LO, Waage A, et al: Magnesium deficiency diagnosed by an intravenous loading test. *Scand J Clin Lab Invest* 52:245, 1992.
231. Ramee SR, White CJ, Svinarich JT, et al: Torsades de pointes and magnesium deficiency. *Am Heart J* 109:164, 1985.
232. Brucato A, Bonati M, Gaspari F, et al: Tetany and rhabdomyolysis due to surreptitious furosemide—importance of magnesium supplementation. *J Toxicol Clin Toxicol* 31:341, 1993.
233. Magnesium in Coronaries (MAGIC) Trial Investigators: Early administration of intravenous magnesium to high-risk patients with acute myocardial infarction in the Magnesium in Coronaries (MAGIC) trial: A randomised controlled trial. *Lancet* 360:1189, 2002.
234. Gullestad L, Oystein DL, Birkeland K, et al: Oral versus intravenous magnesium supplementation in patients with magnesium deficiency. *Magnes Trace Elem* 10:11, 1991.
235. Costello RB, Moser-Veillon PB, DiBianco R: Magnesium supplementation in patients with congestive heart failure. *J Am Coll Nutr* 16:22, 1997.
236. Ross JR, Dargan PI, Jones AL, Kostrzewski A: A case of hypomagnesaemia due to malabsorption, unresponsive to oral administration of magnesium glycerophosphate, but responsive to oral magnesium oxide supplementation. *Gut* 48:857, 2001.
237. Ng LL, Garrido MC, Davies JE, et al: Intracellular free magnesium in lymphocytes from patients with congestive cardiac failure treated with loop diuretics with and without amiloride. *Br J Clin Pharmacol* 33:329, 1992.
238. Ryan MF: The role of magnesium in clinical biochemistry: An overview. *Ann Clin Biochem* 28:19, 1991.
239. Clark B, Brown R: Unsuspected morbid hypermagnesemia in elderly patients. *Am J Nephrol* 12:336, 1992.
240. Wacker WE, Parisi AF: Magnesium metabolism. *N Engl J Med* 278:772, 1968.
241. Cruikshank DP, Pitkin RM, Reynolds WA, et al: Effects of magnesium sulfate treatment on perinatal calcium metabolism. I. Maternal and fetal responses. *Am J Obstet Gynecol* 134:243, 1979.
242. Rizzo MA, Fisher M, Lock P: Hypermagnesemic pseudocoma. *Arch Intern Med* 153:1130, 1993.
243. Morisaki H, Yamamoto S, Morita Y, et al: Hypermagnesemia-induced cardiopulmonary arrest before induction of anesthesia for emergency cesarean section. *J Clin Anesth* 12:224, 2000.
244. Weber C, Santiago R: Hypermagnesemia: A potential complication during treatment of theophylline intoxication with oral activated charcoal and magnesium-containing cathartics. *Chest* 95:56, 1989.
245. Gren J, Woolf A: Hypermagnesemia associated with catharsis in a salicylate-intoxicated patient with anorexia nervosa. *Ann Emerg Med* 18:2, 200, 1989.
246. McGuire JK, Kulkarni MS, Baden HP: Fatal hypermagnesemia in a child treated with megavitamin/megamineral therapy. *Pediatrics* 105:18, 2000.
247. Ashton MR, Sutton D, Nielsen M: Severe magnesium toxicity after magnesium sulphate enema in a chronically constipated child. *BMJ* 300:541, 1991.
248. Collinson PO, Burroughs AK: Severe hypermagnesaemia due to magnesium sulphate enemas in patients with hepatic coma [erratum appears in *Br Med J (Clin Res Ed)* 293:1222, 1986]. *Br Med J (Clin Res Ed)* 293:1013, 1986.
249. Outerbridge EW, Papageorgiou A, Stern L: Magnesium sulfate enema in a newborn. Fatal systemic magnesium absorption. *JAMA* 224:1392, 1973.
250. Castelbaum A, Donofrio PD, Walker FO, Troost BT: Laxative abuse causing hypermagnesemia, quadriparesis, and neuromuscular junction defect. *Neurology* 39:746, 1989.
251. Schelling JR: Fatal hypermagnesemia. *Clin Nephrol* 53:61, 2000.
252. Razavi B, Somers D: Hypermagnesemia-induced multiorgan failure. *Am J Med* 108:686, 2000.
253. Meltzer SJ, Auer J: The antagonistic action of calcium upon the inhibitory effect of magnesium. *Am J Physiol* 21:400, 1908.
254. Porath A, Mosseri M, Harmon I, et al: Dead Sea water poisoning. *Ann Emerg Med* 18:2, 187, 1989.
255. Murthy BV: Hyperkalaemia and rapid blood transfusion. *Anaesthesia* 55:398, 2000.
256. Campieri C, Fatone F, Mignani R, et al: Terminal arrhythmia due to hyperkalemia corrected by intravenous calcium infusion. *Nephron* 47:312, 1987.
257. Lens XM, Montoliu J, Cases A, et al: Treatment of hyperkalaemia in renal failure: Salbutamol v. insulin. *Nephrol Dial Transplant* 4:228, 1989.
258. Blumberg A, Wiedmann P, Ferrari P: Effect of prolonged bicarbonate administration on plasma potassium in terminal renal failure. *Kidney Int* 41:369, 1992.
259. Efstathiadou Z, Bitsis S, Tsatsoulis A: Gastrectomy and osteomalacia: an association not to be forgotten. *Horm Res* 52:295, 1999.
260. Yamaji Y, Hayashi M, Suzuki Y, et al: Thyroid crisis associated with severe hypocalcemia. *Japan J Med* 30:179, 1991.
261. Edwards H, Zinberg J, King TC: Effect of cimetidine on serum calcium levels in an elderly patient. *Arch Surg* 116:1088, 1981.
262. Lin J, Idee JM, Port M, et al: Interference of magnetic resonance imaging contrast agents with the serum calcium measurement technique using colorimetric reagents. *J Pharm Biomed Anal* 21:931, 1999.
263. Hardman KA, Heath DA, Nelson HM: Drug points: hypercalcemia associated with calcipotriol (Dovonex) treatment. *BMJ* 306:896, 1993.
264. Kozeny GA, Barbato AL, Bansal VK, et al: Hypercalcemia associated with silicone-induced granulomas. *N Engl J Med* 311:1103, 1984.
265. Bosch X, Lopez-Soto A, Morello A, et al: Vitamin D metabolite-mediated hypercalcemia in Wegener's granulomatosis. *Mayo Clin Proc* 72:440, 1997.
266. Woywodt A, Schneider W, Goebel U, Luft FC: Hypercalcemia due to talc granulomatosis. *Chest* 117:1195, 2000.
267. Bosch X: Hypercalcemia due to endogenous overproduction of active vitamin D in identical twins with cat-scratch disease. *JAMA* 279:532, 1998.
268. Bendz H, Sjordin L, Toss G, Berglund K: Hyperparathyroidism and long-term lithium therapy: A cross sectional study and the effect of lithium withdrawal. *J Intern Med* 240:357, 1996.
269. McLean TW, Pritchard J: Langerhans cell histiocytosis and hypercalcemia: Clinical response to indomethacin. *J Pediatr Hematol Oncol* 18:318, 1996.
270. Lepre F, Grill V, Ho PWM, Martin TJ: Hypercalcemia in pregnancy and lactation associated with parathyroid hormone-related protein. *N Engl J Med* 328:666, 1993.
271. Fishbane S, Frei GL, Finger M, et al: Hypervitaminosis A in two hemodialysis patients. *Am J Kidney Dis* 25:346, 1995.
272. Westphal SA: Disseminated coccidioidomycosis associated with hypercalcemia. *Mayo Clin Proc* 73:893, 1998.
273. Howard RA, Ashwell S, Bond LR, Holbrook I: Artefactual serum hyperkalemia and hypercalcemia in essential thrombocythemia. *J Clin Pathol* 53:105, 2000.
274. Knox JB, Demling RH, Wilmore DW, et al: Hypercalcemia associated with the use of human growth hormone in an adult surgical intensive care unit. *Arch Surg* 130:442, 1995.
275. Meneghini LF, Oster JR, Camacho JR, et al: Hypercalcemia in association with acute renal failure and rhabdomyolysis.

Case report and literature review. *Miner Electrolyte Metab* 19:1, 1993.

276. Adams JS, Kantorovich V: Inability of short-term, low-dose hydroxychloroquine to resolve vitamin D-mediated hypercalcemia in patients with B-cell lymphoma. *J Clin Endocrinol Metab* 84:799, 1999.

277. Galland L: Magnesium and inflammatory bowel disease. *Magnesium* 7:78, 1988.

278. Lipner A: Symptomatic magnesium deficiency after small-intestinal bypass for obesity. *BMJ* 1:148, 1977.

279. Papazachariou IM, Martinez-Isla A, Efthimiou E, et al: Magnesium deficiency in patients with chronic pancreatitis identified by an intravenous loading test. *Clin Chimica Acta* 302:145, 2000.

280. Eshleman SSH, Shaw LM: Massive theophylline overdose with atypical metabolic abnormalities. *Clin Chem* 36:398, 1990.

Chapter 77

ACID-BASE BALANCE

DAVID KAUFMAN
ANDREW J. KITCHING
JOHN A. KELLUM

KEY POINTS

- *The blood [H^+] and pH are determined by the strong ion difference (SID), the P_{CO_2}, and the total concentration of weak acids, mostly consisting of phosphate and albumin.*
- *Both acidemia and alkalemia have potentially harmful physiologic effects, and the presence of either is related to mortality.*
- *Most acid-base derangements do not benefit from specific correction of the abnormal pH; instead, the intensivist should focus on detecting and treating the underlying condition.*
- *Acid-base disorders are easily characterized using a stepwise approach.*
- *Lactic acidosis is the most important acid-base abnormality in ICU patients. Inadequate tissue oxygenation underlies the lactic acidosis in some patients (acute hemorrhage, critical hypoxemia, cardiogenic shock) but probably does not in others (such as the resuscitated septic patient).*

Acid-base balance and *acid-base disorders* are imperfect terms for the determining factors and disease processes that lead to a particular hydrogen ion concentration [H^+] in the blood. The methodology used routinely to determine an acid-base disorder is accurate in defining the disturbance. This methodology does not, however, reveal the mechanisms that have led to a particular [H^+] in blood. The components of blood that contribute to acid-base balance are

1. Water
2. Strong cations (Na^+, Mg^{2+}, Ca^{2+}, K^+) and strong anions (Cl^-, $lactate^-$)
3. Bicarbonate ion (HCO_3^-)
4. Weak acids and their conjugate bases ($HA + A^- = A_{tot}$) (A_{tot} is the total independent variable, and $HA + A^-$ are dependent variables.)
5. Partial pressure of carbon dioxide (P_{CO_2})
6. Carbonate ion (CO_3^{2-})
7. Hydroxyl ion (OH^-)
8. Hydrogen ion (H^+)

The difference between the strong cations and strong anions (the strong ion difference [SID]), P_{CO_2}, and the total amount of weak acids and their conjugate bases (A_{tot}) are the only independent variables.[1] All the other components are, by definition, dependent, including HCO_3^-, HA, A^-, CO_3^{2-}, OH^-, and H^+. Because the concentrations of each of these six variables are dependent on one or more of the independent variables, we must solve separate equilibrium equations for each. Water itself is minimally dissociated despite the importance of [H^+] and can be considered a constant. The six equations are as follows:

Water dissociation:

$$[H^+] \times [OH^-] = K_1 \times [H_2O] \qquad (77\text{-}1)$$

Weak acid dissociation:

$$[H^+] \times [A^-] = K_2[HA] \qquad (77\text{-}2)$$

Weak acid conservation:

$$[HA] + [A^-] = [A_{tot}] \qquad (77\text{-}3)$$

HCO_3^- formation:

$$[H^+] \times [HCO_3^-] = K_3 \times P_{CO_2} \qquad (77\text{-}4)$$

CO_3^{2-} formation:

$$[H^+] \times [CO_3^{2-}] + K_4 \times [HCO_3^-] \qquad (77\text{-}5)$$

Electrical neutrality:

$$SID + [H^+] - [HCO_3^-] - [A^-] - [CO_3^{2-}] - [OH^-] = 0 \qquad (77\text{-}6)$$

K_1 through K_4 represent constants for the individual reactions. Now that we have six equations and six unknowns, we can arrange any unknown as a fourth-order polynomial and solve the equation. In acid-base balance, the dependent variable in question is [H^+]. Stated less elegantly, there is a unique value for each of the six dependent variables once SID, P_{CO_2}, and A_{tot} are known so that all the equations can be solved simultaneously.

The formula for bicarbonate formation in its most robust form is the familiar Henderson-Hasselbalch equation:

$$pH = pK_a + \log\{[HCO_3^-]/(P_{CO_2} \times 0.03)\} \qquad (77\text{-}7)$$

Since this equation is no more or less correct than any of the other five equations that must be solved simultaneously, there is nothing wrong with using it to determine an acid-base disorder. Indeed, the fact that all three values are readily available from a standard arterial blood gas determination explains the popularity of this equation.

Metabolic Disturbances

By examining Eq. (77-7) it is possible to determine whether an acid-base disturbance is present and whether it is due to respiratory (P_{CO_2}) or metabolic derangements. One might assume, therefore, that pH is determined by the relationship between P_{CO_2} and [HCO_3^-]. This presumption is false. Likewise, solving Eq. (77-2) for [H^+] does not mean that [H^+] is determined by the HA and A^-. In truth, [H^+] and thus pH are determined by P_{CO_2}, SID, and A_{tot}. Since we define respiratory disorders by alterations in P_{CO_2}, metabolic disturbances are brought about by changes in SID and A_{tot}. They are not caused by changes in [HCO_3^-], but rather, changes in [HCO_3^-] occur as a result of the disturbance.

As SID becomes *less* positive, more [H^+] is released into the solution, and acidemia develops. As SID becomes *more* positive, more [H^+] associates with [OH^-], forming water, and alkalemia develops. By contrast, A_{tot}, composed of weak acids, is acidifying. As A_{tot} increases, the pH falls, and as A_{tot} decreases, such as with hemodilution, the pH increases.

Respiratory Disorders

By definition, abnormalities in P_{CO_2} are classified as respiratory disorders. SID (and possibly A_{tot}) is manipulated by the human body to compensate for chronic respiratory disorders, thus maintaining pH within the normal range (7.35–7.45). SID decreases to compensate for a chronic respiratory alkalosis, and SID increases to compensate for a chronic respiratory acidosis. The physiologic determinants of P_{CO_2} are straightforward:

$$P_{CO_2} \propto V_{CO_2}/V_A$$

where V_{CO_2} is CO_2 production and V_A is alveolar ventilation. A change in P_{CO_2} must be explained by one of these factors. Hypercarbia and hypocarbia usually can be explained easily at the bedside.

Acidemia and Alkalemia

Even relative extremes of $[H^+]$ are remarkably well tolerated (e.g., pH 7.1–7.7), at least for the short term, in otherwise healthy individuals. However, some authors have even suggested that acidemia itself may be beneficial to critically ill patients.[2] For example, since acidemia shifts the oxyhemoglobin curve to the right, there is better oxygen delivery under acidemic conditions. Unfortunately, this "benefit" is dubious because acidosis also reduces synthesis of 2,3-diphosphoglycerate (2,3-DPG), and thus chronically, acidosis does not appear to improve oxygen delivery. Acidosis may produce other salutary effects on the circulation that could result in benefit in certain clinical scenarios,[2] but acidosis also produces numerous undesirable effects on various systems (Table 77-1), and we caution against "permissive acidosis."

This is not to say that we believe that correcting an acid-base disorder is always appropriate. Indeed, the existing evidence does not support the use of sodium bicarbonate for the purpose of correcting the pH in most conditions of acute acidosis,[3] and some animal experiments even suggest harm.[4] However, supporting respiratory compensation when feasible and avoiding acidosis when possible seems a prudent course of action in most clinical scenarios. Frequently, when treating critically ill patients, it is easy to blur the lines between supportive measures and therapeutic interventions. Common forms of acidemia may be associated with significant mortality because of the disease processes that underlie them, not necessarily because of the actual $[H^+]$. For instance, bowel infarction is lethal, and only surgical resection is curative. Treating the lactic acidosis without addressing the underlying cause of the lactic acidosis in this scenario is certain to fail. Dissecting out the effects of acidosis itself from the causes that underlie it is difficult in patients. However, acidosis itself has been shown to produce harm in animal models[5–8]— especially in models of sepsis, where decreased survival time and hypotension appear to be attributable to exogenous acid

TABLE 77-1 Potential Clinical Effects of Metabolic Acid-Base Disorders

Metabolic Acidosis	Metabolic Alkalosis
Cardiovascular	**Cardiovascular**
Decreased inotropy	Increased inotropy (Ca^{2+} entry)
Conduction defects	Altered coronary blood flow*
Arterial vasodilation	Digoxin toxicity
Venous vasoconstriction	**Oxygen delivery**
Oxygen delivery	Increased oxy-Hb affinity
Decreased oxy-Hb binding	Increased 2,3-DPG (delayed)
Decreased 2,3-DPG (late)	**Neuromuscular**
Neuromuscular	Neuromuscular excitability
Respiratory depression	Encephalopathy
Decreased sensorium	Seizures
Metabolism	**Metabolic effect**
Protein wasting	Hypokalemia
Bone demineralization	Hypocalcemia
Catecholamine, PTH, and	Hypophosphatemia
aldosterone stimulation	Impaired enzyme function
Insulin resistance	
GI effect	
Emesis	
Electrolytes	
Hyperkalemia	
Hypercalcemia	
Hyperuricemia	

*Animal studies have shown both increased and decreased coronary artery blood flow.
SOURCE: Adapted from Kellum JA: Diagnosis and treatment of acid-base disorders, in Grenvik A, Shoemaker PK, Ayers S, Holbrook (eds): *Textbook of Critical Care*. Philadelphia, Saunders, 1999, Chapter 76, pp 839–853, with permission.

loading.[7,8] Nonetheless, it has yet to be demonstrated that treating acidosis improves outcome.

Specific Metabolic Disorders

To diagnose a disorder leading to a change in SID, an actual accounting of strong ions occurs. A decrease in SID may be brought about by the generation of organic strong anions (e.g., lactate and ketones) or the loss of strong cations paired with weak anions to balance charge. If the patient has diarrhea, he or she is losing $[Na^+]$ and $[HCO_3^-]$; therefore, the $[Cl^-]$ will increase relative to the $[Na^+]$, leading to a decrease in SID and, ultimately, acidosis.

The organs of the gastrointestinal tract are underappreciated regulators of acid-base balance. Their ability to manipulate SID complexly is a direct result of the fact that strong ions are handled differently in different portions of the gastrointestinal tract. Cl^- is pumped into the stomach, reducing SID in the stomach and increasing the $[H^+]$ (decreasing the pH) and, at the same time, causing the alkaline tide in the blood (increasing SID) that occurs at the beginning of a meal when gastric acid secretion is maximal. The *alkaline tide* refers to the Cl^--depleted plasma that leaves the stomach. The elevated SID leads to a decrease in $[H^+]$ (increase in pH). Cl^- is reabsorbed in the duodenum, and plasma $[H^+]$ or pH is restored. Given the combination of Cl^- secretion into the stomach and Cl^- reabsorption in the duodenum, a net balance occurs, and plasma $[H^+]$ or pH is not affected. However, if gastric secretions are removed from the patient by nasogastric (NG) suction or by vomiting, Cl^- cannot be reabsorbed, and SID will increase. Increased SID will lead to a metabolic alkalosis.

The pancreas secretes fluid into the small intestine, which has a SID that is much higher than plasma and very low in $[Cl^-]$. The Cl^--rich plasma leaving the pancreas counteracts the alkaline tide along with Cl^- reabsorption in the duodenum. Large amounts of pancreatic fluid loss will lead to a decrease in plasma SID and an associated acidosis. At the other end of the gastrointestinal (GI) tract, in the large intestine, most of the Cl^- already has been removed in the small intestine, so the only strong ions present are Na^+ and K^+. If large amounts of these strong ions are lost with diarrhea fluid, then the plasma SID will decrease, and acidosis will result. During ischemia to the intestinal tract, significant amounts of lactate can be produced. At physiologic pH, lactate acts as a strong anion and decreases SID, leading to a metabolic acidosis. There is some evidence that the gut may modulate systemic acidosis in experimental endotoxemia by removing anions from the plasma.[9] However, the full capacity of the GI tract to effect acid-base balance is not known. The treatment of metabolic acidosis requires treatment of an underlying disease process and not, strictly speaking, of the acid-base disorder. If the patient developed a lactate acidosis following a seizure, this lactic acidosis would resolve rapidly once the liver metabolized the lactate. Indeed, treatment of acid-base disturbances can lead to severe overshoot alkalosis or acidosis.

Finally, the liver is perhaps the most important abdominal organ involved in the regulation of acid-base balance.[10,11] Hepatic glutaminogenesis is important for systemic acid-base balance and is tightly controlled by mechanisms sensitive to plasma $[H^+]$ and is stimulated by acidosis.[12] Nitrogen metabolism by the liver can produce urea, glutamine, or NH_4^+. Normally, the liver does not release more than a very small amount of NH_4^+ but incorporates this nitrogen into either urea or glutamine. However, the production of urea or glutamine has significantly different effects at the level of the kidney. This is so because glutamine is used by the kidney to generate NH_4^+ and facilitate the excretion of Cl^-. Thus the production of glutamine can be seen as having an alkalinizing effect on plasma pH because of the way in which the kidney uses it. In humans, the liver is also the only organ than synthesizes albumin, the major component of A_{tot}.

Crystalloid Solutions

Manipulating $[H^+]$ in the blood is intellectually easy once one understands the importance of SID but certainly is not of proven benefit. When administered to patients, equimolar concentrations of Na^+ and Cl^- (such as in saline solutions) will increase the $[Cl^-]$ more rapidly than the $[Na^+]$ because $[Na^+]$ is normally much greater than $[Cl^-]$. When this occurs, SID will decrease, and $[H^+]$ will increase. In a test tube, lactated Ringer's solution will behave just like saline because lactate is a strong ion. However, in humans, lactate metabolism is rapid even under conditions of relatively severe hepatic dysfunction. If the liver is functioning and can metabolize lactate, then the unbalanced Na^+ will increase the SID and result in alkalemia. Conversely, if lactate-containing solutions are administered quickly (as in replacement fluid for hemofiltration) and hepatic function is impaired, acidosis

will develop, just as in the case of saline loading, because SID is lowered.

Normal saline (0.9% NaCl) is often blamed for causing a "dilutional" acidosis, but all that is occurring is that $[Na^+]$ is relatively unchanged as the $[Cl^-]$ rises, leading to a decreased SID and hyperchloremic acidosis. Adding 75 mEq/L of $[NaHCO_3]$ to 0.45% saline (77 mEq/L Na^+ and 77 mEq/L Cl^-) will create an isotonic solution that contains half the $[Cl^-]$ (a strong anion) with twice the $[Na^+]$ (strong cation). This solution has a higher SID than normal saline or lactated Ringer's solution and favors alkalemia. Mixing 150 mEq $NaHCO_3$ in 1 L of sterile water increases the SID further and creates an even more potent alkalizing fluid. Again, it is worth emphasizing the need to treat the underlying disorder and not just "correct" the acid-basis disorder.

The Anion Gap and the Strong Ion Gap

The anion gap (AG) was popularized over 30 years ago. Traditionally, it is calculated from the equation $[(Na^+) + (K^+)] - [(Cl^-) + (HCO_3^-)]$ K^+ is often omitted because its plasma concentration is so tightly controlled that there is little variation. However, this is a mistake for two reasons. First, a 2- to 3-mEq difference in the AG may be clinically relevant in some scenarios, and second, techniques used to correct the AG for abnormalities in A_{tot} require a full accounting of other ions. The difference in the gap is made up largely by albumin and, to a lesser extent, phosphate. Other anions, such as sulfate and lactate, normally contribute less than 2 mEq of negative charge, similar in fact to the amount of positive charge contributed by ionized calcium and ionized magnesium. Thus these ions tend to offset each other. Many medical textbooks still report a normal range for the AG of about 12 to 16 mEq (when K^+ is considered). This value, however, is based on older assay methods that were less sensitive for Cl^-; the expected AG using modern analyzers is closer to 8 to 10 mEq. However, many critically ill patients have hypoalbuminemia or hypophosphatemia, and it has been recommended to correct the normal AG for these abnormalities.[10,13] The following formula can be used to estimate the expected "normal" AG for a given patient:

$$AGc = \text{corrected AG} = 2(\text{albumin g/dL}) + 0.5(\text{phosphate mg/dL}) \quad (77\text{-}8)$$

Thus, for a patient with half the normal albumin and phosphate, the AGc should be approximately 5 mEq/dL. If the measured AG is 10 mEq/dL, then there would be 5 mEq/dL of negative charge still unaccounted for—perhaps attributable to lactate, ketoacid anions, or others.

An alternative to using the traditional AG is to focus on SID. By definition, SID must be equal to and opposite of the negative charges contributed by all the anions, including total CO_2. Normally, the plasma SID is strongly positive (between 40 and 42 mEq/L in healthy humans). Since charge must be balanced in any solution (the principle of electrical neutrality), there must be negative charges to balance this positive charge. Total CO_2 and the weak acids (mainly albumin and phosphate) account for the vast majority of this negative charge. These charges are equal to the "buffer base" first mentioned by Singer and Hastings over half a century ago.[14]

Thus, under normal circumstances, SID should equal buffer base. Although hydroxyl ion concentration [OH⁻] is another negative charge, its value is small enough to ignore. Thus total CO_2 + AG = SID.[15,16] This estimate of SID, or buffer base, is termed the *effective SID* (SIDe). Alternatively, the apparent SID (SIDa) can be estimated by the equation

$$SIDa = ([Na^+] + [K^+] + [Ca^{2+}] + [Mg^{2+}]) - ([Cl^-] + [lactate^-])$$

$$(77\text{-}9)$$

Normally, SIDa = SIDe = SID = buffer base. However, if there are unmeasured strong ions (e.g., sulfates or ketoacid anions), then SIDa will be an inaccurate estimate of true SID, and if there are abnormal weak ions (e.g., proteins), then SIDe will be an inaccurate measure of true SID. When SIDa and SIDe are not equal, their difference (SIDa – SIDe) is termed the *strong ion gap* (SIG). The SIG is positive when unmeasured anions exceed unmeasured cations, and the SIG is negative when unmeasured cations exceed unmeasured anions.

Positive-Anion-Gap (SIG) Acidoses

LACTIC ACIDOSIS

In many forms of critical illness, lactate is the most important cause of a metabolic acidosis.[17] Lactate has been shown to correlate with outcome in patients with hemorrhagic[18] and septic shock.[19] Lactic acid traditionally is viewed as the predominant source of metabolic acidosis occurring in sepsis.[20] In this view, lactic acid is released primarily from the musculature and the gut as a consequence of tissue hypoxia. Moreover, the amount of lactate produced is felt to correlate with the total oxygen debt, the magnitude of the hypoperfusion, and the severity of shock.[17] In recent years this view has been challenged by the observations that during sepsis, even with profound shock, resting muscle does not produce lactate. Indeed, studies by various investigators have shown that the musculature actually may consume lactate during endotoxemia.[21–23] Data concerning the gut are less clear. There is little question that underperfused gut can release lactate; however, it does not appear that the gut releases lactate during sepsis if its perfusion is maintained. Under such conditions, the mesentery is either neutral to or even takes up lactate.[21,22] Perfusion is likely to be a major determinant of mesenteric lactate metabolism. In a canine model of sepsis using endotoxin, gut lactate production could not be shown when flow was maintained with dopexamine hydrochloride.[23]

It is interesting to note that studies in animals as well as humans have shown that the lung may be a prominent source of lactate in the setting of acute lung injury.[21,24–26] While studies such as these do not address the underlying pathophysiologic mechanisms of hyperlactatemia in sepsis, they do suggest that the conventional wisdom regarding lactate as evidence of tissue dysoxia is an oversimplification at best. Indeed, many investigators have begun to offer alternative interpretations of hyperlactatemia in this setting,[25–29] including metabolic dysfunction from mitochondrial to enzymatic derangements, which can and do lead to lactic acidosis. In particular, pyruvate dehydrogenase (PDH), the enzyme responsible for moving pyruvate into the Krebs cycle, is inhibited by endotoxin.[30] Catecholamine use, especially epinephrine, also results in lactic acidosis, presumably by stimulating cellular metabolism (e.g., increased hepatic glycolysis), and may be a common source of lactic acidosis in the ICU.[31,32] Interestingly, this phenomenon does not appear to occur with either dobutamine or norepinephrine[32] and does not appear to be related to decreased tissue perfusion.

Although controversy exists as to the source and interpretation of lactic acidosis in critically ill patients, there is no question about the ability of lactate accumulation to produce acidemia. Lactate is a strong ion by virtue of the fact that at a pH within the physiologic range it is almost completely dissociated (i.e., the pK_a of lactate is 3.9; at a pH of 7.4, 3162 ions are dissociated for every one that is not). Because the body can produce and dispose of lactate rapidly, it functions as one of the most dynamic components of the SID. Lactic acid therefore can produce significant acidemia. Virtually anywhere in the body, pH is above 6.0, and lactate behaves as a strong anion. Its generation decreases the SID and results in increased [H⁺].

KETOACIDOSIS

Another common cause of a metabolic acidosis with a positive AG or SIG is ketoacidosis. Ketones are formed by beta-oxidation of fatty acids, a process inhibited by insulin. In insulin-deficient states (e.g., diabetes), ketone formation may increase rapidly. This is so because severely elevated blood glucose concentrations produce an osmotic diuresis, and this may lead to volume contraction. This state is associated with elevated cortisol levels and catecholamine secretion, which further stimulate free fatty acid production.[33] In addition, increased glucagon, relative to insulin, leads to decreased malonyl coenzyme A and increased carnitine palmityl acyl transferase, the combination of which increases ketogenesis.

Ketone bodies include acetone, acetoacetate, and β-hydroxybutyrate. Both acetoacetate and β-hydroxybutyrate are strong anions at physiologic pH (pK_a = 3.8 and 4.8, respectively). Thus, like lactate, their presence decreases the SID and increases the [H⁺]. Ketoacidosis may result from diabetes (DKA) or alcohol (AKA). The diagnosis is established by measuring serum ketones. However, it is important to understand that the nitroprusside reaction used for this measurement only measures acetone and acetoacetate, not β-hydroxybutyrate. The state of measured ketosis depends on the ratio of acetoacetate to β-hydroxybutyrate. This ratio is low when lactic acidosis coexists with ketoacidosis because the reduced redox state of lactic acidosis favors production of β-hydroxybutyrate. In such circumstances, the apparent level of ketosis is small relative to the amount of acidosis and the elevation of the AG. There is also a risk of confusion during treatment of ketoacidosis because ketones, as measured by the nitroprusside reaction, may increase despite resolving acidosis. This occurs as a result of the rapid clearance of β-hydroxybutyrate with improvement in acid-base balance and without change in the measured level of ketosis. Furthermore, ketones may even appear to increase as β-hydroxybutyrate is converted to acetoacetate. Hence it is better to monitor success of therapy by pH and AG or SIG than by the assay of serum ketones.

The acidosis seen in AKA is usually less severe. The treatment consists of fluids and glucose rather than insulin.[34]

TABLE 77-2 Causes of an Increased AG (Na^+-Cl^--HCO_3^-)

Renal failure
Ketoacidosis
  Diabetic
  Alcoholic
  Starvation
  Change in AG (usually small AG)
Lactic acidosis
Toxins
  Methanol
  Ethylene glycol
  Salicylates
  Toluene
Critical illness*
Sodium with weak anions
Decreased cation
  Hypomagnesemia
  Hypokalemia
  Hypocalcemia
Alkalosis

*Unexplained anions have been found in critically ill and injured patients, especially those with sepsis and liver disease. The causative anions have not been identified.

Indeed, insulin is contraindicated because it may cause precipitous hypoglycemia.[35] Thiamine also must be given to avoid precipitating Wernicke's encephalopathy.

RENAL FAILURE

Although renal failure may produce a hyperchloremic metabolic acidosis, especially when chronic, the increase in sulfate and other acids frequently increases the AG and SIG. However, the increase is usually not large. Similarly, uncomplicated renal failure rarely produces severe acidosis except when it is accompanied by high rates of acid generation, such as from hypermetabolism.[36] In all cases, the SID is decreased and is expected to remain so unless some therapy is provided. Hemodialysis will permit the removal of sulfate and other ions and allow normal Na^+ and Cl^- balance to be restored, thus returning the SID to normal (or near normal). However, patients not yet requiring dialysis and those who are between treatments are often given other therapies to increase the SID.

$NaHCO_3$ is used as long as the plasma [Na^+] is not already elevated. Other options include Ca^{2+}, which usually requires replacement anyway. Ca^{2+} replacement cannot increase the SID much given the rather narrow range of ionized Ca^{2+} ($0.975 - 1.125$ mmol/L). Even though Ca^{2+} is a divalent cation, it is unreasonable to expect much effect on the SID by administering Ca^{2+}.

POISONS

Metabolic acidosis with an increased AG and SIG is a major feature of various types of drug and substance intoxications (Table 77-2; see also Chap. 102). Again, it is generally more important to recognize these disorders so that specific therapy can be provided than to treat the acid-base disorder itself.

MISCELLANEOUS AND UNKNOWN

Table 77-2 lists several commonly and not so commonly recognized causes of positive AG metabolic acidosis. It is important to recognize that unexplained anions have been found commonly in the plasma of critically ill and injured patients. The etiology or even identity of these anions has not been established, nor has the clinical significance.

Non–Anion-Gap (Hyperchloremic) Acidoses

Hyperchloremic metabolic acidosis occurs as a result of either the increase in Cl^- relative to strong cations, especially Na^+, or the loss of cations with retention of Cl^-. As seen in Fig. 77-1, these disorders can be separated by history and by examination of the urine [Cl^-]. When acidosis occurs, the normal response by the kidney is to increase Cl^- excretion. Failure to do so identifies the kidney as the source of acidosis. Extrarenal hyperchloremic acidoses occur as a result of exogenous Cl^- loads (iatrogenic acidosis) or because strong cations (Na^+ or K^+) are lost from the lower gastrointestinal tract disproportionally to the loss of strong anions (Cl^-).

FIGURE 77-1 Differential diagnosis for a hyperchloremic metabolic acidosis. *(Used with permission from Kellum JA: Diagnosis and treatment of acid-base disorders, in Grenvik A,*

Shoemaker PK, Ayers S, et al (eds): Textbook of Critical Care. Philadelphia, Saunders, 1999, Chap 76, p 839.)

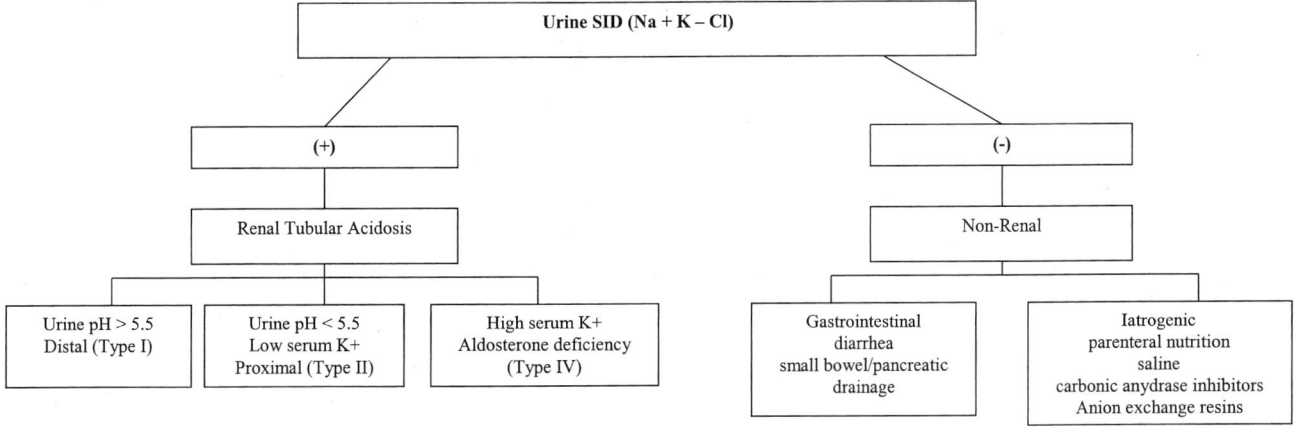

RENAL TUBULAR ACIDOSIS

Examination of the urine and plasma electrolytes and pH and calculation of the urine SIDa allow one to correctly diagnose most cases of renal tubular acidosis (RTA)[37] (see Fig. 77-1). However, caution must be exercised when the plasma pH is greater than 7.35 because this may turn off urine Cl^- excretion. In such circumstances it may be necessary to infuse sodium sulfate or furosemide. These agents stimulate Cl^- and K^+ excretion and may be used to unmask the defect and to probe K^+ secretory capacity.

The mechanisms of RTA are not well established. It is likely that much of the confusion has occurred as a result of attempting to understand the physiology from the point of view of regulating $[H^+]$ and $[HCO_3^-]$. However, as we have discussed, this is simply inconsistent with the principles of physical chemistry. The kidney does not excrete H^+ any more as NH_4^+ than it does as H_2O. The purpose of renal ammoniagenesis is to allow the excretion of Cl^-, which balances the charge of NH_4^+. The defect in all types of RTA is the inability to excrete Cl^- in proportion to Na^+, although the reasons vary by type. Treatment is largely dependent on whether the kidney will respond to mineralocorticoid replacement or there is loss of Na^+ that can be replaced as $NaHCO_3$.

Classic distal (type I) RTA responds to $NaHCO_3$ replacement, and generally 50 to 100 mEq/d is required. K^+ defects are also common in this type of RTA, and K^+ replacement is also required. A variant of the classic distal RTA is a hyperkalemic form, which is actually more common than the classic type. The central defect here appears to be impaired Na^+ transport in the cortical collecting duct. These patients also respond to $NaHCO_3$ replacement. Proximal (type II) RTA is characterized by both Na^+ and K^+ reabsorption defects. The disorder is uncommon and usually part of the Fanconi syndrome, where reabsorption of glucose, phosphate, urate, and amino acids is also impaired. Treatment of this disorder with $NaHCO_3$ is ineffective because increased ion delivery merely results in increased excretion. Thiazide diuretics have been used to treat this disorder with varying success.

Type IV RTA is caused by aldosterone deficiency or resistance. This disorder is diagnosed by the high serum K^+ and low urine pH (< 5.5). Treatment is usually most effective if the cause can be removed. The most common causes are drugs such as nonsteroidal anti-inflammatory agents, heparin, or potassium-sparing diuretics. Occasionally, mineralocorticoid replacement is required.

GASTROINTESTINAL ACIDOSIS

Fluid secreted into the gut lumen contains higher amounts of Na^+ than Cl^-, similar to the differences in plasma. Extremely large losses of these fluids, particularly if volume is replaced with fluids containing equal amounts of Na^+ and Cl^-, will result in a decrease in the plasma $[Na^+]$ relative to $[Cl^-]$ and a decrease in the SID.

IATROGENIC ACIDOSIS

Two of the most common causes of a hyperchloremic metabolic acidosis are iatrogenic, and both are due to administration of chloride. Modern parenteral nutrition formulas contain weak anions such as acetate in addition to Cl^-, and the balance of each anion can be adjusted depending on

the acid-base status of the patient. If sufficient amounts of weak anions are not provided, the plasma $[Cl^-]$ will increase, decreasing the SID and resulting in acidosis. As already discussed, administration of normal saline can cause a decrease in the SID and, subsequently, an acidosis.

METABOLIC ALKALOSIS

Metabolic alkalosis occurs as a result of an increased SID. This may occur secondary to losses of anions (e.g., Cl^- from the stomach) or increases in cations (rare). Metabolic alkaloses can be divided into those in which Cl^- losses are temporary and can be effectively replaced (chloride-responsive) and those in which hormonal mechanisms produce ongoing losses that can, at best, be offset temporarily by Cl^- administration (chloride-resistant) (Fig. 77-2). Similar to hyperchloremic acidosis, these disorders can be distinguished by examination of the urine $[Cl^-]$. Although much more investigation has focused on acidosis, alkalosis appears to be associated with poor prognosis as well. In a prospective study, Anderson and Henrich[38] looked at 409 patients with an arterial pH of greater than 7.48. Of these patients, 213 were medical and 196 were surgical. Overall, hospital mortality was 27.9% and increased as pH values rose, reaching 48.5% when the pH was greater than 7.60. While only 2% had pure metabolic alkalosis, patients at greatest risk were those with a mixed respiratory and metabolic alkalosis, having a mortality of 44.2%.

Chloride-Responsive Disorders

These disorders usually occur as a result of Cl^- losses from the stomach, such as from vomiting or gastric drainage. The treatment involves lowering the SID, by giving NaCl (since serum $[Cl^-]$ will rise greater than serum $[Na^+]$), KCl, or even HCl (which is most potent because it contains only strong anions). Saline plus KCl is usually the treatment of choice because volume depletion usually coexists with these disorders. Volume depletion, in turn, stimulates aldosterone secretion, which results in Na^+ reabsorption and the loss of K^+ and Cl^-.

Diuretics and other forms of volume contraction produce metabolic alkalosis predominantly by stimulating aldosterone, as discussed earlier. However, diuretics also induce K^+ and Cl^- excretion directly, further complicating the problem and inducing metabolic alkalosis more rapidly.

Chloride-Resistant Disorders

These disorders (see Fig. 77-2) are characterized by an increased urine $[Cl^-]$ (>20 mmol/L) and are said to be chloride-resistant because of ongoing Cl^- losses. Most commonly, this occurs as a result of increased mineralocorticoid activity. Treatment requires that the underlying disorder be addressed.

Other Causes of Metabolic Alkalosis

Rarely, an increased SID (and therefore metabolic alkalosis) occurs secondary to cation administration rather than anion depletion. Examples of these disorders include milk-alkali syndrome and intravenous administration of strong cations

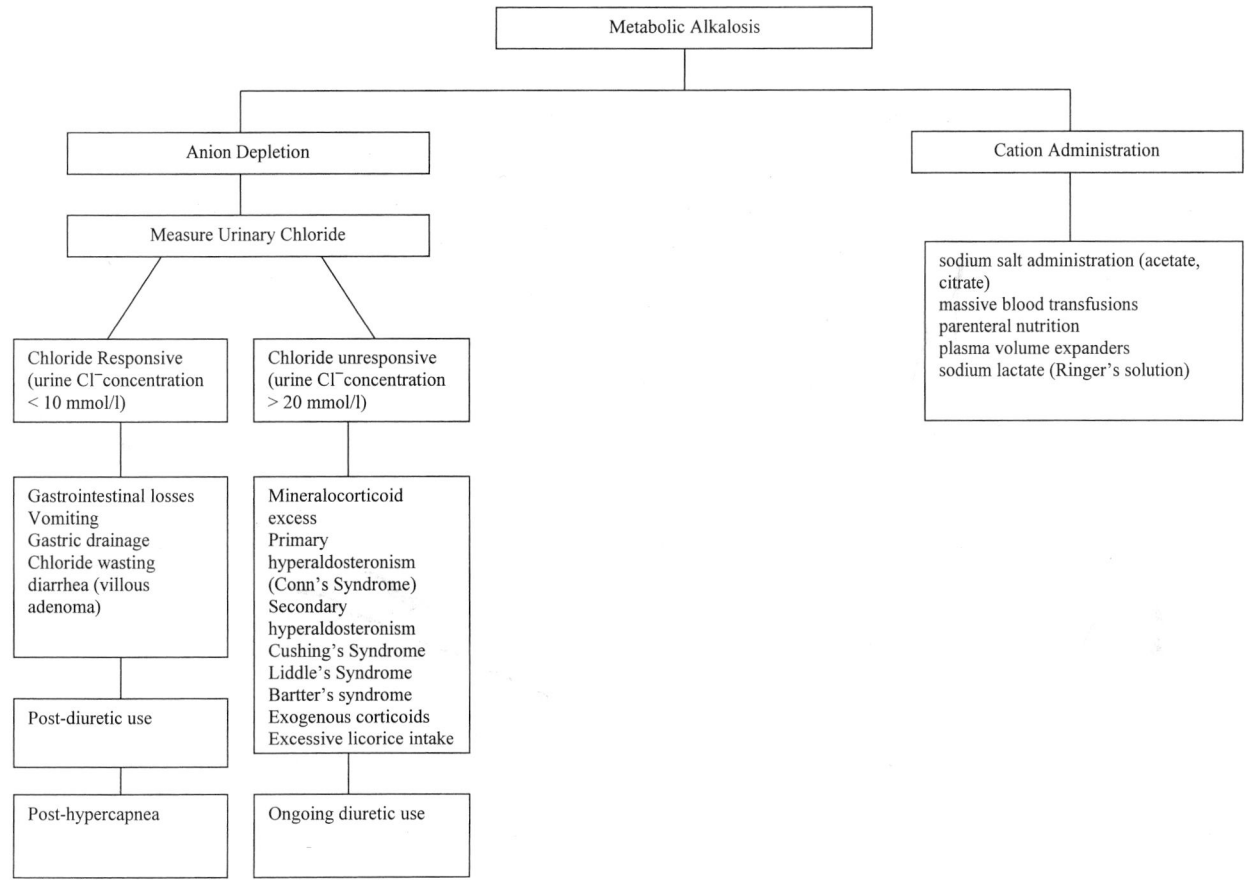

FIGURE 77-2 Differential diagnosis algorithm for metabolic alkalosis (increased SID).

without strong anions. The latter occurs with massive blood transfusion or plasma exchange because Na^+ is given with citrate (a weak anion) instead of Cl^-. Similar results occur when parenteral nutrition formulations contain too much acetate and not enough Cl^- to balance the Na^+ load.

Respiratory Acid-Base Disorders

PATHOPHYSIOLOGY OF RESPIRATORY ACID-BASE DISORDERS

CO_2 production by the body (at 220 mL/min) is equal to 15,000 mM/day of carbonic acid.[39] This compares with less than 500 mM/day (depending on diet) for all nonrespiratory acids, which are managed by the kidney and gut. Pulmonary ventilation is adjusted by the respiratory center in response to signals from P_{CO_2}, pH and P_{O_2}, as well as some from exercise, anxiety, and wakefulness. The normal P_{CO_2} of 40 mm Hg is attained by a precise match of alveolar ventilation to metabolic CO_2 production. P_{CO_2} changes in a "compensatory" ventilatory response to altered arterial pH produced by metabolic acidosis or alkalosis in predictable ways.

DISEASES OF VENTILATORY IMPAIRMENT

As for virtually all acid-base disorders, treatment begins with addressing the underlying disorder. Acute respiratory acidosis can be caused by CNS suppression, neuromuscular disease or impairment (e.g., myasthenia gravis, hypophosphatemia/

hypokalemia), severe mechanical derangements of the chest wall, or airway and parenchymal lung disease (e.g., asthma, acute respiratory distress syndrome [ARDS], etc.). This last category of conditions also produces primary hypoxia, not just alveolar hypoventilation. The two can be distinguished by the alveolar gas equation:

$$P_{A_{O_2}} = P_{I_{O_2}} - P_{CO_2}/R$$

where R is the respiratory exchange coefficient (generally taken as 0.8), $P_{I_{O_2}}$ is the inspired oxygen tension (room air is approximately 150 mm Hg), and $P_{A_{O_2}}$ is the alveolar P_{O_2}. Thus, as P_{CO_2} increases the $P_{A_{O_2}}$ will decrease in a predictable fashion. If the $P_{a_{O_2}}$ is significantly lower than the calculated $P_{A_{O_2}}$, there is a defect in gas exchange.

Chronic respiratory acidosis is caused most often by chronic lung disease (e.g., chronic obstructive pulmonary disease [COPD]) or chest wall disease (e.g., kyphoscoliosis). Rarely, its cause is central hypoventilation or chronic neuromuscular disease.

RESPIRATORY ALKALOSIS

Respiratory alkalosis may be the most frequently encountered acid-base disorder. It occurs in residents at high altitude and in a number of pathologic conditions, the most important of which include salicylate intoxication, early sepsis, hepatic failure, and hypoxic respiratory disorders. Respiratory alkalosis also occurs with pregnancy and with pain or anxiety.

Hypocapnia appears to be a particularly bad prognostic indicator in patients with critical illness.[40] As in acute respiratory acidosis, acute respiratory alkalosis results in a small change in [HCO_3^-], as dictated by the Henderson-Hasselbalch equation. If hypocapnia persists, the SID will begin to decrease as a result of renal Cl^- reabsorption. After 2 to 3 days, the SID will assume a new, lower steady state.[41] Severe alkalemia is unusual in respiratory alkalosis, and management therefore is directed to the underlying cause of the acid-base disorder. Typically, these mild acid-base changes are more important clinically as an alarm than as any threat they pose to the patient.

References

1. Stewart PA: *How to Understand Acid-Base: A Quantitative Acid-Base Primer for Biology and Medicine.* New York, Elsevier, 1981.
2. Laffey JG, Kavanagh BP: Carbon dioxide and the critically ill: Too little of a good thing? *Lancet* 354:1283, 1999.
3. Forsythe SM, Schmidt GA: Sodium bicarbonate for the treatment of lactic acidosis. *Chest* 117:260, 2000.
4. Laffey JG, Engelberts D, Kavanagh BP: Injurious effects of hypocapnic alkalosis in the isolated lung. *Am J Respir Crit Care Med* 162:399, 2000.
5. Pedoto A, Caruso JE, Nandi J: Acidosis stimulates nitric oxide production and lung damage in rats. *Am J Respir Crit Care Med* 159:397, 1999.
6. Pedoto A, Nandi J, Oler A, et al: Role of nitric oxide in acidosis-induced intestinal injury in anesthetized rats. *J Lab Clin Med* 138:270, 2001.
7. Kellum JA: Fluid resuscitation and hyperchloremic acidosis in experimental sepsis: Improved survival and acid-base balance with a synthetic colloid in a balanced electrolyte solution compared to saline. *Crit Care Med* 30:300, 2002.
8. Kellum JA, Song M, Venkataraman R: Effects of hyperchloremic acidosis on arterial pressure and circulating inflammatory molecules in experimental sepsis. *Chest* 125:243, 2004.
9. Kellum JA, Bellomo R, Kramer DJ, Pinsky MR: Splanchnic buffering of metabolic acid during early endotoxemia. *J Crit Care* 12:7, 1997.
10. Kellum JA: Determinants of blood pH in health and disease. *Crit Care* 4:6, 2000.
11. Bourke E, Haussinger D: pH homeostasis: The conceptual change, in Berlin GM (ed): *The Kidney Today: Selected Topics in Renal Science.* Basel, Karger, 1992, p 58.
12. Oliver J, Bourke E: Adaptations in urea and ammonium excretion in metabolic acidosis in the rat: A reinterpretation. *Clin Sci Mol Med* 48: 515, 1975.
13. Figge J, Jabor A, Kazda A, Fencl V: Anion gap and hypoalbuminemia. *Crit Care Med* 26:1807, 1998.
14. Singer RB, Hastings AB: An improved clinical method for the estimation of disturbances of the acid-base balance of human blood. *Medicine* 27:223, 1948.
15. Narins RG, Emmett M: Simple and mixed acid-base disorders: A practical approach. *Medicine* 59:161, 1980.
16. Narins RG, Jones ER, Townsend R, et al: Metabolic acid-base disorders: Pathophysiology, classification and treatment, in Arieff AI, DeFronzo RA (eds): *Fluid Electrolyte and Acid-Base Disorders.* New York, Churchill Livingstone, 1985, p 269.
17. Mizock BA, Falk JL: Lactic acidosis in critical illness. *Crit Care Med* 20:80, 1992.
18. Weil MH, Afifi AA: Experimental and clinical studies on lactate and pyruvate as indicators of the severity of acute circulatory failure (shock). *Circulation* 41:989, 1970.
19. Blair E: Acid-base balance in bacteremic shock. *Arch Intern Med* 127:731, 1971.
20. Madias NE: Lactic acidosis. *Kidney Int* 29:752, 1986.
21. Bellomo R, Kellum JA, Pinsky MR: Visceral lactate fluxes during early endotoxemia in the dog. *Chest* 110:198, 1996.
22. Van Lambalgen AA, Runge HC, van den Bos GC, Thijs LG: Reginal lactate production in early canine endotoxin shock. *Am J Physiol* 254:E45, 1988.
23. Cain SM, Curtis SE: Systemic and regional oxygen uptake and delivery and lactate flux in endotoxic dogs infused with dopexamine. *Crit Care Med* 19:1552, 1991.
24. Brown S, Gutierrez G, Clark C, et al: The lung as a source of lactate in sepsis and ARDS. *J Crit Care* 11:2, 1996.
25. Kellum JA, Kramer DJ, Lee KH, et al: Release of lactate by the lung in acute lung injury. *Chest* 1111:1301, 1997.
26. De Backer D, Creteur J, Zhang H, et al: Lactate production by the lungs in acute lung injury. *Am J Resp Cirt Care Med* 156:1099, 1997.
27. Stacpoole PW: Lactic acidosis and other mitochondrial disorders. *Metab Clin Exp* 46:306, 1997.
28. Fink MP: Does tissue acidosis in spesis indicate tissue hypoperfusion? *Intensive Care Med* 22:1144, 1996.
29. Guitierrez G, Wolf ME: Lactic acidosis in sepsis: A commentary. *Intensive Care Med* 22:6, 1996.
30. Kilpatrick-Smith L, Dean J, Erecinska M, Silver IA: Cellular effects of endotoxin in vitro: II. Reversibility of endotoxic damage. *Circ Shock* 11:101, 1983.
31. Bearn AG, Billing B, Sherlock S: The effect of adrenaline and noradrenaline on hepatic blood flow and splanchnic carbohydrate metabolism in man. *J Physiol* 115:430, 1951.
32. Levy B, Bollaert P-E, Charpentier C, et al: Comparison of norepinephrine and dobutamine to epinephrine for hemodynamics, lactate metabolism, and gastric tonometric variables in septic shock: A prospective, randomized study. *Intensive Care Med* 23:282, 1997.
33. Alberti KGMM: Diabetic emergencies. *Br Med J* 45:242, 1989.
34. Fulop M: Alcoholic ketoacidosis. *Endocrinol Metab Clin North Am* 22:209, 1993.
35. Wrenn KD, Slovis CM, Minion GE, Rutkowski R: The syndrome of alcoholic ketoacidosis. *Am J Med* 91:119, 1991.
36. Widmer B, Gerhardt RE, Harrington JT, Cohen JJ: Serum electrolyte and acid-ase composition: The influence of graded degrees of chronic renal failure. *Arch Intern Med* 139:1099, 1979.
37. Battle DC, Hizon M, Cohen E, et al: The use of the urine anion gap in the diagnosis of hyperchloremic metabolic acidosis. *N Engl J Med* 318:594, 1988.
38. Anderson LE, Henrich WL: Alkalemia-associated morbidity and mortality in medical and surgical patients. *South Med J* 80:729, 1987.
39. Gattinoni L, Lissoni A: Respiratory acid-base disturbances in patients with critical illness, in Ronco C, Bellomo R (eds): *Critical Care Nephrology.* Dordrecht, The Netherlands, Kluwer Academic Publishers, 1998, p 297.
40. Gennari FJ, Kassirer JP: Respiratory alkalosis, in Cohen JJ, Kassirer JP (eds): *Acid-Base.* Boston, Little, Brown, 1982, p 349.
41. Cohen JJ, Madias NE, Wolf CJ, Schwartz WB: Regulation of acid-base equilibrium in chronic hypocapnia: Evidence that the response of the kidney is not geared to the defense of extracellular [H^+]. *J Clin Invest* 57:1483, 1976.

Chapter 78

DIABETIC KETOACIDOSIS, HYPERGLYCEMIC HYPEROSMOLAR NONKETOTIC COMA, AND HYPOGLYCEMIA

JOHN B. BUSE
KENNETH S. POLONSKY

KEY POINTS

- *Diabetic ketoacidosis (DKA), hyperglycemic hyperosmolar nonketotic coma (HHNC), and hypoglycemia are life-threatening disorders of glucose metabolism.*

- *Altered glucose metabolism should be considered in the differential diagnosis of all patients with mental status changes, neurologic deficits, and severe illness.*

- *Therapy of DKA and HHNC requires replacement of deficits of fluids, electrolytes, and insulin.*

- *Mixed-anion-gap acidosis and hyperosmolarity are encountered often in the same patient.*

- *Continuous insulin therapy is essential in DKA.*

- *In DKA and HHNC, careful physical examination and laboratory follow-up with a flow sheet make it possible to prevent the disastrous consequences of aggressive therapy—cerebral edema, pulmonary edema, hypoglycemia, hypokalemia, and hyperchloremic metabolic acidosis.*

- *A search for the underlying cause of metabolic decompensation is required.*

- *Therapy of hypoglycemia requires immediate establishment and maintenance of modest hyperglycemia (glucose concentration above 100 mg/dL or 5.5 mmol/L).*

Diabetes mellitus and its major life-threatening complications—diabetic ketoacidosis (DKA), hyperglycemic hyperosmolar nonketotic coma (HHNC), and hypoglycemia—may precipitate or complicate critical illness. This chapter will focus on the management of DKA because it has been studied more exhaustively and because the same principles are applicable to HHNC. A brief review of the physiology and therapy of hypoglycemia will follow. These conditions have been the subject of other reviews.[1-9a,9b,9c]

Pathophysiology of Diabetic Emergencies

Currently, most patients with diabetes can be classified as having either type 1 diabetes (previously known as *juvenile-onset, ketosis-prone, insulin-dependent,* or *brittle diabetes*) or type 2 diabetes (previously, *adult-onset, non-ketosis-prone, non-insulin-dependent,* or *obesity-related diabetes*). Type 1

diabetes results from the autoimmune destruction of the insulin-secreting β cells in the pancreas, with consequent insulin deficiency. Most persons with type 1 diabetes present in childhood or early adulthood, although well-documented cases also have been described in the geriatric population. Hyperglycemia is usually not present until approximately 90% of insulin secretory capacity is lost. In times of stress (either physiologic or emotional), however, insulin requirements increase and often precipitate metabolic decompensation because of inadequate insulin secretory reserve. Patients with insulin deficiency require insulin therapy for survival. The half-life of insulin in the circulation is 7 minutes, and therapy for insulin deficiency requires continuous delivery of insulin to the circulation by infusion or by diffusion of insulin from depot injections.

The pathophysiology of type 2 diabetes is more heterogeneous. At presentation, persons with type 2 diabetes exhibit both tissue resistance to the action of insulin and a relative deficiency of insulin secretion. Insulin resistance can be overcome only by (1) increasing circulating insulin concentrations, with insulin (often at high doses) or sulfonylureas, (2) imposing calorie restriction, (3) instituting exercise, (4) administering certain antidiabetic medications (metformin and thiazolidine diones), or (5) treating reversible causes of the disease (e.g., obesity; hyperglycemia; sepsis; uremia; catecholamine; excess levels of glucocorticoids, growth hormone, or thyroxine; and antibodies to insulin or to the insulin receptor). Most persons with type 2 diabetes present in middle age and are overweight and sedentary. There is a growing prevalence of the disorder in children and adolescents, as well as a less common familial adolescent form of the disease termed *maturity-onset diabetes of youth* (MODY).

DKA is the life-threatening metabolic consequence of insulin deficiency. Insulin deficiency, in concert with excess secretion of glucagon (primarily), catecholamines, glucocorticoids, and growth hormone, produces hyperglycemia by stimulating glycogenolysis and gluconeogenesis and impairing glucose disposal. As has been elegantly demonstrated by Foster and McGarry,[10] this hormonal milieu also results in lipolysis and unrestrained fatty acid oxidation, producing acetone, β-hydroxybutyrate, and acetoacetate—and thus ketoacidosis.

HHNC is the most severe presentation of a syndrome in which insulin resistance and relative insulin deficiency produce hyperglycemia. The glucose remains largely in the extracellular space and shifts water osmotically from the intracellular compartment. Glucose, water, and salts are filtered at the glomerulus; because the reabsorptive capacity of the renal tubules for glucose has a maximum of approximately 200 mg/min, an osmotic diuresis occurs, with water lost in excess of salts. A vicious cycle of cellular dehydration and diuresis is produced that can only be compensated by adequate fluid intake. With inadequate fluid intake, hyperosmolarity and hypovolemia develop, further increasing insulin resistance and hyperglycemia.

Patients rarely fit purely insulin-deficient or insulin-resistant physiology, particularly when in extremis. Patients with type 1 diabetes whose disease is not well controlled or who are under stress are insulin-resistant. Patients with poorly controlled type 2 diabetes may become insulin-deficient through a process of β-cell exhaustion and present with DKA. In fact, when careful studies of insulin levels, secretory dynamics, and tissue sensitivity are performed, there is considerable overlap between patients with DKA and patients with HHNC. One of the keys to the management of these patients is recognizing the contributions of insulin deficiency and resistance and optimizing each patient's individual therapy.

DKA, HHNC, and Differential Diagnosis

Early in their course, patients with uncontrolled diabetes present with nonspecific complaints. If the disease follows an indolent course over months to years (more common for type 2 than for type 1 diabetes), patients can present with profound wasting, cachexia, and prostration similar in degree to that of patients with long-standing malignancy or chronic infection. With significant physical or emotional stress, sudden metabolic decompensation can occur.[10a] The cases of DKA and HHNC that are missed usually occur in patients with new-onset diabetes. All patients with nonspecific complaints should be questioned about more specific symptoms of diabetes. Polyuria (or at least nocturia) and weight loss are almost always present, although often not reported by the patient. Any patient with severe illness (acute or chronic) or neurologic changes should have glucose and electrolyte levels measured.

HISTORY AND PHYSICAL EXAMINATION

DKA and HHNC are easily recognized, when considered (Table 78-1). In DKA, metabolic decompensation develops over a period of hours to a few days. Patients with severe DKA classically present with lethargy and a characteristic hyperventilation pattern with deep, slow breaths (Kussmaul respiration) associated with the fruity odor of acetone. They often complain of nausea and vomiting; abdominal pain is somewhat less frequent. The abdominal pain can be quite severe and may be associated with distention, ileus, and tenderness without rebound, but it usually resolves relatively quickly with therapy unless there is underlying abdominal pathology. Most patients are normotensive, tachycardic, and tachypneic, with signs of mild to moderate volume depletion. Hypothermia has been described in DKA, and patients with underlying infection may not manifest fever. Cerebral edema does occur.

Patients with HHNC are usually stuporous, with obvious profound dehydration, and may demonstrate focal neurologic deficits, such as Babinski reflexes, asymmetric reflexes, cranial nerve findings, paresis, fasciculations, and aphasia. The syndrome evolves over days to weeks with a progressive decrease in fluid intake and decline in mental status; usually there is no prior history of diabetes. These patients are hypotensive and exhibit normal to depressed ventilation. Hypothermia, again, is common, although cerebral edema is rare.

LABORATORY TESTS AND DIFFERENTIAL DIAGNOSIS

Once DKA or HHNC is considered, the diagnosis can be made quickly with routine laboratory tests. DKA and HHNC need to be differentiated from each other and from the other causes of ketosis and metabolic acidosis. This is often quite difficult;

TABLE 78-1 Signs and Symptoms of Glucose Metabolism Disorders

Uncontrolled diabetes
  Polyuria
  Polyphagia
  Vaginitis
  Nocturia
  Weight loss
  Skin infection
  Thirst
  Blurred vision
  Fatigue
  Polydipsia
  Dizziness
  Malaise
Diabetic ketoacidosis
  Dyspnea
  Normotension
  Hypo- and hyperthermia
  Nausea
  Tachycardia
  Lethargy to coma
  Vomiting
  Tachypnea
  Fruity breath
  Abdominal pain
  Abdominal tenderness
  Orthostasis
  Cerebral edema
Hyperglycemic hyperosmolar nonketotic coma
  Dehydration
  Hypo- and hyperthermia
  Stupor to coma
  Dehydration
  Focal neurologic signs or seizures
  Shallow respiration
  Hypotension to shock

in fact, these disorders often coexist. Table 78-2 and the following discussion are provided to help in making the distinction. Blood and urine glucose and ketone levels can be obtained in minutes using glucose oxidase–impregnated strips and the nitroprusside reaction, respectively.

The sine qua non of HHNC is hyperosmolarity. The osmolarity can be measured by freezing-point depression, or it can be estimated using the following formula:

$$\text{Osmolarity (mOsm/L)} = 2 \times [\text{sodium}] + [\text{glucose}]/18 + [\text{BUN}]/2.8 + [\text{ethanol}]/4.6 \qquad (78\text{-}1)$$

where the concentrations of glucose, blood urea nitrogen (BUN), and ethanol are in milligrams per deciliter, and the concentration of sodium is in milliequivalents per liter. In HHNC, the osmolarity generally is greater than 350 mOsm/L and can exceed 400 mOsm/L. The serum sodium and potassium levels can be high, normal, or low and do not reflect total body levels, which are uniformly depleted. The glucose concentration is usually greater than 600 mg/dL (33.3 mmol/L), and levels over 1000 mg/dL (55.6 mmol/L) are quite common. In pure HHNC, there is usually no significant metabolic acidosis or anion gap. However, severe anion-gap metabolic acidosis of uncertain etiology has been reported in HHNC.[11]

TABLE 78-2 Means of Distinguishing HHNC, DKA, and Other Causes of Metabolic Acidosis

	HHNC	DKA	Lactate	Starvation	Uremia	Rhabdomyolysis	Ethanol	Methanol	Ethylene Glycol	Salicylate
Glucose level	++++	+++	0	0	0	0	−,+	0	0	0,−,+
Ketones	0,+	++++	0	+	0	0	+++	0	0	0,++
pH	0,−	−−−−	−−−−	−	−−	−−−−	−−−	−−−	−−−	−−−
Anion gap	0,+	++++	++++	+	+	+	+++	++	++	++
Osmolarity	++++	++	0	0	+	++	+	++	++	+

NOTE: 0 = normal levels; + = increased levels; − = decreased levels; scale ranges from mild (+, −) to extreme (+ + ++, − − −−).

The sine qua non of DKA is ketoacidosis. As mentioned earlier, two ketoacids are produced in DKA—β-hydroxybutyrate and acetoacetate—as well as the neutral ketone acetone. The nitroprusside reaction commonly used to detect ketone bodies detects acetoacetate much better than acetone and does not react with β-hydroxybutyrate at all. Particularly in severe DKA, β-hydroxybutyrate is the predominant ketone, and it is possible, though unusual, to have a negative serum nitroprusside reaction in the face of severe ketosis. β-Hydroxybutyrate levels can be measured at many centers and commercially, but this service usually is not readily available. Fortunately, there is a readily available index for unmeasured anions in the blood—namely, the anion gap (normally less than 14 mEq/L):

$$\text{Anion gap} = [\text{sodium}] - [\text{chloride}] - [\text{bicarbonate}] \quad (78\text{-}2)$$

Most persons with DKA present with an anion gap greater than 20 mEq/L, and some have an anion gap greater than 40 mEq/L. However, some patients have a hyperchloremic metabolic acidosis without a significant anion gap.[12] Patients with DKA almost invariably have large amounts of ketones in their urine. The serum glucose level in DKA is usually about 500 mg/dL (27.8 mmol/L). However, an entity known as *euglycemic DKA* has been described, particularly in the presence of decreased oral intake or pregnancy, where the serum glucose level is normal or near normal, but the patient requires insulin therapy for the clearance of ketoacidosis.[13] The arterial pH is commonly less than 7.3 and can be as low as 6.5. There is partial respiratory compensation with hypocapnia. Patients are often mildly hyperosmolar, although osmolalities greater than 330 mOsm/kg are unusual without mental status changes.

Not all patients with hyperglycemia and an anion gap metabolic acidosis will have DKA. Lactic acidosis is the most common cause of metabolic acidosis in hospitalized patients and can be seen in uncomplicated diabetes, as well as in DKA and HHNC. Lactic acidosis usually occurs in the setting of decreased tissue oxygen delivery, resulting in the nonoxidative metabolism of glucose to lactic acid. Lactic acidosis complicates other primary metabolic acidoses as a consequence of dehydration or shock. Thus, assessing its relative contribution can be difficult. The presentation is identical to that seen in DKA. In pure lactic acidosis, the serum glucose and ketone levels should be normal, and the serum lactate concentration should be greater than 5 mM. The therapy of lactic acidosis is directed at the underlying cause and at optimizing tissue perfusion.[14]

Starvation ketosis results from inadequate carbohydrate availability, resulting in physiologically appropriate lipolysis and ketone production to provide fuel substrates for muscle. The blood glucose level usually is normal. Although the urine can have large amounts of ketones, the blood rarely does. Usually the arterial pH is normal, and the anion gap is at most mildly elevated.

Alcoholic ketoacidosis is a more severe form of starvation ketosis wherein the appropriate ketogenic response to poor carbohydrate intake is increased through as yet poorly defined effects of alcohol on the liver. Classically, these patients are long-standing alcoholics for whom ethanol has been the main caloric source for days to weeks. The ketoacidosis manifests itself when, for whatever reason, the intake of alcohol and calories decreases. In isolated alcoholic ketoacidosis, the metabolic acidosis is usually mild to moderate in severity. The anion gap is elevated. Serum and urine ketones are always present. However, alcoholic ketoacidosis produces an even higher ratio of β-hydroxybutyrate to acetoacetate than does DKA, and negative or weakly positive serum nitroprusside reactions are common. Respiratory alkalosis associated with delirium tremens, agitation, or pulmonary processes often normalizes the pH but the underlying acidosis should be evident with careful analysis of acid-base status. Usually the patient is normoglycemic or hypoglycemic; sometimes mild hyperglycemia is present. Patients who are significantly hyperglycemic should be treated as if they had DKA. The therapy of alcoholic ketoacidosis consists of administration of thiamine, carbohydrates, fluids, and electrolytes, with special attention to the more severe consequences of alcohol toxicity, alcohol withdrawal, and chronic malnutrition. In more severely ill patients in whom alcoholic ketoacidosis is considered a possibility, there is usually another underlying illness, such as pancreatitis, gastrointestinal bleeding, hepatic encephalopathy, delirium tremens, or infection complicated by coexisting lactic acidosis.[15]

Uremic acidosis is characterized by very large elevations in the BUN level and the creatinine level with normoglycemia. The pH and anion gap are usually only mildly abnormal. The treatment is supportive, with careful attention to fluid and electrolytes until dialysis can be performed. Rhabdomyolysis is a cause of renal failure in which the anion gap can be elevated significantly and acidosis can be severe. There should be marked elevation of creatine phosphokinase (CPK) and myoglobin levels. It should be noted that mild rhabdomyolysis is not uncommon in DKA, but the presence of hyperglycemia and ketonemia leaves no doubt as to the primary etiology of the acidosis.[16]

Toxic ingestions can be differentiated from DKA by history and laboratory investigation. *Salicylate intoxication* can produce an anion-gap metabolic acidosis, usually with a respiratory alkalosis. The plasma glucose level is normal or low and the osmolality normal, and salicylates are detected in the urine or blood. Salicylate uncouples oxidative phosphorylation; consequently, ketonemia and lactic acidosis develop. It should be noted that salicylates can cause a false-positive glucose determination when the cupric sulfate method is used and a false-negative result when the glucose oxidase reaction is used. *Methanol* and *ethylene glycol* also produce an anion gap metabolic acidosis without hyperglycemia or ketones; they need to be kept in mind primarily because they produce an increase in the measured serum osmolality but not in the calculated serum osmolality—an *osmolar gap*. Their serum levels also can be measured. *Isopropyl alcohol* does not cause a metabolic acidosis, but it needs to be borne in mind because it is metabolized to acetone, which can produce a positive result on the nitroprusside reaction commonly used for the detection of ketoacids. Therapy of these intoxications is discussed elsewhere[17-19] (see Chap. 102). Rare cases of anion gap acidoses have been reported with other ingestions, including toluene, iron, hydrogen sulfide, nalidixic acid, papaverine, paraldehyde, strychnine, and isoniazid.

It should be remembered that patients often present with combinations of the preceding conditions. As already noted, DKA not uncommonly appears with hyperosmolarity and coma. HHNC can have mild to moderate ketonemia and acidosis. Alcoholic ketoacidosis can contribute to either DKA or HHNC, and lactic acidosis is common in severe DKA and HHNC. We believe that any patient with hyperglycemia above 250 mg/dL (13.9 mmol/L) and an anion gap metabolic acidosis should be treated according to the general principles outlined below, with special consideration for possible other contributing metabolic acidoses (see Chaps. 77 and 102).

Therapy

The optimal management of DKA and HHNC has been the object of considerable controversy over the past half century. The guidelines we propose rely heavily on prospective studies of DKA treatment by Kitabchi and coworkers[1] and are readily applicable to HHNC. The general approach (Table 78-3) is (1) to provide necessary fluids to restore the circulation, (2) to treat insulin deficiency with continuous insulin, (3) to treat electrolyte disturbances, (4) to follow the patient closely and carefully, and (5) to search for underlying causes of metabolic decompensation.

FLUIDS

Volume contraction is one of the hallmarks of DKA and HHNC. It can contribute to acidosis via lactic acid production, as well as decreased renal clearance of organic and inorganic acids. It contributes to hyperglycemia by decreasing renal clearance of glucose. If decreased tissue perfusion is significant, it causes insulin resistance by decreasing the delivery of insulin to the sites of insulin-mediated glucose disposal—muscle and adipose tissue—as well as by stimulating catecholamine and glucocorticoid secretion. Fluid deficits on the order of 5 to 10 L are common in DKA and HHNC. It should be remembered that the urine produced during the osmotic diuresis of hyperglycemia is approximately half normal with respect to sodium content. Therefore, water deficits are in excess of sodium deficits. Historically, large quantities of isotonic intravenous fluids have been administered rapidly to patients in DKA or HHNC. We tend to be more cautious;

TABLE 78-3 Treatment of Severe Disorders of Glucose Metabolism

Diabetic ketoacidosis
 Fluids (usual deficit, 5–10 L)
  If hypotensive: 1 L normal saline in the first few minutes; repeat as needed to restore the circulation, and consider invasive hemodynamic monitoring
  If normotensive: 1 L 0.45% NaCl in first hour
  In subsequent hours:
   Match urine output with 0.45% NaCl; in addition, provide 100–500 mL/h 0.45% NaCl
   Calculate free water deficit and replace 50% over 12 h with 5% dextrose in water
   After glucose reaches 250 mg/dL (13.9 mmol/L), add dextrose to IV fluids (~100 g/24 h)
 Insulin
  10-unit IV bolus
  0.1 units/(kg · h), IV or IM
  Check glucose hourly, and adjust drip to decrease glucose by 10% or 50 mg/dL (2.8 mmol/L) hourly to a level of 250 mg/dL (13.9 mmol/L)
 Potassium (usual deficit, 200–1000 mEq)
  Establish that the patient is not oliguric
  ECG monitoring for hyperkalemia and hypokalemia
  If hyperkalemic, follow hourly
  If normokalemic, 10–20 mEq/h
  If hypokalemic, 20–40 mEq/h; delay insulin if K < 3.3 mEq/L
  Administer two-thirds as chloride and one-third as phosphate salts
 Bicarbonate
  None is generally indicated
  Consider administering NaHCO₃ 1 mEq/kg IV for pH < 6.9
  May be useful for treatment of hyperkalemia
  Search for underlying cause
  Monitor:
   ECG
   Vital signs
   Hourly: glucose and electrolyte levels
   Every 2–4 h: calcium, magnesium, phosphate
   Every 6–24 h: BUN, creatinine, ketones
Hyperglycemic hyperosmolar nonketotic coma (HHNC)
 HHNC should be treated like DKA, although patients generally will require more fluids and less insulin

for patients with a history of congestive heart failure, chronic or acute renal failure, severe hypotension, or significant pulmonary disease, we give early and frequent consideration to the use of invasive hemodynamic montoring.

When there is physical evidence of dehydration—hypotension, decreased skin turgor, or dry mucous membranes—we generally administer 1 L of normal saline solution over the first few minutes and 200 to 500 mL/h in subsequent hours, until hypotension resolves and an adequate circulation is maintained. If hypotension is severe, with clinical evidence of hypoperfusion, and does not respond to crystalloid, then therapy with colloid is considered, often in combination with invasive hemodynamic monitoring. If there is no hypotension and no concern of renal failure, we administer 1 L of half-normal saline solution over the first hour and 100 to 500 mL/h in subsequent hours.

During that first hour, the results of initial laboratory tests usually are obtained and can be quite helpful in planning further therapy. Despite the excess of water losses over sodium, the measured sodium level is usually low because of the osmotic effects of glucose. These osmotic effects can be corrected using the following simple formula:

Corrected sodium concentration
$$= \text{measured [sodium]} + 0.016 \, ([\text{glucose in mg/dL}] - 100)$$
$$(78\text{-}3)$$

Severe hypertriglyceridemia, which is common in severe diabetes, can cause a false decrease in the serum sodium concentration by approximately 1.0 mEq/L at a serum lipid concentration of 460 mg/dL.[20] An estimated water deficit[21] can be calculated using the corrected sodium concentration:

$$\text{Water deficit in liters} = 0.6 \times (\text{body weight in kg})$$
$$\times (\text{corrected [Na+]} - 140) \div 140 \qquad (78\text{-}4)$$

Using these formulas, a 70-kg patient with a measured sodium level of 140 mEq/L and a glucose level of 1000 mg/dL would have a calculated water deficit of 4.3 L. If the patient is normotensive after the first liter of fluids, we provide generous maintenance fluids while the patient is NPO, replace urinary losses with one-half normal saline solution, and in addition, provide approximately one-half the calculated water deficit as 5% dextrose over the first 12 to 24 hours (using the preceding example, the amount would be 2 L) and the remainder over the subsequent 24 hours. The plan for fluid therapy should be reevaluated continuously in light of the clinical and laboratory response of the patient. Once the serum glucose level reaches 250 mg/dL (13.9 mmol/L), fluids should contain 5% dextrose, and therapy should be aimed at maintaining the serum glucose concentration in the 150 to 250 mg/dL (8.3–13.9 mmol/L) range for 24 hours to allow slow equilibration of osmotically active substances across cell membranes. At least 100 g of dextrose per 24 hours (at least 80 mL/h of 5% dextrose if the patient is NPO) must be given to prevent ketogenesis. In late pregnancy, approximately 100% more carbohydrate may be needed, so 10% dextrose should be used.

The primary goal of fluid therapy is to maintain adequate circulation, and the secondary goal is to maintain brisk diuresis. Beyond that, pulmonary edema, hyperchloremic metabolic acidosis, and a rapid fall in the serum osmolality should be avoided by frequent monitoring of the patient, the glucose level, and the electrolyte levels. It has been demonstrated that fluid administration and subsequent continued osmotic diuresis are responsible for a large portion of the initial decline in glucose during therapy. In general, persons with HHNC present with more profound dehydration and require more intravenous fluids than persons with DKA.

INSULIN

Insulin is the mainstay of therapy of DKA, which is essentially an insulin-deficient state. In the past, high doses of insulin (upwards of 50 units/h) were favored. In more recent studies, low-dose insulin therapy (0.1 unit/kg per hour) has been shown to be equally effective in producing a decrease in serum glucose concentration and effecting clearance of ketones. Furthermore, low-dose therapy results in a dramatic reduction in the major morbidity of intensive insulin therapy—hypoglycemia and hypokalemia.

Studies have also shown that intravenous (IV) insulin is significantly more effective than intramuscular (IM) or subcutaneous (SC) insulin in lowering ketone body concentration over the first 2 hours of therapy. The SC route is inappropriate for critically ill patients because of the possibility of tissue hypoperfusion and the slower kinetics of absorption. Numerous studies attest to the efficacy of IM therapy in severe DKA. In cases where there is insufficient nursing monitoring or IV access to allow for safe IV administration, hourly IM injections of regular insulin is an acceptable substitute. It is important that a needle of adequate length—at least 1.5 inches for adults—be used.

Last, it has been shown that the administration of a 10-unit IV priming dose of insulin, when a patient is being started on insulin therapy (whether IV or IM), significantly improves the glycemic response to the first hour of therapy. The rationale is to fully saturate insulin receptors before continuous therapy is started and thus to avoid the lag time necessary to achieve steady-state insulin levels. It seems to be possible to mix insulin into normal saline solution without adding albumin to prevent adsorption of insulin onto the infusion set. However, the IV tubing should be flushed with the insulin infusate prior to use.

In those rare instances where the glucose level does not decrease by at least 10%, or 50 mg/dL (2.8 mmol/L), in 1 hour, the insulin infusion rate should be increased, and a second bolus of IV insulin should be administered. As the glucose level decreases, it is usually necessary to decrease the rate of infusion. After the glucose level reaches approximately 250 mg/dL (13.9 mmol/L), it is prudent to decrease the insulin infusion rate and to administer dextrose as described under "Fluids" above. It is a common mistake to discontinue IV insulin in response to a falling glucose level. Because of its short half-life, IV insulin should not be discontinued until after SC insulin is initiated. With resolution of ketosis, the rate of insulin administration approaches the physiologic range of 0.5 to 1.0 units/kg per day.

If the patient is not nauseated, early feeding should be considered because it allows more carbohydrates and insulin to be administered, which accelerates the clearance of ketones. When the decision is made to feed the patient, the patient should be switched from IV or IM therapy to SC therapy. SC insulin should be administered before a meal, and the insulin drip should be discontinued approximately 30 minutes later if regular insulin is used, approximately 15 minutes later if a rapid-acting insulin analogue is used, and in 2 hours if only intermediate or long-acting insulin is used. The glucose level should be checked in 2 hours and at least every 4 hours subsequently, until a relatively stable insulin regimen is determined. Early conversion to oral feeding and SC insulin therapy has been associated with shorter length of hospital stay. A proportion of patients with HHNC do not require therapy for their diabetes after hospitalization, and most do not require insulin.

POTASSIUM

Potassium losses during the development of DKA and HHNC are usually quite high (3 to 10 mEq/kg) and are mediated by protein catabolism compounded by hyperaldosteronism and osmotic diuresis. Most persons with DKA or HHNC have normal or even high serum potassium levels at presentation, but the initial therapy with fluids and insulin will cause the serum potassium level to fall. Our approach has been to monitor the electrocardiogram (ECG) for signs of hyperkalemia (peaked T wave, QRS widening) initially and to administer potassium if these signs are absent and the serum potassium level is less than 5.5 mEq/L. If the patient is oliguric, we do not administer potassium unless the serum concentration is less than 4 mEq/L or if there are ECG signs of hypokalemia (U wave)—and even then, only with extreme caution. With therapy of DKA, the potassium level always falls, usually reaching a nadir after several hours. We usually replace potassium at 10 to 20 mEq/h, two-thirds as potassium chloride and one-third as potassium phosphate, and monitor serum levels at least every 2 hours initially, as well as following ECG morphology. Some patients with DKA who have had a protracted course including vomiting present with hypokalemia and acidosis; they may require 20 to 40 mEq/h or more by central line to avoid further decreases in the serum potassium concentration; consideration in these rare cases of delaying the initiation of insulin infusion until potassium concentrations are greater than 3.3 mEq/L may be prudent to avoid precipitating a further decline in serum potassium concentration.

PHOSPHATE

Like potassium, phosphate is depleted in patients with DKA and HHNC. Although patients usually present with an elevated serum phosphate level, the serum level declines with therapy. Although no well-documented clinical benefit of phosphate administration has been demonstrated, most authorities recommend phosphate therapy as above and monitoring for its possible complications—hypocalcemia and hypomagnesemia.

BICARBONATE

The serum bicarbonate level is always low in DKA, but no true deficiency is present because the ketoacid and lactate anions are metabolized to bicarbonate during therapy. The use of bicarbonate in the therapy of DKA is highly controversial; no benefit of bicarbonate therapy has been demonstrated in clinical trials. In fact, in two trials, hypokalemia was more common in bicarbonate-treated patients. There are theoretical considerations against the use of bicarbonate. Cellular levels of 2,3-diphosphoglycerate are depleted in DKA, causing a leftward shift in the oxyhemoglobin dissociation curve and thus impairing tissue oxygen extraction. Acidemia has the opposite effect; therefore, acute reversal of acidosis might decrease tissue oxygen extraction. In addition, there are in vitro data to suggest that pH is a regulator of cellular lactate metabolism and that correction of acidosis could increase lactate production. Most important, bicarbonate administration acutely elevates P_{CO_2}, which may lower intracellular pH. We do not administer bicarbonate routinely, but we understand that other authors advocate its use. Bicarbonate therapy should be restricted to (1) patients with severe acidosis (pH below 6.9), (2) patients with hemodynamic instability in whom the pH is less than 7.1, and (3) patients with hyperkalemia and ECG findings. When bicarbonate is used, it should be used sparingly as a temporizing measure while definitive therapy with insulin and fluids are under way. Approximately 1 mEq/kg of bicarbonate is administered as a rapid infu-

sion over 10 to 15 minutes, with further therapy based on repeat measurement of arterial blood gases every 30 to 120 minutes. Potassium therapy should be considered prior to treatment with bicarbonate because transient hypokalemia is a not uncommon complication of the administration of alkali.

MONITORING

It is possible to manage many cases of mild DKA without ICU admission, depending on staff availability. We routinely admit patients with DKA to the ICU if they have a pH below 7.2. If mental status is compromised, then prophylactic intubation is considered, and nasogastric suctioning is always performed because of frequent ileus and danger of aspiration. Only if the patient cannot void at will is bladder catheterization necessary to follow urine output adequately. ECG monitoring is continuous, with hourly documentation of QRS intervals as well as T-wave morphology. Initially, the levels of serum glucose, electrolytes, BUN, creatinine, calcium, magnesium, phosphate, ketone, lactate, and CPK are measured; liver function tests, urinalysis, ECG, upright chest x-ray, and a complete blood count (CBC) are performed; and arterial blood gases are measured. If there is any concern about possible toxic ingestions, toxicology screening is also performed. Subsequently, glucose and electrolyte levels are measured at least hourly; calcium, magnesium, and phosphate levels are measured every 2 hours; and the levels of BUN, creatinine, and ketones are measured every 6 to 24 hours. This frequency of laboratory analysis generally can be tapered as trends in improvement become clear; glucose monitoring using bedside point-of-care systems can be substituted for laboratory analysis of glucose if appropriate quality assurance and documentation programs are in place once glucose levels are in the 400 to 600 mg/dL (22–33 mmol/L) range. The urine ketone concentration is a more sensitive indicator of ongoing or recurrent hepatic ketogenesis than is the level of serum ketones. It is usually not necessary to routinely monitor arterial blood gases because bicarbonate and the anion gap are relatively good indices of the response to therapy. Monitoring venous pH also has been shown to adequately reflect acidemia and response to therapy. In severely ill patients with obvious underlying disease, the course is often more protracted; when venous access is a problem, early consideration should be given to placement of an arterial line. A flow sheet tabulating these findings, as well as mental status, vital signs, insulin dose, fluid and electrolytes administered, and urine output, allows easy analysis of response to therapy. Once the acidosis begins to resolve and the response to therapy becomes predictable, it is reasonable to curtail laboratory use. The goal should be to rapidly achieve hemodynamic stability and to fully correct DKA in 12 to 36 hours.

THE SEARCH FOR UNDERLYING CAUSES

After the patient is stabilized, a careful history and physical examination and a diagnostic strategy should be aimed at determining the precipitating event. In our practice, the most common cause of DKA is poor compliance with insulin therapy or inadequate outpatient insulin regimens; these causes usually are treated easily. The second most common cause is infection, with urinary tract infection, pelvic inflammatory disease, and respiratory tract infections predominating. It is often difficult to determine initially if the patient is infected. Fever is absent in a significant proportion of patients with diabetic emergencies. The white blood cell count (WBC) is not uncommonly elevated to the range of 20,000/μL or higher, even in the absence of infection.[21] We therefore perform cultures on most patients with DKA or HHNC, and we often treat empirically with antibiotics while awaiting the results of bacterial cultures. Meningitis should be considered in any patient with altered mental status. In this regard, our approach has been to perform lumbar punctures on all patients with meningismus and on patients in whom the change in mental status does not appear to be related to the metabolic insult. The cerebrospinal fluid (CSF) glucose level is not particularly useful in the diagnosis of meningitis in the setting of DKA or HHNC, but a CSF glucose level of less than 100 mg/dL (5.5 mmol/L) is unusual when the serum glucose level is greater than 250 mg/dL (13.9 mmol/L).[22] The relative frequency of sinus infection (the most serious being mucormycosis), foot infection, bacterial arthritis, cholecystitis, cellulitis, and necrotizing fasciitis should be considered. Pneumonia can be difficult to diagnose in patients with dehydration because the alveolar edema fluid, which causes infiltrates on chest x-ray, often is not present but develops along with progressive hypoxia during hydration. To avoid this occurrence, we are particularly judicious with fluid administration in patients we suspect of having pneumonia. Pancreatitis and pregnancy are common precipitants and need to be specially considered in the assessment of abdominal pain, which is extremely common at presentation. Abdominal guarding and tenderness associated with vomiting are seen often. Rebound is present only rarely. These symptoms and findings usually resolve quickly with therapy in the absence of intraabdominal pathology. The serum amylase level is often elevated without pathologic significance, but a high lipase level is usually more specific for a diagnosis of pancreatitis.[23] Acute myocardial infarction and stroke, as well as thromboembolic phenomena, are frequent precipitants and complications of DKA.

Precipitating factors are similar in HHNC, but they are found more commonly and are often more severe. Common associated illnesses are chronic renal insufficiency, pneumonia, gastrointestinal hemorrhage, sepsis (particularly with gram-negative organisms), myocardial infarction, pulmonary embolism, and intracranial events. Burns, hyperalimentation, dialysis, heat stroke, thyrotoxicosis, acromegaly, pancreatitis, and a variety of drugs (mostly diuretics, steroids, and β-blockers) also have been associated.

The more insulin-resistant the patient, the more likely it is that a precipitating cause is present. If a precipitating cause is found, treatment is essential if adequate metabolic control is to be achieved.

COMPLICATIONS AND PROGNOSIS

It should be possible to treat almost all cases of DKA successfully. The most troublesome complication is cerebral edema. It is particularly common in children and can be fatal. In most series, specific causes cannot be assigned, although the use of bicarbonate, more severe DKA, and aggressive hydration, particularly with hypotonic fluids, may contribute.[24]

In 50% of patients who subsequently have a respiratory arrest, there are premonitory symptoms; despite early intervention, only half of such patients avoid severe or fatal brain damage. Cerebral edema is much less common in HHNC but may be associated with decreases in plasma glucose concentration below 250 mg/dL (13.9 mmol/L) during the first day of therapy.[25] Other complications of life-threatening severity that have been reported include the acute respiratory distress syndrome (ARDS) and bronchial mucus plugging.[26–28]

The most common complication of HHNC is death. Female gender, lack of prior knowledge of diabetes, and acute infections are risk factors for the development of HHNC. Despite aggressive therapy, mortality is in the range of 20% to 50% in most recent case series. Prognosis is inversely related to serum osmolality, BUN level, and sodium level, although large differences in values are not apparent between survivors and nonsurvivors.[29] The mortality seems to be in large part a function of the underlying illness and the duration of illness before appropriate medical therapy is instituted. Although complete recovery of neurologic function in survivors is the rule, persistent coma is not infrequent. Arterial and venous thromboembolic events are quite common. Standard prophylactic low-dose heparin administration is certainly a reasonable precaution for patients with HHNC, but currently no indication exists for full anticoagulation.

Recurrent admissions for DKA occur in up to one-third of patients. Ensuring adequate and timely outpatient follow-up and diabetes education will reduce relapses. Patients with frequent DKA are rare and require special consideration of neuropsychological contributors.[30]

Hypoglycemia

Although not a complication of diabetes per se, severe hypoglycemia is a not uncommon complication of its therapy. It also may be a major complication of critical illness—particularly hepatic failure, drug overdose, and sepsis. The serum glucose concentration is very strictly regulated in normal persons, being maintained between approximately 60 and 140 mg/dL (3.3–7.8 mmol/L). The differential diagnosis of hypoglycemia can be divided into fasting and postprandial forms (Table 78-4). Fasting hypoglycemia can result from endocrine disorders, hepatic dysfunction, antibodies to insulin or the insulin receptor, or substrate deficiency. The major endocrine causes are excess secretion of insulin or insulin-like growth factor and deficiency of growth hormone or cortisol. Insulin hypersecretion can be from an insulinoma or from normal islet tissue under pharmacologic stimulation. Certain malignancies, particularly sarcomas, hepatomas, and tumors of the biliary tract, can cause elevated levels of free insulin-like growth factors and can present with hypoglycemia, often in the presence of cachexia. Any cause of severe hepatic dysfunction—toxins, viruses, congestive heart failure, or shock—and enzymatic defects causing decreased gluconeogenesis or glycogen storage diseases can cause hypoglycemia. Hypoglycemia can occur with fasting in alcoholism, pregnancy, or uremia due to substrate unavailability, but otherwise, it occurs only with end-stage protein-calorie malnutrition. Postprandial hypoglycemia can be caused by rapid gastric emptying owing to postoperative changes, or it can

TABLE 78-4 Causes of Hypoglycemia

Fasting hypoglycemia
    Hypersecretion of insulin or increased levels of insulin-like
        growth factors
        Insulinoma
        Nesidioblastosis
        Certain carcinomas (sarcoma, hepatoma, others)
    Hyposecretion of counterregulatory hormones
        Growth hormone deficiency
        Cortisol deficiency
    Hepatic failure
        Toxic (especially alcohol-induced)
        Infectious
        Congestive
        Shock-induced
    Caused by an inborn error of metabolism
    Starvation
    Uremia
    Pregnancy
    Severe protein-calorie malnutrition
    Autoimmune disorder (antibodies to insulin or insulin receptors)
Postprandial hypoglycemia
    Idiopathic
    Alimentary
    Early type 2 diabetes mellitus
Factitious or drug-related hypoglycemia
    Insulin
    Sulfonylureas and other sulfa compounds
    Salicylates
    β-Blockers
    Pentamidine
    Antiarrhythmic agents
    Glucose consumption in test tube by leukocytes

TABLE 78-5 Treatment of Hypoglycemia

Consider the diagnosis
Determine capillary glucose concentration
Confirm with measurement of serum glucose (and insulin,
    C-peptide, and sulfonylurea screen if cause unknown)
Give oral calories if patient is conscious
Reassess; if glucose <100 mg/dL (5.5 mmol/L), *then* administer
    50 mL 50% dextrose
Reassess; if glucose <100 mg/dL (5.5 mmol/L), *then* give infusion
    of 10% dextrose to maintain glucose level > 100 mg/dL
    (5.5 mmol/L)
Reassess; if glucose <100 mg/dL (5.5 mmol/L), *then* give infusion
    of 10% glucose + 100 mg/L hydrocortisone + 1 mg glucagon
Reassess; if glucose <100 mg/dL (5.5 mmol/L), *then* add infusion of
    diazoxide and/or continuous enteral feeding

agnosis in most cases. The various studies that can be used in less obvious cases should be considered only with the help of a specialist and are beyond the scope of this review. Glucose tolerance testing is usually nondiagnostic. A 72-hour fast will produce a diagnosis in the vast majority of patients with fasting hypoglycemia. At a minimum, glucose, insulin, C-peptide, proinsulin, and urine or serum drug screens for oral hypoglycemic agents should be obtained in both the normal and the hypoglycemic state.

TREATMENT

The most critical step in the therapy of hypoglycemia is recognition of its cause, which indicates its likely duration and severity (Table 78-5). If a patient took his or her insulin, forgot to eat breakfast, and subsequently lost consciousness, an ampule of 50% dextrose administered in the field and followed by breakfast almost certainly would be curative. However, if a patient drank a quart of liquor and then made a suicide gesture by taking long-acting oral hypoglycemic agents, aspirin, and β-blockers, then the hypoglycemia is likely to be severe and long-lasting and will require intensive therapy for days. Similarly, patients with hepatic failure will require continuous therapy with hypertonic glucose once hypoglycemia develops and until hepatic function returns. The goal of therapy is to establish and maintain modest hyperglycemia immediately and to monitor blood glucose concentration intensively using hand-held monitors. Seltzer[9] has described a protocol for use in severe hypoglycemia as follows: In the presence of documented hypoglycemia, whether or not the patient responds to 50 mL of 50% dextrose, a continuous infusion of 10% glucose at a rate sufficient to keep the blood glucose level above 100 mg/dL (5.5 mmol/L) should be started. If more than 200 mL/h is necessary to maintain hyperglycemia, then 100 mg hydrocortisone and 1 mg glucagon are added to each liter of 10% dextrose for as long as necessary. Intravenous diazoxide administration to decrease insulin secretion also can be considered. It is important to remember that much more carbohydrate can be delivered enterally than intravenously, and so in extreme cases, jejunal feeding should be considered early. If the patient awakes, a high-carbohydrate diet should be initiated. Progressive hyperglycemia is the signal that therapy can be tapered. With early aggressive therapy, usually coma is reversed and focal deficits resolve over time.

be idiopathic. It has been associated with early type 2 diabetes. Drugs that can cause hypoglycemia include alcohol, insulin, sulfonylureas, salicylates, β-blockers, pentamidine, some antiarrhythmic agents, akee fruit, and the rat poison Vacor.

The symptoms of hypoglycemia initially result from sympathoadrenal responses and consist of palpitations, anxiety, tremulousness, sweating, and hunger. If hypoglycemia progresses, neuroglycopenic symptoms develop. These include headache, nightmares, fatigue, confusion, bizarre behavior, hallucinations, seizures, coma, and focal neurologic deficits. The absolute glucose concentration at which these symptoms develop is highly variable; in part it depends on the rate of fall in glucose concentration. In critically ill patients, symptoms may be obscured by concurrent problems until profound hypoglycemia, with seizures or coma, evolves.

Patients who present with signs and symptoms compatible with hypoglycemia should have their blood glucose concentration measured and glucose administered—by mouth if conscious, intravenously otherwise. The disappearance of symptoms over a period of minutes suggests that hypoglycemia is the likely etiology. IV administration of 50 mL of 50% dextrose will awaken more than 80% of hypoglycemic patients destined for neurologic recovery.

Patients with hypoglycemia should be fully evaluated to determine etiology. A complete history, physical examination, and routine laboratory tests will result in a likely di-

References

1. Kitabchi AE: Low-dose insulin therapy in diabetic ketoacidosis: Fact or fiction? *Diabetes Metab Rev* 5:337, 1989.
2. Krane EJ: Diabetic ketoacidosis. *Pediatr Clin North Am* 34:935, 1987.
3. Brumfield CG, Huddleston JF: The management of diabetic ketoacidosis in pregnancy. *Clin Obstet Gynecol* 27:50, 1984.
4. Board JB, Graber AL, Christman JW, Powers AC: Practical management of diabetes in critically ill patients. *Am J Respir Crit Care Med* 164:1763, 2001.
5. Pope DW, Dansky D: Hyperosmolar hyperglycemic nonketotic coma. *Emerg Med Clin North Am* 7:849, 1989.
6. Maldonado M, Hampe CS, Gaur LK, et al: Ketosis-prone diabetes: Dissection of a heterogeneous syndrome using an immunogenetic and beta-cell functional classification, prospective analysis and clinical outcomes. *J Clin Endocrinol Metab* 88:5090, 2003.
7. Field JB: Hypoglycemia. *Endocrinol Metab Clin North Am* 18:27, 1989.
8. Sherwin RS, Felig P: Hypoglycemia, in Felig P, Baxter JD, Broadus AE, Froliman LA (eds): *Endocrinology and Metabolism.* New York, McGraw-Hill, 1987, p 1179.
9. Seltzer HS: Drug-induced hypoglycemia. *Endocrinol Metab Clin North Am* 18:163, 1989.
9a. Whiteman VE, Homko CJ, Reece EA: Management of hypoglycemia and diabetic ketoacidosis in pregnancy. *Obstet Gynecol Clin North Am* 23:87, 1996.
9b. Kitabchi AE, Umpierrez GE, Murphy MB, et al: Management of hyperglycemic crises in patients with diabetes. *Diabetes Care* 24:131, 2001.
9c. American Diabetes Association. Position statement: Hyperglycemic crises in diabetes. *Diabetes Care* 27(suppl. 1):s94, 2004.
10. Foster DW, McGarry JD: The metabolic derangements and treatment of diabetic ketoacidosis. *New Engl J Med* 309:159, 1983.
10a. Schreiber M, Steele A, Gogven J, et al: Can a severe degree of ketoacidosis develop overnight? *J Am Soc Nephrol* 7:192, 1996.
11. Arieff AI, Carroll HJ: Nonketotic hyperosmolar coma with hyperglycemia: Clinical features, pathophysiology, renal function, acid-base balance, plasma-cerebrospinal fluid equilibria and the effects of therapy in 37 cases. *Medicine* 51:73, 1972.
12. Adrogué HJ, Wilson H, Boyd AE III, et al: Plasma acid-base patterns in diabetic ketoacidosis. *New Engl J Med* 307:1603, 1982.
13. Munro JF, Campbell IW, McCuish AC, Duncan LJP: Euglycaemic diabetic ketoacidosis. *Br Med J* 2:578, 1973.
14. Madias NE: Lactic acidosis. *Kidney Int* 29:752, 1986.
15. Fulop M: Alcoholism, ketoacidosis, and lactic acidosis. *Diabetes Metab Rev* 5:365, 1989.
16. Möller-Petersen J, Andersen PT, Hjörne N, Ditzel J: Nontraumatic rhabdomyolysis during diabetic ketoacidosis. *Diabetologia* 29:229, 1986.
17. Brenner BE, Simon RR: Management of salicylate intoxication. *Drugs* 24:335, 1982.
18. Turk J, Morrell L, Avioli LV (eds): Ethylene glycol intoxication. *Arch Intern Med* 146:1601, 1986.
19. Rich J, Scheife RT, Katz N, Caplan LR: Isopropyl alcohol intoxication. *Arch Neurol* 47:322, 1990.
20. Weisberg LS: Pseudohyponatremia: A reappraisal. *Am J Med* 86:315, 1989.
21. Burris AS: Leukemoid reaction associated with severe diabetic ketoacidosis. *South Med J* 79:647, 1986.
22. Powers WJ: Cerebrospinal fluid to serum glucose ratios in diabetes mellitus and meningitis. *Am J Med* 71:217, 1981.
23. Campbell IW, Duncan LJP, Innes JA, et al: Abdominal pain in diabetic metabolic decompensation. *JAMA* 233:166, 1975.
24. Glaser N, Barnett P, McCaslin I, et al: Pediatric Emergency Medicine Collaborative Research Committee of the American Academy of Pediatrics: Risk factors for cerebral edema in children with diabetic ketoacidosis. *New Engl J Med* 344:264, 2001.
25. Arieff AI: Cerebral edema complicating nonketotic hyperosmolar coma. *Miner Electrolyte Metab* 12:383, 1986.
26. Brun-Buisson CJL, Bonnet F, Bergeret S, et al: Recurrent high-permeability pulmonary edema associated with diabetic ketoacidosis. *Crit Care Med* 13:55, 1985.
27. Brandstetter RD, Tamarin FM, Washington D, et al: Occult mucous airway obstruction in diabetic ketoacidosis. *Chest* 91:575, 1987.
28. Hansen LA, Prakash UBS, Colby TV: Pulmonary complications in diabetes mellitus. *Mayo Clin Proc* 64:791, 1989.
29. Wachtel TJ, Silliman RA, Lamberton P: Predisposing factors for the diabetic hyperosmolar state. *Arch Intern Med* 147:499, 1987.
30. Sobel R, Meyer G, Buse JB: Brittle diabetes, lessons for intensive insulin management. *Pract Diabetol* 13:12, 1994.

Chapter 79

ADRENOCORTICAL INSUFFICIENCY

PAUL E. MARIK
GARY P. ZALOGA

KEY POINTS

- *Activation of the hypothalamic-pituitary-adrenal (HPA) axis with increased glucocorticoid activity is an essential component of the general adaptation to stress.*
- *Mediators released in patients with sepsis may either stimulate or impair the synthesis and action of cortisol via actions on the HPA axis and glucocorticoid receptor.*
- *A random cortisol level in a highly stressed ICU patient is currently the most useful test to assess the integrity of the HPA axis.*
- *A stress cortisol level of less than 25 µg/dL in a highly stressed patient (hypotensive, respiratory failure) is highly suggestive of adrenal failure.*
- *The incidence of adrenal failure may be as high as 60% in patients with septic shock.*
- *All patients with suspected HPA axis dysfunction should be treated with stress doses of hydrocortisone (100 mg q 8 IV) pending the results of diagnostic testing.*
- *A random cortisol level of less than 15 µg/dL or a level of less than 20 µg/dL post low-dose corticotrophin stimulation testing (low-dose ACTH test) in a non-hypotensive patient with unexplained fever, eosinophilia or altered mental status warrants a trial of treatment with stress doses of hydrocortisone.*

The maintenance of life depends on the capacity of the organism to sustain its equilibrium via *allostasis*—the ability to achieve stability through change. Allostasis is critical to survival in stress situations.[1] The three major regulatory systems of the body responsible for allostasis include the central nervous system (CNS), the endocrine system, and the immune system. These three regulatory systems are closely interrelated and orchestrate the stress response. Importantly, activation of the hypothalamic-pituitary-adrenal (HPA) axis with the release of cortisol is the cornerstone of the stress response.

The qualitative and quantitative aspects of the stress response depend on the nature and severity of the stressor and are time-dependent. With mild to moderate short-term stress there is general activation of the CNS, the endocrine system, and the immune system in an attempt to restore homeostasis. However, with severe and/or prolonged stress, this coordinated allostatic response may fail with the ultimate demise of the organism. Teleologically, the latter may be viewed as a mechanism to spare society of those overwhelmed by disease. However, these are the very patients who are treated in ICUs and who are trying to "cheat death."

Cortisol, the primary glucocorticoid hormone in humans, is secreted by the adrenal glands. In healthy, unstressed persons, cortisol is secreted in a diurnal pattern under the influence of corticotropin (ACTH) released from the pituitary gland. Corticotropin secretion, in turn, is under the influence of hypothalamic corticotropin-releasing hormone (CRH), and both hormones are subject to negative-feedback control by cortisol. Aldosterone, the primary mineralocorticoid hormone in the body, is also secreted by the adrenal glands. Aldosterone secretion, however, is regulated primarily by the renin-angiotensin system and potassium levels. Circulating cortisol is bound to corticosteroid-binding globulin, with less than 10% in the free bioavailable form. With acute stress in the form of infection, surgery, trauma, burns, or illness, cortisol production increases by a factor that is roughly proportional to the severity of the stress. The increase in cortisol is due to the increased production of CRH and corticotropin and a reduction in the negative feedback from cortisol. Diurnal variation of cortisol secretion is lost. The increased adrenal glucocorticoid production is associated with a shift away from mineralocorticoid and androgen production (i.e., reprioritization).[2] Indeed, while there is activation of the renin-angiotensin system in an attempt to maintain blood pressure, aldosterone secretion is decreased.[3–6] The dissociation between renin-angiotensin and aldosterone may represent an additional adaptive mechanism designed to promote cortisol production in critically ill patients.[3–6] Sustained high levels of ACTH may explain this finding because in normal subjects ACTH causes a biphasic aldosterone response with an initial increase followed by diminished production.[3–5]

Glucocorticoids exert their effects by binding to and activating a 90-kDa intracellular glucocorticoid receptor (GR) protein.[7] All cells appear to have appreciable levels of GR. The GR is localized in the cytoplasm of the cell and translocates into the nucleus on ligand binding. In the absence of hormone, cytoplasmic GR is associated with a large protein complex that includes heat shock protein 90 (hsp-90) and hsp-56.[8] This protein complex functions to maintain the GR in an inactive conformation that is competent for glucocorticoid binding. When activated by a ligand, GRs bind as dimers to glucocorticoid response elements (GREs) in target genes that then activate or repress transcription of the associated genes. Via this mechanism, glucocorticoids regulate gene transcription in every cell in the body. In addition to increased secretion of cortisol, a number of other mechanisms may increase cellular glucocorticoid activity. An acute decline in the concentration of cortisol-binding globulin, as well as decreased cortisol binding to cortisol-binding globulin, results in an increase in the free biologically active fraction of the hormone.[9–13] In addition, the number of GRs may be upregulated acutely during stress. Sun and colleagues[14] demonstrated increased expression of GR mRNA, increased expression of GRs, and increased binding activity of the GRs in skeletal muscle in a murine cecal ligation and perforation model. In this study, pretreatment of the animals with the GR antagonist RU-38486 prevented the increase in GR protein and mRNA levels seen in sepsis and abolished the sepsis-induced increases in GR binding activity. These data suggest that cortisol may increase synthesis of its own receptor directly via a positive-feedback loop. The collective result of adrenocortical adaptation to severe stress is a dramatic increase in cellular glucocorticoid activity. This activation is an essential component of the general adaptation to illness and stress and contributes to the maintenance of cellular and organ homeostasis. For example, adrenalectomized animals succumb rapidly to hemorrhagic and septic shock, whereas steroid replacement is protective against these challenges.[15,16]

Major Physiologic Actions of Glucocorticoids

In the acutely stressed individual, the metabolic, cardiovascular, and immunologic actions of cortisol play a critical role in mediating the stress response. Glucocorticoids increase blood glucose levels, facilitating the delivery of glucose to cells during acute and chronic stress. Glucocorticoids increase blood glucose concentrations by increasing the rate of hepatic gluconeogenesis and inhibiting adipose tissue glucose uptake.[17] Hepatic gluconeogenesis is stimulated by increasing the activities of phosphoenolpyruvate carboxykinase and glucose-6-phosphatase as a result of binding of glucocorticoids to the GREs of the genes for these enzymes. Glucocorticoids also stimulate free fatty acid release from adipose tissue and amino acid release from body proteins. Proteolysis is activated via glucocorticoid upregulation of the calpain and ubiquitin-proteasome pathways. Major roles of these processes are to supply to the cell energy and substrate that are required for response to stress and repair from injury.

Glucocorticoids are required for normal cardiovascular reactivity to angiotensin II, epinephrine, and norepinephrine, contributing to the maintenance of cardiac contractility, vascular tone, and blood pressure. These effects are mediated partly by the increased transcription and expression of the receptors for these hormones.[18,19] Glucocorticoids are required for the synthesis of N^+,K^+-ATPase and catecholamines. Glucocorticoid effects on the synthesis of catecholamines and catecholamine receptors are partially responsible for the positive inotropic effects of these hormones.[20] Glucocorticoids also decrease the production of nitric oxide and vasodilatory prostaglandins, major vasorelaxants and modulators of vascular permeability.[21–24]

Glucocorticoids possess anti-inflammatory and immunosuppressive effects that are mediated through specific receptor mechanisms.[25–28] Glucocorticoids influence most cells that participate in immune and inflammatory reactions, including lymphocytes, natural killer cells, monocytes, macrophages, eosinophils, neutrophils, mast cells, and basophils. Glucocorticoids decrease the accumulation and function of most of these cells at inflammatory sites. Most of the suppressive effects of glucocorticoids on immune and inflammatory reactions appear to be a consequence of the modulation of production or activity of cytokines (e.g., interleukin 1 [IL-1], IL-2, IL-3, IL-6, interferon-γ [IFN-γ], tumor necrosis factor α [TNF-α]), chemokines, eicosanoids, complement activation, and other inflammatory mediators (e.g., bradykinin, histamine, macrophage migration inhibitory factor). Glucocorticoids control mediator production predominantly through inhibition of transcription factors such as nuclear factor $\kappa\beta$ (NF-$\kappa\beta$).[27,28] This inhibition is mediated by induction of the I-$\kappa\beta\alpha$ inhibitory protein.[29] Glucocorticoids also produce anti-inflammatory effects by enhancing release of anti-inflammatory factors such as IL-1 receptor antagonist, soluble tumor necrosis factor receptor, and IL-10.[30,31] In addition, glucocorticoids block the transcription of mRNA for enzymes required for the synthesis of some mediators (e.g., cyclooxygenase 2, inducible nitric oxide synthase).

Cytokines and the HPA Axis

The HPA axis and the immune response are linked together via a feedback loop in which activated immune cells produce cytokines that signal the brain. Activation of the HPA axis by specific cytokines increases the release of cortisol, which, in turn, feeds back and suppresses the immune reaction (and further cytokine release).[32] IL-1 and IL-6 administered peripherally increase HPA axis activity, increasing levels of CRH, ACTH, and glucocorticoids.[33,34] Cytokines also affect the pituitary and adrenal cortex directly. IL-1, IL-6 and TNF-α stimulate the secretion of ACTH from cultured pituitary preparations, and IL-1 and IL-6 stimulate glucocorticoid production in cultured adrenal preparations.[33,34]

Cytokines, however, also suppress the HPA axis and impair GR function. Whereas acute elevation of IL-6 levels stimulates ACTH release, chronic IL-6 elevation may blunt ACTH release.[35] In addition, TNF-α impairs CRH-stimulated ACTH release,[36,37] and a number of clinical studies have reported inappropriately low ACTH levels in patients with severe sepsis and the systemic inflammatory response syndrome (SIRS).[36,38,39] Indeed, Schroeder and coworkers[40] reported similar circulating levels of ACTH in healthy controls and in patients with severe sepsis. In addition, plasma from patients with septic shock impairs synthesis of corticosteroids by adrenocortical cells.[41–43] TNF-α and corticostatin have been demonstrated to inhibit adrenal gland function.[37,44,45] Corticostatin (defensin) is a peptide produced by immune cells.[46] Concentrations of corticostatin increase over 20-fold in animals with infection but not other forms of stress.[47] TNF-α has been shown to reduce adrenal cortisol synthesis by inhibiting the stimulatory actions of ACTH and angiotensin II on adrenal cells.[44,48,49] Proinflammatory cytokines have been shown to influence the number, expression, and function of GRs. IL-1 has been demonstrated to decrease GR translocation and transcription.[50] The half-life of cortisol has been demonstrated to be prolonged in sepsis; this may reflect a decreased number of GRs or decreased affinity of the receptor for its ligand.[43,51,52] While Sun and colleagues[14] demonstrated increased expression of GRs in skeletal muscle in the early phase of experimental sepsis, Liu and colleagues[53] demonstrated decreased expression of GRs following burn injury. It is particularly noteworthy that in the latter study the decreased expression of GRs was attenuated by treatment with both anti-TNF-α and anti-IL-1 monoclonal antibodies. Ali and colleagues[54] reported a 40% decline in the number of glucocorticoid receptors in the liver of septic rats. The decline in hormone-binding activity was associated with a fall in glucocorticoid receptor mRNA. Decreased affinity of the GR from mononuclear leukocytes of patients with sepsis also has been reported.[55,56] Reduced activity of gluconeogenic enzymes during endotoxemia despite elevated circulating glucocorticoid levels provides further evidence to support impaired intracellular actions of glucocorticoids during sepsis.[57] In total, these data support the idea that mediators released in patients with sepsis may either stimulate or impair the synthesis and action of cortisol via actions on the HPA axis and the GR. The net effect of these opposing actions on the

HPA axis and GR may be time-dependent and in addition depend on the severity of illness and extent of mediator production.

Assessment of Adrenal Function in the Critically Ill

Since there are no clinically useful tests to assess the cellular actions of cortisol (i.e., end-organ effects), the diagnosis of adrenal insufficiency is based on measurement of serum cortisol levels; this has resulted in much confusion and misunderstanding.[39,58–69] Traditionally, the "integrity" of the HPA axis has been assessed by the short corticotropin stimulation test (also known as the *Cosyntropin stimulation test*). This test is usually performed by administering 250 μg of synthetic corticotropin intravenously and obtaining a serum cortisol determination before and 30 and 60 minutes following administration.[58,70] A 30- to 60-minute serum cortisol level below 18 μg/dL or an increase in the cortisol concentration of less than 9 μg/dL has been regarded by many as diagnostic of adrenal insufficiency.[58] However, these criteria were developed to assess adrenal reserve in patients with destructive diseases of the adrenal glands and are based on responses in normal, nonstressed, healthy controls.[58,70] We believe that the standard corticotropin stimulation test lacks sensitivity for the diagnosis of adrenal insufficiency[58,71–74] (Table 79-1).

High doses of corticotropin (e.g., 250 μg) are supraphysiologic (over 1000-fold higher than normal maximal stress ACTH levels).[39,62–65] The very high levels of corticotropin obtained with 250 μg can override adrenal resistance to ACTH and result in a normal cortisol response. Patients with normal responses to high-dose corticotropin may fail to respond normally to stress[61,71] (Fig. 79-1). Owing to the decreased sensitivity of the high-dose ACTH stimulation test (HD-ACTH) for the diagnosis of adrenal insufficiency, many investigators evaluated the use of lower doses of ACTH that approximate stress levels of ACTH (i.e., 1 to 2 μg) for the diagnosis of adrenal insufficiency. A number of studies have demonstrated that a 1-μg dose (LD-ACTH) of corticotropin is more sensitive and specific for diagnosing primary and secondary adrenal insufficiency than the 250-μg dose.[38,71,75–79]

The change in cortisol level following corticotropin stimulation (Δ_{max}) is used by some clinicians to diagnose adrenal insufficiency.[59,63,64,80] However, the Δ_{max} is a measure of adrenal reserve and not adrenal function. The increase in cortisol following administration of corticotropin should not be used as a criterion for the diagnosis of adrenal insufficiency. A maximally stressed patient may be secreting all the cortisol that his or her adrenal glands can synthesize. This patient may have an appropriately high serum cortisol level but be unable to respond further following corticotropin injection (no reserve). For example, a critically ill patient with a basal stress cortisol level of 54 μg/dL that increases to 57 μg/dL with corticotropin does not have adrenal insufficiency. It is the absolute level that is of importance rather than the Δ_{max}. On the other hand, it is clear from a number of studies that impaired response to ACTH (i.e., small Δ_{max}) has prognostic value and generally indicates a poor prognosis. The exact reasons for this are unclear but may relate to high levels of circulating factors that impair adrenal response to maximal stress.

Most important, the administration of exogenous ACTH bypasses the CNS-hypothalamic-pituitary axis and tests the integrity of the adrenal glands directly. It is essential that one evaluate the entire axis because defects in the hypothalamic-pituitary components frequently cause adrenal insufficiency. Endogenous stresses such as hypotension, hypoxemia, fever, and hypoglycemia are superior stimuli for testing the integrity of the HPA axis than is ACTH testing. These endogenous stressors test the function of the entire HPA axis and therefore should be regarded as the "gold standard" for adrenal testing. In other words, the HPA axis evolved to respond to stress and is best evaluated using stress that tests all components of the axis. Many inappropriately assume that the ACTH stimulation test is capable of detecting the presence of adrenal insufficiency because they assume that significant adrenal atrophy has occurred and results in diminished ACTH responsiveness. This concept is flawed for a variety of reasons. First, it takes 1 to 2 weeks for the adrenal gland to atrophy following pituitary removal when all ACTH secretion from the pituitary is lost. Thus the ACTH stimulation test may easily miss acute adrenal insufficiency (the most common form of adrenal insufficiency in critically ill patients). Second, adrenal atrophy may take longer in patients with partial adrenal insufficiency (common in critically ill patients). Third, the response to ACTH may be normal in patients with partial secondary adrenal insufficiency or ACTH resistance. ACTH testing is not required to diagnose adrenal insufficiency in severely stressed patients because the CNS-HPA axis already should be maximally activated. In such patients, a random stress cortisol level provides adequate information on the integrity of the entire HPA axis. In patients in whom the level of stress is less intense (not hypotensive, hypoxemic, or in pain), the LD-ACTH simulation test should be used to assess adrenal reserve (Fig. 79-2). One also may evaluate the pituitary-adrenal axis by administering CRH.[40] This test bypasses the hypothalamus but does require the integrity of the pituitary and adrenal glands. However, the sensitivity and specificity of the test for detecting adrenal insufficiency in critically ill patients have not been determined.

There is much controversy regarding levels of circulating cortisol that are considered to be an adequate response to stress.[58] Many textbooks and published manuscripts state that the normal circulating cortisol response to stress is a level greater than 15 to 20 μg/dL. However, the choice of 15 to 20 μg/dL is based primarily on the response to exogenous high-dose ACTH (250 μg) and the response to insulin-induced hypoglycemia in nonstressed, non-critically ill patients.[70] During surgical procedures such as laparotomy, serum corticotropin and cortisol concentrations rise rapidly,

TABLE 79-1 Causes for Lack of Sensitivity of High-Dose ACTH Stimulation Test for the Diagnosis of Adrenal Insufficiency

Bypasses CNS-hypothalamic-pituitary components of HPA axis

Uses supraphysiologic levels of ACTH

Overrides ACTH resistance

Insensitive for diagnosis of acute adrenal insufficiency; better for detection of chronic adrenal insufficiency

Short-term stimulation may not reflect response to chronic ACTH elevation

May be normal in patients with partial secondary adrenal insufficiency who fail to respond to stress

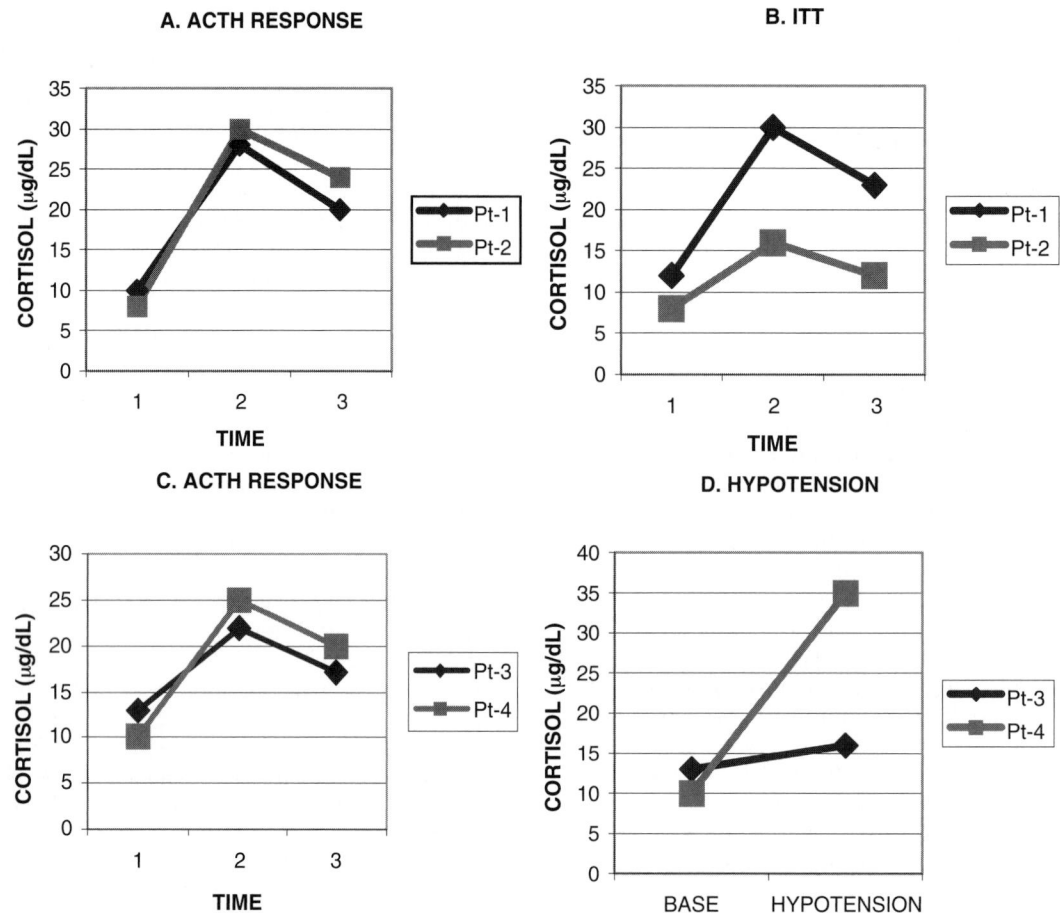

FIGURE 79-1 Discordant cortisol response to ACTH stimulation test and insulin tolerance test (ITT) (*A, B*) and ACTH stimulation test and hypotension (*C, D*). Patients 1 and 2 responded similarly to ACTH, but patient 2 failed to respond adequately to hypoglycemia induced by insulin. Patients 3 and 4 responded similarly to ACTH, but patient 4 failed to respond adequately when he became hypotensive.

peaking in the immediate postoperative period, and then decline to baseline levels over the next 72 hours.[81] The magnitude of the postoperative increase in serum cortisol concentration is correlated with the extent of the surgery, with a peak between 30 and 45 μg/dL in patients undergoing major surgery.[82–87] During severe illness, serum cortisol concentrations tend to be higher than those of patients undergoing major surgery.[81] In patients with multiple trauma, the serum cortisol level remains greater than 30 μg/dL for at least a week, with peak values between 40 and 50 μg/dL.[88] Cortisol levels are increased in critically ill ICU patients, with the highest values being reported in patients with the highest illness severity scores and those with the highest mortality.[89,90] We have found cortisol levels to be elevated in all forms of shock (Fig. 79-3). Interestingly, cortisol levels are significantly lower in patients with septic shock compared with patients with hypovolemic and cardiogenic shock, suggesting the presence of mediators that impair HPA axis function. Overall, the available data suggest that the degree of activation of the HPA axis and elevation in serum cortisol level is related to the severity and duration of the stressor. Animal and human studies demonstrate increasing serum levels of epinephrine and cortisol with increasing severity of stress, with hypotension and sepsis being two of the most intense stressors.[91,92] Based on the available data,[74] we believe that a random cortisol level in

severely stressed patients (e.g., those with hypotension, hypoxemia, burn, high fever, multiple trauma) should be above 25 μg/dL. Higher levels may be appropriate in patients with septic shock due to "tissue cortisol resistance."

The cortisol threshold of 25 μg/dL for an adequate adrenal response to severe stress is supported by two clinical studies that evaluated the hemodynamic response of replacement doses of hydrocortisone in vasopressor-dependent patients. While the hemodynamic response to steroids may be a crude marker of acute adrenal insufficiency, we have no other end-organ or biochemical marker of cellular glucocorticoid activity at this time. Furthermore, this end point has been used in other studies evaluating the role of corticosteroids in vasopressor-dependent patients with sepsis and may serve as a surrogate marker of inadequate glucocorticoid activity during severe illness.[93–96] Rivers and colleagues[97] studied the HPA axis in a group of vasopressor-dependent surgical patients. In a subgroup of patients treated with corticosteroids, the basal serum cortisol concentration was 49 μg/dL in the steroid nonresponders and 20 μg/dL in patients who were weaned from vasopressors within 24 hours of the initiation of steroid treatment. Only one patient in the steroid-responsive group had a baseline serum cortisol level of greater than 25 μg/dL, and only 2 nonresponders had a baseline level of less than 25 μg/dL. In this study, the diagnostic sensitivity

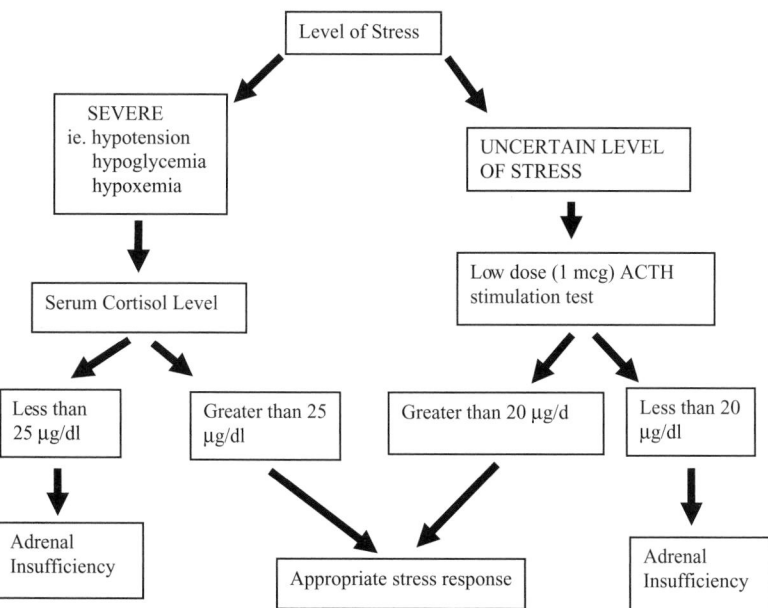

FIGURE 79-2 Evaluation of HPA axis function.

of a threshold of 25 μg/dL was 90%, with a specificity of 92%, a positive predictive value of 60%, and a negative predictive value of 66%. Similarly, we investigated the hemodynamic response following treatment with replacement doses of hydrocortisone in 59 medical patients in septic shock.[71] The baseline serum cortisol level was 14.1 $\pm$ 5.2 μg/dL in the steroid-responsive patients compared with 33.3 $\pm$ 18 μg/dL in the steroid-nonresponsive patients. The sensitivity of a baseline cortisol level of less than 25 μg/dL in predicting steroid responsiveness was 96%, this compared with 22% for the standard HD-ACTH stimulation test. The area under the receiver operating characteristic (ROC) curve of the stress (baseline) cortisol level was 0.84; a stress cortisol level of 23.7 μg/dL had the best discriminating power, with a sensitivity of 86%, a specificity of 66%, a likelihood ratio of 2.6, a positive predictive value of 62%, and a negative predictive value of 88%. Clearly, there is no absolute serum cortisol level that distinguishes an adequate from an insufficient adrenal response.

Based on current evidence, we believe that a random cortisol level should be interpreted in conjunction with the severity of illness, and 25 μg/dL is a useful threshold value for an appropriate response to severe stress (see Fig. 79-2). We believe

that a random cortisol level should be above 25 μg/dL in severely stressed ICU patients with normal adrenal function. It is not necessary to obtain cortisol levels at a specific time of the day because critically ill patients lose the diurnal variation in their cortisol levels.[82] In nonhypotensive critically ill patients, the normal cortisol response (30 to 60 minutes) after 1 to 2 μg corticotropin (LD-ACTH) should be a level greater than 20 μg/dL. We do not recommend performing the unphysiologic high-dose corticotropin stimulation test. Importantly, a random cortisol level of less than 15 μg/dL or a level less than 20 μg/dL post LD-ACTH test in a nonhypotensive critically ill patient with unexplained fever, eosinophilia or, metal status changes may warrant a trial of replacement doses of corticosteroids.

Incidence of Adrenal Insufficiency

The incidence of adrenal insufficiency in critically ill patients is variable and depends on the underlying disease and severity of the illness. The reported incidence varies widely (0% to 77%) depending on the population of patients

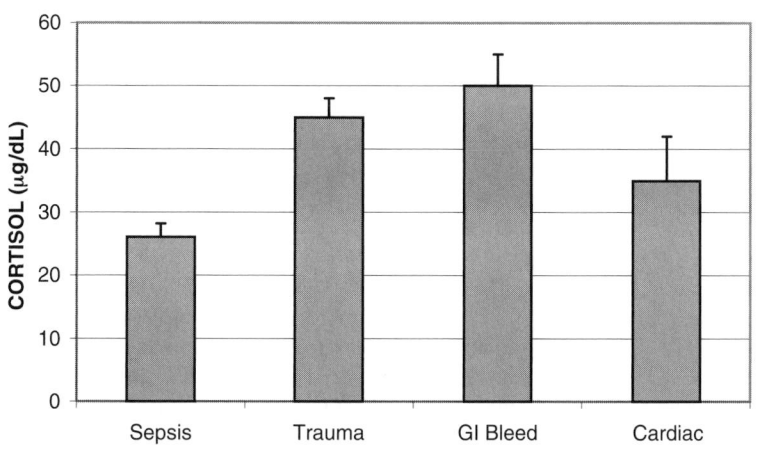

FIGURE 79-3 Cortisol (mean $\pm$ SEM) response to shock in critically ill patients.

studied and the diagnostic criteria used to diagnose adrenal insufficiency.[39,51,62–65,71,97–101] However, the overall incidence of adrenal insufficiency in critically ill patients approximates 30%, with an incidence as high as 50% to 60% in patients with septic shock.[72] The following incidences of adrenal insufficiency apply to patient groups with no previous history suggestive of adrenal insufficiency (e.g., previous use of glucocorticoids). For example, using the criteria cited earlier (stress cortisol level <25 μg/dL), we diagnosed adrenal insufficiency in 36 of 59 (61%) patients with septic shock.[71] Only 5 (9%) of these patients met the "classic criteria" (cortisol level <18 μg/dL 60 minutes after 250 μg corticotropin) for adrenal insufficiency. Rydvall and colleagues[102] reported a 47% incidence of adrenal insufficiency in a general ICU population (using a stress cortisol threshold of 25 μg/dL). Briegel and colleagues[99] reported 13 of 20 (65%) patients with septic shock having a stress cortisol level of less than 25 μg/dL. Sibbald and colleagues[65] reported 20 of 26 (77%) septic patients with stress cortisol levels of less than 25 μg/dL. Moran and colleagues[103] reported a 49% incidence of adrenal insufficiency in patients with septic shock. We reported a 50% to 75% incidence of adrenal insufficiency in critically ill HIV-infected patients.[73]. Interestingly, we found a 0% incidence of adrenal insufficiency in nonhypotensive septic patients, which contrasted with a 61% incidence in septic patients with hypotension.[71] Patients with closed head injury have an incidence of adrenal insufficiency of approximately 15%, whereas patients with cardiogenic shock following myocardial infarction have an incidence of adrenal insufficiency of approximately 5% to 10%. In a subset of patients with acute gastrointestinal hemorrhage and hypotension, we found an incidence of adrenal insufficiency of only 2% to 4%. Unfortunately, the incidence of adrenal insufficiency has not been evaluated reliably in all groups of critically ill patients and clearly varies with the underlying disease.

Clinical Features of Acute HPA Axis Failure

Patients with chronic adrenal insufficiency usually present with a history of weakness, weight loss, anorexia, lethargy, slowed mentation, and general failure to thrive. Some patients complain of nausea, vomiting, abdominal pain, and diarrhea. Clinical signs include orthostatic hypotension and, rarely, hyperpigmentation (primary adrenal insufficiency). Laboratory testing may demonstrate hyponatremia, hyperkalemia, hypoglycemia, and a normocytic anemia.[74,104] This presentation contrasts with the features of acute adrenal insufficiency (Table 79-2). Hypotension refractory to fluids and requiring vasopressors is the most common feature of acute adrenal insufficiency in critically ill patients.[71,74,104] Patients usually have a hyperdynamic circulation, which may compound the hyperdynamic profile of septic patients.[71] However, the systemic vascular resistance, cardiac output, and pulmonary capillary wedge pressure can be low, normal, or high.[72] The variability in hemodynamics reflects the combination of adrenal insufficiency and the underlying disease. Importantly, acute adrenal insufficiency always should be excluded in critically ill patients requiring vasopressor support. CNS dysfunction is common, frequently compounded by the underlying disease. However, adrenal failure may present with altered mental

TABLE 79-2 Symptoms and Signs Suggestive of Hypoadrenalism in Critically Ill Patients

Specific features
- Hypotensive septic patients
- Vasopressor-dependent patients
- Eosinophilia (usually mild)
- Hyponatremia and hyperkalemia
- Hypoglycemia (rare)
- Pituitary deficiencies (gonadotrophin, thyroid, diabetes insipidus)
- Hyperpigmentation (rare)
- Vitiligo (rare)

Nonspecific features
- Weakness, fatigue
- Anorexia, weight loss
- Nausea, vomiting
- Diarrhea
- Anemia
- Metabolic acidosis
- Unexplained fever
- Unexplained mental status changes
- Hyperdynamic circulation

status, particularly unexplained confusion, as the major clinical finding. Lethargy, weakness, anorexia, and abdominal complaints are common. Furthermore, in critically ill patients with unexplained fever, adrenal failure should be excluded. Laboratory assessment may demonstrate eosinophilia and hypoglycemia. Hyponatremia and hyperkalemia are uncommon. Many patients have a mild metabolic acidosis.

Causes of Acute Adrenal Insufficiency in the Critically Ill

Acute adrenal insufficiency (Table 79-3) occurs in patients who are unable to increase their production of cortisol in the face of acute stress. This includes patients with hypothalamic and pituitary disorders (secondary adrenal insufficiency) and patients with destructive diseases of the adrenal glands (primary adrenal insufficiency). Secondary adrenal insufficiency is common in patients who have been treated with exogenous corticosteroids within the past year. Other causes of secondary adrenal insufficiency include pituitary infarction, hypothalamic disease, and sepsis.

Synthetic glucocorticoids are commonly used drugs. The use of these drugs is associated with suppression of the HPA axis. The degree of suppression depends on many factors, including the glucocorticoid potency, the dose, the dosing schedule, and the duration of use. The degree of suppression, however, generally is not predictable in any individual patient.[105] The use of inhaled corticosteroids in asthmatics also has been associated with varying degrees of adrenal suppression.[75,106] Systemic glucocorticoids probably do not cause significant HPA axis suppression when used for less than 5 days. When these drugs are used for between 5 and 30 days, the HPA axis will recover in most patients within 14 days of stopping treatment.[107] However, when used for longer than 30 days, it may take up to a year for the HPA axis to recover. The recovery of the HPA axis can be assessed most reliably by measurement of a random cortisol level in a stressed patient. The degree of adrenal recovery in the

TABLE 79-3 Causes of Adrenal Insufficiency

Primary adrenal insufficiency
Bacterial sepsis/septic shock
    Gram-negative and gram-positive infections
    Tuberculosis
Systemic inflammatory response
HIV infection
Cytomegalovirus infection
Systemic fungal infection (histoplasmosis, cryptococcosis,
    blastomycosis)
Acute adrenal hemorrhage (disseminated intravascular
    coagulation, anticoagulation)
Acute adrenal thrombosis with infarction (antiphospholipid
    antibody syndrome, heparin)
Autoimmune-induced atrophy
Metastatic cancer
Hypothermia
Drugs
    Ketoconazole
    Etomidate
    Metyrapone
    Mitotane
Secondary adrenal insufficiency
Exogenous glucocorticoid use
Sepsis/septic shock
Systemic inflammatory response
Pituitary surgery or irradiation
Pituitary infarction
Pituitary or metastatic tumor
Craniopharyngioma
Infiltrative disease of pituitary or hypothalamus (sarcoidosis,
    histiocytosis)
HIV infection
Head trauma
Drugs
    Megestrol acetate
    Rifampin (increased metabolism)
    Phenytoin (increased metabolism)

unstressed patient can be determined by the response to 1 μg corticotropin.[115] However, it is important to note that supraphysiologic doses of glucocorticoids suppress both CRH production in the hypothalamus and ACTH production in the pituitary gland. This suppression can outlast the duration of adrenal suppression.[108] Therefore, a normal cortisol response to high-dose corticotropin does not predict conclusively a normal response to stress (which involves the hypothalamic-pituitary components of the axis).[109] The properties of the corticosteroids in common use are listed in Table 79-4.

The most common cause of chronic primary adrenal insufficiency (Addison's disease) in the past was tuberculosis, followed by autoimmune disease. However, human immun-odeficiency virus (HIV) infection and other infections in immunosuppressed patients (e.g., tuberculosis, CMV, fungal) are currently the most important causes of primary adrenal insufficiency. The adrenal gland is the endocrine organ most commonly involved in patients with the acquired immunodeficiency syndrome (AIDS).[110–114] Human CMV has been demonstrated in the adrenal glands of 33 to 88 percent of patients who died of AIDS. Less commonly, tubercle bacilli, *Cryptococcus neoformans, Toxoplasma gondii, Histoplasma capsulatum*, lymphoma, hemorrhage, or Kaposi's sarcoma may involve the adrenal gland.[113] In addition, a number of drugs used in patients with HIV infection, most notably ketoconazole and megestrol acetate, can impair adrenal function.[115,116] Although the adrenal gland is commonly affected by opportunistic infections and tumor infiltration in AIDS, adrenal insufficiency in the outpatient setting is uncommon.[113,117] However, these patients may be unable to increase the synthesis of cortisol in the face of stress. Using the revised diagnostic criteria (i.e., stress cortisol level <25 μg/dL), we reported adrenal insufficiency in 75% of critically ill HIV-infected patients who had not been treated with corticosteroids.[73]

Sepsis and the systemic inflammatory response syndrome (SIRS) are the most common causes of adrenal failure in the critically ill. There is increasing evidence of HPA axis insufficiency in critically ill septic patients, which appears to result from circulating suppressive factors released during systemic inflammation.[39,62–65,71,80] It should be emphasized that in most cases adrenal failure results from suppression of the HPA axis and GR expression and is completely reversible, with restoration of normal adrenal function once the patient has recovered from the septic episode.[99] In addition to sepsis, we have noted a high incidence of HPA axis failure in patients with liver failure. The exact cause remains unclear. However, we recommend screening all critically ill cirrhotic patients for adrenal failure.

We have reported three patterns of adrenal insufficiency in patients with septic shock based on their response to low-dose (LD) and high-dose (HD) corticotropin.[71] Forty-two percent of patients failed to respond to both LD and HD corticotropin and most likely represent patients with primary adrenal gland failure. Twenty-eight percent of patients had low stress cortisol levels but responded to both LD and HD corticotropin; we postulate that these patients lacked adequate secretion of CRH or ACTH and represent patients with secondary adrenal insufficiency. In a previous study we demonstrated that 85% of the patients with adrenal insufficiency (baseline cortisol of less than 25 μg/dL) had inappropriately low (<40 pg/mL) ACTH levels.[118] A third group of patients (30%) failed to respond to LD corticotropin but responded normally to HD corticotropin. Due to the ability of pharmacologic doses of corticotropin to produce a normal

TABLE 79-4 Properties of Commonly Used Corticosteroids

Agent	Equivalent Dose, mg	Glucocorticoid Potency	Mineralocorticoid Potency	Duration of Action, h
Dexamethasone	0.75	25	0	72
Methylprednisolone	4	5	0.5	36
Prednisolone	5	4	0.8	24
Prednisone	5	4	0.8	24
Hydrocortisone	25	1	1	8

response, when physiologic stress levels of corticotropin were ineffective, we postulate that this group represents patients with corticotropin resistance. It is possible that these various patterns of HPA axis failure during critical illness represent the differential effects of inhibitory mediators at various levels of the HPA axis.

Adrenal Exhaustion Syndrome

Patients with chronic critical illness may develop adrenal insufficiency while in the ICU. Although not evaluated in prospective trials, we have observed patients who had normal adrenal function when admitted to the ICU but who later developed adrenal insufficiency (e.g., long term ventilated patient with ARDS) (Fig. 79-4). The only apparent cause was a prolonged systemic inflammatory response. The adrenal insufficiency may have resulted from chronic secretion of systemic cytokines and other HPA axis suppressive substances.[119] These patients have a higher mortality compared with patients who maintain adequate cortisol levels (see Fig. 79-4) and illustrate the importance of serial follow-up of adrenal function in long-term critically ill patients.

Prognosis

We believe that there is a bimodal distribution of mortality in relationship to the random cortisol level during sepsis. Patients with low cortisol levels (i.e., <25 µg/dL) who are not treated with corticosteroids and patients with very high levels (i.e., >45 µg/dL) have the highest mortality. This hypothesis may explain the apparent contradictory reports in the literature. Annane and colleagues[59] reported a mean random cortisol level of 34 µg/dL in 189 patients with septic shock, with the nonsurvivors having higher levels than survivors (39 versus 28 µg/dL, respectively). However, in the study by Schroeder and colleagues,[40] the mean random cortisol level

was only 19 µg/dL, with nonsurvivors having a lower cortisol level than survivors (10 versus 17 µg/dL). Most of the patients included in the study by Schroeder and colleagues would have met our criteria for adrenal insufficiency. However, none of the patients was treated with corticosteroids.

Impaired responses to corticotropin and CRH are also associated with increased mortality.[40,103] However, it remains unclear as to whether the impaired response is a direct contributor to the increased mortality or is secondary to hypothalamic-pituitary dysfunction or suppression (i.e., from circulating mediators or elevated cortisol levels).

Treatment of Acute Adrenal Insufficiency

Deficiency of cortisol is associated with increased morbidity and mortality during critical illness. Mckee[68] randomized 18 critically ill patients with adrenal insufficiency to glucocorticoid treatment or placebo. One of eight (13%) steroid-treated patients died compared with 9 of 10 (90%) placebo patients. Evidence for high mortality from adrenal insufficiency in critically ill patients also comes from the report of Ledingham and Watt,[120] who noted increased mortality from use of etomidate (a sedative agent that causes adrenal insufficiency) in multiple-trauma patients (44% etomidate versus 27% other sedatives). The report by Ledingham and Watt emphasizes that even slight impairment of the adrenal response during severe illness can be lethal. Rivers and colleagues[97] reported faster weaning from vasopressors and improved survival in hydrocortisone-treated critically ill patients (79% versus 55%). We found that patients with septic shock and inappropriately low cortisol levels had improved survival when treated with hydrocortisone (65% versus 35%).

Further evidence to support the benefit of glucocorticoid treatment of acute adrenal insufficiency in patients with septic shock comes from the studies of Bollaert and colleagues[94] and Briegel and coworkers.[93] Bollaert and colleagues[94]

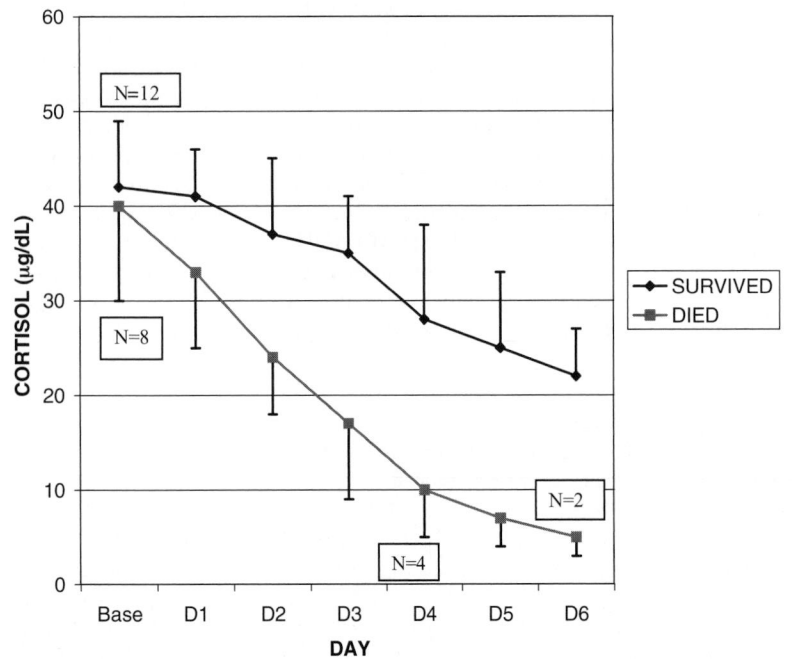

FIGURE 79-4 Adrenal exhaustion syndrome. Daily cortisol levels in a group of patients with sepsis who survived versus died. Cortisol fell to very low levels, which are consistent with adrenal insufficiency in the patients who died.

randomized 41 patients with septic shock to hydrocortisone (100 mg IV every 8 hours) or placebo. Although random cortisol levels were obtained, treatment with hydrocortisone was not stratified based on the levels. However, the glucocorticoid-treated patients had a significantly greater reversal of shock at 7 and 28 days and reduced 28-day mortality (30% versus 70%, $p = 0.09$) compared with the placebo group. Similarly, Briegel and colleagues[93] randomized 40 critically ill septic shock patients to intravenous hydrocortisone or placebo. Hydrocortisone treatment was associated with improved shock reversal and decreased days of vasopressor support. There also was earlier resolution of organ dysfunction, shorter ventilator time, and shorter ICU stay. Annane and colleagues[80,96] randomized 200 septic shock patients to steroid replacement or placebo. There was a significant 30% decrease in death in a subset of the steroid-treated patients. Oppert and colleagues[95] treated 20 septic shock patients with hydrocortisone (10 mg/h for 7 days). Patients with "inadequate" steroid production were weaned from vasopressors significantly faster than patients with "adequate" steroid production. These studies of physiologic stress doses of glucocorticoids administered for many days contrast with earlier studies of high-dose glucocorticoids (i.e., 30 mg/kg methylprednisolone) administered for one to two doses. The short-term pharmacologic dose studies of glucocorticoids failed to report benefit in patients with septic shock.[121,122]

Interestingly, Schelling and colleagues[123] evaluated the effect of hydrocortisone treatment during septic shock on the incidence of posttraumatic stress disorder. The administration of hydrocortisone at stress levels during septic shock reduced the incidence of posttraumatic stress disorder and improved emotional well-being in survivors.

Perioperative Steroid Coverage

The stress of major surgery may precipitate acute adrenal insufficiency in patients with inadequate adrenal reserve (i.e., adrenal crisis). This is especially true in patients with secondary adrenal insufficiency maintained on exogenous glucocorticoids. Prospective, randomized trials have failed to adequately evaluate the dose of glucocorticoid required in various perioperative settings. Thus recommendations for glucocorticoid coverage are based on a risk-benefit evaluation, published studies in the literature, and clinical experience. Importantly, patients with adrenal insufficiency undergoing surgery should receive appropriate stress doses of glucocorticoids before and after surgery. If surgery is prolonged (i.e., >4 to 6 hours), we recommend an additional dose of glucocorticoid during surgery. Patients with a high likelihood of impaired gastric emptying or impaired gut absorption should receive glucocorticoid repletion via the intravenous route until gut function has returned to relatively normal levels. We caution against the use of intramuscular glucocorticoid preparations in patients in whom hypoperfusion of muscle is likely. Patients also should receive sufficient steroid to control their underlying disease (e.g., asthma, autoimmune disease). Minimal doses of glucocorticoid for treatment of patients with suspected adrenal insufficiency based on type of surgery are as follows: First, patients undergoing minor surgery (e.g., hernia repair, laparoscopic cholecystectomy, knee surgery) should receive a minimal dose of 25 mg hydrocortisone equivalent prior to and 8 hours following surgery. This dose may be given orally if gut function is intact or intravenously. If patients demonstrate normal recovery, they may be weaned quickly from steroids or returned to maintenance levels. Second, patients undergoing moderate surgical stress (e.g., open cholecystectomy, partial colon resection, uncomplicated back surgery, hip replacement) should receive 25 to 50 mg hydrocortisone equivalent every 8 hours intravenously for 1 to 2 days. The dose then may be tapered to baseline levels based on clinical response. Third, patients undergoing major surgical stress (e.g., pancreatoduodenectomy, esophagectomy, total colectomy, repair for perforated bowel, cardiopulmonary bypass, ileofemoral bypass) should receive 50 to 100 mg hydrocortisone equivalent every 8 hours intravenously for 2 to 3 days. The dose then can be tapered to baseline doses based on clinical response. Importantly, the dose should be increased to maximal stress doses (100 mg hydrocortisone equivalent every 8 hours intravenously) in patients who remain hypotensive or deteriorate during recovery from surgery.[124]

Therapeutic Approach to Patients with Presumed Adrenal Insufficiency

In patients with severe stress (e.g., hypotension, hypoxemia, pain), a random (stress) serum cortisol level should be obtained (see Fig. 79-2). The patient should be started empirically on hydrocortisone (100 mg IV every 8 hours) pending results of testing. If the serum cortisol level returns less than 25 μg/dL, the hydrocortisone should be continued. In addition, if the patient has improved clinically with hydrocortisone and the cortisol level is greater than 25 μg/dL, we favor continuing the hydrocortisone for a few days (unless there is a specific contraindication). The dose of hydrocortisone should be tapered down toward maintenance doses as the patient's clinical status improves. If the level of stress is uncertain and adrenal insufficiency is suspected, we favor adrenal testing with the low-dose (1 μg) corticotropin stimulation test (see Fig. 79-2). If the corticotropin stimulation test cannot be performed immediately, administer dexamethasone (2 mg) and perform the test within the next 12 hours. Dexamethasone does not significantly crossreact with cortisol in the assay for cortisol and can be given to patients pending adrenal testing.

The currently recommended dosage schedule in adults includes 100 mg hydrocortisone intravenously every 8 hours or 50 mg intravenously every 6 hours.[69,71,80,94,97] While a continuous infusion of hydrocortisone has been recommended, there are no data at this time to suggest that this dosing regimen is more efficacious than intermittent doing. In the study reported by Annane and colleagues,[80] patients were treated with hydrocortisone (50 mg every 6 hours) and fludrocortisone (50 mg daily). However, as demonstrated previously, it appears that low aldosterone levels are part of the "normal" stress response, and there are no data to suggest that fludrocortisone provides any additional benefits over hydrocortisone alone. Furthermore, as illustrated in Table 79-4, hydrocortisone possesses mineralocorticoid activity. When given at high doses (e.g., 200 to 300 mg daily), hydrocortisone has adequate mineralocorticoid activity to treat primary adrenal failure.

Conclusion

HPA axis dysfunction is common in severely ill patients. Even slight impairment of the adrenal response to severe illness can increase morbidity and mortality, and we believe that low serum cortisol levels may be the cause rather than the consequence of poor outcome in these patients. Therefore, a high index of suspicion for adrenal insufficiency is required in all critically ill patients, particularly those with refractory hypotension. All patients with suspected HPA axis dysfunction should be treated with stress doses of corticosteroids pending the results of diagnostic testing.

References

1. Lamas O, Marti A, Martinez JA: Obesity and immunocompetence. *Eur J Clin Nutr* 56(suppl 3):S42, 2002.
2. Parker LN, Levin ER, Lifrak ET: Evidence for adrenocortical adaptation to severe illness. *J Clin Endocrinol Metab* 60:947, 1985.
3. Findling JW, Waters VO, Raff H: The dissociation of renin and aldosterone during critical illness. *J Clin Endocrinol Metab* 64:592, 1987.
4. Zipser RD, Davenport MW, Martin KL, et al: Hyperreninemic hypoaldosteronism in the critically ill: A new entity. *J Clin Endocrinol Metab* 53:867, 1981.
5. Raff H, Findling JW: Aldosterone control in critically ill patients: ACTH, metoclopramide, and atrial natriuretic peptide. *Crit Care Med* 18:915, 1990.
6. Bucher M, Ittner KP, Hobbhahn J, et al: Downregulation of angiotensin II type 1 receptors during sepsis. *Hypertension* 38:177, 2001.
7. Hollenberg SM, Weinberger C, Ong ES, et al: Primary structure and expression of a functional human glucocorticoid receptor cDNA. *Nature* 318:635, 1985.
8. Yang J, DeFranco DB: Assessment of glucocorticoid receptor-heat shock protein 90 interactions in vivo during nucleocytoplasmic trafficking. *Mol Endocrinol* 10:3, 1996.
9. Perrot D, Bonneton A, Dechaud H, et al: Hypercortisolism in septic shock is not suppressible by dexamethasone infusion. *Crit Care Med* 21:396, 1993.
10. Pugeat M, Bonneton A, Perrot D, et al: Decreased immunoreactivity and binding activity of corticosteroid-binding globulin in serum in septic shock. *Clin Chem* 35:1675, 1989.
11. Bonte HA, van den Hoven RJ, van dS, V, Vermes I: The use of free cortisol index for laboratory assessment of pituitary-adrenal function. *Clin Chem Lab Med* 37:127, 1999.
12. Savu L, Zouaghi H, Carli A, Nunez EA: Serum depletion of corticosteroid binding activities, an early marker of human septic shock. *Biochem Biophys Res Commun* 102:411, 1981.
13. Garrel DR: Corticosteroid-binding globulin during inflammation and burn injury: Nutritional modulation and clinical implications. *Horm Res* 45:245, 1996.
14. Sun X, Fischer DR, Pritts TA, et al: Expression and binding activity of the glucocorticoid receptor are upregulated in septic muscle. *Am J Physiol Regul Integr Comp Physiol* 282: R509, 2002.
15. Hinshaw LB, Beller BK, Chang AC, et al: Corticosteroid/antibiotic treatment of adrenalectomized dogs challenged with lethal *E. coli. Circ Shock* 16:265, 1985.
16. Darlington DN, Chew G, Ha T, et al: Corticosterone, but not glucose, treatment enables fasted adrenalectomized rats to survive moderate hemorrhage. *Endocrinology* 127:766, 1990.
17. Pilkis SJ, Granner DK: Molecular physiology of the regulation of hepatic gluconeogenesis and glycolysis. *Annu Rev Physiol* 54:885, 1992.
18. Sakaue M, Hoffman BB: Glucocorticoids induce transcription and expression of the alpha 1B adrenergic receptor gene in DTT1 MF-2 smooth muscle cells. *J Clin Invest* 88:385, 1991.
19. Collins S, Caron MG, Lefkowitz RJ: Beta-adrenergic receptors in hamster smooth muscle cells are transcriptionally regulated by glucocorticoids. *J Biol Chem* 263:9067, 1988.
20. Orlowski J, Lingrel JB: Thyroid and glucocorticoid hormones regulate the expression of multiple Na,K-ATPase genes in cultured neonatal rat cardiac myocytes. *J Biol Chem* 265:3462, 1990.
21. Satoh S, Oishi K, Iwagaki A, et al: Dexamethasone impairs pulmonary defence against *Pseudomonas aeruginosa* through suppressing *iNOS* gene expression and peroxynitrite production in mice. *Clin Exp Immunol Life* 126:266, 2001.
22. Matsumura M, Kakishita H, Suzuki M, et al: Dexamethasone suppresses *iNOS* gene expression by inhibiting NF-$\kappa\beta$ in vascular smooth muscle cells. *Life Sci* 69:1067, 2001.
23. Redington AE, Meng QH, Springall DR, et al: Increased expression of inducible nitric oxide synthase and cyclooxygenase-2 in the airway epithelium of asthmatic subjects and regulation by corticosteroid treatment. *Thorax* 56:351, 2001.
24. Fujii E, Yoshioka T, Ishida H, et al: Evaluation of *iNOS*-dependent and independent mechanisms of the microvascular permeability change induced by lipopolysaccharide. *Br J Pharmacol* 130:90, 2000.
25. Munck A, Naray-Fejes-Toth A: Glucocorticoids and stress: Permisive and suppressive actions. *Ann NY Acad Sci* 746:115, 1994.
26. Fahey JV, Guyre PM: Mechanisms of antiinflammatory actions of glucocorticoids. *Adv Inflamm Res* 2:21, 1981.
27. Barnes PJ, Adcock I: Anti-inflammatory actions of steroids: molecular mechanisms. *Trends Pharmacol Sci* 14:436, 1993.
28. Barnes PJ, Karin M: Nuclear factor-$\kappa\beta$: A pivotal transcription factor in chronic inflammatory diseases. *New Engl J Med* 336:1066, 1997.
29. Auphan N, Didonato JA, Rosette C, et al: Immunosuppression by glucocorticoids: Inhibition of NF-$\kappa\beta$ activity through induction of I-$\kappa\beta$ synthesis. *Science* 270:286, 1995.
30. Barber AEI, Coyle SM, Fischer E, et al: Influence of hypercortosolemia on soluble tumor necrosis factor receptor II aand interleukin-1 receptor antagonist responses to endotoxin iin human beings. *Surgery* 118:406, 1995.
31. van der Poll T, Barber AE, Coyle SM, Lowry SF: Hypercortisolemia increases plasma interleukin-10 concentrations during human endotoxemia—a clinical research center study. *J Clin Endocrinol Metab* 81:3604, 1996.
32. Zaloga GP, Bhatt B, Marik PE: Critical illness and systemic inflammation, in Becker K, Nylen E (eds): *Practice and Principles of Endocrinology and Metabolism.* Philadelphia, Lippincott Williams & Wilkins, 2001, p 2068.
33. Besedovsky HO, del Ray A: Immunoneuroendocrine interactions: Facts and hypotheses. *Endocr Rev* 17:64, 1996.
34. Turnbull AV, Rivier CL: Regulation of the hypothalamic-pituitary-adrenal axis by cytokines: Actions and mechanisms of action. *Physiol Rev* 79:1, 1999.
35. Mastorakos G, Chrousos GP, Weber JS: Recombinant interleukin-6 activates the hypothalamic-pituitary-adrenal axis in humans. *J Clin Endocrinol Metab* 77:1690, 1993.
36. Bateman A, Singh A, Kral T, Solomon S: The immune-hypothalamic-pituitary-adrenal axis. *Endocr Rev* 10:92, 1989.
37. Gaillard RC, Turnill D, Sappino P, Muller AF: Tumor necrosis factor α inhibits the hormonal response of the pituitary gland to hypothalamic releasing factors. *Endocrinology* 127:101, 1990.
38. Richards ML, Caplan RH, Wickus GG, et al: The rapid low-dose (1 microgram) Cosyntropin test in the immediate postoperative period: Results in elderly subjects after major abdominal surgery. *Surgery* 125:431, 1999.
39. Soni A, Pepper GM, Wyrwinski PM, et al: Adrenal insufficiency occurring during septic shock: Incidence, outcome, and relationship to peripheral cytokine levels. *Am J Med* 98:266, 1995.

40. Schroeder S, Wichers M, Klingmuller D, et al: The hypothalamic-pituitary-adrenal axis of patients with severe sepsis: Altered response to corticotropin-releasing hormone. *Crit Care Med* 29:310, 2001.

41. Catalano RD, Parameswaran V, Ramachandran J, Trunkey DD: Mechanisms of adrenocortical depression during *Escherichia coli* shock. *Arch Surg* 119:145, 1984.

42. Keri G, Parameswaran V, Trunkey DD, Ramachandran J: Effects of septic shock plasma on adrenocortical cell function. *Life Sci* 28:1917, 1981.

43. Melby JC, Egdahl RH, Spink WW: Secretion and metabolism of cortisol after injection of endotoxin. *J Lab Clin Med* 56:50, 1960.

44. Jaattela M, Ilvesmaki V, Voutilainen R, et al: Tumor necrosis factor as a potent inhibitor of adrenocorticotropin-induced cortisol production and steroidogenic P450 enzyme gene expression in cultured human fetal adrenal cells. *Endocrinology* 128:623, 1991.

45. Zhu Q, Solomon S: Isolation and mode of action of rabbit corticostatic (antiadrenocorticotropin) peptides. *Endocrinology* 130:1413, 1992.

46. Masera RG, Bateman A, Muscettola M, et al: Corticostatins/defensins inhibit in vitro NK activity and cytokine production by human peripheral blood mononuclear cells. *Regul Pept* 62:13, 1996.

47. Tominaga T, Fukata J, Hayashi Y, et al: Distribution and characterization of immunoreactive corticostatin in the hypothalamic-pituitary-adrenal axis. *Endocrinology* 130:1593, 1992.

48. Natarajan R, Ploszay S, Horton R, Nadler J: Tumor necrosis factor and interleukin-1 are potent inhibitors of angiotenisin II–induced aldosterone synthesis. *Endocrinology* 125:3084, 1989.

49. Jaattela M, Carpen O, Stenman UH, Saksela E: Regulation of ACTH-induced steroidogenesis in human fetal adrenals by rTNF-α. *Mol Cell Endocrinol* 68:R31, 1990.

50. Pariante CM, Pearce BD, Pisell TL, et al: The proinflammatory cytokine, interleukin-1α, reduces glucocorticoid receptor translocation and function. *Endocrinology* 140:4359, 1999.

51. Melby JC, Spink WW: Comparative studies of adrenal cortisal function and cortisol metabolism in healthy adults and in patients with septic shock due to infection. *J Clin Invest* 37:1791, 1958.

52. McCallum RE, Stith RD: Endotoxin-induced inhibition of steroid binding by mouse liver cytosol. *Circ Shock* 9:357, 1982.

53. Liu DH, Su YP, Zhang W, et al: Changes in glucocorticoid and mineralocorticoid receptors of liver and kidney cytosols after pathologic stress and its regulation in rats. *Crit Care Med* 30:623, 2002.

54. Ali M, Allen HR, Vedeckis WV, Lang CH: Depletion of rat liver glucocorticoid receptor hormone-binding and its mRNA in sepsis. *Life Sci* 48:603, 1991.

55. Molijn GJ, Koper JW, van Uffelen CJ, et al: Temperature-induced down-regulation of the glucocorticoid receptor in peripheral blood mononuclear leucocytes in patients with sepsis and septic shock. *Clin Endocrinol* 43:197, 1995.

56. Krasznai A, Aranyi P, Feher T, et al: Alterations in the number of glucocorticoid receptors of circulating lymphocytes in sepsis. *Haematologia* 19:293, 1986.

57. Schuler JJ, Erve PR, Schumer W: Glucocorticoid effect on hepatic carbohydrates metabolism in the endotoxin-shocked monkey. *Ann Surg* 183:345, 1976.

58. Streeten DHP: What test for hypothalamic-pituitary adrenocortical insufficiency? *Lancet* 354:179, 1999.

59. Annane D, Sebille V, Troche G, et al: A three-level prognostic classification in septic shock based on cortisol levels and cortisol response to corticotropin. *JAMA* 283:1038, 2000.

60. Annane D, Bellissant E: Prognostic value of cortisol response in septic shock. *JAMA* 284:308, 2000.

61. Streeten DH, Anderson GH Jr, Bonaventura MM: The potential for serious consequences from misinterpreting normal responses to the rapid adrenocorticotropin test. *J Clin Endocrinol Metab* 81:285, 1996.

62. Beishuizen A, Vermes I, Hylkema BS, Haanen C: Relative eosinophilia and functional adrenal insufficiency in critically ill patients (letter). *Lancet* 353:1675, 1999.

63. Drucker D, McLaughlin J: Adrenocortical dysfunction in acute medical illness. *Crit Care Med* 14:789, 1986.

64. Drucker D, Shandling M: Variable adrenocortical function in acute medical illness. *Crit Care Med* 13:477, 1985.

65. Sibbald WJ, Short A, Cohen MP, Wilson RF: Variations in adrenocortical responsiveness during severe bacterial infections: Unrecognized adrenocortical insufficiency in severe bacterial infections. *Ann Surg* 186:29, 1977.

66. Hampson N, Norkool D: Carbon monoxide poisoning in children riding in the back of pickup trucks. *JAMA* 267:538, 1992.

67. Dennhardt R, Gramm HJ, Meinhold K, Voigt K: Patterns of endocrine secretion during sepsis. *Prog Clin Biol Res* 308:751, 1989.

68. McKee JI, Finlay WE: Cortisol replacement in severely stressed patients (letter). *Lancet* 1:484, 1983.

69. Cooper MD, Stewart PM: Corticosteroid insufficiency in acutely ill patients. *New Engl J Med* 348:727, 2003.

70. Clark PM, Neylon I, Raggatt PR, et al: Defining the normal cortisol response to the short Synacthen test: Implications for the investigation of hypothalamic-pituitary disorders. *Clin Endocrinol* 49:287, 1998.

71. Marik PE, Zaloga GP: Adrenal insufficiency during septic shock. *Crit Care Med* 31:141, 2003.

72. Zaloga GP, Marik P: Hypothalamic-pituitary-adrenal insufficiency. *Crit Care Clin* 17:25, 2001.

73. Marik PE, Kiminyo K, Zaloga GP: Adrenal insufficiency in critically ill HIV-infected patients. *Crit Care Med* 30:1267, 2002.

74. Marik PE, Zaloga GP: Adrenal insufficiency in the critically ill: A new look at an old problem. *Chest* 122:1784, 2002.

75. Broide J, Soferman R, Kivity S, et al: Low-dose adrenocorticotropin test reveals impaired adrenal function in patients taking inhaled corticosteroids. *J Clin Endocrinol Metab* 80:1243, 1995.

76. Mayenknecht J, Diederich S, Bahr V, et al: Comparison of low and high dose corticotropin stimulation tests in patients with pituitary disease. *J Clin Endocrinol Metab* 83:1558, 1998.

77. Rasmuson S, Olsson T, Hagg E: A low dose ACTH test to assess the function of the hypothalamic-pituitary-adrenal axis. *Clin Endocrinol* 44:151, 1996.

78. Tordjman K, Jaffe A, Grazas N, et al: The role of the low dose (1 microgram) adrenocorticotropin test in the evaluation of patients with pituitary diseases. *J Clin Endocrinol Metab* 80:1301, 1995.

79. Abdu TA, Elhadd TA, Neary R, Clayton RN: Comparison of the low dose short Synacthen test (1 microgram), the conventional dose short Synacthen test (250 microgram), and the insulin tolerance test for assessment of the hypothalamo-pituitary-adrenal axis in patients with pituitary disease. *J Clin Endocrinol Metab* 84:838, 1999.

80. Annane D, Sebille V, Charpentier C, et al: Effect of treatment with low doses of hydrocortisone and fludrocortisone on mortality in patients with septic shock. *JAMA* 288:862, 2002.

81. Lamberts SW, Bruining HA, de Jong FH: Corticosteroid therapy in severe illness. *New Engl J Med* 337:1285, 1997.

82. Naito Y, Fukata J, Tamai S, et al: Biphasic changes in hypothalamic-pituitary-adrenal function during the early recovery period after major abdominal surgery. *J Clin Endocrinol Metab* 73:111, 1991.

83. Naito Y, Tamai S, Shingu K, et al: Responses of plasma adrenocorticotropic hormone, cortisol, and cytokines during and after upper abdominal surgery. *Anesthesiology* 77:426, 1992.

84. Karayiannakis AJ, Makri GG, Mantzioka A, et al: Systemic stress response after laparoscopic or open cholecystectomy: A randomized trial. *Br J Surg* 84:467, 1997.

85. Schricker T, Carli F, Schreiber M, et al: Propofol/sufentanil anesthesia suppresses the metabolic and endocrine response during, not after, lower abdominal surgery. *Anesth Analg* 90:450, 2000.

86. Motamed S, Klubien K, Edwardes M, et al: Metabolic changes during recovery in normothermic versus hypothermic patients undergoing surgery and receiving general anesthesia and epidural local anesthetic agents. *Anesthesiology* 88:1211, 1998.

87. Plunkett JJ, Reeves JD, Ngo L, et al: Urine and plasma catecholamine and cortisol concentrations after myocardial revascularization: Modulation by continuous sedation. Multicenter Study of Perioperative Ischemia (McSPI) Research Group, and the Ischemia Research and Education Foundation (IREF). *Anesthesiology* 86:785, 1997.

88. Vermes I, Beishuizen A, Hampsink RM, Haanen C: Dissociation of plasma adrenocorticotropin and cortisol levels in critically ill patients: Possible role of endothelin and atrial natriuretic hormone. *J Clin Endocrinol Metab* 80:1238, 1995.

89. Jurney TH, Cockrell JL Jr, Lindberg JS, et al: Spectrum of serum cortisol response to ACTH in ICU patients: Correlation with degree of illness and mortality. *Chest* 92:292, 1987.

90. Wade CE, Lindberg JS, Cockrell JL, et al: Upon-admission adrenal steroidogenesis is adapted to the degree of illness in intensive care unit patients. *J Clin Endocrinol Metab* 67:223, 1988.

91. Chernow B, Rainey TR, Lake CR: Endogenous and exogenous catecholamines in critical care medicine. *Crit Care Med* 10:409, 1982.

92. Hart BB, Stanford GG, Ziegler MG, et al: Catecholamines: Study of interspecies variation. *Crit Care Med* 17:1203, 1989.

93. Briegel J, Forst H, Haller M, et al: Stress doses of hydrocortisone reverse hyperdynamic septic shock: A prospective, randomized, double-blind, single-center study. *Crit Care Med* 27:723, 1999.

94. Bollaert PE, Charpentier C, Levy B, et al: Reversal of late septic shock with supraphysiologic doses of hydrocortisone. *Crit Care Med* 26:645, 1998.

95. Oppert M, Reinicke A, Graf KJ, et al: Plasma cortisol levels before and during "low-dose" hydrocortisone therapy and their relationship to hemodynamic improvement in patients with septic shock. *Intensive Care Med* 26:1747, 2000.

96. Annane D: Effects of the combination of hydrocortisone-fludrocortisone on mortality in septic shock (abstract). *Crit Care Med* 28(suppl):A46, 2000.

97. Rivers EP, Gaspari M, Abi Saad G, et al: Adrenal insufficiency in high-risk surgical ICU patients. *Chest* 119:889, 2001.

98. Parker LN, Levin ER, Lifrak ET: Evidence for adrenocortical adaptation to severe illness. *J Clin Endocrinol Metab* 60:947, 1985.

99. Briegel J, Scheelling G, Haller M, et al: A comparison of the adrenocorticcal response during septic shock and after complete recovery. *Intensive Care Med* 22:894, 1996.

100. Barquist E, Kirton O: Adrenal insufficiency in the surgical intensive care unit patient. *J Trauma* 42:27, 1997.

101. Schein RMH, Sprung CL, Marcial E: Plasma cortisol levels in patients with septic shock. *Crit Care Med* 18:259, 1990.

102. Rydvall A, Brandstrom AK, Banga R, et al: Plasma cortisol is often decreased in patients in an intensive care unit. *Intensive Care Med* 26:545, 2000.

103. Moran JL, Chapman MJ, O'Fathartaigh MS, et al: Hypocortisolaemia and adrenocortical responsiveness at onset of septic shock. *Intensive Care Med* 20:489, 1994.

104. Oelkers W: Adrenal insufficiency. *New Engl J Med* 335:1206, 1996.

105. Schlaghecke R, Kornely E, Santen RT, Ridderskamp P: The effect of long-term glucocorticoid therapy on pituitary-adrenal responses to exogenous corticotropin-releasing hormone. *New Engl J Med* 326:226, 1992.

106. Kannisto S, Korpi M, Remes K, Voutilainen R: Adreanl suppression, evaluated by a low dose adrenocorticotropin test, and growth in asthmatic children treated with inhaled steroids. *J Clin Endocrinol Metab* 85:652, 2000.

107. Henzen C, Suter A, Lerch E, et al: Supression and recovery of adrenal response after short-term high-dose glucocorticoid treatment. *Lancet* 355:542, 2000.

108. Jasani MK, Boyle JA, Greig WR, et al: Corticosteroid-induced suppression of the hypothalamo-pituitary-adrenal axis: Observations on patients given oral corticosteroids for rheumatoid arthritis. *Q J Med* 36:261, 1967.

109. Krasner AS: Glucocorticoid-induced adrenal insufficiency. *JAMA* 282:671, 1999.

110. Pulakhandam U, Dincsoy HP: Cytomegaloviral adrenalitis and adrenal insufficiency in AIDS. *Am J Clin Pathol* 93:651, 1990.

111. Glasgow BJ, Steinsapir KD, Anders K, Layfield LJ: Adrenal pathology in the acquired immune deficiency syndrome. *Am J Clin Pathol* 84:594, 1985.

112. Welch K, Finkbeiner W, Alpers CE, et al: Autopsy findings in the acquired immune deficiency syndrome. *JAMA* 252:1152, 1984.

113. Grinspoon SK, Bilezikian JP: HIV disease and the endocrine system. *New Engl J Med* 327:1360, 1992.

114. Aron DC: Endocrine complications of the acquired immunodeficiency syndrome. *Arch Intern Med* 149:330, 1989.

115. Sonino N: The use of ketoconazole as an inhibitor of steroid production. *New Engl J Med* 317:812, 1987.

116. Smith GH: Treatment of infections in the patient with acquired immunodeficiency syndrome. *Arch Intern Med* 154:949, 1994.

117. Hofbauer LC, Heufelder AE: Endocrine implications of human immunodeficiency virus infection. *Medicine* 75:262, 1996.

118. Marik PE, Rotella LC, Zaloga GP: Secondary adrenal insufficiency is common in critically ill patients (abstract). *Crit Care Med* 29(suppl):A163, 2001.

119. Zaloga GP: Sepsis-induced adrenal deficiency syndrome. *Crit Care Med* 29:688, 2001.

120. Ledingham IM, Watt I: Influence of sedation on mortality in critically ill multiple trauma patients (letter). *Lancet* 1:1270, 1983.

121. The Veterans Administration Systemic Sepsis Cooperative study Group: Effect of high dose glucocorticoid therapy on mortality in patients with clinical signs of systemic sepsis. *New Engl J Med* 317:659, 1987.

122. Bone RC, Fisher CJ, Clemmer TP, et al: A controlled clinical trial of high-dose methylprednisolone in the treatment of severe sepsis and septic shock. *New Engl J Med* 317:653, 1987.

123. Schelling G, Stoll C, Kapfhammer HP, et al: The effect of stress doses of hydrocortisone during septic shock on posttraumatic stress disorder and health-related quality of life in survivors. *Crit Care Med* 27:2678, 1999.

124. Salem M, Trainsh RE, Bromberg J, et al: Perioperative glucocorticoid coverage: A reassessment 42 years after emergence of a problem. *Ann Surg* 219:416, 1994.

Chapter 80 —————————————————————
THYROID DISEASE
ROY E. WEISS
SAMUEL REFETOFF

KEY POINTS

- *Virtually all patients admitted to an ICU have low levels of serum triiodothyronine (T$_3$), and 30% to 50% have low levels of thyroxine (T$_4$) with normal or low levels of serum thyrotropin (TSH).*

- *Patients who have a T$_4$ level of less than 3.0 μg/dL despite normal levels of T$_4$-binding proteins have a 68% to 84% mortality rate.*

- *T$_3$ is the logical choice for critically ill patients requiring thyroid hormone replacement.*

- *Early intubation and mechanical ventilation are crucial for successful treatment of myxedema coma.*

- *Management of myxedema coma should include administration of glucocorticoids while the adrenal status is being assessed.*

- *Alterations in thyroid function change the metabolism of almost all drugs, and the doses need careful adjustment to prevent drug toxicity or decreased efficacy.*

- *Autonomous hypersecretion and exogenous overdose of thyroid hormone are the most common causes of severe thyrotoxicosis.*

- *Hyperpyrexia and altered mental status are the hallmarks of thyroid storm.*

- *Medical treatment of severe hyperthyroidism usually normalizes circulating thyroid hormone levels in 2 to 3 weeks, except under circumstances of iodine overload, in which case hyperthyroxinemia may persist for months.*

- *Blockade of hormonal secretion is best accomplished by the addition of stable iodine to an antithyroid drug regimen.*

- *In severe thyrotoxicosis, treatment with iopanoic acid (TELEPAQUE) can be lifesaving.*

- *βBlockers prevent thyroid storm in the thyrotoxic patient undergoing surgery, and they may ameliorate cardiovascular dysfunction in thyroid storm, but their side effects often interfere with therapy in the elderly, in patients with asthma, and in patients with cardiomyopathy.*

- *Amiodarone-induced thyrotoxicosis in a critically ill patient should be managed with methimazole (30 to 50 mg/d), potassium perchlorate (500 mg twice a day), and prednisone (30 to 40 mg/d).*

- *After gastric aspiration and lavage, only symptomatic and supportive treatment is needed in cases of levothyroxine overdose.*

- *Neonatal thyrotoxicosis can be life threatening; it is usually caused by transplacental transfer of thyroid-stimulating antibodies. It is transient and requires only short-term treatment.*

Hypothyroidism, Nonthyroidal Illness, and Myxedema Coma

Hypothyroidism is a state of tissue deprivation of thyroid hormone. It is manifested by general reduction of the metabolic rate accompanied by specific symptoms and signs. Usually, hypothyroidism is caused by a decreased supply of thyroid hormone due to one of the following: (1) failure of the gland to synthesize and secrete thyroid hormone, (2) failure of the pituitary to secrete thyrotropin (thyroid-stimulating hormone [TSH]), or (3) hypothalamic disease resulting in a deficiency of thyrotropin-releasing hormone (TRH).

Perhaps the most controversial, if not the most challenging, aspects of thyroidology for the intensivist are how to interpret thyroid function tests in critically ill patients and what to do when the test results are abnormal. Clinically important hypothyroidism in its most severe form usually is seen in patients with primary hypothyroidism who then develop some intercurrent illness; it develops over several weeks and culminates in myxedema coma. Equally challenging are the thyroid function abnormalities seen in patients with concurrent severe illness and the assessment of the thyroid hormone status at the tissue level.

Evaluation of Thyroid Function in Patients with Severe Nonthyroidal Illness Syndrome (NTIS)

DEFINITION OF NONTHYROIDAL ILLNESS SYNDROME

Virtually all critically ill patients have reduced serum levels of triiodothyronine (T$_3$), and approximately 30% to 50% also have low levels of thyroxine (T$_4$), both associated with normal or low serum TSH values.[1] This phenomenon has been termed *low T$_3$ syndrome, nonthyroidal illness* (NTI), or *euthyroid sick syndrome*. Each of these descriptive terms assumes a priori that such patients are euthyroid despite reduced thyroid hormone levels. The condition is not limited to acute illness. Patients with chronic hepatic or renal failure, calorie deprivation, and a variety of other illnesses present similar thyroid hormone profiles.[2] Serum concentrations of both T$_3$ and T$_4$ also are decreased following nonthyroid surgical procedures.[3] In patients with a T$_4$ value of less than 3.0 μg/dL, the mortality rate is 68% to 84%,[4] indicating that a low T$_4$ concentration without a corresponding increase in TSH is a marker for a high risk of death in the critically ill population. To understand this phenomenon and develop a rational basis for treatment, it is useful to review the thyroid physiology, with emphasis on processes occurring in NTI.

THYROID HORMONE PHYSIOLOGY IN CRITICAL ILLNESS (FIG. 80-1)

METABOLISM OF THYROID HORMONE IN PERIPHERAL TISSUES

Ninety percent of the hormone secreted by the thyroid gland is T$_4$, the remainder being T$_3$. Thyroid hormone is metabolized in peripheral tissues by stepwise monodeiodination until the molecule is completely stripped of iodine. This

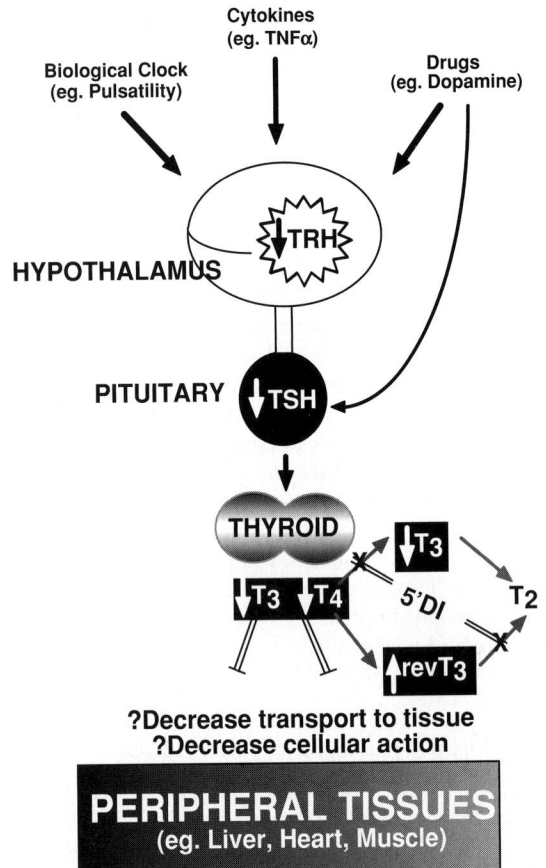

FIGURE 80-1 Physiologic basis for nonthyroidal illness syndrome (NTIS). Diagrammatic representation of the events that may contribute to NTIS, including the effects on the hypothalamus and pituitary and site of thyroid hormone action at the peripheral tissue level. Bold white arrows indicate changes in serum concentrations.

process uses specific enzymes called *deiodinases*. The deiodination of T_4 can take one of two pathways—removal of the iodine from the outer or phenolic ring (5' position), resulting in 3,3', 5-triiodothyronine (T_3) or removal of the iodine from the inner or tyrosyl ring (5 position), yielding 3,3', 5'-triiodothyronine (reverse T_3 [rT_3]). T_3 is the active form of the hormone, whereas rT_3 has no biologic activity. The same enzyme that removes iodine from the 5' position of the T_4 molecule also is responsible for deiodination of the 5' iodine from rT_3. Therefore, reduction in the 5'-deiodinase activity, which is invariably associated with severe illness and malnutrition, not only reduces the serum T_3 level but also increases that of rT_3.

THYROID PHYSIOLOGY IN THE BRAIN IN NTIS

The nature of perturbations of the hypothalamic-pituitary-thyroid axis in critically ill patients is beginning to be understood. The basal TSH values in serum of humans with NTIS can be normal or low, but the response of TSH to TRH usually is attenuated.[2] Stress and malnutrition may be partly responsible. In rats, starvation reduces hypothalamic messenger ribonucleic acid (mRNA) for TRH, reduces portal serum TRH, and lowers pituitary TSH content.[5] Furthermore, low TRH mRNA has been documented in the paraventricular nuclei

of patients with NTIS.[6] One therefore would predict that if diminished TRH is, at least in part, contributing to NTIS and the low thyroid hormone levels, then treatment with TRH should increase the TSH and therefore increase the thyroid hormone levels. In fact, Van den Berghe and colleagues[7] have demonstrated that administration of TRH to patients with NTIS leads to increase in serum TSH, T_3, and T_4 levels. Critically ill patients who eventually will recover from their illness have, as a rule, less impairment of the TSH response to TRH. The mechanism for the reduced TRH production in NTIS is unknown but may be related to cytokines or glucocorticoids. These factors probably are responsible for suppression not only of TRH but also of other hypothalamic factors that may be decreased in NTIS, such as corticotropin-releasing hormone and gonadotropin-releasing hormone.

The preceding, however, does not rule out an effect of NTIS directly on the pituitary. For example, why is serum TSH not elevated when the thyroid hormone levels are low? There is experimental evidence that the pituitary may be "euthyroid" owing to increased pituitary conversion of T_4 to T_3, unlike other tissues.[8]

In addition, drugs commonly administered to ICU patients have inhibitory effects on the hypothalamic and pituitary function. Dopamine is one such drug; it inhibits TSH even when infused at low doses.[9,10]

OTHER ACTIONS OF THYROID HORMONE ON PHYSIOLOGY IN NTIS

Type II pneumocytes, which have been shown to be involved in regulation of lung function, express thyroid hormone receptors on their surfaces.[11] Furthermore, T_3 has been shown to modulate surfactant function during sepsis.[12–14]

Sepsis and multisystem organ failure often are associated with disseminated intravascular coagulation (DIC) and consumption of coagulation inhibitiors such as antithrombin III. Treatment of rats with experimentally induced NTIS with T_3 reduced the sepsis-induced decrease in antithrombin III levels.[15]

INTERPRETATION OF THYROID FUNCTION STUDIES (TABLE 80-1)

The levels of thyroid hormone and TSH are measured in many critically ill patients at some point during the course of hospitalization. Low concentrations of thyroid hormone without an appropriate increase in serum TSH level would, under normal conditions, raise the suspicion of pituitary (secondary) or hypothalamic (tertiary) hypothyroidism. However, in a critically ill patient, the diagnosis of primary hypothyroidism with inadequate pituitary response needs consideration. A modest elevation of serum TSH level without an increase in rT_3 concentration is a strong indicator of primary hypothyroidism. Except in the presence of renal failure, a decreased rT_3 level raises the possibility of hypothyroidism and should prompt a search for the etiology. While these possible diagnoses are being investigated, thyroid hormone replacement and glucocorticoid treatment are indicated. Since results of rT_3 measurement often are not obtained readily, this test is useful in retrospect for ruling out primary endocrine dysfunction and adds little to the decision of initial management of patients. Since only severe primary hypothyroidism requires emergency treatment, its recognition is

TABLE 80-1 Interpretation of Thyroid Function Tests

Diagnosis	T_4 Level	T_3 Level	TSH Level	rT_3 Level
Primary hypothyroidism	↓	↓ or N	↑	↓ or N
Central hypothyroidism	↓	↓	N	↓
NTI	↓ or N	↓	N or ↓	↑ or N

ABBREVIATIONS: ↓, decreased; ↑, increased; N, normal; NTI, nonthyroidal illness.

usually simple because of persistent TSH elevation, a prior history of thyroid disease, and physical findings compatible with hypothyroidism.

TO TREAT OR NOT TO TREAT

Should patients with low serum levels of thyroid hormone in the face of catastrophic NTIS receive hormonal replacement? In order to answer this question, several issues need to be determined: (1) Is the serum TSH level an accurate reflection of the thyroid status of all body tissues, or does it only reflect the status of the pituitary? (2) Are the tissues of the body functionally hypothyroid? and (3) Is the low serum T_3 level an adaptive mechanism for conservation of energy during critical illness? Unfortunately, these questions remain relatively unanswered. In a randomized, prospective study to determine the effect of T_4 treatment in NTIS, 11 patients admitted to an ICU with reduced thyroid hormone levels were treated with intravenous T_4, and 12 served as controls.[16] The study indicated an earlier mortality in the treated group, although the number of survivors was not significantly different between the groups. It was concluded that T_4 therapy was not beneficial, and inhibition of TSH secretion by the administration of T_4 may be detrimental to the recovery of thyroid function. These results have been confirmed in a similar study carried out in an ICU setting.[17] Nevertheless, many physicians understandably find it difficult to withhold treatment in a dying patient with virtually undetectable thyroid hormone levels.

Not only are data on the benefit of thyroid hormone treatment limited, but it is unlikely that an answer regarding the efficacy of this treatment will be forthcoming, given multiple-organ involvement in serious illness and the difficulty of interpreting the effect of thyroid hormone replacement in individuals receiving multiple drugs. Thus the argument centers not only on the question of whether such patients are truly hypothyroid (hence the bias of the term *euthyroid sick*) but also on whether this temporary hypothyroidism may not, in fact, be beneficial. Inhibition of the type I 5'-deiodinase is the principal mechanism that reduces the supply of biologically active thyroid hormone, T_3, to peripheral tissues in the severely ill. Experimental work in a rat model indicates that peripheral tissue hypothyroidism is maintained by an inhibition of the usual compensatory increase in TSH level. This inhibition occurs because normal levels of T_3 are generated in the pituitary gland, which uses a different form of 5'-deiodinase, the type II enzyme, that is actually more active in severe illness.[8,18] Teleologists argue that this mechanism to reduce the delivery of thyroid hormone to peripheral tissues is not accidental and, therefore, that reduced metabolic activity may be beneficial in the face of the increased catabolism characteristic of severe illness. The question is, Does the physician or nature know best? At our institution there is no consensus on this subject.

Recent studies have shown decreased serum T_3 concentrations in patients undergoing cardiopulmonary bypass surgery. T_3 treatment can normalize the serum levels and may increase cardiac output and lower systemic vascular resistance[19]; however, these effects may be negligible.[20]

Table 80-2 may serve as a bedside guide to the intensivist for the selection of patients for thyroid hormone treatment.

WHAT TO TREAT WITH

If the decision is made to treat a sick patient who has reduced thyroid hormone levels, the logical choice is T_3. Administration of T_4 does not change the serum T_3 concentration significantly—it only increases the level of the biologically inactive rT_3. The problem with T_3 treatment is its potential cardiac "toxicity." One possible problem is the proarrhythmogenic effect of T_3 in anesthetized patients; another possible problem is that T_3 may increase the oxygen demand of a myocardium with a fixed coronary artery lesion. T_3 is now available as the product TRIOSTAT; however, the cost of a single day's treatment for myxedema would be in excess of US$3500! Alternatively, a solution of T_3 for intravenous use can be prepared by the hospital pharmacist by dissolving L-T_3 in 0.1 N NaOH, followed by a 10-fold dilution in normal saline containing 2% albumin to a final concentration of 25 μg T_3 per milliliter. The solution is sterilized by a single passage through a 0.22-μm Millipore filter and is stored, for no longer than 1 week, at 4° C, protected from light. The materials for this preparation cost about US$1.

Myxedema Coma

DIAGNOSIS

Myxedema coma is caused by marked and prolonged depletion of thyroid hormone. The cardinal features of myxedema coma are (1) defective thermoregulation to the point of

TABLE 80-2 Indications for Thyroid Hormone Treatment in Patients with Severe NTI

Increased serum TSH concentrations
History of radioactive iodine treatment
Hypothermia
Macroglossia
Goiter
History of thyroid disease
Treatment with thyroid hormone at any time prior to the current illness
Hypercholesterolemia
Hyporeflexia
Unexplained pleural or pericardial effusions
Increased serum creatine phosphokinase level

TABLE 80-3 Common Precipitating Factors of Myxedema Coma

Exposure to cold
Infection
Surgery
Strokes
Occult gastrointestinal bleeding
Trauma
Drug overdose
    Sedatives
    Tranquillizers
    Narcotics
    Anesthetics
Congestive heart failure

TABLE 80-4 Laboratory Findings in Myxedema Coma

Hypoglycemia
Hyponatremia
Hyperkalemia
Hypercortisolemia
Anemia
Leukocytosis with a left shift
Serum creatinine level >2.0 mg/dL
Increased P_{CO_2} in arterial blood
Decreased P_{O_2} in arterial blood

hypothermia, (2) altered mental status to the point of coma, (3) a history or sign (such as a neck scar) of ablative thyroid treatment, and (4) an identifiable precipitating event. The condition is a medical emergency because it is fatal in approximately one-half of cases.[21] This rare entity occurs typically in elderly women with long-standing hypothyroidism who develop an intercurrent illness and lapse into coma or in hypothyroid persons exposed to cold or given tranquilizers, narcotics, or sedatives sufficient to push them to the brink of myxedema coma. Table 80-3 lists events likely to precipitate myxedema coma. The usual features of severe hypothyroidism (myxedema) include dry, coarse skin, scaly elbows and knees, yellowness in the skin without scleral icterus, coarse hair, thinning of the lateral aspect of eyebrows, macroglossia and hoarseness, obtundation, delayed deep tendon reflexes, and hypothermia. When a markedly reduced serum T_4 level and an elevated TSH concentration accompany these signs, the diagnosis is obvious. However, as for thyrotoxic crisis, initiation of treatment should not be delayed until the results of the thyroid function studies are available. Furthermore, because of intercurrent illness, TSH values may not be elevated in proportion to the severity of hypothyroidism. A high index of suspicion in a patient presenting as just described should prompt immediate treatment after a blood sample is taken for laboratory confirmation of the diagnosis.

PULMONARY AND CARDIOVASCULAR COMPLICATIONS

Alveolar hypoventilation is known to occur in myxedema.[22] It is thus not surprising that patients with underlying lung pathology experience worsening of gas exchange. It has been demonstrated that the hypoxic ventilatory drive is depressed in patients with myxedema and that it responds to hormone replacement.[23] The hypercapnic ventilatory response is also significantly depressed, but it does not change with replacement of thyroid hormone. Therefore, a reduced central nervous system (CNS) drive to breathe and decreased respiratory muscle activity are the main reasons for respiratory depression in myxedema coma. Secondary aspiration pneumonia, laryngeal obstruction, and reduced surfactant contribute to lung dysfunction. It is important to be alert to the potential for subtle but progressive aspiration and ventilatory failure.

The cardiovascular complications in myxedema coma are caused by the combination of hypothyroid cardiomyopathy, hypothermia, and hypoxia. Pericardial effusion is al-

most a constant finding, but it rarely leads to tamponade. It is best demonstrated by echocardiography. In patients with long-standing hypothyroidism, hypercholesterolemia may accelerate the progress of atherosclerosis, leading to ischemic heart disease. The reader is referred to the discussion of hypothermia and its cardiovascular complications (see Chap. 110).

The intercurrent illness and decreased food intake caused by the mental obtundation of myxedema may reduce the serum levels of cholesterol and TSH, diminishing their value as indicators of the severity of the myxedema. Patients presenting with a more profound hypothermia have a poor prognosis. The laboratory findings in patients with myxedema coma are listed in Table 80-4.

TREATMENT

THYROID HORMONE

Although severe hypothyroidism, especially in elderly patients, should be treated cautiously, with gradual increments of small doses of thyroid hormone, myxedema coma is an exception to this rule. The immediate threat to life takes precedence over the risks of rapid hormone replacement. The advantage of treating critically ill patients with T_3 as opposed to T_4 was discussed earlier. In hypothyroid patients without major intercurrent illness, T_4 therapy alone may be sufficient to increase the serum T_3 level to normal in 2 to 3 days. This is unlikely to be true in ICU patients with multiple-organ-system failure. The principle of hormonal treatment is to rapidly replenish the extrathyroid pool of thyroid hormone, which consists mainly of hormone bound to serum proteins, and to provide the tissues with their daily requirement of the biologically active hormone. Replenishment is best achieved by the immediate administration of T_4, a hormone with a considerably longer half-life (7 days) and higher affinity for serum proteins than T_3.[22–24] The active form of the hormone, T_3, then can be provided because it is readily available to tissues and carries a smaller risk of accumulating to excessive amounts (owing to a half-life of approximately 1 day).

The average size of the extrathyroid T_4 pool is approximately 800 μg/1.73 m^2.[24–27] On the basis of this estimate and the normal turnover rate of 10% per day, the daily T_4 requirement can be calculated to be, on average, 80 μg (possibly 50 μg in hypothyroidism, owing to a reduced rate of hormone degradation). Intensivists using only T_4 for treatment should give initially 500 μg L-T_4, followed by 50 to 100 μg daily. The serum T_4 concentration should be in the normal range within 24 to 48 hours. Daily electrocardiographic (ECG) monitoring for ischemic changes and continuous monitoring of rhythm are essential.

We prefer a regimen that uses both T_4 and T_3. Following the intravenous loading dose of 500 μg T_4, 25 μg T_3 is given every 6 hours through a nasogastric tube until improvement is noted, and provided the diagnosis has been confirmed by laboratory tests. The dose is then reduced to maintenance level, and the agent is changed to T_4 only after recovery from intercurrent illness.

USE OF STEROIDS

The rate of metabolism of most drugs and natural compounds is markedly reduced in patients with myxedema coma. Therefore, the absolute requirement for steroids is reduced. However, because of the 5% to 10% incidence of associated primary hypoadrenalism, glucocorticoids should be given until evidence for intact adrenal function is secured by the cortisol measurement on the blood sample obtained on admission. The usual dose of hydrocortisone is 50 mg intravenously every 6 hours. The steroid dose then can be tapered rapidly after confirmation of a normal pituitary-adrenal axis. Alternatively, the initial dose can be 2 mg dexamethasone, and a 1-hour adrenocorticotropin hormone (ACTH, cosyntropin) stimulation test can be done on the spot to assess adrenocortical function[26] (see Chap. 79).

SUPPORTIVE CARE

Early intubation and mechanical ventilation are believed to be central for the successful treatment of myxedema coma. Severe hemodynamic collapse in the presence of a large pericardial effusion may necessitate immediate pericardiocentesis. Because hypothyroidism can cause an elevation of the serum creatine phosphokinase (CPK) level, obtaining a baseline value is helpful for follow-up, particularly if a myocardial infarction is later suspected. Moderate elevations of the blood urea nitrogen (BUN) and creatinine levels are not uncommon and are not necessarily indicative of chronic renal failure.

Hypothermia is treated with blankets, letting internal heat generation slowly warm the body.[21] External warming runs the risk of initiating shock by producing peripheral vasodilation in a patient with already reduced cardiac output. Measurement of central venous pressure is useful to guide therapy. Patients with myxedema are rarely volume overloaded, and the use of diuretics runs the risk of further reducing cardiac output. Hyponatremia is best treated by water restriction because the total body sodium content is increased owing to the storage of sodium in glycosaminoglycan, forming the myxedematous accumulation that becomes mobilized with thyroid hormone treatment. Antiulcer prophylaxis is recommended. More important, it should be remembered that hypothyroidism reduces the metabolism of all drugs, and their dosing needs careful adjustment to prevent drug toxicity. Diligent investigation into the precipitating causes should include blood, urine, and sputum cultures, and empirical treatment with antibiotics should be given.

If severe anemia is present, it should be corrected with blood transfusion to increase the oxygen-carrying capacity of the blood. Use of α-adrenergic agents should be avoided because patients are already vasoconstricted.

EFFICACY OF TREATMENT

Assuming that an accurate diagnosis has been made and that proper therapeutic measures have been carried out, how are the patient's progress and the efficacy of treatment followed?

The physician is committed to treat the patient for several days or as long as the serum TSH concentration remains elevated. Reduction of the TSH level is the earliest indicator of a response to thyroid hormone therapy. Irreversible damage to the respiratory centers has been observed, with failure of spontaneous respiration, despite full repletion of thyroid hormone. No laboratory measurements are helpful in assessing the peripheral tissue responses to thyroid hormone in the critical care setting. The ultimate gauge of successful treatment is complete clinical recovery.

Goiter and Acute Airway Obstruction

Large goiters, weighing 150 g or more, can cause some degree of tracheal obstruction, especially if they are substernal in location. In a series of 2908 goiters, only 58 (2.0%) caused tracheal obstruction at presentation. Tracheal compression obstructing up to 75% of the tracheal lumen often remains asymptomatic.[28] Although dyspnea on exertion has been attributed to goiter, the symptoms are often only nocturnal, manifesting as stridor or, when more severe, as sleep apnea. This problem can be confirmed by x-ray views of the trachea at rest and during a reverse Valsalva maneuver and by sleep studies.[29]

Growth of the goiter would have to be extensive to cause direct tracheal compression. In Riedel's struma, there is tracheal cartilage destruction by fibrous invasion, which also can cause bilateral vocal cord paralysis. Several case reports have been published describing the acute presentation of tracheal obstruction associated with goiter.[30,31] Management of these patients is somewhat difficult because emergency tracheostomy may be difficult to perform owing to interference by the thyroid gland. The use of small endotracheal tubes and immediate subtotal thyroidectomy should reduce the need for tracheostomy. It should be noted that subtotal thyroidectomy may not be successful in the presence of tracheomalacia, which may necessitate prosthetic supports.[32] In some instances, a simple division of the thyroid isthmus may be sufficient to relieve the symptoms. Although not particularly useful in the acute care setting, ^{131}I therapy can be effective in the long term in elderly patients with large, compressive goiters.[33]

Thyrotoxicosis

Thyrotoxicosis occurs when the supply of thyroid hormone exceeds the amount needed for normal tissue function. The source of thyroid hormone may be (1) excessive synthesis and secretion of hormone from the thyroid gland in response to either TSH or abnormal thyroid-stimulating substances (usually immunoglobulins), (2) autonomous hormone hypersecretion or abnormal release of preformed hormone, or (3) production of the hormone by an exogenous or ectopic source.[34] Manifestations can be mild or severe depending on the degree of hormone excess and its duration, as well as the presence of intercurrent illness. Aspects related to thyrotoxicosis in the severely ill patient will be the focus of this section.

A few basic facts about thyroid physiology are important for understanding the therapeutic approach to thyroid disorders. Iodine is actively transported into the thyroid gland, where it is covalently bound to tyrosines within the thyroglobulin molecule. The iodinated tyrosines are coupled to form mainly T_4 as well as some T_3. It is in the form of thyroglobulin that the hormone is stored in the colloid of the thyroid follicles. In response to TSH or an abnormal stimulator, thyroglobulin is digested by proteolysis, and the liberated hormone—predominantly T_4—is secreted into the circulation. In the blood, T_4 is transported bound to specific serum proteins. In virtually all peripheral tissues, T_4 derived from blood is converted into the active hormone, T_3, by removal of a single iodine atom from the 5' position in the outer ring of the molecule. This reaction is mediated by a tissue-specific 5'-deiodinase. Removal of iodine from the inner ring yields the inactive form rT_3. Intracellular T_3 binds to nuclear receptors, through which it exerts its effects.

DIAGNOSIS IN THE ICU

Thyrotoxicosis may be manifested by adverse changes in every organ system. Pyrexia, tachycardia, congestive heart failure, oxyhemoglobin desaturation, and hypertension are the hallmarks of thyrotoxic crisis.[35] There also may be involvement of the CNS, ranging from tremulousness to seizures and coma, or involvement of the respiratory system, with tachypnea and respiratory muscle fatigue. Goiter and exophthalmos are as likely to be absent as present. Unfortunately, at the time of presentation in the ICU, most patients with these characteristics have only modest elevations of thyroid hormone concentration in serum (see above). Failure to recognize these symptoms as manifestations of thyrotoxicosis may result in nonspecific treatment, with a resulting risk of morbidity or even death. On the other hand, failure to treat pyrexia as a sign of sepsis or tachycardia as a sign of ischemia or hypoxia could be equally devastating. Stat laboratory measurement of thyroid hormone levels is not always available to provide firm laboratory support for the diagnosis. A 2-hour radioiodine uptake test conceivably could be done at the bedside using a portable gamma counter probe, but it is not practical. Therefore, the preliminary diagnosis of thyrotoxicosis usually is based on a careful history and physical examination. Useful findings are (1) a previous diagnosis and treatment of thyrotoxicosis, (2) presence of exophthalmos, (3) goiter, (4) a history of thyroid hormone ingestion, (5) evidence of previous thyroid surgery, including an anterior neck surgical scar, and (6) recent use of iodine-containing radiologic contrast agents. Such information only supports the possibility that suggestive physical signs may be due to thyrotoxicosis.

PHYSIOLOGIC CONSEQUENCES AND CARDIOVASCULAR COMPLICATIONS

Thyroid hormone exerts its tissue effect both directly by interaction with specific nuclear receptors and indirectly through activation of the sympathoadrenal system. Each of these actions causes unique effects on various tissues. The physiologic basis of the sympathomimetic effect of thyroid hormone is unknown. Table 80-5 summarizes the cardiopulmonary complications of thyrotoxicosis.

Perhaps the most detrimental effect of thyrotoxicosis, which clearly is evident in the more severe state of thyroid storm (see below), is pyrexia. Increased body temperature may be secondary to the increased basal metabolic rate or to actual resetting of hypothalamic thermoregulation. Pyrexia

TABLE 80-5 Cardiopulmonary Complications of Thyrotoxicosis

Increased metabolic demand with increased O_2 consumption and CO_2 production
Respiratory muscle weakness
Increased work of breathing
Hyperdynamic circulation
Potential for high-output heart failure
Potential for myocardial ischemia
Arrhythmias

further increases cardiovascular stress; therefore, reduction of body temperature is an important goal of therapy.

Neurologic complications of severe thyrotoxicosis include neuromuscular disorders of myopathy (present in over 50% of all hyperthyroid patients and classified as severe in 4%),[36] exophthalmic ophthalmoplegia, aggravation of myasthenia gravis, and thyrotoxic periodic paralysis (primarily in Asian men). Except for irritability and tremulousness, the delirium, stupor, coma, and convulsions may be related to the direct action of thyroid hormone on the brain.[37] Thyroid hormone can affect the concentrations and distributions of various neurotransmitters.[38] Hematologic manifestations of thyrotoxicosis[39] are rarely life threatening. It is useful for the intensivist to be aware that hyperthyroidism can cause slight anemia. Anemia may be secondary to hemodilution caused by increased blood volume, but true reduction of red blood cell mass may be caused by reduced iron absorption and vitamin B_{12} deficiency associated with autoimmune reduction of gastric acidity and intrinsic factor. Minimal thrombocytopenia, with rare instances of idiopathic thrombocytopenic purpura, has been reported.[40] Moderate eosinophilia may occur and has been attributed to relative or absolute hypoadrenalism. A variable relative or absolute lymphocytosis may be associated with hyperthyroidism. These manifestations may cloud the picture of a critically ill patient who may have other hematologic perturbations for different reasons.

Hypercalcemia is the most common life-threatening electrolyte abnormality seen in thyrotoxicosis.[39] Severe hypercalcemia (11.8 to 19.2 mg/dL) has been reported in several patients with thyrotoxicosis.[41]

The most notable effect of thyrotoxicosis on the gastrointestinal system is hypermotility with malabsorption.[42] The myopathy of hyperthyroidism may cause weakness of the striated muscles of the pharynx and, perhaps, the smooth muscle of the esophagus. Such patients could have dysphagia and then could aspirate and develop pneumonia.[43] Patients with hyperthyroidism appear to have a higher incidence of gastritis.[44] This association is consistent with the hypergastrinemia seen in thyrotoxic patients.[45] Treatment with H_2 blockers or proton pump inhibitors is indicated.

Rarely, fulminant hepatic necrosis or less severe hepatic injury occurs. Although thyroid hormone has no direct toxic effect on the liver, hyperthermia can result in hepatic failure. In patients receiving propylthiouracil (PTU), drug toxicity is more likely the cause of fulminant hepatic necrosis.[46] Any thyrotoxic patient who presents with jaundice or other signs of hepatic injury should have a thorough evaluation for possible alternative causes of liver damage.

Thyroid Storm

Thyroid storm, or *thyrotoxic crisis*, is a life-threatening though rare complication of severe thyrotoxicosis. The diagnosis is clinical, bearing no direct relation to the absolute levels of thyroid hormones in serum. The cardinal features of thyroid storm are marked tachycardia, hypertension, and widened pulse pressure; hyperpyrexia (usually greater than 38.5° C [101° F]); and altered mental status. In extreme cases, cardio-vascular collapse and shock may be seen. Some investiga-tors contend that abnormal mentation is the most important diagnostic component of thyroid storm.[26] Of course, these clinical features can occur with a multitude of illnesses in the absence of thyrotoxicosis. Some authors propose a "point system" for determining whether a patient's condition repre-sents true storm or severe thyrotoxicosis, but the distinction between these two entities is not useful clinically.[47] A blood sample for measurement of the levels of T_4 or free T_4, or the free T_4 index (FT_4I), and TSH, by a sensitive method, should be obtained immediately in all individuals suspected of hav-ing this disorder. Empirical treatment then should begin. It is prudent to obtain a blood sample for cortisol determina-tion before "stress doses" of steroids are administered for use later in deciding later whether long-term therapy is necessary. Laboratory findings in thyroid storm are listed in Table 80-6.

PRECIPITATING FACTORS

Patients who develop thyroid storm usually have poorly con-trolled thyrotoxicosis; often there is an identifiable precipi-tating factor[26,48] (Table 80-7). In many cases it is difficult to determine whether the intercurrent illness is the cause or the consequence of the thyroid storm.

TREATMENT

To prevent irreversible cardiovascular collapse, the treatment of thyroid storm should take a four-pronged approach: (1) therapy to reduce the serum thyroid hormone levels, (2) ther-apy to reduce the action of the thyroid hormones on periph-eral tissues, (3) therapy to prevent cardiovascular decompen-sation and to maintain normal homeostasis, and (4) treatment of the precipitating event(s).

THERAPY TO REDUCE THYROID HORMONE LEVELS
An antithyroid drug, either PTU or methimazole (MMI), is given to prevent further synthesis of thyroid hormone. These drugs are not available in parenteral form; they can only be given orally or by nasogastric tube. Instances may arise in which these drugs cannot be given even by nasogastric tube—

TABLE 80-6 Laboratory Findings in Thyroid Storm

Elevated levels of T_4 and free T_4
Elevated T_3 level
Hyperglycemia
Leukocytosis with left shift
Anemia
Hypercalcemia
Hypokalemia
Abnormal liver function test findings
Hypercortisolemia

TABLE 80-7 Factors Precipitating Thyroid Storm

Surgery
Infection
Acute psychiatric illness
Congestive heart failure
Diabetic ketoacidosis
Pulmonary embolism
Bowel infarction
Parturition
Trauma
Vigorous palpation of thyroid gland
Withdrawal of antithyroid medication
Drugs
   Sympathomimetic drugs such as pseudoephedrine
   Amiodarone
Radioactive iodide therapy
Iodine-containing contrast agents
"Health food" preparations containing seaweed or kelp

such as, for example, in patients with infarcted bowel. PTU offers a slight advantage over MMI in that, in addition to its inhibitory effect on hormone synthesis, it decreases the con-version of T_4 to T_3 in peripheral tissue. PTU should be given in a dose of 200 to 250 mg every 6 hours, and MMI should be given in a dose of 25 mg every 6 hours. Some authors recom-mend giving an initial PTU loading dose of 600 to 1000 mg, but this strategy has not been proved to be advantageous. An-other regimen that has been reported consists of one 600-mg loading dose of PTU (12 tablets suspended in 90 mL of water) given as a retention enema, followed by 250 mg of PTU every 4 hours plus potassium iodide, 1 g diluted in 60 mL of water, given after the second PTU dose.[49] PTU has an immediate on-set of action for blocking the synthesis of thyroid hormone, but serum levels of thyroid hormone may take several weeks to normalize because of continuing secretion of stored hor-mone. In severe thyrotoxicosis with a decreased glandular content of hormone, a significant decline in serum levels may be observed in a matter of a few days. We usually repeat thy-roid function tests every other day while the patient is acutely ill to help guide management.

Blockade of hormonal secretion usually is best accom-plished by the addition of stable iodine to the antithyroid drug regimen. Iodine can be administered as Lugol's solution or as a saturated solution of potassium iodide (ssKI) (2 drops ev-ery 12 hours) or given by intravenous drip as sodium iodide (0.5 mg every 12 hours). It is important not to give iodide prior to antithyroid drug blockade because new hormone syn-thesis may occur and result in delayed release of hormone. There have been several cases where the use of iodine alone triggered thyroid storm. Administration of antithyroid drugs 1 hour before iodine is given is sufficient to establish blockade of hormone synthesis. A combination of antithyroid drugs and ssKI should decrease the serum T_3 level to the normal range in 1 to 5 days; however, the metabolic response may lag behind by 2 to 3 days.[50] Corticosteroids and propranolol, which also decrease the peripheral conversion of T_4 to T_3, can be used to further reduce the serum T_3 concentration (Tables 80-8 and 80-9).

In the event that antithyroid drugs cannot be used because of a previous history of reactions, such as agranulocytosis or hepatotoxicity, iodine and oral cholecystographic agents may

TABLE 80-8 Mechanisms of Action of Antithyroid Drugs

Mechanism	PTU	MMI	LiCO$_3$	KClO$_4$	ssKI	IOP	β Blocker	Glucocorticoids	Cholestyramine	TBG
REDUCTION OF SERUM HORMONE LEVELS										
Blocking of thyroidal I⁻ uptake	−	−	++	+++	−	−	−	−	−	−
Blocking of T$_4$ synthesis	+++	+++	−	−	−	+	−	−	−	−
Blocking of T$_4$ release	−	−	++	+	+++	+	−	−	−	−
Blocking of T$_4$-to-T$_3$ conversion	++	−	−	−	−	+++	+	+	−	−
Decrease of intestinal absorption of hormone	−	−	−	−	−	−	−	−	+	−
REDUCTION OF ACTION ON PERIPHERAL TISSUES										
Increase of T$_4$ binding to serum protein	−	−	−	−	−	−	−	−	−	+++
Blocking of thyroid hormone receptor	−	−	−	−	−	+	−	−	−	−
Blocking of sympathomimetic activity	−	−	−	−	−	−	+++	+	−	−

ABBREVIATIONS: +, minor effect; ++, moderate effect; +++, strong and principal effect; PTU, propylthiouracil; MMI, methimazole; LiCO$_3$, lithium carbonate; KClO$_4$, potassium perchlorate; ssKI, saturated solution of potassium iodide; IOP, iopanoic acid; TBG, thyroxine-binding globulin.

have to be used alone—the latter in the form of ipodate or iopanoate (iopanoic acid). These agents are strong inhibitors of the 5′ deiodination of thyroid hormones; thus they decrease serum levels of T$_3$ and increase those of rT$_3$.[51] They also bind to the thyroid hormone receptor, but it is unclear whether this results in competitive inhibition of T$_3$ action.[52] These agents have a high iodine content (approximately 60% by weight) and thus also act by releasing iodine in the course of their degradation. As in the case of iodine treatment, their administration in the absence of antithyroid drugs requires careful monitoring of the clinical status. Iopanoic acid (TELEPAQUE) may be given in amounts of 1 to 3 g daily. We have found that 3 g/d often causes diarrhea; this effect can be prevented with no reduction of the drug's therapeutic efficacy by giving 0.5 g three times a day. Alternatively, sodium ipodate (ORAGRAFIN) may be used at a dose of 0.5 mg/d, which can reduce serum T$_3$ by 62% in 1 day.[53,54]

For the rare patient with allergic reactions to both antithyroid drugs and to iodine-containing contrast media, lithium carbonate and perchlorate are alternative drugs. Lithium carbonate can be given in doses of 300 mg every 6 hours, with subsequent adjustments to maintain a serum lithium level of 0.7 to 1.4 mEq/L. Caution should be exercised in patients over 60 years of age. This drug acts by blocking iodide uptake and hormone release by the thyroid gland. Sodium or potassium perchlorate (ClO$_4$) competes with iodide for up-

take by the thyroid gland, ultimately reducing the production of T$_4$. These compounds are not readily available in the United States. Serious side effects, including aplastic anemia and nephrotic syndrome, occur rarely.

Successful reduction of the serum concentration of thyroid hormones by means of plasma exchange has been reported in three patients (two of whom were pregnant).[55,56] Filtration through a resin bed that removes T$_3$ and T$_4$ has been used occasionally.[57] Intravenous administration of thyroxine-binding globulin has been shown experimentally to decrease the transfer of thyroid hormone from blood to tissues.[58]

PREVENTION OF SYSTEMIC DECOMPENSATION

Reduction of the body temperature decreases the demands on the cardiovascular system. Body temperature can be reduced by cooling and by pharmacologic blockade of the thermoregulatory centers. Use of a cooling blanket and ice packs alone will induce shivering; treatment with chlorpromazine, 25 to 50 mg, and meperidine, 25 to 50 mg, intravenously every 4 to 6 hours will decrease the severe shivering and limit further heat generation.[21]

Patients in thyroid storm lose excessive amounts of fluid because of (1) increased insensible water loss associated with hyperthermia and tachypnea, (2) decreased levels of antidiuretic hormone, and (3) vomiting and diarrhea associated with increased intestinal motility. Thus patients may present

TABLE 80-9 Drugs Used in the Treatment of Thyrotoxicosis

Drug	Dose	How Supplied	Adverse Effects
Propylthiouracil	200–250 mg q6h PO	50-mg tablet	Rash, agranulocytosis, hepatic toxicity
Methimazole	25 mg q6h PO	5- and 50-mg tablet	Rash, agranulocytosis, hepatic toxicity
Lithium carbonate	300 mg q6h PO	150-, 300-, and 600-mg tablets	Nausea, vomiting, arrhythmias, pseudotumor cerebri
Lugol's solution	2 drops q12h PO	8-mg iodine drop	Hypersensitivity
ssKI	1 drop q12h PO	50-mg iodide drop	Hypersensitivity
Iopanoic acid	0.5 g tid PO	0.5-g tablet	Abdominal cramps, diarrhea, hypersensitivity, nephrotoxicity
Perchlorate	1.0 g qd	0.5-g tablet (66.7% organically bound)	Aplastic anemia
Propranolol	40 mg q6h PO1 mg slow IVP	10-, 20-, 40-, 60-, and 80-mg tablets; 1-mg/mL vials	Asthma, heart block
Hydrocortisone	100 mg IV piggyback q8h	100-mg vials	Immunosuppression

ABBREVIATIONS: ssKI, saturated solution of potassium iodide.

with either high- or low-output failure, and fluid management may necessitate central venous catheterization to determine filling pressures and guide management. Solutions containing crystalloid (for volume replacement) and dextrose (to replenish hepatic glycogen stores and minimize the breakdown of body protein) are used. Treatment with high doses of propranolol, as discussed below, can make it necessary to use 5% to 10% dextrose solutions. Multivitamins often are administered to replenish the B-complex vitamins.

Treatment of congestive heart failure usually is supportive. While reduction of the high body temperature should be attempted before specific treatment is instituted, the judicious use of inotropic agents and diuretics also should be considered. Since patients are often volume depleted, diuretics should be used carefully and always with meticulous monitoring of intravascular volume. Impending shock should be treated with rapid correction of volume and with inotropic agents, as indicated. Atrial fibrillation is a known complication of thyrotoxicosis. Control of ventricular response can be achieved with β blockers, but conversion to sinus rhythm can be achieved only after the patient is made euthyroid.

Since relative hypoadrenalism is thought to occur in thyroid storm because of accelerated metabolism of glucocorticoids, it is prudent to give 300 mg hydrocortisone intravenously, followed by 100 mg every 8 hours to provide adequate stress levels. In addition, glucocorticoids can be beneficial for their effect in reducing the conversion of T_4 to T_3 in peripheral tissue. Use of parenteral H_2 blockers is indicated to reduce the likelihood of ulcer formation. In thyrotoxicosis, there is rapid clearance of drugs. Therefore, doses of digitalis, insulin, and antibiotics need to be increased to be effective. Two exceptions are adrenergic drugs and anticoagulants.[59] It is necessary to remember to reduce drug doses as the thyrotoxicosis resolves.

REDUCTION OF THYROID HORMONE ACTION ON BODY TISSUES
The effects of thyroid hormone can be reduced by (1) decreasing its conversion to the active form, T_3, (2) counteracting its sympathomimetic effects, (3) displacing it from its receptor, and (4) reducing its transport to tissues.

The oral cholecystographic agents, as discussed earlier, may act in part by displacing T_3 from its site of action at the receptor in cell nuclei. Other analogs of thyroid hormone with reduced thyromimetic activity, which nevertheless compete with thyroid hormone at its site of action, deserve theoretical consideration.[60] The activity of 5'-deiodinase is regulated by the concentration of T_4, as well as by catecholamines and other factors. PTU, glucocorticoids, propranolol, oral cholecystographic agents, and amiodarone also reduce the activity of this enzyme and thus decrease the generation of T_3, resulting in reduction of serum T_3 concentration. Severe acute or chronic nonthyroidal illness also suppresses T_3 generation in peripheral tissues.

β Blockers, which are useful in the preparation of thyrotoxic patients for surgery, should be used with caution in thyroid storm. Whereas surgical stress clearly is related to increased catecholamine levels, and thyroid storm can be prevented by the use of propranolol, it is unclear whether thyroid storm induced by other mechanisms is equally responsive to β blockers. However, when there is evidence of increased

adrenergic activity short of thyroid storm (i.e., no evidence of hyperpyrexia or mental status changes), 1 mg propranolol can be administered by slow intravenous push every 5 minutes until an effect on pulse rate is seen. Usually a total daily dose of 300 to 400 mg oral propranolol is required to achieve effective β blockade in the severely thyrotoxic patient. It appears that younger patients are more susceptible to hyperadrenergic states with more labile courses and do better with β blockers.[21] By contrast, elderly patients may present with "apathetic" thyrotoxicosis without elevation in body temperature and without severe tachycardia. These elderly patients more often experience cardiotoxic effects in response to β blockers. Therefore, β blockers should be used with caution in thyroid storm and in severe thyrotoxicosis, except in the elderly, in asthmatics, and in patients with evidence of dilated cardiomyopathy. When surgery is indicated in such patients, careful titration of the adverse adrenergic cardiovascular effects (tachycardia, large pulse pressure) can be implemented with shorter-duration β blockers (esmolol) preceded by maximal bronchodilator therapy in asthmatic patients or right-sided heart catheterization in elderly patients and those with prior heart failure.

TREATMENT OF PRECIPITATING EVENTS
Without an antecedent history of surgery, any patient with thyroid storm should be suspected of being septic until proven otherwise. Blood, urine, and other body secretions (i.e., ascites or pleural fluid and sputum) should be Gram stained and cultured. Empirical use of broad-spectrum antibiotics is recommended.

In a seriously ill patient in whom an infection or other precipitating cause, such as diabetic ketoacidosis, cannot be identified, pulmonary thromboembolism[61,62] or bowel infarction should be considered.

THYROID STORM IN PREGNANCY
The approach to treatment of thyroid storm in pregnant patients is similar to that outlined earlier. Thyroid storm is clearly a life-threatening condition for the mother. The basic approach to prevent decompensation is aggressive fluid replacement along with treatment of the precipitating event and antithyroid therapy. Because β blockers may have deleterious effects on the fetus at all stages of fetal development, their use must be weighed against maternal safety. While administration of iodide often results in the development of massive fetal goiter, PTU can be given to the toxic pregnant patient with only a small likelihood of adverse effects on the fetus.

Anesthesia and Surgery: Risks and Management in Thyrotoxic Patients

The Swiss surgeon Emil Theodor Kocher (1841–1917), who was the first to operate on hyperthyroid patients, was also among the first to recognize that thyroidectomy carried a high rate of mortality in "unprepared" thyrotoxic patients. The stress of any form of surgery or anesthesia alone could push a mildly decompensated thyrotoxic patient into a thyroid crisis, a life-threatening condition (see above). Therefore, it is important to control thyrotoxicosis prior to surgery. Ideally, the FT_4I should be below the upper limit of normal.

Unfortunately, even in the presence of a rapid turnover rate, thyroxine has a half-life of at least 72 hours, and frequently it takes more than 1 week to achieve a normal FT_4I—an unacceptable wait, especially when the need for surgery is urgent. In such instances, the preoperative therapeutic goal is to prevent the occurrence of thyroid storm. Blocking the effect of thyroid hormone on the sympathetic nervous system, particularly on the heart, is an alternative (if not an ideal) approach to therapy.[63] An arbitrary goal of maintaining a heart rate below 90 beats per minute may not always be achieved in patients who have a pulse rate of 200 beats per minute at the outset. In fact, there are no strict criteria for the response to therapy prior to surgery. Propranolol is the most widely used drug[64–66]; other parenteral preparations are now available, but there is no clear evidence that any of them has advantages over any other. Propranolol, however, has the added effect of decreasing the conversion of T_4 to T_3 in peripheral tissues. This effect may not be shared by other β blockers, such as atenolol. By and large, β blockers have little effect on the serum concentration of T_4 or on the metabolic status of the patient. The combined use of an antithyroid drug (PTU or MMI) and iodide provides the most rapid means of reducing the serum level of thyroid hormone; the antithyroid drug blocks the synthesis of the hormone, and iodide blocks its release. Although the results of determinations of serum thyroid hormone concentrations may not be available on a stat basis, it is important to obtain a blood sample before treatment is initiated.

We would like to discuss three scenarios for the preoperative treatment of thyrotoxic patients. First, consider an ICU patient who is in a septic condition with severe cholecystitis. The presence of thyrotoxicosis has been confirmed by an FT_4I of 21 (normal range = 6 to 10.5) and a TSH level below 0.01 mU/L. A cholecystectomy is planned as the definitive treatment, to take place in approximately 1 week. In this instance, the physician has time to institute therapy aimed at reducing the thyroid hormone concentration and to follow serum hormone levels as guides of therapeutic response. Initiation of PTU, 200 mg every 8 hours given orally or by nasogastric tube, followed by 1 or 2 drops of ssKI twice daily, is the suggested treatment for this patient's thyrotoxicosis. The reason for starting PTU before iodide is to prevent the gland from being flooded with iodide, which has been shown to produce, on occasion, a later exacerbation of thyrotoxicosis. A full discussion of these drugs appears under Thyroid Storm above and in Table 80-4. Thyroid function tests should be performed every 2 days.

Second, consider a 65-year-old woman admitted for semiemergent aortic valvuloplasty for severe aortic stenosis due to rheumatic carditis. She has been noted to be thyrotoxic; recent thyroid function tests revealed an FT_4I of 19 and a TSH level of less than 0.01 mU/L. The valvuloplasty is scheduled for the next morning. While antithyroid drugs and ssKI should be given at the onset, in this case there is little chance for this treatment to reduce the thyroid hormone levels in 24 hours. Propranolol can provide a rapid and effective preparation for surgery.[66] An initial dose of 40 mg every 6 hours is appropriate, to be followed by increments of 20 mg every 6 hours, depending on the response, as judged by the heart rate. Although the usual dose is approximately 40 mg every 6 hours, doses of up to 320 mg/d may be required. Symptoms of tachycardia, anxiety, and sweating should be re-lieved within 12 hours. Intraoperative propranolol may be administered for tachycardia as needed. Propranolol treatment should be resumed within 4 to 6 hours after surgery and maintained for 48 hours. If the patient is unable to take oral medications perioperatively, then propranolol can be administered as a 1.0- to 2.0-mg slow intravenous bolus. On postoperative day 3, the dose of propranolol can be halved; it can be halved again on day 4, and the drug can be discontinued completely on day 5, 6, or 7 depending on the symptoms and the response to continuing antithyroid drug therapy. Propranolol is not indicated in patients with bronchial asthma, advanced grades of heart block, or unstable insulin-dependent diabetes nor in patients taking quinidine or psychotropic drugs that augment adrenergic activity. β Blockers generally are safe and effective in congestive heart failure, when administered with caution, and are useful in correcting the high-output failure of thyrotoxicosis. Three cases have been reported in which thyroid storm followed surgery for which the patient had been prepared with propranolol alone.[67–69]

Third, consider a 25-year-old 38-week primigravida who must undergo emergent cesarean section for fetal distress. The patient is known to have active Graves' disease. She has not been compliant in taking the prescribed PTU and is febrile, tachycardic, and hallucinating. Appropriate preparation for this patient prior to general anesthesia and emergency cesarean section would be intravenous propranolol, 1.0 to 2.0 mg as a slow intravenous bolus. Then 10 to 15 mg propranolol can be added to 500 mL 5% dextrose and infused while the patient's and fetus's heart rates are monitored. Continuation of the propranolol after surgery would be indicated, as discussed earlier. The use of atropine to control bronchial secretions during surgery should be avoided in thyrotoxic patients because of possible exacerbation of the sympathomimetic activity. There are reports of the use of plasma exchange in severe thyrotoxicosis of pregnancy.[54] In summary, euthyroidism can be rapidly accomplished with iopanoic acid and dexamethasone, β-blockers, and, when possible, antithyroid drugs.[69a]

Amiodarone-Induced Thyrotoxicosis

Amiodarone is an iodine-rich antiarrhythmic (37% of its weight is organic iodine). Because of its efficacy, it has become widely used. This has resulted in a significant increase in side effects associated with the drug, such as thyrotoxicosis. Given the patient's underlying cardiac problem that necessitated the use of this drug, the thyrotoxicosis, when it occurs, results in a worsening of the problem. The incidence of amiodarone-induced thyrotoxicosis (AIT) is thought to be higher in individuals with low dietary iodine. Amiodarone also can cause hypothyroidism but usually in populations with relatively high dietary iodine.

The mechanism of AIT is unknown but undoubtedly involves thyroid iodine dysautoregulation and destruction and/or inflammation of the thyroid gland. AIT is classified as types I and II. Type I occurs in structurally abnormal thyroid glands (such as a nodular goiter), and type II occurs in a structurally normal gland.[70] Type I is caused by iodine-induced thyroid hormone synthesis, and type II is believed to be due to a destructive thyroiditis. Treatment of type I and type II AIT in critically ill patients can be a challenge, and often the type of AIT is not apparent at the time of presentation.

The diagnosis is made in a patient who presents with the typical laboratory findings of thyrotoxicosis and a history of being on or recently having been on amiodarone. Owing to accumulation of the drug in fat tissue, it has a long half-life in the body. Laboratory tests such as an elevated spot urinary iodine determination and an ^{123}I uptake test (although the latter is rarely practical in the ICU setting) can be helpful to confirm the diagnosis in a patient who is thyrotoxic and on amiodarone.

The most appropriate treatment of AIT is still to be determined. All agree that amiodarone should be discontinued immediately in all patients, where possible. Two recent investigations have demonstrated that treatment with prednisone or prednisolone was advantageous in resolution of the hyperthyroidism.[71,72] The mechanism of how steroids help may be related to their anti-inflammatory effect during a destructive type II AIT or to the effect on reduction of conversion of T_4 to T_3. A protocol for the treatment of AIT in the ICU is outlined in Fig. 80-2. Briefly, the critically ill patient should be placed on prednisone 30 mg daily, along with an antithyroid drug, PTU 200 mg three times daily or MMI 20 mg twice daily, and potassium perchlorate, 500 mg twice daily. This regimen should continue for 2 weeks, at which time repeat serum FT_4I and FT_3I and urine iodine level should be measured. If the FT_4I and FT_3I both are normal, a rapid taper of the steroid and discontinuation of the potassium perchlorate (because of its poor gastrointestinal tolerance) should be initiated, and management of the antithyroid drug should be as in anyone with hyperthyroidism. If the FT_4I and/or FT_3I are elevated, then the same course of medications should be continued for 2 more weeks, and then remeasurement of the serum thy-

roid hormone and urine iodine levels would be indicated. In circumstances where medication is not an option and the severity of the thyrotoxicosis is causing cardiovascular collapse, patients should be stabilized as much as possible, and emergent thyroidectomy should be considered. Radioactive iodine ablation is rarely an option given the low thyroidal uptake of the isotope.

Levothyroxine Overdose

Levothyroxine (L-T_4) is dispensed commonly and, in the United States, is the fourth most frequently prescribed drug in the 3.05 billion prescriptions written in 2002 (*http://www.rxlist.com/top200.htm*). This wide availability leads to frequent overdoses, with reports of 2000 to 5000 acute toxic exposures annually in this country.[73–75] Despite the high frequency of overdosage, with documented blood levels of T_4 up to 16 times normal, there have been no reported deaths from L-T_4 ingestion.[74] Clearly, patients do become symptomatic, with tachycardia, nervousness, diarrhea, and even seizures, but these symptoms generally are self-limited. In patients suspected (but denying) of having ingested thyroid hormone, the finding of a suppressed serum thyroglobulin level in the presence of a high serum T_4 and/or T_3 level is diagnostic.[76]

The most commonly used thyroid preparation today is synthetic L-T_4, which contains no T_3, in contrast to the thyroid preparations of 20 years ago, which consisted of thyroid gland extracts containing 20% to 30% T_3. Therefore, ingestion of a large quantity of L-T_4 does not cause immediate toxic effects. Symptoms occur after a significant amount of T_4 has been converted to T_3, usually about 24 hours after ingestion. After gastrointestinal decontamination, by induction of vomiting

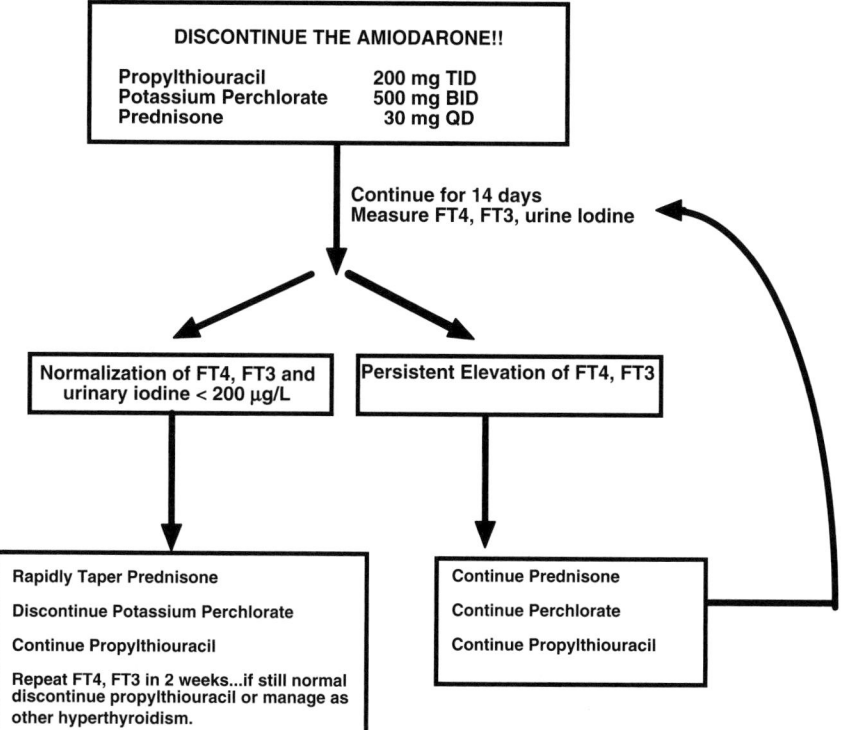

FIGURE 80-2 Proposed protocol for the treatment of critically ill patients with amiodarone-induced hyperthyroidism.

with syrup of ipecac and gastric lavage using charcoal, only symptomatic and supportive treatment is indicated. Recommendations by Lehrner and Weir,[77] based on experience with two patients and review of the literature, are aggressive treatment with (1) gastrointestinal decontamination, (2) cholestyramine to increase fecal elimination of the hormone, (3) prednisone and propylthiouracil, and (4) propranolol. Recently, Gorman and colleagues[74] recommended only gastrointestinal decontamination and propranolol if the patient is markedly symptomatic. They suggested home gastrointestinal decontamination when 0.5 mg L-T$_4$ has been ingested and determination of the serum T$_4$ level for ingestions of roughly 2.0 to 4.0 mg. When we give 1 mg T$_4$ for an absorption test, the serum T$_4$ level increases by only about 2 μg/dL in 8 hours. Therefore, the former guidelines are a bit conservative, and we would recommend that ingestion of over 10 mg in an adult is cause for aggressive treatment. Elderly patients and persons with underlying cardiac disease should be hospitalized for observation if the serum T$_4$ level is high or the patient is symptomatic. Cholestyramine has been used in treating iatrogenic thyrotoxicosis and may shorten the time it takes for the thyroid hormone concentration to normalize.[78] The use of other medical therapy should await the onset of symptoms.

Neonatal Thyrotoxicosis

Neonatal thyrotoxicosis is a rare emergency that is treatable but nevertheless is associated with a 12% to 16% mortality.[79,80] A neonate can present signs of thyrotoxicosis within the first 24 hours of life but usually later if the mother was receiving thyroid-suppressive therapy and when blocking as well as stimulating antibodies are present. Physical findings are goiter, tachypnea, tachycardia, cardiomegaly, hyperkinesis, restlessness, diarrhea, and poor weight gain. Flushing, periorbital edema, and exophthalmos also may be present.

Most infants with neonatal thyrotoxicosis are born to mothers with hyperthyroidism. Neonatal thyrotoxicosis also can occur with no documented maternal thyroid disease and even in the presence of maternal hypothyroidism. In most cases, this disease is caused by transplacental transfer of thyroid-stimulating immunoglobulin.[81] In others, where such a substance cannot be demonstrated in the mother's serum, there may be de novo formation of thyroid-stimulating immunoglobulins in the fetus due to neonatal Graves' disease or autonomous hyperfunction due to an activating mutation in the TSH receptor.[82]

Treatment of neonatal thyrotoxicosis is short term until the placentally transferred immunoglobulins have disappeared. PTU is given at doses of 5 to 10 mg/kg per day in three divided daily doses. Iodide solutions (10% potassium iodide, 76.6 mg/mL) may be given in a dose of 1 drop, or about 4 mg, every 8 hours. High-output congestive heart failure and other sympathomimetic effects can be treated with propranolol, 2 mg/kg per day in two or three divided doses. Caution should be exercised in the use of propranolol because severe bradycardia and hypoglycemia may result.[83] Surgery and radioiodine treatment are required after the initial drug control of thyrotoxicosis in infants with nonautoimmune hyperthyroidism.

Iodide-Induced Thyrotoxicosis (Jodbasedow)

Iodide, in the form of dietary supplements or medication (e.g., antitussive agents, amiodarone, or contrast agents), can induce thyrotoxicosis, especially in patients who are relatively iodide deficient. Treatment requires special considerations because antithyroid drugs alone are slow to act because of a flooded iodine pool. To deplete the gland of iodine, perchlorate must be added to the therapeutic regimen—particularly in amiodarone-induced thyrotoxicosis.[84] Naturally, iodide treatment is not indicated.

Acknowledgment

This work was supported by U.S. Public Health Service Grants DK-02081, DK-15070, and RR-00055.

References

1. Kaptein EM, Weiner JM, Robinson WJ, et al: Relationship of altered thyroid hormone indices to survival in nonthyroidal illnesses. *Clin Endocrinol (Oxf)* 125:565, 1982.
2. Wartofsky L, Burman KD: Alterations in thyroid function in patients with systemic illness: The "euthyroid sick syndrome." *Endocr Rev* 3:164, 1982.
3. Burr WA, Black EG, Griffiths RS, Hoffenber R: Serum triiodothyronine and reverse triiodothyronine concentrations after surgical operation. *Lancet* 2:1277, 1975.
4. Baue AE, Gunther B, Hartl W, et al: Altered hormonal activity in severely ill patients after injury or sepsis. *Arch Surg* 119:1125, 1984.
5. Blake NG, Eckland JA, Foster OJF, Lightman SL: Inhibition of hypothalamic thyrotropin-releasing hormone messenger ribonucleic acid during food deprivation. *Endocrinology* 129:2714, 1991.
6. Fliers E, Guldenaar SEF, Wiersinga WM, Swaab DF: Decreased hypothalamic thyrotropin-releasing hormone gene expression in patients with nonthyroidal illness. *J Clin Endocrinol Metab* 82:4032, 1997.
7. Van den Berghe G, de Zegher F, Baxter RC, et al: Neuroendocrinology of prolonged critical illness: Effects of exogenous thyrotropin-releasing hormone and its combination with growth hormone secretagogues. *J Clin Endocrinol Metab* 83:309, 1998.
8. Lim VS, Passo C, Murata Y, et al: Reduced triiodothyronine content in liver but not pituitary of the uremic rat model: Demonstration of changes compatible with thyroid hormone deficiency in liver only. *Endocrinology* 114:280, 1984.
9. Delatlia D: Dopamine and TSH secretion in man. *Lancet* 2:760, 1877.
10. Scanlon MF, Weightman DR, Shale DJ, et al: Dopamine is a physiological regulator of thyrotrophin (TSH) secretion in normal man. *Clin Endocrinol (Oxf)* 10:7, 1979.
11. Lindenberg JA, Brehier A, Ballard PL: Triiodothyronine nuclear binding in fetal and adult rabbit lung and cultured lung cells. *Endocrinology* 103:1725, 1978.
12. Ksenzenko SM, Davidson SB, Saba AA, et al: Effect of triiodothyronine augmentation on rat lung surfactant phospholipids during sepsis. *J Appl Physiol* 82:2020, 1997.
13. Raafat AM, Franko AP, Zafar R, et al: Effect of thyroid hormone (T$_3$)–responsive changes in surfactant apoproteins on surfactant function during sepsis. *J Trauma* 42:803, 1997; discussion 808.

14. Dulchavsky SA, Ksenzenko SM, Saba AA, Diebel LN: Tri-iodothyronine (T_3) supplementation maintains surfactant biochemical integrity during sepsis. *J Trauma* 39:53, 1995; discussion 57.

15. Chapital AD, Hendrick SR, Lloyd L, Pieper D: The effects of triiodothyronine augmentation on antithrombin III levels in sepsis. *Am Surg* 67:253, 2001; discussion 255.

16. Brent GA, Hershman JM: Thyroxine therapy in patients with severe nonthyroidal illnesses and low serum thyroxine concentration. *J Clin Endocrinol Metab* 62:1, 1986.

17. Arem R, Karlsson F, Depe S: Intravenous levothyroxine therapy does not affect survival in severely ill intensive care unit patients. *Thyroidol Clin Exp* 7:79, 1995.

18. Lim VS, Henriquez C, Seo H, et al: Thyroid function in a uremic rat model: Evidence suggesting tissue hypothyroidism. *J Clin Invest* 66:946, 1980.

19. Klemperer JD, Klein I, Gomez M, et al: Thyroid hormone treatment after coronary-artery bypass surgery. *New Engl J Med* 333:1522, 1995.

20. Bennett-Guerrero E, Jimenez JL, White WD, et al: Cardiovascular effects of intravenous triiodothyronine in patients undergoing coronary artery bypass graft surgery: A randomized, double-blind, placebo-controlled trial. Duke T_3 Study Group. *JAMA* 275:687, 1996.

21. Blum M: Myxedema coma. *Am J Med* 264:432, 1972.

22. Wilson WR, Bedell GN: The pulmonary abnormalities in myxedema. *J Clin Invest* 39:42, 1960.

23. Zwillich CW, Pierson DJ, Hofeldt FD, et al: Ventilatory control in myxedema and hypothyroidism. *New Engl J Med* 292:662, 1975.

24. Holvey DM, Goodner CJ, Nicoloff JT: Treatment of myxedema coma with intravenous thyroxine. *Arch Intern Med* 113:89, 1964.

25. Ingbar SG, Freinkel N: Simultaneous estimation of rates of thyroxine degradation and thyroid hormone synthesis. *J Clin Invest* 34:808, 1955.

26. Nicoloff JT: Thyroid storm and myxedema coma. *Med Clin North Am* 69:1005, 1985.

27. Sterling K, Chodos RB: Radiothyroxine turnover studies in myxedema, thyrotoxicosis and hypermetabolism without endocrine disease. *J Clin Invest* 35:806, 1956.

28. Melliere D, Saada F, Etienne G, et al: Goiter with severe respiratory compromise: Evaluation and treatment. *Surgery* 103:367, 1988.

29. Karbowitz SR, Edelman LB, Nath S, et al: Spectrum of advanced upper airway obstruction due to goiters. *Chest* 87:18, 1985.

30. Torres A, Arroyo J, Kastanos N, et al: Acute respiratory failure and tracheal obstruction in patients with intrathoracic goiter. *Crit Care Med* 11:265, 1983.

31. Tseng KH, Felicetta JV, Rydstedt LL, et al: Acute airway obstruction due to a benign cervical goiter. *Otolaryngol Heat Neck Surg* 97:72, 1987.

32. Geelhoed GW: Tracheomalacia from compressing goiter: Management after thyroidectomy. *Surgery* 104:1100, 1988.

33. Huysmans DA, Hermus AR, Corstens FH, et al: Large, compressive goiters treated with radioiodine. *Ann Intern Med* 121:757, 1994.

34. Ingbar SH: Classification of the causes of thyrotoxicosis, in Ingbar SH, Braverman LE (eds): *The Thyroid*. Philadelphia, Lippincott, 1986, p 809.

35. Tietgens ST, Leinung MC: Thyroid storm. *Med Clin North Am* 79:169, 1995.

36. Kudrjavcev T: Neurologic complications of thyroid dysfunction. *Adv Neurol* 19:619, 1978.

37. Vaccari A: Effects of dysthyroidism on central monoaminergic neurotransmission (review). *Monogr Neural Sci* 9:78, 1983.

38. Adams RD, DeLong GR: The neuromuscular system and brain, in Ingbar SH, Braverman LE (eds): *The Thyroid*. Philadelphia, Lippincott, 1986, p 885.

39. Katz AL, Emmanouel DS, Lindheimer MD: Thyroid hormone and the kidney. *Nephron* 15:223, 1975.

40. Herbert V: The blood, in Ingbar SH, Braverman LE (eds): *The Thyroid*. Philadelphia, Lippincott, 1986, p 878.

41. Parfitt AM, Dent LE: Hyperthyroidism and hypercalcemia. *Q J Med* 39:171, 1970.

42. Sellin JH, Vassilopoulou-Sellin R, Lester R: The gastrointestinal tract and liver, in Ingbar SH, Braverman LE (eds): *The Thyroid*. Philadelphia, Lippincott, 1986, p 871.

43. Sack TL, Sleisenger MH: Effects of systemic and extraintestinal disease on the gut, in Sleisenger MH, Fordtran JS (eds): *Gastrointestinal Disease*. Philadelphia, Saunders, 1989, p 488.

44. Siurala M, Lamberg BA: Stomach in thyrotoxicosis. *Acta Med Scand* 165:181, 1952.

45. Sagara K, Shimada T, Fujiyama S, Sato T: Serum gastrin levels in thyroid dysfunction. *Gastroenterol Jpn* 18:79, 1983.

46. Hanson JS: Propylthiouracil and hepatitis: Two cases and a review of the literature. *Arch Intern Med* 144:994, 1984.

47. Burch HB, Wartofsky L: Life-threatening thyrotoxicosis: Thyroid storm. *Endocrinol Metab Clin North Am* 22:263, 1993.

48. Wartofsky L: Thyrotoxic storm, in Ingbar SH, Braverman LE (eds): *The Thyroid*. Philadelphia, Lippincott, 1986, p 974.

49. Yeung SC, Go R, Balasubramanyam A: Rectal administration of iodide and propylthiouracil in the treatment of thyroid storm. *Thyroid* 5:403, 1995.

50. Wartofsky L, Ransil BJ, Ingbar SH: Inhibition by iodine of the release of thyroxine from the thyroid glands of patients with thyrotoxicosis. *J Clin Invest* 49:78, 1970.

51. Wu S-Y, Chopra IJ, Solomon DH, Johnson DE: The effect of repeated administration of ipodate (oragrafin) in hyperthyroidism. *J Clin Endocrinol Metab* 47:1358, 1978.

52. DeGroot LJ, Rue PA: Roentgenographic contrast agents inhibit triiodothyronine binding to nuclear receptors in vitro. *J Clin Endocrinol Metab* 49:538, 1979.

53. Shen DC, Wu SY, Chopra IJ, et al: Further studies on the long-term treatment of Graves' hyperthyroidism with ipodate: Assessment of a minimal effective dose. *Thyroid* 1:143, 1991.

54. Shen DC, Wu SY, Chopra IJ, et al: Long term treatment of Graves' hyperthyroidism with sodium ipodate. *J Clin Endocrinol Metab* 61:723, 1985.

55. Derksen RHWM, van de Wiel A, Poortman J, et al: Plasma exchange in the treatment of severe thyrotoxicosis in pregnancy (case reports). *Eur J Obstet Gynec Reprod Biol* 18:139, 1984.

56. Schlienger JL, Sapin R, Faradji A: Plasmapheresis induces high reverse T_3 levels in euthyroid and hyperthyroid patients. *Horm Metab Res* 24:46, 1992.

57. Binimelis J, Bassas L, Marruecos L, et al: Massive thyroxine intoxication: Evaluation of plasma extraction. *Intensive Care Med* 13:33, 1987.

58. Wahl R, Schmidberger H, Fessler E, et al: Effects of human thyroxine-binding globulin and prealbumin on the reverse flow of thyroid hormones from extravascular space into the bloodstream in rabbits. *Endocrinology* 124:1428, 1989.

59. Kellett HA, Wyllie AH, Dale AB, et al: Hyperthyroidism due to a thyrotrophin-secreting microadenoma. *Clin Endocrinol* 19:57, 1983.

60. Jorgensen ES: Stereochemistry of thyroxine and analogues. *Mayo Clinic Proc* 39:560, 1964.

61. Giddings NB, Surks MI: Cerebral embolism in atrial fibrillation complicating hyperthyroidism. *JAMA* 240:2567, 1978.

62. Parker JL, Lawson PH: Death from thyrotoxicosis. *Lancet* 2:894, 1974.

63. Toft AD, Irvine WJ, Sinclair I, et al: Thyroid function after surgical treatment of thyrotoxicosis. *New Engl J Med* 298:643, 1978.

64. Crooks JF, Forrest AL, Hamilton WF, Gunn A: Propranolol in the surgical treatment of hyperthyroidism, including severely thyrotoxic patients. *Br J Surg* 68:865, 1981.

65. Haddad HM: Rates of ^{131}I-labeled thyroxine metabolism in euthyroid children. *J Clin Invest* 39:1590, 1960.

66. Lee TC, Coffey RJ, Currier BM, et al: Propranolol and thyroidectomy in the treatment of thyrotoxicosis. *Ann Surg* 195:766, 1982.

67. Eriksson M, Rubenfeld S, Garber A, Kohler P: Propranolol does not prevent thyroid storm. *New Engl J Med* 296:263, 1977.

68. Jackson JA, Smigiel M, Greene JF Jr: Hyperthyroidism due to a thyrotropin-secreting pituitary microadenoma. *Henry Ford Hosp Med J* 35:198, 1987.

69. Jamison M: Postop thyrotoxic crisis in a patient prepared for thyroidectomy with propranolol. *Br J Clin Pract* 33:82, 1979.

69a. Panzer C, Beazley R, Braverman L: Rapid preoperative preparation for severe hyperthyroid Graves' disease. *J Clin Endocrinol Metab* 89:2142, 2004.

70. Martino E, Bartalena L, Bogazzi F, Braverman LE: The effects of amiodarone on the thyroid. *Endocr Rev* 22:240, 2001.

71. Erdogan MF, Gulec S, Tutar E, et al: A stepwise approach to the treatment of amiodarone-induced thyrotoxicosis. *Thyroid* 13:205, 2003.

72. Bogazzi F, Bartalena L, Cosci C, et al: Treatment of type II amiodarone-induced thyrotoxicosis by either iopanoic acid or glucocorticoids: A prospective, randomized study. *J Clin Endocrinol Metab* 88:1999, 2003.

73. Golightly LK, Smolinske SC, Kulig KW, et al: Clinical effects of accidental levothyroxine ingestion in children. *Am J Dis Child* 141:1025, 1987.

74. Gorman GL, Chamberlain JM, Rose SR, Oderda GM: Massive levothyroxine overdose: High anxiety, low toxicity. *Pediatrics* 82:666, 1988.

75. Kulig K, Golightly LK, Rumck BH: Levothyroxine overdose associated with seizures in a young child. *JAMA* 254:2109, 1985.

76. Mariotti S, Martino E, Cupini C, et al: Low serum thyroglobulin as a clue to the diagnosis of thyrotoxicosis factitia. *New Engl J Med* 307:410, 1982.

77. Lehrner LM, Weir MR: Acute ingestion of thyroid hormone. *Pediatrics* 73:313, 1984.

78. Shakir KM, Michaels RD, Hays JH, Potter BB: The use of bile acid sequestrants to lower serum thyroid hormones in iatrogenic hyperthyroidism. *Ann Intern Med* 118:112, 1993.

79. Hollingsworth DR, Mabry CC: Congenital Graves' disease, in Fisher DA, Burrow GN (eds): *Perinatal Thyroid Physiology and Disease.* New York, Raven Press, 1975, p 163.

80. Samuel S, Pildes RS: Neonatal hyperthyroiditis in an infant born to a euthyroid mother. *Am J Dis Child* 121:440, 1971.

81. Singer J: Neonatal thyrotoxicosis. *J Pediatr* 91:749, 1977.

82. Kopp P, Van Sande J, Parma J, et al: Congenital hyperthyroidism caused by a mutation in the thyrotropin-receptor gene. *New Engl J Med* 332:150, 1995.

83. Gardner LI: Is propranolol alone really beneficial in neonatal thyrotoxicosis? *Am J Dis Child* 134:819, 1980.

84. Martino E, Aghini-Lombardi F, Mariotti S, et al: Treatment of amiodarone associated thyrotoxicosis by simultaneous administration of potassium perchlorate and methimazole. *J Endocrinol Invest* 9:201, 1986.

PART IX

GASTROINTESTINAL DISORDERS

Chapter 81
GUT AND HEPATOBILIARY DYSFUNCTION

ELI D. EHRENPREIS
THOMAS D. SCHIANO

KEY POINTS

- *Alterations in gastrointestinal motility occur commonly in critically ill patients.*

- *The small intestine is the site of obstruction in 90% of cases of mechanical bowel obstruction. Pelvic adhesions are the most common cause. Thirty percent of cases require surgery.*

- *Intestinal pseudo-obstruction (nonmechanical bowel obstruction) may present with clinical symptoms that are similar to mechanical obstruction. Treatment includes nasogastric suction, rehydration, and correction of causative factors.*

- *Ogilvie's syndrome (colonic pseudo-obstruction) is characterized by abdominal distension and marked dilation of the cecum and right colon on abdominal x-rays. Treatment with colonoscopic decompression of the right colon is successful in about 60% of patients. Intravenous neostigmine is also effective.*

- *The incidence of diarrhea in the critically ill is greater than 40% and is up to 60% in patients receiving enteral feedings.*

- *Clostridium difficile infections are generally acquired in the hospital in patients receiving broad-spectrum antibiotics. Measurement of C. difficile toxin A or B in the stool by rapid enzyme-linked immunosorbent assay (ELISA) is the most practical method for diagnosis. Treatment consists of metronidazole or vancomycin for 7 to 14 days.*

- *Hyperbilirubinemia is frequently seen in patients with sepsis; cytokines along with bacterial endotoxins impair transport of bile acids at the sinusoidal and canalicular membranes, resulting in cholestasis.*

- *The etiology of total parenteral nutrition (TPN)-associated liver dysfunction appears to be multifactorial. The diagnosis is often made after the exclusion of other causes such as the concurrent use of potentially hepatotoxic medications, biliary obstruction, infections, and underlying intrinsic liver disease.*

- *Critically ill patients have multiple risk factors that predispose to acalculous cholecystitis. Patients often present atypically; unexplained fever and evidence of occult infection may frequently be the only manifestations. Ultrasonography alone is of limited value in diagnosis.*

- *Strong clinical suspicion and early recognition of acalculous cholecystitis are essential. Because of delays in diagnosis, more than 40% of patients develop complicated disease with gangrene, abscess, or perforation of the gallbladder.*

Gastrointestinal (GI) and hepatic dysfunction are common in the critically ill patient, particularly in the setting of multiple organ system failure (MOSF) and the systemic inflammatory response syndrome (SIRS). Many factors are responsible for the pathophysiologic derangements of the GI tract and liver in critically ill patients. Disordered function may be directly related to the precipitating illness of the patient, which can lead to additive morbidity, thus perpetuating a vicious cycle. Management of disordered GI and hepatic function often necessitates aggressive and sometimes invasive diagnostic and therapeutic maneuvers, placing critically ill patients at risk for iatrogenic complications. These conditions may create vexing problems in the ongoing care of patients in the intensive care unit. It is therefore imperative for the clinician to develop a thorough understanding of the pathophysiology of GI and hepatic dysfunction in the critical care patient. This knowledge will permit identification of these conditions and allow for management decisions that are appropriate and timely.

In this chapter, we review the physiology of intestinal motility, and the pathophysiology and clinical features of intestinal obstruction and pseudo-obstruction. We also review the various causes of diarrhea in the critically ill patient, as well as the pathophysiology of bacterial translocation. In addition, the relationship between hepatic dysfunction in the critically ill patient as related to infection and parenteral nutrition will be discussed. The diagnosis and management of acalculous cholecystitis will also be reviewed.

Intestinal Motility

Alterations of intestinal motility are common in the critically ill patient. The following discussion will be restricted to small intestinal and colonic motility, since these are the GI organs most subject to dysfunction in the intensive care setting.

NORMAL FUNCTION OF THE SMALL INTESTINE AND COLON

The contents of the small intestine and colon are subject to complex processing prior to their excretion from the rectum. As GI contents are moved through the stomach and small intestine, mixing and churning result in the reduction in size of individual particles. These smaller particles allow increased exposure of nutrients to the small intestinal mucosa. The contents of the small intestine subsequently undergo nutrient and electrolyte absorption with a net secretion of fluid. The normal transit time of a liquid bolus from the mouth to the ileocecal valve is less than 2 hours, whereas solid substances take up to 8 hours to reach the cecum.[1] The colon functions as a storage organ, with solid contents remaining within the colon for an average of 35 hours prior to excretion.[2] Intraluminal contents undergo solidification as they move from the proximal to distal colon as marked reabsorption of water, sodium, and chloride, and net secretion of potassium, takes place. These processes occur through highly coordinated events with regional differences within portions of the small and large intestine. The control of luminal fluid and electrolyte balance, as well as motility of the small intestine and colon, requires the integration of neuronal, muscular, and endocrine components of these organs.

NEUROANATOMY OF THE SMALL INTESTINE AND COLON

The complexity of intestinal neuroanatomy can be appreciated by the fact that the neuronal density of the gut is

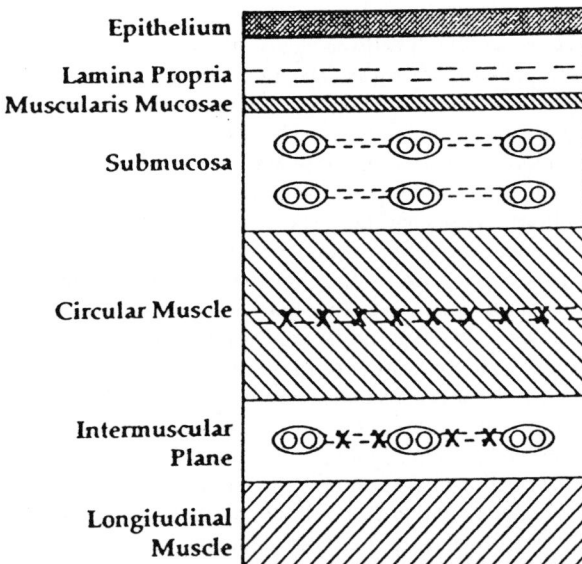

FIGURE 81-1 Schematic representation of a cross-section of the small intestine. Nerve cell bodies are seen within the submucosa (Meissner's plexus) and between the circular and longitudinal muscle layers (Auerbach's plexus). (*Reprinted with permission from Sleisenger MH, Fordtran JS: Gastrointestinal Disease. Philadelphia, Saunders, 1998, p 1438.*)

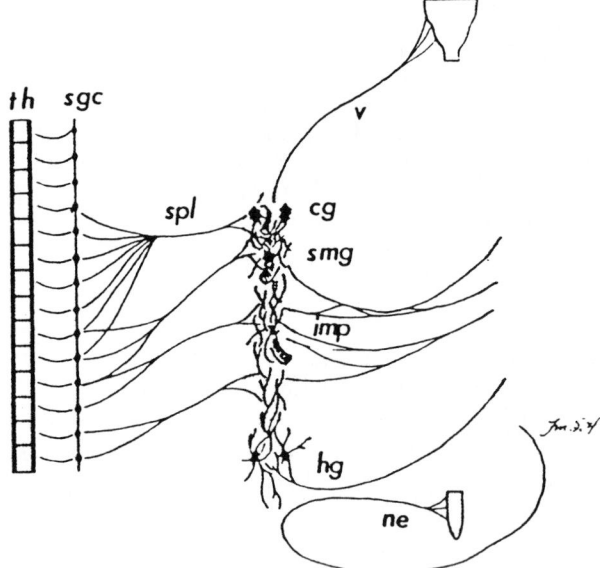

FIGURE 81-2 Diagrammatic representation of autonomic innervation of the colon. Sympathetic preganglionic fibers from the thoracic region of the spinal cord (th) travel to the sympathetic ganglionic chain (sgc). Splanchnic neurons are formed (spl) which travel to prevertebral ganglia (cg, celiac ganglia; smg, superior mesenteric ganglia; imp, intermesenteric plexus; hg, hypogastric ganglia). Postganglionic fibers from these plexuses then travel to submucosal and intramuscular plexuses of the colon. Parasympathetic fibers originate form the medulla and coalesce as the vagus nerve (v) and the pelvic and hypogastric plexuses called the nervi erigentes (ne). (*Reprinted with permission from Berk JE: Gastroenterology. Philadelphia, Saunders, 1985.*)

approximately equivalent to that of the spinal cord. This network of neuronal pathways has been described as the "brain of the gut."[3] The small and large intestine have both intrinsic and extrinsic neuronal components. The intrinsic neurons of the small intestine and colon consist of cell bodies which are located in either the submucosa (Meissner's plexus) or the intermuscular region between the circular and longitudinal muscles of the gut wall (Auerbach's plexus) (Fig. 81-1). Submucosal nerve cell bodies are most prominent in the duodenum and decrease in density in a caudal direction; intermuscular nerve cell bodies are more evenly distributed throughout the GI tract.

The extrinsic intestinal nervous system makes up a significant portion of the autonomic nervous system and consists of parasympathetic and sympathetic branches. The distributions of these pathways are markedly different.[4,5] Parasympathetic motor fibers originating from the medulla coalesce along the vagus nerve. Additional parasympathetic motor axons arise from the sacral portion of the spinal cord and join as the pelvic nerves and hypogastric plexus. The axons of these vagal and sacral parasympathetic plexuses advance directly to the GI tract, where they synapse with cell bodies in the submucosa or intermuscular areas as previously described. Sensory fibers arising from the GI tract that synapse with central nervous system (CNS) ganglia are also present in these plexuses.

Adrenergic pathways start at the thoracolumbar region of the spinal cord. These neurons synapse with ganglia which are located outside the GI tract called the *paravertebral ganglia*. Sympathetic neurons synapse within or pass beyond these ganglia and then form several nerve bundles termed the *splanchnic nerves*. The splanchnic nerves advance to prevertebral ganglia and plexuses located on the aorta and its branches. The prevertebral ganglia include the celiac,

superior mesenteric, inferior mesenteric, intermesenteric, and hypogastric plexuses. Postganglionic axons from these ganglia then travel along the blood vessels to the submucosal and intermuscular plexuses as previously described. Sensory fibers arising from the GI tract are also found within the thoracolumbar sympathetic system (Fig. 81-2). Cholinergic neurons result in stimulation of gut motility by a direct effect on the enteric smooth muscle. Adrenergic neurons cause gut relaxation, primarily by inhibition of cholinergic neurons.[6] Other important enteric neurotransmitters include serotonin, somatostatin, and vasoactive intestinal peptide. For example, stimulation of $5\text{-}HT_4$ (serotonin) receptors promotes intestinal motility and decreases noxious sensations from the gastrointestinal tract.[7] Opioid receptor inhibition also stimulates small intestinal motility and decreases oral-cecal transit time.[8]

MUSCULAR ANATOMY OF THE SMALL INTESTINE AND COLON

Small intestinal and colonic motility are accomplished by contraction of the smooth muscles that make up a portion of the walls of these organs. The muscular portion of the small intestine is divided into an inner circular layer and outer longitudinal layer. In the small intestine and rectum, the longitudinal muscular layer consists of a thick coat which surrounds the entire circumference of these organs. In the colon, the longitudinal muscles are arranged in three bundles, called *teniae coli*, which traverse the colon and then fan out in the rectum. The presence of circular and longitudinal muscle layers in the small and large intestines allows for shortening of intestinal segments when the longitudinal musculature contracts, and narrowing of the intestinal lumen when circular muscles contract.

CLASSIFICATION OF MUSCULAR CONTRACTIONS OF THE GUT

Two main forms of contractions occur in the small intestine. These are called *ring contractions* and *sleeve contractions*. Ring contractions are contractions of circular muscle and result in narrowing of the small intestine lumen. These occur continuously in the fed state, but are intermittent in the fasted state and result in the caudad movement of the intestinal contents. Sleeve contractions are caused by longitudinal muscle contraction. Their primary function is the mixing of small intestinal contents.[5]

Normal motor activity in the small intestine is highly organized. In the fed state, ring contractions moving from the proximal to distal small intestine result in the caudad movement of its contents. Motility in the fasted state is quite complex.[9] The fasted motility pattern occurs 4 to 6 hours after completion of a meal. This pattern consists of three phases (Fig. 81-3). Phase I is a rest phase which makes up about 80% of the entire cycle. Phase II is the beginning of rhythmic ring contractions, which may be solitary or clustered. Phase III consists of maximum ring contractions, also called the *migrating motor complex* (MMC), which begin in the proximal portion of the intestine and move in a distal direction. It is evident that the MMC causes a wave of contractions that sweep along the small intestine.[10] The function of the MMC is the

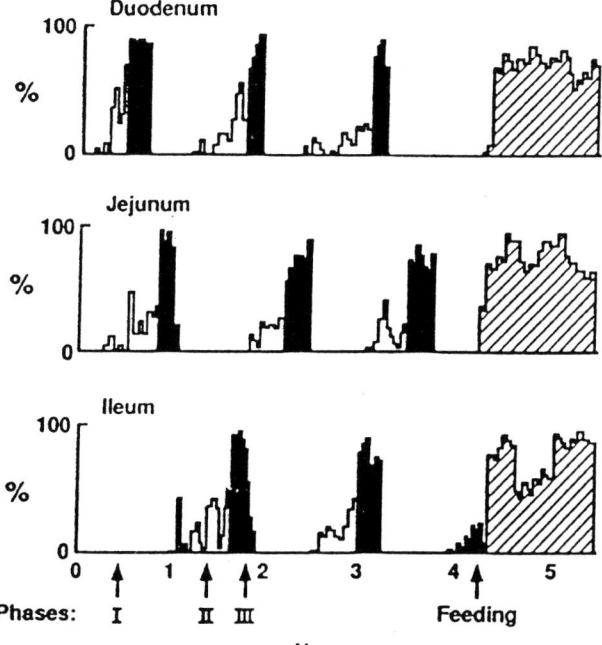

FIGURE 81-3 Normal small intestinal motility. Resting phase I and active phases II (*open bars*) and III (*solid bars*) are shown. After feeding, motility stops periodically, and the fed pattern of motility occurs (*hatched bars*). (*Reprinted with permission from Sleisenger MH, Fordtran JS: Gastrointestinal Disease. Philadelphia, Saunders, 1998, p 1443.*)

emptying of food particles that remain in the small intestine after completion of the fed pattern of motility.

Ring contractions also occur in the colon; sleeve contractions do not. Colonic ring contractions are subdivided into tonic ring contractions and rhythmic ring contractions. Tonic ring contractions are sustained contractions of the circular musculature which form the haustral markings of the colon. The haustra, which divide the colon into individual segments, are stable for long periods. They disappear when mass movement of feces occurs on a periodic basis, then subsequently reappear. Rhythmic ring contractions cause mass movements of fecal material every few hours, as well as continuous caudad and cephalad motion of fecal material. Rhythmic ring contractions cause mixing of the colonic contents.[5]

Unlike the detailed information available on small intestinal motility, the motility patterns of the colon in the fed and fasted state have not been fully elucidated.

Disordered Motility

One of the most common GI abnormalities encountered in the critical care setting is the disruption of normal intestinal motility. Loss of motor function may occur in the small intestine as well as the colon. A variety of terminologies have been used to describe disrupted intestinal motility. *Ileus* is a physiologic term referring to the complete discontinuation of neuromuscular function in the small and large intestine. The term *acute intestinal pseudo-obstruction* refers to nonmechanical causes of small intestinal and colonic dysfunction. *Intestinal obstruction* describes a mechanical blockade of the small or large intestine. *Postoperative ileus* is a term for the normal gut response that occurs for up to 72 hours following abdominal and other types of surgery. Often the clinician will be faced with a diagnostic dilemma in differentiating between mechanical intestinal obstruction, which may require surgical intervention, and pseudo-obstruction, which generally responds to medical therapy.

ACUTE INTESTINAL OBSTRUCTION IN THE CRITICALLY ILL

More than 90% of all cases of mechanical obstruction of the intestine involve the small intestine alone. Intestinal obstruction is generally caused by adhesions within the abdominal and pelvic cavities; hernias, carcinoma, and intestinal volvulus are other less common causes. Intestinal obstruction may also occur as a consequence of congenital anomalies such as intestinal malrotation; inflammatory bowel disease, especially Crohn's disease; intestinal ischemia; or impaction of the intestinal lumen by foreign bodies such as gallstones.[11]

Adhesions develop after abdominal surgery and following prior intra-abdominal sepsis.[12] Intestinal obstruction secondary to adhesions may occur as early as 3 days after the original surgery. However, delayed effects of adhesive small bowel disease are common, with some patients having recurrent bouts of small intestinal obstruction up to 20 years after their initial surgery.[13]

The pathophysiologic consequence of a mechanical small intestinal obstruction is distention of the region of the small intestine proximal to the blockade. High pressures develop within the intestinal lumen that may ultimately compromise the blood flow to affected areas. Bowel edema with fluid secretion into the small intestinal lumen occurs as well. This phenomenon, in conjunction with fluid losses secondary to vomiting, causes fluid and electrolyte derangements. As luminal pressure increases, strangulation of the bowel may occur. Bacterial translocation into the circulatory system with resulting bacteremia as well as perforation, peritonitis, and shock are the sources of mortality associated with this condition.

The clinical presentation of patients with acute intestinal obstruction includes intermittent abdominal pain, nausea, and vomiting. Fever, leukocytosis, and electrolyte disturbances commonly occur. Colicky abdominal pain, distension, and abnormal bowel sounds in a patient with previous abdominal surgery are highly sensitive and specific for the presence of mechanical small intestinal obstruction.[14]

Radiographs of the abdomen with supine and upright views as well as an upright chest x-ray are commonly used to confirm the diagnosis of small intestinal obstruction. Whereas dilated loops of small intestine and colon with the presence of air in the rectum are seen in acute intestinal pseudo-obstruction, mechanical intestinal obstruction is characterized by small intestinal dilation alone without much air in the colon or rectum. Air-fluid levels may be present and represent separation of gas and fluid within fluid-filled, static portions of the small intestine (Fig. 81-4). Absence of

FIGURE 81-4 Radiograph of an acute mechanical small intestinal obstruction showing multiple dilated loops of small intestine. (*Courtesy of Dr. Arunas Gasparaitis.*)

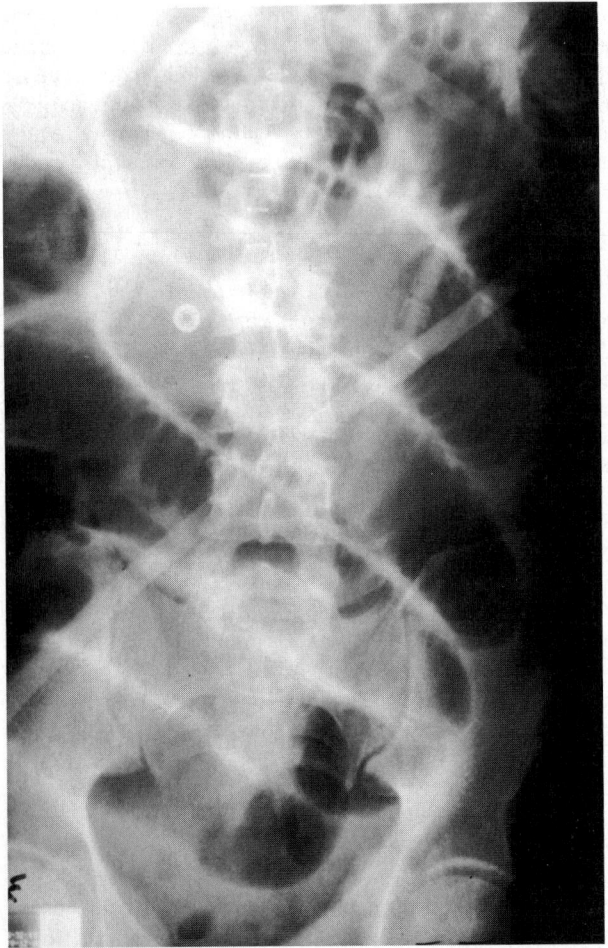

air beyond a dilated segment of the small intestine is seen in a complete small intestinal obstruction. Air under the diaphragm on the upright chest x-ray is indicative of an intestinal perforation.

Computed tomography (CT) scanning with oral contrast has been demonstrated to have better sensitivity in diagnosing complete small intestinal obstruction than plain abdominal radiography.[15] CT with contrast may also be used to pinpoint the location of a mechanical small intestinal obstruction by identifying decompressed bowel that is distal to the obstruction and may be used to diagnose the presence of intestinal ischemia.[16] CT scanning is also used to identify the source of obstruction such as an intra-abdominal or pelvic mass. Small intestinal radiography with contrast may be used to differentiate intestinal obstruction from pseudo-obstruction and for cases not resolving with conservative management. Caution is advised with the use of contrast studies, since barium entering the abdominal cavity through a perforated organ may cause a chemical peritonitis, whereas aspirated water-soluble contrast can result in pneumonitis. The therapeutic role of water-soluble contrast agents for the relief of intestinal obstruction has been investigated and remains controversial.[17]

Partial small intestinal obstruction is initially treated conservatively with nasogastric suction, administration of intravenous fluids, and correction of electrolyte abnormalities. Nasogastric suction is used for bowel decompression. Serial abdominal examinations and x-rays are vital in the ongoing management of partial intestinal obstruction. The development of sepsis, complete obstruction, or clinical signs of perforation are indications for immediate surgery. Nonresolution of partial mechanical small bowel obstruction is another indication for surgery.[18]

Conservative management for partial small intestinal obstruction is effective in about 70% of patients. Patients failing conservative management require laparotomy and lysis of adhesions with resection of nonviable intestine. Hospital mortality for small intestinal obstruction is about 10%. Recurrences are common, and more than 50% of patients undergoing surgery for intestinal obstruction can expect a recurrence during their lifetime.[13]

INTESTINAL PSEUDO-OBSTRUCTION

Intestinal pseudo-obstruction results from disruption of the extrinsic or intrinsic neuronal pathways of the intestine. The mechanism for the development of this disruption varies. In some patients, such as those who have recently undergone abdominal surgery, sympathetic overdrive is present, thus diminishing cholinergic output to the intestine. In others, the direct anticholinergic activity of drugs and neurohumoral mediators inhibits gut function.[19] A variety of conditions may result in acute intestinal pseudo-obstruction (Table 81-1). Small intestinal motility in patients with acute idiopathic intestinal pseudo-obstruction is markedly reduced. For example, manometric studies performed in patients with these disorders show marked abnormalities of the fasted motility pattern, including the MMC.[20]

The clinical symptoms of acute intestinal pseudo-obstruction closely resemble those of mechanical small intestinal obstruction. Most patients have abdominal distention and absence of bowel sounds. Abdominal pain is usual but may not be recognized in the patient who is sedated, delirious,

TABLE 81-1 Common Causes of Acute Intestinal Pseudo-Obstruction

Intra-abdominal
  Surgery (especially abdominal)
  Acute pancreatitis
  Peritonitis
  Retroperitoneal hemorrhage
  Intestinal ischemia
Drugs
  Narcotics
  Anticholinergics
  Cyclic antidepressants
  Antipsychotics
  Clonidine
  Calcium channel blockers
  Ganglionic blockers
Electrolyte abnormalities
  Hypokalemia
  Hypercalcemia
  Hypermagnesemia
Miscellaneous
  Myocardial infarction
  Sepsis
  Shock of any cause
  Bone fractures
  Surgery (postoperative—nonabdominal)
  Vasculitis
  Chronic intestinal motility disorders

or encephalopathic. Vomiting may also be present, placing patients with this condition at risk for aspiration pneumonia.

Treatment consists of correction of electrolyte abnormalities and administration of intravenous fluid. Pharmacologic agents that may be causing or aggravating the condition should be discontinued. Nasogastric suctioning may result in symptomatic improvement and may alter the pathophysiologic consequences of bowel distention in these patients. Limited therapeutic trials of pharmacologic agents for acute intestinal pseudo-obstruction or prolonged postoperative ileus with metoclopramide and erythromycin have shown few beneficial effects.[20] Recent studies of opiate antagonists including methylnaltrexone and alvimopan[21,22] have shown promise as potential therapies for postoperative ileus. Movement of the patient and ambulation when possible are encouraged.

OGILVIE'S SYNDROME: ACUTE COLONIC PSEUDO-OBSTRUCTION

This syndrome, first described by Sir Heneag Ogilvie in 1948, is generally seen in the ICU or in postoperative patients. It is characterized by abdominal distention accompanied by colonic dilation, particularly involving the cecum and right colon. A variety of medical conditions are associated with the development of Ogilvie's syndrome. It is generally accepted that this disorder results from decreased parasympathetic tone to the distal colon from the sacral nerves with normal vagal impulses to the right side of the colon resulting in a pseudo-obstruction of the distal colon with associated proximal colonic dilation.[23] Sympathetic hyperactivity of the right colon has also been postulated as a potential mechanism for the development of this disorder.

The most common medical conditions associated with Ogilvie's syndrome include sepsis, respiratory failure, or-

ganic brain disorders, and malignancy. Trauma to the spine, retroperitoneum, and pelvis, as well as burns, may also result in the development of Ogilvie's syndrome.[24,25] Electrolyte disturbances, including hyponatremia, hypernatremia, hypokalemia, and hypocalcemia, are seen in the majority of patients.[26] A variety of medications have been implicated as potential etiologic agents in Ogilvie's syndrome, including narcotics, phenothiazines, calcium channel blockers, and cyclic antidepressants. For example, in one review of Ogilvie's syndrome, 56% of patients had received opiates on the day of diagnosis, 42% had received phenothiazines, and 15% ingested cyclic antidepressants.[27] Other medications associated with the development of Ogilvie's syndrome include clonidine and anticholinergic agents. Ogilvie's syndrome may also occur in the postoperative period, most commonly after cesarean sections, orthopedic surgery, and urologic procedures.[24]

Physical examination of patients with Ogilvie's syndrome always reveals abdominal distention. Bowel sounds remain present in most patients, but may be hypoactive or high pitched. Leukocytosis may be seen in up to 30% of patients, even prior to the development of associated bowel ischemia or perforation. Abdominal x-rays are the diagnostic test of choice, showing dilation of the cecum, usually with associated dilation of the right colon (Fig. 81-5). A decrease in the gas pattern of the left colon is often seen. At the time of diagnosis of colonic pseudo-obstruction, the transverse diameter of the cecum often measures 9 cm or greater on an unmagnified abdominal film.[28]

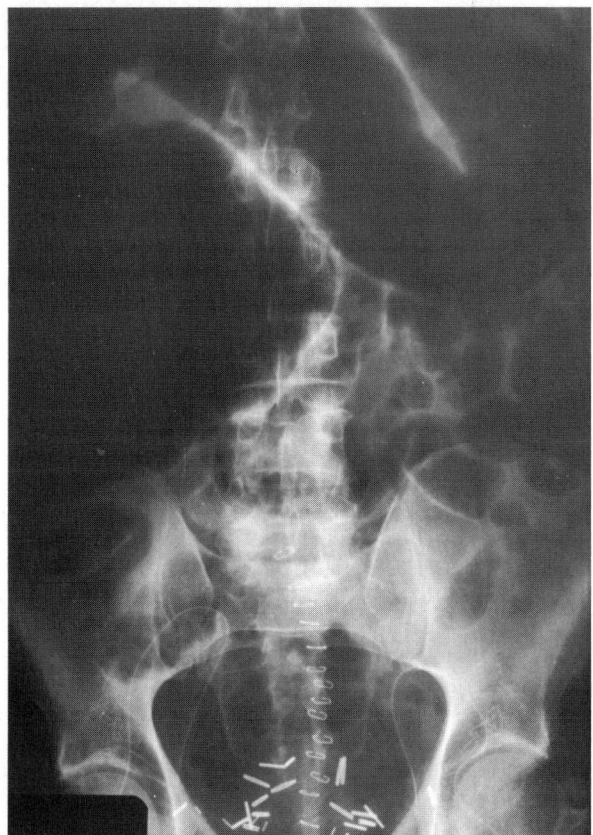

FIGURE 81-5 Plain radiograph of a patient with Ogilvie's syndrome showing massive cecal and transverse colon dilation. (*Courtesy of Dr. Geraldine Newmark.*)

Ogilvie's syndrome may be complicated by ischemia and perforation of the distended cecum. As the colon becomes increasingly enlarged (and its radius of curvature increases), less additional pressure is needed to further distend it, and its wall tension rises dangerously (as described by the law of Laplace).[28] Case series have shown that the spontaneous cecal perforation rate in Ogilvie's syndrome is approximately 13%, and mortality from this occurrence is 43%. However, the absolute cecal diameter does not correlate specifically with the risk of perforation. The duration of cecal dilation and the rate at which it dilates appear to be the most important factors related to perforation.[29]

The goal of therapy for Ogilvie's syndrome is decompression of the colon. Some have advocated an initial conservative approach, including nasogastric suction, intravenous hydration, correction of electrolyte abnormalities, discontinuation of offending medications, and treatment of predisposing medical or surgical conditions.[27] Others suggest early colonoscopic decompression of the cecum and right colon as an effective and safe therapy for the disorder.[26] The colonoscope is advanced to the cecum or the right colon, an often technically challenging procedure because no colonic cleansing preparation is used. Minimal air is insufflated during the procedure to prevent iatrogenic cecal perforation. The reported success rate for initial colonoscopic decompression ranges from 61% to 76%.[23,26] The success rate increases after repeat colonoscopic decompression which is required in 20% to 50% of cases. Complication rates for colonoscopic decompression in Ogilvie's syndrome are modest and range from 0% to 3% in published series. Overall the condition carries a mortality rate of approximately 15% in uncomplicated cases, with patients generally dying from their underlying condition. If bowel becomes ischemic or perforates, mortality increases to about 40% as previously described.[27]

A variety of pharmacologic treatments have been attempted for Ogilvie's syndrome, including cisapride and erythromycin.[30,31] These treatments have been reported as case studies only. Neostigmine, a cholinesterase inhibitor, stimulates neuromuscular activity. Several case studies involving a total of 58 patients have demonstrated the efficacy of neostigmine administered slowly by the intravenous route.[32–34] Most recently, Trevisani and associates treated 28 patients with 2.5 mg neostigmine administered over 3 minutes. Twenty-six patients (93%) had resolution of the condition with therapy.[34] Abdominal cramping, nausea, and diaphoresis were common side effects, although no patients experienced severe bradycardia or cardiovascular collapse, complications that have been described with the use of neostigmine.

Colonoscopic decompression fails in approximately 15% to 20% of patients, even after multiple attempts. These patients require surgical decompression, generally accomplished with a cecostomy and placement of a catheter. A 50% morbidity and 15% mortality is anticipated following cecostomy placement for Ogilvie's syndrome.[29] Complications include pericatheter leakage, superficial wound infections, catheter herniation, catheter dislodgment, and prolonged cecal-cutaneous fistula. Nonetheless, this procedure is reportedly successful in 96% of patients. Occasionally patients will require a colonic resection for treatment of this disorder, with an expected 30% surgical mortality.[27]

TABLE 81-2 Common Causes of Diarrhea in the Critically Ill Patient

Antibiotic effect
Clostridium difficile infection
Medications
    Magnesium-containing antacids
    Sorbitol in suspensions, syrups
    Laxatives
    Others (theophylline, lithium, digoxin, etc)
Enteral feeding
Hypoalbuminemia
Underlying gastrointestinal diseases
    Bacterial overgrowth
    Motility disorders
    Inflammatory bowel disease
    Fecal impaction
    Small intestinal disorders
    Chronic pancreatitis
    Lactose intolerance
Miscellaneous conditions
    Endocrinopathies (i.e., hyperthyroidism)
    Vasculitis
    Ischemia
    Irritable bowel syndrome
    Graft-vs-host disease

Diarrhea in the Critically Ill Patient

The incidence of diarrhea in critically ill patients is greater than 40%.[35] Differentiating between potential causes of diarrhea in these patients is necessary for optimal management of these disorders (Table 81-2). The following discussion will focus on the most common of these conditions.

CLOSTRIDIUM DIFFICILE COLITIS

Clostridium difficile is a fastidious gram-positive spore-forming anaerobe that is toxin-producing. *C. difficile* is found in the colonic flora in up to 3% of the general population. The organism is readily acquired from the environment, and studies have shown that bathrooms, sinks, and floors of hospitals and chronic care facilities often harbor colonies of *C. difficile*.[36] It may persist in the rooms of infected individuals for up to 40 days.[37] Patients are at high risk of developing *C. difficile* colitis after receiving broad-spectrum antibiotics, particularly those with activity against anaerobic organisms. Clindamycin and broad-spectrum cephalosporins are often implicated, but symptomatic *C. difficile* colitis has been described following the administration of almost all currently used antibiotics. Broad-spectrum antibiotics eliminate the normal colonic flora, the majority of which are anaerobic organisms. Preexisting carriage, or more commonly, exposure to environmentally-acquired *C. difficile* results in subsequent colonization, overgrowth, and infection with the toxin-producing organism. Immunosuppressed patients are at particular risk for the development of severe toxic colitis secondary to *C. difficile*. Such patients may develop diffuse colonic involvement with bowel ischemia and perforation.

Symptoms of *C. difficile* colitis include abdominal pain, diarrhea, and fever. Some patients may have neither abdominal pain nor diarrhea, so *C. difficile* colitis should always be considered in the differential diagnosis of patients with occult sepsis.[38] Leukocytosis, electrolyte abnormalities, and hypoalbuminemia may also be present.[39] *C. difficile* is diagnosed by stool examination. Fecal leukocytes are often present. Culturing of *C. difficile* is the gold standard for diagnosing this disorder, but is technically difficult to perform. Measurement for the presence of *C. difficile* toxin A or B by rapid ELISA is the most common method of diagnosis. It has a sensitivity of 86% and specificity of 100%. The cytotoxic assay for toxin B is more sensitive (94% to 100%), but requires a tissue culture laboratory to perform and takes up to 48 hours.[37] Plain radiography or CT imaging may provide clues to the diagnosis (Fig. 81-6A and B). A bedside sigmoidoscopy is useful

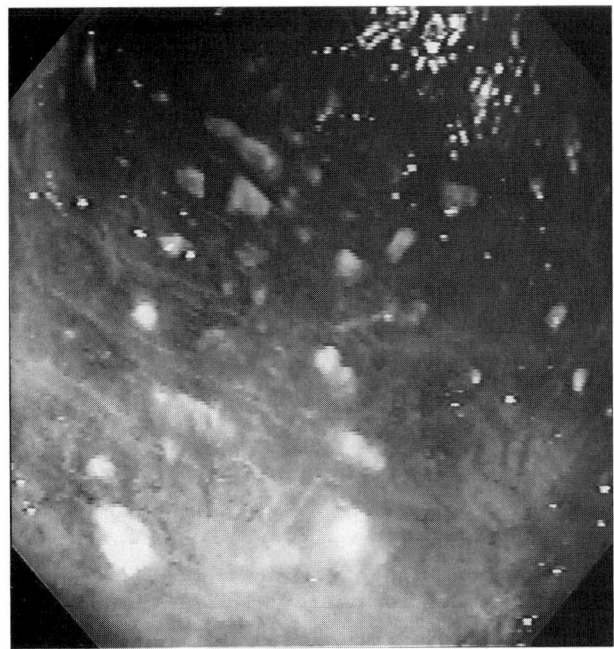

FIGURE 81-7 Endoscopic view of the rectum and sigmoid colon in a patient with pseudomembranous colitis and *Clostridium difficile* infection. Multiple white plaques are seen adherent to the mucosa. (*Courtesy of Dr. Ira Hanan.*)

FIGURE 81-6 *A.* Plain radiograph of the abdomen in a patient with *C difficile* colitis shows mild gaseous distention of the colon associated with moderate haustral thickening ("thumb-printing"). *B.* Unenhanced CT obtained in the same patient on the same day demonstrates thickened colon wall. Note the presence of ascites and subcutaneous edema. (*Courtesy of Ian Boiskin MD.*)

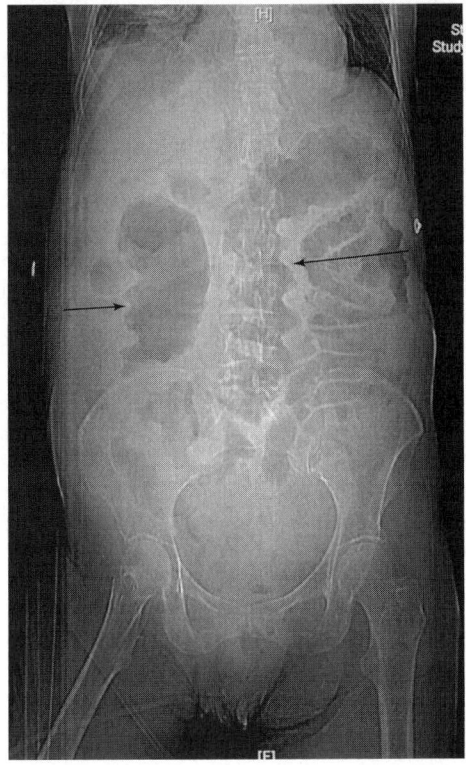

A

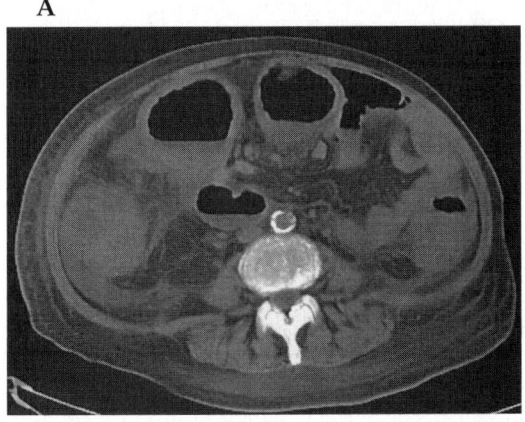

B

for identifying the presence of colitis. If the patient is infected with *C. difficile,* typical pseudomembranes will be seen about 60% of the time (Fig. 81-7).

Treatment for *C. difficile* colitis should be initiated in all patients in whom the toxin has been identified or in whom endoscopic findings suggest this disorder. Broad-spectrum antibiotics should be discontinued if possible. Metronidazole 250 to 500 mg PO qid for 7 to 14 days or vancomycin 125 to 250 mg PO tid for 7 to 14 days is used to eradicate the organism. A high response rate is expected with oral antibiotic therapy, although relapse rates of 15% to 20% following treatment can be expected.[40] Intravenous metronidazole 500 to 750 mg q6h may be used in those patients who cannot tolerate oral antibiotic therapy, but this may not be as effective as oral therapy. For patients who are critically ill due to *C. difficile* colitis, combined therapy with intravenous metronidazole and oral vancomycin may be indicated.[41]

MISCELLANEOUS CAUSES OF DIARRHEA

Patients receiving enteral tube feedings commonly develop diarrhea; the published incidence ranges from 5% to greater than 60%.[31] Diarrhea in these patients can often be attributed to the osmolarity of the feeding solutions. When the rate of administration of enteral feeding is high, the normal mechanisms for fluid and electrolyte reabsorption in the small intestine and colon may be overwhelmed. In other critically ill patients, intestinal wall edema and villous atrophy may be present, resulting in nutrient malabsorption and increased osmotic load to the colon. A number of studies have shown that patients with low serum albumin levels, particularly levels below 2.6 g/dL, are at risk for diarrhea.[42] Finally, altered colonic flora following the administration of broad-spectrum antibiotics results in decreased colonic reabsorption of carbohydrates, which produces an osmotic type of diarrhea as well.

A variety of methods have been suggested to lessen the diarrhea associated with enteral feeding, but these have met with variable success.[43] Current recommendations include decreasing the infusion rate of enteral feedings, adding fiber to enteral formulas, decreasing the osmolality of the feeding solution by diluting it with water, and adding dipeptides and predigested proteins to standard enteral formulas.[44] Lactose-free or reduced-fat-content formulas may benefit occasional patients.

Sorbitol, a common additive in medications that are administered in a liquid or syrup form, may also cause diarrhea. Since sorbitol, a sugar alcohol, is not absorbed in the small intestine, it functions as an osmotic agent in the colon, increasing intraluminal fluid and electrolytes. The sorbitol content of administered medications should be checked in all patients with unexplained diarrhea who are receiving medications in a suspension or syrup form.[45] Magnesium, a common ingredient in antacid preparations, also causes diarrhea. It should also be remembered that many different medications may cause diarrhea in individual patients by a variety of mechanisms. Medications should therefore always be included in the differential diagnosis of diarrhea.

Patients in the ICU may also have diarrhea owing to the presence of preexisting GI illnesses, such as intestinal ischemia, inflammatory bowel disease, small intestinal diseases, and pancreatic insufficiency. Following gastric or small intestinal resections, patients commonly develop diarrhea due to stasis of bowel contents and subsequent bacterial overgrowth, as well as to malabsorption occurring as a direct result of the surgery. Bacterial overgrowth may also occur following prolonged ileus and loss of the MMC, combined with a loss of local immunoglobulin production in the small intestine.

Bacterial Translocation

The gut normally functions as an effective barrier against bacteria and endotoxin present in the intestinal lumen. Some migration of bacteria across the GI mucosa occurs in health, likely contributing to the regulation of local and systemic immunity against the innumerable antigens that contact the intestinal epithelium.[46] In the critically ill patient, however, abnormal intestinal barrier function results in greater transmucosal passage of bacteria and endotoxin. In addition to being a potential source of infection, this bacterial translocation appears to serve as a trigger for the release of cytokines and other cellular mediators that may in turn activate or further perpetuate the inflammatory and hypermetabolic responses to injury. Thus gut dysfunction may play a major role in the initiation and propagation of MOSF.[47]

Components of the physiologic gut barrier include the normal microbial flora, bile salts within the intestinal lumen, the epithelial mucous layer, peristalsis, and an intact local and systemic immune system.[46,48] Normal microbial flora occupy the space closest to the intestinal epithelial cells, thereby limiting attachment to the enterocytes of potentially pathogenic gram-negative enteric bacteria. Oral antibiotics eliminate indigenous microflora and increase the risk of bacterial translocation, an effect which may be seen for prolonged periods

following cessation of antibiotic therapy. *Enterococcus faecalis, Pseudomonas aeruginosa,* and the Enterobacteriaceae appear to translocate in the greatest numbers. H_2 blockers and proton pump inhibitors facilitate upper GI tract bacterial colonization, which may also predispose to translocation. Finally, ileus, hyperosmolar enteral feeding, and TPN all disrupt the normal intestinal microbial flora.[49]

Small amounts of endotoxin normally enter the circulation and appear to play a role in maintaining the reticuloendothelial system in a primed state.[50] Bile salts within the intestinal lumen normally limit endotoxemia by binding intraluminal endotoxin. Loss of bile salts associated with critical illness may allow more endotoxin to reach the portal circulation. In animal models of obstructive jaundice, bacterial overgrowth, which occurs as a consequence of the absence of enteric bile salts, appears to promote bacterial translocation.

Further defense against translocation is provided by the normal mucus layer, which contains immunoglobulin A and other protective substances, as well as normal gut peristalsis, which impedes bacterial penetration of the protective layer of mucus. Translocation appears to become clinically relevant only with failure of local and systemic immunity. Immunosuppressive drugs increase bacterial translocation in animals, indirect evidence that intact systemic immunity may itself limit translocation.[51]

Mucosal atrophy, particularly when it occurs as a consequence of luminal nutrient deprivation, is another predisposing factor. TPN is associated with thinning of the gut mucosa and increased translocation, a consequence that can be prevented by providing nutrition via an enteral rather than intravenous route. Bacterial translocation also more readily occurs in a gut mucosal barrier compromised by ischemia.[52] Hypotension and shock may significantly decrease splanchnic perfusion, resulting in reduced oxygen delivery to the intestinal mucosa and accelerated free radical generation.[46] Lipid peroxidation and cell membrane injury result, leading to ischemia and increased mucosal permeability. Even short periods of hypotension can result in splanchnic ischemia, since splanchnic blood flow is reduced out of proportion to systemic blood flow in models of hypovolemia. This splanchnic ischemia has recently been shown to contribute to the hepatic dysfunction that ultimately occurs over time in critically ill patients. A mismatch between hepatic metabolic demand that appears to be significantly increased in MOSF, and hepatic blood flow may be at the root of this problem.[53]

Protein malnutrition, burns, pancreatitis, inflammatory bowel disease, hemorrhage, systemic infection, any form of shock, abdominal surgery, radiation, trauma, intestinal obstruction, advanced liver disease, and obstructive jaundice all promote bacterial translocation.[52,54–58] Several of these features may interact in critically ill patients to cause infection remote from the GI tract, enteric bacteremia without an identified infectious source, or propagation of systemic inflammation. The presence of two predisposing factors (e.g., treatment with antibiotics in combination with immunosuppressive drugs) appears to synergistically promote systemic spread of translocating bacteria. Intestinal barrier dysfunction and bacterial translocation may thus play a central role in MOSF.[47]

Although it seems clear that the critically ill are predisposed to bacterial translocation, preventive therapy has not been particularly beneficial. Aggressive resuscitation from shock may decrease the chances for translocation. Although TPN has not been proven to predispose to bacterial translocation in humans, enteral feeding is more physiologic and could offset gut barrier failure and thus is always preferred over TPN[56] (see Chap. 11). In rats, use of glutamine in TPN has been shown to minimize intestinal permeability and bacterial translocation caused by trauma and endotoxemia.[59] Selective decontamination of the digestive tract with nonabsorbable antibiotics may decrease bacterial translocation by suppressing potentially pathogenic microorganisms in the oropharynx and upper GI tract. Whereas selective gut decontamination appears to reduce nosocomial colonization, it may or may not have a significant effect on mortality and length of ICU stay.[60–62] In addition, selective gut decontamination may predispose to the development of resistant organisms (see Chap. 43). Improved delineation of the role of bacterial translocation in human critical illness is anticipated.

Hepatobiliary Dysfunction

Patients in the intensive care unit present a difficult challenge when diagnosing and treating complications related to the biliary tract.[63] Laboratory data are often nonspecific in diagnosing biliary tract complications. Gallbladder abnormalities are frequently seen on imaging studies in intensive care patients; therefore their presence does not necessarily indicate acute disease.[64] Because there is often a delay in diagnosing biliary tract disease in these patients, intervention is associated with high morbidity and mortality when compared to the ambulatory setting. Hepatic dysfunction significantly prolongs length of hospital stay and increases mortality in critically ill patients.[65]

CHOLESTASIS OF SEPSIS

Cholestasis results from impaired bile formation or obstruction to bile flow. Biochemically, cholestasis is characterized by a disproportionate increase in serum alkaline phosphatase or bilirubin concentrations relative to aminotransferase elevations. Cholestasis is classified as *intrahepatic* when there is a defect in bile formation at the level of the hepatocyte or *extrahepatic* when there is structural or mechanical impairment to bile flow[66] (Table 81-3).

In the critically ill, cholestasis is at times a manifestation of underlying hepatobiliary disease. Most cholestasis seen in the ICU, however, occurs in the absence of any intrinsic liver disease. Cholestatic jaundice occurring in infected and bacteremic patients, termed the *cholestasis of sepsis*, has been a well-recognized clinical syndrome for two decades.[67,68] Bilirubin levels range typically from 5 to 10 mg/dL, with the conjugated fraction predominating. This suggests that the hyperbilirubinemia seen in sepsis results from impaired bile canalicular secretion.[69,70] Liver biopsy characteristically shows retained bile concretions within bile ductules (Fig. 81-8A and 8B). This histology differs from that seen in patients with biliary obstruction in whom cholestasis is present within both hepatocytes and bile ductules; bile ductular proliferation also occurs in obstructive jaundice (Fig. 81-8C).

Bile formation depends in large part on the ability of hepatocytes to transport bile acids from sinusoidal blood into bile canaliculi against a steep concentration gradient. The

TABLE 81-3 Differential Diagnosis of Cholestasis

Extrahepatic Causes	Intrahepatic Causes
Cholangitis	Medications
Bacterial	Allopurinol
Viral	Amoxicillin/clavulanic acid
Autoimmune	Captopril
Sclerosing cholangitis	Chlorpromazine
Biliary strictures	Estrogens
Choledochal cysts	Erythromycin
Pancreatitis	Flutamide
Neoplasms	Haloperidol
Pancreatic	Hydralazine
Ampullary	Ketoconazole
Bile duct	Phenytoin
Metastatic	Quinidine
Acalculous cholecystitis	Sulfonamides
	Sepsis
	Infiltrative disease
	Sarcoidosis
	Lymphoma/Hodgkin's disease
	Amyloidosis
	Infection
	Mycobacterium avium-intracellulare
	Tuberculosis
	Postoperative jaundice
	Primary biliary cirrhosis
	Sclerosing cholangitis
	Post–liver transplant
	Chronic rejection
	Fibrosing cholestatic hepatitis
	Total parenteral nutrition
	Alcoholic liver disease
	Cholestasis of pregnancy
	Pediatric
	Alagille's syndrome
	Cystic fibrosis
	Biliary atresia

initial step is mediated in part by an active, sodium-driven bile acid uptake system across the sinusoid. An hepatocyte sodium-taurocholate-transporting polypeptide appears to be the major sinusoidal sodium-bile acid cotransporter. Efflux across the canalicular membrane represents the rate-limiting step in the overall transport of bile acids and depends both on a negative membrane potential and on adenosine triphosphate (ATP) hydrolysis.[71] There also appear to be ATP-dependent canalicular transport proteins; endotoxin and certain cytokines released in response to endotoxin may selectively impair these bile acid transporters. Endotoxemia severely impairs the transport of certain bile acids and organic anions at both the sinusoidal and canalicular membranes. As a result of this impaired hepatic bile acid and organic anion transport, bile flow is decreased.[72]

Cholestasis is not restricted to gram-negative sepsis alone, suggesting that nonendotoxin mediators may also impair bile secretion. Tumor necrosis factor-α (TNF-α) inhibits bile acid transport at both the sinusoidal and canalicular membranes. In vivo administration of anti-TNF-α antibody has been shown to prevent endotoxin-induced cholestasis. The end result of this inhibition of bile acid and organic anion transport is that sinusoidal transport may exceed canalicular transport, and potentially toxic compounds may accumulate

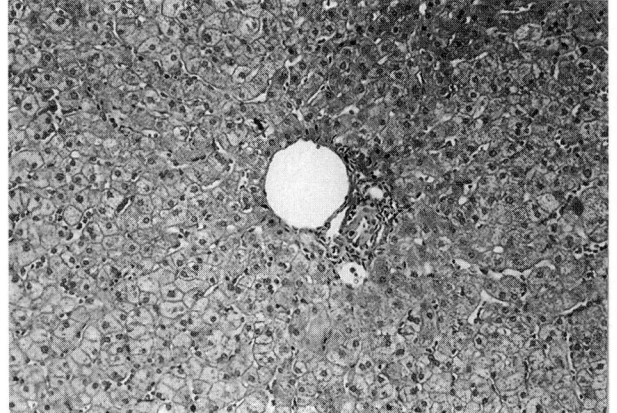

A

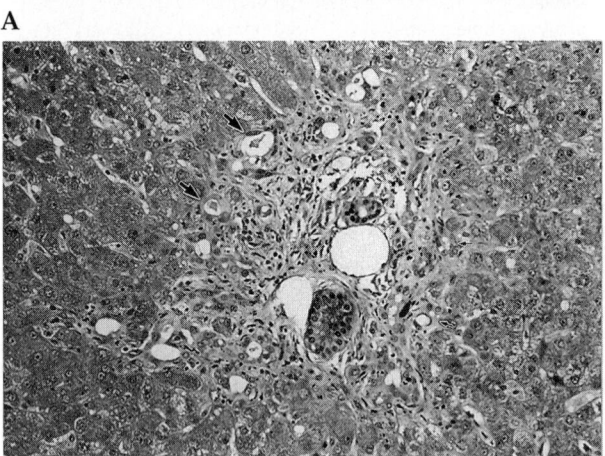

B

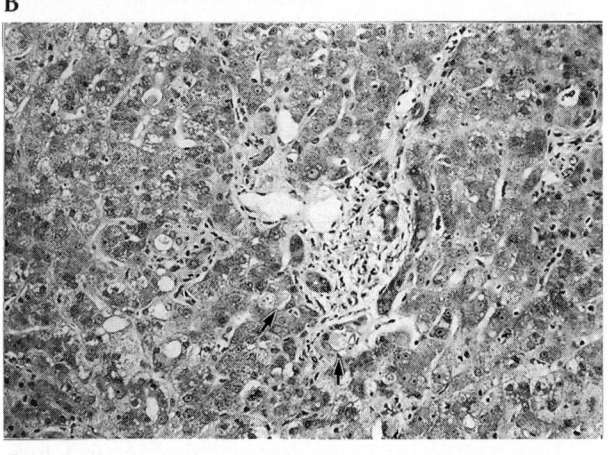

C

FIGURE 81-8 *A.* Photomicrograph of a normal liver demonstrating a central vein and an adjacent portal tract. The liver architecture is well preserved. *B.* In sepsis the portal tract is expanded by a proliferation of bile ductules accompanied by polymorphonuclear leukocytes (*small arrows*). Ductular cholestasis is present (*large arrow*). *C.* In the presence of bile duct obstruction, similar portal tract and bile ductular proliferation occur, but brownish pigment denoting cholestasis is seen in both bile ductules and individual hepatocytes (*arrows*). (*Courtesy of M.I. Fiel, MD.*)

intracellularly.[73] Impaired canalicular bile formation and resulting bile stasis, along with decreased intestinal luminal bile acid concentration, appear to perpetuate a vicious cycle by predisposing to bacterial translocation and further endotoxin absorption.[70,74,75]

When critically ill patients develop elevated serum bilirubin levels, biliary obstruction, viral hepatitis, and drug toxicity[66] should be excluded. As with cases of postoperative jaundice,[76] the etiology of cholestasis is often multifactorial. Hematologic causes of unconjugated hyperbilirubinemia such as hemolysis, multiple blood transfusions, and hematoma resorption should also be sought. Gilbert's syndrome affects approximately 10% of the general population and can present with an isolated unconjugated hyperbilirubinemia.[77] If all these conditions are excluded, infection, whether documented or occult, should be suspected as the cause of hyperbilirubinemia.

HEPATOBILIARY COMPLICATIONS OF TOTAL PARENTERAL NUTRITION

Total parenteral nutrition (TPN) is associated with various catheter-related and metabolic complications (see Chap. 11). In addition, hepatic dysfunction is a common occurrence in many patients.[78] This may result in abnormal liver chemistry tests, and less frequently, in hepatomegaly or jaundice. It is often unclear to what extent other factors such as infection, malnutrition, the concurrent use of potentially hepatotoxic medications, alcoholism, or underlying intrinsic liver disease may contribute to the liver dysfunction.[79]

In adults, modest elevation of serum aminotransferase levels occurs within the first 2 to 3 weeks of initiating TPN. These abnormalities are usually mild and reverse within 10 to 14 days of cessation of TPN. Elevations of serum alkaline phosphatase and bilirubin can occur with more prolonged parenteral nutrition. Since these abnormalities may normalize despite continuance of TPN, they should not be interpreted as evidence of permanent hepatic dysfunction or histologic damage. The early predominant histologic abnormality of the liver is steatosis, which is almost always clinically asymptomatic (Fig. 81-9). Long-term administration of TPN in infants may be accompanied by the development of cirrhosis and chronic liver disease.[78–80] In these infants, chronic liver disease appears to be a direct consequence of prolonged cholestasis. Though once thought to be a rare occurrence, recent studies have shown more adults developing advanced

FIGURE 81-9 Photomicrograph of a liver biopsy specimen from a patient who was given nothing by mouth, after receiving TPN for 1 month. Note the widespread distribution of clear fat vesicles characteristic of hepatic steatosis. (*Courtesy of M.I. Fiel, MD.*)

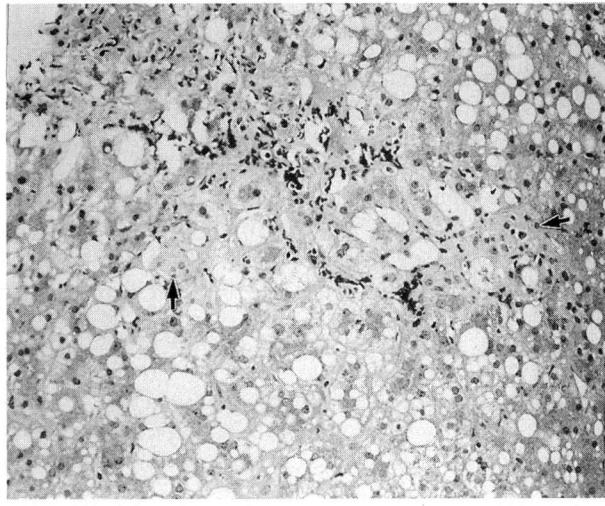

TABLE 81-4 Possible Interrelated Factors Contributing to TPN Hepatotoxicity

Composition of TPN
  Excess glucose (maximal rate of utilization is 4–5 g/kg, beyond which fat synthesis occurs)
  Excess fat calories (hepatic deposition of exogenous fatty acids occurs)
  Imbalance between amino acids and glucose (may impair the hepatic secretion of triglycerides)
  Hypercaloric feeding (may stimulate insulin release which in turn promotes lipogenesis and the
    synthesis of acylglycerol from glucose)
Possible deficiency states
  Selenium
  Carnitine
  Essential fatty acids (impaired lipoprotein formation)
  Glutamine
  Choline
  Vitamin E
  Taurine
Increased bacterial translocation and portal endotoxemia
Toxic amino acid metabolites or bile acids (especially lithocholic acid)
Altered gastrointestinal hormonal milieu
Immaturity of biliary secretory system (pediatric population)
Prolonged fasting
Intestinal stasis and perturbation of the enterohepatic circulation of bile salts (promotes intraluminal
  bile salt deconjugation, leading to increased lithocholic acid production)

liver disease from long-term TPN use.[81] Thus once significant cholestasis has developed, even in adults, TPN should generally be discontinued.

The exact mechanism of TPN-induced liver dysfunction remains unknown but is probably multifactorial in nature. Possible contributing factors are listed in Table 81-4.[78–80] The development of steatosis during TPN appears primarily to be related to the combined effects of excess glucose calories and impaired hepatic triglyceride secretion.[79,82] In addition, lipoprotein synthesis may become impaired and hepatic triglyceride secretion limited when amino acid supplementation is inadequate. Although essential fatty acid deficiency may similarly cause hepatic steatosis, most standard TPN solutions contain all essential amino acids, vitamins, and trace elements, so deficiency states are unlikely to be major contributors to TPN-associated hepatic dysfunction. Bacterial translocation and prolonged fasting may contribute to cholestasis by upsetting the enterohepatic bile salt circulation and affecting biliary secretory capacity. The cholestasis resulting from sepsis itself may be an additive or complicating factor.[72] Patients with TPN-related hepatic dysfunction appear predisposed to infection.

The development of biliary sludge, cholelithiasis, and calculous and acalculous cholecystitis are all increased in patients receiving TPN. Gallbladder sludge is detected in half of patients receiving TPN for a total of 4 to 6 weeks, and in almost 100% of patients after 8 to 13 weeks. TPN-induced gallstones are pigmented and composed primarily of calcium bilirubinate. Gallstone formation may partly relate to prolonged fasting; reduced gallbladder contractility and impaired bile flow result from prolonged use of TPN and may contribute to stone formation. Loss of normal enteral stimulation by oral nutrients also plays a role. Disease or resection of the terminal ileum further promotes the development of cholelithiasis in some patients.[78–80]

Proving TPN-induced hepatobiliary disease is challenging, since this is usually a diagnosis of exclusion. Evaluation in the ICU should include assessment of hepatitis viral serologies; radiologic studies looking for signs of biliary obstruction, liver abscess, or cholecystitis; and a search for systemic infection or hepatotoxic medications. There may be a high incidence of false-positive (nonvisualization) hepato-iminodiacetic acid (HIDA) or diisopropyl iminodiacetic acid (DISIDA) scans related to impaired gallbladder emptying in patients receiving TPN.[78] Liver biopsy may be useful to delineate any intrinsic liver disease contributing to hepatic dysfunction in the critically ill patient, but generally is not required.

If TPN-related liver chemistry abnormalities occur, they will usually normalize with discontinuation of TPN.[78–80] Physicians should avoid using an excess of glucose (>4 to 5 g/kg body weight) or an excess of total calories in TPN. Concurrent use of oral or enteral feeding or discontinuation of TPN may improve gallbladder contractility and decrease the risk of gallstone formation or cholecystitis. Cholecystokinin has been administered periodically to promote gallbladder contractility, though this has not been shown to reliably decrease the formation of gallstones.[78–80] Studies are currently examining the efficacy of ursodiol in preventing the cholestasis associated with prolonged TPN use.[83]

ACALCULOUS CHOLECYSTITIS

Acute cholecystitis may occur at any time in a patient with gallstones but is especially dangerous in patients with chronic debilitating conditions or intercurrent critical illness. Though acalculous cholecystitis comprises only 2% to 15% of all cases of acute cholecystitis, the critically ill appear to be at much greater risk. More than 50% of postoperative cases of acute cholecystitis are of the acalculous form. Risk factors are prevalent in ICU patients and include mechanical ventilation, TPN use, dehydration, use of narcotics, hypotension, chronic renal failure, and massive blood transfusion. Diabetes mellitus, human immunodeficiency virus infection, abdominal vasculitis (such as polyarteritis nodosa), and cardiac surgery are also associated with acalculous cholecystitis. This condition may also occur in trauma and burn patients and following bone marrow transplantation.[63,84–86]

Most patients developing acalculous cholecystitis have no previous history of gallbladder disease and present with atypical clinical manifestations. Abdominal examination is often unreliable owing to the presence of altered mental status, concomitant systemic illness, or recent abdominal surgery. Leukocytosis and hyperbilirubinemia occur commonly but are nonspecific in the setting of critical illness. Unexplained fever or evidence of infection may frequently be the only manifestations of acalculous cholecystitis. Because of the extremely high morbidity and mortality associated with acute acalculous cholecystitis, a high index of suspicion as well as early recognition are of paramount importance. Acalculous cholecystitis occurs commonly enough in critically ill patients that it should be in the differential diagnosis in any septic patient without a clear focus of infection.[63,84]

The etiology of acalculous cholecystitis is not completely understood; one major predisposing factor appears to be biliary stasis. Stasis and gallbladder dysmotility can be precipitated by prolonged fasting, general anesthesia, dehydration, and the use of narcotics. The resultant increase in bile viscosity has been postulated to produce functional cystic duct obstruction, increasing intraluminal gallbladder pressure; it may also render the gallbladder mucosa more susceptible to local injury. Gallbladder ischemia has also been implicated in the development of acalculous cholecystitis. This is supported by the high incidence of gallbladder mucosal necrosis, endothelial dissection, arteriolar thrombosis, gangrene, and perforation noted in autopsy studies. Gallbladder ischemia may occur as a result of low flow states in shock, systemic infection, dehydration, and hypercoagulable disorders. Prolonged mechanical ventilation with positive end-expiratory pressure may result in ischemia by decreasing portal perfusion and by raising hepatic venous and common bile duct pressures.[63,86]

Bedside abdominal ultrasonography is an unreliable routine screening tool for acute acalculous cholecystitis.[87] When present, characteristic findings include pericholecystic fluid, a gallbladder wall thickness greater than 4 mm, subserosal edema, and intramural gas. However, there can be a high false-positive rate in patients receiving TPN and in those with ascites or hypoalbuminemia. HIDA and DISIDA scanning may fail to visualize the gallbladder, implying cystic duct obstruction (Fig. 81-10). False-negative gallbladder scintigraphy is unusual. Neither scintigraphy nor ultrasound can differentiate between calculus and acalculous cholecystitis. Morphine cholescintigraphy is superior to ultrasonography in making a diagnosis. Mariat and associates performed bedside ultrasonography and morphine cholescintigraphy in 28 patients suspected of having acalculous cholecystitis. Sensitivity of ultrasound and scintigraphy was 50% and 67%, specificity was 94% and 100%, positive predictive value was 86% and 100%, and negative predictive value was 71% and 80%, respectively. The probability of disease was 100% with a positive scintiscan regardless of ultrasound results. A positive ultrasound finding was associated with an 86% probability of disease, but with a probability of only 66% with negative scintigraphy results.[88] Diagnostic laparoscopy or laparotomy is a more definitive method of diagnosing cholecystitis but has obvious attendant risks.[89] In some centers, percutaneous cholecystostomy performed by an interventional radiologist provides a less risky means for obtaining bile fluid cultures and decompressing the biliary system,[90] but these

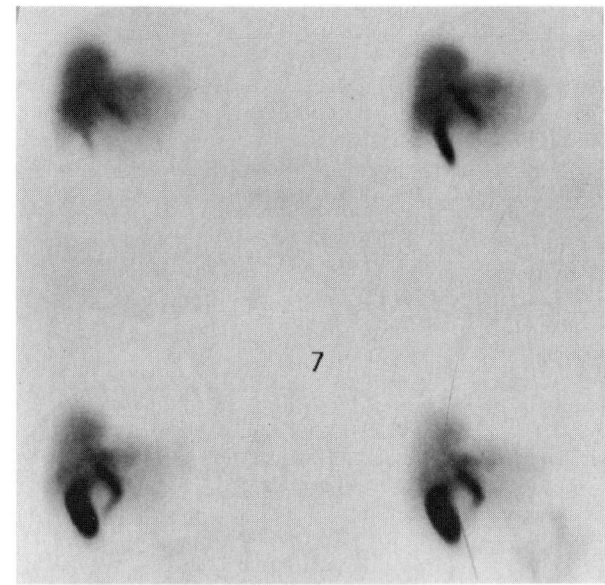

A

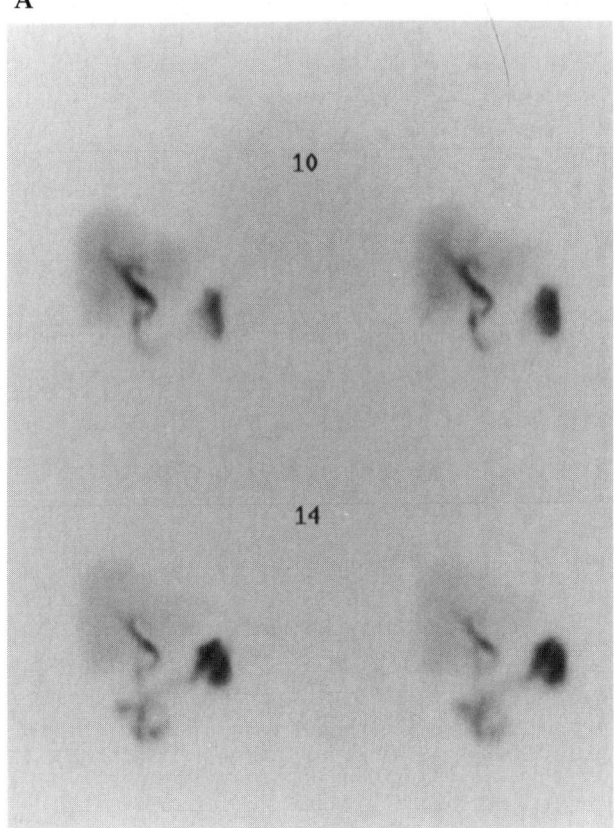

B

FIGURE 81-10 *A.* A normal HIDA scan. Note the appearance (*arrows*) of isotope within the gallbladder within 15 minutes of injection of tracer. *B.* HIDA scan of a 73-year-old man with acalculous cholecystitis. Note the appearance of tracer in the duodenum (*arrows*) and the absence of gallbladder visualization up to 60 minutes after injection of the isotope. (*Courtesy of Richard Gunderman, MD.*)

microbiologic studies may not be sensitive or specific (see Chaps. 89 and 101).

Because of delays in making a diagnosis, more than 40% of patients with acalculous cholecystitis develop complicated disease characterized by gangrene, pericholecystic abscess, or gallbladder perforation. In one series, 40% of patients with acalculous cholecystitis who underwent surgery more than 48 hours after symptom onset developed gallbladder perforation.[63,84–85] The mortality in complicated acalculous cholecystitis may be as high as 75%, with death usually due to MOSF. Once acalculous cholecystitis is recognized, cholecystectomy is the mainstay of treatment. The high incidence of gangrene and perforation makes inspection of the entire gallbladder very important. Cholecystostomy is an option in the critically ill, but this approach risks missing complicated disease and fails to adequately drain the common bile duct in cases of concomitant cholangitis. A cholecystostomy drainage catheter should remain in place for 10 to 14 days to allow maturation of the tract between the gallbladder and the abdominal wall.[90] If rapid clinical improvement does not ensue, open cholecystectomy is indicated. Laparoscopic cholecystostomy and transpapillary endoscopic cholecystostomy have proved to be effective treatment options in some patients.[89,91]

References

1. Jorge JMN, Wexner SD, Ehrenpreis ED: The lactulose hydrogen breath test as a measure of orocecal transit time. *Eur J Surg* 160:409, 1994.

2. Cook IJ, Brooks SJ: Motility of the large intestine, in Feldman M, Friedman LS, Sleisenger MH (eds): *Gastrointestinal and Liver Disease*, 7th ed., Vol. 2. Philadelphia, Saunders, 2002, p 1679.

3. Mayer E, Chang L, Lembo T: Brain-gut interactions: implications for newer therapy. *Eur J Surg Suppl* 582:50, 2001.

4. Roman C, Gonella J: Extrinsic control of digestive tract motility, in Johnson LR (ed): *Physiology of the Gastrointestinal Tract*, 2nd ed., Vol. 1. New York, Raven, 1987, p 507.

5. Andrews JM, Dent J: Small intestinal motor physiology, in Feldman M, Friedman LS, Sleisenger MH (eds): *Gastrointestinal and Liver Disease*, 7th ed. Philadelphia, Saunders, 2002, p 1655.

6. Camilleri M, Coulie B, Tack JF: Visceral hypersensitivity: Facts, speculations and challenges. *Gut* 48:125, 2001.

7. Appel-Dingemanse S: Clinical pharmacokinetics of tegaserod, a serotonin 5-HT(4) receptor partial agonist with promotile activity. *Clin Pharmacokinet* 41:1021, 2002.

8. Yuan CS, Foss JF: Oral methylnaltrexone for opioid-induced constipation. *JAMA* 284:1383, 2000.

9. Husebye E: The patterns of small bowel motility: Physiology and implications in organic diseases and functional disorders. *Neurogastroenterol Motil* 11:141, 1999.

10. Kerlin P, Zinsmeister A, Phillips S: Relationship of motility to flow of contents in the small intestine. *Gastroenterology* 82:701, 1982.

11. Nieuwemhuijzen M, Reijnen MM, Kuijpers JH, van Goor H: Small bowel obstruction after total or subtotal colectomy: A 10-year retrospective review. *Br J Surg* 85:1242, 1998.

12. Landercasper J, Cogbill TH, Merry WH, et al: Long-term outcome after hospitalization for small bowel obstruction. *Arch Surg* 128:765, 1993.

13. Barkhan H, Webster S, Ozeran S: Factors predicting the recurrence of adhesive small bowel obstruction. *Am J Surg* 170:361, 1995.

14. Eskelinen M, Ikonen J, Lipponeu P: Contributions of history taking, physical examination, and computer assistance to diagnosis of acute small bowel obstruction. A prospective study of 1333 patients with acute abdominal pain. *Scand J Gastroenterol* 29:715, 1994.

15. Daneshmand S, Hedley CG, Stain SC: The utility and reliability of computerized tomography scan in the diagnosis of small intestinal obstruction. *Am Surg* 65:922, 1999.

16. Thompson JS: Contrast radiography and intestinal obstruction. *Ann Surg* 236:7, 2002.

17. Choi HK, Chu KW, Law WL: Therapeutic value of gastrograffin in adhesive small bowel obstruction following unsuccessful conservative treatment: A prospective study. Ann Surg 236:1, 2002.

18. Meagher AP, Moller C, Hofmann DC: Non-operative treatment of small bowel obstruction following appendectomy or operation on the ovary or tube. *Br J Surg* 80:1310, 1993.

19. Ogilvy AJ, Smith G: The gastrointestinal tract after anesthesia. *Eur J Anesth* 10(Suppl):35, 1995.

20. Verne G, Sninsky C: Chronic intestinal pseudo-obstruction. *Dig Dis Sci* 13:163, 1995.

21. Kurz A, Sessler DI: Opioid-induced bowel dysfunction: pathophysiology and potential new therapies. *Drugs* 63:649, 2003.

22. Azodo IA, Ehrenpreis ED: Alvimopan. *Curr Opin Investig Drugs* 3:1496, 2002.

23. Jetmore AB, Timmcke AE, Gathright JB, et al: Ogilvie's syndrome: Colonoscopic decompression and analysis of predisposing factors. *Dis Colon Rectum* 35:1135, 1992.

24. Dorudi S, Berry AR, Kettlewell MG: Acute colonic pseudo-obstruction. *Br J Surg* 79:99, 1992.

25. Kadesky K, Purdue GF, Hunt JL: Acute pseudo-obstruction in critically ill patients with burns. *J Burn Care Rehab* 16:132, 1995.

26. Rex DX: Acute colonic pseudo-obstruction (Ogilvie's syndrome). *Gastroenterology* 2:233, 1994.

27. Vanek VW, Al-Salti M: Acute pseudo-obstructions of the colon (Ogilvie's syndrome). An analysis of 400 cases. *Dis Colon Rectum* 29:203, 1986.

28. Johnson CD, Rice RP, Kelvin FM, et al: The radiologic evaluation of gross cecal distension: Emphasis on cecal ileus. *Am J Roentgenol* 145:1211, 1983.

29. Benacci JC, Wolff BG: Cecostomy. Therapeutic indications and results. *Dis Colon Rectum* 38:530, 1995.

30. MacColl C, MacCannell KL, Baylis B, Lee SS: Treatment of acute colonic pseudo-obstruction (Ogilvie's syndrome) with cisapride. *Gastroenterology* 98:773, 1990.

31. Bonacini M, Smith OJ, Pritchard T: Erythromycin as therapy for acute colonic pseudo-obstruction (Ogilvie's syndrome). *J Clin Gastroenterol* 15:169, 1992.

32. Stephenson BM, Morgan AR, Salaman JR, Wheeler MH: Ogilvie's syndrome: A new approach to an old problem. *Dis Colon Rectum* 38:364, 1995.

33. Turegano-Fuentes F, Munoz-Jimenez F, Del Valle-Hernandez E, et al: Early resolution of Ogilvie's syndrome with intravenous neostigmine: A simple, effective treatment. *Dis Colon Rectum* 40:1354, 1997.

34. Trevisani GT, Hyman NH, Church J: Neostigmine: Safe and effective treatment for acute colonic pseudo-obstruction. *Dis Colon Rectum* 43:599, 2000.

35. Kelly TW, Patrick MR, Hillman KM: Study of diarrhea in critically ill patients. *Crit Care Med* 11:7, 1983.

36. Samore MH, Venkaataraman L, DeGirolami PC, et al: Clinical and molecular epidemiology of sporadic and clustered cases of nosocomial *Clostridium difficile* diarrhea. *Am J Med* 100:32, 1996.

37. Hurley BW, Nguyen CC: The spectrum of pseudomembranous colitis and antibiotic associated diarrhea. *Arch Intern Med* 162:2177, 2002.

38. DeMaio J, Bartlett JG: Update on diagnosis of *Clostridium difficile* associated diarrhea. *Curr Clin Top Infect Dis* 15:97, 1995.

39. Kelly CP, LaMont JT: *Clostridium difficile* infection. *Ann Rev Med* 49:375, 1998.

40. Manabe YC, Veneetz JM, Moore RD, et al: *Clostridium difficile* colitis: An efficient clinical approach to diagnosis. *Ann Intern Med* 123:835, 1995.

41. Fekety R: Guidelines for the diagnosis and management of *Clostridium difficile*-associated diarrhea and colitis. *Am J Gastroenterol* 92:739, 1997.

42. Huang TL, Lue MC, Nee YJ, et al: The incidence of diarrhea in patients with hypoalbuminemia due to acute or chronic malnutrition during enteral feeding. *Am J Gastroenterol* 89:376, 1994.

43. Dobb GJ, Towler SC: Diarrhea during enteral feeding in the critically ill: A comparison of feeds with and without fiber. *Intensive Care Med* 16:252, 1990.

44. Heimburger DC, Geels VJ, Bilbery J, et al: Effects of small-peptide and whole-protein enteral feedings on serum proteins and diarrhea in critically ill patients. *JPEN J Parenter Enteral Nutr* 21:162, 1997.

45. Ratnaike RN, Jones TE: Mechanisms of drug-induced diarrhoea in the elderly. *Drugs Aging* 13:245, 1998.

46. Berg RD: Bacterial translocation from the gastrointestinal tract. *J Med* 23:217, 1992.

47. Nieuwenhuijzen GAP, Deitch EA, Goris RJA: Infection, the gut and the development of the multiple organ dysfunction syndrome. *Eur J Surg* 162:259, 1996.

48. Swank GM, Deitch EA: Role of the gut in multiple organ failure: Bacterial translocation and permeability changes. *World J Surg* 20:411, 1996.

49. Wells CL, Maddaus MA, Simmons RL: Proposed mechanism for the translocation of intestinal bacteria. *Rev Infect Dis* 10:958, 1988.

50. Xu D, Oi D, Guillory D, et al: Mechanisms of endotoxin-induced intestinal injury in a hyperdynamic model of sepsis. *J Trauma* 34:676, 1993.

51. Deitch EA, Xu D, Qi L, Berg RD: Bacterial translocation from the gut impairs systemic immunity. *Surgery* 109:269, 1991.

52. Sedman PC, Macfie J, Sagar P, et al: The prevalence of gut translocation in humans. *Gastroenterology* 107:643, 1994.

53. Maynard ND, Bihari DJ, Dalton RN, et al: Liver function and splanchnic ischemia in critically ill patients. *Chest* 111:180, 1997.

54. Cicalese L, Sahai A, Sileri P, et al: Acute pancreatitis and bacterial translocation. *Dig Dis Sci* 46:1127, 2001.

55. Takesue Y, Ohge H, Uemura K, et al: Bacterial translocation in patients with Crohn's disease undergoing surgery. *Dis Colon Rectum* 45:1665, 2002.

56. Moore FA: The role of the gastrointestinal tract in post-injury multiple organ failure. *Am J Surg* 178:449, 1999.

57. Cirera I, Bauer TM, Navasa M, et al: Bacterial translocation of enteric organisms in patients with cirrhosis. *J Hepatol* 34:32, 2001.

58. Kuzu MA, Kale IT, Col C, et al: Obstructive jaundice promotes bacterial translocation in humans. *Hepatogastroenterology* 46:2159, 1999.

59. Ding LA, Li JS: Effects of glutamine on intestinal permeability and bacterial translocation in rats with endotoxemia. *World J Gastroenterol* 9:1327, 2003.

60. Gastinne H, Wolff M, Delatour F, et al: A controlled trial in intensive care units of selective decontamination of the digestive tract with non absorbable antibiotics. *N Engl J Med* 326:524, 1992.

61. Cerra FB, Maddaus MA, Dunn DL, et al: Selective gut decontamination reduces nosocomial infections and length of stay but not mortality or organ failure in surgical intensive care unit patients. *Arch Surg* 127:163, 1992.

62. Henry JA, Hoffman JR: Continuing controversy on gut decontamination. *Lancet* 352:420, 1998.

63. Haun MT: Gallbladder and biliary tact disease in the intensive care unit. *Semin Gastrointest Dis* 14:28, 2003.

64. Boland GW, Slater G, Lu DS, et al: Prevalence and significance of gallbladder abnormalities seen on sonography in intensive care unit patients. *Am J Roentgenol* 174:973, 2000.

65. Harbrecht BG, Zenati MS, Doyle HR, et al: Hepatic dysfunction increases length of stay and risk of death after injury. *J Trauma* 53:517, 2002.

66. Levy C, Lindor KD: Drug-induced cholestasis. *Clin Liver Dis* 7:311, 2003.

67. Franson TR, Hierholzer WJ, LaBrecque DR: Frequency and characteristics of hyperbilirubinemia associated with bacteremia. *Rev Infect Dis* 7:1, 1985.

68. Pirovino M, Meister F, Rubli E, Karlaganis G: Preserved cytosolic and synthetic liver function in jaundice of severe extrahepatic infection. *Gastroenterology* 96:1589, 1989.

69. Moseley RH: Sepsis-associated cholestasis. *Gastroenterology* 112:302, 1997.

70. Moseley RH: Sepsis and cholestasis. *Clin Liver Dis* 3:465, 1999.

71. Müller M, Jansen PLM: Molecular aspects of hepatobiliary transport. *Am J Physiol* 272(*Gastrointest Liver Physiol* 35):G1285, 1997.

72. Moseley RH, Wang W, Takeda H, et al: Effect of endotoxin on bile acid transport in rat liver: A potential model for sepsis-associated cholestasis. *Am J Physiol* 271:G137, 1996.

73. Whiting JF, Green RM, Rosenbluth AB, Gollan JL: Tumor necrosis factor-alpha decreases hepatocyte bile salt uptake and mediates endotoxin-induced cholestasis. *Hepatology* 22:1273, 1995.

74. Szabo G, Romics L, Frendl G: Liver in sepsis and systemic inflammatory response syndrome. *Clin Liver Dis* 6:1045, 2002.

75. Bolder U, Ton-Nu HT, Schteingart CD, et al: Hepatocyte transport of bile acids and organic anions in endotoxemic rats: Impaired uptake and secretion. *Gastroenterology* 112:214, 1997.

76. Molina EG, Reddy KR: Postoperative jaundice. *Clin Liver Dis* 3:477, 1999.

77. Te HS, Schiano TD, Das S, et al: Donor-liver UDP-glucuronsyltransferase-1 A 1 deficiency causing Gilbert's syndrome in liver transplant recipients. *Transplantation* 69:1882, 2000.

78. Chung C, Buchman AL: Postoperative jaundice and total parenteral nutrition-associated hepatic dysfunction. *Clin Liver Dis* 6:1067, 2002.

79. Buchman A: Total parenteral nutrition-associated liver disease. *JPEN J Parenter Enteral Nutr* 26:543, 2002.

80. Sandhu IS, Jarvis C, Everson GT: Total parenteral nutrition and cholestasis. *Clin Liver Dis* 3:489, 1999.

81. Cavicchi M, Beau P, Crenn P, et al: Prevalence of liver disease and contributing factors in patients receiving home parenteral nutrition for permanent intestinal failure. *Ann Intern Med* 132:525, 2000.

82. Briones ER, Iber FL: Liver and biliary tract changes and injury associated with total parenteral nutrition: pathogenesis and prevention. *J Am Coll Nutr* 14:219, 1995.

83. Lazaridis KN, Gores GJ, Lindor KD: Ursodeoxycholic acid mechanisms of action and clinical use in hepatobiliary disorders. *J Hepatol* 35:134, 2001.

84. Ryu JK, Ryu KH, Kim KH: Clinical features of acute acalculous cholecystitis. *J Clin Gastroenterol* 36:166, 2003.

85. Pelinka LE, Schmidhammer R, Hamid L, et al: Acute acalculous cholecystitis after trauma: a prospective study. *J Trauma* 55:323, 2003.

86. Johnson LB: The importance of early diagnosis of acute acalculous cholecystitis. *Surg Gynecol Obstet* 164:197, 1987.

87. Puc MM, Tran HS, Wry PW, Ross SE: Ultrasound is not a useful screening tool for acute acalculous cholecystitis in critically ill trauma patients. *Am Surg* 68:65, 2002.

88. Mariat G, Mahul P, Prev TN, et al: Contribution of ultrasonography and cholescintigraphy to the diagnosis of acute acalculous cholecystitis in intensive care unit patients. *Intensive Care Med* 11:1658, 2000.

89. Yang HK, Hodgson WJ: Laparoscopic cholecystostomy for acute acalculous cholecystitis. *Surg Endosc* 10:673, 1996.

90. Akhan O, Akinci D, Ozmen MN: Percutaneous cholecystostomy. *Eur J Radiol* 229, 1996.

91. Johlin FC, Neil GA: Drainage of the gallbladder in patients with acute acalculous cholecystitis by transpapillary endoscopic cholecystostomy. *Gastrointest Endosc* 39:645, 1993.

Chapter 82

GASTROINTESTINAL HEMORRHAGE

RAM SUBRAMANIAN
TIMOTHY McCASHLAND

KEY POINTS

- *Aggressive intravenous resuscitation with fluids and blood, and airway protection are crucial in the management of the acutely bleeding patient.*

- *Endoscopy should be performed with therapeutic intent for both upper and lower gastrointestinal bleeding.*

- *Pharmacologic therapy should be used as an adjunct to endoscopic therapy.*

- *An early team approach, involving medical, radiologic, and surgical personnel, should be implemented.*

- *In the setting of severe bleeding or bleeding refractory to endoscopic therapy, angiographic and surgical therapies should be instituted promptly.*

Gastrointestinal (GI) hemorrhage continues to be a frequent indication for intensive care management, with over 300,000 hospitalizations reported annually in the United States.[1] Upper GI (UGI) bleeding has continued to predominate, with lower GI (LGI) bleeding constituting approximately 25% of all GI bleeding.[2] Despite improved diagnostic and therapeutic modalities in the last two decades, the mortality rates for upper and lower GI hemorrhage have demonstrated different trends. Mortality from UGI bleeding has remained stable at 10%,[3] and this could be explained by an aging population with a significantly higher GI bleeding mortality due to comorbid conditions.[4] In contrast, the mortality from LGI bleeding has decreased dramatically despite an aging population, and this is probably due to more aggressive diagnostic and therapeutic endoscopic intervention.

The management of GI hemorrhage in the ICU is multidisciplinary, involving the intensivist, gastroenterologist, radiologist, and surgeon. A successful outcome relies on effective fluid resuscitation, maintenance of adequate perfusion pressure, prompt hemostasis, monitoring of end-organ function, and prevention of multiple-organ failure.

Clinical Considerations

PROGNOSTIC FACTORS

Multiple studies focusing primarily on nonvariceal UGI bleeding have been designed to define prognostic factors for GI bleeding and to identify high-risk patients.[5–7] A common and pivotal feature of these studies is the combined use of clinical variables and endoscopic findings to guide risk stratification, thereby stressing the importance of integrating clinical and endoscopic information for optimal decision making. Table 82-1 outlines the clinical and endoscopic indicators associated with an increased risk of rebleeding and higher

mortality. A recent study has identified similar prognostic indicators for LGI bleeding.[8]

INITIAL PRESENTATION

GI bleeding is divided into UGI and LGI bleeding based on its location proximal or distal to the ligament of Treitz at the junction of the duodenum and jejunum. UGI bleeding commonly presents with hematemesis and/or melena, and a nasogastric (NG) lavage that yields blood or coffee-ground material supports the diagnosis. However, it is important to note that a negative or bile-stained NG aspirate (indicating an open pylorus) does not exclude a UGI source because the bleeding may be intermittent.[9] In comparison, hematochezia is usually the presenting sign of an LGI source. These distinctions based on presenting signs are not absolute because melena can be seen with proximal LGI bleeding and hematochezia can be present with massive, brisk UGI bleeding.

INITIAL EVALUATION AND MANAGEMENT

Table 82-2 outlines the initial evaluation and management for GI hemorrhage.

HEMODYNAMIC

Regardless of the etiology and site of GI hemorrhage, the initial management should be directed at maintaining hemodynamic stability by restoring intravascular volume. Intravenous access with two large-bore IV catheters should be maintained at all times. In the presence of hypotension or hypovolemic shock, prompt fluid resuscitation with crystalloids and packed red blood cells is essential. Monitoring end-organ perfusion and preventing ischemic organ injury improves survival. In particular, coronary and renal perfusion should be assessed. An electrocardiogram should be obtained in patients at risk for myocardial ischemia, and renal laboratory parameters and urine output should be followed to assess for possible prerenal azotemia, acute renal failure, and (in cirrhotics) hepatorenal syndrome. In the subset of patients with suspected variceal hemorrhage, central venous pressure (CVP) monitoring may be useful to prevent sustained portal hypertension and recurrent bleeding following fluid replacement; a CVP of less than 10 mm Hg may prevent recurrent variceal bleeding. When left-sided heart failure coexists,

TABLE 82-1 Adverse Clinical and Endoscopic Prognostic Indicators

Clinical indicators
- Age > 60 years
- Severe comorbidities
- Onset of bleeding during hospitalization
- Emergency surgery
- Clinical shock
- Red blood emesis or NG aspirate
- Requiring > 5 U PRBCs

Endoscopic indicators
- Major stigmata: active bleeding, visible vessel, adherent clot
- Ulcer location: posterior duodenal bulb, higher lesser gastric curvature
- Ulcer size > 2 cm in diameter
- High-risk lesions: varices, aortoenteric fistula, malignancy

TABLE 82-2 Initial Management of Gastrointestinal Hemorrhage

Maintain two large-bore IV catheters (14- or 16-gauge peripheral IV/central line)

Fluid resuscitate with crystalloids to maintain hemodynamic stability

Transfuse packed red cells to maintain hematocrit > 30%

Urgent endoscopy with therapeutic intention for refractory hypotension/shock

Acid-suppression therapy with IV H_2RAs or PPIs after endoscopic treatment

Platelet transfusion and fresh frozen plasma/recombinant factor VIIa to correct thrombocytopenia and coagulopathy

ECG in patients at risk for myocardial ischemia

A nasogastric tube should be inserted if patient has hematemesis

CVP or Ppw monitoring may be helpful if variceal bleeding is suspected. A CVP < 10 mm Hg may help prevent recurrent variceal bleeding

Splanchnic vasoconstrictors (octreotide/terlipressin) in variceal bleeding

Empirical antibiotics in variceal bleeding

Consultation with interventional radiology and surgery

monitoring of pulmonary artery wedge pressure (Ppw) may facilitate aggressive fluid resuscitation while reducing the risk of cardiogenic pulmonary edema.

GASTROINTESTINAL/ENDOSCOPIC

Prompt identification and hemostasis of the source of GI hemorrhage are essential in improving patient outcome. In the event that initial fluid resuscitation establishes hemodynamic stability, endoscopy may be performed under stable conditions within the first 24 hours of the bleed. However, emergent endoscopy with therapeutic hemostatic intent should be performed for patients with UGI and LGI hemorrhage who cannot be stabilized hemodynamically with intravascular volume resuscitation and continue to bleed. Multiple studies in UGI bleeding[10,11] and more recent studies in LGI bleeding[12,13] have demonstrated that therapeutic esophagogastroduodenoscopy (EGD) and colonoscopy using hemostatic interventions such as epinephrine injection and electrocautery facilitate early control of bleeding, reduce rebleeding rates, and improve short-term morbidity and mortality. Based on these observations, the 2001 American Society for Gastrointestinal Endoscopy (ASGE) recommendations emphasize the importance of emergent endoscopy with therapeutic intent in the setting of persistent hemodynamic instability.[14,15] Absolute contraindications to endoscopy include suspected GI perforation, acute uncontrolled unstable angina, severe coagulopathy, untreated respiratory decompensation, and severe patient agitation. Apart from perforation, other conditions contraindicating endoscopy can be corrected, following which endoscopy should be performed. In the face of massive exsanguination, emergent surgical intervention (perhaps facilitated by intraoperative endoscopy) should be considered instead of endoscopy.

A potential caveat to emergent endoscopy is the marginally increased risk of complications compared to elective endoscopy, although the development of smaller and more flexible scopes is likely to reduce this risk. A specific risk is perforation, and with regard to upper endoscopy, the anatomically susceptible regions are the cricopharyngeal region at the site of esophageal intubation and the pylorus-duodenum

junction during a blind duodenal intubation. The risk of perforation during emergency EGD can be lowered with pre-endoscopic NG lavage, which facilitates visualization. Recent studies have suggested that the prokinetic agent erythromycin, given as a single intravenous dose of 250 mg prior to EGD, improves visualization and diagnosis.[16]

In the setting of nonvariceal UGI bleeding, acid suppression with histamine receptor antagonists and proton pump inhibitors has shown short-term efficacy only after hemostasis has been achieved using some form of therapeutic endoscopic intervention.[17,18] Therefore, acid suppression may be beneficial in the short-term management of UGI bleeding following endoscopic intervention. In the setting of variceal bleeding, pharmacologic therapy with a splanchnic vasoconstrictor such as octreotide and empiric antibiotic therapy should be initiated.

HEMATOLOGIC

In order to ensure adequate oxygen-carrying capacity in the circulation and to prevent end-organ ischemia, the hematocrit should be maintained above 30%. It should be noted that the initial hematocrit after an acute GI bleed can be misleading because acute hemorrhage produces loss of whole blood, and the hematocrit does not change initially because the initial loss of plasma and erythrocytes is equivalent. Within 24 to 72 hours of the initial bleed, plasma is redistributed from the extravascular to the intravascular space, thus resulting in a dilution of the red cell mass and a fall in the measured hematocrit. Intravenous hydration with crystalloids compounds this dilutional anemia so that red cells should be replaced promptly. In most instances, there is sufficient time to allow typing and cross-matching of red cells; however, in the setting of massive exsanguination, the transfusion of non–cross-matched type-specific blood may be necessary. In the presence of thrombocytopenia, platelets must be transfused to maintain the count above 60,000/μL. Any existing coagulopathy should be corrected with fresh frozen plasma to lower the prothrombin time to within 2 seconds of the normal range. Recent studies have demonstrated the ability of recombinant activated factor VIIa (rFVIIa) to rapidly correct severe coagulopathy in hepatic failure,[19,20] and this agent may assume an important role in the treatment of coagulopathy in the future. During the process of aggressive intravascular volume resuscitation, fluids and blood products should be warmed to prevent the development of a cold coagulopathy, and the core body temperature should be maintained above 35°C (see Chaps. 68 and 69).

PULMONARY

In the presence of active hematemesis, an NG tube should be placed to decrease the risk of aspiration. Endotracheal intubation should be performed for airway protection and to decrease the risk of aspiration in the following situations: (1) in the presence of active hematemesis and decreased mental status, (2) prior to an emergent EGD for active hematemesis, and (3) prior to insertion of an esophageal tamponade tube. In the setting of shock, intubation and full mechanical ventilatory support are indicated to decrease the oxygen consumption of the respiratory apparatus. During the performance of an EGD, significant hypoxemia may occur, especially in elderly patients and in those with moderate to severe obstructive pulmonary disease (defined as a FEV_1/FVC ratio of less than 0.6).[21] Probable causes include hypoventilation due to sedative agents, the partial airway obstruction produced by the endoscope, and aspiration of gastric contents, resulting in bronchospasm and ventilation-perfusion mismatch.

CONSULTATION

Radiology and surgery should be consulted early in the course of management. In the setting of nondiagnostic upper or lower endoscopy, radiologic modalities offer diagnostic and therapeutic options to achieve hemostasis. Emergent surgical intervention is indicated in the exsanguinating patient who may not be stable enough for endoscopic or radiologic evaluation.

When endoscopic evaluation is unable to identify the cause of bleeding, the two diagnostic radiologic modalities available are angiography and radionuclide scans. As outlined later, angiography with embolotherapy or selective infusion of vasoconstrictors offers therapeutic options as well (see Chap. 101).

The angiographic diagnosis of acute arterial hemorrhage is based on visualization of extravasated contrast material in the gastrointestinal lumen. Therefore, it only identifies the bleeding site if active bleeding is occurring when the study is performed. In addition, the rate of bleeding must be brisk, in the range of 0.5 to 1 mL/min. In the case of brisk UGI bleeding, angiography may demonstrate a bleeding site in 75% of patients, with most bleeding episodes originating from a branch of the left gastric artery. In the setting of LGI bleeding, the average diagnostic yield is decreased to about 60%, with diverticular disease and vascular ectasia being the most common findings.

Radionuclide studies occasionally aid in the detection of the bleeding site. The current radionuclide scan of choice is the ^{99m}Tc-pertechnetate-labeled red blood cell scan. The radionuclide scan offers the ability to detect rates of bleeding of less than 0.5mL/min, and the 48-hour stability of the tagged red blood cells allows repeated nuclear imaging for 1 to 2 days following administration of the radionuclide in the setting of intermittent bleeding. However, a positive radionuclide study localizes the bleeding only to an area of the abdomen and cannot define the mucosal location of the bleeding site precisely. Therefore, a positive result should prompt a repeat endoscopy or angiography to localize the bleeding site precisely.

REBLEEDING

In most instances, the presentation of rebleeding is similar to that of the initial episode, and the source is identical to the site of the initial bleed. After hemostasis of the initial bleed following spontaneous cessation or therapeutic intervention, the patient should be monitored closely for rebleeding, especially in the presence of clinical and endoscopic indicators associated with an increased risk of rebleeding (see Table 82-1). Apart from the obvious signs of gastrointestinal blood loss characterized by melena, hematemesis, or hematochezia, more subtle signs of rebleeding may include tachycardia and hypotension owing to a decreasing intravascular volume. Therefore, continuous hemodynamic monitoring should be performed following initial hemostasis, and invasive monitoring with a central venous catheter or an arterial line may be considered for the patient at high risk for rebleeding. A falling serum

hemoglobin concentration on serial measurements may suggest a recurrent bleed. The management of rebleeding should include immediate repeat endoscopic intervention targeted at the initial lesion, followed by radiologic or surgical intervention, if necessary. Specific pharmacologic and endoscopic interventions for long-term secondary prophylaxis against rebleeding will be discussed in the sections that follow.

Upper Gastrointestinal Hemorrhage

With regard to prognosis and treatment, UGI hemorrhage can be divided into (1) variceal hemorrhage and (2) nonvariceal hemorrhage.

Variceal Hemorrhage

Variceal hemorrhage presents as a symptom of decompensated cirrhosis in as many as 50% of patients and accounts for about one-third of all deaths related to cirrhosis. Mortality is related to hepatic disease severity, as defined by the Childs-Pugh classification (Table 82-3), with an overall mortality estimated at 50%. There are two distinct phases in the course of variceal hemorrhage. In the first phase, defined by the initial episode of active hemorrhage, only 50% of patients stop bleeding spontaneously (in contrast to nonvariceal hemorrhage, in which 90% cease spontaneously). The initial bleed is followed by a second phase of an approximately 6-week duration, defined by a high risk of recurrent hemorrhage, with the greatest risk of rebleeding being within the first 48 to 72 hours.

MANAGEMENT

The management of variceal bleeding is outlined in Fig. 82-1. In addition to multiorgan ischemic injury from hypoperfusion, variceal hemorrhage in the setting of cirrhosis predisposes the patient to specific derangements, including hepatic encephalopathy, type 1 hepatorenal syndrome, and systemic infection. These processes contribute to the high mortality associated with variceal bleeding, and therefore,

TABLE 82-3 Childs-Pugh Classification of Hepatic Disease Severity

Parameter	POINTS ASSIGNED		
	1	2	3
Ascites	Absent	Slight	Moderate
Bilirubin (mg/dL)	<2	2–3	>3
Albumin (g/dL)	>3.5	2.8–3.5	<2.8
INR	<1.7	1.8–2.3	>2.3
Encephalopathy	None	Grade 1–2	Grade 3–4

Total Score (Five Parameters)	Childs-Pugh Stage
5–6	A
7–9	B
10–15	C

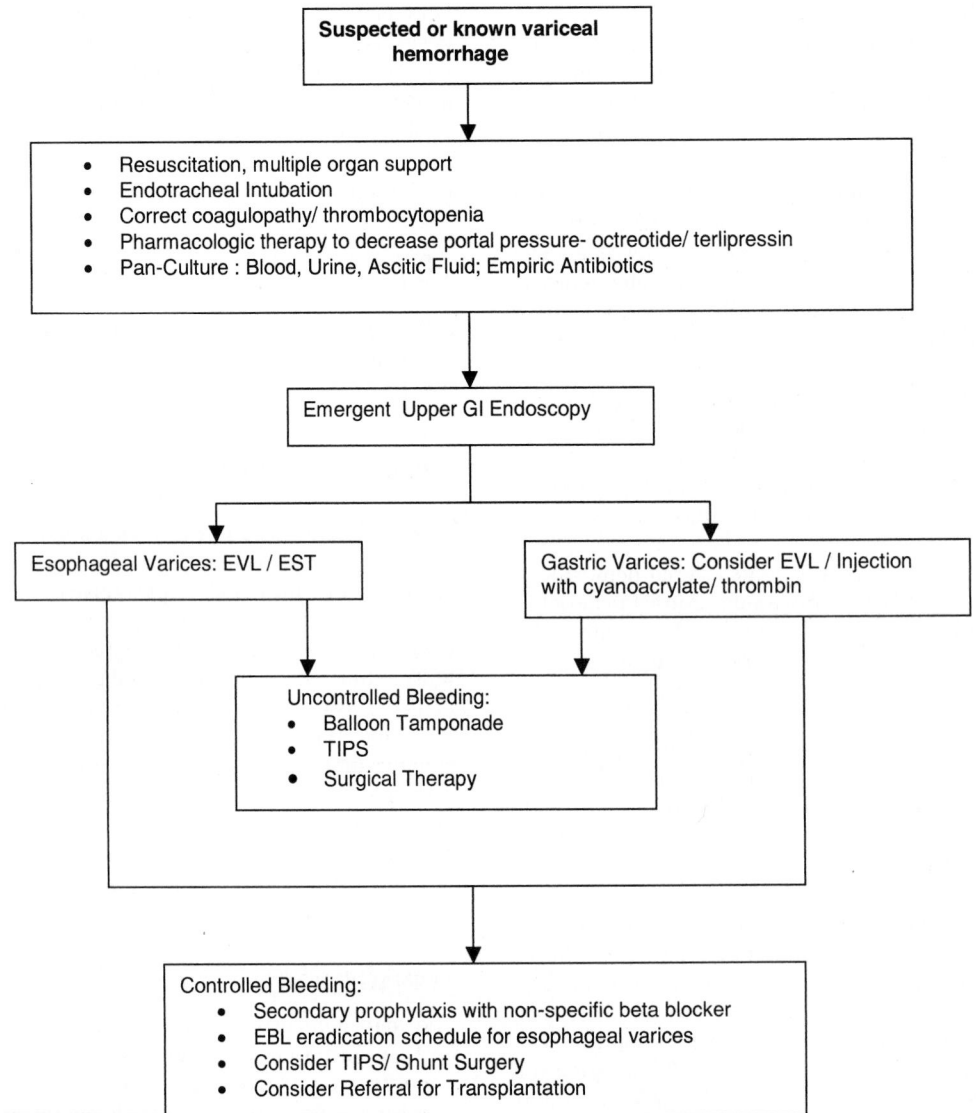

FIGURE 82-1 Management of variceal hemorrhage. EVL, endoscopic variceal band ligation; EST, endoscopic sclerotherapy.

the management should address these issues in addition to achieving hemostasis and hemodynamic stability.

CARDIOPULMONARY

Fluid resuscitation should be aimed at achieving an isovolemic status because this approach prevents persistent portal hypertension and recurrent variceal bleeding.[22] To this end, invasive hemodynamic monitoring with a central venous catheter can be used to guide fluid therapy. In the setting of hypotension that is refractory to fluid resuscitation, a peripheral vasoconstrictor such as norepinephrine should be the vasoactive agent of choice. Agents that have β_2-agonist activity, such as dopamine, should be avoided because they potentially could cause splanchnic vasodilation and therefore worsen the variceal bleed. Splanchnic vasoconstrictors such as octreotide and terlipressin (discussed later) can have a beneficial effect on systemic blood pressure by diverting blood away from the splanchnic circulation. Endotracheal intubation for airway protection is critical, especially in the

setting of encephalopathy, active hematemesis, or emergency endoscopy.

INFECTION

Bacterial infections are common after acute variceal hemorrhage, with the common sites being respiratory, ascitic, and urinary. The presence of infection has been associated with failure to control the initial bleed and an increase in the recurrence of rebleeding, likely owing to the induction of a hyperdynamic circulation and increased portal pressure.[23,24] A meta-analysis of studies regarding the use of prophylactic antibiotics in variceal bleeding suggests that this intervention significantly increases the number of variceal bleeders who do not acquire an infection and improves short-term mortality.[25] Although most of the pertinent studies include a quinolone, the optimal choice and duration of antibiotic therapy have not been defined, and therefore, the choice of empirical antibiotic therapy should be institution-specific. An important consideration is the potential for quinolone resistance in cirrhotic patients who have been on norfloxacin for the prevention of spontaneous bacterial peritonitis (SBP). Prior to initiating antibiotic therapy, blood, urine, and (if indicated) ascitic fluid cultures should be obtained.

HEMATOLOGIC

In addition to fresh frozen plasma, recombinant activated factor VIIa (rFVIIa) is emerging as a procoagulant that can rapidly correct severe coagulopathy associated with decompensated liver disease and promote hemostasis in variceal hemorrhage.[19,20] In a small uncontrolled study of 10 patients,[20] a single dose of 80 μg/kg normalized the prothrombin time in all patients within 30 minutes, and immediate hemostasis was obtained in all patients. Although larger studies are needed to confirm these observations, these initial studies suggest that rFVIIa may assume an important role in the management of acute variceal hemorrhage.

NEUROLOGIC

In the setting of decompensated liver disease, variceal bleeding could induce or exacerbate hepatic encephalopathy (HE). Therefore, in the presence of decreased mental status during variceal bleeding, HE should be considered as a potential etiology in addition to cerebral hypoperfusion, and empirical lactulose therapy via an NG tube or as an enema should be considered (see Chap. 84). Elevated serum ammonia levels may be useful in supporting the diagnosis of HE.

HEMOSTATIC THERAPY

Specific therapies aimed at arresting active bleeding include pharmacotherapy and endoscopic therapy. Multiple studies have proven the increased hemostatic efficacy of combined pharmacotherapy and endoscopic therapy over either treatment alone.

PHARMACOTHERAPY

In the setting of variceal bleeding, pharmacologic agents are aimed at causing splanchnic vasoconstriction and reducing portal hypertension. Empiric pharmacotherapy should be initiated in suspected variceal hemorrhage prior to endoscopic diagnosis and intervention. Selective splanchnic vasoconstriction has the added advantage of diverting blood flow from the splanchnic circulation to the systemic circulation, thereby improving systemic blood pressure. In particular, improved renal perfusion could prevent or ameliorate the hepatorenal syndrome.

The current agent of choice in the United States is the somatostatin analog octreotide. Somatostatin and its analogs inhibit the release of vasodilator hormones such as glucagon, thereby indirectly causing splanchnic vasoconstriction and decreased portal inflow. Although octreotide has a longer half-life than somatostatin, its therapeutic efficacy is obtained only with a continuous infusion; the recommended dose is a 50-μg IV bolus, followed by an infusion of 50 μg/h for 5 days. A recent meta-analysis of trials of octreotide has demonstrated improved control of bleeding compared with other therapies, including the previous agent of choice, vasopressin.[26] Furthermore, the adverse extrasplanchnic vasoconstrictive effects observed with vasopressin, such as myocardial and cerebral ischemia, are not observed with octreotide.

More recently, the long-acting vasopressin analog terlipressin has received a favorable recommendation based on European studies, which report fewer side effects than vasopressin and an efficacy similar to that of octreotide and endoscopic sclerotherapy.[27] In addition, a systematic review comparing trials of terlipressin with other pharmacotherapies identified terlipressin as the only pharmacologic agent that reduced mortality, therefore suggesting that terlipressin may be the future vasoactive agent of choice in acute variceal bleeding.[28] Larger prospective trials are awaited to confirm these encouraging preliminary studies. Terlipressin is currently not available in the United States.

ENDOSCOPIC THERAPY

Following the administration of pharmacotherapy, emergent endoscopy with therapeutic hemostatic intent is imperative. As outlined in Fig. 82-1, endoscopic evaluation can localize the source of the variceal bleed to an esophageal or gastric varix. This is an important distinction because, while esophageal variceal bleeding is amenable to endoscopic therapy, gastric variceal bleeding may require more aggressive salvage measures, as outlined below.

Endoscopic therapy is based on the interruption of blood flow through the venous collateral system lining the distal esophagus and gastric cardia using either stimulation of thrombosis (e.g., sclerotherapy) or immediate occlusion (e.g., band ligation). The two established forms of endoscopic therapy are endoscopic sclerotherapy (EST) and endoscopic variceal band ligation (EVL). While sclerotherapy involves the intravariceal or paravariceal injection of a sclerosant (e.g., sodium morrhuate), band ligation involves the placement of small bands around varices in the distal 5 cm of the esophagus (Fig. 82-2). A meta-analysis has shown that EVL is superior to EST in initial hemostasis, obliteration of varices, rates of recurrent bleeding, complications, and mortality,[29] and EVL is now the endoscopic treatment of choice for acute variceal hemorrhage. However, a technical challenge during use of the band ligator apparatus is the decreased endoscopic field of view in a setting already complicated by active hemorrhage. Therefore, EST may be indicated in the setting of poor initial visualization, followed later by definitive EVL treatment.

GASTRIC VARICES

While the preceding endoscopic interventions are effective in esophageal variceal bleeding, gastric variceal bleeding presents a technical challenge. Gastric varices are located deeper in the submucosa, where EVL and EST are not successful in obtaining sustained hemostasis. Initial studies reporting successful hemostasis with intravariceal injection of cyanoacrylate tissue glue[30] and thrombin[31] suggest novel approaches to endoscopic intervention in gastric variceal bleeding. However, these therapies need further validation. In the setting of gastric variceal bleeding, EVL may be attempted to obtain initial hemostasis. However, given the limited success of endoscopic hemostasis, the emergent application of nonendoscopic interventions should be anticipated, which may include balloon tamponade, transjugular intrahepatic portosystemic shunt (TIPS), and surgery.

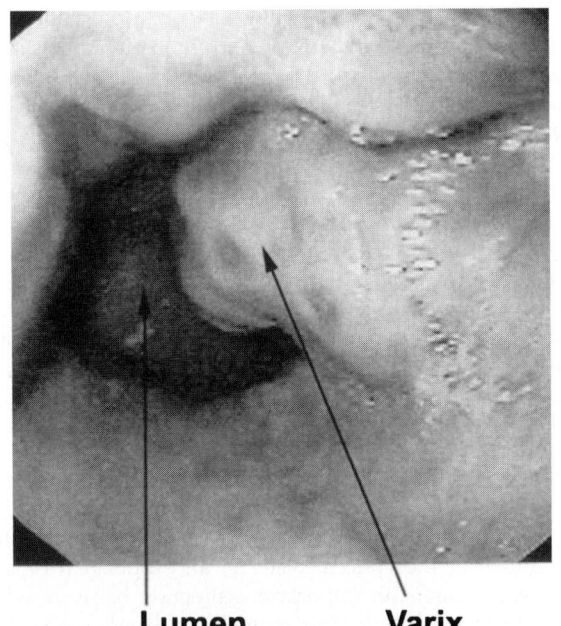

Lumen   **Varix**

A

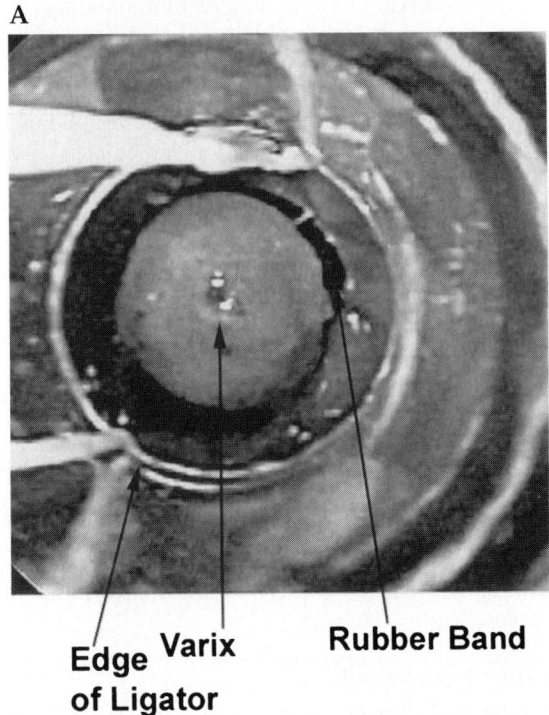

Edge Varix   **Rubber Band**
of Ligator

B

FIGURE 82-2 *A.* Esophageal varix before banding. *B.* Variceal banding viewed through endoscope.

COMPLICATIONS OF ENDOSCOPY

Most complications have been associated with EST, and the advent of variceal band ligation (EVL) has decreased the incidence of complications significantly after therapeutic endoscopy. Following endoscopic intervention, local complications include ulceration, dysmotility, and stricture formation, and regional complications include esophageal perforation and mediastinitis. In addition, both EST and EVL increase the risk of developing portal hypertensive gastropathy (PHG) and its bleeding sequelae because blood is shunted away from

the venous system of the gastroesophageal junction to that of the gastric mucosa. Bleeding from PHG is characterized by a diffuse, slow bleed from the gastric mucosa that typically is not amenable to localized endoscopic therapy.

SALVAGE THERAPY FOR ENDOSCOPICALLY UNCONTROLLED BLEEDING

In the event that hemostasis cannot be achieved by initial endoscopic therapy or there is evidence of rebleeding after initial hemostasis, a repeat trial of endoscopic therapy may be attempted. However, following a second failed endoscopic trial, nonendoscopic interventions need to be implemented emergently. These interventions may include balloon tamponade, TIPS, and surgical therapy.

BALLOON TAMPONADE

Esophageal tamponade tubes (such as the Sengstaken-Blakemore tube) effectively achieve short-term hemostasis by compressing the gastric and distal esophageal mucosa. In most cases, tamponade is effective after inflating only the gastric balloon. Endotracheal intubation is imperative prior to insertion of tamponade tubes to decrease the risk of aspiration. Once the airway is secured, the tube can be passed either nasally or orally to the stomach. The gastric balloon should be inflated only partially (with approximately 30 mL of air) pending radiographic confirmation of correct placement because inadvertent inflation of the balloon in the esophagus can lead to esophageal perforation. Once adequate positioning is ensured, the gastric balloon can be inflated fully according to the manufacturer's recommendations (gastric balloons are inflated to predetermined volumes, whereas the esophageal balloon component is inflated according to pressure). If hemostasis is not achieved by isolated inflation of the gastric balloon, the esophageal balloon can be inflated to 35 mm Hg, a pressure exceeding the intravariceal pressure. Following inflation, traction should be applied to the apparatus at the insertion site to maintain proper positioning. A maximum duration of 48 hours is recommended for variceal compression because prolonged tamponade can lead to esophageal wall ischemia. An NG tube inserted above the esophageal balloon is mandatory to prevent aspiration of oropharyngeal secretions that collect above the inflated apparatus, unless the tube has its own lumen for esophageal suction. A major limitation of tamponade therapy is the high risk of rebleeding following deflation of the balloon. Furthermore, given the serious complications of pulmonary aspiration and esophageal ulceration and perforation, this mode of therapy should be performed by skilled personnel and generally as a temporizing step while planning definitive treatment.

TRANSJUGULAR INTRAHEPATIC PORTOSYSTEMIC SHUNT (TIPS)

Following temporary stabilization with balloon tamponade, further definitive treatment to achieve hemostasis involves the creation of an artificial vascular shunt between the systemic and portal circulation in order to decompress the variceal vasculature. This can be accomplished surgically (discussed below) or via TIPS, which offers a less invasive method for obtaining a vascular shunt. The TIPS consists of an expandable metallic stent placed intrahepatically between portal and hepatic veins using radiologically guided access (see Chap. 101). Traditionally, TIPS has been recommended as secondary prophylactic therapy for variceal bleeding in the setting of mild to moderate liver disease, and advanced cirrhosis has been regarded as a contraindication to TIPS therapy due to increased mortality after TIPS in this setting. However, recent studies with favorable hemostasis and mortality data have supported the use of emergent TIPS as salvage therapy for refractory variceal hemorrhage, even in advanced cirrhosis.[32] Therefore, when variceal hemorrhage is refractory to pharmacologic and endoscopic therapy, urgent TIPS therapy should be considered irrespective of the severity of hepatic disease. The hemodynamic benefits of TIPS therapy can be attributed not only to portal decompression and variceal hemostasis but also to increased venous return due to intravascular mobilization of any existing ascites. Additional beneficial effects of TIPS therapy include treatment of refractory ascites and the hepatorenal syndrome.

SURGICAL THERAPY

Since the advent of TIPS as salvage therapy for refractory variceal hemorrhage, there has been a reduction in the need for surgical intervention. However, shunt surgery for portal decompression is indicated for variceal hemostasis in patients with preserved hepatic synthetic function (i.e., Childs-Pugh A disease).[33] Esophageal transection with or without devascularization may be another surgical option in massive exsanguination refractory to other interventions.

Shunt operations can be divided into (1) nonselective shunts (e.g., portacaval shunts) that decompress the entire portal system and divert all blood flow away from the portal vein and (2) selective shunts (e.g., distal splenorenal shunt) that compartmentalize the portal tree into a decompressed variceal system and a hypertensive superior mesenteric vein that maintains sinusoidal perfusion. A selective shunt is the preferred operation because portacaval shunts significantly alter vascular anatomy and therefore complicate future liver transplant surgery. In addition, emergency portacaval shunts are associated with a higher rate of thrombosis and shunt failure.

Distal esophageal transection in the setting of massive variceal exsanguination may control bleeding, but mortality remains above 80%. Since the transection does not address the underlying portal hypertension, varices recur after a variable period, and rebleeding should be anticipated. Esophageal transection with devascularization of the gastroesophageal junction (Sugiura procedure) may be considered in patients who have an absolute contraindication to shunt surgery, such as extensive thrombosis in the portal venous circulation involving the splenic, superior mesenteric, and portal veins.

Variceal hemorrhage may occur in noncirrhotic patients. Patients with extrahepatic portal hypertension are better operative shunt candidates than cirrhotics. When large gastric varices accompanied by small or absent esophageal varices are identified, splenic or portal vein thrombosis should be considered as a possible etiology rather than cirrhosis. Splenic and portal vein thrombosis may occur in the setting of acute pancreatitis, pancreatic cancer, abdominal trauma, and hypercoagulable states. It is essential to identify this subset of patients with variceal hemorrhage because splenectomy rather than a portosystemic shunt may be curative. Celiac angiography is diagnostic.

SECONDARY PROPHYLAXIS

If successful hemostasis is achieved by any of the interventions just discussed, it is essential that secondary prophylaxis to prevent variceal rebleeding is initiated in the ICU. Once the hemodynamic status is stabilized, nonspecific β-blocker therapy (nadolol 20 to 40 mg/d) should be initiated to decrease portal hypertension. This pharmacologic intervention should be coupled with an endoscopic variceal band ligation schedule as defined by the gastroenterologist because the combination of these therapeutic modalities decreases the risk of variceal recurrence and rebleeding.[34] In addition, the patient should be evaluated for vascular shunt procedures, including TIPS and surgical shunts. Most important, early referral to a transplant center should be initiated to evaluate the patient for liver transplantation.

Nonvariceal Hemorrhage

In contrast to variceal hemorrhage, nonvariceal hemorrhage presents a favorable prognosis. The improved outcome can be attributed to a greater than 90% spontaneous cessation rate of bleeding and to the absence of a predisposition to multiorgan dysfunction that exists in decompensated cirrhosis. As outlined in Table 82-1, multiple studies pertaining to nonvariceal hemorrhage have identified clinical and endoscopic indicators that increase the risk for continued or recurrent bleeding, and therefore predict an adverse prognosis. The remaining mortality rate of 10% is largely due to rebleeding in patients with these factors. The important role of early therapeutic upper endoscopy in achieving hemostasis, reducing rebleeding, and improving short-term morbidity and mortality has been established[10,11] and reiterated in a recent consensus statement addressing the management of nonvariceal bleeding.[11a] Furthermore, with regard to peptic ulcer disease, endoscopic characterization of high-risk ulcer lesions has led to the development of specific endoscopic therapies that have improved hemostatic efficacy and outcome compared with prior medical therapy.[35]

The evaluation and management of nonvariceal hemorrhage are outlined in Fig. 82-3. Following initial hemodynamic, pulmonary, and hematologic management, early upper endoscopic evaluation with therapeutic intent should be conducted. Emergent endoscopy should be pursued in the setting of hemodynamic instability that is refractory to fluid resuscitation. Acid-suppression therapy has demonstrated short-term efficacy only after endoscopic hemostasis has been achieved[17,18] and therefore should be used as an adjunct to endoscopy. Since peptic ulcer disease accounts for the majority of nonvariceal bleeds and has been the focus of therapeutic developments, the different treatment modalities will be discussed in this context. The management of some nonulcer lesions, including stress-related mucosal damage (SRMD), will follow.

PEPTIC ULCER DISEASE (PUD)

ENDOSCOPIC THERAPY

Progress in endoscopic diagnosis and therapy has been due largely to major improvements in endoscopic techniques and equipment. A number of hemostatic endoscopic methods have been developed,[36] but the two used most commonly

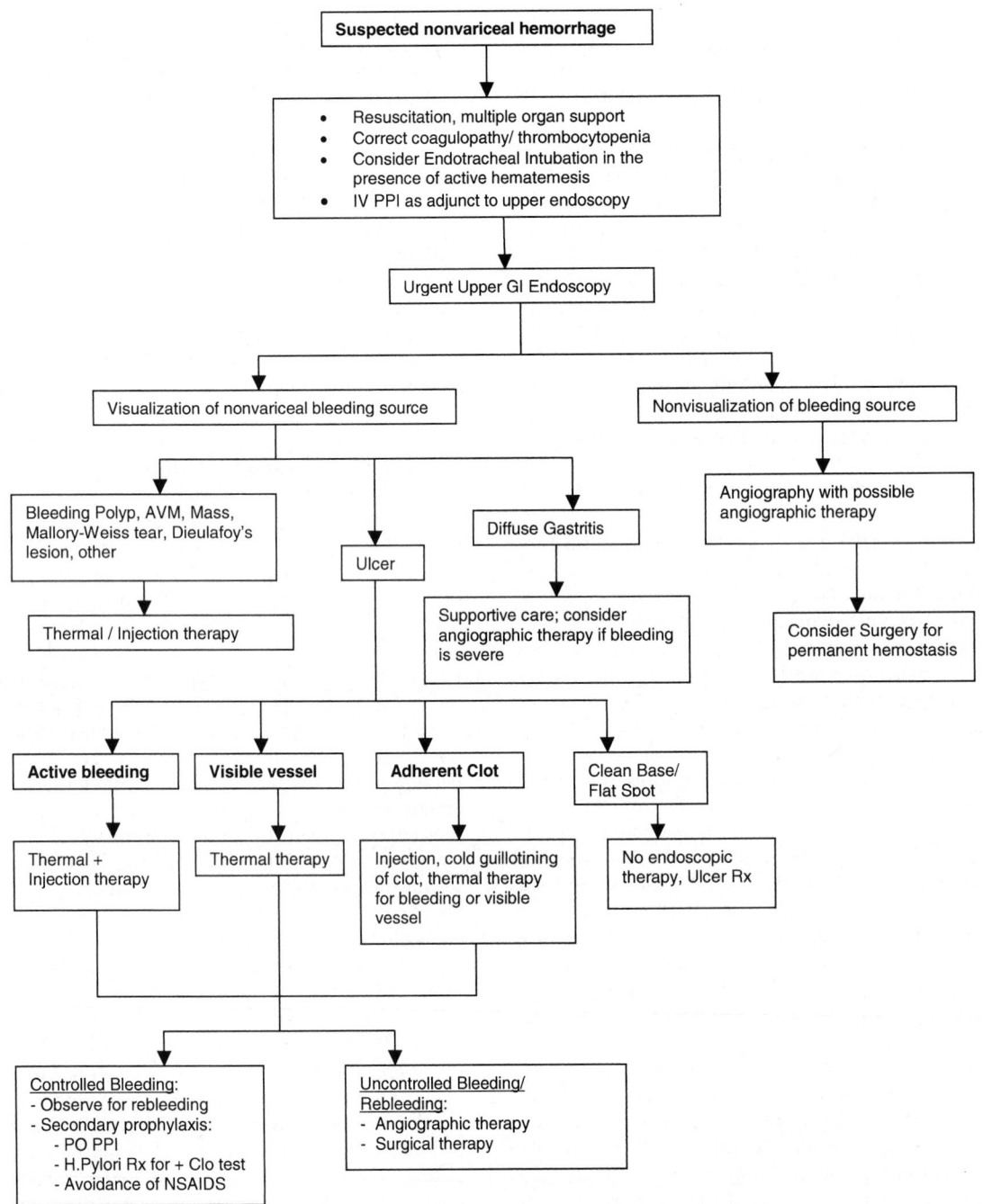

FIGURE 82-3 Management of nonvariceal hemorrhage. Bold entries indicate high-risk lesions

in the United States are contact thermal devices and injection therapy with epinephrine.

Contact Thermal Devices

Thermal therapy is designed to produce coagulation and dehydration in the ulcer base surrounding the bleeding vessel, and this results in constriction and destruction of the submucosal feeding vessels supplying the surface artery. The two types of thermal therapy that have gained popularity are the bipolar probe and the heater probe. Bipolar probes heat contacted tissue by passing electricity via tissue water between positive and negative electrodes located at the tip of the probe.

Once the contact tissue is fully desiccated, electrical conduction ceases, and deeper tissue coagulation is restricted. On the other hand, the heater probe uses a thermocouple at the end of the probe to generate heat, and this process does not depend on tissue water. Therefore, deeper tissue coagulation is achievable despite desiccation, although this increases the risk of perforation.

Injection Therapy

Injection therapy is aimed at causing vasoconstriction and necrosis of the bleeding vessel and surrounding tissue. Injection with epinephrine (1:10,000 dilution in saline) or absolute alcohol has been shown to be effective in achieving acute hemostasis.[37] While epinephrine exerts a vasoconstrictive effect on the vessel, pure ethanol causes dehydration, contraction, and necrosis of the vessel and surrounding tissue. It should be noted that the rebleeding rate is high if epinephrine injection therapy is performed in isolation, and therefore, it should be combined with thermal coagulation therapy. The technique used in injection therapy involves the injection of the agent via an injector catheter in four quadrants within 2 to 3 mm of the active bleeding point in the ulcer base. While the volume of total epinephrine administered can range from 5 to 10 mL, the total volume of ethanol should not exceed 1 mL because extensive ulceration may occur.

Endoscopic Evaluation and Treatment in PUD

As outlined in Fig. 82-3, the endoscopic management of PUD is guided by the characteristics of the ulcer, which defines the lesion as exhibiting "major" or "minor" stigmata of ulcer hemorrhage. The major stigmata consist of (1) active bleeding, (2) a visible, nonbleeding vessel, and (3) an adherent clot, and these three lesions are associated with a high risk of rebleeding and therefore increased short-term mortality. The stigmata associated with a low risk of rebleeding include (1) a clean base and (2) a flat/pigmented spot, and these lesions have a favorable prognosis. Specific endoscopic treatment guidelines have been developed by the ASGE for each of these lesions[14] based on multiple studies addressing the response of these lesions to thermal and injection therapy. These guidelines and subsequent studies have led to the following endoscopic treatment recommendations: (1) combination therapy with injection and thermal coagulation is superior to monotherapy either in active bleeding[38,39] (Fig. 82-4) or for an adherent clot,[40] (2) monotherapy with thermal coagulation is indicated for a nonbleeding visible vessel, and (3) no endoscopic therapy is required for low-risk lesions, which include a clean base and a flat/pigmented spot.

In anticipation of initiating secondary prophylaxis for PUD, the visualization of a duodenal or gastric ulcer should prompt the endoscopist to obtain a gastric antral mucosal biopsy to test for *Helicobacter pylori*. The gastric biopsy may be difficult to perform during the acute phase of the bleeding, and the presence of blood or antiulcer medications may interfere with a biopsy urease test. In the absence of a gastric biopsy, a venous blood sample should be tested for *H. pylori* serology, or stool or breath testing should be performed. Furthermore, a negative gastric antral mucosal biopsy should be confirmed with a serologic test, especially if antiulcer therapy has been initiated prior to the biopsy.

PHARMACOTHERAPY

While intravenous histamine receptor antagonists (H₂RAs) are used commonly in the initial management of PUD bleeding, there is no evidence that this intervention improves short-term outcomes, such as rebleeding rates or transfusion requirements.[41] The concept that more profound acid suppression with proton pump inhibitors (PPIs) will improve short-term outcomes has been investigated, and most studies have shown short-term efficacy of PPIs when administered after successful endoscopic hemostasis.[42,43] Therefore, acid-suppressive therapy in the form of PPIs should be administered as an adjunct to endoscopic therapy and should not be

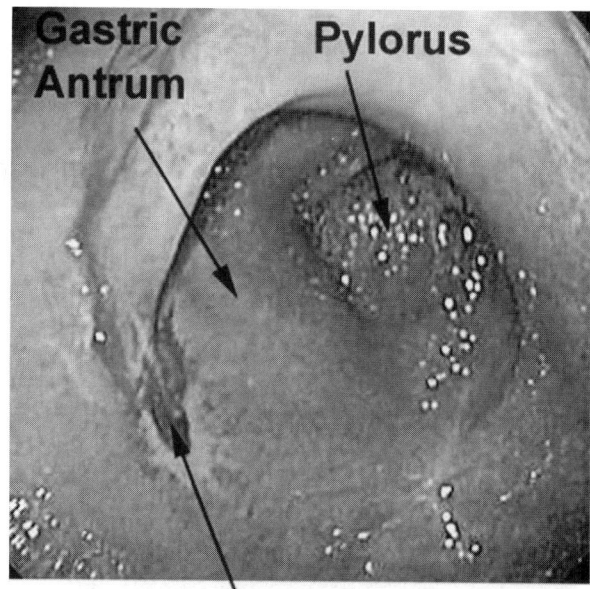

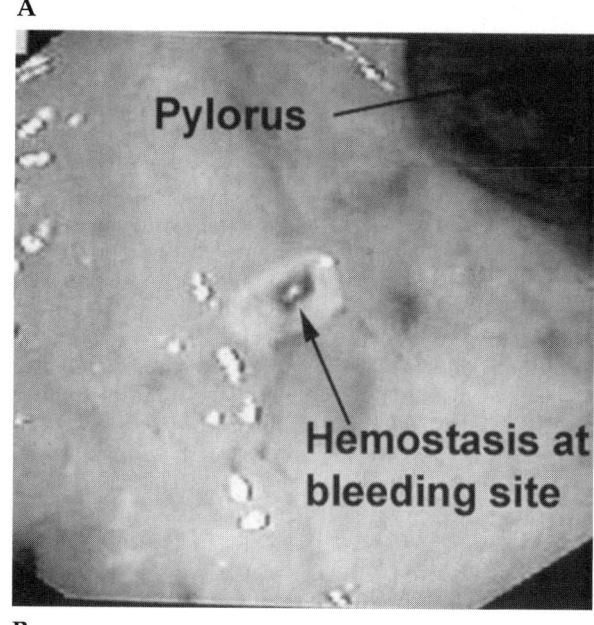

FIGURE 82-4 *A.* Bleeding gastric ulcer prior to therapy. *B.* Successful hemostasis following thermal and injection therapy.

used in lieu of an endoscopic evaluation. Studies comparing intravenous and oral PPI therapy are awaited; however, intravenous PPI therapy may ensure improved bioavailability in the setting of a bleeding gastrointestinal tract. The improved hemostatic efficacy of PPI over H₂RA therapy may be due to the superior ability of PPI therapy to maintain a gastric pH above 6.0 and therefore protect an ulcer clot from fibrinolysis.[44]

Several studies have evaluated the efficacy of the splanchnic vasoconstrictors somatostatin and octreotide in the treatment of acute nonvariceal hemorrhage. A meta-analysis of these studies suggests that somatostatin and octreotide are associated with a reduced risk of continued bleeding and rebleeding in PUD.[45] Therefore, in addition to acid-suppressive therapy, these agents also may be considered as pharmacologic adjuncts to endoscopic therapy.

ANGIOGRAPHY

In most cases of nonvariceal hemorrhage, endoscopic evaluation is able to visualize the bleeding lesion and deliver effective hemostatic therapy. However, in a minority of patients, the bleeding source is not visualized by endoscopy, thereby necessitating angiographic localization. Also, angiography offers the option of hemostatic therapy using arterial vasoconstrictors or embolization; however, this generally is reserved for patients who are poor surgical candidates or for the control of bleeding in an unstable patient awaiting surgery.

Localization

As mentioned previously, angiography can successfully localize brisk UGI bleeding (rate > 0.5 mL/min) in 75% of cases,[46] with most bleeding episodes (85%) originating from a branch of the left gastric artery. The right gastric and short gastric arteries account for the remainder of the sources.

Hemostatic Therapy

UGI arterial bleeding can be controlled by the selective arterial infusion of vasoconstrictors such as vasopressin or embolization of particulate matter. Most studies indicate that selective intraarterial vasopressin is more effective than a peripheral intravenous infusion in achieving hemostasis.[47] Since the vasoconstrictive action of vasopressin is more pronounced on terminal blood vessels such as arterioles, venules, and capillaries, this therapy is more effective in controlling bleeding from such vessels, as in diffuse hemorrhagic gastritis, rather than a duodenal ulcer bleed originating from a large gastroduodenal artery. In the setting of gastric bleeding, therapy appears to be equally effective when administered via the left gastric or celiac artery.[48] A usual therapeutic vasopressin dose is 0.2 unit/min, with a recommended maximum dose of 0.4 unit/min. If hemostasis is achieved, the infusion is continued in the ICU for 24 to 36 hours and then tapered over 24 hours. Rebleeding after cessation of the infusion is a concern[48] and can be treated with repeat vasopressin treatment or embolization.

Embolization therapy uses various substances, most frequently a gelatin sponge (Gelfoam), to selectively embolize the bleeding vessel. Since this technique carries the risk of causing bowel wall ischemia and infarction due to nonspecific embolization, a target vessel must be accessible for selective catheterization of the bleeding site. Necrosis of the stomach, duodenum, gallbladder, liver, and spleen has been documented following nonspecific embolotherapy. Since the duodenum has a dual blood supply from the celiac artery and the superior mesenteric artery, spontaneous infarction of the duodenum is rare. The patient with advanced atherosclerotic vascular disease or with prior gastric surgery involving ligation of collateral vessels is at greater risk of infarction due to a compromised collateral circulation. In view of the higher morbidity associated with embolization therapy, it should be used only after unsuccessful intraarterial vasopressin therapy. Furthermore, embolization therapy should not be followed immediately by vasopressin therapy because this may compromise the collateral circulation, resulting in tissue infarction.

SURGICAL THERAPY

Surgical intervention for bleeding peptic ulcers should be considered in two situations. First, surgery is used to control life-threatening hemorrhage that is refractory to medical and endoscopic intervention. In fact, in patients who have a low operative risk and who have been stabilized effectively to allow surgery, angiographic therapy should not be attempted. Second, surgery should be considered in the patient in whom medical management has failed to heal or prevent recurrence of peptic ulceration, particularly if there have been previous complications attributable to PUD, such as bleeding. The patient who has recurrent hemorrhage owing to noncompliance with maintenance ulcer therapy should be considered for elective surgical therapy once bleeding has stopped. It should be emphasized that surgical morbidity and mortality are greatly reduced when the surgeon operates electively in the nonbleeding patient. Therefore, successful initial hemostasis using endoscopic and pharmacologic therapy is preferable prior to surgical intervention. In the setting of hemorrhage refractory to nonsurgical intervention, stabilization of cardiopulmonary status and optimization of hematologic parameters prepares the patient for emergent surgery and improves postoperative outcome.

The choice of surgical procedure depends on the location of the ulcer and on the stability of the patient. In the patient with an actively bleeding duodenal ulcer undergoing an emergent operation, the bleeding point of the ulcer will be oversewn and truncal vagotomy and pyloroplasty performed. Vagotomy and antrectomy may be considered if the patient has been stabilized adequately. In the setting of exsanguinating hemorrhage, gastric resection may be considered, but this procedure carries a high mortality of approximately 50%.[49] Selective vagotomy with either pyloroplasty or antrectomy, an option in the elective situation, is not advisable in an unstable patient.

Gastric ulcer bleeding is treated with the same approach as a bleeding duodenal ulcer, except that resection is recommended if the situation permits. Partial gastrectomy carries a slightly lower mortality in the setting of gastric ulcer bleeding than when performed for a bleeding duodenal ulcer.[50] Resection for an actively bleeding gastric carcinoma is recommended only when performed electively because it is a prolonged procedure that may be unsuitable for an unstable patient.

Following surgical intervention for bleeding peptic ulcers, mortality approaches 30%, with postoperative wound infection being the major complication.

SECONDARY PROPHYLAXIS

Once successful hemostasis is achieved, secondary prophylaxis is initiated to prevent recurrent ulcer bleeding, especially following nonsurgical hemostatic therapy. If histologic or nonhistologic evaluation for *H. pylori* is positive, appropriate treatment should be initiated because this reduces the long-term (1-year) rate of rebleeding from gastric or duodenal ulcers.[51] In addition, long-term acid suppressive therapy with oral H_2RAs or PPIs is indicated, and nonsteroidal anti-inflammatory drugs (NSAIDs) should be avoided.

MALLORY-WEISS TEAR

Mallory-Weiss tear generally is a self-limited cause of non-variceal bleeding, rarely requiring more than supportive intervention. However, patients with portal hypertension are at increased risk of massive bleeding from Mallory-Weiss tears compared with those with normal portal pressures.[52] In the rare instance of continued bleeding from a Mallory-Weiss tear in a patient without portal hypertension, endoscopic therapy with either thermal coagulation or injection therapy should be attempted prior to surgical oversewing of the lesion. In the presence of portal hypertension, thermal coagulation may worsen the bleeding; therefore, band ligation or sclerotherapy should be performed. Following hemostasis, acid-suppression therapy with H_2RAs or PPIs may be given as adjunctive therapy to accelerate healing.

DIEULAFOY'S LESION

A Dieulafoy's lesion is a dilated aberrant submucosal vessel of unclear etiology that erodes the overlying epithelium in the absence of a primary ulcer. It is usually located along the high lesser curvature of the stomach near the gastroesophageal junction, although it has been found in all areas of the GI tract, including the esophagus and duodenum. Massive bleeding can occur when the eroding submucosal vessel is an artery. The endoscopic treatment of choice is a combination of epinephrine injection therapy and thermal coagulation.[53] Also, endoscopic band ligation has been used successfully to achieve hemostasis in bleeding Dieulafoy's lesions.[54] The risk of rebleeding after endoscopic therapy remains high (up to 40% in some reports) owing to the usually large size of the underlying artery. In the event of rebleeding, repeat endoscopic intervention may be attempted, following which surgical wedge resection of the lesion should be performed to achieve permanent hemostasis.

STRESS-RELATED MUCOSAL DAMAGE (SRMD)

SRMD, also referred to as *stress ulcers* or *stress-related erosive syndrome* (SRES), is the result of multiple-organ-system failure in the critically ill patient. The incidence of hemorrhage due to SRMD appears to be decreasing, probably as a result of significant advances in the intensive care management of the critically ill patient, including optimization of hemodynamic status and tissue oxygenation,[55] and the early initiation of stress ulcer prophylaxis. However, in the event of SRMD-induced hemorrhage, the mortality rate is greater than 30% owing to the difficulty in controlling such bleeding and the poor prognosis of the underlying disease. With regard to etiology, gastric mucosal ischemia secondary to systemic (and splanchnic) hypoperfusion is considered to be the major inciting factor, with acid and pepsin assuming minor roles. Of note, acid and pepsin secretion are normal to low in most critically ill patients, and increased gastric acidity is observed only in patients exhibiting Cushing's ulcers related to central nervous system (CNS) trauma or infection.

Bleeding from SRMD may be *overt* and significant, resulting in hemorrhage and hemodynamic compromise, or *occult* and minimal, detectable only by Gastroccult testing of the gastric contents. Although occult bleeding due to SRMD may occur frequently in critically ill patients, it is of little clinical significance because few of these patients progress to overt bleeding. Multiple studies have attempted to assess the relative importance of the underlying disease processes and biochemical abnormalities in inducing SRMD.[56,57] Two major risk factors identified are coagulopathy and mechanical ventilation for greater than 48 hours.[56] Other suggested risk factors include sepsis, hypotensive shock, acidosis, peritonitis, extensive burns, hepatic failure, and renal failure, with multiple risk factors having an additive effect on the probability of SRMD.

Endoscopically, SRMD may appear as multiple shallow erosions or submucosal hemorrhage during the early stages. After the first several days of the ICU course, SRMD lesions are characterized by multiple, deeper, acute ulcerations, predominantly in the gastric lesser curvature or fundus, and these lesions can erode into the submucosa, causing massive hemorrhage. Bleeding usually manifests as oozing of blood from the margins of these lesions. However, submucosal penetration can cause hemorrhage from a major artery, with the typical endoscopic appearance of an ulcer with a visible vessel.

THERAPY

The mainstay of therapy for SRMD is supportive, with an attempt to reverse the underlying precipitating factors. Acid suppression in the form of intravenous H_2RAs or PPIs may be used as adjunctive therapy to endoscopic or angiographic intervention. The role of endoscopic therapy in SRMD may be limited because the lesions usually are diffuse and not amenable to directed therapy. However, in the setting of a single dominant lesion or a few bleeding lesions, endoscopic therapy may achieve successful hemostasis in 90% of such cases.[58] Therapeutic angiography is recommended for bleeding that is refractory to endoscopic therapy. Both intraarterial vasopressin therapy[59] and embolotherapy[60] are equally successful at controlling hemorrhage without major ischemic complications owing to the rich collateral blood supply of the gastric mucosa. Since the left gastric artery is the source in most cases of SRMD-induced bleeding, this vessel is a convenient target for embolization therapy.

Surgery usually should be avoided because a near-total gastrectomy is required in most instances, and mortality exceeds 50%. Gastrectomy should be undertaken only when massive hemorrhage persists despite nonsurgical therapy in a viable patient with treatable medical problems.

PROPHYLAXIS

Since hemorrhage from SRMD presents a therapeutic challenge and carries a high mortality, much attention has been given to prophylactic therapy. Despite the existence of SRMD in the setting of low or normal acid secretion, prophylaxis has been directed toward acid suppression or neutralization. The superior efficacy of intravenous H_2RAs compared with sucralfate in preventing SRMD has been demonstrated,[61] and therefore, H_2RAs are preferred. Furthermore, prior concerns regarding the increased incidence of nosocomial pneumonia with acid-suppressive therapy has not been observed in subsequent studies. More recently, oral and intravenous PPIs have been added to the regimen of acid-suppressive therapy in the ICU and should assume increasing importance in the prophylaxis of SRMD.

In addition to pharmacologic therapy, adequate nutritional support and, in particular, enteral nutrition have been shown to decrease the incidence of SRMD.[62,63] The prophylactic effect of enteral nutrition is not mediated by an increase in gastric pH and instead may involve an increase in gastric epithelial energy stores, which, in turn, maintain epithelial integrity and prevent necrosis and ulceration. Therefore, the initiation of adequate nutrition support in the critically ill patient, preferably via the enteral route, may play a prophylactic role against SRMD. In the absence of a functional gastrointestinal tract, total parenteral nutrition (TPN), which has demonstrated a protective effect against SRMD, can be considered, although the net effect may be harmful[62] (see Chap. 11).

Lower Gastrointestinal Hemorrhage

LGI bleeding is defined as bleeding originating from a source distal to the ligament of Treitz. Hematochezia is the common presenting sign of LGI bleeding, and the two frequent LGI sources are diverticulosis and angiodysplasia. However, in the patient with hematochezia and hemodynamic compromise, a briskly bleeding UGI source should be included in the differential diagnosis. Studies have indicated that as many as 10% of patients suspected initially to have LGI bleeding ultimately are found to have a UGI source.[64]

In the past decade, technologic advances in endoscopy have greatly improved the diagnostic and therapeutic utility of colonoscopy in LGI bleeding. Traditionally, colonoscopic evaluation in the setting of LGI bleeding was delayed owing to the need for bowel cleansing, the lack of proven diagnostic and therapeutic efficacy, and the fear of increased procedural risks. However, in recent years, several studies have suggested that emergency therapeutic colonoscopy for acute LGI hemorrhage facilitates early control of bleeding, reduces rebleeding and surgical intervention rates, and improves short-term morbidity and mortality.[12,13] Based on these studies, the practice guidelines of the ASGE have emphasized the diagnostic and therapeutic utility of colonoscopy in the early management of LGI bleeding.[15]

The evaluation and management of LGI hemorrhage is outlined in Fig. 82-5. Most patients who experience severe LGI bleeding are elderly, with an average age of 65, and have comorbidities, including cardiac and respiratory disease. Therefore, prompt resuscitative measures aimed at multiple-organ support should be initiated. As mentioned previously, in the setting of hematochezia and hypotension, a UGI source should be considered in the differential diagnosis. The presence of a positive NG aspirate or historical risk factors for UGI bleeding should prompt an emergent EGD. A negative NG aspirate and a clinical suspicion for an LGI source should lead to a diagnostic and potentially therapeutic colonoscopy following a rapid oral purge with polyethene glycol (PEG). In the presence of massive LGI bleeding, immediate angiographic or surgical intervention without endoscopic evaluation is indicated.

The different diagnostic and treatment modalities used in the management of LGI hemorrhage (see Fig. 82-5) are outlined below. In contrast to UGI hemorrhage, a role for adjunctive pharmacotherapy has not been established in LGI bleeding.

COLONOSCOPY

Following the exclusion of a UGI source, an emergent colonoscopy after a rapid oral purge is the initial examination of choice for diagnosis and treatment. Studies have indicated that following colonic cleansing, colonoscopy offers a higher diagnostic yield and a lower complication rate than the traditional angiographic approach.[64,65] An accepted bowel cleansing protocol is 4 L polyethylene glycol (GOLYTELY) given orally or via an NG tube over 2 hours.[64] Metoclopramide (10 mg) is administered at the start of the purge to facilitate intestinal transit and to minimize the risk of emesis. This bowel preparation regimen has not been associated with an increase in the rate of bleeding or rebleeding.[64]

The overall diagnostic yield of emergent colonoscopy in LGI bleeding is 69% to 80%.[64,66] Diverticular bleeding and angiodysplasia are the most common findings in the majority of large series, with colitis (ischemic, inflammatory, or radiation-induced), neoplasia, and anorectal disease being some of the minor etiologies. If an adequate colonoscopic evaluation does not reveal a bleeding source, and an upper endoscopy is negative, a small intestinal etiology should be considered. Intubation of the terminal ileum at the time of colonoscopy may be useful because fresh blood emanating from the ileum may be indicative of small intestinal bleeding. Small bowel evaluation with push enteroscopy, capsule endoscopy, or enteroclysis can be initiated once hemostasis is achieved spontaneously or with nonendoscopic methods. A further discussion regarding the evaluation of small intestinal bleeding will follow.

ENDOSCOPIC THERAPY

The hemostatic techniques used in therapeutic colonoscopy are similar to those used in therapeutic upper endoscopy. Both thermal coagulation and injection therapy with epinephrine have been used successfully to obtain hemostasis in acute LGI bleeding. With further expertise and advances in endoscopic technology, this relatively new field of therapeutic colonoscopy is expected to evolve.

DIVERTICULAR BLEEDING
The endoscopic visualization of a visible vessel or pigmented protuberance within a diverticular segment identifies patients who are at high risk for persistent or recurrent diverticular bleeding.[67] In this setting, thermal coagulation or injection therapy with epinephrine may be used individually or together to achieve successful hemostasis (Fig. 82-6). Studies have suggested that endoscopic hemostasis may prevent recurrent diverticular bleeding and the need for hemicolectomy.[12,15] Therefore, endoscopic therapy offers a viable long-term alternative to surgical therapy for diverticular bleeding in the elderly patient, who may not be an ideal candidate for surgical intervention. However, massive diverticular bleeding may not be amenable to endoscopic therapy because of poor endoscopic visualization or failed endoscopic therapy, thereby necessitating angiographic or surgical therapy.

ANGIODYSPLASIA
Bleeding from angiodysplastic lesions frequently is responsive to endoscopic therapy. These lesions often are located in the cecum and right colon and represent acquired arteriovenous malformations. Successful hemostasis can be achieved

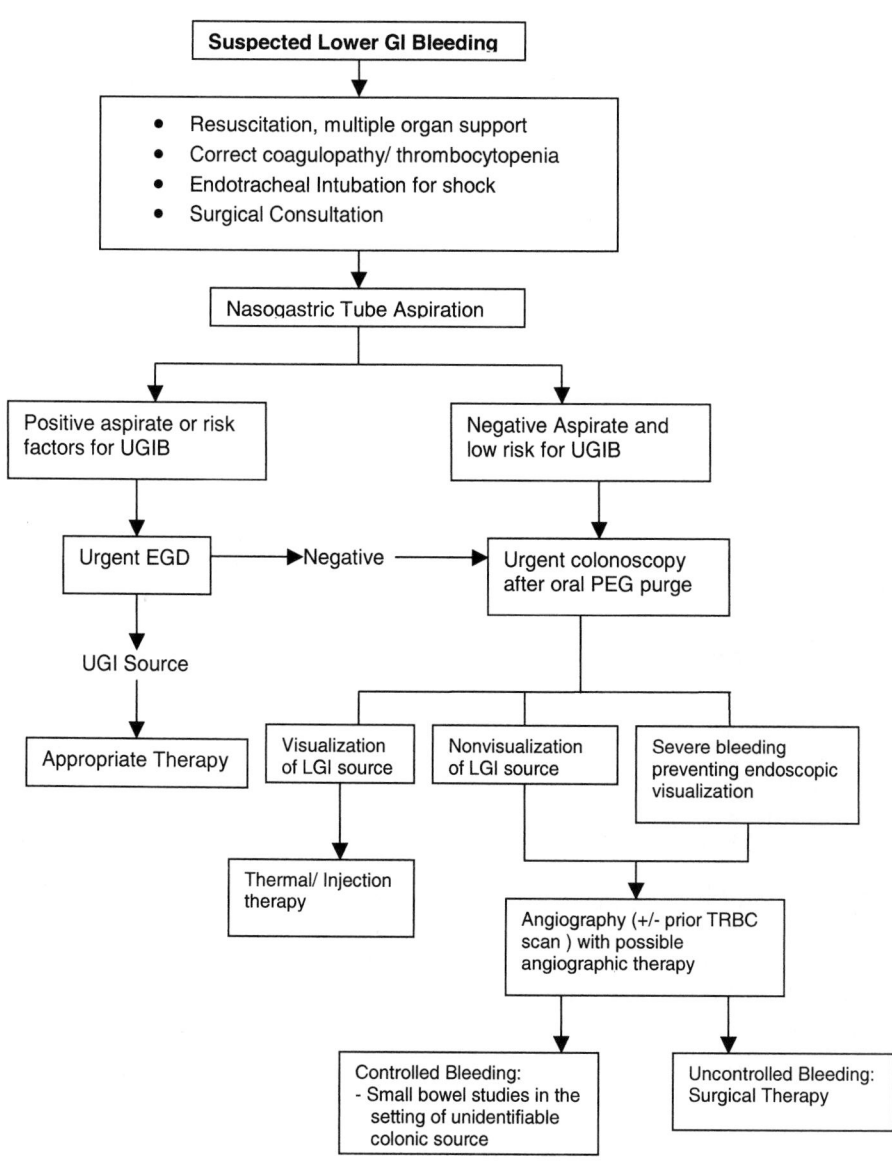

FIGURE 82-5 Management of lower GI hemorrhage. TRBC, tagged RBC; PEG, polyethylene glycol.

with both injection therapy and thermal coagulation.[68] The periphery of the lesion should be treated before the center in order to obliterate the feeder vessels. With respect to thermal coagulation, the recommended power settings are lower than those used for a bleeding peptic ulcer owing to the increased risk of perforation in the right colon.

Additional lesions responsive to thermal and injection therapy include postpolypectomy sites, radiation colitis, and anorectal sources. Noncontact modalities such as the argon-plasma coagulator (APC) have been used effectively in the management of radiation colitis and postpolypectomy bleeding. In addition, a band ligation technique similar to esophageal variceal band ligation can be used to treat bleeding internal hemorrhoids.[69]

RADIONUCLIDE STUDIES

In the event of a negative colonoscopy, a radionuclide scan using ^{99m}Tc-pertechnetate-labeled red blood cells is used frequently to localize the LGI bleeding site prior to subsequent angiographic evaluation. The nuclear scan offers the ability to detect rates of bleeding as low as 0.1 mL/min, and the 48-hour stability of the tagged red blood cells allows repeated imaging during this time period. However, the high sensitivity of radionuclide imaging is offset by its low specificity compared with a positive endoscopic or angiographic examination.[70] A positive radionuclide study localizes the bleeding only to an area of the abdomen and cannot define precisely the mucosal location of the bleeding site. Therefore, a positive scan should be used to direct attention to specific sites of the GI tract that can be examined subsequently by angiography or a repeat endoscopy. Furthermore, surgical intervention should not be based on the results of a radionuclide scan alone but should be guided by accurate angiographic or endoscopic evaluation.

ANGIOGRAPHIC THERAPY

Angiography with therapeutic intent is the appropriate treatment modality in the setting of massive bleeding that precludes colonoscopy or after a nondiagnostic colonoscopy. The overall diagnostic yield of angiography ranges from 40% to 78%, with diverticular disease and angiodysplasia being the

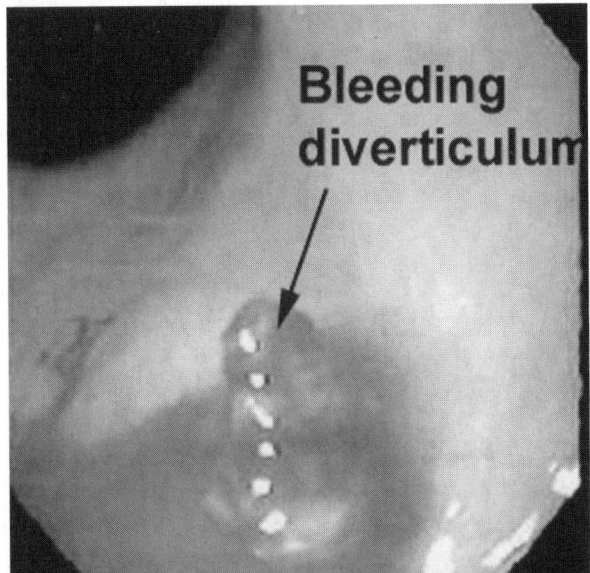

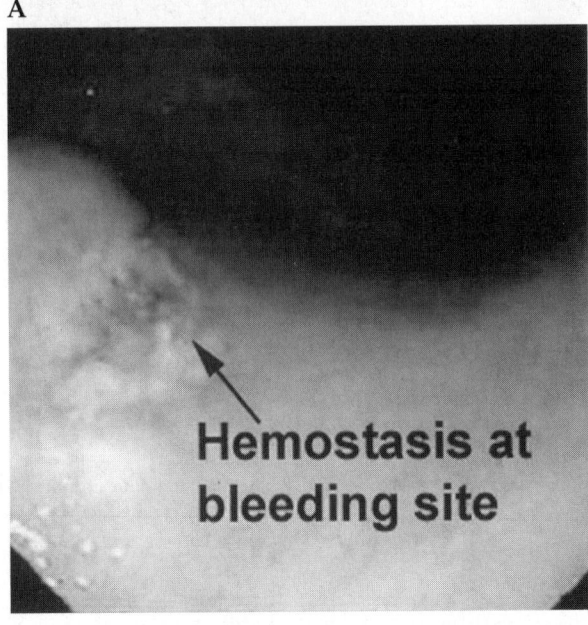

FIGURE 82-6 *A.* Bleeding colonic diverticulum prior to therapy.
B. Successful hemostasis after thermal and injection therapy.

most common findings.[71] In a stable patient, a radionuclide scan is performed often for initial localization prior to angiographic evaluation because the nuclear scan is a more sensitive examination and detects slower rates of bleeding. In the absence of localization via nuclear imaging, the superior mesenteric artery (SMA) is examined first because most diverticular and angiodysplastic bleeds occur in bowel supplied by this artery.[72] If the evaluation of the SMA is negative, the inferior mesenteric and celiac vessels are studied.

The intermittent nature of LGI bleeding in many cases presents a problem for angiographic evaluation and treatment because active bleeding at the time of dye injection is required for a positive examination. Initial angiographic hemostasis using intraarterial vasopressin or embolization ranges from 60% to 100%, although recurrent bleeding may be

as high as 50%, especially following vasopressin therapy.[73] Intraarterial vasoconstrictive therapy with vasopressin is used predominantly in diverticular bleeding and angiodysplasia and is associated with a major complication rate of 10% to 20%, including arrhythmias, ischemia, and pulmonary edema. Transcatheter embolization therapy with various agents, including gelatin sponge and microcoils, may be a more definitive means of controlling hemorrhage but is associated with a risk of intestinal infarction as high as 20%. Attempts to reduce this risk have included the application of a highly selective catheterization technique and the use of a relatively distal site for embolization with temporary occluding agents.[74]

In the event that therapeutic angiography does not achieve permanent hemostasis, emergent surgical therapy is indicated. However, initial angiographic therapy in the actively bleeding patient may achieve temporary hemostasis and hemodynamic stability and thereby allow surgical intervention in a controlled setting with an improved operative mortality.[73]

SURGICAL THERAPY

In the patient presenting with exsanguinating LGI hemorrhage, colonoscopy and angiography should be deferred, and an emergent subtotal colectomy should be performed. In all other cases, surgical therapy should be reserved for hemorrhage that is refractory to nonsurgical interventions. Furthermore, preoperative localization of bleeding is crucial to avoid extensive surgical resection and to ensure that the bleeding is truly arising from the LGI tract.

PREOPERATIVE LOCALIZATION
The role of angiography and colonoscopy in identifying the bleeding site was outlined previously. In addition to angiography and colonoscopy, exploratory laparotomy with intraoperative endoscopy can be used to localize the bleeding source, especially in the small intestine. Intraoperative endoscopy can be performed with oral, rectal, or enterotomy introduction of the endoscope. Following incision of the abdominal wall and exposure of small bowel, the endoscope can be introduced orally. The endoscope, generally a pediatric colonoscope, can be advanced easily to the ligament of Treitz. Subsequently, the entire small bowel is examined by pleating the small bowel over the colonoscope. The endoscopist must limit the amount of air insufflation because excessive distention of the bowel will result in prolonged postoperative ileus. Following inspection of the small bowel to the ileocecal valve, a second inspection is performed as the colonoscope is withdrawn slowly. The surgeon assists the examination by carefully inspecting the serosal side of the bowel for abnormalities, such as a transilluminated angiodysplastic lesion. Alternatively, a sterilized colonoscope may be placed through an enterotomy site in the small bowel and then can be passed proximally and distally into the small bowel to facilitate examination. This approach carries a risk of contamination of the exposed peritoneum. A collaborative effort between the endoscopist and the surgeon is essential for the efficient and safe performance of intraoperative endoscopy.

Once the source of bleeding is localized, a segmental colectomy involving the bleeding lesion can be performed. In a patient with extensive diverticular disease and a localized diverticular bleeding site, a segmental resection eradicating the bleeding site is adequate without the need to resect segments involving nonbleeding diverticula.[73] With respect to angiodysplasia, the presence of cecal angiodysplasia should alert the surgeon to the possibility of angiodysplasia in the distal terminal ileum. It should be noted that angiography that demonstrates cecal angiodysplasia may fail to identify a similar small bowel lesion, and therefore, intraoperative small bowel endoscopy should be used. In addition, when a right hemicolectomy for suspected angiodysplasia is undertaken, resection of the distal 30 to 60 cm of the terminal ileum should be considered.

A subtotal colectomy is indicated for exsanguinating hemorrhage or persistent hemorrhage without an identifiable site of bleeding and involves colonic resection from the cecum to proximal rectum with an ileoproctostomy. This procedure is associated with a high morbidity and mortality, but rebleeding rates are extremely low.[75] Blind segmental resection is contraindicated because this procedure is associated with excessive rates of rebleeding, morbidity, and mortality.[75]

Obscure Bleeding and Small Bowel Evaluation

Occasionally, a patient presenting with acute gastrointestinal bleeding undergoes a nondiagnostic evaluation with endoscopy, radionuclide imaging, and angiography but clinically stabilizes owing to intermittent or permanent cessation of bleeding. In such a situation, emergent surgical exploration and intraoperative endoscopy may not be indicated. Instead, further diagnostic evaluation should be directed specifically at the small bowel, which is the likely source of obscure bleeding in many cases, with angiodysplasia being the most common lesion. Recent advances in endoscopic technology have enabled the gastroenterologist to visualize more distal portions of the small bowel compared with traditional upper endoscopy. These novel endoscopic modalities will be reviewed and will be followed by a discussion of specific lesions associated with obscure bleeding.

NOVEL ENDOSCOPIC MODALITIES

PUSH ENTEROSCOPY
An orally inserted adult/pediatric colonoscope or special enteroscope is passed with or without an overtube as far as possible beyond the ligament of Treitz and allows visualization of the proximal 60 cm of jejunum. The diagnostic yield of this procedure is as high as 50%, with angiodysplasia being the most common lesion.[76] In addition, this technique allows biopsy or therapy of visualized lesions.

SONDE ENTEROSCOPY
This technique should be considered in the setting of a negative push enteroscopy and allows visualization of small bowel distal to the limits of push enteroscopy. During this procedure, a long flexible fiberoptic enteroscope without controls is propelled passively by intestinal peristalsis, allowing a view of the distal small bowel beyond the visualization by push enteroscopy. The endoscopic examination is performed during withdrawal of the instrument. In contrast to push enteroscopy, this technique does not allow biopsy or therapy of visualized lesions, and additional limitations include high equipment costs and a long procedure time.

WIRELESS CAPSULE ENDOSCOPY
This technique has been introduced into clinical practice recently and provides a noninvasive method of examining the entire small bowel via peristaltic propulsion of the endoscopic capsule. The patient swallows a capsule that produces approximately 50,000 images while it traverses the small bowel over 12 to 15 hours. Recent versions of this technique are able to approximate the location of the bleeding lesion within the small bowel. A limitation similar to that for the sonde enteroscopy is the fact that tissue sampling or therapeutic intervention cannot be performed. Experience with this technique is growing rapidly, but extensive studies are yet to be performed.

In addition to the preceding endoscopic modalities, *enteroclysis* radiography can be considered for the evaluation of potential small bowel bleeding sources, although the yield of this test is only about 10%.[77] This study is a double-contrast study performed by passing a tube into the proximal small bowel and injecting barium, methylcellulose, and air. Despite the low sensitivity of this study, it is considered superior to standard imaging using small bowel follow-through.

LESIONS ASSOCIATED WITH OBSCURE BLEEDING

Small intestinal angiodysplasia accounts for the majority of small bowel lesions associated with obscure bleeding. An increased incidence of small bowel angiodyplasia has been reported in patients with end-stage renal disease (ESRD), Von Willebrand disease, and Osler-Weber-Rendu (OWR) syndrome. In the setting of proximal lesions located approximately in the first 60 cm of jejunum, therapeutic push enteroscopy may achieve permanent endoscopic hemostasis. However, more distal lesions are not amenable to endoscopic therapy. In select patient populations, including those with ESRD, Von Willebrand disease, and OWR syndrome, hormonal therapy with estrogen, with or without progesterone, may be useful in controlling bleeding from angiodysplasia.[78] In patients refractory to endoscopic and medical therapy, chronic iron supplementation and periodic transfusions are indicated.

Hemobilia is bleeding from the liver, bile ducts, or pancreas and is characterized by blood emanating from the ampulla of Vater. Hepatic hemobilia usually results from blunt or sharp trauma to the liver. A hepatic artery aneurysm that erodes into the right hepatic or common bile duct produces melena and occasionally presents with right upper quadrant abdominal pain and jaundice. Pancreatic hemobilia is even less common and usually results from pancreatitis-induced pseudoaneurysm formation in the splenic artery. Acquired splenic artery aneurysms may erode into the pancreas, resulting in hemobilia without pancreatitis.

Hemobilia should be suspected when melena occurs in conjunction with jaundice or after blunt trauma or acute pancreatitis. Following a negative forward-viewing upper endoscopy, the endoscopist should examine the duodenal papilla using a side-viewing duodenoscope. Active bleeding or a clot emanating from the papilla may be seen. Alternatively, angiography may reveal active bleeding or associated aneurysms in the hepatic or splenic artery. Angiographic therapy may provide temporary control of hematobilia,[79] but generally definitive surgery is required.

Aortoenteric fistula is a rare development following abdominal vascular surgery involving placement of a synthetic graft. The fistula arises commonly from the proximal anastomosis of the graft and communicates with the fourth portion of the duodenum. Graft infection generally is present and likely plays a role in the pathogenesis of the fistula. Bleeding from aortoenteric fistulas is typically intermittent and profuse. The evaluation of a suspected aortoduodenal fistula should begin with endoscopy. The endoscopist must examine the fourth portion of the duodenum, where bleeding or the graft itself may be seen. If endoscopy fails to identify a fistula, angiography should be performed if clinical suspicion is high. Surgical correction of the fistula, including removal of the graft, is necessary to prevent potential exsanguination.

Meckel's diverticulum should be considered in younger patients presenting with massive bleeding. The diagnosis often is made by a ^{99m}Tc-pertechnetate scan, which has a sensitivity of 75%.[80] Surgical resection of an identified Meckel's diverticulum provides definitive therapy.

References

1. Zimmerman HM, Curfman K: Acute gastrointestinal bleeding. *AACN Clinical Issues* 8:449, 1997.
2. Zuckerman GR, Prakash C: Acute lower intestinal bleeding: I. Clinical presentation and diagnosis. *Gastrointest Endosc* 48:606, 1998.
3. Pitcher JL: Therapeutic endoscopy and bleeding ulcers: Historical overview. *Gastrointest Endosc* 36:S2, 1990.
4. Farrell JJ, Friedman LS: Gastrointestinal bleeding in older people. *Gastroenterol Clin North Am* 29:1, 2000.
5. Kollef MH, O'Brien JD, Zuckerman GR, Shannon W: BLEED: A classification tool to predict outcomes in patients with acute upper and lower gastrointestinal hemorrhage. *Crit Care Med* 25:1125, 1997.
6. Rockall TA, Logan RFA, Devlin HB, Northfield TC: Risk assessment after acute upper gastrointestinal hemorrhage. *Gut* 38:316, 1996.
7. Corley DA, Stefan AM, Wolf M, et al: Early indicators of prognosis in upper gastrointestinal hemorrhage. *Am J Gastroenterol* 93:336, 1998.
8. Strate LL, Orav J, Syngal S: Early predictors of severity in acute lower intestinal tract bleeding. *Arch Intern Med* 163:838, 2003.
9. Cuellar RE, Gavaler JS, Alexander JA, et al: Gastrointestinal tract hemorrhage: The value of a nasogastric aspirate. *Arch Intern Med* 150:1381, 1990.
10. Rollhauser C, Fleischer DE: Ulcers and nonvariceal bleeding. *Endoscopy* 31:17, 1999.
11. Laine L, Peterson WL: Bleeding peptic ulcer. *New Engl J Med* 331:717, 1994.
11a. Barkun A, Bardou M, Marshall JK: Consensus recommendations for managing patients with nonvariceal upper gastrointestinal bleeding. *Ann Intern Med* 139:843, 2003.
12. Jensen DM, Machicado GA, Jutabha R, Kovacs TO: Urgent colonoscopy for the diagnosis and treatment of severe diverticular hemorrhage. *New Engl J Med* 342:78, 2000.
13. Jensen DM, Machicado GA: Colonoscopy for diagnosis and treatment of severe lower gastrointestinal bleeding: Routine outcomes and cost analysis. *Gastrointest Endosc Clin North Am* 7:477, 1997.
14. ASGE Practice Guidelines: An annotated algorithmic approach to upper gastrointestinal bleeding. *Gastrointest Endosc* 53:853, 2001.
15. ASGE Practice Guidelines: An annotated algorithmic approach to acute lower gastrointestinal bleeding. *Gastrointest Endosc* 53:853, 2001.
16. Frossard JL, Spahr L, Queneau PE, et al: Erythromycin intravenous bolus infusion in acute upper gastrointestinal bleeding: A randomized, controlled, double-blind trial. *Gastroenterology* 123:17, 2002.
17. Lau JY, Sung JJ, Lee KK, et al: Effect of intravenous omeprazole on recurrent bleeding after endoscopic treatment of bleeding peptic ulcers. *New Eng J Med* 343:310, 2000.
18. Jensen DM, Cheng S, Kovacs TG, et al: A controlled study of ranitidine for the prevention of recurrent hemorrhage from duodenal ulcer. *New Engl J Med* 330:382, 1994.
19. Ejlersen E, Melsen T, Ingerslev J, et al: Recombinant activated factor VII (rFVIIa) acutely normalizes prothrombin time in patients with cirrhosis during bleeding from oesophageal varices. *Scand J Gastroenterol* 36:1081, 2001.
20. Negrier C, Lienhart A: Overall experience with NovoSeven. *Blood Coagul Fibrinol* 11(suppl 1):S19, 2000.
21. Rostykus PS, McDonald GB, Albert RK: Upper intestinal endoscopy induces hypoxemia in patients with obstructive pulmonary disease. *Gastroenterology* 78:488, 1980.
22. Vlavianos P, MacMathuna P, Williams R, et al: Splanchnic and systemic hemodynamic response to volume changes in patients with cirrhosis and portal hypertension. *Clin Sci* 96:475, 1997.
23. Goulis J, Armonis A, Patch D, et al: Bacterial infection is independently associated with failure to control bleeding in cirrhotic patients with gastrointestinal hemorrhage. *Hepatology* 27:1207, 1998.
24. Goulis J, Patch D, Burroughs A: Bacterial infection in the pathogenesis of variceal bleeding. *Lancet* 353:139, 1999.
25. Bernard B, Cadranel J-F, Valla D, et al: Antibiotic prophylaxis for the prevention of bacterial infections in cirrhotic patients with gastrointestinal hemorrhage: A meta-analysis. *Hepatology* 29:1655, 1999.
26. Corley D, Cello J, Adkisson W, et al: Octreotide for acute esophageal variceal bleeding: A meta-analysis. *Gastroenterology* 120:946, 2001.
27. Escorsell A, Ruiz del Arbol L, Planas R, et al: Multicenter randomized controlled trial of terlipressin versus sclerotherapy in the treatment of acute variceal bleeding: The TEST study. *Hepatology* 32:471, 2000.
28. Ioannou G, Doust J, Rockey DC: *Cochrane Database Syst Rev* 1:CD002147, 2003.
29. Laine L, Cook D: Endoscopic ligation compared with sclerotherapy for treatment of esophageal variceal bleeding: A meta-analysis. *Ann Intern Med* 123:280, 1995.
30. Lo G-H, Lai K-H, Cheung J-S, et al: A prospective, randomized trial of butyl cyanoacrylate injection versus band ligation in the management of bleeding gastric varices. *Hepatology* 33:1060, 2001.
31. Yang WL, Tripathi D, Therapondos G, et al: Endoscopic use of human thrombin in bleeding gastric varices. *Am J Gastroenterol* 97:1381, 2002.
32. Azoulay D, Castaing D, Majno P, et al: Salvage transjugular intrahepatic portosystemic shunt for uncontrolled variceal bleeding in patients with decompensated cirrhosis. *J Hepatol* 35:590, 2001.
33. Henderson J, Nagle A, Curtis S, et al: Surgical shunts and TIPS for variceal decompression in the 1990s. *Surgery* 128:540, 2000.

34. Lo G-H, Lai K-H, Cheng J-S, et al: Endoscopic variceal ligation plus nadolol and sucralfate compared with ligation alone for the prevention of variceal rebleeding: A prospective randomized trial. *Hepatology* 32:461, 2000.

35. Saltzman JR, Zawacki JK: Therapy for bleeding peptic ulcers. *New Eng J Med* 336:1091, 1997.

36. ASGE Technology Status Evaluation Report: Endoscopic hemostatic devices. *Gastrointest Endosc* 54:833, 2001.

37. Kubba AK, Palmer KR: Role of endoscopic injection therapy in the treatment of bleeding peptic ulcer. *Br J Surg* 83:461, 1996.

38. Chung SS, Lau JY, Sung JJ, et al: Randomized comparison between adrenaline injection alone and adrenaline injection plus heat probe treatement for actively bleeding ulcers. *Br Med J* 314:1307, 1997.

39. Jensen DM: Thermal probe or combination therapy for nonvariceal UGI hemorrhage. *Techniques Gastrointest Endosc* 1:107, 1999.

40. Jensen DM, Kovacs TO, Jutabha R, et al: Randomized trial of medical or endoscopic therapy to prevent recurrent ulcer hemorrhage in patients with adherent clots. *Gastroenterology* 123:407, 2002.

41. Collins R, Langman M: Treatment with histamine antagonists in acute upper gastrointestinal hemorrhage: Implications of randomized trials. *New Engl J Med* 313:660, 1985.

42. Lin HJ, Lo WC, Lee FY, et al: A prospective, randomized comparative trial showing that omeprazole prevents rebleeding in patients with bleeding peptic ulcer after successful endoscopic therapy. *Arch Intern Med* 158:54, 1998.

43. Lau JY, Sung JJ, Lee KK, et al: Effect of intravenous omeprazole on recurrent bleeding after endoscopic treatment of bleeding peptic ulcers. *New Engl J Med* 343:310, 2000.

44. Green FW, Kaplan MM, Curtis LE, et al: Effect of acid and pepsin on blood coagulation and platelet aggregation: A possible contributor to prolonged gastroduodenal mucosal damage. *Gastroenterology* 74:38, 1978.

45. Imperiale TF, Birgisson S: Somatostatin or octreotide compared with H$_2$ antagonist and placebo in the management of acute nonvariceal upper gastrointestinal hemorrhage: A meta-analysis. *Ann Intern Med* 127:1062, 1997.

46. Irving JD, Northfield TC: Emergency arteriography in acute gastrointestinal bleeding. *Br Med J* 1:929, 1976.

47. Sherman LM, Shenoy SS, Cerra FB, et al: Selective intra-arterial vasopressin: Clinical efficacy and complications. *Ann Surg* 189:298, 1979.

48. Eckstein MR, Kelemouridis V, Athanasoulis CA, et al: Gastric bleeding: Therapy with intraarterial vasopressin and transcatheter embolization. *Radiology* 152:643, 1984.

49. McArdle CS, Tilney NL: Surgery for peptic ulcer disease: Operative complications and immediate morbidity. *J R Coll Surg Edinb* 21:285, 1976.

50. Foster JH, Hickok DF, Dunphy JE: Factors influencing mortality following emergency operation for massive upper gastrointestinal hemorrhage. *Surg Gynecol Obstet* 117:257, 1963.

51. Laine LA: *Helicobacter pylori* and complicated ulcer disease. *Am J Med* 100:52S, 1996.

52. Schuman BM, Threadgill ST: The influence of liver disease and portal hypertension on bleeding in Mallory-Weiss syndrome. *J Clin Gastroenterol* 18:10, 1994.

53. Steinert D, Masand-Rai A: Successful combination endoscopic therapy for duodenal Dieulafoy's lesion (letter). *Am J Gastroenterol* 91:818, 1996.

54. Matsui S, Kamisako T, Kudo M, et al: Endoscopic band ligation for control of nonvariceal upper GI hemorrhage: Comparison with bipolar electrocoagulation. *Gastrointest Endosc* 55:214, 2002.

55. Haglund U: Stress ulcers. *Scand J Gastroenterol* 175(suppl):27, 1990.

56. Cook DJ, Fuller HD, Guyatt GH, et al: Risk factors for gastrointestinal bleeding in critically ill patients. *New Engl J Med* 330:377, 1994.

57. Zinner MJ, Zuidema GD, Smith PL, et al: The prevention of upper gastrointestinal tract bleeding in patients in an intensive care unit. *Surg Gynecol Obstet* 153:214, 1981.

58. Kovacs TOG, Jensen DM: Therapeutic endoscopy for nonvariceal upper gastrointestinal bleeding, in Taylor MB, Gollan JL, Steer ML, et al (eds): *Gastrointestinal Emergencies*, 2d ed. Baltimore, Williams & Wilkins, 1997, p 181.

59. Baum S: Angiographic diagnosis and treatment of gastrointestinal bleeding, in Baum S, Pentecost MJ (eds): *Abram's Angiography: Interventional Radiology.* Boston, Little, Brown, 1997, p 389.

60. Lederman HP, Schoch E, Jost R, et al: Superselective coil embolization in acute gastrointestinal hemorrhage. *J Vasc Intervent Radiol* 9:753, 1998.

61. Cook D, Guyatt G, Marshall J, et al: A comparison of sucralfate and ranitidine for the prevention of upper gastrointestinal bleeding in patients requiring mechanical ventilation. *New Engl J Med* 338:791, 1998.

62. Pingleton SK, Hadizma S: Enteral alimentation and gastrointestinal bleeding in mechanically ventilated patients. *Crit Care Med* 11:13, 1983.

63. Raff T, Germann G, Hartmann B: The value of early enteral nutrition in the prophylaxis of stress ulceration in the severely burned patient. *Burns* 23:313, 1997.

64. Jensen DM, Machicado GA: Diagnosis and treatment of severe hematochezia: The role of urgent colonoscopy after purge. *Gastroenterology* 95:1569, 1988.

65. Cohn SM, Moller BA, Zieg PM, et al: Angiography for preoperative evaluation in patients with lower gastrointestinal bleeding: Are the benefits worth the risks? *Arch Surg* 133:50, 1998.

66. Rossini FP, Ferrari A, Spandre M, et al: Emergency colonoscopy. *World J Surg* 13:190, 1989.

67. Foutch PG, Zimmerman K: Diverticular bleeding and the pigmented protruberance: Clinical implications, histopathological correlation, and results of endoscopic intervention. *Am J Gastroenterol* 91:2589, 1996.

68. Santos JC, Aprilli F, Guimaraes AS, et al: Angiodysplasia of the colon: Endoscopic diagnosis and treatment. *Br J Surg* 75:256, 1988.

69. Trowers E, Ganga U, Hodges D, et al: Endoscopic hemorrhoidal ligation: Preliminary clinical experience. *Gastrointest Endosc* 48:49, 1998.

70. Dusold R, Burke K, Carpentier W, et al: The accuracy of technetium-99m-labeled red cell scintigraphy in localizing gastrointestinal bleeding. *Am J Gastroenterol* 89:345, 1994.

71. Leitman IM, Paul DE, Shires GT: Evaluation and management of massive lower gastrointestinal hemorrhage. *Ann Surg* 209:175, 1989.

72. Reinus JF, Brandt LJ: Vascular ectasias and diverticulosis: Common causes of lower gastrointestinal bleeding. *Gastroenterol Clin North Am* 23:1, 1994.

73. Browder W, Cerise EJ, Litwin MS: Impact of emergency angiography in massive lower gastrointestinal bleeding. *Ann Surg* 204:530, 1986.

74. Guy GE, Shetty PC, Sharma RP, et al: Acute lower gastrointestinal hemorrhage: Treatment by superselective embolization with polyvinyl alcohol particles. *AJR* 159:521, 1992.

75. Parkes BM, Obeid FN, Sorensen VJ, et al: The management of massive lower gastrointestinal bleeding. *Am Surg* 59:676, 1993.

76. Foutch PG, Sawyer R, Sinowski R: Push enteroscopy for diagnosis of patients with gastrointestinal bleeding of obscure origin. *Gastrointest Endosc* 36:337, 1990.

77. Rex D, Lappas J, Maglinte D: Enteroclysis in the evaluation of suspected small intestinal bleeding. *Gastroenterology* 97:58, 1989.

78. Barkin JS, Ross BS: Medical therapy for chronic gastrointestinal bleeding of obscure origin. *Am J Gastroenterol* 93:1250, 1998.

79. Fagan EA, Allison DJ, Chadwick VS, et al: Treatment of haemobilia by selective embolization. *Gut* 21:541, 1980.

80. Berquist TH, Nolan NG, Stephen DH, et al: Specificity of ^{99m}Tc-pertechnetate in scintigraphy diagnosis of Meckel's diverticulum. *J Nucl Med* 17:465, 1976.

Chapter 83 _____

FULMINANT HEPATIC FAILURE

SANJAY KULKARNI
DAVID C. CRONIN II

KEY POINTS

- *Fulminant hepatic failure (FHF) is defined as the onset of hepatic encephalopathy (HE) within 8 weeks of the onset of liver-related symptoms.*

- *Common complications in patients with FHF include encephalopathy, cerebral edema, cardiovascular instability, renal failure, and infection.*

- *Supportive management of FHF consists of (1) airway protection, (2) intracranial pressure monitoring in the sickest patients, and (3) treatment of complications and vigilance for infection.*

- *Orthotopic liver transplantation (OLT) is the definitive therapy for FHF. Extracorporeal liver support remains investigational.*

Fulminant hepatic failure (FHF) describes a clinical syndrome of progressive hepatocyte necrosis resulting in the dysfunction of virtually every major organ system. Consequently, management of patients with FHF is complicated and unpredictable, where many of the therapies initiated have not been proven effective in controlled clinical trials. Management of this syndrome requires early recognition and treatment of organ system deterioration because overall patient survival is inversely related to the number and extent of extrahepatic organ dysfunction. Therefore, treatment of these organ failures should be highly individualized and tailored toward anticipation and prevention of multisystem organ failure while waiting for recovery of hepatic function or liver transplantation.

Perhaps the most difficult dilemma in treating patients with FHF is the inability to predict which patients will recover adequate liver function and survive an episode of FHF without liver transplantation. Among patients with FHF who have progressed to grade 3 or 4 encephalopathy, expected recovery with medical management alone is approximately 10% to 40%.[1] The advent of liver transplantation has improved survival markedly to 60% to 80% and is currently considered the treatment of choice for progressive FHF.[1] Thus the overall treatment strategy has evolved into early stabilization of the FHF patient, optimization of the patient's general condition, and early and continued evaluation for liver transplantation.

Definitions and Etiology

Trey and Davidson[2] originally proposed the term *fulminant hepatic failure*, which describes a condition of massive hepatic cell necrosis (Fig. 83-1) that is clinically evident by the progression to encephalopathy within 8 weeks of the onset of

jaundice. Since this initial definition, numerous alterations and terms have been proposed that often complicate rather than clarify understanding of this disease process. A more concise definition proposed by O'Grady and colleagues[3] attempts to precisely categorize liver failure into three types based on the time interval between the onset of jaundice and the emergence of encephalopathy: hyperacute (0 to 7 days), acute (8 to 28 days), and subacute (29 days to 12 weeks). The utility of this terminology is supported by the different clinical features and associated mortalities within each category (Table 83-1). Patients with hyperacute FHF tend to have rapidly progressive cerebral edema, to improve with medical management, and to have an overall favorable prognosis. Patients with acute FHF also have rapidly progressive FHF, but they tend to have a worse prognosis without liver transplant. Subacute FHF patients have a lower incidence of cerebral edema but an overall poor prognosis. It is important to distinguish hyperacute and acute FHF from subacute FHF. A recent modification of the nomenclature for liver failure was presented by the International Association for the Study of Liver (IASL) stressing the differences between hyperacute and acute versus subacute liver failure.[4] The modified terminology includes only two groups, acute and subacute liver failure. However, there are temporal subcategories within acute liver failure that include hyperacute (onset less the 10 days), fulminant (onset 10 to 30 days), and acute hepatic failure not otherwise specified (AHF-NOS) that use the time from onset of jaundice to the onset of encephalopathy as the main differentiating feature. Subacute FHF is characterized by persistent, irreversible hepatitis leading to the development of ascites and/or encephalopathy over a protracted period of time (5 to 24 weeks). Wider acceptance of this new classification system will continue when analysis of FHF using this schema becomes more prevalent. Regardless of the classification system used, categorization of FHF is useful for retrospective analyses of patients but does not provide prospective guidelines for initial management. Therefore, all patients should be assumed to have an unpredictable clinical course that may require liver transplantation.

The causes of FHF are numerous and not always known at the time of presentation. Careful history taking from the patient, family, and significant others is mandatory and may provide valuable information for identifying the etiology of FHF. Additionally, certain causes require specific therapies or influence the appropriateness of liver transplantation. In the United States, acetaminophen toxicity has replaced acute viral hepatitis as the most common cause of FHF.[5] Usually, metabolites of acetaminophen are direct hepatotoxins as compared with the hypersensitivity reactions associated with other drugs that cause FHF (e.g., halothane, antidepressants, and nonsteroidal anti-inflammatory drugs). Cellular damage secondary to acetaminophen intoxication is not isolated to the liver and often is associated with other signs of systemic toxicity, most commonly renal dysfunction. In addition to intentional ingestion of large doses of acetaminophen, therapeutic doses of acetaminophen can result in FHF. This therapeutic misadventure occurs when therapeutic doses of acetaminophen undergo rapid conversion to the toxic metabolite at a rate that exceeds the detoxification reaction. The potential for this situation exists in patients

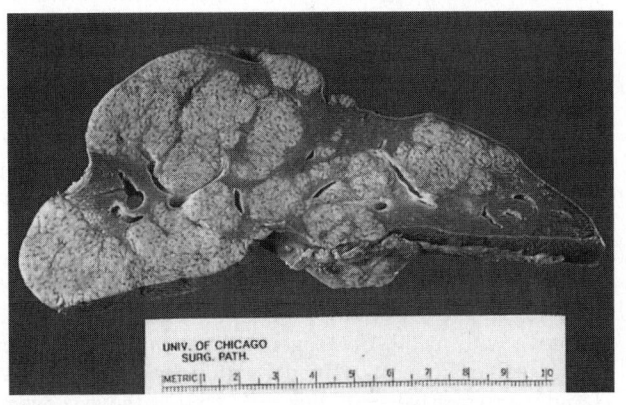

A

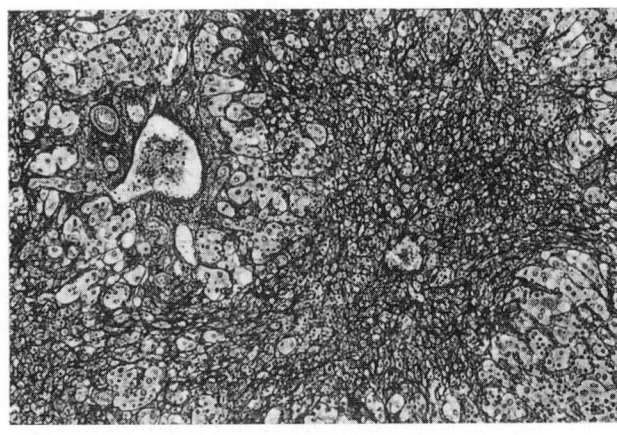

C

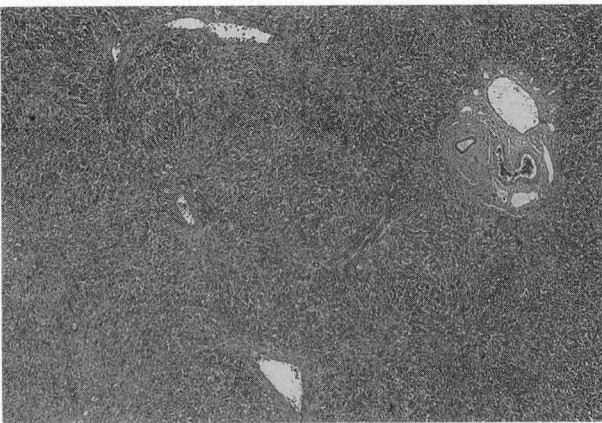

B

FIGURE 83-1 Liver pathology of FHF. *A.* Gross liver section demonstrating regenerative nodules after FHF. *B.* High-power view demonstrating necrosis with lack of hepatocytes and intact portal structures. *C.* High-power view with reticulin stain showing nodular liver regeneration.

with hepatic enzymes that have been induced by exposure to drugs (alcohol, barbiturates, phenytoin, etc.) or in patients with malnutrition resulting in limited detoxification capacity.[6] Of the viral causes of FHF, hepatitis A and hepatitis B are the most common. Hepatitis C infection rarely causes FHF unless coinfection with another hepatitis virus exists.[7] In rare instances, categorized as non-A, non-E hepatitis, no etiologic cause of FHF is clearly evident, but the course is consistent with a viral etiology. Additional causes of FHF are listed in Table 83-2, including rare causes, which always need to be considered, especially when no clear basis for FHF is evident.

TABLE 83-1 Subcategories of FHF

	Hyperacute	Acute	Subacute
Encephalopathy	Yes	Yes	Yes
Onset of jaundice	0–7 days	8–28 days	29–72 days
Cerebral edema	Common	Common	Uncommon
Serum bilirubin	Least elevated	Elevated	Elevated
Prognosis	Intermediate	Poor	Poor

SOURCE: Adapted with permission from O'Grady JG, Schalm SW, Williams R: Acute liver failure: Redefining the syndromes. *Lancet* 342:273, 1993.

TABLE 83-2 Causes of FHF

Viral	HAV, HBV, HCV (usually coinfection), HDV, HEV, HGV
	Herpes simplex virus
	Epstein-Barr virus
Drug toxicity	Acetaminophen
	Halothane, ampicillin-clavulanate, ciprofloxacin, erythromycin, isoniazid, nitrofurantoin, tetracycline, sodium valproate, phenytoin, lovastatin, tricyclic anti-depressants, gold, flutamide, dipyridium, antabuse, cyclophosphamide, methyldioxy-methamphetamine (ecstasy), loratadine, propylthiouracil, troglitazone
Other toxins	*Amanita phalloides*, organic solvents, herbal medicines, bacterial toxins (*Bacillus cereus* and cyanobacteria)
Miscellaneous	Acute Budd-Chiari
	Hepatic ischemia from shock
	Wilson's disease
	Reye's syndrome
	Acute fatty liver of pregnancy
	Heatstroke
	Extensive hepatectomy
	Autoimmune hepatitis
	Lymphoma

Initial Evaluation and Management

INITIAL ASSESSMENT

Patients suspected of having FHF should be managed in a critical care unit associated with an active liver transplant program. A multidisciplinary team composed of critical care specialists, hepatologists, transplant surgeons, and neurointensivists is essential for evaluating the patient and defining a plan of treatment. Ideally, this multidisciplinary care will be provided throughout the ICU admission, and members will participate in the decision making for liver replacement. The diagnosis of FHF is made by careful history, clinical assessment, and biochemical confirmation. A history of preexisting liver disease, toxin exposure (e.g., alcohol, acetaminophen, NSAIDs, etc.), acute viral illness, or a predisposing medical condition should increase suspicion of FHF in a patient presenting with altered mental status, transaminase elevation, and synthetic dysfunction. The latter is best reflected by an elevation in the International Normalization Ratio (INR) of prothrombin time. A rising INR coincident with falling liver transaminases is an ominous sign suggestive of nonrecoverable ongoing hepatic necrosis.

During the initial evaluation, the importance of a detailed history and physical examination cannot be overstated. Interviews with the patient, friends, and family and direct contact with referring physicians may provide insight into the acuity of the illness, social background, and possible coexisting medical conditions that may alter the patient's expected recovery and candidacy for transplantation. Medical records of patients transferred from outside institutions should be reviewed for evidence of administration of sedatives that may have an impact on the initial neurologic examination. Patients with FHF may present with confusion or combative behavior, which is often treated with benzodiazpines or narcotics. Administration of flumazenil or naloxone may be necessary, depending on the amount and type of benzodiazapine or narcotic exposure, to allow for an accurate baseline neurologic evaluation.

MONITORING

The degree of neurologic dysfunction, as measured by encephalopathy grade, should guide the initial level of invasive monitoring. This monitoring strategy is supported by the observation that hemodynamic instability in FHF is usually a late finding and most often occurs among patients in grade 3 or 4 encephalopathy. Large-bore peripheral intravenous lines, a nasogastric tube (or an orogastric tube if there is an uncorrected coagulopathy), a urinary catheter, an electrocardiogram, noninvasive blood pressure monitoring, and pulse oximetery are adequate for patients presenting with grade 1 or 2 encephalopathy. Excessive initial monitoring with invasive catheters is unnecessary and is associated with an increased risk of complications and infection. Among patients with grade 3 or 4 encephalopathy, endotracheal intubation is necessary for maintaining airway patency, oxygenation, and control of respiratory acidosis. Because patients with grade 3 or 4 encephalopathy may become combative and require sedation or have lapsed into coma, intracranial pressure (ICP) monitoring is strongly recommended. Extradural catheter monitoring is preferred in this setting for its safety and ease in placement.[8] This subset of patients

also may benefit from central venous or pulmonary artery monitoring, especially those receiving vasoactive drugs or mannitol to treat intracranial hypertension. Central venous, arterial, and extradural catheters can be inserted safely by experienced staff in the setting of an INR between 2 and 3. The risk of hemorrhage can be reduced further by choosing compressible sites, and using ultrasound guidance for venous and arterial access. For patients with greater degrees of coagulopathy, fresh frozen plasma (FFP) should be given in a limited window during which all necessary invasive procedures are planned. Repeated and intermittent FFP infusion obscures the clinician's ability to assess hepatic synthetic recovery and poses the additional risks of fluid overload and transfusion reaction.

WORKUP

The goal of initial laboratory evaluation is to find the potential causes of FHF, as well as to evaluate other organ system function. On arrival, the patient should have a complete blood count, platelet count, chemistries, liver function tests (albumin, bilirubin, alkaline phosphatase, AST, and ALT), prothrombin time (INR), arterial blood gas, factor V level, blood glucose level, and ammonia level. The preceding tests should be performed on a scheduled basis because clinical deterioration may be swift and unpredictable. Possible causes of FHF are sought through serologic assays for hepatitis A (anti-HAV IgM) and hepatitis B (anti-HBV IgM, HBsAg, HBcAb) and serum assays for ceruloplasmin, iron-binding capacity, toxic substances, and acetaminophen. A right upper quadrant ultrasound is useful in providing information regarding the patency of the hepatic vessels, liver size, presence of acites, and degree of compression of the porta hepatitis by intraabdominal masses. The role for liver biopsy is controversial. Although transjugular liver biopsies can be performed safely, there is little correlation between the extent of hepatic necrosis and the recoverability of the liver likely owing to sampling error. Despite this, liver biopsies are useful in patients for whom the cause of FHF is uncertain, or when lymphoma is a possible cause.

ACETAMINOPHEN INTOXICATION

Patients suspected of acetaminophen intoxication should be treated immediately with oral N-acetylcysteine, a proven free-radical scavenger that improves overall survival among patients with acetaminophen-induced FHF.[9] The biochemical basis for this therapy is that the hepatoxicity induced by acetaminophen is mediated by its metabolite N-acetyl-benzoquinoneimine, which binds sulfhydryl groups in heptocytes.[10] High levels of N-acetyl-benzoquinoneimine deplete glutathione stores, which normally reduce the toxic metabolites of acetaminophen. N-acetylcysteine functions by replenishing stores of intracellular reduced glutathione, thereby detoxifying N-acetyl-benzoquinoneimine. Recently, treatment with N-acetylcysteine also has shown beneficial affects in the overall hemodynamic status of patients with FHF by an undefined mechanism.[11] Regardless of the time elapsed from ingestion, there are significant benefits to giving N-acetylcysteine even 10 to 36 hours after ingestion.[11] Mortality was reduced from 58% to 37%, and significantly fewer patients progressed to grade 3 or 4 encephalopathy. N-Acetylcysteine is given orally in a 5% dextrose solution with a loading dose of 140 mg/kg, followed by 17 doses of 70 mg/kg every 4 hours. The Food and Drug Administration (FDA) has not approved the use of intravenous *N*-acetylcysteine in the United States because of reported anaphylactic reactions and electrocardiographic (ECG) abnormalities. However, in patients who have intractable vomiting, intravenous administration of *N*-acetylcysteine may be the only recourse. One approach is to compound a 3% *N*-acetylcysteine solution dosed intravenously identically to the oral regimen.[12] For patients treated with *N*-acetylcysteine, the INR must be evaluated cautiously because false "improvements" in coagulation have been described.[13]

VIRUS-INDUCED FHF

Virus-induced FHF may present as a rapidly progressive new illness or an acute decompensation superimposed on preexisting liver disease. Regardless, many of these patients will require urgent liver transplantation if criteria for FHF are met. For patients with hepatitis B (with or without hepatitis D coinfection), antiviral therapy may be beneficial. Lamivudine, a nucleoside analog, improves Childs-Pugh status among patients with chronic hepatitis B cirrhosis.[14,15] Experience with its use in the setting of FHF is limited. However, preliminary evidence has demonstrated hepatitis B e-antigen seroconversion in patients with FHF.[16] Although this seroconversion is largely temporary, it suggests significant antiviral activity that may help an acutely decompensated patient with hepatitis B from progressing to FHF. Despite the lack of definitive studies in acute decompensation, we recommend early lamivudine treatment in selected patients given the severity of illness and limited therapeutic options.

Encephalopathy and Cerebral Edema

Central to the care of patients with FHF is the management of encephalopathy and cerebral edema. Starling forces of hydrostatic and osmotic pressure gradients appear to favor cerebral edema in FHF patients.[17] Dysfunction of cerebral blood flow autoregulation, cerebral vasodilation, and a disrupted blood-brain barrier all contribute to the accumulation of interstitial cerebral fluid, resulting in increased ICP. A direct causative relationship between encephalopathy and cerebral edema has not been proven, and in patients with chronic liver failure, worsening encephalopathy is not associated with cerebral edema. In the acute setting, however, cerebral edema clearly is evident in patients with grade 3 or 4 encephalopathy. Progressive cerebral edema leading to uncal herniation and death unfortunately is the end point of many severely ill FHF patients who do not receive a liver transplant.

The extent of cerebral dysfunction should be determined repeatedly through careful neurologic examination. Owing to the limited sensitivity of computed tomography in detecting cerebral edema, repeated clinical evaluations and gradings of encephalopathy are required[18] (Table 83-3). Repeated examinations by the same critical care or neurointensivist staff are optimal because assessment is subjective. Recognizing external factors that can exacerbate encephalopathy is important and probably underemphasized. The most common clinical scenario is that of a combative and confused patient with

TABLE 83-3 Grades of Encephalopathy

Grade	Clinical Examination
1	Confused or altered mood
2	Somnolent or inappropriate behavior, impending stupor
3	Stuporous but arousable or markedly confused behavior
4	Unresponsive or comatose

grade 2 encephalopathy who is treated with sedatives and then appears to progress to grade 3. When sedatives must be given to facilitate care or ensure patient safety, we recommend low-dose, short-acting benzodiazapines (e.g., 0.5 mg IV lorazepam). The mental status then should be assessed carefully and serially during the period of sedation. If sedatives are dosed repeatedly, the safest approach may be to intubate the patient electively and place an extradural monitor. Other external variables that may contribute to worsening encephalopathy include hypoglycemia, hypoxia, electrolyte abnormalities, gastrointestinal bleeding, and sepsis.[19]

Treatments effective in ameliorating the encephalopathy of decompensated cirrhosis, such as selective gut decontamination, lactulose, and dietary nitrogen restriction, have proven ineffective in FHF, and we do not recommend them.

Management of cerebral edema is based on principles of maintaining adequate cerebral perfusion while controlling factors that exacerbate interstitial cerebral fluid accumulation and increases in ICP. Initial measures should include avoidance of unnecessary stimulation, including respiratory suctioning in intubated patients, which may cause acute elevations in ICP. The head of the patient's bed should be elevated to 30 degrees, and the patient's head should be maintained in a neutral position. Simply avoiding, when possible, moving and provoking the patient will stabilize fluctuations in ICP and provide for more consistent assessment. Jugular venous lines risk potential obstruction of cerebral venous outflow, so some have advocated avoiding them, but the risks should be balanced against those of alternate sites (subclavian and bleeding, femoral and infection; see Chap. 12).

Brain blood flow is determined largely by the cerebral perfusion pressure (CPP), a function of mean arterial pressure (MAP) and ICP: CPP = MAP − ICP. At high levels of MAP, hydrostatic forces directly favor interstitial cerebral fluid accumulation. On the other hand, excessive lowering of MAP risks cerebral hypoperfusion if the limits of cerebral autoregulation are breached. Flow sufficiently low to cause brain hypoxia may amplify blood-brain barrier dysfunction.[17] Therefore, optimal CPP is between 60 and 80 mm Hg.

Cerebral capillary osmotic pressure gradients also play an important role in the development of cerebral edema. Blood-brain barrier disruption and elevated serum ammonia levels lead to accumulating cerebral interstitial osmotic forces favoring water efflux into the cerebral interstitium. Approaches to limit this efflux include repair of the blood-brain barrier or increasing the cerebral capillary oncotic pressure. Evidence that the blood-brain barrier can be reconstituted in the setting of FHF is preliminary and involves strategies to reduce serum ammonia levels by continuous venous hemofiltration or by plasma exchange.[20]

The mainstay of current therapy is mannitol, which was the first treatment demonstrated to improve survival in patients with FHF[21] (Fig. 83-2). By increasing cerebral capillary oncotic pressure, mannitol reduces the amount of water efflux into the interstitial space, resulting in lower ICPs. Mannitol (1 g/kg) usually is used in patients who have grade 4 encephalopathy, are intubated, and have appropriate monitoring of central venous pressure (CVP). Hypovolemic hypotension can be avoided by monitoring CVP and serum osmolarity and by ceasing mannitol infusion when osmolality exceeds 320 mOsm/L. In patients with renal failure, mannitol should be used only during continuous renal replacement therapy. In all patients, unnecessary free water should be avoided. Hypovolemia should be corrected using isotonic or hypertonic solutions.

Hyperventilation is no longer advocated to treat intracranial hypertension, except in a crisis (see Chaps. 65 and 93). Although hyperventilation is effective in the short term, tachyphylaxis follows. Moreover, the overall reduction in cerebral blood flow that results from hyperventilation-induced cerebral vasoconstriction may cause further disruption of the blood-brain barrier. The use of barbiturate coma is controversial, but it may be used in patients who have uncontrollable intracranial hypertension, often exacerbated by status epilepticus. Intentional hypothermia, sometimes used in conjunction with barbiturate coma to lower the metabolic demands of the brain, requires continuous electroencephalographic monitoring for titration of barbiturate doses to appropriate levels of sedation. There are many complications associated with barbiturate coma, including persistent post-transplant sedation, myocardial depression, and increased susceptibility to infection.[22] These patients should be placed on empirical prophylactic antimicrobial agents directed toward nosocomial organisms. Despite the risks, coma should be induced with barbiturates on an individualized basis in patients with refractory intracranial hypertension.

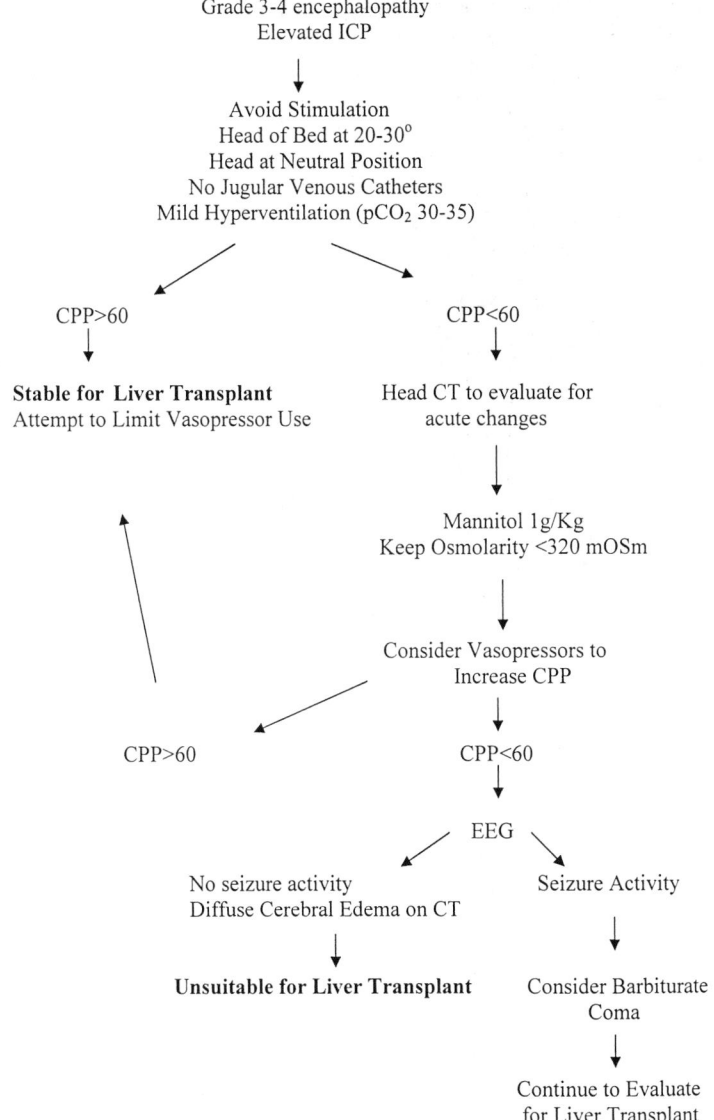

Grade 3-4 encephalopathy
Elevated ICP

Avoid Stimulation
Head of Bed at 20-30°
Head at Neutral Position
No Jugular Venous Catheters
Mild Hyperventilation (pCO$_2$ 30-35)

CPP>60

Stable for Liver Transplant
Attempt to Limit Vasopressor Use

CPP<60

Head CT to evaluate for
acute changes

Mannitol 1g/Kg
Keep Osmolarity <320 mOSm

Consider Vasopressors to
Increase CPP

CPP>60

CPP<60

EEG

No seizure activity
Diffuse Cerebral Edema on CT

Seizure Activity

Unsuitable for Liver Transplant

Consider Barbiturate
Coma

Continue to Evaluate
for Liver Transplant

FIGURE 83-2 Management of intracranial hypertension.

Hemodynamic Management

Progression of FHF may lead to significant hemodynamic instability. Often, the hemodynamic changes resemble those associated with septic shock and include a hyperdynamic heart and a decreased systemic vascular resistance. Episodes of hypotension require aggressive evaluation and correction to prevent cerebral hypoperfusion, worsening injury to the blood-brain barrier, and multisystem organ failure. Although FHF is itself a common cause of hypotension (perhaps mediated by endotoxin[23]), each episode must be evaluated critically in order to recognize new sepsis, hemorrhage, myocardial dysfunction, or arrhythmia.[24]

Contrary to the management of septic shock, aggressive volume resuscitation has undesirable effects in FHF patients. Hypervolemia may contribute to pulmonary and cerebral edema from hydrostatic forces. Therefore, central venous or pulmonary artery monitoring are necessary to guide fluid and vasoactive drug use. When the ICP is being measured, CPP serves as the major parameter for titration of fluid and vasoactive therapy (goal >60 mm Hg) rather than the MAP. N-Acetylcysteine has shown some benefit in hemodynamic stabilization and improved oxygen consumption in FHF patients,[25] but its use has not expanded beyond acetaminophen-induced FHF.

Renal Failure

Acute renal failure is a frequent occurrence in the patients with FHF and is associated with a poor prognosis.[26] The incidence of renal insufficiently approaches 75% among patients with acetaminophen-induced FHF and 30% to 50% among patients with FHF from other causes.[27] Prerenal azotemia, acute tubular necrosis, hepatorenal syndrome, and nephrotoxic drugs may contribute to renal dysfunction and should be treated. One should maintain adequate intravascular volume, avoid and eliminate nephrotoxic agents, and ensure renal perfusion. Difficulties in the management of acute renal failure in the setting of FHF arise when indications for acute hemodialysis are met. Significant fluctuations in hemodynamic pressure and ICP have been demonstrated with intermittent hemodialysis in patients with FHF.[28] For this reason, continuous renal replacement therapies (e.g. CVVHD) are preferred in this setting. Regardless of the method, baseline serum osmolarity should be monitored and maintained under tight control because rapid changes in osmolarity may exacerbate interstitial cerebral edema.

Respiratory Failure

The onset of hypoxic respiratory failure usually is associated with the development of multisystem organ failure and predicts an overall poor prognosis. As an isolated event, hypoxia may be attributed to atelectasis, aspiration, pulmonary hemorrhage, acute respiratory distress syndrome (ARDS), or pneumonia. Diagnostic and therapeutic bronchoscopy generally should be avoided in these patients because of the potential to raise the ICP dramatically.

In patients with significant pulmonary dysfunction, the decision on suitability for liver transplantation is based largely on oxygen requirement and control of sepsis rather than on radiographic appearance. However, the presence of hypoxemia requiring greater than 60% F_{IO_2} is likely to present difficulties with posttransplant management and survivability. During a liver transplant, reperfusion of a donor liver graft may exacerbate underlying pulmonary dysfunction, resulting in immediate right-sided heart failure. In addition, higher levels of positive end-expiratory pressure (PEEP) may reduce portal venous flow to the new graft,[29] provoking hepatoctye dysfunction. Thus preoperative assessment and optimization of respiratory function will have a significant impact on survival of a patient during and following liver transplantation.

Infectious Complications

Patients with FHF have a high incidence of bacterial and fungal infections. Most infections are diagnosed within 72 hours of hospital admission and commonly are localized to the respiratory and urinary tracts. Catheter-related sepsis is also common but usually occurs 72 hours after admission. Cultures often reveal Staphylococcus aureus, Staphylococcus epidermidis, and Candida spp. An analysis of infectious complications among patients with FHF revealed that up to 80% develop bacterial infections, whereas 30% develop fungal infections.[30] In addition, 18% of all patients with FHF ultimately died of infectious-related complications. Prevention, prophylaxis, and early detection are clearly the optimal approaches. Central venous catheters should be inserted using full barrier precautions and maintained with sterile technique (see Chaps. 4 and 12). When line sepsis is suspected, all lines must be removed and (if still necessary) replaced at alternative sites. Urinary catheters can be removed from anuric patients to limit the risk of an ascending urinary tract infection. We recommend prophylactic broad-spectrum antibiotic coverage at the time of hospital admission and adding antifungal coverage if sepsis develops while the patient is on the initial antibiotic regimen. This strategy is unproven and controversial, but it is supported by success in limiting postoperative infectious complications among patients with FHF.[31] Early initiation of prophylactic antibiotic therapy also can be justified on the basis that the development of infection may terminate a patient's candidacy for transplantation, the consequences of which may be lethal.

Systemic infection usually contraindicates transplantation because of the high level of immunosuppression subsequently required. However, this contraindication is not absolute when considering the patient with FHF because recovery depends so heavily on getting a transplant. Thus positive blood, urine, or respiratory cultures are acceptable in a patient urgently needing transplantation so long as there is no associated uncontrollable sepsis with hemodynamic instability. A further difficulty in the patient with FHF is assessing the severity of infection because some consequences of hepatic failure reduce the manifestations of infection (such as a reduced incidence of fever and leukocytosis), whereas others amplify them (such as vasodilatation and hyperdynamic circulation). Proceeding with transplantation in an infected patient with FHF must be a highly individualized decision, with clear delineation of the risk-benefit situation for all involved.

Liver Transplantation

The emergence of liver transplantation for the treatment of FHF has improved survival dramatically and should be considered the primary mode of therapy. Patients with evidence of encephalopathy should be referred to a tertiary care medical center with liver transplant capabilities and should be listed for emergency liver transplantation. The principal clinical dilemma is determining which patients with FHF should undergo liver transplantation and which patients will recover enough of their native livers to allow a reasonable chance of survival without transplantation. Adding to the complexity of decision making, the window of opportunity to benefit from a liver transplant is narrow. Therefore, the longer one waits to assess progress, the greater is the chance of missing the best treatment. One recent study demonstrated that the pretransplant median hospital stay was 3 days, whereas patients who did not receive a transplant died on median hospital day 5.[5] This underscores the need for prognostic indicators capable of predicting survivability of FHF without liver transplantation.

The U.S. Acute Liver Failure Study Group has presented data from 17 tertiary care centers on 308 consecutive patients with FHF.[5] The short-term patient survival was 67%. Twenty-nine percent of patients required liver transplantation, whereas 43% survived without transplantation. The only factor consistently associated with poor outcome was level of encephalopathy at the time of admission. Short-term transplant-free survival varied with the etiology of FHF. Patients with acetaminophen-induced FHF had a 68% survival compared with 25% and 17% for drug reaction and indeterminate-cause FHF, respectively. No consistent patient characteristic could be correlated with survivability without liver transplantation.

Attempts at developing criteria for determining the need for liver transplantation have met with only limited success. The Kings College criteria, developed after retrospective analysis of 580 patients with FHF, uses the following to predict outcome in non-acetaminophen-induced FHF: prothrombin time, age, etiology, time between onset of jaundice and onset of encephalopathy, and bilirubin levels. Criteria for patients with acetaminophen-induced FHF include factor V levels, blood pH, prothrombin time, serum creatinine concentration, and grade of encephalopathy. The Clichy criteria use factor V levels to assess severity of illness. Additional investigators have proposed alternative measurements, including serial prothrombin times,[32] factor VIII/V ratios,[33] serum Gc protein,[34] and Acute Physiology and Chronic Health Evaluation (APACHE) II score. Although both the Kings College and Clichy criteria identify factors that predict poor prognosis, neither provides a clear assessment of which individual patient will survive an episode of FHF without liver transplantation. Moreover, both criteria have failed to predict reproducibly which patients will or will not require liver transplantation.[35,36] Until better prognostic indicators can be developed to ascertain which patients with FHF will recover without liver transplantation, patients must be evaluated on a case-by-case basis.

Other Therapeutic Interventions

The high mortality associated with FHF has prompted the use of many innovative treatments in an effort to improve outcomes. Most of these treatments were embraced initially for their potential but failed in clinical trials. Some of these continue to be of interest for their potential benefit; none, however, are of proven benefit.

HIGH-VOLUME PLASMA EXCHANGE

High-volume plasma exchange is conducted similar to standard plasmapheresis protocols but with exchange volumes in excess of 8 L to improve the clearance of "harmful substances" that accumulate in FHF. The rationale for this approach is to reduce serum ammonia, control coagulopathy, and lower the metabolic demands on the injured liver. High-volume plasma exchange has been shown to reduce serum ammonia levels[37] and improve hemodynamics in the setting of FHF.[38] Although ammonia levels appear to be correlated with severity of encephalopathy, the exact mechanism involved is unknown.[39] In the pediatric population, high-volume plasma exchange has been shown to improve homeostasis and coagulation profiles.[40,41] All the studies have been uncontrolled, and none showed an improvement in overall survival. Randomized, controlled studies are needed before this potential treatment can be advocated.

STEROIDS

Steroid therapy has been tested under controlled conditions and does not confer benefit in clinical course or survival of patients with FHF.[42] Moreover, steroid therapy is ineffective for established cerebral edema.[43] Because steroids probably raise the risk of sepsis while being of no proven benefit, they have no role in the treatment of most FHF patients. One exception is the occasional patient with autoimmune hepatitis, in whom ongoing hepatic inflammation has culminated in FHF. For such patients, steroid therapy is beneficial and can significantly reverse liver failure.[44]

PROSTAGLANDIN E

Prostaglandins E_1 and E_2 (PGEs) have cytoprotective effects and raise hepatic arterial perfusion, both characteristics that could benefit FHF patient survival. However, two clinical trails from Europe and Canada have shown that use of PGEs is not associated with an improved outcome.[45,46] PGEs also may lower MAP, which could compromise CPP in patients with cerebral edema. Thus, until more compelling evidence is available, PGEs cannot be recommended.

AUXILIARY LIVER TRANSPLANTATION

Auxiliary liver transplantation has gained interest in Europe as a potential therapeutic option for FHF.[47] Essentially, a reduced-size liver graft, obtained from living or deceased donors, is transplanted without removal of the recipient's native liver. The potential advantage of this procedure is to provide temporary hepatic function while awaiting recovery of the native liver and then to halt immunosuppression, causing atrophy of the (now redundant) auxiliary liver graft. This approach has not been tested in controlled clinical trials, and it should only be carried out only in highly specialized liver transplant centers with experience in reduced-size and other innovative techniques in liver transplantation.

EXTRACORPOREAL LIVER SUPPORT

Extracorporeal liver-assist devices aim to provide temporary liver function as a bridge to liver transplant or to provide time for recovery of native liver function. There have been many different approaches to supporting liver function extracorporally, including ex vivo whole-organ perfusion,[48] nonbiologic systems using dialysis against charcoal and anion-exchange adsorption (Molecular Adsorbent Recirculating System [MARS][49]), combined nonbiologic-biologic systems that use both synthetic dialysis adsorption and hepatocyte cell mass (HepatAssist[50]), and purely biologic systems that use porcine hepatocytes (AMC Bioreactor[51]) or human hepatoma cell lines (ELAD).[52] Many of these systems continue to be investigational, but some are promising. The combined nonbiologic-biologic system HepatAssist was evaluated in the largest, randomized phase I and II trails reported for extracorporeal liver support systems. A total of 171 patients with FHF ($n = 147$) or primary nonfunction (PNF) ($n = 24$) following liver transplant were randomized to receive standard medical management or medical management with the addition of HepatAssist. Overall, there was no statistically significant survival difference between the groups. However, subgroup analysis demonstrated a significant improvement in outcome following liver transplant in the HepatAssist group and a considerable improvement in a secondary end point (time to death) in patients with acetaminophen toxicity who ultimately underwent liver transplantation. Although extracorporeal liver-assist systems retain promise, they are only available investigationally.

References

1. Caraceni P, Van Thiel DH: Acute liver failure. *Lancet* 345:163, 1995.
2. Trey C, Davidson LS: The management of fulminant hepatic failure, in Popper H, Shaffner F (eds): *Progress in Liver Disease.* New York, Grune and Sratton, 1970, p 282.
3. O'Grady JG, Schalm SW, Williams R: Acute liver failure: Redefining the syndromes. *Lancet* 342:273, 1993.
4. Tandon BN, Bernauau J, O'Grady J, et al: Recommendations of the International Association for the Study of the Liver subcommittee on nomenclature of acute and subacute liver failure. *J Gastroenterol Hepatol* 14:403, 1999.
5. Ostapowicz G, Fontan RJ, Schiodt FV, et al: Results of a prospective study of acute liver failure at 17 tertiary care centers in the United States. *Ann Intern Med* 137:947, 2002.
6. Zimmerman HJ, Maddrey WC: Acetaminophen hepatotoxicity with regular intake of alcohol: Analysis of instances of therapeutic misadventure. *Hepatology* 22:767, 1995.
7. Vento S, Garofano T, Renzini C, et al: Fulminant hepatitis associated with hepatitis A virus superinfection in patients with chronic hepatitis C. *New Engl J Med* 338:286, 1998.
8. Blei AT, Olafson S, Webster S, Levy R: Complications of intracranial pressure monitoring in fulminant hepatic failure. *Lancet* 341:157, 1993.
9. Harrison PM, Keays R, Bray GP, et al: Improved outcome of paracetamol-induced fulminant hepatic failure by late administraion of acetylcysteine. *Lancet* 335:1572, 1990.
10. Slattery JT, Wilson JM, Kalhorn TF, et al: Dose-dependent pharmokinetics of acetaminophen: Evidence of glutathione depletion in humans. *Clin Pharmacol Ther* 41:413, 1987.
11. Harrison PM, Keays P, Bray GP, et al: Improved outcome of paracetamol-induced fulminant hepatic failure by late administration of acetylcysteine. *Lancet* 335:1572, 1990.
12. Yip L, Dar RC, Hurlbut KM: Intravenous adminstration of oral N-acetyl-cysteine. *Crit Care Med* 26:40, 1998.
13. Schmidt LE, Knudsen TT, Dalhoff K, et al: Effect of acetylcysteine on prothrombin index in paracetamol poisoning without hepatocellular injury. *Lancet* 360:1151, 2002.
14. Kapoor D, Guptan RC, Wakil SM, et al: Beneficial effects of lamivudine in hepatitis B virus–related decompensated cirrhosis. *J Hepatol* 33:308, 2000.
15. Yao FY, Bass NM: Lamivudine treatment in patients with severely decompensated cirrhosis resulting from chronic hepatitis B. *J Hepatol* 33:301, 2000.
16. Tsang SW, Chan HL, Leung NW, et al: Lamivudine treatment for fulminant hepatic failure due to acute exacerbation of chronic hepatitis B infection. *Aliment Pharmacol Ther* 15:1737, 2001.
17. Larsen FS, Wendon J: Brain edema in liver failure: Basic physiologic principles and management. *Liver Transplant* 8:983, 2002.
18. Munoz S, Robinson M, Northup B, et al: Elevated intracranial pressure and computed tomography of the brain in fulminant hepatic failure. *Hepatology* 2:209, 1991.
19. Munoz SJ: Difficult management problems in fulminant hepatic failure. *Semin Liver Dis* 13:395, 1993.
20. Sadahiro T, Hirasawa H, Oda S, et al : Usefulness of plasma exchange plus continuous hemofiltration to reduce adverse effects associated with plasma exchange in patients with acute liver failure. *Crit Care Med* 29:1386, 2001.
21. Canalese J, Gimson AES, Davis C, et al: Controlled trial of dexamethasone and mannitol for the cerebral edema of fulminant hepatic failure. *Gut* 23:625, 1982.
22. Forbes A, Alexander G, O'Grady J, et al: Thiopental infusion in the treatment of intracranial hypertension complicating fulminant hepatic failure. *Hepatology* 10:306, 1989.
23. Wilkinson A, Arroyo V, Gazzard S, et al: Relation of renal impairment and haemorrhagic diathesis to endotoxemia in fulminant hepatic failure. *Lancet* 1:521, 1974.
24. Weston M, Talbot I, Howorth P, et al: Frequency of cardiac arrhythmias and other cardiac abnormalities in fulminant hepatic failure. *Br Heart J* 38:1179, 1976.
25. Harrison PH, Wendon JA, Gimson AES, et al: Improvement by acetylcysteine of hemodynamics and oxygen transport in fulminant hepatic failure. *New Engl J Med* 324:1852, 1991.
26. O'Grady J, Alexander G, Hayllar K, et al: Early indicators of prognosis in fulminant hepatic failure. *Gastroenterology* 97:439, 1985.
27. Mas A, Rodes J: Fulminant hepatic failure. *Lancet* 349:1081, 1997.
28. Davenport A, Davidson A, Swindells S, et al: Changes in intracranial pressure during haemofiltration in oliguric patients with grade IV encephalopathy. *Nephron* 53:142, 1989.
29. Brienza N, Revelly JP, Ayuse T, et al: Effects of PEEP on liver arterial and venous blood flows. *Am J Respir Crit Care Med* 152:504, 1995.
30. Rolando N, Harvey F, Brahm J, et al: Prospective study of bacterial infection in acute liver failure: An analysis of fifty patients. *Hepatology* 11:49, 1990.
31. Wiesner R: The incidence of gram-negative bacterial and fungal infections in liver transplant patients treated with selective decontamination. *Infection* 18(suppl 1):519, 1990.
32. Harrison P, O'Grady J, Keays R, et al: Serial prothrombin time as prognostic indicator in paracetamol-induced fulminant hepatic failure. *Br Med J* 301:964, 1990.
33. Bradbery S, Hart M, Bareford D, et al: Factor V and factor VIII ratio as prognostic indicator in paracetamol posioning. *Lancet* 346:646, 1995.
34. Lee W, Galbraith R, Watt G, et al: Predicting survival in fulminant hepatic failure using serum Gc protein concentrations. *Hepatology* 21:101, 1995.
35. Baily B, Amre D, Gaudreault P: Fulminant hepatic failure secondary to acetaminophen poisoning: A systematic review and meta-analysis of prognostic criteria determining the need for liver transplantation. *Crit Care Med* 31:299, 2003.

36. Pauwels A, Mostefa-Kara N, Florent C, et al: Emergency liver transplatation for acute liver failure: Evaluation of London and Clichy criteria. *J Hepatol* 17:124, 1993.

37. Clemmesen J, Kondrup J, Nielsen L, et al: Effects of high-volume plasmapheresis on ammonia, urea, and amino acids in patients with acute liver failure. *Am J Gastroenterol* 96:1217, 2001.

38. Clemmesen J, Larsen F, Ejlersen E, et al: Hemodynamic changes after high-volume plasmapheresis in patients with chronic and acute liver failure. *Eur J Gastroenterol Hepatol* 9:55, 1997.

39. Ong J, Aggarwal A, Krieger D, et al: Correlation between ammonia levels and severity of hepatic encephalopathy. *Am J Med* 114:188, 2003.

40. Singer A, Olthoff K, Haewon K, et al: Role of plasmapheresis in the management of acute hepatic failure in children. *Ann Surg* 234:418, 2001.

41. Mazzoni A, Pardi C, Bortoli M, et al : High-volume plasma exchange: An effective tool in acute liver failure treatment. *Int J Artif Organs* 8:814, 2002.

42. Ware A, Jones RE, Shorey JW, et al: A controlled trial of steroid therapy in massive hepatic necrosis. *Am J Gastroenterol* 62:130, 1974.

43. Canalesse J, Gimson AES, Davis C, et al : Controlled trial of dexamethasone and mannitol for the cerebral edema of fulminant hepatic failure. *Gut* 23:625, 1982.

44. Heneghan MA, McFarlane IG: Current and novel immunosuppressive therapy for autoimmune hepatitis. *Hepatology* 35:7, 2002.

45. Sheiner SB, Sinclair S, Greig P, et al: A randomized, controlled trial of prostaglandin E_2 (E_2) in the treatment of fulminant hepatic failure (FHF). *Hepatology* 16:88A, 1992.

46. Bernuau J, Babany G, Pauwels A, et al: Prostaglandin E_1 (PGE_1) has no beneficial effect in patients with either severe or fulminant hepatitis due to drugs or of undetermined etiology. *Hepatology* 12:373A, 1990.

47. Chenard-Neu MP, Boudjema K, Bernuau J, et al: Auxiliary liver transplantation: Regeneration of the native liver and outcome in 30 patients with fulminant hepatic failure. *Hepatology* 23:1119, 1996.

48. Horslen S, Hammel J, Firstoe L, et al: Extracorporeal liver perfusion using human and pig livers for acute liver failure. *Transplantation* 70:1472, 2000.

49. Awad S, Swaniker F, Magee J, et al: Results of a phase I trial evaluating a liver support device utilizing albumin dialysis. *Surgery* 130:354, 2001.

50. Stevens A, Busutill R, Hans S, et al: An interim analysis of a phase II/III prospective, randomized, multicenter, controlled trial of the HepatAssist bioartificial liver support system for the treatment of fulminant hepatic failure. *Hepatology* 34:299A, 2001.

51. Flendrig L, Calise F, DiFlorio E, et al: Significantly improved survival rime in pigs with complete liver ischemia treated with a novel bioartficial liver. *Int J Artif Organs* 22:701, 1999.

52. Millis JM, Cronin DC, Johnson R, et al : Initial experience with the modified extracorporeal liver-assist device for patients with fulminant hepatic failure: System modifications and clinical impact. *Transplantation* 74:1735, 2002.

Chapter 84 _____

MANAGEMENT OF THE PATIENT WITH CIRRHOSIS

ROHIT SATOSKAR
DAVID T. RUBIN

KEY POINTS

- *Patients with cirrhosis admitted to the ICU are at risk of death due not only to liver disease, but also due to the many complications to which such patients are at risk.*
- *Worsening encephalopathy and loss of the gag reflex are indications for elective intubation in order to forestall potentially catastrophic aspiration or respiratory arrest.*
- *Invasive procedures carry extra risk in cirrhotics. When a procedure must be performed, care should be taken to minimize the likelihood of hemorrhagic complications.*
- *Spontaneous bacterial peritonitis should be considered and excluded in all cirrhotics with fever, encephalopathy, abdominal pain, or sepsis.*
- *Neomycin and metronidazole are superior to lactulose for the treatment of hepatic encephalopathy.*
- *The MELD score is a reliable method for predicting 3-month mortality and is currently used to determine transplant status.*
- *Transplant candidates who are deteriorating from chronic liver disease or its complications should be transferred to a transplant center for management.*

Liver disease in the ICU may be secondary to the acute illness of patients or a complication of chronic disease. The focus of this chapter is to outline issues in the care of those with severe chronic liver disease, namely cirrhosis. Patients with cirrhosis who are admitted to the ICU have a very high risk of death. This stems not only from the underlying liver disease, but also from the complications to which these patients are prone. This chapter discusses the etiology of cirrhosis, the pathophysiology that leads to the complexity in management, common complications of cirrhosis, and a systematic approach to management of the critically ill liver patient. Hospitalized cirrhotic patients are more likely to die or to develop sepsis and respiratory failure than similar patients without cirrhosis. Due to the wide variety of complications and disease manifestations experienced by cirrhotic patients in the intensive care unit, a multidisciplinary approach involving gastroenterologists, hepatologists, intensivists, and transplant physicians must be employed. Particular attention should be given to preventing infection, assuring adequate nutrition and airway protection, and aggressively treating established infection, ascites, electrolyte disturbances, coagulopathy, encephalopathy, and bleeding.

Transfer to ICU

Patients with stable chronic liver disease may suffer from decompensation due to progression of the underlying liver disease or to a comorbid illness that overwhelms the reserve of the diseased liver. Decompensation may be characterized by acute deterioration of otherwise stable clinical parameters such as mental status, coagulation, or hemodynamics. These patients may deteriorate rapidly, and therefore should be monitored closely with a low threshold for transfer to the ICU. Indications for transfer to the ICU include hemodynamic instability, suspected sepsis, decline in mental status, and need for more intensive nursing care.

Etiology

The etiology of cirrhosis can vary greatly (Table 84-1) yet the clinical manifestations and complications due to scarring and fibrosis are similar. Therefore the approach to treatment and management of the cirrhotic is similar no matter what the underlying basis of the liver disease.

Pathophysiology of Portal Hypertension

The majority of complications in patients with cirrhosis arise from hemodynamic changes. The hemodynamic changes seen in cirrhosis can be divided into portal hypertension and a systemic hyperdynamic state. Most cirrhotic patients have increased resistance to portal blood flow as a result of intraparenchymal fibrosis and architectural distortion. In healthy livers, the portal vein comprises approximately two-thirds of the blood flow to the liver, carrying poorly oxygenated but nutrient rich blood from the gut, while the hepatic artery delivers the remaining one-third with primarily oxygen rich blood. The delivered blood enters at the portal triad and subsequently feeds the hepatic sinusoids. The progressive fibrosis associated with many chronic liver diseases eventually results in bridging between portal tracts and subsequent increased resistance to blood flow. As the portocaval gradient increases above the normal range of 2 to 6 mm Hg, collateral blood flow develops that may cause variceal bleeding and encephalopathy.

The hemodynamic state seen in cirrhosis results from decreased effective circulating volume due to massive splanchnic dilation. The forward increase in capillary pressure results in increased lymph oncotic pressure, contributing to production of ascites. The response of the kidneys to arterial underfilling results in activation of the renin-angiotensin system, further contributing to sodium and water retention, and may cause hepatorenal syndrome.

Cirrhosis is also accompanied by systemic circulatory dysfunction, owing largely to splanchnic arterial vasodilation. Nitric oxide (NO), a potent vasodilator elevated in the splanchnic circulation of cirrhotic patients, is thought to reduce the effective arterial blood volume and activate compensatory vasoconstrictors and antinatriuretic factors. Fluid and sodium retention as well as renal dysfunction follow as consequences of arterial underfilling. Hypoalbuminemia and increased splanchnic lymphatic hydrostatic pressure combine with sodium retention to produce ascites and edema.

TABLE 84-1 Causes of Cirrhosis

Alcohol
Chronic viral hepatitis
Chronic biliary obstruction
    Primary biliary cholangitis
    Primary sclerosing cholangitis
    Chronic cholestasis
Autoimmune hepatitis
Metabolic and inherited causes
    Wilson disease
    α_1-Antitrypsin deficiency
    Hemochromatosis
    Glycogen storage diseases
    Cystic fibrosis
Drugs and toxins
    Methotrexate
    Amiodarone
Nonalcoholic steatohepatitis (NASH)
Cryptogenic/idiopathic
Venous outflow obstruction
    Budd-Chiari syndrome
    Veno-occlusive disease
    Severe right-sided heart failure

General Supportive Measures

SURVEILLANCE FOR INFECTION

Infection is common in patients suffering from chronic liver disease. Analysis of 1.7 million patients with cirrhosis from the National Hospital Discharge Summary reveals that patients with cirrhosis are more likely to have hospitalizations associated with sepsis (adjusted relative risk [RR] 2.6) and to die from sepsis (adjusted RR 2.0) than patients without cirrhosis. Other studies have corroborated that patients with cirrhosis who develop bacterial sepsis in the ICU setting are more likely to die than those without cirrhosis.[1] Urinary tract infection is the most frequently encountered, followed by infections of ascites, blood, and the respiratory tract.[2]

The increased incidence of infection leads to both longer hospital stays and increased mortality. While the incidence of infection is elevated in all patients with cirrhosis, patients whose hepatic disease is secondary to alcohol use appear to have an elevated risk.[3] Specific to the ICU setting, the use of invasive monitoring techniques and instrumentation places the patient at even higher risk for introduction of infection.

PATHOPHYSIOLOGY
The propensity for infection in cirrhotic patients is believed due to decreased complement levels, impaired phagocytic activity of macrophages, and impaired neutrophil activity. A prospective study of 49 cirrhotic patients showed that the function of macrophage Fcγ receptors is impaired, resulting in decreased phagocytic ability.[4] The presence of extensive portosystemic collaterals that bypass the reticuloendothelial system, decreased complement levels due to poor hepatic synthesis, and ineffective opsonization may also contribute to the cirrhotic patient's heightened risk of infection.

MANAGEMENT RECOMMENDATIONS
All decompensating patients with cirrhosis should be closely investigated for infection by obtaining cultures of blood, urine, and ascites; analyzing urine and ascitic fluid; examining invasive hardware; and when appropriate, imaging potential sources of sepsis. Patients who exhibit fever or signs of impending sepsis should be treated with broad-spectrum antimicrobial therapy pending confirmation of infection.

AIRWAY PROTECTION

Decompensated cirrhotics often develop airway compromise and respiratory failure. Worsening of hepatic encephalopathy, aspiration, variceal bleeding, and the consequences of sepsis can precipitate respiratory decompensation. Progressively worsening mental status or loss of gag reflex are indications for intubation. Timely elective intubation in such a situation, or prior to high-risk procedures such as endoscopy, can prevent catastrophic respiratory deterioration. Analysis of large numbers of cirrhotic patients has revealed that underlying chronic liver disease places patients at higher risk for acute respiratory failure and resultant death.[5] In addition, cirrhosis is an independent predictor of death in patients who meet criteria for acute respiratory distress syndrome.[6]

COAGULOPATHY

Coagulopathy in patients with chronic liver disease generally arises from low levels of circulating clotting factors secondary to decreased hepatic synthesis. In addition, the risk for bleeding may be increased by underlying malnutrition and vitamin K deficiency as well as thrombocytopenia due to splenic sequestration. All patients with chronic liver disease and an elevated prothrombin time should receive parenteral vitamin K to correct any underlying vitamin K deficiency. In the setting of severe cholestasis, oral vitamin K may be absorbed poorly and unreliably. Great care must be taken when contemplating invasive procedures so that only truly necessary procedures are performed, experienced practitioners are available to perform or supervise them, and that reasonable measures to reduce hemorrhagic risk are taken when practical. Actively bleeding cirrhotics should be transfused with fresh frozen plasma and platelets, guided when possible by measurements of coagulation and platelet count. Since underlying coagulopathy and mechanical ventilation are independent risk factors for gastrointestinal bleeding,[7] our practice is to use H_2 blockers or proton pump inhibitors prophylactically to reduce this risk. Variceal hemorrhage, a catastrophic complication of portal hypertension, is discussed fully in Chap. 82.

NUTRITION

Decreased oral intake as well as underproduction may cause protein calorie malnutrition. The severity of underlying liver disease correlates directly with its degree. In addition, the increasing severity of malnutrition predicts mortality. The majority of cirrhotic patients in the ICU will already have some degree of preexisting malnutrition so that every effort should be made to prevent further deterioration. Unfortunately, even enteral supplementation late in the setting of advanced cirrhosis appears to have no benefit on survival.[8]

TABLE 84-2 Diagnostic Paracentesis

Always Send	Sometimes Send	Rarely Send	Unhelpful
Cell count	Lactate dehydrogenase	Cytology	pH
Culture	Amylase	Triglycerides	Lactate
Total protein	Gram stain	Tuberculosis smear/culture	Tumor markers
Albumin (on first paracentesis)	Glucose	Adenosine deaminase	Cholesterol

Complications of Cirrhosis

ASCITES

The majority of patients with cirrhosis will have ascites at presentation. Ascites can be detected on physical examination using various techniques. In patients with known cirrhosis and a largely distended or tense abdomen, the presence of ascites may be obvious, but in other patients percussion of the abdomen for flank dullness or shifting dullness and the presence of a fluid wave can confirm the diagnosis. However, physical exam is not a sensitive way to determine the presence or absence of a mild or moderate amount of ascites. Ultrasound provides a readily available, quick, and inexpensive way to determine the amount and location of ascites and to facilitate paracentesis. Computed tomography also shows the presence and extent of ascites, but is more cumbersome than ultrasound.

DIAGNOSTIC PARACENTESIS

Examination of ascitic fluid is crucially important in the cirrhotic with new-onset ascites, clinical deterioration, change in mental status, or fever. This procedure can be performed using a commercial kit or by using a 14- to 18-gauge IV catheter. The peritoneal cavity can be entered in the midline (infraumbilical) or in the lower quadrants, taking care to avoid the inferior epigastric vessels and any grossly dilated abdominal wall veins. Ascitic fluid obtained from a diagnostic paracentesis should be sent for cell count, culture, and total protein concentration. Inoculating blood culture bottles at the bedside prior to sending them to the laboratory increases clinical yield.[9] Other tests that may be helpful in selected situations are highlighted in Table 84-2. Large-volume ascites and the presence of a tense abdomen are indications for large-volume paracentesis, especially when the patient's respiratory status is compromised due to the restrictive effect on the diaphragm.

SPONTANEOUS BACTERIAL PERITONITIS

One of the primary reasons to perform diagnostic paracentesis in the ICU is to detect the presence of infection, most importantly spontaneous bacterial peritonitis (SBP). SBP should be suspected in a cirrhotic with fever, abdominal pain, encephalopathy, or acute hemodynamic decompensation. Previous studies have shown that regardless of the reason a patient with cirrhosis requires admission to the hospital, a diagnostic paracentesis will reveal evidence of SBP in 7% to 17%, so any patient with ascites who is transferred to the ICU should be monitored carefully for SBP.[10] Definitive diagnosis of SBP is made by finding >250 polymorphonuclear leukocytes (PMNs)/mm³ on diagnostic paracentesis, as well as a culture positive for a single organism. If only one of the above criteria is met the condition is termed culture-negative neutrocytic ascites or bacterascites, respectively (Table 84-3), but this is generally treated the same as confirmed SBP. Culture of more than one bacterial species should prompt suspicion for secondary peritonitis or perforated viscus. The bacterial pathogens that cause SBP are typically *Escherichia coli* (43%), *Streptococcus* species (23%), or *Klebsiella pneumoniae* (11%). Anaerobic organisms, *Enterococcus* spp., and *Pseudomonas* spp. are rarely involved. Treatment of SBP requires parenteral antibiotics that cover these common pathogens. Those with evidence of SBP should be treated with an intravenous third-generation cephalosporin such as cefotaxime at a dose of 2 g IV every 8 hours.[11] Treatment for 5 days appears equivalent to a longer regimen of 10 days.[12] Evidence also suggests that patients at risk for SBP (i.e., ascitic protein <1 g/dL, gastrointestinal hemorrhage, and previous episode of SBP) should be given prophylaxis with an oral fluoroquinolone.[13] Unfortunately, increasing frequency of quinolone-resistant SBP and gram-positive infection, especially in the ICU setting, may be related to such long-term prophylaxis.[14] Once a particular organism is identified, antibiotic coverage can be narrowed. In patients who do not adequately respond or continue to worsen on empiric antibiotic

TABLE 84-3 Diagnosis of Peritonitis

	Spontaneous Bacterial Peritonitis	Culture-Negative Neutrocytic Ascites	Bacterascites	Secondary Peritonitis
PMN count (cells/mm³)	>250	>250	<250	>250
Culture	Single organism	Negative	Single organism	Multiple organisms
Protein	Usually low	Usually low	Usually low	Usually >1g/dL
LDH	Normal	Normal	Normal	High
Glucose	Normal	Normal	Normal	Low
Treatment	Third-generation cephalosporin	Third-generation cephalosporin	Directed antibiotics	Empiric broad-spectrum antibiotics, surgical intervention

LDH, lactate dehydrogenase; PMN, polymorphonuclear leukocyte.

coverage, the antibiotic regimen should be revised and alternative bases for treatment failure considered.

MANAGEMENT OF ASCITES

Sodium restriction and diuretics are first-line treatments in the management of ascites. Patients should not receive more than 2 g sodium (88 mEq) per day. Optimal treatment usually involves the combination of spironolactone with a loop diuretic. It is our practice to maintain a ratio of 40 mg of oral furosemide to 100 mg of oral spironolactone. In patients with severe liver compromise, spironolactone should only be administered once daily, as the half-life is increased by hepatic insufficiency. These doses can be increased to 160 mg of furosemide and 400 mg of spironolactone daily if the patient has stable renal function. The dose of diuretics should be reduced if the patient develops increasing hyponatremia or worsening renal function.[15]

DIURETIC-RESISTANT AND RECURRENT ASCITES

Repeated large-volume paracentesis of up to 4 to 6 L/day can be performed safely in patients who are diuretic resistant or difficult to control. Postparacentesis circulatory dysfunction, characterized by decreased peripheral vascular resistance, increased plasma renin activity, hyponatremia, and azotemia has been described in patients receiving large-volume paracentesis without volume expansion.[16,17] Paracentesis of 6 L or more should be supplemented by intravenous albumin at 6 to 8 g per liter removed. In patients undergoing paracentesis of less than 6 L, no fluid replacement may be needed or normal saline can be given.[18] Transjugular intrahepatic portosystemic shunting (TIPSS) should be considered for patients who are unable to tolerate diuretics or are diuretic resistant.[19]

COMPLICATIONS OF PARACENTESIS

Paracentesis is considered a relatively safe procedure, with the most common complication being persistent drainage from the abdominal wall. Significant bleeding complications even in patients with thrombocytopenia and coagulopathy are rare, so it is not necessary to routinely administer blood products to all patients.[20] Abdominal wall hematoma and hemoperitoneum occur rarely and may require investigation in patients who develop severe hemodynamic instability after paracentesis.

ELECTROLYTE DISTURBANCES

HYPONATREMIA

Up to 30% of cirrhotic patients with ascites have hyponatremia. Elevated levels and increased half-life of vasopressin contribute to the inability to excrete free water. Even modest decreases in serum sodium may have an adverse effect on hepatic encephalopathy. In general, severe hyponatremia indicates a poor prognosis. The presence of this electrolyte abnormality becomes more important in the ICU when diuretics, fluids for nutrition, or vasopressin analogues are given for sepsis or variceal bleeding. Patients with moderate to severe hyponatremia should be placed on free water restriction with strict monitoring of input and output.[21] Diuretics should be given judiciously and use of vasopressin analogues should be limited. Recent studies of an orally active vasopressin V2 receptor antagonist suggest that this therapy has promise in correcting hyponatremia and fluid overload in this patient population.[22]

HYPERKALEMIA

Widespread use of potassium-sparing diuretics and predisposition to development of renal failure in severe liver disease can cause hyperkalemia. As in any other setting, severe hyperkalemia is a relative emergency and should be managed accordingly. Potassium-sparing diuretics should be discontinued with the knowledge that the half-life of drugs such as spironolactone is increased in the setting of liver disease. Sodium polystyrene compounds may be used cautiously with attention given to further sodium and water retention.[23]

HEPATIC ENCEPHALOPATHY

Cirrhosis is frequently complicated by the presence of hepatic encephalopathy (HE) or portosystemic encephalopathy (PSE). HE can be characterized as a range of neurologic and psychiatric disorders caused by underlying severe liver disease in the absence of other known neurologic disease. In cirrhosis, HE is generally reversible if a precipitant can be determined.

PATHOPHYSIOLOGY

Though HE is commonly recognized clinically, the lack of standardization to describe the syndrome has led to difficulty in determining the pathophysiology and performing valid clinical trials. HE in chronic liver disease likely results from the actions of circulating substances on the brain that are normally cleared by the working liver. Ammonia has long been implicated in the pathogenesis of encephalopathy, though serum levels tend to correlate poorly with grade of encephalopathy. Evidence currently suggests that the astrocyte is a key to the development of hepatic encephalopathy. Astrocytes treated in vitro with ammonia show morphologic changes similar to those seen in vivo in both humans and animals with chronic liver disease and HE. These changes also include alterations seen in Alzheimer's type II astrocytosis. Changes in astrocytes, which normally regulate the extracellular environment and excitability of neurons, result in changes in neurotransmission. Elevated serum ammonia levels decrease glutamate uptake by astrocytes and increase extracellular glutamate concentrations. These changes in glutamate metabolism may be responsible for the disordered neurotransmission seen in HE. Other studies have implicated increased tone at γ-aminobutyric acid (GABA) receptors due to endogenously-derived benzodiazepines in HE. The peripheral-type benzodiazepine (PBR) receptor, located on the outer mitochondrial membrane of astrocytes, has been shown to be upregulated both in postmortem human brains from encephalopathic patients, and in vitro by astrocytes exposed to ammonia. The PBR is intimately involved in regulating synthesis of neurosteroids, which are potent ligands of the GABA-A receptor. Finally, in vitro, astrocytes exposed to elevated manganese levels show similar changes in glutamate uptake to those exposed to ammonia. Interestingly, the increased signal seen on T1 magnetic resonance imaging of the basal ganglia in the majority of cirrhotic patients has been attributed to manganese, and suggests that it has a role in the pathogenesis of HE.[24–27]

CLINICAL MANIFESTATIONS

Due to the lack of standardization in defining and clinically diagnosing HE, a working party was assembled in 1998 and recently published a consensus statement. Type A encephalopathy is defined as that associated with acute liver failure. Type B encephalopathy is that associated with portosystemic bypass in the absence of underlying hepatocellular disease. Type C encephalopathy is that associated with cirrhosis and portal hypertension or portosystemic shunts. Type C hepatic encephalopathy, the focus of this chapter, is further subdivided into minimal, episodic, and persistent. Episodic encephalopathy can further be divided into spontaneous (without a known precipitant), precipitated, and recurrent. Precipitants include drugs that alter mental status, GI bleeding, overdiuresis, azotemia, electrolyte abnormalities, or infection. Recurrent encephalopathy is defined as two or more episodes occurring within 1 year. Minimal encephalopathy is brain dysfunction in the absence of clinical symptoms. Stages of hepatic encephalopathy can range from derangements only detectable by psychometric testing to overt coma. Early findings may include depression, reversal of the sleep-wake cycle, or difficulty concentrating. As encephalopathy worsens, physical signs such as asterixis and "milk-maid's grip" become apparent. Still later, the patient may progress to increasing confusion, obtundation, and overt coma.[28] In the intensive care unit, protection of the airway is most critical in patients entering the later stages of encephalopathy (stages 3 and 4). Patients who have lesser degrees of encephalopathy in the setting of cirrhosis should be treated and offending factors removed to prevent escalation of the problem (Table 84-4).

TREATMENT

The presence of worsening encephalopathy warrants a search for underlying precipitants (Table 84-5). If possible, psychoactive drugs such as narcotics and benzodiazepines should be discontinued immediately. Underlying occult and overt gastrointestinal bleeding and infection should also be ruled out and treated if present. Electrolyte abnormalities should be corrected. Once underlying precipitants have been sought and adequately managed, treatment of hepatic encephalopathy is aimed at reducing further absorption of toxins from the gut. Lactulose, a nonabsorbable disaccharide, can be administered orally every 1 to 2 hours until a bowel movement is produced. At this point, lactulose can be given at regular intervals to produce two to three soft bowel movements per day. Lactulose likely exerts its effects by reducing absorption

TABLE 84-5 Precipitants of Encephalopathy

Narcotics
Benzodiazepines
Alcohol
Gastrointestinal bleeding
Infection (spontaneous bacterial peritonitis, pneumonia, bacteremia)
Dehydration
Overdiuresis
Electrolyte abnormalities
Hepatic decompensation
Increased protein intake
Uremia
Acidosis
Portosystemic shunts
Constipation

of toxins from the gut, both by decreasing transit time through the gut, as well as by altering the luminal pH. The change in pH effectively converts intraluminal ammonia to a quaternary ion and hinders its absorption. Despite the widespread use of lactulose and other nonabsorbable disaccharides for HE, a recent review of 22 trials showed the benefit of these therapies to be mild or nil, and inferior to antibiotics.[29] Therefore if lactulose fails to improve encephalopathy, antibiotics such as neomycin and metronidazole, which presumably alter the gut flora, should be given.[30] More recently, a novel nonabsorbed antibiotic (rifaximin) has been studied in hepatic encephalopathy with encouraging results.[31] Although available in the U.S., this product is not yet FDA-approved for treatment of HE. Based on the "endogenous benzodiazepine" hypothesis of hepatic encephalopathy, the use of flumazenil, a benzodiazepine antagonist, has been studied and may have some beneficial effects in severe HE. A randomized, placebo-controlled study of 527 cirrhotic patients with stage 3 and 4 encephalopathy revealed improvement of both neurologic and electroencephalographic scores after administration of flumazenil with lactulose. Use of flumazenil in unselected patients with hepatic encephalopathy has not been validated.[32]

HEPATORENAL SYNDROME

Renal dysfunction occurs at a high rate in patients with advanced cirrhosis. In the setting of advanced liver disease, hepatorenal syndrome (HRS) is defined as the development of

TABLE 84-4 Stages of Encephalopathy

	Findings	Asterixis	EEG Changes
Stage 0	No detectable changes in personality or behavior	Absent	None
Stage I	Depression, changes in sleep-wake cycle, behavioral changes, inattention, poor concentration	Usually absent	Usually none
Stage II	Mild somnolence or lethargy, inappropriate behavior	Grossly present	Diffuse slowing
Stage III	Increased somnolence, gross disorientation	Present or Absent	Abnormal
Stage IV	Coma	Absent	Abnormal

EEG, electroencephalographic.

renal failure with normal renal histology in the absence of nephrotoxic drugs, sepsis, intrinsic renal disease, and hypovolemia. Hepatorenal syndrome usually occurs in the setting of advanced liver disease with ascites and is often a lethal complication. It occurs in up to 39% of patients with underlying cirrhosis and ascites within 5 years.[33] Hepatorenal syndrome is divided into two types, based on severity of kidney dysfunction. Type I hepatorenal syndrome is rapidly progressive, defined as doubling of the serum creatinine level to >2.5 mg/dL or a 50% reduction in 24-hour creatinine clearance to a level <20 mL/min in less than 2 weeks. Type II HRS progresses slowly and renal function may remain stable for extended periods of time. Precipitants of hepatorenal syndrome may include excessive diuresis, use of prostaglandin inhibitors such as nonsteroidal anti-inflammatory drugs, and large-volume paracentesis or underlying critical illness such as sepsis, hypovolemia, or gastrointestinal bleeding. Severe electrolyte abnormalities (e.g., hyponatremia) and fluid overload are common once renal dysfunction is established, and these must be frequently sought and treated. Medications affected by renal dysfunction may require dose reduction.

PATHOPHYSIOLOGY

The pathogenesis of hepatorenal syndrome appears to be due to severe renal vasoconstriction and decreased renal perfusion. In the peripheral vasodilation model of advanced liver disease, the kidneys perceive a persistent prerenal state and adapt accordingly through vasoconstriction. Activation of the renin-angiotensin system results in increased levels of angiotensin and aldosterone. Levels of antidiuretic hormone and norepinephrine also increase, causing severe renal vasoconstriction. As a consequence, sodium and water retention is exaggerated, exacerbating both ascites and peripheral edema. Early in cirrhosis, the kidneys adapt by overproducing renal prostaglandins, resulting in renal vasodilation and preservation of renal perfusion and function. The importance of prostaglandins in preserving renal function explains the cirrhotic patient's increased sensitivity to the effects of prostaglandin inhibitors such as nonsteroidal anti-inflammatory drugs. As liver disease progresses and splanchnic vasodilation predominates, the heightened effects of potent vasoconstrictors dominate the kidney and override the prostaglandin effect, leading to the hepatorenal syndrome.[34]

DIAGNOSIS

Hepatorenal syndrome is diagnosed in the setting of advanced liver disease by excluding other causes of renal failure. In the ICU, patients may have multiple reasons for renal failure. Other causes need to be systematically excluded prior to delivering a diagnosis of HRS. In diagnosing HRS, underlying intrinsic renal disease should be ruled out by examining urine sediment and imaging the kidneys with ultrasound. Nephrotoxicity due to drugs such as aminoglycosides, cyclosporine, and tacrolimus should also be considered. Hypovolemia can closely mimic HRS and deserves special mention here. Patients should be given a fluid challenge of 1.5 L normal saline with repeat measurement of serum creatinine. No change in the value supports the diagnosis of HRS. Acute tubular necrosis, commonly seen in the critical care setting, can be differentiated from HRS through measurement of the urine sodium. Urine sodium is usually <10 mEq/L in HRS and >20 mEq/L in acute tubular necrosis. In 1998, the International Ascites Club proposed consensus criteria for diagnosis of HRS. In addition to the presence of chronic or acute liver disease with advanced hepatic failure and portal hypertension, major criteria include: (1) serum creatinine >1.5 or creatinine clearance <40 mL/min, (2) absence of shock, bacterial infection, nephrotoxic drugs and fluid losses, (3) no improvement in serum creatinine following withdrawal of diuretics and 1.5 L fluid challenge with normal saline, and (4) proteinuria <500 mg/dL and normal renal ultrasound.[35]

PREVENTION

While prevention of HRS largely depends on the natural history of the underlying liver disease, the setting of spontaneous bacterial peritonitis warrants special consideration. One third of patients with SBP will develop some degree of renal impairment.[36] Recent evidence suggests that intravenous albumin administration during treatment of SBP can prevent development of renal impairment. In a study of 126 patients with cirrhosis and SBP, administration of intravenous albumin along with an antibiotic resulted in a decreased development of renal impairment and decreased mortality. Patients were randomized to receive cefotaxime or cefotaxime plus intravenous albumin (1.5 g/kg on day 1, followed by 1 g/kg on day 3). Rates for development of nonreversible renal impairment during hospitalization were 33% vs. 10% in the antibiotic and antibiotic plus albumin groups, respectively. At 3 months, the mortality rate for the combined treatment group was nearly half that of the antibiotic-alone group.[37]

TREATMENT

Of the complications of cirrhosis, HRS has the worst prognosis. Expected median survival time is 2 weeks and 6 months for type I and II HRS, respectively. Liver transplantation is the only definitive means for reversal and cure of HRS. Unfortunately, in the critically ill, concomitant factors such as sepsis may render the patient unsuitable for transplant. Generally, patients in the ICU with HRS should have aggressive monitoring of fluid balance and weight, as well as evaluation and treatment of electrolyte abnormalities. Fluid overload and refractory ascites are common in patients with HRS. Patients with type I HRS should be managed with fluid restriction to avoid a positive fluid balance. Fluid overload in type II HRS can be managed with diuretics as long as a significant natriuresis is obtained. Potassium-sparing diuretics should be discontinued or used very cautiously in both groups to avoid hyperkalemia. Renal replacement therapy may be needed for patients with severe electrolyte disturbance, fluid overload, or acidosis. Vasoconstrictor therapy has been relatively well studied in the treatment of HRS. The theory behind treatment with vasoconstrictors suggests that administration results in constriction of the dilated splanchnic circulation, alleviating the intense vasoconstriction caused by endogenous vasoconstrictors released by the renal axis. Both vasopressin analogues and α-adrenergic agonists in combination with intravenous albumin have been studied in this setting. Terlipressin, a vasopressin analogue that acts at V1 receptors, when administered with albumin, resulted in improved renal function in 60% of patients, suppression of the renin-angiotensin and sympathetic systems, and a survival advantage in those who responded. Complete responders to terlipressin treatment have a low recurrence rate of HRS. While median survival time is only increased moderately, this may allow enough time for definitive treatment by liver transplantation.[38,39] The use of midodrine, an orally administered α-adrenergic agonist, along with octreotide also improved renal function for a large majority of patients, while octreotide alone seems to have no effect.[40,41] The use of TIPSS appears to improve renal function in patients with both type I and II HRS.[42,43] In type I HRS, TIPSS should be considered in patients who fail to respond to vasoconstrictors. In type II HRS, TIPSS results in decreased progression to type I HRS, improved hemodynamics, and benefit for refractory ascites, but overall survival is unchanged compared to patients managed with repeated paracentesis and intravenous albumin.[43,44]

HEPATOPULMONARY SYNDROME

The relationship between severe liver disease and pulmonary abnormalities has long been recognized. Pulmonary disease secondary to hepatic injury can be divided into hepatopulmonary syndrome (HPS) and portopulmonary hypertension. Hepatopulmonary syndrome, characterized by an increased alveolar-arterial oxygen gradient (A-a)$_{O_2}$, varying degrees of hypoxemia, and pulmonary vasodilation in the setting of liver disease is more common than previously thought. Recent studies suggest that up to 47% of patients with cirrhosis have some degree of pulmonary vasodilation detectable by diagnostic studies.[45] The pathogenesis of the HPS lies in vasodilation of the capillary and precapillary beds of the lung due to increased circulating vasodilators such as nitric oxide (NO) in severe liver disease. In some patients, hypoxemia is seen due to dilation of the pulmonary vasculature that results in right-to-left shunting. In others, ventilation-perfusion mismatch causes hypoxemia, and other theories have been proposed. Clinical manifestations of HPS include platypnea, orthodeoxia, and reduced diffusing capacity for carbon monoxide. Platypnea, defined as dyspnea in the upright position that is relieved by lying supine, and orthodeoxia, which is defined as arterial deoxygenation in the upright position that is relieved by recumbancy, are seen in a majority of patients with severe hypoxemia. In the ICU setting, the importance of HPS lies in the increased mortality of these patients. A recent prospective study of 111 patients with cirrhosis showed that the presence and severity of HPS were independent risk factors for death.[46] HPS is diagnosed by demonstrating an increased age-adjusted (A-a)$_{O_2}$ along with intrapulmonary vascular dilation. Perfusion scanning using technetium 99m-labeled macroaggregated albumin and subsequent demonstration of uptake in the kidneys or brain suggests intracardiac or intrapulmonary shunt. More commonly and easily, the shunt may be demonstrated by contrast echocardiography using microbubbles. The presence of the microbubbles in the left side of the heart after four to six cardiac cycles demonstrates the intrapulmonary shunt.[47] Despite significant ventilation-perfusion mismatch, some cirrhotic patients may not manifest hypoxemia due to increased cardiac output and hyperventilation. This may bear on the cirrhotic patient who becomes critically ill, because as oxygen consumption rises or cardiac output becomes limited, the gas-exchange defect may become manifest.

TREATMENT

Medical therapies in general have proved ineffective for the treatment of HPS. Supplemental oxygen may only temporarily correct the underlying hypoxemia. For many years, hypoxemia has been a contraindication to liver transplantation. Recently, studies showing reversal of the findings of HPS in transplanted patients have resulted in rethinking of this doctrine.[48] As a result, HPS is an indication for orthotopic liver transplantation. However, perioperative complications are frequent in these patients, and at times the resolution of hypoxemia is very protracted, even following successful transplantation. Since the institution of the model for end-stage liver disease (MELD) score in 2002, the United Network for Organ Sharing now reviews cases of hepatopulmonary syndrome for possible assigning of additional points.

PORTOPULMONARY HYPERTENSION

Portopulmonary hypertension is the presence of mean pulmonary pressure >25 mm Hg in the presence of portal hypertension and the absence of left heart failure. The condition is present in 5% to 10% of patients undergoing evaluation for liver transplant. Overall, mortality is greatly increased, with a median survival time of 6 months.[49] Many medical therapies have been tried in the setting of portopulmonary hypertension, yet long-term studies and adequate guidelines are lacking. Intravenous prostacyclin, β-blockers, nitrates, and inhaled NO all show promise in treatment of this condition. Multiple reports show improvement of pulmonary artery pressure (PAP) after liver transplantation, but intraoperative and perioperative mortality is high for patients with a mean PAP >40.[50-52]

LIVER TRANSPLANTATION

Judging expected survival and allocating available donor livers for liver transplantation has historically raised questions rooted in both medicine and ethics. The Child-Turcotte-Pugh (CTP) classification, based on degree of encephalopathy, amount of ascites, serum bilirubin, albumin, and prothrombin time, predicts both survival and surgical risk in cirrhotic patients. Until 2002, the CTP classification was intricately tied to allocation of donor livers. Unfortunately, the classification inherently had values that lacked objectivity in predicting survival. The MELD score was developed prospectively, using methodologically accurate methods and continuous variables, in contrast to the CTP score, and is currently used to stratify potential liver recipients.[53]

MODEL FOR END-STAGE LIVER DISEASE

The model for end-stage liver disease (MELD), a purely objective measurement adopted by the Organ Procurement and Transplantation Network (OPTN) in 2002, has been validated in many studies to predict survival.[54] (Table 84-6). The MELD score is now used as one measure in allocation of donor livers

TABLE 84-6 Calculating the Model for End-Stage Liver Disease (MELD) Score

MELD score = [0.957 $\times$ Log$_e$(creatinine mg/dL)
$\qquad$ + 0.378 $\times$ Log$_e$(bilirubin mg/dL)
$\qquad$ + 1.120 $\times$ Log$_e$(International Normalized Ratio)
$\qquad$ + 0.643] $\times$ 10

Round to the nearest whole number. Laboratory values less than 1 are set to 1 for the purposes of the MELD score calculation. The maximum serum creatinine considered within the MELD score equation is 4 mg/dL.

and has been validated in patients on the transplantation waiting list. The MELD score predicts severity of liver disease based on serum creatinine, serum bilirubin, and International Normalized Ratio. The variable for etiology of liver disease has been omitted in the currently used classification. Three-month mortality with a MELD score <9 is 1.9%. Three-month mortality with a MELD score of ≥ 40 is 71%.[55,56]

References

1. Moreau R, et al: Septic shock in patients with cirrhosis: Hemo-dynamic and metabolic characteristics and intensive care unit outcome. *Crit Care Med* 20:746, 1992.

2. Borzio M, et al: Bacterial infection in patients with advanced cirrhosis: A multicentre prospective study. *Dig Liver Dis* 33:41, 2001.

3. Rosa H, et al: Bacterial infection in cirrhotic patients and its rela-tionship with alcohol. *Am J Gastroenterol* 95:1290, 2000.

4. Gomez F, Ruiz P, Schreiber AD: Impaired function of macrophage Fc gamma receptors and bacterial infection in alcoholic cirrhosis. *N Engl J Med* 331:1122, 1994.

5. Foreman MG, Mannino DM, Moss M: Cirrhosis as a risk factor for sepsis and death: Analysis of the National Hospital Discharge Survey. *Chest* 124:1016, 2003.

6. Monchi M, et al: Early predictive factors of survival in the acute respiratory distress syndrome. A multivariate analysis. *Am J Respir Crit Care Med* 158:1076, 1998.

7. Cook DJ, et al: Risk factors for gastrointestinal bleeding in crit-ically ill patients. Canadian Critical Care Trials Group. *N Engl J Med* 330:377, 1994.

8. Campillo B, et al: Evaluation of nutritional practice in hospitalized cirrhotic patients: Results of a prospective study. *Nutrition* 19:515, 2003.

9. Runyon BA, Canawati HN, Akriviadis EA: Optimization of ascitic fluid culture technique. *Gastroenterology* 95:1351, 1988.

10. Storgaard JS, et al: Incidence of spontaneous bacterial peritonitis in patients with ascites. Diagnostic value of white blood cell count and pH measurement in ascitic fluid. Liver 11:248, 1991.

11. Rimola A, et al: Diagnosis, treatment and prophylaxis of sponta-neous bacterial peritonitis: A consensus document. International Ascites Club. *J Hepatol* 32:142, 2000.

12. Guarner C, Runyon BA: Spontaneous bacterial peritonitis: Patho-genesis, diagnosis, and management. *Gastroenterologist* 3:311, 1995.

13. Choudhury J, Sanyal AJ: Treatment of ascites. *Curr Treat Options Gastroenterol* 6:481, 2003.

14. Fernandez J, et al: Bacterial infections in cirrhosis: Epidemiolog-ical changes with invasive procedures and norfloxacin prophy-laxis. *Hepatology* 35:140, 2002.

15. Moore KP, et al: The management of ascites in cirrhosis: Report on the consensus conference of the International Ascites Club. *Hepatology* 38:258, 2003.

16. Gines P, et al: Randomized comparative study of therapeutic paracentesis with and without intravenous albumin in cirrhosis. *Gastroenterology* 94:1493, 1988.

17. Ruiz-del-Arbol L, et al: Paracentesis-induced circulatory dysfunc-tion: Mechanism and effect on hepatic hemodynamics in cirrhosis. *Gastroenterology* 113:579, 1997.

18. Sola-Vera J, et al: Randomized trial comparing albumin and saline in the prevention of paracentesis-induced circulatory dysfunction in cirrhotic patients with ascites. *Hepatology* 37:1147, 2003.

19. Rossle M, et al: A comparison of paracentesis and transjugular intrahepatic portosystemic shunting in patients with ascites. *N Engl J Med* 342:1701, 2000.

20. Runyon BA: Paracentesis of ascitic fluid. A safe procedure. *Arch Intern Med* 146:2259, 1986.

21. Gines P, et al: Hyponatremia in cirrhosis: From pathogenesis to treatment. *Hepatology* 28:851, 1998.

22. Gerbes AL, et al: Therapy of hyponatremia in cirrhosis with a va-sopressin receptor antagonist: A randomized double-blind mul-ticenter trial. *Gastroenterology* 124:933, 2003.

23. Abbas Z, et al: Factors predicting hyperkalemia in patients with cirrhosis receiving spironolactone. *J Coll Physicians Surg Pak* 13:382, 2003.

24. Butterworth RF: Pathophysiology of hepatic encephalopathy: A new look at ammonia. *Metab Brain Dis* 17:221, 2002.

25. Butterworth RF: Pathogenesis of hepatic encephalopathy: New insights from neuroimaging and molecular studies. *J Hepatol* 39:278, 2003.

26. Norenberg MD: Astroglial dysfunction in hepatic encephalopa-thy. *Metab Brain Dis* 13:319, 1998.

27. Jalan R, Shawcross D, Davies N: The molecular pathogenesis of hepatic encephalopathy. *Int J Biochem Cell Biol* 35:1175, 2003.

28. Ferenci P, et al: Hepatic encephalopathy—definition, nomencla-ture, diagnosis, and quantification: Final report of the working party at the 11th World Congresses of Gastroenterology, Vienna, 1998. *Hepatology* 35:716, 2002.

29. Als-Nielsen B, Gluud LL, Gluud C: Non-absorbable disaccharides for hepatic encephalopathy: Systematic review of randomised tri-als. *BMJ* 328:1046, 2004.

30. Blei AT, Cordoba J: Hepatic encephalopathy. *Am J Gastroenterol* 96:1968, 2001.

31. Mas A, et al: Comparison of rifaximin and lactitol in the treat-ment of acute hepatic encephalopathy: Results of a randomized, double-blind, double-dummy, controlled clinical trial. *J Hepatol* 38:51, 2001.

32. Barbaro G, et al: Flumazenil for hepatic encephalopathy grade III and IVa in patients with cirrhosis: An Italian multicenter double-blind, placebo-controlled, cross-over study. *Hepatology* 28:374, 1998.

33. Gines A, et al: Incidence, predictive factors, and prognosis of the hepatorenal syndrome in cirrhosis with ascites. *Gastroenterology* 105:229, 1993.

34. Gines P, et al: Hepatorenal syndrome. *Lancet* 362:1819, 2003.

35. Arroyo V, et al: Definition and diagnostic criteria of refractory as-cites and hepatorenal syndrome in cirrhosis. International Ascites Club. *Hepatology* 23:164, 1996.

36. Follo A, et al: Renal impairment after spontaneous bacterial peri-tonitis in cirrhosis: Incidence, clinical course, predictive factors and prognosis. *Hepatology* 20:1495, 1994.

37. Sort P, et al: Effect of intravenous albumin on renal impairment and mortality in patients with cirrhosis and spontaneous bacterial peritonitis. *N Engl J Med* 341:403, 1999.

38. Moreau R, et al: Terlipressin in patients with cirrhosis and type 1 hepatorenal syndrome: A retrospective multicenter study. *Gas-troenterology* 122:923, 2002.

39. Ortega R, et al: Terlipressin therapy with and without albumin for patients with hepatorenal syndrome: Results of a prospective, nonrandomized study. *Hepatology* 36(4 Pt 1):941, 2002.

40. Angeli P, et al: Reversal of type 1 hepatorenal syndrome with the administration of midodrine and octreotide. *Hepatology* 29:1690, 1999.

41. Pomier-Layrargues G, et al: Octreotide in hepatorenal syndrome: A randomized, double-blind, placebo-controlled, crossover study. *Hepatology* 38:238, 2003.

42. Guevara M, et al: Reversibility of hepatorenal syndrome by pro-longed administration of ornipressin and plasma volume expan-sion. *Hepatology* 27:35, 1998.

43. Brensing KA, et al: Long term outcome after transjugular in-trahepatic portosystemic stent-shunt in non-transplant cirrhotics with hepatorenal syndrome: A phase II study. *Gut* 47:288, 2000.

44. Gines P, et al: Transjugular intrahepatic portosystemic shunting versus paracentesis plus albumin for refractory ascites in cirrho-sis. *Gastroenterology* 123:1839, 2002.

45. Lange PA, Stoller JK: The hepatopulmonary syndrome. *Ann Intern Med* 122:521, 1995.
46. Schenk P, et al: Prognostic significance of the hepatopulmonary syndrome in patients with cirrhosis. *Gastroenterology* 125:1042, 2003.
47. Krowka MJ, et al: Intrapulmonary vascular dilatations (IPVD) in liver transplant candidates. Screening by two-dimensional contrast-enhanced echocardiography. *Chest* 97:1165, 1990.
48. Taille C, et al: Liver transplantation for hepatopulmonary syndrome: A ten-year experience in Paris, France. *Transplantation* 75:1482, discussion 1446, 2003.
49. Robalino BD, Moodie DS: Association between primary pulmonary hypertension and portal hypertension: Analysis of its pathophysiology and clinical, laboratory and hemodynamic manifestations. *J Am Coll Cardiol* 17:492, 1991.
50. McGilvray ID, Greig PD: Critical care of the liver transplant patient: An update. *Curr Opin Crit Care* 8:178, 2002.
51. Kuo PC, et al: Portopulmonary hypertension and the liver transplant candidate. *Transplantation* 67:1087, 1999.
52. Budhiraja R, Hassoun PM: Portopulmonary hypertension: A tale of two circulations. *Chest* 123:562, 2003.
53. Pagliaro L: MELD: The end of Child-Pugh classification? *J Hepatol* 36:141, 2002.
54. Kamath PS, et al: A model to predict survival in patients with end-stage liver disease. *Hepatology* 33:464, 2001.
55. Wiesner R, et al: Model for end-stage liver disease (MELD) and allocation of donor livers. *Gastroenterology* 124:91, 2003.
56. Malinchoc M, et al: A model to predict poor survival in patients undergoing transjugular intrahepatic portosystemic shunts. *Hepatology* 31:864, 2000.

Chapter 85 _____

ACUTE PANCREATITIS IN THE CRITICALLY ILL

BRYCE R. TAYLOR

KEY POINTS

- *Hypoperfusion injury is the most important of many possible causes of pancreatitis in the ICU setting.*
- *Serial computed tomography is most useful in confirming the diagnosis and in following the inflammatory process.*
- *The likelihood of multisystem failure is high, and preventive measures must be instituted early.*
- *Initial treatment is supportive, with aggressive fluid and electrolyte replacement and close monitoring of hemodynamic, pulmonary, and renal status.*
- *Surgical intervention is indicated for deteriorating patients with a surgically correctable lesion and in patients with complications of the disease, such as major hemorrhage, abscess, or symptomatic pseudocyst.*
- *Close supervision by an experienced abdominal surgeon in collaboration with an intensivist is important in recognizing the indications for surgical exploration.*

Acute pancreatitis can be a frustrating disease to diagnose and treat. Causes are myriad and poorly understood, pathologic variation is great, diagnosis is often difficult, and treatment in most cases is nonspecific and supportive only. Pancreatitis usually presents as a self-limiting disease from which the patient recovers without complication or intervention. In its most severe form (approximately 10% of cases), it is a potentially lethal disease that is complicated by multisystem failure and sepsis, often requires sophisticated intensive care and judiciously timed surgical débridement, and has a mor-

tality rate of up to 30% to 40%.[1–4] Most intensivists therefore are quite familiar with the patient who presents with acute necrotizing pancreatitis and who may occupy a bed for many months, often ultimately dying of septic complications[5] that are generalized or are related to the secondary infection of pancreatic necrosis.[6]

The subject of this chapter is the increasingly recognized entity of acute pancreatitis in the patient who is already critically ill from other causes. Discussion will focus on the associated diseases reported to date, the pathogenesis of this unusual form, its recognition, and its management.

Etiology

Many causes of acute pancreatitis have been recognized, the most common being alcohol and gallstones. Table 85-1 lists the reported causes of acute pancreatitis.

Whatever the initiating cause, the pathogenetic mechanism common to all forms of acute pancreatitis seems to be an intense systemic inflammatory response syndrome (SIRS) caused by the release of activated pancreatic enzymes[7,8] and mediated by cytokines, immunocytes, and the complement system. Inflammatory cytokines (such as tumor necrosis factor) cause macrophages to migrate into tissues distant from the pancreas, including lungs and kidneys. Immunocytes attracted by cytokines released from macrophages release more cytokines, free radicals, and nitric oxide[9,10]; the result is tissue destruction, fluid and electrolyte loss, hypotension, renal and pulmonary complications, late septic complications, and in 20% to 40% of severe cases, multisystem organ failure (MSOF) and death.[11]

The list of illnesses in the critically ill patient that may precede the development of pancreatitis in the ICU is growing (Table 85-2). Why are these seemingly disparate groups of patients all at risk for this apparently unrelated and possibly lethal condition? The answer is not known and may be multifactorial.

In the case of pancreatitis developing after cardiopulmonary bypass, important factors may be microembolism

TABLE 85-1 Acute Pancreatitis—Etiologic Factors

Metabolic	Obstructive Mechanical	Infectious	Idiopathic	Hypoperfusion
Alcohol	Gallstones	Mumps	Familial	Vascular
Hypercalcemia	Afferent loop obstruction	Coxsackie virus infection		PAN[c] and other collagen disorders
Drugs	Duodenal obstruction	*Mycoplasma* infection		Embolic
Hyperlipidemia	Periampullary tumors	Ascariasis[b]		Low-flow states
	Duodenal ulcer	Clonorchiasis[b]		
	Pancreas divisum			
	Trauma			
	Blunt			
	Penetrating			
	Postoperative			
	After ERCP[a]			

[a] Endoscopic retrograde cholangiopancreatography.
[b] May cause pancreatitis by an obstructive mechanism.
[c] Polyarteritis nodosa.

TABLE 85-2 Preexisting Conditions/Procedures

Cardiopulmonary bypass
Cardiac transplantation
Abdominal aortic aneurysm repair
Renal transplantation
Liver transplantation
Shock from any cause
Major upper abdominal surgery

and venous thrombosis,[12,13] a low postoperative flow state, prolonged bypass,[14] intraoperative or postoperative bleeding, hypothermia,[15] and the use of both narcotics and vasopressors.[16] The frequent occurrence of pancreatitis after cardiac transplantation may be related to the effect of heparin on platelet aggregation[17] and to the administration of cyclosporine[18] and prednisone,[19] as well as to the factors suggested for cardiopulmonary bypass. Abdominal aortic aneurysm repair, especially after acute rupture, may produce hypotension, microemboli, and vasoconstriction, resulting in prolonged hypoperfusion of the pancreas.[20]

Pancreatitis developing after renal transplantation may be related to hypercalcemia,[21] specific operative factors, or immunosuppression as for cardiac transplantation. The reasons for severe pancreatitis after liver transplantation may include direct dissection in some cases, blood loss and hypovolemia, or obstruction to pancreatic venous outflow during prolonged venous bypass. One group has suggested that a hepatitis B infectious factor may be involved.[22]

Review of these possible mechanisms for the development of pancreatitis in the critically ill patient seems to confirm *hypoperfusion injury* as a major pathogenetic mechanism. In fact, one group has suggested that a patient in shock from any of a variety of causes (oligemic, cardiogenic, or septic) is at risk of developing pancreatitis.[23] The actual mechanism of this injury, resulting in the release of activated enzymes and an inflammatory response, is not known.

Hypoperfusion may play an important role in the conversion of a less severe, self-limiting pancreatitis into the more lethal necrotizing form, even when the more common etiologic factors, such as alcohol and gallstones, are major contributors in the non-critical-care setting.[24,25]

Many major upper abdominal procedures have been reported to be complicated by pancreatitis, usually as a result of direct dissection or injury of the gland at surgery (see Table 85-2). However, since any patient subjected to a period of hypotension intraoperatively is a candidate for hyperamylasemia, pancreatitis, or both, the cause of pancreatitis in these cases may have been multifactorial rather than purely mechanical, as originally thought.

Diagnosis

Whatever the cause of new pancreatitis in an ICU patient, the physician must diagnose the condition early, attempt to assess the severity of the process, institute appropriate aggressive supportive management, and use judgment in deciding on the timing and type of surgical intervention, if necessary. Most patients improve even if the disease is virtually ignored; those few whose pancreas becomes necrotic and infected need aggressive and timely surgery to avoid MSOF and death.

Clinical signs and symptoms are notoriously variable in patients with pancreatitis,[20] and they are even more difficult to evaluate in the critically ill. The patient may complain of abdominal pain, nausea, and vomiting; often there are nonspecific features such as elevated temperature, leukocytosis, or in more severe cases, unexplained hemodynamic instability and increased fluid requirements without major clinical findings. The serum amylase concentration,[26-28] random urinary amylase concentrations, and the amylase-creatinine clearance ratio may be useful indicators,[29,30] but they are not reliable in all patients. The serum lipase concentration[31] may be a more reliable and specific indicator than the serum amylase level, but its use has not gained wide acceptance. Serum lipase rises somewhat more slowly than amylase, peaks at 24 hours, and normalizes in 1 to 2 weeks.[32] The concentrations of isoamylase,[33] serum elastase, phospholipase A_2, and trypsin have been suggested as tests but have not been practically useful.[34,35]

In addition to clinical evaluation and frequently unreliable biochemical tests, morphologic assessment of the retroperitoneum is necessary. For patients presenting initially with suspected pancreatitis, standard abdominal and chest films usually were obtained routinely to rule out other significant catastrophes, such as perforation and mechanical intestinal obstruction. These films also may suggest pancreatitis by demonstrating pleural effusions, localized jejunal or colonic ileus, the outline of a widened duodenal C loop, pancreatic calcification, associated radiopaque gallstones, or obliteration of psoas shadows and free intraperitoneal fluid. In some cases,[36] laparoscopy may be useful in making a diagnosis of pancreatitis, although early intervention of any kind is to be avoided unless absolutely necessary. However, the increased availability and efficacy of ultrasound and computed tomographic (CT) scanning have made them the mainstays of routine investigation and monitoring of retroperitoneal inflammation.

ULTRASOUND

Ultrasonography is perhaps the most available test and can be carried out at the bedside of an acutely ill patient. It remains the most convenient modality for edematous pancreatitis that responds rapidly to conservative therapy, for suspected biliary pancreatitis with a mild clinical course, and for the monitoring of a retroperitoneal collection or phlegmon for resolution or the development of a pseudocyst.[37] It also has been suggested that Doppler ultrasound may be valuable in detecting pseudoaneurysms 0.1 cm in diameter. However, paralytic ileus and obesity together severely hamper the ultrasonographer's ability to evaluate the retroperitoneum in the acute stages.

The current generation of high-resolution real-time scanners makes it possible to examine in detail the pancreatic gland, its peripancreatic compartments, and the associated biliary tract, with the patient in the semierect, sitting, and supine positions. These maneuvers, unfortunately, may be difficult to perform in a critically ill patient.

The abnormalities detected by ultrasonography are variable. The gland itself may be diffusely enlarged and hypoechoic or have a normal appearance, depending on a number of factors, such as the timing of the study, the presence of underlying chronic disease, and the amount of intrapancreatic fat or hemorrhage. Ductal diameter is similarly variable and may be increased, normal, or decreased. The ultrasonographer is just as interested in the peripancreatic retroperitoneal spaces, looking for evidence of acute fluid collections in the lesser sac, phlegmon, and hemorrhage. It is also possible to detect displacement of the gastrointestinal tract and the presence of intraperitoneal fluid. Fluid collections in the lesser sac usually regress as the clinical picture improves. Those which do not and are surrounded by a dense pseudocapsule legitimately may be termed *chronic pseudocysts* and often are treated by radiologic or surgical intervention.

Critical in the assessment of the retroperitoneum is the detection of scattered pancreatic necrosis and of the involvement of peripancreatic tissues with fat necrosis, hemorrhage, and ultimately, abscess formation; unfortunately, ultrasonography is limited in its ability to define these subtle changes in tissue density.[37]

COMPUTED TOMOGRAPHY

Computed tomography has become the "gold standard" for assessing retroperitoneal morphology, especially in complicated cases, and now is increasingly available in every clinical setting. The procedure in the acutely ill patient may be somewhat inconvenient and cumbersome because of endotracheal intubation, multiple lines, and hemodynamic instability, but these problems are not insurmountable. Images of the retroperitoneum are not compromised by obesity or bowel gas, as they may be with ultrasound.

A mildly inflamed pancreas may show slight diffuse enlargement with irregular borders and patchy densities. Peripancreatic fat may increase in density as it undergoes necrosis. The more severe forms of pancreatitis are accompanied by an increase in peripancreatic inflammatory exudate and intrapancreatic fluid collections. Often the pancreas is markedly enlarged, with irregular fluid collections in the retroperitoneum and poor enhancement in scattered areas within the gland. Unlike ultrasonography, computed tomography is an excellent method for identifying high-density fluid collections in the transverse mesocolon, small bowel mesentery, and pararenal and perirenal spaces[38]; by means of dynamic CT scanning, areas of necrosis in the gland itself may be demonstrated. In sick patients, however, one always must be aware of the potential negative effects of contrast infusion both on the patient and on the pancreatitis.[39]

The critical value of CT scanning is in the detection and follow-up of significant complications. A pancreatic abscess consists of pancreatic necrosis that becomes infected and liquefied; it appears on CT scans as ill-defined or poorly encapsulated fluid collections of different densities, with air bubbles being recognized in about 20% of cases. Pseudoaneurysms also may be detected by CT scanning and, with enhancement, may be highlighted.

Since infusion during CT scanning may present significant risks for the hypovolemic unstable patient, future applications of magnetic resonance imaging (MRI) must be considered in this situation. Currently, however, CT scanning remains the most useful tool for evaluation of retroperitoneal morphology.

SEVERITY OF DISEASE

The intensivist must identify not only the presence of the new condition but also its severity and the likelihood of progression to necrosis and complications. Staging of the acute disease is useful in selecting certain patients for early aggressive supportive therapy, those who may require immediate referral to a specialized center, and those who may be candidates for entry into clinical trials. Ranson's criteria[40] were used extensively in the past, but currently, a number of prognostic scoring systems with clinical, biochemical, and radiologic features are available. The Balthazar score is based primarily on CT findings, focusing on the presence or absence of pancreatic necrosis. It has been suggested that CT scores are more valuable than the Acute Physiologic and Chronic Health Evaluation (APACHE) II score in predicting regional complications associated with pancreatitis.[41] Many use the Atlanta classification, which defines severe acute pancreatitis using features such as clinical presentation, the Ranson criteria, the APACHE II criteria, and evidence of organ failure and anatomic changes. These indicators are directed toward assessing the systemic effects of the disease, and in a critically ill patient, a number of them already may be present before the onset of the pancreatitis.

Numerous blood tests have been suggested as indicators of severity (areas of necrosis within the gland), including the levels of cyclic adenosine monophosphate, albumin, methemalbumin,[42] ribonuclease,[43] C-reactive protein,[44,45] fibrinogen,[34] and urinary trypsinogen-activated polypeptide.[46] Another group has reported that the volume and color of peritoneal aspirate at diagnosis can be useful.[47] None of these tests has proved as accurate, however, as clinical assessment of the patient and serial CT scans of the abdomen, especially in the ICU setting.[48,49] The development of abdominal pain and tenderness, fever, leukocytosis, hemodynamic instability, and CT changes within 1 to 2 weeks of the presumed onset of the pancreatitis provides the best assessment of the severe complications of the disease.

In a patient who is deteriorating or is persistently septic and whose CT scan demonstrates features typical of pancreatic necrosis as listed earlier, percutaneous aspiration of the retroperitoneum with microscopic examination and cultures can be valuable[50–52]; this approach is used frequently in our unit to direct further management.

Treatment

After the patient has been stabilized systemically and the disease has been identified as severe, attention is turned initially to the possible etiologic factors listed in Table 85-1. An ICU patient may develop pancreatitis related to causes other than the described hypoperfusion injury; drugs, gallstones, or other obstructive mechanical factors may be critical. Very frequently, as is the case with gallstone pancreatitis, the disease is short and self-limiting, and in selected patients it can be treated with immediate or delayed endoscopic or surgical intervention as the case demands. The most common scenario is quick resolution of the acute inflammation and a recommendation either for surgery in the same admission if the gallbladder is in situ[53] or for endoscopic sphincterotomy and gallstone removal if the gallbladder was removed previously. In the critically ill person, however, this intervention, unless indicated early by persistent jaundice and acute pancreatitis, should be delayed until after resolution of the primary illness. Some groups, however, advocate routine early endoscopic sphincterotomy and claim modest attendant morbidity.[54–57]

Assuming that the disease in the ICU patient was initiated by a hypoperfusion injury to the gland, however, and that no immediate "corrective" intervention is appropriate, the principles of treatment include careful monitoring, correction of the metabolic and hemodynamic effects of the inflammatory process, respiratory and renal support, nutrition, control of pancreatic enzyme secretion and its sequelae, and prevention and treatment of the local complications of necrotizing pancreatitis. The evaluation and management of such a patient from the outset must be a collaborative effort between the intensivist and an abdominal surgeon experienced in the medical and surgical measures that may become necessary. The decision making with regard to surgery is based to some extent on hard data that can be measured, such as biochemical indicators and radiographs, but it is also based on clinical experience and intuition.[58,59]

MONITORING

The critically ill patient who develops pancreatitis is likely already undergoing hemodynamic monitoring in the ICU setting, with close evaluation of heart rate, arterial blood pressure, hourly urine output, and central venous pressure. Since patients with severe pancreatitis may well have major fluid derangement, renal failure, sepsis, and especially pulmonary complications, a pulmonary artery catheter may be useful for monitoring, but the impact of this device remains controversial.

Frequent determinations of blood counts, blood urea nitrogen (BUN), blood sugar, electrolytes, creatinine, calcium, magnesium, and arterial blood gas levels are useful in detecting deteriorating pulmonary or renal status, the adequacy of treatment, and the evolution of septic complications. In a patient who is slow to respond, serial ultrasound examinations and CT scans especially are critical to the ongoing evaluation of the retroperitoneum.

METABOLIC AND HEMODYNAMIC EFFECTS

The need for volume replacement in patients with severe pancreatitis cannot be overemphasized. Such patients, in effect, have a massive retroperitoneal burn, with ongoing third-space losses in the retroperitoneum, peritoneal cavity, and bowel lumen. Requirements may vary from small amounts to 8 to 10 L of isotonic fluid in the first 24-hour period. In the ICU, especially if the patient has a preexisting brittle cardiovascular status, fluid replacement and its effects may have to be followed even more closely; however, a patient who develops pancreatitis after a cardiopulmonary bypass or cardiac transplantation still requires adequate salt and fluid replacement. Patients who develop hemodynamic instability after appropriate massive fluid administration may benefit from support with vasoactive drugs.

Because hemorrhage can occur as a complication of the retroperitoneal extravasation of proteolytic enzymes, administration of blood may be necessary; for those who develop hypoalbuminemia as a result of significant protein loss, plasma or albumin or both may be indicated.

It should be stressed that the reason why one patient progresses to pancreatic necrosis and/or the development of SIRS and another has a benign, self-limiting course remains a mystery; however, in the usual case of pancreatitis, and especially in a critically ill patient in the ICU, this deterioration may well be exacerbated by hypotension and hypoperfusion related to inadequate attention to volume replacement.

Metabolic abnormalities should be recognized and treated. For example, early fluid management and stabilization usually are sufficient to correct metabolic acidosis. Whether hypocalcemia—even ionized hypocalcemia—should be corrected is controversial, given the central role of elevated intracellular calcium in the pathogenesis of pancreatitis.[60]

RESPIRATORY AND RENAL SUPPORT

Many mechanisms are implicated in the development of typical adult respiratory distress syndrome (ARDS) in this setting. After major heart or transplantation surgery, the patient's pulmonary function already may be compromised by anesthetics, opiates, and pain related to the procedure. In addition, elevation of the diaphragm, pleural effusion, abdominal pain leading to further splinting and atelectasis, and overaggressive fluid replacement may contribute to the respiratory failure. The most important factors may occur in the lung itself, with increased capillary permeability related to serotonin release, breakdown of surfactant by the enzyme phospholipase A released by the necrosing pancreas, or activation of the complement cascade with elaboration of vasoactive prostaglandins and leukotrienes. Whatever the mechanisms, aggressive ventilatory support is required frequently, and this possible need should be anticipated. If the patient was ill previously and develops respiratory insufficiency along with acute pancreatitis or requires multiple operations for complications of the latter, ventilatory support may be prolonged for many weeks. Tracheostomy may become necessary for adequate tracheobronchial toilet or occasionally for protracted ventilation.

No specific renal insult has been recognized in the patient with acute pancreatitis, apart from the secondary effects of volume loss and hypotension. However, as reviewed previously, many patients with ICU-related pancreatitis may have a hypoperfusion injury as a cause; therefore, renal dysfunction may be anticipated in many. Aggressive support with fluids, judicious use of diuretics when fluid has been replaced adequately, and hemodialysis in selected cases of acute tubular necrosis are all part of the therapeutic armamentarium.

One group examining the incidence of pancreatitis in patients undergoing abdominal aortic aneurysm repair found that there was a high correlation of pancreatic injury with ischemic injury to the kidney[23] (acute tubular necrosis), suggesting that the two conditions have similar etiologies and indicating the need for close monitoring of renal function.

NUTRITION

Nutritional support for the seriously ill patient is critical, even though no specific benefit to the patient with an inflamed pancreas has been proven. Most of the conditions listed in Table 85-2 occur in patients at risk for developing pancreatitis; nevertheless, these patients enter the ICU with an expectation of returning to normal feeding within days. The recognition of pancreatitis, however, should carry with it the realization that a prolonged stay is possible. All too often the intensivist withholds total parenteral or enteral nutrition (TPN or EN) until the course of the disease is declared, only to find that after 2 weeks the patient is not improving significantly and now has been starved unnecessarily.

The patient who develops pancreatitis in this setting should be regarded with suspicion, and nutrition should be offered early with an objective of "pancreatic rest." Long-term TPN in a sick, possibly septic patient carries its own frequent complications, among which are line sepsis and opportunistic infections; enteral feeding through a nasojejunal or percutaneous jejunal tube is a valuable adjunct and should, whenever possible, be the feeding method of choice if severe paralytic ileus does not preclude its use.[61–63] Infusion of nutrients into the proximal jejunum bypasses the stimulatory effect of feeding on pancreatic secretion, has fewer complications, is much less costly than TPN, helps maintain mucosal function, and limits absorption of endotoxins and cytokines from the gut.[64–67] The feeding tubes also can be placed via laparoscopy or combined endoscopic and radiologic means.[68]

CONTROL OF PANCREATIC ENZYME SECRETION

Many therapeutic steps have been taken to minimize pancreatic enzyme secretion or limit its effects. Studies to examine the possible benefits in acute pancreatitis of nasogastric suction,[69] anticholinergic agents,[70] H_2-receptor blockers,[71] somatostatin,[72,73] calcitonin,[74] and glucagon[75] have not supported the routine use of these agents.

Similarly, the effects of the proteolytic enzyme inhibitor aprotinin (TRASYLOL),[76,77] the antitrypsin agent ϵ-aminocaproic acid (EACA),[78] and a phospholipase A inhibitor[79] have not been convincingly beneficial. Nasogastric suction is still used routinely, especially in the obtunded patient, to decompress paralytic ileus, control vomiting, perhaps decrease stimulation of the pancreas, and prevent aspiration.

The numerous modalities used and tested in the treatment of the severe form of this disease attest to the failure of most of them to alter the course of the inflammatory process. The mainstay of initial treatment is resuscitation with fluid and electrolytes combined with respiratory and nutritional support, as well as attention to the primary disease state in the case of a critically ill patient. Patients who die from necrotizing pancreatitis, however, do not usually die in the early resuscitation phase, or even in the first 2 weeks, owing to excellent intensive care.

The next step is to evaluate and follow the pathologic process in the retroperitoneum while all supportive measures are continued.

Local Complications of Necrotizing Pancreatitis

At the outset, the clinician must be aware of the pathologic conditions that occur secondarily as a result of acute

pancreatitis. A relatively uncommon but potentially lethal complication is that of intraabdominal hemorrhage requiring immediate intervention.[80] The local complications of necrotizing pancreatitis are pancreatic necrosis, pancreatic abscess, and pseudocyst formation[81]; the process also may have more remote effects, such as formation of multiple intraabdominal collections, colonic perforation,[82] and even gallbladder necrosis[83] and abdominal compartment syndrome.[84] Aggressive early hemodynamic stabilization is probably the only rational way to prevent further hypoperfusion injury to the pancreas and the development of these complications. Institution of peritoneal dialysis via the percutaneous or minilaparotomy route accelerates early improvement in some patients but does not appear to offer any benefit in decreasing the likelihood of complications and death.[85] Patients in whom retroperitoneal necrosis (fat or pancreatic) develops are at high risk for morbidity and death.[6] Those in whom this complication does not develop usually will survive with appropriate supportive measures only.

PANCREATIC AND PERIPANCREATIC NECROSIS

Pancreatic necrosis consists of patchy devitalization of the pancreatic gland; it develops in a few days to weeks after the onset of the inflammatory process. The patient usually has abdominal pain, persistent fever (possibly low grade), and leukocytosis. CT scan with vascular enhancement may demonstrate local or diffuse areas of nonenhancement. Needle aspirates obtained at this stage will show no growth on culture if necrosis is present without infection.

Treatment of this entity is controversial. It is difficult to predict how many cases of pancreatic necrosis (without infection) will resolve spontaneously with simple supportive management and how many will develop sepsis and clearly require débridement. Undoubtedly, the condition does resolve in some patients, who clearly would not benefit from laparotomy. Every pancreatic surgeon has had the experience of extensively débriding sterile retroperitoneal necrosis, subjecting the patient to perhaps many future débridements (which then, of course, involve infected tissue), and wondering whether the original noninfected condition might have resolved spontaneously. In addition, many "sequestrectomies" performed for pancreatic necrosis likely are excisions only of necrotic fat and not of necrotic gland. No comparison of these two pathologic entities in terms of morbidity and mortality has been reported. A retroperitoneum with a well-perfused pancreas surrounded by necrotic fat may carry a different outlook than if the gland itself is compromised. Therefore, removal of uninfected necrotic fat only may be a fruitless and conceivably dangerous exercise.

It has been suggested that infection develops in only 40% of patients with pancreatic and peripancreatic necrosis.[86] Because of this and the aforementioned fear that surgery in the sterile situation actually may cause more harm than good, we tend to avoid major débridement unless sepsis is confirmed. Therefore, if the patient remains stable hemodynamically, has only low-grade fever and leukocytosis, has CT findings that do not suggest extensive glandular necrosis and infection, and has a sterile percutaneous retroperitoneal sample, we continue with supportive management without intervention. However, the patient ultimately may require intervention even in the absence of gross septic parameters simply

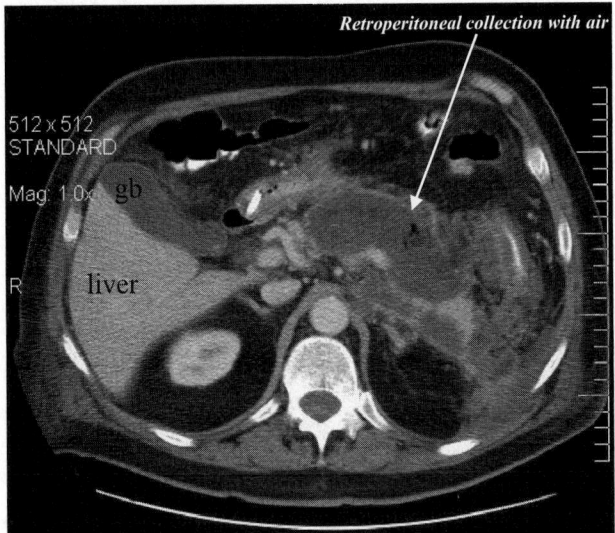

FIGURE 85-1 CT scan of patient with acute alcoholic pancreatitis and evidence of a retroperitoneal collection containing fluid and air bubbles. Aspiration and culture confirmed infection with gram-negative organisms, and the patient was managed eventually with surgical débridement, enteral nutrition, and antibiotic therapy.

because of a prolonged "smoldering" course showing no clinical improvement (Fig. 85-1).

ANTIBIOTIC THERAPY

The role of antibiotics in the patient with pancreatic necrosis or sepsis is similarly controversial.[87–91] Antibiotics are required in patients who have pancreatic necrosis (with or without sepsis), but their purpose is to provide systemic protection rather than local treatment or prophylaxis. Patients with sterile necrosis usually receive broad-spectrum antibiotics for systemic protection while the intensivist monitors the retroperitoneum, although this treatment undoubtedly brings with it a risk of opportunistic infection, such as disseminated candidiasis in the acutely ill host. In recent years, the case for routine antibiotic usage in such patients has strengthened. Certain antibiotics such as imipenem actually penetrate the pancreatic parenchyma, achieving good tissue levels during acute pancreatitis. In several studies, significant reduction in the incidence of septic complications followed the routine use of broad-spectrum antibiotics, but the effect on mortality has been less predictable. One study[92] showed that routine use of imipenem-cilastatin altered the bacteriology in severe acute pancreatitis from predominately gram-negative coliforms to predominately gram-positive organisms without altering the incidence of resistance or fungal superinfection.

Prophylactic antibiotics for the purpose of selective decontamination of the gastrointestinal tract may prevent translocation of bacteria to the inflamed pancreatic bed, presumably from the transverse colon.[93–96] Patients who develop infected necrosis must be treated actively to prevent or manage bacteremia and frequently require surgical débridement and drainage; however, even that approach is being challenged by some anecdotal evidence that antibiotics alone or in conjunction with percutaneous drainage without surgery may be sufficient to treat some patients with aspiration-proven retroperitoneal sepsis.[97–101] This strategy

still may be difficult to accept for those intensivists who have treated patients who developed fatal opportunistic infections in the past after long-term antibiotic therapy.

INFECTED NECROSIS AND PANCREATIC ABSCESS

Some patients with pancreatic and peripancreatic necrosis develop spontaneous infection of the necrotic tissue presumably because of direct contamination by bacteria from the transverse colon. Although some authors do not distinguish between infected necrosis and pancreatic abscess, others differentiate them on the basis of suitability for percutaneous drainage: Infected pancreatic necrosis usually requires extensive surgical débridement and possibly pancreatic resection because of solid necrotic areas, whereas a pancreatic abscess may require just percutaneous drainage if liquefaction has taken place, leaving little solid necrotic tissue.

Notwithstanding the more conservative approach described earlier in selected patients, established sepsis in the retroperitoneum generally requires intervention to avoid the sequelae of systemic infection. This fact has significant implications in the patient who is critically ill from a primary illness. The diagnosis of retroperitoneal sepsis, whether infected pancreatic necrosis or pancreatic abscess, is made by recognition of clinical deterioration, which may be more precipitous than with pancreatic necrosis and may be accompanied by more pronounced fever and leukocytosis, typical CT findings, and a positive percutaneous aspirate.[59,102] When the patient is maintained on broad-spectrum antibiotics (with perhaps decreased immunosuppression in the transplant patient), preparations are made for surgical débridement. Although some cases may be amenable to percutaneous drainage only, as stated previously, in our experience, most require laparotomy.

PRINCIPLES OF SURGICAL DÉBRIDEMENT

The conventional indications for surgery in acute pancreatitis include failure of early medical management, unresolving gallstone pancreatitis, and pancreatic sepsis. In the critical care setting, aggressive supportive care has virtually eliminated the need for early operation. As stated earlier, a persistent gallstone pancreatitis may be treated effectively by early endoscopic sphincterotomy. Therefore, the main indication for surgery in the critically ill patient with pancreatitis is the late development of necrosis or sepsis.[58,59]

Recommended methods of surgical débridement vary considerably, and their description is beyond the scope of this chapter. The principles of the different approaches are similar, however; the critical steps are the recognition of the patient in whom débridement is appropriate and quick execution of the procedure, with excellent anesthesia and postoperative intensive care.

The timing of surgery for pancreatic sepsis is critical,[103] in that early débridement (done usually within 3 weeks of the onset of clinical pancreatitis) may encounter poor demarcation between necrotic and healthy tissue, leading to oozing from partially devitalized tissue after necrosectomy. If a wait can be tolerated by the patient, a late laparotomy (at 3 to 6 weeks) is likely to involve the removal of well-demarcated necrosis (often in a single procedure rather than multiple operations).

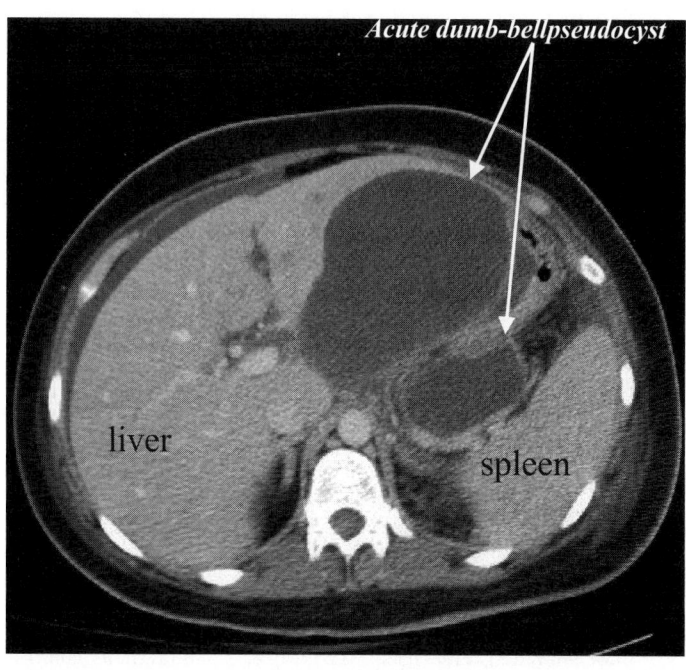

FIGURE 85-2 CT scan of patient with acute pancreatitis and acute pseudocyst formation. The dumbbell-shaped pseudocyst resolved gradually without internal or external drainage.

Surgery should consist of wide débridement of all devitalized peripancreatic fat and pancreatic tissue, followed by adequate dependent drainage, which should be generous enough to allow drainage of thick, purulent, often particulate material.[104,105] Since multiple operations for repeated abdominal toilet sometimes are required, some surgeons have advocated open packing of the abdomen in such cases.[102,106]

Our own preference is for radical excision of all necrotic and infected material followed by generous dependent sump drainage and closure of the abdomen, although some practitioners advocate closed lavage postoperatively.[107] Intubation of the gastrointestinal tract (cholecystostomy, gastrostomy, and jejunostomy were advocated enthusiastically in the past[108]) is to be avoided in this septic setting. Temporary packing of the retroperitoneum and scheduled reoperation occasionally are necessary to control venous oozing from the bed of the necrotic tissue.

The extent of pancreatic resection varies depending on the degree of necrosis of the gland itself. Although some surgeons have recommended routine performance of major pancreatic resection,[109,110] we débride the gland itself only if necessary; only necrotic portions are removed, and major anatomic dissections are avoided, if possible, in these often unstable patients.

The patient who suffers infected pancreatic necrosis and who requires intensive care, often multiple operations, and an extended hospital stay clearly will have a protracted convalescence. However, a recent quality-of-life study[111] found that the survivors of this morbid disease could look forward to good quality of life.

PANCREATIC PSEUDOCYST

With more frequent use of ultrasound and CT scanning in the early stages of pancreatitis, recognition of fluid collections in and around the lesser sac has become the rule rather than the exception. Most collections probably consist of inflammatory exudate, and in fact, most resolve as the pancreatitis settles (Fig. 85-2). The persistence of a lesser sac fluid collection (or of fluid in a variety of areas, such as the peritoneal cavity, the retroperitoneum, or even the mediastinum) implies a communication with a ruptured pancreatic duct system. A collection that develops thick, fibrous walls consisting of the surrounding stomach, colon, and mesentery properly can be termed a *chronic pseudocyst*. Diagnosis of such a condition does not mandate immediate treatment unless the pseudocyst becomes symptomatic, grows quickly, becomes infected, bleeds, or ruptures into the peritoneal cavity or adjacent bowel. In an already sick patient, a quickly enlarging or infected pseudocyst is best treated with percutaneous decompression or endoscopic pseudocyst drainage, whereas immediate surgery is required for bleeding or free rupture. Occasionally, transpapillary stent placement is useful if a direct communication exists between the main pancreatic duct and the pseudocyst.[112] The presence of a large collection does not of itself necessitate percutaneous decompression; in fact, one group found that collections that were drained early had a significantly increased chance of later developing septic complications requiring surgery and a longer hospital stay.[113] It also has been suggested that percutaneous treatment is effective for peripheral collections, whereas more centrally placed collections need operative decompression.[114] Spontaneous rupture into the intestinal tract, a rare occurrence, can be treated expectantly in this setting if the patient is otherwise stable. The uncomplicated pseudocyst that is stable in size and is at least 6 weeks old (to allow the walls to "mature" enough to accept sutures) is conventionally drained internally at laparotomy; in the intensive care situation, percutaneous drainage can be done safely to avoid the dreaded complications, but it must be used with full knowledge that recurrence is frequent.

References

1. Peterson LM, Brooks JR: Lethal pancreatitis, a diagnostic dilemma. *Am J Surg* 137:491, 1979.

2. Trapnell J: The natural history and management of acute pancreatitis. *Clin Gastroenterol* 1:147, 1972.

3. Forsmark CE, Toskes PP: Acute pancreatitis: Medical management. *Crit Care Clin* 11:295, 1995.

4. Bake CC, Huynh T: Acute pancreatitis: Surgical management. *Crit Care Clin* 11:311, 1995.

5. Mann DV, Hershman MJ, Hittinger R, Glazer G: Multicentre audit of death from acute pancreatitis. *Br J Surg* 81:890, 1994.

6. Buchler M, Uhl W, Beger HG: Complications of acute pancreatitis and their management. *Curr Opin Gen Surg* 1:282, 1993.

7. Foitzik T, Hotz HG, Schmidt J, et al: Effect of microcirculatory perfusion on distribution of trypsinogen activation peptides in acute experimental pancreatitis. *Dig Dis Sci* 40:2184, 1995.

8. Fernandez-del Castillo C, Schmidt J, Warshaw AL, Rattner DW: Interstitial protease activation is the central event in progression to necrotizing pancreatitis. *Surgery* 116:497, 1994.

9. Gukovskaya AS, Gukovsky I, Zaninovic V, et al: Pancreatic cells produce, release and respond to tumor necrosis factor-alpha: Role in regulating cell death and pancreatitis. *J Clin Invest* 100:1853, 1997.

10. Norman JG, Fink GW, Franz MG: Acute pancreatitis induces tumor necrosis factor gene expression. *Arch Surg* 130:966, 1995.

11. Keynes M: Heretical thoughts on the pathogenesis of acute pancreatitis. *Gut* 29:1413, 1988.

12. Colon R, Frazier OH, Kahan BD: Complications in cardiac transplant patients requiring general surgery. *Surgery* 103:32, 1988.

13. Feiner H: Pancreatitis after cardiac surgery: A morphologic study. *Am J Surg* 131:684, 1976.

14. Moneta GL, Misbach GA, Ivey TD: Hypoperfusion as a possible factor in the development of gastrointestinal complications after cardiac surgery. *Am J Surg* 149:648, 1985.

15. Mikhailidis DP, Hutton RA, Jeremy JY, Dandona P: Hypothermia and pancreatitis. *J Clin Pathol* 36:483, 1983.

16. Rose DM, Ranson JHC, Cunningham JN, Spencer FC: Patterns of severe pancreatic injury following cardiopulmonary bypass. *Ann Surg* 199:168, 1984.

17. Greenbaum RA, Barradas MA, Mikhailidis DP, et al: Effect of heparin and contrast medium on platelet function during routine cardiac catheterization. *Cardiovasc Res* 21:878, 1987.

18. Grace AA, Barradas MA, Mikhailidis P, et al: Cyclosporine A enhances platelet aggregation. *Kidney Int* 32:889, 1987.

19. Dandona P, Junglee D, Katrak A, et al: Increased serum pancreatic enzymes after treatment with methylprednisolone: Possible evidence of subclinical pancreatitis. *Br Med J* 291:24, 1985.

20. Victor DW, Rayburn JL, McCready RA, Hyde GL: Pancreatitis following aneurysmectomy. *J Ky Med Assoc* 86:285, 1988.

21. Frick TW, Fryd DS, Sutherland DER, et al: Hypercalcemia associated with pancreatitis and hyperamylasemia in renal transplant recipients. *Am J Surg* 154:487, 1987.

22. Alexander JA, Demetrius AJ, Gavaler JS, et al: Pancreatitis following liver transplantation. *Transplantation* 45:1062, 1988.

23. Warshaw AL, O'Hara PJ: Susceptibility of the pancreas to ischemic injury in shock. *Ann Surg* 188:197, 1978.

24. Popper HL, Necheles H, Russell KC: Transition of pancreatic edema to pancreatic necrosis. *Surg Gynecol Obstet* 87:79, 1948.

25. Mithofer K, Fernandez-del Castillo C, Frick TW, et al: Increased intrapancreatic trypsinogen activation in ischemia-induced experimental pancreatitis. *Ann Surg* 221:364, 1995.

26. Read G, Braganza JM, Howat HT: Pancreatitis: A retrospective study. *Gut* 17:945, 1976.

27. Janowitz HD, Dreiling DA: The plasma amylase: Source, regulation and diagnostic significance. *Am J Med* 27:924, 1959.

28. Salt WB, Schenker S: Amylase: Its clinical significance. A review of the literature. *Medicine* 55:269, 1976.

29. Warshaw AL, Fuller AF: Specificity of increased renal clearance of amylase in the diagnosis of acute pancreatitis. *New Engl J Med* 292:325, 1975.

30. Leckie PA, Ferreira P, Debas HT: Assessment of the amylase-creatinine clearance ratio in postoperative patients. *Ann Surg* 192:195, 1980.

31. Lifton LJ, Slickers KA, Pragay DA, Katz LA: Pancreatitis and lipase: A reevaluation with a five minute turbidimetric lipase determination. *JAMA* 229:47, 1974.

32. Frank B, Gottlieb K: Amylase normal, lipase elevated: Is it pancreatitis? A case series and review of the literature. *Am J Gastroenterol* 94:463, 1999.

33. O'Donnell MD, FitzGerald O, McGeeney KF: Differential serum amylase determination by the use of an inhibitor, and design of a routine procedure. *Clin Chem* 23:560, 1977.

34. Bery AR, Taylor TV, Davies GC: Diagnostic tests and prognostic indicators in acute pancreatitis. *J R Coll Surg Edinb* 27:345, 1982.

35. Delcourt A: Controversies in the biological diagnosis of acute pancreatitis, in Hollender LF (ed): *Controversies in Acute Pancreatitis*. New York, Springer-Verlag, 1982, p 38.

36. Kapshitar AV: Laparoscopy in the differential diagnosis of acute disorders of the mesenteric blood circulation and acute pancreatitis. *Klin Khir* 5:17, 1993.

37. Jeffrey RB: Sonography in acute pancreatitis. *Radiol Clin North Am* 27:5, 1989.

38. Balthazar EJ: CT diagnosis and staging of acute pancreatitis. *Radiol Clin North Am* 27:19, 1989.

39. Schmidt J, Hotz HG, Foitzik T, et al: Intravenous contrast medium aggravates the impairment of pancreatic microcirculation in necrotizing pancreatitis in the rat. *Ann Surg* 221:257, 1995.

40. Ranson JHC, Rifkind KM, Turner JW: Prognostic signs and nonoperative peritoneal lavage in acute pancreatitis. *Surg Gynecol Obstet* 143:209, 1976.

41. De Sanctis JT, Lee MJ, Gazelle GS, et al: Prognostic indicators in acute pancreatitis: CT vs APACHE II. *Clin Radiol* 52:842, 1997.

42. Kelly TR, Klein RL, Porquez JM, Homer GM: Methemalbumin in acute pancreatitis: An experimental and clinical appraisal. *Ann Surg* 175:15, 1972.

43. Warshaw AL, Lee KH: Serum ribonuclease elevations and pancreatic necrosis in acute pancreatitis. *Surgery* 86:227, 1979.

44. Buchler M, Malfertheimer P, Schoetensack C: Sensitivity of antiproteases, complement factors and C-reactive protein in detecting pancreatic necrosis. *Int J Pancreatol* 1:227, 1986.

45. Wilson C, Heads A, Shenkin A, et al: C-reactive protein, antiproteases and complement factors as objective markers of severity in acute pancreatitis. *Br J Surg* 76:177, 1989.

46. Neoptolemos JP, Kemppainen EA, Mayer JM, et al: Early prediction of severity in acute pancreatitis by urinary trypsinogen activation peptide: A multicentre study. *Lancet* 355:1955, 2000.

47. McMahon MJ, Pickford IR, Playforth MJ: Early prediction of severity of acute pancreatitis using peritoneal lavage. *Acta Chir Scand* 146:171, 1980.

48. Balthazar EJ, Ranson JHC, Naidich DP: Acute pancreatitis: Prognostic value of CT. *Radiology* 156:767, 1985.

49. Kivisarri L, Somer K, Standertskjold-Nord-Enstam CG: Early detection of acute fulminant pancreatitis by contrast enhanced computed tomography. *Scand J Gastroenterol* 15:633, 1980.

50. Gerzof S, Banks P, Spechler S: Role of guided percutaneous aspiration in early diagnosis of pancreatic sepsis. *Dig Dis Sci* 29:950, 1984.

51. Hill MC, Dach JL, Barkin J: Role of percutaneous aspiration in diagnosis of pancreatic abscess. *AJR* 141:1035, 1983.

52. Karlson KB, Martin EC, Fanuchen EI: Percutaneous drainage of pancreatic pseudocysts and abscesses. *Radiology* 142:619, 1982.

53. Runkel NS, Buhr HJ, Herfarth C: Outcome after surgery for biliary pancreatitis. *Eur J Surg* 162:307, 1996.

54. Welbourn CR, Beckly DE, Eyre-Brook IA: Endoscopic sphincterotomy without cholecystectomy for gallstone pancreatitis. *Gut* 37:119, 1995.

55. Neoptolemos JP, Stonelake P, Radley S: Endoscopic sphincterotomy for acute pancreatitis. *Hepatogastroenterology* 40:550, 1993.

56. Carr-Locke DL: Role of endoscopy in gallstone pancreatitis. *Am J Surg* 165:519, 1993.

57. Fiocca F, Santagati A, Ceci V, et al: ERCP and acute pancreatitis. *Eur Rev Med Pharmacol Sci* 6:13, 2002.

58. McFadden DW, Reber HA: Indications for surgery in severe acute pancreatitis. *Int J Pancreatol* 15:83, 1994.

59. Farthmann EH, Lausen M, Schoffel U: Indications for surgical treatment of acute pancreatitis. *Hepatogastroenterology* 40:556, 1993.

60. Ward JB, Petersen OH, Jenkins SA, Sutton R: Is an elevated concentration of acinar cytosolic free ionised calcium the trigger for acute pancreatitis? *Lancet* 346:1016, 1995.

61. Povoski SP, Nussbaum MS: Nutrition support in pancreatitis: Fertile ground for prospective clinical investigation. *Nutr Clin Pract* 10:43, 1995.

62. Windsor AC, Kanwar S, Li AG, et al: Compared with parenteral nutrition, enteral feeding attenuates the acute phase response and improves disease severity in acute pancreatitis. *Gut* 42:431, 1998.

63. Kalfarentzos F, Kehagias J, Mead N, et al: Enteral nutrition is superior to parenteral nutrition in severe acute pancreatitis: Results of a randomized, prospective trial. *Br J Surg* 84:1665, 1997.

64. Abou-Assi S, O'Keefe SJ: Nutrition support during acute pancreatitis (review). *Nutrition* 18:938, 2002.

65. Eatock FC, Brombacher GD, Steven A, et al: Nasogastric feeding in severe acute pancreatitis may be practical and safe. *Int J Pancreatol* 28:23, 2000.

66. Lange JF, van Gool J, Tytgat GN: The protective effect of a reduction in intestinal flora on mortality of acute haemorrhagic pancreatitis in the rat. *Hepatogastroenterology* 34:28, 1987.

67. Buchman AL, Moukarzel AA, Bhuta S, et al: Parenteral nutrition is associated with intestinal morphologic and functional changes in humans. *J Parenter Enteral Nutr* 19:453, 1995.

68. Mitchell RMS, Byrne MF, Baillie J: Pancreatitis. *Lancet* 361:1447, 2003.

69. Levant JA, Secrist DLM, Resin H: Nasogastric suction in the treatment of alcoholic pancreatitis: A controlled study. *JAMA* 229:51, 1974.

70. Switz DM, Vlahcevic ZR, Farrar JT: The effect of anticholinergic and/or nasogastric suction on the outcome of acute alcoholic pancreatitis: A controlled trial. *Gastroenterology* 68:974, 1975.

71. Meshkinpour H, Molinari MD, Gardner L: Cimetidine in the treatment of acute alcoholic pancreatitis: A randomized, double-blind study. *Gastroenterology* 77:687, 1979.

72. Usadel KH, Leuschner U, Uberla KK: Treatment of acute pancreatitis with somatostatin: A multicenter double-blind trial. *New Engl J Med* 303:999, 1980.

73. Luengo L, Vicente V, Gris F, et al: Influence of somatostatin in the evolution of acute pancreatitis: A prospective, randomized study. *Int J Pancreatol* 15:139, 1994.

74. Goebell H, Ammann R, Herfarth CH: A double-blind trial of synthetic salmon calcitonin in the treatment of acute pancreatitis. *Scand J Gastroenterol* 14:881, 1979.

75. Olazabal A, Fuller R: Failure of glucagon in the treatment of alcoholic pancreatitis. *Gastroenterology* 74:489, 1978.

76. Trapnell JE, Rigby CC, Talbot CH: A controlled trial of Trasylol in the treatment of acute pancreatitis. *Br J Surg* 61:177, 1974.

77. Skyring A, Singer A, Tornya P: Treatment of acute pancreatitis with Trasylol: A report of a controlled clinical trial. *Br Med J* 2:627, 1965.

78. Konttinen YP: Epsilon-aminocaproic acid in the treatment of acute pancreatitis. *Scand J Gastroenterol* 6:715, 1971.

79. Tykka HT, Vaittinen EJ, Mahlberg KL: A randomized, double-blind study using CaNa$_2$ EDTA, a phospholipase A$_2$ inhibitor in the management of human acute pancreatitis. *Scand J Gastroenterol* 20:5, 1985.

80. Tsiotos GG, Munoz Juarez MM, Sarr MG: Intraabdominal hemorrhage complicating surgical management of necrotizing pancreatitis. *Pancreas* 12:126, 1996.

81. Frey CF, Bradley EL, Beger HG: Progress in acute pancreatitis. *Surg Gynecol Obstet* 167:282, 1988.

82. Chartrand-Lefebvre C, Clermont RJ, Heppell J, et al: Necrotic stenosis of the right colon secondary to acute pancreatitis. *Can J Surg* 37:140, 1994.

83. Schein M, Assalia A, Schmulevski P, et al: Infected peripancreatic necrosis causing gallbladder necrosis by direct extension. *HPB Surg* 7:77, 1993.

84. Pupelis G, Austrums E, Snippe K, et al: Clinical significance of increased intraabdominal pressure in severe acute pancreatitis. *Acta Chir Belg* 102:71, 2002.

85. Ranson JHC, Spencer FC: The role of peritoneal lavage in severe acute pancreatitis. *Ann Surg* 187:565, 1978.

86. Berger HG, Krauzberger W, Bittner R: Results of surgical treatment of necrotizing pancreatitis. *World J Surg* 9:972, 1985.

87. Howes R, Zuidema GD, Cameron JL: Evaluation of prophylactic antibiotics in acute pancreatitis. *J Surg Res* 18:197, 1975.

88. Finch WT, Sawyers JL, Schenker SA: A prospective study to determine the efficacy of antibiotics in acute pancreatitis. *Ann Surg* 183:667, 1976.

89. Kim SL, Goldschmid S: Antibiotics in acute pancreatitis: The debate revisited. *Am J Gastroenterol* 90:666, 1995.

90. Trudel JL, Wittnich C, Brown RA: Antibiotics bioavailability in acute experimental pancreatitis. *J Am Coll Surg* 178:475, 1994.

91. Buchler M, Malfertheiner P, Friess H, et al: Human pancreatic tissue concentration of bactericidal antibiotics. *Gastroenterology* 103:1902, 1992.

92. Howard TJ, Temple MB: Prophylactic antibiotics alter the bacteriology of infected necrosis in severe acute pancreatitis. *J Am Coll Surg* 195:759, 2002.

93. Gianotti L, Munda R, Gennari R, et al: Effect of different regimens of gut decontamination on bacterial translocation and mortality in experimental acute pancreatitis. *Eur J Surg* 161:85, 1995.

94. Foitzik T, Fernandez-del Castillo C, Ferraro MJ, et al: Pathogenesis and prevention of early pancreatic infection in experimental acute necrotizing pancreatitis. *Ann Surg* 222:179, 1995.

95. Luiten EJ, Hop WC, Lange JF, Bruining HA: Controlled clinical trial of selective decontamination for the treatment of severe acute pancreatitis. *Ann Surg* 222:57, 1995.

96. Luiten EJ, Hop WC, Lange JF, et al: Controlled clinical trial of selective decontamination for the treatment of severe acute pancreatitis. *Ann Surg* 222:57, 1995.

97. Dubner H, Steinberg W, Hill M, et al: Infected pancreatic necrosis and peripancreatic fluid collections: Serendipitous response to antibiotics and medical therapy in three patients. *Pancreas* 12:298, 1996.

98. Takeda K, Matsuno S, Sunamura M, Kakugawa Y: Continuous regional arterial infusion of protease inhibitor and antibiotics in acute necrotizing pancreatitis. *Am J Surg* 171:394, 1996.

99. Mithofer K, Fernandez-del Castillo C, Ferraro MJ, et al: Antibiotic treatment improves survival in experimental acute necrotizing pancreatitis. *Gastroenterology* 110:232, 1996.

100. Szentkereszty Z, Kerekes L, Hallay J, et al: CT-guided percutaneous peripancreatic drainage: A possible therapy in acute necrotizing pancreatitis. *Hepatogastroenterology* 49:1696, 2002.

101. Adler DG, Chari ST, Dahl TJ, et al: Conservative management of infected necrosis complicating severe acute pancreatitis. *Am J Gastroenterol* 98:98, 2003.

102. Bradley EL: A fifteen-year experience with open drainage for infected pancreatic necrosis. *Surg Gynecol Obstet* 177:215, 1993.

103. Johnson CD: Timing of intervention in acute pancreatitis. *Postgrad Med J* 69:509, 1993.

104. White TT, Heimbach DM: Sequestrectomy and hyperalimentation in the treatment of hemorrhagic pancreatitis. *Am J Surg* 132:270, 1976.

105. Crist DW, Cameron JL: The current management of acute pancreatitis. *Adv Surg* 20:69, 1987.

106. Davidson ED, Bradley EL III: "Marsupialization" in the treatment of pancreatic abscess. *Surgery* 89:252, 1981.

107. Buchler M, Uhl W, Beger HG: Acute pancreatitis: When and how to operate. *Dig Dis* 10:354, 1992.

108. Lawson DW, Daggett WM, Civetta JM: Surgical treatment of acute necrotizing pancreatitis. *Ann Surg* 172:605, 1970.

109. Watts GT: Total pancreatectomy for fulminant pancreatitis. *Lancet* 2:384, 1963.

110. Norton L, Eiseman B: Near total pancreatectomy for hemorrhagic pancreatitis. *Am J Surg* 127:191, 1974.

111. Broome AH, Eisen GM, Harland RC, et al: Quality of life after treatment for pancreatitis. *Ann Surg* 223:665, 1996.

112. Huibregtse K, Schneider B, Vrij AA, et al: Endoscopic pancreatic drainage in chronic pancreatitis. *Gastrointest Endosc* 34:9, 1988.

113. Rattner DW, Legermate DA, Lee MJ, et al: Early surgical débridement of symptomatic pancreatic necrosis is beneficial irrespective of infection. *Am J Surg* 163:105, 1992.

114. Lee MJ, Rattner DW, Legemate DA, et al: Acute complicated pancreatitis: Redefining the role of interventional radiology. *Radiology* 183:171, 1992.

Chapter 86
MESENTERIC ISCHEMIA
DENIS W. HARKIN
THOMAS F. LINDSAY

KEY POINTS

- *Acute mesenteric ischemia is a relatively rare clinical entity, but when diagnosis is delayed, it is almost always fatal; therefore, a high index of suspicion is required, especially in those at high risk: the elderly, those with cardiac dysfunction, patients with diffuse atherosclerosis, and those following aortic and cardiac surgery or arterial catheterization.*

- *The etiology of acute mesenteric ischemia may be embolic, thrombotic, primary vasoconstrictive, or secondary to venous thrombosis. Chronic ischemia is usually due to flow-limiting lesions (stenoses or occlusions) in the presence of inadequate collateralization.*

- *Classic symptoms of acute intestinal ischemia are central abdominal pain (often out of proportion to the benign abdominal examination), weight loss (an important clue even in the acute presentation), bowel emptying, and altered bowel function (vomiting, bloating, constipation, or diarrhea). Once signs of peritonitis or bloody diarrhea present, shock, sepsis, and death almost always follow.*

- *Mesenteric angiography is the investigation of choice, offering diagnostic and therapeutic options, whereas computed tomographic (CT) angiogram and duplex ultrasonography may not be definitive. Frequently, the diagnosis is confirmed only at laparotomy.*

- *Treatment is surgical, with restoration of flow by bypass or embolectomy, resection of nonviable intestine, and liberal use of "second look" laparotomy.*

Acute mesenteric ischemia is a relatively rare but often fatal clinical entity. Although little data exist on its true incidence, data from the Swedish Vascular Registry suggest that it may account for just 1 percent of reconstructions for acute thromboembolism.[1] Contemporary series, however, continue to report a mortality rate of between 32% and 48%.[2,3] Although autopsy studies suggest that atherosclerosis affecting the mesenteric arteries is common (6% to 10%),[4] symptomatic mesenteric occlusive disease is rare. However, of patients presenting with acute mesenteric ischemia, one large series found that 43% had prior symptoms of chronic mesenteric ischemia.[5] The spectrum of mesenteric ischemia includes occlusive disease secondary to atherosclerotic occlusion with thrombosis, embolism, mesenteric venous thrombosis, and nonocclusive mesenteric ischemia due to vasospasm (Table-86-1). At its most florid, it may present with mesenteric infarction, intestinal perforation, and septic circulatory collapse. This relatively rare but often fatal clinical entity must be considered early in the differential diagnosis of any patient with abdominal symptoms or signs but especially those with a history of intestinal angina, peripheral vascular disease, cardiac dysfunction, aortic surgery or recent aortic catherization, hypotension, or prothrombotic state. Noninvasive tests lack

specificity and sensitivity, which indicates that the diagnosis often requires a high index of suspicion, supplemented by a liberal use of diagnostic arteriography (or computed tomographis angiogram) when uncertainty remains. Where doubt exists in the presence of emerging acute abdominal signs or clinical deterioration, diagnostic laparotomy is indicated. This discussion will focus on the etiology, pathophysiology, diagnosis, and management of acute mesenteric ischemia.

Anatomy and Dynamics of the Mesenteric Circulation

The mesenteric circulation is supplied in series by the three major midline branches of the abdominal aorta, namely, the celiac artery, supplying the foregut, hepatic, and splenic beds; the superior mesenteric artery (SMA), supplying the midgut; and the inferior mesenteric artery (IMA) and the internal iliac arteries, supplying the hindgut. An extensive network of actual or potential sites of collateralization exists between individual branch territories and their neighbors, as well as the systemic circulation. The celiac territory may gain supply proximally across the diaphragm from the phrenic and esophageal vessels (that arise from the aorta) and distally from the SMA via the gastroduodenal artery, including the

TABLE 86-1 Potential Causes of Acute Mesenteric Ischaemia

Occlusive disease	
Embolism	Cardiac diseases (atrial fibrillation, post-MI, valvular disease, SBE, dilated left ventricle, myxoma)
	Extracardiac arterial diseases
Arterial thrombosis	Acute on chronic atherosclerosis
	Low cardiac output states
Intrinsic arterial diseases	Occlusive atherosclerosis
	Aortic dissection
	Atherosclerotic aneurysm
	Arteritis and autoimmune diseases
	Fibromuscular dysplasia
Venous thrombosis	Thrombophilia
	Extrinsic compression
Iatrogenic	After aortoiliac surgery
	Catheter related (dissection, embolism)
	Irradiation arteritis
	Vasoconstrictive agents (epinephrine, norepinephrine, dopamine)
Trauma	Penetrating
	Blunt (including deceleration injuries)
Nonocclusive disease	
Shock	Cardiogenic shock
	Hypovolemic shock
	Septic shock
	Neurogenic shock
	Anaphylactic shock
Low cardiac output states	Heart failure
	Arrhythmia
	Acute coronary syndromes
	Pseudocoarctation (aortic dissection)
Pharmacologically induced	Digitalis, vasoactive substances (catecholamines, somatostatin analogues, etc.), ergotism.

ABBREVIATIONS: MI, myocardial infarction; SBE, subacute bacterial endocarditis.

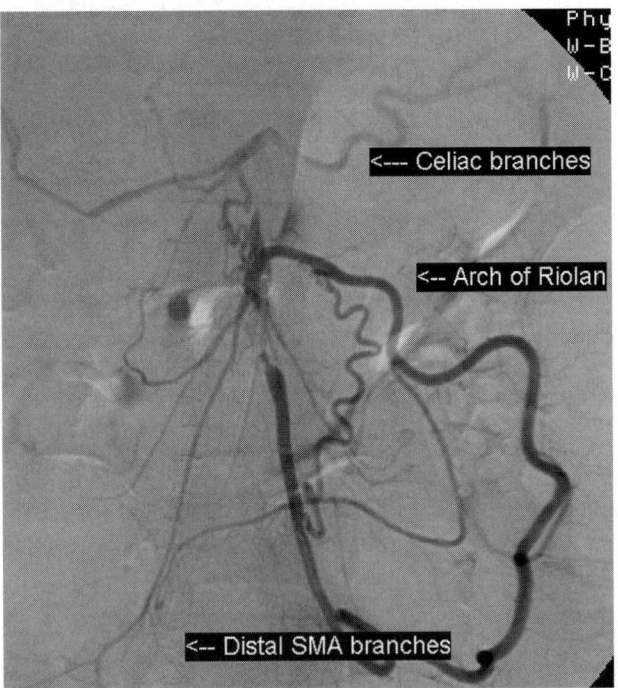

FIGURE 86-1 Late IMA injection demonstrating the IMA to the arch of Riolan, filling the stump of the SMA with its distal branches. Also note filling of hepatic and splenic branches.

superior and inferior gastroduodenal arteries. The SMA territory may be perfused from the celiac artery, as mentioned, or from the IMA territory via the *arch of Riolan*, a collateral that runs in the midmesentery and is fed via the ascending branch of the left colic artery (Fig. 86-1). The IMA territory may collateralize proximally, as described, or distally via the inferior hemorrhoidal arteries from the internal iliac artery. Blood from the pelvis may collateralize to the SMA or above from the communications between the sigmoidal-hemorrhoidal vessels to the marginal artery of Drummond (a collateral that runs within 1 to 2 cm of the mesenteric edge of the bowel) and via the arch of Riolan. Vessel caliber decreases progressively from the main aortic branch to the mesenteric vascular arcades distally, ending with an extensive communicating submucosal vascular plexus. This collateral network explains why many individuals may tolerate chronic occlusion of one or two mesenteric vessels without symptoms, but it also explains why acute-on-chronic occlusion of one branch may lead to a catastrophic loss of intestinal perfusion.

Control of the Mesenteric Circulation

The mesenteric circulation receives approximately 20% to 30% of the cardiac output at rest, which may increase by up to 50% after meals.[6] As such, the mesenteric circulation receives approximately three times more blood per unit weight than most other body tissues. This blood flow is partly to satisfy the absorptive function of the intestine and perfuse the liver via the portal vein, but it also represents a reservoir function from which blood can be mobilized to other sites (vital organs) at times of stress or increased demand. This preferential shunting of blood to vital organs, if acute or severe, can "sacrifice" the mesenteric circulation, leading to low-flow and

ischemic injury. The more metabolically active mucosal layer receives 70% of blood flow, only 30% supplying the muscularis and serosal layers, placing the intestinal mucosa at greatest risk from ischemic injury.[6] Within the intestinal villus, passive exchange of oxygen typically occurs between the afferent arteriole and efferent venule, effectively bypassing the capillary network at the villus tip, a phenomenon called *oxygen countercurrent exchange*. In health, high partial pressures of oxygen ensure that the metabolic needs of the villus mucosa are met despite this shunting, but in deoxygenated states this shunting adversely affects oxygen delivery to the mucosal tip, making it most vulnerable to ischemic injury. A number of extrinsic and intrinsic factors regulate the mesenteric blood flow, leading to a complex interaction between neural, hormonal, and paracrine effectors that regulate the vascular smooth muscle tone in the mesenteric bed and control local blood flow. Vasoactive mediators alter the vascular smooth muscle (VSM) tone of multiple small afferent arterioles, collectively known as *resistance vessels*, changing their cross-sectional area and blood flow (Table 86-2). The interaction between extracellular agonist (first messenger) and VSM receptor leads to accumulation of intracellular second messengers, such as cyclic adenosine monophosphate (cAMP), Ca^{2+}, and cyclic guanosine monophosphate (cGMP). These second messengers directly or indirectly alter the cytosolic concentration of Ca^{2+} and dictate whether VSM contracts.[7] A functioning cardiovascular system is essential because the mesenteric circulation is often sacrificed to maintain blood flow to vital organs at times of detrimental alterations in cardiac output, blood volume, or arterial blood pressure. Increased sympathetic nervous activity associated with cardiogenic, septic, or hypovolemic shock can further compound flow-related ischemia by inducing intense vasocontriction within the mesenteric bed. High-volume hemorrhage (> 35% of blood volume) leads to disproportionate visceral vasoconstriction compared with the reduction in cardiac output.[8] When activated postganglionic sympathetic nerves fibers release norepinephrine, stimulating α_2-adrenergic receptors on VSM of precapillary arterioles (which are the *resistance vessels*), this results in vasoconstriction and reduced intestinal blood flow. Some compensation is provided by the simultaneous stimulation of vasodilatory β_2-adrenergic receptors on VSM by norepinephrine.[9] However the net effect is a rapid reduction in flow followed by a gradual return to prestimulation blood flow levels, a phenomenon known as *autoregulatory escape*. Exogenously administered norepinephrine similarly can cause nonocclusive mesenteric ischemia (NOMI). Parasympathetic nerves induce vasodilation due to the effect of specific neurotransmitters acetylcholine (ACh, increases cGMP and NO), vasoactive intestinal protein (VIP, increases cAMP), and adenosine triphosphate (ATP). Primary sensory nerves also play a role because their activity through C fibers can inhibit sympathetic impulse flow through the spinal cord or sympathetic ganglia. Indeed, direct antidromic vasodilation can occur as C fibers release neuropeptides, including substance P, calcitonin gene–related peptide, and VIP, in response to luminal signals. Humoral (endocrine) messengers also can affect the mesenteric blood flow, most notably adrenal catecholamines in states of systemic stress, shock, or secreting tumor (pheochromocytoma). Similarly vasocontrictive effects are seen with renal-derived angiotensin II in congestive heart failure and pituitary-derived

TABLE 86-2 Potential Vasoactive Mediators of the Enteric Circulation

Mediator	Vasoconstrictors	Vasodilators
Neural	↑ Sympathetic tone (adrenergic)	↓ Sympathetic tone (cholinergic)
	↓ Parasympathetic tone	↑ Parasympathetic tone
	Neuropeptide Y	Substance P
		Vasoactive intestinal peptide (VIP)
		Calcitonin gene-related peptide (CGRPα)
Humoral	Catecholamines (except liver & muscle)	Catecholamines (only liver & muscle)
	Angiotenisin II	Histamine
	Vasopressin	Bradykinin
	Serotonin	Activated complement (C3a, C5a)
	Activated complement (C5a)	Adrenomedullin
Paracrine/	Endothelin-1 (VSM cells)	Endothelium-derived relaxing factor
autocrine	Platelet-activating factor	(EDRF)
	Constrictor prostaglandins ($F_{2\alpha}$)	Endothelium-derived hyperpolarizing
		factor
		Dilator prostaglandins (I_2 or prostacyclin)
		Endothelin-1 (endothelial cells)
Metabolic	↑P_{O_2}	↓P_{O_2}
	↓P_{CO_2}	↑P_{CO_2}
	↑pH	↓pH
	↓ Metabolites (K^+, lactate, adenosine, etc.)	↑Metabolites

vasopressin in shock, respectively. Ingested meals and gastrointestinal luminal peptides stimulate a postprandial increase in mesenteric blood flow. This vasodilatory response is regulated, in part, by the increased metabolic activity in the tissues, leading to local accumulation of vasoactive metabolites such as amines, peptides, prostanoids, and adenosine in the presence of a reduced oxygen concentration. Adenosine itself, increasing as a result of energy-dependent processes, may vasodilate in a paracrine fashion. A number of hormones are also released in response to luminal contents, including gastrin, cholecystokinin, and secretin, with net vasodilatory effects.[10] Somatostatin, released by the mucosal D cells, induces mucosal vasoconstriction, and synthetic analogs (e.g., octreotide) can induce ischemia.

Pathophysiology of Intestinal Ischemia

The unique arrangement whereby the mesenteric blood flow continues in series via the portal vein, supplying much of the metabolic need of the liver, means that oxygen extraction by intestinal tissue remains low at rest. Therefore, intestinal tissues may respond to reduced flow by increasing oxygen extraction from the blood without a requirement for increased blood flow, but this deprives the liver of some of its portal-derived oxygenation, resulting in hepatic ischemia. On a biochemical and microscopic level, acute ischemia of the intestine is characterized by depletion of cellular adenosine triphosphate (ATP), failure of energy-dependent processes (in particular membrane ATPase pumps), cellular swelling, membrane disruption, metabolic arrest, and cell death.[11] Hypoxic conditions themselves favor the conversion of the abundant amounts of xanthine dehydrogenase to xanthine oxidase. Accumulating adenosine is metabolized further to inosine and then hypoxanthine but no further without oxygen. With the reintroduction of oxygen on reperfusion, xanthine oxidase converts hypoxanthine to xanthine, pro-

ducing superoxide (reperfusion tissue injury[12]). Oxygen free-radicals (OFRs), including superoxide anions (O_2^-), hydrogen peroxide (H_2O_2), and hydroxyl radicals (OH^-), arise as by-products of the xanthine–xanthine oxidase system, the mitochondrial electron transport system, and the NADPH oxidase system of infiltrating neutrophils. Endogenous defenses against oxidative injury, including intracellular enzymes (superoxide dismutase, catalase, and glutathione peroxidase) and vitamins (C and E), are overwhelmed by the production of OFRs. The OFRs directly attack cell membranes, inducing lipid peroxidation and synthesis of lipid mediators (thromboxane A_2, leukotiene B_4) and chemotactic peptides (complement component C5a), which promote neutrophil activation and chemotaxis. Sequestration of circulating neutrophils in the microvessels of the intestine begins with constitutively expressed neutrophil L-selectin receptors binding to the postcapillary venule endothelial P-selectin and E-selectin receptors.[13] This is the first phase of neutrophil adhesion, manifested by neutrophil rolling along the venular luminal surface. The second phase of neutrophil adhesion occurs after upregulation of the CD11/CD18 integrins and shedding of L-selectin from the neutrophil surface, caused by release of proinflammatory cytokines, platelet-activating factor (PAF), and eicosanoids from the damaged endothelial cell. This halts neutrophil rolling by providing strong neutrophil–endothelial cell adhesion through the interaction of the CD11b/CD18 integrin with the endothelial receptor, intercellular adhesion molecule 1 (ICAM-1).[14] Finally, neutrophils transmigrate in response to chemotactic stimuli (such as interleukin-8) and binding by platelet–endothelial cell adhesion molecule 1 (PECAM-1). Neutrophils further damage tissue by releasing superoxide anions via the NADPH oxidase system, secreting myeloperoxidase that catalyzes the production of hypochlorous acid (HOCL), and releasing granular enzymes, including elastase, collagenase, and cathepsin G. Many capillaries fail to perfuse on reinstitution of blood flow, the *no-reflow phenomenon*, due to loss of local autoregulation combined with mechanical obstruction of narrowed capillaries by enlarged adherent neutrophils.[15] This results in incomplete and patchy tissue reperfusion, prolonging hypoxia and exposure of the tissues to toxic metabolites. On a microscopic level, complete ischemia causes detectable injury to the superficial part of the mucosa (the villi) within 20 minutes. As the duration of ischemia increases, the villus loss can be complete before the muscular layers are damaged. Patchy cellular necrosis can extend to mucosal sloughing seen clinically as bloody diarrhea. Ultimately, there is transmural infarction, perforation, and septic peritonitis. Prior to reperfusion, metabolic products such as lactate and other acids are not absorbed via the neglible portal circulation but only through the peritoneal surfaces, accounting for the lack of acidosis commonly observed in patients with acute mesenteric ischemia.

Systemic Response to Mesenteric Revascularisation

On reperfusion of the acutely ischemic intestine, local injury can induce a systemic phenomenon as metabolic byproducts of the ischemic process (lactate, H^+, K^+, oxygen reactive species, arachidonic acid derivatives, cytokines, possibly endotoxin, and activated leukocytes) are flushed into the systemic circulation. A systemic inflammatory response syndrome (SIRS) is initiated, triggering the complement and coagulation cascades, elaborating cytokines, and provoking widespread endothelial dysfunction and vital organ injury. Even in those surviving this initial phase of acute gut-derived inflammation, the reperfused but injured intestine can continue to be detrimental to the host. The gastrointestinal tract normally is inhabited by a large collection of gram-negative bacteria. Gut-mucosal barrier disruption after ischemia-reperfusion injury allows translocation of these bacteria.[16,17] The vast hepatic sinusoid network, lined with fixed-tissue macrophages (Kupffer cells), is strategically located to interact with gut-derived endotoxin and contribute to multiple-organ-system failure (MOSF). Noncardiogenic pulmonary edema is well recognized after intestinal ischemia-reperfusion injury.[14,18] Postoperatively, renal and hepatic dysfunction also are common.

Intestinal Ischemia Risk Factors

A number of factors influence the development of and survival from acute mesenteric ischemia. Factors predisposing to occlusive mesenteric ischemia include hypertension, tobacco use, family history of cardiovascular disease, peripheral vascular disease, coronary artery disease, diabetes, congestive heart failure, prior myocardial infarction, cerebrovascular disease, hypercholesterolemia, and atrial fibrillation.[19,20] Nonocclusive mesenteric ischemia results from splanchnic vasoconstriction in response to systemic factors and is associated with acute cardiac dysfunction (myocardial infarction, arrhythmia, left ventricular dysfunction), hypovolemia, and pharmacotherapy.[21] Factors predictive of mortality secondary to intestinal ischemia include advanced age, generally poor health, diagnostic delay, and nonocclusive mesenteric ischemia.[5] Most patients with asymptomatic high-grade

stenosis or occlusions of all three mesenteric trunks will develop symptoms or die during follow-up.[22] Therefore, elective revascularization should be considered if they are fit for surgery.

Clinical Presentation of Mesenteric Ischemia

The classic diagnostic triad for chronic intestinal ischemia includes weight loss, abdominal angina, and altered bowel habit.[4] The acute presentation may be on a background of chronic intestinal angina or de novo in a previously unsuspected individual with symptoms ranging from subtle signs of intraabdominal sepsis to the dramatic acute abdomen.

ACUTE EMBOLIC OBSTRUCTION

Acute embolic obstruction of the SMA is characterized by acute onset of severe central abdominal pain, often associated with nausea, vomiting, and even diarrhea or a bowel movement. Pain often is described as out of proportion to objective findings and is poorly localized until advanced signs of peritonitis ensue. The patient often adopts a chin-to-knees body habitus, initially restless but later lying quiety once peritonitis develops. In the early stages, abdominal examination may be truly unremarkable, perhaps with some diffuse tenderness without localized peritonitis. Development of an ileus or peritoneal findings is a grave sign suggestive of mesenteric infarction. Bloody diarrhea is a late sign associated with mucosal disruption.[20] Initial collapse is not uncommon, but sustained hypotension in the early stages is more likely due to a cardiac than an intestinal cause. Embolic sources, such as arrhythmia (atrial fibrillation), acute myocardial infarction, dilated cardiomyopathy, or a recently instrumented aorta, should be sought.

ACUTE THROMBOTIC OCCLUSION

Thrombotic occlusion occurs often in the setting of chronic symptoms of mesenteric ischemia. When possible, a history of weight loss, intestinal angina, or altered bowel habit should be sought. The presence of chronically developed collaterals may protect against distal ischemia, making the presentation subtle and gradual, with only vague abdominal pain and altered bowel habit initially. However, preexisting atherosclerotic disease in the other major mesenteric trunks will predispose to acute-on-chronic thrombosis of the remaining trunk, critically restricting flow to the entire mesenteric bed and leading to massive mesenteric infarction.

NONOCCLUSIVE MESENTERIC ISCHEMIA

There is increasing awareness of nonocclusive mesenteric ischemia (NOMI). Any systemic hypoperfusion state can threaten the mesenteric territory, with local vasoconstriction leading to a severely reduced mesenteric perfusion. Mesenteric vasoconstriction may be precipitated by a variety of shock states, namely, cardiogenic, septic, hypovolemic, and even anaphylaxis.[23] Furthermore, drugs commonly used to treat acute cardiac dysfunction (digoxin, β blockers) and those employed to support the failing circulation (catecholamines, vasopressin) may exacerbate mesenteric vasoconstriction. Therefore, NOMI should be considered early in any hypotensive patient with suggestive findings.[21] Clinical signs are often vague, with new or persistent ileus, abdominal distention, or sepsis of unknown source. Rectal mucus, melena, or frank blood are nonspecific but may point to bowel ischemia. There may be a role for gastrointestinal balloon tonometry in indentifying patients with or at risk of developing NOMI. Recreational drugs (e.g., cocaine) have been reported recently to cause acute NOMI, and a history should be sought if suspicion arises.[24]

MESENTERIC VEIN THROMBOSIS

Mesenteric vein thrombosis most often results in a delayed presentation, often preceded by several weeks of intermittent abdominal pain and altered bowel habit,[2] but it also can cause acute abdominal signs and fever. It should be suspected in patients with previous abdominal surgery, thrombophilia, prior mesenteric or deep venous thrombosis, cirrhosis, or malignancy.

MISCELLANEOUS CAUSES OF ACUTE MESENTERIC ISCHEMIA

Other pathologic processes occasionally causing acute mesenteric ischemia include aortic surgery (when the IMA is ligated and collateral flow is insufficient[25]), aortic dissection[26] (even when mesenteric vessels are not directly involved, hypotension may combine with pseudocoarctation to provoke ischemia), aortic trauma, mesenteric aneurysm rupture, arteritis, fibromuscular dysplasia (FMD), and extrinsic mechan-

ical vascular obstruction. Acute intestinal ischemia also may arise as a result of extrinsic mechanical compression of the arterial inflow or venous outflow. As low-pressure conduits, veins are most susceptible to extrinsic compression; intramural venous plexi may be obstructed due to wall distention, whereas mesenteric veins may be compressed by tumor, adhesion, volvulus, hernia, or intussusception.

Diagnosis of Acute Mesenteric Ischemia

The single most important factor is clinical suspicion followed by investigation. A delay in diagnosis may be lethal.[20] No single blood marker has proved to be an adequate screening test. Lactic acidosis has poor sensitivity in detecting bowel ischemia. Despite advances with noninvasive radiologic testing, mesenteric angiography remains the definitive test. ACT angiogram may yield similar information while also demonstrating abnormalities of the bowel wall. Even with high-quality imaging studies, laparotomy may be required for definitive diagnosis. A suggested algorithm for the initial approach to a patient with suspected acute mesenteric ischemia is given in Fig. 86-2.

LABORATORY SERUM PARAMETERS

No serum marker has been proven to be sensitive and/or specific enough to confirm reliably the presence or absence of acute mesenteric ischemia. Nevertheless, some are clinically useful. In acute mesenteric ischemia, a leukocytosis is almost invariably present, except in those who are immunocompromised owing to comorbid disease, advanced age,

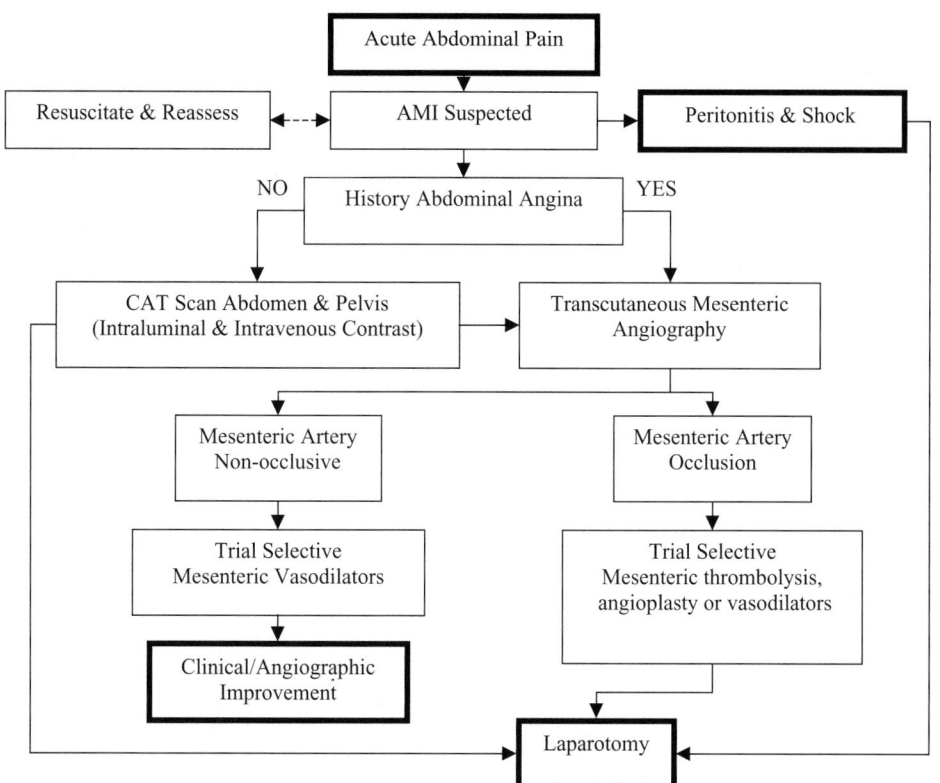

FIGURE 86-2 Algorithm for the diagnosis and investigation of mesenteric ischemia.

corticosteroid treatment, or profound critical illness. A neutrophilia is typical (total white blood cell typically = 16,000 to 30,000/μL), and early white cell forms are common. Platelets typically are reduced. Coagulopathy may be present in advanced mesenteric ischemia with sepsis or perforation. Arterial blood gases frequently are normal initially, but in the later stages, metabolic acidosis and acute hypoxia may supervene. Lactic acidosis is often a late finding. Prerenal azotemia is a grave indicator, signaling hypovolemia, sepsis, nephrotoxic effect, or disseminated intravascular coagulation (DIC). The erythrocyte sedimentation rate (ESR) and later C-reactive protein (CRP) level may rise. Potential alternative serum markers, such as creatinine kinase (CK) BB isoenzyme, lactate dehydrogenase, intestinal isoenzyme of alkaline phosphatase, diamine oxidase, hexosaminidase, and aspartate transferase, have not proved sufficiently sensitive or specific. The most encouraging markers are serum inorganic phosphate,[27] α-glutathione-S-transferase,[28] and D-lactate.[29] Another possible marker is intestinal fatty acid–binding protein (I-FABP), which is currently the focus of a prospective trial.

PLAIN ABDOMINAL RADIOGRAM

Plain abdominal radiographs may reveal supporting information such as heavy calcification of the abdominal vasculature, although this is neither sensitive nor specific. In a retrospective series of 23 patients with acute mesenteric ischemia, 26% had normal plain films. Nonspecific signs of ischemia, such as intestinal dilation or gasless abdomen, may be present, but the greatest value of the abdominal radiograph is in establishing an alternative diagnosis. In the advanced stages of mesenteric ischemia, mural changes such as wall thickening or valvulae conniventes, "thumb printing," or intramural gas (pneumatosis intestinalis) may be present.[30] Intrahepatic portal vein pneumatosis or free intraperitoneal gas also may be seen.

ULTRASOUND

B-mode ultrasonography is quick, readily available, noninvasive, and well tolerated by most patients with abdominal pain. When acute mesenteric ischemia is present, ultrasonography may reveal a thickened (>5 mm) bowel wall and signs of ileus (distended bowel loops and hypoperistalsis). In advanced cases (mesenteric infarction), ultrasound may show intraperitoneal fluid, pneumatosis, or intrahepatic portal venous gas. However, ultrasonography is operator-dependent and may be confounded by the degree of intraluminal intestinal gas or by obesity. For patients with suspected chronic mesenteric ischemia, duplex ultrasonography has become the investigation of choice by many. A peak systolic velocity of greater than 275 cm/s in the SMA or greater than 200 cm/s in the celiac artery or no flow signal (in the SMA or celiac artery) predicts a stenosis of greater than 70% with a sensitivity of 89% and a specificity of 92%.[31]

CT SCAN AND CT-ANGIOGRAM

CT scanning is the radiologic investigation of choice for acute abdominal pain at many centers. Oral contrast enhancement may give better luminal definition but is not used by many centers, especially in the emergency situation. Intravenous contrast enhancement (CT-angiography, CTA) further elabo-

rates the major vessel flow and tissue perfusion (Fig. 86-3). All three mesenteric vessels can be identified and patency assessed by their contrast content. Alternatives to iodinated contrast agents, such as gadolinium, may be used for patients with a contraindication to standard contrast material. Ischemic bowel wall typically is seen as thin and poorly enhanced, more prominent on the antimesenteric border in NOMI. Air may be seen in the bowel wall or the portal vein. Reperfused bowel segments appear enlarged and edematous, often with increased mucosal and submucosal enhancement due to interstitial extravasation of contrast material.[32] With the increased availability of modern multislice helical CT scanners, rapidly acquired high-quality CTA images of the main mesenteric trunks and small collaterals are possible.[64] Compared with mesenteric angiography, CTA may prove safer, cheaper, and better tolerated and result in decreased radiation exposure for both patient and staff.

FIGURE 86-3 *A.* CT slice with SMA almost completely occluded with thrombus. *B.* CT slice that shows SMA without contrast adjacent to portal vein.

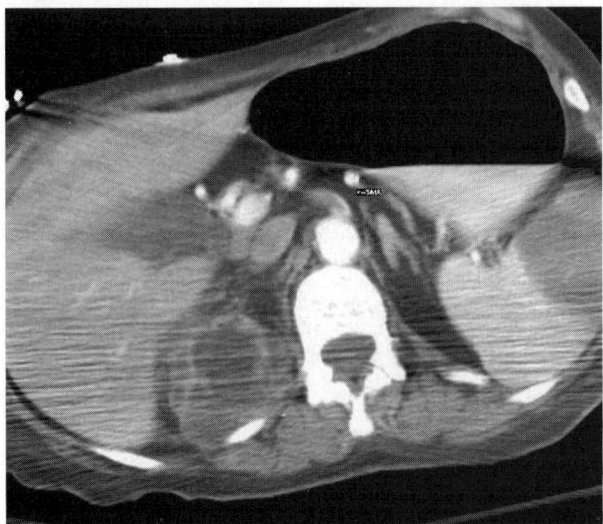

A

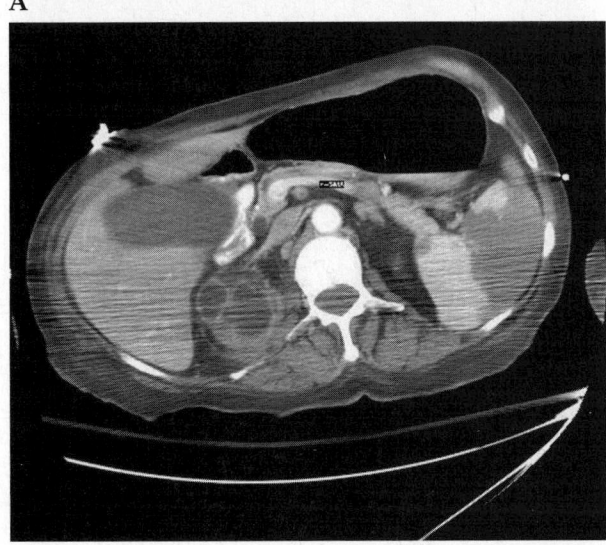

B

MRI AND MR-ANGIOGRAPHY (MRA)

The superior soft-tissue definition and non-contrast-enhanced angiographic ability of MRI give it potential advantages in patients with an acute abdomen.[33] Recent advances in MRA technology and the use of contrast-enhanced (CE) techniques have shortened acquisition times and reduced the impact of motion artifacts, which previously had restricted its use.[34] MRA may prove to be the investigation of choice in chronic mesenteric ischemia, where it has been suggested that CE-MRA is superior to digital subtraction angiography for simultaneous exploration of the abdominal aorta and its major branches, and it can be coupled with measurements of flow and assessment of surrounding soft tissues.[35] However, at present, its use in emergency practice remains experimental.

ANGIOGRAPHY

Mesenteric angiography remains the most specific test for the diagnosis of mesenteric ischemia, giving objective, reproducible evidence and in some instances providing therapeutic catheter-based options.[36] Not only does it identify the location of the flow-limiting lesion, but it also may give information about distal runoff and the extent of collateralization, allowing the most appropriate therapy to be planned. However, it cannot discern whether or not intestinal infarction has occurred, and therefore, treatment always must be planned with full assessment of clinical and laboratory parameters, especially if a catheter-based therapy is planned.[37]

Thrombotic occlusion usually occurs on a background of chronic atherosclerotic disease, where lesions tend to be at or near the ostium, producing an abrupt cutoff of contrast (Fig.-86-4). The chronicity of the atherosclerotic process may be indicated by the presence of multivessel disease or the presence of large collaterals refilling the branch territories distally. One must consider the clinical findings carefully be-

FIGURE 86-4 Angiographic image of elective injection of the IMA with severe origin stenosis.

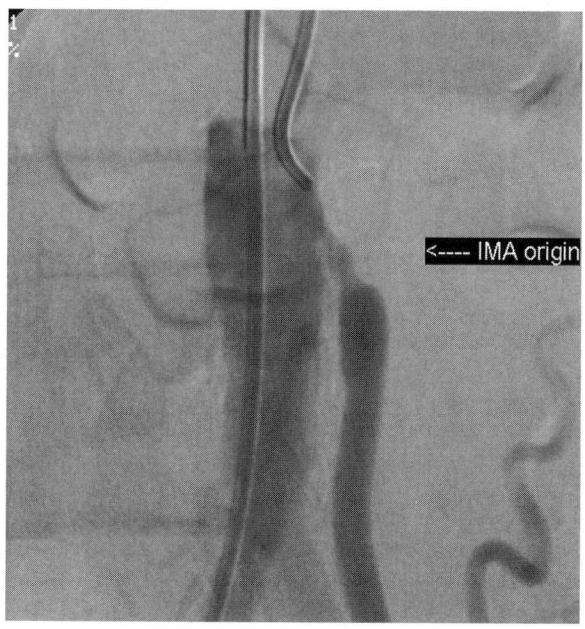

cause chronic mesenteric occlusions are seen in up to 60% of the octogenarian population but cause symptoms in only 5%.

Mesenteric artery emboli present as sharp, rounded filling defects with a typical meniscus sign. Distal vessels may refill through collateral vessels. Emboli typically lodge at the sites of vessel narrowing, such as the origin or a bifurcation. The SMA is affected most often because it is a relatively large vessel with high flow, and its orientation encourages antegrade entry of the embolus. SMA emboli typically occlude the vessel just distal to the middle colic artery origin.

Nonocclusive mesenteric ischemia is typified by diffuse narrowing of the mesenteric artery and its branches, alternating areas of narrowing and dilation of the main trunk and branches ("string of sausages sign"), spasm of the peripheral vascular arcades, impaired filling of intramural vessels, and slow flow with increased reflux of contrast material into the aorta during selective injection. An increase in vessel caliber after transcatheter papaverine injection may clinch the diagnosis. Mesenteric venous thrombosis is seen on the later phase of angiography with contrast stasis and lack of portal venous phase filling.

Management

Initial management includes identifying and correcting immediately any life-threatening hypoperfusion or electrolyte abnormalities while planning further definitive steps toward diagnosis and treatment. Simple airway management with supplemental oxygen by mask, titrated to achieve oxygen saturation above 95%, will suffice in patients who are breathing spontaneously. Obtunded patients typically should be intubated electively, bearing in mind the risk of aspiration owing to gastroparesis and intestinal ileus. A wide-bore nasogastric tube should be placed for intestinal decompression. Acute electrolyte disturbances such as hypokalemia, hypomagnesemia, and hypophosphatemia should be corrected. Broad-spectrum antibiotics (e.g., second-generation penicillin or third-generation cephalosporin, along with anaerobic coverage) should be administered intravenously. Analgesia should not be withheld in the conscious patient. Systemic heparinization is advocated once the diagnosis is strongly suspected, unless there are absolute contraindications. The goal is a partial thromboplastin time (PTT) of greater than 2 times control.

DIAGNOSTIC AND THERAPEUTIC SELECTIVE MESENTERIC ANGIOGRAPHY

Where there is diagnostic doubt in a patient with suspected mesenteric ischemia but stable clinical assessment, diagnostic mesenteric angiography is advocated.[38] Modern catheters and techniques reduce the risks of bleeding, dissection, and embolization. In a well-resuscitated patient, small-volume nonionic contrast and digital subtraction angiography (DSA) limit the risk of nephrotoxicity and contrast reaction. An initial flush aortogram may define the origins of the major vessels and outline possible collateral pathways. Selective mesenteric artery catheterization allows for thorough assessment of individual arterial territories and opens up therapeutic options.[39]

For NOMI, catheter-based therapy is the treatment of choice in the absence of definitive signs of intestinal infarction.[40]

Papaverine (30 to 60 mg/h) is infused selectively into the SMA for a period of 24 hours. Repeat flush angiography should confirm partial or complete resolution of spasm 30 minutes after beginning the infusion and prior to the patient's return to the ICU. Papaverine is a potent phosphodiesterase inhibitor, leading to increased intracellular cAMP and vasodilation.[41] Because of extensive hepatic first-pass metabolism, systemic effects such as hypotension generally are modest. Failure of therapy may be signaled by cardiovascular instability, progression of clinical symptoms or signs, and catheter displacement or blockage.

Occlusive mesenteric ischemia traditionally requires surgery. However, increasing numbers of interventional radiologists are exploring the use of catheter-based therapies as long as there is no frank intestinal infarction. A number of techniques are available for recanalization, including suction clot retrieval, thrombolysis, angioplasty,[42] and stenting.[43] All these techniques remain investigational and should be conducted only in collaboration with an appropriately trained surgeon and an interventional radiologist and with appropriate monitoring and reassessment of the patient.[44] Even when a decision is made to proceed to surgery, continued infusion of papaverine or heparin into the occluded vessel may improve distal circulation and prevent clot propagation pending definitive surgery.

MINIMALLY INVASIVE SURGERY

In the setting of high suspicion of acute mesenteric ischemia, some have advocated laparoscopic assessment of the abdominal contents[45] and have suggested that this can be done safely with high diagnostic accuracy.[46] The minilaparoscopy is being advocated increasingly in the critical care setting where there remains diagnostic doubt in a deteriorating patient, and some have done this safely at the bedside.[47] The generally poor results of open surgery, even in good hands, have encouraged some surgeons to explore less invasive alternatives using laparoscopic techniques. Some practitioners have claimed improved survival and reduced morbidity using this approach, but whether these results in specialized centers can be extended to other settings is unknown.[48]

OPEN SURGERY

Often the definitive assessment and management of acute mesenteric ischemia require open surgery.[49] The surgeon should repeat the abdominal examination once the patient is anesthetized. In the absence of muscle tone and tenderness, new pathology, such as an abdominal mass or aortic aneurysm, may be detected. Adequate exposure generally requires a full midline laparotomy with transperitoneal approach. Although retroperitoneal approaches to the aorta and branches are useful in chronic mesenteric revascularization, they do not allow adequate assessment of intestinal perfusion and viability in the acute setting. The initial aim is to confirm the diagnosis and rule out any major confounding disease. The acutely ischemic intestine may appear remarkably normal prior to infarction and before reperfusion. Changes may be focal, segmental, or global depending on the etiology of the ischemia. The intestine is inspected for loss of sheen, discoloration (gray through black), and lack of peristalsis. SMA thrombosis typically occurs at the origin, so the distri-

bution of ischemia classically involves the entire small bowel and proximal half of the colon. SMA embolism, on the other hand, may spare the right colic branch and proximal jejunum branches if it lodges distal to the origin. However, the clot may lodge at the origin, giving a similar pattern to thrombosis. Microemboli typically disperse and lodge distally, creating patchy areas of ischemia with normal intervening segments. Delicate palpation for arterial pulsation must be carried from the root of the SMA to its mesenteric branches. Visible pulsation may be seen in the mesenteric arterial arcades. More objective assessment by means of sterile Doppler ultrasound probe may reveal an absence of flow in the main branches, arcades, or the intestine itself. Previously used assessment with intravenous fluorescein dye and an ultraviolet lamp is now rarely practiced clinically.[50]

Except in very advanced cases where perforation has occurred or is imminent, revascularization should precede the resection of nonviable bowel. In the presence of frank necrosis, quick segmental resection may be carried out using a gastrointestinal linear stapling device without undue delay of revascularization. On reperfusion, remarkable recovery is often witnessed in seemingly unsalvageable segments, especially important when near-total small bowel resection seems inevitable at first inspection, with the consequent implications of lifelong parenteral nutrition therapy. Caution must be exercised in the setting of an elderly, infirm, or hypotensive patient because the systemic effects of reperfusion of a profoundly ischemic intestine may lead to catastrophic acidosis, hyperkalemia, myocardial depression, and refractory shock. The initial approach to revascularization in most cases is an attempt at embolectomy; if satisfactory antegrade flow cannot be achieved, then one proceeds to mesenteric artery bypass.

SUPERIOR MESENTERIC ARTERY EMBOLECTOMY

The superior mesenteric artery may be exposed and controlled transperitoneally at the base of the transverse mesocolon, where it courses from its midline aortic origin, obscured by the body of the pancreas in its proximal few centimetres, and then rises over the fourth part of duodenum to give off its first branch, the right colic artery, and enter the mesentery. Its localization by palpation may be assisted by sterile Doppler probe in the bulky mesentery. After splitting the mesentery and retroperitoneum in the line of the vessel, it is controlled with vascular loops at the level of its bifurcation. Only minimal dissection of the numerous small perivascular nerves and lymphatics is required. Standard approach is via a tranverse arteriotomy, but longitudinal opening may help if vessel caliber is small or if bypass is to be expected. Proximal embolectomy is carried out first with a balloon catheter (size 3F or 4F). If pulsatile aortic flow is restored, the vessel is reoccluded, and the surgeon proceeds to distal embolectomy.[51] Mesenteric bypass is indicated if there is failure to pass the catheter, inadequate inflow, or a heavily diseased vessel. Distal embolectomy is performed gently manually, guiding the balloon catheter (size 3F) into the major branches, until all thrombus is retrieved and backbleeding is seen. The arterial closure should maintain an adequate lumen and is best achieved with interrupted monofilament sutures, sometimes requiring a patch angioplasty with autologous vein. Restoration of pulsatile flow should be assessed clinically by palpation and visualization of the intestinal perfusion and checked intraoperatively with sterile Doppler probe (at the bowel-intestinal margin) or duplex ultrasound. Spasm is common in the distal vessels and may be relieved by perivascular infusion of papaverine (30 mg).

SUPERIOR MESENTERIC ARTERY BYPASS

Mesenteric artery revascularization is indicated to restore intestinal blood flow if the diagnosis is mesenteric thrombotic occlusion or adequate inflow is not achieved at embolectomy.[1] A number of surgical approaches are available, but in these fragile patients a quick, durable approach is to bring retrograde inflow from the common iliac artery. The choice of inflow vessel is influenced by the quality and patency of the common iliac arteries. Either right or left can provide a suitable graft configuration. Should a vein be chosen secondary to a contaminated field, the left iliac is preferred to avoid potential kinking. If the infrarenal aorta is chosen, a nonocclusive clamp may be used. In the absence of a suitable infrarenal inflow vessel, the supraceliac aorta may be approached through the lesser sac for inflow. The choice of arterial bypass conduit is a matter of debate. Prosthetic material is easy to handle, obviates the need for autologous vein harvest, and reduces operative time. Indeed, even in the presence of moderate contamination, the risks of graft infection remain low when polytetrafluoroethylene (PTFE) or antibiotic-impregnated (rifampin 1 to 60 mg/mL) Dacron is used. In the presence of gross fecal contamination, an autologous vein graft is preferred, the reversed long saphenous vein being most suitable. The inflow anastomosis is classically end to side, and the outflow anastomosis is easiest to construct end to end after division of the superior mesenteric artery or end to side using the anterior arteriotomy employed for thrombectomy.

INTESTINAL VIABILITY

Clinical assessment by an experienced surgeon remains the most widely practiced method to determine intestinal viability. A sensitivity of 82% and a specificity of 91% were achieved using the following factors: presence of visible pulsation in the mesenteric arcades, bleeding, color, and peristalsis.[50] Increasingly, most vascular surgeons now confirm their clinical findings with a sterile Doppler ultrasound flow detector (5 MHz), detecting pulsatile Doppler signals at the mesenteric arcades and intestinal surface. The goal of intestinal resection is to remove areas of nonviable bowel and leave sufficient viable bowel to sustain independent life. In general, if a large segment (>6 ft of small intestine) of obviously viable bowel can be identified, then nonviable segments should be resected liberally. Restoration of continuity is preferred; anastomoses may be hand sewn to preserve more functioning intestine, but a stapler may be quicker. In the presence of gross contamination or doubtful viability, creating a stoma may be considered, but in this setting a "second look" laparotomy (after 18 to 36 hours) would allow adequate resuscitation of the patient and clearer differentiation of bowel viability.[52] In the case where a second look is required, obviously necrotic segments may be resected using a linear gastrointestinal stapling device, and continuity need not be restored, cutting operative

time. A tunneled central venous catheter should be placed at the time of surgery in most of these patients to facilitate long-term parenteral nutrition.

POSTOPERATIVE CARE AND FOLLOW-UP SURVEILLANCE

Postoperative care must be in an intensive care setting if acceptable results are to be achieved in these high-risk patients. Second-look laparotomy should be the rule rather than the exception and, when planned at the initial surgery, must be adhered to despite the patient's clinical course.[19] Reperfusion of the ischemic intestine leads to inflammatory edema of the affected segments, and this, combined with large volumes of intraluminal fluid sequestration, places these patients at risk for developing abdominal compartment syndrome in the postoperative period[53] (see Chap. 42). Beyond basic fluid management and cardiorespiratory support, attention must be given to nutritional support. In the catabolic postoperative recovery phase, demands are increased, often on a background of chronic malnourishment and often compounded by dysfunctional reperfused bowel and short bowel syndromes. After major resections, postoperative parenteral nutrition invariably is required, often for extended periods, because even viable segments often have prolonged absorptive and motility dysfunction for extended periods.[54] Postoperative heparin therapy should be continued in the absence of bleeding diathesis, and oral warfarin should be commenced, with a target International Normailzation Ratio (INR) of 2.0 to 3.0, as soon as oral diet is resumed. In the case of embolic disease, a primary source should be sought by transthoracic or transesophageal echocardiography and full aortic (chest and abdomen) CT scanning.[65] Thoracic aortic mural thrombus is an infrequent cause of emboli that is being recognized with increasing frequency by transesophegeal echocardiography and confirmed by CT scanning.[65] Thrombotic occlusions especially of the mesenteric vein should prompt a thrombophilia evaluation. Secondary prevention strategies such as smoking cessation and dietary and therapeutic lipid

TABLE 86-3 Recent Acute Mesenteric Revascularisation Outcomes

Author	Patients (% acute)	Perioperative Mortality (%)	5-Year (Survival %)
Edwards et al., 2003[54]	76(100)	62	—
Bjorck et al., 2002[1a]	58(100)	43	67
Park et al., 2002[5]	58(100)	32	32[ab]
Endean et al., 2001[2]	58(100)	48	—
Foley et al., 2000[3]	21(100)	24	—
Mamode et al., 1999[57]	57(100)	81	—
Newman et al., 1998[58]	98(100)	60	—
Urayama et al., 1998[59]	34(100)	35	—
Klempnauer et al., 1997[60]	90(100)	66	—
Voltolini et al., 1996[61]	47(100)	72	—
Konturek et al., 1996[62]	28(100)	96	—
Ward et al., 1995[63]	34(100)	45	—
Johnston et al., 1995[56]	9(100)	22	52
Total	668	52	

[a] Multicentre study.
[b] Cumulative 3-year survival.

control may prevent further cerebrovascular and mesenteric vascular events.

Prognosis

Despite numerous advances in the assessment, diagnosis, and treatment of mesenteric ischemia, the mortality rate remains very high even in specialist centres (Table 86-3). Diagnostic delay is perhaps the greatest hurdle to improvement. Most patients who survive the initial perioperative period regain independent living, with results comparable with elective revascularization of chronic mesenteric ischaemia.[55] The sequelae of short-bowel syndrome may necessitate home parenteral feeding for a period in many and for the long term in a third of survivors.[54] Our group has highlighted the need for continued surveillance of mesenteric bypass grafts to improve the secondary patency and avoid recurrent ischemia.[56]

References

1. Bjorck M, Acosta S, Lindberg F, et al: Revascularization of the superior mesenteric artery after acute thromboembolic occlusion. *Br J Surg* 89:923, 2002.
2. Endean ED, et al: Surgical management of thrombotic acute intestinal ischemia. *Ann Surg* 233:801, 2001.
3. Foley MI, et al: Revascularization of the superior mesenteric artery alone for treatment of intestinal ischemia. *J Vasc Surg* 32:37, 2000.
4. Croft RJ, Menon GP, Marston A: Does "intestinal angina" exist? A critical study of obstructed visceral arteries. *Br J Surg* 68:316, 1981.
5. Park WM, et al: Contemporary management of acute mesenteric ischemia: Factors associated with survival. *J Vasc Surg* 35:445, 2002.
6. Chou CC. et al : Localization of mesenteric hyperemia during digestion in dogs. *Am J Physiol* 230:583, 1976.
7. Matheson PJ, Wilson MA, Garrison RN: Regulation of intestinal blood flow. *J Surg Res* 93:182, 2000.
8. Toung T, Reilly PM, Fuh KC, et al: Mesenteric vasoconstriction in response to hemorrhagic shock. *Shock* 13:267, 2000.
9. Donald DE, Shepherd JT: Autonomic regulation of the peripheral circulation. *Annu Rev Physiol* 42:429, 1980.
10. Gallavan RH Jr, Chou CC, Kvietys PR.Sit SP: Regional blood flow during digestion in the conscious dog. *Am J Physiol* 238:H220, 1980.
11. Granger DN, Parks DA: Role of oxygen radicals in the pathogenesis of intestinal ischemia. *Physiologist* 26:159, 1983.
12. Granger DN, McCord JM, Parks DA, Hollwarth ME: Xanthine oxidase inhibitors attenuate ischemia-induced vascular permeability changes in the cat intestine. *Gastroenterology* 90:80, 1986.
13. Parks DA, Shah AK, Granger DN: Oxygen radicals: Effects on intestinal vascular permeability. *Am J Physiol* 247:G167, 1984.
14. Carden DL, Young JA, Granger DN: Pulmonary microvascular injury after intestinal ischemia-reperfusion: Role of P-selectin. *J Appl Physiol* 75:2529, 1993.
15. Jerome SN, Akimitsu T, Korthuis RJ: Leukocyte adhesion, edema, and development of postischemic capillary no-reflow. *Am J Physiol* 267:H1329, 1994.
16. Fine J: The present status of the problem of endotoxin shock. *J Okla State Med Assoc* 59:419, 1966.
17. Bennion RS, Wilson SE, Serota AI, Williams RA: The role of gastrointestinal microflora in the pathogenesis of complications of mesenteric ischemia. *Rev Infect Dis* 6(suppl 1):S132, 1984.
18. Klausner JM, et al: Lower torso ischemia-induced lung injury is leukocyte dependent. *Ann Surg* 208:761, 1988.
19. Levy PJ, Krausz MM, Manny J: Acute mesenteric ischemia: improved results: A retrospective analysis of ninety-two patients. *Surgery* 107:372, 1990.
20. Huang HH, Hu SC, Yen DH, et al: The clinical factors and outcomes in patients with acute mesenteric ischemia in the emergency department. *Acad Emerg Med* 10:499, 2003.
21. Trompeter M, Brazda T, Remy CT, et al: Non-occlusive mesenteric ischemia: Etiology, diagnosis, and interventional therapy. *Eur Radiol* 12:1179, 2002.
22. Thomas JH, Blake K, Pierce GE, et al: The clinical course of asymptomatic mesenteric arterial stenosis. *J Vasc Surg* 27:840, 1998.
23. Lock G, Scholmerich J: Non-occlusive mesenteric ischemia. *Hepatogastroenterology* 42:234, 1995.
24. Sudhakar CB, Al Hakeem M, MacArthur JD, Sumpio BE: Mesenteric ischemia secondary to cocaine abuse: Case reports and literature review. *Am J Gastroenterol* 92:1053, 1997.
25. Valentine RJ, et al: Gastrointestinal complications after aortic surgery. *J Vasc Surg* 28:404, 1998.
26. Muraki SS, Fukada JJ, Morishita KK, et al: Acute type aortic dissection with intestinal ischemia predicted by serum lactate elevation. *Ann Thorac Cardiovasc Surg* 9:79, 2003.
27. Taylor BMJamieson WG, Durand D: Preinfarction diagnosis of acute mesenteric ischemia by simple measurement of inorganic phosphate in body fluids. *Can J Surg* 22:40, 1979.
28. Gearhart SL, et al : Prospective assessment of the predictive value of alpha-glutathione-S- transferase for intestinal ischemia. *Am Surg* 69:324, 2003.
29. Murray MJ, Gonze MD, Nowak LR, Cobb CF: Serum D(−)-lactate levels as an aid to diagnosing acute intestinal ischemia. *Am J Surg* 167:575, 1994.
30. DeLuca SA, Rhea JT: Bowel edema due to acute mesenteric ischemia. *Am Fam Phys* 25:175, 1982.
31. Zwolak RM: Can duplex ultrasound replace arteriography in screening for mesenteric ischemia? *Semin Vasc Surg* 12:252, 1999.
32. Chou CK: CT manifestations of bowel ischemia. *AJR* 178:87, 2002.
33. Hagspiel KD, et al: MR angiography of the mesenteric vasculature. *Radiol Clin North Am* 40:867, 2002.
34. Heiss SG, Li KC: Magnetic resonance angiography of mesenteric arteries: A review. *Invest Radiol* 33:670, 1998.
35. Laissy JP, Trillaud H, Douek P: MR angiography: Noninvasive vascular imaging of the abdomen. *Abdom Imaging* 27:488, 2002.
36. Clark RA, Gallant TE: Acute mesenteric ischemia: Angiographic spectrum. *AJR* 142:555, 1984.
37. Lefkovitz Z, Cappell MS, Lookstein R, et al: Radiologic diagnosis and treatment of gastrointestinal hemorrhage and ischemia. *Med Clin North Am* 86:1357, 2002.
38. Boos S: [Angiography of the mesenteric artery 1976 to 1991: A change in the indications during mesenteric circulatory disorders?] *Radiologe* 32:154, 1992.
39. Morano JU, Harrison RB: Mesenteric ischemia: Angiographic diagnosis and intervention. *Clin Imaging* 15:91, 1991.
40. Kaleya RN, Boley SJ: Acute mesenteric ischemia: An aggressive diagnostic and therapeutic approach. 1991 Roussel Lecture. *Can J Surg* 35:613, 1992.
41. MacCannell KL: Comparison of an intravenous selective mesenteric vasodilator with intraarterial papaverine in experimental nonocclusive mesenteric ischemia. *Gastroenterology* 91:79, 1986.
42. VanDeinse WH, Zawacki JK, Phillips D: Treatment of acute mesenteric ischemia by percutaneous transluminal angioplasty. *Gastroenterology* 91:475, 1986.
43. Rundback JH, et al: Re: Jejunal artery angioplasty and coronary stent placement for acute mesenteric ischemia. *Cardiovasc Intervent Radiol* 23:410, 2000.
44. Senechal Q, Massoni JM, Laurian C, Pernes JM: Transient relief of abdominal angina by Wallstent placement into an occluded superior mesenteric artery. *J Cardiovasc Surg (Torino)* 42:101, 2001.

45. Orlando R III, Crowell KL: Laparoscopy in the critically ill. *Surg Endosc* 11:1072, 1997.

46. Zamir G, Reissman P: Diagnostic laparoscopy in mesenteric ischemia. *Surg Endosc* 12:390, 1998.

47. Gagne DJ, Malay MB, Hogle NJ, Fowler DL: Bedside diagnostic minilaparoscopy in the intensive care patient. *Surgery* 131:491, 2002

48. Regan F, Karlstad RR, Magnuson TH: Minimally invasive management of acute superior mesenteric artery occlusion: Combined urokinase and laparoscopic therapy. *Am J Gastroenterol* 91:1019, 1996.

49. Kazmers A: Operative management of acute mesenteric ischemia, part 1. *Ann Vasc Surg* 12:187, 1998.

50. Bulkley GB, et al: Intraoperative determination of small intestinal viability following ischemic injury: A prospective, controlled trial of two adjuvant methods (Doppler and fluorescein) compared with standard clinical judgment. *Ann Surg* 193:628, 1981.

51. Batellier J, Kieny R: Superior mesenteric artery embolism: Eighty-two cases. *Ann Vasc Surg* 4:112, 1990.

52. Ballard JL, Stone WM, Hallett JW, et al: A critical analysis of adjuvant techniques used to assess bowel viability in acute mesenteric ischemia. *Am Surg* 59:309, 1993.

53. Sullivan KM, Battey PM, Miller JS, et al: Abdominal compartment syndrome after mesenteric revascularization. *J Vasc Surg* 34:559, 2001.

54. Edwards MS, et al: Acute occlusive mesenteric ischemia: Surgical management and outcomes. *Ann Vasc Surg* 17:72, 2003.

55. Cho JS, et al: Long-term outcome after mesenteric artery reconstruction: A 37-year experience. *J Vasc Surg* 35:453, 2002.

56. Johnston KW, Lindsay TF, Walker PM, Kalman PG: Mesenteric arterial bypass grafts: Early and late results and suggested surgical approach for chronic and acute mesenteric ischemia. *Surgery* 118:1, 1995.

57. Mamode N, Pickford I, Leiberman P: Failure to improve outcome in acute mesenteric ischaemia: Seven-year review. *Eur J Surg* 165:203, 1999.

58. Newman TS, Magnuson TH, Ahrendt SA, et al: The changing face of mesenteric infarction. *Am Surg* 64:611, 1998.

59. Urayama H, et al: Acute mesenteric vascular occlusion: Analysis of 39 patients. *Eur J Surg* 164:195, 1998.

60. Klempnauer J, Grothues F, Bektas H, Pichlmayr R: Long-term results after surgery for acute mesenteric ischemia. *Surgery* 121:239, 1997.

61. Voltolini F, Pricolo R, Naldini G, Parziale A: [Acute mesenteric ischemia: Analysis of 47 cases]. *Minerva Chir* 51:285, 1996.

62. Konturek A, Cichon S, Gucwa J, Rogula T: [Acute intestinal ischemia in material of the III Clinic of General Surgery, Collegium Medicum at the Jagellonian University]. *Przegl Lek* 53:719, 1996.

63. Ward D, et al: Improved outcome by identification of high-risk nonocclusive mesenteric ischemia, aggressive reexploration, and delayed anastomosis. *Am J Surg* 170:577, 1995.

64. Laghi A, Iannaccone R, Catalano C, Passariello R: Multislice spiral computed tomography angiography of mesenteric arteries. *Lancet* 358:638, 2001.

65. Bowdish ME, Weaver FA, Liebman HA, et al: Anticoagulation is an effective treatment for aortic mural thrombi. *J Vasc Surg* 36:713, 2002 .

Chapter 87
SPECIAL CONSIDERATIONS IN THE SURGICAL PATIENT
JAMEEL ALI

KEY POINTS

- *The biologic response to surgery results in fluid, electrolyte, and systemic hormonal changes that must be considered in the ICU management of the surgical patient.*

- *Nutritional support of the critically ill surgical patient must involve consideration of the effect of surgical stress on nitrogen balance and on insulin and blood glucose levels.*

- *The hypercoagulable state that follows surgery warrants consideration of prophylaxis against thromboembolic complications, particularly in the ICU patient.*

- *Timely surgical intervention, and treating and preventing hemorrhage and sepsis are crucial in determining outcome in the critically ill.*

- *Surgery increases the demand on the cardiorespiratory system and the likelihood that temporary mechanical ventilatory assistance will be needed.*

- *Pulmonary edema and atelectasis characterize perioperative respiratory failure; hypoventilation and aspiration also contribute.*

- *Where possible a reduction of pulmonary capillary hydrostatic pressure in the perioperative period improves gas exchange by decreasing lung water.*

- *The concept of closing volume and its relationship to functional residual capacity is important in understanding perioperative atelectasis.*

- *Risk factors for perioperative atelectasis include obesity, smoking, advanced age, anesthesia, recumbency, and incisional pain.*

- *Diaphragmatic dysfunction is a major component of perioperative respiratory failure.*

- *Preoperative assessment of respiratory function makes it possible to predict operative risk and to correct abnormalities before operation, particularly in the patient undergoing lung resection.*

- *Early ambulation, physiotherapy, treatment of sepsis and shock, adequate analgesia, and early operative stabilization of fractures are key elements in the treatment and prevention of perioperative respiratory failure.*

The critically ill surgical patient is at risk for developing all of the potential problems that afflict nonsurgical patients in the intensive care unit (ICU). In addition, there are factors unique to the surgical patient that warrant special consideration if management is to be appropriately directed in the ICU environment.

Surgical stress or injury stimulates an orchestrated biologic response[1–4] aimed at preserving the milieu intérieur. This response includes the elaboration of adrenocortical hormones, catecholamines, and glucagon; a decrease in insulin release resulting in hyperglycemia; and the secretion of antidiuretic hormone (ADH) and aldosterone, as well as the release of cytokines and the stimulation of a hypercoagulable state.[5–10] These responses affect the critically ill surgical patient in many ways. Acute fluid and electrolyte shifts may occur, the renal response to volume infusion may be altered, and the catabolic response results in a phase of negative nitrogen balance.[11,12] All these responses vary in intensity, depending on the magnitude and duration of the injury, the adequacy of resuscitation, and the presence of complications such as hemorrhage and sepsis. The increase in metabolic rate increases oxygen requirement and consumption. The management implications of these responses to surgical stress are outlined in the following sections.

Considerations in Critically Ill Surgical Patients

THE ENDOCRINE RESPONSE

The glucagon and insulin response to injury can lead to major changes in glucose metabolism. Hyperglycemia may occur in a patient who has previously demonstrated no evidence of abnormality in glucose levels. This situation may also unmask a latent diabetic state in some patients, as well as complicating the management of already established diabetes mellitus in the critically ill surgical patient. Close monitoring of blood glucose, ketones, electrolytes, and acid-base status is essential for proper management of the surgical patient. Strict control of blood sugar (80 to 110 mg/dL) has been shown to improve outcome in surgical ICU patients,[13] but how to achieve this safely and how low the glucose must be to offer benefit are unknown. Alteration in the glucose content of infused fluids and administration of insulin may be necessary to overcome these responses to surgical stress.

ANTIDIURETIC HORMONE AND ALDOSTERONE

Blood loss, pain related to surgical incisions, fasting prior to surgery, nausea or vomiting, and various drug administrations are only a few of the factors that predispose the surgical patient to release of ADH and aldosterone. The resulting sodium and water retention make it very difficult to monitor the state of hydration of the patient by relying entirely on urine volumes, since these hormones tend to decrease urine output in spite of normovolemia. Other indices of adequacy of perfusion, such as level of consciousness, capillary return, skin warmth, pulse, and blood pressure need to be assessed. In situations in which these indices prove imprecise, central hemodynamic monitoring is required. In addition, the syndrome of inappropriate ADH release (SIADH) is relatively common in the postoperative period, placing patients at risk of water intoxication and severe hyponatremia when even modest water loads are administered. These problems can be largely avoided if treatment is guided by frequent routine monitoring of electrolytes and fluid volume status.

THIRD-SPACE FLUID SEQUESTRATION

Following surgical trauma, occult fluid loss may occur at several sites, including the area of injury, where extravascular fluid may accumulate in the interstitial and intracellular spaces,[14,15] as well as in the retroperitoneal space during intra-abdominal manipulation. In addition, operations involving the gastrointestinal (GI) tract or abnormalities resulting from surgical diseases such as peritonitis may result in decreased motility of the gut and sequestration of large volumes of fluid within the gut lumen, the gut wall, and the entire large surface area of the peritoneal cavity. This type of fluid depletes circulating blood volume and is not easily measured by most available clinical methods. In the patient with compromised cardiorespiratory reserve, close titration of fluid balance is crucial. In such patients, central hemodynamic monitoring may be required in addition to other clinical indices of normal perfusion and volume status.

HYPERCOAGULABLE STATE

The hypercoagulable state resulting from surgical trauma necessitates monitoring of clotting parameters in the surgical patient and the institution of prophylactic measures against thromboembolic sequelae, as outlined in other parts of this text.[8,9] It is important to recognize that virtually every surgical patient is at risk for thromboembolic disease, and some are at extraordinarily high risk. Prophylactic regimens that include the appropriate administration of anticoagulants pose a minor risk of bleeding, but can be employed in most surgical patients.

NUTRITION

Although there is an early phase of negative nitrogen balance following surgical stress, it may be shortened or even aborted by appropriate nutritional support before and immediately after surgery.[16] Early institution of enteric feeding has been shown to be of benefit, including a reduction in septic sequelae, in surgical patients undergoing intra-abdominal procedures.[17] When a prolonged period of gut rest is anticipated, early institution of parenteral nutritional support should be considered to prevent further loss of muscle mass. This measure affects not only the maintenance of muscle mass, but also the maintenance of respiratory function, and thus both dependence on ventilatory support and weaning from mechanical ventilatory assistance.

MAGNITUDE AND DURATION OF SURGICAL INSULT

Since the duration and magnitude of surgical procedures affect the intensity of the metabolic and endocrine response, the aim should be to decrease the magnitude, duration, and frequency of surgical insults to the critically ill patient, particularly patients with poor nutritional and cardiorespiratory reserve. This goal, however, must be considered in the context of the underlying problem. The magnitude and duration of the surgical procedure should not be minimized at the expense of incomplete eradication of a surgical lesion, such as a source of sepsis, since failure to eradicate the septic focus would lead to further complications, such as respiratory failure and dependence on mechanical ventilation in the ICU. In the setting of the multiply-injured patient requiring massive blood transfusions that can lead to hypothermia, coagulopathy, and severe cardiorespiratory and renal compromise, "damage-control laparotomy" or abbreviated laparotomy should be considered. This consists of rapid control of hemorrhage (by ligation of

vessels and packing) and removal of gross contamination followed by temporary closure, which should be followed as soon as possible by more definitive procedures as improvement in the patient's condition in the ICU allows.[18]

AVOIDANCE OF COMPLICATIONS

Hemorrhage is a frequent sequela to many surgical procedures. The resulting hypoperfusion of the myocardium, brain, and kidney produces further dysfunction in the critically ill ICU patient. All of these events result in deterioration of the patient's condition, with a requirement for further supportive measures, prolongation of the ICU stay, and the development of multiple organ failure. Aggressive replacement of lost blood with appropriate fluid resuscitation and correction of the source of any continuing hemorrhage helps minimize these problems.

Sepsis worsens the response to surgery. In addition, cytokine release and the effects of activated macrophages and neutrophils produce a cascade of systemic responses with attendant worsening of respiratory function and predisposition to multiple organ failure.[19] Early identification and drainage of sources of infection, specific antibiotic coverage, careful monitoring of invasive catheters and their removal when intravascular infection may be present, and débridement of areas of serious infection such as gas gangrene and fasciitis, are all necessary to halt this process and prevent further deterioration of the critically ill surgical patient.

INCREASED OXYGEN REQUIREMENTS

The increase in metabolic rate following surgical stress is associated with an increase in oxygen requirement and utilization.[20] In patients with a normal cardiorespiratory reserve, this increased oxygen demand is met without untoward sequelae. However, patients who are nutritionally depleted or whose cardiorespiratory function is already compromised may be unable to meet the increased oxygen demand. The result can be decompensation with anaerobic metabolism, muscle fatigue, and respiratory failure. In the high-risk patient, consideration should be given to providing temporary cardiorespiratory support during the phase of increased oxygen requirement. Such patients may require intubation and mechanical ventilation for short periods until the acute insult has abated.

The increased oxygen requirement of surgery and the postoperative state has caused some authors to recommend measuring and then maximizing oxygen delivery[20] in critically ill patients. Use of invasive hemodynamic monitoring or gastric tonometry allows titration of catecholamine infusions, blood products, or other therapies to increase oxygen delivery to targeted supranormal levels. Many studies supporting this approach were likely flawed by inappropriate methodology, although there is some indication in high-risk surgical patients that outcome can be improved.[21–23]

OTHER CONSIDERATIONS IN THE SURGICAL PATIENT

Pain from surgical incisions may exacerbate the metabolic response to injury and mechanically restrict respiratory function, the latter potentially necessitating mechanical ventilatory assistance. Judicious parenteral analgesia as well as regional, intercostal, and epidural anesthesia may also be useful in these situations.

Neurosurgical patients and those who have suffered head trauma should be monitored closely for signs of increased intracranial pressure. If clinical signs cannot be easily elicited, an intracranial pressure monitoring device should be placed. Apart from the identification of mass lesions that may require evacuation, the mainstay of treatment for these patients is reduction of cerebral edema through the maintenance of cerebral blood flow and oxygenation and the avoidance of hypercapnia (see Chap. 93). The vascular surgery patient requires close monitoring of perfusion, particularly in the arterial territorial distribution of the repaired vessel. Skin temperature, Doppler ultrasound, and digital pressure measurements are required in the ICU setting to identify problems with vascular anastomoses as early as possible and permit early corrective measures. Immediately after surgery carotid artery surgery patients are at higher risk for developing neurologic complications from reocclusion at surgical sites of vascular repair, and careful monitoring of the neurologic status as well as maintenance of adequate oxygenation and perfusion are essential to avoid such complications.

Following GI surgical procedures, the gut should be used early for enteral nutrition whenever appropriate.[17] When that is not possible and a prolonged period of decreased motility is anticipated, intubation and decompression of the GI tract is necessary to prevent distention and to monitor the volume and character of losses. This intervention, together with replacement of measured losses as well as determination of serum electrolytes, allows early identification and correction of abnormalities and the prevention of complications. Patients who develop sepsis following GI surgical procedures should be considered to have a source of that sepsis within the abdomen until proven otherwise. Early aggressive investigation for identifying such a source of sepsis is essential in order to avoid further deterioration in the ICU.

The gut has also been considered to play a major role in the pathogenesis of multiple organ dysfunction syndrome and decontamination of the GI tract has been suggested as a prophylactic measure in this syndrome.[24]

Stress ulcers resulting in GI hemorrhage are a sequela not only of GI surgery, but of other forms of critical illness. As described elsewhere in this text (see Chap. 10), prophylactic measures against stress ulceration directed at decreasing acid injury to the gastroduodenal mucosa are an essential part of the management of critically ill patients.[25]

Perioperative Respiratory Failure

In the period before, during, and after surgical treatment, patients are unusually vulnerable to respiratory failure owing to special manifestations of pulmonary edema, atelectasis, hypoventilation, aspiration, sepsis, and hypotension. Awareness of the factors promoting each of these interrelated processes makes possible an effective prevention program or early diagnosis and treatment of perioperative respiratory failure.

PULMONARY EDEMA

Of the forces in the Starling equation governing transcapillary fluid flux, the ones of particular relevance to surgical patients are microvascular hydrostatic pressure and pulmonary capillary permeability.

MICROVASCULAR PRESSURE

As indicated, secretion of ADH and aldosterone is a major component of the metabolic response to surgery and trauma.[26] Both hormones tend to conserve water and decrease urine output in the postsurgical patient. However, a focus on increasing urine output in the surgical patient by administering large volumes of fluid without regard to this metabolic response could easily result in fluid overload and pulmonary edema, leading to hypoxemia. Guidelines for fluid resuscitation in the perioperative period that focus primarily on urine output and fluid replacements based on empirical values[27] can increase extravascular lung water and predispose the surgical patient to perioperative respiratory failure. Although a young, healthy patient with significant cardiopulmonary reserve will undoubtedly tolerate these insults, an elderly surgical patient with a brittle cardiorespiratory status is more likely to develop respiratory failure unless extreme caution is taken with fluid resuscitation, involving close, constant monitoring of central hemodynamics.

Pulmonary edema occurring in the head-injured patient, or *neurogenic edema*, may be associated with a transient increase in hydrostatic pressure because of intense sympathetic discharge, although it has been suggested that there may be a component of increased capillary permeability as well in this lesion.[28] Therefore, monitoring of pulmonary capillary hydrostatic pressure is important in determining therapeutic approaches to the head-injured patient with pulmonary edema.

High-pressure pulmonary edema does not resolve immediately after vascular pressures are normalized.[29] The implication of this finding is that the timing of the measurement of pulmonary artery wedge pressure (PAWP), which is used as a reflection of capillary hydrostatic pressure, is crucial in determining whether pulmonary edema is considered to be due to high vascular pressures or to an increase in capillary permeability. Ordinarily, the presence of normal or low PAWP in the presence of pulmonary edema would be regarded as evidence of capillary-leak pulmonary edema. However, if the PAWP is measured during the lag phase of resolution of high-pressure pulmonary edema after PAWP has been decreased, then inappropriate therapy directed at capillary leakage may be given, while the role of the cardiogenic edema that is already resolving slowly is overlooked.

Diuretics such as furosemide clear edema by decreasing the central blood volume and pulmonary capillary hydrostatic pressure.[30] However, these agents may produce effects on gas exchange before pulmonary edema has cleared.[31] Accordingly, diuretic therapy and fluid management of the oliguric, hypoxemic perioperative patient may confuse the student of critical care at several levels. First, oliguria in the immediate postoperative period is not necessarily due to reduced blood flow to the renal cortex (prerenal oliguria), so fluid challenges aimed at increasing renal blood flow may not be appropriate in this setting. The consequent increase in pulmonary blood volume and pressure predictably increases pulmonary edema. On the other hand, diuretic therapy in such a patient will increase urine output, even when the oliguria is due to reduced renal blood flow, thereby aggravating the prerenal failure. The best approach to this common perioperative conundrum is to recognize that urine output may be an unreliable index of adequate perfusion in the immediate postoperative period, and to seek other indices of perfusion through careful history-taking, physical examination, and first-hand knowledge of the patient's perioperative course. For example, a prior history of congestive heart failure predicts susceptibility to fluid overload, and thus should slow the physician's hand in administering fluid. Similarly, familiarity with the patient's preoperative blood pressure, heart rate, heart sounds, pulse volume, and digital perfusion allow the discerning physician to detect early signs of hypoperfusion requiring volume replacement. Often, the critical distinction between fluid overload and hypovolemia is not clear even to the astute clinician, and in such cases a low threshold for instituting central hemodynamic measurements is indicated.[32] Once these steps have been taken, fluid can be administered in the setting of low PAWP, low cardiac output, and oliguria in an attempt to return blood flow toward normal without risking edema. An untoward increase in PAWP without much increase in blood flow warrants immediate re-evaluation of the patient's cardiac function, including an electrocardiogram (ECG) and measurement of cardiac enzymes, and administration of vasoactive drug therapy (e.g., dobutamine, 2 to 10 μg/kg per minute), to increase ventricular contractility and output at reduced PAWP.

PULMONARY CAPILLARY PERMEABILITY

A frequent cause of increased capillary permeability and respiratory failure in the surgical patient is unrecognized sepsis, which is commonly seen in the abdomen; this source often requires a surgical or percutaneous radiologic approach. Therefore, a major component of the prevention and treatment of respiratory failure in the surgical patient is the early identification of occult sources of sepsis, aggressive investigation for abdominal causes of sepsis, and the provision of adequate drainage and treatment of septic foci, particularly within the abdomen.

Although both increased microvascular hydrostatic pressure and pulmonary capillary permeability are important factors in the elaboration of extravascular lung water, manipulation of the microvascular pressure (by the use of vasoactive agents and regulation of the state of hydration) is the most direct means of altering pulmonary edema in the surgical patient. A search for a septic focus in the surgical patient is crucial whenever there is evidence of increased capillary permeability. Control of capillary permeability can then be achieved, although only indirectly, by treating the source of sepsis, which may be surgically approachable. The link between sepsis and capillary permeability is thus broken, and the capillary permeability lesion is allowed to resolve with time; its resolution is accompanied by improvement in perioperative respiratory failure. Until the permeability corrects itself, reduction of PAWP to the lowest level associated with adequate peripheral perfusion seems to reduce the edema.[30]

ATELECTASIS

In the normal lung, ventilation and perfusion are not equally matched, because the shape of the thoracic cavity and the descent of the diaphragm result in greater expansion and ventilation of the lower lobes. Also, blood flow is greater in the dependent areas of the lung during spontaneous ventilation and changes with body position. Therefore the normal lung has an average ventilation:perfusion ratio ($\dot{V}/\dot{Q}$) of approximately 0.8. Many factors in the surgical patient reduce this ratio to very low values, causing hypoxemia, and similar factors lead to resorption of alveolar gas behind closed airways or to compression atelectasis.[33,34] This phenomenon of compression atelectasis in the dependent lung is thought to occur within 5 minutes after induction of general anesthesia.

Shunting results from continued perfusion of nonventilated lung units, and the major cause of this imbalance in the surgical patient is perioperative atelectasis, although alveolar edema from fluid overload or capillary leakage could also result in an increase in shunting.

AGE, POSITION, AND AIRWAY CLOSURE

Most surgical patients undergo procedures in the supine position, and we are operating increasingly on elderly patients. Also, one of the major effects of surgery is the pain resulting from surgical incisions. Body position, incisional pain, and age all affect the relationship between the functional residual capacity (FRC) and the closing volume. The FRC has been considered the most important index of mechanical abnormality in the lung because it represents the balance of opposing forces on the rib cage at resting lung volume. The closing volume is the measure of gas in the lung at the time when airway closure begins. When FRC exceeds closing volume, lower airway patency is maintained, while airway closure begins when the FRC falls below the closing volume.[35] FRC falls with age, and in all patients it is lower in the supine position than in the upright position (Fig. 87-1). The commonly used lithotomy position results in a further decrease in FRC relative to closing volume.

When the difference between FRC and closing volume is plotted against the alveolar-arterial oxygen tension gradient $(A-a)_{O_2}$,[36] it is evident that the $(A-a)_{O_2}$ oxygen tension gradient increases as FRC falls below closing volume.

Airway closure tends to occur in the most dependent areas of the lung, and in the supine position, more areas of the lung are dependent, thus predisposing the patient to a greater degree of airway closure and hypoxemia. As indicated above,[33,34] general anesthesia itself may predispose the patient to compression atelectasis in dependent areas of the lung. Also, in both normal individuals and smokers, increasing age is associated with an increase in closing volume, predisposing the patient to airway closure at higher lung volumes.[37] As a group, smokers tend to have higher closing volumes, so that the combination of age and smoking increases the likelihood of significant postoperative hypoxemia. It has generally been accepted that chronic cigarette smoking increases the incidence of postoperative respiratory complications, which may result not only from an alteration in the respiratory defense mechanisms, but also an increase in airway resistance and the work of breathing. It has been demonstrated that cessation of smoking for over 8 weeks is an effective means of decreasing postoperative respiratory complications.[38] Although it has been suggested that abstinence too soon prior to surgery may increase the risk of postoperative pulmonary complications, aggressive counseling for smoking cessation prior to any elective surgical procedure still appears to be the best approach.[39]

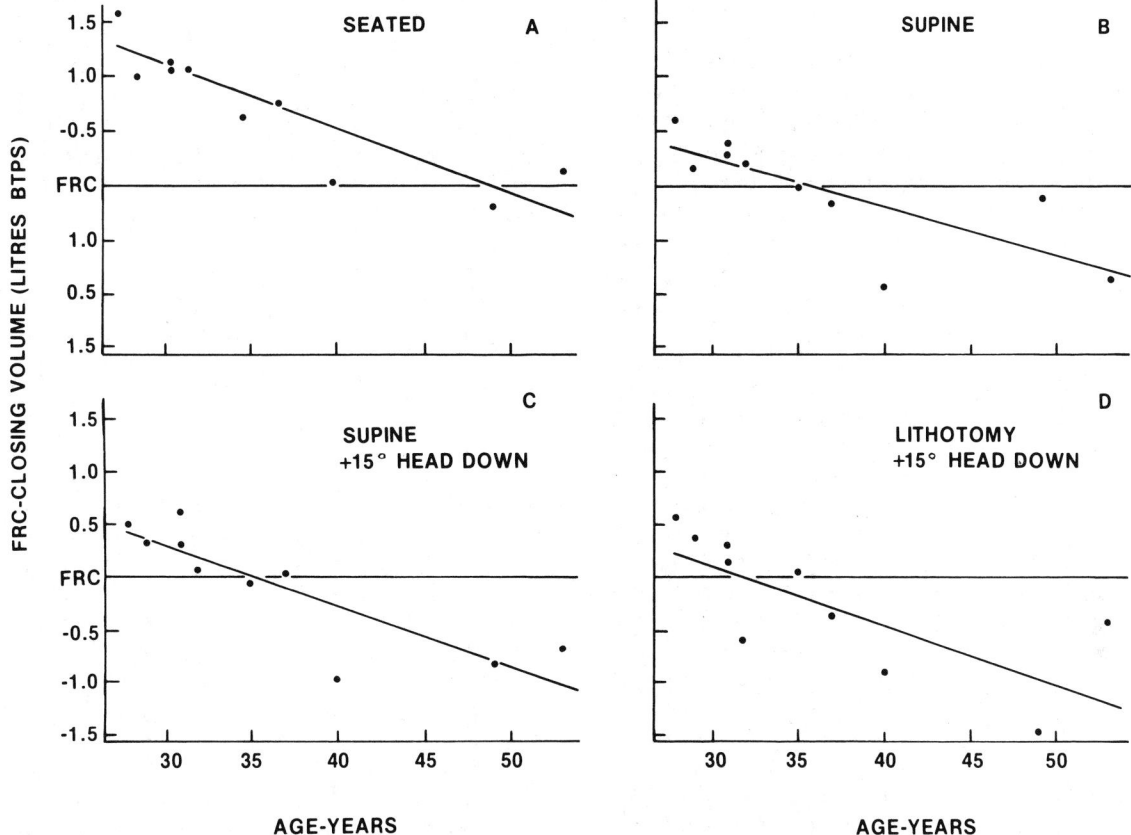

FIGURE 87-1 The difference between FRC and closing volume plotted against age in different surgical positions. Both age and position affect airway closure. (*Reproduced with permission from* *Craig DB, Wahba WM, Don H: Airway closure and lung volumes in surgical positions. Can Anaesth Soc J 18:95, 1971.*)**

Because small airways in the periphery of the lung are not supported by cartilage, they tend to be influenced significantly by changes in pleural pressures. The maintenance of a positive transpulmonary pressure resulting from the negative intrapleural pressure maintains patency of the small airways. Breathing at a reduced FRC, such as occurs with abdominal pain, tends to lead to positive pleural pressures in the dependent areas of the lung, and therefore creates a predisposition to alveolar collapse. Complete collapse results in continued perfusion of nonventilated areas, or shunting; when the airways are merely narrowed, the ventilation:perfusion ratio may be low, which also impairs gas exchange and leads to hypoxemia.

The patient with multiple fractures is at increased risk for developing pulmonary complications, not only from thromboembolic complications, including fat embolism, but also from atelectasis and pneumonia. A major predisposing factor in these patients is the prolonged period of imposed bed rest, particularly in the supine position, with its resultant effect on lung mechanics and lung volumes. Early operative stabilization of fractures in these patients has been shown to decrease pulmonary morbidity[40] because it allows more effective respiratory physiotherapy and early ambulation, as well as frequent changes in body position to minimize dependant alveolar volume loss.

A major cause of morbidity in traumatic quadriplegic patients is respiratory failure secondary to loss of use of the intercostal muscles of respiration.[41] It has been suggested that

the best position for respiratory therapy in these patients is from horizontal to 35° head-up,[42] whereas the maximum FRC is achieved in the 60° to 90° head-up position.

UPPER ABDOMINAL SURGERY AND DIAPHRAGM DYSFUNCTION

Although many of the factors discussed above are present in patients undergoing most surgical procedures, the most serious sequelae are found in patients undergoing upper abdominal procedures. In these patients there is a significant fall in vital capacity (VC) almost immediately postoperatively, within the first 4 hours.[43] There is a slower but definite fall in FRC, which peaks at about 24 hours and is associated with significant hypoxemia. In most patients with no pre-existing lung disease, this effect of upper abdominal intervention on VC and FRC does not result in clinically significant respiratory complications. However, in patients who already have abnormalities of gas exchange, these effects can lead to severe respiratory failure. The postoperative decrease in VC is primarily a restrictive rather than obstructive phenomenon, as evidenced by the maintenance of a normal ratio between the forced expiratory volume at 1 second and the forced vital capacity (FEV_1/FVC).[44] This restriction may be related to incisional pain, which decreases the patient's ability to cough and clear secretions, and eventually leads to an increase in closing volume and a decrease in FRC. If not corrected, a fall in VC results in atelectasis and hypoxemia and a decrease in FRC. To correct this abnormality, transcutaneous electrical nerve stimulation has been used to provide postoperative analgesia after abdominal surgery.[45] Epidural analgesia and intercostal blockade have also been used for this purpose. Although all of these techniques have produced improvements in VC and FRC, none immediately returns VC or FRC to preoperative values. This suggests either that these techniques do not adequately control pain, or that pain is not the only cause of postoperative respiratory dysfunction after upper abdominal surgery.

Patients undergoing upper abdominal operations have a significant decrease in the maximal transdiaphragmatic pressure at FRC, which is not altered by use of epidural analgesia.[46] This finding suggests that the respiratory dysfunction after upper abdominal surgery may result from a primary effect of the procedure on diaphragmatic function. Ford and coworkers showed that there is a switch from predominantly abdominal breathing to rib cage breathing in the postoperative period in patients undergoing upper abdominal surgery (Fig. 87-2).[47] Diaphragmatic dysfunction was similarly identified in an animal model undergoing cholecystectomy.[48] These studies suggest that general anesthesia may not be responsible for the postoperative diaphragmatic dysfunction. Mere traction on the gallbladder in an animal model also produced similar effects on diaphragmatic function.[49]

FIGURE 87-2 **Relationship between the ratio of abdominal to rib cage diameter and time after abdominal surgery. Interrupted lines represent individual patients and the solid line represents the mean values for these four patients. Note the switch from predominantly abdominal breathing preoperatively to rib cage breathing postoperatively.** (*Reproduced with permission from Ford et al.[47]*)

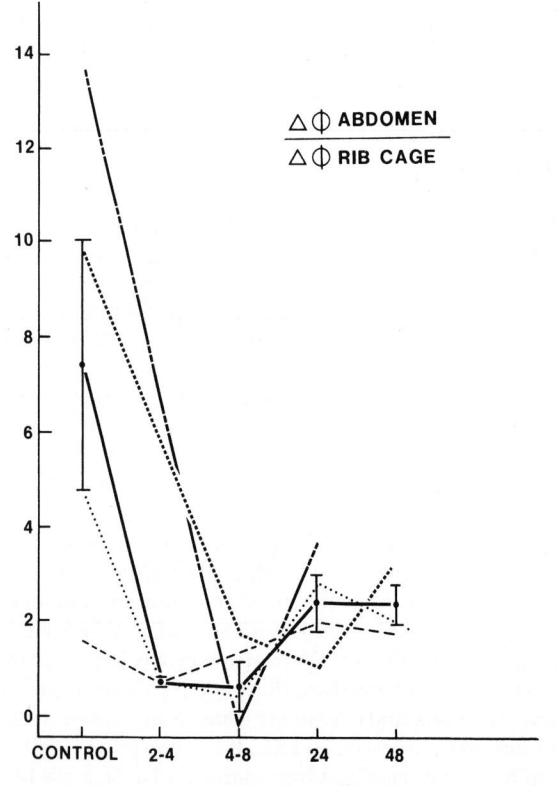

Although open cholecystectomy has been associated with significant depression in postoperative pulmonary function, several reports[50–52] have demonstrated less impairment of postoperative pulmonary function following laparoscopic cholecystectomy. There still is a decrease in FRC immediately after the operation, but it is much smaller and of significantly shorter duration than with the open procedure, and the VC and FRC return to essentially preoperative levels within 24 hours.[52] Therefore from the respiratory standpoint, laparoscopic cholecystectomy is superior to open cholecystectomy and should be the preferred method for critically ill patients requiring this procedure. The increase in intra-abdominal pressure with pneumoperitoneum associated with the laparoscopic procedure has a minimal hemodynamic effect, and in patients with decreased cardiopulmonary reserve may prove significant, warranting close hemodynamic monitoring in the operating room in such patients.[53] As indicated in Chap. 89, less aggressive procedures such as percutaneous drainage of the biliary tract may be indicated in situations in which the patient is too unstable to be taken to the operating room or to be subjected to a general anesthetic.

Apart from the factors identified above, aging has been associated with reduced elastic lung recoil, decreased expiratory flow rate, and diminished airway protective reflexes.[37] Obesity is also a major risk factor for postoperative pulmonary complications, because these patients tend to breathe at reduced lung volumes, so closing volume frequently exceeds FRC, leading to hypoxemia and atelectasis.[53a] The increased work of breathing produced by the increased mass also contributes to respiratory dysfunction. Not only the type of operation, but the location of the incision tends to affect the degree of respiratory impairment seen in the postoperative period.[54] In open cholecystectomy, the subcostal incision tends to produce less impairment than a midline incision. The severity of postoperative lung impairment decreases in the following order: thoracic surgery, upper abdominal surgery, lower abdominal surgery, and superficial surgery (Fig. 87-3).

As pointed out in earlier chapters, shock and pulmonary edema in the form of cardiac failure also affect diaphragmatic function through changes in diaphragmatic force as well as glycogen depletion in diaphragmatic muscle.[55] Table 87-1 summarizes preventive measures as well as some of the factors that reduce the FRC and increase closing volume in the postoperative patient.

ALVEOLAR HYPOVENTILATION

In surgical patients, hypoventilation is characteristically caused by impairment of ventilation resulting from the restrictive effect of painful incisions or peritonitis. It may also result from central nervous system (CNS) depression due to anesthesia, analgesia, or CNS injury. The increased metabolic requirement after injury places a significant demand on the respiratory system. When calories, particularly in the form of carbohydrates, are provided to match this increased energy expenditure, the increase in CO_2 production necessitates a significant increase in ventilation to maintain normocapnia.[56] In surgical patients with significant pulmonary reserve, this added demand can be met without untoward effects. However, in depleted surgical patients with borderline respiratory reserve, this extra demand may precipitate respiratory failure

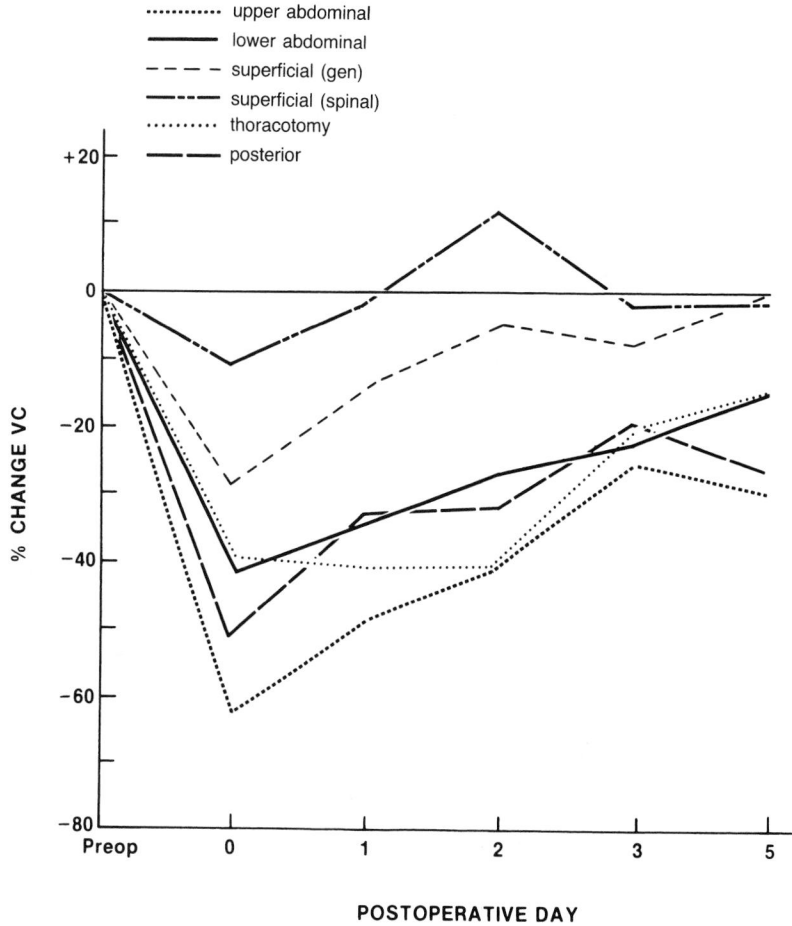

legend:
.... upper abdominal
———— lower abdominal
— — — superficial (gen)
—·—·— superficial (spinal)
············ thoracotomy
— — — posterior

FIGURE 87-3 Postoperative changes in VC for different surgical incisions. Note that the upper abdominal surgery patients have the greatest postoperative depression in VC. (*Reproduced with permission from Ali et al.[43]*)

or lead to other manifestations such as prolonged ventilator dependency.

The respiratory system is protected from sepsis and atelectasis by a respiratory control mechanism that responds to hypoxemia, hypercapnia, acidosis, and the presence of irritating or noxious stimuli in the airway. These mechanisms can be significantly depressed in the postoperative patient as a result of anesthesia or excessive narcotic analgesia. Inhalational anesthetics are known for their respiratory depressive effect, which results in alveolar hypoventilation and a reduced response to carbon dioxide, as well as a blunted response to

hypoxemia and acidosis.[57] In the postoperative period, narcotic analgesics may have undesirable effects. Whereas in optimal doses they decrease abdominal pain and increase the ability to cough and clear secretions, in larger doses they may depress the respiratory center, producing alveolar hypoventilation as manifested by hypercapnia and secondary hypoxemia.

The cough reflex is the main mechanism by which particles are cleared from the upper airway. The cough response is altered not only by anesthesia, but also by narcotic agents. Clearance of particles from the lower airways depends

TABLE 87-1 Perioperative Atelectasis

Component of the Tendency Toward Atelectasis	Promoting Factors	Preventing Factors
Reduced functional residual capacity	Supine position	45° upright position
	Obesity	Alternating postures
	Ascites	Positive end-expiratory
	Peritonitis	pressure
	Upper abdominal incision	Sighs
		Analgesia
Increased closing volume	Age	Preoperative physiotherapy
	History of smoking	Smoking cessation
	Bronchospasm	Bronchodilation
	Airway secretions	Cough, suction, deep breathing
	Pulmonary edema	Avoidance of overhydration

primarily on the mucociliary system, which can be disturbed by several factors in the postoperative period. Anesthetics alter ciliary activity and mucus production which leads to the production of mucus plugs that block the lower airways. In addition, the cellular defense mechanisms of the respiratory system may be altered by anesthetic agents.[58]

ASPIRATION

The supine position and depression of normal protective reflexes during general anesthesia predispose the surgical patient to aspiration of gastric acid, which is one of the major causes of perioperative morbidity and mortality.[59] This event can first produce airway obstruction (from aspirated debris and chemically induced bronchoconstriction), then a chemical burn of the airway (with fluid loss into the injured area), an intense inflammatory response, and finally lung infection. The clinical presentation of patients with gastric acid aspiration varies widely. Very mild cases present only with transient coughing and minimal bronchospasm; the most severe cases exhibit a progressive downhill course characterized by hypovolemia, hypoxemia, and finally fulminant bacterial pneumonia.

The treatment of acid aspiration consists of the following: (1) rapid removal of debris by immediate suction (endotracheal intubation and fiberoptic bronchoscopy may be necessary at this stage); (2) placement of a nasogastric tube to evacuate the stomach and prevent further episodes; (3) oxygen administration and mechanical ventilation if indicated by the degree of respiratory failure; (4) bronchodilator therapy if bronchospasm is significant; (5) maintenance of normovolemia and normal perfusion by monitoring and replacement of lost fluid, as well as vasoactive and inotropic support where necessary; and (6) treatment of pneumonia by appropriate antimicrobial agents on the basis of Gram stain and culture findings. Steroids have not been of any benefit in treating these patients. Preventive measures that can be taken in high-risk patients to prevent the aspiration of low-pH gastric contents include gastric decompression and the use of agents that decrease gastric acid production, although there is evidence that this may predispose to nosocomial pneumonia.[60-62]

PREDICTING AND PREVENTING PERIOPERATIVE LUNG DYSFUNCTION

Many attempts have been made to correct the postoperative abnormalities in lung function, using techniques such as incentive spirometry, intermittent positive-pressure breathing (IPPB), and nasal continuous positive airway pressure (CPAP).[63-65] Although incentive spirometry has been reported to be ineffective in decreasing postoperative pulmonary complications following cardiac and upper abdominal surgery,[64] IPPB, incentive spirometry, CPAP,[65] and physiotherapy generally improve postoperative respiratory function; IPPB offers no advantage over physiotherapy when the latter is maximized in the postoperative period.[66] Although nonyielding abdominal binders have a further restrictive effect on lung volumes postoperatively, the elastic binders may produce some benefit.[67] It must be recognized, however, that none of these methods completely reverses the postoperative respiratory dysfunction.

Attempts have been made to predict postoperative pulmonary morbidity by assessing respiratory mechanics pre-operatively, as well as by identifying risk factors such as age, obesity, smoking, and location of incisions. No individual respiratory parameter predicts respiratory morbidity or mortality in an individual patient. In general, however, the poorer the preoperative respiratory function, the more likely the patient is to have severe postoperative respiratory complications. Based on cumulative experience, the following spirometric criteria for predicting morbidity and mortality in postoperative adult patients have been proposed.[68,69] If the FEV_1 is <1 L, the FVC <1.5 L, the FEV_1/FVC is <30%, or the forced expiratory flow [$FEF_{25\%-75\%}$] is <0.6 L/s, and if the maximum minute ventilation is <50% of the predicted value, then the risk of postoperative pulmonary complications is very high. In patients whose respiratory function is below this threshold, the strategy is to provide treatment that will improve respiratory function to a level above this threshold. Such treatment may involve cessation of smoking, diaphragm muscle conditioning, weight loss, and the treatment of heart failure, fluid overload, and any identifiable reactive airway disease.

A patient who undergoes lung resection is at even greater risk of postoperative pulmonary complication, particularly if the excised lung tissue was functional.[68,69] In these patients, the effect of the lost lung volume must be considered along with the factors discussed above. A quantitative perfusion lung scan can help to predict the postoperative pulmonary spirometric performance of these patients by indicating how much of the lung will remain after the planned procedure. The postoperative FEV_1 is then calculated as the product of the preoperative FEV_1 and the fractional perfusion of the remaining lung. The usual rule for an adult patient is that the operative risk is prohibitive if the predicted postoperative FEV_1 is $\leq$0.8 L. The prediction can be made more accurate by also measuring the diffusing capacity, which is an independent predictor of morbidity and mortality after major lung resection. A useful guideline is to exclude from major lung resection all patients whose diffusing capacity is <60% of the predicted value, even if spirometric values are considered satisfactory.[69] Patients with only slightly impaired pulmonary function (FEV_1 and diffusing capacity $\geq$80% predicted) with no cardiovascular risk factors can undergo pulmonary resections including pneumonectomy without further investigation. For others, exercise testing as well as pulmonary split-function test studies are recommended. The symptom limited cardiopulmonary exercise testing measures the maximum volume of oxygen utilization (V_{O_2}max) as an index of pulmonary and cardiovascular reserve. A V_{O_2}max <10 mL/kg per minute is generally considered a contraindication to any resection, whereas a value >20 mL/kg per minute or >75% of predicted normal is considered safe for major resections. Resections that involve no more than one lobe usually lead to early functional deficit followed by recovery, and permanent loss in pulmonary function is usually <10%. Generally, pulmonary function tests tend to overestimate the functional loss after lung resection.[70] Arterial blood gas criteria may also be used to exclude patients from major lung resection because of the prohibitive risk of postoperative morbidity and mortality. Patients who have a room-air partial pressure of arterial oxygen (Pa_{O_2}) of <50 mm Hg or a partial pressure of carbon dioxide (P_{CO_2}) of >45 mm Hg at rest are considered to have a prohibitive operative risk and should not undergo major pulmonary resection. Other forms of surgical intervention are justifiable in the presence of these blood gas criteria only if they are considered mandatory and lifesaving.

TREATMENT PRINCIPLES FOR PERIOPERATIVE RESPIRATORY FAILURE

At present, no specific therapy exists for underlying diaphragmatic dysfunction. Therefore the principles of respiratory care in the surgical patient are as follows:

1. Maximization of the preoperative respiratory status. Meeting this goal may entail cessation of smoking, diaphragmatic conditioning exercises, reduction in obesity, and treatment of any identified cardiorespiratory disease, including congestive heart failure, bronchopneumonia, or bronchospasm.
2. Aggressive physiotherapy and early ambulation to overcome the effects of the supine position on changes in lung volumes, particularly the relationship between closing volume and FRC. In patients with multiple fractures, early operative stabilization will decrease the period of recumbency.
3. Adequate treatment of sepsis and shock, with recognition of the important role of surgery or interventional radiology in the identification and drainage of areas of sepsis such as intra-abdominal abscesses.
4. Judicious use of intravenous fluids to maintain adequate perfusion while avoiding overhydration and pulmonary edema.
5. Optimal use of analgesics to control pain without producing respiratory depression.
6. Administration of supplemental oxygen to hypoxemic patients to improve arterial oxygenation.
7. Treatment (as specific as possible) of any identifiable cause of hypoxemia; for example, bronchodilator therapy for a patient with bronchospasm, or antibiotic therapy directed against a specific organism isolated in a patient with a pneumonic process.
8. Preoperative pulmonary assessment, especially in patients with poor pulmonary reserve and most especially in those undergoing lung resection. This will allow an assessment of the relative risk of postoperative morbidity.
9. Institution of mechanical ventilation when the above measures fail. Frequently, mechanical ventilation can be avoided if strict attention is paid to preventive measures. Also, vigorous application of these principles immediately after the patient is stabilized can shorten the duration of mechanical ventilation considerably.[71]

References

1. Moore FD: *The Metabolic Care of the Surgical Patient.* Philadelphia, Saunders, 1959, p 1.
2. Bessey PQ, Walters JM, Aoki TJ, Wilmore DW: Combined hormonal infusion simulates the metabolic response to surgery. *Ann Surg* 200:264, 1984.
3. Wilmore DW: Metabolic response to severe surgical illness—overview. *World J Surg* 24:705, 2000.
4. Davies CL, Newman RJ, Molyneaux SK, et al: The relationship between plasma catecholamines and severity of injury in man. *J Trauma* 24:99, 1984.
5. Cafferata HT, Aggeler PM, Robinson AJ, Blaisdell FW: Intravascular coagulation in the surgical patient: Its significance and diagnosis. *Am J Surg* 118:281, 1969.
6. Michie HR, Eberline TJ, Spriggs DR, et al: Interleukin-2 initiates metabolic responses associated with critical illness in humans. *Ann Surg* 208:493, 1988.
7. Blaisdell FW: Acquired and congenital clotting syndromes. *World J Surg* 14:664, 1990.
8. Shackford SR, Moser KM: Deep venous thrombosis and pulmonary embolism in trauma patients. *J Intensive Care Med* 3:87, 1998.
9. Geerts WH, Jay RM, Cokde KI, et al: A comparison of low dose heparin with low molecular weight heparin as prophylaxis against thromboembolism after major trauma. *N Engl J Med* 335:701, 1996.
10. Cinat M, Waxman K, Vaziri ND, et al: Soluble cytokine receptors and receptor antagonists are sequentially released after trauma. *J Trauma* 39:112, 1995.
11. Bessey PQ, Lowe KA: Early hormonal changes affect the catabolic response to trauma. *Ann Surg* 218:476, 1993.
12. Traynor C, Hall GM: Endocrine and metabolic changes during surgery: Anesthetic implications. *Br J Anaesth* 53:153, 1981.
13. Van Den Berghe G, Wouters P, Weekers F, et al: Intensive insulin therapy in critically ill patients. *N Engl J Med* 345:1359, 2001.
14. Roberts JP, Roberts JB, Skinner C, et al: Extracellular fluid deficit following operation and its correction with Ringer's lactate: A reassessment. *Ann Surg* 202:1, 1985.
15. Ali J, Qi W: Fluid and electrolyte deficit with prolonged pneumatic antishock garment application. *J Trauma* 38:612, 1995.
16. Hammarqvist F, Wennerman J, Ali R, et al: Addition of glutamine total parenteral nutrition after elective surgery spares free glutamine in muscle, counteracts the fall in muscle protein synthesis and improves nitrogen balance. *Ann Surg* 209:455, 1989.
17. Moore FA, Feliciano DV, Andrassy RJ, et al: Early enteral feeding, compared with parenteral, reduces postoperative septic complications: the results of a meta-analysis. *Ann Surg* 216:172, 1992.
18. Burch JM, Ortiz VB, Richardson RJ, et al: Abbreviated laparotomy and planned reoperation for critically injured patients. *Ann Surg* 215:476, 1991.
19. Beal AL, Cerra FB: Multiple organ failure syndrome in the 1990s: Systemic inflammatory response and organ dysfunction. *JAMA* 271:226, 1994.
20. Biagorri F, Russell JA: Oxygen delivery in critical illness. *Crit Care Clin* 12:995, 1996.
21. Shoemaker WC, Appel PL, Kram HB, et al: Prospective trial of supranormal values of survivors as therapeutic goals in high risk surgical patients. *Chest* 94:1176, 1988.
22. Guttierez G, Palizos F, Doglio G, et al: Gastric intramucosal pH as a therapeutic index of tissue oxygenation in critically ill patient. *Lancet* 339:195, 1992.
23. Marik PE: Gastric intramucosal pH: a better predictor of multiorgan dysfunction syndrome and death than oxygen derived values in patients with sepsis. *Chest* 104:225, 1993.
24. Meta-analysis of randomized controlled trials of selective decontamination of the digestive tract. Selective Decontamination of the Digestive Tract Trialists' Collaborative Group. *BMJ* 307:525, 1993.
25. Cook DJ, Fuller H, Guyatt GH, et al: Risk factors for gastrointestinal bleeding in critically ill patients. *N Engl J Med* 330:377, 1994.
26. Chung HM, Rudiger K, Schrier RW, Anderson RJ: Postoperative hyponatremia: a prospective study. *Arch Intern Med* 146:333, 1986.
27. Giesecke AH Jr, Egbert LD: Perioperative fluid therapy, in Miller RD (ed): *Crystalloids in Anaesthesia,* 2nd ed. New York, Churchill Livingstone, 1986, p 3132.
28. Colice GL, Matthay MA, Bass E, Matthay RA: Neurogenic pulmonary edema. *Am Rev Respir Dis* 130:941, 1984.

29. Ali J, Duke K: Decreasing hydrostatic pressure does not uniformly decrease high pressure pulmonary edema. *Chest* 91:588, 1987.

30. Wood LDH, Prewitt RM: Cardiovascular management in acute hypoxemic respiratory failure. *Am J Cardiol* 47:963, 1981.

31. Ali J, Wood LDH: Pulmonary vascular effects of furosemide on gas exchange in pulmonary edema. *J Appl Physiol* 57:160, 1984.

32. Matthay MA, Chatterjee K: Bedside catheterization of the pulmonary artery: Risks compared with benefits. *Ann Intern Med* 109:826, 1988.

33. Brismar B, Hedenstierna G, Lundquist H, et al: Pulmonary densities during anesthesia with muscular relaxation—A proposal of atelectasis. *Anesthesiology* 62:422, 1985.

34. Tokics L, Hedenstierna G, Brismar B, et al: Thoracoabdominal restriction in supine men: CT and lung function measurements. *J Appl Physiol* 64:599, 1988.

35. Craig DB, Wahba WM, Don HF, et al: "Closing volume" and its relationship to gas exchange in seated and supine positions. *J Appl Physiol* 31:717, 1971.

36. Alexander JI, Horton PW, Millar WT, et al: The effect of upper abdominal surgery on the relationship of airway closing point to end tidal position. *Clin Sci* 43:137, 1972.

37. Hoeppner VH, Cooper DM, Zamel N, et al: Relationship between elastic recoil and closing volume in smokers and nonsmokers. *Am Rev Respir Dis* 109:81, 1974.

38. Warner MA, Divertie MB, Tinker JH: Preoperative cessation of smoking and pulmonary complications in coronary artery bypass patients. *Anesthesiology* 60:380, 1984.

39. Moores LK: Smoking and postoperative pulmonary complications. An evidence-based review of the recent literature. *Clin Chest Med* 21:139, 2000.

40. Johnson KD, Cadambi A, Seibert AB: Incidence of adult respiratory distress syndrome in patients with multiple musculoskeletal injuries: Effect of early operative stabilization of fractures. *J Trauma* 25:375, 1985.

41. Reines HD, Harris RC: Pulmonary complications of acute spinal cord injuries. *Neurosurgery* 21:193, 1987.

42. Ali J, Qi W: Pulmonary function and posture in traumatic quadriplegia. *J Trauma* 39:334, 1995.

43. Ali J, Weisel RD, Layug AB, et al: Consequences of postoperative alterations in respiratory mechanics. *Am J Surg* 128:376, 1974.

44. Hedenstierna G: Mechanisms of postoperative pulmonary dysfunction. *Acta Chir Scand* 550(Suppl):152, 1989.

45. Ali J, Yaffe C, Serrette C: The effect of transcutaneous electric nerve stimulation on postoperative pain and pulmonary function. *Surgery* 89:507, 1981.

46. Simonneau G, Vivien A, Sartener R, et al: Diaphragm dysfunction induced by upper abdominal surgery. *Am Rev Respir Dis* 128:899, 1983.

47. Ford GT, Whitelaw WA, Rosenal TW, et al: Diaphragm function after upper abdominal surgery in humans. *Am Rev Respir Dis* 127:431, 1983.

48. Road JD, Burgess KR, Whitelaw WA, Ford GT: Diaphragm function and respiratory response after upper abdominal surgery in dogs. *J Appl Physiol* 57:576, 1984.

49. Ford GT, Grant DA, Rideout KS, et al: Inhibition of breathing associated with gall bladder (GB) stimulation in dogs. *J Appl Physiol* 65:72, 1988.

50. Erice F, Fox GS, Salib YM, et al: Diaphragmatic function before and after laparoscopic cholecystectomy. *Anesthesiology* 79:966, 1993.

51. Schulze S, Thorup F: Pulmonary function, pain and fatigue after laparoscopic cholecystectomy. *Eur J Surg* 159:361, 1993.

52. Ali J, Gana T: Lung volumes at 24 hours after laparoscopic cholecystectomy—justification for early discharge. *Can Respir J* 5:109, 1998.

53. Obeid F, Saba A, Fatah J, et al: Increasing intraabdominal pressure affects pulmonary compliance. *Arch Surg* 130:544, 1995.

53a. von Ungern-Sternberg BS, Regli A, Schneider MC, et al: Effect of obesity and site of surgery on perioperative lung volumes. *Br J Anaesth* 92:202, 2004.

54. Ali J, Khan TA: The comparative effects of muscle transection and median upper abdominal incisions on postoperative pulmonary function. *Surg Gynecol Obstet* 148:863, 1979.

55. Roussos C: The failing ventilatory pump. *Lung* 160:59, 1982.

56. Herve P, Simonneau G, Girard P, et al: Hypercapneic acidosis induced by nutrition in mechanically ventilated patients. Glucose vs. fat. *Crit Care Med* 13:537, 1985.

57. Knill RL, Gelb AW: Peripheral chemoreceptors during anesthesia. Are the watch dogs sleeping? *Anesthesiology* 57:151, 1982.

58. Brain JD: Anesthesia and respiratory defense mechanisms. *Int Anesthesiol Clin* 15:169, 1977.

59. Wynne JW, Modell JH: Respiratory aspiration of stomach contents. *Ann Intern Med* 87:466, 1977.

60. Nathens AB, Chu PTY, Marshall JC: Nosocomial infection in the surgical intensive care unit. *Infect Dis Clin North Am* 6:657, 1992.

61. Cook DJ, Laine LA, Guyatt GH, et al: Nosocomial pneumonia and the role of gastric pH: a meta-analysis. *Chest* 100:7, 1991.

62. Du Moulin GC, Paterson DG, Hedley-Whyte J, et al: Aspiration of gastric bacteria in antacid-treated patients: a frequent cause of postoperative colonization of the airway. *Lancet* 1:242, 1982.

63. Celli BR, Rodriguez KS, Snider GL: A controlled trial of intermittent positive pressure breathing, incentive spirometry and deep breathing exercises in preventing pulmonary complications after abdominal surgery. *Am Rev Respir Dis* 130:12, 1984.

64. Overend TJ, Anderson CM, Lucy SD, et al: The effect of incentive spirometry on postoperative pulmonary complications—a systematic review. *Chest* 120:971, 2001.

65. Fagevik OM, Wennberg E, Johnson E, et al: Randomized clinical study of the prevention of pulmonary complications after thoracoabdominal resection by two different techniques. *Br J Surg* 89:1228, 2002.

66. Ali J, Serrette C, Wood LDH, Anthonisen NR: Effect of postoperative intermittent positive pressure breathing on lung function. *Chest* 2:192, 1984.

67. Ali J, Serrette C, Khan TA: The effect of abdominal binders on postoperative pulmonary function. *Infect Surg* 2:875, 1983.

68. Ali MK, Mountain CF, Ewer MS, et al: Predicting loss of pulmonary function after pulmonary resection for bronchogenic carcinoma. *Chest* 77:337, 1980.

69. Ferguson MK, Little L, Rizzo L, et al: Diffusing capacity predicts morbidity and mortality after pulmonary resection. *J Thorac Cardiovasc Surg* 96:894, 1988.

70. Schuurmans MM, Diacon AH, Bolliger CT: Functional evaluation before lung resection. *Clin Chest Med* 23:159, 2002.

71. Hall JB, Wood LDH: Liberation of the patient from mechanical ventilation. *JAMA* 257:1621, 1987.

Chapter 88

PREOPERATIVE ASSESSMENT OF THE HIGH-RISK SURGICAL PATIENT

FERGUS WALSH

JAMEEL ALI

KEY POINTS

- *Perioperative risk assessment by careful history, physical examination, and selective investigation is essential for directing therapy in the high-risk surgical patient.*

- *To decrease mortality and morbidity, cardiac, pulmonary, and endocrine abnormalities must be identified and appropriately managed.*

- *Age >70 years, current or prior angina pectoris, prior myocardial infarction, Q wave on resting electrocardiogram, and cardiac failure are significant clinical risk factors for perioperative cardiac complications.*

- *Perioperative cardiac morbidity can be minimized with pre-emptive medical management which includes the perioperative administration of β-blockers.*

- *Postoperative pulmonary complications can be reduced by aggressive pre- and postoperative care.*

- *Diabetes mellitus, abnormalities in thyroid function, and steroid dependence can significantly influence perioperative morbidity and mortality.*

As indicated in Chap. 87, surgery and anesthesia trigger a host of physiologic responses. In the average otherwise healthy patient these responses result in no major untoward postoperative sequelae. However, in the medically compromised patient the additional burden of surgical stress can prove to be very challenging and sometimes insurmountable. Such patients frequently require detailed evaluation and monitoring in the preoperative as well as postoperative periods in the intensive care unit (ICU) setting. Careful planning of the preoperative assessment and management of identified abnormalities in these patients are crucial to optimize chances of a good postoperative outcome. A major component of this planning involves the assessment of risks for intraoperative and postoperative morbidity. Patients with cardiac, respiratory and endocrine abnormalities pose special risks for postoperative complications. In this chapter we present guidelines for identifying and managing patients at risk of developing postoperative cardiac-, respiratory-, and endocrine-related postoperative morbidity.

Assessment of Cardiac Morbidity for Noncardiac Surgery

CLINICAL ASSESSMENT OF CARDIAC RISK

Over 25% of patients presenting for noncardiac surgery have diagnosed or clinically suspected ischemic heart disease

with increased risk for perioperative complications.[1] The American Society of Anesthesiologists' (ASA) classification of physical status (Table 88-1) is still commonly used as an index of surgical risk.[2] Using multivariate analysis of 1001 consecutive patients presenting for noncardiac surgery, Goldman and associates developed an index for perioperative risk (Cardiac Risk Index; CRI) based on clinical, electrocardiographic (ECG), and routine biochemical parameters (Table 88-2).[3] The strongest predictors of cardiac morbidity were the severity of coronary artery disease, a recent myocardial infarction (MI) and perioperative heart failure. Detsky and coworkers developed a more elaborate scoring system.[4] Such studies suggest an overall perioperative cardiac risk for consecutive patients presenting for noncardiac surgery of 1.4%, and the risk of cardiac death at approximately 1%. However, in patients with previously documented or clinically suspected ischemic heart disease, the rates of perioperative MI (4.1%) and death (1.7%) were markedly higher. The retrospective analysis of 1001 patients from whom the CRI was derived is shown in Table 88-3. Those patients in class IV had a 22% incidence of major cardiac complications and a 56% mortality rate.

Table 88-4 compares the predictive values of the CRI with the ASA scoring system and other noninvasive tests used to assess cardiac risk. Class IV patients were still a high-risk group, but the positive predictive value (PPV) was lower at 0.5.[5] The ASA has a low PPV because of the high number of false-positive results (i.e., although it is sensitive, it is not specific). Although a patient falling into CRI class IV is at high risk, the utility of the test is reduced by its low sensitivity. Only 55% of the patients at risk were in classes III and IV. The sensitivity may be even less when dealing with patients undergoing major vascular surgery.[6]

In summary, generally accepted independent risk factors for perioperative cardiac morbidity include: *age >70 years, current or prior angina pectoris, prior MI, Q wave on resting ECG, and cardiac failure.* It is widely accepted that patients presenting for elective surgery with zero, one to two, or three or more of these clinical markers are at low-, intermediate-, or high-risk respectively, for cardiac complications in the perioperative period. It is clear that patients in the low-risk category may proceed to surgery with an expectation of a low rate of cardiac complications. Similarly, patients deemed to be in the high-risk group may need to proceed to intensive management of their cardiac disease before initiation of the surgery. It is the group of patients in the intermediate-risk category who will benefit most from the investigations described below, in an effort to further elucidate the extent of their underlying

TABLE 88-1 American Society of Anesthesiologists Preoperative Patient Classification

Class	Definition
I	Healthy patient
II	Mild systemic disease
III	Severe systemic disease, limits activity but is not incapacitating
IV	Incapacitating systemic disease which is a constant threat to life
V	Moribund, not expected to survive 24 h with or without operation
E	Added to class if an emergency

TABLE 88-2 Computation of the Cardiac Risk Index

Criteria	Points
1. History	
a. Age >70 years	5
b. Myocardial infarction within previous 6 months	10
2. Physical examination	
a. S_3 gallop or JVD	11
b. Important valvular aortic stenosis	3
3. Electrocardiogram (ECG)	
a. Rhythm other than sinus or PACs on last preop ECG	7
b. >5 PVCs/min documented at any time before operation	7
4. General status	
P_{O_2} <60 or P_{CO_2} >50 mm Hg, K <3.0 or H_{CO_3} <20 mEq/L, BUN >50 or Cr >3.0 mg/dL, abnormal SGOT, chronic liver disease, or bedridden from noncardiac causes	3
5. Operation	
a. Intraperitoneal, intrathoracic, or aortic operation	3
b. Emergency operation	4
Total possible	53

ABBREVIATIONS: BUN, blood urea nitrogen; JVD, jugular venous distention; PAC, premature atrial contraction; P_{CO_2}, partial pressure of carbon dioxide; P_{O_2}, partial pressure of oxygen; PVC, premature ventricular contraction; . SGOT, serum glutamate oxaloacetate transaminase (aspartate aminotransferase).
SOURCE: Reproduced with permission from Goldman et al.[3]

TABLE 88-4 Comparison of Predictors of Cardiac Risk

Risk Index		Reference	PPV	NPV
I.	*Multifactorial Risk Indices*			
	ASA III	4	0.11	0.98
	ASA IV		0.23	0.96
	CRI III		0.21	0.97
	CRI IV		0.77	0.96
	CRI IV	8	0.30	0.98
II.	*Detecting Ischemic Heart Disease*			
	A. Exercise stress testing			
	ECG positive	10	0.32	0.93
	ECG positive	11	0.81	0.91
	Unable to attain HR >100 for >2-min duration	13	0.28	0.92
	B. 24-h Holter monitor—documented ischemia	13	0.38	0.99
	C. DTS	15	0.50	1.00
III.	RF+DTS			
	CRF	17	0.32	0.96
	CRF+DTS		0.42	0.95
	1–2 CRF		0.16	0.97
	1–2 CRF+DTS		0.30	0.97
	3 CRF		0.50	0.89
	3 CRF+DTS		0.64	0.67
	MI within 6 months of operation	22		
	1973–76		0.29	0.95
	1977–82		0.04	0.98

ABBREVIATIONS: ASA, American Society of Anesthesiologists' classification; CRF, clinical risk factors (see text); CRI, Cardiac Risk Index; DTS, dipyridamole-thallium scanning; ECG, electrocardiogram; HR, heart rate; MI, myocardial infarction; NPV, negative predictive value; PPV, positive predictive value; RF risk factor.

cardiac disease and to attempt to quantify the perioperative risks before the commencement of the surgical procedure.

Noninvasive Investigations to Stratify Risk

EXERCISE ELECTROCARDIOGRAM

Exercise ECG (ExECG) is a sensitive marker for subsequent myocardial infarction.[7] Treadmill ExECG, utilized to calculate ventricular response to increasing oxygen demand, has been shown to be a sensitive noninvasive indicator of ventricular performance and predictor of perioperative ventricular failure.[8] The prospective comparative value of ExECG was investigated in over 200 patients deemed to be at intermediate risk of adverse cardiac outcome following noncardiac surgery. Results showed odds ratios (OR) for ST-segment depression of 0.1 mV or greater in the ExECG (OR = 5.2) to be less than a known definite diagnosis of coronary artery

disease (OR = 8.8), but greater than echocardiographic evidence of reduced left ventricular function (OR = 2.0). The combination of clinical variables and ExECG data improved preoperative risk stratification.[9] However, ExECG is rarely practical in critically ill patients.

AMBULATORY ELECTROCARDIOGRAM

Ambulatory electrocardiographic monitoring (AEM) using Holter monitors to detect silent preoperative and perioperative ischemia has been shown to be predictive of postoperative unstable angina, pulmonary edema, and MI.[10] Twenty percent of ischemic events have been shown to occur in the preoperative period, 25% intraoperatively, and 41% postoperatively, with 97% of all events being clinically silent.[11] Silent

TABLE 88-3 Assessment of Cardiac Risk Index in 1001 Patients

Class	Point Total	No or Only Minor Complication (N = 943)	Life-Threatening Complication[a] (N = 39)	Cardiac Deaths (N = 19)
I (N = 537)	0–5	532 (99)[b]	4 (0.7)	1 (0.2)
II (N = 316)	6–12	295 (93)	16 (5)	5 (2)
III (N = 130)	13–25	112 (86)	15 (11)	3 (2)
IV (N = 18)	26	4 (22)	4 (22)	10 (56)

[a]Documented intraoperative or postoperative myocardial infarction, pulmonary edema, or ventricular tachycardia without progression to cardiac death.
[b]Figures in parentheses denote %.
SOURCE: Reproduced with permission from Goldman et al.[3]

ischemic episodes in the preoperative and postoperative periods are associated with perioperative cardiac morbidity; both of these factors are more clearly associated with postoperative MI than intraoperative ischemia. The absence of preoperative ischemia may predict the absence of postoperative MI;[12] however, this has not been a uniform finding.[13]

RADIONUCLIDE SCANNING

Dipyridamole-thallium scanning (DTS) has been shown to be a sensitive predictor of perioperative cardiac complications for patients who cannot exercise.[14] Dipyridamole dilates normal coronary vascular beds and diverts flow away from areas supplied by a stenotic vessel (usually indicative of >70% stenosis), resulting in a perfusion defect. Although DTS has been shown to be highly sensitive and specific in patients presenting for vascular surgery, it has proved less useful when consecutive patients have been studied and all researchers blinded.[15] A similar result was shown when diabetic patients presenting for vascular surgery were evaluated with DTS in addition to clinical risk stratification.[16] A large prospective study of DTS in 2000 vascular patients showed an OR of only 1.95.[17] The authors added that the value of DTS depends on the patient's risk profile (i.e., low-risk patient with positive DTS is a more significant result than a high-risk patient with positive DTS).

Single photon emission tomography (SPECT) may improve accuracy of DTS.[18] However, in patients presenting for abdominal aortic aneurysm surgery, SPECT has not accurately predicted adverse cardiac outcomes.[19] While DTS reflects perfusion defects, a particular form of SPECT imaging (FDG SPECT) allows analysis of myocardial glucose utilization. In a study of 148 patients with ECG and echocardiographic evidence of Q-wave infarction, SPECT diagnosed viable myocardium in 61% of myocardial areas with a Q-wave pattern (i.e., previously deemed to be scar tissue), and 75% of dysfunctional non-Q-wave areas.[20] Therefore, SPECT may have a further role in the evaluation of patients with evidence of myocardial damage.

ECHOCARDIOGRAPHIC IMAGING TECHNIQUES

Transthoracic echocardiography (TTE) provides the clinician with a detailed analysis of ventricular wall motion, ejection fraction, and if present, evidence of left ventricular hypertrophy. Resting TTE is noninvasive and readily applicable to the critically ill patient. Initial investigation of TTE as an assessment tool before noncardiac surgery did not support the routine use of TTE as a preoperative screening tool.[21] However, a larger study showed that when TTE reveals systolic dysfunction in preoperative testing, TTE is associated with an increased OR of postoperative MI (OR = 2.8) and cardiogenic pulmonary edema (OR = 3.2). The authors concluded that in selected intermediate-risk patients, TTE before noncardiac surgery may provide independent information about perioperative cardiac risk.[22]

Dobutamine stress echocardiography (DSE) is echocardiography performed before, during, and after an intravenous infusion of dobutamine. A positive DSE is one that shows ventricular wall motion abnormalities or evidence of ischemia-induced diastolic dysfunction. Initial investigation of DSE to stratify patients at cardiac risk proved superior to DTS.[23] The prognostic value of DSE in comparison to dipyridamole stress echocardiography (DiSE) and DTS was studied in over 2000 patients undergoing major vascular surgery. DSE and DiSE had significantly improved odds ratios for predicting cardiac complications (OR = 9.6 and 37.1, respectively) in comparison to DTS (OR = 1.95). The authors concluded that stress echocardiography effectively stratified patients into low- and high-risk groups regardless of clinical profile. In another study, when preoperative vascular surgery patients were selected to receive DSE according to protocol (one or more clinical risk factors), the prognostic value of DSE was again highlighted.[24] DSE has little prognostic value in low-risk patients, but in the clinically intermediate and high-risk population, DSE may help identify patients in whom cardiac revascularization should be considered before noncardiac surgery.

Clinical Risk Scenarios

RECENT MYOCARDIAL INFARCTION

A history of recent MI remains one of the most significant predictors of perioperative myocardial infarction (PMI). Risk of reinfarction is increased substantially if the infarct occurred within 6 months of proposed surgery. Early studies reported reinfarction rates of 15% if the infarct occurred within 3 to 6 months prior to noncardiac surgery, increasing to 30% if it was within 3 months. Rao and coworkers subsequently studied patients who were aggressively managed in the ICU for up to 96 hours postoperatively. These retrospective data in 733 patients undergoing major noncardiac surgery identified reinfarction rates of 5.7% in patients within 3 months of MI and 2.3% in patients within 6 months of MI.[25]

Patients who have suffered an infarction are frequently assessed by exercise testing or angiography at approximately 6 weeks following infarction, in an effort to provide objective evidence of ongoing ischemia. On the basis of this testing, if patients have good exercise tolerance and are deemed to be at low risk for ongoing ischemia, noncardiac surgery does not necessarily result in increased cardiac morbidity and mortality.[26]

A history of angina was not included in Goldman's original CRI; however, symptoms or signs of ongoing ischemia, whether clinically silent or overt, have been repeatedly shown to be significant predictors of perioperative cardiac events. Based on current knowledge, patients within the first 6 months following MI should all be deemed to be at intermediate risk. These patients will benefit from noninvasive testing to quantify perioperative cardiac risk.

CONGESTIVE HEART FAILURE

Preoperative signs of congestive cardiac failure, a third heart sound, and signs of pulmonary edema are persistently strong predictors of perioperative cardiac morbidity. Left ventricular dysfunction serves as a marker of prior MI, ongoing ischemia, significant valvular disease, or cardiomyopathy. The highest risk for development of perioperative pulmonary edema is among patients >40 years of age who have evidence of cardiac failure preoperatively (approximately 15%, compared to 5% in patients with well-controlled cardiac failure). Patients with no pre-existing diagnosis of cardiac failure have approximately a 2% incidence of developing postoperative pulmonary edema.[27]

AGE

Although multivariate analyses repeatedly show age to be a risk factor, other studies suggest age itself may not be a major risk factor independent of the general health of the patient.[28] However, signs of ischemic heart disease may not be as clinically obvious in the elderly population. One study compared coronary angiography results from 260 elderly (>70 years) patients to 260 control patients (age <60 years). The results for patients with zero, one to two, and three or more clinical markers who exhibited severe stenoses were 17%, 55%, and 85% in the elderly group, in comparison to 14%, 36%, and 68%, respectively, in the control group. Thus the presence of clinical markers of ischemia in the elderly should prompt careful evaluation and a lower threshold for the initiation of noninvasive testing.

DIABETES

Diabetes, like age, may not be an independent risk factor per se. A retrospective multivariate analysis of 282 diabetics who underwent surgery found that the risk of a major cardiac event was related to pre-existing cardiac failure, valvular heart disease, and age >75 years.[29] The age relation may reflect the duration of the diabetes. A large nationally based review of almost 15,000 patients who underwent vascular surgery revealed little influence of diabetes on subsequent cardiac mortality. After controlling for comorbid conditions, procedure type, and diabetic complications, only type 1 diabetics were at increased risk for cardiovascular complications. Neither type 1 nor type 2 diabetes was an independent risk factor for death.[30]

Risk Modification

IMPLEMENTATION OF RECOMMENDATIONS ON PREOPERATIVE TESTING

Recommendations from the American College of Cardiology/American Heart Association (ACC/AHA) have helped refine the clinician's approach to patients with known or suspected ischemic heart disease presenting for major surgery. Previously, 50% to 75% of patients presenting for major vascular surgery were investigated by noninvasive cardiac testing. By comparing historical data from the pre-guideline era (102 patients) and post-guideline implementation (94 patients), one center documented a dramatic reduction in preoperative stress testing (88% to 47%), cardiac catheterization (24% to 11%), and coronary revascularization (25% to 2%).[32] Stress tests were equally distributed between low- and high-risk groups in the pre-guideline era, but were utilized significantly less frequently in the low-risk group in the post-guideline era (31% low-risk, 61% high-risk). As expected, associated costs fell dramatically to 10% of the pre-guideline average, but death (4% vs. 3%) and myocardial infarction rates (7% vs. 5%) were not statistically altered by the reduced number of investigations.[31]

PREOPERATIVE PERCUTANEOUS TRANSLUMINAL ANGIOPLASTY

To date there are no randomized trials demonstrating the effectiveness of preoperative percutaneous transluminal angio-plasty (PTCA) in patients presenting for major surgery with known ischemic heart disease. Elective PTCA carries inherent risks of acute MI (1% to 3%), emergency requirement for coronary artery bypass grafting (CABG) (0.2% to 3%), and in-hospital death (0.5% to 1.4%). The inevitable disruption of the atheromatous plaque in the stable patient may potentially increase the incidence of coronary thrombosis in the setting of major surgery. A retrospective study showed no reduction in perioperative MIs in patients treated with PTCA within 90 days of major surgery, compared to a known coronary artery disease control population.[32] One uncontrolled retrospective study of patients receiving coronary stents before intermediate- or high-risk surgery showed a high rate of perioperative MI (28%), major bleeding (24%), or cardiac death (32%).[33]

PREOPERATIVE CORONARY ARTERY BYPASS GRAFTING

Recommendations for preoperative CABG[34] were based on retrospective data, and either utilized historical controls or did not include the mortality associated with CABG itself. Preoperative prophylactic CABG still remains of unproven benefit. Since the first discernable survival benefit in CABG patients exists at 2 years post-CABG,[35] the relative benefit of preoperative CABG over medical therapy remains unproven.

PERIOPERATIVE BETA-BLOCKADE

Identification of patients at risk for perioperative ischemia facilitates the introduction of perioperative β-blockade. In patients with known reversible ischemia, administration of perioperative β-blockers reduced the MI and death rate from 32% to 12%.[36] This highly significant reduction in cardiac complications probably results from reduction in tachycardia and hypertension. The generalized acceptance of the safety and efficacy of β-blockers has led to calls for their routine use in patients who are at risk for ischemic heart disease. Mangano and coworkers studied 200 patients with known or suspected ischemic heart disease who underwent noncardiac surgery.[37] Patients were randomized to receive atenolol or placebo pre-, intra-, and postoperatively until hospital discharge. In-hospital cardiac mortality was unchanged between groups, but overall mortality was significantly reduced in the three time spans studied: 0 to 6 months following discharge (0% vs. 8%), 0 to 12 months (3% vs. 14%), and 0 to 24 months (10% vs. 21%). In a large group of vascular surgery patients, in the subgroup of patients with fewer than three risk factors (83% of total), patients who received β-blockers had a lower risk of cardiac complications (0.8%) than those not receiving β-blockers (2.3%). The same group reported a 12% incidence of cardiac events in a high-risk vascular surgery population randomized to receive bisoprolol, compared to 32% in patients without β-blockade.[38] They summarized that bisoprolol significantly reduced long-term cardiac death and MI in high-risk patients after major vascular surgery. Despite such widespread recommendations in favor of perioperative β-blockade, the optimal timing for stopping the β-blocker therapy has not been well elucidated. One small series suggested that abrupt withdrawal of β-blockers in the postoperative period may lead to increased postoperative MI (OR = 17.7).[39]

MODIFICATION OF SURGERY

Patients with concomitant unstable angina and recent MI rarely present for noncardiac surgery. However, such patients represent a significant risk for MI and cardiac death. Noncardiac operations in such circumstances should be deferred except in emergency situations. The substitution of major surgery for a minimally invasive approach is frequently impossible and may not lead to an improvement in cardiac risk. In a retrospective review of patients presenting for elective abdominal aortic aneurysm (AAA) repair, similar morbidity and mortality rates were found for an endovascular versus an open approach.[40] While there was a significant increase in preoperative pulmonary compromise in the endovascular group, there were no differences in history and symptoms of ischemic heart disease, blood pressure, lipid profile, or diabetes between groups.

INTENSIVE PERIOPERATIVE MANAGEMENT

The rationale for using aggressive perioperative medical intervention to reduce cardiac risk is compelling. Many of the major cardiac risk factors such as congestive heart failure, myocardial ischemia, and dysrhythmias are detectable and amenable to therapy. The mainstay of intra- and postoperative monitoring for many years has been the pulmonary artery catheter (PAC; see below).

Preoperative ICU admission for investigation and "fine tuning" has been extolled by some centers. The use of such invasive monitoring with aggressive perioperative control of hemodynamics (i.e., admission to the ICU for 72 to 96 hours postoperatively) has been credited for a five- to sevenfold reduction in the reinfarction rate of patients undergoing surgery within 6 months of MI (24 Assessment Section). Precise factors responsible for this reduction are difficult to determine. Others have also reported low perioperative MI rates in high-risk patients when similar pre-, intra-, and postoperative strategies have been employed.[41] However, the better outcomes could be due to factors such as better general medical management of the postinfarct patient prior to surgery, or the administration of β-blockade to the intensively managed patients (not commented upon in earlier papers). Postoperative cardiac morbidity following noncardiac surgery may be predicted. It may be that postoperative cardiac ischemia of long duration rather than the presence of ischemia itself is the factor most significantly associated with adverse cardiac outcome.

Perioperative optimization of oxygen delivery using intravenous fluid and inotropes has been reported to reduce overall mortality in high-risk surgical patients. Landmark papers in the 1980s suggested definitive end points of therapy (so-called "supranormalization"), but these were not specifically described for particular high-risk populations such as septic patients, the elderly, and those with ischemic heart disease. Some authors report higher mortality using an aggressive approach in such patients.[42]

PULMONARY ARTERY CATHETER

The routine use of the pulmonary artery catheter to aid decision making for the high-risk surgical patient has been called into question. A large prospective cohort study of mixed medical and surgical patients in the ICU showed increased mortality, length of ICU stay, and costs associated with use of the PAC.[43] A multicenter randomized trial of the use of the PAC in almost 2000 high-risk patients undergoing elective abdominal, thoracic, vascular, and major orthopedic surgery, showed no benefit to therapy directed by the PAC over standard care.[44] In addition, eight patients in the PAC group showed evidence of pulmonary emboli in comparison to zero in the control patients. This interesting finding prompts even more speculation about the safety of the PAC in surgical patients.

NEWER CARDIAC OUTPUT MONITORS

Such evidence suggests that the PAC may not be an appropriate monitoring tool in the elective surgical population. Newer less-invasive tools have come into clinical use. A central venous catheter capable of continuous measurement of central venous oxygen saturation was used by Rivers and associates to achieve early goal-directed therapy in medical patients, with dramatic improvement in mortality.[45] Another tool that is less invasive than the PAC is the pulse contour cardiac output (PiCCO) monitor. This device requires brachial or femoral arterial cannulation with a specialized arterial catheter containing a thermistor. Using standard cold saline dilution technique, cardiac output analysis and measurement of intrathoracic blood volume (ITBV) and extravascular lung water are possible. Reports suggest that ITBV more reliably predicted cardiac preload than central venous pressure or pulmonary capillary wedge pressure.[46]

TRANSESOPHAGEAL ECHOCARDIOGRAPHY

Transesophageal echocardiography (TEE) is a sensitive marker of myocardial ischemia, often revealing segmental wall motion abnormalities before other signs of ischemia become obvious. TEE has been advocated to detect intraoperative ischemia, and has been shown to have superior sensitivity and specificity (sensitivity 75%, specificity 100%) in comparison to two-lead ECG (sensitivity 56%, specificity 98%) and pulmonary capillary wedge pressure (sensitivity 25%, specificity 93%).[47] A larger study (224 patients) confirms this opinion, finding that TEE is frequently influential in guiding clinical decision making.[48] In comparison to two-lead ECG and PAC, TEE was the most important intraoperative guiding factor in decision making for anti-ischemic therapy (56% of decisions based on TEE), fluid administration (28%), and vasopressor or inotrope administration (16%).

RESOURCE ALLOCATION

If aggressive hemodynamic monitoring in the ICU is responsible for the improved survival of patients with ischemic heart disease following noncardiac surgery, the financial implications are staggering. In Rao's study, more than 1300 ICU days of care were required to bring about a 2.4% reduction in the reinfarction rate. However, if admission criteria were restricted to congestive heart failure, angina plus congestive heart failure, or angina plus hypertension, this would account for almost 80% of the perioperative infarctions, but reduce ICU days to <300. A more recent study found that 77% of postoperative infarctions occurred within 26 hours of surgery, and 100% within 48 hours, suggesting a shorter period of monitoring may be sufficient.

TYPE OF SURGERY: TYPE OF ANESTHETIC

Noncardiac operations may be divided into those that are likely to provoke perioperative ischemia and those that do not increase the risk of ischemia above normal. Major vascular procedures involving aortic cross-clamping and infrainguinal arterial bypass carry a high risk of postoperative ischemia,[49] as do major abdominal and thoracic procedures. Orthopedic procedures such as total hip arthroplasty have a lower incidence of cardiac morbidity, and are deemed intermediate risk. Peripheral nonvascular procedures such as transurethral resection of the prostate, an operation frequently performed in patients with coexisting coronary artery disease, are associated with a low incidence of perioperative MI.[50]

Major surgery is associated with an intense sympathetic and procoagulant response, which may be implicated in the development of myocardial ischemia. These neurohumoral responses to surgery may be diminished with the use of epidural anesthesia and analgesia (EAA) extending into the postoperative period.[51] Stress-mediated release of hormones such as cortisol, antidiuretic hormone, and catecholamines is blunted by epidural anesthesia.[52] In addition, postoperative pain may contribute to tachycardia and resultant subendocardial ischemia. Early studies showed a dramatic reduction in cardiac complications in patients treated with EAA in comparison to general anesthesia (GA) alone.[53] This opinion was further upheld by a large systematic review of relevant trials of epidural or spinal anesthesia vs. GA over the past 30 years, which showed a statistically and clinically significant reduction in mortality and morbidity after surgery.[54] This retrospective work was prospectively tested by a large (915 patients) randomized controlled trial of high-risk surgical patients who either received EAA (intraoperatively and up to 72 hours postoperatively) with GA or GA alone with intraoperative and postoperative opioids as the mainstay of the analgesic regimen.[55] The group observed no reduction in mortality or cardiac morbidity between groups. The only clinical benefit documented was a reduction in postoperative respiratory failure. However, the authors commented that 15 epidurals were required to prevent one episode of respiratory failure. The authors also commented that in no cases were there any serious complications with catheter placement or postoperative problems directly attributable to the placement of the epidural.

RECOMMENDATIONS

Evaluation and treatment of patients presenting for noncardiac surgery requires careful attention to history, functional status, and assessment of clinical evidence of reversible cardiac failure or dysrhythmias, in addition to consideration of the timing and indications for the proposed surgery. There is no doubt that clinical risk factors such as known ischemic heart disease, cardiac failure, age >70 years, and Q waves on a resting ECG are all independently documented to be associated with an increase in perioperative cardiac morbidity. Despite published and validated clinical risk indexes, the clinician will daily assess the patient on the basis of the above criteria, and ascribe the category of low, intermediate, or high risk according to the number of risk factors elucidated.

Following published guidelines and analysis of the literature, it can be recommended that noninvasive cardiac testing will not add to the clinicians knowledge or improve risk stratification in patients with none of the above clinical criteria. Similarly, patients who present a significant clinical risk or who have recently suffered an MI may require interventional cardiology and possible revascularization prior to proposed noncardiac surgery. This high-risk group should be intensively monitored in the perioperative period, including a stay in the ICU for approximately 48 to 72 hours. It is the intermediate-risk group of patients, presenting with one to two clinical risk factors, who will benefit most from noninvasive testing. Current evidence suggests DSE may be superior to DTS, TTE, or ExECG in preoperative cardiac risk stratification. However, DSE is not widely available and requires specialized centers and expertise. Current treatment protocols suggest a significant clinical benefit from the widespread administration of β-blockers to all intermediate- and high-risk patients. Some caution may need to be exercised regarding the duration of dose and discontinuation of the drug. Finally, despite recent negative reports regarding the use of the pulmonary artery catheter, evidence continues to support noninvasive or minimally-invasive perioperative monitoring of high-risk patients following noncardiac surgery.

Assessment of Risk of Postoperative Pulmonary Complications

CLINICAL ASSESSMENT OF PULMONARY RISK

Postoperative alterations in pulmonary physiology predispose to the development of atelectasis (see Chap. 87). Marked decreases in forced expiratory volume in 1 second (FEV_1) and forced vital capacity (FVC) have been documented with serial postoperative pulmonary function tests.[56] A reduction in functional residual capacity (FRC) of approximately 70% of basal values may occur by about 18 hours after surgery, resulting in closure of small airways as FRC approximates closing volume.[57] Progressive loss of functional lung tissue results and intrapulmonary shunting leads to worsening hypoxemia.

Many risk factors for the development of postoperative atelectasis have been highlighted. Each of the following has been shown to predict postoperative atelectasis: preoperative severe bronchitis, FEV_1 more than two standard deviations less than predicted, obesity, malnutrition, abdominal surgery, and age. Analysis of risk factors in a group of 272 patients referred for preoperative assessment concluded that statistically significant predictors of postoperative pulmonary complications were: partial pressure of arterial carbon dioxide (Pa_{CO_2}) ≥ 45 mm Hg (OR = 61.0), FVC ≤ 1.5 L/min (OR = 11.1), maximum laryngeal height ≤ 4 cm (OR = 6.9), forced expiratory time ≥ 9 seconds (OR = 5.7), smoking ≥ 40 pack-years (OR = 5.7), and body mass index (BMI) ≥ 30 kg/m^2 (OR = 4.1).[58]

Bedside pulmonary function tests (PFTs) such as spirometry have been used to identify patients at risk of developing postoperative pulmonary complications, but lack of randomization, selection bias, and retrospective or unblended analysis of outcome invalidate conclusions.[59] Spirometry as a screening procedure for high-risk patients remains unproved and its routine use has been discouraged.[60] The American College of Physicians recommends preoperative pulmonary function testing in the following groups: patients with unexplained dyspnea, patients undergoing high-risk surgery (cardiac, thoracic, and upper abdominal), cigarette smokers, symptoms of dyspnea on exertion, and patients undergoing head and neck or orthopedic surgery with uncharacterized lung disease. All patients undergoing lung resection should have PFTs.[61]

The inability to improve pulmonary function despite adequate therapy may be a more sensitive predictor of postoperative respiratory failure.[62] In a prospective study, those at risk of developing postoperative respiratory failure (defined as ventilator dependent >2 postoperative days) were best identified by the failure of 48 to 72 hours of intensive preoperative preparation to improve FVC, forced expiratory flow over 25% to 75% of the expiratory cycle (FEF_{25-75}), and maximal voluntary ventilation measured over 1 minute (MVV). Five percent of the study group developed postoperative respiratory failure, and all of these patients had an FEF_{25-75} and MVV less than 50% of predicted values, which had not improved with preoperative therapy. The perioperative mortality in this subgroup was 60%.

EVALUATION OF RISK PRIOR TO PULMONARY RESECTION SURGERY

Approximately 80% of patients presenting for lung cancer surgery have concomitant chronic obstructive pulmonary disease (COPD) and 20% to 30% have severe pulmonary dysfunction.[63] Pulmonary resection for lung cancer has been associated with morbidity of 12% to 50% and mortality of 2% to 12%.[64] A more recent retrospective analysis confirms that these figures have not been markedly improved (morbidity 20%, mortality 3%).[65] In addition to the general preoperative preparation of the surgical patient, those patients who will require pulmonary resection must have a preoperative estimation of postoperative pulmonary reserve.

A multifactorial risk index was proposed for patients undergoing thoracic surgery consisting of the Cardiac Risk Index (CRI) and a pulmonary risk index (PRI), known as the cardiopulmonary risk-factor index (CPRI). These pulmonary risk factors had previously been validated as independent risk factors in univariate analysis. The CPRI assesses obesity, cigarette smoking within 8 weeks of surgery, productive cough within 5 days of surgery, FEV_1/FVC <70%, and Pa_{CO_2} >45 mm Hg. Each of these factors was assigned one point. By combining the CRI (0 to 4) and the PRI (0 to 6), patients classified as having a CPRI of 4 or greater were 17 times more likely to develop a postoperative pulmonary complication than patients with a CRPI less than 4.[66]

Guidelines for prediction of outcome following lung resection are generally based on preoperative whole lung function tests.[67] MVV (% of predicted), FEV_1 (liters), and FEV_1 (% of predicted) have been most commonly used. Guideline values for proceeding with pneumonectomy, lobectomy, or wedge/segmental resection are:

- For pneumonectomy MVV >55%, FEV_1 >2 L, FEV_1% >55%;
- For lobectomy MVV >40%, FEV_1 >1 L, FEV_1% 40% to 50%; and
- For wedge/segmental resection MVV >35%, FEV_1 >0.6 L, FEV_1% >40%.

Predicted postoperative FEV_1 has been suggested as a sensitive predictor of postoperative pulmonary complications. For this measurement, FEV_1 and CT calculation of the number of preoperative functioning lung segments are required. Predicted postoperative FEV_1 ($ppoFEV_1$) may then be calculated using the formula:

$$ppoFEV_1 = \text{preoperative } FEV_1/(\text{No. of preop functioning}$$
$$\text{segments} \times \text{No. of postop functioning segments})$$

Studies have suggested that if $ppoFEV_1$ <40% of predicted, this may be a sensitive predictor of prohibitive operative risk and that resection should not be considered. More recent work suggests that a low $ppoFEV_1$ may indeed be a sensitive predictor of postoperative pulmonary complications in lung cancer resection patients, but only in the group without pre-existing COPD. $ppoFEV_1$ was not a significant predictor of postoperative pulmonary complications in patients with a preoperative diagnosis of COPD. This may be due to the fact that while these patients may have been losing lung tissue, a proportionally greater part of it was emphysematous and therefore less involved in gas exchange.[68]

In addition to these standard bedside tests, diffusing capacity (DLCO) may be helpful. If there is evidence of interstitial lung disease on chest x-ray or undue dyspnea on exertion, even if FEV_1 and FVC are normal, a DLCO should be obtained. If preoperative FEV_1 or DLCO is <40% of predicted, these are independent predictors of postoperative pulmonary complications. These patients may benefit from cardiopulmonary exercise testing. This is a sophisticated assessment of cardiopulmonary reserve and allows calculation of maximal oxygen consumption (V_{O_2}max). Risk of perioperative pulmonary complications can be stratified according the V_{O_2}max measured. Patients with a preoperative VO_{2max} >20 mL/kg are not at increased risk of complications; however, patients with V_{O_2}max of <15 mL/kg and <10 mL/kg are at intermediate- and high-risk, respectively, for perioperative pulmonary complications.

RISK MODIFICATION

PREOPERATIVE PREPARATION

Standard preoperative preparation, including the use of intensive chest physiotherapy, bronchodilators, and appropriate use of antibiotics are considered routine practice in an effort to reduce the risks of postoperative pulmonary complications. High-risk patients who were assigned to receive a protocol of intensive pre- and postoperative therapy (including delay of surgery if indicated) had a 22% incidence of postoperative complications, compared to 60% in a group in whom the preoperative preparation was at the discretion of the admitting physician. Aggressive pulmonary therapy resulted in shorter hospital stay despite frequent delays of surgery in the treatment group to improve pulmonary function.[69]

Despite the clinical application of deep breathing exercises, intermittent positive-pressure breathing (IPPB), and incentive spirometry, these treatments have not been shown to be independently successful in the prevention of postoperative pulmonary complications. Incentive spirometry has been shown to be of benefit, but only in high-risk patients. Pre- and postoperative chest physiotherapy per se is of value only in the treatment of established pulmonary atelectasis.

However, high-risk morbidly obese (BMI >40 kg/m^2) patients may benefit significantly from the application of biphasic positive end-expiratory pressure noninvasively and prior to signs of respiratory distress.[70]

CESSATION OF CIGARETTE SMOKING

Continued smoking up to the time of surgery is associated with a significant increase in mortality. Cessation of smoking has been shown to result in a significant increase in FRC and reduced postoperative pulmonary complications. For maximum risk reduction, the patient should stop smoking at least 8 weeks prior to surgery.

SITE OF SURGICAL INCISION

Extremity surgical intervention leads to little alteration in lung volume. However, lower abdominal incision results in a 25% to 30% decrease in FVC and a mild decrease in oxygenation. Upper abdominal and thoracic surgery produces significant impairment of pulmonary ventilation and defense systems independent of the effect of anesthesia.

Maintenance of FVC is essential for effective secretion clearance and is reduced by 50% to 60% immediately following upper abdominal surgery. Gradual restoration of FVC over the next 5 to 7 days is usual. During the first 24 hours after upper abdominal or thoracic surgery, reductions occur in tidal volume (20%) and FRC (70% to 80%) as a result of incision pain and reflex diaphragmatic splinting, resulting in rapid shallow breathing, absence of spontaneous sigh, and chest wall splinting.[71]

Laparoscopic surgery has revolutionized the postoperative care of patients undergoing common surgical procedures such as cholecystectomy and fundoplication. Comparing the open subcostal cholecystectomy to the laparoscopic approach, significant improvements in FVC (52% vs. 73% baseline), FEV$_1$ (53% vs. 72% baseline), and FEF (53% vs. 81% baseline) were documented.[72] A similar comparison of the laparoscopic versus open approach resulted in quicker return of postoperative respiratory mechanics towards but not quite to normal compared to open cholecystectomy.[73] A review of over 300 patients following laparoscopic cholecystectomy showed no major postoperative pulmonary morbidity in the entire group, despite the fact that 45 were deemed to be obese, including 18 who were morbidly obese (BMI >45 kg/m^2).[74]

TYPE OF ANESTHESIA AND ANALGESIA

Repeated attempts to demonstrate a consistent decrease in postoperative pulmonary complications with the use of regional anesthesia alone or in combination with general anesthesia have failed. Anesthetic technique per se is not a significant determinant of postoperative respiratory complications.[75] All forms of regional anesthesia such as epidural local anesthetic, epidural narcotic, intercostal nerve blocks, and paravertebral nerve blocks have beneficial effects on postoperative FEV$_1$, FVC, and partial pressure of arterial oxygen (Pa$_{O_2}$).[76] However, these beneficial effects have not proved to alter outcome in terms of pneumonia, respiratory failure, or death. Perhaps this is because the delayed reduction in FRC, resulting in atelectasis and hypoxemia, remains largely unaffected by the intra- and immediate postoperative analgesic regimens.

Repeated studies of intraoperative positive end-expiratory pressure (PEEP) have failed to show benefit in normal patients; however, the intraoperative application of PEEP 10 cm H$_2$O to morbidly obese patients (BMI >40 kg/m^2) resulted in an improvement in perioperative oxygenation (110 to 130 mm Hg).[77] However, these patients were studied in the early postoperative period and this improvement may not have been maintained.

RECOMMENDATIONS

Although several questions concerning accurate preoperative assessment for prevention of clinically significant pulmonary complications remain unanswered, from available data a few guidelines may be generated. Likely to benefit the patient preoperatively are: cessation of smoking (at least 4 weeks, preferably >8 weeks abstinence), weight loss, and optimization of airway obstruction using bronchodilators. Intraoperative management options that may benefit the patient include: peripheral incision, limiting duration of surgery, endoscopic procedures, and the use of intraoperative PEEP. Postoperatively, good analgesia by the use of regional analgesia and patient-controlled analgesia delivery devices have been shown to be equally effective in reducing morbidity. Postoperative chest physiotherapy has proven value only for the treatment of atelectasis, but is useful as part of a program to encourage deep breathing exercises.

Thyroid Disorders, Diabetes, and Patients on Steroids

HYPERTHYROIDISM

Hyperthyroidism in the surgical patient may significantly alter surgical risk by imposing additional burden on the cardiovascular system.[78,79] Angina pectoris, atrial fibrillation, and cardiac failure may be precipitated, and other abnormalities include hypercalcemia, glucose intolerance, anorexia, myopathy, impaired drug absorption, and coagulation defects.

Preoperative preparation of a hyperthyroid patient includes deferral of elective surgery and optimization of thyroid function where possible. Most patients with hyperthyroidism have Graves disease and should be treated with a combination of antithyroid drugs (such as propylthiouracil and methimazole), iodide solutions, and possibly glucocorticoids to protect against adrenal insufficiency that may be associated with thyrotoxicosis.[80]

Surgical options for the treatment of a patient with Graves disease include subtotal or total thyroidectomy. A recent retrospective analysis of over 1200 patients over a 40-year period suggests that total thyroidectomy is the preferred surgical option for the treatment of Graves disease.[81]

If the surgery is emergent, the mainstay of treatment is perioperative β-blockade to reduce adrenergic thyroxine effects. Traditionally, propranolol has been recommended. However, esmolol may be preferred because of the rapid action and elimination, particularly when hemodynamic instability occurs.[82]

Thyroid storm is fortunately a rare event because of β-blockade prophylaxis, but when it occurs there is still a 40%

mortality rate. Tachydysrhythmias, frequently atrial fibrillation, are seen. Cardioversion is usually unsuccessful. Hyperthermia, hypertension, leukocytosis, and evidence of adrenal insufficiency may occur. Treatment with β-blockade should begin once the diagnosis is suspected. Invasive hemodynamic monitoring should be instituted to guide fluid and electrolyte therapy in the intensive care environment where possible.

HYPOTHYROIDISM

The incidence of hypothyroidism in the general population is 0.5% to 0.8%, increasing to 1% to 3% in patients over 65 years of age. Treatment with lithium or amiodarone, drugs not uncommonly associated with drug-induced hypothyroidism, may alert the clinician to this diagnosis.

Although there are many physical signs of hypothyroidism, the only sign statistically correlated with biochemical abnormalities is the presence of delayed ankle reflexes. Retrospective analysis suggests that postoperative complications are not increased in patients with mild to moderate hypothyroidism, but patients with severe hypothyroidism undergoing surgery are more prone to periods of hypotension, neuropsychiatric disturbance, and intestinal hypomotility.[83] Clinical assessment in addition to serum T_3, T_4, and thyrotropin levels should be used to assess thyroid status.[84]

Patients receiving regular thyroxine replacement, without signs and symptoms of hypothyroidism, can safely withhold oral thyroxine perioperatively for the majority of operations, as the half-life of levothyroxine is 1 week. If parenteral administration is required, thyroxine can safely be given intravenously at half the oral daily dose. Overtly hypothyroid patients undergoing emergency surgery should be treated with thyroxine replacement in addition to hydrocortisone 100 to 300 mg every 8 hours. Elderly patients with a clinical history or suspicion of coronary artery disease require cautious thyroxine replenishment and coadministration of nitrates.[85]

General anesthesia may be associated with profound cardiovascular depression in hypothyroid patients. Special consideration needs to be taken to titrate anaesthetic drugs to avoid this known effect. The use of newer anesthetic monitoring techniques such as bispectral index analysis may help titrate anaesthetic medications.[86]

DIABETES MELLITUS

Diabetes mellitus is the most common endocrine disorder encountered in the perioperative period, since it occurs in almost 5% of the general population.[87] Traditionally, diabetics presented for surgery for limb amputation and wound débridement, but owing to surgical advances in vitrectomy, cataract extraction, renal transplantation, and peripheral vascular repairs, diabetic patients are frequently presenting for preoperative assessment. Type I (insulin-dependent diabetes mellitus) comprises approximately 25% of the diabetic population, and affects a younger population (<35 years) which is prone to perioperative hyperglycemia and ketoacidosis because of inability to secrete insulin. Type II (non-insulin-dependent diabetes mellitus) patients are older and often obese and have a decrease in the number or responsiveness of insulin receptors, together with impaired insulin secretion, features which are accentuated in the perioperative period.[88,89]

The aim of therapy is to avoid excess morbidity and mortality which may be caused or exacerbated by extremes in blood glucose levels, undue protein catabolism, and fluid and electrolyte disturbances.

RISK ASSESSMENT

Although one study showed no difference in mortality and morbidity in vascular surgical patients, it is generally accepted that diabetics encounter increased perioperative morbidity and mortality.[90–92]

A perioperative myocardial infarction rate of 5.2% is reported in diabetics undergoing abdominal aortic reconstruction compared to 2.1% of nondiabetic patients. Inadequate control of blood glucose can lead to ketosis, acidemia, and dehydration. Decreased wound healing occurs at glucose levels greater than 200 mg/dL. Glucose concentrations greater than 250 mg/dL have been shown to impair leukocyte function and exacerbate ischemic brain damage. In addition to the effects of abnormal blood glucose levels, diabetics are at particular risk of atherosclerotic vascular disease, hypertension, and coronary artery disease.

Preoperative clinical markers for increased perioperative complications have been suggested. The presence of congestive cardiac failure, diabetic end-organ failure commonly associated with diabetes, valvular heart disease, and peripheral vascular disease associated with infection are statistically associated with increased mortality. Autonomic neuropathy is found in over 40% of patients presenting for surgery and may alter hemodynamic responses to intubation and surgery.[93,94]

Apart from anesthesia for cataract extraction, choice of anesthetic technique has not been associated with altered outcome.[95] Thoracic epidural and spinal anesthesia techniques are associated with reduced intraoperative catecholamine release. However, to date, no study of exclusively diabetic patients has compared outcome between regional and general anesthesia techniques.

RISK REDUCTION

Preoperative evaluation should include thorough clinical assessment for cardiac, neurologic, and peripheral vascular abnormalities. A careful history for the presence of ischemic heart disease or prior myocardial infarction should be supported by cardiac investigations where appropriate. Glycosylated hemoglobin (HbA_{1c}) levels less than 10% suggest satisfactory glycemic control. Renal failure may be present in up to 35% of diabetic patients upon presentation,[110] and plasma creatinine, urinary sediment examination, and urine analysis for infection should be assessed. Recent evidence that intensive insulin therapy to achieve strict control of blood sugar (80 to 110 mg/dL) improves outcome in nondiabetic surgical ICU patients suggests that general practice (to maintain a blood sugar <200 mg/dL) may be inadequate in the postoperative diabetic.[96]

Nondiabetic patients recovering from surgery commonly show transient hyperglycemia and diminished insulin secretion and end-organ responsiveness in response to increased circulating catecholamines.[97] However, these patients secrete sufficient insulin to suppress lipolysis and ketogenesis. Diabetics present with decreased or absent preoperative insulin secretion and a pre-existing insulin resistance, which serves to worsen the hyperglycemic response to surgery. Decreased peripheral use of glucose results in lipolysis, ketogenesis, possible acidemia, glycosuria, and dehydration.[98]

A variety of insulin regimens have been suggested for the routine perioperative management of diabetics undergoing surgery. No single regimen has proved markedly superior. Currently, perioperative intravenous glucose infusions are recommended, and insulin may be administered via a variety of dosages and routes. Subcutaneous administration of half the regular daily dose before surgery, using a variable-rate glucose infusion to maintain normoglycemia, has proved successful.[99] Mixing insulin, potassium, and 5% or 10% glucose has also been suggested.[100,101] Most authors suggest a variable-rate insulin infusion using an automated syringe device with a simultaneous glucose infusion through an alternative intravenous access.[102,103]

Insulin requirements vary widely in the perioperative patient. The normal state (approximately 0.25 unit of insulin per gram of glucose) is influenced by many factors such as obesity, concomitant glucocorticoid administration, and the septic state, which may increase insulin requirements to as high as 0.4 to 0.8 unit of insulin per gram of glucose. The highest insulin requirements have been observed in patients undergoing CABG (0.8 to 1.2 U/g of glucose).[104]

Recommendations for glucose infusion to prevent catabolism suggest between 5 and 10 g of glucose per hour,[105] although the optimal dose of glucose necessary for prevention of fat and protein catabolism has not been clearly determined. However, clinical experience suggests that most surgical diabetics can be maintained within the normal blood glucose range with an insulin infusion set between 1 and 2 U/h.

Patients receiving total parenteral nutrition, which is generally up to 25% dextrose, usually require an additional 2 to 3 units of insulin per hour. Apart from careful monitoring of blood glucose levels, the patient's overall clinical status (particularly neurologic and hemodynamic) should be closely observed. Avoidance of hypoglycemic episodes while allowing mild hyperglycemia without ketosis is prudent in the diabetic whose blood sugar is extremely difficult to control.

What emerges from all the studies dealing with perioperative diabetes management is that the most important factor in optimal perioperative glycemic control is frequent measurement of blood sugar and appropriate therapeutic interventions by trained staff. Perioperative metabolic management should be planned and coordinated by surgeons, anesthetists, and diabetic care teams in conjunction with the patient when possible. With the exception of type II diabetic patients presenting for minor surgery, all diabetic patients should receive intravenous infusions of glucose with appropriate insulin to achieve normoglycemia until the preoperative regimen is resumed.

GLUCOCORTICOID SUPPLEMENTATION IN CHRONIC GLUCOCORTICOID USERS

Perioperative glucocorticoid supplementation for patients receiving steroid therapy is common. The rationale for its use is the avoidance of hypoadrenalism, resulting in a variety of clinical signs including fever, nausea, dehydration, abdominal pain, hypotension, and shock. Other evidence of hypoadrenalism includes low-voltage complexes on the ECG, hypoglycemia, and eosinophilia. Despite the common use of steroids in hospital patients, the incidence of perioperative adrenal insufficiency is low (0.01% to 0.1%).[106]

Retrospective and prospective data suggest that routine steroid supplementation for all glucocorticoid-treated patients may not be necessary.[107–109] Well-known adverse effects of exogenous glucocorticoids include immunosuppression, exacerbation of osteoporosis, avascular necrosis of the femur, diabetes, peptic ulcer disease, diminished wound healing, and neuropsychiatric disorders.

Daily endogenous cortisol release in normal adults approximates 25 to 30 mg per day at rest. Stressors such as major surgery or critical illness increase endogenous production to 75 to 100 mg per day because of increased secretion of adrenocorticotropic hormone (ACTH) from the anterior pituitary gland. Increased cortisol secretion returns to normal within 24 hours of skin incision in uncomplicated minor surgery.[110]

The clinical rationale for steroid supplementation in the perioperative period is based on the known protracted recovery of the hypothalamus-pituitary-adrenal (HPA) axis following prolonged glucocorticoid administration.[111] However, the stress response observed in perioperative patients results in ACTH levels far in excess of that required for maximal adrenocortical stimulation.[112] A number of studies[113–115] have suggested that patients on chronic steroid therapy undergoing elective major surgery may not require perioperative steroid supplementation in addition to their regular steroid regimen. In a study of 40 renal transplant recipients on chronic prednisone therapy, none of the patients received more than baseline glucocorticoid therapy during admission for surgery or critical illness. Despite biochemical evidence of decreased adrenal response to exogenous ACTH in 67% of the patients, none of the patients exhibited clinically overt hypoadrenalism, and 97% of all patients excreted normal or increased urinary cortisol concentrations during their hospital stay. This suggested that cortisol concentrations were sufficient to meet requirements during the time of stress.[109]

Identification of patients at risk for perioperative hypoadrenalism by history alone is difficult.[113] Functional status of the adrenal gland may be assessed quickly and easily using the 30-minute ACTH test. This is the most effective and convenient tool for perioperative evaluation of HPA function.[116]

Baseline cortisol measurements are taken immediately prior to the intravenous administration of 250 μg of synthetic ACTH. Adequate adrenal function is diagnosed by baseline levels usually above 200 nmol/L, which rises above 500 nmol/L 30 minutes following ACTH administration (see Chap. 79).

Patients who exhibit a subnormal response to ACTH should receive supplemental steroids. Since endogenous cortisol secretion in normal individuals rarely exceeds 200 mg/d, exogenous steroid supplementation should range from 75 to 150 mg per day. To date, no data suggest that supplemental glucocorticoid therapy exceeding this amount is beneficial. Patients on chronic steroid therapy undergoing minor surgery should have their regular steroid dose on the morning of surgery and no additional doses if surgery is uncomplicated. Candidates for major surgery should receive 25 mg hydrocortisone intravenously on induction of anesthesia, and 100 to 150 mg per day over the following 24 to 72 hours. If a patient presenting for surgery is already receiving a maintenance steroid dose greater than the estimated requirement, additional steroid coverage is not necessary.[115]

Clinical and biochemical preoperative assessment of patients on chronic steroid therapy is invaluable in the identification of patients at risk for adrenal insufficiency in the perioperative period. Published recommendations for supplemental steroid coverage should be followed by dosing to physiologic levels. If doubt exists, a preoperative 30-minute ACTH test will clarify the need for perioperative supplemental glucocorticoid administration.

References

1. Report of the American College of Cardiology/American Heart Association Task Force on Practice Guidelines. Guidelines for perioperative cardiovascular evaluation for non-cardiac surgery. *J Am Coll Cardiol* 27:910, 1996.
2. Keats AS: The ASA classification of physical status—a recapitulation (editorial). *Anesthesiology* 49:233, 1978.
3. Goldman L, Caldera DL, Nussbaum SR, et al: Multifactorial index of cardiac index in noncardiac surgical procedures. *N Engl J Med* 297:845, 1977.
4. Detsky AS, Abrams HB, Forbath N, et al: Cardiac assessment for patients undergoing noncardiac surgery. A multifactorial clinical risk index. *Arch Intern Med* 146:2131, 1986.
5. Zeldin RA: Assessing cardiac risk in patients who undergo non-cardiac surgical procedures. *Can J Surg* 27:402, 1984.
6. Jeffrey CC, Kunsman J, Cullen DJ, et al: A prospective evaluation of cardiac risk index. *Anesthesiology* 58:462, 1983.
7. Cutler BS, Wheeler HB, Paraskos JA, et al: Applicability and interpretation of electrocardiographic stress testing in patients with peripheral vascular disease. *Am J Surg* 141:501, 1981.
8. Older P, Smith R, Courtney P, et al: Preoperative evaluation of cardiac failure and ischemia in elderly patients by cardiopulmonary exercise testing. *Chest* 104:701, 1993.
9. Gauss A, Rohm HJ, Schauggelen A, et al: Electrocardiographic exercise stress testing for cardiac risk assessment in patients undergoing non-cardiac surgery. *Anesthesiology* 94:38, 2001.
10. Raby KE, Barry J, Creager MA, et al: Detection and significance of intraoperative and postoperative myocardial ischemia in peripheral vascular disease. *JAMA* 268:222, 1992.
11. Mangano DT, Browner WS, Hollenberg M, et al: Association of perioperative myocardial ischemia with cardiac morbidity and mortality in men undergoing noncardiac surgery. *N Engl J Med* 323:1781, 1990.
12. Garnett RL, MacIntyre A, Lindsay P, et al: Perioperative ischemia in aortic surgery: Combined epidural/general anaesthesia and epidural analgesia vs general anaesthesia and IV analgesia. *Can J Anaesth* 43:769, 1996.
13. Fleischer LA, Rosenbaum SH, Nelson AH, et al: The predictive value of preoperative silent ischemia for postoperative ischemic events in vascular and non-vascular surgical patients. *Am Heart J* 122:980, 1991.
14. Eagle KA, Coley CM, Newell JB et al: Combining clinical and thallium data optimises perioperative assessment of cardiac risk before major vascular surgery. *Ann Intern Med* 110:859, 1989.
15. Mangano DT, London MJ, Tubau JF, et al: Dipyridamole thallium-201 scintigraphy as a preoperative screening test—a re-examination of its predictive potential. *Circulation* 84:493, 1991.
16. Paul SD, L'Italien RC, Hendel RC, et al: Postoperative and late prognosis for diabetics undergoing vascular surgery: Combining clinical evaluation and dipyridamole-thallium improves risk stratification. *J Am Coll Cardiol* 25:367A, 1995.
17. Kertai MD, Boersma E, Sicari R, et al: Which stress test is superior for perioperative risk stratification in patients undergoing major vascular surgery? *Eur J Vasc Endovasc Surg* 24:222, 2002.
18. Hachamovitch R, Berman DS, Kiat H, et al: Exercise myocardial perfusion SPECT in patients without known coronary artery disease, incremental prognostic value and use in risk stratification. *Circulation* 93:905, 1996.
19. Baron JF, Mundler O, Bertrand M, et al: Dipyridamole-thallium scintigraphy and gated radionuclide angiography to assess cardiac risk before abdominal aortic surgery. *N Engl J Med* 330:663, 1994.
20. Schinkel AF, Bax JJ, Elhendy A, et al: Assessment of viable tissue in Q-wave regions by metabolic imaging using single-photon emission computed tomography in ischemic cardiomyopathy. *Am J Cardiol* 89:1171, 2002.
21. Halm EA, Brower WS, Tubau JE, et al: Echocardiography for assessing cardiac risk in patients having non-cardiac surgery. Study of Perioperative Research Group. *Ann Intern Med* 125:433, 1996.
22. Rohde LE, Polanczyk CA, Goldman L, et al: Usefulness of transthoracic echocardiography as a tool for risk stratification of patients undergoing major non-cardiac surgery. *Am J Cardiol* 87:505, 2001.
23. Poldermans D, Arense M, Fioretti PM, et al: Improved cardiac risk stratification in major vascular surgery with dobutamine-atropine stress echocardiography. *J Am Coll Cardiol* 26:648, 1995.
24. Boersma E, Poldermans D, Bax JJ, et al: Predictors of cardiac events after major vascular surgery: Role of clinical characteristics, dobutamine echocardiography and beta-blocker therapy. *JAMA* 285:1865, 2001.
25. Rao TLK, Jacobs KH, El-Etr AA: Reinfarction following anesthesia in patients with myocardial infarction. *Anesthesiology* 59:499, 1983.
26. Rivers SP, Scher LA, Gupta SK, et al: Safety of peripheral vascular surgery after recent myocardial infarction. *J Vasc Surg* 11:70, 1990.
27. Goldman L, Caldera DL, Southwick FS, et al: Cardiac risk factors and complications following non-cardiac surgery. *Medicine* 57:357, 1978.
28. Hosking MP, Warner MA, Lobell CM, et al: Outcomes of surgery in patients 90 years of age or older. *JAMA* 261:1909, 1989.
29. Mackenzie CR, Charlson ME: Assessment of perioperative risk in the patient with diabetes mellitus. *Surg Gynecol Obstet* 167:293, 1988.
30. Current practice in the perioperative evaluation of patients undergoing major vascular surgery: a survey of cardiovascular anesthesiologists. *J Cardiothorac Vasc Anesth* 7:650, 1993.
31. Froehlich JB, Karavite D, Russman PL, et al: American College of Cardiology/American Heart Association preoperative assessment guidelines reduce resource utilization before aortic surgery. *J Vasc Surg* 36:1, 2002.
32. Adverse cardiac outcomes after non-cardiac surgery in patients with prior percutaneous transluminal coronary angioplasty. *Anesth Analg* 89:553, 1999.
33. Catastrophic outcomes of noncardiac surgery soon after coronary stenting. *J Am Coll Cardiol* 35:1288, 2000.
34. Foster ED, Davis KB, Carpenter JA, et al: Risk of non-cardiac operation in patients with defined coronary artery disease: The Coronary Artery Surgery Study (CASS) registry experience. *Ann Thorac Surg* 41:42, 1986.
35. Effect of coronary artery bypass graft surgery on survival: overview of 10 year results from randomised trials by the Coronary Artery Bypass Graft Surgery Trialists Collaboration. *Lancet* 344:563, 1994.
36. Poldermans D, Boersma E, Bax JJ, et al: Bisoprolol reduces cardiac death and myocardial infarction in high-risk patients as long as 2 years after successful major vascular surgery. *Eur Heart J* 22:1353, 2001.
37. Mangano DT, Layug EL, Wallace A, Tateo I: Effect of atenolol on mortality after non-cardiac surgery. Multicenter Study of Perioperative Ischemia Research Group. *N Engl J Med* 335:1713, 1996.

38. The effect of bisoprolol on perioperative mortality and myocardial infarction in high-risk patients undergoing vascular surgery. Dutch Echocardiographic Cardiac Risk Evaluating Applying Stress Echocardiography Study Group. *N Engl J Med* 341:1789, 1999.

39. Shammash JB, Trost JC, Gold JM, et al: Perioperative beta-blocker withdrawal and mortality in vascular surgical patients. *Am Heart J* 141:148, 2001.

40. Analysis of medical factors and outcomes in patients undergoing open versus endovascular abdominal aortic aneurysm repair. *J Vasc Surg* 36:492, 2002.

41. Raby KE, Goldman L, Creager MA, et al: Correlation between perioperative ischemia and major vascular events after peripheral vascular surgery. *N Engl J Med* 321:1296, 1989.

42. Hayes MA, Timmins AC, Yau EHS, et al: Elevation of systemic oxygen delivery in the treatment of critically ill patients. *N Engl J Med* 330:1717, 1994.

43. Connors AFJ, Speroff T, Dawson NV, et al: The effectiveness of right heart catheterisation in the initial care of critically ill patients. *JAMA* 276:889, 1996.

44. Sandham JD, Hull RD, Brant RF, et al: A randomised, controlled trial of the use of pulmonary-artery catheters in high-risk surgical patients. *N Engl J Med* 348:5, 2003.

45. Rivers E, Nguyen B, Havstad S, et al: Early goal-directed therapy in the treatment of severe sepsis and septic shock. *N Engl J Med* 345:1368, 2001.

46. Wiesenack C, Prasser C, Keyl C, et al: Assessment of intrathoracic blood volume as an indicator of cardiac preload: Single transpulmonary thermodilution technique versus assessment of pressure preload parameters derived from a pulmonary artery catheter. *J Cardiothorac Vasc Anesth* 15:584, 2001.

47. Kolev N, Ihra G, Swanevelder J, et al: Biplane transoesophageal echocardiographic detection of myocardial ischemia in patients with coronary artery disease undergoing non-cardiac surgery: segmental wall motion vs. electrocardiography and haemodynamic performance. *Eur J Anaesthesiol* 14:412, 1997.

48. Kolev N, Brase R, Swanevelder J, et al: The influence of transoesophageal echocardiography on intra-operative decision making. A European multicentre study. European Perioperative TOE Research Group. *Anaesthesia* 53:767, 1998.

49. Fleischer LA, Rosenbaum SH, Nelson AH, et al: The predictive value of preoperative silent ischemia for postoperative ischemic cardiac events in vascular and nonvascular surgical patients. *Am Heart J* 122:980, 1991.

50. Ashton CM, Lahart CJ, Wray NP, et al: The incidence of perioperative myocardial infarction with transurethral resection of the prostate. *J Am Geriatr Soc* 37:614, 1989.

51. Tuman KJ, McCarthy RJ, March RJ, et al: Effects of epidural anesthesia and analgesia on coagulation and outcome after major vascular surgery. *Anesth Analg* 73:696, 1991.

52. Kehlet H: Stress response to surgery. Release mechanisms and the modifying effect of pain relief. *Acta Chir Scand* 550(Suppl):22, 1983.

53. Yaeger MP, Glass DD, Neff RK, et al: Epidural anesthesia and analgesia in high-risk surgical patients. *Anesthesiology* 66:729, 1987.

54. Rodgers A, Walker N, Schug S, et al: Reduction of post-operative mortality and morbidity with epidural or spinal anaesthesia: results from overview of randomised trials. *BMJ* 321:1493, 2000.

55. Rigg JR, Jamrozik K, Myles PS, et al: Epidural anaesthesia and analgesia and outcome of major surgery: a randomised trial. *Lancet* 359:1276, 2002.

56. Becquemin JP, Piquet J, Becquemin MH, et al: Pulmonary function after transverse or midline incision in patents with obstructive pulmonary disease. *Intensive Care Med* 11:247, 1985.

57. Craig DB: Postoperative recovery of pulmonary function. *Anesth Analg* 60:46, 1981.

58. McAlister FA, Khan NA, Straus SE, et al: Accuracy of the preoperative assessment in predicting pulmonary risk after nonthoracic surgery. *Am J Respir Crit Care Med* 167:741, 2002.

59. Lawrence VA, Page CP, Harris GD: Preoperative spirometry before abdominal surgery. *Arch Intern Med* 149:280, 1989.

60. De Nino LA, Lawrence VA, Averyt EC, et al: Preoperative spirometry and laparotomy—blowing away dollars. *Chest* 111:1536, 1997.

61. American College of Physicians: Preoperative pulmonary function testing. *Ann Intern Med* 112:793, 1990.

62. Gracey DR, Divertie MB, Didier EP: Preoperative pulmonary preparation of patients with chronic obstructive pulmonary disease. *Chest* 76:123, 1979.

63. Marshall M, Olsen GN: The physiologic evaluation of the lung resection candidate. *Clin Chest Med* 14:305, 1993.

64. Ginsberg RJ, Hill LD, Egan RT, et al: Modern thirty-day mortality for surgical resections in lung cancer. *J Thorac Cardiovasc Surg* 86:654, 1983.

65. Brunelli A, Al Refai M, Monteverde M, et al: Predictors of early mortality after major lung resection in patients with and without airflow limitation. *Ann Thorac Surg* 74:999, 2002.

66. Epstein SK, Faling J, Daly BDT, et al: Predicting complications after pulmonary resection. *Chest* 104:694, 1993.

67. Beckles MA, Spiro SG, Colice GL, et al: The physiologic evaluation of patients with lung cancer being considered for resectional surgery. *Chest* 123(Suppl 1):105S, 2003.

68. Stein M, Cassara EL: Preoperative pulmonary evaluation and therapy for surgery patients. *JAMA* 211:787, 1970.

69. Celli BR, Rodriguez KS, Snider GL: A controlled trial of intermittent positive pressure breathing exercises in preventing pulmonary complications after abdominal surgery. *Am Rev Respir Dis* 130:12, 1984.

70. Ebeo CT, Benotti PN, Byrd RP, et al: The effect of bi-level positive end-expiratory pressure on postoperative pulmonary function following gastric surgery for obesity. *Respir Med* 96:672, 2002.

71. Ford GT, Whitelaw WA, Rosenal TW, et al: Diaphragm function after upper abdominal surgery in humans. *Am Rev Respir Dis* 127:431, 1983.

72. Frazee RC, Roberts JW, Okeson GC, et al: Open versus laparoscopic cholecystectomy: A comparison of postoperative pulmonary function. *Ann Surg* 213:651, 1991.

73. Ali J, Gana T: Lung volumes after laparoscopic cholecystectomy—justification for early discharge. *Can Respir J* 5:109, 1998.

74. Sperlongano P, Pisaniello D, Parmeggiani D, et al: Laparoscopic cholecystectomy in the morbidly obese. *Chir Ital* 54:363, 2002.

75. Peyton P, Myles PS, Silbert BS, et al: Perioperative epidural analgesia and outcome after major abdominal surgery in high-risk patients. *Anesth Analg* 96:548, 2003.

76. Pertunnen K, Nilsson E, Heinonen J, et al: Extradural, paravertebral and intercostal nerve blocks for post-thoracotomy pain. *Br J Anaesth* 75:541, 1995.

77. Pelosi P, Ravangan I, Panigada M, et al: Positive end-expiratory pressure improves respiratory function in obese but not in normal subjects during anesthesia and paralysis. *Anesthesiology* 91:1221, 1999.

78. Woeber KA: Thyrotoxicosis and the heart. *N Engl J Med* 327:94, 1992.

79. Levy GS, Klein I: Catecholamine-thyroid hormone interactions and the cardiovascular manifestations of hyperthyroidism. *Am J Med* 88:642, 1990.

80. Lancefield ML: The surgical patient with thyroid disease, in Goldman DR, Brown FH, Guarnieri DM (eds): *Perioperative Medicine: The Medical Care of the Surgical Patient,* 2nd ed. New York, McGraw-Hill, 1994, p 251.

81. Barakate MS, Agarwal G, Reeve TS, et al: Total thyroidectomy is now the preferred option for the surgical management of Graves' disease. *Aust N Z J Surg* 72:321, 2002.

82. Isley WL, Dahl S, Gibbs H: Use of esmolol in managing a thyrotoxic patient needing emergency surgery. *Am J Med* 89:122, 1990.

83. Landenson PW, Levin AA, Ridgeway EC, et al: Complications of surgery in hypothyroid patients. *Am J Med* 77:261, 1984.

84. Surks MI, Ocampo E: Subclinical thyroid disease. *Am J Med* 100:217, 1996.

85. Pronovost PH, Parris KH: Perioperative management of thyroid disease. *Postgrad Med* 98:83, 1995.

86. Kitamura T, Saijo H, Kameyama R, et al. Efficiency of bispectral index in anesthetic management of a patient with hypothyroidism. *Masui* 50:188, 2001.

87. Milaskiewicj RM, Hall GM: Diabetes and anaesthesia: the past decade. *Br J Anaesth* 68:198, 1992.

88. Campbell PJ, Mandarino L, Gerich J: Insulin response in NIDDM. *Metabolism* 37:15, 1988.

89. Shamoon H, Hendler R, Shearin RS: Synergistic interactions among antiinsulin hormones in pathogenesis of stress hyperglycemia in humans. *J Endocrinol Metab* 52:1235, 1981.

90. Hjortrup A, Sorenson C, Dyremose E, et al: Influence of diabetes mellitus on operative risk. *Br J Surg* 72:783, 1985.

91. Hjortrup A, Sorenson C, Dyremose E, Kehlet H: Morbidity in diabetic and nondiabetic patients after abdominal surgery. *Acta Chir Scand* 151:445, 1985.

92. Fowkes FG, Lunn JN, Farrow SC, et al: Epidemiology in anaesthesia: III. Mortality risk in patients with coexisting disease. *Br J Anaesth* 54:819, 1982.

93. Bourgos LG, Elbert TJ, Assidao C, et al: Increased intraoperative cardiovascular morbidity in diabetics with autonomic neuropathy. *Anesthesiology* 70:591, 1989.

94. Vohra A, Kumar S, Charlton AJ, et al: Effect of diabetes mellitus on the cardiovascular responses to induction of anaesthesia and tracheal intubation. *Br J Anaesth* 71:258, 1993.

95. Barker JP, Robinson PN, Vafidis GC, et al: Metabolic control of non-insulin dependent diabetic patients undergoing cataract surgery: comparison of local and general anaesthesia. *Br J Anaesth* 74:500, 1994.

96. Van den Bergh G, Wouters P, Weekers F, et al: Intensive insulin therapy in the critically ill patient. *N Engl J Med* 345:1359, 2001.

97. Hirsch IB, McGill JB, Cryer PE, et al: Perioperative management of surgical patients with diabetes mellitus. *Anesthesiology* 74:346, 1991.

98. Gavin LA: Perioperative management of the diabetic patient. *Endocrinol Clin North Am* 21:457, 1992.

99. Thomas DJB, Platt HS, Alberti KG: Insulin-dependent diabetes during the perioperative period. *Anesthesia* 39:629, 1984.

100. Alberti KGM, Thomas DJB: The management of diabetes during surgery. *Br J Anaesth* 51:693, 1979.

101. Husband DJ, Thai AC, Alberti KG: Management of diabetes during surgery with glucose-insulin-potassium infusion. *Diabetes Med* 3:69, 1986.

102. Pezzarossa A, Taddei F, Cimicchi MC, et al: Perioperative management of diabetic subjects, subcutaneous versus intravenous insulin administration during glucose-potassium-infusion. *Diabetes Care* 19:722, 1986.

103. Watts NB, Gebhart SS, Clark RV, Phillips LS: Postoperative active management of diabetes mellitus: steady state glucose control with bedside algorithm for insulin adjustment. *Diabetes Care* 10:722, 1987.

104. Gill GV, Sherif IH, Alberti KG: Management of diabetes during open-heart surgery. *Br J Surg* 68:171, 1981.

105. Rosenstock J, Raskin P: Surgery: Practical guidelines for diabetes management. *Clin Diabetes* 5:49, 1987.

106. Alford WC, Meador CK, Mihalevich J, et al: Acute adrenal insufficiency following cardiac surgical procedures. *J Thorac Cardiovasc Surg* 78:489, 1979.

107. Kehlet H, Binder C: Adrenocortical function and clinical course during and after surgery in unsupplemented glucocorticoid-treated patients. *Br J Anaesth* 45:1043, 1973.

108. Symerng T, Karlberg BE, Kagedal B, Schildt B: Physiological cortisol substitution of long-term steroid-treated patients undergoing major surgery. *Br J Anaesth* 53:949, 1981.

109. Bromberg JS, Alfrey EJ, Barker CF, et al: Adrenal suppression and steroid supplementation in renal transplant recipients. *J Transplant* 51:385, 1991.

110. Snow K, Jiang NS, Kao PC, Scheithauer BW: Biochemical evaluation of adrenal dysfunction: the laboratory perspective. *Mayo Clin Proc* 67:1055, 1992.

111. Livanou T, Ferriman D, James VHT: Recovery of hypothalamo-pituitary-adrenal function after corticosteroid therapy. *Lancet* 2:856, 1967.

112. Kehlet H: The stress response to surgery: Release mechanisms and modifying effect on pain relief. *Acta Chir Scand* 550(Suppl):22, 1989.

113. Schlaghecke R, Kormely E, Santen RT, Rudderskamp P: The effect of long term glucocorticoid therapy on pituitary-adrenal response to exogenous corticotropin-releasing hormone. *N Engl J Med* 326:226, 1992.

114. Lindholm L, Kehlet H: Re-evaluation of the clinical value of the 30-minute ACTH test in assessing the hypothalamic-pituitary-adrenocortical function. *Clin Endocrinol* 26:53, 1987.

115. Salem M, Tainsh RE, Bromberf J, et al: Perioperative glucocorticoid coverage. A reassessment 42 years after emergence of a problem. *Ann Surg* 219:416, 1994.

116. Lindholm L, Kehlet H: Re-evaluation of the clinical value of the 30 minute ACTH test in assessing the hypothalamic-pituitary-adrenocortical function. *Clin Endocrinol* 26:53, 1987.

Chapter 89 _____
THE ACUTE ABDOMEN AND INTRA-ABDOMINAL SEPSIS

J.M.A. BOHNEN
R.A. MUSTARD
B.D. SCHOUTEN

KEY POINTS

- *Patterns of presentation of the acute abdomen in the intensive care unit (ICU) may be unusual.*
- *Conjoint evaluation by intensivist, surgeon, and gastroenterologist is frequently needed.*
- *Prompt diagnosis is the key to successful management.*
- *Computed tomography (CT) or ultrasonography should be used liberally in the evaluation of intra-abdominal sepsis.*
- *Complications occur frequently in the postsurgical ICU patient; "stable vital signs" does not imply clinical stability.*
- *Postoperative residual or recurrent intra-abdominal sepsis may not be clinically obvious and may not be demonstrated by a CT scan; cardiorespiratory instability should prompt a high level of suspicion.*
- *The treatment of the febrile postsurgical patient is not simply the administration of further antibiotics.*
- *Acalculous cholecystitis is a treacherous disease which requires urgent treatment; definitive diagnosis is not always possible or necessary before treatment.*

Patients with an "acute abdomen" present challenging problems for surgeons and intensivists. The term *acute abdomen* refers to a patient whose chief presenting symptom is the acute onset of abdominal pain. The vast majority of these patients present in the emergency department and do not require treatment in an ICU. However, the small percentage of patients who do require such treatment constitute a significant fraction of the surgical ICU patients in most general hospitals. Furthermore, the intensivist must be aware that an ICU patient may develop an acute abdomen while being treated for some other condition.

In this chapter, we will first discuss the approach to the ICU patient who develops abdominal pain while undergoing treatment for some other disorder. The bulk of the chapter, however, will be directed to the patient with known intra-abdominal sepsis (IAS) who requires intensive care. Emphasis will be placed on the early diagnosis of intra-abdominal septic complications.

Evaluation of Acute Abdominal Pain in the Intensive Care Unit Patient

The diagnosis of abdominal pain depends heavily on an accurate history and a complete physical examination.[1] Both of these sources of data may be severely limited in the ICU patient. History may be unobtainable because of intubation or a decreased level of consciousness. Physical examination is made difficult by the many tubes emanating from the patient, and may be further compromised by medications such as corticosteroids. Indeed, abdominal pain itself may be masked by narcotics or other painful disease processes. Some physical signs, such as the absence of bowel sounds, which would be considered significant in an otherwise well patient, may not be significant in an ICU patient, in whom multiple extra-abdominal causes of ileus may be present. Hence, in the ICU setting, it is rare that an abdominal complaint comes to light because the patient complains of abdominal pain; rather, the physician usually must infer its presence on the basis of nonspecific findings such as unexplained sepsis, hypovolemia, and abdominal distention.

Table 89-1 provides an abbreviated summary of the many causes of acute abdominal pain. Rather than describing a complete algorithm for the diagnosis of these conditions in ICU patients, we will list some important principles.

1. The patient should be evaluated in the context of the underlying disorder(s). For example, sudden, severe abdominal pain in a patient with congestive heart failure secondary to myocardial infarction is much more likely to be due to mesenteric ischemia than to renal colic.
2. Liberal use should be made of surgical consultants. A patient with significant unexplained abdominal pain lasting more than 4 hours should be seen by a surgeon.
3. CT and ultrasound examination of the abdomen are excellent screening tests for acute abdominal problems in patients in whom the physical examination is unreliable.
4. Laparoscopy, carried out either in the ICU or in the operating room, may be of definite help, particularly in patients suspected of having ischemic bowel or acalculous cholecystitis.[2–4]

In summary, there is no straightforward approach to the ICU patient who develops an acute abdomen. Indeed, the major problem may be simply determining that the patient has an acute abdomen. Successful management of these patients depends on the close collaboration of the intensivist and the surgeon.

The Intensive Care Unit Management of the Patient with an Acute Abdomen

Most patients with an acute abdomen are diagnosed outside the ICU. These patients may require treatment in an ICU for one of four reasons:

1. The patient is very ill but may not require surgical intervention (e.g., severe pancreatitis).
2. The patient requires stabilization prior to operation (e.g., septic shock).
3. The patient has undergone definitive surgical treatment for the acute abdominal disease, but has unrelated medical problems requiring intensive care (e.g., chronic obstructive pulmonary disease [COPD]).

TABLE 89-1 Etiology of Acute Abdominal Pain

Inflammatory disorders (e.g., cholecystitis, diverticulitis, perforated peptic ulcer)
Colic
  Biliary
  Renal
  Intestinal obstruction
Vascular lesions
  Mesenteric ischemia
  Ruptured abdominal aortic aneurysm
  Intra-abdominal or retroperitoneal hemorrhage
Urologic or gynecologic disorders
Medical disorders (e.g., lupus serositis, sickle cell crisis)

4. The patient has undergone definitive surgical treatment and requires intensive care because of the severity of the abdominal pathology or the occurrence of a postoperative complication such as sepsis.

In this chapter we will consider only patients in the fourth group, since the other groups are discussed in other areas of the text. We will primarily consider the ICU management of patients who have undergone treatment of a septic abdominal disease.

A classification of the sources of IAS is given in Table 89-2. Sepsis resulting from disease originating in the pancreas and infections arising in the urinary tract are discussed in other chapters.

The principles of treatment of IAS are well established and are as follows:

1. Prompt diagnosis and resuscitation
2. Prompt treatment of the underlying pathology and mechanical cleansing of the peritoneal cavity
3. Appropriate antibiotic administration
4. Supportive care of the patient
5. Constant vigilance to detect and treat aggressively any complications arising from the underlying disease or its treatment
6. Close collaboration among all physicians caring for the patient

TABLE 89-2 Classification of Intra-Abdominal Sepsis

Primary peritonitis
  Infected ascitic fluid
  Infected peritoneal dialysis catheter
  Miscellaneous (e.g., tuberculosis)
Secondary peritonitis
  Intraperitoneal
    Biliary tree
    Gastrointestinal tract
    Female reproductive system
  Retroperitoneal
    Pancreas
    Urinary tract
  Visceral abscess
    Liver
    Spleen

The importance of prompt diagnosis and treatment cannot be overemphasized. This is one of the few prognostic variables that physicians can control, and prompt treatment has been shown repeatedly to result in decreased mortality.[5–7]

PRIMARY PERITONITIS

Primary peritonitis is a group of diseases characterized by infection in the peritoneal cavity without an obvious source such as a gastrointestinal (GI) tract perforation.[8,9] This most frequently occurs in patients who have ascites secondary to cirrhosis of the liver, congestive heart failure, and renal dialysis, among other disorders. Patients suffering from primary peritonitis rarely require intensive care. However, primary peritonitis may well be present in patients requiring intensive care for other reasons. For example, a cirrhotic patient with portal hypertension and ascites may develop primary peritonitis that precipitates hepatic decompensation, leading to variceal bleeding and hypovolemic shock necessitating ICU admission.

The clinical presentation is usually one of fever and physical signs of peritoneal irritation. However, approximately one third of patients with primary peritonitis have no signs or symptoms of sepsis referable to the abdomen. Diagnosis is based on clinical suspicion, the patient's presentation, and the Gram stain and culture results obtained from ascitic fluid aspiration. Culture of infected ascitic fluid usually yields aerobic enteric organisms; however, approximately 35% of patients with these diseases will have negative ascitic fluid cultures.[9] Blood cultures are also frequently positive in these patients. Primary bacterial peritonitis may be assumed to be present when the ascitic fluid neutrophil count is $>250/\mu L$. The diagnosis may be confirmed in culture-negative patients by the response to appropriate antibiotic treatment, which should be evident within 48 hours and is characterized by both clinical improvement and a decrease in the number of white blood cells present in the ascitic fluid.

It is most important to distinguish primary from secondary bacterial peritonitis. *Secondary bacterial peritonitis* is caused by contamination from the gut lumen, and multiple organisms thus are usually found in the ascitic fluid Gram stain or culture. Patients with secondary bacterial peritonitis are unlikely to respond to antibiotic administration alone, and usually require surgical treatment.

Antibiotic treatment should be initiated on clinical suspicion of primary peritonitis and before final culture and sensitivity results are available. Broad-spectrum treatment with either ampicillin and an aminoglycoside, a third-generation cephalosporin, or ciprofloxacin is usually sufficient. The prognosis of these patients depends almost entirely on the underlying liver disease responsible for the ascites.

Patients who develop peritonitis secondary to an infected peritoneal dialysis catheter may or may not respond to antibiotic treatment (usually instilled into the dialysis fluid). Nonresponse necessitates removal of the catheter and temporary hemodialysis.

BILIARY TRACT SEPSIS

Both sepsis and hyperbilirubinemia are common findings in critically ill patients. When these conditions coexist, the question of biliary tract sepsis arises. However, most jaundiced ICU patients do not have pathology in their biliary tract.[10] Before we discuss biliary tract sepsis, we will briefly outline the approach to the jaundiced patient.

Infection in the biliary tree results in one or more of three rather different clinical entities. Most commonly, infection is only present in the gallbladder and is due to obstruction of the cystic duct by a gallstone. This entity, acute calculous cholecystitis, is usually treated surgically by removal of the gallbladder, and only results in ICU admission if the patient has other major medical problems. Of more relevance to the intensivist are the syndromes of acute cholangitis and acute acalculous cholecystitis.

THE JAUNDICED INTENSIVE CARE UNIT PATIENT

Abnormalities on liver function tests and even clinically evident jaundice are quite common in the ICU patient population. LaMont and Isselbacher, in a classic review article on postoperative jaundice,[10] provide a simple classification, distinguishing jaundice caused by increased pigment load, by impaired hepatocellular function, and by extrahepatic obstruction. The vast majority of ICU patients with abnormal liver function test results represent the first two categories. Exclusion of extrahepatic biliary obstruction is best accomplished[11] by history, physical examination, and routine laboratory tests (i.e., the clinical context) and ultrasonography to look specifically for evidence of bile duct dilation. In certain unusual circumstances,[11] obstructed bile ducts may not be dilated, and clinical suspicion will necessitate direct visualization of the biliary tree with either endoscopic retrograde cholangiopancreatography (ERCP) or percutaneous transhepatic cholangiography (PTC).

ACUTE CHOLANGITIS

Cholangitis is defined as a bacterial infection within bile ducts. It occurs when bacteria are introduced into a partially or totally obstructed duct system. In this situation the bacteria multiply rapidly in the bile and induce an inflammatory reaction around the small biliary radicles in the liver. When the hydrostatic pressure in the ducts exceeds a certain point, bacteria are literally forced out of the bile canaliculi and into the hepatic sinusoids, resulting in systemic bacteremia. The microbiology of this disease is similar to that of peritonitis caused by GI tract perforation. The portal of entry of bacteria into the biliary tree remains a topic of debate.

The clinical presentation is usually obvious, with right upper quadrant abdominal pain, jaundice, and fever (Charcot triad). Patients may be only mildly ill with bactobilia, or critically ill with frank pus under pressure in the biliary tree. Diagnosis may be confirmed with ultrasound, ERCP, or PTC. Treatment consists of biliary decompression and the administration of appropriate broad-spectrum antibiotics to cover aerobic gram-negative rods, anaerobic gram-negative bacilli, and enterococci. Bile and blood for culture are obtained before antibiotics are started (if possible) to be sure the antibiotic coverage is optimal.

These patients may require intensive care if they develop septic shock, either from the disease itself, or from bacteremia induced by an invasive procedure used to diagnose or treat the disease. From the intensivist's point of view, the management is straightforward—support the cardiorespiratory system until the ducts have been decompressed and the patient is hemodynamically stable and ensure that appropriate antibiotics are administered. It must be emphasized that the key to success is adequate biliary decompression. This may be accomplished either surgically (exploration of the common bile duct and insertion of a T tube), endoscopically (insertion of a nasobiliary drain, sphincterotomy and stone extraction, or placement of an internal stent), or percutaneously (placement of a transhepatic external drain). The adequacy of drainage is confirmed by rapid clinical and biochemical improvement (obvious within 24 to 48 hours). A patient with cholangitis who does not improve clinically and may require ongoing cardiopulmonary support must be assumed to have inadequate drainage. In this case, it is essential to image the biliary tree to determine the adequacy of the drainage and to plan for further decompression. It may also be necessary to obtain a CT scan to look for hepatic abscess(es) induced by the cholangitis.

ACALCULOUS CHOLECYSTITIS

This disease is a child of modern intensive care. It was well summarized in a 1978 article by Long and coworkers:

> Acute acalculous cholecystitis is a treacherous and potentially lethal disease. It may occur in patients without known biliary tract disease who are severely compromised by trauma or gastrointestinal dysfunction and require prolonged intensive care. Its onset is insidious, its presenting symptoms are inconstant, and its neglect can lead to necrosis of the gallbladder with sepsis and death.[12]

This disease occurs in approximately 0.5% to 1.5% of long-term (>1 week) ICU patients.[13,14] The etiology of this disease is unknown, and hence there are no known ways to prevent it.[15] It appears that in the occasional critically ill patient the gallbladder wall becomes inflamed and infected with enteric organisms. The cystic duct becomes edematous and occluded, but it is not known whether this event is the cause or a result of the disease. This condition may occur at any time during the patient's ICU stay. In about one-third of patients, the inflammation has induced partial or complete necrosis of the gallbladder by the time of diagnosis.

The real problem with this disease is the difficulty in achieving a definitive diagnosis without resorting to laparotomy or laparoscopy. Attention should be focused on the gallbladder when sepsis or organ failure occurs without a known cause. The patient may have right upper quadrant abdominal tenderness, but an ICU patient can have this sign without cholecystitis. Distention of the liver capsule due to increased venous pressure or sepsis can produce identical physical findings. Liver function tests are not helpful. A biliary radionuclide scan is helpful, in that filling of the gallbladder (perhaps with the aid of morphine-induced spasm of the sphincter of Oddi[16]) implies cystic duct patency, which effectively rules out cholecystitis. The most valuable tests are ultrasonography and CT. Findings of pericholecystic fluid (without ascites), intramural gas, or a sloughed mucosal membrane are virtually diagnostic (Fig. 89-1). Unfortunately, not all patients have these findings.[14] A thick-walled gallbladder is suggestive, unless the patient has generalized edema. Percutaneous bile aspiration for culture has high false-positive and false-negative rates and is therefore not helpful.

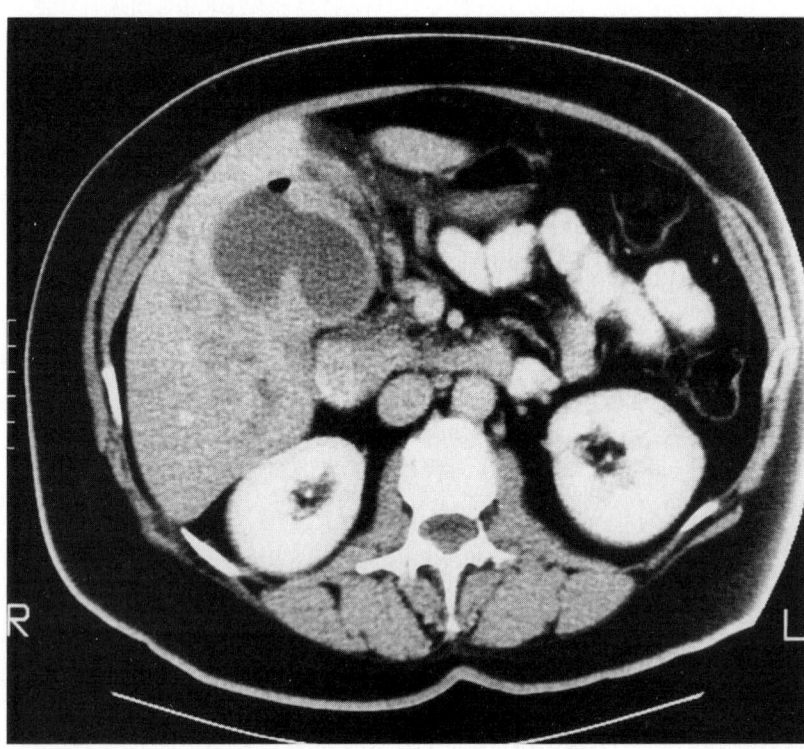

FIGURE 89-1 CT scan diagnostic of acalculous cholecystitis. The patient has an enlarged thick-walled gallbladder with intraluminal gas. The liver around the gallbladder fossa is markedly edematous.

It is our practice to operate on these patients if our clinical index of suspicion is sufficiently high and the patient is deteriorating without obvious cause. About half the patients we operate on for this reason have the disease. These patients are treated with cholecystectomy. In the remaining half, we place a cholecystostomy tube to prevent the disease in the future. To date, direct visualization of the gallbladder in the operating room is the only completely accurate method of diagnosis. This can be carried out under local anesthesia, but this approach seems somewhat pointless in the ventilated patient. In the rare patient who is felt to be "too sick to undergo laparotomy," percutaneous transhepatic drainage of the gallbladder may result in significant clinical improvement.[17] This procedure can be carried out at the bedside under ultrasound guidance. It is our experience, however, that these patients should later undergo cholecystectomy before the drainage tube is removed.

SECONDARY BACTERIAL PERITONITIS

In this section we will discuss the ICU management of patients with secondary bacterial peritonitis, defined as the presence of pus or gastrointestinal contents in the peritoneal cavity.[18] This condition may be either localized (an abscess) or diffuse (generalized peritonitis). Patients with physical signs of peritoneal irritation due to localized gastrointestinal tract infections are discussed elsewhere in this text.

Patients with secondary bacterial peritonitis requiring intensive care constitute a significant fraction both of all surgical ICU admissions and of all patients with peritonitis. For example, at our hospital, 300 patients with generalized peritonitis or abdominal abscess were treated in a recent 5-year period. Of these patients, 107 (mean Acute Physiology and Chronic Health Evaluation [APACHE] II score, 19.3) required posttreatment ventilatory support for an average of 9.6

days (78 treated surgically, 29 treated percutaneously), and 193 (mean APACHE II score, 10.4) did not require ventilation (137 treated surgically, 56 treated percutaneously). Patients requiring postoperative ventilatory support were severely ill and had a 64% mortality rate, compared to patients not requiring such treatment, who had only an 11% mortality rate. Therefore the need for mechanical ventilation may be a marker for general severity of illness, which results in a poor prognosis.

PATHOPHYSIOLOGY AND TREATMENT

Generalized peritonitis is usually caused by either bowel infarction, or more commonly, bowel perforation. Occasionally, generalized bacterial peritonitis results from perforation of an infected gallbladder, infected pancreatic pseudocyst, or other rare disease. We shall restrict our attention in this chapter to the vast majority of cases which are due to gastrointestinal tract perforation.

Patients with generalized peritonitis may become very ill because of the anatomy of the peritoneal cavity. Its large surface area permits massive loss of fluid into the abdomen and rapid absorption of bacteria, endotoxin, and inflammatory mediators into the systemic circulation. The hemodynamic effects of generalized peritonitis have been compared with those of a burn covering 50% of the body surface.

Treatment of this disease is well established.[19] Following rapid fluid resuscitation and the initiation of antibiotic therapy, patients undergo laparotomy to close the perforation (or resect, exteriorize, etc) and to remove as much of the contaminating material and inflammatory exudate as possible. Broad-spectrum antibiotics are used to eliminate residual bacterial contamination after laparotomy and because septicemia is common in these patients. The gold standard in antibiotic therapy is the combination of an aminoglycoside and an antianaerobe agent such as metronidazole or clindamycin. To avoid nephrotoxicity, aminoglycosides should not be given to patients with a significantly decreased glomerular filtration rate (e.g., patients with elevated serum creatinine level, advanced age, or hypotension). In the last 15 years, a plethora of new and very effective antibiotics have appeared.[20,21] Aminoglycosides may be replaced with a third-generation cephalosporin or with ciprofloxacin. Single-agent therapy with a second-generation cephalosporin (cefotetan) is effective for mild to moderate infections. Imipenem should be reserved for severe infections. Since the administration of broad-spectrum antibiotics may lead to systemic candidiasis, pseudomembranous colitis, and the selection of multiply resistant organisms, the drugs should be discontinued as soon as the acute episode of abdominal infection has subsided. Unfortunately, there is no straightforward guide to antibiotic discontinuation. The conventional criteria of clinical improvement, no fever, and no leukocytosis are associated with an exceedingly small rate of relapse of peritoneal infection, but may never be achieved in many ICU patients.[22] In this group, we believe that it is reasonable to stop antibiotics when the patient no longer has physical signs of peritonitis or ileus. If the patient still has fever or leukocytosis, a CT scan should be obtained to rule out intra-abdominal abscess. If no abscess is found, antibiotics can be stopped and a search begun for an extraperitoneal source of infection.

The mortality rate of generalized peritonitis is about 30%. Known prognostic factors include age, pre-existing disease, severity of physiologic derangement at the time of diagnosis, steroid dependency, and peritonitis occurring in the postoperative period.[23] Interestingly, the site of perforation is not a determinant of mortality (with the exception of perforated appendicitis). Perforated peptic ulcers are just as deadly as perforated colons. The cause of death is usually uncontrolled sepsis. Of our 107 ICU patients with peritonitis, 68 died. IAS was considered the main cause in 37 patients (55%) and was a contributing cause in 24 patients (35%). Only 7 patients (10%) suffered a nonseptic death. Essentially all the septic deaths were due to multiple organ dysfunction syndrome (MODS).

It is widely assumed that the cause of MODS in these patients is bacterial infection. (It is also possible that the uncontrolled infections are just another result of MODS caused by an unknown disorder of immune regulation). When considering treatment of these patients, it is helpful to classify the possible anatomic sites of bacterial infection (Table 89-3). At present, we do not have specific treatments for all intra-abdominal sites of infection. The prevention and treatment of infection in fibrin deposits, tissues, or the gut lumen is a very active research field at this time. For example, many postoperative abscesses likely start as small collections of fibrin-encased bacteria. Translocation of bacteria from the gut lumen may be prevented with appropriate enteral nutrition. Interestingly, patients who developed nosocomial pneumonia complicating intra-abdominal sepsis were more likely to die than patients who developed recurrent intra-abdominal infection—perhaps because pneumonia is more difficult to treat than intra-abdominal abscess.[24]

The Intensivist's Role

It is the intensivist's role to support these patients postoperatively and be aware of the possible need for further surgical in-

TABLE 89-3 Anatomic Sites of Bacterial Infection in Postoperative Patients

Intra-abdominal
  Peritoneal fluid
  Peritoneal fibrin
  Extraperitoneal tissues (e.g., hepatic macrophages)
  Visceral abscess
  Within the gastrointestinal tract lumen (bacterial translocation,
    Clostridium difficile colitis)
  Infected prosthetic vascular graft
  Acalculous cholecystitis
Extra-abdominal
  Soft tissue infection
  Pneumonia
  Urosepsis
  Intravascular catheter infection
  Disseminated candidiasis

tervention as well as the potential for a large variety of possible complications. Close collaboration between the intensivist and the surgeon is essential for the optimal management of the patient. Supportive treatment is usually straightforward and includes hemodynamic support (recovering from shock), respiratory support, nutritional support, administration of antibiotics and activated protein C (beginning 12 hours postoperatively in selected patients), and if necessary, renal support with dialysis or hemofiltration. However, complications are many and varied and include complications of the supportive care (e.g., nosocomial infection), complications that may occur in any surgical patient (e.g., pulmonary embolus), and complications that are specific to patients treated surgically for peritonitis. We only consider the latter group of problems (Table 89-4).

These patients must be examined daily by the intensivist as well as the surgeon, with this list of complications in mind. First, all dressings covering the abdomen should be removed and the wound examined. The skin incision is usually packed open at operation to minimize the incidence of

TABLE 89-4 Postoperative Complications Specifically Related to the Surgical Treatment of Peritonitis

Wound complications
  Wound infection
  Necrotizing soft tissue infection
  Fascial dehiscence/evisceration
Gastrointestinal tract complications
  Ileus
  Mechanical obstruction
  Enterocutaneous fistula
  Gastrointestinal bleeding
  Anastomotic disruption or perforation
  Ischemic bowel
  Antibiotic-associated colitis
Complications arising in the peritoneal cavity
  Abscess formation
  Intra-abdominal bleeding
  Compartment syndrome
Miscellaneous
  Postoperative pancreatitis
  Septicemia
  Acalculous cholecystitis

wound infection.[25] Fascial dehiscence may be observed. This complication is not rare and should prompt an immediate surgical consultation. Dehiscence occurred in 17 of our 107 ventilated peritonitis patients. Dehiscence is most common on postoperative days 4 to 8 but may occur at any time. It is heralded by the drainage of serosanguineous fluid through the incision. The diagnosis is confirmed by palpation of the wound (if the skin incision was closed) or the observation of intra-abdominal contents in the wound (if the wound was packed open). The presence of loops of bowel in the wound poses the acute risk of evisceration. In some patients with particularly severe peritonitis, it is not technically possible to reapproximate the fascial edges at the end of the surgical procedure. The surgeon then sutures an artificial mesh or other pliable material to the fascia or skin to prevent postoperative evisceration, and the wound is packed with saline-soaked gauze.[26] These patients are particularly at risk for the formation of enterocutaneous fistulae at the surface of their open wounds, and this complication is easily diagnosed by inspection.[27] Finally, all tubes or drains should be inspected to make sure that they have not been dislodged and are functioning as intended. For example, sump drains should be checked to make sure that the air inlet ports are not occluded.

Second, the intensivist needs to determine whether the gastrointestinal tract is functioning well enough to allow enteral feedings. This is sometimes very difficult to determine in the sedated, ventilated patient, and it is frequently necessary to challenge the patient by starting tube feedings and simply checking the gastric residual volume every 4 hours. As discussed in Chap. 11, enteral feeding is preferred over parenteral feeding in this patient population, if technically feasible. Jejunal feeds are almost always tolerated, even in patients with severe peritonitis. Early enteral feeding may improve outcome.[28]

Third, the intensivist must determine if the patient is septic and if the septic focus is intra-abdominal. The most common IAS complication is abscess formation, which occurred in 21 of the 107 peritonitis patients who required postoperative ventilation in our series. It is often difficult to determine when the patient's original septic response is abating and when a new septic response is being mounted.[29] In general, if the patient is not improving steadily following surgery or if the patient begins to deteriorate in any way, a CT scan of the abdomen should be obtained to identify and localize a possible abscess (Fig. 89-2). However, it is usually not fruitful to scan the patient sooner than 5 to 7 days after laparotomy. Patients in this early postoperative period frequently have multiple intra-abdominal fluid collections, most of which are sterile. The patient who is deteriorating in the first week following surgery for peritonitis and who is thought to have persistent or recurrent peritoneal infection usually requires repeat laparotomy. Beyond this early phase, when abscesses are better formed and sterile collections have been resorbed, percutaneous drainage offers a safe and effective method for the diagnosis and control of abscesses.[30] The tendency to broaden the antibiotic coverage when a patient continues to have fever or develops recurrent fever should be resisted.[31]

Open Abdomen Treatment

In certain circumstances patients with peritonitis require "open abdomen" treatment. The skin and fascia are not closed and evisceration is prevented by suturing an artificial mesh to the fascia or skin. These patients fall into two categories—patients whose fascia could not be closed for technical reasons

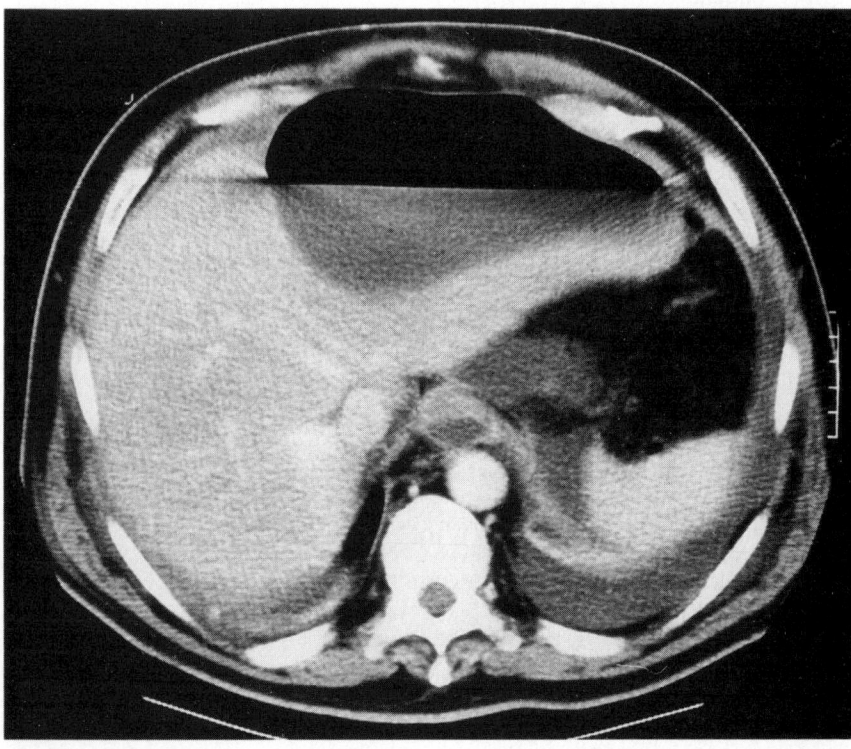

FIGURE 89-2 CT scan demonstrates massive left subphrenic abscess. The patient developed septic shock 11 days after total gastrectomy for adenocarcinoma of the stomach. Following resuscitation in the ICU, this scan was obtained and the abscess was drained percutaneously. The anastomotic leak was later repaired surgically.

TABLE 89-5 Etiology of Hepatic Abscess

Trauma
Perihepatic sepsis
Systemic bacteremia
Portal bacteremia
Cholangitis
Cryptogenic

but who are otherwise stable, and patients whose peritonitis is so severe that in the surgeon's opinion the abdomen should be left open to facilitate repeated laparotomies for peritoneal toilet. The latter group presents a major problem to the intensivist and the ICU nursing staff. These patients undergo laparotomy (through the mesh) every 1 to 3 days until the surgeon feels that the peritoneal cavity is sufficiently clean. Weaning from ventilatory support is almost always impossible until after the last scheduled relaparotomy.[32] Furthermore, during this period of repeated laparotomies, large quantities of proteinaceous fluids are lost through the open abdominal wound, and the patients may therefore require support with plasma as well as aggressive nutritional support. Fortunately, such drastic treatment for peritonitis is rarely required and has not been proved to be more efficacious than conventional management.[33]

VISCERAL ABSCESS

Pyogenic liver abscess is a rare condition that can occur in an ICU patient. Almost any bacterium may be cultured. A wide variety of conditions may give rise to a hepatic abscess (Table 89-5), but it should be noted that at least 20% of cases are cryptogenic.[34]

Patients with hepatic abscess usually present with sepsis associated with right upper quadrant pain and occasionally

with peritoneal findings such as an enlarged liver. Liver function test results are frequently abnormal. The diagnosis is confirmed by CT or ultrasound examination (Fig. 89-3).

The preferred treatment of hepatic abscess is percutaneous drainage for large abscesses. It should be noted that the presence of more than one large abscess does not necessitate open surgical treatment. Antibiotics should be administered as described for patients with peritonitis until culture results are available. This may be the only treatment required for patients with multiple small abscesses, usually secondary to cholangitis, after bile duct drainage has been established.

Splenic abscess formation is rare. It may be due to trauma, direct extension of a septic process such as pancreatic abscess, infection of a splenic infarct, or bacteremia. These patients present with left upper quadrant abdominal pain, left pleural effusion, or sepsis of unknown etiology, and the diagnosis is established by CT or ultrasound examination of the abdomen. The optimal treatment is splenectomy, but percutaneous drainage may be used as a temporizing maneuver.[35]

The Abdomen as a Source of Occult Sepsis

A frequent clinical problem in the ICU is the patient with a septic picture or MODS (or both) with no obvious etiology. Line sepsis, soft tissue infection, foreign body infection, *Candida* septicemia, endocarditis, pneumonia, pseudomembranous colitis, and urosepsis can often be ruled out. Attention then focuses on the abdomen even if the patient had no known pre-existing gastrointestinal pathologic condition. A CT scan of the abdomen is an excellent screening test in this patient group. However, a negative CT scan or ultrasound does not absolutely rule out peritoneal infection.

There are several causes of occult IAS (Table 89-6). Acute acalculous cholecystitis was discussed previously.

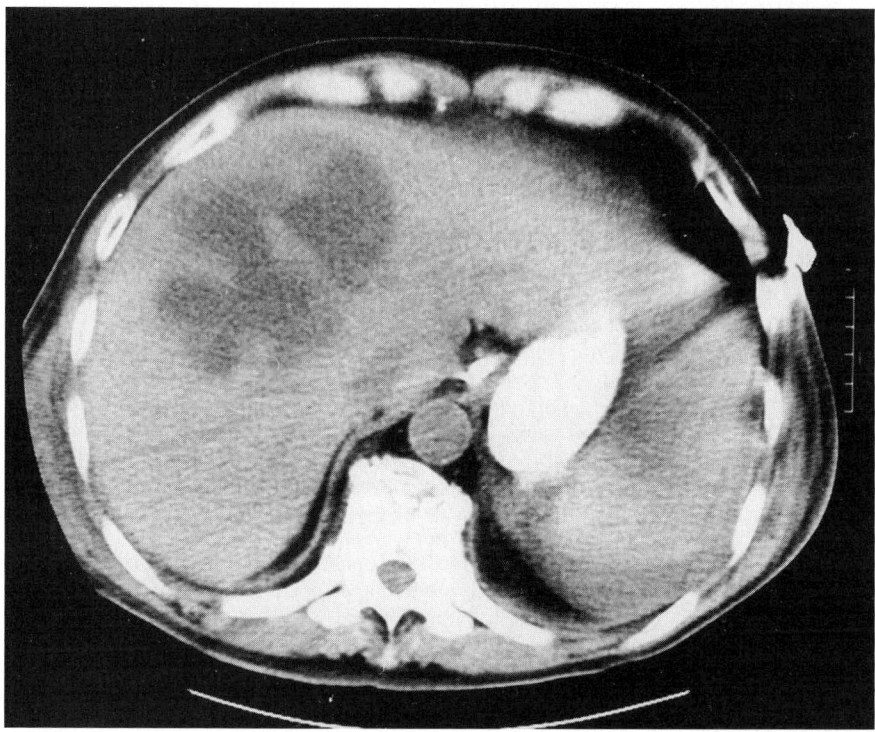

FIGURE 89-3 CT scan demonstrates large pyogenic liver abscess. The patient presented with septic shock and abnormal liver function test results. Following resuscitation in the ICU, an ultrasound examination failed to support the clinical diagnosis of acute cholangitis. This CT scan was therefore obtained, and the abscess was drained percutaneously. No cause for the abscess was found.

TABLE 89-6 Occult Sources of Intra-Abdominal Sepsis

Acalculous cholecystitis
Small intra-abdominal abscess(es)
Ischemic bowel—short segment
Tertiary peritonitis

Intra-abdominal abscesses that are too small to be seen by CT or ultrasound examination or that are hidden between loops of bowel (interloop abscesses) are a second well-recognized cause. These can only be diagnosed by laparotomy prompted by clinical suspicion and exclusion of other causes of sepsis. Rarely, a short segment of ischemic or necrotic bowel may be very difficult to detect. If the segment is in the small bowel, the patient will usually have a clinical picture of mechanical small bowel obstruction. However, if the segment is in the left colon, the patient may have no other obvious symptoms. Colonoscopy is the diagnostic method of choice if this condition is suspected.

Finally, experimental evidence suggests that the gastrointestinal tract itself is the source of systemic endotoxemia or bacteremia in some ICU patients.[36] It has been hypothesized that the patient's initial critical illness may result in increased permeability of the gut mucosa with resulting bacterial translocation, eventually leading to portal vein bacteremia. MODS that is triggered by the initial insult may then be perpetuated by this mechanism. Furthermore, as a result of the use of broad-spectrum antibiotics and potent inhibitors of gastric acid production, blood cultures may grow organisms not usually associated with the gastrointestinal tract, such as *Staphylococcus epidermidis* or *Candida* species. Clearly, diagnosis of this condition (usually called *tertiary peritonitis*) can be made only by exclusion of other causes of sepsis. Treatment (and prevention) consists of stopping all unnecessary antibiotics and initiating enteral feeds if at all possible. Food in the lumen of the gut is a major stimulant of mucosal growth, which preserves mucosal integrity.[37]

When all attempts at determining a definite etiology for the patient's septic state have failed, the intensivist is often tempted to recommend laparotomy as a diagnostic tool. Some have advocated the use of minilaparoscopy in the ICU for diagnosis, but this is rarely, if ever, useful.[37a] Laparotomy in the absence of clinical or laboratory findings pointing to a specific etiology or location of infection is rarely helpful in preventing death.[38] Finally, it must be noted that once MODS is far advanced, even definitive treatment of the underlying intra-abdominal source rarely succeeds in reversing this lethal syndrome.[39–41]

References

1. Silen W: *Cope's Early Diagnosis of the Acute Abdomen,* 18th ed. New York, Oxford University Press, 1991, p 19.
2. Gagne DJ, Malay MB, Hogle NJ, et al: Bedside diagnostic minilaparotomy in the intensive care patient. *Surgery* 131:49, 2002.
3. Walsh RM, Popovich MJ, Hondly J: Bedside diagnostic laparoscopy and peritoneal lavage in the intensive care unit. *Surg Endosc* 12:1405, 1998.
4. Orlando R, Crowell KL: Laparoscopy in the critically ill. *Surg Endosc* 11:1072, 1997.
5. Stephen M, Loewenthal J: Generalized infective peritonitis. *Surg Gynecol Obstet* 147:231, 1978.
6. Bohnen J, Boulanger M, Meakins JL, et al: Prognosis in generalized peritonitis. *Arch Surg* 118:285, 1983.
7. Pitcher WD, Musher DM: Critical importance of early diagnosis and treatment of intraabdominal infections. *Arch Surg* 117:328, 1982.
8. Crossly IR, Williams R: Spontaneous bacterial peritonitis. *Gut* 26:325, 1985.
9. Levison ME, Bush LM: Peritonitis and other intraabdominal infections, in Mandell GL, Douglas RG, Bennett JE (eds): *Principles and Practice of Infectious Diseases,* 3rd ed. New York, Churchill Livingstone, 1990, p 638.
10. LaMont JT, Isselbacher KJ: Current concepts: Postoperative jaundice. *N Engl J Med* 288:305, 1973.
11. Scharschmidt BF, Goldberg HI, Schmid R: Current concepts in diagnosis: Approach to the patient with cholestatic jaundice. *N Engl J Med* 308:1515, 1983.
12. Long TN, Heimbach DM, Carrico CJ: Acalculous cholecystitis in critically ill patients. *Am J Surg* 136:31, 1978.
13. Savino JA, Scalea TM, Del Guercio LRM: Factors encouraging laparotomy in acalculous cholecystitis. *Crit Care Med* 13:377, 1985.
14. Cornwell EE, Rodriguez A, Mirvis SE, et al: Acute acalculous cholecystitis in critically injured patients. *Ann Surg* 210:52, 1989.
15. Parry SW, Pelias ME, Browder W: Acalculous hypersensitivity cholecystitis: Hypothesis of a new clinicopathologic entity. *Surgery* 104:911, 1988.
16. Flanchbaum L, Alden SM, Trooskin SZ: Use of cholescintigraphy with morphine in critically ill patients with suspected cholecystitis. *Surgery* 106:668, 1989.
17. McGahan JP, Lindfors KK: Percutaneous cholecystostomy: An alternative to surgical cholecystostomy for acute cholecystitis? *Radiology* 173:481, 1989.
18. Schein M, Wittmann DH, Wise L, Condon RE: Abdominal contamination, infection and sepsis: A continuum. *Br J Surg* 84:269, 1997.
19. Fry DE: Peritonitis, in Fry DE (ed): *Surgical Infections.* Boston, Little, Brown, 1995, p 227.
20. Bohnen JMA: Antibiotic Therapy for Abdominal Infection. *World J Surg* 22:152, 1998.
21. Mazuski JE, Sawyer RG, Nathans AB, et al: The surgical infection society guidelines on antimicrobial therapy for intra-abdominal infections: An executive summary. *Surg Infect* 3:161, 2002.
22. Stone HH, Bourneuf AA, Stinson LD: Reliability of criterion for predicting persistent or recurrent sepsis. *Arch Surg* 120:17, 1985.
23. Bohnen J, Mustard R, Oxholm S, et al: APACHE II score and abdominal sepsis: A prospective study. *Arch Surg* 3:225, 1988.
24. Mustard RA, Bohnen JMA, Rosati C, Schouten BD: Pneumonia complicating abdominal sepsis: An independent risk factor for mortality. *Arch Surg* 126:170, 1991.
25. Edlich RF, Rodeheaver GT, Thacker JG: Technical factors in the prevention of wound infections, in Howard RJ, Simmons RL (eds): *Surgical Infectious Diseases,* 2nd ed. Norwalk, CT, Appleton & Lange, 1988, p 340.
26. Walsh GL, Chiasson P, Hedderich G, et al: The open abdomen. The Marlex mesh and zipper technique: A method of managing intraperitoneal infection. *Surg Clin North Am* 68:25, 1988.
27. Mastboom WJB, Kuypors HHC, Schoots FJ, et al: Small bowel perforation complicating the open treatment of generalized peritonitis. *Arch Surg* 124:689, 1989.
28. Zaloga GP: Early enteral nutritional support improves outcome: Hypothesis or fact? *Crit Care Med* 27:259, 1999.
29. Machiedo GW, Suval WD: Detection of sepsis in the postoperative patient. *Surg Clin North Am* 68:215, 1988.

30. VanSonnenberg E, Mueller PR, Ferrucci JT: Percutaneous drainage of 250 abdominal abscesses and fluid collections. Part 1: Results, failures, and complications. *Radiology* 151:337, 1984.

31. Rizoli SB, Marshall JC: Saturday night fever: Finding and controlling the source of sepsis in critical illness. *Lancet Infect Dis* 2:137, 2002.

32. Teichmann W, Wittmann DH, Andreone PA: Scheduled reoperations (Etappenlavage) for diffuse peritonitis. *Arch Surg* 121:147, 1986.

33. Bohnen JMA, Mustard RA: A critical look at scheduled relaparotomy for secondary bacterial peritonitis. *Surg Gynecol Obstet* 172:25, 1991.

34. Bowers ED, Doberneck RC: Pyogenic liver abscess and splenic abscess, in Fry DE (ed): *Surgical Infections.* Boston, Little, Brown, 1995, p 297.

35. Gleich S, Wolin DA, Herbsman H: A review of percutaneous drainage in splenic abscess. *Surg Gynecol Obstet* 167:211, 1988.

36. Deitch EA: Does the gut protect or injure patients in the ICU? *Perspect Crit Care* 1:1, 1988.

37. Wilmore DW, Smith RJ, O'Dwyer ST, et al: The gut: A central organ after surgical stress. *Surgery* 104:917, 1988.

37a. Gagne DJ, Malay MB, Hogle NJ, Fowler DL: Bedside diagnostic minilaparoscopy in the intensive care patient. *Surgery* 131:491, 2002.

38. Sinanan M, Maier RV, Carrico CJ: Laparotomy for intraabdominal sepsis in patients in an intensive care unit. *Arch Surg* 119:652, 1984.

39. Norton LW: Does drainage of intraabdominal pus reverse multiple organ failure? *Am J Surg* 149:347, 1985.

40. Darling GE, Duff JH, Mustard RA, et al: Multiorgan failure in critically ill patients. *Can J Surg* 31:172, 1988.

41. Sautner T, Gotzinger P, Redl-Wenzl EM, Dittrich K, et al: Does reoperation for abdominal sepsis enhance the inflammatory host response? *Arch Surg* 132:250, 1997.

Chapter 90

THE TRANSPLANT PATIENT

DAMON C. SCALES
JOHN T. GRANTON

KEY POINTS

- *The critical care of the transplant recipient requires a multidisciplinary approach.*
- *Although some generalizations can be made regarding the management of all transplant patients, organ-specific considerations based on the particular allograft transplanted are often much more important.*
- *Risks and benefits of immunosuppressive therapy must be balanced in transplant recipients. Though immunosuppressive drugs are essential to prevent allograft rejection, they also increase the risk of infection and neoplasm.*
- *All immunosuppressive drugs have side effects and many have important drug-drug interactions that must be recognized by the intensivist.*
- *Rejection of the allograft can be divided into three broad categories: hyperacute, acute, and chronic rejection.*
- *Infections can reactivate in an immunocompromised recipient who has been previously exposed. Alternatively, a naïve recipient may acquire an infection following the transplant of an organ from a seropositive donor.*
- *Infections in transplant recipients can progress rapidly and hence must be promptly recognized and appropriately treated.*
- *Often immunosuppressive therapy must be adjusted or withdrawn in the presence of severe infection.*

This chapter provides a practical approach to the critical care of patients following the most common solid-organ transplant procedures. Important scientific advances have greatly improved our understanding of transplant immunology. Therapies have been developed that markedly decrease the incidence and severity of allograft rejection, and this has resulted in dramatic improvements in the outcomes of transplant recipients (Table 90-1). The major causes of morbidity and death in these patients depend on the time since transplantation. Technical and bacterial infectious complications predominate in the early postoperative period. Chronic rejection remains the major cause of death overall in these patients, occurring months to years after transplantation (Fig. 90-1).

An organ that has been transplanted from one individual to another (of the same species) is called an *allograft*. Although some generalizations can be made regarding the management of all transplant recipients, organ-specific considerations dependent upon the type of allograft that has been transplanted are often much more important. Following a brief introduction covering important aspects of immunosuppressive therapy, allograft rejection, and infectious complications, this chapter has been divided into sections that focus on considerations specific to the organ that has been transplanted.

In this chapter we will not deal with the management of patients following bone marrow transplantation, which is discussed in Chapter 73. Furthermore, as most recipients of kidney transplants now are cared for in step-down units or transplant wards rather than within ICUs, we have chosen to only discuss this procedure when it is performed at the same time as pancreas transplantation.

Immunosuppressive Therapy

The management of all transplant recipients involves a careful balance of the risks and benefits of immunosuppressive therapy. To avoid rejection of the allograft by the recipient's immune system, therapy with immunosuppressive agents is usually required. More than one agent is employed to allow for the targeting of different immunologic effector pathways (Fig. 90-2). As a consequence of the resultant modulation of the immune system's surveillance and response functions, the transplant recipient is placed at risk of developing infections and neoplasms.

Immunosuppressive therapy can be divided into three phases: induction, maintenance, and the treatment of acute rejection. The induction phase commences in the immediate postoperative period and involves intense immunosuppression which usually is continued for 2 to 4 weeks. Although practice at different centers varies, most regimens typically include the use of systemic corticosteroids in conjunction with a calcineurin inhibitor and a proliferation inhibitor (see below).[1] These agents may be started intravenously, but are switched to oral formulations to minimize toxicity once the patient is tolerating and absorbing enteral medications and feeds. To avoid some of the renal toxicity associated with the calcineurin inhibitors, antithymocyte immunoglobulin or anti–interleukin-2-receptor antibodies (IL-2R Abs) may be substituted in the early postoperative period.

The maintenance phase follows the induction period and is heralded by a reduction in the intensity of immunosuppression. Typically the maintenance phase is comprised of the planned regimen that will be used to suppress the immune response to the allograft and thus prevent rejection over a more prolonged period. Most patients will be maintained on either oral prednisone and cyclosporine or tacrolimus,

TABLE 90-1 One- and Five-Year Patient Survival by Organ

Organ Transplanted	1-Year Survival, %	5-Year Survival, %
Kidney		
Cadaveric donor	94.0	79.9
Living donor	97.7	89.7
Pancreas alone	97.8	76.7
Pancreas after kidney	95.4	77.3
Kidney-pancreas	95.1	82.6
Liver		
Deceased donor	86.3	72.4
Living donor	85.2	85.6
Intestine	80.7	48.6
Heart	85.1	69.8
Lung	77.3	42.4
Heart-lung	59.6	48.5

SOURCE: Adapted with permission from United Network for Organ Sharing.[1]

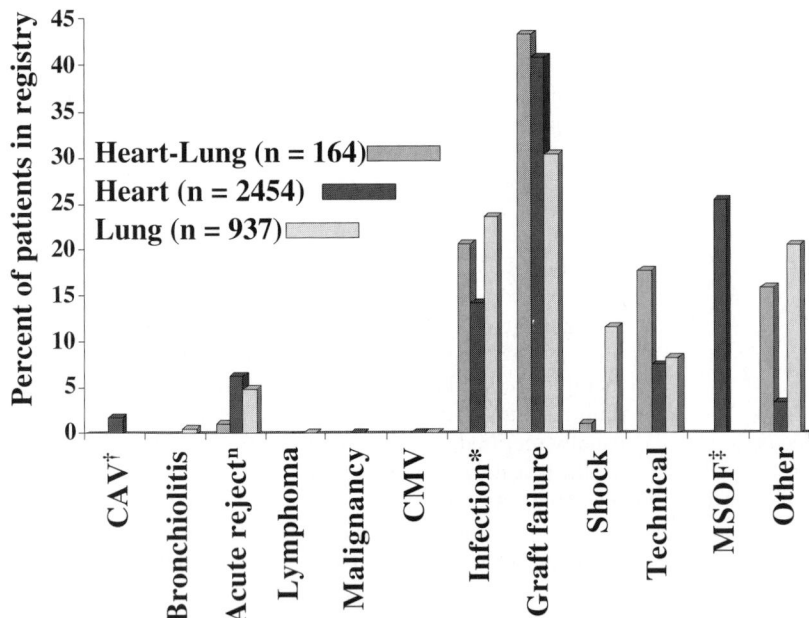

FIGURE 90-1 Graphical presentation of the causes of death in the first 30 days of all patients having had either a heart, heart-lung, or lung transplant who were in the International Society for Heart and Lung Transplantation (ISHLT) registry from the period from January 1992 to June 2002. The graph serves to illustrate the high proportion of deaths from technical problems, infection, and rejection across all types of transplant patients.*Infection relates to non–cytomegalovirus-mediated disease; [†]cardiac, allograft vasculopathy; [‡]multi-system organ failure. Developed using data taken from the ISHLT registry. (*Reproduced with permission from Hertz MI, Mohacsi PJ, Taylor DO, et al: The registry of the International Society for Heart and Lung Transplantation: Introduction to the Twentieth Annual Reports—2003. J Heart Lung Transplant 22:610, 2003.*)

although it appears that in some patients receiving tacrolimus for maintenance the steroid component may be discontinued completely.[2] Azathioprine or mycophenolate mofetil (MMF) are often used during the maintenance phase to permit dose reduction of the other immunosuppressive drugs in order to minimize side effects.

The remaining phase of immunosuppressive therapy is not planned but it is anticipated and involves the treatment of acute rejection. Despite improvements that have been made in immunosuppressive strategies, episodes of acute rejection still commonly occur in the postoperative period, typically between 1 week and 1 year following the operation. Early recognition and prompt treatment of acute rejection is essential if long-term graft function is to be preserved. Treat-

ment involves an intensification of the immunosuppressive regimen, which is usually accomplished through the use of high-dose steroids, short courses of antithymocyte globulin, and increased doses of the other immunosuppressive therapies. Issues pertaining to acute rejection will be discussed in greater detail in the sections dealing with organ-specific considerations.

CALCINEURIN INHIBITORS AND RELATED COMPOUNDS (CYCLOSPORINE, TACROLIMUS, AND SIROLIMUS)

The introduction of cyclosporine was one of the most revolutionary events in the field of transplant medicine,[3] and

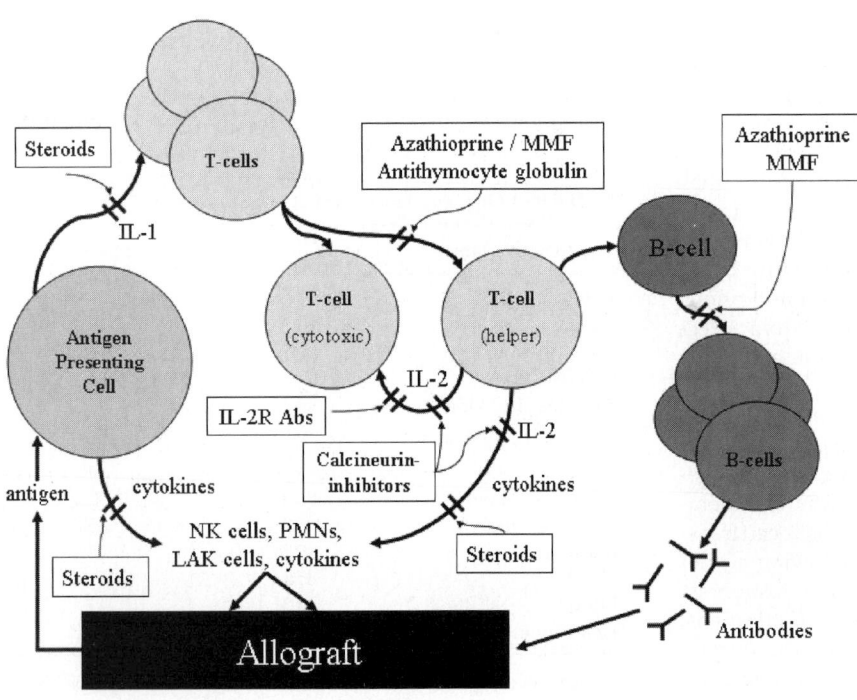

FIGURE 90-2 Sites of action of important immunosuppressive agents used to prevent allograft rejection in transplant recipients (see text for explanation). IL-1, interleukin-1; IL-2, interleukin-2; MMF, mycophenolate mofetil; IL-2R Abs, anti–interleukin-2-receptor antibodies; NK cells, natural killer cells; PMNs, polymorphonuclear neutrophils; LAK cells, lymphokine-activated killer cells.

the drug remains an important component of immunosuppressive regimens used by many institutions. Though in recent years some centers have switched to tacrolimus or sirolimus, two newer immunosuppressive agents, all agents in this class share several features. All provide effective inhibition of T-cell activation by interfering with a receptor on T cells that involves a calcium-dependent signal transduction pathway.

Cyclosporine binds to intracellular cyclophilin, and this complex interacts with calcineurin. Calcineurin is crucial for normal lymphokine gene activation, and its inhibition by cyclosporine consequently interferes with the production of interleukins-2, -3, and -4 (IL-2, IL-3, and IL-4), tumor necrosis factor-α (TNF-α), and other important mediators of inflammation. In turn, specific and potent inhibition of T-cell activation (especially CD4 cells) is achieved. It is important for the intensivist to understand the serious toxicities associated with the use of cyclosporine. The most frequently encountered problem is nephrotoxicity, and in many patients cyclosporine causes a rise in serum creatinine level and a reduction of glomerular filtration rate (GFR). The mechanism of this toxicity is felt to be related to vasoconstriction of the afferent glomerular arteriole.[3] Neurologic complications may be encountered in up to 20% of patients, including tremor, paresthesias, headache, confusion, seizures, and even coma. Other complications include hypertension (which often requires treatment), hyperkalemia, tremor, hirsutism, gingival hyperplasia, and glucose intolerance. Cyclosporine is metabolized by cytochrome P450-3A4 (CYP450-3A4) enzymes. Thus it is important to remember that inhibitors of cytochrome P450 (e.g., erythromycin, fluconazole, diltiazem, and verapamil) will increase serum cyclosporine levels, whereas inducers of these enzymes (e.g., phenobarbital, phenytoin, rifampin, and trimethoprim) will decrease the serum levels (Table 90-2). Previously trough drug concentrations were used to guide therapy. However, more recent recommendations have focused on the use of peak cyclosporine levels to monitor the adequacy of immunosuppression.[4] Ideally the dose of cyclosporine should be titrated using a biological assay or an assessment of the downstream effect of the drug on immune effector function. Such assays are under investigation.

Tacrolimus (formerly FK506) is a macrolide antibiotic with powerful immunosuppressive properties. Its mechanism of action is similar to cyclosporine, but the drug is more potent. Tacrolimus binds to a receptor known as FK-binding protein (FKBP), and suppresses calcineurin-dependent T-cell signaling.[5] Two controlled trials comparing tacrolimus to cyclosporine in liver transplant recipients demonstrated that tacrolimus reduces the incidence of acute rejection, refractory rejection, and chronic rejection[6-8] with similar patient and graft survival. However, the drug has important toxicities. As with cyclosporine, nephrotoxicity is the most troublesome side effect. Important neurotoxicity (seizures, tremor, psychoses, and coma) may also occur with its use. Both tacrolimus and cyclosporine decrease insulin secretion and can lead to hyperglycemia.[9,10] Interestingly, however, in renal transplant recipients who were converted from cyclosporine to tacrolimus, there was an improvement in other cardiovascular risk factors such as blood pressure and lipid profile.[11] The gingival hyperplasia and hirsutism commonly seen with cyclosporine do not occur with tacrolimus. Tacrolimus is also metabolized by CYP450-2A4 enzymes, and the clinician must be cognizant of the effects other drugs will have on its metabolism.

Sirolimus (rapamycin) is a drug related to tacrolimus that binds to FKBP. However, in contrast to tacrolimus it does not interfere with calcineurin activity and consequently does not interfere with the activation of cytokine genes. Its main effects are the inhibition of IL-2 production and the suppression of T-cell proliferation. Side effects include thrombocytopenia, hypercholesterolemia, and hypertriglyceridemia. Compared to cyclosporine and tacrolimus, the drug does not appear to have the same potential to cause renal failure. However, sirolimus may be associated with an increased risk of hepatic artery thrombosis and subsequent allograft loss[12] in liver transplant recipients. There have also been reports of interstitial pneumonitis associated with sirolimus.[13-16] Sirolimus is not recommended in the early postoperative period following lung transplantation, as it has been associated with bronchial anastomotic dehiscence.[17,18]

PROLIFERATION INHIBITORS (AZATHIOPRINE, MYCOPHENOLATE MOFETIL)

The proliferation inhibitors block DNA and RNA synthesis by interfering with normal purine metabolism. Since lymphocytes are unable to salvage purine as efficiently as most other cells, these drugs effectively inhibit lymphocyte proliferation and clonal expansion.

Azathioprine is a purine analogue that is converted in the liver to 6-mercaptopurine and which compromises synthesis of DNA and RNA. Its most important side effect is marrow suppression, and the drug can cause a profound leukopenia. Other important toxicities include hepatotoxicity and rarely fulminant hepatic failure, acute pancreatitis, skin malignancies, and increased susceptibility to infections.

Mycophenolate mofetil (MMF) interferes with purine metabolism as a reversible inhibitor of inosine monophosphate dehydrogenase. It also blocks clonal expansion of B- and T-lymphocytes. Important side effects of MMF include marrow depression (especially leukopenia and thrombocytopenia) and diarrhea. Less common problems include esophagitis, gastritis, and gastrointestinal bleeding. MMF may have an advantage over azathioprine in preventing acute rejection.[19]

TABLE 90-2 Selected Compounds Which Interact with Cytochrome P450 Enzymes to Cause Drug-Drug Interactions with Calcineurin Inhibitors

Inducers of P450 Enzymes (Decrease Serum Levels of Cyclosporine, Tacrolimus, and Sirolimus)	Inhibitors of P450 Enzymes (Increase Serum Levels of Cyclosporine, Tacrolimus, and Sirolimus)
Phenobarbital	Diltiazem
Phenytoin	Verapamil
Rifampin	Erythromycin
Trimethoprim	Clarithromycin
Carbamazepine	Fluconazole
Nafcillin	Itraconazole
	Ketoconazole
	Metoclopramide
	Allopurinol
	Grapefruit juice

Both azathioprine and MMF are now used predominantly as an adjunct to corticosteroid therapy in the maintenance phase of immunosuppression. The major advantage of these drugs is that their use will often enable the doses of corticosteroids and even of the calcineurin inhibitor to be reduced, thus avoiding some of the potential dose-related toxicity associated with these other agents.

ANTILYMPHOCYTE ANTIBODIES

Antibodies directed against lymphocytes were first introduced as an immunosuppressive therapy as antilymphocyte globulin (ALG). This therapeutic agent was created by immunizing animals with human lymphocytes and subsequently purifying the antibody-containing globulin fraction. ALG is very effective at depleting lymphocytes in the peripheral circulation, and quickly became an important component of regimens used for induction of immunosuppression and for the treatment of acute rejection. However, it was subsequently largely replaced by OKT3, a murine monoclonal preparation directed against T lymphocytes which could be used in much smaller doses because of its increased purity. OKT3 binds to the CD3-ε chain present on all human T cells, and causes a rapid clearance of peripheral T cells. Interestingly, it initially causes activation of T cells and the subsequent release of several lymphokines, including IL-2, IL-6, γ-interferon, and TNF. Rabbit antithymocyte globulin and to a lesser extent equine antithymocyte globulin are currently the antilymphocyte antibody preparations used most frequently by most centers.[1]

The antilymphocyte preparations are used primarily in the induction phase, and they have been shown to have higher success rates than steroids for the treatment of acute rejection.[20] When administered for this latter problem, prompt resolution of the rejection episode is usually observed. However, these preparations have significant toxicity. Fever is almost always observed at the time of infusion. Nonetheless, the importance of careful surveillance for infectious complications cannot be understated, as these therapies significantly attenuate the normal host immune response. The inflammatory response due to lymphokine production that is often seen with the initiation of therapy usually responds to corticosteroids, antihistamines, and acetaminophen.[21] Serum sickness has been observed with repeated use of these preparations. Furthermore, when these agents (especially OKT3) are administered more than once, the patient may develop antibodies directed against the globulin preparation that can substantially limit its efficacy. Long-term use is also associated with increased risk of viral infections (particularly cytomegalovirus) and posttransplant malignancy. Other less common complications of therapy include seizures (especially when concomitant hypocalcemia is present) and the acute respiratory distress syndrome (ARDS), possibly due to increased pulmonary capillary permeability arising from lymphokine stimulation.

SYSTEMIC CORTICOSTEROIDS

Systemic corticosteroids remain a key component of each phase of immunosuppression, and are received by over 95% of patients with pancreas, heart, lung, and heart-lung transplants.[1] They have multiple effects on the immune response. Importantly, steroids block T-cell proliferation and IL-2 synthesis. The phagocytic function of macrophages is inhibited, and in high doses corticosteroids prevent neutrophil degranulation.

Though they effectively attenuate the immune response and help prevent allograft rejection, corticosteroids also significantly increase the recipient's susceptibility to infection. In particular, viral and fungal infections appear to be highly associated with the use of corticosteroids. An important consideration is that steroids can also mask the typical signs of infection. For example, patients on high doses of these medications may not present with signs of peritonitis despite having intra-abdominal infections. As transplant patients typically remain on steroids chronically, the possibility of adrenal suppression and even overt adrenal insufficiency must be considered if these medications are discontinued. Despite their widespread use and important role in most immunosuppressive regimens, corticosteroids are associated with many of the significant side effects encountered by transplant patients. Insulin resistance is common, and the use of oral hypoglycemic agents and often insulin may be required. Both cyclosporine and tacrolimus affect insulin release and can induce insulin resistance, and may contribute to the hyperglycemia.[22–25] Increased sodium and water retention induced by steroids may aggravate posttransplant hypertension. Impaired wound healing has been well documented with the use of corticosteroids, and consequently these drugs may contribute to the development of postoperative surgical complications. Steroids are associated with increased risk of gastrointestinal hemorrhage, and thus most patients will be placed on routine stress ulcer prophylaxis, usually with either a histamine (H$_2$)-antagonist or a proton pump inhibitor. Long-term use of steroids often leads to osteopenia, overt osteoporosis, and fractures. Aseptic necrosis is a dreaded complication of steroid use that can occur at any time following the institution of therapy. Skin changes and fat redistribution are common. Steroids are also associated with mood changes and rarely even frank psychoses. Because of the significant side effects associated with steroid use, most maintenance immunosuppressive regimens now include antiproliferation inhibitors such as azathioprine or MMF to facilitate the early reduction of the corticosteroid dose.

NEW AGENTS

Recently, there has been increased use of anti–interleukin-2 receptor antibodies (basiliximab, daclizumab) during the induction phase.[1] Both agents bind to the α-chain of the IL-2 receptor, and competitively inhibit IL-2–induced proliferation of active T cells. The advantage of these compounds is that they are not associated with the toxicity produced by antilymphocyte preparations. Their use has been shown to decrease the rate of acute rejection following kidney[26,27] and heart transplantation.[28]

Rejection

Rejection of the allograft can be divided into three broad categories: hyperacute, acute, and chronic rejection. Hyperacute rejection is mediated by preformed antibodies directed against donor antigens, and occurs immediately following the transplant operation. Matching of donor and recipient major blood group type (A, B, O) essentially eliminates this class of rejection, which can have devastating consequences.

Immunosuppressive therapy is generally ineffective at treating this cause of graft failure, and retransplantation of the organ may be the only possible recourse to prevent death.

Acute rejection is much more commonly encountered, occurring in 20% of kidney-pancreas transplants, 30% of liver transplants, and 40% of lung and heart transplants during the first year.[1] Usually rejection does not manifest until the first several days following the transplant procedure. It occurs as the result of cell-mediated immunity, and it generally responds well to escalation of the immunosuppressive regimen.

Chronic rejection tends not to develop during the initial stay in the ICU, but patients may require ICU care as a result of the sequelae of the chronic inflammation and fibrosis that is the hallmark of this complication. Manifestations of chronic rejection are organ specific. In liver transplant recipients, it is characterized by the "vanishing-bile-duct syndrome," whereas bronchiolitis obliterans is the scourge that faces lung transplant recipients and is the leading cause of late death in these patients. Premature and accelerated atherosclerosis of the coronary arteries characterizes chronic rejection in heart transplant recipients.

Infectious Complications

Prior to the transplant procedure, it is important to know whether or not the transplant recipient has been exposed to common infections that can cause serious morbidity in the postoperative period when immunosuppressive therapies are instituted. Patients are routinely screened for antibodies to cytomegalovirus (CMV), Epstein-Barr virus (EBV), herpes viruses, hepatitis B and C viruses, human immunodeficiency virus (HIV), *Toxoplasma*, and tuberculosis exposure via skin testing. These infections can reactivate in an immunosuppressed recipient who has been previously exposed. Alternatively, a naïve recipient may acquire an infection following the transplant of an organ from a seropositive donor.

Because of the considerable morbidity associated with these infections, most transplant patients will receive prophylactic therapy if they are seronegative for any of these agents. If not already done preoperatively, transplant recipients can be vaccinated with killed vaccines in the postoperative period. Vaccination still confers some protection despite the attenuated humoral response in these patients.

In the early posttransplant period, however, bacterial and fungal infections predominate and are a frequent cause of morbidity and mortality (see Fig. 90-1). Since the regimens used for immunosuppression are similar for all solid-organ transplants, the recipients of such transplants will be susceptible to similar infectious agents. Specifically, using relatively high doses of calcineurin inhibitors such as cyclosporine or tacrolimus in combination with high doses of corticosteroids places the recipient at high risk of early infectious complications. This intensity of immunosuppression amplifies the risk of infection faced by all critically-ill patients.

Opportunistic infections can develop through three general mechanisms. A virulent pathogen may be acquired from the environment (e.g., pneumococcal pneumonia, *Aspergillus* infections, etc), an endogenous but latent organism may become reactivated (e.g., tuberculosis, herpes viruses, etc.), or there may be invasion of an endogenous organism (e.g., *Candida*, enteric bacteria, etc.) into a normally sterile site. Several authors have proposed an approach that classifies the most likely infectious complications according to the time that has elapsed since the original procedure (Fig. 90-3).[29,30]

INFECTIONS OCCURRING IN THE FIRST POSTTRANSPLANT MONTH

In the first month after transplantation most infections will be similar to those encountered following any major surgery, including bacterial or candidal infections involving the lungs, urinary tract, surgical wound, or indwelling catheters. Consequently, efforts should be made to remove all vascular-access catheters and drains as soon as possible. As with any critically-ill patient, strategies to facilitate liberation from mechanical ventilation should be employed. The high level of immunosuppression during the induction phase significantly contributes to the development of infections during this time period, but usually the state of immunosuppression has not been of sufficient duration to allow many of the opportunistic infections that become so problematic in subsequent months to develop.[31] Occasionally infections may be transmitted to the recipient by the allograft itself. The presence of bacteremia, fungemia, or active infection in a donor is generally considered a contraindication to organ donation given the associated high probability that infection will be transmitted to the host. Cultures obtained at the time of implantation (e.g., via bronchoscopic-guided lung lavage) may be used to guide treatment. Typically most centers employ prophylactic antibiotic strategies to empirically treat the microbes that are transplanted into the recipient. The choice of prophylactic antibiotics varies and usually reflects differences in the center's bacterial ecology. Parenteral, oral, topical, and inhaled medications are often used alone or in combination.

Similarly, any untreated infection that is present in the recipient at the time of the transplant may become a devastating problem following the initiation of immunosuppressive therapy. As a result, any active infection in a potential recipient is generally considered to be an absolute contraindication to transplant surgery.

INFECTIONS OCCURRING BETWEEN 1 AND 6 MONTHS POSTTRANSPLANT

Following the first month, the recipient is at risk for infections due to several viral infections that would normally be suppressed by an intact immune response. Particularly problematic are infections due to CMV, EBV, other herpes viruses, hepatitis B and C viruses, and HIV. Screening for these viruses is usually performed in both the donor and recipient prior to the transplant procedure, and pre-emptive therapy is often employed. Infection with HIV has traditionally been considered an absolute contraindication to transplantation. However, recently some experts have argued that asymptomatic HIV-positive patients should no longer be excluded from consideration for transplant of solid organs, citing the substantially improved survival of HIV carriers following the introduction of highly active antiretroviral therapy.[32–34]

The sustained immunosuppression used in the induction phase and early maintenance phase leads to an increased risk of opportunistic infections. Infections due to *Pneumocystis carinii*, *Aspergillus*, *Listeria monocytogenes*, and tuberculosis become important considerations. Most transplant

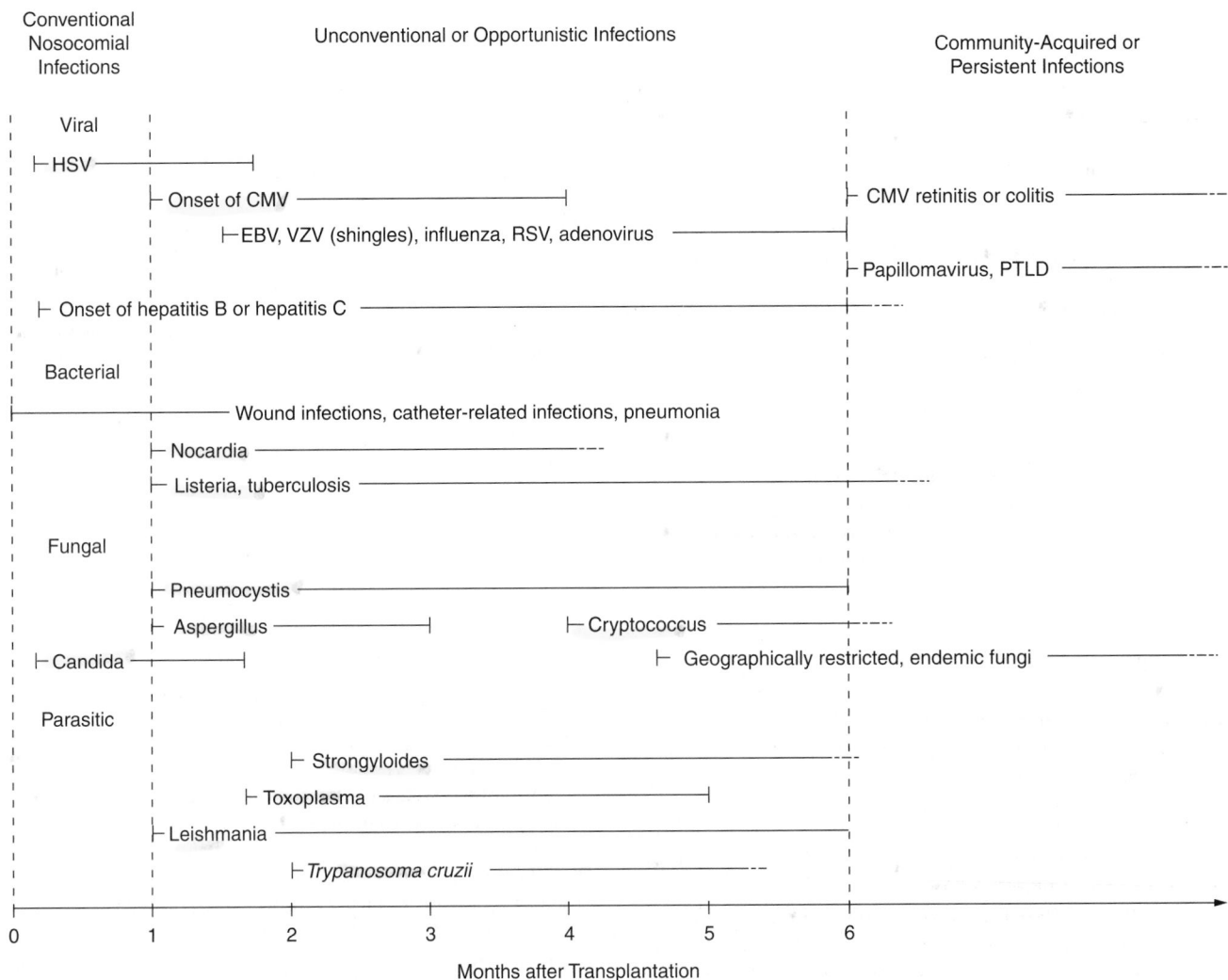

FIGURE 90-3 Usual sequence of infections after organ transplantation. Zero indicates the time of transplantation. Solid lines indicate the most common period for the onset of infection; dotted lines and arrows indicate periods of continued risk at reduced levels. HSV, herpes simplex virus; CMV, cytomegalovirus; EBV, Epstein-Barr virus; VZV, varicella-zoster virus; RSV, respiratory syncytial virus; PTLD, posttransplantation lymphoproliferative disease. (*Reproduced with permission from Fishman et al.[29]*)

programs routinely provide recipients with trimethoprim-sulfamethoxazole (TMP-SMX) to reduce the risk of *Pneumocystis carinii* infection. Should a transplant patient develop *Pneumocystis carinii* pneumonia, the treatment of choice is intravenous TMP-SMX. Pentamidine can be used as an alternative, but it is associated with a greater incidence of toxicity and side effects, and is generally considered to be less effective therapy. In patients who have a positive purified protein derivative tuberculosis skin test (>5 mm induration[35]) or who are at high-risk for reactivation of latent tuberculosis infection, prophylactic therapy with isoniazid for 9 to 12 months should be considered.[35,36] *Aspergillus* infections are most problematic for lung transplant recipients, but they can develop in any patient who has undergone solid-organ transplantation and is receiving chronic immunosuppressive therapy. The treatment of choice is amphotericin; liposomal preparations of amphotericin are available that are associated with less nephrotoxicity, but these are much more expensive. More recently caspofungin the first in a new class of antifungal

agents (echinocandins) has been shown to be active against *Aspergillus* species.[37–39] Although its role in treating immunosuppressed transplant patients has not been systematically evaluated, there is at least one suggestion that its antifungal effects (tested in vitro) may be enhanced in patients who are receiving concomitant calcineurin inhibitors.[40] Voriconazole, a newer azole anti-fungal agent, has demonstrated better outcomes and fewer side effects in comparison to amphotericin in patients with bone marrow transplantation.[40a] Experience in patients with solid organ transplantation is growing.

INFECTIONS OCCURRING MORE THAN 6 MONTHS POSTTRANSPLANT

Severe infections occurring more than 6 months following the transplant procedure may necessitate ICU admission. Most commonly these infections are similar to those experienced by the general community and involve the respiratory tract.[29] Other problems developing in this time frame include the progression of underlying infection with hepatitis B or C, CMV, EBV, and human papillomavirus. There is also a continued risk for the opportunistic infections that develop after the first posttransplant month (discussed above) during this time period, and careful surveillance for their occurrence must be maintained.

INFECTION DUE TO CYTOMEGALOVIRUS

The most important and the most common viral infection for all solid-organ transplant recipients is CMV infection. Once an individual is infected by this herpes virus, they will be infected for life, though the virus generally remains in a latent or dormant phase. Recipients who are seronegative for CMV that receive an allograft from a seropositive donor are at greatest risk of developing symptomatic illness, including tissue-invasive disease from primary infection. Patients who are already seropositive for CMV prior to the procedure (indicating past exposure and latent infection) are at risk for reactivation following the initiation of immunosuppressive therapy. Superinfection by a new strain of CMV contracted from the allograft of a CMV-seropositive donor can also occur. Strategies to prevent CMV infection are usually based on the recipient's relative risk of developing infection, with those who are recipient-negative, donor-positive and recipient-positive, donor-negative (in the case of lung transplantation) receiving the more intense regimens.[41] The monitoring of CMV antigenemia or viral load using polymerase chain reaction may be a component of these regimens, and may be used to guide duration of prophylaxis and provide evidence of infection or emergence of a resistant strain.[42]

The spectrum of disease caused by CMV infection among transplant recipients is quite variable.[43] Infection can be completely asymptomatic or can be associated with an acute flu-like or mononucleosis-like illness characterized by fever and myalgias. The virus can cause bone marrow suppression and consequently leukopenia and thrombocytopenia. Infection of the allograft can cause organ-specific inflammation resulting in acute hepatitis, pneumonitis, myocarditis, nephritis, or pancreatitis, depending on the organ that was transplanted.[31] Active CMV infection is also associated with the development of other opportunistic infections, likely due to CMV-mediated immune defects, and consequently it should be considered whenever an unusual infection (such as *Pneumocystis carinii* pneumonia or invasive aspergillosis) develops.[29] Acute rejection has been associated with CMV infection. However, the role of CMV infection in contributing to chronic rejection is likely much more important. It has been associated with the development of bronchiolitis obliterans in lung transplant patients, the vanishing-bile-duct syndrome in recipients of liver allografts, and in premature and accelerated atherosclerosis of the coronary arteries following heart transplantation.[29] Though posttransplant lymphoproliferative disease is usually associated with EBV infection, active CMV infection has also been implicated as a risk factor for its development.[44–46]

Treatment of CMV infection generally consists of intravenous ganciclovir for 2 to 4 weeks. Confirmation that CMV viremia has resolved should be sought before therapy is discontinued. In the near future ganciclovir use may be replaced or consolidated with the use of newer oral analogues, especially for long-term regimens.[47,48] Occasionally a CMV iso-

late will be resistant to ganciclovir, and intravenous foscarnet must be used despite its increased toxicity.

ORGAN-SPECIFIC INFECTIOUS CONSIDERATIONS

LIVER TRANSPLANT RECIPIENTS

Bacterial infections are frequent among liver transplant patients, and the source is most often intra-abdominal.[49] Recognizing that overgrowth of pathogenic aerobic bacteria from the gastrointestinal tract may contribute to the development of many of these infections, some experts have recommended that oral selective bowel decontamination be started 3 days prior to the transplant operation.[31] Though this approach may decrease the relative incidence of gram-negative infections in the first month, selective bowel decontamination has not been adopted by all transplant programs.[50,51] Recent evidence suggests that this therapy only leads to a substitution for infections caused by gram-negative bacilli and *Candida* species with infections due to gram-positive organisms, and yet it is associated with a substantially increased cost.[52]

Transient biliary tree infection and subsequent bacteremia may occur following biliary tree manipulation (T-tube manipulation, cholangiography, etc). This has prompted many experts to advocate the use of pre-emptive systemic antibiotics around the time of such procedures.[31]

Liver disease resulting from hepatitis B or C infection remains one of the most common indications for liver transplant. The reactivation of these viruses in the recipient and resultant allograft infection remains a major challenge. Most patients who are seropositive for hepatitis B will receive hepatitis B immunoglobulin (HBIg) and lamivudine to suppress replication of the virus in the postoperative setting. These therapies are generally continued indefinitely, and have resulted in allograft and patient survival rates similar to those of patients not infected with hepatitis B.[53] Recipients who are positive for hepatitis C virus prior to transplant have also been shown to have poorer graft and patient survival rates.[54] However, no antiviral regimens have yet been shown to be effective at improving outcomes for these patients following orthotopic liver transplantation.[55]

Infections due to *Candida* are particularly common in liver transplant recipients, and the most common source is the gastrointestinal tract. Risk factors for these infections include concomitant CMV infection, retransplantation, the presence of choledochojejunostomy, and the use of OKT3 immunosuppression. The use of a regimen of oral selective bowel decontamination that includes an antifungal agent has already been discussed, and certainly this intervention decreases the incidence of candidal infections. There is evidence that the routine pre-emptive use of oral fluconazole (100 mg/d[56] to 400 mg/d[57]) or liposomal amphotericin B[58,59] after liver transplant is effective at reducing the incidence of these infections. However, some have cautioned that routine prophylaxis may encourage the emergence of resistant candidal strains, and have suggested that only high-risk patients be targeted for therapy.[60]

LUNG TRANSPLANT RECIPIENTS

Following lung transplantation, patients are at risk for all of the infections that plague individuals with a chronically immunosuppressed state. However, the incidence of infection in these patients is much higher than that reported for recipients of other solid organs, presumably due to the exposure of the allograft to the external environment.[61,62] The development of CMV infection can cause significant morbidity and can increase transplant-related mortality, especially if new infection develops in a seronegative recipient who has received an allograft from a seropositive donor. Seropositive recipients can also be reinfected by a new strain of CMV, but these infections tend not to be as severe. Treatment consists of intravenous ganciclovir, and many centers will routinely use this agent as prophylaxis against CMV infection if either the donor or the recipient is seropositive.

Aspergillus is an organism that frequently colonizes the airways of lung transplant recipients, but may also lead to clinically important infections. Oral itraconazole or inhaled or intravenous amphotericin are usually effective therapies. In its most severe form, invasive aspergillosis and disseminated disease are associated with high mortality rates. The bronchial anastomosis is particularly vulnerable to infection with this organism, though the airways may become more diffusely affected, and mucosal edema, ulceration, and formation of pseudomembranes may occur.[61] Patients with septic lung disease (cystic fibrosis or bronchiectasis) are a unique group and have a very high risk of early infection. These patients' airways are typically highly colonized. Despite efforts to sterilize the trachea and major bronchi in the perioperative period, secretions originating from these recipients' upper airways and proximal lower airways likely contaminate the transplanted lungs. Consequently most centers employ an antibiotic strategy to deal with these colonizing organisms, which are typically *Staphylococcus aureus*, nontuberculosis mycobacteria, *Pseudomonas* species, or enteric gram-negative bacilli. Owing to longstanding antibiotic pressure these organisms are often highly resistant to first-line agents, and can be difficult to treat if an infection becomes established. In particular *Burkholderia cepacia* is a dreaded colonizer that represents a major threat for some centers caring for cystic fibrosis patients.[63] Indeed, patients with cystic fibrosis complicated by *B. cepacia* infection have a worse outcome than their counterparts without this infection.[64,65] *Aspergillus* lung infection may also be more common in patients transplanted for cystic fibrosis.[66]

Defining the etiology of new or progressive airspace opacities in the perioperative lung transplant period is a frequent dilemma. Airspace disease may represent reperfusion injury (see below), volume overload, acute lung injury, early rejection, or infection.[67] Computed tomographic (CT) scanning of the chest and bronchoscopic sampling of the distal airways is often required to rule out an infectious cause. A trial of diuresis or placement of a pulmonary arterial flotation catheter may be required to evaluate the contribution of volume overload to the opacities. The role of lung biopsy in establishing the cause of radiographic worsening is controversial. Transbronchial lung biopsy may lack sufficient sensitivity in the perioperative setting.[68] However, the utility of open lung biopsy (OLB) is variable,[69,70] and hence it should be carefully considered if the etiology of the lung infiltrates remains uncertain. In one retrospective series of 48 open biopsies from 42 patients, 32 (67%) of the biopsies confirmed the clinicians' initial suspicions and prompted the initiation of "new therapy" in 30 (71%) of the patients.[69] A new diagnosis was made following 14 of the biopsies (29%). Only two patients (4% of all OLBs) had a nondiagnostic OLB. Four biopsies (8% of all

OLBs), including the two nondiagnostic OLBs, did not result in any change in therapy. Complications of the procedure were rare, though three (7%) patients developed an air leak which persisted more than 7 days. In contrast an earlier report of 38 biopsies (representing 32 patients) found that early open lung biopsies (performed <45 days after transplant) were not useful, and resulted in a change in therapy for only 1 of 11 cases.[70]

HEART TRANSPLANTATION

Most heart transplant recipients will receive intravenous ganciclovir for 3 to 4 weeks as prophylactic therapy if they are seropositive for CMV before transplantation. If a seronegative recipient receives an allograft from a seropositive donor, they are given prophylactic therapy for 12 weeks following the procedure.[71]

Infective endocarditis is an infrequent complication following heart transplantation, usually developing on the supravalvular suture line. Antibiotic prophylaxis is generally recommended for heart transplant recipients prior to dental, gastrointestinal, or genitourinary tract surgery.[72]

Organ-Specific Considerations

LIVER TRANSPLANTATION

THE PROCEDURE

During orthotopic liver transplantation, the native organ is removed and replaced by a cadaveric liver. Extracorporeal venovenous bypass is often used during the procedure to decompress the systemic and splanchnic venous systems. Although this may help preserve hemodynamic stability during the operation and decrease intraoperative bleeding problems, potential complications include intraoperative air embolism[73,74] and thromboembolism. The biliary tract will be reconstructed either by creating an end-to-end anastomosis of the donor and recipient common ducts (using a T-tube stent) or by connecting the donor's common duct to the recipient's jejunum. Anastomoses are created between the native and allograft cava (supra- and infrahepatic), portal veins, and hepatic arteries. Removal of the venous clamps leads to reperfusion of the organ, and this will often be associated with hemodynamic instability, coagulopathy, and electrolyte abnormalities (particularly hyperkalemia).

Recently, there have been a growing number of patients who undergo living-donor transplants. In Asia, almost all liver transplant procedures have involved living donors.[75] In this procedure, the right hepatic lobe from a donor with a compatible blood type is implanted into the recipient following hepatectomy of the diseased organ. Along with an often substantially reduced waiting time for the procedure, living related transplants may also allow for better selection of healthy donors (and consequently donor organs) and a considerably decreased cold ischemia time. The elective nature of the procedure also enables potential recipients to be medically stabilized preoperatively. The major disadvantage is the small but significant risk of complications for the donor. Biliary complications may occur in up to 6% of donors,[76] and other complications of abdominal surgery such as wound infection may develop; the reported mortality of donors following living-donor liver transplant is 0.28%.[75] One study suggests that in the United States approximately 99% of living donors are genetically or emotionally related to the recipient,[76] creating important ethical and psychosocial challenges.

POSTOPERATIVE CONSIDERATIONS
Mechanical Ventilation

Most patients will require mechanical ventilation for the first 24 to 48 hours following the liver transplant procedure. Extubation should not be considered until there is evidence that the allograft is functioning properly and the patient's level of arousal is sufficient to allow for adequate airway protection. This latter consideration is especially important given that anesthetic agents and sedating medications may be cleared more slowly from the circulation by the newly transplanted liver. The need for reintubation in liver transplant patients has been associated with poorer outcomes and even increased mortality.[77] However, there is mounting evidence to support the notion that attempts at early extubation of liver transplant recipients may reduce ICU utilization. Selection of suitable candidates seems crucial.[78–82]

Monitoring of Liver Function

The function of the new allograft should be assessed in the same manner that liver function is assessed in any patient. Coagulopathy is often present in the immediate postoperative period, but should correct soon after the transplant. The prothrombin time (PT) or International Normalized Ratio (INR) should be followed closely. Administration of fresh frozen plasma will interfere with the ability to monitor these parameters. Consequently some programs avoid the transfusion of coagulation factors unless necessitated by bleeding complications.

Glucose should be monitored frequently during the ICU stay as liver failure will often result in refractory hypoglycemia. Conversely, the use of corticosteroids may lead to insulin resistance and hyperglycemia, which should be treated appropriately. Bilirubin often remains elevated for many days following the transplant, but should be followed closely as abrupt changes may herald complications involving the biliary tree or the vascular supply to the liver. Serum lactate levels are frequently elevated immediately following the operation, but if the graft is functioning properly they should return to normal within a few days.

Serum transaminase levels (AST/ALT) are usually measured postoperatively; these usually rise in the first 2 to 3 days following the procedure, but then can be expected to normalize. Similar to changes in bilirubin levels, abrupt changes or progressive elevations of these enzymes may also signify complications and mandate further evaluation.

Fluids and Hemodynamics

Physiologic derangements following liver transplantation are common. Intraoperative blood and fluid loss may be considerable. The use of aprotinin during the operation has been advocated by some as a means to reduce blood loss.[83–85] Interestingly, several studies also report decreased vasopressor requirements in patients who receive this therapy intraoperatively.[86,87] Its use has also been associated with an improvement in renal function.[88] However, this initial enthusiasm for aprotinin therapy needs to be tempered by concerns regarding a possible increased potential for thrombembolism.[89,90]

Following the operation, patients may lose significant amounts of fluid and protein via the abdominal drain, especially if massive ascites was present preoperatively owing to advanced cirrhosis and decompensated liver disease. These latter patients are at particularly high risk of developing intravascular volume depletion, and they must be monitored carefully and treated aggressively. Serial hematocrit determinations should be measured (usually every 4 to 6 hours) to ensure that significant bleeding is not present. It should be noted that the hyperdynamic circulatory state that characterizes liver dysfunction will often persist in the postoperative period, making interpretation of hemodynamic measurements difficult. An increased cardiac output with decreased systemic vascular resistance is often observed. Although aggressive fluid resuscitation is indicated to treat intravascular volume depletion, it should also be noted that patients are at particularly high risk of cardiopulmonary complications following liver transplantation.[91] Electrolyte abnormalities, particularly hyponatremia, are often observed. Overly aggressive treatment of derangements of sodium can precipitate the osmotic demyelination syndrome (formerly called central pontine myelinolysis).

Particular care is required for the patient who has significant preoperative portopulmonary hypertension. These patients will often encounter pulmonary hemodynamic instability and may have increased cardiopulmonary mortality, especially if the preoperative mean pulmonary artery pressure is greater than 35 mm Hg.[92] Invasive hemodynamic monitoring with a pulmonary artery catheter should be considered to guide therapy in these patients. Specific pulmonary vasodilators such as inhaled nitric oxide or nebulized prostaglandins may be required in the setting of right ventricular dysfunction in order to preserve cardiac output.

A system for classifying patients based on their anticipated need for fluid and electrolyte replacement has been proposed[93] and advocated by several experts.[94] Such an approach may be practically useful in that it creates a framework to understand the hemodynamic considerations for a given patient (Table 90-3). According to this classification, a patient with class I liver disease can be expected to have a normal postoperative response to intravenous fluid therapy. Patients with class II or III liver disease will have more ascites,

TABLE 90-3 Classification of End-Stage Liver Disease Severity for the Purposes of Intensive Care Unit Management

Class	Hyperdynamic Circulation	Hyponatremia	Malnutrition	Portopulmonary Hypertension	Cardiac Dysfunction
I	−	−	−	−	−
II	+	+/−	−	−	−
III	++	++	−	−	−
IV	++	++	+	+	+

SOURCE: Adapted with permission from Lowell et al[93] and McGilvray et al.[94]

leading to greater fluid and protein loss from the abdominal drain, and can be anticipated to need more fluids postoperatively and careful monitoring of electrolytes. Patients with class IV disease require the closest monitoring and may benefit from insertion of a pulmonary artery catheter to assist with the management of the portopulmonary hypertension and cardiac dysfunction that is often present.

Postoperative Renal Dysfunction

Following the liver transplant procedure renal dysfunction is frequently observed, and postoperative renal failure can be severe enough to require renal replacement therapy in up to one third of patients. However, kidney function generally improves, and only 5% of patients require chronic hemodialysis following liver transplant.[95]

The most common precipitant is intravascular volume depletion resulting in prerenal azotemia. However, nephrotoxicity due to the immunosuppressive drugs is also common. The development of hepatorenal syndrome occurs in 7% to 15%[94,96] of patients with cirrhosis, and is commonly observed following orthotopic liver transplant. It is likely that strategies aimed at preventing hepatorenal syndrome are the most effective. Thus care should be taken to promptly treat bleeding insults and to avoid intravascular volume depletion. When CT scanning or other imaging techniques are being considered, the use of intravenous contrast dye should be avoided if possible. If intravenous contrast is required for proper imaging (and the benefits outweigh the risks of the test), consideration should be given to the use of acetylcysteine if renal function has not completely returned to normal, in order to protect the kidney from further insult and contrast nephropathy.[97] Terlipressin (a long-acting vasopressin analogue) has been reported to be successful in improving urine output in cirrhotic patients with hepatorenal syndrome.[98,99] The relative contribution of albumin coadministration to the success of this pharmacologic strategy has been evaluated and supports the notion that maintenance of intravascular volume is integral in the treatment of these patients.[100] One study also advocates the addition of acetylcysteine to mitigate the potential ischemic nephropathy that may result from the vasoconstrictive effects of terlipressin on the kidney.[99] The role of terlipressin in patients with established hepatorenal failure following transplantation has not been systematically evaluated. Indeed, in theory, liver transplantation should correct hepatorenal failure.[101,102]

Primary Graft Nonfunction

Primary graft nonfunction refers to a failure of the transplanted liver early in the postoperative period. The characteristics of this devastating complication include minimal bile output, refractory coagulopathy, progressive elevation of transaminases, acidosis, hypoglycemia, and cerebral edema. The incidence of this dreaded complication is likely only between 3% and 5%,[103,104] but the associated mortality rate may be higher than 20%.[105–107]

Several considerations exist if the graft fails to work postoperatively. The possibility of vascular complications should be entertained and excluded with Doppler ultrasonography.[108] Investigations to detect severe infection or acute rejection should be initiated. If all these tests fail to elucidate the cause of graft failure, primary graft nonfunction is the likely cause.

Vascular Complications

The incidence of vascular complications following liver transplant ranges from 8% to 14%.[109,110] These develop most commonly on the first postoperative day, but may occur up to several weeks following the surgery.[108] Thombosis is the most common early complication, and stenosis and pseudoaneurysm formation generally develop later in the patient's course. The presentation of hepatic artery thrombosis has been associated with hepatic artery reconstruction with an interposition graft to the supraceliac aorta.[111] Despite reassurances, some concerns about an increased risk of hepatic artery thrombosis with the use of sirolimus remain.[112] The clinical picture of this complication can vary from the asymptomatic rise in liver enzymes to fulminant hepatic failure. Urgent laparotomy and revision of the hepatic artery anastomosis is required if this complication develops, and unfortunately retransplantation is often necessary if hepatic necrosis has occurred.

Portal vein thrombosis develops less frequently and may present more insidiously. Ascites may be seen to develop or worsen, and variceal bleeding (usually from pre-existing varices) may ensue. Thrombectomy and anastomotic revision can be successful if this complication is diagnosed early.

Biliary Leaks

Biliary complications occur in approximately 15% of patients following orthotopic liver transplantation.[113] Of these, bile leak is the most common early complication. Symptoms are nonspecific, and can include fever, abdominal discomfort, and signs of peritoneal irritation. Though ultrasound may demonstrate an intra-abdominal fluid collection, cholangiography will provide a definitive diagnosis. Endoscopic insertion of biliary stents can sometimes provide satisfactory results, but surgical repair of the leak may be required.

Biliary strictures and stones typically appear later in the postoperative period. Obstructions usually can be managed endoscopically[114] or through the use of interventional radiology techniques, but surgical correction is sometimes necessary. Strictures typically develop at the anastomotic site, and are likely the result of local ischemia. These may present as cholestasis or possibly as overt cholangitis. Balloon dilation of the stricture with or without stent placement usually is successful treatment, but surgical revision and even retransplantation may be required.

Intra-Abdominal Infections

Intra-abdominal infections ranging from local abscess formation to overt peritonitis can occur following liver transplantation. Development of these complications should always lead the clinician to suspect that a leak has occurred from the biliary anastomosis or from the jejunojejunostomy; correction of these problems will often require laparotomy and surgical repair. However, abscesses can usually be treated with CT-guided drainage and subsequent serial CT scans to ensure that the collection has been adequately drained.

Rejection

Rejection of the hepatic allograft is usually not seen until about 1 to 2 weeks following the procedure, and most often manifests as fever, right upper quadrant pain, and reduced bile pigment and volume. However, the most sensitive marker of early rejection is a rise in serum transaminase

(AST/ALT) levels and bilirubin. A rise in total white blood count may also develop. The most important consideration when elevation of these serum enzymes occurs early in the postoperative course is the exclusion of one of the various mechanical complications (such as vascular compromise, biliary obstruction, and primary graft nonfunction). After the biliary tree and vascular structures have been imaged using ultrasonography, a liver biopsy will help confirm the diagnosis of acute rejection. As is the case in any solid-organ transplant recipient, treatment of acute rejection should be aggressive and must be instituted promptly. For liver transplant recipients, therapy usually involves antithymocyte globulin and increased or pulsed doses of methylprednisolone.

The management of chronic rejection of the transplanted liver usually does not involve the intensivist, but occasionally these patients may require ICU admission. Chronic rejection of the liver presents clinically as progressive cholestasis and histologically with mononuclear infiltration of the allograft, vascular abnormalities, and fibrosis. These findings are most commonly seen as part of the vanishing-bile-duct syndrome; treatment is often unsuccessful and may require retransplantation.

LUNG TRANSPLANTATION

THE OPERATION

While combined heart-lung transplantation is still performed for patients with Eisenmenger syndrome and complex congenital cardiac defects that cannot be easily repaired at the time of the lung transplant, most patients will undergo either bilateral or single-lung transplantation. Bilateral lung transplantation is the preferred procedure for patients with septic pulmonary disorders such as cystic fibrosis and bronchiectasis. In contrast, single-lung transplantation can be performed in patients with chronic obstructive pulmonary disease (COPD) and idiopathic pulmonary fibrosis. The observation that right ventricular dysfunction generally improves in patients with pulmonary hypertension following single- or double-lung transplantation[115] has obviated the need for performing combined heart-lung transplantation in this group of patients.

During single-lung transplantation, sequential anastomoses are performed to attach the donor and recipient mainstem bronchus and pulmonary artery. The donor left atrial cuff and pulmonary veins are then attached to the recipient's left atrium. In a similar manner, bilateral lung transplantation is performed as two sequential single-lung transplant procedures. Most patients can be supported intraoperatively through the ventilation of a single lung while surgery is performed on the contralateral side. Consequently, cardiopulmonary bypass is generally only required if profound hypoxia is encountered.

COMPLICATIONS
Ischemia-Reperfusion Injury

Since hyperacute rejection (due to ABO mismatch) has become extremely rare, the earliest serious complication of the lung transplant operation is ischemia-reperfusion (IR) injury (also called primary graft failure or pulmonary reimplantation response). IR injury is a syndrome of severe allograft dysfunction characterized histologically by marked alveo-

lar damage which manifests clinically as severe pulmonary edema. The incidence of this complication ranges from 10% to 20%, depending on the reporting center and the definition used,[116–118] and when severe, it is associated with a very poor prognosis; as many as 41% of affected patients may die.[117] A recent study also suggests that IR injury may be associated with the development of bronchiolitis obliterans later in the patient's course.[119] Most series of patients with IR injury demonstrate that recipients will develop pulmonary infiltrates on chest x-ray during the first 3 days following transplantation.[120] When entertaining this diagnosis, it is essential that the clinician perform a careful evaluation to exclude other possible complications. Confirmation should be sought that a donor-recipient cross-match (hyperacute rejection) has not occurred, that bacterial pneumonia has not developed (negative cultures from bronchoalveolar lavage), and that pulmonary venous return is not compromised owing to technical problems with the left atrial anastomosis (transesophageal echocardiography should be performed to ensure adequate blood flow through pulmonary veins). Invasive monitoring with a pulmonary catheter will help exclude volume overload or cardiogenic pulmonary edema. Transbronchial biopsy may be required to rule out the possibility of acute rejection. Treatment of IR injury is similar to the management of ARDS. Extending the results of trials of mechanical ventilation in patients with ARDS we recommend that lung-protective ventilation strategies with low tidal volumes be employed, with the use of sufficient positive end-expiratory pressure (PEEP) to reduce the fraction of inspired oxygen to acceptable levels.[121] Since IR is characterized by increased alveolar capillary permeability, care must be taken to provide judicious fluid management. Some success at attenuating the injury from IR has been observed with the administration of prostaglandin E$_1$, though this may lead to hypotension owing to the effects of the drug on the systemic vasculature. Inhaled nitric oxide (NO) has been advocated as a means to both treat and prevent IR injury. Initial preclinical and uncontrolled clinical studies of inhaled NO suggest that administration prior to IR injury may improve graft function.[122–126] However, a recent controlled study of NO administered 10 minutes after reperfusion failed to show any benefit in terms of graft function.[127] NO has also been used to improve oxygenation and reduce pulmonary arterial pressures in patients with oxygenation and vasomotor dysfunction after lung transplantation.[128–130] If inhaled NO is used for its pulmonary vasodilatory properties and to decrease ventilation/perfusion mismatch, it should be understood that these effects should be seen within minutes of the institution of this therapy. Daily measurements of methemoglobin levels are required. If one extrapolates from studies of NO use in acute lung injury, the effects of NO on lung function are likely short lived.[131] Consequently the rationale for long-term use of NO is unclear. Furthermore, the benefit of therapy is often difficult to assess owing to the development of rebound during attempts to withdraw NO therapy.[123] We often employ sildenafil to prevent such rebound associated with withdrawal of NO therapy in these patients.[132]

Following single-lung transplantation, IR injury will often compromise lung function in the allograft. To avoid exposing the native lung (which is often emphysematous and prone to hyperinflation) to potentially injurious high airway pressures and alveolar overdistention, independent lung ventilation is often used. If conventional ventilation is causing overexpansion of the native lung leading to an increase in its pulmonary vascular resistance, blood may be preferentially shunted to the compromised graft. Independent lung ventilation involves the use of a double-lumen endotracheal tube (avoiding intubation of the transplanted bronchus), and enables each lung to be ventilated with different airway pressures and tidal volumes. This strategy can dramatically improve ventilation-perfusion ($\dot{V}/\dot{Q}$) mismatch. In the extreme case, the native lung may become sufficiently overdistended to cause mediastinal shift and lead to hypotension as a result of compromised venous return or cardiac tamponade.[133] Other measures that can ameliorate the $\dot{V}/\dot{Q}$ mismatch and other sequelae of native lung overexpansion include the positioning of the patient in a lateral decubitus position to direct the allograft superiorly (to preferentially perfuse the native lung) and the use of lower tidal volumes. The use of this latter strategy often comes at the expense of a mild respiratory acidosis. Rarely, lung reduction surgery performed on the native emphysematous lung may be required if the overdistension of this lung remains a problem.[134,135]

Airway and Mechanical Complications

Although the incidence of airway and other mechanical complications has decreased,[136] it is important for the intensive care physician to have an understanding of these problems. Bronchial dehiscence is an infrequent yet potentially devastating complication. It may manifest within a few days of the operation and is usually heralded by persistent or large air leaks from thoracostomy tubes, but may present as pneumomediastinum with or without mediastinitis, pneumopericardium, or empyema. Usually the complication results from ischemia and necrosis at the anastomosis suture line. Although most cases can be managed conservatively by decompressing the large extrapulmonary air collections, bronchoscopic débridement and even bronchial stenting may be required to ensure airway patency. Complete dehiscence of the anastomosis mandates surgical correction or retransplantation.

Bronchial strictures leading to airway stenosis and compromise are sequelae of bronchial dehiscence and/or ischemia, but usually do not develop until several weeks following the transplant procedure. Strictures typically arise in the mainstem bronchus at or just distal to the anastomosis. Ischemic injury to the bronchi may also lead to bronchomalacia, which is characterized by weakened cartilage that is prone to (expiratory) dynamic collapse. Permanent stenting is the preferred approach to this problem. More commonly patients develop inspissation of secretions in the bronchi that cannot be cleared. This may manifest as areas of airspace disease on chest x-ray, atelectasis, or a worsening in oxygenation. In this setting, bronchoscopy is valuable to both establish the cause and clear the retained secretions.

Extracorporeal Membrane Oxygenation

Extracorporeal membrane oxygenation (ECMO) has been used with success to support patients with severe graft dysfunction resulting from ischemia-reperfusion injury. This therapy has generally been used only once conventional strategies to improve oxygenation have failed. Mechanical support is employed in some centers to treat patients with moderate to severe IR injury. ECMO employs a membrane with a large surface area through which oxygen and carbon dioxide may passively diffuse to equalize their respective concentration gradients in the patient's blood. This exploits the notion that resting the lung will allow time for the graft to overcome the initial IR insult. At present a systematic evaluation of this treatment is lacking and experience is restricted to case series and registry databases.[137]

Acute Rejection

Acute rejection may occur while the transplant recipient is being cared for in the ICU, and generally occurs within the first 100 days. The signs are nonspecific, and thus it is important to differentiate the bilateral airspace infiltrates that characterize this complication from those caused by infections. Other features are also unreliable discriminators, and include low-grade fever, impaired oxygenation, and leukocytosis. Findings on chest radiography other than alveolar infiltrates include nodular or interstitial opacities and pleural effusions; after the first month acute rejection is often undetectable radiologically.[138] Routine bronchoscopy has become widely accepted as a means of differentiating infection from rejection. Bronchoalveolar lavage or protected-specimen brushing of the airways can exclude any important infection, whereas transbronchial lung biopsy (with at least five pieces of alveolated parenchyma, each containing bronchioles and more than 100 air sacs) can confirm rejection. Treatment of acute rejection entails the use of high-dose parenteral steroids (i.e., methylprednisolone 10 to 15 mg/kg daily), which usually provide a good response, though biopsy-proven rejection may persist in up to one third of patients.[61]

A detailed discussion of the problem of chronic rejection is beyond the scope of this chapter. However, intensivists may encounter these individuals who develop chronic airflow limitation (usually more than 6 months following the transplant) that is characterized histologically as bronchiolitis obliterans. Although aggressive immunosuppression is often employed, the prognosis for posttransplant bronchiolitis is still poor, with 2-year mortality rates approaching 40%.[139,140] The definitive treatment remains retransplantation.

HEART TRANSPLANTATION

THE OPERATION

Although other variations have been described, the standard approach for heart transplantation involves the creation of four separate anastomoses between the recipient atria and great vessels and the atria and great vessels of the donor heart (the biatrial technique). There has been renewed interest in bicaval and pulmonary vein to pulmonary vein anastomoses, and the bicaval technique has now been recommended by many experts.[141]

THE IMMEDIATE POSTOPERATIVE PERIOD

The care of the heart transplant recipient is similar in many respects to the care of patients who have undergone aortocoronary bypass and other cardiac operations involving cardiopulmonary bypass. The heart is denervated during the transplant procedure, and frequently a junctional rhythm develops, requiring atrial pacing and possibly isoproterenol infusion. Owing to this denervation, the transplanted heart will also have an altered physiologic response to stress. The heart becomes dependent on circulating catecholamines rather than direct sympathetic stimulation, and consequently increases in heart rate and contractility in response to stress will occur more slowly. Changes in cardiac output become much more dependent on changes in stroke volume, which are in turn mediated by changes in venous return. Sinus bradycardia is the most common dysrhythmia present following heart transplantation, and usually lasts less than a week. Isoproterenol is frequently used for both its chronotropic and inotropic properties, and is typically titrated to achieve a heart rate between 90 and 100 beats per minute. As already mentioned, temporary atrial pacing may be required. If the recipient's native atrial appendage and sulcus terminalis including the sinoatrial (SA) node are preserved during the surgical procedure, two P waves may be seen on the postoperative electrocardiogram (one from the donor heart and one from the recipient's SA node). Other atrial dysrhythmias are frequently seen and include atrial fibrillation and flutter in 15% to 20% of patients.[142]

Nearly all patients will have a pulmonary artery catheter in place for hemodynamic monitoring following the operation to help guide fluid and vasoactive management. Generally, the goal is to keep both the central venous pressure (CVP) and the pulmonary capillary wedge pressure (PCWP) <10 mm Hg if possible, though these goals should be individualized, and the management should be guided by the clinical picture and not purely based on hemodynamic measurements. Consequently intravenous fluids are used sparingly and aggressive diuresis is continued postoperatively. However, the denervated heart will not be able to respond acutely to hypovolemia with reflex tachycardia, and adequate preload must be present to maintain stroke volume and to preserve blood pressure. A decreased cardiac output can be supported with inotropes (dobutamine or milrinone), but transient support with intra-aortic balloon counterpulsation may be required. If the cardiac output acutely deteriorates, urgent echocardiography should be obtained to exclude the possibility of tamponade and to evaluate left and right ventricular dysfunction. Left ventricular function of the allograft may also be reduced and a restrictive physiology may be observed if there has been prolonged ischemic time and poor myocardial preservation. Other causes of ventricular dysfunction should be sought such as acidemia, hypovolemia, hypoxemia, and medications. Systemic vascular resistance can be decreased following the procedure, and should be supported with vasopressors.

PULMONARY HYPERTENSION

If significant pulmonary hypertension was present before the transplant procedure, it may also persist in the postoperative period. This increase in right ventricular afterload can generate significant strain on the newly transplanted right ventricle (which is accustomed to pumping against a normal mean pulmonary artery pressure). Tricuspid regurgitation is often present following the transplant (especially if the biatrial technique was used), and this may be exacerbated by increased right ventricular strain. Through its effects as a pulmonary vasodilator, isoproterenol can often reduce the right ventricular afterload that is frequently present. However, when significant pulmonary hypertension persists postoperatively, intravenous nitroglycerine, nitroprusside, and prostaglandin E may be required. If vasodilators are used in this setting, systemic infusion of α-agonists such as norepinephrine or phenylephrine may be needed to support the systemic arterial pressure. Inhaled nitric oxide offers the advantage of reducing pulmonary vascular resistance while causing minimal systemic side effects and without increasing shunting.[143–147] Routine measurement of methemoglobin level is required when nitrate-containing pulmonary vasodilators are employed. Recently, sildenafil, a cyclic guanosine monophosphate (cGMP)-specific phosphodiesterase type 5 inhibitor has been used with success for persistent pulmonary hypertension, and to prevent rebound after withdrawal of inhaled NO.[132] Owing to the expense associated with the use of inhaled NO, other inhaled therapies have been evaluated (NO donors and prostaglandin analogues) and appear to be of equal benefit.[148–151] However, the half-lives of these medications mandate repeated dosing.

RIGHT AND LEFT VENTRICULAR ASSIST DEVICES

Patients with failing hearts are frequently bridged to transplantation using mechanical cardiac assist devices. Both left (LVAD) and right (RVAD) ventricular assist devices are used.[152,153] Preliminary reports suggest that although mechanical devices may be associated with more serious adverse effects, they may be superior to medical therapy alone in supporting the patient to transplantation.[154] The role of ventricular assist devices in right ventricular failure or primary graft failure following transplantation is evolving. A report from New York reviewed one institution's experience with assist devices in 462 transplants. Of the 20 patients diagnosed with primary cardiac graft dysfunction, 11 received RVAD, 4 required LVAD, 3 received biventricular support, and 2 were treated with intra-aortic balloon counterpulsation.[155] This group with primary graft dysfunction tended to have longer ischemic times and developed early noncardiac organ dysfunction, which was the primary mode of death in the nonsurvivors. Forty-five percent were weaned from mechanical support; the mean duration of support was 114.7 $\pm$ 207 hours (median = 54 hours). The 2-year survival in this group with primary graft dysfunction was 67% compared to 79% in the entire cohort. The authors reported that ventricular recovery within 96 hours was associated with better early survival.

REJECTION

Though immunosuppressive regimens have improved the impact of episodes of acute rejection on graft function and overall survival among heart transplant recipients, this complication still is responsible for 7% of deaths within the first 30 days of the procedure.[156] Most episodes of acute rejection are asymptomatic and are diagnosed on routine endomyocardial biopsy. When symptoms are present, they are often nonspecific and may include fever, malaise, hypotension, congestive heart failure, or reduced exercise tolerance and fatigue. Consequently, surveillance for rejection through the use of endomyocardial biopsy has become standard practice. When performed by an experienced operator, this procedure is associated with a morbidity of less than 1% and a procedure-related mortality of less than 0.2%.[157,158] The most concerning complication of this procedure is cardiac perforation with acute pericardial tamponade or injury to the tricuspid valve. Typically biopsies (with multiple sampling) are performed 5 to 7 days following the transplantation and then twice weekly for the first 2 months.

Once rejection is diagnosed histologically, imaging to assess cardiac function should be obtained (two-dimensional echocardiography or multiple-gated acquisition).[141] Mild rejection in the absence of cardiac dysfunction is usually treated conservatively with an increase in the dose of immunosuppressive agents. If moderate rejection or left ventricular dysfunction is present, the episode of rejection should be treated using high-dose pulsed steroids with or without cytolytic therapy (antithymocyte globulin or OKT3). Repeat endomyocardial biopsy should always be performed to assess the response to therapy.

Chronic rejection in the cardiac allograft typically manifests as aggressive and premature coronary artery disease. This complication usually develops months to years after the procedure, and usually will not involve the intensivist. In contrast to classic coronary artery disease, transplant-associated coronary artery disease is generally more diffuse, involving all the vessels of the heart including the arteries, veins, and great vessels. Because the allograft is denervated, classic angina only develops in a minority of patients, and coronary artery disease more typically presents with "angina-equivalent" symptoms such as dyspnea.

KIDNEY-PANCREAS TRANSPLANTATION

THE OPERATION
Kidney-pancreas transplantation is almost exclusively performed on patients with end-stage kidney disease secondary to diabetes mellitus.

POSTOPERATIVE CARE
Following kidney-pancreas transplantation many patients will not require ICU admission, and can be extubated before leaving the recovery room. However, ICU admission may be necessary for these patients because of pre-existing medical problems, due to difficulties encountered during the operation, or owing to complications that develop in the postoperative period.

The most common initial complication following the transplant of a kidney is oliguric or nonoliguric acute tubular necrosis (ATN) resulting from ischemic-preservation injury to the renal allograft. Care must be taken in this setting to avoid hypovolemia which can lead to prerenal azotemia and exacerbate the ATN. Urine output following the transplant procedure is usually high (800 to 1000 mL/h) and should be associated with a decline in creatinine; a lower urine output in the immediate postoperative period may herald graft dysfunction. Fluid management can often be facilitated through the use of a pulmonary artery catheter for hemodynamic monitoring. If oliguria develops, the urinary catheter should be flushed to ensure patency, especially if hematuria has been observed. Duplex sonography or radionuclide renal imaging should be considered to exclude the possibility of vascular thrombosis. If these interventions fail to elucidate the cause of the oliguria, the most likely remaining explanation is ATN and ischemic-preservation injury.

Following combined kidney-pancreas transplantation patients are at risk of developing metabolic derangements, and are particularly prone to developing hyper- or hypoglycemia. Usually a continuous intravenous infusion of insulin is started intraoperatively and continued through the postoperative period. A glucose-containing maintenance infusion should also

be used to protect against the development of hypoglycemia. Care should be taken to avoid mixing medications in glucose-containing solutions, as these will provide boluses of glucose that can aggravate the control of blood sugar levels.

REJECTION
The diagnosis of rejection in recipients of pancreas transplants is often challenging. Overt hyperglycemia does not occur until approximately 80% to 90% of the allograft has been destroyed, and consequently by the time clinical evidence of rejection is present it is often too late for therapy to be effective. For this reason, diagnosis of pancreatic rejection is usually made by inference after diagnosing rejection in a kidney allograft. This likely explains the improved graft survival in recipients of combined kidney-pancreas transplants as compared to patients who only receive a pancreas transplant; in the former group rejection is likely diagnosed and treated at a much earlier stage. In contrast, rejection of a renal allograft is usually suspected when the serum creatinine rises by more than 10%. If another cause of renal dysfunction (such as prerenal azotemia, pyelonephritis, etc) is not readily apparent, kidney biopsy should be performed. This procedure is relatively safe and will enable treatment of rejection to be instituted early and promptly. Recent reports suggest that use of the renal arterial resistance index[159] or DNA microarray profiling[160] may become important methods for diagnosing rejection in the renal allograft in the future.[161]

Other Management Issues Involving Solid Organ Transplant Recipients

THE DEVELOPMENT OF LUNG INFILTRATES IN THE TRANSPLANT PATIENT

A frequently encountered problem following the transplant procedure is the development of lung infiltrates. Though pneumonia is common, there are a variety of other conditions that cause a similar appearance on chest radiography and must be considered. These include congestive heart failure, atelectasis, ARDS, aspiration, and transfusion-related acute lung injury. In the lung transplant recipient, IR injury or rejection of the allograft also have a nonspecific appearance on chest radiography. Thus it is important that the clinician have an approach to the patient who develops lung infiltrates.

Because pulmonary infections may progress rapidly in the immunocompromised host, empiric antimicrobial therapy should be started promptly if pneumonia is suspected. Usually the patient will have other signs of infection such as fever or leukocytosis, but these findings will not always be present, depending on the degree of immunosuppression. Usually there is increased quantity and purulence of sputum or secretions from the endotracheal tube. If possible, respiratory secretions should be cultured prior to the initiation of empiric antibiotics. Invasive tests such as bronchoalveolar lavage or protected brush specimen obtained through bronchoscopy may be useful to optimize culture yield and ensure that appropriate antibiotic therapy is chosen.[162] If culture results are negative, the empiric antibiotics should be discontinued, as the continued use of inappropriate therapy may increase antimicrobial resistance.

Pneumonia in transplant patients may be caused by a variety of organisms, including gram-negative aerobes, fungi, *Legionella*, *P. carinii*, and viruses (especially CMV). Consequently, broad-spectrum therapy should be initiated when infection is suspected, but treatment should be changed to an appropriate agent with the narrowest spectrum of activity possible once susceptibilities of the causative organism are known. Initial therapy should have activity against *Pseudomonas* and other gram-negative organisms as well as gram-positive bacteria. Appropriate choices would include ceftazidime, piperacillin-tazobactam, or meropenem or imipenem. Consideration should be given to also including trimethoprim-sulfamethoxazole (TMP-SMX) to treat possible *P. carinii*, ganciclovir to treat CMV infection, and a macrolide to treat *Legionella*, if infection with any of these organisms is suspected.

THE TRANSPLANT PATIENT WITH DECREASED LEVEL OF CONSCIOUSNESS

A frequently encountered postoperative problem in the transplant recipient is the development of a decreased level of consciousness. When this occurs, a systematic evaluation is required to ensure that the etiology is correctly identified and appropriately treated. Distinguishing between structural problems and metabolic or drug-induced disturbances is often useful. Though the former are less common, the development of any localizing neurologic findings suggests a structural lesion and mandates CT or MRI examination. Stroke can occur in the perioperative period, and may be ischemic or embolic in nature. Perioperative cardioembolic stroke is more commonly seen following heart transplantation, and can be the result of intracardiac or aortic thrombosis. Intracranial bleeding usually occurs following hemorrhagic transformation of an ischemic infarct or a central nervous system infection. Liver transplant patients commonly develop coagulopathy, and this likely explains the relatively higher incidence of intracranial hemorrhage seen in this group.[163] Air embolism has been described in liver transplant recipients,[164–168] especially following venovenous bypass, and in cardiac and lung transplant recipients.[73,74]

Metabolic derangements leading to alterations in mental status are commonly encountered by transplant recipients. Electrolyte and glucose abnormalities are often present and should be corrected. However, care is required to avoid overly aggressive and rapid correction of sodium problems, which can precipitate central demyelination syndromes following treatment of hyponatremia or cerebral edema following treatment of hypernatremia. When present, renal failure and associated uremic encephalopathy may contribute to abnormal mentation. Hepatic encephalopathy is common in liver transplant patients and should be treated in the same manner as for all patients with liver disease. Hypoxia and hypotension can both cause a decreased level of consciousness, but are usually easily recognized.

Drug-induced depression of the central nervous system (CNS) is common. Clearance of the anaesthetic agents used during the transplant procedure may take longer in the transplant recipient, especially following liver or kidney transplantation. Narcotic analgesics, benzodiazepines, and other CNS depressants are frequently required following transplantation, and these agents may accumulate and lead to decreased arousal. Importantly, both cyclosporine and tacrolimus are associated with neurologic toxicity and can even lead to coma.[169,170] Serum levels of these agents must be monitored carefully, and if no other explanation for the decreased level of consciousness can be found the drugs must occasionally be held or discontinued. The use of tacrolimus and cyclosporine has also been linked to the development of thrombotic thrombocytopenic purpura and the hemolytic uremic syndrome, which can have neurologic manifestations.[171–173] A very rare but potentially devastating complication of transplantation that leads to severe CNS depression is the hyperammonia syndrome.[174–177] This syndrome is characterized by tremulousness progressing to seizures, coma, brain edema, and death. Severe elevations in serum ammonia will be present despite normal or only minimally elevated liver enzymes and normal indices of hepatic function. The syndrome appears to develop in individuals with abnormalities or deficiencies of enzymes in the urea cycle. Therapy consists of minimizing amino acid intake (especially parenteral), and treatments that enhance or increase elimination of nitrogenous waste products.[176,177]

Systemic infections can be associated with severe encephalopathy. However, when caring for a transplant patient, the intensivist must have a heightened suspicion for infections that involve the CNS. When these infections develop in the early postoperative period, they are usually related to nosocomial or donor-related organisms.[178,179] Meningeal signs may be lacking in the transplant recipient, and so lumbar puncture with cerebrospinal fluid analysis should be considered if CNS infection is suspected and empiric therapy should be instituted promptly.

A rare but important cause of decreased level of consciousness or coma in the transplant recipient is nonconvulsive status epilepticus. Indeed, seizures may be the most common neurologic complication for all solid-organ transplant recipients.[179] These may be precipitated by electrolyte and metabolic disturbances (especially of sodium and glucose), drugs (cyclosporine, tacrolimus, OKT3, antibiotics, etc) or drug withdrawal, CNS infections, or intracranial lesions (stroke, hemorrhage, abscess, etc). Evaluation should include CT scan and electroencephalogram, and treatment should be focused on correcting the underlying problem if possible, and treatment with benzodiazepines. Since many transplant patients are hypoalbuminemic, when therapy with phenytoin is employed it is necessary to calculate the unbound fraction of the drug to avoid potential toxicity. Valproate is not commonly used because of its potential for myelosuppression and hepatotoxicity.[179]

Role of the Intensivist

The very nature of transplant medicine mandates the adoption of a multidisciplinary approach to patient care. As such, one of the most important roles the intensivist can assume is to coordinate the management of the patient and to act as an intermediary between the numerous specialists and professionals involved in the case. The transplant surgeon and the transplant team will need to be frequently consulted and kept informed of changes in the patient's status in order for appropriate modifications to the immunosuppressive regimen to be made or surgical intervention provided if necessary.

The needs of the transplant recipient are often quite complex, and the intensivist must frequently coordinate the involvement of other professionals, including dieticians, physiotherapists and occupational therapists, respiratory therapists, pharmacists, and nurses. It is usually the intensivist who will liaise with the patient's family and identify important psychosocial issues. Often the need to involve the social worker, psychiatrist, and chaplaincy is identified by the intensivist. Thus the critical care of the transplant patient requires the intensivist to be an expert in acute physiology and to have an understanding of the important medical issues facing the recipient, but also requires someone who can coordinate other professionals involved in the patient's care, and identify the medical and social needs of both the patient and family. It is only through such a multidisciplinary approach, coordinated by the intensivist, that transplant patients will achieve good outcomes.

References

1. United Network for Organ Sharing: 2002 Annual Report of the U.S. Organ Procurement and Transplantation Network and the Scientific Registry of Transplant Recipients: Transplant Data 1992–2001. Rockville, MD, Department of Health and Human Services/Health Resources and Services Administration/Office of Special Programs/Division of Transplantation, p 1.

2. Eason JD, et al: Steroid-free liver transplantation using rabbit antithymocyte globulin and early tacrolimus monotherapy. *Transplantation* 75:1396, 2003.

3. Kahan BD: Cyclosporine. *N Engl J Med* 321:1725, 1989.

4. Grant D, et al: Peak cyclosporine levels (Cmax) correlate with freedom from liver graft rejection: results of a prospective, randomized comparison of Neoral and Sandimmune for liver transplantation (NOF-8). *Transplantation* 67:1133, 1999.

5. Gummert JF, Ikonen T, Morris RE: Newer immunosuppressive drugs: a review. *J Am Soc Nephrol* 10:1366, 1999.

6. Mayer AD, et al: Multicenter randomized trial comparing tacrolimus (FK506) and cyclosporine in the prevention of renal allograft rejection: A report of the European Tacrolimus Multicenter Renal Study Group. *Transplantation* 64:436, 1997.

7. Randomised trial comparing tacrolimus (FK506) and cyclosporin in prevention of liver allograft rejection. European FK506 Multicentre Liver Study Group. *Lancet* 344:423, 1994.

8. A comparison of tacrolimus (FK 506) and cyclosporine for immunosuppression in liver transplantation. The U.S. Multicenter FK506 Liver Study Group. *N Engl J Med* 331:1110, 1994.

9. First MR, et al: Posttransplant diabetes mellitus in kidney allograft recipients: Incidence, risk factors, and management. *Transplantation* 73:379, 2002.

10. Ericzon B, et al: Glucose metabolism in liver transplant recipients treated with FK 506 or cyclosporin in the European multicentre study. *Transpl Int* 7(Suppl 1):S11, 1994.

11. Artz MA, et al: Improved cardiovascular risk profile and renal function in renal transplant patients after randomized conversion from cyclosporine to tacrolimus. *J Am Soc Nephrol* 14:1880, 2003.

12. Liver Transplantation—Excess Mortality, Graft Loss, and Hepatic Artery Thrombosis (HAT) with Sirolimus. Letter from Wyeth to the U.S. Food and Drug Association, 2002.

13. Morelon E, Stern M, Kreis H: Interstitial pneumonitis associated with sirolimus therapy in renal-transplant recipients. *N Engl J Med* 343:225, 2000.

14. Morelon E, et al: Characteristics of sirolimus-associated interstitial pneumonitis in renal transplant patients. *Transplantation* 72:787, 2001.

15. Henry MT, Newstead CG: Sirolimus: another cause of drug-induced interstitial pneumonitis. *Transplantation* 72:773, 2001.

16. Lennon A, et al: Interstitial pneumonitis associated with sirolimus (rapamycin) therapy after liver transplantation. *Transplantation* 72:1166, 2001.

17. King-Biggs MB, et al: Airway anastomotic dehiscence associated with use of sirolimus immediately after lung transplantation. *Transplantation* 75:1437, 2003.

18. Letter from Wyeth Medical Affairs to Health Care Providers. Warning regarding bronchial anastomotic dehiscence including fatal cases, 2003.

19. Meier-Kriesche HU, et al: Long-term use of mycophenolate mofetil is associated with a reduction in the incidence and risk of late rejection. *Am J Transplant* 3:68, 2003.

20. A randomized clinical trial of OKT3 monoclonal antibody for acute rejection of cadaveric renal transplants. Ortho Multicenter Transplant Study Group. *N Engl J Med* 313:337, 1985.

21. Chatenoud L, Ferran C, Bach JF: The anti-CD3-induced syndrome: A consequence of massive in vivo cell activation. *Curr Top Microbiol Immunol* 174:121, 1991.

22. Dmitrewski J, et al: Metabolic and hormonal effects of tacrolimus (FK506) or cyclosporin immunosuppression following renal transplantation. *Diabetes Obes Metab* 3:287, 2001.

23. Yoshida EM, et al: Post-transplant diabetic ketoacidosis—a possible consequence of immunosuppression with calcineurin inhibiting agents: a case series. *Transpl Int* 13:69, 2000.

24. Polastri L, et al: Secretory defects induced by immunosuppressive agents on human pancreatic beta-cells. *Acta Diabetol* 39:229, 2002.

25. Fuhrer DK, Kobayashi M, Jiang H: Insulin release and suppression by tacrolimus, rapamycin and cyclosporin A are through regulation of the ATP-sensitive potassium channel. *Diabetes Obes Metab* 3:393, 2001.

26. Adu D, et al: Interleukin-2 receptor monoclonal antibodies in renal transplantation: meta-analysis of randomised trials. *BMJ* 326:789, 2003.

27. Vincenti F, et al: Interleukin-2-receptor blockade with daclizumab to prevent acute rejection in renal transplantation. Daclizumab Triple Therapy Study Group. *N Engl J Med* 338:161, 1998.

28. Beniaminovitz A, et al: Prevention of rejection in cardiac transplantation by blockade of the interleukin-2 receptor with a monoclonal antibody. *N Engl J Med* 342:613, 2000.

29. Fishman JA, Rubin RH: Infection in organ-transplant recipients. *N Engl J Med* 338:1741, 1998.

30. Rubin RH, et al: Infection in the renal transplant recipient. *Am J Med* 70:405, 1981.

31. Villacian JS, Paya CV: Prevention of infections in solid organ transplant recipients. *Transpl Infect Dis* 1:50, 1999.

32. Halpern SD, Ubel PA, Caplan AL: Solid-organ transplantation in HIV-infected patients. *N Engl J Med* 347:284, 2002.

33. Roland ME, Havlir DV: Responding to organ failure in HIV-infected patients. *N Engl J Med* 348:2279, 2003.

34. Calabrese LH, et al: Successful cardiac transplantation in an HIV-1-infected patient with advanced disease. *N Engl J Med* 348:2323, 2003.

35. Targeted tuberculin testing and treatment of latent tuberculosis infection. Official statement of the American Thoracic Society was adopted by the ATS Board of Directors, July 1999. *Am J Respir Crit Care Med* 161:S221, 2000.

36. Soave R: Prophylaxis strategies for solid-organ transplantation. *Clin Infect Dis* 33(Suppl 1):S26, 2001.

37. Pacetti SA, Gelone SP: Caspofungin acetate for treatment of invasive fungal infections. *Ann Pharmacother* 37:90, 2003.

38. Pound MW, Drew RH, Perfect JR: Recent advances in the epidemiology, prevention, diagnosis, and treatment of fungal pneumonia. *Curr Opin Infect Dis* 15:183, 2002.

39. Letscher-Bru V, Herbrecht R: Caspofungin: the first representative of a new antifungal class. *J Antimicrob Chemother* 51:513, 2003.

40. Kontoyiannis DP, et al: Combination of caspofungin with inhibitors of the calcineurin pathway attenuates growth in vitro in *Aspergillus* species. *J Antimicrob Chemother* 51:313, 2003.

40a. Herbrecht R, Denning DW, Patterson TF, et al: Voriconazole versus amphotericin B for primary therapy of invasive aspergillosis. *N Engl J Med* 347:408, 2002.

41. Kusne S, Shapiro R, Fung J: Prevention and treatment of cytomegalovirus infection in organ transplant recipients. *Transpl Infect Dis* 1:187, 1999.

42. Peggs KS, Preiser W, Kottaridis PD, et al: Extended routine polymerase chain reaction surveillance and pre-emptive antiviral therapy for cytomegalovirus after allogeneic transplantation. *Br J Haematol* 111:782, 2000.

43. Rubin RH: Cytomegalovirus in solid organ transplantation. *Transpl Infect Dis* 3(Suppl 2):1, 2001.

44. Manez R, et al: Factors associated with the development of post-transplant lymphoproliferative disease (PTLD) in Epstein-Barr virus (EBV)-seronegative adult liver transplant recipients. *Transpl Int* 7(Suppl 1): S235, 1994.

45. Walker RC, et al: Pretransplantation assessment of the risk of lymphoproliferative disorder. *Clin Infect Dis* 20:1346, 1995.

46. Tzakis AG: Cytomegalovirus prophylaxis with ganciclovir and cytomegalovirus immune globulin in liver and intestinal transplantation. *Transpl Infect Dis* 3(Suppl 2):35, 2001.

47. Squifflet JP, Legendre C: The economic value of valacyclovir prophylaxis in transplantation. *J Infect Dis* 186(Suppl 1):S116, 2002.

48. Batiuk TD, Bodziak KA, Goldman M: Infectious disease prophylaxis in renal transplant patients: A survey of U.S. transplant centers. *Clin Transplant* 16:1, 2002.

49. Rubin RH: Prevention of infection in the liver transplant recipient. *Liver Transpl Surg* 2(5 Suppl 1):89, 1996.

50. Cuervas-Mons V, et al: Bacterial infections in liver transplant patients under selective decontamination with norfloxacin. *Transplant Proc* 21:3558, 1989.

51. Emre S, et al: Selective decontamination of the digestive tract helps prevent bacterial infections in the early postoperative period after liver transplant. *Mt Sinai J Med* 66:310, 1999.

52. Zwaveling JH, et al: Selective decontamination of the digestive tract to prevent postoperative infection: A randomized placebo-controlled trial in liver transplant patients. *Crit Care Med* 30:1204, 2002.

53. Lo C, et al: Prophylaxis and treatment of recurrent hepatitis B after liver transplantation. *Transplantation* 75(3 Suppl):S41, 2003.

54. Forman LM, et al: The association between hepatitis C infection and survival after orthotopic liver transplantation. *Gastroenterology* 122:889, 2002.

55. Nair S, et al: Treatment of recurrent hepatitis C in liver transplant recipients: Is there any histologic benefit? *Liver Transpl* 9:354, 2003.

56. Lumbreras C, et al: Randomized trial of fluconazole versus nystatin for the prophylaxis of *Candida* infection following liver transplantation. *J Infect Dis* 174:583, 1996.

57. Winston DJ, Pakrasi A, Busuttil RW: Prophylactic fluconazole in liver transplant recipients. A randomized, double-blind, placebo-controlled trial. *Ann Intern Med* 131:729, 1999.

58. Tollemar J, et al: Liposomal amphotericin B prevents invasive fungal infections in liver transplant recipients. A randomized, placebo-controlled study. *Transplantation* 59:45, 1995.

59. Tollemar J, et al: Prophylaxis with liposomal amphotericin B (AmBisome) prevents fungal infections in liver transplant recipients: Long-term results of a randomized, placebo-controlled trial. *Transplant Proc* 27:1195, 1995.

60. Husain S, et al: Changes in the spectrum and risk factors for invasive candidiasis in liver transplant recipients: Prospective, multicenter, case-controlled study. *Transplantation* 75:2023, 2003.

61. Arcasoy SM, Kotloff RM: Lung transplantation. *N Engl J Med* 340:1081, 1999.

62. Maurer JR, et al: Infectious complications following isolated lung transplantation. *Chest* 101:1056, 1992.

63. Husain S, Singh N: *Burkholderia cepacia* infection and lung transplantation. *Semin Respir Infect* 17:284, 2002.

64. Charman SC, et al: Assessment of survival benefit after lung transplantation by patient diagnosis. *J Heart Lung Transplant* 21:226, 2002.

65. Egan TM, et al: Long term results of lung transplantation for cystic fibrosis. *Eur J Cardiothorac Surg* 22:602, 2002.

66. Helmi M, et al: *Aspergillus* infection in lung transplant recipients with cystic fibrosis: risk factors and outcomes comparison to other types of transplant recipients. *Chest* 123:800, 2003.

67. Chan KM, Allen SA: Infectious pulmonary complications in lung transplant recipients. *Semin Respir Infect* 17:291, 2002.

68. Burns KE, Johnson BA, Iacono AT: Diagnostic properties of transbronchial biopsy in lung transplant recipients who require mechanical ventilation. *J Heart Lung Transplant* 22:267, 2003.

69. Weill D, et al: The utility of open lung biopsy following lung transplantation. *J Heart Lung Transplant* 19:852, 2000.

70. Chaparro C, et al: Role of open lung biopsy for diagnosis in lung transplant recipients: ten-year experience. *Ann Thorac Surg* 59:928, 1995.

71. van der Bij W, Speich R: Management of cytomegalovirus infection and disease after solid-organ transplantation. *Clin Infect Dis* 33(Suppl 1):S32, 2001.

72. Dajani AS, et al: Prevention of bacterial endocarditis. Recommendations by the American Heart Association. *JAMA* 277:1794, 1997.

73. Tingleff J, Joyce FS, Pettersson G: Intraoperative echocardiographic study of air embolism during cardiac operations. *Ann Thorac Surg* 60:673, 1995.

74. McCarthy PM, et al: Air embolism in single-lung transplant patients after central venous catheter removal. *Chest* 107:1178, 1995.

75. Trotter JF, et al: Adult-to-adult transplantation of the right hepatic lobe from a living donor. *N Engl J Med* 346:1074, 2002.

76. Brown RS Jr, et al: A survey of liver transplantation from living adult donors in the United States. *N Engl J Med* 348:818, 2003.

77. Glanemann M, et al: Incidence and indications for reintubation during postoperative care following orthotopic liver transplantation. *J Clin Anesth* 13:77, 2001.

78. Mandell MS, et al: Reduced use of intensive care after liver transplantation: influence of early extubation. *Liver Transpl* 8:676, 2002.

79. Mandell MS, et al: Reduced use of intensive care after liver transplantation: patient attributes that determine early transfer to surgical wards. *Liver Transpl* 8:682, 2002.

80. Glanemann M, et al: Postoperative tracheal extubation after orthotopic liver transplantation. *Acta Anaesthesiol Scand* 45:333, 2001.

81. Neelakanta G, et al: Early tracheal extubation after liver transplantation. *J Cardiothorac Vasc Anesth* 11:165, 1997.

82. Mandell MS, Lockrem J, Kelley SD: Immediate tracheal extubation after liver transplantation: Experience of two transplant centers. *Anesth Analg* 84:249, 1997.

83. Findlay JY, et al: Aprotinin reduces red blood cell transfusion in orthotopic liver transplantation: A prospective, randomized, double-blind study. *Liver Transpl* 7:802, 2001.

84. Molenaar IQ, et al: Aprotinin in orthotopic liver transplantation: Evidence for a prohemostatic, but not a prothrombotic, effect. *Liver Transpl* 7:896, 2001.

85. Rentoul TM, Harrison VL, Shun A: The effect of aprotinin on transfusion requirements in pediatric orthotopic liver transplantation. *Pediatr Transplant* 7:142, 2003.

86. Findlay JY, Kufner RP: Aprotinin reduces vasoactive medication use during adult liver transplantation. *J Clin Anesth* 15:19, 2003.

87. Molenaar IQ, et al: Reduced need for vasopressors in patients receiving aprotinin during orthotopic liver transplantation. *Anesthesiology* 94:433, 2001.

88. Molenaar IQ, et al: The effect of aprotinin on renal function in orthotopic liver transplantation. *Transplantation* 71:247, 2001.

89. Molenaar IQ, Porte RJ: Aprotinin and thromboembolism in liver transplantation: Is there really a causal effect? *Anesth Analg* 94:1367, 2002.

90. Fitzsimons MG, Peterfreund RA, Raines DE: Aprotinin administration and pulmonary thromboembolism during orthotopic liver transplantation: report of two cases. *Anesth Analg* 92:1418, 2001.

91. Levy MF, et al: Readmission to the intensive care unit after liver transplantation. *Crit Care Med* 29:18, 2001.

92. Krowka MJ, et al: Pulmonary hemodynamics and perioperative cardiopulmonary-related mortality in patients with portopulmonary hypertension undergoing liver transplantation. *Liver Transpl* 6:443, 2000.

93. Lowell JA, Shaw BW Jr: Critical care of liver transplant recipients, in Maddrey WC, Schiff ER, Sorrell MF (eds): *Transplantation of the Liver*. Philadelphia, Lippincott, Williams & Wilkins, 2001, p 385.

94. McGilvray ID, Greig PD: Critical care of the liver transplant patient: an update. *Curr Opin Crit Care* 8:178, 2002.

95. Cardenas A, et al: Hepatorenal syndrome. *Liver Transpl* 6(4 Suppl 1):S63, 2000.

96. Seu P, et al: The hepatorenal syndrome in liver transplant recipients. *Am Surg* 57:806, 1991.

97. Tepel M, et al: Prevention of radiographic-contrast-agent-induced reductions in renal function by acetylcysteine. *N Engl J Med* 343:180, 2000.

98. Solanki P, et al: Beneficial effects of terlipressin in hepatorenal syndrome: a prospective, randomized placebo-controlled clinical trial. *J Gastroenterol Hepatol* 18:152, 2003.

99. Sen S, Mookerjee RP, Jalan R: Terlipressin-induced vasoconstriction reversed with N-acetylcysteine: a case for combined use in hepatorenal syndrome? *Gastroenterology* 123:2160, 2002.

100. Ortega R, et al: Terlipressin therapy with and without albumin for patients with hepatorenal syndrome: results of a prospective, nonrandomized study. *Hepatology* 36:941, 2002.

101. Blendis L, Wong F: The natural history and management of hepatorenal disorders: From pre-ascites to hepatorenal syndrome. *Clin Med* 3:154, 2003.

102. Moreau R: Hepatorenal syndrome in patients with cirrhosis. *J Gastroenterol Hepatol* 17:739, 2002.

103. Fernandez-Merino J, Nuno-Garza J, Lopez-Hervas P, et al: Influence of ischemia and surgery times on development of primary dysfunction liver transplant in patients. *Transplant Proc* 35:1439, 2003.

104. Bennett-Guerrero E, Feierman DE, Barclay GR, et al: Preoperative and intraoperative predictors of postoperative morbidity, poor graft function, and early rejection in 190 patients undergoing liver transplantation. *Arch Surg* 136:1177, 2001.

105. Pokorny H, Gruenberger T, Soliman T, et al: Organ survival after primary dysfunction of liver grafts in clinical orthotopic liver transplantation. *Transpl Int* 13 Suppl 1:S154, 2000.

106. Lerut J, Laterre PF, Roggen F, et al: Adult hepatic retransplantation. UCL experience. *Acta Gastroenterol Belg* 62:261, 1999.

107. Brokelman W, Stel AH, Ploeg RJ: Risk factors for primary dysfunction after liver transplantation in the University of Wisconsin solution era. *Transplant Proc* 31:2087, 1999.

108. Kok T, et al: Routine Doppler ultrasound for the detection of clinically unsuspected vascular complications in the early postoperative phase after orthotopic liver transplantation. *Transpl Int* 11:272, 1998.

109. Pungpapong S, et al: Cigarette smoking is associated with an increased incidence of vascular complications after liver transplantation. *Liver Transpl* 8:582, 2002.

110. Cavallari A, et al: Treatment of vascular complications following liver transplantation: multidisciplinary approach. *Hepatogastroenterology* 48:179, 2001.

111. Stange BJ, et al: Hepatic artery thrombosis after adult liver transplantation. *Liver Transpl* 9:612, 2003.

112. Trotter JF: Sirolimus in liver transplantation. *Transplant Proc* 35:S193, 2003.

113. Fleck A, et al: Biliary tract complications after orthotopic liver transplantation in adult patients. *Transplant Proc* 34:519, 2002.

114. Park JS, et al: Efficacy of endoscopic and percutaneous treatments for biliary complications after cadaveric and living donor liver transplantation. *Gastrointest Endosc* 57:78, 2003.

115. Ritchie M, et al: Echocardiographic characterization of the improvement in right ventricular function in patients with severe pulmonary hypertension after single-lung transplantation. *J Am Coll Cardiol* 22:1170, 1993.

116. de Perrot M, et al: Ischemia-reperfusion-induced lung injury. *Am J Respir Crit Care Med* 167:490, 2003.

117. King RC, et al: Reperfusion injury significantly impacts clinical outcome after pulmonary transplantation. *Ann Thorac Surg* 69:1681, 2000.

118. Schulman LL: Perioperative mortality and primary graft failure. *Chest* 114:7, 1998.

119. Fiser SM, et al: Ischemia-reperfusion injury after lung transplantation increases risk of late bronchiolitis obliterans syndrome. *Ann Thorac Surg* 73:1041, 2002.

120. Kundu S, Herman SJ, Winton TL: Reperfusion edema after lung transplantation: Radiographic manifestations. *Radiology* 206:75, 1998.

121. Ventilation with lower tidal volumes as compared with traditional tidal volumes for acute lung injury and the acute respiratory distress syndrome. The Acute Respiratory Distress Syndrome Network. *N Engl J Med* 342:1301, 2000.

122. Bacha EA, et al: Lasting beneficial effect of short-term inhaled nitric oxide on graft function after lung transplantation. Paris-Sud University Lung Transplantation Group. *J Thorac Cardiovasc Surg* 112:590, 1996.

123. Ardehali A, et al: A prospective trial of inhaled nitric oxide in clinical lung transplantation. *Transplantation* 72:112, 2001.

124. Bacha EA, et al: Inhaled nitric oxide attenuates reperfusion injury in non-heartbeating-donor lung transplantation. Paris-Sud University Lung Transplantation Group. *Transplantation* 63:1380, 1997.

125. Date H, et al: Inhaled nitric oxide reduces human lung allograft dysfunction. *J Thorac Cardiovasc Surg* 111:913, 1996.

126. Fukahara K, et al: Inhaled nitric oxide after lung ischemia reperfusion: effect on hemodynamics and oxygen free radical scavenger system. *Eur J Cardiothorac Surg* 11:343, 1997.

127. Meade MO, et al: A randomized trial of inhaled nitric oxide to prevent ischemia-reperfusion injury after lung transplantation. *Am J Respir Crit Care Med* 167:1483, 2003.

128. Adatia I, et al: Inhaled nitric oxide in the treatment of postoperative graft dysfunction after lung transplantation. *Ann Thorac Surg* 57:1311, 1994.

129. Della Rocca G, et al: Hemodynamics during inhaled nitric oxide in lung transplant candidates. *Transplant Proc* 29:3367, 1997.

130. Fiser SM, et al: Early intervention after severe oxygenation index elevation improves survival following lung transplantation. *J Heart Lung Transplant* 20:631, 2001.

131. Sokol J, Jacobs SE, Bohn D: Inhaled nitric oxide for acute hypoxemic respiratory failure in children and adults. *Cochrane Database Syst Rev* 1:CD002787, 2003.

132. Atz AM, Wessel DL: Sildenafil ameliorates effects of inhaled nitric oxide withdrawal. *Anesthesiology* 91:307, 1999.

133. Chakinala MM, Kollef MH, Trulock EP: Critical care aspects of lung transplant patients. *J Intensive Care Med* 17:8, 2002.

134. Venuta F, et al: Thoracoscopic volume reduction of the native lung after single lung transplantation for emphysema. *Am J Respir Crit Care Med* 157:292, 1998.

135. Anderson MB, et al: Volume reduction surgery in the native lung after single lung transplantation for emphysema. *J Heart Lung Transplant* 16:752, 1997.

136. Meyers BF, et al: Lung transplantation: A decade of experience. *Ann Surg* 230:362, 1999.

137. Bohn D: Extracorporeal life support in heart and lung transplantation. *Semin Thorac Cardiovasc Surg Pediatr Card Surg Annu* 4:94, 2001.

138. Millet B, et al: The radiographic appearances of infection and acute rejection of the lung after heart-lung transplantation. *Am Rev Respir Dis* 140:62, 1989.

139. Date H, et al: The impact of cytolytic therapy on bronchiolitis obliterans syndrome. *J Heart Lung Transplant* 17:869, 1998.

140. Ross DJ, et al: FK 506 "rescue" immunosuppression for obliterative bronchiolitis after lung transplantation. *Chest* 112:1175, 1997.

141. Ross H, et al: 2001 Canadian Cardiovascular Society Consensus Conference on cardiac transplantation. *Can J Cardiol* 19:620, 2003.

142. Little RE, et al: Arrhythmias after orthotopic cardiac transplantation. Prevalence and determinants during initial hospitalization and late follow-up. *Circulation* 80(5 Pt 2):III140, 1989.

143. Ardehali A, et al: Inhaled nitric oxide for pulmonary hypertension after heart transplantation. *Transplantation* 72:638, 2001.

144. Auler JO Jr, et al: Low doses of inhaled nitric oxide in heart transplant recipients. *J Heart Lung Transplant* 15:443, 1996.

145. Kieler-Jensen N, Lundin S, Ricksten SE: Vasodilator therapy after heart transplantation: effects of inhaled nitric oxide and intravenous prostacyclin, prostaglandin E_1, and sodium nitroprusside. *J Heart Lung Transplant* 14:436, 1995.

146. Mosquera I, et al: Pulmonary hypertension and right ventricular failure after heart transplantation: usefulness of nitric oxide. *Transplant Proc* 34:166, 2002.

147. Pielstickler EJ, Martinez FJ, Rubenfire M: Lung and heart-lung transplant practice patterns in pulmonary hypertension centres. *J Heart Lung Transplant* 20:1297, 2001.

148. Sablotzki A, et al: Iloprost improves hemodynamics in patients with severe chronic cardiac failure and secondary pulmonary hypertension. *Can J Anaesth* 49:1076, 2002.

149. Wittwer T, Franke U, Wahlers T: Impact of aerosolized prostacyclin analog for severe pulmonary hypertension in thoracic organ transplantation. *J Thorac Cardiovasc Surg* 124:211, 2002.

150. Haraldsson A, Kieler-Jensen N, Ricksten S: Inhaled prostacyclin for treatment of pulmonary hypertension after cardiac surgery or heart transplantation: a pharmacodynamic study. *J Cardiothorac Vasc Surg* 10:864, 1996.

151. Stobierska-Dzierzek B, Awad H, Michler RE: The evolving management of acute right-sided heart failure in cardiac transplant recipients. *J Am Coll Cardiol* 38:923, 2001.

152. Aaronson KD, et al: Left ventricular assist device therapy improves utilization of donor hearts. *J Am Coll Cardiol* 39:1247, 2002.

153. Richenbacher WE, et al: Surgical management of patients in the REMATCH trial. *Ann Thorac Surg* 75:S86, 2003.

154. Jaski BE, et al: Cardiac transplant outcome of patients supported on left ventricular assist device vs. intravenous inotropic therapy. *J Heart Lung Transplant* 20:449, 2001.

155. Kavarana MN, et al: Mechanical support for the failing cardiac allograft: a single-center experience. *J Heart Lung Transplant* 22:542, 2003.

156. Hosenpud JD, et al: The Registry of the International Society for Heart and Lung Transplantation: eighteenth Official Report—2001. *J Heart Lung Transplant* 20:805, 2001.

157. Billingham ME: Diagnosis of cardiac rejection by endomyocardial biopsy. *J Heart Lung Transplant* 1:25, 1982.

158. Reitz BA, et al: Diagnosis and treatment of allograft rejection in heart-lung transplant recipients. *J Thorac Cardiovasc Surg* 85:354, 1983.

159. Radermacher J, Mengel M, Ellis S, et al: The renal arterial resistance index and renal allograft survival. *N Engl J Med* 349:115, 2003.

160. Sarwal M, Chua MS, Kambham N, et al: Molecular heterogeneity in acute renal allograft rejection identified by DNA microarray profiling. *N Engl J Med* 349:125, 2003.

161. Marsden P: Predicting outcomes after renal transplantation—new tools and old tools. *N Engl J Med* 349:182, 2003.

162. Fagon JY, et al: Invasive and noninvasive strategies for management of suspected ventilator-associated pneumonia. A randomized trial. *Ann Intern Med* 132:621, 2000.

163. Wijdicks EF, et al: Intracerebral hemorrhage in liver transplant recipients. *Mayo Clin Proc* 70:443, 1995.

164. Wong AY, O'Regan A, Irwin MG: Venous air embolism during liver transplantation. *Anaesth Intensive Care* 29:668, 2001.

165. Olmedilla L, et al: Fatal paradoxical air embolism during liver transplantation. *Br J Anaesth* 84:112, 2000.

166. Thiery G, et al: Paradoxical air embolism during orthotopic liver transplantation: Diagnosis by transoesophageal echocardiography. *Eur J Anaesthesiol* 16:342, 1999.

167. Souron V, et al: Venous air embolism during orthotopic liver transplantation in a child. *Can J Anaesth* 44:1187, 1997.

168. Murakawa M, et al: Prevention of venous air embolism related to veno-venous bypass during orthotopic liver transplantation. *Anesthesiology* 76:662, 1992.

169. Mueller AR, et al: Severe neurotoxicity after liver transplantation: association between FK 506 therapy and hepatitis C virus disease. *Transplant Proc* 26:3131, 1994.

170. Mueller AR, et al: Neurotoxicity after orthotopic liver transplantation. A comparison between cyclosporine and FK506. *Transplantation* 58:155, 1994.

171. Masterson R, et al: Sirolimus: a single center experience in combination with calcineurin inhibitors. *Transplant Proc* 35:S99, 2003.

172. Evens AM, et al: TTP/HUS occurring in a simultaneous pancreas/kidney transplant recipient after clopidogrel treatment: evidence of a nonimmunological etiology. *Transplantation* 74:885, 2002.

173. Chiurchiu C, Ruggenenti P, Remuzzi G: Thrombotic microangiopathy in renal transplantation. *Ann Transplant* 7:28, 2002.

174. Yoshida EM, et al: Hyperammonemia after heart-lung transplantation. *Gastroenterology* 112:2162, 1997.

175. Lichtenstein GR, et al: Fatal hyperammonemia following orthotopic lung transplantation. *Gastroenterology* 112:236, 1997.

176. Rueda JF, Caldwell C, Brennan DC: Successful treatment of hyperammonemia after lung transplantation. *Ann Intern Med* 128:956, 1998.

177. Berry GT, et al: Successful use of alternate waste nitrogen agents and hemodialysis in a patient with hyperammonemic coma after heart-lung transplantation. *Arch Neurol* 56:481, 1999.

178. Conti DJ, Rubin RH: Infection of the central nervous system in organ transplant recipients. *Neurol Clin* 6:241, 1988.

179. Pless M, Zivkovic SA: Neurologic complications of transplantation. *Neurology* 8:107, 2002.

Chapter 91 —————————————

CARE OF THE MULTIORGAN DONOR

F. D'OVIDIO
D. MCRITCHIE
S. KESHAVJIE

KEY POINTS

- *Increasingly successful solid organ transplantation has increased the need for organ donors.*
- *Maximizing organ procurement and expanding donor acceptance criteria should decrease the organ shortage.*
- *Aggressive ongoing critical care of the multiorgan donor is essential to improve organ retrieval and posttransplant graft performance.*
- *Understanding the process of brain death is essential for directing donor treatment strategies to ensure preservation and function of donor organs.*
- *The goals of management of the multiorgan donor are to maximize organ function by maintaining organ perfusion and oxygenation, and to promptly recognize and treat potential complications such as hypotension, dysrhythmia, pulmonary edema, massive diuresis, coagulopathy, hypothermia, and sepsis.*

Organ transplantation has evolved rapidly from the first early successes to the current widespread use of donated organs for the treatment of end-stage kidney, liver, heart, and lung failure.[1] The success of solid organ transplantation has increased the need for an expanded supply of organ donors. In response to this need, the age limit for cadaveric donors has been increased, and donors over the age of 50 years are now routinely used. The use of organs from living related donors, living unrelated donors, and non–heart-beating donors (those declared dead on the basis of cardiopulmonary criteria) has also increased. Nevertheless, there has been a progressively widening gap between the number of patients waiting for transplants and the number of transplantations performed. The number of patients on the national waiting list was 25% higher than the number of transplantations in 1988.[2] According to the United Network for Organ Sharing (UNOS), as of April 24, 2003, the number of patient registrations was 81,208, with the majority of patients in the 18- to 64-year age range. In 2002 a total of 24,847 transplants were performed, thus the number of patients on the waiting list was about 325% higher than the number of transplanted patients.[3]

In the past 10 years, the waiting list has increased 229%, and waiting list deaths have increased 192%. In contrast, during this same time period, the number of cadaveric organ donors has increased only 32%, with donors younger than 50 years of age increasing only 10.3%. The largest increase in cadaveric donors has been in donors older than 50 years of age (135%). One consequence of the increased proportion of older and more diverse donors has been the increase in organs discarded after they had been procured.[3]

The relevance of a properly functioning transplanted organ cannot be overemphasized and is clearly crucial for the success of transplantation of organs requiring immediate function such as the heart and lung. Temporary failure of the liver, kidneys, and pancreas may be tolerated with supportive measures such as hemodialysis and pharmacologic interventions. Early graft failure accounts for approximately 30% of all deaths of cardiac and lung recipients, and the deaths of 30% of liver and 5% of renal recipients.[4]

At a time when transplant surgeons are facing an increasing number of deaths on the waiting list, and as the size of the list continues to grow, there has never been a greater need to utilize a higher percentage of older or otherwise marginal donors, minimize the incidence of primary graft nonfunction, and develop organ donor management strategies that continue to increase the number of organs available for transplant.[3,4–6]

To increase the number of transplantable organs, UNOS created the Critical Pathway for the Organ Donor, a blueprint of an organ donor's treatment plan. The Critical Pathway is a concise, one-page document designed to help critical care staff and procurement coordinators understand and follow the steps required for effective donor management.[3]

After brain death has been declared in potential organ donors and consent is given for donation, donors need to be medically managed to keep their organs viable until organ recovery can occur. The Critical Pathway describes optimal care for the organ donor and maps the process to improve the outcome for successful organ transplantation. The Pathway promotes collaboration between organ procurement coordinators and critical care staff, and delineates roles to prevent duplication of effort or confusion.

Recent studies have shown that the Critical Pathway, which has been endorsed by four major transplantation associations, significantly increased the number of organs procured and transplanted from brain-dead donors.[3,5,6] There is no sacrifice in the quality of the transplanted organs or an increase in donor management time.

The two most limiting factors in organ donation today are: (1) failure to identify patients that are potential organ donors and lack of referral of those patients to the organ procurement organization, and (2) refusal of patients' families to consent to donation. A proactive donor detection program maintained by well-trained transplant coordinators, the introduction of systematic death audits in hospitals combined with a positive social atmosphere, appropriate management of mass media relations, and appropriate economic reimbursement for the hospitals are the measures advocated by the Spanish model, which has resulted in the highest continuous increase by far in cadaveric organ donation within a large country, reaching 32.5 organ donors per million population in 2001.[7]

Once a patient has been identified as a potential organ donor, the critical pathway should be initiated by contacting the local organ procurement organization to make the referral. Referral is critical; if this does not occur the opportunity for donation may be lost entirely. Organ procurement organization staff may wish to be notified as the condition of the patient deteriorates even before brain death occurs. Most often, the organ procurement organization can quickly do a preliminary assessment to determine whether the patient is a potential candidate for organ donation. If the patient is not a candidate, there is no need to discuss the option of donation with the patient's family members, and the pathway is stopped. Furthermore, if family members broach the subject of organ donation, a clear answer can be provided as to why the patient is not a candidate for donation, and any confusion can be avoided. Even if a patient is not a candidate for organ donation, the family may have other options to consider, such as donations of eyes, skin, bone, and heart valves.[8]

Referral systems should be automatic and simple. Donors are lost when hospital staff with limited knowledge of the acceptance criteria for organ donors inappropriately rule out potential organ donors as medically unsuitable. Retrospective reviews of the records of patients who have died while in the hospital indicate that a surprising number of potential donors were never evaluated by organ procurement organization staff for this reason. The reasons given for the determination of unsuitability, if any reason is noted in the chart, are many, and include age, use of vasoactive drugs, disease (i.e., diabetes), cardiopulmonary resuscitation, and positive cultures. Any patient with a significant and potentially life-threatening injury to the head, whether caused by trauma, an intracerebral hemorrhage, or an anoxic event, should be referred to the organ procurement organization as early as possible for evaluation as a potential organ donor. This practice allows the organ procurement organization to evaluate the situation and apprise staff members early on about whether the patient is a potential donor or not. Currently, only a few medical contraindications to donation are absolute, including:

- Transmissible infectious disease that will adversely affect the recipient (i.e., human immunodeficiency virus (HIV) infection, active viral hepatitis B, encephalitis of unknown cause, prion disease, malaria, and disseminated tuberculosis)
- Active visceral or hematologic malignant neoplasm
- Characteristics that indicate the organ is unlikely to function

Indeed, the only typical feature of a potential donor today is brain death, and with the increased use of non–heart-beating donors in the United States, even brain death is not necessarily typical anymore.

Early referral is also key to success in recovering transplantable organs for potential recipients. If an organ procurement organization receives a referral from the critical care staff well after brain death has occurred, decreases in end-organ function will already have taken place. If the organ procurement organization is called in only well after the signs of brain death are present, the donor who might have had 5 to 7 organs suitable for donation and transplantation may by that time have only 1 or 2 suitable organs. It has been questioned whether it is reasonable to expect nurses and physicians to keep pace with all of the changes taking place in organ donation, and thus systems have been developed and implemented, sometimes required by law, that do not rely on hospital staff to screen potential donors.[9]

Declaration of Brain Death

The introduction of successful kidney transplantation in the 1950s led to the concept of the use of organs from "heart-beating cadavers." The clinical findings of "brain death" were first described by French investigators Mollaret and Gaulon

in 1959, describing patients on ventilators who have loss of neurologic function after persistent deep coma and loss of spontaneous ventilation; they first called this condition "coma depassé" to denote neurologic damage beyond coma, but they did not equate this entity with death itself.[10] In 1968, the Ad Hoc Committee of the Harvard Medical School to Examine the Definition of Brain Death was created to standardize the definition of brain death and resolve some of the growing controversies surrounding organ procurement for transplantation from heart-beating donors. The resolutions from this committee are known as the Harvard Criteria of Brain Death. The reasons for this redefinition of death, according to the aforementioned Committee, were the need to bring relief to the families of the sick, free up beds in the intensive care units, and remove the grounds for objecting to the obtaining of organs for transplantation.[11]

Two criteria were considered for determining brain death: either the irreversible loss of all of the functions of the entire brain, including the brain stem, or the irreversible loss of the functions of the brain stem only.

The concept of brain death continues to be a topic of international debate among medical clinicians, anthropologists, philosophers, and ethicists. Much of this discussion is the result of the awareness of continuing technological advances, neurodiagnostic developments, and clinical insight. This ongoing dialogue can be viewed as a dynamically developing process of achieving a multidisciplinary consensus that is responsive to a continually changing technological environment.[11,12]

It has been argued that brain death, either when referring to the entire brain or to the brain stem alone, is a concept without a precise clinical or pathologic basis, and for this reason, the criteria employed in its diagnosis are somewhat arbitrary. It has also been said that it is difficult or almost impossible to have diagnostic standards for a condition that has never been adequately defined.[12]

Evidence-based guidelines for determining the brain-death criteria in the United States are based on the Report of the Medical Consultants on the Diagnosis of Death to the President's Commission on the Study of Ethical Problems in Medicine and Biomedical and Behavioral Research of 1981.

The President's Commission requires loss of brain stem function, loss of cortical function, and that the condition is irreversible. Although the guidelines reflect generic, scientifically based recommendations, adaptation of certain details may vary across practice settings and states according to variations in institutional policy and local legislation.[11–13] The full description of the diagnosis of brain death is explained further in chapter 67.

Request for Consent

Refusal by the family to provide consent for donation is the most common reason that organs of medically suitable potential donors are not recovered. According to estimates, 35% of the medically suitable organ donors do not donate because the family of the potential donor refuses to consent to donation. Hospitals with low donation rates were more likely to have staff members who perceived dealing with a potential donor as time-consuming and burdensome, and who were uncomfortable with how their hospital handled donation. The role that personal attitudes play in the ability of staff members to handle donation is unclear. Staff members in hospitals with high donation rates have a more positive personal attitude toward donation than do staff members in hospitals with low donation rates; however, a positive personal attitude does not correlate with the ability to approach families about donation.[9]

Another situational variable that has a marked influence on donation rates is the timing of the request (i.e., when the request is made relative to when the family is informed of the death). Research clearly shows that inappropriate timing of the request (i.e., informing the family of the death and requesting donation at the same time) is a formula for family refusal. Families need time to acknowledge the death before they are approached about donation. Consent rates have been shown to increase from 18% to 60% if there was a delay between death and the request for donation. Ensuring that this delay occurs is referred to as "decoupling" of the request. The timing of the request has been evaluated in numerous studies, and all the researchers have reached the same conclusion: that decoupling the request leads to improved donation rates. However, despite vigorous attempts by the organ donation community to educate critical care staff, and by the health care community about the importance of decoupling the request, a significant number of requests are still "coupled."[9,14]

Unfortunately, current medical school curricula generally lack training on how to break bad news and inform of death. It is important that the word "dead" should be pronounced and not avoided. At the brain death declaration, the main task of the intensive care unit staff is not that of obtaining consent for organ removal, but rather counseling and helping the family to cope with the grieving process. Minimizing the family's distress is the focus of care and is an essential prerequisite for a subsequent organ donation request.[10]

Unrestricted visits to the potential donor should not only be permitted, but actively encouraged. All the family's questions about brain death must be answered unhurriedly by the staff, and the right words should be used in front of a warm cadaver with a heart that is still beating. For example, it is better to use terms which strengthen the certainty of the death, such as "no, he does not breathe, but the ventilator forces the air into the lungs," or "yes, the heart is still pumping the blood, and it will do so for some hours more because it is artificially stimulated and this is why the skin is warm." No mention about organ donation should be raised before the concept of brain death is comprehended and the death is accepted by the family. The staff should refer to the dead patient using the past tense; as soon as family members begin to talk of him or her using "was," the acceptance of death becomes clear. The physician who is in charge of the intensive care unit should only discuss brain death with the family. The discussion relating to organ donation should be introduced by the transplant coordinator so that there is a clear distinction between the two functions (i.e., treatment of the patient and preparation for donation). The request should be made by the transplant coordinator in a positive way. It should be proposed as an option that the hospital offers the family for helping other patients, rather than an apologetic or indifferent businesslike gesture. Those who have difficulty in requesting consent should delegate the task to more confident staff. The family must never be forced into making a hasty decision, and it is always advisable to let them take their time and discuss the matter among themselves

and with other members of the family before asking again. Often an initial refusal turns into a convinced consent over the course of two or three meetings. While a firm refusal must be respected, hesitation can easily lead to authorization if the subject of the urgent need of organs for many patients, as a life-saving procedure or a dialysis-relieving therapy, is raised tactfully. The consent process for organ and tissue donation should not only be considered a necessity, but also a family's right.[9]

Obtaining consent for organ donation from families is enhanced by:

- Allowing time for families to accept death
- Having someone who is an expert in donation consent approach the family
- Approaching the family in a private, quiet area in an unhurried manner
- Involving nursing and the organ procurement organization staff in the coordination of the entire consent and donation process

Evaluation of a Potential Donor

Once consent for organ donation is given, a thorough evaluation is conducted. The organ procurement coordinator collaborates with the critical care nurse to obtain the necessary history and results of diagnostic tests. The donor's chart is reviewed for prehospital and emergency department entries for details of the events leading to admission. The duration of "downtime" (cardiopulmonary arrest) and cardiopulmonary resuscitation, vital signs, drugs administered, and obvious signs of chest and abdominal trauma are noted. If an old chart or the patient's primary physician is available, a pertinent medical history is obtained.

Completing a battery of laboratory tests in a timely manner will expedite organ placement and decrease the time required for donor management. A blood sample is also obtained from the donor, to perform bacteriologic and serological screening for infectious disease. This serological sample is usually sent to a central laboratory that performs such testing on a 24-hour basis; however, once the sample arrives at the laboratory, it usually takes about 6 hours for the results to be determined. Usually, the donation coordinator is aware of the serological results as the offers for organ-specific recovery are made.

The organ procurement coordinator reviews a comprehensive medical and social history with the appropriate family members or significant others. Donors are screened for a number of factors, including but not limited to, any history or treatment of heart disease, hypertension, chest pain, or diabetes; use of tobacco, drugs, and alcohol; and high-risk behaviors for transmission of human immunodeficiency and hepatitis viruses. Pertinent family history is reviewed also. The organ procurement coordinator does a complete physical examination of the donor, paying close attention to any finding that may influence organ integrity. The transplant surgeons determine the suitability of the donor with respect to the transplantable organs.[8–10]

SCREENING FOR INFECTIOUS AGENTS

Serological screening for HIV, human T lymphotropic virus (HTLV), hepatitis B virus (HBV), hepatitis C virus (HCV), and cytomegalovirus (CMV) is routinely performed along with screening for *Treponema* antigen (syphilis) and for *Toxoplasma*.

The presence of an active viral infection in the form of encephalitis or meningitis, varicella-zoster virus infection, or HIV infection is an absolute contraindication to organ donation because of the hazard that each of these clinical situations pose to the allograft recipient.

Isolated hepatitis B surface antibody positivity usually implies previous vaccination. Hepatitis B surface antigen (HBsAg) positivity reflects the presence of viral DNA in the blood that is related to current hepatitis B infection or a remote infection that has not cleared. These donors have contagious hepatitis B and will transmit the disease to the recipients unless the recipient has neutralizing antibodies due to previous exposure or vaccination. Patients who have acute hepatitis infection develop antibodies to the core antigen early in the course of the disease. Donors who are core antibody–positive should be considered infectious because they may be convalescing from acute infection. If both surface and core antibodies are positive, then the patient has recovered from hepatitis B and demonstrates immunity. Nevertheless, liver recipients from these donors are at significant risk for the development of acute hepatitis B infection, as opposed to the recipients of the other organs. Organs from these core-positive donors are generally reserved for patients with a documented response to the hepatitis B vaccine.[15]

All hepatitis C antibody-positive donors should be considered infectious. The hazard of HCV transmission from a previously infected organ donor is a concern for all allograft recipients. Approximately 5% of all organ donors are positive for antibody to HCV. The presence of antibody to HCV is indicative of HCV infection, because antibody to HCV appears in peripheral blood within 2 months of HCV exposure. Most organ procurement organizations have adopted a policy of screening organ donors for antibody to HCV. IgG antibody to HCV does not protect against donor organ contamination; however, it is also important to emphasize that detection of antibody to HCV by serological screening of the donor is not predictive of HCV transmission.

Although a positive screening result does not necessarily rule out organ donation, a selective strategy of reserving organs from HCV-positive donors for recipients with previous HCV exposure and detectable antibody to HCV can be applied. Transplantation of a liver from a donor positive for antibody to HCV to a recipient positive for antibody to HCV does not appear to cause increased morbidity or mortality. Transplantation of an HCV-positive heart or lung allograft when a HCV-negative recipient's life is in danger may be the only alternative to immediate death.[16,17] Kidney recipients who are hepatitis C positive can shorten their time on the waiting list by accepting a kidney from a HCV-positive donor. Table 91-1 shows the relative risk of viral transmission for hepatitis B and C viruses.[17]

Transplantation of an organ from a CMV-positive donor can result in subsequent reactivation of latent virus and replication in the immunosuppressed host. The specific CMV serological status of the donor and recipient has implications for prophylaxis, the highest-risk group being CMV-seronegative recipients of CMV-seropositive donor organs (i.e., the so-called primary infection group).

Nevertheless, transplantation of organs from CMV-seropositive donors has not been considered an absolute contraindication for transplantation, because the high seroprevalence of the virus among the general population makes it impractical to rule out such donors. Furthermore, recent evidence suggests that even mismatches between CMV-positive donors and CMV-negative recipients can be successfully overcome by strategies aimed at prophylaxis for CMV infection.

Over 95% of potential adult donors are seropositive (IgG antibody) for Epstein-Barr virus (EBV); thus serological screening of organ donors for EBV is not routinely performed. However, primary EBV infection (i.e., transplantation of an organ from an EBV-seropositive donor to an EBV-seronegative recipient) is associated with an increased risk of

TABLE 91-1 Risk of Hepatitis Viral Transmission

Donor serology	HBsAb+ recipient	HBsAb−recipient
HBsAg+	Liver: Insufficient data Non-liver: Insufficient data	Liver: High Non-liver: High
HBcAb+	Liver: Low – Moderate[a] Non-liver: Very low	Liver: Moderate to High Non-liver: low
HCVAb+	HCVAb+ recipient Liver: High[b] Non-liver: Insufficient data[c]	HCVAb−recipient Liver: High Non-liver:High

[a] Data indicate that the risk of viral transmission may be lower for recipients who are immune from previous HBV infection (HBsAb+/HBcAb+) compared to recipients who are immune from vaccination (HBsAb+/HBcAb−).
[b] Although there is evidence that the donor virus is transmitted to the recipient, repopulation after liver transplantation occurs with approximately even frequency by donor or recipient strain. Available data indicate *no* increase in short (1-year) and medium (5-year) term mortality and morbidity (incidence, timing, or severity of liver disease) is associated with transplantation of a liver from a HCVAb+ donor vs. a liver from an HCV Ab−donor into a hepatitis C+ recipient.
[c] There are insufficient data regarding persistence of donor vs. recipient virus strains after transplantation to determine the true incidence of viral transmission. Available data indicate that transplantation of a kidney from an HCVAb+ donor has *no* adverse impact on graft and patient survival (5 years) or the recipient's HCV disease compared to a kidney from an HCVAb-donor.
ABBREVIATIONS: HBsAb, hepatitis B surface antibody; HBcAb, hepatitis B core antibody; HBsAg, hepatitis B surface antigen; HCVAb, hepatitis C virus antibody; HCV, hepatitis C virus.
SOURCE: Reproduced with permission from Rosengard et al.[17]

posttransplant lymphoproliferative disease. Therefore, recognition of this mismatch in a potential allograft recipient known to be EBV-negative may be important prognostic information. Currently, there is no effective means of preventing this complication.

The detection of antibody to treponemal antigen is not a contraindication to organ procurement, but it is a contraindication to tissue procurement. A standard course of penicillin therapy would provide sufficient antibiotic coverage to prevent syphilitic complications in an allograft recipient.

The possible transmission of the protozoan *Toxoplasma gondii* is a concern, especially for heart allograft recipients, because of the predilection of this parasite for muscle tissue. Organ procurement from seropositive donors is not contraindicated; however, the detection of seropositivity means that the recipient may be placed at high risk. Fortunately, the use of trimethoprim-sulfamethoxazole as prophylaxis for *Pneumocystis carinii* infection prevents transmission of *T. gondii*.[16]

Regional directives will need to be implemented as necessary with regard to novel infectious agents carrying alarming epidemic/pandemic life-threatening potential. Recently regions of North America have been faced with two relatively new entities, West Nile virus and the severe acute respiratory syndrome (SARS). Organ donors should be tested for evidence of both West Nile virus viremia by polymerase chain reaction (PCR) and early antibody response (IgM) to West Nile virus. If either test is positive the potential donor is to be deemed ineligible for organ donation.

SARS screening is currently conducted by using a specifically directed series of questions on the donor medical and social history questionnaire. This investigates the donor institution's category of contamination as determined by the infection control officer at that institution; the donor's clinical history relative to the last 10 days prior to donor assessment with regard to signs or symptoms associated with SARS; and epidemiologic links related to direct contact with SARS risk or travel to an area listed in the current Travel Health Advisory.[18]

DONOR-RELATED MALIGNANCIES

Transmission of donor malignancies is rare, with 18 cases from 34,933 cadaver donors and 3 cases from 32,052 living donors being reported to UNOS from 1994 through 2001. Donors with past histories of certain types of cancers may be considered as donors, including certain types of primary central nervous system (CNS) tumors. Risks of cancer transmission from donors with a history of nonmelanoma skin cancer and selected cancers of the CNS appear to be small. When considering organ use from donors suffering from intracranial malignancies, there are a number of general guidelines. Most important is to consider the known biologic behavior of various CNS neoplasms and their propensity to spread outside of the cranial vault. Repeated craniotomies as well as ventriculoperitoneal or ventriculojugular shunts have been associated with increased risk of metastasis.[17,19–21]

Risks of tumor transmission with certain other types of cancer may be acceptable, particularly if the donor has a long cancer-free interval prior to organ procurement, while certain other cancers pose a high transmission risk. Tumors that pose a high transmission risk include choriocarcinoma, melanoma,

TABLE 91-2 Relative Risk of Central Nervous System Tumor Transmission

Lowest risk
  Benign meningiomas
  Pituitary adenomas
  Acoustic schwannomas
  Craniopharyngiomas
  Astrocytoma (grade I)
  Epidermoid cysts, colloid cysts
  Low-grade oligodendromas
  Gangliogliomas, gangliocytomas
  Pineocytomas, ependymomas
  Well-differentiated teratomas
  Papillomas
  Hemangioblastomas
Moderate risk
  Astrocytoma (grade II)
  Gliomatosis cerebri
Highest risk
  Anaplastic astrocytoma (grade III)
  Glioblastoma multiforme
  Medulloblastoma
  Anaplastic oligodendroglioma
  Pineoblastomas
  Chordomas
  Malignant ependymomas
  Primary cerebral lymphomas

SOURCE: Reproduced with permission from Rosengard et al.[17]

lymphoma, and carcinoma of the lung, colon, breast, kidney, and thyroid.

A list has been developed outlining the relative risks of CNS tumor transmission from cadaver donor to allograft recipient (Table 91-2).

CARDIAC EVALUATION

An initial electrocardiogram (ECG) should be obtained on every potential cardiac donor, and additional ECGs should be obtained when changes in heart rhythm occur. ECG changes may be temporary and related to alterations in sympathetic output. Nonspecific ST-segment and T-wave changes, prolonged QT intervals, and T-wave inversion are common. Tachycardia is common and may be caused by diabetes insipidus, diuresis, hemorrhage, vasopressor therapy, or electrolyte disturbances. ECGs are evaluated for signs of acute myocardial injury.[8]

A transthoracic or transesophageal echocardiogram may be obtained to evaluate motion of the heart wall and valve function, estimate ejection fraction, and to detect a pericardial effusion. Transient changes that do not preclude heart donation include a stunned myocardium or myocardial depression related to acidosis and hypoxemia. If the causes of the changes are reversible, the heart may still be successfully transplanted. Although echocardiography is effective in screening for anatomic abnormalities of the heart, the use of a single echocardiogram to determine the physiologic suitability of a donor is not supported by clinical evidence. An alternative approach, using a pulmonary artery catheter to guide the physiologic assessment and management of ventricular dysfunction, has been used with success in the United Kingdom.

TABLE 91-3 Heart Donor Criteria

Criteria	Modification(s)
Age	Donors >55 may be used selectively, though coexisting LVH and longer ischemic times may increase recipient mortality risks
Size	Despite an increased risk associated with small donors, a normal-sized adult male (>70 kg) donor is suitable for most recipients
LVH	Mild LVH (wall thickness <13 mm by echocardiography and no LVH by ECG criteria) does not preclude recovery, particularly with shorter ischemic times
Valvular lesions	Certain lesions, such as mild or moderate mitral or tricuspid regurgitation, or a normally functioning bicuspid aortic valve may be amenable to repair prior to transplantation
Congenital lesions	Certain lesions, such as a secundum type ASD, may be amenable to repair
Coronary angiography	a. Male donor age 35–45 years and female donor age 35–50 years: perform angiography if there is a history of cocaine use or ≥3 risk factors for CAD b. Male donor age 46–55 years and female donor age 51–55 years: angiography recommended c. Age >55 years: angiography strongly recommended
CAD	Donor hears with mild coronary artery disease should be considered for recipients with relatively urgent need

ABBREVIATIONS: ASD, atrial septal defect; CAD, coronary artery disease; ECG, electrocardiographic; LVH, left ventricular hypertrophy.
SOURCE: Reproduced with permission from Rosengard et al.[17]

Assessment and management of donor left ventricular dysfunction offers the greatest potential to increase heart donor utilization. Strong evidence indicates that younger hearts with left ventricular dysfunction can recover normal function over time in the donor and after transplantation into a recipient. Metabolic abnormalities, anemia, and excessive doses of inotropes should be corrected prior to obtaining an echocardiogram. Aggressive donor management, including pulmonary artery catheterization and hormonal resuscitation, should be performed in donors with an initial left ventricular ejection fraction less than 45%. Table 91-3 shows the heart donor criteria recently modified to potentially expand the available pool of cardiac donors.[17]

PULMONARY EVALUATION

The suitability of donor lungs for transplantation is determined with several diagnostic tests. A chest radiograph should be interpreted by a radiologist or qualified physician. A complete history of the donor's treatment while in the hospital, including the use of vasopressors and results of arterial blood gas analyses, are shared with centers considering the transplantation of lungs. Smoking history should be reported, along with the results of Gram stains of sputum (a specimen for detection of yeasts and fungi is desirable), and a description of the sputum characteristics. In addition, a bronchoscopic examination is performed to assess for signs of aspiration, and to document evidence of a foreign body or presence of blood or other material entering the lower airways from above. It also allows assessment of the character and amount of secretions in the lung and provides microbiologic specimens. A bronchoscopic examination will also promote pulmonary stability in the donor by removing airway secretions that may have accumulated. Blood gases are repeated every 3 hours to assess the results of interventions and to determine trends. Repeat pulmonary recruitment maneuvers are performed to optimize ventilation-perfusion matching.

Wider application of broader criteria for donor selection and procurement is possible and can clearly increase the size of the donor pool. If uniform multidisciplinary donor management protocols were developed, increased lung utilization would follow. Table 91-4 shows the current criteria that are used to determine the suitability of a cadaver lung donor. The Lung Transplant Working Group proposed the new criteria to include virtually any donor up to the age of 65 years, in the absence of significant lung injury from smoking, and absence of cancer with metastatic potential.[8,17,22,23]

In an effort to augment the donor pool, criteria have been loosened with the retrieval of organs from donors with greater smoking histories, infiltrates on radiography, or marginal gas exchange. Because these previously-considered marginal donors, or more appropriately termed "extended" donors, are now being used *any* potential brain-dead patient without obvious contraindication to cadaveric donation should be referred to appropriate local organ procurement agencies for final determination of suitability.[17,23]

TABLE 91-4 Lung Donor Criteria

- P_{O_2}:$F_{I_{O_2}}$ ratio >300, $F_{I_{O_2}}$ = 1.0, PEEP = 5 cm H_2O
- Clear chest x-ray
- Age <55 years
- Absence of major chest trauma
- Absent aspiration, sepsis, or purulent secretions
- Smoking history of <20 pack-years
- No history of malignancy

ABBREVIATIONS: $F_{I_{O_2}}$, fraction of inspired oxygen; PEEP, positive end-expiratory pressure; P_{O_2}, partial pressure of oxygen.

TABLE 91-5 Marginal Cadaver Kidney Donors

Donor Condition	Donor age categories				
	<10	10–39	40–49	50–59	≥60
CVA + HTN + Creat >1.5				•	•
CVA + HTN				•	•
CVA + Creat >1.5				•	•
HTN + Creat >1.5				•	•
CVA					•
HTN					•
Creatinine >1.5					•
None of the above					•

ABBREVIATIONS: Creat > 1.5, creatinine > 1.5 mg/dL; CVA, cerebrovascular accident was cause of death; HTN, history of hypertension; •, marginal donors.
SOURCE: Reproduced with permission from Rosengard et al.[17]

RENAL EVALUATION

The discard rate of kidneys procured from cadaveric donors in the U.S. has been increasing to an alarming level of more than 15% of those kidneys recovered for transplantation. Approximately 50% of kidneys from cadaveric donors over 60 years of age (older-age donors) are not transplanted due to donor quality.

The renal system in a cadaveric donor undergoes a number of physiologic changes that are influenced dramatically by both the medical therapies used to prevent brain death and by brain death itself. The results of basic renal function tests such as measurement of serum levels of creatinine and urea nitrogen and urinalysis should be reviewed to provide a profile of renal system function in the donor since admission. When kidney donors are evaluated, the effect of hemoconcentration on the results of these studies should always be considered. Elevated levels of serum creatinine and urea nitrogen and atypical urinalysis findings may suggest that renal function was compromised. The relative risk of dialysis after transplantation is 1.5 times greater in recipients of kidneys from donors >55 years of age vs. those who are <55. Table 91-5[17] shows the latest approved expanded kidney donor criteria, based on the relative risk >1.7 of having a graft failure for donors older than 50 years of age with at least two of the following factors: creatinine >1.5 mg/dL, a cerebrovascular accident (CVA) as a cause of death, and hypertension, as compared to a reference group of nonhypertensive donors between the ages of 10 and 39 whose cause of death was not CVA, and whose creatinine was <1.5 mg/dL.[1,8,17]

LIVER EVALUATION

The assessment of a donor liver before transplantation has been the subject of much research; however, clinically one still relies on a subjective interpretation of donor data and the macro- and microscopic appearance of the liver to decide whether to use the graft. More reliable predictors of graft function are required. Significant efforts have been made to try to assess donor grafts by evaluating different aspects of liver function, including the ability of the liver to synthesize proteins, metabolize drugs, secrete bile, produce high-energy phosphates, and by following the levels of markers of microvascular injury. To date, many donor organs that were previously not considered suitable for transplantation, "marginal" grafts, are now being used in selected circumstances. The marginal donors are identified based on demographic, clinical, laboratory, and histologic data. This includes donor age >70 years or <3 months, donor body weight over 100 kg, moderate or severe macrovesicular fat infiltration of the liver, and abnormal liver function tests. Serum aspartate aminotransferase (AST) >160 IU/L, serum sodium >160 mmol/L, donor stay in intensive care of more than 5 days, significant periods of hypotension (<60 mm Hg systolic BP for more than 30 minutes associated with a rise in serum AST), and significant systemic infection are all parameters considered to define marginal grafts. Important in the assessment of potential grafts is the presence of hepatic steatosis: increased donor age, obesity, and a history of high alcohol intake have all been associated with fatty infiltration.

Donor selection remains highly subjective, and in the absence of reliable laboratory tests the decision whether to use a marginal graft is left to the judgment of the transplant surgeon. The definition of what constitutes a "marginal" or "extended" graft will continue to vary between centers until reliable parameters are available for prospectively predicting early graft function.[17,24,25]

Donor Management

Specific donor management may only begin after the diagnosis of brain death has been firmly established. Brain death is a catastrophic event associated with significant disturbances to many organ systems (Table 91-6).[15] Table 91-7 summarizes the key points of donor management (which are discussed in the following paragraphs) based on the current recommendations.[3,17,27]

Understanding and management of these changes is essential for optimal preservation of organs for transplantation.[8,10,15] In general, there should be a shift in emphasis from more focused cerebral resuscitation, to optimization of oxygen delivery to other organs and tissues. This shift of management may only begin after consent has been obtained from the family. Routine care with frequent turning, protection of the eyes, frequent airway suctioning, physiotherapy to prevent atelectasis and pneumonia, gastric decompression, and limited exposure to prevent hypothermia are important aspects of this regimen. Intensive nursing care is needed, with a 1:1 or even 2:1 nurse:patient ratio.[10]

Successful transplantation of organs from donors is dependent on adequate resuscitation. Potential donors manifest profound hemodynamic and metabolic abnormalities, which can result in a loss of valuable organs. Autonomic instability and hypotension occur in approximately 80% of donors. Even with aggressive management as many as 25% of potential organ donors are lost due to hemodynamic instability. Even more organs are lost as a consequence of the high doses of vasopressors required to maintain adequate perfusion of the brain-dead organ donor.

Hypovolemia from osmotic agents given to treat high intracranial pressure, poorly treated diabetes insipidus, and traumatic blood loss all may contribute to hypotension. A sudden increase in intracranial pressure may cause hypotension and severe bradyarrhythmias because of

TABLE 91-6 Physiologic Changes Associated with Brain Death

Neurologic
  Increased intracranial pressure, herniation
Cardiopulmonary
  Hypertension followed by hypotension
  Tachycardia
  Bradycardia
  Arrhythmias (premature ventricular beats, asystole)
  Myocardial dysfunction
  Myocardial ischemia
  Increased pulmonary artery pressures
  Pulmonary edema
  Cardiac arrest
Endocrine and metabolic[a]
  Decreased aerobic metabolism
  Increased anaerobic metabolism
  Decreased circulating pituitary hormones
  Diabetes insipidus
  Electrolyte disturbances
    Hypernatremia
    Hypokalemia
    Hypomagnesemia
    Hypocalcemia
    Hypophosphatemia
    Hyperglycemia
Hematologic
  Coagulopathy
  Disseminated intravascular coagulation
  Factor and platelet dilution
Other
  Hyperthermia followed by hypothermia

[a] Other than antidiuretic hormone, the exact hormones that become deficient is controversial.
SOURCE: Reproduced with permission from Tuttle-Newhall et al.[15]

parasympathetic stimulation from dural stretch, which is encountered after failure of the Cushing reflex, which causes severe systemic hypertension as a final effort to maintain cerebral perfusion in the face of drastically elevated intracranial pressure. As the vagal cardiomotor centers become ischemic, termination of parasympathetic activity occurs with resulting unopposed sympathetic stimulation. This marked increase in vascular resistance may lead to myocardial ischemia.[10,13]

Animal models have demonstrated profound systemic and pulmonary vasoconstriction with a massive systemic increase in catecholamine levels, termed the *autonomic storm*. This autonomic storm is followed by a transient shift of systemic intravascular fluid volume to the lungs. Cardiac output decreases and left atrial pressure may exceed pulmonary artery pressure. This may result in capillary wall disruption and leakage of protein-rich fluid into the pulmonary interstitium, resulting in pulmonary edema (also referred to as "neurogenic pulmonary edema").[10,13]

A second major injury is the derangement of the hypothalamic-hypophyseal axis, with the associated changes in circulating plasma hormones. The loss of hypothalamic influence and sympathetic tone is characterized by a progressive decrease in serum norepinephrine and a decrease in systemic vascular resistance. This is analogous to a high cervical spinal cord transection. As a result, most potential organ donors require vasoactive agents to maintain blood pressure. The hypothalamic-pituitary axis dysfunction leads to neurogenic diabetes insipidus and a marked decrease in levels of

thyroid hormone and cortisol in animal models. In the clinical setting the role these endocrine abnormalities play in the status of donors may vary among donors.[4,8,10,13]

Since the most crucial factor in determining optimal organ viability is the maintenance of adequate systemic perfusion pressure, invasive monitoring is recommended given the complex physiologic changes that are associated with brain death. This is particularly true if the heart and lungs are being considered for donation. Cautious repeated fluid challenges are administered until 10 cm H_2O central venous pressure (CVP) is reached (assuming positive end-expiratory pressure [PEEP] = 5 cm H_2O), thereafter aiming for the lowest CVP that maintains urine output and adequate perfusion pressure maintaining the CVP at 6 to 8 mm Hg. Crystalloid, colloid solutions, and blood products may be infused as indicated. Systolic blood pressure should not be allowed to fall below approximately 90 mm Hg. Red blood cells must be used to maintain a hemoglobin of at least 10 g/dL. Severe coagulopathy should be treated before organ procurement using appropriate blood component therapy. Low doses of dopamine or dobutamine at 2 to 10 μg/kg per minute are traditionally used, although arginine vasopressin at 0.5 to 4.0 U/h is an increasingly favored alternative. The systemic vascular resistance should be kept between 800 and 1200 dynes/s per cm². If necessary, a combination of these drugs, each in the lower dosage range, often produce the best results, while maintaining at least 1 mL/kg per hour of urine output. Reduced diuresis despite adequate perfusion pressure can be increased by mannitol administration, at the dosage of 0.25 g/kg as an intravenous bolus. Fluid resuscitation therapy should be guided by data from a central venous catheter or a pulmonary artery catheter, with euvolemia (not hypervolemia) being the target of volume replacement therapy.

Dysrhythmias are quite common and should be treated aggressively. Persistent bradycardia is treated by isoproterenol infusion or even pacing. Minute ventilation should be adjusted to keep the CO_2 and pH in a mild respiratory alkalosis. It is better to reduce the frequency of ventilation rather than tidal volume in order to prevent the development of atelectasis. PEEP is optimized and is regulated to maintain 95% oxygen saturation, and if possible the F_{IO_2} should be no higher than 50%. Peak inspiratory pressures (PIP) are also important because high pressure results in barotrauma and impaired venous return to the heart, thereby compromising cardiac output. Pressure control modes of ventilation may be preferable for the minimization of these risks. Ideally PEEP is maintained at <7.5 and PIP at <30 cm H_2O. Bronchoscopy may be necessary for pulmonary toilet, to collect samples for microbiology, and to reinflate atelectatic regions of the lung, thereby decreasing shunting. Bronchodilators should be administered. Continuous full monitoring is of course essential.

Maintenance of normal acid base balance in organ donors is often difficult. Partial pressure of arterial carbon dioxide (P_{CO_2}) should be maintained in the normal range and optimum pH is between 7.35 and 7.45. Glucose consumption is also decreased and parenteral or enteral nutrition must be decreased to around 50% to avoid hyperglycemia and unnecessary metabolic workload. Ongoing nutrition must be maintained, as it is associated with improved graft function, particularly for the liver graft. In the liver, glycogen stores are depleted within 12 hours of brain death, with suggested reduced resistance of the graft to ischemia. Persistent

TABLE 91-7 Important Aspects of Donor Management

1. The airway
Perform bronchoscopy
Use frequent suctioning and aspiration precautions
Use albuterol therapy for wheezing (may improve lung fluid clearance)

2. Mechanical ventilation
Adequate oxygenation:
$P_{O_2} > 100$ mm Hg, $F_{IO_2} = 0.40$ or O_2 saturation $>95\%$
Adequate ventilation:
Maintain tidal volume 10-12 mL/kg
PEEP + 5 cm H_2O
Keep peak airway pressures <30 mm Hg
Maintain a mild respiratory alkalosis (pH 7.35–7.45 and P_{CO_2} 30–35 mm Hg)

3. Monitoring
Central venous line
Arterial line and pulse oximetry
Pulmonary artery catheter desirable for rational use of inotropes,
pressors and fluids

4. Fluid management
Judicious fluid resuscitation to achieve the lowest CVP/PCWP consistent with adequate urine output
and blood pressure to ensure end-organ perfusion (*euvolemia not hypervolemia*)
Maintenance CVP 6–8 mm Hg, PCWP 8–12 mm Hg
Urine output 1 mL/kg per hour
Colloid as the fluid of choice for volume resuscitation
Albumin with normal PT, PTT; fresh frozen plasma with coagulopathy
Hemoglobin >10g/dL or hematocrit ≥30%
Electrolytes
Maintain Na^+ <150 mEq/dL
Maintain K+ >4.0 mEq/dL
Correct acidosis with sodium bicarbonate and mild to moderate hyperventilation
(P_{CO_2} 30–35 mm Hg)

5. Hemodynamic management
Donor resuscitation as outlined above to attain:
BP ≥90 or MAP ≥60 mm Hg
SVR 800–1200 dyn/s per cm^2
Cardiac index 2.4 L/min per m^2
Dopamine or dobutamine dose <10μg/kg per minute
Arginine vasopressin: 1 unit bolus, then 0.5–4.0 U/h drip

6. Hormonal resuscitation
Methylprednisolone: 10–15 mg/kg bolus (repeat q24h prn)
Arginine vasopressin: titrate to BP
Insulin: drip at a minimum rate of 1 U/h (titrate blood glucose to 120–180 mg/dL)
Triiodothyronine (T_3): 4μg bolus; 3μg/h continuous infusion

7. Early echocardiogram for all cardiac donors
Insert pulmonary artery catheter to monitor patient management (placement of the PAC is particularly relevant in patients with an EF <45% or on high-dose inotropes)
If EF <45%, need to optimize hemodynamic and hormonal management and then reassess

ABBREVIATIONS: CVP, central venous pressure; EF, ejection fraction; F_{IO_2}, fraction of inspired oxygen; MAP, mean arterial pressure; PEEP, positive end-expiratory pressure; P_{CO_2}, partial pressure of carbon dioxide; PCWP, pulmonary capillary wedge pressure; P_{O_2}, partial pressure of oxygen; PT, prothrombin time; PTT, partial thromboplastin time; SVR, systemic vascular resistance.

hyperglycemia despite reduced glucose administration can be treated with insulin. Loss of the hypothalamic-pituitary axis can result in diabetes insipidus. Associated electrolyte abnormalities are hypernatremia, hypocalcemia, hypokalemia, hypophosphatemia, and hypomagnesemia. In addition, the variety of strategies used to treat intracranial pressure may exaggerate the hypernatremic state. Aggressive correction of the electrolyte state should be performed and levels should be checked every 4 hours in order to prevent development of

lethal dysrhythmias, myocardial dysfunction, and rhabdomyolysis. Sodium levels should be kept <155 mEq/dL, as liver primary graft nonfunction has been associated with hypernatremia. The diagnosis of central diabetes insipidus is easily made when more than 4 mL/kg per hour of dilute urine is produced while the serum sodium is above 145 mmol/L. Hypotonic fluids can be used to restore intravascular volume with a simple volume-for-volume replacement of the urine. Development of hyperglycemia may be caused by the dextrose or glucose in the hypotonic intravenous fluids; but on the other hand, it will help restore glycogen liver reserves in a setting of inadequate nutritional support. More practical is to use desmopressin (DDAVP) in a loading dose of 8 ng/kg, followed by an infusion of 4 ng/kg per hour and a reassessment and titration up or down every 30 minutes; alternatively, a 1-μg bolus every 2 hours can be used as long as the urine output remains >300 mL/h. DDAVP has a longer half-life and minimal vasopressor activity (2000:1) as compared to arginine vasopressin. Arginine vasopressin is particularly useful in hypotensive patients in a continuous infusion of aqueous vasopressin at the dosage of 0.5 U/hr, which can be titrated as necessary by monitoring the urine output. A relatively small percentage of organ donors are resistant to aqueous vasopressin. In these cases desmopressin acetate should be considered.

Warmed intravenous fluid, heated humidified oxygen, and warming blankets may need to be used to limit hypothermia. The core temperature should be maintained above 35°C. Hypothermia contributes to donor hemodynamic instability, myocardial depression, severe dysrhythmias, and coagulopathy, and may even cause cold diuresis and also predispose to sepsis. It is much better to prevent hypothermia, because once it has occurred it may be difficult to correct.

The recognition of the metabolic derangements following brain death, including autonomic storm and hypothalamic-pituitary axis dysfunction, has highlighted the need for hormonal resuscitation as an integral part of the donor management protocol.[3–6,8,26–29]. The recommended hormonal resuscitation consists of methylprednisolone in a 10–15 mg/kg bolus; triiodothyronine in a 4-μg bolus followed by a continuous infusion of 3 μg/h; arginine vasopressin in a 1-unit bolus, then a continuous infusion at 0.5 to 4 U/h, titrated to a systemic vascular resistance of 800 to 1200 dynes/s per cm^2; and insulin 1 U/h titrated to maintain blood sugar at 120 to 180 mg/dL.[6] The use of steroids is based on the intensive effort to increase the number of usable lungs given the low recovery rate of lungs from potential donors. Retrospective studies have repeatedly showed that high-dose steroid administration improved oxygenation in the brain-dead donor and was associated with increased rates of successful donation.[30,31]

Though initial evidence showed that vasopressin used with epinephrine maintains hemodynamic stability and tissue viability, its implementation was not adopted universally. Rather DDAVP was used, with the assumption that the effectiveness of arginine vasopressin was related to its treatment of the diabetes insipidus that is commonly found in organ donors. DDAVP is an analogue that is highly selective for the vasopressin V$_2$-receptor subtype that is found in the renal collecting ducts, and has no vasopressor activity in humans, which is mediated by V$_1$-receptors on vascular smooth muscle. Arginine vasopressin was in fact abandoned due to concerns that the vasoconstrictive effect could be harmful for donor organs. This resulted in unnecessarily excessive fluid resuscitation with crystalloid, colloid, and blood products, along with higher doses of vasopressor agents with widely recognized adverse effects. Many transplant centers consider a donor heart to be unsuitable if dopamine requirements exceed 10 to 15 μg/kg per minute, because at such doses it can also affect both kidney and liver.[27]

Hemodynamic instability has also been suggested to be a consequence of diminished levels of circulating thyroxin, leading to reduced myocardial energy stores and a shift from aerobic to anaerobic metabolism, with the subsequent accumulation of lactate. These observations were initially described in animal studies, and the administration of thyroid hormone replacement to human brain-dead donors has shown improvement in the cardiovascular status of donors, with reduction in the inotropic support, particularly in hemodynamically unstable organ donors. This benefit is most pronounced in cardiac transplantation and heart graft function.[26]

Considerable debate is ongoing regarding the role of thyroid hormone therapy in the management of organ donors. Several studies have shown no correlation between thyroid hormone levels and hemodynamic status. Some observed no beneficial effect and a trend toward worsening metabolic acidosis following thyroid hormone administration. Contrarily, the implementation of the three-hormone resuscitation therapy, with methylprednisolone, arginine vasopressin, and triiodothyronine or levothyroxin, has been associated with an increased number of transplanted hearts and improved short-term graft function.[26,27] The selection of donors who are predicted to benefit from hormonal resuscitation has been outlined. After conventional management to adjust volume status, anemia, and metabolic abnormalities, the recommendation is that an echocardiogram be obtained to rule out structural abnormalities and document the ejection fraction. If the ejection fraction is <45%, a pulmonary artery catheter is placed and hormonal resuscitation is instituted. Subsequent cardiac function can be monitored using the pulmonary artery catheter.

References

1. Gridelli B, Remuzzi G: Strategies for making more organs available for transplantation. *N Engl J Med* 343:404, 2000.
2. Hauptman PJ, O'Connor KJ: Procurement and allocation of solid organs for transplantation. *N Engl J Med* 336:4422, 1997.
3. www.unos.org/resources/donorManagement.asp?index=2
4. Novitzky D: Donor management: state of the art. *Transplant Proc* 29:3773, 1997.
5. Rosendale JD, Chabalewski FL, McBride MA, et al: Increased transplanted organs from the use of a standardized donor management protocol. *Am J Transplantation* 2:761, 2002.
6. Rosendale JD, Kauffman MH, McBride M, et al: Aggressive pharmacologic donor management results in more transplanted organs. *Transplantation* 75:482, 2003.
7. Matesanz R: Factors influencing the adaptation of the Spanish Model of organ donation. *Transpl Int* 16:736, 2003.
8. Holmquist M, Chabalewski F, Blount T, et al: A critical pathway: guiding care for organ donors. *Crit Care Nurse* 19:84, 1999.
9. Ehrle RN, Shafer TJ, Nelson KR: Referral, request and consent for organ donation: best practice and blue print for success. *Crit Care Nurse* 19:21, 1999.
10. Sarti A: Organ donation. *Paediatr Anaesth* 9:287, 1999.
11. Karakatsanis KG, Tsanakas JN: A critique on the concept of brain death. *Issues Law Med* 18:127, 2002.
12. Truog RD: Is it time to abandon brain death? *Hastings Cent Rep* 27: 29, 1997.
13. Razek T, Olthoff K, Reilly PM: Issues in potential organ donor management. *Surg Clin North Am* 80:1021, 2000.
14. Gortmaker SL, Beasley CL, Sheehy E, et al: Improving the request process to increase family consent for organ donation. *J Transpl Coord* 8:210, 1998.

15. Tuttle-Newhall JE, Collins BH, Kuo PC, Schoeder R: Organ donation and treatment of the multi-organ donor. *Curr Probl Surg* 40:266, 2003.

16. Delmonico FL: Cadaver donor screening for infectious agents in solid organ transplantation. *Clin Infect Dis* 31:781, 2000.

17. Rosengard BR, Feng S, Alfrey EJ, et al: Report of the Crystal City meeting to maximize the use of organs recovered from the cadaver donor. *Am J Transplant* 2:701, 2002.

18. www.giftoflife.on.ca

19. Kauffman MH, McBride MA, Cherikh WS, et al: Transplant tumor registry: Donor related malignancies. *Transplantation* 74:358, 2002.

20. Kauffman MH, McBride MA, Delmonico FL: First Report of the United Network for Organ Sharing Transplant Tumor Registry: Donors with a History of Cancer. *Transplantation* 70:1747, 2000.

21. Kauffman MH, McBride MA, Cherikh WS: Transplant tumor registry: Donors with central nervous system tumors. *Transplantation* 73:579, 2002.

22. Chakinala MM, Kollef MH, Trulock EP: Critical care aspects of lung transplant patients. *J Intensive Care Med* 17:8, 2002.

23. Gabbay E, Williams TJ, Griffiths AP, et al: Maximizing the utilization of donor organs offered for lung transplantation. *Am J Respir Crit Care Med* 160:265, 1999.

24. Melendez HV, Rela M, Murphy G, et al: Assessment of graft function before liver transplantation: quest for the lost ark?. *Transplantation* 70:560, 2000.

25. Jimenez Romer, Moreno Gonzalez E, Colina Ruiz F, et al: Understanding marginal liver grafts. *Transplantation* 68:469, 1999.

26. Rosendale JD, Kauffman MH, McBride MA, et al: Hormonal resuscitation yields more transplanted hearts with improved early function. *Transplantation* 75:1336, 2003.

27. Zaroff JG, Rosengard BR, Amstrong WF, et al: Consensus Conference Report. Maximizing use of organs recovered from the cadaver donor: cardiac recommendations. *Circulation* 106:836, 2002.

28. Chen JM, Cullinane S, Spainer TB, et al: Vasopressin deficiency and pressor hypersensitivity in hemodynamically unstable organ donors. *Circulation* 100(Suppl II):244, 1999.

29. Salim A, Vassiliu P, Velmahos GC, et al: The role of thyroid hormone administration in potential organ donors. *Arch Surg* 136:1377, 2001.

30. Follette DM, Rudich S, Babcock WD: Improved oxygenation and increased lung donor recovery with high dose steroid administration after brain death. *J Heart Lung Transplant* 17:423, 1998.

31. McElhinney DB, Khan J, Babcock WD, et al: Thoracic organ donor characteristics associated with successful lung procurement. *Clin Transplant* 15:68, 2001.

Chapter 92

PRIORITIES IN MULTISYSTEM TRAUMA

JAMEEL ALI

KEY POINTS

- *To improve survival, injury management must be prioritized in the multiply injured patient.*
- *The order of priority among injuries is related to time and degree of life threat posed by each injury.*
- *Immediate priority is given to airway control and to maintenance of ventilation, oxygenation, and perfusion.*
- *Cervical spine protection is crucial during airway intubation.*
- *A trauma team leader is important to coordinate management in the multiply injured patient.*
- *Complete familiarity with techniques for airway control, chest decompression, and the establishment of intravenous access is essential in management of multiple trauma.*
- *Complete in-depth assessment of the multiply injured patient is required only after immediately life-threatening injuries have been treated.*
- *Repeated assessment is necessary to diagnose and treat injuries that are not obvious on initial presentation.*

Mortality from multiple injuries follows a trimodal distribution.[1,2] The first peak represents death occurring at the scene and results from such injuries as cardiac rupture or disruption of the major intrathoracic vessels, and severe brain injury that is incompatible with survival. Death from such injuries occurs within minutes of the traumatic event and medical intervention is usually futile. The second peak in mortality following multiple injuries occurs from minutes to a few hours after the event. Mortality during this phase is related to injuries that are immediately life-threatening, such as airway compromise, tension pneumothorax, and cardiac tamponade. This is also a period during which simple appropriate resuscitative measures can significantly affect the outcome. The third peak occurs as a result of complications of the injury, such as sepsis or multiple-system organ failure.[3] However, mortality in this third phase can also be significantly affected by the type of intervention during the second phase. The intensivist dealing with the multiple trauma patient is very likely to be involved in the institution of resuscitative measures during the second phase as well as the management during the third phase of the complications of the injury or complications arising from inadequate treatment. Many of the chapters in this text deal with the complications of trauma, such as sepsis and multiple organ failure. This chapter will deal with treatment priorities during the second peak of the trimodal distribution of trauma-related mortality.

Blunt trauma from motor vehicle collision is the most frequent cause of injuries in general. This type of impact usually results in injuries to many different parts of the body simultaneously. Figure 92-1 shows the distribution of motor vehicle driver injuries over a 2-year period at Sunnybrook Health Science Centre in Toronto, Canada, where 338 drivers with 2566 injuries were treated. Head and neck injuries were the most frequent, occurring at a frequency of 1.88 per patient, and the overall frequency of injuries was 7.6 per patient.

When faced with multisystem injury, the intensivist must prioritize treatment according to the threat to the patient's survival.[4] Prioritization of assessment and intervention requires a coordinated team approach. Where personnel are available from different specialties, it is of paramount importance that the entire resuscitative effort be coordinated through an identified team leader. This very simple decision should be made prior to institution of therapy and can be critical to the outcome in the patient with multisystem trauma. The team leader, who may be an intensivist, must be completely familiar with a wide variety of injuries and the relative threat they pose to life in order to prioritize intervention and direct personnel appropriately.

Certain fundamental concepts underlie the approach to resuscitation of the multiply injured patient. The most important of these is that immediately life-threatening injuries should be treated as they are identified. Therefore, assessment and resuscitation must proceed simultaneously. The initial goal in managing the trauma patient is to provide adequate oxygenation and perfusion. This goal is achieved by approaching assessment and treatment so that abnormalities in the injured patient that affect oxygenation and perfusion take top priority. It is also of prime importance to recognize findings that suggest a need for emergent surgical intervention.

Priorities

The order of priorities is a key feature for successful management of the multiply injured patient and should adhere to the following sequence:

1. Establishment of the airway and of oxygenation and ventilation with cervical spine control
2. Control of hemorrhage
3. Maintenance of adequate perfusion
4. Identification and correction of neurologic abnormalities
5. Total exposure of the patient to allow complete assessment while preventing hypothermia by minimizing the duration of this exposure
6. Temporary stabilization of fractures
7. Detailed systematic assessment and provision of definitive care

In the Advanced Trauma Life Support (ATLS) course for physicians,[1] steps 1 to 5 constitute the Primary Survey, during which immediately life-threatening injuries are identified by adhering to the sequence ABCDE, where A stands for *a*irway, B for *b*reathing, C for *c*irculation and hemorrhage control, D for neurologic *d*isability, and E for *e*xposure.

The basis for this order of priorities is the degree to which abnormalities in the different systems threaten the life of the patient. Adherence to this order allows assessment and resuscitation to occur simultaneously, because injuries will be identified in the order in which they are likely to threaten the patient's life. Although the patient with multiple fractures

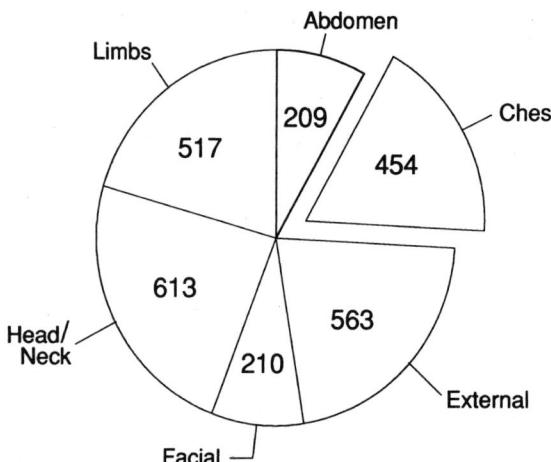

FIGURE 92-1 Injuries in 338 motor vehicle drivers (total = 2566 injuries). As indicated in the text, most of these patients had injuries to the head and neck area, and the average number of injuries per patient was 7.6.

requires treatment of these fractures, apart from hemorrhage control associated with the fractures, such treatment should take lower priority compared to treatment of abnormalities affecting the airway or respiratory status.

Complete evaluation requires assessment of the entire front and back of the patient, necessitating full exposure. Once this assessment is completed, the patient should again be covered to minimize heat loss and the risk of hypothermia.

AIRWAY, OXYGENATION, VENTILATION, AND CERVICAL SPINE CONTROL

The most frequent cause of airway obstruction in the multiply injured patient is loss of tone of the muscles supporting the tongue, either because of hypoperfusion of the brain from hypovolemic shock or because of central nervous system (CNS) injury. As outlined in Chaps. 15 and 35, the simple maneuvers of chin lift and jaw thrust move the mandible forward. Because the tongue muscles are attached to the mandible, these actions move the tongue anteriorly and open the upper airway. It is essential in the trauma victim to inspect the oropharynx to ensure that there is no foreign material (including vomitus) in the pharynx that will occlude the airway. Quick observation of the patient's nares and mouth and listening for unobstructed passage of air through the upper airway, together with inspection for the presence of foreign objects in the oropharynx, are all very simple maneuvers that should be undertaken in the initial care of the multiply injured patient. The patient who is fully conscious, vocalizing and breathing adequately, and who is not in shock does not require an artificial airway.

The underlying principle of establishing an airway in the trauma victim is to institute the simplest technique that allows effective oxygenation and ventilation. Over 90% of patients do not require endotracheal intubation. Measures short of endotracheal intubation include the insertion of oropharyngeal or nasopharyngeal tubes. However, when endotracheal intubation is necessary, it should be performed promptly and expeditiously. Prolonged unsuccessful attempts at endotracheal intubation without oxygenation and ventilation should be avoided. Mask ventilation with oxygen and an oropharyn-

geal airway should be performed intermittently to avoid hypoxia during prolonged attempts at endotracheal intubation. All multiply injured patients should have oxygen administered by the most appropriate means as early as possible. A pulse oximeter should be attached to monitor O_2 saturation, which should be maintained at 95% or greater.

In very rare circumstances, the patient's airway may not be patent and it may be impossible to establish an airway nasally or orally. In such situations, cricothyroidotomy is required. This procedure should only be done when an airway cannot be established by other, nonsurgical means. The landmarks for the cricothyroid membrane are indicated in Fig. 92-2. A cricothyroidotomy may be done using a large-bore needle or scalpel, the former method being preferable in children under 8 years of age because the cricoid cartilage is essential to the stability of the upper airway of infants and young children. A 14-gauge needle and cannula may be inserted through the cricothyroid membrane for temporary oxygenation, but this is not a very efficient means of ventilation. To maximize oxygenation and avoid hypercapnia, the needle cricothyroidotomy should be followed by tracheostomy in an operating room under ideal circumstances if a surgical airway is still required. The placement of the cricothyroidotomy needle allows approximately 30 to 45 minutes of adequate oxygenation without severe hypercapnia. The surgical cricothyroidotomy is preferable and more effective in adults. A transverse skin incision is made directly over the cricothyroid membrane, and after the subcutaneous structures are reflected, the cricothyroid membrane is identified and incised transversely. A pair of forceps is then inserted to spread the opening, and a tube of appropriate caliber, usually a 6F or 7F tracheostomy or endotracheal tube, is inserted through the opening and secured.[5]

Many techniques for establishing an artificial airway are associated with risks of cervical spine injury. Awareness of these risks during airway intubation is crucial in preventing spinal cord injury in the multiply injured patient. Inappropriate manipulation of the cervical spine during airway intubation could convert an unstable cervical spine injury without neurologic deficit into one with permanent neurologic deficits, including paraplegia, quadriplegia, and even

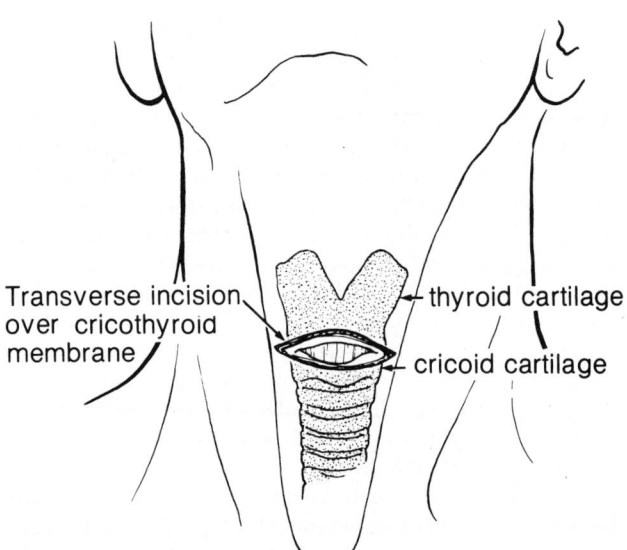

FIGURE 92-2 Landmarks for cricothyroidotomy.

death. In a patient who is unconscious or who is suspected of having a cervical spine injury, the neck should not be flexed, extended, or rotated. In-line immobilization with the neck in the neutral position should be maintained while the airway is secured. If the patient is conscious and breathing, then a blind nasotracheal intubation may be attempted with cricoid pressure anteriorly. If the patient is apneic, then orotracheal intubation with in-line cervical immobilization will have to be attempted. Failure or inability to secure the airway by nonsurgical means in a patient who requires a definitive airway necessitates cricothyroidotomy. Where fiberoptic bronchoscopy is immediately available, it may be used to facilitate endotracheal intubation. All unconscious patients or patients suspected of cervical spine injury should have a lateral cervical spine x-ray done as a minimum, and all seven cervical vertebrae and the superior aspect of the first thoracic vertebra should be clearly visualized. Failure to visualize all these vertebrae should necessitate other views of the spine, including a swimmer's view. An open-mouth anteroposterior odontoid and anteroposterior x-ray view of the cervical spine should also be done. If there is doubt as to the presence of a cervical spine injury, the neck should be immobilized with a semirigid cervical collar and computed tomography (CT) is performed to assess the integrity of the cervical spine. If the patient is awake and alert and has no cervical pain or tenderness or other abnormality on physical examination, then the cervical collar may be removed after adequate cervical spine x-rays. In the presence of clinical signs of spinal cord injury, the cervical spine is considered to be abnormal even if the cervical spine x-ray appears normal. In selected patients who have not had a period of unconsciousness or another painful distracting injury, and are alert and have no clinical evidence of cervical spine injury, x-rays of the cervical spine may be omitted and the cervical collar removed.[6,7]

Adequacy of ventilation is quickly assessed by observation of the chest for asymmetrical or paradoxical movement, followed by quick auscultation and percussion to determine whether there is any hyperresonance or dullness to suggest pneumothorax or hemothorax. Deviation of the trachea suggests the presence of a pneumothorax or hemothorax, but this finding is not always evident. Although one may confirm the diagnosis of a simple traumatic pneumothorax with an upright chest x-ray, suspicion of a tension pneumothorax requires immediate decompression, without prior x-ray confirmation. Further examination of the chest should be conducted to determine the presence of other life-threatening thoracic injuries, such as cardiac tamponade, open pneumothorax, flail chest, ruptured thoracic aorta, and massive hemothorax (see Chap. 95).

ADEQUACY OF PERFUSION

After airway control, oxygenation, and adequate ventilation have been secured, the next priority is maintenance of adequate perfusion. The most common source of hypoperfusion in the multiply injured patient is hemorrhage. Its clinical presentation will depend on such factors as the patient's age, as well as the duration and magnitude of the hemorrhage. The presence of a normal or even elevated blood pressure, particularly in the young patient, does not rule out blood loss. The physiologic response to hypovolemia includes sympathetic discharge with vasoconstriction and tachycardia, which

will tend to maintain the blood pressure. Older patients tend to manifest hypotension much earlier in the course of hypovolemia. Therefore, other signs of hypoperfusion should be sought in assessing the trauma patient. The location and character of the pulse, the skin color, and capillary refill time are all signs that are immediately accessible to the examining physician and should be used in determining adequacy of perfusion. Failure to palpate a radial pulse may signify hypotension of the order of 70 to 80 mm Hg. Tachycardia with cool extremities suggests hypoperfusion from hemorrhage until proven otherwise. Hemorrhage may be subdivided into classes I to IV,[1] each class having an associated clinical response, as indicated in Table 92-1. The patient who has a normal heart rate with a strong, bounding radial pulse, warm skin, and a capillary refill time of less than 2 seconds would be considered not to have lost any significant volume of blood, and the degree of deviation from these clinical parameters would correlate with the magnitude of blood loss.

Although the most common cause of hypoperfusion in trauma patients is hemorrhage, other causes, such as tension pneumothorax, cardiac tamponade, myocardial contusion, open pneumothorax, and flail chest must be considered. Hypoperfusion in the trauma patient first requires a search for a source of hemorrhage, which should be immediately controlled. Any external source of hemorrhage should be controlled by direct pressure, without resorting to blind application of clamps or tourniquets. Improving the hemodynamic status should be the next goal. This should be accomplished by appropriate fluid replacement through at least two large-bore intravenous catheters (14 to 16 gauge minimum). It is very helpful to establish multiple IV catheters, not only to facilitate rapid volume infusion, but to ensure that an IV line will still be available if one of the catheters becomes disconnected, plugged, or otherwise nonfunctional. In the adult, the preferred peripheral percutaneous intravenous site is in the forearm or the antecubital vein. Failure to establish intravenous access through these routes should prompt establishment of intravenous access by other routes such as the internal jugular or subclavian vein in the neck or femoral vein in the groin using the Seldinger technique. Venous cutdown of the saphenous vein at the ankle or the antecubital vein or the femoral vein at the groin are other approaches, but are now seldom necessary because of the success in establishing access through the other nonsurgical routes. The route will depend on the experience and skill of the physician. Placement of central lines should always be followed by a chest x-ray as soon as feasible, not only to confirm proper location of the catheter, but also to check for the presence of pneumothorax or hemothorax. Because these lines are placed under less than ideal conditions, the risk of septic complications is high, and the lines should be replaced later under more sterile conditions. In children under age 6 years, the intraosseous route should be attempted before proceeding to the central venous routes. With specially designed devices the intraosseous route is also possible in adults but is seldom required.[8] As a rule, it is best to avoid placing IV catheters in limbs that have major soft tissue or bony injuries. The intensivist must be completely familiar with the usual sites for venous access and also be prepared to proceed to venous cutdown where percutaneous techniques are not successful. Venous access should be achieved promptly, since cannulation

TABLE 92-1 Clinical Classification of Shock in a 70-kg Male

Criterion	Class I	Class II	Class III	Class IV
Blood loss (mL)	Up to 750	750–1500	1500–2000	≥2000
Blood loss (% blood volume)	Up to 15	15–30	30–40	≥40
Pulse rate (beats per minute)	<100	>100	>120	≥140
Blood pressure	Normal	Normal	Decreased	Decreased
Pulse pressure (mm Hg)	Normal or increased	Decreased	Decreased	Decreased
Capillary refill test	Normal	Positive	Positive	Positive
Respiratory rate	14–20	20–30	30–40	>35
Urine output (mL/h)	≥30	20–30	5–15	Negligible
CNS (mental status)	Slightly anxious	Mildly anxious	Anxious and confused	Confused or lethargic
Fluid replacement (3:1 rule)	Crystalloid	Crystalloid	Crystalloid + blood	Crystalloid + blood

NOTE: The clinical signs of shock are very subtle for class I and II hemorrhage, but it is crucial to make the diagnosis at this stage before deeper levels of shock ensue. This is ensured by prompt fluid resuscitation. When crystalloid is used to replace estimated blood loss, a very rough guide is the 3:1 rule, according to which the estimated amount of blood lost should be replaced by three times as much crystalloid to produce a similar effect on vascular volume. This rule is only a guideline, however, and the adequacy of perfusion should be the end point for determining adequacy of fluid resuscitation.
ABBREVIATION: CNS, central nervous system.
SOURCE: Reproduced from the Committee on Trauma, American College of Surgeons.[1]

of the veins becomes more difficult as shock continues, owing to venoconstriction and venous spasm.

In the course of establishing IV access, blood is drawn for complete blood count, cross-matching of blood, coagulation, and toxicology screens. Prior to the availability of blood products, it is essential to maintain adequate perfusion, as judged by clinical indicators, including blood pressure, pulse, status of the neck veins, and urinary output. In most circumstances, there is sufficient time to obtain the patient's blood type. However, if after approximately 2 to 3 L of crystalloid have been given, the patient's vital signs do not normalize or normalize only temporarily, and typed blood is not available, then emergency blood (group O) will be required for resuscitating the patient. Packed cells in the amount of anywhere from 4 to 10 U should be ordered for resuscitating the patient with major hemorrhage.

If there is no obvious external source of hemorrhage, bleeding from pelvic or extremity fractures should be sought. Failure to demonstrate blood loss in these areas suggests that the blood loss is in either the thorax or the abdomen. Most sources of thoracic hemorrhage can be identified by a combination of physical examination and chest x-ray. Therefore by a process of elimination it is usually possible to determine the source of the hemorrhage. If the areas identified earlier do not represent the source of hemorrhage, the most likely source is intra-abdominal. If the patient shows signs of continued hemorrhage with only a transient response or failure to respond to volume infusion, laparotomy may be required for the identification and control of intra-abdominal hemorrhage. In some cases in which there is an obvious source of blood loss such as an extremity fracture, there may still be uncertainty regarding possible concurrent intra-abdominal hemorrhage. In these situations, ultrasonography, diagnostic peritoneal lavage, or CT of the abdomen (see Chap. 95) is helpful in determining whether or not there is an intra-abdominal source of hemorrhage.[9,10]

As indicated earlier, other causes of hypoperfusion should be sought in the trauma patient by assessing for such signs as those of cardiac tamponade, myocardial contusion, and tension pneumothorax, with prompt institution of corrective measures.[11] These intrathoracic causes of hypoperfusion are discussed in Chap. 95.

In patients sustaining major blood loss, end points of resuscitation and the volume of infused fluids should be based on the rapidity with which such patients can be taken to the operating room for definitive control of hemorrhage. In patients without major head injury, particularly those with penetrating torso trauma, borderline hypotension in the range of 90 mm Hg systolic should be the goal in preparation for the operating room, since massive volume infusion towards normalization of the hemodynamic status could aggravate blood loss.[12,13]

In evaluating the patient's response to volume infusion, it is important to recognize that massive blood loss may trigger a vagally mediated bradycardia, and that in these circumstances the absence of tachycardia does not represent adequate volume resuscitation.[14] When one is judging the amount of fluid required and the requirement for blood, a useful guideline is that if blood pressure has not approached normalcy after infusion of 50 mL/kg of crystalloid, then blood administration should be considered.[15] As indicated earlier, if type-specific blood is not available, then emergency type O packed red blood cells may be used. Because one of the most common causes of hypothermia and its complications is the rapid infusion of cold solutions in the resuscitation of trauma patients, techniques for warming both the patient and the infused fluid must be employed.[16,17] In addition to electrocardiographic monitoring and continued assessment of vital signs, core temperature monitoring is therefore important, using a device that is capable of reading temperatures at hypothermic levels.

Although volume deficit is the major cause of hypoperfusion in the trauma patient, failure to respond to adequate volume infusion may represent cardiovascular decompensation. If such causes as cardiac tamponade or tension pneumothorax have been ruled out as the cause of this cardiovascular decompensation, consideration should be given to the use of inotropes and vasoactive agents to support the circulation in these circumstances. Such intervention is accomplished with close hemodynamic monitoring, as outlined in earlier chapters.

In situations in which the hypoperfused patient fails to respond to massive fluid infusion and there is no obvious nonhemorrhagic source of the hypoperfusion, emergency thoracotomy[18,19] may be required. This allows (1) identification and treatment of pericardial tamponade, (2) internal cardiac massage, (3) identification and control of intrathoracic hemorrhage, and (4) cross-clamping of the thoracic aorta to maintain cerebral perfusion and coronary blood flow while decreasing bleeding from a subdiaphragmatic source. Emergency thoracotomy also allows the diagnosis and treatment of air embolism, which is discussed in Chap. 95.

NEUROLOGIC STATUS

Following control of the respiratory and circulatory status, attention is directed at assessment and management of the neurologic status. The hallmark of CNS injury is a change in the level of consciousness. Therefore it is essential that the level of consciousness be defined, so that repeated assessment will detect any changes over time. The Glasgow Coma Scale score (GCS; see Chaps. 67 and 93) is the generally accepted means of establishing this level of consciousness in the trauma patient.

The brain is very sensitive to hypoxia and hypoperfusion, and one of the most common causes of a depressed level of consciousness in the multiply injured patient is uncorrected hypovolemia resulting in hypoperfusion and cerebral hypoxia. Therefore, overall resuscitative measures aimed at maintaining vascular volume and arterial oxygenation are of prime importance in the treatment of a patient with a possible head injury. Volume restriction as a primary goal, with the aim of decreasing intracranial pressure and cerebral edema, is inappropriate in the hypovolemic head-injured patient. In fact this approach is more likely to aggravate the head injury and increase cerebral edema and intracranial pressure. The key features of initial assessment and resuscitation of the brain-injured patient are to prevent secondary brain injury due to hypoperfusion and hypoxemia, control of cerebral edema, and identification and evacuation of significant mass lesions based on careful clinical and CT scan assessment under the guidance of a qualified neurosurgeon. The detailed assessment and management of such patients is discussed in Chap. 93.

FRACTURE STABILIZATION

Although the most dramatic injury in the multiply injured patient is frequently the mangled limb resulting from major fractures, fractures as such do not pose an immediate threat to life, and therefore are generally lower in our list of management of priorities. However, the secondary effects of fractures may have high priority. For instance, massive hemorrhage associated with a fracture will require direct control of the hemorrhage where possible, aggressive early fluid resuscitation, reduction of the fracture, and in the case of massive hemorrhage from pelvic fractures, the use of such techniques as external fixation. Time is also of the essence in the management of fractures when there is interference with the blood supply to the limb, as from spasm of the blood vessels or direct injury to the blood vessels adjacent to the fracture. Early assessment of neurovascular integrity and the correction of any abnormality are essential in the management of fractures to ensure limb salvage and to prevent rhabdomyolysis and compartment syndrome. Limb ischemia associated with the fracture should be initially treated by reduction of the fracture and immobilization. If this maneuver fails to restore perfusion, early

angiographic assessment should be undertaken. To improve the chances of saving the limb, the period of limb ischemia should be less than 4 to 6 hours. Therefore all efforts should be made to obtain early angiography and definitive repair of the vascular injury associated with a fracture. The possibility of compartment syndrome should be kept in mind, particularly after perfusion has been re-established to a previously ischemic limb. Definitive management of the fracture itself is discussed in Chap. 96.

DETAILED SYSTEMATIC ASSESSMENT AND DEFINITIVE CARE

Once the initial rapid assessment and resuscitation of the patient has been completed, a more in-depth assessment is conducted systematically, beginning with the head and ending with the lower extremities. The multiply injured patient must be completely undressed so that a complete physical examination can be done. This includes assessment of the back and requires careful log-rolling of the patient to visualize the back while protecting the spinal column. X-rays of the thoracolumbar spine should be considered in unconscious patients or those with major torso trauma with or without neurologic deficit, and in those in whom the mechanism of injury suggests the possibility of spinal column injury. Until adequate radiologic assessment is complete, these patients should be moved with caution by log-rolling, and any rotation, flexion, or extension of the thoracolumbar spine should be avoided.

All multiply injured patients should have (1) large-bore intravenous access, (2) a nasogastric tube to decompress the stomach and monitor for evidence of upper gastrointestinal hemorrhage (unless contraindicated, as discussed below), and (3) a transurethral Foley catheter for monitoring urine output, unless contraindicated by the presence of a urethral injury. Patients in whom urethral injury may be present include those with a major pelvic fracture, perineal and scrotal ecchymosis, or bleeding through the urethral meatus, and those in whom a high-riding, boggy prostate is found on rectal examination. If these signs are present, a urethrogram should be performed; only if the results are normal should the Foley catheter be inserted per urethra. The presence of a cribriform plate fracture is a relative contraindication to insertion of a nasogastric tube.[20,21] Gastric decompression in this situation should be achieved by orogastric intubation.

If a rectal examination has not already been conducted to rule out a urethral injury prior to the insertion of a urethral catheter, it should be done as part of the complete assessment. The rectal examination not only assesses the integrity of the rectum, but provides information on the presence of blood in the gastrointestinal tract, the possibility of extrarectal pelvic injury (bony as well as soft tissue, e.g., injury of the prostatic urethra), and the presence of rectal sphincter tone, which may be abnormal in patients with spinal cord injury. During this phase of the assessment, potentially life-threatening injuries or injuries that are likely to produce morbidity and require correction on a nonurgent basis are detected. If the techniques of inspection, percussion, palpation, and auscultation are used appropriately, injuries such as simple pneumothoraces, uncomplicated fractures, and soft tissue wounds are detected and managed.

Reduction and stabilization of uncomplicated fractures are conducted once the life-threatening injuries have been treated. The tetanus immunization status of the patient should be determined, and appropriate prophylactic measures instituted. The trauma flow sheet should be completed, and the use of agents such as tetanus toxoid should be clearly documented and must be available for continued reference during the patient's stay in the ICU. It is at this point that subspecialty services such as plastic surgery and otolaryngology may be consulted.

Repeated examination of the trauma patient is important so injuries that are not obvious at presentation may be diagnosed and treated appropriately. The mechanism of the injury should be carefully noted in the history, and a high index of suspicion is required so that occult injuries are not missed. Patients who are relatively stable but who have been involved in a collision in which there is an associated fatality must be monitored very carefully in an ICU setting, since it must be assumed that they were exposed to the same force and energy transfer as the dead victim. Such patients may have temporarily contained hematomas in the spleen, liver, or retroperitoneum or around major vascular structures. These patients can decompensate abruptly with sudden spontaneous hemorrhage. Slowly progressive tachycardia, hypotension, a fall in hemoglobin concentration, or any worsening of abdominal findings, such as increasing pain or signs of peritoneal irritation, should warrant aggressive investigation and consideration of intervention, including surgical exploration. For these high-risk patients, approximately 4 to 6 U of blood should be available at all times in the early phase of treatment. An unexplainable fall in hemoglobin concentration must be considered a sign of continued hemorrhage, and any sudden increase in heart rate or decrease in blood pressure must be considered signs of major hemorrhage. The source of this hemorrhage should be identified promptly and treated appropriately. A more subtle sign of impending hemodynamic instability is a progressive decrease in urine output despite volume replacement that appears to be adequate in relation to the recognized injuries. Deterioration in the respiratory status should prompt assessment for the presence of a pneumothorax, lung contusion, or another type of subtle injury, such as a ruptured esophagus with pleural effusion that may present later in the patient's course. Delayed cardiac decompensation without obvious blood loss should warrant investigation for myocardial contusion, cardiac tamponade, or tension pneumothorax. The latter condition may develop on institution of positive pressure ventilation in a patient who sustained a simple pneumothorax which was not treated by tube thoracostomy. As discussed in Chaps. 42 and 95, the clinical presentation and operative findings may suggest the possible development of traumatic abdominal compartment syndrome in the ICU, prompting decompression of the abdominal cavity to improve the patient's cardiorespiratory and hemodynamic status.[22] Respiratory deterioration may also occur in spontaneously breathing patients who sustained a rupture of the diaphragm and in whom the abdominal viscera at first remained in the abdominal cavity but later migrated above the diaphragm, causing respiratory compromise. For these reasons, continuous close monitoring in an ICU setting is crucial to improving survival of the multiply injured patient.

X-rays are obtained as indicated. In most multiply injured patients, these will include cervical spine x-rays if there is any suggestion of cervical spinal injury, a chest x-ray, and an x-ray of the pelvis. Other radiologic investigations will be undertaken as indicated by the assessment, such as the presence of deformity in an extremity warranting x-ray to confirm a fracture.

Deciding on Surgical Intervention

One of the most important decisions to be made in the emergency management of the trauma patient is whether or not surgical intervention is necessary. If the decision based on the initial assessment is that surgery is not warranted, then continued observation in an intensive care setting is necessary for most multiply injured patients. This approach, combined with a high index of suspicion, will minimize the risk of overlooking occult injuries, such as a subcapsular hepatic hematoma in a patient who is stable initially, which carries the potential for major sudden hemorrhage and hypovolemic shock.

In considering the need for surgical intervention, the common emergency indications are for thoracic, abdominal, and intracranial injuries. For thoracic injuries, this includes an uncontrollable pneumothorax representing a major airway laceration, a massive hemothorax usually representing laceration of a systemic artery (e.g., intercostal or internal mammary) or central pulmonary vessel, a widened mediastinum or other sign of aortic disruption, or signs of a ruptured esophagus, cardiac tamponade, or air embolism. The hypovolemic patient who suddenly becomes asystolic or suffers electromechanical dissociation is also a candidate for emergency thoracotomy. The details of assessment and management of these indications for thoracic surgery are considered in Chap. 95. The indications for laparotomy in the multiply injured patient are signs of peritoneal penetration, perforation, or hemorrhage in general; these are discussed in more detail in Chap. 95.

The indication for surgical intervention in head injuries is usually a change in level of consciousness in the presence of a mass lesion requiring evacuation or placement of an intracranial pressure monitoring device (see Chap. 93).

Acknowledgment

The author acknowledges the assistance of Sunnybrook Studios of the Sunnybrook and Women's College Health Science Centre, Toronto, for preparation of the illustrations.

References

1. Committee on Trauma, American College of Surgeons: *Advanced Trauma Life Support Manual.* Chicago, American College of Surgeons, 2002, p 5.
2. Trunkey DD: Trauma. *Sci Am* 249:28, 1983.
3. Rixen D, Siegel JH, Friedman HP: Sepsis/SIRS. Physiologic classification, severity stratification, relation to cytokine elaboration, and outcome prediction in posttrauma critical illness. *J Trauma* 41:581, 1996.
4. Melio FR: Priorities in the multiple trauma patient. *Emerg Med Clin North Am* 16:28, 1998.
5. Narrod JA, Moore EE, Rosen P: Emergency cricothyrostomy, technique and anatomical considerations. *J Emerg Med* 2:443, 1985.

6. Roth BJ, Martin RR: Roentgenographic evaluation of the cervical spine: a selective approach. *Arch Surg* 129:643, 1994.

7. Roberge RJ, Wears RC, Kelly M, et al: Selective application of cervical spine radiography in alert victims of blunt trauma: a prospective study. *J Trauma* 28:784, 1988.

8. Sawyer RW, Bodai BI, Blaisdell FW, et al: The current status of intraosseous infusion. *J Am Coll Surg* 179:353, 1994.

9. Rozycki GS, Ochsner MG, Schmidt JA, et al: A prospective study of surgeon-performed ultrasound as the primary adjuvant modality for injured patient assessment. *J Trauma* 39:492, 1995.

10. Rozycki GS, Ballard RB, Feliciano DV, et al: Surgeon performed ultrasound for the assessment of truncal injuries: lessons learned from 1,540 patients. *Am Surg* 228:557, 1998.

11. Petre R, Chilcott M: Current concepts: Blunt trauma to the heart and great vessels. *N Engl J Med* 336:626, 1997.

12. Bickell WH, Wall MJ Jr, Pepe PE, et al: Immediate vs delayed fluid resuscitation for hypotensive patients with penetrating torso injuries. *N Engl J Med* 331:1105, 1994.

13. Burris D, Rhee P, Kaufman C, et al: Controlled resuscitation for uncontrolled hemorrhagic shock. *J Trauma* 46:216, 1999.

14. Demetriades D, Chan LS, Bhasin P, et al: Relative bradycardia in patients with traumatic hypotension. *J Trauma* 45:534, 1998.

15. Rush BF Jr, Richardson JD, Bosomworth P, Eiseman B: Limitations of blood replacement with electrolyte solution: A control clinical study. *Arch Surg* 98:49, 1969.

16. Gentilello L, Cobean RA, Offner PJ, et al: Continuous arteriovenous rewarming: Rapid reversal of hypothermia in critically ill patients. *J Trauma* 32:316, 1992.

17. Gentilello LM: Temperature associated injuries and syndromes, in Mattox KL, Feliciano DV, Moore EE (eds): *Trauma*, 4th ed. New York, McGraw Hill, 2000, p 1153.

18. Baxter BT, Moore EE, Moore JB, et al: Emergency department thoracotomy following injury: Critical determinants for patient salvage. *World J Surg* 12:671, 1988.

19. Rhee PM, Acosta J, Bridgeman A, et al: Survival after emergency department thoracotomy: review of published data from the past 25 years. *J Am Coll Surg* 190:288, 2000.

20. Bouzarth WF: Intracranial nasogastric tube insertion. *J Trauma* 18:319, 1978 (editorial).

21. Fremstad JD, Martin GH: Lethal complication from insertion of nasogastric tube after severe basilar skull fracture. *J Trauma* 18:820, 1978.

22. Chang MC, Miller PR, D'Agostino R, et al: Effects of abdominal decompression on cardiopulmonary function and visceral perfusion in patients with intraabdominal hypertension. *J Trauma* 44:440, 1998.

Chapter 93

HEAD INJURY AND INTRACRANIAL HYPERTENSION

RICHARD J. MOULTON
LAWRENCE H. PITTS

KEY POINTS

- *Secondary brain injury from hypoxia and ischemia should be prevented by appropriate airway ventilatory and fluid management in all comatose patients.*

- *In appropriately selected patients aggressive monitoring and treatment of intracranial pressure is warranted.*

- *Early identification and evacuation of operable intracranial hematomas can be life-saving.*

- *Change in the level of consciousness is one of the hallmarks of brain injury. Its recognition through careful history, physical examination, and close monitoring is therefore essential.*

- *Prophylaxis and aggressive treatment of seizures following head injury must be instituted.*

- *Maintenance of normal fluid and electrolyte balance and early provision of enteral nutrition is necessary.*

- *Risk of central nervous system infection is reduced by surgical débridement and restoration of dural integrity in cases of open cranial injury.*

- *Systemic sepsis often complicates recovery and should be diagnosed and treated aggressively.*

Epidemiology and Etiology of Head Injury

The incidence of head injury in the United States is approximately 200 to 400 per 100,000 population per year. Similar incidence rates have been documented for other countries. Male-to-female incidence ratios vary between 2:1 and 3:1, and incidence peaks in the second and third decades of life.[1] Patients with severe head injuries—i.e., those admitted in coma, with a Glasgow Coma Scale score (GCS) of 8 (Table 93-1)[2,3]—constitute a minority of head-injured patients admitted to hospital, but account for most of the morbidity and mortality (Fig. 93-1). Hospitals with a large primary care population see relatively fewer severely head-injured patients than do those functioning primarily as tertiary referral centers.

The most common cause of closed head injury is road traffic collisions. These include injuries to vehicle occupants, pedestrians, motorcyclists, and bicyclists. Falls are the next most common cause of injury. Gunshot injuries are a major cause of penetrating head injury in the United States and account for up to 44% of head injuries in some series.[1] Etiology varies considerably with local patient demographics and proximity to major highways, among other factors, and the resulting case mix will vary from center to center in terms of intracranial hematoma incidence, mean patient age, and consequently outcome from injury. Younger adults are more often involved

in vehicular trauma, and there is a lower incidence of intracranial mass lesions in this patient population. Older patients are more often injured as a result of falls and have a higher incidence of mass lesions. At an equivalent depth of coma, both increasing age and presence of intracranial hematomas predispose patients to a poorer outcome.

Intoxication with alcohol or other agents is a significant factor in all causes of injury and across virtually all age groups except the very young and very old. Depending on etiology, 10% to 50% of our patients were obviously intoxicated at admission (Fig. 93-2).

The social and economic costs of head injury are enormous. Severe injury carries a high mortality, and patients who survive severe and moderate injuries may remain substantially disabled for years after the injury. The persistent effects of head injury on personality and mentation may be devastating for both patients and their families.

Pathophysiology of Craniocerebral Trauma

ACCELERATION-DECELERATION INJURY

Injury to the brain is produced by energy transfer to the cranium and its contained structures. In blunt injury, angular acceleration-deceleration forces cause shear strains within the cerebral parenchyma, which in turn are responsible for the characteristic diffuse axonal injury. The force may be applied directly to the head (i.e., impact injury) or indirectly via the body (i.e., impulse injury). The physiologic hallmark of diffuse injury to the brain is loss of consciousness. *Concussion* is a brief loss of consciousness without obvious sequelae. *Coma* is defined as a state of unconsciousness in which the patient does not open the eyes, follow commands, or utter any recognizable words. The severity of diffuse brain injury may be gauged by the depth and duration of coma or the duration of posttraumatic amnesia. The duration of both coma and posttraumatic amnesia can be judged only in retrospect, so the depth of coma as quantified by the GCS has been widely

TABLE 93-1 The Glasgow Coma Scale Score

Finding	Score
Eye opening	
Spontaneous	4
To voice	3
To pain	2
None	1
Verbal response	
Oriented	5
Confused speech	4
Inappropriate words	3
Incomprehensible sounds	2
None	1
Motor response	
Obeys commands	6
Localizes pain	5
Withdraws	4
Abnormal flexion	3
Extension	2
None	1

SOURCE: Reproduced with permission from Teasdale et al[2] and Jennett et al.[3]

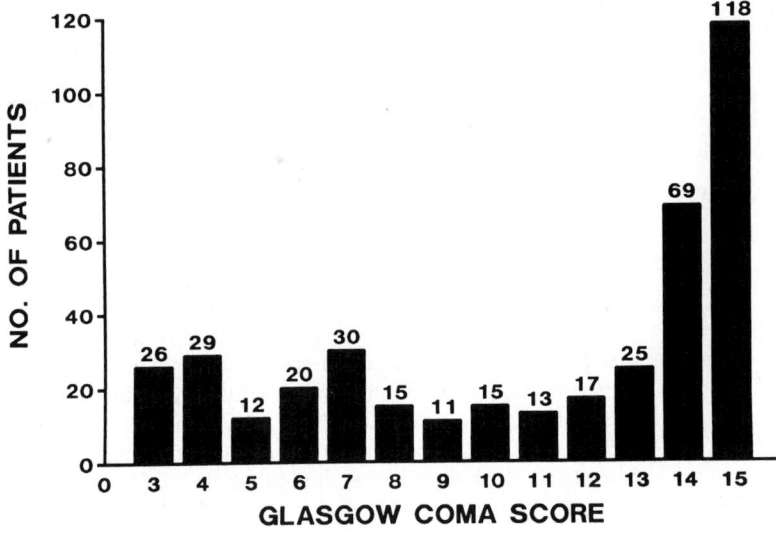

FIGURE 93-1 Distribution of head injury severity (measured by the Glasgow Coma Scale score at admission) in 400 consecutive admissions to a tertiary care hospital neurosurgical unit.

adopted as the most convenient measure of injury severity. With severe and prolonged coma, the patient may reach a state characterized by observable periods of eye opening and sleep without appreciation of the environment or of people or objects in it. This has been called the *persistent vegetative state*.

Acceleration-deceleration injury occurring as a result of impact or impulse mechanisms may produce gross disruption of brain tissue (laceration and/or contusion), diffuse axonal injury, or both. The characteristic histologic findings of diffuse injury consist of axon retraction balls (the pathologic marker of axonal separation) and microglial stars. Experimental evidence, and more recently human postmortem material, have shown that axon retraction balls develop over hours from initially intact axons.[4] Hemorrhagic lesions of the an-

terior corpus callosum may be seen on careful postmortem examination or may be apparent on computed tomography (CT) scans, as may small punctate hemorrhages deep in the hemispheres or small amounts of blood in the ventricular system (Fig. 93-3). For a given force, the greatest degree of injury occurs in the white matter of the hemispheres, and the brain stem is less severely injured.

Laceration/contusion of the brain surface may underlie the site of a blow (coup contusion), but more typically is found on the orbitofrontal surface of the frontal lobes and/or the anterior portion of the temporal lobes, remote from the site of the blow (contrecoup injury; Figs. 93-4 and 93-5). To-and-fro motion of the brain over the uneven surfaces of the anterior and middle fossae has been postulated as the underlying mechanism of contrecoup contusion. Cavitation of the brain

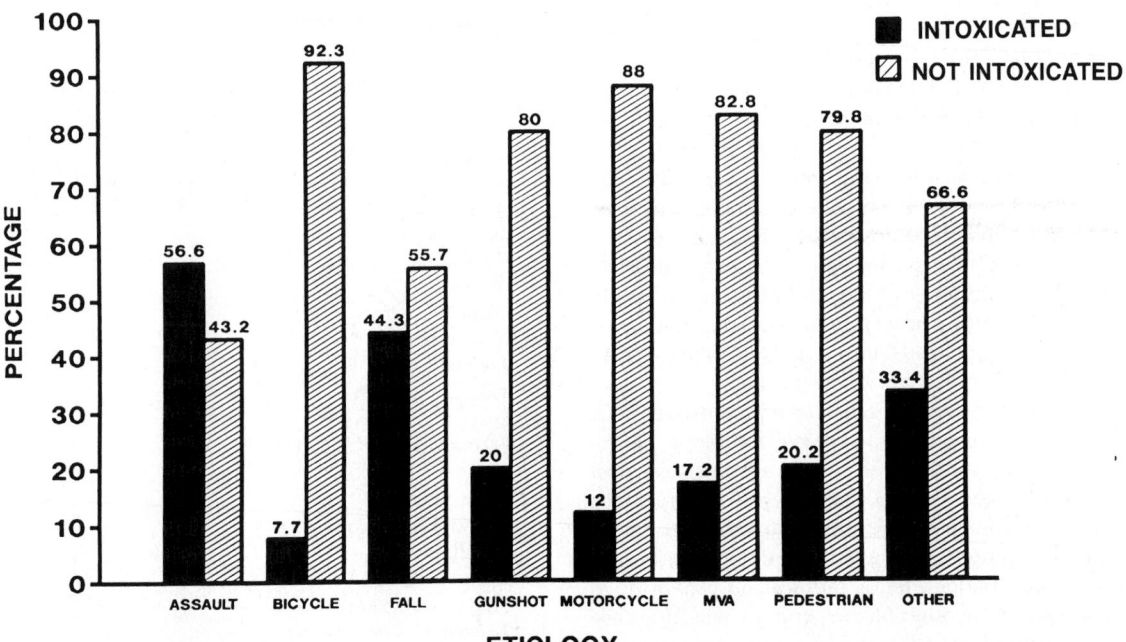

FIGURE 93-2 Proportional incidence of alcohol intoxication by injury etiology in 400 consecutive head injury patients. MVA, injuries to motor vehicle occupants.

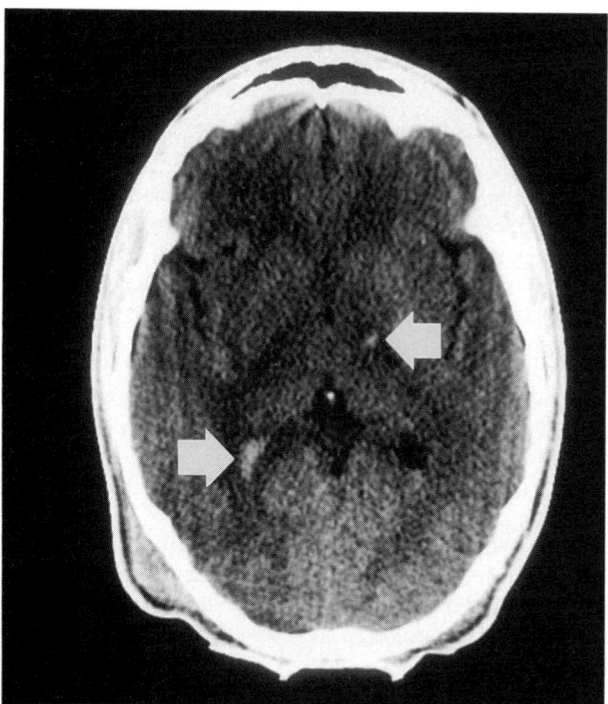

FIGURE 93-3 CT scan of a 16-year-old patient with a typical diffuse head injury. The patient's GCS at admission to hospital was 4. There is a small amount of blood in the trigone and occipital horn of the right lateral ventricle (*lower arrow*). There is a small punctate hemorrhage in the left internal capsule (*upper arrow*).

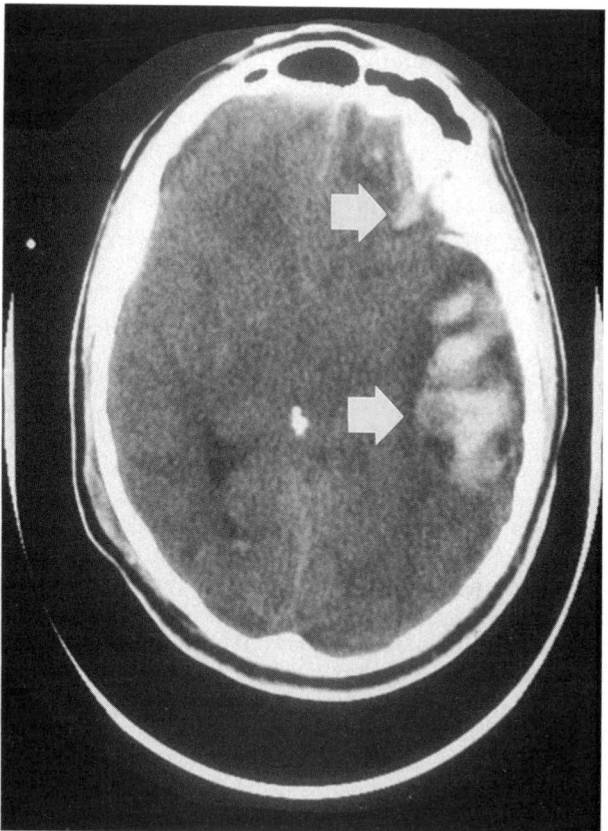

FIGURE 93-4 CT scan of a 50-year-old man injured in a fall. There is a large mixed-density lesion in the left temporal lobe (*lower arrow*) and a similar, smaller lesion in the left orbitofrontal cortex (*upper arrow*). The appearance is typical of cerebral contusions.

produced by the rapid acceleration of the skull away from the brain at contusion sites is an alternate hypothesis. Both cerebral parenchyma and blood vessels are disrupted at the sites of contusion, and the bleeding may be sufficient to produce a subdural hematoma, a large confluent intracerebral hematoma, or both.

In addition to the disruption of cerebral parenchyma, direct impact injury may disrupt the skull and meninges or their blood vessels. Skull fractures are of importance primarily because they may trigger epidural bleeding, provide a portal of entry for infective organisms if compound (either directly or indirectly via the middle ear or paranasal sinuses), or lacerate the meninges and underlying brain if depressed fragments are present. Cranial nerves may be injured as they exit the skull base, and fractures involving the petrous temporal bone may injure the auditory and/or vestibular end organs, or disrupt the ossicles of the middle ear.

PENETRATING INJURY

Penetrating injury produces direct disruption and laceration of brain tissue. In low-velocity injuries (stab wounds or impalements), damage is confined to the directly disrupted tissue. There is often no loss of consciousness. In missile injuries, cavitation occurs along the track of the missile, and depending on the size and velocity of the missile, disruption of surrounding cerebral tissue is often widespread and severe. Both high- and low-velocity penetrating injuries disrupt the overlying skin, skull, and meninges of the brain, thereby allowing contamination of cerebrospinal fluid (CSF) or brain with infective microorganisms.

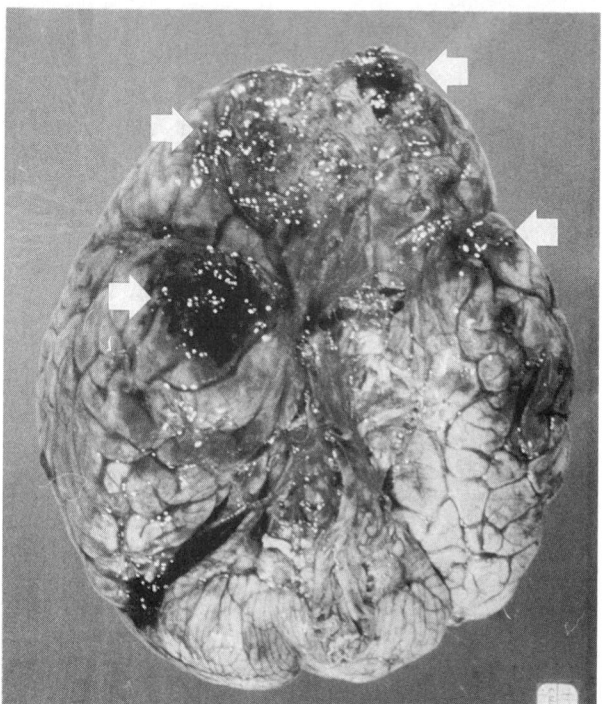

FIGURE 93-5 Pathologic specimen showing asymmetric hemorrhagic contusions of both temporal lobes (*lower arrows*) and both frontal poles (*upper arrows*). These are the usual locations of cerebral contusions.

SECONDARY INJURY TO THE BRAIN

Direct and immediate disruption of the brain tissue by blunt or penetrating trauma constitutes primary injury. Unfortunately, despite encouraging results in the elucidation of the mechanism of primary impact injury and the development of potential neuroprotective therapies in the experimental laboratory over the last decade and a half, effective treatment for primary impact injury still eludes us. Large multicenter trials of pharmacologic agents (including antioxidant drugs and excitatory amino acid antagonists) and hypothermia have failed to yield positive clinical results.[5] Clinical management of patients with traumatic brain injury continues to be grounded in the successful prevention, detection, and treatment of secondary insults to the injured brain. These secondary processes may be initiated at the time of injury or at any subsequent time, and these may aggravate existing injury to the brain. Secondary injuries include intracranial bleeding, hypoxia, ischemia, raised intracranial pressure (ICP), infection, and electrolyte and metabolic disturbances.[6] The incidence of secondary injury generally increases with the severity of the primary injury, although the relationship is not completely congruent. Patients with devastating primary injuries may initially have very little secondary injury. Conversely, patients with little primary injury may die or be crippled as a result of an enlarging intracranial hematoma. Clinically, the neurologic disturbance produced by primary injury is maximal at onset and then lessens or remains stable. By contrast, secondary injuries produce worsening of the patient's clinical neurologic status as their effects are added to those of the primary injury. Of considerable importance is the fact that secondary injuries are treatable and/or preventable.

Intracranial hematomas occur between the skull and dura mater (epidural; Fig. 93-6), between the dura mater and brain (subdural; Fig. 93-7), or within the substance of the brain (intracerebral; Fig. 93-8). As intracranial hematomas enlarge, they produce compression and shifting of the adjacent brain. This enlargement produces rapid and large increases in ICP as the volume-buffering capacity of the cranial contents is exhausted (see below). Hypoxia may occur as the result of central depression of respiration consequent to loss of consciousness, chest injury, aspiration of gastric contents, neurogenic pulmonary edema, or any combination of the above.

Evidence of ischemia is frequently found at autopsy following blunt head injury.[7] Focal ischemia may occur at the site of contusions or may be the result of vasospasm induced by traumatic subarachnoid hemorrhage. Global ischemia may be induced by systemic hypotension or reduction in cerebral perfusion pressure secondary to increased ICP.[8] Systemic hypotension at the time of admission to hospital has been shown to increase the mortality from severe head injury by approximately 150%.[9]

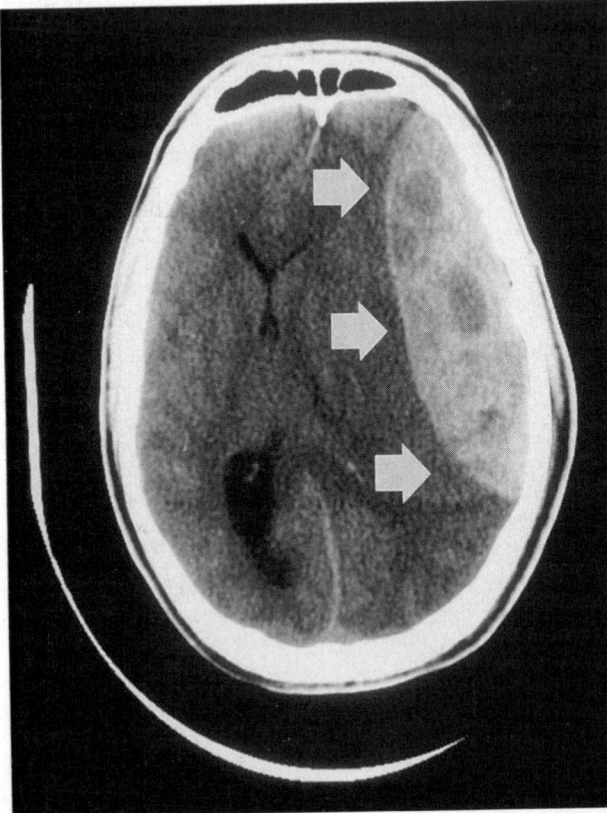

FIGURE 93-6 CT scan of a large acute epidural hematoma (*arrows*). Epidural (or extradural) hematomas have a convex medial border, which produces the lens shape that distinguishes epidural from subdural hematomas.

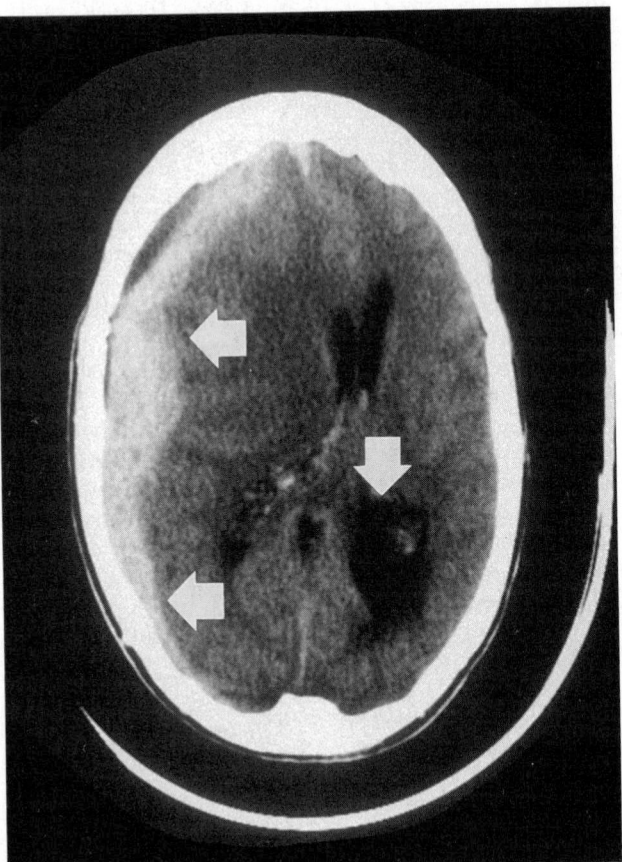

FIGURE 93-7 CT scan of a large acute subdural hematoma (*horizontal arrows*). The hematoma spreads over the entire convexity of the hemisphere, so that the medial border of the hematoma is concave. Note also the large amount of midline shift. The occipital horn of the left lateral ventricle is acutely enlarged as a result of trapping of CSF by ventricular distortion and obstruction of CSF flow (*vertical arrow*).

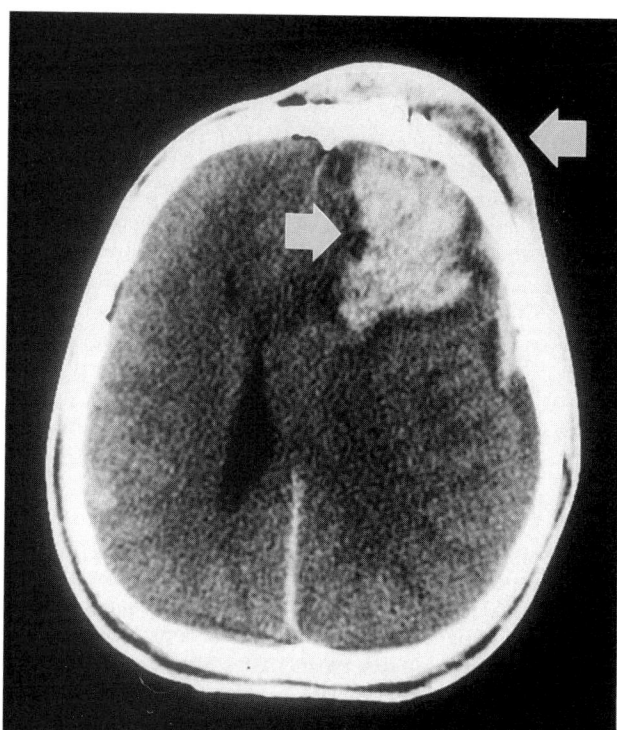

FIGURE 93-8 CT scan of a confluent traumatic intracerebral hematoma in the left frontal lobe of a patient struck by a motor vehicle (*lower arrow*). There is overlying scalp swelling and contusion at the site of the blow to the head (*upper arrow*).

Infection may be local (e.g., meningitis or brain abscess) or systemic. The former occurs when the integrity of the meninges is compromised as a result of penetrating injuries or compound fracture of the vault or skull base. Meningitis or ventriculitis may be iatrogenic, as a result of insertion of ICP-monitoring apparatus. Systemic infection typically involves the lungs or genitourinary tract. Systemic sepsis often causes neurologic deterioration that may improve with resolution of the infection. The accompanying hyperthermia often aggravates existing ICP problems.

Electrolyte disorders are common in patients with moderate and severe head injuries. The most frequent is the syndrome of inappropriate antidiuretic hormone secretion (SIADH). Serum sodium may fall significantly, and deterioration in patients' neurologic status usually occurs at levels below 120 to 125 mEq/L. Diabetes insipidus usually occurs in more severe injuries, often as a preterminal event in patients with progressive rostrocaudal neurologic deterioration caused by uncontrollable ICP elevation. In a much smaller number of patients, diabetes insipidus may be the result of focal injury to the hypothalamic-pituitary axis.

Severe head injury induces a state of catabolism with net excretion of nitrogen similar to that seen in other injuries. Catecholamine-induced tachycardia, increased blood pressure, and increased cardiac output are common. Myocardial ischemia may occur as a result of closed head injury.[10]

Abnormalities of blood coagulation are known to occur as a result of brain injury and are predictive of a poor outcome.[11] The reported incidence of coagulopathy depends to a certain extent on the diligence with which this entity is sought; its presence is often obscured by that of other potential causes of coagulation disturbance, such as massive transfusion in the multiply injured patient. Delayed and recurrent hematomas, including those related to placement of ventricular catheters, have been described in patients with disseminated intravascular coagulation.[12] In patients in whom a bleeding diathesis is known or suspected, it is preferable to use a subarachnoid bolt or epidural transducer rather than a ventricular catheter for ICP monitoring when there is a high likelihood of increased ICP (e.g., in the presence of a mass lesion). In patients who are known to have a low risk of raised ICP (i.e., those with normal CT scans), monitoring can be deferred until the coagulation abnormality is reversed.

INTRACRANIAL PRESSURE

Over the past 15 years, monitoring and control of ICP have been hallmarks of aggressive management of traumatic brain injury, and their use has been increasingly common in management of other cerebral disorders such as subarachnoid hemorrhage (SAH), intracerebral hematoma (ICH), brain tumors and liver disease. ICP monitoring and control are routine features of intensive care in most major neurosurgical centers and are done commonly in community hospitals. Although level one evidence of their efficacy is lacking, there is a substantial body of data to support their use and growing application.[13–16] Consensus guidelines derived by a panel of experts in the care of neurotrauma patients recommend the use of ICP monitoring in severely head-injured patients.[17] In this chapter, ICP monitoring will be discussed in the context of traumatic brain injury, but the techniques of monitoring and treatment are equally applicable to other conditions.

Since Lundberg[18] described ICP monitoring in 1960, its use in adults has been mainly in patients with severe head injury, both because of the large number of such patients and because intracranial hypertension is common when the injury is severe. We cannot tell whether a bad outcome in an individual patient results directly from the head injury, with brain swelling and increased ICP being epiphenomena, or whether it stems from secondary brain injury caused by cranial hypertension. In the first case, no remedy is possible. Most neurosurgeons assume and hope that the second case is actually present—i.e., that intracranial hypertension is adding to brain injury—and believe that ICP elevations should be detected and controlled. Any experienced neurosurgeon can relate anecdotes of cases in which detection and treatment of elevated ICP reversed neurologic deterioration and contributed to a good outcome. For example, detection of a delayed expanding intracranial hematoma by observation of rising ICP can lead to more prompt, and possibly life-saving, clot removal.

ICP is the pressure measured from some intracranial site and is generally recorded in millimeters of mercury. The site of measurement is usually in the cerebral ventricles or in the subdural or epidural space, or rarely in the brain parenchyma. While the brain is reasonably plastic, and the ICP measured at one place within the skull reflects fairly well the pressure at any other place, pressure gradients may develop across semirigid dural partitions in the skull when pathology is localized in one compartment (e.g., supratentorial vs. infratentorial). The combination of brain shift from focal masses, high intracranial pressure, and pressure gradients across dural and bony partitions (i.e., falx cerebri, tentorium, and foramen magnum) causes brain tissue to herniate from compartments with higher pressure to compartments with lower pressure. The most important of these cases is transtentorial herniation, signaled by the presence of an ipsilateral dilated and fixed or sluggishly reactive pupil. Intracranial hypertension is clearly potentially injurious. While the precise point at which ICP should be considered abnormal is not agreed upon and undoubtedly varies among different pathologies, ICP levels above 20 or 25 mm Hg that have been present for 10 to 15 minutes generally are considered pathologic and treatment is recommended.[17]

Cerebral perfusion pressure (CPP) represents the difference between mean arterial pressure (MAP) and ICP (CPP = MAP − ICP). In normal brain, cerebral blood flow (CBF) remains fairly constant at around 50 mL/100 g brain tissue per minute as long as cerebral autoregulation is intact—i.e., cerebral vessels change their diameter and resistance with pressure changes, so that a constant CBF is maintained as long as CPP is about 50 to 150 mm Hg. If MAP falls substantially or ICP rises substantially, then CPP falls too low to be corrected by autoregulation, and cerebral ischemia results. In cases of uncontrolled ICP, the terminal event is usually an increase of the ICP to a level at or slightly above the MAP. In severe head injury, there is some evidence of an autoregulatory breakpoint at a perfusion pressure of about 70 mm Hg.[19] In the case of marginal CPPs of around 50 to 60 mm Hg, one must remember that the focal CPP can be lower than the overall CPP if there are focal brain lesions, and a more generous CPP of 70 to 80 mm Hg may be necessary to prevent focal ischemia. A treatment protocol has been proposed (supported by uncontrolled data) wherein the emphasis on treatment resides primarily on elevating and maintaining the CPP above 70 mm Hg, often with systemic vasopressors with less emphasis on managing ICP in isolation.[20] A more recent review of ICP and CPP data from a large clinical trial in head injury suggests that it is ICP alone, rather than CPP, that is the more critical variable in determining outcome.[21] A randomized prospective trial of ICP- vs. CPP-targeted treatment showed a reduction in episodes of jugular venous oxygen desaturation (a surrogate measure for cerebral ischemia), but failed to show any beneficial effect on overall neurologic outcome. Furthermore, there was a fivefold increase in the incidence of acute respiratory distress syndrome in the CPP-targeted treatment group.[22]

One particularly dangerous situation for patients with severe head injury is when the hemisphere subjacent to a large subdural or epidural hematoma undergoes massive swelling after the hematoma is removed. The mass effect of the hematoma undoubtedly causes severe unilateral ischemia, but this effect is dramatically worsened by the hypoxia or hypotension that are present in about half the patients who develop this particularly severe postoperative complication. Even if ICP is normal shortly after the initial operative procedure, intracranial hypertension occurs in virtually all of these patients and may be uncontrollable and fatal in a high percentage.[23]

A small percentage of patients with intracranial hematomas develop delayed traumatic hematomas not seen on the initial CT scan, some after previous surgery for extracerebral hematomas and sometimes more than a day after injury.[24] ICP monitoring and recognition of intracranial hypertension can lead to earlier repeat CT and earlier identification and removal of clots than can reliance on the neurologic

examination alone,[25] although earlier clot removal has an uncertain effect on outcome.[26]

Management of Acute Head Injury

As may be inferred from the discussion of pathology and pathophysiology presented earlier, the management of head injury during the acute period is based primarily on the timely diagnosis and treatment of secondary insults to the injured brain. In the continued absence of effective drugs or other treatment strategies to reverse the pathophysiologic changes of diffuse axonal injury, management of the primary injury consists of providing the best possible physiologic milieu to permit unimpeded recovery of sublethally injured neurons.

DIAGNOSIS

Diagnosis in closed head injury is based on history, physical examination, and radiologic investigation. The relevant facts to be ascertained from the history are the mechanism of injury, whether there was any initial loss of consciousness, and whether the level of consciousness has improved or deteriorated since the injury. This last item is of paramount importance, since worsening of the patient's neurologic state subsequent to injury always implies the presence of secondary injury to the brain. Patients who have talked at some point after injury and who subsequently lapse into unconsciousness almost invariably are harboring an intracranial hematoma. One should determine whether or not there has been any witnessed seizure activity, since seizures may produce transient profound deterioration in the level of consciousness that may mimic that induced by an expanding intracranial hematoma.

Neurologic examination consists of two components: determination of the level of consciousness and identification of any focal deficits to aid in lesion localization and the measurement of severity. Determination of the level of consciousness is the single most important measure to be taken following traumatic brain injury and is best accomplished by use of the Glasgow Coma Scale (GCS). Although the scores in the three response categories of the GCS are frequently summed for convenience, more information is conveyed by reporting them separately. The motor score from the patient's "best" side is used if there is a discrepancy in response between sides. Intubation may be designated by a "T" for the verbal response score. In patients with a disturbed level of consciousness, the scope of the traditional neurologic examination is severely limited because of its considerable dependence on patient cooperation. In unconscious patients, crude localization may be achieved by observing discrepancies between sides in the patient's motor response to pain. Evidence of brain stem dysfunction should be sought; the common measures are pupillary reaction to light, oculocephalic responses (doll's-eye movements) or oculocaloric responses, and corneal reflexes. Doll's-eye testing should be deferred until the cervical spine is known to be intact, and oculocaloric testing should not be carried out in the presence of a ruptured tympanic membrane. Unless there has been local ocular trauma, the presence of unilateral pupillary dilation and unreactivity implies the presence of a mass lesion, and urgent diagnosis and evacuation of the mass are essential. This is particularly important in cases of unwitnessed unconsciousness, and investigation of metabolic causes of coma should be deferred until a CT scan has been obtained.

Another relevant aspect of the physical examination is examination of the head for signs of trauma. These include bruising or laceration of the face and scalp; open skull fractures; hemotympanum and bruising over the mastoid process (Battle sign), indicating fracture of the petrous temporal bone; and periorbital hematoma (raccoon eye), indicating fracture of the floor of the anterior fossa. One should also look for signs of CSF leakage from the nose or ears. CSF may be mixed with blood; if the draining fluid forms a target shape on a piece of filter paper, the presence of CSF is indicated. Biochemical determination of the presence of CSF is usually not possible because of the difficulty in collecting a sufficient volume of the draining fluid.

CT is essential to the proper management of unconscious head-injured patients. It makes it possible to diagnose all types of intracranial hematoma and to determine their location and the extent of the mass effect they produce (measured by the displacement of the septum pellucidum from the midline). The scan should be obtained as soon as the patient is stable and any more urgent management priorities have been addressed. It is occasionally necessary to forego CT to deal with life-threatening injuries to other systems or because there would be an unacceptably long wait for a scan in a patient with a high likelihood of having an intracranial surface clot. Unconscious patients should have radiologic assessment of the cervical spine to the level of T1 to rule out cervical fracture. In the absence of x-ray evidence of an intact cervical spine, one must presume there is a fracture and continue to immobilize the head and spine until appropriate x-rays are obtained and the necessary treatment instituted.

Magnetic resonance imaging (MRI) has been used on a limited basis with head-injured patients. MRI is better than CT at detecting some types of small extra-axial fluid collections and parenchymal injuries. However, it offers no advantage in detecting hematomas requiring surgical treatment, and the difficulties inherent in having to exclude metallic objects from the scan environment render the technique somewhat impractical in the acute posttrauma setting. A potential application is the improved identification of parenchymal changes following mild and moderate head injury that have been shown to correlate with the neuropsychologic sequelae of head injury.[27,28]

PREOPERATIVE MANAGEMENT

In the initial phase of head injury management, the usual diagnostic and treatment priorities for the management of trauma patients are followed. Establishment of an adequate airway is of paramount importance in unconscious patients. All patients with a GCS ≤8 should have endotracheal or nasotracheal intubation and mechanical ventilation, regardless of whether other indications for intubation are present or not. Direct laryngoscopy can raise ICP dramatically, potentially worsening cerebral ischemia. Intubation should be performed by experienced personnel and after appropriate premedication (see Chap. 35).[29] Nasotracheal intubation should be avoided in patients with signs of basal skull fracture. Patients should be hyperventilated to a modest degree (partial pressure of carbon dioxide [P_{CO_2}] 30 to 35 mm Hg) to reduce raised ICP. Patients with a clear-cut deterioration in neurologic status should be given mannitol in a dose of approximately

1 g/kg body weight. Contraindications to the use of mannitol are hypotension, anuria, and severe congestive heart failure. Corticosteroids are of no benefit in reducing ICP in head injury, and their use has been abandoned in most centers. As soon as other management priorities have been dealt with, the patient should undergo CT.

Mild therapeutic hypothermia was first proposed as a treatment for brain trauma in the late 1950s. Hypothermia can lower ICP, alter chemical pathways that could contribute to injury, and modulate apoptosis. In 2001 the results of a large multicenter trial were published, demonstrating that hypothermia (target = 33°C) was not effective in improving functional outcome at 6 months, even though ICP was better controlled.[30] A more recent study raises again the possibility that hypothermia may confer benefit. Patients with severe head injury (GCS score ≤8) who continued to have intracranial hypertension (ICP >20 mm Hg) despite standard resuscitation, attention to the adequacy of CPP, surgery (when indicated), sedation, mannitol, therapeutic paralysis, and pentobarbital infusion, were cooled to 32°C.[31] Hypothermia was maintained for at least 24 hours or until slow rewarming did not cause the ICP to rise (mean duration of cooling = 4.8 days). Hypothermic subjects were less likely to die (62% vs. 72%), but only a small subgroup of patients with a GCS of 5 to 6 accounted for the majority of the response difference (12/25 hypothermia subjects survived vs. 6/25 control subjects). Given these conflicting data, as well as the fact that hypothermia is potentially harmful, leading to hypovolemia, hypotension, and electrolyte disturbances, this intervention should be considered investigational.

OPERATIVE MANAGEMENT

INTRACRANIAL HEMATOMA

The cornerstone of acute head injury management is the rapid diagnosis and prompt surgical evacuation of intracranial hematomas. Twenty-five to fifty percent of patients rendered comatose as a result of acute head injury have an operable intracranial hematoma.[3,6,14,32,33] Approximately 20% of patients with intracranial hematomas have an extradural hematoma, and the rest have hemispheric acute subdural hematomas, significant brain contusions, or both.[6,32,33] Traumatic hematomas in the posterior fossa are unusual. The diagnosis is ordinarily made by CT. Surgical evacuation is then accomplished via craniotomy, with wide exposure and evacuation of the hematoma and coagulation of sources of hemorrhage. Rarely, when there is clear-cut evidence of neurologic deterioration with progression to signs of uncal herniation (i.e., pupillary dilation), it is necessary to proceed directly to operation, bypassing CT. The other circumstance in which exploratory burr holes may be necessary is in comatose patients with signs of brain stem compromise who must be taken to the operating room for life-threatening systemic injuries without benefit of a CT scan. An alternate strategy in these patients is twist-drill air ventriculography in the operating room. The standard landmarks are used for cannulation of the frontal horn of the lateral ventricle. Once the ventricle is cannulated, 4 to 8 mL of air is introduced into the ventricles, and a brow-up anteroposterior skull film is obtained. The presence of a mass lesion is inferred from shift of the ventricular system (Fig. 93-9).

The frequent coexistence of acute subdural hematomas and temporal and/or frontal cortical laceration/contusion dictates

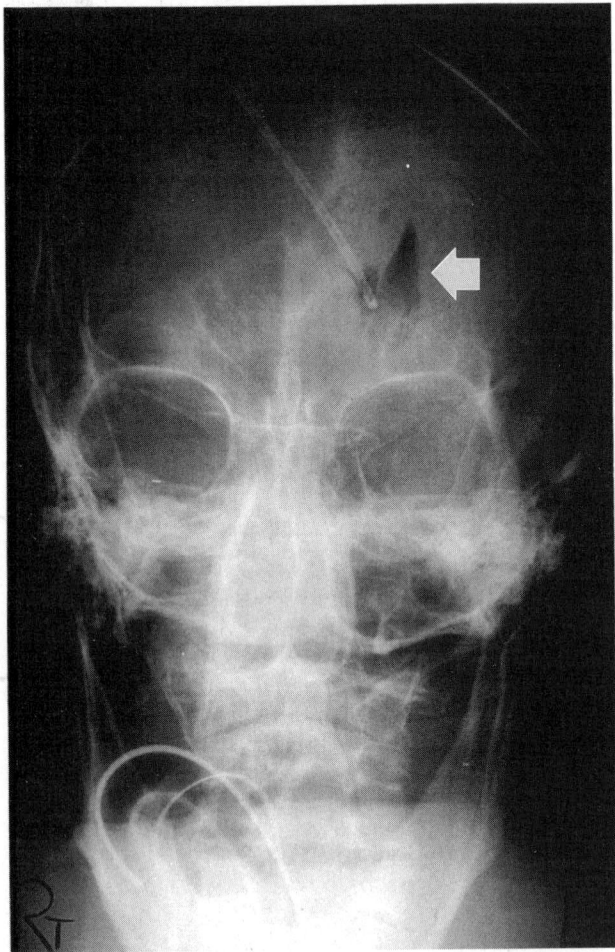

FIGURE 93-9 Air ventriculogram done in the operating room in a multiply injured patient. Air (4 mL) was injected into the ventricular catheter and an anteroposterior skull film obtained. The displacement of the frontal horns of the ventricles (*arrow*) away from the midline toward the left side indicates a mass lesion on the right side. Subsequent craniotomy revealed a large right frontal intracerebral hematoma.

the necessity of a wide operative exposure, allowing access to both the frontal and temporal lobes, as well as the medial convexity adjacent to the sagittal sinus, where there may be torn bridging veins (Fig. 93-10). The operative approach to an isolated extradural hematoma may be more circumscribed. Contusions of the frontal and temporal lobes, or confluent blood clots producing a midline shift greater than 5 mm, should be evacuated operatively through the standard large flap. Often, removal of the contused brain must be accompanied by formal frontal or temporal lobectomy to provide adequate internal decompression in the face of a traumatized, swollen brain. In this circumstance, the question of whether or not to leave out the craniotomy bone flap (or remove it later) to provide more room for the swollen brain has engendered some controversy. The prevailing view is that this measure does not improve the functional outcome. It is probable, however, that poor outcomes with this procedure are usually due to the fact that the patient had overwhelming primary injury, and that decompressive craniectomy may be useful in patients in whom the degree of primary injury is compatible with a reasonable neurologic outcome.

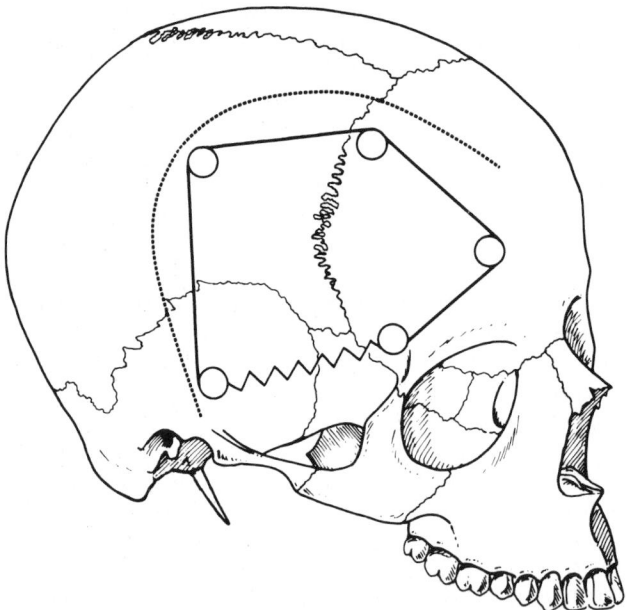

FIGURE 93-10 Diagram of the operative exposure for the removal of a traumatic intracranial hematoma. The skin incision is shown with the dotted line. The skull flap is outlined with a solid line. The exposure permits access to the major portion of the hemisphere convexity, as well as sufficient access for débridement/lobectomy of the frontal or temporal lobes.

At the conclusion of the evacuation of a hematoma, an ICP monitoring device is placed in almost all cases. The exceptions are patients whose level of consciousness was only mildly depressed preoperatively (GCS >10), and in whom the brain is not significantly contused or swollen at the time of operative exposure. The techniques and indications for ICP monitoring will be discussed.

PENETRATING INJURY

The same principles of prompt evacuation of intracranial hematomas and débridement of contused brain apply to penetrating injuries. The other indication for operating on compound lesions is the restoration of the integrity of the dura and overlying tissues to prevent bacterial infection of CSF (i.e., meningitis) or cerebral parenchyma (brain abscess). Accessible indriven bone fragments should all be removed, as well as underlying hematoma and devitalized brain. It is not necessary to attempt to remove inaccessible missile or bone fragments from the depths of the missile tract. Prophylactic antibiotics are used to reduce the incidence of delayed infection in cases of penetrating injury. Broad-spectrum coverage with antibiotics capable of crossing the blood-brain barrier should be used.[34]

BASAL SKULL FRACTURE

A special case of compound injury is the basal skull fracture with leakage of CSF through the paranasal sinuses or into the mastoid air cells, middle ear, and external ear or pharynx. CSF otorrhea almost always stops spontaneously, and surgical repair of the leak is rarely necessary. Rhinorrhea is more likely to continue, and the continued presence of a CSF fistula will eventually lead to meningitis. Surgical repair of an anterior fossa fistula may be undertaken early when there is an obvious bony disruption of the anterior fossa floor, often coincident with complex facial fractures. In this case, repair of the CSF leak is undertaken at the time of facial reconstructive surgery. In cases of persistent CSF leak without obvious bony disruption, the site of the fistula may sometimes be localized with coronal CT cuts through the anterior fossa following the instillation of water-soluble radiographic contrast material into the CSF. Investigation of persistent CSF leakage should be deferred until the patient is stable with respect to both ICP and coexisting systemic injuries. Occasionally, bilateral anterior fossa exploration is necessary in the face of persistent CSF rhinorrhea for which the site cannot be identified radiologically.

There is considerable debate about the merits of prophylactic antibiotics for CSF rhinorrhea and otorrhea. Unfortunately, there are no good clinical studies to support either their use or their abandonment, and this remains largely a matter of personal preference. We do not use prophylactic antibiotics for CSF leakage in our unit for fear of selecting for multiply resistant organisms. When there is established infection, the diagnosis and treatment are the same as for meningitis of any cause. Operative repair of the dural fistula should not be undertaken until the infection has been cleared with appropriate antibiotic therapy.

CRITICAL CARE MONITORING

Monitoring of the head-injured patient is designed to detect and treat secondary injuries before they further compromise the injured brain. Ideally one would like to monitor neurologic function, cerebral blood flow and cerebral metabolism, intracranial pressure, and those systemic parameters required for the maintenance of adequate perfusion and oxygenation of the brain. Measurement of all these parameters is possible, but cerebral blood flow and cerebral metabolism are difficult to measure, and the ideal situation described here is rarely practiced.

CLINICAL EXAMINATION

Monitoring of neurologic function is most commonly and simply carried out by means of hourly repetition of the abbreviated version of the neurologic examination described earlier, in the section on diagnosis. Any deterioration in the patient's neurologic status should trigger an investigation for treatable causes. Neuromuscular blocking agents used to treat raised ICP or respiratory problems make it impossible to conduct a meaningful neurologic examination. In addition, these drugs are associated with numerous complications and may be associated with a worse outcome in head-injured patients.[35] When neuromuscular blocking agents are given, only the pupillary responses are available as a means of assessment. Because significant deterioration in the patient's neurologic function may occur before pupillary changes are evident, ICP monitoring becomes essential to provide some information about the status of the patient. Although ICP is not a measure of neurologic function per se, many of the pathologic processes that endanger the head-injured patient in the early phase after injury manifest themselves with raised ICP in addition to neurologic deterioration. In a patient who is pharmacologically paralyzed for ICP control, paralysis should be allowed to wear off at intervals of 12 to 24 hours so that a neurologic assessment may be carried out. Occasionally the effects of reversal of ICP are intolerable, and reversal

is not possible. A potential alternative to clinical neurologic monitoring is electrophysiologic measurement of neurologic function. The common techniques are electroencephalography (EEG) and evoked potentials (EPs).

Electroencephalography

EEG recordings in comatose patients typically show slowing of the background frequencies; in most cases there is a correlation between the degree of slowing and the depth of coma. Conventional strip-chart EEG is impractical because of the amount of data generated. Various methods of data compression have evolved, the most common being fast Fourier transformation of the EEG. Fourier transformation yields quantitative frequency and amplitude data from the EEG, and is well suited to detecting long-term trends in the background frequencies and to performing quantitative analysis of such trends. Recognition of specific patterns (e.g., seizure spikes) is sacrificed. Survival from head injury has been correlated with a return of higher-frequency activity in the first week after injury.[36]

Evoked Potentials

EPs have been demonstrated to be particularly useful in predicting outcome from head injury. The single most useful measure is the somatosensory evoked response,[37] although combinations of EPs (somatosensory, auditory, and visual) yield the highest prognostic accuracy.[38] Deterioration in serially measured EPs, occurring as a result of secondary injury to the brain, have been shown to correlate with poor patient outcome.[39] In the past, EPs have been used primarily in an intermittent manner for determination of prognosis. With further technologic improvements and increased automation of data collection, these techniques may see more widespread use for continuous monitoring in an ICU setting.

ICP Monitoring

Numerous reports suggest a beneficial effect of ICP monitoring and treatment of intracranial hypertension, although there are no controlled trials to support this. In a group of patients with GCS scores of 3, 4, or 5, the mortality rate was 39% when ICP was monitored and 67% when it was not; however, the patients were not randomly allocated to the two groups.[40] In another series, using patients evaluated in sequential time periods with slightly different treatment protocols, the mortality rate fell from 46% to 33% when ICP was rigorously controlled below 15 mm Hg.[14] In as many as 75% of patients who die after head injury, there is pathologic evidence of intracranial hypertension as measured by medial temporal lobe necrosis, secondary brain stem damage, or cerebral ischemic changes.[41] These and other reports have convinced most neurosurgeons that ICP monitoring is appropriate in patients with traumatic coma.

Elevated ICP clearly correlates with a poor outcome in head-injured patients. In one series of patients with severe head injury, 74% of the patients whose ICP remained below 20 mm Hg had a satisfactory outcome, while only 55% of the patients who required therapy to control ICP to this level had a similar outcome. Of the patients whose ICP could not be controlled, 92% died, and only 3% had a satisfactory outcome.[32] In another series, the number of patients who died or remained institutionalized more than doubled when ICP was higher than 15 mm Hg (57% versus 23%) than when it remained below that level.[42] In addition to its effects on survival, intracranial hypertension affects brain function in survivors. Neuropsychologic assessment done 1 year after severe head injury revealed that hyperemia during the acute phase correlated better with poor intellectual and memory function than did low-flow states, and that patients who had experienced intracranial hypertension had more memory deficits than those whose ICP had remained normal.[43]

A variety of monitoring techniques have been used over the past 30 years. Lundberg first used a ventriculostomy coupled to a fluid-filled manometer.[18] This system was cumbersome and carried a considerable risk of causing infection. As electronic transducers became available, closed monitoring systems came into use. Although a few implantable transducers have been used experimentally, they are not in regular clinical use today. The two most common ICP monitoring systems used now are fluid-filled catheters and rigid bolts[44] attached to an electromechanical transducer or a fiberoptic system that detects deflection of a sensing mirror to measure ICP.[45] The former devices are generally less expensive, but are prone to blockage and may require more experience on the part of the clinician to keep them functioning optimally. The latter may provide more accurate data for longer periods without the need for intervention by doctors or nurses. The fluid-filled systems may be more appropriate in hospitals where ICP monitoring is common and is applied in several patients simultaneously; in such settings, medical personnel become familiar with the system and can recognize and correct problems as they arise. The fiberoptic systems may be more appropriate for facilities where fewer patients require ICP monitoring.

We currently use either subdural or intraventricular catheters for monitoring ICP, which we place either in the operating room at the time of surgery or at the bedside in the ICU (Fig. 93-11). We prefer an intraventricular position, so that CSF can be drained when necessary to lower ICP. An intraventricular catheter can be placed through a craniotomy opening in the operating room or by twist-drill ventriculostomy in the

operating room or ICU when the ventricles seem to be large enough to permit entry. When the ventricles are compressed by brain swelling, we prefer to use a subdural catheter, which can only be placed in the operating room. (Because a twist-drill hole is perpendicular to the skull and brain, it precludes catheter insertion parallel to the inner table of the skull over the brain surface.) Placement of an ICP device requires meticulous sterile technique; if any part of the system is contaminated during insertion or attachment, it must be discarded and replaced. Intracranial infection is a devastating complication when added to the brain dysfunction for which monitoring is required. ICP monitors should be placed by neurosurgeons, since they are most familiar with manipulating brain tissue and are least likely to induce brain hemorrhage, a risk that is always present and that can be fatal. Epidural catheters must be placed through a burr hole in the operating room and are used less frequently than subdural or intraventricular monitors.

We attach the ICP catheter to pressure transducers connected to monitors, which provide continuous digital and waveform displays of ICP as well as of arterial, central venous, or pulmonary vascular pressures as needed in either the operating room or the ICU. The data can be sampled by a central ICU computer so that these and other parameters can be analyzed over a few hours or days. Usually a good pressure tracing is easily recognized, having a regular pulse pressure of 3 to 7 mm Hg (the pulse pressure can be greater at elevated ICP). The ICP baseline gently drifts up and down with respiratory or ventilatory excursions as intrathoracic pressure changes cause slight alterations in the intracranial venous pressure and ICP. A flat ICP tracing cannot be interpreted; a grave error in ICP monitoring is accepting a meaningless digital readout number as the actual ICP when the tracing clearly does not reflect a valid waveform. A flat tracing usually is due to blockage by blood or brain occluding the catheter tip or to a kink somewhere along the catheter. After the extracranial portion of the monitor is inspected for proper placement, it may be necessary to inject a small amount (0.25 mL initially) of an irrigating solution to clear the catheter tip; a larger amount, even only 1 mL, can markedly increase ICP when the brain is tight. It is helpful to turn the system stopcock from the injection position back to the monitoring position *while the irrigant is being injected.* If the stopcock is turned after the injection is completed, brain under pressure may immediately occlude the catheter tip when the injection pressure is stopped. Even if a catheter reoccludes and produces a flat waveform, a valid estimate of the ICP usually can be made. After a small amount of irrigant is injected, the ICP will be briefly elevated and have large pulse pressures, but will drift asymptotically toward the true ICP before becoming a flat line again.

The ICP catheter and transducer are filled with an antibiotic solution containing gentamicin, 1 mg/mL, which is stable in solution for 4 to 6 days and has wide antibacterial activity. It is important to maintain a closed system as much as possible; this requires tight connections throughout the monitoring system. It is imperative that no CSF leak around the catheter; any such leakage greatly increases the risk of infection. If leakage is noted, a new purse-string suture must be placed around the catheter's exit from the scalp. If the monitoring device is sufficiently flexible, it should be brought out through a stab wound a short distance from the incision made to insert it to further reduce infection risk. Our intracranial infection rate

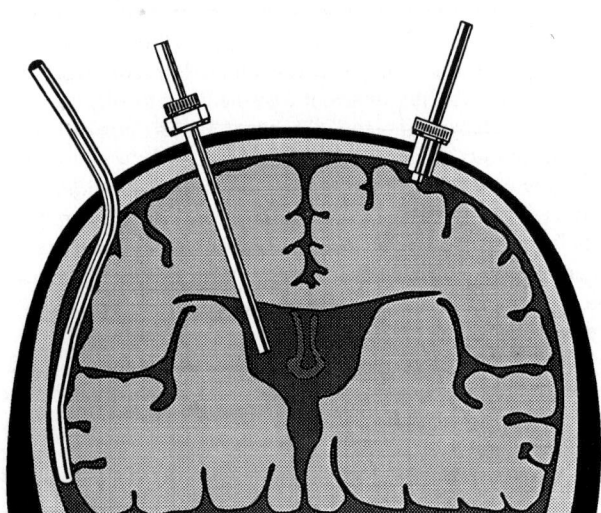

FIGURE 93-11 Schematic drawing of a coronal section of the brain, showing (left to right) the placement of a subdural flexible catheter, an intraventricular catheter, and a rigid subarachnoid bolt.

for treatment of a variety of open or penetrating brain injuries is <2%, so the infection rate attributable to ICP monitoring is extremely low. Infection rates vary from 0.7% to 6.3% in other series using different devices.[46,47] In 378 patients, several different fluid-filled systems for monitoring ICP were compared regarding their tendency to become blocked or infected. The rigid Richmond bolt[42] became occluded 16% of the time; subdural or intraventricular catheters became blocked only 3% of the time, but the intraventricular catheters were associated with complications of infection or intracerebral hemorrhage, and led the authors to recommend the subdural catheter as the best of the methods.[48] However, intraventricular catheters allow withdrawal of CSF, which can be a critical method of ICP control. Some prefer to measure the change in ICP produced by withdrawal of a measured volume (ΔV) of CSF to determine the intracranial compliance ($\Delta V/\Delta ICP$); we have not found this additional measurement to provide a sufficient increment in useful data to warrant the time and risk involved.

Blood Flow and Metabolic Rate

Cerebral blood flow and cerebral metabolism have been measured in a number of units engaged in clinical research. The common techniques rely on measurement of washout curves from the brain of nitrous oxide or radioactive xenon. The equipment and techniques for conducting CBF measurements are complicated and expensive, and this fact has discouraged widespread adoption of these methods. Furthermore, in the case of xenon CBF measurement, the number of studies that can be carried out in a given patient is limited by radiation safety concerns. The incidence of ischemic levels of blood flow is highest within 12 hours of severe injury, and blood flow usually increases to normal levels by 24 hours.[49] Knowledge of CBF may be useful in identifying patients in whom hyperemia is contributing substantially to increased ICP, and thus to determine if treatment with hyperventilation may be used safely. CBF, the cerebral metabolic rate for oxygen (CMR_{O_2}), and the arterial-jugular oxygen content difference (AVD_{O_2}) are related by the following equation:

$$CMR_{O_2} = (AVD_{O_2} \times 3\ CBF)/100$$

When CMR_{O_2} is relatively constant, AVD_{O_2} varies inversely with CBF; therefore, it has been suggested that AVD_{O_2} could be used as an index of the adequacy of cerebral blood flow.[50] The jugular oxygen content may be measured by advancing a central venous catheter rostrally in the internal jugular vein upward to the base of the skull. The normal AVD_{O_2} is 4 to 9 vol%. Higher values indicate increased oxygen extraction and potential ischemia. More recently, fiberoptic catheters have been developed that will give a continuous readout of jugular venous oxygen saturation. Episodes of desaturation have been correlated with a poor outcome.[51,52]

Hemodynamics

Hemodynamic monitoring in the acute phase of head injury management should include arterial pressure monitoring and detailed measurement of fluid input and output. When repeated large doses of mannitol are administered, invasive hemodynamic monitoring may be necessary to maintain an accurate assessment of intravascular volume status in the face of massive diuresis and consequent fluid replacement (see below).

MEDICAL MANAGEMENT

MANIPULATING INTRACRANIAL PRESSURE

The medical management of acute head injury focuses primarily on the detection and treatment of raised intracranial pressure. Although the ICP is less than 10 mm Hg in normal individuals, 20 to 25 mm Hg is generally accepted as the point at which ICP requires treatment in head injury patients. Transient elevations above this level are common when patients are restless or coughing; therefore, persistence of the ICP elevation for 5 to 10 minutes in a nonagitated patient should be observed before treatment is initiated. In all cases, a cause for the elevation should be sought. There may be a problem with ventilation or obstruction of jugular venous return. Unless contraindicated by other injuries, patients should be positioned head-up 30° with the neck neutral between flexion and extension. If the ICP elevation persists after adequacy of ventilation and unimpeded jugular venous return have been assured, it is incumbent on the physician to rule out a surgically treatable cause of the ICP elevation with a CT scan. In cases of unoperated cerebral contusion, an increase in ICP may signify the need for surgical evacuation of the contused brain.[53]

Once it has been determined that the ICP increase has no surgically treatable cause, management depends on pharmacologic reduction of ICP and manipulation of the patient's P_{CO_2}. If the patient is not ventilated, intubation and mechanical ventilation should be instituted with moderate hyperventilation (i.e., P_{CO_2} 30 to 34 mm Hg). Hyperventilation to levels of 25 mm Hg or below has been shown to have an adverse effect on outcome.[54] If the patient is already ventilated, sedation with morphine or an analog should be given. The anesthetic agent propofol has come into increasing use for this indication. A recent randomized clinical trial has shown that it is safe and efficacious for sedation of intubated and ventilated head-injured patients.[55] If this measure is insufficient to reduce the ICP, then pharmacologic paralysis should be induced. In patients who are febrile, reduction of the core temperature to 37°C or lower by means of a cooling blanket frequently results in reduction of raised ICP. Often these measures alone are sufficient.

If the ICP elevation persists, and there is a ventricular drain in place, intermittent drainage of CSF may be instituted. It may be necessary to repeat drainage several times an hour. Continuous drainage should not be used, because drainage will often cease as the ventricles undergo progressive compression, and during ventricular drainage the ICP is not being measured. One is then in the unfortunate situation of not reducing the ICP and not being aware of the true ICP. If ventricular drainage is not feasible or effective, then mannitol must be used.

Mannitol, an osmotic diuretic, is the single most useful pharmacologic agent in the management of raised ICP following head injury. The dosage is 0.5 to 1.0 g/kg of a 20% solution infused as a bolus. Typically, the effects of mannitol on ICP will last from 2 to 6 hours, depending on the severity of the underlying pathologic process. Mannitol may be administered repeatedly as long as the serum osmolarity does not exceed 320 mOsm/L. At osmolarities greater than this, the effectiveness of the drug is reduced, and there is an increasing risk of renal toxicity.[56] With frequent repeated doses of mannitol and the consequent diuresis, the patient may become systemically dehydrated, resulting in hypotension and increased serum osmolarity. Systemic dehydration is not necessary to achieve reduction in ICP. Therefore, the excess urine loss caused by mannitol should be replaced. The amount and type of replacement fluid should be calibrated to maintain high normal intravascular volume, a serum osmolarity of <320 mOsm/L, and normal serum electrolytes. With this regimen, it may be possible to give mannitol at intervals of 2 hours for several days at a time using aggregate volumes of 2 to 3 L of mannitol per day.

Furosemide can be used to reduce intracranial hypertension and probably works by inducing diuresis, increasing intravascular oncotic pressure, removing brain water, and possibly reducing CSF production.[57] The combination of mannitol and furosemide may be more effective in lowering ICP than either drug alone. This synergistic effect is not from an altered renal excretion of mannitol; furosemide may help to sustain the elevated serum osmolarity induced by mannitol, or may sustain the osmotic gradient across the blood-brain barrier induced by mannitol.[57] However, some caution is advised, since the combined use of mannitol and furosemide can cause rapid dehydration, hypotension, and a reduced CPP with the risk of brain ischemia.

In situations in which the combination of measures listed above is insufficient to control ICP, or where mannitol can no longer be used because of extant or incipient renal failure, pentobarbital may be a useful adjunct in the management of ICP.[58] It is not a first-choice agent, since it is clearly less effective than mannitol in lowering raised ICP,[59] may cause harmful cardiovascular side effects, and has no demonstrated protective effects on the brain when administered prophylactically to head-injured patients with or without raised ICP.[60] The dose regimen varies in the published literature, and pentobarbital may be given by bolus infusion or by drip. A typical approach is to administer a bolus of 10 mg/kg over 30 minutes, followed by a continuous infusion at 1 to 3 mg/kg per hour. The end point of administration is reduction of ICP or an unacceptable decrease in arterial blood pressure. Adequate hemodynamic monitoring (i.e., an arterial line and central venous catheter) must be in place before pentobarbital is given, and adequate intravascular volume should be assured prior to administration. Infusion of norepinephrine or other vasoactive agents is often necessary to maintain an adequate arterial pressure. Administration of high doses of pentobarbital will result in pupillary dilation and unreactivity, so that no clinical neurologic examination is possible. Brain stem auditory evoked responses (BAEPs) are preserved, and their recording may be a useful adjunct to the management of patients in barbiturate coma.[61]

The medical management of intracranial hypertension after head injury is generally successful in the vast majority of patients with severe head injury.[58,62,63] In one series, when standard medical management was unsuccessful, pentobarbital coma was induced, but it only controlled intracranial hypertension in about 30% of these patients. A subtemporal decompression was then performed, resulting in a significant further reduction in ICP and a 60% survival, compared with <20% survival when subtemporal decompression was not done.[62] Other surgical options available for the treatment of refractory ICP include subfrontal decompressive craniectomy, removal of an existing bone flap, or internal decompression by removal of a swollen or damaged frontal or temporal lobe. The controversy surrounding decompressive craniectomy has been alluded to above. These surgical adjuncts perhaps deserve consideration for a very small number of head-injured patients who do not respond to other avenues of ICP control. We have used surgical management in young patients with refractory ICP who have a reasonable potential for neurologic recovery (i.e., GCS ≥7).

MANAGEMENT OF SEIZURES

Seizures may aggravate an existing brain injury; therefore, their prompt treatment is essential. Factors that increase the risk of late epilepsy include severe injuries, intracranial hematomas, and the presence of seizures early after injury. Ordinarily, patients in these risk categories are given prophylactic phenytoin at the time of admission, and the medication is continued for 6 to 12 months, depending on the injury type and on whether or not any seizures have occurred. Prophylactic anticonvulsants have only been shown to be effective in the early posttraumatic period.[64] A discussion of acute seizure management is provided elsewhere in this text (see Chap. 64).

NUTRITION

The caloric requirements imposed by a head injury are comparable to those of a burn covering 20% to 40% of the body surface area. The requirements are increased by motor posturing and reduced by barbiturate coma or muscle relaxants. Enteral feeding via nasogastric tube is usually possible and is certainly desirable early after injury, unless there has been major abdominal trauma, in which case parenteral alimentation may be used. Although the nitrogen loss resulting from a severe head injury may be mitigated by early feeding, it may not be possible to reverse it consistently.[65]

FLUID AND ELECTROLYTES

SIADH is usually successfully managed by restricting free water intake to 1 liter or less per 24 hours. Demeclocycline may be a useful adjunct when the syndrome persists beyond a few days. Hypertonic saline (3%) is occasionally necessary to correct profound hyponatremia in the presence of serious neurologic symptoms (e.g., seizures). Diabetes insipidus may be managed with desmopressin acetate (DDAVP). The dosage is 1 to 2 μg (0.25 to 0.5 mL) intravenously two to four times daily as necessary to control urine output. Serum and urine osmolarity and electrolyte measurements are necessary to distinguish true diabetes insipidus from excessive diuresis caused by mobilization of fluids used during resuscitation or as a result of the use of mannitol for control of ICP.

REHABILITATION

Attention to the rehabilitation needs of the patient should begin on or shortly after admission to the critical care unit. In the early days after admission, this consists of proper positioning, regular turning, skin care, and movement of patients' limbs through their full range to minimize or prevent late joint contractures and skin decubiti, either of which may significantly retard recovery; more active rehabilitation begins once consciousness has been regained. Sensory stimulation programs to facilitate the return of normal consciousness are attractive in theory, but they have not been tested by randomized clinical trials. As the patient's level of consciousness improves, the goals of rehabilitation therapy change from maintenance of normal limb posture and movement to the retraining of simple and then progressively more complex physical and mental activities. Although at this time the patient will normally be out of the ICU, it is important that these measures be initiated in the ICU.

Outcome from Traumatic Brain Injury

The mortality from severe head injury varies from 30% to just over 50% in most published series.[3,6,14,32,33,40] Factors associated with a decreased likelihood of survival are low GCS, advanced age, the presence of significant intracranial hematomas, and the presence of significant systemic injuries in addition to the head injury. Approximately 50% of patients dying from head injury do so from uncontrollable ICP, and this occurs early in the patient's course. In 30% to 60%, there is a good outcome or moderate disability. In contrast, the number of patients with a good outcome or moderate disability following hypoxic-ischemic coma was 13% in one large series.[66] In addition to those patients who die, small numbers will be left in a persistent vegetative state or alert but totally dependent. The numbers of such patients have not been increased in those series of patients in which mortality was reduced by early aggressive management of head injury.[6] Recovery may continue for up to 18 to 24 months after head injury, although the most significant gains are made during the first 6 months.[3]

References

1. Frankowski RF, Annegers JF, Whitman S: Epidemiological and descriptive studies. Part 1: The descriptive epidemiology of head trauma in the United States, in Becker DP, Povlishock JT (eds): *Central Nervous System Trauma Status Report.* Bethesda, MD, National Institute of Neurological and Communicative Disorders and Stroke, National Institutes of Health, 1985, p 33.
2. Teasdale G, Jennett B: Assessment of coma and impaired consciousness: A practical scale. *Lancet* 2:81, 1974.
3. Jennett B, Teasdale G, Galbraith S, et al: Severe head injury in three countries. *J Neurol Neurosurg Psychiatry* 40:291, 1977.
4. Povlishock JT: Pathobiology of traumatically induced axonal injury in animals and man. *Ann Emerg Med* 22:980, 1993.
5. Narayan RK, Michel ME et al: Clinical trials in head injury. *J Neurotrauma* 19:503, 2002.
6. Becker DP, Miller JD, Ward JD, et al: The outcome from severe head injury with early diagnosis and intensive management. *J Neurosurg* 47:491, 1977.
7. Graham DI, Adams JH, Doyle D: Ischaemic brain damage in fatal non-missile head injuries. *J Neurol Sci* 39:213, 1978.
8. Bouma GJ, Muizelaar JP: Cerebral blood flow in severe clinical head injury. *New Horiz* 3:384, 1995.
9. Chesnut RM, Marshall LF, Klauber MR, et al: The role of secondary brain injury in determining outcome from severe head injury. *J Trauma* 34:216, 1993.
10. Robertson CS, Clifton GL, Taylor AA, Grossman RG: Treatment of hypertension associated with head injury. *J Neurosurg* 59:455, 1983.
11. Olson JD, Kaufman HH, Moake J, et al: Incidence and significance of hemostatic abnormalities in patients with head injuries. *Neurosurgery* 24:825, 1989.
12. Kaufman HH, Moake JL, Olson JD, et al: Delayed and recurrent intracranial hematomas related to disseminated intravascular clotting and fibrinolysis in head injury. *Neurosurgery* 7:445, 1980.
13. Brajtbord D, Parks RI, Ramsay MA, et al: Management of acute elevation of intracranial pressure during hepatic transplantation. *Anesthesiology* 70:139, 1989.
14. Saul TG, Ducker TB: Effect of intracranial pressure monitoring and aggressive treatment on mortality in severe head injury. *J Neurosurg* 56:498, 1982.
15. Potter D, Peachey T, Eason J, et al: Intracranial pressure monitoring during orthotopic liver transplantation for acute liver failure. *Transplant Proc* 21:3528, 1989.
16. Takeuchi S, Koike T, Sasaki O, et al: Intracranial extradural pressure monitoring after direct operation on ruptured cerebral aneurysms. *Neurosurgery* 24:878, 1989.
17. Consensus Statement: Guidelines for the management and prognosis of severe traumatic brain injury. *J Neurotrauma* 17:451, 2000.
18. Lundberg N: Continuous recording and control of ventricular fluid pressure in neurosurgical practice. *Acta Psychiatr Neurol Scand* 36(Suppl 149):1, 1960.
19. Chan KH, Miller JD, Dearden NM, et al: The effect of changes in cerebral perfusion pressure upon middle cerebral artery blood flow velocity and jugular bulb venous oxygen saturation after severe brain injury. *J Neurosurg* 77:55, 1992.
20. Rosner MJ, Rosner SD, Johnson AH: Cerebral perfusion pressure: management protocol and clinical results. *J Neurosurg* 83:949, 1995.
21. Juul N, Morris GF, Marshall SB, et al: Intracranial hypertension and cerebral perfusion pressure: influence on neurological deterioration and outcome in severe head injury. *J Neurosurg* 92:1, 2000.
22. Robertson CS, Valadka AD, Hannay HJ, et al: Prevention of secondary ischemic insults after severe head injury. *Crit Care Med* 27:2086, 1999.
23. Lobato RD, Sarabia R, Cordobes F, et al: Posttraumatic cerebral hemispheric swelling. Analysis of 55 cases studied with computerized tomography. *J Neurosurg* 68:417, 1988.
24. Soloniuk D, Pitts LH, Lovely M, Bartkowski H: Traumatic intracerebral hematomas. Timing of appearance and indications for operative removal. *J Trauma* 26:787, 1986.
25. Bullock R, Golek J, Blake G: Traumatic intracerebral hematoma—which patients should undergo surgical evacuation? CT scan features and ICP monitoring as a basis for decision making. *Surg Neurol* 32:181, 1989.
26. Gentleman D, Nath F, Macpherson P: Diagnosis and management of delayed traumatic intracerebral haematomas. *Br J Neurosurg* 3:367, 1989.
27. Snow RB, Zimmerman RD, Gandy SE, Deck MDF: Comparison of magnetic resonance imaging and computed tomography in the evaluation of head injury. *Neurosurgery* 18:45, 1986.
28. Levin HS, Amparo E, Eisenberg HM, et al: Magnetic resonance imaging and computerized tomography in relation to the neurobehavioral sequelae of mild and moderate head injuries. *J Neurosurg* 66:706, 1987.
29. Abrams KJ: Airway management and mechanical ventilation. *New Horiz* 3:479, 1995.
30. Clifton GL, Miller ER, Choi SC, et al: Lack of effect of induction of hypothermia after acute brain injury. *N Engl J Med* 344:556, 2001.
31. Polderman KH, Tjong Tjin Joe R, Peerdeman SM, et al: Effects of therapeutic hypothermia on intracranial pressure and outcome in patients with severe head injury. *Intensive Care Med* 28:1563, 2002.
32. Miller JD, Butterworth JF, Gudeman SK, et al: Further experience in the management of severe head injury. *J Neurosurg* 54:289, 1981.

33. Marshall LF, Smith RW, Shapiro HM: The outcome with aggressive treatment in severe head injuries. Part 1: The significance of intracranial pressure monitoring. *J Neurosurg* 50:20, 1979.

34. Guidelines Authors: Management and prognosis of penetrating brain injury. *J Trauma* 51(Suppl): S34, 2001.

35. Hsiang JK, Chesnut RM, Crisp CB, et al: Early, routine paralysis for intracranial pressure control in severe head injury: Is it necessary? *Crit Care Med* 22:1471, 1994.

36. Steudel WI, Kruger J: Using the spectral analysis of the EEG for prognosis of severe brain injuries in the first post-traumatic week. *Acta Neurochir* 28(Suppl):40, 1979.

37. Lindsay KW, Carlin J, Kennedy I, et al: Evoked potentials in severe head injury—analysis and relation to outcome. *J Neurol Neurosurg Psychiatry* 44:796, 1981.

38. Narayan RK, Greenberg RP, Miller JD, et al: Improved confidence of outcome prediction in severe head injury. *J Neurosurg* 54:751, 1981.

39. Newlon PG, Greenberg RP, Hyatt MS, et al: The dynamics of neuronal dysfunction and recovery following severe head injury assessed with serial multimodality evoked potentials. *J Neurosurg* 57:168, 1982.

40. Bowers SA, Marshall LF: Outcome in 200 consecutive cases of severe head injury treated in San Diego County: A prospective analysis. *Neurosurgery* 6:237, 1980.

41. Graham DI, Lawrence AE, Adams JH, et al: Brain damage in nonmissile head injury secondary to high intracranial pressure. *Neuropathol Appl Neurobiol* 13:209, 1987.

42. Marshall LF, Smith RW, Rauscher LA, Shapiro HM: The outcome with aggressive treatment in severe head injuries. Part II. *J Neurosurg* 50:20, 1979.

43. Uzzell BP, Obrist WD, Dolinskas CA, Langfitt TW: Relationship of acute CBF and ICP findings to neuropsychological outcome in severe head injury. *J Neurosurg* 65:630, 1986.

44. Vries JK, Becker DP, Young HF: A subarachnoid screw for monitoring intracranial pressure. Technical note. *J Neurosurg* 39:416, 1973.

45. Ostrup RC, Luerssen TG, Marshall LF, Zornow MH: Continuous monitoring of intracranial pressure with a miniaturized fiberoptic device. *J Neurosurg* 67:206, 1987.

46. Narayan RK, Kishore PRS, Becker DP, et al: Intracranial pressure: To monitor or not to monitor? Review of our experience with severe head injury. *J Neurosurg* 56:650, 1982.

47. Rosner MJ, Becker DP: ICP monitoring: Complications and associated factors. *Clin Neurosurg* 23:494, 1976.

48. North B, Reilly P: Comparison among three methods of intracranial pressure recording. *Neurosurgery* 18:730, 1986.

49. Bouma GJ, Muizelaar JP, Choi SC, et al: Cerebral circulation and metabolism after severe traumatic brain injury: The elusive role of ischemia. *J Neurosurg* 75:685, 1991.

50. Obrist WD, Langfitt TW, Jaggi JL, et al: Cerebral blood flow and metabolism in comatose patients with acute head injury. *J Neurosurg* 61:241, 1984.

51. Sheinberg M, Kanter M, Robertson CS, et al: Continuous monitoring of jugular venous oxygen saturation in head-injured patients. *J Neurosurg* 76:212, 1992.

52. Robertson CS, Gopinath SP, Goodman JC, et al: SjvO2 monitoring in head-injured patients. *J Neurotrauma* 12:891, 1995.

53. Galbraith S, Teasdale G: Predicting the need for operation in the patient with an occult traumatic intracranial hematoma. *J Neurosurg* 55:75, 1981.

54. Muizelaar JP, Marmarou A, Ward JD, et al: Adverse effects of prolonged hyperventilation in patients with severe head injury: A randomized clinical trial. *J Neurosurg* 75:731, 1991.

55. Kelly DF, Goodale DB, Williams J, et al: Propofol in the treatment of moderate and severe head injury: a randomized, prospective double-blinded pilot trial. *J Neurosurg* 90:1042, 1999.

56. Becker DP, Vries JK: The alleviation of increased intracranial pressure by the chronic administration of osmotic agents, in Brock M, Dietz H (eds): *Intracranial Pressure: Experimental and Clinical Aspects.* New York, Springer-Verlag, 1972, p 309.

57. Roberts PA, Pollay M, Engles C, et al: Effect on intracranial pressure of furosemide combined with varying doses and administration of mannitol. *J Neurosurg* 66:440, 1987.

58. Wilberger JE, Cantella D: High-dose barbiturates for intracranial pressure control. *New Horiz* 3:469, 1995.

59. Schwartz ML, Tator CH, Rowed DW, et al: The University of Toronto head injury treatment study: A prospective, randomized comparison of pentobarbital and mannitol. *Can J Neurol Sci* 11:434, 1984.

60. Ward JD, Becker DP, Miller JD, et al: Failure of prophylactic barbiturate coma in the treatment of severe head injury. *J Neurosurg* 62:383, 1985.

61. Newlon PG, Greenberg RP, Enas GG, Becker DP: Effects of therapeutic pentobarbital coma on multimodality evoked potentials recorded from severely head-injured patients. *Neurosurgery* 12:613, 1983.

62. Gower DJ, Lee KS, McWhorter JM: Role of subtemporal decompression in severe closed head injury. *Neurosurgery* 23:417, 1988.

63. Rosner MJ, Daughton S: Cerebral perfusion pressure management in head injury. *J Trauma* 30:933, 1990.

64. Temkin NR, Dikmen SS, Wilensky AJ, et al: A randomized, double-blind study of phenytoin for the prevention of post-traumatic seizures. *N Engl J Med* 323:497, 1990.

65. Clifton GL, Robertson CS, Grossman RG, et al: The metabolic response to severe head injury. *J Neurosurg* 60:687, 1984.

66. Levy DE, Coronna JJ, Singer BH, et al: Predicting outcome from hypoxic-ischemic coma. *JAMA* 253:1420, 1985.

Chapter 94

SPINE INJURIES
G. E. JOHNSON

KEY POINTS

- *Management of life-threatening injuries takes priority over management of spinal injuries.*
- *In the multiple-trauma setting, spinal injury should be assumed to be present pending appropriate assessment.*
- *Spinal injuries must be considered unstable until they are evaluated thoroughly.*
- *Vertebral injuries must be assessed in terms of the potential to create early neurologic injury or late deformity.*
- *Spinal cord injury is minimized or prevented by limiting the secondary ischemic phase and maintaining appropriate spinal immobilization.*
- *Complete spinal cord injuries have no potential for functional recovery. Incomplete injuries have recovery potential, which must be maximized.*
- *Considerations in rehabilitation must be initiated at the outset.*

Severely injured patients frequently require ICU admission preoperatively and more commonly postoperatively for monitoring and assessing for change that may require intervention, including surgery. It is estimated that approximately 20% of patients sustaining multiple injuries have associated spinal column trauma that may be the prime reason for ICU admission. More commonly, ICU admission is necessitated by the more immediately life-threatening injuries, and the spinal injury then could be missed or management delayed, leading to significant morbidity or even death. The intensivist plays an important role in determining outcome in these injuries by having a high index of suspicion based on awareness of the mechanisms of spinal injuries and their clinical features. This chapter reviews (1) the mechanism, classification, and clinical picture of spinal injuries and (2) the principles of management of vertebral and spinal neurologic injuries to enable the intensivist to optimize ICU management and recognize the need for early orthopedic and/or neurosurgical consultation.

It is extremely important in the management of multiply injured patients that longer-term rehabilitation considerations not be forgotten because this may result in serious chronic disability. The possibility of cervical spine injury must be considered in anyone who has suffered significant injuries to the face or head, especially those who are unconscious from trauma.[1] However, patients who are at risk on the basis of preexisting abnormalities of the cervical spine (e.g., ankylosing spondylitis and congenital anomalies) may suffer serious neck injury as a result of what might appear to be trivial trauma. Knowledge of the mechanism of injury is helpful in considering the possibility of spinal injury (e.g., fractures at the thoracolumbar junction associated with falls from a height).

Anatomy

The vertebral column consists of three components (Fig. 94-1)[2]:

1. The anterior column, consisting of the anterior two-thirds of the vertebral body, disk, and annulus and the anterior longitudinal ligament
2. The middle column, consisting of the posterior one-third of the vertebral body, disk, and annulus and the posterior longitudinal ligament
3. The posterior column, consisting of the pedicles, laminae, facets, capsule, and the interspinous and supraspinous ligaments

An injury is considered to be stable if only one of the columns is involved and if the injury does not pose a risk of damage to neural structures. Any injury resulting in damage to two or more columns or risking neurologic injury (i.e., damage to the middle column) is considered to be unstable. A great variety of forces or combinations of forces may be applied to the vertebral column (e.g., flexion, extension, flexion-rotation, shear, axial load). The effect of the application of these forces to the vertebral column depends on (1) the magnitude and direction of the force and (2) the underlying anatomy.

A flexion force applied to the cervical spine may result in a pure soft tissue ligamentous injury and dislocation because of the relatively horizontal alignment of the facets. A similar force applied to the lumbar spine most commonly would result in fracture because of the vertical orientation of the facets. An exception is ankylosing spondylitis, where the force is dissipated across the vertebral column, much as it would be in a long bone.[3]

Classification of Vertebral Injuries

CERVICAL

UPPER CERVICAL SPINE
Because of the unique anatomy of the occipital-atlantoaxial complex, applied forces result in characteristic injury patterns, as described below.

Jefferson's Fracture
This is a four-part fracture of the ring of the atlas (C1) caused by axial loading (e.g., a fall on the vertex of the skull). If the combined lateral displacement of the lateral masses exceeds 7 mm, disruption of the transverse ligament has occurred, indicating a greater degree of instability[4] (Fig. 94-2*A*). This injury must be differentiated on a lateral x-ray view from a stable fracture involving only the posterior arch of C1 caused by extension (see Fig. 94-2*B*).

Atlantoaxial Instability (C1 and C2)
SAGITTAL A gap greater than 4 mm between the anterior arch of the atlas and the odontoid is due to insufficiency of the transverse ligament. This condition may result from trauma or inflammatory erosion (e.g., rheumatoid arthritis).

ROTATIONAL This injury is a subluxation of variable degree, recognized by asymmetry of the gap between the lateral

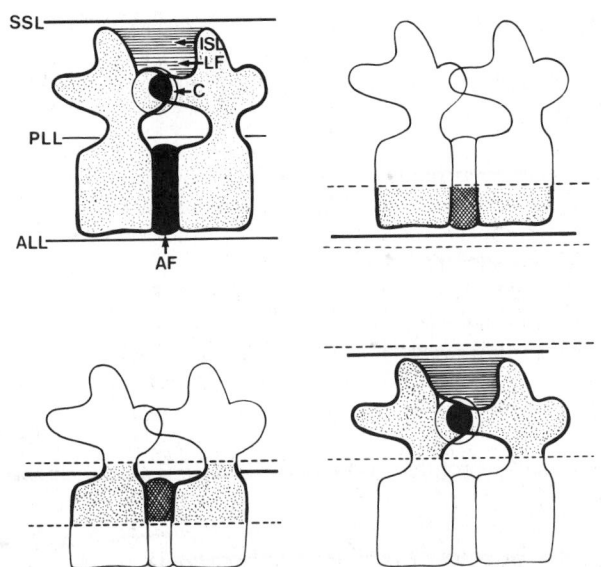

FIGURE 94-1 The anterior, middle, and posterior columns are illustrated. SSL, supraspinous ligament; ISL, interspinous ligament; LF, ligamentum flavum; C, capsule; PLL, posterior longitudinal ligament; AF, annulus fibrosis; ALL, anterior longitudinal ligament. (*Used with permission from Denis.*[2])

aspect of the odontoid and the lateral mass of C1 on each side and also a decreased joint space between the lateral masses of C1 and C2.

FIGURE 94-2 *A.* AP tomogram confirming an unstable Jefferson's fracture with avulsion of the transverse ligament from the lateral

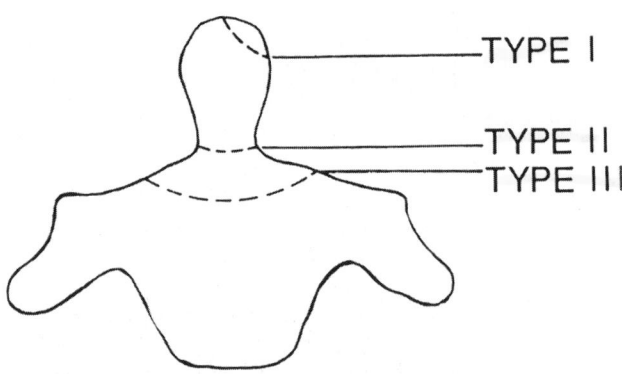

FIGURE 94-3 Fractured odontoid. (*Used with permission from Anderson and D'Alonzo.*[5])

Fractures of the Odontoid

Shear forces in the sagittal plane cause these fractures. The level of the fracture is variable and has been classified by Anderson and D'Alonzo[5] into three types (Fig. 94-3).

Hangman's Fracture

This injury is a traumatic spondylolisthesis of C2–C3. It is a bipedicle fracture of C2, usually from an extension force, with anterior displacement of the body of C2 on C3. There is a low incidence of neurologic injury.

LOWER CERVICAL SPINE

These injuries are classified on the basis of the force applied to the neck, as described below.[5]

mass of C1. *B.* Lateral view showing fracture of the posterior arch of C1 (*arrow*).

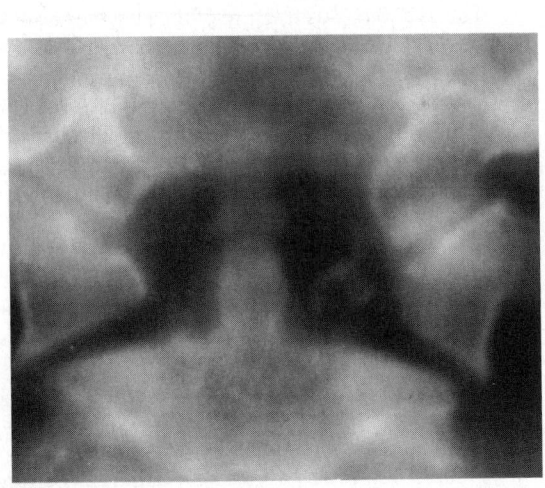

A

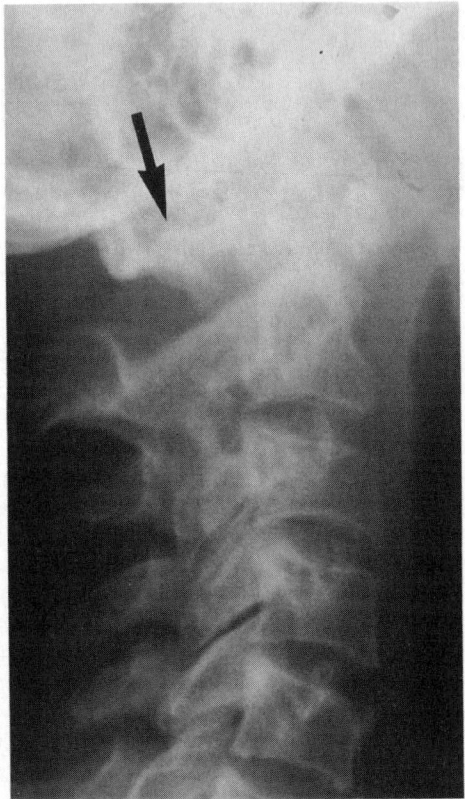

B

Flexion

The applied force may be either compressive or distractive.

COMPRESSIVE   The force acting through the anterior column results in fracture of the vertebral body. The extent of the injury varies from stable minor wedging of the anterior vertebral body only, with no neurologic loss, to marked intrusion into the neural canal, with frequent severe neurologic loss. There is usually associated facet subluxation and instability (e.g., teardrop and quadrangular fractures).

DISTRACTIVE   The applied force begins posteriorly, involving the posterior ligamentous complex and, if severe, may involve all three vertebral column components. The extent of the injury varies from relatively stable subluxation through unilateral and bilateral facet dislocations to a complete vertebral body dislocation. The extent and frequency of neurologic injury usually are in proportion to the vertebral injury, but the initial displacement of the vertebrae may have been much more severe than that seen on x-ray.

Extension

The applied force may also be compressive or distractive.

COMPRESSIVE   This type of force results in fractures through the laminae, which may be sheared off. These fractures can be unilateral or bilateral, and at the extreme, there may be displacement of the vertebral body anteriorly and severe instability. However, since the laminae are sheared off, there may be little intrusion into the neural canal, so the extent of neurologic injury may be less severe than the vertebral injury (Fig. 94-4).

FIGURE 94-4 Compressive extension fracture dislocation of C6–C7. There is dislocation of the facets, but since the spinous process and lamina were sheared off (*arrow*), there was minimal neural canal encroachment, and the patient suffered only bilateral C7 root injury.

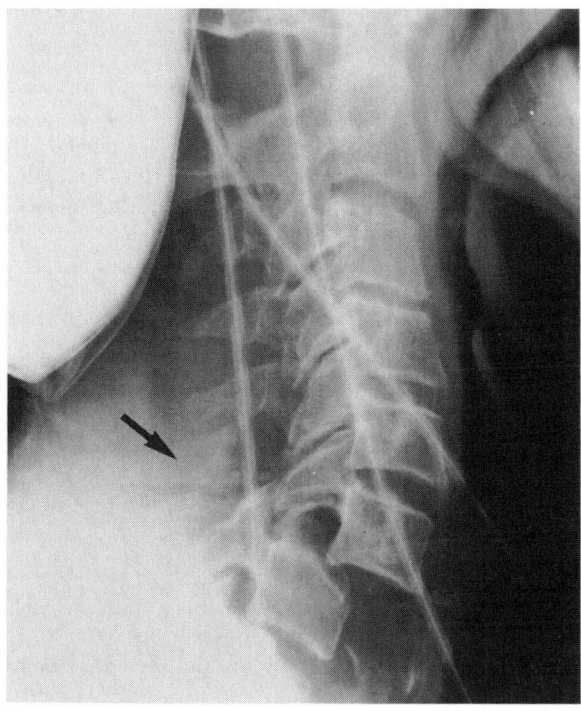

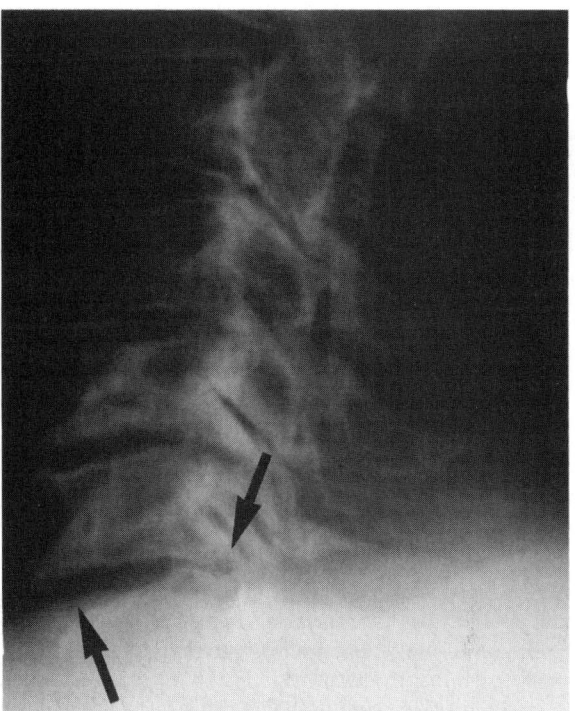

FIGURE 94-5 Distractive extension injury with severe preexisting osteoarthritis of the cervical spine. The disk space is opened anteriorly (*arrow*). Posterior osteophytes encroach on the neural canal, and there is a myelographic block (*arrow*).

DISTRACTIVE   There is failure of the anterior column (anterior longitudinal ligament and disk) in tension, and therefore, the anterior column is usually stable in flexion. In young individuals, this condition may be missed easily clinically and radiologically and is associated with a low incidence of neurologic involvement. However, in the elderly with associated preexisting degenerative changes, there may be avulsion of bony spurs from the anterior vertebral body. The cervical spinal cord may be pinched between osteophytes on the posterior vertebral body and infolded ligamentum flavum posteriorly, typically resulting in incomplete injury (usually central cord syndrome; Fig. 94-5).

Vertical Compression

Axial load causes centrifugal displacement and intrusion into the neural canal and subsequent serious neurologic injury.

Lateral Flexion

This results in compression and fracturing of the lateral mass and also frequent contralateral ligament disruption. It is usually associated with nerve root injury on the compression side.

THORACOLUMBAR

Since the underlying anatomy in the thoracic and lumbar spine is similar, the mechanistic classification proposed by Denis[2] is helpful.

COMPRESSION

This is usually stable and only involves the anterior column, so there is a low incidence of neurologic injury.

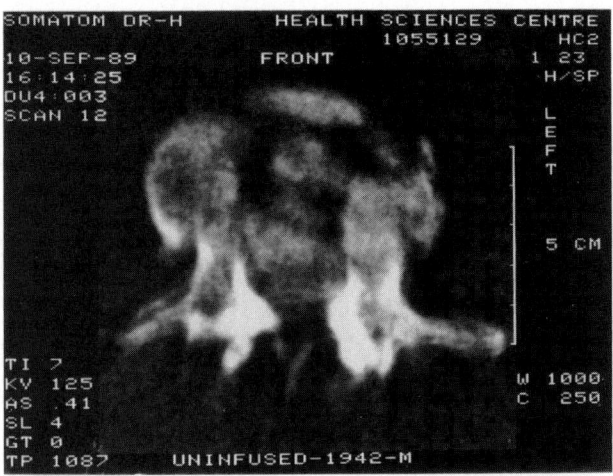

FIGURE 94-6 CT scan showing nearly total encroachment on the neural canal.

BURST

This condition results from axial load forces and results in major injury to the centrum of the vertebral body and intrusion of bone into the neural canal (Fig. 94-6), often associated with lateral displacement of the pedicles and a vertical fracture of the laminae. There frequently is associated neurologic injury.

SEAT-BELT TYPE (CHANCE FLEXION-DISTRACTION)

This injury is caused by a severe flexion force with the axis of rotation anterior to the vertebral body, resulting in failure of all three columns in tension. The pattern can involve various combinations of bony and ligamentous injury. There is minimal encroachment into the neural canal, and the most common neurologic injury involves the nerve root exiting beneath an involved pedicle and may be unilateral or bilateral.

FRACTURE DISLOCATIONS

These injuries usually are caused by a combination of forces (flexion, rotation, and shear) and result in translation of the vertebrae and severe neurologic loss.

The Neurologic Injury

Nerve tissues can be injured by stretching, compression, and laceration. Physical disruption of the spinal cord results in complete, irreversible loss of function. However, autopsy examination of the spinal cord in patients who clinically had a complete injury showed the spinal cord frequently to be structurally intact but to exhibit fibrous and cystic degeneration resembling end-stage ischemic changes.[6] Experimentally, in drop-weight tests, the initial finding is hemorrhage into the gray matter of the central cord, which may coalesce and form a central hematomyelia, surrounding edema, and increased interstitial pressure and local ischemia, as evidenced by a severe decrease in oxygen tension and an increased lactic acid concentration.

A second ischemic phase begins shortly afterward and may persist for more than 24 hours, involving both gray and white matter and spreading both proximally and distally from the site of injury.[7,8] The mechanism for this secondary vascular injury may be local high concentrations of norepinephrine[10–12]

or other vasoactive amines. In addition to vascular injury, direct axonal injury would result in permanent functional loss due to the limited ability of central axons to recover.

It has been shown clearly that the effect of injury is directly related to the magnitude of the force and the duration of its application.[13,14] Since the initial force cannot be changed, we can only prevent further force application first by immobilizing the unstable area and then by relieving the continued compression through early reduction of displaced bony fragments and disks.

SPINAL SHOCK AND SPINAL CORD INJURIES

The direct force applied to the spinal cord results in a physiologic block to conduction (called *spinal shock*), which is recognized clinically as complete cessation of all neurologic function—motor, sensory, and autonomic—below the level of the injury. In slight injuries, this phase lasts only minutes, but in more severe injuries, it may last weeks. During this phase, predictions of neurologic recovery should be avoided.

The *pattern of spinal cord injury* is determined clinically when the patient is out of spinal shock.

COMPLETE CORD INJURY

Clinically, in cases of complete cord injury, there is no voluntary movement and no sensation, but spinal reflexes are present or exaggerated.

INCOMPLETE CORD INJURY

Some recognized forms of incomplete cord injury are listed below.

Anterior Cord Syndrome

This syndrome is characterized by complete motor loss below the level of injury and loss of light touch sensation but preservation of position, vibration, and deep touch sensation. This pattern is caused by anterior compression of the spinal cord, which injures the lateral corticospinal and spinothalamic tracts but spares the posterior tracts.

Central Cord Syndrome

Clinically, this injury is marked by disproportionate loss of motor power in the upper extremities, with less severe loss in the lower extremities. Sensation is variably altered. This pattern is caused by central hemorrhage in the cord, which affects the lower motor neurons and decussating tracts but spares the lateral corticospinal tracts.

Brown-Séquard Syndrome

Rarely, this syndrome is seen as a pure injury with blunt trauma, but it also may be seen in penetrating injuries. Motor power is lost on the ipsilateral side, and pain and temperature sensations are lost on the contralateral side, up to one or two segments below the level of the injury.

POSTERIOR CORD SYNDROME

This rare condition results in loss of position sense.

CAUDA EQUINA SYNDROME

The degree of neurologic loss with this syndrome varies greatly, depending on the extent of nerve root damage. The motor and sensory loss is symmetric, and there may be loss of bladder and bowel control.

ROOT LOSS

A few specific vertebral injuries are associated with loss of function of individual nerve roots. For example, a C5–C6 unilateral facet dislocation may cause ipsilateral C6 root injury. In a seat-belt injury, it is not uncommon that the nerve root exiting below the affected pedicle either unilaterally or bilaterally may be injured.

CLINICAL ASSESSMENT

Assessment of patients specifically for possible spinal injury begins after general assessment and resuscitative measures have been carried out. The patient must have an intact airway, adequate ventilation and circulation, and control of hemorrhage.

A history of the mechanism of injury is helpful in anticipating the type of injury. Other important information includes a history of previous neurologic abnormalities. Observations by the patient, witnesses, or the primary care giver of the occurrence of transient or persistent weakness or sensory changes or loss of bladder function related to the injury are very helpful.

On examination, any evidence of head or facial trauma, such as bruises, lacerations, or abrasions, can suggest the direction of an applied force. Especially important is any asymmetry of head position and tenderness along the sternomastoids. In a patient with an injured cervical cord, the arms may be held in the typical position of shoulder abduction and elbow flexion of a C5 quadriplegic. An ominous sign of neurologic loss is the presence of a paradoxical pattern of respiration. Priapism in a male patient with an injured cervical cord indicates loss of thoracolumbar sympathetic outflow. Examination of the trunk may show bruises or abrasions of the shoulders, the periscapular area, or the buttocks, suggesting a rotatory or flexion force to the spine.

A detailed neurologic examination then should be performed; it is recorded on a flow sheet to allow for serial examinations. Standardized methods of scoring for neurologic deficits have been developed that are extremely useful making neurologic assessments more consistent and reliable.[15,16]

The patient, wearing a cervical collar and held with gentle manual traction, may be carefully logrolled to allow examination of the back for tenderness, malalignment of the spinous processes, or a boggy gap in the supraspinous ligament, suggesting disruption of the posterior column (Fig. 94-7). While the patient is turned, sensation in the perianal area and rectal examination to include resting tone and voluntary contraction should be performed, along with testing of the bulbocavernosus reflex (Fig. 94-8).

RADIOLOGIC EXAMINATION

In multiple-trauma patients, the initial films are the scout lateral cervical spine film and an anteroposterior (AP) view of the chest and pelvis. Other, more detailed films are obtained on the basis of the clinical findings. In addition to the configuration and alignment of the vertebral bodies, the general alignment of the facets, the posterior vertebral bodies, and the interspinous distances, the specific points to observe on each film are listed in Table 94-1.

Following these x-rays, further detail may be required, and the following techniques are helpful. Since they require move-

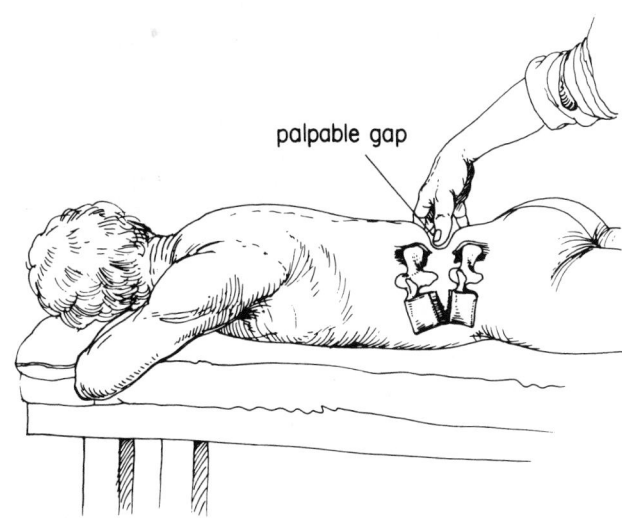

FIGURE 94-7 A palpable gap between the spinous processes indicating complete disruption of the supraspinous and infraspinous ligaments and severe posterior column injury. *(Used with permission from Hoppenfield S: Orthopaedic Neurology. Philadelphia, Saunders.)*

ment or turning of the patient, they should be done only when no instability has been demonstrated on plain films.

CERVICAL SPINE
Swimmer's View
This view helps to visualize the cervicothoracic junction but is difficult to interpret and may show only gross malalignment.

Oblique and Pillar Views
These views are used to show the facets and lateral masses, respectively, and can be obtained with minimal movement of the patient.

FIGURE 94-8 Bulbocavernosus reflex produced by stimulation of the dorsum of the glans penis resulting in anal sphincter contraction. *(Used with permission from Hoppenfield S: Orthopaedic Neurology. Philadelphia, Saunders.)*

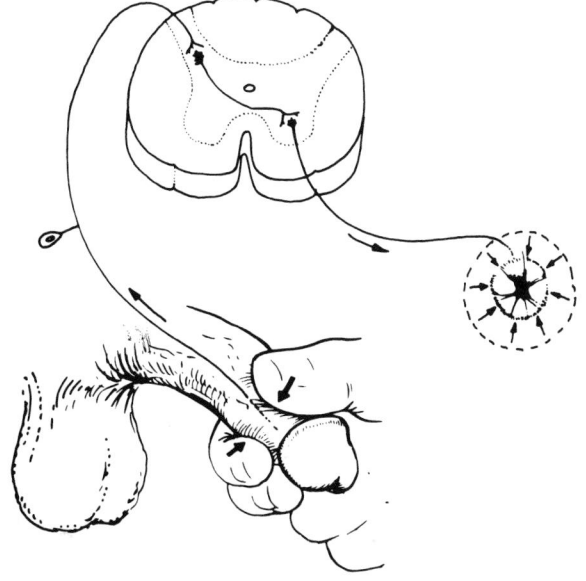

TABLE 94-1 Radiologic Evaluation of Spine Injuries

Location of Injury	Lateral	Anteroposterior
Cervical spine	Adequacy of the film (top of T1 should be visible)	
	Retropharyngeal swelling at C3 (>3 mm) and C6 (>15 mm)	
Upper	Odontoid	(Through-mouth)
	Gap from anterior arch to odontoid <4 mm	Odontoid
		Interval between odontoid and the lateral mass of C1
		General alignment occipital condyle to the lateral mass of C1, and C1–C2
		C1–C2 Joint space
Lower (C3–C7)	Disc space height	Fracture of lateral mass
	Compression or avulsion of the anterior vertebral body	Abrupt change in alignment of the spinous processes
	Widening or asymmetry of interspinous distance	
Thoracic and lumbar spine	Vertebral body configuration especially of the posterior wall	Vertebral body height
	Pedicles	H-shape of the lamina
		Interpedicular distance
		Interspinous distance

Oblique Lumbar View

This view shows the lamina, pars interarticularis, and facets.

Conventional Tomography

This technique considerably improves detail and helps to show difficult areas (e.g., the cervicothoracic junction). It always should be done in two planes (AP and lateral) and requires turning of the patient; therefore, this technique is being replaced by computed tomography.

Computed Tomography

Computed tomography (CT) is a very valuable modality and requires only a single transfer of the patient, which can be done on the spine board or patient mobilizer. Routine, coronal, and sagittal reconstructions should be obtained. It is important that this examination be coordinated with other disciplines so that the patient with known or suspected spinal injury can have the appropriate areas examined at the same time as examination for other injuries (e.g., head, intrathoracic, intraabdominal).

Myelography

Myelography is indicated only under the following conditions:

1. The extent of the neural injury cannot be explained on the basis of the findings from plain films or CT.
2. Progressive neurologic loss occurs in the absence of severe encroachment on the neural canal, suggesting that the loss is ischemic in nature.
3. It is necessary to demonstrate possible dural defects or avulsed nerve roots.

Magnetic Resonance Imaging (MRI)

MRI has been used to assess the degree of soft tissue and ligamentous injury in the spine, looking for potentially unstable injury, particularly in the cervical spine. Overall, the results have not shown much advantage compared with conventional films and CT. There is a tendency to overcall significant injury. MRI does have a very high negative predictive value for significant soft tissue injury but is of uncertain positive predictive value and specificity.[17] This modality offers clear imaging of the acute injury to the spinal cord as well as of late changes, such as the development of traumatic syringomyelia. Rizzolo and colleagues[18] emphasized its usefulness in the unconscious or uncooperative patient in whom disk material must be removed before reduction is attempted.

CLEARING OF THE CERVICAL SPINE

Occasionally, when routine films are negative and a ligamentous injury to the cervical spine is suspected, flexion and extension films are indicated. They must be done only actively and, therefore, in an awake patient with medical supervision. Other methods for assessing the potential for unstable skeletal injuries in the unconscious patient include passive flexion extension using the image intensifier.[19] This can be done by experienced personnel when good visualization of the entire cervical spine can be obtained by passively flexing and extending the patient through an arc of about 30 degrees of flexion and extension.[20] MRI, when performed within 48 hours, also may be helpful.

Pitfalls in the Assessment of Spinal Injuries

ANKYLOSING SPONDYLITIS

The fracture may not be seen initially. The patient should be managed as having an unstable injury until further investigations (tomograms, bone scan) are performed.[3]

MULTIPLE NONCONTIGUOUS INJURIES

It is becoming more common for patients to have more than one spinal fracture at nonadjacent levels, especially in high-velocity injuries. The primary injury is considered to be the one associated with neurologic deficit. This is most often in the upper thoracic level. When a fracture in the spine is diagnosed, the entire spine should be x-rayed.[21]

UNCONSCIOUS OR HEAD-INJURED PATIENTS

The absence of symptoms and/or a compromised neurologic examination in these patients makes assessment very difficult.

Management of Spinal Injuries

IMMEDIATE

PREHOSPITAL
Multiple-trauma victims and patients with spinal injuries, especially spinal injuries involving neurologic loss, should be taken directly to a level 1 tertiary care center if they are physiologically stable and if the transport time is reasonable. Major trauma-receiving centers must have a formal team designated for the management of spinal injuries.[22]

PRIORITIES
The presence of a spinal injury, although serious and carrying a risk of severe late disability, does not alter the priorities of ensuring a clear airway, adequate ventilation, and adequate circulation.

OTHER TREATMENT MEASURES
Trauma patients with suspected or proven spinal injuries must continue to be immobilized or logrolled as indicated until definitive care is instituted. Temporary immobilization of the cervical spine is accomplished by appropriate application of a cervical collar. A long spine board should be used for transporting the patient. It is important that this initial assessment and resuscitation be expedited to avoid prolonged pressure on areas such as the occiput, sacrum, and heels.

It is imperative that adequate perfusion with well-oxygenated blood be maintained to the injured spinal cord, and therefore, supplemental oxygen is given by facemask to maintain a Pa_{O_2} of at least 100 mm Hg. Other measures, as outlined below, are used to maintain a blood pressure of at least 100 mm Hg systolic.

Other general measures that should be instituted in the emergency department include insertion of intravenous lines, a nasogastric tube, and a Foley catheter.

As soon as the patient arrives in the emergency department, the spine injury team should be notified. That team then may supervise the spinal aspects of overall patient management and participate in decision making. Patients requiring manipulation for reduction of the spine should be managed where they can be monitored carefully and have easy access to x-ray facilities for serial films. Spine injury patients with other multiple trauma, all patients with high spinal cord injuries (above C5), and patients who have low cervical or thoracic cord injury as well as with significant preexisting disease are best treated initially in the intensive care setting until stabilized.[23]

Management of Complications of Spinal Injuries

NEUROGENIC SHOCK

Patients with neurogenic shock, particularly those with injuries above the level of T6, will be hypotensive and bradycardic owing to the combination of (1) loss of thoracic sympathetic outflow, vasodilatation, and pooling of blood and (2) relative predominance of vagal stimulation to the heart. In the absence of associated hypovolemia, the patient should be given a maintenance crystalloid infusion. If tissue perfusion is inadequate and/or the response to infusion is unsatisfactory, the patient should be investigated for concealed bleeding. Central lines are indicated, and monitoring of central venous pressure is used to gauge further fluid resuscitation. Extremes of crystalloid administration to maintain a normal pressure should be avoided, and colloids should be given as a volume expander, as repeated challenges. A persistently low perfusion pressure despite adequate fluid resuscitation warrants consideration of small doses of vasopressors.[24,25]

RESPIRATORY

Respiratory complications after cervical spinal cord injury occur in 60% of patients. The single most significant determining factor is the severity of the spinal cord injury.[26] Respiratory complications[27] are greatest in cervical cord injuries in which the patient has lost intercostal function and the abdominal muscle function needed to support a vigorous cough. The phrenic nerve is involved in lesions above C5. In lesions below C5, with a functioning diaphragm and accessory muscles and in the absence of lung injury or preexisting disease, most patients can support satisfactory ventilation. There is a tendency, even with good general care, for ventilatory function to deteriorate by the third or fourth day because of fatigue and retained secretions, and intubation and ventilation may be required early. While the patient is being ventilated, the position of the cervical vertebrae can be maintained by traction, giving access to the chest for therapy. Once the respiratory compromise has stabilized and weaning can begin, it is advantageous to immobilize the cervical spine in a halo vest (Fig. 94-9). The vest restricts access to the chest and increases chest wall stiffness.

FIGURE 94-9 Halo vest.

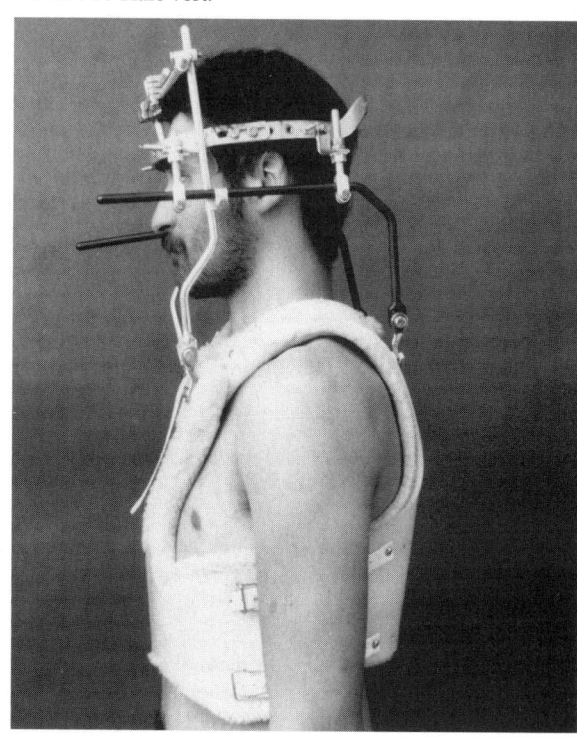

However, the upright or semiupright position facilitates diaphragmatic excursion, improving functional residual capacity,[28] especially in patients lacking intercostal function. While the patient is in neurogenic shock, postural hypotension will not allow maintenance of the upright position.

CARDIAC

Acute spinal cord injury may be associated with pulmonary edema. This usually occurs early, possibly owing to massive sympathetic outflow, increased afterload, and a predisposition to dysrhythmia.[29,30] A persistent feature following acute spinal cord injury above the T6 level is hypotension and bradycardia, even after administration of enough fluid and colloid to fill the venous capacitance vessels. These problems may respond to atropine (0.2 to 0.4 mg); if hypotension persists, vasopressors may be required.

GASTROINTESTINAL

Almost every patient with spinal cord injury and most patients with significant fractures of the thoracic or lumbar spine in the absence of neurologic injury will have a transient ileus, and a nasogastric tube should be inserted.

THROMBOEMBOLIC PREVENTION

Approximately 50% of patients with spinal cord injuries develop deep vein thrombosis.[31] Prophylaxis with low-dose heparin appears ineffective. Better methods include adjusted-dose heparin, low-molecular-weight heparin, low-dose heparin plus electrical stimulation of the calf, and low-dose heparin plus graduated stockings plus intermittent pneumatic compression; these measures should be continued for 6 to 12 weeks.[32]

SKIN CARE

Avoidance of decubitus ulceration depends on meticulous attention to frequent turning and protection of pressure points. This regimen is made easier by the use of special mechanized beds for turning (e.g., Stoke-Mandville bed).

NUTRITION

Following acute spinal cord injury, the patient becomes catabolic.[33] To minimize this effect and encourage early rehabilitation, early alimentation is encouraged as soon as the ileus resolves. If the gut cannot be used for a long period, then parenteral nutrition should be considered.

MANAGEMENT OF THE NEUROLOGIC INJURY

Decision making is based on accurate neurologic assessment initially, serial examinations, and accurate documentation. In the presence of neurologic injury, the two fundamental principles of management are

1. *Provision of an adequate perfusion pressure and well-oxygenated blood.* The patient must not be allowed to become hypotensive or hypoxic.
2. *Decompression.* The degree of injury and, conversely, the ability of the spinal cord to recover vary according to the magnitude of the applied force and the duration of compression. Decompression of the injured cord must be achieved as quickly as possible, usually by reduction of displaced fracture fragments by either closed means (e.g., halo traction, postural reduction on bolsters) or open ones.

The adequacy of decompression must be proven radiologically.

Principles of Surgical Management

1. Decompression should be performed from the direction of encroachment on the neural canal (anterior or posterior).
2. The adequacy of decompression should be proven intraoperatively by direct visualization or myelography or postoperatively by CT.
3. Following decompression, a stable construct must be achieved by internal stabilization.[34]

Indications for surgical decompression of spinal cord and cauda equina or root injuries are as follows:

1. *Progressive neurologic loss.* This development is seen clinically as either an ascending level of neurologic loss or progression from incomplete to complete injury. Not infrequently, the neurologic level rises by one segment in the very early stages following injury. This event is due to ischemia, and subsequently, the neurologic loss usually recedes to the original level.
2. *Failure or anticipated failure of nonoperative decompression* (owing to retained bone or disk fragments). Generally, the reduction seen on plain x-rays represents the residual encroachment on the neural canal. Only in 3% of cases is there residual soft-tissue compression.
3. *Incomplete cord and/or cauda equina lesions with residual compression.*

In the following situations, surgical decompression will be of no benefit or may even be harmful:

1. A complete spinal cord lesion in a patient out of spinal shock
2. Progressive neurologic loss due to ischemia, with no blockage or significant residual compression, as seen on myelography

TECHNIQUES OF SPINAL CORD DECOMPRESSION

Anterior decompression of the cervical spinal cord[35] is the technique of choice in the following injuries:

1. Axial load (burst) fractures
2. Cervical disk injuries
3. Distractive extension injuries with residual neural canal encroachment by posterior vertebral body osteophytes

Extremely complex patterns of fractures and fracture dislocations (e.g., quadrangular,[36] teardrop,[37] compressive extension) may be treated by a combination of anterior and posterior approaches.

The most common type of injury to the upper thoracic spine that may require decompression is a fracture dislocation that is extremely unstable and difficult to reduce nonoperatively. When decompression is indicated, the reduction can best be performed posteriorly, followed by stabilization using a segmental spinal instrumentation technique. New developments in instrumentation such as hook rods, pedicle screws, cages, and anterior plating systems have made it possible to achieve neural decompression, as well as a high degree of stability and correction of deformity, while also limiting the extent of the fusion.

For fracture dislocations, surgical decompression can be performed by laminectomy, clearing residual bone from within the neural canal followed by reduction and stabilization using pedicle screw or hook rod systems.

Burst fractures of the thoracolumbar spine usually can be decompressed posteriorly by pedicle screw distraction (ligamentotaxis) if done within 4 to 5 days of the injury. Anterior corpectomy and reconstruction are another option in the situation of severe canal encroachment or if residual neural compression persists after a posterior procedure.[38]

ADJUNCTIVE TECHNIQUES TO REDUCE SPINAL INJURY

The secondary ischemia following initial spinal cord injury is a major contributor to further neurologic damage and functional loss. Attention has been paid to understanding the pathophysiology of this process in order to identify ways to minimize its effect.[39] Despite initial enthusiasm, many modalities, such as spinal cord cooling, hyperbaric oxygen, mannitol, and dimethylsulfoxide (DMSO), have not been shown to be effective.

STEROIDS

The glucocorticoids (e.g., dexamethasone) are presumed to act by decreasing the effect of norepinephrine, stabilizing cell membranes, preventing release of lysosomal enzymes, inhibiting complement activation, and reversing the sodium and potassium electrolyte imbalance that results from tissue edema and necrosis.[40] Experimentally, controversy exists regarding the effectiveness of steroids. Clinically, Bracken and colleagues[41] have indicated that the administration of methylprednisolone, 30 mg/kg within 8 hours of injury, followed by infusion of 5.4 mg/kg per hour for 23 hours resulted in improvement in neurologic function. A further study[42] suggested that there was improved motor outcome when methyprednisolone was initiated earlier than 3 hours and for 24 hours or between 3 and 8 hours for 48 hours. However, functional outcome was not improved. Review of the data leaves unsolved issues.[43–45]

Since complications may be associated with the use of steroids,[46] administration of these agents on an ad hoc basis is discouraged. The spine injury team should adopt a policy with respect to the use of steroids, standardizing dosage, time of administration, and duration of treatment.

Management of the Vertebral Injury

When considering the bony injury, the principles of fracture management (reduction, maintenance, and mobilization) apply. These goals may be accomplished nonoperatively. With failed closed reduction, inability to maintain position, or the desire for early mobilization, an open reduction and internal stabilization are indicated. Stable fractures of the cervical or thoracolumbar spine can be mobilized early with limited use of an orthosis for pain relief.

In the cervical spine, unstable fractures that do not require reduction may be managed in an orthosis only (e.g., a nondisplaced type III fracture of the odontoid), but careful

TABLE 94-2 Halo Vest Management of Cervical Injuries

Suitable	Unsuitable
Fracture of the odontoid of types II and III	Axially unstable fractures (e.g., Jefferson's)
Hangman's fracture	Primarily ligamentous injuries (e.g., distraction flexion causing unilateral and bilateral facet dislocations)
Minimal compression-flexion injuries	
Fracture of the lateral mass	Obesity
	Noncompliant patient
	Multiple-level injuries

monitoring is necessary to demonstrate that the position is maintained. When a reduction is necessary, halo traction should be used so that once the fracture is reduced, the patient can be mobilized in a halo vest (see Fig. 94-9). The initial enthusiasm regarding the ability of the halo vest to control unstable cervical injuries has been challenged.[47] Patient selection criteria for halo vest management are outlined in Table 94-2.

When open reduction and internal stabilization are indicated, the fracture pattern must be analyzed carefully in preoperative planning to make sure that the force causing the injury will be neutralized so that sufficient stability will be achieved that minimal, if any, external support will be required. Using modern implant techniques, this result is for the most part achievable.[48,49]

In fractures of the thoracic and lumbar spine, similar principles may be applied. Unstable fractures not requiring reduction may be treated with bed rest and logrolling for 2 to 3 weeks, followed by a well-fitted, rigid polypropylene brace. Closed postural reduction of some minimally displaced thoracolumbar fractures can be achieved by positioning the patient on corrective bolsters and careful logrolling until sufficient bony healing has occurred to allow mobilization in an orthosis. However, this approach requires skilled personnel in specialty units. With the advent of much-improved techniques of stabilization, there is an increased emphasis on health care costs and earlier mobilization, and thus there is an increasing trend toward early surgical stabilization.[50,51] However, careful attention must be given to achieving sufficient stability to allow early mobilization.[52–54]

Pitfalls in the Management of Spinal Cord Injury

HYPOTHERMIA

Hypothermia is a particularly important problem in patients with cervical or high thoracic cord injuries. The patient is unable to produce vasoconstriction because of loss of the thoracic sympathetic outflow and also is unable to shiver to maintain core temperature. This results in hypotension and bradycardia. The temperature must be monitored carefully, and the patient must be kept covered or warmed by radiant heaters.

AUTONOMIC DYSREFLEXIA

This potentially dangerous complication occurs in patients with spinal cord injuries above the T6 level at any time after the stage of spinal shock. The presenting symptoms are quite variable, the most consistent being hyperhidrosis, headache, and vasodilatation above the level of the neurologic loss with nasal stuffiness. Paroxysmal hypertension is the cardinal sign; bradycardia is present inconsistently. The usual precipitating events are distention or manipulation of the bladder or rectum or intraabdominal pathology. These stimuli result in massive reflex sympathetic outflow, causing hypertension and reflex bradycardia and vasodilatation in the part of the body above the level of the spinal cord lesion. Immediate management should consist of placing the patient in an upright position and removing the stimulus, e.g., by bladder decompression. Vasodilator therapy may be required for severe hypertension.[55]

THE SWOLLEN LIMB

The neurologically impaired patient may present at any time after the injury with a painless swollen limb. The differential diagnosis includes fracture, venous thrombosis, and myositis ossificans. Myositis ossificans is a frequent occurrence in association with spinal cord injury. In total joint arthroplasty, the use of indomethacin may decrease the occurrence and severity of this complication, but the usefulness of this agent is unproven in spinal injuries. Physiotherapy to maintain range of motion should be reduced but probably not discontinued.

Considerations in Rehabilitation

Many assessment tools are available for documenting neurologic status after acute spinal cord injury, such as the Frankel scale and the American Spinal Injury Association (ASIA) scale. A practical method of determining function is incorporated in the Functional Independent Measure (FIM), which is a combination of a neurologic assessment and an assessment of the ability to perform various self-care activities. Restoration of the highest possible level of function in the patient with a spinal injury begins with initial management. Since function is related directly to the level of neurologic injury, preservation of even a single nerve root or segment, especially in the cervical cord, may make the difference between independence and the need for attendant care. For example, a C7 quadriplegic with strong active elbow extension can do transfers from bed to chair and chair to toilet and can live independently with some assistance at home. A C6 quadriplegic with good shoulder muscles and some active wrist extension is capable of independent feeding and grooming because of a fairly strong tenodesis grip. The patient can turn independently in bed, assist with transfers, operate a regular wheelchair, and even operate a car with hand controls. By contrast, a patient with a C5 injury is capable of very limited self-care, cannot turn in bed, and can only use an electric wheelchair.

Maintaining range of movement of joints that can be moved actively is essential to achieving maximum function. This is also important in joints that have lost active movement because flexion contractures of hips and knees interfere severely with independent transfers.

In some instances, it may be advantageous to leave an imbalance of certain muscle groups in order to facilitate function. For example, some tightness of the long finger flexors will improve the grip in patients dependent on the tenodesis effect for grasping objects.

Active therapy must begin during the phase of spinal shock and continue as the patient passes into the stages of spasticity.

References

1. Frankel HL, Rozycki GS, Ochsner MG, et al: Indications for obtaining surveillance thoracic and lumbar spine radiographs. *J Trauma* 37:673, 1994.
2. Denis F: The three column spine and its significance in the classification of acute thoracolumbar spine injuries. *Spine* 8:817, 1983.
3. Hunter T, Dubo H: Spinal fractures complicating anklyosing spondylitis. *Arthritis Rheum* 26:751, 1983.
4. Spence KF, Decker S, Sell KW: Bursting atlantal fracture associated with rupture of the transverse ligament. *J Bone Joint Surg* 52A:543, 1970.
5. Anderson LD, D'Alonzo RT: Fractures of the odontoid process of the axis. *J Bone Joint Surg* 56A:1663, 1974.
6. Allen RL, Ferguson RL, Lehman TR, et al: A mechanistic classification of closed, indirect fractures and dislocations of the lower cervical spine. *Spine* 7:1, 1982.
7. Tator CH: Acute spinal cord injury: A review of recent studies of treatment and pathophysiology. *Can Med Assoc J* 107:143, 1972.
8. De la Torre JC: Spinal cord injury: Review of basic and applied research. *Spine* 6:315, 1981.
9. Tator CH, Rivlin AS, Lewis AJ, et al: The effect of acute spinal cord injury on axonal counts in the pyramidal tract of rats. *J Neurosurg* 61:118, 1984.
10. Osterholm JL, Mathews GJ: Altered norepinephrine metabolism following experimental spinal cord injury: 1. Relationship to hemorrhagic necrosis and post-wounding neurological defects. *J Neurosurg* 36:386, 1972; 2: Protection against traumatic spinal cord hemorrhagic necrosis by norepinephrine synthesis blockade with alpha methyl tyrosine. *J Neurosurg* 36:395, 1972.
11. De la Torre JC, Johnson CM, Harris LH, et al: Monoamine changes in experimental head and spinal cord trauma: Failure to confirm previous observations. *Surg Neurol* 2:5, 1974.
12. Naftchi NE, Demeny M, DeCrescito V, et al: Biogenic amine concentrations in traumatized spinal cords of cats. *J Neurosurg* 40:52, 1974.
13. Rivlin AS, Tator CH: Effect of duration of acute spinal cord compression in a new acute cord injury model in the rat. *Surg Neurol* 10:38, 1978.
14. Tator CH, Rowed DW: Current concepts in the immediate management of acute spinal cord injuries. *Can Med Assoc J* 121:1453, 1979.
15. American Spinal Injury Association/International Medical Society of Paraplegia: *Internal Standards for Neurological and Functional Classification of Spine Cord Injury,* rev ed. Chicago, American Spinal Injury Association, 1996.
16. El Masry WS, Tsubo M, Katon S, et al: Validating of the American Spinal Injury Association (ASIA) motor score and the National Acute Spinal Cord Injury Study (NASCIS) motor score. *Spine* 21:614, 1996.
17. Benzel EC, Hart BL, Ball PA, et al: Magnetic resonance imaging for the evaluation of patient with occult cervical spine injury. *J Neurosurg* 85:824, 1996.
18. Rizzolo SJ, Vaccaro AR, Cotler JM: Cervical spine trauma. *Spine* 19:2288, 1994.
19. Davis JW, Parks SN, Detlefs CL, et al: Clearing the cervical spine in obtunded patients: The use of dynamic fluoroscopy. *J Trauma* 39:435, 1995.
20. Grossman MD, Reilly PM, Gillett T, Gillett D: National survey of the incidence of cervical spine injury and approach to cervical spine clearance in US trauma centers. *J Trauma* 47:684, 1999.

21. Powell JN, Waddell JP, Tucker WS, et al: Multiple level noncontiguous spinal fractures. *J Trauma* 29:1146, 1989.

22. Donovan WH, Carter RE, Bedbrook GM, et al: Incidence of medical complications in spinal cord injury: Patients in specialized compared with non-specialized centres. *Paraplegia* 22:282, 1984.

23. Hadley MN: Guidelines for management of acute cervical spinal injuries: Chap 7: Management of acute spinal cord injuries in an intensive care unit or other monitored setting. *Neurosurgery* 50:51, 2000.

24. King BS, Gupta R, Narayan RK: The early assessment and intensive care unit management of patients with severe traumatic brain and spinal cord injuries. *Surg Clin North Am* 80:855, 2000.

25. Vale, FL, Burns J, Jackson AB, Hadley MN: Combined medical and surgical treatment after acute spinal cord injury: Results of a prospective pilot study to asess the merits of aggressive medical resuscitation and blood pressure management. *J Neurosurg* 87:239, 1997.

26. Lemons VR, Wagner FC: Respiratory complications after cervical spinal cord injury. *Spine* 19:2315, 1994.

27. Tator CH, Duncan EC, Edmond, VE, et al: Complications and costs of management of acute spinal cord injury. *Paraplegia* 31:700, 1993.

28. Ali J, Qi W: Pulmonary function and posture in traumatic quadriplegia. *J Trauma* 39:334, 1995.

29. Albin MS, Buregin L, Wolf S: Brain and lungs at risk after cervical spinal cord transection. *Surg Neurol* 24:191, 1985.

30. Evans DF, Kobrine AL, Rizzoli HV: Cardiac arrhythmias accompanying acute compression of the spinal cord. *J Neurosurg* 52:52, 1980.

31. Merli GJ, Crabbe S, Paluzzi RG, et al: Etiology, incidence, and prevention of deep vein thrombosis in acute spinal cord injury. *Arch Phys Med Rehabil* 74: 1199, 1993.

32. Green D, Chen D, Chmiel JS: Prevention of thromboembolism in spinal cord injury: Role of low molecular weight heparin. *Arch Phys Med Rehabil* 75:290, 1994.

33. Rodriguez DJ, Benzel EC, Clevenger FW: The metabolic response to spinal cord injury. *Spinal Cord* 35:599, 1997.

34. White AA, Manohan M, Panjabi D: The role of stabilization in the treatment of cervical spine injuries. *Spine* 9:512, 1984.

35. Aebi M, Hohler J, Zach GA, et al: Indication, surgical technique, and results of 100 surgically treated fractures and fracture dislocations of the cervical spine. *Clin Orthop* 203:244, 1986.

36. Favero KJ, Van Peteghem PK: The quadrangular fragment fracture: Roentgenographic fractures and treatment protocol. *Clin Orthop* 239:40, 1989.

37. Schneider RC, Kahn EA: Chronic neurologic sequelae of acute trauma to the spine and spinal cord: 1. The significance of the acute flexion or "tear-drop" fracture dislocation of the cervical spine. *J Bone Joint Surg* 38A:985, 1956.

38. Ghanayem AJ, Zdeblick TA: Anterior instrumentation in the management of thoracolumbar burst fractures. *Clin Orthop* 335:89, 1997.

39. Amar PA, Levy ML: Pathogenesis and pharmacological strategies for mitigating secondary damage in acute spinal cord injury. *Neurosurgery* 44:1027, 1999.

40. Ducker TB, Zeidman SM: Spinal cord injury: The role of steroid therapy. *Spine* 19:2281, 1994.

41. Bracken MB, Shepard MJ, Collins WF, et al: A randomized controlled trial of methylprednisolone or naloxone in the treatment of acute spinal cord injury: Results of the Second National Acute Spinal Cord Injury Study (NASCIS-2). *New Engl J Med* 322:1405, 1990.

42. Bracken MB, Shepard MJ, Holford TR, et al: Administration of mehylprednisolone for 24 or 48 hours of tirilazad mesylate for 48 hours in the treatment of acute spinal cord injury: Results of the Third National Acute Spinal Cord Injury Randomized Controlled Trial-National Acute Spinal Cord Injury Study. *JAMA* 277:1597, 1997.

43. Coleman WP, Benzel D, Cahill DW, et al: A critical appraisal of the reporting of the National Acute Spinal Cord Injury Studies (II and III) of methylprednisolone in acute spinal cord injury. *J Spinal Disord* 13:185, 2000.

44. Hurlbert RJ: The role of steroids in acute spinal cord injury: An evidence-based analysis. *Spine* 26(suppl):S39, 2001.

45. Short DJ, El Masry WS, Jones PW: High-dose methylprednisolone in the management of acute spinal cord injury: A systematic review from a clinical perspective. *Spinal Cord* 38:273, 2000.

46. Wing PC, Nance P, Connell DG, Gagnon F: Risk of avascular necrosis following short-term megadose methylprednisolone treatment. *Spinal Cord* 36:633, 1998.

47. Whitehill R, Richman JA, Glaser JA: Failure of immobilization of the cervical spine by the halo vest. *J Bone Joint Surg* 68A:326, 1986.

48. Aeibi M, Zuber K, Marchesi D: Treatment of cervical spine injuries with anterior plating. Indications, techniques and results. *Spine* 16:S38, 1991.

49. Fehlings MG, Cooper PR, Errico TJ: Posterior plates in the management of cervical spine instability: Long-term results in 41 patients. *J Neurosurg* 81:341, 1994.

50. Rechtine G, Cahill D, Chrin A: Treatment of thoracolumbar trauma: Comparison of complications of operative versus non-operative treatment. *J Spinal Disord* 12:406, 1999.

51. Knight R, Stornelli D, Caan D, et al: Comparison of perative versus nonoperative treatment of lumbar burst fractures. *Clin Orthop* 293:112, 1993.

52. Luque ER, Cassis N, Ramirez-Wiella C: Segmental spinal instrumentation in the treatment of fractures of the thoracolumbar spine. *Spine* 7:312, 1982.

53. Dick W: The "fixateur interne" as a versatile implant for spine surgery. *Spine* 12:882, 1987.

54. Gertzbein SD, Court-Brown C: Decompression and circumferential stabilization of unstable spinal fractures. *Spine* 13:892, 1988.

55. Jant MJ, Freehafer AA, Hazel C, et al: Autonomic dysreflexia: A cause of morbidity and mortality in orthopedic patients with spinal cord injury. *Clin Orthop* 169:151, 1982.

Chapter 95 _____

TORSO TRAUMA

JAMEEL ALI

KEY POINTS

- *Consideration of abdominal and thoracic injuries as one complex torso trauma is a useful treatment strategy.*
- *Prioritization of intervention in torso trauma is based on the relative threat to life from specific injuries.*
- *In managing torso trauma, the surgeon must be prepared to explore the chest and/or abdomen because the source of instability frequently is not obvious.*
- *The major decision in assessing the traumatized abdomen is to recognize the need for surgical exploration.*
- *In general, indications for surgical intervention in abdominal trauma are perforation, penetration, and hemorrhage.*
- *An organ-specific diagnosis is not necessary to establish the need for laparotomy in trauma.*
- *Ultrasound, peritoneal lavage, and computed tomographic (CT) scan are important tools in assessing the traumatized abdomen when physical examination alone is unreliable.*
- *Most thoracic injuries can be managed appropriately by simple measures aimed at correcting thoracic sources of hypoperfusion and hypoxemia.*
- *Emergency thoracotomy should be considered in the unstable patient who has a potentially correctable source of instability in the thorax.*

Injuries involving the chest and abdomen may be considered as a single complex torso trauma. The rationale for this point of view is based on several factors. The configuration of the diaphragm and its attachment to the rib cage result in marked variability in its position with respiration and thus in demarcation of the thoracic and abdominal cavities. It is not unusual for the diaphragm to traverse distances of over 15 cm between the inspiratory and expiratory phases of respiration. The diaphragm may be at the level of the nipple line during full expiration and well below the costal margin during full inspiration, with corresponding shifts of the abdominal and thoracic contents (Fig. 95-1). This phenomenon, together with the variable trajectory of objects or forces after penetrating the torso, makes it virtually impossible in many instances to determine on the basis of the external point of impact or penetration whether intrathoracic or intraabdominal injury has been sustained. The concept of torso trauma ensures that injuries in one cavity will not be overlooked while injuries in the other are being managed.[1,1a,1b]

As outlined in Chap. 92, the initial approach in trauma management is to secure the airway, to maintain respiration, and to identify and control hemorrhage and institute immediate fluid resuscitation as required. Definitive management of intraabdominal or thoracic injury may be necessary as part of this resuscitative phase, particularly if the source of instability is major hemorrhage in the thoracic or abdominal cavity. Al-

though it may be possible to identify a specific source in the thorax or abdomen for the abnormal hemodynamics in the trauma patient, it is frequently impossible to be absolutely certain of such a source. Therefore, a decision has to be made to approach the hemodynamically abnormal patient through either a laparotomy or a thoracotomy if a source outside the thorax or abdomen has been ruled out. With this approach, one must be prepared to stop exploration of one cavity when it becomes obvious that the source of the hemodynamic abnormality is in the other.

Classification of Torso Trauma

Generally, torso trauma may be classified into two broad groups: penetrating and blunt. As indicated earlier, any penetrating missile entering inferior to the nipple line can produce diaphragmatic, intrathoracic, or abdominal injuries. Similarly, blunt injuries may disrupt intrathoracic contents as well as intraabdominal contents either directly or indirectly through fractures of the lower ribs, which then puncture intraabdominal organs such as the spleen, liver, and stomach.

A more clinically applicable method of classifying torso trauma involves two categories. The first category consists of injuries that are immediately life threatening and thus require immediate intervention because of cardiorespiratory or hemodynamic compromise. The other category includes injuries in a relatively hemodynamically normal patient. These latter injuries are considered to be potentially life threatening because, if left unattended, they eventually may threaten the patient's survival.

Occasionally, neck injuries, particularly the penetrating type, may involve intrathoracic structures. In addition to causing vascular injury (which may present with hemorrhage or ischemic sequelae), injury to the thoracic duct (resulting in chylothorax), or violation of the pleura (resulting in pneumothorax), penetrating neck wounds may affect any of the intrathoracic structures, depending on the trajectory of the offending weapon.

The neck traditionally is divided into three anatomic regions for the purposes of categorizing penetrating wounds. Zone I extends from the cricoid to the clavicle, zone II from the cricoid to the angle of the mandible, and zone III lies between the angle of the mandible and the base of the skull.

Penetrating wounds of the neck should be explored in the operating room under sterile conditions with adequate anesthetic support. A preoperative plain x-ray of the neck if the patient is stable could provide information such as depth of penetration and the presence of air in the tissues, hematoma, airway deviation, etc. Impaling objects should be removed only in the operating room with vascular equipment available and a securely controlled airway in place. Although there is reasonably good agreement that zone III injuries should be investigated with angiography, the use of angiography and other diagnostic modalities in zone II injuries is controversial because this area can be assessed thoroughly and more easily through direct surgical exploration in the operating room. Diagnostic modalities include angiography, endoscopy, contrast radiography, and computed tomography (CT).[2]

A nasogastric tube should be inserted in the operating room, preferably after the airway is securely controlled by

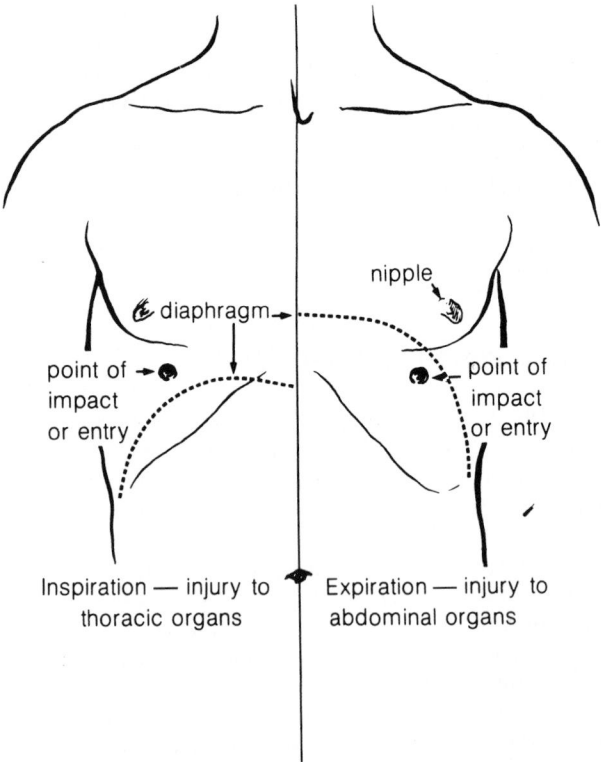

FIGURE 95-1 The rationale for regarding torso trauma as a unified entity. A blunt or penetrating impact at a given level of the chest wall may cause either intraabdominal or intrathoracic injury depending on the trajectory of the missile and/or the position of the diaphragm.

endotracheal intubation, because retching during the insertion of such a tube could lead to clot dislodgment, hemorrhage, and airway compromise. The possibility of intrathoracic injury always should be considered in patients with penetrating neck wounds. The chest therefore should be prepared and draped adequately in the event that thoracic exploration is necessary for repair of intrathoracic injury or possible vascular control for vascular injuries in the neck.

Thoracic Injuries Requiring Immediate Intervention

Although thoracic injury frequently is associated with trauma-related deaths, less than 10% of blunt chest injuries and only 15% to 30% of penetrating chest injuries require open thoracotomy.[3] Lifesaving skills for dealing with thoracic trauma generally are within the scope of most practicing intensivists. Of the injuries that require open surgical intervention, most do not require the expertise of a trained thoracic surgeon. From the intensivist's standpoint, resuscitative measures are aimed at correcting hypoxemia and maintaining normal hemodynamic status. These two aims are achieved by techniques for establishing patency of the airway[3,4] (see Chap. 35), chest decompression for evacuating fluid or air, pericardiocentesis, and vascular access for fluid administration.

In addition to upper airway obstruction, which is discussed in Chap. 34 and poses an immediate threat to life, the following thoracic injuries require immediate intervention[4–6]:

1. Tension pneumothorax
2. Open pneumothorax
3. Cardiac tamponade
4. Massive hemothorax
5. Massive pneumothorax
6. Traumatic air embolism
7. Flail chest

Since all of these conditions require immediate intervention, the intensivist who sees such patients must be prepared to institute therapy before any other physician is available. To guide appropriate intervention, a brief description of the pathophysiology, diagnosis, and treatment principles for each of these conditions follows. In all cases, the airway must be secured and adequate intravenous (IV) access established.

TENSION PNEUMOTHORAX

This lesion arises when a one-way valve mechanism exists after chest wall or lung injury. Gas enters the pleural space but has no escape, and with each subsequent respiratory cycle, there is increased intrapleural pressure and gas accumulation. This increased tension causes the ipsilateral lung to be compressed and displaced to the opposite side. With the resulting mediastinal shift, there is not only compromise of ventilation and gas exchange but also kinking of the major veins at the thoracic inlet of the neck and at the diaphragmatic entrance of the inferior vena cava, thus compromising venous return to the heart. Continued shift of the mediastinum eventually compresses the contralateral lung as well, producing further ventilatory compromise. This combination of hypoperfusion and hypoxemia can be lethal, and immediate treatment is required. The diagnosis is suspected in a patient who presents with chest trauma, tachypnea, severe dyspnea, decreased air entry, and hyperresonance on the affected side and, sometimes, a clinically detectable shift of the trachea to the opposite side with hypotension.

The treatment is immediate decompression of the pleural space, which is accomplished initially by inserting a large-bore needle or incising with a scalpel down through the chest wall into the pleural space at the second intercostal space in the midclavicular line or the fourth to fifth intercostal space just anterior to the midaxillary line. If a plunger syringe is used with the needle, an immediate spontaneous rise of the plunger in the barrel will be seen. Similarly, when the scalpel enters the pleural space, there is a massive loud decompression of the pleural space, followed by immediate respiratory improvement. Either procedure should be followed by formal insertion of a chest tube. Briefly, the technique of chest tube insertion requires an incision down to the pleura in the fourth to fifth intercostal space just anterior to the midaxillary line. The large-bore chest tube (F32 to F36) is inserted directly with a clamp after verification with finger palpation that the pleural space has been entered and there are no pleural adhesions (Fig. 95-2). When needle decompression is performed prior to insertion of the chest tube, the needle may be inserted through the finger portion of a glove so that air may exit but not enter

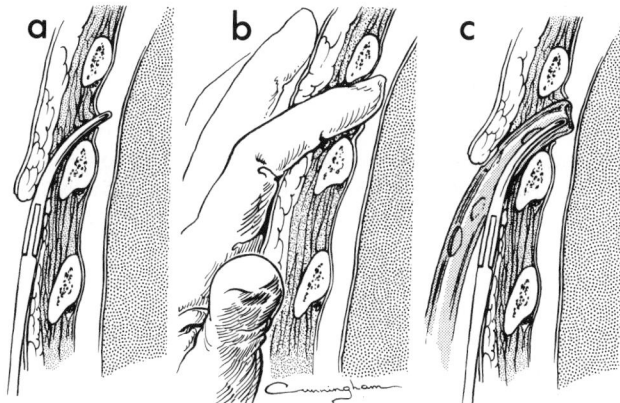

FIGURE 95-2 Technique of chest tube insertion. The incision is made 2 cm below the chosen interspace, and the clamp (*A*) followed by the finger (*B*) is inserted into the pleural space above the upper border of the rib. The tube is inserted and directed with the Kelly clamp (*C*). The tube is then gently directed posteriorly and toward the apex.

the pleural space from the atmosphere (Fig. 95-3). Once the chest tube is inserted, it is connected to an underwater seal system with the option of applying suction. Figure 95-4 illustrates the classic chest tube drainage system. However, commercially available prepackaged chest tube drainage systems are available that operate on the same principles.

OPEN PNEUMOTHORAX

In open pneumothorax, there is free communication through a chest wall wound between the pleural space and the atmosphere. Entry of air with each respiratory cycle results in progressive collapse of the ipsilateral lung. The larger the defect in the chest wall, the greater is the rate at which pleural air accumulates, and the more rapid is the collapse of the ipsilateral lung. This pathophysiology is similar to that in tension

FIGURE 95-3 Needle decompression of the pleural space. Use of the finger portion of a glove prevents air from entering the pleural space.

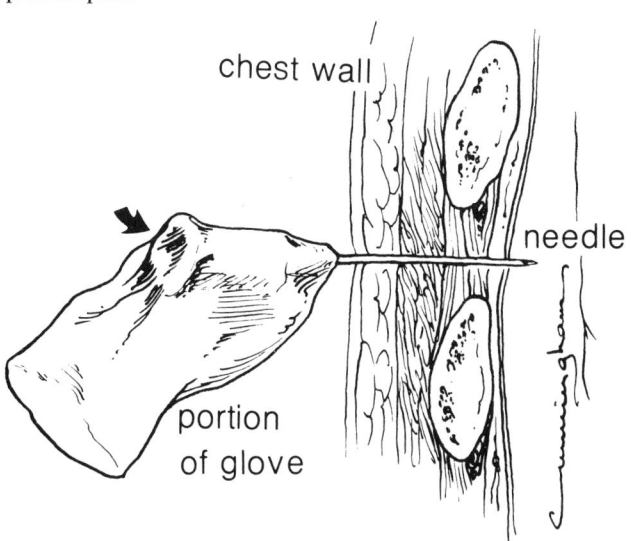

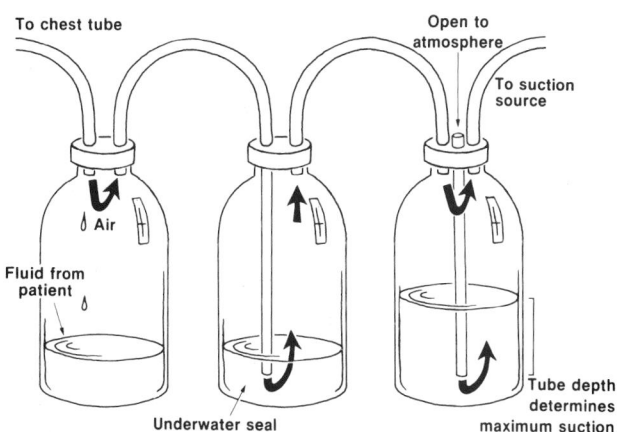

FIGURE 95-4 Chest drainage collection systems.

pneumothorax because collapse of the lung and shift of the mediastinum to the opposite side will cause hypoxemia and decreased venous return. The diagnosis usually is obvious, with a visible open wound in the chest wall and a characteristic loud noise created from atmospheric air entry into the pleural space.

The first principle in treating this injury is occlusion of the open wound. This usually can be accomplished with an occlusive gauze dressing (Fig. 95-5). Larger defects will require much larger dressings, and major defects that cannot be occluded readily by dressing technique will require support of the patient with endotracheal intubation and positive-pressure ventilation until formal surgical repair of the chest wall defect can be accomplished. After the opening in the chest wall is occluded, a chest tube should be inserted through a separate opening, as indicated earlier. Figure 95-5 shows a

FIGURE 95-5 Temporary occlusive dressing for open pneumothorax. This dressing allows egress of air but prevents entry of air into pleural space.

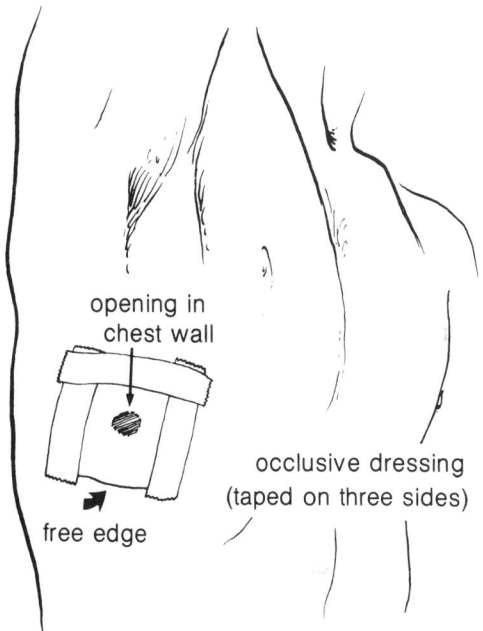

technique whereby an occlusive dressing can be applied that allows decompression of the pleural space as well as occlusion of the opening. The nonpermeable dressing is applied over the opening and secured on all but one side. This allows egress of air from the pleural space but prevents air from entering the pleural space.

CARDIAC TAMPONADE

Cardiac tamponade occurs when fluid accumulation in the pericardial sac interferes with cardiac filling. Elevated pericardial pressure decreases transmural filling pressures of the cardiac chambers, resulting in diminished filling and stroke volume of the right and the left side of the heart. Cardiac output falls, with an attendant decrease in systolic blood pressure and pulse pressure.

The diagnosis of cardiac tamponade is one that requires a high index of suspicion and should be considered in any patient who has blunt or penetrating trauma to the chest and is hypotensive without any obvious signs of blood loss. The classic triad described by Beck of hypotension, elevated venous pressure, and muffled heart tones is not always present or easily discernible.[7] The status of the neck veins is particularly important in distinguishing hypotension caused by hypovolemia from that caused by cardiac tamponade. In the former case, the neck veins are flat, whereas in the latter, they are distended. However, a struggling or straining patient may produce misleading bulging of the neck veins, which must be taken into consideration. An increase in pulsus paradoxus (the difference in systolic blood pressure between inspiration and expiration) above 10 mm Hg suggests the diagnosis of cardiac tamponade. However, in the emergency setting it may be difficult to quantitate the degree of pulsus paradoxus. During arterial pressure transduction in the ICU, it is possible to measure pulsus paradoxus accurately. The physician should note the difference between systolic blood pressure during inspiration and expiration. The pressure waveform will exhibit a lower peak level in inspiration, with higher peak levels in expiration. The difference between the two peaks is the pulsus paradoxus. The degree of pulsus paradoxus may be determined at the bedside by listening for the first set of sounds with the sphygmomanometer slowly deflating. The first set of sounds represents the systolic blood pressure on expiration. As the pressure in the cuff is slowly released, the gaps in systolic blood pressure sounds between inspiration and expiration disappear, and there is an increased frequency of sounds heard with the stethoscope. The difference between the initial pressure and the pressure when the gaps in sounds have disappeared is the degree of pulsus paradoxus. Since distended neck veins and hypotension are present in both tension pneumothorax and cardiac tamponade, differentiation between these two conditions is important but at times difficult. The physician must rely on evidence of hyperresonance and decreased breath sounds that will suggest tension pneumothorax. If a search for these signs still leaves doubt, the patient should be treated first for possible tension pneumothorax by insertion of a needle in the pleural space. This step can be performed quickly and will give the diagnosis as well as be therapeutic for a tension pneumothorax. Once tension pneumothorax is ruled out, one should proceed to treatment for cardiac tamponade if signs of circulatory compromise persist. If immediately available in the emergency setting, epigastric placement of an ultrasound probe is also helpful in diagnosing hemopericardium.[8]

Although performance of a subxiphoid pericardial window in the relatively stable patient is acceptable, the initial treatment of cardiac tamponade consists of prompt pericardiocentesis.[9] This usually is performed with a 16- to 18-gauge needle that is at least 6 in long, incorporates a catheter, and is attached to a 50-mm empty syringe with a three-way stopcock. If time permits, the skin below the xiphoid process is anesthetized, and an electrocardiographic lead is attached to the hub of the needle as the needle is inserted below the skin at roughly a 45-degree angle and advanced cephalad toward the tip of the left scapula.[3,9] Gentle aspiration is maintained as the needle is advanced. A sense of "give" may be noted as the needle enters the pericardial sac. Nonclotting blood aspirated at this time confirms a pericardial position of the needle. If the needle is advanced into the myocardium, an injury pattern is seen on the electrocardiogram (ECG) monitor. If this is noted, the needle should be withdrawn slightly and then aspirated coincident with return to the previous baseline ECG tracing. Other ECG patterns, including premature ventricular contractions, may occur when the needle contacts the myocardium.

Although the pericardial sac can accommodate large volumes of fluid when the fluid accumulates chronically, in acute pericardial tamponade, a volume as small as 100 mL can compromise cardiac function significantly. Similarly, withdrawal of as little as 20 to 50 mL of blood from the pericardial sac results in significant improvement in hemodynamic status.[10] Apart from the signs noted earlier that suggest successful aspiration of the pericardial sac, recovery of blood that immediately clots in the syringe, particularly if the patient's hemodynamic status does not improve, should raise the concern that the needle has penetrated the heart and that intracardiac rather than pericardial blood is being aspirated. As pericardiocentesis is being conducted, the operating room (OR) should be prepared; whether pericardiocentesis fails or succeeds and results in stabilization of the hemodynamic status, it should be followed by formal thoracotomy and repair of the lacerated heart.[10–13] This usually is conducted through an anterolateral thoracotomy incision in the fifth intercostal space. However, a median sternotomy is an alternate route. When the thoracic cavity is entered, the pericardium is identified, and a longitudinal incision is made in it, care being taken to avoid transection of the phrenic nerve. Blood is aspirated, and the laceration in the heart is identified and controlled quickly by digital pressure. With finger control of the bleeding point, interrupted sutures are placed and secured with Teflon pledgets to repair the laceration, and the pericardium is then resutured, with a small opening (approximately 1 cm) left to prevent reaccumulation of blood in the pericardial sac. Other reported techniques for repair of the cardiac laceration include temporary Foley catheter insertion into the cardiac wound, followed by inflation of the balloon of the catheter and repair of the laceration. Skin staples also may be used to close the cardiac wound. In very rare circumstances, the laceration involves the coronary arteries. Formal repair of the artery will require heart-lung bypass and may be accomplished in the acute setting if the resources are immediately available. If the patient's condition stabilizes and the bleeding and laceration have been controlled, then definitive therapy for the coronary artery laceration may be pursued subsequently on a semielective basis. In placing sutures for the cardiac repair, care should be taken to avoid incorporating and ligating coronary arteries.

MASSIVE HEMOTHORAX

Although most patients with traumatic hemothorax are relatively stable and do not require immediate surgical intervention, a few present with massive intrathoracic hemorrhage. This condition requires prompt diagnosis and immediate treatment to ensure survival. The mechanism of injury may be blunt or penetrating and generally involves disruption of a major central vascular structure or laceration of a systemic artery such as an intercostal artery or internal mammary artery. Intrathoracic hemorrhage usually arises from parenchymal lesions of the lung and stops spontaneously, particularly with reexpansion of the lung. The patient with massive intrathoracic hemorrhage presents initially with severe hypotension from blood loss and later with hypoxemia from collapse of the lung caused by the mass effect of the blood in the involved thoracic cavity.[14] Apart from severe hypotension and tachycardia, these patients demonstrate dullness to percussion and decreased air entry on the involved side and a shift of the mediastinum to the opposite side. The central venous pressure or jugular venous pressure is usually low, but it may be elevated in the unusual circumstance that a mass effect from the blood contained in the thorax produces a mechanical obstruction to venous inflow into the chest.

The diagnosis is confirmed and treatment instituted by insertion of a large-bore chest tube, through which a large volume (frequently close to 2000 mL) of blood drains immediately, to be followed by a continuous drainage of blood at rates approximating 100 mL/h. If either of these conditions is present, the patient is considered to have a massive hemothorax requiring surgical intervention. These should not be considered absolute indications for thoracotomy but merely guidelines. The most important indicator of whether or not surgical intervention is necessary is whether the patient's hemodynamics improve significantly and remain so after chest decompression and with fluid resuscitation. If bleeding continues at a rapid rate, or if the patient's hemodynamic status cannot be normalized with rapid infusions of blood and crystalloid, surgical intervention is warranted. The involved chest is opened through a posterolateral incision. Once the blood has been evacuated from the pleural space, a search is made for the bleeding point. It is frequently necessary to clamp the hilum of the lung temporarily and to release it intermittently in order to identify the area of bleeding, which is repaired by direct suture. Occasionally, massive hemorrhage necessitates resection of the involved lung, which should be accomplished quickly using staple devices. Very occasionally, the bleeding is from a ruptured thoracic aorta. Usually patients with free bleeding into the thoracic cavity from a ruptured aorta exsanguinate at the scene or immediately thereafter. However, in certain instances, it is possible to salvage some of these patients by clamping the aorta proximal and distal to the laceration and expeditiously repairing the laceration or inserting an aortic graft prosthesis.[4,15,16] If available, a preheparinized shunt may be of use in these circumstances to bypass the lacerated area of the aorta and maintain perfusion of the distal aorta and spinal cord while the repair is

undertaken.[17] Occasionally, access to the bleeding source will require extension of the unilateral thoracotomy incision into the opposite chest by transection of the sternum and ligation of the internal mammary arteries.

The Massively Bleeding Patient

As indicated previously, it is not always possible to determine precisely whether massive bleeding arises from a thoracic or an abdominal source. Therefore, it is crucial that the entire abdomen and chest be prepared and draped for exposure in the OR. In these circumstances, if the bleeding is into the right chest and the apparent site of impact or penetrating injury is in the lower right chest below the nipple line, laparotomy through an upper midline incision should be conducted because the source of the hemorrhage is usually a liver injury with penetration of the right hemidiaphragm. Where ultrasound assessment is immediately available, this may allow more precise location of the source of the hemorrhage and thus guide the location of the incision in the abdomen or thorax. Failure to reveal an abdominal source of hemorrhage at laparotomy will necessitate an anterolateral thoracotomy on the right side, which usually will reveal lacerated intercostal arteries, which should be identified and ligated. As indicated earlier, injuries to the low-pressure pulmonary vasculature usually are not associated with massive hemorrhage, and the bleeding stops spontaneously, particularly with reexpansion of the lung and decompression of the pleural space. If the impact is to the right upper chest or to any portion of the left chest, then massive hemorrhage should be treated by anterolateral thoracotomy on the bleeding side, and the incision should be extended as necessary to obtain control of the bleeding site. Occasionally, bleeding into the chest arises from a penetrating injury to the base of the neck. In these circumstances, the chest should be opened through a median sternotomy, with the option of extending laterally into the chest as well as above the clavicle to convert the incision to a trapdoor type of exposure. The median sternotomy under these circumstances allows better exposure of the vascular structures of the base of the neck than would be available through an anterolateral thoracotomy.[18]

MASSIVE PNEUMOTHORAX AND AIRWAY INJURY

Most patients with traumatic pneumothoraces present with signs characteristic of a pneumothorax but without any major degree of hemodynamic compromise, and the pneumothorax responds very promptly to chest tube insertion. Occasionally, however, the pneumothorax persists despite adequately functioning large-bore chest tubes and is accompanied by massive subcutaneous emphysema and continued hypoxemia and respiratory instability. The patient usually also has some degree of hemoptysis, which may be evidenced by blood draining through the endotracheal tube if the patient has been intubated, as is often the case. This scenario suggests the presence of a large airway laceration and requires immediate surgical intervention.

The patient is immediately placed on 100% oxygen. If time allows, bronchoscopy should be performed to identify the level of the lacerated airway. However, thoracotomy is warranted even if the lesion is not identified or there is insufficient time to perform bronchoscopy. It is essential that one be certain that the chest tubes are functioning adequately in these circumstances, and if mechanical problems are ruled out, the patient should be taken to the OR promptly. Occasionally, for a right-sided bronchial leak, insertion of a balloon-tipped catheter down the right mainstem bronchus may allow ventilation of the normal left lung after the right bronchus is occluded by inflation of the balloon. This measure temporarily stabilizes the patient by decreasing the air leak on the involved side. It is technically very difficult to accomplish, however, and should not take priority over getting the patient to the operating room as quickly as possible. For a left-sided bronchial tear, the endotracheal tube may be directed into the right mainstem bronchus and the cuff of the endotracheal tube inflated. This would allow ventilation of the right lung until the left lung lesion has been repaired.[19] In the OR, a double-lumen tube, if available, will allow selective ventilation of the normal lung. At surgery, the lesion is identified and repaired directly. If there is massive destruction of the airway with failure to achieve an anastomosis or a high risk of subsequent stenosis of the airway, lung resection should be considered.[20]

TRAUMATIC AIR EMBOLISM

The exact incidence of this entity in patients with multiple injuries is not known. However, to make the diagnosis, a very high index of suspicion must be maintained, and this diagnosis should be suspected in any patient with sudden cardiovascular collapse who demonstrates a neurologic deficit after chest injury, especially if these signs occur with the initiation of positive-pressure ventilation.[21] In most cases, the diagnosis of traumatic air embolism is made at thoracotomy that is conducted on the basis of sudden collapse of a patient who has sustained major chest trauma. Occasionally, these patients may be quite stable initially, only to develop a focal neurologic deficit suddenly with cardiovascular collapse immediately after being placed on positive-pressure ventilation. Another sign suggestive of the diagnosis is the presence of bubbles within arterial blood drawn by arterial puncture, usually for blood gas analysis. It must be recognized, however, that the most common cause of air bubbles in the syringe is a loosely fitting syringe connector; this must be ruled out prior to making the diagnosis. Occasionally, air may be seen in the retinal arteries on funduscopic examination as well.

An anterolateral thoracotomy should be performed on the side of the penetrating injury or on the left side if no penetration is apparent. On entry into the thoracic cavity, prevention of further embolization is accomplished by cross-clamping of the pulmonary hilum. An 18-gauge needle should be used for venting the most anterior surfaces of the left atrium, left ventricle, and ascending aorta. This maneuver is followed by compressing the root of the aorta between the thumb and index finger, which are placed in the transverse sinus. Massaging the heart should drive air bubbles out of the coronary microvasculature. Maintenance of a high systemic blood pressure, with α agonists if necessary, should help to force trapped air from the heart and brain through the microvasculature into the venous circulation. With reestablishment of cardiac activity, the left-sided chambers and the aorta should be vented once more. Attention is then directed to the pulmonary lesion, which will require repair by direct suture, lobectomy, or pneumonectomy as necessitated by the nature of the injury.

FLAIL CHEST

This condition arises whenever a portion of the chest wall becomes completely discontinuous from the rest of the rib cage. It usually results from blunt chest trauma in which several adjacent ribs are fractured on both sides of the sternum or, at least, at two locations on each of the ribs involved. This leads to a free-floating segment of the chest wall that positions itself in response to changes in pleural pressure rather than to the mechanical positions of the rest of the chest wall. The result is paradoxical movement of this portion of the chest wall. During spontaneous breathing, the flail segment moves inward with the negative pleural pressure of inspiration and moves outward with expiration. The diagnosis frequently is missed initially if one relies entirely on the detection of paradoxical movement of the chest wall because muscle spasm and pain restrict movement of the chest wall and make it very difficult to detect the paradoxical movement. This is particularly true in injuries involving the posterior thorax, where the muscle mass makes it even more difficult to detect paradoxical movement. Also, if the patient has been intubated and positive-pressure ventilation is instituted, paradoxical movement of the chest wall will not be seen. The presence of multiple adjacent rib fractures involving the same rib in different segments on chest x-ray would suggest the presence of flail chest even if it is not apparent clinically. The degree of pulmonary and hemodynamic disability that arises is related to the extent of the flail, the degree of underlying lung contusion, and the restrictive effect of chest wall pain from the multiple fractures. There is, therefore, a wide spectrum of presentation of patients with flail chest.

In the severely hypoxemic patient with a large flail and/or hemodynamic instability, immediate endotracheal intubation and positive-pressure ventilation are indicated, with prompt chest tube insertion on the involved side to prevent a tension pneumothorax from developing on institution of positive-pressure ventilation. Patients who are able to maintain adequate oxygenation and ventilation with supplemental oxygen may be maintained without mechanical ventilation and endotracheal intubation, particularly if adequate pain control can be achieved. This may require frequent or continuous intravenous analgesia in the form of titrated fentanyl, morphine, or other agents. In other circumstances, epidural or, less preferably, intercostal blockade with long-acting local anesthetic agents may be used to control the pain. With adequate analgesia, it is possible to avoid endotracheal intubation and mechanical ventilation in most patients with flail chest.[22]

Emergency thoracotomy is not required for treating flail chest. Also, mechanical fixation of the rib fractures usually is not necessary. There is still controversy as to whether formal thoracotomy and mechanical fixation of the fractured ribs should be considered at all in these patients.[23] However, in situations where thoracotomy is required for other reasons, it may be appropriate to reduce and plate the fractures involved.

If a decision is made to ventilate the patient with a flail chest, the timing of weaning will not necessarily depend on disappearance of the paradoxical movement of the chest wall. Rather, weaning from the respirator may be initiated when the gas exchange abnormality associated with the underlying lung contusion is resolved. In fact, frequently these patients are weaned completely off respiratory support (with adequate pain control) when the lung contusion clears, even when residual paradoxical movement remains apparent for several weeks. A potential disadvantage of the nonsurgical and conservative nonventilating approach to flail chest is the acceptance of a high degree of ultimate chest wall deformity. However, these chest wall abnormalities are of questionable significance in terms of producing a long-term restrictive defect in these patients.

Other Chest Injuries

Although the following chest injuries do not immediately threaten life, early diagnosis and treatment are essential to prevent significant morbidity and later mortality:

1. Lung contusion
2. Blunt cardiac injury
3. Aortic rupture
4. Esophageal disruption
5. Diaphragmatic rupture
6. Rib fractures
7. Simple hemopneumothorax

A very brief discussion of the pathophysiology, diagnosis, and treatment of these entities follows.

LUNG CONTUSION

This lesion results from direct trauma to the lung parenchyma, usually by a blunt mechanism, although it can occur from penetrating injuries as well. There is a wide spectrum of severity, ranging from very minor localized hemorrhage into the lung parenchyma to complete obliteration of an entire lung or even bilateral involvement. This injury is missed often because the respiratory failure that develops is not immediately evident, and indeed, chest films may be completely normal initially. It is essential, therefore, that the diagnosis be considered whenever there is significant direct injury to the chest wall. Initially, there may be chest pain and minimal dyspnea or hypoxia. However, within hours there may be slow deterioration in gas exchange and a progressive development of radiologic densities on chest x-ray. As pointed out earlier, there may or may not be an associated flail chest.

The treatment is selective and is based on the degree of respiratory impairment.[24] When the gas exchange abnormality is minimal and oxygenation and ventilation can be maintained without endotracheal intubation, close attention to fluid balance is required. However, fluid should not be restricted in a patient with lung contusion if fluid resuscitation is required in a hemodynamically abnormal patient. Close, continuous monitoring of the hemodynamic and respiratory status is essential; if there is no major hemodynamic or respiratory compromise, the patient will not require mechanical ventilation. The criteria for initiation of mechanical ventilation are outlined in earlier chapters, but certain associated disorders increase the likelihood that mechanical ventilation will be needed. These include preexisting chronic respiratory failure and associated abdominal, thoracic, or central nervous system injuries.

BLUNT CARDIAC INJURY

This lesion probably occurs much more commonly than was suspected previously because of the subtle nature of its pre-

sentation among other associated injuries.[4,25] It usually results from blunt trauma to the sternum, most commonly caused by steering wheel impact. In fact, whenever a fractured sternum is diagnosed in chest trauma, one must assume an underlying myocardial contusion. The patient's symptoms frequently are clouded by associated chest wall contusion and other causes for chest wall discomfort and cardiorespiratory dysfunction. The diagnosis is suggested by the presence of ECG abnormalities, serial elevations in the level of the creatine kinase MB isoenzyme, or abnormalities found by two-dimensional echocardiography. However, myocardial enzymes do not contribute significantly to the diagnosis or management in this injury.[26] Although cardiac troponins usually are helpful in the diagnosis of myocardial infarction, the levels obtained following trauma are too inconclusive to allow a diagnosis of blunt cardiac injury and provide no additional information beyond that available by electrocardiography. ECG abnormalities may vary from few to multiple premature ventricular contractions, persistent tachycardia, dysrhythmias such as atrial fibrillation, bundle branch block, ST-segment changes, or even changes indistinguishable from those of acute myocardial infarction. None of these tests is specific for blunt cardiac injury.

Because of the nature of this entity and its propensity for certain life-threatening dysrhythmias, consideration should be given to monitoring these patients in an ICU environment. Oxygen should be administered, pain should be treated with parenteral analgesics, and the patient should be treated in the same way as for myocardial ischemia, as outlined in other chapters of this book. The indications for inotropic agents, vasoactive drugs, and other forms of cardiac support are comparable with those for any patient with myocardial ischemia. Most patients with minor degrees of contusion do not require ICU admission.

AORTIC RUPTURE

Traumatic disruption of the thoracic aorta frequently is lethal.[16] In patients who reach the hospital alive, the rupture tends to be located at the point of fixation of the aorta just distal to the origin of the left subclavian artery at the ligamentum arteriosum, which represents the junction between a relatively fixed and mobile portion of the vessel. Therefore, the mechanism is a shear force, commonly seen with acceleration-deceleration injuries, although a sudden increase in intraluminal hydrostatic pressure may play a role in its pathogenesis. Aortic rupture at other sites near the root of the aorta usually results in death at the scene. In patients who survive the initial injury, the hematoma is contained by an intact adventitial layer. Because of the possibility of free rupture and exsanguination whenever this diagnosis is suspected, investigations and treatment should be prompt. Although several radiologic signs are described (such as widened mediastinum, fractures of the first and second ribs, obliteration of the aortic knob, deviation of the trachea to the right, presence of a pleural cap, elevation and rightward shift of the right mainstem bronchus, depression of the left mainstem bronchus, and obliteration of the space between the pulmonary artery and the aorta), frequently the only suggestive sign is a widening of the mediastinum on the plain chest film (Fig. 95-6). Other suggestive signs are the presence of a thoracic bruit or a discrepancy in blood pressure between the upper and lower limbs or between the right and left upper limbs. Placement

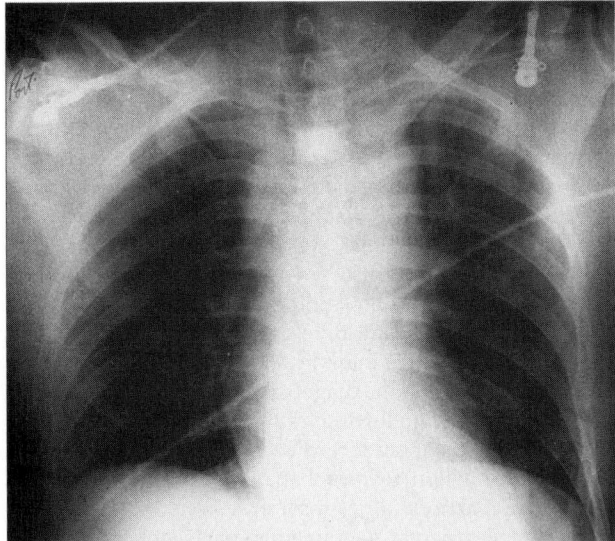

A

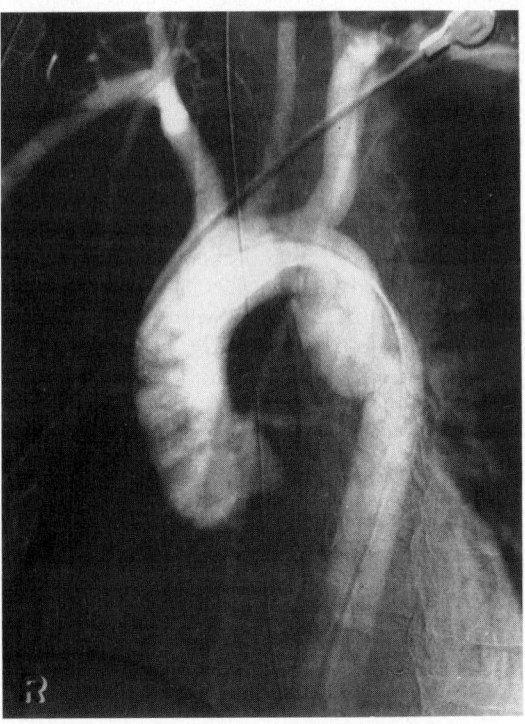

B

FIGURE 95-6 Ruptured thoracic aorta. *A.* **Chest film showing widened mediastinum.** *B.* **Aortogram from the same patient showing lacerated aorta.**

of a nasogastric tube may highlight the degree of esophageal deviation and hematoma size on the chest film. Since most chest x-rays in traumatized patients are done in the supine position, the size of the mediastinum is exaggerated, and consequently, this diagnosis is considered in a large percentage of patients who do not actually have a traumatic aortic rupture. However, because of the lethal nature of this disease, it seems justified to pursue further imaging whenever aortic rupture is seriously suspected.[27]

Spiral computed tomography (CT) is recommended in the presence of suspected mediastinal widening, and if this is

totally normal, then further imaging is not warranted.[28,29] If the CT scan is questionable or suspicious, then an aortogram should be obtained. In any event, most surgeons still insist that angiography be performed prior to surgery.

The use of transesophageal echocardiography[30,31] also has given excellent results in the diagnosis of aortic rupture, and in some centers it has virtually replaced angiography because of its accuracy and relative noninvasiveness, but there still remains a worrisome incidence of false positivity with this diagnostic tool.

The approach to management of the patient with aortic rupture is early surgical repair unless contraindicated by significant associated life-threatening injuries such as major head injuries. Resection with placement of a prosthetic graft frequently is necessary, although direct repair without the use of a prosthetic graft is sometimes possible. As soon as immediate life-threatening injuries have been addressed, the aortic lesion should be treated surgically. If surgical treatment is delayed because of associated major injuries, then treatment and close monitoring in the ICU with afterload reduction, β blockade, and maintenance of borderline hypotension are appropriate.[32]

ESOPHAGEAL DISRUPTION

The most common cause of esophageal rupture is iatrogenic injury during endoscopic maneuvers. However, this injury may result from both penetrating and blunt injury. A severe blow to the upper abdomen in the presence of a closed glottis can result in a sudden increase in intraesophageal pressure with rupture. The resulting tear allows leakage of gastric contents into the mediastinum, causing severe mediastinitis.

The patient presents with severe retrosternal chest pain and very soon develops profound hypotension and tachycardia. Frequently, pneumothorax or hemothorax is evident without a rib fracture, and if a chest tube is inserted, particulate matter may appear in the drainage. The drainage of pleural fluid with a very low pH and a high amylase content also should suggest the diagnosis. Other radiologic signs include the presence of mediastinal air. The diagnosis may be confirmed by gastrograffin swallow or esophagoscopy.

Treatment consists of massive infusion of crystalloid to maintain euvolemeia, antibiotic coverage, and early thoracotomy with repair of the lesion. If the diagnosis is made late in the onset of the disease, direct repair of the laceration may not be possible, and esophageal diversion techniques may become necessary as part of the surgical therapy. This may require the formation of an esophagostomy in the neck, as well as a gastrostomy, pleural drainage through chest tubes, and parenteral nutrition and antibiotic therapy.[33]

DIAPHRAGMATIC RUPTURE

Lacerations of the diaphragm may occur from blunt and penetrating injuries, and the injury may originate from either the thorax or the abdomen. The injury is diagnosed most frequently on the left side but may occur with equal frequency on the right side. Penetrating injuries tend to be small and sharply demarcated, whereas blunt injuries often result in large, irregular lacerations with herniation of intraabdominal contents into the chest.[34]

The diagnosis is missed frequently because of misinterpretation of the chest film, often thought to represent an elevated left hemidiaphragm, gastric dilatation, or loculated hemopneumothorax or hematoma. The placement of a nasogastric tube with its location above the diaphragm after entry into the stomach suggests the diagnosis.

Depending on the degree to which abdominal contents herniate into the thoracic cavity, the symptoms may be very minimal or very significant.[35–37] A patient with blunt chest or abdominal trauma who exhibits sudden deterioration in respiratory status when intraabdominal pressure is increased should be considered as having a ruptured diaphragm. This was noted frequently when the abdominal compartment of the pneumatic antishock garment was used in the past. During peritoneal lavage, drainage of lavage fluid through a chest tube that is in place also indicates that diaphragmatic rupture is present.

The urgency of treatment depends on the degree to which the patient's hemodynamic and respiratory status is compromised. In most instances, an isolated diaphragmatic hernia can be repaired within several hours of admission, after the patient is resuscitated. Repair is done through a midline upper abdominal incision. This approach allows complete examination of the abdominal cavity. The hernia can be reduced quite easily and the repair conducted from within the abdomen. Associated injuries, such as splenic rupture, also can be treated easily during the laparotomy. If the diagnosis is made several weeks after the injury, then it is preferable to approach the lesion through a thoracotomy because any intraabdominal injury would have declared itself already; also, it will be much easier to reduce the hernia from within the thoracic cavity. Although laparoscopy increases the risk of tension pneumothorax in the presence of a diaphragmatic rupture, recent reports have suggested that this technique may be employed cautiously in the diagnosis and treatment of diaphragmatic rupture when the laparoscope is used in assessment of the traumatized abdomen.[38–40]

RIB FRACTURES

Rib fractures are very common with chest injuries. Frequently they are missed on x-ray examination unless special rib views are taken. However, the diagnosis is suspected when there is localized chest wall pain. The diagnosis is also suggested when one is able to elicit crepitus over the fracture site or auscultate a "click" with inspiration over the fracture site. Tenderness on compression of the chest wall is also suggestive of rib fractures.

The treatment of rib fractures consists of analgesics, which may be administered orally, parenterally, or epidurally, depending on the degree of discomfort and the number of ribs involved. In the ICU setting, parenteral analgesics or regional blocks are preferable. Generally, the fractured ribs do not require any specific treatment. However, in the setting of a patient with preexisting pulmonary dysfunction, the restriction produced by fractured ribs can make the difference between normal gas exchange and severe respiratory failure. Maintenance of adequate respiratory function therefore is the mainstay of treatment in these patients.

SIMPLE HEMOPNEUMOTHORAX

In contrast to a tension pneumothorax, the simple hemopneumothorax usually is diagnosed by a combination of physical examination and chest x-ray. Although it has been suggested

recently that small pneumothoraces may be treated by close monitoring in the ICU without chest tube insertion, generally, if a hemothorax or pneumothorax is noted following trauma, a chest tube is inserted regardless of the size of the air or blood collection. This measure allows decompression of the pleural space, as well as monitoring of the drainage from the pleural space. It is particularly important that chest tube decompression of the pleural space be secured before mechanical ventilation is instituted or a general anesthetic administered.

Abdominal Injuries

GENERAL PRINCIPLES

Apart from patients with pericardial tamponade or traumatic air embolism, any hemodynamically compromised patient with torso trauma in whom adequately functioning chest tubes demonstrate no free pleural blood or continued major air leakage must be considered to have an intraabdominal source of blood loss until another cause is proven. Hence, when the decision is unclear in an unstable patient with torso trauma, the combination of physical examination, chest x-ray, and chest tube insertion frequently will allow one to determine whether the lesion is located in the chest. With a negative chest film and no chest tube drainage in the absence of cardiac tamponade or air embolism, laparotomy frequently is required in the unstable patient with torso trauma.

In the OR, all such patients should have the entire abdomen and chest prepared and draped. They also should receive preoperative antibiotics that will cover aerobic gram-negative and anaerobic organisms. It is crucial that the antibiotics be administered before the incision is made in order to minimize septic complications.[41] If there is no fecal contamination in the peritoneal cavity, the antibiotics may be stopped within 24 hours. However, in the presence of contamination, antibiotic administration should be continued until the temperature is normal and there is no leukocytosis. An increase in the temperature and white blood cell (WBC) count after antibiotics are stopped suggests residual sepsis, which often is in the form of an undrained intraabdominal abscess.

A generous upper midline incision extending from the xiphoid process to just below the umbilicus is the exposure of choice because most of the lesions producing instability arise from injuries to the upper abdominal contents. This incision can be extended easily up into the chest through lateral thoracotomy or a median sternotomy or extended into the lower abdomen for lower abdominal injuries. Occasionally, the history suggests an isolated lower abdominal injury, and in this circumstance, a lower midline incision beginning at the umbilicus may be undertaken.

Prior to laparotomy, the surgeon need only decide that surgical intervention is necessary; a specific diagnosis is not necessary. In deciding on laparotomy, one looks for the signs of penetration, perforation, or hemorrhage. Penetration of the peritoneum in stab wounds is diagnosed by exploration of the abdominal wound under local anesthesia with good lighting; if it is determined that the peritoneum has been violated, in most instances laparotomy is performed. This approach has been questioned, and peritoneal lavage has been conducted in conjunction with exploration of the wound to determine the need for laparotomy on a more selective basis.[42,43] In these circumstances, demonstration of violation of the peritoneum and positive peritoneal lavage are used as indications for laparotomy. All bullet wounds to the abdomen are treated by laparotomy,[44] although a selective approach based on careful scanning of the abdomen to identify tangential nonpenetrating wounds has been reported. The signs of perforation are abdominal pain, tenderness, guarding, and rigidity. Signs of hemorrhage also may present with signs of peritoneal irritation, shoulder tip pain, or variable degrees of hemodynamic instability.

On entry into the peritoneal cavity, the presence of dark blood usually suggests a liver injury, whereas bright red blood suggests an arterial source of bleeding. Rapid evisceration of the small intestine and liberal use of packs wherever blood is accumulating allow identification of the source of blood loss. Concentration on the first site of bleeding should be avoided. The lesions should be approached in order of severity; i.e., the areas that are bleeding most briskly should be treated first.

In general, findings on physical examination determine the need for surgical intervention. There are situations, however, in which the signs may be equivocal or impossible to elicit in the unstable patient. In these circumstances, ultrasound,[45] peritoneal lavage, and CT[46] are all very helpful in determining the need for laparotomy.

Massive intraabdominal hemorrhage may require thoracotomy to allow clamping of the supradiaphragmatic aorta for temporary control of intraabdominal hemorrhage and the maintenance of perfusion to the brain and myocardium.[47,48] Prompt laparotomy after aortic clamping would allow identification and control of intraabdominal hemorrhage before release of the aortic clamp. In many instances, aortic clamping also may be achieved through a laparotomy with compression and/or clamping of the infradiaphragmatic abdominal aorta.

ROLE OF PERITONEAL LAVAGE, CT, AND ULTRASOUND IN ASSESSING ABDOMINAL TRAUMA

Diagnostic peritoneal lavage, ultrasound, and CT are all useful diagnostic tools in assessing the traumatized abdomen. These modalities are all very sensitive for the detection of hemoperitoneum. Of the three modalities, CT is the most specific.[46] However, it requires transporting the patient to the CT suite and is relatively costly and time-consuming. Its main use, therefore, is in relatively stable patients, particularly those who are already having CT for another indication, such as possible head injury. The main advantages of ultrasound are its rapidity, sensitivity, noninvasiveness, and portability. Where emergency ultrasound assessment is available (focused assessment for the sonographic examination of the trauma patient [FAST]), this is preferred and superior to diagnostic peritoneal lavage, but like all imaging techniques, is not sufficiently sensitive to be used in isolation to make judgments regarding the need for surgery.[48a] With proper training of personnel, FAST can be very accurate in detecting hemoperitoneum, even when conducted and interpreted by nonradiologists.[45,49] Like other investigative tools, peritoneal lavage, ultrasound, and CT should be used only if the results will affect the decision on whether to perform a laparotomy. If there is an obvious need for laparotomy, then these modalities are not indicated.

INDICATIONS

1. When there are equivocal abdominal findings. Certain conditions, such as fractures of the lower ribs, pelvis, or lumbar spine, may produce abdominal signs that are difficult to separate from those injury due to intraabdominal structures.
2. When abdominal findings are impossible to elicit (e.g., when pain perception is abnormal, such as with severe head injury, drug intoxication, or spinal cord injuries).
3. When there may be long periods during which the patient is unavailable for repeated physical examination and observation, such as during lengthy surgical procedures.
4. When there is an obvious source of hemorrhage, such as a pelvic or extremity fracture, which could account for hypotension, but when simultaneous intraabdominal bleeding is also a possibility.

CONTRAINDICATIONS

An absolute contraindication to diagnostic peritoneal lavage is an already identified indication for laparotomy. Relative contraindications to diagnostic peritoneal lavage include previous abdominal operations with scars in the abdomen, morbid obesity, a preexisting coagulopathy, and advanced pregnancy. An incision may be made above the umbilicus in advanced pregnancy or distant from prior surgical wounds, and the open technique may be used if necessary. Otherwise, the closed Seldinger technique for insertion of the peritoneal catheter is acceptable.[50] There are virtually no contraindications to ultrasound assessment of the traumatized abdomen except an obvious need for laparotomy on the basis of clinical examination alone. The relative contraindication to CT is instability of the patient that makes transfer to the CT suite unsafe.

TECHNIQUES FOR CT, ULTRASOUND, AND DIAGNOSTIC PERITONEAL LAVAGE

CT

Whenever possible, CT of the abdomen should be conducted with oral, intravenous, and rectal contrast agents to enhance specificity. This approach allows assessment not only for solid-organ injury and hemoperitoneum but also for injury of hollow organs.

Ultrasound Examination for Fluid

The ultrasound probes are placed in four locations[45]:

1. Right upper quadrant—Morison's pouch
2. Epigastric area (pericardial)
3. Left upper quadrant (perisplenic)
4. Suprapubic area—pouch of Douglas

FAST detects blood in the pericardial sac as well as the perihepatic, splenoral, and pelvic regions of the abdomen.

Open Peritoneal Lavage

The urinary bladder and stomach should be decompressed by urinary catheter and nasogastric tube, respectively. The abdomen should be surgically prepared with an antiseptic solution, and local anesthetic should be infiltrated below the umbilicus in the midline if the patient perceives pain. The skin is incised in the midline, and an opening is made that permits visualization of the subcutaneous tissue and fascia. After hemostasis in the skin and subcutaneous tissue has been ensured, the fascia is incised, and the peritoneum is grasped with clamps. A purse-string suture is then inserted in the peritoneum, and an opening is made for insertion of the peritoneal dialysis catheter into the peritoneal cavity. The catheter is directed toward the pelvis, connected to a syringe, and aspirated. If no gross blood or obvious enteric contents are aspirated, 10 mL/kg of Ringer's lactate or normal saline is allowed to drain by gravity into the peritoneal cavity. The abdomen is palpated and agitated gently to distribute the fluid throughout the peritoneal cavity. After approximately 5 to 10 minutes, the fluid is siphoned off and examined.

Closed Diagnostic Peritoneal Lavage (Seldinger Technique)

In the closed technique[50] of diagnostic peritoneal lavage, preparation of the patient is similar. After a puncture wound is made through the skin with a scalpel, a needle with a guidewire is inserted into the subcutaneous tissue, fascia, and peritoneum. A peritoneal lavage catheter then is introduced over the guidewire and directed toward the pelvis, after ensuring that bowel has not been penetrated by the needle by aspirating and examining for bowel liquid contents or gas.

Semiclosed Peritoneal Lavage Technique

In this technique, an incision is made down to the fascia, which is grasped and then punctured. The catheter is then introduced through the opening in the fascia.

Interpretation of Diagnostic Peritoneal Lavage

1. Aspiration of more than 5 mL of gross blood or obvious enteric contents signifies a positive peritoneal lavage.
2. A positive result is also suggested when newsprint cannot be read through the IV tubing containing the drained fluid.
3. The fluid is sent for microscopic analysis, and the following criteria are used for positivity: more than 10^5 red blood cells (RBCs) per microliter, more than 500 WBCs per microliter, or the presence of bacteria, vegetable fibers, etc. on Gram stain. Lower counts also are used in special circumstances, such as the selective approach to laparotomy in penetrating wounds.[51]

With use of these criteria, the peritoneal lavage findings are falsely negative in approximately 2% of patients, and these patients usually have isolated injuries of the pancreas, duodenum, diaphragm, small bowel, or bladder.[52] Retroperitoneal injuries are missed frequently by peritoneal lavage.

SELECTING THE DIAGNOSTIC MODALITY IN BLUNT ABDOMINAL TRAUMA

Hemoperitoneum is the major indication for laparotomy in blunt abdominal trauma. Therefore, a diagnostic technique other than physical examination that detects hemoperitoneum accurately, quickly, noninvasively, and with minimal cost, such as ultrasound, appears most attractive. However, there is still a role for other modalities, such as diagnostic peritoneal lavage and CT,[53] in the assessment of the patient sustaining blunt abdominal trauma. If the ultrasound examination is negative, the patient may be followed clinically without the need for CT or diagnostic peritoneal lavage. With an equivocal ultrasound examination in a stable patient, CT should be done. An unstable patient with an equivocal ultrasound examination should either have a diagnostic

peritoneal lavage or be taken directly to the OR. When the ultrasound examination in a stable patient is positive for hemoperitoneum and a more specific diagnosis is desired, CT should be conducted. CT is particularly useful in patients who have hemoperitoneum with solid-organ injury that may be treated nonoperatively. Use of this approach significantly reduces the frequency with which CT is necessary as a screening tool for hemoperitoneum. The unstable patient in whom ultrasound examination is positive for hemoperitoneum generally requires laparotomy.

Specific Abdominal Injuries—Diagnosis and Management Principles

Although the nonsurgeon intensivist does not need detailed knowledge of the surgical management of specific intraabdominal injuries, some familiarity with the diagnostic and management principles to be applied in the surgical treatment of specific intraabdominal organ injuries is likely to improve the confidence with which these patients are managed in the ICU.

Penetrating abdominal injury differs significantly from nonpenetrating injury. Penetrating injury may result from stab wounds or wounds from other sharp objects or from bullet or shotgun wounds. Stab wounds tend to be the least serious, in that they involve organs only within the short trajectory of the weapon, and unless the stab wound impales a major vessel directly, major hemorrhage is not as likely as in other forms of penetrating or blunt abdominal injury. Patients with stab wounds require exploration of the wound to determine whether the peritoneum has been violated. If the peritoneum has been violated, a decision has to be made to proceed with formal laparotomy unless one is prepared to use peritoneal lavage as an adjunctive test in determining whether laparotomy should be conducted.[42] Although a selective approach using imaging such as CT and MRI to identify tangential nonpenetrating wounds that would not require laparotomy is suggested, generally, all bullet and shotgun wounds to the abdomen require laparotomy.[44] These missile injuries usually result in damage to more than one organ. Since kinetic energy transfer is affected most significantly by missile velocity ($K = 1^1/_2MV^2$), low-velocity missiles tend to produce limited surrounding injury, whereas high-velocity missiles produce greater damage. Organ involvement, therefore, is very unpredictable because of the variable trajectory and wide variable area of dissipated energy. A straight line joining the points of entry and exit usually does not represent the pathway of the missile. In shotgun injuries, much less damage is inflicted when the injury occurs from far range rather than close range.

The crushing force produced by blunt injuries results in very irregular lacerations. Multiple injuries are also common. Diagnosis and therapy are more challenging and should be more aggressive with blunt injury. Hemorrhage, devitalization of tissue, morbidity, and mortality are all increased in blunt injury compared with penetrating injuries of the abdomen.

The frequency of organ involvement in penetrating trauma is also different from that in blunt trauma to the abdomen. In penetrating trauma, the organs involved, in order of frequency, are the liver, small bowel, stomach, colon, major vessels, and retroperitoneum. In blunt injuries, the solid organs—the spleen, kidney, and liver—are damaged most often, followed by the intestines.[54]

STOMACH INJURIES

The diagnosis of stomach injury is suggested by epigastric pain and pain at the shoulder tip if there is free perforation. Usually there is very minimal hemorrhage, and the patient's hemodynamic status is not particularly affected. Upright chest x-ray reveals free air under the diaphragm. The diagnosis also may be suggested by bloody aspirate from the nasogastric tube.

The surgical treatment of stomach injuries is straightforward and involves débridement of devitalized tissue and usually primary suture or anastomosis if resection is required for wide areas of devitalization. It is essential that the entire stomach, including the posterior wall, is visualized to minimized missed injuries.

DUODENAL INJURIES

These injuries are seen often in association with other injuries, and the second portion of the duodenum is involved most commonly. Because the duodenum is a retroperitoneal structure, frank peritonitis is a very late sign, and the diagnosis is made only with a very high index of suspicion based on the mechanism of injury. A useful sign is the identification of retroperitoneal air on a plain film of the abdomen (Fig. 95-7). Occasionally, a free perforation of the first portion of the duodenum produces pneumoperitoneum and can be identified on an upright chest film.

In the surgical treatment of injuries to the duodenum, complete mobilization and visualization of the entire duodenum are crucial. Patients with intramural hematomas of the duodenum may present with vomiting and symptoms of gastric outlet obstruction; radiologic examination of the stomach and duodenum with contrast agents reveals the presence of an intramural hematoma. If this is the only injury, treatment can be conservative, with nasogastric suctioning and intravenous fluids until the hematoma resolves. If the lesion is found at laparotomy, the hematoma is evacuated easily through an incision in the duodenal wall.[55] The principle of treatment is to débride the area of injury, removing all devitalized tissue. If, after this is accomplished, the edges of the duodenum can be approximated without undue tension, primary suture closure is appropriate. The defect also may be closed by a serosal patch from adjacent small bowel or a resection and end-to-end anastomosis. When these techniques are not possible, then roux-en-Y anastomosis between the duodenal ends and the small bowel needs to be conducted. When there is concern about the duodenal closure, it is wise to place a duodenal catheter, brought out as a tube duodenostomy. If the anastomosis is not secure, the resulting duodenal fistula will be controlled and can be treated by observation and parenteral nutrition until the fistula tract matures, after which the duodenal tube is removed.[56,57] Severe duodenal injuries require pyloric exclusion procedures in which the gastric contents are diverted through a gastrojejunostomy.[58]

PANCREATIC INJURIES

Injuries to the pancreas usually result from blunt trauma and are caused by impact of the pancreas against the vertebral column. Diagnosis is often difficult because the retroperitoneal

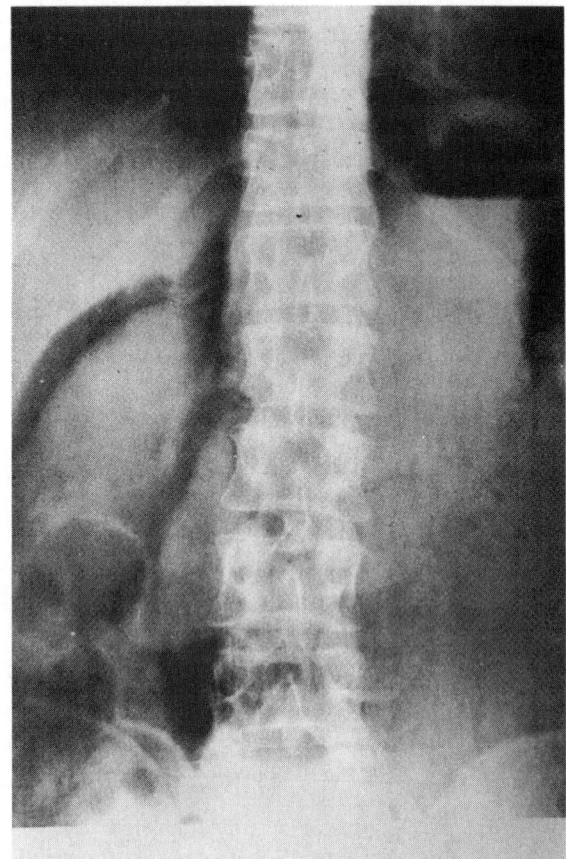

A

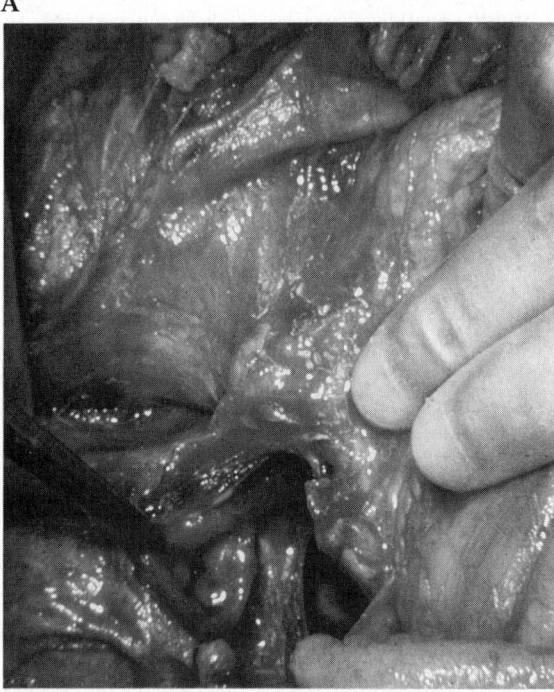

B

FIGURE 95-7 Ruptured duodenum. *A.* Plain radiograph showing retroperitoneal air around the right kidney. *B.* Transected duodenum found at laparotomy on the same patient.

position of this organ prevents early physical signs of peritoneal irritation. Frequently, the diagnosis is made at laparotomy for other associated conditions. However, the diagnosis is suggested by an increase in the serum amylase level. If the diagnosis is suspected and findings on physical examination are minimal, upper gastrointestinal radiographic studies with gastrograffin may demonstrate a widening of the duodenal loop. CT of the abdomen allows assessment of the retroperitoneum and pancreatic area for evidence of retroperitoneal hematomas or even ductal injury. Peritoneal lavage frequently is negative in the presence of severe retroperitoneal pancreatic injuries.

Treatment of these injuries depends largely on whether or not the pancreatic duct has been violated. In simple contusions of the pancreas, drainage of the area is all that is required after mobilization of the pancreas and full inspection to rule out any associated ductal injury. Any devitalized area should be débrided, and bleeding points should be controlled by direct suture ligations combined with cautery.

Ductal injury usually is identified during laparotomy. However, in exceptional circumstances where endoscopic retrograde pancreatography (ERP) is immediately available in an otherwise stable patient, this may allow assessment of ductal integrity prior to the laparotomy.[59] When the duct has been injured, there is often a mixture of pancreatic fluid and blood over the surface of the pancreas, which should be exposed for complete inspection. Although ductal injury involving the body and tail of the pancreas may be treated by transection and anastomosis of the ends of the duct to the small bowel, this injury is treated more appropriately by distal pancreatic resection without an enteroanastomosis. When the head of the pancreas is involved, a roux-en-Y anastomosis of the distal pancreatic segment is advisable.[60] This type of injury usually is a combined pancreaticoduodenal injury and may require a Whipple procedure (pancreaticoduodenectomy). This procedure carries a high mortality and should be conducted only when more conservative measures are unsuccessful.[61,62] An alternative approach to combined pancreaticoduodenal injury is the diverticulization procedure, in which the pylorus is closed internally, and a gastrojejunostomy is constructed with an added option of drainage of the duodenum through a tube duodenostomy after repair of the duodenal injury and wide drainage of the pancreas. The entire area is drained, with drains placed around the peripancreatic and duodenal area and exiting posteriorly.[63] It should be emphasized that pancreaticoduodenal resection should be a last resort because of the high associated mortality. Less aggressive treatment should be instituted initially if possible.[39] Even though this approach is more likely to result in complications such as pancreatic abscess, the overall mortality is still less with drainage than with resection.

Postoperatively, patients with pancreatic injury are at risk for development of complications such as pancreatic abscess and pseudocyst. The former is suggested by a continued septic course with the development of a peripancreatic mass, which is identified by CT. This lesion requires drainage and antibiotic coverage.

The complication of pancreatic pseudocyst results from pancreatic secretions and debris in the lesser sac. Symptoms may be those of a mass effect and may include gastric outlet obstruction with vomiting. The presence of a symptomatic mass in these patients requires decompression of the pseudocyst. However, if the pseudocyst is not symptomatic, it may be observed for up to 6 weeks, at which time, if there are no signs of spontaneous decrease in size, it should be drained. There is much controversy as to whether drainage should be conducted internally or externally. If the external route is chosen, percutaneous drainage may be done under ultrasound or CT guidance. In any event, if this technique is attempted and the catheter is incapable of draining the very thick secretions, internal drainage should be performed via pseudocystgastrostomy or cystenterostomy.[64] Apart from the mass effect of the pseudocyst, these patients require frequent monitoring of the serum amylase level, which often remains elevated during the active phase when the pseudocyst is enlarging. Percutaneous drainage also is unlikely to be effective when the pseudocyst is multiloculated.

INTESTINAL INJURIES

Acceleration-deceleration injuries are most likely to occur at points of fixation of the bowel, e.g., the ligament of Treitz, the ileocecal junction, and the rectosigmoid area. Blowout perforations of the small bowel, however, can occur at any site. Another mechanism for bowel perforation and injury is related to the lap seat belt. The presence of contusion on the abdominal wall from a lap seat belt often makes it difficult to assess the abdomen for signs of peritoneal irritation. In these circumstances, ultrasound or CT examination of the abdomen is quite helpful in determining whether or not there is a seat belt type of related intestinal injury. The presence of peritoneal signs will necessitate laparotomy. A high index of suspicion and aggressive investigation using ultrasound and CT are required to minimize missed small bowel injuries because these injuries occur frequently in the setting of other associated injuries.[65–67]

Treatment of injuries to the small bowel involves débridement of devitalized tissue and control of any associated bleeding points with primary suture. Devitalized areas may require formal resection of segments of bowel; this is usually followed by primary anastomosis with excellent results. The treatment of injuries to the colon depends on the time elapsed between injury and surgery, the degree of contamination, the stability of the patient, and the presence of associated injuries. If there is minimal gross contamination, the operation is being performed within 3 to 4 hours of the injury, and the patient is not in shock, primary anastomosis may be conducted safely. Devitalization of a large portion of the right colon often necessitates resection of the ileum and ascending colon with an ileocolic anastomosis. Left colonic lesions are more likely to be associated with frank fecal spillage. However, if there is very minimal spillage and no evidence of continued hemorrhage or associated injury, even these injuries may be treated by primary closure.[68] Whenever there is doubt, however, the safest technique for treating left-sided colonic injuries is the fashioning of a colostomy together with repair of the laceration and irrigation of the peritoneal cavity. In situations where the lacerated bowel can be exteriorized, the resection may be performed and the ends of the bowel brought out as a proximal defunctioning colostomy and a mucous fistula. This technique is preferable to a defunctioning colostomy and Hartmann's procedure (oversewing of the rectal stump in the pelvis), which is associated with greater difficulty in subsequent reanastomosis of the large bowel.

Injuries to the rectum should be assessed in the operating room and frequently require general anesthesia with a proctosigmoidoscopic (preferably flexible) assessment to determine whether or not the anorectum has been perforated. Because of the propensity for major septic complications, particularly in the multiply injured patient, patients with possible perforating rectal injuries should be treated by a proximal defunctioning colostomy and the fashioning of a mucous fistula through which a catheter can be inserted for performing complete rectal washout.[69] The irrigation of the rectum is conducted with the anus being held dilated. The perirectal space is then drained with appropriately placed drainage tubes. Once the gross fecal contents have been irrigated, the rectal mucosa and major lacerations should be repaired and the sphincter muscles reapproximated with interrupted sutures. This approach in the acute phase prevents retraction of the transected sphincter muscles, which makes later repair and maintenance of continence very difficult. Failure to adhere to the system of drainage, irrigation, and proximal defunctioning colostomy can lead to a protracted septic course with multiorgan failure and death from rectal injuries. A patient with a rectal injury with gross fecal contamination in the perineal area may require reexploration if the he or she continues to run a septic course in the ICU.

As indicated in Chapter 89, the abdomen remains a frequent source of sepsis in surgical patients in the ICU setting. These complications arise primarily after operations on the bowel, so any traumatized patient who has had bowel lesions treated surgically and who remains septic should be considered as having an intraabdominal source for that sepsis. This requires intensive investigation using modalities such as CT scan and ultrasound; drainable lesions may be treated by percutaneous techniques under CT or ultrasound guidance. When such techniques are contraindicated or are likely to be ineffective, or when the source is not obvious despite investigations, laparotomy may be necessary to identify and treat septic complications. With the availability of sophisticated technology in the form of CT and ultrasound investigations, it is usually possible to make a diagnosis prior to laparotomy, and only under very unusual circumstances is the lesion not identified prior to laparotomy.

One of the common areas of sepsis in patients with a perforated bowel is wound infection. Although the incisions in these patients frequently are left packed and open, in some instances the wound is closed primarily. The possibility of suppuration in the wound always should be considered at the first sign of sepsis, and the wound should be opened for diagnosis as well as treatment.[70]

LIVER INJURIES

Although liver injuries may occur from both blunt and penetrating trauma, patients with blunt injury to the liver tend to have a higher morbidity and mortality because of the irregular type of laceration and the involvement of an entire lobe or frequently both lobes of the liver. The signs of liver injuries are very nonspecific, and the diagnosis frequently is made only at laparotomy, the patient presenting with signs of intraabdominal hemorrhage. Liver hemorrhage is sometimes the chief cause of a patient presenting in hemorrhagic shock. Although diagnostic peritoneal lavage for hemorrhage may suggest liver injuries, it is not as specific as CT or ultra-

sound and is indicated in the hemodynamically compromised patient when FAST is not available or the patient cannot be transferred safely to the CT suite. Otherwise, these injuries are very clearly outlined by CT or ultrasound examination of the abdomen. Other signs that suggest the possibility of liver injuries include bruising of the lower chest, particularly on the left side; contusions over the upper abdomen; fractured lower ribs: an elevated hemidiaphragm; and increased size of the liver shadow on plain films of the abdomen. The usual indication for surgery in a patient with liver injury is intraabdominal hemorrhage.[71]

Although reported mortality rates from major liver trauma vary from 20% to 60%, most of the deaths are due to severe associated injuries, particularly of the head and thorax. When death is attributed to the liver injury itself, it is usually secondary to uncontrollable hemorrhage and later in the course is due to sepsis and multiorgan failure. Careful surgical technique and postoperative management of these patients will decrease the morbidity and mortality. The objectives of surgical management of liver injuries are (1) control of hemorrhage, (2) removal of nonviable tissue, and (3) provision of adequate drainage.

Exposure must be adequate, which necessitates a midline upper abdominal incision with the ability to extend into the chest. The liver itself should be mobilized completely by transection of the triangular ligaments, as well as the falciform ligament, with care taken to secure the inferior phrenic artery. The operative strategy should allow exposure of all structures that are likely to be injured or have an impact on management of the injury, including the vena cava and other retroperitoneal structures, and the surgeon must be prepared to perform the Kocher maneuver, right medial visceral rotation (Cattel and Braasch maneuver)[72] and left medial visceral rotation (Mattox maneuver).[73]

CONTROL OF HEMORRHAGE

In most instances, once the peritoneal blood has been aspirated, a nonbleeding hepatic laceration is identified. Such lacerations require drainage and no further surgical exploration. If hepatic bleeding is still active at the time of laparotomy, then the initial maneuver is to pack the liver area very tightly with dry gauze and continue with the remainder of the laparotomy for approximately 15 minutes. This allows time for stabilization of the patient's hemodynamic status, as well as time for replacement of fluid deficits. If, on removal of the pack, the bleeding has stopped, as is frequently the case, then the treatment is drainage of the perihepatic space. Failure to control bleeding by this technique necessitates clamping the portal triad, examining the wounds to determine the source of hemorrhage, and direct suture ligation of the bleeding points. Intermittent release of the clamp will allow examination for hemostasis. Hepatic artery ligation may be of benefit in some patients, although its effectiveness has been questioned.[74] When bleeding arises from the retrohepatic vena cava, as evidenced when clamping of the portal triad fails to control the bleeding, it is necessary to rotate the liver medially and visualize the retrohepatic vena cava. Earlier reports have suggested the use of intracaval shunts to assist in preserving a dry field so that the injured hepatic veins and retrohepatic vena cava may be identified and repaired.[75] However, recent data have shown a very high mortality associated with the use of the intracaval shunts, and aggressive hepatic packing has been an alternative that results in a better outcome.[76,77] In extreme circumstances, complete vascular isolation of the liver by also clamping the suprahepatic and infrahepatic vena cava may be successful, although this maneuver frequently results in cardiac arrest in the already hypovolemic patient. Bleeding from through-and-through penetrating wounds of the liver also can be tamponaded by insertion of inflatable devices directly into the hepatic wound.[78] In some instances, formal resection of liver tissue is required to control hemorrhage, particularly when there is major devitalization of liver tissue. This measure usually does not require formal anatomic lobectomy but instead consists of resectional débridement of the bleeding, devitalized liver tissue as demarcated by the edges of the laceration itself. The bare area of the liver is then treated with suture ligature, cautery, and the application of microfibrillar collagen or other types of topical hemostatic agents. In some instances, the patient may lose several units of blood as well as have other injuries that require attention. In addition, with the massive blood transfusions, the patient may show signs of coagulopathy. In such instances, it is advisable to pack the liver temporarily, close the abdominal wound, and correct the coagulopathy in the ICU with the hope of stabilizing the patient. The patient may then be taken back to the OR in 48 hours for removal of the pack, after which the bleeding will have either ceased or decreased considerably, allowing formal treatment of the bleeding source.[79]

DAMAGE-CONTROL SURGERY

Patients presenting with major liver injury frequently sustain other intraabdominal, thoracic, extremity, and head injuries. Such patients pose a great challenge to the surgeon and anesthetist. Massive blood transfusions with hemodynamic and respiratory compromise are seen in such patients, who become hypothermic, hypocoagulapathic, acidotic, and hypoperfused. These responses are not entirely confined to the patient with major liver injuries but also accompany other injuries to the chest and abdomen. In these circumstances, operative strategy should be directed at temporarily controlling hemorrhage and contamination by the most expeditious means and allowing the patient to return to the ICU setting, where the cardiorespiratory, renal, metabolic, hypocoagulable, and hypothermic states can be monitored and corrected before returning the patient to the OR for more definitive surgical care. In the setting of abdominal injuries, this involves control of hemorrhage by packing and ligation of vessels without attempts at formal repair, as well as ligation and temporary stapling of injured bowel ends with evacuation of intestinal contents by suction, followed by temporary rapid skin closure of the abdomen. Similar damage-control techniques for thoracic injuries, including tractotomy and quick stapling of vascular and bronchial structures, allow the patient to return to the ICU environment for correction of these immediately life-threatening abnormalities before being returned to the OR for formal, definitive surgical repair of the injuries.[79–82]

RESECTION OF DEVITALIZED TISSUE

Formal hepatic lobectomy is seldom necessary for trauma. Resection usually is confined to removal of frankly nonviable tissue. The area for resectional débridement usually is well demarcated by the nature of the liver laceration itself. Manual compression is maintained on the liver while the resection is conducted to control hemorrhage. Intermittent packing and

compression of the liver are required to allow volume resuscitation of the patient during the procedure.

DRAINAGE

The lacerated liver continues to drain bile, blood, and tissue fluid for a considerable period postoperatively. Accumulation of this fluid in the peritoneal cavity is prevented by appropriately functioning peritoneal drains. T-tube drainage of the common bile duct is not required unless there is a central ductal injury requiring surgical repair or unless the common bile duct is enlarged because of previous pathology.

During the postoperative period, these patients frequently run a febrile course, which makes it difficult to determine whether or not there is underlying sepsis. Therefore, antibiotics frequently are administered in the immediate perioperative period. With major hepatic resection, glucose infusions are required to treat hypoglycemia, and hypoalbuminemia needs to be treated temporarily with plasma and albumin infusions until the nutritional status of the patient is improved. Coagulation defects are treated with fresh frozen plasma, vitamin K supplements, and platelets when indicated. Most of these patients also develop some degree of jaundice, which usually is transient but may last from several days to several weeks. Because many of the signs indicated earlier are common in uncomplicated liver injuries, the presence of septic complications may go unnoticed. Frequent radiologic investigation and monitoring of the WBC count are necessary, and baseline estimate of these parameters would allow one to determine whether the patient is progressing satisfactorily or not. A patient whose bilirubin level and WBC count are decreasing but who suddenly shows an increase in serum bilirubin level or has a spike in temperature should be investigated carefully for a source of sepsis in the abdomen. Another complication that may arise in hepatic injury is hemobilia, which may present with upper gastrointestinal hemorrhage, as evidenced by hematemesis or blood-stained nasogastric drainage. This lesion requires immediate investigation in the form of hepatic angiography and CT or ultrasound examination. Once the source of the intrahepatic hemorrhage is identified, hepatic artery embolization or balloon tamponade is a viable option for controlling the hemobilia[83] before formal hepatic resection is considered.

SPLEEN INJURIES

Injuries to the spleen should be suspected in patients who present with left upper quadrant pain, especially in the presence of left lower rib fractures. There may be associated shoulder tip pain on the left side. A frequent mode of presentation, however, is a patient with signs of massive intraperitoneal hemorrhage requiring immediate laparotomy for hemorrhagic shock. In situations where the signs are equivocal, ultrasound examination may be diagnostic. CT of the abdomen in an otherwise stable patient also will identify splenic injury. Most patients who are able to maintain adequate hemodynamics with minimal requirements for blood transfusions, particularly children, can be treated conservatively without the need for laparotomy.[84] Such patients should be monitored very closely in the ICU setting for signs of continued blood loss and requirement for continued fluid infusions. Although imaging techniques have been attempted to identify splenic injury patients that will require surgical intervention, the most important determinant of the need for surgical intervention remains the hemodynamic status of the patient and the requirement for continued fluid infusion.[85] Where the patient's condition allows, angiography can identify bleeding vessels that may be embolized to control bleeding from the traumatized spleen.[86] Currently, nearly all children and 50% to 80% of adults with blunt hepatic or splenic injuries are treated without laparotomy.[87] Whenever there is a suggestion of associated injury or there is an acute splenic injury in an adult who is severely compromised hemodynamically, laparotomy is advised.

At laparotomy, the aim should be to control hemorrhage, with splenic salvage if possible. In order to assess the splenic injury adequately, complete mobilization and delivery of the spleen into the wound are necessary. Superficial supcapsular tears of the spleen may be treated by initial packing for approximately 15 minutes. Failure to control the hemorrhage by this means will necessitate such techniques as the application of microfibrillar collagen or fine sutures. Identifiable bleeding points are coagulated as well as suture ligated, particularly when bleeding points occur near the hilum of the spleen. Ligation of the short gastric vessels in certain instances also will arrest splenic hemorrhage. In some instances, a lacerated portion of the spleen may be excised, with suturing of the remainder of the spleen with large chromic sutures with Teflon pledgets for securing the sutures. When multiple lacerations are evident, it is possible to control the hemorrhage by placing the spleen in a net of Dexon mesh, which can be tightened to produce compression and control of hemorrhage.[88] If control of hemorrhage by a combination of these techniques is impossible, then splenectomy should be conducted. Also, if the patient remains unstable from other major injuries and bleeding from the spleen is a major problem, splenectomy should be conducted most expeditiously to decrease the operating time and improve the patient's chances of survival.

Postsplenectomy patients are very prone to septic complications, particularly from infections associated with the encapsulated pneumococcous, *Haemophilus influenzae,* and *Neisseria meningitidis.* Prior to discharge from the unit, these patients should be vaccinated against these organisms. Patients also should be warned that any infective process is cause for seeking medical attention because of the increased risk of overwhelming sepsis in splenectomized patients.[89] One of the areas of concern in monitoring patients after splenectomy in the ICU is the frequent occurrence of leukocytosis and thrombocytosis. This situation makes monitoring for intraabdominal sepsis difficult, and one has to follow the WBC count until it plateaus. A deviation or a sudden increase from a plateau high WBC count could be considered evidence of occult sepsis. In patients who are in the ICU for prolonged periods with platelet counts above $10^6/\mu L$, consideration should be given to prophylactic anticoagulation to prevent thrombotic complications.

INJURIES TO THE EXTRAHEPATIC BILIARY TRACT

These injuries are relatively infrequent. Common bile duct injuries commonly involve the other structures in the porta hepatis, with frequently associated injury to the liver, duodenum, or other structures in the abdomen. Vascular injuries isolated to the porta hepatis are relatively rare and carry a very high mortality rate. If a porta hepatis injury is suspected,

the Pringle maneuver would allow better identification of the injury with dissection of the structures of this area. Vascular injuries take priority over duct injuries because of the immediate threat to survival posed by massive hemorrhage. If the portal vein is the source of the hemorrhage, then attempts should be made to repair this by lateral venorrhaphy, resection, and anastomosis or interposition grafting. Portal systemic shunting usually results in severe encephalopathy in previously healthy patients with normal hepatic flow and should be avoided if possible. Common hepatic artery injury should be repaired where possible; otherwise, ligation may be performed as a last resort.[90,91]

Common bile duct injuries that involve less than 50% of the circumference of the duct should be treated by débridement and primary closure with a stent (a ureteric stent or T-tube) exiting away from the anastomosis. If more than 50% of the circumference of the bile duct is involved, then there is an over 50% rate of late stricture that diminishes to about 5% if a biliary enteric anastomosis is performed.

Injuries to the gallbladder should be treated by cholecystectomy unless the patient's hemodynamic status is precarious, when a cholecystostomy may be performed as a temporizing measure.[92,93]

RETROPERITONEAL HEMORRHAGE

Frequently, hemorrhage in the retroperitoneal space is identified at laparotomy. This problem can be very difficult to treat, and when possible, preoperative investigation including x-ray of the pelvis, CT scan, or angiography will allow consideration of specific diagnostic possibilities and a more directed surgical approach. When the patient is taken to the OR prior to any of these investigations because of instability, however, a decision needs to be made regarding proper treatment of the retroperitoneal hemorrhage.

Division of the retroperitneum into three zones may be used to guide therapeutic decisions (zone 1, central; zone 2, lateral; zone 3, pelvic). In general, hemorrhage that is associated with a major pelvic fracture and confined to the pelvis or originating in the pelvis should be treated without exploration unless either there is a penetrating injury that is likely to involve the iliac vessels or the hematoma is pulsatile.[94,95] Exploration of such retroperitoneal hematomas usually results in massive uncontrollable hemorrhage when the source is the pelvic fracture. This type of hemorrhage often is best treated by external fixation of the fractured pelvis and blood transfusions. Angiography is required when hemorrhage is continuing with a view to embolizing any identifiable bleeding artery. The mainstay of controlling hemorrhage from pelvic fractures, however, is immediate stabilization of the pelvis to prevent undue motion of the fracture fragments, and this is accomplished most expeditiously by external fixator application.[96]

Apart from hematomas arising from the pelvis, hematomas that are not pulsatile or expanding and that are located in the lateral retroperitoneal spaces (zone 2) also should be left unexplored, and further investigation should be done postoperatively in the form of contrast-enhanced CT scan and angiography as indicated. If the lesion is expanding or pulsatile, the retroperitoneal space has to be explored to identify the bleeding source and control it. Temporary control of an infradiaphragmatic source of hemorrhage can be achieved by thoracotomy and clamping of the supradiaphragmatic aorta.[47] However, when the hematoma or bleeding does not extend to the aortic hiatus, temporary control may be achieved within the abdomen by compressing the aorta at the diaphragmatic crura. This compression can be done by an assistant's hand, an aortic compressor, or a sponge stick. By incising the peritoneum and mobilizing and displacing the esophagus, a clamp also may be applied directly to the aorta to achieve temporary control of intraabdominal hemorrhage.[97]

A retroperitoneal hematoma that is centrally located (zone 1) in the midabdomen represents possible injury to the pancreas and major retroperitoneal vessels. These hematomas require exploration with a view to determining the extent of the injury and, in the case of the pancreas, to determine whether the pancreatic duct has been violated. The lesion is then treated as outlined earlier for pancreatic trauma. Surgical exposure strategies are as outlined previously to allow adequate visualization of retroperitoneal structures as well as vascular control.

Occasionally, retroperitoneal hemorrhage, particularly in the pelvis, cannot be controlled by surgical means, and one has to resort to packing of the retroperitoneal space and closure of the abdomen with a view to exploring the patient within 48 hours, hopefully after cessation of the bleeding. These patients require very close observation in the ICU with correction of any coagulopathy, acidosis, hemodynamic derangement, and hypothermia.[66]

GENITOURINARY INJURIES

Although hematuria is absent in 5% to 10% of patients with genitourinary trauma,[98] it still is a most important sign of genitourinary injury. The patient frequently has sustained blunt or penetrating injury to the flank or diffuse transfer of force to the abdomen. Occasionally, there is a direct penetrating injury into the bladder or kidney. Penetrating injury resulting in ureteric lacerations is very rare, and where possible, these injuries are repaired by débridement, primary repair, and stenting. Although in the past traumatic hematuria of any degree has been investigated with IV pyelography, a more selective approach is more appropriate. This change in approach has resulted from the low yield of IV pyelography in all patients with trauma; also, in the presence of hematuria, the yield in terms of positive lesions identified varies from 15% to 60%.[99] Most of the injuries discovered (65% to 70%) are considered minor, involving a parenchymal laceration or contusion that does not require surgical intervention. Major parenchymal laceration through the corticomedullary junction and often into the collecting system usually causes gross hematuria and represents 10% to 15% of renal injuries.[100] The remainder of renal injuries are associated with a shattered kidney or renal pedicle injury. These considerations, together with the cost of the procedure, as well as the incidence of allergic reaction (5.7%), including anaphylaxis, renal failure, and death (0.0074%), have led to a change in the approach to hematuria in the assessment of genitourinary trauma. In most instances, the major cause of death from genitourinary trauma is the associated injuries, and the investigation using IV pyelography has had very little effect on management or outcome in general.

Microhematuria without shock has not been shown to be associated with lesions requiring surgical intervention, whereas gross hematuria or microhematuria with shock or a major abdominal injury has been associated with lesions requiring surgery in up to 10% of cases.[99,100] Penetrating renal injuries are associated with lesions requiring surgery both with and without hematuria.[100] On the basis of these observations, IV pyelography should not be routine in abdominal trauma.[101] Also, if the patient is having a CT scan of the abdomen for another reason, or if there is only microhematuria without shock or any evidence of severe injury, IV pyelography is not recommended. The IV pyelogram, however, is helpful in the following circumstances: (1) if a CT scan is not being done and there is gross hematuria or microhematuria with shock, (2) if there is hematuria in the presence of a major abdominal injury, or (3) if there is a penetrating injury and the trajectory suggests the possibility of renal injury, even without hematuria. One other relative indication for IV pyelography is if the patient is unstable but hematuria is present; if time allows, a one-shot IV pyelography may be conducted to assess the functioning of both kidneys in the event that nephrectomy may be required during laparotomy.

The main indication for surgical intervention in renal trauma is an injury with major hemorrhage such that the patient's hemodynamic stability cannot be maintained with rapid transfusion of crystalloid and blood. Otherwise, most patients with renal trauma are treated nonoperatively (Fig. 95-8) at first. They should be observed very closely in an ICU setting for any deterioration in hemodynamic status suggesting continued major hemorrhage that requires surgical intervention. If there is failure to visualize both kidneys on IV pyelography, then contrast-enhanced CT or angiography should be conducted to determine the extent of the injury producing nonfunctioning of the kidneys.

The main principle in surgical treatment of kidney injury is to control hemorrhage while preserving kidney function; this is best achieved by exploring the kidney only in selected patients in whom there is an expanding of pulsatile hematoma or signs of urine extravasation. In order to ensure adequate hemorrhage control, the renal vascular pedicle should be isolated first and secured to allow occlusion if this becomes necessary. If after attempts at repair or partial nephrectomy there is still massive bleeding after release of renal pedicle occlusion, then nephrectomy becomes necessary, especially in the unstable patient who is known to have a contralateral normal kidney.

Hematuria also may result from injury to the bladder, and the suspicion of bladder injury should be investigated by cystography, at least three views being taken with the bladder both filled and emptied to determine whether or not there is any extravasation of bladder contents. Retrograde cystography has been reported to be more accurate in diagnosing bladder injuries than the spiral CT.[102] Extraperitoneal bladder rupture may be treated by catheter drainage alone, whereras intraperitoneal bladder rupture usually warrants open laparotomy with débridement and formal repair of the laceration.[103,104]

Although in most multiply injured patients urinary catheterization per urethra is routine for monitoring the urine volume and consistency as a reflection of the hemodynamic status, there are certain contraindications to catheterization per urethra. Blood at the urethral meatus or the presence of scrotal or perineal hematomas with a large, high-riding, boggy prostate may signal injury to the urethra; these findings

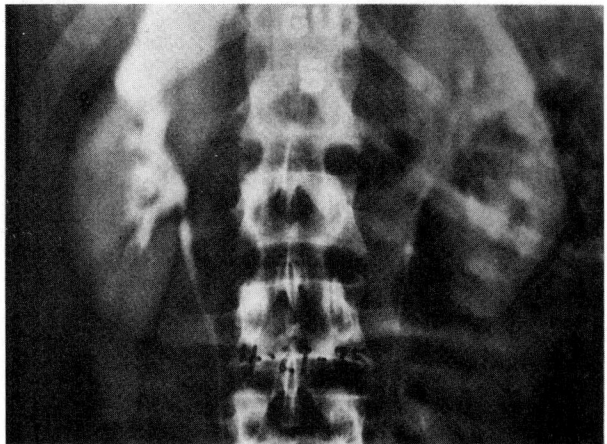

A

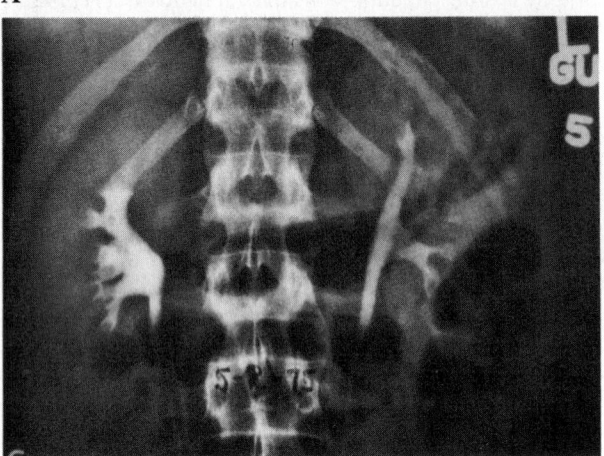

B

FIGURE 95-8 Spontaneous resolution of renal injury. *A.* **Intravenous pyelogram showing extravasation of contrast material immediately after blunt trauma with hematuria.** *B.* **Repeat intravenous pyelogram after 5 days of observation shows no extravasation.**

necessitate a urethrogram to exclude urethral laceration prior to transurethral placement of a Foley catheter. Urethral rupture necessitates urologic consultation and treatment.

Postoperative care of these patients requires maintenance of renal perfusion; thus careful attention to maintenance of hemodynamic stability is important. In addition, maintenance of good urinary output and close monitoring of the degree of hematuria, as well as the volume of urine, are required in the ICU setting. An occult injury to the genitourinary tract with extravasation of urine that is left undiagnosed is another means by which a multiple-trauma patient may develop septic complications in the ICU. This type of complication is diagnosed by ultrasonography or CT and is treated by drainage of the urinoma with or without repair of the source of the urinoma.

TRAUMATIC ABDOMINAL COMPARTMENT SYNDROME

Although the deleterious effects of increased intraabdominal pressure have been identified prior to the twentieth century,[105] improvements in prehospital care and the rapid-

ity with which multiply injured patients are taken to the OR room have led to an increased recognition of the syndrome caused by acute increases in intraabdominal pressure (see Chap. 42) because this syndrome is more likely to occur in the presence of multiple major intraabdominal injuries resulting in severe blood loss, massive fluid requirements, and prolonged surgery. Previously, most of these patients would not survive to reach the operating room. The *traumatic abdominal compartment syndrome* may be defined as the adverse clinical consequences of an acute increase in intraabdominal pressure following trauma. The generally accepted parameters for defining this syndrome include an increase in intraabdominal pressure above 20 cm H_2O, peak airway pressure of greater than 40 cm H_2O, oxygen saturation of less than 90% on 100% oxygen, and oxygen delivery index of less than 600 mL/m^2 per minute, as well as oliguria of less than 0 .5 mL/kg per minute.[106] The condition is diagnosed usually at the end of a surgical procedure when attempts are made to close the abdomen or early in the postoperative period of the massively injured patient, although it may occur in patients with major intraabdominal hemorrhage or retroperitoneal hemorrhage prior to surgical intervention. The source of the increased intraabdominal pressure is usually edema, blood accumulation, or distention of the hollow viscera. Prevention of this syndrome therefore is achieved by minimizing intraabdominal edema through decreasing the period of hypotension, minimizing manipulation of the bowel, limiting the duration of surgical procedures, adequate control of hemorrhage, and appropriate decompression of the gastrointestinal tract.[107]

In the setting of hemodynamically compromised patients requiring massive blood transfusions leading to hypocoagulability states, acidosis, and hypothermia, major definitive surgical procedures should be postponed in order to eliminate factors that predispose to increases in intraabdominal pressure. The concept of damage-control laparotomy is therefore an important consideration in this setting.[79-81]

The increase in intraabdominal pressure affects virtually all systems in the body,[108,109] including a decrease in cardiac output from the decrease in venous return arising from compression of the vena cava, decreased renal perfusion, decreased myocardial perfusion, and increased airway pressure resulting in inability to mechanically ventilate and maintain oxygenation of the patient—all of which are associated with a poor outcome unless the increase in intraabdominal pressure is treated promptly by abdominal decompression. In the OR, apart from the practice of damage-control laparotomy, if on attempting formal closure of the abdomen there is major increase in intraabdominal pressure, as reflected by an extraordinary increase in airway pressures with difficulty in ventilating the patient, the formal closure should be aborted. In these circumstances, the abdominal contents are contained by using temporary devices such as plastic bags sutured to the edges of the skin. In some instances, skin closure without fascia closure may be possible without a major increase in intraabdominal pressure. The patient is returned to the ICU for stabilization, monitoring, and correction of associated abnormalities. With improvement in these parameters and signs of reduction in the intraabdominal pressure, the patient is returned to the OR for further surgical intervention, which may allow either primary closure of the fascia with skin closure or the use of mesh for closing the fascia followed by skin closure or skin grafts later on. Other more elaborate techniques of abdominal wall closure are required in the long term for these patients.[110,111]

Apart from recognition of this entity in the OR, it may develop slowly or abruptly without previous surgery (e.g., the patient with major retroperitoneal hemorrhage from a pelvic fracture) or in the postoperative period during the patient's ICU stay. In a patient in whom this syndrome is likely to develop, close monitoring of airway pressures, hemodynamics, renal perfusion, gas exchange, and intraabdominal pressure is required. A simple means of monitoring intraabdominal pressure is by attaching a three-way stopcock to the side tubing of a Foley catheter after instilling 50 to 100 mL of sterile saline into the bladder through the catheter. On clamping the Foley catheter tubing distal to the three-way stopcock, the stopcock is opened to a manometer that is zeroed at the level of the symphysis pubis.[112]

The mainstay of treatment of patients with this traumatic abdominal compartment syndrome is immediate abdominal decompression, which can be performed in the ICU. Without decompression, mortality is prohibitive and arises from the development of cardiopulmonary failure, renal failure, hepatic failure, and bowel ischemia.

Patients at particularly high risk of developing this entity include those with massive retroperitoneal hematomas from conditions such as pelvic fractures and those with major intraabdominal hemorrhage requiring prolonged operative procedures, the use of massive amounts crystalloids and blood transfusions leading to hypothermia and hypocoagulable states. Treatment should be directed at correction and prevention of these precipitating factors. A high index of suspicion should be maintained in order to predict the onset of this condition so that preventive measures and early diagnosis will result in prompt abdominal decompression.

Acknowledgment

We acknowledge the assistance of Sunnybrook Studios of the Sunnybrook and Women's College Health Science Centre, Toronto, for preparation of the illustrations.

References

1. Moore JB, Moore EE, Thompson JS: Abdominal injuries associated with penetrating trauma in the lower chest. *Am J Surg* 140:724, 1980.

1a. Wanek S, Mayberry JC: Blunt thoracic trauma. *Crit Care Clin* 20:71, 2004.

1b. Todd SR: Critical concepts in abdominal injury. *Crit Care Clin* 20:119, 2004.

2. Jurkovich GJ, Zingarelli W, Wallace J, et al: Penetrating neck trauma: Diagnostic studies in the asymptomatic patient. *J Trauma* 25:819, 1985.

3. Committee on Trauma, American College of Surgeons: *Advanced Trauma Life Support Manual*. Chicago, American College of Surgeons, 2002.

4. Pretre R, Chilcott M: Current concepts: Blunt trauma to the heart and great vessels. *New Engl J Med* 336:626, 1997.

5. Mattox KL: Indications for thoracotomy: Decding to operate. *Surg Clin North Am* 69:47, 1989.

6. Mattox KL: Thoracic injury requiring surgery. *World J Surg* 7:47, 1982.

7. Fowler NO: Physiology of cardiac tamponade and pulsus paradoxus in cardiac tamponade. *Mod Concepts Cardiovasc Dis* 47:109, 1978.

8. Rozycki GS, Feliciano DV, Schmidt JA, et al: The role of surgeon-performed ultrasound in patients with possible cardiac wounds. *Ann Surg* 223:737, 1996.

9. Spodick DH: Acute cardiac tamponade: Pathologic physiology, diagnosis and management. *Prog Cardiovasc Dis* 10:64, 1967.

10. Kilpatrick ZM, Chapman CB: On pericardiocentesis. *Am J Cardiol* 16:722, 1965.

11. Pories WJ, Guadiani VA: Cardiac tamponade. *Surg Clin North Am* 55:573, 1975.

12. Mattox KL, Beal AC Jr, Jordan GL Jr, et al: Cardiorrhaphy in the emergency centre. *J Thorac Cardiovas Surg* 68:886, 1974.

13. Mitchell ME, Muakkassa FF, Poole GV, et al: Surgical approach of choice for penetrating for cardiac wound. *J Trauma* 34:17, 1993.

14. Ali J, Qi W: Effectiveness of chest tube clamping in massive hemothorax. *J Trauma* 38:59, 1995.

15. Mattox KL, Holtzman M, Pickard LR, et al: Clamp/repair: A safe technique for treatment of blunt injury to the descending thoracic aorta. *Ann Thorac Surg* 40:456, 1985.

16. Hunt JP, Baker CC, Lentz CW, et al: Thoracic aorta injuries: Management and outcome of 144 patients. *J Trauma* 40:547, 1996.

17. Wolfe WG, Klainman LA, Sabiston DC Jr: Heparin coated shunts for lesions of the descending thoracic aorta. *Arch Surg* 112:1481, 1977.

18. Demetriades D, Asensio JA, Valmahos G, et al: Complex problems in penetrating neck trauma. *Surg Clin North Am* 76: 661, 1996.

19. Barone JE, Pizzi WF, Nealon TF: Indications for intubation in blunt chest trauma. *J Trauma* 26:334, 1986.

20. Symbas PN: Cardiothoracic trauma. *Curr Probl Surg* 28:747, 1991.

21. King MW, Aitchison JM, Nel JP: Fatal air embolism following penetrating lung trauma: An autopsy study. *J Trauma* 24:753, 1984.

22. Shackford SR, Virgilio RW, Peters RM: Selective use of ventilator therapy in flail chest injury. *J Thorac Cardiovasc Surg* 81:194, 1981.

23. Trinkle JF, Richardson RD, Franz JL, et al: Management of flail chest without mechanical ventilator. *Ann Thorac Surg* 19:355, 1975.

24. Richardson JD, Adams L, Flint LM: Selective management of flail chest and pulmonary contusion. *Ann Surg* 196:481, 1982.

25. Tenzer ML: The spectrum of myocardial contusion: A review. *J Trauma* 25:620, 1985.

26. Biffl WL, Moore FA, Moore EE, et al: Cardiac enzymes are irrelevant in the patient with suspected myocardial contusion. *Am J Surg* 169:523, 1994.

27. Marnocha KE, Maglinte DDT, Woods J: Blunt chest trauma and suspected aortic rupture: Reliability of chest radiograph findings. *Ann Emerg Med* 14:644, 1985.

28. Dyer DS, Moore EE, Mastek MF, et al: Can chest CT be used to exclude aortic injury? *Radiology* 213:195, 1999.

29. Gavant ML, Menke PG, Fabian TC, et al: Blunt traumatic aortic rupture: Detection with helical CT of the chest. *Radiology* 197:125, 1995.

30. Smith MD, Cassidy JM Souther S, et al: Transesophegeal echocardiography in the diagnosis of traumatic rupture of the aorta. *New Engl J Med* 332:356, 1995.

31. Kearney PA, Smith AW, Johnson SB, et al: Use of transesophageal echocardiography in the evaluation of traumatic aortic injury. *J Trauma* 34:696, 1993.

32. Fabian TC, Davis KA, Gavant ML, et al: Prospective study of blunt aortic injury: Helical CT is diagnostic and anti hypertensive therapy reduces rupture. *Ann Surg* 227:606, 1998.

33. Ajalal GM, Mulder DG: Esophageal perforations: The need for an individualized approach. *Arch Surg* 119:1318, 1984.

34. Brasel KJ, Borgstrom DC, Meyer P, Weigelt JA: Predictors of outcome in blunt diaphragm rupture. *J Trauma* 41:484, 1996.

35. Ali J, Qi W: The influence of intermittent positive pressure ventilation on the cardiorespiratory dynamics of diaphragmatic rupture with gastric herniation. *Can J Surg* 36:417, 1993.

36. Ali J, Qi W: The cardiorespiratory effect of increased intraabdominal pressure in diaphragmatic rupture. *J Trauma* 33:233, 1992.

37. Ali J, Qi W: The effect of positive airway pressure and intraabdominal pressure in diaphragmatic rupture. *World J Surg* 16:1120, 1992.

38. Ivatury RR, Simon RJ, Stahl WM: A critical evaluation of laparoscopy in penetrating abdominal trauma. *J Trauma* 34:822, 1993.

39. Rossi P, Mullins D, Thal E: Role of laparoscopy in the evaluation of abdominal trauma. *Am J Surg* 166:707, 1993.

40. Fabian TC, Croce MA, Stewart RM, et al: A prospective analysis of diagnostic laparoscopy in trauma. *Ann Surg* 217:557, 1993.

41. Oreskovich MR, Dellinger EP, Lennard ES, et al: Duration of preventive antibiotics administration for penetrating abdominal trauma. *Arch Surg* 117:200, 1982.

42. McAlvanak MJ, Shaftan GW: Selective conservatism in penetrating abdominal wounds: A continuing re-appraisal. *J Trauma* 18:206, 1978.

43. Oreskovich MR, Carrico CJ: Stab wounds of the anterior abdomen: Analysis of a management plan using local wound exploration and quantitative peritoneal lavage. *Ann Surg* 198:411, 1993.

44. Moore EE, Moore JB, VanDuzer-Moore S: Mandatory laparotomy for gunshot wounds penetrating the abdomen. *Am J Surg* 140:847, 1980.

45. Rozycki GS, Ochsner MG, Schmidt JA, et al: A prospective study of surgeon performed ultrasound as the primary adjuvant modality for injured patient assessment. *J Trauma* 39:492, 1995.

46. Liu M, Lee C, Veng F: Prospective comparision of diagnostic peritoneal lavage, computed tomographic scanning and ultrasonography for the diagnosis of blunt abdominal trauma. *J Trauma* 35:267, 1993.

47. Ledgerwood AM Kazmers M, Lucas CE: The role of thoracic aortic occlusion for massive hemoperitoneum. *J Trauma* 16:610, 1976.

48. Millikan JS, Moore EE: Outcome of resuscitative thoracotomy and descending aortic occlusion performed in the operating room. *J Trauma* 24:387, 1984.

48a. Soffer D, McKenney MG, Cohn S, et al. A prospective evaluation of ultrasonography for the diagnosis of penetrating torso injury. *J Trauma* 56:953, 2004.

49. Ali J, Rozycki GS, Campbell JP, et al: Trauma ultrasound workshop improves physician detection of peritoneal and pericardial fluid. *J Surg Res* 61:275, 1996.

50. Howdieshell TR, Osler RM, Demarest GB: Open versus closed peritoneal lavage with particular attention to time, accuracy and cost. *Am J Emerg Med* 7:367, 1989.

51. Feliciano DV, Bitondo-Dyer CG: Vagaries of the lavage white blood cell count in evaluating abdominal stab wounds. *Am J Surg* 168:680, 1994.

52. Fischer RP, Beverlin BC, Engrav LH: Diagnostic peritoneal lavage: Fourteen years and 2586 patients later. *Am J Surg* 136:701, 1978.

53. Rozycki GS, Shackford S: Ultrasound, what every surgeon should know. *J Trauma* 40:1, 1996.

54. Blaisdell FW, Trunkey DD: *Abdominal Trauma.* New York, Thieme-Stratton, 1982, p 11.

55. Fullen WD, Selle JG, Whitely DH, et al: Intramural duodenal hematoma. *Ann Surg* 179:549, 1974.

56. Shorr RM, Greaney GC, Donovan AJ: Injuries of the duodenum. *Am J Surg* 154:193, 1987.

57. Cogbill TH, Moore EE, Feliciano DV, et al: Conservative management of duodenal trauma: A multicentre perspective. *J Trauma* 30:1469, 1990.

58. Degiannis E, Krawczykowski D, Velmahos GC, et al: Pyloric exclusion in severe penetrating injuries of the duodenum. *World J Surg* 17:751, 1993.

59. Stone A, Sugawa C, Lucas C, et al: The role of endoscopic retrograde pancreatography (ERP) in blunt abdominal trauma. *Am J Surg* 56:715, 1990.

60. Cogbill TH, Moore EE, Kashuk JL: Changing trends in the management of pancreatic trauma. *Ann Surg* 187:555, 1978.

61. Feliciano DV, Martin JD, Cruse PA, et al: Management of combined pancreaticoduodenal injuries. *Ann Surg* 205:673, 1987.

62. Mckone TK, Bursch LR, Schoelten DJ: Pancreaticduodenectomy for trauma: A lifesaving procedure. *Am Surg* 54:361, 1988.

63. Vaughan GD III, Frazier OH, Graham DY, et al: The use of pyloric exclusion in the management of severe duodenal injuries. *Am J Surg* 134:785, 1977.

64. Bradley EL III, Clements JL Jr, Gonzalez AC: The natural history of pancreatic pseudocysts: A unified concept of management. *Am J Surg* 137:135, 1979.

65. Wisner DH, Chun V, Blaisdel FW: Blunt intestinal injury: Key to diagnosis and management. *Arch Surg* 125:1319, 1990.

66. Sherck J, Shatney C, Sensaki K, et al: The accuracy of computer tomography in the diagnosis of blunt small bowel perforation. *Am J Surg* 168:670, 1994.

67. Hackam D, Ali J, Jastaniah S: Effects of other intraabdominal injuries on the diagnosis management and outcome of small bowel trauma. *J Trauma* 49:606, 2000.

68. Stone HH, Fabian TC: Management of perforating colon trauma: Randomisation between primary closure and exteriorization. *Ann Surg* 190:430, 1979.

69. Trunkey DD, Haves RJ, Shires FT: Management of rectal trauma. *J Trauma* 13:411, 1973.

70. Cohn SM, Giannotti G, Ong W, et al: Prospective randomized trial of two wound management strategies for dirty abdominal wound. *Ann Surg* 233:409, 2001.

71. Ali J: Abdominal trauma with special reference to hepatic trauma. *Can J Surg* 21:512, 1978.

72. Cattel RB, Braasch RW: A technique for the exposure of the third and fourth parts of the duodenum. *Surg Gynecol Obstet* 111:379, 1960.

73. Mattox KL, McCollum DB, Jordan GL Jr, et al: Management of upper abdominal vascular trauma. *Am J Surg* 128:183, 1974.

74. Moore FA, Moore EE, Seagraves A: Non-resectional management of major hepatic trauma. *Am J Surg* 150:725, 1985.

75. Schrock TR, Blaisdell FW, Mathewson C Jr: Management of blunt trauma to the liver and hepatic veins. *Arch Surg* 96:698, 1968.

76. Feliciano DV, Mattox KL, Jordan GL Jr: Intra-abdominal packing for control of hepatic hemorrhage: A reappraisal. *J Trauma* 21:285, 1981.

77. Pachter HL, Knudson MM, Esrig B, et al: Status of nonoperative management of blunt hepatic injuries in 1995: A multicenter experience with 404 patients. *J Trauma* 40:31, 1996.

78. Poggetti RS, Moore EE, Moore FA, et al: Balloon tamponade for bilobar transfixing hepatic gunshot wounds. *J Trauma* 33:694, 1992.

79. Shapiro MB, Jenkins DH, Schwab CW, et al: Damage control: Collective review. *J Trauma* 49:969, 2000.

80. Moore EE, Thomas G: Orr Memorial Lecture: Staged laparotomy for the hypothermia acidosis and coagulopathy syndrome. *Am J Surg* 172:405, 1996.

81. Hirshberg A, Wall MJ Jr, Mattox KL: Planned reoperation for trauma: A two-year experience with 124 consecutive patients. *J Trauma* 37:365, 1994.

82. Wall MJ Jr, Hirshberg A, Mattox KL: Pulmonary tractotomy with selective vascular ligation for penetrating injuries to the lung. *Am J Surg* 168:665, 1994.

83. Neilson ML, Mygind T: Selective arterial embolization in trauma hemobilia. *World J Surg* 4:357, 1980.

84. Wesson DE, Filler RM, Ein SH, et al: Ruptured spleen—when to operate? *J Pediatr Surg* 16:324, 1981.

85. Smith JS, Cooney RN, Mucha P: Nonoperative management of the ruptured spleen: A revalidation of criteria. *Surgery* 120:745, 1996.

86. Sclafani SJA, Shaftan GW, Scalea TM, et al: Nonoperative salvage of computed tomography–diagnosed splenic injuries: Utilization of angiography for triage and embolization for hemostasis. *J Trauma* 39:818, 1995.

87. Powell M, Courcoulas A, Gardner M, et al: Management of blunt splenic trauma, significant differences between adults and children. *Surgery* 122:654, 1997.

88. Delany HM, Porreca F, Mitscido S, et al: Splenic capping: An experimental study of new techniques for splenorrhaphy using polyglycolic acid mesh. *Ann Surg* 196:187, 1982.

89. Francke EL, Neu HC: Postsplenectomy infection. *Surg Clin North Am* 61:135, 1981.

90. Busutti RW: Management of blunt and penetrating trauma to the porta hepatis. *Ann Surg* 191:641, 1980.

91. Sheldon GF, Lim RC, Yee ES, et al: Management of injuries to the porta hepatis. *Ann Surg* 202:539, 1985.

92. Ivatury RR, Rohman M, Nallathambi M: The morbidity of injuries of the extrahepatic biliary system. *J Trauma* 25:967, 1985.

93. Soderstrom CA, Naekawa K, Du Priest RW Jr: Gall bladder injuries resulting from blunt abdominal trauma. *Ann Surg* 193:60, 1987.

94. Ryan W, Snder W III, Bell J, et al: Penetrating injuries of the iliac vessels: Early recognition and management. *Am J Surg* 144:642, 1982.

95. Patel KR, Kulkarni S, Semel L, et al: Abdominal vascular trauma. *Contemp Surg* 30:13, 1987.

96. Mucha P Jr, Farnell MB: Analysis of pelvic fracture management. *J Trauma* 24:379, 1984.

97. Veth FJ, Gupta S, Daly V: Technique for occluding the supraceliac aorta through the abdomen. *Surg Gynecol Obstet* 151:427, 1980.

98. Bright TC, White K, Peters PC: Significance of hematuria after trauma. *J Urol* 120:445, 1978.

99. Thomason RB, Julian JS, Mortellar HC, et al: Microscopic hematuria after blunt trauma—is pyelography necessary? *Am Surg* 55:145, 1989.

100. Mee SL, McAninch JW, Robinson AL, et al: Radiographic assessment of renal trauma: A 10-year prospective study of patient selection. *J Urol* 141:1095, 1989.

101. Carlin BF, Resnick MI: Indications and technique for urologic evaluation of the trauma patient with suspected urologic injury. *Semin Urol* 13:9, 1995.

102. Haas CA, Brown SL, Spirnak JP: Limitation of routine spiral computerized tomography in the evaluation of the bladder trauma. *J Urol* 162:51, 1999.

103. Carroll PR, Mc Aninch JW: Major bladder tauma: Mechanism of injury and a unified method of diagnosis and repair. *J Urol* 132:254, 1984.

104. Volpe MA, Pachter EM, Scalea TM, et al: Is there a difference in outcome when treating traumatic intraperitoneal bladder rupture with or without a suprapubic tube? *Clin Urol* 161:1103, 1999.

105. Emerson H: Intraabdominal pressures. *Arch Intern Med* 7:754, 1911.

106. Meldrum DR, Moore EE, Moore FA, et al: Prospective characterization and selective management of the abdominal compartment syndrome. *Am J Surg* 174:667, 1997.

107. Burch JM, Moore EE, Moore FA, et al: The abdominal compartment syndrome. *Surg Clin North Am* 76:833, 1996.

108. Barnes CE, Laine GH, Giam PY, et al: Cardiovascular responses to elevation of intraabdominal hydrostatic pressure. *J Appl Physiol* 248:R208, 1985.

109. Diebel LN, Wilson RF, Dulchavsky SA, et al: Effect of increased intraabdominal pressure on hepatic arterial, portal venous and hepatic microcirculatory blood flow. *J Trauma* 33:279, 1992.

110. Fabian TC, Croce MA, Pritchard FE, et al: Planned ventral hernia: Staged management for abdominal wall defects. *Ann Surg* 219:643, 1994.

111. Wittman DH, Iskander G: Compartment syndrome of the abdominal cavity: State of the art review. *J Intensive Care Med* 15:210, 2001.

112. Kron IL, Harman PK, Stanton PN: The measurement of intraabdominal pressure as a critiria for abdominal reexploration. *Ann Surg* 199:28, 1984.

Chapter 96 ───────────────────
PELVIC RING INJURIES AND EXTREMITY TRAUMA

A. S. L. LIEW

KEY POINTS

- *Hemorrhage from pelvic injuries is underestimated frequently, leading to delayed diagnosis and treatment.*
- *Pelvic ring injuries frequently are associated with other significant injuries resulting in major morbidity and mortality.*
- *Management of pelvic injuries initially requires hemorrhage control and volume resuscitation.*
- *Temporary external fixation is a key element in the initial control of hemorrhage from pelvic fractures.*
- *Extremity fractures, though frequently not life threatening, require accurate diagnosis and appropriate management to prevent significant morbidity.*
- *Complications of extremity injuries, such as compartment syndrome and neurovascular compromise, can best be avoided by a high index of suspicion, careful assessment, and institution of appropriate preventive measures.*
- *Knowledge of the mechanism of injury is crucial in predicting the type and severity of extremity injuries.*

Pelvic Ring Injuries

Patients sustaining major pelvic and extremity trauma frequently are managed in the ICU setting. These patients may present with significant hemodynamic abnormality owing to their associated injuries, and this can be compounded by inadequate resuscitation resulting from underestimation of the volume of blood loss associated with such injuries. The following information is provided to assist the intensivist in understanding extremity and pelvic ring injuries, thus allowing early diagnosis with prompt and appropriate management aimed at preventing major morbidity and mortality.

Significant force is required to sustain an injury to the pelvic ring. In various epidemiologic studies, mortality rates of up to 25% have been reported, depending on the pattern and severity of the pelvic injury.[1,2] While the direct cause of death is usually attributed to a head or thoracic injury,[3] pelvic bleeding significantly contributes to this high rate of mortality. There is an increased risk of mortality in association with open pelvic fractures, a high injury severity score (ISS), or concomitant head, thoracic, abdominal, or neurologic injury.[4]

When the body is subjected to such forces, other injuries are very common. On presentation to the hospital, 15% of patients with pelvic ring injuries are hemodynamically unstable, 66% have a closed head injury, 25% have a thoracic injury, 20% have an abdominal injury, 20% have a urologic injury, and 8% have a lumbosacral injury.[3] A team approach is required to treat trauma victims adequately, including the

trauma team leader, surgical team (general, thoracic, orthopedic, and neurosurgery), and intensivist.

ANATOMY

The pelvis is composed of the two innominate bones (hemipelvis) and the sacrum joined anteriorly by the pubic symphysis and posteriorly by the anterior and posterior sacroiliac ligaments, as well as the interosseous sacroiliac ligaments. Within the pelvic floor, the pelvis is further reinforced by the sacrospinous and sacrotuberous ligaments, as well as the muscles and fascia of the pelvic floor (Fig. 96-1).

Running over the sacral ala and into the pelvis are the common iliac artery and vein, bifurcating to the internal and external iliac vessels above and below the pelvic brim, respectively. These vessels run close to the innominate bones, thus making them vulnerable to injury with any disruption of the pelvic ring. In particular, there is a plexus of veins running along the walls of true pelvis below the pelvic brim that is commonly disrupted by pelvic injuries, contributing to the rapid venous blood loss seen with these injuries (Fig. 96-2).

Arterial injuries are less common, accounting for 20% of pelvic exsanguinating deaths.[5] The arteries most at risk are the internal pudendal, superior gluteal, obturator, and lateral sacral arteries, usually as they exit the pelvis or at a branching or tethering point within the pelvis.

The bladder lies directly behind the pubic symphysis, with the urethra exiting inferiorly, making both these structures vulnerable to injury. Similarly, the sigmoid colon and rectum are vulnerable as they run along the posterior pelvis and through the pelvic floor.

The lumbar and lumbosacral plexi composed of the ventral nerve roots also lie against the posterior pelvis, and the resulting peripheral nerves, particularly the sciatic nerve, can be injured as they exit the pelvis. The sacral nerve roots are particularly vulnerable with injuries that involve a fracture through the sacral foramen.

MECHANISM AND INJURY CLASSIFICATION

The mechanism of injury is an important part of the presenting history in that it can be used to predict what type of pelvic injury has been sustained, as well as the pattern of associated head, thoracic, abdominal, and extremity injuries.[2] For example, in motor vehicle crashes, side impacts are more likely to result in a pelvic ring injury than a frontal impact.[6] Associated injuries that can be expected with a side impact include a closed head injury, cervical spine injury, rib fractures with pneumo- or hemothorax, splenic or liver laceration, lateral compression pelvic injury, and ipsilateral extremity fractures. A fall from a height has a pattern of injury including closed head injury, shearing injuries of the great vessels in the thorax, spinal burst fractures, vertical shear injuries of the pelvis, femoral neck fractures, and other lower extremity fractures.

Several pelvic fracture classifications exist to assist in deciding the appropriate treatment. The Young-Burgess classification stratifies the injury first by mechanism, i.e., anteroposterior compression (APC), lateral compression (LC), vertical shear (VS), and combined, and then subclassifies by severity of injury (Fig. 96-3). Higher grades of injury within each mechanistic subclass usually require operative fixation. The Tile classification stratifies the injury first by resulting stability,

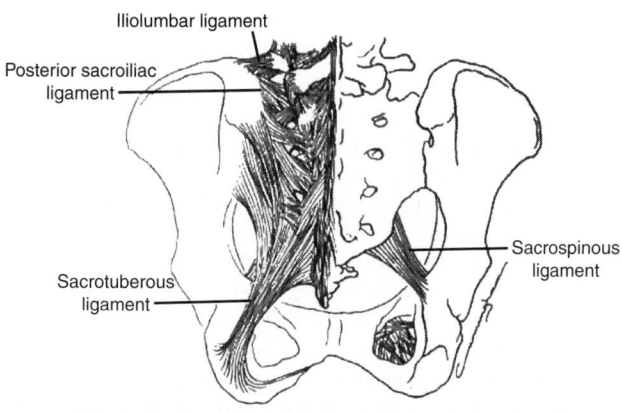

FIGURE 96-1 The bony and ligamentous anatomy of the posterior pelvis. (From Tile M, Hearn T: Biomechanics, in Tile M (ed): *Fractures of the Acetabulum*, 2nd ed. Baltimore, Williams & Wilkins, 1995, p 23.)

i.e. stable (A), rotationally unstable only (B), and vertically and rotationally unstable (C), and then subclassifies by pattern of injury (Table 96-1). Type B and C injuries usually require operative fixation. Both these commonly used classification systems have their merit, in that they communicate information about the pattern of injury, functional stability, and appropriate treatment.

Acetabular fractures are not uncommon in association with pelvic fractures. For the most part, they are also associated with similar visceral injuries as pelvic fractures. The classification system is descriptive in nature and also can be used to predict concomitant injuries; however, this is beyond the scope of this book.

CLINICAL ASSESSMENT

A pelvic ring injury should be suspected if there is any visible swelling, ecchymosis, or compound wounds around the pelvis. Scrotal or labial swelling and ecchymosis, i.e., bleeding from the urethral meatus, vagina, or rectum, are also good clinical signs of pelvic injury. Obvious rotational deformity or shortening of the lower extremities also may be indicative of injury.

The pelvis should then be assessed by manual palpation of tenderness anywhere around the pelvic ring. Next, the clinical stability should be tested by anterior compression of the pelvis at the anterosuperior iliac spines, followed by lateral compression of the iliac wings. Any gross motion that is felt indicates an unstable pelvic ring injury.

The peripheral pulses should be palpated, and a detailed neurologic examination of the lower extremities should be recorded to document the baseline function and to determine whether a peripheral nerve versus nerve root is involved in the injury.

RADIOGRAPHIC ASSESSMENT

The routine anteroposterior (AP) pelvis film obtained during the advanced trauma life support (ATLS) resuscitation is adequate to correctly identify 90% of pelvic ring injuries.[7] Virtually any clinically relevant pelvic instability can be identified. Indicators of instability include greater than 5 mm of displacement of the posterior elements in any plane and greater than 2.5 cm of widening of the pubic symphysis, avulsion fractures of the ischial spines or tuberosities, and avulsion fractures of the L5 transverse process. Additional inlet and outlet radiographs are helpful to assess AP displacement and superior migration of the hemipelvis, respectively.

For sacral fractures and subtle sacroiliac joint disruptions, the CT scan can further delineate fracture displacement.

MANAGEMENT

The most important aspect of management of the patient with a pelvic ring injury is the resuscitation as per the ATLS

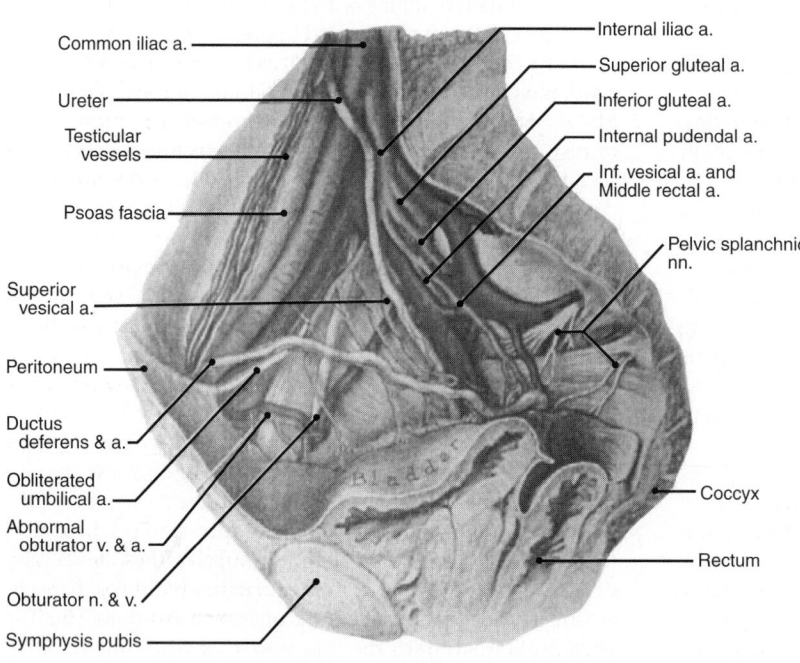

FIGURE 96-2 The vascular anatomy of the pelvis. (From Moore KL: *Clinically Oriented Anatomy*, 2nd ed. Baltimore, Williams & Wilkins, 1985, p351.)

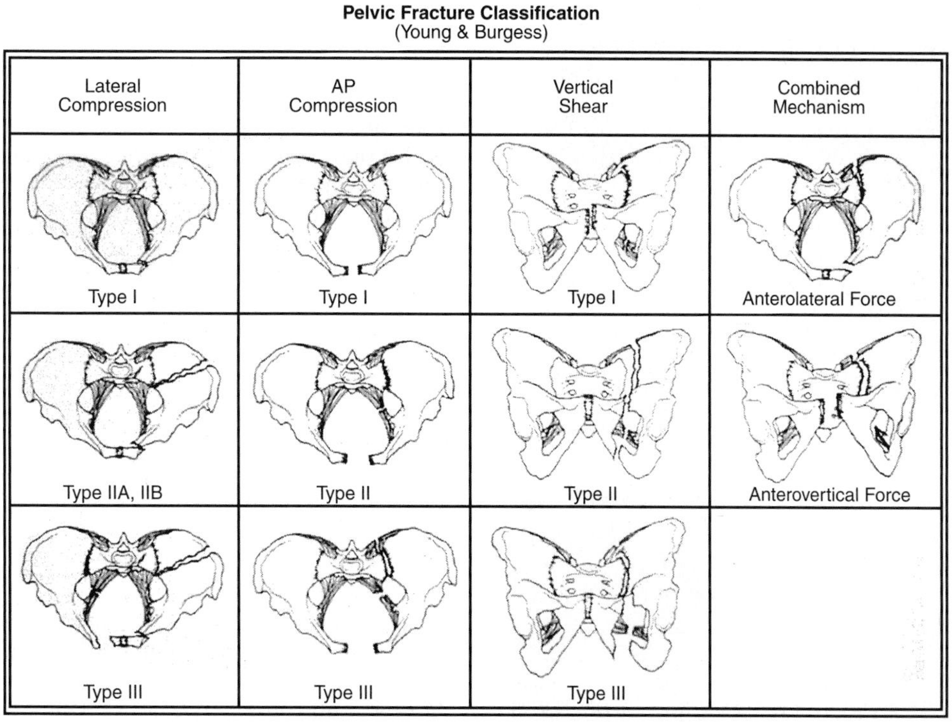

Pelvic Fracture Classification
(Young & Burgess)

Lateral Compression	AP Compression	Vertical Shear	Combined Mechanism
Type I	Type I	Type I	Anterolateral Force
Type IIA, IIB	Type II	Type II	Anterovertical Force
Type III	Type III	Type III	

FIGURE 96-3 Young-Burgess pelvic fracture classification. (From Bosse MJ: The acute management of pelvic ring injuries, in Levine AM (ed): *Orthopaedic Knowldge Update Trauma*, 1st ed. American Academy of Orthopaedic Surgeons, 1996, p 220.)

protocol.[8] During the circulatory assessment, the presence of other thoracic, abdominal, or extremity sources of blood loss should be ruled out. Massive fluid replacement, including transfusions, may be necessary.

Initial stabilization of the pelvis is important to minimize or decrease bleeding from the pelvis and to stabilize intrapelvic vascular clots.[9,10] Historically, military antishock trousers (MAST) were used for this, but they have been found to contribute to decreased ventilatory ability and lower extremity compartment syndrome.[11] Recently, it has been found that simply wrapping and tying a sheet around the pelvis can effectively provide initial provisional stability.[12] A simple two-pin anterior external fixator or the pelvic C-clamp can be applied quickly to the anterior pelvis in the emergency room and provide adequate stability. Caution should be exercised in using the pelvic C-clamp posteriorly because improper pin placement can easily result in visceral, neurologic,

or arterial injury. There is a greater margin of safety if the technique is applied using fluoroscopic assistance.[13,14]

The next priority is the identification and treatment of all significant sources of bleeding. If the patient is responding to the fluid resuscitation and becomes hemodynamically stable, other imaging, such as contrast-enhanced CT scanning, can be used to further delineate other sources of blood loss. Angiography for pelvic bleeding is indicated if there is ongoing unaccountable blood loss after provisional stabilization of the pelvis with an external fixator. It has been shown to be an effective way to rule out and treat arterial sources of hemorrhage in the pelvis.[15,16]

In the face of exsanguinating hemorrhage from venous pelvic bleeding not controllable by obtaining mechanical stability, open packing of the pelvis may be considered as a last resort; however, mortality rates are extremely high.

Provisional stabilization while the patient is being optimized in the ICU includes external fixation for unstable injuries, as well as skeletal traction on the lower extremity if there is associated vertical instability of the pelvis.[17]

Definitive stabilization usually requires internal fixation, provided there are no contraindications to surgery. The ideal time for this is when the patient is stable and systemically optimized. Fixation usually includes SI screws for posterior injuries[18] and open reduction and internal fixation or percutaneous screws for anterior injuries (Fig. 96-4). The use of external fixation and traction for routine injuries treatable with open reduction and internal fixation is not advised[19,20] because this usually compromises mobilization of the patient and increases the risk of associated problems of prolonged bed rest, including pneumonia, venous thromboembolism, and decubitus skin ulceration, as well as an increased mortality rate.

TABLE 96-1 Classification of Pelvic Fractures

Type A—stable
  A1 Avulsion fractures
  A2 Isolated fractures of the iliac wing, undisplaced ring fractures
  A3 Transverse fractures of the sacrum and coccyx

Type B—vertically stable, rotationally unstable
  B1 Open book injury
  B2 Lateral compression injury
  B3 Bilateral partially stable injuries

Type C—vertically and rotationally unstable
  C1 Fracture of the ilium
  C2 Fracture or fracture-dislocation of the sacroiliac joint
  C3 Fracture of the sacrum

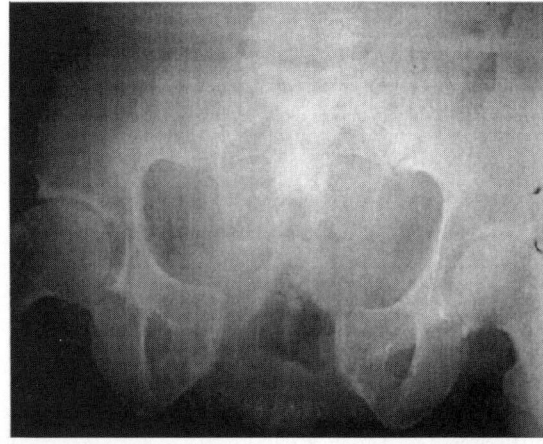

A

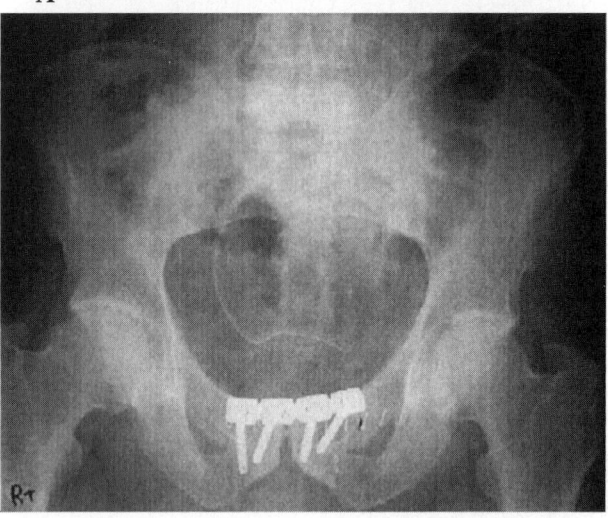

B

FIGURE 96-4 *A.* 46-year old man in motor vehicle accident sustains an APC type II pelvic injury with hemodynamic instability on presentation. *B.* Definitive fixation of the pelvis after provisional reduction and fluid resuscitation.

COMPLICATIONS

Other complications may arise as a direct result of the pelvic ring injury. Massive blood loss and hemodynamic instability as described earlier are the most acute issues to be managed. Injuries to the gastrointestinal and urologic systems, vaginal tears, and skin degloving can cause significant problems if not managed properly in the acute setting.

Laceration of the colon or rectum results in fecal contamination of the peritoneal and retroperitoneal space. If left untreated, this results in abdominal or pelvic sepsis. The clinical diagnosis can be made with the finding of blood per rectum or on rectal examination. Rectal tears also can be palpated in the digital rectal examination and visualized by flexible proctosigmoidoscopy. Treatment consists of provisional external fixation of the pelvis, laparotomy with defunctioning colostomy, wide drainage and irrigation of the perirectal space, and repeated débridements until the pelvis and abdomen are clean. Definitive internal fixation may be considered at this time.

Injuries to the bladder and urethra are also very common, especially with high-grade anteroposterior compression or vertical shear injuries. The physical findings of blood at the urethral meatus and high-riding or mobile prostate with perineal ecchymosis suggest the diagnosis. This is confirmed with a retrograde urethrogram. Intraperitoneal bladder rupture should be repaired, whereas extraperitoneal ruptures may be treated by drainage only. Urethral tears should be stented, if possible, by a catheter. A defunctioning suprapubic catheter followed by delayed repair may be necessary with complete or complicated urethral tears. Once it is ensured that the pelvic contents are sterile, internal fixation of the pelvis may follow.

A laceration of the vagina should be suspected if there is blood in the perineum. This can occur with pelvic ring injuries with greater degree of displacement anteriorly. A bimanual and culposcopic examination to palpate and visualize the tear will confirm this. In general, these lacerations may be débrided and repaired and usually do not require a laparotomy. Timely repair has been seen to decrease the incidence of pelvic abscesses and infection.[21]

The soft tissue envelope around the pelvis is contused frequently; any laceration should be considered a possible open wound communicating with the pelvic ring injury. The Morel-Lavallee lesion is a closed lateral skin degloving injury that occurs most commonly with lateral compression injuries. This is apparent clinically by a large subcutaneous hematoma and lateral pelvic ecchymosis. There is an increased risk of cellulitis, as well as deep wound infection. They should be treated as open wounds, with serial débridements as necessary.[22]

The patient with a pelvic ring injury is at high risk of developing a deep vein thrombosis (DVT) owing to the injury itself, the often-accompanying lower extremity injury, immobilization, and altered coagulation profile secondary to transfusions of blood products. Prophylaxis is required, both mechanically and pharmacologically, in the absence of contraindications. Mechanical methods include intermittent pneumatic compression devices and graduated compression stockings if there are no extremity injuries that prevent the application of these devices. Pharmacologic prophylaxis, such as subcutaneous low-molecular-weight heparin, should be administered routinely, except when contraindicated by active bleeding or intracranial neurologic injury. The presence of a DVT in the lower extremities can be detected by venous duplex ultrasound. Intrapelvic DVTs are best detected by venography or magnetic resonance angiography; ultrasound is not a reliable modality in this situation.[23] There is a very high rate of embolism of intrapelvic clots; therefore, treatment is imperative. If anticoagulation is contraindicated owing to ongoing bleeding or upcoming major surgery, an inferior vena cava filter should be placed.

Extremity Trauma

Extremity trauma is very common, occurring in up to 75% of patients with multisystem and pelvic ring injuries.[1] Established patterns of injury are seen with common mechanisms, such as head-on and side-impact motor vehicle collisions, a pedestrian struck by a vehicle, and falls from a height. The

TABLE 96-2 Gustilo-Anderson Open Fracture Classification

Type I: Low-velocity injuries less than 1 cm long, usually compound from within, with minimal soft-tissue injury or comminution of the fracture.

Type II: Lacerations more than 1 cm long, with minimal to moderate soft-tissue crushing.

Type III: High-velocity injuries with severe crushing and the presence of skin flaps.

    IIIA: No soft tissue loss

    IIIB: Soft-tissue loss with periosteal stripping

    IIIC: Associated vascular injury requiring repair

extremity injuries include injuries to the bones, joints, soft tissues, vascular system, and peripheral nerves.

Head-on motor vehicle collisions often result in a closed head injury, flexion-distraction injuries of the spine, intraabdominal injuries, posterior element acetabular fractures, hip fracture dislocations, bilateral femur and tibia fractures, and posterior knee dislocation with associated popliteal artery injury. Lateral-impact collisions and pedestrian injuries also have their own distinct patterns. Falls from a height frequently result in head injury; thoracic vascular shear injuries; abdominal visceral lacerations; spinal burst fractures; vertical shear injuries of the pelvis; and lower extremity fractures, including femoral neck and shaft fractures; tibial plateau, shaft, and pilon fractures; and calcaneal fractures. Although every patient should be examined thoroughly for all injuries, these patterns help to direct the focus of assessment to the most likely areas of injury.

FRACTURE ASSESSMENT

In general, all fractures need to be assessed for specific findings aside from the underlying fracture or dislocation. Excessive bleeding from fractures or vascular, neurologic, and soft tissue envelope injuries should be assessed, as well as the presence of compartment syndrome and open fractures.

Subtle injuries require palpation of each bone and motion of each joint. Even then, serial examinations several days after the initial injury may be required to detect all injuries. Any suspected areas should be imaged with radiographs in orthogonal planes.

Open fractures are graded by the system of Gustilo and Anderson[24,25] (Table 96-2).

TREATMENT

Although the initial fracture care usually is done in the emergency department, occasionally patients will be admitted to the ICU before any treatment can be initiated. After the initial assessment, any wounds should be flushed with saline and covered with a sterile dressing. Gross limb deformity and joint dislocations should be reduced and splinted and the neurovascular examination repeated. All musculoskeletal injuries should be imaged, and repeat fracture reductions or reductions of dislocations may be performed at this time as necessary. The patient should be prepared for operative intervention if a vascular injury, open fracture, irreducible dislocation, or compartment syndrome is detected.

In the case of open fractures, intravenous antibiotics should be administered, with gram-positive coverage for all compound fractures and with the addition of gram-negative and anaerobic coverage for contaminated wounds. The patient's tetanus status should be determined, and tetanus toxoid and immunoglobulin should be administered as required (Table 96-3).

All compound fractures should be treated with urgent irrigation and débridement within 8 hours, followed by provisional or definitive fixation, depending on the condition of the soft tissue envelope and the amount of wound contamination. Gustilo-Anderson type I, II, and IIIA fractures can be treated with irrigation and débridement and immediate definitive fixation, followed by serial débridements every 48 hours until the wound is clean. Type IIIB injuries usually require provisional external fixation and serial débridements until the wound is clean enough for definitive fixation and soft tissue coverage. For type IIIC injuries, the most pressing concern initially is reestablishment of perfusion to the extremity. After provisional fixation and vascular repair, serial débridements again may be required before definitive fixation can be performed, with soft tissue coverage as necessary. Prophylactic fasciotomies are frequently required to prevent reperfusion compartment syndrome. There is an increased risk of infection and nonunion with increasing grade of injury.

If the patient has not been optimized or there is some other delay postponing definitive treatment, provisional treatment of the fractures by splints, traction, or external fixation may be necessary. In addition, prophylaxis for DVT should be initiated, as discussed earlier. Attention to the skin, especially in dependent areas such as the sacrum, heels, and posterior

TABLE 96-3 Tetanus Immunization Schedule

History of Absorbed Tetanus Toxoid, Number of Doses	Non-Tetanus-Prone Wounds		Tetanus-Prone Wounds	
	Td[a]	TIG[b]	Td	TIG
Unknown or less than three	Yes	No	Yes	No
Three or more[c]	No[d]	No	No[e]	No

[a] Td: Tetanus and diphtheria toxoids absorbed—for adult use. For children under 7 years old, diphtheria and pertussis (dPT) (Td, if pertussis vaccine is contraindicated) is preferred to tetanus toxoid alone. For persons 7 years old and older, Td is preferred to tetanus toxoid alone.

[b] TIG: Tetanus immune globulin—human.

[c] If only three doses of fluid toxoid have been received, a fourth dose of toxoid, preferably an absorbed toxoid, should be given.

[d] Yes, if more than 10 years since last dose.

[e] Yes, if more than 5 years since last dose. (More frequent boosters are not needed and can accentuate side effects.)

scalp, should be maintained, with frequent log-rolling and skin care to avoid the development of decubitus ulcers.

Definitive fixation of most fractures allows greater ease of mobilization for general care and pulmonary toilet. Early mobilization and physical therapy also prevent the development of joint contractures and muscle atrophy, resulting in a faster recovery and reduced morbidity. DVT prophylaxis should be maintained during the postoperative period until the patient is mobilizing well independently.

COMPLICATIONS

Blood loss from fractures alone can be enough to cause hemodynamic instability. Even without a significant arterial laceration, femur fractures can result in blood loss of up to 2 units, tibia fractures 1 unit, and pelvic and acetabular fractures 4 units or more. Aggressive fluid resuscitation must be maintained while reassessing for other causes of hemodynamic instability. With increasing swelling of the extremities from fracture bleeding, there must be a high index of suspicion for compartment syndrome.

VASCULAR INJURY

The vascular status of each limb must be assessed by checking for the presence and quality of peripheral pulses, as well as the perfusion of the tissues distal to the zone of injury. Blunt or nonpenetrating vascular injuries often are associated with traction or avulsion injuries, fractures, and dislocations. It is important to assess the entire peripheral vasculature if there are multiple ipsilateral injuries, such as concomitant femur and tibia fractures. Knee dislocations and tibia fractures have the highest incidence of arterial injury, followed by femur fractures and traction injuries to the shoulder girdle. An abnormal vascular examination may be due to vascular spasm, external compression, intimal tear, or disruption of the artery itself. If the vascular examination is abnormal before or after gross realignment of fractures and reduction of dislocations, further investigation with an ankle-brachial index, angiogram, or magnetic resonance angiography is indicated to determine the nature of the injury. External compression of the artery usually can be relieved by reduction of the fracture or dislocation, and vascular spasm usually resolves after reduction as well.

Penetrating injuries such as gunshot and knife wounds also have a high incidence of vascular injury. All structures in the path of the projectile should be assessed from entry to exit wounds, including a generous surrounding area of collateral damage.

If the limb remains dysvascular, urgent operative intervention is required because muscle necrosis begins after 6 hours of warm ischemic time.[26] The sequence of events for vascular repair usually begins with provisional fracture stabilization with an external fixator or rapid internal fixation followed by the establishment of a provisional shunt to restore perfusion.[27] Definitive vascular repair, ideally with an end-to-end anastamosis or saphenous vein graft, if necessary, then can be performed, followed by definitive fracture fixation.[26] Reperfusion edema and compartment syndrome are common; thus a prophylactic fasciotomy usually is indicated. Wound coverage by skin graft or free flap can be achieved after the wound has undergone serial débridements to minimize the risk of wound infection and sloughing of the graft[28] (Fig. 96-4).

NEUROLOGIC INJURY

If the patient is awake and cooperative, a detailed neurologic examination of each extremity should be done, with particular attention distal to the zone of injury. If the patient cannot participate in the examination, general observations of gross limb movements and reaction to pain stimulus help to establish baseline function. Most peripheral nerve injuries are neuropraxias, which begin to recover spontaneously over 6 to 12 weeks. The progress of recovery can be monitored with serial nerve conduction studies. In the situation of penetrating injuries or dissection for open reduction and internal fixation of fractures, the nerve may be explored to assess for injury. If it is found to be lacerated, direct primary repair is indicated once the wound is clean.[29]

With or without nerve repair, it is important to splint the extremity in a functional position of rest, with occupational and physical therapy involvement to maintain motion of the affected joints. Muscle stimulators also may be beneficial to decrease the rate of atrophy of the affected muscles. If acute repair or grafting has been performed, the extremity should be splinted in a resting position temporarily (1 to 2 weeks) to allow the repair to begin to heal and then gradually mobilized to prevent arthrofibrosis and contractures.

COMPARTMENT SYNDROME

Increased compartment pressures result from intercompartmental edema and bleeding associated with fractures or vascular injury. The increase in pressure causes a compressive occlusion of capillary venules, stopping capillary flow and perfusion of tissues, the most sensitive of which are the muscles and nerves. Because the compressive phenomenon affects the microvasculature, distal pulses usually are maintained during this process.[30]

Clinically, compartment syndrome is manifested by the "five P's". In order of clinical relevance, these are pain out of proportion to the injury,[31] pain with passive stretching of the affected muscles, paresthesia (numbness) involving the nerves within and distal to the compartment, powerlessness (weakness) of the muscles within the compartment, and a pulseless extremity (which may not necessarily ever happen). If left untreated, the muscles and nerves undergo necrosis, resulting in ischemic contractures and loss of sensation or painful paresthesias, leaving the limb with very poor function.

The most common sites affected are the lower leg, in association with tibia fractures, and the forearm, in association with radius and ulna fractures. Compartment syndrome also can occur in the thigh, buttock, upper arm, hand, and foot.[32,33]

Early recognition is mandatory either clinically, as described earlier, or by compartment pressure monitoring. A compartment pressure greater than 30 mm Hg or within 30 mm Hg of the diastolic pressure is diagnostic for compartment syndrome. It may be necessary to rely on pressure monitoring if the patient is obtunded, there are significant distracting injuries, or the clinical examination is unreliable (psychiatric conditions, intoxication, etc).

The initial treatment includes elevation of the limb to the level of the heart and release of all circumferential or compressive dressings. If there has been no improvement within 1 hour, a fasciotomy is required. If in doubt, it is far better to perform a fasciotomy because the consequences of untreated compartment syndrome are extremely debilitating and usually permanent. Owing to the typical amount of swelling with these injuries, the wound usually cannot be closed and requires coverage with a skin graft several days after release.[34]

FAT EMBOLISM SYNDROME

Fat embolism syndrome (FES) encompasses the respiratory, neurologic, and other systemic sequelae of the embolism of fat from the marrow space of long bones. It occurs in up to 2% of isolated long bone fractures and up to 10% of multiply injured patients. The most significant feature of FES is the potentially severe respiratory effects, which may result in adult respiratory distress syndrome (see Chap. 27). It usually occurs within 1 to 3 days following injury, and the clinical presentation includes the following: lethargy, disorientation, and irritability with the appearance of petechiae on the trunk and in the axillary folds, conjunctiva, and fundi in 50% of cases. Blood tests may demonstrate anemia and thrombocytopenia, and examination of the urine may show lipiduria.

The diagnosis of FES can be made on major and minor criteria. The major criteria include respiratory insufficiency, central neurologic impairment, and petechial rash. The minor criteria include tachycardia, fever, retinal fat emboli, lipiduria, anemia, and thrombocytopenia.[35]

Once the patient becomes hypoxemic, supportive measures are all that can be done, including positive end-expiratory pressure (PEEP) and lung-protective ventilation. The most significant treatment aspect of FES is prevention. Early long bone fracture fixation has been shown to be a key factor,[36] particularly with tibia and femur fractures. Aggressively fluid resuscitation and maintaining an adequate circulatory volume also have been shown to be protective. Despite aggressive management, the mortality rate of full-blown FES is up to 15%; thus the importance of early fracture fixation is critical.

References

1. Gokcen EC, Burgess AR, Siegel JH, et al: Pelvic fracture mechanism of injury in vehicular trauma patients. *J Trauma* 36:789, 1994.

2. Whitbeck MG Jr, Awally HJ II, Burgess AR: Innominosacral dissociation: Mechanism of injury as a predictor of resuscitation requirements, morbidity, and mortality. *J Orthop Trauma* 11:82, 1997.

3. Burgess AR, Eastridge BJ, Young JW, et al: Pelvic ring disruptions: Effective classification system and treatment protocols. *J Trauma* 30:848, 1990.

4. McMurty R, Walton D, Dickinson D, et al: Pelvic disruption in the polytraumatized patient: A management protocol. *Clin Orthop* 151:22, 1980.

5. Brown JJ, Greene FL, McMillin RD: Vascular injuries associated with pelvic fractures. *Am Surg* 50:150, 1984.

6. Pattimore D, Thomas P, Dave SH: Torso injury patterns and mechanisms in car crashes: An additional diagnostic tool. *Injury* 23:123, 1992.

7. Young JWR, Burgess AR (eds): *Radiologic Management of Pelvic Ring Fractures: Systematic Radiographic Diagnosis.* Baltimore, Urban & Schwarzenberg, 1987.

8. Mears DC, Rubash HE (eds): *Pelvic and Acetabular Fractures.* Thorofare, NJ, Slack, 1986, p 163.

9. Grimm MR, Vrahas MS, Thomas KA: Pressure-volume characteristics of the intact and disrupted pelvic retroperitoneum. *J Trauma* 44:454, 1998.

10. Ghanayem AJ, Wilber JH, Lieberman JM, Motta AO: The effect of laparotomy and external fixator stabilization on pelvic volume in an unstable pelvic injury. *J Trauma* 38:396, 1995.

11. Templeman D, Lang R, Harms B: Lower-extremity compartment syndromes associated with use of pneumatic antishock garments. *J Trauma* 27:79, 1987.

12. Routt MLC Jr, Falicov A, Woodhouse E, Schildhauer TA: Circumferential pelvic antishock sheeting: A temporary resuscitation aid. *J Orthop Trauma* 16:45, 2002.

13. Heini PF, Witt J, Ganz R: The pelvic C-clamp for the emergency treatment of unstable pelvic ring injuries: A report on clinical experience of 30 cases. *Injury* 27(suppl 1):SA38, 1996.

14. Ganz R, Krushell RJ, Jakob RP, Kuffer J: The antishock pelvic clamp. *Clin Orthop* 267:71, 1991.

15. Velmahos GC, Toutouzas KG, Vassiliu P, et al: A prospective study on the safety and efficacy of angiographic embolization for pelvic and visceral injuries. *J Trauma* 53:303, 2002.

16. Cook RE, Keating JF, Gillespie I: The role of angiography in the management of haemorrhage from major fractures of the pelvis. *J Bone Joint Surg* 84B:178, 2002.

17. Reimer BL, Butterfield SL, Diamond DL, et al: Acute mortality associated with injuries to the pelvic ring: The role of early patient mobilization and external fixation. *J Trauma* 35:671, 1993.

18. Routt ML Jr, Simonian PT, Mills WJ: Iliosacral screw fixation: Early complications of the percutaneous technique. *J Orthop Trauma* 11:584, 1997.

19. Kellam JF: The role of external fixation in pelvic disruptions. *Clin Orthop* 241:66, 1989.

20. Matta JM, Saucedo T: Internal fixation of pelvic ring fractures. *Clin Orthop* 242:83, 1989.

21. Niemi TA, Norton LW: Vaginal injuries in patients with pelvic fractures. *J Trauma* 25:547, 1985.

22. Hak DJ, Olson SA, Matta JM: Diagnosis and management of closed internal degloving injuries associated with pelvic and acetabular fractures: The Morel-Lavallee lesion. *J Trauma* 42:1046, 1997.

23. Montgomery KD, Potter HG, Helfet DL: Magnetic resonance venography to evaluate the deep venous system of the pelvis in patients who have an acetabular fracture. *J Bone Joint Surg* 77A:1639, 1995.

24. Gustilo RB, Anderson JT: Prevention of infection in the treatment of one thousand and twenty-five open fractures of long bone. *J Bone Joint Surg Am* 58:453, 1976.

25. Gustilo RB, Mendoza RM, Williams DN: Problems in the management of type III (severe) open fractures: A new classification of type III open fractures. *J Trauma* 24:742, 1984.

26. Gates JD: The management of combined skeletal and arterial injuries of the lower extremity. *Am J Orthop* 24:76, 1995.

27. Miller HH, Welch CS: Quantitative studies on time factor in arterial injuries. *Ann Surg* 130:428, 1949.

28. Wagner WH, Calkins ER, Weaver FA, et al: Blunt popliteal artery trauma: One hundred consecutive injuries. *J Vasc Surg* 7:736, 1988.

29. Tupper JW, Crick JC, Matteck LR: Fascicular nerve repairs: A comparative study of epineurial and fascicular (perineurial) techniques. *Orthop Clin North Am* 19:57, 1988.

30. Mubarak SJ, Hargens AR, Owen CA, et al: The wick catheter technique for measurement of intramuscular pressure. *J Bone Joint Surg* 58A:1016, 1976.

31. Gulli B, Templeman D: Compartment syndrome of the lower extremity. *Orthop Clin North Am* 25:677, 1994.

32. Halpern AA, Green R, Nichols T, et al: Compartment syndrome of the interosseous muscles. *Clin Orthop* 140:23, 1979.

33. Bonutti PM, Bell GR: Compartment syndrome of the foot. *J Bone Joint Surg* 68A:1449, 1986.

34. Matsen FA, Winquist RA, Krugmire RB: Diagnosis and management of compartmental syndromes. *J Bone Joint Surg* 62A:286, 1980.

35. Gurd AR: Fat embolism: An aid to diagnosis. *J Bone Joint Surg* 52B:732, 1970.

36. Riska EB, Vonbonsdorff H, Hakkinen S, et al: Primary operative fixation of long bone fractures in patients with multiple injuries. *J Trauma* 17:111, 1977.

Chapter 97

ELECTRICAL TRAUMA

LAWRENCE J. GOTTLIEB
RAPHAEL LEE

KEY POINTS

- *Aggressive and prolonged life support maneuvers should be performed as necessary on all electrical injury patients in the first few hours.*

- *All patients are to be considered to have multisystem injuries, including cervical spine fracture, until such injuries are eliminated diagnostically.*

- *Intravenous fluid resuscitation should not be underestimated.*

- *Most patients should be monitored for cardiac dysrhythmias for 24 to 48 hours after injury, particularly if electrocardiographic abnormalities were present or persist.*

- *The preservation of renal function depends largely on adequate volume resuscitation. If urine is visibly discolored by myoglobin, then renal function may depend on supplemental therapies.*

- *The neurologic examination should be monitored carefully for seizure activity, which should be treated if it develops.*

- *Early recognition and decompression of compartment syndromes are critical for maximizing extremity salvage and long-term function.*

- *Adequate wound care necessitates complete débridement of nonviable tissue followed by wound closure as expeditiously as possible.*

Electrical shock is one of the leading causes of work-related injury, comprising 7% of all workplace fatalities. Typical victims of high-voltage electrical injury are young industrial workers or linemen usually between the ages of 20 and 34 years, with 4 to 8 years experience on the job. Immediate death can result from cardiac dysrhythmia, central respiratory arrest, or asphyxia due to tetanic contraction of the muscles of respiration. If victims survive the initial cardiopulmonary or central nervous system (CNS) insult, they then may face potential limb- and life-threatening sequelae from cutaneous injury, internal tissue destruction, and organ system dysfunction. The distribution of the tissues and organs damaged depends on the path of the injury current. Frequently, the injury is complicated by associated blunt trauma when the patient falls from a height or is thrown by the force of the electric current.

When the voltage is less than 1000 V, direct mechanical contact usually is required for electrical contact. For high voltages (>1000 V), arcing usually initiates the electrical contact. Most electrical injuries are due to low-voltage (<1000 V) electrical shock. Whereas low-voltage shocks carry a significant risk of electrocution-induced cardiac arrest, high-voltage shock injury is characterized by extensive tissue damage rather than electrocution. Approximately 3% to 4% of all U.S. hospital burn unit admissions are for electrical injury, mostly a result of high-voltage (>1000 V) shocks.

The duration of contact with the high-voltage power source and the distribution of electric current are important factors in the magnitude of the injury. If the contact is brief (i.e., <0.5 s), cell damage can occur through nonthermal components of electrical injury, called *electroporation*.[1] If the contact is longer, both heating caused by electrical conduction (joule heating) and electroporation play important roles. Prolonged contact can lead to thermal burning of tissues in the current path. The electric current distribution across the tissues between the surface contact points depends on the electrical conductivity of the various tissues and on the variation in electrical field intensity. Usually, current density is greatest at the contact points. Once the current travels away from the contact points into the subcutaneous tissues, the tissues with the least electrical resistance, i.e., muscle, nerve, and blood vessels, will have the largest current densities and will experience the most rapid heating.[2]

Many cells, such as muscle and nerve cells, use electrical signals to control their function. The application of weak electrical fields from a nonphysiologic source can interfere with cell function and, if the field is strong enough, cause direct cell damage. Electricity at frequencies below 1 MHz may produce tissue injury primarily by permeabilizing cell membranes, electroconformational denaturation of cell membrane proteins, and thermal denaturation of tissue proteins. Factors that determine the anatomic pattern, extent of tissue injury, and relative contribution of heat versus direct electrical damage include the amount of current, the anatomic location, and the contact duration. The type of clothing, use of protective gear, and the power capability of the electrical source also contribute to the wide range of clinical manifestations observed in electrical shock victims.

At the commercial frequency of 60 Hz, the threshold for human perception of a current passed hand to hand is approximately 1.0 mA. As the current reaches 16 mA, the muscles in the arm develop involuntary spasms. Within 10 to 100 milliseconds of the onset of the current (the excitation-contraction response time of human skeletal muscles), muscles located in the current path will contract. If the hand is holding the conductor at that time, the strong forearm flexor muscles will contract, causing the victim to grasp the conductor strongly and thus maintaining contact uncontrollably with the current source. This is called the *no-let-go phenomenon*. Alternatively, if the victim is close to but not touching the conductor at the time of current passage, the strong muscle contractions generally propel the person away from the contact. Judging from eyewitness reports, the latter phenomenon may be more common. In addition, a very high-energy electrical arc can produce a strong thermoacoustic blast force leading to significant barotrauma.

When a current of 60 mA or greater traverses the mediastinum, there is enough depolarization of myocardial membranes to cause cardiac arrhythmias, particularly if induced during early myocardial repolarization. When the current amplitude reaches 1500 mA through the upper extremity, skeletal muscle and peripheral nerve cells are damaged by electrical forces, independent of heat. Smaller currents, in the range of 200 to 500 mA, can generate enough joule heating to cause tissue damage if the duration of current passage is sufficient. The rise in serum creatine phosphokinase (CPK) levels that results may be a useful prognostic indicator.[3]

While the spectrum of electrical injury ranges from minor cutaneous trauma to severe multisystem injury, the

TABLE 97-1 Criteria for Admission of Electrically Injured Victims to the ICU

Any the following qualify a patient for admission to an ICU:

1. Thermal injury (arc or flash) to greater than 20% of the body surface area
2. Thermal injury (arc or flash) to hands, feet, face, or perineum
3. Suspicion of inhalation injury or upper airway swelling
4. Evidence or suspicion of direct electrical contact with more than 100 V and more than 200 mA across the body (or at least one limb)
5. History of loss of consciousness
6. Abnormal neurologic examination findings (central or peripheral)
7. Cardiac dysrhythmia (at the scene or in the emergency room)
8. Abnormal electrocardiogram
9. History of cardiopulmonary arrest (at the scene or in the emergency room)
10. Evidence or suspicion of developing increased muscle compartment pressure
11. CPK level greater than 400 units/L
12. Pigments (hemochromogens) in urine
13. History of blunt trauma associated with electrical injury (e.g., a fall or being thrown from a power source)
14. Signs of visceral injury

victims of high-voltage electrical injury are usually the patients who are admitted to a critical care unit (Tables 97-1 and 97-2).

Initial Evaluation

On arrival at a critical care facility, the ABC's of trauma (airway, breathing, and circulation) are assessed, and appropriate therapeutic maneuvers are initiated. Cardiopulmonary resuscitation (CPR) is initiated or continued, as needed, and routine advanced trauma life support (ATLS) procedures and protocols are performed. Life support activities should be continued for a prolonged period because complete functional recovery after lengthy resuscitatory efforts has been well documented.[4] Precise time limits for the continuation of life support have not been elucidated.

After the patient is stabilized, a complete history should be obtained, if possible, and a careful physical examination should be performed. Witnesses and family members often give pertinent information regarding the accident, as well as

TABLE 97-2 Criteria for Transfer Out of the ICU

All the following criteria need to be met for safe transfer at 48 hours:

1. Thermal injury on less than 20% of the body surface area
2. No evidence of inhalation injury or upper airway edema
3. Neurologic stability
4. No cardiac dysrhythmia for 24–48 hours or cardiac rhythm stability documented by serial ECGs
5. Hemodynamic stability for 24–48 hours
6. Normal acid-base balance
7. Compartment syndrome diagnostically excluded or appropriately treated
8. Peak CPK serum level less than 400 units/L in first 48 hours[a]
9. Clearance of urinary pigments (hemochromogens)

[a]See Ahrenholz et al.[3]

significant medical history. On physical examination, particular attention should be paid not only to the sites of electrical contact but also to other areas of significant patient complaint. It is a misnomer to refer to electrical "entry" and "exit" sites. When the electrical source is an alternating current (e.g., a home 60-Hz electrical socket), any point of physical contact will carry the current in and out of the body at 120 times per second. The location of surface contact points, which usually are full-thickness burns, allows the physician to establish the most likely pathway of the current and the region(s) of potential tissue damage. Obvious cutaneous injury is usually only the tip of a large soft tissue injury (iceberg theory). During resuscitation, electrical trauma victims frequently require large volumes of isotonic intravenous fluids, in excess of calculated needs. These large fluid requirements are due to considerable third-space losses secondary to deep or occult tissue damage. Unlike purely thermal burn injuries, resuscitation formulas such as the Parkland formula are not helpful guides to fluid management. Isotonic fluids should be given liberally, with the initial goal of resuscitation being a urine output of between 0.5 and 1 mL/kg per hour. Any electrolyte abnormalities should be quickly corrected. If hemochromogens (such as myoglobin or free hemoglobin) are found in the urine, the rate of fluid administration is increased to achieve a goal of a urine output of 1.5 to 2.0 mL/kg per hour. Mannitol infusion may aid in maintaining high urine flow. The recommended dosage is 12.5 g administered as an intravenous bolus. If hemochromogens persist in the urine after mannitol bolus therapy, then a mannitol infusion should be started at the rate of 12.5 g/h continuously until the urine clears. Careful observation of electrolytes is required when a patient is treated with continuous mannitol infusion. Other therapies include alkalinization of the urine (to pH > 6.5) with bicarbonate to prevent precipitation of urine myoglobin in the renal collecting system. Loop diuretics rarely, if ever, should be used to improve urine output. Reliable large-bore intravenous access is essential, as well as arterial blood pressure monitoring and a urinary catheter. A pulmonary artery catheter is not essential in most patients, but it may be helpful in those with significant left ventricular dysfunction if the volume status cannot be ascertained on clinical grounds.

Victims of electrical trauma should be viewed as potentially having multiple traumatic injuries. A large percentage of high-voltage electrical trauma patients have either fallen from a height or been thrown by the force of the electric current. Cervical spine as well as other orthopedic injuries should be suspected and sought, and therapy should be initiated as appropriate. A falling hematocrit or hemodynamic instability must be investigated thoroughly. Changes found by the mental status examination must be explained. An unstable level of consciousness cannot be attributed to changes secondary to electricity until any systemic hypoperfusion or surgically correctable head trauma has been eliminated. The initial physical examination also should include a careful evaluation and documentation of both the central and peripheral nervous systems. A paralyzed ventilated patient may need electroencephalographic (EEG) monitoring to assess seizure control. The manifestation of neurologic deficits may be delayed, so these evaluations should be repeated daily.

Appropriate tetanus prophylaxis is provided, as delineated by the American College of Surgeons Committee on Trauma guidelines. Antistreptococcal and anticlostridial antibiotics should be administered prophylactically in patients with significant soft tissue injuries. Appropriate evaluation and management of corneal injury and tympanic membrane rupture should be instituted.

CARDIAC

Lethal ventricular dysrhythmias are a major cause of immediate death from electrical injury. If an initial dysrhythmia is corrected and the patient is stabilized hemodynamically, recurrence of a potentially fatal dysrhythmia is unusual unless a cardiac pathology exists. As stated earlier, it is important to remember that electrical injury victims who require CPR because of a dysrhythmia should be given prolonged ACLS because reports of complete functional survival after significant periods of CPR do exist.[4]

Close to 50% of patients exhibit electrocardiographic (ECG) changes or rhythm disturbances after injury. The most common ECG alterations are nonspecific ST-T-wave changes and sinus tachycardia, which usually revert with time. Most dysrhythmias are transient, and therapeutic intervention is rarely needed. The difficulty lies in identifying the existence of new myocardial damage and determining its physiologic significance. Some patients may suffer long-term damage to the conductive system.[4a]

The usual clinical diagnostic criteria for myocardial infarction include ECG changes and elevation of cardiac isoenzyme levels in a setting compatible with myocardial ischemia. These pieces of evidence are not reliable, however, in the circumstance of electrical injury. ECG abnormalities after electrical trauma are common, temporary, and usually physiologically insignificant. The levels of the CPK MB isoenzymes may be elevated owing to large-scale muscle damage and may give a false impression of myocardial damage.[5] Clinical symptomatology of cardiac ischemia, which is subjective at the best of times, usually is not helpful in the face of multisystem electrical trauma. The technetium-99m pyrophosphate scan also has been used to try to identify myocardial damage. However, transmural myocardial damage is rare, and this test does not assess nontransmural injury accurately. Since diagnostic tests are not helpful and significant myocardial injury historically is known to be unlikely, aggressive volume resuscitation and surgical intervention should proceed as required. The exception to this principle is the patient who has been hemodynamically unstable as a result of congestive heart failure, malignant dysrhythmia, or clinically obvious myocardial ischemia.

The evaluation of these patients includes daily ECGs for 3 days following injury, as well as serial cardiac isoenzyme determinations. The results of these tests are interpreted in light of the clinical situation. It has been suggested that not all patients need to have continuous cardiac monitoring after injury unless they have a history of (1) loss of consciousness, (2) recurrent dysrhythmia in the field or emergency room, (3) abnormal ECG on admission, or (4) other injuries that necessitate cardiac monitoring.[6]

RENAL

Renal dysfunction occurs in approximately 10% of patients who suffer high-voltage electrical trauma. The most frequent cause of renal dysfunction, and the most easily treated, is hypovolemia. A common mistake is to grossly underestimate the volume requirements in electrically injured patients. The extent of soft tissue damage and the resulting third-space losses are not always immediately apparent, so fluid resuscitation may be inadequate. Intravascular volume depletion can lead to a decrease in the renal blood flow, which leads to decreasing glomerular filtration rate, renal cortical ischemia, and acute tubular necrosis. Aggressive volume replacement is therapeutic by restoring the circulating plasma volume. The goal for urinary output is 0.5 to 1 mL/kg per hour.

The precipitation of intravascular hemochromogens in the renal tubules is another cause of renal dysfunction. Hemochromogens can be visualized in the urine in approximately 25% of patients with electrical injuries. The responsible pigments are myoglobin, secondary to rhabdomyolysis, and free hemoglobin, from lysed red blood cells. The detrimental effect of pigments deposited in the tubules is thought to increase with hypovolemia, which further underscores the need for adequate fluid resuscitation.

The best prophylactic and therapeutic regimen to prevent renal toxicity secondary to hemochromogen deposition is to maintain adequate intravascular volume and high urine output. This is accomplished with lactated Ringer's solution and mannitol infused hourly in 12.5-g increments. The resulting solute diuresis must be monitored carefully to prevent intravascular volume depletion and electrolyte abnormalities. In the presence of urine pigments, the goal is to create a flow of urine of at least 1 to 2 mL/kg per hour.

Myoglobin is much more soluble and less likely to be retained by the kidney when the urine is alkaline. Some contend that the provision of adequate resuscitation and a solute diuresis will automatically create a urine pH that is clinically therapeutic. However, others recommend maintaining a urinary pH of greater than 6.5 by adding sodium bicarbonate to the intravenous fluids. This treatment is continued until urinary myoglobin has cleared, which may take from 48 to 60 hours. There is evidence that bicarbonate also participates in the solute diuresis; hence its value may be twofold.[8] If the urine does not clear of hemochromogens within 24 hours and the serum levels of CPK isoenzymes continue to rise, then a source of undetected muscle ischemia or myonecrosis should be sought actively. Careful, repeated physical examination, specifically looking for areas of swelling and tenderness, should be performed. Technetium-99m nuclear scanning may be helpful in localizing areas of ischemic muscle, although its lack of specificity may lead to false-positive results.[8a] Xenon 131 scanning and arteriography have both been shown to be generally unhelpful in localizing areas of muscle ischemia or myonecrosis. Magnetic resonance imaging (MRI) provides a reliable method of evaluating edematous muscle. When occult muscle ischemia is discovered, surgical decompression or débridement may or may not lead to functional recovery of that muscle group but may alleviate the systemic problems related to toxic effects of injured or dying muscle.

PULMONARY

There are relatively few pulmonary complications that are characteristic of electrical injury. Acute ventilatory failure secondary to electrical injury is usually related to CNS injury or to chest wall impairment. Depressed respiratory drive due to CNS damage may lead to respiratory failure, necessitating mechanical ventilation. The chest wall and the muscles of respiration may be injured directly, compromising neuromuscular efficiency and leading to the need for ventilatory support.

Long-term pulmonary sequelae such as pneumonia or effusion are treated as in any other injury. There are isolated reports of current-induced bronchopleural fistula, but in most cases the need for ventilatory support is not due to current injury to the pulmonary parenchyma.

When the transient path of the current passes through the pharynx, significant upper airway swelling may develop. All patients at risk should undergo serial examinations of the upper airway by fiberoptic endoscopy and should be intubated prophylactically if hypopharyngeal edema is found.

GASTROINTESTINAL

Abdominal complications following electrical trauma are relatively infrequent. Most often gastric atony and adynamic ileus are seen. These complications usually resolve with nasogastric suction, intravenous fluid administration, nutrition, and time. More serious complications, such as gastrointestinal bleeding, acalculous cholecystitis, and rupture of colon, gall bladder, and other organs, have been reported. It is difficult to know whether all these processes are due to electricity or to the stresses of severe shock and systemic illness. If a contact point on the abdomen has caused a full-thickness burn, the wound should be excised surgically. If this wound includes the posterior fascia of the abdominal wall, then formal exploratory celiotomy should follow. Intraabdominal pathology may be present even without abdominal wall injuries, however. Systemic signs of sepsis or changes on serial physical examination of the abdomen should alert the clinician to intraabdominal pathology. White blood cell counts, liver function tests, amylase and lipase determinations, and examination of the abdomen by ultrasound, computed tomography (CT), MRI, and peritoneal lavage may be required in making the correct diagnosis and directing therapy. Virtually any abdominal catastrophe can be caused by electrical current, and thus the physician must be alert and respond appropriately to subtle clinical changes in abdominal signs and symptoms.[9] If intraabdominal injury is not suspected, then enteral feedings should be instituted within 6 hours of admission, if possible.

NEUROLOGIC

It is possible for any aspect of the human nervous system to be affected by high-voltage trauma. Neurologic deficits may appear in either the central or peripheral nervous system. Evidence of injury may be immediate or delayed. Finally, the duration of neurologic deficit ranges from transient to permanent.[9a]

Neurologic changes often are poorly described and documented when they do occur, and hence evaluation of retrospective data is difficult. Immediate neurologic deficits occur in more than 40% of patients. The most common symptom is loss of consciousness. This occurs in up to 65% of symptomatic patients and usually resolves without permanent sequelae. However, long-term complaints include headache, dizziness, vertigo, and seizure activity, as well as psychosocial behavioral disorders such as impotence and personality changes.

Spinal cord injuries can have acute or delayed presentations. Acute neurologic deficiencies can demonstrate a frighteningly complete motor and sensory loss. Yet acute deficits have a tendency to resolve over hours or days. Delayed spinal cord symptomatology is much more ominous and less likely to resolve. The pathophysiology of these delayed findings is not well understood.[10]

Peripheral nerve injuries account for 5% to 23% of all posttraumatic neurologic sequelae. The most common injury is to the median nerve, followed by the ulnar, radial, and peroneal nerves. In the acutely damaged edematous arm and hand, immediate operative decompression of the carpal tunnel, cubital tunnel, and Guyon's canal is urgent if peripheral neuropathy develops. Following appropriate release, signs of acute peripheral nerve compression should dissipate if thermal injury to the nerve has not occurred.

EXTREMITY AND WOUND

Care of the extremity and the wound caused by electrical trauma will be discussed concurrently. The rationale behind this approach is that the attempted salvage of the extremity, particularly the arm and hand, best demonstrates the principles of maximal tissue preservation with optimal residual function.

After life-threatening emergencies are addressed, attention should be turned to assessing the soft tissue injury. The injury always should be suspected of being more extensive than it initially appears because visible cutaneous injury is only a portion of the total tissue destruction. Compartment syndromes are a common manifestation of the electrically traumatized extremity. Within minutes after injury, tissue edema begins to increase owing to increased vascular permeability and release of intracellular contents into the extracellular space. Pain with passive movement is an early finding. Tense compartments may be recognized by palpation, but compartment pressure should be documented.

Compartment fluid pressures in excess of 30 mm Hg are abnormal and indicate the need for decompressive fasciotomy. Measurement of pressure in smaller compartments such as that of the intrinsic muscles of the hand is notoriously unreliable. Exploration of the fascial compartments of the acutely swollen hand should be performed empirically whenever high-voltage trauma involves the hand and there is a high index of suspicion of compartment syndrome. Fasciotomy of any fascially bound muscle group may salvage an otherwise moribund muscle. Complete release may be facilitated by incising the epimysium of each muscle. All nonviable skin is débrided. Deciding which tissue is irretrievably injured and requires débridement is often a difficult problem. We define healthy muscle as that which is of normal color and contracts with electrocautery stimulation. All noncharred nerves and tendons are preserved, as is marginal muscle when intermixed with healthy muscle.

It is at this point in management that controversy exists. The most widely practiced surgical approach is to reinspect the wound and débride obviously necrotic tissue every 48 hours.[11] Between débridements, one must be careful to avoid tissue drying or desiccation. Typically, allograft is applied to decompressed exposed, viable muscle, and a topical antimicrobial is applied to marginal tissue. Closure is usually delayed until the wound is in bacteriologic balance and is free of all dead or marginal tissue. Whether a finding of additional nonviable tissue at each of the serial débridements represents *progressive necrosis* or *progressive recognition* of fatally damaged tissue remains an unresolved question.

Based on the hypothesis that marginally viable tissue is potentially salvageable if covered acutely with well-vascularized tissue, another more aggressive therapeutic regimen exists for selected patients. After decompression of tense compartments, obviously nonviable muscle and skin is débrided. Exposed, devascularized tendons and nerves, as well as marginal muscle, are covered acutely with well-vascularized tissue. Consideration is given to replacement of injured major arteries and veins with healthy vein grafts before they rupture or thrombose. Owing to the limited availability of suitable local tissue, distant flaps or microvascular free tissue transfers are generally used for coverage.[12]

The decision to salvage an injured extremity must involve careful weighing of the potential morbidity and mortality. A cold, insensate, stiff extremity will be less useful to the patient than a functional prosthesis. This decision of whether to attempt salvage or to amputate should be made as soon as possible, thereby minimizing the risks as well as the physical and psychological efforts invested in salvaging an extremity that eventually will be amputated.

Lightning Injury

Injuries due to lightning are often fatal, and the pathophysiology is relatively complex.[12a] Lightning injury is a powerful manifestation of arc-mediated electrical contact. Arcing occurs when the voltage gradient in air exceeds 2 million V/m. The arc consists of a hot ionized gas of subatomic particles that is highly conductive. Peak lightning currents reach into the range of 30,000 to 50,000 A for a duration of 5 to 10 microseconds. Lightning arc temperatures reach up to 30,000 K, which generates thermoacoustic blast waves commonly called *thunder*. Peak blast pressures reach 4 or 5 atm in the immediate vicinity of a lightning strike and up to 1 or 2 atm 1 m away. Clearly, substantial barotrauma can result. Lightning produces a high transient electrical field and resulting magnetic field. Because of its high-frequency characteristics, the electrical field only penetrates the outer surface of the body, but the huge magnetic field can penetrate throughout. Victims of direct lightning strikes experience a multimodal injury. Superficial burns on the skin represent the current path along the skin surface. The intense brief shock pulse seems to arrest all electrophysiologic processes. The victim appears lifeless. Prolonged CPR may be necessary. Muscle and nerve necrosis is rare in survivors. Deeper injury results when the victim is in contact with a large conducting object such as a truck or fence that has been struck by lightning, which then will discharge over several milliseconds through the victim.

Hundreds of fatalities occur in the United States alone each year as a result of lightning injury.[13] Delay in resuscitation is the most common cause of death. Bystanders usually are afraid to touch the victim while precious minutes pass. However, unless the victim is on an insulating platform, there is no residual electric charge on the body after several milliseconds. When needed, CPR should be given without hesitation. Victims should be cared for in an ICU until life-threatening CNS and cardiac injuries are ruled out. Late neurologic and ophthalmologic sequelae often develop. Treatment of lightning injury should follow the guidelines given for major electrical trauma. In addition to the electrical effects, one may expect tissue injury from the electrothermal-acoustic shock waves that also occur.

Survivors of lightning injury are not likely to be the victims of a direct hit. Rather, they are likely to have been in the vicinity of the hit and to have experienced surface burns and arc effects.

Late Sequelae of Electrical Injury

The late sequelae of electrical injury generally result from the acute loss or damage of tissue. The extent of tissue damage may not be recognized acutely. Neuromuscular problems usually are due to muscle fibrosis and peripheral neuropathies coupled with loss of tissue from débridements and joint stiffness. Sensorimotor neuropathies, paresthesias, dysesthesias, and reflex sympathetic dystrophy may manifest long after the wounds have healed. Severely injured victims may require functional muscle and nerve reconstruction, as well as correction of scar contractures. Cold intolerance may persist for up to 2 to 3 years, and growth disturbances producing skeletal deformities in children are frequent long-term sequelae.

There are also late sequelae of electrical trauma in which the etiology is unknown. Cataracts occur in 1% to 2% of victims even though the current path did not necessarily involve the head and neck. A full spectrum of central neurologic disorders has been described as late sequelae of electric shock. Persistent peripheral neurologic, psychological, and neurocognitive problems often require detailed evaluation and therapeutic intervention. Although unusual, paraplegia and quadriplegia may manifest up to 5 years after the injury.

Rehabilitation into society and gainful employment are the ultimate objectives of the care of these patients. Subtle mental status and personality changes may have a severe effect on the patient's motivation and participation in the rehabilitation program that is crucial to optimal function.[14] Workforce reentry should be guided by consultation with the employer, the patient, coworkers, and an experienced occupation medicine and rehabilitation team.[14a]

References

1. Block TA, Aarsvold JN, MatthewsKL, et al: Non-thermally mediated muscle injury and necrosis in electrical trauma. *J Burn Care Rehabil* 16:581, 1995.
2. Lee RC: Electrical and lightning injuries, in Braunwald et al (eds): *Harrison's Principles of Internal Medicine*, 15th ed. New York, McGraw-Hill, 2001.
3. Ahrenholz DH, Schubert W, Solem LD: Creatine kinase as a prognostic indicator in electrical injury. *Surgery* 104:741, 1988.
4. Taussig HB: Death from lightning and the possibility of living again. *Ann Intern Med* 68:1345, 1968.
4a. Robinson NM, Chamberlain DA: Electrical injury to the heart may cause long-term damage to conducting tissue: A hypothesis and review of the literature. *Int J Cardiol* 53:273, 1996.
5. McBride JW, Labrosse KR, McCoy HG: Is serum creatine-kinase-MB in electrically injured patients predictive of myocardial injury. *JAMA* 255:764, 1986.
6. Purdue GF, Hunt JL: Electrographic monitoring after electrical injury: Necessity or luxury. *J Trauma* 26:2, 1986.

7. Better OS, Stein JH: Early management of shock and prophylaxis of acute renal failure in traumatic rhabdomyolysis. *New Engl J Med* 322:825, 1990.

8. Zagaer RA: Studies of mechanism and protective maneuvers in myoglobinuric acute renal injury. *Lab Invest* 60:619, 1989.

8a. Fleckenstein JL, Chason DP, Bonte FJ, et al: High-voltage electrical injury: Assessment of muscle viability with MR imaging and Tc-99m pyrophosphate scintigraphy. *Radiology* 195:205, 1995.

9. Miller FE, Peterson D, Miller J: Abdominal visceral perforation secondary to electrical injury: Case report and review of the literature. *Burns* 12:505, 1986.

9a. Cooper MA: Emergency care of lightning and electrical injuries. *Semin Neurol* 15:268, 1995.

10. Lee RC, Cravalho EG, Burke JF (eds): *Electrical Trauma: The Pathophysiology, Manifestations, and Clinical Management.* Cambridge, England, Cambridge University Press, 1991.

11. Artz CP: Electrical injury simulating crush injury. *Surg Gynecol Obstet* 125:1316, 1967.

12. Gottlieb LJ, Saunders J, Krizek TJ: Surgical technique for salvage of electrically damaged tissue, in Lee RC, Cravalho EG, Burke JF (eds): *Electrical Trauma: Pathophysiology.* Cambridge, Emgland, Cambridge University Press, 1990.

12a. O'Keefe Gatewood M, Zane RD: Lightning injuries. *Emerg Med Clin North Am* 22:369, 2004.

13. Monafo WW, Freedman BM: Electrical and lightning injury, in Boswick JA Jr (ed): *The Art and Science of Burn Care.* New York, Aspen Publications, 1987.

14. Rosenberg DB, Nelson M: Rehabilitation concern in electrical burn patients: A review of the literature. *J Trauma* 28:808, 1988.

14a. Cochran A, Edelman LS, Saffle JR, et al: Self-reported quality of life after electrical and thermal injury. *J Burn Care Rehabil* 25:61, 2004.

Chapter 98 _____

BURNS: RESUSCITATION PHASE (0 TO 36 HOURS)

ROBERT H. DEMLING
LESLIE DESANTI

KEY POINTS

- *A burn patient is a trauma patient; therefore, other injuries should be expected and sought.*

- *Endotracheal tubes should be large enough to allow ventilation and pulmonary toilet.*

- *Hypothermia is a major concern, and early, aggressive attempts at prevention are required.*

- *Modification of the standard lactated Ringer's resuscitation is often necessary in the massive burn or inhalation injury patient or in the very young and old. Additions of colloid, blood, and inotropes are often very useful in restoring hemodynamic stability. Fluid formulas should not be rigid.*

- *It is important to watch for local perfusion problems and chest wall restriction caused by the burn.*

- *The burn itself is a low priority for initial care.*

Care of the burn patient has improved dramatically over the past 10 to 15 years, resulting in a marked decrease in mortality and morbidity, as well as improved functional outcome. The major reason for this improvement is the multidisciplinary approach by a team that has the clinical decision-making skills, experience, and scientific background to render care in a manner that avoids the predictable pitfalls while also maintaining critical care monitoring. A burn center is the best environment to provide this care.

The burn patient's condition changes dramatically over the course of the injury. The initial postburn period is character-ized by cardiopulmonary instability caused by fluid shifts and direct smoke injury to the airways. With the onset of in-tense wound inflammation, immunosuppression, and infec-tion, physiologic and metabolic parameters change substan-tially from those seen initially. Treatment therefore must be based on a clear understanding of these changes over time.[1,2] This discussion thus will be divided into three time periods—the initial resuscitation period (0 to 36 hours; this chapter), the early postresuscitation period (2 to 6 days; Chap. 99), and the inflammation-infection period, which is usually most evident after the first week (Chap. 100).

Monitoring requirements are no different from those for any other ICU patient. However, vascular access is much more of a problem, and noninvasive measures are often all that are available. A typical burn unit has a procedure room for wound care and often an operating room, but wound care in the ICU is very feasible and actually essential in the unsta-ble patient. Hyperbaric oxygen chambers are not a necessary component and are really only indicated in patients with such severe carbon monoxide exposure that the cytochrome sys-tem is saturated with carbon monoxide, which is not read-ily displaced with 100% oxygen alone (see Chap. 102). It is safe to say that 99% of patients with major burns and some degree of carbon monoxide inhalation do not benefit from hyperbaric oxygen. The secret to a successful patient out-come, however, remains in the knowledge base, judgment, and decision-making skills of the personnel, not in the exter-nal environment.[1,2]

Cardiopulmonary instability characterizes the resuscita-tion phase. Life-threatening airway and breathing problems are major concerns at this time, with carbon monoxide poison-ing, upper airway edema, and the immediate effect of smoke inhalation injury being the most common. The initial phase is also characterized by hypovolemia because plasma volume is lost into the burn tissue. The burn itself is of less immediate concern, with initial treatment of pulmonary and circulatory abnormalities taking first priority. Any early management er-ror will lead to a dramatic increase in morbidity and mortality during the subsequent injury phases. It is of critical impor-tance to remember that the burn patient is a trauma patient with the potential for many other injuries. The standard ap-proach to trauma resuscitation therefore must be followed, including assessment for cervical spine and head injuries, pulmonary and abdominal trauma, fractures, and so on.[2a] Management of these problems is the same as in the nonburn patient.

Airway and Pulmonary Abnormalities

Abnormalities of ventilation and oxygenation are common in the immediate postburn period.[2b] Several fairly distinct critical disease processes must be recognized and managed aggressively.[3] The first three are associated with the inhala-tion injury complex and are presented below in the approxi-mate order in which symptoms will develop (carbon monox-ide toxicity, upper airway obstruction, and chemical burn to the lung). These sections are followed by discussions of lung changes due to the skin burn and, finally, of the effects of impaired chest wall compliance.

SMOKE INHALATION INJURY COMPLEX

Pulmonary insufficiency caused by the inhalation of heat and smoke is the major cause of mortality among fire victims, ac-counting for over 50% of fire-related deaths.[4,5] The exposure time, concentration of fumes, elements released, and degree of accompanying body burn are critical variables in determin-ing outcome.

CARBON MONOXIDE AND CYANIDE TOXICITY
Carbon monoxide, a by-product of incomplete combustion, is one of the leading causes of death in fires. Hydrogen cyanide is also a well-recognized cause of morbidity and mortality, especially with burning of synthetics such as polyurethane.

Symptoms of carbon monoxide toxicity usually are not present until the carboxyhemoglobin concentration exceeds 15%. Symptoms are those of decreased tissue oxygenation, with the initial manifestations being neurologic. Cyanide tox-icity presents in a very similar fashion, with severe metabolic acidosis and obtundation. Diagnosis, however, is more dif-ficult because measurement of cyanide levels is not always readily available or very reliable. Normal levels are less than

0.1 mg/L (even in smokers). A level near 1 mg/L is lethal. Neurologic dysfunction also can be caused by factors other than carbon monoxide toxicity, such as alcohol or drug intoxication or blunt head trauma. A toxicology screen therefore is warranted. The indications for obtaining a computed tomographic (CT) scan of the head are the same as for other trauma patients.

The persistence of a metabolic acidosis in a patient with adequate volume resuscitation and cardiac output suggests that oxygen transport and use are being impaired by carbon monoxide or cyanide. Pa_{O_2} can remain relatively normal because the chemical alteration of hemoglobin by carbon monoxide will not affect the amount of oxygen dissolved in arterial plasma. A high carboxyhemoglobin level also indicates a significant smoke exposure and, therefore, a chemical burn to the airways. Treatment of carbon monoxide toxicity is covered more fully elsewhere in this text; briefly, it consists of the early displacement of carbon monoxide from hemoglobin by administration of 90% to 100% oxygen (see Chap. 102). Treatment of cyanide toxicity involves restoration of hepatic blood flow to clear the cyanide. In addition, sodium nitrite is given, followed by sodium thiosulfate. Hyperbaric oxygen is best used in patients who show severe neurologic compromise with a high carboxyhemoglobin level (>50%) but no major burns and who are not responding to high-flow oxygen. The vast majority of patients can be managed successfully using simply 90% to 100% oxygen.

UPPER AIRWAY OBSTRUCTION FROM AIRWAY EDEMA
Heat produces an immediate injury to the airway mucosa, resulting in edema, erythema, and ulceration. Although these mucosal changes may be present anatomically shortly after the burn, physiologic alterations will not be present until the edema is sufficient to produce clinical evidence of impaired upper airway patency. This may not occur for 12 to 18 hours. The presence of a body burn magnifies the effects of airway injury in direct proportion to the size and depth of the skin burn. The massive amount of fluid administered is in part responsible. A face or neck burn will accentuate these problems by producing marked anatomic distortion and, in the case of a deep neck burn, external compression of the larynx. The airway edema and the external burn edema have a parallel time course so that by the time symptoms of airway edema develop, external and internal anatomic distortion is extensive. The local edema usually resolves in 4 to 5 days.

Inspection of the oropharynx for soot or evidence of a heat injury should be routine in every burn victim. Numerous techniques have been used in further assessing the degree of injury and in determining the need for endotracheal intubation. Fiberoptic bronchoscopy or laryngoscopy will show whether physical evidence of pharyngeal or laryngeal mucosal injury is present. Laryngoscopy will demonstrate the presence of mucosal irritation at and above the cords and provide information about the need for endotracheal intubation.[4,5] Unfortunately, unless serial studies are performed, none of these tests can predict the severity of subsequent airway compromise accurately because the edema progresses during the first 18 to 24 hours. Repeated examinations for airway compromise are feasible in patients without facial burns. However, in the presence of a large burn, it is best to proceed with intubation if there is any concern.

An early decision regarding the need for airway intubation is crucial. When there is doubt, it is safer to intubate. A patient with a significant inhalation injury and deep facial burns usually should be managed by early endotracheal intubation. There are many other indications for intubation in burn patients besides airway edema, such as hemodynamic instability and impaired consciousness. A large orotracheal tube (at least 7 mm in internal diameter) should be used in adults because very thick secretions develop. If the initial tube is too small, it will be dangerous to change once massive facial

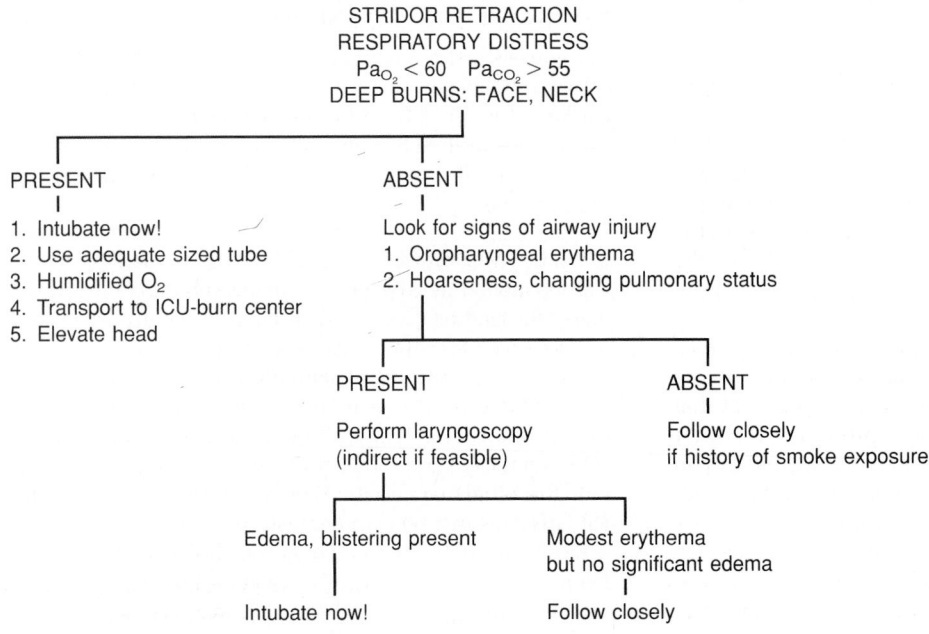

FIGURE 98-1 Initial assessment of airway (for the decision of whether or not to intubate).

TABLE 98-1 Toxic Elements in Housefire Smoke

Gas	Source	Effects
Carbon monoxide	Any organic matter	Tissue hypoxia
Nitrogen dioxide	Wallpaper, wood	Bronchial irritation, dizziness, pulmonary edema
Hydrogen chloride (from phosgene)	Plastics (polyvinyl chloride)	Severe mucosal irritation
Hydrogen cyanide	Wool, silk, nylons (polyurethane)	Headache, respiratory failure, coma
Benzene	Petroleum plastics	Mucosal irritation, coma
Aldehydes	Wood, cotton, paper	Severe mucosal damage, extensive lung damage
Ammonia	Nylon	Mucosal irritation

and airway edema develops. An algorithm for this approach is presented in Fig. 98-1.

CHEMICAL BURNS OF THE UPPER AND LOWER AIRWAYS

Toxic gases contained in smoke, as well as carbon particles coated with irritating aldehydes and organic acids, can injure both upper and lower airways (Table 98-1). The location of injury will depend on the duration of exposure, the size of the particles, and the solubility of the gases.

Breath holding and laryngospasm are protective mechanisms against excessive exposure in the conscious patient. The unconscious patient, however, loses this protection and sustains more severe injury to the lower airways. Information regarding loss of consciousness at the scene should be sought in the history.

Symptoms may well be absent on admission, with the true magnitude of injury becoming evident only after 24 to 48 hours. Early symptoms usually consist of wheezing and bronchorrhea. This intense initial bronchorrhea caused by irritation of the airway mucosa in combination with increased oral and nasal secretions can give the false appearance of fulminant pulmonary edema. Soot in the lung secretions is certain evidence of smoke exposure but is not always present.

Early bronchospasm and bronchiolar edema initiated by the irritant gases cause a marked decrease in dynamic lung compliance with increased work of breathing. Impaired clearance of secretions will accentuate this problem.

Impairment of gas exchange is due to ventilation/perfusion ($\dot{V}/\dot{Q}$) mismatching related to airway injury rather than to alveolar edema.[6-8] A body burn markedly potentiates the inhalation-induced lung dysfunction caused by chemical injury. The combination of a major burn and smoke inhalation is more lethal than either injury alone.

Initial treatment of this component consists of an aggressive approach to upper airway maintenance and pulmonary support that includes maintenance of small-airways patency and removal of soot and mucopurulent secretions. Careful, well-monitored fluid resuscitation is necessary to avoid accentuation of the process. The addition of positive end-expiratory pressure (PEEP) frequently is necessary to maintain small-airways patency and an adequate functional residual capacity (FRC), assisting in holding the edematous airway open until edema resolves. Endotracheal in-

tubation and PEEP have been reported to decrease the rate of early pulmonary death after severe burns and smoke inhalation.[9]

Beginning about 18 to 24 hours after a burn, increasing airway resistance is often due to bronchiolar edema and airway plugging rather than to bronchospasm. The associated impairment of gas exchange often responds to further increases in PEEP in addition to bronchodilator administration. The injured airway mucosa frequently becomes colonized with bacteria. Prophylactic antibiotic administration only selects for resistant organisms and therefore is not indicated. Corticosteroids increase morbidity and mortality in the presence of a body burn and are, therefore, contraindicated.[10]

IMPAIRED CHEST WALL COMPLIANCE

Respiratory excursion can be impaired markedly by a burn to the chest wall, especially a circumferential third-degree burn.[11,12] The loss of chest wall compliance increases the work of breathing. Symptoms may not be evident until edema formation peaks. The first clinical evidence of chest wall restriction is often labored breathing, followed by rapid respiratory deterioration, particularly in the patient who is not receiving ventilatory support. Clearance of secretions can be impaired owing to the inability to generate enough hyperinflation to cough well.

Treatment involves surgical decompression or escharotomy of the chest wall. Longitudinal incisions placed in the midaxillary lines should be connected across the lower chest wall. Bleeding usually is controlled easily if the incisions stay within the margins of the third-degree burn because the dermal vessels are thrombosed. The incision must extend into the subeschar area to allow adequate chest wall expansion. Escharotomies usually are not required in a second-degree burn unless the edema is so massive that the burned skin is tight. (This approach is diagrammed in Fig. 98-2.)

Restoration and Maintenance of Hemodynamic Stability

Massive fluid shifts occur during the resuscitation phase of burn injuries and can lead to severe impairment in oxygen

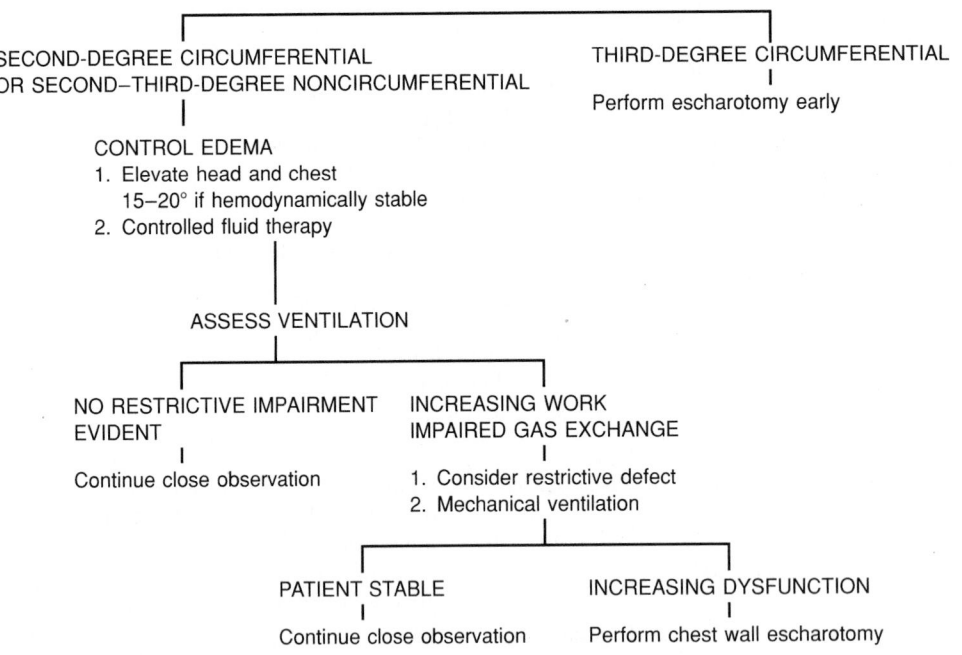

FIGURE 98-2 Treatment of chest wall burn.

delivery to tissues. An understanding of these early fluid shifts is necessary to avoid hemodynamic instability and to initiate appropriate treatment.

PATHOPHYSIOLOGY OF BURN SHOCK

With a major burn, intravascular volume is lost into burned tissue as well as nonburned tissue. Increased vascular permeability, the increased osmotic forces in burned tissue, and cellular swelling contribute.[14] The most pronounced shift occurs in the first several hours as a result of the increased protein permeability and the apparent increase in burn tissue osmotic pressure.[15] The fluid and protein shifts are the greatest in the first several hours because of the combined effect of increased permeability and an imbalance of osmotic forces. Subsequently, the quantity of edema depends on the adequacy of the fluid resuscitation. Severe hypoproteinemia also occurs as a result of the loss of protein into the wound. The major protein losses occur in the first 6 to 8 hours, during the period of peak fluid loss. Plasma proteins can decrease to less than 50% of normal. Resolution of edema depends on restoration of lymphatic pa-

tency, which may take a number of days to weeks. Edema in deeper burns resolves more slowly than in superficial burns.

Generalized tissue edema in nonburned tissues is evident in patients with burns covering more than 30% of the total body surface area (TBS). The edema appears to be due, at least in part, to the low protein content.[16]

Cardiac output is depressed initially, primarily as a result of hypovolemia. Afterload is also increased owing to a marked increase in systemic vascular resistance (SVR) elicited by vasoactive mediators such as catecholamines. A decrease in cardiac contractility[17] is most evident in third-degree burns covering more than 40% of the TBS and is probably due to myocardial edema rather than to a circulating factor. All these contributors to impaired perfusion are summarized in Fig. 98-3.

MANAGEMENT OF THE CIRCULATION

INTRAVENOUS ACCESS

A peripheral vein catheter through nonburned tissue is the preferred route for fluid administration. A central line or

FIGURE 98-3 Causes of decreased oxygen delivery to tissues after a burn injury.

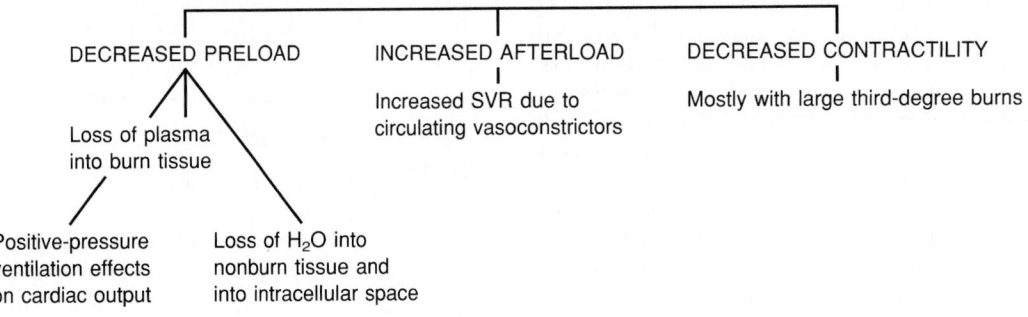

pulmonary artery line, preferably through nonburned tissue, is needed only occasionally to monitor the patient during the initial resuscitation period and is removed as soon as it is no longer needed.

Monitoring lines are required primarily for elderly patients or patients with severe heart disease. Because of the high infection rate, an intravenous catheter should not be placed through burn tissue unless no other possible route exists. Some centers rotate central line sites regularly (e.g., every 3 days) to minimize the risk of catheter sepsis, but any benefits may be offset by the risks of repeated procedures.

WHAT TO MONITOR

No one parameter of perfusion in a burn patient is a completely reliable indicator of tissue oxygenation (perfusion). The increased sympathetic tone characteristic of this early period makes arterial pressure an insensitive measure of volume status. However, a minimum perfusion pressure—e.g., a mean arterial pressure of more than 85 mm Hg—must be maintained.

Tachycardia is inevitable owing to hypovolemia and catecholamine release. In most patients, a pulse rate of less than 120 beats per minute usually indicates adequate volume, whereas a pulse rate of more than 130 beats per minute usually indicates that more fluid is needed.

Renal blood flow is another reflection of the adequacy of systemic perfusion during this early phase of injury. A urine output of 0.5 to 1 mL/kg per hour normally reflects adequate renal blood flow, assuming that there are no factors such as hyperglycemia, mannitol, or alcohol to alter the relationship between renal perfusion and urine output. A value greater than 1.0 mL/kg per hour usually means that too much fluid is being given and that excess edema therefore is being produced.

The measurement of base deficit is extremely useful for the assessment of tissue oxygenation. A base deficit during this phase usually reflects impaired tissue oxygenation due to hypovolemia or carbon monoxide (or cyanide) toxicity, and a progressive decrease in base deficit is a very sensitive indicator of the adequacy of restoration of perfusion.

Burn patients are very prone to hypothermia during this early period, especially with infusion of cool fluids. A decrease in temperature will lead to further hemodynamic instability and impaired perfusion. The external environment must be altered to allow for maintenance of a normal temperature (37 to 37.5° C) for this period.

The filling pressures in a large burn at this stage are usually low even with adequate fluid resuscitation because the rate of fluid loss increases markedly with small rises in capillary pressure. Use of an arbitrary filling pressure as an end point of resuscitation should be avoided.

Only older patients with massive burns or smoke inhalation are typically monitored with a central catheter. Hypoperfusion is almost always due to hypovolemia. Measurement of the mixed venous oxygen tension, however, can assist greatly in this determination.

CHOICE OF RESUSCITATION FLUID

In general, fluids that contain at least as much salt as is present in plasma are appropriate in resuscitation.[16a] Restoration of sodium lost into the burn is essential. Flu-

ids should be free of glucose (except in the treatment of small children) because glucose intolerance characteristically is present. Blood volume can be restored more effectively as the leakage decreases at about 24 to 36 hours. Volume infusion above the amount necessary for adequate perfusion can accentuate edema-related complications markedly.

Crystalloid

Crystalloid, in particular lactated Ringer's solution, is the most popular resuscitation fluid in the United States. The amount of isotonic crystalloid required in the first 24 hours is adjusted on the basis of the parameters used to monitor the adequacy of resuscitation (see below). If a hypertonic solution is used, the serum sodium level should not be allowed to exceed 160 mEq/L.[15]

Colloid

Since nonburned tissue appears to regain normal permeability very shortly after injury, and since hypoproteinemia may accentuate the edema in nonburned tissue, protein restoration beginning at about 8 to 12 hours with 6% albumin seems appropriate if edema in noninjured tissue and total fluid requirements are to be minimized. The use of fresh frozen plasma should be reserved for correction of documented clotting abnormalities.

Hetastarch, a 6% starch solution, has colloid properties similar to those of a 6% protein solution and generates an oncotic pressure comparable with that of protein. The molecules are much larger than those of most dextrans, and vascular clearance therefore is much slower. As with dextran, volumes exceeding several liters can lead to clotting abnormalities and to the potential for immune dysfunction from reticuloendothelial blockade.

Blood

Because there is no early red blood cell deficit with a burn alone (unless severe hemolysis occurs), blood replacement usually is not needed.

RATE OF INFUSION

An initial rate can be estimated using the size of the burn (combined second and third degree) relative to the TBS and body weight:

24-h volume in mL (of which half is given in the first 8 h)

$$= 4 \text{ mL} \times \% \text{ TBS burned} \times \text{body weight in kg}$$

However, the volume of fluid required is that necessary to maintain perfusion. Any formula is only an initial guide. Approximately half the fluid requirements for the first 24 hours need to be given in the first 8 hours. Beginning at 8 to 10 hours, an attempt should be made to decrease the rate of fluid administration gradually to the lowest level that maintains adequate perfusion.

INDICATION FOR INOTROPIC SUPPORT

Inotropic support to supplement fluids is indicated if adequate perfusion cannot be maintained without excessive fluid administration. In contrast to nonburned patients, it is very difficult to increase preload to values above normal levels in order to increase cardiac output in burned

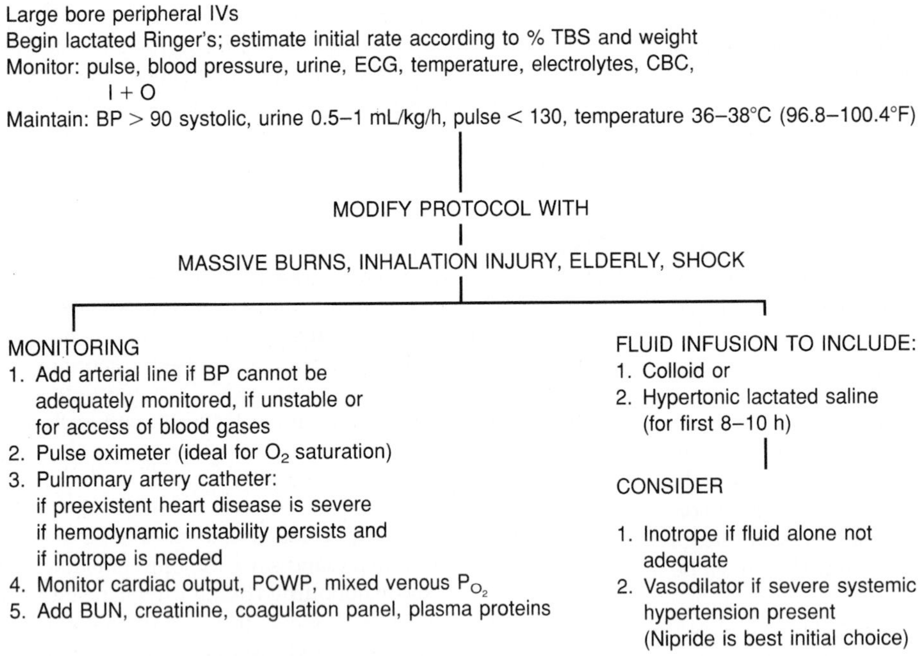

Large bore peripheral IVs
Begin lactated Ringer's; estimate initial rate according to % TBS and weight
Monitor: pulse, blood pressure, urine, ECG, temperature, electrolytes, CBC,
I + O
Maintain: BP > 90 systolic, urine 0.5–1 mL/kg/h, pulse < 130, temperature 36–38°C (96.8–100.4°F)

MODIFY PROTOCOL WITH

MASSIVE BURNS, INHALATION INJURY, ELDERLY, SHOCK

MONITORING
1. Add arterial line if BP cannot be
   adequately monitored, if unstable or
   for access of blood gases
2. Pulse oximeter (ideal for O_2 saturation)
3. Pulmonary artery catheter:
   if preexistent heart disease is severe
   if hemodynamic instability persists and
   if inotrope is needed
4. Monitor cardiac output, PCWP, mixed venous P_{O_2}
5. Add BUN, creatinine, coagulation panel, plasma proteins

FLUID INFUSION TO INCLUDE:
1. Colloid or
2. Hypertonic lactated saline
   (for first 8–10 h)

CONSIDER

1. Inotrope if fluid alone not
   adequate
2. Vasodilator if severe systemic
   hypertension present
   (Nipride is best initial choice)

FIGURE 98-4 Treatment summary (0 to 24 hours) for maintaining hemodynamic stability. All patients had burns of more than 20% of the TBS.

patients. Hemodynamic management is summarized in Fig. 98-4.

Hematologic Changes

A number of hematologic disorders are seen after major burns.[18] Hemolysis occurs commonly after deep third-degree burns or any prolonged exposure to a heat source. In addition, red blood cell fragility is increased markedly. Increased cell wall lipid peroxidation is evident, and fragmented cells are seen often on smears. The injured red blood cells will have a markedly shortened life span, leading to an anemia beginning in the first week. Red blood cell hematopoiesis is also markedly impaired and remains so until the burn is closed, resulting in a persistent anemia. A leukocytosis is also characteristic during this early phase. A marked consumption of platelets, fibrinogen, and plasminogen is seen in the burn wound, as well as a marked depletion of hemostatic components. A hypercoagulable state may be seen in the initial period in moderate burn injuries. A hypocoagulable state, resulting from depletion of clotting factors, is seen frequently with massive burns. Thrombocytopenia also will be evident in the latter group. It most likely results from the tremendous stimulus to clotting created by the large area of injured collagen tissue.

Assessment of the Burn Itself

ANATOMY AND FUNCTION OF THE SKIN

The skin is the largest organ of the body, ranging in area from 0.25 m^2 in newborns to over 2 m^2 in adults. It consists of two layers, epidermis and dermis (or corium). The outermost cells of the epidermis are dead cornified cells that act as a tough protective barrier against the environment. The second, thicker layer, the corium (0.06 to 0.12 mm thick), is composed chiefly of fibrous connective tissue. The dermis contains the blood vessels to the skin and the epithelial appendages of specialized function. The nerve endings that mediate pain are also found in the dermis. Partial-thickness injuries are extremely painful because the nerve endings are exposed. Full-thickness burns usually are anesthetic because the nerves have been destroyed by heat. The skin is also the barrier that prevents loss of body fluids through evaporation and limits the loss of body heat. In addition, the skin is the primary protective barrier against penetration of microorganisms into the subdermal tissues. Loss of this function results in increased risk of invasive infection.

DEPTH OF BURN INJURY

Traditionally, burn depth has been classified in degrees of injury based on the amount of epidermis and dermis injured. At present, depth is estimated by physical appearance, pain, and skin texture or pliability. A *first-degree burn* involves only the thin outer epidermis and is characterized by erythema and mild discomfort, healing rapidly.

Second-degree burns are defined as those in which the entire epidermis and variable portions of the dermis are destroyed. A *superficial second-degree burn* involves heat injury to the upper third of the dermis. The microvessels perfusing this area are injured, and permeability is increased, resulting in the leakage of large amounts of plasma into the interstitium. This fluid lifts off the thin, heat-destroyed epidermis, causing blister formation. Despite loss of the entire basal layer of the epidermis, a burn of this depth will heal in 7 to 14 days.

A *deep dermal* (or *deep second-degree*) burn extends well into the dermal layer, and fewer viable epidermal cells remain. Therefore, reepithelialization is extremely slow, sometimes requiring months. The wound surface usually is red, with white areas in deeper parts. Because the remaining blood supply is marginal, there is a high probability that the tissue damage will deepen with time.

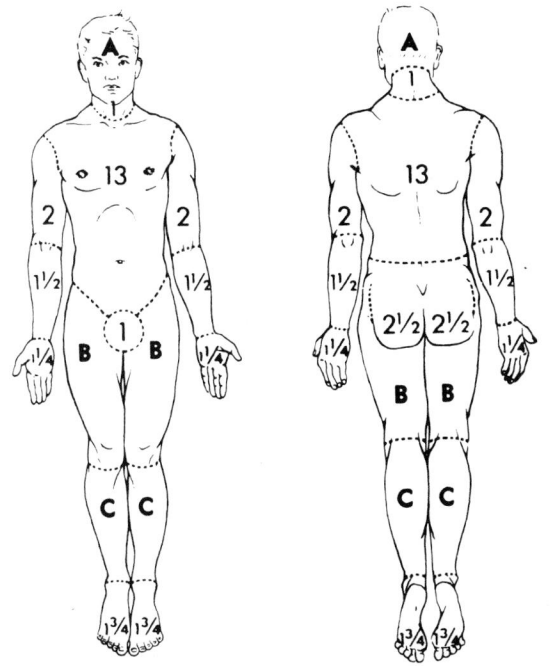

Relative Percentages of Areas Affected by Growth

Area	Age		
	10	15	Adult
A = half of head	5½	4½	3½
B = half of one thigh	4¼	4½	4¾
C = half of one leg	3	3¼	3½

FIGURE 98-5 Lund and Browder method of calculating the percentage of the body surface area burned.

A *full-thickness* (or *third-degree*) *burn* occurs with destruction of the entire epidermis and dermis, leaving no residual epidermal cells to repopulate the burned area. The portion of the wound not closed by wound contraction will require skin grafting. The exact depth of many deep burns cannot be defined on first appearance. A zone of ischemia is present between the dead superficial tissue and the deeper living tis-

sue. This marginally viable tissue can be readily converted to nonviable tissue by infection or a further decrease in blood flow.

SEVERITY OF INJURY

The size of the burn is defined as a percentage of the TBS. A useful initial guide is the *rule of nines*, which divides the body into areas that each represent 9% of the TBS. The head and each arm are considered 9% of the total, whereas the chest and abdomen, the back, and each lower extremity are considered to be 18% of the TBS. However, the Lund and Browder chart (Fig. 98-5) is more accurate and should be used for more precise calculation. The surface area of the body involved, the depth and location of injury, the patient's age, and the presence of associated injuries determine morbidity and mortality.[1] Age and the presence of associated injury appear to be the most significant parameters affecting the chance of survival (Table 98-2).

Treatment

The early treatment focuses on neutralizing the source of burn injury, avoiding excess heat loss, determining the extent of injury, cleaning and débriding the wound, controlling infection, and maintaining tissue perfusion.

AVOIDING EXCESS HEAT LOSS

With a deep burn, the barrier to evaporative water loss is markedly impaired. As a consequence, the barrier to heat loss is also impaired, a fact that is extremely important to recognize in the resuscitation period. Heat loss can be decreased by closing the wound under dressings, thereby limiting air movement and decreasing the air-to-wound temperature gradient. Therefore, the burn is only cooled initially to neutralize excessive heat and to control pain in superficial second-degree burns covering less than 15% of the TBS.[21] Patients with major burns must be placed in a warmed external environment to minimize heat loss. Wound débridement and washing should not be initiated on a large burn until the external temperature is controlled.[19]

TABLE 98-2 Data Obtained from Specialized Burn Facilities: Mean Survival Rate (%) According to Age and Burn Size

% TBS Burned[a]	AGE (YEARS)						
	0–1	2–4	5–34	35–49	50–59	60–74	>75
0–10	>95	>95	>95	>95	>95	95	90
10–20	95	>90	>95	>90	>85	80	50
20–30	90	90	95	90	75	50	25
30–40	75	80	90	80	60	30	<10
40–50	70	85	80	80	70	20	<5
50–60	60	80	85	70	40	15	<5
60–70	50	70	75	70	50	<10	0
70–80	40	60	60	50	40	<10	0
80–90	30	45	45	40	10	0	0
90–100	0	30	30	15	0	0	0

[a] Combined second-degree and third-degree burns.

TABLE 98-3 Standard Burn Categorization

Critical burns
1. Second-degree burns involving >30% TBS
2. Third-degree burns involving >10% TBS
3. Burns complicated by respiratory tract injury or fractures or involving critical areas such as the face, hands, feet, or perineum
4. High-voltage electrical burns
5. Lesser burns in patients with significant preexisting disease

Moderate burns
1. Second-degree burns involving 15%–30% TBS (but not involving the face, hands, feet, or perineum)
2. Third-degree burns involving 2%–10% TBS (but not involving the face, hands, feet, or perineum)

Minor burns
1. Second-degree burn involving <15% TBS
2. Third-degree burns involving <2% TBS

DETERMINING THE EXTENT OF INJURY

The wound can be categorized on the basis of size, depth, age, and other complicating factors. Table 98-3 presents the standard categorization used by the American Burn Association.

CONTROLLING INFECTION

The management of the burn wound itself depends on the status of initial cardiopulmonary function. Adequate control of the airway, maintenance of adequate gas exchange,

and restoration of fluid loss must precede attempts at wound cleaning and débridement. Initial débridement consists of the elimination only of superficial, easily removed dead tissue; once this is accomplished, control of potential infection in the injured tissue is the next priority. Tetanus prophylaxis is necessary. Numerous studies have demonstrated that prophylactic systemic antibiotics in patients with either minor or major burns are of no benefit in decreasing the rate of wound infection.[22]

The recommendation for the use of topical antibiotics is based on the fact that nonviable tissue is present and will act as a nidus for infection and on the lack of effectiveness of systemic antibiotics.

IMPAIRED DISTAL PERFUSION AND NEED FOR ESCHAROTOMY

As subeschar edema develops under the burn tissue, pressure increases. This development is of particular concern in extremities with a circumferential burn, where the increasing pressure cannot be dissipated by expansion of neighboring tissue. The pressure impedes blood flow. Perfusion to the distal extremity must be monitored closely. Pain and color are unreliable indicators of perfusion in the presence of a burn. The use of a Doppler flowmeter is the most practical means of assessing perfusion. Decreasing distal flow with a proximal deep burn is also an indication for escharotomy. Wound management is summarized in Fig. 98-6.

FIGURE 98-6 Treatment summary (0 to 24 hours). Wound management.

1. Assure adequate ventilation and perfusion
2. Remove heat source and any constricting items
3. Cool water for small second degree burns only
4. Assess depth and size—"rule of nines"
5. Tetanus prophylaxis

PATIENT NOT STABLE
1. Remove clothing
2. Cover with warm dry dressing
3. Wait until ABC's controlled to initiate aggressive wound care
4. Do not put in hydrotherapy tank or move away from adequate monitoring

PATIENT REASONABLY STABLE
1. Maintain warm external temperature during wound cleaning
2. Use adequate pain control (small doses IV narcotics for major burn)
3. Chlorhexidine wash: dilute contents of one packet in 1–2 quarts warm (85–90°F, 29.4–32.2°C) H$_2$O
4. Remove dirt, loose skin May leave large blisters intact

SUPERFICIAL SECOND-DEGREE BURN

WOUND RELATIVELY CLEAN
1. Can use petrolatum gauze with dressing
2. Consider temporary skin substitutes: Biobrane
3. Elevate burned extremity: bacitracin
4. Perineum, feet: use Silvadene

WOUND DIRTY
1. Use topical antibiotic: Silvadene 1st choice
2. Elevate burned extremity

DEEP BURN
1. Use topical antibiotic cream: Silvadene 1st choice
2. Closed dressing technique exception: face, perineum
3. Monitor perfusion to distal extremity

THIRD-DEGREE BURN
1. Use topical antibiotic cream Silvadene: if wound not grossly infected; Sulfamylon for small to moderate size infected burn
2. Parenteral antibiotics if infected, not for prophylaxis
3. Closed dressing technique except: face, perineum
4. Monitor perfusion: may need escharotomy

References

1. Sheridan R: Burns. *Crit Care Med* 30:500, 2002.

2. Hill A, Germa F, Boyle J: Burns in older people: Outcomes and risk factors. *J Am Geriatr Soc* 50:1912, 2002.

3. Darling GE, Keresteci MA, Ibanez D, et al: Pulmonary complications in inhalation injuries with associated cutaneous burn. *J Trauma* 40:83, 1996.

4. Demling R: Anabolic inhalation injury. *New Horizons* 1:422, 1993.

5. Alarie Y: Toxicity of fire smoke. *Crit Rev Toxicol* 32:259, 2002.

6. Bard F, Barriot P, Toffis V, et al: Elevated blood cyanide concentrations in victims of smoke inhalation. *New Engl J Med* 325:1761, 1991.

7. Willey-Courand D, Harris R, Gabetti G., et al: Alterations in regional ventilation perfusion and shunt after smoke inhalation by PET. *J Appl Physiol* 93:1115, 2002.

8. Demling R, Lalonte C, Youn Y, Picard L: Effect of graded increases in smoke inhalation injury on the early systemic response to a body burn. *Crit Care Med* 23:171, 1995.

9. Ventilatory support following burns and smoke inhalation injury. *Respir Care Clin North Am* 3:21, 1997.

10. Robinson W, Hudson L, Riem M, et al: Steroid therapy following isolated smoke injury. *J Trauma* 22:876, 1982.

11. Hobson K, Young K, Cirauto A, et al: Release of abdominal compartment syndrome improves survival in patients with burn injury. *J Trauma* 53:1129, 2002.

12. Pruitt B, Dowling J, Monerref J: Escharotomy in early burn care. *Arch Surg* 96:502, 1968.

13. Jin L, LaLonde C, Demling RH: Lung dysfunction after thermal injury: Relationship to prostanoid and oxygen radical release. *J Appl Physiol* 61:103, 1986.

14. Demling RH: Fluid resuscitation after major burns. *JAMA* 250:1438, 1983.

15. Guha SC, Kinsky MP, Button B, et al: Burn resuscitation: Crystalloid versus colloid versus hypertonic saline hyperonicotic colloid in sheep. *Crit Care Med* 24:1849, 1996.

16. Fitzpatrick J, Croffe W: Diagnosis and treatment of inhalation injuries. In Herdon D (ed): *Total Burn Care*. Philadelphia, Saunders, 2001, p 232.

17. Carleton SC: Cardiac problems associated with burns. *Cardiol Clin* 13:257, 1995.

18. Shankar R, Amin C, Gamelli R: Hematologic, hematopoetic and acute phase response, in Herndon D (ed): *Total Burn Care*. Philadelphia, Saunders, 2002, p 331.

19. Wallace B, Caldwell F, Cone J: The interrelationship between wound management, thermal stress, energy metabolism and temperature profiles of patients with burns. *J Burn Care Rehabil* 15:499, 1994.

20. Murphy K, Lee J, Herndon D: Current pharmacotherapy for the treatment of severe burns. *Exp Opin Pharmacother* 4:369, 2003.

21. Shirans K, Vaughan G, Mason A, Pruitt B: Update on current therapeutic approaches in burns. *Shock* 5:4, 1996.

Chapter 99 _____
BURNS: POSTRESUSCITATION PHASE (DAYS 2 TO 6)

ROBERT DEMLING
LESLIE DESANTI

KEY POINTS

- *Pulmonary problems must be controlled during this period to allow for an aggressive surgical excisional approach.*
- *Fluid management changes dramatically to a strategy of replacing evaporative water losses.*
- *Postburn anemia will develop and necessitate increased blood transfusions.*
- *Monitoring must be primarily noninvasive to avoid line sepsis.*
- *Nutritional support should begin at this point, using enteral alimentation.*
- *Controlled surgical excisions should begin as soon as the patient is hemodynamically stable, to avoid having extensive burns still in place when the infection-inflammation phase begins.*

The early postresuscitation phase is a period of transition from the ebb, or shock, phase to the flow, or hypermetabolic, phase. Major cardiopulmonary and wound changes occur that alter patient care substantially from that given during resuscitation. In general, cardiopulmonary stability is optimal during this period because wound inflammation and infection have not yet developed. Early wound excision and grafting are initiated during this period because operative risks, especially blood loss and septicemia, are substantially less than after inflammation and infection develop.

Pulmonary Abnormalities

Five major abnormalities impair pulmonary function during this period: (1) continued upper airway obstruction, (2) decreased chest wall compliance, (3) tracheobronchitis, (4) pulmonary edema, and (5) lung dysfunction induced by surgery (and anesthesia). Upper airway and facial edema caused by the heat-induced tissue and mucosal damage begins to resolve between days 2 and 4. The decision to extubate (Fig. 99-1) is a difficult one because there is no good test for determining the adequacy of airway patency.[1,2] Laryngoscopy to determine the presence of cord edema is helpful, as is deflation of the cuff to determine if air moves around the tube. The impaired compliance of the chest wall caused by deep burns is improved, but certainly not eliminated, by escharotomy. Early excision of the full-thickness wound can improve chest wall motion by removing both edema and noncompliant tissue.

The chemical burn to the airways results in a spectrum of clinical manifestations during this period. At the very least, mucosal irritation will persist for several days and cause bronchorrhea, cough, and increased mucus production. The damaged ciliary function of the airways leads to a high risk for infection, manifested first (in the next 3 to 4 days) by a bacterial tracheobronchitis that is often followed by bronchopneumonia. Bacterial colonization is inevitable. If infection can be controlled and secretions cleared, the acute process will resolve over the next 7 to 10 days. However, the risk of infection persists for several weeks, extending well into the inflammation period. The treatment of lung dysfunction during this phase is summarized in Fig. 99-2. The clearance of soot, mucopurulent exudate, and sloughing mucosa is essential to avoid progression of the lung injury.

Infection surveillance is crucial during this early period in order to detect bacterial bronchitis before pneumonia develops. Unlike typical bronchopneumonia, presenting with a localized infiltrate, the entire tracheobroncheal tree becomes colonized with pathogens, and the resulting infection is often a diffuse bronchopneumonia. Sputum smears and monitoring of the character of the sputum are useful as early guides. Systemic antibiotics are not given prophylactically but are initiated when a bacterial tracheobronchitis becomes evident. This approach is summarized in Fig. 99-3.

Repeated excision and grafting procedures, especially on large body burns, usually result in a situation in which the patient either is recovering from an inhalational anesthetic or is awaiting surgery. Most general anesthetics cause deterioration in an already marginal respiratory status and put the patient at further increased risk for pneumonia and respiratory failure during the subsequent phase of injury. Muscle relaxants compound this problem.

Maintaining Hemodynamic Stability

PATHOPHYSIOLOGIC CHANGES

FLUID LOSSES

Evaporation from the surface of the burn becomes a major source of water loss that persists until the wound is closed. This loss is related to the water vapor pressure at the surface.[4] A reasonable estimate of loss can be obtained from the following formula, where TBS is the total body surface area:

$$\text{Evaporative water loss in mL/h} = (25 + \% \text{ of TBS burned})$$
$$\times (\text{TBS in m}^2)$$

Red blood cell mass can decrease markedly during this period because of breakdown and decreased production of red blood cells.[5,6] Lipid peroxidation of the red blood cell membrane after burn injury is well described. The hematocrit characteristically falls to between 30% and 35% or lower several days after the burn injury. Besides increased red blood cell breakdown, there is decreased red blood cell production by the bone marrow—an effect characteristic of any chronic injury state. Red blood cell production does not return to normal until after the wound is closed.

FLUID GAINS

Intravascular fluid is gained during the postresuscitation period as a result of absorption of edema. Edema resorption is much more rapid in the case of superficial burns where lymphatics are intact and begins at about day 2 or 3. Edema

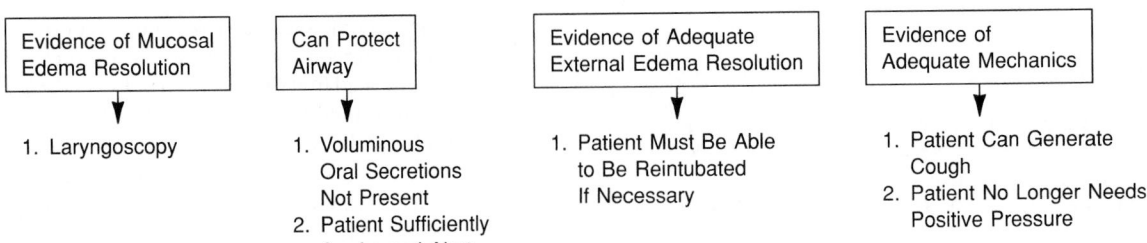

FIGURE 99-1 Criteria for deciding when to extubate a patient. All these criteria should be met to ensure safe extubation.

resorption is much slower after full-thickness injury because of the lack of local lymphatics and venules. However, the magnitude of tissue edema is not a valid reflection of the circulating volume and never should be used to judge the correct rate of fluid replacement.

SYSTEMIC METABOLIC CHANGES AND CIRCULATORY RESPONSES

The ebb, or hypometabolic, phase characteristic of the initial burn shock period begins to change into the flow, or hypermetabolic, phase over the next 3 to 5 days.[7,8] Tachycardia, ranging from modest to significant (100 to 120 beats per minute), is seen frequently and results partly from persistent elevation of catecholamine levels. Systemic vascular resistance begins to decrease. The vasodilatation results in an increase in the capacity of the vascular space and, therefore, an increased need for colloid and red blood cells.

Oxygen consumption usually peaks 5 to 7 days after the burn.[7] The transition to the flow state also initiates an increase in body temperature, which increases further with the release of pyrogens from the burn wound. The characteristic increase in body temperature by 1 to 2°F makes it more difficult to diagnose infection. Patients with subclinical glucose intolerance (typically obese or elderly patients) may develop hyperglycemia, especially with a large burn. Increased catabolism leads to increased urea production, especially if inadequate

glucose calories are being provided. The rate of body protein loss is massive as a result of the increased levels of catecholamines and cortisol, as well as inflammatory cytokines, which markedly stimulate gluconeogenesis using protein as a substrate.[9,10] Decreased levels of human growth hormone and testosterone amplify the catabolism.[11] A total of 20% to 30% of calories come from proteins, as opposed to the protein sparing, which occurs in starvation, where fat is the main fuel. Loss of the amino acid glutamine is particularly pronounced because it is used heavily as a fuel source by the gut as well as a precursor for the antioxidant glutathione.[12] Muscle losses of a kilogram a day are common with large burns. Over a 10-day period, 10% to 15% of body protein stores can be lost, resulting not only in muscular weakness, including weakness of the intercostal muscle and diaphragm, but also in decreased wound healing and immune function. Because of the large increase in oxidant release due to inflammation, the levels of endogenous antioxidants fall rapidly, increasing the risk of further oxidant injury and generalized organ dysfunction.[13]

HEMODYNAMIC MANAGEMENT

Understanding the physiologic and metabolic changes during this period is the key to successful management. The major decisions relate to fluid therapy and the ongoing assessment of the adequacy of perfusion.

FIGURE 99-2 Summary of treatment of pulmonary abnormalities from 36 hours to 6 days after the burn injury.

Airway Maintenance

1. Maintain Artificial Airway Until Face and Neck Edema and Intraoral Swelling Have Adequately Resolved
2. Laryngoscopy or Bronchoscopy Prior to Tube Removal

Maintain Pulmonary Toilet

1. Do Not Underestimate Inhalation Injury
2. Avoid Airway Plugging from Inhalation Injury; Vigorous Cough, Suctioning, Bronchoscopy in Selected Patients
3. Aggressive Chest Physiotherapy
4. Avoid Nosocomial Pneumonia

Maintain Adequate Gas Exchange

1. Avoid Pulmonary Edema from Volume Overload
2. Aggressively Treat CHF (May Need Inotropes)
3. Avoid Hypoventilation (Especially Prevalent in Perioperative Period)
4. Consider Partial Mechanical Ventilation, Especially with Frequent Operative Interventions

Maintain Infection Control

1. Primary Therapy Is Pulmonary Toilet
2. Initiate Antibiotics with Early Evidence of Bacterial Tracheobronchitis

Increased Airway Resistance (Edema)	Increased Secretions; Bacterial Colonization
1. Continuous Positive Airway Pressure (CPAP) to Increase FRC 2. Consider Bronchodilators 3. Avoid CHF, Volume Overload	1. Aggressive Pulmonary Toilet (Postural Changes Extremely Important) 2. Infection Surveillance; Daily Sputum Smear; Assess for Antibiotic Use

Note: Do *Not* Produce Hypovolemia in an Attempt to Correct Airway Edema

FIGURE 99-3 Treatment of tracheobronchial injuries.

SELECTION OF FLUID

A common error is continued infusion of isotonic crystalloid during a period when major losses of sodium do not occur. A 5% glucose-containing solution with a low sodium content and an increased potassium content is the primary replacement fluid for evaporative and urinary losses during this period. Initiation of nutrition is also essential, preferably by the enteral route. To restore blood volume and maintain the protein binding required for predictable pharmacokinetics, protein losses should be replaced. A serum albumin level of 2.5 g/dL is a reasonable goal. It is also frequently necessary to replace red blood cells. The hematocrit should be kept at least at a level of 30% to optimize delivery of oxygen to tissues. Hemodynamic management is summarized in Fig. 99-4.

WHAT TO MONITOR

Assessment of the adequacy of perfusion, tissue oxygenation, and fluid and electrolyte balance can be difficult during this period of evolving hemodynamics. Oxygen consumption increases gradually with the transition from the ebb state to the flow state. The absolute value of body weight cannot be used to reflect blood volume during this transition. However, if weight is increasing, excess fluid (and salt) is probably being given. One should anticipate a gradual increase of 1 to $2°F$ in body temperature over normal; this increase is due to hypermetabolism. Further increases are common with wound manipulation.

Care of the Burn Wound

The wound undergoes dramatic changes during this period as inflammation develops. In addition, wound colonization and the potential for wound infection increase. This process of deepening of the burn (called *wound conversion*) is seen most commonly in deep second-degree burns and can occur even with optimal management. Processes such as wound

FIGURE 99-4 Maintenance of hemodynamic stability from 36 hours to 6 days after the burn injury.

All Major Burns
1. Infuse Glucose (5%–10%) in Low-Salt Crystalloid to Replace Evaporative Loss Minus Gain from Edema Resorption 2. Replace Plasma Protein Losses with Albumin >2.5 g/dL; Be Careful If Patient is Already Hypervolemic 3. Assure Adequate O_2 Delivery; Maintain O_2 SAT ≥95%, HCT >30, Cardiac Output >1.5 Times Normal 4. Begin Nutritional Support (Calories and Proteins); Can Use Peripheral Vein and Enteral Route Instead of Central Line 5. Monitor Pulse, B.P., T°, Urine, Body Wt., I & O, ECG, Acid-Base Balance, Electrolytes, CBC, BUN, Creatinine, Albumin 6. Maintain Urine Output >0.5 mL/kg per h 7. Maintain T° >37.5°C

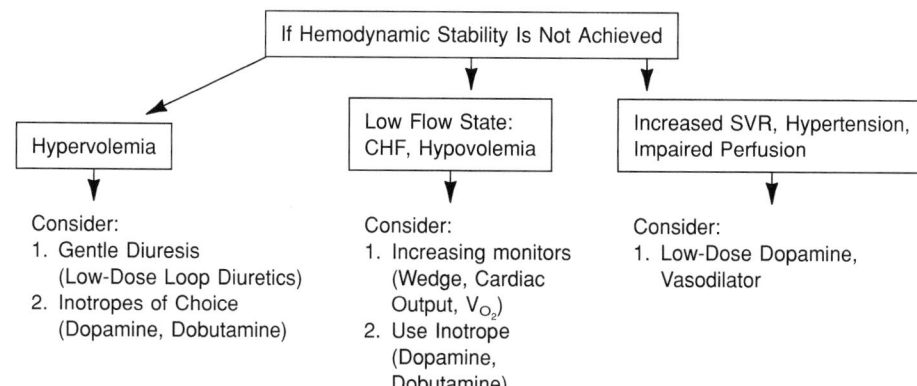

If Hemodynamic Stability Is Not Achieved		
Hypervolemia	Low Flow State: CHF, Hypovolemia	Increased SVR, Hypertension, Impaired Perfusion
Consider: 1. Gentle Diuresis (Low-Dose Loop Diuretics) 2. Inotropes of Choice (Dopamine, Dobutamine)	Consider: 1. Increasing monitors (Wedge, Cardiac Output, V_{O_2}) 2. Use Inotrope (Dopamine, Dobutamine)	Consider: 1. Low-Dose Dopamine, Vasodilator

desiccation, hypovolemia, increased tissue pressure, and hypothermia all can accentuate the potential for conversion. The most common cause, however, is local infection.

PATHOPHYSIOLOGIC CHANGES IN THE BURN WOUND

Intense inflammation is seen at about 7 to 10 days in deep burns. The rate of onset of inflammation depends on the blood flow to the wound, with inflammation occurring more rapidly in more superficial burns. A marked increase in wound vascularity is also seen. As wound blood flow increases, so do water loss and heat loss. Heat and water losses are further accentuated by the increase in core temperature that develops with the onset of hypermetabolism.[14]

MANAGEMENT OF BURN WOUND INFECTION

PATHOGENESIS OF BURN WOUND INFECTION

With loss of the outer skin barrier, bacteria can populate the burn wound.[15] Most of these early colonizing bacteria are

TABLE 99-1 Effects of a Major Burn on the Immune System

Effects of impaired cell-mediated immunity:
Altered skin test reactivity (anergy)
Increased allograft survival
Decreased T cell response to mitogen
Decreased T cell numbers and response to antigen
Increase in suppressor relative to helper T cells
Effects of impaired neutrophil function:
Decreased chemotaxis
Decreased phagocytosis
Decreased bacterial killing
Effects of alterations in humoral defenses:
Decreased immunoglobulins
Decreased fibronectin
Decreased primary antibody response

endogenous, originating from the heat-injured skin (especially hair follicles, glands, and so on), the nares and oropharynx, and the perineal and stool microflora. In addition, systemic host defenses are significantly impaired after a major burn[17] (Table 99-1). Movement of organisms via hand contact,

FIGURE 99-5 General principles of burn excision.

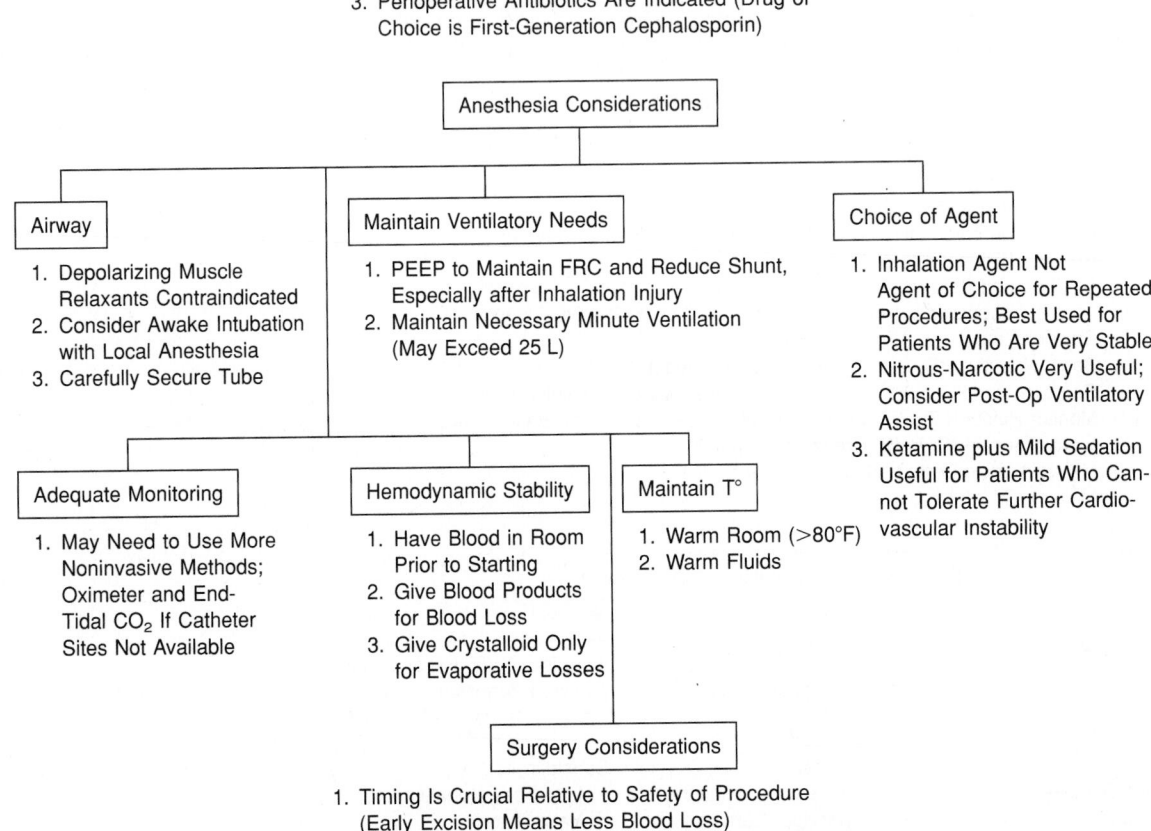

by patient and by personnel, from area to area on the patient—or between patients—is the major factor leading to bacterial contamination of the wound.

USE OF TOPICAL ANTIBIOTICS

The mainstay of infection control is the use of topically applied antibiotics. Silver sulfadiazine is the most common and least toxic. Mafenide is more potent and is reserved for the treatment of deep infections because of its toxicity (carbonic anhydrase inhibitor).[14,15]

DIAGNOSIS OF WOUND INFECTION

In order to assess the wound for infection, a definition of infection must be well understood. Burn wounds are never sterile, even in the presence of topical agents or systemic antibiotics. The presence of bacteria on the wound surface or in the nonviable tissue is called *colonization*. *Infection* of the wound (or *local wound sepsis*), in contrast, indicates invasion of the underlying viable tissue. As infection progresses, the viable tissue and its blood vessels are invaded, and sepsis develops.[14]

The clinical diagnosis of wound infection is difficult. Fever, leukocytosis, tachycardia, and intermittent temperature spikes are seen characteristically in the burn patient with or without infection. Wound purulence is a reliable indicator of infection only if the purulence is in the subeschar space.[11]

The organism most often involved in wound infection, particularly in the first week, is *Staphylococcus aureus*.[14,15] Infection with gram-negative organisms is more evident after the first week. *Pseudomonas aeruginosa* is present on the wounds of approximately 25% of burn patients. Enterococci and *Candida albicans* are now seen with increasing frequency, each being found in the wounds of about 50% of burn patients.

A reliable method of diagnosing a burn wound infection is bacterial analysis of a full-thickness wound biopsy.[14,16] It has been established that 10^5 organisms per gram of tissue is the bacterial load that is preinvasive and indicates infection and the need for systemic antibiotics.

EARLY WOUND EXCISION AND GRAFTING

Early excision and grafting should be considered for all burns that will not heal by primary intention within 3 weeks. Full-thickness burns require grafting unless they are smaller than 3 to 4 cm in diameter. The more rapidly the wound is closed, the better. At least in theory, burns covering less than 30% of the TBS can be closed rapidly because adequate donor sites are available. Larger burns are more difficult, if not impossible, to graft early. Deep partial-thickness burns are also difficult to assess clearly as regards time to healing. Considerable judgment and assessment skills, therefore, are essential (Fig. 99-5).

PAIN AND STRESS CONTROL

Management of pain and anxiety is of extreme importance and should begin soon after the burn injury to avoid accentuation of the stress response to injury, with further catabolism. Since pain and stress are present at all times and are amplified by wound management, a continuous background use of narcotics—often patient-regulated or continuously infused kind—is used. Low doses of benzodiazepines are also used. Burn patients are very prone to the extrapyramidal side effects of phenothiazines.[15,19,20] In many cases, the dosages of all drugs must be increased because of rapid drug clearance when the patient is in the hypermetabolic state.[23]

References

1. Demling R, Read T, Lind L, et al: Incidence and morbidity of extubation failure in surgical intensive care patients. *Crit Care Med* 16:573, 1988.
2. Ruo L, Cioffi W, Mason A, et al: Improved survival of burned patients with inhalation injury. *Arch Surg* 128:772, 1993.
3. Demling R, Crawford G, Lind L, et al: Restrictive pulmonary dysfunction caused by the grafted chest and abdominal burn. *Crit Care Med* 16:743, 1988.
4. Lamke L: Evaporative water loss from normal and burnt skin. *Scand J Plast Reconstr Surg* 5:17, 1971.
5. Deitch E, Sittig K: A serial study of the erythropoetic response to thermal injury. *Ann Surg* 217:293, 1993.
6. Shankav R, Amin C, Gamelli R: Hematopoietic and acute phase response. In Herdon D (ed): *Total Burn Care,* Philadelphia Saunders, 2001, p 331.
7. Tredget E, Yu Y: The metabolic effects of thermal injury. *World J Surg* 16:68, 1992.
8. Demling R, Seigne P: Metabolic management of patients with severe burns. *World J Surg* 24:673, 2000.
9. Gore D, Chinkis D, Hart D, et al: Hyperglycemia exasce> rbates muscle protein catabolism in burn injured patients. *Crit Care Med* 30:2438, 2002.
10. Foex BA, Shelly MP: The cytokine response to critical illness. *J Accid Emerg Med* 13:154, 1996.
11. Jeevanandam M, Ramas L, et al: Decreased growth hormone levels in the catabolic phase of severe injury. *Surgery* 111:495, 1992.
12. Gore D, Jahoor F: Glutamine kinetics in burn patients: comparison with hormonal stress in volunteers. *Arch Surg* 129:1318, 1994.
13. Latha B, Baber M: The involvement of free radicals in burn injury: A review. *Burns* 27:309, 2001.
14. Gore D, Chinkes D, Sanford A, et al: Influence of fever on the hypermetabolic response in burn injured patients. *Arch Surg* 38:169, 2003.
15. Heggars J, Hawkins H, Edgar P: Treatment of infection in burn, in Herndon D (ed): *Total Burn Care.* Philadelphia, Saunders, 2002, p 120.
16. Demling RH: Infection following burns, in Hoeprich P (ed): *Infectious Diseases,* 4th ed. Philadelphia, Lippincott, 1989, p 1424.
17. Garrison JL, Thomas F, Cunningham P: Improved large burn therapy with reduced mortality following an associated septic challenge by early excision and skin allografting using donor-specific tolerance. *Transplant Proc* 27:1416, 1995.
18. Hart D, Wolf S, Chinkes D, et al: Effects of early excision and aggressive enteral feeding on hypermetabolism, catabolism and sepsis after severe burn. *J Trauma* 54:755, 2003.
19. Carrougher G, Ptacek J, Sharar S, et al: Comparison of patient satisfaction and self-reports of pain in adult burn injured patients. *J Burn Care Rehabil* 24:1, 2003.
20. Hedderich R, Ness T: Analgesia for trauma and burns. *Crit Care Clin* 15:167, 1999.

BURNS: INFLAMMATION-INFECTION PHASE (DAY 7 TO WOUND CLOSURE)

ROBERT DEMLING
LESLIE DESANTI

KEY POINTS

- *This period is characterized by hypermetabolism and sepsis syndrome owing to wound inflammation.*
- *Adequate nutritional support is critical to attenuate the rate of catabolism.*
- *Enteral nutrition should begin by 3 days, and 80% of nutritional needs should be met by 7 days.*
- *Inappropriate use of systemic antibiotics is common during this period because infection is overdiagnosed.*
- *During this period, wound manipulation and operative procedures must be limited because of wound colonization and hypervascularity.*
- *Pulmonary complications are the most common cause of mortality during this period; general anesthesia and transport are high-risk periods.*
- *Anemia is characteristic of this period because of decreased red blood cell production and continued red blood cell losses.*
- *A close working relationship with the patient is the key to control stress.*
- *Pain and stress management are major problems often necessitating extensive use of narcotics, sedatives, and antipsychotic drugs.*

The interval from day 7 after a burn to wound closure is the most complicated phase of management of a large burn. The systemic effects of burn wound inflammation alter the function of all organ systems and magnify any preexisting organ dysfunction—especially cardiopulmonary dysfunction. There is marked catabolism with loss of body protein, especially from muscle but also from viscera, that can lead to organ dysfunction. The increase in metabolic rate resulting from hormonal response to the inflammatory process leads to a marked increase in O_2 consumption and CO_2 production. The burn wound is now colonized with bacteria, and wound sepsis is a prominent concern. The hyperdynamic hypermetabolic state makes it increasingly difficult to diagnose wound and lung infection.

Pulmonary Abnormalities

Pulmonary problems remain a major cause of morbidity and mortality during this phase.[1,2] Respiratory failure and

pneumonia surpass burn wound sepsis as causes of mortality. The burn patient is especially prone to pulmonary infection after smoke inhalation. In addition, the hypermetabolic state produces a marked increase in O_2 consumption and CO_2 production at a time when respiratory function may be seriously impaired by pneumonia, pulmonary edema, or muscle weakness. Burn patients with the combination of inhalation injury and a major body burn have the greatest risk of pneumonia, with a rate approaching 50%. The high incidence is a result of the presence of virulent organisms in the ICU environment and the immunosuppressed state of burn patients. Ciliary action is injured directly by heat and by chemicals in inhaled smoke and often does not regenerate adequately, contributing further to the risk of retention of contaminated secretions and development of pneumonia. Since eradication of an established pneumonia in a burn patient is very difficult, prevention is of primary importance.[3]

When using antibiotics, it is important to remember that the dosages of most antimicrobials required to obtain adequate levels are much higher in hypermetabolic burn patients.[4] If continued intubation is expected for weeks, conversion to a tracheostomy in the first week will greatly assist the clearance of secretions. The tracheostomy should not be placed through burned tissue. If the neck is burned, early excision and grafting are indicated. The tracheostomy can be performed through the skin graft.

The increase in O_2 consumption and CO_2 production during this period imposes increased demand on the respiratory system relative to that seen in the previous periods.[5,6] A 50% to 100% increase in CO_2 production will be seen with burns in excess of 50% of total body surface (TBS). In addition, the severe catabolism initiated by the inflammatory response can lead to weakness of the respiratory muscles.

Protection of the lungs against processes that would impair their function is the best form of support. Controlling edema and infection, maintaining nutrition, and providing for adequate rest, as well as respiratory muscle exercise, are key components. CO_2 production should be limited by avoiding excess carbohydrate calories and controlling hyperthermia. Partial ventilatory support via a tracheostomy may be useful, especially if recovery is not anticipated for several weeks.

Hemodynamic and Metabolic Support

A good understanding of the metabolic and physiologic changes is necessary to determine fluid, electrolyte, and nutrient requirements.

FLUID, PROTEIN, AND RED BLOOD CELL LOSSES

Evaporative water losses remain increased until the wound is closed. Even after closure, evaporative losses through the grafted wound are much higher than through normal skin. Increased water intake is essential to compensate for this loss, which can be 2 to 4 L/d. Protein losses from wound exudation and from bleeding persist until wound closure.

THE HYPERMETABOLIC-CATABOLIC STATE

The host response to a severe burn is an amplification of the fright-flight reaction. The insult (afferent arc) leads to the release of inflammatory cytokines that activate a very

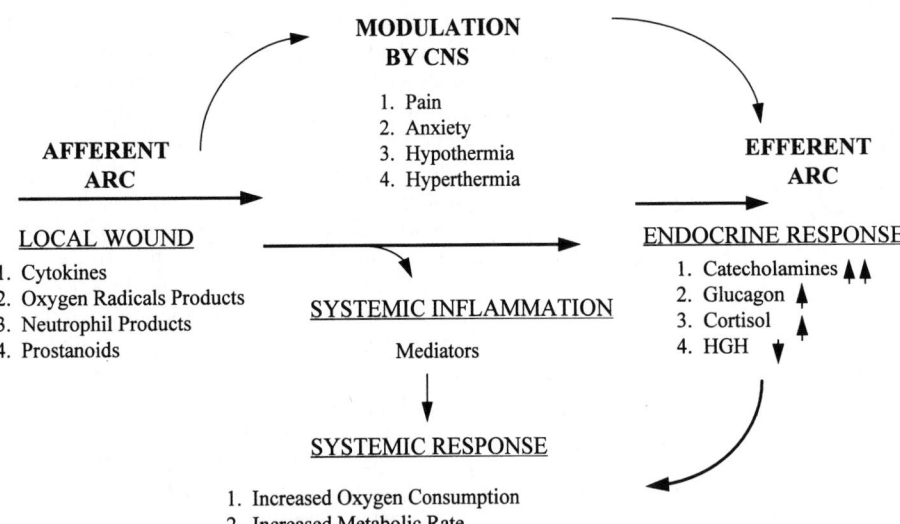

STRESS RESPONSE TO INJURY

FIGURE 100-1 The host response to a severe burn.

abnormal hormonal response led by a marked increase in catecholamines and other hormones (efferent arc) that produce a hypermetabolic-catabolic state (Fig. 100-1 and Table 100-1). Oxygen consumption can double during this period because of the abnormal endocrine environment. Any added central nervous system (CNS) stress such as pain will further amplify the catechol-induced process.

Hepatic gluconeogenesis is intensely stimulated, and body protein is broken down rapidly to provide amino acids for carbohydrate substrate.[6-9] The amino acids are released mainly from muscle as alanine for liver glucose formation and glutamine. Glutamine from muscle is exported in large quantities for use as fuel for the gut, as well as a precursor for the endogenous antioxidant glutathione. As opposed to starvation, where 85% of calories come from fat, protein is not spared for use for fuel, and muscle is lost rapidly.

Optimal nutrition attenuates the process and decreases net protein losses by about 50%, but catabolism still outweighs anabolism because the catabolic hormones predominate and the anabolic hormones, especially growth hormones, are decreased. Morbidity from rapid protein depletion can occur in days to weeks after injury rather than after months, as seen with starvation alone (Fig. 100-2). Oxidants released by the generalized inflammation produce direct cell damage, especially because endogenous antioxidant levels are decreased. The direct cell injury and loss of cellular protein can result in progressive multiple-organ dysfunction.

The wound or focus of inflammation develops a high blood flow owing to demand for substrate caused by inflammatory mediators that produce local vasodilatation. This blood flow, which steals from the systemic circulation, can lead to a systemic O_2 debt. The wound consumes large quantities of energy during the healing process both by inflammatory cells and by fibroblast collagen formation. The wound uses glucose as its primary fuel for ATP but does so in an anaerobic fashion despite oxygen availability. Lactate is returned to the liver to re-form glucose. Gluconeogenesis also employs skeletal muscle amino acids, primarily alanine.

The size of the wound or focus of inflammation corresponds with the magnitude of the stress response. In addition, the wound becomes the preferred consumer of amino acids obtained from muscle until 20% of muscle is lost, at which time both muscle and wound compete equally. With a 30% loss of muscle, the wound now receives less protein substrate than muscle, and poor healing becomes evident as the body attempts to restore lean body mass before a lethal fall[10] (Fig. 100-3).

TREATMENT

CONTROLLING THE STRESS RESPONSE

It is not necessary that the "stress response" go unchecked. The underlying disease process and the degree and time course of the calorie and protein depletion can be modulated by (1) controlling the source of the stress response and

TABLE 100-1 The Hormonal and Metabolic Response to Burn

	Hormone Levels	Gluconeogenesis	Lipolysis	Proteolysis
Catechols	↑↑↑	↑↑↑	↑↑↑	↑↑
Cortisol	↑↑	↑↑	↓	↑↑
Glucagon	↑	↑↑	—	↑
Insulin	↑	↓	↓	↓↓

DAILY POST INJURY CATABOLISM

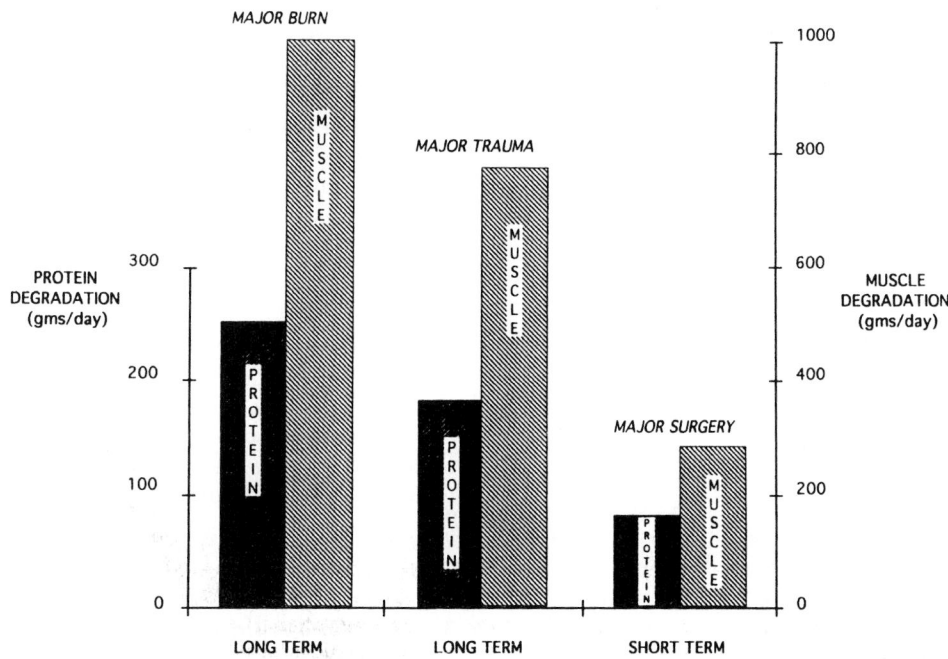

FIGURE 100-2 Daily catabolism following major injury.

(2) increasing the process of anabolism through nutrition, nutritional adjuvants, and increased muscle activity.

The hypermetabolic-catabolic state is driven by the presence of an injury, infection, or ischemia and resulting inflammation. Therefore, control of the source of the systemic response is critical[11] (Table 100-2). Aggressive surgical control of the focus, which is usually devitalized tissue such as burn eschar, is essential to minimize the degree and time course of the response. Both local ischemia and systemic oxygen debt are strong stimuli to continued inflammation and further catechol and cortisol release. The increase in cortisol requirements may not be able to be maintained. Liberal use of analgesics, anxiolytic drugs, and other methods to control psychological stress are required. A relative adrenal insufficiency has been reported with increasing frequency, especially in the elderly burn patient, requiring additional cortisol.[12] A controlled

PRIORITY FOR PROTEIN INTAKE
VS.
LOSS OF LEAN TISSUE

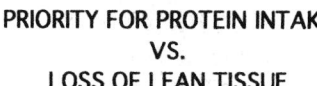

FIGURE 100-3 The wound healing rate progressively decreases as the muscle loss increases.

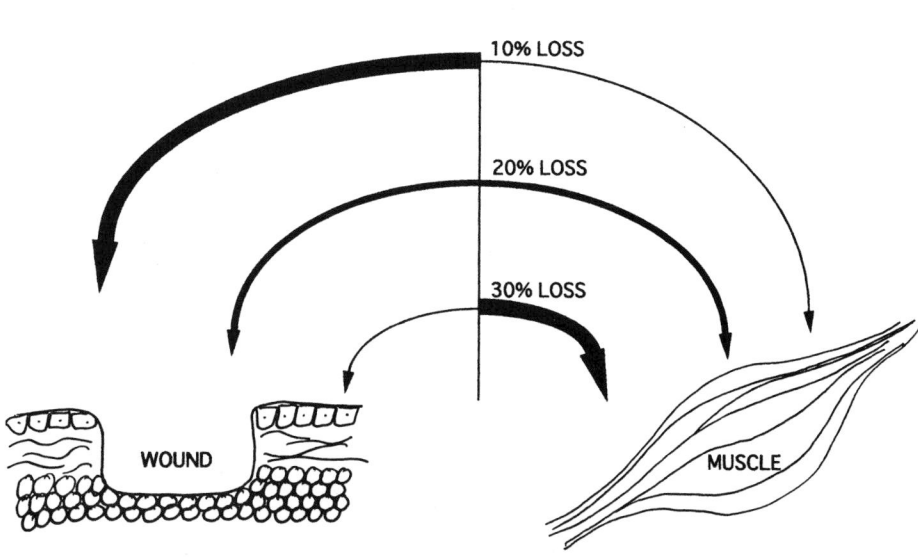

TABLE 100-2 Controlling the Source of the Stress Response

By removing dead tissue, draining infection, and decreasing inflammation and mediator changes in metabolism

By maintaining optimum blood volume thereby avoiding ischemia-induced catechol release

By controlling secondary stresses, e.g., pain, anxiety, which also increase catechol release

β blockade has been shown to decrease the degree of postburn catabolism significantly.[13] Optimizing tissue perfusion is essential.

NUTRITION

It is expected that nutritional support has been started in the early postresuscitation period; however, this support will require adjustment during this period of increasing metabolic activity. The first requirement is an estimation of energy requirements; this is followed by an organized approach to nutrient delivery, tailoring the proportions of carbohydrate, protein, and fat to the individual patient's needs. The use of indirect calorimetry and estimating nutrient needs based on burn size are the most common approaches used.[8,11]

The nutrition support should begin by the end of the resuscitation period. The enteral route is preferred because nutrient utilization clearly is improved over the parenteral route, and the gut integrity is maintained.[11] In general, the caloric requirements for burns of 30% of TBS or greater are 30 to 35 cal/kg per day based on formulas or direct measurements.

Nutrient Mix

Increased *carbohydrate* (CHO) calories (60% of total) are used to try to control the rate of gluconeogenesis, decreasing proteolysis. Excess CHO, however, is deleterious, leading to hyperglycemia, fat formation, and additional carbon dioxide. *Fat* calories (30% of total) are also given. Endogenous fat stores are also used. However, fat will not spare protein loss. Excess fat is also deleterious, being a substrate for immunosuppressive mediators.[11]

Protein Requirements

Protein requirements are two to three times the recommended daily allowance, 1.5 to 2.0 g/kg of body weight per day. The increased protein intake will decrease the net nitrogen (N) losses. Protein supplements usually are necessary to achieve this intake because tube feedings or regular food is not sufficiently protein-rich. Supplements must contain protein of high biologic value, a standard measure of the percentage of the protein amino acids that can be absorbed and used. Egg albumin has a 91% value compared with casein, which is 56% (Table 100-3).

Glutamine, the most common circulatory and intracellular amino acid, is depleted rapidly after a burn and needs to be replaced for glutathione synthesis.[12] Since glutamine represents

TABLE 100-3 Biologic Value of Common Proteins

Protein	Percent of N Retained for Protein Synthesis
Egg albumin	91
Beef muscle	67
Casein	56

over 30% of the amino acid used in catabolism and protein loss exceeds 100 g/d, replacement with 30 to 40 g will attenuate the deficiency state. Soluble glutamine is now available for oral use or via tube feedings (Cambridge Nutraceuticals, Boston, Mass.). Glutamine is also known to stimulate release of human growth hormone, adding to its anticatabolic effects.[13]

Vitamin and Mineral Requirements

Vitamins and minerals are consumed at a rapid rate and should be given at a dose of 10 times the Recommended Daily Allowance (RDA).[11] Well-accepted daily doses include vitamin A, 10,000 to 15,000 units; vitamin C, 1 g; vitamin E, 500 to 1000 IU; selenium 100 μg; carotene 50 mg; and zinc sulfate, 220 mg bid.

Use of Anabolic Agents

Increasing the patient's anabolic activity has been shown to further attenuate net catabolism[15,16] during the stress phase and to increase muscle restoration in the recovery phase. Currently, only two agents are available—human growth hormone and the testosterone analog oxandrolone.

HUMAN GROWTH HORMONE   This agent has been shown to increase healing rate, muscle mass, nitrogen retention, and survival in burn patients when given parenterally in doses of 5 to 10 times that normally produced (0.8 mg/d).[14] The major complication is hyperglycemia.

OXANDROLONE (OXANDRIN)   Oxandrolone, a 17-hydroxyl-17-methyl ester of testosterone, is the anabolic steroid that is approved by the Food and Drug Administration (FDA) for restoration of muscle loss after severe trauma, burns or major surgical procedures, or infections.[17] The anabolic effect is primarily on muscle (or lean body mass).[15,16]

Clinical trials on a variety of burn patient populations from children to the elderly have demonstrated significant decrease in lean mass loss during the catabolic state and a marked increase in the rate of lean mass restoration. Oxandrolone (BTG Pharmaceuticals, Iselin, New Jersey) is the only steroid in which a carbon atom in the phenanthrene nucleus has been replaced by another element, namely, oxygen. This alteration appears to be responsible for its potent anabolic activity—5 to 10 times that of methyl testosterone. In addition, its androgenic effect is considerably less than testosterone, thereby minimizing the complication of excess androgen activity common to other testosterone derivatives. The drug is given orally with 99% bioavailability. It is protein-bound in plasma with a biologic half-life of 9 hours. The compound is excreted unchanged primarily by the kidney with minimal hepatic metabolism and therefore results in minimal to no hepatic toxicity. No significant complications have been reported.

INFECTION AND SEPSIS

Sepsis is the leading cause of morbidity and mortality during this period. The most common sites of infection in the burn patient are the lungs, the burn wound, and vascular catheters.[18] Intraabdominal processes, in particular, cholecystitis, are uncommon but are well recognized as sources of sepsis in critically ill patients.

Appropriate antibiotic dosing is a crucial aspect of management. Because of the hypermetabolic state, as well as the loss of antibiotics from the wound, the burn patient generally requires a larger total antibiotic dose and increased frequency

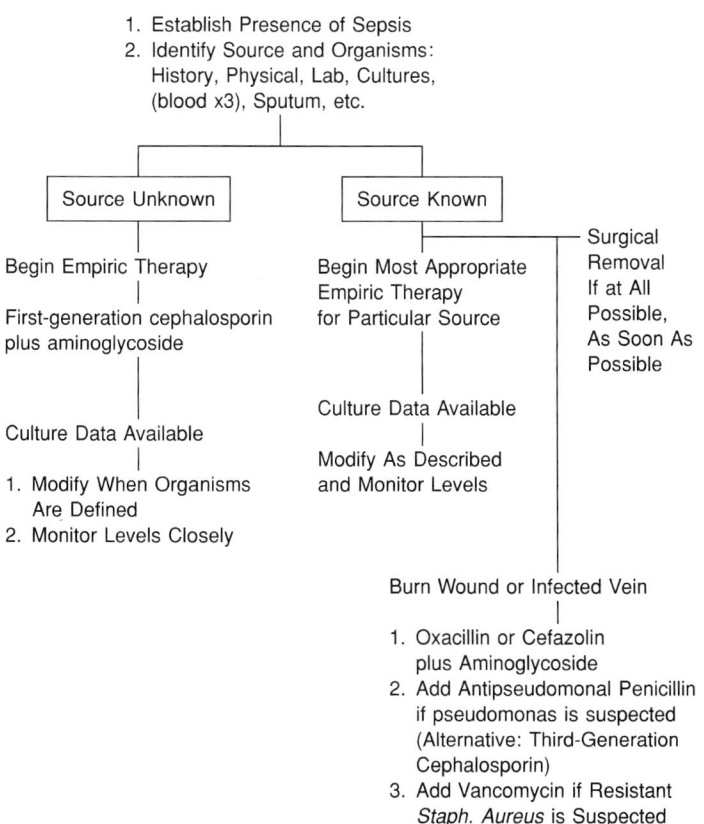

1. Establish Presence of Sepsis
2. Identify Source and Organisms:
   History, Physical, Lab, Cultures,
   (blood x3), Sputum, etc.

Source Unknown

Begin Empiric Therapy

First-generation cephalosporin
plus aminoglycoside

Culture Data Available

1. Modify When Organisms
   Are Defined
2. Monitor Levels Closely

Source Known

Begin Most Appropriate
Empiric Therapy
for Particular Source

Culture Data Available

Modify As Described
and Monitor Levels

Surgical
Removal
If at All
Possible,
As Soon As
Possible

Burn Wound or Infected Vein

1. Oxacillin or Cefazolin
   plus Aminoglycoside
2. Add Antipseudomonal Penicillin
   if pseudomonas is suspected
   (Alternative: Third-Generation
   Cephalosporin)
3. Add Vancomycin if Resistant
   Staph. Aureus is Suspected
4. Consider Candida (or Other Fungi)
   and Need for Amphotericin

FIGURE 100-4 Approach to the burn patient with sepsis.

of doses to maintain adequate levels. This increased requirement is well documented for the aminoglycosides. Renal impairment may mandate lower doses. Monitoring antibiotic levels is the only valid approach to the use of systemic antibiotics in major burn patients.

Because of the immunocompromised nature of the burn patient, as well as the use of topical and systemic antibiotics, fungal sepsis—especially caused by *Candida albicans*—is relatively common. The prodrome is often more subtle than with other microorganisms, with patients appearing more chronically ill and just "not doing well."

As with any form of sepsis, the removal or control of the septic focus is of primary importance. Débridement should be performed gently to unroof pockets of infection and allow for better local wound and topical antibiotic care. Large excisions often are poorly tolerated during this period because of dissemination of infection and blood loss.[18] The approach to infection is summarized in Fig. 100-4.

References

1. Sheridan R, Ryan C, Yin L, et al: Death in the burn unit: Sterile multiple organ failure. *Burns* 24:307, 1998.
2. Park G, Park J, Jeong D, Jeong S: Prolonged airway and systemic inflammatory reactions after smoke inhalation. *Chest* 123:473, 2003.
3. Wilkinson R, Fishman J: Effect of thermal injury with *Pseudomonas aeruginosa* infection on pulmonary and systemic bacterial clearance. *J Trauma* 47:912, 1999.
4. Murphy K, Lee J, Herndon D: Current pharmacotherapy for the treatment of severe burns. *Exp Opin Pharmacother* 4:369, 2003.
5. Tredget E, Yu Y: The metabolic effects of thermal injury. *World J Surg* 16:68, 1992.
6. Dickerson R: Estimating energy and protein requirements of thermally injured patients: Art or science. *Nutrition* 18:439, 2002.
7. Cumming J, Purdue G, Hunt J, O'Keefe G: Objective estimates of the incidence and consequences of multiple organ dysfunction and sepsis after burn trauma. *J Trauma* 50:510, 2001.
8. Wray C, Mammen J, Hasselgren P: Catabolic response to stress and potential benefits of nutrition support. *Nutrition* 18:971, 2002.
9. Hasselgren P: Catabolic response to stress and injury: Implications for regulation. *World J Surg* 29:1452, 2002.
10. Moore FD: *Metabolic Care of the Surgical Patient.* Philadelphia, Saunders, 1959.
11. Hart D, Wolf S, Chinkes D, et al: Effect of early excision and aggressive enteral feeding on hypermetabolism, catabolism and sepsis after severe burn. *J Trauma* 54:755, 2003.
12. Bershwizen A, Thijs L: Relative adrenal failure in intensive care: An identifiable problem requiring treatment. *J Clin Endocrinol Metab* 15:513, 2001.
13. Herndon DN, Hart DW, Wolfe SE, et al: Reveral of catabolism by beta-blockade after severe burns. *New Engl J Med* 345:1223, 2001.
14. Lai S, Wolf S, Herndon D: Growth hormone, burns and tissue healing. *Growth Horm IGF Res* 10:39, 2002.
15. Demling R, DeSanti L: The beneficial effects of the anabolic steroid oxandrolone in the geriatric burn population. *Wound* 15:54, 2003.
16. Demling R, DeSanti L: Oxandrolone, an anabolic steroid significantly increases the rate of weight gain in the recovery phase after major burns. *J Trauma* 43:47, 1997.
17. Fox M, Minor A: Oxandrolone: A potent anabolic steroid. *J Clin Endocrinol Metab* 22:21, 1962.
18. Heggers J, Hawkins H, Edgar P: Treatment of infection in burns, in Herndon D (ed): *Total Burn Care,* 2d ed. London, Elsevier, 2002, p 120.

Chapter 101

INTERVENTIONAL RADIOLOGY

JENNIFER E. GOULD
DANIEL PICUS

KEY POINTS

- *Availability of appropriately trained interventional radiologists is an important component of ICU patient care.*
- *Interventional radiologic techniques may be prophylactic (e.g., use of vena caval interruption to prevent pulmonary embolism), diagnostic (e.g., angiography in gastrointestinal hemorrhage), or therapeutic (e.g., drainage of abscess, control of gastrointestinal hemorrhage through embolotherapy or vasoconstrictor infusion, creation of transjugular intrahepatic portosystemic shunts [TIPS], or retrieval of a foreign body).*
- *Interventional radiologic techniques are as effective as many open surgical techniques but carry lower morbidity and mortality in the ICU patient.*
- *Interventional radiologic techniques should be considered in ICU patients when the risk of more invasive procedures is greater and the outcome is not predictably better.*
- *Appropriate ICU monitoring devices and support systems (oxygen, suction, ventilation, ICU-type personnel) must be available in the radiology suite for safe management of ICU patients.*

Interventional radiology encompasses a wide variety of percutaneous procedures that use one or more imaging modalities to guide the placement of needles, guidewires, and catheters. The choice of fluoroscopy, ultrasound (US), and/or computed tomography (CT) depends on the patient, the clinical circumstances, and the procedure. Many of these procedures are performed as an alternative or adjunct to surgery because they are less invasive and carry a lower overall morbidity and mortality as compared with the comparable surgical intervention. This fact is particularly important in ICU patients, who frequently are poor surgical candidates and for whom procedures carry a higher-than-average risk owing to associated comorbidities. Furthermore, while many surgical procedures require general anesthesia or deep conscious sedation, interventional radiology procedures typically can be performed with mild to moderate levels of conscious sedation and/or local anesthesia, further reducing the risk, the length of the procedure, and the need to consult the anesthesiology service for assistance.

When and Where to Perform the Procedure

Deciding when and where to perform an interventional radiologic procedure is often a difficult decision requiring close communication and cooperation between the critical care and interventional staffs. The interventional radiologist should be consulted early to allow adequate time for a meaningful exchange between the two services.

In general, working with "stable" patients is preferable, although not always possible. In certain situations, it is better to proceed with an examination despite patient instability. For instance, in a patient with gastrointestinal (GI) bleeding, instability may indicate active bleeding, and immediate angiography during ongoing bleeding is necessary to identify the source. If the patient is stabilized first, the opportunity to locate the bleeding site may be lost. Nevertheless, despite the need for prompt treatment, the appropriate venous lines, oxygen support, monitoring devices, and fluid resuscitation and blood product administration should be initiated prior to any interventional procedure.

The risks in complex interventional procedures are minimized and the success enhanced when the patient is transported to the special procedures suite. Although CT and US are useful for some nonvascular procedures, fluoroscopic guidance is required for all vascular interventions and many nonvascular procedures. Portable fluoroscopy units are available in most ICUs, but these units have several disadvantages. They are cumbersome to use, have no radiographic shielding, and restrict imaging to a small area of the body.

A few interventional procedures can be performed at the bedside with US guidance. US units are mobile, inexpensive, and allow cross-sectional imaging. This particular approach is useful for straightforward percutaneous procedures such as fluid aspiration, abscess drainage, biopsy, or cholecystostomy tube insertion. The limitations of US guidance include the need for direct contact between the US transducer and the skin and the need for a "window" without intervening bowel gas, bone, surgical dressings, or open wounds.

Despite the ability of US to provide portable guidance, many biopsies and drainage procedures preferably are performed with CT. CT provides a detailed display of the entire fluid collection and its relationship to surrounding structures, allowing precise planning of the safest percutaneous access route. Oral and intravenous contrast agents can be administered in circumstances that require differentiation among a fluid collection, bowel, and nearby vascular structures. Unlike US, CT is not limited by overlying dressings, wounds, or ostomy devices.

Preprocedure Evaluation and Preparation

It is necessary to obtain coagulation parameters prior to most interventions. The risk of procedure related hemorrhage is reduced when laboratory prothrombin time (PT) and platelet counts are within the normal reference ranges. In emergent situations, a PT of less than 20 seconds (International Normalization Ratio [INR] < 3.0) and a platelet count greater than 50,000/μL are acceptable for most vascular procedures. In nonvascular procedures, a PT of less than 16 seconds (INR <2.0) and a platelet count greater than 100,000/μL generally are required. If an emergent procedure is needed and the PT is elevated, fresh frozen plasma should be administered. When platelet counts are low, platelet transfusions can be administered just prior to the procedure to raise values to an acceptable level. Heparin infusions should be discontinued 2 to 4 hours before procedures. For emergent vascular studies, an arterial sheath can be left in place and subsequently removed when PT values decrease to acceptable levels.

An estimated 5% to 12% of patients receiving high-osmolality contrast agents and 0.5% to 3.0% of patients receiving newer low-osmolality contrast agents experience some type of acute adverse reaction. In patients at high risk for iodinated contrast anaphylaxis (asthma, severe allergies, or history of a previous reaction to a contrast agent), when possible, corticosteroid premedication should be administered to prevent or reduce the severity of any potential reaction. Prednisone 50 mg orally (or its equivalent intravenous dose) may be administered every 6 hours starting at least 12 hours (optimally 24 to 36 hours) before the procedure.[1]

Many patients in the ICU suffer from acute and/or chronic renal failure. Intravascular contrast agents are excreted renally, and therefore, adequate renal function is necessary to reduce the risk of contrast nephropathy. This risk cannot be overemphasized because radiocontrast nephropathy is associated with prolonged hospitalizations and higher rates of morbidity and in-hospital mortality.

There is no absolute creatinine value above which contrast agents should not be administered, but the risk of contrast nephropathy is increased in the setting of impaired renal function (serum creatinine > 1.5 mg/dL), diabetes mellitus, age over 60 years, dehydration, multiple myeloma, concomitant nephrotoxic medication administration, severe hypertension or cardiovascular disease, hyperuricemia, use of high-osmolar contrast agents, use of large volumes of contrast material in a short time period, or recent exposure to a large contrast load. Intravascular contrast administration typically is contraindicated in renal failure patients for whom renal function is expected to return unless evaluation of a life-threatening problem necessitates proceeding in spite of the risk of temporary or permanent renal dysfunction.

If a contrast study is necessary, hydration before and after the procedure and the use of low-osmolality contrast agents are the most important factors in reducing the rate of nephrotoxicity.[1a] Recently, investigative work has centered on use of two drugs to preserve renal function. Several studies have documented a reduction in the rise in creatinine levels and an increase in creatinine clearance with the use of oral or intravenous *N*-acetylcysteine in patients with stable moderate renal insufficiency.[2,3] Unfortunately, the results with this agent have been mixed, and some data suggest that it may be useful only for subsets of patients with lesser degrees of renal dysfunction who receive low to moderate doses of contrast material.[4]

Another agent undergoing active investigation is fenoldopam, a selective dopamine receptor agonist with renoprotective properties. Fenoldopam is administered by continuous IV infusion before, during, and after the procedure and is titrated to blood pressure. Although results have been mixed, some researchers have documented preservation of renal blood flow as well as lower rates of creatinine elevation and renal failure than hydration alone.[5–7]

In addition, several interventional radiology procedures can be performed with alternative contrast agents that reduce the amount of intravascular contrast material required or eliminate the need for it altogether. Carbon dioxide and gadolinium each have been used successfully in insertion of inferior vena caval filters.[6–8] Transjugular intrahepatic portosystemic shunts (TIPS), which typically use carbon dioxide for transhepatic retrograde portal venography, also have been created successfully with carbon dioxide alone.

Carbon dioxide gas is an effective negative contrast agent that displaces the blood volume during injection and then is excreted rapidly from the lungs through respiration.[8,9] This agent is particularly useful because it has no dose limitations and no allergic reactions and is of low cost. Unfortunately, it usually is injected by hand, and contamination by room air must be avoided. Carbon dioxide is contraindicated for arteriography of the thoracic aorta, cerebral arteries, or upper extremity arteries owing to the risk of neurologic symptoms from "vapor lock," which can obstruct flow within a vessel and cause distal ischemia.

Gadolinium, typically known for its use in magnetic resonance imaging (MRI), can be used in high doses for fluoroscopic vascular imaging and some genitourinary and biliary procedures. Its use is limited by the maximal approved dose (0.3 to 0.4 mmol/kg), its high expense, and its poor radiopacity. However, its safety profile is high for all vascular applications, and it has low rates of nephrotoxicity and anaphylaxis. It is used typically in conjunction with carbon dioxide, and in some cases it can be mixed with iodinated contrast agents to reduce the dose of iodinated agents administered.[10–12]

Monitoring the Patient in Interventional Radiology

Interventional suites should simulate the ICU environment to allow close patient monitoring during all procedures.

EQUIPMENT

All interventional radiology suites should be equipped with basic patient monitoring equipment, including electrocardiography (ECG), noninvasive blood pressure monitoring devices (preferably automated), and pulse oximetry devices. Pulse oximetry is useful for documenting a patient's baseline respiratory status and monitoring the effects of sedation with narcotic analgesics. It is also useful to have devices that record hemodynamic information. A standard emergency "crash" cart, defibrillator, and backboard always should be available for cardiopulmonary resuscitation, and all special procedure suites should be equipped with a reliable source of oxygen and suction.

PERSONNEL

ICU patients require constant nursing care while in the interventional suite. Most radiology departments employ nurses who are specially trained to care for patients during special procedures. However, the ICU patient generally has particular needs, and an ICU-trained nurse who can provide continuity of care should accompany the patient to the radiology department and be responsible for monitoring the patient, recording vital signs, and administering medications.

In general, an ICU physician need not accompany patients to the interventional radiology suite. However, this decision depends on the patient's condition and the complexity of the procedure and should be made on a case-by-case basis.

Nonvascular Interventional Radiology Procedures

PERCUTANEOUS ABSCESS DRAINAGE (PAD)

INDICATIONS AND PATIENT SELECTION

Fever in ICU patients is very common. Abscess formation, particularly in postoperative patients, is frequently the cause. Although small abscesses often respond to antibiotics alone, larger collections are best treated with drainage—especially when symptoms such as sepsis, pain, and/or visceral compression are present. In the past 10 to 15 years, percutaneous abscess drainage (PAD) has all but replaced surgical drainage as the treatment of choice for abscesses and other problematic fluid collections (e.g., biloma, urinoma).[13,14] PAD is less invasive and maintains the integrity of surrounding structures and overlying skin, thus reducing morbidity and saving time and expense. PAD also makes nursing care easier because drainage systems are closed, and there is no extensive surgical wound or need for frequent dressing changes. Drainage of sterile collections typically is not necessary unless there is a concern for infection or the collection is causing symptoms such as pain or visceral compression.

PAD is most successful when the fluid collection is well defined, unilocular, and free flowing (Fig. 101-1 *A − C*). These characteristics are found in more than 90% of intraabdominal collections. PAD also may be helpful in less favorable situations (e.g., multilocular, necrotic debris), particularly when the patient is a high surgical risk. In such circumstances, PAD may improve the patient's condition so that a more definitive surgical drainage can be performed later. The only absolute contraindication to PAD is the lack of a safe access route. This rarely is a problem when CT guidance is used. Fluid collections deep within the pelvis may require transrectal or transvaginal drainage routes using special ultrasound probes for guidance.

TECHNIQUE

The most important step in PAD is planning the access route. This is done following review of all the pertinent imaging studies. In general, the shortest, straightest tract is the best approach, but care must be taken to avoid adjacent bowel, pleura, and major blood vessels.

Antibiotics selected to cover the likely microorganisms should be initiated as soon as an abscess is suspected by imaging and always prior to intervention because manipulation of the cavity and its contents may result in bacteremia or spillage into sterile cavities.

Diagnostic aspiration sometimes is performed first with a 20- to 22-gauge needle. The position of the needle is confirmed with US or CT, and the fluid is aspirated for culture and diagnosis. A small volume of contrast material can be injected to define the cavity. If the decision is made to drain the fluid, the collection can be accessed and drained using either an over-the-wire (Seldinger) or trocar (one-step) technique. The size of the drain ranges from 10F to 20F and depends on the type and viscosity of fluid obtained on aspiration. The catheter is then secured to the skin with a suture, allowing easy access for local skin care and reducing the risk of tube dislodgment.

When the catheter is in place, the collection may be aspirated completely, and the catheter is then connected to gravity drainage. When subsequent drainage has decreased, follow-up imaging should be obtained to ensure complete evacuation. If residual fluid or additional loculated collections are identified and drainage is incomplete, repositioning the catheter or placing a second drain may be necessary. For complex collections, dilute streptokinase or tissue-type plasminogen activator (t-PA) may be instilled into the cavity to chemically disrupt loculations and optimize drainage. Typically, percutaneously placed catheters are left to gravity drainage, but on occasion, they are connected to low intermittent suction. With empyema or infected intrathoracic collections, the drainage catheters are placed to Pleurovac or water-seal suction devices identical to standard thoracostomy tubes.

IMMEDIATE POSTPROCEDURE CARE

The output of the drainage catheter should be monitored and recorded carefully. The catheter is left in place as long as it continues to drain, which usually requires 3 to 10 days, although longer periods may be necessary for large or complicated collections or when a fistula is present. Antibiotic coverage should be modified after culture and sensitivity results are obtained from the initial aspirate.

Percutaneous catheters are irrigated only when material is too viscous to drain spontaneously. When necessary, it should be done with 5- to 10-mL aliquots of sterile saline. Fluid should be injected into the catheter and then allowed to drain on its own. Vigorous suction generally draws debris into the catheter that can obstruct the lumen. If the catheter occludes, fails to drain easily, or drains significantly around the tube, it may need to be exchanged for a larger one. This is a relatively quick and simple procedure but does require fluoroscopic guidance. When a culture-proved sterile collection is encountered, early tube removal is warranted to prevent secondary infection.

Once effective drainage has been established, the patient's condition should improve within 24 to 48 hours. Incomplete drainage should be suspected when the patient remains febrile or the white blood cell count remains elevated. In these cases, follow-up CT should be obtained promptly and additional drainage catheters placed as needed. If the drainage first tapers and then increases abruptly, a fistula may be present. Injection of contrast media through the catheter under fluoroscopic observation usually demonstrates the communication. When a fistula is present, PAD can still be successful but may require extended drainage with complete bowel rest. If present, obstruction distal to the fistula also should be corrected.

RESULTS AND COMPLICATIONS

PAD compares favorably with surgical treatment in overall success, duration of drainage, and recurrence rates.[13] Between 70% and 90% success rates have been reported and depend on abscess location and complexity, patient immunocompetency, and subsequent fistula formation. Failed or prolonged PAD is caused most often by an unrecognized fistula or an undrained collection. Premature withdrawal of the drainage catheter or attempts at draining a relatively solid collection (e.g., necrotic tumor, pancreatic phlegmon) are also causes of failed PAD.

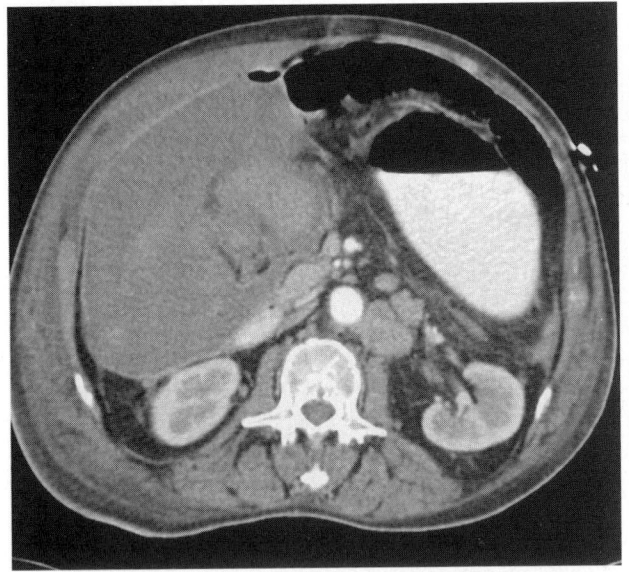

A

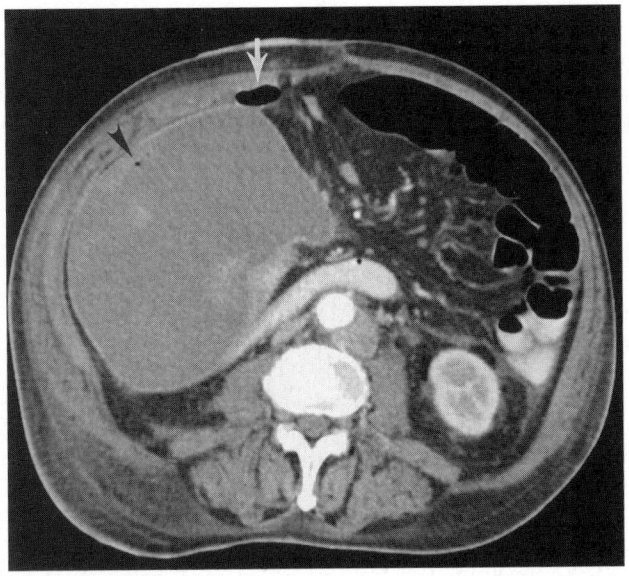

B

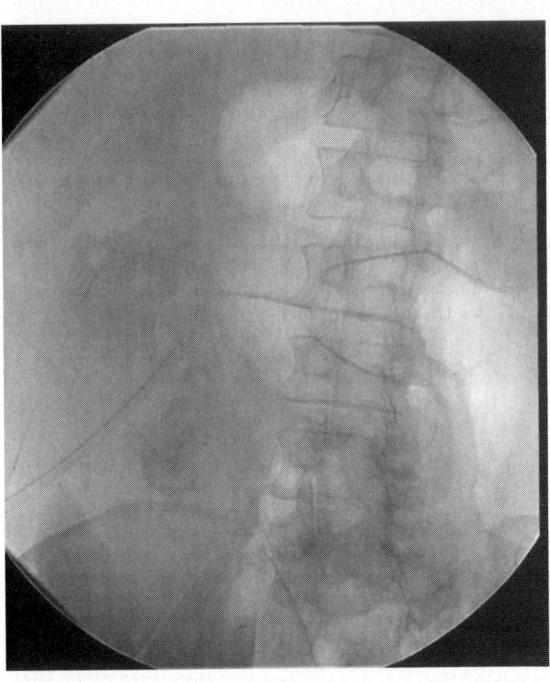

C

FIGURE 101-1 This patient was status post total colectomy and ileostomy and developed fevers and an elevated white blood cell count. *A, B*. CT demonstrates a large, well-defined, rim-enhancing collection in the right abdomen with high-density contents suggesting a postoperative hematoma. Foci of gas within the collection (*black arrowhead*) and small amounts of peritoneal gas (*white arrow*) are of concern for anastomotic dehiscence or bowel perforation. Thickening and edema in the right abdominal wall soft tissues suggest cellulitis as well. *C*. Fluoroscopic image showing large-diameter drainage catheter insertion.

Overall complication rates for PAD range from 10% to 15%, with serious complications accounting for less than 5% of cases.[13,14] Minor complications include transient bacteremia, skin infection, and minor bleeding. Major complications include hemorrhage requiring transfusion, sepsis, and bowel perforation. The recurrence rate following PAD is approximately 5%. These statistics compare favorably with the surgical literature, which reports mortality rates of 10% to 20% and recurrence rates of 15 to 30%.

PERCUTANEOUS CHOLECYSTOSTOMY

INDICATIONS AND PATIENT SELECTION

Elective cholecystectomy in an otherwise healthy patient is a safe procedure with an operative mortality rate of less than 0.5%. Morbidity and mortality rates increase dramatically in ICU patients with multiorgan compromise, sepsis, diabetes, and/or immunosuppression and in the elderly. Historically, critically ill patients have been treated with operative cholecystostomy until they were stable enough to undergo elective cholecystectomy.

Percutaneous cholecystostomy has emerged as an alternative to standard surgical therapy.[15–19] A very important advantage to the newer approach is that it can be done at the patient's bedside without an incision using only local anesthesia.

Indications for percutaneous cholecystostomy include acute calculus or acalculous cholecystitis in a patient who is too ill to withstand surgical cholecystectomy. In calculous disease, the gallbladder can be removed electively when the patient's condition stabilizes. An alternative to operative cholecystectomy is percutaneous stone removal or dissolution therapy via the existing cholecystostomy tract. This is especially useful in patients who remain poor surgical candidates after transfer from the ICU.[11]

Acute acalculous cholecystitis is increasingly recognized in ICU patients. Its diagnosis is difficult to establish despite the use of US. US is extremely accurate in identifying cholelithiasis but is less reliable in diagnosing acute acalculous cholecystitis, with reported accuracy rates of 50% to 60% (Fig. 101-2*A − C*). Nuclear medicine hepatobiliary scans are useful in evaluating cystic duct patency, but false-positive rates are in the range of 25% to 30%. Generalized hepatocellular dysfunction, prolonged total parenteral nutrition, sepsis, and fasting all predispose to false-positive hepatobiliary scans.

In patients with acalculous cholecystitis, percutaneous cholecystostomy can confirm the diagnosis and serve as definitive therapy. Prompt decompression can result in dramatic symptomatic relief. Typically, the cystic duct opens eventually, allowing tube removal without requiring a formal cholecystectomy.

TECHNIQUE

In unstable patients, percutaneous cholecystostomy can be done at the patient's bedside with portable US guidance. Transhepatic access to the gallbladder is preferred to decrease the risk of bile spillage into the peritoneal cavity. A 22-gauge needle is advanced into the gallbladder, and bile is aspirated (see Fig. 101-2*D*). Since Gram stain and culture results of the bile are helpful but not sensitive (30% to 50%), a cholecystostomy tube is inserted at the time of initial aspiration. Negative Gram stain and cultures do not exclude the diagnosis of acute cholecystitis. After aspiration, either a Seldinger or a trocar technique can be used to place a retention catheter for drainage (see Fig. 101-2*E*, *F*). If the procedure is guided by fluoroscopy, contrast agent injection is used to confirm catheter position. Care should be taken not to overdistend an acutely inflamed gallbladder.

IMMEDIATE POSTPROCEDURE CARE

Catheters are left to drain by gravity. When the cystic duct is obstructed, the gallbladder normally produces 50 to 70 mL of clear mucus daily. Larger volumes of bilious drainage indicate cystic duct patency. Very large volumes persisting may indicate common duct obstruction as well.

After the patient's condition stabilizes, the cholecystostomy tube is injected under fluoroscopy to evaluate for stones in the gallbladder, cystic duct, or common bile duct. If no stones are seen and contrast material flows freely into the duodenum, the tube can be capped and subsequently removed as early as 10 to 14 days following placement, when a mature tract has formed.

RESULTS AND COMPLICATIONS

Percutaneous cholecystostomy placement is technically successful in over 95% of patients.[18] In a study by Boland and colleagues,[19] approximately 60% of patients demonstrated clinical improvement following cholecystostomy in the setting of sepsis with suggestive US findings of a gallbladder source. Interestingly, up to 20% to 30% of patients will not have acute cholecystitis. This confirms the difficulty in diagnosing acute cholecystitis in critically ill patients. Percutaneous cholecystostomy still is helpful in these patients because it excludes the diagnosis of acute cholecystitis and avoids unnecessary surgery.

With proper technique, complications are few. Bile peritonitis is avoided by decompressing the gallbladder rapidly through the transhepatic route and by carefully performing cholangiography with fluoroscopic guidance. Sepsis, hemobilia, and vagal reactions all have been reported in less than 5% of patients.

PERCUTANEOUS NEPHROSTOMY

INDICATIONS AND PATIENT SELECTION

Percutaneous nephrostomy (PCN) is a standard interventional radiologic procedure.[20] Obstruction of the renal collecting system can be secondary to any number of causes ranging from stone disease to malignancy. ICU patients with fever and documented urinary tract obstruction are at high risk for pyonephrosis and urosepsis. In these situations, percutaneous nephrostomy can be a lifesaving procedure. Percutaneous drainage has become the treatment of choice for initial decompression of an infected collecting system, whatever the underlying etiology. Surgical alternatives are used only rarely in the treatment of renal infection. PCN is safe, but for critically ill patients on ventilators, placing them in the prone position can be difficult.

An obstructed collection system can be diagnosed by any number of imaging modalities. US is portable and readily identifies hydronephrosis (Fig. 101-3*A*, *B*). It is a good first-choice examination, especially when the patient's creatinine concentration is elevated and a genitourinary source is suspected. When the source of underlying sepsis is uncertain, CT evaluation may identify unsuspected hydronephrosis. Although contrast administration is preferable, it is not mandatory for diagnosing an obstructed system.

In patients with urosepsis/pyonephrosis, PCN can confirm the diagnosis and act as the initial therapy until the patient is stabilized (see Fig. 101-3*C*). Prompt decompression can result in rapid improvement in the patient's overall condition, and in some cases (e.g., fungal infection), medication can be infused into the collecting system as part of a therapeutic regimen. When renal calculi are present, the nephrostomy tract ultimately can be used for percutaneous nephrolithotomy after the initial infection has resolved. In this latter situation, care must be taken in placement of an appropriate access site for subsequent tract dilatation and stone removal.

TECHNIQUE

PCN insertion preferably is done in the interventional suite with the patient placed in the prone or semiprone position. Preprocedure antibiotics aimed at treating typical infectious organisms are necessary. As with other nonvascular interventional radiology procedures, the renal collecting system is accessed initially with a 22-gauge needle under US guidance, and fluid is aspirated for microbiologic evaluation. Contrast material and air are then instilled into the collecting system, and a posterior calyx is chosen and accessed with an 18-gauge needle. A guidewire is then advanced into the system, the tract is dilated, and a self-retaining drain is positioned into the renal pelvis. Aspirated samples are sent routinely for microbiologic studies. Contrast agent injection is

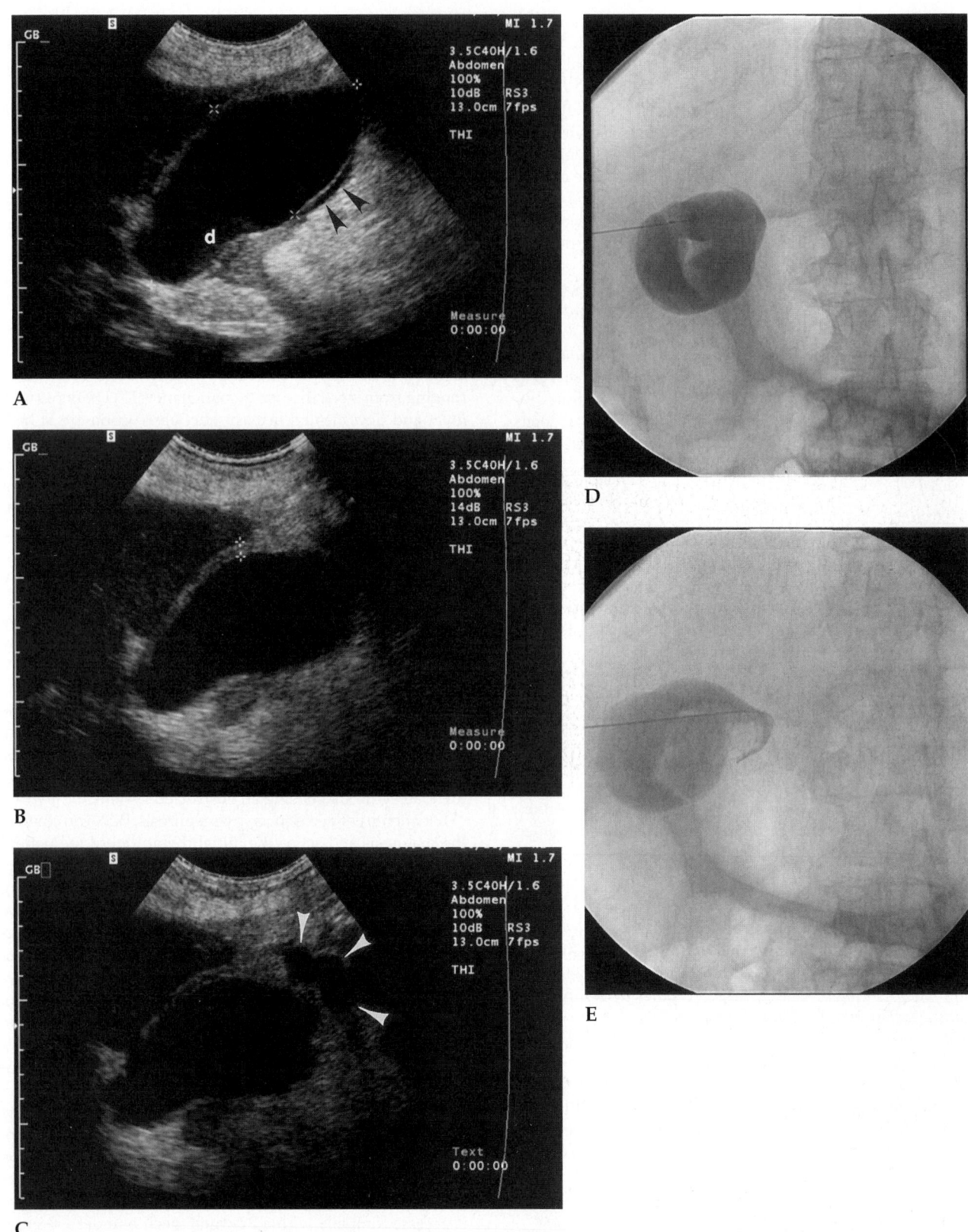

FIGURE 101-2 This elderly woman recently underwent endoscopic removal of a common bile duct stone. Owing to continued symptoms, an ultrasound was obtained. *A.* Sonographic imaging demonstrates an enlarged, distended gallbladder with a small amount of pericholecystic fluid (*black arrowheads*) and echogenic debris (*d*) but no calculi. *B.* Gallbladder wall thickening is present (normal < 3 mm). The wall measures 5.9 mm. *C.* A small inflammatory fluid collection is present adjacent to the gallbladder (*white arrowheads*). Under US, a needle was inserted into the gallbladder. *D.* Fluoroscopy of contrast injection reveals filling of the gallbladder with no filling of the cystic duct, indicating cystic duct obstruction. Using a Seldinger technique, (*E*) a guidewire was coiled within the gallbadder, and

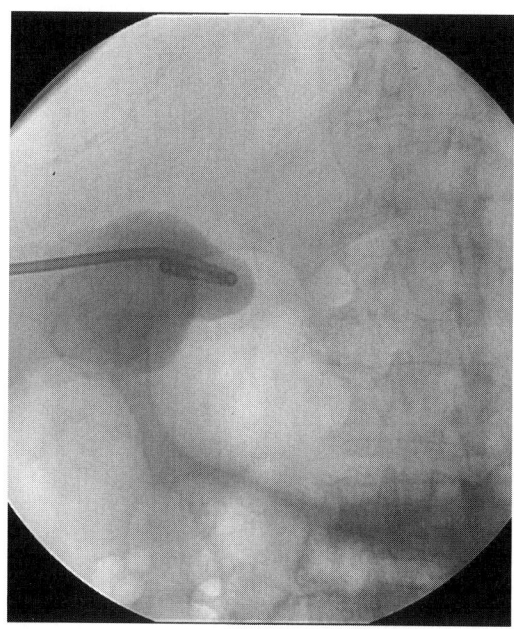

F

FIGURE 101-2 (Continued) (*F*) a locking-loop catheter was inserted.

mandatory to confirm tube placement, and drainage is then left to gravity. In pyonephrosis or suspected infection, manipulations should be minimized to prevent bacteremia/sepsis.

IMMEDIATE POSTPROCEDURE CARE

Daily fluid input and urine and PCN output should be recorded. Tube output should reflect the output of the kidney drained. In patients with infection, broad-spectrum antibiotics should be continued and tailored to the offending organism when culture and sensitivity reports are available.

When the patient stabilizes, the fever resolves, and the white blood cell count returns to normal, a formal nephrostogram should be done to identify the cause of the obstruction. External decompression should be continued until the infection clears and obstruction is relieved. In cases of stone disease, either extracorporeal shock wave lithotrypsy or percutaneous nephrolithotomy can be performed as the definitive procedure. In patients with ureteral obstruction relating to neoplastic, inflammatory, or iatrogenic causes, an internal ureteral stent may be inserted to restore antegrade flow to the bladder. In situations when internal stenting is not feasible or practical, external drainage can be continued indefinitely.

RESULTS AND COMPLICATIONS

Technical success for emergent PCN placement is in excess of 95%.[20] This is particularly true when a dilated collecting system is encountered.

Major complications of percutaneous nephrostomy insertion are uncommon, with urosepsis, hydro/pneumothorax, and hemorrhage requiring transfusion occurring in less than 6% of patients.[16] Urosepsis is minimized by limiting catheter manipulation after the urinary system is accessed. A pneumothorax is a rare complication (<1%) that occurs most commonly when the route of entry is above the eleventh or twelfth rib.

Vascular Interventional Radiology Procedures

GI BLEEDING: DIAGNOSIS AND TREATMENT

Interventional radiology plays an important role in the diagnosis and treatment of GI bleeding.[21-36] The overall management of GI hemorrhage is discussed elsewhere (see Chap. 82). This section will focus on angiographic localization and treatment of upper and lower GI bleeding.

INDICATIONS AND PATIENT SELECTION

GI bleeding typically occurs intermittently, not continuously. Angiography should be performed during active bleeding because often the only angiographic abnormality to guide treatment is the presence of contrast agent extravasation. Unfortunately, the clinical determination of active bleeding can be difficult. A decline in the hematocrit reflects previous bleeding, and large quantities of blood can accumulate within the intestines and slowly be expelled over hours following a bleeding event. Therefore, hemodynamic parameters such as tachycardia and hypotension often are the most accurate indicators of *active* bleeding.

Fortunately, the widespread use of endoscopy and nuclear medicine bleeding scans has improved the ability to document active bleeding and localize the source. Endoscopy should be the initial diagnostic modality in the workup of GI hemorrhage, particularly in the upper tract where it also may be therapeutic. Even if the source is not visualized, secondary findings usually can confirm the presence of active bleeding.

Nuclear medicine bleeding scans with technetium-labeled red blood cells are most useful in the evaluation of bleeding distal to the ligament of Treitz. Radionuclide studies can confirm active bleeding and localize intermittent lower intestinal hemorrhage because the radiopharmaceutical can be monitored for up to 24 hours. These studies are noninvasive and can be performed portably in the ICU. Angiography, on the other hand, is an invasive test that requires transport to the special procedures suite. For diagnosis, there must be active bleeding during the 10-second angiographic injection at a rate sufficient for detection. It is estimated that a bleeding rate of at least 0.5 mL/min is needed for angiographic visualization, whereas a rate of only 0.1 mL/min is required for radionuclide localization.

Preprocedure assessment includes confirmation of probable active bleeding and an estimation of the rate and severity of the bleeding. It is important to document the presence of known cardiovascular disease that would preclude vasoconstrictor administration and establish if there is a history of intestinal or intraabdominal vascular surgeries that may have altered the vascular anatomy. Resuscitation with blood products should be ongoing. In particular, accurate assessment of the coagulation profile is necessary because all endovascular therapies rely on normal coagulation to form a stable clot. A treatment plan should be selected prior to angiography, and surgical consultation should be sought early because failure

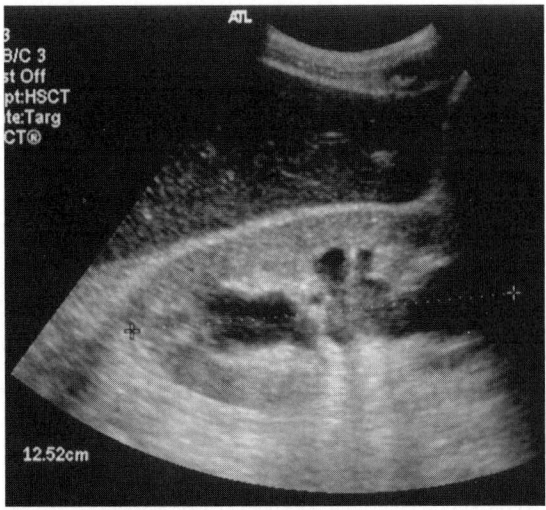

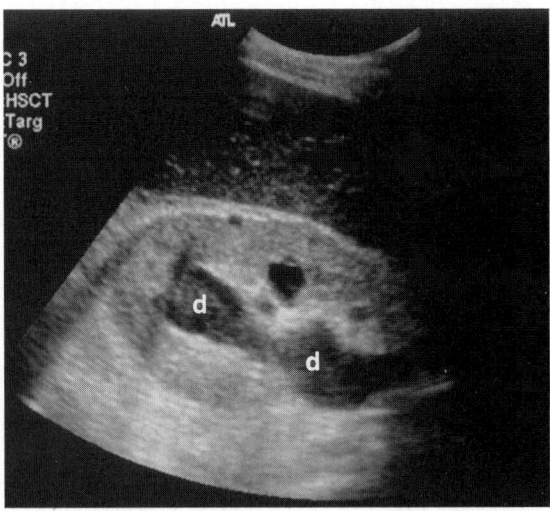

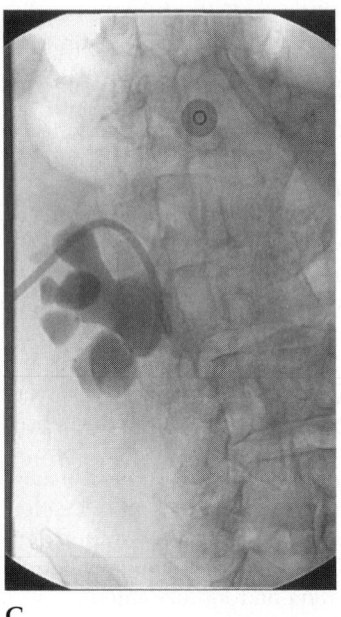

FIGURE 101-3 This elderly man with a history of bladder cancer presented with a fever and an elevated white blood cell count. *A.* US of the right kidney demonstrates a normal-size kidney with hydronephrosis. *B.* Echogenic debris is present within the collecting system (*d*). In a patient with clinical signs of infection, this debris must be presumed to represent infection. *C.* Percutaneous nephrostomy was performed. Grossly purulent material was aspirated and sent for culture. Contrast injection demonstrates the dilated pelvicalyceal system.

to control bleeding by endovascular methods may necessitate emergent surgery.

TECHNIQUE

Once active bleeding is confirmed and angiography is deemed beneficial, the patient should be transported promptly to the angiographic suite. Portable fluoroscopy units are inadequate for these complex examinations.

In upper GI bleeding, initial celiac axis and subsequent selective left gastric and gastroduodenal arteriography are performed. In lower GI bleeding, the superior and inferior mesenteric arteries, as well as the celiac artery, must be studied. The nuclear medicine bleeding scan is useful to guide selective injections.

The diagnosis of active bleeding is confirmed by identifying extravasated contrast material within the bowel lumen (Fig. 101-4*A*). In suspected lower intestinal bleeding, bladder catheterization is important so that extravasated contrast material is not obscured in the lower pelvis and rectum.

Transcatheter embolization or selective intraarterial vasoconstrictor infusion techniques are endovascular alternatives to surgery in these critically ill patients. Therapy is individualized to the patient's overall medical condition, the cause and location of the bleeding, and the experience of the interventional radiologist.

For lower GI bleeding, the nonoperative therapy of choice traditionally has been selective vasoconstrictor infusion. However, embolotherapy, which has long been valuable in

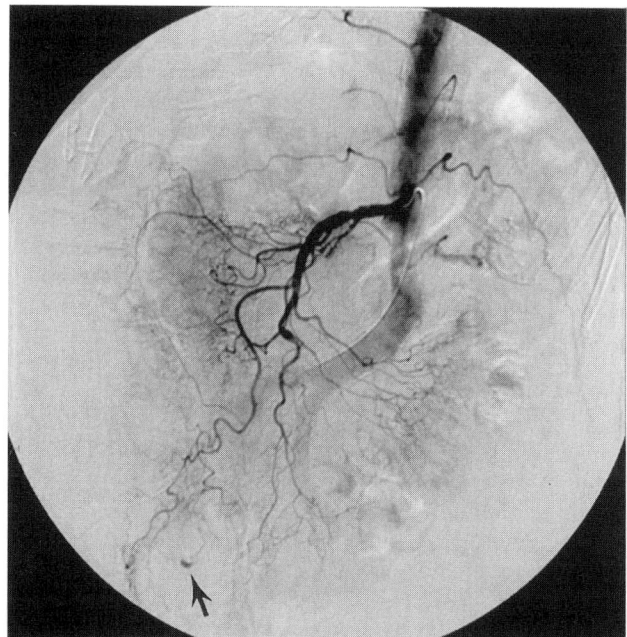

A

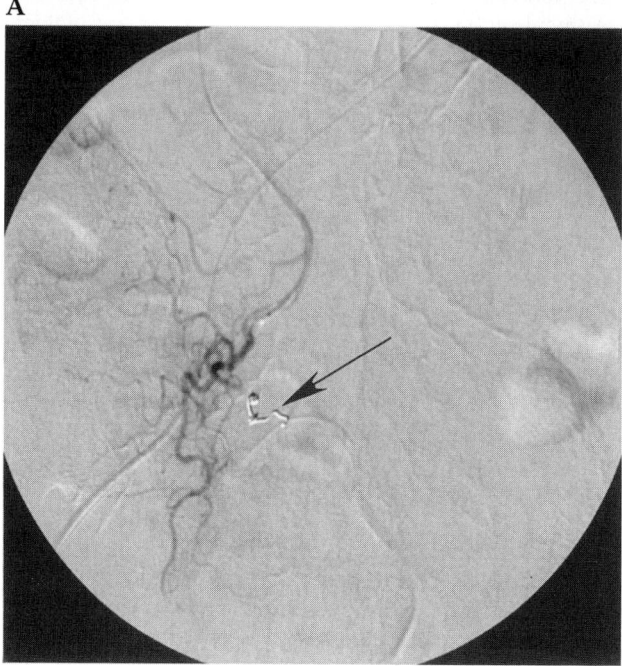

B

FIGURE 101-4 **This elderly woman presented with severe lower GI bleeding.** *A.* **Digitial substraction angiography with selective injection of the superior mesenteric artery demonstrates a focus of contrast extravasation (*short arrow*) within the ileocolic region.** *B.* **After coil embolization (*long arrow*) of the bleeding vessel, repeat contrast injection demonstrates occlusion of the coiled vessel and no further extravasation.**

upper GI bleeding, is being chosen more frequently in the treatment of lower GI bleeding as well. Embolotherapy typically has been considered safe in the upper GI tract owing to its rich collateral arterial network. Embolization of the lower GI tract, with its lesser degree of collateralization, raised con-

cerns for precipitating bowel ischemia and infarction, suppositions that were proven true in the past.[21–23] However, with the development of microcatheters, there is renewed interest in embolization as the primary treatment for lower GI tract bleeding. Microcatheters allow selective catheterization of a peripheral bleeding vessel, thus limiting the region of intestine affected by embolization. Superselective embolization is proving to have high technical success rates with lower rebleeding rates than vasopressin infusion and low rates of ischemia and infarction[25,26] (see Fig. 101-4*B*). When superselective catheterization is not possible, vasoconstrictor infusion remains the best endovascular therapy.

Vasopressin is a potent vasoconstrictor that is the pressor component of the active hormone of the posterior pituitary gland. It produces constriction of the splanchnic vascular bed and contraction of the smooth muscle of the gut. Direct intraarterial injection of vasopressin results in fewer systemic side effects than intravenous administration because a lower dose is required.

Vasopressin therapy is started immediately after selective angiography with direct infusion into the major artery supplying the bleeding site. In an area with a dual blood supply (e.g., the duodenum), vasopressin must be infused through both vascular beds (celiac and superior mesenteric artery) and is less effective. Initial infusion rates generally range from 0.1 to 0.4 unit/min, with angiography repeated at 20-minute intervals to assess the vasoconstrictive effect. If the bleeding stops, the patient is returned to the ICU on a continuous infusion. If bleeding persists, the vasopressin infusion is increased. In general, an infusion of more than 0.4 unit/min results in significantly more systemic side effects. Therefore, if bleeding is not controlled at 0.4 unit/min, alternative therapies should be considered.

The vasopressin infusion is continued for 12 to 24 hours and then tapered gradually over 24 to 48 hours while the patient's condition is monitored carefully. An infusion of saline for the final 12 to 24 hours is helpful in the event of rebleeding. If rebleeding does occur, vasopressin infusion can be repeated.

Transcatheter embolotherapy carries a higher rate of success without rebleeding and eliminates the need for prolonged indwelling arterial catheters. In some cases, embolotherapy serves as definitive treatment of bleeding. Embolotherapy is most helpful in areas with rich collateral arterial networks (i.e., esophagus, stomach, duodenum, and rectum), where multiple blood supplies minimize the risk of ischemic injury. As discussed earlier, because of the high success rates without rebleeding, embolization is being selected more frequently as therapy for bleeding in the small intestine and colon, regions without the same degree of collateralization. Owing to the risk of ischemia and infarction, embolotherapy typically should be avoided in the postoperative gut, especially near anastomoses.

Multiple agents have been used for embolization in the GI tract, and the agent of choice varies by bleeding location and experience of the operator. Surgical gelatin (Gelfoam), polyvinyl alcohol (Ivalon), and microcoils all have been used with success. Gelfoam and coils are the most commonly used agents. Many authors favor Gelfoam because it is a resorbable agent that provides temporary occlusion (approximately 5 to 10 days), allowing the bowel lesion to heal. Injected as particles intermixed with contrast material, it carries a small risk of nontarget embolization. Many authors prefer coil embolization because, when superselective catheterization is possible, the coils can be deployed precisely without affecting nearby vessels.

Certain locations are best treated using a particular agent. For example, the left gastric artery can be embolized with Gelfoam for treatment of a Mallory-Weiss tear, even when endoscopy has suggested a bleeding site near the gastroesophageal junction but angiography has failed to document active extravasation. Coil embolization of this vessel should be avoided because permanent occlusion would preclude treatment via this vessel should rebleeding occur. The morbidity of Gelfoam embolization of the left gastric artery is extremely low, and the method decreases rebleeding. In contrast, coils are much preferred in the small bowel and colon because they can be deployed precisely with permanent occlusion of the bleeding vessel.

IMMEDIATE POSTPROCEDURE CARE

Embolotherapy and vasoconstrictive infusions both work by decreasing the pulse pressure at the bleeding site. This allows hemostasis and healing of the bleeding lesion. This approach requires a functioning hemostatic mechanism. Frequently, patients with massive GI bleeding have multisystem organ failure or sepsis or have received many units of transfused blood. Any of these can result in an underlying coagulopathy, which should be corrected as rapidly as possible.

Patients on vasopressin infusion must be monitored carefully. During the initial infusion, many patients experience abdominal cramps secondary to the effects on intestinal smooth muscle. This may result in dramatic emptying of accumulated blood from the bowel. If cramps fail to subside within 30 to 60 minutes, or if they recur, significant gut ischemia may be present. The vasopressin dose should be decreased slowly until the pain is relieved. Patients also should be monitored carefully for signs of myocardial and peripheral ischemia, dysrhythmia, and hyponatremia secondary to the antidiuretic effect of vasopressin. Hyponatremia and decreased urine output usually are treated easily with diuretics.

RESULTS AND COMPLICATIONS

Results with transcatheter therapy for acute GI bleeding are highly variable depending on several factors, including the underlying medical condition, the cause of bleeding, and the bleeding site. In our experience, patients with extensive multisystem organ failure and GI bleeding rarely benefit from intervention. Unfortunately, it is difficult to determine beforehand which individuals may benefit.

In patients without multisystem organ failure, control of upper GI bleeding with embolotherapy usually is successful in 70% to 80% of cases.[28,30] In lower GI bleeding, vasopressin infusion is effective in 60% to 90% of patients, but the overall recurrence rate can be as high as 40%. Despite rebleeding, these patients can benefit from this temporary control, allowing elective surgical intervention under more favorable conditions. Embolization for lower GI tract bleeding has resulted in clinical success rates of 60% to 100%, with recent series limited to the colon reporting greater than 85% success. Rebleeding rates following embolization are approximately 10%.[24]

Complications of embolotherapy in the upper GI tract are rare[28] owing to the rich collateral network around the stomach and duodenum that protects against infarction. Care must be taken in postoperative patients, in whom collateral vessels have been ligated. Backflow of embolic material into the liver and spleen occurs occasionally and generally is well tolerated. Clinically significant hepatic or splenic infarctions are rare.

Complications of vasopressin treatment typically are related to diffuse vasoconstriction, which results in significant ischemia to the heart or extremities. Other complications include dysrhythmia and hyponatremia. Thrombosis of the femoral or visceral arteries may result from prolonged placement of the intraarterial catheter. Significant complications related to catheter-directed vasopressin therapy are infrequent, generally less than 10%.[31]

Despite multiple scintigrams, endoscopies, and/or arteriograms, some patients with lower GI tract hemorrhage will have no bleeding site identified. For this subset with obscure bleeding, elective arteriography is indicated to evaluate for the presence of a structural abnormality that may bleed intermittently and guide surgical resection of this offending lesion.[32] In addition, heparin, intraarterial vasodilators, and/or intravenous or intraarterial thrombolytics have been administered in an attempt to provoke bleeding. Several studies have evaluated one or a combination of these agents and have documented a contribution to detection and treatment of bleeding in between 20% and 50% of patients without any adverse events or complications.[33–36] Thus the diagnostic yield of provocative arteriography may be somewhat disappointing, but for a subset of patients with chronic, repetitive, nonlocalized bleeding, it may serve a role when all other measures have failed.

TRANSJUGULAR INTRAHEPATIC PORTOSYSTEMIC SHUNT

INDICATIONS AND PATIENT SELECTION

Patients with portal hypertension represent a diverse group in the ICU. Typically, patients fall into one of two broad categories with respect to their symptoms. The most urgently ill are those with uncontrollable bleeding from esophagogastric varices. The second group, consisting of those with fluid management problems, includes patients with intractable ascites, hydrothorax, or hepatorenal syndrome.

Portal hypertension with variceal bleeding is a special form of upper GI hemorrhage that requires a different approach than arterial bleeding. Endoscopy with sclerotherapy/banding remains the initial diagnostic and therapeutic procedure of choice. However, endoscopic treatment is not always successful, and recurrent bleeding occurs in about 30% to 50% of patients.

Portal hypertension with ascites or hydrothorax typically is managed with diuretics and paracentesis/thoracentesis. However, when the fluid reaccumulates in a short time period requiring frequent repeat percutaneous removal or therapy results in the development of renal failure, electrolyte imbalances, or encephalopathy, alternate therapy may need to be employed.

Historically, the definitive therapeutic intervention was the surgical creation of a shunt from the high-pressure portal system to the central circulation, allowing decompression of the portal system. Interventional radiologists now play a significant role in the treatment of these complex patients with percutaneous creation of transjugular intrahepatic portosystemic shunts (TIPS).[37–41] TIPS is a percutaneous portocaval shunt through the liver parenchyma connecting a portal vein and a hepatic vein. Its function is identical to a surgically created portosystemic shunt, but morbidity and mortality are reduced markedly with this less invasive alternative.

Indications for TIPS include multiple episodes of esophagogastric variceal hemorrhage refractory to sclerotherapy, presence of gastric varices in the absence of splenic vein thrombosis, intractable ascites, hepatic hydrothorax, hepatorenal syndrome, Budd-Chiari syndrome, and preoperative portal decompression in patients awaiting liver transplantation.

Preprocedure evaluation includes a determination of the indication and urgency for TIPS, review of hepatic imaging, and assessment of patient candidacy. Patients with decompensated portal hypertension typically are very sick, and for some, TIPS will improve their symptomatology and may be lifesaving. However, for others, TIPS may result in fulminant liver failure, new or worsening encephalopathy, or premature death. Several parameters have been used in an attempt to stratify patient risk and predict survival after TIPS. The Child-Pugh classification considers the presence and degree of ascites and encephalopathy, as well as the serum bilirubin and albumin concentrations and the INR. A newer measurement, the MELD score, is a mathematical model based on the serum creatinine and bilirubin concentrations, the INR, and the etiology of the underlying liver disease. Although neither can predict survival with complete accuracy, recent data support that the MELD score is a better predictor of 3-month outcome than the Child-Pugh score[37] and that a MELD risk score less than 1.8 is associated with improved survival.[38]

Fluid resuscitation to treat ongoing bleeding and correction of an existing coagulopathy are critical prior to and during the procedure. For patients with ascites, paracentesis just prior to the procedure can facilitate safe creation of a TIPS. Finally, for some patients, general anesthesia may be necessary and helpful because many of these patients have low baseline blood pressures that preclude sedation at levels necessary to provide patient comfort.

TECHNIQUE

Prior to TIPS placement, it is useful to confirm portal vein patency. This is typically done by US evaluation or other noninvasive imaging but, if necessary, can be determined via superior mesenteric arteriography. In the emergent situation, this preprocedure imaging may not be feasible.

When the decision to perform a TIPS procedure has been made, the patient is transported to the interventional suite. The right internal jugular vein is accessed, and a venous sheath is inserted into the right atrium. The right hepatic vein is catheterized. Wedged hepatic venography typically is performed using carbon dioxide. This gas diffuses rapidly through the liver retrogradely, providing an image of the portal vein and its branches. Using this venogram for guidance, a needle is directed through the hepatic parenchyma into the portal vein. Pressure measurements between the portal vein and the right atrium are obtained, and the portosystemic gradient is calculated. Direct portal venography is then performed to document the anatomy and the presence of varices (Fig. 101-5*A*). The newly created tract is dilated and held open by one or more self-expanding metal stents. After stent placement, pressures are again obtained to confirm reduction of the portosystemic gradient, and venography is

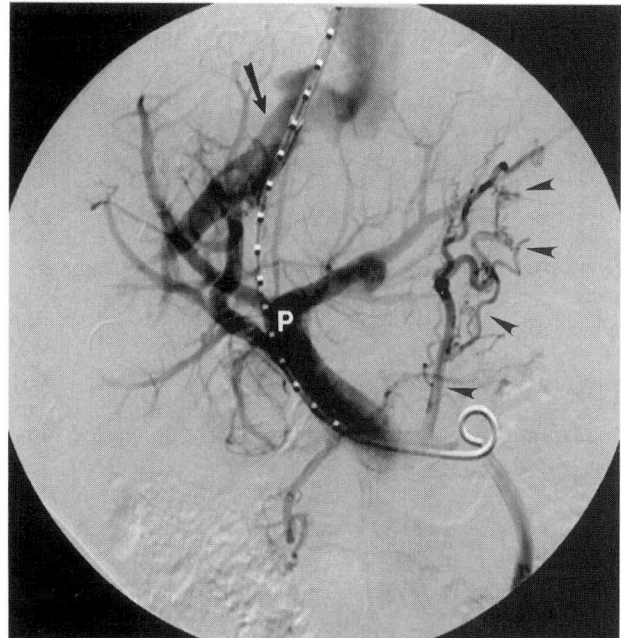

A

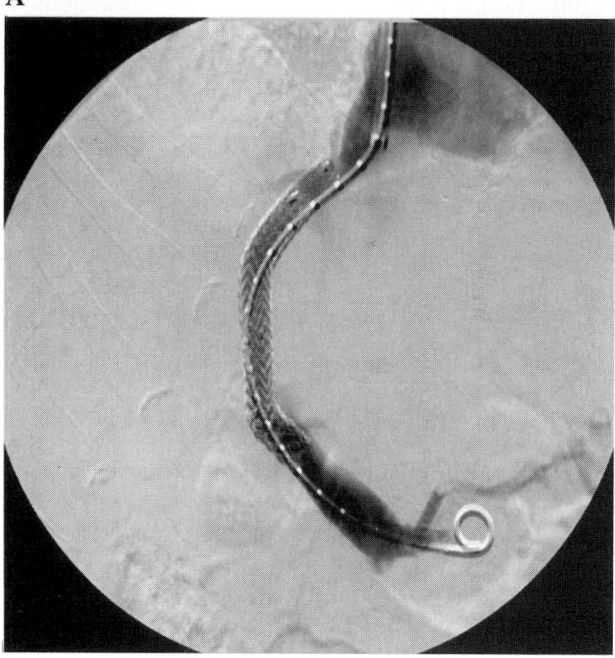

B

FIGURE 101-5 This 40-year-old woman with a history of cirrhosis due to ethanol abuse developed intractable ascites not responsive to medical management. Creation of a transjugular intrahepatic portosystemic shunt (TIPS) was requested. *A.* Initial venography after passage of a needle through the hepatic parenchyma from the right hepatic vein (*arrow*) into a portal vein (*P*) demonstrates filling of varices (*arrowheads*). *B.* Following TIPS creation, contrast agent injection demonstrates brisk flow through the shunt and no filling of the varices.

performed to document stent patency and assess the degree of variceal filling (see Fig. 101-5*B*). A gradient of less than 12 mm Hg is desired because pressure gradients above this level are associated with recurrent variceal hemorrhage. If initial shunt placement is unsuccessful at reducing the gradient adequately and varices continue to opacify, variceal embolization with Gianturco coils or ethanol injection can be performed as an adjunct.

IMMEDIATE POSTPROCEDURE CARE

Following portal decompression and stabilization, patients should be monitored carefully for at least 24 hours and should continue to receive any needed blood products. A color duplex US of the shunt, as well as the hepatic and portal veins, should be obtained the following day to assess adequacy of flow through the shunt and to provide a baseline for subsequent follow-up.

RESULTS AND COMPLICATIONS

Technical success of TIPS placement is greater than 90% when the portal vein is patent. TIPS have been created in the presence of a thrombosed portal vein, but technical success rates are lower. Primary shunt patency at 6 months ranges from 75% to 90%,[39,40] with recurrent bleeding occurring in 4% to 17%. A 30-day mortality rate of approximately 15% and a 6-month mortality rate of 30% have been reported. The overall mortality rate varies by the Child-Pugh classification and patient stability at the time of the shunt procedure. A series by Encarnacion and coworkers[41] broke down the cumulative 30-day survival rates for Child-Pugh classes A and B (91%) and class C (71%). These figures compare favorably with surgically placed portosystemic shunts in terms of overall morbidity and mortality and the length of postprocedure survival. In terms of rebleeding, the recurrence rate is lower with TIPS when compared with sclerotherapy. It is, of course, understood that many of the patients undergoing percutaneous shunt creation have failed sclerotherapy.

TIPS creation has been very successful in acutely relieving portal hypertension and variceal bleeding, but shunt stenosis may occur in up to 70%.[40] Routine surveillance with Doppler US is necessary to identify shunt problems requiring further venographic examination and intervention. TIPS venography and revision can be performed on an outpatient basis in most cases.

Complications of TIPS include neck hematoma, liver capsule puncture with or without abdominal hemorrhage, encephalopathy, hemobilia, or worsening liver failure. Occasionally, patients develop multisystem organ failure with no evident source of sepsis. This may emphasize the importance of a functioning liver for the modulation of systemic inflammation.

BRONCHIAL ARTERY EMBOLIZATION

Life-threatening hemoptysis, although uncommon, is associated with an exceedingly high mortality rate (50% to 70%) in patients treated by conservative means (see Chap. 41). Since the early 1970s, interventions in the management of massive hemoptysis have gravitated toward transcatheter embolization. The mortality rate for surgery in the setting of acute hemorrhage remains high (33%). Embolization can act as palliative therapy or can temporize patients until surgery is feasible.[44–47]

INDICATIONS AND PATIENT SELECTION

Massive hemoptysis is defined as bleeding in excess of 300 mL during a 24-hour period. However, smaller amounts may be life threatening due to airway compromise, so intervention may be indicated with lesser amounts of hemorrhage.

Bleeding arises from the systemic circulation (bronchial arteries and transpleural collaterals) in about 95% of patients. Chronic inflammatory diseases such as tuberculosis, bronchiectasis, aspergillosis, and cystic fibrosis and neoplastic diseases such as bronchogenic carcinoma all may predispose to bronchial bleeding. In about 5% of patients, hemoptysis relates to lesions of the pulmonary arterial circulation (Rasmussen/mycotic aneurysm or pulmonary arteriovenous fistula). A particular cause of massive hemoptysis in the ICU patient is an iatrogenic injury of the pulmonary artery following pulmonary artery catheter insertion. Both systemic and pulmonary arterial causes of hemoptysis are amenable to transcatheter embolization.

Attempts to localize or lateralize the bleeding to one or more lobes should be undertaken prior to angiography. Chest radiography, chest CT, and/or bronchoscopy can be used. Bronchoscopy has long been considered the primary method of diagnosis and localization, but CT has proven to be very helpful in preprocedure evaluation.[44] CT has higher rates of localization, may detect causative vascular lesions, may suggest a specific diagnosis, and may identify bronchial and nonbronchial systemic feeder arteries.[45,46] Protective measures prior to transport to angiography include insertion of a double-lumen endotracheal tube to allow selective ventilation and protection of the contralateral lung and/or insertion of a balloon occlusion catheter at the bleeding site to tamponade the source until embolization.

TECHNIQUE

As with other complicated vascular diagnostic and therapeutic interventional radiologic procedures, patients must be transported to the angiographic suite for optimal angiographic imaging and intervention.

There is marked variability in bronchial arterial anatomy, so evaluation begins with a nonselective descending thoracic aortogram. After anatomic mapping, selective arteriography is performed in the bronchial artery corresponding to the radiographic and/or bronchoscopic abnormality. In situations where the underlying process is related to chronic inflammation, transpleural collateral vessels from the subclavian, axillary, internal mammary, intercostal, and phrenic arteries may be recruited. Depending on the location of the bleeding site, evaluation of one or more of these potential pathways via selective arteriography may be necessary.

Unlike arteriographic evaluation of GI bleeding, extravasation of contrast material is not identified commonly. Angiography more often will reveal a hypertrophied and abnormal bronchial artery with neovascularity, hypervascularity, aneurysm formation, or shunting of blood into the pulmonary artery or vein. Prior to transcatheter embolization, the diagnostic arteriogram must be reviewed carefully for the presence of arterial branches supplying the spinal cord. This anatomic configuration occurs more commonly on the right, where 90% of patients have a common bronchial-intercostal artery trunk, 5% to 10% of which have branches supplying the spinal cord. Embolization should not be performed if a spinal branch could be embolized inadvertently as well. In some cases, the selective catheter or a coaxial microcatheter can be advanced beyond a spinal branch origin, allowing safe embolization. If no abnormal bronchial or other systemic transpleural collateral source is found, pulmonary arteriography should follow.

For bronchial and nonbronchial systemic sources of massive hemoptysis, polyvinyl alcohol foam (Ivalon) and gelatin sponge (Gelfoam) are the embolic agents used most commonly. In selected cases of hemoptysis secondary to an arteriovenous malformation (AVM) arising from the pulmonary artery, coils or detachable balloons can be used to occlude the large single feeding vessel with good results. This latter situation is seen more commonly in patients with hereditary hemorrhagic telangiectasia, where multiple AVMs may be present.

IMMEDIATE POSTPROCEDURE CARE

As with any embolization procedure performed to treat bleeding, patients should be monitored closely over at least 24 hours for signs of rebleeding. Considering the potential risk of nontarget embolization to the spinal cord, neuromuscular checks should be obtained at frequent intervals following embolization.

RESULTS AND COMPLICATIONS

Bronchial artery embolization for the immediate control of massive hemoptysis is successful in more than 75% of patients, with recurrence of bleeding in approximately 20%.[46,47] In one report, embolization was unsuccessful and hemoptysis continued to death in approximately 9% of patients.[47] Long-term success rates are lower, likely owing in part to progression or continuation of the underlying disease. Recurrent bleeding following embolization may be the result of partial embolization, recanalization, revascularization by collateral channels, inadequate treatment, development of systemic nonbronchial collaterals, or progression of the lung disease. Repeat embolization has been shown to improve outcomes in patients with recurrent hemoptysis, particularly when repeat embolization entails embolization of previously overlooked supplying vessels.[47] It is important to note that bronchial artery embolization should be considered a palliative, not a curative, procedure. It allows time to plan elective surgery or to treat the patient with antimicrobials.

Procedure-related complications of diagnostic arteriography are uncommon but include chest pain due to transient ischemia, temporary dysphagia due to embolization of esophageal branches, and arterial dissection. A rare additional risk is transverse myelitis following contrast agent injection into a spinal artery, particularly ionic agents. The major feared complication of bronchial artery embolization is spinal cord ischemia due to inadvertent embolization of one or more spinal arteries. Careful evaluation for bronchial or intercostal arteries that provide branches to the anterior spinal artery is critical because embolization should be avoided in such situations.

FOREIGN BODY RETRIEVAL AND CATHETER REPOSITIONING

INDICATIONS AND PATIENT SELECTION

ICU patients often require one or more intravascular infusion catheters and/or monitoring devices. On occasion, catheters are malpositioned or fractured and may lodge in the vascular system—usually the central veins, heart, or pulmonary arteries. This typically occurs during catheter introduction or repositioning and rarely is related to a defect in the material itself. Other types of intravascular foreign bodies may include broken pacemaker leads or migrated caval filters.

The presence of an intravascular foreign body usually is an indication for its removal. Complications have been reported in up to 70% of patients in whom catheter fragments were left in place.[48] Major complications of a retained catheter fragment include vascular or cardiac perforation, sepsis, dysrhythmia, and pulmonary embolism. The medicolegal implications also should be considered.

TECHNIQUE

Percutaneous retrieval of the intravascular foreign body is the treatment of choice. It generally can be accomplished without an incision or general anesthesia. The alternative is a major surgical procedure that can pose high risks. Standard monitoring is necessary, with special attention to ECG monitoring given the risk of inducing arrhythmias when manipulating catheters or fragments within the heart.

Access into the vascular system typically is chosen to facilitate easy, minimally traumatic removal. A venogram is performed to confirm the intravascular position of the fragment and to select a suitable site of engagement. A number of retrieval devices are available, but the snare device is selected most commonly. Once the fragment has been engaged and trapped, it is pulled taut and folded on itself so that it can be withdrawn at the venous access site. Rarely, a surgical cutdown is necessary if the fragment is large or not pliable. Alternative retrieval devices include baskets, graspers, and balloon catheters.

A number of maneuvers can redirect malpositioned central venous catheters. When standard replacement is unsuccessful at the patient's bedside, fluoroscopic guidance can facilitate repositioning. Prior to catheter manipulation, venography should be performed to define the anatomy and document any potential problems or occlusions. In many cases, redirection under direct visualization is all that is required. In other cases, the venous system can be entered from a separate site and the end of the catheter snared and pulled into the desired orientation.

RESULTS AND COMPLICATIONS

Percutaneous foreign body retrieval is very effective, with success rates ranging from 80% to 95%.[49] Unsuccessful retrieval often is due to the lack of a free end to grasp, incorporation of the fragment into the vessel wall, or location in an extravascular compartment.

Complications of percutaneous retrieval and catheter repositioning are rare. Transient dysrhythmias can occur during catheter manipulation within the heart. Most resolve by withdrawing all devices from the heart. If the foreign body is firmly adherent to the endothelium, endocardium, or a cardiac valve, traction must be applied gently to avoid vascular damage.

PERCUTANEOUS CAVAL FILTER PLACEMENT

INDICATIONS AND PATIENT SELECTION

Pulmonary embolism is a common cause of morbidity and mortality in the ICU patient. Anticoagulation with intravenous heparin, oral warfarin, or subcutaneous low-molecular-weight heparin remains the first-line therapy for treatment. However, in some patients, anticoagulation is contraindicated or ineffective. This has led to the development of a number of mechanical devices to "filter" emboli from the pelvis and lower extremities.[50–58]

Until the mid-1980s, these devices required a surgical cut-down in the internal jugular vein owing to the large size of the deployment sheath. In recent years, the profile of caval filters has decreased from 24F (Greenfield filter) to between 6F and 12F, making percutaneous placement feasible. This approach is convenient and can be combined with pulmonary arteriography and/or central venous catheter insertion.

As insertion techniques evolved over the past 10 years, many new devices have been developed. Several excellent reviews of caval filters are available.[51–53] Currently, a number of permanent low-profile caval filters are available for patient use in the United States. These include the Titanium Greenfield, Bird's Nest, VenaTech, Simon Nitinol, TrapEase, Optease, and Gunther tulip vena caval filters.

Temporary or retrievable filters are the newest development in caval filtration devices. Temporary filters remain tethered to a transcutaneous catheter or wire at the insertion site so that early removal can be accomplished to prevent infection. Retrievable filters are designed with a hook at one end that can be engaged using a snare device, allowing removal through a long sheath. The Gunther tulip and TrapEase vena caval filters have been deployed and retrieved successfully, although each is approved by the Food and Drug Administration (FDA) for permanent deployment only, and this represents an off-label use of these products[52,53] (Fig. 101-6). Retrieval within 10 to 14 days of insertion is recommended owing to "endothelialization" of the filter legs and the potential for vein damage with later removal. Venography is required at the time of retrieval to ensure the absence of thrombus within or around the filter because removal of the filter would result in dislodgment of this clot and pulmonary embolism.

Indications for caval filter placement generally fall into three categories: (1) contraindication to or complication of anticoagulation in a patient with documented pulmonary emboli, (2) recurrent pulmonary embolism despite anticoagulation, and (3) prophylaxis. Although the first two are well-accepted indications, prophylaxis is controversial.[53] Indications for prophylactic vena caval interruption have become more liberal as the procedure has become simpler and safer and retrievable filters have been developed. Nevertheless, many physicians remain unfamiliar with filter placement or consider it too invasive for common use. Caval filtration is greatly underused in the management of critically ill patients.

Prophylactic filter placement (in addition to heparin therapy) is warranted in patients with proven venous thromboembolism and cardiovascular compromise or severe chronic obstructive pulmonary disease, as well as in all patients with free-floating pelvic thrombi. In addition, prophylactic caval filter placement should be considered in certain high-risk surgical (orthopedic, trauma, neurosurgical) and oncology patients. If retrievable filters become more accepted and gain FDA approval, prophylactic filter placement may become more common.

TECHNIQUE

Inferior vena caval filter placement generally requires transport to the interventional radiology suite. Rarely, in highly unstable patients, filter placement may be done at the bedside with portable fluoroscopy equipment. However, the lack of high-quality fluoroscopy equipment makes performance of an adequate inferior vena cavagram difficult (see below).

The femoral approach generally is preferred for percutaneous caval filter placement because it is easily accessible. The internal jugular approach may have advantages in patients with extensive pelvic and caval thrombosis, tortuous iliac veins, or multiple femoral lines.

An inferior vena cavagram should be performed before filter deployment to demonstrate the level of the renal veins, the presence of thrombus in the inferior vena cava, the diameter of the inferior vena cava, and the presence of congenital venous anomalies. After the inferior vena cavagram is performed, the puncture site is dilated to a suitable size, and a sheath is placed. The filter is introduced through the sheath and discharged below the renal veins. Infrarenal placement is preferred to maintain renal vein patency in the event of caval thrombosis. If thrombus extends to the level of the renal veins, suprarenal filter placement may be used.[53] A follow-up cavagram is done to document filter placement.

IMMEDIATE POSTPROCEDURE CARE

The patient should be kept at bed rest with close observation of the puncture site for 4 to 6 hours. If indicated, heparin can be restarted immediately after local hemostasis is obtained. Continued heparin therapy can be helpful to prevent extension of thrombus in the legs or pelvis.

RESULTS AND COMPLICATIONS

The reported rate of recurrent pulmonary emboli varies with each particular filter design but ranges from 0.5% to 3%. In most cases, however, documentation of recurrent pulmonary emboli is difficult to obtain.

Complications of inferior vena cava filter placement include caval thrombosis, filter migration, and trauma at the insertion site. Caval thrombosis varies with filter design and ranges from 2% to 9%. In recent years, the currently available filters have been modified such that filter migration is a rare event.

A potential complication with the percutaneous approach is puncture-site thrombosis. Significant access-site thrombosis with the newer low-profile filters ranges from 2% to 10%, with an overall (nonocclusive and occlusive) thrombosis frequency of up to 35%. Between 4% and 6% of patients display clinical symptoms.[58]

CATHETER-DIRECTED FIBRINOLYTIC THERAPY

Local catheter-directed fibrinolytic therapy is an important addition to the nonsurgical treatment of acute and subacute arterial occlusion. Catheter-directed fibrinolytic infusions infuse the thrombus directly and therefore concentrate the fibrinolytic agent's action at the site of the vascular occlusion. This is favored over systemic therapy because it permits lower doses and minimizes systemic side effects.[59–64]

INDICATIONS AND PATIENT SELECTION

Catheter-directed fibrinolytic therapy achieves the best results with acute thrombosis. Therefore, the best indication is thrombosis that occurs during angiography or angioplasty. The arterial catheter is already in place, and the clot is fresh.

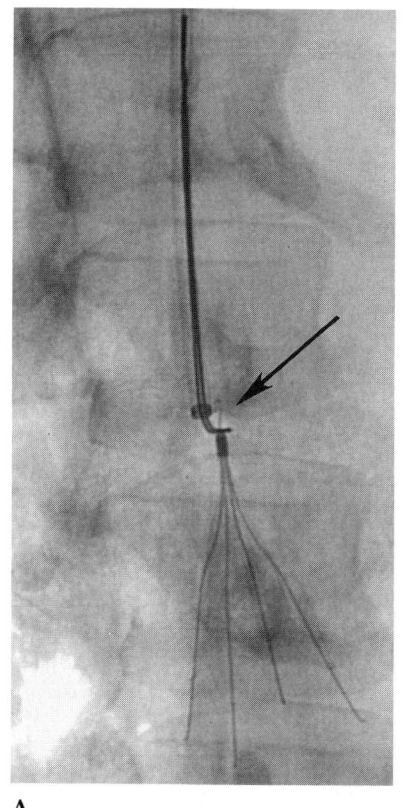

A

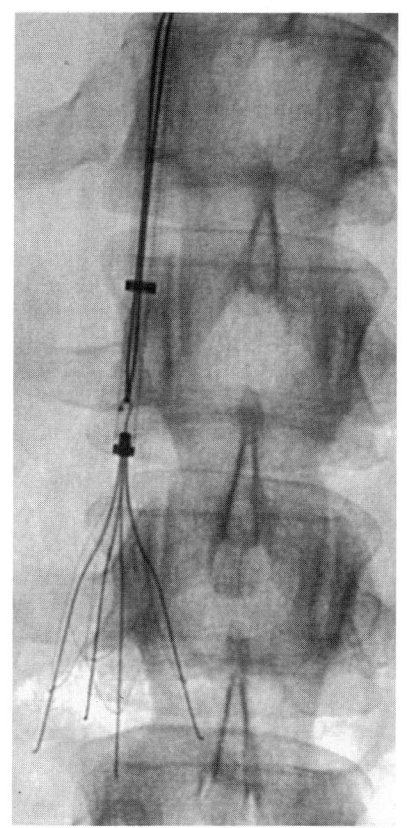

B

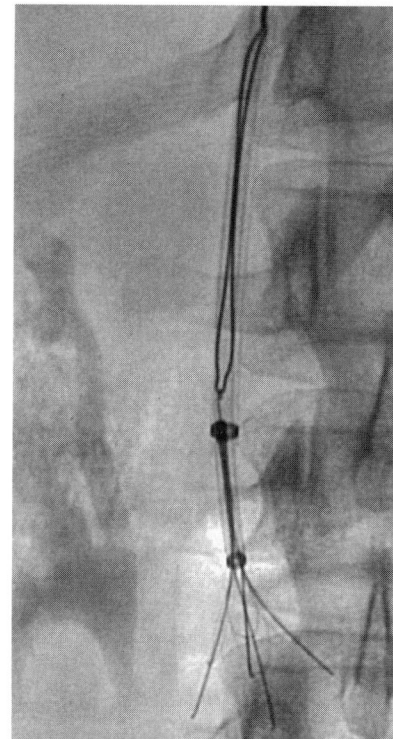

C

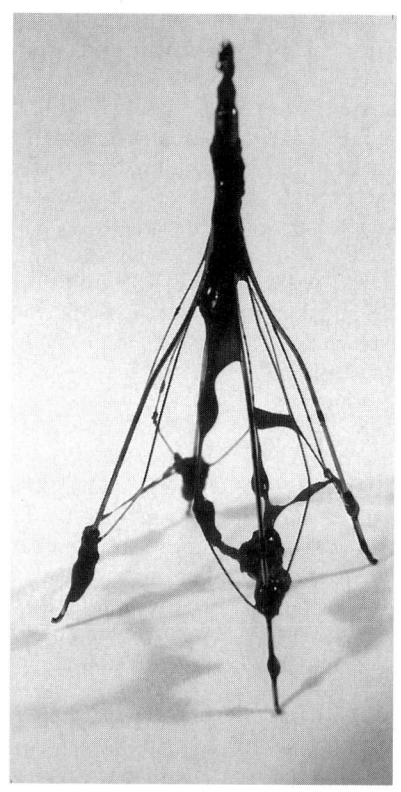

D

FIGURE 101-6 Retrieval of a Gunther tulip inferior vena caval filter. *A.* Fluoroscopy demonstrates a long vascular sheath through which a snare device is used to engage the hook of the filter (*arrow*). *B.* The hook is engaged and the sheath advanced over the snare and hook. *C.* As the sheath is further advanced over the filter, the legs collapse and pull away from the vessel wall. *D.* The filter is covered with fibrinous debris and blood clot.

Fibrinolytic therapy also is beneficial in native-artery and bypass-graft occlusions. Thrombosis in these cases usually is a manifestation of underlying stenotic disease. Frequently, these stenoses can be treated with interventional radiologic techniques such as angioplasty, sparing the patient a surgical bypass. Although the exact age of the clot can be difficult to determine, best results are seen with occlusions that are less than 6 to 10 weeks old.

Another indication for fibrinolytic therapy is embolic occlusion. In large-vessel emboli (e.g., femoral or brachial artery), a surgical Fogarty embolectomy is extremely effective. Small-vessel emboli, however, are difficult to remove mechanically owing to vessel size, so catheter-directed fibrinolysis frequently is the best treatment available.

Despite the effectiveness of fibrinolytic therapy, not all patients are candidates. Patients with acute thrombosis and limb-threatening ischemia should be treated with surgery because catheter-directed thrombolysis is a slow process, requiring 12 or more hours of treatment for reperfusion. In addition, although the fibrinolytic agent is directed into the clot, a significant amount of it enters the systemic circulation as it diffuses through the clot. Therefore, patients at risk of significant bleeding are not candidates. Specifically, contraindications to thrombolysis include recent intracranial, thoracic, or abdominal surgery; recent GI bleeding; recent stroke or known intracranial neoplasm; recent major trauma; current pregnancy; severe hypertension; known bleeding diathesis; and infected thrombus.

TECHNIQUE

In catheter-directed fibrinolytic therapy, the goal is to deliver the drug directly into the thrombus in order to activate plasminogen bound to the fibrin clot directly without activating significant amounts of circulating plasminogen. Various coaxial catheters and multisidehole catheters are available that allow maximum permeation of the fibrinolytic agent into the thrombus. Typically, the infusion catheter is placed through an arterial sheath that facilitates the catheter exchanges necessary for repeat arteriograms.

After a complete diagnostic arteriogram, a multisidehole catheter is embedded into the thrombus and the infusion started. Traditionally, urokinase was the agent of choice. However, when sales of urokinase were suspended in 1998 owing to production problems, several other fibrinolytic agents, including tissue-type plasminogen activator (t-PA) and recombinant tissue-type plasminogen activator (rt-PA), became more widely used. Streptokinase, the first lytic agent used, is currently in disfavor because of its antigenicity and inferior results in clinical studies.[60] Although urokinase has now returned to the American market, its use remains limited in some areas because of cost.

No standard doses for these agents have been agreed on. Most involve a steady infusion over a period of hours with or without a loading dose. For urokinase, a typical protocol is to lace the clot with 250,000 units and then initiate infusion with 250,000 units/h for 2 hours. After the initial high-dose infusion, the dose is decreased to 80,000 to 100,000 units/h for the duration of the therapy, which may last up to 24 to 36 hours. A recent review of rt-PA indicates that protocols for rt-PA have been more variable, with both weight-based and non-weight-based dosing, dosing with or without an initial bolus, and/or the use of high-dose short-duration pulse-spray thrombolysis.[59] Typical doses range from 0.02 to 0.1 mg/kg per hour for weight-based and 0.25 to 10 mg/h for non-weight-based regimens to a maximum of 100 mg.

IMMEDIATE POSTPROCEDURE CARE

Patients undergoing catheter-directed fibrinolytic infusions are placed in the ICU. The puncture site, the affected extremity, and the patient's bleeding parameters are monitored frequently. Patients are kept at strict bed rest, with frequent Doppler examinations of the ischemic extremity.

Low-dose intravenous heparin (500 to 1000 units/h) is frequently instilled through a sheath to decrease the incidence of pericatheter thrombosis (see below). Anticoagulation with heparin also is helpful to prevent rebound thrombosis after the fibrinolytic infusion is completed.

Laboratory monitoring tests should include baseline fibrinogen, partial thromboplastin time, and hematocrit. Every 4 hours, the fibrinogen level should be checked to monitor for systemic effects of the fibrinolytic agent. If the fibrinogen level falls below 100 mg/dL, the infusion should be slowed or discontinued. Experience has shown that a fibrinogen level below 100 mg/dL is associated with a significantly increased incidence of remote bleeding.[60] However, fibrinogen levels rarely fall this low during catheter-directed urokinase infusions.

Periodic angiographic follow-up is essential and must be performed in the angiographic suite. High-quality fluoroscopic observation is necessary to evaluate progression of lysis. Frequently, the position of the catheter must be changed to keep it embedded in clot.

Successful lysis generally is achieved after 12 to 18 hours of infusion. At that point, underlying stenotic lesions are treated with angioplasty, and the catheter is removed. If no progress is noted over 6 to 12 hours, the infusion is stopped. It is critical that all decisions regarding institution of fibrinolytic therapy, continuation of the therapy, and termination of the infusion be made in conjunction with the vascular surgeon caring for the patient.

RESULTS AND COMPLICATIONS

A successful fibrinolytic infusion generally is one that yields either complete lysis or lysis with significant clinical improvement. Success rates reported in the literature vary from 40% to 90%, with an average of 60% to 70%[61,62] Comparison of various series and fibrinolytic agents is extremely difficult because of heterogeneous patient populations and protocols. Several studies, however, have evaluated the effectiveness of catheter-directed fibrinolysis versus surgery. The Rochester study found similar limb salvage rates for both groups (82%) but improved overall survival in the thrombolysis group at 1 year (84% versus 58% for surgery, $p = 0.01$).[63] The Surgery versus Thrombolysis for Ischemia of the Lower Extremity (STILE) trial comparing thrombolysis (urokinase or rt-PA) and surgery found no difference in morbidity or mortality between the two groups based on intent to treat but noted better amputation-free survival for the thrombolysis patients at 6 months (85% versus 62% for surgery, $p = 0.01$) and reduction in the extent of surgery needed for patients with acute limb ischemia, whereas patients with chronic limb ischemia had lower amputation rates with surgery (4% versus 14% for lysis).[47] Generally, success correlates best with age of the thrombus and status of the distal runoff vessels.

Complications are related primarily to bleeding. Most bleeding occurs at arterial puncture sites and is relatively minor. However, life-threatening bleeding at remote sites (intracranial, gastrointestinal, retroperitoneal) has been reported and can result in significant morbidity. When serious bleeding occurs, therapy should be discontinued unless the bleeding can be controlled by manual compression. Fresh frozen plasma can be given to replace coagulation factors. Significant bleeding generally is reported in 10% to 12% of patients. The risk of bleeding increases with the length of infusion, so the duration of the infusion should be kept under 24 hours if possible. In addition, bleeding risk increases when fibrinogen levels drop below 100 mg/dL, and the infusion should be reduced or stopped if levels fall. Finally, the use of systemic heparin adds to the risk of bleeding. Therefore, the partial thromboplastin time should be monitored carefully when concomitant heparin therapy is given.

Patients may experience dramatic worsening of their ischemic symptoms during the fibrinolytic infusion. This "trashing" of the extremity is usually due to fragmentation of the thrombus and distal embolization. Generally, the symptoms will resolve rapidly by continuing the fibrinolytic infusion and treating the patient with narcotic analgesia. Surgery usually is ineffective for such embolization. However, if significant clinical deterioration persists longer than an hour, angiography should be repeated, and emergent surgery should be considered.

Pericatheter thrombosis is an occasional problem that usually is caused by poor blood flow along the path of the catheter. To prevent this, the intravascular length of catheter must be kept to a minimum, and the smallest possible catheter system should be used. Pericatheter thrombosis can be minimized by using low-dose systemic heparin.

References

1. McClennan BL: Adverse reaction to iodinated contrast media recognition and response. *Invest Radiol* 29:S46, 1994.
1a. Mueller C, Buerkle G, Buettner HJ, et al: Prevention of contrast media-associated nephropathy: Randomized comparison of 2 hydration regimens in 1620 patients undergoing coronary angioplasty. *Arch Intern Med* 162:329, 2002.
2. Kay J, Chow WH, Chan TM, et al: Acetylcysteine for prevention of acute deterioration of renal function following elective coronary angiography and intervention. *JAMA* 289:553, 2003.
3. Baker CSR, Wragg A, Kumar S, et al: A rapid protocol for the prevention of contrast-induced renal dysfunction: The RAPPID study. *J Am Coll Cardiol* 41:2114, 2003.
4. Boccalandro F, Amhad M, Smalling RW, et al: Oral acetylcysteine does not protect renal function from moderate to high doses of intravenous radiographic contrast. *Cathet Cardiovas Intervent* 58:336, 2003.
5. Madyoon H: Clinical experience with the use of fenoldopam for prevention of radiocontrast nephropathy in high-risk patients. *Rev Cardiovasc Med* 2(suppl 1):S26, 2001.
6. Kini A, Sharma S: Managing the high-risk patient: experience with fenoldopam, a selective dopamine receptor agonist, in prevention of radiocontrast nephropathy during percutaneous coronary intervention. *Rev Cardiovasc Med* 2(suppl 1):S19, 2001.
7. Tumlin JA, Wang A, Murray PT, et al: Fenoldopam mesylate blocks reductions in renal plasma flow after radiocontrast dye infusion: A pilot trial in the prevention of contrast nephropathy. *Am Heart J* 143:894, 2002.
8. Boyd-Kranis R, Sullivan KL, Eschelman DJ, et al: Accuracy and safety of carbon dioxide inferior vena cavography. *J Vasc Intervent Radiol* 10:1183, 1999.
9. Dewald CL, Jensen CC, Park YH, et al: Vena cavography with CO_2 versus with iodinated contrast material for inferior vena cava filter placement: A prospective evaluation. *Radiology* 216:752, 2000.
10. Kaufman JA, Geller SC, Bazari H, et al: Gadolinium-based contrast agents as an alternative at vena cavography in patients with renal insufficiency: Early experience. *Radiology* 212:280, 1999.
11. Spinosa DJ, Hagspiel KD, Angle JF, et al: Gadolinium-based contrast agents in angiography and interventional radiology: Uses and techniques. *J Vasc Intervent Radiol* 11:985, 2000.
12. Spinosa DJ, Matsumoto AH, Hagspiel KD, et al: Gadolinium-based contrast agents in angiography and interventional radiology. *AJR* 173:1403, 1999.
13. Van Sonnenberg E, Mueller PR, Ferrucci JT: Percutaneous drainage of 250 abdominal abscesses and fluid collections. *Radiology* 151:337, 1984.
14. Gerzof SG, Johnson WC, Robbins AH, et al: Expanded criteria for percutaneous abscess drainage. *Arch Surg* 120:227, 1985.
15. Van Sonnenberg E, D'Agostino HB, Casola G, et al: Interventional radiology in the gallbladder: Diagnosis, drainage, dissolution, and management of stones. *Radiology* 174:1, 1990.
16. Werbel GB, Nahrwold DL, Joehl RJ, et al: Percutaneous cholecystostomy in the diagnosis and treatment of acute cholecystitis in the high-risk patient. *Arch Surg* 124:782, 1989.
17. McGahan JP, Lindfors KK: Acute cholecystitis: Diagnostic accuracy of percutaneous aspiration of the gallbladder. *Radiology* 167:669, 1988.
18. McGahan JP, Lindfors KK: Percutaneous cholecystostomy: An alternative to surgical cholecystostomy for acute cholecystitis. *Radiology* 173:481, 1989.
19. Boland GW, Lee MJ, Leung J, et al: Percutaneous cholecystostomy in critically ill patients: Early response and final outcome in 82 patients. *AJR* 163:339, 1994.
20. Lee WJ, Patel U, Patel S, Pillari GP: Emergency percutaneous nephrostomy: Results and complications. *J Vasc Intervent Radiol* 5:135, 1994.
21. Mitty HA, Efremidis S, Keller RJ: Colonic stricture after transcatheter embolization for diverticular bleeding. *AJR* 133:519, 1979.
22. Shenoy SS, Satchidanand S, Wesp EH: Colonic ischemic necrosis following therapeutic embolization. *Gastrointest Radiol* 6:235, 1981.
23. Rosenkrantz H, Bookstein JJ, Rosen RJ, et al: Postembolic colonic infarction. *Radiology* 142:47, 1982.
24. Peck DJ, McLoughlin RF, Hughson MN, et al: Percutaneous embolotherapy of lower gastrointestinal hemorrhage. *J Vasc Intervent Radiol* 9:747, 1998.
25. Funaki B, Kostelic JK, Lorenz J, et al: Superselective microcoil embolization of colonic hemorrhage. *AJR* 177:829, 2001.
26. Bandi R, Shetty PC, Sharma RP, et al: Superselective arterial embolization for the treatment of lower gastrointestinal hemorrhage. *J Vasc Intervent Radiol* 12:1399, 2001.
27. Lang EV, Picus D, Marx MV, et al: Massive upper gastrointestinal hemorrhage with normal findings on arteriography: Value of prophylactic embolization of the left gastric artery. *AJR* 158:547, 1992.
28. Keller FS: Nonoperative management of gastrointestinal hemorrhage. *Semin Intervent Radiol* 5:1, 1988.
29. Darcy M: Treatment of lower gastrointestinal bleeding: Vasopressing infusion versus embolization. *J Vasc Intervent Radiol* 14:535, 2003.
30. Goldman ML, Land WC, Bradley EL, et al: Transcatheter therapeutic embolization in the management of massive upper gastrointestinal bleeding. *Radiology* 120:513, 1976.

31. Walker TG, Waltman AC: Vasoconstrictive infusion therapy for management of arterial gastrointestinal hemorrhage. *Semin Intervent Radiol* 5:18, 1988.

32. Rollins ES, Picus D, Hicks M, et al: Angiography is useful in detecting the source of chronic gastrointestinal bleeding of obscure origin. *AJR* 156:385, 1991.

33. Malden ES, Hicks ME, Royal HD, et al: Recurrent gastrointestinal bleeding: Use of thrombolysis with anticoagulation in diagnosis. *Radiology* 207:147, 1998.

34. Ryan JM, Key SM, Dumbleton SA, Smith TP: Nonlocalized lower gastrointestinal bleeding: Provocative bleeding studies with intraarterial tPA, heparin, and tolazoline. *J Vasc Intervent Radiol* 12:1273, 2001.

35. Koval G, Benner KG, Rosch J, Kozak BE: Aggressive angiographic diagnosis in acute lower gastrointestinal hemorrhage. *Dig Dis Sci* 32:248, 1987.

36. Mernagh JR, O'Donovan N, Somers S, et al: Use of heparin in the investigation of obscure gastrointestinal bleeding. *Can Assoc Radiol J* 52:232, 2001.

37. Salerno F, Merli M, Cazzaniga M, et al: MELD score is better than Child-Pugh score in predicting 3-month survival of patients undergoing transjugular intrahepatic portosystemic shunt. *J Hepatol* 36:494, 2002.

38. Ferral H, Vasan R, Speeg KV, et al: Evaluation of a model to predict poor survival in patients undergoing elective TIPS procedures. *J Vasc Intervent Radiol* 13:1103, 2002.

39. Coldwell DM, Ring EJ, Rees CR, et al: Multicenter investigation of the role of transjugular intrahepatic portosystemic shunt in management of portal hypertension. *Radiology* 196:335, 1995.

40. Miller-Catchpole R: Transjugular intrahepatic portosystemic shunts (TIPS): Diagnostic and therapeutic technology assessment (DATTA). *JAMA* 273:1824, 1995.

41. Encarnacion CE, Palmaz JC, Rivera FJ, et al: Transjugular intrahepatic portosystemic shunt placement for variceal bleeding: Predictors of mortality. *J Vasc Intervent Radiol* 6:687, 1995.

42. Naidich DP, Funt S, Ettenger NA, et al: Hemoptysis: CT-bronchoscopic correlations in 58 cases. *Radiology* 177:357, 1990.

43. Tak S, Ahluwalia G, Sharma SK, et al: Haemoptysis in patients with a normal chest radiography: Bronchoscopy-CT correlation. *Australas Radiol* 43:451, 1999.

44. McGuinness G, Beacher JR, Harkin TJ, et al: Hemoptysis: Prospective high-resolution CT/bronchoscopic correlation. *Chest* 105:1155, 1994.

45. Roberts AC: Bronchial artery embolization therapy. *J Thorac Imaging* 5:60, 1990.

46. Uflacker R, Kaemmerer A, Picon PD, et al: Bronchial artery embolization in the management of hemoptysis: Technical aspects and long-term results. *Radiology* 157:637, 1985.

47. Kato A, Kudo S, Matsumoto K, et al: Bronchial artery embolization for hemoptysis due to benign diseases: Immediate and long-term results. *Cardiovasc Intervent Radiol* 23:351, 2000.

48. Fisher RG, Ferreyro R: Evaluation of current techniques for nonsurgical removal of intravascular iatrogenic foreign bodies. *AJR* 130:541, 1978.

49. Uflacker R, Lima S, Melichar AC: Intravascular foreign bodies: Percutaneous retrieval. *Radiology* 160:731, 1986.

50. Schmidt GA, Hall JB: Pulmonary embolism: Beyond anticoagulation. *Intensive Crit Care Dig* 8:3, 1989.

51. Grassi CJ: Iinferior vena caval filters: Analysis of five currently available devices. *AJR* 156:813, 1991.

52. Dorfman GS: Percutaneous inferior vena caval filters. *Radiology* 174:987, 1990.

53. Kinney TB: Update on inferior vena cava filters. *J Vasc Intervent Radiol* 14:425, 2003.

54. Nutting C, Coldwell D: Use of a TrapEase device as a temporary caval filter. *J Vasc Intervent Radiol* 12:991, 2001.

55. Millward SF, Bhargava A, Aquino J, et al: Gunther tulip filter: Preliminary clinical experience with retrieval. *J Vasc Intervent Radiol* 11:75, 2000.

56. Tobin KD, Pais SO, Austin CBP: Reevaluation of indications for percutaneous placement of the Greenfield filter. *Invest Radiol* 24:115, 1989.

57. Orsini RA, Jarrell BE: Suprarenal placement of vena caval filters: Indications, techniques, and results. *J Vasc Surg* 1:124, 1984.

58. Hicks ME, Middleton WD, Picus D, et al: Incidence of local venous thrombosis following Bird's Nest IVC filter placement. *J Vasc Intervent Radiol* 1:63, 1990.

59. Semba CP, Murphy TP, Bakal CW, et al: Thrombolytic therapy with use of alteplase (rt-PA) in peripheral arterial occlusive disease: review of the clinical literature. *J Vasc Intervent Radiol* 11:149, 2000.

60. Marker VJ, Sherry S: Thrombolytic therapy: Current status. *New Engl J Med* 318:1512, 1585, 1988.

61. Durham JD, Geller SC, Abbott WM, et al: Regional infusion of urokinase into occluded lower-extremity bypass grafts: Long-term clinical results. *Radiology* 172:83, 1989.

62. Klatte EC, Becker GJ, Holden RE, et al: Fibrinolytic therapy. *Radiology* 159:619, 1986.

63. Ouriel K, Shortell CK, DeWeese JA, et al: A comparison of thrombolytic therapy with operative revascularization in the initial treatment of acute peripheral arterial ischemia. *J Vasc Surg* 19:1021, 1994.

64. STILE Investigators: Results of a prospective, randomized trial evaluating surgery versus thrombolysis for ischemia of the lower extremity: STILE trial. *Ann Surg* 220:251, 1994.

PART XI

SPECIAL PROBLEMS
IN CRITICAL CARE

Chapter 102

TOXICOLOGY IN ADULTS

THOMAS CORBRIDGE
PATRICK MURRAY
BABAK MOKHLESI

KEY POINTS

General Measures

- *Supportive measures supercede other considerations in the management of the poisoned patient. After addressing the ABCDs of life support, the focus can switch to confirmation of intoxication and targeted therapy.*

- *Administer a "cocktail" of oxygen, dextrose, thiamine, and naloxone to patients with depressed mental status.*

- *An increase in anion gap, osmolal gap, or arterial saturation gap should raise the suspicion of intoxication.*

- *An osmolal gap of large magnitude (>25 mOsm) suggests methanol or ethylene glycol poisoning; however, serious intoxication with either agent can occur without increasing the osmolal gap. Serum levels of these alcohols should be measured when clinical features are suggestive.*

- *Carbon monoxide and methemoglobin elevate the arterial oxygen saturation gap. These toxins interfere with oxygen binding to hemoglobin and decrease oxygen content without lowering the Pa_{O_2}. Oxygen saturation measured by pulse oximetry is falsely high in this setting.*

- *Toxicology screening can provide direct evidence of intoxication, but it rarely impacts initial management.*

- *Poison control center consultation is advised to determine appropriate laboratory testing and patient disposition and treatment. The emergency phone number is 1-800-222-1222.*

- *Gastric lavage only improves outcome in obtunded patients if performed within 1 hour of ingestion (this time may be extended in poisonings that delay gastric emptying). Risks of lavage preclude its use in nontoxic ingestions, subtoxic amounts of a toxic ingestion, ingestion of caustic liquids, and when the toxin is no longer expected to be in the stomach. The airway must be protected prior to lavage.*

- *Activated charcoal should be administered for most oral ingestions after the airway has been protected.*

- *Whole-bowel irrigation with a polyethylene glycol electrolyte solution is indicated for iron overdose, ingestion of sustained-release tablets, and "body packing" with illicit drugs.*

- *Urinary alkalinization enhances excretion of nonpolar weak acids. Urinary acidification augments excretion of nonpolar weak bases, but is generally not recommended.*

Acetaminophen

- *All overdose cases should be screened for acetaminophen poisoning.*

- *The antidote, n-acetylcysteine (NAC), should be started within 8 hours of ingestion to decrease the risk of hepatotoxicity. The Rumack-Matthew nomogram allows for stratification of selected patients into categories of probable, possible, and no hepatic toxicity.*

Alcohols

- *Metabolic acidosis with an elevated anion gap and/or the presence of an osmolal gap are classic in methanol and ethylene glycol poisoning.*

- *Features of methanol poisoning include inebriation, optic papillitis, and pancreatitis. Treatment with fomepizole or ethanol inhibits metabolism by alcohol dehydrogenase to the toxic metabolite formic acid. Dialysis is indicated in severe cases.*

- *Features of ethylene glycol poisoning include inebriation, acute renal failure, crystalluria, and myocardial dysfunction.*

- *Treatment with fomepizole or ethanol inhibits metabolism by alcohol dehydrogenase to toxic metabolites (oxalic and glycolic acids). Dialytic removal of ethylene glycol and its metabolites is indicated in severe poisonings.*

- *Isopropanol causes hemorrhagic gastritis, ketonemia, and ketonuria, but not acidosis. Fomepizole and ethanol are not indicated because metabolites are nontoxic. Dialysis is effective in severe cases.*

Barbiturates

- *Hypothermia, hypotension, bradycardia, flaccidity, hyporeflexia, coma, and apnea are features of barbiturate overdose. Severe overdose can mimic death.*

- *Supportive measures include gastric emptying and activated charcoal. Alkalinization of the urine increases elimination of phenobarbital, but not other barbiturates, and may aggravate pulmonary edema. Of disputed importance, hemoperfusion may be considered in severe cases.*

Benzodiazepines

- *Supportive measures, gastric emptying, activated charcoal, and flumazenil treat benzodiazepine overdose.*

- *Flumazenil reverses sedation but may increase the toxicity of coingested drugs. Flumazenil should be avoided in patients taking benzodiazepines therapeutically and in benzodiazepine-addicted patients.*

- *There is no role for forced diuresis, dialysis, or hemoperfusion in benzodiazepine overdose.*

Beta-Blockers

- *Cardiovascular manifestations of overdose are treated with fluids, vasopressors, atropine, electrical pacing, and glucagon.*

- *Glucagon effectively reverses myocardial depression and bradycardia.*

Calcium Channel Blockers

- *Hypotension is treated first with fluids and calcium chloride. Glucagon may decrease vasopressor requirements.*

Carbon Monoxide

- *Exposure to smoke, poorly ventilated charcoal or gas heaters, and automobile exhaust are responsible for most poisonings.*

- *Carbon monoxide poisoning can present with myocardial ischemia, arrhythmias, mental status changes, headache, and generalized weakness.*

- *Prompt oxygen therapy is crucial.*

- Pulse oximetry is unreliable in detecting carboxyhemoglobin; pulse oximetry overestimates oxyhemoglobin by the amount of carboxyhemoglobin present; saturation by pulse oximetry may be normal despite elevated carboxyhemoglobin.
- The use of hyperbaric oxygen is controversial. Patients with potentially life-threatening exposures should receive hyperbaric therapy if it is readily available and other life-threatening conditions do not preclude its use.
- Delayed neurologic sequelae may occur in survivors.

Cocaine

- Cocaine is often mixed with other substances of abuse.
- Cocaine causes acute coronary syndromes, hypertensive crisis, seizures, rhabdomyolysis, intracranial hemorrhage, pneumomediastinum, and respiratory failure.
- Agitation and hyperthermia should be treated rapidly with benzodiazepines and cooling strategies. Paralysis is occasionally required.
- Benzodiazepines are first-line therapy for hypertensive crisis. Refractory patients should receive an α-adrenergic antagonist. Nonselective β-blockers (eg, propranolol) should not be used alone to treat hypertension because of the potential for unopposed α-adrenergic stimulation. Labetalol is controversial. Selective β-blockers do not aggravate hypertension but may cause hypotension.
- Acute coronary syndromes should be treated with nitrates and benzodiazepines. Refractory patients should receive α-adrenergic antagonists. Nonselective β-blockers are contraindicated; selective β-blockers do not aggravate hypertension, but may induce hypotension.

Cyanide

- Features of cyanide poisoning depend on the amount and rate of cyanide absorption. Patients who are asymptomatic after inhalation generally do not require treatment. Oral ingestion causes progressive symptoms over minutes to hours.
- Sodium nitroprusside infusions can cause cyanide and thiocyanate poisoning.
- Symptoms include anxiety, dyspnea, headache, confusion, tachycardia, and hypertension. High concentrations of cyanide cause stupor or coma, seizures, fixed and dilated pupils, hypoventilation, hypotension, arrhythmias, and cardiopulmonary collapse.
- In addition to supportive measures and oxygen, several antidotes are available: amyl and sodium nitrite, sodium thiosulfate, hydroxycobalamin, and dicobalt ethylenediamine tetraacetic acid (EDTA).

Cyclic Antidepressants

- Patients with anticholinergic, neurologic, or cardiac toxicity (including QRS prolongation ≥100 ms) require monitoring.
- Neurologic deterioration is often abrupt and unpredictable.
- Acidemia potentiates toxicity. Therapeutic alkalemia with sodium bicarbonate or hyperventilation is beneficial.
- Lidocaine should be used for ventricular arrhythmias resistant to sodium bicarbonate. Procainamide is contraindicated.

Digoxin

- Features of digitalis intoxication include fatigue, gastrointestinal symptoms, neurologic disturbances (blurred vision, visual color changes, headache, dizziness, and delirium), and cardiac arrhythmias (supraventricular tachycardia with AV block). Significant overdose may cause hyperkalemia.
- Supportive therapy includes rapid correction of arrhythmogenic metabolic disturbances, particularly hypokalemia if present. Hyperkalemia requires treatment unless Fab therapy is immediately available.
- Immunotherapy with digoxin-specific antibody Fab fragments is indicated for severe intoxications.
- Gastrointestinal decontamination measures include gastric lavage and activated charcoal. Hemodialysis removes only small amounts of total body digitalis, but may be indicated for correction of hyperkalemia or other acid-base derangements in renally impaired patients.
- Electrical cardioversion of a digitalis toxicity–induced arrhythmia should be reserved as a last resort, using the minimum effective energy level.

Gamma Hydroxybutyrate

- Depressed mental status, emesis, bradycardia, hypotension, and respiratory depression are features of GHB overdose.
- Treatment is mainly supportive.
- In cases of alleged sexual assault, GHB can be identified by analysis of hair, blood, and urine in selected laboratories.

Lithium

- Most cases of intoxication, associated with levels above 1.5 mEq/L, are caused by unintentional overdose during chronic therapy.
- High levels of lithium decrease the anion gap.
- Severe poisoning causes coma, seizures, and cardiovascular instability.
- Treatment includes seizure control and vasopressors for hypotension refractory to fluids. Gastric emptying should be performed initially. Oral charcoal is of little benefit. Whole-bowel irrigation is important with sustained-release preparations.
- Lithium is the prototypical dialyzable intoxicant.

Methemoglobinemia

- Hereditary methemoglobinemia (e.g., hemoglobin M or cytochrome b5 reductase deficiency) is generally insignificant and does not require treatment. Acquired and potentially life-threatening methemoglobinemia can occur after oxidant drug or toxin exposure.
- Methemoglobinemia decreases oxyhemoglobin saturation and blood oxygen carrying capacity by decreasing available hemoglobin and shifting the oxyhemoglobin dissociation curve to the left.
- Symptoms of moderate methemoglobinemia include dyspnea, headache, and weakness. Confusion, seizures, and death can occur with levels >60%.
- Co-oximetry measures methemoglobin saturation. Standard pulse oximetry registers falsely high in patients with methemoglobinemia. Arterial blood gases typically demonstrate a normal Pa_{O_2} and a normal calculated oxygen saturation.
- Treatment of methemoglobinemia consists of oxygen, methylene blue, and exchange transfusion.

Opioids

- *The triad of miosis, respiratory depression, and coma suggests opioid intoxication.*
- *Naloxone reverses sedation, hypotension, and respiratory depression. The initial dose is 0.4 mg IV or 0.8 mg IM or SC. Lower doses should be given to opioid-dependent patients and when there is a concurrent stimulant overdose. Larger initial doses may be required when there is abuse of naloxone-resistant opioids. Lack of response to 6 to 10 mg of naloxone generally excludes opioid toxicity.*

Organophosphate and Carbamate Insecticides

- *Organophosphates are irreversible inhibitors of acetylcholinesterase (AChE); carbamates reversibly inhibit AChE.*
- *Signs of cholinergic poisoning include salivation, lacrimation, urination, diarrhea, gastrointestinal cramping and emesis (SLUDGE). Muscle fasciculations, coma, and seizures also occur.*
- *Respiratory failure results from muscle weakness, bronchorrhea, depressed respiratory drive, and bronchoconstriction.*
- *The level of red blood cell cholinesterase helps diagnose organophosphate poisoning.*
- *Treatment includes supportive measures, atropine, and oximes.*

Phencyclidine

- *PCP intoxication incites bizarre behavior, violence, agitation, euphoria, and lethargy, as well as stupor and coma that may last for days. Additional features include fever, tachycardia, hypertension, leukocytosis, renal failure, intracranial hemorrhage, and rhabdomyolysis.*
- *Pinpoint pupils in an agitated patient suggests PCP intoxication.*
- *Haloperidol is the drug of choice to treat PCP psychosis. Benzodiazepines expedite control of the difficult patient.*

Salicylates

- *The Done nomogram for predicting salicylate toxicity is of limited use in current practice.*
- *Salicylate poisoning causes respiratory alkalosis and metabolic acidosis; the latter is more prominent in children.*
- *Manifestations of chronic ingestion may be subtle and occur at relatively low serum salicylate levels.*
- *Acidemia favors tissue penetration of salicylates; urinary alkalinization enhances renal clearance; hypokalemia must be corrected to succeed in urinary alkalinization; carbonic anhydrase inhibitors should not be used to alkalinize urine.*
- *Seizures, coma, refractory acidosis, and high serum salicylate levels are indications for hemodialysis.*

Selective Serotonin Reuptake Inhibitors

- *In combination with a number of drugs, SSRIs may cause serotonin syndrome. Toxic combinations may not be evident for days to weeks.*
- *Features of serotonin syndrome include confusion, agitation, shivering, flushing, hyperthermia, tachycardia, disseminated intravascular coagulation, convulsions, coma, muscle rigidity, myoclonus, hyperreflexia, involuntary movements, autonomic instability, nausea, diarrhea, orthostatic hypotension, rhabdomyolysis, hyponatremia, and SIADH. Trazodone, which is also an α-adrenergic blocker, causes hypotension.*
- *Treatment is supportive. Gastric emptying and activated charcoal are effective. Serotonin antagonists have not been studied adequately in controlled trials.*

Theophylline

- *Clinical features of theophylline toxicity are cardiovascular, metabolic, and neurologic.*
- *Tachyarrhythmias are common at plasma levels >20 mg/L.*
- *Metabolic abnormalities include hypokalemia, hypomagnesemia, hyperglycemia, hypophosphatemia, hypercalcemia, and respiratory alkalosis.*
- *Uncontrolled seizures cause hyperthermia and rhabdomyolysis.*
- *For any plasma level, chronic intoxication causes more severe clinical sequelae.*
- *Extracorporeal removal by "in-series" hemodialysis and hemoperfusion is indicated for severe intoxications.*

Envenomations

- *The majority of poisonous snake bites in the United States involve the Crotalidae or pit viper family of snakes (e.g., rattlesnakes, copperheads, and water moccasins).*
- *Treatment of rattlesnake bite consists of immobilizing the bitten extremity and placing a loose-fitting tourniquet proximal to the bite to impede venom spread. Surgical consultation may be required for local wound management.*
- *Unstable patients should be treated with equine Crotalidae antivenin.*
- *In North America, only the widow spiders (Latrodectus species) and the recluse spiders (Loxosceles species) are medically important.*
- *Features of black widow spider bite include local pain and erythema followed by muscle cramps and fasciculations that may generalize to the abdomen, back, and chest. Hypertension, tachycardia, tremor, fever, agitation, diaphoresis, and nausea are common.*
- *Treatment of black widow spider bite consists of supportive measures, analgesia, calcium, methocarbamol, and in severe cases, equine-derived antivenin.*
- *Recluse spider bite (loxoscelism) is characterized by localized swelling, erythema, and formation of bullae, often forming a "bull's eye" lesion with central necrosis. Some patients develop fever, myalgias, headache, and nausea. Rare patients develop intravascular hemolysis, disseminated intravascular coagulopathy, acute renal failure, and the acute respiratory distress syndrome. Treatment is supportive; antivenin is not available.*

In their 2001 annual report, the American Association of Poison Control Centers reported 2,267,979 human toxic exposure cases. Three percent of these cases, or more than 69,000 patients, required critical care. There were 1074 fatalities, occurring most commonly after intentional overdose.[1]

Intentional overdose or accidental exposure may be the chief complaint at the time of emergency department evaluation, but not all patients provide this information, particularly when toxin or trauma clouds mental status. In these cases signs and symptoms may be attributed to another disorder and poisoning remains obscure. In hospital, inappropriate drug dosing or unforeseen drug interactions may lead to toxic side effects.

Classic features of overdose, referred to as a toxidrome, help establish a diagnosis, but signs and symptoms may be nonspecific or lacking altogether, as in the early stages of acetaminophen overdose. The protean manifestations of intoxication mandate a high index of suspicion in critically ill patients.

Treatment of the poisoned patient often occurs before a diagnosis has been established. Most important in this regard are standard supportive measures. The ABCDs (airway, breathing, circulation, and differential diagnosis) come first while efforts ensue to confirm intoxication and initiate targeted therapy.

In this chapter we will review (1) initial supportive efforts, (2) diagnosis of poisoning and drug overdose, (3) techniques to limit drug absorption and enhance drug elimination, and (4) specific treatments of the most commonly encountered drugs, toxins, and envenomations seen in the intensive care unit.

Initial Supportive Measures

Primary physician responsibilities are to identify and treat life-threatening problems. The ABCDs of life support should be addressed as in any medically unstable patient, but for the first time, the 2000 version of the American Heart Association guidelines included a separate section on resuscitating the poisoned patient.[2] Recommendations provided in these guidelines are discussed in this chapter.

With cervical spine precautions in place (unless trauma has been reasonably excluded) airway patency must be established. In obtunded patients, obstruction by the tongue is treated initially with a jaw-thrust maneuver, followed by either placement of an oral airway, nasal trumpet, or endotracheal tube. The choice of airway depends on the level of obtundation, the vigor of protective reflexes, the degree of respiratory depression, and initial response to pharmacologic therapy (Table 102-1). In nonintubated patients, the left side down, head-down position allows the tongue to drop forward and decreases risk of aspiration of oral secretions and stomach contents.

Patients with an adequate airway and intact protective reflexes may not require intubation (even if they are lethargic), particularly if treatment improves mental status. Intubation is indicated when a patient is unable to protect the airway or maintain respirations. Intubation protects the airway and decreases but does not eliminate the risk of aspiration, which occurs in approximately 11% of comatose patients with drug overdose.[3–5] Intubation further allows for administration of high concentrations of oxygen and assisted ventilation.

Selected causes of hypoxemia in drug overdose and toxic ingestion are listed in Table 102-2. Hypoxemia must be corrected quickly to avoid anoxic brain injury, myocardial ischemia, and arrhythmias. In some poisonings (eg, carbon monoxide, cyanide, and methemoglobinemia), a fraction of inspired oxygen (F_{IO_2}) of 1.0 is therapeutic, whereas in paraquat poisoning and bleomycin toxicity oxygen potentiates lung injury.

The clinician should choose a ventilator mode with which she or he is familiar and which achieves the greatest degree of synchrony between patient and machine. The initial ventilator mode should provide adequate back-up minute ventilation (which can be achieved with either assist control or synchronized intermittent mandatory ventilation). If intubation is performed solely to protect the airway or to provide supplemental oxygen, the endotracheal tube may be connected to a T-tube. Positive end-expiratory pressure (PEEP) recruits atelectatic and fluid-filled alveoli and may decrease ventilator-induced lung injury in selected patients. PEEP should be used cautiously in hypotensive patients to avoid decreasing cardiac preload. Low levels of pressure support ventilation (5 to 8 cm H_2O) help overcome endotracheal tube resistance and may decrease inspiratory work of breathing.

Circulatory manifestations of drug overdose are common and varied. Bradycardia and/or atrioventricular (AV) block can result from cholinergic excess (e.g., with organophosphate, carbamate, physostigmine, and digoxin toxicity), sympatholytic drugs (e.g., β-blockers, clonidine, and opioids), membrane-depressant agents (e.g., type 1a and 1c antiarrhythmic drugs, quinidine, and cyclic antidepressants), calcium channel blockers, and lithium overdose (Table 102-3). Bradycardia can also occur from a reflex response to

TABLE 102-1 Initial Pharmacologic Treatment of Patients with Altered Mental Status

Drug	Dose	Comment
Oxygen	Titrate to Sp_{O_2} >92%; F_{IO_2} 1.0 for carbon monoxide and cyanide toxicity	Oxygen may increase risk of pulmonary toxicity in paraquat intoxication
Dextrose	50 mg IV	Antidote for oral hypoglycemic or insulin overdose
Thiamine	100 mg IV	Used to prevent Wernicke encephalopathy; rare anaphylactoid reactions have been reported
Naloxone	0.2–0.4 mg IV initial dose; if no clinical response after 2–3 minutes, an additional 1–2 mg IV may be administered to a total dose of 10 mg; higher doses may be required in meperidine or propoxyphene overdose; in opioid-addicted patients, lower doses (0.1–0.2mg) may help without causing drug withdrawal	Short duration of action (approximately 20–60 minutes) requires repeat dosing or continuous infusion

TABLE 102-2 Selected Causes of Hypoxemia in Drug Overdose and Toxic Ingestion

Cause	Drugs/Toxins
Hypoventilation	Alcohols
	Barbiturates
	Benzodiazepines
	Botulinum toxin
	Cyclic antidepressants
	Neuromuscular blockade
	Opioids
	Sedative-hypnotics
	Snake bite
	Strychnine
	Tetanus
Aspiration	Drugs/toxins depressing mental status
Pneumonia	Drugs resulting in aspiration;
	IV drug abuse with pulmonary seeding of infectious agents;
	Inhalation injury interfering with lung protective mechanisms
Cardiogenic pulmonary edema	Antiarrhythmics
	β-Blockers
	Cyclic antidepressants
	Verapamil
Inert gases	Methane
	Nitrogen
	Propane
Noncardiogenic pulmonary edema	Cocaine
	Ethylene glycol
	Hydrocarbons
	Inhalation injury
	Opioids
	Phosgene
	Paraquat
	Salicylates
Bronchospasm	β-Blockers Cocaine Heroin
	Organophosphates
	Drugs resulting in aspiration
	Drugs associated with myocardial depression (cardiac asthma)
Alveolar hemorrhage	Cocaine
Pneumothorax	Cocaine
	IV drug abuse with aberrant venipuncture or bullous lung disease
Cellular hypoxia	Carbon monoxide
	Cyanide
	Hydrogen sulfide
	Methemoglobinemia
	Sulfhemoglobinemia

TABLE 102-3 Selected Drugs/Toxins Causing Tachycardia and Bradycardia

Tachycardia	Bradycardia
Amphetamines	Antiarrhythmics (types 1a and 1c)
Anticholinergics	β-Blockers
Antihistamines	Calcium channel blockers
Caffeine	Carbamates
Carbon monoxide	Clonidine
Clonidine	Cyclic antidepressants
Cocaine	Digoxin
Cyanide	Lithium
Cyclic antidepressants	Metoclopramide
Drug withdrawal	Opioids
Ephedrine	Organophosphates
Hydralazine	Phenylpropanolamine
Hydrogen sulfide	Physostigmine
Methemoglobinemia	Propoxyphene
Phencyclidine (PCP)	Quinidine
Phenothiazines	
Pseudoephedrine	
Theophylline	
Thyroid hormone overdose	

vagolytic, so further administration of atropine beyond this dose is unlikely to be beneficial. An exception to this tenet is cholinergic poisoning, in which extremely high doses of atropine may be required to increase heart rate and dry secretions. In selected overdoses, antidotes are available for treatment of bradycardia: calcium chloride for calcium channel blocker toxicity; glucagon in β-blocker overdose; sodium bicarbonate in cyclic antidepressant overdose; naloxone in opioid overdose; and digoxin-specific antibodies in digoxin toxicity. Refractory and symptomatic bradycardia or heart block is an indication for transcutaneous or transvenous pacing or infusion with dopamine or epinephrine. If transcutaneous pacing is used successfully, a prophylactic transvenous pacemaker is not recommended because the wire may trigger ventricular arrhythmias.[2]

Table 102-3 includes selected drugs and toxins causing tachycardia. Sinus tachycardia and supraventricular arrhythmias commonly result from sympathetic overstimulation (e.g., with cocaine, theophylline, amphetamines, or phencyclidine) or inhibition of parasympathetic tone (e.g., with cyclic antidepressants, phenothiazines, or antihistamines). Anxiety, hypovolemia, hypoxemia, myocardial infarction, hyperthermia, infection, and pregnancy are in the differential diagnosis. Treatment of sinus tachycardia should be aimed at correcting the underlying cause. In the setting of stimulant intoxication, sedation with benzodiazepines is usually sufficient. β-Blockade can be helpful in the setting of excessive sympathetic stimulation and myocardial ischemia; however, nonselective β-blockers should not be used alone to treat cocaine toxicity because of the potential for unopposed α-adrenergic stimulation. In anticholinergic intoxication, physostigmine decreases heart rate by increasing acetylcholine concentration at myoneural junctions; however, the potential for physostigmine to worsen cardiac conduction disturbances precludes its use in most cases of cyclic antidepressant overdose.

Drugs such as cocaine, caffeine, and amphetamines cause ventricular arrhythmias through sympathomimetic effects.

α-adrenergic-induced hypertension (e.g., phenylpropanolamine).

The differential diagnosis of bradycardia includes hypoxemia, myocardial infarction, hyperkalemia, hypothermia, hypothyroidism, and intracranial hypertension. If bradycardia persists despite correction of hypoxemia or hypothermia and is hemodynamically significant, atropine 0.5 to 1.0 mg IV should be given and repeated every 5 to 10 minutes until a therapeutic response has been achieved or adverse drug effects appear. Three milligrams of atropine is fully

Membrane depressants such as cyclic antidepressants are arrhythmogenic by prolonging depolarization and negative inotropy. Drugs which prolong the QT interval (e.g., amiodarone, astemizole, terfenadine, cyclic antidepressants, quinidine, procainamide, and disopyramide) may induce polymorphic ventricular tachycardia or torsades de pointes. Drug-induced torsades de pointes is treated by correction of risk factors (hypokalemia, hypomagnesemia, and hypoxemia), magnesium supplementation (even when serum concentrations are normal), and overdrive pacing by electrical stimulation or isoproterenol.[2]

Treatment of ventricular tachycardia and ventricular fibrillation is similar to that recommended in advanced cardiac life support. However, important exceptions pertain to cyclic antidepressant overdose.[6] These patients should immediately receive hypertonic sodium bicarbonate (1 to 2 mEq/kg IV bolus) aiming for a serum pH of 7.5 to 7.55. In intubated patients, hyperventilation achieves alkalemia without the need to deliver a large sodium load, but hypertonic sodium usually provides greater benefit. Lidocaine is the drug of choice when ventricular arrhythmias are refractory to sodium bicarbonate.[6] Class 1a antiarrhythmics (e.g., procainamide) are contraindicated in cyclic antidepressant overdose because of added cardiac toxicity. Anecdotal reports have also suggested a primary role for phenytoin; however, convincing data are not available to support the use of phenytoin in the setting of cyclic antidepressant overdose as either a prophylactic or therapeutic drug.[7,8] Physostigmine should not be used in cyclic antidepressant overdose because of possible worsening of cardiac conduction disturbances.

Based on limited data in humans and animals and extensive unpublished experience, the expert panel on toxicologic-oriented advanced life support suggests a primary role for sodium bicarbonate and lidocaine in cocaine-associated ventricular tachycardia and ventricular fibrillation.[6,9–12] In making these recommendations the panel did take into account studies in animals showing that lidocaine worsened seizures and widened the QRS complex in the setting of cocaine toxicity.[6]

Cardioversion or defibrillation is appropriate for pulseless patients with drug-induced ventricular tachycardia (VT) or ventricular fibrillation (VF). Whether epinephrine should be used in this setting is unknown; if used, the working group of the AHA recommends increasing the interval between doses and avoidance of high-dose epinephrine.[2] This group also recommends more prolonged cardiopulmonary resuscitation (CPR) in poisoning cases because of anecdotal reports of good neurologic recovery after 3 to 5 hours of CPR.[2,13,14]

A variety of mechanisms are responsible for hypotension in drug overdose: hypovolemia, cardiac arrhythmias, systemic vasodilation and myocardial depression. An initial strategy of rapid fluid administration (e.g., 1 L normal saline over 30 minutes) is appropriate in most cases, although caution is warranted in the setting of pulmonary edema or poor cardiac contractility (e.g., in verapamil overdose). Cardiac arrhythmias and hypothermia should be corrected and antidotes administered if appropriate. Hypotension refractory to the above measures should be treated with vasopressors. Dopamine (5 to 20 μg/kg per minute IV) stimulates α, β, and dopaminergic receptors to increase heart rate, blood pressure, and cardiac output in most patients. In patients with tachyarrhythmias or ventricular fibrillation, agents with weak β_1-activity

(norepinephrine) or no β-receptor activity (phenylephrine) are preferred. Norepinephrine and phenylephrine are preferred in cyclic antidepressant overdose because cyclic antidepressants deplete presynaptic catecholamine stores, limiting the effectiveness of dopamine.[15–17] In contrast, in the presence of cocaine, dopamine and other vasopressors may trigger an exaggerated response caused by inhibition of catecholamine reuptake; in the presence of monoamine oxidase inhibitors an exaggerated response occurs because of inhibition of catecholamine degradation. An enhanced hypertensive response to phenylephrine can occur in anticholinergic overdose because anticholinergics interfere with phenylephrine-induced reflex bradycardia. Vasopressor agents should not be used in the setting of ergot derivative toxicity because of the potential for severe and sustained vasoconstriction.

Hypertension with tachycardia occurs in the setting of (1) sympathomimetic drugs (amphetamines, cocaine, lysergic acid diethylamide [LSD], marijuana, monoamine oxidase inhibitors, and phencyclidine [PCP]); (2) anticholinergics (antihistamines, atropine, cyclic antidepressants, and phenothiazines); and (3) withdrawal from nicotine, alcohol, and sedative-hypnotics. Hypertension with reflex bradycardia occurs in ergot derivative, methoxamine, phenylephrine, and phenylpropanolamine toxicity.

Treatment of hypertension depends on the chronicity and severity of hypertension and on the response to initial supportive efforts (e.g., agitated patients often respond well to benzodiazepines alone). When hypertension is severe in the setting of chronic hypertension, lowering diastolic blood pressure by 20% or to approximately 100 to 110 mm Hg is recommended. In the absence of prior hypertension, diastolic blood pressure may be lowered safely into the normal range. Drug-induced hypertension refractory to benzodiazepines should be treated with a short-acting agent such as nitroprusside. Phentolamine is effective in the setting of α-adrenergic stimulation from phenylephrine, phenylpropanolamine, or cocaine. Labetalol in carefully titrated doses is a third-line agent. Nonselective β-blockers are contraindicated because they may worsen α-adrenergic-induced hypertension.[2,18]

"COMA COCKTAIL"

A "cocktail" of oxygen, dextrose, thiamine, and naloxone should be administered to patients with depressed mental status (see Table 102-1). These relatively innocuous drugs are helpful diagnostically and therapeutically. Although not well supported in the literature,[19] thiamine is administered to prevent Wernicke-Korsakoff syndrome. This disorder is characterized by ocular disturbances (nystagmus and weak external rectus muscles), ataxia, and deranged mental status (confusion, apathy, drowsiness, and confabulation). Tachycardia, hypotension, electrocardiographic abnormalities, and cardiovascular collapse also occur. Thiamine is particularly important in the nutritionally depleted alcoholic receiving intravenous glucose. Glucose further depletes thiamine and may precipitate or worsen Wernicke-Korsakoff syndrome. There are no compelling data to support the practice of withholding dextrose until thiamine has been administered.[19]

A blood dipstick test can be used to detect severe hypoglycemia. However, a normal value for glucose by dipstick does not exclude a low serum level, thereby warranting treatment in all patients with normal or low values. If the dipstick reading is high, it is reasonable to wait for serum confirmation of hyperglycemia. There is concern that overadministration of dextrose may cause harm by increasing serum osmolality or extending ischemic stroke, but this has not been well supported in the literature.[19]

Naloxone is an opioid antagonist with no opioid agonist properties. It can rapidly reverse opioid-induced coma, hypotension, respiratory depression, and analgesia.[20] Naloxone is administered intravenously, intramuscularly, or subcutaneously. The initial dose is 0.4 mg IV or 0.8 mg IM or SC. Lower doses (0.1 to 0.2 mg) are preferred in opioid-dependent patients to avoid severe withdrawal.[6] A low dose is also appropriate when concurrent stimulant use is suspected.[6,19]

The goal is to restore airway reflexes and adequate ventilation, not complete arousal. Abrupt withdrawal may increase the risk of arrhythmias, agitation, and acute pulmonary edema.[2,21] If naloxone does not produce a clinical response after 2 to 3 minutes, an additional 1 to 2 mg IV may be administered to a total dose of 6 to 10 mg. In general, a lack of response to 6 to 10 mg of naloxone is required to exclude opioid toxicity.[6] Even higher doses may be required to antagonize the effects of meperidine, propoxyphene, diphenoxylate, methadone, and pentazocine.[22] Continuing naloxone beyond a total dose of 10 mg is reasonable if there is a suspicion of opioid overdose and a partial response has been achieved.

In general, opioid antagonism occurs within minutes of naloxone administration and lasts for 1 to 2 hours. The effects of naloxone do not last as long as those of heroin or methadone, so repeat boluses may be required every 20 to 60 minutes to maintain an adequate clinical response. Alternatively, a continuous naloxone infusion may be started (0.4 to 0.8 mg/h, or two thirds of the initial dose needed to achieve a response per hour IV).

Consider flumazenil if benzodiazepine overdose is highly suspected or confirmed and benzodiazepines have not been prescribed for a potentially life-threatening condition (such as status epilepticus or raised intracranial pressure). In the setting of long-term benzodiazepine use, flumazenil may result in severe withdrawal or seizures.[23,24] In a rat model of combined cocaine-diazepam poisoning, flumazenil precipitated seizures and increased mortality.[25]

Seizures may occur in the setting of cyclic antidepressant coingestion; however, prospective data demonstrate that cautious administration of flumazenil is safe in this setting.[26] Flumazenil is effective in improving mental status in patients with suspected drug overdose and depressed mental status; however, it does not decrease the cost or number of major diagnostic and therapeutic interventions.[27]

Flumazenil is generally not recommended as a routine diagnostic or therapeutic agent in patients with depressed mental status.[2] Still, flumazenil can be useful to distinguish benzodiazepine overdose from mixed-drug intoxication or non–drug-induced coma, and it may improve clinical status. The recommended initial dose of flumazenil is 0.2 mg (2 mL) IV over 30 seconds. A further 0.3-mg (3-mL) dose can be given over 30 seconds if the desired clinical effect is not seen within 30 seconds. Additional 0.5-mg doses can be administered over 30 seconds at 1-minute intervals as needed to a total dose of 3 mg. Flumazenil dosed beyond 3 mg generally does not provide additional benefit. Patients should be monitored for resedation, particularly in cases involving high-dose or long-acting preparations or when there has been long-term use of benzodiazepines.

When mental status changes persist, other conditions should be considered. These include subdural or epidural hematoma, intracerebral hemorrhage, embolic stroke, abnormalities of sodium and other electrolytes, hypoxemia, hypothyroidism, liver or renal failure, central nervous system infection, seizures, and significant alterations in temperature. A head CT scan should be performed early in the course of an obtunded patient, and there should be a low threshold to perform lumbar puncture.

THE AGITATED OR SEIZING PATIENT

Agitated, violent, or acutely psychotic patients unresponsive to verbal counseling and a calm environment require pharmacologic treatment and/or physical restraints to establish adequate control and enhance patient and staff safety. A common error in the management of the agitated patient is to delay treatment, allowing patients to harm themselves and others. Causes of agitation other than drug overdose should be considered: drug withdrawal, head trauma with subdural hematoma, intracerebral hemorrhage, meningitis, hypoglycemia, thyrotoxicosis, pheochromocytoma, malignant hypertension, hyperthermia, and acute psychiatric illnesses.

Haloperidol (1 to 5 mg IM or IV) may be repeated every 30 to 60 minutes to a total dose not exceeding 100 mg/d. Debilitated and elderly patients should receive lower doses, and care must be taken in patients with cardiovascular disease to avoid hypotension and arrhythmias. Haloperidol prolongs the QT interval and therefore must be used cautiously (and with continuous monitoring) in the presence of other QT-prolonging drugs. Haloperidol lowers the seizure threshold and can cause neuroleptic malignant syndrome, tardive dyskinesia, and extrapyramidal symptoms (which may be treated with benztropine 1 to 4 mg PO). Haloperidol also has anticholinergic effects that are undesirable in anticholinergic overdose. Adding a benzodiazepine (e.g., lorazepam 1 mg) to each dose of haloperidol may accelerate control of the difficult patient.

Seizures are a common cause of drug-related morbidity and mortality. Multiple drugs and toxins (Table 102-4) cause them, but other etiologies such as CNS infection, stroke, head trauma, and severe metabolic disturbance must be considered in the differential diagnosis. A brief seizure that is temporally

TABLE 102-4 Common Drugs and Toxins Causing Seizures

Amphetamines
Antihistamines/decongestants
Antipsychotics
Caffeine/theophylline
Carbamates
Carbon monoxide
Cocaine
Cyclic antidepressants
Ethylene glycol
Isoniazid
Lead
Lidocaine
Lithium
Methanol
Organophosphates
Phencyclidine (PCP)
Salicylates
Withdrawal from alcohol or sedative-hypnotics

related to drug ingestion (e.g., cocaine) may be observed without further evaluation, provided the patient is alert and has a normal neurologic exam. Recurrent seizures should raise suspicion of body packing (which may be evaluated by abdominal imaging and digital and visual search of body cavities). Status epilepticus should be treated with a benzodiazepine IV followed by a barbiturate (amobarbital or phenobarbital) if necessary. Phenytoin is less likely to be of benefit in cocaine or caffeine/theophylline overdose. Patients who continue to seize despite adequate treatment with a benzodiazepine and barbiturate should be considered for paralysis to prevent hyperthermia and rhabdomyolysis. Paralysis requires continuous electroencephalographic (EEG) monitoring to follow seizure activity.

ALTERATIONS IN TEMPERATURE

Drugs and toxins have the potential to alter body temperature through a number of mechanisms (Table 102-5). Hypothermia is caused by peripheral vasodilation, inhibition of shivering, depression of metabolic activity, and exposure to a cold environment. Hyperthermia occurs when there is excessive heat generation from seizures, muscle rigidity, increased metabolic rate, or decreased sweating. Hyperthermia also occurs when drugs alter hypothalamic activity or a patient loses consciousness in a hot environment.

The differential diagnosis for hypothermia includes infection, hypoglycemia, CNS injury, and hypothyroidism. For hyperthermic patients consider infection, thyrotoxicosis, environmental heat stroke, and drug withdrawal.

Extreme temperatures must be treated aggressively to minimize life-threatening complications.[28] Specifics regarding complications and treatment of hypo- and hyperthermia are included in Chaps. 110 and 111. Two of the more notable life-threatening hyperthermic disorders are neuroleptic malignant syndrome and malignant hyperthermia. Neuroleptic malignant syndrome occurs in patients taking antipsychotic medications or withdrawing from levodopa. Clinical features include hyperthermia, muscle rigidity, mental status changes, rhabdomyolysis, and metabolic acidosis. Treatment consists of immediate administration of bromocriptine. Malignant hyperthermia is an inherited disorder characterized by hyperthermia, rigidity, and metabolic acidosis. It occurs in response to certain anesthetic agents and is treated with dantrolene.

TABLE 102-5 Selected Drugs Affecting Temperature

Hypothermia	Hyperthermia
Alcohols	Amphetamines
Barbiturates	Anticholinergics
Cyclic antidepressants	Antihistamines
Hypoglycemic agents	Cocaine
Opioids	Cyclic antidepressants
Phenothiazines	Drug withdrawal
	Lysergic acid diethylamide (LSD)
	Monoamine oxidase inhibitors
	Malignant hyperthermia
	Neuroleptic malignant syndrome
	Phencyclidine (PCP)
	Phenothiazines
	Salicylates
	Serotonin syndrome

TABLE 102-6 Clinical Features Mandating Consideration of Toxic Ingestion

Past history of drug overdose or substance abuse
Suicidal ideation or prior suicide attempt
History of other psychiatric illness
Agitation
Stupor or coma
Delirium or confusion
Seizures
Muscle rigidity
Dystonia
Cardiopulmonary arrest
Unexplained cardiac arrhythmia
Hyper/hypotension
Ventilatory failure
Aspiration
Bronchospasm
Liver failure
Renal failure
Hyper/hypothermia
Rhabdomyolysis
Elevated osmolal gap
Elevated anion gap acidosis
Elevated oxygen saturation gap
Hyper/hypoglycemia
Hyper/hyponatremia
Hyper/hypokalemia
Polypharmacy

Diagnosis of Toxic Ingestion

HISTORY AND PHYSICAL EXAMINATION

Clinical features mandating consideration of drug overdose or poisoning are listed in Table 102-6. Whenever possible, a careful history should be elicited from the patient to identify potential drugs or toxins, the timing and amount of drugs taken, and the clinical course. Information should be sought regarding prescription medications, over-the-counter drugs, and illicit substances. Friends, relatives, and other involved health care providers (including paramedics) should be questioned, and medications available to or in the vicinity of the patient should be identified. The pharmacy on the medication label should be called to determine the status of all prescription medications. Information gathered might prove unreliable or incomplete, particularly in cases of attempted suicide or illicit drug abuse, but it may also favorably impact care.[29]

Physical examination is directed toward evaluation and support of airway patency, respiration, and circulation (see above), followed by rapid assessment of mental status, temperature, pupil size, muscle tone, reflexes, skin, and peristaltic activity. In cases of a single or dominant exposure, the examination may reveal signs of a toxic syndrome (or toxidrome). A *toxidrome* is a pattern of signs and symptoms that suggests a specific class of poisoning. Common toxidromes are listed in Table 102-7.

When initial signs and symptoms are less specific, we find it useful to categorize patients as physiologically depressed (Table 102-8) or agitated and hyperadrenergic (Table 102-9). This categorization narrows the list of possible ingestions and impacts initial treatment strategies (see below). When

TABLE 102-7 Common Toxidromes

Toxidrome	Features	Drugs	Drug Treatment
Anticholinergic "Hot as a hare, dry as a bone, red as a beet, mad as a hatter"	Mydriasis Blurred vision Fever Dry skin Flushing Ileus Urinary retention Tachycardia Hypertension Psychosis Coma Seizures Myoclonus	Antihistamines Atropine Baclofen Benztropine Cyclic antidepressants Phenothiazines Propantheline Scopalamine	Physostigmine (do not use in cyclic antidepressant overdose because of potential worsening of conduction disturbances) Sodium bicarbonate in cyclic antidepressant overdose
Cholinergic *"SLUDGE"*	*Salivation* *Lacrimation* *Urination* *Diarrhea* *GI cramps* *Emesis* *Wheezing* *Diaphoresis* *Bronchorrhea* *Bradycardia* *Miosis*	Carbamate Organophosphates Physostigmine Pilocarpine	Atropine Pralidoxime for organophosphates
β-Adrenergic	Tachycardia Hypotension Tremor	Albuterol Caffeine Terbutaline Theophylline	β-Blockade (caution in asthmatics)
α-Adrenergic	Hypertension Bradycardia Mydriasis	Phenylephrine Phenylpropanolamine	R Treat hypertension with phentolamine or nitroprusside; not with β-blockers alone
Both β-and α-adrenergic	Hypertension Tachycardia Mydriasis Diaphoresis Dry mucous membranes	Amphetamines Cocaine Ephedrine Phencyclidine Pseudoephedrine	Benzodiazepines
Sedative-hypnotic	Stupor and coma Confusion Slurred speech Apnea	Anticonvulsants Antipsychotics Barbiturates Benzodiazepines Ethanol Meprobamate Opiates	Naloxone for opioids Flumazenil for benzodiazepines Urinary alkalinization for phenobarbital
Hallucinogenic	Hallucinations Psychosis Panic Fever Mydriasis Hyperthermia	Amphetamines Cannabinoids Cocaine Lysergic acid diethylamide (LSD) Phencyclidine (PCP) (may present with miosis)	Benzodiazepines Haloperidol
Extrapyramidal	Rigidity/tremor Opisthotonos Trismus Hyperreflexia Choreoathetosis	Haloperidol Phenothiazines	Diphenhydramine Benztropine
Narcotic	Altered mental status Slow respirations Miosis Bradycardia Hypotension Hypothermia Decreased bowel sounds	Dextromethorphan Opioids Pentazocine Propoxyphene	Naloxone
Serotonin	Irritability Hyperreflexia Flushing Diarrhea Diaphoresis Fever Trismus Tremor Myoclonus	Fluoxetine Meperidine Paroxetine Sertraline Trazodone	Benzodiazepine

TABLE 102-8 Selected Drugs Causing a Depressed Physiologic State

Sympatholytics
   Adrenergic blockers
   Antiarrhythmics
   Antihypertensives
   Antipsychotics
   Cyclic antidepressants
Cholinergics
   Bethanecol
   Carbamates
   Nicotine
   Organophosphates
   Physostigmine
   Pilocarpine
Sedative-hypnotics
   Alcohols
   Barbiturates
   Benzodiazepines
   Ethchlorvynol
Narcotics
   Analgesics
   Antidiarrheal agents
Other
   Carbon monoxide
   Cyanide
   Hydrogen sulfide
   Hypoglycemic agents
   Lithium
   Salicylates

TABLE 102-9 Examples of Drugs/Toxins Causing an Agitated Physiologic State

Sympathomimetics
   Adrenergic agonists
   Amphetamines
   Caffeine
   Cocaine
   Ergot alkaloids
   Monoamine oxidase inhibitors
   Theophylline
Anticholinergics
   Antihistamines
   Antiparkinsonian drugs
   Antipsychotics
   Antispasmodics
   Cyclic antidepressants
   Cyclobenzaprine
Drug withdrawal
   β-Blockers
   Clonidine
   Ethanol
   Opioids
   Sedative-hypnotics
Hallucinogens
   Lysergic acid diethylamide
   Marijuana
   Mescaline
   Phencyclidine
Other
   Thyroid hormones

TABLE 102-10 Common Drugs/Toxins Causing Delirium and Confusion

Alcohol/drug withdrawal
Anticholinergics
Antihistamines
Carbon monoxide
Cimetidine
Heavy metals
Lithium
Salicylates

confusion or delirium are primary, drugs listed in Table 102-10 deserve consideration.[30] Note that certain drugs, such as anticholinergics, present variably with stupor, coma, agitation, confusion, or delirium, depending on the timing, dose, and host factors.

Drugs affecting the autonomic nervous system (Table 102-11) alter pupil size. Combining the patient's physiologic state (i.e., agitated or depressed) with pupil size provides for rapid assessment of the dominant ingestion. For example, the constellation of agitation, tachycardia, and pinpoint pupils is suspicious for phencyclidine intoxication; lethargy and pinpoint pupils is characteristic of narcotic overdose.

Pupil reactivity and nystagmus are additional useful signs. In anticholinergic intoxication, pupils dilate and generally do not react to light, whereas in cocaine intoxication, dilated pupils usually respond to light. Alcohols, cholinergics, lithium, carbamazepine, phenytoin, and barbiturates cause horizontal gaze nystagmus. Phencyclidine, phenytoin, and barbiturates cause horizontal, vertical, or rotatory nystagmus.

Selected drugs and toxins affecting muscle tone and movement are listed in Table 102-12.[28,30] Dystonic reactions characterized by torticollis, tongue movements, and trismus are classic in haloperidol, phenothiazine, or metoclopramide overdose. Dyskinesias (e.g., myoclonus, hyperkinetic activity, and repetitive activity) are seen with anticholinergics, PCP, and cocaine. Muscle rigidity with hyperthermia is characteristic of neuroleptic malignant syndrome, malignant hyperthermia, PCP intoxication, and black widow spider bite.

LABORATORY EVALUATION

Clinical laboratory data include assessment of the "three gaps of toxicology": the anion gap, the osmolal gap, and the arterial oxygen saturation gap. Unexplained widening of

TABLE 102-11 Selected Drugs Affecting Pupil Size

Miosis	Mydriasis
Barbiturates	Amphetamines
Carbamates	Anticholinergics
Clonidine	Antihistamines
Ethanol	Cocaine
Isopropyl alcohol	Cyclic antidepressants
Organophosphates	Dopamine
Opioids (meperidine may cause mydriasis)	Drug withdrawal
	Glutethimide
Phencyclidine (PCP)	Lysergic acid diethylamide (LSD)
Phenothiazines	Monamine oxidase inhibitors
Physostigmine	
Pilocarpine	

TABLE 102-12 Selected Drugs and Toxins Affecting Muscle Tone

Dystonic Reactions	Dyskinesias	Rigidity
Haloperidol	Anticholinergics	Black widow spider bite
Metoclopramide	Cocaine	Malignant hyperthermia
Phenothiazines	Phencyclidine	Neuroleptic malignant syndrome

SOURCE: Adapted with permission from Olson et al.[30]

these gaps should raise the possibility of drug overdose or toxic ingestion.

ANION GAP

The *anion gap* (AG) refers to the difference between one measured cation (Na^+) and two measured anions (mainly Cl^- and HCO_3^-):

$$AG = [Na^+] - [Cl^-] - [HCO_3^-]$$

with a normal value of approximately 12 ± 4 mEq/L.[31–34]

The presence of an anion gap indicates that there are more unmeasured anions than cations, since total serum cations equals total serum anions. *Unmeasured cations* include potassium, magnesium, and calcium, totaling about 11 mEq/L under normal conditions. The concentration of *unmeasured anions*, including mainly albumin, sulfates, phosphates, and organic acids, is about 23 mEq/L (and thus the difference of approximately 12 mEq/L).[35] It follows that the presence of hypoalbuminemia requires a downward adjustment of the expected normal anion gap: the anion gap falls 2.5 mEq/L for every 1 g/L decrease in plasma albumin concentration.[36]

The anion gap increases through three possible mechanisms: a decrease in unmeasured cations, an increase in unmeasured anions, or a laboratory error in measurement of Na^+, Cl^- or HCO_3^-. An increase in anion gap resulting from decreased unmeasured cations is rare but may occur in severe potassium, calcium, or magnesium depletion. The most common cause of an elevated anion gap is an increase in unmeasured anions. This includes accumulation of organic acids, as in lactic acidosis or ketoacidosis, or accumulation of the anions of organic acids such as sulfate and phosphate in uremia. Common causes of an elevated anion gap are listed in Table 102-13.

Toxic ingestions may increase unmeasured anions and elevate the anion gap (e.g., ethylene glycol elevates the anions glycolate and lactate). An elevated anion gap mandates

TABLE 102-13 Common Causes of an Elevated Anion Gap

Lactic acidosis
Uremia
Sepsis
Rhabdomyolysis
Ketoacidosis
  Diabetic
  Alcoholic
  Starvation
Toxic ingestions
  Ethylene glycol
  Methanol
  Paraldehyde
  Salicylate
Metabolic alkalosis with volume depletion

TABLE 102-14 Selected Drugs Associated with an Elevated Anion Gap Metabolic Acidosis

Amiloride	Ketamine
Ascorbic acid	Metformin
Carbon monoxide	Methanol
Chloramphenicol	Niacin
Colchicine	Nitroprusside
Cyanide	NSAIDs
Dapsone	Papaverine
Epinephrine	Paraldehyde (hippuric acid)
Ethanol	Phenformin
Ethylene glycol	Propofol
Formaldehyde	Salicylates
Hydrogen sulfide	Terbutaline
Iron	Tetracycline (outdated)
Isoniazid	Toluene (hippuric acid)
	Verapamil

ABBREVIATION: NSAIDs, nonsteroidal anti-inflammatory drugs.

consideration of toxic ingestion, even in the presence of ketones or lactate, which can occur with toxic ingestion.[37,38] Drugs associated with an elevated anion gap are included in Table 102-14.

Rarely, toxic ingestion decreases the anion gap (<6 mEq/L). Causes of decreased anion gap are listed in Table 102-15. Note the presence of lithium on this list.

OSMOLAL GAP

Certain drugs and toxins of low molecular weight (Table 102-16) produce a discrepancy between measured and calculated plasma osmolality, commonly referred to as the *osmolal gap* (osmolal gap equals measured minus calculated osmolality). The plasma osmolal gap can thus be used to detect the presence of these toxins in the blood. Normal plasma osmolality, determined by the millimolar concentrations of major solutes in plasma, is approximately 285 to 295 mOsm and is calculated as:

$$\text{Calculated osmolality} = 2[Na^+] + [BUN]/2.8 + [glucose]/18 + [ethanol]/4.6$$

where Na^+ (in mmol/L) is multiplied by two to account for accompanying anions (chloride and bicarbonate), and the concentrations of BUN (blood urea nitrogen) and glucose

TABLE 102-15 Causes of Decreased Anion Gap

Increased unmeasured cation
  Hyperkalemia
  Hypercalcemia
  Hypermagnesemia
  Acute lithium intoxication
  Elevated IgG (myeloma; cationic paraprotein)
Decreased unmeasured anion
  Hypoalbuminemia
Drugs
  Bromide
  Iodide
  Lithium
  Polymyxin B
  Tromethamine
Analytical artifact
  Hypernatremia (>170 mEq/L)
  Hyperlipidemia

TABLE 102-16 Drugs/Toxins Associated with an Elevated Osmolal Gap

Ethanol (if not included in the formula)
Ethylene glycol/glycolaldehyde
Glycerol
Glycine
Intravenous immunoglobulin (maltose)
Isopropanol/acetone
Mannitol
Methanol/formaldehyde
Propylene glycol
Radiocontrast media
Sorbitol

are divided by 2.8 and 18, respectively, to convert mg/dL to mmol/L. Dividing ethanol concentration by 4.6 accounts for the effect of a measured plasma ethanol concentration (in mg/dL) on calculated plasma osmolality. Of note, spuriously low serum sodium values (pseudohyponatremia) due to hyperlipidemia or hyperproteinemia may indicate the presence of a factitious osmolal gap.

Methanol and ethylene glycol are unique in producing both severe metabolic acidosis with elevated anion gap and an elevated osmolal gap. Isopropanol intoxication can elevate the osmolal gap and cause ketonemia and ketonuria (owing to its metabolism to acetone) without elevation of the anion gap or acidosis. Through CNS and cardiac effects, isopropanol may cause respiratory acidosis and lactic acidosis, respectively.

Caution must be used when interpreting the osmolal gap. First, measurement of osmolality by vapor pressure osmometry does not detect volatile alcohols such as ethanol and methanol (but does detect ethylene glycol); freezing point depression osmometry does measure these solutes.[39,40] Although 10 mOsm is often used as the upper limit of normal, osmolal gaps may range from −9 mOsm to +5 mOsm in normal individuals (using the standard formula for calculations).[41] Thus, an osmolal gap of 10 mOsm in a patient whose baseline value is −2 mOsm could represent the presence of significant amounts of low-molecular-weight substances (e.g., ethylene glycol level over 70 mg/dL).[42,43] In one study the range of osmolal gaps measured in 300 consecutive patients presenting to Bellevue Hospital in New York (with indications for measurement of electrolytes and ethanol) was −2 ± 6 mOsm using the standard formula, including the contribution of measured ethanol concentrations.[44] Large variations existed in the range of osmolal gap that was very dependent on the equation used. Because of the large range of values, the authors noted that small osmolal gaps in no way exclude the possibility of toxic alcohol ingestion. Furthermore, as ethylene glycol/glycoaldehyde and methanol/formaldehyde are metabolized, the osmolal gap may decrease into the normal range in the continued presence of toxic metabolites. By contrast, concurrent ethanol ingestion may prevent early development of metabolic acidosis, so that the presence of an osmolal gap greater than expected from the measured ethanol level may be the only clue to the presence of a non-ethanol alcohol.[45] Lactic acidosis and ketoacidosis have also been reported to cause elevation of the osmolal gap.[46] Finally, chronic (but not acute) renal failure is a cause of increased osmolal gap, a phenomenon corrected by dialysis.[47]

In summary, the presence of an elevated anion gap metabolic acidosis, even in the presence of an apparent clinical explanation, warrants consideration of intoxication. The additional presence of an elevated osmolal gap, particularly of large magnitude (>25 mOsm), is indicative of methanol or ethylene glycol intoxication (see below). The converse is not true, in that serious intoxications with either agent can occur in the absence of a documented increased osmolal gap. Thus measuring serum levels of these alcohols is important in any patient in whom inebriation, acidosis, or other clinical features suggest intoxication with these agents.

OXYGEN SATURATION GAP

An elevated arterial oxygen saturation gap is defined by a >5% difference between saturation calculated from an arterial blood gas and saturation measured by co-oximetry. Elevated oxygen saturation gap is seen in carbon monoxide poisoning and with methemoglobinemia. These toxins interfere with oxygen binding to hemoglobin and thereby significantly decrease oxygen content without lowering arterial oxygen pressure (Pa_{O_2}). *It is important to note that oxygen saturation measured by pulse oximetry is falsely high in these settings.* Hydrogen sulfide and cyanide interfere with cellular utilization of oxygen, leading to an abnormally high venous oxygen saturation and "arteriolization" of venous blood.

ADDITIONAL LABORATORY TESTS

Additional useful laboratory data include: urine ferric chloride analysis, which provides rapid evidence of salicylate or phenothiazine intake; a pregnancy test in women of childbearing age; and abdominal radiography, which may detect retained pills (such as iron pills). Sustained-release preparations may be detected more easily through digital enhancement of the radiograph.[48]

TOXICOLOGY SCREENING

Toxicology screening provides direct evidence of ingestion, but it rarely impacts initial management; supportive measures should never await results of such analysis. In Brett's review of 209 cases of intentional drug overdose,[49] toxicology analysis supported the clinical suspicion in 47% of cases. Clinically unsuspected drugs were detected in 27% of cases, but unexpected findings altered management in only three cases. Kellerman and coworkers reviewed urine toxicology screens in 361 of 405 consecutive ED patients with suspected drug overdose.[50] Management changes followed drug screening in only 16 (4.4%) of cases.

Toxicology screening confirms the presence of a drug and provides grounds for treatment with a specific antidote or method for enhancing elimination. Toxicology screening also identifies drugs that should be quantitated to guide subsequent management.[51] If at all possible, samples should be collected before administration of medications that might confuse toxicologic analysis.

Understanding the limitations of toxicology screening is important, including which drugs are (and which drugs are not) included in routine screening panels. These panels are institutionally variable. Most institutions offer urine screening for commonly abused drugs only, preferring to send more extensive screening panels to outside laboratories. Other institutions routinely perform extensive urine and blood analysis

TABLE 102-17 Drugs Commonly Included in Urine Substances of Abuse Screens (Available in 30 Minutes)

Amphetamines
Barbiturates
Benzodiazepines
Cannabinoids
Cocaine
Opioids
Phencyclidine (PCP)

on all patients in selected categories (e.g., trauma patients). Urine screens used in the ED are aimed at detecting six or seven of the most commonly abused drugs (Table 102-17). Results are generally available in 30 minutes. Approximately 60 drugs are included in the expanded screening panel (Table 102-18), the results of which should be available in 2 to 3 hours. Table 102-19 lists some drugs not included in routine drug screening.

Toxicologic screening of blood is generally not additive to comprehensive urine testing,[52] although rarely blood analysis is useful in acute cases when the drug or toxin is not yet detectable in urine (particularly in anuric or oliguric patients). Quantitative blood analysis of suspected drugs can be useful for diagnostic and therapeutic reasons, particularly in overdoses involving alcohols, acetaminophen, salicylates, and cyclic antidepressants. A strong argument can be made for checking acetaminophen levels in all cases of suspected intoxication given the subtle manifestations of early poisoning and the importance of targeted therapy.

Poison Control Centers

Poison control centers provide 24-hour emergency and technical information by telephone to anyone concerned with drug overdose or toxic ingestion. These centers are staffed variably by nurses, pharmacists, pharmacologists, and physicians trained in clinical toxicology. The staff provides information regarding substance identification, drug interactions, adverse drug reactions, and management of poisoned patients. These centers maintain current references and information about toxins or drugs specific to certain areas, including information about street drug activity.

Poison control center consultation is strongly advised to help determine appropriate laboratory testing, patient disposition, and treatment, including the need for a specific antidote or method to enhance drug elimination. Information provided by regional poison control centers may be more accurate than advice provided by local EDs.[53] The national toll-free emergency phone number is 1-800-222-1222.

Detoxification

GASTRIC EMPTYING

Gastric emptying is achieved by gastric lavage (GL) or syrup of ipecac. Ipecac is useful for certain ingestions in pediatric patients, but it is contraindicated in poisoning with corrosives, petroleum products, antiemetics, and strychnine. There is little role for ipecac in hospital because delayed use is of

TABLE 102-18 Drugs Commonly Included in Urine Toxicology Screens (Available in 2–3 Hours)

Acetaminophen
Amoxapine
Barbiturates other than phenobarbital
Benzodiazepine metabolites
   Chlordiazepoxide
   Diazepam
   Flurazepam
   Oxazepam
Cannabinoids (marijuana)
Carbamezepine
Chlorpromazine
Cimetidine
Codeine
Cocaine metabolites
Desiprimine
Dextromethorphan
Diphenhydramine
Doxepin
Doxylamine
Ephedrine
Erythromycin
Glutethimide
Guaifenesin
Hydrocodone
Hydromorphone
Imipramine
Lidocaine
Meperidine
Meprobamate
Methadone
Methamphetamine
Methaqualone
Morphine
Nortryptyline
Opiates
Orphenadrine
Pentazocine
Phenacetin
Phencyclidine
Phenethylamine
Phenmetrazine
Phenobarbital
Phentermine
Phenothiazine metabolites
   Prochlorperazine
   Promethazine
   Trifluoperazine
   Trimeprazine
   Triflupromazine
Phenylpropanolamine
Propranolol
Propxyphene
Pseudoephedrine
Pyrilamine
Quinine
Strychnine
Temazepam
Terpin hydrate
Trazodone
Triamterene
Trimethoprim
Trimethobenzamide
Trimipramine
Tripelennamine

TABLE 102-19 Drugs/Toxins *Not* Commonly Included in Toxicology Screens

Antiarrhythmic agents
Bromide
Cyanide
Digitalis
Ethylene glycol
Hypoglycemic agents
Lithium
Lysergic acid diethylamide (LSD)
Methanol
Monoamine oxidase inhibitors
Serotonin reuptake inhibitors
Theophylline

questionable efficacy and it is contraindicated in obtunded patients.[54,55]

GL is advocated in the initial management of many orally ingested agents. However, risk-benefit analysis casts doubt as to the appropriateness of GL in many situations. The risks associated with GL (including aspiration, arrhythmias, and stomach perforation) preclude its use in patients who have ingested a nontoxic substance or a nontoxic amount of a toxic substance. Additionally, GL should not be performed when the toxin is no longer expected to be present in the stomach. Examples include patients who have vomited extensively prior to admission, patients who present several hours after ingesting an agent that does not decrease gut motility, and patients who have taken agents that are readily absorbed from the gastrointestinal tract.

To minimize risk, experienced personnel should perform GL lavage in a facility where resources are available to manage complications. Nonintubated patients must be alert and have adequate pharyngeal and laryngeal protective reflexes. In semicomatose patients, GL should be performed after intubation. Intubation for the sole purpose of GL is reasonable only if there is a high likelihood that a highly lethal agent remains in the stomach.

The usual teaching is to empty the stomach of alert patients (who are expected to remain alert), with GL within 1 hour of ingestion of potentially dangerous amounts of a toxic substance.[56] In obtunded patients, GL results in a more satisfactory clinical outcome only if performed within 1 hour of ingestion.[57] Although controversial, this time limit may be extended to 12 hours in cases of poisoning with agents that delay gastric emptying such as cyclic antidepressants, opioids, or salicylates. In cases of ingestion of a caustic liquid like kerosene or its derivatives, GL should be avoided because of the risk of aspiration-induced lung injury.

Prior to inserting a large-bore gastric tube (Ewald tube), the mouth should be inspected for foreign material and equipment should be readied for suctioning. Large gastric tubes (37F to 40F) are less likely to enter the trachea than smaller nasogastric tubes, and are necessary to facilitate removal of gastric debris. Once the tube has been passed with the help of patient swallowing, proper position is confirmed by aspirating acidic stomach contents and auscultating the left upper abdominal quadrant during insufflation of air. Stomach contents should be retained for analysis. Lavage is performed by instilling 200-mL aliquots of warmed tap water until there is clearing of aspirated fluid. Tap water is preferred over normal saline because it avoids unnecessary salt loading, and neither irrigant significantly alters blood cell concentrations or electrolyte concentrations.[58] After clearing, the Ewald tube may be replaced by a nasogastric tube for intermittent suctioning and/or administration of activated charcoal.

ACTIVATED CHARCOAL

Charcoal is a by-product of the combustion of various organic compounds such as wood, coconut parts, bone, sucrose, rice, and starch. It is activated by removing materials previously absorbed by a process that involves steam heating and chemical treatment, thereby increasing the surface area available for absorption. The result is a powerful nonspecific adsorbent that irreversibly binds intraluminal drugs and interferes with their absorption. Activated charcoal (AC) also decreases serum drug levels in some cases by creating a favorable diffusion gradient between blood and gut, referred to as *gastrointestinal dialysis*.[59]

Activated charcoal should be administered in a timely fashion after gastric emptying (if performed) because efficacy decreases with time.[60] It should not be given to stuporous, comatose, or convulsing patients unless an endotracheal tube protects the airway and a gastric tube is in place to administer the charcoal. Gastric stapling is a risk factor for emesis and aspiration in patients treated with single or repeated doses of AC.[61] Aspiration of this particulate has been associated with pneumonia[62] (including fungal pneumonia),[63] bronchiolitis obliterans,[64] acute respiratory distress syndrome,[65] and death.[66]

Activated charcoal is generally given as a single dose. The dose is based on patient weight (1 g/kg added to 4 parts water to form an aqueous slurry). Mixing AC with juice may improve patient acceptance of this black and gritty adsorbent.

Multiple-dose AC can enhance the elimination of selected toxins that have been absorbed.[67] This may occur through interruption of the enterohepatic/enterogastric circulation of drugs or through the binding of drugs that diffuse from the circulation into the gut lumen (so called gastrointestinal dialysis). However, multiple-dose AC is of limited use because the toxin must have a low volume of distribution, low protein binding, prolonged elimination half-life, and low pK_a (negative logarithm of the acid ionization constant), which maximizes transport across mucosal membranes into the gastrointestinal tract.[68] Based on experimental and clinical studies, it should be considered only in life-threatening ingestions of selected drugs: carbamazepine, dapsone, phenobarbital, quinine, or theophylline.[69]

In a recent review, the American Academy of Clinical Toxicologists reported that multidose AC increases drug elimination, but has not been shown to reduce morbidity and mortality in controlled trials.[69] The optimal dose and frequency of administration of AC following the initial dose has not been established. Most experts recommend a dose not less than 12.5 g/h.[70] After the initial dose of 1 g/kg, AC may be administered at 0.5 g/kg every 2 to 4 hours for at least 3 doses. Multiple doses should be used with caution in patients with decreased bowel sounds, abdominal distension, and emesis.

Combining AC with a cathartic may facilitate evacuation of the toxin and avoids constipation. Preparations for coadministration with AC include 1 to 2 mL/kg of a 70% solution of sorbitol titrated to several loose stools over the first day of treatment. An alternative is to use 2 to 3 mL/kg of a 10% solution of magnesium sulfate PO, but magnesium-based cathartics may lead to magnesium accumulation in the setting of renal failure, and sodium-based products carry the risk of exacerbating hypertension or congestive heart failure. If aspirated, oil-based cathartics may produce lipoid pneumonia.

The efficacy of adding a cathartic to AC is unclear. Keller and colleagues demonstrated that AC with sorbitol decreased absorption of salicylates compared to AC alone.[71] McNamara and colleagues found no benefit to adding sorbitol to a simulated acetaminophen overdose.[72] Catharsis has not been shown to decrease morbidity, mortality, or hospital length of stay, and it is not recommended for routine use in combination with AC by the American Academy of Clinical Toxicology.[73,74]

WHOLE-BOWEL IRRIGATION

Whole-bowel irrigation (WBI) with a polyethylene glycol electrolyte solution (e.g., GoLYTELY) 1 to 2 L/h by mouth or nasogastric tube may clear tablets or packages from the gastrointestinal tract. Irrigation is generally continued until the rectal effluent is clear or there is radiographic evidence of clearance. The efficacy of WBI has not been established in controlled trials, but it is reasonable to consider its use in iron and lithium overdose (situations in which AC is ineffective), ingestion of sustained-release tablets, and in cases of "body packing" with packages of illicit drugs. Contraindications to WBI include ileus, gastrointestinal hemorrhage, and bowel perforation.

FORCED DIURESIS AND URINARY PH MANIPULATIONS

We do not recommend forced diuresis by volume loading and diuretic administration, which is intended to augment elimination of renally excreted toxins through inhibition of tubular reabsorption. This regimen is of unproven benefit and has the potential to compromise fluid and electrolyte homeostasis.[75–78] The minimum criteria for augmented clearance of a drug by forced diuresis are that the substance normally undergoes extensive tubular reabsorption and that renal excretion becomes the major route of elimination under conditions of forced diuresis. It is notable that if tubular reabsorption is pH sensitive, then increased urine flow does not significantly increase urinary drug elimination when added to alkaline or acid diuresis (see below).[79]

Therapeutic manipulation of urinary pH can enhance elimination of some intoxicants. Most drugs are weak acids or bases and are present in both ionized and nonionized fractions in serum and glomerular filtrate. Normally, passive renal tubular reabsorption of the nonionized lipid-soluble fraction of such drugs occurs by nonionic diffusion; this process is accentuated by the progressive tubular reabsorption of water and solutes as the glomerular filtrate traverses the nephron, resulting in an increasing filtrate/serum concentration gradient which favors drug reabsorption. Back-diffusion of some acidic and basic drugs from renal tubular lumen to the peritubular fluid and capillaries can be decreased by manipulation of urinary pH to create more of the ionized (less lipid-soluble) salt of the drug. Urinary alkalinization is expected to augment excretion of nonpolar weak acids with pK_a values between 3 and 7.5 (Table 102-20), because these drugs

TABLE 102-20 Toxins Eliminated by Manipulation of Urinary pH

Alkaline Urine	Acid Urine
2,4 Dichlorophenoxyacetic acid	Amphetamines
Fluoride	Bismuth
Isoniazid	Ephedrine
Mephobarbital	Flecainide
Methotrexate	Nicotine
Phenobarbital	Phencyclidine
Primidone	Quinine
Quinolone antibiotics	
Salicylic acid	
Uranium	

become more dissociated as urinary pH rises, resulting in ion trapping of the drug in the tubular lumen.[79] (The *dissociation constant*, pK_a, of a drug refers to the pH at which the compound is equally ionized and unionized.) Because the limits of urinary pH are 4.5 to 7.5 under conditions of enhanced alkalinization and acidification, elimination of very strong (pK_a <3) or very weak (pK_a >8) acids is unaltered by urinary pH manipulation. Other acidic or basic drugs do not undergo renal tubular absorption regardless of urinary pH since they are polar in their nonionized form (e.g., gentamicin). Urinary alkalinization (pH >7) is usually achieved by administration of intravenous sodium bicarbonate (1 to 2 mEq/kg every 3 to 4 hours); this may be administered as two 50-mL ampules of 8.4% sodium bicarbonate (each containing 50 mEq of $NaHCO_3$) per liter of 5% dextrose in water infused at 250 mL/h.[80] Complications of this therapy include alkalemia (particularly in the presence of concurrent respiratory alkalosis), volume overload, hypernatremia, and hypokalemia. It is particularly important to avoid hypokalemia, which prevents excretion of alkaline urine by promoting distal tubular potassium reabsorption in exchange for hydrogen ion. Accordingly, bicarbonate administration in the presence of significant hypokalemia will not achieve an alkaline urine, yet increases the risk of alkalemia. Since urinary alkalinization can cause hypokalemia (caused by alkalemia-induced intracellular potassium shift and by increased urinary potassium losses with alkaline diuresis), addition of potassium chloride to the bicarbonate infusion is commonly required and may be considered prophylactically.[78] We do not recommend the use of acetazolamide to induce alkaline diuresis. This therapy causes metabolic acidosis, which can further complicate management, particularly in the case of salicylate intoxication (where acidemia increases CNS entry of the drug).

Urinary acidification (pH <5.5) likewise increases renal clearance of some nonpolar weak bases (see Table 102-20), with pK_a values between 6 and 12. These drugs include PCP (pK_a 8.5) and amphetamines (pK_a 9.9).[79] Again, elimination of very weak (pK_a <6) or very strong (pK_a >12) nonpolar bases is less affected by urinary pH changes. Arginine or lysine hydrochloride or ammonium chloride is most commonly used for urinary acidification. However, this therapy is generally not recommended because of the potential for urinary acidification to exacerbate myoglobinuric renal tubular injury. Also, systemic acidosis must be carefully controlled to avoid additive effects with toxin-induced metabolic or respiratory acidosis.

EXTRACORPOREAL REMOVAL OF TOXINS

In some instances, treatment of an intoxicated patient with supportive measures, decontamination, and acceleration of renal drug elimination does not alter the course of events to optimize outcome. Application of extracorporeal drug removal (ECR) techniques may be life-saving for such patients, although clear proof that ECR favorably alters the course of any intoxication is generally lacking.[81] Application of ECR for any intoxication is based on critical appraisal of both the clinical status of the patient and of current available data on the prognosis and treatment of the intoxication. In general, ECR should be considered when (1) supportive care fails to stabilize the patient's clinical status; (2) the intoxication is projected to undergo delayed or insufficient clearance because of renal, hepatic, or cardiac dysfunction; (3) the intoxicating agent produces toxic metabolites; or (4) delayed toxicity is characteristic of the intoxication.[76–78,81–83] In addition to these general considerations, specific clinical features or serum drug levels may indicate the necessity for ECR. Finally, physicochemical properties of the intoxicant, and its pharmacokinetic behavior in overdose (which may differ from the agent's pharmacokinetic properties in the therapeutic range), also dictate the feasibility of ECR and the choice of method. Three methods for ECR are generally available: (1) dialysis (usually hemodialysis rather than peritoneal dialysis); (2) hemoperfusion; and (3) hemofiltration. Rarely, other techniques such as plasmapheresis and exchange transfusion are considered for specific intoxications; these will not be further discussed here.

HEMODIALYSIS

Hemodialysis (HD) is the treatment of choice for ECR of very few intoxicants, because hemoperfusion (HP) provides superior drug extraction in most cases in which ECR is considered. Hemodialysis is still preferred to HP for removal of substances that are particularly dialyzable (see below), especially in the presence of metabolic acidosis, renal failure, dialyzable toxic metabolites, or other HD indications. Hemodialysis removes water-soluble unbound (free) solutes that are small enough to pass through the pores of the semipermeable dialysis membrane, which separates the patient's blood from the countercurrent flow of the dialysis bath fluid (which is discarded as effluent dialysate following passage through the dialyzer). Solute transport, including transfer of drugs, toxins, or metabolites, occurs by diffusion down the blood-to-dialysis bath concentration gradient, which is maintained by countercurrent flow of dialysate. In addition to low molecular weight and water solubility, both low protein binding and a small volume of distribution are necessary characteristics of a substance that is readily cleared by HD.[84–88]

Criteria for potential dialyzability include:

1. *Water solubility:* Water-soluble substances cross dialysis membranes more readily than lipid-soluble agents (drugs or metabolites).
2. *Low molecular weight:* Traditionally, a substance is described as small enough to be significantly removed by hemodialysis when it has a molecular weight of <500 daltons (Da). More recently, high-flux dialysis membranes with increased porosity and surface area have been introduced. Such membranes are capable of removing drugs with weights in the middle-molecule range, up to 5000 Da. For example, vancomycin has a molecular weight of 1500 Da, but is significantly cleared by HD with a high-flux membrane.[87,89,90]

3. *Protein binding:* Low protein binding (<90%) facilitates drug removal by hemodialysis, since only unbound drug is free to cross the hemodialysis membrane; for example, for a drug which is 90% protein-bound, hemodialytic removal of 50% of free drug only reduces its concentration in blood passing through the dialyzer by 5%.
4. *Volume of distribution (Vd):* This is the theoretical volume into which the intoxicant is distributed. As a general rule, substances with a Vd of <250 L (approximately 3 to 4 L/kg) are potentially significantly cleared by hemodialysis. Conversely, hemodialytic removal of substances with a larger Vd is generally insignificant in comparison to the total body load of the substance, which often equilibrates too slowly with the vascular space to allow significant removal. In fact, most substances substantially removed by HD have a smaller Vd of 1 L/kg (Table 102-21).
5. *Intrinsic clearance of the substance:* Most drugs have a hemodialysis clearance of 5 to 100 mL/min; if a patient's clearance of a substance exceeds 500 to 700 mL/70 kg per minute, hemodialysis is unlikely to significantly augment the substance's clearance.[89] It is important to note that the clearance of a drug at toxic levels may be significantly less than that reported within the therapeutic range, because of saturable hepatic metabolism at high drug concentrations (concentration-dependent kinetics) or intoxication-induced renal, hepatic, or cardiac dysfunction. Furthermore, there is usually a paucity of information regarding the production and relative clearance (intrinsic versus extracorporeal) of toxic metabolites.

Complications of HD include:

1. Intravenous access complications: If possible, temporary vascular access should be placed in the femoral vein to minimize the potential for serious complications (pneumothorax, central vessel or nerve injury, or catheter-induced arrhythmia). Vascular access should also be removed as soon as possible (but not before the period for potential development of rebound intoxication has passed) to minimize the potential for access infection or thrombosis.
2. Hypophosphatemia: In patients without concomitant renal failure and hyperphosphatemia, the dialysis bath should be supplemented with phosphorus to prevent severe dialysis-induced hypophosphatemia. Addition of 1.3 mmol/L of phosphorus to the dialysis bath should prevent hypophosphatemia.
3. Alkalemia: Since the usual dialysis bath bicarbonate (buffer) concentration is 35 to 38 mEq/L, severe alkalemia can result from hemodialysis against a standard bath in the absence of associated acidosis (particularly in the presence of hyperventilation or emesis-induced metabolic alkalosis). If the predialysis plasma bicarbonate concentration is 28 mEq/L or higher, then the bath bicarbonate concentration must be lowered to 15 to 28 mEq/L.
4. Disequilibrium syndrome: Acute neurologic deterioration caused by large, rapid changes in cerebral tissue osmolality may occur in an acutely uremic patient who receives a prolonged initial session of intensive hemodialysis for

TABLE 102-21 Extracorporeal Removal (ECR) of Selected Intoxicants: Pharmacokinetic Considerations

Intoxicant	Molecular Weight (Da) Protein Binding (%) Vd (L/kg)	Endogenous Clearance (mL/min per kg)	Serum Level for ECR[a]	Removal Techniques
Acetaminophen	151 0–25 1.0	5.0		HP[b]
Aminoglycosides	>500 <10 0.3	1.5		HD + HP
Carbamazepine	236 74 1.4	1.3		HP[b]
Digoxin	765 20–30 6.0–12.0	0.88 CrCl + 0.33)± 52%		HP (digoxin)[b] HF or plasmapheresis (Fab)[b]
Ethylene glycol	62 0 0.6	2.0	50–100 mg/dL	HD
Isopropanol	60 0 0.6	0.5	400 mg/dL	HD
Lithium	7 0 0.8	0.35	2.5 mEq/L	HD
Methanol	32 0 0.6	0.7	50–100 mg/dL	HD
Phenobarbital	232 24 0.54	0.06	10 mg/dL	HP > HD[b]
Phenytoin	252 90[d] 0.64	V_m 5.9/K_m 5.7[c]		HP[b]
Procainamide/NAPA	272/ 16/10 1.9/1.4	8.0/3.0	20 mg/L	HD (procainamide) HP (NAPA)[b]
Salicylate	138 50–90 0.2	0.88	80–100 mg/dL	HD
Theophylline	180 56 0.5	0.65	30–40 μg/mL	HP > HD
Valproic acid	144 90–95[e] 0.22	0.11		HD + HP[b]

ABBREVIATIONS: CrCl, creatinine clearance; HD, hemodialysis; HF, hemofiltration; HP, hemoperfusion; NAPA, N- acetyl-procainamide; Vd, volume of distribution.
[a] Approximate levels: use of ECR usually based upon clinical criteria.
[b] ECR use controversial.
[c] Saturable metabolism:Michaelis-Menten kinetics.
[d] Decreased in uremia and hypoalbuminemia.
[e] Decreases at levels above 90–100 (g/mL).

drug removal. High-sodium dialysis bath and intravenous mannitol may be useful prophylactically in blunting large acute transcellular water shifts caused by HD removal of uremic toxins.

5. System saturation: This is not possible using standard hemodialysis, because of maintenance of the concentration gradient for diffusion by countercurrent flow (blood versus dialysate), except when a sorbent dialysis system is used. This system is inappropriate for extracorporeal removal of an intoxicant, since the sorbent cartridge used to regenerate new dialysis solution from dialysate may become saturated and cease to function. If such a system is the only available option, frequent cartridge changes will be required.

6. Other: Hypotension is a potential adverse effect of HD (or HP), particularly if this therapy is instituted in an already unstable patient, though hemodynamic compromise is less likely if not actively removing plasma volume (by ultrafiltration). Finally, air embolism is an extremely rare consequence of HD.

PERITONEAL DIALYSIS

Intoxicant removal across the peritoneal membrane is generally only one-eighth to one-fourth as efficient as hemodialysis, even when maximizing solute exchange volume and frequency. This technique is therefore never the preferred method for extracorporeal drug removal, unless other considerations supervene (e.g., use as an adjunctive measure or in the absence of available HD or HP).

HEMOPERFUSION

Hemoperfusion (HP) is defined as direct contact of blood with a sorbent system.[82,91] Currently available systems perfuse a cartridge packed with coated AC (carbon). Blood perfusing such a cartridge is exposed (via a highly porous coating) to a large sorbent surface area, thus maximizing drug adsorption. Activated charcoal adsorbs both water-soluble and lipid-soluble substances and can remove essentially all of an adsorbing substance from blood perfusing the cartridge. Thus it is not unusual to achieve drug clearances of 200 to 400 mL/min, particularly early in the treatment period, before cartridge saturation begins. Polymer coating reduces adsorption of larger compounds (>3500 Da). The drug adsorption process competes with plasma proteins and tissue stores to greatly augment removal of bound drug beyond the level achievable by HD.

Complications of HP include:

1. *Cartridge saturation:* The extraction ratio (EX) of a substance by HP (or HD) is the amount of the solute removed as a fraction of the maximum it is theoretically possible to remove: $EX = (A - V)/A$, where A and V are the cartridge inlet and outlet blood concentrations, respectively. This ratio declines during an HP treatment session as the cartridge becomes saturated; as noted above, this occurs during HD only if a sorbent-based dialysis system is used.
2. *Hematologic:* Thrombocytopenia commonly occurs due to platelet adsorption, inducing up to a 30% decrement in platelet count, which usually recovers within 24 to 48 hours. Leukopenia and coagulation factor depletion also occur, to a lesser extent.
3. *Metabolic:* Cartridge adsorption can cause hypoglycemia and hypocalcemia.
4. *Technical:* Access complications can occur as for HD. Hypothermia is an additional risk, because HP pumps do not warm blood as the HD apparatus does. Particle embolization (prevented by a filter in the line returning effluent blood to the patient) and development of pyrogenic reactions are of largely historic interest at this point.

Most drugs are extractable by HP, which is particularly suitable for extracorporeal removal of toxins that are of high molecular weight, highly protein-bound, or lipid-soluble. Drugs poorly extracted by HP include heavy metals (lithium and bromide), some alcohols (ethanol and methanol), carbon monoxide, and some illicit drugs (cocaine, phencyclidine, and others). Efficacy of intoxicant removal is diminished for substances with a large Vd (i.e., highly lipid-soluble and/or extensively tissue-bound), which may be more effectively removed by hemofiltration.

TABLE 102-22 Antidotes

Drug/Poison	Antidotes
Acetaminophen	Acetylcysteine
Anticholinergics	Physostigmine
Anticholinesterases	Atropine
Benzodiazepines	Flumazenil
β-Blockers	Glucagon
Black widow spider bite	Equine-derived antivenin
Calcium channel blockers	Calcium chloride, glucagon
Carbon monoxide	Oxygen
Coral snake (Eastern and Texas) bite	Equine-derived antivenin
Cyanide	Amyl nitrite, sodium nitrite, sodium thiosulfate, hydroxycobalamin
Digoxin	Digoxin-specific antibodies
Ethylene glycol	Ethanol, 4-methylpyrazole
Heavy metals (arsenic, copper, gold, lead, mercury)	Dimercaprol, Ethylenediamine tetra-acetic acid (EDTA), penicillamine
Hypoglycemic agents	Dextrose, glucagon
Iron	Deferoxamine mesylate
Isoniazid	Pyridoxine
Methanol	Ethanol, folic acid, 4-methylpyrazole
Methemoglobinemia	Methylene blue
Opioids	Naloxone
Rattlesnake bite	Equine-derived antivenin

HEMOFILTRATION

Hemofiltration (HF) achieves drug removal by convection, transporting drugs and other solutes through a highly porous membrane by bulk flow with filtered plasma water. Such membranes are generally permeable to substances with weights of up to 6000 Da, including virtually all drugs, and in some cases HF membranes are permeable to substances weighing up to 20,000 Da.[92–94] There are increasing numbers of case reports of extracorporeal intoxicant removal using hemofiltration, by either the arteriovenous (continuous arteriovenous hemofiltration; CAVH) or venovenous (continuous venovenous hemofiltration; CVVH) method.[95,96] Hemofiltration is potentially useful for removal of substances with a large Vd, slow intercompartmental transfer, or avid tissue binding. Specific highly porous HF cartridges are also particularly useful for removal of large-molecular-weight solutes or complexes, such as combined digoxin-Fab fragment complexes or deferoxamine complexes with iron or with aluminum. CAVH also has the advantage that trained personnel can perform this technique without the assistance of a pump.

ANTIDOTES

An antidote is any substance that increases the mean lethal dose of a toxin, or that can favorably affect the toxic effects of a poison.[97] Table 102-22 lists antidotes for specific drugs/poisons.

Indications for ICU Admission

In the current healthcare environment, the practice of routinely admitting poisoned patients to the medical intensive care unit or a cardiac monitored bed is being questioned. In one retrospective study, Brett and colleagues identified several factors that predicted the need for ICU admission: partial pressure of arterial carbon dioxide (Pa_{CO_2}) $\geq$45 mm Hg, the need for intubation, seizures, QRS duration $\geq$0.12 seconds, second- or third-degree atrioventricular block, cardiac arrhythmias, systolic blood pressure <80 mm Hg, and unresponsiveness to verbal stimuli.[98] If none of these factors was present, no ICU interventions (intubation, vasopressors, antiarrhythmics, dialysis, or hemoperfusion) were required. Other considerations include a Glasgow Coma Scale score <12, progressive metabolic acidosis, and a cyclic antidepressant or phenothiazine overdose with signs of anticholinergic cardiac toxicity.[99,100] Cyclic antidepressants in particular may cause delayed cardiac toxicity.[101] Severe hyperkalemia, extreme body temperatures, and need for continuous infusion of naloxone are also reasons to admit to an ICU. Often, staffing issues including the availability of a "sitter" in cases of attempted suicide, have an important impact on the disposition of the patient.

Specific Intoxications

ACETAMINOPHEN

In 2001, alone or in combination with other drugs, acetaminophen accounted for over 112,000 exposures, making it the most common pharmaceutical overdose reported to poison control centers. Approximately 60,000 of these cases were treated in health care facilities; 12,744 patients received n-acetylcysteine (NAC); 2257 had major complications; 238 died.[1]

The evolution of acetaminophen toxicity is often divided into four phases.[102,103] Phase I refers to the first 24 hours after ingestion. During this period, acetaminophen is absorbed and metabolized, glutathione stores are depleted, and hepatotoxicity begins. Patients are alert but may experience nausea, vomiting, anorexia, malaise, pallor, or diaphoresis. These nonspecific signs and symptoms create the potential for a missed diagnosis. Furthermore, when acetaminophen is combined with another drug such as codeine or oxycodone, the effects of the other drug may further mask the initial subtle manifestations of acetaminophen poisoning.

Phase II occurs 24 to 72 hours after untreated ingestion. During this period, patients may develop right upper quadrant pain and minor abnormalities of liver function consisting of elevation of hepatic enzymes, prothrombin time, and bilirubin. Phase III (72 to 96 hours after untreated ingestion) is characterized by continued hepatic necrosis, hepatic encephalopathy, disseminated intravascular coagulation, and jaundice. Liver function abnormalities typically peak during phase III. It is not unusual for serum aspartate aminotransferase levels to rise to 10,000 IU/L or higher. Extreme elevation of alanine aminotransferase may also be seen. Rare phase III sequelae include hemorrhagic pancreatitis, myocardial necrosis, and acute renal failure.[103] Phase IV takes place 4 days to 2 weeks after ingestion. During this period, the patient may die, fully recover without chronic liver disease, or undergo emergent liver transplantation. Some patients with untreated acetaminophen poisoning exhibit a pattern of rising prothrombin time, ammonia, and bilirubin, as levels of hepatic enzymes decline, indicating fulminant hepatic necrosis.

A product of normal acetaminophen metabolism is responsible for hepatotoxicity. As acetaminophen is metabolized by the cytochrome P-450 mixed oxidase system, a toxic product (possibly N-acetyl-p-benzoquinone imine or NAPQI)[104] is rapidly detoxified by hepatic intracellular glutathione. In overdose cases, glutathione is depleted, allowing the toxic metabolite to combine with hepatic cell proteins and cause centrilobular necrosis with periportal sparing. Local production of NAPQI makes the liver the primary target, but other organs can be affected as indicated above.

It follows that a relationship exists between plasma levels of acetaminophen and the potential for toxicity. The Rumack-Matthew nomogram (Fig. 102-1) for acetaminophen poisoning allows stratification of patients into categories of probable hepatic toxicity, possible hepatic toxicity, and no hepatic toxicity, based on the relationship between acetaminophen level and time after ingestion.[105] The lower line of this nomogram, which defines serum levels 25% below those expected to cause hepatotoxicity, is generally used to guide treatment.

There are several limitations to the use of the Rumack-Matthew nomogram. First, note that a serum level obtained prior to 4 hours postingestion is not interpretable because of ongoing absorption and distribution of the drug, and patients in phases II to IV may have trivial or undetectable serum concentrations despite a potentially lethal dose. Second, the nomogram is less predictive in chronic ingestion or use of an extended-release preparation. For extended-release preparations serial acetaminophen levels should be drawn every 4 to 6 hours after ingestion and plotted on the Rumack-Matthew nomogram. If any point is above the lower line, an entire course of the antidote NAC is indicated. Third, the nomogram does not take into account at-risk populations. Acute ingestion of 7.5 to 10 g is potentially hepatotoxic in normal adults; however, the risk of toxicity increases in alcoholics, individuals who are malnourished, patients with induced cytochrome P-450 enzymes, and patients with low glutathione stores at baseline (as may be seen with recent subtoxic acetaminophen use).[106] In such cases doses as low as 4 to 6 g may be toxic. In this situation, NAC should be considered even if the serum level falls below the lower line. Fourth, accurate risk assessment requires an accurate time of ingestion, which is not always attainable. A 1- to 2-hour difference easily moves the borderline patient above or below the treatment line. Based on these limitations, Bond and Lite reported that the Rumack-Matthew nomogram could not be used for risk assessment in 44% of hospitalized patients and 83% of patients who suffered severe hepatic injury.[107]

Treatment of acetaminophen overdose should be initiated during phase I. Gastric lavage is indicated in patients seen within 1 hour of ingestion. Children at home may be given ipecac. Activated charcoal may be administered even though it has the potential to partially adsorb orally administered NAC. Activated charcoal reduces the number of patients reaching toxic serum levels after ingesting more than 10 g of acetaminophen and presenting within 24 hours of ingestion, and may reduce the need for a full treatment course of NAC and hospital length of stay.[108] When AC and NAC are used simultaneously, they should be administered 2 hours apart to minimize interaction. Hemoperfusion effectively accelerates

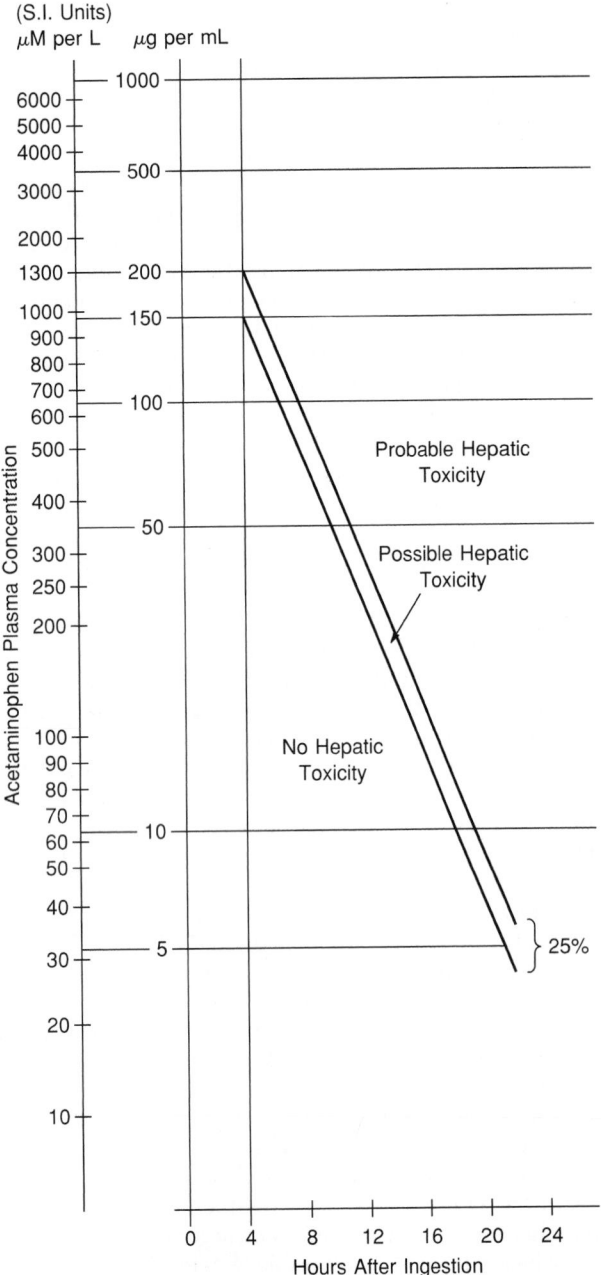

FIGURE 102-1 The Rumack-Matthew nomogram for predicting acetaminophen hepatoxicity. This nomogram allows for stratification of patients into categories of probable hepatic toxicity, possible hepatic toxicity, and no hepatic toxicity, based on the relationship between acetaminophen level and time after ingestion. When this relationship is known, n-acetylcysteine (NAC) therapy is indicated for acetaminophen levels above the lower nomogram line. NAC should also be given if there is >5 μg/mL acetaminophen and an unknown time of ingestion (but <24 hours), and if there is a history of overdose and a serum acetaminophen level is not immediately available. Serum levels obtained prior to 4 hours postingestion are uninterpretable because of ongoing absorption and distribution of the drug. (*Reproduced with permission from Rumack BH: Acetaminophen overdose in children and adolescents. Pediatr Clin North Am 33:691, 1986.*)

removal of acetaminophen from the blood; however, benefit has not been demonstrated in controlled trials. This technique may prove helpful in patients with high acetaminophen levels presenting late in the course of intoxication.[103]

All patients with probable or possible hepatic toxicity based on the Rumack-Matthew nomogram (i.e., all patients with serum acetaminophen levels above the lower line) should receive NAC to replete glutathione stores. NAC should also be given if there is >5 μg/mL acetaminophen and an unknown time of ingestion (but <24 hours), evidence of hepatotoxicity, or if a serum acetaminophen level is not immediately available. In this latter situation, the antidote may be discontinued if the acetaminophen level is found to be at a nontoxic level according to the nomogram. Importantly, NAC should be considered in at-risk patients even if levels are nontoxic.

The effectiveness of NAC depends on the time of administration. It is almost 100% effective when administered within the first 8 to 10 hours. Efficacy decreases over time, but there is still benefit for up to 24 hours.[109] NAC may even improve outcome when it is administered after the onset of fulminant hepatic failure.[110] In the setting of liver failure, NAC lowers the incidence of hepatic encephalopathy and improves oxygen transport and consumption.[111,112]

The oral loading dose of NAC is 140 mg/kg. This is followed by a dose of 70 mg/kg every 4 hours for 17 doses. There are limited data supporting shorter treatment courses in selected patients. Woo and colleagues conducted a retrospective, observational case study of short-course treatment in acute overdose with acetaminophen levels in the toxic range.[113] Patients received an oral loading dose of 140 mg/kg NAC followed by 70 mg/kg every 4 hours until the serum acetaminophen level was undetectable. Of the 75 patients, 25 (33.3%) were treated for less than 24 hours. The mean duration of therapy was 31 ± 16 hours. The incidence of hepatotoxicity was low and comparable to patients treated in the standard way. Protocols using a 20-hour IV course and a 48-hour IV course have also been shown to be safe and effective.[114,115] NAC is prepared using the standard 10% (100 mg/mL) or 20% (200 mg/mL) formulations diluted to a 5% solution in juice. If vomiting interferes with oral NAC use, the dose should be repeated along with an antiemetic such as metoclopramide or ondansetron. Occasionally, a nasogastric tube is necessary. Intravenous administration of NAC using the same dose and dosing schedule may be beneficial in patients unable to tolerate the oral preparation. When administered intravenously, a micropore filter should be used to decrease the risk of adverse reactions.

Fatal outcomes in acetaminophen overdose are associated with late presentation, high coma grade, prothrombin time >100 seconds, pH <7.30, creatinine >300 μmol/L, cerebral edema, and sepsis.[116,117] When poor prognostic features are present, liver transplantation is often considered, but whether to perform liver transplantation is a difficult decision. An accurate assessment of prognosis at the time of admission to the ICU would help to apply this therapy to the appropriate patient population. To this end, investigators from King's College Hospital Liver Unit demonstrated that an Acute Physiology and Chronic Health Evaluation (APACHE) II score >15 provided an accurate assessment of hospital mortality and identified patients in need of transplantation in the setting of acetaminophen-induced liver failure.[118]

TABLE 102-23 Toxic Alcohols: Clinical Features and Management

Sources	Distinguishing Features	Pharmacokinetic/ Pharmacodynamic Parameters	Specific Treatment
Methanol (Metabolites: Formaldehyde, Formic Acid, Lactic Acid)			
Antifreeze	Optic papillitis	Lethal serum level: 80–100 mg/dL	Charcoal (<1–2 h after ingestion)
		Lethal dose: 150–240 mL of a 40% solution	Ethanol, 4-methylpyrazole
Solvent	Pancreatitis	Peak conc.: 30–90 min	Consider bicarbonate infusion
		Vd: 0.6 L/kg	Folate 50–70 mg IV q4h × 24 h
Fuel		Excretion: 90–95% saturable hepatic metabolism; 5–10% unchanged renal	HD until serum level <20 mg/dL for:
		Half-life is dose dependent:	1. Serum level >50 mg/dL
		Mild intoxication: 14–20 h	2. Eye involvement
		Severe intoxication: 24–30 h	3. Altered mental status
		With ethanol: 30–35 h	4. Ingestion of >30 mL
		Ethanol + HD: 2.5 h	5. Elevated formic acid level
			6. Refractory metabolic acidosis
Ethylene Glycol (Metabolites: Glycoaldehyde, Glycolic Acid, Oxalic Acid)			
Antifreeze	Acute renal failure	Lethal serum level: 19.2 mg/dL	GL (<1–2 h after ingestion)
		Lethal dose: 100 mL	Ethanol, 4-methylpyrazole
Solvent	Crystalluria	Peak conc.: 1–4 h	Thiamine 100 mg IM qid
		Vd: 0.6 L/kg	Pyridoxine 500 mg IM qid
	Wood light: urinary fluorescene	Excretion: hepatic metabolism	Consider bicarbonate infusion
	Myocardial dysfunction	Half-life:	Consider calcium administration
		Untreated: 3–8.5 h	Consider forced diuresis
		With ethanol: 10–102 h	HD until serum level 20 mg/dL for:
		Ethanol + HD: 2.5–3 h	1. Serum level >50 mg/dL
			2. End-organ damage
			3. Refractory metabolic acidosis
Isopropanol (Metabolite: Acetone)			
Rubbing alcohol	Hemorrhagic gastritis	Lethal serum level: 400 mg/dL	Supportive care
		Lethal dose: 150–240 mL of 40% solution (highly variable)	GL (<1–2 h after ingestion)
Solvents			Ethanol not indicated (nontoxic metabolites)
	Ketonemia	Peak conc.: <2 h	
De-icers		Vd: 0.6 L/kg	HD for:
	Ketonuria	Excretion: 50–80% hepatic metabolism; 20–50% unchanged renal	1. Serum level >400 mg/dL
			2. Shock
		Half-life: Untreated: 2.5–3 h	3. Prolonged coma
	No acidosis or hyperglycemia		4. Hepatic or renal insufficiency

ABBREVIATIONS: GL, gastric lavage; HD, hemodialysis; Vd, volume of distribution.

ALCOHOLS

Clinical features of ethylene glycol, methanol, and isopropanol poisoning are listed in Table 102-23. Ethylene glycol is an odorless and sweet tasting fluid that is found in antifreeze, de-icers and industrial solvents. Blue or green fluorescent dye is added to some (e.g., antifreeze) but not all products to identify leaks, allowing for evidence of poisoning by urinary fluorescence under a Wood lamp. Methanol is colorless and odorless but has a bitter taste. It is present in many paint removers, gas-line antifreeze, windshield washing fluid, and solid canned fuel. Isopropanol is a colorless and bitter tasting alcohol. It has the smell of acetone or alcohol and is found in rubbing alcohol, skin lotions, hair tonics, aftershave, de-icers, and glass cleaners.

A history of ingestion or inebriation that is not explained by a blood ethanol level suggests toxic alcohol poisoning. Metabolic acidosis with an elevated anion gap and an elevated osmolal gap are cardinal features of methanol and ethylene glycol poisoning, but poisoning can occur without either.[119,120] Isopropanol elevates the osmolal gap but does not cause metabolic acidosis.[121]

Ethylene glycol is metabolized by alcohol dehydrogenase to glycoaldehyde and glycolic acid, and then to glyoxylic acid and oxalic acid. Accumulation and precipitation of oxalic acid and calcium oxalate in renal tubules produces calcium oxalate crystals that are present in the urine in 50% of cases.[122] Ingestion of as little as 100 mL can be lethal in an adult patient.

Ethylene glycol poisoning has a triphasic clinical course: stage 1 (30 minutes to 12 hours postingestion) consists of inebriation, ataxia, seizures, variable levels of elevated anion gap metabolic acidosis with Kussmaul breathing, elevated osmolal gap, crystalluria, and hypocalcemia. Cerebral edema causes coma or death. Symptoms may be delayed if there is concurrent ethanol consumption, which competes for alcohol dehydrogenase and limits conversion of ethylene glycol to its toxic metabolites.

Stage 2 (12 to 24 hours) is dominated by myocardial dysfunction with high- or low-pressure pulmonary edema. Myocardial dysfunction or respiratory failure causes death in this stage. Stage 3 (2 to 3 days) is dominated by acute renal failure due to acute tubular necrosis with an element of tubular obstruction from calcium oxalate precipitation.[68,123,124] Late (6 to 18 days) neurologic sequelae have also been described in survivors.[125–128]

Methanol is metabolized by alcohol dehydrogenase to formaldehyde, which is metabolized to formic acid by aldehyde dehydrogenase. Formic acid is the primary toxin responsible for metabolic derangements and ocular disturbances. Intoxication can occur orally, by inhalation, or by absorption through skin. As little as 30 mL causes significant morbidity; 150 to 240 mL of 40% solution can be lethal. Methanol causes an initial period of headache, inebriation, dizziness, ataxia, and confusion. As formic acid accumulates (6 to 72 hours), the anion gap elevates and the optic nerve swells. Decreased visual acuity and blindness are classic features of this poisoning. Pancreatitis also occurs.[129,130] As in ethylene glycol poisoning, symptoms of methanol poisoning may be delayed by concurrent ethanol use.

Treatment of ethylene glycol and methanol poisoning is similar.[131] Inhibiting the formation of toxic metabolites by alcohol dehydrogenase and/or urgent dialytic removal of these alcohols and their metabolites are the cornerstones of therapy. Supportive measures include gastric lavage in the first hour postingestion. Bicarbonate infusion may be necessary to improve metabolic acidosis, but has not been shown to improve outcome. Hypocalcemia and hypoglycemia should be corrected. In methanol intoxication, folate is important in the metabolism of formic acid to CO_2 and water; in ethylene glycol poisoning, pyridoxine and thiamine are important in the metabolism of glycolic acid.

Fomepizole (4-methylpyrazole) inhibits alcohol dehydrogenase; ethanol prolongs the half-life of methanol and ethylene glycol by competing for alcohol dehydrogenase. Of the two, fomepizole is preferred because it does not exacerbate the inebriated state or require blood monitoring.[132,133] The protocol consists of a 15 mg/kg IV loading dose followed by a 10 mg/kg IV bolus every 12 hours. After 48 hours, the bolus dose should be increased to 15 mg/kg every 12 hours to account for enhanced fomepizole metabolism. For both ethylene glycol and methanol, patients are treated until serum levels fall below 20 mg/dL. Hemodialysis can be performed concurrently with fomepizole if clinically indicated. In ethylene glycol poisoning, hemodialysis is indicated when serum levels are greater than 50 mg/dL, when there is significant and refractory metabolic acidosis, or when there is evidence of end-organ damage. In methanol poisoning, hemodialysis is indicated if serum methanol levels are above 50 mg/dL, a lethal dose of methanol has been ingested, or there is significant and refractory metabolic acidosis or evidence of end-organ damage.

Ethanol can be administered orally or intravenously aiming for a level of 100 to 200 mg/dL. One protocol for therapeutic ethanol administration to such patients is as follows:[134]

Loading dose: 0.6 g/kg ethanol IV
Maintenance dose:

Nonalcoholic patient: 66 mg/kg per hour ethanol by continuous IV infusion
Alcoholic patient: 154 mg/kg per hour ethanol by continuous IV infusion
Patients receiving HD: double continuous infusion rate

Intravenous ethanol is supplied as a 10% solution in 5% dextrose, containing 10 g of ethanol per 100 mL of solution. Blood ethanol levels should be maintained in the target range during hemodialysis by either dialysis bath supplementation with 200 mg/dL ethanol, or doubling the dose of intravenous ethanol infusion.[134–140]

A high index of clinical suspicion is necessary to identify methanol- or ethylene glycol–intoxicated patients. Early institution of measures to inhibit metabolism by alcohol dehydrogenase of either substance to its toxic metabolites (formic acid from methanol, oxalic and glycolic acids from ethylene glycol) and urgent dialytic removal of the alcohol and its metabolites are of paramount importance in optimizing outcome. We also recommend alcohol dehydrogenase inhibition and prophylactic hemodialysis in any intoxicated patient with an unexplained elevation of the plasma osmolal gap, especially if serum levels are not immediately available. Further complicating matters, intoxication with diethylene glycol, which is undetected by assessment for serum ethylene glycol, but is associated with elevation of the osmolal gap and development of metabolic acidosis and acute renal failure, responds to inhibition of alcohol dehydrogenase and dialytic therapy. It is thus conceivable that an inebriated patient presenting with an elevated osmolal gap but negative serum levels for ethanol, methanol, and ethylene glycol, might benefit from empiric inhibition of alcohol dehydrogenase and hemodialysis.

Isopropanol is metabolized by alcohol dehydrogenase to acetone, which is excreted through the kidneys and breath, creating a sweet smell. Clinical features of poisoning include ketonemia, ketonuria, lack of an elevated anion gap or metabolic acidosis, an elevated osmolal gap, and hemorrhagic gastritis.[135] A serum isopropanol level confirms the diagnosis. Supportive measures are usually sufficient in the treatment of these patients. Gastric lavage can be helpful if performed in the first hour postingestion. Hemodialysis is indicated when lethal doses have been ingested (150 to 240 mL of 40% to 70% solution), or when lethal serum levels are detected (400 mg/dL). Refractory shock and prolonged coma are other indications for dialysis.[135] Fomepizole is not indicated.

AMPHETAMINES

Common amphetamine and amphetamine-like prescription drugs include methylphenidate, dextroamphetamine, and pemoline, used primarily for narcolepsy and attention-deficit disorder; and various anorectic medications used for weight loss, including diethylpropion and phentermine.

Illicit drugs include methamphetamine, an addictive stimulant that is made in small laboratories. Street methamphetamine is referred to by many names, such as "speed" and "meth." When it is inhaled in powder form or by smoking it is referred to as "crank," "crystal," or "ice." Over the past decade methamphetamine use has increased rapidly in the United States.[141] Ecstasy or "XTC" is the street name for 3,4-methylenedioxymethamphetamine or MDMA. Ecstasy use has become common among teenagers and young adults, particularly at "rave" parties.

Amphetamines exert their toxicity via central nervous system stimulation, peripheral release of catecholamines, inhibition of reuptake of catecholamines, or inhibition of monoamine oxidase. They generally have a low therapeutic index. In overdose, they cause confusion, tremor, anxiety, agitation, and irritability. Additional features include mydriasis, tachyarrhythmias, myocardial ischemia, stroke, hypertension, hyperreflexia, hyperthermia, rhabdomyolysis, renal failure, coagulopathy, and seizures. Hepatotoxicity requiring liver transplantation has been reported with ecstasy abuse.[142] Death may result from arrhythmias, status epilepticus, intracranial hemorrhage, or aspiration pneumonitis.

Treatment is supportive, including maintenance of the airway and mechanical ventilation if necessary. Hypertension generally responds to systemic vasodilation with phentolamine or nitroprusside. Tachyarrhythmias may respond to esmolol or propranolol. Benzodiazepines, droperidol, or a phenothiazine are indicated for agitation.

Gastric lavage is helpful if performed within 1 hour of ingestion and AC should be administered promptly to adsorb remaining drug. Ipecac-induced emesis is not recommended because of the risk of abrupt onset of seizures and risk of aspiration. Elimination of amphetamines may be enhanced by forced-acid diuresis; however, acidification of the urine may increase risk of nephrotoxicity when there is myoglobinuria. Dialysis and hemoperfusion are not effective. In hyperthermic patients, the role of dantrolene is controversial, particularly due to its potential for hepatotoxicity.[143,144]

BARBITURATES

Clinical manifestations of mild to moderate barbiturate overdose include reduction in the level of consciousness, slurred speech, and ataxia. In higher doses, barbiturates cause hypothermia, hypotension, bradycardia, flaccidity, hyporeflexia, coma, and apnea. Patients with severe overdose may appear to be dead, including absence of EEG activity.

Cardiovascular depression is caused by a combination of decreased arterial tone and myocardial depression, leading to a high filling pressure, low cardiac output, and hypotension. Respiratory depression with hypercarbia and hypoxemia are common. In deep coma, the usual acid-base disturbance is a mixed respiratory and metabolic acidosis. Patients completely unresponsive to painful stimuli tend to be significantly more acidemic and hypoxemic than those who show some response, a finding that is not explained by differences in alveolar ventilation.[145] Hypoxemia may be aggravated by ventilation/perfusion mismatch and/or increased capillary permeability with development of the acute respiratory distress syndrome, possibly related to aspiration pneumonitis. Local tissue hypoxia resulting from vascular stasis and arterial hypoxemia may contribute to the development of barbiturate-related skin blisters, which commonly develop over areas of increased pressure.[146]

The diagnosis of sedative overdose is generally made on clinical grounds. Confirmation of barbiturate ingestion is readily available by routine urine toxicology screening. Blood levels are generally available and correlate with the severity of clinical findings; however, they rarely affect management.

As in all toxic ingestions, treatment of barbiturate overdose starts with supportive measures. There is no antidote. Gastric lavage is useful in acute massive overdose; ipecac-induced vomiting should be considered immediately after ingestion, particularly in children. Activated charcoal (AC) decreases further drug absorption and increases drug elimination,[147–149] but may not alter clinical course.[150] Multidose AC may be useful in life-threatening overdoses.[151]

Alkalinization of the urine (pH >7.5) increases the elimination of phenobarbital, but not other barbiturates, and may aggravate pulmonary edema.[152] Forced alkaline diuresis may be sustained by dopamine hydrochloride,[153] but this is generally not required or recommended. Charcoal hemoperfusion is indicated in severe poisoning characterized by prolonged coma or refractory hypotension, although its role is disputed.[154–156]

When mental status changes persist, other conditions should be considered and excluded: head trauma with subdural or epidural hematoma, intracerebral hemorrhage, embolic stroke, electrolyte abnormalities, hypoxemia, hypothyroidism, liver or renal failure, central nervous system infection, seizures, and significant alterations in temperature.

BENZODIAZEPINES

Benzodiazepines enhance the inhibitory effects of the neurotransmitter γ-aminobutyric acid (GABA), causing generalized depression of the central nervous system. Symptoms in overdose range from slurred speech and lethargy to respiratory arrest and coma, depending on the dose and compound ingested. In general, patients in coma from benzodiazepine poisoning are hyporeflexic with small to midposition pupils.

The diagnosis of benzodiazepine overdose depends on a history of ingestion or a high index of suspicion for drug overdose, combined with compatible clinical features. Confirmation of exposure is available by urine toxicology screening.

Treatment of benzodiazepine overdose consists of initial supportive measures, gastric emptying in acute ingestions, activated charcoal,[157] and flumazenil. There is no role for forced diuresis, dialysis, or hemoperfusion.

Flumazenil, a specific benzodiazepine antagonist, is useful in reversing sedation in patients undergoing procedures and in patients who have taken an intentional benzodiazepine overdose. Its effect on reversal of respiratory depression is less clear.[158,159] Judicious use of flumazenil provides diagnostic information, because flumazenil does not antagonize the CNS effects of alcohol, barbiturates, cyclic antidepressants, or narcotics.

Flumazenil should be considered if benzodiazepine overdose is highly suspected or confirmed and benzodiazepines have not been prescribed for a potentially life-threatening condition.[160] However, the risks and benefits of flumazenil compared to supportive measures alone are not clear. Flumazenil may cause severe withdrawal or seizures in dependent patients, and in an animal model of combined cocaine-diazepam poisoning, flumazenil precipitated seizures and increased mortality. Seizures may also occur in combined cyclic antidepressant-benzodiazepine overdose; however, cautious administration of flumazenil in this setting is likely to be safe.

Flumazenil is not a recommended component of the "coma cocktail."[2] Still, in selected cases it may help to distinguish benzodiazepine overdose from mixed-drug intoxication or non–drug-induced coma, and it improves the clinical status of patients with benzodiazepine overdose. The recommended initial dose of flumazenil is 0.2 mg (2 mL) IV over 30 seconds. A further 0.3-mg (3 mL) dose can be given over 30 seconds if the desired clinical effect is not seen within 30 seconds. Additional 0.5-mg doses can be administered over 30 seconds at 1-minute intervals as needed to a total dose of 3 mg. Flumazenil dosed beyond 3 mg generally does not provide additional benefit.[161] Patients should be monitored for resedation. Resedation usually occurs within 0.5 to 3.0 hours after the first flumazenil dose.[162] In some cases repeat doses of flumazenil or a continuous infusion (0.1 to 0.5 mg/h) is necessary.[162] Hepatic dysfunction significantly changes the pharmacokinetic profile of flumazenil, requiring downward adjustment in dosage.[163]

Naloxone may partially reverse the antianxiety effects of benzodiazepines,[164] but it does not significantly alter motor or respiratory effects.[165,166]

When mental status changes persist, other conditions should be considered. These include subdural or epidural hematoma, intracerebral hemorrhage, embolic stroke, abnormalities of sodium and other electrolytes, hypoxemia, hypothyroidism, liver or renal failure, central nervous system infection, seizures, and significant alterations in temperature. A head CT scan should be performed early in the course of an obtunded patient, and there should be a low threshold to perform lumbar puncture.

BETA-BLOCKERS

Clinical features of β-blocker overdose depend on the drug type, amount and timing of overdose, coingestions, and comorbidities. The diagnosis is usually established on clinical grounds; blood levels are available but do not correlate well with severity.[167] Risk factors for cardiovascular morbidity include coingestion of another cardioactive drug and a β-blocker with myocardial membrane-stabilizing activity (acebutolol, betaxolol, pindolol, or propranolol).[168] Most patients develop β-blocker toxicity within 4 hours of ingestion.[169] Asymptomatic patients with a normal electrocardiogram after 6 hours generally do not require ICU monitoring.[169]

Cardiovascular complications of β-blockers include hypotension, bradycardia, atrioventricular block, and congestive heart failure and pulmonary edema. Hypotension is mainly due to decreased myocardial contractility rather than bradycardia. Other clinical manifestations of overdose are bronchospasm, hypoglycemia, hyperkalemia, lethargy, stupor, coma, and seizures. The risk of seizure is highest with propranolol, particularly when the QRS complex is >100 ms.[170] In a large retrospective review of 52,156 cases of β-blocker overdose, there were 164 deaths.[171] Propranolol was responsible for the greatest number of toxic exposures (44%) and implicated as the primary cause of death in a disproportionately higher percentage of fatalities (71%).

Treatment of β-blocker toxicity is largely supportive. Induced emesis is contraindicated because of the risk of sudden cardiovascular collapse.[170] Gastric lavage may help if the procedure is undertaken within 60 minutes of ingestion. Single-dose AC is recommended; there is no clear role for multidose AC.

Cardiovascular manifestations are treated with fluid resuscitation, vasopressors, atropine, electrical pacing, and glucagon. Glucagon effectively reverses myocardial depression and bradycardia. Its positive inotropic and chronotropic effect is mediated through adenyl cyclase, which increases cyclic adenosine monophosphate and intracellular calcium influx.[172] Improvements in bradycardia and hypotension occur within a few minutes and may preclude the need for high-dose catecholamine infusion.[173] Glucagon is given as bolus of 5 to 10 mg IV over 1 minute followed by an infusion of 1 to 10 mg/h. Dilution in saline or dextrose as opposed to the diluent provided by the manufacturer, which contains 2 mg of phenol per 1 mg of glucagon, is recommended to avoid phenol toxicity. The use of an insulin-glucose infusion for β-blocker toxicity may prove to be superior to glucagon alone; this strategy is under investigation.[174]

CALCIUM CHANNEL BLOCKERS

Calcium channel blockers (CCBs) selectively inhibit the movement of calcium ions through the membrane of cardiac and vascular smooth muscle during the slow inward phase of excitation-contraction. These agents have varying degrees of cardiovascular effects. Verapamil is more of a negative inotrope; nifedipine has more vasodilatory effects. Verapamil and diltiazem depress the sinus node and slow conduction through the atrioventricular node. The most common cardiovascular effect is hypotension, which generally occurs within 6 hours of CCB overdose (except with sustained-release preparations, in which toxicity may not be evident for 12 hours). Hypotension is mainly secondary to peripheral vasodilation as opposed to myocardial depression. Conduction abnormalities are worsened with concurrent β-blocker ingestion and existing cardiovascular disease.[175] Nausea, vomiting, hyperglycemia, confusion, lethargy, and coma have all been attributed to CCB overdose. Seizures are uncommon.

Gastric lavage may be useful for up to 8 hours after ingestion of a sustained-release preparation. Whole bowel irrigation has similarly been used for sustained-release preparations.[176] Multidose activated charcoal and hemodialysis are not indicated. However, charcoal hemoperfusion may have a role in verapamil overdose in the setting of hepatic dysfunction.[177]

Hypotension is treated first with fluids and vasopressors. For refractory hypotension, calcium chloride infusions (1 to 3 g by slow IV push) are recommended.[6] Additional calcium infusions (by bolus or constant infusion) are warranted in patients who demonstrate a transient response to the initial calcium infusion. Calcium gluconate (2 to 3 g total or 0.2 to 0.5 mL/kg of a 10% solution every 15 to 20 minutes to a total of 4 doses) has also been recommended.[178,179] Glucagon, given as a bolus of 5 to 10 mg IV over a minute followed by an infusion of 1 to 10 mg/h, may decrease vasopressor requirements.[173,180] Recently, several investigators have reported successful reversal of refractory shock in CCB toxicity with hyperinsulinemia-euglycemia therapy by continuous infusion of insulin and glucose.[181,182] Larger trials are needed to confirm its safety and efficacy.

CARBON MONOXIDE

Carbon monoxide (CO) is a nonirritating, colorless, tasteless, and odorless gas formed by incomplete combustion of carbon-containing materials (complete oxidation produces carbon dioxide). Poisoning occurs in the setting of smoke inhalation, attempted suicide from automobile exhaust, and poorly ventilated charcoal and gas stoves. Rarely, CO is generated during hepatic metabolism of dichloromethane, a component of paint and varnish removers. Carbon monoxide is a common cause of death by poisoning in the United States.[183]

Carbon monoxide binds to hemoglobin with an affinity that is 240 times greater than oxygen. Fetal hemoglobin binds carbon monoxide to an even greater degree, placing the fetus at particularly high risk during CO exposure. Carboxyhemoglobin (HbCO) decreases oxyhemoglobin saturation and blood oxygen-carrying capacity, in a way that is analogous to anemia (a HbCO concentration of 50% effectively lowers hemoglobin concentration by half). However, CO poisoning causes significantly more toxicity than similar degrees of anemia because in CO poisoning (1) HbCO shifts the oxyhemoglobin dissociation curve to the left, interfering with off-loading of oxygen in peripheral tissues; (2) CO reacts with myoglobin to form carboxymyoglobin; (3) CO blocks myoglobin-facilitated diffusion of oxygen (particularly in tissues rich in myoglobin), as well as myoglobin-mediated oxidative phosphorylation, resulting in impaired cardiac contractility; (4) CO inhibits enzymes of the mitochondrial electron-transfer chain, further interfering with cellular function; and (5) CO binds and inhibits various intracellular enzymes including cytochrome P-450 and NADPH reductase.[184,185] Tissues with high oxygen consumption (namely, heart and brain) are particularly vulnerable to toxic effects.

The severity of CO poisoning depends on the concentration of CO, duration of exposure, and minute ventilation. Carboxyhemoglobin levels do not correlate well with clinical severity of CO poisoning. Generally, mild exposures (HbCO 5% to 10%) cause headache and mild dyspnea. These concentrations may be seen in heavy smokers and commuters on busy highways and are generally well tolerated, even in the presence of documented coronary artery disease and ventricular ectopy.[186] Carboxyhemoglobin concentrations between 10% and 30% cause headache, dizziness, weakness, dyspnea, and irritability. These concentrations may cause angina and myocardial infarction even in young and otherwise healthy patients.[187] Exposures to >50% HbCO result in coma, seizures, cardiovascular collapse, and death.

Ten to thirty percent of survivors of CO poisoning develop delayed neurologic sequelae (DNS) of hypoxic brain injury.[188,189] Clinical manifestations of DNS are variable, including persistent vegetative state, parkinsonism, memory deficits, behavioral changes, and hearing loss. Neurologic sequelae cannot be predicted by severity of carboxyhemoglobin exposure, age, method of exposure (accidental or intentional), or results of early neuroimaging (which may be normal or show low-density lesions in the globus pallidus or deep white matter changes).[190]

The diagnosis of CO poisoning is often made on clinical grounds in the setting of smoke inhalation or attempted suicide. However, the diagnosis can be missed if the history is incomplete and the clinical presentation is nondescript. There should be a high index of suspicion, particularly during cold weather months in patients with myocardial ischemia/infarction, cardiac arrhythmias, mental status changes, headache, and generalized weakness. Rarely, cherry-red skin discoloration reflecting high venous saturation (arteriolization of venous blood) provides an additional clue. Failure to diagnose CO may have disastrous consequences for the patient and other members of an affected household.

Laboratory confirmation of elevated HbCO is available by co-oximetry. Pulse oximetry is unreliable in detecting HbCO because it cannot distinguish carboxyhemoglobin from oxyhemoglobin. Pulse oximetry overestimates oxyhemoglobin by the amount of HbCO present, and may be in the normal range despite high concentrations of HbCO.[191] Arterial blood gases typically demonstrate a normal P_{O_2}, contrasting with low oxyhemoglobin saturation by co-oximeter, and metabolic acidosis. Of note, patients with suspected CO poisoning can be screened by analysis of venous blood because venous HbCO levels accurately predict arterial blood levels.[192]

Treatment of CO poisoning consists of immediate removal of the patient from the exposure and administration of 100% supplemental oxygen. Breathing 100% oxygen reduces the half-life of HbCO from 5 to 6 hours on room air to 40 to 90 minutes. Breathing oxygen that contains 4.5% to 4.8% carbon dioxide allows for a greater minute ventilation while maintaining normocapnia and further accelerates CO clearance. In one study of seven healthy volunteers, this method decreased the half-life of CO from 78 ± 24 minutes to 31 ± 6 minutes compared to 100% O_2 at resting minute ventilation.[193] Hyperbaric oxygen (HBO) (2.8 atmospheres) further decreases the half-life of HbCO to 15 to 30 minutes.

The role of HBO, which can result in arterial oxygen tensions greater than 2000 mm Hg and oxygen tensions in tissue approaching 400 mm Hg, is debated.[194] Several nonrandomized studies have demonstrated that HBO improves acute and delayed effects of CO poisoning.[195] One trial in 343 patients comparing HBO with 100% normobaric oxygen (NBO) delivered outside a hyperbaric chamber in patients without loss of consciousness showed no significant difference between groups in acute or delayed symptoms of CO poisoning.[196] Another unblinded study comparing HBO with 100% NBO in 65 patients without loss of consciousness demonstrated significantly fewer patients with DNS in the HBO group (0% versus 23%).[197] HBO has also been found to be beneficial in patients (n = 26) with loss of consciousness.[198] Another study comparing HBO with 100% NBO delivered in a hyperbaric chamber (i.e., blinded) in CO-poisoned patients with and without loss of consciousness showed no difference in the development of delayed neurologic sequelae, and that "normal neuropsychologic and functional outcomes are possible after severe CO poisoning without the use of HBO therapy."[199] In a recent double-blind, randomized trial, patients (76 in each group) with symptomatic CO poisoning were assigned to three HBO sessions within 24 hours or one NBO treatment plus two sessions of normobaric room air. Cognitive sequelae were less frequent in the HBO group at 6 weeks and 12 months.[200] In this study, the presence of cerebellar dysfunction before treatment was associated with the occurrence of cognitive sequelae.

Although the use of HBO remains controversial, we believe that patients with potentially life-threatening exposures should receive at least one HBO treatment (if hyperbaric capability is readily available). Particularly controversial is whether a patient with severe CO poisoning should be transferred solely for the purpose of HBO, a problem that may be solved by refinement of portable HBO chambers.[201] Also controversial is the relative efficacy of single versus multiple

HBO treatments.[202,203] Since CO poisoning may occur with other life-threatening injuries (e.g., burns or other trauma), the judgment to utilize HBO must take into consideration the patient's stability and the ability to monitor and treat during HBO therapy.

COCAINE

Cocaine may be snorted nasally, inhaled orally, or used intravenously. Body packers swallow multiple wrapped packages of cocaine in an attempt to smuggle the drug across national borders; body stuffers swallow or conceal wrapped packets of cocaine in various body cavities when law enforcement agents approach. Freebase cocaine is prepared for smoking by dissolving cocaine salt in an aqueous alkaline salt solution and then extracting the freebase form with a solvent such as ether. Heat is often used to speed this process, creating a fire hazard. The preferred freebase preparation for smoking is crack cocaine, which is a more potent, rapidly absorbed, water-soluble alkaloid form of the drug.

Cocaine is often mixed with other substances of abuse including heroin ("speedball"), phencyclidine, and various sympathomimetic drugs used to treat nasal congestion.[204] In the presence of ethanol, cocaine is transesterified in the liver to cocaethylene, which has similar properties to cocaine but a longer half-life. Cocaethylene is a myocardial depressant capable of reducing stroke volume and arterial pressure while increasing pulmonary artery wedge pressure. Cocaethylene also prolongs QRS and QTc intervals.[205] Individuals combine cocaine and ethanol to achieve a more pronounced and prolonged euphoria, but this combination is more toxic than either drug alone.

Toxic effects of cocaine stem from excessive central nervous system stimulation and inhibition of neuronal uptake of catecholamines. The result is generalized sympathetic overstimulation similar to that of amphetamine intoxication. Onset and duration of symptoms depend on route of administration, dose, and patient tolerance. Smoking and intravenous use produce symptoms within 1 to 2 minutes; oral use delays onset of symptoms by 20 to 30 minutes. The half-life of cocaine is approximately 60 minutes.

Common central nervous system manifestations include euphoria, anxiety, agitation, psychosis, and delirium. Rarely, cocaine-induced ischemic cerebral infarction is mistaken for a psychiatric condition.[206] Seizures are generally short-lived and self-limited unless there is ongoing drug absorption (as in body packers or body stuffers) or other central nervous system pathology. Several mechanisms are likely responsible for more serious central nervous system complications. A sudden rise in systemic arterial pressure may cause intracerebral hemorrhage and subarachnoid hemorrhage,[207] particularly in association with an underlying aneurysm or arteriovenous malformation. Vasospasm, vasculitis, myocardial infarction with cardiac arrhythmias, and increased platelet aggregation may further trigger ischemic events.[208] Benign angiopathy of the CNS has also been reported.[209] In most cases, the time interval between drug abuse and the cerebrovascular event is less than 3 hours.[210]

Cardiovascular manifestations of cocaine abuse include chest pain, myocardial ischemia and infarction, sudden death, arrhythmias, congestive heart failure, pulmonary hyperten-sion, endocarditis, and aortic dissection.[211–214,144] Common findings include a significant increase in heart rate and mean arterial blood pressure consistent with sympathetic stimulation combined with a fall in ejection fraction as determined by two-dimensional echocardiography.[215] The pathogenesis of these cardiovascular complications has not been fully explained, but may be related to a combination of the sympathomimetic and membrane effects (sodium and potassium channel blockade) of cocaine.

The mechanism by which cocaine induces myocardial ischemia remains controversial. Most prior studies have postulated that cocaine-induced coronary vasoconstriction limits myocardial oxygen. Platelet aggregation and increased myocardial oxygen requirements may fuel the imbalance between supply and demand. Asymptomatic cocaine abusers have been reported to have left ventricular hypertrophy, segmental wall motion abnormalities, ST-T wave changes, pathologic Q waves, and increased QRS voltage on electrocardiogram.[216]

Baseline electrocardiographic changes complicate decisions regarding the need to hospitalize patients with cocaine-associated chest pain. Studies have yielded conflicting data regarding the incidence of myocardial infarction in cocaine abusers, and there are no clinical parameters that reliably identify patients at very low risk for myocardial infarction. These considerations mandate that all patients with cocaine-associated chest pain are evaluated for myocardial infarction.[217] Furthermore, cocaine-related mental status changes may interfere with patient reporting of cocaine-associated chest pain.[218]

Patients with cocaine-associated chest pain often continue to use cocaine after discharge. Cardiac stress tests or cardiac angiography may not be necessary for patients in whom myocardial infarction has been ruled out and who do not continue to have chest pain; such patients appear to have a low risk for subsequent myocardial infarction and death. Instead, efforts should emphasize cessation of cocaine abuse.[219]

Respiratory complications of cocaine include status asthmaticus,[220] upper airway obstruction (stridor),[221] pulmonary hypertension,[222] barotrauma, pulmonary edema, and alveolar hemorrhage.[223] Not uncommonly, crack cocaine causes an acute pulmonary syndrome characterized by dyspnea, diffuse infiltrates, and hemoptysis.[224] The severity of respiratory complications ranges from mild dyspnea to severe respiratory failure requiring intubation and mechanical ventilation.

Another severe manifestation of cocaine abuse is rhabdomyolysis.[225] Creatine kinase levels are often over 10,000 U/L on presentation, with values reported as high as 85,000 U/L.[226] There is often concurrent hyperthermia, tachycardia, muscle rigidity, disseminated intravascular coagulation, hepatic dysfunction, and renal failure.[225,226] Cocaine also has a direct toxic effect on muscles.

Cocaine-induced hyperthermia resembles neuroleptic malignant syndrome;[227] both are characterized by a decrease in the number of dopamine receptors or depletion of dopamine. Contributors to hyperthermia include agitation and adrenergic stimulation causing vasoconstriction.

Rare cocaine-associated complications include ischemic colitis,[228] renal infarction,[229] nasal septal perforation, and localized areas of skin necrosis due to accidental subcutaneous injection. Intranasal use of cocaine has been associated with sinusitis and botulism;[230] botulism also occurs with skin wounds.[231] In addition, the behavioral effects of cocaine increase the likelihood of violent fatal injuries.[232]

Treatment of cocaine intoxication starts with the ABCDs of resuscitation and treatment of seizures, hyperthermia, and agitation. For orally ingested drug, AC should be given to decrease drug absorption. Gastric lavage and ipecac-induced vomiting are not recommended because of the risk of seizures and subsequent aspiration. In body packers whole bowel irrigation with a polyethylene glycol electrolyte solution (e.g., GoLYTELY) 1 to 2 L/h is recommended until the rectal effluent clears and there is no radiographic evidence of retained drug condoms (Fig. 102-2).[233] For this purpose, abdominal ultrasound, a CT scan with contrast or a small bowel follow-through contrast study is more sensitive and specific than routine abdominal radiographs.[234] Contraindications to whole-bowel irrigation include ileus, gastrointestinal hemorrhage, and bowel perforation. Polyethylene glycol electrolyte solutions may also displace cocaine from AC.[235] Surgical removal of retained packages may be required, particularly if there is bowel obstruction or package perforation.[236] Endoscopic approaches risk packet rupture and are not recommended. Neither dialysis nor hemoperfusion effectively removes cocaine.

Perhaps the most important treatment strategy in cocaine intoxication is rapid treatment of agitation and hyperthermia. Along these lines, patient cooling, benzodiazepines, and occasionally muscle relaxation improve outcome,[237] although there are concerns that benzodiazepines may enhance cocaine-induced hyperactivity.[238] For purposes of patient sedation, haloperidol has not been shown to be of benefit,[237] and few data are available regarding a possible role for barbiturates.

First-line treatments of cocaine-associated chest pain are nitrates and benzodiazepines.[2,6,239,240] Use of an α-adrenergic receptor blocker such as phentolamine is recommended in patients refractory to nitrates and benzodiazepines.[6,241] Non-selective β-blockers should not be used alone to treat cocaine toxicity because of the potential for unopposed α-adrenergic stimulation and potentiation of coronary vasoconstriction.[242] Propranolol worsens outcome in an animal model;[243] esmolol produces an inconsistent antihypertensive response and may cause hypertension or hypotension.[244] The use of labetalol is controversial.[6] Labetalol blocks both α- and β-adrenergic receptors and may reverse cocaine-induced hypertension, but there are data that show that it is ineffective in cocaine-induced coronary vasoconstriction.[245]

The role of thrombolytic therapy remains unclear in patients with cocaine-associated acute myocardial infarction. Intracoronary administration of thrombolytics has been recommended over peripheral administration in refractory cases, but further studies addressing safety and efficacy are needed before firm recommendations can be made.[6,246] Thrombolytics are contraindicated in uncontrolled hypertension, aortic dissection, and intracerebral hemorrhage.

Treatment of respiratory complications is supportive. Oxygen is delivered to improve arterial oxygen saturation; continuous positive airway pressure or positive end-expiratory pressure may decrease intrapulmonary shunting in patients with diffuse lung disease. Inhaled bronchodilators and corticosteroids are indicated for cocaine-associated bron-

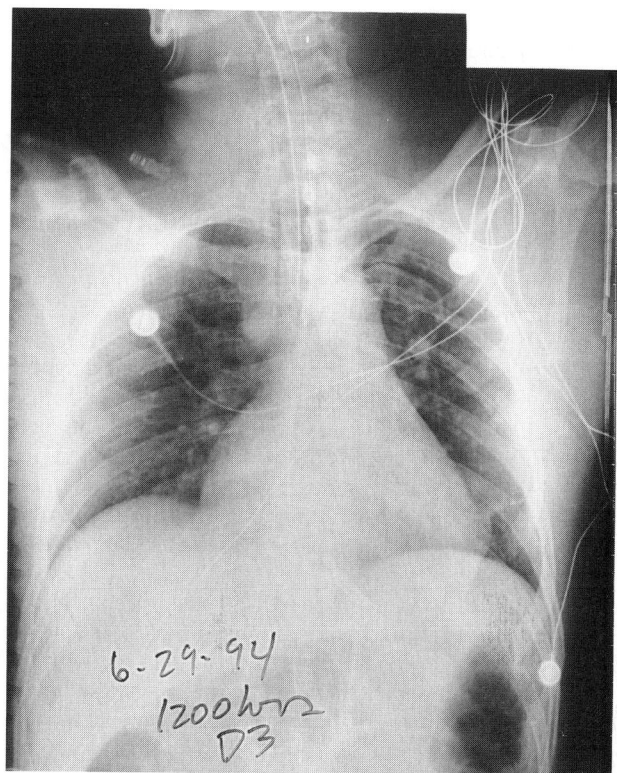

A

B

FIGURE 102-2 A chest radiograph (*A*) and an abdominal CT scan with oral contrast (*B*) in a patient "body packing" cocaine. Note the presence of multiple densities in the stomach visible on the abdominal CT scan consistent with partially filled bags of cocaine, and that these bags are barely visible (if at all) in the left upper quadrant on the plain film.

chospasm. Tube thoracostomy may be required for pneumothorax; pneumomediastinum is watched expectantly.

CYANIDE

Cyanide is found in a variety of synthetic and natural substances: plastics, glue removers, wool, silks, nylons, and various seeds and plants. Poisoning occurs through a number of mechanisms including (1) ingestion (e.g., the cassava-based foodstuff "gari"[247] or tainted over-the-counter preparations[248]); (2) inhalation of hydrogen cyanide gas (HCN), a combustion by-product of cyanide-containing products; (3) sodium nitroprusside infusion; and very rarely (4) absorption of cyanide-containing solutions or gas through skin.

Cyanide is a rapidly-acting poison that binds to cellular cytochrome oxidase and interferes with aerobic oxygen utilization. Once ingested, it is detoxified by enzymatic conversion to the less toxic, renally excreted metabolite thiocyanate. The most important enzyme for cyanide conversion is rhodenase (a sulfur transferase), which forms thiocyanate in the presence of sulfane sulfur. This reaction occurs in liver, although the kidney also contains high concentrations of rhodenase. Serum albumin plays an important role in cyanide detoxification because it is a readily available source of sulfane sulfur and it has sulfurtransferase activity. A small amount of cyanide is also detoxified by the vitamin B_{12} precursor hydroxycobalamin. This agent binds cyanide to form nontoxic cyanocobalamin.

Clinical manifestations of cyanide poisoning depend upon the amount and rate of cyanide absorption. Patients who are asymptomatic after inhalation (which is associated with immediate absorption) do not require treatment and can be discharged after a short period of observation. Patients who ingest cyanide orally may present with progressive symptoms over minutes to hours. Oral ingestion on an empty stomach with low pH results in the rapid generation of HCN from potassium and sodium salts (KCN and NaCN). Oral ingestion into a full and alkaline stomach delays generation of HCN, resulting in progressive symptoms over 1 to 2 hours. Ingestion of plants containing cyanogenic glycosides also causes delayed and progressive toxicity.

At low concentrations, cyanide acts as a respiratory and central nervous system stimulant. Clinical manifestations include anxiety, dyspnea, headache, confusion, tachycardia, and hypertension. At higher concentrations, patients may develop stupor or coma, seizures, fixed and dilated pupils, hypoventilation, hypotension, bradycardia, heart block and ventricular arrhythmias. Patients with massive ingestion present in coma and cardiopulmonary collapse. Survival in these cases depends on the success of cardiopulmonary resuscitation, with survivors at great risk of permanent sequelae of anoxic brain injury.[249,250]

The diagnosis of cyanide poisoning is usually made on clinical grounds, often in the setting of smoke inhalation injury, where combined carbon monoxide and cyanide toxicity occurs. Highly suggestive is the rapid onset of coma, seizures, and cardiopulmonary dysfunction. Lactic acidosis and an elevated mixed venous oxyhemoglobin saturation provide evidence for the blocking of aerobic oxygen utilization.[251] Elevated venous oxyhemoglobin is further demonstrated by arteriolization of retinal veins on funduscopic examination or venous blood on venipuncture. The bitter almond scent of HCN may also be detected.

Short-term high-dose sodium nitroprusside therapy (>10 μg/kg per minute) may result in acute cyanide poisoning characterized by anxiety, agitation, tachycardia, myocardial ischemia, metabolic acidosis, hyperventilation, seizures, and paradoxical hypertension (or difficulty in lowering blood pressure). Cyanide poisoning is uncommon at nitroprusside infusion rates less than 10 μg/kg per minute; however,

toxicity has been reported at an infusion rate of 4 μg/kg per minute after 3 hours of therapy.[252] Prolonged nitroprusside infusion increases the risk of thiocyanate toxicity. Thiocyanate levels should be followed in these cases, particularly when there is renal dysfunction. Thiocyanate levels greater than 50 to 100 mg/L cause confusion, somnolence, and seizures.[252]

When clinical features of cyanide poisoning are present, treatment should proceed before confirmation of the diagnosis by determination of whole blood cyanide levels. The laboratory should be notified prior to drawing the blood, since special instructions may be required to measure this unstable compound. Whole blood levels greater than 0.5 to 1.0 mg/L are considered toxic.[253] Smokers may have cyanide levels nearing 0.1 mg/mL.

Treatment begins by identifying and treating life-threatening problems. Survival depends on prompt and successful CPR.[254] Oxygen therapy at 100% fraction of inspired oxygen (F_{IO_2}) is effective in cyanide poisoning and should be administered immediately.[255–258] Hyperbaric oxygen is of unproven benefit in cyanide poisoning (in part because of the time element involved).[259]

Several antidotes are available to treat cyanide poisoning. Amyl and sodium nitrite induce formation of methemoglobin. Cyanide has a high affinity for the ferric iron contained in methemoglobin, thereby rendering methemoglobin an effective scavenger of unbound cyanide. Amyl nitrite is administered by inhalation of crushable ampules. Ampules are inhaled for 15 to 30 seconds; effects last approximately 2 to 3 minutes. This therapy can be used in spontaneously breathing patients and in patients receiving ventilatory support by face mask or endotracheal tube until administration of sodium nitrite. Sodium nitrite is administered intravenously at a dose of 300 mg over 3 minutes to convert hemoglobin to methemoglobin. Half this dose may be repeated after 2 hours if there is persistent toxicity and a tolerable degree of methemoglobinemia. Conversion of 25% to 30% of hemoglobin to methemoglobin effectively treats cyanide poisoning,[260] although in usual practice, methemoglobin levels generally remain less than 20%.[261] Induction of methemoglobinemia of course has several disadvantages, including the reduction of circulating hemoglobin available for oxygen transport (which may be further aggravated by concurrent carboxyhemoglobinemia in the setting of smoke inhalation) and the risk of hemolysis in glucose-6-phosphate dehydrogenase (G6PD) deficient patients.[262] In one study evaluating serial cyanide, methemoglobin, and carbon monoxide levels in seven critically ill smoke inhalation patients receiving sodium nitrite, peak measured methemoglobin levels did not occur until a mean of 50 minutes following administration of sodium nitrite.[261] The total oxygen-carrying capacity reduced by the combination of carboxyhemoglobin and methemoglobin was never more than 21% (range = 10% to 21%). Of note, methylene blue should be avoided to treat methemoglobinemia because it will release free cyanide.

Sodium thiosulfate is safe and effective in cyanide poisoning. It acts as a sulfur donor to rhodenase and other sulfurtransferases thereby enhancing conversion of cyanide to thiocyanate.[263,264] The dose is 12.5 g IV (50 mL of a 25% solution) over 10 minutes. Half this dose may be repeated in 2 hours for persistent toxicity. Coadministration of thiosulfate with nitroprusside (in a ratio of 1:10 thiosulfate to nitroprusside) effectively eliminates the possibility of cyanide intoxication without altering the efficacy of nitroprusside.[265] Treatment with sodium thiosulfate can cause thiocyanate toxicity, particularly in the setting of renal insufficiency. Fortunately, thiocyanate is readily dialyzable.

Hydroxycobalamin is a cyanide antidote capable of reducing red blood cell and plasma cyanide concentrations. Little is known, however, about the safety, efficacy, and pharmacokinetics of hydroxycobalamin in human cyanide poisoning. Acute allergic reactions have been reported,[266] and hydroxycobalamin may interfere with several chemistry methodologies affecting measurement of aspartate aminotransferase, total bilirubin, creatinine, magnesium, and iron.[267] In healthy adult smokers, hydroxycobalamin 5 g IV resulted in transient reddish discoloration of skin, mucous membranes, and urine, slight elevation in blood pressure, and a decrease in heart rate.[268] It did, however, decrease whole blood cyanide levels by 59% and increase urinary cyanide excretion. As with thiosulfate, coadminstration of hydroxycobalamin (25 mg/h IV) with nitroprusside may protect against nitroprusside-induced cyanide toxicity.[269,270] The currently recommended dose of hydroxycobalamin in acute cyanide poisoning is 4 to 5 g IV administered as a one-time dose.[270–272]

Intravenous dicobalt ethylenediamine tetraacetic acid (EDTA) is a potent cyanide antidote. When cyanide binds to cobalt a stable and nontoxic compound is formed. The initial dose is 300 to 600 mg IV over 1 minute, followed by an additional 300 mg if the patient fails to improve. Side effects from EDTA include cardiac arrhythmias, hypotension, nausea, vomiting, and severe allergic reactions.[273]

Additional treatment strategies include removal and isolation of all contaminated clothing. Health care workers should avoid contact with cyanide-containing solutions and vapors. Gastric emptying is recommended for acute ingestions, followed by AC. Induced emesis is not recommended because of the risk of rapid cyanide-induced deterioration in clinical status (and subsequent risk of aspiration). There is no role for hemodialysis or hemoperfusion except to clear high levels of thiocyanate.

CYCLIC ANTIDEPRESSANTS

Cyclic antidepressant drugs (including the tricyclics, tetracyclics, bicyclics, and monocyclics) are among the most commonly encountered causes of self-poisoning.[2] Tricyclic antidepressants include amitriptyline, desipramine, doxepin, imipramine, nortriptyline, protriptyline, and amoxapine. In overdose, these drugs primarily affect the central nervous and cardiovascular systems. Lesser effects are seen in the gastrointestinal tract. Central nervous system toxicity results from anticholinergic effects and inhibition of neural reuptake of norepinephrine or serotonin. Cardiovascular manifestations stem from anticholinergic effects, inhibition of neural uptake of norepinephrine or serotonin, peripheral α-adrenergic blockade, and membrane depressant effects. Most patients develop symptoms within the first 6 hours after ingestion or not at all.

Clinical presentation is divided into anticholingeric effects, cardiovascular effects, and seizures. Mydriasis, blurred vision, fever, dry skin and mucous membranes, lethargy, delirium, coma, tachycardia, ileus, myoclonus, and urinary retention are manifestations of anticholinergic toxicity. These symptoms are described by the common mnemonic: "hot as a hare, dry as a bone, red as a beet, mad as a hatter."

Cardiovascular effects consist of sinus tachycardia with prolongation of the QRS, QTc, and PR intervals. Occasionally, sinus tachycardia with QRS prolongation is difficult to distinguish from ventricular tachycardia. Torsades de pointes is rare. Various forms of atrioventricular block may accompany cyclic antidepressant overdose. Right bundle-branch block is common.

A maximal limb-lead QRS interval longer than 0.10 second reliably predicts serious intoxication (except in cases of amoxapine overdose) requiring monitoring until resolution.[274] QRS duration <0.1 second is rarely associated with arrhythmias or seizures. Patients with QRS >0.10 second are at risk for seizures and arrhythmias. In one prospective trial seizures occurred at any QRS duration ≥0.10 second, but ventricular arrhythmias were seen only with a QRS duration ≥0.16 second.[274] Serum drug levels in this study did not predict complications.

Hypotension is relatively common (although hypertension also occurs). It results from venodilation and decreased myocardial contractility. In severe cyclic antidepressant overdose, hypotension may be refractory to fluid administration and vasopressors and associated with pulmonary edema.

Seizures are common in cyclic antidepressant overdose. They may be short-lived and self-limited or prolonged and refractory to treatment. Neurologic deterioration may be abrupt and unpredictable. A "downward spiral" occurs when seizures or arrhythmias cause metabolic acidosis. Metabolic acidosis increases the fraction of free drug and enhances drug toxicity.

The diagnosis of cyclic antidepressant overdose depends on a history of ingestion or a high index of suspicion and compatible clinical features. Cyclic antidepressant overdose should be considered in all patients with QRS prolongation. Confirmation of cyclic antidepressant exposure is rapidly available by urine toxicology screening.

Treatment of cyclic antidepressant overdose starts with identifying and treating life-threatening problems. Sodium bicarbonate (1 to 2 mEq/kg IV) is indicated if there is widening of the QRS interval to decrease the fraction of free drug. Sodium bicarbonate should be continued until there is narrowing of the QRS interval or serum pH exceeds 7.5 to 7.55. In intubated patients, hyperventilation can achieve the same target pH, but hypertonic sodium usually provides greater benefit.[6] The electrocardiogram (ECG) should be followed closely in all cases for 48 to 72 hours.[275] In general patients should remain in an ICU for 12 hours after discontinuation of all therapy and be asymptomatic with a normal ECG and pH before transfer.[276,276a]

Lidocaine is the drug of choice when ventricular arrhythmias are refractory to sodium bicarbonate.[6] Class 1a antiarrhythmics (e.g., procainamide) are contraindicated in cyclic antidepressant overdose because of added cardiac toxicity. Anecdotal reports have also suggested a primary role for phenytoin; however, convincing data are not available to support the use of phenytoin in the setting of cyclic antidepressants as either a prophylactic or therapeutic drug. Physostigmine should not be used in cyclic antidepressant overdose because of possible worsening of cardiac conduction disturbances.

Hypotension refractory to sodium bicarbonate should be treated with vasopressors. A pulmonary artery catheter rarely helps direct therapy and may be arrhythmogenic.

Norepinephrine and phenylephrine are the preferred vasopressors because cyclic antidepressants deplete presynaptic catecholamine stores, limiting the effectiveness of dopamine. Dopamine and other vasopressors may cause an exaggerated vasopressor response in the presence of cyclic antidepressants because of inhibition of catecholamine reuptake. An enhanced hypertensive response to phenylephrine can be also seen in anticholinergic overdose because anticholinergics interfere with phenylephrine-induced reflex bradycardia.

Seizures should be treated with intravenous diazepam or lorazepam. Phenytoin may be administered cautiously in refractory cases. Paralysis may be indicated when seizures are refractory (as may be seen in amoxapine overdose) to control temperature and muscle breakdown. After paralysis, an EEG monitor should be placed to guide subsequent therapy.

Because delayed gastric emptying is extremely common, gastric lavage may be considered during the first 12 hours after a large ingestion. Syrup of ipecac is contraindicated in cyclic antidepressant overdose because patients may suddenly seize or develop a lethal arrhythmia at any time after dosing. Single-dose AC is effective, although anticholinergic-induced ileus increases risk of charcoal-induced bowel obstruction. Because these drugs are lipid-soluble and protein-bound, dialysis and hemoperfusion are not effective.

GAMMA-HYDROXYBUTYRATE

Gamma-hydroxybutyrate (GHB), also known as "liquid ecstasy," "liquid G," "date-rape drug," or "fantasy," has become a popular drug of abuse among young individuals. In the 1980s, the drug was promoted to bodybuilders as a growth hormone stimulator and muscle-bulking agent. Recreationally, it was claimed to cause euphoria without a hangover and to increase sensuality and disinhibition. In 1990 GHB was banned outside of clinical trials approved by the FDA. However, products such as Revivarant, containing a precursor of GHB (gamma-butyrolactone), continued to be available until a recent ban by the federal government.[277,278]

GHB is derived from γ-aminobutyric acid (GABA) and is thought to function as an inhibitory transmitter through specific brain receptors for GHB and possibly through GABA receptors.[279] GHB increases stage IV of non–rapid eye movement sleep (slow-wave deep sleep).[280] In narcoleptics it decreases cataplexy, sleep paralysis, hallucinations, and daytime sleep attacks.[281] Clinical manifestations of GHB depend on the dose ingested. Regular use causes tolerance and dependence, and abrupt discontinuation can result in delirium and psychosis.[282] Low doses of GHB can induce a state of euphoria. Higher doses can cause coma and death.[283] Emesis, bradycardia, hypotension, and respiratory acidosis have all been described.[284]

Treatment of GHB poisoning is mainly supportive. It is important to keep in mind that coingestions are common, especially with ethanol and amphetamines.[284] Mechanical ventilation may be required for brief periods, as most patients regain consciousness spontaneously within 5 hours.[284]

Yates and Viera have described two patients with GHB overdose who awoke in less than 5 minutes after a single dose of physostigmine.[285] Whether physostigmine will prove to be useful in this setting is unclear since rapid recovery is the norm and there are risks in its use, particularly when there is coingestion of a cyclic antidepressant.

Normal toxicologic screens do not include GHB. However, when documentation is important in cases of sexual assault, GHB can be detected in urine and blood by special laboratories using gas chromatography-mass spectroscopy.[286,287] GHB can also be detected by hair analysis.[288]

DIGOXIN

Digitalis is a cardiac glycoside clinically used for treatment of systolic myocardial dysfunction and supraventricular arrhythmias. Two formulations are commercially available: digoxin and digitoxin. These compounds differ importantly in their routes of metabolism: digoxin depends upon renal excretion (60% to 70% unchanged, including filtration and some tubular secretion), whereas digitoxin is hepatically metabolized (to form renally excreted metabolites, including digoxin). They share the important property of prolonged half-life (42 hours for digoxin, 7 days for digitoxin). Digoxin is extensively tissue bound (mostly in muscle), resulting in a massive apparent volume of distribution (4 to 7 L/kg). Digoxin intoxication may occur accidentally during chronic therapy. Diminished clearance because of renal insufficiency, which often increases half-life to 80 to 180 hours, is the most common precipitant of such episodes. Drug interactions may also elevate digoxin levels by impairing renal excretion (e.g., verapamil, other calcium channel blockers, quinidine, or cyclosporine) or hepatic biotransformation (e.g., cyclosporine, verapamil, other calcium channel blockers, or amiodarone), or decreasing digoxin tissue binding and Vd (e.g., quinidine). Finally, increased oral bioavailability because of antibiotic-induced sterilization of digoxin-metabolizing gut flora may also precipitate digoxin toxicity.[289] Variability between digoxin preparations is no longer a major problem.[290] Digitalis may also be ingested in toxic amounts as an unsuspected component of herbal preparations[291] or as a deliberate self-overdose.

The clinical manifestations of digitalis intoxication include fatigue, gastrointestinal symptoms (anorexia, nausea, vomiting, diarrhea, and abdominal pain), neurologic disturbances (blurred vision, visual color changes, headache, dizziness, and delirium), and cardiac arrhythmias (including any category, classically supraventricular tachycardia with AV block). Massive digoxin overdose also causes hyperkalemia, because of inhibition of cellular Na-K-ATPase function. Plasma digoxin levels correlate generally with therapeutic and toxic effects, but interindividual variability in response to a particular digoxin level is common.[292–294] In addition, several factors aside from excess total body digoxin can precipitate digitalis toxicity, even in the therapeutic range, by increasing myocardial digitalis sensitivity. Such factors include hypokalemia, hypomagnesemia, myocardial disease, old age, hypothyroidism, and a variety of other metabolic disturbances (hypoxemia, acid-base abnormalities, hypercalcemia, and hypernatremia). More commonly, digitalis intoxication during chronic therapy results from renal insufficiency or drug interactions (see above).

To be most informative, a digoxin level should be taken when steady-state conditions are in effect. This occurs after approximately 1 week when renal function is normal. The timing of blood sampling is also crucial. To allow time for distribution a sample should be obtained at least 6 hours after the last dose. Based on data demonstrating benefit of low serum digoxin concentrations in heart failure,[295] many laboratories have lowered the therapeutic range for digoxin to 0.5 to 1.0 ng/mL.

Supportive therapy of overdose includes rapid correction of arrhythmogenic metabolic disturbances, particularly hypokalemia. As noted above, hyperkalemia may also require treatment unless Fab therapy is immediately available. Severe bradyarrhythmias that are unresponsive to atropine may require electrical pacing. Ventricular tachycardia should be treated with lidocaine or phenytoin. Electrical cardioversion of any digitalis toxicity–induced arrhythmia should be reserved as a last resort, using the minimum effective energy level.

Gastrointestinal decontamination measures should include emesis or lavage and should be followed by activated charcoal. Charcoal doses may be repeated to minimize enterohepatic recirculation of active digitalis metabolites; orally administered cholestyramine has also been used for this purpose. Timely elimination of digoxin may be difficult to achieve in the face of significant renal insufficiency. Hemodialysis or hemoperfusion can remove only small amounts of total body digitalis (because of extensive tissue binding), but HD may still be indicated for correction of hyperkalemia or other acid-base derangements in renally impaired patients. Fortunately, immunotherapy with digoxin-specific antibody Fab fragments is widely available. These sheep-derived antibodies bind intravascular digoxin, also competitively removing digoxin bound to cellular Na-K-ATPase sites.[296–298] Indications and protocol for Fab therapy are contained in Table 102-24.

Following intravenous administration, plasma free digoxin levels and toxic effects (hyperkalemia and arrhythmia) decrease almost immediately, and the Fab fragments and bound digoxin are eliminated by glomerular filtration (Fab molecular weight is 50,000 Da). Standard digoxin levels can be misleading after treatment. Fab fragments have also been successfully used to treat digoxin toxicity in patients with renal insufficiency, including chronic hemodialysis patients; the potential late complication of rebound intoxication because of impaired Fab-digoxin complex excretion is not commonly seen even in such circumstances.[299] Nevertheless, monitoring of free (rather than total) plasma digoxin levels, and consideration of follow-up plasmapheresis to remove Fab-digoxin complexes has been advocated to prevent late rebound toxicity in renal failure patients.[300]

LITHIUM

Lithium (Li) is used for treatment of bipolar affective disorders. Chronic use is associated with development of nephrogenic diabetes insipidus, renal insufficiency, hypothyroidism, and leukocytosis. Lithium has a low therapeutic index (target range = 0.5 to 1.25 mEq/L). Most cases of intoxication, associated with levels above 1.5 mEq/L, are caused by unintentional overdose during chronic therapy. Volume depletion (aggravated by underlying diabetes insipidus) and renal insufficiency are the common precipitants of lithium overdose. Li is a low-molecular-weight monovalent cation (7 Da), has a small volume of distribution (0.66 L/kg), and is eliminated by glomerular filtration. Li has a prolonged elimination half-life that is increased by advancing age, renal insufficiency, and duration of therapy: 18 hours in adults with normal renal function; up to 36 hours in the elderly; and increased up to twofold in chronically treated subjects.[301] Lithium is predominantly (80%) reabsorbed in the proximal renal tubule, and the other 20% of filtered load is excreted. Any stimulus which augments proximal tubular sodium reabsorption tends to cause increased Li reabsorption in parallel and may precipitate Li intoxication; volume depletion, congestive heart failure, cirrhosis, and other salt-avid states all reduce Li clearance

TABLE 102-24 Indications and Protocol for Digoxin Immune Fab Therapy (Digibind)

Indications	Dose Estimate (# Vials) Based on Serum Steady State Digoxin Levels[a]	Approximate Digibind Dose for Treatment of a Single Large Ingestion[b]
1. Severe ventricular arrhythmias	# Vials = (serum digoxin level in ng/mL) (weight in kg)/100	# Vials = (total digitalis body load in mg)/(0.5 mg digitalis bound/vial)[c]
2. Progressive, atropine unresponsive bradyarrhythmias		
3. Ingestion of >10 mg of digoxin in adults	Examples: for a 70-kg adult: Serum concentration (ng/ml) #Vials	Examples: Quantity of 0.25-mg tabs ingested (80% bioavailable) #Vials
4. Steady-state concentration >10 mg/mL	1 1 2 2	
5. Progressive potassium elevation or potassium >5 mEq/L	4 3 8 6 12 9 16 11 20 14	25 10 50 20 75 30 100 40

[a]Six vials is usually adequate to reverse most cases of chronic toxicity.
[b]Twenty vials is usually adequate to treat acute ingestions of unknown quantity.
[c]Each vial of Digibind contains 38 mg of purified digoxin-specific Fab fragments which will bind 0.5 mg of digoxin or digitoxin.
SOURCE: Adapted with permission from the *Physicians' Desk Reference*, Montvale, NJ, Medical Economics, 1996, p 1091.

in this manner, independently of effects on glomerular filtration rate. Deliberate acute lithium overdose by ingestion with suicidal intent also commonly occurs.[302]

Serum levels following acute Li ingestion correlate poorly with intracellular Li levels and clinical symptoms. A closer correlation exists between serum levels and clinical symptoms in chronic and acute-on-chronic intoxications. Thus severe toxicity may occur at lower serum levels in the setting of chronic Li ingestion than following acute ingestion without previous use.

Clinical manifestations of overdose are primarily neurologic. Clinical features of mild (1.5 to 2.5 mEq/L) and moderate (2.5 to 3.5 mEq/L) intoxication include nausea, vomiting, diarrhea, weakness, and neurologic dysfunction (confusion, tremor, nystagmus, dysarthria, ataxia, and other signs of cerebellar dysfunction), and choreiform and Parkinsonian movements reflecting basal ganglia involvement. Severe toxicity (>3.5 mEq/L) is characterized by worsening neurologic dysfunction (seizures and coma) and cardiovascular instability (sinus bradycardia and hypotension). Decreased serum anion gap (<6 mEq/L, because of excess cation) is an interesting consequence of severely elevated (>3.5 mEq/L) Li levels. Both hypothermia and hyperthermia have been reported to occur in Li-intoxicated patients. Acute overdose has a 25% mortality, and 10% of survivors have permanent neurologic deficits.

Treatment of Li intoxication is guided by a combination of clinical features and serum levels. Supportive care includes seizure control and use of vasopressors for hypotension refractory to fluids. Gastrointestinal decontamination following excessive lithium ingestion is the subject of a number of in vitro and animal research projects and is particularly important because sustained-release preparations are usually involved. Induction of emesis or gastric lavage should be performed initially. Oral activated charcoal is ineffective in preventing Li absorption, because it adsorbs Li poorly.[303–305] However, it is not harmful in this setting, and should be administered to limit absorption of other potential ingested poisons. Animal and in vitro studies suggest that oral sodium polystyrene sulfonate (Kayexalate) impairs absorption of ingested Li,[304] and that a form of gastrointestinal dialysis using multiple doses also lowers serum Li levels, but this therapy is unproven in human subjects.[306] Polyethylene glycol whole bowel irrigation has also been used to limit absorption of an acute overdose of sustained-release lithium in normal volunteers.[307] Elimination of Li is enhanced by volume loading (with normal saline) of hypovolemic patients, but this therapy has limited efficacy after normovolemia has been restored and risks precipitating hypernatremia in the presence of excessive ongoing water losses because of underlying diabetes insipidus. Lithium is the prototypical dialyzable intoxicant, owing to its hydrophilicity, low molecular weight, complete absence of protein binding, small apparent volume of distribution (0.66 L/kg, reflecting distribution in the total body water space), and prolonged half-life.

HD indications include: (1) Serum level >4 mEq/L; (2) serum level >2.5 mEq/L with symptoms or renal insufficiency (the latter making timely endogenous clearance unlikely); (3) serum level <2.5 mEq/L but following a large ingestion, so that rising levels are anticipated; (4) serum level <2.5 mEq/L if levels not anticipated to be <0.6 mEq/L at 36 hours after ingestion (this assessment is made by plotting three or more 2-hourly Li levels on a log-linear scale to estimate half-life). HD (clearance 70 to 170 mL/min) is preferred to peritoneal dialysis (clearance 15 mL/min, compared to 10 to 40 mL/min by renal excretion in normal subjects).[301,302,308] Rebound increase of serum levels often occurs several hours after dialysis; this phenomenon is mostly attributable to slow extracellular transfer of intracellular lithium,[301,309] although delayed absorption from slow-release preparations may also be contributory.[310] Prolonged dialysis (8 to 12 hours) with a large surface area dialyzer is generally performed initially, with repetition as needed for levels in excess of 1.0 at 6 to 8 hours after treatment. Alternatively, there are advocates of the use of continuous arteriovenous or venovenous hemofiltration/hemodialysis (14 to 44 hours) to attain both dialytic clearance of extracellular Li and effective mobilization and removal of intracellular stores,[95,96] but the obtained clearances of 20.5 to 62 mL/min (highest with continuous venovenous hemodialysis) were inferior to reported results with standard HD. Rebound of serum Li levels was prevented by prolonged therapy in the latter report,[96] even in chronic intoxications, suggesting some utility in such cases. Acute hemodialysis followed by a period of continuous venovenous hemodialysis to prevent rebound is a potentially useful combination approach.

METHEMOGLOBINEMIA

Reduced (Fe^{2+}) hemoglobin (ferrihemoglobin) is capable of binding oxygen; oxidized (Fe^{3+}) hemoglobin (methemoglobin or ferrihemoglobin) is not. In health, a small amount of methemoglobin is formed by auto-oxidation of circulating red blood cells continuously exposed to high concentrations of oxygen. Reduced cytochrome $b5$ reacts with circulating methemoglobin to restore hemoglobin and oxidized cytochrome $b5$. The red cell enzyme NADH-cytochrome $b5$ reductase (methemoglobin reductase) is responsible for regenerating reduced cytochrome $b5$, thereby ensuring insignificant concentrations of methemoglobin in circulating blood.[311]

Hereditary methemoglobinemia develops when circulating methemoglobin cannot be reduced (e.g., hemoglobin M) or there is a deficiency in red cell cytochrome $b5$ reductase. These hereditary conditions are of little clinical significance and usually do not require treatment, although individuals with cytochrome $b5$ reductase deficiency and G6PD deficiency are at increased risk of developing acquired methemoglobinemia. Acquired methemoglobinemia, which can be life threatening, occurs in the setting of oxidant drugs or toxin exposure (Table 102-25). Many of these drugs, such as commonly used analgesics, sulfonamides, sulfones, and local anesthetics, are derivatives of aniline, originally called "blue oil" which may beget "blue people" (those with methemoglobinemia).[312] Aniline drugs, particularly if taken in combination, are the most common cause of methemoglobinemia today.[312]

Methemoglobinemia decreases oxyhemoglobin saturation and blood carrying capacity in a way that is analogous to carbon monoxide poisoning. Not only does 50% methemoglobinemia effectively decrease hemoglobin concentration by half, methemoglobinemia also shifts the oxyhemoglobin dissociation curve to the left, thereby interfering with off-loading of oxygen in peripheral tissues. In mild methemoglobinemia (<15% of the total hemoglobin) patients

TABLE 102-25 Selected Drugs/Toxins Associated with Acquired Methemoglobinemia

Acetanilid
Amyl nitrite
Butyl nitrite
Bromates
Aniline dyes
Benzocaine
Bupivacaine
Chlorates
Chloroquine
Dapsone
Flutamide
Herbicides
Isobutyl nitrite
Isosorbide dinitrate
Lidocaine
Loxosceles gaucho venom
Methyl nitrite
Metoclopramide
Nitric oxide
Nitroethane
Nitrobenzene
Nitroglycerin
Nitroprusside
Pesticides
Petrol octane booster
Phenacetin
Phenazopyridine
Potassium ferricyanide
Prilocaine
Primaquine
Pyridium Plus
Silver nitrate
Sodium chlorite
Sodium nitrite
Sulfonamides

generally remain asymptomatic despite exam evidence of cyanosis. One possible exception is the patient with critical coronary artery disease, who may develop angina or myocardial infarction in the presence of mild functional anemia. Higher methemoglobin concentrations result in dyspnea, headache, and weakness. Severe methemoglobinemia (>60%) causes confusion, seizures, and death.

Laboratory confirmation of elevated methemoglobin is available by co-oximetry, which directly measures oxygen saturation and methemoglobin saturation. Of note, the antidote methylene blue (see below) causes falsely elevated methemoglobin levels by co-oximetry (a dose of 2 mg/kg methylene blue gives a falsely elevated methemoglobin level of 15%).[313] Pulse oximetry is unreliable in patients with methemoglobinemia. Pulse oximeter saturation may fall, but it is falsely high in patients with methemoglobinemia and falsely low after methylene blue.[314–316] Another clue is the finding of chocolate-colored venous blood.[317]

Treatment of methemoglobinemia starts with supportive measures and removal of the inciting drug or toxin. This may involve removal of contaminated clothing, washing of contaminated skin, gastric emptying, and AC, depending on the nature of the intoxication. Methylene blue, a dye capable of reversing drug- or toxin-induced methemoglobinemia by increasing conversion of methemoglobin to hemoglobin,

should be considered in symptomatic patients. A dose of 1 to 2 mg/kg (0.1 to 0.2 mL/kg of a 1% solution) IV administered over 5 minutes generally results in a significant reduction in methemoglobin level within 30 to 60 minutes. A repeat dose of methylene blue may be given after 60 minutes if needed. Additional doses may be required in patients who have taken a long-acting oxidant drug such as dapsone; however, higher doses of methylene blue may paradoxically increase oxidant stress and methemoglobinemia. Contraindications to methylene blue include G6PD deficiency (in which methylene blue may trigger hemolytic anemia), renal failure (because the antidote is renally excreted), and reversal of nitrite-induced methemoglobinemia during treatment of cyanide poisoning.[318] Failure to respond to methylene blue suggests cytochrome *b*5 reductase deficiency, G6PD deficiency, or sulfhemoglobinemia. Additional therapies of possible value in severe conditions include exchange transfusion and hyperbaric oxygen.

OPIOIDS

Opioid stimulation of opiate receptors causes generalized depression of the central nervous system. Symptoms in cases of overdose range from lethargy to respiratory arrest and coma, depending on the dose, agent ingested, and patient tolerance. The majority of deaths occur in chronic abusers of IV heroin.[319,320] Ethanol appears to enhance the acute toxicity of heroin and may contribute to deaths in infrequent users of heroin with low tolerance to its acute toxic effects.[321]

Opioids cause respiratory failure through a number of mechanisms such as alveolar hypoventilation, aspiration, and acute noncardiogenic pulmonary edema (which occurs most notably with heroin).[322] Noncardiogenic pulmonary edema often occurs after successful resuscitation and administration of naloxone, which itself has been reported to induce pulmonary edema in certain individuals. By inhalation, heroin may trigger an acute exacerbation of asthma.[323,324]

Other features of opioid intoxication include hypotension, bradycardia, decreased gut motility, rhabdomyolysis, muscle flaccidity, hypothermia, and seizures. Seizures are most common with propoxyphene[325] and meperidine. The meperidine metabolite normeperidine may cause seizures in the therapeutic dosing range, particularly if there is renal insufficiency.[326]

Pupils are commonly small or pinpoint-sized and respond to naloxone; however, the lack of miosis does not rule out opioid poisoning, as coexisting toxins or other conditions such as anoxic brain injury may influence pupil size.

The diagnosis of opioid overdose depends on a history of ingestion or a high index of suspicion for drug overdose, combined with compatible clinical features. The combination of a Glasgow Coma Scale score ≤12 with one of the following: respiratory rate ≤12, miotic pupils, or circumstantial evidence of drug use, has a sensitivity of 92% and a specificity of 76% for opioid overdose.[327] Rapid response to naloxone corroborates the diagnosis, which can be confirmed by urine or blood toxicology screening. However, certain opioids such as fentanyl are not detected by routine urine toxicology screening.[328]

Treatment of opioid overdose involves initial supportive measures and naloxone (see below). Gastric emptying may be helpful acutely, but extreme care must be taken not to empty the stomach in lethargic or comatose patients unless the airway has been adequately protected. Although gastric lavage is most useful when it is performed within 1 hour of ingestion, this time limit may be extended several hours because of decreased gut motility. Activated charcoal should be administered once the airway has been protected;[329] there is a small risk of small-bowel obstruction in the setting of decreased bowel motility.[330] There is no role for forced diuresis, dialysis, or hemoperfusion.

Naloxone, a specific opioid antagonist with no opioid agonist properties, reverses opioid-induced sedation, hypotension, and respiratory depression. The initial dose is 0.4 mg IV or 0.8 mg IM or SC. Endotracheal administration has been described.[331] Lower doses should be given to opioid-dependent patients and when there is a concurrent stimulant overdose. Larger initial doses may be required when there is abuse of naloxone-resistant opioids. If naloxone does not produce a clinical response after 2 to 3 minutes, an additional 1 to 2 mg IV may be administered to a total dose of 10 mg. In general, a lack of response to 6 to 10 mg naloxone is required to exclude opioid toxicity; rarely doses >10 mg are required to antagonize the effects of propoxyphene, diphenoxylate, methadone, and pentazocine. Continuing naloxone beyond a total dose of 10 mg is reasonable if there is a very high index of suspicion for opioid overdose or a partial response has been achieved. In general, opioid antagonism occurs within minutes of naloxone administration and lasts for 1 to 3 hours. Repeat boluses may be needed every 20 to 60 minutes to maintain an adequate clinical response. Alternatively, a continuous naloxone infusion may be used (0.4 to 0.8 mg/h, or two thirds of the initial dose needed to achieve a response, given each hour intravenously).

Noncardiogenic pulmonary edema may be initially difficult to distinguish from aspiration pneumonitis with the acute respiratory distress syndrome; however, improvement is generally more rapid in opioid-induced pulmonary edema. Supplemental oxygen, positive end-expiratory pressure, and mechanical ventilatory support may all be required to achieve adequate arterial oxygen saturation.[322] Since central venous pressure is low, diuresis may aggravate hypotension.

Seizures unresponsive to naloxone may be treated with intravenous diazepam or lorazepam. Refractory seizures suggest either body packing or a secondary process.

ORGANOPHOSPHATE AND CARBAMATE INSECTICIDES

Most insecticides in the United States are organophosphates or carbamates. Organophosphates act as irreversible acetylcholinesterase (AChE) inhibitors. Carbamates are reversible AChE inhibitors. Insecticides can be absorbed through the mouth, skin, conjunctiva, gastrointestinal tract, or respiratory tract. Toxicity occurs within 12 to 24 hours after exposure from excess acetylcholine at neural end-plates due to inhibition of AChE.[332]

The diagnosis of organophosphate poisoning is made on clinical grounds and by measurement of cholinesterase activity in the blood. The history may suggest attempted suicide, accidental ingestion, industrial/agricultural exposure, or rarely ingestion of contaminated food.[333,334] Emergency department personnel have also been inadvertently poisoned through contact with poisoned patients.[335] The signs and symptoms of poisoning by both classes of insecticides are

TABLE 102-26 Classification of Signs and Symptoms of Acute Organophosphate Poisoning

Muscarinic	Nicotinic	Central
Salivation	Fasciculations	Anxiety
Lacrimation	Paresis/paralysis	Confusion
Urination	Hypertension	Seizures
Diarrhea	Tachycardia	Psychosis
GI cramps		Ataxia
Emesis		
Blurred vision		
Miosis		
Bradycardia		
Wheezing		

virtually identical except that carbamates do not readily cross the blood-brain barrier to cause CNS toxicity. Clinical features include miosis (85%), vomiting (58%), excessive salivation (58%), respiratory distress (48%), abdominal pain (42%), depressed mental status (42%), and muscle fasciculations (40%).[336] In one large study, tachycardia occurred more often than bradycardia (21% versus 10% of cases). In early poisoning, there is a transient period of intense sympathetic tone causing tachycardia, followed by heightened parasympathetic tone and bradycardia, heart block, and ST- and T-wave abnormalities.[336] An odor of garlic may be noted from the breath or sweat.

Clinical features of organophosphate poisoning result from overstimulation of muscarinic, nicotinic, and central receptors (Table 102-26). Muscarinic overstimulation results in sustained toxicity characterized by the mnemonic SLUDGE (salivation, lacrimation, urination, diarrhea, gastrointestinal cramps, and emesis). Blurred vision, miosis, bradycardia, and wheezing are also muscarinic effects. Nicotinic effects are less sustained and characterized by fasciculations, muscle weakness (that can progress to paralysis), hypertension, and tachycardia. Organophosphates penetrate the blood-brain barrier to cause anxiety, confusion, psychosis, seizures, and ataxia.

The two principal cholinesterases are RBC cholinesterase (also called acetylcholinesterase or AChE), which is present in red blood cells and nerve endings, and pseudocholinesterase (PChE), which is found primarily in liver and serum. Carbamates and organophosphates inhibit both. Clinical toxicity is due primarily to inhibition of AChE, but PChE is more readily quantified. Levels may not correlate with the severity of poisoning.[337] A falsely low PChE may be seen in liver disease, anemia and malnutrition, and as a normal genetic variant (familial succinylcholine sensitivity). Normal levels of enzyme activity do not exclude poisoning because of wide variations in normal levels. In the absence of a baseline AChE level, serial measurement helps confirm the diagnosis.[338]

During initial patient stabilization, attention should be paid to the respiratory status. Bronchoconstriction, excess secretions, muscle weakness and an altered mental status all increase the risk of respiratory failure requiring intubation and mechanical ventilation. In agricultural exposures it is extremely important to remove all contaminated clothing and cleanse hair and skin thoroughly to decrease skin absorption. Health care workers must protect themselves from accidental exposure by wearing appropriate gloves and gowns. Activated charcoal is indicated to limit further absorption. Gastric lavage may be useful if done immediately after ingestion.

Symptomatic patients should receive atropine immediately. Treatment should not await results of AChE or PChE levels. Atropine competitively blocks acetylcholine at muscarinic receptors but has no effect on nicotinic receptors. Thus atropine should not worsen fasciculations, hypertension, or tachycardia. Atropine crosses the blood-brain barrier and can cause CNS toxicity that is difficult to distinguish from organophosphate toxicity. In this situation, glycopyrrolate (which does not penetrate the CNS) is a reasonable alternative to atropine.[339] The dose of atropine required to achieve atropinization (mydriasis, dry mouth, and tachycardia) varies depending on the severity of poisoning. Doses of up to 40 mg/d are not uncommon. If atropinization occurs after 1 to 2 mg of atropine, the diagnosis of acetylcholinesterase inhibitor poisoning should be questioned. The initial dose of atropine is 2 mg IV followed by 2 mg every 15 minutes until adequate atropinization has occurred.

Pralidoxime (2-PAM) reverses nicotinic and muscarinic effects of organophosphate poisoning by reactivating AChE and protecting the enzyme from further inhibition. In carbamate poisoning, pralidoxime is generally not needed because of the more rapid resolution of symptoms and reversible nature of enzyme inhibition. Moreover, pralidoxime may enhance carbaryl (or Sevin, a carbamate insecticide) toxicity.[340] To be effective pralidoxime should be given within the first 6 hours of poisoning (although treatment in the first 24 to 48 hours may still be effective), prior to irreversible phosphorylation of cholinesterase (a process referred to as "aging"). After this critical period, restoration of normal cholinesterase function requires regeneration of the enzyme, a process that may take weeks to complete. Antimuscarinic effects allow for atropinization more quickly, and with lower doses of atropine. The initial dose of pralidoxime is 1 to 2 g IV given over approximately 10 to 20 minutes. Clinical response should be evident within 30 minutes. If there is no improvement in fasciculations or weakness the dose may be repeated once. A continuous infusion is then administered at a rate of 200 to 500 mg/h, titrated to achieve the desired effect. Continuous infusion of pralidoxime may be necessary for over 24 hours, depending on the half-life and lipid solubility of the poison, after which the dose may be gradually reduced and stopped while the patient is observed for signs of recurrent muscle weakness.

PHENCYCLIDINE

Phencyclidine (PCP) or "angel dust" is a dissociative anesthetic agent that is similar in many ways to ketamine. It decreases the perception of pain and has variable anticholinergic, opioid, dopaminergic, CNS stimulant, and α-adrenergic effects. PCP is usually smoked; however, it can also be nasally snorted, orally ingested, or intravenously injected. PCP is often mixed with other substances including ethanol, marijuana, and LSD. The long-term outlook for chronic abusers is characterized by unemployment, financial dependence on others, and repeated need for hospitalization.[342]

Persons intoxicated with PCP may demonstrate fluctuating, bizarre, and violent behavior that occasionally lasts for days following exposure.[343,344] In one study of 1000 patients evaluated in the ED for PCP intoxication, violence was present in 35% of cases, bizarre behavior in 29%, and agitation in 34%.[345] Forty-six percent of patients were alert and oriented; others demonstrated alterations in mental status ranging from lethargy to coma. Nystagmus (vertical or horizontal) and hypertension occurred in 57% of cases. Diaphoresis, hypersalivation, bronchospasm, and urinary retention occurred in less than 5% of cases. Grand mal seizures, muscle rigidity, dystonic reactions, catalepsy and athetosis occurred but were rare. Twenty-eight cases (2.8%) were apneic, and three cases (0.3%) presented in cardiac arrest. Hypoglycemia and elevated serum CPK, uric acid, and SGOT/SPGT were common. Rhabdomyolysis results in renal failure in 50% of cases.[346] Other features of PCP intoxication include self-inflicted injuries, aspiration pneumonia, hypertensive crisis, and intracranial and subarachnoid hemorrhage.[347-349]

The diagnosis of PCP intoxication is usually made on clinical grounds (fluctuating behavior, signs of sympathomimetic overstimulation, and vertical nystagmus). Particularly suggestive is the finding of pinpoint pupils in an agitated patient. Confirmation of PCP exposure is available through qualitative urine screening. PCP levels do not correlate with the severity of the clinical findings.[345]

Treatment of PCP intoxication involves initial supportive measures aimed at identifying and treating life-threatening problems. Few data are available regarding safety and efficacy of gastric emptying in PCP toxicity; however, this strategy is unlikely to be of significant benefit in patients presenting more than 1 hour after oral ingestion, and gastric emptying carries significant risk. Ipecac-induced vomiting should be avoided because of the risk of wide fluctuations in mental status, and the placement of a nasogastric tube may result in extreme agitation. Activated charcoal is effective in reducing intoxication. Acidifying the urine with NH_4Cl and diuresis enhances drug elimination.[350-352] However, the benefits of urinary acidification are small,[353] and urinary acidification may exacerbate myoglobinuric renal failure. Therefore urinary acidification is not recommended for routine use in PCP overdose. Neither hemoperfusion nor dialysis effectively eliminates PCP because of its large volume of distribution.

Violent or acutely psychotic patients unresponsive to verbal feedback and reduction in environmental stimuli require immediate pharmacologic treatment or physical restraints to establish adequate patient and staff safety. A common error in the management of the agitated patient is to delay treatment, allowing patients to harm themselves or others; another error is premature discharge of PCP-intoxicated patients after they demonstrate a period of normal behavior. Haloperidol appears to be the drug of choice to treat PCP psychosis.[354] Haloperidol (2 to 5 mg IM) may be repeated every 30 to 60 minutes to a total dose not exceeding 100 mg. Haloperidol prolongs the QT interval and therefore should be used with continuous monitoring. In addition, haloperidol lowers the seizure threshold and is associated with neuroleptic malignant syndrome, tardive dyskinesia, and the development of extrapyramidal symptoms. Adding a benzodiazepine (e.g., lorazepam 1 mg) to each dose of haloperidol may expedite control of the difficult patient. Data are limited regarding the use of chlorpromazine and opioids in PCP psychosis.[355] Other causes of agitation including head trauma, intracerebral or subarachnoid hemorrhage, CNS infection, thyrotoxicosis, pheochromocytoma, hyperthermia, and acute psychiatric illnesses should be considered.

Hypertension often responds to haloperidol or benzodiazepine therapy. In cases of severe hypertension, nitroprusside or labetalol may be required. β-Blockers should be avoided as sole drugs because of the risk of worsening hypertension as β_2 sites are blocked.

SALICYLATES

Acetylsalicylic acid or aspirin is converted rapidly to salicylic acid, its active moiety. Salicylic acid is readily absorbed from the stomach and small bowel. At therapeutic doses, it is metabolized by the liver and eliminated in 2 to 3 hours. Chronic ingestion can increase the half-life to more than 20 hours.[356] Overdose can be accidental or deliberate, acute or chronic. A number of over-the-counter combination formulations and herbal remedies contain salicylates. The use of alternate analgesics, child-resistant containers, and package size restrictions has decreased the incidence of poisoning.[357,358]

Therapeutic serum levels of salicylates are 10 to 30 mg/dL. Clinical features of intoxication occur in most individuals with serum levels above 40 to 50 mg/dL; in chronic intoxication, severe poisoning occurs at lower serum levels (particularly in elderly patients). In toxic amounts, salicylates are metabolic poisons that affect a number of organ systems by uncoupling oxidated phosphorylation and interfering with the Krebs cycle.[359]

Minor intoxication causes tinnitus, vertigo, nausea, vomiting, and diarrhea. More significant ingestions cause acid-base disturbances. Respiratory alkalosis is caused by direct central ventilatory stimulation. Organic acids (including lactate and ketoacids) accumulate with uncoupling of oxidative phosphorylation to cause an elevated anion gap metabolic acidosis. Salicylic acid itself contributes only minimally to the measured anion gap (only 3 mEq/L with a 50-mg/dL level). Adults commonly present with respiratory alkalosis or combined metabolic acidosis and respiratory alkalosis.[360,361] Children may develop pure metabolic acidosis. Severe poisoning also causes noncardiogenic pulmonary edema, mental status changes, seizures, coma, gastrointestinal bleeding, liver failure, renal failure, and death.[362] Low cerebrospinal fluid glucose is a characteristic finding.[362]

Thisted and colleagues reported the clinical findings in 177 consecutive admissions to an ICU with acute salicylate poisoning.[363] Neurologic abnormalities occurred in 61% of cases, acid-base disturbances in 50%, pulmonary complications in 43%, coagulation disorders in 38%, fever in 20%, and hypotension in 14%. In a separate 2-year review of salicylate deaths in Ontario, 31.4% of patients were dead on arrival.[364] ICU mortality has been reported to be 15%.[363] The clinical features of salicylate intoxication are reviewed in Tables 102-27 and 102-28.

The lethal adult dose is approximately 10 to 30 g (35 tablets or more). Lethality correlates poorly with serum levels. The Done nomogam may be of little value, particularly if the time of ingestion is incorrectly estimated, more than a single dose is taken, or an enteric-coated preparation is used.[356,365,366] These caveats hold particularly true for chronic salicylism, which commonly occurs unintentionally in elderly patients receiving long-term analgesic therapy.[367] These patients are more likely to present with CNS injury[368] or noncardiogenic pul-

TABLE 102-27 Clinical Findings in 177 Patients Admitted to an ICU with Acute Salicylate Poisoning

Clinical Signs	Percent
Neurologic abnormalities (depressed consciousness)	61
Acid-base disturbances	50
Pulmonary complications	43
Coagulation disorders	38
Hyperpyrexia	20
Circulatory disorders (hypotension)	14
Electrocardiographic abnormalities (Wide QRS, first- and second-degree atrioventricular block, ventricular arrhythmias)	10
Renal abnormalities (oliguria)	7

SOURCE: Reproduced with permission from Thisted et al.[363]

monary edema;[369] isolated mild elevation of the prothrombin time is another telltale sign. Salicylate ingestion is usually diagnosed by serum level measurements, which are less helpful in chronic intoxication. Urine tests with Phenistix or ferric chloride can also be used to detect salicylate poisoning.[370]

Optimal management of a salicylate-intoxicated patient requires appreciation of the toxicokinetics of ingestion and the importance of serum pH in determining disposition of this drug. At therapeutic levels, salicylic acid is 90% protein-bound. Most (75%) is partially glycinated in the liver to form salicyluric acid, a less toxic and more water-soluble renally excreted metabolite. Proximal organic anion secretion, rather than glomerular filtration, is normally responsible for the bulk of salicylate excretion, since salicylate is a highly protein-bound drug; and pH-dependent nonionic back-diffusion from the tubular lumen occurs at alkaline urine pH. At toxic levels, however, only 50% of salicylic acid is protein-bound, so that (with increased tissue distribution) the customary metabolic pathway via salicyluric acid becomes saturated, and elimination half-life increases from 3 to 12 hours to 15 to 30 hours.

Supportive care includes empiric administration of dextrose to treat low CSF glucose level. Treatment of an acute ingestion starts with gastric lavage and AC. These strategies are not helpful in chronic salicylism, although there is debate regarding the efficacy of multidose AC.[371]

The extent of tissue distribution of absorbed salicylate is influenced by plasma pH. For instance, CNS toxicity may

TABLE 102-28 Clinical Features of Salicylate Intoxication

Mild to Moderate	Severe
Headache	Lethargy
Dizziness	Hallucinations
Tinnitus	Delirium
Deafness	Seizures
Hyperventilation	Coma
Nausea	Respiratory alkalosis
Vomiting	Metabolic acidosis
Vasodilation	Gastrointestinal bleeding
Tachycardia	Hypotension
	Pulmonary edema
	Cerebral edema
	Hypoglycemia
	Hyperpyrexia
	Renal and liver failure

TABLE 102-29 Indications for Hemodialysis in Salicylate Intoxication

Serum level: >120 mg/dL acutely, or >100 mg/dL 6 h after
    ingestion
Volume overload
Noncardiogenic pulmonary edema
Renal failure precluding bicarbonate therapy
CNS toxicity: coma or seizures
Refractory acidosis
Deteriorating course
Chronic ingestion

TABLE 102-30 Selected Drugs That Increase Risk of Serotonin Syndrome in Patients Taking Selective Serotonin Reuptake Inhibitors

Almotripan
Buspirone
Caffeine
Cocaine
Dextromethorphan
"Ecstasy" (3,4-methylenedioxymethamphetamine; MDMA)
Eletriptan
Ergotamine
Frovatriptan
L-tryptophan
Linezolid
Lithium
Monoamine oxidase inhibitors
Meperidine
Methylphenidate hydrochloride
Mirtazapine
Naratriptan
Nefazodone
Rizatriptan
Sumatriptan
Tramadol
Trazodone
Tricylic antidepressants
Venlafaxine
Zolmitriptan

be ameliorated by administration of bicarbonate to raise plasma pH to 7.45 to 7.5 (of course, such therapy may be contraindicated in the presence of alkalemia caused by salicylate-induced hyperventilation). Systemic alkalinization has the additional salutary effect of augmenting renal salicylate excretion. Raising urinary pH from 6.1 to 8.1 results in an over 18-fold increase in renal clearance by preventing nonionic tubular back-diffusion.[372] This decreases the half-life of salicylates from 20 to 24 hours to <8 hours. To accomplish urinary alkalinization, it is vital to avoid hypokalemia that prevents excretion of alkaline urine by promoting distal tubular potassium reabsorption in exchange for hydrogen ion. Forced diuresis appears not to add additional clearance to such therapy and tends to precipitate volume overload. Treatment with acetazolamide has also been used to induce alkaline diuresis, but we do not recommend this approach because "overshoot" acidemia may increase drug entry into the CNS and salicylate toxicity.

Indications for hemodialysis are listed in Table 102-29.[356,365] They include a serum level >120 mg/dL acutely, >100 mg/dL 6 hours postingestion, refractory acidosis, coma, seizures, noncardiogenic pulmonary edema, and renal failure. In chronic overdose, hemodialysis may be necessary for symptomatic patients with serum levels over 60 mg/dL.[373]

SELECTIVE SEROTONIN REUPTAKE INHIBITORS

The SSRIs, which include sertraline, citalopram, nefazodone, venlafaxine, paroxetine, fluoxetine, escitalopram, trazodone, and fluvoxamine, are noncyclic antidepressant agents that selectively inhibit the presynaptic neural uptake of serotonin.[374] These drugs are indicated for treatment of patients with affective disorders. They are relatively nontoxic when taken alone, but when taken in combination with a number of other drugs (listed in Table 102-30), there is the potential for excessive stimulation of 5-HT1A and 5-HT2 receptors and development of the serotonin syndrome.[375–380] Because of the long half-life of some of these drugs, toxic combination therapy may not be apparent for days to weeks.

Features of the serotonin syndrome include various combinations of confusion, agitation, coma, shivering, flushing, hyperthermia, diaphoresis, mydriasis, tachycardia, disseminated intravascular coagulation, convulsions, muscle rigidity, myoclonus, hyperreflexia, involuntary movements, autonomic instability, nausea, diarrhea, orthostatic hypotension, and rhabdomyolysis, which may not develop until 6 to 12 hours after overdose.[28,375,378] Trazodone, which also acts as an α-adrenergic blocker, may cause a hypoten-

sive response. Other findings include hyponatremia and SIADH.[381,382] Death is rare.

The diagnosis of serotonin syndrome should be considered in any patient with compatible clinical features, particularly if there is a history of depression. Blood levels are not helpful because the syndrome is a result of increased concentrations at nerve endings.

Treatment of serotonin syndrome starts with identifying and treating life-threatening problems. Gastric emptying should be considered in patients with acute ingestion. Ipecac-induced vomiting may be useful in the early management of children outside the hospital setting. Activated charcoal with a cathartic should be administered. Dialysis and hemoperfusion are not effective. Prognosis is generally good in mild cases, with resolution within 24 to 36 hours with supportive therapy alone. In severe cases, anecdotal reports suggest that serotonin antagonists (methysergide and cyproheptadine) may be beneficial.[383] Chlorpromazine, diphenhydramine, and benzodiazepines have also been used to treat serotonin syndrome.[384,385]

THEOPHYLLINE

Theophylline has a low therapeutic index, with a recommended therapeutic range of plasma levels between 10 and 20 mg/L. Toxicity can occur in the therapeutic range, but is more frequently associated with plasma levels >20 mg/L. Intoxication may result from either acute massive ingestion or chronic overmedication. The latter scenario may result from diminishing theophylline clearance on a stable chronic regimen. Drug interactions, smoking cessation, congestive heart failure, and hepatic dysfunction all diminish theophylline clearance. Chronic intoxication is associated with more severe clinical sequelae at any given plasma level due to larger body stores.[386,387]

Clinical features of theophylline toxicity are neurologic, cardiovascular, and metabolic.[388] Seizures occur at lower serum levels in chronic intoxication than in acute overdose.[389] For reasons unknown, seizures occur several hours after peak serum levels in acute intoxication. Uncontrolled seizures can lead to hyperthermia and rhabdomyolysis. Tachyarrhythmias, both supraventricular and ventricular, are common at theophylline levels of 20 to 30 mg/L;[390] cardiovascular collapse can occur at levels over 50 mg/L. Metabolic abnormalities include hypokalemia, hypomagnesemia, hyperglycemia, hypophosphatemia, hypercalcemia, and respiratory alkalosis.[391]

Initial treatment should include gastric lavage and activated charcoal. Emesis is contraindicated because of the risk of seizures. Since theophylline undergoes enterohepatic circulation, multidose AC can enhance elimination.[69]

Seizures should be treated with benzodiazepines. Refractory seizures are an indication for the addition of phenobarbital or other antiepileptics. Phenytoin can worsen theophylline-induced seizures and should be avoided.[392,393] Supraventricular tachyarrhythmias are best controlled by a cardioselective β-blocker (metoprolol or esmolol), but these must be used with care in patients with underlying obstructive airways disease and not at all in patients who are actively wheezing. Calcium channel blockers may be useful in supraventricular tachycardia.[394,395] However, hypotension due to β_2-adrenergic stimulation should be treated with fluids and phenylephrine. Interestingly, refractory hypotension has been treated with a nonselective β-blocker such as esmolol.[396–398] Lidocaine and other standard agents are suitable for therapy of ventricular arrhythmias. Electrolyte repletion may be required.

Patients presenting with seizures or arrhythmias are candidates for extracorporeal drug removal (ECR). Other indications are a plasma level >100 mg/L at 2 hours after initial charcoal therapy, a level >50 mg/L in chronic ingestion, a 2-hour level >35 mg/L associated with clinical instability (shock), and a high risk of adverse outcome and/or prolonged intoxication. High-risk characteristics include: (1) chronic intoxication; (2) intolerance of oral charcoal; (3) impaired theophylline metabolism (congestive heart failure, cirrhosis, or severe hypoxemia [P_{O_2} <40 mm Hg]); (4) susceptibility to cardiovascular toxicity (elderly or coronary artery disease), seizures (epilepsy or coingestion of other convulsant drugs), or respiratory failure (severe pulmonary disease).

Extracorporeal therapy is best achieved by use of "in-series" hemodialysis (HD) and hemoperfusion (HP).[389,399,400] The physical and disposition characteristics of theophylline allow fairly effective clearance by HD, which has an extraction ratio (ER) of 0.5, achieving a clearance of up to 150 mL/min at a 300 mL/min blood flow rate. HP is more effective, with ERs of 0.6 to 0.9, allowing clearance twice that of HD. Cartridge replacement is required every 2 hours during isolated HP, because of adsorption saturation and declining ER (0.99 at initiation of therapy, decreasing to 0.5 by 2 hours). Placement of a hemodialyzer in series proximal to the HP cartridge in the extracorporeal circuit delays development of system saturation, adds additional clearance by HD, and allows for more rapid correction of metabolic derangements. Peritoneal dialysis does not add to endogenous clearance, even though

this is low in nonsmokers (0.7 to 1.0 mL/min). Continuous extracorporeal therapies are of some utility and are indicated only in the absence of available HD or HP. Other techniques such as plasmapheresis and exchange transfusion have been successfully used in pediatric patients.

ENVENOMATIONS

SNAKE BITE

The majority of poisonous snake bites in the United States involve the Crotalidae (pit viper) family of snakes (e.g., rattlesnakes, copperheads, and water moccasins) in the southwest, west, and southeast. Pit vipers are named for a small pit between their eyes and nostrils. Large venom glands located in the temporal region result in a triangular shaped head; a horny rattle on the tail is vibrated when the rattlesnake is agitated.

Most bites involve native, noncaptive snakes, and are considered accidental. Accidental bites are more common in the summer months, in the afternoon or evening, and during recreational activities.[401] Young men are the most frequent victims.

Rattlesnakes strike when they are disturbed. Telltale fang marks appear as paired puncture wounds or lacerations a few millimeters deep, although atypical wounds consisting of single or multiple puncture sites or scratches are also seen. Twenty-five percent of bites do not result in envenomation (i.e., "dry bites"); half of all bites result in minimal or no envenomation.[401,402] Dry bites are generally benign, although there is potential for infection due to bacteria in the snake's mouth or on the victim's skin. When envenomation occurs, a variety of toxic proteins and enzymes are introduced into the victim that are capable of producing serious local and systemic reactions. Local effects develop within minutes and consist of stinging, burning, swelling, erythema, ecchymosis, and hemorrhagic blebs. Extremities swell over the next several hours, occasionally resulting in compartment syndrome. Facial bites with severe local swelling may obstruct airways.[403] Systemic effects of rattlesnake venom include fever, nausea, vomiting, delirium, seizures, muscle cramps, jaundice, disseminated intravascular coagulation, acute renal failure, and shock. Death is rare but may occur hours to days after envenomation. Of note, the Mojave rattlesnake is unique in causing minimal local tissue damage and serious delayed systemic effects.

Treatment of rattlesnake bite consists of splinting and immobilizing the bitten extremity at heart level to slow the spread of venom.[404] A loose fitting tourniquet should be placed above the bite site to impede lymph flow and rate of venom spread. Surgical consultation should be obtained for management of serious wounds. Débridement of necrotic wounds may be necessary. If compartment syndrome is suspected, tissue pressure should be measured. Surgery should be reserved only for severe and refractory cases and may not improve outcome.[405] Tetanus prophylaxis should be provided.

Rapid volume infusion is indicated in the initial management of hypotensive patients. Several liters of isotonic fluid may be required. One animal study suggests that in severe cases colloid infusion is more effective than crystalloid.[406] Patients with significant envenomations with progressive local or systemic effects should be considered for specific treatment with equine-derived Crotalidae antivenin. Antivenin is a lyophilized protein product derived from horses immunized with venom pooled from several members of the Crotalidae family of snakes. Prior to antivenin administration, patients should be skin tested with a 1:10 dilution of antivenin (or per instructions in the commercially available antivenin kit). Patients with a positive skin test should be reconsidered for supportive care only; however, in the setting of severe envenomation, diluted antivenin may still be administered slowly after pretreatment with diphenhydramine and corticosteroids. This situation mandates large-bore IV access and epinephrine at the bedside in anticipation of anaphylaxis. A negative skin test is reassuring but does not exclude the possibility of anaphylaxis or the need for close monitoring and bedside availability of antihistamines and epinephrine. Antivenin is dosed by vial. Minimal envenomations with progressive symptoms can be treated effectively with five vials. Severe envenomations with hypotension and coagulopathy should receive 15 to 20 vials as guided by the instructions in the antivenin kit.[407] Most patients respond to the initial antivenin infusion, but some patients require additional infusions every few hours. Patients should be monitored closely for immediate hypersensitivity reactions and delayed hypersensitivity reactions (i.e., serum sickness) which commonly occur 5 to 14 days later. Of note, commercially available equine antivenin is also available for eastern coral snake (*Micrurus fulvius*) and Texas coral snake (*Micrurus fulvius tenere*) envenomation.

SPIDER BITE

In North America, only the widow spiders (*Latrodectus* species) and the recluse spiders (*Loxosceles* species) are medically important. The female black widow spider (*Latrodectus mactans*) has a shiny black body approximately 1 cm in diameter with a red hourglass mark on the abdomen. This spider, which favors woodpiles, dimly lit sheds, greenhouses, basements, and outdoor toilets, is most often encountered during the summer months. It bites aggressively to introduce potent venom into its victim. Envenomation results in local pain and erythema followed by muscle cramps and muscle fasciculations near the bite site. Painful cramps may generalize to the abdomen, back, and chest, mimicking myocardial infarction or an acute surgical abdomen.[284] Cramps may last for several days. Hypertension, tachycardia, tremor, fever, agitation, diaphoresis, and nausea are also common. Rarely, black widow spider bite results in hypertensive crisis or cardiopulmonary arrest. Treatment of black widow spider bite consists of general supportive measures combined with adequate analgesia and sedation. Intravenous calcium and methocarbamol effectively treat muscle cramps. Rare patients with significant signs and symptoms not responding to conservative measures should be considered for specific treatment with equine antivenin. As with other equine-derived antivenins, skin testing should be performed prior to antivenin administration, and precautions should be taken for anaphylaxis.[284]

Recluse spider bite (loxoscelism) is characterized by pain and burning at the bite site followed by localized swelling, erythema, and formation of bullae. A bull's eye–shaped lesion ranging from 1 to 5 cm may develop, consisting of an erythematous or hemorrhagic center, surrounded by a blanched ring that is enclosed in an ecchymotic ring. Central necrosis may develop and last for weeks to months. Some patients develop systemic symptoms including fever, myalgias, headache, and nausea. Rare patients develop intravascular hemolysis, disseminated intravascular coagulation, acute renal failure, and the acute respiratory distress syndrome. Treatment of loxoscelism is largely supportive. Cool compresses have been recommended for the bite site. Systemic steroids and dapsone have been advocated in severe cases, but convincing evidence supporting the use of these agents is lacking, and they should be considered experimental. Antivenin is not currently available.

References

1. Litovitz TL, Klein-Schwartz W, Rodgers GC, et al: 2001 Annual Report of the American Association of Poison Control Centers Toxic Exposure Surveillance System. *Am J Emerg Med* 20:391, 2002.
2. Emergency Cardiac Care Committee and Subcommittee, American Heart Association. Part 8-Advanced Challenges in the ECC: Section 2—Toxicology in the ECC. *Circulation* 108:1223, 2000.
3. Roy TM, Ossorio MA, Cipolla LM, et al: Pulmonary complications after tricyclic antidepressant overdose. *Chest* 96:852, 1989.
4. Aldrich T, Morrison J, Cesario T: Aspiration after overdosage of sedative or hypnotic drugs. *South Med J* 73:456, 1980.
5. Marik PE: Aspiration pneumonitis and aspiration pneumonia. *N Engl J Med* 344:665, 2001.
6. Albertson TE, Dawson A, de Latorre F, et al: Tox-ACLS: Toxicologic oriented advanced cardiac life support. *Ann Emerg Med* 37:S78, 2001.
7. Mayron R, Ruiz E: Phenytoin: Does it reverse tricyclic-antidepressant-induced cardiac conduction abnormalities? *Ann Emerg Med* 15:876, 1986.
8. Callaham M, Schumaker H, Pentel P: Phenytoin prophylaxis of cardiotoxicity in experimental amitriptyline poisoning. *J Pharmacol Exp Ther* 245:216, 1988.
9. Kerns W, Garvey L, Owens J: Cocaine-induced wide complex dysrhythmia. *J Emerg Med* 15:321, 1997.
10. Wang RY: pH-dependent cocaine-induced cardiotoxicity. *Am J Emerg Med* 17:364, 1999.
11. Beckman KJ, Parker RB, Hariman RJ, et al: Hemodynamic and electrophysiological actions of cocaine: effects of sodium bicarbonate as an antidote in dogs. *Circulation* 83:1799, 1991.
12. Shih RD, Hollander JE, Burstein JL, et al: Clinical safety of lidocaine in patients with cocaine-associated myocardial infarction. *Ann Emerg Med* 26:702, 1995.
13. Ramsay ID: Survival after imipramine poisoning. *Lancet* 2:1308, 1967.
14. Southall DR, Kilpatrick SM: Imipramine poisoning: survival of a child after prolonged cardiac massage. *BMJ* 4:508, 1974.
15. Teba L, Schiebel F, Dedhia HV, et al: Beneficial effect of norepinephrine in the treatment of circulatory shock caused by tricyclic antidepressant overdose. *Am J Emerg Med* 6:566, 1988.
16. Vernon DD, Banner W Jr, Garrett JS, et al: Efficacy of dopamine and norepinephrine for treatment of hemodynamic compromise in amitriptyline intoxication. *Crit Care Med* 19:544, 1991.
17. Buchman AL, Dauer J, Geiderman J: The use of vasoactive agents in the treatment of refractory hypotension seen in tricyclic antidepressant overdose. *J Clin Psychopharmacol* 10:409, 1990.
18. Ramoska E, Sacchetti AD: Propranolol-induced hypertension in treatment of cocaine intoxication. *Ann Emerg Med* 14:1112, 1985.

19. Hoffman RS, Goldfrank LR: The poisoned patient with altered consciousness: Controversies in the use of a "coma cocktail." *JAMA* 274:562, 1995.

20. Handal KA, Schauben JL, Salamone FR: Naloxone. *Ann Emerg Med* 12:438, 1983.

21. Schwartz JA, Koenigsberg MD: Naloxone-induced pulmonary edema. *Ann Emerg Med* 16:1294, 1987.

22. Goldfrank LR: The several uses of naloxone. *Ann Emerg Med* 30:105, 1984.

23. Longmire AW, Seger DL: Topics in clinical pharmacology: Flumazenil, a benzodiazepine antagonist. *Am J Med Sci* 306:49, 1993.

24. Mordel A, Winkler E, Almog S, et al: Seizures after flumazenil administration in a case of combined benzodiazepine and tricyclic antidepressant overdose. *Crit Care Med* 20:1733, 1992.

25. Derlet RW, Albertson TE: Flumazenil induces seizures and death in mixed cocaine-diazepam intoxications. *Ann Emerg Med* 23:494, 1994.

26. Weinbroum A, Rudick V, Sorkine P, et al: Use of flumazenil in the treatment of drug overdose: A double-blind and open clinical study in 110 patients. *Crit Care Med* 24:199, 1996.

27. Barnett R, Grace M, Boothe P, et al: Flumazenil in drug overdose: randomized, placebo-controlled study to assess cost effectiveness. *Crit Care Med* 27:10, 1999.

28. Hadad E, Weinbroum AA, Ben-Abraham R: Drug-induced hyperthermia and muscle rigidity: a practical approach. *Eur J Emerg Med* 10:149, 2003.

29. Wright N: An assessment of the unreliability of the history given by self-poisoned patients. *Clin Toxicol* 16:381, 1980.

30. Olson KR, Pentel PR, Kelley MT: Physical assessment and differential diagnosis of the poisoned patient. *Med Toxicol* 2:52, 1987.

31. DuBose TD, Cogan MG, Rector FC: Acid-base disorders, in Brenner BM (ed): *Brenner and Rector's The Kidney*, 5th ed. Philadelphia, Saunders, 1996, p 1805.

32. Rose BD: Metabolic acidosis, in Rose BD, Post TW (eds): *Clinical Physiology of Acid-Base and Electrolyte Disorders*, 5th ed. New York, McGraw-Hill, 2001, p 579.

33. Narins RG, Krishna GG, Yee J, et al: The metabolic acidoses, in Narins RG (ed): *Maxwell and Kleeman's Clinical Disorders of Fluid and Electrolyte Metabolism*, 5th ed. New York, McGraw-Hill, 1994, p 85.

34. Winter SD, Pearson R, Gabow PA, et al: The fall of the serum anion gap. *Arch Intern Med* 150:311, 1990.

35. Oh MS, Carroll HJ: Current concepts: The anion gap. *N Engl J Med* 297:814, 1977.

36. Gabow PA: Disorders associated with an altered anion gap. *Kidney Int* 27:472, 1985.

37. Gabow PA, Clay K, Sullivan JB, et al: Organic acids in ethylene glycol intoxication. *Ann Intern Med* 105:16, 1986.

38. Leatherman J, Schmitz PG: Fever, hyperdynamic shock, and multiple-system organ failure. A pseudo-sepsis syndrome associated with chronic salicylate intoxication. *Chest* 110:1391, 1991.

39. Walker JA, Schwartzbard A, Krauss EA, et al: The missing gap: A pitfall in the diagnosis of alcohol intoxication by osmometry. *Arch Intern Med* 146:1843, 1986.

40. Sweeney TE, Beuchat CA: Limitations of methods of osmometry: Measuring the osmolality of biological fluids. *Am J Physiol* 264:R469, 1993.

41. Glasser L, Sternglanz PD, Combie J, et al: Serum osmolality and its applicability to drug overdose. *Am J Clin Pathol* 60:695, 1973.

42. Glaser DS: Utility of the serum osmolal gap in the diagnosis of methanol or ethylene glycol ingestion. *Ann Emerg Med* 27:343, 1996.

43. Trummel J, Ford M, Autin P: Ingestion of an unknown alcohol. *Ann Emerg Med* 27:368, 1996.

44. Hoffman RS, Smilkstein MJ, Howland MA, et al: Osmol gaps revisited: normal values and limitations. *J Toxicol Clin Toxicol* 31:81, 1993.

45. Ammar KA, Heckerling PS: Ethylene glycol poisoning with a normal anion gap caused by concurrent ethanol ingestion: importance of the osmolal gap. *Am J Kidney Dis* 27:130, 1996.

46. Schelling JR, Howard RL, Winter SD, et al: Increased osmolal gap in alcoholic ketoacidosis and lactic acidosis. *Ann Intern Med* 113:580, 1990.

47. Sklar AH, Linas SL: The osmolal gap in renal failure. *Ann Intern Med* 98:481, 1983.

48. Tillman DJ, Ruggles DL, Leikin JB: Radiopacity study of extended-release formulations using digitalized radiography. *Am J Emerg Med* 12:310, 1994.

49. Brett AS: Implications of discordance between clinical impression and toxicology analysis in drug overdose. *Arch Intern Med* 148:437, 1988.

50. Kellerman AL, Fihn SD, LoGerfo JP, Copass MK: Impact of drug screening in suspected overdose. *Ann Emerg Med* 16:1206, 1987.

51. Gibb K: Serum alcohol levels, toxicology screens, and use of the breath alcohol analyzer. *Ann Emerg Med* 15:349, 1986.

52. Mahoney JD, Gross PL, Stern TA, et al: Quantitative serum toxic screening in the management of suspected drug overdose. *Am J Emerg Med*. 8:16, 1990.

53. Wigder HN, Erickson T, Morse T, et al: Emergency department poison advice telephone calls. *Ann Emerg Med* 25:349, 1995.

54. Merigan KS, Woodard M, Hedges JR, et al: Prospective evaluation of gastric emptying in the self-poisoned patient. *Am J Emerg Med* 8:479, 1990.

55. Vale JA, Meredith TJ, Proudfoot AT: Syrup of ipecacuanha: Is it really useful? *Br Med J* 293:1321, 1986.

56. Vale JA: American Academy of Clinical Toxicology, European Association of Poison Control Centres and Clinical Toxicologists. Position Statement: gastric lavage. *J Toxicol Clin Toxicol* 35:711, 1997.

57. Kulig K, Bar-Or D, Cantrill SV, et al: Management of acutely poisoned patients without gastric emptying. *Ann Emerg Med* 14:562, 1985.

58. Rudolph JP: Automated gastric lavage and a comparison of 0.9% normal saline solution and tap water irrigant. *Ann Emerg Med* 14:1156, 1985.

59. Levy G: Gastrointestinal clearance of drugs with activated charcoal. *N Engl J Med* 307:676, 1982.

60. Chyka PA, Seger D: Position Statement: single-dose activated charcoal. American Academy of Clinical Toxicology, European Association of Poisons Centres and Clinical Toxicologists. *J Toxicol Clin Toxicol* 35:721, 1997.

61. Varga DW, Roy TM, Ossorio MA: Gastric stapling: a significant risk factor in the treatment of tricyclic antidepressant overdose. *J Ky Med Assoc* 87:501, 1989.

62. Givens T, Holloway M, Wason S: Pulmonary aspiration of activated charcoal: A complication of its misuse in overdose management. *Pediatr Emerg Care* 8:137, 1992.

63. George DL, McLeod R, Weinstein RA: Contaminated commercial charcoal as a source of fungi in the respiratory tract. *Infect Control Hosp Epidemiol* 12:732, 1991.

64. Elliott CG, Colby TV, Kelly TM: Charcoal lung. Bronchiolitis obliterans after aspiration of activated charcoal. *Chest* 96:672, 1989.

65. Harris CR, Filandrinos D: Accidental administration of activated charcoal into the lung: aspiration by proxy. *Ann Emerg Med* 22:1470, 1993.

66. Menzies DG, Busuttil A, Prescott LF: Fatal pulmonary aspiration of oral activated charcoal. *Br Med J* 297:459, 1988.

67. Bradberry SM, Vale JA: Multiple-dose activated charcoal: a review of relevant clinical studies. *J Toxicol Clin Toxicol* 33:407, 1995.

68. Krenzelok EP, Leikin JB: Approach to a poisoned patient. *Dis Mon* 42:513, 1996.

69. Vale JA, Krenzelok EP, Barceloux GD, et al: Position statement and practice guidelines on the use of multi-dose activated charcoal in the treatment of acute poisoning. American Academy of Clinical Toxicology; European Association of Poisons Centres and Clinical Toxicologists. *J Toxicol Clin Toxicol* 37:731, 1999.

70. Ilkhanipour K, Yealy DM, Krenzelok EP: The comparative efficacy of various multiple-dose activated charcoal regimens. *Am J Emerg Med* 10:298, 1992.

71. Keller RE, Schwab RA, Krenzelok EP: Contribution of sorbitol combined with AC in prevention of salicylate absorption. *Ann Emerg Med* 19:654, 1990.

72. McNamara RM, Aaron CK, Gembroys M, et al: Sorbitol catharsis does not enhance efficacy of charcoal in a simulated acetaminophen overdose. *Ann Emerg Med* 17:243, 1988.

73. Krenzelok EP, Keller R, Stewart RD: Gastrointestinal transit times of cathartics combined with charcoal. *Ann Emerg Med* 14:1152, 1985.

74. Barceloux D, McGuigan M, Hartigan-Go K: Position statement: cathartics. American Academy of Clinical Toxicology; European Association of Poisons Centres and Clinical Toxicologists. *J Toxicol Clin Toxicol* 35:743, 1997.

75. Snodgrass WR, Klaasen CD, Amdur MO, Doull J: Clinical toxicology, in *Casarett and Doull's Toxicology: The Basic Science of Poisons*, 5th ed. New York, McGraw-Hill, 1995, p 969.

76. Pond SM: Diuresis, dialysis, and hemoperfusion: Indications and benefits. *Emerg Med Clin North Am* 2:29, 1984.

77. Pond SM: Principles of techniques used to enhance elimination of toxic compounds, in Goldfrank LR, Flomenbaum NE, Lewin NA, et al (eds): *Goldfrank's Toxicologic Emergencies*, 5th ed. Norwalk, CT, Appleton & Lange, 1994, p 77.

78. Winchester JF: Active methods for detoxification, in Haddad LM, Winchester JF (eds): *Clinical Management of Poisoning and Drug Overdose*, 2nd ed. Philadelphia, Saunders, 1990, p 174.

79. Rowland M, Tozer TN: Elimination, in *Clinical Pharmacokinetics: Concepts and Applications*, 3rd ed. Baltimore, Williams & Wilkins, 1995, p 156.

80. Ismail N, Becker BN: Common poisoning and drug overdose, in Jacobson HR, Striker JE, Klahr S (eds): *The Principles and Practice of Nephrology*, 2nd ed. St Louis, Mosby, 1995, p 726.

81. Garella S: Extracorporeal techniques in the treatment of exogenous intoxications. *Kidney Int* 33:735, 1988.

82. Winchester JF: Use of dialysis and hemoperfusion in treatment of poisoning, in Daugirdas JT, Ing TS (eds): *Handbook of Dialysis*, 2d ed. Boston, Little, Brown, 1994, p 569.

83. Pond SM: Extracorporeal techniques in the treatment of poisoned patients. *Med J Aust* 154:617, 1991.

84. Gwilt PR, Perrier D: Plasma protein binding and distribution characteristics of drugs as indices of the dialyzability. *Clin Pharmacol Ther* 24:154, 1978.

85. Blye E, Lorch J, Cortell S: Extracorporeal therapy in the treatment of intoxication. *Am J Kid Dis* 3:321, 1984.

86. Tilstone WJ, Winchester JF, Reavey PC: Pharmacokinetic concepts. The use of pharmacokinetic principles in determining the effectiveness of removal of toxins from blood. *Clin Pharmacokinet* 4:23, 1979.

87. Alexander DP, Gambertoglio JG: Drug overdose and pharmacologic considerations in dialysis in Cogan MG, Garovoy MR (eds): *Introduction to Dialysis*. New York, Churchill Livingston, 1985, p261.

88. Aronoff GR, Brier ME: Prescribing drugs for dialysis patients, in Henrich WL (ed): *Principles and Practice of Dialysis*, 3rd ed. Philadelphia, Lippincott Williams & Wilkins, 2004, p 147.

89. DeSoi CA, Sahm DF, Umans JG: Vancomycin elimination during high-flux hemodialysis: kinetic model and comparison of four membranes. *Am J Kid Dis* 20:354, 1992.

90. Touchette MA, Patel RV, Anandan JV, et al: Vancomycin clearance by high-flux polysulfone hemodialysis membranes in critically ill patients with end-stage renal disease. *Am J Kid Dis* 26:469, 1995.

91. Winchester JF, Kriger FL: Hemoperfusion, in Jacobson HR, Striker JE, Klahr S (eds): *The Principles and Practice of Nephrology*, 2nd ed. St Louis, Mosby, 1995, p 721.

92. Golper TA, Wedel SK, Kaplan AA, et al: Drug removal by continuous arteriovenous hemofiltration: Theory and clinical observations. *Int J Artif Organs* 8:307, 1985.

93. Golper TA: Drug removal during continuous renal replacement therapies. *Dial Transplant* 22:185, 1993.

94. Reetze-Bonorden P, Bohler J, Keller E: Drug dosage in patients during continuous renal replacement therapy: Pharmacokinetic and therapeutic considerations. *Clin Pharmacokinet* 24:362, 1993.

95. Bellomo R, Kearly Y, Parkin G, et al: Treatment of life-threatening lithium toxicity with continuous arterio-venous hemodiafiltration. *Crit Care Med* 19:836, 1991.

96. Leblanc M, Raymond M, Bonnardeaux A, et al: Lithium poisoning treated by high-performance continuous arteriovenous and venovenous hemodiafiltration. *Am J Kid Dis* 27:365, 1996.

97. Collee GG, Hanson GC: The management of acute poisoning. *Br J Anesth* 70:562, 1993.

98. Brett AS, Rothschild N, Gray R, et al: Predicting the clinical course of intentional drug overdose: Implications for the use of the intensive care unit. *Arch Intern Med* 147:133, 1987.

99. Kulling P, Persson H: The role of the intensive care unit in the management of the poisoned patient. *Med Toxicol* 1:375, 1986.

100. Hamad AE: Predicting the need for medical intensive care monitoring in drug-overdosed patients. *J Intensive Care* 15:321, 2000.

101. Callaham M: Admission criteria for tricyclic antidepressant ingestion. *West J Med* 137:425, 1982.

102. Linden CH, Rumack BH: Acetaminophen overdose. *Emerg Med Clin North Am* 2:103, 1984.

103. McBride PV, Rumack BH: Acetaminophen intoxication. *Semin Dial* 5:292, 1992.

104. Corcoran GB, Mitchell JR, Vaishnav YN, et al: Evidence that acetaminophen and N-hydroxyacetaminophen form a common arylating intermediate, N-acetyl-p-benzoquinoneimine. *Mol Pharmacol* 18:536, 1980.

105. Rumack BM, Matthew M: Acetaminophen poisoning and toxicity. *Pediatrics* 55:871, 1975.

106. Whitcomb DC, Block GD: Association of acetaminophen hepatotoxicity with fasting and ethanol abuse. *JAMA* 272:1845, 1994.

107. Bond GR, Lite LK: Population-based incidence and outcome of acetaminophen poisoning by type of ingestion. *Acad Emerg Med* 6:1115, 1999.

108. Buckley NA, Whyte IM, O'Connell DL, et al: Activated charcoal reduces the need for N-acetylcysteine treatment after acetaminophen (paracetamol) overdose. *J Toxicol Clin Toxicol* 37:753, 1999.

109. Smilkstein MJ, Knapp GL, Kulig KW, et al: Efficacy of oral n-acetylcysteine in the treatment of acetaminophen overdose. Analysis of the national multicenter study (1976–1985). *N Engl J Med* 319:1557, 1988.

110. Keays R, Harrison PM, Wendon JA, et al: Intravenous acetylcysteine in paracetamol-induced fulminant hepatic failure: A prospective controlled trial. *Br Med J* 303:1026, 1991.

111. Harrison PM et al: Improved outcome of paracetamol-induced fulminant hepatic failure by late administration of acetylcysteine. *Lancet* 335:1572, 1990.

112. Harrison PM et al: Improvement by N-acetylcysteine of hemodynamics and oxygen transport in fulminant hepatic failure. *N Engl J Med* 324:1852, 1991.

113. Woo OF et al: Shorter duration of oral N-acetylcysteine therapy for acute acetaminophen overdose. *Ann Emerg Med* 35:363, 2000.

114. Prescott LF, Illingworth RN, Critchley JA, et al: Intravenous N-acetylcysteine: The treatment of choice for paracetamol poisoning. *BMJ* 2:1097, 1979.

115. Smilkstein MJ, Bronstein AC, Linden C, et al: Acetaminophen overdose: a 48-hour intravenous N-acetylcysteine treatment protocol. *Ann Emerg Med* 20:1058, 1991.

116. Mutimer DJ, Ayres RC, Neuberger JM, et al: Serious paracetamol poisoning and the results of liver transplantation. *Gut* 35:809, 1994.

117. O'Grady JG, Alexander GJ, Hayllar KM, et al: Early indicators of prognosis in fulminant hepatic failure. *Gastroenterology* 97:439, 1989.

118. Mitchell I, Bihari D, Chang R, et al: Earlier identification of patients at risk from acetaminophen-induced acute liver failure. *Crit Care Med* 26:279, 1998.

119. Ammar KA, Heckerling PS: Ethylene glycol poisoning with a normal anion gap caused by concurrent ethanol ingestion: Importance of the osmolal gap. *Am J Kid Dis* 27:130, 1996.

120. Walker JA, Schwartzbard A, Krauss EA, et al: The missing gap: a pitfall in the diagnosis of alcohol intoxication by osmometry. *Arch Intern Med* 146:1843, 1986.

121. Halperin ML, Goldstein MB: Metabolic acidosis, in Halperin ML, Goldstein MB (eds): *Fluid, Electrolyte, and Acid-Base Physiology: A Problem-Based Approach*, 2nd ed. Philadelphia, Saunders, 1994, p 67.

122. Jacobsen D, McMartin KE: Antidotes for methanol and ethylene glycol poisoning. *Clin Toxicol* 35:127, 1997.

123. Gabow PA: Ethylene glycol intoxication. *Am J Kid Dis* 11:277, 1988.

124. Wine H, Savitt D, Abuelo JG: Ethylene glycol intoxication. *Semin Dial* 7:338, 1994.

125. Palmer BF, Eigenbrodt EH, Henrich WL: Cranial nerve deficit: A clue to the diagnosis of ethylene glycol poisoning. *Am J Med* 87:91, 1989.

126. Mallya KB, Mendis T, Guberman A: Bilateral facial paralysis following ethylene glycol toxicity. *Can J Neurol Sci* 13:340, 1986.

127. Gabow PA: Ethylene glycol intoxication. *Am J Kid Dis* 11:277, 1988.

128. Wine H, Savitt D, Abuelo JG: Ethylene glycol intoxication. *Semin Dial* 7:338, 1994.

129. Kruse JA: Methanol poisoning. *Intensive Care Med* 18:391, 1992.

130. Hantson P, Mahieu P: Pancreatic injury following acute methanol poisoning. *J Toxicol Clin Toxicol* 38:297, 2000.

131. Brent J: Current management of ethylene glycol poisoning. *Drugs* 61:979, 2001.

132. Brent J, McMartin K, Phillips S, et al: Fomepizole for the treatment of ethylene glycol poisoning. *N Engl J Med* 340:832, 1999.

133. Brent J, McMartin K, Phillips S, et al: Fomepizole for the treatment of methanol poisoning. *N Engl J Med* 344:424, 2001.

134. McCoy HG, Cipolle RJ, Ehlers SM, et al: Severe methanol poisoning: application of a pharmacokinetic model for ethanol therapy and hemodialysis. *Am J Med* 67:804, 1979.

135. Lacouture PG, Wason S, Abrams A, Lovejoy FH: Acute isopropyl alcohol intoxication: Diagnosis and management. *Am J Med* 75:680, 1983.

136. Parry MF, Wallach R: Ethylene glycol poisoning. *Am J Med* 57:143, 1974.

137. Peterson CD, Collins AJ, Himes JM, et al: Ethylene glycol poisoning: pharmacokinetics during therapy with ethanol and hemodialysis. *N Engl J Med* 304:21, 1981.

138. Baud FJ, Gaillot M, Astier A, et al: Treatment of ethylene glycol poisoning with intravenous 4-methylpyrazole. *N Engl J Med* 319:97, 1988.

139. Rosansky SJ: Isopropyl alcohol poisoning treated with hemodialysis: kinetics of isopropyl alcohol and acetone removal. *J Toxicol Clin Toxicol* 19:265, 1982.

140. Sabeel AI, Kurkus J, Lindholm T: Intensified dialysis treatment of ethylene glycol intoxication. *Scand J Urol Nephrol* 29:125, 1995.

141. Richards JR, Bretz SW, Johnson EB, et al: Methamphetamine abuse and emergency department utilization. *West J Med* 170:198, 1999.

142. Jones AL, Simpson KJ: Mechanisms and management of hepatotoxicity in ecstasy (MDMA) and amphetamine intoxications. *Aliment Pharmacol Ther* 12:129, 1999.

143. Watson JD, Ferguson C, Hinds CJ, et al: Exertional heat stroke caused by amphetamine analogues. Does dantrolene have a place? *Anaesthesia* 48:1057, 1993.

144. Denborough MA, Hopkinson DC. Dantrolene and "ecstasy." *Med J Aust* 166:165, 1997.

145. Sutherland GR, Park J, Proudfoot AT: Ventilation and acid-base changes in deep coma due to barbiturate or tricyclic antidepressant poisoning. *Clin Toxicol* 11:403, 1977.

146. Raymond LW: "Barbiturate blisters" in a case of severe hypoglycaemic coma. *Lancet* 2:764, 1972.

147. Boldy DA, Vale JA, Prescott LF: Treatment of phenobarbitone poisoning with repeated oral administration of activated charcoal. *Q J Med* 61:997, 1986.

148. Goldberg MJ. Berlinger WG: Treatment of phenobarbital overdose with activated charcoal. *JAMA* 247:2400, 1982.

149. Berg MJ, Berlinger WG, Goldberg MJ, et al: Acceleration of the body clearance of phenobarbital by oral activated charcoal. *N Engl J Med* 307:642, 1982.

150. Pond SM, Olson KR, Osterloh JD, et al: Randomized study of the treatment of phenobarbital overdose with repeated doses of activated charcoal. *JAMA* 251:3104, 1984.

151. Vale JA, Krenzelok EP, Barceloux GD, et al: Position statement and practice guidelines on the use of multi-dose activated charcoal in the treatment of acute poisoning. American Academy of Clinical Toxicology; European Association of Poisons Centres and Clinical Toxicologists. *J Toxicol Clin Toxicol* 37:731, 1999.

152. Linton AL, Luke RG, Briggs JD: Methods of forced diuresis and its application in barbiturate poisoning. *Lancet* 2:377, 1967.

153. Costello JB, Poklis A: Treatment of massive phenobarbital overdose with dopamine diuresis. *Arch Intern Med* 141:938, 1981.

154. Lorch JA, Garella S: Hemoperfusion to treat intoxications. *Ann Intern Med* 91:301, 1979.

155. Lindberg MC, Cunningham A, Lindberg NH: Acute phenobarbital intoxication. *South Med J* 85:803, 1992.

156. Jacobsen D, Wiik-Larsen E, Dahl T, et al: Pharmacokinetic evaluation of haemoperfusion in phenobarbital poisoning. *Eur J Clin Pharmacol* 26:109, 1984.

157. Bouget J, Breurec JY, Baert A, et al: Value of charcoal by oral route in patients admitted to emergency department for voluntary absorption of benzodiazepines (French). *J Toxicol Clin Exp* 9:287, 1989.

158. Gross JB, Blouin RT, Zandsberg S, et al: Effect of flumazenil on ventilatory drive during sedation with midazolam and alfentanil. *Anesthesiology* 85:713, 1996.

159. Shalansky SJ, Naumann TL, Englander FA: Effect of flumazenil on benzodiazepine-induced respiratory depression. *Clin Pharmacol* 12:483, 1993.

160. The Flumazenil in Benzodiazepine Intoxication Multicenter Study Group: Treatment of benzodiazepine overdose with flumazenil. *Clin Ther* 14:978, 1992.

161. Spivey WH, Roberts JR, Derlet RW: A clinical trial of escalating doses of flumazenil for reversal of suspected benzodiazepine overdose in the emergency department. *Ann Emerg Med* 22:1813, 1993.

162. Weinbroum A, Halpern P, Geller E: The use of flumazenil in the management of acute drug poisoning—a review. *Intensive Care Med* 17(Suppl 1):S32, 1991.

163. Hoffman EJ, Warren EW: Flumazenil: A benzodiazepine antagonist. *Clin Pharmacol* 12:641; quiz 699, 1993.

164. Handal KA, Schauben JL, Salamone FR: Naloxone. *Ann Emerg Med* 12:438, 1983.

165. Agmo A, Galvan A, Heredia A, et al: Naloxone blocks the antianxiety but not the motor effects of benzodiazepines and pentobarbital: Experimental studies and literature. *Psychopharmacology* 120:186, 1995.

166. Forster A, Morel D, Bachmann M, et al: Respiratory depressant effects of different doses of midazolam and lack of reversal with naloxone—a double-blind randomized study. *Anesth Analg* 62:920, 1983.

167. Love JN: Beta-blocker toxicity: a clinical diagnosis. *Am J Emerg Med* 12:356, 1994.

168. Love JN, Howell JM, Litovitz TL, et al: Acute beta blocker overdose: factors associated with the development of cardiovascular morbidity. *J Toxicol Clin Toxicol* 38:275, 2000.

169. Love JN: Beta blocker toxicity after overdose: when do symptoms develop in adults? *J Emerg Med* 12:799, 1994.

170. Reith DM, Dawson AH, Epid D, et al: Relative toxicity of beta blockers in overdose. *J Toxicol Clin Toxicol* 34:273, 1996.

171. Love JN, Litovitz TL, Howell JM, et al: Characterization of fatal beta blocker ingestion. A review of the American Association of Poison Control Centers data from 1985 to 1995. *J Toxicol Clin Toxicol* 35:353, 1997.

172. Lipski JL, Kaminsky D, Donoso E, et al: Electrophysiological effects of glucagon on the normal canine heart. *Am J Physiol* 222:1107, 1972.

173. Love JN, Sachdeva DK, Bessman ES, et al: A potential role for glucagon in the treatment of drug-induced symptomatic bradycardia. *Chest* 114:323, 1998.

174. Kerns W, Schroeder D, Williams C, et al. Insulin improves survival in a canine model of acute beta-blocker toxicity. *Ann Emerg Med* 29:748, 1997.

175. Kerns W, Kline J, Ford MD: Beta-blocker and calcium channel blocker toxicity. *Emerg Med Clin North Am* 12:365, 1994.

176. Buckley NA, Dawson AH, Howarth DM, et al: Slow release verapamil poisoning: Use of polyethylene glycol whole-bowel lavage and high-dose calcium. *Med J Aust* 158:202, 1993.

177. Rosansky SJ: Verapamil toxicity—treatment with hemoperfusion. *Ann Intern Med* 114:340, 1991.

178. Kenny J: Treating overdose with calcium channel blockers. *BMJ* 308:992, 1994.

179. Luscher TF, Noll G, Sturmer T, et al: Calcium gluconate in severe verapamil intoxication. *N Engl J Med* 330:718, 1994.

180. Papadopoulos J, O'Neil MG: Utilization of a glucagon infusion in the management of a massive nifedipine overdose. *J Emerg Med* 18:453, 2000.

181. Yuan TH, Kerns WP, Tomaszewski CA, et al: Insulin-glucose as adjunctive therapy for severe calcium channel antagonist poisoning. *J Toxicol Clin Toxicol* 37:463, 1999.

182. Boyer EW, Shannon M: Treatment of calcium-channel blocker intoxication with insulin infusion. *N Engl J Med* 344:1721, 2001.

183. Cobb N, Etzel RA. Unintentional carbon monoxide-related deaths in the United States, 1979 through 1988. *JAMA* 266:659, 1991.

184. Wittenberg BA, Wittenberg JB: Effects of carbon monoxide on isolated heart muscle cells. *Res Rep Health Eff Inst* 62:1, 13, 1993.

185. Taitelman U, Schmidt GA: Inhaled toxins, in Hall JB, Schmidt GA, Wood LDH (eds): *Principles of Critical Care.* New York, McGraw-Hill, 1992, p 2117.

186. Dahms TE, Younis LT, Wiens RD, et al: Effects of carbon monoxide exposure in patients with documented cardiac arrhythmias. *J Am Coll Cardiol* 21:442, 1993.

187. Birky MM, Clarke FB: Inhalation of toxic products from fires. *Bull N Y Acad Med* 57:997, 1981.

188. Sawa GM, Watson CPM, Terbrugge K, et al: Delayed encephalopathy following carbon monoxide intoxication. *Can J Neurol Sci* 8:77, 1981.

189. Choi IS: Delayed neurologic sequelae in carbon monoxide intoxication. *Arch Neurol* 40:433, 1983.

190. Tom T, Abedon S, Clark RI, et al: Neuroimaging characteristics in carbon monoxide toxicity. *J Neuroimaging* 6:161, 1996.

191. Buckley RG, Aks SE, Eshom JL, et al: The pulse oximetry gap in carbon monoxide intoxication. *Ann Emerg Med* 24:252, 1994.

192. Touger M, Gallagher EJ, Tyrell J: Relationship between venous and arterial carboxyhemoglobin levels in patients with suspected carbon monoxide poisoning. *Ann Emerg Med* 25:481, 1995.

193. Takeuchi A, Vesely A, Rucker J, et al: A simple "new" method to accelerate clearance of carbon monoxide. *Am J Resp Crit Care Med* 161:1816, 2000.

194. Tibbles PM, Edelsberg JS: Hyperbaric-oxygen therapy. *N Engl J Med* 334:1642, 1996.

195. Tibbles PM, Perrotta PL: Treatment of carbon monoxide poisoning: A critical review of human outcome studies comparing normobaric oxygen with hyperbaric oxygen. *Ann Emerg Med* 24:269, 1994.

196. Raphael JC, Elkharrat D, Jars-Guincestre MC, et al: Trial of normobaric and hyperbaric oxygen for acute carbon monoxide intoxication. *Lancet* 2:414, 1989.

197. Thom SR, Taber RL, Mendiguren II, et al: Delayed neuropsychologic sequelae after carbon monoxide poisoning: prevention by treatment with hyperbaric oxygen. *Ann Emerg Med* 25:474, 1995.

198. Ducasse JL, Celsis P, Marc-Vergnes JP: Non-comatose patients with acute carbon monoxide poisoning: Hyperbaric or normobaric oxygenation? *Undersea Hyperb Med* 22:9, 1995.

199. Weaver LK, Hopkins RO, Larson-Lohr V: Neuropsychologic and functional recovery from severe carbon monoxide poisoning without hyperbaric oxygen therapy. *Ann Emerg Med* 27:736, 1996.

200. Weaver LK, Hopkins RO, Chan KJ, et al: Hyperbaric oxygen for acute carbon monoxide poisoning. *N Engl J Med* 347:1057, 2002.

201. Shimada H, Morita T, Kunimoto F, et al: Immediate application of hyperbaric oxygen therapy using a newly devised transportable chamber. *Am J Emerg Med* 14:412, 1996.

202. Gorman DF, Clayton D, Gilligan JE, et al: A longitudinal study of 100 consecutive admissions for carbon monoxide poisoning to the Royal Adelaide Hospital. *Anaesth Intensive Care* 20:311, 1992.

203. Raphael J-C, Elkharrat D, Jars-Guincestre M-C, et al: Trial of normobaric and hyperbaric oxygen for acute carbon monoxide intoxication. *Lancet* 1:1414, 1989.

204. Cregler LL, Mark H: Medical complications of cocaine abuse. *N Engl J Med* 317:1495, 1986.

205. Wilson LD, Henning RJ, Suttheimer C, et al: Cocaethylene causes dose-dependent reductions in cardiac function in anesthetized dogs. *J Cardiovasc Pharmacol* 26:965, 1995.

206. Reeves RR, McWilliams ME, Fitz-Gerald M: Cocaine-induced ischemic cerebral infarction mistaken for a psychiatric syndrome. *South Med J* 88:352, 1995.

207. Nolte KB, Brass LM, Fletterick CF: Intracranial hemorrhage associated with cocaine abuse: a prospective autopsy study. *Neurology* 46:1291, 1996.

208. Daras M, Tuchman AJ, Koppel BS, et al: Neurovascular complications of cocaine. *Acta Neurol Scand* 90:124, 1994.

209. Martin K, Rogers T, Kavanaugh A: Central nervous system angiopathy associated with cocaine abuse. *J Rheumatol* 22:780, 1995.

210. Lalouschek W, Schnider P, Aull S, et al: Cocaine abuse—with special reference to cerebrovascular complications (German). *Wiener Klinische Wochenschrift* 107:516, 1995.

211. Chang RA, Rossi NF: Intermittent cocaine use associated with recurrent dissection of the thoracic and abdominal aorta. *Chest* 108:1758, 1995.

212. Willens HJ, Chakko SC, Kessler KM: Cardiovascular manifestations of cocaine abuse. A case of recurrent dilated cardiomyopathy. *Chest* 106:594, 1994.

213. Billman GE: Cocaine: A review of its toxic actions on cardiac function. *Crit Rev Toxicol* 25:113, 1995.

214. Mouhaffel AH, Madu EC, Satmary WA, et al: Cardiovascular complications of cocaine. *Chest* 107:1426, 1995.

215. Fraker TD Jr, Temesy-Armos PN, Brewster PS, et al: Interaction of propranolol, verapamil, and nifedipine on the myocardial depressant effect of cocaine. *J Cardiovasc Pharmacol* 25:579, 1995.

216. Chakko S, Myerburg RJ: Cardiac complications of cocaine abuse. *Clin Cardiol* 18:67, 1995.

217. Hollander JE, Hoffman RS, Gennis P, et al: Prospective multicenter evaluation of cocaine-associated chest pain. Cocaine Associated Chest Pain (COCHPA) Study Group. *Acad Emerg Med* 1:330, 1994.

218. Trabulsy ME: Cocaine washed out syndrome in a patient with acute myocardial infarction. *Am J Emerg Med* 13:538, 1995.

219. Hollander JE, Hoffman RS, Gennis P, et al: Cocaine-associated chest pain: One-year follow-up. *Acad Emerg Med* 2:179, 1995.

220. Averbach M, Casey KK, Frank E: Near-fatal status asthmaticus induced by nasal insufflation of cocaine. *South Med J* 89:340, 1996.

221. Silverman RS, Lee-Chiong TL Jr, Sherter CB: Stridor from edema of the arytenoids, epiglottis, and vocal cords after use of free-base cocaine. *Chest* 108:1477, 1995.

222. Yakel DL Jr, Eisenberg MJ: Pulmonary artery hypertension in chronic intravenous cocaine users. *Am Heart J* 130:398, 1995.

223. Albertson TE, Walby WF, Derlet RW: Stimulant-induced pulmonary toxicity. *Chest* 108:1140, 1995.

224. Forrester JM, Steele AW, Waldron JA, et al: Crack lung: An acute pulmonary syndrome with a spectrum of clinical and histopathologic findings. *Am Rev Resp Dis* 142:462, 1990.

225. Daras M, Kakkouras L, Tuchman AJ, et al: Rhabdomyolysis and hyperthermia after cocaine abuse: A variant of the neuroleptic malignant syndrome? *Acta Neurolog Scand* 92:161, 1995.

226. Roth D, Alarcon FJ, Fernandez JA, et al: Acute rhabdomyolysis associated with cocaine intoxication. *N Engl J Med* 319:673, 1988.

227. Daras M, Kakkouras L, Tuchman AJ, et al: Rhabdomyolysis and hyperthermia after cocaine abuse: A variant of the neuroleptic malignant syndrome? *Acta Neurol Scand* 92:161, 1995.

228. Sanjuanbenito Dehesa A, Fernandez Cebrian JM: Ischaemic colitis induced by cocaine abuse. *Br J Surg* 82:138, 1995.

229. Goodman PE, Rennie WP: Renal infarction secondary to nasal insufflation of cocaine. *Am J Emerg Med* 13:421, 1995.

230. Kudrow DB, Henry DA, Haake DA, et al: Botulism associated with *Clostridium botulinum* sinusitis after intranasal cocaine abuse. *Ann Intern Med* 109:984, 1988.

231. MacDonald KL, Rutherford GW, Friedman SM, et al: Botulism and botulism-like illness in chronic drug abusers. *Ann Intern Med* 102:616, 1985.

232. Marzuk PM, Tardiff K, Leon AC, et al: Fatal injuries after cocaine use as a leading cause of death among young adults in New York City. *N Engl J Med* 332:1753, 1995.

233. Hoffman RS, Smilkstein MJ, Goldfrank LR: Whole bowel irrigation and the cocaine body-packer: A new approach to a common problem. *Am J Emerg Med* 8:523, 1990.

234. Hierholzer J, Cordes M, Tantow H, et al: Drug smuggling by ingested cocaine-filled packages: conventional x-ray and ultrasound. *Abdominal Imaging* 20:333, 1995.

235. Makosiej FJ, Hoffman RS, Howland MA, et al: An in vitro evaluation of cocaine hydrochloride adsorption by activated charcoal and desorption upon addition of polyethylene glycol electrolyte lavage solution. *J Toxicol Clin Toxicol* 31:381, 1993.

236. Glass JM, Scott HJ: "Surgical mules": The smuggling of drugs in the gastrointestinal tract. *J Roy Soc Med* 88:450, 1995.

237. Catravas JD, Waters IW: Acute cocaine intoxication in the conscious dog: studies on the mechanism of lethality. *J Pharmacol Exp Ther* 217:350, 1981.

238. Thiebot MH, Kloczko J, Chermat R, et al: Enhancement of cocaine-induced hyperactivity in mice by benzodiazepines: Evidence for an interaction of GABAergic processes with catecholaminergic neurons? *Eur J Pharmacol* 76:335, 1981.

239. Brogan WC 3rd, Lange RA, Kim AS, et al: Alleviation of cocaine-induced coronary vasoconstriction by nitroglycerin. *J Am Coll Cardiol* 18:581, 1991.

240. Hollander JE: The management of cocaine-associated myocardial ischemia. *N Engl J Med* 333:1267, 1995.

241. Hollander JE, Carter WA, Hoffman RS: Use of phentolamine for cocaine-induced myocardial ischemia. *N Engl J Med* 327:361, 1992.

242. Lange RA, Cigarroa RG, Flores ED, et al: Potentiation of cocaine-induced coronary vasoconstriction by beta-adrenergic blockade. *Ann Intern Med* 112:897, 1990.

243. Smith M, Garner D, Niemann JT: Pharmacologic interventions after an LD50 cocaine insult in a chronically instrumented rat model: are beta-blockers contraindicated? *Ann Emerg Med* 20:768, 1991.

244. Sand IC, Brody SL, Wrenn KD, et al: Experience with esmolol for the treatment of cocaine-associated cardiovascular complications. *Am J Emerg Med* 9:161, 1991.

245. Boehrer JD, Moliterno DJ, Willard JE, et al: Influence of labetalol on cocaine-induced coronary vasoconstriction in humans. *Am J Med* 94:608, 1993.

246. Hollander JE, Burstein JL, Hoffman RS, et al: Cocaine-associated myocardial infarction. Clinical safety of thrombolytic therapy. Cocaine Associated Myocardial Infarction (CAMI) Study Group. *Chest* 107:1237, 1995.

247. Akintonwa A, Tunwashe OL: Fatal cyanide poisoning from cassava-based meal. *Hum Exp Toxicol* 11:47, 1992.

248. Logan B, Howard J, Kiesel EL: Poisonings associated with cyanide in over the counter cold medication in Washington State, 1991. *J Forensic Sci* 38:472, 1993.

249. Yen D, Tsai J, Wang LM, et al: The clinical experience of acute cyanide poisoning. *Am J Emerg Med* 13:524, 1995.

250. Salkowski AA, Penney DG: Cyanide poisoning in animals and humans: A review. *Vet Hum Toxicol* 36:455, 1994.

251. Yeh MM, Becker CE, Arieff AI: Is measurement of venous oxygen saturation useful in the diagnosis of cyanide poisoning? *Am J Med* 93:582, 1992.

252. Benowitz NL: Nitroprusside, in Olson KR (ed): *Poisoning and Drug Overdose*, 2nd ed. Norwalk, CT, Appleton & Lange, 1994, p 231.

253. Blanc PD: Cyanide, in Olson KR (ed): *Poisoning and Drug Overdose*, 2nd ed. Norwalk, CT, Appleton & Lange, 1994, p 145.

254. Taitelman U: Acute cyanide poisoning, in Hall JB, Schmidt GA, Wood LDH (eds): *Principles of Critical Care*. New York, McGraw-Hill, 1992, p 2125.

255. Way JL, Gibbon SL, Sheehy M: Cyanide intoxication: Protection with oxygen. *Science* 152:210, 1966.

256. Cope C: The importance of oxygen in the treatment of cyanide poisoning. *JAMA* 12:109, 1961.

257. Isom GE, Way JL: Effect of oxygen on cyanide intoxication. VI. Reactivation of cyanide-inhibited glucose metabolism. *J Pharmacol Ther* 1:235, 1974.

258. Isom GE, Way JL: Effects of oxygen on the antagonism of cyanide intoxication-cytochrome oxidase, in vivo. *Toxicol Appl Pharmacol* 65:250, 1982.

259. Litovitz TL, Larkin RF, Myers RAM: Cyanide poisoning treated with hyperbaric oxygen. *Am J Emerg Med* 1:99, 1983.

260. Way JL, End E, Sheehy MH, et al: Effects of oxygen on cyanide intoxication. IV. Hyperbaric oxygen. *Toxicol Appl Pharmacol* 22:415, 1972.

261. Kirk MA, Gerace R, Kulig KW: Cyanide and methemoglobin kinetics in smoke inhalation victims treated with the cyanide antidote kit. *Ann Emerg Med* 22:1413, 1993.

262. Hoffman RS, Sauter D: Methemoglobinemia resulting from smoke inhalation. *Vet Hum Toxicol* 31:168, 1989.

263. Westley J, Adler H, Westley L, Nishida C: The sulfur transferases. *Fund Appl Toxicol* 3:337, 1983.

264. Robin ED, McCauley R: Nitroprusside-related cyanide poisoning. Time (long past due) for urgent, effective interventions. *Chest* 102:1842, 1992.

265. Hall VA, Guest JM: Sodium nitroprusside-induced cyanide intoxication and prevention with sodium thiosulfate prophylaxis. *Am J Crit Care* 1:19, 1992.

266. Posner MA, Tobey RE, McElroy H: Hydroxycobalamin therapy in of cyanide intoxication in guinea pigs. *Anesthesiology* 2:157, 1976.

267. Curry SC, Connor DA, Raschke RA: Effect of the cyanide antidote hydroxocobalamin on commonly ordered serum chemistry studies. *Ann Emerg Med* 24:65, 1994.

268. Forsyth JC, Mueller PD, Becker CE, et al: Hydroxocobalamin as a cyanide antidote: Safety, efficacy and pharmacokinetics in heavily smoking normal volunteers. *J Toxicol Clin Toxicol* 31:277, 1993.

269. Zerbe NF, Wagner BK: Use of vitamin B_{12} in the treatment and prevention of nitroprusside-induced cyanide toxicity. *Crit Care Med* 21:465, 1993.

270. Keller KH: Hydroxycobalamin, in Olson KR (ed): *Poisoning and Drug Overdose*, 2nd ed. Norwalk, CT, Appleton & Lange, 1994, p 344.

271. Houeto P, Borron SW, Sandouk P, et al: Pharmacokinetics of hydroxocobalamin in smoke inhalation victims. *J Toxicol Clin Toxicol* 34:397, 1996.

272. Houeto P, Hoffman JR, Imbert M, et al: Relation of blood cyanide to plasma cyanocobalamin concentration after a fixed dose of hydroxocobalamin in cyanide poisoning. *Lancet* 346:605, 1995.

273. Nagler J, Provoost RA, Parizel G: Hydrogen cyanide poisoning: Treatment with cobalt EDTA. *J Occup Med* 6:414, 1978.

274. Boehnert MT, Lovejoy FH Jr: Value of the QRS duration versus the serum drug level in predicting seizures and ventricular arrhythmias after an acute overdose of tricyclic antidepressants. *N Engl J Med* 313:474, 1985.

275. Stern TA, O'Gara PT, Mulley AG, et al: Complications after overdose of tricyclic antidepressants. *Crit Care Med* 13:672, 1985.

276. Callaham M: Admission criteria for tricyclic antidepressant ingestion. *West J Med* 137:425, 1982.

276a. Callaham M: Epidemiology of fatal tricyclic antidepressant ingestion: implications for management. *Ann Emerg Med* 14:1, 1985.

277. Anonymous: Adverse events associated with ingestion of gamma-butyrolactone—Minnesota, New Mexico and Texas 1998–1999. *MMWR Morb Mortal Wkly Rep* 48:137, 1999.

278. Anonymous: Placement of gamma-butyrolactone in List 1 of the Controlled Substances Act [21 U.S.C. 802(34)]. Drug Enforcement Administration, Justice. Final rule. *Fed Regist* 65:1645, 2000.

279. Tunnicliff G: Sites of action of gamma-hydroxybutyrate (GHB)—a neuroactive drug with abuse potential. *J Toxicol Clin Toxicol* 35:581, 1997.

280. Van Cauter E, Plat L, Scharf MB, et al: Simultaneous stimulation of slow wave sleep and growth hormone secretion by gamma-hydroxybutyrate in normal young men. *J Clin Invest* 100:745, 1997.

281. Lammers GJ, Arends J, Declerck AC, et al: Gammahydroxybutyrate and narcolepsy: A double-blind placebo-controlled study. *Sleep* 16:216, 1993.

282. Dyer JE, Roth B, Hyma BA: Gamma-hydroxybutyrate withdrawal syndrome. *Ann Emerg Med* 37:147, 2001.

283. Davis LG: Fatalities attributed to GHB and related compounds. *South J Med* 92:1037, 1999.

284. Chin RL, Sporer KA, Cullison B, et al: Clinical course of gamma-hydroxybutyrate overdose. *Ann Emerg Med* 31:716, 1998.

285. Yates SW, Viera AJ: Physostigmine in the treatment of gamma-hydroxybutyric acid overdose. *Mayo Clinic Proc* 75:401, 2000.

286. ElSohly MA, Salamone SJ: Prevalence of drugs used in cases of alleged sexual assault. *J Anal Toxicol* 23:141, 1999.

287. LeBeau MA, Montgomery MA, Miller ML, et al: Analysis of biofluids for gamma-hydroxybutyrate (GHB) and gamma-butyrolactone (GBL) by headspace GC-FID and GC-MS. *J Anal Toxicol* 24:421, 2000.

288. Kalasinsky KS, Dixon MM, Schmumk GA, et al: Blood, brain, and hair GHB concentrations following fatal ingestion. *J Forensic Sci* 46:728, 2001.

289. Lindenbaum J, Rund DG, Butler VP: Inactivation of digoxin by the gut flora: Reversal by antibiotic therapy. *N Engl J Med* 305:789, 1981.

290. Huffman DH, Azarnoff DL: Absorption of orally given digoxin preparations. *JAMA* 222:957, 1972.

291. Centers for Disease Control and Prevention: Deaths associated with a purported aphrodisiac, New York City, February 1993–May 1995. *JAMA* 274:1828, 1995.

292. Beller GA, Smith TW, Abelmann WH, et al: Digitalis intoxication: A prospective clinical study with serum level correlations. *N Engl J Med* 284:989, 1971.

293. Lewis RP: Clinical use of serum digoxin concentrations. *Am J Cardiol* 69:97G, 1992.

294. Smith TW: Digitalis toxicity: Epidemiology and clinical use of serum concentration measurements. *Am J Med* 58:470, 1975.

295. Adams KF, Gheorghiade M, Uretsky BF, Patterson JH, et al: Clinical benefits of low serum digoxin concentrations in heart failure. *J Am Coll Cardiol* 39:946, 2002.

296. Antman EM, Wenger TL, Butler VP, et al: Treatment of 150 cases of life-threatening digitalis intoxication with digoxin-specific Fab antibody fragments. Final report of a multicenter study. *Circulation* 81:1744, 1990.

297. Smith TW, Butler VP, Haber E, et al: Treatment of life-threatening digitalis intoxication with digoxin-specific Fab antibody fragments. *N Engl J Med* 307:1357, 1982.

298. Saluk Martiny S, Phelps SJ, Massey KL: Treatment of severe digitalis intoxication with digoxin-specific antibody fragments: A clinical review. *Crit Care Med* 16:629, 1988.

299. Ujhelyi MR, Robert S, Cummings DM, et al: Influence of digoxin immune Fab therapy and renal dysfunction on the disposition of total and free digoxin. *Ann Intern Med* 119:273, 1993.

300. Rabetoy GM, Price CA, Findlay JW, Sailstad JM: Treatment of digoxin intoxication in a renal failure patient with digoxin-specific antibody fragments and plasmapheresis. *Am J Nephrol* 10:518, 1990.

301. Okusa MD, Crystal LJT: Clinical manifestations and management of acute lithium intoxication. *Am J Med* 97:383, 1994.

302. Amdisen A: Clinical features and management of lithium poisoning. *Med Toxicol* 3:18, 1988.

303. Favin FD, Klein-Schwartz W, Oderda GM, Rose SR: In vitro study of lithium carbonate absorption by activated charcoal. *Clin Toxicol* 26:443, 1988.

304. Linakis JG, Lacouture PG, Eisenberg MS, et al: Administration of activated charcoal or sodium polystyrene sulfonate (Kayexalate) as gastric decontamination for lithium intoxication: an animal model. *Pharmacol Toxicol* 65:387, 1989.

305. Watling SM, Gehrke JC, Zumwalt R, Pribble J: In vitro binding of lithium using the cation exchange resin sodium polystyrene sulfonate. *Am J Emerg Med* 13:294, 1995.

306. Linakis JG, Eisenberg MS, Lacouture PG, et al: Multiple-dose sodium polystyrene sulfonate in lithium intoxication: an animal model. *Pharmacol Toxicol* 70:38, 1992.

307. Smith SW, Ling LJ, Halstenson CE: Whole-bowel irrigation as a treatment for acute lithium overdose. *Ann Emerg Med* 20:536, 1991.

308. Jaeger A, Sauder P, Kopferschmitt T, et al: When should dialysis be performed in lithium poisoning? A kinetic study in 14 cases of lithium poisoning. *Clin Toxicol* 31:429, 1993.

309. Clendeninn NJ, Pond SM, Kaysen G, et al: Potential pitfalls in the evaluation of the usefulness of hemodialysis for the removal of lithium. *J Toxicol Clin Toxicol* 19:341, 1982.

310. Friedberg RC, Spyker DA, Herold DA: Massive overdoses with sustained-release lithium carbonate preparations: Pharmacokinetic model based on two case studies. *Clin Chem* 37:1205, 1991.

311. Mansouri A, Lurie AA: Concise review: methemoglobinemia. *Am J Hematol* 42:7, 1993.

312. Fairbanks VF: Blue gods, blue oil, and blue people. *Mayo Clin Proc* 69:889, 1994.

313. Blanc PD: Methemoglobinemia, in Olson KR (ed): *Poisoning and Drug Overdose,* 2nd ed. Norwalk, CT, Appleton & Lange, 1994.

314. Reider HU, Frei FJ, Zbinden AM, et al: Pulse oximetry in methaemoglobinaemia. Failure to detect low oxygen saturation. *Anaesthesia* 45:56, 1990.

315. Watcha MF, Connor MT, Hing AV: Pulse oximetry in methemoglobinemia. *Am J Dis Child* 143:845, 1989.

316. Barker SJ, Tremper KK, Hyatt J: Effects of methemoglobinemia on pulse oximetry and mixed venous oximetry. *Anesthesiology* 70:112, 1989.

317. Donnelly GB, Randlett MS: Methemoglobinemia. *N Engl J Med* 343:337, 2000.

318. Keller KH: Methylene blue, in Olson KR (ed): *Poisoning and Drug Overdose,* 2nd ed. Norwalk, CT, Appleton & Lange, 1994, p 351.

319. Sporer KA: Acute heroin overdose. *Ann Intern Med* 130:584, 1999.

320. Darke S, Zador D: Fatal heroin overdose: A review. *Addiction* 91:1675, 1996.

321. Ruttenber AJ, Kalter HD, Santinga P: The role of ethanol abuse in the etiology of heroin-related death. *J Forensic Sci* 35:891, 1990.

322. Sternbach G: William Osler: narcotic-induced pulmonary edema. *J Emerg Med* 1:165, 1983.

323. Cygan J, Trunsky M, Corbridge T: Inhaled heroin-induced status asthmaticus. *Chest* 117:272, 2000.

324. Krantz A, Hershow RC, Prachand N, et al: Heroin insufflation as a trigger for patients with life-threatening asthma. *Chest* 123:510, 2003.

325. Ng B, Alvear M: Dextropropoxyphene addiction: a drug of primary abuse. *Am J Drug Alcohol Abuse* 19:153, 1993.

326. Hershey LA: Meperidine and central neurotoxicity. *Ann Intern Med* 98:548, 1983.

327. Hoffman JR, Schriger DL, Luo JS: The empiric use of naloxone in patients with altered mental status: a reappraisal. *Ann Emerg Med* 20:246, 1991.

328. Schwartz JG, Garriott JC, Somerset JS, et al: Measurements of fentanyl and sufentanil in blood and urine after surgical application. Implication in detection of abuse. *Am J Forensic Med Pathol* 15:236, 1994.

329. Boehnert MT, Lewander WJ, Gaudreault P, et al: Advances in clinical toxicology. *Pediatr Clin North Am* 32:193, 1985.

330. Merriman T, Stokes K: Small bowel obstruction secondary to administration of activated charcoal. *Aust N Z J Surg* 65:288, 1995.

331. Tanberg D, Abercrombie D. Treatment of heroin overdose with endotracheal naloxone. *Ann Emerg Med* 11:443, 1982.

332. Namba T, Nolte CT, Jackrel J, et al: Poisoning due to organophosphate insecticides. Acute and chronic manifestations. *Am J Med* 50:475, 1971.

333. Sungur M, Guven M: Intensive care management of organophosphate insecticide poisoning. *Crit Care* 5:211, 2001.

334. Wu ML, Deng JF, Tsai WJ, et al: Food poisoning due to methamidophos-contaminated vegetables. *J Toxicol Clin Toxicol* 39:333, 2001.

335. Geller RJ, Singleton KL, Tarantino ML, et al: Nosocomial poisoning associated with emergency department treatment of organophosphate toxicity—Georgia, 2000. *J Toxicol Clin Toxicol* 39:109, 2001.

336. Hayes MM, Van der Westhuizen NG, et al: Organophosphate poisoning in Rhodesia. A study of the clinical features and management of 105 patients. *S Afr Med J* 54:230, 1978.

337. Nouira S, Abroug F, Elatrous S, et al: Prognostic value of serum cholinesterase in organophosphate poisoning. *Chest* 106:1811, 1994.

338. Coye MJ, Barnett PG, Midtling JE, et al: Clinical confirmation of organophosphate poisoning by serial cholinesterase analyses. *Arch Intern Med* 147:438, 1987.

339. Bardin PG, Van Eeden SF: Organophosphate poisoning: Grading the severity and comparing treatment between atropine and glycopyrrolate. *Crit Care Med* 18:956, 1990.

340. Lieske CN, Clark JH, Maxwell DM, et al: Studies of the amplification of carbaryl toxicity by various oximes. *Toxicol Lett* 62:127, 1992.

341. Miller NS, Gold MS, Millman R: PCP: A dangerous drug. *Am Fam Physician* 38:215, 1988.

342. Wright HH, Cole EA, Batey SR, et al: Phencyclidine-induced psychosis: Eight-year follow-up of ten cases. *South Med J* 81:565, 1988.

343. Isaacs SO, Martin P, Washington JA Jr: Phencyclidine (PCP) abuse. A close-up look at a growing problem. *Oral Surg Oral Med Oral Pathol* 61:126, 1986.

344. Poklis A, Graham M, Maginn D, et al: Phencyclidine and violent deaths in St. Louis, Missouri: A survey of medical examiners' cases from 1977 through 1986. *Am J Drug Alcohol Abuse* 16:265, 1990.

345. McCarron MM, Schulze BW, Thompson GA, et al: Acute phencyclidine intoxication: incidence of clinical findings in 1000 cases. *Ann Emerg Med* 10:237, 1981.

346. Akmal M, Valdin JR, McCarron MM, et al: Rhabdomyolysis with and without acute renal failure in patients with phencyclidine intoxication. *Am J Nephrol* 1:91, 1981.

347. Eastman JW, Cohen SN: Hypertensive crisis and death associated with phencyclidine poisoning. *JAMA* 231:1270, 1975.

348. Bessen HA: Intracranial hemorrhage associated with phencyclidine abuse. *JAMA* 248:585, 1982.

349. Boyko OB, Burger PC, Heinz ER: Pathological and radiological correlation of subarachnoid hemorrhage in phencyclidine abuse. Case report. *J Neurosurg* 67:446, 1987.

350. Lyddane JE, Thomas BF, Compton DR, et al: Modification of phencyclidine intoxification and biodisposition by charcoal and other treatments. *Pharmacol Biochem Behav* 30:371, 1988.

351. Perez-Reyes M, Di Guiseppi S, Brine DR, et al: Urine pH and phencyclidine excretion. *Clin Pharmacol Ther* 32:635, 1982.

352. Domino EF, Wilson AE: Effects of urine acidification on plasma and urine phencyclidine levels in overdosage. *Clin Pharmacol Ther* 22:421, 1977.

353. Cook CE, Brine DR, Jeffcoat AR, et al: Phencyclidine disposition after intravenous and oral doses. *Clin Pharmacol Ther* 31:625, 1982.

354. Giannini AJ, Loiselle RH, DiMarzio LR, et al: Augmentation of haloperidol by ascorbic acid in phencyclidine intoxication. *Am J Psychiatr* 144:1207, 1987.

355. Giannini AJ, Loiselle RH, Price WA, et al: Chlorpromazine vs. meperidine in the treatment of phencyclidine psychosis. *J Clin Psychiatr* 46:52, 1985.

356. Done AK: Salicylate intoxication. *Pediatrics* 26:800, 1960.

357. Chan TY: Improvements in the packaging of drugs and chemicals may reduce the likelihood of severe intentional poisonings in adults. *Hum Exp Toxicol* 19:387, 2000.

358. Hawton K, Townsend E, Deeks J, et al: Effects of legislation restricting pack sizes of paracetamol and salicylate on self poisoning in the United Kingdom: before and after study. *BMJ* 322:1203, 2001.

359. Temple AR: Acute and chronic effects of aspirin toxicity and their treatment. *Arch Intern Med* 141:364, 1981.

360. Eichenholz A, Mulhausen RO, Redleaf PS: Nature of acid-base disturbance in salicylate intoxication. *Metabolism* 12:164, 1963.

361. Gabow PA, Anderson RJ, Potts DE, Schrier RW: Acid-base disturbances in the salicylate-intoxicated adult. *Arch Intern Med* 138:1481, 1978.

362. Hill JB: Salicylate intoxication. *N Engl J Med* 288:1110, 1973.

363. Thisted B, Kantz T, Strom J, et al: Acute salicylate self-poisoning in 177 patients treated in ICU. *Acta Anesth Scand* 31:312, 1987.

364. McGuigan MA: A two-year review of salicylate deaths in Ontario. *Arch Intern Med* 147:510, 1987.

365. Goldfrank LR, Bresnitz EA, Hartnett L, Flomenbaum NE: Salicylates, in Goldfrank LR, Flomenbaum NE, Lewin NA, et al (eds): *Goldfrank's Toxicologic Emergencies*, 4th ed. Norwalk, CT, Appleton & Lange, 1990, p 261.

366. Dugandzic RM, Tierny MG, Dickenson GE, et al: Evaluation of the validity of the Done nomogram in the management of acute salicylate intoxication. *Ann Emerg Med* 18:1186, 1989.

367. Anderson RJ, Potts DE, Gabow PA, et al: Unrecognized adult salicylate intoxication. *Ann Intern Med* 85:745, 1976.

368. Greer HD, Ward HP, Corbin KB: Chronic salicylate intoxication in adults. *JAMA* 193:85, 1965.

369. Heffner JE, Sahn SA: Salicylate-induced pulmonary edema. *Ann Intern Med* 95:405, 1981.

370. Gabow PA: How to avoid overlooking salicylate intoxication. *J Crit Illness* 1:77, 1986.

371. Kirshenbaum LA, Mathews SC, Sitar DS, et al: Does multiple-dose charcoal therapy enhance salicylate excretion? *Arch Intern Med* 150:1281, 1990.

372. Prescott LF, Balali-Mood M, Critchley JAJH, et al: Diuresis or urinary alkalinisation for salicylate poisoning? *Br Med J* 285:1383, 1982.

373. Garella S: Extracorporeal techniques in the treatment of exogenous intoxications. *Kidney Int* 33:735, 1988.

374. Corkeron MA: Serotonin syndrome—a potentially fatal complication of antidepressant therapy. *Med J Aust* 163:481, 1995.

375. Power BM, Hackett LP, Dusci LJ, et al: Antidepressant toxicity and the need for identification and concentration monitoring in overdose. *Clin Pharmacokinet* 29:154, 1995.

376. Graber MA, Hoehns TB, Perry PJ: Sertraline-phenelzine drug interaction: A serotonin syndrome reaction. *Ann Pharmacother* 28:732, 1994.

377. Nemeroff CB, DeVane CL, Pollock BG: Newer antidepressants and the cytochrome P450 system. *Am J Psychiatr* 153:311, 1996.

378. Bodner RA, Lynch T, Lewis L, et al: Serotonin syndrome. *Neurology* 45:219, 1995.

379. Karle J, Bjorndal F: Serotonergic syndrome in combination therapy with lithium and fluoxetine. *Ugeskrift for Laeger* 157:1204, 1995.

380. Bastani JB, Troester MM, Bastani AJ: Serotonin syndrome and fluvoxamine: A case study. *Nebr Med J* 81:107, 1996.

381. Taylor IC, McConnell JG: Severe hyponatraemia associated with selective serotonin reuptake inhibitors. *Scott Med J* 40:147, 1995.

382. Goldstein L, Barker M, Segall F, et al: Seizure and transient SIADH associated with sertraline. *Am J Psychiatr* 153:732, 1996.

383. Lappin RI, Auchincloss EL: Treatment of the serotonin syndrome with cyproheptadine. *N Engl J Med* 331:1021, 1994.

384. Chan BS, Graudins A, Whyte IM, et al: Serotonin syndrome resulting from drug interactions. *Med J Aust* 16:523, 1988.

385. Gillman PK: Serotonin syndrome treated with chlorpromazine. *J Clin Psychopharm* 17:128, 1997.

386. Olson KR, Benowitz NL, Woo OF, et al: Theophylline overdose: Acute single ingestion versus chronic repeated overmedication. *Am J Emerg Med* 3:386, 1985.

387. Shannon M: Predictors of major toxicity after theophylline overdose. *Ann Intern Med* 119:1161, 1993.

388. Sessler CN: Theophylline toxicity and overdose: Predisposing factors, clinical features, and outcome of 116 consecutive cases. *Am J Med* 88:567, 1990.

389. Benowitz NL, Toffelmire EB: The use of hemodialysis and hemoperfusion in the treatment of theophylline intoxication. *Semin Dial* 6:243, 1993.

390. Sessler CN, Cohen MD: Cardiac arrhythmias during theophylline toxicity. A prospective continuous electrocardiographic study. *Chest* 98:672, 1990.

391. Hall KW, Dobson KE, Dalton JG, et al: Metabolic abnormalities associated with intentional theophylline overdose. *Ann Intern Med* 101:457, 1984.

392. Hoffman A, Pinto ED, Gilhar D: Effects of pretreatment with anticonvulsants on theophylline-induced seizures in the rat. *J Crit Care* 8:198, 1993.

393. Delanty N, Vaughan CJ, French JA: Medical causes of seizures. *Lancet* 352:383, 1998.

394. Greenberg A, Piraino BH, Kroboth PD: Severe theophylline toxicity. Role of conservative measures, antiarrhythmic agents, charcoal hemoperfusion. *Am J Med* 76:854, 1984.

395. Marchlinski FE, Miller JM: Atrial arrhythmias exacerbated by theophylline. Response to verapamil and evidence for triggered activity in man. *Chest* 88:931, 1985.

396. Kearney TE, Manoguerra AS, Curtis GP, et al: Theophylline toxicity and the beta-adrenergic system. *Ann Intern Med* 102:766, 1985.

397. Kempf J, Rusterholtz T, Ber C, et al: Haemodynamic study as guideline for the use of beta blockers. *Intensive Care Med* 22:585, 1996.

398. Seneff M, Scott J, Friedman B, et al: Acute theophylline toxicity and the use of esmolol to reverse cardiovascular instability. *Ann Emerg Med* 19:671, 1990.

399. Hootkins R, Lerman MJ, Thompson JR: Sequential and simultaneous "in series" hemodialysis and hemoperfusion in the management of theophylline intoxication. *J Am Soc Nephrol* 1:923, 1990.

400. Okada S, Teramoto S, Matsuoka R: Recovery from theophylline toxicity by continuous hemodialysis with filtration. *Ann Intern Med* 133:922, 2000.

401. Plowman DM, Reynolds TL, Joyce SM: Poisonous snakebite in Utah. *West J Med* 163:547, 1995.

402. Cold BS, Dart RC, Barish RA: Bites of venomous snakes. *N Engl J Med* 347:347, 2002.

403. Lewis JV, Portera CA Jr: Rattlesnake bite of the face: Case report and review of the literature. *Am Surg* 60:681, 1994.

404. Dart RC, Russell FE: Animal poisoning, in Hall JB, Schmidt GA, Wood LDH (eds): *Principles of Critical Care*. New York, McGraw-Hill, 1992, p 2163.

405. Stewart RM, Page CP, Schwesinger WH, et al: Antivenin and fasciotomy/debridement in the treatment of severe rattlesnake bite. *Am J Surg* 158:543, 1989.

406. Schaeffer RC Jr, Carlson RW, Puri VK, et al: The effects of colloidal and crystalloidal fluids on rattlesnake bite venom shock in the rat. *J Pharmacol Exp Ther* 206:687, 1978.

407. Davidson TM, Schafer SF: Rattlesnake bites. Guidelines for aggressive treatment. *Postgrad Med* 96:107, 1994.

Chapter 103

CRITICAL CARE PHARMACOLOGY

VIDYA KRISHNAN
THOMAS CORBRIDGE
PATRICK MURRAY

KEY POINTS

- *Critical care therapeutics should be individualized to maximize therapeutic effect while minimizing the potential for adverse drug reactions.*
- *The appropriate loading dose is determined primarily by the volume of distribution of the drug in the patient.*
- *The maintenance dose is proportional to the clearance and the desired steady-state plasma concentration.*
- *Elimination half-life is inversely proportional to clearance and directly proportional to volume of distribution.*
- *Steady-state conditions are obtained after the passage of three to five half-lives.*
- *Prospective consideration of possible drug-patient, drug-disease, and drug-drug interactions minimizes the potential for undertreatment or adverse drug reactions.*
- *Therapeutic drug monitoring may follow purely pharmacodynamic parameters or additionally use plasma levels to calculate pharmacokinetic parameters.*
- *Therapeutic drug monitoring attempts to ensure adequate therapy and to prevent, detect, and appropriately report adverse drug reactions.*
- *Systemwide changes in management of critically ill patients, including physician order entry systems and dedicated intensivists and pharmacists, can potentially decrease the incidence of adverse drug reactions.*

Individualization of critical care therapeutics through the application of pharmacologic principles is intended to reconcile important features of ICU management including polypharmacy, altered drug disposition, and cost considerations, in the design of a rational drug regimen. Critically ill patients routinely receive multiple medications, and the potential for adverse drug reactions (ADRs), particularly drug-drug interactions, increases in proportion to the number of agents received. Furthermore, physiologic changes resulting from critical illness may alter several aspects of drug disposition in a manner that is often difficult to predict based on available information. Finally, rational critical care therapeutics is a major component of providing cost-effective critical care, because of the substantial fraction of the average hospital pharmacy budget consumed by critical care therapeutic agents.

Individualization of pharmacotherapy attempts to avoid ADRs caused by drug overdosage or undertreatment, including ADRs caused by drug-disease, drug-drug, and drug-patient interactions. Correct drug dosing is frequently complicated in critical illness by alterations in bioavailability, volume of distribution, and elimination.[1] Errors in choosing a

therapeutic regimen are frequently poorly tolerated by these patients; rapid efficacy may be necessary for survival, but physiologic reserve may also be inadequate to withstand the effects of drug intoxication. Concentrating efforts on optimal dosing of drugs that have a low therapeutic index (low ratio of toxic to therapeutic plasma level) is therefore particularly important. Consideration of pharmacokinetic (PK) and pharmacodynamic (PD) principles, and their application to design an approximate patient model for individualized therapeutics, should precede addition of any new drug to an ICU patient's regimen. Furthermore, the dynamic physiology of these patients mandates frequent reassessment of the accuracy of this model, updating drug regimens as required. Therapeutic drug monitoring is used to titrate therapy with drugs that have both a low therapeutic index and readily measurable plasma concentrations that are proportional to drug effects (therapeutic and toxic). Finally, any change in the status of an ICU patient must be considered to be potentially the result of an adverse drug reaction, especially in the absence of a clear-cut explanation.

Pharmacokinetic and Pharmacodynamic Principles

Pharmacokinetics is the study of drug movement through the body,[2–7] encompassing all aspects of drug disposition ("what the body does to the drug"), including (1) entry, (2) distribution, and (3) elimination. The three most important quantifiable PK parameters considered in evaluating the disposition of a drug are therefore (1) bioavailability (fraction of administered dose reaching the systemic circulation), (2) volume of distribution, and (3) clearance (elimination by biotransformation and/or excretion). Pharmacokinetic models divide the body into one or more compartments (see below), so that drug disposition may be described by a series of mathematical equations. *Pharmacodynamics* refers to the relationship of drug movement to pharmacologic response ("what the drug does to the body"). The relationship between PK data and the PD phenomenon of drug effect is based on the drug-receptor complex theory, which states that there is a correlation between drug concentrations in the plasma and at the receptor site, and that drug effect is proportional to the extent of drug-receptor complex formation.

BIOAVAILABILITY

The fraction of administered drug reaching the systemic circulation is termed its *bioavailability*. Intravascular injection generally results in 100% bioavailability. Other parenteral routes (intramuscular, subcutaneous, transdermal, intraperitoneal, and inhalational) and enteral (oral, through enteral feeding tubes, and rectal) of administration often achieve bioavailability which is both less complete and less predictable, although selected agents administered by the sublingual, inhalational, and other routes may undergo extensive and rapid absorption. Formulation properties (e.g., elixir vs. tablet) and the physicochemical properties (e.g., lipid solubility and degree of ionization at gastric pH) of the administered drug can substantially affect systemic bioavailability, particularly following enteral administration. Enterally administered agents, except drugs administered by sublingual or rectal routes, are uniquely subjected to the potential influence of first-pass (presystemic) metabolism of drug by gut flora and by intestinal and liver enzymes (see below), which tends to decrease the systemic bioavailability of the parent compound.[4,6,8] Presystemic metabolism may result in the production of metabolites that are inactive (e.g., most propranolol metabolites), or active (4-hydroxypropranolol from propranolol, morphine from codeine, or enalaprilat from enalapril) following enteral substrate administration. Agents requiring metabolism to an active metabolite to elicit pharmacologic response, such as enalapril and codeine, are commonly referred to as *prodrugs*. Locally administered drugs (e.g., intraperitoneal antibiotics for peritonitis or intraocular β-blocking agents for glaucoma) are intended for local effects, but it is important to remember the potential systemic absorption and systemic effects of these drugs. In addition to the factors that determine extent of absorption, drug formulation can be manipulated to alter the rate of drug absorption (e.g., standard-release vs. extended-release preparations), which will in turn potentially blunt the peak drug concentration obtained after drug administration. Important considerations in choosing the route of drug administration in the critically ill patient will be further discussed below.

DRUG DISTRIBUTION AND ELIMINATION

The simplest compartmental PK model describes the body as a single homogenous compartment. An amount or dose of drug (D) is administered intravenously, instantaneously distributed into a space of volume (Vd), and the immediate serum or plasma concentration (C) measured. Given these simplifications, the volume of this theoretical compartment Vd (the apparent volume of distribution) may be calculated: Vd = D/C, since C = D/Vd. By assuming instantaneous distribution and concentration sampling (before any elimination has occurred), this model describes the theoretical volume into which the administered drug must be distributed in order to produce the observed drug concentration (Fig. 103-1*A*). The volume of distribution of most drugs does not usually correspond to a physiologic volume (such as the extracellular fluid volume [0.2 L/kg] or total body water space [0.5 to 0.7 L/kg]), but is often many times larger than the total body volume; drugs with a large volume of distribution are usually characterized by low plasma protein binding, high lipid solubility, and extensive tissue binding.

Drugs whose disposition may be described by a one-compartment kinetic model exhibit log-linear plasma concentrations as a function of time, thus exhibiting "simple" or "linear" pharmacokinetics (see Fig. 103-1*B*). Since the absolute rate of drug elimination is a linear function of its plasma concentration, and the fraction of drug eliminated per unit time is constant, a "first-order" kinetic model applies. Following a single intravenous bolus (and assumed instantaneous complete distribution), plasma drug concentration declines owing to a first-order elimination process (biotransformation and/or excretion), so that a semilogarithmic plot of the logarithm of plasma drug concentration (log Cp) versus time yields a linear graph. Back-extrapolation of this graph to time zero permits estimation of the plasma drug concentration immediately following the bolus (Cp₀), and thus an estimate of Vd, since Vd = D/C. The slope of this plot is called the elimination rate constant k (or k_e).

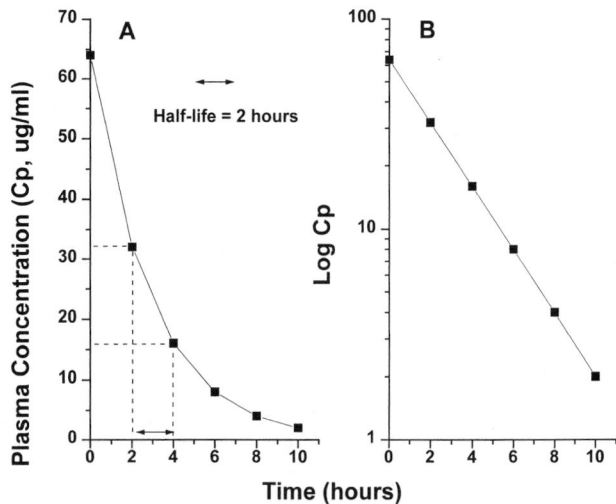

FIGURE 103-1 Linear pharmacokinetic profile with a single-compartment model. *A* depicts the plasma concentration (Cp, μg/mL) versus time (hours) curve following intravenous administration of an 800-mg drug dose to a 100-kg adult. The first plasma sample, obtained 2 hours after bolus administration, contains a measured drug concentration of 32 mg/mL. Subsequent samples reveal that the plasma drug concentration declines by 50% every 2 hours, consistent with an elimination half-life of 2 hours. *B* shows the semilog plot of the same data plotted in panel *A*. Log transformation of the plasma concentration values yields a linear plot, consistent with first-order elimination. Back-extrapolation to time 0 suggests that the plasma concentration at this time was 64 μg/mL (Cp₀); assuming instantaneous complete distribution, Vd is estimated (Vd = dose/Cp₀ = 800 mg divided by 64 μg/mL = 12.5 L, or 0.125 L/kg). The slope (k_e) of the log-linear plot is 0.3465 h^{-1}, consistent with the known half-life ($t_{1/2}$) of 2 hours (k_e= 0.693/$t_{1/2}$). Clearance (CL) may be estimated using the equation CL = k_e × Vd = 0.3465 × 12.5 = 4.33 L/h = 72 mL/min.

The kinetics of drug elimination by this first-order process are described by the equation:

$$Cp_{(T2)} = Cp_{(T1)}e^{-k(T2-T1)}$$

where $Cp_{(T2)}$ and $Cp_{(T1)}$ are the plasma drug concentrations at later and earlier measurement points, respectively; T2 − T1 is the time elapsed between these two time points; and k is the elimination rate constant (in units of time^{-1}).

The elimination half-life ($t_{1/2}$) of the drug, which is the amount of time required for the plasma drug concentration to decrease by 50%, can be determined from the elimination rate constant by the equation:

$$t_{1/2} = 0.693/k_e$$

Using the above equation, it can be shown that the drug concentration declines by 50% during each half-life, so that little of the bolus dose remains after four to five half-lives (Table 103-1). Alternatively, if a drug is eliminated by a *saturable* process, elimination may become saturated at high concentration, so that kinetics become zero-order (a constant *amount* of drug, rather than a constant *fraction*, is eliminated per unit time). The half-life of elimination of such agents is concentration-dependent, because of *capacity-limited* (saturable) clearance, and PK assessment requires the use of

TABLE 103-1 Number of Half-Lives Required to Eliminate a Drug Bolus by a First-Order Process

Number of Half-Lives	Percentage of Original Concentration
0	100.0
1	50.0
2	25.0
3	12.5
4	6.25
5	3.125

TABLE 103-2 Number of Half-Lives Required to Attain Steady-State Plasma Concentration (Cp$_{ss}$)

Number of Half-Lives	Percentage of Cp$_{ss}$, %
0	0.0
1	50.0
2	75.0
3	87.5
4	93.75
5	96.875

Michaelis-Menten kinetics. Small dose escalations may result in disproportionately large plasma concentration increments when the maximum metabolic capacity is exceeded. Ethanol, phenytoin, and salicylic acid are examples of drugs with capacity-limited clearance, and many other agents develop saturation of metabolic pathways in overdose (see Chap. 102).

If the same drug given above as a bolus to estimate simple (single-compartment) PK parameters is instead administered as a continuous intravenous infusion, and the rate of infusion exceeds the rate of simultaneous (first-order) elimination, then the plasma drug concentration will increase as accumulation occurs. Eventually, since the amount of drug excreted per unit time increases with increasing plasma drug concentration, the elimination rate becomes equal to the rate of administration; the plasma drug concentration at this time, which from then onward remains constant (unless the rates of administration or elimination change), is termed the *steady-state concentration* (Cp$_{ss}$) (Fig. 103-2, upper panel). Accumulation of an agent exhibiting linear pharmacokinetics proceeds in a fashion which is the mirror image of its elimination following a single intravenous bolus (Table 103-2). Accumulation of intermittently administered drugs differs from constant intravenous infusion only in the presence of peak and trough plasma drug concentration fluctuations; steady-state still develops over the same number of half-lives, with peak-

to-trough fluctuations around a mean Cp$_{ss}$ (see Fig. 103-2, lower panel). Therefore one can use the concept of half-life to estimate the time to attainment of a steady-state plasma drug level (and pharmacologic effect) following initiation of therapy, and to offset of drug effect following discontinuation of the agent, regardless of the dosing regimen in use.

The conceptually simple linear PK profile of a drug that fits a single-compartment model is actually inadequate to fully describe the disposition of most drugs. Multicompartmental models more accurately describe the rate and extent of drug shifts between these spaces, requiring multiple slope calculations to include the effects of intercompartmental distribution and elimination from the body (Fig. 103-3).[3] Such models divide the body into a *central* (the blood volume and highly perfused tissues, Vd$_c$) and one or more *peripheral* or *tissue* (fat, muscle, or skin) compartments. The final volume

FIGURE 103-3 Schematic representation of a two-compartment pharmacokinetic model. A variable fraction (F, bioavailability) of administered dose (D) reaches the systemic circulation and is then distributed. Initial distribution occurs into the vascular space and rapidly perfused tissues, comprising the central or initial compartment (Vd$_c$). Subsequently, further distribution into the peripheral or tissue compartment (Vd$_t$) occurs, at a rate quantified by the *distribution* half-life ($\alpha t_{1/2}$). During and after the initial distribution period, drug is eliminated by metabolism and/or excretion. Following complete distribution to Vd$_t$, the rate of plasma drug concentration decline is quantified by the *terminal* or *elimination* half-life ($\beta t_{1/2}$), which is directly proportional to Vd$_t$ and inversely proportional to clearance (CL).

FIGURE 103-2 Drug administration by continuous intravenous infusion (*upper panel*) or intermittent intravenous bolus (*lower panel*). Attainment of steady-state plasma concentration (Cp$_{ss}$) occurs after three to five half-lives, regardless of the dosing regimen. Peak and trough fluctuations around Cp$_{ss}$ are aimed to each be within the therapeutic range (therapeutic but subtoxic plasma levels).

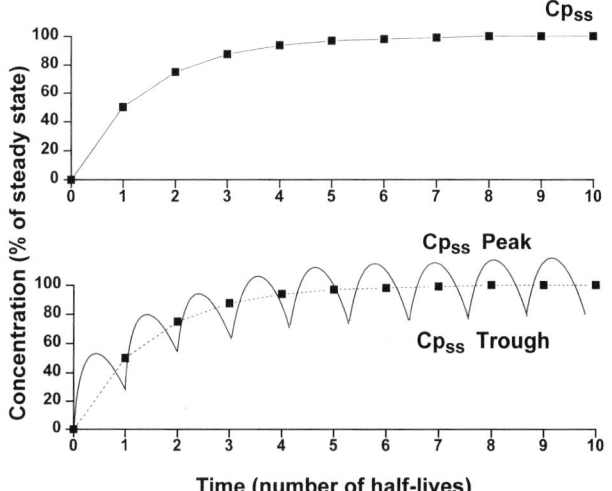

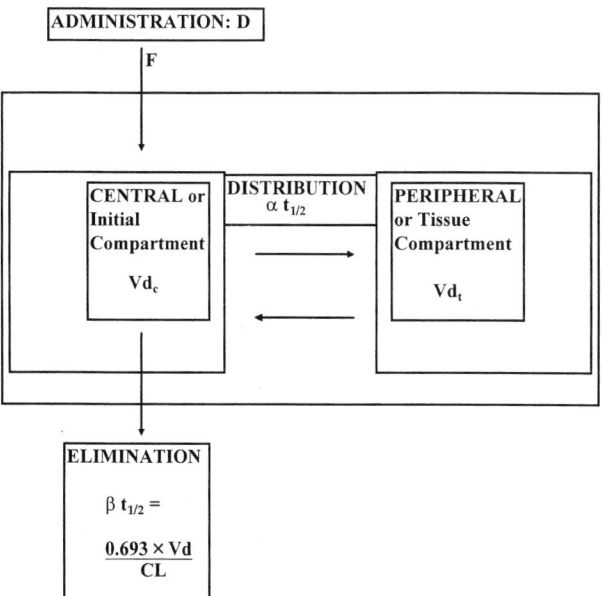

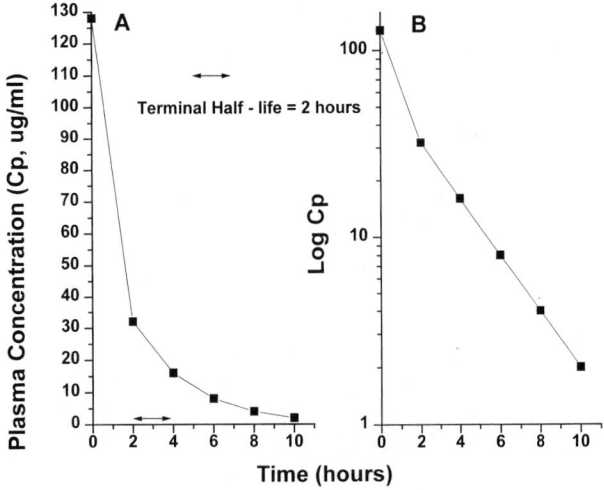

FIGURE 103-4 Linear pharmacokinetic profile with a two-compartment model. *A.* When earlier plasma samples are obtained following repetition of the same drug administration procedure described in Fig. 103-1, it is apparent that in fact this drug is distributed into two compartments rather than a single space. The earliest plasma sample, obtained *immediately* after administration of the drug bolus, contains 128 μg/mL (Cp$_0$) of the drug; the initial volume of distribution is thus 6.25 L or 0.0625 L/kg. By 2 hours postinjection this has declined to 32 μg/mL, as found in the Fig. 103-1 protocol; subsequently the plasma concentration declines as in Fig. 103-1. *B.* Log transformation of the plasma concentration values now reveals multiexponential kinetics, with two distinct slopes, indicating a more rapid early decline owing to a combination of drug distribution and simultaneous elimination, followed by a second phase owing to elimination only (postdistribution).

of distribution (Vd$_{tot}$) reflects the sum of central and tissue compartments. Vd$_c$ is calculated by measuring the instantaneous plasma concentration (Cp$_0$) after an intravenous drug dose is administered (Fig. 103-4*A*), then Vd$_{tot}$ is calculated by back-extrapolation from the *elimination* phase of the plasma concentration versus time curve to the y-axis (concentration) at zero time (see Fig. 103-4*B*). The two-compartment model also involves consideration of another aspect of drug distribution: the rate of distribution of drug from the central to the final volume of distribution is quantified by the *distribution half-life* ($\alpha t_{1/2}$), although some of the decline in plasma drug concentration during this period often is due to simultaneous drug elimination during the initial distribution phase. The *elimination half-life* ($\beta t_{1/2}$) corresponds to the half-life considered using a single-compartment approach.

Despite these refinements, the principles of linear pharmacokinetics hold for most agents in practice. Thus from a semilog plot [log concentration (y) versus time (x)], the slope is k$_e$ (the elimination rate constant) following full distribution (Vd$_{tot}$), and the rate of drug clearance (CL) is based on the balance of distribution and excretion rates:

$$CL = -k_e \times Vd_{tot}(min^{-1} \cdot mL)$$

It is often incorrectly assumed that CL may be calculated from this equation. In fact, both CL and Vd$_{tot}$ are quantified to determine k$_e$. In other words, CL and Vd$_{tot}$ determine k$_e$: CL is a physiologic value, a measurement of the volume of plasma from which a substance is completely cleared per unit time (in units of volume per unit time, usually milliliters per minute); Vd$_{tot}$ is a theoretical volume determined by a post-distribution plasma concentration measurement; thus k$_e$ is a derived variable, and the rate of elimination may thus be considered to reflect the balance of drug distribution to tissues and drug elimination from the body,[9] so that it is useful to consider this relationship as follows:

$$k_e = CL/Vd_{tot}$$

and, since

$$t_{1/2} = 0.693/k_e$$

then

$$t_{1/2} = (0.693 \times Vd_{tot})/CL$$

In other words, the elimination half-life of drug is prolonged by a large volume of distribution or low clearance value, and shortened by limited distribution or a vigorous clearance process.[6] The measured clearance of a substance (CL$_{TOT}$) usually represents the algebraic sum of several clearance processes; in many cases, this may be represented as follows:

$$CL_{TOT} = CL_{renal} + CL_{hepatic} + CL_{other}$$

For most drugs, it is appropriate to consider the magnitude of each of these component processes and the effects of the altered physiology of critical illness on their relative importance in achieving clearance of parent drug and metabolites. Clearance of any agent by an eliminating organ is proportional to, but cannot exceed, blood flow to the eliminating organ: CL = Q $\times$ (C$_A$ − C$_V$), where Q is organ blood flow, and C$_A$ and C$_V$ are the drug concentrations in the arterial and venous blood supplies to the eliminating organ, respectively. These and other PK parameters relevant to the individualization of critical care drug therapeutics will be discussed below.

PHARMACODYNAMIC MODELING

It is a basic tenet of the above approach that pharmacologic response is proportional to plasma drug concentration. Four additional determinants of pharmacologic response merit emphasis in this regard: (1) the "effect site" concept, (2) the importance of the free (unbound) plasma drug concentration, (3) interindividual variability in drug response, and (4) dose-dependent alterations in receptor activation and pharmacologic effect.

EFFECT SITE

The *effect site* concept was introduced to more completely describe the relationship of drug disposition to pharmacologic response. This term refers to the tissue compartment containing the receptors that must be bound in order to elicit drug effect.[10] If the effect site is located in a rapidly perfused compartment (Vd$_c$), then intravenous drug administration will elicit immediate pharmacologic response. The antiarrhythmic effect of lidocaine is an example of such behavior, and thus initial serum lidocaine levels correlate directly with drug effect. In fact, the well-established practice of empirically administering additional lidocaine boluses following an initial load is based on the necessity of maintaining adequate serum levels, which tend to decline as the drug distributes into other tissues or is eliminated.[3,11] The distribution half-life ($\alpha t_{1/2}$) of lidocaine is only 8 minutes (see Fig. 103-3), so the plasma level following an initial bolus may decline to subtherapeutic levels before a simultaneously administered continuous infusion results in drug accumulation sufficient to attain the desired steady-state plasma level (Cp_{ss}). By contrast, plasma digoxin levels do not correlate with drug effect until the postdistribution phase (2 to 4 hours following an IV bolus), because distribution to tissues is required for binding to the target tissue receptors. The usual total digoxin loading dose of 1 mg is generally administered in smaller fractions (typically 0.5 mg first, with 0.25 mg following at 6 and 12 hours later), because the full effects of each loading dose fraction cannot be assessed until tissue distribution has occurred, at which time the loading procedure can continue, if it is necessary and safe to do so.

FREE OR UNBOUND PLASMA DRUG CONCENTRATION

Only free (unbound) drug is available for receptor binding, so that alterations in plasma protein binding may profoundly affect the interpretability of measured total (free plus bound) plasma drug concentrations. For example, plasma protein binding of phenytoin is diminished by either hypoalbuminemia or uremia, the former owing to lesser absolute availability of albumin binding sites, and the latter thought to be a result of competitive occupancy of these sites by "uremic substances." As a result of this phenomenon, total plasma phenytoin concentrations are often misleading in such patients. Phenytoin is normally 90% plasma protein-bound, so that the usual total plasma concentration range is 10 to 20 mg/L, and the free level is 1 to 2 mg/L. If plasma albumin is decreased from 4 g/dL to 2 g/dL, then an apparently therapeutic total plasma phenytoin level of 16 mg/L may be associated with a toxic free phenytoin level of over 7 mg/L; this is because the unbound or free fraction increases from the customary 10% toward 50%. It is therefore wise to monitor plasma free phenytoin levels in patients with hypoalbuminemia or renal insufficiency.

INTERINDIVIDUAL RESPONSE VARIABILITY (SENSITIVITY)

Another point to note is the variability between individual responses to a given plasma drug level; sensitivity to drug action may differ between individuals or groups. For example, elderly subjects are more sensitive to the sedative effects of benzodiazepines (and many other sedatives) than younger subjects;[12] American subjects of Chinese descent are twice as sensitive as American white men to the β-blocking effects of propranolol;[13] black subjects are less sensitive to the vasodilatory effect of isoproterenol than are white Americans.[14] Recent evidence implicates pharmacogenomics as the cause of variability of drug effect between races, and even individuals within races.[15]

DOSE-DEPENDENT EFFECTS

The predominant drug-receptor complex mediating a drug's effect may change according to drug concentration, resulting in variable pharmacologic responses at different plasma levels. For example, dopamine predominantly activates dopaminergic receptors (and causes mesenteric and renal vasodilation) only at infusion rates of up to 2 μg/kg per minute. β_1-Adrenergic (inotropic) and α-adrenergic (vasoconstrictor) activation occur at doses as low as 2 to 4 μg/kg per minute and 5 to 10 μg/kg per minute, respectively; as a result, the hemodynamic effect of dopamine infusion changes with increasing dose.[15] Despite such concerns, we expect the attainment of drug levels in the usual therapeutic range to elicit the desired effect in most patients.

Most drugs used in the ICU are dosed according to broadly applicable population-based PK and PD parameters and titrated to pharmacologic response only if this is readily quantifiable, rather than being subjected to rigorous PK modeling with therapeutic drug level monitoring. The latter approach is applied to drugs that have a low therapeutic index and plasma drug concentrations that correlate with drug effect. The intermediate-complexity approach of monitoring physiologic parameters (PD monitoring) of drug effect is more readily applied in the ICU (and operating room) than in other patient care settings because of the routine use of monitoring devices. Sedation, neuromuscular paralysis, seizure suppression, diuretic agent action, and the effects of cardiovascular drugs (antiarrhythmic, chronotropic, inotropic, vasodilator, and vasoconstrictor actions) and bronchodilators are commonly assessed in this fashion, in conjunction with formal PK monitoring using drug levels for appropriate agents.

What follows is a framework for drug administration based upon physiologic modeling of the patient and application of known drug characteristics to this patient model, in order to optimize ICU therapeutics and minimize the potential for iatrogenic adverse events. Furthermore, this approach includes routine surveillance to prevent adverse drug reactions, and to assess the potential for such a phenomenon to be the underlying cause of a change in patient status.

Individualization of Drug Therapy in the ICU: An Approach to Rational Drug Dosing in Critically Ill Patients

The PK and PD principles outlined above may be applied routinely to attempt optimal design of drug regimens for ICU patients. As shown in Fig. 103-5, focused consideration of PK and PD parameters to answer a series of questions can provide a framework for therapeutic individualization. Individualization of drug therapy requires consideration of the effects of multiple factors responsible for variability in drug response (aside from disease severity); these include: (1) drug-patient interactions (including body habitus, age, gender, and race); (2) drug-disease interactions; and (3) drug-drug interactions. This approach only yields an approximation of ideal therapeutics, because information addressing drug disposition in this population is often incomplete, and its interpretation is further complicated by the dynamic physiology of critical illness. This method simply attempts to maximize the potential for rational therapy based upon available information. As a result, any drug regimen in critically ill patients requires early and frequent reassessment. The customary prudent approach to drug dosing in settings in which altered disposition is anticipated but poorly quantifiable, embodied in the phrase "start low and go slow," is generally inappropriate in this setting, in which immediate therapeutic effect may be vital. Nevertheless, a rational approach to critical care therapeutics should

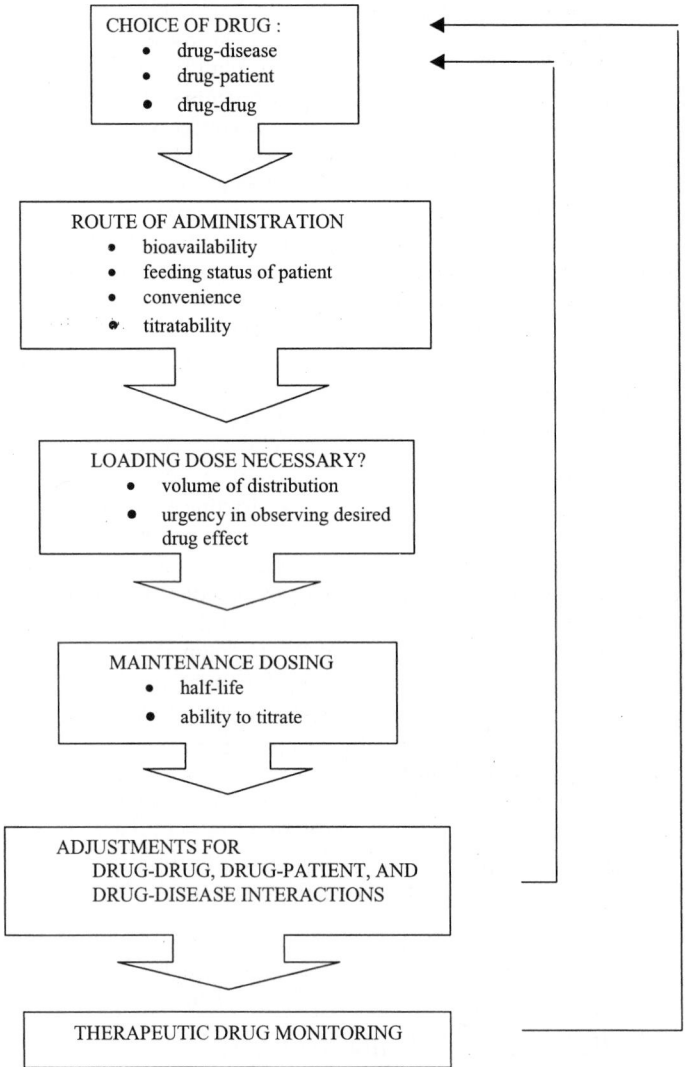

FIGURE 103-5 Flowchart for a suggested method of design for a rational drug dosing regimen. This illustration serves to depict the process of drug prescription and dosing as a perpetual cycle of actions. Individualization of drug therapy involves careful consideration of the patient's unique clinical status for each step along the path of drug prescription and dosing. The initial choice of drug, route of administration, loading dose, and maintenance dose calculations involve consideration of desired drug effects, titratability, and convenience. Modifications of the dosing regimen may be required to accommodate the individual characteristics of the patient, including allergies, age, sex, and race; potential drug-drug interactions; and potentially confounding disease states. Once a drug regimen is designed and implemented, therapeutic drug monitoring is indicated to ensure adequate drug effect and to minimize potential adverse events. The results of therapeutic drug monitoring may indicate the need for further modification of the drug regimen.

reduce the incidence of iatrogenic pharmacotherapeutic complications of critical illness.

The key principles underlying this approach, which relates PK parameters to choices of drug regimen, may be summarized as follows:

1. The appropriate loading dose is determined by estimation of the volume of distribution of the agent in the patient; the regimen for administering this dose is chosen based upon the desired effect site and the distribution half-life for the agent.
2. The maintenance dose is chosen to equal the elimination rate of the agent at steady state (the product of $CL \times Cp_{ss}$).
3. Steady-state plasma drug level and stable drug effect are not obtained until three to five half-lives (see Table 103-2 and Fig. 103-2) have passed.
4. Many adverse drug reactions are predictable and preventable by individualization of therapeutics and by consideration of known or potential drug interactions.

Patient characteristics are used to estimate physiologic and pathophysiologic variables affecting drug disposition. Several patient characteristics should be routinely consid-

ered, including age, gender, drug allergies, body habitus, volume status, plasma protein concentrations, and parameters of organ function (gastrointestinal tract, circulatory, renal, and liver function).

Age, gender, body habitus, and volume status are variables used to estimate expected parameters of drug disposition, based upon population PK/PD data. For most dosing calculations, the lesser of lean (or ideal) and actual body weight is used. Lean body weight (LBW) is calculated from the patient's height: For males, LBW (kg) = $50 + (2.3 \times$ each inch above 5 feet). For females, LBW (kg) = $45.5 + (2.3 \times$ each inch above feet). Some drugs are dosed according to actual weight or to patient body surface area, the latter obtainable from published nomograms using height and weight.

Using these data, we approach the design of individualized drug therapy for ICU patients as follows:

ROUTE OF DRUG ADMINISTRATION

Oral bioavailability of the agent may be inadequate to achieve systemic effect owing to luminal conditions (alkaline pH or tube feeds) or first-pass metabolism (by luminal bacteria, intestinal enzymes, or hepatic enzymes). Intravenous drug administration is often preferred in the ICU, even for administration of highly bioavailable drugs, for several reasons. Rapid onset and offset of effect may be desirable to rapidly initiate therapy, while retaining the capacity for titration. Gastrointestinal dysfunction (ileus or bowel wall edema) may also result in unpredictable drug delivery by the enteral route, although there is no evidence (in subjects with decompensated congestive heart failure, renal failure, or cirrhosis) that this theoretical concern is actually relevant.[17] Formulation properties (e.g., extended-release preparations) do not affect the extent of absorption, but rather the rate of absorption and potentially the peak drug concentration after each dose.

LOADING DOSE

Many therapies initiated in the ICU are intended to have a rapid onset of effect. Whether administered by continuous intravenous infusion or by intermittent intravenous bolus or oral dosing, plasma drug concentration and therapeutic effect will not reach steady-state levels until three to five half-lives have passed; such a delay may be unacceptable, particularly for drugs which have a prolonged half-life (which may be a normal feature of a drug's disposition [e.g., digoxin], or caused by organ dysfunction and impaired elimination [e.g., aminoglycosides with renal failure]). Conversely, drugs that have a very short half-life (e.g., nitrovasodilators, esmolol, atracurium, and propofol) may achieve a rapid therapeutic effect when administered by infusion but without a loading bolus, since three to five half-lives pass in a matter of minutes. Administration of a loading dose, calculated as follows, rapidly achieves the desired target level (but does not alter the time required to attain steady-state conditions):

$$\text{Loading dose} = Vd \times Cp$$

where Cp is the desired plasma concentration.

The appropriate loading dose is primarily determined by the distribution characteristics of the drug (Vd) and the body habitus and volume status of the patient. Usual volume of distribution values are readily available for most drugs; however, the effects of alterations in body habitus, nutrition, and volume status are much more difficult to quantify. Estimates of drug distribution characteristics are further confounded in critically ill patients by dynamic hypercatabolic losses of fat and lean body mass, accompanied by massive third-space volume retention or intravascular volume depletion, often associated with development of hypoalbuminemia and relative hyperglobulinemia. Following a period of marked positive fluid balance in a hospitalized patient, the weight increment may be used to estimate the total body water increase. Otherwise, estimates of altered body water content are usually empiric, although therapeutics in some specific disease states have been studied in sufficient detail to provide useful information. For example, a decreased aminoglycoside loading dose is required in volume-depleted acute renal failure. Furthermore, "uremic substances" that accumulate in renal failure appear to displace some drugs from tissue-binding sites, thus reducing their Vd regardless of volume status. As a result, the appropriate digoxin loading dose is decreased by 50% in the presence of renal failure; Vd is also decreased for methotrexate and insulin in renal failure patients. Conversely, edematous states such as sepsis,[18,19] cirrhosis, nephrosis, and

congestive heart failure often increase Vd. Determination of the ideal or lean body weight is difficult in the presence of obesity, cachexia, or combinations of the above factors, such as in a typical hypercatabolic patient with sepsis, acute renal failure, and postresuscitation volume overload. Loading dose regimens may also be altered based upon the relationship between the desired onset of effect to the distribution pattern at the effect site, as discussed above in contrasting the standard loading dose regimens for lidocaine and digoxin.

Volume of distribution for a given drug is reported in units of volume per weight in a normal patient. In the critically ill patient, the alterations in weight and body fluid compartments will alter the distribution of the drug. A reasonable approach to approximate these alterations in the calculation of the loading dose of hydrophilic drugs is to adjust the normal volume of distribution in proportion to the estimation of the patient's water compartment. It is reasonable to assume that water comprises approximately 10% of adipose tissue weight (estimated as actual body weight minus lean body weight). Additionally, the net weight gain secondary to fluid resuscitation will contribute to the volume of distribution for water-soluble drugs. Mathematically, we can express this by the following:

$$
\begin{aligned}
\text{Adjusted Vd} = {} & (\text{Vd based on ideal body weight}) \\
& + (10\% \text{ of adipose tissue weight}) \\
& + (\text{net weight gain from fluid resuscitation})
\end{aligned}
$$

MAINTENANCE DOSE

ADMINISTRATION REGIMEN

In the critical care setting, the administration regimen usually consists of a choice between intermittent intravenous bolus therapy and continuous intravenous infusion. Factors considered in this decision include: drug characteristics (half-life and therapeutic index), patient characteristics, the desired pharmacologic effect, and cost/staffing considerations. When drugs with a low therapeutic index are dosed intermittently, the fluctuations (peak-to-trough) of plasma concentration may require formal monitoring of plasma concentrations and PK parameter estimates to ensure adequate therapy without toxicity. Administration by infusion eliminates the peak-to-trough plasma concentration fluctuations associated with intermittent parenteral boluses, which may be accompanied not only by failure to achieve continuous therapeutic effect, but also by activation of rebound counterregulatory effects during trough periods (negating prior and subsequent drug action). Continuous intravenous infusion may thus improve therapeutic efficacy of some agents. Loop diuretic agent infusions have been reported to augment sodium excretion compared to equivalent intermittent dosing, probably because of a combination of effects: increased cumulative renal tubular diuretic agent exposure (the product of time and concentration) and avoidance of periods of physiologic rebound salt conservation.[20,21] Since diuretic effect onset is delayed when using only continuous intravenous infusion (until drug accumulates; see Fig. 103-2), the ideal regimen to maximize natriuresis may include an initial bolus dose to achieve the required luminal threshold drug concentration and induce immediate natriuresis. Likewise, gastric acidity is also far better controlled by continuous intravenous infusion of H_2 blockers than by equivalent intermittent dosing.[22]

Continuous infusion of short-acting agents may also be desirable to allow titration of effect; nitrovasodilators, esmolol, propofol, and atracurium may be used for optimal control of vasodilation, β-blockade, sedation, or neuromuscular paralysis, respectively. It is widely assumed that continuous infusion of agents that have a short elimination half-life guarantees rapid reversal of drug effect following cessation of the infusion, but various factors may retard offset of effect, as is the case for reversal of sedation using agents administered by continuous infusion.[23,24] Potential explanations for such alterations in drug disposition or response during continuous infusion compared to intermittent bolus therapy include compartmentalized tissue distribution, accumulation of active metabolites, or saturation of clearance mechanisms. Intermittent bolus administration titrated to specific sedation parameters is less likely than continuous infusion to result in undetected drug or metabolite accumulation if excretory mechanisms deteriorate or become saturated, unless a routine assessment of time to awakening is performed daily in patients receiving continuous infusion. Clinically, it has been shown that daily interruption of sedation of mechanically ventilated patients results in decreased duration of ventilation, likely due to the minimization of drug accumulation.[25] Conversely, tolerance to the effects of several drugs (a pharmacodynamic phenomenon) occurs if a drug-free interval cannot be included in the administration regimen, requiring escalating dosages of agents such as nitroglycerin, dobutamine, and opiate analgesics to maintain a therapeutic effect. Finally, the convenience for nursing staff of administering agents by continuous infusion rather than intermittent bolus translates into decreased staffing expenditures.

CLEARANCE

Clearance includes all processes that eliminate the drug from the body—both excretion and biotransformation. Because the total body clearance of a drug involves the actions of multiple organ systems, the estimation of the predominant rate of elimination and route of elimination is often complicated, and warrants further discussion.

What is the Predicted Elimination Rate of the Drug?

The predicted elimination of the drug usually corresponds to the drug administration regimen that elicits an optimal therapeutic response in most subjects. Agents with a low therapeutic index may be subjected to therapeutic drug monitoring, aiming for a maintenance dose equaling the product of $CL \times Cp_{ss}$. The desired Cp_{ss} is selected based on the therapeutic response required (e.g., target plasma lidocaine level for suppression of ventricular arrhythmias) and the clearance rate is estimated based on published data (usually obtained from healthy patients). At steady state, the rate of administration (Ra) equals the rate of excretion (Re). Ra is dose (mg) divided by interval (minutes), and Re is CL (mL/min) $\times$ Cp_{ss} (mg/mL).

What are the Predominant Routes of Elimination of the Parent Drug and Its Metabolites (Particularly Those that Are Pharmacologically Active or Toxic)?

Renal insufficiency (Table 103-3), hepatic disease (Table 103-4), or circulatory dysfunction (Table 103-5) may affect clearance of parent drug or metabolites. There are several well-known examples of drugs with metabolites that are phar-

TABLE 103-3 Effects of Renal Failure on Drug Disposition and Effect

Bioavailability
Absorption of specific drugs may impaired by increased gastric pH (because of gastric urease-produced ammonia), chelation by orally-administrered phosphate-binding agents, or by bowel wall edema. Conversely, bioavailability may be increased by uremia-induced impairment of first-pass metabilism. Uremic effects on intestinal motility (ileus) affect the rate, rather than the extent, of drug absorption, unless emesis result in loss of ingested drug.

Protein binding
Binding of acidic drugs to albumin is decreased, because of competition with accumulated organic acids, and because of uremia-induced structural changes in albumin, which decrease drug-binding affinity (e.g., barbiturates, cephalosporins,. penicillins, phenytoin, salicylate, sulfonamides, valproate, warfarin).

Volume of distribution
Vd may be altered in the presence of renal failure. Drugs which are acidic, are highly protein-bound, and have a small volume of distribution are likely to be significantly affected. Other drugs may also be affected (e.g., aminoglycosides [volume status effects]), digoxin (displacement from tissue sites by ["uremic substances"]).

Biotransformation
Nonrenal (i.e., hepatic) clearance may be impaired. This phenomenon is best characterized in chronic renal insufficiency (rather than acute renal failure), affecting oxidative metabolism (phase I enzymes). Conversely, phenytoin clearance is augmented.

Excretion
Drugs which are more than 30% eliminated unchanged in the urine are likely to have significantly diminished CL in the presence of renal insufficiency. This results in a prolonged half-life for elimination of drugs such as digoxin, aminoglycosides, insulin, and others. The renal excretory route may assume increased importance in clearance of some drugs in the presence of hepatic impairment. Other drugs have toxic or active metabolites requiring renal elimination (Table 103-6). If dialysis or hemofiltration is required, drug removal may be significant.

Pharmacodynamic effects
Some drugs, such as sedative agents, may have enhanced effect in combination with the uremic milieu. Electrolyte abnormalities and acidosis may alter affects of drugs such as antiarrhythmic agents.

macologically active or even toxic. Accumulation of active or toxic metabolites in the presence of renal failure is probably the most common clinical scenario in which this feature of drug disposition is important (Table 103-6). Nonrenal (usually hepatic) elimination of parent drug or metabolites has been increasingly documented to be quantitatively important in subjects with renal impairment (as discussed below). Likewise, renal drug or metabolite elimination assumes an increased role in subjects with liver disease.

Is a Dose Reduction or Escalation Required, Owing to Impaired (Renal, Hepatic, or Circulatory Dysfunction) or Augmented (Induction of Metabolism or Extracorporeal Drug Removal) Clearance of the Drug or Its Metabolites?

As outlined below, glomerular filtration rate (GFR) may be estimated routinely to a reasonable approximation, and the

TABLE 103-4 Effects of Liver Dysfunction on Drug Disposition and Effect

Bioavailability

Drugs which undergo extensive first-pass metabolism may have a significantly higher oral bioavailability in cirrhotics than in normal subjects. Impaired drug absorption because of bowel wall edema has not been found in studies of cirrhotic subjects. GI hypomotility may delay peak response to enterally-administered drugs in these patients.

Protein binding

Hypoalbuminemia or altered glycoprotein levels may significantly affect the fractional protein binding of acidic or basic drugs, respectively. Monitoring of free drug levels may be indicated. In addition, drug-drug interactions by displacement from plasma protein binding sites may become important when biotransformation is concomitantly impaired.

Volume of distribution

Altered plasma protein concentrations may affect the extent of tissue distribution of drugs which are normally highly protin-bound. The presence of significant edema and ascites may alter she Vd of highly water-soluble agents (e.g., aminoglycosides).

Biotranformation

The presence of cirrhosis may result in some decrease in drug clearance, though not predictably so. Specific information regarding use of each agent prescribed in patients with a type and severity of liver disease similar to the patient in question should be sought, if possible.

Excretion

Renal elimination of drug or metabolites may be impired by concomitant renal insufficiency, which may be unsuspected based upon a "inappropriately" low serum creatinine in patients with severe liver disease.

Pharmacodynamic effects

Sedative effects (and side effects) of drugs may be augmented in patients with liver disease.

TABLE 103-5 Effects of Congestive Heart Failure (CHF) on Drug Disposition and Effect

Bioavailability

Impaired drug absorption because of bowel wall edema. Passive hepatic congestion may alter first-pass metabolism. Peripheral edema inhibits absorption of nonintravenous parenteral routes.

Protein binding

Protein amount and function is altered to the extent that renal and liver function is compromised with circulatory failure. In addition, competitive binding of plasma proteins may accur with common CHF therapy agents (e.g., furosemide).

Volume of distribution

The presence significant edema and pulmonery edema may alter the Vd of highly water-soluble agents (e.g., aminoglycosides).

Biotransformation

Hypoperfusion of liver may alter drug metabolizing enzyme function, especially with flow-dependent drugs (e.g., lidocaine).

Extretion

Renal elimination is decreased to extent that reanal and liver function are compromised by circulatory dysfunction; hepatic elimination is limited in flow-dependent drugs (e.g., lidocaine).

Pharmacodynamic effects

Increased sinsitivity to negative inotropes at therapeutic doses. Increased arrhythmic potential with antiarrhythmic drugs. Patients with CHF are more prone to contrast nephropathy.

TABLE 103-6 Selected Drugs Which Have Active Metabolites Requiring Renal Excretion

Drug	Metabolite
Acebutolol	N-Acetylacebutolol
Allopurinol	Oxypurinol
Atracurium	Laudanoside
Azathioprine	Mercaptopurine
Cimetidine	Cimetidine sulfoxide
Cyclophosphamide	4-Hydroxycyclophosphamide, others
Digitoxin	Digoxin
Disopyramide	Mono-N-desisopropyldisopyramide (MND)
Flecainide	Meta-O-Dealkylflecainide
Hydroxyzine	Cetirizine
Ifosfamide	4-Hydroxyifosfamide, others
Meperidine	Normeperidine
Metoprolol	α-Hydroxymetoprolol
Morphine	Morphine-6-glucuronide
Nitroprusside	Thiocyanate
Pancuronium	3-OH-pancuronium
Procainamide	N-Acetyl-procainamide (NAPA)
Propafenone	5-Hydroxypropafenone
Propoxyphene	Norpropoxyphene
Sulfonamides	Acetyl- metabolites
Tolbutamide	Hydroxy- and carboxy-tolbutamide
Vecuronium	3-Desacetylvecuronium

SOURCE: Modified with permission from Brater.[38]

effects of renal dysfunction on drug clearance may be estimated with some degree of precision (see Table 103-3). The effects of varying levels and etiologies of hepatic and circulatory dysfunction (see Tables 103-4 and 103-5) on drug disposition are far more difficult to predict. Estimation of renal and hepatic clearance functions and factors that alter drug metabolism and excretion will be further discussed below. Biliary, pulmonary, cutaneous, and extracorporeal elimination may be important for clearance of some specific agents and will not be discussed in detail here. For further information regarding drug clearance by extracorporeal devices, see Chap. 102; as a general rule, an increase in drug clearance by 30% or more is regarded as significant. Dialyzability by hemodialysis (HD) or peritoneal dialysis is suggested by water solubility, low molecular weight (<500 Da; up to 5000 Da with high-flux membranes), low protein binding (<90%), small volume of distribution (Vd <1 L/kg), and a low intrinsic clearance (<500 mL/70 kg per minute).[3] HD clearance is additionally affected by the porosity and surface area of the membrane used, and the blood pump and dialysate flow rates. Drug clearance by hemofiltration (slow continuous ultrafiltration, continuous arteriovenous hemofiltration, or continuous venovenous hemofiltration) may be achieved by either transmembrane sieving (convection) or membrane drug adsorption (e.g., it requires 20 mg of aminoglycosides such as gentamicin or tobramycin, which are polycationic, to saturate each new AN69 hemofilter, which is anionic); the addition of diffusive clearance by use of countercurrent dialysate flow (continuous arteriovenous hemodiafiltration or continuous venovenous hemodiafiltration) augments small-solute clearance (since the capacity of these substances to cross the membrane is limited by the concentration gradient, not particle size). Data regarding altered drug disposition (changes in Vd or clearance) induced by extracorporeal membrane oxygenation (ECMO) or plasmapheresis are available only for agents which have been specifically studied (e.g., aminoglycosides, opiates, and phenytoin), and in the case of ECMO, studies have been performed almost exclusively in pediatric patient populations.

RENAL EXCRETION

Renal clearance of drugs or metabolites is usually achieved by glomerular filtration, and diminished clearance owing to renal insufficiency is therefore proportional, caused by a decline of GFR. Renal blood flow (RBF) averages approximately 1300 mL/min, which is about 20% to 25% of cardiac output. Renal plasma flow (RPF, 650 mL/min) is about 50% of RBF, and 20% of RPF undergoes glomerular filtration, so that GFR averages 130 mL/min. The remaining 80% of RPF circulates in peritubular capillaries, where constituents may be secreted into or reabsorbed from renal tubules. Only 1.8 L of urine is produced from the 190 L per 24 hours of daily glomerular filtrate (130 mL/min × 1440 minutes), because water and most solutes are predominantly reabsorbed (e.g., the fractional excretion of sodium in a stable subject is 1%, thus 99% of filtered sodium is reabsorbed).

Glomerular filtration of plasma constituents is primarily limited by size ($\leq$50,000 Da), water solubility, plasma protein binding (only free drug is filtered), and volume of distribution (extensively tissue-bound substances are less likely to be renally excreted).[4,6] Some drugs also undergo significant renal tubular secretion or reabsorption (passive or active). Passive reabsorption of weak acids or bases from the renal tubular lumen may be influenced by urinary alkalization or acidification, respectively. Active tubular secretion by proximal tubular cationic or anionic pumps may be subject to competitive inhibition, resulting in decreased renal clearance and prolonged plasma half-life of the lower affinity substance. For example, probenecid inhibits tubular penicillin secretion, prolonging penicillin elimination half-life. Similarly, trimethoprim and cimetidine inhibit renal tubular creatinine secretion, reducing creatinine clearance and elevating serum creatinine, without affecting actual GFR (see below).

The plasma clearance of creatinine (creatinine clearance; CrCl) provides a close approximation of GFR, because creatinine is produced from muscle at a constant rate and freely filtered (it has a molecular weight of 113 Da, is water soluble, and is not protein bound). The amount of creatinine filtered (the product of the GFR and the plasma creatinine, PCr) is (theoretically) equal to the amount of creatinine excreted during the same period (the product of the urine creatinine concentration UCr, and the urine flow rate V); thus, GFR = (UCr × V)/PCr. Measurement of CrCl requires a timed urine collection to quantify the urinary excretion rate and a midpoint plasma creatinine sample (PCr). CrCl normally slightly overestimates GFR because some plasma creatinine is also secreted by renal tubules, augmenting the measured clearance value beyond that due to filtration. This effect is magnified with the development of progressive glomerular disease, as hypersecretion of creatinine by remnant tubules accounts for an increasing fraction of declining serial CrCl values.[26] In critically ill patients, collection of a urine sample during a period of stable renal function with a steady plasma creatinine value may not be possible; short (0.5- to 4-hour) collections have been used in an attempt to overcome this problem. Inulin

clearance more closely approximates GFR, but is impractical for clinical use, since determination requires inulin infusion, and the assay is difficult to perform. Other clearance techniques are equally impractical for routine clinical use, and more complex devices measuring real-time changes in renal function are not widely available for clinical applications at this time.[27]

The steady-state serum creatinine concentration is commonly applied to the Cockcroft-Gault formula to estimate GFR, without urinary collection, because of the relationship between patient age and weight (muscle mass), serum creatinine value, and CrCl.[28] For males:

$$CrCl \ (mL/min) = \frac{(140 - age) \ (weight \ in \ kg)}{72 \times SCr_{ss}}$$

For females multiply the above value by 0.85.

Confounding factors include: requirement of a steady-state serum creatinine value (SCr_{ss}), estimation of ideal body weight, the empiricism of the age and gender estimates used in development of the formula,[29–31] and the effects of some medications on tubular creatinine secretion.[32] It is particularly difficult to account accurately for the effects on the estimated GFR calculation of diminished muscle mass (and thus creatinine generation) in the elderly, or in patients with cirrhosis, spinal cord injury, cachexia, or other causes of muscle wasting. Nevertheless, a rough estimate of the current GFR is obtained and should be used to guide dosing calculations.[33–35] In fact, one study found that this formula, using a "corrected" serum creatinine concentration of 1 mg/dL in cachectic patients, provided a more accurate GFR estimate in critically ill patients than either short (half-hour) or long (24-hour) creatinine clearance measurements.[35] The Modification of Diet in Renal Disease (MDRD) Equation offers another method to approximate GFR; the equation is found to be more accurate than the Cockcroft-Gault equation and takes into account more clinical factors, such as serum albumin and blood urea nitrogen, that likely reflect the patient's clinical status more accurately, but is much more complicated to use.[36] Websites are available (such as www.nephron.com) to facilitate the use of the MDRD Equation. Another interesting and accurate approach uses measured aminoglycoside clearance, which occurs entirely by glomerular filtration, as a surrogate measurement of GFR.[37]

Following GFR estimation, dosage is usually adjusted based upon published criteria for the agent in question. These maintenance dose adjustments for renal insufficiency are made as follows:[38–41]

$$\text{Patient's estimated GFR/normal GFR} \times 100$$
$$= \text{dose adjustment, \%}$$

(i.e., percentage increase in interval or percentage decrease in dose). The dosing interval may be increased (interval extension), the size of individual doses decreased (dose reduction), or a combination of both approaches may sometimes be necessary.

For the interval extension method, the usual size dose is given, but the intervals between individual doses are lengthened. This method is useful for drugs characterized by long plasma half-lives in the presence of renal impairment and a wide therapeutic range. This approach is convenient but results in large plasma concentration fluctuations between peak and trough levels; in drugs with a low therapeutic index, toxic or subtherapeutic levels may result. For example, aminoglycosides are ideally suited to such a dosing strategy: The peak plasma concentration correlates with therapeutic efficacy, but trough levels must be monitored and kept low to minimize toxicity.

Alternatively, in drugs with a low therapeutic index, and those for which a constant level is preferred, the size of individual doses is reduced. This achieves a more constant plasma concentration, with less peak-trough fluctuation; however, increased toxicity because of higher average trough levels may result. For example, antiseizure drugs must be dose-adjusted in this fashion.

In the presence of renal insufficiency, hepatic metabolism accounts for the bulk of nonrenal elimination of drugs that are normally renally excreted. Hepatic biotransformation of some drugs is altered in patients with renal insufficiency; the cause of this phenomenon is unknown. Most available data come from studies of patients with chronic renal insufficiency, including those with end-stage renal disease.[39] Unfortunately, the effect of acute renal failure on hepatic drug biotransformation is little studied, and specific studies in this population have yielded some unexpected results. Normally, about 30% of vancomycin is cleared by nonrenal routes (approximately 40 mL/min). Nonrenal vancomycin clearance is decreased to 6 mL/min in patients with chronic renal failure on maintenance dialysis. The elimination pattern in acute renal failure (ARF) is more complex. Nonrenal elimination is approximately halved early in the course of ARF (16 to 17 mL/min), and decreases to values closer to those of subjects with chronic renal insufficiency (CRI) (10 mL/min) after 1 week of ARF.[43] This phenomenon requires an appropriate dosage adjustment, which is facilitated in this case by the routine availability of plasma level monitoring. Conversely, nonrenal clearance of imipenem in acute renal failure is nearly double that found in chronic renal insufficiency (95 mL/min vs. 51 mL/min), approaching that found in patients with normal renal function (130 mL/min; comprising over half of normal total clearance of approximately 230 mL/min). As a result, the total clearance of imipenem in anuric ARF patients is 108 mL/min, compared with 64 mL/min in CRI, and 230 mL/min in normal subjects. Therefore, the daily dose requirement is appropriately reduced from 2000 to 4000 mg/d hours in normal subjects to 1847 mg/d in ARF patients—a near doubling of the dose that would be administered based on CRI data (1111 mg/d).[44] In this case, the risk of seizure because of impaired clearance and imipenem accumulation is balanced against the risk of undertreatment, but accurate dosing would not be achieved based solely on clearance data from CRI patients, and plasma drug levels are not routinely available for clinical use in most institutions. Acute renal failure data should be used whenever possible; absent this information, CRI data must be used, but with an appropriate cautionary approach.

HEPATIC BIOTRANSFORMATION

Most drugs are lipophilic, so that they tend to be reabsorbed across renal tubular or intestinal membranes following glomerular filtration or biliary excretion, respectively. These drugs must therefore undergo biotransformation to more polar/hydrophilic compounds to allow urinary or

TABLE 103-7 Selected Cytochrome P450 Inhibitors and Inducers

Inhibitors	Inducers
Amiodarone	Anticonvulsants
Celecoxib	Carbamazepine
Cimetidine	Phenobarbital
Erythromycin	Phenytoin
Ethanol (acute intoxication)	Cigarette smoking
Fluconazole	Corticosteroids
Fluoxetine	Prednisone
Isoniazid	Dexamethasone
Itraconazole	Ethanol (chronic use)
Ketoconazole	Grape fruit juice
Neuroleptics	Omeprazole
Oral contraceptives	Pioglitazone
Psoralen dermatologics	Rifampin
Quinidine	
Quinolone antibiotics	
Selective serotonin reuptake inhibitors	
Ticlopidine	
Tricyclic antidepressants	

biliary excretion. Drug biotransformation reactions are classified as phase I (functionalization reactions, exposing or introducing a functional group), or phase II (biosynthetic) reactions. Phase I reactions are predominantly oxidations, reductions, and hydrolysis reactions, and are usually catalyzed by enzymes of the cytochrome P450 (CYP450) system, located in the endoplasmic reticulum (Tables 103-7, 103-8, and 103-9). Phase II reactions are conjugations, catalyzed by a variety of (mainly cytosolic) enzymes, which covalently link the parent drug or metabolite to a variety of compounds. Biliary excretion of a conjugated compound may result in enterohepatic recirculation of the parent compound if intestinal flora cleave the conjugate bond. Both phase I and II reactions generally

TABLE 103-8 Low Therapeutic Index Drugs Cleared by Cytochrome P450 Oxidation

Anesthetic agents	Enflurane
	Halothane
	Isoflurane
	Methoxyflurane
	Sevoflurane
Antiarrhythmic drugs	Amiodarone
	Flecainide
	Lidocaine
	Mexiletine
	Propafenone
	Quinidine
Anticonvulsants	Carbamazepine
	Phenobarbital
	Phenytoin
β-Adrenergic receptor blockers	Carvedilol
	Metoprolol
	Timolol
Immunosuppressive/antineoplastic drugs	Cyclophosphamide
	Cyclosporine
	Etoposide (VP16)
	Ifosfamide
	Tacrolimus (FK506)
Oral anticoagulant	Warfarin
Bronchodilator	Theophylline

TABLE 103-9 Cytochrome P450 Classes: Selected Substrates, Inhibitors, and Inducers

Isozymes	Substrates	Inhibitors and Inducers

CYP1A2	Amitryptiline
	Antipyrine
	Caffeine
	Clomipramine
	Clozapine
	Cyclobenzaprine
	Dapsone (minor)
	Estradiol
	Haloperidol
	Imipramine (also 2C9 & 3A4)
	Mexiletine
	Naproxen
	Ondansetron (minor)
	Propranolol
	Tacrine
	Theophylline
	Warfarin (minor)
	Verapamil
	Zolmitriptan
		Inhibitors
		  Amiodarone
		  Cimetidine
		  Ciprofloxacin (all quinolones)
		  Ticlopidine
		Inducers
		  Broccoli, Brussels sprouts
		  Char-grilled meats
		  Cigarette smoking
		  Insulin
		  Nafcillin
		  Omeprazole

CYP2B6	Buproprion
	Cyclophosphamide
	Efavirenz
	Ifosfamide
	Methadone
		Inhibitors
		  Orphenadrine
		  Thiotepa
		  Ticlopidine
		Inducers
		  Phenobarbital
		  Phenytoin
		  Rifampin

CYP2C	Amitriptyline
	Carbamazepine
	Celecoxib
	Chlorguanide
	Clomipramine (minor)
	Cyclophosphamide
	Diazepam
	Diclofenac
	Glimepiride
	Glipizide
	Glyburide
	Ibuprofen
	Ifosfamide
	Imipramine (minor)
	Indomethacin
	Irbesartan
	Lansoprazole (most proton
	pump inhibitors)
	Losartan
	Mefenamic acid
	(S)-Mephenytoin
	(R)-Mephobarbital
	Naproxen
	Nelfinavir
	Omeprazole
	Phenytoin
	Piroxicam, other oxicam drugs
	Progesterone
	Propranolol
	Rosiglitazone
	Tolbutamide
	Torsemide
	(S)-Warfarin
	Zafirlukast (2C9)
		Inhibitors
		  Amiodarone
		  Chlorguanide
		  Fluconazole
		  Fluvastatin
		  Fluvoxamine
		  Isoniazid
		  Itraconazole
		  Ketoconazole
		  Lovastatin
		  Omeprazole
		  Ritonavir
		  Simvastatin
		  Sulfaphenazole
		Inducers
		  Carbamazepines
		  Norethindrone
		  Phenobarbital
		  Prednisone
		  Rifabutin
		  Rifampin

TABLE 103-9 (*continued*)

CYP2D6	Amitryptiline	**Inhibitors**
	Amphetamines	Amiodarone
	Carvedilol	Cimetidine
	Chlorpromazine	Fluconazole
	Clomiprarnine (major)	Fluoxetine
	Clonazepine (minor)	Fluphenazine
	Codeine	Fluvoxamine
	Debrisoquine	Haloperidol
	Despiramine	Ketoconazole
	Dexotromethorphan	Paroxetine
	Dihydrocodeine	Propafenone
	Dolasetron	Quinidine
	Flecainide	Quinine
	Fluoxetine	Ritonavir
	Haloperidol	Sertraline
	Hydrocodone	**Inducers**
	Imipramine	Dexamethasone
	Lidocaine	Rifabutin
	Loratadine (minor)	Rifampin
	Metoclopramide	
	Metoprolol	
	Mexiletine	
	Nortryptiline	
	Ondansetron	
	Penbutolol	
	Perphenazine	
	Phenacetin	
	Propafenone	
	Propranolol	
	Risperidone	
	Ritonavir (minor)	
	Tamoxifen	
	Thiorizadine	
	Timolol	
	Tramadol	
	Tropisetron	
	Venlafaxine	
	Verapamil	
	Zuclopenthixol	
CYP2E	Acetaminophen (2E1)	**Inhibitors**
	Chlorzoxazone (2E1)	Cimetidine (2E1)
	Ethanol (2E1)	Disulfiram (2E1)
	Flurane anesthetics (2E1):	Isoniazid (2E1)
	Enflurane	**Inducers**
	Halothane	Ethanol (2E1)
	Isoflurane	Isoniazid
	Methoxyflurane	
	Sevoflurane	
	Theophylline (2E1 minor)	
CYP3A	Alfentanil (3A4)	**Inhibitors**
	Alprazolam	Amiodarone
	Amiodarone	Cimetidine (3A4)
	Amlodipine	Ciprofloxacin
	Astemizole	Clarithromycin
	Buspirone	Clotrimazole
	Carbamazepine (3A4)	Delavirdine
	Cisapride	Diltiazem
	Clarithromycin	Erythromycin
	Clotrimazole	Fluconazole (3A4)
	Clozapine	Fluvoxamine
	Codeine (minor)	Grapefruit juice (naringin)
	Cortisol	Indinavir
	Cyclobenzaprine	Itraconazole (3A4)
	Cyclophosphamide	Ketoconazole (3A4)

(continued)

TABLE 103-9 (*continued*)

Cyclosporine	Metronidazole
Dapsone (3A4)	Miconazole
Dexamethasone	Nefazodone (3A4)
Digitoxin	Norfloxacin
Diltiazem (3A4)	Quinidine (3A4)
Erythromycin	Ritonavir
Ethinyl estradiol (3A4)	Saquinivir
Ethosuximide	Sertraline (3A4)
Etoposide (VP16)	Troleandomycin
Felodipine (3A4)	Verapamil
Granisetron	**Inducers**
Hydrocortisone	Carbamazepine
Imipramine (3A4)	Dexamethasone (3A4)
Indinavir	Efavirenz
Lansoprazole	Pentobarbital
Lidocaine (3A4)	Phenobarbital
Loratadine (major)	Phenylbutazone (3A4)
Losartan	Phenytoin
Lovastatin (3A4)	Pioglitazone
Methadone	Rifabutin
Midazolam (3A4)	Rifampin (3A4)
Nelfinavir	St. John's wort
Nefedipine (3A4)	Troglitazone
Nisoldipine (3A4)	
Ondansetron	
Paclitaxel	
Progesterone (3A4)	
Quinidine (3A4)	
Rifabutin	
Ritonavir	
Salmeterol	
Saquinavir	
Simvastatin	
Sirolimus (rapamycin)	
Tacrolimus (FK506)	
Tamoxifen (3A4)	
Teniposide	
Terfenadine (3A4)	
Testosterone (3A4)	
Tirilazad	
Triazolam (3A4)	
Troleandomycin	
Verapamil	
Vinblastine	
Vindesine	
(R)-Warfarin (3A4)	
Zatosetron	

The information in this table was provided in part by Roger P. Dean, PharmD, University of Chicago Hospitals.

result in a loss of pharmacologic activity, although more active metabolites are less commonly produced. Hepatic drug metabolism is functionally characterized by two patterns of clearance, which may be flow-limited or capacity-limited. The hepatic extraction ratio (ER) is derived as follows: $ER = (C_A - C_V)/C_A$, where C_A and C_V are the drug concentration in hepatic arterial (or portal venous) and hepatic venous blood, respectively. The hepatic ER is low for capacity-limited drugs (which have saturable biotransformation pathways) and high for flow-limited drugs (the liver essentially metabolizes any drug delivered, a process limited only by drug-delivering blood flow).

The bulk of drug biotransformation is performed by hepatic enzymes, and the remainder by renal tubular, intestinal, cutaneous, and pulmonary enzymes. The CYP450 system, comprising at least 12 families (in humans) of heme-containing endoplasmic reticulum enzymes, is the major catalyst of hepatic drug biotransformation reactions (see Table 103-9).[5,45–48] Three families (CYP1, CYP2, and CYP3) are responsible for essentially all drug biotransformations, through phase I (primarily oxidative) reactions. Cytochrome P450 nomenclature is based on amino acid sequence homology. Families (designated by numbers, such as CYP3) contain at least 40% homology; subfamilies (designated by capital letters, such as CYP3A) are over 55% homologous; individual P450 enzymes are again designated by Arabic numerals (for example, CYP3A4). The CYP3A subfamily accounts for over 50% of phase I drug metabolism, predominantly by the

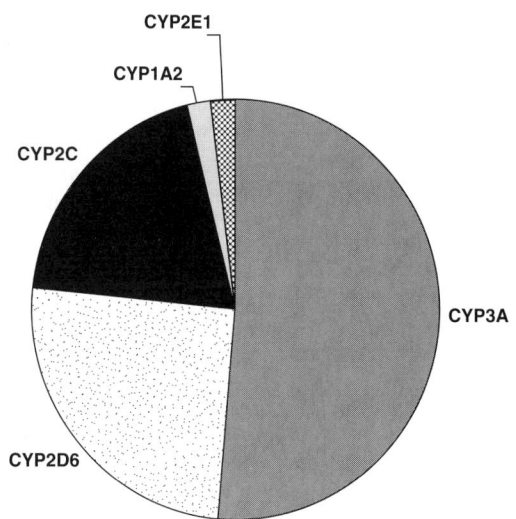

FIGURE 103-6 The proportion of drugs metabolized by the major cytochrome P450 enzymes. (*Reproduced with permission from Benet et al.[5]*)

CYP3A4 subtype. Most other drug biotransformations are performed (in decreasing order of frequency) by CYP2D6, CYP2C, CYP2E1, and CYP1A2 (Fig. 103-6).[5] More than one enzyme may metabolize a particular drug, but metabolism of many drugs is dependent upon a single enzyme. Since the CYP450 nomenclature is based on structural criteria, rather than biotransformation function, isozymes of a particular class often lack any common substrates.

Phase II (conjugation) reactions form a covalent linkage between a drug's functional group and one of a number of compounds: glucuronic acid, sulfate, glutathione, acetate, or amino acids. These conjugates are highly polar, usually inactive, and undergo urinary or fecal excretion.[46,49]

Drug biotransformation may be enhanced or impaired by multiple factors, including age, gender, enzyme induction or inhibition (see Table 103-7), pharmacogenetics, and the effects of hepatic dysfunction or other disease states (including those which decrease hepatic perfusion). Conditions that impair drug biotransformation may result in type A adverse drug reactions, caused by accumulation of toxic concentrations of parent drug or metabolites (see section on adverse drug reactions, below).

EFFECTS OF AGE

CYP1A2 activity is increased in children compared to adults, causing the well-known increased theophylline dosage requirements in this population.[50,51] Similarly, CYP3A4 activity appears to decline in the elderly compared to younger adults,[52–54] although age-related declines in hepatic size, hepatic blood flow, or drug binding and distribution may underlie this phenomenon, because in vitro enzyme activity is unchanged with age.[55]

EFFECTS OF GENDER

Differences in pharmacokinetic and pharmacodynamic properties of drugs between men and women are more commonly being recognized. These differences can sometimes have major clinical impact, or be as subtle as gender-related differences in metabolism of specific stereoisomers of a particular drug formulation. Differences in rate of absorption and

extent of first-pass metabolism have been reported for some drugs, including ondansetron[56] and zolmitriptan,[57] but these generally lack major clinical significance. Gender differences in volume of distribution, after adjustment for weight effects, have also been identified for a number of drugs. Theophylline exhibits a smaller volume of distribution in females compared to males,[58] as do the fluoroquinolones.[59] Possible explanations include differences in body composition between men and women, physiologic changes associated with menstrual cycles, and differences in plasma protein binding secondary to hormonal characteristics. Gender differences in drug elimination have been studied in hepatic and renal processes. Clinically significant differences were predominantly linked to gender-specific expression of metabolic enzymes (e.g., CYP3A4 and CYP1A2); gender differences in renal handling of drugs tend to be clinically silent. Pharmacodynamic variability in humans is more difficult to measure, because the measured parameters can often be subjective, such as pain or depression. Nonetheless, relevant gender differences have been identified. Women treated with thrombolytics after a myocardial infarction are more likely to experience intracranial hemorrhage. Other examples include drugs involved in glucose management and arrhythmia treatment.

PHARMACOGENETICS

Many adverse drug reactions which were formerly termed idiosyncratic are now recognized to be caused by genetic polymorphisms of expression (through autosomal recessive traits) of genes involved in drug disposition and effects, including the hepatic drug metabolizing enzymes (phase I or phase II) in particular individuals and racial groups, which have been most well-studied[16,61–64] (see Table 103-9; Tables 103-10 and 103-11). The identified polymorphisms of these metabolic enzymes differ in their rate of metabolism: "extensive metabolizers" are the common wild-type phenotype, "poor metabolizers" exhibit a decreased rate of substrate metabolism, and the rare "ultra-rapid metabolizers" display an increased rate of substrate metabolism. The incidence of expression of the different phenotypes varies by race and ethnic group. The effect of racial origin on drug metabolism is receiving increasing attention in the drug development process,[13,65–67] although it must be remembered that pharmacogenetic factors controlling drug disposition and response vary not only according to race and gender, but also between individuals of the same race and gender.

CYP2D6 Polymorphism

The most common P450 polymorphism in Caucasians is of CYP2D6 expression. CYP2D6 is responsible for metabolism of approximately 30 to 40 commonly used drugs, about half of which are psychoactive agents (antidepressants, including all tricyclic antidepressants [TCAs] and selective serotonin reuptake inhibitors [SSRIs], and antipsychotics, including haloperidol[68]); other substrates include β-blockers (all except atenolol and sotalol, which are renally excreted, not metabolized), other antiarrhythmic drugs, and codeine. Approximately 7% to 10% of the Caucasian population, 2% to 5% of Africans, but only rare Asian subjects lack expression of this enzyme and are poor metabolizers of CYP2D6 substrates.[66] Such patients are prone to develop profound bradycardia during standard β-blocker therapy or severe drowsiness when receiving psychoactive drug therapy; in each case the adverse

TABLE 103-10 Phase II Drug Metabolizing Enzymes: Substrates and Polymorphisms

Polymorphism	Examples
"Slow" acetylation	*N-acetylation polymorphism.* Slow acetylators have deficient N-acetylatransferase activity (NAT-2).
	Incidence of slow acetylators : 50%–60% (Caucasian and African Americans; southern Indians); 5%–20% (Chinese, Japanese, Eskimos)
	Incidence increased in HIV patients (thus sulfa reactions are more common)
	Slow acetylators have increased risk of (1) isoniazid-induced peripheral neuropathy, and possibly hepatotoxicity; (2) drug-induced lupus: hydralazine, procainamide; (3) sulfonamide hypersensitivity: deficient hydroxylamine metabolite detoxification; (4) sulfasalazine-induced hemolysis
Dihydropyrimidine dehydrogenase deficiency	*Dihydropyrimidine dehydrogenase polymorphism.* 3%–4% taking 5-fluorouracil (5-FU) have defident metabolism, and develop severe toxicity (myelosuppression, etc).
Glucuronidation deficiency	*UDP-glucuronyltransferase polymorphism.* Deficiency of hepatic UDP-glucuronyltransferase activity manifests as two syndromes of impaired bilirubin conjugation: Gilbert's (2%–12% of population) and Crigler-najjar (<1%) syndromes.
	Potential but undocumented effects on metabolism of heavily glucuronidated drugs (acetaminophen; HIV drugs; oncologic agents).
Glucose-6-phosphate-dehydrogenase deficiency	*G-6-PD deficiency.* Occurs in approximately 20% of African-American males; less frequent in females. Since erythrocytes from these patients are susceptible to oxidative stress, they are prone to develop hemolytic anemia induced by antimalarials (chloroquine, mefloquine, primaquine), probenecid, nitrofurantoin, sulfa drugs (sulfamethoxazole, dapsone), sulfonylurea hypoglycemic agents (chlorpropamide, tolbutamide)
Glutathione transferase deficiency	*Glutathione-s-transferase polymorphism.* Absent activity of GSTM1 (50% Caucasians, 30% African-Americans) and/or GSTT1 (15% Caucasians, 24% African-Americans) impairs clearance of electrophilic toxins.
	Increased vulnrability to acetaminophen, metronidazole, and nitrofurantoin toxicity, because of depletion of mitochondrial glutathione stores.
Atypical pseudocholinesterase	*Pseudocholinesterase polymorphism.* Subjects have impaired hydrolysis of succinylcholine, resulting in prolonged paralysis following use of this agent; incidence is 1 in 2500 people.
Thiopurine methylation deficiency	*Thiopurine methyltransferase polymorphism.* Deficient (heterozygotes: 11%) or absent (homozygotes: 1 in 300) s-methylation of thiopurine drugs: azathioprine and 6-mercaptopurine, resulting in development of profound leukopenia with standard doses.
Atypical alcohol and aldehyde dehydrogenase activities	*Alcohol dehydrogenase activity.* Five-to six fold more rapid alcohol dehydrogenase activity is found in the majority of Japanese subjects (compared to Caucasians), resulting in acute symptoms following consumption of low doses of ethanol, because of rapid aldehyde production.
	Aldehyde dehydrogenase deficiency. Up to 50% of Asian and Native American subjects develop a disulfiram-like reaction (profound nausea and emesis) following ethanol consumption, because of deficient conversion of aldehyde to acetate. This enzyme also participtes in conversion of cyclophosphamide and ifosfamide to active metabolites (after cytochrome P450 oxidation).

event is caused by accumulation of the parent drug. Conversely, these individuals derive little analgesic effect from codeine, which must be metabolized by CYP2D6 to its more potent metabolite morphine to achieve therapeutic efficacy. Quinidine, fluoxetine, and amiodarone are potent inhibitors of CYP2D6 activity, and convert genetically extensive metabolizers to phenotypically poor metabolizers of CYP2D6 substrates.

CYP2C19 Polymorphism

The most prevalent P450 polymorphism in Asians is of CYP2C19 expression; 15% to 27% of Asians but only 3% to 5%

TABLE 103-11 Prevalence of Phase I and II Enzyme Polymorphisms by Race

	Polymorphism Phenotype	Overall U.S. Population	White	Black	Asian
CYP2D6	Poor	10%	5%–10%	0–20%	1%
	Ultrarapid	6%	1%–10%	2%	0–2%
CYP2C9	Poor	1%	0.2%–1%	Not determined	2%–3%
	Ultrarapid	Not identified	—	—	—
CYP2C19	Poor	4%–5%	3%–6%	4%	8%–23%
	Ultrarapid	Not identified	—	—	—
Dihydropyrimidine dehydrogenase	Poor	0–1%			
	Ultrarapid	Not identified	—	—	—
Plasma Pseudocholinesterase	Poor	<1%	0–1%	Not determined	Not determined
	Ultrarapid	Not identified	—	—	—
N-acetyltransferase	Poor		40%–70%	50%–60%	10%–20%
	Ultrarapid	Not identified	—	—	—
Thiopurine methyltransferase	Poor	0–3%	0.33%	Not determined	0.04%
	Ultrarapid	Not identified	—	—	—
UDP-glucuronosyltransferase	Poor	10%–15%	10.9%	Not determined	3%–5%
	Ultrarapid	Not identified	—	—	—

of Caucasians lack expression of this isozyme and are poor metabolizers of substrates such as S-mephenytoin, phenytoin itself, diazepam, and omeprazole.[67] Poor metabolizers of CYP2C19 have a better response to omeprazole in eradication of *Helicobacter pylori* than do extensive metabolizers. However, prolonged (>1 year) exposure to high serum omeprazole levels is more likely to cause cobalamin deficiency and result in neuropsychiatric and hematologic side effects.[69]

CYP2C9 Polymorphism
The incidence of CYP2C9 polymorphism is up to 20% in black patients, but only 1% in Caucasians; important substrates include S-warfarin, phenytoin, diclofenac (and other hepatically metabolized nonsteroidal anti-inflammatory drugs [NSAIDs]), glipizide, and losartan. Fluconazole at usual therapeutic doses is a powerful CYP2C9 inhibitor. Clinically useful laboratory studies are being developed to determine CYP2C9 phenotype and guide therapy of drugs with narrow therapeutic indices, such as warfarin and phenytoin.

CYP2E1 Polymorphism
CYP2E1 metabolizes acetaminophen and many volatile anesthetics and is induced by isoniazid and ethanol. Interestingly, 2.4% of Caucasians and 10% of subjects with alcoholic liver disease have a CYP2E1 rapid metabolizer phenotype and metabolize CYP2E1 substrates to a greater extent than most of the general population.

CYP3A Polymorphism
The CYP3A family of enzymes displays a wide range of expression of activity for each enzyme in normal populations, contributing to the difficulty in identifying clinically significant polymorphisms. Additionally, substrates of the CYP3A family enzymes often are metabolized in a multigenic pathway. Many common substrates are metabolized by both CYP3A4 and CYP3A5; the relatively common CYP3A5 poor-metabolizer phenotype may then be clinically obscured by this dual pathway. The role of the CYP3A4 enzyme in drug elimination is further complicated by the presence of

polymorphisms that alter the rate of metabolism of some substrates but not others.[70] The clinical implications of these polymorphisms remain unclear.

Phase II Enzyme Polymorphisms
A genetic polymorphism for acetylation of procainamide, hydralazine, isoniazid, and sulfa drugs (see Table 103-10) underlies the "slow acetylator" phenotype seen in over 50% of American blacks and whites but only 10% of Asian individuals. Many other phase II reactions are subject to pharmacogenetic variation[56] (see Table 103-10), resulting in polymorphic expression of the metabolic capacity for specific agents. Examples include glucuronidation (Gilbert syndrome), and the activities of glutathione-S-transferase (acetaminophen metabolism), thiopurine methyltransferase (azathioprine metabolism), glucose-6-phosphate-dehydrogenase (quinine-induced hemolysis), pseudocholinesterase (prolonged paralysis following succinylcholine), and dihydropyrimidine dehydrogenase (5-fluorouracil toxicity).

ENZYME INDUCTION AND INHIBITION
Common substrates of the P450 enzyme responsible for metabolism of a particular drug may be inhibitors or inducers of its metabolism and therefore create the potential for drug interactions (see Tables 103-7 and 103-9). Substances that are not substrates of a P450 isozyme may also be inhibitors or inducers of its activity (e.g., fluconazole and CYP2C9, quinidine and CYP2D6). The potential for such an interaction is increasingly predictable, and consequent overdosage or underdosage preventable, owing to identification of the specific P450 isozyme responsible for drug metabolism in recent product package inserts and other standard sources (see section on general drug information reference texts, below). For example, since both cyclosporine and tacrolimus (formerly FK506) are metabolized by CYP3A4, biotransformation of both agents is predictably affected by known inhibitors and inducers of this enzyme (see Table 103-9). Ketoconazole is a particularly potent inhibitor of CYP3A4 and has been used to deliberately lower cyclosporine dosage requirements as a

cost-saving measure.[71,72] By contrast, phenobarbital induces cyclosporine metabolism to such an extent that concomitant use of these agents is not advisable; likewise, therapeutic cyclosporine levels are difficult to maintain during rifampin therapy. Inducers and inhibitors of phase II enzymes have been less extensively characterized, but some clinical applications of this information have emerged; for example, phenobarbital is used to induce glucuronyl transferase activity in icteric neonates, and both phenobarbital and valproate have been used to modulate chemotherapeutic agent glucuronidation and toxicity.[73]

EFFECTS OF DISEASE STATES

Critical illness routinely alters all the physiologic processes involved in drug disposition. It would be surprising if drug disposition and/or response were not significantly altered in such patients. Unfortunately, most data regarding drug disposition in critically ill patients must be extrapolated from other populations; clearly, such information must be interpreted with extreme caution.

EFFECTS OF CIRCULATORY DYSFUNCTION

The effects of congestive heart failure (CHF) on drug disposition are the best-studied examples of alterations of drug absorption, distribution, and elimination associated with circulatory insufficiency (see Table 103-5). Secondary decrements in hepatic and renal blood flow result in impaired clearance of some drugs excreted by these routes. Clearance of hepatically eliminated drugs is more likely to be impaired by CHF if their metabolism is flow-limited (i.e., characterized by a high extraction ratio, such as lidocaine). It is doubtful that most such information, even from populations with decompensated CHF, is applicable to the setting of cardiogenic shock. Even fewer data are available regarding disposition of most agents in patients with hypovolemic or septic shock, or even sepsis syndrome without frank hypoperfusion. Just as is the case in CHF, septic hypoperfusion may disproportionately involve the renal or splanchnic circulations, resulting in impairment of renal or hepatic perfusion to a degree that would not be expected based upon global hemodynamic data. Furthermore, experimental evidence suggests that endotoxemia impairs hepatic drug metabolizing-enzyme function[74] and that nitric oxide probably mediates much of this inhibition.[75]

Effects of Liver Disease

The effects of hepatic disease on PK and PD parameters of drug disposition are much more difficult to predict than the consequences of renal disease, based on data available for most agents.[76,77] Standard indices of hepatic function, such as the clinical features and biochemical values comprising the Child or Child-Turcotte scores, do not correlate even qualitatively with the capacity of the diseased liver to biotransform xenobiotics.[78] Activity of particular cytochrome P450 isozymes or conjugating enzymes may be decreased, preserved, or even increased in the presence of different liver diseases at various stages of severity.[17,77,79] Most data suggest that cirrhosis variably affects the hepatic content and activity of particular cytochrome 450 isozymes; contents of CYP3A are not demonstrably changed, CYP1A2 and CYP2E1 activities are decreased, and CYP2C activity may even be increased (as is tolbutamide clearance in cirrhosis).[77] In addition, the presence of gastrointestinal hypomotility, hypoalbu-

minemia, increased or decreased plasma glycoprotein levels, ascites/edema, and altered hepatic blood flow may all alter drug absorption, distribution, elimination, and effects unpredictably (see Table 103-4). Gastric hypomotility does not alter bioavailability; rather it delays absorption and reduces the peak plasma level. Altered levels of the major drug-binding plasma proteins in cirrhosis or other forms of liver dysfunction have complex secondary effects. The frequent presence of hypoalbuminemia decreases binding of acidic drugs, such as phenytoin. Production of α_1-acid glycoprotein, which binds many basic drugs (e.g., lidocaine and quinidine), is impaired by severe cirrhosis but increased by inflammatory states (it is an acute-phase reactant). The importance of decreased plasma protein binding (caused by decreased binding protein levels or by displacement by a competing substance) is determined by the hepatic extraction ratio of the drug, and the presence or absence of concomitant impairment of hepatic biotransformation capacity (caused by disease or by competition with an interacting agent). Changes in protein binding do not alter clearance of high-extraction (flow-limited) drugs, but if hepatic metabolism of a low-extraction (capacity-limited) drug is impaired and protein binding of the drug is also decreased, then the plasma free drug level will increase.[80] Renal elimination of drugs or metabolites (inactive, active, or toxic) is also commonly impaired in patients with cirrhosis by the associated decrement in glomerular filtration rate, which is often unappreciated because of the poor correlation between plasma creatinine values and GFR in cirrhotic subjects.[16] Finally, liver disease patients appear to have increased sensitivity to many drugs or their metabolites; some of this phenomenon is attributable to synergistic sedation (a PD phenomenon), although many such instances are probably caused by unrecognized accumulation of active or toxic metabolites or abnormally increased CNS distribution (e.g., increased blood-brain barrier permeability to cimetidine in cirrhosis).[81]

In practice, the presence of hepatic dysfunction should prompt a thorough drug regimen re-evaluation to examine all disposition parameters.[17,76,78,82] Useful data may be available regarding the effects of cirrhosis on clearance of the agent, permitting an appropriate dose reduction. More commonly, the only information available details the predominant route of drug elimination. In either case, careful dose titration upward from a dose lower than normal is obviously the prudent approach; however, such a cautious approach may not be consistent with the rapid therapeutic effect desired in critically ill patients. Dose reduction is most likely to be necessary when a drug which usually undergoes extensive first-pass metabolism is enterally administered in the presence of liver disease severe enough to impair hepatic clearance of the agent; in such a situation, both increased oral bioavailability and decreased clearance tend to increase plasma drug levels:

$$Cp_{ss} = (\text{bioavailability} \times \text{maintenance dose})/(\text{dosing interval} \times \text{clearance})$$

Careful therapeutic monitoring of agents that have a low therapeutic index (see Table 103-8), using plasma levels if these are clinically available, represents the optimal approach in cases in which impaired clearance is suspected. Otherwise, monitoring of physiologic parameters during graded upward dose titration may be the best available option. It is important to remember that, because of impaired elimination and the resultant prolongation of half-life, achievement of steady-state plasma drug levels and corresponding maximal effect will be correspondingly delayed. Failure to wait for achievement of steady-state conditions prior to dose escalation may result in drug accumulation to toxic levels. Important drug interactions are also more likely to occur in the presence of impaired drug elimination "reserve," so that increased vigilance regarding potential protein-binding or hepatic biotransformation interactions is warranted in the presence of liver disease (see below).

HALF-LIFE

When clearance is diminished, elimination half-life increases proportionately, as does the time required to achieve steady-state plasma levels (three to five half-lives). The appropriate time for assessment of full pharmacologic effect and measurement of levels may thus be markedly delayed. For example, the elimination half-life of digoxin is normally 20 hours, but increases to 1 week with end-stage renal disease (ESRD); an ESRD patient discharged from the hospital with a plasma level within the therapeutic range 1 week after starting maintenance therapy with 0.25 mg per day of digoxin will probably subsequently develop digitalis toxicity.

CONSIDERATION OF POTENTIAL DRUG-DRUG INTERACTIONS

Drug-drug interactions may occur owing to alterations in drug disposition (PK interactions), or drug effect (PD interactions).[4,83,84] PK interactions occur through effects on four drug disposition mechanisms: (1) gastrointestinal absorption, (2) drug distribution, (3) hepatic metabolism, and (4) renal excretion. These categories will be further discussed below. PD interactions occur by three basic mechanisms: (1) pharmacologic interactions, usually based on binding of an antagonist to the target receptor mediating drug effect (e.g., use of a nonselective β-blocker such as propranolol in a patient requiring inhaled nebulized β-agonist therapy for bronchospasm); (2) physiologic interactions, such as the additive effects of multiple sedatives or vasodilators, or the opposing effects of warfarin and vitamin K on coagulation factor synthesis; and (3) drug-induced changes in the intracellular milieu resulting in altered effects of other agents (the best such example is the precipitation of digitalis toxicity by loop diuretic–induced hypokalemia and hypomagnesemia). It is worth emphasizing the fact that individual sensitivity to drug effect (e.g., sedative effects in the elderly) may predispose particular patients to suffer the consequences of PD drug interactions more readily than others. Prevention of PD drug interactions is best accomplished through a basic understanding of the mechanism of action, common side effects, and population-specific issues (if any) pertinent to any drug prescribed.

PK interactions are the subject of many exhaustive compendia, but a few general principles are required to interpret such information. In order for a reported PK drug interaction to be of clinical significance, three criteria should be fulfilled.[5,38] First, one of the drugs involved must have a low therapeutic index, so that an alteration in its disposition results in either toxic or subtherapeutic effect (there are important exceptions to this rule). Second, the drug disposition parameter alteration should be on the order of 30% or more, because changes of lesser magnitude are unlikely to be of clinical importance. Finally, only reports in humans should be considered definite, since animal studies of drug disposition do not always accurately reflect human processes. Conversely, the absence of reported data from animal studies does not preclude drug interactions in humans, particularly with respect to newer agents undergoing wide use for the first time.

ABSORPTION

Most such interactions affect the rate rather than the extent of absorption, so that the magnitude and timing of peak plasma drug level is altered, but the fraction absorbed (and thus bioavailability) is unchanged. Interaction mechanisms include physicochemical complexing (e.g., tetracycline and milk products); gastric pH changes (e.g., failure to absorb ketoconazole when gastric pH is made alkaline by coadministration of antisecretory agents); alterations in gastrointestinal motility; effects on gastrointestinal mucosa or flora (e.g., increased digoxin levels after antibiotic therapy; see Chap. 102); changes in mesenteric blood flow; and finally changes in first-pass metabolism (e.g., cyclosporine with ketoconazole[71,72,85]).

DISTRIBUTION

Altered drug binding because of displacement by another agent is of far lesser importance as a source of drug interaction than is generally appreciated. In fact, drug displacement from binding sites simply makes more free drug available for excretion or biotransformation.[84] The net effect on plasma levels of active drug is thus usually negligible, unless clearance of the displaced drug is also impaired because of organ dysfunction or the inhibition of drug metabolism or excretion by the displacing agent itself.

HEPATIC METABOLISM

Inducers and inhibitors of hepatic biotransformation are important causes of drug interactions. This is well illustrated by considering common interactions with the enzyme predominantly responsible for cyclosporine metabolism, underlining the importance of considering drug interactions when adding new agents to a patient's drug regimen. Cyclosporine, a potent immunosuppressive drug used in the prevention of allograft rejection, is metabolized by the CYP3A4 enzyme in both the liver and small intestine. Modulation of the pharmacokinetics of cyclosporine has been reported with a large number of drugs. For example, ketoconazole is known to be a potent inhibitor of CYP3A4, and therefore both increases oral bioavailability and reduces the rate of elimination of the drug, increasing blood cyclosporine levels. This predictable interaction can be used favorably to minimize the cost of therapy by decreasing the necessary dose of cyclosporine by co-administration with the cheaper drug, ketoconazole. More commonly, drug interactions result in unfavorable outcomes. Inadvertent co-administration of cyclosporine with a CYP3A4 inducer, such as troglitazone (now removed from the market) or rifampin, can result in rapid drug elimination (a state similar to the previously described "ultra-rapid metabolizer" phenotype) and subtherapeutic cyclosporine levels, with subsequent potential rejection of the transplanted organ.[87]

There are numerous clinically important examples of such interactions involving the other P450 isozymes also. Theophylline is metabolized by CYP1A2; theophylline toxicity may be precipitated by addition of the quinolone antibiotic ciprofloxacin (an inhibitor of CYP1A2) or by smoking cessation (because of withdrawal of the CYP1A2-inducing effect of cigarette smoking), unless theophylline dosage is reduced appropriately. Only one dose of quinidine (a CYP3A4 substrate) is required to convert a normal, extensive metabolizer of CYP2D6 substrates (including numerous β-blockers, antidepressants, and antipsychotic agents) into a poor metabolizer of these agents. Inhibition of drug biotransformation activity by a drug which is not a substrate of the impaired enzyme is not uncommon: quinidine is a powerful CYP2D6 inhibitor and CYP3A4 substrate; fluconazole is also a CYP3A4 substrate but impairs phenytoin and warfarin metabolism by CYP2C enzymes, in addition to competitive inhibition of metabolism of other CYP3A substrates. Such instances reinforce the need to examine both the known and potential interactions of each additional agent with those in the patient's current regimen.

Finally, agents that diminish hepatic blood flow (vasopressors and cimetidine) may impair clearance of high-extraction drugs such as lidocaine and propranolol.

RENAL EXCRETION

Drug interactions can affect glomerular filtration, tubular secretion, or tubular reabsorption (active or passive). It is obvious that agents that impair or augment glomerular filtration tend to cause a corresponding change in excretion of drugs eliminated by this route, such as aminoglycosides. Active tubular drug secretion is performed primarily by two groups of proximal tubular pumps: an anion pump (which secretes organic acids) and a cation pump (which secretes organic bases). Competitive inhibition of the anion pump by probenecid impairs elimination of penicillin, thus prolonging the half-life of this organic acid. Methotrexate is another anion secreted by this pump, and subject to the same interaction. Cimetidine and trimethoprim inhibit cationic pump secretion of procainamide and some other cationic drugs. Digoxin undergoes distal tubular secretion by a third pump system, which is inhibited by multiple drugs, including quinidine, amiodarone, spironolactone, and several calcium channel blockers; this is the mechanism partly responsible for the elevation of serum digoxin levels routinely encountered following combination of these agents with digitalis therapy. Finally, as discussed in Chap. 102, alterations in urinary pH alter passive distal tubular reabsorption of weak acids and bases, including drugs such as salicylic acid and phenobarbital (a basic drug).

THERAPEUTIC DRUG MONITORING

Most drugs are dosed according to population-based PK/PD data. In most cases, critical care therapy is initiated in this fashion, but may be monitored and titrated using readily available pharmacodynamic parameters (sedation, analgesia, paralysis, hemodynamic data, cardiac rhythm, and electroencephalography). Selected agents, usually those with a low therapeutic index, are additionally monitored and dose-adjusted using plasma drug levels and calculations of individual drug disposition parameters. Whether monitored using pharmacodynamic indexes alone, or more precisely with the addition of PK data, ongoing attempts to optimize

therapeutics should minimize the occurrence of inadequate therapy or adverse drug reactions (ADR).

Appropriate direct therapeutic drug monitoring involves consideration of many variables. The form of drug measured is important, especially in drugs with high plasma-protein binding. Because only the free fraction of the drug is clinically active, the useful plasma test is one that accurately reflects the free fraction. For example, phenytoin is highly albumin-bound. In the setting of critical illness, hypoalbuminemia, malnutrition, or cirrhosis, total phenytoin levels may be low, while free phenytoin levels are likely to be in the therapeutic range. The timing of plasma drug testing is also important. In drugs such as aminoglycosides, peak and trough levels need to be monitored, since peak levels reflect therapeutic efficacy and trough levels are monitored to ensure adequate drug clearance and to avoid drug accumulation.

Drug regimen adjustment may be precipitated by multiple intercurrent factors, including changes in volume status; alterations (worsening or improvement) in gastrointestinal tract or circulatory, renal, or liver function; the application of extracorporeal therapies which impact drug disposition; and potential drug interactions or other ADRs associated with addition of new agents. Finally, any change in patient status should be considered a potential ADR, and this possible diagnosis assessed using available resources. If an ADR is strongly suspected, this should be reported to the appropriate institutional and extramural authorities, and management altered accordingly.

ADVERSE DRUG REACTIONS

Drug prescribing intended to achieve beneficial therapeutic effects is necessarily accompanied by the possibility of eliciting an unintended adverse drug reaction (ADR). ADRs are common in the ICU, where multiple drugs are administered to unstable patients who commonly are unable to give a complete medical history and manifest altered drug disposition parameters (including metabolism and excretion). ADRs present diagnostic and therapeutic problems that complicate ICU admission, increasing morbidity, mortality, and length of stay.[89]

To minimize ADRs, all drugs prescribed by a critical care physician should be reviewed (prior to administration) by the critical care nurse and pharmacist for potential errors including patient identity, known patient allergies, correct dosing, and potential drug-drug interactions. Most preventable ADRs involve (1) prescribing a drug despite a documented allergy to the medication ordered or to a cross-reactive agent; (2) the use of anticoagulants or thrombolytic agents; (3) failure to appropriately monitor and adjust low-therapeutic-index drug administration using plasma drug concentration analysis; and (4) failure to adjust the regimen for administration of renally eliminated drugs in the presence of renal dysfunction.[81] Accordingly, we advocate a daily review of all medications given to each ICU patient, focusing on the following issues: (1) drug-patient interactions, including known drug allergies; (2) drug-disease interactions, including presence and severity of organ dysfunction, and appropriate dosing adjustments; (3) potential drug-drug interactions; (4) the possibility of an ADR causing any new corporeal dysfunction; and (5) discontinuation of all unnecessary drugs, in an ongoing attempt to simplify and rationalize therapy. The importance of minimizing the number of drugs prescribed is demonstrated by the fact that there is a 40% probability of developing an ADR when more than 15 drugs are given to a hospitalized patient, compared to a 5% ADR probability when receiving fewer than 6 medications.[90]

Adverse drug reactions may be classified as type A (an exaggerated pharmacologic effect related to high drug concentration), or type B (an idiosyncratic reaction).[61] Increasingly, reactions formerly classified as idiosyncratic (type B) have been shown to be type A reactions based on polymorphic expression of metabolizing enzyme activity and impaired drug metabolism and target effect. Individuals deficient in activity of the necessary metabolizing enzyme develop ADRs caused by accumulation of previously undocumented toxic metabolites; for example, sulfonamide hypersensitivity has been linked to an increase in prevalence of the "slow acetylator" phenotype, and defective detoxification of hydroxylamine metabolites.[91,92] Other idiosyncratic phenomena, such as halothane hepatitis and carbamazepine reactions, may also be caused by defective metabolism.[92]

The diagnosis of an ADR requires a high index of suspicion that signs or symptoms may be drug-related. Distinguishing between an ADR and manifestations of other diseases can be challenging, particularly in critically ill patients with a myriad of problems.

Identification of a temporal relationship between drug initiation and onset of signs or symptoms is useful, but not always possible. For example, supraventricular tachycardia after initiation of theophylline, wheezing after β-blocker administration, or seizures during meperidine therapy may each be caused by, aggravated by, or unrelated to drug effects. Furthermore, patients may develop a type A adverse drug reaction in the ICU when elimination of an agent, which they have received chronically prior to hospitalization, is subject to a drug-disease interaction (e.g., theophylline toxicity precipitated by development of congestive heart failure), or drug-drug interaction (e.g., theophylline toxicity caused by concurrent ciprofloxacin administration). In the absence of another convincing etiology, discontinuation or dose reduction of the suspected drug is indicated. Subsequent improvement in signs or symptoms is presumptive evidence of an ADR; of note, ADRs precipitated by agents with long half-lives may require a longer period for resolution. The degree of certainty in ADR diagnosis increases if rechallenge with the suspected drug leads to reappearance of the presumed ADR; however, readministration of drug for this purpose is not recommended unless the information is crucial for subsequent patient management and alternative drugs are not available. If an idiosyncratic or allergic type reaction is suspected, drug readministration may be hazardous. Prior to considering rechallenge, appropriate consultation is suggested, to evaluate viable alternative therapies, the potential for challenge-induced anaphylaxis, possible desensitization procedures (if any), and formulation of a comprehensive treatment protocol to manage any adverse sequelae of re-exposure to the agent.

Identifying the culprit drug in patients receiving multiple medications can be challenging. The most likely offender should be either dose-reduced or discontinued (as appropriate based on the suspicion of a dose-dependent versus an idiosyncratic/allergic phenomenon), while less likely candidate drugs are continued. If the suspected reaction does not improve, remaining drugs may be discontinued sequentially,

beginning with the most likely candidate. In a patient suffering a severe reaction, all medications should be stopped if possible. A common example in the ICU is the patient who develops thrombocytopenia while receiving prophylactic therapy with an H_2 blocker and subcutaneous heparin. In this situation, thrombocytopenia frequently represents a manifestation of disease, particularly if hemodynamic instability is present, and not an ADR. Nevertheless, in the presence of severe or progressive thrombocytopenia, an ADR should be considered and medication adjustments made. Heparin use correlates most firmly with drug-induced thrombocytopenia, and this agent should be discontinued first.[93] H_2 blockers (and indeed most other drugs used in the ICU) are not responsible for the majority of cases of thrombocytopenia and may be continued if clinically important.[93] In patients with critical thrombocytopenia, however, risk-benefit analysis supports discontinuation of both drugs pending further evaluation, which may include assay for antiplatelet antibodies (drug-specific tests are possible).

Numerous published tables list drugs associated with ADRs.[90,94] These lists are merely suggestive that a sign or symptom may be drug-related. They include both well-documented and poorly-documented drug reactions and are clearly not all inclusive. The absence of a drug from a particular category does not exclude the possibility of drug reaction, since there is always a first identified or reported reaction, especially during the initial period of postmarketing surveillance following approval and release of a new drug for widespread use. In the absence of a simple, dedicated, and exhaustive source of information about ADRs specific to critical care, most clinicians rely on their institution's hospital drug information service, and various library and Internet resources.[95] It is important to become familiar with these resources and to utilize government and pharmaceutical industry information services to aid in evaluating potential ADRs. Appropriate information resources include the following:

GENERAL DRUG INFORMATION REFERENCES

1. *Physicians' Desk Reference.* Medical Economics Company, Inc. (annual editions).
2. *American Hospital Formulary Service Drug Information.* Bethesda, MD, American Society of Health-Systems Pharmacists, Inc. (annual editions).
3. *Drug Facts and Comparisons.* Philadelphia, Lippincott. Phone: 1-800-232-0554 for product information (updated monthly).
4. Hansten PD, Horn JR: *Drug Interactions Analysis and Management.* Applied Therapeutics, Inc. (updated quarterly).
5. Tatro DS (ed): *Drug Interaction Facts.* St Louis, Lippincott (updated quarterly).
6. medicine.iupui.edu/flockhart/ (updated periodically).

DRUG INTERACTION SOFTWARE
SUBSCRIPTION SERVICES

Most institutions utilize one or more computer software programs available by subscription, such as ePocrates Rx Pro, to help identify drug interactions. These programs are continuously in development, and to date no system has been demonstrated to be superior to an experienced clinician in identifying drug interactions. Barriers to the development of drug-drug interaction (DDI) detection software for widespread use include difficulty of portability and integration into existing hospital computer systems, development and maintenance of the knowledge base, and establishment of formal methodology of evaluation of these systems. Nonetheless, existing available software are a good initial step toward decreasing ADRs due to drug-drug interactions.

DEDICATED ICU INTENSIVISTS AND PHARMACISTS

Many studies have investigated the benefits of a dedicated team of professionals in the ICU, with the team led by a physician with specialized training in critical care medicine.[96,97] This advantage is theorized to be a result of specialized training in particular issues that arise in critically ill patients, a broader perspective of issues that pertain to critically ill patients, and improved continuity of care. In fact, the Leapfrog Initiative—a coalition of some of the nation's largest employers, such as General Electric and General Motors—has identified this as one of the three changes that they believe would most improve safety.[98] This same rationalization can be used to justify the role of a dedicated ICU pharmacist. The traditional role of a pharmacist to accept and clarify orders and dispense medications is antiquated. Having a pharmacist who participates in clinical rounds as a full member of the patient care team in the ICU can significantly decrease ADRs and decrease costs of hospitalization as compared to pharmacist review alone.[99] The benefits may be explained by improved communication between the health care professionals, optimization of therapy, and improved monitoring and management of adverse drug events. For example, for the treatment of an infection in a critically ill patient, the ICU pharmacist may contribute specialized knowledge in selecting the narrowest-spectrum antibiotic, in selecting an appropriate drug to minimize antibiotic resistance based on patterns of organism resistance in the hospital, in minimizing potential adverse drug reactions, and in selecting the most cost-effective agent. Barriers to implementing the dedicated ICU pharmacist model include the initial investment of money and time to create a new staff position, but these initial costs are likely to be easily overcome by savings in drug costs and prevention of adverse drug events.

COMPUTERIZED ORDER SCREENING SYSTEMS

Computerized screening of medication orders at the time of prescription data entry is performed in many acute care practice settings. Such programs allow for real-time checks for potential drug interactions with the patient, disease states, or other drugs. Physician order entry (POE) systems also obviate potential medical errors due to illegible handwriting or transcription errors. Common problems with these programs include a lack of primary literature referencing, routine detection of insignificant interactions, and a significant lag time between introduction of a new drug and interaction data updates. Physicians with minimal technological expertise may also be hesitant to use such technology. Nonetheless, POE systems are another change that the Leapfrog Initiative has identified that may contribute to significant reduction in ADRs.

REPORTING UNUSUAL OR NEW DRUG INTERACTIONS

Medwatch is a voluntary program sponsored by the Food and Drug Administration for reporting adverse events and problems with drugs and other products regulated by this agency. Although it is not a direct information source, contributed data collectively provide continuous new drug information.

Medwatch is a major component of the FDA's postmarketing drug product surveillance and has identified ADRs that were not apparent during preapproval clinical trials (e.g., cardiotoxic effects of astemizole). Reports are encouraged even if the practitioner is not certain the product caused the event and whether or not all details are available. The program utilizes a consolidated reporting form (FDA form 3500), which may be submitted by mail or facsimile. Reports can also be sent by computer modem or by phone 24 hours a day 7 days a week. For more information or to report quality problems call 1-800-FDA-1088.

DRUG MANUFACTURER INFORMATION

The package insert which accompanies all products contains FDA-approved information regarding the known properties and appropriate use of the drug. Contact information (including toll-free telephone numbers) for pharmaceutical companies can also generally be found in this insert or other package labeling or through the hospital drug information center. Pharmaceutical manufacturing companies usually have drug information support services that can provide up-to-date information pertinent to their products. Manufacturers are required to perform postmarketing surveillance of their products and to collect information about drug interactions and other ADRs.

COMPUTERIZED RESOURCES IN THE ICU

Application of computer technology to medical care can improve efficacy and decrease errors at every step of drug administration. Computers can serve as a repository for references. Availability of textbooks, journals, review services and formularies may be valuable at the time of drug prescription. While availability of all references by print may be prohibitive, online references are easily accessible, such as Medline (National Library of Medicine, United States), MDConsult (LLC Ltd Liability Co., DE), Physician Drug References,[100] and UptoDate (UptoDate Inc., DE), to name a few.

Most institutions in the United States use computers to store patient medical records. A step further in the integration of computer technology into medical practice is patient information capture. Real-time capture of patient data, such as vital signs, pulse oximetry, and laboratory results, aids in the dissemination of information and more informed decisions for drug prescription and drug effect monitoring. Therapeutic drug monitoring can be more effectively regulated with integration of patient data and drug administration.

Recent advances in handheld devices make all of the aforementioned systems even more convenient and portable. Software for handheld devices, such as Epocrates Rx (Epocrates, Inc., CA) and Medcalc for example, allow for quick and convenient references for patient data interpretation. While computer technology continues to advance, the major barriers to incorporation of these systems into the medical practice include the initial costs of the computer devices and software, the time to install the appropriate software, the education and willingness of health care professionals to use the technology available, and the real possibility of technical malfunction. Future trends in computer technology in the ICU involve expert systems that can simulate human judgment to aid in diagnostic and therapeutic decision making, and data mining that can analyze large amounts of data to recognize relationships that have not been otherwise discovered.

References

1. Bodenham A, Shelly MP, Park GR: The altered pharmacokinetics and pharmacodynamics of drugs commonly used in critically ill patients. *Clin Pharmacokinet* 14:347, 1988.
2. Nightingale CH, Carver P: Basic principles of pharmacokinetics. *Clin Lab Med* 7:267, 1987.
3. Winter ME: Basic principles, in Koda-Kimble MA, Young LY (eds): *Basic Clinical Pharmacokinetics*, 3rd ed. Vancouver, WA, Applied Therapeutics, 1994, p 12.
4. Rowland M, Tozer TN: *Clinical Pharamcokinetics: Concepts and Applications,* 3rd ed. Philadelphia, Lea and Febiger, 1995, p 35.
5. Benet LZ, Kroetz DL, Sheiner LB: Pharmacokinetics: The dynamics of drug absorption, distribution, and elimination, in Hardman JG, Gilman AG, Limbird LI (eds): *Goodman & Gilman's The Pharmacological Basis of Therapeutics*, 9th ed. New York, McGraw-Hill, 1996, p 3.
6. Pratt WB: The entry, distribution, and elimination of drugs, in Pratt WB, Taylor P (eds): *Principles of Drug Action,* 3rd ed. New York, Churchill Livingstone, 1990.
7. Neubig RR: The time course of drug action, in Pratt WB, Taylor P (eds): *Principles of Drug Action,* 3rd ed. New York, Churchill Livingstone, 1990, p 48.
8. Pond SM, Tozer TN: First-pass elimination: Basic concepts and clinical consequences. *Clin Pharmacokinet* 9:1, 1984.
9. Gibaldi M, Koup JR: Pharmacokinetic concepts—drug binding, apparent volume of distribution and clearance. *Eur J Clin Pharmacol* 20:299, 1981.
10. Sheiner LB, Stanski DR, Vozeh S, et al: Simultaneous modeling of pharmacokinetics and pharmacodynamics: Application to d-tubocurarine. *Clin Pharmacol Ther* 25:358, 1979.
11. Stargel WW, Shand DG, Routledge PA, et al: Clinical comparison of rapid infusion and multiple injection methods for lidocaine loading. *Am Heart J* 102:872, 1991.
12. Reidenberg MM, Levy M, Warner H, et al: Relationship between diazepam dose, plasma level, age, and central nervous system depression. *Clin Pharmacol Ther* 23:371, 1978.
13. Zhou H-H, Koshakji RP, Silberstein DJ, et al: Racial differences in drug response: Altered sensitivity to and clearance of propanolol in men of Chinese descent as compared to American whites. *N Engl J Med* 320:565, 1989.
14. Lang CC, Stein CM, Brown RM, et al: Attenuation of isoproterenol-mediated vasodilatation in blacks. *N Engl J Med* 333:155, 1995.
15. Weinshilboum R: Genomic medicine: Inheritance and drug response. *N Engl J Med* 348:529, 2003.
16. Murray P, Wylam ME: Dopamine, dobutamine, and dopexamine, in Leff AR (ed): *Pulmonary and Critical Care Pharmacology and Therapeutics.* New York, McGraw-Hill, 1996, p ???.
17. Brater DC: Pharmacokinetics and pharmacodynamics in cirrhosis, in Epstein M (ed): *The Kidney in Liver Disease,* 4th ed. Philadelphia, Hanley & Belfus, 1996, p ???.
18. Summer WR, Michael JR, Lipsky JJ: Initial aminoglycoside levels in the critically ill. *Crit Care Med* 11:948, 1983.
19. Marik PE: Aminoglycoside volume of distribution and illness severity in critically ill septic patients. *Anaesth Intensive Care* 21:172, 1993.
20. Martin SJ, Danziger LH: Continuous infusion of loop diuretics in the critically ill: A review of the literature. *Crit Care Med* 22:1323, 1994.
21. Rudy DW, Voelker JR, Greene PK, et al: Loop diuretics in chronic renal insufficiency: A continuous infusion is more efficacious than bolus therapy. *Ann Intern Med* 115:360, 1991.
22. Ballesteros MA, Hogan DL, Koss MA, Isenberg JI: Bolus or intravenous infusion of ranitidine: Effects on gastric pH and acid secretion. *Ann Intern Med* 112:334, 1990.
23. Kress JP, O'Connor MF, Pohlman AS, et al: Sedation of critically ill patients during mechanical ventilation: A comparison of propofol and midazolam. *Am J Respir Crit Care Med* 153:1012, 1996.
24. Pohlman AS, Simpson KP, Hall JB: Continuous intravenous infusions of lorazepam versus midazolam for sedation during mechanical ventilatory support: A prospective, randomized study. *Crit Care Med* 22:1241, 1994.
25. Kress JP, Pohlman AS, O'Connor MF, Hall JB: Daily interruption of sedative infusions in critically ill patients undergoing mechanical ventilation. *N Engl J Med* 342:1471, 2000.
26. Shemesh O, Golbetz H, Kriss JP, Myers BD: Limitations of creatinine as a filtration marker in glomerulopathic patients. *Kidney Int* 28:830, 1985.
27. Rabito CA, Panico F, Rubin R, et al: Noninvasive, real-time monitoring of renal function during critical care. *J Am Soc Nephrol* 4:1421, 1994.
28. Cockroft DW, Gault MH: Prediction of creatinine clearance from serum creatinine. *Nephron* 16:31, 1976.
29. Gault MH, Longerich LL, Harnett JD, Weslowski C: Predicting glomerular function from adjusted creatinine. *Nephron* 62:249, 1992.
30. Luke DR, Halstenson CE, Opsahl JA, Matzke GR: Validity of creatinine clearance estimates in the assessment of renal function. *Clin Pharmacol Ther* 48:503, 1990.
31. Lindeman RD: Assessment of renal function in the old: Special considerations. *Clin Lab Med* 13:269, 1993.
32. Ducharme MP, Smythe M, Strohs G: Drug-induced alterations in serum creatinine concentrations. *Ann Pharmacother* 27:622, 1993.
33. Martin C, Alaya M, Bras J, et al: Assessment of creatinine clearance in intensive care patients. *Crit Care Med* 18:1224, 1990.
34. Robert S, Zarowitz BJ: Is there a reliable index of glomerular filtration rate in critically ill patients? *Ann Pharmacother* 25:169, 1991.
35. Robert S, Zarowitz BJ, Peterson EL, Dumler F: Predictability of creatinine clearance estimates in critically ill patients. *Crit Care Med* 21:1487, 1993.
36. Levey AS, Bosch JP, Lewis JB, et al: A more accurate method to estimate glomerular filtration rate from serum creatinine: A new prediction equation. Modification of Diet in Renal Disease Study Group. *Ann Intern Med* 130:461, 1999.
37. Zarowitz BJ, Robert S, Peterson EL: Prediction of glomerular filtration rate using aminoglycoside clearance in critically ill medical patients. *Ann Pharmacother* 26:1205, 1992.
38. Brater DC: Dosing regimens in renal disease, in Jacobson HE, Striker GA, Klahr S (eds): *The Principles and Practice of Nephrology,* 2nd ed. St. Louis, Mosby-Year Book, 1995, p 15.
39. Bennett WM, Aronoff GR, Golper TA, et al: *Drug Prescribing in Renal Failure: Dosing Guidelines for Adults,* 3rd ed. Philadelphia, American College of Physicians, 1994, p 38.
40. Swan SK, Bennett WM: Drug dosing guidelines in patients with renal failure. *West J Med* 156:633, 1992.
41. Shuler C, Golper TA, Bennett WM: Prescribing drugs in renal disease, in Brenner BM (ed): *The Kidney,* 5th ed. Philadelphia, Saunders, 1996, p 51.
42. Touchette MA, Slaughter RL: The effects of renal failure on hepatic drug clearance. *Ann Pharmacother* 25:1214, 1991.
43. Macias WL, Mueller BA, Scarim SK: Vancomycin pharmacokinetics in acute renal failure: Preservation of nonrenal clearance. *Clin Pharmacol Ther* 50:688, 1991.
44. Mueller BA, Scarim SK, Macias WL: Comparison of imipenem pharmacokinetics in patients with acute or chronic renal failure treated with continuous hemofiltration. *Am J Kidney Dis* 21:172, 1993.
45. Wrighton SA, Stevens JC: The human hepatic cytochromes p450 involved in drug metabolism. *Crit Rev Toxicol* 22:1, 1992.
46. Tukey RH, Johnson EF: Molecular aspects of regulation and structures of the drug-metabolizing enzymes, in Pratt WB,

Taylor P (eds): *Principles of Drug Action,* 3rd ed. New York, Churchill Livingstone, 1990, p 56.

47. Watkins PB: Drug metabolism by cytochromes p450 in the liver and small bowel. *Gastroenterol Clin North Am* 21:511, 1992.

48. Spinler SA, Cheng JWM, Kindwall KE, Charland SL: Possible inhibition of hepatic metabolism of quinidine by erythromycin. *Clin Pharmacol Ther* 57:89, 1995.

49. Alvares AP, Pratt WB: Pathways of drug metabolism, in Pratt WB, Taylor P (eds): *Principles of Drug Action,* 3rd ed. New York, Churchill Livingstone, 1990, p 40.

50. O'Malley K, Crooks J, Duke E, Stevenson IH: Effect of age and sex on human drug metabolism. *Br Med J* 3:607, 1971.

51. Masimirembwa CM, Beke M, Hasler JA, et al: Low CYP 1A2 activity in rural Shona children of Zimbabwe. *Clin Pharmacol Ther* 57:25, 1995.

52. May DG, Porter GR, Branch RA: Frequency distribution of dapsone N-hydroxylase, a putative probe for P4503A4 activity, in a white population. *Clin Pharmacol Ther* 55:492, 1994.

53. Lown K, Kolars J, Turgeon K, et al: The erythromycin breath test selectively measures P450IIIA in patients with severe liver disease. *Clin Pharmacol Ther* 51:229, 1992.

54. Lown KS, Thummel KE, Benedict PE, et al: The erythromycin breath test predicts the clearance of midazolam. *Clin Pharmacol Ther* 57:16, 1995.

55. Hunt CM, Westerkam WR, Stave GM: Effect of age and gender on the activity of human hepatic CYP3A. *Biochem Pharmacol* 44:275, 1992.

56. Jann MW, ZumBrunnen TL, Tenjarla SN, Ward ES Jr, Weidler DJ: Relative bioavailability of ondansetron 8-mg oral tablets versus two extemporaneous 16-mg suppositories: formulation and gender differneces. *Pharmacotherapy* 18:288, 1998.

57. Seaber E, On N, Dixon RM, et al: The absolute bioavailability and metabolic disposition of the novel antimigraine compound zolmitriptan (311C90). *Br J Clin Pharmcol* 43:579, 1997.

58. Loi CM, Parker BM, Cusack B, Vestal RE: Aging and drug interactions. III. Individual and combined effects of cimetidine and cimetidine and ciprofloxacin on theophylline metabolism in helathy male and female nonsmokers. *J Pharmacol Exp Ther* 280:627, 1997.

59. Reigner BG, Welker HA: Factors influencing elimination and distribution of fleroxacin: metaanalysis of individual data from 10 pharmacokinetic studies. *Antimicrob Agents Chemother* 40:575, 1996.

60. Schwartz JB, Capili H, Daugherty J: Aging of women alters S-verapamil pharmacokinetics and pharmacodynamics. *Clin Pharmacol Ther* 55:509, 1994.

61. Lennard MS: Genetically determined adverse drug reactions involving metabolism. *Drug Safety* 9:60, 1993.

62. Tucker GT: Clinical implications of genetic polymorphism in drug metabolism. *J Pharm Pharmacol* 46(Suppl 1):417, 1994.

63. Vessel ES: Therapeutic lessons from pharmacogenetics. *Ann Intern Med* 126:653, 1997.

64. Nebert DW, Weber WW: Pharmacogenetics, in Pratt WB, Taylor P (eds): *Principles of Drug Action,* 3rd ed. New York, Churchill Livingstone, 1990, p 60.

65. Tseng C-Y, Wang S-L, Lai M-D, et al: Formation of morphine from codeine in Chinese subjects of different CYP2D6 genotypes. *Clin Pharmacol Ther* 60:177, 1996.

66. Relling MV, Cherrie J, Schell MJ, et al: Lower prevalence of the debrisoquin oxidative poor metabolism phenotype in American black versus white subjects. *Clin Pharmacol Ther* 50:308, 1991.

67. Flockhart DA: Drug interactions and the cytochrome p450 system: The role of cytochrome p450 2C19. *Clin Pharmacokinet* 29:45, 1995.

68. Lerena AL, Alm C, Dahl ML, et al: Haloperidol disposition is dependent on debrisoquine hydroxylation phenotype. *Ther Drug Monit* 14:92, 1992.

69. Sagar M, Janczewska I, Ljungdahl A, et al: Effect of CYP2C19 polymorphism on serum levels of vitamin B-12 in patients on

long-term omeprazole treatment. *Aliment Pharmacol Ther* 13:453, 1999.

70. Evans WE, McLeod HL: Drug therapy: Pharmacogenomics—drug disposition, drug targets, and side effects. *N Engl J Med* 348:538, 2003.

71. Keogh A, Spratt P, McCosker C, et al: Ketoconazole reduces the need for cyclosporine after cardiac transplantation. *N Engl J Med* 333:628, 1995.

72. Gomez DY, Wacher VJ, Tomlanovich SJ, et al: The effects of ketoconazole on the intestinal metabolism and bioavailability of cyclosporine. *Clin Pharmacol Ther* 58:15, 1995.

73. Gupta E, Wang X, Ramirez J, Ratain MJ: Modulation of glucuronidation of SN-38, the active metabolite of irinotecan, by valproic acid and phenobarbital. *Cancer Chemother Pharmacol* 39:440, 1997.

74. Shedlofsky SI, Israel BC, McClain CJ, et al: Endotoxin administration to humans inhibits hepatic cytochrome p450-mediated drug metabolism. *J Clin Invest* 94:2209, 1994.

75. Muller CM, Scierka A, Stiller RL, et al: Nitric oxide mediates hepatic cytochrome p450 dysfunction indued by endotoxin. *Anesthesiology* 84:1435, 1996.

76. Morgan DJ, McLean AJ: Clinical pharmacokinetic and pharmacodynamic considerations in patients with liver disease. *Clin Pharmacokinet* 29:370, 1995.

77. Murray M: P450 enzymes. Inhibition mechanisms, genetic regulation and effects of liver disease. *Clin Pharmacokinet* 23:132, 1992.

78. Williams RL: Drug administration in hepatic disease. *N Engl J Med* 309:1616, 1983.

79. Huet P-M, Villeneuve J-P: Determinants of drug disposition in patients with cirrhosis. *Hepatology* 3:913, 1983.

80. Wilkinson GR, Shand DG: Commentary: A physiological approach to hepatic drug clearance. *Clin Pharmacol Ther* 18:377, 1975.

81. Schentag JJ, Cerra FB, Calleri GM, et al: Age, disease, and cimetidine disposition in healthy subjects and chronically ill patients. *Clin Pharmacol Ther* 29:737, 1981.

82. Bass NM, Williams RL: Guide to drug dosage in hepatic disease. *Clin Pharmacokinet* 15:396, 1988.

83. Rudy AC, Brater DC: Drug interactions, in Chernow B (ed): *The Pharmacologic Approach to the Critically Ill Patient,* 3rd ed. Baltimore, Williams & Wilkins, 1994, p 15.

84. Wright JM: Drug interactions, in Melmon KL, Morrelli HF, Hoffman BB, Nierenberg DW (eds): *Melmon and Morrelli's Clinical Pharmacology: Basic Principles in Therapeutics,* 3rd ed. New York, McGraw-Hill, 1992, p 21.

85. Kolars JC, Awni WM, Merion RM, Watkins PB: First-pass metabolism of cyclosporine by the gut. *Lancet* 338:1488, 1991.

86. MacKichan JJ: Protein binding drug displacement interactions: Fact or fiction? *Clin Pharmacokinet* 16:65, 1989.

87. Kaplan B, Friedman G, Jacobs M, et al: Potential interactions of troglitazone and cyclosporine. *Transplantation* 65:1399, 1998.

88. Thompson D, Oster G: Use of terfenadine and contraindicated drugs. *JAMA* 275:1339, 1996.

89. Pearson TF, Pittman DG, Longley JM, et al: Factors associated with preventable adverse drug reactions. *Am J Hosp Pharm* 51:2268, 1994.

90. Wood AJJ: Adverse reactions to drugs, in Isselbacher KJ, Braunwald E, Wilson JD, et al (eds): *Harrison's Principles of Internal Medicine,* 13th ed. New York, McGraw-Hill, 1994, p 25.

91. Cribb AE, Lee BL, Trepanier LA, Speilberg SP: Adverse reactions to sulphonamide and sulphonamide-trimethoprim antimicrobials: Clinical syndromes and pathogenesis. *Adverse Drug React Toxicol Rev* 15:9, 1996.

92. Rieder MJ: Immunopharmacology and adverse drug reactions. *J Clin Pharmacol* 33:316, 1993.

93. Bonfiglio MF, Traeger SM, Kier KL, et al: Thrombocytopenia in intensive care patients: a comprehensive analysis of risk factors in 314 patients. *Ann Pharmacother* 29:835, 1995.

94. Albertson TE, Foulke GE, Tharratt S, Allen R: Pharmacokinetics and iatrogenic drug toxicity in the intensive care unit, in Hall JB, Schmidt GA, Wood LDH (eds): *Principles of Critical Care*, 1st ed. New York, McGraw-Hill, 1992, p 2061.

95. Bates DW, Gawande AA: Improving safety with information technology. *N Engl J Med* 348:2526, 2003.

96. Pronovost PJ, Waters H, Dorman T: Impact of critical care physician workforce for intensive care unit physician staffing. *Curr Opin Critical Care* 7:456, 2001.

97. Goh AY, Lum LC, Abdel-Latif ME: Impact of 24 hour critical care physician staffing on case-mix adjusted mortality in paediatric intensive care. Lancet 357:445, 2001.

98. Shaprio JP: Industry preaches safety in Pittsburgh. *US News World Rep* 56, 2000.

99. Anderson JG, Jay SJ, Anderson M, Hunt TJ: Evaluating the capability of information technology to prevent adverse drug events: A computer simulation approach. *J Am Med Inform Assoc* 9:479, 2002.

100. *Physicians' Desk Reference 2003*. Edition 57, PDR/Medical Economics Company, 2002, p 5.

Chapter 104

RHEUMATOLOGY IN THE ICU

WALTER G. BARR
JOHN A. ROBINSON

KEY POINTS

- *Most ICU admissions for rheumatology patients are prompted by infection.*

- *New-onset rheumatic diseases rarely prompt ICU admission in the absence of a revealing prodrome.*

- *In most patients without a previously established collagen vascular disease, suspected vasculitis will be explained by an alternative diagnosis.*

- *Immunoserologic assessment of critically ill patients is a double-edged sword providing both enlightenment and misleading shadows. All immunoserologic testing must be interpreted with a thorough understanding of the patient's clinical condition.*

- *Inability to assign specific diagnostic labels to patients with severe life-threatening immunoinflammatory disease should not delay therapeutic intervention.*

- *Not all ischemic skin lesions that appear to be vasculitis are. Pseudovasculitis of various causes should always be part of the differential diagnosis.*

- *Empiric trials with corticosteroids can be a rational approach to patient care when such trials are carried out appropriately.*

- *Acute organic brain syndrome without focal neurologic deficits or evidence of systemic vasculitis is unlikely to be secondary to vasculitis.*

- *Fever in patients with collagen vascular disease should be presumed infectious if accompanied by chills, leukocytosis with a left shift, or hypotension.*

- *Patients who have been treated with significant doses of corticosteroids within the past year may require empiric replacement therapy during critical illness or surgical procedures until adrenal insufficiency can be excluded.*

Rheumatologists seldom lend their expertise to the medical ICU. The tempo and level of intensity of most rheumatic disorders are more suited to outpatient management. Nonetheless, approximately 10% to 25% of all rheumatic disease patients visiting the emergency department require hospitalization and up to one-third of these patients will require intensive care.[1] Patients with rheumatic diseases admitted to the medical ICU most often have problems not directly related to their primary illness. Sepsis, massive gastrointestinal bleeding, and myocardial infarcts may arise secondary to treatment. The major direction of care in these circumstances often comes from the intensivist. Circumstances do arise that require the unique insight of the experienced clinical rheumatologist, who at times must direct the management of a disease-specific complication. Just as often the rheumatologist is asked to address a diagnostic dilemma spawned by puzzling clinical and laboratory data. This chapter addresses the more common issues that prompt the rheumatologist and the intensivist to collaborate.

Rheumatic Disease–Specific Intensive Care Scenarios

SYSTEMIC LUPUS ERYTHEMATOSUS

FEVER: IS IT THE LUPUS?

Fever in the patient with lupus presses the clinician for an urgent answer to the question: Is this caused by lupus activity or infection? Fever is a common finding in active systemic lupus erythematosus (SLE) and follows no specific curve or pattern.[2] It may respond to the usual antipyretics or require corticosteroids. Single-daily-morning dose prednisone may not control late afternoon or evening fevers. Leukocytosis and increased bands on peripheral smear are strong presumptive evidence for infection, as is the presence of shaking chills. Complement proteins or components, including C3 and C4, are acute-phase reactants and usually rise with infection. Low levels of complement occur in some but not all patients with active lupus. Using discriminant analysis, Inone and colleagues[3] showed that 95% of 74 febrile episodes could be correctly classified as to the cause of fever when a combination of white blood count (low in SLE, normal to high with infection) and α_2-globulin levels (high with SLE, normal with infection) are used as variables.

In the ICU setting, the febrile patient with SLE is probably best considered infected and treated with broad-spectrum antibiotics pending results of cultures.[4] Infection is most likely to be caused by nonopportunistic organisms, and coverage for gram-positive and gram-negative aerobes represents adequate empirical therapy when no obvious source has been recognized. Systemic infections with *Salmonella*, endocarditis involving lupus-related valvular lesions, and pneumococcal sepsis in the splenectomized (surgical or autosplenectomy) are among the infections that have special significance for lupus patients.

MYOCARDIAL INFARCT IN THE LUPUS PATIENT: IS IT VASCULITIS?

Myocardial infarction makes a major contribution to excessive mortality in SLE. Mortality data suggest a bimodal distribution with many late deaths in SLE secondary to ischemic heart disease. The primary cause of ischemic heart disease in lupus is atherosclerosis. Autopsy studies in young women with lupus with death from any cause show an excessive incidence of atherosclerosis in comparison to age-matched females.[5] The cause of accelerated atheroma is not totally clear, but inflammation of the vascular endothelium due to chronic immune complex disease compounded by the effects of corticosteroids probably is the major contributing factor.

Vasculitis in SLE may affect any organ including the heart. Most patients with coronary artery vasculitis have evidence of vasculitis in other organs. Serologic evidence of active lupus and markers of systemic inflammation including low hemoglobin and albumin are likely to be present. Acute therapy would include high-dose corticosteroids (see below). In the face of widespread vasculitis, additional intervention with parenteral immunosuppressives, B-cell–depleting biopharmaceuticals, and plasmapheresis may be indicated.

Another potential cause of myocardial ischemia is coronary thrombosis secondary to antiphospholipid syndrome.[6] Treatment is anticoagulation with heparin. Thrombolytic therapy has been successfully used in some patients with antiphospholipid syndrome.[7]

Corticosteroids are potentially hazardous, and high doses may predispose to ventricular rupture. Therefore corticosteroids should not be used in the absence of reasonable clinical suspicion for coronary vasculitis. If the lupus patient is in apparent clinical remission without evidence of widespread vasculitis, treatment should be the same as that for the non-lupus patient. Early cardiac catheterization may help clarify the nature of the vascular disease.

RENAL FAILURE: IS IT TREATABLE LUPUS NEPHRITIS?

In patients with SLE in the ICU, renal insufficiency may be caused by a variety of factors, including drugs, especially non-steroidal anti-inflammatory drugs (NSAIDs), hypovolemia, sepsis, or previous renal disease.[8] In some cases, active lupus nephritis is a contributing factor. A careful examination of the urinary sediment is the most critical diagnostic tool. Protein-uria, casts, and red blood cells indicate glomerulitis. Lupus patients with active nephritis are most often hypertensive. Significant renal lupus (other than membranous disease) is often associated with low complement levels and elevation of anti-DNA antibody.

In a patient with a creatinine level above 4.0 mg/dL who has been adequately hydrated, has been divorced from nephrotoxic drugs, and shows evidence of active glomerulitis, the question arises: Is more aggressive immunosuppression desirable? The answer to this question depends on the degree of potential disease reversibility. A renal biopsy can help clarify this issue. The presence of significant chronic disease should dampen enthusiasm for aggressive therapy. Review of old records can be enlightening if long-standing loss of renal function is documented.

Clinicians have become increasingly aware that immuno-suppression in the lupus patient with advanced renal disease can be more hazardous than progression to complete renal failure. Patients with lupus tolerate dialysis in a fashion comparable to other patients, and results of renal transplantation are favorable.[9] Paradoxically, patients with lupus who develop chronic renal failure often enjoy an amelioration of extrarenal symptoms.[10] A few patients have recovered sufficient renal function to allow withdrawal from dialysis. For all these reasons, the overzealous administration of immunosuppression in patients with lupus and advanced renal disease is to be discouraged.

RESPIRATORY FAILURE AND LUNG INFILTRATES: IS IT LUPUS PNEUMONITIS?

Respiratory failure in the patient with SLE is an ominous development. A paradigm of a compromised host is a patient with lupus who is on high-dose corticosteroid therapy. The usual opportunistic pulmonary infections need to be urgently excluded by bronchoalveolar lavage, bronchoscopic transbronchial biopsy, or open lung biopsy. If no superimposed infections or embolic etiology can be found and treated, lupus-related respiratory failure remains a diagnosis of exclusion and can be caused by either lupus pneumonitis or diffuse pulmonary hemorrhage. Acute lupus pneumonitis may occur as an initial manifestation of SLE and is characterized by fever, tachypnea, and hypoxemia, which may be ac-companied by cough, pleuritic chest pain, and hemoptysis.[11] Radiologic findings are highly variable but usually bilat-eral and at least bibasilar. This diagnosis is not only one of exclusion; it unfortunately still rests solely on clinical suspicion.

The other SLE-related cause of respiratory failure is diffuse alveolar pulmonary hemorrhage.[12] Although invasive *Aspergillus* or tuberculosis can erode a pulmonary vessel and cause hemorrhage, gross hemoptysis, when present, usually indicates alveolar hemorrhage. Hemoptysis is not usually seen in lupus pneumonitis; unfortunately, this finding is present in <50% of patients with alveolar hemor-rhage. Blood or hemosiderin-laden macrophages found during bronchoscopy in a patient without heart failure can be helpful findings but are nonspecific. The presence of thrombocytopenia is not helpful, but bleeding sufficient to cause acute respiratory failure most invariably causes an acute drop in hematocrit. In fact, treatment should not be delayed in order to distinguish between lupus pneumonitis and lupus-associated hemorrhage, because mortality is extremely high in either syndrome and treatment strategies are similar.

Pulmonary hypertension, sometimes severe, is frequently present. Cardiac filling pressures, in contrast to B-type natriuretic peptide determinations, can occasionally be helpful discriminators to exclude acute cardiogenic pulmonary edema. Pulmonary artery thrombosis masquerading as massive pulmonary emboli can occur in patients with pulmonary hypertension or thrombotically active anticardiolipin (ACL) antibodies.

The mortality of lupus pneumonitis is high, and treatment should be aggressive. Individual preferences will dictate modes of therapy, since no consensus exists on either the etiology of the syndrome or effective treatment. Pulse methyl-prednisolone, usually 500 to 1000 mg intravenously given for 3 to 5 days, or bolus cyclophosphamide at 0.5 to 1.0 g/m^2 has been used. Uncontrolled studies of plasmapheresis for alveolar hemorrhage in SLE do not reveal striking therapeutic efficacy. In the absence of alternate therapy with proven effect, plasmapheresis may be useful as a temporizing measure during the induction period required for the optimal effects of immunosuppressive agents like cyclophosphamide.[13]

BRAIN DYSFUNCTION: IS IT LUPUS?

A patient with acute, severe neurologic deficits and a history of SLE or a clinical syndrome and laboratory evidence suggestive of systemic vasculitis presents a diagnostic and therapeutic dilemma for the critical care clinician. In the vast majority of instances, involvement of the central nervous system (CNS) in SLE occurs as an organic brain syndrome or seizures in young females with active multisystem disease. Patients with organic brain syndromes manifest psychosis usually early after the onset of SLE. A common dilemma is to differentiate between steroid-induced pseudo-organic brain syndromes and those owing to active SLE. Interleukin-6 (IL-6) levels are markedly increased in the CSF of patients with active CNS SLE. Minimal, if any, IL-6 should be present in the CSF of patients with steroid-induced psychosis, and IL-6 may prove very helpful in differentiating between drug-induced CNS changes and active SLE. Early-onset development of psychosis while on low doses of corticosteroids and fulminant progression usually characterize the CNS disease caused by SLE.[14] Depressive syndromes with or without auditory, visual, or even olfactory hallucinations in a patient on a dose of corticosteroids usually higher than 0.5 mg/kg per day are usually drug-induced. Because there is little evidence that high-dose corticosteroids ameliorate the CNS manifestations of SLE, rapid reduction of corticosteroid dosage is usually the simplest and most direct clinical strategy when a quandary exists as to whether CNS dysfunction is drug-induced.

Lupus-induced seizures are usually grand mal but can be very pleomorphic and usually occur in patients with active SLE.[15] Rapidly progressive, multisystem SLE that is further complicated by early onset of a seizure syndrome usually portends a poor outcome. The development of a seizure disorder in a patient with a long history of inactive SLE or in a patient with SLE entering remission is usually caused by something else. There is also little clinical evidence that high-dose corticosteroids alone influence the course of seizure disorders in SLE, and these patients should be aggressively treated with conventional anticonvulsive therapy. A difficult but critical differentiation must be made in SLE patients with CNS findings, anemia, and thrombocytopenia. The latter findings, while very common in active SLE, coupled with peripheral blood smear evidence of microangiopathy, point instead to thrombotic thrombocytopenic purpura (TTP) (see Chap. 70). Case reports suggest that TTP and SLE can co-occur, and the differentiation between the two diseases is vital since the treatment of life-threatening TTP is plasma exchange and not concomitant pulse methylprednisone, alkylating agents, and/or plasmapheresis that many rheumatologists, in spite of unproven benefit, will resort to in the setting of fulminant CNS SLE.

Three other CNS manifestations of SLE can be puzzling. A small subset of patients with SLE who have taken NSAIDs, especially ibuprofen, will develop a meningitis-like picture that is characterized by fever, severe headache, nuchal rigidity, and cerebrospinal fluid neutrophilia or pleocytosis.[16] In an immunosuppressed patient, these findings prompt consideration of both common and unusual bacterial and fungal etiologies. The entire syndrome will remit rapidly once the drug is discontinued.

Migraine headaches, some of spectacular intensity, are frequent in SLE.[17] They usually respond to increases in corticosteroid dosage.

Actual paralysis is uncommon in SLE. Rare instances of transverse myelitis occur in the context of active SLE, and myelopathy may rarely be the presenting symptom of lupus. Until recently this was thought to be secondary to necrotizing vasculitis in the spinal arteries. It is likely, however, that many instances have been secondary to thrombosis associated with high titers of IgG ACL antibodies.[18] This differentiation may be important because the primary treatment of this syndrome is not aggressive immunomodulation of SLE, but appropriate anticoagulation.

Some investigators have reported elevated serum levels of anti-ribosomal P antibodies in patients with lupus-induced depression or psychosis. Other studies have not confirmed the association of these antibodies with psychosis.

SCLERODERMA

PULMONARY HYPERTENSION

The emergence of effective therapeutic options has given the detection of pulmonary vascular disease a new sense of urgency. The exact prevalence of pulmonary hypertension in scleroderma is unknown. Hospital-based studies would suggest the number to be in the 10% to 15% range.[19] There are generally two settings in which it is identified. In patients with limited cutaneous systemic sclerosis (*c*alcinosis, *R*aynaud's phenomenon, *e*sophageal motility disorders, *s*clerodactyly, and *t*elangiectasia [CREST] variant of scleroderma) it occurs classically as an isolated phenomenon in the absence of pulmonary fibrosis. This generally occurs in the second decade of disease or later. Patients who fall into the second major category of scleroderma, diffuse disease, may develop pulmonary hypertension as the result of advanced pulmonary fibrosis. In both settings the vascular disease is characterized by bland endothelial proliferation and vascular occlusion. The vasculopathy of scleroderma is not characterized by an inflammatory infiltrate and is not treated with corticosteroids or immunosuppression in the manner that typifies the treatment of lupus vasculitis.

Early symptoms of pulmonary hypertension are exertional breathlessness, but later symptoms are likely to provoke admission to the medical ICU or critical care unit (CCU). These include near-syncope or syncope with exertion and right ventricular angina or heart failure. Scleroderma patients, especially those at greatest risk for pulmonary hypertension, are now screened yearly or every few years using Doppler echocardiography. Confirmation of diagnosis demands a right heart catheterization, which provides additional important information about pulmonary capillary wedge pressure and cardiac output.

The treatment of pulmonary hypertension in the context of scleroderma is similar to that in idiopathic and familial pulmonary hypertension.[20] Anticoagulation, diuretics, digoxin, and supplemental oxygen form the basic management program. A small subset of patients may benefit from calcium channel blockers. Two exciting breakthroughs have substantially changed the quality of life of these patients for the better. Parenteral epoprostenol was initially viewed as a bridge to transplant, but some patients have elected to continue the drug as a chronic maintenance therapy. The emergence of a broad-spectrum endothelin receptor antagonist in the form of bosentan now offers the option of oral therapy to patients with moderately severe disease.[20] End-stage pulmonary hypertension may require heart-lung transplantation. Traditionally scleroderma patients have been considered poor candidates for transplantation. However, a recent report of 12 patients with scleroderma-associated pulmonary artery hypertension who underwent transplantation suggests similar beneficial outcomes compared to those with other acquired lung diseases.[21]

Other less common causes of pulmonary hypertension should not be overlooked in scleroderma patients, including recurrent thromboembolic disease. This may be a particular problem in patients with antiphospholipid antibodies.

HYPERTENSIVE RENAL CRISIS

Until recently, hypertensive renal crisis in patients with scleroderma was the major cause of mortality. The advent of angiotensin-converting enzyme (ACE) inhibitors thrust pulmonary disease into the role of leading cause of death in scleroderma. Nonetheless even recent studies of patients with scleroderma renal crisis suggest a continued high mortality rate in this subset of patients.[22] Therefore strategies for prevention of scleroderma renal crisis are crucial. Scleroderma renal crisis typically develops in patients with diffuse cutaneous disease and rarely in patients with limited cutaneous disease or CREST.[23] At its onset patients experience a marked increase in blood pressure that may be accompanied by abnormalities of urinary sediment (erythrocytes and protein) and the peripheral blood smear (fragmented cells) and thrombocytopenia. Headache, visual disturbance, congestive heart failure, and mental status dysfunction may accompany the hypertension.

The pathogenesis of hypertensive renal crisis is complex and involves a very high renin state. Although combinations of older antihypertensive agents were occasionally successful, the advent of ACE inhibitors has revolutionized the outlook for this problem. Rheumatologists have a low threshold for using these agents in scleroderma patients and typically initiate them at the first diagnosis of hypertension.

In the setting of acute hypertensive renal crisis, larger doses of ACE inhibitors should be used. Although captopril, enalapril, and newer ACE inhibitors have all been used, some prefer captopril because the dose can be adjusted more flexibly. Angiotensin receptor blockers, calcium channel blockers, prostacyclin, and endothelin receptor antagonists have all been suggested as adjunctive therapy for patients refractory to maximum doses of ACE inhibitors.[24]

Some patients may progress to complete renal failure despite blood pressure control. Continued use of ACE inhibitors and dialysis may be required for months prior to recovery of renal function. Such improvement can continue for up to 2 years.

Progressive renal failure can occur in the absence of significant hypertension in as many as 10% of patients with scleroderma renal crisis. Microangiopathic changes may be seen on peripheral smear. Treatment with ACE inhibitors is indicated for this normotensive subset of patients.

POLYMYOSITIS/DERMATOMYOSITIS

DIAGNOSIS IN THE ICU

Very ill patients in the ICU may be weak and have elevations of creatine phosphokinase (CPK). Such clinical data prompt speculation about the presence of immune-mediated myositis. The most common presentation of polymyositis is the insidious onset of proximal muscle weakness, at times associated with myalgia. The acute development of de novo polymyositis in the ICU is unlikely. Similarly, acute fulminant disease requiring ICU admission with subsequent diagnosis is uncommon. Nonetheless, patients with undiagnosed polymyositis may be discovered in the ICU following admission for another reason (e.g., aspiration pneumonia). More likely is the presence of weakness (usually generalized) in combination with a spurious or nonimmune cause of CPK elevation. Intramuscular injections and myonecrosis during severe episodes of hypotension are common causes of increased CPK levels in critically ill patients. ICU-acquired myopathy can usually be distinguished from polymyositis by clinical history. Critical illness myopathy is usually characterized by normal or modestly elevated serum CPK levels.[25]

The skin lesions of dermatomyositis are so highly characteristic as to be diagnostic of dermatomyositis when accompanied by weakness and an elevated CPK value. Nearly all patients with active polymyositis will display an elevated CPK or aldolase level, although occasional patients will have normal muscle enzymes.[26] A unilateral electromyogram (EMG) can provide supportive evidence for the presence of myopathy and identify a biopsy site. Fibrillation potentials suggest active inflammation. A bedside EMG can be done in the ICU, although technical artifact may complicate the interpretation. Magnetic resonance imaging (MRI) may also confirm the presence of inflammatory muscle disease, but is generally impractical for ICU patients.

The EMG should be done unilaterally because EMG needle artifact may be confused with muscle inflammation histologically. Because polymyositis/dermatomyositis is a symmetrical disease, the corresponding maximally affected muscle group can be biopsied on the opposite side. Open biopsy can be done at the bedside, preferably by an experienced surgeon to ensure proper handling of muscle tissue. Needle biopsy of muscle using a Polley-Bickel needle is advocated by some and appears suitable for providing confirmation of active muscle inflammation.

RESPIRATORY FAILURE

Patients with polymyositis/dermatomyositis may develop respiratory failure secondary to muscle weakness involving the diaphragm, intercostals, and accessory muscles. If pharyngeal muscles are involved, acute respiratory failure may be precipitated by aspiration pneumonia. Patients with respiratory failure have a poor prognosis.[27] Some patients with dermatomyositis and this type of profound weakness harbor an underlying malignancy. Such patients are notably refractory to treatment.

Steroids are the mainstay of acute management of inflammatory myositis. Prednisone, 1 to 2 mg/kg per day or its approximate intravenous equivalent of methylprednisolone (in single or divided doses) may be given. In the ventilator-dependent patient, a short trial of pulse steroids may be justified—500 to 1000 mg methylprednisolone intravenously every day for 3 days. Improvement in respiratory muscle strength can be judged by a rise in the maximal inspiratory pressure. Intravenous immunoglobulin (IVIg) is another option for the acute management of the severely ill patient refractory to therapy with corticosteroids.[28] Second-line agents in polymyositis/dermatomyositis include methotrexate, azathioprine, and cyclophosphamide. Azathioprine is not useful in the acute setting owing to slow onset of action. Methotrexate is most commonly used after corticosteroids. In the ICU setting the intravenous route of administration may be preferred; the dose is 25 to 75 mg intravenously weekly.

Uncontrolled trials with plasmapheresis and combination plasmapheresis and leukocytapheresis have reported benefits and may be considered in refractory patients.[29,30] However, a randomized double-blind trial comparing plasmapheresis, leukapheresis, and sham pheresis in 39 patients with polymyositis and dermatomyositis showed comparable improvements in the three treatment groups.[31] The role for therapeutic pheresis in patients refractory to conventional therapy seems limited.

RHEUMATOID ARTHRITIS

METHOTREXATE PNEUMONITIS

Oral low-dose methotrexate given intermittently emerged as the major therapeutic innovation in the treatment of rheumatoid arthritis (RA) during the 1980s. In the era of biological therapies methotrexate continues to be the gold standard of RA therapy and a frequent adjunct to cytokine-directed therapy. Methotrexate therapy is both highly effective and generally well tolerated. A major, albeit uncommon, toxicity is an acute pneumonitis characterized by dyspnea and nonproductive cough.[32,33] Fever is a frequent accompaniment.[34] Diffuse alveolar and interstitial infiltrates are present at diagnosis or appear within days. Opportunistic infections mimicking this syndrome have only rarely been reported.[35] According to one study risk factors for the development of methotrexate-induced lung injury include elderly patients, diabetes, and underlying rheumatoid pleuropulmonary disease.[36] Patients suffer profound hypoxemia. They appear extremely ill, and deaths have been reported. The mechanism is unclear but is presumed to be a hypersensitivity reaction to the drug. Some patients have been rechallenged without developing the syndrome while others have relapsed.

Diagnosis depends on the above clinical scenario developing in a patient taking methotrexate at any dose. Duration of treatment prior to symptoms has been variable. Bronchoscopy with brushings and biopsy shows nonspecific inflammation, and bronchoscopy's main justification is to rule out an opportunistic infection. Because these are rare, it is not unreasonable to forego bronchoscopy initially. Open-lung biopsy is usually unnecessary.

Treatment includes O_2, withdrawal of drug, and corticosteroids. Some have argued that steroids are not critical to recovery. The usual dose is prednisone 1 mg/kg per day or its equivalent in single or divided doses. Most patients will show signs of recovery within a week. Eventually, recovery is typically near complete.

CERVICAL SPINE SUBLUXATION

Arthritis commonly affects the cervical spine in rheumatoid arthritis, with estimates as high as 80% of patients. Subluxation of vertebrae secondary to ligamentous laxity may occur at single or multiple levels. Anterior atlantoaxial subluxation of C1 on C2 is the most frequent cervical abnormality and is particularly dangerous because of the capacity of the odontoid process (or dens) of C2 to compress the anterior spinal cord with motion. Thus sudden hyperextension of the neck during intubation could result in quadriplegia. In reality such occurrences are rare. The explanation may in part include the fact that progressive resorption of the dens often accompanies the most severely unstable necks. Symptomatic patients can be diagnosed with MRI or a myelogram. However, some dramatic subluxations on MRI are not accompanied by neurologic signs or symptoms. Flexion and extension films of the cervical spine may show dynamic instability and subluxation of C1 on C2. There are few data about the specificity or sensitivity of such films to predict a cervical cord catastrophe. Clearly, caution should be exercised in the intubation of patients with rheumatoid arthritis and neck disease; if time allows, nasotracheal or fiberoptically guided endotracheal intubation is preferred. However, when the risk of delayed intubation is sufficiently great, the procedure should not be delayed for radiographic studies, because the risk of cord catastrophe is quite low. Cervical instability is a problem that attends advanced destructive rheumatoid arthritis. Early aggressive treatment of RA patients with disease-modifying therapy has dramatically reduced the prevalence of this problem.[37]

OUTCOMES OF PATIENTS WITH RHEUMATOLOGIC DISEASES IN THE INTENSIVE CARE UNIT

Mortality rates for patients with systemic rheumatic diseases admitted to the ICU is high.[38] This is perhaps not unexpected when consideration is given to a typical scenario of a chronically ill patient with multiple impaired organs, a disordered immune system, treatment with chronic immunosuppression, and admission to the ICU with infection. Reported ICU mortality rates for patients with rheumatic disease are higher than would be predicted using the Acute Physiology, Age, and Chronic Health Evaluation II or simplified acute physiology score II (SAPS).[39,40] Factors associated with poor outcome include higher SAPS II scores, poor health status prior to admission, duration of rheumatic disease, corticosteroids and immunosuppressive drugs, renal failure, coma, and acute respiratory distress syndrome. The overall ICU mortality rate for patients with rheumatic disease ranges from 30% to 60%.[38] Mortality rates are higher for patients admitted because of infection compared to those admitted for exacerbation of rheumatic disease.[39,40] Since infection may cause two-thirds of ICU admissions among patients with rheumatic disease, aggressive intense therapy of the febrile patient with broad-spectrum antibiotic coverage is appropriate.

Perplexing Cases: Is This a Rheumatic Disease?

FEVER OF UNDETERMINED ORIGIN: RHEUMATIC CAUSES

The traditional definition of a fever of undetermined origin (FUO) depicts a patient with a significant fever of 6 weeks' or greater duration and no definable cause. In actual practice, depending on the impatience of the attending physician, FUO usually becomes the working diagnosis within 3 to 14 days after a fruitless search for classic causes of pyrexia. The most common causes by far of FUO are occult infection, drugs, and occasionally malignancy. After those are excluded, one must consider a limited array of rheumatic diseases that could be present in a febrile patient with protracted fever. Rheumatic disorders may account for 10% of cases of FUO. Because rheumatoid arthritis, scleroderma and its variants, dermatomyositis, polymyositis, and polymyalgia rheumatica are not usual causes of significant fever, they need not be strongly considered.

SLE can present with high fevers, either spiking or relatively constant, and leukopenia, hypoalbuminemia, anemia, and an elevated erythrocyte sedimentation rate (ESR), but few other overt clinical signs of lupus such as rash or serositis, polyarthritis, or active urinary sediment. Since SLE is readily diagnosed serologically, it represents a small fraction of FUO patients. Most systemic necrotizing vasculitides will be evident after examination of the skin, chest radiograph, and urinary sediment. Myocardial dysfunction, age, and demographics of the patient with fever may point to either Kawasaki's disease or Lyme disease as the source, and acute valvular dysfunction is being increasingly recognized in SLE and may be the clue to acute rheumatic fever in an adult.[41] An extremely high ESR is a nonspecific laboratory clue in FUO, but antibodies to relevant specific antinuclear or streptococcal disorders provide supportive evidence.

A most vexing diagnosis to pin down is that of adult Still's disease. These patients will have relentless spiking fevers, at times a history of FUO in childhood, leukocytosis, mild to moderate hepatic enzyme changes, and an occasional truncal rash.[42] Polyarthritis or arthralgias are not a constant feature early in this syndrome. Hepatosplenomegaly and lymphadenopathy are common. Rarely, acute pericarditis with tamponade or myocarditis with respiratory failure may complicate the course of adult Still's disease.

In the final analysis, treatment may have to be based on the supposition that the patient has relentless, immunologically driven, noninfectious inflammation that evades specific diagnosis. Blanket suppression of cytokines and white blood cell responses by corticosteroids may be necessary. The steroid dose is tailored to control fever and normalize the acute-phase response. NSAIDs may provide a less potent but possibly better tolerated alternative strategy.

MULTIPLE AUTOANTIBODIES AND MULTISYSTEM INFLAMMATORY DISEASE: WHAT NAME DO I GIVE IT?

The collagen-vascular diseases are characterized by the presence of sterile inflammation in multiple organs and multiple autoantibodies.[43] The prototype disease is SLE, which is characterized by the widest clinical and serologic spectrum. Other diseases include scleroderma, Sjögren's syndrome, polymyositis dermatomyositis, rheumatoid arthritis, and syndromes with overlapping features (overlap syndrome or undifferentiated connective tissue disease). One subset of the latter group has been called *mixed connective tissue disease* (MCTD). The clustering of clinical features and the nature and diversity of autoantibodies may strongly suggest one disorder rather than another, but the overlap of clinical, serologic, and pathologic features among these diseases is great. This can lead to considerable consternation for clinicians. Debates about whether a given patient has SLE, primary Sjögren's syndrome, MCTD, or another overlap syndrome are tiring, usually unresolvable, and generally irrelevant. The therapy for the immunologically active phase of these disorders is not disease-specific. The absence of a consensus label should not delay therapeutic efforts.

THE ELDERLY PATIENT WITH AN ELEVATED SEDIMENTATION RATE: IS THIS TEMPORAL ARTERITIS?

Within the ICU, advanced age, elevation of the ESR, anemia, and various nonspecific clinical features—chiefly fever—may converge to raise the question of temporal arteritis. Temporal arteritis is a granulomatous vasculitis that affects those over age 60 (mean age 70) and has a proclivity to affect extracranial vessels and branches of the aorta. Myriad uncommon clinical features may develop, but headache, polymyalgia rheumatica, visual disturbance, scalp tenderness, and jaw claudication are the common fingerprints of this disease. Treatment is highly effective with prednisone in doses of 40 to 60 mg/d.[44]

The onset of this disease is typically insidious, and its complications rarely prompt admission to the ICU. Therefore, the question is more commonly framed in terms of whether the patient has developed new-onset temporal arteritis in the ICU (probably not) or have it as a comorbid state at admission? History and old records are critical in this regard.

Physical examination is unreliable. Temporal artery biopsy is the gold standard, although sensitivity varies with the institution. A classical clinical scenario that includes headache, visual symptoms, jaw claudication, scalp tenderness, and polymyalgia rheumatica may be sufficiently compelling to prompt treatment. Usually the situation is murkier. There is no substitute for the temporal artery biopsy, which can be done under local anesthesia with little morbidity. A sufficiently large piece (4 to 5 cm) should be obtained and adequate cuts done for pathology. Contralateral biopsy is done routinely by some if a first biopsy is negative. That decision will be influenced by the details of the clinical scenario and the risk of an empiric trial with steroids. A negative biopsy in a marginal clinical situation is reasonable grounds to withhold therapy.

ABDOMINAL PAIN AND ELEVATED ERYTHROCYTE SEDIMENTATION RATE: IS THIS VASCULITIS?

The clinical presentation of acute abdominal pain is constrained to a limited number of clinical findings, regardless of cause. Unfortunately, there is nothing unique about massive gastrointestinal bleeding or the development of an acute abdomen when a patient has a high ESR and vasculitis is the etiology.

If the patient is already known to have systemic vasculitis, and this is usually the case when the gut becomes involved, the differential diagnosis of the acute abdomen and elevated ESR is a bit more simple. Here, early gastroduodenoscopy and colonoscopy with biopsy and perhaps vascular contrast studies may be necessary. MRI can assess arterial wall thickening, and in large-vessel vasculitis magnetic resonance angiography correlates well with conventional angiography. In the rare situation when a patient with no or relatively limited vasculitic findings in skin and renal and pulmonary systems develops fulminant vasculitis of the bowel, diagnosis may remain elusive until arteriography or surgical exploration. Patients on high-dose corticosteroid therapy for pre-existing systemic vasculitis may develop small-bowel or colonic ischemia or perforation with relatively few physical findings, even in the face of profound intra-abdominal sepsis.

Unusual causes of acute abdominal pain in patients with systemic vasculitis include hepatic infarctions, especially in SLE and polyarteritis, which can mimic many other intraperitoneal acute events. In this situation, hepatic computed tomography (CT) or MRI imaging is helpful. Massive bleeding can occur in most forms of systemic vasculitis, especially Henoch-Schönlein purpura, polyarteritis, and mixed cryoglobulinemia. Diarrhea and profound protein-losing enteropathy and acute bowel obstruction secondary to adhesive serositis have occurred rarely in SLE. There is nothing unique about acute pancreatitis in the patient with SLE; appropriate biochemical and imaging assessment will confirm this diagnosis.

The proper perspective must be maintained when the clinician attempts to make the diagnosis of systemic vasculitis involving the gut by analysis of small bowel or colonic tissue, since <50% of endoscopically obtained biopsies will be helpful in the diagnosis.[45] Although careful circumspection should be exercised before embarking on exploratory laparotomy in patients with SLE or other vasculitis with abdominal pain and suspected perforation, one should err on the side of surgical exploration. More than one-half the patients with SLE and an acute abdomen will die.[46] Surgical exploration will correctly identify the major pathophysiology of the syndrome and dictate appropriate management. Increasing availability of laparoscopes with enhanced optics may obviate the need for laparotomy. The vast majority of patients with polyarteritis nodosa who develop an acute abdomen usually die from extensive bowel ischemia, infarction, and perforation unless early surgical intervention is done. The contemporary use of alkylating agents, corticosteroids, and other aggressive therapies may reduce this highly fatal complication in this group of vasculitides.

In summary, any patient with vasculitis, especially one with SLE, who develops an acute abdomen is in dire jeopardy. Routine clinical, laboratory, and radiology assessments are not usually helpful. Early endoscopy, biopsy, arteriography in selected instances, and ultimately early surgical exploration are usually necessary.

LUNG INFILTRATES IN RENAL FAILURE: IS THIS AN IMMUNE-MEDIATED PULMONARY-RENAL SYNDROME?

When a patient, usually but not always a young male, has abnormalities of renal function and then develops increasing shortness of breath, hemoptysis, and bilateral diffuse infiltrates, an immune-mediated pulmonary-renal syndrome should be strongly considered and ruled out as soon as possible. The clinician must be wary because the symptoms can occur in reverse; that is, increasing compromise of pulmonary function may precede significant changes in renal function.

Hemoptysis has many causes in patients with renal failure. Some examples would include SLE, Wegener's granulomatosis, advanced cardiac failure, microscopic polyangiitis, infection, and rapidly progressive glomerulonephritis. The latter disease in actuality is probably one end of the spectrum of a group of diseases mediated by antibodies to epitopes common to both alveolar and glomerular basement membranes (GBM).[47] In its classical expression, anti-GBM disease is called *Goodpasture's syndrome.*

Most diseases with pulmonary and renal manifestations can be distinguished from the immune-mediated pulmonary renal syndromes by their unique extrarenal characteristics. Once they are excluded, one is then confronted with a patient with glomerulonephritis and pulmonary hemorrhage. The diagnosis of the pulmonary-renal syndrome rests on establishing the presence of anti–basement membrane antibodies in the peripheral blood or in situ deposition in a renal biopsy. Characteristic histologic findings in the renal biopsy are those of a diffuse proliferative necrotizing glomerulitis highlighted by a somewhat unique characteristic of rather exuberant crescent formation. Although not well documented by contemporary clinical studies, immunohistologic analysis of tissue obtained by the transbronchial route has not been helpful in most instances.[48] The diagnosis of an antibody-mediated pulmonary-renal syndrome is important because efficacious therapy exists, especially when initiated early in the disease course. Alveolar GBM antibodies can be rapidly removed by vigorous plasmapheresis, and then B-cell clones with basement membrane specificities can be suppressed or clonally eliminated with cytoreductive therapy.[49] The efficiency of GBM antibody removal can be monitored easily by sequential

GBM antibody assays. The antibody-mediated pathogenesis of Goodpasture's disease is beyond doubt and makes this syndrome a logical candidate for B-cell attrition with the chimeric monoclonal anti-CD20 antibody rituximab.[50] The approach to a patient in the ICU with hemoptysis and renal failure should include close attention to maintenance of adequate pulmonary function, rapid acquisition of tissue (either renal or pulmonary or both), and appropriate immunopathologic analysis of any and all biopsy specimens in parallel with serologic assays for circulating GBM antibodies.

CNS DYSFUNCTION: IS THIS CEREBRAL VASCULITIS?

Patients with or without connective tissue disease and nonspecific markers of systemic inflammation who develop signs of brain dysfunction are routinely suspected of having CNS vasculitis. Often the likelihood is considered low but addressed in the interest of being thorough.

Rarely does CNS vasculitis cause psychosis or coma without focal neurologic signs. Primary angiitis of the CNS, particularly in early stages, is an exception, but would not be expected to show signs or symptoms of multisystem disease or coma that would prompt ICU admission. Finding focal deficits on examination is problematic in the comatose or disoriented patient. A skilled neurologist can contribute more than imaging techniques. MRI and CT scanning may reveal a lesion suggesting an ischemic event. While no pattern is specific for vasculitis, a completely normal MRI makes the diagnosis less likely. Angiography is the gold standard, although in small-vessel vasculitis angiography may be nondiagnostic. Access to angiography can be problematic for the critically ill ICU patient. Leptomeningeal biopsy is the gold standard for diagnosis of granulomatous angiitis of the CNS, an important subset of CNS vasculitis. An empiric trial with steroids may be appropriate.

HYPERSENSITIVITY VASCULITIS: WHAT IS THE CAUSE?

The most common form of cutaneous vasculitis in any setting is leukocytoclastic vasculitis (LCV), often referred to as *hypersensitivity vasculitis* and recognized clinically as palpable purpura. The palpability of these lesions is caused by inflammatory infiltrates. Other less common expressions include *bullous disease* and *cutaneous ulcers.* The lesions have a tendency to occur in dependent areas and in ambulatory patients are found in the legs and buttock area. Localization may be atypical in bedridden ICU patients. By far the most common cause of new-onset LCV in the ICU patient is drugs. Any drug may be implicated, but thiazides, sulfa drugs, and penicillins are common offenders. Clues to nondrug causes would include significant digital involvement including associated nailbed infarcts, ulcerative lesions, significant glomerular inflammation, and any other evidence of extracutaneous vasculitis such as mononeuritis multiplex.

The presence of cryoglobulins or low complement levels suggests a nondrug cause. Skin biopsy can be done early but usually adds no additional diagnostic information. Predominant lymphocytic infiltration may help to support a diagnosis of drug-induced disease.[51] Immunofluorescence on biopsied tissue is rarely helpful, but the presence of IgA is supportive of a diagnosis of Henoch-Schönlein purpura.[52] Progression to major vasculitis does not predictably occur, but hypersensitivity vasculitis may be the presenting manifestation of a major systemic vasculitis such as Wegener's granulomatosis or Churg-Strauss vasculitis. Therapy may be restricted to withdrawal of the most likely offending drug. Refractory cases have been managed with prednisone (0.5 mg/kg per day), colchicine (0.6 mg twice daily), dapsone (150 mg/d), and rarely cytotoxic agents or azathioprine. Topical therapy adds little in the absence of skin breakdown. Complete resolution may take weeks.

HEPATITIS C VIRUS INFECTION

A significant number of patients with hepatitis C virus (HCV) infection can develop urticaria, livedo reticularis, leukocytoclastic vasculitis, and membranoproliferative glomerulonephritis. The syndrome is mediated by HCV-driven formation of cryoglobulins that act as immune complexes. Indeed, it is highly likely that almost all patients previously diagnosed as idiopathic mixed cryoglobulinemia with vasculitis were actually patients with HCV. High titers of rheumatoid factors and hypocomplementemia strongly support the diagnosis. Treatment is directed at control of viral replication in the liver and attenuation of immune complex activity by plasmapheresis and cyclophosphamide. Until the role of B cells in defense against HCV is better understood, the temptation to deplete antibody-producing cells with anti-CD20 monoclonals should be approached with caution.

ISCHEMIC DIGITS: IS THIS VASCULITIS?

Patients in the ICU may develop ischemic digits. Contributing factors include hypotension, use of radial arterial lines, and vasoconstrictors. Often the issue of vasculitis is raised.

Single extremity involvement speaks strongly against systemic vasculitis as the cause. Similarly, isolated toe involvement is more likely to be caused by a combination of noninflammatory vascular disease and diminished blood flow owing to hypotension, vasoconstrictors, or cholesterol emboli. The latter may shower from the aorta and create a pseudovasculitic picture, particularly after anticoagulation therapy is initiated or following instrumentation of the aorta.[53] Extreme symmetry of lesions with all digits involved is more suggestive of a generalized low-flow state than vasculitis.

Clues to vasculitis as the cause of digital ischemia include the coexistence of a disease associated with digital vasculitis such as SLE or scleroderma, random involvement of multiple limbs, the presence of nailbed infarcts, and other associated cutaneous markers specific to vasculitis such as palpable purpura. Likewise, extracutaneous markers of vasculitis including glomerulitis and patchy neurologic deficits would enhance suspicion for that diagnosis.

Male patients with a history of heavy smoking should be suspected of Buerger's disease (thromboangiitis obliterans). Patients with lupus and other connective tissue diseases who have ischemic digits may have thrombotic complications secondary to ACL antibody and not true vasculitis.[54]

Biopsy of ischemic digits is usually impractical and potentially hazardous. The necessity to amputate a gangrenous digit should prompt careful instruction to the surgeon to be sure to biopsy the digital artery immediately proximal to the gangrene. In this setting angiography often reveals nonspecific findings of small-vessel disease, but may suggest emboli,

and at times reveal the source such as a subclavian plaque. An angiographic pattern suggestive of Buerger's disease has been described.[55]

LUNG INFILTRATES AND ELEVATED SEDIMENTATION RATE: IS THIS VASCULITIS?

Elevated ESRs frequently become laboratory aberrations looking for a disease state. The unwary clinician may let an elevated ESR be the driver for a costly and unrewarding workup. Once it is known that a patient has an elevated ESR and the usual causes for this nonspecific laboratory abnormality have been reasonably excluded, the impulse is to link any and all remaining clinical abnormalities to the abnormal ESR. Unexplained pulmonary infiltrates, a common finding in critically ill patients, are good examples that provoke the question: Is this a pulmonary vasculitis? Common sense should prevail and dictate that the diagnosis of pulmonary vasculitis as a principal entity should be one of exclusion. If a young female on corticosteroids with a fever, rash, alopecia, and pericarditis develops a pulmonary infiltrate, she should be considered to have an infectious disease or pulmonary embolism until otherwise proved. If a previously bedridden patient with advanced rheumatoid arthritis suddenly develops pulmonary infiltrates and hypoxemia, the etiology should be considered embolic until proved otherwise. If a patient with advanced scleroderma that includes the proximal gut develops pulmonary infiltrates, aspiration pneumonia should be strongly considered. Conversely, one can approach the patient with pulmonary infiltrates and an elevated ESR in reductionist fashion.

If a careful search for extrapulmonary evidence of vasculitis is not rewarding, it will be highly unlikely that primary pulmonary vasculitis is present, since vasculitis very rarely involves only the pulmonary tree. There are unusual instances when vasculitis can be isolated to the pulmonary tree in a systemic rheumatic disease. Rarely, patients with ACL antibodies may develop pulmonary infiltrates secondary to in situ pulmonary artery thrombosis and/or pulmonary embolism. These patients will simulate a primary vasculitic pulmonary picture, but the primary therapy is anticoagulation. The proclivity of lung infections (especially bacterial) to generate positive anti-neutrophil cytoplasmic antibodies (ANCA) can create a diagnostic quandary when the question of Wegener's granulomatosis is raised.

Interpretation of Rheumatology Laboratory Abnormalities in the ICU

ERYTHROCYTE SEDIMENTATION RATE

The ESR is an indirect determination of the acute phase response and may be elevated in the setting of infection or active rheumatic disease. Values are higher for women and the elderly. Although the exact appropriate adjustments for age and sex are not certain, a common rule used to calculate a "normal" ESR in patients over 40 is divide the age by 2 and add 10 if the patient is female.

The presence of monoclonal proteins, polyclonal hypergammaglobulinemia, hyperfibrinogenemia, and alterations in size, shape, and number of red blood cells will influence the ESR. ESR rises during normal pregnancy and should not be used to monitor rheumatic diseases under these circumstances. The ESR increases in end-stage renal failure of whatever cause and is not indicative of an underlying rheumatic disorder.[56] Parallel confirmation of a normal C-reactive protein level often clarifies the noninflammatory origin of the elevated ESR. The level of the rise in ESR correlates imperfectly with disease activity and may at times be normal in patients with active rheumatoid arthritis or SLE. Patients with a markedly elevated ESR (MESR) are those with values >100 mm/h. These patients deserve special attention because such elevations are unlikely to be explained by age or normal physiologic state and are a more reliable sickness indicator. The illnesses associated with MESR include infection, malignancy, rheumatic disorders such as vasculitis, connective tissue disease, rheumatoid arthritis, and temporal arteritis, as well as end-stage renal failure, nephrotic syndrome, and other inflammatory diseases such as hepatitis and colitis. In most series looking at MESR, 3% to 10% of patients will have no diagnosis to explain the abnormal laboratory value.[57] Some of these patients will eventually reveal an underlying pathology, whereas others will demonstrate spontaneous improvement in the ESR.

In the ICU, the ESR is likely to be elevated for multiple reasons. An MESR should not prompt an unreasonable search for vasculitis or other concurrent rheumatic disease, particularly in the presence of renal failure and nephrotic syndrome.

C-REACTIVE PROTEIN

The availability of rapid, reproducible, high-sensitivity, low-cost assays for C-reactive protein (CRP) in many circumstances obviate a clinician's reliance on the vagaries of the ESR to detect inflammation. CRP is an acute phase serum protein that acts as a surrogate for the proinflammatory interleukin IL-6. Serum/plasma levels of CRP are tightly linked not only to the absolute level of IL-6, but also to the rise and fall of the cytokine. Sequential CRP determinations, in contrast to the slowly responsive ESR, can provide a more accurate assessment of inflammatory changes in response to therapy. CRP determination is most helpful in assigning a noninflammatory cause to a markedly abnormal ESR. An example would be a patient with a monoclonal protein without infection, who could have an ESR of 100 but a normal CRP. The latter alleviates concern that significant inflammation may be part of the clinical picture.

Several cautions apply to the interpretation of CRP levels. Although there are weak correlations between CRP levels and age and gender, they are less marked than the same variables and the ESR. CRP also varies directly with body mass index. The very new ultrasensitive CRP assays have not only changed the normal ranges, but are expressed in markedly different concentrations that can be very confusing to the unwary.

The bottom line for the critical care clinician might be that significant elevations of CRP usually signal the presence of clinically relevant inflammation, and the absence of a high CRP helps in excluding it.

ANTINUCLEAR ANTIBODIES

The presence of antinuclear antibodies (ANA) in high titer provides presumptive evidence for the presence of collagen vascular disease, and in particular, SLE (Table 104-1). Lower levels of ANA can be nonspecific, possibly normal, and at times explained by age, prior drug therapy, or a first-degree relative with lupus. Low levels of ANA in the elderly can be particularly misleading in the presence of an age-related elevation of the ESR. It has been estimated that 15% to 25% of normal, healthy individuals over the age of 60 will have circulating ANA.[58] These data are confounded by a small but definite incidence of new cases of SLE among the elderly.

Screening ANA is typically done by a standard, indirect immunofluorescence technique. The test is now performed most commonly on HEp-2 cells and is sensitive for detecting the presence of SLE and other collagen vascular diseases, but as noted above, the test is hindered by the lack of specificity. Interest in specific ANA has spawned a long and at times confusing list of tests of variable utility. A brief overview of the most useful specific ANA tests follows.

ANTICENTROMERE ANTIBODY

This antibody to the kinetochore of chromosomes is detected by recognition of a particular speckled pattern of immunofluorescence on HEp-2 cells. It is, in general, the only pattern detected on screening ANA useful for diagnostic purposes. The antibody is found most commonly in the limited cutaneous variant of scleroderma (CREST). In this subset of patients, the test has been positive in 44% to 98% of those tested.[59,60] Less commonly, it may be seen in diffuse scleroderma and primary biliary cirrhosis with or without evidence of scleroderma.

ANTIBODIES TO DNA

Antibodies to DNA fall into two major categories by virtue of reacting to antigenic determinants on the phosphate deoxyribose backbone of the DNA helix or determinants on the nucleotide bases. The former represent antibodies to native double-stranded DNA while the latter react with single-stranded DNA.

Antibodies to single-stranded DNA are more common and are found across a spectrum of rheumatic and nonrheumatic disorders. They are of no practical clinical utility. Antibodies to double-stranded DNA are useful since they have great specificity for SLE and are found in 60% to 70% of patients with that disease.[43,61] In many, but not all lupus patients, levels of anti-DNA antibody will correlate positively with disease activity. Low levels of this antibody have occasionally been found in other connective tissue diseases.

ANTIBODIES TO Sm

This antibody is named after a patient ("Smith") in whom it was first described. The antibody has high specificity for SLE and is rarely found in patients with other connective tissue diseases. Sensitivity is only about 30% for SLE. Sm is not to be confused with an antibody to smooth muscle (SM), which is not a marker for collagen vascular disease, but is found in patients with chronic liver disease. There is no specific clinical profile of Sm-positive patients with SLE. Titers are not useful for assessment of disease activity.

ANTIBODIES TO nRNP

Antigenic determinants for nuclear ribonucleoprotein (nRNP) may occur in a molecular complex with Sm, and antibodies to Sm and RNP are often found in the same patient. Antibodies to nRNP may be seen in SLE, scleroderma, or overlap syndromes. The presence of overlapping clinical features and high titers of antibody to RNP defines a clinical

TABLE 104-1 Serologic Tests in Rheumatic Diseases

Antibody	Disorder
Tests with high specificity[a] for collagen vascular disease:	
Anti-native DNA	SLE
	Rarely anything else
Anti-Sm (Smith)	SLE
Anti-Ro (SS-A)	Congenital heart block
	Antinuclear antibody-negative lupus
	Subacute cutaneous LE
	Primary Sjögren syndrome
	SLE
Anticentromere	Limited cutaneous variant of scleroderma (CREST)
Anti-Scl-70 (topoisomerase I)	Diffuse scleroderma, less commonly CREST
Antineutrophil cytoplasmic antibody	Wegener's granulomatosis
	Microscopic polyangiitis
	Idiopathic crescentic glomerulonephritis
Anti-ribonucleoprotein	SLE
	Mixed connective tissue disease
	Undifferentiated connective tissue disease
Anti-La (SS-B)	SLE
	Primary Sjögren syndrome
Tests with low specificity for collagen vascular disease:	
Antinuclear antibody	SLE
	Other autoimmune diseases
	Normals (usually low titer)
	Drug-induced
	Aging
Rheumatoid factor	Rheumatoid arthritis
	Mixed cryoglobulinemia
	Aging
	Subacute bacterial endocarditis
	Any cause of chronic antigenic stimulation
Anticardiolipin antibody	Anticardiolipin antibody syndrome
	Normals
	Viral illness
	SLE
	Other autoimmune diseases

[a] Unlikely to be found in normals, with aging, or as a nonspecific immune response to infection.
CREST (syndrome), calcinosis, Raynaud's phenomenon, esophageal motility disorders, sclerodactyly, and telangiectasia; LE, lupus erythematosus; SLE, systemic lupus erythematosus.

subset of patients referred to as those with mixed connective tissue disease (MCTD).

ANTIBODIES TO SS-A/Ro AND SS-B/La

These antigens were originally described in patients with Sjögren's syndrome (SS) and SLE. They are RNA-protein conjugates. SS-A and Ro have antigenic identity, as do SS-B and La. The *Ro* and *La* refer to the antigen as localized to the cytoplasm, whereas *SS-A* and *SS-B* are nuclear antigens.

The presence of SS-B/La may be seen in SLE or Sjögren's syndrome, and in most assays is measured along with SS-A/Ro. The Ro antibody has been described in 60% of so-called ANA-negative SLE. Anti-Ro antibody is also highly prevalent in the setting of congenital heart block and neonatal SLE.[62] In those cases, the antibody is found in mother and child. Other clinical scenarios associated with anti-Ro antibody include subacute cutaneous lupus and C2 deficiency. Anti-Ro antibody occurs in 25% to 40% of unselected patients with SLE.

The major indications for ordering these tests are: in a setting in which SLE is strongly suspected but the screening ANA is negative, congenital heart block, neonatal lupus, and the initial evaluation of a patient with a positive ANA.

ANTIBODIES TO SCL-70 (TOPOISOMERASE I)

Antibodies to Scl-70 are directed toward DNA topoisomerase I and inhibit its function.[63] They are found in 20% to 40% of patients classified as diffuse systemic sclerosis, and less commonly in patients with limited cutaneous disease or CREST. Determination of this antibody is part of the evaluation of patients suspected of having scleroderma.

ANTINEUTROPHIL CYTOPLASMIC AUTOANTIBODIES

The detection of antibodies directed against neutrophil cytoplasmic components now offers a useful serologic tool for the diagnosis and management of a group of disorders characterized by systemic necrotizing vasculitis and glomerulonephritis.[64,65] These disorders include Wegener's granulomatosis, microscopic polyangiitis, Churg-Strauss syndrome, and idiopathic crescentic glomerulonephritis. The renal lesions in these disorders have in common necrotizing vascular injury and a paucity of immune deposits.

Antineutrophil cytoplasmic autoantibodies (ANCA) are found in 90% of patients with active, generalized Wegener's granulomatosis and 60% to 70% of those with limited disease. The titer often parallels disease activity and may be helpful in distinguishing a disease flare from intercurrent infection or other morbidity in patients with Wegener's granulomatosis. ANCA can be found in 80% of patients with active pauci-immune necrotizing and crescentic glomerulonephritis, which is one of the major causes of rapidly progressing glomerulonephritis.

Two specific patterns of ANCA have been identified and are referred to as *cytoplasmic ANCA* (C-ANCA) and *perinuclear ANCA* (P-ANCA). In general, patients with Wegener's granulomatosis have demonstrated C-ANCA, whereas those with idiopathic crescentic glomerulonephritis have demonstrated P-ANCA.[66] P-ANCA has been reported with other forms of systemic vasculitis, including microscopic polyangiitis and Churg-Strauss vasculitis. P-ANCA has also been observed in patients with ulcerative colitis and Crohn's disease.

The clinical scenarios that warrant measurement of ANCA are patients with known or suspected Wegener's granulomatosis or other small-vessel vasculitis and patients with rapidly progressing glomerulonephritis. These antibodies have also been occasionally identified in Takayasu's disease, SLE, relapsing polychondritis, and Behçet's disease.

ANTIBODIES IN POLYMYOSITIS/DERMATOMYOSITIS

In general, serologic testing has been of little practical value in the diagnosis and management of patients with polymyositis or dermatomyositis. Recently, the emergence of a family of autoantibodies that are found nearly exclusively in patients with myositis, known as myositis-specific autoantibodies or MSA, has focused interest on the role of humoral immunity in this disease. MSA are usually directed against intracellular, intracytoplasmic antigens involved in protein synthesis. Specific ANA have been identified in patients with these diseases and are available commercially. The exact role of these antibodies in the management of patients is unclear, but identification of these antibodies may be useful in patients who represent a diagnostic dilemma.

Jo-1 antibody is the most common of the MSA and belongs to a family of autoantibodies known as antisynthetases. It can be found in 15% to 40% of patients with polymyositis, and less commonly in dermatomyositis. The presence of the antibody highly correlates with associated interstitial lung disease. Antibodies to the nuclear antigen Mi occur in about 5% of patients with dermatomyositis and rarely in polymyositis. MSA titers have not proved useful in monitoring the course of patients with polymyositis or dermatomyositis. Specific MSA may prove to define unique clinical and immunogenetic groups that represent separate but related diseases. Antibody to PM-1 or PM-Scl defines a small subset of polymyositis patients (10%), half of whom will have accompanying features of scleroderma. Occasionally, patients with scleroderma and no myositis will have this antibody.

RHEUMATOID FACTOR

Rheumatoid factors (RFs) are autoantibodies, predominantly IgM isotype, that are directed against multispecies antigenic determinants on the heavy chain of IgG. They are nonspecific, rarely diagnostic, and almost never useful in the critical care setting. These autoantibodies can be found in normals and many disease states and have a prevalence that varies directly with age and gender (female preponderance). RFs can arise as an epiphenomenon during acute illness or chronic antigenic stimulation of almost any cause. They are present,

sometimes in significant titer, in bacterial endocarditis, granulomatous diseases, and most rheumatic diseases at some point in time. The presence of RFs, occurring in tandem with significant decreases of serum complement components C3 and C4, may provide a diagnostic clue in rarely encountered clinical syndromes such as rheumatoid vasculitis with cryoglobulins or hepatitis C–associated mixed cryoglobulinemia and vasculitis. These syndromes can present with gastrointestinal tract involvement and hemorrhage, compromised renal function or progressive peripheral neuropathy, and skin ulceration. The recognition of these vasculitic syndromes mandates aggressive intervention with cytoreductive therapy—usually cyclophosphamide and therapeutic plasmapheresis.[67,68]

COMPLEMENT LEVELS

In theory, the detection of direct (classic) complement pathway activation by the measurement of serum C3 and C4 levels should provide the clinician with laboratory support for using treatment protocols that suppress the sequelae of complement activation. A prototype disease where C3 and C4 changes should be helpful is SLE. Unfortunately, there is an imperfect correlation between clinical activity of any disease, especially SLE, and decreased C3 and C4 levels. In fact, reliance upon conventional measurements of serum C3 and C4 assays, which supposedly detect immune complex complement activation in the patient, can inappropriately drive therapy decisions toward the use of immunosuppressives or corticosteroids when they are not indicated.[69]

Moreover, C3 synthesis is increased by acute inflammation of any cause, serving as a classic acute-phase reactant. It is easy to visualize a scenario in which a patient with SLE being treated with corticosteroids who has increased consumption of C3 secondary to immune complex formation and deposition may develop secondary bacterial infection, which stimulates the production of C3 in its role as an acute-phase reactant. The end result will be a normal serum level of C3, which may engender a false sense of security with regard to SLE disease activity. Conversely, the significantly reduced synthesis of C3 in many hepatic diseases is reflected in low plasma levels that can be misinterpreted. Plasma C4 is a more sensitive indicator of direct pathway activation, but for many of the same reasons that relate to C3 determinations, a decreased C4 level should never be the sole determinant of intervention with potent immunosuppressive therapy. Patients with SLE or overlap variants may have heterozygous or homozygous defects in C4 production. These patients will always have low C4 levels, regardless of disease activity.

ICU patients admitted with either meningococcemia or gonococcemia provide one of the rare reasons for the determination of total hemolytic complement level. This assay serves as a screening test that depends on the functional presence of all individual complement components. A significant decrease in hemolytic activity may identify patients with terminal complement component deficiency who are at high risk for recurrent bacteremia. Such patients may require fresh frozen plasma in conjunction with antibiotic therapy and should be immunized with meningococcal vaccine prior to discharge.

In summary, conventional measurements of serum complement levels are not helpful in predicting activation in this complex system. When sensitive assays for activation peptides or complement activation complexes become available, assessment of the complement pathway may become more clinically relevant.

CRYOGLOBULINS

Cryoglobulins are monoclonal, oligoclonal, or polyclonal immunoglobulins with a thermal propensity for precipitation at decreased temperatures and subsequent resolubilization with warming. In the vast majority of instances, they occur as acute or chronic phase reactants during bacterial or viral infections and many rheumatic disease syndromes. Plasma cryoglobulins, especially when assessed as cryocrits, are very nonspecific and may simply reflect ongoing antibody formation and subsequent complexing with antigen; indeed, they have been termed "the poor man's immune complex assay." Abnormal elevations of the ESR can be masked by some cryoglobulins that form gels at ambient temperatures and impede the rate of erythrocyte descent. Pseudoleukocytosis can occur when automated cell-counting procedures count crystallized cryoproteins as white blood cells. Pseudohypogammaglobulinemia and pseudothrombocytosis have also been reported. Almost all patients with cryoglobulin-mediated immune complex syndromes have active HCV infection that should be aggressively treated. Cryoglobulin-mediated vasculitis should be followed in terms of its clinical activity; clinicians should not rely on cryocrit decreases during therapy. Falls in cryocrits may be misleading because cryoproteins, even at extremely low levels in plasma, can be highly efficient complement activators.

ANTICARDIOLIPIN ANTIBODIES

The anticardiolipin (ACL) antibodies belong to a family of antiphospholipid antibodies (APLA), including those responsible for the lupus anticoagulant (LA), the biologic false-positive test for syphilis, and anti-B$_2$-glycoprotein-I antibodies. These antibodies often, although not always, occur together. The clinical syndromes associated with these antibodies belong to a growing list that can be explained largely by the capacity of these antibodies to induce thrombosis in the venous and arterial circulation. Thrombocytopenia and recurrent fetal loss are the other major consequences of APLA. The combination of APLA and one or more of these clinical features has been termed the "antiphospholipid antibody syndrome."[70]

Chronic false-positive serologic tests for syphilis are associated with autoimmune disease, notably SLE, and are found with increased frequency in patients with ACL and LA activity. Lupus anticoagulants are IgG or IgM antibodies that prolong phospholipid-dependent tests in vitro by interference with the calcium-dependent binding of prothrombin (factor II) and factor Xa to phospholipids, thus inhibiting the generation of prothrombinase. This usually results in prolongation of the activated partial thromboplastin time (APTT) with or without slight prolongation of the prothrombin time (PT).[54] LA is a common cause of prolongation of the PTT, but not the only cause. Most patients with LA do not have SLE.

Usually ACL antibodies are detected in an enzyme-linked immunosorbent assay (ELISA) using bovine cardiolipin as substrate. These are the most commonly detected antiphospholipid antibodies. They are generated transiently in the course of acute infections including mycoplasma and gram-negative infections. These antibodies are usually of the IgM isotype and are not associated with thrombosis. IgM ACL as

well as the LA may be induced by a variety of drugs including phenothiazines, procainamide, phenytoin, hydralazine, quinidine, and streptomycin. These antibodies are most often not associated with thrombotic events, but exceptions to this rule occur. Antibodies to B$_2$-glycoprotein-1 in the absence of phospholipids can be measured on oxidized polystyrene plates. These antibodies are more specific for the diagnosis of APLA syndrome than the anticardiolipin test.

ACL antibodies are noted in 2.5% of the general population.[54] For most of these patients, the antibodies have no clinical significance. The risk of thrombosis and fetal loss has been generally associated with higher levels of antibody and the IgG isotype. Unfortunately, exceptions occur. Thus the presence of ACL antibody should not in itself prompt therapeutic intervention.

A myriad of neurologic events including stroke, transient ischemic attacks, and amaurosis fugax have been associated with the presence of LA and ACL antibody. Their presence should be suspected in patients who have no risk factors for thrombosis or who have associated autoimmune disease or suggestive screening laboratory abnormalities, including prolonged PTT or false-positive serologic tests for syphilis. Skin lesions secondary to LA and ACL include gangrene, hemorrhage, and purpura. Necrosis may mimic vasculitis.

The vasculopathy of APLA syndrome is not vasculitis, but primarily thrombosis of large or small arteries or veins. Steroids may normalize the LA but have little impact on ACL antibody levels. Treatment for major thrombotic complications of this syndrome is heparin or enoxaparin and warfarin. Steroids are indicated for associated clinical features related to systemic inflammation.

Rarely patients may present with evidence of widespread vascular occlusion and multiorgan failure occurring concurrently or over a short period of time related to antiphospholipid antibodies. Kidneys, bowels, lungs, brain, and heart are frequently involved. This so-called catastrophic antiphospholipid syndrome (CAPS) is associated with significant morbidity and mortality in spite of empiric therapy with corticosteroids, anticoagulation, and apheresis.[72] CAPS needs to be distinguished from thrombotic thrombocytopenia purpura (TTP) and diffuse intravascular coagulation. Precipitating events, such as infection, trauma, surgical procedures, or reduction in anticoagulation therapy, may contribute to the development of CAPS.[73]

Use of Corticosteroids, Immunosuppressives, and Anti-inflammatory Drugs in the Critically Ill Patient

CORTICOSTEROIDS

Corticosteroids have potent immunosuppressive and anti-inflammatory properties that, in combination with rapid onset of action, make them the drugs of choice for the initial therapy of most acute, life-threatening rheumatic disorders. Even low doses of prednisone (<10 mg/d) have potent anti-inflammatory effects and are highly effective in patients with rheumatoid arthritis.

For purposes of controlling inflammation and immunomodulation, "short-acting" glucocorticoids with little or no mineralocorticoid activity are preferred. The oral drug of choice is prednisone, which is converted to prednisolone in the liver. Whereas active liver disease impairs that conversion, it appears to be offset sufficiently by decreased rate of elimination of prednisolone to eliminate the need to preferentially use prednisolone in patients with cirrhosis or active liver disease. The intravenous drug of choice is methylprednisolone. The dose equivalency is 4 mg methylprednisolone to 5 mg prednisone.

The dose of prednisone or methylprednisolone is largely empiric. For serious, life-threatening problems, 1 mg/kg per day of prednisone is a good starting point. Dividing the dose into a twice-a-day or other dose-divided schedule may increase efficacy (as well as toxicity) and is recommended by some for initial therapy. Extremely large doses of intravenous methylprednisolone (500 to 1000 mg) daily have been used for brief periods (3 to 5 days) with variable success in a variety of clinical settings, mostly in the context of SLE. In vitro studies suggest that such large doses may produce a qualitatively different response in lymphocyte function.[74] Unique side effects to this form of therapy, including sudden overwhelming sepsis and sudden death, are rare. This form of therapy is generally reserved for patients who have failed conventional high-dose therapy with corticosteroids with or without another immunosuppressive agent.

Patient response to corticosteroids varies. Failure to respond is likely a result of the nature and severity of the disease. The effectiveness of glucocorticoids may be reduced by simultaneous use of other drugs that induce hepatic microsomal enzyme activity, such as phenytoin, barbiturates, and rifampin. Bioavailability of prednisone may be reduced by antacids sometimes prescribed for concurrent use. Cortisol and its synthetic derivatives are bound to corticosteroid-binding globulin and albumin. The bound steroid is not active. Increased frequency of prednisone side effects has been observed at low serum albumin levels, probably reflecting an increase in the unbound, active fraction of the drug.

Patients who have a positive purified protein derivative (PPD) test about to undergo corticosteroid therapy (particularly with doses of prednisone of 20 mg/d or greater) should be considered for isoniazid (INH) prophylaxis (300 mg/d orally). The reported risk of reactivation ranges from low in asthmatics to higher in the elderly and in patients immunosuppressed by virtue of other drugs or their primary disease. The patient with a positive PPD and either a normal chest x-ray or a single calcified nodule probably does not require prophylaxis.[76] If the patient has significant impairment of the immune system or the chest film shows fibronodular scarring, the risk is enhanced considerably, and prophylaxis with INH is advisable.[77]

Steroid therapy suppresses cutaneous delayed hypersensitivity responses by inhibiting recruitment of macrophages to the skin test site. This phenomenon is reversible on stopping the drug. In one study, treatment with 10 mg prednisone daily totally inhibited cutaneous tuberculin sensitivity in both active and inactive cases of tuberculosis, with a mean reversion time of 13.6 days and reconversion time of 6 days following discontinuation of the drug.

Acute adrenocortical insufficiency may occur in critically ill patients who have been treated with chronic glucocorticoid therapy. On the basis of available data, any patient who has received a glucocorticoid at a dose equivalent to 20 to 30 mg prednisone daily should be suspected of having hypothalamic-pituitary-adrenal (HPA) axis suppression.[78] At doses closer to but above the physiologic range, a month is probably the minimum duration required for HPA suppression. Patients receiving the equivalent replacement doses of steroid (5 mg prednisone) as single morning dose therapy are at low risk of iatrogenic adrenal insufficiency. In the absence of hemodynamic instability, these patients do not require full "stress dose" replacement therapy. An adrenocorticotropic hormone stimulation test can resolve the question of adrenal suppression, but the clinical reality usually dictates empirical coverage with "stress doses" of corticosteroids. This can be accomplished with 100 mg hydrocortisone intravenously every 8 hours. This is approximately the equivalent of 75 mg prednisone. Higher doses are not necessary and are potentially more hazardous.

Use of corticosteroids on alternate days is associated with some decrease in chronic drug morbidity. In the urgent setting of the critically ill patient, the greater effectiveness of daily or split daily doses of steroids recommends such a dosing schedule.

IMMUNOSUPPRESSIVES

CYCLOPHOSPHAMIDE

Cyclophosphamide is an alkylating agent with broad immunosuppressive properties. It is generally embraced as the drug of choice for suppression of progressive, life-threatening autoimmune disease unresponsive to corticosteroids alone. Effectiveness has been reported in a broad spectrum of collagen vascular diseases and primary vasculitides, including SLE, Wegener's granulomatosis, polyarteritis nodosa, and polymyositis/dermatomyositis.

Cyclophosphamide causes broad suppression of B- and T-cell function and acts as a potent inhibitor of antibody production. Anti-inflammatory effects have also been described.

The drug is rapidly absorbed orally. It is inert until metabolized in the liver. Extravasation of the drug is not caustic to soft tissues. Sixty percent of the drug is excreted in the urine in the form of active metabolites. Impaired excretion of these active metabolites because of renal insufficiency can potentiate the therapeutic and toxic effects of a given dose of drug.

The drug can be given orally, usually at a dose of 2 mg/kg per day, or intravenously. To circumvent toxic effects associated with chronic drug exposure, intravenous bolus cyclophosphamide therapy has become an increasingly popular alternative at doses of 0.5 to 1.0 g/m². The onset of immunosuppressive activity of cyclophosphamide is estimated at 10 to 14 days following initiation of therapy. Although unproved in rigorous clinical trials, there is an operational principle that immunosuppression can be achieved more rapidly with intravenous bolus therapy. Hence bolus cyclophosphamide is most often given in the setting of progressive life-threatening disease requiring immunosuppression. A major short-term side effect of bolus therapy is a predictable white blood cell count nadir 7 to 10 days after drug infusion. Leukocyte count levels typically recover in 2 to 3 days. However, if the patient has a concurrent bacterial infection during the nadir period, the consequences of even transient profound neutropenia can be disastrous. Gross hematuria may signal the development of hemorrhagic cystitis or bladder malignancy. Bladder problems are related to duration of therapy and total cumulative dose administered. Many of the other side effects of therapy with cyclophosphamide are related to chronic use, including gonadal suppression, oncogenesis, pulmonary interstitial fibrosis, and hypogammaglobulinemia.

One report suggests that bolus cyclophosphamide is less effective than oral cyclophosphamide in patients with Wegener's granulomatosis.[71] This study raises questions about the predicted superiority of bolus cyclophosphamide in all clinical situations.

AZATHIOPRINE

Azathioprine is a commonly used immunomodulating drug with mild to moderate immunosuppressive properties that may in large part be explained by a preferential reduction of natural killer cells. Onset of action is slow, probably taking months. It is often used concurrently with corticosteroids in patients requiring unacceptably high doses of steroids, to reduce the steroid dose. Azathioprine is not the drug of choice when significant immunosuppressive effect is needed on an urgent basis. Risk for infection is modest in the absence of leukopenia.

Azathioprine is metabolized in the liver to the active metabolite, 6-mercaptopurine, a purine analogue. The drug interferes with purine biosynthesis and is ultimately metabolized by xanthine oxidase. Administration of allopurinol, which inhibits xanthine oxidase, to a patient on a stable dose of azathioprine may result in a fatal drug overdose. The azathioprine dose should be reduced by 50% to 75% in the presence of allopurinol.

Dose range for this drug is 1 to 3 mg/kg per day. The drug is primarily metabolized in the liver, but the need for dose adjustment in the presence of liver disease is variable and may be unnecessary. Drug half-life can increase in renal failure but may not prove clinically significant. Cautious observation for the development of cytopenia is indicated in the presence of hepatic or renal failure. The drug is well absorbed orally and may be given intravenously in doses equivalent to the oral form.

MYCOPHENOLATE MOFETIL

Mycophenolate mofetil (MMF) interferes with de novo purine synthesis by inhibiting inosine monophosphate dehydrogenase. Nonlymphocytic cells recycle purine precursors through salvage pathways and are not dependent on de novo purine synthesis, in contrast to proliferating T and B lymphocytes, which are completely dependent on the de novo pathway. This difference confers selectivity on MMF and makes it an attractive choice for preventing allograft rejection. MMF is rapidly supplanting azathioprine in multiagent immunosuppressive protocols used in heart, lung, and renal transplantation. The conventional daily dose of MMF is usually 2.0 g and greater therapeutic effects are not usually found with higher doses. Mild reversible leukopenia and mild gastrointestinal side effects have occurred with MMF, and dose adjustments should be made when a patient has a glomerular filtration rate less than 25% of predicted value. There is a low incidence of opportunistic infection that can be directly attributed to MMF when used at less than 3 g daily. In most clinical scenarios, plasma levels of its active metabolite, mycophenolic acid, do not need to be monitored to achieve therapeutic effects. Based on its selectivity, ease of administration, and low side-effect profile, there is increasing interest in using MMF for the treatment of patients with autoimmune diseases.

METHOTREXATE

Although methotrexate was introduced for the treatment of rheumatoid arthritis more than 30 years ago, several open trials in the early 1980s resulted in renewed interest in this drug. Low-dose oral methotrexate has now replaced gold as the remitting agent of first choice in rheumatoid arthritis for many rheumatologists. The drug is accepted as effective in psoriatic arthritis and Reiter's syndrome as well as polymyositis. Experience is being gained with its use in SLE and scleroderma. Use of methotrexate in the critically ill rheumatic disease patient is currently limited to patients with polymyositis/dermatomyositis that is refractory to corticosteroids.

Methotrexate is a folic acid analogue and the major folic acid antagonist in clinical use. The drug is absorbed after oral ingestion but with significant variability. More predictable serum levels can be achieved by intramuscular or intravenous administration. High-dose methotrexate can alter antibody production and cellular immunity. Low-dose oral methotrexate (25 mg/wk or less), as used in rheumatoid arthritis, may be mainly anti-inflammatory or directly inhibiting to synovial lining cells.

Low-dose methotrexate is given in rheumatoid arthritis in initial doses of 5.0 to 10 mg and may be gradually increased to levels of 25 mg/wk. Methotrexate for rheumatic disorders is delivered on a weekly basis. This regimen is associated with less toxicity than when the drug is given more frequently, particularly hepatotoxicity. Most patients will respond at doses between 10 and 20 mg weekly. Intravenous methotrexate for myositis is given in doses ranging from 25 to 75 mg weekly. A dose of 1 mg/kg per week has been used in childhood dermatomyositis/polymyositis.[79] Such a dose calculation may be a reasonable first approach in the treatment of adults.

Adverse reactions forcing discontinuation of the drug in short-term trials with rheumatoid arthritis occur in 5% to 31% of patients. Most toxicity is relatively minor and associated with advanced age, malnutrition, and impaired renal function. Nausea, vomiting, oral ulcers, rash, leukopenia, thrombocytopenia, and pancytopenia all may occur. Cirrhosis may occur in some patients treated for long periods and appears to be related to cumulative dose and probably the nature of the underlying disease being treated. The risk is asserted to be greater in psoriatic arthritis than rheumatoid arthritis. Ethanol potentiates the hepatotoxicity of methotrexate. Pretreatment screening for hepatitis B and C is usually done. Baseline liver biopsy is not indicated in the absence of risk factors for existing liver disease. The concurrent use of other antifolates (e.g., sulfonamides) increases toxicity. Pancytopenia has been reported in some patients receiving methotrexate and trimethoprim-sulfamethoxazole together. Patients with ascites and large effusions are at greater risk for methotrexate toxicity. Folic acid, 1 mg daily, has been recommended as a means of preventing adverse reactions and particularly hematologic side effects in patients treated for rheumatoid arthritis.[80] The use of folic acid does not appear to significantly reduce effectiveness of the drug. In serious episodes of pancytopenia, leucovorin may be used.

Toxicities of particular concern in ICU patients include leukocytoclastic vasculitis, which has been reported with high-dose therapy used to treat osteogenic sarcoma as well as low-dose therapy for rheumatoid arthritis. Opportunistic infections with herpes zoster and *Pneumocystis carinii* have been reported even with low-dose methotrexate, although they are uncommon. Finally, an acute hypersensitivity pneumonitis as discussed earlier occurs infrequently but may result in profound hypoxemia.

CALCINEURIN INHIBITORS

The emergency use of cyclosporine and tacrolimus outside the setting of clinical transplantation will be rare. Their role in the urgent therapy for fulminant psoriasis and inflammatory bowel disease has been superseded by the availability of anti–tumor necrosis factor (TNF)-α biopharmaceuticals. The mechanism of action and dosing intricacies of both drugs are very similar. There is an accelerating trend favoring the use of tacrolimus in organ transplantation because the incidence of hypertension, hyperlipidemia, and nephrotoxicity appear to be less than with cyclosporine. If rapid achievement of therapeutic blood levels is needed, continuous intravenous administration of the calculated daily dose is required. The intravenous route is mandatory in children and patients with hypermotile or maladsorptive gastrointestinal disease. In a critically ill patient, maintenance of therapeutic plasma levels of a calcineurin inhibitor requires intensive monitoring of trough drug levels and frequent dose adjustments. A disparate group of commonly used drugs affect calcineurin inhibitor metabolism and eternal vigilance is required to prevent sudden decreases to subtherapeutic levels or increases that are nephrotoxic. The volume-depleted patient is especially susceptible to renal failure caused by either calcineurin inhibitor. Acute, severe gouty arthropathy is extremely common in patients being treated with cyclosporine.

HIGH-DOSE INTRAVENOUS GLOBULIN

Intravenous infusion of pooled IgG antibodies from large numbers of normal volunteers activates a diverse spectrum of immunomodulatory effects. The primary mechanism may be mediated by downregulation of Fc receptors on neutrophils and macrophages and inhibition of B-cell antigen receptors, but cytokine, idiotypic, and major histocompatibility antibodies may play a role also.[86] The spectrum of immunomodulation provides a rationale for the use of intravenous immunoglobulin (IVIg) in the treatment of life-threatening vasculitic syndromes of unknown etiology. IVIg can also be useful in patients who require immunosuppression or modulation, but cannot tolerate cyclophosphamide because their bone marrow is suppressed or hypoplastic.

High-dose intravenous antibody therapy may be indicated for therapy-resistant immune-mediated thrombocytopenia associated with significant bleeding, especially gastrointestinal bleeding, or when there is a need to either transiently elevate platelets or prolong the half-life of transfused platelets prior to splenectomy.[75] These modified, biologically active immunoglobulins are given at approximately a 0.4-g/kg dose and followed by platelet transfusions as indicated. Imaginative uses of these expensive biologics are frequent, usually in disease settings where all else has failed. Appropriate clinical trials are needed before their widespread use. There are few safety issues with the use of IVIg, but several instances of large vein thrombosis at the site of IVIg infusion have been reported.

The theoretical risk of generating anaphylatoxins or other complement-derived vasoactive mediators during rapid infusion of modified immunoglobulin preparations has been overstated.

ANTI-INFLAMMATORY AGENTS

NONSTEROIDAL ANTI-INFLAMMATORY DRUGS

The NSAIDs generally have little role to play in the management of patients in the ICU. Ulcerogenesis, hemostatic defects, and impairment of renal function converge as a group of notably unfriendly toxic effects for the critically ill patient. In general, corticosteroids are usually a safer alternative when an anti-inflammatory agent is necessary in the ICU. For instance, corticosteroids in low doses can be used to control symptomatic synovitis in the rheumatoid patient and are considerably less hazardous than NSAIDs. Moderate-dose oral, parenteral, or intra-articular steroids may be used for gout.

The emergence of drugs that selectively block the cyclooxygenase isoform COX-2, an inducible isoenzyme involved in inflammation, has created a safer class of NSAID. Selective COX-2 inhibitors including celecoxib, rofecoxib, and valdecoxib have been associated with a reduction in major gastrointestinal complications when compared to traditional NSAIDs. They are not renal sparing and do not appear to be safe in patients with aspirin-sensitive asthma. Nonetheless, because of the absence of platelet effect and lower GI toxicity they would be preferred agents if an NSAID was required. The concurrent use of a proton pump inhibitor to further reduce the risk of GI toxicity would seem prudent in the critically ill patient.

COX-2 drugs have recently been implicated in an increased risk of myocardial infarction and stroke. The story is unfolding as this book goes to press.

COLCHICINE

Colchicine is a plant-derived alkaloid that exerts a complex array of physiologic changes in the neutrophil. This appears to explain its therapeutic benefit in the acute phases of crystalline-induced arthritis, especially gout. Since it is not ulcerogenic and has no effect on platelet function it would seem to have advantages in the treatment of the medical ICU patient. However, because the therapeutic dose is close to the toxic dose there is substantial risk of inducing vomiting or diarrhea in a patient population not well suited to withstand additional stress. While the intravenous preparation of colchicine is associated with less gastrointestinal toxicity, it is associated with more systemic toxicity and occasionally death. Risk factors for toxicity with intravenous colchicine include renal and hepatic insufficiency, advanced age, volume depletion, and underlying cytopenia. The use of intravenous colchicine should be avoided in critically ill patients.

BIOLOGICAL AGENTS

Tumor Necrosis Factor-α Inhibition

The selective targeting of the proinflammatory cytokine TNF-α has produced a therapeutic revolution in rheumatology. While most widely used in the management of the synovitis of rheumatoid arthritis, these agents have been widely applied to a variety of immune-mediated disorders including psoriatic arthritis, ankylosing spondylitis, Behçet's disease, and sarcoidosis. Three commercial products are available, including two monoclonal antibodies (infliximab [chimeric] and adalimumab [humanized]) and one recombinant TNF receptor Fc fusion protein (etanercept). There is an emerging consensus that the antibodies may be more effective in the non-RA patients, but perhaps not without additional toxicity. In general, these drugs are extremely well tolerated and are neither renal toxic or marrow suppressing. They can reactivate granulomatous infections, notably tuberculosis. They must be used cautiously in patients with chronic or recurrent infection. They should be discontinued in the setting of serious infection or sepsis. There is currently no established indication to begin TNF-directed therapy in critically ill patients. The observations that such therapy can benefit patients with refractory Wegener's granulomatosis and Behçet's disease with progressive visual loss suggest scenarios in which initiation of TNF-directed therapy might begin in the ICU.

Interleukin-1 Inhibition

The currently available therapy directed against the pivotal proinflammatory cytokine IL-1 is anakinra. It is a recombinant human IL-1 receptor antagonist. While moderately effective for rheumatoid arthritis, it has not been nearly as effective as the TNF-α drugs. Although it is associated with fewer serious infections than TNF-directed therapy, when they are used in combination the increased risk of serious infection outweighs any additional therapeutic benefit.

B-CELL DEPLETION

Rituximab is a chimeric (mouse/human) monoclonal antibody that targets the CD20 molecule on B cells. CD20 is unique to B cells and is a stable transmembrane marker expressed during all stages of their maturation. The monoclonal antibody depletes B cells by activating apoptosis signals and complement and Fc receptor cytotoxicity.[87] Rituximab has an extensive history of effective use in B-cell lymphomas, and this bioengineered smart bomb has a surprisingly low number of significant side effects that can be characterized as constitutional symptoms of fever, chills, and rare hypotension attributable to cytokine release. All of the latter are most frequently experienced on the first infusion and are probably much more common in lymphoma patients with a large lymphocyte burden. The ability to selectively target and destroy B cells has generated tremendous interest in the rheumatologic community because rituximab offers a novel way to treat autoantibody-mediated autoimmune diseases like SLE, myasthenia gravis, autoimmune hemolytic anemia, and Goodpasture's syndrome.[82] In critically ill patients who cannot tolerate or have failed alkylating agent therapy, rituximab offers the option of definitive suppression of autoantibody production. The creative use of rituximab in autoimmune disease will be limited only by the imagination of the rheumatologist, and the reality is that widespread off-label use is already in progress. However, it is doubtful that many of its diverse applications will be confirmed by appropriate clinical trials. In theory, the focused destruction of B cells should culminate eventually in hypogammaglobulinemia and put the patient at high risk for bacterial infection. However, this has not been the case in most patients with lymphoma who are treated with the standard protocol of two to six weekly infusions of 375 mg/m^2. The treatment of patients with an autoimmune disease like SLE and the nephrotic syndrome may be a different situation since significant hypogammaglobulinemia requiring monthly replacement with IVIg has been reported. Careful monitoring of serum immunoglobulin

levels at least in these patients is warranted over the 6- to 9-month period of rituximab-induced depletion.

Therapeutic Pheresis in the Critically Ill Patient with Rheumatic Disease

PLASMAPHERESIS

Therapeutic plasmapheresis can effect rapid removal of circulating antigens, immune complexes, pathologic antibodies, and circulating cytokines, and improvement in the function of the fixed monocyte system. Plasmapheresis should be considered for patients with fulminant vasculitis of any cause, drug-resistant thyroid storm, selected poisonings, and a subset of life-threatening pulmonary-renal syndromes. Because cyclophosphamide has at least a 7- to 14-day window prior to a therapeutic effect, plasma exchange can be efficacious as a temporizing measure in many syndromes that will ultimately require cytoreductive therapy. Plasma exchange is also the treatment of choice for patients with thrombotic thrombocytopenic purpura (TTP), acutely deteriorating myasthenia gravis, and rapidly progressive or severe inflammatory peripheral neuropathies. Therapeutic apheresis may also provide an immediate clinical response in some patients with fulminant SLE with severe CNS dysfunction. Cryoglobulinemia with deteriorating renal or nervous system disease and hyperviscosity syndrome are other disorders for which plasmapheresis may play an important therapeutic role.

The procedure has a wide margin of safety when contemporary machines are used. At any point in time the amount of extracorporeal volume is much less than when the patient is exchanged with equipment that requires centrifuge bowl separation of blood components. Still, patients with decreased effective plasma volume or significant coronary artery disease remain at risk with all plasma-separation technologies available and must be closely monitored during the procedure. The frequency of exchange can be based on the isotype of the putative pathogenic antibody involved and the known kinetics of IgG clearance. Ultimately, however, the frequency and amount of exchange depends on the clinical status of the patient. Plasma volume varies with the height, size, sex, and hematocrit; nomograms are available that should be used for effective calculation if the apheresis machine itself does not calculate the values automatically. A 1.0 plasma volume exchange will remove approximately 65% of intravascular IgG from a patient and 1.5 plasma volume exchange 78% to 80% of IgG. Larger volume removals are associated with increased time on the machine, increased citrate toxicity, and most importantly, only very small incremental increases in IgG removal. A common rationale used to determine the frequency of plasmapheresis is based on "resting" the patient on alternate days to allow re-equilibration between extravascular and intravascular IgG. TTP and hyperviscosity syndromes, in which plasma volumes are expanded and the proteins generating hyperviscosity are predominantly within the intravascular space, can be effectively treated by aggressive and daily higher volume exchanges.

Patients with severe hepatic disease cannot metabolize citrate rapidly, and plasma exchanges should be done at the lowest possible citrate:plasma ratio. Serious side effects of citrate-induced hypocalcemia are extremely rare when volume is replaced with calcium-spiked 5% albumin. Fresh frozen plasma should never be used for routine replacement unless the patient has TTP, concomitant severe clotting factor deficiencies, or will be undergoing major surgery within the next 24 to 48 hours. Temporary decreases in several clotting factors during plasma removal, reflected by changes in the PT and APTT, are usually transient and not of clinical concern unless the patient has significant associated hemostatic deficiencies or severe hepatic dysfunction.

Because many patients in ICUs will not have suitable antecubital venous access or will be unable to provide arm pumping to generate sufficient venous flow during an apheresis procedure, dual-lumen polyurethane dialysis apheresis catheters are usually placed in a central vein and will provide high-flow access. If subclavian or internal jugular catheters are used, the return port should be in the cava, since relatively undiluted citrated blood has on rare occasion been thought to precipitate arrhythmias. Most patients undergoing plasma exchange do not require intravenous antibody replacement after each apheresis procedure. Exceptions to this rule are patients with hypoproteinemic states, especially the nephrotic syndrome, those with active infection, and those undergoing intensive, daily, high-volume therapeutic aphereses.

A standard rule for apheresis treatment of patients with autoaggressive syndromes, especially those with autoimmune antibody production, is that plasma exchange alone, although an effective temporizing measure, will ultimately not be efficacious and theoretically could be deleterious to the patient unless the apheresis treatment is closely linked to the use of an alkylating agent. The theory behind coupled therapy is straightforward.[82] Reduction in levels of pathogenic antibody, regulatory antibody, and regulatory cytokines can induce proliferation of B cells and possibly also T cells. Proliferating cells then become susceptible to alkylation, and either clonal abortion or anergy occurs when cyclophosphamide is given. The dose of cyclophosphamide ranges from 500 mg to 1 g/m^2 in 5% dextrose and water over a period of 30 to 60 minutes. Premedication for nausea is given routinely but may be unnecessary in some patients. The alkylating treatment can be given immediately after the last plasmapheresis and up to 48 hours thereafter. Protocols for the frequency of apheresis, at least in the treatment of SLE, vary widely but usually encompass an induction period of five to seven exchanges of 1.0 to 1.5 plasma volume over 7 to 10 days until approximately 250 mL plasma per kilogram have been removed from the patient. This induction period is followed by some form of immunosuppressive therapy, usually cyclophosphamide.[83]

PROTEIN A COLUMNS

Protein A absorption columns provide on-line removal of IgG antibody and circulating immune complexes; they have the benefit of returning most other plasma components to the patient. Protein A pheresis has been sporadically effective in drug-resistant idiopathic thrombocytopenic purpura and cancer chemotherapy–associated TTP/hemolytic uremic syndrome.[84] Angiotensin-converting enzyme inhibitors should be discontinued prior to the procedure. The efflux of activated inflammatory and vasoactive mediators generated from plasma by the protein A silica absorption vehicle can cause transient shaking, chills, fever, and hypotension.

This usually occurs at the end or after the termination of the procedure.

LEUKAPHERESIS

Leukapheresis can be performed efficiently on centrifuge belt machines and is highly effective in reducing peripheral blast counts to levels that are less threatening to maintenance of adequate microcirculation and more amenable to chemotherapy. Combination leukaplasmapheresis has been performed in patients with scleroderma and polymyositis/dermatomyositis that was refractory to conventional management.

Empirical Therapy for Suspected Rheumatic Disease

In puzzling cases the rheumatologist may discern from the nuances of the clinical examination, serologic testing, and invasive procedures that the patient has rheumatic disease. Sometimes the rheumatologist, like the intensivist, cannot make a definite diagnosis, yet confronts a critically ill patient who *may* have a rheumatic disease. The clinical status of such patients is usually at an unacceptable plateau or even more likely deteriorating. Should that patient be given empiric therapy? Recognition of our shortcomings in diagnosis and the inability of some patients to tolerate a critical invasive test recommends such a course in selected patients.

Prior to initiation of empirical therapy, it is helpful to ask a series of related questions:

1. Has infection been reasonably excluded? Infection and cancer most commonly mimic rheumatic disease. Since empiric therapy usually implies immunosuppressive drugs, most commonly corticosteroids, infection must be ruled out. Here the emphasis should be on *reasonably* making such an assessment. Endless sets of blood cultures should not delay a difficult decision.
2. What do I suspect the patient may have? It should be possible to formulate a plausible if unprovable diagnostic hypothesis. Such a hypothesis is critical to the rest of the experiment. If it is impossible to generate a "working diagnosis," it is doubtful that the therapeutic trial will work. Autopsy study of these patients is likely to reveal cancer or no diagnosis.
3. What is adequate therapy for this suspected diagnosis? Treatment for a suspected diagnosis ranges from adequate to aggressive. In the absence of a definite diagnosis, it is reasonable to choose a level of therapeutic intensity that is usually adequate for the suspected disorder. Aggressive treatment approaches to an unconfirmed illness create another set of confounding variables and may place the patient at a further disadvantage.
4. What will I use as my parameters to judge therapeutic success? Empiric therapy should proceed with a clear understanding of the yardsticks that will measure therapeutic responsiveness. These parameters can then be rigorously monitored. Furthermore, blind spots in the baseline data can be addressed before therapy is begun.
5. What is the duration of a reasonable trial for this disorder? Agreement on the duration of a therapeutic trial should precede its initiation. Failure to develop such an end point can result in excessively long and risky therapy on the one

hand, or a course that falls short of an adequate trial on the other. Furthermore, spontaneous improvement or improvement in response to other therapies may result in prolonged and unnecessary treatment.

The clinician needs to be vigilant about the risks associated with any trial of empiric therapy. However, after addressing the above questions, such a trial may represent both rational and compassionate care.

References

1. Janssen NM, Karnad DR, Guntupalli KK: Rheumatologic diseases in the intensive care unit: Epidemiology, clinical approach, management, and outcome. *Crit Care Clin* 18:729, 2002.
2. Wallace DJ: The clinical presentation of systemic lupus erythematosus, in Wallace DJ, Han BH (eds): *Dubois' Lupus Erythematosus*, 6th ed. Philadelphia, Lippincott Williams & Wilkins, 2002, p 622.
3. Inoue T, Takeda T, Koda S, et al: Differential diagnosis of fever in systemic lupus erythematosus using discriminant analysis. *Rheum Int* 5:69, 1986.
4. Iliopoulos AG, Tsokos GC: Immunopathogenesis and spectrum of infections in systemic lupus erythematosus. *Semin Arthritis Rheum* 25:318, 1996.
5. Haider TS, Roberts WC: Coronary arterial disease in systemic lupus erythematosus—quantification of degrees of narrowing in 10 necropsy patients. *Am J Med* 70:775, 1981.
6. Asherson RA, Kham Ashta MA, Baguley E, et al: Myocardial infarction and antiphospholipid antibodies in SLE and related disorders. *Q J Med* 73:1103, 1989.
7. Julkunen H, Hedman C, Kauppi M: thrombolysis for acute ischemic stroke in primary antiphospholipid syndrome. *J Rheumatol* 24:181, 1997.
8. Boumpas DT, Austin HA, Fessler BJ, et al: Systemic lupus erythematosus: Emerging concepts. Renal, neuropsychiatric, cardiovascular, pulmonary, and hematologic disease. *Ann Intern Med* 122:940, 1995.
9. Stone JH: End-stage renal disease in lupus: Disease activity, dialysis, and outcome of transplantation. *Lupus* 7:654, 1998.
10. Cheigh JS, Stenzek KH, Rubin AL, et al: Systemic lupus erythematosus in patients with chronic renal failure. *Am J Med* 75:602, 1983.
11. Lawrence EC: Systemic lupus erythematosus and the lung, in Lahita RG (ed): *Systemic Lupus Erythematosus*. New York, Wiley, 1987, p 691.
12. Zamora MR, Warner ML, Tuder R, et al: Diffuse alveolar hemorrhage and systemic lupus erythematosus. New York, Wiley, 1987, p 691.
13. Millman RP, Cohen TB, Levinson AI, et al: SLE complicated by acute pulmonary hemorrhage: Recovery following plasmapheresis and cytotoxic therapy. *J Rheumatol* 8:1021, 1981.
14. Fessler BJ, Boumpas DT: Severe major organ involvement in systemic lupus erythematosus. Diagnosis and management. *Rheum Dis Clin North Am* 21:81, 1995.
15. McCune WJ, Golbus J: Neuropsychiatric lupus. *Rheum Dis Clin North Am* 14:149, 1988.
16. Widener HL, Littman DH: Ibuprofen induced meningitis in systemic lupus erythematosus. *JAMA* 239:1062, 1978.
17. Brandt KD, Lessell S: Migrainous phenomena in systemic lupus erythematosus. *Arthritis Rheum* 21:7, 1978.
18. Harris EN, Gharavi AE, Hughes GRV: Anti-phospholipid antibodies. *Clin Rheum Dis* 11:591, 1985.
19. Denton CP, Black CM: Pulmonary vascular involvement in systemic sclerosis, in Clements PJ, Furst DE (eds): *Systemic Sclerosis*, 2nd ed. Philadelphia, Lippincott Williams & Wilkins, 2004, p 184.
20. Rubin LJ, Badesch DB, Barst RJ, et al: Bosentan therapy for pulmonary arterial hypertension. *N Engl J Med* 346:896, 2002.
21. Kobo M, Vensak J, Dauber J, et al: Lung transplantation in patients with scleroderma. *J Heart Lung Transplant* 120:1547, 2001.
22. DeMarco PJ, Weisman, MH, Seibold JR, et al: Predictors and outcomes of scleroderma renal crisis: The high-dose versus low-dose d-penicillamine in early diffuse systemic sclerosis trial. *Arthritis Rheum* 46:2983, 2002.
23. Steen VD: Scleroderma renal crisis. *Rheum Dis Clin North Am* 29:315, 2003.
24. Rhew EY, Barr WG: Scleroderma renal crisis: New insights and developments (review). *Curr Opin Rheumatol* 6:129, 2004.
25. Marinelli WA, Leatherman JW: Neuromuscular disorders in the intensive care unit. *Crit Care Clin* 18:915, 2002.
26. Bohan A, Peter JB, Bowman RL, Pearson CM: A computer assisted analysis of 153 patients with polymyositis and dermatomyositis. *Medicine* 56:255, 1977.
27. Medsger TA, Robinson H, Masi AT: Factors affecting survivorship in polymyositis: A life table study of 124 patients. *Arthritis Rheum* 14:249, 1971.
28. Catoggio LJ: Management of inflammatory muscle disease, in Hochberg MC, Silman AJ, Smolen JS et al (eds): *Rheumatology*, 3rd ed. Edinburgh, Mosby, 2003, p 1555.
29. Dau PC: Plasmapheresis in idiopathic inflammatory myopathy: Experience with 35 patients. *Arch Neurol* 38:544, 1981.
30. Cecere FA, Spiva DA: Combination plasmapheresis leukocytapheresis for the treatment of dermatomyositis polymyositis. *Plasma Ther Transfus Technol* 3:401, 1982.
31. Miller FW, Leitman SF, Cronin ME, et al: Controlled trial of plasma exchange and leukapheresis in polymyositis and dermatomyositis. *N Engl J Med* 326:1380, 1992.
32. Sostman HD, Matthay RA, Putman CE, Walker Smith GJ: Methotrexate-induced pneumonitis. *Medicine (Baltimore)* 55:371, 1976.
33. Cottin V, Tebib J, Massonet B, et al: Pulmonary function in patients receiving long-term low-dose methotrexate. *Chest* 109:933, 1996.
34. Battistone MJ, Williams HJ. Disease-modifying antirheumatic drugs 3: Methotrexate, in Hochberg MC, Silman AJ, Smolen JS et al (eds): *Rheumatology*, 3rd ed. Edinburgh, Mosby, 2003, p 417.
35. Perrquet JL, Harrington TM, Davis DE: *Pneumocystis carinii* following methotrexate therapy for rheumatoid arthritis [letter]. *Arthritis Rheum* 16:1291, 1983.
36. Alarcon GS, Kremer JM, Macaluso M, et al: Risk factors for methotrexate-induced lung injury in patients with rheumatoid arthritis: A multicenter, case-control study. *Ann Intern Med* 127:356, 1997.
37. Neva MH, Kauppi MJ, Kautiainen H, et al: Combination drug therapy retards the development of rheumatoid atlantoaxial subluxations. *Arthritis Rheum* 43:2397, 2000.
38. Janssen NM, Karnad DR, Guntupalli KK: Rheumatologic diseases in the intensive care unit: Epidemiology, clinical approach, management, and outcome. *Crit Care Clin* 18:729, 2002.
39. Godeau B, Mortier E, Roy PM, et al: Short and long term outcomes from patients with systemic rheumatoid diseases admitted to intensive care units: A prognostic study of 181 patients. *J Rheumatol* 24:1317, 1997.
40. Pourrat O, Bureau JM, Hira M, et al: Outcomes of patients with systemic rheumatic disease admitted to intensive care units: A retrospective study of 39 cases. *Rev Med Interne* 21:147, 2000.
41. Pope RM: Rheumatic fever in the 1980s. *Bull Rheum Dis* 38:1, 1989.
42. Elkon KB, Hughes GR, Bywaters EG, et al: Adult onset Still's disease: Twenty year follow-up and further study of patients with active disease. *Arthritis Rheum* 25:647, 1982.
43. Moder KG: Use and interpretation of rheumatologic tests: A guide for clinicians. *Mayo Clin Proc* 71:391, 1996.
44. Hunder GG: Giant cell (temporal) arteritis. *Rheum Dis Clin North Am* 16:399, 1990.

45. Camilleri M, Pusey CD, Chadwick VS, Rees AJ: Gastrointestinal manifestations of systemic vasculitis. *Q J Med* 52:141, 1983.

46. Zizic TM, Classen JN, Stevens MB: Acute abdominal complications of systemic lupus erythematosus and polyarteritis nodosa. *Am J Med* 73:525, 1982.

47. Johnson JP, Moore J, Austin HA, et al: Therapy of antiglomerular basement membrane antibody disease: Analysis of the prognostic significance of clinical, pathologic and treatment factors. *Medicine* 64:219, 1985.

48. Dweik RA, Arroliga AC, Cash JM: Alveolar hemorrhage in patients with rheumatic disease. *Rheum Dis Clin North Am* 23:395, 1997.

49. Johnson JP, Whitman W, Briggs WA, Wilson CB: Plasmapheresis and immunosuppressive agents in anti-basement membrane antibody-induced Goodpasture's syndrome. *Am J Med* 64:354, 1978.

50. Arzoo K, Sadeghi S, Liebman HA: Treatment of refractory antibody mediated autoimmune disorders with an anti-CD20 monoclonal antibody (Rituximab). *Ann Rheum Dis* 61:922, 2002.

51. Massa MC, Su WPD: Lymphocytic vasculitis: A clinical pathologic study. *J Cutaneous Pathol* 11:132, 1984.

52. Van Hale HM, Gibson LE, Schroeter AL: Henoch-Schönlein vasculitis: Direct immunofluorescence study of uninvolved skin. *J Am Acad Dermatol* 15:665, 1986.

53. Sigal LH: Pseudovasculitis syndromes, in McCarty DJ (ed): *Arthritis and Allied Conditions*, 11th ed. Philadelphia, Lea & Febiger, 1989, p 1189.

54. Bowles CA: Vasculopathy associated with the antiphospholipid antibody syndrome. *Rheum Dis Clin North Am* 16:471, 1990.

55. Joyce JW: Buerger's disease (thromboangiitis obliterans). *Rheum Dis Clin North Am* 16:471, 1990.

56. Bathon J, Graves J, Jens P, et al: The erythrocyte sedimentation rate in end-stage renal failure. *Am J Kidney Dis* 10:34, 1987.

57. Connelly CS, Panush RS: Markedly elevated sedimentation rates: What is their clinical significance?, in *Postgraduate Advances in Rheumatology*. Berryville, Virginia, Forum Medicum, 1990, p IV.

58. Recker DP, Klippel JH: Perplexing antinuclear antibody syndrome (PANAS), in *Postgraduate Advances in Rheumatology*. Berryville, Virginia, Forum Medicum, 1989, p IV.

59. Cattogio LJ, Bernstein RM, Black CM, et al: Serologic markers in progressive systemic sclerosis: Clinical correlations. *Ann Rheum Dis* 42:23, 1983.

60. Chorzelski TP, Jablonska S, Beutner EH, et al: Anticentromere antibody: An immunological marker of a subset of systemic sclerosis. *Br J Dermatol* 113:381, 1985.

61. Harmon CE: Antinuclear antibodies in autoimmune disease. *Med Clin North Am* 69:547, 1985.

62. Ramsey-Goldman R, Hom D, Deng J-S, et al: Anti-SS-A antibodies and fetal outcome in maternal systemic lupus erythematosus. *Arthritis Rheum* 29:1269, 1986.

63. Jarzabek-Chorzelska M, Blaszczyk M, Jablonska S, et al: Scl 70 antibody—a specific marker of systemic sclerosis. *Br J Dermatol* 115:393, 1986.

64. Falk RJ, Jennette JC: Anti-neutrophil cytoplasmic autoantibodies with specificity for myeloperoxidase in patients with systemic vasculitis and idiopathic necrotizing and crescentic glomerulonephritis. *N Engl J Med* 318:1651, 1988.

65. Schnabel A, Hauschild S, Gross WL: Anti-neutrophil cytoplasmic antibodies in generalized autoimmune diseases. *Int Arch Allergy Immunol* 109:201, 1996.

66. Specks U, DeRemee RA: Granulomatous vasculitis. *Rheum Dis Clin North Am* 16:377, 1990.

67. Scott DG, Bacon PA: Intravenous cyclophosphamide plus methylprednisolone in treatment of systemic rheumatoid vasculitis. *Am J Med* 76:377, 1984.

68. Geltner D, Kohn RW, Gorevic P, Franklin EC: The effect of combination therapy (steroids, immunosuppressives, and plasmapheresis) on 5 mixed cryoglobulinemia patients with renal, neurologic, and vascular involvement. *Arthritis Rheum* 24:1121, 1981.

69. Frank MM: Complement: A brief review. *J Allergy Clin Immunol* 84:411, 1989.

70. Ames PR, Pyke S, Iannaccone L, Brancaccio V: Antiphospholipid antibodies, haemostatic variables and thrombosis—a survey of 144 patients. *Thromb Haemost* 73:768, 1995.

71. Hoffman, GS, Leavitt RY, Fleischer TA, et al: Treatment of Wegener's granulomatosis with intermittent high-dose intravenous cyclophosphamide. *Am J Med* 89:403, 1990.

72. Asherson RA: The catastrophic antiphospholipid syndrome. *J Rheumatol* 19:508, 1992.

73. Westney GE, Harris EN: Catastrophic antiphospholipid syndrome in the intensive care unit. *Crit Care Clin* 18:805, 2002.

74. Kimberly RP: Pulse methylprednisolone in SLE. *Clin Rheum Dis* 8:261, 1982.

75. National Institutes of Health Consensus Conference: Intravenous immunoglobulin: Prevention and treatment of disease. *JAMA* 264:3189, 1990.

76. Sahn SA, Lakshiminarayan W: Tuberculosis after corticosteroid therapy. *Br J Dis Chest* 70:195, 1976.

77. Iseman MD: Tuberculosis prophylaxis during corticosteroid therapy—reply. *JAMA* 258:263, 1987.

78. Behrens TW, Goodwin JS: Glucocorticoids, in McCarty DJ (ed): *Arthritis and Allied Conditions*, 11th ed. Philadelphia, Lea & Febiger, 1989, p 604.

79. Fischer TJ, Rachelefsky GS, Klein RB, et al: Childhood dermatomyositis and polymyositis—treatment with methotrexate and prednisone. *Am J Dis Child* 133:386, 1979.

80. Morgan SL, Baggott JE, Vaughn WH, et al: The effect of folic acid supplementation on the toxicity of low dose methotrexate in patients with rheumatoid arthritis. *Arthritis Rheum* 33:9, 1990.

81. Silverman GJ, Weisman S: Rituximab therapy and autoimmune disorders: prospects for anti-B cell therapy. *Arthritis Rheum* 48:1484, 2003.

82. Schroeder JO, Euler HH, Loffler H: Synchronization of plasmapheresis and pulse cyclophosphamide in severe systemic lupus erythematosus. *Ann Intern Med* 107:344, 1987.

83. Barr WG, Hubbell EA, Robinson JA: Persistently active systemic lupus erythematosus treated with intermittent plasmapheresis and bolus cyclophosphamide, in Oda T, Shiokawa Y, Inque N (eds): *Proceedings of the 1st International Congress of the World Apheresis Association*. Cleveland, ISAO Press, 1987, p 696.

84. Snyder HW, Mittelman A, Cochran SK, et al, and PROSORBA Clinical Trial Group: Successful treatment of cancer chemotherapy-associated thrombotic thrombocytopenic purpura hemolytic uremic syndrome (TTP HUS) with protein A immunoadsorption. Presented at the American Society of Hematology, Boston, November 28–December 4, 1990.

85. Kobo M, Vensak J, Dauber J, et al: Lung transplantation in patients with scleroderma. *J Heart Lung Transplant* 120:1547, 2001.

86. Kazatchkine MD, Kaveri SV: Immunomodulation of autoimmune and inflammatory diseases with intravenous immune globulin. *N Engl J Med* 345:747, 2001.

87. Johnson PWM, Glennie MJ: Rituximab: Mechanisms and applications. *Br J Cancer* 85:1619, 2001.

Chapter 105 _____

CRITICAL ILLNESS IN PREGNANCY

MARY E. STREK
MICHAEL O'CONNOR
JESSE HALL

KEY POINTS

- *Understanding the normal physiology of pregnancy is essential to evaluate the adequacy of cardiopulmonary function in the critically ill gravid woman.*

- *Pregnancy results in an increased cardiac output, which in late pregnancy may be diminished in the supine position by vena caval compression from the enlarged uterus.*

- *The reduced functional residual capacity (FRC) and increased oxygen consumption noted in normal pregnancy increase the risk of hypoxemia during intubation or hypoventilation.*

- *Hyperventilation during pregnancy results in a primary respiratory alkalosis and a compensatory metabolic acidosis with the following typical arterial blood gas values: P_{O_2} >100 mm Hg, P_{CO_2} 27 to 32 mm Hg, and serum bicarbonate concentration 18 to 21 mEq/L.*

- *Fetal viability depends on adequate oxygen delivery. As a result of the dilutional anemia of pregnancy, cardiac output becomes the critical determinant of fetal oxygen delivery and must be maintained.*

- *Hemorrhage in pregnancy may be massive and require extraordinary fluid resuscitation.*

- *Vasoactive drugs should be used with caution in the pregnant patient, since they may reduce uterine blood flow.*

- *Control of increased afterload may require intravenous agents: Sodium nitroprusside should be used only for imminently life-threatening conditions, since cyanide toxicity may result in fetal injury or demise. Nicardipine is an intravenous calcium channel blocker that is preferable to nitroprusside, and experience with labetalol, a combined alpha-beta blocker, is growing and promising.*

- *Preeclampsia is a multisystem disorder characterized by hypertension, central nervous system dysfunction, coagulopathy, pulmonary edema, renal failure, and liver function abnormalities.*

- *Cardiopulmonary resuscitation must be modified in pregnancy and includes emergent cesarean section in selected patients.*

- *Pregnancy may represent a state of increased risk of pulmonary edema formation; acute hypoxemic respiratory failure is most often due to tocolytic therapy, and if due to tocolytics, usually resolves with supportive care.*

- *Successful management of critical illness in pregnancy requires continuous integration of the intensive care team with obstetric and neonatal consultants; mechanisms should exist for emergent involvement of the appropriate personnel.*

Pregnancy greatly complicates critical illness, since assessment, monitoring, and treatment must take into account both maternal and fetal well-being. Knowledge of the normal changes in maternal respiratory, cardiac, and acid-base physiology in pregnancy is essential to distinguish between adaptive and pathologic changes.

This chapter begins with an overview of the changes in cardiovascular, respiratory, renal, and gastrointestinal physiology in normal pregnancy. Next, the determinants of fetal oxygen delivery are reviewed. The remainder of the chapter focuses on the disorders that can result in critical illness in pregnancy and the appropriate management of each. Finally, the importance of acid-base homeostasis, prophylaxis to prevent gastrointestinal bleeding, and early nutrition are discussed.

In many ways our understanding of the complex interaction between disease state and maternal/fetal physiology is incomplete. Thus we rely on an approach that assumes that measures that optimize maternal well-being are usually best for the fetus as well. Nonetheless, throughout critical illness, monitoring and management decisions must take into account fetal as well as maternal parameters. That is best achieved by expanding the typical critical care team consisting of nurse, respiratory therapist, and intensivist to include obstetrician and neonatologist as well.

Physiology of Pregnancy

ADAPTATION OF THE CIRCULATION

In pregnancy, numerous circulatory adjustments occur that ensure adequate oxygen delivery to the fetus (Table 105-1). Early in pregnancy maternal blood volume increases, reaching a level 40% above baseline by the thirtieth week.[1–3] This increase is due both to a 20% to 40% increase in the number of erythrocytes and a larger 40% to 50% increase in plasma volume. A mild dilutional anemia results, with a decrease in hematocrit of about 12%.[1,2] The magnitude of the increase in blood volume is greater with multiple births. This extracellular volume expansion is associated with parallel decreases in colloid osmotic pressure and serum albumin concentration; both indices reach a plateau at 26 weeks, although there is a further decline in colloid osmotic pressure immediately postpartum.[2] The extracellular volume expansion is caused by activation of the renin-angiotensin system with increased aldosterone production and results in mild peripheral edema in 50% to 80% of normal pregnancies.[1,2]

Coincident with the change in maternal blood volume is a 30% to 50% increase in cardiac output, most of which occurs in the first trimester and continues throughout gestation.[4–6] The augmented cardiac output results from an increase in heart rate, and to a lesser degree stroke volume, with heart rate reaching a maximum of 15 to 20 beats per minute above resting nonpregnant levels by weeks 32 to 36.[5,7] The increase in stroke volume is due both to an increase in preload caused by augmented blood volume and to a decrease in afterload caused by a 20% to 30% fall in systemic vascular resistance (SVR). The fall in SVR is attributed both to arteriovenous shunting through the low-resistance uteroplacental bed and vasodilation that may result from decreased vascular responsiveness to endogenous pressors and/or increased synthesis of vasodilators. Some studies suggest that since left ventricular end-diastolic pressure remains normal despite a rise in left ventricular end-diastolic volume,[4,7] ventricular

TABLE 105-1 Circulatory Changes in Pregnancy

Parameter	Direction	Time Course
Heart rate	↑	First and second trimesters
Blood pressure	↓	Falls in first and second trimesters; returns to baseline in third trimester
Cardiac output	↑	Progressive increases throuhout pregnancy to as much as 50% above baseline value by the 24th week
Stroke volume	↑	Increase peaks at 16–24 weeks
Systemic vascular resistance	↓	Reaches nadir by mid-pregnancy: 20%–30% decline from baseline
Pulmonary vascular resistance	↓	20%–30% decrease

diastolic compliance may be increased. Others have postulated a decrease in ventricular compliance based on studies demonstrating increased left ventricular wall thickness and mass.[5,6] While some authors have suggested that left ventricular performance improves during pregnancy;[1] recent studies have noted no increase in ejection fraction as calculated from echocardiography.[4,6] The exact contributions of increased heart rate and stroke volume, loading conditions, and ventricular performance to the increase in flow have not been conclusively determined.

During the course of pregnancy, cardiac output becomes more dependent upon body position, since the gravid uterus can cause significant obstruction of the inferior vena cava with reduced venous return. This effect is most notable in the third trimester. Vena caval obstruction is maximal in the supine position and much less pronounced in the left lateral decubitus position.[1] During labor, uterine contraction can increase cardiac output 10% to 15% over resting pregnant levels by increasing blood return from the contracting uterus.[2,8] This effect on cardiac output, however, may be tempered by blood loss during delivery.

Blood pressure decreases early in pregnancy owing to peripheral vasodilation as noted above. The peak decreases in systolic and diastolic pressures average 5 to 9 and 6 to 17 mm Hg, respectively, and occur at 16 to 28 weeks.[9] Blood pressure then increases gradually, returning to prepregnancy levels shortly after delivery. A review of hypertension in pregnancy suggests that diastolic pressures of 75 mm Hg in the second trimester and 85 mm Hg in the third trimester should be considered the upper limits of normal.[9]

The normal adaptation of the circulatory system to pregnancy results in a physiologic third heart sound in the majority of pregnant patients. The chest radiograph reveals an enlarged cardiac silhouette. As will be discussed below, right ventricular, pulmonary artery, and pulmonary artery wedge pressures are unchanged from prepartum values in the healthy pregnant woman.[10]

ADAPTATION OF THE RESPIRATORY SYSTEM

Oxygen consumption increases 20% to 35% in normal pregnancy;[11,12] during labor there is a further rise in oxygen consumption.[13] The increase in oxygen consumption occurs because of fetal and placental needs, as well as maternal requirements resulting from increases in cardiac output and work of breathing.[12] Increased oxygen consumption is associated with a 34% to 50% increase in carbon dioxide produc-

tion by the third trimester, necessitating an increase in minute ventilation that begins in the first trimester and peaks at 20% to 40% above baseline at term.[2,14] Alveolar ventilation is increased above the level needed to eliminate carbon dioxide, and partial pressure of carbon dioxide (P_{CO_2}) falls to a level of 27 to 32 mm Hg throughout pregnancy. The augmented alveolar ventilation is attributed to respiratory stimulation due to increased levels of progesterone, and results from a 30% to 35% increase in tidal volume (from 450 to 600 mL) while respiratory rate is unchanged.[2,11,15] Renal compensation results in a maternal pH that is only slightly alkalemic, in the range of 7.40 to 7.45, with serum bicarbonate decreasing to 18 to 21 mEq/L[11] (Table 105-2).

Maternal arterial partial oxygen pressure (P_{O_2}) is increased throughout pregnancy, to greater than 100 mm Hg, by virtue of augmented minute ventilation, but this increase does not significantly increase oxygen delivery. Mild hypoxemia and an increased alveolar-to-arterial oxygen gradient [$(A\text{-}a)_{O_2}$] may occur in the supine position.[16] This likely results from airway narrowing or closure with resultant ventilation-perfusion mismatch related to a further decrease in the already reduced difference between functional residual capacity (FRC) and closing capacity that occurs in gravid individuals (see below).[17] Whenever possible, arterial blood gas samples should be obtained in the seated position to avoid confounding effects from the mild positional hypoxemia of pregnancy (see Table 105-2).

FRC decreases progressively (10% to 25% at term) as a result of increased abdominal pressure from the enlarged uterus, which results in diaphragmatic elevation and decreased chest wall compliance.[2,15] Expiratory reserve volume (ERV) and residual volume are decreased during the second half of pregnancy.[15] Total lung capacity decreases minimally

TABLE 105-2 Typical Arterial Blood Gas Values

	P_{O_2}	P_{CO_2}	pH	$(A\text{-}a)_{O_2}$	S_{O_2},%
Nonpregnant	98	40	7.40	2	98
Term pregnancy, seated	101	28	7.45	14	98
Term pregnancy, supine	95	28	7.45	20	97

NOTE: $(A\text{-}a)_{O_2}$ is the difference between the predicted alveolar P_{O_2} and the measured arterial P_{O_2}, assuming a respiratory quotient of 0.8. Normally this value is <10 mm Hg. S_{O_2} is the saturation of hemoglobin with oxygen.
SOURCE: Reproduced with permission from Schmidt GA, Hall JB: Pulmonary diseases in pregnancy, in Barron W, Lindheimer M (eds): *Medical Disorders during Pregnancy*, 2nd ed. St. Louis, Mosby Year-Book, 1995, p 169.

because the function of the diaphragm and thoracic muscles is unimpaired, and widening of the thoracic cage results in an increased inspiratory capacity.[11,15] Vital capacity remains unchanged during pregnancy. Diffusing capacity is unchanged or slightly increased early in pregnancy and then decreases to normal or slightly below normal after the first trimester.[18] Airway closure may occur near or above FRC in some women late in pregnancy.[17,18] As discussed above, airway closure may be responsible, at least in part, for the positional hypoxemia noted late in pregnancy. The decreased FRC, when combined with the increased oxygen consumption found in pregnancy, makes the pregnant woman and fetus more vulnerable to hypoxia in the event of hypoventilation or apnea. This is an important consideration during endotracheal intubation.

Despite increases in levels of many hormones known to affect smooth muscle, the function of large airways does not appear to be altered in pregnancy. Forced expiratory volume in 1 second (FEV_1), the ratio of FEV_1 to forced vital capacity (FVC), and specific airways conductance are unchanged during pregnancy. The fact that flow-volume loops are also unaffected by pregnancy is further evidence of normal airway function.[19] Lung compliance is unchanged.

RENAL AND GASTROINTESTINAL ADAPTATION

Renal blood flow increases during the first and second trimesters to 60% to 80% above prepregnancy levels and then declines during the third trimester.[2] The glomerular filtration rate rises early in pregnancy to 50% above baseline at 12 to 16 weeks and remains increased during pregnancy.[20] This change means that serum creatinine during pregnancy (0.5 to 0.7 mg/dL) is somewhat lower than baseline. Therefore creatinine levels that would be normal in a nonpregnant patient can indicate renal dysfunction in pregnant patients.

Lower esophageal sphincter tone decreases during the first trimester of pregnancy and remains low until near term, perhaps as a result of increased plasma progesterone levels.[2] The gravid uterus displaces the stomach, further reducing the effectiveness of the gastroesophageal sphincter. Basal gastric acid secretion and pH remain unchanged during pregnancy.[21] Labor and narcotic analgesics given during labor delay gastric emptying time, significantly increasing the risk of aspiration.

FETAL OXYGEN DELIVERY

Oxygen delivery to the fetal tissues depends on the oxygen content of uterine artery blood, as determined by maternal P_{O_2}, hemoglobin concentration and saturation, and uterine artery blood flow.[2] As discussed above, the small increases in arterial P_{O_2} attributable to hyperventilation have little effect on oxygen content, since maternal hemoglobin saturation is only marginally increased. However, the anemia of pregnancy reduces the oxygen content significantly, and thus the critically ill gravid patient is more dependent than the nonpregnant individual on cardiac output for maintenance of oxygen delivery.

Numerous factors affect uterine artery blood flow. The uterine vasculature is maximally dilated under normal conditions and therefore is unable to adapt to stress by increasing flow through local vascular adjustment.[22] This assertion is supported by investigations in a gravid ewe model of progressive anemia in which the hematocrit was lowered from 31% to 8%.[23] There was no augmentation of flow to either the

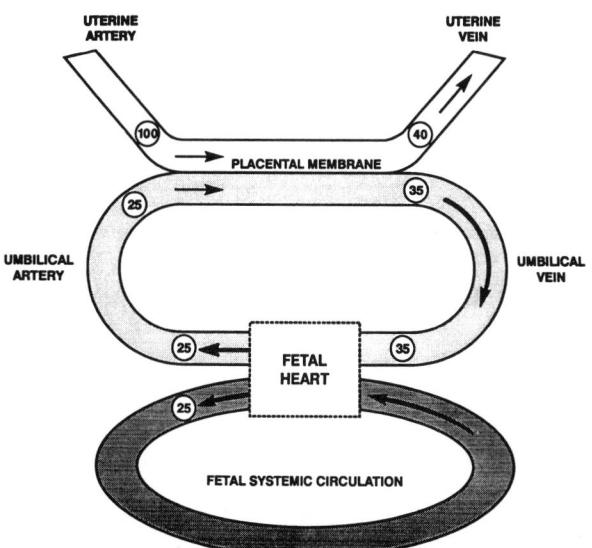

FIGURE 105-1 Maternal-fetal oxygen transfer. The circled numbers represent approximate values of the partial pressure of oxygen in mm Hg. (*Reproduced with permission from Lapinsky et al.[2]*)

uterine or the placental beds, and consequently there was a progressive decline in oxygen delivery to the fetus. This finding suggests that the uterine bed is not readily able to increase fetal oxygen delivery by vascular autoregulation. Fetal oxygen delivery can be decreased by uterine artery vasoconstriction. Exogenous or endogenous sympathetic stimulation and maternal hypotension elicit uterine artery vasoconstriction. In addition, maternal alkalosis causes uterine artery vasoconstriction.[2] The latter effect may be compounded by the resulting leftward shift of the maternal oxyhemoglobin saturation curve, which increases oxygen affinity, thereby reducing the P_{O_2} in the uterine artery and decreasing the gradient that drives oxygen across the placenta.

In the placenta, a concurrent exchange mechanism driven by the difference in oxygen tension between maternal and fetal blood results in the transfer of oxygen from the maternal to the fetal circulation (Fig. 105-1).[2] Complete equilibration does not occur, so the umbilical venous blood going to the fetus has a lower oxygen tension than the blood in the uterine vein. The oxygenated umbilical venous blood, which has a P_{O_2} of 30 to 40 mm Hg, combines with deoxygenated fetal inferior vena caval blood, resulting in a fetal arterial P_{O_2} of 20 to 25 mm Hg.[2] In spite of the low umbilical vein and fetal arterial P_{O_2} values, compensatory mechanisms maintain fetal oxygen delivery, and fetal oxygen content is relatively high. At all levels of P_{O_2}, fetal hemoglobin has a higher affinity for oxygen than maternal hemoglobin, being 80% to 90% saturated at a P_{O_2} of 30 to 35 mm Hg.[2] In addition, the fetus has a higher hemoglobin concentration (150 g/L) than does the adult and has a high systemic cardiac output, with both left and right ventricles delivering blood to the systemic circulation. Studies indicate that fetal tissue hypoxia does not occur until levels of hypoxemia are reached that would be catastrophic by adult criteria. Brief reductions by up to 50% in uterine blood flow are well tolerated in animal models.[2] In a primate model of asphyxia, brain injury did not occur until fetal P_{O_2} fell to 9 to 14 mm Hg.[24] Protective responses to hypoxic stress also exist at the level of the fetal circulation. A reduction in oxygen supply by >50% in a sheep preparation caused some fetal tissues to shift to anaerobic metabolism, and the fetal cardiac output was redirected to the brain, heart, and adrenal glands.[25] When fetal oxygen content is reduced by more than 75%, the oxygen supply is inadequate to most of the organism, including the central nervous system. Irreversible brain damage begins after 10 minutes without oxygen.[2] This fact suggests that compensatory mechanisms, such as redistribution of fetal blood flow to vital organs, decreased oxygen consumption in response to hypoxic stress, and the successful prolonged dependence of certain tissue beds on anaerobic metabolism may occur.

In summary, during pregnancy oxygen delivery to maternal and fetoplacental tissue beds is highly dependent on adequate blood flow and maternal oxygen content. Maternal oxygen consumption increases progressively during gestation and rises further in labor. In late pregnancy or near term, the fetoplacental unit is unable to increase oxygen delivery by local vascular adjustment. The fetus, however, is protected from hypoxic insult by the avidity of fetal hemoglobin for oxygen relative to maternal hemoglobin, the high fetal hemoglobin content, the high fetal cardiac output, and the autoregulatory responses of the fetal circulation in response to hypoxic insult. These general physiologic characteristics of pregnancy have the following implications for management of critical illness:

1. Assessment of the adequacy of maternal blood flow must be made with an understanding that baseline flow is substantially increased, with further increases during active labor or with fever, infection, or pain.
2. Diminished placental blood flow represents a threat to fetal well-being and viability, especially if superimposed on maternal anemia, hypoxemia, or both. Maternal hypoxemia can be particularly damaging if it elicits vasodilation of nonplacental beds, as this results in redistribution of blood flow from the fetoplacental unit.
3. The delivery of oxygen to the fetoplacental unit can be optimized by maintaining or restoring adequate circulating volume and cardiac function, giving blood transfusions to increase oxygen carrying capacity, by putting the mother in the left lateral decubitus position to improve maternal cardiac output, and by giving supplemental oxygen to increase maternal oxygenation.
4. Delivery of the fetus may be the best option if gestational age permits. However, since labor represents a tremendous aerobic load for the mother, the team must judge whether labor should be avoided or postponed during periods of critical illness in which oxygen delivery is marginal.
5. One effective way to reduce aerobic requirements in the critically ill gravid patient is to assume the work of breathing in evolving respiratory failure. Thus early elective intubation and mechanical ventilation may be beneficial in selected patients.
6. Fetal monitoring is at present an inexact and evolving science and should be performed in conjunction with the obstetric team. Measurement of fetal heart rate is a useful but nonspecific indicator of well-being and a late sign of inadequate oxygen delivery. It is most accurate after 32 weeks of gestation and is best used as a screening tool. Although continuous transcutaneous P_{O_2} measurement is feasible in the fetus, the results are difficult to interpret, and

TABLE 105-3 Maternal Mortality[a] in the United States, 1991–1999

Cause	Percentage
Embolism	19.6
Hemorrhage	17.2
Hypertensive disease	15.7
Infection	12.6
Cardiomyopathy	8.3
Cerebrovascular accident	5.0
Anesthetic complications	1.6
Other[b]	19.2

[a] Direct maternal deaths.
[b] The majority of the other maedical conditions were cardiovascular, pulmonary, and neurologic problems.
SOURCE: From *MMWR*.[26]

the low baseline value does not provide a wide margin for identifying evolving hypoxia. Fetal acid-base status can be measured by means of scalp blood sampling if membrane rupture and cervical dilation have occurred. A pH less than 7.2 suggests physiologic depression of the fetus.[2] In general, the routinely obtained parameters of oxygen delivery and acid-base status in the mother are the best measures of the adequacy of oxygen delivery for both the fetus and the mother.

Circulatory Disorders of Pregnancy

In pregnancy, circulatory impairment may be life-threatening, given the dependence of the mother and fetus on cardiac output for oxygen delivery. In the next section, common causes of hypoperfusion, such as hemorrhage, cardiac dysfunction, aortic dissection, trauma, and sepsis, are discussed. The pathophysiology and treatment of preeclampsia, which may occur as a result of uteroplacental hypoperfusion, is also explored. Venous thromboembolic disease in the setting of pregnancy is addressed in Chap. 27. Together these disorders account for a significant percentage of maternal deaths related to pregnancy (Table 105-3).[26] Finally, modifications of cardiopulmonary resuscitation algorithms that are necessary in pregnancy are considered.

HYPOPERFUSED STATES

The initial approach to the critically ill hypoperfused gravida is to distinguish between low-flow states caused by inadequate circulating volume, cardiac dysfunction, or trauma, and high-flow states such as septic shock, while taking into account the physiologic alterations associated with pregnancy. Most often the state of perfusion of the critically ill gravid patient can be determined by bedside assessment. Occasionally, the adequacy of intravascular volume remains unclear despite a careful history, physical examination, and review of routine laboratory data. Other patients are encountered who have obvious ventricular failure requiring the use of vasoactive drugs or respiratory failure requiring careful fluid management. In these instances right heart catheterization should be considered (Table 105-4), although a survival benefit from this invasive procedure has not been confirmed in obstetric patients.[27] When this procedure is necessary in a pregnant patient, a subclavian or internal jugular approach should be used. Femoral vein catheterization is relatively

TABLE 105-4 Relative Indications for Right Heart Catheterization

Routine operative or labor/delivery monitoring for:
    Severe pulmonary hypertension
    Significant valvular heart disease
    New York Heart Association class III or IV congestive heart failure
Hypertension or preeclampsia comlicated by:
    Pulmonary edema
    Heart failure
    Oliguric renal failure
Shock, if :
    Etiology is obscure
    Volume resuscitation fails
    Central venous pressure is elevated
    Vasoactive drugs are required
Acute respiratory failure that is:
    Accompanied by shock
    Requires mechanical ventilation and positive end-expiratory
        pressure
    Accompanied by pulmonary edema of unknown etiology

contraindicated because of the obstruction of the vena cava by the uterus and the possible need for emergent delivery. In the healthy pregnant woman, right ventricular, pulmonary artery, and pulmonary capillary wedge pressures are unchanged from prepartum values.[2,10] As discussed above, cardiac output is increased, and SVR and pulmonary vascular resistance are decreased during pregnancy (see Table 105-1). Assessment of left and right ventricular hemodynamics by echocardiography was shown to correlate with pulmonary artery catheter results in a heterogeneous group of critically ill obstetric patients.[28] Thus in centers with sophisticated echocardiography techniques this may provide an alternative to invasive monitoring.

HEMORRHAGIC SHOCK
The common causes of hemorrhagic shock in pregnancy are listed in Table 105-5. When hemorrhage occurs in pregnancy, it can be massive and swift, necessitating immediate intervention. It is the second leading cause of both maternal death and admission to the ICU.[26,29] Antepartum hemorrhage is most often caused by premature separation of the normal placental attachment site (abruptio placentae), disruption of an abnormal placental attachment (placenta previa), and spontaneous uterine rupture.

Abruptio placentae occurs in 1 of every 77 to 250 pregnancies, with an increased incidence in patients with hypertension (half from chronic hypertension, half from preeclampsia), high parity, cigarette smoking, cocaine use, and previous abruption.[30–33] Maternal mortality, usually from postpartum hemorrhage, ranges from 0% to 5.2%, while fetal mortality is higher (between 5% and 36%).[30] The cause of the premature

placental separation is not well understood, but the initiating event may be a rupture of the spiral arterioles with formation of a hematoma, which then separates the placenta from its site of attachment.[31] The severity of maternal blood loss is correlated with the extent and duration of abruption and fetal demise. Blood loss averages 2 to 3 L when abruption results in fetal death, and much of this blood can remain concealed within the uterus.[30] Maternal complications include acute renal failure and disseminated intravascular coagulation (DIC), which occurs in up to 30% of patients with fetal death.[2,30] Patients may initially present with painful vaginal bleeding and be misdiagnosed as having premature labor. The diagnosis is made using a combination of clinical information and ultrasound.

Placenta previa occurs in approximately 1 of 200 pregnancies and only infrequently causes massive hemorrhage because near-universal ultrasound examination during pregnancy leads to identification prior to delivery. Nonetheless, if vaginal examination results in disruption of the placenta over the cervical os, or if trophoblastic tissue invades the myometrium (placenta previa et accreta), the patient is at risk for massive hemorrhage at delivery.[31] Placenta previa is more common in multiparas with prior cesarean delivery and in cigarette smokers.[3,32,34] Fetal mortality is low, but it can be much higher if maternal shock occurs.

Uterine rupture occurs in approximately 1 of 2000 pregnancies.[31] The most common setting in which rupture occurs spontaneously is the multipara with protracted labor. Other risk factors include prior cesarean section, operative (assisted) vaginal delivery, and use of uterotonic agents.[34] In overt rupture, peritoneal signs may be observed. Nonetheless, substantial blood loss can occur in the absence of significant physical findings.

Common causes of postpartum hemorrhage include uterine atony, surgical obstetric trauma, uterine inversion, retained placental tissue, and coagulopathies due to DIC from amniotic fluid embolism, fetal death, and saline solution abortion.[2,3] Uterine atony occurs after prolonged labor, overdistention of the uterus from multiple gestation or hydramnios, abruptio placentae, oxytocin administration, or cesarean section, or as a result of retained intrauterine contents or chorioamnionitis. Hemorrhage from surgical obstetric trauma may be due to cervical or vaginal lacerations or uterine incision for cesarean section.

Management
Patients at increased risk of bleeding should be identified early, so that intravenous access and blood typing can be achieved ahead of time. When massive hemorrhage occurs, the initial management of the patient is similar to that of the nonpregnant patient, and two or three large-bore (16-gauge

TABLE 105-5 Etiology of Hemorrhagic Shock in Pregnancy

Early	Late (Third Trimester)	Postpartum
Trauma	Trauma	Uterine atony
Ectopic or abdominal pregnancy	Placenta previa or abruptio placentae	Surgical trauma
Abortion	Uterine rupture	Uterine inversion
DIC	DIC	DIC
Hydatidiform mole	Marginal sinus rupture	Retained placenta

ABBREVIATION: DIC, disseminated intravascular coagulation.

or larger) venous catheters should be inserted. Immediate volume replacement with crystalloid should be instituted until blood is available, and supplemental oxygen should be administered. It is beneficial to position the patient in the left lateral decubitus position to prevent vena caval obstruction from worsening the reduction in venous return that results from massive hemorrhage. Fetal monitoring is important, as fetal distress in the setting of obstetric hemorrhage indicates hemodynamic compromise.[2]

If shock is not immediately reversed by volume resuscitation or is accompanied by respiratory dysfunction, elective intubation and mechanical ventilation is indicated, since hypoxemia superimposed on a low-flow state is particularly injurious to fetus and mother. Blood replacement with packed red blood cells should begin immediately. Massive obstetric hemorrhage is one setting in which initial resuscitation may require the use of unmatched type-specific blood until more complete cross-matching can be accomplished (see Chap. 68). Because critical illness in pregnancy is frequently associated with DIC, massive bleeding should prompt an evaluation for coagulopathy. If the peripheral blood smear, platelet count, prothrombin time (PT), partial thromboplastin time (PTT), or fibrinogen level suggests excessive factor consumption (DIC), measurement of plasma levels of fibrin degradation products and specific factors should be performed (see Chap. 69). Measurement of factor VIII levels is inexpensive and can be accomplished more quickly than a full DIC screen. Massive blood loss can result in a dilutional coagulopathy with secondary thrombocytopenia which needs to be corrected with appropriate blood product replacement.

Uterine atony is routinely treated with uterine massage, draining the bladder, and intravenous oxytocin.[2,34] Oxytocin can cause hyponatremia by virtue of its antidiuretic effect. Alternatively, prostaglandin analogues such as carboprost tromethamine can be used to improve uterine contraction and decrease bleeding.[2,34] Side effects include hypertension, bronchoconstriction, and intrapulmonary shunt with arterial oxygen desaturation. Ergot preparations such as methyl-ergonovine have been associated with cerebral hemorrhage and are contraindicated if the patient is hypertensive. Ultrasonography is used to diagnose retained intrauterine products of conception that require curettage. Embolization of the hypogastric, internal pudendal, or uterine artery with slowly absorbable gelatin sponge can sometimes control hemorrhage and allow subsequent recanalization of the embolized vessel.[35] Surgical exploration to repair lacerations, ligate arteries, or remove the uterus is necessary in some cases.

CARDIAC DYSFUNCTION

Hypoperfusion from cardiac dysfunction is most often caused by congestive heart failure due to either preexisting myocardial or valvular heart disease, or to a cardiomyopathy arising de novo. However, the prevalence of heart disease during pregnancy is low, but its presence increases the likelihood of maternal and fetal morbidity and mortality. Patients with Eisenmenger syndrome, cyanotic congenital heart disease, or pulmonary hypertension have a high mortality rate (33% to 40%) during pregnancy.[36] A recent study of 599 pregnancies in Canadian women with either congenital or acquired heart disease (40% had valvular heart disease) identified risk factors for adverse outcomes.[37] Pulmonary edema, arrhythmia, stroke, or cardiac death complicated 13% of pregnancies. Pre-

dictors of maternal cardiac complications included prior cardiac events, poor functional class (New York Heart Association class III or IV) or cyanosis, left heart obstruction (aortic or mitral stenosis), and left ventricular systolic dysfunction. Adverse outcomes (<1% mortality) occurred in 27% of those with one risk factor and 62% of those with two or more risk factors. Neonatal complications (2% mortality) occurred in 20% of pregnancies and were associated with poor functional class or cyanosis, left heart obstruction, anticoagulation, smoking, and multiple gestation.

Prior subclinical heart disease may manifest itself for the first time during pregnancy owing to the physiologic changes of pregnancy described earlier. Peripartum cardiomyopathy (1 of every 1300 to 4000 deliveries) first presents in the last month of pregnancy or the first 6 months after parturition.[38] Postulated risk factors include black race, older age, twin gestations, multiparity, anemia, preeclampsia, and postpartum hypertension. Bacterial endocarditis rarely complicates pregnancy, most often occurring in patients with preexisting cardiac abnormalities, although infection of previously normal valves has been reported in pregnancy, particularly in patients with a history of intravenous drug use.[39] Myocardial infarction is extremely uncommon during pregnancy but should be considered in the hypoperfused patient with chest pain. Maternal mortality is high in patients delivering within 2 weeks of infarction.[40] There is an increased incidence of aortic dissection during pregnancy, perhaps related to the increase in shear stress on the aorta from the increased heart rate and stroke volume associated with pregnancy and hormonal factors.[40] Risk factors include hypertension, older age, multiparity, trauma, Marfan syndrome, Ehlers-Danlos syndrome, coarctation of the aorta, and bicuspid aortic valve. Aortic dissection presents most commonly during the third trimester, often as a tearing interscapular pain. Pulse asymmetry or aortic insufficiency may be noted on examination.

Management

It is essential to determine the cause of the underlying cardiac dysfunction and hypoperfusion. The chest radiograph may suggest the diagnosis; mediastinal widening is often noted in patients with aortic dissection. Echocardiography can help determine the volume status and detect valvular abnormalities, myocardial dysfunction, or ischemia. Transesophageal echocardiography and magnetic resonance imaging are the most sensitive and specific tests for detecting aortic dissection, although computed tomography of the chest is often done first given its ready availability.[40] Once the cause of cardiac dysfunction is determined, the initial management of the hypoperfused cardiac patient should focus on volume status, and hypovolemia should be excluded as a cause of the low-flow state. As discussed above (see Table 105-4), right heart catheterization may be helpful in this regard, as well as in the further management of cardiogenic shock. Metabolic disturbances can worsen ventricular function in patients with a cardiomyopathy; therefore hypocalcemia, hypophosphatemia, acidosis, and hypoxemia should be avoided. Vasoactive drugs are reserved for situations in which hypovolemia has been corrected and maternal perfusion remains inadequate. If cardiogenic shock persists despite an adequate preload, dobutamine is the drug of choice. However, it should be reserved for life-threatening conditions because at least in animal models, it reduces placental blood flow.[41] Infusion of dopamine in low doses [2 to 3 μg/(kg · min)] has been advocated to preserve splanchnic and renal perfusion. Its use in pregnancy has been limited, and recent studies demonstrated that it does not benefit critically ill patients with sepsis syndrome.[42] Accordingly, we do not advocate its routine use in the critically ill pregnant patient, but it may be useful in treating oliguria associated with preeclampsia (see below). When cardiogenic shock is complicated by pulmonary edema, parenteral furosemide should be given; right heart catheterization may help to titrate therapy.

When cardiogenic shock persists despite inotropic drug support, afterload reduction with nicardipine should be considered.[43] Intravenous sodium nitroprusside or nitroglycerin are second-line agents and when used the dose and duration of therapy should be minimized, and oral agents such as hydralazine or labetalol should be substituted as soon as possible to avoid nitroprusside toxicity. Angiotensin-converting enzyme inhibitors are absolutely contraindicated during pregnancy, because they have been found to cause fetal growth retardation, oligohydramnios, congenital malformations, and anuric renal failure in human neonates exposed in utero, as well as neonatal death.[44]

The hemodynamic alterations of labor and delivery, superimposed on those of pregnancy, make this an especially dangerous time for women with cardiac disease. The optimal method of delivery is an assisted vaginal delivery in the left lateral decubitus position.[38] Epidural anesthesia will ameliorate tachycardia in response to pain, and its vasodilatory actions may be of benefit in patients with congestive heart failure.[1] Since decreased SVR may lead to further decompensation in patients with aortic stenosis, hypertrophic cardiomyopathy, or pulmonary hypertension, general anesthesia may be preferred in these patients.[1] The current consensus is that cesarean section should be reserved for cases with obstetric complications or fetal distress, although with improved surgical techniques and close hemodynamic monitoring, cesarean sections may be safer than in the past.[1] Invasive monitoring may be required to follow shifts in volume status that occur from the tremendous "autotransfusions" produced by each uterine contraction and the blood loss that occurs with delivery.

TRAUMA

Death from trauma is a leading cause of nonobstetric maternal mortality. During pregnancy, hypoperfusion and shock may occur as a result of injury from motor vehicle accidents, falls, and assaults.[45] The gravid woman is at greater risk of hemorrhage after trauma, as blood flow to the entire pelvis is increased. Some injuries are unique to pregnancy, including amniotic membrane rupture, abruptio placentae, uterine rupture, premature labor, and fetal trauma.[45] In a series of patients with blunt abdominal trauma in late pregnancy, the most serious complications were placental abruption and uterine rupture and preterm labor was the most common.[46] Rapid deceleration injury can cause abruptio placentae (20% to 40% of major injuries) as a result of deformation of the elastic uterus around the less elastic placenta. In most cases, vaginal bleeding will be present when abruption has occurred, although there are reports of occult abruption without vaginal bleeding following traumatic injury.[46] Abruption can be complicated rapidly by DIC; therefore coagulation profiles should be monitored in all severely injured gravid patients.

The cephalad displacement of abdominal contents in pregnancy increases the risk of visceral injury from penetrating trauma of the upper abdomen including splenic rupture. The urinary bladder is a target for injury because it is displaced into the abdominal cavity beyond 12 weeks of gestation.

The physiologic changes of pregnancy may make evaluation and treatment of the gravid trauma patient more difficult. Borderline tachycardia and supine hypotension (from obstruction of the vena cava by the uterus in late pregnancy) may be caused by pregnancy itself and thus may not indicate significant blood loss. Clinical signs of hypovolemia are not observed in trauma victims until intravascular volume is reduced by 15% to 20%. When hypovolemia is clinically evident in gravid patients, it signifies enormous blood loss because of the expanded blood volume associated with pregnancy. Pregnancy may mask findings of peritoneal irritation. In one series of 12 gravid patients undergoing peritoneal lavage for evaluation of blunt abdominal trauma, only 2 of the patients exhibited abnormal abdominal signs or symptoms.[47] Nonetheless, 8 had positive lavage with confirmation of intra-abdominal bleeding or injury at laparotomy.

Blunt trauma rarely causes fetal injuries. Fetal skull fracture occurs most often in the third trimester, when the engaged fetal head is at risk of injury from maternal pelvic fractures.[45] The risk of fetal death depends on the severity of maternal injury and hemodynamic compromise and on the extent of injury to the fetus.[2] Maternal shock, pelvic fractures, severe head injury, and hypoxemia all increase the risk of fetal demise.

Management

Initially, maternal cardiopulmonary function and the extent of injury should be assessed. If required, emergent intubation should be performed by a skilled individual because of the increased risk of aspiration during pregnancy. Since maternal shock is a major cause of fetal demise, ensuring the adequacy of the maternal circulation is paramount. If significant hemorrhage is obvious, aggressive fluid replacement, as discussed above for hemorrhagic shock, is appropriate. Once the cervical spine is cleared, the patient should be placed in the left lateral position. Pelvic examination should be performed, provided there is no overt vaginal bleeding, to look for blood, urine, and amniotic fluid. Nitrazine paper can identify amniotic fluid and confirm rupture of the amniotic membranes. The diagnosis of pelvic or abdominal injury can usually be made by ultrasonography, computed tomography, or lavage.[47–49] Because needle paracentesis is difficult to perform in the second and third trimesters, open peritoneal lavage is advised for assessing severe blunt abdominal trauma and confirming that intraperitoneal fluid noted on imaging studies is hemorrhagic. Once the mother is stabilized, cardiotocographic monitoring, including Doppler measurement of fetal cardiac activity and measurement of uterine activity, should be performed for 4 hours after the injury. When used in trauma patients who are beyond the twentieth week of pregnancy, cardiotocographic monitoring can identify placental abruption, fetal distress, and uterine contractions.[45] Fetomaternal hemorrhage—that is, blood loss from the fetal to the maternal circulation—may be identified by the Kleihauer-Betke test, which identifies fetal hemoglobin in red blood cells. Rh sensitization of Rh-negative patients, neonatal anemia, fetal cardiac arrhythmias, and fetal exsanguination are potential complications of fetomaternal hemorrhage.[45] Maternal Rh sensitization can be prevented by administration of $Rh_O(D)$ immune globulin.

If maternal death occurs despite aggressive resuscitation and the fetus is alive and undelivered, a postmortem cesarean section should be considered. A review of over 150 cases revealed that the outcome was significantly related to the length of time between maternal death and delivery and to the gestational age of the fetus.[50]

SEPTIC SHOCK

Sepsis is another important cause of hypoperfusion in pregnancy, accounting for 13% of maternal deaths in the United States in the 1990s.[26] The diagnosis of sepsis in the febrile gravid patient can be obscured by the normal hemodynamic changes of pregnancy (i.e., increased cardiac output and decreased SVR). An awareness of the usual settings and patients at risk for sepsis will increase the chance of recognizing this life-threatening state. Animal data suggest pregnancy may cause increased vulnerability to the systemic effects of bacteremia and endotoxemia.[51] In addition, pregnant patients have an increased susceptibility to infection with *Listeria monocytogenes* and disseminated herpesvirus, varicella, and coccidioidomycosis infections, perhaps owing to a decreased cell-mediated immune response during pregnancy.[2]

The common causes of sepsis in pregnancy include septic abortions, antepartum pyelonephritis, chorioamnionitis, and postpartum infections (puerperal sepsis) (Table 105-6).[52] Septic abortion is more often seen in countries where access to abortion is limited. Chorioamnionitis or intra-amniotic infection complicates up to 1% of all pregnancies. It occurs most commonly after prolonged rupture of membranes or prolonged labor, or after invasive procedures such as amniocentesis or cervical cerclage, but occasionally it reflects hematogenous spread from maternal bacteremia.[53] Patients present with fever, tachycardia (both maternal and fetal), uterine tenderness, and foul-smelling amniotic fluid.

Sepsis in obstetric patients usually occurs postpartum. Clinical settings that increase the risk of postpartum sepsis include cesarean section, prolonged rupture of membranes, and prior instrumentation of the genitourinary tract.[52,54] Infection usually occurs at the placental site, resulting in endometritis. Patients with endometritis may present with fever, abdominal pain and tenderness, and purulent lochia. Episiotomy sites and cesarean section incisions are less common sources of postpartum infection. Rarely, life-threatening wound infection with group A streptococci results in necrotizing fasciitis, while *Clostridium* species may cause gas gangrene of the uterus.[2,52] The bacteria that must be considered include *Staphylococcus aureus* and *S. epidermidis*; groups A, B, and D streptococci; *Escherichia coli*; *Proteus mirabilis*; *Enterobacter* spp.; *Klebsiella* spp.; *Pseudomonas* spp.; anaerobic streptococci and *Bacteroides* spp.; and *Clostridium perfringens* (Table 105-7).[52] Rarely, toxic streptococcal syndrome may occur as a result of infection with pyrogenic exotoxin A–producing group A streptococci in patients with necrotizing fasciitis or may unexpectedly follow an uncomplicated pregnancy and delivery.[2] Patients present with an influenza-like prodrome and gastrointestinal symptoms followed by shock and multiple organ system dysfunction. If a patient deteriorates while receiving appropriate antibiotic therapy, surgical exploration with possible hysterectomy are indicated.[2]

The hemodynamic profile in septic shock is similar to that of the nonpregnant septic patient.[54] In a study by Lee and colleagues of 10 obstetric patients with septic shock, right heart catheterization of the 8 surviving patients revealed a high cardiac index and heart rate with a low blood pressure and a decreased systemic vascular resistance index (SVRI). Analysis of left ventricular function curves revealed that 50% of the patients had evidence of myocardial depression despite an increased cardiac index. The greatest improvement in SVRI occurred in the eight surviving women; their initial SVRI was 885 ± 253 dyne $\cdot$ s/(cm$^5 \cdot$ m^2), and it rose to 1672 ± 413 dyne $\cdot$ s/(cm$^5 \cdot$ m^2) following resolution of their hyperdynamic state. It is important to remember that pregnancy itself results in a 25% decrease in vascular resistance from the prepregnancy level of 900 to 1500 dyne $\cdot$ s/cm^5, a decrease in blood pressure, and a 20% increase in heart rate. Thus three useful signs of sepsis—tachycardia, hypotension, and low systemic vascular resistance—must be interpreted with caution in the gravid patient, particularly in the third trimester. However, a rapid

---

TABLE 105-6 Bacterial Infections Associated with Sepsis in Pregnancy and after Parturition

Obstetric
   Postpartum endometritis
   Chorioamnionitis (intra-amniotic infection)
   Septic abortion
   Septic pelvic thrombophlebitis
   Antepartum pyelonephritis
Nonobstetric
   Appendicitis
   Cholecystitis
   Pyelonephritis
   Pneumonia
Invasive procedures
   Abdominal wall or perineal incisions (necrotizing fasciitis)
   Amniocentesis/chorionic villus sampling (septic abortion)
   Infected cerclage (chorioamnionitis)

SOURCE: Reproduced with permission from Fein et al.[52]

TABLE 105-7 Pathogens Responsible for Severe Sepsis in Obstetric Patients

Gram-negative rods
   E. coli
   Klebsiella-Enterobacter spp.
   Proteus spp.
   Serratia spp.
   Pseudomonas spp.
   Haemophilus influenzae
Anerobes
   Clostridium perfringens
   Fusobacterium spp.
   Bacteroides spp.
   Peptostreptococcus
Gram-positive cocci
   Streptococci, groups A, B, and D
   Pneumococcus
   Staphylococcus

NOTE: Infectious but nonbacterial pathogens (viruses, fungi, and mycoplasma) seem to be rare for extrapulmonary infections.
SOURCE: Reproduced with permission from Fein et al.[52]

change in hemodynamic parameters suggests infection. Complications of sepsis in pregnancy include pulmonary capillary leakage with subsequent acute respiratory distress syndrome (ARDS) and DIC.[54]

Management

The septic gravid patient requires thorough culturing and evaluation of pelvic sites. Empiric antibiotic therapy, designed to cover what is typically a polymicrobial infection involving gram-positive, gram-negative, and anaerobic organisms, as discussed above, should be given until specific bacteriologic cultures are available. Reasonable regimens to cover the above organisms should include at least two antibiotics such as clindamycin and a third-generation cephalosporin; in certain patients it is necessary to expand the initial regimen to include a semisynthetic penicillin, an aminoglycoside, or another broad-spectrum agent.[52] If possible, however, it is best to avoid aminoglycosides in patients with sepsis antepartum, because these agents can be ototoxic and nephrotoxic to the fetus. Chorioamnionitis associated with sepsis is unlikely to respond to antibiotic therapy alone, and delivery of the fetus is required.[2] Postpartum deterioration in septic patients receiving adequate antibiotic coverage suggests a localized abscess, a resistant organism, or septic pelvic thrombophlebitis.[2] Surgical drainage of appropriate pelvic and abdominal sources, with possible hysterectomy, may be required, particularly in patients with myometrial microabscesses or gas gangrene from clostridial species. Computed tomography or magnetic resonance imaging of the pelvis may help in the diagnosis of septic pelvic thrombophlebitis, which is treated with antibiotics and anticoagulation.[2] Venous ligation or surgical excision is sometimes required.

Patients who have evidence of adequate tissue perfusion and oxygen delivery may not require fluid or vasoactive drugs for the treatment of tachycardia and moderate hypotension. Lactic acidosis or end-organ dysfunction is an indication for volume resuscitation, but given the risk of precipitating low-pressure pulmonary edema, right heart catheterization may be helpful to allow titration of volume therapy. Mechanical ventilatory support should be instituted if needed. If hypoperfusion persists despite volume replacement, the use of vasoactive agents such as dobutamine to increase forward flow may be of value in patients who have markedly abnormal ventricular performance. Since there are no clear benefits from inotropic agents in patients with high-flow states whose cardiac function is near normal, these drugs should be withdrawn if adverse effects are noted. Elevated temperature should be controlled with acetaminophen and a cooling blanket, because fever is detrimental to the fetus. The role that vasopressin might play in the pregnant patient with septic shock remains undefined, but institution of an infusion at 40 mU/h is reasonable in the patient with refractory shock.

Naloxone has not proven useful in septic shock, and recent trials of immunotherapeutic agents directed against bacterial antigens or exotoxins have to date not added to the armamentarium available to treat these patients.[55] As in the nonpregnant septic patient, corticosteroids should be given if adrenal insufficiency is documented.[56] The corticotropin stimulation test may be difficult to interpret in the pregnant woman because baseline cortisol may be elevated in pregnancy and stimulation tests have not been studied in this population.

Recombinant protein C has not been systematically evaluated in pregnant patients and it is impossible to make informed commentary on its risk/benefit profile in this setting. At present, the essentials of treatment are early appropriate antibiotics, surgical treatment if necessary, and meticulous supportive care.

PREECLAMPSIA

Preeclampsia is a unique disorder of pregnancy that complicates 5% to 10% of all pregnancies, accounting for a substantial proportion of obstetric ICU admissions (38% in a recent series in the United States) and 10% to 15% of maternal deaths.[3,26,57] It occurs most often in nulliparous women after the twentieth week of gestation, typically near term, and may even occur postpartum. It is characterized by hypertension, proteinuria, and generalized edema; however, these features may be mild and may not occur simultaneously, making the diagnosis of early disease difficult in some cases. Hyperuricemia is also present in almost all cases of preeclampsia and may be useful in differentiating preeclampsia from both preexisting chronic hypertension and gestational hypertension.[44] Multiple other organ systems may be involved, as discussed below. Risk factors for the development of preeclampsia, besides the primigravid state, include both preexisting and gestational hypertension, maternal or paternal family history of preeclampsia, preexisting renal disease, diabetes mellitus, multiple gestation, hydatidiform mole, and antiphospholipid antibody syndrome.[2,58] Preeclampsia may progress to a convulsive and potentially lethal phase, termed *eclampsia*, without warning. Eclampsia occurs in more than 0.2% of all deliveries, with an incidence of 1.5% in twin deliveries.[59] An especially fulminant complication of preeclampsia is the HELLP syndrome (*h*emolysis, *e*levated *l*iver enzymes, and *l*ow *p*latelets), which occurred in 0.3% of deliveries in one large clinical series.[60] Maternal and fetal morbidity and mortality are significant if eclampsia or the HELLP syndrome develops or if preeclampsia develops prior to 34 weeks of gestation.[44] In one large study of women with eclampsia, perinatal mortality was 8.6%, with placental abruption accounting for four of the six perinatal deaths; there were no maternal deaths.[59] In a recent review of women with HELLP syndrome, perinatal mortality was 12.6%.[60] While there were no maternal deaths, life-threatening complications such as placental abruption often with associated DIC, pulmonary edema, and ARDS, cerebral hemorrhage, and hepatic hematoma occurred in 10.3% of patients.

Although the exact etiology of preeclampsia is unknown, nearly all maternal organ systems are affected. The common pathologic feature is vascular endothelial damage that may be due to mediator release as a result of placental ischemia.[61] Maternal vascular endothelial dysfunction results in increased loss of fluid from the intravascular compartment, increased sensitivity to pressor agents and activation of the coagulation cascade.[62] Increased endothelin production and decreased release of nitric oxide may also be important in the development of this disorder.[63] The reduction in placental perfusion and increased circulating concentrations of markers of endothelial activation and intravascular coagulation occurs before the onset of clinical disease.[9,62] Cardiac output and plasma volume are reduced in preeclampsia, while SVR is increased.[44] In one study, right heart catheterization of 44 untreated preeclamptic patients revealed low normal right atrial and pulmonary capillary wedge pressures (Ppw), a reduced cardiac output, and a markedly elevated systemic vascular resistance.[9] A study of 41 preeclamptic patients found that the majority of the patients had a normal Ppw, normal to high cardiac index, and upper normal to moderately elevated SVR compared to historical controls.[64] The eight patients with pulmonary edema had a high wedge pressure.

Preeclampsia may be mild or severe. Markers of disease severity that should alert the physician to an increased risk of complications include systolic or diastolic blood pressures of ≥160 and ≥110 mm Hg, respectively (especially after 24 hours of hospitalization), proteinuria ≥2 g in 24 hours or ≥100 mg/dL in a random specimen, oliguria, or pulmonary edema.[2,9] Especially worrisome symptoms and signs in any patient with preeclampsia include headache, blurred vision, scotomata, altered consciousness, clonus, epigastric or right upper quadrant pain, increasing serum creatinine level, consumptive coagulopathy with thrombocytopenia and/or microangiopathic hemolytic anemia, and even mildly elevated values on liver function tests.[2,9]

Maternal complications of severe preeclampsia include seizures (eclampsia); cerebral hemorrhage or edema; renal dysfunction; pulmonary edema; placental abruption with DIC; the HELLP syndrome; and hepatic infarction, failure, subcapsular hemorrhage, or rupture.[44,65] The etiology of eclamptic seizures is presumed to be related to cerebral vasospasm, ischemia, or edema and hypertensive encephalopathy.[2] Although the risks of eclampsia are higher when the above markers of disease severity are present, in one large clinical series 20% of eclamptic patients had a blood pressure below 90 mm Hg or no proteinuria prior to experiencing convulsions.[44] Though it is rare, cerebral edema is a cause of death in patients with preeclampsia. It may result from severe hypertension and large volumes of fluid administered to treat the oliguria and decreased plasma oncotic pressure frequently noted in preeclampsia.[66] Renal dysfunction may result from intravascular volume depletion, renal ischemia, and glomerular disease characterized by swollen glomerular endothelial cells known as glomeruloendotheliosis.[20,67] Acute renal failure is rare and most often is seen in patients with the HELLP syndrome, placental abruption, massive hemorrhage, or coagulopathy.[2] Pulmonary edema is uncommon, having an incidence of 2.9% in patients with severe preeclampsia.[68] Contributing factors include increased left ventricular afterload, myocardial dysfunction, decreased colloid osmotic pressure, vigorous fluid therapy, and in some cases increased capillary permeability.[2] It most commonly occurs after parturition. In a subgroup of patients, antepartum pulmonary edema develops.[69] These patients are typically obese and chronically hypertensive with secondary left ventricular hypertrophy. The increased intravascular volume of pregnancy and the hemodynamic derangements of preeclampsia cause diastolic dysfunction with an elevated Ppw and pulmonary edema.

The HELLP syndrome is characterized by multiorgan dysfunction arising from an endothelial abnormality with secondary fibrin deposition and organ hypoperfusion.[2] A microangiopathic hemolytic anemia and consumptive coagulopathy develop. When DIC occurs, it is often in the setting of placental abruption, sepsis, or fetal demise.[2] The liver involvement is characterized by periportal or focal parenchymal necrosis with elevated liver function tests. Intrahepatic hemorrhage or subcapsular hematoma occurs in 2% of patients and may progress to hepatic rupture.[60,65]

The HELLP syndrome occurs in 4% to 20% of patients with preeclampsia.[61] There is an increased incidence in white women and in one series 45% of the patients were multiparous.[2,60] Patients are more often preterm than those with uncomplicated eclampsia. In up to 30% of patients, the HELLP syndrome develops after parturition; typically it appears within 48 hours, but it has been reported up to 7 days postpartum. Presenting symptoms are usually nonspecific, the most common being malaise, epigastric or right upper quadrant pain, nausea, vomiting, and edema. Patients less frequently present with jaundice, gastrointestinal bleeding, or hematuria. Signs and symptoms of preeclampsia may be mild or absent upon initial presentation. Complications include acute renal failure, ARDS, hemorrhage, hypoglycemia, hyponatremia, and nephrogenic diabetes insipidus. Fetal growth restriction and prematurity are the major causes of perinatal morbidity and mortality. Maternal mortality ranges from 0% to 24%, with higher perinatal mortality (8% to 60%).

Laboratory values that suggest the diagnosis include:[61] (1) hemolysis demonstrated by an abnormal peripheral smear; (2) increased levels of bilirubin (≥1.2 mg/dL) or lactate dehydrogenase (≥600 U/L); (3) increased liver enzyme levels with an elevated serum level of glutamic oxaloacetic transaminase (≥70 U/L); and (4) thrombocytopenia with a platelet count of <100,000/μL. Isolated thrombocytopenia that progresses may be one of the first clues to the diagnosis.

Management

The principles of management of preeclampsia include early diagnosis, close medical observation, and timely delivery. Delivery is curative in most cases. The differential diagnosis of preeclampsia includes thrombotic thrombocytopenic purpura (TTP), hemolytic uremic syndrome (HUS), acute fatty liver of pregnancy, and idiopathic postpartum renal failure (Table 105-8) (see Chap. 70). Once the diagnosis is made, further management is based on an evaluation of the mother and fetus. Mild preeclampsia may be managed on an outpatient basis if hypertension is mild, the fetus is doing well, and compliance is good.[44] The patient will require close monitoring, since this condition can worsen suddenly. The presence of symptoms and proteinuria increases the risk of placental abruption and eclampsia. These patients and those with disease progression should be hospitalized and observed closely. In patients who have mild preeclampsia at term and have a favorable cervix, labor should be induced. There is no consensus regarding the utility of bed rest, antihypertensive therapy, or anticonvulsant prophylaxis in this group of patients. Based on a number of clinical trials, there is no clear benefit to antihypertensive drug treatment in women with mild gestational hypertension or preeclampsia.[44]

Because severe eclampsia can progress rapidly, delivery is recommended in these patients. Immediate delivery is appropriate when there are signs of impending eclampsia, multiorgan involvement, or fetal distress, and in patients who are more than 34 weeks pregnant.[44] Early in gestation, conservative management with close monitoring to improve neonatal survival and morbidity may be appropriate in selected cases at tertiary perinatal centers. The objective of antihypertensive

TABLE 105-8 Differential Diagnosis of Characteristic Features of Preeclampsia and Its Complications

Feature	Pregnancy-Specific	Nonspecific
Hypertension	Preeclampsia	Essential hypertension
	Preeclampsia superimposed on chronic hypertension	Secondary hypertension (renal, pheochromocytoma)
	Transient hypertension	
Thrombocytopenia	Preeclampsia	TTP
	HELLP syndrome	ITP
	Acute fatty liver of pregnancy	Sepsis
Elevated liver enzymes	Preeclampsia	Viral hepatitis
	HELLP syndrome	Drug-induced hepatitis
	Acute fatty liver of pregnancy	
	Cholestasis of pregnancy	
Renal dysfunction	Preeclampsia	Sepsis
	Acute fatty liver of pregnancy	Hypovolemia/hemorrhage
	Idiopathic postpartum renal failure	TTP/HUS
Pulmonary edema	Preeclampsia	Valvular heart disease
	Peripartum cardiomyopathy	Ischemic heart disease
	Tocolytic pulmonary edema	ARDS
	Amniotic fluid embolism	

ABBREVIATIONS: ARDS, acute respiratory distress syndrome; HELLP, hemolysis, elevated liver enzymes, low platelets; HUS, hemolytic uremic syndrome; ITP, idiopathic thrombocytopenic purpura; TTP, thrombotic thrombocytopenic purpura.
SOURCE: Reproduced with permission from Lapinsky et al.[2]

therapy is to prevent cerebral complications such as encephalopathy and hemorrhage. A sustained diastolic blood pressure of 110 mm Hg or greater should be treated to keep the mean arterial pressure between 105 and 126 mm Hg and the diastolic pressure between 90 and 105 mm Hg. While hydralazine 5 mg IV every 20 minutes to a total dose of 20 mg has been the traditional treatment, blood pressure control in the ICU setting is best obtained with either intravenous labetalol or nicardipine.[43] A loading dose of labetalol 20 mg is recommended, followed by either repeated incremental doses of 20 to 80 mg at 10- to 15-minute intervals or an infusion starting at 1 to 2 mg/min and titrated up until the target blood pressure is achieved.[43] Since calcium channel blockers may be potentiated by magnesium infusion, care should be taken to avoid hypotension when the two medications are used together.[3] Acute nicardipine infusion can induce severe maternal tachycardia.[70] (Table 105-9). *Nitroprusside is relatively contraindicated, and angiotensin-converting enzyme inhibitors are absolutely contraindicated, in pregnancy.* Diuretics should be used with caution, as they may aggravate the reduction in intravascular volume that is often seen in preeclampsia. Volume expansion may decrease SVR and improve oliguria; however, the increased risk of pulmonary or cerebral edema makes fluid administration difficult without a right heart catheter in place.[3,71] Antihypertensive therapy has no effect on the progression of disease and does not prevent complications such as HELLP.

Magnesium sulfate prophylaxis has been shown to be better than placebo, phenytoin, or nimodipine in the prevention of eclampsia.[72–74] In a recent large study, magnesium sulfate was superior to both phenytoin and diazepam for the treatment and prevention of recurrent convulsions in women with eclampsia.[75] Magnesium sulfate should be given to all women with either preeclampsia or eclampsia and for a minimum of 24 hours postpartum. Aspirin has no role in the treatment of preeclampsia.

The preeclamptic patient with oliguria may benefit from judicious volume loading and low-dose dopamine therapy.[76] Invasive monitoring is recommended to prevent pulmonary and cerebral edema. Pulmonary edema is managed conventionally. Patients with delayed postpartum resolution of the HELLP syndrome with persistent thrombocytopenia, hemolysis, or organ dysfunction may benefit from plasmapheresis with fresh frozen plasma.[2,77] Many of these patients may actually have TTP or HUS, which can be difficult to distinguish from the HELLP syndrome. In two studies, administration of corticosteroids resulted in improved maternal platelet counts and liver function test results and in a trend toward better

TABLE 105-9 Drugs Used in the Management of Acute Hypertensive Crises in Pregnancy

Drug	Regimen
Nicardipine	5 mg/h increasing the infusion rate by 2.5 mg/h every 5 min (to a maximum of 15 mg/h)
Hydralazine	Initial dose: 5 mg IV bolus; then 5–10 mg every 20–30 min; side effects include tachycardia and headache
Labetalol	Small IV boluses, initially 20-mg, followed by 20 mg to 80 mg, given every 10–20 min until blood pressure is controlled or total dose is 300 mg; can use continuous infusion of 1–2 mg/min titrated up until blood pressure is controlled.
Diazoxide	For use in refractory patients; given in 30-mg miniboluses every 5 min
Sodium nitroprusside	May be used in standard doses [initially 0.25 μg/(kg. min)] for a short period (30 min) in acute crises; potential for fetal cyanide toxicity.

SOURCE: Reproduced with permission from Lapinsky et al[2] and Varon et al.[43]

fetal outcome.[78] No significant effect in delaying delivery was noted. Management of intrahepatic hemorrhage with subcapsular hematoma includes administration of blood products, delivery, and control of liver hemorrhage.[65] Embolization of the hepatic artery is often successful, but evacuation of the hematoma and packing of the liver may be required.

CARDIOPULMONARY RESUSCITATION

Pregnancy can interfere with the performance of adequate cardiopulmonary resuscitation (CPR). If cardiopulmonary arrest occurs, the physiologic changes of pregnancy must be taken into account when performing CPR, including the increased metabolic rate and cardiac output and decreased oxygen reserve typical of the pregnant patient. The gravid uterus may impede venous return and distal arterial perfusion by compressing the inferior vena cava and aorta. In late pregnancy, the gravid uterus acts like an abdominal binder; the resulting elevation of intrathoracic pressure may limit the ability to create forward flow during CPR.

These considerations have prompted some pregnancy-specific modifications of the usual approach to CPR.[79,80] The key modification is that the pregnant patient should receive standard CPR while in the left lateral decubitus position to decrease aortocaval compression by the uterus. That can be accomplished by using a table that provides a lateral tilt, by placing a wedge under the patient's right hip, or by manually displacing the uterus to the left.[2] Otherwise, standard resuscitative measures using currently approved protocols should be followed. Defibrillation (after removal of fetal monitoring devices to prevent arcing) and pharmacologic therapy should be employed as clinically indicated.

If standard closed-chest CPR cannot generate a pulse, especially in late pregnancy, open-chest massage and emergency cesarean section should be considered. In one case report, the mother could not be resuscitated until the fetus was delivered; both subsequently survived.[81] To facilitate this plan, obstetric, internal medicine, and anesthesiology staff need to be apprised early of any acute deterioration in the circulation of a critically ill gravida. Delivery within 4 to 5 minutes of the arrest will improve the chance of a good outcome for both mother and fetus.[79]

Respiratory Disorders of Pregnancy

During pregnancy, ventilatory failure may occur as a result of a chronic lung disease such as cystic fibrosis or asthma and may require mechanical ventilation. A more common cause of respiratory compromise in pregnant women is acute hypoxemic respiratory failure related to amniotic or venous air embolism, tocolytic-induced pulmonary edema, aspiration, or pneumonia. This section focuses on the management of both ventilatory and hypoxemic respiratory failure in the gravid patient.[82]

VENTILATORY FAILURE

With improved medical care, patients with chronic lung diseases such as cystic fibrosis are surviving to childbearing age, presenting new management problems for the intensivist. Asthma, however, remains the most common pulmonary problem encountered in pregnancy, affecting 1% to 4% of all gravidas. When these conditions require mechanical support,

ventilator management necessitates careful attention to the special needs of mother and fetus.

MECHANICAL VENTILATION

If ventilatory failure is imminent, intubation and mechanical ventilation should be performed electively. The indications for intubation and mechanical ventilation are not significantly changed by pregnancy, although the normal P_{CO_2} of 27 to 32 mm Hg during pregnancy should be considered when deciding on mechanical ventilation.[3] Several difficulties in airway management should be anticipated in the critically ill pregnant patient (Table 105-10). Pharyngeal, laryngeal, and vocal cord edema are common, and the highly vascular upper airway may bleed from even minor intubation-related trauma.[83] Relatively small endotracheal tubes (6- to 7-mm diameter) may be necessary, and nasotracheal intubation is best avoided because of this upper airway narrowing.[2] There may be an increased risk of aspiration during pregnancy because of delayed gastric emptying, increased intra-abdominal pressure from compression by the gravid uterus, and diminished competence of the gastroesophageal sphincter.[84] Use of cricoid pressure to minimize the risk of pulmonary aspiration is recommended. Approximately 40% of maternal deaths associated with general anesthesia in England and Wales from 1976 to 1978 were related to difficulties with endotracheal intubation.[85] Control of the airway should be achieved in an early and elective fashion by a skilled individual. Noninvasive mask ventilation for acute respiratory failure has not been studied in pregnancy. In the awake patient needing temporary ventilatory assistance, noninvasive positive pressure ventilation is a reasonable first step. Theoretical limitations to this therapy include pregnancy-related upper airway edema and increased risk of aspiration.

The initial ventilator settings should be aimed at achieving eucapnia, which in this patient population is a P_{CO_2} of 28 to 35 mm Hg. Respiratory alkalosis should be avoided, since studies in animal models suggest that hyperventilation can reduce fetal oxygenation and decrease uteroplacental flow.[2,86] Alkalosis can usually be avoided with tidal volumes in the range of 10 mL/kg and respiratory rates of 15 to 18 breaths per minute (bpm). In the asthmatic patient (see below), the use of a lower tidal volume and respiratory rate minimizes the adverse effects of intrinsic positive end-expiratory pressure (PEEP) (see Chap. 38).

The patient with acute pulmonary edema (see below) should be ventilated with a small tidal volume (4 to 6 mL/kg) and a high respiratory rate (24 to 30 bpm).[87] While recent studies of nonpregnant adults managed with mechanical ventilation for ARDS have shown improved survival when low (~6 mL/kg) tidal volumes were used—even if this was associated with hypercapnia—the safety of this permissive hypercapnia in pregnancy remains to be determined. In one animal model, acute hypercapnia during mechanical ventilation was associated with fetal distress. During any mechanical ventilatory period, continuous fetal monitoring should be conducted, usually accomplished by heart tone determination,

TABLE 105-10 Problems with Airway Management in Pregnancy

Upper airway edema
Diminished airway caliber
Propensity for hemorrhage
Increased risk of aspiration

and if acute ventilatory changes are associated with any evidence of challenge to the fetus, they should be avoided. It is important to note that pregnancy, particularly in the third trimester, can result in significant chest wall stiffness resulting from the gravid uterus, and high airway pressures may not signal lung stiffness or overdistension per se. Taken together, these observations would suggest an approach to acute hypoxemic respiratory failure in pregnancy that would begin with careful fetal monitoring, instituting low tidal volumes, avoiding acute rises in partial arterial pressure of carbon dioxide (Pa_{CO_2}) and increasing tidal volume if they occur in association with fetal distress, and allowing plateau airway pressures to be somewhat higher than the 30 cm H_2O often recommended for individuals without such abdominal distension.

When a diffuse lung lesion is present and toxic levels of oxygen would be needed, sufficient PEEP should be imposed to correct arterial hypoxemia at a nontoxic fraction of inspired oxygen (Fi_{O_2} <0.6). In the pregnant patient, we aim to keep the Pa_{O_2} >90 mm Hg, a value higher than that used in the nonpregnant patient, to prevent fetal distress. To minimize the decrease in venous return that occurs with positive pressure ventilation, it is important that the pregnant patient be managed in a lateral position whenever possible. Measures to avoid atelectasis in the ventilated gravid patient include PEEP, sighs, and alternating the position between left lateral and right lateral.

In patients with severe lung lesions requiring toxic concentrations of oxygen and high levels of PEEP, and in patients with hemodynamic instability, muscle relaxation and sedation will decrease oxygen consumption and assist in stabilization. Nondepolarizing neuromuscular blocking agents including cisatracurium, pancuronium, vecuronium, and atracurium, produce no adverse fetal effects with short-term use.[2] Of these, cisatracurium is preferred because it does not depend on renal or hepatic function for elimination. Benzodiazepines may increase the risk of cleft palate and other major birth defects when used early in pregnancy, although this has not been conclusively demonstrated. If enzodiazepines are necessary for sedation, the lowest dose and shortest duration of use are recommended. Propofol, pregnancy category B hypnotic agent (see Chap. 14), may be considered, however no data exist on its use in the first or second trimesters in humans. Narcotic analgesics such as morphine sulfate and fentanyl may be used safely during pregnancy. These agents all cross the placenta; therefore if given near the time of delivery, immediate intubation of the neonate may be required.

Fetal viability can be maintained throughout pregnancy with mechanical ventilation, even when maternal death occurs. Mechanical ventilation is most appropriate when instituted early in the course of progressive ventilatory failure, to stabilize mother and fetus and then permit identification of reversible factors to allow either safe withdrawal of mechanical support or controlled delivery. These complex decisions are best made in collaboration with the critical care physician, obstetrician, and neonatologist.

CHRONIC LUNG DISEASE
Most chronic pulmonary diseases that can result in ventilatory failure, such as cystic fibrosis, kyphoscoliosis, neuromuscular diseases, pulmonary fibrosis, and chronic obstructive pulmonary disease (COPD), are uncommon in pregnant women. Despite the increased ventilatory demands that oc-

cur in pregnancy, ventilatory failure is rare. In one study, several women with a preconception vital capacity of 40% to 70% predicted due to lung resection or collapse for tuberculosis, carried their pregnancy to term and had few respiratory symptoms.[88] Although several authorities suggest that a vital capacity of at least 1 L is essential for a safe and successful pregnancy,[89] one patient has been reported to have completed pregnancy with a vital capacity of only 0.8 L (25% of predicted) and a P_{CO_2} of 45 mm Hg.[90] Thus severe reduction in lung volume to a level that would represent impairment of ventilatory function in a nonpregnant individual does not in itself preclude a successful conception and pregnancy.

Patients with severe restrictive lung disease and progressive ventilatory insufficiency during pregnancy may benefit from nocturnal positive pressure ventilation and oxygen administration. One patient with severe kyphoscoliosis and a forced vital capacity of 580 mL, a P_{O_2} of 59 mm Hg, and a P_{CO_2} of 52 mm Hg at 25 to 28 weeks of gestation avoided mechanical ventilation by using nocturnal positive pressure ventilation with a tight-fitting mask during weeks 28 to 30 of pregnancy, until delivery could be accomplished by cesarean section.[91] This approach may be applicable to other pregnant patients with chronic ventilatory impairment. Pulse oximetry should be used to screen patients with marginal ventilatory function for nocturnal hypoxemia.

ASTHMA
The course of asthma during pregnancy is variable: In approximately 35% of pregnant asthmatic women the asthma does not change; in 36% it improves; and in 28% it worsens.[92] Patients with more severe asthma are more likely to experience worsening of their asthma during pregnancy. Asthma typically worsens during the second and third trimester with improvement during the last month of pregnancy. Adverse maternal outcomes in pregnant women with asthma have been noted including preterm labor, pregnancy-induced hypertension and preeclampsia, chorioamnionitis, and cesarean delivery. Adverse fetal outcomes include preterm birth and infants small for gestational age.[93] Treatment of the gravid patient with asthma by a specialist reduces the likelihood of preterm birth, low birth weight infants, and perinatal mortality, suggesting that control of asthma and prevention of acute exacerbations are crucial to a good outcome.[94,95]

Management
The management of the pregnant patient with status asthmaticus is similar to that of the nonpregnant patient, with a few exceptions.[2] Even the usually mild hypoxemia seen in asthma should be treated aggressively in the gravid patient because it is detrimental to the fetus. Oxygenation therefore should be assessed even in mild attacks. Since the baseline P_{CO_2} is decreased in pregnancy and probably falls further with an acute asthma attack, an arterial blood gas determination that shows a P_{CO_2} of >35 mm Hg during status asthmaticus should alert the clinician to impending ventilatory failure. However, experience with nonpregnant patients with status asthmaticus and mild hypercapnia has suggested that many can be managed without mechanical ventilatory support.

Most drugs used to treat asthma are considered safe for use during pregnancy.[94,95] Inhaled bronchodilators are standard therapy. A study of inhaled β-agonists in 259 pregnancies (most subjects used metaproterenol) noted no difference in the incidence of congenital malformations, premature births, low birth weight, poor Apgar scores, or perinatal mortality when compared with asthmatic subjects not using inhaled bronchodilators.[96] Use of parenteral β-agonists is generally limited to situations in which inhaled agents have been ineffective, since epinephrine causes vasoconstriction of the uteroplacental circulation in animal studies, and there is one report of an increased incidence of congenital malformations in humans who used this drug in the first trimester, and terbutaline may inhibit labor and cause pulmonary edema if given near term.[3] Inhaled corticosteroids have been shown to decrease the incidence of asthma attacks and hospital readmissions in studies of pregnant women with asthma.[87] Budesonide is the inhaled corticosteroid of choice with triamcinolone being absolutely contraindicated due to cleft palate formation in rabbits. Oral corticosteroids have been associated with a twofold increase in the incidence of preeclampsia, and in one study an increased risk of cleft palate (0.4% absolute incidence). Systemic corticosteroids remain recommended therapy for the treatment of acute asthma exacerbations and patients with severe asthma.[97] Although there is a risk of causing fetal adrenal insufficiency, this is a rare occurrence. Heliox, a low-density mixture of helium and oxygen, may decrease the work of breathing and preclude intubation and mechanical ventilation when given to subjects in status asthmaticus (see Chap. 40). Despite isolated reports of congenital cardiovascular anomalies in infants born to asthmatic women taking theophylline, it has an extensive safety record in pregnancy, with the only fetal risk being neonatal theophylline toxicity when the drug is given at the time of delivery.[3] Pregnancy decreases theophylline clearance in the third trimester, so dose adjustment may be necessary.[83]

ACUTE HYPOXEMIC RESPIRATORY FAILURE

Pregnancy creates an increased susceptibility to acute hypoxemic respiratory failure caused by a variety of disorders, including those that result in pulmonary edema, such as amniotic fluid embolism, β-adrenergic tocolytic therapy, and aspiration (Table 105-11). Other causes of hypoxemic respiratory failure include venous air embolism and respiratory infections.

AMNIOTIC FLUID EMBOLISM

Amniotic fluid embolism occurs in 1 of every 8000 to 80,000 pregnancies, and is estimated to account for over 10% of peripartum maternal deaths.[98] The mortality rate is very high (80% to 90%) with many of the deaths occurring within 1 hour of the onset of symptoms.[98,99]

The two most important risk factors are advanced maternal age (mean = 32 years) and multiparity. Other, less well established risk factors include amniotomy, cesarean section, insertion of intrauterine fetal or pressure monitoring devices, and term pregnancy in the presence of an intrauterine device. The use of uterine stimulants, tumultuous labor, excessive fetal size, and intrauterine fetal death have not been substantiated as important risk factors.[83] It is important to note that while most cases occur during labor and delivery, amniotic fluid embolism may be associated with uterine manipulation during first- and second-trimester abortions or trauma and has been reported to occur spontaneously at 20 weeks of gestation.[100]

The classic presentation of amniotic fluid embolism, seen in more than 50% of cases, is the abrupt onset of severe dyspnea, tachypnea, and cyanosis during labor or soon after delivery, frequently in association with cardiovascular collapse, hypoxemia, and seizures.[100] Shock and bleeding each are the initial presentation in 10% to 15% of cases. Bleeding secondary to DIC occurs in up to 50% of patients who survive the first 30 to 60 minutes. Most of the remaining patients will have evidence of DIC on laboratory tests. Amniotic fluid embolism is frequently complicated by pulmonary edema; it was found in 70% of the cases on chest radiograph.[100]

TABLE 105-11 Differential Diagnosis of Acute Respiratory Distress in Pregnancy

Disorder	Distinguishing Features	Chest Radiograph
Venous thromboembolism	Evidence of DVT, pleuritic chest pain, positive V/Q scan, leg Dopplers, angiogram	Normal/atelectasis/effusion
Amniotic fluid embolism	Hemodynamic collapse, seizures, DIC	Normal/pulmonary edema
Pulmonary edema secondary to preeclampsia	Hypertension, proteinuria	Pulmonary edema
Tocolytic pulmonary edema	Tocolytic adminstration, rapid improvement	Pulmonary edema
Aspiration pneumonitis	Vomiting, reflux, fever	Focal infiltrate/pulmonary edema
Peripartum cardiomyopathy	Gradual onset, cardiac gallop	Cardiomegaly, pulmonary edema
Pneumomediastinum	Occurs during delivery, subcutaneous emphysema	Pneumomediastinum, subcutaneous air
Air embolism	Profound hypotension, cardiac murmur	Normal/pulmonary edema
Other: asthma, pneumonia, cardiac disease, ARDS	AS for nonpregnant patient	As for nonpregnant patient

ABBREVIATIONS: ARDS, acute respiratory distress syndrome; DIC, disseminated intravascular coagulatoin; DVT, deep venous thrombosis, V/Q, ventilation-perfusion.
SOURCE: Reproduced with permission from Lapinsky et al.[2]

The mechanisms of respiratory and circulatory failure in amniotic fluid embolism remain controversial. Amniotic fluid and particulate matter (lanugo hairs, meconium, fat, or fetal squames) may enter the maternal venous circulation via endocervical veins or uterine tears or at the placental site itself.[11] In some animal studies, filtered amniotic fluid has been found to be relatively innocuous in less than massive amounts. This finding suggests that cellular and other debris present in the fluid embolism may either mechanically obstruct the maternal pulmonary vasculature, leading to the development of pulmonary hypertension, or trigger a maternal systemic reaction. Others believe that vasoconstrictor arachidonic acid metabolites present in the amniotic fluid itself may elicit pulmonary hypertension.[83] Circulatory failure has been ascribed to various pathophysiologic processes, and these may vary over time. Initially, acute right heart strain from acute pulmonary hypertension may occur. Acute elevation of pulmonary artery and central venous pressures with subsequent hypotension have been observed in animal models of amniotic fluid embolism.[100] Elevation of Ppw, minimal increase in the pulmonary vascular resistance, and depressed left ventricular performance have been observed in human patients with amniotic fluid embolism, suggesting that left ventricular dysfunction contributes to circulatory collapse.[99] In addition, a component of pulmonary capillary leakage must exist, as severe pulmonary edema occurs at a Ppw <19 mm Hg.[99]

Management

The treatment of patients with amniotic fluid embolism and cardiovascular collapse is supportive and is aimed at ensuring adequate oxygenation, stabilizing the circulation, and controlling bleeding. The initial management should include intubation, administration of 100% oxygen, and mechanical ventilation with a small tidal volume (4 to 6 mL/kg) and rapid rate (24 bpm). Early sedation and muscle relaxation may allow complete rest of the respiratory muscles and confer hemodynamic stability. PEEP is then added to achieve a Pa_{O_2} of >90 mm Hg at an FI_{O_2} <0.6. Pulmonary artery catheterization allows measurement of the cardiac output and Ppw, which can be used to guide hemodynamic adjustments aimed at minimizing Ppw (to reduce vascular leak) while providing an adequate cardiac output. Pulmonary arterial blood can be examined cytologically for evidence of abnormal amniotic fluid components—fetal squamous cells, lanugo hairs, etc. However, demonstration of these amniotic fluid elements in the maternal pulmonary circulation is not sufficient to make this diagnosis, since small numbers of fetal squamous cells have been observed in patients without clinical evidence of amniotic fluid embolism.[82] Vasoactive drugs are frequently necessary to reverse hypotension. Once DIC is established, factor replacement and heparin therapy, which are controversial, should be undertaken only in conjunction with a hematology consultant.[30] Intravenous corticosteroid therapy has been reported to be of benefit in limited case reports.[101]

TOCOLYTIC THERAPY

Pulmonary edema associated with β-adrenergic agents given to inhibit preterm labor is seen in as many as 4.4% of patients receiving these drugs.[102] Most of the reported cases have resulted from use of intravenous β-mimetics such as ri-

todrine, terbutaline, isoxuprine, and salbutamol. There is an increased incidence in women with multiple gestations, concurrent infection, and those receiving corticosteroid therapy.[3] Most women have intact membranes at the time of presentation. Pulmonary edema typically develops during tocolytic therapy or within 24 hours after the discontinuation of these drugs. When pulmonary edema develops postpartum, the vast majority of cases are encountered within 12 hours of delivery.[102]

The pathogenesis of this disorder remains unknown. Pulmonary edema has never been associated with similarly high doses of β-adrenergic agonists during the treatment of asthma. Therefore, some alteration related to pregnancy may predispose women to this complication. Left ventricular function was normal in those patients assessed with echocardiography and invasive monitoring.[102] The observation that Ppw is normal in most patients who have pulmonary artery catheters placed has led to speculation that these drugs or occult infection produce a pulmonary capillary leak.[3,102] Several facts suggest that increased circulatory volume may also play a major role: (1) large volumes of crystalloid are often given in response to the reflex tachycardia resulting from sympathomimetic drugs; (2) the intravascular volume expansion and reduced colloid oncotic pressure characteristic of pregnancy increase susceptibility to hydrostatic edema; (3) sodium and water excretion may be impaired in the supine pregnant patient; (4) tocolytic agents may increase arginine vasopressin secretion and thus impair water balance; and (5) the response to diuresis is prompt in these patients.[102]

Most patients complain of chest discomfort and dyspnea, manifest tachypnea, have tachycardia with crackles on lung auscultation, and have pulmonary edema on chest radiography (Table 105-12). A positive fluid balance is often noted in the hours to days preceding the onset of symptoms. In the largest collected series, the mean arterial P_{O_2} when breathing room air was 50.4 ± 2.9 mm Hg with a P_{CO_2} of 28.1 ± 2.1 mm Hg.[102] The history and clinical findings should help in distinguishing this disorder from acute thromboembolic disease, acid aspiration, and amniotic fluid embolism.

Management

The course of this disease is usually benign, and invasive hemodynamic monitoring is usually not required. In a large series there were only two maternal deaths (3%); fetal survival was 95%.[102] Treatment should consist of discontinuation of tocolytic therapy, oxygen administration, and diuresis. Response is usually rapid, with resolution of tachypnea and hypoxemia often occurring within hours.

ASPIRATION

Aspiration is an uncommon but well-described and ominous complication of the peripartum period.[84] Factors that increase the risk of aspiration in the pregnant woman

---

TABLE 105-12 Features of Tocolytic-Induced Pulmonary Edema

Most common cause of pulmonary edema in pregnancy
Associated with β-adrenergic agonist use
Dyspnea, tachypnea, and crackles are typical
Occurs <24 hours after tocolytic agents are stopped
Responds promptly to oxygen and diuretics

include the increased intragastric pressure that results from external compression by the enlarged uterus, relaxation of the lower esophageal sphincter due to progesterone, delayed gastric emptying during labor, and depressed mental status and vocal cord closure from analgesia. Injury due to aspiration of gastric contents is related to the volume of aspirated material, its acidity, the presence of particulate material, the bacterial burden of the aspirated material, and host resistance to subsequent infection. The early injury is a chemical pneumonitis, the severity of which is determined primarily by the acidity and volume of the aspirate. Diffuse lung injury with the development of ARDS may occur early in the course. A late complication of aspiration is the evolution to bacterial pneumonia, which tends to be focal and polymicrobial and occurs 24 to 72 hours after the event.

Management

Prevention of this dread complication should be the primary goal of all physicians assessing and managing the patient's airway. Once aspiration has occurred, treatment is supportive and is similar to that for the nonpregnant individual, as discussed elsewhere in this text (see Chap. 51). Antibiotics should be given only if bacterial pneumonia develops.

VENOUS AIR EMBOLISM

Although a rare occurrence, venous air embolism may account for 1% of all maternal deaths.[103] It occurs during normal labor, delivery of women with placenta previa, criminal abortions using air, orogenital sex, and insufflation of the vagina during gynecologic procedures.[103] Air is thought to enter subplacental venous sinuses, then to embolize through the venous circulation, and finally to obstruct pulmonary blood flow when it reaches the right ventricle. Two other mechanisms may be important in the pathophysiology of this disorder—the obstruction of pulmonary arterioles by fibrin microemboli and the recruitment and activation of polymorphonuclear leukocytes by aggregated proteins; both the fibrin microemboli and the aggregated proteins would be produced by the turbulent air-blood interface. Symptoms include cough, dyspnea, dizziness, tachypnea, tachycardia, and diaphoresis. Sudden hypotension is usually followed by respiratory arrest. A mill wheel murmur or bubbling sound is occasionally heard over the precordium. Right heart strain, ischemia, and arrhythmias have been noted on the electrocardiogram. Patients who survive the initial cardiopulmonary collapse may develop noncardiogenic pulmonary edema.

Management

When venous air embolism is suspected, the patient should be placed immediately in the left lateral decubitus position to direct the air embolus away from the right ventricular outflow tract. The patient should be ventilated with 100% oxygen in an effort to decrease the size of the embolus by removing nitrogen.[103] Hyperbaric therapy has been an effective way to treat air embolism in diving medicine. Anticoagulation with heparin to treat fibrin microemboli and administration of high-dose corticosteroids to decrease pulmonary edema formation have been proposed, but their usefulness in this disorder remains untested.[103]

TABLE 105-13 Bacteriology of Pneumonia in Pregnancy (in Decreasing Order of Frequency)

Pneumococcus
Haemophilus influenzae
No pathogen identified (common finding in most studies)
"Atypical pneumonia" agents
   Legionella species
   Mycoplasma pneumoniae
   Chlamydia pneumoniae (TWAR agent)
Viral agents
   Influenza A virus
   Varicella zoster virus
Aspiration
Fungi

SOURCE: Reproduced with permission from Rodrigues et al.[104]

RESPIRATORY INFECTIONS

The incidence of pneumonia in pregnancy may be increasing, reflecting a decline in the general health of a segment of the population of childbearing women and infection with human immunodeficiency virus (HIV).[104] In a large retrospective review of pneumonia during pregnancy, pneumonia complicated 1 out of every 1287 deliveries.[105] The incidence may be even higher in urban areas, with one study reporting pneumonia in 1 of every 367 deliveries at a large city hospital. Obstetric complications included preterm labor in 44% and preterm delivery in 36% in one large study of pneumonia during pregnancy.[105] In addition, 20% of the cases had respiratory failure requiring mechanical ventilation; maternal mortality was 4%, while fetal mortality was 12%. Underlying maternal disease, such as the acquired immunodeficiency syndrome (AIDS) and cystic fibrosis, were associated with maternal medical complications and preterm delivery. The spectrum of organisms that causes bacterial pneumonia is similar to that in the nonpregnant population (Table 105-13).[83,104] An increased incidence of influenza pneumonia was noted among pregnant patients during the 1918–1919 and 1957–1958 influenza pandemics. Autopsy reports noted the cause of death as respiratory insufficiency from fulminant influenza pneumonia rather than from secondary bacterial infection as is usually the case in the nonpregnant population.[103] However, pregnancy has not been demonstrated to be a risk factor for severe influenza infection except during those pandemic years. Primary infection with varicella zoster virus progresses to pneumonia more often in adults than in children. Some investigators have noted an increased rate of progression to pneumonia and an increased mortality in pregnant patients, but the validity of this claim has not been proved conclusively. Coccidioidomycosis is the fungal infection most commonly associated with increased risk of dissemination during pregnancy, especially if it is contracted in the third trimester or immediately postpartum.[104] The decreased cell-mediated immunity thought to occur during pregnancy may predispose the pregnant patient to disseminated varicella and coccidioidomycosis. Infection with *Mycobacterium tuberculosis* during pregnancy occurs. Whether pregnancy adversely influences the course of active tuberculosis is a matter of debate.[106] It is clear that with appropriate chemotherapy, the prognosis for pregnant women with tuberculosis is excellent. There is no evidence for increased activation of quiescent disease during pregnancy. In vivo studies suggest that pregnancy does not affect the response to tuberculin skin testing, and this test can be performed safely during pregnancy.[106] Maternal and fetal mortality from advanced tuberculosis was high in the era before effective chemotherapy. At present, the outcome for mother and child is excellent except in rare cases of congenital or neonatal tuberculosis.

HIV infection in the pregnant patient is complicated by the risk of perinatal transmission to the fetus, preterm delivery, and opportunistic infection, especially pneumonia.[107] Testing for HIV infection and antiretroviral therapy to prevent vertical transmission are currently the standard of care in the pregnant patient. *Pneumocystis carinii* pneumonia (PCP) may complicate pregnancy and may be especially virulent in this setting. It is the most common cause of AIDS-related death in pregnant women in the United States, with respiratory failure requiring mechanical ventilation occurring in 59% of patients and with a mortality rate of 50%.[108] Fetal mortality is also high and appears to be worse if PCP occurs during the first or second trimester. The clinical presentation is not altered by pregnancy.

Management

The choice of antibacterial agents to treat pneumonia during pregnancy should take account of potential fetal toxicity. The penicillins, cephalosporins, and erythromycin (except for the estolate, which increases the risk of cholestatic jaundice in pregnancy) are considered safe.[103,104] Tetracycline and chloramphenicol are contraindicated, and sulfa-containing regimens should be avoided near term except for the treatment of PCP, as discussed below.[83,104] Amantadine has been shown to be teratogenic at very high but not at lower doses in animals; its use has not been studied in pregnant women.[103] Favorable results have been obtained using acyclovir to treat pregnant women with varicella pneumonia.[83] No teratogenic effects have been noted in animal studies of acyclovir.[103] It is important to initiate therapy with acyclovir early to affect outcome favorably. Thus acyclovir should be started at the first sign of respiratory system involvement in pregnant patients with cutaneous varicella infection.[103] Amphotericin B should be used to treat disseminated coccidioidal infections in pregnancy. Fluconazole and likely other azole antifungals are teratogenic and best avoided.[109] No adverse effects on the fetus have been reported for amphotericin. Active tuberculosis during pregnancy should be treated with isoniazid, rifampin, and ethambutol plus pyridoxine until drug susceptibility testing is complete.[110] All three of these medications cross the placenta, but none has been shown to have teratogenic effects. In patients with sensitive organisms, isoniazid and rifampin should be continued for 9 months. Although pyrazinamide is recommended for routine use in pregnant women by the World Health Organization, in which case the treatment duration is shortened to 6 months, the drug has not been routinely used in the United States due to lack of data regarding safety. Streptomycin is the only antituberculosis drug with documented harmful effects on the human fetus and it should not be used during pregnancy.[110] PCP should be treated with trimethoprim-sulfamethoxazole.[104] Treatment with trimethoprim-sulfamethoxazole, compared with other therapies, may result in improved outcome.[108] Corticosteroids are added if clinically indicated as for the nonpregnant patient.[104]

Other Disorders of Pregnancy

ACUTE RENAL FAILURE

The incidence of acute renal failure associated with pregnancy is between 0.02 and 0.05%.[20] The differential diagnosis of acute renal failure in pregnancy can be found in Table 105-14.[2] As discussed above, acute renal failure may complicate preeclampsia, the HELLP syndrome, and acute fatty liver of pregnancy. Acute tubular necrosis may occur from hemorrhage or sepsis. Acute cortical necrosis is associated with placental abruption, septic abortion, prolonged intrauterine retention of a dead fetus, hemorrhage, and amniotic fluid embolism.[20] Acute oliguric renal failure necessitating dialysis typically results. Arteriography may demonstrate loss of the cortical circulation, and renal biopsy can confirm the diagnosis. While renal function often improves, end-stage renal failure is the eventual outcome.[20] Idiopathic postpartum acute renal failure is an unusual complication of pregnancy and may occur days to weeks after a normal pregnancy and delivery.[20] The etiology is unknown. The disorder may be a variant of HUS or TTP, since it is clinically and pathologically similar to these entities although without hemolysis or thrombocytopenia, and many patients respond to treatment with prednisone administration and plasmapheresis.[2] In general, the treatment of acute renal failure in pregnancy is similar to that in the nonpregnant patient, with supportive care and dialysis as necessary. Renal dysfunction associated with preeclampsia and the HELLP syndrome should respond to delivery of the fetus, while TTP and HUS require plasmapheresis with fresh frozen plasma.[77]

ACUTE LIVER FAILURE

Acute liver failure is an uncommon complication of pregnancy.[65] The differential diagnosis and characteristics of liver diseases in pregnancy can be found in Table 105-15.[78] In pregnancy, de novo liver function test abnormalities are

---

TABLE 105-14 Differential Diagnosis of Acute Renal Failure in Pregnancy and the Postpartum Period

Prerenal
  Hemorrhage
  Hyperemesis gravidarum
Renal
  Acute tubular necrosis (secondary to sepsis, hemorrhage, placental abruption, intrauterine fetal death, etc)
  Bilateral renal cortical necrosis (secondary to abruption, hemorrhage, preeclampsia, septic abortion, etc)
  Preeclampsia
  HELLP syndrome
  Acute fatty liver of pregnancy
  HUS/TTP
  Idiopathic postpartum renal failure
  Acute glomerulonephritis (e.g., lupus flare precipitated by pregnancy)
Postrenal
  Gravid uterus
  Nephrolithiasis

ABBREVIATIONS: HELLP, hemolysis, elevated liver enzymes, low platelets; HUS, hemolytic uremic syndrome; TTP, thrombotic thrombocytopenic purpura.
SOURCE: Reproduced with permission from Lapinsky et al.[2]

TABLE 105-15 Characteristics of Liver Diseases in Pregnancy

Disease	Symptoms	Jaundice	Trimester	Incidence in Pregnancy	Laboratory Values[a]	Adverse Effects
Hyperemesis gravidarum	Nausea, vomiting	Mild	1 or 2	0.3%–1.0%	Bilirubin <4 mg/dL, ALT <200 U/L	Low birth weight
Intrahepatic cholestasis of pregnancy	Pruritus	In 20%–60%, 1–4 weeks after pruritus starts	2 or 3	0.1%–0.2% in U.S.	Bilirubin <6 mg/dL, ALT <300 U/L, increased bile acids	Stillbirth, prematurity, bleeding, fetal mortality 3.5%
Biliary tract disease	Right upper quadrant pain, nausea, vomiting, fever	With CBD obstruction	Any	Unknown	If CBD stone, increased bilirubin and GGT	Unknown
Drug-induced hepatitis	None, or nausea, vomiting, pruritus	Early (in cholestatic hepatitis)	Any	Unknown	Variable	Unknown
Acute fatty liver of pregnancy	Upper abdominal pain, nausea, vomiting, confusion late in disease	Common	3	0.008%	ALT <500 U/L, low glucose, DIC in >75%, increased bilirubin and ammonia late in disease	Increased maternal mortality (≤20%) and fetal mortality (13%–18%)
Preeclampsia and eclampsia	Upper abdominal pain, edema, hypertension, mental status changes	Late, 5%–14%	2 or 3	5%–10%	ALT <500 U/L (unless infarction), proteinuria, DIC in 7%	Increased maternal mortality (~1%)
HELLP syndrome	Upper abdominal pain, nausea, vomiting, malaise	Late, 5%–14%	3	0.1% (4%–12% of women with preeclampsia)	ALT <500 U/L, platelets <100,000/μL, hemolysis, increased LDH, DIC in 20%–40%	Increased maternal mortality (1%–3%) and fetal mortality (35%)
Viral hepatitis	Nausea, vomiting, fever	Common	Any	Same as in general population	ALT greatly increased (>500 U/L), increased bilirubin, DIC rare	Maternal mortality increased with hepatitis E

ABBREVIATIONS: ALT, alanine aminotransferase; CBD, common bile duct; DIC, disseminated intravascular coagulation; GGT, γ-glutamyl transferase; HELLP, hemolysis, elevated liver enzymes, and low platelets; LDH, lactate dehydrogenase.
SOURCE: Reproduced with permission from Knox et al.[78]

uncommon and occur in less than 5% of pregnancies in the United States.[65] Serum alkaline phosphatase increases during the first 7 months of pregnancy peaking at two to four times normal at term. As discussed above, serum albumin concentrations decrease in pregnancy. Levels of serum aminotransferases and bilirubin are unchanged in normal pregnancy.

Liver failure rarely complicates preeclampsia and the HELLP syndrome; subcapsular hematoma and rupture are more common complications, as discussed above. Acute fatty liver of pregnancy is estimated to occur in 1 of 13,000 deliveries.[65] Risk factors include male fetus, multiple gestations, and a first pregnancy. Mean onset is at 36 weeks' gestation, although the disorder can be seen as early as 26 weeks and postpartum. Patients present with nonspecific symptoms such as headache, nausea and vomiting (70%), right upper quadrant or epigastric pain (50% to 80%), malaise, and anorexia.[78] The onset of acute fatty liver of pregnancy may be similar to the onset of preeclampsia, with peripheral edema, hypertension, and proteinuria. Jaundice may follow 1 to

2 weeks later. Cholestasis with mild-to-moderate elevations in serum aminotransferases are the rule. Ultrasound may show increased echogenicity. Computed tomographic abdominal scans are more sensitive and may demonstrate decreased attenuation, although this imaging exposes the fetus to significant radiation. Liver biopsy is sometimes necessary to make the diagnosis but must be undertaken with caution because these patients often have a coagulopathy. The biopsy is characterized by microvesicular fatty infiltration detected only on frozen sections.[65] Acute fatty liver of pregnancy progresses to fulminant hepatic failure complicated by encephalopathy, renal failure, pancreatitis, hemorrhage, DIC, seizures, coma, and death.[78] Because deterioration may occur rapidly, expectant management is generally not advised. The treatment is delivery of the fetus. Jaundice, liver dysfunction, and DIC may worsen for a few days after delivery but then should improve. Maternal and fetal mortality has improved with early delivery and is less than 20%. Full maternal recovery is to be expected. Because long-chain 3-hydroxyacyl-coenzyme

dehydrogenase deficiency in the fetus has been reported to be associated with acute fatty liver of pregnancy in seven of ten women in a recent study, infants may have hypoglycemia, hypotonia, acute or chronic skeletal and cardiac muscle dysfunction, and sudden infant death syndrome.

Maintenance of the Internal Environment

While early mortality can be reduced in the critically ill gravid patient by the therapies outlined above, malnutrition, nosocomial infection, and gastrointestinal hemorrhage often complicate a prolonged ICU stay and account for much of the later morbidity and mortality. Several of these issues are discussed below with the aim of establishing the best milieu for recovery from critical illness.

ACID-BASE STATUS

As previously discussed, pregnancy results in a compensated respiratory alkalosis in which P_{CO_2} and bicarbonate concentration average 30 mm Hg and 18 to 20 mEq/L, respectively. During labor this respiratory alkalosis worsens because of maternal hyperventilation. Nonetheless, current evidence suggests that the resulting alkalemia is not clinically relevant. In one study, fetal oxygen delivery was not impaired when mothers hyperventilated in labor, as fetal P_{O_2} decreased by only 4 mm Hg despite significant increases in maternal and fetal plasma pH.[111] Fetal compensation may result from the facts that the alkalosis-induced leftward shift of the fetal hemoglobin saturation curve may preserve fetal oxygen-carrying capacity and that carbon dioxide diffuses rapidly across the placenta, allowing quick reestablishment of acid-base homeostasis. Unlike spontaneous hyperventilation, however, respiratory alkalosis from excessive mechanical ventilation can cause fetal asphyxia in animal models as a result of decreased uteroplacental blood flow.[86] Furthermore, maternal metabolic alkalosis has been shown in animal models to significantly decrease placental blood flow and fetal carotid P_{O_2}.[112] Since severe respiratory and metabolic alkaloses in the critically ill are often a result of medical treatment—excessive mechanical ventilation, nasogastric suction, diuretic use, and corticosteroid administration—close monitoring of maternal acid-base status should allow prevention or early correction of the alkalosis.

Acidosis may be detrimental to the fetus and should be avoided. Decreased ventilation, with elevation of P_{CO_2} even to prepregnancy levels, will result in respiratory acidosis. Early intubation and mechanical ventilation are indicated in gravidas before hypercapnia and severe respiratory acidosis develop.

Maternal metabolic acidosis occurs in normal labor and delivery, presumably as a result of hyperventilation and other muscle activity.[113] Lactic acid is produced, and these maternal fixed acids pass rapidly to the fetus. In early labor, fetal pH averages 7.30 and P_{CO_2} averages 45 mm Hg, with a fall in pH to 7.20 immediately after delivery.[114] The pH falls owing to a metabolic acidosis, which resolves over the first 60 minutes of neonatal life. When a maternal metabolic acidosis develops as a result of illness, treatment should be directed at the underlying process after it is determined whether the anion gap is normal or increased. The use of bicarbonate to correct

pH is controversial for both pregnant and nonpregnant patients, as is discussed in Chap. 77. When bicarbonate is given, serum carbon dioxide levels rise, and carbon dioxide diffuses rapidly across the placenta. The rise in fetal bicarbonate levels is slower, because this charged species equilibrates more slowly across the placenta. Thus infused bicarbonate may increase acidosis intracellularly or in fetal tissue beds. For this reason, if correction of an underlying acidosis or delivery are likely to be achieved within hours, treatment with bicarbonate is not recommended. Controlled mechanical ventilation to correct metabolic acidosis is indicated when the patient cannot generate sufficient respiratory compensation or the work of breathing will further aggravate the acidosis. This measure should make it possible to provide enough ventilation to minimize acidosis.

PREVENTION OF GASTROINTESTINAL HEMORRHAGE

Pregnancy is not known to result in abnormal gastric acid secretion or to increase the vulnerability of the upper gastrointestinal mucosa to ulceration, but critical illness is often complicated by gastric erosion and severe bleeding. A number of interventions are currently used as prophylaxis against this common complication.

Antacids and sucralfate act by mixing with and neutralizing the gastric contents or by directly coating the gastric mucosa. Because the enlarging uterus may divide the stomach into antral and fundal pouches, complete mixing of gastric contents is unlikely.[115] Therefore these agents may fail to provide prophylaxis against gastric ulceration. Histamine-receptor blockers such as cimetidine and ranitidine are category B medications, as are the proton pump inhibitors, and are the medications of choice in pregnant critically ill patients to reduce the risk of gastrointestinal hemorrhage.

NUTRITION

Total parenteral nutrition (TPN) has been used in pregnant patients for extended periods for disorders such as inflammatory bowel disease, esophageal stricture, and malignancy. Its use in acute malnutrition associated with critical illness is less well described.[116] Animal studies find that the mother is favored over the fetus during starvation, and in human beings maternal body stores are maintained at the expense of fetal growth during semistarvation.[3] For these reasons, aggressive and early nutritional support should be instituted. Patients who have not resumed normal oral intake within 3 days of the onset of critical illness should receive nutritional support. The gut should be used if possible, and feedings given as a bolus by nasogastric tube or as infusions by a soft duodenal feeding tube. Caloric requirements during pregnancy are close to 40 kcal/(kg/d). Sepsis, trauma, burns, and recent surgery are likely to increase this requirement. If severe liver disease is not present, it is recommended that 1.5 g/(kg/d) of protein be given and that approximately 20% of calories be provided as lipids. A variety of enteral feeding supplements can meet these goals at tolerable infusion rates. Finally, electrolyte disorders are common in these patients, and careful attention must be paid to serum calcium, phosphate, and magnesium levels, with additional supplements given as necessary.

TABLE 105-16 Safety of Drugs Used in the ICU, according to the FDA Classification of Drug Safety in Pregnancy

Categories A and B	Category C	Categories D and X
Acyclovir	Albuterol	ACE inhibitors
Amphotericin	Atracurium	Acetylsalicylic acid
Cephalosporins	Atropine	Aminoglycosides
Cimetidine	Bretylium	Benzodiazepines
Clindamycin	β-Blockers	Midozolam
Erythromycin	Bupivacaine	Phenytoin
Glycopyrrolate	Dantrolene	Tetracyclines
Insulin	Digoxin	Warfarin
Lidocaine	Haloperidol	
Magnesium sulfate	Inotropes	
Meperidine	Flumazenil	
Methyldopa	Fluconazole	
Metronidazole	Furosemide	
Naloxone	Heparin	
Penicillins	Hydralazine	
Propofol	Labetalol	
Ranitidine	Meperidine	
Terbutaline	Nifedipine	
	Nitroglycerine	
	Nitroprusside	
	Pancuronium	
	Prednisone	
	Procainamide	
	Suxamethonium	
	Thiopental	
	Vecuronium	
	Vancomycin	

NOTE: Column 1 (categories A and B) represents drugs for which no fetal risk has been demonstrated in human and/or animal studies in the first trimester. Column 2 (category C) represents drugs for which animal studies have demonstrated adverse effects, or for which inadequate data exists. These may be used for clear indications where the benefit justifies the potential risks. Column 3 (categories D and X) represents drugs for which evidence of human fetal risks exist. Category D drugs may be used in exceptional circumstances for serious diseases where the expected benefit outweighs the risks.

Classification of some drugs differs in different reference. The physician should weigh the available evidence, or lack thereof, before using any drug in a pregnant woman. This table serves only as a general guide to the method of classification of drug safety in pregnancy.

SOURCE: From Lapinsky et al.[2]

ABBREVIATION: ACE, angiotensin-converting enzyme.

Patients who do not tolerate enteral feeding will require TPN. The same guidelines for total calories and for the distribution of calories among lipids, carbohydrates, and protein can be used. There is a theoretical concern that the use of intravenous fat emulsions in pregnancy could result in placental infarction due to fat emboli.[117] However, this complication has not been reported and fat emulsions are used in our institution.

FDA DRUG CLASSIFICATION

Since pregnant patients being treated for critical illness may require multiple pharmacologic interventions, intensivists in the United States should be aware of the Food and Drug Administration use-in-pregnancy ratings. Commonly prescribed medications in the intensive care unit are listed in Table 105-16. Category A drugs are those that have undergone adequate controlled studies in pregnant women and have not demonstrated a risk to the fetus. Category B drugs

are those with no evidence of fetal risk in human beings (if animal studies demonstrate risk, human findings do not, or if human studies are inadequate, animal findings are negative). Category C agents are those in which risk cannot be ruled out (human studies are lacking, and animal studies are either positive for fetal risk or lacking; still, potential benefits may outweigh risk). Category D includes agents with positive evidence of fetal risk by virtue of investigational or postmarketing human data (still, in critical illness potential benefits may outweigh risks). Category X includes drugs contraindicated in pregnancy.

References

1. Sullivan JM, Ramanathan KB: Management of medical problems in pregnancy—Severe cardiac disease. *N Engl J Med* 313:304, 1985.
2. Lapinsky SE, Kruczynski K, Slutsky AS: Critical care in the pregnant patient. *Am J Respir Crit Care Med* 152:427, 1995.
3. Rizk NW, Kalassian KG, Gilligan T, Druzin MI, Daniel DL: Obstetric complications in pulmonary and critical care medicine. *Chest* 110:791, 1996.
4. Capeless EL, Clapp JF: Cardiovascular changes in early phase of pregnancy. *Am J Obstet Gynecol* 161:1449, 1989.
5. Mabie WC, DiSessa TG, Crocker LG, et al: A longitudinal study of cardiac output in normal human pregnancy. *Am J Obstet Gynecol* 170:849, 1994.
6. Mesa A, Jessurun C, Hernandez A, et al: Left ventricular diastolic function in normal human pregnancy. *Circulation* 99:511, 1999.
7. Robson SC, Hunter S, Boys RJ, et al: Serial study of factors influencing changes in cardiac output during human pregnancy. *Am J Physiol* 256:H1060, 1989.
8. Robson SC, Dunlop W, Boys RJ, et al: Cardiac output during labor. *Br Med J* 295:1169, 1987.
9. Barron WM, Murphy MB, Lindheimer MD: Management of hypertension during pregnancy, in Laragh JH, Brenner BM (eds): *Hypertension: Pathophysiology, Diagnosis, and Management*. New York, Raven, 1990, p 1.
10. Clark SL, Cotton DB, Lee W, et al: Central hemodynamic assessment of normal term pregnancy. *Am J Obstet Gynecol* 161:1439, 1989.
11. Weinberger SE, Weiss ST, Cohen WR, et al: State of the art: Pregnancy and the lung. *Am Rev Respir Dis* 121:559, 1980.
12. Pernoll ML, Metcalfe J, Schlenker TL, et al: Oxygen consumption at rest and during exercise in pregnancy. *Respir Physiol* 25:285, 1975.
13. Gemzell CA, Robbe H, Stern B, Ström G: Observations on circulatory changes and muscular work in normal labour. *Acta Obstet Gynecol Scand* 36:75, 1957.
14. Rees GB, Pipkin FB, Symonds EM, et al: A longitudinal study of respiratory changes in normal human pregnancy with cross-sectional data on subjects with pregnancy-induced hypertension. *Am J Obstet Gynecol* 162:826, 1990.
15. Cugell DW, Frank NR, Gaensler EA, et al: Pulmonary function in pregnancy. I. Serial observations in normal women. *Am Rev Tuberc* 67:568, 1953.
16. Awe RJ, Nicotra MB, Newsom TD, et al: Arterial oxygenation and alveolar-arterial gradients in term pregnancy. *Obstet Gynecol* 53:182, 1979.
17. Craig DB, Toole MA: Airway closure in pregnancy. *Can Anaesth Soc J* 22:665, 1975.
18. Elkus R, Popovich J: Respiratory physiology in pregnancy. *Clin Chest Med* 13:555, 1992.
19. Baldwin GR, Moorthi DS, Whelton JA, et al: New lung functions and pregnancy. *Am J Obstet Gynecol* 127:235, 1977.

20. Dafnis E, Sabatini S: The effect of pregnancy on renal function: Physiology and pathophysiology. *Am J Med Sci* 303:184, 1992.

21. Van Thiel DH, Gavaler JS, Joshi SN, et al: Heartburn of pregnancy. *Gastroenterology* 72:666, 1977.

22. Assali NS: Dynamics of the uteroplacental circulation in health and disease. *Am J Perinatol* 6:105, 1989.

23. Edelstone DI, Paulone ME, Maljovec JJ, et al: Effects of maternal anemia on cardiac output, systemic oxygen consumption, and regional blood flow in pregnant sheep. *Am J Obstet Gynecol* 156:740, 1987.

24. Adamsons K, Myers RE: Perinatal asphyxia—Causes, detection and neurologic sequelae. *Pediatr Clin North Am* 20:465, 1973.

25. Peeters LLH, Sheldon RE, Jones MD, et al: Blood flow to fetal organs as a function of arterial oxygen content. *Am J Obstet Gynecol* 135:637, 1979.

26. Chang J, Elam-Evans LD, Berg CJ, et al: Pregnancy-related mortality surveillance—United States, 1991–1999. *Morb Mortal Wkly Rep* 52:1, 2003.

27. Nolan TE, Wakefield ML, Devoe LD: Invasive hemodynamic monitoring in obstetrics. A critical review of its indications, benefits, complications, and alternatives. *Chest* 101:1429, 1992.

28. Belfort MA, Rokey R, Saade GR, et al: Rapid echocardiographic assessment of left and right heart hemodynamics in critically ill obstetric patients. *Am J Obstet Gynecol* 171:884, 1994.

29. Hazelgrove JF, Price C, Pappachan VJ, et al: Multicenter study of obstetric admissions to 14 intensive care units in southern England. *Crit Care Med* 29:770, 2001.

30. Finley BE: Acute coagulopathy in pregnancy. *Med Clin North Am* 73:723, 1989.

31. Hayashi RH: Hemorrhagic shock in obstetrics. *Clin Perinatol* 13:755, 1986.

32. Naeye RL: Abruptio placentae and placenta previa: Frequency, perinatal mortality, and cigarette smoking. *Obstet Gynecol* 55:701, 1980.

33. Slutsker L: Risks associated with cocaine use during pregnancy. *Obstet Gynecol* 79:778, 1992.

34. Roberts WE: Emergent obstetric management of postpartum hemorrhage. *Obstet Gynecol Clin North Am* 22:283, 1995.

35. Gilbert WM, Moore TR, Resnik R, et al: Angiographic embolization in the management of hemorrhagic complications of pregnancy. *Am J Obstet Gynecol* 166:493, 1992.

36. Reimold SC, Rutherford JD: Valvular heart disease in pregnancy. *N Engl J Med* 349:52, 2003.

37. Siu SC, Sermer M, Coleman JM, et al: Prospective multicenter study of pregnancy outcomes in women with heart disease. *Circulation* 104:515, 2001.

38. Beus E, Mook WNKA, Ramsay G, et al: Peripartum cardiomyopathy: a condition intensivists should be aware of. *Intensive Care Med* 29:167, 2003.

39. Cox SM, Hankins GDV, Leveno KJ, Cunningham FG: Bacterial endocarditis: A serious pregnancy complication. *J Reprod Med* 33:671, 1988.

40. Mabie WC, Freire CMV: Sudden chest pain and cardiac emergencies in the obstetric patient. *Obstet Gynecol Clin North Am* 22:19, 1995.

41. Fishburne JI, Meis PJ, Urban RB, et al: Vascular and uterine responses to dobutamine and dopamine in the gravid ewe. *Am J Obstet Gynecol* 137:944, 1980.

42. Olson D, Pohlman A, Hall JB: Administration of low dose dopamine to nonoliguric patients with sepsis syndrome does not raise intramucosal gastric pH nor improve creatinine clearance. *Am J Respir Crit Care Med* 154:1664, 1996.

43. Varon J, Marik PE: The diagnosis and management of hypertensive crises. *Chest* 118:214, 2000.

44. Sibai BM: Treatment of hypertension in pregnant women. *N Engl J Med* 335:257, 1996.

45. Pearlman MD, Tintinalli JE, Lorenz RP: Blunt trauma during pregnancy. *N Engl J Med* 323:1609, 1990.

46. Williams JK, McClain L, Rosemurgy AS, et al: Evaluation of blunt abdominal trauma in the third trimester of pregnancy: Maternal and fetal considerations. *Obstet Gynecol* 75:33, 1990.

47. Rothenberger DA, Quattlebaum FW, Zabel J, et al: Diagnostic peritoneal lavage for blunt trauma in pregnant women. *Am J Obstet Gynecol* 129:479, 1977.

48. Ma OJ, Mateer JR, DeBehnke DJ: Use of ultrasonography for the evaluation of pregnant trauma patients. *J Trauma* 40:665, 1996.

49. Goldman SM, Wagner LK: Radiologic management of abdominal trauma in pregnancy. *Am J Roentgenol* 166:763, 1996.

50. Weber CE: Postmortem cesarean section: Review of the literature and case reports. *Am J Obstet Gynecol* 110:158, 1971.

51. Beller FK, Schmidt EH, Holzgreve W, et al: Septicemia during pregnancy: A study in different species of experimental animals. *Am J Obstet Gynecol* 151:967, 1985.

52. Fein AM, Duvivier R: Sepsis in pregnancy. *Clin Chest Med* 13:709, 1992.

53. Gibbs RS, Duff P: Progress in pathogenesis and management of clinical intraamniotic infection. *Am J Obstet Gynecol* 164:1317, 1991.

54. Lee W, Clark SL, Cotton DB, et al: Septic shock during pregnancy. *Am J Obstet Gynecol* 159:410, 1988.

55. Sibbald WJ, Vincent JL: Roundtable conference on clinical trials for the treatment of sepsis. *Crit Care Med* 23:394, 1995.

56. Cooper MS, Stewart PM: Corticosteroid insufficiency in acutely ill patients. *N Engl J Med* 348:727, 2003.

57. Afessa B, Green B, Delke I, et al: Systemic inflammatory response syndrome, organ failure, and outcome in critically ill obstetric patients treated in an ICU. *Chest* 120:1271, 2001.

58. Pipkin FB: Risk factors for preeclampsia. *N Engl J Med* 344:925, 2001.

59. Sibai BM, McCubbin JH, Anderson GD, et al: Eclampsia. I. Observations from 67 recent cases. *Obstet Gynecol* 58:609, 1981.

60. Gilson G, Golden P, Izquierdo L, Curet L: Pregnancy-associated hemolysis, elevated liver functions, low platelets (HELLP) syndrome: An obstetric disease in the intensive care unit. *J Intensive Care Med* 11:173, 1996.

61. Mushambi MC, Halligan AW, Williamson K: Recent developments in the pathophysiology and management of preeclampsia. *Br J Anaesth* 76:133, 1996.

62. Roberts JM: Prevention or early treatment of preeclampsia. *N Engl J Med* 337:124, 1997.

63. Boccardo P, Soregaroli M, Aiello S, et al: Systemic and fetal-maternal nitric oxide synthesis in normal pregnancy and preeclampsia. *Br J Obstet Gynaecol* 103:879, 1996.

64. Mabie WC, Ratts TE, Sibai BM: The central hemodynamics of severe preeclampsia. *Am J Obstet Gynecol* 161:1443, 1989.

65. Wolf JL: Liver disease in pregnancy. *Med Clin North Am* 80:1167, 1996.

66. Benedetti TJ, Quilligan EJ: Cerebral edema in severe pregnancy-induced hypertension. *Am J Obstet Gynecol* 137:860, 1980.

67. Krane NK: Acute renal failure in pregnancy. *Arch Intern Med* 148:2347, 1988.

68. Sibai BM, Mabie BC, Harvey CJ, et al: Pulmonary edema in severe preeclampsia-eclampsia: Analysis of thirty-seven consecutive cases. *Am J Obstet Gynecol* 156:1174, 1987.

69. Mabie WC, Ratts TE, Ramanathan KB, et al: Circulatory congestion in obese hypertensive women: A subset of pulmonary edema in pregnancy. *Obstet Gynecol* 72:553, 1988.

70. Aya AGM, Mangin R, Hoffet M, et al: Intravenous nicardipine for severe hypertension in pre-eclampsia—effects of an acute treatment on mother and fetus. *Intensive Care Med* 25:1277, 1999.

71. Linton DM, Anthony J: Critical care management of severe pre-eclampsia. *Intensive Care Med* 23:248, 1997.

72. The MAGPIE Trial Collaborative Group: Do women with preeclampsia, and their babies, benefit from magnesium sulphate? The MAGPIE Trial: a randomized placebo controlled trial. *Lancet* 359:1877, 2002.

73. Lucas MJ, Leveno KJ, Cunningham FG: A comparison of magnesium sulfate with phenytoin for the prevention of eclampsia. *N Engl J Med* 333:201, 1995.

74. Belfort MA, Anthony J, Saade GR et al: A comparison of magnesium sulfate and nimodipine for the prevention of eclampsia. *N Engl J Med* 348:4, 2003.

75. The Eclampsia Trial Collaborative Group: Which anticonvulsant for women with eclampsia? Evidence from the Collaborative Eclampsia Trial. *Lancet* 345:1455, 1995.

76. Kirshon B, Lee W, Mauer MB, Cotton DB: Effects of low-dose dopamine therapy in the oliguric patient with preeclampsia. *Am J Obstet Gynecol* 159:604, 1988.

77. Sibai BM, Kustermann L, Velasco J: Current understanding of severe preeclampsia, pregnancy-associated hemolytic uremic syndrome, thrombotic thrombocytopenic purpura, hemolysis, elevated liver enzymes, and low platelet syndrome, and postpartum acute renal failure: different clinical syndromes or just different names? *Curr Opin Nephrol Hypertension* 3:436, 1994.

78. Knox TA, Olans LB: Liver disease in pregnancy. *N Engl J Med* 335:569, 1996.

79. Emergency Cardiac Care Committee and Subcommittees, American Heart Association: Guidelines for cardiopulmonary resuscitation and emergency cardiac care: Special resuscitation situations. *JAMA* 268:2242, 1992.

80. Lee RV, Rodgers BD, White LM, et al: Cardiopulmonary resuscitation of pregnant women. *Am J Med* 81:311, 1986.

81. DePace NL, Betesh JS, Kotler MN: 'Postmortem cesarean' section with recovery of both mother and offspring. *JAMA* 248:971, 1982.

82. Deblieux PM, Summer WR: Acute respiratory failure in pregnancy. *Clin Obstet Gynecol* 39:143, 1996.

83. Noble PW, Lavee AE, Jacobs MM: Respiratory diseases in pregnancy. *Obstet Gynecol Clin North Am* 15:391, 1988.

84. Baggish MS, Hooper S: Aspiration as a cause of maternal death. *Obstet Gynecol* 43:327, 1974.

85. Tomkinson J, et al: *Report on Confidential Enquiries into Maternal Deaths in England and Wales 1976–1978.* London, Her Majesty's Stationery Office, Department of Health and Social Security, Report on Health and Social Subjects No. 26, 1982, p 1.

86. Levinson G, Shnider SM, deLorimier AA, et al: Effects of maternal hyperventilation on uterine blood flow and fetal oxygenation and acid-base status. *Anesthesiology* 40:340, 1974.

87. Campbell LA, Klocke RA: Update in nonpulmonary critical care. *Am J Respir Crit Care Med* 163:1051, 2001.

88. Gaensler EA, Patton WE, Verstraeten JM, et al: Pulmonary function in pregnancy: III. Serial observations in patients with pulmonary insufficiency. *Am Rev Respir Dis* 67:779, 1953.

89. King TE: Restrictive lung disease in pregnancy. *Clin Chest Med* 13:607, 1992.

90. Hung CT, Pelosi M, Langer A, et al: Blood gas measurements in the kyphoscoliotic gravida and her fetus: Report of a case. *Am J Obstet Gynecol* 121:287, 1975.

91. McKim DA, Dales RE, Lefebvre GG, et al: Nocturnal positive-pressure nasal ventilation for respiratory failure during pregnancy. *Can Med Assoc J* 139:1069, 1988.

92. Gluck JC, Gluck PA: The effect of pregnancy on the course of asthma. *Immunol Allergy Clin North Am* 20:729, 2000.

93. Liu S, Wen SW, Demissie K et al: Maternal asthma and pregnancy outcomes: a retrospective cohort study. *Am J Obstet Gynecol* 184:90, 2001.

94. Schatz M: Interrelationships between asthma and pregnancy: A literature review. *J Allergy Clin Immunol* 103:S330, 1999.

95. National Asthma Education Program Working Group on Asthma and Pregnancy: *Management of Asthma during Pregnancy.* Bethesda, National Heart, Lung and Blood Institute, National Institutes of Health, 1993, p 1.

96. Schatz M, Zeiger RS, Harden KM, et al: The safety of inhaled β-agonist bronchodilators during pregnancy. *J Allergy Clin Immunol* 82:686, 1988.

97. American College of Obstetricians and Gynecologists, and American College of Allergy, Asthma and Immunology: The use of newer asthma and allergy medications during pregnancy. *Ann Allergy Asthma Immunol* 84:475, 2000.

98. Masson RG: Amniotic fluid embolism. *Clin Chest Med* 13:657, 1992.

99. Clark SL, Montz FJ, Phelan JP: Hemodynamic alterations associated with amniotic fluid embolism: A reappraisal. *Am J Obstet Gynecol* 151:617, 1985.

100. Clark SL: Amniotic fluid embolism. *Clin Perinatol* 13:801, 1986.

101. Dashow EE, Cotterill R, Benedetti TJ, et al: Amniotic fluid embolus: A report of two cases resulting in maternal survival. *J Reprod Med* 34:660, 1989.

102. Pisani RJ, Rosenow EC: Pulmonary edema associated with tocolytic therapy. *Ann Intern Med* 110:714, 1989.

103. Hollingsworth HM, Pratter MR, Irwin RS: Acute respiratory failure in pregnancy. *J Intensive Care Med* 4:11, 1989.

104. Rodrigues J, Niederman MS: Pneumonia complicating pregnancy. *Clin Chest Med* 13:679, 1992.

105. Madinger NE, Greenspoon JS, Ellrodt AG: Pneumonia during pregnancy: Has modern technology improved maternal and fetal outcome? *Am J Obstet Gynecol* 161:657, 1989.

106. Vallejo JG, Starke JR: Tuberculosis and pregnancy. *Clin Chest Med* 13:693, 1992.

107. Sperling RS, Stratton P, et al: Treatment options for human immunodeficiency virus-infected pregnant women. *Obstet Gynecol* 79:443, 1992.

108. Ahmad H, Mehta N, Manikal VM, et al: *Pneumocystis carinii* pneumonia in pregnancy. *Chest* 120:666, 2001.

109. Galgiani JN, Ampel NM, Catanzaro A, et al: ISDA practice guidelines for the treatment of coccidioidomycosis. *Clin Infect Dis* 30:658, 2000.

110. American Thoracic Society, Centers for Disease Control and Prevention, and the Infectious Diseases Society of America: Treatment of Tuberculosis. *Am J Respir Crit Care Med* 167:603, 2003.

111. Miller FC, Petrie RH, Arce JJ, et al: Hyperventilation during labor. *Am J Obstet Gynecol* 120:489, 1974.

112. Ralston DH, Shnider SM, deLorimier AA: Uterine blood flow and fetal acid-base changes after bicarbonate administration to the pregnant ewe. *Anesthesiology* 40:348, 1974.

113. Albright GA, Ferguson JE, Joyce TH, et al: *Anesthesia in Obstetrics: Maternal, Fetal, and Neonatal Aspects.* Boston, Butterworth, 1986, p 41.

114. Eguiluz A, López Bernal A, McPherson K, et al: The use of intrapartum fetal blood lactate measurements for the early diagnosis of fetal distress. *Am J Obstet Gynecol* 147:949, 1983.

115. Holdsworth JD, Johnson K, Mascall G, et al: Mixing of antacids with stomach contents. *Anaesthesia* 35:641, 1980.

116. Lee RV, Rodgers BD, Young C, et al: Total parenteral nutrition during pregnancy. *Obstet Gynecol* 68:563, 1986.

117. Heller L: Parenteral nutrition in obstetrics and gynecology, in Greep JM, et al (eds): *Current Concepts in Parenteral Nutrition.* The Hague, Martinus Nijhoff, 1977.

Chapter 106

ANAPHYLACTIC AND ANAPHYLACTOID REACTIONS

JONATHAN MOSS
PAUL-MICHEL MERTES

KEY POINTS

- *Mast cells or basophils release mediators of anaphylactic and anaphylactoid reactions as a result of direct drug actions or interaction of antigen with mast cell or basophil immunoglobin E.*

- *Agents that commonly cause hypersensitivity reactions are antibiotics, blood products, radiocontrast media, muscle relaxants, colloids, preservatives, protamine, and latex.*

- *Histamine, eosinophilic chemotactic factor of anaphylaxis, slow-reacting substance of anaphylaxis, platelet-activating factor, prostaglandins, and kinins are the six major pharmacologic mediators known to be released in anaphylactic and anaphylactoid reactions.*

- *Symptoms caused by these mediators are usually immediate but may be delayed by 2 to 15 minutes or, in rare cases, by as long as 2.5 hours after the parenteral injection of antigen.*

- *Because this reaction includes vasodilation and translocation of fluid from capillaries and postcapillary venules (resulting in loss of fluid and colloid from intravascular spaces), effective plasma volume and systemic vascular resistance is decreased, which can lead to shock.*

- *The sine qua non of anaphylaxis is severe cardiovascular or respiratory compromise; most conscious patients sense impending doom before the clinical event occurs.*

- *Tryptase is helpful in distinguishing between anaphylactic and anaphylactoid reactions.*

- *Although various drugs are used to treat anaphylactic and anaphylactoid reactions, discontinuation of the offending drug, maintenance of the airway, administration of oxygen, blood volume expansion, and administration of titrated doses of epinephrine (very large doses may be needed) are the mainstays of therapy.*

- *Anaphylactic and anaphylactoid reactions are acute, potentially fatal events, but their morbidity and mortality rates can be decreased by preparation, drills such as those done for cardiopulmonary resuscitation, and prompt recognition and aggressive treatment.*

Life-threatening hypersensitivity or pseudoallergic reactions to exogenously derived and administered agents in critical care environments can be, and usually are, treated successfully by a prepared intensivist.[1] These reactions are anaphylactic if immune mediated and anaphylactoid if chemically mediated. Data from multicenter studies of perioperative patients show an incidence of life-threatening reactions of 1 in 5000 anesthetics, half of which are immune mediated.

Although chemically mediated reactions may be much more common, they usually are less severe.[2] Rapid recognition and treatment of such reactions can prevent much of the morbidity and mortality that would otherwise occur.

Life-Threatening Hypersensitivity Reactions

Anaphylaxis is a life-threatening allergic, immune-mediated reaction. The term *allergic* applies to immune-mediated reactions, as opposed to those caused by pharmacologic idiosyncrasy, direct toxicity, drug overdose, or drug interactions.[3] Anaphylactoid reactions produce the same clinical syndrome but are not immune mediated. Interaction of antigen with mast cell immunoglobin (Ig) E or direct drug actions cause mast cells to release mediators of anaphylactic and anaphylactoid reactions (Fig. 106-1). Vasoactive mediators of these reactions include histamine, eosinophilic chemotactic factor of anaphylaxis (ECF-A), slow-reacting substance of anaphylaxis (SRS-A; a mixture of three leukotrienes, including a potent coronary vasoconstrictor), platelet activating factor (PAF), kinins, and prostaglandins (see Fig. 106-1). Symptoms usually occur within 15 minutes of parenteral injection of the causative agent, although they may be delayed. The net effect of these agents is a marked decrease in systemic vascular resistance and the leakage of fluid from the capillaries and postcapillary venules. This excessive vasodilation and reduction in effective plasma volume can result in shock. Thus, volume replacement and administration of epinephrine are therapeutic mainstays. Common causes of such reactions are antibiotics, blood products, muscle relaxants, colloids, preservatives, latex, protamine, and radiocontrast medium.

Incidence and Prevalence

Anaphylactic and anaphylactoid reactions to drugs and adjuvants represent an important component of iatrogenic pathology responsible for significant morbidity, mortality, and medical care costs.[4,5] However, there is no existing comprehensive epidemiologic study of drug allergy in the general population because many reactions attributed to allergic events are not intensively investigated. Also, many authentic allergic events are not reported. However, several series from different countries have estimated the incidence of anaphylaxis during anesthesia[6–17] to be between 1 in 10,000 to 1 in 20,000.[9,12] Despite the fact that these reactions are witnessed and occur in a monitored setting, they have a mortality rate ranging from 3.5%[18] to 4.7%[19] even when appropriately treated.[9,12]

Skin testing overestimates the incidence of reactions. Although the occurrence of these events is well documented, the prevalence of sensitization to anesthetic drugs in the overall population remains poorly defined. For example, there is a 9.3% prevalence of sensitivity to neuromuscular blocking agents in the general population,[20] based on skin test positivity and/or detection of specific IgE to quaternary ammonium ions, although anaphylaxis to neuromuscular blocking agents occurs in only 1 in 6500 anesthetics.[9] Similarly, the prevalence of latex sensitization, a major cause of anaphylaxis during anesthesia, depends on the population studied. It ranges from 1% to 6.6% in the general population,[21,22] reaching 15.8% in

DIAGNOSIS AND MANAGEMENT OF CRITICAL ILLNESS

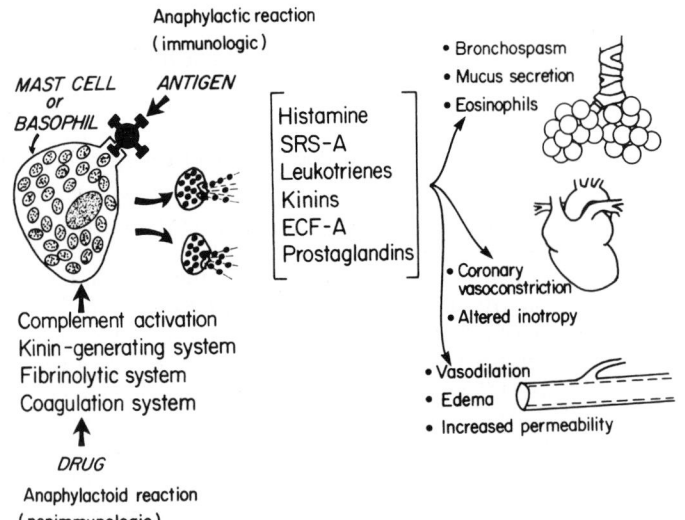

FIGURE 106-1 Summary of the pathophysiologic changes in anaphylactic and anaphylactoid reactions. *Top.* **Anaphylactic reactions. The allergen enters the body and combines with immunoglobulin E antibodies on the surface of mast cells and basophils. The mast cells and basophils degranulate, releasing mediators (histamine, slow-reacting substance of anaphylaxis, leukotrienes, kinins, eosinophilic chemotactic factor of anaphylaxis, prostaglandins, platelet activating factor, and others). The release of these substances is associated with some of the signs and symptoms of anaphylaxis: bronchospasm; pharyngeal, glottic, and pulmonary edema; vasodilation; hypotension; decreased cardiac contractility and arrhythmias; subcutaneous edema; and urticaria.** *Bottom.* **Anaphylactoid reactions. The offending agent enters the body and works by nonimmunologically activating systems that cause degranulation of mast cells and basophils. These systems include the complement system, the coagulation and fibrinolytic systems, and the kinin-generating system. Activation of these systems can result in the release from basophils and mast cells of the same mediators as in anaphylaxis and in a syndrome that is clinically indistinguishable from anaphylaxis.**

an anesthesiology staff.[23] However, this IgE-dependent sensitivity does not necessarily indicate that an allergic reaction will occur in case of exposure to latex.

Clinical Presentation

The end-organ effects of different mediators produce the clinical syndrome of anaphylaxis. In a sensitized individual, the onset of the signs and symptoms caused by these mediators is usually immediate but may be delayed by 2 to 15 minutes or, in rare cases, by as long as 2.5 hours after the parenteral injection of antigen (Fig. 106-2).[24] After oral administration, manifestations occur at unpredictable times. True anaphylaxis requires immune-mediated release of some or all of the above vasoactive mediators. In contrast, other mechanisms can liberate the vasoactive substances that produce this clinical syndrome. Patients with anaphylactic or anaphylactoid reactions may manifest some or all of the signs and symptoms described in the following sections.[24,25]

FIGURE 106-2 Interval between exposure and reaction to the allergen in 43 cases of anaphylactic death. (*Adapted with permission from Delage and Irey.*[35])

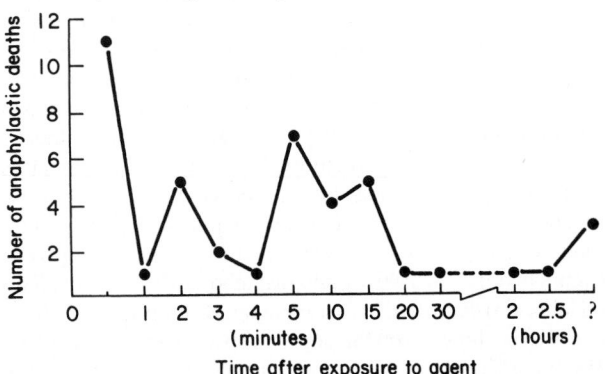

RESPIRATORY SYSTEM

Awake patients may complain of nasal stuffiness or itching, difficulty in breathing, or retrosternal tightness. Coughing, wheezing, tachypnea, laryngeal stridor, and cyanosis are other manifestations, as are acute respiratory distress and pharyngeal, epiglottic, or glottic edema. Respiratory symptoms under anesthesia occur but represented 75% of mortality rate in one series.[25a]

CARDIOVASCULAR SYSTEM

Conscious patients may complain of dizziness. They may also complain of chest tightness, sometimes due to myocardial ischemia. Electrocardiographic changes can vary from tachyarrhythmias and nonspecific changes of the ST segment or T wave, to ventricular fibrillation, electromechanical dissociation, and asystole. In anesthetized patients, hypotension, tachycardia, and cardiovascular collapse are the hallmarks of these reactions.

SKIN

Complaints range from itching, warmth, and minor swelling of the face or an extremity to itching of the eyes and nonpitting deep edema in the cutaneous tissue. Patients may manifest the characteristic urticaria or flare of histamine release. However, cutaneous manifestations alone may not be a harbinger of more severe reactions. The myorelaxant atracurium, known to stimulate histamine release, causes a skin rash in about 33% of patients. Antihistamines completely abolish the skin rash. However, the cutaneous manifestation is independent of hemodynamic effects or plasma histamine levels. Thus, the risk-benefit relation of discontinuing the use of a drug that induces a rash should be considered if that drug represents a needed therapy.[26] Conversely, even in severe reactions, cutaneous manifestations may not be present in many instances.

Other Manifestations

Perhaps most impressive in the awake patient is the expression of a sense of doom. Most conscious patients experiencing an anaphylactic or anaphylactoid reaction who were attended by the authors said something like "I feel horrible" or "I'm going to die" before any hemodynamic or pulmonary symptoms or signs were evident.

An anaphylactic or anaphylactoid reaction may involve any combination of these symptoms; however, the sine qua non of anaphylaxis is severe cardiovascular or respiratory compromise. Because this reaction includes vasodilation and translocation of fluid from capillaries and postcapillary venules (resulting in loss of fluid and colloid from intravascular spaces), there is a reduction in effective plasma volume and systemic vascular resistance followed by shock. Thus, fluid resuscitation is a first priority in treating this syndrome.

The most severe life-threatening reactions result from laryngeal edema, bronchospasm, and vascular collapse, which are probably end-organ responses to the release of vasoactive substances. The full variety of vasoactive mediators of anaphylactic and anaphylactoid reactions is not known. However, an understanding of the known pharmacologic mediators responsible for the clinical manifestations provides a rationale for therapy of anaphylaxis.

Mediators of Anaphylactic Reactions

HISTAMINE

Histamine is a low-molecular-weight amine that is stored predominantly in tissue mast cells and circulating basophils. It dilates capillaries and venules and promotes vascular permeability. Its actions on the histamine H_1 and H_2 receptors are thought to be responsible for decreased systemic vascular resistance and increased permeability in venules.[27] Through H_1-mediated effects on vascular smooth muscle, histamine is also a potent coronary vasoconstrictor.[28] Vascular responses of vasodilation and local cutaneous reactions (wheal and flare) are mediated by H_1 and H_2 receptors. H_2 receptors mimic β-adrenergic receptors in molecular biology function and role, and mediate chronotropic responses. Histamine has a complex array of effects on the vasculature, depending on the presence or absence of vascular endothelium. It is important to note that histamine is a potent constrictor if the endothelium is damaged.

EOSINOPHILIC CHEMOTACTIC FACTOR OF ANAPHYLAXIS

ECF-A, an acidic peptide with a molecular weight of 500 to 600, is stored in mast cell granules. It is chemotactic for eosinophils. The exact role of the eosinophil in the allergic response is unclear. During phagocytosis, eosinophils release histaminase, phospholipase D, and arylsulfatase, enzymes that can inactivate histamine and SRS-A.

PLATELET ACTIVATING FACTOR

PAF, acetyl glyceryl ether phosphorylcholine, causes platelet aggregation and bronchoconstriction, increases vascular permeability, and modulates leukocyte function.

LEUKOTRIENES

Leukotrienes are synthesized in response to antigens and are not stored intracellularly. Products of the oxidative metabolism of arachidonic acid through the lipooxygenase pathway, leukotrienes were once known as SRS-A (leukotrienes C_4, D_4, and E_4).[29] End-organ effects include potent constriction of bronchial smooth muscle. On a molar basis, leukotrienes are 4000 times more potent than histamine in causing bronchoconstriction in normal human beings. Other systemic effects of leukotrienes include cutaneous inflammation, chemotaxis of polymorphonuclear leukocytes, and promotion of lysosomal enzyme release from leukocytes.

PROSTAGLANDINS

Prostaglandins are unsaturated fatty acids that are synthesized at the time of the inflammatory stimulus. Like leukotrienes, they are products of the metabolism of arachidonic acid, but through the cyclooxygenase pathway. Their biologic activities are specific to the target organ on which they act. Prostaglandins are potent mediators of the inflammatory response and can increase capillary permeability and result in bronchospasm, pulmonary hypertension, and peripheral vasodilation.

KININS

Kinins are low-molecular-weight peptides that enhance capillary permeability, dilate certain blood vessels, contract certain smooth muscles, and are perhaps leukotactic. Bradykinin is a potent stimulus for the release of nitric oxide from vascular endothelium. Several processes independent of IgE can generate kinins.

Mediators of Anaphylactoid Reactions

There are multiple processes by which biologically active mediators can be generated to produce an anaphylactoid reaction.

Histamine, and to a lesser extent other vasoactive mediators described above, can be liberated independently of immune reactions to produce an almost identical clinical syndrome. Mast cells (usually derived from connective tissue) and basophils release histamine in response to chemicals or drugs.[30] Activation of the blood coagulation and fibrinolytic systems, the kinin-generating sequence, or the complement cascade can produce the same inflammatory substances as are produced in an anaphylactic reaction (see Fig. 106-1).

When given rapidly in large doses, morphine and meperidine can cause histamine release,[31] resulting in an anaphylactoid reaction. Such large doses are rarely administered fast enough to cause histamine release except when given to induce anesthesia. Sedative doses of opioids or slowly administered anesthetic doses usually do not cause the release of appreciable quantities of histamine. Radiographic contrast medium, *d*-tubocurarine, and vancomycin can also trigger histamine liberation and produce anaphylactoid reactions.[32] Interestingly, small variations in molecular structure can markedly alter histamine-releasing potential. Cisatracurium, the R-cis,R'-cis isomer of atracurium, is one of 10 isomers present in the commercial form of atracurium. It is only one-eighth as likely to cause histamine release as is the mixture.

However, the actual mechanisms for non–immune-mediated histamine release are not completely understood. Why some patients are prone to histamine release in response to drugs is unknown.

Common Causes of Anaphylactic and Anaphylactoid Reactions in the Critical Care or Operating Room Environment

NEUROMUSCULAR BLOCKING AGENTS

Neuromuscular blocking agents are responsible for up to 70% of anaphylactic reactions during general anesthesia.[33] In France in 1996, the incidence of anaphylaxis was estimated at 1 in 6500 anesthetics involving a muscle relaxant[9] and occurred whether or not the agents cause chemically mediated reactions. In most series, succinylcholine appears to be most frequently involved, although variations in practice patterns account for some differences. In the most recent French series, rocuronium, a steroidal relaxant devoid of chemically mediated histamine release, was the primary drug responsible for reactions.[10] Because the main antigenic determinants in the generation of specific IgE antibodies are substituted ammonium ions,[34] an 80% cross-reactivity between the different muscle relaxants is observed by skin tests. Cross-reactivity explains why many patients may exhibit allergic symptoms on first exposure to a neuromuscular blocking agent.[35] Details for skin testing of these agents are included in a recent article by Laxenaire et al[10] (Fig. 106-3).

ANTIBIOTICS

Although allergic reactions to β lactams are the most common cause of anaphylactic reactions in the population at large, they occur far less frequently in the operating room (12% of events). These reactions, classifiable as immediate or nonimmediate, can be produced by the four classes of β lactams (penicillins, cephalosporins, carbapenems, and monobactams), which share a common β-lactam ring structure. Cross-reactivity among cephalosporins and between cephalosporins and penicillins can occur.[36]

Immediate reactions (type I or mediated by IgE), usually within the first hour after drug administration, are characterized by diffuse erythema, pruritus, urticaria, angioedema, rhinitis, bronchospasm, hyperperistalsis, hypotension, cardiac arrhythmias, and anaphylactic shock alone or in combination. Anaphylaxis occurs in about 0.004% to 0.015% of penicillin[37] and 0.001% to 0.1% of cephalosporin[36] treatments. The fatality rate from shock after administration of penicillin is 0.0015% to 0.002%. Despite the fact that penicillin-induced anaphylaxis is rare, this drug remains the most common cause of anaphylaxis in human beings, accounting for approximately 75% of anaphylactic deaths in the United States each year.[38,39]

In many cases, a detailed history of a patient's reaction to penicillin may allow clinicians to exclude true penicillin allergy, thus allowing these patients to receive the drug.[40] Skin tests are the quickest and most reliable method for demonstrating the presence of β-lactam–specific IgE antibodies. Using the suspected β lactams themselves (in particular cephalosporins) in addition to penicillin major and minor determinants as test agents is highly desirable. Patients with a compelling history of type I penicillin allergy who require penicillin should undergo skin testing. Those with a negative skin test result can take penicillin without serious sequelae.[41] Only 10% to 20% of patients reporting a history of penicillin allergy are truly allergic when skin testing is performed. Conversely, many patients with positive skin tests have only vague penicillin allergy histories.[42]

Although serum-specific IgE assays can be used as complementary tests, negative test results should be interpreted in light of the time elapsed from the last exposure to the suspected β lactam because in vivo and in vitro test sensitivity decreases over time. In some diagnostic workups, patients with a strong history of type I β-lactam allergy and negative skin and in vitro tests undergo a controlled administration of the suspected β lactam.[41]

Strategies for dealing with penicillin-allergic patients are evolving and are institution specific. Patients who are allergic to penicillin have been reported to have a 5% to 30% incidence of cross-reactivity to cephalosporins. The recent trend in the United States is to use cephalosporins without a convincing history of penicillin allergy[36,41] because alternative antibiotics can cause severe anaphylactoid reactions. For example, chemically mediated red-man syndrome manifested as hypotension and flushing[3,43] occurs with rapid vancomycin administration.[44]

HYPNOTICS

The incidence of anaphylactoid reactions with thiopental is estimated to be 1 in 30,000.[33] Most of the generalized reactions are linked to direct leukocyte histamine release.

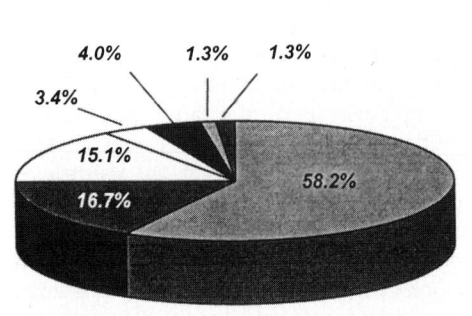

■ Neuromuscular blocking agents (n = 306)
■ Latex (n = 88)
□ Antibiotics (n = 79)
□ Hypnotics (n = 18)
■ Colloids (n = 21)
■ Opioïds (n = 7)
■ Other agents (n = 7)

FIGURE 106-3 Agents involved in anaphylactic reactions observed during anesthesia in France between January 1, 1999 and December 31, 2000 (526 reactions). (*Reproduced with permission from Mertes et al.[73]*)

However, there is evidence for IgE-mediated anaphylactic reactions based on skin tests and specific IgE assay.[45]

Ever since Cremophor EL has been discontinued as a solvent for some non-barbiturate hypnotics, many previously reported anaphylactoid reactions have disappeared. Although less frequent, anaphylaxis to all induction agents has been observed.[46,47] However, in recent studies, induction agents caused only 3.7% of all anaphylactic cases during anesthesia.[10]

OPIOIDS

Although patients often relate anaphylactic reactions to opiates, immunologically mediated reactions to morphine, codeine phosphate, meperidine, fentanyl and its derivatives are quite rare, occurring only once in 100,000 to 200,000 anesthetics.[33] Because of the direct histamine-releasing properties and frequent non–histamine-related cutaneous manifestations, there is significant over-reporting of allergy to opiates. Most opioids (with the possible exception of the fentanyl family) may cause direct release of histamine, urticaria along the vein of administration, and vasodilation. Bronchospasm and angioedema have not been reported, even when large doses of these agents were used for anesthesia before cardiac procedures.[48] Codeine has been implicated in several cases of anaphylactoid reactions, but in all of the reported instances, more than one drug was used simultaneously. An anaphylactoid reaction to morphine and an inordinate sensitivity to histamine release have been reported, but skin testing in this patient produced negative results.[49]

Radiocontrast Medium

Anaphylactoid reactions during infusion of radiocontrast material occur in 1% to 2% of procedures.[50] Although the mechanism of such reactions remains unknown, anaphylactic treatment may diminish them. When repeated infusions of radiocontrast materials were given to patients with a history of an immediate anaphylactoid reaction to them, the incidence of repeat reactions was 17% to 35%. Pretreatment with prednisone, diphenhydramine, and ephedrine significantly decreased repeat reactions in these at-risk patients. Steroid pretreatment should be given at least 12 hours before administration of the contrast agent.

Local Anesthetics

True allergy to the para-aminobenzoic ester agents, such as procaine, is well documented, but documented allergic reactions to the amide local anesthetics are rare.[51] Methylparaben, a derivative of para-aminobenzoic acid and a preservative used in many multidose vials of local anesthetics, may well be the offending agent in anaphylactic reactions. With a true allergy to one amide local anesthetic agent, a potential for cross-reactivity exists. Although skin testing is used to identify safe local anesthetic agents, there is no support for applying this technique to humans. Clinical history appears to be a good discriminator. Most "reactions" in the dental chair appear to result from anxiety or epinephrine responses. For example, in a series of 71 patients who gave a history of possible allergic reaction to local anesthetics, only 15% had had history

TABLE 106-1 Incidence of Anaphylactoid Reactions to Colloid Volume Expanders

Colloid	Incidence (%)
Plasma protein	
Plasma protein derivative	0.019
Human serum albumin	0.011
Dextran	
Dextran 60/75	0.069
Dextran 40	0.007
Starch	
Hydroxyethyl starch	0.085

SOURCE: Adapted with permission from Ring and Messmer.[54]

of clinical manifestations of a hypersensitivity response (i.e., urticaria, wheezing, or facial swelling).[52]

Volume Expanders

COLLOID

Anaphylactoid reactions to the clinically used colloids have been studied extensively in Europe (Table 106-1).[53,54] Because of kinin contaminants, the purified protein fractions are associated with a higher incidence of reactions than are other colloids. The complex polysaccharides can activate the complement system. These reactions do not depend on prior sensitization. The reported incidence of anaphylactoid reactions after purified protein fractions varies from 0.007% to 0.085%.

BLOOD PRODUCTS

Transfusion reactions can be classified as hemolytic or nonhemolytic. Hemolytic reactions result from ABO-antigen–incompatible transfusions in which IgG or IgM antibodies from the donor or recipient react with red blood cells, complement is fixed and activated, cells are destroyed, and complement anaphylatoxins are released.[55] Urticaria, hypotension, and bronchospasm may accompany activation of the clotting cascade. In a sedated and/or paralyzed patient, bleeding or severe hypotension may be the only sign of a transfusion reaction. The most common allergic reactions to transfusions are nonhemolytic, febrile reactions from leukoagglutinins. Unlike red blood cells, leukocytes and platelets contain HLA antigens of the human histocompatibility system. Antibodies of the IgG or IgM class to these antigens are known as *leukoagglutinins*. The precise relation of leukoagglutinins to anaphylactoid reactions remains unclear. Transfusion-related acute lung injury is produced by leukoagglutinin reactions.[3] Patients who lack serum IgA will generate antibodies to IgA and may have a severe anaphylactoid reaction with transfusion of IgA-replete normal blood.[56] In most cases of transfusion reaction, the magnitude of cell lysis, hypotension, bronchospasm, and increased capillary permeability probably relates directly to the rate and extent of complement activation.

PROTAMINE

Many case reports and studies have provided evidence that protamine reversal of the effects of heparin can cause a severe, life-threatening reaction with generation of anaphylatoxins (C5a) and thromboxane.[57] Multiple mechanisms have been implicated in protamine reactions, including mechanisms that are immune mediated, mechanisms that are mediated otherwise, and mechanisms that combine immune-mediated and vasoactive-mediated reactions when vasoactive substances are displaced by protamine. Because protamine is a histone derived from salmon sperm, antigenic crossover with fish allergy is possible. Diabetics who have received protamine zinc insulin (25 U contains 0.7 mg protamine) appear to have an increased incidence of this reaction and of antibodies to protamine.[57,58] More than one mechanism may be involved; production of C5a anaphylatoxins by any mechanism generates thromboxane A_2, which causes pulmonary vasoconstriction, bronchoconstriction, and systemic hypotension. Substitutes for heparin and protamine are being developed, so that patients with known risk factors will be able to undergo safe cardiopulmonary bypass. Until then, dose modification, the use of hexadimethrine (Polybrene) for heparin reversal (obtained by an investigational drug request from the Food and Drug Administration) or ancrod for "anticoagulation" remain options.

LATEX

Allergy to latex has been increasingly recognized as an important cause of allergy in anesthesia and critical care.[59] Although latex allergy was first described in urologic patients in 1983, the role of latex as an allergen in the perioperative period was not described until 1988. Latex allergy currently represents 12% of life-threatening events, according to one recent French study.[60] This true allergy should be distinguished from the cutaneous reactions to the products of vulcanization. It is important to note that, in the same study population, latex allergy was largely unreported in a previous 5-year period. Approximately 1% of the general population has the IgE antibody to latex (vs. 8% of surgeons or nurses), but it is unclear whether the increase in latex allergy is related to the more widespread use of latex since the epidemic of acquired immunodeficiency syndrome or to prior lack of recognition of the allergy.[61–63] Clearly, some instances of allergy attributed to drugs were latex allergies. The first documented case of fentanyl allergy was reexamined and found to be an allergy to latex.[64]

Because of the ubiquity of latex in the operating room and intensive care units, allergies to latex are frequently difficult to distinguish from allergies to drugs. Epidemiologic studies report that patients with multiple latex exposures and a history of atopy are at particular risk. In a population of children with meningomyelocele and other midline disorders, antibodies to latex were detected in more than 35%. In the operative setting, this allergy typically occurs some 30 minutes after induction and is characterized by cutaneous, respiratory, and hemodynamic disturbances. This timing distinguishes latex allergy from reaction to induction agents. Diagnosis of this disorder can be made by radioallergosorbent test or enzyme-linked immunosorbent assay, with approximately 90% sensitivity and with specificity ranging from 60% to 90%.

Protocols for the management of patients with known or suspected latex allergy have been developed, but they are frequently difficult to carry out in the critically ill patient. Aside from the use of nonlatex gloves, masks, and catheters, exceptional vigilance must be paid to percutaneous and inhalational sources of latex.[65] In addition, cross-reactivity with ethylene oxide, often used to sterilize instruments, has been reported.

Anaphylaxis: Prevention, Recognition, and Treatment

There seems to be good evidence that preoperative preparation and physician training can decrease morbidity and mortality rates from anaphylaxis. The French Society of Anesthesiologists has suggested a comprehensive strategy for such preoperative evaluations.[33] An aggressive preoperative evaluation to identify patients at risk for latex allergy significantly decreased the frequency of these reactions in France. An allergic history is important, particularly for latex allergy.

The introduction of chymopapain into the armamentarium for treating herniated nucleus pulposus was highly instructive about prophylaxis and treatment of anaphylactic reactions. Before the introduction of IgE screening, a relatively high incidence (0.3% to 2%) of anaphylactic reactions was associated with chymopapain administration. Although now infrequently used, its introduction prompted a new prospective study of anaphylaxis. From the release of chymopapain by the Food and Drug Administration in November 1982 until September 1983, the incidence of anaphylactic reactions was similar to that in the phase II trial (i.e., approximately 0.4% in men and 1.3% in women for the first 30,000 patients treated).[66] Then the incidence decreased significantly (to 0.25% in men and 0.7% in women). The mortality rate from chymopapain anaphylaxis also decreased from 2 of 13 to 3 of 252. We believe that improved survival rate is attributable to awareness of the pathophysiology of such reactions, vigilance during administration of the drug, and pretreatment of the patient with H_1 and H_2 antihistamines. *Although prophylactic administration of antihistamines did not significantly decrease the overall rate of anaphylaxis, it significantly decreased mortality rate attributable to anaphylactic reactions.* Alternatively, increased physician awareness and treatment of anaphylaxis may be a significant factor in the decrease in mortality rates.

A subject of some interest is whether the patient with an atopic history is at special risk. It now appears that a history of generalized allergy does not predispose to anaphylactoid or anaphylactic reaction in the perioperative period. Thus, limiting histamine-releasing drugs in this population does not seem justified by current evidence. Populations at risk appear to be better categorized by concurrent illness. Older patients or those with myocardial ischemia present a special problem. They are at greater risk of complications than are other patients from pretreatment (especially vigorous hydration and steroid administration) and therapy for anaphylactic reactions. The possibility of triggering anaphylactic or anaphylactoid reactions in this group should be weighed against the clinical advantage of these drugs.

Aside from preoperative assessments, pretreatment with antihistamines remains an option for patients at risk. One might consider giving patients H_1- and H_2-receptor antagonists for 16 to 24 hours before exposure to a suspected allergen or agent known to cause histamine release. Some experts argue that large doses of steroids (2 g hydrocortisone) should also be administered to women before exposure to agents associated with a high incidence of anaphylactic or anaphylactoid reactions.[67]

The treatment plan for an anaphylactic or anaphylactoid reaction should be reviewed with other physicians and nurses caring for the patient, and, if anticipated, specific tasks should be assigned in advance (e.g., who starts the second

TABLE 106-2 Possible Therapy for a 70-kg Individual in the Event of an Anaphylactic or Anaphylactoid Reaction

A. Pretreatment
  1. Consider desensitization
  2. Administer 50 mg diphenhydramine q 6 h for 24 h, and either 300 mg cimetidine q 6 h for 24 h, or 150 mg ranitidine q 9–12 h for 24 h; and 2 g hydrocortisone IV 1–6 h before anticipated exposure
  3. Establish large-bore IV line and prehydrate patient with maintenance fluid plus perhaps an additional 500 mL
B. Plan for the worst and assign tasks in advance (e.g., who starts extra IV line, who turns patient, who gets crash cart, who draws blood for blood gas measurement)
C. Initial therapy
  1. Stop administration of allergen
  2. Maintain airway with 100% O_2
  3. Stop negative inotropic and vasodilating agents
  4. Expand blood volume
  5. If indicated, administer 0.05–0.1 mg epinephrine (0.5–1 mL of 1:10,000 solution) q 1–5 min up to a total of 1–2 mg over 1 h or more often, if needed
D. Secondary therapy (if indicated)
  1. Administer antihistamines (50 mg diphenhydramine, 300 mg cimetidine)
  2. Administer inhaled β_2-adrenergic agents for bronchospasm
  3. Administer drip infusion of catecholamines
  4. Administer steroids (2 g hydrocortisone IV)
E. Evaluate airway for edema before extubating the trachea

ABBREVIATIONS: IV, intravenous; q, every.

intravenous infusion, who turns the patient supine). The fact that the chance of a serious reaction is slight does not justify lack of planning. If the worst is routinely expected and planned for, the rate of adverse outcomes of anaphylactic and anaphylactoid reactions is likely to decrease.

Although various drugs are used to treat anaphylactic and anaphylactoid reactions, discontinuation of the offending drug, maintenance of the airway, administration of oxygen, blood volume expansion, and administration of epinephrine are the mainstays of therapy (Table 106-2). These procedures are necessary to treat the sudden hypotension and hypoxia that result from vasodilation, increased capillary permeability, and bronchospasm. Establishing a plan beforehand for the successful therapy for these reactions will diminish the risk of unfavorable outcomes. Although a dogmatic treatment protocol is not warranted by the data, data are consistent enough to justify a proposed treatment protocol. Anaphylactic and anaphylactoid reactions are triggered by different mechanisms, but the mediators released and the treatment for these severe reactions are indistinguishable.

Identifying the Agent Involved

Testing for allergic reactions and the diagnosis of allergic disorders begins with a symptom history and physical examination, although many individuals will deny prior exposure. Thus, 20% of patients with allergies to neuromuscular blockers have not received these drugs previously. In addition, a time frame for reaction after the injection of the incriminated drug is very helpful. In chymopapain allergy, 90% of reactions were manifest within 10 minutes on the day of administration. When more than one drug has been injected or absorbed over a short period, a diagnostic strategy based on laboratory tests on samples taken during and shortly after the reaction and on tests carried out days to weeks later may be helpful. Early tests are mainly designed to determine whether or not an allergic mechanism is involved, whereas delayed testing attempts to identify the responsible drug.

TRYPTASE

Tryptase levels acquired during or immediately after a reaction can be helpful in determining whether the reaction is immunologically mediated. Mast cells activated during an IgE-mediated hypersensitivity reaction release proteases such as tryptase and prestored histamine and newly generated vasoactive mediators. Because tryptase content in basophils is 300- to 700-fold less than in mast cells in humans, tryptase levels in serum are a marker for systemic mast cell activation. Although it can be marginally elevated in different situations,[68] an elevated serum tryptase concentration above 25 μg/L strongly suggests an anaphylactic mechanism.[69,70]

Although a negative tryptase test does not completely rule out anaphylaxis, a 2-year survey of anaphylactoid reaction during anesthesia conducted in France between 1999 and 2000 confirmed its utility in clinical practice. There has been the suggestion that tryptase can distinguish between anaphylactic and anaphylactoid reactions, based on the observation that rapid infusion of vancomycin leads to a 40-fold increase in histamine levels without a change in tryptase.[71] The elevated histamine levels persist even when patients are pretreated with oral or intravenous H_1/H_2 antagonists, although the accompanying hypotension is attenuated, confirming the vancomycin reaction as chemically mediated.[72] A contrasting view emerged from a study demonstrating that pharmacologic concentrations of vancomycin can release histamine in isolated mast cell preparations. The most recent epidemiologic evidence demonstrates that an elevated tryptase is a reliable, although imperfect, sign of an immunologic reaction (Fig. 106-4).

The sensitivity of tryptase measurements for the diagnosis of anaphylaxis was estimated at 64%, the specificity at 89.3%, the positive predictive value at 92.6%, and the negative predictive value at 54.3%.[73] Peak serum tryptase levels are found between 30 and 60 minutes, and optimum sampling is 1 hour after the start of the reaction. The biological half-life of tryptase is estimated at 2 hours; therefore, increased levels can sometimes be detected for 1 to 6 hours or longer after the onset of anaphylaxis. Increased tryptase levels in sera after death suggest systemic anaphylaxis as a cause of death.[74]

Skin Testing

Skin testing is one of the most frequently used primary confirmatory tests for allergen-specific IgE antibody in the diagnosis of human allergic disease, although its reliability somewhat depends on which class of drug is being tested.

Application of an allergen extract to the skin may be accomplished through a prick puncture or an intradermal injection. Control tests using saline (negative control) and codeine or histamine (positive control) must accompany skin tests to determine whether or not the skin is able to release histamine and react to it. In the prick test, allergen is introduced into the epidermis by means of a puncture. The immediate reaction (wheal and erythema) is read at 15 to 20 minutes. A prick test is considered positive when the diameter of the wheal is at

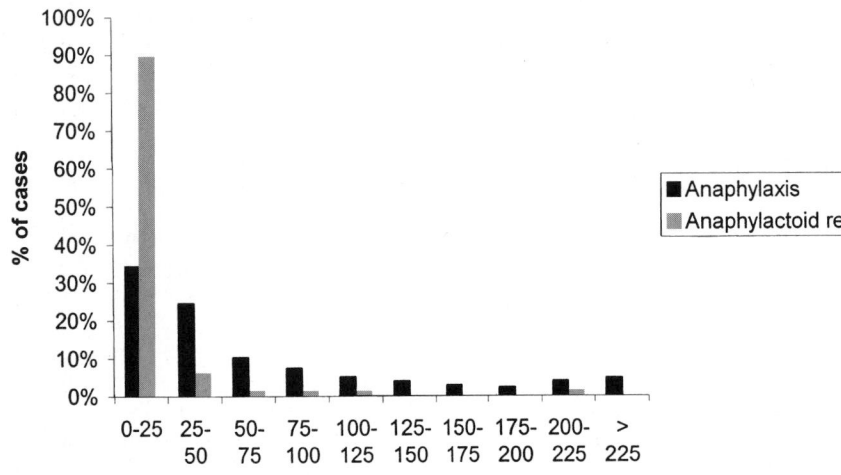

■ Anaphylaxis
■ Anaphylactoid reactions

FIGURE 106-4 Tryptase levels for anaphylactic and anaphylactoid reactions. The percentage of cases that are of anaphylactic or anaphylactoid origin is presented at a predefined tryptase level. At levels lower than 25 μg/mL, both types of reactions can occur, but anaphylactoid reactions predominate. For patients exhibiting levels higher than 25 μg/mL, the etiology is far more likely to be anaphylactic.

least equal to half of that produced by the positive control and at least 3 mm larger than the negative control. Alternatively, allergen (0.01 to 0.05 mL) can be administered intracutaneously through a 26- to 27-gauge needle. In a skin test titration, the same volume of 10-fold serial dilutions of an allergen extract is injected. The objective of skin test titration is to determine the concentration of an extract that produces a wheal or erythema of a defined diameter (e.g., diameter of the wheal is at least twice that of the injection wheal).

Several factors may contribute to the variability of skin test results, including the individual's biologic responsiveness, the technique used to perform the test, the reagents (stability, vehicle, allergen concentration, and purity), and the method used to evaluate skin reactions. Despite the problems of possible false-positive and false-negative results, prick tests in case of suspected latex allergy and prick and intradermal tests in case of drug allergy are advised.[33,75] Recent guidelines concerning the maximal concentration to be used during skin testing for the diagnosis of anaphylaxis during anesthesia have been reported.[10] Although some controversy on the validity of skin test persists, the development of such standardized diagnostic protocols should facilitate interpretation.

Radioallergosorbent Test

Allergen-specific IgE antibody is also an important confirmatory test in the diagnosis of type 1 hypersensitivity reactions. The radioallergosorbent test was the first assay reported for the detection of allergen-specific IgE antibodies. This assay is a noncompetitive solid phase immunoradiometric assay. The allergosorbent assay is prepared by covalently coupling allergen onto cyanogen bromide-activated cellulose disks that are then incubated with the patient's serum. The amount of bound immunospecific IgE is determined by incubation with radioiodinated antihuman IgE Fc. Bound radioactivity is proportional to the amount of allergen-specific IgE in the initial patient's serum and is compared with an IgE antibody reference serum. This early allergen-specific IgE antibody assay was followed by second-generation assays with new matrix materials such as the cellulose sponge used in the Pharmacia CAP system, various polyclonal and monoclonal anti-IgE detection antibody combinations, and non-isotopic labels. Automation has improved assay precision and reproducibility.

Despite promising results as in the case of sensitization to neuromuscular blocking agents,[76–78] when maximal clinical sensitivity is needed, as in the case of drug allergies, intradermal skin tests are preferred. IgE antibody serologic results are viewed as complementary to skin tests.[76]

In Vivo Provocation

In rare instances, in vivo provocation tests may be performed to confirm the identity of an allergen that may be clinically necessary. These tests place the patient at some risk for a reaction because they involve a direct allergen challenge. Therefore, their indication will ultimately depend on whether one can identify a substitute therapy for the putative allergen.

If a patient must receive a drug that is likely to trigger an anaphylactic or anaphylactoid reaction, several steps should be taken. First, an allergist should be consulted. Second, repeated injections of small amounts of antigen or offending hapten may be given because this procedure decreases the amount of specific IgE antibody produced and may stimulate T-suppressor cells. At the same time, this procedure usually increases the amount of competitive IgG antibody (i.e., blocking antibody). Blocking antibody can compete with IgE for receptors on the surface of basophils and mast cells to decrease the mediators released from these cells. Third, small amounts of drug are injected, for example, 5 mg of lidocaine intravenously. This "test dose" hypothesis is verified by the chymopapain experience. Fourth, these tests are done in the post-anesthesia care unit or other setting where resuscitation equipment is available.

Treatment and Initial Therapy

1. Discontinue suspected allergen. This step prevents further recruitment of mast cells and release of mediators.
2. Maintain airway and administer 100% oxygen. Bronchospasm, pulmonary hypertension, and pulmonary capillary leakage may cause severe mismatching of ventilation and perfusion.[79] These changes can persist for several hours during anaphylactic reactions, producing hypoxemia. Therefore, the airway should be maintained, and supplemental oxygen (we recommend 100% oxygen)

should be administered until the situation improves. Intubation of the trachea should be considered, if it has not already been done.

3. Discontinue all sedative, vasodepressing agents. Agents that may have negative inotropic properties or that may decrease systemic vascular resistance should be discontinued because they may contribute to decreased vascular compensation and often interfere with the body's compensatory response to cardiovascular problems. Thus, we believe that these agents should be discontinued to avoid hypotension.

4. Expand blood volume. Because up to 40% of intravascular volume is rapidly lost into the interstitial spaces in an acute anaphylactic reaction during anesthesia,[80] effective therapy consists of rapid replacement of blood volume.[81] Rapid fluid loss and successful treatment with fluid replacement have been documented in the case of an anaphylactic reaction observed incidentally by transesophageal echocardiography.[82] Evidence does not indicate that colloid is more effective than crystalloid. Rapid administration of 1 to 2 L of lactated Ringer's solution or normal saline is important in the initial therapy for these reactions. Further blood volume expansion may be necessary, if hypotension persists.

5. Administer epinephrine. Epinephrine is a mainstay of therapy in acute anaphylaxis for several reasons. Its α_1-adrenergic effects make it useful for treating hypotension. Its β_2-adrenergic effects inhibit bronchoconstriction and the release of mediators from stimulated mast cells or basophils by stimulating the production of intracellular cyclic adenosine monophosphate.[83] For hypotension, 0.05 to 0.1 mg of epinephrine (0.5 to 1 mL of a 1:10,000 solution) should be given initially as an intravenous bolus and repeated every 1 to 5 minutes up to 0.015 mg/kg (or 10 mL of a 1:10,000 solution) for a 70-kg patient, as needed. In cardiac arrest or with a total loss of blood pressure or pulse, full cardiopulmonary resuscitative doses of epinephrine are indicated (0.01 mg/kg, not to exceed 1.0 mg total) in addition to rapid volume expansion. Larger, even massively larger, doses have been needed when titrated to effect, but we do not recommend them as initial doses, because hypertension and tachycardia resulting in myocardial cell death have been reported in such situations. Intramuscular or subcutaneous administration of epinephrine may be unreliable in a hypotensive patient who requires immediate therapy. Interactions with propranolol are possible, and care must be taken not to overdose the patient with epinephrine to the point of severe hypertension (unopposed α-adrenergic effects) and its consequence. Overdose can occur in the absence of propranolol. The major threat from chronic β-adrenergic blockade appears to be that responses to epinephrine may be insufficient to terminate the reaction, and increased doses of epinephrine may be required.[84] We believe that any amount of epinephrine is appropriate when titrated to effect; the doses indicated above provide a starting point.

Secondary Treatment

If the above treatment does not resolve symptoms and signs, additional treatment with antihistamines, aminophylline, catecholamines, corticosteroids, calcium, and endotracheal intubation may be indicated.

ANTIHISTAMINES

Histamine is one of the major mediators of the acute manifestations of anaphylactic and anaphylactoid reactions. Because the vasodilatory effects are mediated by H_1 and H_2 receptors, both types of receptor site must be blocked if all potentially harmful cardiovascular effects of histamine are to be antagonized. Studies in which patients were pretreated before histamine release demonstrate that adverse cardiopulmonary responses can be blunted or prevented when H_1- and H_2-receptor antagonists are used.[85] Although histamine is only one of the mediators released in anaphylactic and anaphylactoid reactions, it may account for many of the initial adverse manifestations. No clinical evidence indicates that administration of antihistamines is effective in treating anaphylaxis once mediators have been released. Administration of antihistamines is therefore recommended only as secondary treatment in acute reactions. (Suggested doses are 1 mg/kg diphenhydramine or 0.1 mg/kg chlorpheniramine as the H_1 blocker and 4 mg/kg cimetidine as the H_2 blocker.)

CATECHOLAMINES

INHALED β_2 AGONIST

If bronchospasm persists (and hemodynamic function is stable), terbutaline or albuterol may be administered as a bronchodilator.

INTRAVENOUS ISOPROTERENOL

If bronchospasm persists, isoproterenol may be useful as a pure β-adrenergic agonist and bronchodilator. This drug may also prove useful when combined with epinephrine in the patient taking β-adrenergic receptor blocking drugs. The β_2-adrenergic effects of isoproterenol cause vasodilation and possible hypotension, especially in patients already experiencing vasodilation or depletion of blood volume. Tachycardia is another possible unwanted effect. Because isoproterenol dilates the pulmonary artery, it may be useful for treating the increased pulmonary vascular resistance of severe anaphylactic reactions when oxygenation is a problem or right ventricular dysfunction occurs (but see Chap. 26 for cautions in this regard). (Starting doses for persistent bronchospasm are 0.5 to 1 μg/min per 70 kg.)

INTRAVENOUS EPINEPHRINE

When hypotension and bronchospasm persist, an intravenous epinephrine drip may be given after blood volume has been expanded and epinephrine boluses have been administered. The starting dose of epinephrine is 1 to 2 μg/min per 70 kg and should be titrated to the desired effect.

INTRAVENOUS NOREPINEPHRINE (LEVOPHED)

Blood pressure can be maintained in a hypotensive patient with norepinephrine until adequate volume expansion has been achieved. Although α-adrenergic drugs may theoretically potentiate the release of mediators, hypotension is deleterious to cerebral and coronary perfusions and must be treated aggressively.

STEROIDS

Corticosteroids should be given in severe reactions, such as shock with refractory bronchospasm and hypotension; there is no evidence to suggest an appropriate dose or preparation.[68,86] We believe 2 g of hydrocortisone phosphate (or its equivalent) is appropriate for severe cardiopulmonary dysfunction. Large doses of methylprednisolone (35 mg/kg) have been shown to inhibit complement-induced polymorphonuclear cell aggregation and lysosomal enzyme release in vitro. Corticosteroids may decrease release of vasoactive mediators and metabolites of arachidonic acid in anaphylaxis by stabilizing membrane phospholipids or by generating macrocortin, which inhibits phospholipid turnover.

AIRWAY EVALUATION

If laryngeal edema occurs in anaphylactic reactions, swelling can persist.[87] In such instances, the larynx can be examined on extubation.

CALCIUM

Because release of mediators is a calcium-dependent process, theory and experimental evidence indicate that administration of calcium may worsen an anaphylactic condition.[88]

Other Immunologic Considerations

Further study is necessary to confirm the effects of trauma and sedative-hypnotics on immunity and the mechanism of this alteration. For now, we know that the perioperative period interferes with innate immunity (e.g., by mucous and skin membrane transgressions), but the effect of alteration of acquired immunity is not clear.

Follow-up

An integral part of therapy is to communicate effectively to patients when an agent is responsible for a true allergic event, and to identify the responsible agent. Although anaphylactic reactions in the perioperative period remain uncommon, there has been a significant tendency to attribute perioperative hemodynamic and respiratory compromises to an anaphylactic origin without appropriate testing. *In our preoperative clinics, there is a 200-fold over-reporting by patients of anaphylaxis to opiates or local anesthetics.* It is important, medicolegally and for patient safety reasons, that patients be fully aware which agents are implicated.

References

1. Levy JH, Roizen MF, Morris JM: Anaphylactic and anaphylactoid reactions. A review. *Spine* 11:282, 1986.
2. Lorenz W, Duda D, Dick W, et al: Incidence and clinical importance of perioperative histamine release: Randomised study of volume loading and antihistamines after induction of anaesthesia. Trial Group Mainz/Marburg. *Lancet* 343:933, 1994.
3. Levy JH: *Anaphylactic Reactions in Anesthesia and Intensive Care*, 2nd ed. Boston, Butterworth-Heinemann, 1992.
4. Einarson TR: Drug-related hospital admissions. *Ann Pharmacother* 27:832, 1993.
5. Vervloet D, Durham S: Adverse reactions to drugs. *BMJ* 316:1511, 1998.
6. Laxenaire MC, Moneret-Vautrin DA, Boileau S, Moeller R: Adverse reactions to intravenous agents in anaesthesia in France. *Klin Wochenschr* 60:1006, 1982.
7. Laxenaire MC: Drugs and other agents involved in anaphylactic shock occurring during anaesthesia. A French multicenter epidemiological inquiry. *Ann Fr Anesth Reanim* 12:91, 1993.
8. Laxenaire MC: Substances responsible for peranesthetic anaphylactic shock. A third French multicenter study (1992–94). *Ann Fr Anesth Reanim* 15:1211, 1996.
9. Laxenaire MC: Epidémiologie des réactions anaphylactoïdes peranesthésiques. Quatrième enquête multicentrique (juillet 1994–décembre 1996). *Ann Fr Anesth Reanim* 18:796, 1999.
10. Laxenaire M, Mertes PM, Group d'Etudes des Reactions Anaphylactoides Peranesthesiques: Anaphylaxis during anaesthesia. Results of a two-year survey in France. *Br J Anaesth* 87:549, 2001.
11. Fisher MM, More DG: The epidemiology and clinical features of anaphylactic reactions in anaesthesia. *Anaesth Intensive Care* 9:226, 1981.
12. Fisher MM, Baldo BA: The incidence and clinical features of anaphylactic reactions during anesthesia in Australia. *Ann Fr Anesth Reanim* 12:97, 1993.
13. Clarke RS: Epidemiology of adverse reactions in anaesthesia in the United Kingdom. *Klin Wochenschr* 60:1003, 1982.
14. Clarke RS, Watkins J: Drugs responsible for anaphylactoid reactions in anaesthesia in the United Kingdom. *Ann Fr Anesth Reanim* 12:105, 1993.
15. Watkins J: Adverse anaesthetic reactions. An update from a proposed national reporting and advisory service. *Anaesthesia* 40:797, 1985.
16. Watkins J: Adverse reaction to neuromuscular blockers: Frequency, investigation, and epidemiology. *Acta Anaesthesiol Scand* 102:6(suppl), 1994.
17. Galletly DC, Treuren BC: Anaphylactoid reactions during anaesthesia. Seven years' experience of intradermal testing. *Anaesthesia* 40:329, 1985.
18. Currie M, Webb RK, Williamson JA, et al: The Australian Incident Monitoring Study. Clinical anaphylaxis: An analysis of 2000 incident reports. *Anaesth Intensive Care* 21:621, 1993.
19. Mitsuhata H, Matsumoto S, Hasegawa J: The epidemiology and clinical features of anaphylactic and anaphylactoid reactions in the perioperative period in Japan. *Masui* 41:1664, 1992.
20. Porri F, Lemiere C, Birnbaum J, et al: Prevalence of muscle relaxant sensitivity in a general population: Implications for a preoperative screening. *Clin Exp Allergy* 29:72, 1999.
21. Turjanmaa K, Reunala T: Incidence of positive prick test to rubber protein. *Contact Dermatitis* 23:279, 1990.
22. Porri F, Lemiere C, Birnbaum J, et al: Prevalence of latex sensitization in subjects attending health screening: Implications for a perioperative screening. *Clin Exp Allergy* 27:413, 1997.
23. Konrad C, Fieber T, Gerber H, et al: The prevalence of latex sensitivity among anesthesiology staff. *Anesth Analg* 84:629, 1997.
24. Smith PL, Kagey-Sobotka A, Bleecker ER, et al: Physiologic manifestations of human anaphylaxis. *J Clin Invest* 66:1072, 1980.
25. Austen KF: Systemic anaphylaxis in the human being. *N Engl J Med* 291:661, 1974.
25a. Fisher MM, Baldo A: The incidence and clinical features of anaphylactic reactions during anaesthesia in Australia. *Ann Fr Anesth Reanim* 12:97, 1993.
26. Doenicke A, Moss J, Lorenz W, et al: Are hypotension and rash after atracurium really caused by histamine release? *Anesth Analg* 78:967, 1994.
27. Plaut M: Histamine, H1 and H2 antihistamines, and immediate hypersensitivity reactions. *J Allergy Clin Immunol* 63:371, 1979.

28. Bristow MR, Ginsburg R, Harrison DC. Histamine and the human heart: The other receptor system. *Am J Cardiol* 49:249, 1982.

29. Goetzl EJ: Mediators of immediate hypersensitivity derived from arachidonic acid. *N Engl J Med* 303:822, 1980.

30. Lorenz W, Doenicke A, Schöning B, et al: The role of histamine in adverse reactions to intravenous agents, in Thornton JA (ed): *Adverse Reactions to Anaesthetic Drugs.* Amsterdam, Elsevier/North-Holland Biomedical, 1981.

31. Rosow CE, Moss J, Philbin DM, et al: Histamine release during morphine and fentanyl anesthesia. *Anesthesiology* 56:93, 1982.

32. Moss J, Rosow CE, Savarese JJ, et al: Role of histamine in the hypotensive action of *d*-tubocurarine in humans. *Anesthesiology* 55:19, 1981.

33. Mertes PM, Laxenaire MC: Allergic reactions occurring during anaesthesia. *Eur J Anaesthesiol* 19:240, 2002.

34. Baldo BA, Fisher MM: Substituted ammonium ions as allergenic determinants in drug allergy. *Nature* 306:262, 1983.

35. Delage C, Irey NS: Anaphylactic deaths: A clinicopathologic study of 43 cases. *J Forensic Sci* 17:525, 1972.

36. Kelkar PS, Li JT: Cephalosporin allergy. *N Engl J Med* 345:804, 2001.

37. Idsoe O, Guthe T, Willcox RR, de Weck AL: Nature and extent of penicillin side-reactions, with particular reference to fatalities from anaphylactic shock. *Bull World Health Organ* 38:159, 1968.

38. Joint Task Force on Practice Parameters, American Academy of Allergy, Asthma and Immunology, American College of Allergy, Asthma and Immunology, and the Joint Council of Allergy, Asthma and Immunology.:The diagnosis and management of anaphylaxis. *J Allergy Clin Immunol* 101:S465, 1998.

39. Neugut AI, Ghatak AT, Miller RL: Anaphylaxis in the United States: an investigation into its epidemiology. *Arch Intern Med* 161:15, 2001.

40. Romano A, Mayorga C, Torres MJ, et al: Immediate allergic reactions to cephalosporins: cross-reactivity and selective responses. *J Allergy Clin Immunol* 106:1177, 2000.

41. Salkind AR, Cuddy PG, Foxworth JW: The rational clinical examination. Is this patient allergic to penicillin? An evidence-based analysis of the likelihood of penicillin allergy. *JAMA* 285:2498, 2001.

42. Solensky R, Earl HS, Gruchalla RS: Penicillin allergy: Prevalence of vague history in skin test-positive patients. *Ann Allergy Asthma Immunol* 85:195, 2000.

43. Newfield P, Roizen MF: Hazards of rapid administration of vancomycin. *Ann Intern Med* 91:581, 1979.

44. Renz C, Lynch J, Thurn J, Moss J: Histamine release during rapid vancomycin administration. *Inflamm Res* 47:S69, 1998.

45. Fisher MM, Ross JD, Harle DG, Baldo BA: Anaphylaxis to thiopentone: An unusual outbreak in a single hospital. *Anaesth Intensive Care* 17:361, 1989.

46. Laxenaire MC, Mata-Bermejo E, Moneret-Vautrin DA, Gueant JL: Life-threatening anaphylactoid reactions to propofol (Diprivan). *Anesthesiology* 77:275, 1992.

47. Fisher M, Baldo BA: Anaphylaxis during anaesthesia: Current aspects of diagnosis and prevention. *Eur J Anaesthesiol* 11:263, 1994.

48. Lowenstein E, Hallowell P, Levine FH, et al: Cardiovascular response to large doses of intravenous morphine in man. *N Engl J Med* 281:1389, 1969.

49. Fahmy NR: Hemodynamics, plasma histamine, and catecholamine concentrations during an anaphylactoid reaction to morphine. *Anesthesiology* 55:329, 1981.

50. Greenberger PA, Patterson R, Tapio CM: Prophylaxis against repeated radiocontrast media reactions in 857 cases: Adverse experience with cimetidine and safety of beta-adrenergic antagonists. *Arch Intern Med* 145:2197, 1985.

51. Fisher MM, Pennington JC: Allergy to local anaesthesia. *Br J Anaesth* 54:893, 1982.

52. Incaudo G, Schatz M, Patterson R, et al: Administration of local anesthetics to patients with a history of prior adverse reaction. *J Allergy Clin Immunol* 61:339, 1978.

53. Ring J, Stephan W, Brendel W: Anaphylactoid reactions to infusions of plasma protein and human serum albumin. *Clin Allergy* 9:89, 1979.

54. Ring J, Messmer K: Incidence and severity of anaphylactoid reactions to colloid volume substitutes. *Lancet* 1:466, 1977.

55. Barton JC: Nonhemolytic, noninfectious transfusion reactions. *Semin Hematol* 18:95, 1981.

56. Schmidt AP, Taswell HF, Gleich GJ: Anaphylactic transfusion reactions associated with anti-IgA antibody. *N Engl J Med* 280:188, 1969.

57. Stoelting RK: Allergic reactions during anesthesia. *Anesth Analg* 62:341, 1983.

58. Stewart WJ, McSweeney SM, Kellett MA, et al: Increased risk of severe protamine reactions in NPH insulin-dependent diabetics undergoing cardiac catheterization. *Circulation* 70:788, 1984.

59. Ownby D: An overview of the clinical problems related to latex allergy, in *International Latex Conference: Sensitivity to Latex in Medical Devices.* Washington, DC, US Food and Drug Administration, 1992.

60. Agre K, Wilson RR, Brim M, et al: Chymodiactin postmarketing surveillance. Demographic and adverse experience data in 29,075 patients. *Spine* 9:479, 1984.

61. Arellano R, Bradley J, Sussman G: Prevalence of latex sensitization among hospital physicians occupationally exposed to latex gloves. *Anesthesiology* 77:905, 1992.

62. Turjanmaa K, Reunala T: Healthcare workers: A risk group for latex allergy, in *International Latex Conference: Sensitivity to Latex in Medical Devices.* Washington, DC, US Food and Drug Administration, 1992.

63. Lagier F, Vervloet D, Lhermet I, et al: Prevalence of latex allergy in operating room nurses. *J Allergy Clin Immunol* 90:319, 1992.

64. Zucker-Pinchoff B, Chandler MJ: Latex anaphylaxis masquerading as fentanyl anaphylaxis: Retraction of a case report. *Anesthesiology* 79:1152, 1993.

65. Holzman R, Sethna N: Latex-allergic patients and the operating room: Preoperative profile and response to a latex-safe environment, in *International Latex Conference: Sensitivity to Latex in Medical Devices.* Washington, DC, US Food and Drug Administration, 1992.

66. Moss J, Roizen MF, Nordby EJ, et al: Decreased incidence and mortality of anaphylaxis to chymopapain. *Anesth Analg* 64:1197, 1985.

67. Schreiber AD: Clinical immunology of the corticosteroids. *Prog Clin Immunol* 3:103, 1977.

68. Veien M, Szlam F, Holden J, et al: Mechanisms of nonimmunological histamine and tryptase release from human cutaneous mast cells. *Anesthesiology* 92:1074, 2000.

69. Laroche D, Vergnaud MC, Sillard B, et al: Biochemical markers of anaphylactoid reactions to drugs. Comparison of plasma histamine and tryptase. *Anesthesiology* 75:945, 1991.

70. Fisher MM, Baldo BA: Mast cell tryptase in anaesthetic anaphylactoid reactions. *Br J Anaesth* 80:26, 1998.

71. Renz CL, Laroche D, Thurn JD, et al: Tryptase levels are not increased during vancomycin-induced anaphylactoid reactions. *Anesthesiology* 89:620, 1998.

72. Renz CL, Thurn JD, Finn HA, et al: Antihistamine prophylaxis permits rapid vancomycin infusion. *Crit Care Med* 27:1732, 1999.

73. Mertes PM, Laxenaire MC, Alla F: Anaphylactic and anaphylactoid reactions occurring during anesthesia in France in 1999–2000. *Anesthesiology* 99:536, 2003.

74. Pumphrey RS, Roberts IS: Postmortem findings after fatal anaphylactic reactions. *J Clin Pathol* 53:273, 2000.

75. Hamilton RG, Adkinson NF Jr: Clinical laboratory assessment of

IgE-dependent hypersensitivity. *J Allergy Clin Immunol* 111:S687, 2003.

76. Gueant JL, Mata E, Monin B, et al: Evaluation of a new reactive solid phase for radioimmunoassay of serum specific IgE against muscle relaxant drugs. *Allergy* 46:452, 1991.

77. Fisher MM, Baldo BA: Immunoassays in the diagnosis of anaphylaxis to neuromuscular blocking drugs: The value of morphine for the detection of IgE antibodies in allergic subjects. *Anaesth Intensive Care* 28:167, 2000.

78. Guilloux L, Ricard-Blum S, Ville G, Motin J. A new radioimmunoassay using a commercially available solid support for the detection of IgE antibodies against muscle relaxants. *J Allergy Clin Immunol* 90:153, 1992.

79. Pavek K, Wegmann A, Nordström L, et al: Cardiovascular and respiratory mechanisms in anaphylactic and anaphylactoid shock reactions. *Klin Wochenschr* 60:941, 1982.

80. Fisher M: Blood volume replacement in acute anaphylactic cardiovascular collapse related to anaesthesia. *Br J Anaesth* 49:1023, 1977.

81. Fisher MM: The management of anaphylaxis. *Med J Aust* 1:793, 1977.

82. Beaupre PN, Roizen MF, Cahalan MK, et al: Hemodynamic and two-dimensional transesophageal echocardiographic analysis of an anaphylactic reaction in a human. *Anesthesiology* 60:482, 1984.

83. Winslow CM, Austen KF: Enzymatic regulation of mast cell activation and secretion by adenylate cyclase and cyclic AMP-dependent protein kinases. *Fed Proc* 41:22, 1982.

84. Jacobs RL, Rake GW Jr, Fournier DC, et al: Potentiated anaphylaxis in patients with drug-induced beta-adrenergic blockade. *J Allergy Clin Immunol* 68:125, 1981.

85. Philbin DM, Moss J, Akins CW, et al: The use of H1 and H2 histamine antagonists with morphine anesthesia. A double-blind study. *Anesthesiology* 55:292, 1981.

86. Halevy S, Altura BT, Altura BM: Pathophysiological basis for the use of steroids in the treatment of shock and trauma. *Klin Wochenschr* 60:1021, 1982.

87. James LP Jr, Austen KF: Fatal systemic anaphylaxis in man. *N Engl J Med* 270:597, 1964.

88. Tanz RD, Kettelkamp N, Hirshman CA: The effect of calcium on cardiac anaphylaxis in guinea pig Langendorff heart preparations. *Agents Actions* 16:415, 1985.

Chapter 107 _____

DERMATOLOGIC CONDITIONS

MARIO E. LACOUTURE
MICHAEL JUDE WELSCH
ANNE E. LAUMANN

KEY POINTS

- *In a patient with a dermatologic condition, observation and description of the lesions (morphology, distribution, and texture) are important for developing a differential diagnosis.*

- *Mucous membranes (oral, ocular, nasal, genital, and perianal) should be examined in all patients.*

- *The skin may provide clues to an underlying, life-threatening condition, such as endocarditis, graft-versus-host disease, bacterial sepsis, toxic shock syndrome, systemic vasculitis, or complications from the human immunodeficiency virus.*

- *Drug-related dermatoses are prevalent in the intensive care unit. Clues to diagnosis include a rapidly developing eruption; generalized, symmetrical, predominantly truncal distribution; maculopapular, urticarial, or acneiform morphology; and accompanying pruritus.*

- *Extensive skin disease can cause important fluid, electrolyte, and protein losses and predisposes the patient to life-threatening infections.*

Basics of Dermatology

APPLICATION OF STRUCTURE AND FUNCTION TO DERMATOSES

The basic anatomy of the skin is described in Fig. 107-1. The skin is a complex organ whose major function is to provide a barrier against the environment. Other major functions include temperature regulation and sensation. The skin is divided into three major layers: epidermis, dermis, and subcutaneous tissue. The outermost layer of the epidermis, the stratum corneum, is composed of dead, anucleate keratinocytes and serves as the first and major physical barrier. The stratum granulosum and stratum spinosum lie below the stratum corneum and are composed of keratinocytes in the process of differentiation. They are derived from the bottom layer of the epidermis, the basal cell layer. The epidermis is connected to the dermis by a complex of proteins and adhesion molecules in the basement membrane zone. Nutrients and products of metabolism are exchanged in the superficial and deep vascular networks located in the dermis. The dermis also contains nerve endings and supporting structures such as sebaceous glands, eccrine sweat glands, and hair follicles.

Alteration of any layer or structure of the skin can result in primary dermatologic disease. Often the skin is secondarily affected in underlying comorbid conditions and may serve as a window to internal disease processes. The stratum corneum can be damaged in the intensive care setting by tape, electrocardiographic leads, defibrillator devices, dry environments, pressure, or adhesives. Alteration may impair barrier resistance to infectious agents or allow passage of antigens to deeper layers of the skin. Preparing the skin for invasive procedures with topical solutions exposes the patient to potential sensitizers. Metabolically active cells in the suprabasal layers are susceptible to inflammatory and cytotoxic reactions from medications and toxins. Disruption in cell adhesion clinically manifests as blisters and may result from medications, toxins, pressure, extremes in temperature, or autoimmune diseases. Infections and inflammatory processes can occur at any level or in any structure, leading to conditions such as impetigo, folliculitis, cellulitis, fasciitis, or vasculitis.

BASIC MORPHOLOGIC APPROACH AND DESCRIPTIONS

When approaching a patient with skin disease, careful observation, palpation, and description are critical for developing a differential diagnosis. The morphology, or type, of lesion may be flat (macule), elevated (papule, nodule, plaque, cyst, vesicle, bulla, pustule, or hyperkeratosis), or depressed (ulcer or atrophy; Table 107-1). Shape, margination (well or poorly defined borders), and arrangement of the lesions are important. Color may be white (leukoderma or hypomelanosis); red (erythema), pink, violaceous (purple), brown (hypermelanosis or hemosiderin), black, blue, gray, or yellow. Particular attention should be paid to the distribution of the eruption (e.g., localized, systemic, truncal, acral, unilateral, or intertriginous). Palpation will help determine consistency, temperature, mobility, tenderness, and depth of lesion. When various lesions are present, one should attempt to determine the primary lesion.

Clinical history is essential. Symptoms (fever, malaise, arthralgias, myalgias, etc.) must be questioned, especially cutaneous symptoms (pruritus, pain, tenderness, burning, or stinging). Time course of the skin lesions should be determined, with particular attention to medication history (prescription and nonprescription, oral, topical, and alternative). Common diagnostic aids in dermatology are skin biopsy for hematoxylin and eosin or other special staining, direct immunofluorescence (DIF), or culture; potassium hydroxide preparation (for dermatophytic infections); mineral oil mounts (for scabies); Gram stain (for bacterial infections); fluid cultures; and Tzanck smears (for herpes simplex and varicella zoster virus infections).

TABLE 107-1 Basic Morphologic and Descriptive Terminology

Macule	Flat lesion of variable size
Papule	Elevated lesion less than 0.5 cm diameter
Plaque	Elevated lesion greater than 0.5 cm diameter
Nodule	Elevated, palpable lesion greater than 0.5 cm diameter
Vesicle	Fluid filled lesion less than 0.5 cm diameter
Bullae	Fluid filled lesion greater than 0.5 cm diameter
Pustule	Pus-filled lesion
Ulcer	Depressed lesion with loss of epidermis and variable levels of dermis
Wheal	Evanescent pale-red papule or plaque

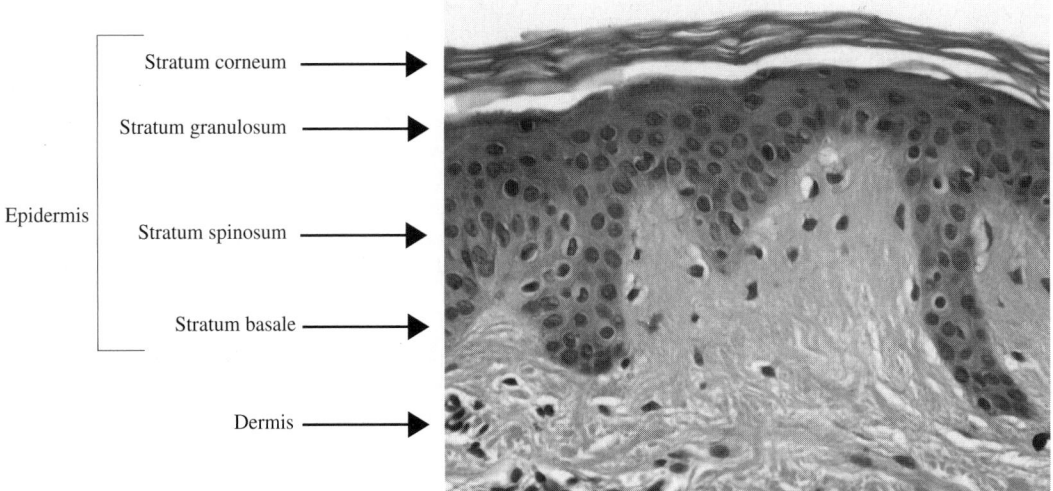

FIGURE 107-1 Structure of normal skin.

Dermatoses Precipitated by Drugs

EPIDEMIOLOGY AND PROBABILITY OF ADVERSE DRUG REACTIONS

The World Health Organization (WHO) defines an adverse drug reaction (ADR) as any noxious, unintended, and undesired effect of a drug that occurs at diagnostic, prophylactic, or therapeutic doses used in humans.[1] This definition excludes untoward events due to noncompliance or errors in drug administration, therapeutic failures, intentional and accidental poisoning, and drug abuse. A meta-analysis of 39 prospective studies covering 32 years reported a 10.9% incidence of ADR in admitted hospital patients and a 4.7% incidence for patients admitted because of serious ADR.[2] In addition, fatal ADR ranked "between the fourth and sixth" leading causes of death in the United States in 1994, exceeding deaths due to pneumonia and diabetes.[2] The rate and severity of preventable ADRs in intensive care units (ICUs) is nearly twice that in non-ICUs,[3] and ADRs are responsible for lengthening the stay in medical and surgical ICUs.[4] It has been estimated that ADRs cost a 700-bed teaching hospital $5 million to $6 million a year[5] and $1.56 billion to $4 billion for all hospitals in the United States.[6,7]

Cutaneous ADRs (CADRs) are the most common type of ADR and occur in 2% to 3% of hospitalized patients.[8] One in 1000 patients has a serious CADR,[9] representing approximately 3% of all disabling injuries in hospitalized patients.[10]

Many commonly used drugs have reaction rates exceeding 1%.[11] The numbers of CADR may be higher in the ICU setting owing to the critical and compromised nature of the patient compounded by the multiplicity of drugs. Several factors influence the probability of a drug producing an adverse reaction: the size of the compound (larger compounds are more likely to act as haptens), drug-drug interactions (altered metabolism and protein displacement), the route of delivery (intravenous administration increases the incidence of reactions), and patient factors such as renal function, alcohol use, hepatic function, and severity of concomitant disease.[12,13] However, a recent nested case-control study showed severity of illness and length of stay as the only

relevant risk factors.[14] A review of nine articles studying rates of CADR found that antibiotics (e.g., amoxicillin, penicillin, fluoroquinolones, sulfonamides, and cephalosporins), nonsteroidal anti-inflammatory agents (NSAIDs), and other analgesics were the leading culprits.[11] Another study found that antiepileptics (e.g., phenytoin and carbamazepine) were also common causal agents. The following medications only rarely cause CADR: digoxin, acetaminophen, meperidine, aminophylline, diphenhydramine, bisacodyl, prochlorperazine, spironolactone, prednisone, thiamine, ferrous sulfate, atropine, morphine, insulin, and spironolactone.

AN APPROACH TO CUTANEOUS ADVERSE DRUG REACTIONS

Cutaneous eruptions are the most frequent ADR in hospitalized patients, accounting for 97.5% of cases in a prospective study by Thong et al.[15] Maculopapular or morbilliform exanthems (Fig. 107-2, Plate 107-2) and urticaria are responsible for 95% and 5% of CADRs, respectively.[11] Onset of the exanthem is usually within 1 week of administration, with the notable

FIGURE 107-2 Maculopapular or morbilliform eruption. This is the most common presentation of a cutaneous adverse drug reaction. (Collection of Dr. Mario Lacouture.) See Plate 107-2.

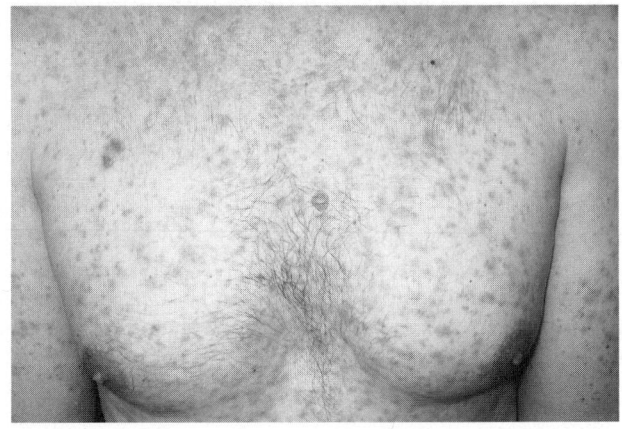

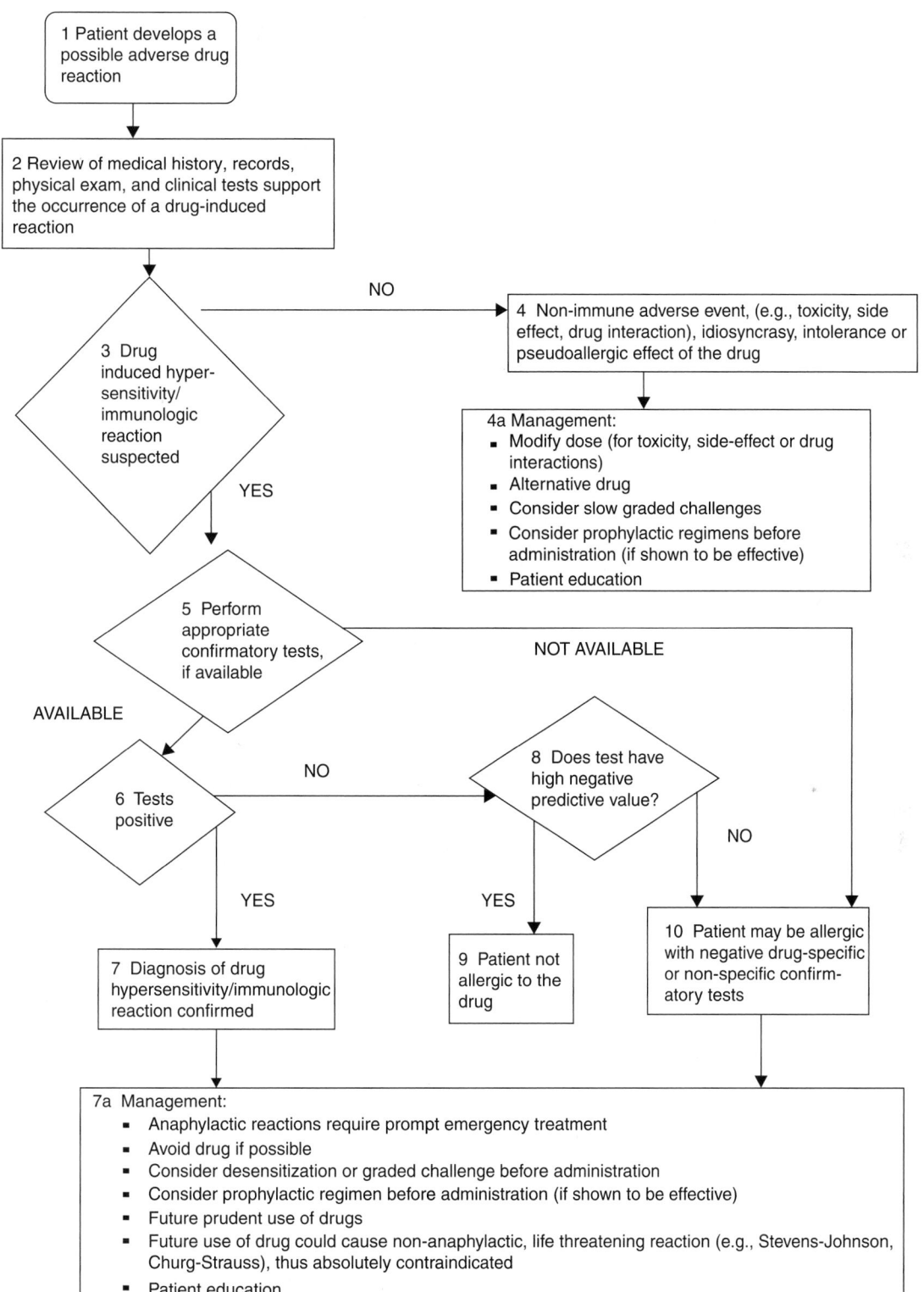

FIGURE 107-3 Algorithm for the management of adverse drug reactions. Adapted from Joint Task Force on Practice Parameters, the American Academy of Allergy, Asthma and immunology. Executive summary of disease management of drug hypersensivity: A practice parameter. Ann Allergy Asthma Immunol 83:665, 1999. Used with permission.

exceptions of antibiotics and allopurinol. Clues to recognizing a CADR include a rapidly developing rash, with an onset temporally related to the administration of a drug. Medical history, physical examination, and laboratory findings may provide clues, although an extensive laboratory workup is usually unnecessary for diagnosis (Fig. 107-3). Identifying the causative agent in the ICU setting may be problematic due to the concurrent administration of multiple drugs and the inability of patients to recall important facts. Hence, all medical records and family members or close contacts should be

TABLE 107-2 Indicators that an Adverse Drug Reaction May Become Serious

Cutaneous Findings	Systemic Findings
Confluent erythema	High fever (>40°C)
Rash or edema involving the face	Lymphadenopathy
Tender skin lesions	Joint pain
Palpable purpura	Dyspnea, wheezing,
Necrotizing skin lesions	hypotension
Vesicles/bullae	**Laboratory Findings**
Positive Nikolsky's sign*	Abnormal liver function tests
Mucous membrane erosions	Lymphocytosis with atypia
Urticaria	Eosinophilia (>1000/mm^3)
Tongue edema	

*Outer layer of epidermis separates readily with lateral pressure.
SOURCE: Ref. 9.

questioned. Important information includes (1) time of onset and course of the reaction; (2) dosage and time of initiation and/or discontinuation of any medications (including over-the-counter and alternative products); (3) the patient's previous exposure to this or other related medications; (4) any previous history of ADR, its management, and any measures taken to prevent future ADRs; (5) the patient's medical problems; and (6) any physical and/or laboratory abnormalities present with the ADR, with special attention to organ system(s) involved. Clues to diagnosis include (1) an eruption that develops very rapidly; (2) a generalized, symmetrical, predominantly truncal distribution; (3) an exanthematous (maculopapular), urticarial, fixed drug, or acneiform morphology; and (4) accompanying pruritus. Other less common drug-associated morphologies are lichenoid, photosensitive, vasculitic, or lupus-like patterns. With all this information in hand and knowing the reaction rate of various medications, identification of the cause of an eruption becomes more likely.

Despite the benign nature of the overwhelming majority of CADRs, it important to evaluate for increasing liver or renal dysfunction and for signs suggesting progression to severe skin disease (Stevens-Johnson syndrome [SJS] or toxic epidermal necrolysis [TEN]). Signs indicative of serious skin problems include mucosal involvement, blistering lesions, and a positive Nikolsky sign (Table 107-2).

CLASSIFICATION OF CUTANEOUS ADVERSE DRUG REACTIONS

The classification of CADRs can be problematic, largely due to the lack of data on molecular mechanisms underlying these reactions. The most widely used classification scheme for ADR was devised by Rawlins and Thomson[12] (Table 107-3): type A reactions are related to the pharmacologic effects of the drug, are consequently predictable, and occur with great frequency; type B reactions are unrelated to the pharmacologic actions of the drug and are therefore unpredictable and uncommon; type C reactions result from long-term use of a drug; and type D reactions relate to carcinogenicity and teratogenicity of a drug. Type A reactions are the most common (80%) and can occur at any dose. Type B reactions occur in susceptible individuals (6% to 10%) a few days after administration or with reexposure and are independent of dose. Type B comprises drug intolerance, idiosyncratic reactions, and allergic or hypersensitivity reactions (those having a well-defined immunologic mechanism). Allergic reactions can be catego-

TABLE 107-3 Classification of Cutaneous Adverse Drug Reactions (CADR)

Type A reactions (common, predictable)
- Toxicity or overdose (hepatic failure with high-dose isotretinoin)
- Side effects (dry skin with topical retinoids)
- Drug interaction (increased coumadin bleeding when a macrolide is administered)

Type B reactions (uncommon, unpredictable)
- Idiosyncratic reaction (the very rare cholestatic liver dysfunction occurring after 3–4 weeks of oral terbinafine therapy)
- Immunologic reactions
  Type I (immediate, IgE-mediated): anaphylaxis
  Type II (cytotoxic, IgG, complment-mediated): hemolysis
  Type III (immune complex): serum sickness
  Type IV (delayed-type hypersensitivity): contact dermatitis

Type C reactions
- Long-term use (blue discoloration with the use of hydroxychloroquine)

Type D reactions
- Carcinogenic or teratogenic effects (squamous cell carcinoma after ultraviolet A radiation therapy)

SOURCES: References 12, 16.

rized further into those that are mediated by drug-specific antibodies or drug-specific T lymphocytes. These include the four mechanisms identified in the Gell and Coombs classification: immediate, cytotoxic, immune complex, and delayed hypersensitivity.[16] Allergic CADRs are characterized by occurrence in a subset of people who have had a previous exposure to the same or similar drug. The reactions often develop rapidly with reexposure and produce clinical syndromes that are commonly associated with immunologic reactions. These may include systemic manifestations such as hepatitis, fever, and eosinophilia, which have been found in 30% of hospitalized patients with drug reactions, particularly in those induced by allopurinol or anticonvulsants.

Anaphylaxis and urticaria are Gell-Coombs type I (immediate) hypersensitivity reactions. They usually occur within 1 hour of drug administration, although they may occur as late as 72 hours. These reactions are mediated by immunoglobulin (Ig) E antibodies specific to the causative drug, found on mast cells and peripheral blood basophils, and occur more frequently with parenteral administration. Urticaria may occur in the setting of the systemic manifestations of anaphylaxis, which comprise angioedema with laryngeal edema, bronchospasm, hypotension, diffuse erythema, hyperperistalsis, cardiac arrhythmias, and pruritus (see Chap. 106). Drug-induced anaphylaxis occurs in 1 of 2700 hospitalized patients and is most frequently induced by β-lactam antibiotics (including penicillin), radiocontrast medium, intravenous anesthetic drugs, aspirin, other NSAIDs, and opiates. In the United States, the most common cause of anaphylaxis is penicillin, accounting for 75% of 500 to 1000 anaphylactic deaths in 1 year.[17] Urticarial lesions are pruritic, erythematous or white, nonpitting, round or oval edematous papules or plaques surrounded by a clear or red halo, usually at different stages of formation. Penicillins, sulfonamides, and NSAIDs are the most common causal medications.[18] Angioedema refers to the same pathophysiologic process as urticaria with transudation of interstitial fluid into the dermis or hypodermis. Treatment of urticaria consists of discontinuation of the offending drug and the administration of oral antihistamine H_1 blockers. These include diphenhydramine, hydroxyzine, and the nonsedating agents, loratadine, cetirizine, and fexofenadine. If anaphylaxis develops, emergency treatment is instituted with intramuscular or subcutaneous epinephrine, high-flow oxygen and airway management, intravenous diphenhydramine, steroids, fluids, vasopressors, and cardiopulmonary resuscitation, as needed. Skin testing with the offending agent is usually positive in IgE-mediated reactions.

Cytotoxic (type II) reactions are mediated by IgG and complement, usually occur longer than 72 hours after drug exposure, and manifest as increased clearance of red blood cells and platelets by the lymphoreticular system. Skin testing is not useful.

Type III reactions are serum sickness-like reactions, in which IgG and/or IgM immune complex deposition leads to diffuse tissue injury. Common clinical findings include fever, urticaria (often figurate or polycyclic), angioedema, malaise, arthralgias (particularly of the hands and feet with swelling), lymphadenopathy, and occasionally nephritis or endocarditis, usually starting after 1 to 3 weeks of drug administration. There is an associated eosinophilia. Heterologous antisera, xenogeneic antibodies, and drugs with a low molecular weight (e.g., penicillin) are common triggers. Systemic steroids are often used to treat this reaction, although large-scale controlled clinical trials are lacking.

Allergic contact dermatitis is the most common type IV, delayed-type hypersensitivity reaction, usually caused by topically applied medications. Sensitization is required and usually occurs over 5 to 7 days, after which the reaction can be elicited by topical or systemic administration of the same or a structurally similar agent. This means that a previous exposure is necessary, although a reaction may appear de novo after several days of contact with the offending agent. A pruritic, erythematous, vesicular, scaly eruption occurs at the site of contact, which, with time, may become lichenified (thickened with accentuation of skin markings) related to rubbing or scratching.

Diagnostic tests for CADR may be useful to determine the causative agent, the type of reaction, and the prognosis. Skin testing may be performed by a prick or intradermal administration of the suspected drugs to determine the presence of drug-specific IgE antibodies (type I Gell-Coombs reactions). Penicillin, muscle relaxants, and barbiturates are amenable to this type of testing because their epitopes are known. In some institutions, allergists and immunologists are able to purify the offending epitopes from other drugs. Medicines that undergo significant metabolism and those with undefined epitopes cannot be tested. An in vitro test to study the presence of circulating drug-specific IgE antibodies is the radioallergosorbent test. Penicillin, insulin, thiopental, protamine, latex, chymopapain, and selected muscle relaxants can be tested by radioallergosorbent test, with variable consistency.

When ADRs are mediated by drug-specific T cells (type IV; e.g., contact dermatitis), patch testing is a useful adjunct. It is performed by applying predetermined dilutions of the compound on intact skin for different periods and assessing for erythema, edema, or vesiculation, all indicative of specific T-cell reactivity. A skin biopsy aids in clarifying the pathophysiology of a reaction, for example, by the demonstration of immune complexes, leukocytoclastic vasculitis, or tissue eosinophilia. However, the biopsy often does not help in establishing whether or not the cutaneous reaction is drug induced. Blood eosinophil counts have been regarded as an indicator of ADR; however, recent studies have shown that this criterion carries a low sensitivity (22% to 36%, depending on arbitrarily defined cutoff rates), making routine eosinophil testing unhelpful.[19] Serum tryptase levels are useful in reactions caused by diffuse mast cell (anaphylactic or anaphylactoid) activation, especially when hemodynamic changes are present. Tryptase is a protease stored in the granules of mast cells and released with mast cell activation. Levels should be obtained within 2 hours of initiation of the episode. Serum tryptase concentrations are recommended over serum histamine concentrations due to the greater stability of tryptase.[20]

The clinical usefulness of in vitro diagnostic tests to detect the presence of drug-specific antibodies capable of eliciting basophil histamine release, lymphocyte blast transformation, or complement activation remains to be proven. These tests carry a low sensitivity, are currently used mainly as research tools, and therefore are not recommended for routine clinical use.

Despite the high prevalence of ADR to sulfonamides in the general population (3%) and those infected with the human immunodeficiency virus (HIV; 60%), there are no reliable diagnostic tests available for clinical use. If, however, there is certainty that a sulfa drug has caused a CADR, desensitization protocols have been developed for patients with the acquired immunodeficiency syndrome that allow for sulfonamide administration during treatment and prophylaxis of opportunistic infections.[21]

Despite the different proposed mechanisms, overlap is common, and one cannot infer the pathogenesis of an eruption by its morphology or causative drug alone. The diagnosis of a drug-related dermatosis encompasses a complex mental algorithm of probability, time and causality, alternative diagnoses, and plausibility.

CHEMOTHERAPY-INDUCED DERMATOSES

Cancer patients may be affected by cutaneous reactions of diverse etiologies, including infections, paraneoplastic pemphigus, dermatomyositis, graft-versus-host disease (GVHD), nutritional deficiency, metastases, cutaneous neoplasms, radiation reactions, and administration of chemotherapeutic agents.

The most common CADR to chemotherapeutic agents is alopecia (hair loss), which may present as anagen (hair growth phase) or telogen (hair resting phase) effluvium.[22] Anagen effluvium is usually caused by antineoplastic agents, which weaken the hair shaft, resulting in severe hair loss apparent 1 to 2 months after therapy. Telogen effluvium occurs secondary to acute physical or psychological stress, malnutrition, or drugs. Spontaneous regrowth with drug discontinuation is the norm for both types of alopecia. The most common causative agents include vincristine, cyclophosphamide, doxorubicin, daunorubicin, dactinomycin, and paclitaxel. Treatments are rarely successful. The effectiveness of 2% minoxidil has been inconsistent.[23,24]

Adverse effects in the oral mucosa occur in 40% of patients as a result of direct drug toxicity or indirectly via effects on the

TABLE 107-4 Antidotes used in chemotherapeutic agent extravasation

Agent	Antidote
Anthracycline	Topical DMSO
Mitomycin	Topical DMSO
Vinca alkaloid	Hyaluronidase (ICA)
Mechlorethamine	Sodium thiosulfate (ICA)
Dacarbazine	Sodium thiosulfate (ICA)
Cisplatin	Sodium thiosulfate (ICA)

DMSO, dimethylsulfoxide; ICA, intracutaneous administration.
SOURCE: Reference 22.

bone marrow. Stomatitis is a frequent complication leading to erythema, edema, ulceration, pain, burning, and xerostomia. It is particularly common in individuals who are younger than 20 years, who have prior oral disease, or who have hematologic malignancies. Common culprits include topotecan, methotrexate, fluorouracil, doxorubicin, docetaxel, daunorubicin, dactinomycin, and bleomycin. Healing occurs within 2 to 3 weeks. Treatment consists of adequate oral hygiene and the use of topical agents such as attapulgite, magnesium/aluminum hydroxide, diphenhydramine elixir, benzocaine, and viscous lidocaine.

Candidiasis, with its white, adherent velvety plaques, and varicella zoster virus may also affect the inside of the mouth. Herpes simplex usually affects the vermilion border of the lips, but in the immunosuppressed may cause indolent intraoral ulcers.

Intravenous administration of chemotherapeutic agents may result in extravasation into surrounding tissues. Severity depends on type, quantity, and concentration of drug,[25] and disabling sequelae are uncommon. Agents may be irritants (e.g., bleomycin, carboplatin, cyclosphamide, doxorubicin, etoposide, fluorouracil, paclitaxel, or vinblastine), which cause sclerosis, hyperpigmentation, and tenderness along the vein, or vesicants (e.g., bleomycin, carmustine, cisplatin, doxorubicin, etoposide, fluorouracil, melphalan, mechlorethamine, mitomycin, paclitaxel, vinblastine, or vincristine), which cause burning, necrosis, and ulceration. Treatment consists of discontinuing the infusion, elevating the affected extremity, and applying local heat or cold. Heat should not be applied when extravasation of vinca alkaloids occurs because this may cause ulceration.[26] Surgical debridement and skin grafting may be needed in persistent ulcers. Antidotes are also recommended (Table 107-4).

Localized or diffuse hyperpigmentation is a common CADR, as a result of melanin, carotene, hemoglobin, or other pigment. Characteristic gingival bands occur with cisplatin; horizontal hyperpigmented bands on blond hair (flag sign) with methotrexate; flagellate streaks of hyperpigmentation with bleomycin; pigmented nail bands with bleomycin, cytarabine, cyclophosphamide, daunorubicin, doxorubicin, fluorouracil, hydroxyurea, idarubicin, mitomycin, tegafur, or vinblastine; and mucosal hyperpigmentation with busulfan, fluorouracil, tegafur, doxorubicin, hydroxyurea, cisplatin, or cyclophosphamide.[22]

Another well-described ADR to chemotherapeutic agents is acral erythema, occurring in 6% to 24% of patients,[27] mainly those treated with cytarabine, doxorubicin, and fluorouracil. This painful eruption consists of diffuse erythema and edema on the palms and soles. This resolves with exfoliation within 4 weeks of discontinuing the drug. It needs to be differentiated from acute GVHD in the appropriate clinical setting. Treatment is supportive, with elevation, cold compresses, analgesics, and pyridoxine 150 mg each day.[28]

ANTICOAGULANT-INDUCED DERMATOSES

Adverse reactions to anticoagulants can be localized or diffuse and mediated by various mechanisms. Unfractionated heparin, low-molecular-weight heparins, and vitamin K antagonists are drugs used routinely in the treatment and prophylaxis of thromboembolic disease. In addition to the well-known ADRs such as an increased bleeding tendency, these agents may cause CADR which necessitate institution of alternative therapies.

Heparin is a mucopolysaccharide that can induce various ADRs, including immediate reactions (e.g., urticaria, asthma and anaphylaxis), delayed-type reactions (e.g., erythematous plaques, skin necrosis, a generalized eruption, and thrombocytopenia).[29] Delayed-type reactions manifest as erythematous, vesicular, or pruritic plaques at the injection site within 2 to 5 days of therapy, whereas heparin-induced skin necrosis develops between 5 and 10 days of therapy. Cutaneous reactions have also been described related to the use of low-molecular-weight heparins and heparinoids.[30] In patients with skin necrosis, heparin must be discontinued due to the increased risk of developing heparin-induced thrombocytopenia II.[31] These patients usually have significant concurrent illnesses but no coagulation abnormalities. Histology shows fibrin deposition in venules and capillaries in the dermis and hypodermis, with necrosis. Intracutaneous testing is useful for the diagnosis of delayed reactions (erythematous plaques at heparin injection sites) but is contraindicated in the presence of skin necrosis. A positive skin test has been associated with heparin-induced IgG antibodies. There may be cross-reactivity between unfractionated heparin and low-molecular-weight heparins and heparinoids. Rates of 50% and 30%, respectively, have been reported.[32] Therefore, treatment consists of discontinuing heparin and administering one of the newly developed direct thrombin inhibitors (argatroban and lepirudin) to provide protection during warfarin initiation.

Warfarin, a racemic mixture of R and S enantiomers, inhibits the vitamin K–dependent clotting factors II, VII, IX, and X; it also inhibits the anticoagulant proteins C and S, thereby causing a transient hypercoagulable state.[33] On rare occasions, skin necrosis, which is potentially fatal (15% of cases), occurs with initiation of therapy before full anticoagulation is achieved. Three to 10 days after starting therapy, pain precedes the appearance of ill-defined erythematous plaques, which progress into edematous, blue-black plaques with hemorrhagic bullae in the center. The lesions necrose, leaving central eschars. Necrosis commonly affects the breasts, abdomen, and thighs in females and the abdomen and thighs in males. Histopathology shows fibrin occluding dermal and hypodermal veins, with diffuse necrosis.[34] This occurs more commonly in women. Other risk factors include a large loading dose, protein C deficiency, and the presence of the factor V Leiden mutation. Treatment consists of discontinuation of warfarin and administration of intravenous heparin. Some investigators have reported success with the use of protein C concentrate, prostacyclin, and factor VII.[35] Lesions are treated as any other skin ulcer; however, when they

TABLE 107-5 Commonly Used Herbal Remedies and Reported Adverse Reactions

Name of Plant/Constituent	Adverse Effect	Alleged Indications
Flavonoids	Hemolytic anemia chronic diarrhea, nephropathy, colitis	Antioxidant, edema
Germander	Hepatotoxicity	Choleretic, antiseptic, weight loss
Valerian root, skullcap, chaparral	Hepatotoxicity	Antioxidant
Momordica charantia	Hepatotoxicity	Diabetes
Sauropus androgynus	Bronchiolitis abliterans	Weight loss
Chinese herbal preparations		
Aconite	Arrythmias, abdominal pain	Various
Aristolochia fangchi/pistolochia	Nephrotoxicity	Weight loss
Jin Bu Huan	Hepatotoxicity	Sedative, analgesic
Bajiaolian	Hepatotoxicity	Eczema
Syo-saiko-to	Hepatotoxicity	Cold, liver disease
Shiitake mushroom	Dermatitis	Immunostimulant
Kombucha mushroom	Hepatotoxicity	Cancer, hair growth
Tripterygium wilfordii hook F	Lupus nephritis	Antiinflamatory
"Eternal life" tea	Hepatotoxicity	Variable
Ginseng	Mania, SJS, bleeding	Stimulant
Siberian ginseng	Increases digoxin levels	Stimulant
Ma Huang	Psychosis	Stimulant
Agnus castus	Increases risk of miscarriage	Gynecologic diseases
Guar gum	Intestinal obstruction, death	Weight loss
Licorice root	Hypokalemia, hypertension, arrythmias, edema	Various
Sparteine	Shock	Weight loss
Salicylates in oil of wintergreen, eamphor, peppermint, menthol eucalyptus	Salicylism	
Aloe, cascara, frangula, rhubarb senna	Colorectal Cancer	Laxatives
Capsaicin	Gastric Cancer	
Ayurvedic remedies	Heavy metal poisoning	Various
Pyrrolizidine alkaloids*	Hepatotoxicity	Various
St John's Wort (Hypericum perforatum)	↑ Sensitivity to sunlight, radiation therapy	Depression
Ginko biloba	Hematoma, hyphema	Dementia, pain
Ginseng	Bleeding	Various (mood, HTN)
Ginger	Inhibit coagulation	Motion sickness, vertigo
Echinacea	Hepatotoxicity	Immunostimulant (colds)

*Present in comfrey and other plants (e.g., borage, senecio, coltsfoot).
SOURCES: References 38, 43.

are extensive, surgical debridement, grafting, or occasionally amputation may be necessary to prevent the development of infection and sepsis. In one review, surgical treatment was found to be necessary in more than 50% of cases.[36]

ADVERSE REACTIONS TO ALTERNATIVE DRUGS

Botanical products are classified as dietary supplements. As such, they are exempt from the stringent evaluation and regulatory processes that drugs have to undergo to show efficacy, safety, and quality.[37,38] Although not allowed to make specific health claims, the manufacturers of these remedies are permitted to state they maintain good health. Herbal remedies account for a $1.5 billion per year industry in the United States, and it is estimated that 33% of Americans use these remedies, especially women and people of high socioeconomic status.[39] Eighty percent of the world population uses herbal remedies. In Taiwan, herbal remedies ranked third among culprits for ADR in a study of 2695 patients admitted to the medicine ward.[40] In a Hong Kong study, 0.2% of all admissions were due to adverse reactions to Chinese herbal drugs.[41] Another

survey found that 8% of 400 users of complementary medicine experienced adverse herbal reactions (AHRs).[42]

It is not uncommon for patients admitted to the ICU to have been taking herbal medicines, or "supplements." Contrary to popular belief, herbal products may result in clinically significant adverse reactions and herbal-drug interactions, which may alter diverse organ systems and drug metabolism (Table 107-5).

In addition to AHRs due to the major compounds present, contaminants are a significant source of adverse reactions. Contamination of herbal remedies is abundant, due in part to lack of regulation. Lead, arsenic, and other heavy metals have been found in numerous herbal remedies. Autoimmune thrombocytopenia has been reported in a patient receiving kelp tainted with arsenic. In addition, some remedies have been found to contain traditional drugs, such as aspirin, paracetamol, mefenamic acid, diazepam, and triamcinolone, with corresponding adverse reactions.

There are some herbal remedies not yet reported to cause adverse reactions: camomile (anti-inflammatory), garlic (cholesterol lowering, and antihypertensive, although it may

TABLE 107-6 Interactions Between Herbal Products and Drugs

Name of Botanical Constituent/Drug	Effect
Shankhapushi/Phenytoin	Decreases phenytoin levels
Grapefruit juice/Cyclosporin, Ca channel blockers	Increases levels
Chinese herbal:danshen, MS oil/warfarin	Coagulation abnormality
Glycyrrhizin*/Prednisone	Altered prednisolone metabolism
St John's Wort/SSRIs	Serotonin syndrome (sweating, hyperreflexia, and shivering); seizures; coma
Kava-Kava/SSRIs	Serotonin syndrome (sweating, hyperreflexia, and shivering); seizures; coma
Garlic/anticoagulants	↑bleeding
Ginger/anticoagulants	↑bleeding
Ginko biloba/anticoagulants	↑bleeding
Ginseng/anticoagulants	↑bleeding
Echinacea/ketoconazole/phenytoin	Hepatotoxicity

*Found in licorice and the following Chinese herbs: Sho-saiko-Tok, Sai-boku-To, and Sairei-To.
SSRIs, selective serotonin re-uptake inhibitors (paroxetine, trazodone, sertalin).
SOURCES: References 38, 43.

cause a contact dermatitis when topically applied), *Ginkgo biloba* (increases blood flow), peppermint (analgesic), Sabal (anti-inflammatory), and saw palmetto (antiandrogenic, estrogenic, anti-edema). Underreporting is prevalent; therefore, it should not be assumed that these medicines are free of adverse reactions.

Similarly, interactions with traditional drugs are a significant cause of concern in individuals taking herbal remedies concurrently with traditional medicines[43] (estimated at 18% of the population; Table 107-6). Components in herbal remedies such as St. John's Wort and Kava-Kava, used for depression and anxiety, respectively, have been shown to inhibit monoamine oxidase activity. Interactions with drugs affecting the metabolism of neuroactive amines, such as the selective serotonin-reuptake inhibitors, are a potential problem. Therefore, coffee, tea, and foods containing tyramine (aged cheese, soy sauce, smoked meats, bananas, and avocados) should be avoided.

Because many of the mechanisms underlying AHR are unclear, a careful history and evaluation is necessary. In addition, because the half-life of many of these components is not known, they should be discontinued immediately on admission to the hospital or the critical care unit.

VASOPRESSIN-INDUCED SKIN NECROSIS

Vasopressin, a nonselective vasoconstrictor, is used in the treatment of vasodilatory septic shock, hypotension unresponsive to catecholamines,[44] and variceal hemorrhage.[45] Uncommon adverse reactions to large-dose (0.2 to 0.4 U/min), centrally administered vasopressin include cardiac arrhythmias, ischemia, infarction, and bowel ischemia.[46] When peripheral intravenous administration is used, accidental extravasation of the drug may result in skin necrosis and gangrene. This CADR may occur even at small doses (0.04 U/min) or when small quantities that are undetectable by the occlusion pressure monitor infiltrate the tissue. Interestingly, this skin necrosis does not occur with large-dose subcutaneous administration, as performed for diabetes insipidus. Treatment consists of stopping the vasopressin infusion, surgically débriding the ischemic tissue, and applying wet dressings or grafting. Administration through a central venous

catheter is encouraged, even for small doses, to minimize the occurrence of this adverse reaction.

Diffuse ischemic skin lesions, defined as new areas of mottled or livid skin, have been found to occur in approximately 30% of patients during infusion of arginine-vasopressin, an alternative powerful vasopressor agent that is increasingly used in catecholamine-resistant vasodilatory shock. Sepsis and arterial occlusive disease are predisposing factors. These lesions, often seen on the limbs and trunk but also on the tongue, may lead to gangrene, necessitating débridement and amputation.[47]

Severe Cutaneous Adverse Drug Reactions

STEVENS-JOHNSON SYNDROME AND TOXIC EPIDERMAL NECROLYSIS

CADRs are classified by the WHO as severe when they are life-threatening, require hospitalization, or lead to permanent disability. Stevens-Johnson Syndrome (SJS) (Fig. 107-4,

FIGURE 107-4 Stevens-Johnson syndrome/toxic epidermal necrolysis. Erosive involvement of lips and oral mucosa. (*Courtesy Dr. Iris K. Aronson collection.*) See Plate 107-4.

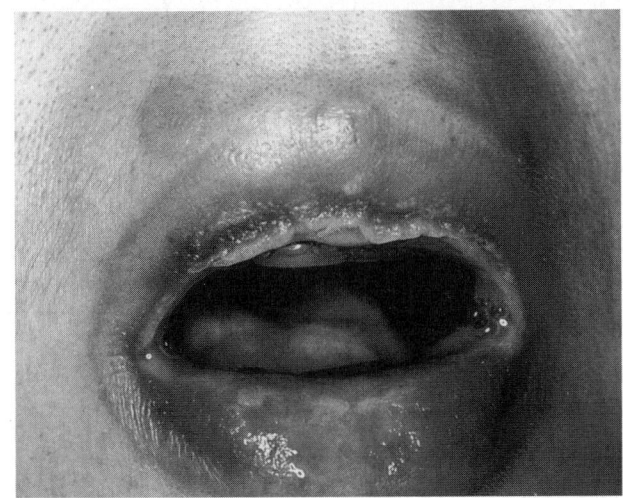

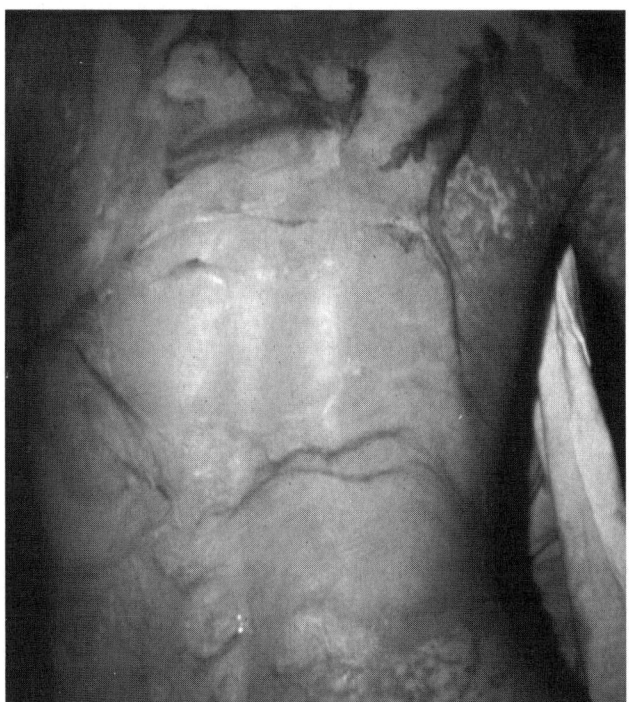

FIGURE 107-5 Toxic epidermal necrolysis: >30% of the body surface area involved. Necrotic epidermis sloughs, revealing moist, bright red dermis. *(Courtesy Dr. Iris K. Aronson collection.)* **See Plate 107-5.**

Plate 107-4) and toxic epidermal necrolysis (TEN) (Fig. 107-5, Plate 107-5) are rare, serious CADRs, with calculated incidences of 1 to 6 and 0.4 to 1.2 cases per million person-years, respectively.[48] SJS and TEN are histopathologically identical diseases that are differentiated by the extent of epidermal detachment: less than 10% in SJS, 10% to 29% in transitional SJS/TEN, and greater than 30% in TEN. In addition to the hypersensitivity syndrome/drug reaction with eosinophilia and systemic symptoms, SJS and TEN constitute the major groups of severe CADRs[49] (Table 107-7).

Fever, sore throat, cough, and burning eyes may precede painful skin eruptions resembling burns for 1 to 3 days. Lesions usually appear within 3 weeks of drug administration

and begin as irregularly defined, painful erythematous macules with purpuric centers that tend to coalesce. Within a few hours or days, blisters appear and epidermal detachment extends over the body. Lesions in the mucosae are characteristic, occasionally preceding skin lesions by several days. However, initial presentation of SJS and TEN may be very similar to less serious CADR, that is, a maculopapular rash. Involvement of the epithelium of the trachea, bronchi, or gastrointestinal tract increases morbidity rate.

TEN is the most severe form of drug eruption known, with a mortality rate of approximately 30%.[50] Mortality is mainly a result of respiratory complications or sepsis. Prognosis is influenced by age (>60 years), the presence of comorbidities, sepsis, and extent of body surface area involved.[9,50,51] TEN is caused almost exclusively by medications, although it may be a manifestation of severe acute GVHD.[52] The implicated medication is usually started within 3 weeks of the eruption. An increased risk for SJS and TEN has been found with the use of the following drugs: anticonvulsants (phenytoin, valproic acid, phenobarbital, and carbamazepine), antibiotics (sulfonamides and aminopenicillins), NSAIDs (oxicam derivatives), chlormezanone, allopurinol, and, interestingly, corticosteroids.[48] Drugs with long-half lives, known to be frequent culprits, have been associated with higher fatality rates.[53] TEN occurs more frequently in HIV-infected individuals, especially those receiving sulfonamides and/or nevirapine. This may be related to the concurrence of the glutathione S-transferase M1 null and the slow acetylator genotypes.[54] Precipitation of SJS and TEN by infectious agents is much less common. Infection with *Mycoplasma pneumoniae* is the best documented[55] (Table 107-8).

The pathogenesis of SJS and TEN remains unclear. Humoral and cell-mediated cytotoxicities, drug metabolites, and apoptotic mechanisms have been implicated, with inconsistent data. Experimental data suggest that activation of Fas (CD95) through its ligand, FasL (CD95L), results in caspase-mediated keratinocyte apoptosis, possibly an important pathophysiologic mechanism in TEN.[56] Fas (CD95) is a cell surface receptor expressed on keratinocytes and most cells and can be activated by FasL, which is expressed by natural killer cells and activated T lymphocytes.[57] FasL can also exist in a soluble form (sFasL), capable of inducing apoptosis.[58] Soluble FasL results from metalloproteinase-mediated cleavage

TABLE 107-7 Classification of Severe Cutaneous Adverse Drug Reactions

	SJS	TEN	Hypersensitivity/DRESS
Mucous membrane	>90%	>90%	<30%
BSA involvement[a]	<10%	>30%	<10%
Erosions	Several sites	Several sites	Mouth and lips
Detachment of epidermis	Yes	Yes	No
Hyperkeratosis/desquamation	No	No	Usual
Neutropenia	No	30%	No
Eosinophilia	No	No	90%
Atypical lymphocytes	No	No	30–40%
Respiratory tract	Bronchial erosions/ARDS	Bronchial erosions/ARDS	Interstitial pneumonitis
Liver	Hepatitis 10%	Hepatitis 10%	Hepatitis 60%
Heart	No	No	Myocarditis
Lymph node enlarged	No	No	Usual

[a] When detachment involves 10%–29% of BSA, we classify the case as SJS-TEN overlap. ARDS, adult respiratory distress syndrome; BSA, Body surface area; DRESS, drug reaction with eosinophilia and systemic symptoms; SJS, Stevens-Johnson syndrome; TEN, toxic epidermal necrolysis.
SOURCE: References 49.

TABLE 107-8 Fcctors Associated with SJS and TEN

Drugs	**Infections** (isolated cases)
Antibiotics	Mycoplasma Peumoniae
• Sulfonamides	Histoplasmosis
• Aminopenicillins	Hepatitis A
• Cephalosporins	Epstein-Barr virus
• Quinolones	Coxsackievirus B5
Anticonvulsants	Milker's nodules
• Phenobarbital	Yersiniosis
• Phenytoin	Adenovirus
• Valproic acid	Gram-negative septicemia
• Carbamazepine	
NSAIDs	
• Proxicam	
• Tenoxicam	
Allopurinol	
Chlormezanone	
Graft-versus-host disease	

SJS, Stevens-Johnson syndrome; TEN, toxic epidermal necrolysis.
SOURCE: References 9, 52.

of cell surface FasL and stimulation of peripheral blood mononuclear cells by an offending drug results in upregulated sFasL expression. Sera from SJS and TEN patients can induce Fas-FasL–mediated keratinocyte apoptosis in vitro and contain elevated concentrations of sFasL when compared with control patients.[59]

Initially, patients develop pain, tenderness, or a burning sensation in the skin. These symptoms often begin abruptly and are associated with fever and general malaise. Over the next 1 to 3 days, ill-defined erythematous macules or a diffuse erythema develop over the trunk and extremities. As the red areas enlarge, central dusky necrotic sites develop with subsequent bullae formation. Bullae result from edema occurring beneath the necrotic epidermis. As the disease progresses, sheets of full-thickness epidermis slough off, revealing dark red, moist dermis (resembling severe second-degree burns). The Nikolsky sign (separation of the skin with lateral traction) is positive and an important diagnostic clue.

Mucous membrane involvement occurs in 85% to 95% of patients and may be the presenting sign.[60] The oropharynx and conjunctivae are most affected, resulting in severe erosions and pain. Keratitis, ocular erosions, and symblepharon may result in blindness. Dysuria is a sign of urethral involvement. Erosions in the lower respiratory tract and the intestine have also been described.[61]

Hematologic studies may show anemia, eosinophilia, neutropenia, lymphopenia, thrombocytopenia, and an elevated erythrocyte sedimentation rate. Lymphopenia is seen early in the course of disease in up to 90% of cases and is a result of depletion of CD4 T lymphocytes. Neutropenia is seen in up to 30% of cases and carries a poor prognosis.[62] Serum chemistries show evidence of extensive fluid and protein loss, hypoalbuminemia, and hypocalcemia.[63] Taking a small piece of tender erythematous skin for frozen section may help make a rapid diagnosis. This will show the level of the separation within the skin and, in TEN, reveals full-thickness necrosis of the epidermis, with an intact dermis with little or no inflammation. Alternatively, a skin biopsy in an area immediately adjacent to and overlapping a blister may be sent for routine histology. The irregular presence of necrotic keratinocytes

along the dermal-epidermal junction is a hallmark of early lesions, whereas diffuse epidermal necrosis with subepidermal clefting is present in late lesions. There is minimal dermal inflammation. Immunofluorescence findings are nondescript, with no significant complement or antibody deposition, suggesting that cell-mediated cytotoxicity is an important mechanism.

The clinical differential diagnosis includes staphylococcal scalded skin syndrome, acute GVHD, scarlet fever, erythema multiforme, and pemphigus vulgaris. In all these cases, full-thickness epidermal necrosis is rare (except in GVHD, in which epidermal necrosis is accompanied by an abundant lymphocytic infiltrate).

Erythema multiforme (previously referred to as erythema multiforme minor), is an acute, self-limited reaction characterized by asymptomatic, annular erythematous, or urticarial plaques with central areas of blistering and necrosis, resulting in the so-called target lesions. Lesions usually develop on the extensor surfaces of the extremities and mucosae and cover less than 10% of the body surface area. Outbreaks last for 1 to 4 weeks. Relapses are frequent. It is associated with recurrent herpes simplex virus infections in the great majority of cases and with *M. pneumoniae* infection in a smaller subset.

Treatment for SJS and TEN includes pain management and prompt withdrawal of any agents that are not essential for the maintenance of life. This latter has been shown to decrease mortality rate in TEN by about 30% per day, despite some progression of the mucocutaneous involvement.[64] Fluid resuscitation, treatment of infections, and meticulous skin and eye care are most appropriately managed in an isolation room in a burn unit, where the staff is trained in topical wound and skin care. Severe airway involvement may necessitate intubation and ventilation. An ophthalmologic consultation should be obtained to assess eye involvement, which is usually treated with topical antibiotics and lubricants. If symblepharon occurs, early lysis must be performed. Fluid and electrolyte imbalances are related to the percentage of body surface area involved; however, fluid loss tends to be less than in severe burn patients. Topical therapy includes gentle debridement of necrotic skin followed by the application of nonadherent dressings to the areas of skin erosion, a wrapping of a thin silver-impregnated dressing, and an outer linen covering to hold all in place. Antibiotic ointments are widely used, although their value is unproved. It is important to avoid the sulfonamide derivatives (silver sulfadiazine cream, topical mafenide acetate, and ophthalmic sodium sulfacetamide) because of potential significant absorption and the possibility of inducing SJS.[65] A variety of other dressings may be used to decrease fluid loss and pain and promote wound healing, and may be useful adjuncts to therapy. These include porcine xenografts[66] and synthetic dressings such as Omniderm, OpSite, Vigilon, Mepitel, and Biobrane. Systemic antibiotics should be used only when there is documented infection or neutropenia.

The use of corticosteroids and immunosuppressive agents in the treatment of TEN is controversial. The rationale for such an approach is based on the assumption that TEN is an immune-mediated event. There are no case-controlled studies supporting the use of corticosteroids; however, several case reports have advocated their use.[67,68] In most cases in which steroids were found effective, they were started very early in the course of the disease. More recent literature has indicated a higher mortality rate, increased time to recovery, and increased length of hospital stay in patients treated with systemic corticosteroids.[69,70] Patients undergoing long-term glucocorticoid therapy who develop TEN may have a delay in onset, but the severity of disease is unaffected.[71] Based on this information, corticosteroids should not be used routinely in TEN and should only be considered in patients who present early in the course of disease. Intravenous immunoglobulin therapy in TEN aims to decrease Fas-mediated keratinocyte apoptosis by sequestering Fas available for binding to CD95. Four nonrandomized, uncontrolled studies have shown that large-dose intravenous immunoglobulin decreases mortality rate and progression of TEN,[72–75] whereas one prospective study showed no benefit.[49] Hence, there is no consensus, and controlled, randomized trials are needed. The use of plasmapheresis and immunosuppressive drugs remains controversial due to the lack of strong clinical data.

HYPERSENSITIVITY SYNDROME/DRUG REACTION WITH EOSINOPHILIA AND SYSTEMIC SYMPTOMS

A severe hypersensitivity syndrome consisting of fever, rash, lymphadenopathy, and variable organ (usually liver) involvement may appear after several weeks of drug ingestion. When associated with eosinophilia and systemic symptoms, the term *drug reaction with eosinophilia and systemic symptoms* is used (see Table 107-7). The most common precipitants are the aromatic anticonvulsants (e.g., phenytoin, phenobarbital, and carbamazepine). Faulty metabolism of these drugs is thought to precipitate the disease process, which has also been associated with the initiation or reactivation of infection with human herpes virus type 6.[76] There is a 75% incidence of cross-reactivity between these anticonvulsants; therefore, once one of these drugs has caused a reaction, further exposure to any of them should not be attempted. Other medications known to cause this syndrome include dapsone, sulfonamides, allopurinol and minocycline.[77]

The cutaneous component of this ADR varies from a maculopapular eruption to frank erythroderma. Discontinuation of the offending agent and the administration of moderate to large doses of systemic steroids are the treatments of choice and have shown benefit in multiple case reports. Supportive care, similar to that for SJS and TEN, in an ICU or burn unit, must be instituted when life-threatening visceral manifestations are present, whereas topical steroids alone may be sufficient for mild disease.

Medical Dermatoses

PEMPHIGUS VULGARIS

Pemphigus vulgaris (PV) is an autoimmune, mucocutaneous, blistering disease characterized by an intraepidermal split that results in superficial flaccid bullae. Autoantibodies directed against intercellular adhering junction antigens lead to bullae formation. Circulating IgG directed toward intercellular desmogleins 3 and 1, which interact with plakoglobin in the dense plaque of the desmosome, can be detected in the serum and skin biopsies from perilesional skin.[78,79] The stimulus for the circulating autoantibodies is unknown. PV has been described in association with autoimmune diseases, malignancy, and medications.[80] The medications most often cited

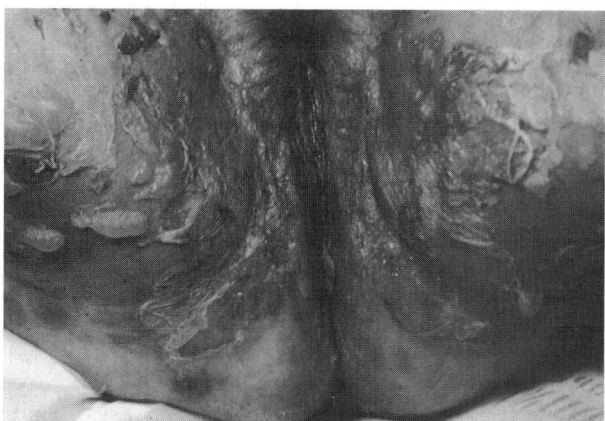

FIGURE 107-6 Pemphigus vulgaris. Flaccid, superficial bullae which rupture easily leaving superficial erosions. (*Courtesy Dr. Anne Laumann collection.*) See Plate 107-6.

have thiol groups in their molecules, such as penicillamine and captopril.[81] PV occurring in association with an underlying neoplasm is termed paraneoplastic pemphigus. Paraneoplastic PV is seen primarily with lymphomas. Patients develop flaccid bullae on normal or slightly erythematous skin. The bullae rupture easily, leaving superficial and crusted erosions (Fig. 107-6, Plate 107-6). The presence of Nikolsky's sign (lateral extension of an intraepidermal split with application of pressure to small intact bullae) is a characteristic feature. Blisters may occur anywhere on the body, with a predilection for the trunk, groin, scalp, and face. Mucous membrane involvement is characteristic. The oral mucosa is involved in more than 95% of patients and is the initial manifestation in up to 70%.[82] Intact bullae are rarely seen due to their superficial location. PV occurs primarily in the middle and older age groups.

The diagnosis of PV is made using routine (hematoxylin and eosin) dermatopathologic analysis of a biopsy from the border of an active lesion in addition to direct immunofluorescence (DIF: patient's skin and anti-immunoglobulin) of a biopsy specimen from perilesional skin and indirect immunofluorescence (IIF) of a serum sample (patient's serum incubated with monkey esophagus and then with anti-immunoglobulin). Histologic examination shows loss of adhesion between keratinocytes (acantholysis) above the basal layer, resulting in an intraepidermal split. DIF reveals IgG and complement deposition between keratinocytes within the epidermis. IIF reveals intercellular IgG deposition on monkey esophagus. The IIF titer may be quantified and loosely reflects disease activity.

Before the advent of corticosteroids, PV carried a high mortality rate. At present, patients are typically started on doses of at least 1 to 2 mg/kg per day of prednisone to halt progression of the disease. Azathioprine may be started concurrently at a dose of 50 to 100 mg/day. The dose is calculated based on the red blood cell concentration of thiopurine methyltransferase, an enzyme involved in the metabolism of the thiopurine drugs, because low concentrations of this enzyme may lead to serious side effects, such as excessive myelosuppression, and high concentrations may lead to rapid metabolism of azathioprine and potential underdosing.[83] Immunosuppressants should be initiated early in the course of the disease to allow time for their immunosuppressant

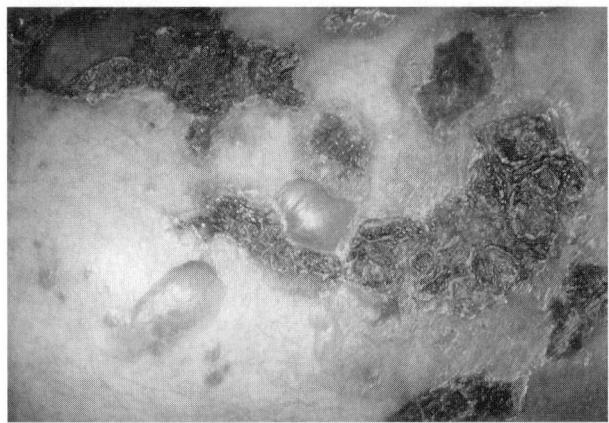

FIGURE 107-7 Bullous pemphigoid. Tense bullae arising on an erythematous plaque. *(Courtesy Dr. Anne Laumann collection.)* See Plate 107-7.

actions to take effect as this may take up to 6 weeks. Current therapeutic regimens also include parenteral gold, dapsone, plasmapheresis, intravenous immune globulin, and other immunosuppressant agents, such as cyclosporine, cyclophosphamide, and mycophenolate mofetil.[84,85]

BULLOUS PEMPHIGOID

Bullous pemphigoid (BP) is a self-limited autoimmune blistering disease characterized by tense, subepidermal bullae (Fig. 107-7, Plate 107-7). Autoantibodies develop to portions of the hemidesmosome complex in the basement membrane zone. The resulting disruption in adhesion leads to a subepidermal split from the dermis. These antigens are identified by their molecular weights, 230 kDa (BPAGI) and 180 kDa (BPAG2). Table 107-9 lists the characteristics that distinguish BP from PV.

BP has an estimated incidence rate of 7 per million per year. It occurs equally in men and women usually between 60 and 80 years of age. Approximately 50% of treated patients will go into remission within 2.5 to 6 years of onset of disease; however, individuals may have active disease for as long as 10 years. There is a predilection for tense blisters on normal or erythematous skin to occur in the groin, axillae, and flexu-

ral areas. Nikolsky sign is negative. Mucous membranes are involved in approximately 20% of patients. In addition to the bullae, patients may have urticarial weals and serpiginous erythematous plaques. Lesions heal without scarring, although there may be significant pigmentary change.[86]

Histopathologic sections show a split between the epidermis and the dermis, with an infiltrate consisting predominantly of eosinophils. Lymphocytes and neutrophils may also be present in the superficial and deep dermis. DIF of perilesional skin shows a linear deposition of IgG and complement along the basement membrane zone. Although the titer does not reflect disease activity, indirect immunofluoresence (IIF) studies show circulating antibasement membrane zone IgG antibodies in 70% to 80%.[87]

Corticosteroids, at smaller doses ($\leq$1 mg/kg per day) than those used for pemphigus vulgaris (PV), have been the mainstay of treatment for widespread disease. Localized or mild disease may respond to antibiotics at anti-inflammatory doses such as tetracycline 1 to 3 g/day or erythromycin 1 to 3 g/d with nicotinamide 1 g three times daily and/or high-potency topical steroids. Other therapies include dapsone and immunosuppressants such as azathioprine, cyclophosphamide, chlorambucil, mycophenolate mofetil, and methotrexate.[88]

PSORIASIS

Psoriasis is a chronic, recurrent skin condition that affects 1% to 3% of the population. Both sexes are equally affected. Well-defined circular or oval plaques with adherent silver scale characterize the lesions. Lesions have a predilection for extensor surfaces, especially the knees, elbows, scalp, and the superior end of the gluteal fold. Psoriatic lesions often develop at sites of physical trauma such as scratched areas, surgical incisions, and tape removal. This finding is referred to as the Köbner phenomenon. Initial psoriatic episodes that may occur 2 to 3 weeks after a streptococcal infection sometimes appear as widespread, asymptomatic, small red papules with a silvery scale. This is called guttate psoriasis and usually resolves over 2 to 3 months with no specific treatment. Drugs may also precipitate or exacerbate preexisting psoriasis. Well-known culprits include the withdrawal of systemic or strong topical steroids or other immunosuppressive agents and the administration of β blockers, antimalarials, or lithium.

TABLE 107-9 Comparison of Pemphigus Vulgaris and Bullous Pemphigoid

	Pemphigus Vulgaris	Bullous Pemphigoid
Age at onset	40–60 y	50–80 y
Clinical appearance	Superficial *flaccid* bullae erosions	Large *tense* bullae, urticarial wheals and serpigenous plaques
Nikolsky sign	Positive	Negative
Mucous membrane involvement	$\geq$95% (often is initial sign of disease)	$\leq$20%
Histology	Intraepidermal split	Subepidermal split
Direct immunofluorescence	IgG and complement (C3) deposition between keratinocytes	Linear deposition of IgG and C3 along basement membrane zone
Antigen	Desmoglein 3 (130 kDa), plakoglobin (85 kDa)	BP Ag I (230 kDa), BP Ag II (180 kDa)
Course	Mild to severe, may require large doses of steroids to control	Mild, tends to respond readily to systemic steroids

ABBREVIATION: Ag, antigen; BP, bullous pemphigoid; IgG, immunoglobulin G.

Alcohol abuse and HIV infection are associated with extensive and resistant psoriasis.[89]

Many clinical variants of psoriasis exist. Generalized pustular psoriasis, also referred to as von Zumbusch psoriasis, is a rare but serious variant that is characterized by diffuse pustules on erythematous plaques. Erythematous skin rapidly develops crops of pustules that coalesce to form "lakes of pus." Nails, palms, and soles are often affected. Fever, hypocalcemia, and leukocytosis may accompany the outbreak. The average age of onset is 50 years, with no sexual predilection. Precipitating factors include drugs, infection, pregnancy, exertion, and menstruation. The differential diagnosis in a patient with diffuse pustules and fever includes infection, drug reaction, acute generalized exanthematous pustulosis, pustular psoriasis, and subcorneal pustular dermatosis.[90,91]

Psoriasis may be treated initially with a variety of topical medications. These include corticosteroids, calcipotriene, tar, anthralin, and topical retinoids. These agents are used as monotherapy or in combination. Systemic drugs are reserved for extensive or disabling disease and include methotrexate, cyclosporine, and oral retinoids. Ultraviolet (UV) light therapy is often used in combination with topical and/or systemic agents. UV light therapy has been a mainstay of treatment for years. This includes natural sunshine, broadband UVB (280 to 320 nm), UVA (320 to 400nm), and a single-wavelength light narrowband UVB (311 nm). Psoralen, a photosensitizer, is used to potentiate the UVA effects in a regimen called PUVA. Acitretin, a systemic retinoid, may be used alone or in combination with phototherapy. Biologic therapy that targets specific cytokines and intercellular adhesion molecules has recently been introduced. At the time of writing three of these agents have been approved by the Food and Drug Administration for the treatment of psoriasis. Alefacept is a recombinant protein containing human leukocyte function-associated antigen 3 and human IgG1. IG binds to CD2 on memory-effector cells. Efalizumab is a humanized monoclonal antibody to CD11a, a subunit of LFA-1. IG inhibits trafficking of T-cells to the skin and T-cell reactivation in the skin. Etanercept is a soluble recombinant human tumor necrosis factor 2 receptor that binds the circulating inflammatory stimulator tumor necrosis factor 2. Each is administered parenterally using unique dosing regimens.[92,93] The long-term affects of these therapies are not yet known. Acitretin, narrowband UVB, PUVA, methotrexate, and cyclosporine have been used effectively in the treatment of generalized pustular psoriasis.[94]

ERYTHRODERMA

Erythroderma or *exfoliative dermatitis* is a descriptive term for a clinical condition characterized by total body diffuse erythema and scaling (Fig. 107-8, Plate 107-8). The skin is initially red and warm. Scaling and exfoliation, often accompanied by fever, chills, and lymphadenopathy, follow. The percutaneous absorption barrier is lost and blood flow to the skin increases, which may lead to serious complications such as hypoalbuminemia, peripheral edema, loss of muscle mass, and high-output cardiac failure, with as much as 8% of the total cardiac output being directed at the inflamed cutaneous vasculature. Causes of exfoliative dermatitis include inflammatory conditions, drug eruptions, cutaneous T-cell lymphoma, and systemic neoplasms (Table 107-10). Common inflammatory

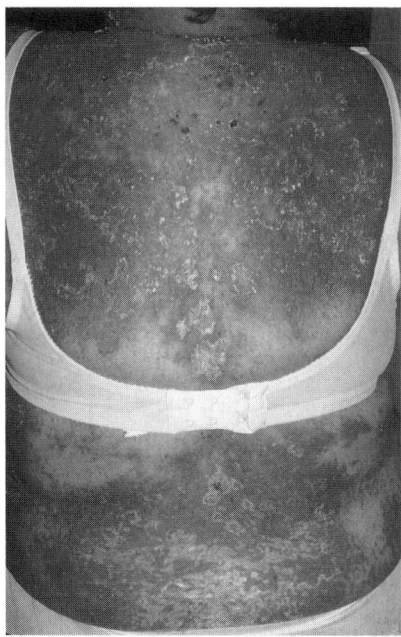

FIGURE 107-8 Erythroderma. Generalized erythema, edema, and scaling. *(Courtesy Dr. Anne Laumann collection.)* **See Plate 107-8.**

conditions include psoriasis, atopic dermatitis, contact dermatitis, and pityriasis rubra pilaris. Antiepileptic medications (carbamazepine, phenobarbital, or phenytoin), antihypertensive medications (captopril or chlorothiazide), antibiotics (cephalosporins, dapsone, isoniazid, or minocycline), and calcium channel blockers have been associated with exfoliative erythroderma.[95] Lymphomas and hematologic malignancies are common systemic neoplasms that may cause erythroderma. Sézary syndrome is the leukemic form of cutaneous T-cell lymphoma, which is characterized by circulating atypical lymphocytes with hyperconvoluted nuclei (Sézary cells). These atypical cells are identified on blood smear or in skin biopsies. Internal malignancies occasionally cause erythroderma.

The erythrodermic patient should be monitored with specific attention to fluid and electrolyte balance, temperature regulation, and nutritional status. Skin biopsy may help identify the underlying cause of the dermatosis and thus direct specific treatment. Initial management includes the use of medium potency topical steroid ointments covered with a

TABLE 107-10 Differential Diagnosis of Erythroderma

Atopic dermatitis
Contact dermatitis
Graft-versus-host disease
Lymphoma:
  Cutaneous T-cell lymphoma
  Sézary syndrome
Leukemia
Psoriasis
Pityriasis rubra pilaris
Seborrheic dermatitis
Toxic epidermal necrolysis (early)
Toxic shock syndrome
Streptococcal toxic shock syndrome

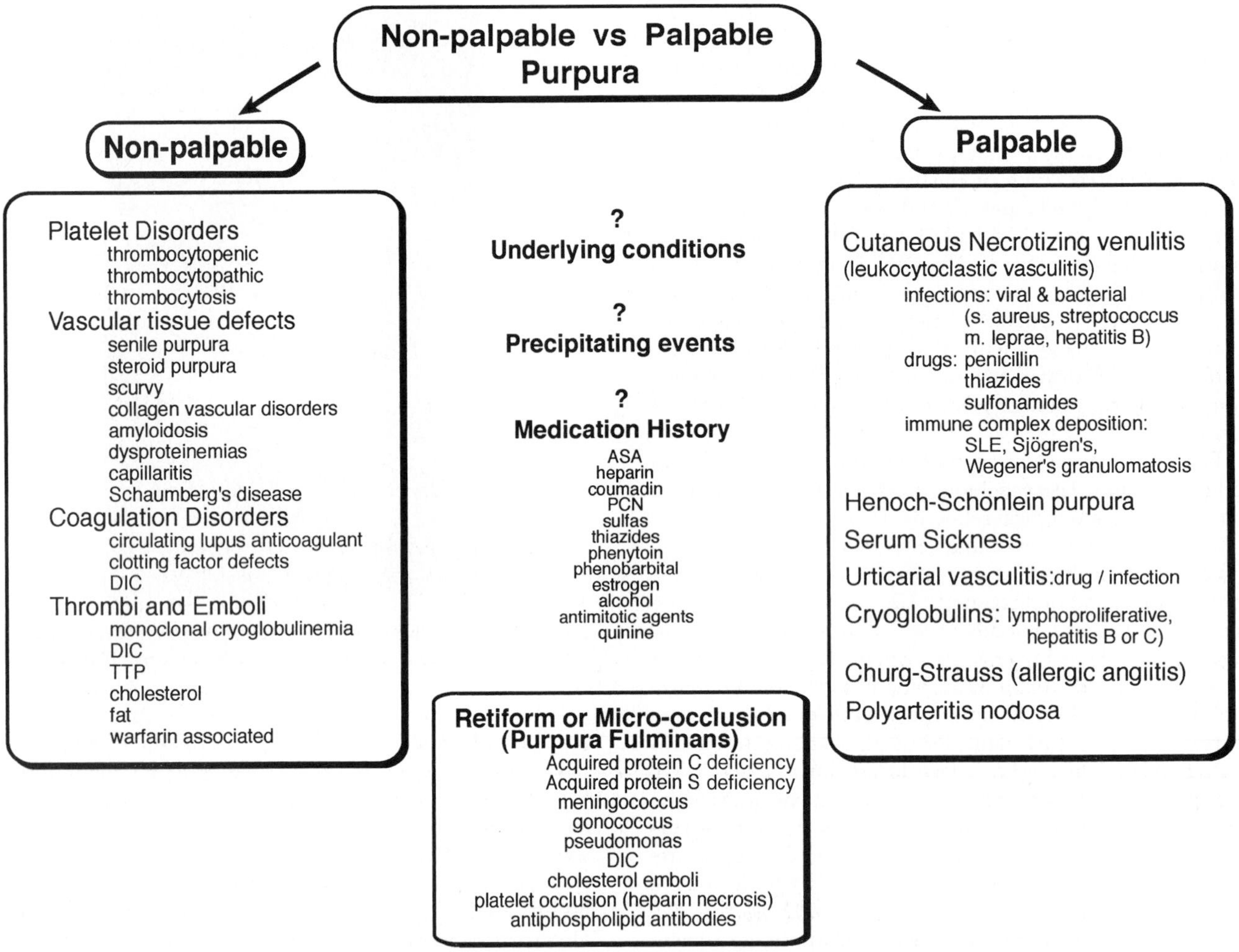

FIGURE 107-9 An approach to purpura. DIC, disseminated intravascular coagulation; TTP, thrombotic thrombocytopenia purpura; ASA, aspirin; PCN, penicillin; SLE, systemic lupus erythematosus.

bland ointment, such as zinc oxide ointment and wrapped with clean cloths, or topical steroids applied directly under a plastic sauna suit. It is important to avoid topical irritant agents, such as tar-containing ointments. Wet dressings may help weeping or crusted areas. Pruritus and anxiety typically respond to the sedating antihistamines. Alternatively, doxepin at doses of 25 to 50 may be given at bedtime.

PURPURA

Purpura is a clinical term that represents the extravasation of blood into surrounding tissues.[96] Purpura is a common skin condition that has many causes. An approach to the patient with purpura focusing on the dermatologic decision-making algorithm is discussed (Fig. 107-9). The type of lesion depends on the depth of the vascular plexus involved, the size of the vessel injury, precipitating factors, and coextravasated circulating substances. Visual and tactile assessments of a lesion are crucial. Lesions are placed into two main categories, palpable or nonpalpable (Fig. 107-10, Plate 107-10). The patient's underlying conditions, potential precipitating events, current and past laboratory values, and medication history are analyzed.

Nonpalpable (macular), nonblanching purpura arises from simple hemorrhage into tissue. The dermal vascular network consists of superficial and deep vascular plexuses. The superficial plexus possesses arteriovenous loops that ascend into the dermal papilla. Petechiae are lesions smaller than 0.2 cm in diameter that result from superficial vascular hemorrhage. Larger areas are termed *ecchymoses*. Nonpalpable purpura is most commonly attributed to fragility of the vascular tissue or defects in hemostasis. Examples include actinic or solar purpura (owing to the age-related loss of collagen in the basement membrane of blood vessels) and purpura secondary to systemic corticosteroids (related to inhibition of lysyl oxidase that is required for synthesis of type IV collagen, the principal collagen associated with blood vessel basement membrane integrity). Cutaneous amyloid, primary or secondary resulting from myeloma, may be deposited in endothelial cells.[97] Deposition results in vascular fragility so that nonpalpable lesions representing common bruises, sometimes called *pinch purpura*, may occur after minor trauma. This occurs mainly on the face, especially periorbitally. Other common causes of flat purpura include platelet disorders (thrombocytopenia, thrombocytopathia, and thrombocytosis), disseminated intravascular coagulation (DIC), and warfarin-associated necrosis. If the diagnosis cannot be made on clinical grounds, a skin biopsy may be helpful. Flat purpura in neutropenic patients is approached as if it were palpable purpura, because these patients are unable to mount the appropriate

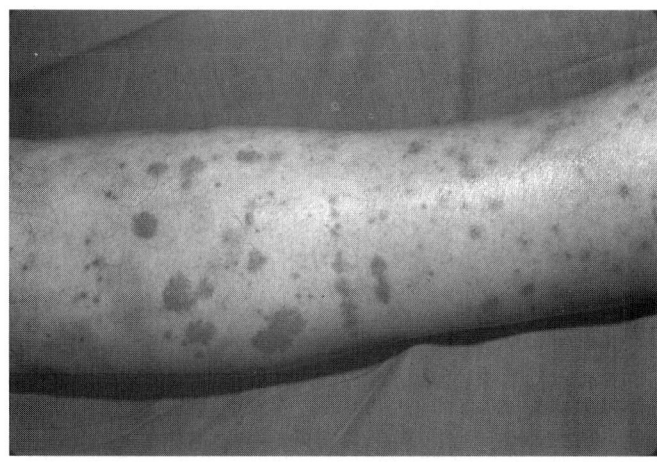

FIGURE 107-10 Palpable purpura (leukocytoclastic vasculitis). Erythematous to violaceous plaques on the lower extremity, which do not blanch with pressure. *(Courtesy Dr. Denise Rubenstein collection.)* **See Plate 107-10.**

immune response to cause dermal inflammation. In such patients, biopsy is important to assist with diagnosis.

Palpable purpura indicates underlying vasculitis (also called *cutaneous necrotizing venulitis* or *leukocytoclastic vasculitis*). For the first 24 to 48 hours, the lesions are a deep erythematous color that eventually becomes violaceous. The pathologic process results from segmental vascular inflammation, swelling and necrosis of endothelial cells, and neutrophilic infiltration of vessel walls with fragmentation of nuclei.

As outlined in Fig. 107-9, many factors may lead to vasculitic injury. Precipitating factors include infections, drugs, autoimmune diseases, and immunoglobulin-mediated complement activation. Common infectious agents include *Staphylococcus aureus*, hepatitis B, and hepatitis C. Drugs commonly associated with vasculitis include ampicillins, thiazides, phenytoin, sulfa-containing compounds, allopurinol, hydralazine, and propylthiouracil.

Workup includes identification of a potential primary cause and evaluation for systemic involvement. In addition to a biopsy, a complete blood count, chemistry panel, liver function tests, urinalysis, stool guaiac, hepatitis B and C viral serologies, cryoglobulins, and complement levels are evaluated. Antinuclear antibody titers are evaluated in patients with suspected connective tissue diseases. In patients with a fever and heart murmur, blood cultures and echocardiography should be performed.[98]

Retiform purpura is referred to as *purpura fulminans*, a pattern usually indicative of micro-occlusion. In contrast to inflammatory purpura, this type immediately manifests as violaceous purpura that may or may not be palpable. Lesions appear abruptly and display a retiform or jagged edge, sometimes blending into a livedo pattern at the periphery. The major causes of micro-occlusive disease include disseminated intravascular coagulation, meningococcemia, acquired protein C or S deficiency, warfarin-induced skin necrosis, antiphospholipid antibody syndrome, sepsis of various causes, cryoglobulinemia, cryofibrinogenemia, paroxysmal nocturnal hemoglobinuria, and cholesterol emboli.[99]

GRAFT-VERSUS-HOST DISEASE (GVHD)

GVHD is a complex syndrome which occurs after allogeneic bone marrow transplantation. The skin is often the first and is the most frequent organ involved. Biopsy may help distinguish GVHD from other causes of erythema such as drug eruptions or viral exanthems. Acute GVHD usually occurs between days 10 and 30 after transplantation, but may appear at anytime.[100]

Skin changes consist of a generalized morbilliform eruption progressing to extensive redness, blistering, or skin necrosis. The earliest sign is pruritus and tenderness of the palms and soles, with reddening of the dorsal aspects of the fingers and periungual skin. Diffuse erythema of the hands and feet soon follows. In addition, the ears are commonly affected. Unusual clinical patterns may be seen due to the polymorphous nature of this disease. Confluence of lesions occurs on the trunk as the disease progresses. Blisters (with a positive Nikolsky sign) and generalized desquamation portend a poor prognosis. The palmar and plantar erythemas of acute GVHD need to be differentiated from those of palmar-plantar erythrodysesthesia due to chemotherapeutic agents. This syndrome may occur with GVHD or in similar clinical situations. The erythrodysesthesia begins as spotty erythema on the thenar and hypothenar eminences and progresses to severe pain and swelling.

The original grading system for GVHD was described in 1974 and is still in use today.[101] Several features of GVHD are recognized: (1) 72% of transplanted patients develop clinically recognizable GVHD; (2) an increase in the serum aspartate aminotransferase concentration is related to the onset or worsening of the skin erruption; (3) cutaneous symptoms precede systemic involvement by 2 to 3 days; and (4) the severity of GVHD does not correlate with the underlying disease process, the conditioning regimen, or the day of onset after grafting. The initial management strategy when GVHD is suspected includes obtaining a skin biopsy to look for the characteristic changes. Unfortunately, the diagnostic yield of skin biopsies for GVHD is only 50% to 65%. When biopsies show nonspecific changes, additional biopsies are recommended in 24 to 48 hours. Tissue cultures to look for bacteria, mycobacteria, and fungi should be performed in febrile patients.

Factors associated with a high risk of developing GVHD include an HLA mismatch, an unrelated donor, older age of the recipient or donor, a sex mismatch, T-cell replete grafts, donor allosensitization, regimen toxicity, and compromised delivery of GVHD prophylaxis.[102] splenectomy, bone marrow cell dose, and ABO match. Polymorphism of minor determinants such as the adhesion molecule CD31 may account for the risk of GVHD between HLA identical donor and transplant recipients.[103] Future testing for minor and major determinants may help decrease the risk and severity of GVHD.

GVHD has also been described after autologous and syngeneic transplantation. This phenomenon has stimulated much interest because it indicates that factors other than donor reactivity against recipient antigens may be involved in allogenic GVHD. In autologous GVHD, only the skin is involved, and lesions typically resolve within 7 days. The combination of total body irradiation (which causes failure of the peripheral autoregulatory mechanisms) and cyclosporine (which blocks clonal deletion of autoreactive T cells that escape from the thymus) are believed to be important factors.[104] Treatment for acute GVHD includes modifying the original immunosuppressive prophylactic regimen (cyclosporine, tacrolimus, or mycophenolate mofetil) and adding methylprednisolone at 2 mg/kg. Treatment protocols differ and may include anti-thymocyte globulin, intravenous immunoglobulin (IVIG), and monoclonal antibodies. Topical treatment is mainly supportive, with emollients and topical steroids. Erythrodermic and severe blistering patients deserve close monitoring and aggressive immunosuppression. Other therapies reported to be beneficial in the treatment of GVHD include ultraviolet light therapy (PUVA, broad band or narrow band UVB) extracorporeal photochemotherapy (photopheresis), pentoxifylline, and thalidomide.

Dermatoses Precipitated by Infection

BACTERIAL INFECTIONS

Infectious organisms can involve the skin via a primary or secondary route. Primary infections begin as a localized exogenous invasion that can spread superficially or invade to the deeper subcutaneous tissue, depending on host and virulence factors. Secondary infections occur by hematogenous dissemination of the organism or portions of the organism and may be accompanied by immune complex deposition.

IMPETIGO

Impetigo is a primary bacterial infection that occurs in two forms: impetigo contagiosa (caused by staphylococci and, less commonly, streptococci), and bullous impetigo (caused by a toxin released from *S. aureus*). Impetigo usually appears on exposed areas such as the face and extremities in children, the elderly, and the immunosuppressed. Impetigo begins as an erythematous plaque with scattered vesicles that subsequently rupture to form honey-colored crusts. The infection often begins after minor trauma allows bacterial invasion of the superficial epidermis. Constitutional symptoms are generally absent but regional lymphadenopathy is common. Bullous impetigo is characterized by large flaccid bullae that have a positive Nikolsky sign. Bullous impetigo is caused by a toxin-producing strain of phage group II *S. aureus*. Bullous impetigo may be considered a localized form of staphylococcal scalded skin syndrome.

The diagnosis of impetigo is made based on clinical findings. Culture and sensitivity may be useful to confirm the diagnosis or when resistant or nephritogenic strains are suspected. Anti-DNAase B and antihyaluronidase titers rise significantly after streptococcal skin infection, but there is no change in the antistreptolysin titer.[105] Bullous impetigo is a toxin-mediated process and culture of blister fluid is often

negative. Serious secondary infections related to pyoderma include osteomyelitis, septic arthritis, and pneumonia.

The prevalence of erythromycin-resistant streptococci and staphylococci has been increasing in recent years, so erythromycin is no longer a treatment of choice. Treatment includes room temperature tap water compresses in conjunction with topical mupirocin or a β-lactamase–resistant penicillin (dicloxacillin or cloxacillin) or a first-generation cephalosporin (cephalexin). Azithromycin may be given to penicillin-allergic patients. Up to 15% of individuals, usually children between the ages of 2 and 4 years, with impetigo caused by a group A streptococcal nephritogenic strain (usually M-49 serotype) develop acute poststreptococcal glomerulonephritis 1 to 5 weeks (median = 10 days) after infection. Occasionally, a group C streptococcus is involved.[106] The overall incidence of nephritis related to impetigo is 2% to 5%. The use of antibiotics does not appear to decrease the incidence of poststreptococcal glomerulonephritis, despite prompt clinical and bacteriologic responses.[107]

NECROTIZING FASCIITIS

Necrotizing fasciitis (NF) is a rapidly progressive suppurative bacterial infection of the superficial and deep fascia that, if left unchecked, progresses to gangrene, sepsis, and death (see Chap. 55). Classically, this has been associated with group A streptococcus alone or with concomitant facultative and anaerobic bacteria (clostridium, bacteroides, Enterobacteriaceae, *Vibrio* species, and non–group A streptococci).[108]

NF occurs in adults of any age who may be otherwise healthy. Predisposing factors include any condition that may cause a break in the skin, such as varicella, cuts, burns, surgical procedures, and child birth. Diseases such as diabetes and cirrhosis, immunosuppression, and drugs such as infliximab may also increase the risk of infection.[109] The patient's use of NSAIDS may delay diagnosis and allow for rapid progression of infection owing to attenuation of the early inflammatory host response and alteration of the humoral immune response.[110]

Patients present with skin erythema, edema, warmth, and tenderness often localized to one limb. Other areas such as the face are affected less often.[111] Within 24 hours there is rapid spread proximally and distally along the limb, and there may be a bluish necrotic hue and bullae appearing within the affected area. The key features that distinguish NF from cellulitis are rapid spread and significant tenderness.

The diagnosis of NF is primarily clinical. Computed tomography or magnetic resonance imaging may help locate the site and extent of infection. In mixed anaerobic infections, plain radiographs may detect gas in the soft tissues. In evaluation of a swollen painful extremity, compartment pressure measurements may be useful. If pressures are elevated (>40 mm Hg), immediate fasciotomy is indicated. A superficial skin biopsy does not aid in the diagnosis. Tissue sampling that extends to the fascia is required.

Surgical debridement or incisional drainage is essential for treatment. Concomitant treatment with antibiotics should not delay surgical management. Antibiotics alone are ineffective owing to the amount of vascular occlusion in the affected area and to the slower growth rate of streptococci in large inocula.[112] After debridement, tissue should be Gram stained and cultured for aerobes and anaerobes. Empiric antibiotic therapy includes penicillin and/or clindamycin.

TOXIC SHOCK SYNDROME

Toxic shock syndrome (TSS) is characterized by fever, shock, desquamating rash, and multiorgan system failure in association with toxins mediated from group A streptococcal or *S. aureus* infections. Streptococcal TSS (STSS) is seen most often in association with soft tissue infection, including necrotizing fasciitis (NF). The syndrome appears to be mediated by one or more of the streptococcal pyrogenic exotoxins (types A, B, or C). Type A exotoxin has the most potent inflammatory and cytotoxic properties and is most closely associated with STSS.[113] These toxins may act as superantigens by directly linking the major histocompatibility complex of antigen presenting cells to the V-β portion of the T-cell receptor, thus bypassing the limiting step of antigen processing and resulting in massive T-cell activation.[114] Up to 80% of patients with this syndrome present with soft tissue infections.[115] Other access sites include the mucous membranes, such as the vagina, intravenous drug use, and burn wounds.[116,117] In patients with no identifiable portal of entry, seeding of infection is thought to occur by a transient bacteremia originating in the pharynx. Symptomatic sore throat may occasionally precede STSS. Patients, who tend to be young and in good health, present with influenza-like symptoms (fever, myalgias, malaise, headache, nausea, vomiting, or diarrhea) often in conjunction with pain and erythema of an area such as an extremity. Approximately 20% of patients will develop a generalized blanching erythema that desquamates at days 7 to 14.[118]

The criteria for diagnosis of STSS are presented in Table 107-11. Laboratory data that support the diagnosis of STSS include a normal or moderately elevated white blood cell count with a profound left shift, azotemia, hypocalcemia, hypoalbuminemia, thrombocytopenia, hematuria, and an elevated creatine kinase. It is interesting to note that evidence of renal impairment precedes hypotension in approximately 50% of patients at the time of admission to the hospital and develops in all others within 4 to 8 hours after admission.

TSS caused by *S. aureus* begins with a scarlatiniform eruption. There may be flexural accentuation, erythema and edema of the palms and soles, hyperemia of the conjunctivae and mucous membranes, and a strawberry tongue.[119] In contrast to STSS, which tends to present with a localized soft tissue infection, signs of infection are often absent in TSS mediated by *S. aureus*–producing toxin. Both syndromes tend to occur in young healthy adults, but TSS may be associated with staphylococcal overgrowth of occluded mucosal surfaces (e.g., superabsorbent tampons or nasal gauze packing).

Treatment of STSS and TSS consists of supportive care, vasopressors, and antibiotics. Adequate antimicrobial coverage for *Staphylococcus* and *Streptococcus* should be initiated with clindamycin alone or in combination with penicillin.[120] Treatment with intravenous γ globulin may be considered in patients who present hypotensive and with a cellulitis.[121] Hyperbaric O_2 and plasmapheresis have also been used in STSS.[41,122]

STAPHYLOCOCCAL SCALDED SKIN SYNDROME

Staphylococcal scalded skin syndrome (SSSS; Fig. 107-11, Plate 107-11) is a desquamative exanthem that occurs in conjunction with infection of toxin-producing *S. aureus* phage group II types 3A, 3C, 55, and 71.[123] The desquamation is mediated by exfoliative toxins A and B.[124] Most patients are younger than 5 years, and adults are only rarely affected. The major risk factors for developing SSSS in adults are renal failure (owing to decreased filtration of toxin), hematologic malignancies, and immunosuppression. The concurrent use of NSAIDs may predispose to SSSS.[125]

Several factors make SSSS an important consideration in the ICU setting. Nasal carriage of *S. aureus* is three times higher in hospital personnel and dialysis patients than in the general population. Approximately 6% of the coagulase-positive *S. aureus* strains randomly isolated from hospitalized patients are toxigenic. Patients in the ICU may be immunosuppressed and/or have renal failure, thereby increasing their risk for acquiring SSSS.

The disease process is similar to bullous impetigo but is generalized rather than localized. Patients may have a preceding upper respiratory infection with rhinorrhea, pharyngitis, and conjunctivitis. The exanthem begins abruptly with diffuse tender erythema and subsequent superficial desquamation. The erythematous skin has a rough sandpaper-like texture often accentuated in the flexural and periorificial area. Because the split occurs in the granular layer (superficial) of the epidermis), intact bullae are rarely seen although when present, the Nikolsky sign may be positive. The skin appears bright pink, moist, and eroded skin after desquamation. The clinical presentation sometimes may be difficult to separate from that of toxic epidermal neurolysis (TEN).

Cultures are taken from all orifices (eye, nose, throat, vagina, and rectum) and blood. The diagnosis of SSSS is supported by the isolation of *S. aureus*. Rapid distinction from TEN may be made by frozen section of the exfoliated skin and histopathologic examination to determine the level of cleavage. Biopsy at the border of a blister and normal skin should also be sent for routine processing. Cultures from blisters are negative owing to the toxin-mediated nature of the disease.

Treatment of SSSS requires appropriate antibiotics and vigilant monitoring of fluids and electrolytes. Antibiotic choice usually includes penicillinase-resistant semisynthetic penicillins (nafcillin, methicillin, or dicloxacillin) or a

---

TABLE 107-11 Definition of Streptococcal Toxic Shock Syndrome (Proposed)

Isolation of group A streptococci from a normally sterile site[a] (e.g., blood, pleural fluid, cerebrospinal fluid, tissue biopsy) or from nonsterile site[b] (e.g., oral, vaginal, and rectal mucosa).

Systolic blood pressure < 90 mm Hg in adults

At least two of the following

Renal impairment

Disseminated intravascular coagulation

Elevated liver enzymes

Adult respiratory distress syndrome

Generalized cutaneous erythema

Severe soft tissue inflammation and necrosis.

[a] Definite case

[b] Probable case

SOURCE: Adapted from the Working Group on Severe Streptococcal Infections. Defining the group A streptococcal toxic shock syndrome. Rationale and consensus definition. *JAMA* 269:390, 1993.

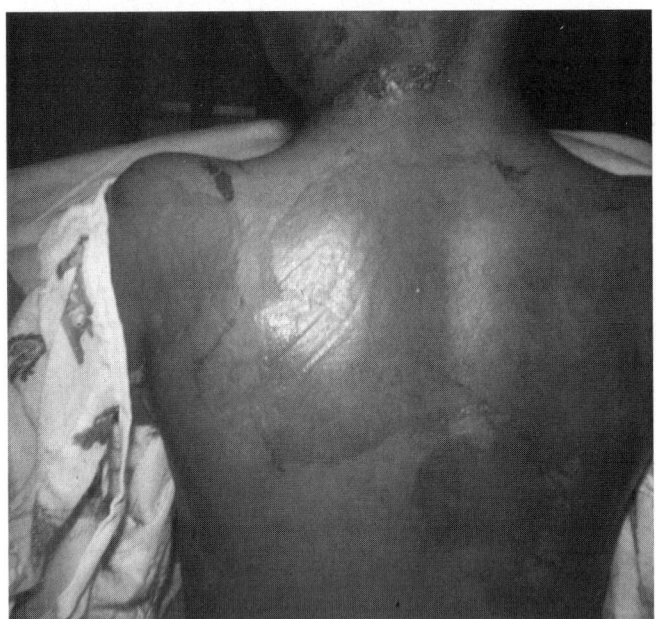

FIGURE 107-11 Staphylococcal scalded skin syndrome. Superficial desquamation of non-necrotic epidermis. (Courtesy Dr. Denise Rubenstein collection.) See Plate 107-11.

first-generation cephalosporin. Monotherapy is usually adequate because multiresistant strains of *S. aureus* are rarely encountered among the toxigenic strains. Adjunctive measures include the application of bland lubricants for the patient's comfort. Healing occurs in 7 to 10 days.

PSEUDOMONAS BACTEREMIA

Different skin manifestations of pseudomonas bacteremia have been described. These have been divided into four categories.[126] The first is ecthyma gangrenosum, which is characterized by a localized, erythematous, tender plaque or bulla that subsequently develops central necrosis leaving a gangrenous eschar with an erythematous annular border. The lesions can occur anywhere but are usually found in the anogenital region, buttocks, or axilla.[127] Ecthyma gangrenosum occurs in approximately 5% of patients with pseudomonas bacteremia and has been described in association with localized pseudomonas infection without bacteremia. The second category includes vesicles or bullae that can occur anywhere and may occur singly or in clusters. These lesions frequently become hemorrhagic and take on the appearance of ecthyma gangrenosum lesions when ruptured. The third category is a cellulitis with a sharply demarcated border. This contrasts with cellulitis caused by staphylococcal or streptococcal infection, which tends to have ill-defined borders. The fourth category of lesion are small pink, round plaques or subcutaneous nodules that are concentrated on the trunk and proximal extremities. The nodules are considered a form of nodular cellulitis and, when incised and drained, grow *Pseudomonas aeruginosa* in culture. *Pseudomonas aeruginosa* bacteremia carries a high mortality rate and treatment should be initiated early. This requires dual therapy with an aminoglycoside in conjunction with ticarcillin, piperacillin, ceftazidime, or imipenem.

VIBRIO VULNIFICUS BACTEREMIA

Vibrio vulnificus is a gram-negative rod that is found in salt water and in shellfish. The main portals of entry in humans are via ingestion (gastroenteritis) or direct inoculation into the skin (cellulitis). There may be an associated septicemia. The other *Vibrio* species (e.g., cholerae and parahaemolyticus) primarily cause gastroenteritis. *Vibrio vulnificus* infection is seen most commonly in association with underlying hepatic disease (cirrhosis or fatty liver), diabetes mellitus, chronic renal insufficiency, or underlying immune suppression. Most of the case reports in the United States involve patients with cirrhosis who injured themselves while in salt water or who ate raw oysters.[128]

A patient will present with an erythematous painful swollen limb with overlying hemorrhagic bullae and fever. Thirty-three percent of patients are in shock within 12 hours of presentation. The incubation period after ingestion is 4 to 96 hours. There may be a history of an abrasion occurring while in salt water or the recent ingestion of raw shellfish. The presence of hemorrhagic bullae overlying a cellulitis with the appropriate clinical history is highly suspicious for *V. vulnificus* septicemia. The clinical picture may be very similar to that of NF.

Aspiration of blister fluid for Gram stain and culture is essential, and biopsy for culture may be useful. Elevated creatine phosphokinase levels are often present in this condition and in STSS. This is in contrast to the normal creatine phosphokinase levels usually found in the less rapidly progressive conditions of cellulitis and erysipelas, and may be a helpful distinguishing feature.[129] The laboratory should be alerted when *Vibrio* infection is suspected so that the material is set up for culture on thiosulfate-citrate-bile salt-sucrose agar. On thiosulfate-citrate-bile salt-sucrose agar, *V. vulnificus* yields large green colonies within 24 hours of aerobic incubation.[130]

Fortunately, *V. vulnificus* is sensitive to most antibiotics. Because of the high mortality and morbidity rates, effective treatment includes early search for and recognition of the infection, aggressive antibiotic therapy, supportive care, and, in cases of wound infections, débridement.[131] Empiric therapy includes doxycycline or minocycline with an aminoglycoside or cephalosporin.

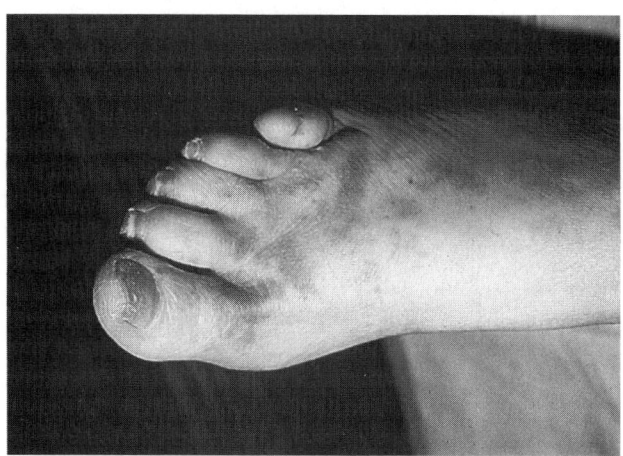

FIGURE 107-12 Meningococcemia. Purpuric lesions with irregularly angulated borders. See Plate 107-12.

MENINGOCOCCEMIA

Acute infection with the gram-negative diplococcus *Neisseria meningitidis* is associated with characteristic cutaneous findings, which may aid in the early diagnosis of this rapidly fatal disease. Characteristic findings are petechiae, ecchymoses, or palpable purpura. Petechiae may be preceded by an urticarial, rubella-like, papular, or generalized scarlatiniform eruption for 2 days. Petechiae may have a smudged appearance and tend to be concentrated on the trunk, proximal extremities, and mucosal surfaces (Fig. 107-12, Plate 107-12). The number of petechiae correlates with the degree of thrombocytopenia and is indistinguishable from other causes of petechiae such as diffuse intravascular coagulation (DIC). A late finding may be hemorrhagic vesicles or bullae centrally located within a purpuric patch. Patients with deficiency of late-acting complement factors (C5 to C8) are at particular risk for severe or recurrent meningococcal infections.[132]

The purpura seen in meningococcemia is mediated by two events. The first is thrombosis precipitated by meningococcus, fibrin, and leukocytes with a corresponding leukocytoclastic vasculitis. Thrombi are concentrated in the lung, skin, spleen, heart, and liver. The second is DIC precipitated by meningococcal endotoxin.[133] Fibrin thrombi within a vessel and a corresponding vasculitis are seen on histology.

The diagnosis is aided by a skin smear for Gram stain and biopsy for culture. Blood polymerase chain reaction is a sensitive test for confirming meningococcal disease.[134] Mortality rates are high and fewer than 30% with septic shock survive. Mortality rate is higher with increasingly extensive skin hemorrhage (purpura fulminans). Prompt antibiotic treatment is essential to decrease mortality rate, and drotrecogin-alpha (recombinant human activated protein C) may be particularly valuable. High-dose penicillin is still the drug of choice despite evidence of some less susceptible strains of meningococcus.[135] Cefotaxime and ceftriaxone have the advantages of being safe with a rapid onset of action and also being excellent antibiotics for *Streptococcus pneumoniae* and *Haemophilus influenza*, pending confirmatory diagnosis. Chloramphenicol is an acceptable alternative in penicillin-allergic patients.

The differential diagnosis of the purpuric lesions of meningococcemia includes gonococcemia, rickettsial infec-

tion, allergic vasculitis, bacterial endocarditis (with *S. aureus* or viridans streptococci), and DIC. Patients with gonococcemia usually have an associated arthritis and tenosynovitis with a very few scattered petechiae, each surmounted by a tiny pustule occurring in an acral distribution. Symmetric petechiae of the palms and soles are highly suggestive of Rocky Mountain spotted fever (infection with *Rickettsia rickettsii*).

INFECTIVE ENDOCARDITIS

The most common cutaneous finding in patients with infective endocarditis is petechiae. Petechiae are found in approximately 30% of patients and may be secondary to microemboli; however, bacteria are rarely cultured from skin specimens. Petechiae may appear on conjunctiva, buccal mucosa, palate, and retina (Roth spots). Petechiae on fingers or nail beds manifest as red to brown streaks termed *splinter hemorrhages*. Splinter hemorrhages are also seen in the elderly or related to trauma. The lesions are most suggestive of infective endocarditis when they occur on the proximal nail beds.

Petechiae occurring on the palms and soles with a nodular character are termed *Janeway lesions* (Fig. 107-13, Plate 107-13). Janeway lesions are characteristically nontender.[136] The lesions result from septic emboli consisting of bacteria, neutrophilic infiltration, and subcutaneous hemorrhage. Janeway lesions persist for several days and occur commonly in staphylococcal endocarditis. Osler nodes are small (2 to 15 mm) painful nodules.[137] The lesions are commonly found on the pads of the fingers, toes, or thenar eminences. They tend to occur in crops, are frequently multiple and evanescent, and disappear within hours to days. Osler nodes are seen in 5% to 15% of patients with streptococcally induced infective endocarditis but may also be seen in systemic lupus erythematosus, endocarditis due to fungal or gram-negative bacilli, typhoid fever, gonococcemia, and on the arms of patients with cannulated radial arteries. Microscopic examination shows microemboli in adjacent arterioles. Janeway lesions and Osler nodes resolve with appropriate antibiotic therapy. Clubbing of the digits is a nonspecific finding found in 10% to 20% of cases of infective endocarditis, especially when the disease is of long duration.

FIGURE 107-13 Subacute bacterial endocarditis. Nontender, purpuric macules with irregular borders scattered on the toes (Janeway lesions). See Plate 107-13.

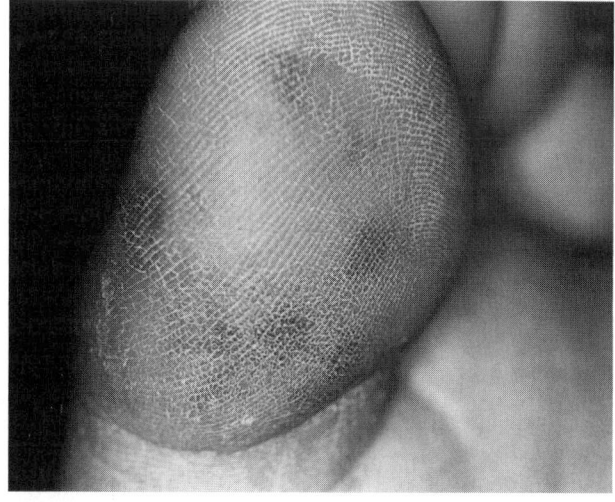

Viral Infections

HERPES SIMPLEX

Cutaneous herpes infection is associated with herpes simplex virus (HSV) types 1 and 2 that can occur on any cutaneous area. In general, HSV-1 causes orofacial infection and HSV-2 causes anogenital infection, although this distinction is changing with HSV-1 causing up to one-third of new genital infections. HSV-2 genital infection recurs six times more frequently than HSV-1 genital infection.[138] Any stress on the immune system increases the likelihood of expression of HSV in a previously infected individual. The classic appearance of recurrent HSV infection is a cluster of vesicles or shallow erosions over the lips, genitals, and lumbosacral region (Fig. 107-14, Plate 107-14). It is not uncommon for the vesicles to go undetected, so the patient presents with punched-out erosions or shallow ulcerations. In the ICU, recurrent infections are extremely common and related to the stress of illness or the degree of immunosuppression. The patient may not have been aware of any previous outbreaks, but in the immunosuppressed, if early lesions go undetected, large, erosive areas of ulceration may occur. Chronic perianal HSV ulcers are easily mistaken for decubitus ulcers. Scalloped borders and small circular ulcerations at the periphery of the ulcer may be helpful distinguishing signs.

Rapid diagnosis in 30 minutes to 2 hours may be done by DIF on cells that have been smeared on a glass slide with saline and dried or by direct fluorescent antibody (DFA) testing with monoclonal antibodies on cultured specimens.[139,140] This highly sensitive test distinguishes HSV-1 from HSV-2. Bedside diagnosis is aided by performing a Tzanck smear. The vesicle is unroofed, and the base of the lesion is scraped with a blade. The scraping is spread evenly on a glass slide and then allowed to air dry or is fixed with alcohol. The slide is then stained with Giemsa, Toluidine blue, or Diff-Quik stain and examined for multinucleated giant and/or balloon cells. If no vesicles are present, a scraping from a moist erosion may be helpful (crusted lesions generally will not yield a positive result). An early vesicle should be chosen for biopsy

to avoid secondary changes that might obscure the characteristic features. These include an intraepidermal bulla with ballooning degeneration of keratinocytes at the base of the vesicle. Balloon cells develop intracellular edema and subsequently break their desmosomal attachment to adjacent cells and float up into the bulla cavity. These cells are often multinucleated (2 to 15 nuclei) and correspond to the multinucleated giant cells seen on the Tzanck smear. Culture of the vesicle fluid will allow identification of HSV or varicella zoster virus (VZV). HSV usually grows within 48 hours in tube cell cultures, whereas VZV may take 7 to 14 days to grow. Antibodies to HSV are found in 50% to 90% of adults. Testing is generally unhelpful for a diagnosis of a particular outbreak. The presence of IgM or a fourfold or greater rise in IgG titer reflects recent infection. The presence of IgG indicates prior exposure.

All HSV and VZV infections encountered in the ICU should be treated promptly with an antiviral agent such as acyclovir, famciclovir, or valacyclovir usually intravenously, although the medications are effective orally. These medications are converted to triphosphorylated purine analogues via viral thymidine kinase and host cell enzymes. Acyclovir triphosphate is an inhibitor and a substrate for viral DNA polymerase and becomes incorporated into the growing DNA chain. Acyclovir triphosphate lacks a hydroxyl group in the 3' position and further chain synthesis is halted. In the setting of immunosuppression, strains of acyclovir-resistant HSV and VZV have developed. Resistance occurs when viral thymidine kinase no longer phosphorylates acyclovir (or famciclovir). Foscarnet is a second-line agent for treatment of HSV and VZV in cases where resistance occurs. Foscarnet attaches to the pyrophosphated binding sites of viral DNA and RNA polymerases, causing reversible inhibition of enzyme activity. Foscarnet does not require viral thymidine kinase for activation. Foscarnet is administered intravenously at a dose of 60 mg/kg twice daily or 40 mg/kg three times daily. HSV and VZV resistance to acyclovir can be determined in the laboratory.[141]

Local care consists of 0.5% silver nitrate or Burrow compresses applied for 20 minutes three to four times daily to alleviate swelling, inflammation, maceration, and crusting of extensive erosions. Topical acyclovir in general is not useful but may speed the healing of erosive HSV in immunosuppressed individuals. Topical penciclovir applied every 2 hours for 4 days has been shown to decrease clinical healing time by about 1 day in primary infections.

An important complication of HSV infection is eczema herpeticum. This is disseminated cutaneous HSV infection that occurs in patients with an underlying dermatitis such as atopic dermatitis, seborrheic dermatitis, contact dermatitis, or Darier disease. Patients present with diffuse crusting that may or may not be preceded by typical herpetic lesions. Intact vesicles are rarely seen. Diffuse eczema herpeticum is a severe and potentially life-threatening condition that may require therapy with intravenous acyclovir.[142]

VARICELLA ZOSTER

The varicella zoster virus belongs to the herpesvirus family (DNA-enveloped viruses). Varicella (chicken pox) is the primary disease, and zoster (shingles) is a recrudescence of the latent form. Primary infection occurs via aerosolized

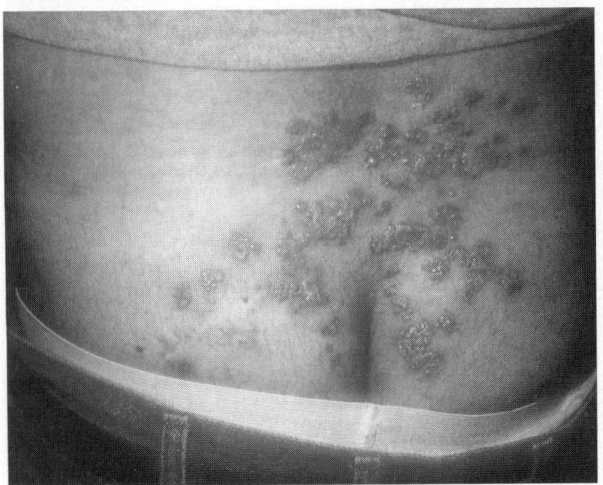

FIGURE 107-14 Severe recurrent herpes simplex infection associated with systemic steroid administration. Grouped vesicles and pustules on an erythematous base. *(Courtesy Dr. Anne Laumann collection.)* **See Plate 107-14.**

respiratory droplets (most common) or direct contact with vesicle fluid. After primary infection, the virus lies dormant in the dorsal root ganglion until reactivation occurs. Reactivation results in spread of the virus down the nerve root, causing pain, erythema, and vesicles in a dermatomal distribution.

The classic cutaneous finding in varicella is a generalized eruption of discrete vesicles, each on an erythematous base ("dew-drop on a rose petal"). These appear after an average incubation period of 14 days (range = 9–21 days) and are usually seen in association with prodromal symptoms of fever and malaise. The patient is contagious from 2 days before the eruption until all lesions have crusted. The vesicles first appear on the trunk and spread to the extremities. Lesions commonly occur in the mouth and vagina and tend to rupture rapidly, leaving small ulcers (aphthae). The cutaneous lesions progress from an erythematous papule to a vesicle to a hemorrhagic crust. There may be lesions at various stages of development at any one time. Varicella infection in adults and the immunosuppressed can be life-threatening. The most common complication is varicella pneumonia. Pneumonia generally appears 1 to 6 days after the onset of the rash. The symptoms may be out of proportion to chest radiographic findings. Encephalitis may be seen in patients with a persistent viremic state and appears to correspond to direct infection of the central nervous system. An immune complex vasculitis may lead to pancreatitis, myocarditis, arthritis, and palpable purpura.

Herpes zoster presents with a prodrome of intense pain affecting a dermatome before the onset of an erythematous, urticarial plaque in which the characteristic vesicles are seen. The eruption is generally unilateral, but spread across the midline and "spillover" into adjacent dermatomes may be seen. After several days the vesicles appear purulent or hemorrhagic. A crust subsequently forms. Occasionally, the only symptom is unilateral severe pain because the associated rash does not occur or goes undetected.

The most common dermatomes affected are in the thoracic (55%) and trigeminal (15% to 20%) distribution. Varicella zoster rarely occurs distal to the elbows or knees. Involvement of the eye is caused by infection of the ophthalmic branch of the trigeminal nerve. This may lead to conjunctivitis, keratitis, and iridocyclitis. The nasociliary branch innervates the tip and side of the nose. This branch also supplies the globe of the eye. Vesicles occurring in this area (Hutchinson sign) may be a clue to potential eye involvement. Ophthalmologic consultation is mandatory.

In patients who are immunosuppressed, disseminated herpes zoster may occur. The rash is initially limited to a few contiguous dermatomes and spreads to involve large areas of the body over several days. Patients should receive full doses of intravenous antiviral therapy.

Varicella zoster and HSV infection are diagnosed by Tzanck smear, histology, culture, DIF, and DFA. Tzanck smear and histology do not distinguish between VZ and HSV. Culture will identify the virus but may be delayed up to 14 days. DIF or DFA is recommended when rapid diagnosis is required.

SMALLPOX (VARIOLA)

The WHO declared the world free of smallpox in 1980. The last case of naturally acquired smallpox occurred in Somalia in 1977 and the last case in the United States occurred in 1949. The threat of smallpox as a potential agent of terror has brought the disease back into focus (see Chap. 61). The cause is one of two Orthopoxviridae, variola major or variola minor. We have not seen the natural disease for more than 25 years, so the following description is based on old experience. The disease is spread through droplets during face-to-face contact by coughing or by contact with body fluids such as vesicle or conjunctival fluid, urine, or saliva. It enters the body through the respiratory tract.[143] Infectiousness starts 1 day before the onset of the rash, peaks during the first week of the rash, and continues until the lesions are completely healed across. Incubation time is typically 7 to 17 days. Malaise, fever, and backache are followed by the exanthem in 2 to 4 days. Case fatality rate may be as high as 60% in an unvaccinated population with variola major and is due to pulmonary edema from heart failure.

The Center for Disease Control and Prevention (http://www.bt.cdc.gov/agent/smallpox/index.asp) has defined three major criteria for smallpox: (1) febrile prodrome occurring 1 to 4 days before rash onset, fever with a temperature higher than 101°F, and at least one of the following: prostration, headache, backache, chills, vomiting, or severe abdominal pain; (2) classic smallpox lesions consisting of deepseated, firm, round, well-circumscribed vesicles or pustules that may become umbilicated or confluent; and (3) all lesions are in the same stage of development on any one part of the body, such as the face or the arm. Minor criteria include: (1) a centrifugal distribution of lesions with a predilection for the face and distal extremities; (2) lesions first appearing on the oral mucosa/palate, face, or forearms; (3) a toxic- or moribund-appearing patient; (4) slow evolution of lesions from macules to papules to pustules, with each stage lasting 24 to 48 hours; and (5) lesions on the palms and soles. The lesions scab at about 9 days and often leave pink, depressed pock marks that become permanent scars. The presence of many confluent or hemorrhagic lesions is correlated with the severity of the disease and portends a poor prognosis.

Varicella is the most likely condition to be confused with smallpox. The lesions of varicella are more superficial and are not preceded by a prodrome. They appear in crops, evolve rapidly, and have different stages of evolution, with papules, vesicles, and erosions appearing on any individual body segment at the same time. Other conditions to consider include disseminated herpes zoster, molluscum contagiosum, bullous impetigo, morbilliform drug eruptions, contact dermatitis, erythema multiforme, Stevens-Johnson syndrome, enteroviral infections, especially hand-foot-and-mouth disease, disseminated herpes simplex, scabies, and insect bites including flea bites.

No curative treatment is known for smallpox. Supportive care and treatment of secondary infections, often staphylococcal, are mainstays of therapy. Vaccination within 4 days of exposure may prevent or lessen the severity of the illness. Vaccinia immune globulin, which is in limited supply but can be obtained from the Centers fro Disease Control and Prevention, may be helpful if given early enough. There is no experience with antiviral agents.

HEPATITIS C VIRUS

Infection with the hepatitis C virus (HCV) is associated with several dermatologic conditions. These include vasculitis (secondary to cryoglobulinemia), porphyria cutanea tarda, lichen planus, polyarteritis nodosa (rare), and generalized pruritus (common). Necrolytic acral erythema is associated with acute hepatitis C.

Two types of vasculitis have been associated with hepatitis C: leukocytoclastic vasculitis (which affects postcapillary venules) and necrotizing arteritis (which affects arteries in the subcutaneous tissue). The vasculitis is secondary to a mixed cryoglobulinemia. Palpable purpura, urticarial weals, or livedo reticularis (a mottled net-like pattern of blue-brown macules) characterize the vasculitis. The prevalence of mixed cryoglobulinemia in HCV-positive patients is 2% to 5% and is probably twice this in patients with hepatitis C–related chronic active hepatitis. Leukocytoclastic vasculitis may be the presenting sign of HCV infection. Rheumatoid factor is an extremely sensitive serologic marker for mixed cryoglobulinemia in HCV-infected patients.

Porphyria cutanea tarda (PCT) is a rare disease that is characterized by a defect in the enzyme uroporphyrinogen decarboxylase, which is essential to the production of protoporphyrin. Protoporphyrin is the precursor of heme, which is an important component of hemoglobin, myoglobin, cytochromes, peroxidases, and catalases. Two types of PCT exist: acquired and familial (autosomal dominant). Acquired PCT has been classically associated with liver disease. HCV may be the factor that links PCT and liver disease. The prevalence of HCV may be as high as 95% in patients with acquired PCT. The cutaneous manifestations of PCT include bullae and hyperpigmentation over sun-exposed areas of the body. Scarring, milia, and hypertrichosis, often seen on the sides of the face, develop as lesions resolve. The bullae of PCT are induced by visible light in the 400- to 410-nm wavelength (Soret band).[144]

A 24-hour collection of urine will show elevated levels of uroporphyrin and coproporphyrin. Quick screening for excess urinary porphyrins using a Woods lamp (blue light) on an acidified urine sample will demonstrate a characteristic coral-pink fluorescence.

Skin biopsy of a bulla shows characteristic histologic findings of a subepidermal separation of the epidermis from the dermis, with festooning of the dermal papillae into the base of the bulla related to the presence of hyaline-like material around the blood vessels and in the upper dermis. Laboratory data demonstrate excess total body iron stores.

The treatment of PCT is focused on decreasing the patient's iron load. Periodic phlebotomy to maintain a hemoglobin level of 10 g/dL or until the serum iron drops to 50 to 60 μg/dL. In cases in which phlebotomy is contraindicated or ineffective, small doses of chloroquine (125 mg twice weekly) may be effective. The response of PCT in patients treated with pegylated interferon α and ribavirin for hepatitis C has not been determined.

Lichen planus (LP) is an inflammatory cutaneous eruption characterized by purple-violaceous, polygonal, pruritic papules that have a predilection for the flexor surfaces of the forearms and wrists. Mucosal involvement manifests as a lacy white reticulate pattern on the buccal mucosa and gingiva. The prevalence of hepatitis C in patients with LP is variably estimated to be from 4% to 38%. LP also may occur secondary to medications such as thiazide diuretics, β blockers, gold, and antimalarials. Most cases are idiopathic.[145,146]

Other skin manifestations are a consequence of treatment with interferon α. These include erythema at injection sites, transient alopecia, excessive skin dryness, and sweating. Psoriasis may flare, and cutaneous necrosis has occurred due to the accidental injection of interferon α into an artery. There appears to be a high incidence of lichenoid cutaneous reactions with the combination of interferon α and ribavirin.

HUMAN IMMUNODEFICIENCY VIRUS

The cutaneous manifestations of HIV infection are protean. An acute nonspecific exanthem in association with influenza-like symptoms is seen in up to 66% of patients soon after initial infection. Subsequent cutaneous manifestations of HIV can be divided into three broad categories: inflammatory, infectious, and malignant.[147]

The most common inflammatory cutaneous manifestation of HIV-1 infection is seborrheic dermatitis. Seborrheic dermatitis is characterized by erythema and greasy scales over the scalp, eyebrows, nasolabial folds, chin, chest, and groin areas. The etiology of seborrheic dermatitis is unclear, but infection with the yeast *Pityrosporum ovale* has been proposed as the underlying cause. Psoriasis is also commonly seen in HIV-1 infection. Psoriasis is characterized by erythematous, well-demarcated plaques with a silvery scale that has a predilection for the extensor surfaces of the extremities, scalp, and trunk. Psoriasis may be seen alone or in association with Reiter syndrome (classic triad of conjunctivitis, urethritis, and arthritis). The rash associated with Reiter syndrome is also referred to as *keratoderma blenorrhagicum* (psoriasis of the soles) and *balanitis circinata* (psoriasis of the glans penis). The initial lesions are dull red macules that become papular and pseudovesicular. The roofs thicken to form hyperkeratotic plaques, and scaly collarettes may be seen. The mature lesions may stand out 1 cm or so from the skin. Reiter syndrome may be a reaction pattern seen in association with gastrointestinal infection (*Salmonella*, *Shigella*, or *Yersinia*) or *Chlamydia* infections.

The infections seen in patients with HIV-1 range from common conditions that take on a more aggressive and recalcitrant course (common warts, molluscum contagiosum, herpes simplex (HSV), varicella zoster, candidiasis, and dermatophyte infections) to rare conditions seen more commonly in the immunocompromised host (*Mycobacterium tuberculosis*, atypical mycobacteria, *Mycobacterium avium intracellulare*, *Cryptococcus neoformans*, and deep fungal infections). Infectious diseases may have atypical appearances. The classic flesh-colored papules with central umbilication seen in molluscum contagiosum closely resemble the cutaneous manifestations of *C. neoformans* and histoplasmosis. Chronic cutaneous ulceration may be the result of an underlying infection such as HSV, bacteria, fungus, mycobacteria, and atypical mycobacteria. Oral hairy leukoplakia (OHL; secondary to Epstein-Barr virus) and mucous membrane candidiasis are commonly seen. White plaques of OHL appear on the sides of the tongue, and the white patches due to colonization by *Candida albicans* may occur on any mucosal surface. Rubbing the white plaques removes candidal colonies, but OHL lesions are adherent.

The most common malignancies seen in association with HIV-1 infection are Kaposi's sarcoma (KS) and lymphomas. KS is almost always associated with human herpes virus 8 infection, although other factors, such as immunosuppression, may be necessary for its induction. HIV-associated KS is seen almost exclusively in homosexual males. It is rarely seen in patients who contracted the virus by nonsexual means. Cutaneous findings in KS vary from violaceous macules to plaques or nodules. Lesions may appear anywhere and at any time during the course of HIV infection. They tend to be symmetrically distributed, form oval patches along skin tension lines, and are often seen on the palate and tongue.[148] Individuals with HIV have a 200-fold increased risk of non-Hodgkin's lymphoma compared with the general population. Most of these lymphomas are of the B-cell variety and are associated with aggressive disease. The pathogenesis is not known but probably involves HIV, immune dysfunction, cytokine dysregulation, and other viral antigens (e.g., human herpes virus 8 and Epstein-Barr virus). Extranodal disease is the norm, and skin involvement is not unusual. Clinically, this includes variably distributed erythematous to flesh-colored papules or nodules.[149]

Fungal Infections

SUPERFICIAL FUNGAL INFECTIONS

Fungi are ubiquitous. Geophilic fungi inhabit soil and are frequently isolated from the hair of small wild animals and birds. Zoophilic fungi are parasitic on animals, whereas anthropophilic fungi primarily live on human beings. Dermatophytes are specialized saprophytic fungi that use keratin and establish an equilibrium with the host, causing an ongoing toxic or allergic reaction. Yeasts are unicellular fungi. Dermatophytes (*Epidermophyton*, *Microsporum*, and *Trichophyton*) and yeasts (*Candida* species and *Pityrosporum*) cause superficial fungal infections. Dermatophyte infection may occur on any cutaneous surface including the hair and nails. Classic lesions are polycyclic, erythematous, scaling and have central clearing and a raised border. Pruritus is common. A raised, pustular, boggy inflammatory lesion is more likely to occur when a zoophilic fungus causes a human infection (e.g., a kerion in the scalp caused by *Microsporum canis*). Infections are named according to site of infection: tinea capitis (scalp and hair), tinea manuum (hand), tinea corporis (body), tinea cruris (groin), and tinea unguium (nail). All these conditions are common. For instance, tinea capitis occurs predominantly in prepubertal inner city children with a classroom prevalence rate 15% or higher in some areas, and toenail onychomycosis is variously estimated to have prevalence rates of 2% to 13% in the United States population, 15% to 20% in persons 40 to 60 years old, and higher than 50% in persons older than 70 years.

A bedside diagnosis can be made by demonstrating septate hyphae in potassium hydroxide mounts of scales or in material obtained from debris under an infected nail. The addition of chlorazol black E may enhance the visibility of the hyphae.[150] Culture for accurate identification of a fungus may be done on Sabouraud dextrose agar with cycloheximide and chloramphenicol. The fungus may take 4 weeks to grow. For more rapid confirmation that a dermatophyte is present, dermatophyte test medium (turns red by 2 weeks when a dermatophyte is present) is often used. This test does not allow separation of one dermatophyte species from another.

Twice-daily topical treatment with allylamines (naftifine or terbinafine) or imidazoles (ketoconazole, econazole, or clotrimazole) is usually curative for skin infections. Despite a relative lack of sensitivity of trichophyton tonsurans, the common

cause of tinea capitis, to oral griseofulvin, this agent is still in general use for scalp and hair infections. It is likely that one of the newer oral agents (e.g., terbinafine) will soon become the preferred treatment. Topical therapy has only limited success for nail involvement. A 3- or 4-month course of oral terbinafine or pulsed itraconazole is necessary to clear toenails. Fingernails require only 6 weeks of oral therapy. Other possible agents include fluconazole and ketoconazole.[151,152] Primary cutaneous infection with *C. albicans* occurs in moist, warm environments such as intertriginous areas. Patients develop bright red, moist plaques with satellite pustules. The differential diagnosis includes dermatophyte infection, erythrasma (caused by *Corynebacterium minutissimum*), seborrheic dermatitis, and psoriasis. The diagnosis is supported by the typical pseudohyphae on potassium hydroxide mount or culture.

During the past two decades, the incidence of candidemia in patients in ICUs has soared from 1.5 to 60 infections per 10,000 adult ICU admissions and from 23 to 123 infections per 10,000 neonatal ICU admissions. Even with antifungal therapy, the mortality rate approaches 30%. Most cases occur in patients who have central venous lines placed. *Candida* species on the skin of the patient or caregivers can insinuate their way into these catheters, adhere to the inside of the tubing, and form biofilms.[153] Disseminated candidiasis presents with the characteristic cutaneous finding of widespread papules and pustules. In neutropenic patients with candidiasis, the skin lesions may not develop until the white count begins to recover.[154] Neutropenia and immunosuppression are the greatest risk factors for disseminated candidiasis. The differential diagnosis includes steroid-induced acne, which may develop in conjunction with chemotherapy. In steroid acne, the pustules arise from the hair follicle, are all in the same stage of development, and tend to concentrate on the face, shoulders, and upper trunk.

Diagnosis can be attempted by culturing the blood, the pustule contents, or tissue obtained from a skin biopsy, but the yield may be as low as 50%. Biopsy specimens may be stained with periodic acid-Schiff (PAS) or silver methenamine stain to visualize yeast forms. There is a need for better technology to identify disseminated candidiasis. Detection of anti-*Candida* antibodies, *Candida* metabolites, *Candida* DNA or the release of β glucan into the blood have not proved to be of general clinical use thus far.[155]

Colonization with *Pityrosporum ovale* or *orbiculare* may cause the very common tinea versicolor or it may lead to *Pityrosporum folliculitis*. Tinea versicolor presents with hypo- or hyperpigmented, regularly colored tan macules superimposed with a very fine scale, often on the upper trunk and limbs. It is seen in adolescents and young to middle-age adults. Typical hyphae and spores ("spaghetti and meatballs") are seen on potassium hydroxide mounts. Treatment with topical antifungals, such as selenium sulfide or ketoconazole, is effective, but the pigmentary change may persist for some months. Recurrence is common.

Pityrosporum folliculitis presents with asymptomatic or slightly itchy follicular papules and pustules on the face, chest, and back of mainly young women. Predisposing factors include antibiotic ingestion, steroid treatment, diabetes, Hodgkin disease, and living in the tropics, where men and women are equally affected. The involvement of the periphery of the face, the nape of the neck, the lower trunk, buttocks, and thighs distinguishes this infection from acne vulgaris. Resolution follows the use of topical antifungals as for tinea versicolor or the use of oral ketoconazole and topical keratolytic agents.

DEEP FUNGAL INFECTIONS

Deep cutaneous fungal infections are uncommon in the immunocompetent host. Opportunistic infections occur in patients who are immunocompromised by malignancies, systemic agents, or medical conditions, including the acquired immunodeficiency syndrome. Hematogenous seeding to the skin from the lung is the most common route for aspergillosis, histoplasmosis, blastomycosis, cryptococcosis, and zygomycosis (including the frequently fatal infections caused by *Mucorales*).[156] Direct inoculation may occur but is less common. Lesions present as inflammatory plaques, ulcerations, nodules, and papules. Differentiation cannot be made on clinical grounds alone. Umbilicated papules resembling lesions of molluscum contagiosum are characteristically seen in disseminated cryptococcosis, but they have also been reported in disseminated aspergillosis and histoplasmosis. Biopsy and culture of the lesions is imperative. Under the microscope with the appropriate stains, rounded refractile spherical cells with broad-based buds are seen in blastomycosis (potassium hydroxide mounts of pus smears), macrophages containing tiny yeast-like spores in histoplasmosis (hematoxylin and eosin, Gram stain, or a Giemsa stain), round to ovoid spores usually with large capsules in cryptococcosis (India ink mounts of pus smears), branching septate hyphae in aspergillosis (hematoxylin and eosin, PAS or silver methenamine stains), and vascular invasion by very large, long, nonseptate hyphae in mucormycosis (hematoxylin and eosin, PAS, or silver methenamine stains). Systemic treatment with itraconazole, fluconazole, amphotericin B, or caspofungin is required to control each of these diseases, as is extensive debridement of all necrotic tissue.[157]

Selected Dermatoses

MILIARIA

Miliaria, sometimes referred to as heat rash, is caused by obstruction of the eccrine (sweat) ducts at a variety of levels causing sweat retention. Miliaria can be classified into three groups, based on the levels of ductal obstruction: miliaria crystalline, miliaria rubra, and miliaria profunda.[157]

Miliaria crystallina (also known as sudamina), presents as crops of 1 to 2 mm asymptomatic, clear fluid-filled vesicles ("dew drops") on the skin, which develop after an episode of increased termperature (e.g., fever, increased ambient temperature), or after increased sweating (e.g., fever or drug-induced), increased ambient humidity (particularly in babies and the bedridden).

Miliaria rubra (also known as prickly heat) represents the same pathologic process o sweat duct obstruction and sweat retention, but in the stratum granulosum, resulting in 1–2 mm paroxysmally pruritic or stinging erythematous papules or macules. This type of miliaria is characteristic of hot and humid climates, affecting up to 30% of the population. Resolution of lesions is followed by variable periods of anhidrosis. The eruption often occurs on the trunk and neck, but it ca occur

anywhere except the face and volar areas. Treatment consists of reducing the ambient temperature and humidity, and emollient application. When there is bacterial overgrowth, miliaria pustulosa may occur.[158]

Miliaria profunda (also known as mamillaria) is less frequent than the other types, and is characterized by asymptomatic 1 to 3 mm pink papules usually located on the trunk, that result from sweat duct obstruction at or below the dermal-epidermal junction. This type of miliaria results from multiple episodes of miliaria rubra, as occurs in tropical climates. It may lead to extensive anhidrosis, predisposing the individual to malaise, dyspnea, tachycardia, hyperpyrexia, heat exhaustion, and in prolonged cases, to tropical anhidrotic asthenia.[159]

DRY SKIN

Xerosis (dry skin, asteatosis) is one of the most common dermatologic conditions, and is characterized by a dry, scaly noncompliant, and rough appearance of the skin. Although most individuals will experience some degree of xerosis, prevalence increases with age (>75% of individuals over 64).[160] Most commonly affected areas are the hands, the shins, the posterior upper arms, and the back.

In spite of its generally benign course, systemic causes must be taken into consideration, especially if the condition is severe and associated with inflammation: malignancies (usually lymphoproliferative), renal disease (uremic frost), obstructive biliary disease, hypothyroidism, drugs (lithium, isotretinoin), chronic diseases, and malnutrition leading to hypovitaminosis. Aggravating factors such as cold, dry, windy climates, air-conditioning, as well as organic solvents, harsh detergents, excessive bathing, or hot baths result in decreased water content in the stratum corneum and an increase in transepidermal water loss (TEWL). Erythema and pruritis are indicators of inflammation, present when the condition is sever. Rubbing and scratching can lead to dermatitis or thickened skin with accentuated markings (lichenification).

Treatment consists in restoring the epidermal water barrier, in order to minimize TEWL.[162] This can be achieved by avoiding aggravating factors (see above), only using emollient soaps or soap substitutes, and lipid-based agents (e.g., emollients) that reduce water evaporation (petrolatum, mineral oil, dimethicone, cyclomethicone); humectant agents that attract water into the stratum corneum (glycerin, propylene glycol, urea, sodium lactate, sorbitol). In addition, skin roughness can be decreased with the use of the keratolytic alpha- or beta-hydroxy acids.

PRESSURE ULCERS

Continuous pressure over a bony site obstructs microcirculation, leading to tissue ischemia and necrosis. Pressure ulcers result, constituting a major problem in the ICU, with reported incidences of 1% to 56% and prevalences of 14% to 41%, which are two- to threefold higher than in other hospitalized patients.[158,159] Altered circulation and ventilation and the use of vasoactive drugs may decrease peripheral oxygen delivery to tissues, thereby increasing the risk of pressure ulcers. The development of pressure ulcers leads to increased mortality rates, costs, and lengths of hospital stays.

A National Pressure Ulcer Advisory Panel in 1998 developed the most widely used staging system of pressure ulcers.[160] It encompasses four grades.

STAGE I

A stage I pressure ulcer is an observable pressure-related alteration of intact skin whose indicators, as compared with the adjacent or opposite area on the body, may include changes in one or more of the following: skin temperature (warmth or coolness), tissue consistency (firm or boggy feel), and/or sensation (pain, itching). The ulcer appears as a defined area of persistent redness in lightly pigmented skin, whereas the ulcer may appear with persistent red, blue, or purple hues in darker skin tones.

STAGE II

A stage II ulcer is defined as partial-thickness skin loss involving epidermis, dermis, or both. The ulcer is superficial and presents clinically as an abrasion, blister, or shallow crater.

STAGE III

Stage III ulcer is characterized by full-thickness skin loss involving damage to, or necrosis of, subcutaneous tissue that may extend down to, but not through, underlying fascia. The ulcer presents clinically as a deep crater with or without undermining of adjacent tissue.

STAGE IV

This ulcer is characterized by full-thickness skin loss with extensive destruction, tissue necrosis, or damage to muscle, bone, or supporting structures (e.g., tendon, joint capsule). Undermining and sinus tracts also may be associated with stage IV pressure ulcers.

Given the right set of circumstances, pressure ulcers can develop within 2 to 6 hours. Many risk factors have been described in the literature, but the risk assessment scales have not been specific for the ICU.[161] Notwithstanding the limitations of the studies, risk factors include the duration of previous surgeries and number of operations, preoperative protein and albumin concentrations, skin moisture, use of inotropic drugs, fecal incontinence or diarrhea, altered circulatory status, diabetes mellitus, decreased mobility, and a high score on the Acute Physiology and Chronic Health Evaluation II (APACHE II). Preventive strategies should be implemented from the moment of entry into the ICU. These include the use of risk assessment scales, repositioning the patient every 2 hours, provision of dynamic or static support surfaces that redistribute pressure, and proper nutrition.[162] A critical aspect of the topical treatment is the maintenance of a moist environment. This can be achieved by the use of any one of many different dressings: transparent films, hydrocolloids, alginates, foams, hydrogels, or hydrofibers marketed for pressure ulcer care. These dressings require few changes, so they result in less need for nursing care, faster healing, and decreased infection. Gauze dressings, particularly wet to dry dressings, are to be avoided because they allow the wound to dry and, as such, slow healing.[163] Surgery may be attempted for recalcitrant, full-thickness ulcers. However, recurrence rates are high.

References

1. World Health Organization: *International Drug Monitoring: The Role of the Hospital.* Technical Report Series. Geneva, World Health Organization, 1966.
2. Lazarou J, Pomeranz BH, Corey PN: Incidence of adverse drug reactions in hospitalized patients. A meta-analysis of prospective studies. *JAMA* 279:1200, 1998.
3. Cullen DJ, Sweitzer BJ, Bates DW, et al: Preventable adverse drug events in hospitalized patients: A comparative study of intensive care and general units. *Crit Care Med* 25:1289, 1997.
4. Vargas E, Terleira A, Hernando F, et al: Effect of adverse drug reactions on length of stay in surgical intensive care units. *Crit Care Med* 31:694, 2003.
5. Gruchalla RS: Clinical assessment of drug-induced disease. *Lancet* 356:1505, 2000.
6. Classen DC, Pestonik SL, Evans RS, et al: Adverse drug events in hospitalized patients: Excess length of stay, extra costs, and attributable mortality. *JAMA* 277:301, 1997.
7. Bates DW, Spell N, Cullen DJ, et al: The costs of adverse drug events in hospitalized patients. *JAMA* 277:307, 1997.
8. Bigby M, Jick S, Jick H, Arndt K: Drug-induced cutaneous reactions: A report from the Boston Collaborative Drug Surveillance Program on 15438 consecutive inpatients, 1975 to 1982. *JAMA* 256:3358, 1986.
9. Roujeau JC, Stern RS: Severe adverse cutaneous reactions to drugs. *N Engl J Med* 331:1272, 1994.
10. Leape LL, Brennan TA, Laird N, et al: The nature of adverse events in hospitalized patients: results of the Harvard Medical Study II. *N Engl J Med* 324:377, 1991.
11. Bigby M: Rates of cutaneous reactions to drugs. *Arch Dermatol* 137: 765, 2001.
12. Rawlins M, Thompson J: Mechanisms of adverse drug reactions, in Davies D (ed): *Textbook of Adverse Drug Reactions,* 4th ed. Oxford, Oxford University Press, 1991.
13. Hurwitz N: Admissions to hospital due to drugs. *Br Med J* 1(643):539, 1969.
14. Bates DW, Miller EB, Cullen DJ, et al: Patient risk factors for adverse drug events in hospitalized patients. ADE Prevention Study Group. *Arch Intern Med* 159:2553, 1999.
15. Thong BY, Leong KP, Tang CY, Chng HH: Drug allergy in a general hospital: Results of a novel prospective inpatient reporting system. *Ann Allergy Asthma Immunol* 90:342, 2003.
16. Gell PGH, Coombs RRA: Classification of allergic reactions responsible for clinical hypersensitivity and disease, in Gell PGH, Coombs RRA, Hachmann PJ (eds): *Clinical Aspects of Immunology.* Oxford, Blackwell Scientific Publications, 1975, p 761.
17. Neugut AI, Ghatak AT, Miller RL: Anaphylaxis in the United States: an investigation into its epidemiology [review]. *Arch Intern Med* 161:15, 2001.
18. Shipley D, Ormerod AD: Drug-induced urticaria. Recognition and treatment. *Am J Clin Dermatol* 2:151, 2001.
19. Berman B, Villa AM: Is eosinophilia helpful in diagnosing drug eruptions? *SkinMED* 1:147, 2002.
20. Schwartz LB, Metcalfe DD, Miller JS, et al: Tryptase levels as an indicator of mast-cell activation in systemic anaphylaxis and mastocytosis. *N Engl J Med* 316:1622, 1987.
21. Tilles SA: Practical issues in the management of hypersensitivity reactions: sulfonamides. *South Med J* 94:817, 2001.
22. Susser WS, Whitaker-Worth DL, Grant-Kels JM: Mucocutaneous reactions to chemotherapy. *J Am Acad Dermatol* 40:367, 1999.
23. Rodriguez R, Machiavelli M, Leone B, et al: Minoxidil (Mx) as a prophylaxis of doxorubicin-induced alopecia. *Ann Oncol* 5:769, 1994.
24. Duvic M, Lemak NA, Valero V, et al: A randomized trial of minoxidil in chemotherapy-induced alopecia. *J Am Acad Dermatol* 35:74, 1996.

25. Davis M, DeSantis D, Klemm K: A flow sheet for follow-up after chemotherapy extravasation. *Oncol Nurs Forum* 22:979, 1995.

26. Bertelli G, Gozza A, Forno GB, et al: Topical dimethylsulfoxide for the prevention of soft tissue injury after extravasation of vesicant cytotoxic drugs: A prospective clinical study. *J Clin Oncol* 13:2851, 1995.

27. Baack BR, Burgdorf WH: Chemotherapy-induced acral erythema. *J Am Acad Dermatol* 24:457, 1991.

28. Vukelja S, Baker W, Burris H, et al: Pyridoxine therapy for palmar-plantar erythrodysesthesia associated with Taxotere. *J Natl Cancer Inst* 85:1432, 1993.

29. Grassegger A, Fritsch P, Reider N: Delayed-type hypersensitivity and cross-reactivity to heparins and danaparoid: A prospective study. *Dermatol Surg* 27:47, 2001.

30. Harenberg J, Hoffmann U, Huhle G, et al: Cutaneous reactions to anticoagulants. Recognition and management. *Am J Clin Dermatol* 2:69, 2001.

31. Warkentin TE: Heparin-induced skin lesions. *Br J Haematol* 92:494, 1996.

32. Harenberg J, Huhle G, Wang L, et al: Association of heparin-induced skin lesions, intracutaneous tests, and heparin-induced IgG. *Allergy* 54:473, 1999.

33. Gelwix TJ, Beeson MS: Warfarin-induced skin necrosis. *Am J Emerg Med* 16:541, 1998.

34. Faraci PA, Deterling RA Jr, Stein AM, et al: Warfarin induced necrosis of the skin. *Surg Gynecol Obstet* 146:695, 1978.

35. Scarff CE, Baker C, Hill P, Foley P: Late-onset warfarin necrosis. *Australas J Dermatol* 43:202, 2002.

36. Cole MS, Minifee PK, Wolma FJ: Coumarin necrosis-a review of the literature. *Surgery* 103:271, 1988.

37. Barnes J: Quality, efficacy and safety of complementary medicines: Fashions, facts and the future. Part II: Efficacy and safety. *Br J Clin Pharmacol* 55:331, 2003.

38. Ernst E: Harmless herbs? A review of the recent literature. *Am J Med* 104:170, 1998.

39. Eisenberg DM, Kessler RC, Foster C, et al: Unconventional medicine in the United States. Prevalence, costs, and patterns of use. *N Engl J Med* 328:246, 1993.

40. Lin SH, Lin MS: A survey on drug-related hospitalization in a community teaching hospital. *Int J Clin Pharmacol Ther Toxicol* 31:66, 1993.

41. Chan TYK, Chan AYW, Critchley JAJH: Hospital admissions due to adverse reactions to Chinese herbal medicines. *J Trop Med Hyg* 95:296, 1992.

42. Abbot NC, White AR, Ernst E: Complementary medicine. *Nature* 381:361, 1996.

43. Meredith MJ: Herbal nutriceuticals: A primer for dentists and dental hygienists. *J Contemp Dent Pract* 2:1, 2001.

44. Kahn JM, Kress JP, Hall JB: Skin necrosis after extravasation of low-dose vasopressin administered for septic shock. *Crit Care Med* 30:1899, 2002.

45. Sirinek KR, Levine BA: High-dose vasopressin for acute variceal hemorrhage. Clinical advantages without adverse effects. *Arch Surg* 123:876, 1988.

46. Korenberg RJ, Landau-Price D, Penneys NS: Vasopressin-induced bullous disease and cutaneous necrosis. *J Am Acad Dermatol* 15(2 pt 2):393, 1986.

47. Dünser MW, Mayr AJ, Tür A, et al: Ischemic skin lesions as a complication in catecholamine-resistant vasodilatory shock: Incidence and risk factors. *Crit Care Med* 31:1394, 2003.

48. Roujeau JC, Kelly JP, Naldi L, et al: Medication use and the risk of Stevens-Johnson syndrome or toxic epidermal necrolysis. *N Engl J Med* 333:1600, 1995.

49. Bachot N, Roujeau JC: Physiopathology and treatment of severe drug eruptions. *Curr Opin Allergy Clin Immunol* 1:293, 2001.

50. Murphy JT, Purdue GF, Hunt JL: Toxic epidermal necrolysis. *J Burn Care Rehabil* 18:417, 1997.

51. Ducic I, Shalom A, Rising W, et al: Outcome of patients with toxic epidermal necrolysis syndrome revisited. *Plast Reconstr Surg* 110:768, 2002.

52. Becker DS: Toxic epidermal necrolysis. *Lancet* 351:1417, 1998.

53. Garcia-Doval I, LeCleach L, Bocquet H, et al: Toxic epidermal necrolysis and Stevens-Johnson syndrome. Does early withdrawal of causative drugs decrease the risk of death? *Arch Dermatol* 136:323, 2000.

54. Wolkenstein P, Mitrofanoff M, Lantieri L, et al: Prospective evaluation of detoxification pathways as markers of cutaneous adverse reactions to sulphonamides in AIDS. *Pharmacogenetics* 10:821, 2000.

55. Tay YK, Huff JC, Weston WL: Mycoplasma pneumoniae infection is associated with Stevens-Johnson syndrome, not erythema multiforme (von Hebra). *J Am Acad Dermatol* 35(5 pt 1):757, 1996.

56. Nagata S: Apoptosis by death factor. *Cell* 88:355, 1997.

57. Iwai K, Miyawaki T, Takizawa T, et al: Differential expression of bcl-2 and susceptibility to anti-Fas-mediated cell death in peripheral blood lymphocytes, monocytes, and neutrophils. *Blood* 84:1201, 1994.

58. Tanaka M, Suda T, Haze K, et al: Fas ligand in human serum. *Nat Med* 2:317, 1996.

59. Abe R, Shimizu T, Shibaki A, et al: Toxic epidermal necrolysis and Stevens-Johnson syndrome are induced by soluble fas ligand. *Am J Pathol* 162:1515, 2003.

60. Roujeau JC, Guillaume JC, Fabre JP, et al: Toxic epidermal necrolysis (Lyell syndrome), Incidence and drug etiology in France, 1981–1985. *Arch Dermatol* 126:37, 1990.

61. Roupe G, Ahlmen M, Fagerberg B, et al: Toxic epidermal necrolysis with extensive mucosal erosions of the gastrointestinal and respiratory tracts. *Int Arch Allergy Appl Immunol* 80:145, 1986.

62. Westly ED, Wechsler HL: Toxic epidermal necrolysis. Granulocytic leukopenia as a prognostic indicator. *Arch Dermatol* 120:721, 1984.

63. Parsons JM: Toxic epidermal necrolysis. *Int J Dermatol* 31:749, 1992.

64. Garcia-Doval I, LeCleach L, Bocquet H, et al: Toxic epidermal necrolysis and Stevens-Johnson syndrome. Does early withdrawal of causative drugs decrease the risk of death? *Arch Dermatol* 136:323, 2000.

65. Frenia ML, Schauben P: Use of silver sulfadiazine in Stevens-Johnson syndrome. *Ann Phramacother* 28:736, 1994.

66. Heimbach DM, Engrav LH, Marvin JA, e tal: Toxic epidermal necrolysis. A step forward in treatment. *JAMA* 257:2171, 1987.

67. Fine JD: Management of acquired bullous skin diseases. *N Engl J Med* 333:1475, 1995.

68. Stables GI, Lever RS: Toxic epidermal necrolysis and systemic corticosteroids. *Br J Dermatol* 128:357, 1993.

69. Rzany B, Mockenhaupt M, Baur S, et al: Epidemiology of erythema exudativum multiforme majus, Stevens-Johnson syndrome, and toxic epidermal necrolysis in Germany (1990–1992): Structure and results of a population-based registry. *J Clin Epidemiol* 49:769, 1996.

70. Halebian PH, Madden MR, Finklestein JL, et al: Improved burn center survival of patients with toxic epidermal necrolysis managed without corticosteroids. *Ann Surg* 204:503, 1986.

71. Guibal F, Bastuji-Garin S, Chosidow O, et al: Characteristics of toxic epidermal necrolysis in patients undergoing long-term glucocorticoid therapy. *Arch Dermatol* 131:669, 1995.

72. Viard I, Wehrli P, Bullani R, et al: Inhibition of toxic epidermal necrolysis by blockade of CD95 with human intravenous immunoglobulin. *Science* 282:490, 1998.

73. Stella M, Cassano P, Bollero D, et al: Toxic epidermal necrolysis treated with intravenous high-dose immunoglobulins: Our experience. *Dermatology* 203:45, 2001.

74. Prins C, Kerdel FA, Padilla RS, et al, for the TEN-IVIG Study Group: Treatment of toxic epidermal necrolysis with high-dose

intravenous immunoglobulins: Multicenter retrospective analysis of 48 consecutive cases. *Arch Dermatol* 139:26, 2003.

75. Trent JT, Kirsner RS, Romanelli P, Kerdel FA: Analysis of intravenous immunoglobulin for the treatment of toxic epidermal necrolysis using SCORTEN: The University of Miami experience. *Arch Dermatol* 139:39, 2003.

76. Descamps V, Valance A, Edlinger C, et al: Association of herpes virus 6 infection with drug reaction with eosinophilia and systemic symptoms. *Arch Dermatol* 137:301, 2001.

77. Gruchalla RS: Allergic disorders 10. Drug allergy. *J Allergy Clin Immunol* 111(suppl):S548, 2003.

78. Diaz LA, Giudice GJ: End of the century overview of skin blisters. *Arch Dermatol* 136:106, 2000.

79. Amagai M, Tsunoda K, Zillikens D, et al: The clinical phenotype of pemphigus is defined by the anti-desmoglein profile. *J Am Acad Dermatol* 40:167, 1999.

80. Kurzock R, Cohen PR: Mucocutaneous paraneoplastic manifestations of hematologic malignancies. *Am J Med* 99:207, 1995.

81. Ruocco V, Sacerdoti G: Pemphigus and bullous pemphigoid due to drugs. *Int J Dermatol* 30:307, 1991.

82. Scully C, Paes De Almeida O, et al: Pemphigus vulgaris: The manifestations and long-term management of 55 patients with oral lesions. *Br J Dermatol* 140:84, 1999.

83. Snow JL, Gibson LE: The role of genetic variation in thiopurine methyltransferase activity and the efficacy and/or side effects of azathioprine in dermatologic patients. *Arch Dermatol* 131:193, 1995.

84. Bystryn JC, Jiao D, Natow S: Treatment of pemphigus with intravenous immunoglobulin. *J Am Acad Dermatol* 47:358, 2002.

85. Nousari HC, Griffin WA, Anhalt GJ: Successful treatment for bullous pemphigoid with mycophenolate mofetil. *J Am Acad Dermatol* 39,497, 1998.

86. Cotell S, Robinson ND, Chan LS: Autoimmune blistering skin diseases. *Am J Emerg Med* 18:288, 2000.

87. Cohen LM, Skopicki DK, Harrist TJ, Clark WH Jr: Noninfectious vesiculobullous and vesiculopustular diseases, in Elder D, Elenitsas R, Jaworsky C, Johnson B Jr (eds): *Lever's Histopathology of the Skin*, 8th ed. Philadelphia, Lippincott Williams & Wilkins, 1997, p 227.

88. Wojnarowska F, Kirtschig G, Highet AS, et al: Guidelines for the management of bullous pemphigoid. *Br J Dermatol* 147:214, 2002.

89. Smith KE, Fenske KA: Cutaneous manifestations of alcohol abuse, *J Am Acad Dermatol* 43(1 pt 1):1, 2000.

90. Spencer JM, Silvers DN, Grossman ME: Pustular eruption after drug exposure: Is it pustular psoriasis or a pustular drug eruption? *Br J Dermatol* 130:514, 1994.

91. Zelickson BD, Muller SA: Generalized pustular psoriasis. A review of 63 cases. *Arch Dermatol* 127:1339, 1991.

92. Weinberg JM, Tutrone WD: Biologic therapy for psoriasis: The tumor necrosis factor inhibitors-infliximab and etanercept. *Cutis* 71:25, 2003.

93. Weinberg JM, Tutrone WD: Biologic therapy for psoriasis: The T-cell-targeted therapies-efalizumab and alefacept. *Cutis* 71:41, 2003.

94. Roenigk HH Jr: Acitretin combination therapy. *J Am Acad Dermatol* 41:S18, 1999.

95. Karakayli G, Beckham G, Orengo I, Rosen T: Exfoliative dermatitis. *Am Fam Phys* 59:625, 1999.

96. Lotti T: The purpuras. *Int J Dermatol* 33:1, 1994.

97. Touart DM, Sau P: Cutaneous deposition diseases. Part 1. *J Am Acad Dermatol* 39:149, 1998.

98. Fiorentino DF: Cutaneous vasculitis. *J Am Acad Dermatol* 48:311, 2003.

99. Piette WW. Hematologic diseases, in Freedberg IM, Wolff K, Austen KF, et al (eds): *Dermatology in General Medicine*, 5th ed. New York, McGraw-Hill, 1993, p 1867.

100. Horn TD: Graft-versus-host disease, in Freedberg IM, Wolff K, Austen KF, et al (eds): *Dermatology in General Medicine*, 5th ed. New York, McGraw-Hill, 1993, p 1426.

101. Glucksberg H, Storb R, Fefer A, et al: Clinical manifestations of graft-versus-host disease in human recipients of marrow from HLA-matched sibling donors. *Transplantation* 18:295, 1974.

102. Anasetti C: Advances in the prevention of graft-versus-host disease after hematopoietic cell transplantation. *Transplantation* 77:79, 2004.

103. Behar E, Chao NJ, Hiraki, et al: Polymorphism of adhesion molecule CD31 and its role in acute graft-versus-host disease. *New Engl J Med* 334:286, 1996.

104. Vogelsang G, Hess A: Graft versus host disease: New directions for a persistent problem. *Blood* 84:2061, 1994.

105. Lee PK, Weinberg AN, Swartz MN, Johnson RA: Pyodermas: *Staphylococcus aureus*, streptococcus, and other gram-positive bacteria, in Freedberg IM, Wolff K, Austen KF, et al (eds): *Dermatology in General Medicine*, 5th ed. New York, McGraw-Hill, 1993, p 2183.

106. Bisno AL, Brito MO, Collins CM: Molecular basis of group A streptococcal virulence. *Lancet Infect Dis* 3:191, 2003.

107. Bisno AL, Stevens DL: Streptococcal infections of skin and soft tissues. *N Engl J Med* 334:240, 1996.

108. Seal DV: Necrotizing fasciitis. *Curr Opin Infect Dis* 14:127, 2001.

109. Chan ATY, Cleeve V, Daymond TJ: Necrotizing fasciitis in a patient receiving infliximab or rheumatoid arthritis. *Postgrad Med* 78:47, 2002.

110. Stevens DL: Invasive group A streptococcus infections. *Clin Infect Dis* 14:2, 1992.

111. Nouraei SA, Hodgson EL, Malata CM: Cervicofacial. *J Wound Care* 12:147, 2003.

112. Guiliano A, Lewis F Jr, Hadley K, Blaisdell FW: Bacteriology of necrotizing fasciitis. *Am J Surg* 134:52, 1977.

113. Musser JM, Hauser AR, Kim MH, et al: *Streptococcus pyogenes* causing toxic-shock-like syndrome and other invasive diseases: clonal diversity and pyrogenic exotoxin expression. *Proc Natl Acad Sci USA* 88:2668, 1991.

114. Llewelyn M, Cohen J: Superantigens: microbial agents that corrupt immunity. *Lancet Infect Dis* 2:156, 2002.

115. Stevens DL, Tanner MH, Winship J, et al: Severe group A streptococcal infections associated with a toxic shock-like syndrome and scarlet fever toxin A. *N Engl J Med* 321:1, 1989.

116. Schlievert PM, Bohach GA, Ohlendorf, et al: Molecular structure of staphylococcus and streptococcus superantigens. *J Clin Immunol* 15:4S, 1995.

117. Bohach GA, Fast DJ, Nelson RD, Schlievert PM: Staphylococcal and streptococcal pyrogenic toxins involved in toxic shock syndrome and related illnesses. *Crit Rev Microbiol* 17:251, 1989.

118. Reingold AL, Hargrett NT, Shands KN, et al: Toxic shock syndrome surveillance in the United States, 1980–1981. *Ann Intern Med* 96:875, 1982.

119. Manders SM: Toxin-mediated streptococcal and staphylococcal disease. *J Am Acad Dermatol* 39:383, 1998.

120. Wolf JE, Rabinowitz LG: Streptococcal toxic shock-like syndrome. *Arch Dermatol* 131:73, 1995.

121. Feingold DS, Weinberg AN: Group A streptococcal infections. *Arch Dermatol* 132:67, 1996.

122. Hoeper MM, Abou-Rebyeh F, Athman C, Schwarz A: Plasmapheresis in streptococcal toxic shock syndrome. *Crit Care Med* 29:2399, 2001.

123. Cribier B, Piemont Y, Grosshans E: Staphylococcal scalded skin syndrome in adults. *J Am Acad Dermatol* 30:319, 1994.

124. Cribier B, Piemont Y, Grosshans E: Staphylococcal scalded skin syndrome in adults. *J Am Acad Dermatol* 30:319, 1994.

125. Khuong MA, Chosidow O, El-Soln N, et al: Staphylococcal scalded skin syndrome in an adult: Possible influence of

non-steroidal anti-inflammatory drugs. *Dermatologica* 186:153, 1993.

126. Forkner CE, Frei E III, Edgcomb JH, Utz JP: Pseudomonas septicemia. Observations on twenty-three cases. *Am J Med* 25:877, 1958.

127. Bodey GP, Jadeja L, Elting L: Pseudomonas bacteremia. Retrospective analysis of 410 episodes. *Arch Intern Med* 145:1621, 1985.

128. Hlady WG, Klontz KC: The epidemiology of *Vibrio* infections in Florida, 1981–1993. *J Infect Dis* 173:1176, 1996.

129. Nakafusa J, Misago N, Miura Y, et al: The importance of serum creatine phosphokinase level in the early diagnosis, and as a prognostic factor, of *Vibrio vulnificus* infection. *Br J Dermatol* 145:280, 2001.

130. Bisharat N, Agmon V, Finkelstein R, et al: Clinical, epidemiological and microbiological features of *Vibrio vulnificus* bio group 3 causing outbreaks of wound infection and bacteraemia in Israel. Israel Vibrio Study Group. *Lancet* 354:1421, 1999.

131. Kumamoto KS, Vukich DJ: Clinical infections of *Vibrio vulnificus*: A case report and review of the literature. *J Emerg Med* 16:61, 1998.

132. Spencer LV, Callen JP: Cutaneous manifestations of bacterial infections. *Dermatol Clin* 7:579, 1989.

133. Holland PC, Thompson D, Hancock S, Hodge D: Calciphylaxis, proteases, and purpura: an alternative hypothesis for the severe shock, rash, and hypocalcemia associated with meningococcal septicemia. *Crit Care Med* 30:2757, 2002.

134. Hackett SJ, Carrol ED, Guiver M, et al: Improved case confirmation in meningococcal disease with whole blood TaqMan PCR. *Arch Dis Child* 86:449, 2000.

135. Trotter CL, Fox AJ, Ramsay ME, et al: Fatal outcome from meningococcal disease—an association with meningococcal phenotype but not with reduced susceptibility to benzylpenicillin. *J Med Microbiol* 51:855, 2002.

136. Cardullo AC, Silvers DN, Grossman ME: Janeway lesions and Osler's nodes: A review of histopathologic findings. *J Am Acad Dermatol* 22:1088, 1990.

137. Yee J, McAllister CK: Osler's nodes and the recognition of infective endocarditis: A lesion of diagnostic importance. *South Med J* 80:753, 1987.

138. Whitley RJ, Kimberlin DW, Roizman B: Herpes simplex viruses. *Clin Infect Dis* 26:541, 1998.

139. Giamarellou H, Antoniadou A: Antipseudomonal antibiotics. *Med Clin North Am* 85:19, 2001.

140. Zirn JR, Tompkins SD, Huie C, Shea CR: Rapid detection and distinction of cutaneous herpesvirus infections by direct immunofluorescence. *J Am Acad Dermatol* 33:724, 1995.

141. Balfour HH Jr, Benson C, Braun J, et al: Management of acyclovir-resistant herpes simplex and varicella-zoster virus infections. *J Acquir Immune Defic Syndr* 7:254, 1994.

142. Brown TJ, McCrary M, Tyring SK: Antiviral agents: non-antiviral drugs. *J Am Acad Dermatol* 47:581, 2002.

143. Diven DG: An overview of poxviruses. *J Am Acad Dermatol* 44:1, 2001.

144. Fargion S, Piperno A, Cappellini MD, et al: Hepatitis C virus and porphyria cutanea tarda: evidence of a strong association. *Hepatology* 16:1322, 1992.

145. Bonkovsky HL, Mehta S: Hepatitis C: A review and update. *J Am Acad Dermatol* 44:159, 2001.

146. Pawlotsky JM, Dhumeaux D, Bagot M: Hepatitis C virus in dermatology. A review. *Arch Dermatol* 131:1185, 1995.

147. Garman ME, Tyring SK: The cutaneous manifestations of HIV infection. *Dermatol Clin* 20:193, 2002.

148. Geraminejad P, Memar O, Aronson I, et al: Kaposi's sarcoma and other manifestations of human herpes virus 8. *J Am Acad Dermatol* 47:641, 2002.

149. Gates AE, Kaplan LD: Biology and management of AIDS-associated non-Hodgkin's lymphoma. *Hematol Oncol Clin North Am* 17:821, 2003.

150. Lawry MA, Haneke E, Strobeck K, et al: Methods for diagnosing onychomycosis. *Arch Dermatol* 136:1112, 2000.

151. Brennan B, Leyden JJ: Overview of topical therapy for common superficial fungal infections and the role of new topical agents. *J Am Acad Dermatol* 36:3, 1997.

152. Vander Straten M, Gannoum MA, Hossain MA: Cutaneous infections: Dermatophytosis, onychomycosis, and tinea versicolor. *Infect Dis Clin North Am* 17:87, 2003.

153. Stephenson J: Can a common medical practice transform *Candida* infections from benign to deadly? *JAMA* 286:2531, 2001.

154. Roth JS, Grossman ME: Cutaneous lesions of disseminated candidiasis. *N Engl J Med* 330:1650, 1994.

155. Ostrosky-Zeichner L, Rex JH, Bennet J, Kullberg B: Deeply invasive candidiasis. *Infect Dis Clin North Am* 16:821, 2002.

156. Gonzalez G, Rinaldi M, Sugar AM: Zygomycosis. *Infect Dis Clin North Am* 16:895, 2002.

157. Welsh O, Schimid-Grendelmeier P, Stingl P, et al: Tropical dermatology. Part II. *J Am Acad Dermatol* 46:748, 2002.

158. Keller BP, Wille J, van Ramshorst B, van der Werken C: Pressure ulcers in intensive care patients: a review of risks and prevention. *Intensive Care Med* 28:1379, 2002.

159. Lyder CH: Pressure ulcer prevention and management. *JAMA* 289:223, 2003.

160. National Pressure Ulcer Advisory Panel: Available at: http://www.npuap.org. Accessed June 2, 2004.

161. Fife C, Otto G, Capsuto E, et al: Incidence of pressure ulcers in a neurologic intensive care unit. *Crit Care Med* 29:283, 2001.

162. Hunt J: Application of a pressure area risk calculator in an intensive care unit. *Intensive Crit Care Nurs* 9:226, 1993.

163. Colwell JC, Foreman MD, Trotter JP: A comparison of the efficacy and cost effectiveness of two methods of managing pressure ulcers. *Decubitus* 6:28, 1993.

Chapter 108

SICKLE CELL DISEASE

GREGORY J. KATO
MARK T. GLADWIN

KEY POINTS

- *Sickle cell disease causes a chronic hemolytic anemia associated with acute and chronic vaso-occlusion.*

- *Baseline hemodynamic and laboratory values in patients with sickle cell disease can be confused with sepsis.*

- *Serum creatinine levels of 1 to 1.5 mg/dL often indicate significant renal dysfunction.*

- *The most common intensive care management problems in patients with sickle cell disease include the acute chest syndrome, very severe anemia, sepsis, stroke, priapism, and splenic sequestration.*

- *Secondary pulmonary hypertension occurs in 30% of patients with sickle cell disease, often unrecognized.*

- *Red cell transfusion is an important treatment for most patients with sickle cell disease requiring intensive care management.*

- *Rapid exchange transfusion is indicated for central nervous system events, serious respiratory disease, or multiorgan failure.*

- *Transfusion management in patients with sickle cell disease requires investigation of alloimmunization history.*

- *Preoperative red cell transfusion and detailed supportive care are advisable for significant surgery in patients with sickle cell disease.*

Sickle cell disease is a highly prevalent disease in the United States, affecting 1 in 500 African American infants. It is common in individuals of African, Caribbean, Mediterranean, Arab, and other Middle Eastern descent. It is a genetic disorder with an autosomal recessive inheritance pattern. Sickle cell disease is often called "the first molecular disease" because the biochemical alteration in sickle hemoglobin described by Linus Pauling in 1948 was one of the first lesions identified at the molecular level for a human disease. Sickle hemoglobin forms rod-like polymers in deoxygenated red cells in areas of the circulation, with low oxygen tension, acidosis, or hyperosmolarity. Sickle hemoglobin polymerization causes a host of secondary molecular and cellular changes, many of which impair blood flow and contribute to tissue damage. The microcirculation can be acutely or chronically impaired in virtually any organ in the body, resulting in the characteristic crisis pattern of intermittent pain and acute organ injury superimposed on the gradual development of chronic organ failure.

Despite the early progress in a molecular understanding of sickle cell disease, its treatment remained largely palliative for many decades. In recent years, the longevity of patients with sickle cell disease has been prolonged by the institution of prophylactic penicillin treatment and immunization to decrease mortality rate from pneumococcal sepsis. Chronic transfusion therapy for selected patients has improved outcome, and acute transfusion therapy is the central intervention for most complications requiring admission to the intensive care unit (ICU). Hydroxyurea, the first treatment approved by the Food and Drug Administration for sickle cell disease, decreases disease severity and mortality rate.[1,2] Most recently, new paradigms have emerged regarding the pathophysiology of secondary complications of sickle cell disease, with much of this involving impairment of normal intravascular signaling via the nitric oxide (NO) pathway[3–5] (Fig. 108-1). These new paradigms have triggered a wave of research seeking to translate these basic science advances into clinical practice.[6] This chapter reviews general aspects of the genetics and pathophysiology of sickle cell disease, common clinical problems with an emphasis on those faced in a critical care setting, and contemporary therapeutic approaches to these complications of sickle cell disease.

General Background

In 1910, James Herrick first reported the observation of sickle-shaped red cells from the blood of an anemic Chicago dental student from Grenada. Subsequently, in 1949, Linus Pauling and his colleagues demonstrated a difference in the electrophoretic pattern of sickle hemoglobin compared with normal hemoglobin and introduced the label of "molecular disease." Marotta and colleagues in 1977 showed that the hemoglobin alteration was due to a single nucleotide change in the gene encoding the β subunit of hemoglobin A.

Genetics and Epidemiology

Sickle cell disease is inherited in a classic Mendelian autosomal recessive pattern, with homozygous individuals demonstrating complications of hemolytic anemia and impaired microvascular blood flow. Usually the heterozygous carrier state, sickle trait, is completely asymptomatic, although rarely vaso-occlusive events, splenic infarction, renal papillary necrosis, or sudden death can occur, usually under high-altitude hypoxic conditions. Several other mutant β-globin alleles can induce sickling disorders when inherited in combination with the sickle trait, the most common of which are β thalassemia and hemoglobin C. Although the homozygous state typically results in severe disease, the sickle trait appears to confer resistance to severe malaria, leading to an evolutionary selection for this carrier state in geographic regions with a high prevalence of malaria.[7] The sickle trait allele appears to have independently arisen at least three times in Africa and once in the Arab-Indian region. Migration from these regions has brought sickle cell disease to all parts of the world, particularly the Caribbean, Mediterranean, and the North and South American regions. Some variation in disease severity has been attributed to distinct haplotypes surrounding these alleles; additional polymorphisms in several other genes appear to modify disease severity, including those affecting expression of the α- and β-globin (thalassemia mutations) and γ-globin (fetal hemoglobin) genes.

Homozygous sickle cell disease is also referred to as *SS disease* or *sickle cell anemia*, to distinguish it from *hemoglobin SC disease*, a compound heterozygous combination of sickle trait and hemoglobin C trait. Hemoglobin SC disease is clinically similar in scope to SS, but hemoglobin SC disease on average presents milder or less frequent vaso-occlusive

CHRONIC COMPLICATIONS

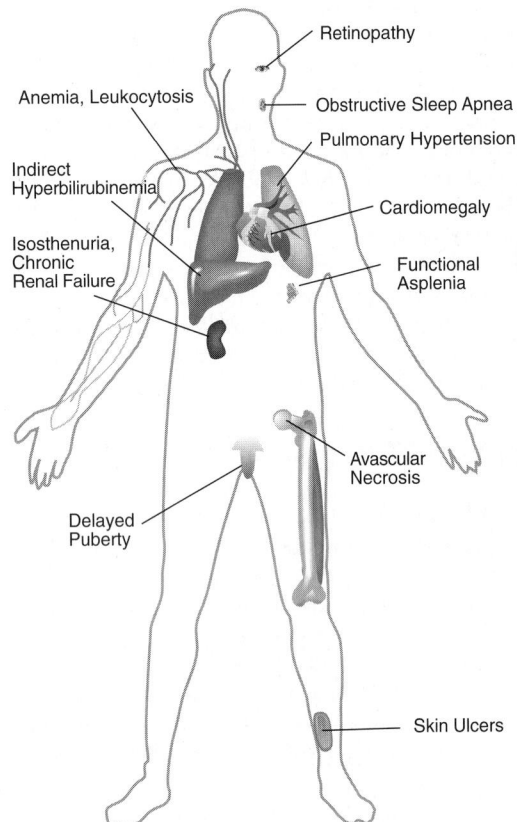

ACUTE COMPLICATIONS

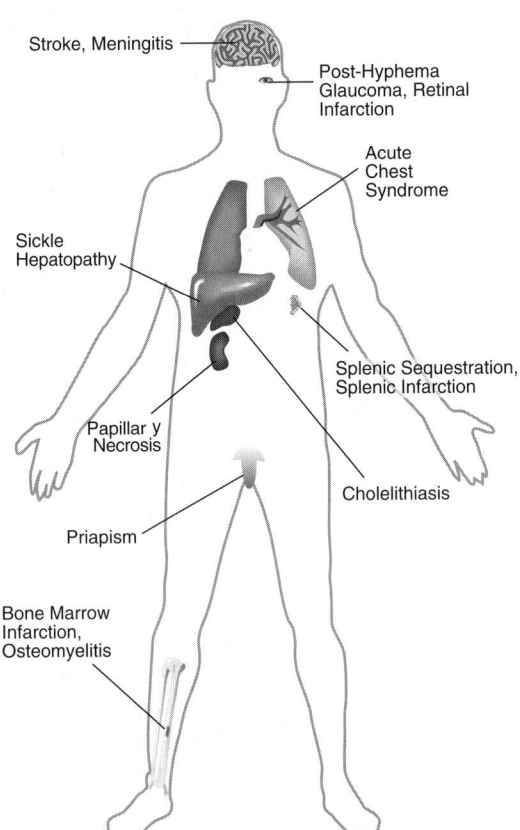

FIGURE 108-1 Chronic and acute complications of sickle cell disease. Sepsis is an additional potential acute complication of sickle cell disease.

complications. The spectrum of SC disease overlaps considerably with SS. Another compound heterozygous form of sickle cell disease is that of S-β-thalassemia. A combination of a β-globin S allele with a nonexpressing β-globin allele, called *S-β⁰-thalassemia*, results in production of only hemoglobin S, and the clinical phenotype closely resembles SS. If the thalassemia allele of β globin permits partial expression of a normal β-globin protein, the combination is called *S-β⁺-thalassemia*, and like hemoglobin SC, the disease tends to be milder. There are several additional combinations of the β-globin S allele with rare variant hemoglobins that can result in different severities of sickle cell disease.

Pathophysiology

The single nucleotide mutation in the sixth codon of the β-globin gene changes the corresponding amino acid in β globin from valine to glutamic acid. This induces a conformational change in the hemoglobin tetramer that renders it susceptible to polymerization with deoxygenation in hypoxic, hyperosmolar, or acidic regions of the circulation. The rod-like polymer bundles distort the red cell membrane into the characteristic sickle shape. Intracellular hemoglobin S polymerization and "sickling" are associated with a complex combination of pathophysiologic changes (Table 108-1 and Fig. 108-2). It is likely that adhesion of erythrocytes and leukocytes to endothelial receptors such as vascular cellular

adhesion molecule 1 (VCAM-1) combines with physical rigidity and distortion ("sickling") of the red blood cells to occlude the microvascular circulation. Additional involved cell adhesion molecules include intercellular adhesion molecule 1, E selectin, and P selectin. The resulting tissue ischemia-reperfusion drives tissue and organ injury, generalized inflammation, and ultimately produces tissue infarction. These pathophysiologic events produce clinical and biochemical perturbations, such as fever and leukocytosis, which can mimic sepsis. Tissue ischemia and infarction produce severe pain attacks called *acute pain crisis* or *vaso-occlusive crisis* (VOC) and specific end-organ pathophysiology, such as the acute chest syndrome (ACS), an acute lung injury syndrome similar to acute respiratory distress syndrome (ARDS), discussed in greater detail below.

Steady-state sickle cell disease is characterized by intense inflammation that accelerates during VOC, likely secondary to nearly constant tissue ischemia-reperfusion. This is illustrated by frequent fever during VOC and the ACS and by increased leukocyte, platelet, and endothelial cell activation, with increased circulating mediators and markers of oxidant stress and inflammation. Examples of these inflammatory markers include elevated levels of C-reactive protein, cytokines (tumor necrosis factor α, interleukin 1β, and granulocyte-macrophage colony-stimulating factor), chemokines (interleukin 8), integrins ($\alpha_4\beta_1$), selectins (E and P), adhesion molecules (VCAM-1 and intracellular adhesion molecule 1), markers of oxidant stress and inflammation

TABLE 108-1 Pathogenesis of Sickle Cell Anemia

Mechanism	Modifying factors
RBC sickling	
Hemoglobin polymerization (crystal-solution equilibrium)	Hemoglobin deoxygenation-degree and duration of hypoxia
	Hemoglobin concentration-cellular dehydration
	Inversely proportional to hemoglobin F concentration
RBC interactions with vascular endothelial cells	Supporting evidence
Disturbance of vasoregulation	Transcriptional induction of endothelial cell genes encoding endothelin 1, a potent vasoconstrictor, after contact with sickled RBCs
	Endothelin 1 levels are elevated during VOC and ACS
	Cell-free plasma hemoglobin impairs nitric oxide bioavailability
Activation of the coagulation system	Central nervous system vascular thrombosis
	Pulmonary in situ thrombosis and thromboembolia from distant sources
	Elevated whole blood tissue factor procoagulant activity
Increased adhesion of RBCs and WBCs to vascular endothelium	Increased expression of adhesion molecules results in RBC-endothelial cell adhesion and endothelial cell damage
	Association between clinical severity and in vitro adhesion of sickled RBCs to endothelial cells
	Increased expression of adhesion molecules after activation by inflammatory cytokines (TNF α and IL-1 β)
	Reticulocyte integrin complex, $\alpha_4\beta_1$, binds to plasma fibronectin and endothelial cell VCAM-1
	Sickle red blood cell CD36 and endothelial cell CD36 bind to thrombospondin secreted by activated platelets
	Increased numbers of circulating microvascular endothelial cells in sickle cell disease, particularly during VOC
	Increased endothelial cell activation as evidenced by increased ICAM-1, VCAM-1, E selectin, P selectin

ABBREVIATIONS: ACS, acute chest syndrome; ICAM-1, intercellular adhesion molecule 1; IL-1β, interleukin 1β; RBC, red blood cell; TNFα, tumor necrosis factor α; VCAM-1, vascular cellular adhesion molecule 1; VOC, vaso-occlusive pain crisis; WBC, white blood cell.

(isoprostanes and tyrosine nitration), and vasoconstrictors (endothelin 1).[4,5]

Associated with this inflammation is a state of endothelial dysfunction, with impaired NO bioavailability. Strong evidence points to intravascular consumption of NO by cell-free plasma hemoglobin liberated from red cells by intravascular hemolysis and by radical-radical inactivation reactions with superoxide produced by xanthine oxidase.[8,9] Impairment of NO signal transduction leads to many adverse consequences, including increased inflammation and impaired microcirculatory blood flow.[10,11] It may also lead to platelet activation and acute and chronic pulmonary hypertension.[12,13]

Baseline Physiology

Sickle cell disease is fundamentally a severe hemolytic anemia. This is characterized by a normocytic, normochromic anemia with reticulocytosis at baseline. Characteristic laboratory profiles for patients with SS and SC without hydroxyurea treatment are presented in Table 108-2. Hemolysis is mostly but not exclusively extravascular and is due primarily to mechanical injury and destruction of erythrocytes rendered rigid by intracellular hemoglobin S polymerization. Baseline

leukocytosis is commonly present and should not necessarily be construed as evidence of infection. Nucleated red blood cells commonly are miscounted in the complete blood count as white cells, although the overall counting error is usually relatively small. The diminished oxygen-carrying capacity due to chronic anemia is compensated by increased cardiac output (Table 108-3). Cardiomegaly and biventricular chamber dilation due to constant increased cardiac output are common (Table 108-4). Splenic dysfunction due to subclinical infarction is almost universal by late childhood in patients with homozygous sickle cell disease; on computed tomography, the spleen appears typically as a small calcified mass (Fig. 108-3). As discussed below, patients with SC disease or S thalassemia may retain their spleens and present with acute splenic sequestration or infarction. Likewise, gradual infarction of the renal medulla by adolescence leads to isosthenuria (iso-osmolar urine), with increased urination because of diminished urinary concentrating capacity, mimicking a nephrogenic diabetes insipidus phenotype. Aside from increasing maintenance fluid requirements, these changes mean that urine specific gravity is not closely indicative of hydration status. The increased cardiac output and higher plasma content of each milliliter of blood present the renal glomeruli with a volume of plasma per minute up to twice

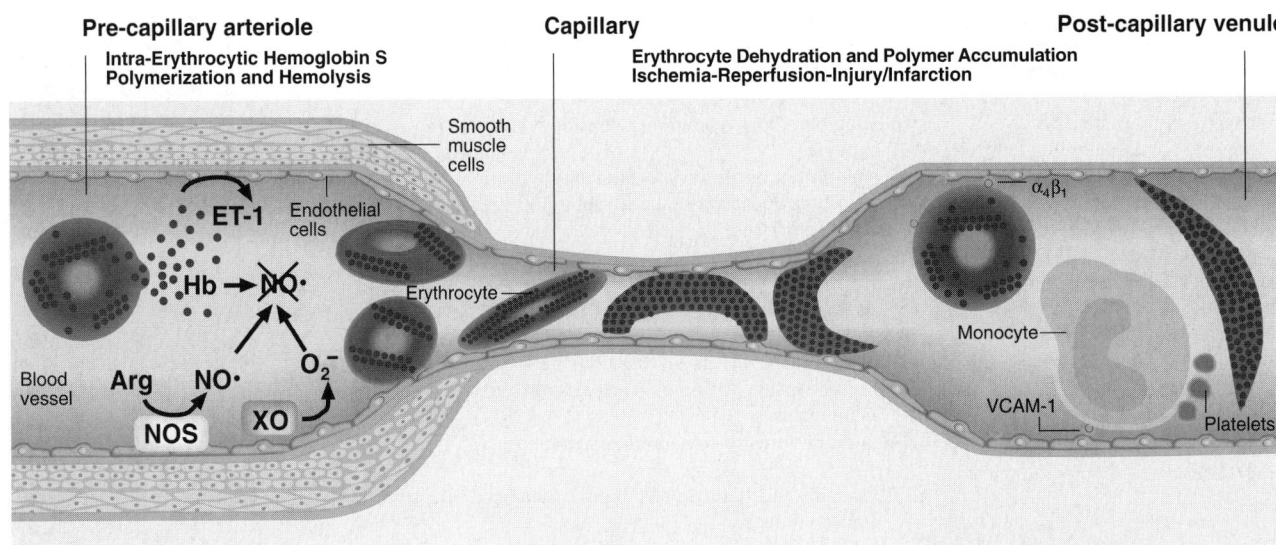

Pre-capillary arteriole
Intra-Erythrocytic Hemoglobin S Polymerization and Hemolysis

Capillary
Erythrocyte Dehydration and Polymer Accumulation Ischemia-Reperfusion-Injury/Infarction

Post-capillary venule

Vascular instability due to:
• Inactivation of NO• and induction of Endothelin-1 by cell free hemoglobin
• Inactivation of NO• by superoxide generated by xanthine oxidase

Pre-capillary vascular obstruction due to rigid erythrocytes

Inflammation-induced adhesion of sickle erythrocytes, leukocytes platelet-monocyte aggregates mediated through VCAM-1 and other adhesion molecules

FIGURE 108-2 Model of pathophysiology of sickle cell disease. This model reflects a summary of pathophysiologic events for which there is substantial supportive evidence. Nitric oxide (NO·) is normally synthesized from L-arginine by isoforms of NO synthase (NOS). Recent findings have implicated vascular instability due to inactivation of endogenous NO by free plasma hemoglobin released from lysed red cells and by superoxide (O_2^-) generated possibly by xanthine oxidase (XO), which is strongly expressed in the plasma of patients with sickle cell disease. NO deficiency leads to vasoconstriction and inflammation. Cell-free hemoglobin also induces the expression of endothelin 1 (ET-1), an extremely potent vasoconstrictor. The best characterized mechanism of vaso-occlusion occurs due to extensive hemoglobin S polymerization, leading to dense, poorly compliant red cells that cannot readily traverse capillaries. More recent evidence has indicated the adhesion of immature red cells and leukocytes to cell adhesion molecules (*green arcs*) expressed on endothelial luminal surfaces of postcapillary venules in response to NO deficiency, tumor necrosis factor α and other inflammatory cytokines, commonly found to be in patients with sickle cell disease. Activated monocytes and platelet-monocyte aggregates have been described in patients with sickle cell disease, and these appear to secrete inflammatory cytokines. The resulting sluggish flow of desaturated red cells in the venules may promote sickling, leading to multifactorial vaso-occlusion.

TABLE 108-2 Ranges of Laboratory Values in Normal Adults with Sickle Cell Disease[a]

Parameter	SS	SC	General Population
Oxygen saturation (%)	95.4 ± 3.3	98.3 ± 1.2	95–98
Leukocyte count (K/μm^3)	11.3 ± 3.2	8.7 ± 4.0	4.5–11.0
Hemoglobin (g/dL)	8.3 ± 1.1	11.6 ± 1.2	M: 13.5–17.5
			F: 12.0–16.0
Platelets (K/μm^3)	401 ± 119	268 ± 117	150–450
Urea nitrogen (mg/dL)	9 ± 6	9 ± 5	6–20
Creatinine (mg/dL)	0.7 ± 0.3	0.8 ± 0.2	0.7–1.2
Alkaline phosphatase (U/L)	115 ± 91	95 ± 51	25–100
Bilirubin, total (mg/dL)	3.5 ± 1.8	1.7 ± 1.1	0.3–1.2
Bilirubin, direct (mg/dL)	0.5 ± 0.3	0.4 ± 0.6	0–0.2
Lactate dehydrogenase (U/L)	437 ± 154	247 ± 80	208–378
Ferritin (ng/mL)	656 ± 1058	253 ± 395	M: 20–250
			F: 10–120
Iron (μg/dL)	94 ± 41	87 ± 57	M: 65–175
			F: 50–170
Transferrin (mg/dL)	215 ± 57	249 ± 46	200–400

[a] Ranges are mean ± standard deviation for sickle cell patients not on hydroxyurea treatment.[50] Laboratory values are included only for those common tests in which sickle cell patient values often differ from the general population. Additional data are available from the cooperative study.[51] The ranges for the general population are adapted from other sources.[52]

ABBREVIATIONS: F, female; M, male; SC, hemoglobin sickle cell disease; SS, homozygous sickle cell disease.

SOURCES: Gladwin et al,[50] West et al,[51] and Elm.[52]

TABLE 108-3 Echocardiographic Measurements in Adults with Sickle Cell Disease with or without Pulmonary Hypertension[a]

Parameter	Without Pulmonary HTN	With Pulmonary HTN	Normal Range
LA size (mm)[b]	39 ± 5	45 ± 8	<40
LV size (mm)[b]	37 ± 7	40 ± 7	37–56
RA area (cm²)[b]	17 ± 4	20 ± 5	<18
Ejection fraction (%)	61 ± 5	60 ± 9	55–74
Systolic blood pressure (mm Hg)[b]	119 ± 15	129 ± 21	90–135
Diastolic blood pressure (mm Hg)	67 ± 11	68 ± 13	50–90
Mean arterial pressure (mm Hg)[c]	85 ± 11	88 ± 15	70–105
Tricuspid regurgitant jet velocity (m/s)	2.0 ± 0.4	2.8 ± 0.3	<2.5
Systolic pulmonary artery pressure, estimated (mm Hg)	26 ± 6	42 ± 8	19–37

[a] Ranges are mean ± standard deviation.
[b] $p \leq 0.05$ for pulmonary hypertension vs. no pulmonary hypertension.
[c] $1/3 \times$ systolic blood pressure $+ 2/3 \times$ diastolic blood pressure.
ABBREVIATIONS: HTN, hypertension; LA, left atrial; LV, left ventricular: RA, right atrial.
SOURCE: Gladwin et al.[50]

that of patients without sickle cell disease. This leads to baseline glomerular hyperfiltration (up to 200 mL/min) and a low baseline serum creatinine range of approximately 0.5 to 0.6 mg/dL (see Table 108-2). Serum creatinine levels above this level actually imply renal insufficiency. A serum creatinine level of 1.0 mg/dL may often be associated with other consequences of renal insufficiency, such as hyperkalemia, hyperuricemia, and increased anemia due to a partial defect in erythropoietin secretion. Importantly, these features of renal insufficiency may arise even when the glomerular filtration rate may be in the 80-mL/min range.

These baseline physiologic perturbations result in a hyperdynamic cardiovascular state with relatively low blood pressure, low systemic and pulmonary vascular resistances, high cardiac output. and renal hyperfiltration (see Tables 108-3 and 108-4). These findings are similar to other high cardiac output states such as pregnancy and thyrotoxicosis. These hemodynamic parameters combined with significant baseline inflammation in patients with sickle cell disease, characterized by leukocytosis and increased serum ferritin, often can be mistaken for sepsis in the absence of a true infectious insult (see Table 108-4).

Common Clinical Problems

Common and significant clinical problems in patients with sickle cell disease are summarized in Fig. 108-1.

VASO-OCCLUSIVE PAIN CRISIS

VOC is perhaps the most characteristic manifestation of sickle cell disease. These severe painful attacks, most commonly affecting the extremities and back, result from acutely impaired microvascular blood flow. Most commonly affected are bones, due primarily to ischemia and infarction of the bone marrow and inflammation of the periosteum, with intense bone pain due to the resulting edema and tissue swelling in the inelastic compartment of the bone marrow medulla. Most often, pain affects the lumbosacral vertebrae and the long bones, although any bone may be affected. Joint effusions of the elbows and knees are common. At times, especially in children, there is difficulty in distinguishing painful crisis from osteomyelitis. The mainstays of treatment for pain crisis are analgesics, in particular nonsteroidal anti-inflammatory drugs and opioids. Correction of dehydration or hypoxemia is important, as is careful monitoring for development of ACS (see below). Clinicians frequently undertreat the severe pain of sickle cell crisis. Opioid tolerance due to recurrent or chronic opioid treatment may dramatically increase the dosage required in individual patients. There is little, if any, risk for developing opioid dependency with short courses of large-dose opioids for VOC.

STROKE

Ischemic stroke is a frequent complication of sickle cell disease, occurring at any age, but mainly in children. This topic is discussed in detail below in the section on special problems in the ICU.

EYE DISEASE

A proliferative retinopathy develops in 10% of patients with SS disease and at least twice as often in patients with

TABLE 108-4 Cardiac Catheterization Data for Adults with Sickle Cell Disease[a]

Parameter	Without Pulmonary HTN	With Pulmonary HTN
Pulmonary artery systolic (mm Hg)	30.3 ± 5.77	54.3 ± 12.26
Pulmonary artery diastolic (mm Hg)	11.7 ± 4.86	25.2 ± 7.72
Pulmonary artery mean (mm Hg)	17.8 ± 4.86	36.0 ± 7.78
Cardiac output (L/min)	8.62 ± 3.03	8.60 ± 1.76
Pulmonary capillary wedge pressure (mm Hg)	10.6 ± 3.82	16.0 ± 5.87
Pulmonary vascular resistance (dynes/s/cm⁻⁵)	57	162

[a] Ranges are mean ± standard deviation.
SOURCE: Castro et al.[15]

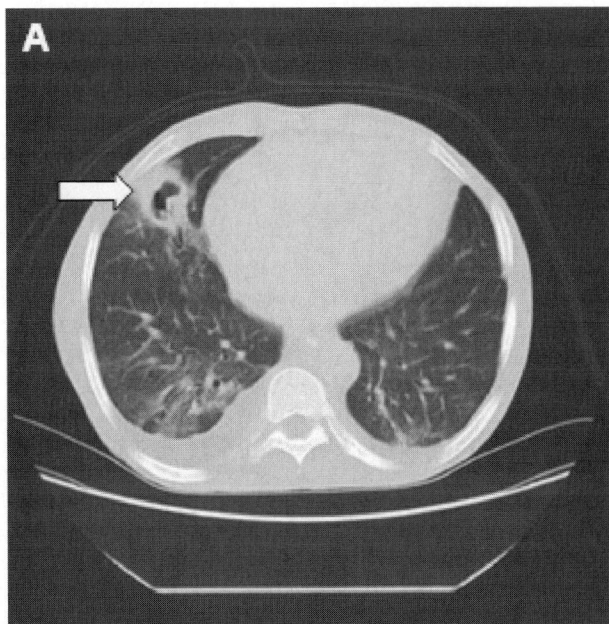

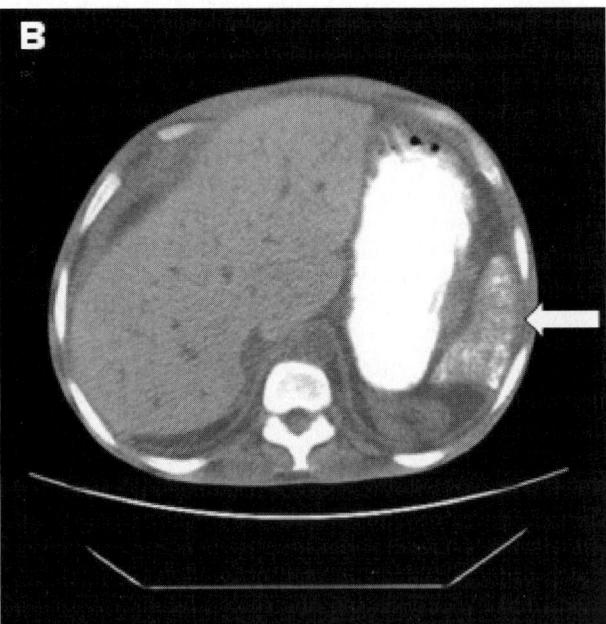

FIGURE 108-3 Sickle cell disease injury to soft tissues. *A.* Lung cavitation resulting from previous acute chest syndrome, causing infarction and necrosis of a subsegmental region of the left middle lobe. The cavitary lesion (*arrow*) has an inflammatory wall that subsequently resolved after antimicrobial therapy.

B. The calcified, atrophic spleen (*arrow*) is visible on an abdominal scan from the same patient. This is typical in adults with homozygous sickle cell disease. The stomach is visualized by oral contrast material.

SC disease. This chronic complication may be treated with laser photocoagulation. Two acute complications present ophthalmologic emergencies. The first is vision loss due to acute occlusion of the central retinal artery. This may resolve with emergency exchange transfusion before retinal infarction occurs. The second emergency is traumatic hyphema in a patient with sickle cell disease or sickle trait. The environment of the anterior chamber of the eye promotes sickling, and this can readily cause acute glaucoma. Evacuation of the blood should be undertaken for hyphema without delay to avoid vision loss.[14]

LUNG DISEASE

Sickle cell disease is associated with a high incidence of acute and chronic lung complications. The ACS is a lung injury syndrome and, in cases of extensive lung involvement, is similar to ARDS. It is defined by a new pulmonary infiltrate secondary to alveolar consolidation, not atelectasis, in a patient with sickle cell disease accompanied by chest pain, fever, tachypnea, wheezing, or cough. It is caused frequently by pulmonary fat embolism syndrome from severe vaso-occlusion of the bone marrow or by an excessive pulmonary inflammatory response to common respiratory pathogens. Its pathogenesis and treatment are discussed in detail in the section on special ICU problems. Chronic complications can include the development of restrictive lung disease, pulmonary fibrosis, or pulmonary hypertension, with the latter occurring in up to 30% of adults with sickle cell disease.[15] Pulmonary hypertension appears to be the most serious risk factor for early mortality in adult patients with sickle cell disease and, in the past, may have been under-recognized by clinicians. Reactive airway disease or asthma occurs with increased frequency in children with sickle cell disease.[16]

HEART DISEASE

Although vaso-occlusion of the coronary microcirculation can produce myocardial infarction, acute wall motion abnormalities, and cardiac enzyme release, coronary atherosclerosis is essentially nonexistent in patients with sickle cell disease for reasons that are poorly understood, possibly owing to low levels of low-density lipoprotein cholesterol, early mortality of males, and increased heme oxygenase activity. Cardiomegaly and biventricular chamber dilation are nearly universal due to a long-term high cardiac output state as compensation for severe chronic anemia. High-output cardiac failure, diastolic dysfunction, and pulmonary hypertension are common cardiac complications of sickle cell disease (see Tables 108-3 and 108-4).

HEPATOBILIARY

Up to 42% of patients with sickle cell disease have calcium bilirubinate gallstones by age 18 years, although only a fraction of these patients are symptomatic. Stones develop due to the very high rate of bilirubin excretion in bile as a breakdown product of hemoglobin turnover. In cases of acute cholecystitis, awaiting its resolution decreases perioperative complications. Acute vaso-occlusion in the liver can cause pain, elevated transaminases, and extreme hyperbilirubinemia, generally responding well to supportive care. Rarely, the liver may acutely sequester peripheral blood cells, clinically analogous to splenic sequestration syndrome (see Special Problems in the ICU).

SPLENIC

Nearly all patients with sickle cell disease develop progressive loss of splenic function secondary to its microvascular vaso-occlusion and infarction, beginning at birth and complete by age 10 years. This manifests primarily as a marked susceptibility to sepsis and meningitis due to encapsulated organisms, particularly in children younger than 5 years. The incidence of serious infection is dramatically decreased by penicillin prophylaxis and immunization against *Haemophilus influenzae* and *Streptococcus pneumoniae*. However, splenic dysfunction still causes a modest lifelong risk of overwhelming sepsis. The spleen is atrophic and nonfunctional in 98% of adults with SS sickle cell disease (see calcified spleen in Fig. 108-3B). A dramatic acute complication of sickle cell disease is splenic sequestration crisis, described in detail in the section on special problems in the ICU. This complication occurs frequently in pediatric patients with functioning spleens, primarily young children with homozygous SS disease, and adults with hemoglobin SC sickle cell disease or S-β^+-thalassemia because approximately 50% of these patients retain their spleen into adulthood. It is conceivable that hydroxyurea therapy in children with sickle cell disease might lead to prolongation of splenic function.

RENAL

Isosthenuria develops in most patients by age 10 years, with increasing maintenance fluid and sodium requirements. Hematuria due to papillary necrosis is an occasional complication, usually self-resolving. A nephropathy with nephrotic-grade proteinuria can frequently progress to uremia. Early signs include the normally low serum creatinine exceeding 0.6 mg/dL, progressively severe anemia, and a rise in the serum uric acid level. Angiotensin-converting enzyme inhibitors can decrease proteinuria and potentially slow progression of renal insufficiency. Uremia has been treated with dialysis and with renal transplantation.

SKELETAL

Bone marrow infarcts are frequent causes of pain. These may be detected on magnetic resonance imaging or radionuclide imaging with technetium sulfur colloid, although it is not normally clinically helpful to ascertain these by imaging. The heads of the femur and humerus are susceptible to avascular necrosis, a potential source of constant pain and disability. Ischemic bone becomes susceptible to bacterial osteomyelitis. *Staphylococcus aureus* is the most common organism in sickle cell osteomyelitis episodes. *Salmonella* species are frequently encountered, which very rarely cause bone sepsis in patients without sickle cell disease. Joint effusions and occasionally hemarthrosis may be seen adjacent to infarcted bones. Septic arthritis is seen less commonly.

SKIN

Leg ulcers, a clinical feature of this and other hemolytic disorders, are usually limited to adolescence and adulthood. They heal very slowly and can cause very severe pain. They rarely develop acute cellulitis. They are best treated with scrupulous wound care.

Special Problems in the ICU

The demographics of adult patients with sickle cell disease admitted to the medical ICU at a single institution over a

TABLE 108-5 Demographics of MICU Admissions for Patients with SCD[a]

SCD hospitalizations resulting in MICU admission (range)	1.5–2.9%
MICU stay, days (mean ± standard deviation)	5.0 ± 6.5
MICU mortality rate	13%
MICU diagnosis:	
Acute chest syndrome (including pneumonia)	43%
Severe anemia	36%
Sepsis	20%
Pulmonary hypertension	9%
Left heart failure	4%
Multiorgan failure	3%

[a]Chart survey between 1983 and 1994 at Howard University Hospital in Washington, DC.
ABBREVIATIONS: MICU, medical intensive care unit; SCD, sickle cell disease.
SOURCE: Castro and Adams.[49]

10-year span are presented in Table 108-5. Specific issues in management of patients with sickle cell disease admitted to the ICU are discussed in detail below.

ACUTE CHEST SYNDROME

The ACS of sickle cell disease is an all-inclusive lung injury syndrome, akin to ARDS. The largest clinical study of ACS defined ACS on the basis of the finding of a new pulmonary infiltrate involving at least one complete lung segment that was consistent with the presence of alveolar consolidation but excluding atelectasis. In addition, the case definition required chest pain, a temperature higher than 38.5°C, tachypnea, wheezing, or cough. [17] Implicit in this definition is the acknowledgment that lung injury from a wide variety of causes can induce pulmonary microvascular sickling to a greater or lesser extent.

Identified etiologies of the ACS include infection, vascular infarction, and fat emboli (Table 108-6). Vichinsky and colleagues found that infections account for about one-half of cases with identified etiologies, with identified pathogens in order of frequency: *Chlamydia*, *Mycoplasma*, respiratory syncytial virus, *Staphylococcus aureus*, *Streptococcus pneumoniae*, and Parvovirus (Table 108-7). Approximately one-third of cases were presumed due to pulmonary infarction from vaso-occlusion.[17] Some of these cases may have resulted from pulmonary atelectasis due to hypoventilation caused by painful infarction of ribs or vertebrae. Localized hypoxemia due to ventilation-perfusion mismatch of any cause may result in intrapulmonary sickling and vaso-occlusion (see Table 108-6).

Fat embolism appears to play a large role in episodes of ACS developing after the onset of a pain crisis. In the study by Vichinsky et al, oil droplets in pulmonary macrophages were found in bronchoalveolar lavage fluid from approximately one-sixth of all cases, indicative of fat embolism.[18] The mechanism appears to involve infarction of bone marrow, with sloughing of fat droplets from necrotic marrow into the venous circulation, resulting in pulmonary fat emboli resembling those classically seen in patients with femur and pelvic fractures after trauma (Figs. 108-4 and 108-5). Serum levels of secretory phospholipase A$_2$ rise before the clinical onset of ACS associated with painful crisis.[19] This enzyme can hydrolyze phospholipids into potent inflammatory mediators

TABLE 108-6 Pathogenesis of the Acute Chest Syndrome

Mechanism	Supporting Evidence			
Bone infarction leads to atelectasis and regional hypoxia	Rib, vertebral, and sternal bone infarctions result in pain, hypoventilation, atelectasis, and subsequent hypoxia			
	Incentive spirometry decreases radiographic atelectasis in patients with sickle cell anemia and VOC			
Fat emboli	Evidence of bone marrow embolization found in 9%–75% of autopsy series			
	Lipid-laden alveolar macrophages can be recovered from 20%–60% of patients with ACS; $sPLA_2$ levels are elevated in ACS; $sPLA_2$ may liberate free fatty acids from bone marrow lipid, releasing arachidonic acid and promulgating inflammation			
Infection	Microbiological, serologic, or PCR evidence of pathogens[a]			
	Pathogen	Episodes	Pathogen	Episodes
	Chlamydia pneumoniae	29%	*Haemophilus influenzae*	2%
	Mycoplasma pneumoniae	20%	Cytomegalovirus	2%
	Respiratory syncytial virus	10%	Influenza A virus	2%
	Staphylococcus aureus	5%	*Legionella pneumophila*	2%
	Streptococcus pneumoniae	4%	*Escherichia coli*	1%
	Mycoplasma hominis	4%	Epstein-Barr virus	1%
	Parvovirus	4%	Herpes simplex virus	1%
	Rhinovirus	3%	Pseudomonas species	1%
	Parainfluenza virus	2%	Miscellaneous	6%
Vascular occlusion	Increased adherence of erythrocytes to endothelial cells			
	In animal models, regional pulmonary hypoxia results in entrapment of sickle erythrocytes			
	Vascular obstruction indicated by ventilation/perfusion scan			
	Pulmonary emboli documented by autopsy series			
Vascular injury and inflammation	Endothelin 1 levels are elevated during VOC and ACS			
	Elevated levels of inflammatory mediators such as $sPLA_2$			
	Clinical progression to adult respiratory distress syndrome (noncardiogenic pulmonary edema)			

[a] From Vichinsky et al.[17]

ABBREVIATIONS: ACS, acute chest syndrome; $sPLA_2$; secretory phospholipase A_2; PCR, polymerase chain reaction; VOC, vaso-occlusive pain crisis.

such as free fatty acids and lysophospholipids. Liberation of arachidonic acid may lead to production of leukotrienes, thromboxanes, and prostaglandins, all of which mediate inflammation and affect endothelial function. Inflammation leads to endothelial cell surface expression of cell adhesion molecules, especially VCAM-1. Expression of VCAM-1 may be further increased by depletion of NO and its precursor arginine, which normally suppress VCAM-1 expression.[20,21] This receptor, normally involved in the recruitment of inflammatory cells, may bind erythrocytes and leukocytes, contributing to pulmonary vaso-occlusion. This pulmonary microvascular obstruction worsens ventilation-perfusion mismatch, thereby aggravating hypoxemia, which increases sickling and leads

TABLE 108-7 Causes of Acute Chest Syndrome[a]

Cause	Cases with Identified Etiology
Fat embolism	16%
Chlamydia	13%
Mycoplasma	12%
Virus	12%
Typical bacteria	8%
Mixed infections	7%
Legionella	1%
Miscellaneous infections	1%
Infarction	30%

[a] Only those cases with complete analysis for the indicated potential infectious causes by culture, serology, and polymerase chain reaction are reported. Cases without any defined infectious etiology were presumed to be due to infarction without infection.

SOURCE: Vichinsky et al.[17]

to a vicious cycle (see Fig. 108-5). The ACS can evolve to a common end point of acute lung injury resembling that of ARDS, regardless of the initial etiology.[22]

The clinical severity of ACS is highly variable. Common physical findings include fever, tachypnea, rales, and wheezing. Laboratory findings often include leukocytosis, an acute decrease in hemoglobin level (~1.6 g/dL), and hypoxemia. Pulmonary infiltrates are often found in the upper lobes in children and lower lobes in adults. Multilobar disease suggests a worse prognosis. In addition to a new pulmonary infiltrate or consolidation, pleural effusions develop in up to half of the episodes during the course of hospitalization (see Fig. 108-4). In the study by the National Acute Chest Syndrome Study Group, 22% of ACS episodes in adults and 10% of episodes in children required management with mechanical ventilation. Risk factors for requiring mechanical ventilation were decreased platelet count ($<200,000/mm^3$), multilobar disease, a history of cardiac problems, and neurologic complications. Total mortality rates were 9% in adults but lower than 1% in children. Other than pain (especially abdominal pain), the most common complications are neurologic (11% of episodes), including seizures or stroke. Cardiac, gastrointestinal, or renal complications are infrequent. Mean duration of hospitalization was 10.5 days, as compared with 3 to 4 days for uncomplicated ACS.[17]

Treatment of ACS involves careful supportive care, empiric antibiotic therapy, and transfusion therapy (Table 108-8). Pain should be treated aggressively, and often patient-controlled analgesia is best. Relief of chest pain may improve tidal volume and improve oxygenation, although it is important to avoid excessive sedation and respiratory suppression.

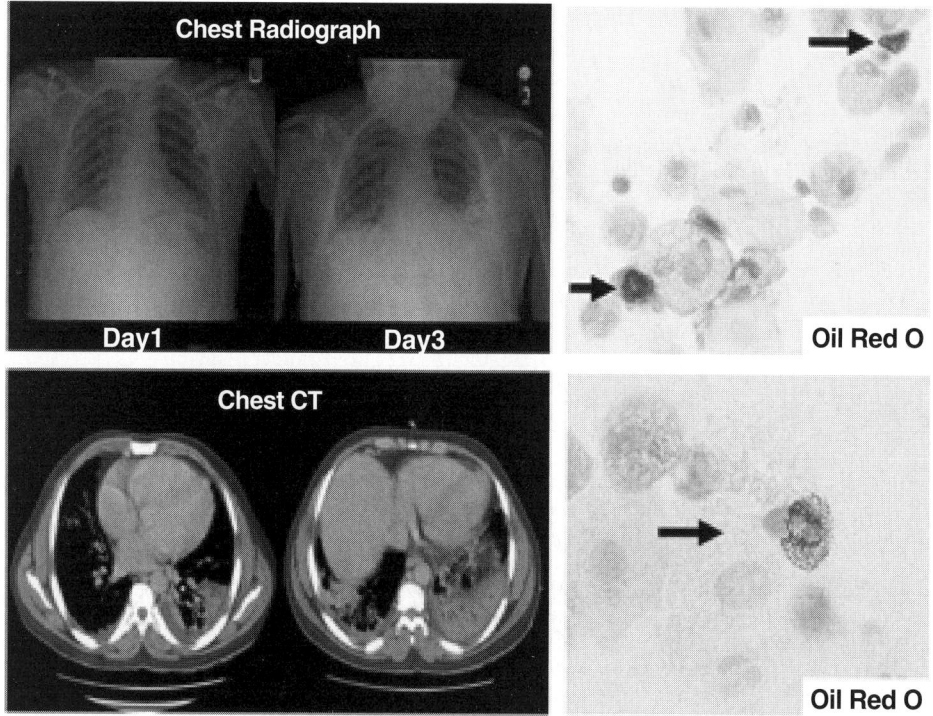

FIGURE 108-4 Acute chest syndrome of sickle cell disease. A 27-year-old male with sickle cell disease presented with fever, shortness of breath, and vaso-occlusive crisis with left chest wall pain. A chest radiograph on day 3, initially normal on day 1, demonstrates the development of a bilateral lower lobe infiltrate and bilateral pulmonary volume loss. Chest computed tomographic images on day 3 show bilateral basilar infiltrates, with dense consolidation of left lower lobe, and small bilateral pleural effusions. Micrographs after oil red O staining (which stains fat red) of specimens obtained by bronchoalveolar lavage showed lipid-laden macrophages consistent with the acute chest syndrome caused by bone marrow fat embolism to lung. *(Haley M, Gladwin MT, unpublished observations.)*

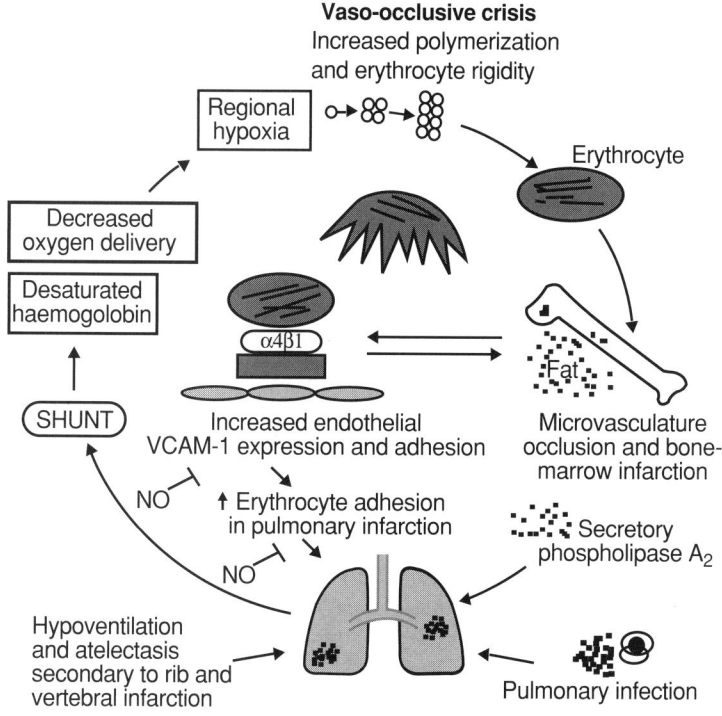

Acute chest syndrome

FIGURE 108-5 Model of acute chest syndrome pathophysiology. Vaso-occlusive crisis mediated though increased polymerization of hemoglobin S, erythrocyte rigidity, deformation, mechanical obstruction, and blood cell adherence to vascular cell adhesion molecule 1 (VCAM-1) leads to infarction of a variety of tissues, most characteristically the marrow of bones, causing severe bone pain. In some cases, fat droplets from necrotic marrow appear to slough into the venous circulation of the bone medulla, where the droplets embolize to the pulmonary circulation and increase the amount of secretory phospholipase A_2 in blood plasma. Hydrolysis of these fat emboli releases proinflammatory free fatty acids that can induce VCAM-1 expression in the pulmonary microvasculature, leading to adhesion of red and white blood cells. The pulmonary microvascular occlusion can lead to ventilation-perfusion mismatch, generalized hypoxemia, and increased systemic hemoglobin S polymerization. Alternatively, the cycle may be initiated by hypoventilation due to chest wall pain, causing localized hypoxia and pulmonary microvascular hemoglobin S polymerization, or by a pulmonary infection, which generates local hypoxia with shunting and inflammation to induce VCAM-1. The cycle may be broken by exchange transfusion or possibly by glucocorticoids. The potential therapeutic effect of inhaled nitric oxide on ventilation-perfusion matching, which decreases pulmonary artery pressure and inhibits adhesion events, is currently being studied. *(Reproduced with permission from Gladwin and Rodgers.[22])*

TABLE 108-8 Therapy of the Acute Chest Syndrome of Sickle Cell Disease

Judicious hydration
  1–1.5 times daily requirement; fluid restriction may be indicated in patients with severe acute chest syndrome and capillary leak
  or in renal insufficiency
Oxygen
  Indicated to maintain adequate oxygenation; does not offer benefit for vaso-occlusive crisis in the absence of hypoxemia
Pain management
  Mild pain
    Oral codeine, acetaminophen or ibuprofen
  Moderate to severe pain
    Medication can be administered on a fixed time schedule with interval analgesics to obtain adequate pain control (see Table
      108–9)
    Consider patient controlled analgesia (see Table 108–10)
Prevent atelectasis
  Incentive spirometry: 10 maximum inspirations q 2 h while awake
Empiric antibiotics
  Cephalosporin to cover *Streptococcus pneumoniae*
  Include macrolide or quinolone for coverage of atypical pathogens *Chlamydia pneumoniae* and *Mycoplasma pneumoniae*
  Cultures should include nasal washings for viral pathogens (influenza, respiratory syncytial virus, adenovirus, parainfluenza
    virus, cytomegalovirus, and parvovirus)
Diagnose and treat reactive airways disease
    Consider occult lack of positive end-expiration pressure and its complications
Consider exchange transfusion or simple transfusion (see Table 108–12)
Inhaled nitric oxide
  May prove efficacious but cannot be recommended routinely at this time

Incentive spirometry also helps to reduce atelectasis. Because an infectious etiology in practice can rarely be ruled out, initial management should include empiric antibiotic coverage for *Chlamydia pneumoniae*, *Mycoplasma pneumoniae*, and *Streptococcus pneumoniae*, frequently encountered organisms in ACS.[17] Commonly a third-generation cephalosporin is combined with a macrolide or quinolone antibiotic. Patients may respond to inhaled bronchodilator therapy, especially if they have a history of reactive airway disease.[16]

Pulse oximetry is a useful tool to monitor the severity of hypoxemia. Due to difficulties in interpretation caused by sickle cell disease, the data from pulse oximetry is only approximate.[23–25] Pulse oximetry while the patient is on room air should be followed, with consideration of arterial blood gas sampling while the patient is on room air if the oxygen saturation is below 92%. An increase in the alveolar-arterial oxygen gradient is the best predictor of ACS severity. The magnitude of the gradient and rate at which it develops determine the need for ICU admission, emergency transfusion, and aggressive respiratory support.[26]

Transfusion therapy is an important consideration in any case of ACS. Simple transfusion of 2 to 4 U of packed red blood cells should be considered early when ACS is diagnosed. Simple transfusion appears to be as effective as a more complete red blood cell exchange, but hemoglobin must be maintained below 10 g/dL.[27] This is usually possible because hemoglobin levels decrease during ACS. In the event of rapid progression of respiratory distress, more severe hypoxemia, multilobar disease, or requirement for mechanical ventilation, exchange transfusion is more definitive and the current standard of care (see section on transfusion therapy). Simple transfusion can be performed as a temporizing maneuver until manual or automated exchange transfusion can be performed.

Other treatments for ACS have been reported in the literature. Dexamethasone pulse therapy (0.3 mg/kg intravenously every 12 hours in four doses) has been reported to be effective in decreasing the severity of ACS in children. However, the rate of rebound pain or ACS progression when dexamethasone is stopped may exceed 25%, thus preventing widespread acceptance of this treatment.[28] Our own anecdotal experience indicates that a steroid taper does not alleviate this rebound. Dexamethasone may be useful in clinical settings in which transfusion therapy is not available or as a temporizing measure pending definitive therapy with exchange transfusion. Two case series have suggested that inhaled NO might provide clinical benefit, but this cannot be recommended without further clinical investigation in patients with sickle cell disease.[28a,28b]

PULMONARY HYPERTENSION

This frequent but previously underreported complication of sickle cell disease is associated with a high mortality rate. In a current prospective study of the prevalence and severity of pulmonary hypertension in adult patients with sickle cell disease, our group found a prevalence of 33%, and affected patients had a significantly lower survival rate at 21 months of follow up than did patients with sickle cell disease without pulmonary hypertension.[28c] A retrospective analysis suggested a 2-year mortality rate of 50%, comparable to that of primary pulmonary hypertension.[15] Sudden death from sickle cell disease may be linked to pulmonary hypertension. Severity of pulmonary hypertension in patients with sickle cell disease in steady state is mild to moderate and associated with a high cardiac output and low pulmonary vascular resistance compared with control subjects with sickle cell disease without pulmonary hypertension (see Tables 108-3 and 108-4). In our experience, pulmonary vasculature remains vaso-responsive to prostacyclin and NO in approximately 80% of patients.

Our data indicated that endogenous NO is consumed in the plasma of patients with sickle cell disease by the cell-free hemoglobin liberated from red cells by intravascular hemolysis.[8] The increase in plasma hemoglobin commonly observed during VOC may heighten NO consumption during crisis and cause decompensation of previously moderate pulmonary hypertension. This is exacerbated by an apparent depletion of the substrate for NO synthesis, the amino acid L-arginine.[29,30] Elevated plasma levels of endothelin 1, an extremely potent vasoconstrictor, are found in patients with sickle cell disease during VOC, potentially increasing pulmonary artery pressures in VOC.

SEPSIS AND MENINGITIS

Due primarily to splenic dysfunction, patients with sickle cell disease are at particular risk for sepsis. Children younger than 6 years are at greatest risk, especially for meningitis. Advances in immunizations are improving these risks, but these patients remain at higher risk for sepsis and meningitis than the general population. Although sepsis and meningitis may be caused by any organisms pathogenic in the general population, patients with sickle cell disease are particularly susceptible to infection with encapsulated organisms, especially *Streptococcus pneumoniae*. This organism may be resistant to β-lactam antibiotics due to long-term penicillin prophylaxis or recurrent courses of empiric antibiotics. Empiric antibiotic coverage with ceftriaxone or cefotaxime should be considered for fever in children younger than 6 years and in patients of all ages who appear toxic or have fever with high-grade leukocytosis. These antibiotics have rarely been associated with immune-mediated hemolytic anemia, and appropriate caution and monitoring should be undertaken. Cerebrospinal fluid pleocytosis or strongly suspected bacterial meningitis should be treated initially with vancomycin in addition to large doses of ceftriaxone or cefotaxime. Antimicrobial management of ACS was discussed earlier.

STROKE

Approximately 7% of patients with sickle cell disease will develop clinically detected cerebral infarction, with much of this risk occurring in early childhood. Young children are at risk of ischemic stroke, with a peak incidence between ages 2 and 5 years, and another peak is seen in adults older than 53 years.[31] These strokes are commonly in large vessel distributions, in contrast to the microvascular infarcts incurred in other organs. The infarctions are commonly multifocal and can be clinically overt or subclinical in nature. Population screening with transcranial Doppler ultrasonography is performed prospectively to identify those at high risk for strokes because prophylactic transfusion therapy can prevent these strokes. Patients at risk are those with time-averaged mean blood flow velocity over 200 cm/second in the internal or middle carotid arteries.[32] Clinical strokes can manifest during acute illness or as isolated neurologic events. Children with acute neurologic events should be rapidly assessed clinically for the likelihood of ischemic stroke versus bacterial meningitis, with the latter normally presenting with features of sepsis. Ischemic clinical stroke mandates rapid treatment with exchange transfusion to limit the extent of the infarction and prevent recurrences. Emergency exchange transfusion should be considered in children with sickle cell disease and acute neurologic disability even before neuroimaging studies. Without continued chronic transfusion, two of three patients

will have a recurrence. The required duration of long-term transfusion remains unclear, although most children with stroke are transfused into adulthood. Issues in stroke in sickle cell disease have recently been reviewed.[33]

Hemorrhagic stroke predominates over nonhemorrhagic stroke in adults with sickle cell disease, primarily during the third decade.[31] They are usually intracerebral hemorrhages but may occur as subarachnoid hemorrhages, with the latter often following rupture of aneurysms. Hemorrhages occur apparently due to chronic vasculopathy, and there is no published evidence to indicate whether or not its course is modified by transfusion therapy. Unfortunately, there is a dearth of published experience to guide therapy in these patients, and treatment is largely supportive, with consideration of exchange transfusion. Surgical intervention may be indicated for aneurysms.

SPLENIC SEQUESTRATION AND INFARCTION

Splenic sequestration involves acute engorgement of the spleen, presumably due to obstruction of its venous outflow by sickled erythrocytes.[34] The volume of blood acutely sequestered from the circulation can cause severe anemia and life-threatening hypotension. Because most patients with homozygous sickle cell disease have splenic atrophy by age 10 years due to gradual microinfarction, this complication occurs only in those patients with significant residual splenic parenchyma, namely young children with sickle cell disease and individuals at all ages with less severe sickling syndromes, such as hemoglobin SC disease and hemoglobin S-β-thalassemia. Splenic sequestration when acute and severe should be treated with rapid red cell transfusion, analogous to the treatment of acute severe traumatic blood loss. Overtransfusion should be avoided because, during resolution, sequestered red cells can be abruptly released, potentially causing hyperviscosity. When this syndrome occurs in adolescents or adults with hemoglobin SC disease, it may be associated with acute splenic infarction. This clinically impressive syndrome can present with very high-grade fever, extraordinary splenic pain and tenderness, and enormous splenomegaly. Sonography or computed tomography may depict inhomogeneity representative of hemorrhagic infarction, which should be differentiated from possible splenic abscess. Patients with acute splenic infarction can be managed medically with transfusions and supportive care.[35]

Recurrence of splenic infarction indicates a risk of multiple future recurrences, and some have recommended splenectomy. If this is done, it should probably be done electively after medical management and clinical resolution of the acute episode to avoid undue operative risk.

PRIAPISM

Priapism refers to pathologically prolonged erection of the penis, which is often extremely painful.[36] Although its pathophysiologic mechanism remains to be elucidated, it seems likely that penile venous outflow is obstructed by sickled erythrocytes. Case reports of many therapeutic approaches have been proposed based on experience in limited numbers of patients, but these have rarely proved to be of benefit in larger clinical experiences. The most widely recommended acute treatment for severe episodes is exchange transfusion, although evidence of its efficacy is limited. Therapies of questionable value have included adrenergic agonists, nitrates, and a surgical approach known as a Winter shunt. Only one therapy has shown some benefit in a relatively large single-institution study involving percutaneous drainage and irrigation of the corpus cavernosum initiated within 3 hours of onset.[37] The value of this approach has not been validated in other institutions, but it may have the clearest evidence of benefit in absence of a well-established standard of care. One very interesting, counterintuitive approach has been reported. Sildenafil, normally used clinically to treat erectile dysfunction, given in single 50-mg doses as needed, rapidly relieved several episodes of priapism in three patients with sickle cell disease.[38] Because of the possibility that this drug might also be capable of inducing priapism, its use cannot be recommended until further research is conducted.

PERIOPERATIVE MANAGEMENT

Patients with sickle cell disease have a high risk of perioperative complications, with 10% to 50% developing a VOC or ACS postoperatively. Careful preoperative anesthesiology consultation should be undertaken. Many sickle cell centers have traditionally performed serial transfusion or exchange transfusion preoperatively with a goal of preventing postoperative complications by reducing the hemoglobin S fraction to less than 30%, with a final total hemoglobin level of at least 10 gm/dL. A randomized study by Vichinsky et al showed that preoperative simple transfusion with a goal of raising the total hemoglobin concentration to 10 gm/dL, without a specific goal for hemoglobin S percentage, has similar efficacy. However, this study included predominantly patients with less invasive surgical procedures, such as tympanostomy tube placement or laparoscopic cholecystectomy. Some centers still prefer to perform exchange transfusion before major surgery in patients with sickle cell disease, although many transfuse less aggressively. A careful risk-benefit evaluation must be applied to each case, especially in patients with a history of red blood cell alloimmunization.

Supportive care should include careful attention to avoiding dehydration, overhydration, deoxygenation, vascular stasis, low temperature, acidosis or infection. The operating room should be kept warm, and warming devices should be used for the patient. Oxygenation status should be closely monitored intraoperatively and postoperatively, and incentive spirometry should be prescribed postoperatively. The literature regarding perioperative management of patients with sickle cell disease has been reviewed in more detail by Marchant and Walker.[39]

Treatments

OXYGEN AND FLUIDS

Because hypoxemia and dehydration can trigger sickling, it is important to prevent these from developing. Contrary to traditional teaching in many medical training programs, there is no indication of benefit from aggressive hydration in patients who are not dehydrated or from oxygen therapy in the absence of hypoxemia. Excessive fluid resuscitation may even compromise some older patients who have some degree of congestive heart failure or renal insufficiency.

ANALGESICS

At times, acetaminophen can suffice for mild pain. More severe pain often requires addition of an oral opioid analgesic such as codeine, hydromorphone, morphine, or oxycodone; morphine and oxycodone are available as short-acting or sustained-release preparations (Table 108-9). Severe pain episodes are best treated with intravenous opioids, usually morphine or hydromorphone, with considerable added convenience to patient and clinician when administered via a patient-controlled analgesia pump (Table 108-10). Patients with severe pain may also benefit from the parenteral nonsteroidal anti-inflammatory drug ketorolac, although questions have been raised about potential impairment of renal blood flow. Ketorolac also presents a risk of gastrointestinal hemorrhage, particularly if used for 5 days or longer. We recommend that nonsteroidal anti-inflammatory agents be withheld in patients with sickle cell disease with pulmonary hypertension or serum creatinine level above 0.8 mg/dL. Clinicians should consider the baseline narcotics the patient is using for determining an adequate dose of narcotics. Opioid tolerance due to previous chronic or frequent opioid administration may be an indication for much larger doses of opioids for acute pain control. Elderly or debilitated patients may require smaller doses of opioids to reduce toxicity. Opioid therapy may result in constipation, nausea, or pruritus. A laxative such as Senokot should be administered prophylactically. Nausea may be treated with diphenhydramine, hydroxyzine, promethazine, ondansetron, or dolasetron. Pruritus may be treated with diphenhydramine or hydroxyzine. Very severe pruritus may respond to naloxone

TABLE 108-9 Parenteral Analgesics Commonly Used in Painful Crisis of Sickle Cell Disease[a]

Class	Agent	Adult Dose	Pediatric Dose	Notes
NSAID	Ketorolac	30 mg IV q 6 h	0.5 mg/kg IV q 6 h	After 3 d, change to oral ibuprofen due to risk of gastrointestinal bleeding; omit in patients with known pulmonary hypertension
Opioid	Morphine	5–20 mg IV q 3 h	0.1–0.2 mg/kg IV q 3–6 h	Usually use morphine as opioid except in cases of previous morphine intolerance
	Hydromorphone	1–4 mg IV q 3–6 h	0.015–0.03 mg/kg IV q 3–6 h	

[a]Most patients will require midrange doses. Use a lower dose range in elderly or debilitated patients or consider an upper dose range in opioid-tolerant patients. Highly tolerant patients at times may require even larger doses than the ranges listed. The use of meperidine is generally discouraged, due to seizures occasionally seen as a complication of its use. Most patients can obtain satisfactory analgesia with morphine or hydromorphone. Opioid-induced side effects often require medical management (see text).
ABBREVIATIONS: IV, intravenously; NSAID, nonsteroidal anti-inflammatory drug.

TABLE 108-10 Approaches for Patient-Controlled Analgesia[a]

Agent	ADULT DOSE		PEDIATRIC DOSE	
	Continuous	Demand	Continuous	Demand
Morphine	1–2 mg/h	1–2 mg	0.01–0.03 mg/kg per hour	0.01–0.03 mg/kg
Hydromorphone	0.2–1 mg/h	0.2–1 mg	0.003–0.005 mg/kg per hour	0.003–0.005 mg/kg

[a] In adults and children, common parameters include 6- to 10-minute lockout, limited to five demand doses per hour. Meperidine should never be administered by continuous infusion. Most patients will require midrange doses. Use a lower dose range in elderly or debilitated patients or consider an upper dose range in highly opioid-tolerant patients. Highly tolerant patients at times may require even larger doses than the ranges listed. Opioid-induced side effects often require medical management (see text).

1 μg/kg per hour as a continuous intravenous infusion. This small dose can block opioid receptors associated with pruritus without blocking those associated with analgesia. Detailed recommendations for analgesia in patients with sickle cell disease have been published.[40]

INCENTIVE SPIROMETRY

Bedrest during a pain crisis may lead to pulmonary atelectasis. This can trigger ACS (see below). Bedside incentive spirometry during pain crisis has been shown to prevent the development of pulmonary infiltrates.

TRANSFUSION

Although there is probably no indication for treatment of the acute pain crisis, most other acute serious complications of sickle cell disease can be stabilized through the use of transfusions to diminish the percentage of circulating hemoglobin S. Table 108-11 lists indications for transfusion therapy. It is clear from reviewing this list that almost any patient who requires an ICU visit is likely to require a simple or exchange transfusion. As such, the intensivist must be well versed in the indications, complications, and pitfalls of transfusion therapy in this population.

Patients with sickle cell disease have severe chronic anemia, and they generally tolerate transient episodes of at least a 20% decrease in their baseline hemoglobin level quite well, if the reticulocyte count remains high. Knowledge of a given patient's baseline parameters can help to determine the need for transfusion for exacerbation of anemia. The most severe and life-threatening anemia and reticulocytopenia occurs during aplastic crisis resulting from infection with the parvovirus

B19, otherwise known as erythema infectiosum, fifth disease, or slapped-cheek disease. Life-threatening anemia and hypovolemia due to splenic sequestration are other such indications, discussed in more detail below.

There are several important transfusion issues unique to patients with sickle cell disease to consider. First, transfused red cells should be negative by Sickledex or another rapid screening test to exclude blood from sickle trait donors. Second, the detailed red cell phenotype should be ascertained in the blood bank, particularly for patients who will be chronically transfused, such as children with a new stroke. This permits more directed management of alloimmunization to red cell antigens, although the actual approach is controversial. The rate of alloimmunization to red cell antigens in patients with sickle cell disease is 18% to 36%, most often involving the D, C, and E antigens in the Rh system and less often the Kell, Kidd and Duffy blood groups. This is attributable in large part to discrepancy in allele frequency between these patients of African descent and the blood pool from donors of mostly European descent. One workshop report has recommended the use of red cell units prophylactically matched to prevent sensitization to the Rh antigens D, C, and E and the Kell antigen K.[41] However, others have advocated matching these antigens only after the patient has become immunized to antigens.[42] The high rate of alloimmunization in patients with sickle cell disease promotes a higher incidence (3%) of delayed hemolytic transfusion reactions. These are defined as premature clearance of transfused red cells, usually several days after transfusion. In some cases, the hemoglobin level may decrease to below the pretransfusion level, with the immune reaction to transfused cells apparently generalizing to also involve the patient's

TABLE 108-11 Acute Indications for Transfusion in Patients with Sickle Cell Disease

Indication	Transfusion Form
Severe anemia associated with high output cardiac failure, dyspnea, postural hypotension, angina, or cerebral dysfunction	Simple
Sudden reduction in hemoglobin concentration (splenic or hepatic sequestration, aplastic crisis)	Simple
Acute or suspected stroke	Exchange
Multiorgan failure syndrome	Exchange
Acute chest syndrome with severe hypoxia	Exchange
Acute chest syndrome with acute anemia	Simple
Preoperative preparation, hemoglobin SS	Simple
Preoperative preparation, hemoglobin SC, major surgery	Partial exchange
Acute severe priapism	Exchange

ABBREVIATIONS: SC, hemoglobin sickle cell disease; SS, homozygous sickle cell disease.

own red cells, a phenomenon that has been called "bystander hemolysis."

Because of this complication, it is critical to obtain a transfusion antibody history from blood banks where a patient was previously transfused. Over several months, alloantibody titers to red blood cell antigens may become undetectable on a routine type and cross-match but remain capable of mediating a transfusion reaction. The resulting delayed transfusion reaction in an acutely ill hospitalized patient can be catastrophic, with hemoglobin levels decreasing to 2 to 3 g/dL.

Simple transfusion is sufficient for correcting severe anemia, but exchange transfusion can more rapidly dilute sickle hemoglobin to less than 40% of circulating hemoglobin, which is desirable in acute life-threatening sickle cell complications, in particular stroke, ACS, and multiorgan failure syndrome. Exchange transfusion may be accomplished rapidly and isovolumetrically by erythrocytapheresis, when this procedure is available (Table 108-12). This requires upper extremity veins sufficient for two large-bore needles, placement of a Quinton or similar apheresis, or hemodialysis venous catheter in a central vein (femoral, internal jugular, or subclavian). Alternatively, manual exchange transfusion may be performed by using one of several protocols, with a goal of replacing 70% of the sickle red cell mass with transfused red cells. One simplified approach for adults is presented in Table 108-12. Another approach useful in children and adults is to exchange the red cell mass twice, as calculated below:

$$\text{volume transfused} = \frac{2\times(\text{patient hematocrit, decimal, not \%})\times(\text{patient weight in kg})\times(70\text{ mL/kg})}{\text{average hematocrit of transfused packed red blood cells, usually }0.55}$$

This volume may be transfused while whole blood is being withdrawn from a high-flow site, often an arterial or central venous line. The transfusion may be accomplished as rapidly as the inflow and outflow catheters allow, as long as care is taken to maintain balanced hourly inflow and outflow rates for the duration of the procedure. If the hemoglobin level exceeds 10 gm/dL or hematocrit exceeds 30% during the first half of the exchanged volume, the red cell hourly infusion rate should be halved, and the reduced red cell rate replaced with normal saline, so that the hourly inflow rate continues to equal the outflow rate. The final target hemoglobin level should be 10 gm/dL. Higher hemoglobin levels can cause hyperviscosity problems at the microvascular level in patients with sickle cell disease.

HYDROXYUREA

This agent was first widely used to treat chronic myeloid leukemia and has found a place in the prophylactic treatment of sickle cell disease. At least in adults with more severe than average sickle cell disease, it decreases the incidence of significant pain episodes, ACS, and transfusions by approximately 50% and significantly prolongs lifespan. Its favorable effects are mediated through its elevation of fetal hemoglobin, which inhibits sickle hemoglobin polymerization. Its use may be complicated by myelosuppression, and administration is commonly interrupted during sepsis or serious infection, although it is unclear whether this is truly necessary in the absence of drug-induced neutropenia. Hydroxyurea is contraindicated in pregnancy due to its potential teratogenicity, and a potential carcinogenic effect after long-term use has not been completely excluded.

GLUCOCORTICOIDS

Methylprednisolone (15 mg/kg per day intravenously IV in two doses) and dexamethasone (0.3 mg/kg every 12 hours intravenously in four doses) have produced statistically significant improvements in painful crisis and ACS, respectively, but this treatment is troubled by significant rebound symptoms in at least 25% of patients. The partial success of these

TABLE 108-12 Exchange Transfusion in Sickle Cell Disease

Indications
  Patients with extensive pulmonary infiltrates (especially multilobar)
  Rapidly progressive respiratory disease
  Signs of respiratory distress
  Pa_{O_2} <60 mm Hg in an adult breathing supplemental oxygen (70 mm Hg for children) or a decrease >25% from baseline in a patient with known hypoxemia.
  Patient requiring ICU admission for ACS
  Before major surgery (controversial)
  Priapism and other severe symptoms.
Goals
  Increase hematocrit to 10 gm/dL (do not exceed 12 g/dL to avoid hyperviscosity)
  Decrease percentage of hemoglobin S to <30% (i.e., replace >70% of red cell mass)
Methods of exchange transfusion
  Exchange transfusion is preferred if there is concern about volume overload, initial hemoglobin is >9–10 g/dL, or a significant rapid reduction in hemoglobin S is required (which is often the case in the ICU)
  Remove 500 mL of whole blood from an arterial line or freely flowing venous line while infusing into another venous line simultaneously; repeat until the goals are met
  Alternatively, remove 500 mL of blood, infuse 500 mL of normal saline, remove another 500 mL of blood, then transfuse 2 U of packed red cells; repeat until the goals are met
  Automated apheresis devices can also be used; a typical adult will require 6–8 U of blood for apheresis exchange

ABBREVIATIONS: ACS, acute chest syndrome; ICU, intensive care unit; Pa_{O_2}, arterial pressure of O_2.

agents indicates the probable role that inflammatory pathways play in acute vaso-occlusive phenomena.

INVESTIGATIONAL

Inhaled NO at 80 ppm for 4 hours produces a trend toward significant improvement in the duration of crisis and pain scores in a preliminary study in children with VOC.[43] Case reports have documented its effect on increasing arterial oxygenation and decreasing pulmonary pressures during the ACS.[28a,28b] Its use in secondary pulmonary hypertension in sickle cell disease is being studied. The natural NO donor L-arginine often is depleted from the blood of patients with sickle cell disease in crisis, and its supplementation is being evaluated.[44] Inhibitors of the red cell Gardos channel enhance water transport into normally dehydrated sickle cells, thereby decreasing hemoglobin S polymerization, and these are in clinical trial.[45] Poloxamer 188 (Flocor) is a rheological agent that has shortened the duration of VOC under some circumstances.[46]

References

1. Charache S, Terrin ML, Moore RD, et al: Effect of hydroxyurea on the frequency of painful crises in sickle cell anemia. Investigators of the Multicenter Study of Hydroxyurea in Sickle Cell Anemia. *N Engl J Med* 332:1317, 1995.
2. Steinberg MH, Barton F, Castro O, et al: Effect of hydroxyurea on mortality and morbidity in adult sickle cell anemia: Risks and benefits up to 9 years of treatment. *JAMA* 289:1645, 2003.
3. Reiter CD, Gladwin MT: An emerging role for nitric oxide in sickle cell disease vascular homeostasis and therapy. *Curr Opin Hematol* 10:99, 2003.
4. Frenette PS: Sickle cell vaso-occlusion: multistep and multicellular paradigm. *Curr Opin Hematol* 9:101, 2002.
5. Stuart MJ, Setty BN: Hemostatic alterations in sickle cell disease: relationships to disease pathophysiology. *Pediatr Pathol Mol Med* 20:27, 2001.
6. Steinberg MH, Brugnara C: Pathophysiological-based approaches to treatment of sickle cell disease. *Annu Rev Med* 54:89, 2003.
7. Aidoo M, Terlouw DJ, Kolczak MS, et al: Protective effects of the sickle cell gene against malaria morbidity and mortality. *Lancet* 359:1311, 2002.
8. Reiter CD, Wang X, Tanus-Santos JE, et al: Cell-free hemoglobin limits nitric oxide bioavailability in sickle-cell disease. *Nat Med* 8:1383, 2002.
9. Aslan M, Ryan TM, Adler B, et al: Oxygen radical inhibition of nitric oxide-dependent vascular function in sickle cell disease. *Proc Natl Acad Sci USA* 98:15215, 2001.
10. Gladwin MT, Schechter AN, Ognibene FP, et al: Divergent nitric oxide bioavailability in men and women with sickle cell disease. *Circulation* 107:271, 2003.
11. Stuart MJ, Setty BN: Sickle cell acute chest syndrome: pathogenesis and rationale for treatment. *Blood* 94:1555, 1999.
12. Loscalzo J: Nitric oxide insufficiency, platelet activation, and arterial thrombosis. *Circ Res* 88:756, 2001.
13. Jison ML, Gladwin MT: Hemolytic anemia-associated pulmonary hypertension of sickle cell disease and the nitric oxide/arginine pathway. *Am J Respir Crit Care Med* 168:3, 2003.
14. Cohen SB, Fletcher ME, Goldberg MF, et al: Diagnosis and management of ocular complications of sickle hemoglobinopathies: Part V. *Ophthalmic Surg* 17:369, 1986.
15. Castro O, Hoque M, Brown BD: Pulmonary hypertension in sickle cell disease: Cardiac catheterization results and survival. *Blood* 101:1257, 2003.
16. Minter KR, Gladwin MT: Pulmonary complications of sickle cell anemia. A need for increased recognition, treatment, and research. *Am J Respir Crit Care Med* 164:2016, 2001.
17. Vichinsky EP, Neumayr LD, Earles AN, et al: Causes and outcomes of the acute chest syndrome in sickle cell disease. National Acute Chest Syndrome Study Group. *N Engl J Med* 342:1855, 2000.
18. Vichinsky E, Williams R, Das M, et al: Pulmonary fat embolism: a distinct cause of severe acute chest syndrome in sickle cell anemia. *Blood* 83:3107, 1994.
19. Styles LA, Schalkwijk CG, Aarsman AJ, et al: Phospholipase A2 levels in acute chest syndrome of sickle cell disease. *Blood* 87:2573, 1996.
20. Stuart MJ, Setty BN: Acute chest syndrome of sickle cell disease: new light on an old problem. *Curr Opin Hematol* 8:111, 2001.
21. Morris CR, Vichinsky EP, Van Warmerdam J, et al: Hydroxyurea and arginine therapy: Impact on nitric oxide production in sickle cell disease. *J Pediatr Hematol Oncol* 25:629, 2003.
22. Gladwin MT, Rodgers GP: Pathogenesis and treatment of acute chest syndrome of sickle-cell anaemia. *Lancet* 355:1476, 2000.
23. Ortiz FO, Aldrich TK, Nagel RL, et al: Accuracy of pulse oximetry in sickle cell disease. *Am J Respir Crit Care Med* 159:447, 1999.
24. Fitzgerald RK, Johnson A: Pulse oximetry in sickle cell anemia. *Crit Care Med* 29:1803, 2001.
25. Blaisdell CJ, Goodman S, Clark K, et al: Pulse oximetry is a poor predictor of hypoxemia in stable children with sickle cell disease. *Arch Pediatr Adolesc Med* 154:900, 2000.
26. Emre U, Miller ST, Rao SP, et al: Alveolar-arterial oxygen gradient in acute chest syndrome of sickle cell disease. *J Pediatr* 123:272, 1993.
27. Vichinsky EP: Current issues with blood transfusions in sickle cell disease. *Semin Hematol* 38:14, 2001.
28. Bernini JC, Rogers ZR, Sandler ES, et al: Beneficial effect of intravenous dexamethasone in children with mild to moderately severe acute chest syndrome complicating sickle cell disease. *Blood* 92:3082, 1998.
28a. Atz AM, Wessel DL: Inhaled nitric oxide in sickle cell disease with acute chest syndrome. *Anesthesiology* 87:988, 1997.
28b. Sullivan KJ, Goodwin SR, Evangelist J, et al: Nitric oxide successfully used to treat acute chest syndrome of sickle cell disease in a young adolescent. *Crit Care Med* 27:2563, 1999.
28c. Gladwin MT, Sachdev V, Jison M, et al: Pulmonary Hypertension as a Risk Factor for Death in Patients with Sickle Cell Disease. *N Engl J Med* 350:886, 2004.
29. Morris CR, Morris SM, Hagar W, et al: Arginine therapy: A new treatment for pulmonary hypertension in sickle cell disease? *Am J Respir Crit Care Med* 168:63, 2003.
30. Morris CR, Kuypers FA, Larkin S, et al: Arginine therapy: A novel strategy to induce nitric oxide production in sickle cell disease. *Br J Haematol* 111:498, 2000.
31. Ohene-Frempong K, Weiner SJ, Sleeper LA, et al: Cerebrovascular accidents in sickle cell disease: rates and risk factors. *Blood* 91:288, 1998.
32. Adams RJ, McKie VC, Hsu L, et al: Prevention of a first stroke by transfusions in children with sickle cell anemia and abnormal results on transcranial Doppler ultrasonography. *N Engl J Med* 339:5, 1998.
33. Prengler M, Pavlakis SG, Prohovnik I, et al: Sickle cell disease: The neurological complications. *Ann Neurol* 51:543, 2002.
34. Emond AM, Collis R, Darvill D, et al: Acute splenic sequestration in homozygous sickle cell disease: Natural history and management. *J Pediatr* 107:201, 1985.
35. Yeung KY, Lessin LS: Splenic infarction in sickle cell-hemoglobin C disease. Demonstration by selective splenic arteriogram and scintillation scan. *Arch Intern Med* 136:905, 1976.
36. Emond AM, Holman R, Hayes RJ, et al: Priapism and impotence in homozygous sickle cell disease. *Arch Intern Med* 140:1434, 1980.

37. Mantadakis E, Cavender JD, Rogers ZR, et al: Prevalence of priapism in children and adolescents with sickle cell anemia. *J Pediatr Hematol Oncol* 21:518, 1999.

38. Bialecki ES, Bridges KR: Sildenafil relieves priapism in patients with sickle cell disease. *Am J Med* 113:252, 2002.

39. Marchant WA, Walker I: Anaesthetic management of the child with sickle cell disease. *Paediatr Anaesth* 13:473, 2003.

40. Platt A, Eckman JR, Beasley J, et al: Treating sickle cell pain: an update from the Georgia comprehensive. *J Emerg Nurse* 28:297, 2002.

41. Telen MJ: Principles and problems of transfusion in sickle cell disease. *Semin Hematol* 38:315, 2001.

42. King KE, Ness PM: Treating anemia. *Hematol Oncol Clin North Am* 10:1305, 1996.

43. Weiner DL, Hibberd PL, Betit P, et al: Preliminary assessment of inhaled nitric oxide for acute vaso-occlusive crisis in pediatric patients with sickle cell disease. *JAMA* 289:1136, 2003.

44. Morris CR, Morris SM, Jr., Hagar W, et al: Arginine therapy: A new treatment for pulmonary hypertension in sickle cell disease? *Am J Respir Crit Care Med* 168:63, 2003.

45. Stocker JW, De Franceschi L, McNaughton-Smith GA, et al: ICA-17043, a novel Gardos channel blocker, prevents sickled red blood cell dehydration in vitro and in vivo in SAD mice. *Blood* 101:2412, 2003.

46. Orringer EP, Casella JF, Ataga KI, et al: Purified poloxamer 188 for treatment of acute vaso-occlusive crisis of sickle cell disease: A randomized controlled trial. *JAMA* 286:2099, 2001.

Chapter 109

THE OBESITY EPIDEMIC AND CRITICAL CARE

BRIAN GEHLBACH
JOHN P. KRESS

KEY POINTS

- *Morbid obesity presents unique cardiorespiratory challenges in the intensive care unit and frustrates the delivery of routine care. Whether or not obesity itself influences the outcome of critical illness is unclear.*

- *Morbid obesity leads to heart disease through a number of diverse mechanisms. Therefore, a high index of suspicion for its presence is warranted in the critically ill patient.*

- *An increased risk of venous thromboembolism in obesity merits an aggressive approach to prophylaxis.*

- *Cor pulmonale occurs in individuals with nocturnal and diurnal hypoxemia related to the obesity hypoventilation syndrome or coexisting obstructive sleep apnea and obstructive lung disease.*

- *Although simple obesity has relatively minor effects on pulmonary function, morbid obesity may be associated with reductions in forced vital capacity, forced expiration volume in 1 second, and total lung capacity. An increase in mid to late expiratory flow may be seen.*

- *Morbid obesity is associated with a significant increase in the percentage of oxygen consumption attributable to the work of breathing. This decreased respiratory reserve results in a predisposition to the development of respiratory failure even after trivial insults.*

- *Atelectasis is common in the morbidly obese postoperative patient and, in addition to any accompanying sleep-disordered breathing, may lead to respiratory failure. Although conclusive data are lacking, the early use of noninvasive ventilation in the high-risk postoperative patient may prevent the development of respiratory failure.*

- *Intubation of the morbidly obese patient may be technically challenging because of poor visibility of the glottis and decreased oxygen stores in alveoli from a reduced functional residual capacity.*

- *Morbidly obese patients should be ventilated in the upright or semi-upright position to improve respiratory system compliance and reduce the work of breathing. Positive end-expiratory pressure between 8 and 15 cm H_2O may be necessary to prevent atelectasis.*

- *Because the compliance of the chest wall is diminished in morbid obesity, a high plateau pressure does not necessarily indicate alveolar overdistention. When using low tidal volume ventilation in the management of the acute respiratory distress syndrome, a plateau pressure of 35 to 40 cm H_2O may be acceptable in some patients.*

- *Ultrasound guidance may be useful in establishing vascular access in the morbidly obese patient.*

- *Numerous unpredictable alterations in pharmacokinetics have been described in obesity. Reference to published guidelines for*

individual drugs and close monitoring of clinically available serum drug levels are recommended.

- *Attempts by clinicians to accelerate a program of weight loss during the course of critical illness are misguided and may interfere with immune function, wound healing, and respiratory muscle strength. Carefully balanced hypocaloric regimens may be safe.*

An ever-increasing percentage of the inhabitants of developed countries is obese or overweight. This trend includes men and women and spans all age groups, including children. Obesity is associated with diabetes mellitus, cardiovascular disease, hypertension, and cancer and confers a reduced life expectancy, particularly in younger and severely obese individuals. Extreme obesity is frequently associated with life-threatening cardiopulmonary disease and presents substantial obstacles to the delivery of routine care. We present a summary of the challenges inherent in the care of the morbidly obese critically ill patient and highlight physiological principles important to the care of such patients.

The Obesity Epidemic

DEFINING OBESITY

Due to the impracticality of determining body fat composition in the clinical setting, obesity is typically defined as excessive weight relative to body surface area as determined by calculation of the body mass index (BMI), calculated as weight in kilograms divided by height in square meters. The correlation between BMI and obesity in most middle-age adults is very good, although using BMI as a proxy for body fat is misleading in individuals engaged in weight training who have increased muscle mass, and when significant edema is present. The World Health Organization and National Institutes of Health recommend the following definitions of overweight and obesity: overweight is defined as a BMI greater than 25 kg/m^2, obesity is defined as a BMI greater than 30 kg/m^2, and morbid obesity is defined as a BMI greater than 40 kg/m^2. Some authorities have extended the definition of morbid obesity to individuals with a BMI greater than 35 kg/m^2 if they have serious medical comorbidities.

THE MAGNITUDE OF THE PROBLEM

Data from the 1999–2000 National Health and Nutrition Examination Survey show a continued increase in the prevalence of overweight and obesity in the United States over the past 15 years. Relative to the 1988–1994 survey, the prevalence of overweight individuals has increased from 55.9% to 64.5%, obesity has increased from 22.9% to 30.5%, and morbid obesity has increased from 2.9% to 4.7%.[1] Non-Hispanic black women have the highest prevalence of obesity and overweight, but increases were found across all ethnic groups and in men and women. Perhaps of greatest concern is an increase in the prevalence of overweight and obesity among children, particularly Mexican American and non-Hispanic black adolescents.[2,3]

There are many potential explanations for the increasing number of persons who are overweight or obese. Technologic advances have decreased the cost of food production, thereby making food more affordable, and decreased the energy expended by the typical worker.[4] Leisure time is increasingly dominated by sedentary activities such as watching television or using the computer. Television viewing is associated with increased food intake and a decrease in metabolic rate even when compared with other sedentary activities such as reading or sewing.[5] The risks of obesity and type II diabetes mellitus have been positively correlated with the amount of television watched,[6] and children randomized to an intervention discouraging television viewing had significant reductions in relative BMI compared with controls.[7] Other possible explanations for the obesity epidemic include an increased percentage of meals eaten outside the home, the serving of larger portions at commercial establishments, and the widespread consumption of diets low in vegetables and fibers and high in refined sugars. Individual susceptibility to these influences is poorly understood but likely includes a genetic component.

Unfortunately, the obesity epidemic is not confined to highly developed countries. The World Health Organization estimates that 1 billion people worldwide are overweight or obese. Worse, most indications are that the epidemic has not yet peaked: obesity is increasing in prevalence in developing countries coincident with decreased physical activity and the replacement of traditional fruits and whole grains in the diet with calorie-dense, processed foods.

Physiologic Effects of Morbid Obesity

Obesity is associated with a shortened life expectancy, particularly in severely obese younger individuals.[8] This section summarizes important physiologic derangements associated with obesity, with an emphasis on those germane to the care of the morbidly obese critically ill patient.

CARDIOVASCULAR EFFECTS

The risk of death from cardiovascular disease rises steeply above a BMI of 30 kg/m^2.[9] There are several mechanisms through which obesity can cause cardiovascular disease. First, obesity increases the risk of coronary atherosclerosis by inducing several risk factors in parallel. For example, obesity is associated with hypertension, insulin resistance, dyslipidemia, and coagulation abnormalities, which separately and collectively promote the development of cardiovascular disease.

There are other mechanisms through which obesity causes heart disease. Obesity may impair cardiac function through chronic pressure and volume overload.[10] Cardiac output is increased in obesity as a result of increased extracellular volume and increased blood flow to most tissue beds. This increased cardiac output is associated with increased preload and cardiac dilatation, with the subsequent development of eccentric left ventricular hypertrophy. This chronic volume-overloaded state, when combined with increased left ventricular afterload from concurrent hypertension, may result in marked left ventricular hypertrophy. Over time, left ventricular hypertrophy leads to impaired ventricular filling and diastolic heart failure. Systolic heart failure may result from ischemic heart disease, microvascular disease from diabetes mellitus, longstanding hypertension, or, in severe, longstanding obesity, a decrease in mid-wall fiber shortening and ejection fraction.[9]

Pulmonary hypertension with right ventricular hypertrophy and dilation may accompany obesity. When not caused by left ventricular failure, pulmonary hypertension in these patients typically arises from conditions that cause nocturnal and diurnal hypoxemia. A relatively common presentation of this problem is that of the patient with obstructive sleep apnea who has coexisting chronic obstructive pulmonary disease. Cor pulmonale may also develop in patients with the obesity hypoventilation syndrome (OHS). This poorly understood disorder is associated with daytime hypercapnia and hypoxemia, with the latter arising from alveolar hypoventilation and poor ventilation of the basal lung due to airway closure and atelectasis. Hypercapnia and hypoxemia elicit pulmonary vasoconstriction. Eventually, this may lead to vascular remodeling with resulting irreversible pulmonary hypertension and cor pulmonale. Individuals with the OHS frequently, but not always, have coexisting obstructive sleep apnea.

Plasminogen activator inhibitor I and fibrinogen levels are elevated in most patients with obesity, suggesting a role for hypercoagulability and impaired fibrinolysis in cardiac and cerebrovascular diseases. Elevated proinflammatory cytokines, for example, interleukin 6 and C-reactive protein, potentially indicate the presence of a low-grade inflammatory state in this condition.[9]

What are the clinical implications of this susceptibility to such a range of cardiovascular disorders? First, the intensivist caring for the morbidly obese patient should have a high index of suspicion for the presence of ischemic heart disease from coronary artery or microvascular disease. Second, abnormal cardiac function, diastolic or systolic, may be present, even if other risk factors for heart disease are absent. Particular sensitivity to changes in intravascular volume may result. Third, pulmonary hypertension and right ventricular failure should be suspected when obstructive lung disease and/or daytime hypoxemia or hypercapnia are present. The diagnosis of these conditions is complicated by poor sensitivity of physical examination and transthoracic echocardiography in morbidly obese individuals. In selected patients, transesophageal echocardiography or invasive hemodynamic monitoring may be necessary.

PULMONARY EFFECTS

MECHANICS OF THE RESPIRATORY SYSTEM
The effect of obesity on pulmonary function varies considerably between individuals, ranging from trivial to profound impairment, but generally increases in severity with the BMI.[11,12] The overall compliance of the respiratory system is reduced, mildly so in simple obesity and as low as 45% of normal in patients with OHS. Some studies have suggested that decreased chest wall compliance from the mechanical effect of adipose tissue on the thoracic cage is the principal cause of this abnormality, whereas other investigators have implicated reduced lung compliance as an additional factor, probably from a decrease in functional residual capacity. Airway resistance has been found to be increased, and a reduction in mid to late expiratory flows has been noted; because the ratio of forced expiratory volume in 1 second (FEV$_1$) to forced vital

capacity (FVC) is typically normal or even elevated in obesity, a reduction in small airway caliber is likely responsible.

PULMONARY FUNCTION

The most frequent abnormality in pulmonary function in obesity is a decrease in the expiratory reserve volume attributable to cephalad displacement of the diaphragm by adipose tissue. In severely obese individuals and in those with the OHS, total lung capacity and vital capacity may be reduced. In such patients, the residual volume may actually be increased relative to total lung capacity because of small airway closure and gas trapping. This is supported by the finding of larger total lung capacity by body box plethysmography than by helium dilution.[13] Similarly, spirometry is typically normal in simple obesity, whereas severely obese individuals or those with the OHS may exhibit reductions in FEV_1 and FVC, even though the ratio of these two variables is preserved or even increased.

Why do some individuals exhibit diminished pulmonary function and/or the OHS, whereas comparably overweight individuals may be little affected? Some, but not all, data suggest that the distribution of body fat may be an important determinant of pulmonary function; simply put, adipose tissue that is more centrally located is more likely to negatively influence pulmonary function. There are also important differences in respiratory muscle strength between patients with simple obesity and those with the OHS, with the latter exhibiting decreased inspiratory muscle strength. Weakness may be considered absolute, a result of mechanical disadvantage from diaphragm malposition, and relative, when the increased work of breathing from morbid obesity is considered (see below).

GAS EXCHANGE

Morbid obesity causes closure of small peripheral airways in the dependent regions of the lung, resulting in mismatching of ventilation and perfusion.[14] The result may be a widened alveolar to arterial oxygen gradient and mild to moderate hypoxemia that worsens in the supine position. Severe hypoxemia may be present in individuals with the OHS because of the additional contribution of hypoventilation. The diffusing capacity for carbon monoxide is typically normal and may be elevated when indexed to alveolar volume.

CONTROL OF BREATHING

Ventilatory drive is increased in simple obesity as assessed by the mouth occlusion pressure and diaphragm electrical activity in response to carbon dioxide inhalation. In contrast, mouth occlusion pressure response to carbon dioxide is reduced in OHS compared to normal individuals and to patients with simple obesity. Diaphragm electrical activity in response to carbon dioxide is inappropriately low in OHS.

PERIOPERATIVE AND OTHER PULMONARY CONSIDERATIONS IN OBESITY

The reduced functional residual capacity associated with severe obesity encroaches on the closing capacity, the lung volume at which small airways in the lung bases begin to close. This places severely obese patients at significant risk for atelectasis in the perioperative period, particularly where upper abdominal or thoracic operations are concerned. Hypoxemia may result and may be marked in the setting of a relatively unremarkable chest radiograph. Pulmonary embolism should always be considered in the differential diagnosis of such patients. Treatment involves adequate analgesia, avoidance of oversedation, early mobilization, and vigorous pulmonary toilet. Sleep-disordered breathing may worsen in the postoperative period, thereby increasing the risk of respiratory failure. Early application of noninvasive ventilation may decrease the incidence of postoperative pulmonary complications. The risk of aspiration of gastric contents is generally felt to be increased in obesity, and efforts to minimize this occurrence should be taken at the time of intubation (see below).

Not surprisingly, the risk of obstructive sleep apnea increases significantly with obesity, to as high as 40% when the BMI exceeds 40 kg/m². Patients who successfully lose a significant amount of weight, usually via surgical approaches to weight reduction, may exhibit significant improvements in lung volumes, gas exchange, and work of breathing, and sleep-disordered breathing may improve or even resolve.

OTHER EFFECTS OF OBESITY

An intriguing association between obesity and progressive renal insufficiency is becoming apparent.[10,15] Obesity is associated with increased renal blood flow, glomerular filtration rate, and microalbuminuria. Glomerular hyperfiltration may subsequently lead to glomerular sclerosis in a manner analogous to diabetes, even in obese patients without this diagnosis. Several potential mechanisms for this process have been suggested, ranging from hyperleptinemia to insulin resistance to a chronic state of low-grade inflammation induced by obesity. Apart from the direct effects of obesity on the kidney, a significant proportion of cases of end-stage renal disease may be attributable to the diabetes and hypertension associated with obesity.

The risk of venous thromboembolism is greatly increased in obese patients (BMI > 30 kg/m²). Inactivity, venous stasis, and hypercoagulability likely contribute to this risk. The risk of death from cancer is substantially increased in individuals with a BMI greater than 40 kg/m².[16]

Management of Respiratory Failure

PATHOPHYSIOLOGY OF RESPIRATORY FAILURE IN MORBID OBESITY

Morbidly obese patients may be particularly susceptible to respiratory failure. Under normal conditions, very little (<5%) of the body's total oxygen consumption (V_{O2}) is attributable to the work of breathing. Emphysema and other forms of chronic lung disease increase the oxygen consumed by the respiratory muscles (V_{O2RESP}) by increasing the load on the respiratory muscles. In such conditions, the strength of the respiratory system may be just adequate for the load on the system, and further insults, however trivial, may provoke respiratory failure.

Evidence suggests that morbidly obese patients may be similarly compromised. Baseline V_{O2RESP} averaged 16% in a group of morbidly obese (average BMI = 53 kg/m²) patients scheduled for gastric bypass surgery.[17] Further, obesity is associated with a disproportionate rise in V_{O2RESP} for a given increase in minute ventilation, similar to emphysema.[18] Together these data suggest reduced respiratory reserve in morbid obesity, thereby increasing the risk of respiratory failure even from seemingly trivial insults (e.g., viral infection or, particularly in the postoperative patient, atelectasis) in a manner analogous to emphysema or other chronically compensated forms of respiratory failure.

EVALUATION OF RESPIRATORY FAILURE

The evaluation of morbidly obese patients with critical illness and with respiratory failure, in particular, is challenging. Physical examination is difficult, and chest radiography is commonly unhelpful. Computed tomography or other similar diagnostic studies are impossible if the patient exceeds the weight limit or width of the scanner table. Even when such studies are possible, there are enormous technical and safety challenges that accompany the transfer of such patients throughout the hospital. Frequently, diagnoses must by necessity be made on the basis of other clinical criteria.

The diagnosis of pulmonary edema is often frustrated by uncertainty regarding the presence of edema on the chest radiograph. Soft tissue shadows on portable chest radiographs are often difficult to distinguish from airspace edema. When suspected, other clinical signs may assist in making a diagnosis. For example, abundant frothy secretions from the endotracheal tube commonly accompany pulmonary edema. Analysis of the protein content of the initial secretions may permit a distinction between high- and low-pressure edema, as the latter is associated with a protein content greater than one-half that of serum.[19] Measurement of a frankly elevated pulmonary capillary wedge pressure usually indicates that pulmonary edema is present. Similarly, pulmonary edema may be diagnosed in the patient with hypoxemia refractory to high-flow oxygen who also has an elevated right atrial pressure and abnormal left ventricular systolic or diastolic function, although this approach also makes an inference that pulmonary edema necessarily results from abnormal pump function. Acute lung injury may be diagnosed on the basis of appropriate setting (e.g., aspiration after the administration of sedation) and hypoxemia refractory to high-flow oxygen. Although differentiating this condition from atelectasis can be difficult, noting abundant protein-rich endotracheal secretions may be helpful.

Pulmonary embolism is another serious condition that is particularly difficult to diagnose in the morbidly obese patient. Computed tomography of the chest and pulmonary angiography may be technically unfeasible. Serial lower extremity Doppler examinations should be performed, although pulmonary embolism is not disproved solely through this approach. A normal D-dimer as determined by enzyme-linked immunosorbent assay reliably excludes the diagnosis, but such a result is unlikely in the critically ill population, given the multitude of conditions associated with elevations in D-dimer levels. Echocardiography may suggest the diagnosis by demonstrating acute right heart dysfunction, but this finding lacks specificity given the range of disorders precipitating respiratory failure (e.g., acute lung injury or severe, untreated sleep disordered breathing) that cause this. Because there are no good data to guide the clinician, our approach is

to initiate therapeutic anticoagulation in the setting of significant pulmonary hypertension (mean pulmonary artery pressure >40 mm Hg), if acute right heart dilation without another satisfactory cause is present, or when historical features (e.g., acute onset of chest pain and dyspnea) suggest the diagnosis.

MANAGEMENT OF RESPIRATORY FAILURE

Noninvasive positive pressure ventilation has several potential benefits in the initial management of morbidly obese patients with respiratory failure, including unloading the respiratory muscles, decreasing atelectasis, and treating any underlying sleep-disordered breathing. It may also have a role in preventing respiratory complications in the postoperative period. Joris et al demonstrated the utility of noninvasive positive pressure ventilation in reducing the postoperative decrease in FVC and FEV_1 when applied to morbidly obese patients in the first 24 hours after gastroplasty.[20] We recommend the early use of noninvasive positive pressure ventilation in morbidly obese patients who have developed respiratory failure. Extubation to noninvasive ventilation may also be considered for morbidly obese patients at high risk for respiratory failure after thoracic or abdominal surgery, although this approach is unproven. Noninvasive ventilation is discussed in greater detail in Chap. 33.

Intubation of the morbidly obese patient can be problematic.[21] The view afforded the operator may be suboptimal because of extensive soft tissue in the hypopharynx. Reduced functional residual capacity from morbid obesity and from sedation diminishes the oxygen stores available for the patient during apnea. The risk of aspiration of gastric contents may be increased in this population, and obese patients should be considered to have "full stomachs" during airway manipulation. For these reasons, we recommend that intubation be performed in the presence of an experienced operator, if possible. Once the decision has been made to intubate, appropriate planning should commence without delay. Early planning allows for the consultation of an experienced operator and an opportunity to perform an awake intubation, with or without fiberoptic assistance. If the patient is too unstable to attempt this, we recommend the routine use of cricoid pressure to minimize the risk of aspiration.

Several factors promote the development of atelectasis in the morbidly obese patient who is intubated for respiratory failure. These include the supine position, administration of sedatives and narcotics, and translaryngeal intubation. As a result, extremely obese patients frequently require increased levels of positive end-expiratory pressure to prevent atelectasis and maintain adequate oxygenation, even in the absence of acute lung injury. In our experience, a positive end-expiratory pressure of 8 to 15 cm H_2O is frequently necessary. Because of atelectasis, significant hypoxemia may be present at the time that the patient is otherwise ready to sustain spontaneous breathing. Extubation to noninvasive positive pressure ventilation (NIPPV) may facilitate this transition and may maintain upper airway patency when residual sedation promotes obstructive respiratory events, although the routine use of NIPPV for post-extubation respiratory failure cannot currently be supported.[21a] If possible, morbidly obese patients should be ventilated and undergo spontaneous breathing trials in the reverse Trendelenburg position, a maneuver that improves respiratory system compliance by shifting the abdominal contents off the chest wall.

Lung protective ventilatory strategies are challenging to apply in the morbidly obese patient with acute lung injury because of the difficulty in diagnosing alveolar overdistension in this population. The plateau pressure represents the pressure required to inflate the lung against the elastic recoil of the lung and chest wall. Because the compliance of the chest wall is diminished in morbid obesity, a high plateau pressure does not necessarily indicate alveolar overdistension. Thus, when using low tidal volume ventilation in the management of acute lung injury or the acute respiratory distress syndrome, the delivery of a tidal volume of 6 mL/kg *ideal body weight* may result in a plateau pressure easily exceeding 30 cm H_2O but not necessarily overdistend alveoli. Given the lack of convincing utility of pressure-volume curves in the management of acute lung injury, we do not advocate their use in such cases. We recommend measurement of the plateau pressure in the upright or semi-upright position to minimize the contribution of increased intraabdominal pressure from obesity and at times accepting an arbitrarily higher plateau pressure, for example, up to 35 to 40 cm H_2O in the extremely obese patient, if necessary.

TRACHEOSTOMY

Although firm data are lacking, we have found early tracheostomy to be useful in the management of many morbidly obese patients with respiratory failure. We recommend that consideration be given to early tracheostomy in the following settings: (1) when severe obstructive sleep apnea that is refractory to medical therapy is present, (2) when long-term nocturnal ventilation for the treatment of obesity hypoventilation syndrome is planned, and (3) when the course of recovery is expected to be prolonged.

Other Problems in the Delivery of Critical Care

ESTABLISHING VASCULAR ACCESS

Establishing intravenous access may be particularly difficult in the morbidly obese patient, beginning with the frequent inability to place a peripheral intravenous line. The increased distance from skin to blood vessel makes any attempt to cannulate a central vein more difficult, and the sharp angle required, particularly to enter the subclavian vein, may make it impossible for the operator to pass the wire and/or dilator. In some patients, the needle and the introducer may be too short for the subclavian site. The femoral site should be used as a last resort because of the increased risk of infection and thrombosis associated with this site; in addition, this site is frequently inaccessible because of intertrigo. The internal jugular vein is therefore generally the site of choice for extremely obese patients, even with the difficulties imposed by a short, thick neck.

There is very little information regarding the practice of central venous catheterization in the morbidly obese. Because bedside ultrasound has been shown to decrease the risk of in-

sertion complications in high-risk patients,[22] we recommend its use in the morbidly obese patient with poor landmarks.

NUTRITIONAL SUPPORT

Critically ill obese patients exhibit less lipolysis and fat oxidation than nonobese subjects.[23] This decreased ability to mobilize fat increases protein breakdown to fuel gluconeogenesis and, hence, ensure adequate carbohydrates for energy. An increased risk for protein malnutrition results, with potentially detrimental effects on immune function, wound healing, and lean muscle mass. Thus, the clinician should avoid the temptation to starve the patient in a misguided attempt to accelerate a program of weight loss during the course of critical illness. In contrast, several trials of carefully controlled hypocaloric nutritional support in which adequate protein was supplied demonstrated that chronically critically ill patients receiving such a regimen had nitrogen balance comparable to those patients receiving conventional total parenteral nutrition.[24]

We recommend the provision of not less than 60% of the measured energy expenditure with 1.5 to 2.0 g /kg ideal body weight as protein, or less if renal insufficiency is present, to ensure adequate carbohydrates for energy and prevent protein malnutrition. Indirect calorimetry should be used to guide nutritional support because of the unreliability of conventional equations in this setting.

DRUG DOSING

Different alterations in pharmacokinetics have been described in obese patients.[25] In general, the volume of distribution for drugs with greater lipophilicity is increased. There are notable exceptions, however, thus illustrating the importance of other factors, such as plasma protein binding, in the distribution of drugs. Some studies have shown an increase in protein binding of some drugs because of increased levels of α_1-acid glycoprotein in obesity, whereas other studies have shown decreased protein binding related to elevated triglycerides, lipoproteins, cholesterol, and free fatty acids.[23] Variable alterations in enzymatic and antioxidant systems have been described, and increased and decreased renal clearance rates have been found.

This tremendous intersubject variability, combined with important differences between drugs make generalizations about the dosing of individual medications impossible. Drugs with a narrow therapeutic window such as theophylline and digoxin may confer toxicity when dosed according to total body weight. Reference to published guidelines for individual drugs is recommended, as is close monitoring of clinically available serum drug levels. Because of data indicating an increased volume of distribution and prolonged half-life for midazolam in obese subjects and an apparent lack of accumulation for propofol when given as a general anesthetic, we prefer propofol as a continuous intravenous sedative, when this method of administration is indicated.[26,27] A strategy to prevent any potential accumulation of this sedative or the accompanying analgesic is still desirable, whether it be by daily interruption of continuous intravenous sedation or conversion to a validated regimen of intermittent sedative administration.

MINIMIZING COMPLICATIONS OF CRITICAL ILLNESS

Because of the significantly elevated risk of venous thromboembolism in obesity, we recommend an aggressive approach to prophylaxis. Unfortunately, data on this subject are lacking, and a survey of surgeons who perform bariatric surgery showed wide variation in practice.[28] Without good data to guide the clinician, we suggest the joint use of pneumatic compression boots and increased-dose subcutaneous heparin (7500 U twice per day).

Most studies suggest that the risk of aspiration of gastric contents is increased in the obese patient due to increased intraabdominal pressure and the high volume and low pH of gastric contents in such patients. This has implications not only for intubation (see above) but also for routine nursing and feeding. We recommend that all morbidly obese patients be fed and nursed in the semi-upright position.

NURSING ISSUES

The patient should be nursed in the semi-upright position to improve respiratory function and decrease the risk of aspiration. Special beds are available that accommodate extremely large patients. Hoists can be obtained that assist in lifting and turning the patient. The services of a lift team, if available, should be employed whenever moving the patient to minimize the risk of injury to staff members. Careful attention to the development of bed sores should be paid, because of patient immobility and the difficulty of examining and moving the patient.

Weight Loss

Recovery from critical illness related to morbid obesity provides an opportunity to engage the patient in a long-term plan to achieve weight loss. Referral to a weight-loss specialist is indicated. In addition to dietary counseling and physical activity (insofar as possible), available medical therapies include a variety of appetite-suppressant and anti-absorptive medications. Unfortunately, although short-term success is frequent, significant long-term weight loss is uncommon in this population. Therefore, careful consideration should be given to the option of surgical therapy for obesity. Currently favored techniques such as the Roux-en-Y gastric bypass and the biliopancreatic diversion with duodenal switch combine gastric restriction with different degrees of malabsorption. Improvement in or resolution of insulin resistance, obstructive sleep apnea, hypertension, left ventricular systolic dysfunction, and left ventricular hypertrophy have been reported.[29] Properly selected patients have a low ($\leq 1\%$) perioperative mortality rate, although anemia and vitamin deficiency are common in the first year after the procedure. Mean excess weight loss exceeded 50% at 14 years after surgery in a large cohort of patients who had undergone gastric bypass.[30] A randomized trial comparing open versus laparoscopic Roux-en-Y gastric bypass surgery demonstrated less deterioration in pulmonary function postoperatively when using the laparoscopic approach.[31] Noninvasive positive pressure ventilation may be useful in preventing postoperative respiratory failure in patients with marginal pulmonary function.

Until a large trial comparing medical with surgical approaches to morbid obesity is performed, we believe that properly motivated morbidly obese patients who have failed nonsurgical attempts at weight loss should be considered for bariatric surgery. Careful preoperative evaluation is necessary to exclude patients in whom the potential benefit is exceeded by the risk (e.g., older patients with cor pulmonale).

Does Obesity Influence the Outcome of Critically Ill Patients?

Obesity has obviously detrimental effects on health across many domains, including an increase in the rate of malignancies and an increase in mortality rate. The influence of obesity on outcome of patients undergoing intensive care is less clear. Whereas some investigators have found an increased mortality rate with morbid obesity,[32] others have not.[33] Conceivably, increased nutritional reserve could provide a protective effect from overweight in the setting of prolonged critical illness, although further studies are needed to reconcile the different reports of outcome from the studies to date.

References

1. Flegal KM, Carroll MD, Ogden CL, Johnson CL: Prevalence and trends in obesity among US adults, 1999–2000. *JAMA* 288:1723, 2002.
2. Ogden CL, Flegal KM, Carroll MD, Johnson CL: Prevalence and trends in overweight among US children and adolescents, 1999–2000. *JAMA* 288:1728, 2002.
3. Strauss RS, Pollack HA: Epidemic increase in childhood overweight, 1986–1998. *JAMA* 286:2845, 2001.
4. Mitka M: Economist takes aim at "big fat" US lifestyle. *JAMA* 289:33, 2003.
5. Ainsworth BE, Haskell WL, Leon AS, et al: Compendium of physical activities: Classification of energy costs of human physical activities. *Med Sci Sports Exerc* 25:71, 1993.
6. Hu FB, Li TY, Colditz GA, et al: Television watching and other sedentary behaviors in relation to risk of obesity and type 2 diabetes mellitus in women. *JAMA* 289:1785, 2003.
7. Robinson TN: Reducing children's television viewing to prevent obesity: A randomized controlled trial. *JAMA* 282:1561, 1999.
8. Flegal KM, Carroll MD, Ogden CL, Johnson CL: Prevalence and trends in obesity among US adults, 1999–2000. *JAMA* 288:1723, 2002.
9. Schunkert H: Obesity and target organ damage: The heart. *Int J Obesity* 26(suppl 4):S15, 2002.
10. Hall JE, Crook ED, Jones DW, et al: Mechanisms of obesity-associated cardiovascular and renal disease. *Am J Med Sci* 324:127, 2002.
11. Koenig SM: Pulmonary complications of obesity. *Am J Med Sci* 321:249, 2001.
12. Unterborn J: Pulmonary function testing in obesity, pregnancy, and extremes of body habitus. *Clin Chest Med* 22:759, 2001.
13. Rubinstein I, Zamel N, DuBarry L, Hoffstein V: Airflow limitation in morbidly obese, nonsmoking men. *Ann Intern Med* 112:828, 1990.
14. Douglas FG, Chong PY: Influence of obesity on peripheral airways patency. *J Appl Physiol* 33:559, 1972.
15. de Jong PE, Verhave JC, Pinto-Sietsma SJ, Hillege HL: Obesity and target organ damage: The kidney. *Int J Obesity* 26:S21, 2002.

16. Calle EE, Rodriguez C, Walker-Thurmond K, Thun MJ: Overweight, obesity, and mortality from cancer in a prospectively studied cohort of U.S. adults. *N Engl J Med* 348:1625, 2003.

17. Kress JP, Pohlman AS, Alverdy J, Hall JB: The impact of morbid obesity on oxygen cost of breathing at rest. *Am J Respir Crit Care Med* 160:883, 1999.

18. Kaufman BJ, Ferguson MH, Cherniack RM: Hypoventilation in obesity. *J Clin Invest* 38:500, 1959.

19. Fein A, Grossman RF, Jones JG, et al: The value of edema fluid protein measurement in patients with pulmonary edema. *Am J Med* 67:32, 1979.

20. Joris JL, Sottiaux TM, Chiche JD, et al: Effect of bi-level positive airway pressure (BiPAP) nasal ventilation on the postoperative pulmonary restrictive syndrome in obese patients undergoing gastroplasty. *Chest* 111:665, 1997.

21. Ogunnaike BO, Jones SB, Jones DB, et al: Anesthetic considerations for bariatric surgery. *Anesth Analg* 95:1793, 2002.

21a. Esteban A, Frutos-Vivar F, Ferguson ND, et al: Noninvasive positive-pressure ventilation for respiratory failure after extubation. *N Engl J Med* 350:2452, 2004.

22. Randolph AG, Cook DJ, Gonzales CA, Pribble CG: Ultrasound guidance for placement of central venous catheters: A meta-analysis of the literature. *Crit Care Med* 24:2053, 1996.

23. Marik P, Varon J: The obese patient in the ICU. *Chest* 113:492, 1998.

24. Mechanick JI, Brett EM: Nutrition support of the chronically critically ill patient. *Crit Care Clin* 18:597, 2002.

25. Blouin RA, Warren GW: Pharmacokinetic considerations in obesity. *J Pharm Sci* 88:1, 1999.

26. Greenblatt DJ, Abernathy DR, Locniskar A, et al: Effect of age, gender, and obesity on midazolam kinetics. *Anesthesiology* 61:27, 1984.

27. Servin F, Farinotti R, Haberer JP, Desmonts JM: Propofol infusion for maintenance of anesthesia in morbidly obese patients receiving nitrous oxide. *Anesthesiology* 78:657, 1993.

28. Wu EC, Barba CA: Current practices in the prophylaxis of venous thromboembolism in bariatric surgery. *Obes Surg* 10:7, 2000.

29. Brolin RE: Bariatric surgery and long-term control of morbid obesity. *JAMA* 288:2793, 2002.

30. American Society for Bariatric Surgery: Rationale for the surgical treatment of morbid obesity, 2001. Available at: http://www.asbs.org./html/rationale/rationale.html. Accessed June 2, 2004.

31. Nguyen NT, Lee SL, Goldman C, et al: Comparison of pulmonary function and postoperative pain after laparoscopic versus open gastric bypass: A randomized trial. *J Am Coll Surg* 192:469, 2001.

32. El-Solh A, Sikka P, Bozkanat E, et al: Morbid obesity in the medical ICU. *Chest* 120:1989, 2001.

33. Tremblay A, Bandi V: Impact of body mass index on outcomes following critical care. *Chest* 123:1202, 2003.

Chapter 110 _____

HYPOTHERMIA

NICOLA A. HANANIA
JANICE L. ZIMMERMAN

KEY POINTS

- *Accidental hypothermia results from the unintentional decrease in core body temperature to lower than 35°C (95°F) and can be classified as mild (32.2°C to 35°C, or 90°F to 95°F), moderate (28°C to 32.2°C, 82°F to 90°F), or severe (<28°C, 82°F).*

- *Although hypothermia from environmental exposure is very common, several medical conditions may also predispose to hypothermia necessitating hospitalization and admission to the intensive care unit.*

- *Individuals at highest risk for hypothermia include the homeless, the mentally ill, trauma victims, outdoor workers, those at the extremes of age, those with serious underlying medical conditions, and those with ethanol or drug intoxication.*

- *Several organ systems are affected by hypothermia: clinical manifestations depend on the underlying cause and core body temperature. Below 30°C (86°F), shivering ceases, level of consciousness progressively declines, and cardiac arrhythmias become more common.*

- *In the initial stages, wet clothing should be removed promptly, continued heat loss must be prevented, and the underlying illness should be identified and treated.*

- *Rewarming is the primary treatment for moderate to severe hypothermia. For patients with a core body temperature above 32°C (90°F), passive and active external rewarming and supportive therapies are preferred; for patients with lower temperatures and those with hemodynamic instability, active core rewarming using body cavity lavage or extracorporeal blood warming may be considered.*

- *In addition to rewarming, all patients with hypothermia need continuous monitoring of cardiac status, intensive fluid resuscitation, and circulatory support.*

Hypothermia is defined as a core body temperature lower than 35°C (<95°F). The severity of hypothermia is indicated by the degree to which the core body temperature is lowered and is classified as mild, moderate, or severe. Several medical conditions may increase the risk of hypothermia. Individuals at the extremes of age are at greatest risk. Risk of death from hypothermia is related to age, preexisting illnesses, nutritional status, and alcohol and drug intoxication.[1] In cases of severe hypothermia, prompt intervention with rapid rewarming is crucial and may be life saving. This chapter discusses the pathophysiology, risk factors, clinical diagnosis, and management of hypothermia. The use of hypothermia as a treatment, such as after cardiac arrest, is covered in Chap. 16.

Regulation of Body Temperature

Body temperature is closely regulated through a balance between heat production and heat dissipation.[2] The majority of endogenous heat production results from metabolic activity in the heart and liver. The skin accounts for 90% of heat loss and the lungs contribute the rest. Radiation cooling is the primary method of thermal load dissipation. The preoptic nucleus of the anterior hypothalamus is the thermal control center, which maintains body temperature at a given set value. In response to a decrease in core body temperature, the hypothalamus initiates mechanisms to conserve heat by cutaneous vasoconstriction and stimulation of muscular activity in the form of shivering.[2,3] In a conscious individual, the appreciation of cold induces the individual to exercise, wear more clothes, or move to a warmer environment.

As the core temperature decreases below 35°C (95°F), the coordinated systems responsible for thermoregulation begin to fail because the physiologic responses to minimize heat loss are very limited.[4] *Primary hypothermia (accidental hypothermia)* refers to a spontaneous decrease of core body temperature, usually as result of exposure to cold environments without adequate protection. Environmental hypothermia results from a combination of heat loss by convection (degree of wind exposure), conduction, and radiation to the surrounding ambient air. *Secondary hypothermia* represents a complication of an underlying disorder. Some of the disorders and conditions that may predispose an individual to hypothermia by decreasing heat production, increasing heat loss, or interfering with the central or peripheral control of thermoregulation are listed in Table 110-1.[1–9]

Epidemiology

From 1979 through 1995, 12,368 deaths were reported in the United States for which hypothermia was the underlying cause (an annual average of 723 and a rate of 0.3 deaths per 100,000 population).[10] Approximately half of the deaths from hypothermia occurred in persons older than 65 years; the annual death rate from hypothermia in this age group was 1.2 per 100,000. The age-adjusted death rate for men was almost triple that for women. In addition, for persons older than 65 years, the death rate for men and women of black and other races was much higher than that for white men and women.[11] Race-specific differences may reflect differences in socioeconomic determinants for factors that are important in the prevention of hypothermia, such as access to protective clothing, shelter, and medical care. Hypothermia may occur in any climate and during any season of the year. Hypothermia is most common among the elderly, the homeless or mentally ill, trauma victims, outdoor workers, children, and individuals with certain medical conditions as mentioned above.

Clinical Presentation

DIAGNOSIS

Historical facts do not always suggest hypothermia. When exposure to cold is obvious by history, the diagnosis is simple. Measurement of core body temperature is important in diagnosis of less overt presentations. Core temperature is best measured by using a cold-recording rectal probe thermometer capable of measuring temperatures as low as 25°C (77°F). Clinical manifestations differ with the severity of hypothermia, which is classified based on core temperature as mild

TABLE 110-1 Causes of Hypothermia

Mechanism	Clinical Disorder
Decreased heat production	Endocrinologic failure
	Hypopituitarism
	Hypoadrenalism
	Hypothyroidism
	Insufficient fuel
	Extreme exertion
	Hypoglycemia
	Malnutrition
	Neuromuscular inefficiency
	Age extremes
	Impaired shivering
	Inactivity
Increased heat loss	Environmental exposure
	Induced vasodilation
	Drugs, including alcohol
	Toxins
	Skin disorders
	Burns
	Psoriasis
	Exfoliative dermatitis
	Iatrogenic
	Cold infusion
	Emergent deliveries
Impaired thermoregulation	Peripheral failure
	Neuropathies
	Spinal cord transection
	Diabetes
	Central failure
	Metabolic
	Drugs: barbiturates, tricyclic antidepressants, sedatives, alcohol
	Trauma
	Cerebrovascular accident (CVA), subarachnoid bleed
	Parkinsonism
	Hypothalamic dysfunction
	Multiple sclerosis
	Anorexia nervosa
Miscellaneous	Sepsis
	Pancreatitis
	Carcinomatosis
	Uremia
	Vascular insufficiency

(35°C to 32.2°C, 95°F to 90°F), moderate (<32.2°C to 28°C, <90°F to 82°F), and severe (<28°C, <82°F).[2,3,5,7,12,13] This classification has implications for management because appropriate treatment depends on severity of the disorder, as described below. The onset of hypothermia is often insidious. Initial symptoms may be vague and include hunger, nausea, dizziness, chills, pruritus, or dyspnea. Extremity stiffness, weakness, and shivering may also be prominent. As core body temperature decreases, many patients no longer complain of cold, shivering disappears at temperatures below 32°C (<90°F), and muscles become rigid.[5,14] At this point, the level of consciousness becomes markedly altered and systemic manifestations are readily evident. A severely hypothermic victim has a markedly decreased metabolic rate. As a consequence, the cerebral ischemic tolerance during cardiocircu-

latory arrest is considerably longer in contrast with the normothermic state.[5,15,16] Therefore, one has to be very careful in assessing brain death while a patient remains hypothermic. Low temperatures cause the myocardium to become irritable and cardiovascular abnormalities are common.[15] These may include initial tachycardia followed by progressive bradycardia with an increase in systemic vascular resistance. Arrhythmias are common at core temperatures below 32°C (90°F), and ventricular fibrillation may occur spontaneously when the temperature is below 28°C (82°F).[14] Systemic blood pressure is often decreased in patients with severe hypothermia. Other clinical manifestations of hypothermia are listed in Table 110-2.

LABORATORY EVALUATION

Initial laboratory evaluations should be obtained to assess metabolic status and organ dysfunction. Recommended tests include blood glucose, electrolytes, renal and hepatic functions, complete blood count, and coagulation profile. Arterial blood gases should be obtained, and correction for temperature is not necessary.[5,17,18] Electrolytes, hematocrit, and coagulation status change with rewarming, so frequent monitoring is necessary. Other laboratory tests such as thyroid function studies, cardiac isoenzymes, toxicologic screen, and cultures should be used selectively based on the clinical history and examination. Chest and abdominal radiographs should be obtained with the need for other radiographs dictated by the clinical situation. The following are common laboratory findings in patients with hypothermia.

ARTERIAL BLOOD GASES
Typically, pH values increase as body temperature decreases (0.0147 and 1°C). Arterial pressures of O_2 and CO_2 also decrease with a decrease in temperature (7.2% and 4.4% and 1°C decrease in temperature), and the oxyhemoglobin dissociation curve is shifted to the left. However, because all arterial blood gas samples are warmed to 37°C (98.6°F) before values are measured, simply comparing uncorrected values measured at 37°C with the normal reference values at 37°C yields an accurate interpretation. Respiratory acidosis and metabolic acidosis are common findings in patients with moderate and severe hypothermia.[17]

COMPLETE BLOOD COUNT
An increase in hematocrit secondary to decrease in plasma volume is common (2% for each 1°C decrease in temperature). White blood cell and platelet counts may decrease as temperature decreases.[2,5]

COAGULATION PROFILE
A physiologic increase in coagulation occurs with hypothermia, and disseminated intravascular coagulation may occur with rewarming. Prolonged bleeding and clotting times are common. Prothrombin time and partial thromboplastin time may initially appear normal despite the presence of clinical coagulopathy because the values are measured after warming the blood sample to 37°C. Blood viscosity may be exacerbated in patients with cryoglobulinemia or cryofibrinogenemia, which is more common in elderly patients.

TABLE 110-2 Clinical Manifestations of Hypothermia

System	Mild Hypothermia	Moderate Hypothermia	Severe Hypothermia
CNS	Confusion, slurred speech, impaired judgment, amnesia	Lethargy, hallucinations, loss of pupillary reflex, EEG abnormalities	Loss of cerebrovascular regulation, decline in EEG activity, coma, loss of ocular reflex
CVS	Tachycardia, increased cardiac output and systemic vascular resistance	Progressive bradycardia (unresponsive to atropine), decreased cardiac output and BP, atrial and ventricular arrhythmias, J (Osborn) wave on ECG	Decline in BP and cardiac output, ventricular fibrillation ($<28°C$) and asystole ($<20°C$)
Respiratory	Tachypnea, bronchorrhea	Hypoventilation (decreased rate and tidal volume), decreased oxygen consumption and CO_2 production, loss of cough reflex	Pulmonary edema, apnea
Renal	Cold diuresis	Cold diuresis	Decreased renal perfusion and GFR, oliguria
Hematologic	Increased hematocrit and decreased platelet, white blood cell count, coagulopathy, and DIC		
GI	Ileus, pancreatitis, gastric stress ulcers, hepatic dysfunction		
Metabolic endocrine	Increased metabolic rate, hyperglycemia	Decreased metabolic rate, hyper- or hypoglycemia	
Musculoskeletal	Increased shivering	Decreased shivering ($<32°C$, 90°F), muscle rigidity	Patient appears dead, "pseudo-rigor mortis"

ABBREVIATIONS: BP, blood pressure; CNS, central nervous system; CVS, cardiovascular septem; DIC, disseminated intravascular coagulation; ECG, electrocardiogram; EEG, electroencephalogram; GFR, glomerular filtration rate; GI, gastrointestinal.

SERUM ELECTROLYTES
Recurrent evaluation of electrolytes is essential during rewarming because no consistent effect is present. Hypo- and hyperkalemia may complicate the course of hypothermia and either should be promptly corrected.

SERUM UREA NITROGEN AND CREATININE
These are almost always elevated because of decreased urinary clearance and decreased renal perfusion.

BLOOD GLUCOSE
Especially when core body temperature is above 30°C (86°F), acute hypothermia may be associated with an initial elevation of blood glucose due to catecholamine-induced glycogenolysis, whereas subacute and chronic hypothermia produce glycogen depletion with subsequent hypoglycemia. Nevertheless, hypoglycemia is one of the most common causes of mild hypothermia in a hospitalized patient.

OTHER LABORATORY ABNORMALITIES
Hyperamylasemia is common and may be related to a preexisting pancreatitis or pancreatitis induced by hypothermia. Hyperamylasemia correlates with the severity of hypothermia and with mortality rate. Variable elevation in creatine phosphokinase levels may reflect underlying rhabdomyolysis.

ELECTROCARDIOGRAPHIC ABNORMALITIES
PR, QRS, and QT intervals may be prolonged. When body temperature decreases below 33°C (91.4°F), the J (Osborn) wave may be noted as a positive deflection in the left ventricular leads at the junction of the QRS and ST segments in 25% to 30% of patients.[2,19–21] The presence of this wave is not pathognomonic and has no prognostic implication (Fig. 110-1).

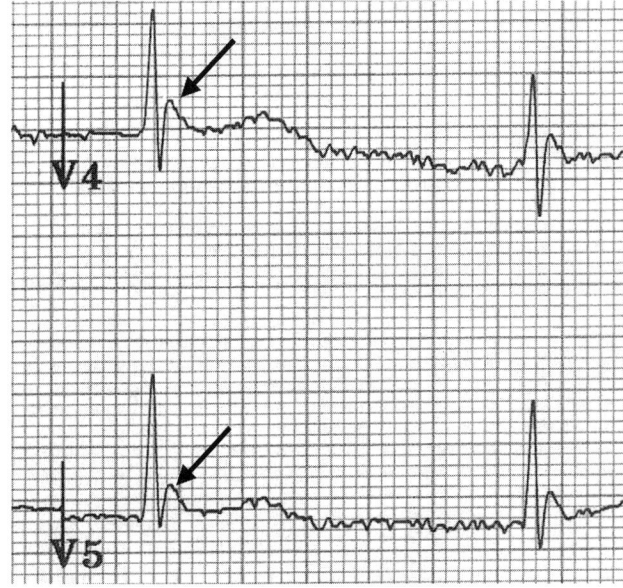

FIGURE 110-1 The J (Osborn) wave (*arrows*) **appears on electrocardiograms of approximately 80% of hypothermic patients. In general, the amplitude and duration of the Osborn wave are inversely related to core temperature.**

Management

The severity of hypothermia, clinical findings, and comorbid conditions of the patient are important factors for determining the aggressiveness of resuscitation techniques (Fig. 110-2). Actions in all patients should include prompt removal of wet clothing, protection against continued heat loss, continuous monitoring of cardiac status, and avoidance of rough movement and excess activity, which can precipitate ventricular fibrillation.[20–25] Patients received in the hospital with moderate or severe hypothermia should be resuscitated until adequate rewarming has occurred or efforts are deemed unsuccessful.[13,23,24]

INITIAL STABILIZATION

Hypothermia should be confirmed by an accurate assessment of core temperature with a low reading thermometer. A rectal temperature is most practical, even though it may lag behind core changes. The probe should be inserted to an adequate depth but avoid cold fecal material. An esophageal temperature is an alternative to monitoring of rectal temperature, but readings may be falsely elevated in the intubated patient ventilated with warmed gas. In patients with moderate to severe hypothermia, temperature should be assessed continuously. The reliability of tympanic temperature devices has not been established in hypothermia.[5] Other vital signs may be difficult to evaluate, but evidence of a spontaneous pulse or blood pressure should be aggressively sought. The use of a Doppler ultrasound device may be necessary. Pulse oximetry is unlikely to be accurate in the setting of hypothermia and poor perfusion.

Supplemental oxygen should be administered pending assessment of oxygenation. Endotracheal intubation is indicated unless the patient is alert and has intact airway reflexes. Orotracheal intubation is preferred due to the risk of traumatic bleeding with the nasal route. However, muscle rigidity of the jaw in moderate to severe hypothermia may preclude use of the oral route. Neuromuscular blockers are unlikely to be effective at temperatures below 30°C (86°F) and should be avoided. Topical vasoconstrictors and the use of a smaller endotracheal tube may facilitate blind nasotracheal intubation in the patient with some spontaneous respirations. Intubation is unlikely to induce dysrhythmias in hypothermic patients.[8]

A nasogastric or orogastric tube should be placed in patients with moderate or severe hypothermia to relieve gastric distention. A urinary catheter is also essential to monitor urine output and assess volume resuscitation efforts. Peripheral

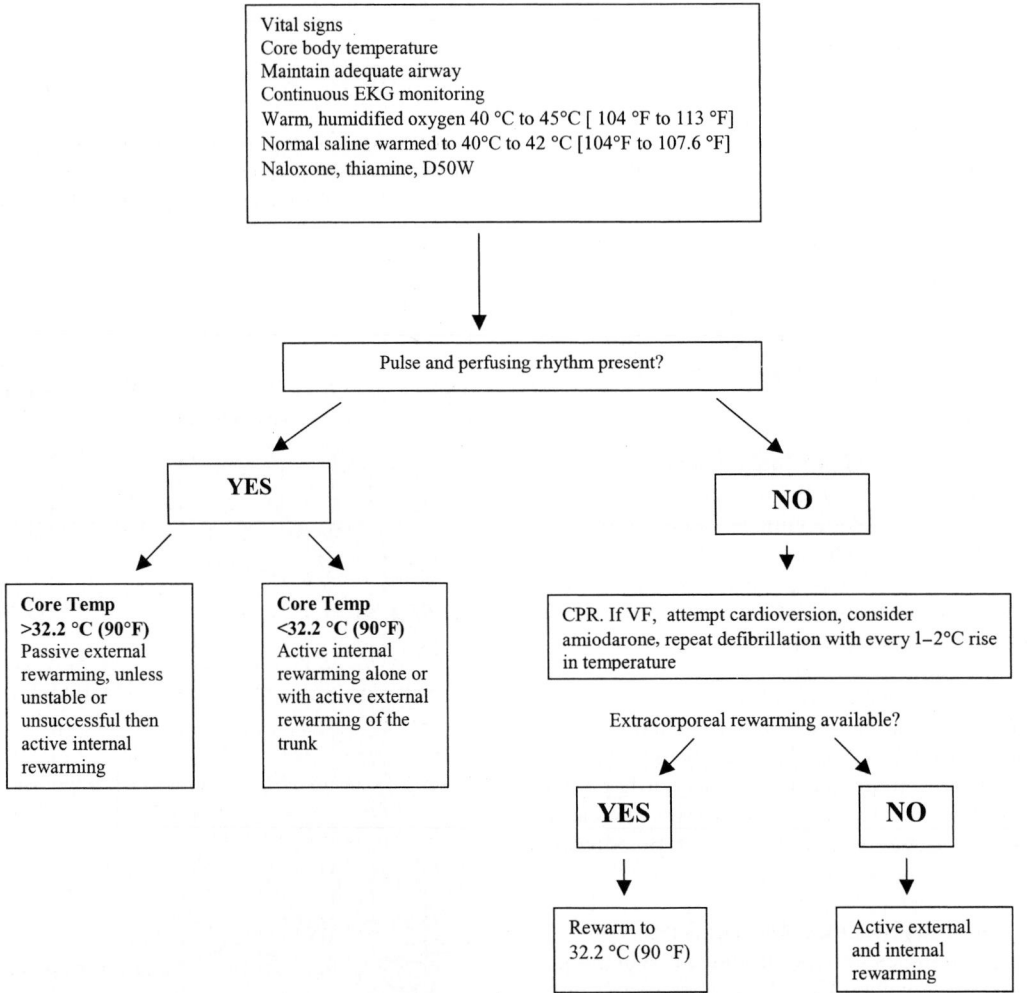

FIGURE 110-2 A systematic approach to a patient with hypothermia.

venous catheters are preferred over central venous access due to the potential to precipitate dysrhythmias. Needle electrodes are preferred for electrocardiographic monitoring. Intraarterial catheters for pressure monitoring should be used selectively. Pulmonary artery catheters are avoided due to potential dysrhythmias and the risk of vascular perforation. After rewarming, invasive monitoring may be warranted in complicated cases. Patients with moderate or severe hypothermia should be handled gently because movement and manipulation may precipitate dysrhythmias. Associated conditions requiring urgent intervention, such as traumatic injuries, hypoglycemia, or endocrinologic insufficiency, should be sought.

VOLUME RESUSCITATION

Patients with moderate or severe hypothermia are volume depleted and require rapid assessment of volume status and administration of fluids. A reasonable approach is to administer a 250- to 500-mL fluid challenge of warmed 5% dextrose in normal saline until further evaluation can be completed. During rewarming, increased fluid requirements are often necessary to prevent or treat hypotension. It has been recommended that lactated Ringer solution be avoided due to decreased ability of the liver to metabolize lactate.

In moderate or severe hypothermia, intravenous fluids heated to 40°C to 42°C (104°F to 107.6°F) should be administered. Heated intravenous fluids add little heat (unless very large volumes are infused) but do avoid the cooling effect of fluid therapy. Crystalloids can be heated in a microwave or commercial fluid warmer and should be mixed adequately before administration. Conductive heat loss can be minimized by using short segments of intravenous tubing and administering fluid as intermittent boluses.[26] Alternatively, fluids can be heated to higher temperatures (60°C, 140°F) when long lengths of tubing cannot be avoided.

Hemoconcentration is usually present in the severely hypothermic patient. A low initial hematocrit suggests acute hemorrhage or preexisting anemia. Occasionally, transfusion of packed red blood cells may be necessary as part of acute resuscitation. Different blood warming devices are available to deliver warm red cell products. The patient should be monitored closely for clinical signs of fluid overload during rewarming.

CIRCULATORY SUPPORT

Cardiopulmonary resuscitation is indicated in any patient with moderate to severe hypothermia in whom no pulse is present after appropriate evaluation or who has a nonperfusing rhythm such as ventricular fibrillation or asystole. The patient with a bradycardic pulse does not require pharmacologic manipulation of heart rate. Chest wall compressions are difficult and require more force in the hypothermic patient due to decreased chest wall elasticity. Frequent change of personnel performing chest compressions is necessary to prevent fatigue and ineffectiveness.

Initial defibrillation should be attempted for ventricular fibrillation or ventricular tachycardia without a pulse, although attempts may be unsuccessful at temperatures below 30°C to 32°C (86°F to 90°F). If initial defibrillation is unsuccessful, rewarming is instituted and defibrillation is attempted again after every 1°C to 2°C increase in temperature or when core temperature rises above 30°C to 32°C. Antiarrhythmic and vasoactive drugs are usually ineffective at temperatures below 30°C (86°F). These drugs should be avoided until rewarming to above 30°C (86°F), and then the lowest effective dose should be used. Excessive administration of resuscitation drugs may result in toxicity with rewarming due to altered metabolism.

Most hypothermia-induced dysrhythmias will convert spontaneously with rewarming. Atrial fibrillation is seen frequently and does not usually require specific treatment because the ventricle generally responds slowly. The best approach to ventricular dysrhythmias has not been determined. Bretylium tosylate has been effective in animal studies but is not currently used in resuscitation.[27,28] Lidocaine appears to be less effective, and procainamide may increase the incidence of ventricular fibrillation. The effects of amiodarone in hypothermic patients have not been evaluated. The optimal dose and infusion rate of bretylium and other vasoactive drugs are unknown in severe hypothermia.

Hypotension should be treated initially with volume replacement. Vasopressor agents have minimal effect on constricted vessels in moderate or severe hypothermia but may increase the risk of dysrhythmias.

REWARMING METHODS

Although rewarming is the primary treatment for moderate or severe hypothermia, controversy exists as to the optimal method, duration, and rate of rewarming. No controlled studies comparing rewarming methods exist, and rigid treatment protocols cannot be recommended. Rapid rates of rewarming have not proved to improve outcome in patients with severe hypothermia. The clinical circumstances, availability of resources, and advantages and disadvantages of available methods should be taken into account when selecting specific interventions for the patient.[3,5–7,13,14,18,23,29]

PASSIVE EXTERNAL REWARMING

Passive external rewarming involves covering the patient with an insulating material to prevent further heat loss. This method is the treatment of choice for most patients with mild hypothermia and is used as an adjunct in patients with moderate or severe hypothermia. Patients must be able to generate heat to rewarm themselves. Rewarming rates with passive external rewarming in mild hypothermia vary between 0.5°C to 2.0°C per hour.[4]

ACTIVE REWARMING

Active rewarming involves the transfer of exogenous heat to the patient by using external or internal techniques. Indications for active rewarming include cardiovascular instability, poikilothermia (<32°C), inadequate rewarming with other methods, endocrinologic insufficiency, and traumatic peripheral vasodilation (i.e., spinal core injury). Patients with endocrinologic diseases may have insufficient glycogen stores or insufficient endogenous thermogenesis.

ACTIVE EXTERNAL REWARMING

Different methods have been used for active external rewarming (AER), including immersion in a 40°C bath, warming blankets, heating pads, radiant heat, and forced air rewarming.

Indications for use of these devices remain controversial. Concerns have been raised regarding AER because vasodilation in the extremities may facilitate transport of colder peripheral blood to the warmer core, thereby lowering the core temperature ("afterdrop"). Peripheral vasodilation may also potentially worsen hypotension. Immersion in a warm water bath can impede monitoring and active resuscitation. Thermal injury can occur with heating pads, warming blankets, and radiant heat sources. The most practical technique for AER is forced air rewarming, which transfers heat convectively and prevents heat loss. These devices are usually readily available from postoperative care units. They enable greater contact of warm air with the patient's body than traditional warming blankets. Successful use of forced air as the primary rewarming method in patients with severe hypothermia with and without cardiac arrest has been reported.[30] Additional forced air warming systems are being evaluated.[31]

Warming rates of 1°C to 2.5°C per hour have been reported with AER after accidental hypothermia without any evidence of afterdrop.[30,32] Circulatory problems may be minimized if AER is applied only to the trunk. Truncal AER may be combined successfully with other methods of active core rewarming such as warmed intravenous fluids and heated humidified oxygen. The advantages of AER are ease of institution, availability, low cost, and noninvasiveness.

ACTIVE CORE REWARMING

Numerous alternatives are available for active core rewarming. Airway rewarming using heated humidified oxygen is relatively simple to institute and should be a part of management of most patients with moderate or severe hypothermia.[33] The delivery of heated oxygen is more effective through an endotracheal tube than by mask. Oxygen should be warmed to 40°C to 45°C (104°F to 113°F) through modification of humidifier devices.[34] A rewarming rate of 1°C to 2.5°C per hour can be expected.[5] Although there are several proposed advantages of airway rewarming that include decreased respiratory heat loss, increased heat donation to the respiratory tract, and direct heat transfer to the hypothalamus, brain stem, and medulla, its efficacy remains equivocal.[35]

Heated irrigation has been used to transfer heat from fluids to internal areas with a variety of techniques. Peritoneal dialysis or lavage is probably the most widely recognized method of heated irrigation. Peritoneal dialysis can deliver fluid heated to 40°C to 45°C (104°F to 113°F) to the peritoneal cavity with flow rates of approximately 6 L/h. Potential advantages of this technique are hepatic rewarming, use during chest compressions, and the capability to simultaneously provide renal replacement when a dialysate is used. Rewarming rates average 1°C to 3°C per hour.[4] This technique is not routinely advocated for stable patients but may be considered in combination with other rewarming methods for the patient with no evidence of perfusion.

Closed thoracic lavage also has been proposed for treatment of hypothermia.[36–38] This technique uses a large thoracostomy tube inserted into the anterior second or third intercostal space in the midclavicular line. A second tube is inserted in the posterior axillary line in the fifth or sixth intercostal space. Sterile normal saline heated to 40°C to 42°C (104°F to 107.6°F) is infused through the anterior tube and

allowed to drain passively from the posterior tube. This technique may have the advantage of warming the heart and great vessels. However, clinical experience is limited. Mediastinal irrigation and myocardial lavage could be considered in patients with severe hypothermia and no spontaneous perfusion. These techniques require expertise for thoracotomy and clinical experience is limited.

Irrigation of the stomach, bladder, or colon has limited utility because the surface area available for heat transfer is small. In addition, gastric lavage may predispose to aspiration and must be discontinued during chest compressions. Special double lumen esophageal tubes or modified Sengstaken tubes have had limited evaluation and use.[39,40] These techniques are warranted only if no other methods are available for rewarming.

Four methods are available for extracorporeal blood rewarming. These include hemodialysis, arteriovenous rewarming, venovenous rewarming, and cardiopulmonary bypass (CPB). Hemodialysis uses a two-way flow catheter with percutaneous cannulation of a single vessel. The femoral vein is preferred over the subclavian vein to avoid myocardial irritation with the guidewire. This technique may be most appropriate in the patient without severe hemodynamic instability, although it has been used in unstable patients.[41,42] Hemodialysis may be the preferred rewarming method when hypothermia is associated with severe renal dysfunction or intoxication with dialyzable substances. Relatively new alternatives to hemodialysis are arteriovenous and venovenous rewarming.[43] These techniques use countercurrent fluid warming. Arteriovenous techniques depend on the patient's blood pressure to support flow, whereas venovenous techniques use a roller pump.

CPB using standard access through the femoral artery or femoral vein is the most invasive and labor-intensive technique for rewarming.[44] It has the advantages of providing complete hemodynamic support during rewarming and rapid rewarming rates.[15] Core temperature can increase 1°C to 2°C every 3 to 5 minutes with femoral flow rates of 2 to 3 L/min.[4] Unfortunately, CPB may require considerable time to institute and is not available in all institutions. Systemic anticoagulation may be contraindicated in trauma victims or contribute to hypothermic coagulopathy. Heparin-bonded tubing, portable circuits, and methods using venovenous access may overcome some of these problems.[45,46] These advances have allowed the institution of CPB in emergency departments and intensive care units.[47] Long-term outcomes of patients with severe hypothermia treated with CPB have been favorable.[48]

FUTURE TECHNIQUES

Techniques such as the use of very high-temperature intravenous fluids and diathermy are being explored for the treatment of moderate or severe hypothermia. Intravenous fluids heated to 65°C (149°F) have been used in animal studies and resulted in rewarming rates of 2.9°C to 3.7°C per hour with minimal intimal injuries.[49,50]

Diathermy involves the conversion of energy waves into heat. Ultrasound or low-frequency microwave radiation can deliver large amounts of heat to deep tissues. Although animal studies are promising, further investigation is needed to determine optimum clinical use.[4,35]

SUPPORTIVE CARE

Numerous complications are associated with moderate and severe hypothermia and should be anticipated by the clinician. Continuous monitoring and frequent reassessment of metabolic and hemodynamic parameters are essential to successful outcome. Rhabdomyolysis is frequent and may result in electrolyte disturbances and renal dysfunction. Compartment syndromes may become apparent several days after initial treatment. Acute respiratory distress syndrome, acute tubular necrosis, and disseminated intravascular coagulation may require intensive interventions.

Prognosis

The prognosis for hypothermia is improved by prompt recognition of the clinical presentation and institution of appropriate management strategies.[51] The risk of death from hypothermia is related to age, preexisting illnesses, nutritional status, and alcohol and drug intoxication. Outcome from severe hypothermia is difficult to predict. Mortality rates vary in several cohorts between 40% and 75%.[18] Clearly, resuscitation will be successful only if cardiac arrest is due to hypothermia and not a consequence of anoxia or other injuries. Underlying diseases, precipitating events, and duration and severity of exposure are important factors to be considered.[52] Although the treatment dictum has been that "no one is dead until warm and dead," clinical judgment is necessary for determining the most appropriate treatment and termination of efforts.[18] Proposed indicators of prognosis on arrival include severe hyperkalemia (>10 mEq/L), which may indicate death before severe hypothermia, a venous pH below 6.5, and severe coagulopathy.[33,53]

Prevention

Many episodes of severe hypothermia may be preventable by implementing public health strategies that include education programs targeting high-risk individuals such as the elderly and the homeless. Specific preventive measures include wearing adequate protective clothing, maintaining fluid and calorie intake, avoiding fatigue, ensuring heated shelter, and avoiding excessive alcohol consumption. Emergency departments and intensive care units should be prepared to manage victims with hypothermia especially in the winter months. Social services should be adequately staffed to provide counseling and shelter to homeless persons during periods of extreme cold. Family members, home health care workers, and social service providers should closely monitor the elderly and patients with medical conditions that may predispose to hypothermia.

References

1. Koutsavlis AT, Kosatsky T: Environmental-temperature injury in a Canadian metropolis. *J Environ Health* 66:40, 2003.
2. Schneider SM, Danzl DF: Hypothermia: from recognition to rewarming. *Emerg Med Rep* 13:1, 1992.
3. Bangs CC: Hypothermia and frostbites. *Emerg Med Clin North Am* 2:475, 1984.
4. Danzl DF, Pozos RS, Hamlet MP: Accidental hypothermia, in Auerbach PS (ed): *Wilderness Medicine.* St Louis, Mosby, 1995, p 51.
5. Danzl DF, Pozos RS: Accidental hypothermia. *N Engl J Med* 331:1756, 1994.
6. Jacobsen TD, Krenzelok EP, Shicker L, Weiner SL: Environmental emergencies. *Disease-A-Month* 43:809, 1997.
7. Lee-Chiong TL, Stitt JT: Disorders of temperature regulation. *Compr Ther* 21:697, 1995.
8. Danzl DF, Pozos RS, Auerbach PS, et al: Multicenter hypothermia survey. *Ann Emerg Med* 16:1042, 1987.
9. Petty KJ. Hypothermia, in Fauci AS, Braunwald E, Isselbacher KJ, et al (eds): *Harrison's Principles of Internal Medicine, vol 1,* 14th ed. New York, McGraw-Hill, 1998, p 97.
10. Center for Disease Control: Hypothermia-related deaths—January 1996—December 1997, and United States, 1979–1995. *MMWR* 47:1037, 1998.
11. Center for Disease Control: Hypothermia-related deaths—Virginia, November 1996–April 1997. *MMWR* 46:1157, 1997.
12. Jolly T, Ghezzi KT: Accidental hypothermia. *Emerg Med Clin North Am* 10:311, 1992.
13. Weinberg AD: Hypothermia. *Ann Emerg Med* 22(pt 2):370, 1993.
14. Bartley B, Crnkovich DJ, Usman AR, Carlson RW: How to recognize hypothermia in critically ill patients. *J Crit Care Illness* 11:118, 1996.
15. Antretter H, Dapunt OE, Bonatti J: Management of profound hypothermia. *Br J Hosp Med* 54:215, 1995.
16. Silfvast T, Pettila V: Outcome from severe accidental hypothermia in Southern Finland—A 10-year review. *Resuscitation* 59:285, 2003.
17. Delaney KA, Howland MA, Vassallo S, Goldfrank LR: Assessment of acid-base disturbances in hypothermia and their physiologic consequences. *Ann Emerg Med* 18:72, 1989.
18. Larach MG: Accidental hypothermia. *Lancet* 345:493, 1995.
19. Patel A, Gestos JP, Moussa G, et al: The Osborn wave of hypothermia in normothermic patients. *Clin Cardiol* 17:273, 1994.
20. Gussak I, Bjerregaard P, Egan TM, et al: ECG phenomenon called the J wave. History, pathophysiology, and clinical significance. *J Electrocardiogr* 28:49, 1995.
21. Solomon A, Barish RA, Browne B, et al: The electrocardiographic features of hypothermia. *J Emerg Med* 7:169, 1989.
22. Kloeck W, Cummins RO, Chamberlain D, et al: Special resuscitation situations: An advisory statement from the International Liaison Committee on resuscitation. *Circulation* 95:2196, 1997.
23. Braun R, Krishel S: Environmental emergencies. *Emerg Med Clin North Am* 15:451, 1997.
24. Lazar HL: The treatment of hypothermia. *N Engl J Med* 337:1545, 1997.
25. Bartley B, Crnkovich DJ, Usman AR, Carlson RW: Techniques for managing severe hypothermia. *J Crit Illness* 11:123, 1996.
26. Handrigan MT, Wright RO, Becker BM, et al: Factors and methodology in achieving ideal delivery temperatures for intravenous and lavage fluid in hypothermia. *Am J Emerg Med* 15:350, 1997.
27. Murphy K, Nowak RM, Tomlanovich MC: Use of bretylium tosylate as prophylaxis and treatment in hypothermic ventricular fibrillation in the canine model. *Ann Emerg Med* 15:1160, 1986.
28. Orts A, Alcaraz C, Delaney KA, et al: Bretylium tosylate and electrically induced cardiac arrhythmia during hypothermia in dogs. *Am J Emerg Med* 10:311, 1992.
29. Gentilello LM: Advances in the management of hypothermia. *Surg Clin North Am* 75:243, 1995.
30. Koller R, Schnider TW, Neidhart P: Deep accidental hypothermia and cardiac arrest—Rewarming with forced air. *Acta Anaesthesiol Scand* 41:1359, 1997.

31. Goheen MSL, Ducharme MB, Kenny GP, et al: Efficacy of forced-air and inhalation rewarming by using a human model for severe hypothermia. *J Appl Physiol* 83:1635, 1997.

32. Steele MT, Nelson MJ, Sessler DI, et al: Forced air speeds rewarming in accidental hypothermia. *Ann Emerg Med* 27:479, 1996.

33. Lloyd ELI: Accidental hypothermia treated by central rewarming through the airway. *Br J Anaesth* 45:41, 1973.

34. Slovis CM, Bachvarov HL: Heated inhalation treatment of hypothermia. *Am J Emerg Med* 2:533, 1984.

35. Giesbrecht GG, Bristow GK: Recent advances in hypothermia research. *Ann NY Acad Sci* 813:663, 1997.

36. Hall KN, Syverud SA: Closed thoracic cavity lavage in the treatment of severe hypothermia in human beings. *Ann Emerg Med* 19:204, 1990.

37. Iversen RJ, Atkin SH, Jaker MA, et al: Successful CPR in a severely hypothermic patient using continuous thoracostomy lavage. *Ann Emerg Med* 19:1335, 1990.

38. Winegard C: Successful treatment of severe hypothermia and prolonged cardiac arrest with closed thoracic cavity lavage. *J Emeg Med* 15:629, 1997.

39. Kristensen G, Gravesen H, Benveniste D, Jordening H: An oesphageal thermal tube for rewarming in hypothermia. *Acta Anaesthesiol Scand* 29:846, 1985.

40. Ledingham IM, Routh GS, Douglas IHS, MacDonald AM: Central rewarming system for treatment of hypothermia. *Lancet* 1:1168, 1980.

41. Hernandez E, Praga M, Alcazar JM, et al: Hemodialysis for treatment of accidental hypothermia. *Nephron* 63:214, 1993.

42. Brodersen HP, Meurer T, Bolzenius K, et al: Hemofiltration in severe hypothermia with favorable outcome. *Clin Nephrol* 45:413, 1996.

43. Gentilello LM, Cobean RA, Offner PJ, et al: Continuous arteriovenous rewarming: Rapid reversal of hypothermia in critically ill patients. *J Trauma* 32:316, 1992.

44. Vretenas DF, Urschel JD, Parrott JCW, Unruh HW: Cardiopulmonary bypass resuscitation for accidental hypothermia. *Ann Thorac Surg* 58:895, 1994.

45. Waters DJ, Belz M, Lawse D, Ulstad D: Portable cardiopulmonary bypass: Resuscitation from prolonged ice-water submersion and asystole. *Ann Thorac Surg* 57:1018, 1994.

46. Gregory JS, Bergstein JM, Aprahamian C, et al: Comparison of three methods of rewarming from hypothermia: Advantages of extracoporeal blood warming. *J Trauma* 31:1247, 1991.

47. Ireland AJ, Pathi VL, Crawforn, Colquhoun IW: Back from the dead: extracorporeal rewarming of severe accidental hypothermia victims in accidental emergency. *J Accid Emerg Med* 14:255, 1997.

48. Walpoth BH, Walpoth-Aslan BN, Mattle HP, et al: Outcome of survivors of accidental deep hypothermia and circulatory arrest treated with extracorporeal blood rewarming. *N Engl J Med* 337:1500, 1997.

49. Fildes J, Sheaff C, Barrett J: Very hot intravenous fluid in the treatment of hypothermia. *J Trauma* 35:683, 1993.

50. Sheaff CM, Fildes JJ, Keogh P, et al: Safety of 65°C intravenous fluid for the treatment of hypothermia. *Am J Surg* 172:52, 1996.

51. Mair P, Kornberger E, Furtwaengler W, et al: Prognostic markers in patients with severe accidental hypothermia and cardiocirculatory arrest. *Resuscitation* 27:47, 1994.

52. Danzl DF, Hedges JR, Pozos RS, et al: Hypothermia outcome score: development and implications. *Crit Care Med* 17: 227, 1989.

53. Schaller M-D, Fischer AP, Perret CH: Hyperkalemia: a prognostic factor during acute severe hypothermia. *JAMA* 264:1842, 1990.

Chapter 111
HYPERTHERMIA

JANICE L. ZIMMERMAN
NICOLA A. HANANIA

KEY POINTS

- *Heat stroke is distinguished from less severe forms of environmental hyperthermia by higher body temperature and the presence of severe central nervous system dysfunction.*

- *Classic (nonexertional) heat stroke affects the elderly and the chronically ill and is associated with high morbidity and mortality rates.*

- *Exertional heat stroke affects younger individuals who exercise in hot environments, and it develops over a short period.*

- *Immediate conductive or evaporative cooling should be instituted for heat stroke victims with a core temperature above 41°C.*

- *Malignant hyperthermia is a rare syndrome of hyperthermia, muscle contractions, and cardiovascular instability triggered by succinyl choline and inhaled anesthetics.*

- *Management of malignant hyperthermia includes the prompt recognition of the syndrome, discontinuation of the inciting drug, administration of dantrolene, and supportive care.*

- *Neuroleptic malignant syndrome is an idiosyncratic reaction to neuroleptic drugs characterized by hyperthermia, muscle rigidity, alterations in mental status, autonomic dysfunction, and rhabdomyolysis.*

- *Treatment of neuroleptic malignant syndrome includes discontinuation of the triggering drug, administration of dantrolene for muscle rigidity and hyperthermia, administration of dopaminergic drugs such as bromocriptine and amantadine, and supportive care.*

Hyperthermia is defined as a core body temperature above 38.2°C (101.8°F) and is commonly present in patients in the intensive care unit. In most cases, hyperthermia is a consequence of the presence of pyrogens that reset the hypothalamic thermoregulatory mechanism to a higher temperature.[1] This response, referred to as *fever*, is part of the individual's immune response to infection, malignancy, inflammation, or autoimmune disease.

The disorders discussed in this chapter, environmental hyperthermia, malignant hyperthermia, and the neuroleptic malignant syndrome, are not part of the body's immune response and result from a failure of homeostatic thermoregulatory mechanisms. Prompt recognition and appropriate treatment of these syndromes are critical to prevent irreversible cellular and organ injury.

Environmental Hyperthermia

PATHOPHYSIOLOGY

Environmental hyperthermia is related to endogenous heat production, high ambient temperatures, and/or high humidity. Humans produce approximately 50 to 60 kcal/m² per hour of heat, or approximately 100 kcal/hour.[2] Minimal activity can increase heat production two- to fourfold, and strenuous exercise may increase heat production as much as 20 times the baseline level. Normally, most heat loss (50% to 70%) occurs from the skin and lungs through radiation in neutral environments. Conduction of heat through direct contact with cooler objects or loss of heat due to convection accounts for a smaller percentage of heat loss. Evaporation of sweat from the skin is a major mechanism of heat loss in a warm environment.

The preoptic nucleus of the anterior hypothalamus receives information from temperature-sensitive receptors in the skin, viscera, and great vessels and initiates physiologic responses to temperature increases. Increased temperatures result in cutaneous vasodilation, decreased muscle tone, and increase in sweating. As ambient temperature nears 37°C (98.6°F), the body relies primarily on evaporation of sweat as a cooling mechanism. Evaporation can result in the loss of 580 kcal/L of evaporated sweat. Conditions of high humidity (>75%) impair the loss of heat through evaporation and increase the risk of heat injury.

An acute phase inflammatory response may cause or contribute to the pathophysiology of heat stroke. Increased concentrations of endotoxin, tumor necrosis factor, soluble tumor necrosis factor receptor, and interleukin 1 have been demonstrated in patients with classic heat stroke (CHS).[3,4] Interleukin 6 and nitric oxide metabolite concentrations correlate with the severity of illness. Endothelial cell activation or injury is suggested by findings of increased concentrations of circulating intracellular adhesion molecule 1, endothelin, and von Willebrand factor antigen.[5] Altered expression or blocked activity of protective heat shock proteins may also contribute to injury in heat stroke.[6]

PREDISPOSING FACTORS

Environmental hyperthermia results from increased heat production and/or decreased heat loss (Table 111-1). Environmental heat stress includes high heat and humidity that contribute to heat production and limit heat loss. Numerous drugs interfere with the thermoregulatory process. Sympathomimetic drugs, such as amphetamines, cocaine, phencyclidine, ecstasy and ephedrine, increase muscle activity and heat production and may also disrupt hypothalamic regulatory mechanisms.[7] Drugs with anticholinergic effects, such as cyclic antidepressants, antihistamines, and antipsychotics, inhibit cholinergically mediated sweating and disrupt hypothalamic function. Ethanol may contribute to heat stroke by several mechanisms: vasodilation resulting in heat gain from the environment, impaired perception of the environment, and diuresis. β-Adrenergic blockers may impair the cardiovascular compensation of increased output needed to compensate for cutaneous vasodilation and decrease cutaneous blood flow. Patients with stroke or head injury may also have impaired regulatory mechanisms. Dehydration by itself has been documented to increase core body temperature. Obese individuals have a lower ratio of body surface area to mass than do the nonobese, which limits radiant heat loss. Loss of apocrine sweat glands due to skin conditions such as burns or scleroderma is a much less common risk factor for heat injury. Factors that increased the risk of death in the July 1995

TABLE 111-1 Predisposing Factors for Heat Stroke

Increased Heat Production	Decreased Heat Loss
Environmental heat stress	Environmental heat stress
Exertion	Cardiac disease
Fever	Peripheral vascular disease
Hypothalamic dysfunction	Dehydration
Drugs (sympathomimetics)	Anticholinergic drugs
Hyperthyroidism	Obesity
	Skin disease
	Ethanol
	β Blockers

heat wave in Chicago included being confined to bed due to medical problems and living alone.[8]

SPECTRUM OF HEAT INJURY

The most commonly described types of heat injury include heat cramps, heat exhaustion, and heat stroke. Heat cramps are unlikely to result in the need for critical care. Heat cramps usually occur in individuals who work or exercise for long periods in hot environments, sweat heavily, and consume large quantities of hypotonic fluid.[9] Heat cramps often occur after exertion in abdominal, thigh, and calf muscles. The etiology is thought to be due to shifts of electrolytes and water between intracellular and extracellular spaces. Many patients experiencing heat cramps never present for medical care. Management includes rest and hydration (intravenously or orally) with a salt solution.

Heat exhaustion also does not usually require intensive care, but it is an important syndrome to distinguish from heat stroke. It may complicate other critical illness such as myocardial infarction and stroke. Patients with heat exhaustion usually experience salt or water depletion as a result of heat stress. Temperatures can be mildly elevated (<40°C), but other clinical manifestations are nonspecific. Patients may complain of malaise, weakness, irritability, nausea, vomiting, and heat cramps. Although patients may have headache and/or mild confusion, severe disturbances of central nervous system (CNS) function are not present. Tachycardia and orthostatic hypotension may suggest significant dehydration. Treatment includes rest in a cool environment and fluid replacement based on clinical and laboratory parameters.

Heat stroke is the syndrome most likely to require intensive care, and it results from failure of normal homeostatic thermoregulatory mechanisms. The diagnosis of heat stroke requires a history of exposure to a heat load (external or internal), severe CNS dysfunction, and elevated temperature (usually >40°C, or >104°F). The absolute temperature may not be critical because cooling measures are often instituted before the patient is admitted to a health care facility. An alternative definition for heat stroke has been proposed that takes into account the current understanding of the pathophysiology: "A form of hyperthermia associated with a systemic inflammatory response leading to a syndrome of multiorgan dysfunction in which encephalopathy predominates."[6] The presence of severe CNS abnormalities distinguishes heat stroke from less severe forms of heat injury such as heat exhaustion. The absence of sweating is not a useful diagnostic criterion. If the history is inadequate, other disorders associated with hyperthermia must be considered in the differential diagnosis, such as infection, hypothalamic injury, thyrotoxicosis, neuroleptic malignant syndrome, and malignant hyperthermia.

HEAT STROKE SYNDROMES

Two syndromes of heat stroke occur: classic (nonexertional) heat stroke (CHS) and exertional heat stroke (EHS). CHS typically affects elderly individuals with underlying chronic illness and tends to occur when environmental heat stress is maximal for several days. This syndrome usually develops over several days and results in significant dehydration and absence of sweating.

EHS typically occurs in young, healthy individuals such as amateur athletes and military recruits who exercise in hot environments. This syndrome occurs sporadically depending on initiation of significant activity in a hot environment. These individuals usually have no chronic illness and are more likely to be nonacclimated individuals. Exertional heat stroke can occur over a short period. Dehydration may be mild, and approximately 50% of individuals will have profuse sweating on presentation.

CLINICAL MANIFESTATIONS

Heat stroke is a multisystemic disorder, and the manifestations in an individual depend on rapidity of onset, severity of exposure (temperature and duration), and comorbid conditions.[10] CNS dysfunction may range from bizarre behavior, delirium, and confusion to decerebrate rigidity, cerebellar dysfunction, seizures, and coma. Cerebellar abnormalities are often the first to appear and the last to resolve. These changes are potentially reversible, although permanent deficits such as cerebellar dysfunction, hemiparesis or dementia can occur. Lumbar puncture in patients with heat stroke may reveal increased protein, xanthochromia, and lymphocytic pleocytosis.

Tachycardia is an almost universal cardiovascular finding in heat stroke unless the patient is receiving β-adrenergic blockers or calcium channel blockers. Tachycardia occurs in response to peripheral vasodilation and the need for increased cardiac output. Supraventricular tachycardia and atrial fibrillation may also occur. The systemic vascular resistance is usually low unless severe hypovolemia is present.[11] Compensatory vasoconstriction occurs in the splanchnic and renal vascular beds. If the patient is unable to increase cardiac output, hypotension develops. Reversible myocardial dysfunction has been described in heat stroke,[12] and a variety of electrocardiographic changes have been described, including conduction defects, prolonged QT interval, nonspecific STT changes, and STT changes consistent with myocardial ischemia.[13] Additional physical examination findings may include ileus, gastric distension, diarrhea, decreased muscle tone, and tachypnea.

LABORATORY FINDINGS

The acid-base status in patients with heat stroke may be difficult to predict. Tachypnea may result in significant respiratory alkalosis, but most patients also have a metabolic lactic acidosis.[10,14,15] The etiology of the lactic acidosis differs with the type of heat stroke syndrome. In CHS, lactic acidosis more commonly results from hypoperfusion and is often mild. In EHS, lactate is produced as a consequence of anaerobic muscle metabolism and acidosis may be severe. Hypoglycemia may be present in patients with EHS due to increased glucose use and impaired hepatic gluconeogenesis. Rhabdomyolysis with elevation of creatine kinase and renal failure occur more commonly with EHS. Renal failure occurs in approximately 25% of patients with EHS and 5% of patients with CHS. Renal injury may be due to myoglobinuria, direct thermal parenchymal damage, or decreased renal blood flow due to hypotension. Hematologic effects of heat stroke include leukocytosis and hypocoagulability that may progress to disseminated intravascular coagulation (DIC). Coagulation abnormalities may peak hours to days after heat injury.[10] Hepatic heat injury results in elevation of bilirubin and transaminase levels. Electrolyte concentrations are variable in heat stroke.[14] Hyperkalemia can result from rhabdomyolysis, but hypokalemia occurs more commonly. Hypocalcemia can occur, particularly with rhabdomyolysis, but usually does not require specific therapy.

TREATMENT OF HEAT STROKE

In addition to resuscitative measures, immediate cooling should be instituted for any patient with a temperature above 41°C (>105.8°F). Diagnostic testing such as computed tomography should be performed after cooling. Two methods of cooling have been used: conductive cooling and evaporative cooling. Although specific methods are promoted by individual clinicians, definitive human studies are lacking and the optimal cooling method remains controversial. Available resources and personnel may dictate the exact method used. Most patients can be effectively cooled in 30 to 45 minutes with either technique.

Direct cooling by enhancing conduction of heat from the body is accomplished by immersion of the patient in cold water. Skin massage to counter cutaneous vasoconstriction in the limbs has been recommended. Shivering can result in an undesirable increase in heat production, and chlorpromazine has been recommended to prevent this response. However, chlorpromazine may lower the seizure threshold and impair sweating. This method requires considerable staff time and may interfere with other resuscitative measures such as intubation and intravenous access. Variants of this method include ice-water soaks and application of ice packs to the axillae, groin, and neck, where the great vessels are closer to the skin surface. A protocol used by the U.S. Marine Corps training base for EHS has been described as follows[16]:

- A stretcher holding the victim is placed on top of a bathtub containing water and ice.
- One liter of normal saline is administered intravenously as a bolus.
- Sheets are dipped into the ice water and used to cover and drench the patient.
- Ice is added to the top of the sheet for further cooling and skin is massaged is improve skin blood flow.
- The head is constantly irrigated with more ice water and a fan is directed at the patient.

Evaporative cooling is a widely used cooling method based on a body cooling unit developed in the Middle East for treatment of individuals with heat stroke during the annual pilgrimage to Mecca.[17] Optimum cooling was achieved with unclothed volunteers suspended on a net sprayed with 15°C water and warm air at 30°C to 35°C (at the skin surface). A practical adaptation for hospital use is to place the unclothed patient on a stretcher and spray with warm (not cold) water. High-flow air currents are created with the use of fans to enhance evaporative cooling. This method allows personnel to institute other resuscitative measures while cooling occurs.

Other cooling methods such as peritoneal lavage, iced gastric lavage, or cardiopulmonary bypass have not been effectively tested in humans. Dissipation of heat by lavage of body cavities is limited by the small surface area available for conductive heat transfer. Gastric lavage may also predispose to aspiration. Antipyretics are not indicated, and dantrolene is ineffective.[18]

A thermistor probe (esophageal or rectal) should be used for monitoring core temperature during cooling efforts. Cooling should be stopped at 38.0°C to 38.8°C (100.4°F to 102°F) to prevent hypothermic overshoot. Continued monitoring is needed to detect a subsequent increase in core temperature. In addition to cooling, many patients will require intubation for airway protection. Supplemental oxygen should be instituted for all patients. The type and quantity of intravenous fluids should be individualized based on an assessment of electrolytes, volume status, and urine output. Overaggressive hydration during cooling may result in cardiac decompensation, especially in the elderly as vasodilation corrects. Significant rhabdomyolysis indicates the need to achieve urine outputs of 100 to 200 mL/hour with fluid therapy. Hypotension usually responds to fluid administration and cooling as peripheral vasodilation decreases. Vasopressor agents may result in vasoconstriction and an undesirable decrease in heat exchange. Invasive hemodynamic monitoring may be warranted in patients with refractory hypotension or suspected cardiac impairment. Significant electrolyte abnormalities should be corrected and monitored closely. Benzodiazepines should be used to control any seizure activity. Bleeding secondary to DIC may require transfusion of fresh-frozen plasma and/or platelets.

OUTCOME FROM HEAT STROKE

The survival rate from heat stroke approaches 90% with appropriate management. However, morbidity rate is related to the duration of hyperthermia and to underlying conditions. Advanced age, severe hypotension, coagulopathy, hyperkalemia, acute renal failure, and prolonged coma are associated with a poor prognosis.[14] Elevated lactate levels are associated with a poor prognosis in CHS but not in EHS.[19] In a retrospective study, rapid cooling (<1 hour) was associated with decreased mortality rate.[20]

Malignant Hyperthermia

Malignant hyperthermia (MH) is an inherited drug- or stress-induced hypermetabolic syndrome characterized by hyperthermia, muscle contractures, and cardiovascular instability. The incidence of MH in patients who receive anesthesia with a triggering agent varies in different populations and age groups. The incidence in adults is approximately 1 in 20,000 to 50,000. The syndrome is genetically transmitted as an autosomal dominant trait. Although a similar syndrome in swine is caused by a single-point mutation of the ryanodine receptor, MH in humans is believed to result from a more heterogeneous group of mutations. The syndrome results from defects in calcium transport in skeletal muscle. The primary defects are postulated to be impaired reuptake of calcium into the sarcoplasmic reticulum, enhanced release of calcium from the sarcoplasmic reticulum, and a defect in the calcium-mediated excitation-contraction coupling mechanism. The resultant intracellular hypercalcemia leads to hypermetabolism.

Diagnostic testing for susceptibility to MH is problematic. Currently, a muscle biopsy sample from the patient is exposed in vitro to halothane and caffeine in selected laboratories.[21–23] The muscle of an affected individual contracts rather than relaxes in the presence of caffeine or halothane. A normal contracture test does not completely rule out the possibility of MH susceptibility, but no alternate tests are available. This limitation of the test probably reflects the heterogeneous nature of the underlying mutations.

TRIGGERS OF MALIGNANT HYPERTHERMIA

Halothane and succinylcholine have been implicated in most reported cases of MH. The combination of the two agents is more commonly involved than either agent alone. Additional potentiating agents include potent inhalational anesthetics, ethanol, caffeine, sympathomimetics (vasopressors), parasympathomimetics (atropine), cardiac glycosides, and quinidine analogues. Less commonly, MH can be precipitated by infection, physical or emotional stress, anoxia or high ambient temperatures. Nondepolarizing neuromuscular blockers, etomidate, nitrous oxide, ketamine, opiates, barbiturates, benzodiazepines, propofol, and local anesthetics are considered safe in patients with MH.

CLINICAL MANIFESTATIONS

Manifestations of MH usually occur within 30 minutes of the initiation of anesthesia in 90% of cases. However, the syndrome may occur at any time during anesthesia and the recovery period. The spectrum of presentations ranges from minor symptoms to a fulminant crisis. A clinical grading scale has been devised for diagnosis of MH but is not readily applicable at the bedside, and required data may not be available.[24] Muscle rigidity begins in muscles of the extremities or the chest. In patients receiving succinylcholine, the stiffness most commonly begins in the jaw. The development of masseter muscle rigidity after administration of a neuromuscular blocker should be considered an early sign of possible MH.[25,26] In the North American MH Registry, masseter muscle rigidity was the first sign in 30% of likely cases.[27] However, muscle rigidity may not be present in all cases. Monitoring of arterial blood gases or end-tidal CO_2 levels by capnography may detect an increase in CO_2 that may be the earliest sign of MH. Tachycardia is an early, although nonspecific, sign. Hypertension and mottling of the skin also occur. The increase in temperature usually occurs later but is followed rapidly by metabolic acidosis, ventricular arrhythmias, and hypotension. Temperature may increase as rapidly as 1°C every 5 minutes. Laboratory abnormalities include increased levels of sodium, calcium, magnesium, potassium,

phosphate, creatine kinase, and lactate dehydrogenase and the presence of myoglobinuria. Lactate levels increase, and arterial blood gases indicate hypoxemia and hypercapnia if minute ventilation is constant.

TREATMENT

Once the diagnosis of MH is considered, the inciting drug should be discontinued immediately and the patient should be ventilated with 100% O_2. The most effective and safe therapy is dantrolene, a drug that blocks calcium release from the sarcoplasmic reticulum without inhibiting its reuptake.[28] Uncoupling of the excitation-contraction mechanism in skeletal muscle decreases thermogenesis. Dantrolene should be administered by rapid intravenous push at a dose of 2.5 mg/kg and repeated every 5 minutes as needed until the symptoms subside or the maximum dose of 10 mg/kg has been reached. Dantrolene is poorly water soluble and using 40°C water as the diluent may facilitate reconstitution.[29] A decrease in muscle rigidity should be evident within minutes. Subsequent doses of 1 mg/kg every 4 to 6 hours should be continued for 36 to 48 hours. If dantrolene is ineffective or slowly effective, evaporative or conductive cooling can also be used. Calcium channel blockers are of no benefit in MH and should not be used to treat arrhythmias. Sodium bicarbonate administration is often recommended to treat the acidosis, but evidence of efficacy is lacking. Urine output, vital signs, and blood gases should be monitored to guide ventilation and fluid therapy. A urine output of 100 to 200 mL/hour may be needed for treatment of rhabdomyolysis and myoglobinuria. Significant hyperkalemia should be treated with intravenous insulin and glucose. The coagulation profile should be followed to assess for the presence and severity of DIC.

OUTCOMES AND PREVENTION OF MALIGNANT HYPERTHERMIA

Several measures can be taken to prevent the occurrence of MH or limit the severity of the syndrome. The preoperative history may suggest a family history of anesthetic problems or neuromuscular disorders. Known MH triggers should be avoided in known susceptible individuals. Temperature and end-tidal CO_2 monitoring should be used during all general anesthesia procedures lasting longer than 30 minutes. Masseter muscle rigidity and increases in heart rate, CO_2 levels, and temperature should be evaluated as possible signs of MH. Dantrolene should be readily available in adequate doses. Prophylactic administration of dantrolene is not recommended.

The Malignant Hyperthermia Association of the United States provides a hot line for assistance in managing MH (1-800-MH-HYPER, 1-800-644-9737, or 1-315-464-7079 if outside the United States). The organization also maintains a Web site with useful information online (www.mhaus.org).

The mortality rate from MH, which was 50% to 70% decades ago, has decreased to lower than 10% because it is more appropriately recognized and treated. Death may result early in the clinical course from hyperkalemia, acidosis, or hypotension. Later deaths are often related to DIC, renal failure, and multiple organ dysfunction.

Neuroleptic Malignant Syndrome

Neuroleptic malignant syndrome (NMS) is an idiosyncratic reaction, usually to neuroleptic drugs, characterized by hyperthermia, muscle rigidity, mental status changes, autonomic dysfunction, and rhabdomyolysis. It may occur in up to 1% of all patients on neuroleptic agents and affects males more than females and the young more than the old.[30] The pathogenesis of NMS is unknown but is thought to be related to CNS dopamine-2 receptor antagonism or dopamine deficiency in the basal ganglia and hypothalamus resulting in altered temperature set point.[31]

TRIGGERS OF NEUROLEPTIC MALIGNANT SYNDROME

Most cases of NMS have been associated with high-potency neuroleptics such as haloperidol and thiothixene. However, the list of potential triggers includes butyrophenones (e.g., haloperidol), phenothiazines (e.g., chlorpromazine and fluphenazine), thioxanthenes (e.g., thiothixene), dopamine-depleting agents (e.g., tetrabenazine), dibenzoxazepines (e.g., loxapine), and withdrawal of levodopa/carbidopa or amantadine. The newer atypical antipsychotic drugs such as clozapine, risperidone, olanzapine, ziprasidone and quetiapine have also been reported to induce NMS. NMS can be associated with antiemetics (prochlorperazine), peristaltic agents (metoclopramide), anesthetics (droperidol), and sedatives (promethazine).[32] Rechallenge with the inciting drug may not result in recurrence of NMS. Other factors suggested to contribute to the development of NMS include lithium therapy, ambient heat, dehydration, psychomotor agitation, and underlying brain injury.[33,34]

CLINICAL MANIFESTATIONS

NMS usually occurs 3 to 9 days after initiating a neuroleptic agent or changing the dose. The reaction is not related to dose and may occur after a single dose. The syndrome may last for a period of 1 to 3 weeks, especially with depot drug forms. A similar onset occurs with dose reduction or withdrawal of dopaminergic agents in patients with Parkinson disease. The onset of symptoms can be insidious or fulminant. Symptoms often begin with mental status changes followed in sequence by muscle rigidity, hyperthermia, and autonomic dysfunction, but variability exists.[35] Hyperthermia is universally present, and the average maximum temperature is 39.9°C (103.8°F).[36,37] However, NMS has been reported to occur without temperature elevation.[38] Autonomic dysfunction includes tachycardia, diaphoresis, blood pressure instability, and arrhythmias. Autonomic dysfunction may precede changes in muscle tone. A general increase in muscle tone, "lead pipe" rigidity, or tremors occurs in more than 90% of patients. Early manifestations of changes in muscle tone include dysphagia, dysarthria, or dystonia that may be mistaken for extrapyramidal side effects of the drug. Altered mental status occurs in 75% of patients and can range from agitation to coma. The rigidity, tremors, and confusion of NMS may be attributed to the underlying disease in patients with Parkinson disease and delay the diagnosis. Rhabdomyolysis occurs frequently.

TABLE 111-2 Diagnostic Criteria for Neuroleptic Malignant Syndrome[a]

Major criteria
Fever
Muscle rigidity
Elevated creatine kinase
Minor criteria
Tachycardia
Abnormal blood pressure
Tachypnea
Altered consciousness
Diaphoresis
Leukocytosis

[a] Diagnosis of neuroleptic malignant syndrome is suggested by presence of all three major criteria or two major criteria with four minor criteria.
SOURCE: Mann et al.[42]

Laboratory findings include elevated creatine kinase levels and myoglobinuria. White blood cell counts are often increased (10,000 to 40,000/mm^3) and may demonstrate a left shift.[30] DIC has also been reported. Volume depletion or renal injury from rhabdomyolysis results in elevated levels of serum urea nitrogen and creatinine. Significant rhabdomyolysis may lead to serious electrolyte abnormalities.

Various diagnostic criteria have been proposed (Table 111-2), but NMS remains a clinical diagnosis based on exposure to neuroleptic agents or other dopamine antagonists in association with characteristic clinical manifestations.

TREATMENT OF NEUROLEPTIC MALIGNANT SYNDROME

Recommendations for treatment of NMS are based primarily on case reports and retrospective analyses because no controlled trials have been conducted in humans and no animal model exists. The patient should be admitted to an intensive care unit, and the precipitating medication should be discontinued. Treatment then involves three aspects: stopping thermogenesis, repletion of dopamine in the CNS, and general support.[32] Specific therapy should be individualized to each patient. The Neuroleptic Malignant Syndrome Information Service (www.nmsis.org) maintains a hotline for medical professionals (1-888-667-8367) if assistance is needed. Dantrolene is the most effective agent for decreasing muscle rigidity and temperature, although its role in NMS is less well defined than in MH. It can be given in the same doses as described for MH. Neuromuscular blockers and sedation may be infrequently needed for rigidity refractory to dantrolene. Dopamine agonists have been reported to have beneficial effects in NMS,[39,40] but results have been inconsistent.[41] These drugs include bromocriptine (2.5 to 5 mg orally three times daily, <30 mg/day), amantadine (100 mg orally three times daily), and levodopa/carbidopa. In severe cases, use of all three dopamine agonists may be considered. Benzodiazepines (lorazepam 1 to 2 mg every 8 hours) may be helpful in catatonia and for control of agitation. Electroconvulsive therapy has been used successfully in NMS, but indications are not well established. It may be considered when the clinical presentation overlaps with lethal catatonia.[32,42] Supportive therapy is crucial to successful management of NMS because patients typically die of complications such as arrhythmias or aspiration. Intravascular volume should be optimized to replace increased insensible losses and maintain renal blood flow and urine output. Tachycardia and hypertension may respond to β blockers. External cooling may be required, and prophylaxis for venous thromboembolism should be instituted. Complications may include respiratory failure, cardiovascular collapse, renal failure, arrhythmias, or thromboembolism. Mortality rates are lower than 10% if recognition is prompt and appropriate treatment provided.

References

1. Marik PE: Fever in the ICU. *Chest* 117:855, 2000.
2. Knochel JP, Reed G: Disorders of heat regulation, in Kleeman, CR Maxwell MH, Narwin RG (eds): *Clinical Disorders of Fluid and Electrolyte Metabolism*. New York, McGraw-Hill, 1987.
3. Bouchama A, Al-Sedairy S, Siddiqui S, et al: Elevated pyrogenic cytokines in heatstroke. *Chest* 104:1498, 1993.
4. Hammami MM, Bouchama A, Al-Sedairy S, et al: Concentrations of soluble tumor necrosis factor and interleukin-6 receptors in heatstroke and heatstress. *Crit Care Med* 25:1314, 1997.
5. Bouchama A, Hammami MM, Haq A, et al: Evidence for endothelial cell activation/injury in heatstroke. *Crit Care Med* 24:1173, 1996.
6. Bouchama A, Knochel JP: Heat stroke. *N Engl J Med* 346:1978, 2002.
7. Marzuk PM, Tardiff K, Leon AC, et al: Ambient temperature and mortality from unintentional cocaine overdose. *JAMA* 279:1795, 1998.
8. Semenza JC, Rubin CH, Falter KH, et al: Heat-related deaths during the July 1995 heat wave in Chicago. *N Engl J Med* 335:84, 1996.
9. Noakes TD: Fluid and electrolyte disturbances in heat illness. *Int J Sports Med* 19(suppl 2):5146, 1998.
10. Dematte JE, O'Mara K, Buescher J, et al: Near-fatal heat stroke during the 1995 heat wave in Chicago. *Ann Intern Med* 129:173, 1998.
11. Dahmash NS, Al-Harthi SS, Akhtar J: Invasive evaluation of patients with heat stroke. *Chest* 103:1210, 1993.
12. Rousseau J-M, Villevieille T, Schiano P, et al: Reversible myocardial dysfunction after exertional heatstroke. *Intensive Care Med* 27:328, 2001.
13. Akhtar MJ, Al-Nozha M, Al-Harthi S, Nouh MS: Electrocardiographic abnormalities in patients with heat stroke. *Chest* 104:411, 1993.
14. Tucker LE, Stanford J, Graves B, et al: Classical heatrstroke: Clinical and laboratory assessment. *South Med J* 78:20, 1985.
15. Bouchama A, De Vol EB: Acid-base alterations in heatstroke. *Intensive Care Med* 27:680, 2001.
16. Gaffin SL, Gardner JW, Flinn SD: Cooling methods for heatstroke victims. *Ann Intern Med* 132:678, 2000.
17. Weiner JS, Khogali M: A physiological body-cooling unit for treatment of heat stroke. *Lancet* 1:507, 1980.
18. Bouchama A, Cafege A, Devol EB, et al: Ineffectiveness of dantrolene sodium in the treatment of heatstroke. *Crit Care Med* 19:176, 1991.
19. Hart GR, Anderson RJ, Crumpler CP, et al: Epidemic heat stroke: Clinical characteristics and course of 28 patients. *Medicine* 61:189, 1982.
20. Vicario SJ, Okabajue R, Halton T: Rapid cooling in classic heatstroke: Effect on mortality rates. *J Emerg Med* 4:394, 1986.
21. European Malignant Hyperpyrexia Group: A protocol for the investigation of malignant hyperpyrexia. *Br J Anaesth* 56:1267, 1984.
22. Larach MG: Standardization of the caffeine halothane muscle contracture test. *Anesth Analg* 69:511, 1989.
23. Melton AT, Martucci RW, Kien ND, Gronert GA: Malignant hyperthermia in humans—standardizaton of contracture testing protocol. *Anesth Analg* 69:437, 1989.
24. Larach MG, Localie AR, Allen GC, et al: A clinical grading scale to predict malignant hyperthermia susceptibility. *Anesthesiology* 80:771, 1994.
25. O'Flynn R, Shutack J, Rosenberg H, Fletcher J: Masseter muscle rigidity (MMR) and malignant hyperthermia susceptibility (MHS): An update on management and diagnosis. *Anesthesiology* 77:A917, 1992.
26. Ellis FR, Hopkins PM, Halsall PJ, Christian AS: Masseter muscle spasm and the diagnosis of malignant hyperthermia susceptibility. *Anesth Analg* 75:143, 1992.
27. Rosenberg H: Malignant hyperthermia. Available at: www.mhaus.org. Accessed June 3, 2004.
28. Kolb ME, Horne ML, Martz R: Dantrolene in human malignant hyperthermia. *Anesthesiology* 56:254, 1982.
29. Mitchell LW, Leighton BL. Warmed diluent speeds dantrolene reconstitution. *Can J Anesth* 50:127, 2003.
30. Pelonero AL, Levenson JL, Pandurangi AR: Neuroleptic malignant syndrome: A review. *Psychiatr Serv* 49:1163, 1998.
31. Mann SC, Caroff SN, Lazarus A: Pathogenesis of neuroleptic malignant syndrome. *Psychiatr Ann* 21:175, 1991.
32. Caroff SN, Mann SC, Campbell EC: Neuroleptic malignant syndrome. *Adverse Drug React Bull* 209:799, 2001.
33. Naganuma H, Fijii I: Incidence and risk factors in neuroleptic malignant syndrome. *Acta Psychiatr Scand* 90:424, 1994.
34. Viejo LF, Morales V, Puñal P, et al: Risk factors in neuroleptic malignant syndrome. A case-control study. *Acta Psychiatr Scand* 107:45, 2003.
35. Velamoor VR, Norman RMG, Caroff SN, et al: Progression of symptoms in neuroleptic malignant syndrome. *J Nerve Ment Dis* 182:168, 1994.
36. Kurlan R, Hamill R, Shoulson I: Neuroleptic malignant syndrome. *Clin Neuropharmacol* 7:109, 1984.
37. Caroff SN, Mann SC: Neuroleptic malignant syndrome. *Med Clin North Am* 77:185, 1993.
38. Peiris DTS, Kuruppuarachchi KALA, Weerasena LP, et al: Neuroleptic malignant syndrome without fever: A report of three cases. *J Neurol Neurosurg Psychiatry* 69:277, 2000.
39. Rosenberg MR, Green M: Neuroleptic malignant syndrome: Review of response to therapy. *Arch Intern Med* 149:1927, 1989.
40. Sakkas P, Davis JM, Hua J, et al: Pharmacotherapy of neuroleptic malignant syndrome. *Psychiatr Ann* 21:157, 1991.
41. Shalev A, Hermesh H, Munitz H: Mortality from neuroleptic malignant syndrome. *J Clin Psychiatry* 50:18, 1989.
42. Mann SC, Caroff SN, Bleier HR, et al: Electroconvulsive therapy of the lethal catatonia syndrome: Case report and review. *Convuls Ther* 1990; 6:239.

Chapter 112 _____

DIVING MEDICINE AND NEAR DROWNING

CLAUDE A. PIANTADOSI
STEVEN D. BROWN

KEY POINTS

- *Immersion and diving produce physiologic effects from increased hydrostatic pressure and its effects on the behavior of gases.*

- *When diving with compressed air or other breathing gases, the body takes up extra nitrogen or other inert gas, which must be allowed to leave through the lungs gradually to avoid decompression sickness (DCS). DCS occurs when gas comes out of solution and forms bubbles in body tissues, which causes pain or neurologic symptoms by obstruction of blood flow and initiation of secondary inflammatory events.*

- *DCS is treated by prompt administration of high-flow O_2 and hydration. Oxygen recompression therapy is definitive treatment for symptom resolution and avoiding recurrence, even if delayed 1 or 2 days.*

- *Arterial gas embolism is usually the result of pulmonary overpressurization during ascent from diving with compressed gas and may occur at shallow depths. Arterial gas embolism is the second leading cause, after drowning, of fatalities in recreational diving.*

- *Near drowning (ND) is caused by asphyxia underwater, which may or may not be associated with aspiration. The primary injuries are to the brain, heart, lungs, and kidneys.*

- *In young adults, ND is often associated with drug or alcohol ingestion and may be accompanied by traumatic injuries.*

- *ND may be complicated by acute respiratory distress syndrome; its onset may be delayed or aggravated by aspiration of gastric contents or other foreign debris and pneumonia.*

- *ND may be complicated by pneumonia (or sepsis) caused by unusual pathogens present in contaminated water. Prophylactic antibiotic treatment is not indicated.*

Recreational activities involving water are enjoyed by millions of swimmers, boaters, and divers of all ages with various degrees of physical skill and judgment. However, the water environment is deceptively hazardous, and too often, swimmers or divers venture into peril with deadly results. In many situations, they ignore their physical limitations or impair their faculties with alcohol or other drugs. In other situations, such as with young children, the encounter with water is unsupervised or unexpected and frequently results in death by drowning. There are millions of recreational divers and many more recreational swimmers in the United States, which translates to thousands of diving accidents, drowning, and near drowning (ND) episodes each year. The exact number of such aquatic incidents and their effect on the health care system are difficult to estimate, but there may be more than 80,000 episodes per year in the United States. Victims often survive the incident only to die hours or days later in the hospital. Thus, the intensive care specialist should be knowledgeable about the clinical consequences and management of diving accidents and ND.

The Physics of Underwater Environments

Underwater environments produce physiologic changes as a result of the direct effects of increased hydrostatic pressure and its effects on the physical behavior of gases. Pressure is measured in units of force per area, which is expressed commonly in several convenient forms (Table 112-1). The pressure of the atmosphere at sea level is approximately 760 mm Hg (14.7 pounds per square inch). Underwater, the pressure of the water changes directly with depth, and this pressure must be added to atmospheric pressure to obtain total pressure, usually expressed in atmospheres absolute (ATA). Table 112-1 shows that a seawater column 33 ft deep (fsw) exerts a pressure equivalent to 1 atmosphere at sea level. Thus, a diver immersed at 33 fsw is exposed to a total pressure of 2 ATA.

When diving with compressed breathing gases, for the diver to inhale, the inspired gas pressure must be increased in proportion to the absolute pressure. Therefore, a larger number of gas molecules must be contained in the lungs (or other gas-filled body cavities) to maintain constant volume at a given temperature. The relation of pressure (P), volume (V), temperature (T) to number of moles of gas (n) is described by the *ideal gas law*:

$$PV = nRT \qquad (112\text{-}1)$$

where R is the universal gas constant. The ideal gas law gives rise to the special gas laws important in diving. Three relevant special gas laws in which one of the three variables is held constant are shown in Table 112-1. In diving the most important of these is the Boyle law, which explains the need to equilibrate pressure inside gas-containing spaces in the body, such as the middle ear space and lungs, to avoid barotrauma of descent (e.g., ear squeeze) or ascent (e.g., gas embolism).

Air and other breathable gases are mixtures of different molecules in which the total pressure is equal to the sum of the partial pressures of each gas. This expresses the Dalton law of partial pressures, which means that each gas in a mixture behaves as though it alone occupies the entire space. The uptake of gases by tissue is determined primarily by diffusion of gas from the alveolar spaces into blood and by transport of gas to tissues by the circulation (perfusion). The amount of a gas dissolved in liquid at any temperature, such as blood or tissues of the body at 37°C (98.6°F), is also proportional to its partial pressure (Henry law). The gas concentration in tissue at equilibrium is related to the partial pressure of the gas multiplied by its solubility coefficient. The physiologic effects of diving gases, such as nitrogen narcosis or the risk of decompression sickness (DCS), generally correlate with the partial pressure of the gas in the tissues of the body.

Immersion and Breath-Hold Diving

Water immersion produces adjustments by the respiratory, cardiovascular, renal, and endocrine systems.[1] Immersion produces three main physiologic effects: a decrease in thoracic gas volume, an increase in cardiac output, and a diuresis, which may lead to dehydration. These responses are caused

TABLE 112-1 Pressure Equivalents and Gas Laws

Condition	Pressure fsw	mm Hg	psig	ATA
Sea level	0	760	0	1.0
Sea water	33	1520	14.7	2.0
Sea water	66	2280	29.4	3.0
Sea water	330	8360	147.0	11.0

Boyle law $P_1V_1 = P_2V_2$
Charles law $V_1/T_1 = V_2/T_2$
Gay Lussaac law $P_1/T_1 = P_2/T_2$

ABBREVIATIONS: ATA, atmosphere absolute (depth in ATA = [fsw + 33]/33); fsw, feet sea water; psig, pounds per square inch gauge, (a pressure gauge at sea level reads zero).

by hydrostatic pressure and the high density of water relative to air. During immersion, the blood vessels outside the thorax are supported by water, and an upright body is exposed vertically to a hydrostatic pressure gradient. The pressure around the body compresses the abdomen relative to the thorax, thereby causing negative pressure breathing (approximately −20 cm H_2O). The diaphragm is displaced upward, which decreases thoracic gas volume and expiratory reserve volume. The pressure gradient across the diaphragm, coupled to a hydrostatic decrease in venous capacitance in the legs, increases the volume of blood in the thorax, including the heart, by about 20%. Blood volume may be increased further by arterial vasoconstriction if the water is cooler than the thermoneutral point (~34°C, 93.2°F).

During immersion, cardiovascular distention activates mechanoreceptors that normally respond to hypervolemia. The apparent hypervolemia is detected in the hypothalamus via vagal afferents and leads to an immersion response. This response consists of diuresis and natriuresis, which have time profiles that suggest they operate by different mechanisms. Peak diuresis occurs rapidly (1 to 2 hours), whereas peak natriuresis occurs later (4 to 5 hours). Immersion diuresis but not natriuresis can be prevented by fluid restriction and vasopressin administration. The distention of the heart correlates with urinary sodium excretion. The mechanism of the immersion response is suppression of antidiuretic hormone release, also known as the *Gauer-Henry response*. The mechanism of natriuresis is related to a decrease in tubular reabsorption of sodium and not to an increase in filtered sodium. Natriuresis involves aldosterone suppression via decreased renin-angiotensin activity, increased release of atrial natriuretic factor, release of renal prostaglandins, and decreased renal sympathetic activity.

The increase in thoracic blood volume in immersion distends the heart and enhances ventricular diastolic filling (preload), which increases cardiac output.[2] Cardiac output increases almost entirely due to an increase in stroke volume, which may double. The elevated cardiac output is sustained and not accompanied by an increase in oxygen consumption.

Immersion has important implications for the physiology of the breath-hold.[3] In a breath-hold maneuver, the lungs are a reservoir for the exchange of O_2 for CO_2. During breath-hold in air, mean alveolar partial pressure of O_2 (P_{O_2}) decreases linearly as a function of the decrease in the mixed venous P_{O_2}. As alveolar P_{O_2} decreases, body O_2 consumption eventually decreases and anaerobic metabolism increases. CO_2 enters the lungs in proportion to pulmonary blood flow and the gradient

for CO_2 diffusion between mixed venous and alveolar partial pressure of CO_2 (P_{CO_2}). The CO_2 transfer rate is high initially but then decreases because the diffusion gradient decreases as alveolar P_{CO_2} approaches the mixed venous P_{CO_2}. Further CO_2 production increases mixed venous P_{CO_2}, which causes alveolar P_{CO_2} to increase again. When the rising P_{CO_2} causes breathing to resume, the break point is reached. The time to the break point can be extended by maneuvers that lower P_{CO_2} or raise P_{O_2} such as hyperventilation or O_2 breathing. Hyperventilation does not increase the body's O_2 store appreciably because the increase in alveolar P_{O_2} resulting from a decrease in alveolar P_{CO_2} increases blood O_2 content only slightly. Thus, hyperventilation extends breath-hold time, but profound hypoxia may develop before the CO_2 reaches the break point.

Alveolar gas exchange during breath-holding is altered by underwater descent when thoracic compression decreases lung volume and the partial pressures of O_2, CO_2, and N_2 increase in the lungs (Fig. 112-1). On descent, alveolar O_2 and CO_2 concentrations decrease because of greater transfer of those gases to pulmonary capillary blood in relation to inert gas (N_2). Alveolar P_{O_2} increases during breath-hold diving compared with simple breath-holding (due to the increase in ambient pressure) and the transfer of CO_2 during early descent is opposite normal, that is, CO_2 moves from alveoli to pulmonary capillary blood. During ascent, the lung re-expands and alveolar P_{O_2} and P_{CO_2} decrease (as pressure decreases). Near the surface, the alveolar P_{O_2} may be almost as low as mixed venous P_{O_2}. In strenuous dives, expansion of hypoxic alveoli during ascent may result in reverse O_2 transfer from mixed venous blood to alveoli (see Fig. 112-1). Carbon dioxide retained in the blood during the dive also leaves during ascent as alveolar P_{CO_2} decreases. Carbon dioxide elimination continues after the dive, in addition to the small amount of N_2 that entered the blood during the dive.

Hyperventilation before breath-hold diving is a dangerous way to extend the dive. During the dive, compression of the lungs causes the alveolar P_{O_2} to increase. Thus, the primary signal to return to the surface is the P_{CO_2}. When the diver hyperventilates before the dive, the arterial P_{CO_2} begins at a lower level, and the time to the breath-hold break point is extended. However, alveolar O_2 concentration decreases to lower levels during the longer dive, and life-threatening hypoxia may occur as the diver approaches the surface. Loss of consciousness by this mechanism, known as *shallow water blackout*, causes many drowning episodes.

The body's response to breath-hold diving can be modified by a diving response induced by apnea and facial immersion,

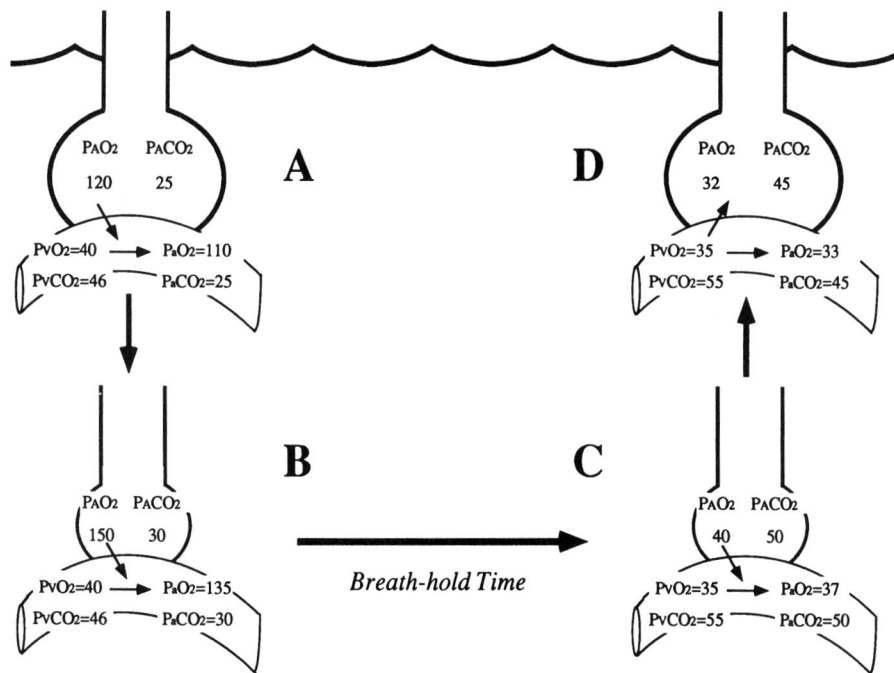

FIGURE 112-1 Mechanism of shallow water blackout. All values are expressed in millimeters of mercury. *A.* The breath-hold diver hyperventilates before the dive. *B.* At depth, arterial partial pressures of CO_2 (Pa_{CO_2}) and O_2 (Pa_{O_2}) increase as the alveoli are compressed by hydrostatic pressure. *C.* At the end of the breath-hold dive, CO_2 increases toward the break point, and the diver begins to ascend. Note the decreased Pa_{O_2} and Pa_{O_2} at this point. *D.* When approaching the surface, Pa_{CO_2} and Pa_{O_2} decrease as the alveoli reexpand; O_2 leaves the pulmonary capillaries and enters the alveoli. This may result in profound hypoxemia and produce unconsciousness.

particularly in cold water. This diving response, manifested primarily as bradycardia, is most pronounced in young children. The diving response has been interpreted as an O_2-conserving response that redistributes blood flow from organs resistant to hypoxia to organs with continuous O_2 needs such as heart and brain. This interpretation is controversial for humans, although a diving response may contribute to survival of children resuscitated successfully after submersion in cold water.

Diving with Compressed Gases

The limitations of breath-hold diving are precluded by underwater breathing apparatuses that provide the diver with a continuous supply of breathing gas at any depth. In shallow water, for instance, 0 to 135 fsw, diving is usually carried out by using compressed air because it is inexpensive and readily available, even at remote locations. Air divers are usually free swimming, that is, they use a self-contained underwater breathing apparatus (SCUBA). The maximum safe depths are considered to be 135 fsw for SCUBA divers and approximately 200 fsw for divers tethered to a safety line.[4] Safety concerns are brought about by three factors: nitrogen narcosis, safe decompression, and oxygen toxicity. The problems of greatest importance to the intensive care specialist are caused by decompression and are discussed below. The other problems are covered in standard textbooks on diving medicine.

To dive beyond the practical range of compressed air, special gas mixtures, such as helium-oxygen (heliox) or oxygen-enriched air (nitrox) must be supplied. In heliox operations, inspired oxygen pressure is usually maintained at a constant 0.4 to 1.0 ATA, and the helium may be recycled by gas reconditioning equipment. Surface-supplied heliox diving is expensive but effective and relatively safe to depths of 400 fsw. Most dives deeper than 400 fsw require saturation of the diver with inert gas at the approximate working depth of

the dive. Divers can live and work for weeks after saturation and then undergo a single slow decompression.

PRINCIPLES OF DECOMPRESSION

The use of compressed gases in diving produces physiologic problems during ascent because of the escape of inert gas from tissues. Elimination of inert gas from the body as the pressure decreases during ascent from diving or to altitude is known as *decompression*. The rate of uptake or elimination of inert gases from the body after a change in pressure is determined primarily by gas solubility in blood and tissue, blood flow, and the volume of tissue. Inert gas exchange usually follows an exponential function with respect to time. Tissues that behave this way are perfusion limited, and the characteristics of their inert gas exchange are defined by a half-time. Because the body tissues receive different amounts of blood flow and nitrogen is more soluble in fatty tissues, half-times for different tissues vary considerably. The principle of multiple tissues was used to calculate the first safe decompression tables, with the assumption that gas bubbles and, hence, DCS would occur only if the tissues were supersaturated to allow a nitrogen partial pressure of about twice the absolute pressure. Modern decompression tables are still based on multiple parallel exponential models, but other concepts have been used with success.[5] The variable that most affects inert gas uptake and elimination is tissue perfusion, but diffusion may limit tissue gas exchange under some conditions. Diffusion limitation may occur if the rate of inert gas exchange by perfusion is extremely rapid, if tissue perfusion is very low, or if a tissue barrier such as capillary endothelium has a high diffusion resistance.

Diffusion also may be important when two adjacent tissues have very different rates of perfusion. In such conditions, elimination of inert gas from the faster tissue may allow more inert gas to diffuse from the slower tissue. Thus, a faster tissue may remain supersaturated for longer than expected.

Diffusion is also important after gas bubbles have formed in a tissue during decompression. Gas bubbles contain large amounts of N_2 gas that can be removed by perfusion only after the N_2 diffuses back into the tissue. The rate at which N_2 diffuses away from a gas bubble is determined by the bubble surface area, the intrabubble pressure, and the difference in partial pressure between bubble and tissue.

During decompression, bubbles form in specific places in the body called *nucleation sites*. Microscopic gas nuclei remain stable for a long time at hydrophobic sites in the body and grow into bubbles during decompression. The number of nucleation sites and their location and propensity to form macroscopic bubbles differ according to physiologic conditions. For example, exercise may increase the number of bubbles formed by *tribonucleation*, a mechanism whereby large negative pressures can generate bubbles by traction between surfaces lubricated by a liquid, such as joints. Bubbles created by tribonucleation may arise from preexisting gas nuclei or by de novo formation.

DECOMPRESSION SICKNESS

There is little doubt that gas bubbles cause DCS, but some bubbles are clinically silent. However, there is uncertainty about the exact mechanisms of bubble growth and precisely how bubbles trigger the diverse features of DCS. The factors that govern bubble formation in "aqueous" tissues have been used to develop tables for safe decompression. Decompression tables usually assume that DCS will not occur unless the inert gas tension exceeds some threshold of critical supersaturation. The assumption of such a threshold conflicts with data indicating that DCS occurs as a stochastic event.[6] Therefore, even appropriate use of well-tested decompression tables or a decompression computer is associated with a finite risk of DCS for dives of approximately 25 fsw or deeper. However, most serious cases of DCS are due to omitted decompression.

The clinical manifestations of DCS are attributed to growth of bubbles in body tissues. Primary sites of bubble growth are the joint spaces, tendon sheaths, and periarticular tissues, including peripheral nerves. Bubbles in these locations produce pain that is known as *type I DCS*, or *bends*. Bubbles also form in the spinal cord and other areas of the central nervous system. This is called *type II* or *serious DCS*. Other serious forms of DCS involving the audiovestibular system (staggers) and pulmonary system (chokes), although relatively rare, also occur. The common clinical manifestations of DCS are presented in Table 112-2.

DCS in military and commercial divers occurs with a predominance of type I symptoms. Altitude bends, or dysbarism, is generally accompanied by mild to moderate type I DCS. Tunnel workers have a reported incidence of DCS of 0.7% to 1.5%, primarily consisting of type I symptoms of the knee and lower leg.[7] In contrast, some survey data have suggested a predominance of type II symptoms in recreational divers.[8] The reasons for this difference in DCS in recreational diving are not clear, although underreporting of type I DCS and overdiagnosis of type II DCS are likely. In some cases, long delays in the diagnosis and treatment of type I DCS may allow more severe manifestations to evolve. Recreational divers are more likely to omit decompression than are professional divers, thus increasing the probability of serious DCS.

TABLE 112-2 Clinical Manifestations of DCS

Type I (mild DCS)
  Limbs
    Pain (bends), niggles, lymphatic obstruction, numbness, and paresthesias usually involving the large joints, e.g., shoulders, elbows and knees
  Skin
    Mottling, itching, rash, pallor, urticaria, edema
Type II (serious DCS)
  CNS
    Brain
      Headache, seizures, loss of consciousness, visual disturbances, hemiparesis, aphasia, tremor, ataxia (staggers)
    Spinal cord
      Low back or pelvic girdle pain, paraparesis, urinary retention, incontinence
    Audiovestibular DCS
      Tinnitus, vertigo, nystagmus, decreased hearing, nausea and vomiting
  Cardiopulmonary DCS (chokes)
      Dyspnea, cough, wheezing, hemodynamic collapse

ABBREVIATIONS: CNS, central nervous system; DCS, decompression syndrome.

One of the most serious forms of DCS is spinal paralysis.[9] Spinal cord DCS is not fully understood, but in some animals the injury has been related to intravascular bubbles that form in the low-pressure, epidural venous plexus of the spinal cord.[10] Because of its slow blood flow, the plexus is susceptible to bubble formation. Bubble-induced thrombi can obstruct venous outflow, leading to ischemic injury of the spinal cord. Despite evidence for bubble formation in the spinal venous plexus, intravascular formation of bubbles appears to be otherwise uncommon. Most intravascular bubbles probably originate at the tissue-blood interface and stream into the circulation to be absorbed by the lungs. Bubbles arising in the body of the spinal cord (autochthonous) have also been implicated in the etiology of spinal DCS.[11]

Once bubbles enter the circulation, surface activity at the blood-to-bubble interface produces changes in blood proteins. These include complement activation, activation of coagulation and fibrinolysis, platelet and neutrophil aggregation and destruction, and release of inflammatory mediators. Precise roles for these events have not been determined in DCS pathogenesis.

If a large number of bubbles is released into the venous system during decompression, they may obstruct the pulmonary circulation and cause sore throat, cough, chest pain, and shortness of breath. This syndrome, known as *the chokes*, if untreated, may lead to cardiovascular collapse and death. Some bubbles may also cross pulmonary capillaries as small gas emboli or pass into the arterial circulation through right-to-left cardiac shunts, for example, patent foramen ovale (PFO).[12] However, PFO is present in about 20% of normal individuals, and its presence probably leads to more severe rather than more frequent episodes of DCS.[13]

Divers with the chokes develop symptoms minutes to hours after decompression, which may be progressive. Physical examination reveals tachypnea, tachycardia, crackles, wheezing, cyanosis, and gasping in severe cases. The chest radiograph may show diffuse pulmonary infiltrates similar to acute respiratory distress syndrome (ARDS). Should bubbles pass into the arterial circulation, neurologic findings may appear, primarily involving cerebral symptoms and signs. Arterial blood-gas determinations often show hypoxemia and respiratory alkalosis.

PULMONARY BAROTRAUMA

Pulmonary barotrauma of ascent, also known as *pulmonary overpressurization*, is a potentially serious consequence of failure of expanding gas in the lung to escape from alveoli. Overstretching of lung regions may rupture acini or alveoli and cause pulmonary interstitial emphysema. Disruption of the pulmonary parenchyma may cause mediastinal or soft tissue emphysema, pneumopericardium, pneumothorax, or arterial gas emboli (AGE). Pulmonary overinflation occurs during ascent while diving with compressed breathing gases. It is most likely to occur with breath-holding, loss of consciousness underwater, or airway obstruction that traps gas. Pulmonary overinflation also may occur after explosive decompression of aircraft at altitude.

Lung rupture during ascent also depends on physiologic factors such as pulmonary compliance, transpulmonary pressure, and lung volume. Airway closure and air trapping induced by immersion in the upright position may increase the risk of lung overstretching during ascent.[14] Once alveolar pressure becomes positive by about 100 cm H_2O to that at the mouth, the lung will rupture. During breath-holding at total lung capacity (TLC), the difference between alveolar and ambient pressure is approximately 50 cm H_2O. Thus, hydrostatic pressure outside the body during ascent must decrease another 50 cm H_2O for the lung to rupture. Assuming a compliance of the lung and chest wall at a TLC of 15 mL/cm H_2O, lung volume during ascent must increase by 15 mL × 50 cm H_2O, or 750 mL, before the lung ruptures. Using the Boyle law (see Table 112-1), an approximate depth can be determined from which a diver must ascend for pulmonary rupture during a breath-hold at TLC. At the surface, P_1 = 1.0 ATA; suppose V_1 = 7000 mL. Then, V_2 = 7000 − 750, or 6250 mL. Therefore,

$$(1.0)\ (7000\ \text{mL}) = P_2\ (6250\ \text{mL}) \tag{112-2}$$

and

$$P_2 = (1.0)\ (7000/6250) = 1.12\ \text{ATA, or 4.0 ft} \tag{112-3}$$

This calculation illustrates why pulmonary overinflation and AGE occur in shallow water during rapid ascent. The calculation also points out that relative volume changes are greatest at low hydrostatic pressures.

Venous and Arterial Gas Embolism

Venous gas emboli (VGE) occur fairly often in compressed gas diving and in diverse clinical settings (see Chap. 27). Asymptomatic venous bubbles occur often in divers during and after decompression. In clinical settings, even careful intravenous infusion of solutions or contrast materials may be accompanied by VGE. If a small volume of gas enters the circulation, such emboli are usually clinically silent. VGE thus create injurious consequences in four situations: (1) obstruction of the heart or major vessels by gas, (2) arterialization of bubbles across the pulmonary vasculature, (3) arterialization of bubbles across a PFO, and (4) physical interactions between air and blood. When venous gas bubbles enter the arterial system, even a small amount of gas can produce substantial morbidity or death.[15,16]

The lungs effectively filter VGE larger than about 20 μm in diameter;[17] this size barrier is not absolute because bubbles of 500 μm may cross the lung in some cases. VGE spillover through the pulmonary system has been demonstrated in animals such as dogs, in which spillover to the pulmonary veins occurred at an intravenous air bubbling rate of 0.3 mL/kg per minute.[15] The VGE crossover rate and passage size increases in the setting of a large difference between pulmonary arterial and pulmonary venous pressures. Pulmonary arterioles constrict in response to VGE and pulmonary arterial pressures increases.[18] As more VGE mechanically obstruct the vasculature, the gradient of pulmonary arterial versus venous pressure increases, thereby decreasing the filtering effectiveness of the pulmonary capillaries and allowing VGE to pass.[19] Anatomic intrapulmonary shunting also decreases the filtering efficiency of the lungs.

Paradoxical air embolism may occur when VGE are arterialized via a PFO in divers or patients.[11] Detection of PFO by echocardiography relies on gas microbubbles for ultrasonic contrast. Right-to-left atrial crossover of these bubbles is variable and may require Valsalva or other special maneuver to increase right atrial pressure. Bubble crossover also may occur spontaneously during some phases of the cardiac cycle.[20] The probability of paradoxical gas embolism increases in patients who develop pulmonary hypertension and vascular obstruction from VGE.

VGE also become physiologically significant when a large quantity of gas obstructs major vessels at the level of the pulmonary vasculature or the heart. In the heart, gas churned to foam obstructs inflow and outflow and diminishes cardiac output. In addition to obstructing the pulmonary vasculature, venous gas triggers pulmonary arterial constriction, bronchospasm, and dyspnea.[21]

Physical interactions at the blood-bubble interface complicate mechanical obstruction of the circulation and amplify the physiologic effects of small volumes of intravenous gas. The blood-bubble interface stimulates biochemical events associated with release of multiple inflammatory mediators with subsequent damage to the vascular endothelium. Noncardiogenic pulmonary edema may develop quickly as extravasated fluid floods alveoli and may progress to ARDS.[22] Compressed gas divers have long recognized a similar sequence of events as the syndrome of chokes.[23]

AGE may occur in diving by VGE that cross into the arterial circulation or by gas entering the left heart after pulmonary overpressurization. AGE is second to drowning as the leading cause of fatal accidents in SCUBA diving. The most common source of AGE in divers is pulmonary barotrauma. Similar events may occur in patients on mechanical ventilation who require high airway pressures for ventilation. Pulmonary overdistention, which produces AGE in divers or ventilated patients, may not produce other evidence of barotrauma such as pneumothorax, pneumomediastinum, or pneumopericardium. Gas in vessels is not detected reliably by radiography, and the diagnosis is suggested by clinical evidence of end-organ damage, primarily ischemia of the brain or heart.[24] Therefore, procedures to document the presence of air may delay treatment of a critically ill patient. Appropriate management of AGE begins with heightened suspicion of the problem in an appropriate setting.

Like VGE, AGE obstruct, induce vasoconstriction, activate coagulation, complement, and neutrophils and aggregate platelets. This leads to release of mediators of inflammation that activate and may subsequently damage vascular endothelium. Even minor AGE have the potential for permanent injury and should never be regarded as benign, but the severity of injury in general appears to be related to the volume of intravascular gas. In the heart, the myocardial response to AGE is similar to coronary insufficiency of any etiology. Ventricular arrhythmias and ST-segment elevation or depression are common and may lead to infarction.[25,26] Cerebral manifestations of AGE are similar to those of thromboembolism and include focal neurologic deficits, loss of consciousness, seizures, and death. The distinction between AGE and VGE may become blurred clinically because the possibility of arterial spillover is difficult to exclude, and either event may be heralded by cardiovascular collapse.

Divers who have AGE are most often inexperienced and frequently arrive suddenly at the surface after diving. They may cry out, indicating a rapid ascent with a closed glottis, or they may surface unconscious. AGE are complicated occasionally by pneumothorax or pneumomediastinum and accompanied by clinical signs of pulmonary barotrauma, such as mediastinal crunch (Hamman sign), subcutaneous air, or tension pneumothorax. The onset of AGE is quite sudden, virtually always within 15 minutes of surfacing, and presents with symptoms of brain ischemia, which may be progressive. Initial symptoms of AGE appearing more than 1 hour after ascent should not be attributed to AGE but to serious DCS, ND, or stroke. Common clinical findings of AGE include headache, confusion, nausea, vomiting, blindness, hemiparesis, seizures, and unconsciousness. Chest pain, hemoptysis, and shortness of breath may also occur. Laboratory abnormalities may include elevated serum creatine kinase levels, signifying injury to skeletal and cardiac muscle.[27]

Therapy of Arterial Gas Embolism and Decompression Sickness

ADJUNCTIVE THERAPY

The management of VGE or AGE begins with identifying the problem and preventing additional emboli. In VGE of any etiology, a "mill wheel" murmur produced by air in the right ventricle may be audible with a stethoscope.[28] Positioning the patient in the left lateral decubitus and Trendelenburg position in an effort to avoid PFO crossover and brain emboli is traditional clinical practice for AGE and serious DCS.[28,29] The Trendelenburg position has been proposed to reduce cerebral bubble diameter by increasing hydrostatic pressure in the cranium; however, animal studies have suggested that positioning efforts are not efficacious because blood flow rather than buoyancy of the bubble determines the course of air emboli.[29,30] Further, Trendelenburg positioning has been associated in animals with increased cerebral edema. Ventilation with 100% O_2 helps correct hypoxemia and increases the diffusion gradient for nitrogen out of the bubbles, causing them to shrink.[31,32] Vasopressors and antiarrhythmic agents may

be required for hypotension and ventricular arrhythmias associated with AGE. Lidocaine at 2 to 4 mg/min intravenously after a 1-mg/kg loading dose ameliorates cerebral injury after experimental cerebral AGE.[33]

Adjunctive therapy for AGE and serious DCS, other than oxygen and lidocaine, consists of correction of hemoconcentration with intravenous fluids and management of complications.[34,35] Parenteral corticosteroids such as dexamethasone, 4 mg every 6 hours, have been recommended to decrease cerebral or spinal cord edema after AGE and serious DCS, but evidence demonstrating efficacy in either situation is lacking. Stress ulceration may occur after AGE, and prophylaxis for this complication should be used routinely. Because of blood-bubble physical interactions discussed earlier, treatment of cerebral AGE with heparin was once recommended, but has not proved efficacious, and is associated with hemorrhage into areas of cerebral infarction induced by the air embolus.[33] However, heparin prophylaxis of deep venous thrombosis and pulmonary emboli should be given for spinal cord DCS because of immobility of the patient.

RECOMPRESSION THERAPY

Gas bubbles in tissue or circulation slowly resolve spontaneously, but the rate at which they are removed can be enhanced greatly by oxygen breathing and recompression. Recompression and hyperbaric oxygen (HBO) administration are primary therapy for DCS and AGE.[34] Bubble resolution is related to size and the partial pressure difference between the bubble and tissue. This partial pressure difference is due to the inherent unsaturation of venous blood that results from the difference in solubility of CO_2 and O_2 in body tissues. CO_2 is 20 times more soluble than is O_2 in tissues. As O_2 is consumed, it is replaced by CO_2 from substrate oxidation at a ratio of about 0.8 mol of CO_2 for each mole of O_2. Thus, O_2 entering tissue at an arterial P_{O_2} of 100 mm Hg leaves the venous capillary at a P_{O_2} of 40 mm Hg. In contrast, CO_2 enters at 40 mm Hg and leaves at only 46 mm Hg. The remaining gas pressure in tissues is primarily N_2, which is inert and has the same partial pressure at equilibrium, 573 mm Hg, on both sides of the circulation. Therefore, the sum of partial pressures in the venous system is 54 mm Hg less than in the arterial system. This "oxygen window" provides a pressure gradient to eliminate N_2. As a gas pocket or bubble collapses from removal of O_2 by metabolism, the internal partial pressure of N_2 (P_{N_2}) increases above tissue P_{N_2} because total pressure in the bubble remains in equilibrium with ambient pressure. In this way, N_2 is gradually absorbed. The oxygen window can be expanded during and after decompression and during recompression by administration of high values of P_{O_2}, which decreases tissue P_{N_2} and increases the partial pressure gradient for N_2 between bubble and tissue. Immediate O_2 administration at the scene of a diving accident before recompression therapy is clearly beneficial in the management of DCS and AGE.

Different recompression schedules are effective for AGE and DCS if treatment is begun promptly. Recompression tables that use HBO and minimal recompression are the treatment of choice. U.S. Navy Treatment (USNT) Table 6, which uses intermittent HBO at a maximum depth of 2.8 ATA (60 fsw), is a standard for primary DCS and for recurrent symptoms.[4] Recurrent or persisting symptoms should be retreated with USNT Table 6 once a day or with USNT

Table 5 twice a day; in general, a point of diminishing returns is reached after a small number (approximately six to eight) treatments. Persistent bladder and bowel dysfunction or neuromuscular weakness also may respond to saturation therapy (e.g., USNT Table 7), if resources and expertise are available for conducting prolonged treatments.[4] In some cases of DCS, oxygen recompression is not available, and air recompression tables must be used. Air treatment tables are longer and less effective than HBO tables and are more likely to produce DCS in the chamber attendants. Recompression presents several logistical challenges for the intensive care team.[36]

HBO is also used to treat AGE and clinically serious VGE on the basis of the following rationale. First, an increase in ambient pressure compresses the gas and increases the ratio of surface area to volume of the bubble, thus improving nitrogen diffusion from the bubble. Second, greater oxygen tension in the blood increases the nitrogen gradient across the blood-bubble interface. Third, the amount of O_2 physically dissolved in plasma during HBO ($\sim$6 mL O_2/dL of plasma at 2.8 ATA) may avert or reverse ischemia if plasma streaming occurs around emboli, which obstruct erythrocyte flow.

The optimal depth and duration of HBO treatment of AGE are still debatable. Experience by the U.S. Navy with air embolism after military diving accidents led to the development of USNT Table 6A, which uses initial recompression of the patient breathing air to an equivalent pressure of 165 fsw (6 ATA) followed by prompt decompression to 60 fsw (2.8 ATA), when the patient breathes 100% O_2. The chamber is then decompressed slowly to the surface while the patient breathes O_2 in cycles alternating with air. The intent of the initial, deep compression in USNT Table 6A is reduction of emboli size to 55% of their original diameter (assuming spherical geometry). This approach may be appropriate for very recent AGE or when the quantity of intravascular gas is very large. Deep compression on air, however, may actually allow nitrogen into the emboli so that they are larger after decompression than before compression. This problem can be circumvented in part by having the patient breathe a mixture of 50% O_2 and 50% N_2 during compression to decrease the driving force of N_2 into the emboli. Of note, recent experience using USNT Table 6 to treat air embolism suggests that equally good results are obtained when using USNT Table 6 at 2.8 ATA. This compresses the emboli to about 70% of their original diameter and expedites release of nitrogen. USNT Table 6, originally designed for the treatment of type II DCS, is more amenable to hospital-based chambers and is particularly well suited to critically ill patients with AGE at sea level pressure. Like DCS, recurrent or persisting symptoms of gas embolism may respond to daily USNT Table 6 treatments until no further improvement is noted.

Many hospitals may not have the experience or equipment to manage critically ill patients in a hyperbaric chamber. In that case, the patient may require transfer to a suitably equipped facility. This can be accomplished by ground or air transportation as long as the aircraft can be pressurized to 1 ATA or safely fly below 1000 ft of altitude to avoid further enlargement of gas emboli.

The best responses to therapy for AGE and serious DCS occur with prompt treatment. However, even recompression therapy delayed as long as 12 to 24 hours may be useful for both conditions.[37] Advice from a diving medicine physician concerning diving-related injuries is available 24 hours a day by calling the Divers Alert Network (919- 684-8111. The Divers Alert Network is a nonprofit organization that collects and disseminates information on diving safety and related injuries and is associated with the Center for Hyperbaric Medicine at Duke University Medical Center.

Near Drowning

PATHOPHYSIOLOGY

The consequences of ND are primarily those of asphyxia. When effective gas exchange ceases, the individual presents the consequences of hypoxia and hypercapnia. Excellent summaries of the demographics and emergency response to ND are available and are not covered here.[38–40] This section summarizes the pathogenesis of ND injury of the frequently injured systems supported in the intensive care unit (ICU): lungs, brain, heart, and kidneys.

LUNG

The pathogenesis of lung injury in ND is initiated by upper airway obstruction when fresh water (FW) or sea water (SW) contacts the respiratory tract mucosa and provokes laryngospasm. Laryngospasm is a protective response provided the duration of hypoxemia is limited by a brief immersion time. Approximately 10% to 15% of individuals with ND aspirate trivial amounts of water, but some of these individuals develop sufficient O_2 deprivation to produce hypoxic encephalopathy or ventricular arrhythmia due directly to laryngospasm.[41] Aspiration of SW and FW also induces mechanical airway obstruction with a small airway component. Small airway obstruction is aggravated by bronchoconstriction, mucosal edema, and plugging by water and suspended debris such as algae, diatoms, sand, mud or by teeth and gastric contents.[42]

Aspiration of even small quantities of water immediately decreases lung compliance and creates persistent areas of low ventilation-perfusion ratio and shunt.[42,43] Therefore, aspiration of water may produce a longer lasting hypoxemia than laryngospasm alone. Some of the mechanisms of the early changes in pulmonary gas exchange have been elucidated in animals and are attributable, in general, to loss of surfactant or its activity, damage to the alveolar epithelium and capillary endothelium, and alveolar flooding. In human beings, vomiting and aspiration of stomach contents during ND is common and aggravates mucosal and alveolar epithelial injury.

The combination of alveolar flooding, loss of surfactant or its function, atelectasis, and alveolar damage may give rise to progressive hypoxemia from intrapulmonary shunting, which in severe cases may reach 70% of the cardiac output.[42,44] In about 40% of individuals with ND, the injury culminates in ARDS hours to days after the episode.[45,46] Hypoxemia usually necessitates treatment with supplemental oxygen at high inspired O_2 fraction, which may superimpose pulmonary oxygen toxicity on ARDS. Fortunately, ARDS, which develops after ND, is more likely to be reversible than ARDS from other causes.[46]

BRAIN

ND is the second leading cause of brain death, after trauma, in children admitted to a pediatric ICU.[47] Brain injury pathogenesis in ND is that of global anoxia or severe hypoxia.

Prolonged anoxia or hypoxia produces diffuse neuronal damage that, if severe, compromises the function of the blood-brain barrier, leading to cerebral edema. As edema develops, intracranial pressure (ICP) may increase, further decreasing brain perfusion, exacerbating intracellular hypoxia, and, in severe cases, causing uncal herniation. Profound increases in ICP are infrequent after ND but tend to appear more than 24 hours after resuscitation of patients who already show evidence of neurologic dysfunction.[46] There is some evidence that the increase in ICP indicates severity of neuronal injury rather than being a major contributor to the insult.[46,48]

The difference between ND and anoxic brain injury of other etiologies involves the potential mitigating effects of the diving reflex and hypothermia.[49] In human beings, the diving reflex is not well developed and most apparent in young children exposed to cold water.[49,50] ND in cold water leading to rapid hypothermia slows cerebral metabolism, thereby postponing the deleterious effects of anoxia.[51] These factors are associated with a better prognosis after an apparently severe ND episode.[50–52]

HEART

The most important cardiac effects of ND are atrial and ventricular arrhythmias, in particular ventricular fibrillation.[53] Studies of drowning in animals have demonstrated hemolysis and rapid shifts in blood electrolyte composition after instillation of FW and SW into the lungs. These responses correlated with the occurrence of ventricular arrhythmias. However, human studies have not confirmed significant electrolyte changes even in patients with ventricular fibrillation,[54] except for drowning in Dead Sea waters, which have a much higher mineral content than other SW. Individuals with ND in the Dead Sea develop hypernatremia, hyperchloremia, hypermagnesemia, and hypercalcemia more than 24 hours after exposure because electrolytes are absorbed from the gastrointestinal tract after swallowing large amounts of water during the episode.[52]

ND in human beings differs from that in animal studies primarily because humans rarely aspirate enough water to produce significant electrolyte changes.[54] Human pathologic studies after SW or FW drowning have demonstrated cardiac myocyte hypercontraction and hypereosinophilic sarcomeres. These pathologic changes are characteristic of catecholamine excess and suggest that intense adrenergic stimulation contributes to the arrhythmias after ND.[55] Thus, the etiology of ventricular fibrillation in human beings is most likely related to hypoxia, respiratory and metabolic acidosis, and catecholamine excess. A review of cases of children with brain death has demonstrated myocardial infarction to be commonly associated with ND.[56]

KIDNEY

The incidence of renal insufficiency after ND is unknown but is reported far less frequently than lung, brain, or cardiac injury. The renal complication cited most often is oliguria attributable to acute tubular necrosis,[57] probably caused by hypoxemia and hypotension. Infrequently, ND may be complicated by rhabdomyolysis and hemolysis with disseminated intravascular coagulation.[58,59] Hemolysis and disseminated intravascular coagulation also may contribute to acute tubular necrosis. Although patients with acute renal failure after

ND may require transient dialysis, recovery of adequate renal function can be expected in most patients.

MANAGEMENT

GENERAL MEASURES

ND in adults and adolescents is associated with several predisposing factors and complicating injuries, which are easily overlooked in the unconscious, critically ill ND patient. They must be considered in each case because they may affect the treatment and prognosis of the patient.

Alcohol and other drugs that alter the central nervous system are commonly implicated in adult ND.[60] Sedatives and alcohol in particular may complicate the patient's initial ICU course by exacerbating hypothermia and hypotension and impairing mental status and respiratory drive. Levels of toxic drugs and blood alcohol should be measured in complicated patients admitted to the ICU.

Other predispositions to ND include unrelated pathologic events in otherwise unimpaired adult swimmers. Myocardial infarction, cardiac arrhythmias, seizures, subarachnoid hemorrhage, and AGE in the SCUBA diver have been implicated in many ND episodes.[60] These events may require extraordinary diagnostic efforts in the immediate postresuscitation environment of the ICU. Electrocardiography should be obtained routinely because the heart is a target organ for hypoxemia in patients with ND. Serial measurements of cardiac enzymes in ND are useful for confirming the diagnosis of myocardial infarction when electrocardiographic changes are nondiagnostic. Acute intracranial hemorrhage or status epilepticus may need to be ruled out in patients whose course is complicated by neurologic dysfunction. Recompression and HBO therapy should be considered for ND in SCUBA divers with unexplained obtundation, coma, or other neurologic deficit (see section on VGE and AGE).

Injuries to the spine and skull are common in patients with ND. These occur most often when a swimmer dives into shallow water and strikes the head on the bottom or on a submerged object.[60] A common scenario involves a motor vehicle accident that leaves the passenger submerged in a body of water. Burst fractures of the cervical vertebrae resulting in tetraplegia have been reported in these settings. In addition, skin, middle ear, or sinus trauma sustained during ND may serve as portals of entry for infection.[61]

ICU MANAGEMENT

The ND patient should be placed in an ICU for respiratory insufficiency, after cardiac arrest or arrhythmia, and for altered mental status. Clinically, the patient may exhibit cyanosis, tachycardia, hypo- or hypertension, hypothermia, respiratory distress with frothy, blood-tinged sputum, diffuse crackles, and wheezing on examination. Initial laboratory evaluation often shows a metabolic acidosis (caused by lactic acid) and hypoxemia on arterial blood-gas analysis. Serum electrolytes, with the exception of a decreased bicarbonate concentration, are rarely perturbed significantly.[62] However, ND in industrial fluids or the Dead Sea can perturb serum electrolytes. As an example, a 28-year-old male developed severe hypercalcemia after a ND incident in an industrial vessel with oil-well drilling fluid that contained calcium salts.[63] Hypoglycemia is common.[64] Hemolysis and rhabdomyolysis, if seen, tend to occur early in the clinical course unless they are the result

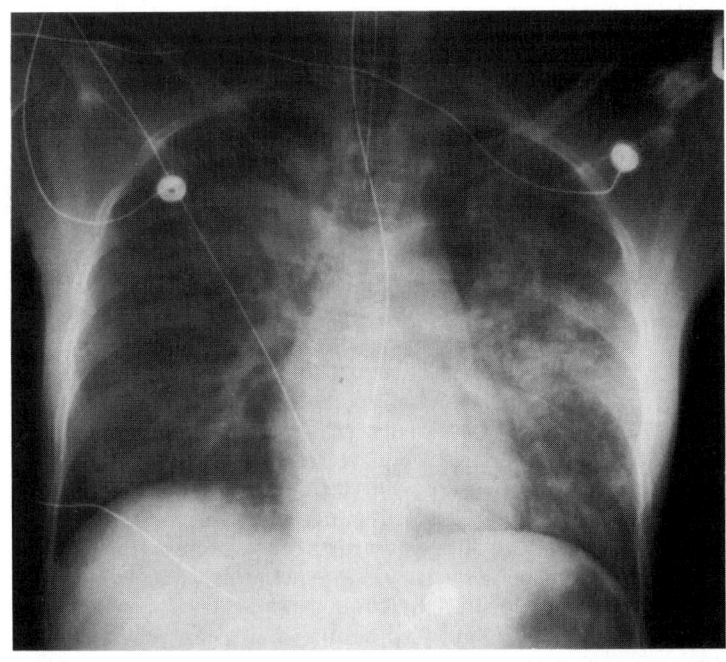

FIGURE 112-2 Chest radiograph 2 hours after an episode of near drowing shows typical patchy infiltrates.

of late sepsis. Electrocardiographic abnormalities include evidence of ischemia or injury and ventricular and atrial arrhythmias. Initial chest radiographic findings range from patchy infiltrates to diffuse airspace disease (Fig. 112-2). Progressive increase in parenchymal infiltrates over hours to days is not unusual.

RESPIRATORY CARE

Mechanical ventilation can be a challenge in the severely injured ND patient. Atelectasis and pulmonary edema with intrapulmonary shunting are encountered in all types of ND. ARDS can develop with poor lung compliance that should be treated, like all cases of ARDS, with normal tidal volume ventilation (6mL/kg ideal body weight; see Chap. 38). These conditions can be further complicated by the presence of foreign bodies in the airways. Heavy sedation or muscle relaxants are best avoided in ND patients because the drugs impair the clinician's ability to follow the neurologic examination. However, careful use of these agents may improve mechanical ventilation by synchronizing the patient with the ventilator or decreasing airway pressures and the risk of barotrauma. The advantages of positive end-expiratory pressure in decreasing intrapulmonary shunt can be dramatic in severe hypoxemia after ND. Treatment of children with ARDS after ND with artificial surfactant did not improve outcome but did improve pulmonary function modestly.[65]

Respiratory insufficiency in ND may be complicated by factors other than atelectasis and intrapulmonary shunt. Airway obstruction may occur as bronchospasm or from a foreign body. Bronchodilator therapy may benefit the patient with diffuse wheezing. Patients with localized atelectasis that fails to improve with effective ventilation or those who exhibit localized wheezing should undergo fiberoptic bronchoscopy to exclude or remove a foreign body.

Many ND accidents occur in water contaminated with human or animal waste or naturally containing pathogenic bacteria or fungi. The lung is the most common portal of entry for a wide variety of these organisms. Infection is heralded by

fever 2 to 7 days after the event and should prompt sputum and blood cultures before initiation of antibiotic therapy.[66] Prophylactic antibiotic coverage has not improved outcome after ND, and routine use of antibiotics is not indicated. Reported infections are presented in Table 112-3. Awareness of infection by more unusual organisms is crucial because they may have specific culture requirements not offered routinely in many hospital microbiology laboratories.[61]

TABLE 112-3 Microbial Isolates Associated with Infection in Individuals After Near Drowning[a]

	Type of Water	Reference
Bacteria		
Klebsiella oxytoca	FW	64, 58
Herellea spp.	FW	55
Neiserria meningitidis	FW	55
Pseudomonas aeruginosa	FW	64
Listeria monocytogenes	FW	64
Plesiomonas shigelloides	FW	64
Edwardsiella tarda	FW	64
Chromobacterium violaceum	FW	81
Aeromonas hydrophila	SW, FW	64, 58
Escherichia coli	SW, FW	64, 58
Proteus mirabilis	SW, FW	58, 64
Staphylococcus aureus	SW, FW	64, 65
Neiserria mucosus	Brackish	66
Pseudomonas putrefaciens	SW	58, 65
Francisella philomiragia	SW	63
Vibrio parahemolyticus	SW	58
Fungus		
Pseudoallescheria boydii	FW	64
Aspergillus fumigatus	FW	67, 64

[a] Organisms isolated from sputum or blood of clinically infected ND victims soon after admission. This list does not include organisms recovered from infected wounds.

ABBREVIATIONS: FW, fresh water; SW, sea water.

TABLE 112-4 Classification of Individuals After Near Drowning and Initial Resuscitation

Category A	Awake, fully conscious
Category B	Blunted consciousness, stuporous but arousable
Category C	Comatose
C.1	Decorticate posturing
C.2	Decerebrate posturing
C.3	Flaccid

BRAIN RESUSCITATION

Brain resuscitation measurements after ND are controversial. The debate is complicated by the diverse parameters that influence brain injury and recovery, including age, water temperature and submersion time (or period of asphyxia), coexisting injuries, and preexisting disease.[67] The matter is complicated further by anecdotes of complete or nearly complete neurologic recovery in association with specific therapeutic modes after prolonged immersion. The initial prognostic uncertainties about brain recovery after ND mandate a full effort at cardiopulmonary resuscitation, including correction of hypothermia.[68]

Classification of neurologic status 1 to 2 hours after resuscitation allows assessment of prognosis. A system with reasonable discrimination for outcome in humans classifies patients after resuscitation into three categories, as listed in Table 112-4.[50,51]

The best discrimination for outcome using this system has been found in children in whom all category A and B patients (n = 57) recovered completely. Level C patients (n = 39) had 33.3% and 23.9% cerebral morbidity rates (mortality rate + morbidity rate = 56.2%), with the lowest survival rate in the C.3 group.[51] In another series of patients that included 52 adults, the category A patients recovered completely, and two adults and one child in level B eventually succumbed to barotrauma or other complications.[50] Eight of 11 (73%) adult and 8 of 18 (44%) child category C patients recovered completely in that series.

Use of a brain resuscitation regimen known as HYPER (hyperhydration, hyperpyrexia, hyperexcitability, and hyperrigidity) suggested that a larger fraction of seriously injured ND children had complete recovery.[51] The acronym addressed the overhydration, fever, excitability, and muscular rigidity noted in some patients. These findings were thought to affect outcome adversely, and aggressive therapy was recommended to minimize them.

HYPER therapy consists of systemic corticosteroids, osmotic diuretics, hyperventilation, barbiturate coma, and muscle relaxants administered to minimize cerebral edema and decrease ICP. Controlled hypothermia (32°C, 89.6°F) to decrease neuronal metabolism also was advocated.[52] ICP monitoring is necessary to guide such aggressive therapy. The rationale for HYPER therapy was based on the idea that control of ICP would minimize neuronal damage after diffuse anoxia. However, the increase in ICP that develops 24 to 48 hours after ND may be a result of severe neuronal injury rather than its cause.

Critical reviews and subsequent experience with HYPER therapy failed to confirm its efficacy and highlighted its potentially detrimental effects.[41,46,68] A retrospective review of 40 ND patients from the same institution that reported the original experience with HYPER found increased incidences of sepsis and multiple organ failure in patients treated with hypothermia.[67] This may result from cold-induced immune suppression (including neutropenia) complicated by cold-induced bronchorrhea and decreased mucociliary clearance.[67]

Corticosteroids have no proved benefit in decreasing brain edema associated with trauma, intracerebral hemorrhage, or stroke. In the absence of convincing evidence that corticosteroids increase edema and, hence, ICP and that decreased ICP improves neurologic outcome after ND, these agents should be avoided because they are immunosuppressive and predispose to infection and gastric ulceration.[69] Although hypothermia and barbiturates can decrease ICP in some circumstances, their use has not been demonstrated to improve neurologic outcome. Attempts to decrease ICP by use of osmotic agents also have not been shown to improve neurologic outcome after ND and may induce hyperosmolarity and renal insufficiency. Mild hyperventilation is a comparably benign intervention to decrease ICP temporarily, and ICP monitoring may help direct therapy in the subset of ND patients with increased ICP and poor prognosis. More recent experience with aggressive cerebral monitoring and resuscitation of the ND patient has shown no benefit.[70]

PROGNOSIS

Overall, about 80% of child and adult ND victims recover completely, 8% to 10% survive but with brain damage, and 10% to 12% die. About 90% of category A and B and approximately 50% of category C patients survive with full recovery, whereas 10% to 23% of the later group survive but have permanent neurologic sequelae.[45,46,50,54] Thus, respiratory insufficiency in the absence of sepsis or infection is seldom the cause of death in ND patients in hospitals with modern intensive care capabilities.

Many parameters such as serum electrolytes, arterial blood-gas and pH values, electroencephalographic findings or clinical features (body temperature, absence of pupillary response, cardiac arrest, duration of submersion, and resuscitative efforts), and cross-brain oxygen content differences[71] have been examined for use as indicators of prognosis. None is sufficiently discriminating to guide early therapy. Conversely, the presence of cardiac arrest and absence of spontaneous respirations after resuscitation are ominous signs associated with permanent neurologic impairment or death.[68] In a retrospective review of 44 ND children, all survivors who regained good neurologic function, were awake with purposeful motion 24 hours after the incident.[72]

Therapeutic Lung Lavage

Therapeutic flooding of the whole lung is a form of controlled ND used for many years to treat alveolar filling diseases including lipoid pneumonia, cystic fibrosis, and pulmonary alveolar proteinosis (PAP). Whole lung lavage is currently used primarily for PAP, a rare diffuse lung disease of unknown etiology.[73] In PAP, a combination of lipoproteins and noninflammatory cellular debris accumulates in the alveoli and creates a physiologic picture of low ventilation-perfusion ratio that may progress to severe shunting and refractory hypoxemia. The disease affects men twice as often as women and begins commonly in the fourth to sixth decade of life. Occasional onset in childhood is also well documented. Approximately 33% of patients with PAP spontaneously remit, 33% do not progress, and 33% progress to pulmonary fibrosis that may be fatal.

Indications for whole lung lavage include resting hypoxemia, for instance, less than 90% hemoglobin oxygen saturation or arterial desaturation with routine activities. The frequency of need for lavage is variable; some patients require only one, whereas others require the procedure every few months for extended periods. Therapeutic whole lung lavage with warm saline is more effective for physical removal of the debris than segmental lavage via a bronchoscope in patients with PAP. The efficiency of protein clearance is increased by manual percussion of the chest during the emptying phases of the lavage but not by additives such as proteolytic enzymes or heparin in the lavage fluid.[74] Complications of the procedure include inadvertent flooding of the contralateral lung, hypoxemia, arrhythmias, hydropneumothorax (<5%), and bronchitis or pneumonia (<5%).[75,76]

TECHNIQUE

Whole lung lavage should be performed under general anesthesia by an experienced team. Standard monitoring during the procedure includes pulse oximetry, electrocardiography, blood pressure by indwelling radial artery catheter, core temperature, and volume of exchange in and out of the lung.[74,77] The trachea and left main bronchus are intubated with a dual-lumen endotracheal tube (Fig. 112-3). Although intubation of the left main bronchus is technically more difficult than that of the right main bronchus, the longer left mainstem before the first bifurcation provides better mechanical stability of the dual-lumen tube and less chance of bronchial obstruction. Proper placement of the tube is crucial for success in separating the lungs for independent lavage and ventilation. Tube placement is verified anatomically by fiberoptic bronchoscopy and functionally by auscultation and inflation of one lung to 50 cm H_2O to ensure that the contralateral main bronchus has been isolated. This is accomplished by connecting the appropriate bronchial tube to a connecting tube to a beaker of saline and observing for bubbles. Although a few

FIGURE 112-3 Schematic drawing of left main bronchus intubation with a dual-lumen endotracheal tube (Broncho-Cath, Mallinckrodt).

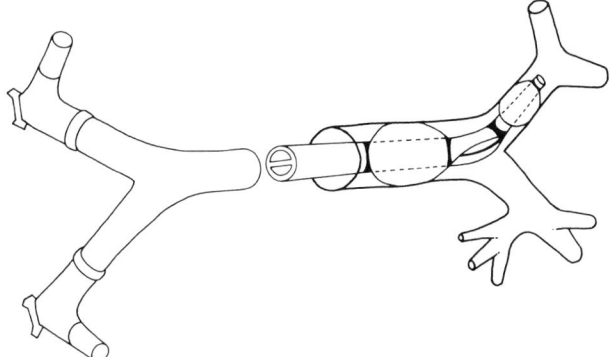

bubbles are seen initially from compression by the pressurized lung, persisting bubbles indicate a leak and incomplete separation of the lungs.

Some patients with PAP are referred for lavage with advanced lung disease and severe hypoxemia despite supplemental O_2. In these cases, the procedure may be performed in a large hyperbaric chamber by a team composed of an anesthesiologist, a pulmonologist, a nurse and a physical therapist. This permits HBO to be used to maintain adequate arterial oxygenation during the procedure, if necessary.[78]

In many patients with PAP, hypoxemia worsens during the lavage procedure, particularly during the emptying phases of the lavage. This occurs because pulmonary blood flow to the lavaged lung increases when the hydrostatic compression of the pulmonary capillaries is alleviated by lung emptying. Therefore, it is useful to simulate the emptying phase of the lavage before the procedure by ventilating the lung to be lavaged with 6% O_2 (approximate mixed venous P_{O_2}) and the other lung with 100% O_2 for 5 minutes. Hemoglobin saturation is monitored by pulse oximetry, and an arterial P_{O_2} at the nadir of the response is used to confirm the level of hypoxemia. Hemoglobin saturations below 85% ($P_{O_2} < 55$ mm Hg) during this maneuver indicate that lavage will be more safely performed under hyperbaric conditions (1.2 to 2.8 ATA).

The first phase of the procedure is to wash N_2 out of the lungs by ventilating the patient with 100% O_2. This prevents relatively insoluble and non-metabolizable N_2 from creating an "air lock" in the lavaged lung. The lung is then flooded with normal saline at 37°C (98.6°F) at a rate based on one-half the patient's O_2 uptake (1 to 2 mL O_2/kg body weight per minute) through a tube connected to a reservoir of saline 45 to 50 cm above the mid-axillary line. Prior lung volume measurements are used to estimate the volume of fluid that the lung will hold. If HBO is required, compression begins during flooding as the hemoglobin saturation decreases. Compression of the chamber continues until hemoglobin saturation can be maintained at 90%.

After filling the lung, the hemithorax is percussed vigorously as 400 to 500 mL of fluid is drained by gravity into a graduated receiver 40 to 45 cm below the patient. Some investigators have advocated nearly complete emptying of the lung with each aliquot, but smaller tidal aliquots minimize the hypoxemia associated with the emptying phases of the lavage.[77,78] After emptying, repeated tidal aliquots of saline are instilled and emptied until the effluent is nearly clear to inspection. This usually requires 10 to 25 L of fluid per lung. The efficiency of this method with respect to yield of wet debris is comparable to that achieved with nearly complete emptying of the lung (Fig. 112-4). Afterward, the lung is drained and suctioned before reinflating with 100% O_2 and administration of positive end-expiration pressure. The availability of HBO allows the patient after one lung lavage to remain well oxygenated during the contralateral procedure. Hence, both lungs can be lavaged in sequence on the same day. This allows a single period of general anesthesia and a shorter hospitalization for the patient. Some institutions require a 2- to 4-day recovery period after one lavage before performing the procedure on the second lung. After the procedure, the patient is weaned rapidly from 10 cm H_2O positive end-expiration pressure and a high inspired O_2 fraction in the ICU and usually can be extubated within 12 hours.

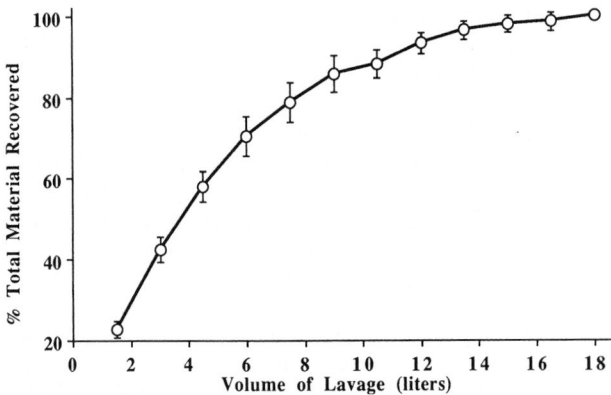

FIGURE 112-4 Cumulative recovery of wet debris in lavage fluid compared with lavage volume in six patients with alveolar proteinosis. Approximately 95% of the debris is recovered within 12 to 15 L of lavage. *(Data courtesy Dr. Alexander Spock, Department of Pediatrics, Duke University Medical Center, Durham, North Carolina.)*

References

1. Epstein M, De Nunzio A, Ramachandran M: Characterization of the renal response to prolonged immersion in normal man: Implication for an understanding of the circulatory adaptation to manned space flight. *J Appl Physiol: Resp Environ Exercise Physiol* 49:184, 1980.
2. Lin YC: Circulatory functions during immersion and breath-hold dives in humans. *Undersea Biomed Res* 11:123, 1984.
3. Stolp BW, Lundgren CEG, Piantadosi CA: Diving and Immersion, in Crystal RG, West JB, Weibel ER, Barnes PJ (eds): *The Lung: Scientific Foundations.* New York, Raven Press, 1996.
4. Department of the US Navy: *U.S. Navy Diving Manual, vols 1 and 2,* 4th revised ed. Flagstaff, Arizona, Best Publishing Company, 2001.
5. Vann RD, Thalmann ED: Decompression physiology and practice, in Bennett PB, Elliott DH (eds): *The Physiology and Medicine of Diving,* 4th ed. London, WB Saunders, 1993, p 376.
6. Weathersby PK, Homer LD, Flynn ET: On the likelihood of decompression sickness. *J Appl Physiol* 57:815, 1984.
7. Lam TH, Yau KP: Manifestations and treatment of 793 cases of decompression sickness in a compressed air tunneling project in Hong Kong. *Undersea Biomed Res* 15:377, 1988.
8. *Report on Decompression Illness, Diving Fatalities and Project Dive Exploration.* Durham, North Carolina, Divers Alert Network, 2002, p 22.
9. Hallenbeck JM, Bove AA, Elliott DH: Mechanism underlying spinal cord damage in decompression sickness. *Neurology* 25:308, 1975.
10. Leitch DR, Hallenback JM: Neurological forms of decompression sickness, in Shilling CW, Carlston CB, Mathias RA (eds): *The Physician's Guide to Diving Medicine.* New York, Plenum Press, 1984, p 326.
11. Francis TJR, et al: Is there a role for the autochthonous bubble in the pathogenesis of spinal cord decompression sickness? *Neuropathol Exp Neurol* 47:475, 1988.
12. Moon RE, Camporesi EM, Kisslo JA: Patent foramen ovale and decompression sickness in divers. *Lancet* 1:513, 1989.
13. Cantais E, Louge P, Suppini A, et al: Right-to-left shunt and risk of decompression illness with cochleovestibular and cerebral symptoms in divers: Case control study in 101 consecutive dive accidents. *Crit Care Med* 31:84, 2003.
14. Dahlback GO, Lundgren CEG: Pulmonary air-trapping induced by immersion. *Aerospace Med* 43:768, 1972.
15. Katz J, Leiman BC, Butler BD: Effects of inhalation anaesthetics on filtration of venous gas emboli by the pulmonary vasculature. *Br J Anaesth* 61:200, 1988.
16. Thalmann ED: Principles of U.S. Navy recompression treatments for decompression sickness, in Moon RE, Sheffield PJ (eds): *Treatment of Decompression Illness.* 45th Workshop of the Undersea and Hyperbaric Medical Society. Kensington, Maryland, Undersea and Hyperbaric Medical Society, 1996, p 75.
17. Butler BD, Hills BA: The lung as a filter for microbubbles. *J Appl Physiol* 47:537, 1979.
18. Neuman TS, Spragg RG, Wagner PD, et al: Cardiopulmonary consequences of decompression stress. *Respir Physiol* 41:143, 1980.
19. Butler BD, Katz J: Vascular pressures and passage of gas emboli through the pulmonary circulation. *Undersea Biomed Res* 15:203, 1988.
20. Black S, Cucchiara RF, Nishimur RA, et al: Parameters affecting occurrence of paradoxical air embolism. *Anesthesiology* 71:235, 1989.
21. Ence TJ, Gong H Jr: Adult respiratory distress syndrome after venous air embolism. *Am Rev Respir Dis* 119:1033, 1979.
22. Lamm WJE, Luchtel D, Albert RK: Sites of leakage in three models of acute lung injury. *J Appl Physiol* 64:1079, 1988.
23. Zwirewich CV, Muller NL, Abboud RT, et al: Noncardiogenic pulmonary edema caused by decompression sickness: Rapid resolution following hyperbaric therapy. *Radiology* 163:81, 1987.
24. Marini JJ, Culver BH: Systemic gas embolism complicating mechanical ventilation in the adult respiratory distress syndrome. *Ann Intern Med* 110:699, 1989.
25. Hadjimiltiades S, Goldbaum TS, Mostel E, et al: Coronary air embolism during coronary angioplasty. *Catheter Cardiovasc Diagn* 16:164, 1989.
26. Kanter AS, Stewart BF, Hampson NB: Myocardial infarction during scuba diving: A case report and review. *Am Heart J* 130:1292, 1995.
27. Smith RM, Neuman TS: Elevation of serum creatine kinase in divers with arterial gas embolization. *N Engl J Med* 330:19, 1994.
28. Gottlieb JD, Ericsson JA, Sweet RB: Venous air embolism: A review. *Anesth Analg* 44:773, 1965.
29. Butler BD, Laine GA, Leiman BC, et al: Effect of the Trendelenburg position on the distribution of arterial air emboli in dogs. *Ann Thorac Surg* 45:198, 1988.
30. Mehlhorn U, Burke EJ, Butler BD, et al: Body position does not affect hemodynamic response to venous air embolism in dogs. *Anesth Analg* 79:734, 1994.
31. Butler BD, Luehr S, Katz J: Venous gas embolism: Time course of residual pulmonary intravascular bubbles. *Undersea Biomed Res* 16:21, 1989.
32. Annane D, Troche G, Delisle F, et al: Effects of mechanical ventilation with normobaric oxygen therapy on the rate of air removal from cerebral arteries. *Crit Care Med* 22:851, 1994.
33. Dutka AJ: A review of pathophysiology and potential application of experimental therapies for cerebral ischemia to the treatment of cerebral arterial gas embolism. *Undersea Biomed Res* 12:403, 1985.
34. Moon RE: Treatment of diving emergencies. *Crit Care Clin* 15:429, 1999.
35. Moon RE (ed): *Adjunctive Therapy for Decompression Illness. Report of the DCI Adjunctive Therapy Committee of the Undersea and Hyperbaric Medical Society.* Kensington, Maryland, Undersea and Hyperbaric Medical Society, 2003.
36. Tetzlaff K, Shank ES, Muth CM: Evaluation and management of decompression illness-intensivist's perspective. *Intensive Care Med* 29:2128, 2003.
37. Bitterman H, Melamed Y: Delayed hyperbaric treatment of cerebral air embolism. *Isr J Med Sci* 29:22, 1993.
38. Shepherd S: Immersion injury: Drowning and near drowning. *Postgrad Med* 85:183, 1989.
39. Shaw KN, Briede CA: Submersion injuries: Drowning and near-drowning. *Emerg Med Clin North Am* 7:355, 1989.

40. Modell JH: Drowning. *N Engl J Med* 328:253, 1993.

41. Modell JH: Near drowning. *Circulation* 74(suppl IV):27, 1986.

42. Colebatch HJH, Halmagyi DFJ: Lung mechanics and resuscitation after fluid aspiration. *J Appl Physiol* 16:684, 1961.

43. Modell JH, Moya F: Effects of volume of aspirated fluid during chlorinated fresh water drowning. *Anesthesiology* 7:662, 1966.

44. Lheureux P, Vincent JL, Brimioulle S: Fulminant pulmonary edema after near-drowning: Remarkably high colloid osmotic pressure in tracheal fluid. *Intensive Care Med* 10:205, 1984.

45. Kaukinen L: Clinical course and prognostic signs in near drowning patients. *Ann Chir Gynaecol* 73:34, 1984.

46. Oakes DD, Sherck JP, Maloney JR, et al: Prognosis and management of victims of near-drowning. *J Trauma* 22:544, 1982.

47. Staworn D, Lewison L, Marks J, et al: Brain death in pediatric intensive care unit patients: Incidence, primary diagnosis, and the clinical occurrence of Turner's triad. *Crit Care Med* 22:1301, 1994.

48. Sarnaik AP, Preston G, Lieh-Lai M, et al: Intracranial pressure and cerebral perfusion pressure in near-drowning. *Crit Care Med* 13:224, 1985.

49. Siebke H, Breivik H, Rod T, et al: Survival after 40 minutes' submersion without cerebral sequelae. *Lancet* 1:1275, 1975.

50. Modell JH, Graves SA, Kuck EJ: Near-drowning: Correlation of level of consciousness and survival. *Can Anaesth Soc* 27:211, 1980.

51. Conn AW, Montes JE, Barker GA, et al: Cerebral salvage in near-drowning following neurological classification by triage. *Can Anaesth Soc J* 27:201, 1980.

52. Yagil Y, Stalnikowicz R, Michaeli J, et al: Near drowning in the Dead Sea. *Arch Intern Med* 145:50, 1985.

53. Sarnaik AP, Vohra MP: Near-drowning: Fresh, salt, and cold water immersion. *Clin Sports Med* 5:33, 1986.

54. Modell JH, Graves SA, Ketover A: Clinical course of 91 consecutive near-drowning victims. *Chest* 70:231, 1976.

55. Karch SB: Pathology of the heart in drowning. *Arch Pathol Lab Med* 109:176, 1985.

56. Doroshow RW, Ashwal S, Saukel GW: Availability and selection of donors for pediatric heart transplantation. *J Heart Lung Transplant* 14:52, 1995.

57. Neale TJ, Dewar JM, Parr R, et al: Acute renal failure following near drowning in salt water. *N Z Med J* 97:319, 1984.

58. Ports TA, Deuel TF: Intravascular coagulation in fresh-water submersion. *Ann Intern Med* 87:60, 1977.

59. Agar JWM: Rhabdomyolysis and acute renal failure after near-drowning in cold salt water. *Med J Aust* 161:686, 1994.

60. Manolios N, Mackie I: Drowning and near-drowning on Australian beaches patrolled by life-savers: A 10-year study, 1973–1983. *Med J Aust* 148:165, 1988.

61. Sims JK, Enomoto PI, Frankel RI, et al: Marine bacteria complicating seawater near-drowning and marine wounds: A hypothesis. *Ann Emerg Med* 12:212, 1983.

62. Modell JH, Davis JH, Giammona ST, et al: Blood gas and electrolyte changes in human near-drowning victims. *JAMA* 203:99, 1968.

63. Fromm RE: Hypercalcemia complicating an industrial near-drowning. *Ann Emerg Med* 20:669, 1991.

64. Boles JM, Mabille S, Scheydecker JL, et al: Hypoglycemia in salt water near-drowning victims. Correspondence. *Intensive Care Med* 14:30, 1988.

65. Perez-Benavides F, Riff E, Franks C: Adult respiratory distress syndrome and artificial surfactant replacement in the pediatric patient. *Pediatr Emerg Care* 11:153, 1995.

66. Wenger JD, Hollis DG, Weaver RE, et al: Infection caused by *Francisella philomiragia* (formerly *Yersinia philomiragia*). *Ann Intern Med* 110:888, 1989.

67. Bohn DJ, Biggar WD, Smith CR, et al: Influence of hypothermia, barbiturate therapy, and intracranial pressure monitoring on morbidity and mortality after near-drowning. *Crit Care Med* 14:529, 1986.

68. Anonymous: Advanced challenges in resuscitation. Submersion or near drowning. *Resuscitation* 46:273, 2000.

69. Modell JH: Treatment of near-drowning: Is there a role for H.Y.P.E.R. therapy? *Crit Care Med* 14:593, 1986.

70. Lavelle JM, Shaw KN: Near drowning: Is emergency department cardiopulmonary resuscitation or intensive care unit cerebral resuscitation indicated? *Crit Care Med* 21:368, 1993.

71. Connors R, Frewen TC, Kissoon N, et al: Relationship of cross-brain oxygen content difference, cerebral blood flow, and metabolic rate to neurologic outcome after near-drowning. *J Pediatr* 121:839, 1992.

72. Bratton SL, Jardine DS, Morray JP: Serial neurologic examinations after near drowning and outcome. *Arch Pediatr Adolesc Med* 148:167, 1994.

73. Claypool WD, Rogers RM, Matuschak GM: Update on the clinical diagnosis, management, and pathogenesis of pulmonary alveolar proteinosis (phospholipidosis). *Chest* 85:551, 1984.

74. Selecky PA, Wasserman K, Benfield JR, et al: The clinical and physiological effect of whole-lung lavage in pulmonary alveolar proteinosis: A ten-year experience. *Ann Thorac Surg* 24:451, 1977.

75. Hudes ET, Bradley JW, Brebner J: Hydropneumothorax—An unusual complication of lung lavage. *Can Anaesth Soc J* 33:662, 1986.

76. Ramirez-RJ: Alveolar proteinosis: Importance of pulmonary lavage. *Am Rev Respir Dis* 103:666, 1971.

77. Smith LJ, Ankin MG, Katzenstein AL, et al: Management of pulmonary alveolar proteinosis: Clinical conference in pulmonary disease from Northwestern University McGaw Medical Center, Chicago. *Chest* 78:765, 1980.

78. Jansen HM, Zuurmond WA, Roos CM, et al: Whole-lung lavage under hyperbaric oxygen conditions for alveolar proteinosis with respiratory failure. *Chest* 91:829, 1987.

INDEX

Page numbers followed by f indicate figures; page numbers followed by t indicate tables.